PRINCIPLES OF

AMBULATORY MEDICINE

FIFTH EDITION

PRINCIPLES OF

AMBULATORY MEDICINE

FIFTH EDITION

Editors

L. Randol Barker, M.D., Sc.M.
Professor of Medicine
The Johns Hopkins University School of Medicine
Co-Director, Division of General Internal Medicine
Johns Hopkins Bayview Medical Center
Baltimore, Maryland

John R. Burton, M.D.
Mason F. Lord Professor of Medicine
Director, Division of Geriatric Medicine and Gerontology
The Johns Hopkins University School of Medicine
Director, Division of Geriatric Medicine
Johns Hopkins Bayview Medical Center
Baltimore, Maryland

Philip D. Zieve, M.D.
Professor and Chairman
Department of Medicine
The Johns Hopkins University School of Medicine
Johns Hopkins Bayview Medical Center
Baltimore, Maryland

Associate Editor
Thomas E. Finucane, M.D.
Associate Professor of Medicine
Johns Hopkins University School of Medicine
Baltimore, Maryland

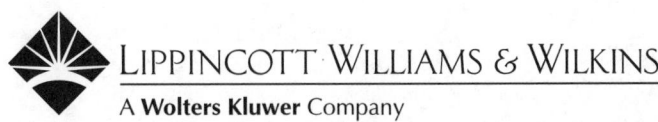

LIPPINCOTT WILLIAMS & WILKINS
A **Wolters Kluwer** Company

Philadelphia • Baltimore • New York • London
Buenos Aires • Hong Kong • Sydney • Tokyo

Editor: Jonathan W. Pine, Jr.
Managing Editor: Leah Ann Kiehne Hayes
Marketing Manager: Daniell T. Griffin
Production Coordinator: Peter J. Carley
Project Editor: Jeffrey S. Myers
Design Coordinator: Mario Fernandez
Illustration Planner: Graphic World, Inc.
Typesetter & Digitized Illustrations: Graphic World, Inc.
Printer & Binder: World Color, Inc.

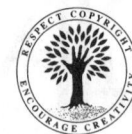
First Edition 1982
Second Edition 1986
Third Edition 1991
Fourth Edition 1995

Library of Congress Cataloging-in-Publication Data

Principles of ambulatory medicine / editors, L. Randol Barker, John R.
   Burton, Philip D. Zieve : associate editor, Thomas E. Finucane. —
   5th ed.
       p.   cm.
   Includes bibliographical references and index.
   ISBN Q-683-30352-X
   1. Family medicine.   2. Ambulatory medical care.   I. Barker, L.
Randol (Lee Randol), 1939   II. Burton, John R. (John Russell), 1937–   .
III. Zieve, Philip D., 1932–   .
   [DNLM: 1. Ambulatory Care.   WX 205 P957 1999]
RC46.P894   1999
616—dc21
DNLM/DLC
for Library of Congress   97-40570
                                                                        CIP

To purchase additional copies of this book, call our customer service department at **(800) 638-0672** or fax orders to **(800) 447-8438.** For other book services, including chapter reprints and large quantity sales, ask for the Special Sales department.

Canadian customers should call **(800) 665-1148,** or fax **(800) 665-0103.** For all other calls originating outside of the United States, please call **(410) 528-4223** or fax us at **(410) 528-8550.**

                                                         99   00   01
                                      3   4   5   6   7   8   9   10

PREFACE TO THE FIFTH EDITION

This book is directed to physicians who care for ambulatory adult patients. The purposes of the book are *(a)* to provide an in-depth account of the evaluation, management, and long-term course of those common clinical problems that are addressed in the ambulatory setting, and *(b)* to provide guidance for recognizing those problems that require either referral for specialized care or hospitalization and for appreciating the expected course of those problems.

Three principles have guided the preparation of each edition of *Principles of Ambulatory Medicine.*

1. Physicians working in a busy practice need to know about *probabilities* related to the occurrence, course, evaluation, and treatment of their patients' problems.
2. The patient makes most decisions in ambulatory care, and the quality of those decisions depends on *the doctor–patient relationship and patient education.*
3. The physician and the patient should incorporate *a preventative point of view* into all actions taken to address the patient's health.

The first four chapters describe the following general approaches for applying these principles in patient care: making decisions on the basis of evidence, developing a therapeutic doctor–patient relationship, using patient-centered patient education, and integrating prevention into practice.

In planning the scope of the book, the editors have selected those conditions that most office-based internists and family practitioners encounter in caring for adult patients from the general population. Updating and revising this edition has been based on evidence from recent clinical trials, on current consensus-based recommendations for many conditions, and on the comments of those who have used the book. Bold print (general references) and bold numerals (specific references) denote at the end of each chapter the published clinical trial reports, meta-analyses, and consensus-based recommendations that have guided the writing of the chapter.

Principles of Ambulatory Medicine is extensively cross-referenced to both avoid redundancy and facilitate access to useful information contained elsewhere in the book. In addition, for easy reference, the key topics in each chapter are presented in outline form at the beginning of the chapter.

CONTRIBUTORS

Unless otherwise indicated, hospital appointments are at Johns Hopkins Bayview Medical Center, Baltimore, Maryland, and faculty appointments are at The Johns Hopkins University School of Medicine.

Frank C. Arnett, Jr., M.D.
Professor of Internal Medicine
University of Texas-Houston Health
  Science Center
Houston, Texas

L. Randol Barker, M.D., Sc.M.
Professor of Medicine
Co-Director, Division of General Internal
  Medicine

William H. Barker, M.D.
Associate Professor of Preventive
  Medicine and Gerontology
University of Rochester Medical Center
Rochester, New York

Linda F. Barr, M.D.
Assistant Professor of Medicine
Division of Pulmonary and Critical Care
  Medicine
Assistant Professor of Oncology

John G. Bartlett, M.D.
Professor of Medicine
Chief, Division of Infectious Diseases
The Johns Hopkins Hospital

William E. Beatie, M.D.
Assistant Professor of Orthopedic Surgery

Jeffrey S. Bender, M.D., F.A.C.S.
Associate Professor of Surgery
Chief, General Surgery

Richard G. Bennett, M.D.
Associate Professor of Medicine

George E. Bigelow, Ph.D.
Professor of Behavioral Biology
Director, Behavioral Pharmacology
  Research Unit

Marc R. Blackman, M.D.
Professor of Medicine
Chief, Division of Endocrinology and
  Metabolism
Program Director, General Clinical
  Research Center
The Johns Hopkins Bayview Medical
  Center

David G. Borenstein, M.D.
Clinical Professor of Medicine
The George Washington University
  Medical Center
Washington, D.C.

Gary R. Briefel, M.D.
Associate Professor of Medicine
Director of Hemodialysis

M. Janette Busby-Whitehead, M.D.
Associate Professor of Medicine
University of North Carolina School
  of Medicine
Chapel Hill, North Carolina

Ronald P. Byank, M.D.
Associate Professor of Orthopaedic
  Surgery

Hugh Calkins, M.D.
Associate Professor of Medicine
Division of Cardiology
The Johns Hopkins Hospital

Nisha Chandra Strobos, M.D.
Professor of Medicine
Director, Coronary Care Unit

Lawrence J. Cheskin, M.D.
Associate Professor of Medicine
Director, Division of Digestive Diseases
Associate Professor of International
  Health
The Johns Hopkins University, School
  of Public Health

Karan A. Cole, Sc.D.
Assistant Professor of Medicine

Andrea M. Corse, M.D.
Assistant Professor of Neurology
The Johns Hopkins Hospital

Vanessa E. Cullins, M.D., M.P.H.
Assistant Professor of Obstetrics
  and Gynecology

J. Raymond DePaulo, Jr., M.D.
Professor of Psychiatry
The Johns Hopkins Hospital

Mark D. Duncan, M.D.
Assistant Professor of Surgery
Section of Surgical Sciences

Christopher J. Earley, M.D., Ph.D.
Assistant Professor of Neurology

Lori Fantry, M.D., M.P.H.
Assistant Professor of Internal Medicine
University of Maryland School
  of Medicine
Baltimore, Maryland

Michael I. Fingerhood, M.D.
Assistant Professor of Medicine

Thomas E. Finucane, M.D.
Associate Professor of Medicine

John A. Flynn, M.D.
Assistant Professor of Medicine
Clinical Director, Division of General
  Internal Medicine
The Johns Hopkins Hospital

Steve N. Georas, M.D.
Assistant Professor of Medicine
Division of Pulmonary and Critical Care

Sheldon H. Gottlieb, M.D.
Associate Professor of Medicine
Clinical Chief, Division of Cardiology

Robert I. Gregerman, M.D.
Professor of Medicine
University of Texas Health Science Center
  at San Antonio
Research Director
Geriatric Research, Education, and
  Clinical Center
Audie L. Murphy Hospital Division
South Texas Veterans Health Care System
San Antonio, Texas

Richard J. Gross, M.D., F.A.C.P, Sc.M.
Assistant Professor of Medicine
Division of General Internal Medicine

S. Mitchell Harman, M.D.
Associate Professor of Medicine
Chief, Section of Endocrinology
Gerontology Research Center
National Institute on Aging

David B. Hellmann, M.D.
Mary Betty Stevens Professor of Medicine

Janet Horn, M.D., M.S.
Associate Professor of Medicine

George R. Huggins, M.D.
Professor and Chairman of Obstetrics
  and Gynecology

Constance J. Johnson, M.D.
Associate Professor of Neurology

Calvin E. Jones, M.D.
Associate Professor of Surgery
Chief, Division of Vascular Surgery

Peter W. Kaplan, M.B., B.S., F.R.C.P.
Associate Professor of Neurology
Chairman, Department of Neurology

Philip O. Katz, M.D., F.A.C.P., F.A.C.G.
Associate Professor of Medicine
Alleghany Unviersity of the Health
    Sciences
Medical College of Pennsylvania–
    Hahnemann School of Medicine
Philadelphia, Pennsylvania

James P. Keogh, M.D.
Associate Professor of Medicine,
    Epidemiology and Preventive Medicine
University of Maryland, School of
    Medicine
Baltimore, Maryland

David E. Kern, M.D., M.P.H.
Associate Professor of Medicine
Co-Director, Division of General Internal
    Medicine

Frederick T. Koster, M.D.
Professor of Internal Medicine
University of New Mexico Health
    Sciences Center
Albuquerque, New Mexico

Phillip D. Kramer, M.D.
Assistant Professor of Neurology
    and Otolaryngology
The Johns Hopkins Hospital

Edward S. Kraus, M.D.
Associate Professor of Medicine
Division of Nephrology
Medical Co-Director, Kidney Transplant
    Program

Ralph W. Kuncl, M.D., Ph.D.
Professor of Neurology
The Johns Hopkins Hospital

Bruce S. Lebowtiz, D.P.M.
Director, Podiatry Clinic
Department of Orthopedic Surgery

Frederick A. Lenz, M.D.
Professor of Neurosurgery

Mark C. Liu, M.D.
Associate Professor of Medicine

Douglas K. MacLeod, D.M.D.
Department of Dentistry
Wake Medical Center
Raleigh, North Carolina

Esteban Mezey, M.D.
Professor of Medicine

Patrick A. Murphy, M.D.
Professor of Medicine and Microbiology
Chief, Infectious Diseases Division

David N. Neubauer, M.D.
Assistant Professor of Psychiatry
Director, Acute Psychiatric Unit
Associate Director, Johns Hopkins Sleep
    Disorders Center

John K. Niparko, M.D.
Professor of Otolaryngology, Head and
    Neck Surgery
Director, Division of Otology and
    Neurotology
The Johns Hopkins Hospital

Nathaniel F. Pierce, M.D.
Professor of Medicine

Michael J. Purtell, M.D., Ph.D.
Assistant Professor of Medicine
Division of Hematology and Oncology

Peter V. Rabins, M.D., M.P.H.
Professor of Psychiatry
Department of Psychiatry and Behavioral
    Sciences

Cynthia Rand, Ph.D.
Associate Professor of Medicine

Stephen G. Reich, M.D.
Associate Professor of Neurology
Director, Movement Disorders Clinic
The Johns Hopkins Hospital

John C. Roberts, M.D.
Attending Physician
Madrona Medical Group
Bellingham, Washington

Robert P. Roca, M.D., M.P.H.
Associate Professor of Psychiatry
Director
Geriatrics Services and General Hospital
    Programs
The Sheppard Pratt Health System
Baltimore, Maryland

Anne Marie Rompalo, M.D., Sc.M.
Associate Professor of Medicine
Medical Director
Centers for Disease Control and
    Prevention HIV and STD Prevention
    Training Center
Baltimore City Health Department
Baltimore, Maryland

Kevin A. Rossiter, M.D.
Assistant Professor of Medicine

David A. Sack. M.D.
Professor of International Health

Andrew P. Schachat, M.D.
Professor of Ophthalmology

Larry N. Scherzer, M.D., M.P.H., Sc.D.
Assistant Professor of Pediatrics
University of Connecticut
Farmington, Connecticut
Chief of Pediatrics
Northeast Permanente Medical Group
East Hartford, Connecticut

Chester W. Schmidt, Jr., M.D.
Professor and Chairman of Psychiatry

Marvin M. Schuster, M.D.
Professor of Medicine and Psychiatry
Director, Motility Center
Marvin M. Schuster Center for Digestive
    and Motility Disorders

Stephen D. Sears, M.D., M.P.H.
Senior Vice President Medical
    Administration
Maine General Medical Center
Augusta, Maine

Edward P. Shapiro, M.D.
Professor of Medicine
Director, Cardiac Non-Invasive Service

Stephen Sisson, M.D.
Assistant Professor of Medicine
The Johns Hopkins Hospital

Gardner W. Smith, M.D.
Professor Emeritus of Surgery
Past Chairman
Section of Surgical Sciences

Philip L. Smith, M.D.
Professor of Medicine
Instructor of Anesthesiology
Director, Johns Hopkins Sleep Disorders
    Center

David A. Spector, M.D.
Associate Professor of Medicine
Chief, Division of Renal Medicine

Robert J. Spence, M.D.
Associate Professor of Surgery
Johns Hopkins School of Medicine
Chief of Plastic Surgery

**Kerry J. Stewart, Ed.D., F.A.C.S.M.,
    F.A.A.C.V.P.R.**
Associate Professor of Medicine
Division of Cardiology
Director, Cardiac Rehabilitation and
    Prevention

Ray E. Stutzman, M.D.
Associate Professor of Urology
Director of Outpatient Urology
The Johns Hopkins Outpatient Center

Alexander S. Townes, M.D., F.A.C.P.
Professor of Medicine
Vanderbilt University School of Medicine
Chief of Staff
Veterans Administration Medical Center
Nashville, Tennessee

Peter V. Vaitekevicius, M.D.
Assistant Professor of Medicine

Martin D. Valentine, M.D.
Professor of Medicine

Larry Waterbury, M.D.
Associate Professor of Medicine and
    Oncology
Chief, Hematology-Oncology Division

Peter White, Jr., M.D.
Assistant Professor of Medicine and
  Oncology

S. Elizabeth Whitmore, M.D.
Assistant Professor of Dermatology

Fredrick M. Wigley, M.D.
Professor of Medicine
Chief, Division of Rheumatology

Robert A. Wise, M.D.
Professor of Medicine
Interim Director, Division of Pulmonary
  and Critical Care Medicine

Scott M. Wright, M.D.
Assistant Professor of Medicine

Philip D. Zieve, M.D.
Professor of Medicine
Chairman, Department of Medicine

Acknowledgments

The Editors wish to acknowledge the helpful suggestions of many colleagues, both generalists and specialists, who provided feedback on the third edition and who reviewed chapters for the fourth and fifth editions. Two persons, Mrs. Carole Messman and Ms. Susan McFeaters, provided excellent administrative and typographic assistance throughout the preparation of all five editions of this book.

CONTENTS

Section 9:   Musculoskeletal Problems   889

Section 10:   Metabolic and Endocrinologic Problems   1021

Section 11:   Neurologic Problems   1199

Section 12:   Selected General Surgical Problems   1329

Section 13:   Gynecologic Problems   1421

Section 14:   Problems of the Eyes and Ears   1459

Section 15:   Miscellaneous Problems   1497

Index   1565

Issues of General Concern in Ambulatory Medicine

C H A P T E R   1

Ambulatory Care, Evidence-Based Medicine, and Other Core Proficiencies for Ambulatory Practice

L. RANDOL BARKER, MD
JOHN C. ROBERTS, MD

The fundamental tenet of this book is that ambulatory care has distinctive characteristics that should shape physicians' approaches to patients. This chapter describes the domain of ambulatory care in the United States. It also addresses in detail the evidence-based practice of medicine, and it describes briefly other proficiencies that are central to ambulatory medicine.

DOMAIN OF AMBULATORY CARE

Who are the physicians providing ambulatory care? What patients visit physicians in their offices? What problems do these patients present to their physicians? What ambulatory care is provided for these problems? To answer these questions, the United States National Ambulatory Medical Care Survey (NAMCS), started in 1973, has collected information periodically from a representative sample of physicians' offices.

Office-Based Generalist Physicians

Table 1.1 shows the distribution by physician specialty of the nearly 670 million office visits to physicians in the United States during 1991. Of these visits, approximately 15% were to internists and 25% were to general/family practitioners, the groups of generalists to whom this book is directed primarily.

Ambulatory Patients

The NAMCS *definition of an ambulatory patient* is "an individual presenting for personal health services who is neither bedridden nor currently admitted to any health care institution." A critical expansion of this definition is that ambulatory or homebound patients (or members of their households) have most of the responsibility for carrying out their own care: They must administer most or all treatments, must monitor symptoms and functional status, must adapt activity to the constraints imposed by illness, and must decide how to deal with new problems when they arise. These characteristics have important implications for the care of ambulatory patients, as discussed below.

The age and sex distribution of the patients who visit internists and general/family practitioners is shown in Table 1.2. Approximately 60% of visits to all generalists are made by female patients. The principal differences shown in Table 1.2 are that adolescents and young adults account for a larger proportion of visits to general/family practitioners than to internists, and that visits by older patients make up a larger proportion of the practice of internists.

Problems of Ambulatory Patients

What types of problems are seen in ambulatory practice? Physicians participating in NAMCS were asked to name the principal reasons (using the International Classification of Diseases) for the visits by patients. Table 1.3 lists the most common responses given by internists and general/family practitioners, respectively.

Ambulatory Care

The NAMCS *defines ambulatory care* as "health services rendered to individuals under their own cognizance, any time when they are not in a hospital or other health care institution." In 1989, the annual number of office visits by adults to all types of physicians ranged from 1.9 for people 19 to 24 years old to 5.9 for people aged 75 and over.

Table 1.4, from the 1989 NAMCS report, shows the frequency of the therapeutic services that are most commonly provided or ordered at ambulatory visits by internists and general/family practitioners: medications and counseling. The table also shows the frequency distributions of visit duration, visit status of

Table 1.1. Number, Percentage Distribution, and Annual Rate of Office Visits by Physician Specialty and Professional Identity: United States, 1991

Physician Specialty	Number of Visits (Thousands)	Percent Distribution	Number of Visits per 100 Persons per Year[a]
All Visits	669,689	100.0	269.3
General and family practice	164,857	24.6	66.3
Internal medicine	102,923	15.4	41.4
Pediatrics	74,646	11.1	30.0
Obstetrics and gynecology	56,834	8.5	22.9
Ophthalmology	41,207	6.2	16.6
Orthopedic surgery	35,932	5.4	14.4
Dermatology	29,659	4.4	11.9
General surgery	21,285	3.2	8.6
Otolaryngology	19,101	2.9	7.7
Psychiatry	15,720	2.3	6.3
Urological surgery	12,758	1.9	5.1
Cardiovascular diseases	11,629	1.7	4.7
Neurology	6,798	1.0	2.7
All other specialties	76,341	11.4	30.7
Professional Identity			
Doctor of osteopathy	46,727	7.0	18.8
Doctor of medicine	622,962	93.0	250.5

From National Ambulatory Medical Care Survey. Hyattsville, MD: National Center for Health Statistics, 1991.

[a] Based on US Bureau of the Census estimates of the civilian noninstitutionalized population of the United States as of July 1, 1991.

Table 1.2. Distribution of Visits to General and Family Physicians and to Internists by Age and Sex of Patient: United States, 1989

Age and Sex of Patient	Percentage Distribution (Rounded)	
	Internal Medicine	General and Family Practice
All ages	100	100
Under 15 years	2	16
15–24 years	6	11
25–44 years	24	29
45–64 years	29	23
65–74	20	12
75 years and over	19	9
Female	58	61
Male	42	39

From National Ambulatory Medical Care Survey. Hyattsville, MD: National Center for Health Statistics, 1989.

Table 1.3. Reasons for Ambulatory Visits to Generalists: United States, January to December 1985

	25 Most Common Reasons (by ICD-9-CM Categories)	
Rank	Internists: Reason for Visit	General and Family Practitioners: Reason for Visit
1	Essential hypertension	Essential hypertension
2	Diabetes mellitus	General medical examination
3	Other forms of chronic ischemic heart disease	Acute upper respiratory infections
4	Acute upper respiratory infections	Diabetes mellitus
5	General medical examination	Normal pregnancy
6	Osteoarthrosis and allied disorders	Suppurative and unspecified otitis media
7	General symptoms	Acute pharyngitis
8	Chronic airway obstruction	Bronchitis
9	Asthma	Chronic sinusitis
10	Bronchitis	Certain adverse effects not elsewhere classif.
11	Neurotic disorders	Health supervision of infant or child
12	Angina pectoris	Sprains and strains
13	Chronic sinusitis	Others disorders of urethra and urinary tract
14	Acute pharyngitis	Obesity and other hyperalimentation
15	Cardiac dysrhythmias	General symptoms
16	Other disorders of soft tissue	Contact dermatitis and other eczema
17	Symptoms involving respiratory system	Neurotic disorders
18	Heart failure	Osteoarthrosis and allied disorders
19	Peripheral enthesopathies	Other and unspecified arthropathies
20	Other and unspecified arthropathies	Other disorders of soft tissues
21	Diseases of esophagus	Other noninfectious gastroenteritis
22	Other noninfectious gastroenteritis	Asthma
23	Other disorders of urethra and urinary tract	Sprains and strains of sacroiliac region
24	Allergic rhinitis	Acute tonsillitis
25	Hypertensive heart disease	Disorders of external ear

From National Ambulatory Medical Care Survey. Hyattsville, MD: National Center for Health Statistics, 1985.

patients, and disposition. The majority of visits (70%) included prescribing or providing medication. A significant part of the visit was devoted to counseling for approximately 40% of visits. At about 60% of visits to internists and 55% of visits to general/family practitioners, the patient had been seen before for the same problem. At all other visits the patient was new to the physician (approximately 15% of visits) or was an old patient with a new problem (25 to 30% of visits).

In addition to office visits, *telephone encounters and house calls* are important in the care of ambulatory patients. Telephone encounters enable physicians and patients to handle many problems efficiently; they constitute approximately 25% of all patient contacts for internists and 19% for family physicians (4). Home visits are helpful for providing care to patients who are too frail to make office visits or for learning facts about patients' home conditions that may facilitate management of their problems at future office visits.

Self-Care and Alternative Care

Before making visits to physicians, patients usually attempt to diagnose and treat their own symptoms. Approximately one third of Americans also seek help each year from practitioners outside the mainstream of medicine (6).

Studies of self-care show that at any one time, approximately 30% of persons are taking nonprescribed medications or are engaged in self-care for a problem for which they have not consulted a physician (10). The frequency distribution of conditions managed by self-care was estimated by Fry (9) on the basis of many years of general practice in a community well known to him: 25% upper respiratory infections, 20% musculoskeletal symptoms, 20% emotional problems, 10% acute gastrointestinal symptoms, 5% skin rashes, and 20% miscellaneous other symptoms.

The time interval between the onset of a new problem and the decision to go to a physician (i.e., the duration of self-care) is shown for a number of common conditions in Table 1.5, adapted from NAMCS data.

Table 1.4. Distribution of Visits to Office-Based Generalists by Selected Therapeutic Services Ordered or Provided, Duration of Visits, Visit Status, and Disposition, United States 1989

	Percentage of Visits	
	To Internists	To General and Family Practitioners
Selected Therapeutic Services[a]		
≥1 Medications ordered or provided	75.4	70.7
Counseling advice		
Diet, weight reduction	21.1	14.3
Smoking cessation	3.2	3.7
HIV transmission	0.3	0.1
Breast self-examination	2.1	1.7
Psychotherapy	1.9	1.4
Other counseling	21.1	23.9
No counseling	61.2	63.0
Duration of Visit		
0 min (no face-to-face encounter with physicians)	1.7	1.9
1–5 min	5.0	8.7
6–10 min	20.2	30.4
11–15 min	39.1	32.4
16–30 min	27.1	24.0
More than 30 min	6.8	2.7
Visit Status of Patient		
New patient	15.7	14.5
Old patient, new problem	25.0	30.1
Old patient, old problem	59.4	55.4
Disposition of Visit		
No follow-up planned	6.8	11.5
Return at specified time	65.3	54.1
Return if needed	19.7	30.3
Telephone follow-up planned	8.0	3.3
Referral to other physician	4.6	3.6
Admit to hospital	1.0	0.5

From National Ambulatory Medical Care Survey. Washington, DC: Department of Health and Human Services, 1989.

[a] Total exceeds 100% because more than one service reported for many visits.

Not surprisingly, patients with lacerations, symptoms of acute infections, and new chest pain presented within 1 to 6 days, whereas those with subacute problems (headache or back pain) tended to present after at least 1 week of self-care.

Self-care before professional care is an important way in which the patient, not the physician, makes the decisions in the domain of ambulatory medicine. The patient's primary role in carrying out the plan of care after visiting a physician has already been emphasized in the expanded definition of the ambulatory patient given previously. These two features confirm the primacy of the patient's actions in influencing the course of events in ambulatory medicine.

The Temporal Dimension of Ambulatory Medicine

The information from NAMCS contained in Tables 1.1 to 1.5 does not illuminate the longitudinal nature of ambulatory care. Table 1.6 shows the 5-year profile of care for an elderly woman. This patient's story illustrates each of the following important questions, for which only the passage of time provided the answers:

- *What is the significance of a recent symptom* (e.g., the temporal headache for 1 year reported in 1975, subsequently not a serious problem)?
- *What is the advisability of initiating a referral for a problem* (e.g., cataract problem identified but asymptomatic in 1975, evaluated when more symptomatic in 1978 and classified as not mature)?
- *How well will the patient adhere to recommended treatment* (e.g., the digoxin prescribed in 1975 for heart failure, taken reliably for 5 years)?
- *What is the impact of a new treatment on the patient's health* (e.g., adding a diuretic in 1978; heart failure gradually improved during the month after diuretic)?
- *What is the impact of intercurrent medical problems on the patient's usual activities?* (The answer to this question varied over time depending on intercurrent problems: During the 5 years the patient's ambulation deteriorated greatly; however, other valued activities, such as crocheting and canning, did not.)

Table 1.5. Percentage Distribution of New Problem Office Visits by Time Since Onset of Complaint or Symptom, According to Selected Principal Reasons for Visit: United States, January to December 1977

		Time Since Onset of Complaint or Symptom					
Principle Reason for Visit	Total	1 Day	1–6 Days	1–3 wk	1–3 mo	>3 mo	Not Applicable
All new problem visits	100.0	8.2	37.3	15.6	10.3	13.9	14.8
Symptoms of throat	100.0	6.9	77.9	10.6	2.3	1.9	0.4
Cough	100.0	3.3	73.0	18.6	2.9	2.1	0.2
Head cold, upper respiratory tract infection	100.0	6.2	72.5	16.5	3.0	1.1	0.7
Fever	100.0	17.6	76.4	4.7	0.2	1.0	
Headache	100.0	5.1	35.6	19.0	16.5	19.7	3.2
Back symptoms	100.0	6.5	37.6	26.4	11.8	16.2	1.5
Chest pain	100.0	7.6	45.8	22.6	9.3	13.6	1.2
Laceration, upper extremity	100.0	70.4	15.4	7.8	3.0	2.1	1.3

From National Ambulatory Medical Care Survey, 1977, Summary. Hyattsville, MD: National Center for Health Statistics.

Table 1.6. Profile of 5 Years in the Care of an Elderly Patient (each problem *italicized*)

Feature	1975	1976	1977	1978	1979
Encounters	Initial visit, 4 office visits, many phone calls	3 office visits, many phone calls	5 office visits, 2 hospital admissions, 1 home visit, many phone calls	4 office visits, many phone calls	4 office visits, many phone calls
Principal medical problems	*Acute myocardial infarction* (mild congestive heart failure; digitalized; home management by patient's choice)	Stable (digoxin)	Stable (digoxin)	Congestive heart failure (diuretic added)	Stable (digoxin, diuretic)
	Degenerative joint disease (knees for years; cervical spine for years)	Waxes and wanes (aspirin, Motrin)	Same (coated aspirin)	Same (coated aspirin)	Same (coated aspirin)
	Temporal headaches for 1 year (erythrocyte sedimentation rate 30)	Rarely	Rarely	Rarely	Rarely
	Hearing loss (ear, nose, and throat examination: senile high frequency deficit, no prescription)	Stable	Stable	Stable	Stable
	Bilateral cataracts	Stable	Stable	Referred (not mature)	Stable
	Leukoplakia, mouth (biopsy: not malignant)	Stable	Stable	Stable	Referred for change in appearance (biopsy: not malignant)
	Hematocrit 35 (guaiac-negative)	Stable	Stable	Stable	Stable
	Constipation (for years)	Waxes and wanes (OTC laxative as needed)	Stable. Same (OTC laxative as needed)	Same (OTC laxative as needed and stool softener)	Same (OTC laxative as needed and stool softener)
		Leg cramps (quinine at bedtime)	Minimal (quinine at bedtime)	Same (quinine at bedtime)	Same (quinine at bedtime)
		Left cerebral *transient ischemic attack*	*Left CVA* (hospital, physical therapy)	Stable (right hemiparesis)	Recurrent left CVA (home management)
			Dog bite (cellulitis)	No recurrence	No recurrence
			Rectal bleeding (hospital, negative workup)	No recurrence	No recurrence
			Dysuria (culture negative)	*Family* (temporarily "exhausted" (Visiting Nurses Association)	Family doing well
				Painful toe	Persists (codeine)
				Appetite lost temporarily	No recurrence
Overall profile	87-year-old widow living with daughter's family, ambulatory and independent in the home, mentally intact, crochets and cans food; weight 166; multiple medical problems identified at initial visit (above)	88 years old, status the same; weight 160; 2 new problems (above)	89 years old, ambulation with walker assistance after CVA; weight 151; 4 new problems (above), hospitalized twice	90 years old, status the same; weight 140; 3 new problems (above)	91 years old; ambulation more impaired after second CVA; mentally intact, crochets and cans food; weight 139; no new problem

OTC, Over-the-counter; *CVA,* cerebrovascular accident.

- *What is the impact of the patient's illness on family members in the same household?* (The answer also varied over time; "exhaustion" at one point did not predict transfer to a long-term care facility.)

Goals of Ambulatory Care

Patient Expectations

The goals of ambulatory care are determined by the expectations of patients who are residing in the community. When they make office visits for stated medical reasons, ambulatory patients are ultimately seeking help to maintain or resume valued activities. Depending on the severity of their medical problems, they may be greatly, moderately, or not at all constrained from attaining these expectations. But by virtue of living in the community, they are dealing with these expectations daily, in contrast to hospitalized patients for whom these expectations must await return to home.

Implications for Practice

To determine how any patient is doing, it is helpful to be aware of that person's particular expectations and how well he or she is meeting them. This usually involves learning about the makeup of the patient's current household and the patient's usual role in the family, the patient's occupation and level of formal education, and valued activities. It is also helpful to be aware of the developmental tasks that may be relevant to a patient's family. Tasks that are typical of the various stages in the life cycle of a family are listed in Table 1.7.

Table 1.7. Factors to Consider in the Family Life Cycle State of One's Patient

Family Life Cycle States	Developmental Tasks
Leaving home	Differentiate self in relation to family
	Develop intimate peer relationships
	Establish oneself in work
Couples and pairing	Form a committed relationship
	Realign relationships with extended family to include partner
Pregnancy and childbirth	Make room for children in the family
	Become parents while remaining spouses
Family with young children	Form a parent team
	Negotiate relationships with extended family to include parenting and grandparenting roles
Family with adolescents	Shift parent–child relationship to permit adolescent to move in and out of system
Adulthood and middle years	Refocus on marital and career issues
	Deal with disabilities and death in grandparents
	Deal with own aging and mortality
Graying of the family	Maintain functioning in face of physiologic decline
Death and grieving	Deal with loss of spouse, siblings, and peers
	Prepare for own death

Adapted from Carter CA, McGoldrick M, eds. The family life cycle: a framework for family therapy. New York: Gardner Press, 1980.

The significance of this information can be illustrated by a common example: a middle-aged man who has had an uncomplicated myocardial infarction. After 3 months, the patient might be assessed as "status post–myocardial infarction—doing well." If he has resumed work and other valued activities, then he is probably "doing well." If he is not back at work, is financially stressed, and his wife reports that he has become irritable, then he is not doing well and the situation requires evaluation.

Awareness of a patient's life circumstances is also important in preventive care (see Chapter 2), in which the patient's degree of wellness rather than degree of illness is assessed. Assessing wellness means learning whether a patient engages in health-promoting behaviors and determining what health risks the patient has. For example, a 45-year-old mother who is happily married, free of chronic disease, has stopped smoking, has had periodic negative Pap smears, and drinks alcohol only socially would be assessed as very well. If everything were the same but she smoked two packs of cigarettes daily, she would be assessed as only moderately well because of the major risk posed by heavy tobacco exposure. If she were recently divorced, had stopped seeing friends, and was smoking and drinking heavily, she would be assessed as not very well, even though she might not complain of any particular symptoms or have objective evidence of any disease.

PRACTICING EVIDENCE-BASED MEDICINE

Doctors are increasingly being called on by society to provide both scientifically sound and cost-effective medical care. These pressures have given rise to the term *evidence-based medicine* (EBM). EBM focuses on issues integral to day-to-day patient care: diagnosis, prognosis, treatment, compliance, assessment of risks, prevention, and management of the increasing amount of medical information that confronts doctors. More directly, evidence-based medicine is the conscientious, explicit, and judicious use of current best evidence in making decisions about the care of individual patients (11).

Evidence-based decision making is especially important in ambulatory practice because this is the setting where patients are most likely to present with undifferentiated problems. It is also the setting where most clinical decisions are made.

The Diagnostic Process

Four Ways that Clinicians Formulate a Diagnosis

Diagnostic assessment begins the moment one meets a patient. Behavioral scientists have described at least four ways that clinicians formulate diagnoses:

- *Pattern recognition:* Many diagnoses are made instantly because physicians have learned to recognize patterns specific to certain diseases, such as the face of the patient with Down's syndrome and the elbows of the patient with psoriasis. The certainty of these types of diagnosis is so great that further testing often is unnecessary.

- *Algorithm:* Algorithms are growing more common as a result of the growth of clinical practice guidelines, which, when grounded scientifically, can be extremely helpful. The drawbacks of algorithms are that they must be constructed before a patient is seen, and they must account for every possibility in a workup. For example, the algorithm for polycythemia must consider cigarette smoking, high-altitude living, and other causes, as well as polycythemia vera.

- *Exhaustion:* As Sackett has pointed out (see *Clinical Epidemiology,* in "General References"), medical students should both be taught how to do a complete history and physical examination, and once they have mastered the components, be taught never to do one. However, on occasion, clinicians do resort to comprehensive histories and examinations, as much to buy time to think as to uncover hidden disease.

- *Hypothesis–deduction:* On most occasions, physicians diagnose by forming hypotheses and testing them, as is done in scientific experimentation. Upon hearing that a patient has chest pain, one builds a short list of hypotheses, then invites a further description, then asks focused questions that help confirm or rule out the hypotheses. The questions in the interview and each maneuver in the examination are as much diagnostic tests as the electrocardiogram and the chest radiograph. Studies of physicians' behavior reveal that the short list of hypotheses usually does not exceed three or four diagnoses. Typically, new hypotheses are added as others are discarded, but the eventual goal is to narrow the list and reduce the uncertainty about which diagnosis is most likely. Studies of physicians in ambulatory practice show that hypotheses were generated, on average, 28 seconds into the interview and that correct diagnoses of standard problems were made 6 minutes into 30-minute workups; the correct diagnoses were made in 75% of the encounters (2).

The hypothesis–deduction model reveals a truth common to all methods of diagnosis: A doctor can rarely be absolutely certain of any diagnosis. Physicians live with uncertainty, and the role of all diagnostic tests—the interview, the physical examination, the laboratory evaluation, trials of empiric treatments, allowing time to pass (expectant observation)—is to narrow the uncertainty enough to place a diagnostic label on a patient. How narrow the uncertainty must be depends on the physician's and patient's tolerances of uncertainty, the severity of the suspected disease, the treatability of the suspected disease, and the benefits and risks of possible treatments.

Steps in the Hypothesis–Deduction Process

Evidence shows that clinicians implicitly use common sense and their medical knowledge to reach a diagnosis with adequate certainty. Explicitly, the diagnostic process follows certain steps:

Step 1: Form a hypothesis and estimate its likelihood. The estimate of likelihood is called the *pretest probability* (or *prior probability*), which simply represents the estimate of prevalence of the disease in a group of people similar to the patient at hand. Each hypothesized diagnosis and the estimate of its likelihood comes initially from evidence collected during the interview and physical examination and from one's fund of knowledge from sources such as other patients, colleagues, textbooks, and journals.

Step 2: Decide how certain the diagnosis must be. If the hypothesized disease is easily and safely treated, one might have to be less certain than if the disease has an ominous prognosis or demands complex, risk-laden treatment. For example, a 75% certainty that a patient has streptococcal pharyngitis might be enough for one to prescribe an antibiotic, whereas one would want a much higher level of certainty before diagnosing and treating a patient with suspected leukemia. If one is above the threshold for a hypothesized disease (e.g., over 75% for streptococcal pharyngitis), then further tests are unnecessary and treatment is prescribed. Conversely, if one is adequately certain that a patient does not have a hypothesized disease (e.g., 90% certainty that a patient does not have streptococcal pharyngitis), then no further tests are required and the patient is reassured. However, if the level of uncertainty remains between these two extremes, further testing (e.g., a throat culture) can help move one toward one extreme or the other.

Step 3: Choose a diagnostic test. Which test to choose depends on many factors: its safety, its *accuracy* (e.g., how closely an observation or a test result reflects the true clinical state of a patient), how easily it can be done, its costs, and not least, a patient's own preferences and values regarding tests, especially those that carry risks. When considering a test, one needs to reflect on each of these factors. Critical appraisal of reported studies of tests includes the steps listed in Table 1.8. When selecting a test for a patient, the crucial questions to ask are: "Will the results of the test change my plan?" and "Will my patient be better off from having the test?" *(the utility of the test).* If the answer to these is "no," the test does not need to be recommended.

Table 1.8. Guidelines for Assessing a Study of a Diagnostic Test

Has there been an independent blind comparison with a gold standard?

Has the test been evaluated in a *sample of patients* that included an appropriate spectrum of disease (mild and severe, treated and untreated) plus patients with different but commonly confused disorders?

Was the *setting* for the evaluation adequately described?

Have the *reproducibility* of the test result (precision) and its interpretation (observer variation) been determined?

Has the term *normal* been defined sensibly?

Have the *tactics of the test* been described well enough for you to apply it in your practice?

Has the *utility* of the test been determined? (Were the patients better off for having the test?)

Adapted from Sackett DL, Haynes RB, Guyatt GH, Tugwell P. Clinical epidemiology: a basic science for clinical medicine. 2nd ed. Boston: Little Brown, 1991.

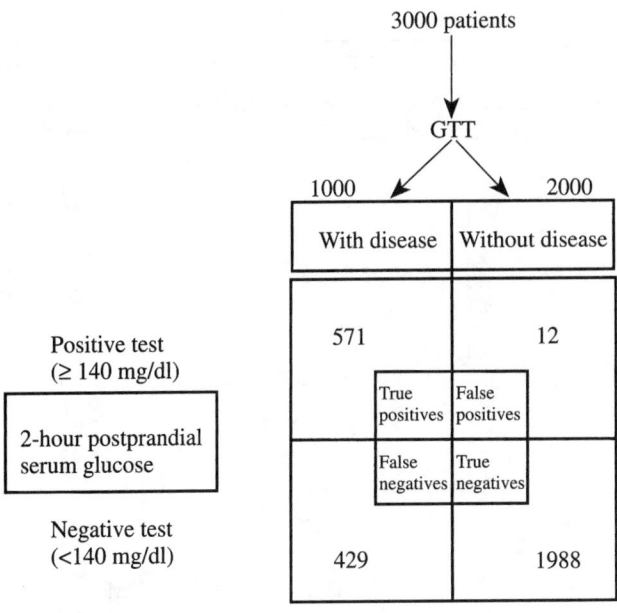

Sensitivity = $\dfrac{TP}{TP+FN}$ Specificity = $\dfrac{TN}{TN+FP}$

= $\dfrac{571}{571+429}$ = $\dfrac{1988}{1988+12}$

= .571   = .994

Figure 1.1. Test performance determined by research. Researcher identifies diseased and nondiseased patients using a gold standard, and wants to know the performance characteristics (sensitivity and specificity) of a new test. *Example:* Diabetes, using glucose tolerance test *(GTT)* as gold standard and 2-hour postprandial glucose as screening test for diabetes.

Step 4: Be aware of the test's performance characteristics. Every test has a certain sensitivity and specificity for every disease it tests for. For example, if one is checking for anemia caused by hemolysis, a hematocrit is very sensitive but not very specific. However, if one is trying simply to diagnose anemia, the same test becomes 100% specific because anemia is defined as a low hematocrit.

Sensitivity and *specificity* have become common terms in medical discussion, but they are commonly misunderstood. The 2 × 2 table in Figure 1.1 reveals much about these and other terms. A fundamental fact about sensitivity and specificity is that they are determined by researchers, not clinicians. Researchers study groups of patients with or without disease, and they go about measuring how well tests perform when applied to those two known groups. The sensitivity of a test (the *true positive rate*) is the number of study subjects with a disease who have a positive test divided by all study subjects with disease. The specificity of a test (the *true negative rate*) is the number of study subjects without disease who have a negative test divided by all those without disease. "Diseased" and "not diseased" are labels that reflect a best test or a definition of a certain disease: the so-called *gold standard.* For pulmonary embolus, the gold standard remains the pulmonary angiogram. For angina, there is no sure test, so a case definition becomes the gold standard. Skepticism must be used in considering gold standards. For example, the oral cholecystogram was once the gold standard by which gallbladder ultrasonography was tested for use in the diagnosis of cholelithiasis; however, ultrasonography seemed to be a poor test, not because of problems with the new test, but because the gold standard was itself a poor test, as was later shown.

Sensitivity and specificity are not static properties of a test. As the cutoff is made more abnormal, a test's sensitivity (and false-positive rate) decreases, while its specificity (and false-negative rate) increases. This principle is illustrated for progressively more abnormal blood glucose levels used in the 1960s to screen for diabetes (Table 1.9). This illustration matches the common-sense conclusion that as a patient's test result becomes more abnormal, one can be more certain that a patient has disease—although never fully certain. Using the data in Table 1.9, if one selects a very high glucose value for the cutoff between normal and abnormal, many people with diabetes will remain undiagnosed (i.e., the sensitivity will be low). Conversely, when one decides to label patients diabetic based on single marginally elevated blood glucose values, one will not miss much disease, but will risk falsely labeling many without diabetes (i.e., the specificity will be low). This example illustrates how a physician can interpret test results flexibly, taking into consideration the severity of disease, the potential risks and benefits of treatment, and changing information about risks and benefits of treatment. The glucose values that are now recommended for diagnosing impaired glucose tolerance (see Table 72.3) and frank diabetes mellitus (see Table 72.3) illustrate the use of these principles by a national standard-setting organization.

Step 5: Determine a posttest probability of disease. In contrast to the researcher, who determines the sensitivity and specificity of a test by applying the test to groups of patients who have disease (to determine sensitivity) or do not have disease (to determine specificity), a *clinician begins with the result of a test* and asks "Does my patient have disease or not?" or "What is the *posttest probability* (also called *predictive value*) that my patient has (or does not have) disease?" Posttest probability takes into account the performance characteristics (sensitivity and specificity) of the test *and* the pretest (prior) probability of disease in a group of patients like one's own patient. A *positive predictive value* is the probability of disease in a given patient who has an abnormal test result. A *negative predictive value* is the probability of not having the disease when the patient's test result is normal.

Published information is available about predictive values of some tests in subgroups of patients with selected characteristics. Examples are published findings useful for making decisions in patients with varying pretest probabilities of having deep vein thrombosis (Doppler ultrasound; see Chapter 52) or renovascular hypertension (captopril renal scan; see Chapter 62). If there is no information on patients comparable to one's own patient, it is possible to

Table 1.9. Tradeoff Between Sensitivity and Specificity When Diagnosing Diabetes

Blood Glucose Level 2 hr After Eating (mg/100 mL)	Sensitivity (%)	False-Negative Rate (1 – Sensitivity) (%)	Specificity (%)	False-Positive Rate (1 – Specificity) (%)	Positive Likelihood Ratio (Sensitivity ÷ False-Positive Rate)	Negative Likelihood Ratio (False-Negative Rate ÷ Specificity)
70	98.6	1.4	8.8	91.2	1.1	0.16
80	97.1	2.9	25.5	74.5	1.3	0.11
90	94.3	5.7	47.6	52.4	1.8	0.12
100	88.6	11.4	69.8	30.2	2.9	0.16
110	85.7	14.3	84.1	15.9	5.4	0.17
120	71.4	28.6	92.5	7.5	9.5	0.31
130	64.3	35.7	96.9	3.1	20.7	0.37
140	57.1	42.9	99.4	0.6	95.2	0.43
150	50.0	50.0	99.6	0.4	125	0.50
160	47.1	52.9	99.8	0.2	236	0.53
170	42.9	57.1	100	0	>1000	0.57
180	38.6	61.4	100	0	>1000	0.64
190	34.3	65.7	100	0	>1000	0.66
200	27.1	72.9	100	0	>1000	0.73

Adapted from Diabetes Program Guide, Public Health Service Publication No. 506, 1960.
Note that as sensitivity increases, so does false-positive rate.

compute the posttest probability. One must begin with a reasonable estimate of the pretest probability of disease. The determination is made using *Bayes' theorem*, which can be summarized as

Posttest probability of disease given
a positive test =
Pretest probability × Performance of the test

The Bayes calculation can be made formally, as illustrated in Figure 1.2. Alternatively, if one thinks in terms of the *odds of disease being present,* it is easy to estimate the posttest odds of disease using *likelihood ratios* (LR). These combine the relationships of sensitivity and specificity into a single number. The *positive likelihood ratio* is the sensitivity divided by the false-positive rate, and the *negative likelihood ratio* is the false-negative rate divided by the specificity (see calculated LRs for different cutoff points to screen for diabetes in Table 1.9).

For example, suppose one is faced with a patient who is a 65-year-old obese man with increasing nocturia and with two brothers who have diabetes. Knowing that the baseline prevalence (pretest probability) of diabetes at this age has been estimated to be 20%, one might use the additional information from this patient to revise that probability to, perhaps, 33% or an odds of 1 in 2 or 0.50 [Odds = Probability ÷ (1 – Probability)]. A fasting serum glucose is drawn and is reported as 120 mg/100 mL. If one considers this level as a positive test,

Posttest odds of diabetes = Pretest odds × LR+ =
Pretest odds × (0.714 ÷ 0.075) =
0.50 × 9.5 = 4.75

So the patient has nearly a 5:1 odds of having diabetes after this one test. A second test with the same result would move those odds toward 45:1, or a probability of approximately 98% [Probability = Odds ÷ (1 + Odds)]. (The actual odds would not reach 45:1 because the two tests are not truly independent.) A nomogram that allows one to avoid converting probabilities to odds is shown in Figure 1.3. As shown in

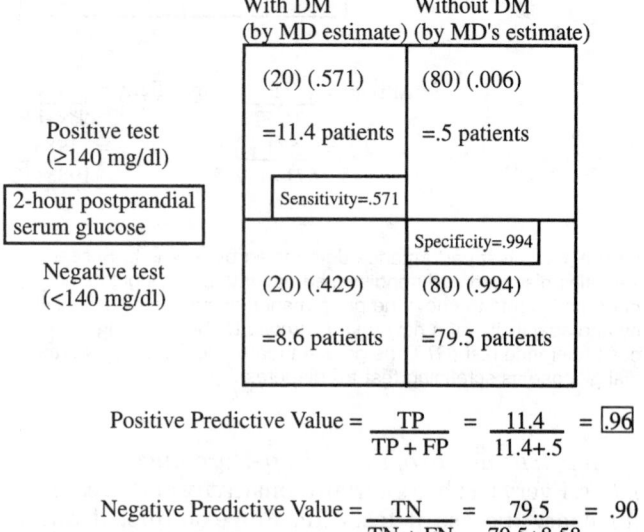

Figure 1.2. Test use performed by the clinician. Clinician knows the results of a test in a patient and the performance characteristics of the test, and needs to know whether a patient has a disease. *Example:* Middle-aged obese man with new onset of increased thirst and two first-degree relatives with Type 2 diabetes. First, clinician estimates, based on history, a pretest probability of diabetes of 20% (clinician's pretest estimate of patient not having diabetes is 80%). Two-hour postprandial glucose is measured and returns at 145 mg/dL. Clinician uses test characteristics from Figure 1.1. Therefore, posttest probability of diabetes, given a 2-hour postprandial glucose level of 145 (i.e., above 140), is 96%. (Posttest probability of no diabetes, given a 2-hour postprandial glucose level below 140, is 90%).

this example, likelihood ratios can be used easily with serial testing, which is why the use of two serial tests of serum glucose is recommended to confirm a diagnosis of diabetes in such a patient.

Treatment

Once a tentative diagnosis is made, treatment often becomes the focus of care, although diagnosis is constantly revisited in longitudinal care. Before embarking on a treatment plan, one must decide on the goals of treatment (to cure, delay complications, prevent further deterioration, relieve acute distress, reassure, or comfort). Clearly, more than one goal may be chosen. For example, when diagnosing and treating Type 2 diabetes, one may seek to cure (counseling weight loss), delay or prevent complications (teaching bodily hygiene and seeking tight glucose control), relieve acute distress (listening to the patient's fears), reassure (that diabetes is a treatable disease), and comfort (reassuring the patient that he will not be abandoned).

Once the goals have been set, treatments are chosen. Unfortunately, many treatments have never been tested scientifically to answer the questions of interest to physicians and their patients (e.g., probability of benefit, size of benefit, onset time and duration of response, or frequency of complications of treatment), and many aspects of treatment are difficult to measure through scientific experiments. These situations are changing as drugs and procedures are being increasingly subjected to clinical trials, measures of quality of life are being included in evaluation of therapies, and the

effects of cognitive therapy (e.g., counseling and reassurance) are being measured.

The *clinical trial* is the current standard for assessing drugs and therapeutic procedures. Clinical trials often are called *randomized double-blinded controlled trials,* or RCTs. This latter term is somewhat of a misnomer in the real world. For example, randomization from a population (done to ensure that treatment and control groups have equal chances of having similar traits, not to ensure that the two groups are the same) is difficult to accomplish in a real world, where patients are free to join or refuse to join a clinical trial and where money to support research is limited. A trial that is double-blinded, meaning that neither the patient nor the researcher knows who is receiving the experimental treatment, is seldom truly blind. For example, a trial of β-blockers against placebo for hypertension cannot be truly blinded because patients and doctors can measure pulse rates. Nonetheless, the clinical trial is the least biased method currently available for researchers to test how well drugs and other interventions work in ideal situations *(efficacy)* and in the real world *(effectiveness).* Table 1.10 lists guidelines that clinicians can use when assessing the results of a trial for use in their practice. Two important questions to ask of a clinical trial that reports benefits to treated subjects are: "Were measures of patient health (e.g., morbid events or functional status), not just surrogate end points (e.g., reduction of blood pressure), reported?" and "Was all-cause mortality, not just mortality due to the disease in question (e.g., colon cancer), reported?"

Researchers often report *relative risk reduction* (RRR) of treatment or *relative risk* (RR) of adverse events. Although these can be useful, they can be misleading when applied to individual patients. For example, it has been estimated that the relative risk of primary pulmonary hypertension (PPH) developing from a fenfluramine-type anorectic drug is approximately 6.3 (1). However, when looking at the general population's risk, PPH remains a very rare event (i.e., the *absolute risk* is very small), even among people taking the drug.

One can usually extract clinically helpful information by carefully reading the original report of a clinical trial. Subsequent reviews often leave out important clinical data that are provided in original studies. *Number needed to treat* (or *number needed to test* or *number needed to treat to cause harm*) is a very useful

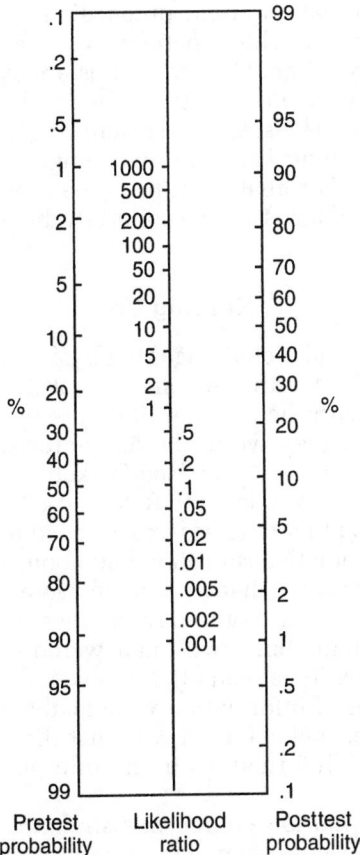

Figure 1.3. Nomogram for interpreting test results using likelihood ratios. *Example from text:* Patient with a pretest probability of having adult onset diabetes equal to 20%. Two-hour postprandial blood glucose measurement of 145 mg/dL (from published reports) gives a likelihood ratio of 95. A posttest probability (positive predictive value) is thus 96%. (Adapted from Fagan TJ. Nomogram for Bayes' theorem. N Engl J Med 293:257, 1975.)

Table 1.10. Guidelines for Assessing a Study of Therapy (Clinical Trials)

Was the assignment of patients to treatments really randomized?
Were all clinically relevant outcomes reported?
Were the study patients recognizably similar to your own?
Were both statistical and clinical significance considered?
Is the therapeutic maneuver feasible in your practice?
Were all patients who entered the study accounted for at its conclusion? (i.e., was an intention-to-treat analysis used?)

Adapted from Sackett DL, Haynes RB, Guyatt GH, Tugwell P. Clinical epidemiology: a basic science for clinical medicine. 2nd ed. Boston: Little Brown, 1991.

Table 1.11. Use of Data to Estimate Clinical Consequences of Treatment from Data from an Original Article: The Diabetes Control and Complications Trial

Occurrence of Neuropathy at 5 yr Among Type 1 Diabetic Patients		RRR	ARR	NNT to Benefit One Patient
CER: Usual Insulin	EER: Intensive Insulin	(CER − EER) ÷ CER	CER − EER	1 ÷ ARR
9.6%	2.8%	(9.6% − 2.8%) ÷ 9.6% = 71%	9.6 − 2.8% = 6.8%	1 ÷ 6.8% ≈ 15 patients, for 5 years, with intensive treatment

From The Diabetes Control and Complications Trial Research Group. The effect of intensive treatment of diabetes on the development and progression of long-term complications in insulin-dependent diabetes mellitus. N Engl J Med 329:977–986, 1993.

ARR, Absolute risk reduction; *CER,* control event rate; *EER,* experimental event rate; *NNT,* number needed to treat; *RRR,* relative risk reduction.

concept in practice, and it can be estimated from original reports. An example is the report of Diabetes Control and Complications Trial (5), which reported the clinical results of "tight control" of glucose among patients with Type 1 diabetes. In considering progression to neuropathy, the researchers reported a relative risk reduction of 71% among those using "tight control" (three or more insulin injections per day or use of an insulin pump) compared with those receiving "usual care" (one to two insulin injections per day). This also can be expressed as a relative risk of 3.4 of complications for those in usual care compared with tight control [RR = 1 ÷ (1 − RRR)]. But in analyzing the data that the researchers used, *one can estimate how many patients one would need to treat with intensive insulin therapy to prevent one case of neuropathy.* Table 1.11 explains this estimate. In this example, one would have to aggressively treat about 15 patients with Type 1 diabetes for 5 years to prevent one case of neuropathy. Similarly, one can estimate the number needed to treat to produce one episode of severe hypoglycemia, which is a problem with tight glucose control.

Prognosis

Often, the information that is most important to a patient who has a new diagnosis is the prognosis ("What is going to happen to me?"). In choosing therapy, one decides what one can do for the patient's disease. Prognosis addresses *what one will tell the patient.* Yet predicting what will happen to a particular patient is usually not possible. Thus, clinicians use probabilities to predict the future course of disease. For probabilities, they turn to familiar sources: recollections from other patients, colleagues, textbooks, and journals.

Prognosis can be addressed in two ways: *natural history* of a disease and *clinical course* of a disease. Because few diseases today progress without medical intervention, less is being learned about natural history and more is being learned about clinical course. For example, the natural history of diabetes in the late 20th century is unknown because virtually no diagnosed patients go without some type of therapy. But through dozens of studies, more is known about the course of treated diabetes (13).

Table 1.12. Guidelines for Assessing a Study of Prognosis (cohort studies)

Was an inception cohort assembled?
Was the referral pattern described?
Was complete follow-up achieved?
Were objective outcome criteria developed and used?
Was outcome assessment blind?
Was adjustment for extraneous prognostic factors carried out?

Adapted from Sackett DL, Haynes RB, Guyatt GH, Tugwell P. Clinical epidemiology: a basic science for clinical medicine. 2nd ed. Boston: Little Brown, 1991.

Most information about prognosis comes from *cohort studies,* in which patients with a disease are followed over time. Cohort studies are simple in design, yet they are often costly in time and money. They are fraught with biases, such as sampling bias, in which a group of patients being followed might not represent all patients. For that reason, guidelines have been recommended for assessing cohort studies (Table 1.12).

Keeping Up

One of the major challenges to physicians is keeping up to date. One author estimated that if doctors tried to keep up with the medical literature by reading one article a day, they would be 55 centuries behind in their reading after 1 year (see Sackett et al., *Clinical Epidemiology,* in "General References"). A seminal study showed that whereas experienced physicians in ambulatory practice said they had about two clinical questions per week that went unanswered, when they were shadowed in day-to-day practice, they actually found they had about two unanswered questions for every three patients seen (3). Moreover, they said their main sources of information were textbooks and journals, but their behavior showed that they got most of their clinical information from colleagues and drug detailers.

Each information source has strengths and weaknesses. Colleagues may be as misinformed as the questioner. Drug detailers have a product to sell, making them biased. Textbooks may be out of date, sometimes by as much as a decade. Traditional reviews fail to give important data that clinicians can apply to their own patients. Traditional continuing medical educa-

Table 1.13.   Usefulness of Information Sources Commonly Used by Doctors

Information Source	Relevance	Validity	Work	Usefulness
Evidence-based, regularly updated textbook	High	High	Low	High
Systematic journal review	High	High	Low	High
Portable summary of systematic reviews	High	High	Low	High
Internet in 10 years' time	High	High	Low	High
Drug reference book	High	Moderate	Low	High or moderate
ACP Journal Club, Evidence-Based Medicine— forerunners of systematic abstract journals	Moderate	High	Low	High or moderate
Colleagues	High	Moderate	Low	High or moderate
Standard textbook	High	Low	Low	Moderate
Standard journal review	High	Moderate	Low	Moderate
Collections of systematic reviews, such as Cochrane library	Moderate but rising rapidly	High	High but should fall	Moderate
Free medical newspapers	High	Low	Low	Moderate
Continuing medical education, lectures	Moderate	Moderate	Low	Moderate
Continuing medical education, small groups	High	Moderate	Moderate	Moderate
Consensus statements	Moderate	Moderate	Low	Moderate
Clinical guidelines	Moderate	Moderate	Low	Moderate
Online searching	Moderate	High	High	Moderate
Journal articles	Low	High	High	Low
Drug advertising	Moderate	Low	Low	Low
Drug company representatives	High	Low	Low	Low
Mass media	Low	Low	Low	Low
Internet now	Low	Low	High	Low

From Smith R. What clinical information do doctors need? BMJ 313:1062–1068, 1996.

Table 1.14.   Elements of an Information Plan

Browse at least one general journal regularly.
Maintain surveillance on new information.
Establish reliable ways of looking up common facts.
Identify a set of ways to look up obscure facts.
Develop critical appraisal skills.
Set aside high-quality time regularly to deal with information needs.
Invest time to discover new sources of useful information.

From Fletcher RH, Fletcher SW. Keeping clinically up-to-date. J Gen Intern Med 12(2):S5, 1997.

tion courses have been shown to have virtually no effect on practice. Journals are difficult to use. Smith (12) suggests an equation for assessing the usefulness of various information sources:

$$\text{Usefulness of medical information} = (\text{Relevance} \times \text{Validity}) \div \text{Work to access}$$

Table 1.13 gives this author's usefulness ratings for each of the information sources that is currently available to clinicians for decision making. Others have suggested the strategy for keeping up with information that is summarized in Table 1.14 (7).

OTHER CORE PROFICIENCIES FOR AMBULATORY PRACTICE

Information such as that provided by the National Ambulatory Medical Care Survey (see above) and the approaches to decision making in the preceding section have implications for other core proficiencies needed in the practice of ambulatory medicine. These include proficiency in clinical pharmacology, communication with patients, record keeping, coordination of care, discharge planning, and cost containment.

Clinical Pharmacology

Clinical pharmacology is the source for the many details needed for appropriate prescribing of medications. Apart from the impact of a medication on a patient's condition, it is important to be aware of the following aspects of each drug that one prescribes:

- *Practical information about initiating the drug:* appropriate starting dosage and schedule; modifications in dosage and schedule dictated by patient age, concurrently administered drugs, and the presence of diseases affecting drug metabolism; time interval for the effect of the drug to be apparent; duration of a course of the drug (when not a maintenance drug); how to assess the impact of the drug; potential interaction with other drugs the patient is taking; the approximate cost to the patient of the drug; and whether the patient can afford it
- *The major side effects of the drug:* when to anticipate them and how to detect and manage them
- *The major reasons for inadequate response to a drug:* nonadherence, insufficient dosage of drug, antagonism of the drug by patient behavior or concurrent drugs, and primary refractoriness to the drug; how to recognize and manage each of these problems
- *Practical information about adjusting the dosage:* minimum and maximum dosages that can be tried and the time intervals that are appropriate for adjusting dosages and assessing impact

Because administering or prescribing of medications is the single most common action taken by generalists in ambulatory practice (Table 1.4), access to this practical information is particularly important.

Communication and Patient Education

As stated earlier, the goals of care in ambulatory medicine are derived from the patient's expectations for activities in the community. The attainment of these goals depends on a process in which the patient has the major responsibility for carrying out the plan of care. Given this central characteristic of ambulatory medicine, proficiency in interpersonal communication and patient education is fundamental to helping patients select, concur in, and adhere to appropriate care. In recent years, these proficiencies have been delineated more explicitly, and a growing number of investigations confirm the positive impact of effective communication and patient education on patient care (see Chapters 3 and 4).

Documentation of Care

The ambulatory care records of patients should be structured in a manner that facilitates the recording and accessing of important information, both by the patient's primary care physician and by cross-covering and consultant physicians. A well-structured primary care record includes the following components:

- *A primary care front sheet* (see example in Fig. 1.4) that includes a social profile (information about living situation, marital status, family makeup, occupation, education, social and recreational environment), a problem list that is prominently displayed and facilitates awareness of the patient's problems, and other information that should be readily findable such as the patient's allergic history, past hospitalization and operations, and the status of advance directives
- *A medication/nondrug therapy flow sheet and a clinical/laboratory flow sheet* that is prominently displayed and makes important past and current information accessible for decision making
- *A preventive care profile and flow sheet* that documents the patient's risk factors and promotes the appropriate provision of periodic preventive care (see example, Fig. 2.3)
- Concise, well-organized visit and *telephone encounter notes* that document, by problem, data, and thinking (assessment/plan)
- Dividers, color-coded forms, and *standardized locations for various types of information* such as consultant's letters and laboratory reports, to increase the accessibility of clinical data

To document patient education, prescriptions, and work slips, it is helpful to use forms that make duplicates for mounting in the patient's record.

Coordination of Care

Another proficiency important in ambulatory medicine is skill in coordinating the patient's care. Coordination of care refers to referral for and interpretation of the services that a patient may need or receive. The availability of many diagnostic and consultative services requires generalists to be prudent in recommending them and in using the information they provide and to be aware of the cost of a service, the nature of the experience the patient will undergo, and the likelihood that the service will be of value to the patient.

The services recommended for patients may involve permanent, temporary, or partial transfer of responsibility for the patient's care (e.g., to a surgeon), or they may be strictly consultative, meaning that they provide information to be used by the referring physician (ranging from diagnostic test results to a consultant's suggestions).

The following general guidelines are important in coordinating the care of a patient who is referred for services by others:

- Whenever referring a patient for a service, provide the necessary information to the person who will provide the service. For example, there should be a clear documentation of what laboratory test is required or of the facts generally needed by consultants Table 1.15).
- Ensure that the patient understands the reason for services that are recommended, arrange to obtain information promptly after a service has been performed, and ensure that the patient learns, as soon as is appropriate, the meaning of this information.

Patients sometimes obtain services for medical problems without referral by their personal physician. These most often include visits to emergency departments, to specialists such as ophthalmologists, or to alternative practitioners (6). Being aware of these visits is another way in which generalists coordinate their patients' care. When they obtain services elsewhere, patients can play an essential role by requesting that information be sent to their personal physicians.

Discharge Planning

Admission of the patient to the hospital may follow 0.5 to 1% of office visits to generalists (Table 1.4). For these admissions and other admissions by surgeons and specialists, hospital discharge usually means the return of the patient to ambulatory care by the patient's primary physician. Each of the generic proficiencies described earlier is especially important when patients make the transition from dependence on hospital personnel to dependence on themselves or their families for the management of their medical problems.

Table 1.15.   Information that Subspecialty Consultants Generally Need from the Referring Physician

The specific reason for the consultation
Relevant current medical problems
Relevant current medications
Relevant diagnostic tests already completed
What the patient has been told about the referral
The patient's attitude about the problem (if relevant)
Patient's address or telephone number

Name _Doe, Jane_

Chart # _-_   FSK # _-_

Address _-_

DOB _1920_   Telephone #   H _000-000_   W _-_

Chesapeake Physicians, P.A.

PRIMARY CARE FRONT SHEET

Primary Provider _Jones_

Advance Directives   ☑ LW   ☑ DPA

Other: _(both completed 1990)_

Allergic / Drug Reactions (Year)

☐ None Known

Penicillin (hives 1968)

_____

_____

Social Profile

Marital Status _widow (2/83)_   Lives With _2 daughters_

Occupation _Retired munitions plant worker - 1950s - 1976_   Religion _Catholic_

Highest Education _High School_   Permanent Impairments _None_

Other (children, support system, activities, major life events) _2 daughters, 6 grandchildren, bowls, walks dog, active in church_

Operations and Hospitalizations (Year)

1. _Hysterectomy 1968_
2. _Carpal Tunnel Release 1975_
3. _Pneumonia 1976_
4. _____
5. _____
6. _____
7. _____
8. _____
9. _____
10. _____
11. _____
12. _____

☐ T&A ( )   ☐ Appx ( )
☐ GB ( )   ☐ TURP ( )
☒ Hys (1968)   ☐ ^B_LSO ( )
☐ BTL ( )   ☐ Vas ( )

(over for guidelines and abbreviations)

Problem List

Onset	First Note	#	Problem & Comments (Key Tests / Consults)
		1	HM (Health Maintenance)
?	'76	2	COPD FEV-1/FVC $^{1.3}$/1.9
1940's	'76	3	Smoker - stopped 1977
?	'76	4	Mitral Valve Prolapse Echo 1976
'83	'83	5	Prolonged Grief p̄ Husband ↓
'83	'83	6	Stress Incontience → learned self-control
?	'83	7	Immature Cataracts - Ophth 1983
?	'85	8	Alcoholism → Recovering; in AA since 1986

9003A (7/92)   ☐ Check if Problem List continued on reverse side

Figure 1.4.   Example of a primary care front sheet for an office record.

Beginning with the implementation of the federal prospective payment systems in the 1980s and continuing with the growth of managed care in the 1990s, very short hospital stays have become the norm in the United States. This situation has drawn attention to the elements of effective discharge planning, such as ensuring good understanding of the plan of care by patients and their families, ensuring that a concise discharge summary goes promptly to the physician(s) or settings responsible for postdischarge care, and using home health services or other community-based services to help patients accomplish care previously carried out during prolonged hospital stays.

Cost Containment and Managed Care

Because of the extraordinary increase in available medical services in the past three decades and because of the parallel increase in the cost and the use of these services, cost containment in medical care is generally recognized as a national imperative. *Managed care*—that is, health care in which delivery and financing are organized by the same entity—has emerged as a major strategy for containing costs. Managed care plans make a variety of arrangements with physicians, whom they either employ directly (in staff-model HMOs) or contract with (in group-model, network-model, and independent practice association–model HMOs) (8). Invariably, plans expect evidence-based care and encourage or impose gatekeeping by generalist physicians.

The goals of containing costs while providing high-quality care have critical implications for generalist physicians in office practice, for it is they who coordinate much of the medical care provided in our society. Physicians can address these goals in a number of ways:

- Taking a history carefully and allowing some time to pass before embarking on an extensive diagnostic workup of a new symptom
- Keeping well informed about the impact on health outcomes of costly diagnostic procedures and therapies
- Avoiding additional tests that will not alter one's decisions
- Devoting sufficient time to educating patients about their conditions (especially about conditions that often lead to inappropriate and costly doctor shopping by the patient)
- Prescribing only necessary medications and selecting the least expensive preparations
- Using home health services and other community services to forestall the need for hospital admission or to shorten length of hospitalization

In past decades, third-party reimbursement patterns promoted excessive use of laboratory tests and costly procedures, and they provided little incentive for physicians to engage in the inquiry, observation, counseling, and critical thinking about decisions that would have obviated much inappropriate use of health services. To the extent that managed care plans reward physicians for these cognitive services—and do not overburden them with administrative hurdles—these plans have the potential to both promote the health of patients and reduce the unnecessary use of costly technical services.

General References*

ACP Journal Club. Philadelphia: The American College of Physicians, since 1991.

Evidence-Based Medicine. Philadelphia: The American College of Physicians, since 1995.
> Two journals published every 2 months. One-page critical assessments of recent articles on therapy, diagnosis, prognosis, and etiology. Both cover the disciplines of internal medicine. EBM also covers pediatrics and the major disciplines of surgery.

Fletcher RH, Fletcher SW, Wagner EH, eds. Clinical epidemiology: the essentials. 3rd ed. Baltimore: Williams & Wilkins, 1996.
> All important points are simply and accurately illustrated. The book focuses on study design and its importance to the clinician, with special attention to newer developments such as meta-analysis and clinical guideline development.

Fry J, Light D, Rodnick J, Orton P. Reviving primary care: a US–UK comparison. New York: Radcliffe Medical Press, 1995.
> Analysis of the revival of primary care in both the United States and the United Kingdom. It addresses the resurgence of interests in primary care, the strengths of the discipline, and the weaknesses that remain to be addressed.

Griner PF, Mayewski RJ, Mushlin AI, Greenland P. Selection and interpretation of diagnostic tests and procedures. Ann Intern Med 94:553, 1981.
> Lucid guidelines for appropriate use of diagnostic tests (special supplementary issue).

Kassirer JP, Kopelman RI, eds. Learning clinical reasoning. Baltimore: Williams & Wilkins, 1991.
> The authors examine how physicians think and sometimes err in diagnostic logic.

The National Ambulatory Medical Care Survey. Periodic publications issued by the Department of Health and Human Services. Washington, DC.
> Nationwide study of a probability sample of office-based physicians from all medical specialty areas, using physician- and patient-generated information to delineate the ambulatory care activities of physicians and patients, started 1973.

Panzer RJ, Black ER, Griner PF. Diagnostic strategies for common medical problems. Philadelphia: American College of Physicians, 1991.
> Forty-one contributors take on 47 common problems in internal medicine, from pharyngitis to cancer, and apply clinical epidemiologic principles to them.

Phillips CL, ed. Logic in medicine. 2nd ed. Belfast: BMJ Publishing Group, 1996. (Distributed in the *US by the American College of Physicians.*)
> A British book that looks at the philosophical underpinnings of why doctors behave as they do. It does not address day-to-day practice, but it is an excellent review for those who seek the deeper meanings of physicians' behavior as they work with patients.

Sackett DL, Haynes RB, Guyatt GH, Tugwell P. Clinical epidemiology: a basic science for clinical medicine. 2nd ed. Boston: Little, Brown, 1991.
> Based on the evidence-based medicine curriculum at McMaster University, this book uses the same principles to demonstrate that clinical epidemiology is truly a bedside (office) science.

Sackett DL, Richardson WS, Rosenberg W, Haynes RB. Evidence-based medicine: how to teach and practice EBM. New York: Churchill Livingstone, 1997.

---

*Bold print (general references) and bold numerals (specific references) denote published controlled clinical trials, meta-analyses, or consensus-based recommendations.

A pocket handbook that helps learners (students or experienced physicians) to take patient problems, develop answerable questions, efficiently search out evidence, and assess whether the current evidence is adequate to direct practice.

Starfield B. Primary care: concept, evaluation, and policy. New York: Oxford University Press, 1992.

Comprehensive monograph that defines primary care, describes in detail its components, reviews the evidence of effectiveness of primary care in the United States and in 10 other countries, and delineates options for expanding the role of primary care in the United States.

Web site of the Centre for Evidence-Based Medicine, Oxford, England (http://cebm.jr2.ox.ac.uk/).

A core Web site for EBM. It includes numerous tools to practice EBM, databases of current clinical evidence, links to evidence-based journals and Internet-based journals, and links to other EBM sites, such as the Cochrane Collaboration, the NHS Centre for Reviews and Dissemination at the University of York, and McMaster University's EBM site.

Specific References

1. Abenhaim L, Moride Y, Brenot F, et al. Appetite-suppressant drugs and the risk of primary pulmonary hypertension. N Engl J Med 335:609–616, 1996.
2. Barrows HS, Norman GR, Neufeld VR, Feightner JW. The clinical reasoning of randomly selected physicians in general medical practice. Clin Invest Med 5:49, 1982.
3. Covell DG, Uman CG, Manning PR. Information needs in office practice: are they being met? Ann Intern Med 103:596–599, 1985.
4. Curtis P: The practice of medicine on the telephone. J Gen Intern Med 3:294, 1988.
5. The Diabetes Control and Complications Trial Research Group. The effect of intensive treatment of diabetes on the development and progression of long-term complications in insulin-dependent diabetes mellitus. N Engl J Med 329:977–986, 1993.
6. Eisenberg DM, Kessler RC, Foster C, et al. Unconventional medicine in the United States. N Engl J Med 328:246, 1993.
7. Fletcher RH, Fletcher SW. Evidence-based approach to the medical literature. J Gen Intern Med 12(2):S5, 1997.
8. Gold MR, Hurley R, Lake T, et al. A national survey of the arrangements managed-care plans make with physicians. N Engl J Med 333:1678–1683, 1995.
9. Fry J. Common diseases: their nature, incidence and care. 2nd ed. Philadelphia: JB Lippincott, 1979.
10. Kohn R, White KL, eds. Health care. New York: Oxford University Press, 1976.
11. Sackett DL, Rosenberg WM, Gray JAM, et al. Evidence-based medicine: what it is and what it isn't. BMJ 312:71–72, 1996.
12. Smith R. What clinical information do doctors need? BMJ 313:1062–1068, 1996.
13. Wang PH, Lau J, Chalmers TC. Meta-analysis of effects of intensive blood-glucose control on late complications of type I diabetes. Lancet 341:1306, 1993.

CHAPTER 2

Preventive Medicine in Ambulatory Practice

DAVID E. KERN, MD, MPH
SCOTT M. WRIGHT, MD

Prevention has become a central part of patient care. Medical organizations, government agencies, insurance companies, and patients themselves increasingly expect physicians to offer preventive services. In fact, physicians are in an important position to help reduce the burden of disease that affects society and its members. Evidence suggests that a doctor's advice is the single most influential factor in patients' decisions to reduce their risk of future disease (17,28). Increasingly, physicians are being trained to interpret risks to health, to effectively communicate this information to patients, and to assist patients in desired behavior changes.

Three characteristics distinguish preventive from curative care:

1. The physician, not the patient, usually initiates preventive care.
2. Preventive care aims to protect health prospectively. This is even so when health may mean, for a chronically ill patient, a sedentary existence at home rather than admission to a hospital or nursing home for preventable worsening of his or her illness.
3. In preventive care, the physician must be more certain that an intervention is effective than in the care of established disease or symptomatic conditions. Uncertainty is inherent in medicine. When an ill patient seeks treatment, the physician often must

make a best guess regarding treatment. In prevention, however, when the patient is usually healthy, there is an ethical obligation for the physician to have a high degree of certainty that any suggested intervention is likely to result in more good than harm (13).

Several considerations underlie the importance of prevention in routine office practice: (*a*) Approximately 50% of mortality from the 10 leading causes of death in the United States can be traced to alterable behavior (lifestyle) (10). (*b*) Early detection and treatment of a number of common disorders, such as breast cancer, cervical carcinoma in situ, and hypertension, effectively reduce mortality and morbidity from these conditions. (*c*) Although infectious diseases have, to a large extent, been controlled in developed countries by public health measures, including immunization, outbreaks continue to occur, especially among the poor, elderly, and immunocompromised. For example, tuberculosis is reemerging as a major cause of death, and influenza remains a major preventable cause of death (24). (*d*) The value of a comprehensive approach to prevention is suggested by the reduction in maternal and perinatal deaths that has been attributable to prenatal care (5,8). In addition, a comprehensive, preventive approach to care has been shown to reduce mortality, acute hospitalizations, and nursing home placement in high-risk elderly patients, while improving their functional status and morale (4,25,31,32).

TERMINOLOGY

Depending on when the effort is made, prevention can be divided into three stages (Fig. 2.1). *Primary prevention* prevents the disease from occurring. For example, smoking cessation decreases the likelihood that a person will develop coronary artery disease or lung cancer. Immunization against various infectious diseases also is primary prevention. *Secondary prevention* detects disease once it has begun but before it has appeared clinically. Breast examinations, Pap smears, and fecal blood tests to identify occult malignancies (in which early intervention may lead to better outcomes) represent secondary prevention. *Tertiary prevention* seeks to stop further complications after a disease has become clinically evident. Cholesterol reduction and

β-blockers given after myocardial infarction represent tertiary prevention.

Although conceptually useful, the distinctions between primary, secondary, and tertiary prevention can become blurred in clinical practice. The early detection and treatment of asymptomatic hypertension, for example, would be considered secondary prevention if one considers hypertension a disease and considers congestive heart failure, stroke, and renal failure complications of that disease. On the other hand, hypertension can be considered a risk factor for congestive heart failure, stroke, and renal failure, so that detection and treatment of hypertension to prevent these diseases from occurring can be considered primary prevention. Smoking cessation, as another example, represents primary prevention in the healthy patient but tertiary prevention in the patient with atherosclerotic cardiovascular or chronic obstructive pulmonary disease.

Several other terms are relevant to the practice of prevention. *Screening* is the process of identifying patients with unrecognized diseases or risk factors by the application of examinations, tests, or other procedures. A positive test is usually not diagnostic, but requires further testing. *Mass screening* is screening applied to a large group, and *multiphasic screening* is simultaneous screening for various diseases, such as blood pressure and cholesterol measurement done at health fairs. *Case finding* occurs in a physician's practice when the clinician screens for disease unrelated to the symptom for which the patient has come.

EVALUATING PREVENTIVE MEASURES FOR USE IN AMBULATORY PRACTICE

The first step in integrating preventive care into office practice is deciding which measures to offer patients routinely. In deciding which measures to recommend, one should consider (*a*) the burden of suffering attributable to each preventable condition, in terms of its prevalence and severity; (*b*) the availability of effective screening tests; (*c*) the efficacy, cost-effectiveness, and complications of treatment; and (*d*) the usefulness of each measure in office practice (Table 2.1). Recommendations that are periodically published by organizations such as the United States Preventive Services Task Force, Canadian Task Force on the

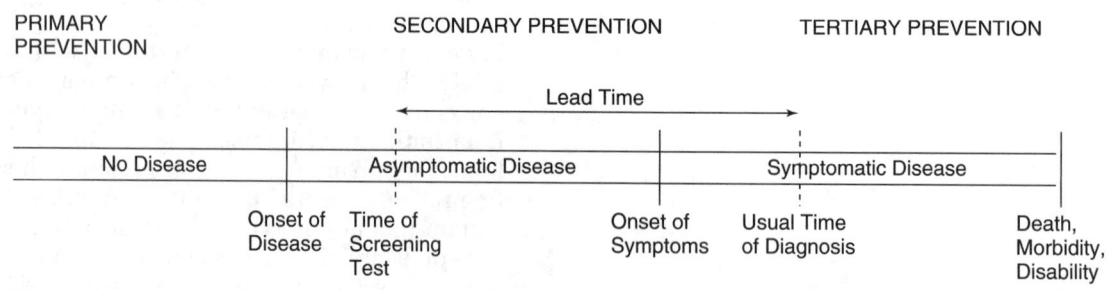

Figure 2.1. Primary, secondary, and tertiary prevention in the spectrum of a disease (see text for definitions).

Table 2.1. Questions to Ask in Evaluating
a Recommended Preventive Measure

What Is the Burden of Suffering Attributable to the Targeted Condition?
What is the prevalence and/or incidence of the condition?
What is the size of the attributable morbidity?
What is the mortality rate?

Do Efficacious Screening Tests Exist?
Do they have acceptable sensitivity, specificity, and predictive value?[a]
Are they reliable?[a]
Are they practical and reasonably priced?
Are the side effects of screening acceptable?

Is Preventive Intervention Efficacious in Research Settings?
Is the intervention efficacious in study groups?
Are compliance levels in study situations acceptable?
Are side effects acceptable?
Is intervention in the asymptomatic stage more beneficial than intervention after onset of symptoms?

Would Use of the Measure be Effective in Routine Office Practice?
Have suitable field trials been conducted?
Is the measure effective in reducing morbidity and mortality in non-study situations?
Are the compliance levels in nonstudy situations acceptable?
Are side effects in nonstudy situations acceptable?
What are the reliability, sensitivity, specificity, and predictive value of screening tests in one's own setting?[a]
Is the measure cost-effective?

[a]See Chapter 1 for a discussion of reliability, sensitivity, specificity, and predictive value.

Periodic Health Examination, the American Cancer Society, the American College of Physicians, the American Medical Association, the Centers for Disease Control and Prevention (CDC), and others can be consulted. For some measures, however, the recommendations are conflicting. The reports of the United States Preventive Services Task Force and the Canadian Task Force are firmly grounded in clinical epidemiology and provide the most scientific, least biased framework to date for evaluating which preventive health measures should be included in routine care (see "General References").

In evaluating a given measure, it is important to be aware of certain terms, concepts, pitfalls, and special considerations. The terms *sensitivity, specificity, prevalence,* and *predictive value,* which help define the value of a screening test, are defined in Chapter 1. *Efficacy* describes how well a test or maneuver performs under ideal circumstances. *Effectiveness* describes how well a test or maneuver performs under real-world circumstances. The effectiveness of a test or maneuver is usually somewhat less than its efficacy. *Efficiency* describes how well the test or maneuver optimizes the use of limited resources. A *risk factor* is anything that, if present, increases the likelihood of disease. The proportion of a specific disease that can be accounted for by a risk factor is called the *attributable risk.*

Lead time (Fig. 2.1) is the period between the early detection of disease and its usual time of diagnosis. In the evaluation of the efficacy of early detection and treatment, lead time must be subtracted from overall survival time in screened patients to avoid *lead time bias.* Otherwise, early detection might increase the duration of patients' awareness of their disease without reducing morbidity or mortality. Numerous cancer screening procedures have been thought to improve survival until lead time was addressed (1). A related bias in screening is *length-time bias* (also called length bias, time-linked biased sampling, and length-biased sampling). Most types of tumors have variable rates of growth. Screening tests may selectively find slow-growing tumors, which have long presymptomatic stages and better prognoses, but miss fast-growing cancers, which have short presymptomatic stages, develop and become clinically manifest between screening intervals, and have worse prognoses. Thus, survival is better for patients detected by screening because of the characteristics of the tumor (less aggressive, lower grade), and not because of the screening. *Selection bias* occurs when patients undergoing a preventive measure differ from those with whom they are compared in a manner that affects the likelihood of their developing disease or the natural history of their disease, once acquired. Volunteers, for example, may have more healthful lifestyles than those who do not volunteer. In the absence of randomized assignment to preventive care and control groups, these types of biases are difficult to avoid.

The process of screening itself can cause morbidity, independent of any physical complications from the screening test. If a disease is rare or if the screening test does not have a high specificity (see Chapter 1), a screening campaign will result in people being labeled as having a disease, when they are in fact healthy *(false positives),* thereby causing suffering in the absence of disease. Thus, it is usually important to follow positive screening tests with more specific diagnostic tests, which themselves may carry risks. If a screening test does not have a high sensitivity (see Chapter 1), some patients with the disease may be inappropriately reassured that they are healthy *(false negatives)* and may not seek care promptly when they become symptomatic. Even when a test correctly identifies patients with a disease, evidence suggests that undue suffering can occur from the *labeling* effect (11,12,27). For example, one study showed that absenteeism from work increased after workers were found to be hypertensive (12). A disadvantage of mass screening is that a significant proportion of labeled people will not seek follow-up with a physician. Physicians can minimize problems of labeling by (*a*) confirming that a problem is present, usually through repeated or additional observations; (*b*) taking time to explain the meaning of a problem to a patient and answering his or her questions (effective patient education); (*c*) screening only for conditions for which early detection is likely to benefit the patient; and (*d*) ensuring follow-up.

Caution should be used in adopting recommendations or guidelines that are based on proof of efficacy in highly controlled situations. Costs and conditions may be different in office practice. For example, before deciding to screen for carotid artery disease, it is important to know the level of expertise and complication rate associated with carotid endarterectomy at one's institution. Before recommending routine sigmoidoscopy to all patients over the age of 50 (a recommendation based on less than conclusive evidence in study situations), the clinician should assess the cost, availability of diagnostic services, and complication rates in the local setting. Although colon perforation rates of less than 1 per 1000 examinations have been reported among trained gastroenterologists, the rates for trained and untrained generalists have not been established.

Despite these precautions, there is sufficient evidence to support the integration of a number of primary and secondary preventive measures into office practice. Failure to do so reflects an inadequacy in the provision of primary care.

COMPONENTS OF PREVENTIVE CARE

General Examination and Baseline Data

Most physicians perform a baseline general examination (history, physical, and selected laboratory tests) for some or all of their ambulatory patients. In addition, some physicians update all or part of this examination on a periodic basis. As contrasted to the provision of selected preventive care measures discussed below, no firm scientific evidence links most of the general examination to reductions in morbidity and mortality. However, most clinicians would agree that knowledge of a patient's past hospitalizations and operations; past and present illnesses; medication and allergic history; and diet, habit, social, and family history is indispensable to the provision of effective preventive, symptomatic, and curative care. Periodic general examinations are sometimes required and may be of use for people upon whom others' lives depend (e.g., airline pilots).

Provision of Selected Measures for Asymptomatic Patients (Primary and Secondary Preventive Care)

It is generally recommended that physicians offer asymptomatic patients certain preventive care measures, selected on the basis of their likely benefits versus harm (see above and Table 2.1). Preventive measures that are often considered for inclusion in the care of asymptomatic nonpregnant adults are summarized in Table 2.2. For each preventive measure, the table provides the following information:

1. The *patient population* to which the measure should be applied (age, sex, risk status)
2. Recommended *time interval between preventive interventions*
3. *Quality of the evidence* regarding the effectiveness of the intervention, classified using a rating system (I–III) adapted by the United States Preventive Services Task Force (USTF) and the Canadian Task Force (CTF) on the Periodic Health Examination from one originally developed by the Canadian Task Force:

   I. Evidence obtained from at least one properly randomized controlled trial
  II-1. Evidence obtained from well-designed controlled trials without randomization
  II-2. Evidence obtained from well-designed cohort or case-control analytic studies, preferably from more than one center or research group
  II-3. Evidence obtained from comparison between times or places (CTF) or from multiple time series (USTF) with or without the intervention. Dramatic results in uncontrolled experiments (such as the results of the introduction of penicillin treatment in the 1940s) could also be regarded as this type of evidence.
  III. Opinions of respected authorities, based on clinical experience, descriptive studies, or reports of expert committees

4. *Strength of the recommendation* for including or excluding the preventive measure in the care of asymptomatic patients, classified using a rating system (A–E) developed by the Canadian Task Force on the Periodic Health Examination and adapted by the U.S. Preventive Services Task Force
  A. There is good evidence to support the recommendation that the condition be specifically considered in a periodic health examination.
  B. There is fair evidence to support the recommendation that the condition be specifically considered in a periodic health examination.
  C. There is insufficient evidence to recommend for or against the inclusion (USTF) or poor evidence regarding the inclusion or exclusion (CTF) of the condition in a periodic health examination, but recommendations may be made on other grounds.
  D. There is fair evidence to support the recommendation that the condition be excluded from consideration in a periodic health examination.
  E. There is good evidence to support the recommendation that the condition be excluded from consideration in a periodic health examination.
  In determining the strength of recommendation, special emphasis was placed on the strength of the evidence regarding the effectiveness of preventive intervention, but consideration was also given to the burden of suffering caused by the target condition and to the characteristics of the intervention (e.g., cost, invasiveness, complications).

5. *Location of additional information elsewhere in this book*

The preventive measures summarized in Table 2.2 pertain to average and high-risk asymptomatic adults. Factors that may dictate expanded or more limited surveillance for the individual patient may not be included. A characteristic that should always be considered when planning preventive care, for example, is the expected longevity of an individual patient. Thus, a 55-year-old male patient with inoperable lung cancer should receive influenza and pneumococcal vaccines, but should not receive most of the other preventive care

Table 2.2. Preventive Measures to Consider in the Care of Asymptomatic Nonpregnant Adults

Preventive Measure	Patient Population (Age, Sex, Risk Status)	Time Interval	Quality of Evidence Regarding Effectiveness of Intervention	Strength of Recommendation	Chapter to See for Details
Good Evidence to Include					
Blood pressure	All M, F	1–2 yr	1,[a] III[b]	A,[a] B[b]	62
Cervical cytology (Pap test)	All F, onset of sexual activity or age 18 (whichever comes earlier) to age 60 or 70 (assuming past normal cytology)	1 yr × 2, then 3 yr[d]	II-2,[a,b] II-3[a]	A,[a] B[b]	95
Folate prophylaxis	F, previously affected pregnancy (neural tube deficit) or planning pregnancy	Beginning 1–3 months before conception through 1st trimester	I,[a,b] II-2[a,b]	A[a,b]	93
	F, capable of pregnancy	Ongoing	II-2[a,b]	A,[b] B[a]	93
Gonococcal culture, screening	High-risk M, F[e]	Discretionary	II-2,[a,b] III[a]	A,[b] B[a]	27, 94
Hepatitis B vaccination	All young adults not previously immunized and high-risk M, F of all ages[f]	3 doses, at 0, 1, and 6 months	I,[a] II-3[a]	A[a]	32, 43
HIV antibody testing	High-risk M, F[g]	Discretionary	I,[a,b] II-2[a]	A[a,b]	34
Influenza vaccination	All M, F ≥65; High-risk M, F of all ages[h]; Health providers for high-risk patients	1 year	I,[a] II-2[a,b]	A,[a] B[b]	32
Mammography, with (preferable) or without clinical breast examination by physician	All F 50–69	1–2 yr	I,[a,b] II-2[a]	A[a,b]	89
Measles, mumps, rubella (MMR) vaccination (live)	All M and nonpregnant F born after 1956 who lack evidence of immunity to measles[i]	Once	I[a]	A[a]	32
Pneumococcal vaccination	High-risk M, F[j] (see below for others)	Once	I,[a,b] II-2[a,b]	A,[b] B[a]	32
Smoking/tobacco use, counseling	All M, F	1–5 yr	I,[a,b] II-2[a]	A[a,b]	20
Syphilis (serology), screening	High-risk M, F[e]	Discretionary	II-3[a]	A[a]	30, 94
Tetanus/diphtheria vaccination	All M, F	10–30 yr (boosters), primary series at 0, 2, and 6–14 months if not previously immunized	I,[a] II-3[a]	A[a]	32
Tuberculin skin test	High-risk M, F	Discretionary	I,[a,b] II-2[b]	A[a,b]	29, 34
Travel to developing countries: immunization, prophylactic medications, counseling regarding preventive health practices	At-risk M, F	Varies	Varies with specific measure	A[c]	33
Fair Evidence to Include					
Alcohol use, screening, with counseling of patients with problem drinking and counseling/referral of alcohol dependent patients	All M, F	Discretionary	I,[a,b] II-2[a]	B[a,b]	21
Birth control counseling to reduce unwanted pregnancies	All sexually active M, F of childbearing age, especially adolescents	Discretionary	II-3[a,b]	B[a,b]	93

Continued

Table 2.2—*continued.* Preventive Measures to Consider in the Care of Asymptomatic Nonpregnant Adults

Preventive Measure	Patient Population (Age, Sex, Risk Status)	Time Interval	Quality of Evidence Regarding Effectiveness of Intervention	Strength of Recommendation	Chapter to See for Details
Chlamydia screening	High-risk F[l]	Discretionary, recommend at time of Pap smears[c]	I,[a,b] II-2,[a,b] III[a]	B[a,b]	27, 94
Cholesterol, nonfasting total cholesterol levels with further evaluation and treatment of those found to be hypercholesterolemic[m]	All M 35–65 All F 45–65	5 yr	I,[a,b] II-2,[a] III[b] II-2[a]	B,[a,b] C[b] B[a]	75
Colorectal cancer screening					
Fecal occult blood testing	All M, F >40–50	1 yr	I,[a,b] II-1,[a] II-2[a]	B,[a] C[b]	38
Sigmoidoscopy		3–10 yr	II-2,[a,b] II-3[a]	B,[a] C[b]	
Dietary					
Limit dietary fat	All M, F	Ongoing	I,[a,b] II-2,[a,b] II-3[a]	A,[a] B[b]	75
Limit dietary cholesterol	All M, F	Ongoing	II-2[a]	B[a]	75
Increase fruits, vegetables, grain products containing fiber	All M, F	Ongoing	II-2,[a,b] II-3[a]	B[a]	39, 75
Maintain caloric balance through diet and exercise	All M, F	Ongoing	II-2[a]	B[a]	—
Maintain adequate calcium intake	All M, F	Ongoing	I,[a] II-1,[a] II-2,[a] II-3[a]	B[a]	74, 77
Dietary counseling by					
Specially trained educators	All M, F	Discretionary, follow-up important	I[a,b]	B[a]	—
Primary care physician	All M, F	Discretionary, follow-up important	III[a]	B,[b,n] C[a,b,o]	—
Hearing impairment, screening	All M, F >65	Discretionary	I,[a,b] III[a,b]	B[a,b]	96
Hormone replacement therapy, counseling[p]	Perimenopausal and postmenopausal women	Discretionary	I,[a,b] II-2[a,b]	B[a,b]	74, 77
Pneumococcal vaccination	All M, F ≥65 (see above for others)	Once	I,[b] II-2,[a,b] II-3[b]	B,[a] C[b]	32
Rubella vaccination (or MMR); or rubella antibody screening and vaccination of those susceptible[q]	All nonpregnant F of childbearing age without documentation of previous rubella vaccination (age ≥1)	Once	II,[b] II-2[a]	B[a,b]	32
Seat belt use, counseling	All M, F	Discretionary	II-1,[a] II-3[a,b]	B[a,b]	—
Skin inspection to detect skin cancer	High-risk M, F[r]	Discretionary	II-3,[a,b] III[a]	B,[b] C[a]	100
Visual acuity testing	All M, F >65	Discretionary	II-2,[b] II-3[a]	B[a,b]	97
Insufficient Evidence to Include or Exclude					
Abdominal aortic aneurysm, screening Physical examination Ultrasonography	All M, F ≥60	Discretionary	II-2,[a,b] III[b]	C[a,b]	87
Aspirin therapy for the primary prevention of cardiovascular disease	All M 40–84 All F 50–84	Not applicable	I[a,b] II-2[a,b]	C[a,b] C[a,b]	52, 57
Bicycle helmets[s]	All M, F	Discretionary	I,[a,b] III[a]	C[a,b]	—
Bone densitometry	Postmenopausal F	Discretionary	II-2,[a,b] III[b]	C,[a] D[b]	74, 77

Preventive Measure	Patient Population (age, sex, risk status)	Time Interval	Quality of Evidence Regarding Effectiveness of Intervention	Strength of Recommendation	Chapter to See for Details
Breast self-examination, teaching/encouraging	All F ≥20	1 month	I,[a] II-2,[a,b] III[a]	C[a,b]	89
Carotid artery stenosis, screening					
Auscultation	All M, F >40–60 or at high risk for atherosclerotic cardiovascular disease	Discretionary	I,[a] II-2,[a] III[b]	C,[a] D[b]	83
Auscultation or ultrasound			I,[a] II-2[a]	C[a]	
Dementia (cognitive impairment) screening	All M, F ≥65–75	Discretionary	II-2,[b] III[a,b]	C[a,b]	17
Dental hygiene, physician screening (for periodontal disease) or counseling (regarding brushing, flossing, fluoride, diet, and regular dental visits)[t]	All M, F	Discretionary	III[a,b]	C[a,b]	101
Depression, screening	All M, F	Discretionary	I,[a,b] II-1[a]	C,[a] D[b]	17
Diabetes mellitus, screening (with plasma glucose or glycosylated hemoglobin)	All M, F	Discretionary	II-2[a,b]	C,[a] D[b]	72
Domestic violence, screening	All F and elderly	Discretionary	II-3,[a] III[a,b]	C[a,b]	21
Driving while impaired by alcohol or drugs, counseling	All M, F	Discretionary	III[a]	C[a,b]	21, 22
Drug abuse, screening	All M, F	Discretionary	III[a]	C[a]	22
Electrocardiography, resting or exercise	All M, F ≥50	Discretionary	II-2[a]	C[a]	57
Exercise, inquiry and counseling (to promote physical activity, which is associated with decreases in premature mortality, cardiovascular disease, obesity, osteoporosis, and improvements in self-esteem, stress management, lipoprotein levels, and physical fitness)	All M, F	Discretionary	I,[a] II-2,[a] III[b]	C[a,b]	6, 58, 74–76
Falls prevention, counseling[u]	All M, F ≥70–75	Discretionary	I,[a] III[b]	C[a,b]	6
Firearms at home, counseling[v]	All M, F	Discretionary	III[a,b]	C[a,b]	—
Mammography, with (preferable) or without clinical breast examination by physician	All F 40–49 All F ≥70	1–2 yr	I,[a,b] II-3[a] I,[a] II-3,[a] III[a]	C,[a] D[b] C[a]	89
Obesity					
Screening (weight and height measurement)	All M, F	Discretionary	I,[a,b] II-2,[a,b] II-3[a]	C,[b] B[a]	76
Counseling			II-2[b]	C[b]	
Sexually transmitted diseases, counseling	All sexually active M, F	Discretionary	I,[a] II-2[a]	C[a]	27, 34, 94
Thyroid function tests (TSH) or clinical examination to diagnose occult hyper- and hypothyroidism	All F, postmenopausal	Discretionary	I,[a,b] II-3,[a] III[a,b]	C[a,b]	73
Tonometry and ophthamoscopy to detect glaucoma	All M, F ≥40	Discretionary	I,[a,b] II-2,[a,b] III[a,b]	C[a,b]	98

Continued

Table 2.2—*continued.* **Preventive Measures to Consider in the Care of Asymptomatic Nonpregnant Adults**

Preventive Measure	Patient Population (age, sex, risk status)	Time Interval	Quality of Evidence Regarding Effectiveness of Intervention	Strength of Recommendation	Chapter to See for Details
Fair to Good Evidence to Exclude					
Lung cancer screening					
Chest radiograph	All smoking M, F	4 months–1 yr	I,[a,b] II-1,[a] II-2[a]	D,[a] E[b]	56
Sputum cytology		4 months	I,[a,b] II-1,[a] II-2[a]	D[a,b]	
Gonococcal culture	All sexually active M, F	Discretionary	II-2,[b] III[a]	D[a,b]	27, 94
Electrocardiography, resting	All M, F ≤50	Discretionary	III[a]	D[a]	57
Prostate cancer screening, digital rectal examination	All M ≥40–50	1 yr	II-2,[a,b] II-3[b]	D,[a] C[b]	49
prostate specific antigen (PSA), prostate acid phosphatase, transrectal ultrasound, or magnetic resonance imaging (MRI) to detect prostate cancer		1–2 yr	I,[a] II-2,[a] II-3,[b] III[a]	D[a,b]	

This table is organized into four major categories, based on the *strength of the recommendation* for including or excluding a preventive measure, as rated by the U.S. Preventive Services Task Force (USTF) and the Canadian Task Force on the Periodic Health Examination (CTF) (see text for explanation of ratings). When ratings differ between the USTF and CTF, a preventive measure is placed in one of the four categories based upon its highest rating. Preventive measures are listed in alphabetical order under each category.

[a] Rated by the USTF. See text for explanation of ratings.

[b] Rated by the CTF. See text for explanation of ratings.

[c] Rated by the authors on the basis of USTF, CTF, or other reports.

[d] Recommended intervals vary. When screening is initiated it is often recommended that the first two to three smears be obtained 1 yr apart to compensate for possible physician error in collection or laboratory error. The best tradeoff between yield and use of resources for the general population seems to occur at a screening interval of 3 yr. Risk factors such as early onset of sexual intercourse, history of multiple sexual partners, and low socioeconomic status may warrant more frequent testing. More frequent intervals are recommended for HIV-infected patients (currently every 6 months until two successive normals, then every yr).

[e] High-risk groups include persons with multiple sexual partners or a partner with multiple sexual contacts, sexual contacts of persons known to have a sexually transmitted disease, persons with repeated episodes of gonorrhea, and prostitutes.

[f] High-risk groups include homosexually active men, injection drug users and their sex partners, persons who have a history of sexual activity with multiple partners in the previous 6 months or who have recently acquired another sexually transmitted disease, international travelers to countries where HBV is of high or intermediate endemicity, and persons in health-related jobs with frequent exposure to blood or blood products.

[g] High-risk groups include homosexual and bisexual men, prostitutes and their sex partners, injection drug users and their sex partners, people with sexually transmitted diseases, people who received blood products between 1978 and 1985, sexual contacts of HIV-positive people, and people from countries with a high prevalence of HIV infection.

[h] High-risk groups include residents of chronic care facilities and other institutions and persons with chronic cardiopulmonary disorders, metabolic diseases (including diabetes mellitus), hemoglobinopathies, immunosuppression, or renal dysfunction.

[i] Evidence of immunity can include receipt of two doses of live vaccine after first birthday, laboratory evidence of immunity, or physician-diagnosed disease. Contraindicated in immunosuppressed and pregnant patients. Women should be advised not to become pregnant for 1–3 months after vaccination. Patients vaccinated before 1967 are likely to have received inactivated vaccine or have been vaccinated before the age of 12 months. Two doses may be required ≥1 month apart to ensure long-term efficacy.

[j] High-risk groups include patients with sickle cell disease, patients postsplenectomy; institutionalized patients ≥50, people in epidemic or endemic settings. Antibody levels may fall after 5 yr, and revaccination at 5-yr intervals is recommended by the Advisory Committee on Immunization Practices (ACIP) of The Centers for Disease Control and Prevention (see Chapter 32).

[k] High-risk groups include household/close contacts of patients with tuberculosis (e.g., staff members of tuberculosis clinics, homeless shelters); recent immigrants from countries with high tuberculosis prevalence; migrant workers and other populations with high prevalence of tuberculosis; residents of nursing homes, correctional institutions, and homeless shelters; persons with certain underlying medical disorders (e.g., HIV infection); alcoholics; and injection drug users.

[l] High-risk group includes sexually active female ≤25; new sexual partner; multiple sexual partners; history of sexually transmitted disease; cervical friability, ectopy, or mucupurulent discharge; unmarried status; inconsistent use of barrier contraceptives; other settings where prevalence is known to be high.

[m] Because of biologic variation and measurement error, two blood tests are often recommended to provide a more accurate measure for classification of risk. When total cholesterol concentration is >200–240 mg/dL (>5.2–6.2 mmol/L), a fasting determination of total cholesterol, triglyceride, and HDL-cholesterol levels with calculation of LDL-cholesterol level is recommended to more precisely determine risk and direct treatment (see Chapter 75).

[n] General dietary advice on fat and cholesterol intake, M 30–69 (CTF).

[o] General dietary advice on fat and cholesterol intake, all others (CTF).

[p] Patients should receive information on the benefits and risks of hormonal therapy. Concerns about actual and potential complications of treatment prevented a higher level recommendation. The presence of postmenopausal symptoms, a high risk of fracture (thin, Caucasian, premature or surgical menopause), the absence of a uterus, and potential cardiovascular/lipoprotein benefits increase the likelihood of benefit in individual patients. Hormonal replacement therapy is contraindicated in patients with breast cancer. See Chapters 74 and 77 for details.

[q] For prevention of congenital rubella. Contraindicated in immunosuppressed and pregnant patients. Women should be advised not to become pregnant for 1–3 months after vaccination.

[r] High-risk groups defined as persons of high risk for cancer of skin, such as outdoor workers, and those in contact with polycyclic aromatic hydrocarbons.

[s] Efficacy of physician counseling unproven. There is good (A) evidence, based on level II-2 and II-3 evidence, to support wearing approved helmets.

[t] Efficacy of physician screening or counseling to change behaviors has not been adequately evaluated. There is fair (B) to good (A) evidence, however, based on level I, II-1, and II-2 evidence to support water fluoridation, tooth brushing with fluoride-containing toothpaste, and professionally applied topical fluorides (for high-risk patients) to prevent caries, and to support regular brushing and flossing, professional scaling and prophylaxis, and use of chlorhexidine or listerine oral rinses as an adjunct to tooth cleaning to prevent gingivitis/periodontal disease.

[u] Efficacy of physician counseling to patients to address risk factors for falls unproven. There is good (A) to fair (B) evidence, based on I, II-1, and II-2 level evidence, to support multidisciplinary assessment and intervention to prevent falls in the elderly.

[v] Efficacy of physician counseling is unproven. There is fair (B) evidence, based on level II-2, II-3, and III evidence to support removal of guns from or safe storage of guns in the home (USTF).

appropriate for his age and sex. On the other hand, a 50-year-old male patient who has survived an uncomplicated myocardial infarction at the age of 48 has a reasonable life expectancy and should be offered all of the preventive care appropriate for his age group. Another characteristic that may influence decisions about preventive care is the presence of certain diseases. For example, in the presence of hereditary polyposis or ulcerative colitis, endoscopic screening should be encouraged because of the increased risk of colorectal cancer.

Preventive Care for Established Conditions (Tertiary Preventive Care)

Preventing complications of chronic diseases is a major part of office practice. By careful practice of tertiary prevention, physicians may minimize or postpone the poor outcomes of diabetes mellitus, congestive heart failure, degenerative joint disease, and other conditions. Of course, appropriate preventive care for an established disease depends on the disease and the patient. Examples include appropriate education and monitoring of foot care and screening for retinopathy in diabetic patients, taking steps to enhance compliance and prevent rehospitalization in a poorly compliant elderly patient with congestive heart failure, prescribing aspirin and controlling cholesterol in a hypercholesterolemic patient after myocardial infarction, and providing short-term counseling for a survivor of a myocardial infarction who is showing early symptoms of depression. The strategies for optimal preventive management of established conditions are discussed in later chapters.

Extending Prevention to the Family and the Community

Physicians should extend preventive care beyond the individual when this is appropriate. In some instances, preventive treatment should be recommended for members of a *patient's family and other close contacts.* Immunoglobulin prophylaxis for the family of a patient with infectious hepatitis A and treatment of sexual contacts of patients with sexually transmitted diseases are classic examples. In other situations, the physician should recommend evaluation of the relatives of patients with certain chronic diseases that show a tendency to occur in families. For example, relatives of patients with familial hypercholesterolemia should have plasma lipid levels determined, and routine screening should be encouraged for at-risk relatives of patients with breast and colon cancers.

Prevention should be extended to the *community at large* when a *notifiable communicable disease* is diagnosed in an individual patient (Table 2.3). Similarly, any suspected *occupational disease* in an individual worker should be reported to local health authorities. Such reporting may be critical in protecting the health of other workers in that environment (see Chapter 7).

More emphasis is being placed on this *social role of the doctor.* Although doctors are bound to protect confidentiality, some states and some courts have ruled that society's welfare occasionally outweighs the patient's right to privacy. Some states now require reporting of all patients with newly diagnosed human immunodeficiency virus (HIV) infection, and some protect physicians who break confidentiality to notify exposed individuals at risk. Most courts agree that doctors are bound to notify individuals when patients make threats to harm them. Primary care physicians should become acquainted with local and state rules regarding reporting.

Finally, some practices are situated to address the *preventive care needs of defined populations and not just the patients who visit the practice.* Examples of defined populations might be all enrollees in a managed care plan assigned to one's practice or people living in a geographic area related to one's practice. Increasingly, practices are being encouraged to develop processes by which the health problems and preventive care needs of such defined populations can be systematically identified and addressed. This approach to health care, called *community-oriented primary care,* combines principles of primary care medical practice, clinical epidemiology, and public health (26). Increasing computerization, health care databases, and opportunities for the linkages of databases are enhancing the feasibility of such approaches. However, limited financial support is an important current barrier to widespread implementation.

PUTTING PREVENTION INTO PRACTICE

Physician Performance

Despite sound evidence that supports the routine provision of selected preventive measures, studies show that physicians often fail to provide them (7,19,21,30). This is so even in academic centers (14,16,22,35). Results from the CDC's 1992 National Health Interview Survey illustrated that Pap tests were obtained within the last 3 years for 67% of eligible women, clinical breast examinations in 50% within the last 1 year, mammography in 36% within the last year, and fecal occult blood testing in 14% within the last year (33). Although these rates represent an improvement from the last time this data was collected (1987), the results are still far short of the national health objectives for the year 2000 (33).

Barriers to Optimal Performance

Only recently has organized medicine begun to emphasize prevention as an integral part of adult medical care. Favorable physician attitudes toward prevention have been shown to be important predictors of performance (7). Noncoverage of preventive services by fee-for-service insurance companies has created a financial barrier for many patients. However, this barrier is rapidly decreasing, as increasing numbers of patients enter HMO or managed care practices and as increasing numbers of private insurers decide to

Table 2.3. Reportable Diseases and Conditions[a]

Acquired immunodeficiency syndrome (AIDS) and symptomatic human immunodeficiency virus (HIV) infection[b]
Amebiasis
Animal bites[c]
Anthrax[b,c]
Botulism[b,c]
Brucellosis[b]
Cancer, most types
Chancroid
Chlamydia trachomatis, genital infection[b]
Cholera[b,c]
Coccidiomycosis[b]
Congenital rubella syndrome[b,c]
Congenital syphilis[b]
Cryptosporidiosis[b]
Diphtheria[b,c]
Encephalitis[b]
Encephalitis, postinfectious[b]
Escherichia coli 0157:H7
Gonocorrhea[b]
Haemophilus influenzae, invasive disease[b,c]
Hantavirus pulmonary syndrome
Hemolytic-uremic syndrome, postdiarrheal
Hepatitis A
Hepatitis B
Hepatitis C/non-A, non-B
HIV infection, pediatric (age <13)[b]
Kawasaki syndrome
Legionellosis[b]
Leprosy (Hansen disease)[b]
Leptospirosis
Lyme disease[b]
Malaria[b]
Measles (rubeola)[b,c]

Meningitis (viral, bacterial, parasitic, and fungal)
Meningococcal disease[b,c]
Mumps (infectious parotitis)[b]
Mycobacteriosis, other than tuberculosis and leprosy
Occupational disease
Pertussis[b,c]
Pertussis vaccine adverse reactions
Plague[b,c]
Poliomyelitis, paralytic[b,c]
Psittacosis[b]
Rabies, human or animal[b,c]
Rocky Mountain spotted fever[b]
Rubella (German measles)[b,c]
Salmonellosis[b]
Septicemia in newborns
Shigellosis[b]
Streptococcal disease, invasive, group A[b]
Streptococcal toxic shock syndrome[b]
Streptococcus pneumoniae, drug resistant[b]
Syphilis[b]
Tetanus[b]
Toxic shock syndrome[b]
Trichinosis[b]
Tuberculosis[b]
Tularemia[b]
Typhoid fever[b,c]
Varicella (chickenpox)[d]

An outbreak of disease of known or unknown etiology that may be a danger to public health[c]
A single case of a disease of known or unknown etiology that may be a danger to public health
An unusual manifestation of a communicable disease

[a]Determined at the state and federal levels. Reportable to local health department. This list was developed based on information obtained from the Maryland Department of Health and Mental Hygiene and Department of the Environment; and from Summary of Notifiable Diseases, United States, 1995, MMWR 45(53):i-64, 1996. Other disease may be reportable in other states.

[b]Notifiable Diseases, United States (reported by state or local health departments to the Centers for Disease Control and Prevention, Atlanta, Georgia).

[c]Reportable immediately by telephone to the local health department.

[d]Although varicella is not a nationally notifiable disease, the Council of State and Territorial Epidemiologists recommends reporting of cases of this disease to the CDC.

pay for preventive service. The promotion of guidelines by special interest medical groups for the provision of innumerable preventive services has been overwhelming and confusing to practicing physicians and the public alike, because the guidelines are often short-lived, conflicting, and based on incomplete analysis and inadequate evidence. The publishing of guidelines based on clearly defined rules of evidence by the United States Preventive Services Task Force and the Canadian Task Force on the Periodic Health Examination has helped alleviate the situation (see above and Table 2.2). Despite the guidelines, some practicing physicians choose not to follow them because they disagree with the recommendations (36,37). Also, as was shown in a study of one family practice setting, implementation of all relevant USTF recommendations would still present a formidable challenge to most practices: 15.4 risk factors, 13 screening recommendations, 10.5 counseling recommendations, and 1.1 immunization recommendations per adult patient (23). Perhaps the most important barriers to providing preventive services are physicians' time limitations and the failure of physicians to organize their practices for the efficient, reliable provision of selected indicated preventive services.

Improving Performance in One's Practice

It is generally agreed that preventive care must be planned carefully if it is to be offered routinely and effectively to patients in a busy office practice. First, agreed-upon and feasible guidelines must be developed that outline which measures are to be offered to which patients. Second, a plan must be developed to implement the guidelines.

The guidelines can be made accessible to physicians by posting them, in abbreviated form, for quick reference in each examining and consulting room (Fig. 2.2). Including health maintenance as a problem at the top of each patient's problem list (see Fig. 1.4) and including a risk profile on the front sheet or on a preventive care profile (Fig. 2.3) in the chart of each patient are methods of cueing physicians to provide indicated preventive care. Maintenance of a preventive care flow sheet (Fig. 2.3) will help the physician efficiently determine which measures are due and which have already been done. Otherwise, much time may be spent trying to retrieve relevant information that has become buried in the text of the chart. Office computers can be programmed or available computer software can be used to produce preventive care reminders for each visit, which can then be attached to each patient's chart

(3,18,20,21). Nurses (6) or midlevel practitioners also can be trained to monitor and provide preventive care within the office. Audit and feedback can result in improvements in physician performance that can be transferred from one setting to another and persist after cessation of the intervention (14,15,35). Financial reimbursement in fee-for-service settings and financial incentives in managed care settings may also motivate improved physician performance (9).

Although it is desirable to schedule special time for a baseline history and physical examination for patients new to a practice, ongoing preventive care is best incorporated into routine office visits. This is so because few visits to the doctor are purely preventive and because attendance rates are lower for preventive than for problem-based visits (29). For otherwise healthy patients who see their physicians infrequently, however, health maintenance visits should be scheduled and appointment reminders sent to increase attendance rates.

Motivating Patients

Unfortunately, simply recommending a preventive measure to a patient is not sufficient to ensure compliance. When the preventive measure involves an unpleasant procedure (e.g., sigmoidoscopy or pelvic examination) or requires active participation (e.g., collection and return of stool samples or the long-term taking of medication), poor compliance is likely. It is most likely to be a problem when the preventive intervention requires a major change in behavior on the part of the patient (e.g., dietary change or smoking cessation).

Motivating patients to comply with recommendations requires considerable skill on the part of the physician. Increasing patients' knowledge and understanding is a necessary but often insufficient prerequisite for behavioral change. Important additional ingredients for success include the establishment of a trusting, friendly, and supportive patient–physician relationship (see Chapters 3 and 4), involvement of patients in planning and monitoring their own health maintenance plan (see Chapter 4), use of motivational and behavioral strategies to enhance compliance (see Chapters 4 and 20), and the promotion of healthy, positive beliefs, attitudes, values, and self-perceptions in one's patients (see Chapter 4). Patients who have confidence and truly believe that they can affect their health are more likely to do so than those who do not. This perceived self-efficacy or expectation for success may be the best predictor of whether patients will initiate and persist in an activity (2,34). It should be remembered that a patient's motivation to comply may be different from the physician's motivation in wanting them to comply. For example, patients tend to be less impressed than physicians with long-term and more impressed with short-term benefits. Accordingly, the physician should stress the factors that seem to motivate the patient. Conversations related to prevention provide opportunities for patients to share their life goals with physicians and may increase the satisfaction of both with the doctor–patient relationship.

JOHNS HOPKINS BAYVIEW MEDICAL CENTER
GUIDELINES FOR ROUTINE HEALTH MAINTENANCE OF NONPREGNANT ADULTS

	INTERVAL	PATIENTS		INTERVAL	PATIENTS
BASELINE DATA			**PHYSICAL EXAM**		
Complete H&P	Baseline	All	Blood pressure	At least q2yr	All
			Breast examination	q1yr	All F ≥40
					(↑ risk, younger)
			Hearing	Discretionary	↑ risk (all ≥65)
LIFESTYLE, COUNSELING			Height	Once	All
Advance directives	Once, w.f/up	All	Weight	q1–2yr	All
Alcohol/drug use	q1–5yr	All			
Birth control	q1–5yr	Childb. age	**LABORATORY/PROCEDURES**		
Exercise	q1–5yr	All	Chlamydia	At time of Pap	All F ≤25, ↑ risk
Hormone replacement	Once	All F postmenop	Cholesterol (nonfast)	q5yr	All M 35–65
Sexual practices	Discretionary	All			All F 45–65
Tobacco use	q1–5yr	All	Fecal Occult Blood	q1yr	All ≥50 (↑ risk ≤50)
			GC culture, cervix	q1yr	↑ risk F
IMMUNIZATIONS			HIV antibody	Discretionary	↑ risk M, F
Hepatitis B vac.	Once (0, 1, 6 m)	↑ risk (all <25)	Mammogram	q1–2yr	All F 50–69
Influenza vac.	q1yr	↑ risk (all ≥65)			↑ risk ≥35
Measles vac. (MMR)	2 doses ≥1 month apart	All born after 1957	Pap (pt w/o cervix)	1 yr ×2, then	All F 18–60
Pneumococcal vac.	Once	↑ risk (all ≥65)		q3yr, after 2 nl	
	Booster q5yr	↑ risk	PPD	Discretionary	↑ risk
Rubella vac. (MMR)	2 doses ≥1 month apart	F childb. age	Sigmoidoscopy	q5–10yr	All ≥50 (↑ risk ≤50)
Tet/diphth toxoid	Primary (0, 1, 6–14 m)	All	STS	Discretionary	↑ risk
	Booster q10yr	All			
PREVENTION FLOW SHEET		All			
PROBLEM LIST		All			

Figure 2.2. Sample of abbreviated preventive care standards available as wallet-size cards and posted in each examining room in the medical clinic. (Johns Hopkins Bayview Medical Center, Baltimore, MD.)

Johns Hopkins Bayview Physicians, P.A.

PREVENTIVE CARE PROFILE
&
FLOW SHEET
(over for guidelines)

Patient Name __Jane Doe__

Chart # __01-23-45__

Date of Birth: __2/23/44__

BASELINE HISTORY & PHYSICAL (Dates Performed _____5/94_____)

FAMILY HISTORY (Dates Performed _____)

ASHD : N☐ Y☑ (__fa d. MI 67__) Other: _____

Breast Ca : N☐ Y☑ (__mo d. 74__) _____

Colon Ca : N☐ Y☑ (__ma uncle d. 68__) _____

HABIT HISTORY (Dates Performed __5/94, 5/95, 5/97__)

Smoking : N☑ Y☐ (__1 PPD, stopped 1994__) Seatbelt : N☐ Y☑ (_____)

ETOH : N☐ Y☑ (_____) Sexual Activity: ☐ Never ☐ Past, Currently Inactive ☑ Active

CAGE : __0__ of 4 (_____) If Active: ☑ 1 partner ☐ > 1 partner (past 1 year)

Birth Control/Safe Sex Method: __NA__ or ☐ None

Drug Use : N☑ Y☐ (_____)

Exercise : N☐ Y☑ (__walks 3-5 x/week__ / __stationary bike 3 x/wk__) Other : _____

OCCUPATIONAL HAZARDS (& Date) _____

YEAR	1994	1995	1996	1997	1998					

PHYSICAL EXAM (Date / Results)

Breast Exam	5/24 NL	6/5 NL	5/2 NL	6/20 NL						
Rectal Exam	5/24			10/15						
Hearing	NL			NL						
Vision/Glaucoma	14/94		9/96							
Dental	5/24 +brush +floss 10/1 Dentist	10/95 Dentist	11/96 Dentist	10/97 Dentist						

LABORATORY (Date / Results)

Cholesterol	5/94 176									
Hemoccult	5/94 ⊖ x3	6/95 ⊖ x3	6,8/96 No return	6/97 ⊖ x3						
Mammogram	6/94 ⊖	2/95 ⊖	6/96 ⊖	2/97 ⊖						
PAP	5/94 NL			10/97 NL						

IMMUNIZATION (Date)

Influenza										
Pneumococcal										
Tetanus/Diphtheria	5/94									
MMR										
Hepatitis B										

3003A
(8/95)

Figure 2.3. Sample preventive care flow sheet. (Johns Hopkins Bayview Physicians, PA.)

The U.S. Preventive Services Task Force recommends the following strategies for promoting behavioral change:

1. Match the teaching to the patient's perceptions. It is important to understand the patient's beliefs and concerns and to focus the teaching accordingly (e.g., "What gets in the way of your exercising regularly?"). The same "sales pitch" will not work on everyone.

2. Fully inform patients about the purposes and expected effects of an intervention (e.g., a cholesterol lowering medication) and when to expect the effects.

3. Be specific and suggest small changes rather than large ones (e.g., walking for more than 20 minutes three or more times per week, reading labels for fat or salt content when shopping, or not cooking with salt).

4. When possible, add new behaviors rather than eliminating established ones (e.g., suggesting that sexually promiscuous patients always use condoms rather than promoting abstinence).

5. Use the power of the profession. A direct simple message such as "I want you to stop smoking" may be effective simply because it is coming from a physician.

6. Try to get an explicit commitment from the patient as to how they will achieve mutually agreed-upon health goals.

7. Use a combination of strategies. Interventions that use more than one strategy are most likely to be successful.
8. Involve the entire office staff; a team approach can facilitate improved patient education.
9. Use available resources, such as voluntary health organizations (e.g., the American Diabetes Association) and patient support groups (e.g., a smoking cessation group).
10. Monitor progress through follow-up contact.

Mechanical aids may assist this process. Printed education materials can provide information on preventive care measures for patients. Easy-to-use forms for recording and monitoring their own preventive care may promote patients' involvement in their own care, thereby prompting patients to achieve and physicians to address recommended preventive measures.

General References*

Canadian Task Force Publications

The Canadian Task Force on the Periodic Health Examination. **The Canadian guide to clinical preventive health care.** Ottawa: Minister of Supply and Services Canada, Canada Communication Group, 1994.
> Critical evaluations of 81 preventive measures and recommendations regarding their use in periodic health examinations.

Canadian Task Force on the Periodic Health Examination. **Periodic health examination, 1994 update: 2. Screening strategies for colorectal cancer.** Can Med Assoc J 150(12):1961–1970, 1994.
> Revised recommendations on the effectiveness of screening for colorectal cancer in asymptomatic patients over 40 years of age.

Canadian Task Force on the Periodic Health Examination. **Periodic health examination, 1994 update: 3. Primary and secondary prevention of neural tube defects.** Can Med Assoc J 1994;151:159–166, 1994.

Canadian Task Force on the Periodic Health Examination. **Periodic health examination, 1994 update: 4. Secondary prevention of elder abuse and mistreatment.** Can Med Assoc J 151:1413–1420, 1994.

Canadian Task Force on the Periodic Health Examination. **Periodic health examination, 1995 update: 3. Screening for visual problems among elderly patients.** Can Med Assoc J 152(8):1211–1222, 1995.

Davies HD, Wang EEL. **Canadian Task Force on the Periodic Health Examination. Periodic health examination, 1996 update: 2. Screening for chlamydial infections.** Can Med Assoc J 154(11):1631–1644, 1996.

Johnson K, The Canadian Task Force on the Periodic Health Examination. **Periodic health examination, 1995 update: 1. Screening for human papillomavirus infection in asymptomatic women.** Can Med Assoc J 152:483–493, 1995.

Lewis DW, Ismail AI. **Canadian Task Force on the Periodic Health Examination. Periodic health examination, 1995 update: 2. Prevention of dental caries.** Can Med Assoc J 152:835–846, 1995.
> For more information, call 613-731-9331, or Nadine Wathen 519-685-4929, ext. 2327; e-mail cwathen@julian.uwo.ca.

United States Preventive Services Task Force Publications

Guide to clinical preventive services: report of the United States Preventive Services Task Force. 2nd ed. Baltimore: Williams & Wilkins, 1996.
> Reviews of 70 preventive measures that include Task Force recommendations, recommendations of others, analysis of the

---

burden of suffering caused by the condition being considered, efficacy of screening tests, evidence of effectiveness of preventive intervention, discussion, and references. In-depth reviews of specific measures have also been published.
> For more information, contact Dr David Atkins at 301-594-4015; e-mail datkins@ahcpr.gov.

Other Publications

ACP Task Force on Adult Immunization and Infectious Diseases Society of America. Guide for adult immunization. 3rd ed. Philadelphia: American College of Physicians, 1994.
> Guidelines for adult immunization developed by a task force composed of representatives from the American College of Physicians, the Infectious Diseases Society of America, and the Centers for Disease Control and Prevention. The guidelines are said to be based on critical reviews of the epidemiologic and immunologic evidence. Rationales for the guidelines are provided, and selected references are provided. The book contains several useful appendices including a summary of recommendations, list of available immunobiologic agents according to product name and manufacturer, school and college immunization requirements by states, addresses and telephone numbers of each state and territorial health department, sources for vaccine information, model forms for recording immunizations, and information about the reporting of adverse reactions.

Elster AB, Kuznets NJ. **AMA guidelines for adolescent preventive services (GAPS).** Baltimore: Williams & Wilkins, 1994.
> Guidelines for the preventive care of adolescents developed by the American Medical Association, with the assistance of a national scientific advisory board. The recommendations represent expert opinion, based on targeted literature reviews. They are based on less explicit criteria, and appear less evidence-based, than the guidelines developed by the Canadian and US Task Forces.

Health information for international travel. Published yearly by the Centers for Disease Control (CDC), United States Department of Health and Human Services.
> This monograph provides up-to-date and comprehensive information on immunization requirements and health recommendations for international travelers. For general information or specific questions, see the CDC's Web site at http://www.cdc.gov or by phone at 404-639-3311 (general number) or 404-332-4555 (voice information system).

Morbidity and Mortality Weekly Report. Atlanta: Centers for Disease Control, U.S. Department of Health and Human Services.
> A weekly report containing very current information about disease incidence (e.g., regional incidence of influenza) and updated recommendations for disease prevention (including immunizations). Printed and distributed by the Massachusetts Medical Society, CSPO Box 9120, Waltham, MA 02254-9120. Also see Summary of Notifiable Diseases, United States 1995.

Woolf SH, Jonas S, Lawrence RS, eds. Health promotion and disease prevention in clinical practice. Baltimore: Williams & Wilkins, 1996.
> Multiauthor book that focuses on the practical implementation of preventive measures in office practice, with numerous examples, sample forms, tables, and lists of resources.

Specific References

1. Bailar JC III, Smith EM. Progress against cancer? N Engl J Med 314:1226, 1986.
2. Bandura A. Self-efficacy; toward a unifying theory of behavior change. Psychol Rev 84:191, 1977.
3. Burack RC, Gimotty PA, George J, et al. Promoting screening mammography in inner-city settings: a randomized controlled trial of computerized reminders as a component of a program to facilitate mammography. Med Care 32(6):609, 1994.
4. Burns R, Nichols LO, Graney MJ, Cloar FT. Impact of continued geriatric outpatient management on health outcomes of older veterans. Arch Intern Med 155:1313–1318, 1995.
5. Committee to Study the Prevention of Low Birth Weight. Preventing low birth weight. Washington, DC: Institute of Medicine, National Academy Press, 1985;132.

---

*Bold print (general references) and bold numerals (specific references) denote published controlled clinical trials, meta-analyses, or consensus-based recommendations.

6. Davidson RA, Fletcher SW, Retchin S, Duh S. A nurse-initiated reminder system for the periodic health examination. Implementation and evaluation. Arch Intern Med 144:2167, 1984.

7. Dietrich AJ, Goldberg H. Preventive content of adult primary care. Do generalists and subspecialists differ? Am J Public Health 74:223, 1984.

8. Fiscella K. Does prenatal care improve birth outcomes? A critical review. Obstet Gynecol 85(3):468, 1995.

9. Gold MR, Hurley R, Lake T, et al. A national survey of the arrangements managed-care plans make with physicians. N Engl J Med 333:1678, 1995.

10. Hamburg DA, Elliott GR, Parron DL, eds. The contribution of behavior to the burden of illness. In: Health and behavior, frontiers of research in the behavior sciences. Washington, DC: Institute of Medicine, National Academy Press, 1982;33.

11. Hampton ML, Anderson J, Lavizzo BS, Bergman AB. Sickle-cell nondisease: a potentially serious public health problem. Am J Dis Child 128:58, 1974.

12. Haynes RB, Sackett DL, Taylor DW, et al. Increased absenteeism from work after detection and labeling of hypertensive patients. N Engl J Med 299:741, 1978.

13. Holland WW. Screening: reasons to be cautious. BMJ 306:1222, 1993.

14. Kern DE, Harris WL, Boekeloo BO, et al. Use of an outpatient medical record audit to achieve educational objectives: changes in residents' performance over six years. J Gen Intern Med 5:218, 1990.

15. Korn JE, Schossberg LA, Rich EC. Improved preventive care following an intervention during an ambulatory care rotation: carryover to a second setting. J Gen Intern Med 3:156, 1988.

16. Kosecoff J, Fink A, Brook RH, et al. General medical care and the education of internists in university hospitals: an evaluation of the Teaching Hospital General Medicine Group Practice Plan. Ann Intern Med 102:250, 1985.

17. Li VC, Coates TJ, Ewart CK, Kim YJ. The effectiveness of smoking cessation advice given during routine medical care: physicians can make a difference. Am J Prev Med 3:81, 1987.

18. Litzelman DK, Dittus RS, Miller HE, Tierney WM. Requiring physicians to respond to computerized reminders improves their compliance with preventive care protocols. J Gen Intern Med 8:311, 1993.

19. Lurie N, Manning WG, Peterson C, et al. Preventive care: do we practice what we preach? Am J Public Health 77:801, 1987.

20. McDonald CJ, Sui LH, Smith DM, et al. Reminders to physicians from an introspective computer medical record. A two-year randomized trial. Ann Intern Med 100:130, 1984.

21. McPhee SJ, Bird JA, Fordham D, et al. Promoting cancer prevention by primary care physicians: results of a randomized controlled trial. JAMA 266:538, 1991.

22. McPhee SJ, Richard RJ, Solkowitz SN. Performance of cancer screening in a university general internal medicine practice: comparison with the 1980 American Cancer Society guidelines. J Gen Intern Med 1:275, 1986.

23. Meddar JD, Kahn NB Jr, Susman JL. Risk factors and recommendations for 230 adult primary care patients, based on US Preventive Services Task Force guidelines. Am J Prev Med 8:150, 1992.

24. Moran WP, Nelson K, Wofford JL, et al. Increasing influenza immunization among high risk patients: education or financial incentive? Am J Med 101(6):612, 1996.

25. Naylor M, Brooten, Jones R, et al. Comprehensive discharge planning for the hospitalized elderly: a randomized trial. Ann Intern Med 120:999–1006, 1994.

26. Nutting PA, Green LA. Community-oriented primary care. In: Rakel RE, ed. Textbook of family practice. 5th ed. Philadelphia: WB Saunders, 1995;225.

27. Quill TE, Lipkin M Jr, Greenland P. The medicalization of normal variants. The case of mitral valve prolapse. J Gen Intern Med 3:267, 1988.

28. Russell MAH, Wilson C, Taylor C, Baker CD. Effects of general practitioners' advice against smoking. BMJ 2:231, 1979.

29. Sackett DL, Snow JC. The magnitude of compliance and noncompliance. In: Haynes RB, Taylor DW, Sackett DL, eds. Compliance in health care. Baltimore: Johns Hopkins University Press, 1979;11.

30. Smith HE, Herbert CP. Preventive practice among primary care physicians in British Columbia: relation to recommendations of the Canadian Task Force on the Periodic Health Examination. Can Med Assoc J 149(12):1795, 1993.

31. Stuck AE, Siu AL, Wieland GD, et al. Comprehensive geriatric assessment: a meta-analysis of controlled trials. Lancet 342:1032–1036, 1993.

32. Stuck AE, Aronow HU, Steiner A, et al. A trial of annual in-home comprehensive geriatric assessments for elderly people living in the community. N Engl J Med 333:1184–1189, 1995.

33. Trends in cancer screening: United States, 1987 and 1992. MMWR 45(3):57, 1996.

34. Wilson GT. Cognitive factors in life style changes: a social learning perspective. In: Davidson PO, Davidson SM, eds. Behavioral medicine: changing health lifestyles. New York: Brunner/Mazel, 1980.

35. Winickoff RN, Coltin KL, Morgan MM, et al. Improving physician performance through peer comparison feedback. Med Care 22:527, 1984.

36. Woo B, Woo B, Cook EF, et al. Screening procedures in the asymptomatic adult. Comparison of physician's recommendations, patients' desires, published guidelines, and actual practice. JAMA 254:1480, 1985.

37. Zyzanski SJ, Stange KC, Kelly R, et al. Family physicians' disagreement with the US Preventive Services Task Force recommendations. J Fam Pract 39(2):140, 1994.

C H A P T E R 3

The Doctor–Patient Relationship*

L. RANDOL BARKER, MD

Each doctor–patient relationship is established through person-to-person interactions in which the physician's goals are to obtain accurate and critical information from the patient and reach a valid formulation of the patient's problem or status, to provide information and ensure that the patient comprehends it, to arrive at plans with which the patient concurs, to promote patient adherence to agreed-on plans, to attain patient satisfaction with the relationship, and to alleviate the patient's symptoms. Achievement of these goals depends equally on the physician's knowledge of medicine, respect for the patient's participation in the interaction, and skills in communication and patient education. This chapter and Chapter 4 ("Patient Education, Behavior Change, and Compliance") address the latter two issues.

DOCTOR–PATIENT RELATIONSHIP

Types of Relationships

Our society's concept of the doctor–patient relationship has evolved through the years. In 1951 Parsons described the patient's role as essentially passive (10).

*Edward Bartlett, PhD, and Archie S. Golden, MD, contributed to this chapter in previous editions of this book.

Later Szasz and Hollender (19) outlined the following three types of interactions between physician and patient: the *active–passive relationship,* in which the physician has all authority (similar to Parson's conceptualization); the *guidance–cooperation relationship,* in which the physician still is somewhat authoritarian and the patient cooperates; and *mutual participation,* in which there is active collaboration between patient and physician and patients assume more responsibility for their care. The consumer movement of the 1960s and 1970s promoted the mutual participation relationship between doctors and patients (13).

In the past decade the general term *patient-centeredness* has been introduced to emphasize the primacy of the patient in the mutual participation model. Authors have pointed out that *the several facets of patient-centeredness include* the following (8,16,18):

- The reframing of the physician's goals, which became to learn and value the patient's personal illness story and to reach agreement with the patient on the meaning of the illness and on the management plan
- The grounding of current law in the concept of patient autonomy
- The inclusion of the patient's perspective as a fundamental component of quality assessment
- The importance of each of these factors for planning physician education and research

Ethical Aspects of the Relationship

The mutual participation model is central to *the principles of medical ethics that have been delineated in the past two decades* (1). These principles define a doctor–patient relationship in which the physician respects the sanctity of the individual person and believes that that person's goals should be the basis for medical decisions. In practice, these principles require that physicians learn what their patients' expectations and goals are and that patients (or their surrogates) participate as fully as possible in decisions about their health care. Such participation requires several conditions: that the patient be competent to consider a specific decision; that the patient receive sufficient information regarding available options, demonstrate comprehension of that information, and be given sufficient time to consider the options; and that the patient's decision be voluntary, that is, free from constraints imposed by the interests of other persons. Additional ethical principles that are critical in a respectful doctor–patient relationship are truthfulness and protection of confidentiality.

Adherence to each of the principles of patient-centered medical ethics is not always possible or appropriate in ambulatory practice. For example, although patients generally want to be well informed, many still prefer to have their physician recommend choices for them (5). In addition, a physician's personal beliefs and standards of practice must be considered. If a patient requests a course of action that is contrary to the physician's beliefs or standards or endangers others, the physician must indicate this to the patient and, if the patient's wishes cannot be accommodated, the physician should transfer care to another physician or to the court system. Challenging situations such as these are not uncommon in ambulatory practice (3).

For situations that involve patient behaviors that may harm others, patient competence, truth telling, and confidentiality, a doctor–patient relationship that has been developed over time may make both prevention and resolution of problems more feasible (e.g., an elderly patient may agree to discontinue driving and propose satisfactory alternatives in the context of a trusting relationship).

Problems caused by *external factors,* particularly the ground rules governing services covered under managed care plans, may also be amenable to resolution through the doctor–patient relationship. Ensuring that patients are informed about HMO processes and guidelines and offering other options when patients make unreasonable requests are examples of ways to include the patient in addressing such externally imposed challenges (see "Managed Care and the Doctor–Patient Relationship," below).

Involvement with Family Members and Significant Others

Commonly, a spouse, family members, or friends—especially those who are close to the patient during a period of illness—want to know about the patient's condition, are affected by the patient's illness, and may play an important role in determining the course of the illness. Developing a relationship with those close to the patient is therefore a predictable and important aspect of the care of many patients. A physician's involvement with others may range from the brief exchanges that occur at the beginning or end of office visits to interactions during a planned family meeting. The skills for use in the traditional physician–patient dyad, described below, are the skills appropriate when others are included.

Special considerations for relating to family members and friends include recognizing the impact on the patient's illness of patient–family dynamics and physician–family dynamics; avoiding breach of confidentiality by ensuring that the patient consents and, when feasible and appropriate, meeting with others in the presence of the patient; learning about and acknowledging the distress that the patient's illness has caused for those close to the patient; and providing information and engaging in problem solving that will facilitate the roles of others in promoting the patient's health. Details about the positive and negative influences of family on a patient's health are found in Chapter 4 (under "Social Support").

Planned Family Meetings

There are a number of situations when it is helpful to convene the members of a patient's family and, at times, others such as a nurse or social worker. Common examples include diagnosis of and plans for addressing a terminal illness; poor control of chronic illness; decisions regarding a long-term care plan; substance abuse (see "Family Intervention," Chapter 21); and marital or sexual difficulties or other family dysfunction (see "Family Counseling," Chapter 11). Table 3.1 describes specific tasks that one should consider when planning and conducting a family meeting.

Sociocultural Diversity and the Doctor–Patient Relationship

A classic paper published in 1978 points out that there are usually differences in the ways in which a physician and patient think about and respond to the patient's medical problems (7). The sources of these differences range from the unique ideas of individual patients to ideas and barriers that come from the social or cultural groups to which patients belong. The late 20th-century changes in the racial, national, and ethnic composition of the United States, summarized in Table 3.2, indicate that patients with diverse cultural traditions are likely to make up a substantial proportion of the patients in the practice of most physicians.

In a number of ways, the effectiveness of a doctor–patient relationship may be enhanced, or diminished, depending on physician awareness of and response to differences between patient and physician. General approaches that can enhance the relationship are the following:

- Learning and inquiring explicitly about the beliefs and behaviors of the sociocultural group to which one's patient belongs (Common sources of group-determined beliefs and behaviors are religious tenets related to illness, traditional roles of family members in medical decisions, the use of folk healers, and unique concerns related to sexual orientation.)
- Recognizing and reflecting about one's own biases and emotional reactions toward cultural and individual differences
- Ensuring that a translator is present when there is a language barrier
- Ensuring that patients who are illiterate have access to someone, ideally a family member, who can read information that is important to the patient's medical care
- Learning and explicitly inquiring about patients' explanatory models for their illnesses

Patients' explanatory models for their illnesses address the same issues as physicians' explanatory models: etiology, name of the illness, pathophysiology ("what is wrong"), expected course, treatment, and response to treatment (7). Often, there are differences in the two models, based on the difference in perspective of patients and physicians (Table 3.3). Both parties may inhibit the development of an effective relationship: physicians, by focusing only on abstract disease formulations to address each of the above issues, and patients, by dwelling on their own formulation of what is wrong and resenting their physician's apparent

Table 3.1. Tasks to Consider for Planning and Conducting a Family Meeting

Premeeting Tasks
Clarify the rationale for the meeting.
Establish which family members, friends, or professionals should attend.
Set up the appointment, specifying the planned duration, location.
Develop a strategy for conducting the meeting, including specific questions, observations, or tasks that will facilitate addressing the purpose of the meeting.

The Five Phases of a Family Meeting
Phase 1: Socialize (approximately 5 minutes)
Greet each person attending the meeting.
Introduce the purpose for the meeting, and talk briefly with each family member about themselves, their work, their relation to the patient, etc.
Phase 2: Set the goals (approximately 5 minutes)
Ask the group, "What would you like to make sure we accomplish today?"
Restate each goal so it is clear, concise, and realistic; propose any important goals that the family has not mentioned.
Set priorities among the goals.
Phase 3: Discuss the illness or issue (approximately 15 minutes)
Elicit each participant's view of the illness or issue. Ask about past experiences or recent changes that could have an impact on the issue of concern, such as moves, occupational changes, other illness, or deaths. Observe repetitive family interactional patterns. Final plans should not go against these patterns, unless specifically negotiated.
Encourage the patient and family to ask questions.
Ask how the family has dealt with similar illness or issues in the past.
Phase 4: Identify resources and ideas (approximately 10 minutes)
Identify family strengths and resources of all kinds.
Identify medical resources and community resources.
Phase 5: Establish a plan (approximately 10 minutes)
Include resources and ideas that family members have suggested.
Negotiate a formal or an informal contract with the family. Have each person state what he or she will do.
Discuss any referrals, if relevant, at this point.
Offer to write down key information for family members.
Ask for any final questions.
Summarize the plan.
Thank everyone for coming and participating in the meeting.

Postmeeting Tasks
Write up a report of the meeting, including the attendance, the problem list, a global assessment of individual and family functioning, the family's strengths and resources, and the plan (e.g., both the medical regimen and the roles to be played by the patient and family members).

Adapted from McDaniel S, Campbell T, Seaburn D. Family oriented primary care: a manual for medical providers. New York: Springer-Verlag, 1990.

Table 3.2. Composition of United States Population, 1990, and Percentage Change, 1980–1990

Population	U.S. Population, 1990		% Increase from 1980
	No.	%	
Total	248,709,873	100	10
Race[a]			
White	199,686,060	83	6
African American	29,968,060	12	13
Native American	1,959,234	1	38
Asian and Pacific Islander	7,273,662	3	108
All other	9,804,847	4	45
Hispanic origin[b]	22,354,059	9	53

From the Bureau of the Census, Economics and Statistics Administration, US Department of Commerce. Press releases on 1990 Census data, April 1991, CB91-100, and June 1991, CB91-215.

[a]Race does not denote any clear-cut definition of biologic stock but rather is a self-classification by people to the race with which they most closely identify.

[b]Hispanic origin denotes origination of Spanish-speaking people from the Caribbean, Central or South America, Spain, or elsewhere. It is distinct from race; thus, persons of Spanish or Hispanic origin may be of any race.

inattention to that formulation. By inviting patients to describe their own explanatory models (and, at times, learning of conflicting beliefs about the illness held by others close to the patient), then coming up with mutually acceptable ways of accounting for and ad- dressing the illness, physicians are more likely to help patients who bring strongly held personal or cultural beliefs to the encounter.

The fund of useful information about relationships with patients from diverse social and cultural back- grounds is growing rapidly as the composition of the United States evolves (see "General References").

Managed Care and the Doctor–Patient Relationship

The ways in which managed care may affect the doctor–patient relationship have received much atten- tion recently. Table 3.4 contains a summary assessment of potential improvements and threats to the relation- ship that are associated with managed care. The au- thors considered the impact on factors (the six Cs) key to the relationship: patient *choice,* physician *compe- tence,* doctor–patient *communication,* physician *com- passion* for the patient, *continuity* of physician(s), and the *avoidance of conflict* of interest (4).

Shorey has captured much about the change that managed care has brought to the doctor–patient re- lationship: From the need to build trust in the context of a dyad (physician and patient), physicians need

Table 3.3. Summary of Common Differences in Explanatory Models Between Western-Trained Physicians and Traditional Ethnic Patients

Aspect of Model	Western Physician	Ethnic Patient
Etiologic Beliefs		
Social causes of illnesses	Usually limited to stress model or attributed to paranoia	Many social indiscretions can cause illness; blaming of self or others for symptoms is common
Environmental causes of illnesses	Exposure to known pathogens, toxins, and social stress may cause symptoms	"Hot–cold" imbalance in the body caused by dietary indiscretions or drafts may cause symptoms
Belief that conditions of the blood cause illness	Limited to specific hematologic disorders or hypertension	Many "conditions" of blood can cause illness (e.g., "too thick," "too slow," "too little")
Symptom Interpretation and Presentation		
Altered states of consciousness (trance, visions, etc.)	Usually considered abnormal	Often considered normal, desirable
Attitudes toward pain expression	Stoicism expected unless complaints are congruent with clear organic pathology	Either total stoicism or emotional expression of pain is healthy and expected
Focus on physical symptoms (somatization)	May be considered as a psychiatric syndrome	Expected, proper way of expressing distress
Treatment Expectations		
Who is the patient?	Individual is the focus of decision making and care	Family must be involved in decision making
Beliefs about self-medication and alternative practitioners	Considered potentially dangerous, undesirable	Common

From Johnson TM, Hardt EJ, Kleinman A. Cultural factors in the medical interview. In: Lipkin M Jr, Putnam SM, Lazare A, eds. The medical interview: clinical care, education, and research. New York: Springer-Verlag, 1995.

now to inspire trust in a context (managed care) in which they (physicians) value dyadic relationships but also consider the health of all patients in their panels (15). Demystifying this new context, for both patients and physicians, is recommended as the best starting point for building relationships in managed care. A number of other authors have written helpful analyses of this topic (see *Managed Care and the Physician–Patient Relationship,* in "General References").

COMMUNICATION

The Three Functions of the Medical Interview

The following three functions, delineated by Lazare, Putnam, and Lipkin (9), are widely accepted as ways to describe what happens in medical interviews:

- *Determining and monitoring the nature of the patient's problems*
- *Developing, maintaining, or concluding the therapeutic relationship*
- *Carrying out patient education and implementing a treatment plan*

One or more of these three functions is central to all studies of doctor–patient communication and to each set of skills used in doctor–patient interactions.

Importance of Effective Communication

The importance of effective communication has been confirmed in a variety of studies of the doctor–patient relationship. A large body of published research has shown that effective communication skills are correlated with obtaining valid information, getting patients to disclose fully the reasons for visits, reporting satisfaction with the physician, attaining patient adherence to medical regimens, and reducing risk of being sued for malpractice (see *The Medical Interview,* in "General References"). A smaller body of literature also exists in which experimental studies, using control and intervention subjects, have documented the impact of effective communication skills on patient outcomes including emotional health, symptom resolution, patient function, blood pressure and glucose control, and pain control (17).

Although gathering and providing of information may appear to be the primary reason for direct communication with patients, the *therapeutic nature of the interaction* is perhaps the factor that is most important to the health of the patient. As summarized by Reiser and Schroder (14):

Repeatedly, physicians will feel the power of something intangible, yet unmistakable, in the nature of the doctor–patient relationship that helps a sick person to get better. It is hard to overestimate the potency and curative potential of this very unique and special relationship. For all our technical advances, this relationship remains one of medicine's most powerful therapeutic tools.

Or, as Balint put it in describing his classic studies, "By far the most frequently used drug in general practice was the doctor" (2). The skills that establish the therapeutic nature of *every* medical encounter are described here and in Chapter 4. Chapter 11 describes the important phenomenon of transference and additional skills that are useful when the primary purpose of the encounter is to deal with psychosocial problems.

Communication During Ambulatory Encounters

The quality of communication during an ambulatory encounter is determined by the way that both parties think about the encounter in advance and by the communication skills used during the encounter. The latter can be seen as skills that are useful for organizing the flow of the visit and skills that are useful throughout the visit.

Recognizing What the Patient Experiences

An interaction with a patient is likely to be more effective when, as much as possible, one recognizes the feelings and concerns that patients may bring to visits. As discussed under "Sociocultural Diversity," this may include being aware of traditional beliefs and behaviors of patients from diverse cultural backgrounds (7).

What It Is Like for a Patient to Go to a Doctor. "Expectant trust" (see Chapter 11) describes the general way in which patients think about a visit to the doctor (6). They may come with anxieties concerning what the doctor will find wrong with them, they may come expecting the doctor to solve a broad array of problems, or they may have any of a number of other types of expectations of the visit. Patients know that

their doctors have busy schedules, and some may be reluctant to ask what they think the doctor will regard as trivial questions. Social distance often exists between doctor and patient, and the combination of this and the physician's special knowledge gives the physician considerable authority. As a result, patients may be reluctant to contradict or correct their physicians' statements, may block or misrepresent their thoughts or feelings to provide answers they think the physician wants to hear, and may not ask for clarification despite being confused by medical terminology. During the physical examination, some patients feel embarrassment at being exposed, and this may further inhibit disclosure of important concerns. Predictably, most patients, even those who have had a long-standing relationship with their physician, experience some of these types of discomfort during an office visit, and it can help to ask oneself, "If I were this patient, how would I be feeling during this visit?" It is equally telling to ask oneself, after a visit, "If I were that patient, how would I be feeling about the visit when I have reached home?"

As discussed under "Challenging Situations" and "Physician Self-Care," physicians also bring expectations and vulnerabilities to encounters with patients. Awareness of these factors can be seen as an important

Table 3.4.   The Effects of Managed Care on the Physician–Patient Relationship

Potential Improvements	Potential Threats
CHOICE	
Expanded choice of managed care plans, particularly in areas with low managed care penetration	"Cherry picking" increasing the number of uninsured Americans
Expanded choice of preventive and pediatric services	Employers restricting patients' choice of managed care plans and physicians
	Price competition forcing patients to choose between continuing with their current physicians or switching to a cheaper plan
	Financial failures of managed care plans forcing change in managed care plan without choice
	Restrictions by managed care plans of choice of specialists and particular services
COMPETENCE	
Development and use of measures to assess quality of physicians and managed care plans	Underuse of specialists and specialized facilities
Greater use of preventive medical care	Unreliable and non–risk-adjusted quality measures providing a distorted view of competence
COMMUNICATION	
Increased number of generalists and primary care providers	Productivity requirements creating shorter office visits, reduced telephone access, and other access barriers to physicians
Creation of physician–nonphysician provider teams to provide a broader range of providers knowledgeable about the patient's condition	Advertising creating inflated patient expectations
COMPASSION	
	Less time for interaction with patients during stressful decisions
CONTINUITY	
	Price competition forcing patient choice of continuity at a higher price vs the cheapest plan
	"Deselection" of physicians disrupting existing physician–patient relations
	Frequent changes by employer of managed care plans forcing changes of physician
(NO) CONFLICT OF INTEREST	
	Linking physician salary incentives and bonuses to reduce use of tests and procedures for patients

From Emanuel EJ, Dubler NN. Preserving the physician–patient relationship in the era of managed care. JAMA 273:323–329, 1995.

skill that may determine the quality of communication during a visit.

Rapport. A component of communication that especially facilitates disclosure of concerns by patients and readies them to make decisions is the development and maintenance of rapport. Rapport is a feeling that one has of being with a friend. Rapport is present when, often through previous experience with a physician, the patient feels trust. Two phenomena during first or repeat encounters that usually foster rapport are the feeling by the patient that he or she is *respected* and that the physician has *empathy* for him or her (see "Noting and Addressing Emotions," below).

Skills for Organizing the Flow of the Visit

Given the limited time available for ambulatory visits, it is helpful to have a scheme for organizing the flow of a visit. The scheme described here emphasizes patient-centered skills useful for each of the stages of a visit. The section after this one describes skills that may be helpful in any part of the visit.

Planning the Visit

It is helpful to review critical information about a patient before conducting the visit. This can be done before seeing the patient or just after the greeting ("Before we start, let me take a minute to get right up to the date with what is in your chart"). This planning ensures that one knows information that will help set the agenda for the visit, and it limits greatly the need to look through the chart in the presence of the patient.

Opening the Interaction

In *greeting* a patient, shaking the patient's hand, using the patient's name, and if it is a first visit, introducing oneself all make the patient feel welcome. The first few moments of first or second encounters are crucial because the physician and the patient are sizing up one another, and nonverbal behavior takes precedence over what is being said. Both physician and patient are paying attention to physical features, type of handshake, voice tone and pitch, age, dress, and overall demeanor.

The *seating arrangement* of the office can affect the development of rapport. When the patient's and the physician's chairs are arranged so that the two are facing one another, without the full breadth of a desk interposed, some patients are less intimidated than when facing a physician across a desk.

Exploratory Information Gathering

For gathering information about a patient's problems, it helps to begin with an *exploratory approach* and to ensure that the patient knows that this is one's intent. Exploratory interviewing combines *open-ended phrasing of questions and allowing a patient to respond without being interrupted.* An exploratory approach is the most efficient way to learn what the patient knows, and it indicates interest in the patient

from the outset. Asking the patient "How have you been doing since your last visit?" is an appropriate open-ended question for a planned follow-up visit. For a new-patient visit, or a visit requested by the patient, one will want to explore the reason for the visit by saying "Please tell me what brings you in today." This type of phrasing provides an opportunity for the patient to describe the reasons for the visit and does not imply that there is a problem.

Agenda Setting. In response to the opening inquiry, an example of the patient response might be "Well, I haven't been doing so well lately. My shoulder has been giving me a problem." Before exploring the first problem mentioned, it is helpful to establish whether there are any other problems that will be addressed at the visit. If one assumes that the patient wishes to discuss only one problem and proceeds to explore that problem, the patient may mention other problems whenever there is an opportunity, often when one is preparing to close the visit. This dilemma can usually be avoided by inviting patients to name each of their concerns at the outset, naming one's own concerns (e.g., "I also want to get up to date on your smoking"), and restating the issues to be addressed during the visit. If too many issues are identified, it is appropriate to ask, "Which problems seem to be bothering you the most?" and mutually to prioritize those issues to be addressed at the visit.

Getting the Patient's Story. After agreement on the agenda for the visit, one continues to explore the problems one at a time. "Tell me about the shoulder pain" would be a clear invitation to the patient to describe the problem in his or her own words. When patients give the history in their own words, the length of the interview does not increase (11) and they are more likely to explain why a problem concerns them (e.g., "With spring coming, I'm thinking that I might have to give up tennis altogether because of the pain").

If an exploratory approach is maintained, a patient's medical problem usually emerges as part of a meaningful personal story (16). For example, the patient's concern that a shoulder pain means that he or she will never play tennis again may be founded in the experience of the patient's father years before—a personal story that would clarify the importance of the symptom to the patient and would be crucial to consider in the closing part of the visit (see below). In addition to bringing out important information, an interview that allows emergence of a patient's personal story invariably contributes to the development of the rapport described earlier.

Exploratory questions can be used throughout the interaction. When the patient produces information that needs clarifying, additional exploratory questions are helpful to establish a common meaning. For example, if the patient has named "constipation" as a new concern, it helps to explore what this means to the patient (e.g., "What do you mean by constipation?"). One may discover that the patient has a bowel movement every other day and yet believes that this means constipation.

Clarifying and Hypothesis Testing

Not visible to the patient, but constantly operating during an interview, is hypothesis testing by the physician. Because exploratory inquiry rarely provides all of the information needed to evaluate a problem, it is usually necessary to use focused questions to fill in gaps and narrow the differential diagnosis. Table 3.5 lists generic information that is important in assessing most problems.

Direct questions are questions phrased to clarify specific facts, such as "When did you first notice the pain?" or "What words would you use to describe the pain?" or "Can you show me with your hand where the pain is?" When seeking such specific information, it is important to *avoid asking leading questions*—questions that tend to elicit predetermined answers, usually in the form of a simple "yes" or "no." An example would be the following question, presumably related to a hypothesis that has occurred to the physician: "You don't have the pain every day, do you?" This leading question gives the message to the patient that the physician does not expect the pain to occur every day. Patients who are somewhat passive may agree to whatever their physician suggests, even if the answer is inaccurate. Once a patient has responded inaccurately, the patient may become distracted and forget to report important information.

When a patient cannot provide needed information, it helps sometimes to offer a number of *choices from which to select*. For example, if the patient reports chest pain but is unable to provide accurate information about whether the pain radiates, one might ask "Does the pain seem to go anywhere else, such as to your back, one of your arms, your neck, or your legs?" While the physician may have an idea of the likely response, this will not be obvious to the patient because the patient is given several choices. This is contrasted with a question such as "Does the pain move to your left arm?" which is a somewhat leading question, giving the patient the impression that this is the correct answer.

A patient will at times give a vague, aggregate description of an episodic symptom. In this situation, it is helpful to have the patient *describe in detail a single episode:* "Tell me about the last time you felt the nausea and crampy pain," for example. This technique clarifies the nature of the symptoms and, importantly, it often brings to light social or environmental factors important to the problem (e.g., "Well, the last bad headache was Saturday . . . yeah, my teenage son had stayed out all night").

When asking direct questions, it is important to *ask only one question at a time* and to phrase each question so that it refers to one piece of information. Thus, when the patient responds, one knows what the patient is referring to. For example, to questions such as "Are you having any problems sleeping or eating?" or "Are you constipated or do you have diarrhea?" a positive response may not reveal which is the problem. Conversely, a negative response may refer to only one of these problems.

While responding to questions, the *patient may give verbal cues* related to the discussion or concerning other issues that need exploration. At times, it is appropriate to pursue a verbal cue when it is mentioned; at other times it is more appropriate to acknowledge it and let the patient know that one will return to it later. If a verbal cue is pertinent to the present discussion, it is helpful to repeat the patient's words or to explore what the patient means. For example, in response to a question about pain, a patient may respond "Well, it seems to have gotten worse lately, but maybe it's just my nerves." Here, an appropriate response would be an open-ended question such as "Your nerves?" or "What do you mean?" An example of a verbal cue that one would explore separately would be the following response to a question about sleep quality in a patient with pain: "Sometimes I wake up in the middle of the night, but it isn't because of the pain." Depending on the hypothesis that one is testing regarding the patient's pain, it might be more appropriate to pursue the sleep problem later in the interaction.

A patient's *nonverbal cues* may provide important information. A patient's *vocal message*—including the pitch, tone, and tempo—may confirm or contradict the content of the patient's verbal message. Nonverbal cues also include *body language*. Elements of body language that can be observed are the patient's sitting position (e.g., sitting on the edge of the chair suggests apprehension, facing away from the physician suggests mental discomfort), head position (e.g., held back in defiance, anxiety, or fear, or held down or turned away in sadness, shame, or denial), facial expression (eyes, eyebrows, and forehead show the greatest range of emotions, including surprise, fear, anger, happiness, disgust, sadness), hands (wringing or rubbing of hands can show anxiety, clenched fists may signify anger), and arms and legs (crossing of the legs, and especially the arms, can signify resistance or defensiveness). At times, incongruity between what the patient says and the patient's voice quality or body language is the only indicator of an important problem that the patient is hesitant to disclose.

Table 3.5. Generic Information Important in Assessing Most Problems

Chronology of symptoms:
  Onset of problem: since when?
  Frequency
  Duration of an episode
  Temporal trend: unchanging, better, worse
  Past history of similar problem: when, etc.?
Quality of symptoms:
  Severe to not severe
  Quality consistent or variable
  Location, radiation (if pertinent)
  Patient's own words to describe quality
Description of one episode (for recurring symptom)
Associated additional symptoms
Factors, circumstances that aggravate symptoms
Factors, circumstances that alleviate symptoms
Remedies or measures tried
Impact of symptoms on valued activities
Patient's explanatory model for symptoms
Fears or concerns caused by symptoms

Carrying Out Patient Education and Choosing a Treatment Plan

Telling the patient one's formulation of a medical problem and reaching consensus on next steps are the final steps in an ambulatory encounter. Because ambulatory patients are by definition quite autonomous, the skills needed in these steps are uniquely important in ambulatory care. Chapter 4 ("Patient Education, Behavior Change, and Compliance") describes in detail the principles and skills for addressing this part of the visit.

At the close of a visit, it is important to accomplish a number of concrete tasks:

- Schedule a follow-up visit at a mutually agreed-to interval.
- Instruct the patient to phone back (or tell the patient that you or someone from the office will phone) when this is indicated.
- Reemphasize one's interest in the patient. Actions such as shaking the patient's hand or touching the patient on the shoulder, using the patient's name, ensuring that the patient has one's professional card, and encouraging telephone contact for interval problems convey to the patient one's interest.

Skills Useful Throughout the Visit

A number of communication skills, described here, may be useful in any part of an ambulatory visit.

Providing "Road Signs"

Providing understandable "road signs" helps patients participate effectively in the visit. This includes *using orienting and transitional statements* to ensure that the patient understands when the focus of the interview is changing (e.g., "At this point, I would like to learn more about your day-to-day activities"); naming, then addressing, *one problem or issue at a time* (e.g., "Now, about your shoulder pain . . ." or "The medicine that I will prescribe . . ."); *summarizing and checking periodically* (e.g., "So far, what I understand about your trouble sleeping is that . . ."), which lets patients know that one has heard what they said and gives them the chance to clarify or expand on important information; and using *vocabulary consistent with the patient's background* and avoiding formulations that may confuse the patient (e.g., telling a patient that test results are "negative" may convey to the patient that something is wrong).

Noting the Patient's Educational Needs

Patient education can be addressed most efficiently by *ascertaining the patient's educational needs throughout the interview*—by hearing or asking what the patient knows or wants to know about issues as they come up—but *deferring the process of providing information and working out a plan* to the latter part of the visit. It helps to provide a road sign (e.g., "When we finish up your visit, we will go over several things you can do to lose the weight you have

gained"). (See details in the schemes described in Chapter 4.)

Using Eye Contact

The eyes are a primary medium of expression and often tell more about a person's message than words. Maintaining eye contact and communicating with eyes at the same level as the patient's (e.g., both parties seated) are basic to patient comfort. Looking at one's watch or at the chart while discussing a patient's problem may indicate to a patient that the physician is not listening, is not interested, or is too busy to answer questions that a patient may already be reluctant to ask. Although eye contact is one of the best methods for conveying interest, staring can be uncomfortable and should be avoided.

Noting and Addressing Emotions

Predictably, patients experience one or more emotions when they are preparing for, engaging in, and recalling visits to the doctor. During visits, patients may or may not disclose their feelings. A number of communication skills can facilitate disclosure of emotions and help in addressing emotions (Table 3.6). Three basic reasons for addressing emotions are that patients usually feel better when they know that the physician is aware of their feelings; patients may be more able to concentrate and make decisions after an emotional state such as anxiety, sadness, or anger has been addressed even briefly; and expressing emotions may be therapeutic for a patient.

Skills Related to Physical Examination and Documentation

Physical Examination

Appropriate communication during the physical examination includes describing what one is doing, obtaining further history when examining the location of a symptom, and avoiding the tendency to give important information (diagnosis and plan) during the physical examination or when the patient is getting dressed; in both instances the patient is distracted and cannot be expected to focus on the physician's message or to formulate questions as well.

Note Taking

Dictating or writing a visit note can be done in a way that does not diminish rapport with the patient. It is helpful to point out that one will be making a few notes during the visit. It is equally helpful to suspend the interaction briefly while focusing on one's note, as this is a time that requires thought as well as writing or dictating.

Challenging Situations

All physicians have been faced with difficult patients in medical practice. Patients may be difficult to care for because of their style of communicating, because of the overwhelming nature of their problems,

Table 3.6. Skills for Addressing a Patient's Emotions

Skills for Facilitating Disclosure of Feelings
Explicitly ask or encourage patient to express/clarify feelings/concerns.
  Restate patient's words about how he/she feels (e.g., "You feel down . . . ?" repeated immediately after the patients says these words).
  Probe feelings that seem to be just under the surface (e.g., "How do you feel about . . .? I notice you're getting tearful").
  Clarify or check feelings that patient has disclosed (e.g., "Let me see if I can better understand what you are feeling").
Allow patient to express feelings/concerns.
  Be attentive, do not interrupt.
  Allow silence while patient prepares response or experiences emotional reaction.

Skills for Responding to and Supporting Patient
Convey concern for and interest in the patient.
  Explicitly by saying so (e.g., "My concern is to get you well.").
  Implicitly by remaining attentive, facilitating disclosure, indicating that patient has been heard (e.g., by mentioning aspects of patient's life
    so that patient realizes he or she is known as a unique person or by changing facial expression and vocal tone).
Communicate understanding of patient's feelings (empathize).
  Name patient's feelings/situation (e.g., "Sounds as if you are pretty angry").
  Check accuracy of naming (e.g., "Is this the way you experience it?").
  Use facilitative utterances (e.g., lower voice, use appropriate utterances such as "uh huh" that indicate that the patient is being
    attended to).
Legitimize patient's feelings/thoughts/actions: Indicate that patient's emotions/thoughts/actions are understandable and "normal" under the
    circumstances (e.g., "It's understandable that you feel this way," "Many would have done as you did.").
Convey respect for the patient's efforts, ideas: Compliment patient for whatever patient is doing well or plans to do (e.g., "Your decision to
    join Weight Watchers sounds good to me," "I can see that you have given a lot of thought to . . .").
Respond nonjudgmentally: Do not impose own bias, values, or assumptions on patient actions.
  Nonverbally: Maintain interest, do not give negative message (e.g., nodding head disapprovingly, sighing in frustration, when a patient
    reports noncompliance).
  Verbally: Do not imply that patient is "bad" (e.g., "Didn't you realize that if you ate crabs you'd put yourself into heart failure again?").
Respond nondefensively.
  Do not respond to patient anger or criticism by defense of performance but acknowledge anger/criticism and try to address the reasons
    for the patient's behavior and concerns.
  Admit mistakes, apologize when appropriate, be open to considering second opinions, avoid self-righteousness.
Use self-disclosure effectively: Reveal information about self, when appropriate, to convey support, empathy to patient (e.g., "I felt the same
    way after I lost my mother.").
Assure partnership/support: Make statements, using the first person, that assure support to the patient and convey the sense of partnership
    (e.g., "I will be with you throughout this illness.").

because of their failure to adhere to appropriate treatment or behavior, because they present psychosocial distress through somatic symptoms, because they do not respond positively to the physician's efforts, or because they have lifelong maladaptive personalities. Approaches to dealing with situations that may be difficult for physicians are covered in Section 2 of this book ("Psychiatric and Behavioral Problems") and in chapters describing patients who are noncompliant (Chapter 4); adolescent and geriatric patients (Chapters 5 and 6); patients who have illnesses that create major psychosocial stress, such as cancer (Chapter 8), human immunodeficiency virus (HIV) infection (Chapter 34), diabetes (Chapter 72), or epilepsy (Chapter 80); and patients who are recuperating from myocardial infarction (Chapter 58) and stroke (Chapter 83).

Physicians occasionally react negatively to difficult patients and situations. Often, these reactions are evoked by patients' feelings that seem to be directed personally at the physician; at times they are caused by recapitulation of aspects of the physician's own relationships (see discussion of countertransference, Chapter 11). Table 3.7 summarizes common negative reactions of physicians and strategies for dealing with these reactions. Most of the strategies require one to take time for self-exploration, one of several strategies that physicians identify as healthy adaptations to stress (see "Physician Self-Care," next section).

PHYSICIAN SELF-CARE

An unstated assumption about the doctor–patient relationship is that a physician is always ready to respond with skill and concern to a patient's distress. Because of the extraordinary needs of sick patients and the demands of running a practice, most physicians are at risk of experiencing excessive stress themselves, beginning during training and spanning their professional careers. Substance abuse, mental illness, family dysfunction, and loss of satisfaction are well-recognized accompaniments of physician stress. To counterbalance the risk of excessive stress and to increase the likelihood that they will be skillful, caring, and satisfied in their professional relationships, physicians need to address the care of themselves.

When asked about their healthy approaches to stress, physicians identify the following personal strategies, each of which should be available to most physicians (12).

Values clarification and time management. This strategy, although it is implicitly present in each person's life, can be especially helpful when it is undertaken explicitly by professionals such as physicians, whose working days often bring more demands than they can reasonably meet. The process of thinking about and writing down one's core values can help to identify activities that do or do not reflect those core values and to rearrange one's priorities. A common

Table 3.7. Common Negative Responses of Physicians to Difficult Patients and Strategies to Cope with These Responses

Physician's Emotional or Behavioral Reaction	Coping Strategies[a]
Avoidance	Analyze why; attempt to understand and master feelings that lead to avoidance; stay with the patient; discuss with colleagues.
Identification with patient	Recognize, avoid tendency to deny seriousness of disease or to give way to despair; stay with the patient.
Hostility/rejection	Acknowledge and analyze; do not attempt to like the unlikable patient; use behavioral approaches; if situation is intolerable, transfer patient to another physician.
Feelings of impotence, inadequacy (e.g., in caring for dying patient)	Discover areas in which help and comfort can be rendered, both physical and emotional; be realistic about limitations to medicine; give the patient time to go through the stages of bereavement.
Feelings of loss of control or threatened authority	Acknowledge and analyze; be realistic about personal limitations and actual range of influence and authority; be aware that patient's need for control over his or her own body may conflict with physician's urge to control the situation.
Frustration, confusion, uncertainty about dealing with the patient; coping strategies not effective	Request psychiatric consultation/referral.
Anxiety, guilt, frustration about meeting patient's recognized emotional needs	Allocate time realistically according to need; request consultation/referral.

From Gorlin R, Zucker HD. Physicians' reaction to patients. N Engl J Med 308:1059, 1983.
[a]See also skills in Table 3.6 and Psychosocial Treatment Techniques in Chapter 11.

example of the impact of value clarification would be the decision of an overcommitted professional to say no to, to delegate, or to discontinue low-priority activities so that more time can be allocated to valued family activities and personal life.

Self-awareness and sharing feelings with others. These strategies may be important for addressing predictable stressful situations, which range from patient care encounters that evoke negative responses (Table 3.7) to family tension caused by the demands of one's professional life. One may incorporate these strategies by reserving time to reflect privately or to write a personal journal and, if one has a group of like-minded colleagues, by scheduling regular meetings at which to share in confidence one another's dilemmas and joys (20) and to better recognize feelings and responses such as those listed in Table 3.7. The latter strategy is especially helpful for dealing with the negative effects of reflecting alone on stressful issues.

Personal health care. The strategies in this section can be seen as ways to promote and protect one's mental well-being. It is equally important for physicians to identify goals for their physical health and to address these goals with concrete measures such as exercising regularly, getting adequate sleep, avoiding harmful health habits, selecting and visiting a personal physician, and taking sick time when they are not well enough to work.

The 1997 paper by Novack et al provides extensive information related to physician self-awareness and self-care.

General References*

The American Academy on Physician and Patient (AAPP).
> National organization that offers a wide variety of courses and learning materials (including quarterly journal Medical Encounter on the doctor–patient relationship). Address: 6728 Old McLean Village Drive, McLean, VA 22101-3906. Phone 703-556-9222.

---

*Bold print (general references) and bold numerals (specific references) denote published controlled clinical trials, meta-analyses, or consensus-based recommendations.

American College of Physicians ethics manual. 2nd ed. Ann Intern Med 111:245, 317, 1989; 3rd ed. Ann Intern Med 117:949, 1992.
> Helpful descriptions and discussions of ethical principles governing physician–patient, physician–physician, and physician–society relationships.

Cross-cultural medicine. West J Med 139(6), 1983.

Cross-cultural medicine: a decade later. West J Med 157(3), 1992.
> Two special issues, covering major problems that are generic to cross-cultural medicine in the United States and containing articles on most of the major immigrant populations in the United States.

Lipkin M, Putnam SM, Lazare A. The medical interview: a textbook on medical interviewing. New York: Springer-Verlag, 1994.
> Multiauthored text with extensively referenced chapters on all of the uses of the interview in medical practice and research supporting them.

Novack DH. Therapeutic aspects of the clinical encounter. J Gen Intern Med 2:346, 1987.
> Thorough, well-referenced review, focusing largely on ordinary medical encounters.

Novack DH, Suchman AL, Clark W, Epstein RM, et al. Calibrating the physician: personal awareness and effective patient care. JAMA 278(6):502–509, 1997.
> Extensively referenced paper covering the following four core topics: physician's beliefs and attitudes, physician's emotional responses in patient care, challenging clinical situations, and physician self-care.

Quill TE. Recognizing and adjusting to barriers in doctor–patient communication. Ann Intern Med 111:51, 1989.
> Delineates common barriers and practical ways to address them.

Smith RC, Hoppe RB. The patient's story: integrating the patient- and physician-centered approaches to interviewing. Ann Intern Med 115:470, 1991.
> Well-referenced description, with concrete illustrations, of ways to ensure active patient involvement in an exploratory interview.

vom Eigen KA, Inui TS. Special issue: medical care and the physician–patient relationship. Med Encounter 13(2), 1997.
> Thoughtful essays by 10 authors on the challenges that managed care brings to the doctor–patient relationship.

Specific References

1. Arnold R, Forrow L, Barker LR. Medical ethics and doctor–patient communication. In: Lipkin M, Putnam SM, Lazare A, eds. The medical interview: a textbook on medical interviewing. New York: Springer-Verlag, 1994.
2. Balint M, ed. His patient and the illness. New York: International University Press, 1972.

3. Connelly JE, DalleMura S. Ethical problems in the medical office. JAMA 260(6):812, 1988.
4. Emanuel EJ, Dubler NN. Preserving the physician–patient relationship in the era of managed care. JAMA 273:323–329, 1995.
5. Ende J, Kazis L, Ash A, Moskowitz MA. Measuring patients' desire for autonomy. J Gen Intern Med 4:23, 1989.
6. Frank JD. The influence of patients' and therapists' expectations on the outcome of psychotherapy. Br J Med Psychol 41:349, 1968.
7. Kleinman A, Eisenberg L, Good B. Culture, illness, and care: clinical lessons from anthropologic and cross-cultural research. Ann Intern Med 88:251, 1978.
8. Laine C, Davidoff F. Patient-centered medicine. JAMA 275:152–156, 1996.
9. Lazare A, Putnam SM, Lipkin M Jr. Three functions of the medical interview. In: Lipkin M Jr, Putnam SM, Lazare A, eds. The medical interview: clinical care, education, and research. New York: Springer-Verlag, 1995.
10. Parsons T. The social system. New York: Free Press, 1951.
11. Putnam SM, Stiles WB, Jacab MC, James SA. Teaching the medical interview, an intervention study. J Gen Intern Med 3:38, 1988.
12. Quill TE, Williamson PR. Healthy approaches to physician stress. Arch Intern Med 150:1857, 1990.
13. Reeder LC. The patient–client as a consumer: some observations on the changing professional–client relationship. J Health Soc Behav 13:406, 1972.
14. Reiser DE, Schroder AK. Patient interviewing: the human dimension. Baltimore: Williams & Wilkins, 1980.
15. Shorey JM. Research in doctor–patient communication within a managed care era: a physician's perspective. Med Encounter 13(2), 1997.
16. Smith RC, Hoppe RB. The patient's story: integrating the patient- and physician-centered approaches to interviewing. Ann Intern Med 115:470–477, 1991.
17. Stewart MA. Effective physician–patient communication and health outcomes: a review. Can Med Assoc J 152(9):1423, 1995.
18. Stewart M, Brown JB, Weston WW, et al. Patient-centered medicine: transforming the clinical method. Beverly Hills, CA: Sage, 1995.
19. Szasz T, Hollender MH. A contribution to the philosophy of medicine: the basic models of the doctor–patient relationship. Arch Intern Med 97:585, 1956.
20. Williamson PR. Support groups: an important aspect of physician education (editorial). J Gen Intern Med 6:179, 1991.

C H A P T E R 4

Patient Education, Behavior Change, and Compliance

DAVID E. KERN, MD
KARAN A. COLE, ScD

One meaning of the word *doctor* is "teacher." Teaching is an important physician function that can help patients understand their conditions, relieve anxieties, and enhance compliance with treatment regimens. Most of the elements of communication during a visit, described in Chapter 3, contribute to the process of patient education, a process that depends as much on developing trust, identifying the patient's information needs and psychosocial context, and involving the patient in developing a plan as on the giving of information.

The goals of this chapter are to review fundamental educational and behavior change principles, describe factors that influence patient compliance with medical recommendations, and based on this information, describe effective, practical approaches to patient education and behavior change.

PATIENT EDUCATION

Definition

Patient education can be defined as *a patient learning experience during which the physician or teacher uses a combination of educational needs assessment and instructional, behavioral, motivational/empowerment, mechanical, and practice operations interventions that influence the patient's knowledge, attitudes, and health behaviors. Health behaviors* encompass a wide range of activities that relate to health, including seeking health advice; keeping health care appointments; taking medications; undertaking recommended preventive measures; modifying existing patterns of eating, exercising, or substance use; and solving problems. Patient education sometimes is completed during one physician–patient interaction, but more often is *an ongoing process that occurs over the course of several visits.*

The Doctor–Patient Relationship

Patient education takes place in the context of a doctor–patient relationship, which influences the nature of the educational process. As discussed in Chapter 3, the relationship between physician and patient can be conceptualized in a spectrum that ranges from active–passive to mutual participation. In an *active–passive* relationship, the physician as expert is responsible for explaining and prescribing and the patient is responsible for following orders. This type of relationship presumes an *authoritative approach* to patient education and behavior change. In a *mutual participation* relationship, the patient and physician actively collaborate, and patients take more responsibility for their care. This type of relationship assumes that most patients are capable of participating with the physician in the development of their own management plans. It incorporates an *empowerment approach* to patient education and behavior change, during which the physician facilitates patient involvement in goal identification, problem solving, and planning (22,58). Patients bring to this process their expertise with respect to themselves: their experience, beliefs, values, goals, daily routines, social setting, perceived educational needs, and expectations. Physicians assume the role of mentor, consultant, and expert in medical knowledge.

Effective patient education does not involve the exclusive use of either an authoritative or an empowerment approach. Actually, the two approaches are at opposite ends of a continuum. Often, approaches are combined, and the balance of authoritative and empowerment approaches within a given physician–patient interaction is determined by physician attitude and skill, patient attitude and skill, and patient need.

EDUCATIONAL AND BEHAVIOR CHANGE PRINCIPLES

An effective approach to patient education and behavior change requires an understanding of certain principles that guide the assessment of educational needs and the planning of educational interventions. These principles relate to learning and the adoption of new behaviors. An understanding of these principles helps physicians identify factors that need to be assessed and to choose strategies when creating an educational intervention.

Adult Learning

As people age, they become less dependent and more *self-directed* (8,20,42). They are more likely to make changes and to learn when they perceive a need or desire to do so than when they are told to do so. They *prefer to be actively, rather than passively, involved* with their learning. They tend to be *problem-oriented* rather than subject-oriented. And increasingly with age, they define themselves by their *experience*. A physician who defines a goal and management strategy for a patient, therefore, is less likely to be successful than one who pursues a more *learner-centered* approach. The latter physician starts with the patient's perceived needs and expectations, then develops, with the patient, achievable goals and management strategies that take account of the patient's past experience, expectations, and strengths, and that address barriers through problem solving.

Single Versus Multilevel Interventions

Clinical experience and research support the principle that *knowledge is necessary, but not sufficient,* when patients are expected to make lifestyle changes. Such changes may range from fitting a medication regimen into a patient's daily routine to altering longstanding patient habits such as overeating and smoking. *Educational interventions that are targeted at several levels, including knowledge, attitudes, behavior, and environment, are most effective.* Studies of the impact of patient education on a number of conditions confirm this principle (5,10,33,49,50,56,57,69).

Readiness for Change

Patient readiness for change predicts patients' success in achieving behavioral change (54). There are *five stages of readiness for change* (Fig. 4.1). They include *precontemplation, contemplation, action, maintenance,* and *relapse.* A patient may move through this cycle many times before successfully eliminating an old habit or adopting a new habit.

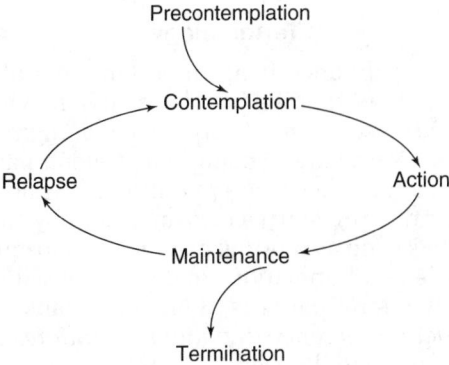

Figure 4.1. The readiness for change cycle.

Successfully identifying the stage of readiness for change helps the physician in identifying appropriate strategies. If a patient has not even considered a specific behavior change, such as stopping smoking (precontemplative), the goal might be to pursue strategies that would help the patient move toward contemplation, such as the exploring the reasons why the patient might want to stop smoking. If the patient is contemplating a behavior change, the goal might be to begin to identify potential facilitators or barriers to achieving that change. In the action phase, specific goal setting and anticipatory problem solving would occur. In the maintenance and relapse phases, reactive problem solving is appropriate.

Self-Efficacy

According to social learning theory (3), the strongest factor in predicting whether a behavior occurs is the level of self-efficacy, or the individual's *confidence in performing a behavior.* Numerous studies have identified the relationship between self-efficacy and behavior and demonstrate the effectiveness of interventions targeted toward increasing an individual's self-efficacy (67).

Locus of Control

Individual beliefs regarding who controls one's health status reflect a patient's orientation to control. These include internal locus of control, external locus of control, and chance locus of control (73). Patients' perceptions of locus of control, self-efficacy, and behavioral change are complexly interrelated, and to a significant degree are specific to a given situation (61,72). A patient's beliefs about locus of control are relevant in that they help determine whether an authoritative or empowerment approach will be most effective.

Patients who believe that their health is a consequence of their own efforts have an *internal locus of control.* These patients prefer to take a high level of responsibility for their health care; for them, a collabo-

rative doctor–patient relationship and an empowerment approach to patient education and behavior change are most appropriate.

Patients who believe that their health is a consequence of others' efforts, particularly of physician efforts, have an *external locus of control.* These patients prefer explicit directions from their physician; and an active–passive doctor–patient relationship, an authoritative approach to patient education, and behavioral change are most appropriate.

Finally, patients who have a *chance locus of control* believe that health-related outcomes are determined by fate and are therefore uncontrollable. When this belief is inappropriate to the situation (e.g., in uncontrolled hypertension), the physician may wish to explore and address the belief.

Health Beliefs and Explanatory Models

Most patients come to the doctor with their own ideas about their health and health problems, which are grounded in their own experiences, social interactions, and culture. Their *explanatory models* may include ideas about etiology, pathophysiology, susceptibility, severity, prognosis, treatment, and prevention (39). Social scientists have described a *health belief model* that consists of five categories of beliefs and has been shown to influence a patient's health-related behavior (37). The categories of patient beliefs in this model are (*a*) *severity of a disease,* condition, or consequences of not changing one's behavior; (*b*) one's *vulnerability or susceptibility to* the disease, condition, or the consequences of certain behaviors; (*c*) the *effectiveness of* the therapy or change in behavior; (*d*) the *benefits* of therapy or change in behavior; and (*e*) *potential risks* of the therapy or change in behavior.

Physicians who provide explanations and negotiate management plans that make sense in the context of patients' own health belief systems are more likely to satisfy patients and influence their behavior (68). Likewise, the degree to which patients and physicians are able to achieve congruence of beliefs about causality and treatment predicts patient satisfaction and patient compliance with treatment recommendations (24,25,69,70).

Intention to Comply

The relationship between patient intention to comply and health behavior is straightforward and is often a consequence of earlier mentioned principles. Patients who are ready to make a behavior change, have high self-confidence in their ability to make the change, agree with the explanation provided by the physician, and believe they will experience benefits if they make the behavior change and experience consequences if they do not, are likely to have a greater intention to comply than patients who do not have these characteristics. Also, patients who have been part of the process of decision-making are more likely to have a greater intention to comply than those who have simply been told to make a change.

Empowerment

Ambulatory patients are responsible for implementing most management strategies developed in physicians' offices. To implement a management plan, not only do patients have to be ready for it, believe it is in their best interest, and believe that they can accomplish it; they also have to do it. Empowerment is the facilitation of active self-management by patients. The more complex and behaviorally demanding a management plan, the greater the challenge for the patient who must integrate it into the demands of day-to-day living. Some patients are more prepared to meet such challenges than others. Many patients fail if provided only with a general directive, but not with the specific information and skills necessary to achieve it. Patients are more likely to successfully implement challenging management plans when their needs have been assessed and when attention has been paid to the knowledge, attitudes, and skills that underlie relevant motivation, goal-setting, behavioral change, problem solving, stress management, coping, and the development of social support (see "Assessment" and "Intervention" later in this chapter).

Social Support

Within the coping appraisal model (45), social support is defined as external resources that, when cognitively appraised, assist the efforts of the patient to manage internal and external demands. A substantial body of literature explores the primary effects of social support in preventing illness. In addition, there is a documented positive relationship between social support and compliance with medical recommendations (6), myocardial infarction readjustment (7,9), smoking cessation (14). The existence of a marriage partner has been shown to positively affect health outcomes (74).

It has also been shown that the *quality,* as well as the quantity, of support is important. An unsatisfying marriage may be worse than no marriage for health outcomes (15). The overinvolvement of spouses, characterized as misguided helping, can have negative effects (16,17). Patients whose family members exhibit a harmful behavior that the patient is trying to change, such as smoking or eating a high-fat diet, have a particularly difficult time changing that behavior. On the other hand, if family members can be enlisted to support patients in facilitative and positive ways, patients are more likely to make a change.

Therefore, assessment of the quality as well as the quantity of social support is an important step in developing an educational intervention. No matter how many potential supports are available, patients need to be asked for their own perception of these because the available supports may not be resources but actually barriers to behavioral change.

PATIENT COMPLIANCE

Terminology

Patient compliance is an important goal of patient education. It is defined *as the extent to which the patient adheres to medical advice or agreed-upon treatment plans.* Patient compliance encompasses taking medications, keeping appointments, undertaking recommended preventive measures, and, with respect to activities such as dieting, exercising, substance use, and problem-solving styles, changing possibly deep-seated behavioral patterns. Some clinicians favor the term *patient adherence* to *patient compliance,* but the latter is more widely used.

Noncompliance can be caused by a failure to understand instructions, *noncomprehension,* or can exist in the presence of adequate understanding.

Noncompliance should be viewed as a neutral term. It describes one aspect of patient behavior that may be either appropriate or inappropriate to the patient's best interests. For example, it may be appropriate for a patient with mild chronic obstructive pulmonary disease to be noncompliant in taking a regularly prescribed medicine, such as theophylline, if it causes more distress (e.g., nausea) than relief. On the other hand, it would be inappropriate for a patient with severe hypertension to stop taking antihypertensive medication because of denial of the medical problem. It should be recognized that responsibility for noncompliant behavior may rest with the physician. For example, it is not valid to blame noncompliant patients for failure to understand instructions or to realize the importance of therapy when there has been ineffective communication by the physician.

Importance

Problems Caused by Noncompliance

Patient noncompliance is important from at least three perspectives: individual patient care, public health efforts, and economic consequences.

First, patient noncompliance with efficacious regimens may thwart the goals of both physician and patient in preventing illness, reducing suffering, improving functional status, and increasing longevity. If physicians are unaware of their patients' noncompliance, they may falsely attribute poor outcomes to inadequate dosage, failure of the regimen itself, or incorrect diagnosis. Any of these conclusions could lead to inappropriate action by the physician. Thus, medication might be changed or dosage might be increased, or new diagnoses might be entertained and the patient subjected to unnecessary procedures and testing.

Second, noncompliance may increase the cost and reduce the effectiveness of preventive measures such as screening, immunization, and disease control programs. For example, a screening program that identifies undiagnosed hypertension is less effective and costs more for each hypertensive complication prevented if the dropout rate after screening is high or compliance with medication is low.

Third, noncompliance with indicated medical regimens has been shown to increase medical costs for active problems by increasing hospitalization rates for cardiac and other patients, contributing to the need for nursing home placement in the elderly, and increasing use of outpatient services, including emergency room care (62).

Prevalence of Noncompliance

The high prevalence of noncompliance underscores the importance of the problem. Reported noncompliance rates must be viewed critically and compared with caution because of differences in definition from study to study. Nevertheless, the results of extensive reports are almost unanimous in identifying noncompliance, variably defined, as extremely prevalent. Rates vary from less than 10% to more than 90%, depending on the setting. Because of previous dropouts, cross-sectional studies of patients taking medication chronically tend to underestimate noncompliance, but even then the prevalence of noncompliance is often in the 20 to 70% range. Among newly diagnosed hypertensives, for example, in classic community-based studies, up to 50% failed to follow through with referral advice, more than 50% of those who began treatment dropped out by 1 year, and only about two-thirds of those who stayed under care consumed enough prescribed medications to achieve adequate blood pressure reduction (32).

Lack of comprehension of a regimen is a common cause of noncompliance. Unfortunately, most studies do not separate noncomprehension from volitional noncompliance, but where studied, noncomprehension has been shown to be responsible for 20 to 70% of objectively measured noncompliance.

ASSESSMENT

Importance

Patient education can be conceptualized as successive cycles of assessment and intervention (Fig. 4.2). The effectiveness of an educational intervention depends on the accuracy of the educational assessment as well as the physician's skill in using instructional, behavioral, motivational/empowerment, mechanical, and practice operations strategies (see "Intervention"). *Patient education, therefore, should begin with an*

assessment of (*a*) background information that defines the patient's educational needs and relates to compliance, and (*b*) the patient's current health-related behaviors, such as medication taking and nondrug treatments. The knowledge gained from such an assessment permits one to focus an educational intervention in a manner that is likely to be both efficient and effective.

Knowing or Obtaining Background Information

There are multiple factors to consider before making an educational diagnosis and developing an educational intervention. These can be classified as those related to the patient, the disease, the treatment, the environment, or the doctor–patient relationship. Most are associated with patient compliance (Table 4.1). Knowledge of this background information about a patient makes it possible to individualize an explanation or a management plan in a way that is likely to be effective.

Patient Characteristics

It is important to assess a patient's *knowledge, attitudes, and beliefs* about a condition and its management. As distinguished from disease, which is an objective entity based on the presence of independently verifiable findings, a patient's explanation and experience of illness is a subjective state that is shaped by personal, interpersonal, and cultural factors. It is the patient's perceptions of an illness and its treatment (see "Health Beliefs and Explanatory Models" earlier in this chapter) that correlate with compliance rather than the objective realities. An extreme example occurs in patients who deny illness. Thus, patients who have had a myocardial infarction, who answer "no" or "maybe" rather than "yes" when asked whether they have experienced a heart attack, are less likely to comply with physicians' instructions for decreased activity and reduced cigarette smoking (19).

Patients often have their own *models of disease and treatment.* If this model conflicts with the regimen prescribed for the patient, noncompliance may follow. For example, the commonly held perception of hypertension as an intermittent, symptomatic, stress-related condition encourages an erratic approach to medication taking. Some patients with clearly diagnosable soft tissue injuries may think that their evaluation was incomplete without a radiograph and therefore mistrust the physician's diagnosis. Ethnic concepts of disease and treatment can also conflict with the physician's approach to diagnosis and management and result in noncompliance. Such concepts are more prevalent among ethnic group members who experience a language barrier, are generationally close to immigration, live in segregated neighborhoods, are lower in education level and socioeconomic class, and experience barriers to receiving personalized medical care—that is, those who are least integrated into the mainstream culture. For example, some patients might change physicians or refuse treatment if they are told

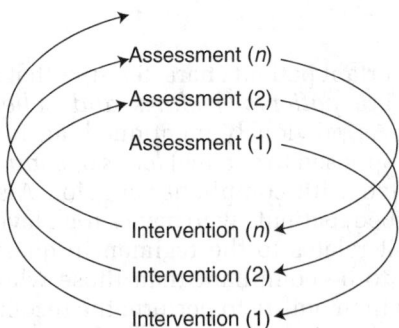

Figure 4.2. The assessment–intervention spiral.

Table 4.1. Assessment: Factors Associated with Compliance

Patient Characteristics
Personal knowledge, attitudes, and beliefs, including
  Explanatory model, fears, concerns
  Past experience
  Locus of control: internal or external vs. chance
  Readiness for change
  Perceived self-efficacy
  Intention to comply
Cultural/ethnic models of disease and treatment
Value systems: personal and cultural/ethnic
Self-care/self-management skills
Ability to pay for treatment
Previous or concurrent compliance
Psychologic factors (e.g., immaturity, impulsivity, paranoia, hostility, fear of dependence, denial, commitment to a bad decision, type A personality)

Disease Features
Symptomatic vs. asymptomatic condition
Comorbid conditions
  Cognitive impairment
  Psychiatric illness (e.g., depression, mania, schizophrenia, paranoia, antisocial or paranoid personality disorders)
  Alcoholism/drug addiction

Treatment Factors
Complexity of treatment regimen (number of medicines or treatments, frequency of dosage or treatment)
Duration of therapy
Requirement for significant behavior change
Side effects, actual and perceived
Expense (to patient)

Environmental Factors
Family/social support
Cultural norms
Residential stability
Experience of similar illness among family/friends
Individual vs. block appointments[a]
Convenience (location, quality of transportation, flexibility and accessibility of appointment times)[a]
Waiting time[a]
Referral to specific doctors rather than clinics[a]
Communication skills of support staff (respectfulness, friendliness, caring)[a]

Doctor–Patient Relationship
Effective communication of information and instructions
Explanations that make sense from patient's perspective
Doctor–patient congruence in understanding of problem and its management
Fulfillment of patient's expectations; address of patient's concerns
Patient participation/involvement in development of treatment plan
Empathetic understanding by physician
Positive, friendly, confident approach by physician
Transference/countertransference reactions
Patient trust, confidence in physician
Patient satisfaction
Level of physician supervision
Continuity of provider

[a]Refers to appointment keeping.

they have both "high blood pressure" and a "low blood count" (anemia). According to some folk beliefs these diagnoses are mutually exclusive, so the physician making them may be regarded as untrustworthy.

Self-care and self-management skills are important factors that vary among patients and should similarly be assessed. These include general problem-solving, decision-making, and coping skills, as well as condition-specific skills such as changing wound dressings, self-monitoring of blood pressure and blood sugar, and the mixing and injecting of insulin.

Other important patient characteristics that are often overlooked are *patients' feelings and beliefs about themselves.* As previously mentioned, an internal or external (as opposed to chance) *locus of control* is usually associated with compliant behavior. Also previously described, patients who have a high level of *self-efficacy,* as it relates to the regimen in question, are more likely to be compliant than those who are not confident in their ability to perform the recommended behavior. Patients' *readiness for change,* as well as their *intention to comply,* are usually found to be associated with compliance. *Other feelings,* such as dislike of taking medication, the desire not to depend on or be controlled by others, and the need to be seen by self or others as normal, may also interfere with compliance.

Patients' *value systems* may be congruent with or conflict with those of physicians, and affect compliance. For example, an elderly patient may prefer to accept an increased risk of death rather than endure an inconvenient, impersonal hospitalization that separates him from home and family.

Surprisingly, *sociodemographic variables* such as age, sex, race, education, occupation, income, and marital status usually do not correlate with compliance behavior. However, elderly patients have been shown to have difficulty in opening childproof medication containers, and they may be at increased risk for noncomprehension. *Inability to pay* for visits, medication, or transportation can be an important barrier to compliance for some patients. In some studies, older age, retired status, married status, patient initiation (as opposed to provider initiation) of an appointment, and third-party payment, prepayment, or lack of copayment have been associated with improved appointment keeping behavior, whereas lower education, lower socioeconomic status, and language barriers have been negatively correlated with appointment keeping.

Previous or concurrent compliance with one aspect of treatment usually correlates with adherence to other aspects of the regimen.

Psychologic factors, such as immaturity, impulsivity, hostility, fear of dependence, denial, commitment to a bad decision, and type A personality have been found to correlate with noncompliance in some studies. Moreover, some patients who come to physicians are experiencing considerable anxiety, which may interfere with cognitive functioning, of which comprehension is one element. Other patients may experience a period of grief in reaction to a diagnosis, such as diabetes or coronary artery disease, and such grief interferes with their ability to master the demands of a new treatment regimen. Understanding may be further hampered by the tendency of many patients, such as blue-collar workers, to ask few questions of their physicians even when they desire information (30).

Disease Features

Patients who are *experiencing symptoms* such as pain, lethargy, and palpitations are more likely than asymptomatic patients to respond to treatment recommendations, especially if the symptoms are relieved by the treatment. On the other hand, patients may be so overwhelmed and debilitated by their symptoms that they may be unable to follow through with aspects of the regimen.

Comorbidity may either create problems for patients or provide the patient with a set of self-management skills that are easily applied. A patient with hypertension and diabetes, for example, who has recently had a myocardial infarction, may either have trouble following recommendations because of the multiple de-

mands or may actually have an easier time as the result of having learned self-management skills with the hypertension and diabetes. Patients with certain *psychiatric illnesses,* such as depression, mania, schizophrenia, paranoia, or antisocial or paranoid personality disorders, tend to be less compliant. Factors that affect the patient's *ability to comprehend,* or to organize and initiate deliberate behavior, such as a language barrier, dementia, or mental retardation, should be expected to decrease compliance. *Alcoholism and drug addiction* tend to correlate highly with noncompliance.

Treatment Factors

The *complexity of the medical regimen* correlates inversely with compliance. Compliance decreases as the number of medications or the number of daily doses per medication increases. Unsynchronized schedules (e.g., one drug every 4 hours and another every 6 hours) should also be expected to affect compliance adversely. *The duration of therapy* and the *requirement for significant behavioral change* (e.g., weight reduction or smoking cessation) are negatively correlated with compliance. *Side effects of medications* may result in noncompliance when they cause significant symptoms or interfere with an important function in the individual's life (e.g., impotence secondary to an antihypertensive drug in a young, sexually active man). *Medication class* is related to compliance, with seemingly more important drugs (e.g., cardiac and diabetic agents—more than 70% compliance in cross-sectional studies) resulting in higher compliance rates than seemingly less important medicines (e.g., antacids, sedatives, and drugs prescribed for symptomatic relief—less than 50% compliance) (13,34–36). The reason for these differences is unknown and could conceivably be due either to sound patient judgment or to increased physician emphasis, supervision, and teaching. The relationship between independently audited medication need and compliance remains unexplored. Other aspects of the treatment regimen that may influence compliance include *delayed or not obvious benefits of the therapy,* the *degree of lifestyle interference,* and *expense* (to the patient).

Environmental Factors

Patients who have stable *support systems* and stable *family situations* tend to be more compliant. A spouse's concern about a patient's illness can encourage compliance with medication taking, appointment keeping, and prescribed behavior changes (e.g., diets and smoking cessation). Advice and reinforcement from other family, friends, and lay practitioners can also encourage compliance. Nursing and office staff may promote compliance by demonstrating enthusiasm and positive attitudes about patients' adherence to a treatment regimen. On the other hand, an overly protective family member can sabotage a plan for progressive return to normal function. Disinterested or poorly informed family members or friends may actually discourage patient compliance with a treatment plan.

Family dysfunction or high levels of dependence on the patient, such as when a patient is a caretaker, can create a burden that makes compliance more difficult.

The *cultural norms* of social class, ethnicity, family, age, and sex are also important. Adherence to these norms is likely to supersede adherence to the norms of the medical profession when the two are in conflict.

It should be remembered that patients' *previous experiences of similar disease* among relatives or friends can profoundly affect their beliefs about their own illnesses, and influence their health-related behaviors.

Appointment keeping is positively correlated with *appointment scheduling systems* that reduce waiting time, give individual rather than block appointments, minimize the time between scheduling and the actual appointment date, and make referrals to specific doctors rather than to clinics. *Convenience* in terms of location or hours of operation of a physician's practice and support staff who are respectful, friendly, and helpful may also encourage appointment keeping and discourage dropouts.

Doctor–Patient Relationship

Establishment of a good doctor–patient relationship is well recognized as an important determinant of patient compliance. Although *effective communication* is a prerequisite to the establishment of such a relationship and affects health care outcomes (29,40,66,70) as well as compliance (1,24,25,31,48,59,63,68,70), studies show that physicians commonly communicate poorly with their patients (21,23,41,68). The necessary skills (see Chapter 3) can be learned and are being taught with increasing frequency in medical schools, residencies, and continuing education courses (41).

Effective transfer of information is important (47,49) because patients must understand their regimen before they can be expected to comply with it (see "Instructional Strategies" later in this chapter). Because the patient may already have some ideas and concerns about his or her problems, *explanations that justify a treatment regimen, correct or accommodate misconceptions, and make sense to the patient* are most likely to promote compliance.

Other features of the communication process that correlate with patient compliance include *fulfillment of patient expectations* (requires detection of and attention to the patient's underlying concerns); physician *friendliness*; a *positive, confident approach* on the part of the physician; physician *response to patient complaints; encouragement of patient questions;* a *supportive, nonjudgmental method of eliciting and responding to patient admissions of noncompliance;* communication to the patient of a genuine and accurate *empathetic understanding* of the patient's perspective and feelings; *encouragement of patients to become actively involved* in their own care; *active patient participation* as opposed to physician dominance; *negotiation rather than dictation of a treatment plan; identification and resolution of barriers to compliance;*

congruence between patient and physician in their understanding of a problem and its management; *physician effort to motivate* the patient; and *patient satisfaction* (24,25,29,31,40,59,63,64,68,70).

Transference, or the subconscious redirection to one person of feelings and attitudes toward others (e.g., parents or authority figures), may further influence patients' relationships to their physicians. Depending on their nature, transference reactions, which are based on previous experiences, can promote compliance (e.g., the patient who finds it rewarding to please authority figures) or impede it (e.g., the patient who distrusts authority figures). *Countertransference,* the redirection toward the patient of previously developed physician attitudes and feelings, can also be detrimental or beneficial to the doctor–patient relationship (see Chapter 11).

Close supervision of the patient by the physician (or an assistant) has proved a consistent and significant correlate of compliance with therapeutic regimens. In most studies, *continuity in provider care* has also contributed.

Many of the above features contribute to the development of *patient trust in the physician,* and trust is one of the most important factors in any approach to helping people change. Because a key element of trust is self-disclosure and because self-disclosure exposes the patient to possible rejection, ridicule, shame, or exploitation, the importance of eliciting and responding to admissions of noncompliance in a nonjudgmental manner, in the context of a positive and supportive relationship, is clear.

Some practitioners prefer patients who do not ask too many questions and who simply follow instructions. Although this active–passive relationship may be appropriate for some patients, to be effective with other ambulatory patients, physicians must enter into a relationship of *mutual participation* in which they listen to, educate, and negotiate with patients (28,29,40). Such an approach need not be time-consuming. It is the quality of the interaction, not the amount of time spent, that correlates with compliance and satisfaction (21,41).

Methods for Assessing Background Information

Much of the information detailed previously may already be known to the physician who has an ongoing relationship with a patient. *Review of the primary care and other front sheets* (see Chapter 1) in a well-maintained patient record is an efficient method of obtaining relevant information. A *focused medical and social history* can also elicit important background information. Whenever patients present with new problems or difficulty managing old ones, it is helpful to *inquire about their understanding, beliefs, feelings, and readiness for change related to the problem, and their expectations for the physician–patient encounter.* The information-gathering skills described in Chapter 3 and demonstrated in the following examples pertain to this task.

EXAMPLES

Doctor: Mrs. Smith, tell me your understanding of hypertension . . . what it is and how it should be treated. (understanding)

or

Doctor: Mr. Jones, it seems like you have been troubled by this back pain for some time now. What would you most like me to do for you today? (expectations)

or

Doctor: Ms. Jackson, tell me how you feel about stopping smoking? (readiness for change)

Some patients may not expect, or may feel awkward about, such open inquiry about their opinions. They may be embarrassed to reveal their ideas or fear being ridiculed for them by the physician. Therefore, they may initially avoid answering the questions. In these situations, it is helpful to be gently persistent while conveying genuine interest in and respect for the patient.

EXAMPLE

Doctor: Mr. Johnson, you seem worried about you sore throat. What do you think might be causing it?

Patient: I don't know. That's what I came here for . . . to find out. (possible avoidance)

Doctor: Well, I have some ideas, but its also helpful for me to hear about my patients' concerns so I can make sure I address them. (gentle persistence)

Patient: Well, I really don't know. I just wanted to make sure it wasn't something serious, since it's been hanging on. You know I'm a smoker, and so was my dad. He died of throat cancer.

Doctor: Well, that's a very understandable concern. (nonjudgmental, supportive, and respectful response)

Result: The doctor proceeds to explain that there is no reason to suspect cancer on the basis of the history or physical examination, and uses the opportunity to explore the patient's readiness to stop smoking.

Assessing Health-Related Behaviors

Knowledge of a patient's current health-related behaviors, including lifestyle patterns and compliance with prescribed medications and nondrug regimens, is a prerequisite to evaluating the effectiveness of current regimens and to determining whether there is a need for behavioral change or reinforcement. This section focuses on the assessment of patient compliance with recommended treatment, although some of the methods that are discussed (asking, outcomes, observations) are relevant to the assessment of any health-related

behavior. Subsequent chapters address the measurement of some specific health-related behaviors (Chapters 20 and 21 on substance use, Chapter 58 on exercise, Chapter 76 on obesity) and problem-solving styles (Chapters 10, 11, and 14).

Explicit assessment of compliance is important because studies have shown that physicians are poor at subjectively predicting compliance behavior in their patients, sometimes performing no better than expected by chance (11,12,27,53). There are several approaches to assessing compliance-related behaviors in patients (Table 4.2). Because each method has some limitations, it is often necessary to use more than one method to arrive at a reasonably valid estimate of such behaviors in an individual patient.

Asking

The simplest and most practical method of assessing health-related behavior is to ask the patient. Self-reports of noncompliance with prescribed or desired regimens are generally valid, although the degree of noncompliance tends to be underestimated. There is even some evidence that patients who admit to being noncompliant may be more amenable to intervention than those who do not (38).

Because only about 40 to 80% of patients admit to noncompliance with a prescribed regimen, self-reports cannot be relied on. In studies of various patient populations, reported compliance rates almost always overestimate true compliance rates.

The manner of asking influences the accuracy of patient response. Certain interview methods can provide reasonably valid estimates of patient compliance (65). It is generally agreed that patients should be questioned about compliance in an *open-ended, facilitative, nonthreatening, nonjudgmental, yet detailed and specific* way. Questioning should continue until the patient has provided information about what medicines are being taken and how often, how often doses are missed, and what nonpharmacologic modes of treatment are being used. Patients should be specifically asked about compliance on the day of and the day preceding their visit. (For example, some diabetic patients routinely omit all drugs, including insulin, at the time of a morning visit; *24-hour recalls* are more accurate than general reports, which tend to be idealized.) Using such techniques, the physician will identify 50% or more of patients who are not complying with a prescribed regimen (and all of those who do not

Table 4.2. Assessment: Health-Related Behaviors

Asking: open-ended, facilitative, nonjudgmental, detailed, and specific questioning of patient or family regarding nonpharmacologic as well as medication-taking health-related behaviors; 24-hour recalls (see text example)
Frequency of patient-requested prescription renewals or medication counts
Inspection of all pill bottles
Drug assays
Achievement of expected therapeutic and physiologic outcomes (e.g., blood pressure, weight, heart rate)
Review of longitudinal relationship between therapeutic and outcome measures
Direct observation by physician or staff (office or hospital)
Observations reported by others (e.g., family, visiting nurses)

comply because they do not understand the regimen). Sensitivity can be increased by asking family or household members.

EXAMPLE: INEFFECTIVE METHOD

Doctor: Now, Mrs. Smith, are you taking your medications as prescribed? (judgmental and leading question, which permits a yes/no and promotes a yes answer; confines response to medications).

Patient: Yes, every day.

Result: The doctor raises dosage or adds new medication because her blood pressure is still not adequately controlled. The patient becomes frustrated.

EXAMPLE: EFFECTIVE METHOD

Doctor: Now, Mrs. Smith, can you tell me what you are doing to control your blood pressure? (open-ended; nonjudgmental; focuses responsibility on patient; does not confine response to medications)

Patient: Well, I've stopped adding salt to my food and have pretty much cut out all salted snacks. I do occasionally have a frozen dinner when I'm alone. And, of course, I'm taking the medication.

Doctor: Uh, huh . . . (facilitative)

Patient: Yes, that blue pill.

Doctor: And how are you taking it? (directive, not leading)

Patient: Twice a day.

Doctor: Any other medications? (directive, not leading)

Patient: No. I stopped the fluid pill when we started the blue one.

Doctor: And did you take the blue one this morning? (directive)

Patient: No, I never take my medicine the day I come to the office!

Doctor: What about yesterday? (directive, not leading)

Patient: Yes . . . at least in the morning. Yesterday afternoon was so hectic! You know how busy my days are!

Doctor: I guess it's hard to take that afternoon dose? (facilitative, empathetic, nonjudgmental)

Patient: Yes, because my schedule varies so much.

Doctor: What did you decide about starting on an exercise program? (directive, nonjudgmental, focuses responsibility on the patient)

Patient: Thought about it, but haven't done anything yet. Do you really think it's important?

Result: The doctor congratulates (positively reinforces) the patient on salt restriction, tailors a medication regimen to the patient's schedule, explains why she should take her medication on the day of an office visit, provides more information on the value of regular exercise, and provides written instructions/contract to which both agree. The doctor decides not to restart the diuretic because of the patient's compliance with salt restriction and the lack of a blood pressure reading reflecting the effect of the current medication regimen. If the dietary history had been less convincing or the patient had gained weight, the patient might have been asked for a 24-hour diet recall (which is more accurate than general questioning) on this and subsequent visits.

Medication Counts

Medication counts (pill counts) are a form of indirect behavioral monitoring that provides a more objective measure of compliance with a prescribed regimen than does simply asking patients. They have been used to demonstrate the lack of reliability of patient-reported compliance. Results are usually expressed in terms of percentages. The ability to measure sequential behavior depends on the use of short intervals between counts, which is usually not feasible. Although more accurate than reported compliance, medication counts also have limitations. If patients are suspicious of being monitored, they can remove medicines from containers without ingesting them. Overestimates of compliance can also occur if other people are using medicine from the same container. Compliance may be underestimated if the patient is using two or more medication containers but makes only one available for counting. Furthermore, many patients do not bring their medication containers with them to the physician's office, despite reminders. Finally, some patients might take offense at having their medications counted, resulting in deterioration of the physician–patient relationship.

The medication count can be approximated by the more practical and less intrusive method of prescribing quantities of medication that should be consumed within a reasonable interval of time, and then observing the *frequency with which prescription renewals are requested.*

Ingenious medication dispensers have been devised that monitor not only the amount but also the regularity with which medicine is removed (18). They are emerging as a new gold standard of compliance assessment but are used primarily in research trials, are expensive, and are not generally available for use in clinical practice.

Assays

Another objective method of estimating *compliance with a prescribed medication regimen* involves testing drug levels in blood, urine, breath, or saliva. Drug levels have been shown to correlate with compliance determined by other methods as well as by outcome. Marked variation in drug levels may reflect inconsistencies in medication taking. Monitoring drug levels and relaying results to the patient may also improve compliance.

However, there are limitations to the method. Assays can be expensive. For accurate assessment, multiple measurements are required over an extended period. There is the possibility that if patients know they are being monitored, they may take medicine immediately before the collection of specimens but not at other times. More important may be differences in drug absorption, distribution, metabolism, and excretion among individuals, making it impossible in the individual patient to decide whether a low level represents noncompliance or inadequate dosage. The absence of any drug in the specimen suggests noncompliance, assuming the specimen has been collected appropriately. The physician should have a working knowledge of the pharmacokinetics of the medicine being assayed so that the collection of specimens can be timed correctly. Compliance with short-acting drugs, which are rapidly cleared from the blood and excreted, is difficult to monitor by assay techniques because of the difficulty in collecting specimens at appropriate times. Finally, assays are not available for many medications.

Assays can also be used to assess *abstention* from alcohol, drugs, and smoking (see Chapters 20–22).

Outcomes

Another objective but more indirect method of estimating compliance with a specific regimen is to *monitor expected therapeutic or physiologic outcomes.* For example, blood pressure can be followed in a patient taking antihypertensive medication, weight in a patient on a weight reduction diet, and pulse rate in a patient prescribed a β-blocker. *Review of the longitudinal relationship between* a specific *therapeutic regimen and outcome* measures can provide clues to noncompliance (e.g., review may disclose widely varying blood pressures on a constant regimen). Such a review can be expedited by the presence and maintenance of a treatment versus outcome flow sheet.

Many of the limitations of drug assays also affect assessment of outcome, which can be influenced by variations in drug bioavailability, absorption, distribution, and excretion; multiple measurements are required. Furthermore, other factors can influence outcome. For example, a reduction in stress may lower blood pressure, or the presence of concomitant heart disease might be responsible for bradycardia.

Observation

An additional approach to assessing health-related behaviors is to *observe patients directly, or indirectly through others.* Family, household members, or visiting nurses can sometimes provide reliable information on medication taking and other health-related behaviors.

An extension of this approach involves the comparison of *drug levels or outcomes of therapy during observed versus unobserved periods of a targeted behavior such as medication consumption.* Observations and measurements can be accomplished either in the office, at home, or during hospitalization, depending on the pharmacokinetics of a medication, insurance coverage, and the availability of home care resources. A specific example of this methodology is the 5-hour office blood pressure check in patients who have resistant hypertension, during which the patients take their medication under supervision, then have their blood pressures measured at regular intervals for several hours (4).

Inspection of all pill bottles is a commonly used and important form of observation. When the patient appears confused or is unable to provide sufficient information, having him or her bring all medication containers to the office (for both prescribed and over-the-counter medications) may provide invaluable information. For example, it may be discovered that a patient is still taking a discontinued medication or is taking two different preparations of the same drug. Selected patients should be encouraged to bring their medication containers with them at every visit.

INTERVENTION

Overall Strategy

Once an educational assessment has been made, the physician is well-positioned to help the patient acquire the information, attitudes, skills, and behaviors needed to deal with the medical problem. It is helpful to keep in mind the elements in the overall strategy summarized in Table 4.3 and described here when designing and implementing an educational intervention for a given patient.

- Whenever possible, *ground the educational intervention in a doctor–patient relationship that promotes patient trust in the physician* (see "Doctor–Patient Relationship," earlier in this chapter, and Chapter 3 for the characteristics of and methods for developing such a relationship). The successful past management of problems will also enhance trust in the physician.
- *Target the intervention to:*
  - Address the stage of the patient's readiness to change, which has been identified as part of the educational assessment process described earlier (see "Educational and Behavioral Change Principles and Background Information" and Fig. 2.1).
  - *Meet the patient's educational needs,* which have been identified using assessment approaches described earlier (see "Background Information").
- *Develop specific measurable objectives* that can be used to focus the educational strategies. Then, the numerous instructional, behavioral, and motivational/empowerment strategies and mechanical aids discussed below can be viewed as a menu of options that can be used to help achieve the objectives.

EXAMPLES

Between this visit and the next, the patient will comply with a mutually agreed-upon medication regimen.

By the end of this visit, the patient will be reassured that her malaise and weight loss are unlikely to be caused by cancer (her fear), and will entertain the possibility of depression as a cause.

- *Prioritize and limit the objectives and material to be covered* at each interaction, so that they do not

---

Table 4.3.   Intervention: General Principles

Start with a doctor–patient relationship that promotes patient trust in the physician.
Target the educational intervention to:
　address patient identified readiness to change (Fig. 4.1); and
　meet the patient's specific educational needs.
Use specific measurable objectives to focus each interaction; use instructional, behavioral, and motivational/empowerment strategies and mechanical aids as a menu of options to achieve objectives.
Prioritize and limit objectives and material to be covered at each interaction.
Remain patient-centered and interactive.
Avoid premature education before relevant information has been collected and synthesized.
Check for patient comprehension and agreement.

overwhelm the patient and can be accomplished within available time limits.

- *Remain patient-centered* (e.g., by accommodating or addressing the patient's routines, beliefs, values, and expectations) *and interactive* throughout the educational intervention. This permits the physician to continually adapt educational strategies to meet patient needs. It enhances patient understanding, retention, and compliance with treatment regimens and agreed-upon lifestyle changes.
- *Avoid premature education.* Except for simple responses to answerable questions, it is generally preferable to provide patient education *after* relevant historical and physical examination data have been collected, information synthesized, an educational assessment made, and a tentative plan formulated. Premature education can result in the giving of misinformation, which will later have to be corrected. It can be ineffective or inefficient if it is not based on adequate assessment or not appropriately focused and prioritized. It is also inefficient because it provides information early in an encounter that will usually be repeated at the close of the encounter.
- *Check for patient comprehension and agreement* with explanations and management plans. Checking helps the physician gauge the success of an intervention.

EXAMPLES

Doctor: I know we covered a lot today. It would help if you could tell me in your own words what you are going to do between now and the next visit.

or

Doctor: Last visit we discussed treatment options for your angina. I also gave you a handout on angina. I wonder what your thoughts are now on the options and my recommendations?

Adherence to these components of an overall strategy should enhance patient understanding, compliance, and satisfaction.

Specific educational/behavior change methods are discussed later in this chapter. They should be viewed as a menu of options that can be used in implementing the overall strategy discussed above and summarized in Table 4.3.

Efficacy of Educational/Behavior Change Interventions

Educational/behavior change interventions can be classified as instructional, behavioral, motivational/empowerment, or practice operations strategies, or mechanical aids. Successful interventions have increased compliance rates by less than 10% to almost 70%, averaging between 25 and 30% (percentage change equals percentage of compliant patients in the experimental group minus percentage of compliant patients in the control group). When studied, compliance-improving interventions have also been shown to have favorable cost–benefit ratios (62). A combination of instructional and behavioral/motiva-

tional interventions is more effective than instruction alone.

Instructional Strategies

Some sort of explanation or communication of information is a part of almost every doctor–patient interaction. Sometimes the explanation is an end in itself (e.g., explaining to a patient the expected course of a condition for which there is no treatment or clarifying a patient's unfounded fears about a laboratory test). In other situations it promotes compliance by providing patients with a rationale for treatment and clarifying a treatment regimen (47,49). The patient education content related to specific problems and diagnostic procedures is described in later chapters of this book, often in brief "Patient Experience" sections. Instructional strategies that enhance understanding, retention, and compliance are displayed in Table 4.4 and discussed next.

Information is most effective when it is *targeted* to the needs of the patient, provides an *explanatory framework* understandable and acceptable to the patient, and *addresses misconceptions and potential barriers* to compliance. The use of *medical jargon should be avoided,* and the *use of language should be tailored to the educational and cultural background* of the patient.

To improve retention, verbal instructions should be *clear, concise, and explicit,* with *important features emphasized and repeated* (46). When there is a large or complex body of information to be conveyed, it is helpful to break it down into *understandable categories,* as in "I am going to tell you what I think is causing your symptoms, what tests I am going to suggest, and the treatment that should help you. Now, what I think is causing these symptoms . . . " This technique has been shown to improve retention of information when compared with a less organized recitation of facts (46).

Because patient factors such as anxiety and reluctance to ask questions may interfere with understanding, it is useful to *check for patient receipt, understanding, and retention* of the essentials of the information

Table 4.4.   Intervention: Instructional Strategies

Target information to meet educational needs.
   Provide explanatory framework understandable and acceptable to patient.
   Address misconceptions, fears, and barriers.
Use language appropriate to educational and cultural background of patient; avoid medical jargon.
Use verbal communication methods that increase understanding and retention.
   Be clear
   Be concise
   Be explicit
   Repeat important content
   Categorize
   Use dialog, as opposed to monolog
Test for comprehension.
Give written instructions.
Give printed educational material.

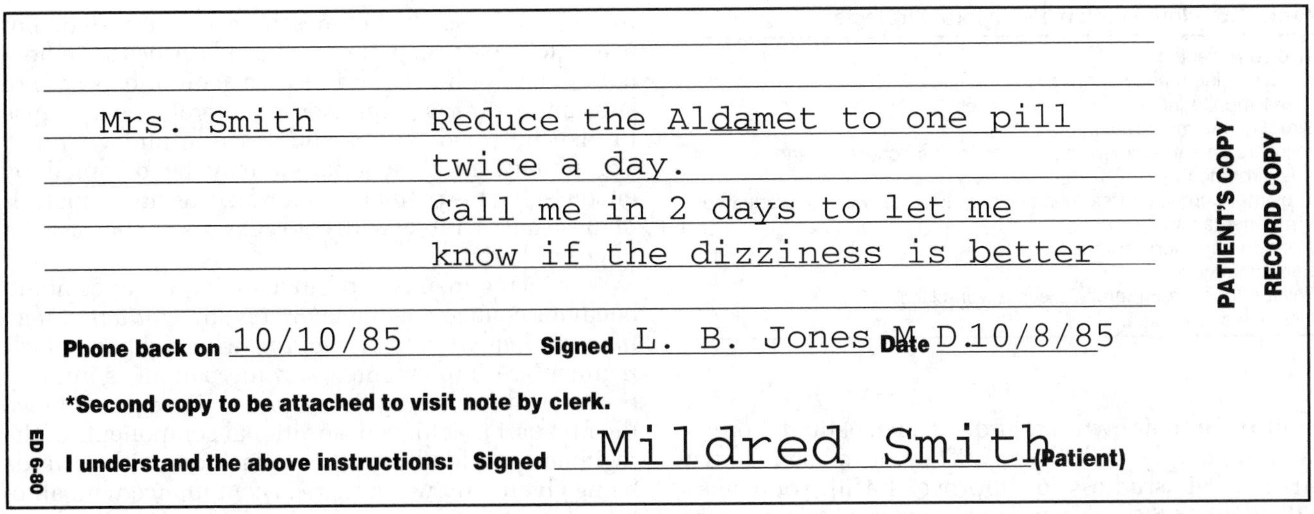

Mrs. Smith   Reduce the Aldamet to one pill twice a day.
Call me in 2 days to let me know if the dizziness is better

PATIENT'S COPY RECORD COPY

Phone back on 10/10/85   **Signed** L. B. Jones M. D. **Date** 10/8/85

*Second copy to be attached to visit note by clerk.

ED 6-80   **I understand the above instructions: Signed** Mildred Smith **(Patient)**

Figure 4.3. Examples of written instructions for a patient (form makes a copy for the patient's folder). (Courtesy of Johns Hopkins Bayview Medical Center, Baltimore, MD.)

that has been communicated. Furthermore, because it has been found that patients tend to recall the diagnosis better than the treatment plan (46), it is important to ascertain retention of the essentials of the treatment plan; for example, for a streptococcal throat infection, determine whether the patient understands that penicillin will be taken for a full 10 days (not the exact dosage or schedule, which will be transcribed onto the pill bottle). In order not to offend the patient when checking for comprehension, it is helpful to use an approach such as, "We covered a lot today, and I'm not sure whether I have explained things clearly. It would help me if you would tell me what you understand to be the plan," rather than directly ordering the patient, "Now tell me what the plan is."

An *interactive* as opposed to monolog approach to communicating information encourages patients to ask questions and have their questions answered. It permits ongoing targeting of the educational message and assessment of patient understanding. It should also increase retention.

Written instructions further enhance compliance (47) and are an important adjunct to verbal instruction. They can be documented on self-duplicating forms (Fig. 4.3). The duplicate portion can be attached to a visit note or a specially constructed educational flow sheet for documentation and future reference. Medication charts are specialty formatted written instructions that can be used to enhance compliance with prescribed medications (55). Legible written or printed instructions provide a remedy for forgetfulness, and can be reviewed at leisure in the less stressful environment of the patient's home.

Because it usually requires time to make sense out of information about one's condition (e.g., newly diagnosed hepatitis), because patients retain only about one-half of the essential information communicated at a visit (21,46), and because doctor–patient communication is usually focused and time-limited, *printed educational materials* can be used to reinforce and expand on what the patient is told. When printed materials are given to a patient, the physician can personalize them by underlining important points, writing down additional important information, and by writing the day's date on it. A large collection of printed educational handouts is available in the periodically updated book by Griffith (see "General References"). Condition-specific publications that are widely available (e.g., from the American Heart Association or National Cancer Institute) are cited in later chapters of this book.

Behavioral Strategies

Communication of information is necessary but often insufficient to ensure the adoption and maintenance of health-related behaviors by a patient. This is particularly true in the setting of chronic disease, probably because most patients have already learned their prescribed regimen and have learned something about their disease. Behavioral strategies (Table 4.5) are strategies that attempt to directly influence the adoption or maintenance of certain behaviors. Strategies that incorporate various combinations of patient involvement, alterations in the treatment regimen (simplification, tailoring, shaping), use of behavioral stimuli and reinforcers, and supervision have been shown to improve patient compliance with chronic therapy. Patient involvement, simplification and tailoring of the treatment regimen, and supervision also enhance compliance with short-term therapeutic regimens.

Mechanisms of *enhancing patient involvement* include facilitating patient question asking, negotiating a treatment plan with patients (rather than dictating treatment plans to patients), signing contracts with patients, and encouraging patient self-monitoring, such as the measuring of glucose levels or taking of blood pressures at home. All increase patient respon-

Table 4.5. Intervention: Behavioral Strategies

Involve patients in:
   developing management plan.
   self-monitoring.
Simplify treatment regimen.
Tailor treatment regimen to fit patient's characteristics and
   environment.
Implement complex treatment regimen in a stepwise or graduated
   manner (shaping).
Manage behavioral stimuli (cues).
Use reinforcers.
Enlist support from family, friends, workplace.
Increase supervision.

sibility for their own care and enhance patient motivation to comply with therapy. They have been shown in several studies to improve health outcomes (28,29,40,43,66). Self-monitoring may also move patients from precontemplation to contemplation to action in the readiness to change cycle (Fig. 4.1), and motivate problem solving in cases of noncompliance.

Simplification of the treatment regimen refers to minimizing the number of medications, minimizing the duration of treatment (for short-term regimens), minimizing the frequency of dosing (e.g., once instead of three times daily), and synchronizing the dosing (e.g., three medicines twice daily instead of one medicine twice daily, the second medicine three times daily, and the third medicine four times daily). The less complex the regimen, the greater the compliance rate. This is a particularly important strategy because of both its effectiveness and its ease of implementation.

Tailoring is a process whereby the therapeutic regimen is fitted to the patient's characteristics and environment. Effective tailoring requires knowledge of patients as persons—their beliefs, lifestyles, social and family support systems, and specifically, any barriers to compliance. Forgetful patients may benefit from linking medication taking or prescribed activities to daily routines such as eating meals, brushing teeth, getting up in the morning, or going to bed at night. In addition, medication should be kept available where it is taken (e.g., at the breakfast table). If possible, patients should avoid taking medication at times of the day when their activities are variable or when they are likely to be distracted (e.g., at work). Other examples of tailoring include involving patients who like to be in control in planning and monitoring their own therapy, substituting liquid medication in patients who have difficulties swallowing tablets or capsules, increasing supervision and peer support for patients who are having difficulty on their own following a desired regimen (e.g., a weight reduction diet), and recommending exercise programs that can be incorporated into the schedules of extremely busy, time-pressured patients and that eliminate travel, waiting time, and the need for special scheduling. The physician needs to search specifically for barriers that interfere with compliance. When cost is a factor, less expensive regimens can be prescribed or financial assistance sought. When a patient's health belief or ethnic model of disease

interferes, it can sometimes be accommodated. For example, Hispanic patients who subscribe to the hot–cold theory of health and disease avoid the use of hot substances during pregnancy and therefore may refuse to take hot medications such as iron and vitamins. Compliance in this situation may be obtained by encouraging the patient to neutralize the hot properties of these medications with cool substances such as fruit juices or herb teas.

When a regimen is particularly complex or difficult, behavior change may be facilitated by *graduated regimen implementation* or *shaping,* whereby parts of the regimen are implemented and the patient is initially rewarded for adhering to only part of the regimen. Once the first part is achieved, additional components of the regimen are added in stepwise fashion, with rewards being given only when there is compliance with all of the components that have been implemented.

In addition to adjusting the therapeutic regimen to meet the patient's needs, the patient and physician can work together to identify and manage *behavioral stimuli (cues)* and reinforcers that promote or diminish desired behaviors. Watching television, for example, may be an environmental cue for patients who have learned the habit of eating when they watch television, even when they are not hungry. To eliminate this behavior, the physician and patient might reach an agreement whereby a patient eats only at the dining room table with the television off. Another behavioral cue might be the presence of cigarettes or a friend smoking. In preparation for a smoking cessation effort, a patient might want to remove all cigarettes from her house or to negotiate an agreement with her friend to refrain from smoking in her presence. Patient involvement is critical because almost all environmental stimuli exist in the patient's environment outside the physician's office and because something that might work from the physician's perspective might not work at all for the patient. Involvement of family and friends can be helpful in supporting the management of behavioral cues in the patient's environment. Alternatively, family and friends may be a barrier if they refuse to cooperate.

Reinforcement consists of feedback that can either promote or discourage specified behaviors. Feeding back to the patient results of drug level assays and therapeutic outcomes (e.g., decrease in blood pressure, cholesterol, or weight) are examples of physician controlled reinforcers. Together with the patient, the physician can identify already existing reinforcers, support or initiate those that promote, and attempt to eliminate or diminish those that discourage desired behaviors. Because positive feedback is more effective than punishment in helping patients adopt new behaviors, measures and outcomes that indicate compliance with desired behaviors should be praised, otherwise rewarded, or viewed by the patient as rewards in themselves. When measures or outcomes suggest noncompliance, the problem should be discussed. Rewards should be appropriate to the goals (e.g., eating an ice cream cone would be an inappropriate reward for having followed a diet), and can be increased as the patient gets closer to achieving the goals.

Education and use of family, friends, and employers may be required to optimize rewards for desired behaviors or to reduce the rewards for undesired behaviors at home and in the community. Two common examples for such an intervention are reversal of reinforced psychosocial disability in the physically capable patient after myocardial infarction and maintenance of abstention in the detoxified alcoholic patient.

Increased supervision is a specific form of stimulus management and reinforcement that has been shown to improve compliance. It includes the scheduling of more frequent provider–patient contacts, the use of reminders, the use of drug assays, and the eliciting of family or community support to assist in administering and monitoring treatment. For example, the physician may request more frequent blood pressure values in a hypertensive patient. The blood pressures can be taken either by a nurse at the physician's office, a nurse at work, a family member, or the patient. The direct supervision of medication administration is an option that is especially helpful for ensuring compliance in situations where compliance is known to be low, such as patients who are forgetful or unreliable, or have impaired intellectual or psychologic functioning (e.g., patients with alcoholism, dementia, or schizophrenia). Examples include the use of a single intramuscular long-acting penicillin rather than 10 days of an oral preparation, intermittent supervised oral antituberculosis therapy, and long-acting parenteral drugs in the ambulatory management of schizophrenia.

Motivation and Empowerment Strategies

Compliance tends to decay toward baseline after the cessation of many successful interventions. One explanation for the failure of most compliance-improving interventions to have enduring impact is their reliance on actions and supports *external* to the patient. Based on reviews of the relevant compliance, psychologic, sociologic, and behavioral literature, DiMatteo and DiNicola and Meichenbaum and Turk (see "General References") suggest *approaches that promote internalization of the patient's motivation and ability to comply.* These approaches include helping patients to adopt new beliefs, attitudes, or values; setting agreed-upon goals; enhancing patients' perceptions of their self-efficacy; and facilitating new skill development in patients (Table 4.6).

Patients may have to adopt new beliefs, attitudes, or values and abandon others. Because physicians are the major source of health information for most Americans (21), they can assist in this process. They are more likely to succeed if they have earned the patient's trust and if they incorporate empowerment strategies of involving the patient in setting goals, solving problems, and planning for the intervention (see "Doctor–Patient Relationship" earlier in this chapter). As previously mentioned, the first step in promoting change in health attitudes is to explore patients' present knowledge, beliefs, attitudes, and values, as well as their social and cultural norms. Education about their diseases and regimens can then be tailored to correct misconceptions, fill in gaps in their knowledge bases, provide explanations that are understandable and acceptable to patients, and motivate them in the context of their value systems. Simply taking time for discussion will raise the salience in the patient's mind of the issue being discussed. Threat or fear messages can motivate behavioral change but should not be too strong (can cause patient denial or paralysis) or too weak. Furthermore, they should be combined with a positive message about a feasible (for the patient) and effective therapeutic regimen. Because patients are often more present-oriented than future-oriented, short-term as well as long-term benefits of any regimen should be stressed. Because behavior can influence attitudes, as well as vice versa, the practitioner should point out the patient's own behaviors that support the attitude being promoted. One can help integrate the new attitude into the patient's total system of beliefs by noting how it correlates with other beliefs the patient has. One can also note how it adheres to cultural and social norms. Of course, new attitudes and beliefs need positive reinforcement, as previously discussed.

The *setting of agreed-upon goals* can be motivational and provide direction for the patient. Patient involve-

Table 4.6. Intervention: Motivation and Empowerment Strategies

Help patients adopt appropriate new beliefs, attitudes and values.
   Target education to fill in gaps in knowledge base, correct misconceptions, provide explanations that are understandable and acceptable to patients, and motivate patients in the context of their value systems.
   Use fear and benefit messages appropriately (relevant, accurate, connected to treatment plan that is effective and feasible for patient).
   Point out current/past patient beliefs, attitudes, behaviors that are congruent with the desired new beliefs, attitudes, and values.
Set agreed-upon goals.
Enhance patient self-perceptions (self-efficacy, locus of control).
   Project a positive attitude about patient's abilities to change.
   Emphasize past and present behaviors that demonstrate self-control.
   Help patients take credit for changes that have been accomplished.
   Reframe "failures" as successes.
Facilitate new skill development.
   Involve the patient in the development of management strategies.
   Facilitate problem solving by the patient.
   Facilitate the development of specific, achievable behavioral objectives by the patient.
   Facilitate the development of self-monitoring skills.

ment in, and preferably initiation of, goal setting is a crucial component of this step. For goals to be most effective, they must be "owned" by the patient. Goals should be set at two levels. The first level is long-term, such as, "I want to quit smoking in 6 months." The second level is short-term, or proximal goals. These goals refer to the specific actions that will be required to meet the long-term goal, such as, "I will begin using Nicorette gum at a 4-mg dosage next Monday, and I will reduce this to 2 mg in 1 month." These are actually more helpful to the patient in that they are easier to achieve and can be measured more directly. They should be specific, measurable, realistic, and achievable in order to be effective. Having a patient sign a contract can further increase the likelihood of success.

Patients with unhealthy *self-perceptions* or perceived low *self-efficacy* may need to be convinced that they can indeed effect a change in their lives (a process sometimes called *cognitive restructuring*). The physician can help by emphasizing the patient's past and present behaviors that demonstrated self-control, by enhancing the patient's feelings of responsibility for accomplished changes, by pointing out inaccuracies in the patient's negative self-perceptions, and by having and projecting a positive attitude to the patient about his or her ability to change.

EXAMPLES

Doctor: On one hand, you say you have no self-control. On the other, you tell me you stopped smoking for the entire period of your second pregnancy. That demonstrates to me that you can exhibit tremendous self-control.

Doctor: Two months ago you told me that you would never be able to manage insulin. Now you are monitoring your own blood sugars and calling me to propose changes in your insulin schedule. What does that tell you about yourself?

Patients and their physicians often view partial successes as failures (e.g., the patient who has started drinking or smoking after a period of abstinence, the patient who has cut caffeine intake in half). In the office, physicians can promote patients' self-esteem and sense of self-efficacy by *reframing* these *"failures" as successes,* as important steps along the way to accomplishing important health goals.

EXAMPLE

Doctor: It's great you were able to stop smoking for a month! That really increases your chances of being able to quit for good. Did you know that most people who stop smoking require more than one attempt?

In addition, patients can learn how to shift their own self-perceptions during vulnerable moments at home, when negative thoughts may interfere with following through with a plan. In anticipation, patients can be asked about potential "sticking points." In response to having experienced these sticking points, they can be encouraged to reflect on and contrast their thoughts during the times they have been successful versus the times they have not. Using these awarenesses, they can reframe a failure into a partial success in the moment,

or can use positive self-statements that have been previously effective (e.g., "I can do this"). Patients can take this one step further by *posting positive statements or images as reminders* where they can often see them or where they are likely to be tempted to not follow through with a treatment plan. Family members can be enlisted to be a verbal source of the positive statements or to help patients reframe their negative thoughts. However, it is essential that patients consider this as helpful and not as overinvolvement or an attempt by the family to control their behaviors.

New skills can also be taught to patients, an empowerment approach that enhances their ability, as well as motivation, to initiate and maintain compliance with difficult regimens. Patients can learn problem-solving skills by analyzing, with the physician, the health problem, treatment alternatives, and the advantages and disadvantages of potential actions. They can participate in the development of overall treatment goals. They can be tutored in developing specific, feasible, and measurable behavioral objectives for themselves, and in breaking down large tasks into several small, manageable steps. When patients have adopted new attitudes, beliefs, or behaviors, they can be taught to anticipate and prepare themselves for likely challenges.

EXAMPLES

Doctor to the recovering alcoholic: What challenges do you expect to your new sobriety? How are you going to handle it when people try to get you to drink at your niece's wedding this weekend?

Doctor to the hypertensive patient who is sensitive to being viewed as ill by others: How are you going to respond when one of your colleagues at work sees you taking your medication and says "Oh, you have to take medicine now! What's wrong with you?"

Patients can also be taught to analyze and learn from past failures to enhance the likelihood of future success.

EXAMPLES

Doctor: Why has it been difficult for you to take the second dose?

Doctor: Exactly how did it occur, when you started smoking again? What does that tell you?

Doctor: If you could overcome that problem, your chances for success would be really high! Any ideas?

Efforts to help patients adopt appropriate health-promoting beliefs, attitudes, values, skills, and behaviors can be integrated into ongoing care and should usually span several office visits. *Referral to supportive groups* that expose patients to others with similar problems (e.g., asthma, postmyocardial infarction, ostomy, and mastectomy groups; Alcoholics Anonymous; or Weight Watchers) is an important adjunct to management. Once patients have experienced success in implementing changes in one health-related behavior, their sense of efficacy increases, and they are more likely to be successful in changing other behaviors.

Mechanical Aids

Compliance with therapeutic regimens can also be improved by the use of a number of mechanical aids. These include well-labeled medication containers (51), medication charts (55), pill calendars (devices on which patients keep track of their medication taking), special pharmaceutical packaging designed to aid memory (e.g., the packaging of birth control pills), and pill dispensers (devices that can be purchased for laying out medications in advance by day and, when necessary, by time of day). Well-designed forms can promote the use and effectiveness of written instructions (Fig. 4.3) (55) and the compliance of patients with self-monitoring (e.g., by providing patients with flow sheets for recording blood pressures or blood sugars, and asking the patients to bring the sheets with them to the next visit).

Compliance with Appointment Keeping

A number of factors have been shown to improve appointment keeping by patients (48). Table 4.7 lists the strategies that can be used to improve patient compliance with appointment keeping.

Telephone and mail reminders, in which patients receive messages several days before their scheduled visits informing them of the dates and times of their appointments or messages inviting patients to reschedule after missed appointments, have consistently improved compliance, usually in the range of 10 to 20%. The impact of the reminders may attenuate over time, however (26), and it may be possible to discontinue reminders without a subsequent increase in missed appointments (52). Wording of the message may be influential. In one study of high-risk patients (44), postcards with a persuasive educational message resulted in a significantly higher compliance rate for influenza vaccination than those with a neutral message simply announcing the availability of the vaccine.

The introduction of *individual instead of block appointment systems* and the *substitution of a single for multiple providers* have resulted in decreased waiting time and improved appointment keeping. Individual appointment systems give each patient a precise time for an appointment; block systems schedule several or all patients for the same time, usually at the beginning of office hours.

Techniques that the physician can use to improve appointment keeping for individual patients include logically *"bridging" to* the next visit by discussing its purpose with the patient (e.g., monitoring for recurrence, review of test results, decision about therapy), *negotiating a visit interval* that is mutually acceptable, *tailoring the appointment time* to the patient's needs, *obtaining a verbal agreement* from the patient to follow through, and *scheduling the appointment* instead of asking the patient to call for an appointment. Bridging and scheduling have been tested in one successful clinical trial (71).

Because *missed appointments* could presage dropouts from treatment, the charts or names of these patients should be reviewed daily by the patient's physician or a nurse familiar with the patient. When indicated, the patient can be contacted by telephone, letter, or postcard. This review method will help prevent dropouts for patients given a follow-up appointment at the time of the previous visit, but will fail to identify dropouts who were instructed to call for their next appointments.

If referral is required, *educating the patient about the purpose of referral, minimizing the elapsed time* between the referral and the referral appointment, providing secretarial assistance to *facilitate scheduling and transportation,* and *referring the patient to a specific physician* and not simply to a specialty group or clinic have also been shown to improve appointment keeping for diagnostic studies and specialty consultations.

Combining Strategies (Case Example)

Strategies that combine two or more methods are generally much more effective than single interventions (5,33,69). For example, such combination strategies have been shown to improve compliance in patients with asthma (2), congestive heart failure (56,57), diabetes (10), and hypertension (50), and after myocardial infarction (1). In the latter study, patient involvement was accomplished by having patients set their own goals and monitor their own behavior. Frequent contact with the physician allowed reinforcement, modification of goals on a negotiated basis, and discussion of problems with the regimen. Involvement of the spouse led to increased supervision. In the asthma study, compliance and functional status was better after 1 year in a group of patients with asthma who received an instructional workbook, one-on-one counseling, self-monitoring, and an asthma support group, and who were asked to identify an asthma control partner, than in a group given standard informational pamphlets on asthma.

The following is an example of how instructional, behavioral, and motivational/empowerment strategies can be integrated into a visit (continuation of a previous example).

Table 4.7. Intervention: Improving Compliance with Appointment Keeping

Logically "bridge" to the next appointment.
Negotiate appointment time and interval with patient.
Refer to specific doctors rather than to clinics.
Educate patient about purpose of referral.
Reach agreement with or obtain verbal committment from patient.
Schedule appointment for patient rather than having patient call for one.
Use individual, as opposed to block, appointment systems.
Minimize waiting time.
Use telephone or mailed reminders.
Establish review system for missed appointments.

Doctor: Well, Mrs. Smith, your blood pressure is 150/100 today, which is better than when we started but not as low as we'd like it. Do you remember the goal we agreed upon? (We implies shared responsibility. Doctor focuses patient on a specific measurable objective and points out that some progress has been made.)

Patient: I believe it was under 140 on the top and under 90 on the bottom.

Doctor: Right. What do you think you could do to bring it down further? (Doctor further involves and transfers responsibility to the patient.)

Patient: Well, as you said, part of the problem with today's blood pressure could be my not taking the medicine this morning. So I'll be sure to take it from now on, on the days I come to see you. Also I've been thinking about enrolling at the athletic club. I like dancing. The club has convenient hours and is on my way to work. I'd prefer not to take any more medicines.

Doctor: The athletic club is an excellent idea. Regular exercise not only has a direct effect that lowers blood pressure, but it might also indirectly lower your pressure by helping you to lose weight. (Doctor provides positive reinforcement and notes an added benefit that relates to another goal the patient has for herself.)

Patient: That would be nice.

Doctor: I am concerned though about the difficulty you have getting the second dose of medication into your schedule. Blood pressure pills work best when you can take them almost 100% of the time. (Doctor provides a rationale for this concern.) Would dinner be a good time for you? (Doctor initiates negotiation process)

Patient: My meal times are irregular and I don't always eat at home.

Doctor: How about bedtime?

Patient: Sometimes I'm so exhausted, I just fall to sleep while I'm reading, before I've brushed my teeth or anything. Don't you have a pill that can be taken just once a day?

Doctor: As a matter of fact, that's a possibility. When would you take it?

Patient: With my morning coffee. I never miss that!

Doctor: Fine, I'll give you a prescription for a pill that you can take once a day with your morning coffee, 100% of the time, even the mornings you come to my office. Is that a deal? (repetition and emphasis to increase retention)

Patient: Yes! (solution and verbal contract achieved through tailoring and negotiation)

Doctor: The side effects for this medicine are the same as for the other. Since you experienced none with the other, you should tolerate this one well.

Patient: Good.

Doctor: Together with the salt restriction and exercise program, this medicine alone may be enough to control your blood pressure. (Doctor provides further motivation for salt restriction and exercise.) Of course, we'll start with a low dosage, so we may have to increase it. Can you come back in 2 weeks?

Patient: How about 2 months?

Doctor: Well, I'd really like to see you more often until your blood pressure is controlled. Of course, if you monitored your own blood pressure at home, you could call the results in to me and there would be less need for frequent office visits. (The doctor prefers not to yield on the follow-up interval and uses the opportunity to motivate the patient to become further involved in her own management and to create a new environmental reinforcer.)

Patient: How can I do that?

(Doctor proceeds (*a*) to explain the process of getting a blood pressure cuff, coming to the office to have it checked, and learning how to use it; (*b*) to test the patient for her understanding of her responsibilities; (*c*) to get her verbal commitment; and (*d*) to write down for her the new management plan.)

FOLLOW-UP

Education can involve the adoption of new beliefs, attitudes or values, the development of a patient's sense of self-efficacy, the development of a patient's self-management skills, the setting of agreed-upon goals, the adoption of new or cessation of old behaviors, and the maintenance of successfully changed behaviors (e.g., the taking of a chronic medication or the cessation of smoking). In the process, patients move forward in the readiness for change cycle (Fig. 4.1). Sometimes, as in the case of diabetes, the required cognitive and behavioral changes are both numerous and complex (see Chapter 72) and are best implemented in incremental steps (see above) over the span of several visits. Commonly, patients successfully implement only part of a prescribed or agreed-upon regimen. Often periods of successful implementation are followed by periods of relapse (Fig. 4.1). Therefore, *follow-up is a crucial component of patient education.* Repetitive cycles of assessment and intervention (Fig. 4.2) are associated with increased success in helping patients adopt and maintain healthy behaviors, and should therefore be integrated into ongoing care. The following example illustrates this principle.

A patient with hypertension, diabetes, and hypercholesterolemia was also a heavy smoker. Over the course of 2 years, he gradually succeeded in accepting and understanding his medical conditions; reliably taking his antihypertensive, oral hypoglycemic, and lipid-lowering medications; altering his diet to one low in cholesterol, saturated fats, salt, and concentrated sweets; inspecting his feet regularly; and having yearly eye examinations. Initially, however, he was very resistant to the suggestion that he stop smoking (*precontemplation stage*). However, his doctor listed smoking as a problem on his medical problem list and let him know that smoking cessation was probably the single most effective thing he could do to improve his health (*instruction*). On successive visits, she explored with him his feelings about smoking, the pros and cons of his stopping, the barriers to his stopping (*assessment, raising the problem to the level of contemplation*), and the role of nicotine use in smoking cessation (*instruction*). She expressed confidence in his ability to stop when he was ready, and indicated her interest in helping him (*promotion of his sense of self-efficacy and support*). She checked on his smoking behavior and readiness to stop periodically (*maintenance of contemplation*). He made one attempt to stop after 2 years (*action*) and succeeded for 2 months, but then resumed smoking during a period of stress at work (*relapse*). His doctor congratulated him on his success and told him that it proved he was capable of quitting. She noted that most patients who successfully quit require more than one attempt (*reframing a "failure" as a success*). Two months later, after discussing his brother's death of a myocardial infarction with his doctor *(additional stimulus that moved patient back from a contemplation phase into an action phase),* the patient set a quit date, removed all cigarettes from his home and work environment, elicited support for his quitting from family and friends, and planned for his responses to stressful situations. With the additional help of a nicotine patch and periodic encouragement from his doctor, he succeeded in stopping for good.

ETHICAL CONSIDERATIONS

It has been suggested that the following three conditions be met before attempting to improve compliance: (*a*) the diagnosis should be correct, (*b*) the therapy should be proven efficacious and benefits should outweigh adverse effects, and (*c*) the patient should be an informed and willing partner in the compliance-improving intervention (60).

Although the first two conditions are probably applicable to interventions directed toward populations, they may be too rigid for application to individual patients. In some circumstances, it may be reasonable to prescribe an efficacious treatment as a therapeutic trial when the diagnosis is in question. Furthermore, many treatments have not been unequivocally proven to be efficacious, although some evidence supports their usefulness. The physician is justified in encouraging the use of such therapies in an attempt to determine whether they relieve symptoms or improve functional status. How else will the physician know whether a given antiarrhythmic or analgesic, for example, is effective for a given patient?

In individual practice, therefore, the first two conditions might be replaced with the following requirements: (*a*) that the therapy be rational and based on sound medical knowledge, and (*b*) that the potential risks of therapy be less than the likely benefits.

The third condition is that of an informed and willing partner in the compliance-improving intervention. In medical practice one may encounter patients who understand their regimen but fail to comply against their own best interest. Is the physician justified in increasing supervision or attempting to elicit familial support to improve compliance, without obtaining explicit consent from the patient? On one hand, the patient has come to the doctor's office, voluntarily entered into the patient–physician relationship, and accepted a prescribed regimen, suggesting implicit consent. On the other hand, the patient is willfully noncomplying, suggesting a rejection of the regimen at some level. The dilemma may be somewhat artificial because most compliance-improving strategies require participation of the patient and, therefore, implicit consent. Going beyond the patient–physician relationship to enroll family help, however, requires consideration of the patient's feelings with respect to this intervention. Some patients are mentally or psychologically impaired in their ability to understand or make sound decisions regarding their situations. An example might be the symptomatic schizophrenic patient who fails to comply in taking oral antipsychotic medication, when introduction of long-acting parenteral therapy could reduce symptoms, rate of relapse, and rehospitalization. There are no definitive guidelines in these situations, but the following suggestions may be helpful:

- The physician should attempt to determine the patient's own best interest, considering not only the disease but also the patient's desires, values, psychologic makeup, and social environment, and should use this information as a guide to action.
- The physician should weigh the relative benefits versus risks of intervention (self-monitoring of blood pressure in some individuals, for example, might markedly increase their anxiety).
- The physician should respect the patient's autonomy and legal rights.
- When patients are incapable of understanding or making reasonable decisions related to their situation, the physician should consult with responsible family members or guardians before deciding on a course of action. (See Chapter 10 for determination of mental competence.)
- In particularly difficult situations, the physician should seek advice from others.

Finally, there is the question of where the patient's responsibilities begin and those of the physician end. Is the physician ethically bound to use educational strategies that diminish noncompliance and to identify and treat noncompliance when it compromises the health of one's patient? Once a patient–physician relationship has been established, it is certainly the physician's responsibility to work with the patient to improve the patient's health status to the best of the physician's ability, taking into consideration the severity of the problem, economic constraints, time constraints, and competing obligations to other patients. To achieve this end a physician should use not only the traditional methods of diagnosis, treatment, and instruction of patients but, when appropriate, interventions that improve compliance as well.

PRACTICE OPERATIONS

Patient education and compliance can be enhanced not only through doctor–patient communication, but also through the implementation of effective practice operations. *Nurses* often have considerable interest in patient education, and involving them in this effort can save physician time and enhance the effectiveness of care. Many office practices involve the nurse in educating patients about preventive measures such as immunizations, breast cancer screening, and family planning, and in working with patients newly diagnosed with such chronic illnesses as diabetes mellitus, asthma, and hypertension. In these instances, it is important to agree in advance what aspects of patient education will be covered by the nurse and which will be covered by the physician.

Mailing information to patients about the results of tests can be incorporated into office procedures. Depending on the situation, one may include additional material (e.g., information about dietary changes indicated by a test result).

A collection of preselected *printed patient educational materials* can be maintained in an office file and distributed at the discretion of the physician or nurse.

A certain amount of general patient education can be promoted in the *waiting room* by setting up a *pamphlet rack* containing 10 to 15 of the most commonly applicable printed materials. These might include pamphlets on smoking cessation, weight reduction, low-salt diets, exercise, and other topics of interest to patients and their families. Some practices have found it helpful to have a *bulletin board* with newspaper clippings about current health topics.

Other possibilities include the delivery of *health messages to patients on telephone hold, practice newsletters, audiovisual materials,* and *computerized interactive programs.*

Volunteer patients followed regularly in one's practice who have successfully managed their chronic illness can serve as important resources to patients newly diagnosed with the same condition.

As already mentioned, *telephone or mailed reminders, accessible individualized appointment systems,* and the implementation of a *review process for missed appointments* are operational measures that promote appointment keeping and prevent dropouts.

Finally, *medical records and related forms* can be structured in ways that promote patient education and physician monitoring of patient compliance. As mentioned earlier, *self-duplicating forms for written instructions* (Fig. 4.3) facilitate the provision of written instructions to the patient and follow-up by the physician at the next visit. *Preprinted forms* can be used to facilitate or to assist the physician in the mailing of diagnostic test results to patients. A *flow sheet that chronologically aligns chronic medications and non-drug therapy with clinical and laboratory data* facilitates review of the relationship between a specific therapeutic regimen and related clinical/laboratory parameters. A *method for keeping track of prescription renewals* can be incorporated into the patient record, such as the attachment of duplicate copies of all written prescriptions to a flow-carrier sheet. Such a method allows the physician to ascertain quickly when the patient is due for a refill. It is especially helpful when prescriptions are filled by more than one physician.

General References*

Cramer JA, Spiker B, eds. Patient compliance in medical practice and clinical trials. New York: Raven Press, 1991.
    Recent text on compliance. Special emphasis on microelectronic monitors for measuring compliance, what we have learned from them, and the practical and conceptual issues related to compliance and clinical trials.

---

*Bold print (general references) and bold numerals (specific references) denote published controlled clinical trials, meta-analyses, or consensus-based recommendations.

Cross-cultural medicine. West J Med 139(6), 1983.
Cross-cultural medicine: a decade later. West J Med 157(3), 1992.
    Two special issues covering major problems that are generic to cross-cultural medicine in the United States, containing articles on most of the major immigrant populations in the United States.
DiMatteo MR, DiNicola DD. Achieving patient compliance: the psychology of the medical practitioner's role. New York: Pergamon, 1982.
    Important contribution that describes an in-depth social-psychologic approach to the understanding, prevention, and management of noncompliant behavior.
Griffith HW. Instructions for patients. 5th ed. Philadelphia: WB Saunders, 1994.
    Soft-bound collection of one- to two-page instructions, which can be reproduced for individual patients, on over 200 conditions. Includes anatomic sketches of most organ systems, useful for instructing patients.
Grueninger UJ, Duffey FD, Goldstein MG. Patient education in the medical encounter: how to facilitate learning, behavioral change, and coping. In: Lipkin M, Putnam SM, Lazare A, eds. The medical interview: clinical care, education, and research. New York: Springer-Verlag, 1994;122–133.
    Useful chapter, built on Proschaska's readiness-to-change cycle, that addresses cognitive, attitudinal, skill, coping/planning, and social support approaches to learning and behavioral change. Other chapters in this well referenced, multiauthor text address issues relevant to patient education, behavior change, and compliance, such as negotiation, barriers to effective communication, cultural factors, and bilingual interviews.
Harwood A. Ethnicity and medical care. Cambridge, MA: Harvard University Press, 1981.
    Useful reference on ethnic health beliefs and practices.
Haynes RB, Taylor DW, Sackett DL, eds. Compliance in health care. Baltimore: Johns Hopkins University Press, 1979.
    Excellent comprehensive reference with annotated bibliography.
Lassiter SM. Multicultural clients: a professional handbook for health care providers and social workers. Westport, CT: Greenwood, 1995.
    Useful, concise, practical reference on many ethnic groups living in the United States.
Meichenbaum D, Turk DC, eds. Facilitating treatment adherence: a practitioner's guidebook. New York: Plenum, 1987.
    A book, written by two leading clinical researchers in cognitive-behavioral therapy, that provides a useful analysis of the compliance literature. It is clinically oriented and full of suggestions for the health care provider on how to increase patient compliance by enhancing the doctor–patient relationship and by use of effective patient education, behavioral modification, and motivational strategies.
Sackett DL, Haynes RB, Guyatt GH, Tugwell P. Helping patients follow the treatments you prescribe. In: Clinical epidemiology: a basic science for clinical medicine. 2nd ed. Boston: Little, Brown, 1991;249–281.
    Fun, very practical clinical epidemiologic approach to evaluating and improving patient compliance.

Specific References

1. Baile WF, Engel BT. A behavioral strategy for promoting treatment compliance following myocardial infarction. Psychosom Med 40:413, 1978.
2. Bailey WC, Richards JM Jr, Brooks CM, et al. A randomized trial to improve self-management practices of adults with asthma. Arch Intern Med 150:1664, 1990.
3. Bandura A. Self-efficacy theory: toward a unifying theory of behavior change. Psychol Rev 84:191, 1977.
4. Barker LR. Five-hour blood pressure check to assess hypertension not responding to conventional therapy. Md Med J 35:94, 1986.
5. Bartlett EE. The contribution of consumer health education to primary care practice: a review. Med Care 18:862, 1980.

6. Becker MH, Green LW. A family approach to compliance with medical treatment: a selective review of the literature. Int J Health Educ 18(3):173, 1975.

7. Ben-Sira Z, Eliezer R. The structure of readjustment after heart attack. Soc Sci Med 30(5):523, 1990.

8. Brookfield S, ed. Self-directed learning: from theory to practice. San Francisco: Jossey-Bass, 1985.

9. Burgess AW, Lerner DJ, D'Agostino RB, et al. A randomized control trial of cardiac rehabilitation. Soc Sci Med 24(4):359, 1987.

10. Campbell EM, Redman S, Moffitt PS, Sanson-Fisher RW. The relative effectiveness of educational and behavioral instruction programs for patients with NIDDM: a randomized trial. Diabet Educ 22:379, 1996.

11. Caron HS. Patient's cooperation with a medical regimen: difficulties in identifying the noncooperator. JAMA 203:120, 1968.

12. Charney E, Bynum R, Eldredge D, et al. How well do patients take oral penicillin? A collaborative study in private practice. Pediatrics 40:189, 1967.

13. Closson R, Kikuwago C. Noncompliance with drug class. Hospitals 49:89, 1975.

14. Cohen S, Lichtenstein E. Partner behaviors that support quitting smoking. J Consult Clin Psychol 58(3):304, 1990.

15. Coyne JC, Delonges A. Going beyond social support: the role of social relationships in adaptation. J Consult Clin Psychol 54(4):454, 1986.

16. Coyne JC, Ellard JH, Smith DAF. Social support, interdependence, and the dilemmas of helping. In: Sarason BR, Sarason IG, Pierce G, eds. Social support: an interactional view. New York: John Wiley & Sons, 1990;129–149.

17. Coyne JC, Worthan C, Lehman D. The other side of support: emotional overinvolvement and miscarried helping. In: Gottlieb B, ed. Social support: formats, process and effects. Newbury Park, CA: Sage, 1988;305–330.

18. Cramer JA, Mattson RH, Prevey ML, et al. How often is medication taken as prescribed? A novel assessment technique. JAMA 261:3273, 1989.

19. Croog SH, Shapiro DS, Levine S. Denial among heart patients: an empirical study. Psychosom Med 33:385, 1971.

20. Cross KP. Adults as learners. San Francisco: Jossey-Bass, 1988.

21. DiMatteo MR, DiNicola DD. Practitioner–patient relationships: the communication of information. In: DiMatteo MR, DiNicola DD, eds. Achieving patient compliance, the psychology of the medical practitioner's role. New York: Pergamon, 1982;29–67.

22. Feste C, Anderson RM. Empowerment: from philosophy to practice. Patient Educ Couns 26:139, 1995.

23. Fletcher C. Listening and talking to patients. I. The problem. BMJ 281:845, 1980.

24. Francis V, Korsch BM, Morris MJ. Gaps in doctor–patient communication: patients' response to medical advice. N Engl J Med 280:535, 1969.

25. Garrity TF. Medical compliance and the clinician–patient relationship: a review. Soc Sci Med 15E:215, 1981.

26. Gates SJ, Colborn DK. Lowering appointment failures in a neighborhood health center. Med Care 14:263, 1976.

27. Gilbert JR, Evans CE, Haynes RB, Tugwell P. Predicting patient compliance with a regimen of digoxin therapy in family practice. Can Med Assoc J 123:119, 1980.

28. Golin CE, DiMatteo MR, Gelberg L. The role of patient participation in the doctor visit: implications for adherence to diabetes care. Diabetes Care 19:1153, 1979.

29. Greenfield S, Kaplan SH, Ware JE, et al. Patients' participation in medical care: effects on blood sugar control and quality of life in diabetes. J Gen Intern Med 3:448, 1988.

30. Hackett TP, Cassem NH. White-collar and blue-collar responses to heart attack. J Psychosom Res 20:85, 1976.

31. Hall JA, Roter DL, Katz NR. Meta-analysis of provider behavior in medical encounters. Med Care 26:657, 1988.

32. Haynes RB, Mattson ME, Chobanian AV, et al. Management of patient compliance in the treatment of hypertension. Report of the NHLBI Working Group. Hypertension 4:415, 1982.

33. Haynes RB, McKibbon K, Kanani R. Systematic review of randomized trials of interventions to assist patients to follow prescriptions for medications. Lancet 348:383, 1996.

34. Hemminki E, Heikkila J. Elderly people's compliance with prescriptions, and quality of medication. Scand J Soc Med 3:87, 1975.

35. Hulka B, Kupper L, Cassel J, et al. Medication use and misuse: physician–patient discrepancies. J Chronic Dis 28:7, 1975.

36. Inui TS, Carter WB, Pecoraro RE, et al. Variations in patient compliance with common long term drugs. Med Care 18:986, 1980.

37. Janz NK, Becker MH. The health belief model: a decade later. Health Educ Q 11(1):1, 1984.

38. Johnson AL, Taylor DW, Sackett DL, et al. Self-recording of blood pressure in the management of hypertension. Can Med Assoc J 119:1034, 1978.

39. Johnson TM, Hardt EJ, Kleinman A. Cultural factors and the medical interview. In: Lipkin M Jr, Putnam SM, Lazare A, eds. The medical interview: clinical care, education and research. New York: Springer-Verlag, 1995;153.

40. Kaplan SH, Greenfield S, Ware JE. Assessing the effects of physician–patient interactions on the outcomes of chronic disease. Med Care 27:S110, 1989.

41. Kern DE, Grayson M, Barker LR, et al. Residency training in interviewing skills and the psychosocial domain of medical practice. J Gen Intern Med 4:421, 1989.

42. Knowles MS. Introduction: the art and science of helping adults learn. In: Knowles MS, ed. Andragogy in action. San Francisco: Jossey-Bass, 1984;6–21.

43. Lahdensuo A, Haahtela T, Herrala J, et al. Randomized comparison of guided self-management and traditional treatment of asthma over one year. BJM 312:748, 1996.

44. Larson EB, Bergman J, Heidrich F, et al. Do postcard reminders improve influenza vaccination compliance? A prospective trial of different postcard cues. Med Care 20:639, 1982.

45. Lazarus RS, Folkman S. Stress, appraisal and coping. New York: Springer, 1984.

46. Ley P. Memory for medical information. Br J Soc Clin Psychol 18:245, 1979.

47. Ley P. Cognitive variables and non-compliance. J Compliance Health Care 1:171, 1986.

48. Macharia WM, Leon G, Rowe BH, et al. An overview of interventions to improve compliance with appointment keeping for medical services. JAMA 267:1813, 1992.

49. Mazzuca SA. Does patient education in chronic disease have therapeutic value? J Chronic Dis 35:521, 1982.

50. Morisky DE, Levine DM, Green LW, et al. Five year blood pressure control and mortality following health education for hypertensive patients. Am J Public Health 73:153, 1983.

51. Morrow D, Leirer V, Sheikh J. Adherence and medication instructions: review and recommendations. J Am Geriatr Soc 36:1147, 1988.

52. Morse DL, Coulter MP, Nazarian LF, et al. Waning effectiveness of mailed reminders on reducing broken appointments. Pediatrics 68:846, 1981.

53. Mushlin A, Appel FA. Diagnosing potential noncompliance: physicians' ability in a behavioral dimension of care. Arch Intern Med 137:318, 1977.

54. Prochaska JO, DiClemente CC, Norcross JC. In search of how people change: applications to addictive behaviors. Am Psychol 47:1102, 1992.

55. Raynor DK, Booth TG, Blenkinsopp A. Effects of computer generated reminder charts on patients' compliance with drug regimens. BMJ 306:1158, 1993.

56. Rich MW, Beckham V, Wittenberg C, et al. A multidisciplinary intervention to prevent the readmission of elderly patients with congestive heart failure. N Engl J Med 333:1190, 1995.

57. Rich MW, Gray DB, Beckham RN, et al. Effort of a multidisciplinary intervention on medication compliance in elderly patients with congestive heart failure. Am J Med 101:270, 1996.

58. Rodwell CM. An analysis of the concept of empowerment. J Adv Nurs 23:305, 1996.

59. Rost K, Carter W, Inui T. Introduction of information during the initial medical visit: consequences for patient follow through with physician recommendations for medication. Soc Sci Med 28(4):315, 1989.

60. Sackett DL. Introduction. In: Sackett DL, Haynes RB, eds. Compliance with therapeutic regimens. Baltimore: Johns Hopkins University Press, 1976;4.

61. Schapiro DH Jr, Swartz CE, Astin JA. Controlling ourselves, controlling our world: psychology's new role in understanding positive and negative consequences of seeking and gaining control. Am Psychol 51:1213, 1996.

62. Smith M. The cost of noncompliance and the capacity of improved compliance to reduce health care expenditures. In: Improving medication compliance, proceedings of a symposium. National Pharmaceutical Council, 1985;35.

63. Squier RW. A model of empathetic understanding and adherence to treatment regimens in practitioner–patient relationships. Soc Sci Med 30:325, 1990.

64. Steele DJ, Blackwell B, Gutmann MC, Jackson TC. Beyond advocacy: a review of the active patient concept. Patient Educ Couns 10:3, 1987.

65. Steele DJ, Jackson TC, Gutman MC. Have you been taking your pill? The adherence monitoring sequence in the medical interview. J Fam Pract 30(3):294, 1990.

66. Stewart MA. Effective physician–patient communication and health outcomes: a review. Can Med Assoc J 152:1423, 1995.

67. Strecher VJ, Devellis BM, Becker MH, Rosenstock IM. The role of self-efficacy in achieving health behavior change. Health Educ Q 13:73–91, 1986.

68. Svarstad BL. Physician–patient communication and patient conformity with medical advice. In: Mechanic D, ed. The growth of bureaucratic medicine. New York: Wiley, 1976;243.

69. Theis SL, Johnson JH. Strategies for teaching patients: a meta-analysis. Clin Nurs Spec 9:100, 1995.

70. Uhlmann RF, Inui TS, Pecoraro RE, Carter WB. Relationship of patient request fulfillment to compliance, glycemic control, and other health care outcomes in insulin-dependent diabetes. J Gen Intern Med 3:458, 1988.

71. Waggoner DM, Jackson EB, Kern DE. Physical influence on patient compliance: a clinical trial. Ann Emerg Med 10:348, 1981.

72. Wallston KA. Hocus-pocus, the focus isn't strictly on locus: Rotter's social learning theory modified for health. Cognitive Res Ther 16:183, 1992.

73. Wallston KA, Wallston BS, DeVillis R. Development of the multidimensional health locus of control scales. Health Educ Monogr 6:160, 1978.

74. Williams RB, Barefoot JC, Califf RM, et al. Prognostic importance of social and economic resources among medically treated patients with angiographically documented coronary artery disease. JAMA 267(4):520, 1992.

CHAPTER 5

Adolescent Patients: Special Considerations

LARRY N. SCHERZER, MD

From a developmental perspective, adolescence is a time of dynamic changes, with tremendous physical, sexual, psychologic, and intellectual growth. This chapter describes the normal changes and the major problems associated with each of these four spheres of development and delineates practical approaches to the office care of the adolescent patient.

ADOLESCENT MORTALITY AND MORBIDITY

Adolescence should be the healthiest period of life; morbidity and mortality rates are low compared with other age groups, but the absolute number of adolescents who die or have chronic illnesses is considerable. Because the number of productive years at stake for a teenager with a significant illness is large, adolescent health is a special priority.

Accidents are by far the leading cause of death among adolescents and young adults. The victims of accidental death usually have bypassed preventive measures, and in many instances, behavioral problems underlie those deaths. For example, alcohol is implicated in more than 50% of automobile accidents, and there may be an element of suicidal intent in some of them.

The second and third leading causes of death in older adolescents (and an important problem in young adolescents) are *homicide* and *suicide,* problems that are discussed later in this chapter.

The fourth leading cause of death among adolescents and young adults is *neoplasia.* The most common diagnoses are acute leukemia (both lymphocytic and myelogenous), lymphomas (including non-Hodgkin's lymphoma and Hodgkin's disease), central nervous system tumors (especially supratentorial and infratentorial gliomas), bone tumors (especially osteogenic sarcomas and Ewing's sarcomas), and solid organ tumors (especially of genital organs).

As medical treatment improves, conditions that were previously fatal in childhood are being seen frequently in adolescents and young adults. It is common for patients with cystic fibrosis, nephritis, congenital heart disease, and leukemia to survive into adolescence and young adulthood.

Most visits to a physician by adolescents are for preventive care or minor problems (Table 5.1). However, a number of more severe medical problems are limited chiefly to the adolescent period or are problems of adulthood that begin during adolescence (Table 5.2). The data in Tables 5.1 and 5.2 do not depict the significant distress that many adolescent patients (and their physicians) experience. This distress is often related to the pressures unique to the several chronological stages of adolescence.

The *young teen* (11 to 15 years old), who typically has special concern over physical development, may have anxieties about mutilation and death. Hostility toward an illness may be expressed in a fantasy of invincibility, leading to an uncooperative, noncompliant patient. Other young adolescents become greatly depressed by their illnesses and become annoying, complaining, whiny patients, often regressing to a childlike dependence on adult caretakers.

The *middle adolescent* (14 to 19 years old) who is seriously ill suffers from the loss of valued contact with friends and schools. Illness may interrupt important aspirations and shatter dreams. Body image is at a critical developmental stage in midadolescence, and the teen may be more worried about a cosmetic defect resulting from an illness than about the disease or its therapy. Such fears must be faced early and dealt with honestly.

The *older adolescent* (18 to 21 years old) shares many adult concerns. For example, the patient may express anxiety over the cost of an illness, the length of hospitalization, and the burdens these place on the family.

PHYSICAL DEVELOPMENT

Normal Patterns and Concerns

Physical maturation is an important feature of the second decade of life. Although the rate and the timing

Table 5.1. Number of Office Visits Made by Adolescents and Percentage Distribution by the 15 Most Common Diagnoses (by ICD-9-CM Categories), According to Age: United States, 1985[a]

Principal Diagnosis[b]	No. of Visits (Thousands)	Percentage Distribution	Principal Diagnosis[b]	No. of Visits (Thousands)	Percentage Distribution
11–14 yr			**15–20 yr**		
Total	58,996	100.0	Total	39,637	100.00
General medical examination	1,433	7.40	Normal pregnancy	3,391	8.56
Acute pharyngitis	709	3.66	Diseases of sebaceous glands	2,487	6.27
Acute upper respiratory infections of multiple or unspecified sites	637	3.29	General medical examination	1,942	4.90
Certain adverse effects, not elsewhere classified	555	2.87	Acute upper respiratory infections of multiple or unspecified sites	1,169	2.95
Allergic rhinitis	553	2.86	Acute pharyngitis	1,105	2.79
Health supervision of infant or child	527	2.72	Other diseases caused by viruses and chlamydias	965	2.43
Contact dermatitis and other eczema	475	2.46	Allergic rhinitis	803	2.03
Suppurative and unspecified otitis media	473	2.44	Disorders of refraction and accommodation	722	1.95
Other diseases caused by viruses and chlamydias	459	2.37	Suppurative and unspecified otitis media	668	1.68
Disorders of refraction and accommodation	458	2.37	Acute tonsillitis	585	1.48
Diseases of sebaceous glands	401	2.07	Other disorders of urethra and urinary tract	547	1.38
Curvature of spine	311	1.61	Contact dermatitis and other eczema	535	1.35
Acute tonsillitis	308	1.59	Contraceptive management	510	1.29
Streptococcal sore throat and scarlet fever	300	1.55	Certain adverse effects, not elsewhere classified	483	1.22
Asthma	297	1.53	Specific investigations and examinations	464	1.17
All other diagnoses	11,464	59.21	All other diagnoses	23,208	58.55

[a]From Nelson C. Office visits by adolescents: National Ambulatory Medical Care Survey, 1985. Advance Data from Vital and Health Statistics of the National Center for Health Statistics, No. 196, April 11, 1991.

[b]Based on Public Health Service and Health Care Finance Administration. International classification of diseases. 9th revision, clinical modification (ICD-9-CM). Washington, DC: Public Health Service, 1980.

Table 5.2. Selected Medical Problems Limited to Adolescence or Persisting into Adulthood

Limited Chiefly to Adolescence	Chronic Problems that May Begin in Adolescence
Slipped epiphysis	Obesity
Distortion of body image	Hypertension
Delinquency[a]	Diabetes mellitus
Anorexia nervosa	Hypercholesterolemia
Primary amenorrhea	Duodenal ulcer
School or learning problems[b]	Inflammatory bowel disease
	Irritable bowel syndrome
	Dental caries
	Drug abuse
	Alcoholism
	Personality disorders
	Somatization disorder
	Depressive neurosis

[a]May begin earlier.
[b]Often develop earlier.

of maturation may vary, they follow the hormonal changes of puberty in a given individual.

A notable *growth spurt* occurs during the adolescent years, with a 20 to 25% increase in height over 2 to 3 years. This spurt usually occurs earlier in the female than in the male (as does sexual maturation).

During puberty, there is an average twofold increase in both lean and nonlean body mass. The ratio of lean to nonlean body mass is greater in males than in females. Fat accumulation tends to be greatest when growth ceases and may extend into adulthood.

The *musculoskeletal system* has special characteristics during adolescence. To accommodate growth, the ligaments and tendons become lax and elastic, often giving the teen a slouched-over appearance. Similarly, there is an increase in skeletal growth, particularly in long bones, and metaphyseal–epiphyseal junctions remain soft. Thus, the actively growing teen, who may not have developed muscle mass to correspond to skeletal growth, may be prone to some special injuries, particularly joint dislocations and fractures along epiphyseal plates.

As with all areas of development, the adolescent may have particular concerns about growth and weight. The principal reason for this is that adolescents often base judgment of each other's adequacy and acceptability on size or (for males) on athletic ability, and adult criteria of social status based on other standards (or prejudices) are less important.

Children called "squirt" or "runt" are given various types of parental advice, much of it unhelpful. Some children adapt by engaging in an activity in which height is unimportant (e.g., debating, chess, fencing, swimming, or body building). Occasionally, normal children with a familial basis for their short stature require psychologic counseling to promote effective adaptation to their stature. Some teens who are very sensitive about height and strength limitations may try radical and potentially harmful solutions such as self-injections of purported growth stimulants.

The concern of the adolescent about height may be generalized to many other aspects of appearance, in-

cluding body habitus, beauty (or lack of beauty), and skin condition. It is important to recognize when concern about body image is the patient's primary concern and to provide reassurance that he or she is medically and biologically normal. The physician can promote such reassurance by suggesting books in which the adolescent can learn more about normal growth (see "General References").

Short Stature

Short stature is discussed under "Short Stature and Delayed Sexual Maturation."

Obesity

A practical definition of *obesity* is a weight of 20% or more over ideal body weight (see also Chapter 76). This can be estimated by determining the weight that corresponds to the growth chart height percentile for the age and sex of the child and dividing this into the actual weight (Fig. 5.1). A result of greater than 1.2 would be suspect. This ratio should be compared with the clinical appearance of the child because the fat distribution changes at puberty in boys, when extra weight may be transformed into musculature, and in girls, who normally increase their storage of fat. Obesity remains a clinical diagnosis. Adolescent obesity is usually caused by overeating. Most estimates place the prevalence between 4 and 10%, with the highest frequency among lower socioeconomic groups. Often, obesity begins in early childhood but becomes a concern in adolescence because of desires to conform to peer standards.

Obese teens should be screened for other cardiovascular risk factors, such as positive family history, high blood pressure, elevated serum cholesterol or triglyceride, diabetes mellitus, and smoking. If multiple risk factors are present, the patient should be monitored more frequently and risk modification should be encouraged.

To treat adolescent obesity successfully, the teen must be motivated to accept the physician's assessments and recommendations. Often, the patient has attempted to cope with the problem by him- or herself. Certain fad diets, such as fasting and water diets, may yield rapid weight loss but will deplete the strength of the child. Generally, because no modification of long-term eating habits is attempted, the weight is regained upon cessation of the diet. Occasionally, serious biological complications are associated with prolonged adherence to highly restrictive diets. Macrobiotic diets have been associated with symptoms of protein and vitamin deficiencies and liquid protein diets have cardiotoxic effects that have resulted in deaths (see details in Chapter 76). Severely calorie-restricted diets lead to a cessation of linear growth and may cause menstrual irregularities.

Medications are of no value in weight control. In particular, amphetamines and methamphetamines are contraindicated because of their potential for abuse.

Surgical treatment (e.g., jejunoileal bypass or gastric stapling) of obesity is rarely indicated, particularly in the adolescent years.

One is left with methods of dietary control by modification of eating habits and by increasing exercise, together with moderate calorie restriction. These methods, although successful for some, are not successful for all. Often, the teen who wants to diet is well motivated, if for personal and emotional reasons rather than for reasons of health. A group meeting of obese teens provides a nucleus of peer support, with an opportunity for mutual discussions of problems of dieting and appetite control that may not be aired in a brief office visit. Such a group may also help alleviate home pressures. Parental coercion and control of diet in the context of a normally antagonistic parent–teen relationship may result in an angry, rebellious youngster who is gaining rather than losing weight.

For overweight young to mid-adolescents a reasonable goal is to maintain their current body weight because excess caloric restriction may result in a loss of lean body weight. For the late adolescent, the goal may be weight loss. For all obese patients, one wishes to achieve a change in long-term eating patterns.

Some adolescents overeat because of unresolved psychologic difficulties. If there are expressions of problems in peer, school, or parental relationships, these should be explored further. However, obesity alone is not an indication of psychopathology.

Anorexia Nervosa and Bulimia

Anorexia nervosa is an uncommon but serious disorder of growth in adolescents. It is marked by extreme loss of appetite and weight (at least 15% of the baseline weight) that is not attributable to a medical or psychiatric illness ordinarily associated with weight loss (i.e., inflammatory bowel disease or a major affective disorder). Patients characteristically exhibit an intense fear of becoming obese and, even when very thin, have a distorted body image, so they still consider themselves overweight (Table 5.3).

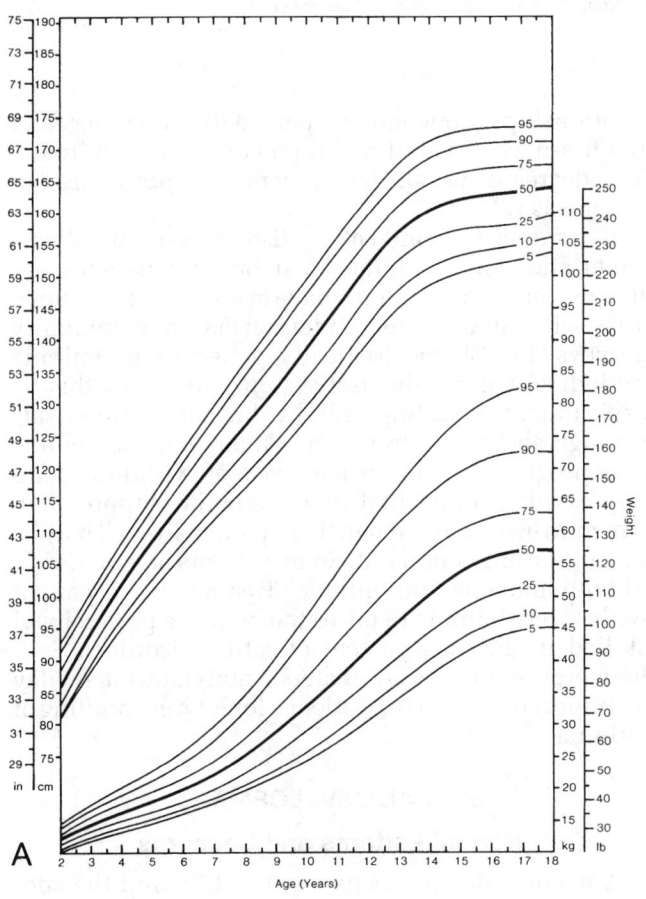
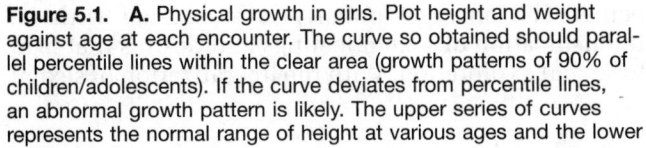
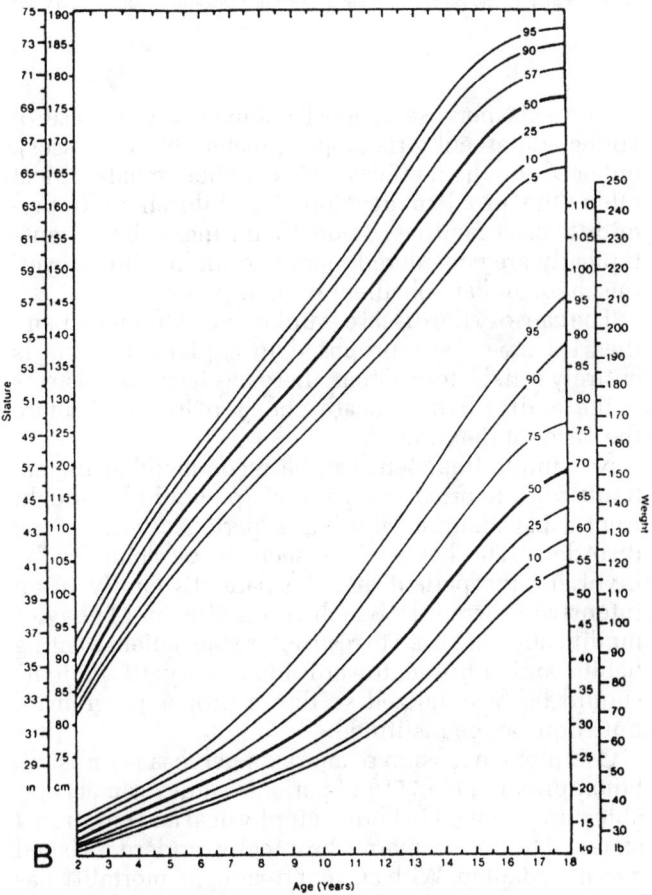

Figure 5.1. A. Physical growth in girls. Plot height and weight against age at each encounter. The curve so obtained should parallel percentile lines within the clear area (growth patterns of 90% of children/adolescents). If the curve deviates from percentile lines, an abnormal growth pattern is likely. The upper series of curves represents the normal range of height at various ages and the lower series of curves, the normal range of weight at various ages. (From National Center for Health Statistics. NCHS growth charts, 1976. Monthly vital statistics report, vol. 25, no. 3, suppl. [HRA] 76-1120. Rockville, MD: Health Resources Administration, June 1976.) **B.** Physical growth in boys.

Table 5.3. DSM-IV Criteria for Diagnosing Eating Disorders

Anorexia Nervosa	Bulimia Nervosa

1. Refusal to maintain body weight at or above a minimally normal weight for age and height (e.g., weight loss leading to maintenance of body weight less than 85% of that expected; or failure to make expected weight gain during period of growth, leading to body weight less than 85% of that expected)
2. Intense fear of gaining weight or becoming fat, even though underweight
3. Disturbance in the way in which one's body weight or shape is experienced, undue influence of body weight or shape on self-evaluation, or denial of the seriousness of the current low body weight
4. In postmenarchal females, amenorrhea (i.e., the absence of at least three consecutive menstrual cycles). (A woman is considered to have amenorrhea if her periods occur only following hormone, e.g., estrogen, administration.)
	1. Recurrent episodes of binge eating. An episode of binge eating is characterized by both of the following:
	  a. Eating, in a discrete period of time (e.g., within any two-hour period), an amount of food that is definitely larger than most people would eat during a similar period of time and under similar circumstances,
	  b. A sense of lack of control over eating during the episode (e.g., a feeling that one cannot stop eating or control what or how much one is eating)
	2. Recurrent inappropriate compensatory behavior in order to prevent weight gain, such as self-induced vomiting, misuse of laxatives, diuretics, or other medications; fasting; or excessive exercise.
	3. The binge eating and inappropriate compensatory behaviors both occur, on average, at least twice a week for three months.
	4. Self-evaluation is unduly influenced by body shape and weight.
	5. The disturbance does not occur exclusively during episodes of anorexia nervosa.

Specify Type: **Restricting type:** During the episode of anorexia nervosa, the person does not regularly engage in binge eating or purging behavior (i.e., self-induced vomiting or the misuse of laxatives or diuretics). **Binge eating/purging type:** During the episode of anorexia nervosa, the person regularly engages in binge eating or purging behavior (i.e., self-induced vomiting or the misuse of laxatives or diuretics).	**Specify Type:** **Purging type:** The person regularly engages in self-induced vomiting or the misuse of laxatives or diuretics. **Nonpurging type:** The person uses other inappropriate compensatory behaviors, such as fasting or excessive exercise, but does not regularly engage in self-induced vomiting or the misuse of laxatives or diuretics.

From Diagnostic and Statistical Manual of Mental Disorders. 4th ed. (DSM-IV). Washington, DC: American Psychiatric Association, 1994.

Anorexia nervosa is most commonly a disease of young adolescent girls (approximately 90% of cases), but occasionally it affects males or older females. Most often, the problem develops in children of upper-middle-class families. Before their illness, the patients typically are considered model children who do well in school and are obedient to their parents.

The cause of the disease is unknown. Although many theories have been proposed to explain it, none is entirely satisfactory. Often, there has been some stress in the family (divorce, death, change of location) before the onset of the illness.

No simple treatment can be recommended for patients with anorexia nervosa. Help should be sought from a psychiatrist who has experience with eating disorders. The best results seem to be achieved by involving the patient and the patient's family in an intensive program in which counseling and behavior modification are used to restructure the patient's eating habits and attitude toward food. Very ill patients should be hospitalized so that a proper program of nutrition can be instituted.

Complete remission of anorexia nervosa is unusual, but approximately 75% of patients achieve an acceptable improvement in both their physical and emotional states. The rest remain chronically undernourished and maladapted. With current treatment, mortality has been reduced to 2 to 8%. Cause of death is equally attributable to overt suicide and medical complications of starvation. Poor prognosis has been associated with long duration of illness, disturbed parent–child relationships, concomitant personality disorder, and the presence of vomiting (more common in bulimia). The degree of weight loss generally is not related to prognosis (7).

Bulimia is a second eating disorder seen in adolescents and young adults. Most bulimic patients are female; bulimic symptoms have been reported by up to 10% of young women interviewed in community surveys (13). Characteristically, patients with bulimia periodically gorge themselves, only to follow this by self-induced vomiting and by further self-reprisals through abstinence from food (Table 5.3). As the disease progresses, patients may become withdrawn and depressed, leading to further appetite suppression. Amenorrhea is common in these patients, and it may be the presenting complaint. Some patients have a history of both anorexia and bulimia. Treatment of a patient with severe bulimia requires the help of a professional skilled in the management of eating disorders. Self-help groups such as Overeaters Anonymous may play an important role in the patient's long-term handling of bulimia.

SEXUAL DEVELOPMENT

Normal Patterns and Concerns

A major difference between the child and the adolescent is the development of the teen into a sexual being. The onset of puberty is associated with an intensification of sexual feelings and desires that lead to sexual exploration. With the liberalization of sexual mores in recent years, the problems of adolescent pregnancy and venereal diseases have grown to epidemic proportions.

The *staging of physical sexual development* of adolescents established by Tanner is a widely accepted method of following the physical changes of puberty (Tables 5.4 and 5.5 and Fig. 5.2).

As the adolescent enters puberty, he or she also assumes a role as a sexual being who must begin to meet expectations of society, family, and peer group and who is pushed into sexual propriety and conformity. These expectations are transmitted to the teen by multiple messages that are often conveyed poorly, and many teens remain ignorant and insecure about sexual issues.

Early adolescence is characterized by a bisexual period, in which close friendships are formed with members of the same sex but heterosexual attitudes develop. Young teens often develop best-buddy relationships. These relationships may even be physically intimate, but they are not considered characteristic of adult homosexuality. However, the teen (particularly male) may fear being a homosexual, and the frequent name calling of this period (in which people are called "gay" or "queer" with little provocation) may be taken too seriously. Boys who have developed noticeable gynecomastia may be particularly confused about their sexual identity. Such boys need to be reassured of the normality of these concerns. Masturbation tends to be a frequent practice in this period, and there may be associated guilt that increases as the sex drive stimulates the teen to continue the practice. Again, where appropriate, problems associated with masturbation should be met with reassurance of its normality.

In mid to late adolescence, dating and heterosexual activities begin in earnest. By age 15, one in four females and one in three males have had sexual intercourse (1). Often, teens rush into sexual activity before they fully understand their own feelings about it. It is often part of the dating relationship—a prerequisite to communication, rather than vice versa. It may be part of thrill-seeking behavior for some teens, and others use it to escape from loneliness and depression.

Short Stature and Delayed Sexual Maturation

A common problem that comes to the attention of physicians is the teenager with short stature or delayed puberty. These two symptoms are often interrelated, and the medical investigation is similar, so they are discussed together. However, the presence of one does not necessarily indicate a problem with the other.

Most of these patients simply are at one end of the spectrum of normal development (6). Many teenage boys may not appreciate the fact that some people fall into the 10th percentile of a normal curve, and they may not accept a cursory dismissal of their concerns about size. Some may be helped by looking at normal growth curves that indicate the predicted ultimate height for people in their percentile (Fig. 5.1). Patients may need detailed discussion to comprehend fully and to cope with normal findings.

Table 5.4. Typical Progression of Female Adolescent Sexual Development (see also Fig. 5.2)

Stage 1
There is no pubic hair present, and there is no breast development.
The ovaries have begun to enlarge. The external genitalia are preadolescent or those of a child.

Stage 2
Breast bud formation usually begins before pubic hair growth. A small mound is formed by the elevation of the breast and papilla. Areolar diameter increases. The adolescent height spurt begins, and there is an acceleration in the deposition of total body fat. The adult female habitus emerges as the breasts enlarge and the hips widen.

Stage 3
There is further spread of pubic hair and further enlargement of breasts and areola, with no separation of their contours. The vagina enlarges and the vaginal epithelium, responding to estrogen stimulation from the maturing ovaries, increases in thickness, with considerable deposition of glycogen. The height spurt usually reaches a peak early in stage 3, before menarche.

Stage 4
If menarche has not occurred late in stage 3, it should occur during stage 4. Axillary hair appears just before or after menarche, usually in early stage 4. There is a projection of the areola and papilla to form a secondary mound above the level of the breast. The areolar mound may be absent (25% of females). The breasts and pubic hair progress. The ovaries continue to enlarge. Ovulation may occur just after menarche, but it is usually delayed until stage 5.

Stage 5
Pubic hair and breast development resemble those of the adult female; the areola has recessed to the general contour of the breast. Height increase has decelerated since menarche; height may increase 2 to 4 inches after menarche. By 2 years after menarche, regular ovulation may be expected.

Stage 6
In 10% of females there is a further spread of pubic hair.

From Tanner JM. Growth at adolescence. New York: Appleton-Century-Crofts, 1966.

Table 5.5.   Typical Progression of Male Adolescent Sexual Development

Stage 1
The male has no pubic hair or increase in size of the penis.
This describes the male as a preadolescent or child. However, the testes are beginning to mature. Usually there is considerable acceleration in height and weight gain along with changes in body composition (especially more body fat).

Stage 2
There is early growth of the testes and scrotum before pubic hair appears. The height spurt accelerates; the male physique begins to change as fat and muscle are added, and the areola of the breast increases in size and darkens slightly.

Stage 3
There is further enlargement of the testes and scrotum, enlargement of the penis (mainly in length), and spreading and darkening of the pubic hair. Facial hair first appears at the corners of the upper lip. The height spurt accelerates further; there is broadening of the shoulders relative to the hips and generalized increased molding of the body, with considerable increase in muscle mass relative to fat. Hair appears in the perineum. Facial expression is significantly altered and appears more adult. The cartilage of the larynx enlarges, and the voice may begin to deepen. There is transient gynecomastia with slight projection of the areola.

Stage 4
Axillary hair first appears. There is continued enlargement of the scrotum, testes, and penis (the last, mainly in breadth). The pubic hair begins to appear adult. Facial hair is still limited to upper lip and chin. The first ejaculation, indicating considerable growth of the prostate gland, occurs early in stage 4. Sebaceous glands are approaching adult size and function. The voice deepens further.

Stage 5
Genital size and pubic hair distribution are adult in appearance. Hairs are present on the sides of the face. Gynecomastia has disappeared. The height spurt has decelerated and the physique is that of the mature male.

Stage 6
Some adolescents have a further spread of pubic hair up the linea alba, which may be described as stage 6. This later development, often not reached until the early twenties, occurs in 80% of males.

From Tanner JM. Growth at adolescence. New York: Appleton-Century-Crofts, 1966.

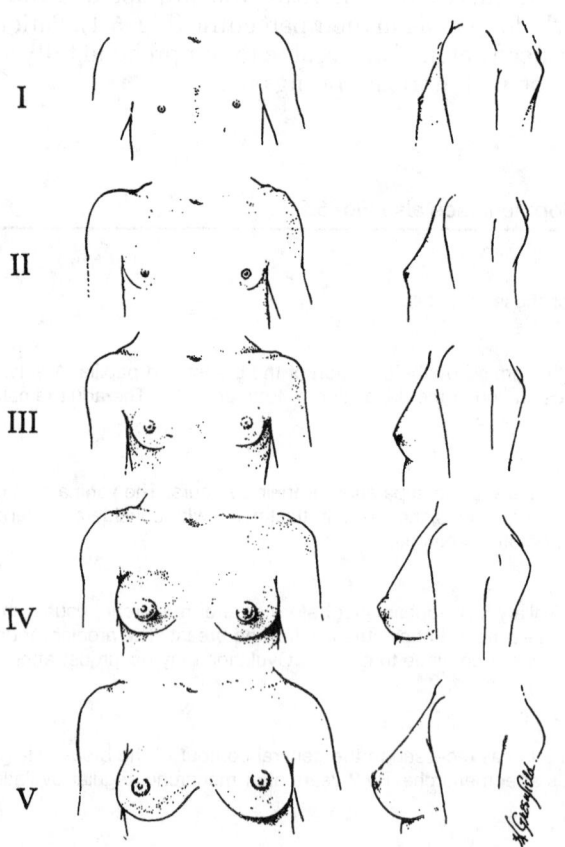

Figure 5.2. Diagrammatic representation of Tanner stages I to V of human breast maturation. (Adapted from Marshall WA, Tanner JM. Variations in pattern of pubertal changes in girls. Arch Dis Child 44:291, 1969.)

Assessment of short stature and delayed puberty by the generalist consists of the following steps:

1. A history of the onset of puberty and of the height of siblings, parents, and grandparents should be obtained. In particular, a history of several short family members (males under 5'6", females under 5'0") should be noted.
2. Growth records of the patient should be reviewed. Heights and weights should be plotted on an appropriate growth curve (Fig. 5.1). If a child has followed a single curve throughout life, a significant metabolic reason for this short stature is unlikely. However, if there is a falling away from a growth line, a metabolic problem is more likely.
3. The medical history should be reviewed, including a prenatal and neonatal history. A history of operations, head injuries, or chronic medical conditions that could predispose the patient to failure to thrive should be noted. If the child had a low birth weight, a review of underlying factors may disclose a possible chromosomal abnormality or toxic exposure (e.g., maternal cigarette smoking or alcohol use) that could produce long-term growth delay.
4. A developmental and psychosocial history may indicate possible familial problems or emotional neglect that could predispose to constitutional growth delay (so-called psychosocial dwarfism).
5. Inquiries into the teen's general health and daily habits may reveal problems needing investigation, such as poor appetite, frequent infections, drug abuse, chronic abdominal pain, or general fatigue and listlessness.

A *physical examination* is essential, including an accurate height and weight and Tanner stage assessment (Tables 5.4 and 5.5). If the testes are softening and show enlargement or if breast budding is present, there usually will be a normal sexual development. Unusual facies or ears, unusual hand creases, clinodactyly (deviation or deflection of the fingers), obesity, or delayed intellectual development may suggest a recognizable hereditary syndrome.

The initial *laboratory investigation* should include urinalysis; measurement of serum urea nitrogen, creatinine, and electrolytes; and radiographs of the hands and wrists to assess skeletal growth.

More specific laboratory investigations may be suggested by the history and physical examination. Examples are thyroid enlargement (testing for hypothyroidism); normal physical examination and appearance but markedly short stature that is falling away from growth lines (testing for growth hormone deficiency); girls with delayed puberty, heights under the 3rd percentile, associated with a short, webbed neck, a systolic murmur, or widely spaced nipples (buccal smears performed to rule out Turner's syndrome, i.e., X-O chromosomes); and striking pubertal delay without a history of similar delay in other family members (testing for gonadal failure including measurement of serum follicle-stimulating and luteinizing hormones, estradiol or testosterone, and urinary 17-ketosteroids and 17-hydroxysteroids; vaginal smear for maturation index and buccal smear for sex chromatin analysis or blood chromosome analysis).

Definitive diagnosis and planning for adolescents with suspected endocrine, metabolic, genetic, or psychologic reasons for maturation delay require referral to an appropriate specialist. Patients with hereditary disorders may benefit from genetic counseling, particularly those who will be unable to bear children (e.g., patients with Turner's syndrome). The availability of biosynthetic growth hormone has raised possibilities for the management of teens with familial short stature. It is unclear whether growth hormone will increase the final adult height of normal children, although for some the rate of growth increases. Weighed against its questionable efficacy, growth hormone treatment is very expensive (often costing $5000 to $10,000 per year).

Sexually Transmitted Disease

Sexually transmitted diseases (STDs) are epidemic in 15- to 19-year-olds. For example, more than 500,000 adolescents contract gonorrhea each year (1). The high frequency of STDs is partially caused by more casual attitudes toward sex, with frequent changes of sex partners. Sex education programs have had little impact on the problem. Fear of infection apparently does not deter some teens, who seem irresponsible, impulsive, and emotionally insecure, and who appear to have little respect for others. Often, parents fail to provide basic information about sex and the risks of infection and pregnancy that accompany it.

In most states, adolescents have a legal right to receive treatment for STDs without the parents' knowledge; it is important to be receptive to the teen seeking treatment. Visits for treatment should also be used to explain the mechanism of acquiring venereal infection and to explain and encourage the use of condoms to prevent reinfection. The diagnosis and treatment of various STDs are discussed elsewhere in this book (see Chapters 27 and 94).

The high rates of sexual intercourse and adolescent pregnancy in the 1980s and 1990s have raised concerns about acquisition of infection with the human immunodeficiency virus (HIV) in this age group. Given the long incubation period of HIV infection, data showing that 21% of all acquired immunodeficiency syndrome (AIDS) cases occur in people 20 to 25 years of age suggest strongly that adolescence is an important period of acquisition of HIV infection (5). Other data suggest that a frequent route of spread of the virus in adolescence is by heterosexual transmission, rather than intravenous drug abuse, blood products, or homosexual contacts. Furthermore, many cases of HIV infection in infants may be linked to maternal acquisition of the virus during adolescence. It is imperative that teenagers, especially sexually active teens, be counseled about high-risk behaviors that may expose them to HIV infection and about safe sex practices. This information and details about the ambulatory care of HIV-infected patients are described in Chapter 34.

Pregnancy

By age 18, 1 in 4 female adolescents has had a pregnancy, and this number increases to more than 4 in 10 by age 20. Each year more than a million women under the age of 20 become pregnant, half of them out of wedlock (1). Many of these pregnancies are associated with serious medical risks for the mother and the fetus. Mothers under 14 have particularly high risks of toxemia, anemia, prematurity, infants with low birth weight, prolonged labor, and postpartum complications. Many of these problems can be prevented by good obstetric care, so that the first goal in adolescent pregnancy should be early diagnosis and entry into a comprehensive treatment program.

There are multiple social and behavioral reasons for the high number of teenage pregnancies. For many adolescents, pregnancy may be part of a maladaptive attempt to solve psychologic issues, such as independence from a clinging mother or manipulation of a boyfriend. Such patients may have previously engaged in other maladaptive activities, such as drug abuse or delinquency. They may also be ignorant about methods and availability of birth control (see Chapter 93).

The teenager herself may be ambivalent about her pregnancy. Often, the manipulations that led to the pregnancy (e.g., the promise of a prolonged relationship) have not succeeded and the patient feels abandoned. Furthermore, the pregnancy may result in hostility from the family when the teenager is in greatest need of help from her parents.

Clearly, the teenager about to make important decisions about herself and her pregnancy needs counseling. It can be provided by her primary physician or, commonly, by a staff member of a counseling agency such as Planned Parenthood. In either case, the patient's primary physician should be aware of programs in the community, including public schools that accommodate the needs of teenagers who choose to have their babies, and should be available for any problems that a pregnant teenager may wish to discuss. In many states, adolescents have the right to treatment for pregnancy-related events, including abortion, without parental consent or knowledge. If the teenager decides to continue with the pregnancy, she should be prepared to assume a parenting role. Furthermore, she should be educated about future pregnancies and given medical assistance for the pediatric care needed for her infant. If possible, day-care, vocational, and educational services should be available for the mother so that she may continue her education after the birth of her child. As an integral part of counseling, a stable, caring person should be identified (a parent, if possible) who can assist the teen emotionally and financially and who can help her see the future for herself and her baby in a realistic manner.

Rape

Rape is a sexual act, usually intercourse, with a nonconsenting victim. The most common type of adolescent rape has been called acquaintance rape, and it is probable that most instances are never reported. Acquaintance rape occurs when the victim is sexually misused by a boyfriend during a date or by a casual friend, or when a trusting teen accompanies her friends to a strange place where she is gang raped.

Teens, in exploring sexuality, may not have set limits to their petting, or if limits have been set unilaterally, they may afford little protection for the victim, especially when the assailant is an adolescent for whom limit setting has not been successful in other areas. Some teens may also, in their uncertainty, present themselves in provocative, pseudomature ways (e.g., by wearing clothing that may be viewed as sexually inviting by male acquaintances).

There is a tendency in dealing with adolescent rape victims to imply that the victim may have invited the assault. This viewpoint inappropriately diverts attention from the fact that rape should always be treated as a very serious problem for the victim who reports it.

Initial care for the rape victim should be handled by a physician, with follow-up by a rape counseling service if one exists in the community. Often, a physician who is already acquainted with the patient can provide the best care.

There are several important considerations in caring for the rape victim:

- Rape is a crime of violence, not a sexual act.
- Above all else, the adolescent reporting rape has usually had a very frightening experience and needs short-term counseling either by her regular physician (see Chapter 11) or, ideally, through the auspices of a rape victim's support program. She will usually have a number of questions about the physical meaning of her experience, and it is important to ensure that she obtains answers to them.
- She should be examined carefully for evidence of trauma, both to the pelvic organs and to the rest of her body, and the information should be carefully recorded.
- She must decide whether she wishes to report the rape to the police. In this instance, it is essential to obtain a wet and fixed smear of the vaginal contents as early as possible to confirm the presence of spermatozoa.
- Most rape victims will need ongoing counseling by their physician or a counselor for a number of months to discuss persisting anxieties and questions.
- When it is not possible to exclude (by identifying and testing the rapist) exposure to HIV, the rape victim should be offered surveillance for HIV infection following a protocol similar to that described in Chapter 34 for accidental needle sticks in health care personnel.
- If sexual intercourse occurred within 72 hours of the examination, the rape victim should be offered emergency STD prophylaxis and contraception.
  - *STD prophylaxis* in adolescents and adults following sexual assault:
    - Ceftriaxone 125 mg intramuscularly in a single dose, *plus*
    - Metronidazole 2 g orally in a single dose, *plus*
    - Doxycycline 100 mg orally twice a day for 7 days.
    - Consider Hepatitis B vaccination if nonimmune.
  - *Pregnancy prophylaxis* (emergency contraception) in adolescents and adults following sexual assault:
    - Norgestrol or levonorgestrol plus ethinyl estradiol pills (oral contraception pills) within 72 hours of assault and again 12 hours later.

Brand	Color	First Dose	Second Dose
Ovral	White	2 pills	2 pills
Lo/Ovral	White	4 pills	4 pills
Levlen	Light orange	4 pills	4 pills
Nordette	Light orange	4 pills	4 pills
Tri-Levlen	Yellow	4 pills	4 pills
Triphasil	Yellow	4 pills	4 pills

- Serum pregnancy test should be obtained and proven negative. If a woman is pregnant, there is a risk of fetal urogenital malformations if emergency contraception fails.
- Nausea is a common side effect of treatment.
- Informed consent should be obtained.

PSYCHOSOCIAL DEVELOPMENT

Normal Patterns and Concerns

The major psychosocial developmental task for the adolescents as adulthood approaches is to increase independence from their parents and to establish a positive identity congruent with social norms.

In early adolescence, the young teen is faced with the dilemma of seeking independence from parents while at the same time relying on them for emotional and physical support. The conflict over independence is evidenced by contradiction and ambivalence. For example, a teen may refuse to listen to parents' suggestions about study habits, but blame mediocre grades on the fact that the parents did not help with homework assignments.

As teens enter middle and late adolescence, they demonstrate a remarkable resourcefulness in coping with anxiety over separation and in learning more mature behavior. Much assistance comes through peer relationships. Teens support each other by experimenting with adult roles that mirror societal expectations of behavior; a sense of moral responsibility begins to take shape. In this period, individual identity tends to be blunted by the seeking of independence from the family. Peers tend to look alike, dress alike, date alike, and experiment with drugs and sex alike. Later, as teens address their concerns about careers, a greater differentiation of personalities takes shape and individual identities emerge.

Normal development also requires the example of secure, healthy parents in an environment in which the teen can feel secure. Thus, parents who are preoccupied with their own psychologic problems at work, in their marriage, or with their own families may have difficulties helping and coping with the development of their adolescent offspring. Often such parents have not previously succeeded at their own adolescent tasks and so are unable to proceed with the task of adulthood—they have not developed the ability for intimacy, close personal feelings, the sharing of feelings and thoughts with others, and adhering to reasonable limits.

One clear fact about adolescent development is that its *emotional course is variable,* even among normal adolescents. The idea that adolescence is usually a time of crisis, in which persistent neurotic behavior is essential for development of a personal identity, has not been borne out by longitudinal research. On the other hand, it has been found that at least 20% of first-year college students have psychologic problems, usually personality disorders of the compulsive, schizoid, or passive–aggressive type expressed as difficulties in academic, social, and psychosexual functioning (8). Furthermore, adolescents are more likely than people in other age groups to be hospitalized for psychiatric conditions (2). A longitudinal study of teenage boys (12) points out that achievement of identity is a long-term process. Subjects were first studied in the first year of high school and were followed for 7 years. At the end of this interval, most subjects had yet to consolidate their identities to the point where they could develop an intimate relationship, one of the best indicators of progress to adulthood. Despite this, self-satisfaction and parental satisfaction were the norm. For many, adolescence is a crisis but an internalized, noiseless one.

Generally the teen must succeed in the other spheres of development to meet tasks in the psychosocial sphere successfully. In children with retardation, physical disabilities, or chronic illness, the dependence–independence struggle may persist, impairing the development of self-esteem needed to develop a sense of identity.

Juvenile Delinquency

Juvenile delinquency is a legal term for youthful behavior that violates the law and would be adjudicated and punished if it had been committed by an adult. It is a major social problem and is sometimes brought to the attention of the practitioner, who is asked whether there is an underlying psychologic cause for the delinquent behavior. To deal with this issue, it is necessary to distinguish between three broad categories of delinquency, described by Weiner (14) as sociologic delinquency, characterologic delinquency, and neurotic delinquency.

Sociologic delinquency refers to illegal acts organized by a subcultural group (i.e., street gang). The delinquent acts are adaptive in that the teen receives the approval of his or her peers. The following four features of the clinical history suggest sociologic delinquency: first, the delinquent acts are performed with valued companions, rather than alone or with strangers; second, these teens see themselves as accepted and integral members of their peer group and rarely exhibit feelings of alienation or inadequacy; third, sociologic delinquents give little evidence of neurotic symptom formation or basic character flaws; and fourth, these delinquents often have had supportive family relationships during early childhood, although there may have been more recent problems that have led to their current activities. Often, involvement in other positive group activities changes the delinquent orientation of these teens.

Characterologic delinquents reflect a basically antisocial attitude toward life. Their acts do not evoke in them any guilt or remorse. Such teens are often loners who have not established a strong relationship of basic trust in their life. Their history suggests a series of problems, with a flurry of destructive acts such as fighting, fire setting, and cruelty to animals preceding their more destructive delinquent activity. Such children often require long-term psychiatric treatment. Chapter 14 provides additional details about the course and management of patients with an antisocial personality.

The *neurotic delinquent* commits destructive acts as an atypical (for him or her) behavior pattern to illustrate and emphasize certain needs. These acts may reflect feelings of being ignored by family or peers or indicate that the teen is suffering from some form of psychologic distress, most often depression. The acts are committed in such a way that the teen is caught in the process or gives himself or herself away soon after; generally, if concealment of illegal acts is repetitive and successful, a neurotic basis of the delinquency is unlikely. There is rarely a history of early behavioral problems, and typically the delinquent has enjoyed a loving relationship with parents and family members. Occasionally, however, some recent family stress may trigger the delinquent act. In general, neurotic delinquency may be treated through short-term counseling (see Chapter 11).

Substance Abuse

Although substance abuse, including tobacco use, is a major problem of adult life, it often begins during the adolescent years (see statistics in Table 22.2). By age 11, 1 in 5 adolescents has smoked cigarettes and approximately 1 in 11 adolescents has had his or her first drink of alcohol; by the age of 15, 1 in 7 adolescents smokes on a daily basis and more than 1 in 3 adolescents has drunk excessively at least once (1). Experimenting with substances of abuse may be viewed as a rite of passage bridging the gap between childhood and adulthood or as a condition for belonging to peer groups or organizations. Advertising or exposure to images that appear to link the use of cigarettes and alcohol to life successes, popularity, and sex can be important inducements for adolescents to try alcohol or tobacco. A major concern is to identify the adolescent abuser—one whose life is being disrupted by aberrant activities. This teenager is most likely to continue to abuse alcohol or drugs in adult life.

The routine evaluation of a teen should include questioning about the use of alcohol and of drugs. Substance use should be explored using nonthreatening questions such as those listed in Table 5.6. The presence of drug abuse and its impact on a teenager can also be uncovered by asking the parents questions such as those in Table 5.7. If the use of a substance is excessive and hazardous, factors that might have led to abuse should be explored. Drugs and alcohol are often abused as a response to some psychosocial problem, and it is only by identifying the problem that the abuse may be stopped. Lecturing on the dangers of alcohol, drugs, or tobacco seems to have little impact on adolescents.

Occasionally, the serious abuser of hazardous substances develops physiologic symptoms that are dramatic enough to come to the physician's attention. Hospitalization for observation is almost always indicated for the teenager presenting with drug intoxication, even if emergency room evaluation indicates that

Table 5.6. Sample Questions Concerning Drug Use for Adolescents

I know that many schools have drug problems. Does your school have such a problem?

Do most of your friends drink alcohol or smoke marijuana at parties?

Do any of your friends use drugs other than alcohol or marijuana?

Where do most young people obtain drugs?

Do you smoke cigarettes? How many per day?

Have you ever tried alcohol? Marijuana? Other drugs?

Have you ever been ill as a result of using drugs or drinking?

Have you ever been in trouble with the law as a result of drugs or alcohol?

Do your parents know that you've used alcohol or _____?

What would (did) they say?

Have you ever worried about your alcohol or _____ use?

Have you ever been drunk or stoned and driven a car (or motorcycle)?

From Schonberg SK, ed. Substance abuse: a guide for health professionals. Elk Grove Village, IL: American Academy of Pediatrics, 1988.

there are no immediate medical risks. The possibility of attempted suicide may be real and must be explored. Even if this is not a factor, there is still concern about the teen's ability to control his or her own drug abuse behavior.

How to intervene in teenage drug abuse behavior is a difficult question. Practical approaches to patients with substance abuse are contained in Chapters 20 ("Tobacco Use and Dependence"), 21 ("Alcoholism and Associated Problems"), and 22 ("Illicit Use and Abuse of Drugs and Substances").

Depression and Suicide

A behavioral hallmark of adolescents is mood shifts, from the peaks of elation to the depths of despair. Depressive symptoms are normal parts of psychosocial development. The quest for identity is balanced by a sense of loss once independence is achieved. Similarly, rejections by peers (e.g., first loves) may be felt very deeply. It is not unusual, as part of these depressions, for the adolescent to contemplate suicide. More than one in four adolescents in grades 9 through 12 has thought seriously about suicide and one in twelve adolescents has actually attempted suicide (1).

Mattsson (10) describes *five depressive states of adolescence.*

- Normal depressive mood swings represent transient reactions to personal disappointments or family difficulties. They rarely affect other life functions.
- Acute depressive reactions are more severe states, often lasting weeks or months. They are normal reactions, similar to states of grief (see Chapter 19), often related to separation or loss of a close friend, relative, or teacher.
- The adolescent who does not successfully work through grief, and who becomes increasingly depressed and incapacitated by loss, suffers from a depressive neurosis. Such teens withdraw from their normal functioning, are chronically sad, and begin to

entertain suicidal ideation. This is a fairly severe level of depression and demands professional intervention.

- The masked depressions of adolescence can be viewed as a subgroup of the depressive neuroses. Such teens cannot tolerate their painful feelings and express them through a variety of somatic or behavioral complaints. They may be frequent visitors to the primary care physician, suffering from ill-defined, atypical symptoms without a clear organic basis. Their behavior may include overeating, delinquent acts, exhibitionist acts resulting in accidental self-destruction, and drug and alcohol abuse.
- Psychotic depressive disorders are marked by impaired reality testing, thought disorders, paranoia, and suicidal intention, in addition to depressive symptomatology.

Primary care physicians are sometimes asked to evaluate depressed or suicidal adolescents. In taking the history, one should try to uncover recent events that may have precipitated the depressive disorder: any long-standing family, school, or peer problems; possibilities of organic brain disease or drug abuse that may mimic depressive symptoms; symptoms of cognitive or reality disturbances, suggesting a psychosis; and symptoms suggesting a masked depres-sion. Openness in inquiry about depression usually puts the adolescent at ease and conveys that the physician truly understands what he or she may be feeling. A physical examination helps to rule out physical problems, and communication with the school may provide additional observations about the teen's current level of functioning.

Adolescents with depressive symptoms need some counseling. If one believes medication is necessary and is unfamiliar with the use of psychoactive drugs in adolescents, conjoint treatment with a psychiatric consultant may prove helpful. Patients with long-standing depressive symptoms, which suggest thought disturbances, and possible suicide attempts should be referred for psychiatric intervention. Additional details about the office assessment and management of depression are contained in Chapter 15.

INTELLECTUAL DEVELOPMENT

Normal Patterns and Concerns

In adolescence, a major change occurs with respect to education and intellect. Schools differentiate students, placing them into vocational or academic tracks. The emphasis shifts from the learning of tasks (e.g., basic reading, writing, and arithmetic) to the

Table 5.7. Questions for Interviewing the Parents of the Adolescent Suspected of or Known to Be Abusing Drugs or Alcohol

1. Does your son/daughter spend many hours alone in his/her bedroom apparently doing nothing?
2. Does your son/daughter resist talking to you or persistently isolate himself/herself from the family?
3. Has your daughter's/son's taste in music had a dramatic change to hard rock music?
4. Has there been a definite change in your son's/daughter's attitude at school? With his/her friends? At home?
5. Has your daughter/son shown recent pronounced mood swings with increased irritability and angry outbursts?
6. Does your son/daughter always seem to be unhappy and less able to cope with frustration than he/she used to be?
7. Has your daughter's/son's personality changed from being a considerate and caring person to being selfish, unfriendly, and unsympathetic?
8. Does your son/daughter always seem to be confused or "spacey"?
9. Have money or valuable articles recently disappeared from your home?
10. Has your daughter/son begun to neglect household chores or homework?
11. Has there been a change in your son's/daughter's friends from age-appropriate friends to older, "unacceptable" associates?
12. Has there been a change in your daughter's/son's appearance (i.e., sloppy dress and poor grooming and hygiene)?
13. Have there been excuses and alibis made, and has there been lying in order to avoid confrontation or not to get caught?
14. Do you feel you have lost control of your son/daughter?
15. Has your daughter/son begun lying in order to cover up sources of money and possessions?
16. Have there been episodes of "ditching" or "skipping" school? Has your son/daughter lied to cover up bad report cards?
17. Have there been stealing, shoplifting, or encounters with the police?
18. Has your daughter/son become a "con artist"?
19. Have you noticed a marked increase in your son's/daughter's interest in drugs, drug literature, and the drug "culture" (i.e., clothing and accoutrements, paraphernalia, belt buckles, and tee shirts with a drug theme)?
20. Has your daughter/son recently quit a sport or dropped out of school clubs or social groups, stopped music lessons, quit the band or orchestra, or lost interest in a hobby?
21. Has there been a deterioration of school performance, frequent truancy, or conflict with coaches or teachers?
22. Do you feel your daughter/son has become untrustworthy, insincere, and distrustful ("paranoid")?
23. Has he/she become unpredictable or rebellious?
24. Has your son/daughter been verbally abusive to you or your spouse?
25. Has your daughter/son been physically abusive to you or your spouse?
26. Has your son/daughter tried to introduce any of your other children to drugs or alcohol?
27. Has your daughter/son talked about suicide or running away?
28. Is your son/daughter more argumentative lately? Does he/she tend to blame others for his/her problems?
29. Is there a paranoid flavor to all of your daughter's/son's relationships with adults, siblings, and authority figures?

From Schonberg SK, ed. Substance abuse: a guide for health professionals. Elk Grove Village, IL: American Academy of Pediatrics, 1988.

accumulation of facts and the ability to think abstractly. As teens prepare for college, learning becomes a competitive task. Career choices become limited as an individual's abilities and talents become manifest. Upon entering college, a greater amount of independence and responsibility is expected. Symbolically, the university begins to resemble the workplace in terms of both potential rewards and potential pressures.

Scholastic Failure

Academic achievement is strongly related to parental aspirations, socioeconomic status, and intellectual ability. Occasionally, a child cannot meet parental expectations, and the resultant crisis may lead to a visit to the physician. Failure in school may also be a symptom of a physical impairment, mental retardation, specific learning disabilities, or emotional stress. By making an accurate diagnosis of the underlying problem, a caring practitioner can help such children.

First, a history is necessary to determine the nature of the school difficulties. When did they begin? Has educational achievement been a problem throughout a school career, as with a global intellectual deficit, or is it specific to certain subjects or tasks, as with learning disorders? Is there a family history of poor school performance, as is seen with familial dyslexics? How does the teen act with family and peers? Is there evidence of disturbed behavior outside school, as with emotional disorders? Is the family structure stable, or has there been separation, divorce, or death of a parent or grandparent? Is there evidence of substance abuse or physical abuse on the part of the teen or a member of the family? Is there daytime hypersomnolence that suggests a sleep disorder? What has the family done to try to work through problems?

Second, a physical examination, including neurologic examination, is indicated, with emphasis on signs of minimal cerebral dysfunction, such as difficulty with right–left discrimination or spatial orientation, or overt signs of cerebral palsy (3). In such patients there may be suggestions of a neurologic problem in the medical history, the birth may have been abnormal, or the patient may have shown hyperactivity or attention deficits as a child. Vision testing and office assessment for slight or moderate hearing loss (see Chapter 96) are also particularly important.

Third, some specific intelligence testing is indicated. Children with mental retardation tend to show low intelligence quotient (IQ) scores, and achievement tests show a delay of several grades in math and reading levels. Children with dyslexia have a normal IQ but show a wide scatter of scores on subtests, indicating a nonglobal deficit. Achievement tests may also show a difference between abilities in reading and mathematics.

Some learning problems may appear late in a school career (9). The recent criticism of the ability of some college students to write well has given credence to the notion of expressive language disorders, which may not become manifest until adolescence. Some people with fine perceptual problems may not reveal difficulties until geometry or drafting is studied in high school.

In 1974 Congress passed Federal Law 94-142, ensuring a free, appropriate educational placement for all children up to age 21. Thus, adolescents with specific learning problems, retardation, or emotional difficulties are entitled to be placed in a classroom setting where they will learn. The physician who suspects an unrecognized problem in one of these spheres may help by referring the teen and the teen's parents for evaluation, usually available through the school or the local education system. Unfortunately, problems remain unrecognized for many children and, out of frustration, they drop out of school.

Attention Deficit/Hyperactivity Disorder

Attention deficit/hyperactivity disorder (AD/HD) may be one of the most common disorders of childhood, with prevalence rates ranging from 3 to 5% of prepubertal children. Although data on prevalence in adolescents and adults are limited, long-term follow-up studies show that critical symptoms of AD/HD—(a) impairment of attention and regulation of activity and (b) impulse control—often persist into adulthood, and many adults with AD/HD remain distractible, impulsive, inattentive, and disruptive throughout life. Adolescents with AD/HD may have impaired school performance, limited participation in extracurricular activities, increased risk of delinquency, and harmful social relationships and family interactions. In adults, AD/HD is often linked with psychiatric illness, incarceration, job failures, marital discord, and divorce (4).

AD/HD is diagnosed by recognizing the presence of several of its hallmark symptoms (Table 5.8). The diagnostic challenge in adolescents and adults is to detect the more subtle presentations of symptoms in these stages of life. For example, in teens and adults, symptoms of hyperactivity may be confined to fidgetiness or an inner feeling of jitteriness or restlessness. Current nomenclature differentiates AD/HD into three types: predominantly impulsive, predominantly inattentive, and combined.

The physical examination usually is noncontributory in diagnosing AD/HD, but may be useful to rule out other conditions that are characterized by hyperactivity or short attention spans (see below). In teens, it is helpful to examine results of intellectual testing and academic achievement testing. A symptom checklist (Connors scale, Child Behavior Checklist) that can be completed by teachers and parents

Table 5.8.   Diagnostic Criteria for Attention Deficit/Hyperactivity Disorder

A. Either 1. or 2.
  1. Six (or more) of the following symptoms of **inattention** have persisted for at least 6 months to a degree that is maladaptive and incon-
     sistent with developmental level.
     Inattention
     a. Often fails to give close attention to details or makes careless mistakes in schoolwork, work, or other activities.
     b. Often has difficulty sustaining attention in tasks or play activities.
     c. Often does not seem to listen when spoken to directly.
     d. Often does not follow through on instructions and fails to finish schoolwork, chores, or duties in the workplace (not because of op-
        positional behavior or failure to understand instructions).
     e. Often has difficulty organizing tasks and activities.
     f. Often avoids, dislikes, or is reluctant to engage in tasks that require sustained mental effort (such as schoolwork or homework).
     g. Often loses things necessary for tasks or activities (e.g., toys, school assignments, pencils, books, or tools).
     h. Is often easily distracted by extraneous stimuli.
     i. Is often forgetful in daily activities.
  2. Six (or more) of the following symptoms of **hyperactivity–impulsivity** have persisted for at least 6 months to a degree that is mal-
     adaptive and inconsistent with developmental level.
     Hyperactivity
     a. Often fidgets with hands or feet or squirms in seat.
     b. Often leaves seat in classroom or in other situations in which remaining seated is expected.
     c. Often runs about or climbs excessively in situations in which it is inappropriate (in adolescents or adults, may be limited to subjec-
        tive feelings of restlessness).
     d. Often has difficulty playing or engaging in leisure activites quietly.
     e. Is often "on the go" or often acts as if "driven by a motor."
     f. Often talks excessively.
     Impulsivity
     a. Often blurts out answers before questions have been completed.
     b. Often has difficulty awaiting turn.
     c. Often interrupts or intrudes on others (e.g., butts into conversations or games).
B. Some hyperactive–impulsive or inattentive symptoms that caused impairment were present before age 7 years.
C. Some impairment from the symptoms is present in two or more settings (e.g., at school [or work] and at home).
D. There must be clear evidence of clinically significant impairment in social, academic, or occupational functioning.
E. The symptoms do not occur exclusively during the course of a pervasive developmental disorder, schizophrenia, or other psychotic disor-
   der and are not better accounted for by another mental disorder (e.g., mood disorder, anxiety disorder, dissociative disorder, or a person-
   ality disorder).
Diagnosis is:
Attention deficit/hyperactivity disorder, combined type if both criteria A1 and A2 are met for the past 6 months.
Attention deficit/hyperactivity disorder, predominantly inattentive type if criterion A1 is met but criterion A2 is not met for the past
   6 months.
Attention deficit/hyperactivity disorder, predominantly hyperactive–impulsive type if criterion A2 is met but criterion A1 is not met for
   the past 6 months.
For individuals (especially adolescents and adults) who currently have symptoms that no longer meet full criteria, "in partial remission"
   should be specified.

From Diagnostic and Statistical Manual of Mental Disorders. 4th ed. (DSM-IV). Washington, DC: American Psychiatric Association, 1994.

is also helpful to identify and quantify symptoms that teens may be demonstrating in their classrooms and homes.

AD/HD in adolescence may be associated with several comorbid conditions, such as learning disabilities, depression, substance abuse, and alcoholism, and may also be confused with other conditions that have hyperactivity as a feature, such as hyperthyroidism, Gilles de la Tourette syndrome, adjustment or oppositional disorders, affective disorders with manic features, social or personality difficulties, and medication-induced attention problems (e.g., substance abuse). These patients have difficulty in the workplace, in school, and in social relations. They have more cognitive difficulties, poor performance in school, and significant difficulties with social skills and appropriate behavior. As a result, they tend to be underachievers with personalities that may be intrusive, immature, or negative.

Treatment

AD/HD is treated best with a multimodal combination of medication and counseling. It is estimated that 70 to 80% of children and 60% of adults are aided by medication, with improvement in academic and social behaviors and a reduction of disruptive and negative behaviors. Most patients with AD/HD are treated pharmacologically with psychostimulant medications, such as methylphenidate or dextroamphetamine, although a small number respond well to antidepressant agents, such as desipramine. Medication should be used on school or work days and other days where focus and attention may be needed (e.g., for long-distance drives). Medication should be prescribed to cover learning and work-related needs, such as homework and examination preparation times. With short-acting stimulant medications such as methylphenidate, holiday periods off medication may be permitted. Counseling interventions include psychoeducational

Table 5.9. Medications for Attention Deficit Disorder with Hyperactivity (AD/HD) in Adolescents and Adults

Drug	Available Strengths (mg)	Dosage	Comments
Methylphenidate (Ritalin)	Tabs: 5, 10, 20 Slow-release tabs: 20 (8-hr duration)	Initial: 0.25 mg/kg/dose given with breakfast and lunch Maintenance: 1–2 mg/kg/24 hr Maximum: 60 mg daily	Begin with initial dose. May double dosage weekly until desired clinical effect is achieved or maintenance dosage is reached. Stop if no improvement in 1 month. May give after-school dose for homework. Use cautiously in pts with HTN, epilepsy. Contraindicated in pts with glaucoma, Gilles de la Tourette syndrome, MAO inhibitor use. Commonly causes insomnia, anorexia.
Dextroamphetamine (Dexedrine)	Tabs: 5, 10 Elixir: 5 mg/5 mL Sustained-release caps: 5, 10, 15 Caps: 15	Initial: 10 mg/24 hr in morning Maximum: 60 mg daily	Begin with initial dose. May increase by 10 mg/wk until maximum dose. Same guidelines as methylphenidate. Side effects more common than with methylphenidate because of longer duration of action.
Desipramine (Norpramine)	Tabs: 10, 25, 50, 100, 150	Initial: 10 mg/24 hr in morning Maximum: 100 mg daily	Begin at lowest dose for adolescent. Increase according to tolerance and response. Usual dosage 25–50 mg/day for adolescents. Must obtain ECG when using medication to look for signs of prolongation of QRS and QT intervals. For this reason, a poor choice in patients with cardiovascular disease, congenital heart disease, hypertension, etc. Occasional behavioral side effects noted, especially if manic–depressive illness not recognized. May cause leukopenia, especially during febrile illness.

counseling, behavioral management, school-based interventions, family therapy, and social competence training. Practical information regarding these medications is summarized in Table 5.9.

APPROACH TO THE ADOLESCENT PATIENT IN THE OFFICE SETTING

When interviewing teens, it is helpful to keep in mind that the transitional nature of adolescence makes it a time of great experimentation and risk taking (see sections on "Sexual Development" and "Substance Abuse," above).

Each adolescent approaches the developmental pressures of this period of life with his or her particular skills and emotions. From a health perspective, adolescents can be responsible partners in maintaining their well-being and complying with medical care, or they can be infantile, dependent, uncommunicative, aggressive, or irresponsible. It is important to interview adolescents in private. Adolescents need to feel that they are the patient and that their problems are being listened to and taken seriously. It is often useful to talk to the parents separately as well.

Interviewing the Patient

Some adolescent patients are difficult to interview. An uncommunicative patient may have been sent to a physician involuntarily or may lack verbal skills needed for coherence. One must be verbally active with such patients and watch for any nonverbal cues to use

as wedges in trying to get the patient to speak. Examples of nonverbal cues are a look of interest or initiation of eye contact when a subject is mentioned that the patient would like to discuss, a clenched fist when an anger-provoking subject is raised, and frequent position change and fidgeting when the patient is anxious about a specific subject or about the visit to the physician in general. Because adolescents are often reticent about their major concerns, open-minded invitations to share information (e.g., "Is there anything else you wanted to talk about?") should be included in each office contact. The initial comprehensive interview may require several sessions. At the first visit, warmth and interest in the adolescent may open the way to better communication in future sessions.

Some adolescents respond more honestly to *written questionnaires* rather than interviews. It may be a useful strategy to preface an interview with a form questionnaire for both the adolescent and the parent. As part of this questionnaire, ground rules can be outlined, such as assurances of confidentiality. In general, an adult-oriented questionnaire, with reviews of systems, is not appropriate for younger teens and should be reserved for teens aged 18 years or older. The questionnaire should not take the place of the personal interview but can guide the interview to address issues of concern of the patient in greater detail.

Many adolescents continue to go to a pediatrician for medical care until they enter college, take a job, or marry. Because of this long-term association, their relationship may be almost like that of a parent and child: warm, intense, and comradely. These feelings cannot be transferred easily to a new physician, and it is unwise to attempt to transfer them.

Physicians can most effectively surmount problems in communicating with adolescents by explaining their modus operandi in advance, emphasizing that they will be primarily the adolescent's physician, rather than an agent of the patient's parents, as had been the case previously. The adolescent should also be encouraged to initiate patient–doctor contacts, guard against paternalistic advice giving, and avoid showing disapproval or surprise when the adolescent attempts to impress one with tales of sexual exploits or the use of vulgar language. *Sexuality* is an important topic to address with teens, but one should not impose judgment on a teen's sexual activities, gender preferences, or other characteristics. Instead, one should address how a teen's sexuality may create health risk and focus screening and health education efforts on these risks.

It is wise to *establish certain ground rules* with adolescents. Patient–doctor confidentiality, for example, can be assured to adolescents only insofar as they do not reveal that they are contemplating harmful acts, such as running away or committing suicide. However, certain privileged communications should be kept confidential from parents. In particular, adolescent minors have the right to be seen for sexually transmitted diseases or for sex offense–related examinations without the prior consent of a parent. The teen may also wish to keep some health-related or emotional problems, such as drug experimentation, from a parent's knowledge.

Interviewing the Parents

Whenever possible, parents should be involved with and concerned about the health of the teen. A separate interview with parents, immediately before or after the examination, may prove helpful and can emphasize particular concerns downplayed or denied by the patient. The parents of adolescent patients may be useful in providing emotional support and ensuring compliance with therapy; therefore, informing them about the adolescent's problems and needs is important.

Some parents ask physicians to take on the role of health educator or counselor for their adolescent child. Usually, these requests are for anticipatory guidance about birth control or drug usage. At times, the physician is asked to help the teen work through an upcoming family crisis, such as divorce, serious illness, or death. Often, adolescents welcome the opportunity to discuss these issues in private. Their knowledge in these areas is often found wanting, and a sensitive physician may help the adolescent grasp realities and make intelligent decisions. A number of books on these subjects are directed to an adolescent and young adult audience, and it may be useful to make these titles available (see "General References").

Parents often have questions about specific adolescent behavior. A particular episode or issue may come to the parents' attention, and they may ask the physician whether they should exert control over it. In such instances, one should not offer specific advice but should try to discern any moral or behavioral conflicts between the parents and the adolescent. When the parents' behavior is inconsistent with the parents' own stated values, adolescents often act in opposition to those values. Miller (11) suggests that parents are not helped in this instance by being told how to behave. Advice either increases the parents' uncertainty when faced with later difficulties or implies that the parents' own opinions are inappropriate. Adolescents probably turn out mentally healthier when presented with models of adult behavior with which their parents are comfortable, whether consistent with societal norms or not. However, parents must be prepared to make allowances so that their children have freedom to make their own mistakes. Family counseling is a technique that a general physician can use when several members of a household are involved (see Chapter 11).

Health Assessment and Preventive Care

The initial interview(s) should be comprehensive enough to ensure that the adolescent is meeting *appropriate developmental tasks*. Inquiries should be made into teenagers' relationships and functioning with their families, at school, and with peers. It is important to determine whether teenagers are establishing positive personal identities (Do they have hobbies? Do they voice their own opinions? Can they choose their own friends or must friends be approved by the parents? Do they have plans for the future?), whether they are accepting their sexuality and adjusting to adult sexual roles (Do they date? Are they sexually active? Do they have a knowledge of contraception? Is contraception used?), whether they are establishing independence from the family (Do they drive? Do they earn money on their own? What sort of hours do they keep?), whether they are working toward a career (What are their plans after high school? What subjects in school do they like? What are their grades? Do they plan to go to college? Are their goals realistic and are they supported by the family?), whether they have established good health habits (What are their views about nutrition? Have they experimented with alcohol, tobacco, or other recreational drugs? What drugs? Have they ever been drugged or high when driving or when attending school?), and whether affective swings are interfering with functioning (Do they often feel down? What makes them happy? Have sad feelings ever made them consider harming themselves?).

As part of the *review of systems before examination*, a self-administered medical questionnaire may be useful and time-saving. Such a questionnaire should be brief, with language simple enough to be understood by teens with poor reading skills. Positive answers must be explored further.

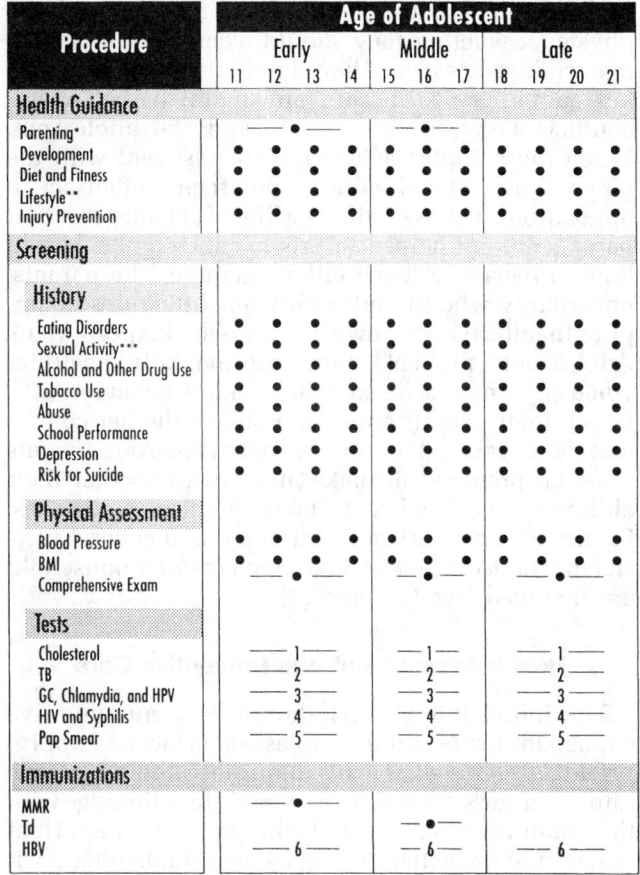

Procedure	Age of Adolescent										
	Early				**Middle**			**Late**			
	11	12	13	14	15	16	17	18	19	20	21
Health Guidance											
Parenting*		•			•						
Development	•	•	•	•	•	•	•	•	•	•	•
Diet and Fitness	•	•	•	•	•	•	•	•	•	•	•
Lifestyle**	•	•	•	•	•	•	•	•	•	•	•
Injury Prevention	•	•	•	•	•	•	•	•	•	•	•
Screening											
History											
Eating Disorders	•	•	•	•	•	•	•	•	•	•	•
Sexual Activity***	•	•	•	•	•	•	•	•	•	•	•
Alcohol and Other Drug Use	•	•	•	•	•	•	•	•	•	•	•
Tobacco Use	•	•	•	•	•	•	•	•	•	•	•
Abuse	•	•	•	•	•	•	•	•	•	•	•
School Performance	•	•	•	•	•	•	•	•	•	•	•
Depression	•	•	•	•	•	•	•	•	•	•	•
Risk for Suicide	•	•	•	•	•	•	•	•	•	•	•
Physical Assessment											
Blood Pressure	•	•	•	•	•	•	•	•	•	•	•
BMI	•	•	•		•	•		•	•	•	•
Comprehensive Exam				•		•		•			
Tests											
Cholesterol		— 1 —			— 1 —			— 1 —			
TB		— 2 —			— 2 —			— 2 —			
GC, Chlamydia, and HPV		— 3 —			— 3 —			— 3 —			
HIV and Syphilis		— 4 —			— 4 —			— 4 —			
Pap Smear		— 5 —			— 5 —			— 5 —			
Immunizations											
MMR		— • —									
Td						— • —					
HBV		— 6 —			— 6 —			— 6 —			

1. Screening test performed once if family history is positive for early cardiovascular disease or hyperlipidemia.
2. Screen if positive for exposure to active TB or lives/works in high-risk situation, (e.g., homeless shelter, jail, health care facility).
3. Screen at least annually if sexually active.
4. Screen if high-risk for infection.
5. Screen annually if sexually active or if 18 years or older.
6. Vaccinate if high-risk for hepatitis B infection.
* A parent health-guidance visit is recommended during early and middle adolescence.
** Includes counseling regarding sexual behavior and avoidance of tobacco, alcohol, and other drug use.
*** Includes history of unintended pregnancy and STD.

Figure 5.3. Preventive health services for adolescents by age and procedure. (American Medical Association. AMA guidelines for adolescent preventive services [GAPS]: recommendations and rationale. Baltimore: Williams & Wilkins, 1994.)

A *physical examination* should be performed in the absence of parents. Teenage girls examined by male physicians may be more comfortable with a female adult in the room with them. Some parts of the physical examination occasionally omitted by physicians but essential for adolescent patients include blood pressure measurement and examination of the entire integument, the spine (for scoliosis), and the external genitalia (for signs of venereal disease and for assessment of sexual development using Tanner's staging [Tables 5.4 and 5.5]). All sexually active adolescent girls should have a pelvic examination, including gonorrheal cultures and a Pap smear (see Chapter 95). If one is uncomfortable doing this examination, the teen should be referred to a gynecologist (preferably female) who is used to dealing with adolescents.

There are *several important adjuncts to the physical examination of the healthy adolescent.* These include testing for myopia and hyperopia (using a Snellen chart) and screening for deafness (by pure tone audiometry). Adolescence is a period marked by noise pollution, in the form of loud music that can cause permanent damage to the eighth nerve (see Chapter 96). Adolescents who have difficulty in school should be screened for learning disorders. Having a teenager read a newspaper paragraph out loud or do some simple arithmetic may reveal a previously undetected learning disability.

Laboratory screening tests for healthy adolescents are remarkably few. Screening for anemia with a hematocrit or hemoglobin determination may be limited to menstruating young women. Tuberculosis screening with purified protein derivative (PPD) should be performed only if there are family or community risk factors. Screening for hyperlipidemia is controversial during adolescence. The chance of diagnosing a problem severe enough to require pharmacologic therapy is small, whereas the benefits of a diet low in total fat and cholesterol may be universal. The decision to screen adolescents may be influenced by family history of myocardial infarction or stroke under the age of 55, or by personal opinion about whether an abnormal lipid profile may influence a patient's dietary practices. Urinalysis, blood chemistry screens, chest radiographs, and electrocardiograms are not indicated in healthy adolescents.

Recommended Preventive Services

Figure 5.3 summarizes the consensus AMA Guidelines for Adolescent Preventive Services (GAPS). Some offices find it useful to keep this table, as a prompt and for documenting completed actions, in the records of adolescent patients (1).

Examining the Adolescent Athlete

The examination of adolescent athletes requires an evaluation of their health and consideration of their functional ability, growth, and maturation. The purpose of the *preparticipation health evaluation* is to identify medical conditions that might preclude safe and effective athletic participation, including those that might become worse by participation in sports activities. A brief screening questionnaire (Table 5.10) along with information already known to the physician will identify most conditions that may disqualify an adolescent from participation in various types of sports (Table 5.11).

As athletes become more experienced, the most commonly encountered problems are residuals of previous sports injuries, most of them musculoskeletal problems. Common exercise-related musculoskeletal injuries that can be managed in the office are described in Chapter 67.

Table 5.10.   Sports Participation Health History

This evaluation is only to determine readiness for sports participation. It should not be used as a substitute for regular health maintenance exams.

Name _____ Grade _____ Sports _____

	YES	NO
1. Have you ever had an illness that		
a. required you to stay in the hospital?	_____	_____
b. lasted longer than a week?	_____	_____
c. caused you to miss 3 days of practice or a competition?	_____	_____
d. is related to allergies? (i.e., hay fever, hives, asthma, insect stings)	_____	_____
e. required an operation?	_____	_____
f. is chronic? (i.e., asthma, diabetes)	_____	_____
2. Have you ever had an injury that		
a. required you to go to an emergency room or see a doctor?	_____	_____
b. required you to stay in the hospital?	_____	_____
c. required x-rays?	_____	_____
d. caused you to miss 3 days of practice or a competition?	_____	_____
e. required an operation?	_____	_____
3. Do you take any medication or pills?	_____	_____
4. Have any members of your family under age 50 had a heart attack or heart problems, or died unexpectedly?	_____	_____
5. Have you ever		
a. been dizzy or passed out during or after exercise?	_____	_____
b. been unconscious or had a concussion?	_____	_____
6. Are you unable to run ½ mile (2 times around the track) without stopping?	_____	_____
7. Do you		
a. wear glasses or contacts?	_____	_____
b. wear dental bridges, plates, or braces?	_____	_____
8. Have you ever had a heart murmur, high blood pressure, or a heart abnormality?	_____	_____
9. Do you have any allergies to any medicines?	_____	_____
10. Are you missing a kidney?	_____	_____
11. When was your last tetanus booster?	_____	
12. For Women		
a. At what age did you experience your first menstrual period?	_____	
b. In the last year, what was the longest time you have gone between periods?	_____	

EXPLAIN ANY "YES" ANSWERS

Signature of parent _____

Signature of athlete _____

Date _____

INTERIM HEALTH HISTORY

This form should be used during the interval between participation evaluations. Positive responses should prompt a physical exam.

1. Over the next 12 months, I wish to participate in the following sports:

   a. _____

   b. _____

   c. _____

   d. _____

2. Have you missed more than 3 consecutive days of participation in usual activities because of an injury this past year? YES_____ NO_____

3. Have you missed more than 5 consecutive days of participation in usual activities because of an illness, or have you had a medical illness diagnosed that has not resolved in the past year?

   YES_____ NO_____

   If yes, please indicate type of illness:_____

   _____

4. Have you had a seizure or concussion, or been unconscious for any reason in the last year?
   YES_____ NO_____

5. Have you had surgery or been hospitalized in this past year? YES_____ NO_____
   If yes, please indicate:

   a. Reason for hospitalization _____

   b. Type of surgery _____

6. List all medications you are currently taking and what condition the medication is for.

   a. _____

   b. _____

   c. _____

   d. _____

7. Are you worried about any problem or condition at this time? YES_____ NO_____

   If yes, please explain: _____

   _____

Signature of athlete _____

Signature of parent _____

Date _____

From Committee on Sports Medicine and Fitness, American Academy of Pediatrics. Sports medicine: health care for young athletes. 2nd ed. Elk Grove Village, IL: American Academy of Pediatrics, 1991.

Table 5.11.   Medical Conditions and Sports Participation

Condition	May Participate?	Explanation[b]
Atlantoaxial instability	Qualified yes	Condition common with Down's syndrome. Athlete needs evaluation to assess risk of spinal cord injury during sports participation.
Bleeding disorder	Qualified yes	Athlete needs evaluation.
Cardiovascular diseases[a]		
Carditis	No	Carditis may result in sudden death with exertion.
Hypertension	Qualified yes	With essential hypertension, avoid weight and power lifting, body building, and strength training. Those with secondary hypertension or severe essential hypertension need evaluation.
Congenital heart disease	Qualified yes	Those with mild forms may participate fully. Those with moderate or severe forms, or who have undergone surgery, need evaluation.
Arrhythmia	Qualified yes	Athlete needs evaluation because some types require therapy or make certain sports dangerous, or both.
Mitral valve prolapse	Qualified yes	Those with symptoms (chest pain, symptoms of possible arrhythmia) or evidence of mitral regurgitation on physical examination need evaluation. All others may participate fully.
Heart murmur	Qualified yes	If the murmur is innocent, full participation is permitted. Otherwise, the athlete needs evaluation.
Cerebral palsy	Qualified yes	Athlete needs evaluation.
Diabetes mellitus	Yes	All sports can be played with proper attention to diet, hydration, and insulin therapy. Particular attention is needed for activities that last 30 min or more.
Diarrhea	Qualified no	Unless disease is mild, no participation is permitted because diarrhea may increase the risk of dehydration and heat illness. See "Fever."
Eating disorders		
Anorexia nervosa	Qualified yes	These patients need both medical and psychiatric assessment before participation.
Bulimia nervosa		
Eyes: functionally one-eyed athlete, loss of any eye, detached retina, previous eye surgery or serious eye injury	Qualified yes	A functionally one-eyed athlete has a best-corrected visual acuity of less than 20/40 in the worse eye. These athletes would suffer significant disability if the better eye were seriously injured, as would those with loss of an eye. Some athletes who have undergone eye surgery or had a serious eye injury may have an increased risk of injury because of weakened eye tissue. Availability of eye guards approved by the American Society of Testing Materials (ASTM) and other protective equipment may allow participation in most sports, but this must be judged on an individual basis.
Fever	No	Fever can increase cardiopulmonary effort, reduce maximum exercise capacity, make heat illness more likely, and increase orthostatic hypotension during exercise. Fever may rarely accompany myocarditis or other infections that make exercise dangerous.
Heat illness, history of	Qualified yes	Because of the increased likelihood of recurrence, the athlete needs individual assessment to determine the presence of predisposing conditions and arrange a prevention strategy.
HIV infection	Yes	Because of the apparent minimal risk to others, all sports may be played that the state of health allows. In all athletes, skin lesions should be properly covered, and athletic personnel should use universal precautions when handling blood or body fluids containing visible blood.
Kidney, absence of one	Qualified yes	Athlete needs individual assessment for contact/collision and limited contact sports.
Liver, enlarged	Qualified yes	If the liver is acutely enlarged, participation should be avoided because of the risk of rupture. If the liver is chronically enlarged, individual assessment is needed before collision/contact or limited contact sports are played.
Malignancy	Qualified yes	Athlete needs individual assessment.
Musculoskeletal disorders	Qualified yes	Athlete needs individual assessment.
Neurologic conditions		
History of serious head or spine trauma, severe or repeated concussions or craniotomy	Qualified yes	Athlete needs individual assessment for collision or limited contact sports and for noncontact sports if there are deficits in judgment or cognition. Recent research supports a conservative approach to management of concussion.
Convulsive disorder, well controlled	Yes	Risk of convulsion during participation is minimal.
Convulsive disorder, poorly controlled	Qualified yes	Athlete needs individual assessment for collision or limited contact sports. Avoid the following noncontact sports: archery, riflery, swimming, weight or power lifting, strength training, or sports involving heights. In these sports, occurrence of a convulsion may be a risk to self or others.
Obesity	Qualified yes	Because of the risk of heat illness, obese athletes need careful acclimatization and hydration.
Organ transplant recipient	Qualified yes	Athlete needs individual assessment.
Ovary, absence of one	Yes	Risk of severe injury to the remaining ovary is minimal.
Respiratory		
Pulmonary compromise including cystic fibrosis	Qualified yes	Athlete needs individual assessment, but generally all sports may be played if oxygenation remains satisfactory during a graded exercise test. Patients with cystic fibrosis need acclimatization and good hydration to reduce the risk of illness.
Asthma	Yes	With proper medication and education, only athletes with the most severe asthma must modify their participation.
Acute upper respiratory	Qualified yes	Upper respiratory obstruction may affect pulmonary function. Athlete needs individual assessment for all but mild disease. See "Fever."

Table 5.11—*continued.*   Medical Conditions and Sports Participation

Condition	May Participate?	Explanation[b]
Sickle cell disease	Qualified yes	Athlete needs individual assessment. In general, if status of the illness permits, all but high-exertion collision/contact sports may be played. Overheating, dehydration, and chilling must be avoided.
Sickle cell trait (AS)	Yes	It is unlikely that athletes with sickle cell trait have an increased risk of sudden death or other medical problems during athletic participation except during the most extreme conditions of heat, humidity, and possibly increased altitude. These patients, like all athletes, should be carefully conditioned, acclimatized, and hydrated to reduce any possible risk.
Skin: boils, herpes simplex, impetigo, scabies, molluscum contagiosum	Qualified yes	While the patient is contagious, participation in gymnastics with mats, martial arts, wrestling, or other collision/contact or limited contact sports is not allowed. Herpes simplex virus is probably not transmitted via mats.
Spleen, enlarged	Qualified yes	Patients with acutely enlarged spleens should avoid all sports because of risk of rupture. Those with chronically enlarged spleens need individual assessment before playing collision/contact or limited contact sports.
Testicle, absent or undescended	Yes	Certain sports may require a protective cup.

From Andrews JS. Making the most of the sports physical. Contemp Pediatr 14(3):183–205, 1997; and American Academy of Pediatrics, Committee on Sports Medical Fitness. Medical conditions affecting sports participation. Pediatrics 94(5):757, 1994.

[a]Cardiac causes of sudden death in sports: hypertrophic cardiomyopathy, aortic rupture secondary to Marfan's syndrome, congenital coronary artery anomalies, atherosclerotic coronary artery disease, and aortic stenosis. Most are rarely diagnosed during routine physical examination, although presence of marfanoid body habitus or characteristic heart murmur could aid early detection. Examiner needs to be alert to patients with positive family histories of early heart disease, hyperlipidemia, early sudden death, and Marfan's syndrome.

[b]"Needs evaluation" means that a physician with appropriate knowledge and experience should assess the safety of a given sport for an athlete with the listed medical condition. Unless otherwise noted, this is because of the variability of the severity of the disease or the risk of injury among specific sports.

General References*

American Academy of Pediatrics. Sports participation examination (Chapter 4). In: Dyment PG, ed. Sports medicine: health care for young athletes. 2nd ed. Elk Grove Village, IL: American Academy of Pediatrics, 1991.

American Academy of Pediatrics, Committee on Sports Medicine Fitness. Medical conditions affecting sports participation. Pediatrics 94(5):757, 1994.

   Comprehensive references on sports medicine for children and adolescents.

American College of Physicians. Position paper: Health care needs of the adolescent. Ann Intern Med 110:930, 1989.

   Consensus recommendations, with references, for internists.

American Medical Association. **AMA guidelines for adolescent preventive services (GAPS): recommendations and rationale.** Baltimore: Williams & Wilkins, 1994.

   A set of 24 guidelines, by an expert panel, addressing recommendations for the delivery of health services, health guidance, screening, and immunizations for adolescents.

D'Angelo JD, Farrow J. Clinical problems in adolescent medicine. J Gen Intern Med 4:64, 1989.

   Brief review of selected problems of adolescents (growth and development, substance abuse, eating disorders, sexual problems, and violence).

Erickson EH. Identity, youth and crisis. New York: WW Norton, 1968.

   The most widely used theoretical model of adolescent psychosocial development.

McAnarney ER, Kreipe RE, Orr DP, Comerci GD. Textbook of adolescent medicine. Philadelphia: WB Saunders, 1992.

   An excellent comprehensive textbook with large sections on practice applications, psychologic issues, and medical problems as they present and are managed in teens.

Schomberg SK, ed. Substance abuse: a guide for health professionals. Elk Grove Village, IL: American Academy of Pediatrics, 1988.

   A comprehensive review of the substance abuse problem in adolescents.

Tanner JM. Growth at adolescence. 2nd ed. Springfield, IL: Charles C Thomas, 1962.

A classic system for describing the physiologic changes of adolescents.

Books and Materials that May Be Helpful for Adolescents to Read

Pamphlets such as the following titles are available from the American Academy of Pediatrics, Division of Publications, 141 Northwest Point Boulevard, P.O. Box 927, Elk Grove Village, IL 60009-0927.

- *Better Health Through Fitness*
- *Important Information for Teens Who Get Headaches*
- *Acne Treatment and Control*
- *Making the Right Choice: Facts Young People Need to Know About Avoiding Pregnancy*
- *Striving: Coping with Adolescent Depression and Suicide*

Bell R, ed. Changing bodies, changing lives. New York: Random House, 1988.

Otis CL, Goldingay R. Campus health guide. The college student's handbook for healthy living. New York: College Entrance Examination Board, 1989.

   A guide for teens living away from home for the first time.

Ropes E, ed. The kids book of divorce. Boulder, CO: Louis Publishing, 1982.

Resources for Parents

Alexander-Roberts C. ADHD and teens: a parent's guide for making it through the tough years. Dallas: Taylor, 1995.

   A learning tool to help parents understand the heightened difficulties of transition faced by teens with AD/HD.

Dinkmeyer D, McKay GD. Parenting teenagers: systematic theory for parenting of teens. Circle Pines, MN: American Guidance Service, 1990.

   A STEP guide with helpful exercises and improvement insights regarding communication skills for parents with teens in trouble.

Elkind D. Parenting your teenager. New York: Ballantine, 1993.

   A set of columns and contributions to Parents Magazine. Strong on normal development and everyday problems of normal teens.

Fenwick E, Smith T. Adolescence: the survival guide for parents and teenagers. New York: DK Publishing, 1996.

   A good general sourcebook, including teen milestones, talking to teens, and helping teens deal with their growing independence.

---

*Bold print (general references) and bold numerals (specific references) denote published controlled clinical trials, meta-analyses, or consensus-based recommendations.

Philadelphia Child Guidance Center. Your child's emotional health: adolescence. New York: Macmillan, 1995.

> Directive style to help parents deal with a number of common teen issues.

Weiss L. Give your ADD teen a chance. A guide for parents of teenagers with attention deficit disorder. Colorado Springs: Pinon, 1996.

Specific References

1. American Medical Association. AMA guidelines for adolescent preventive services (GAPS): recommendations and rationale. Baltimore: Williams & Wilkins, 1994.
2. Burns BJ, Taube CA. Mental health service for adolescents: assessment background paper for US Congress, Office of Technology Assessment. In: Adolescent health I: summary and policy options. OTA-H-468. Washington, DC: US Government Printing Office, 1991.
3. Desmond MM, Volderman AL, Fisher ES. Assessment of learning competence during the pediatric examination. Curr Prob Pediatr 8:2, 1978.
4. Fargason RE, Ford CV. Attention deficit hyperactivity disorder in adults: diagnosis, treatment and prognosis. South Med J 87:302, 1994.
5. Hein K. Commentary on adolescent acquired immune deficiency syndrome: the next wave of the human immunodeficiency virus epidemic? J Pediatr 114:144, 1989.
6. Kogut MD. Growth and development in adolescents. Pediatr Clin North Am 20:789, 1973.
7. Kreipe RE. Eating disorder among children and adolescents. Pediatr Rev 16:370, 1995.
8. Kysar JR, Zaks MS, Schuchman HP, et al. Range of psychological functioning in normal late adolescents. Arch Gen Psychiatry 21:515, 1969.
9. Levine MD, Zallen BG. The learning disorders of adolescence: organic and non-organic failure to thrive. Pediatr Clin North Am 31:345, 1984.
10. Mattsson A. Adolescent depression and suicide. In: Hockelman RA, Blatman S, Bounell PA, et al, eds. Principles of pediatrics. New York: McGraw-Hill, 1978.
11. Miller D. Adolescent crisis: challenge for patient, parent, and internist. Ann Intern Med 79:435, 1973.
12. Offer D, Marcus D, Offer JL. A longitudinal study of normal adolescent boys. Am J Psychiatry 126:917, 1970.
13. Pope HG, Hudson JI, Yurgelun-Todd D. Anorexia nervosa and bulimia among 300 suburban women shoppers. Am J Psychiatry 141:292, 1984.
14. Weiner IB. Delinquent behavior. In: Psychological disturbance in adolescence. New York: Wiley, 1992.

C H A P T E R 6

Geriatric Medicine: Special Considerations*

THOMAS E. FINUCANE, MD

Geriatrics is formed from two Greek roots meaning "old age" and "healing" or "physician." Related words are *gerontology,* which refers generally to the study of aging, and *iatrogenic,* which literally means "caused by a physician or healer."

Ambulatory adult medicine in the United States is already geriatric medicine to a great extent, and it is

---

*John R. Burton, MD, contributed to this chapter in previous editions. Jane L. Marks, RN, MS, contributed to the urinary incontinence portion of this chapter.

likely to become increasingly geriatric in the next several decades. These observations result from two distinct phenomena. First, at every age life expectancy is increasing. In 1980 a 65-year-old American could expect on average to live 16.4 years. By 1991 a full year had been added to that life expectancy. In the same interval, a 75-year-old individual's life expectancy increased from 10.4 to 11.1 years and in 1991 the average number of years of life remaining to an 85-year-old individual was 5.3. These "oldest old," over age 85, are a special challenge to society as a whole and to physicians in particular: As a group, they are exceedingly frail, requiring a great deal of medical and social support. They are predominantly women and the difference in life expectancy between African Americans and whites has been practically eliminated. Of people 65 years old in 1980, 25% are expected to survive to age 90. In 50 years, more than 40% will survive to age 90, based on moderate assumptions about mortality rates (29).

The second important phenomenon is the postwar baby boom of children born between 1945 and 1965. From 2010 to 2030, the U.S. population aged 65 to 84 will increase 80%, whereas the population under 65 will increase only 7%. Thereafter, boomers will become old-old, above age 85. In 1990 there were 3 million old-old Americans. In 2010 there will be 6 million, and in 2050, 19 million people will be over age 85 (29).

The challenge for physicians will be sharpened by two additional effects: the rates of disability and poverty among the elderly. The percentage of people who need assistance with everyday activities rises steeply with age. Among the "young-old," aged 65 to 75 years, approximately 10% require assistance, whereas among the old-old, nearly half do. These figures are higher for African-American and Hispanic elders. Large numbers of caregivers will be needed, but in 1990 approximately one-fourth of boomers remained childless. Defining poverty in the United States is arbitrary, but 1992 Census Bureau data showed that 10% of men and 20% of women aged 75 and over were poor. Of African Americans over age 75, 35% of men and 43% of women were poor, and of Hispanics, 19% of men and 32% of women were poor. The rate for all U.S. children was 22%. These demographic changes are not limited to the United States or developed countries. In 1993 and 1994, the number of people over age 65 in the world increased by 1000 per hour, with nearly two-thirds of the increase occurring in developing countries (29).

The elderly are at increased risk of prolonged catastrophic illness. Consequently, ethical issues surrounding limitations of therapy are often a central part of clinical decision making. Care of the old, and especially the very old, requires special awareness of the progressive socioeconomic and physiologic vulnerability of old age. More than knowledge of specific disease states, awareness of the extreme frailty of the very old defines clinical geriatrics.

PUBLIC POLICY

Medicare

The structure of Medicare—benefits, copayments, and eligibility—may change dramatically in the near future. Some predictions envision bankruptcy in 2002 and health care reform is constantly debated. As of now, Medicare eligibility is not means-tested. Eligibility depends on age or other qualifying condition (e.g., end-stage renal disease) but not on income. In general, Part A pays institutions for hospital inpatient care, brief posthospital care (whether institutional or provided by a home health agency), and Medicare hospices. Part B pays physicians and providers of outpatient services such as independent laboratory, mental health services, and rehabilitation services. Durable medical equipment is also covered by Part B.

Medicare was originally intended as hospital insurance for the elderly, regardless of income, covering a period of acute illness and subsequent convalescence. Medicare's hospice benefit was a radical change in philosophy: Patients in hospice will not improve. In 1996 Medicare indicated that it would cover inpatient hospital admission for symptom palliation in terminally ill patients, a further evolution of the program (7). Long-term care remains beyond Medicare's purview, however. Chronically ill patients in nursing homes are generally not covered. Short-term stays for rehabilitation after hospitalization are reimbursed, but Medicare coverage ends, as a rule, once the patient stops improving.

Medicare also pays for some preventive services, such as influenza and pneumococcal vaccine, screening mammograms every 2 years, and screening Pap smears every 3 years. These benefits may also change as part of health care reform.

Medicaid

To be eligible for Medicaid, it is necessary, but not sufficient, to be impoverished and age is unimportant. Less than half of poor Americans are covered by Medicaid. Most Medicaid dollars are spent on long-term care in nursing homes, and about half of nursing home revenue comes from Medicaid. Eligibility for nursing home placement is defined by the states, and depends on functional disability and medical illness. Medicaid pays for nursing home care only if the person is indigent. Thus, a person with assets may qualify in one of two ways. He or she may spend the assets on nursing home care until impoverished or divest the assets by giving them to adult children, for example. Rules about divestment are changing, but a "lookback" period is common: Any assets given away in the last 30 months, for example, may be counted as current assets. This topic of divestment is extremely divisive: It is mainly the well-off who can plan ahead to this extent. Because Medicaid is defined on a state-by-state basis, within broad federal guidelines, and because the program is in a state of rapid flux, this chapter cannot provide specific advice about nursing home placement and Medicaid eligibility.

Home Health Care

Part A Medicare certifies home health agencies and pays them for in-home care, primarily by nurses and aides. In keeping with Medicare philosophy, the program was intended to facilitate hospital discharge planning and to manage episodes of acute illness at home, thus preventing some admissions. From 1988 to 1994, home health agency reimbursements grew from $2 billion to almost $13 billion. Although the intent of the home health care program was to provide a substitute for or adjunct to acute hospital care, 61% of all visits were to enrollees receiving services for 6 months or more, and geographic areas with high use rates of home care do not have lower rates of hospitalization or shorter lengths of stay. The need for chronic care among community-dwelling elderly, along with several other factors, simply was not foreseen in the original design of Medicare (56).

Public policy about medical care of the elderly, especially the poor and frail elderly, is in flux. Out-of-pocket and government expenses are rising. Many different legislative initiatives are in various stages of development, and underlying problems are enormous. Costs are high and are rising. Substantial change is possible in the near future.

GENERAL ISSUES

Evaluating Older Patients

Several aspects of clinical evaluation deserve emphasis.

Old records should be obtained before the first visit, when possible. If not, they should be requested at the first visit. A patient's medical records invariably contain useful information. Patients should routinely bring all of their medications, including over-the-counter medications, to appointments.

Bright, direct light is often uncomfortable for patients with cataracts. Prolonged sitting on a backless examining table or in a chilly room can be uncomfortable. Making a patient comfortable probably improves the quality of the history. For patients with presbycusis, it is more important to face the patient and speak slowly and clearly than it is to speak loudly. Also, the practitioner should have an assistive listening device (see Chapter 96) available for use by the patient when needed. Patients with marked kyphosis can often lie down more comfortably if a rolled-up sheet is placed on the pillow under the occiput.

Some form of mental status examination should be included in the initial evaluation of every older patient (see Chapter 17). Clinicians' judgment has been shown to be insensitive in detecting mild cognitive impairment (35). Cognitive impairment is extremely common, with prevalence rates of 30 to almost 50% among the very old (13). It is now common that symptoms of

disease in the elderly may be absent, atypical, or ignored by the physician. Subtle deterioration of cognitive or functional capacity may be the only indication of a serious pathologic condition.

In general, more time is needed for evaluation of an elderly patient than for a younger patient. The former often has multiple problems, including sensory and mobility impairments, that require a slower evaluation. Diagnostic testing should be highly selective. Stressful tests (which may include radiographic studies for a frail person with a mobility disorder) should have an expected therapeutic implication and should be explained thoroughly to the patient and, where applicable, the caregiver. Extensive evaluation may require several visits. The highly streamlined evaluations so characteristic of modern medicine are simply too stressful for many ill elderly patients. Empathy and compassion are essential in high-quality care for a frail, older patient. Several 30- or 60-minute visits may be more easily tolerated than a single longer encounter, provided it is not too difficult for the patient and family to come to the office. However, too short an encounter (e.g., 10 to 20 minutes) is disappointing, inadequate for proper care, and difficult for many elders.

Decisions About Limiting Therapy

For some people a prolonged interval of chronic illness and dependency before death is undesirable. Above some threshold of suffering and incapacity, many would choose to limit treatment that will prolong life but not restore health, and in its *Cruzan* decision the United States Supreme Court assumed a constitutional right to decline life-sustaining treatment. For patients who lack the cognitive capacity to accept or decline, however, decisions about limiting treatment are extremely controversial.

Advance directives are intended to allow a patient to state in advance wishes about medical care in the event of subsequent incapacitation. Laws vary from state to state, but the directives take two general forms. The first is exemplified by the *living will:* A patient states what treatments should or should not be withheld in the event of incapacity. *This type of directive is often limited.* In many states it becomes effective only when the patient is terminally ill. The second form of advance directive names an agent or proxy who will represent the patient if he or she becomes incapacitated. These directives are called *durable powers of attorney for health care.* Requirements for witnesses and notarization, acceptability of directives from other states, determination of patient capacity to make decisions, and other technical aspects vary from state to state. Use of advance directives has been officially encouraged by the federal government since the implementation of the Patient Self-Determination Act in 1991 (36). Evidence for the effectiveness of advance directives is uncertain.

Making decisions for the many patients who are incapacitated and who have left no advance directives is even more difficult. For these often vulnerable people, careful therapeutic restraint, in the minds of some, closely resembles neglect. States vary widely in how they use the family guidance. In the *Cruzan* decision, the Supreme Court ruled that families have no constitutional right to direct the limitation of life-sustaining treatment for an incapacitated adult. Furthermore, as with the abortion question, some people have strong beliefs about the definition and value of life and about the need to protect it in any circumstance. As Ms. Cruzan lay dying in a persistent vegetative state, for example, people associated with Operation Rescue maintained a vigil outside her nursing facility and at one point stormed the clinic in an attempt to reattach her feeding tube (57).

Hospital administrators are generally familiar with pertinent local laws. For the primary physician three general points are worth emphasis.

First, there is no perfect protection from liability. Physicians have been taken to court because they have withdrawn therapy from an incompetent patient at the family's unanimous request. Under almost identical circumstances, physicians have been sued because they have refused to discontinue therapy.

Second, the process of planning with capable patients, in the presence of the family when indicated, is at least as important as the product of the planning session. Informed consent, or informed refusal, is as fundamental here as in any other area of medical care.

Third, a unanimous consensus among family and involved health care workers is the surest method of avoiding litigation when making decisions about incapacitated elderly patients.

Functional Assessment and Disability

The traditional problem-oriented approach to medical care focuses primarily on medical diagnoses. Functional assessment is intended to measure the impact of disease and aging on a patient's ability to care for him- or herself, to live in the community, and to accomplish goals that are meaningful on the patient's terms. Problems in constructing valid and useful measures have been carefully described (15). The *Barthel Index* is significantly correlated with recovery from stroke and location after discharge. Poor performance of the Katz *activities of daily living (ADLs)* (Table 6.1) correlates with mortality, nursing home placement, and inadequate recovery from hip fracture (31,38). In addition, dependency in ADLs is part of the determination of nursing home eligibility and has been an entry criterion for many proposed long-term care plans in the debate over health care reform. Despite this, physicians caring for ambulatory patients often underestimate or overlook important disabilities in their patients (6). *Instrumental activities of daily living* require a higher level of function. Inability to travel outside the home, shop, prepare meals, do housework, or handle finances indicates a different degree of frailty (16). Investigations of the assessment, natural history, demography, impact of disability, and of interventions to prevent disability are elegantly summarized (18).

Table 6.1. Areas and Levels of Assessment in the Katz Index of Independence in Activities of Daily Living

Bathing:	_____	Receives no assistance
	_____	Receives assistance in bathing only one part
	_____	Receives assistance in bathing more than one part
Dressing:	_____	Gets clothes and dresses without assistance
	_____	Needs assistance in tying shoes only
	_____	Needs assistance greater than above or stays undressed
Toileting:	_____	Needs no assistance
	_____	Needs assistance only in getting to toilet room or in cleaning self
	_____	Does not go to toilet room
Transferring:	_____	Needs no assistance from another person
	_____	Needs assistance with transferring
	_____	Does not get out of bed
Continence:	_____	Continent
	_____	Occasional accident
	_____	Needs supervision, uses catheter, or is incontinent
Feeding:	_____	Needs no assistance
	_____	Needs assistance in cutting meat or buttering bread
	_____	Needs more assistance or is tube or intravenously fed

From Katz S, Ford AB, Moskowitz RW, et al. Studies of illness in the aged: the index at ADL: standardized measures of biological and psychosocial function. JAMA 185:94, 1963.

GERIATRIC ASSESSMENT

Comprehensive geriatric assessment is a multidisciplinary (usually), multidimensional (always) assessment of frail elderly patients and their support systems. It is occasionally confused with functional assessment, described in the previous section. Although it has received a great deal of favorable attention, geriatric assessment lacks a precise definition and data supporting its usefulness are sketchy. The referral source and initial characteristics of patients, the nature of intervention (e.g., whether inpatient, in the office, or in the home, and whether consultation or ongoing therapy), and the measured outcomes vary from study to study.

There is no doubt that certain frail, elderly patients and their companions would benefit from assessment by a careful and competent social worker or a nurse who has the time and desire to teach, or perhaps a visit with a pharmacist, nutritionist, or therapist. On the other hand, it is difficult to imagine how this multidisciplinary approach would cause a 50% reduction in mortality in treated subjects compared with randomized controls in 1 year, as reported in a prominent article on inpatient geriatric assessment (50). A subsequent large, randomized study of inpatients from the same institution showed no clinically meaningful difference on any of the measured outcomes (48). A randomized outpatient study showed no effect on survival (11). Medicare currently does not provide specific compensation for multidisciplinary comprehensive geriatric assessment.

Assessment of elderly patients in their homes has definite benefits. Studies of case-finding and surveillance (43), postdischarge assessment (24), and pharmacy assessment (10) done in the home have demonstrated significantly improved outcomes.

DRUG USE IN THE ELDERLY

Elderly Americans take large numbers of drugs. Although some drugs are clearly beneficial, many others have little or no evidence of efficacy. Risks to the elderly patient from imprecise drug use can be substantial. In a British study, psychiatrist, patient, and caregiver were asked in the clinic and the general practitioner was interviewed about the patient's medication regimen. At a home visit later in the same week, patient and caregiver were questioned again. Most physicians, patients, and caregivers could not recount what the patient actually was taking (1). In an epidemiologic study in the United States, 87% of independent elderly were taking at least one over-the-counter medication and 6% were taking five or more (53). A useful clinical strategy is to insist that all medication, including over-the-counter drugs, be brought to each visit and then to consider the justification for each drug.

Studies of drug disposition in the elderly demonstrate wide heterogeneity in several important physiologic functions. Although drug absorption is unimpaired in general, distribution within the body compartments may be different in older than in younger subjects. Muscle mass, bone mass, body water, and some serum proteins are lower and body fat higher in older subjects. Hepatic drug clearance, in simplest terms, depends on hepatic blood flow, serum protein binding, and the intrinsic capacity of the hepatocyte mass. The first two of these factors may decrease with age, resulting in impaired drug metabolism in some patients. Glomerular filtration rate (GFR) can fall approximately 30% from the third decade to the eighth. The fall in GFR may not be accompanied by a rise in serum creatinine because muscle mass is falling concomitantly. Because of variability among subjects, prediction of drug levels from dosage is unreliable.

In many cases, very low dosages of medication may be effective, such as 12.5 mg of hydrochlorothiazide per day and beginning dosages of 0.25 mg haloperidol or 10 mg imipramine or nortriptyline per day. Unless the clinical situation requires otherwise, drugs should be started at low dosages in the elderly and titrated carefully upward during frequent early follow-up. Drug levels, when available, are useful in monitoring the patient.

New drugs pose particularly serious risks for the elderly. In general the FDA approves new drugs after safety has been demonstrated in small trials (32). Once the drugs are released, however, they are often used widely by the frail elderly, and serious but uncommon toxicities become apparent. Benoxaprofen (Oraflex), zomepirac (Zomax), suprofen (Suprol), nomifensine (Merital), and temafloxacin (Omniflox) have been heavily promoted and then withdrawn from the market after reports of serious injury or death of patients. Encainide and flecainide, both of whose advertising campaigns initially referred specifically to their safety, doubled the death rate in patients taking these drugs for asymptomatic ventricular arrhythmias after myocardial infarction. Tramadol (Ultram) and Zolpidem (Ambien) are more recent examples of drugs whose early advertising campaigns touted safety, but that later demonstrated unexpected toxicities. New drugs should be tried carefully in older patients only after all more standard drugs have been tried and have failed. Older drugs have more well-established safety profiles and are generally less expensive. Prescribing a new drug means entering a patient into the postmarketing surveillance phase. Claims about the safety or the lack of side effects of newly released drugs should be viewed as advertising techniques.

Some specific drugs selected because of their widespread use in the elderly are considered here.

Oral Hypoglycemic Drugs

The FDA requires that all of these drugs, including the new ones, be labeled with a Special Warning about the possibility of increased risk of cardiovascular mortality, although the findings of the study on which this warning is based remain highly controversial. Further study has not convincingly demonstrated reduction in the microvascular complications of diabetes mellitus as a result of the use of these agents. No study has shown reduction in risk of blindness, renal failure, amputation, or death as a result of treating elderly diabetic patients with oral agents. Moderate control of hyperglycemia may result in symptomatic improvement in some patients. Oral hypoglycemic drugs are discussed fully in Chapter 72. Finally, hypoglycemia is a particular concern in elderly patients who are treated with these agents and with insulin.

Major Tranquilizers

These drugs are associated with increased risk of falls, hip fracture (47), and tardive dyskinesia. They are sometimes efficacious in treating the behavioral complications of dementia. Of 100 demented patients treated with neuroleptics, 18 could be expected to benefit beyond placebo, according to a meta-analysis. No one neuroleptic has been shown to be more effective than another (51). If these drugs are prescribed, evidence of good effect should be sought. If they provide nothing more than sedation (assuming sedation is desirable), other drugs should be used instead, such as short-acting benzodiazepines. The use of psychoactive drugs in the elderly is discussed fully in Chapter 17.

Nonsteroidal Anti-Inflammatory Drugs

For treatment of inflammatory conditions, nonsteroidal anti-inflammatory drugs (NSAIDs) are excellent drugs. When they are used as analgesia for noninflammatory chronic pain, their considerable toxicities may outweigh their benefit. Current users of NSAIDs are almost five times more likely to have a fatal upper gastrointestinal hemorrhage when compared with former users or subjects who have never used them (20). The cited study suggests that frail, elderly white women are especially at risk. Renal and central nervous system (CNS) toxicities are well known (see Chapter 70 for a full discussion on NSAIDs). In many cases of pain without underlying inflammation, acetaminophen may have a superior risk–benefit profile. In middle-aged women with osteoarthritis of the knee, for example, 4 g of acetaminophen daily was as good as low-dosage (1200 mg daily) or high-dosage (2400 mg daily) ibuprofen for pain relief (3).

Cold Remedies

There is no cure for the common cold, but there is a multimillion-dollar market in remedies. Common treatments bring the risk of antihistaminic or narcotic sedation, sympathomimetic stimulation, or a combination of the two. Substantial amounts of alcohol are often included: Vicks NyQuil is 50 proof, for example. Many common combinations are irrational, even contradictory. Clinicians should discourage their elderly patients, who are likely to be susceptible to anticholinergic and sympathomimetic effects, from buying these nostrums, many of which contain a variety of useless ingredients. However, they will be working against a mammoth advertising campaign as they do so. The use of zinc and chromium as treatment for the common cold is discussed in Chapter 28.

Drug–Drug Interactions

Elderly patients who take many medications are at high risk for drug–drug interactions. Selegiline (Eldepryl) taken with a selective serotonin reuptake inhibitor can cause delirium and death. Terfenadine (Seldane) taken with certain antifungal or antibiotic medicines can lead to ventricular arrhythmia and death. An industry publication has compiled 1231 pages of drug–drug interactions and 250 pages of side effects (44). Physicians should become familiar with and use a small number of medications.

NEGLECT AND ABUSE IN THE ELDERLY

Most dependent elderly live in the community and are cared for by relatives. In most of these cases, excellent, loving care is provided. In some cases, however, there is frank abuse or neglect and in some the situation is ambiguous. The number of older Americans who are abused is likely to increase for a variety of reasons, including the national trend toward smaller families and the rapidly increasing numbers of the very old, who are no longer wage earners and are more likely to be frail and dependent. Clear-cut examples of physical and emotional violence, sexual abuse, and harmful neglect against frail elderly people have been reported.

Definition of abuse can be difficult, in large part because the victims are presumably competent adults who choose to continue the relationship leading to putative abuse. Neglect is also often difficult to define, especially in a relationship in which the caregiver has no legally defined responsibility. Furthermore, some situations offer only tragic options. If a single working mother cares for her demented mother who repeatedly wanders or urinates in closets, is it abuse if the daughter uses physical restraints? Suppose neither mother nor daughter will accept a nursing home and employment of professional caregivers is not financially feasible.

Diagnosis is difficult because both abuser and victim may deny or minimize abuse. Therefore, diagnosis is often inferential. Treatment may be problematic in all but extreme cases. Remedies might include an alternative environment that is healthful, supportive, and acceptable to the victim, or the provision of services that can relieve a stressed caregiver. Such treatment is often unavailable. Risk factors for abuse are shown in Table 6.2 (8,30).

Clinicians may be reluctant to become involved in a situation in which there is little reward, poor reimbursement, and potential liability. State statutes vary in defining the physician's liability. The Council on Scientific Affairs of the American Medical Association has published a useful report on this subject. The report outlines several strategies for prevention and intervention (8). The full report may be obtained by writing to the Council on Scientific Affairs, AMA, 535 N. Dearborn St., Chicago, IL 60610. In severe cases, however, legal advice should be sought and state and local agencies such as Adult Protective Services should be involved.

FALLS

The risk of frequent or severe falls accompanies many geriatric syndromes. Etiology is often multifactorial and hard to define. Caregivers, the environment, medications, sensory impairment, dementia, and deconditioning—as well as specific neurologic, cardiovascular, or musculoskeletal diseases—often contribute to the problem. Falls are common in the elderly and often have serious consequences, including death.

Progress in research about falls has been steady. More risk factors have been identified, such as impaired cognition, abnormal reaction to a push, history of

---

Table 6.2. Risk Factors for Elder Abuse

Victim Characteristics
Lives with related relative, not spouse
Severely demented
Behavior problem
Medically ill

Abuser
Has provided long-term care
Stressed significantly by care of the victim
Under severe external stress
Abused as a child
Expresses frustration
Uses recreational drugs, including alcohol

palpitations, abnormal stepping, slow timed chair stands, decreased arm strength, vision or hearing impairment, and high anxiety or depression scores (55). Perhaps most important, interventions designed to reduce falls have been successful. Exercise programs, particularly those including balance exercise, reduce risk of falls by 10 to 17% (12). An intervention targeting four specific risk factors in a vulnerable population reduced falls during 1 year of follow-up from 47 to 35%. The risk factors are postural hypotension, use of sedatives, use of four or more prescription medications, and impairment in arm or leg strength or range of motion, transfer skills, or gait skills (54). Falls in elderly outpatients are carefully reviewed by King and Tinetti (34).

NUTRITION

For a variety of reasons, precise definition of dietary requirements for ambulatory elderly people is difficult. The elderly are physiologically and metabolically an extremely diverse group with a variety of illnesses, taking a variety of medicines. Absorptive function in the aging gut is poorly studied. However, recommended daily allowances (RDAs) for the elderly are extrapolated from data collected in studies of younger people. RDAs based on age alone are imprecise. More complicated calculations will probably replace them.

Two general principles have been demonstrated. First, most elderly Americans who seek medical attention are not undernourished. Second, desirable body weight for the elderly may be somewhat heavier than previously determined on the basis of insurance company tables of mortality and body mass index (BMI). These tables do not consider age. Based on independent analysis of insurance company data, Andres (2) has calculated mortality ratios in various age groups according to BMI. This analysis suggests that the BMI associated with the lowest mortality rate varies with age. The older the age group, the higher the best BMI. For example, the BMI associated with the lowest mortality among 25-year-old men is 21.4. For a 6-footer, this corresponds to a weight of 158 lb. For a 65-year-old man, the best BMI is 26.6, 196 lb for the same 6-footer. Roughly speaking, these tables allow a gain of approximately 1 pound per year throughout adult life. Several studies of long-term weight change tend to confirm that modest weight gain during adult life is associated with lower mortality (52). These tables do not apply to patients with diseases that are related to weight. For patients with Type 2 diabetes mellitus, hypertension, and hyperlipidemia, weight loss is often an essential part of treatment.

The pattern of body fat distribution has been shown to be associated with several important diseases and with mortality. High waist-to-hip circumference ratio has been shown to be more strongly associated with death than is BMI in women (see Chapter 76) (17).

A variety of psychosocial factors (e.g., isolation, alcoholism, depression, low income) and physiologic changes (e.g., diminished taste and smell sensation,

dental problems, dementia, dysphagia, acid peptic disease) may contribute to a diminished intake of nutritious meals. Although difficult to demonstrate except in extreme cases, malnutrition may occur in these situations. The effects of multivitamin supplements are unknown. Several trials of vitamin supplementation have shown no benefit (26,46). Although risks are low when vitamins are taken in moderation, costs can be high.

Weight loss can result from a variety of causes, some trivial and some lethal. In general, the known causes of weight loss can be classified as decreased intake, reduced absorption, and increased use. Involuntary weight loss can be troubling in the elderly. In 25% of cases no cause is discovered despite intensive evaluation. Almost all of the remaining causes can be found with a careful history and physical examination and judicious use of the laboratory. In the elderly, decreased intake should be carefully sought. The search for malignancy during a careful history and physical examination and the exclusion of hyperthyroidism with appropriate laboratory investigation are also an important part of the evaluation.

ELDERLY DRIVERS

Increasing interest has focused on the risks generated by elderly drivers. Risk factors have been identified. Impaired copy design on the Mini Mental State Examination, walking less than a block per day, and foot and leg abnormalities (toe deformities, bunions, knee contractures, slowed toe tapping, or impaired toe walk) all predicted adverse outcomes (40). The use of long-acting benzodiazepines has been associated with an increased risk of motor vehicle crash among the elderly (25). Whether 90-year-old drivers are more dangerous than 16-year-old drivers and when the freedom to drive should be coercively limited are complex questions. Medical, legal, and ethical considerations interact, and laws vary from state to state. The American Geriatrics Society and the American Association of Retired Persons cosponsor 55 Alive/Mature Drivers Program. Information is available at AARP 55 Alive, 601 E. Street N.W., Washington, DC 20049.

A 90-year-old driver in the year 2000, born when cars were a novelty, will probably be different from a 90-year-old driver in 2030.

EXERCISE AND THE ELDERLY

Benefits from exercise are now incontrovertible and include improvements in bone density, sleep (33), risk of falls (45), disability and pain from knee arthritis (12), cardiovascular risk factors and disease (41), and rate of disability (19). Even low levels of exercise confer benefit. The value of exercise testing for apparently healthy elderly patients who want to begin an exercise program is uncertain. A combined American College of Cardiology/American Heart Association Practice Guideline gives a Class II-b recommendation ("usefulness/efficacy is less well established by evidence/opinion") for the use of exercise testing to evaluate asymptomatic men over age 40 and women over 50 who plan to start vigorous exercise (23). The American College of Sports Medicine (ACSM) recommends testing for elderly patients planning a program of vigorous but not moderate exercise. The ACSM defines moderate exercise as "exercise intensity well within the individual's current capacity [that] can be comfortably sustained for a prolonged period of time, i.e., 60 minutes, slow progression, and generally non-competitive." Vigorous exercise is "enough to represent a substantial challenge and which would ordinarily result in fatigue within 20 minutes." Risks from false-positive test results and low risk of moderate exercise in general are mentioned in both sets of guidelines. Patients with risk factors for or with established cardiovascular disease require careful evaluation, and perhaps in part for legal reasons, a stress test should be considered. The adage for medications applies here as well: Start low, go slow. Two guidelines may be useful. First, the pace of walking should be slow enough that the elderly person can converse comfortably. Second, competition between walkers should be specifically discouraged. Malls are good places to walk.

HOSPITALIZATION

In planning a course of care for a sick elderly patient, hospitalization is often an option. However, the incidence of adverse events in hospitalized patients is well documented, and elderly patients are at particular risk. Patients over age 65 have more than twice the risk of adverse effects compared with those 16 to 44 and have the highest rates of adverse effects caused by negligence among all age groups (4). Rates for every category of non–procedure-related adverse event are highest in patients over age 65 (37). The effects of prolonged immobilization on ventilation, bone metabolism, plasma volume, and muscle strength, as well as the risks of sensory deprivation, physical restraints, and sensory deprivation have been well described (9). Bed sores, diminished functional status, nosocomial infection, delirium, malnutrition from hospital diets, and trauma are all further risks of hospitalization. Efforts to take care of many moderately ill elderly patients at home are likely to develop further. This trend is independent of payer considerations.

URINARY INCONTINENCE

Although urinary incontinence is an important and embarrassing problem for elderly patients, they often do not report it and physicians often fail to ask about it (21). In this chapter urinary incontinence is defined as a situation in which a patient gets wet with urine involuntarily, and the wetness is a problem for the person or caregivers. Urinary incontinence can be costly and humiliating, and it is a common reason for placing a community-dwelling elder in a nursing home.

In the ambulatory elderly, urinary incontinence should generally be evaluated and treated by the primary care physician. It is often multifactorial in origin and can be improved significantly with conservative measures. Treatment should be guided by an understanding of the pathophysiology, but it often remains empiric. In some cases, urinary incontinence has been shown to improve or resolve spontaneously. Referral to a geriatrician, urologist, or gynecologist should be a last resort.

Pathophysiology

The bladder is innervated by an autonomous spinal reflex arc that can be modulated effectively by the cerebral cortex, permitting the patient, under normal circumstances, to empty the urinary bladder in a socially acceptable fashion. Spontaneous contraction of the detrusor muscle usually occurs when the urinary bladder fills to approximately 150 to 250 mL; under normal circumstances most people can suppress this urge to void. Conditioning by chronic high- or low-volume voiding can change the bladder capacity substantially in either direction.

The anatomy and neuroanatomy of the bladder and its sphincters are the subject of intense study. In simple terms, urine flows when intravesical pressure exceeds the pressure in the urethra. Determinants of these two pressures are complex, but two basic principles help guide the evaluation. First, just as injuries to nerves innervating skeletal muscles can be divided into upper and lower motor neuron damage on the basis of clinical examination, the pattern of neurogenic incontinence can be divided into spastic and flaccid varieties. Second, autonomic innervation of the lower tract can be simplified to the following mnemonic: *Sympathetics* lead to *storage*. Thus, adrenergic blockers and cholinergic agonists promote emptying, and anticholinergics, as well as adrenergic agonists, interfere with emptying. The situation is considerably more complex than this, of course. For example, coordination of detrusor and sphincter is often disrupted, and the resulting detrusor–sphincter dyssynergia is a common finding on invasive testing of the elderly. At present, however, therapies are still imprecise enough that the above generalizations can be useful.

Clinical Approach

The first step in approaching a patient with urinary incontinence is to establish the diagnosis. This requires asking the patient, often in a variety of ways, because the modesty of many patients may interfere with reporting of symptoms. On the basis of history alone, classification of incontinence is possible. Five types of urinary incontinence can be identified: *acute, urge, stress, overflow,* and *functional*. Each has characteristic pathophysiology, clinical presentation, and treatment, but commonly, as with many geriatric syndromes, more than one cause contributes, and the syndrome is amenable to multiple small, nontoxic interventions.

Acute Urinary Incontinence

Four general types of problems can produce an acute and often treatable syndrome. The first is a diminished will or ability to use the toilet. Delirium, depression, and sedation by medicines are common causes. Causes of functional incontinence often may be relevant here as well. Second, local perineal problems can lead to incontinence. Symptomatic urinary tract infection (but not asymptomatic bacteriuria), stool impaction, and perhaps atrophic urethritis accompanying vaginitis are examples. Third, drugs such as potent diuretics or those with autonomic side effects can cause incontinence. A fairly common example is an elderly man who catches a cold and has overflow incontinence 2 days later because he has taken over-the-counter "decongestants" (adrenergics) and antihistamines (with anticholinergic properties). Fourth, and least commonly, syndromes that produce polyuria can overwhelm an older person's ability to use the toilet properly and stay dry. Treatment, when possible, is generally obvious once the cause is identified.

Urge Incontinence

Urge incontinence is identified when a patient has the sensation that voiding is imminent, but the warning is too brief to allow reaching the toilet and a variable, but often a large amount of urine is spilled. This has also been called a *spastic neurogenic bladder,* referring to a pattern of upper motor neuron dysfunction. When the bladder stretches, sensory information is delivered, but inhibition of the stretch reflex is inadequate and voiding occurs. This syndrome is often seen in patients with dementia and stroke, who of course may also be slow to respond to the sensation.

Stress Incontinence

The cause of stress incontinence generally is *sphincter incompetence,* often caused by problems with the pelvic floor, especially in postmenopausal or multiparous women, or by damage to the sphincter itself in men who have had urologic surgery. Sudden increases in intra-abdominal pressure, as with increased muscle tone during coughing, sneezing, or lifting, are transmitted to the bladder lumen, and the sphincter is incapable of preventing urine leakage. Small amounts of urine are generally spilled simultaneously with the activity that increased intra-abdominal pressure. In the elderly, stress incontinence often occurs with urge incontinence. If there is a delay in leakage after activity, an uninhibited bladder contraction may have been provoked by the activity; this is an additional pattern of mixed incontinence called *stress-induced urge incontinence.*

Overflow Incontinence

When bladder pressure remains low or outlet pressure remains high, the bladder may distend and spill small, or sometimes large, amounts of urine. Low pressures in the bladder are often caused by lower motor neuron disease, commonly diabetes mellitus, and this situation may be called flaccid neurogenic bladder. High outlet pressures are usually caused by prostatic hyperplasia in men.

Functional Incontinence

Functional incontinence is diagnosed when environmental factors interact with a patient's inability, or occasionally unwillingness, to use a toilet. In the extreme case, a normal person suffers functional incontinence if given diuretics and then restrained in a chair. As a rule, however, functional incontinence is again mixed; the patient has some problem voiding (typically urge with or without stress incontinence), and the environment is not well suited to accommodating that problem.

Evaluation

History

Classification of urinary incontinence is often possible after the history. If the problem is of recent onset, or has worsened recently, a search for reversible causes may lead to cure. New medications, symptoms of infection or irritation, and changes in cognitive or physical capacity should be sought.

The pattern of chronic urinary incontinence is generally recognizable from the history, as described earlier in this chapter. Figure 6.1 shows examples of bladder records for two patients, one with urge and one with stress incontinence. Specific descriptions of accidents are recorded and can be reviewed with the patient. These records may also be useful in helping to plan a regimen of timed voidings as described in the "Therapy" section later in this chapter. Symptoms of partial outlet obstruction, neurologic disease, depression, gait problems, and descriptions of physical barriers in the home should be sought.

Examination

Evidence of neurologic disease, gait problems, and depression are important in planning treatment. *Digital rectal examination* is necessary to diagnose fecal impaction and, in men, prostatic enlargement. For women, a *pelvic examination* should be done to look for a relaxation (e.g., cystocele) or atrophic vaginitis. It is also necessary to test for *urinary sphincter adequacy.* This may be accomplished by having the patient, while in the lithotomy position, cough after her bladder is full. If urinary sphincter insufficiency is present, a small urine leak will result. If the patient has a leak after coughing and surgery can reasonably be considered, a Bonney's test may be performed: Incontinence as a result of cough is prevented by lifting the urethra and base of the bladder with the tips of two fingers placed in the vagina, just lateral to, and not obstructing, the urethra. Although the predictive value of the test is controversial, correction of incontinence by this maneuver correlates generally with a good surgical outcome, if sphincter insufficiency is the only pattern of incontinence that is identified. If the patient did not have an incontinent episode in the lithotomy position, she should be asked to stand while properly draped, holding an absorbent pad over her urethra, and to

Bladder Record

Name_____   Date_____

Instructions: 1. In the first column, mark the time every time you void.
2. In the second or third column, mark every time you accidentally leaked urine.
3. Write "dry" if no accident occurred in the 2-hour interval.

Time Interval	Urinated in Toilet	Leaking Accident	or	Large Accident	Reason for Accident
6–8 AM	✓				
8–10 AM					
10–12 AM	✓				
12–2 PM					
2–4 PM	✓	✓			Running water
4–6 PM					
6–8 PM				✓	Waited too long
8–10 PM	✓				
10–12 PM				✓	Running water
Overnight					

Number of pads used today: _____

Comments: _____

Exercises: _____

_____

A   _____

Total: _____

Figure 6.1. A. Bladder record from patient with urinary incontinence: uninhibited bladder.

cough. This maneuver may precipitate an episode of stress incontinence.

After the patient has voided completely, it is important to carefully evaluate bladder emptying. Identification of enlarged postvoid residual volume is a key decision point in the treatment algorithm. Bladder emptying may be evaluated by the performance of a postvoid catheterization or by a portable bladder scanner.

Patient Experience. Catheterization may be performed simply by obtaining a catheterization kit, which contains all of the materials necessary (cleansing solutions, a catheter, sterile gloves, collection containers, and lubricant). After preparation of the urethral meatus, the sterile catheter is inserted gently into the bladder. In male patients, the shaft of the penis must be extended and lifted in a cephalad direction to align the urethra with the bladder outlet. The urine volume is measured and the catheter is removed. When catheterization is properly performed, the incidence of infection is less than 1% and only 3 to 4% of patients—usually males—experience mild discomfort, typically a burning sensation. This discomfort may be minimized by carefully inserting a well-lubricated catheter and thoroughly explaining the procedure to the patient before its performance.

A portable bladder scanner (using ultrasound technology) is a safe and simple device that can be used reliably to evaluate bladder volume noninvasively, if one of the office staff is trained to use it.

If the postvoiding residual volume is greater than 100 mL of urine, overflow incontinence may be present; this is a special concern with very large residual volumes (more than 200 mL). Analysis of the urine,

Bladder Record

Name_____ Date_____

Instructions: 1. In the first column, mark the time every time you void.
2. In the second or third column, mark every time you accidentally leaked urine.
3. Write "dry" if no accident occurred in the 2-hour interval.

Time Interval	Urinated in Toilet	Leaking Accident	or	Large Accident	Reason for Accident
6–8 AM	✓	✓			Fast walking
8–10 AM	✓				
10–12 AM	✓				
12–2 PM					
2–4 PM	✓				
4–6 PM		✓			Coughed
6–8 PM	✓				
8–10 PM		✓			Sneezed
10–12 PM	✓				
Overnight					

Number of pads used today: _2_____

Comments: _____

_____

Exercises: _____

_____

B _____

Total: _____

Figure 6.1—*continued*. **B.** Bladder record from patient with urinary incontinence: sphincter insufficiency. (Patient data courtesy of Kathryn L. Burgio, PhD, Gerontology Research Center, National Institute on Aging, Baltimore, MD. Bladder record from Whitehead WE, Burgio KL, Engel BT. Behavioral methods in the assessment and treatment of urinary incontinence. In: Brocklehurst JC, ed. Urology in the elderly. New York: Churchill Livingstone, 1984;81.)

both microscopically and by dipstick, can be accomplished on the urine specimen obtained by the catheterization and is helpful in evaluating for an infection or in suggesting less common diagnoses. Gross hematuria may suggest a tumor, for example.

An additional technique useful in the evaluation of selected patients is simple cystometry. This procedure requires recording the volume while filling the bladder incrementally with sterile water through a catheter and subsequently measuring the voided volume. It can easily be performed by a nurse or physician following the guidelines established by Ouslander et al. (42). The procedure is helpful when the patient's history is unclear or suggests a mixed disorder. It also ensures that the test for stress incontinence is performed when the bladder is full, thus increasing validity. Also, involuntary contractions are easily seen using this technique, and when these occur at a low volume (e.g., less than 250 mL), urge incontinence is suggested.

Referral

Patients with large postvoid residual volumes (more than 200 mL) should generally be referred to a urologist or gynecologist because cystoscopy and cystometrographic studies are often necessary to classify precisely the voiding disorder and to plan for definitive therapy. In elderly patients with other patterns of incontinence, cystometrographic study has not been found to be useful. When the pattern of incontinence strongly suggests urge incontinence (large-volume accidents, often occurring within moments of the first urge to void), for example, further evaluation is usually not indicated because at present these patients are not surgical candidates. In contrast, elderly women with pure stress incontinence may be surgical candidates. Urodynamic studies are necessary when surgery is considered to be certain no other pattern of incontinence is present simultaneously (such presence would predict a much less favorable surgical outcome). Surgical success in correcting stress incontinence is dramatic in younger women. With endoscopic suspension of the bladder neck, a procedure with less operative stress than with earlier operations, elderly women with pure stress incontinence may be helped. The physician should refer the patient to a geriatrician with special interest in incontinence or to a urologist or gynecologist when basic therapies (see the "Therapy" section that follows) have failed, if there is doubt about the cause of the incontinence, or if there is concern about a serious underlying problem (e.g., a bladder or prostate tumor or the cauda equina syndrome).

Therapy

It is most important to recognize that small therapeutic gains often are extremely important to an elderly patient (a fundamental precept of geriatric medicine). Cure is not always accomplished, but if incontinent episodes can be minimized, the patient and caregiver may express considerable satisfaction. Furthermore, nonsurgical, nonpharmacologic therapies have a dramatic success rate in ambulatory patients.

The bladder record (see Fig. 6.1) may provide an important clue to the treatment (as well as the cause) of the incontinence. For example, the physician might advise avoiding situations that increase the urge to void (as in the patient who comments that incontinence occurs only when drinking warm milk or listening to running water). Also, the willingness with which the patient uses the bladder record provides insight about the likelihood that a program of education will be successful.

Educational Programs

An education program is an important first step in the treatment of any patient with stress, urge, or functional patterns of incontinence who is not significantly demented. The initial focus should be on a thorough explanation of the mechanisms of incontinence and reassurance that a great deal can be done by the patient to avoid the problem. Having the patient void at timed intervals permits the beginning of a *behavioral modification program*. The patient learns to empty the bladder by the clock, before a bladder volume is achieved that results in spontaneous detru-

sor contraction, although this also will help those patients with stress or functional incontinence as well. Occasionally, when asked to void at 2-hour intervals (following the pattern on the bladder record, Fig. 6.1), a patient with urge incontinence will become continent. If that happens the patient who stays on a fixed intake of fluid can increase the interval between voidings by 30 to 60 minutes every week or so until incontinence recurs. Then, by continuing to void by the clock (at the longest interval without incontinence), the patient may achieve acceptable continence.

For patients who are not severely demented and who have a pattern of stress incontinence, the mechanism of sphincter insufficiency should be explained. The patient should learn to avoid increasing abdominal pressure while the bladder is full and to perform the exercises described in the following paragraphs to strengthen the sphincter. The patient should be taught to avoid consuming a large volume of fluid 2 to 6 hours before being in a situation without easy access to a toilet.

Pelvic muscle exercises help many women and men with stress incontinence. Pelvic exercise may be initiated by asking the patient to contract the anal sphincter during a digital rectal examination. Identifying the correct muscles can best be achieved during the initial examination by asking the patient to contract around the finger during the digital rectal examination. If the patient has difficulty identifying the correct muscles, prompting with instruction that these are the muscles that contract to avoid expelling flatus will often facilitate understanding. It is important to instruct patients to relax all other muscles and breathe deeply while focusing on contracting only the pelvic muscles. After this step has been accomplished, the patient should be given an exercise regimen to follow at home. Initially, the patient is asked to contract the pelvic muscles for short intervals (hold until the count of 3), then relax for the same interval. Patients should repeat this contraction/relaxation cycle 15 times, three sessions per day. For each session, the patient should be instructed to either sit, stand, or lie comfortably to be able to identify the correct muscles in all positions. In time, the patient should increase the contraction/relaxation phase to the count of 10, thus strengthening the pelvic muscles that support the ureteral sphincter. As he or she gains confidence, the patient should be instructed to contract the sphincters whenever abdominal pressure is increased (e.g., in anticipation of a cough, a sneeze, or a quick movement). This educational program has effectively cured or significantly improved approximately 80% of nondemented ambulatory patients with incontinence (5).

In those with urge incontinence, pelvic muscle exercises should be combined with an attempt to have the patient relax at the very first sense of an urge. This takes some effort because patients may have become conditioned to move quickly toward a lavatory, thus inadvertently increasing abdominal and bladder pressure. The patient, once relaxed, can contract the pelvic muscles until the contraction subsides and then walk slowly to a lavatory to void.

Biofeedback techniques (forms of educational therapy) are highly effective in treating elderly men and women with incontinence from sphincter insufficiency or from an uninhibited bladder. Severe dementia precludes this technique, which requires learning skills. Referral to a geriatric center offering this therapy should be considered when educational methods or drug therapy (described in the next section) have failed to achieve adequate control. Simply stated, biofeedback is an educational method using the feedback (usually visual) to the patient of physiologic signals and simultaneously using this information to teach the patient how to control various muscle groups involved in achieving continence. Usually three to six 30- to 40-minute sessions are required to teach a patient how to achieve continence using biofeedback. In addition, low-voltage electric stimulation of perianal or vaginal bladder inhibitory reflexes has been shown to markedly improve continence (14). Electrical functional stimulation was designed to facilitate the identification of the correct muscles needing strengthening and voluntary control in patients with weak pelvic musculature. The goal is to have patients learn without stimulation to contract the appropriate muscles actively and voluntarily. Patients are instructed in this procedure and then can use a commercially available stimulation device (e.g., Microgyn II, In Care Medical Products, a division of Hollister Inc., or Restore Unit 200, Interactive Medical Technologies) to continue the therapy at home. A geriatric medicine, urologic, or gynecologic continence program should be consulted about the use of this safe, effective, inexpensive, and well-tolerated technique.

Some elderly patients have difficulty opening their garments to void. Replacing buttons and zippers with Velcro fasteners (easily done by a tailor) will save time and may avoid an accident. Similarly, a lavatory should be conveniently accessible. Men with symptoms of obstruction should be taught to take their time while voiding to empty as completely as possible.

Two especially valuable resources are available to patients with urinary incontinence and both should be recommended to every patient with this problem. *Staying Dry: A Practical Guide to Bladder Control* is a short, practical book written in lay language and is a valuable resource (published by the Johns Hopkins University Press, 701 West 40th St., Baltimore, MD 21211, telephone 410-516-6900; paperback copies are available from the publisher or a bookstore for approximately $13.00). *HIP Resource Guide and Newsletter* is available for a few dollars from Help for Incontinent People (HIP, P.O. Box 544, Union, SC 29739, telephone 803-579-7990). The *HIP Resource Guide* provides information about incontinence, available products for use, and accessible services to guide patients.

The physician may wish also to order supplies of *Urinary Incontinence in Adults: Consumer Version* (AHCPR Pub. No. 92-0040) and *Caregiver Guide* for the office to give to patients with incontinence and their caregivers. These short booklets provide important, easily understood information. An accompanying booklet, *Clinical Practice Guidelines, Urinary Incontinence in Adults: Update* (AHCPR Pub. No. 96-0862) and a *Quick Reference Guide* (AHCPR 90-0041) are also available as resources for the physician. (Both can be ordered from the U.S. Department of Health and Human Services Clearing House; write to AHCPR Publications, P.O. Box 8547, Silver Spring, MD 20907, telephone 800-358-9295.)

Drug Therapy

Although many drugs are promoted as effective in the treatment of urinary incontinence, currently only a few have been adequately studied and shown to be effective in the treatment of elderly patients.

Estrogen. For female patients with atrophic vaginitis, estrogen replacement may improve continence. Atrophic vaginitis may be diagnosed during the pelvic examination and if there is doubt on inspection, a therapeutic trial still may be beneficial. A course of estrogen therapy should be tried if the patient has no contraindication to this hormone (see Chapter 77). If the patient is willing to try vaginal cream, a topical estrogen such as Premarin may be the best first step, although severe atrophy may interfere with absorption. A 1-month trial should be adequate; if there is significant improvement, the physician should discuss with the patient the possibility of long-term estrogen therapy. For many patients symptoms can be controlled by applying topical estrogen once or twice a week. Topical estrogen therapy does have a systemic effect, and the complications (e.g., uterine cancer, especially when unopposed by progestins) should be considered. Some patients may be unwilling or unable to use vaginal estrogen cream. In such cases, a 1-month trial of an oral estrogen (e.g., Premarin, 0.625 mg every day) is appropriate. If successful, long-term administration may be tried. The lowest effective dosage of estrogen should be used, and cycling with a progestin (e.g., Provera) should be considered. Such a regimen, described fully in Chapter 77, minimizes or eliminates the risk of uterine cancer previously associated with unopposed continuous estrogen therapy. The many other benefits of estrogen in postmenopausal women are discussed in Chapter 77.

Oxybutynin. Oxybutynin (Ditropan, 5-mg tablets or liquid), an anticholinergic, is effective in patients with an uninhibited bladder (urge incontinence). It probably works by increasing bladder capacity. Oxybutynin is administered orally at a dosage of one 5-mg tablet three times a day. In frail elderly patients the drug should be started at a lower dosage: 2.5 mg (one-half tablet or appropriate volume of the liquid preparation) once or twice a day, then advanced to a maximum of 5 mg three times a day or until either an acceptable response or a significant side effect is seen. Also, patients in a scheduled toileting program during the day may benefit from a small dose of oxybutynin at night if incontinence is a problem during sleep. It is effective in approximately 50% of patients, but the side effects of dry mouth, blurred vision, abdominal cramps, urinary retention, or constipation are encountered in nearly 50%; also, 20% of patients taking higher dosages stop the drug because of intolerance. A trial of this drug for 7 to 10 days may be considered. Long-term studies with this agent are not available. Nevertheless, when symptoms of urgency are present and educational programs (described earlier in this chapter) have not been adequately effective and, in women, when no response to estrogen is seen, a trial of oxybutynin should be considered.

Imipramine. Imipramine (Tofranil, 10-mg and 25-mg tablets), an agent with anticholinergic and α-agonist properties, has also been shown to be effective in some elderly patients with sphincter insufficiency (stress) or an uninhibited bladder (urge). It is the only antidepressant adequately studied for this effect. The drug probably works via its anticholinergic activity, by increasing bladder capacity and increasing sphincter tone. It should be begun at 10 mg orally every night, then increased every third night to a maximum of 150 mg/night or until side effects occur. Drug levels are useful at higher dosages in older or smaller patients or those with renal impairment. The most common side effects are postural hypotension, urinary retention, constipation, dizziness, and mucous membrane dryness. Although the drug may be partially effective in 50 to 60% of patients, more than half experience some side effects and approximately 20% discontinue the medication because of intolerance. Because of its side effects, careful telephone follow-up may be needed.

α-Agonists. Some patients with stress incontinence may benefit from α-agonists, which are thought to increase the tone of the urethral sphincter. Sustained-release phenylpropanolamine (e.g., Profen-LA 25 to 100 mg daily or twice daily) is the best studied. Side effects, including palpitation, nervousness, dry mucous membranes, urinary retention, or hypertension, limit its use in many, especially older patients.

Other Medications. Calcium channel blockers (e.g., nifedipine) and NSAIDs (e.g., Indocin) are being studied but have not yet been fully evaluated. Flavoxate has been shown to be ineffective.

Garments and Catheters

Increasingly comfortable briefs are available to avoid embarrassing incontinent accidents, (e.g., Attends, Proctor and Gamble; Asorb-fil, Sears; Curity, Kendall-Futro; Depends, Kimberly-Clark; Oripride, Weyerhaeuser; Suretys, ICD Industries; or Tranquility, Devilbiss) are available from pharmacies, medical supply stores, or large catalog stores. The cost of such garments is surprisingly high (e.g., approximately $950 per year with a requirement of four pads per day) and they never should be prescribed as the initial approach. For men there are also comfortable (day and night) condom catheter kits (e.g., United Weimer Urinal, United Medical), drip urinals, or supporters with absorbent liners, generally for less than $75. However, if the patient frequently manipulates the external catheter, urinary tract infection is a common complication, and in that instance it is probably wise to use a diaper. External catheter systems for women are available (e.g., from

Hollister, 800-323-4060 in the United States, except 800-942-1141 in Illinois). Although these devices have improved considerably, their application requires a large degree of dexterity and commitment. More information about available urinary incontinence products can be obtained from the *HIP Resource Guide* (described under "Educational Programs" earlier in this chapter).

Indwelling urinary catheters have no place in the treatment of urinary incontinence, except in rare instances (e.g., when there is secondary skin maceration, pressure sore development, caretaker exhaustion, or terminal illness). In these cases the catheter should be used as briefly as possible. Intermittent self-catheterization is a useful technique for patients with an atonic bladder and overflow incontinence. However, the patient or the caretaker must be able and willing to perform the procedure several times a day. When this procedure is considered, it is usually best to refer the patient and caretaker to a urologist or geriatrician with a special interest in incontinence for education, unless the general physician or a staff member is experienced in educating others in its performance. Since the introduction of improved and smaller catheters and intermittent catheterization, a chronic indwelling suprapubic catheter is rarely used today. Such a catheter adds no benefit in the reduction of the incidence of renal infection, sepsis, or other complications.

Surgical Innovations

Surgical techniques of creating artificial urinary bladder sphincters—some of which are simple, requiring only the suburethral injection of collagen (28)—are gaining clinical applicability, but it is still uncertain which candidates will benefit most; a geriatrician with expertise in treating incontinent patients or a urologist should be consulted, initially by telephone, to help determine which patients might be candidates for such procedures.

PREVENTIVE GERIATRICS

Rowe and Kahn distinguish usual from successful aging (49). In a group of usual aging Americans, for example, bone and muscle mass fall and glucose tolerance worsens with age. However, regular exercise is associated with improved glucose metabolism, increased bone mass, and muscle strength and thus modifies "usual" aging.

Data show that although elderly women visit physicians more often, they are less likely to have a pelvic examination and Pap smear and less likely than younger women to be diagnosed with uterine, ovarian, or cervical cancer in a localized (and potentially curable) stage (22). The prevalence of abnormal Pap smears among elderly women was 13.5 per 1000 in one study, and the death rate from cervical cancer is highest in women over 65 (39). Chapter 95 provides guidelines for gynecologic cancer screenings.

A discussion of the controversy concerning screening for prostate disease in men is provided in Chapter 49.

Although available data do not permit clear-cut recommendations, most authorities believe that the well elderly should receive periodic testing similar to that of younger patients (see Chapter 2). Elderly patients with marked cognitive impairment or severe chronic disease make up a separate group of patients for whom the value of screening is particularly uncertain.

Screening for and treating hyperlipidemia in elderly patients is a controversial topic discussed in Chapter 75.

Screening methods for visual loss and hearing loss are discussed in Chapters 98 and 96, respectively.

In patients at high risk for vertebral compression or hip fracture and for those with established kyphosis, a survey of the house for environmental hazards is recommended; such patients also should not lift heavy objects, including grandchildren. Prevention of falls is discussed earlier in this chapter. Treatment of osteoporosis is discussed in Chapter 74.

The benefits of discontinuing cigarette smoking among the elderly are probably substantial. Although several studies of smoking cessation among the elderly show little effect on primary prevention of coronary heart disease, in those with established disease, smoking cessation reduces the risk of myocardial infarction and death (27). Cessation is a key step in the primary prevention of lung and other cancers and the primary or secondary prevention of obstructive lung disease, peripheral vascular disease, and peptic ulcer disease. A full discussion of strategies for smoking cessation is presented in Chapter 20.

The routine use of aspirin and, in women, estrogens in old age is under considerable scrutiny (see Chapters 52 and 77, respectively). Both of these agents may provide valuable benefits to certain elderly people, but each has associated risks. Immunization information is provided in Chapter 32.

PRERETIREMENT COUNSELING AND PLANNING

Several problems of the elderly can be minimized if they are anticipated and planned for well in advance. Books are available to help the older person in planning (see "General References"), and large corporations, senior citizen centers, and several colleges offer courses in preretirement counseling and planning. The American Association of Retired Persons (AARP) has a wide range of materials to assist in such planning. (Information is available by writing to the AARP Fulfillment Department, 601 E Street N.W., Washington, DC 20049.) Important topics for the older person to consider are anticipated economic changes, preparation of wills and estate planning, changes in tempo and nature of activities, the importance of developing hobbies and activities for leisure time, health care resources, and systems of health care and social support. As noted under "Decisions about Limiting Therapy," advance directives guiding medical therapy

in the event of debilitating illness can be extremely valuable and are important for every adult to consider. A useful publication on the Medicare insurance program, *Your Medicare Handbook,* is available to patients and physicians. (It may be obtained from the Superintendent of Documents, U.S. Government Printing Office, Washington DC 20402, telephone 202-783-3238.) This concise booklet explains services and provides definitions of terms used by Medicare (e.g., skilled nursing facility care). An understanding of the Medicare program is important for every elderly citizen. However, Medicare covers only 44% of total health expenditures for the elderly, so the aging patient and his or her family will need sound advice to plan properly for potential health care needs. The physician should encourage young elderly patients to investigate all of these resources before they attain the age at which frailty is more common.

SPECIAL HOUSING AND OTHER COMMUNITY-BASED PROGRAMS

Housing programs primarily for the elderly are increasingly available. Many states or local governments have developed programs in which, in the setting of a congregate facility, support services such as eating programs or housekeeping are provided. These programs may be called *sheltered housing* or *elder housing* and are generally available only to people who are able to satisfy an economic means test. Information regarding such programs can be obtained through the state or regional office on aging.

Continuing care retirement communities are increasingly available. These require that an elder move (usually while still functionally independent) to a community that provides a variety of resources and usually includes primary medical care, access to nursing home care and personal care, and meal and social programs. Several types of retirement communities exist. Some provide comprehensive services including nursing home and medical service, meals, and programs for an inclusive entrance and monthly fee. Others provide only housing and access to additional services that may be purchased on an a la carte basis. Cost varies tremendously. Patients who ask about entering such a community should be advised to carefully analyze the services included in the fee, review the record of the community with the state office on aging, and review the contract with a lawyer before agreeing to sign it. Some people are exuberant about such retirement communities, arguing that they provide excellent socialization and the reassurance that providing care, in the event of dependency, will never be a direct burden to one's family. Others reject these arguments, claiming that these retirement communities are simply ghettos for the frail elderly. Because of the expense, only a small portion of the elderly population could ever consider such an option.

In part because of the high cost of community care retirement communities, programs are being developed to provide similar support services while patients remain in their own homes. Such programs, typically called *social health maintenance organizations* or *life care at home programs,* are still experimental. One such model, OnLok, developed in the late 1970s in San Francisco, is now being replicated at a number of sites around the country. This *Program for All-Inclusive Care for the Elderly (PACE)* provides comprehensive care on a capitated basis featuring adult medical day-care and, in many sites, special housing programs.

Medical and social day-care centers are available in many communities. The state, county, or city area office of aging will have information about these programs. Generally such programs provide an opportunity for daytime socialization or medical care and surveillance. Importantly, they also provide an opportunity for caregivers to have a respite from their care responsibilities. Unfortunately, medical day-care programs are not covered by most private insurance programs or Medicare (except for those who receive it under a Medicare/Medicaid waiver, e.g., via PACE). Medicaid does provide reimbursement for medical day-care services in some states but it is means-tested. For others, medical day-care is an out-of-pocket expense that, although expensive, is usually about half the cost of nursing home care. Social day-care programs are more accessible but usually require that a person be functionally totally independent. Social day-care programs (as opposed to medical day-care) are often sponsored by churches, local government, or other organizations, which usually help offset the cost.

OTHER IMPORTANT PROBLEMS OF THE ELDERLY PATIENT

The following problems are discussed in detail elsewhere in this book: constipation (Chapter 39), diverticular disease (Chapter 41), musculoskeletal problems (Section 9), menopause (Chapter 77), osteoporosis (Chapter 77), hearing loss (Chapter 96), skin problems (Chapter 100), dental problems (Chapter 101), disorders of the feet (Chapter 102), hypertension (Chapter 62), cataracts and macular degeneration (Chapter 97), psychiatric illnesses of old age such as dementia and delirium (Chapter 17), depression (Chapter 15), bereavement (Chapter 19), and urinary problems such as infection (Chapter 27) and retention (Chapter 49).

General References*

Cassel CK, Cohen HJ, Larson EB, et al, eds. Geriatric medicine. 3rd ed. New York: Spring-Verlag, 1997.

Hazzard WR, Bierman EL, Blass JP, et al, eds. Principles of geriatric medicine and gerontology. 3rd ed. New York: McGraw-Hill, 1994.

Jahnigen DW, Schrier RW, eds. Geriatric medicine. 2nd ed. Cambridge: Blackwell Science, 1996.

Three comprehensive texts.

*Bold print (general references) and bold numerals (specific references) denote published controlled clinical trials, meta-analyses, or consensus-based recommendations.

Specific References

1. Anderson DN, Prunty N, Partridge M, et al. Does anyone know what medication the patient should be taking? Int J Geriatr Psychiatry 9:573, 1994.
2. Andres R. Mortality and obesity: the rationale for age-specific height–weight tables. In: Hazzard WR, et al, eds. Principles of geriatric medicine and gerontology. New York: McGraw-Hill, 1990.
3. Bradley JD, Brandt KD, Katz BP, et al. Comparison of an antiinflammatory dose of ibuprofen, an analgesic dose of ibuprofen and acetaminophen in the treatment of patients with osteoarthritis of the knee. N Engl J Med 325:87, 1991.
4. Brennan TA, Leape LL, Laird NM, et al. Incidence of adverse events and negligence in hospitalized patients: results of the Harvard Medical Practice Study I. N Engl J Med 324:370, 1991.
5. Burton JR, Pearce KL, Burgio KL, et al. Behavioral training for urinary incontinence in elderly ambulatory patients. J Am Geriatr Soc 36:693, 1988.
6. Calkins DR, Rubenstein LV, Cleary PD, et al. Failure of physicians to recognize functional disability in ambulatory patients. Ann Intern Med 114:451, 1991.
7. Cassel CK, Vladeck BC. ICD-9 code for palliative or terminal care. N Engl J Med 335:1232, 1996.
8. Council on Scientific Affairs, American Medical Association. Elder abuse and neglect. JAMA 257:966, 1987.
9. Creditor MC. Hazards of hospitalization of the elderly. Ann Intern Med 118:219, 1993.
10. Der EH, Rubenstein LZ, Choy GS. The benefits of in-home pharmacy evaluation for older persons. J Am Geriatr Soc 45:211, 1997.
11. Epstein AM, Hall JA, Besdine R. The emergence of geriatric assessment units: the new technology of geriatrics. Ann Intern Med 106:299, 1987.
12. Ettinger WH, Burns R, Messier SP, et al. A randomized trial comparing aerobic exercise and resistance exercise with a health education program in older adults with knee osteoarthritis: the Fitness, Arthritis and Seniors Trial (FAST). JAMA 277:25, 1997.
13. Evans DA, Funkenstein HH, Albert MS, et al. Prevalence of Alzheimer's disease in a community population of older persons: higher than previously reported. JAMA 262:2551, 1989.
14. Fall M, Illston LH, Miller NA. Electric stimulation: a physiological approach to treatment of urinary incontinence. Urol Clin North Am 18:393, 1991.
15. Feinstein AR, Josephy BR, Wells CK. Scientific and clinical problems in indexes of functional disability. Ann Intern Med 105:413, 1986.
16. Fillenbaum GG. Screening the elderly: a brief instrumental activities of daily living measure. J Am Geriatr Soc 33:698, 1985.
17. Folsom AR. Body fat distribution and 5-year risk of death in older women. JAMA 269:483, 1993.
18. Fried LP, Guralnik JM. Disability in older adults: evidence regarding significance, etiology, and risk. J Am Geriatr Soc 45:92, 1997.
19. Fries J, Singh G, Morfeld D, et al. Running and the development of disability with age. Ann Intern Med 121:502, 1994.
20. Griffin MR, Ray WA, Schaffner W. Non-steroidal anti-inflammatory drug use and death from peptic ulcer in elderly persons. Ann Intern Med 22:82, 1988.
21. Grimby A, Milson I, Molanter U, et al. The influence of urinary incontinence on the quality of life of elderly women. Age Aging 22:82, 1993.
22. Grover SA, Cook EF, Adam J, et al. Delayed diagnosis of gynecologic tumors in elderly women: relation to national medical practice patterns. Am J Med 86:151, 1989.
23. Guidelines for exercise testing and prescription, American College of Sports Medicine. 4th ed. Philadelphia: Lea & Febiger, 1991.
24. Hansen FR. Geriatric follow-up by home visits after discharge from hospital: a randomized controlled trial. Age Ageing 21:445, 1992.

25. Hemmelgarn B, Suissa S, Huang A, et al. Benzodiazepine use and the risk of motor vehicle crash in the elderly. JAMA 278:27, 1997.
26. Hennekens CH, Buring JE, Manson JE, et al. Lack of effect of long-term supplementation with beta carotene on the incidence of malignant neoplasms and cardiovascular disease. N Engl J Med 334:1145, 1996.
27. Hermanson B, Omenn GS, Kormal RA, et al. Beneficial six-year outcome of smoking cessation in older men and women with coronary artery disease: results from the CASS registry. N Engl J Med 319:1365, 1988.
28. Herschorn S, Radomski SB, Steele DJ. Early experience with intraurethral collagen injections for urinary incontinence. J Urol 148:1797, 1992.
29. Hobbs FB, Damon BL. U.S. Bureau of the Census. Current Population Reports, Special Studies, P23-190, 65+ in the United States. Washington, DC: US Government Printing Office, 1996.
30. Jones J, Dougherty J, Schelble D, et al. Emergency department protocol for the diagnosis of geriatric abuse. Ann Emerg Med 17:1006, 1988.
31. Katz S, Stoud MW. Functional assessment in geriatrics: a review of progress and directions. J Am Geriatr Soc 37:267, 1987.
32. Kessler DA. The regulation of investigational drugs. N Engl J Med 3(20):81, 1989.
33. King AC, Oman RF, Brassington GS, et al. Moderate-intensity exercise and self-rated quality of sleep in older adults. JAMA 277:32, 1997.
34. King MB, Tinetti ME. Falls in community-dwelling older persons. J Am Geriatr Soc 43:1146, 1995.
35. Klein LE, Tovs RP, McArthur J, et al. Diagnosing dementia: univariate and multivariate analysis of the mental status examination. J Am Geriatr Soc 1985;33:483, 1985.
36. LaPuma J, Orentlicher D, Moss RJ. Advance directives on admission: clinical implications and analysis of the Patient Self Determination Act of 1990. JAMA 266:402, 1991.
37. Leape LL, Brennan TA, Laird N, et al. The nature of adverse events in hospitalized patients: results of the Harvard Medical Practice Study II. N Engl J Med 324:377, 1991.
38. Lichtenstein MJ, Federspiel CF, Schaffner W. Factors associated with early demise in nursing home residents: a case-control study. J Am Geriatr Soc 33:315, 1985.
39. Mandelblatt J, Bopaul I, Wistreich M. Gynecologic care of elderly women: another look at Papanicolaou smear testing. JAMA 256:367, 1986.
40. Marottoli RA, Cooney LM Jr, Wagner DR, et al. Predictors of automobile crashes and moving violations among elderly drivers. Ann Intern Med 121:842, 1994.
41. National Institutes of Health. Physical activity and cardiovascular health. JAMA 276:241, 1996.
42. Ouslander JG, Leach GE, Staskin DR. Simplified tests of lower urinary tract function in the evaluation of geriatric urinary incontinence. J Am Geriatr Soc 37:706, 1989.
43. Pathy MS, Bayer A, Harding K, et al. Randomised trial of case finding and surveillance of elderly people at home. Lancet 340:890, 1992.
44. PDR guide to drug interactions, side effects, indications, contraindications. Montvale, NJ: Medical Economics Company, 1997.
45. Province MA, Hadley EC, Hornbrook MC, et al. The effects of exercise on falls in elderly patients a preplanned meta-analysis of the FICSIT trials. JAMA 273:1341, 1995.
46. Rapola JM, Virtamo J, Ripatti S, et al. Randomized trial of α-tocopherol and β-carotene supplements on incidence of major coronary events in men with previous myocardial infarction. Lancet 349:1715, 1997.
47. Ray WA, Griffin MR, Schaffner W, et al. Psychotropic drug use and the risk of hip fracture. N Engl J Med 316:363, 1987.
48. Reuben D, Borok G, Wolde-Tsadik GD, et al. A randomized trial of comprehensive geriatric assessment in the care of hospitalized patients. N Engl J Med 332:1345, 1995.
49. Rowe JW, Kahn RL. Human aging: usual and successful. Science 237:143, 1987.
50. Rubenstein LZ, Josephson KR, Wieland GD, et al. Effectiveness of a geriatric evaluation unit: a randomized clinical trial. N Engl J Med 311:1664, 1984.
51. Schneider LS, Pollock VE, Lyness SA. A meta analysis of controlled trials of neuroleptic treatment in dementia. J Am Geriatr Soc 38:553, 1990.
52. Shimokata H, Andres R, Coon PJ, et al. Studies in the distribution of body fat II: longitudinal effects of change in weight. Int J Obesity 13:455, 1989.
53. Stoehr GP, Ganguli M, Seaberg EC, et al. Over-the-counter medication use in an older rural community: the MoVIES Project. J Am Geriatr Soc 45:150, 1997.
54. Tinetti ME, Baker DI, McAvav G, et al. A multifactorial intervention to reduce the risk of falling among elderly people living in the community. N Engl J Med 331:821, 1994.
55. Tinetti ME, Inouye SK, Gill TM, et al. Shared risk factors for falls, incontinence, and functional dependence: unifying the approach to geriatric syndromes. JAMA 273:1348, 1995.
56. Welch HG, Wennberg DE, Welch WP. The use of Medicare home health care services. N Engl J Med 335:324, 1996.
57. Woman in right-to-die case succumbs. *Washington Post,* December 7, 1990:A3.

CHAPTER 7

Occupational and Environmental Disease

JAMES P. KEOGH, MD

This is an era characterized by widespread proliferation of new and potentially toxic chemicals and exposure to novel forms of energy. These hazardous exposures are encountered in homes, schools, the general environment, and especially the workplace. The extent to which such exposures may be causing health problems is a grave concern. Few communities in the United States have escaped public concern over the health hazards of pesticide spraying, asbestos in school buildings, contaminated drinking water, electromagnetic radiation, or toxic waste disposal.

This chapter provides an overview of how environmental diseases occur and outlines an approach for recognizing and addressing them. It emphasizes the workplace, where environmentally induced illness is most commonly recognized. Each year in the United States more than 100,000 people die and more than 400,000 become ill as a direct result of occupational disease. Hazardous exposures and resulting illness also occur in the home or community environment.

The same principles that apply to workplace exposure apply to home and community exposure as well.

VITAL ROLE OF PRIMARY PRACTITIONERS

Primary practitioners are often the first professionals to recognize the hazards of occupational exposure and to document the link between their patients' illnesses and their patients' work. The task of controlling the hazards usually involves public health specialists, but it is vitally important that primary practitioners take the time to report and follow up suspected occupational diseases.

Although the United States has for three decades had the Occupational Safety and Health Administration (OSHA) to ensure workplace safety, there are only enough inspectors to visit every workplace once every 200 years. Every year still brings efforts in Congress to weaken the program that does exist. Locked fire exits, exploitation of immigrants, child labor, and sweatshop conditions persist 60 years after the New Deal took steps to abolish them. Most workers are unaware of their right to request investigation of potential hazards at work, and concerns for job security deter them from raising complaints about safety with supervisors. Inspectors who do visit workplaces usually lack medical training, so they often focus on safety rather than on health issues. Public health surveillance of occupational and environmental disease has been improved in the past decade by the efforts of the National Institute for Occupational Safety and Health (NIOSH) working with state health agencies, but it remains limited in scope and coverage. For all these reasons, if a patient has an occupational health problem or is exposed to a dangerous situation at work, his or her physician may be the single most important factor in protecting the patient's and the community's health.

PATHOGENESIS OF OCCUPATIONAL DISEASE

The pathogenesis of occupational disease is complex and involves not only the interaction between the host and a toxic exposure, but also a complex set of social interactions.

Toxin–Host Interaction

For an occupational disease to occur, there must be a triad consisting of a toxic agent, a host, and an environment in which the host is exposed. The illness that may result depends on the toxic properties of the substance or energy source, its route of entry, the dosage received by the host, and the susceptibility of the host to the toxin.

Toxic agents can be inhaled, ingested, or absorbed through the skin. With *inhalation,* the dosage received depends on whether the substance is present as a fume or a dust. Deposition of dust in the lungs depends to a great extent on particle size and distribution because smaller particles can more easily enter the alveoli and become trapped. The concentration of the substance in the air (which is related to room ventilation, temperature, and humidity), the rate at which the worker is exercising and breathing, protective factors such as special clothing or respirator use are other factors that affect the likelihood of illness.

Once the toxic substance is absorbed there may be an instantaneous effect (as in the case of carbon monoxide poisoning), a brief latent period (as in the case of occupational asthma), or a latent period of years or decades (as in the pneumoconioses). A brief, high-dose exposure may cause serious illness and death and be easy to recognize. Prolonged exposure to a low dosage of a toxin may not cause symptoms at the outset but may produce disease years later.

Impact of Economic and Social Factors

Thousands of new chemicals are introduced into industrial processes every year; few have been tested to determine their potential toxicity. Even when toxicologic screening tests are done on a compound, they may not predict human disease. Despite the implementation of the Toxic Substances Control Act (TOSCA), which gave EPA authority to require pretesting of chemicals, in too many cases the hazard of a chemical is recognized only after an outbreak of illness. Economic factors play a major role in determining how safe a workplace is. Industrial hygiene programs to monitor exposure are common only in the largest plants. Important decisions, such as improving ventilation or decreasing exposure to noise, may involve significant expense. Workers may be reluctant to complain about working conditions for fear of losing their jobs. This is especially likely during periods of high unemployment, when acceptance of unpleasant and potentially unhealthy working conditions may be the price of having a job. Even when workers are strongly organized, the desire for a safer workplace may be balanced by a concern that increased production costs may result in the decision of a company to relocate its plant to areas where unions are less effective or do not exist. Such anxieties have been heightened by the passage of the North American Free Trade Agreement (NAFTA) and the globalization of manufacturing. These trends persist in America in the 1990s despite the fact that weaker enforcement of safety rules has made workplaces more dangerous and has had negative economic effects. Stringent health and safety regulations, with strong enforcement, can put competitors on a more equal footing and protect responsible businesses from being undercut by irresponsible ones.

DIAGNOSING WORK-RELATED DISEASE

Although episodes of illness caused or exacerbated by the patient's work are often seen in ambulatory practice, they often are not recognized as such. Misdiagnosing an occupational disease means that the patient does not benefit from correct diagnosis and management, and there is no correction of the poor working conditions that may subsequently injure others or even result in death. Two cases illustrate these points:

CASE STUDY: A TEENAGER WITH BRONCHITIS

An 18-year-old woman complained to her physician of a severe cough and some wheezing. The physician treated her with erythromycin and fluids and advised her to stay in bed for a few days. She recovered and returned to work feeling well. Several days later she had a severe recurrent cough with wheezing and dyspnea and saw her physician again. The physician again prescribed erythromycin and rest. She remained off work for a week. She felt better and returned to work. After 2 days she became extremely short of breath and was brought to the emergency room. She had severe bronchospasm and was admitted, improving on bronchodilators and corticosteroids after a few days. An occupational history on admission disclosed that her work involved grinding drill bits made of tungsten carbide containing a small amount of *cobalt,* a known pulmonary sensitizer. Once the patient was sensitized, each fresh exposure to the dust caused symptoms after a shorter incubation period. Had the first physician considered the diagnosis of extrinsic asthma and inquired about occupational exposures, the patient's subsequent deterioration could have been prevented.

CASE STUDY: A MAN WITH SEVERE ABDOMINAL PAIN

A 28-year-old man presented to the emergency room of a community hospital with a chief complaint of severe abdominal pain. There was significant abdominal tenderness with a question of guarding. He reported having seen his family physician on two occasions during the preceding 2 weeks, with severe cramping pain felt around the umbilicus. His physician had prescribed an H_2 blocker and tried to schedule a gastroenterologic consult, which the patient had not set up because of difficulties with his work schedule. The pain that had been intermittent had now become constant, more in the lower quadrants, and more severe for over 6 hours. Blood work showed a normal amylase and a leukocytosis. A surgical consultant suggested the possibility of an appendiceal abscess but believed that the patient was stable enough to await the results of a computerized tomography (CT) scan. A gastroenterologist was consulted, and was the first physician to take an occupational history. The patient had been a painter for several years and was currently working for a contractor repainting the elaborate metal cornices of a building. For more than a month he had been using a vibrating tool to remove old paint and this created a lot of dust. He did not know whether lead was in the paint. The gastroenterologist suggested a *blood lead level* and watchful waiting. The CT scan was normal and the blood lead level was elevated. Several coworkers were also poisoned and the patient's son had an elevated lead level from the contaminated work clothes his father had brought home.

To avoid the pitfalls these cases demonstrate, the following three strategies are fundamental in evaluating a patient:

- Ask every patient about his or her job.
- Consider the possibility that the patient's illness is related to the work or home environment.
- Follow up on one's suspicions. Others may be in danger.

Taking an Occupational History

Inquiring about a patient's job not only helps identify occupational disease, but also provides other information useful in caring for a patient. Clearly the physical demands of the job are important when advising a patient about a health problem such as coronary artery disease or diabetes mellitus. Knowing the patient's work schedule is also important because shift work affects medication schedules, diet, and family life. Medications can dramatically affect the patient's comfort or safety at work (e.g., diuretics in an interstate truck driver or antihistamines in an iron worker). Financial and psychologic stress may result from lay-offs, whereas regular overtime may bring about chronic fatigue and psychological problems of its own. Usually, a brief discussion of the current job, including a brief description of how the patient spends the working day, is sufficient. This rarely takes more than 3 minutes. The major points to cover in this inquiry are summarized in Table 7.1.

When some aspect of the medical or occupational history has raised suspicions of a work-related condition, further questioning flows naturally. The inquiry should focus on a temporal relationship between symptoms and possible exposure, exposure to an agent known to cause disease, or a pattern of similar illness among coworkers. Because every patient, every job, and every medical presentation is different, there is no single way of taking a history. If the patient uses jargon or job titles that are unfamiliar, it is important to ask for clarification.

The screening history sometimes reveals the need to take a *lifelong work history.* An account of the previous jobs and exposures is especially important when the patient has a chronic illness or the possibility of work-related neoplasia. In such cases, the following approach is recommended (it may save time to have the patient bring this information, written out, to a follow-up visit after the initial evaluation):

1. Begin with parents' jobs and childhood exposures.
2. Review each of the patient's jobs in chronological order.

3. Elicit relevant aspects of each period of employment (Table 7.1).

Diseases that Are Commonly Related to Work

The occupational diseases that physicians encounter depend on the industry in the immediate vicinity and the demographic makeup of their practice. For example, practitioners caring for the elderly may see retired workers with previous exposure in all types of industry. Any organ system can be affected by hazardous exposures. Table 7.2 lists clinical problems grouped according to the organ system affected.

Dermatitis and pneumoconiosis are the most commonly reported occupational illnesses. This probably reflects both true incidence (skin and pulmonary epithelium are most in contact with the outside environment) and the greater likelihood of recognition of these disorders as being occupational in origin.

The number of chemicals that are toxic to the liver and kidney is so great that a careful exposure history should be taken from all patients with unexplained hepatitis and hepatic or renal failure. Many chemicals can affect the gastrointestinal tract and cause functional disturbances that may be misdiagnosed as peptic disease or irritable bowel syndrome.

Low-level exposure of the respiratory organs to a variety of substances may result in the production of nonspecific upper respiratory syndromes that the patient may describe as an intractable cold or as sinus trouble.

Although occupational diseases sometimes present with striking and unusual signs (e.g., acro-osteolysis in vinyl chloride workers or nasal septal perforation in patients exposed to chromates), more commonly they present with the vague systemic symptoms typical of early intoxication.

A few specific clinical situations should always raise the consideration of an occupational or environmental cause:

Any unexplained change in personality or behavior. Poisoning with mercury, lead, pesticides, and a wide variety of other central nervous system toxins may present this way.

New onset of asthma. Because of the time lapse when an immunologic mechanism is involved, wheezing and dyspnea may not be noted until after the workday is over.

Any case of pulmonary fibrosis. A prolonged latent period between exposure and disease onset means that abnormalities that appear on radiographs may result from a job the patient had decades ago.

Peripheral neuropathy. A toxic neuropathy may be recognizable by an unusual pattern of presentation, but in most cases only careful history taking will reveal the cause.

Overuse syndromes in the extremities. Tendonitis, epicondylitis, and shoulder bursitis often are the result of a pattern of overuse. This can result from occupational or recreational activities. When they are work related, modification of the job is essential.

Table 7.1.   Components of an Occupational History

Description of the Job
Physical exertion
Body mechanics
Pace of work
Repetitive tasks
Job stress

Exposure to Hazards
Risk of trauma
Noise and vibration
Heat and cold
Ionizing and nonionizing radiation
Dusts, fumes, mists
Contamination of skin and clothing

Protective Measures
Ventilation and respiratory protection
Protective clothing
Medical surveillance

Effects of Exposure
Temporal relationship of any symptoms to work (e.g., relationship to time of day, day of week, change of symptoms on vacation, weekends)
Similar symptoms in coworkers

Table 7.2.   Common Medical Problems with Examples of Environmental Causes

Clinical Problem	Causative Agent	Clinical Problem	Causative Agent
SKIN		Ataxia, tremor, spasticity	Manganese
Cyanosis	Methemoglobin formers		Organic lead compounds
	Aniline		Organic tin compounds
	Anisidine, *ortho-* and *para-* isomers	Hyperreflexia, micrographia	Mercury
	Dimethylaniline		DDT
	Dinitrobenzene, all isomers	Peripheral neuropathy	Peripheral neurotoxins
	Dinitrotoluene		Acrylamide
	Monomethylaniline		Arsenic and compounds
	p-Nitroaniline		Calcium arsenate
	Nitrobenzene		Carbon disulfide
	p-Nitrocholorobenzene		*n*-Hexane
	Nitrogen trifluoride		Lead and inorganic lead compounds
	Nitrotoluene		Dimethylaminopropionitrile
	Perchloryl fluoride		Lucel-7 (2-*t*-butylazo-2-hydroxy 5-methyl hexane)
	n-Propyl nitrate		Mercury
	Tetranitromethane		Methyl bromide
	o-Toluidine		Methyl butyl ketone
	Xylidine		Thallium, soluble compounds
Contact dermatitis	Many chemicals with irritant or sensitizing properties		2,4,6-Trinitrotoluene
Chronic eczematous dermatitis	Solvents		Tri-*o*-cresyl phosphate
	Detergents		
Folliculitis	Oil exposure	**HEARING**	
	Grease exposure	Decreased acuity and tinnitus	Noise exposure especially above 85 decibels
Acne	Polychlorinated biphenyls	Acoustic neuritis	Aniline
	Chlorinated naphthalenes		Arsenic
	Paraffin		Carbon monoxide
	Coal tar		Hypoxia
	Dioxin		Lead
Photosensitization	Coal tar		Organic mercury
	Pitch		Phosphorus
	Asphalt		Sodium nitrate
	Anthracene	Otitis externa	Contamination of earplugs used for noise protection
	Creosote		
	Fluorescein	Ear pain	Acute shifts in pressure
	Phenanthrene		
Granulomas	Beryllium	**RESPIRATORY**	
Corns	Asbestos	Nasal septal perforation	Chromic acid and other chromates
	Fiberglass		
Punctate ulcers	Chromic acid	Laryngeal carcinoma	Asbestos
Painful burns	Hydrofluoric acid (deep pain out of proportion to appearance of burn)	Laryngitis, bronchitis tracheitis, pneumonitis	Many irritants including
			Ammonia
Skin cancer	Soots		Chlorine
	Tars		Oxides of nitrogen
	Arsenic		Ozone
	Coke oven emissions		Phosgene
	Cutting oils		Sulfur dioxide
	Sunlight		Vanadium pentoxide
			Mercury
NERVOUS SYSTEM			Manganese
Central Effects			Cadmium dust
Altered consciousness	Hundreds of chemicals have CNS-depressant properties and other CNS effects	Bronchiolitis obliterans	Nitrogen dioxide
		Allergic alveolitis	Many different antigens
Headaches	Carbon monoxide	Bagassosis	*Thermoactinomyces vulgaris* and *Micropolyspora* sp.
	Nitrites		
	Nitrates	Bird-breeder's lung	Avian proteins
	Alcohols	Byssinosis	Cotton, flax, and soft fiber hemps
	Lead		
	Organic lead compounds	Cheese-washer's lung	*Penicillium caseil*
	Methemoglobin formers (see under "Cyanosis")	Detergents	*Bacillus subtilis*
		Farmer's lung	*Micropolyspora faeni* and *Thermoactinomyces vulgaris*
Behavioral change	Mercury		
	Lead	Feathers	Feather proteins
	Carbon disulfide	Furrier's lung	Keratinized particles of hair
	Carbon monoxide	Malt-worker's lung	*Aspergillis clavatus*
	Methyl chloride	Maple bark-stripper's disease	*Cryptostroma corticale*
	Methyl bromide	Paprika-splitter's lung	*Mucor stolinifer*

Table 7.2—_continued._   Common Medical Problems with Examples of Environmental Causes

Clinical Problem	Causative Agent	Clinical Problem	Causative Agent
RESPIRATORY—cont'd		Hepatomegaly	Hepatotoxins
Bronchospasm	Pulmonary sensitizers		Acetylene tetrabromide
	Castor bean pomace		Carbon disulfide
	Cobalt, metal fume, and dust		Carbon tetrachloride
	Enzymatic detergents		Chlorodiphenyl
	Grain dusts		Chloroform
	Maleic anhydride		p-Dichlorobenzene
	Methylene bisphenyl isocy-anate		Dimethylacetamide
			Dimethylformamide
	Methyl isocyanate		Dioxane
	Nickle, metal		Ethylene chlorohydrin
	p-Phenylenediamine		Ethylene dibromide
	Phthalic anhydride		Ethylene dichloride
	Platinum salts		Hexachloronaphthalene
	Polyvinyl chloride (fume from heated film: meat-wrapper's asthma)		Kepone
			Nitroethane
			Octachloronaphthalene
	Toluene 2,4-diisocyanate		Pentachloronaphthalene
	Tungsten carbide		Picric acid
	Western red cedar		Tetrachloroethane
	Plicatic acid		Tetrachloroethylene
Pulmonary fibrosis	Asbestos		Tetrachloronaphthalene
	Silica		Trichloronaphthalene
	Beryllium		2,4,6-Trinitrotoluene
	Talc	Jaundice	Hepatotoxins (see above)
	Coal dust		Hemolytic agents
	Cobalt		Arsine
	Hematite		Butyl cellosolve
	Kaolin		Naphthalene
Benign pneumoconiosis depos-its in lung without fibrosis	Aluminum powder		Phenylhydrazine
	Barium		Stibine
	Graphite	Angiosarcoma of liver	Vinyl chloride
	Iron oxide	Abdominal pain	Antimony
	Tin		Arsenic
	Cerium oxide		Bromine
	Silver		Cadmium
	Titanium		Lead
Pleural effusion	Asbestos		Mercury
	Paraquat		Nicotine
	Talc		Organophosphates
			Thallium
GASTROINTESTINAL			Many other chemicals when ingested
Gingivitis and gum pigmentation	Mercury		
	Lead		
	Bismuth	**CARDIOVASCULAR SYSTEM**	
Dental erosion	Acetic acid	Myocardial damage	Antimony
	Hydrochloric acid		Arsine
	Lactic acid		Carbon disulfide
	Nitric acid		Cobalt
	Nitrogen dioxide	Ischemic disease	Nitroglycerin
	Sulfuric acid		Nitroglycol
Tongue paresthesias	Furfural		Other vasodilating nitrates
	Rotenone	Hypertension	Noise exposure
	Cresol		Aminopyridine
Green tongue	Vanadium		Arsenic
Nausea and vomiting	Many chemicals including		Barium
	CNS depressants		Boron hydride
	Cholinesterase inhibitors		Carbon disulfide
	Methemoglobin formers		Cobalt
Constipation	Lead		Diphenyl
	Barium sulfate		Lead
	Thallium		Mercury
	Tellurium		Thallium
	Vanadium		
	Fluorides		

Table 7.2—*continued.*   Common Medical Problems with Examples of Environmental Causes

Clinical Problem	Causative Agent	Clinical Problem	Causative Problem
CARDIOVASCULAR—cont'd		**REPRODUCTIVE ABNORMALITIES**	
Vasospastic disorders "White finger"	Vibrating tools	Female sterility	Lead
		Male sterility	Glycolethers
Raynaud's phenomenon	Vinyl chloride		Carbon disulfide
			Dibromochloropropane (DBCP)
GENITOURINARY			Lead
Renal disease	Nephrotoxins		Microwaves to testes (radar workers)
	4-Aminodiphenyl		Stilbestrol
	Cadmium		
	Carbon disulfide	**HEMATOLOGIC PROBLEMS**	
	Carbon tetrachloride	Anemia	Lead
	Chloroform		Hemolytic agents
	Dioxane		Arsine
	Ethylene chlorohydrin		Butyl cellosolve
	Ethylene dibromide		Naphthalene
	Lead		Phenylhydrazine
	Mercury		Stibine
	Oxalic acid		Marrow depressants
	Picric acid		Benzene
	Tetrachloroethane		Dinitrophenol
	2,4,6-Trinitrotoluene		Tetryl
	Turpentine		2,4,6-Trinitrotoluene
	Uranium		
Renal carcinoma	4-Aminodiphenyl	Leukemia	Benzene
	Auramine		Radiation
	Benzidine		Styrene-butadiene
	β-Naphthylamine		Ethylene oxide
	4-Nitrodiphenyl		
	Magenta	**MUSCULOSKELETAL**	
Urinary retention	Dimethylaminopropionitrile	Osteonecrosis	Phosphorus
		Osteomalacia	Cadmium
		Osteosclerosis	Fluorine
		Acro-osteolysis	Vinyl chloride

Hearing loss. Noise-induced hearing loss occurs gradually and usually in older workers, so it is rarely recognized in time to prevent severe damage.

Inability to conceive. More and more compounds that affect the reproductive system and cause sterility are being identified.

Lung cancer. Exposures to asbestos and cigarette smoke are very common throughout the United States. Other lung carcinogens may be important in certain parts of the country.

Other cancers. Specific carcinogens are identified in Table 7.3.

Determining Work Relatedness

The key to identifying occupational disease is to be sure that a toxic or environmental etiology is at least considered. In addition, the patient should always be asked, "Do you think this problem could have anything to do with your work?" and, "Does anyone else at work have this same problem?" Very often, if there is a connection, the patient will be able to identify it.

If neither the physician nor the patient knows whether a syndrome is occupational in origin, resources are available that identify toxic causes of a given symptom complex, toxic exposures of given occupations, and the potential hazards of exposure to given substances (Table 7.4).

FOLLOW-UP OF OCCUPATIONAL DISEASE

Physician's Role

If there is suspicion that a patient became ill from an occupational exposure, it is the physician's responsibility to follow up. Not only does diagnosing an occupational disease affect therapy and eligibility for compensation for a patient, but it may indicate that the health of others is also in danger. Often physicians overcome their own uneasiness about a patient's job by advising the patient to change jobs. Then, instead of the potentially hazardous job being made safe, another unsuspecting person is brought in to take the risk.

In some circumstances, occupational disease is recognized but the original hazard has been eliminated (e.g., in a patient with asbestosis who worked in a now-closed shipyard). Even in these circumstances, former coworkers need to be informed of the risk resulting from previous exposure.

It is not necessary to wait for absolute proof of etiology before beginning an investigation of a possible workplace hazard. The least severely affected member of a group of workers may be the one who seeks attention. Moreover, for most occupationally induced diseases, proof of a relationship rests on epidemiologic data rather than on diagnostic study of the individual patient. Often the most practical way to learn whether a patient's problems are caused or exacerbated by his or her occupation is to find out whether coworkers are similarly affected.

Investigative and Enforcement Agencies

State Level

Many states have a health department unit for investigation of occupational disease. Some states require physicians to report all cases of suspected occupational disease. Such laws should and probably will become more widespread. Reporting any suspected occupational disease problem to the local health department can be the first step in follow-up. In many states, the National Institute of Occupational Safety and Health (NIOSH) assists the health department in surveillance and control of specific occupational diseases.

Federal Level

If there is difficulty in clarifying the potential relationship of illness to environment or if the concerns raised are not addressed by a specific OSHA regulation (see below), it may be helpful to request assistance from NIOSH. This institute is the part of the United States Public Health Service (USPHS) Centers for Disease Control and Prevention that conducts research on occupational disease. An employer, union, or any three employees can request a formal health hazard evaluation (HHE) of a workplace. Furthermore, NIOSH now has educational resource centers (where consultants are available to help physicians, employers, and workers) available in each region of the United States. These centers can provide literature searches and information on available publications and current areas of research and can refer a physician to others who are experts in the field. Access to regional centers can be provided by the central office.

In addition to its investigative function, NIOSH can assist a physician directly in investigating a patient's exposure. Its clearinghouse responds to practitioners' inquiries with information about the hazards of par-

Table 7.3. Cancers Known to Be Caused by Environmental Agents

Site/Cell Type	Toxic Agent	Industry/Occupation
Liver/hemangiosarcoma	Vinyl chloride monomer	Vinyl chloride polymerization industry
	Arsenical pesticides	Vintners
Nose	Hardwood dusts	Woodworkers, cabinet and furniture makers
	Radium	Radium chemists and processors, dial painters
	Chromates	Chromium producers, processors, users
	Nickel	Nickel smelting and refining
	Unknown agent	Boot and shoe industry
Larynx	Asbestos	Asbestos product manufacture, shipbuilding, construction and maintenance work
Lung	Asbestos	Asbestos product manufacture, shipbuilding, construction and maintenance work
	Coke oven emissions	Topside coke oven workers
	Radon daughters	Uranium and fluorspar miners
	Chromates	Chromium producers and processors, users
	Nickel	Nickel smelters, processors, and users
	Arsenic	Smelters
	Silica	Foundries, abrasive blasting
	Mustard gas	Mustard gas formulators
	Bis(chloromethyl) ether, chloromethyl methyl ether	Ion exchange resin makers, chemists
Pleura and peritoneum/mesothelioma	Asbestos	Asbestos product manufacture, shipbuilding, construction and maintenance work
Bone	Radium	Dial painters, radium chemists and processors
Scrotum	Mineral/cutting oils	Automatic lathe operators, metalworkers
	Soots and tars, tar distillates	Coke oven workers, petroleum refiners, tar distillers
Bladder	Benzidine, α- and β-naphthylamine, auramine, magenta, 4-aminobiphenyl, 4-nitrophenyl	Rubber and dye workers
Esophagus	Asbestos	Asbestos product manufacture, shipbuilding, construction and maintenance work
Stomach	Asbestos	Asbestos product manufacture, shipbuilding, construction and maintenance work
Colon	Asbestos	Asbestos product manufacture, shipbuilding, construction and maintenance work
Kidney	Coke oven emissions	Coke oven workers
Hematopoietic/lymphoid leukemia, acute	Unknown	Rubber industry
	Ionizing radiation	Radiologists
Myeloid leukemia, acute	Benzene	Refining, chemical, and manufacturing industries
	Ionizing radiation	Radiologists
Erythroleukemia, acute	Benzene	Refining, chemical, and manufacturing industries

Table 7.4. How to Determine the Potential Hazards of an Exposure

Identify the Chemical *Shortcut:* Call your local poison center for help	• Employers are required to provide Material Safety Data Sheets (MSDS) on all materials containing potentially hazardous chemicals. Check with the manufacturer, using the phone numbers on the MSDS. • For energy exposure, ask employer about equipment specifications or measurements of wavelength and intensity.
Clarify Potential Health Effects *Shortcut:* Call the NIOSH or ATSDR helplines NIOSH: 513-533-8326 ATSDR: 404-488-4100	• Use one of the general references listed at the end of this chapter for an overview. • Use your medical library or Grateful Med to access Medline and Toxnet at the National Library of Medicine to check newer information.
Synthesize Information *Shortcut:* Involves a consultant through AOEC AOEC: 202-347-4976	• Organize what you have learned from patient history about the exposure: identity of the chemical or mixture, source and wavelength of the energy source, intensity, duration, and time course of exposure. Compare this to dosages known to cause human health effects, animal effects.

ticular trades and toxic substances. (Physicians can contact NIOSH at 513-533-8326.)

Enforcement Agencies

Although health departments generally have authority to investigate occupational diseases, regulation of workplace conditions is usually the responsibility of a separate state agency or the local OSHA office in the United States Department of Labor (telephone number is listed under *United States Government, Labor Department, OSHA*). When a state takes over OSHA enforcement, its regulations are required to be as strict as the federal regulations. In every state, every employer is obligated to report workplace injuries and illness to OSHA.

If other workers may be in imminent danger of being made ill, the physician should communicate this urgently to OSHA to request an immediate investigation. In most cases OSHA enforcement officers can determine easily whether regulations are being violated at a workplace, and they provide a follow-up report to the referring physician. In some cases, the inspection may suggest that the patient's illness was job related, but that at the time of the inspection no specific OSHA regulation was being violated. If a continuing hazard does exist, OSHA can force changes by invoking the employer's general duty to maintain a safe workplace. Especially in these situations, physicians may need to be patient but persistent to see that appropriate action is taken.

The Mine Safety and Health Agency (MSHA) is the specific federal agency with responsibility for safety inspection and enforcement of occupational health standards for the mining industry.

Consultants

Consultants who are particularly knowledgeable about specific problems are increasingly available to help practicing physicians. *Poison centers* through their national network of contacts can usually identify an appropriate expert for telephone consultation about an acute problem. *The Association of Occupational and Environmental Clinics* (AOEC), a national network of primarily university-based clinics, can be contacted to identify resources available in most parts of the United States (telephone 202-347-4976).

WORKER'S COMPENSATION

Every state has a worker's compensation act that provides a system to pay for medical expenses related to occupational disease and injury and for employees' lost earnings. These acts were passed to provide a no-fault system of compensating workers injured on the job and to provide employers with a statutory protection from being sued for negligence by their employees.

Although this system sometimes works well for on-the-job injuries, it does not respond well to the needs of a worker with an occupational disease. Here the burden of proof that the disease is work related falls on the worker, and the process of obtaining compensation is often slow and difficult. Because most small employers insure themselves with an insurance company, the insurer may delay action on a claim even when the employer believes the illness was caused by the job. Usually the worker can obtain legal assistance without having to pay an attorney directly, because provision is made for cases to be taken on a contingency basis (i.e., the attorney receives no fee unless the claim is upheld; then the attorney receives a fixed percentage). Because illness claims are usually complex, the worker will often need a lawyer.

If a physician concludes or even strongly suspects that a patient has an illness caused or made worse by his or her job, the patient should be encouraged to file for worker's compensation (through the employer, the worker's compensation local office, or his or her lawyer).

If a claim is pursued and won (even though it takes time), the patient is usually guaranteed lifetime *medical coverage from worker's compensation funds for that illness.* Compensation may lift some of the financial burdens from the patient and his or her family, particularly in cases of chronic or fatal diseases.

To some extent worker's compensation has failed

because of inadequate physician diagnosis and follow-through. For example, a 1980 Department of Labor survey showed that only 3% of workers disabled by occupational respiratory disease were receiving compensation. The remaining 97% who were not receiving worker's compensation were living on social security or welfare. Their medical bills were being paid by health insurance, Medicare, or state welfare funds. Thus, most economic and social costs of industrial disease are borne not by the companies that may have acted irresponsibly but by the victims and the taxpayers, including businesses that are trying to protect their employees properly.

Physicians are often reluctant to become involved with worker's compensation, feeling that a claim may tie them up in court. This is an unsubstantiated fear because the medical record usually provides sufficient medical evidence and the physician does not have to appear at the hearing. If the record does not provide adequate information, the attorneys involved are almost always willing to take a statement at the physician's convenience.

PART-TIME OCCUPATIONAL HEALTH PHYSICIAN

A primary care practitioner may become involved in a workplace at the invitation of the employer or the union representing the employees. Many small- and medium-sized workplaces need the assistance of part-time physicians to conduct effective programs to detect and prevent occupational disease. A physician who takes on an occupational health role should become thoroughly acquainted with the goals and procedures of the proposed program, as well as the applicable regulations. Table 7.5 lists the principal responsibilities that an occupational physician might be asked to assume and the sources of regulations that guide these

physician responsibilities. The American College of Occupational and Environmental Medicine (ACOEM) sponsors regular training sessions to keep its members and interested physicians up to date in these roles.

Many physicians in occupational medicine regard themselves as responsible to the management of the company that pays them, rather than to the patients they serve. In some instances, physicians have withheld information from patients about work-related diseases. In other cases, physicians modify their therapy for illnesses and injuries to meet the needs of production rather than the needs of the patient. This role of the company physician as servant of management rather than of the patient has had tacit acceptance in the past. In the last decade the ACOEM, composed principally of industry-employed physicians, has called for adherence to ethical practice, and many abuses have been ended. Today, physicians who practice as plant physicians differently from the way they practice in their own offices may face professional discipline and malpractice suits. Table 7.6 summarizes the principal ethical responsibilities of an occupational health physician.

PHYSICIANS AND HEALTH CARE INSTITUTIONS AS EMPLOYERS

Promulgation of the OSHA Blood-Borne Pathogens Standard has reminded physicians and health care organizations of their responsibilities to those they employ and supervise. Most hospitals and state and local medical societies have available information and instructional material to simplify compliance with the requirements for protective equipment, immunization, and education. The basic components of universal precautions to protect health workers from infected body fluids are summarized in Table 34.16; postexpo-

Table 7.5. Responsibilities for the Part-Time Occupational Health Physician

Responsibilities	Regulations to Be Familiar With	Source of Information and Training
Preplacement and fitness-for-duty examinations	Americans with Disabilities Act Federal Aviation Administration, Department of Transportation (DOT) requirements	Equal Employment Opportunity Commission *Technical Assistance Manual* ACOEM training courses[a]
Testing for substance abuse	DOT regulations	Medical review officer course[a] Substance-specific regulations
Surveillance	OSHA regulations	
Care of injured or ill workers	Worker's compensation procedures for one's state Rules governing access to medical records	

[a]American College of Occupational and Environmental Medicine (telephone 708-228-6850).

Table 7.6. Ethical Responsibilities of the Occupational Health Physician

The primary responsibility of the physician is to the individual patient, no matter who is paying the bill.
The physician may reveal nothing to others, including management, about the patient without his or her permission. Reports should be limited to a statement about the patient's illness to work and any specific limitations of activity.
The physician must acquire all available information about the workplace that may be relevant to a patient's health.
Everything that the physician learns or may deduce about the safety of the workplace must be explained to those whose health may be affected.
The physician should report occupational disease to the local health department or state OSHA.
The physician should not take sides in any dispute between the management, the workers, or the government, but should only provide accurate information and honest opinion to all concerned.

sure actions to address the risk of acquiring hepatitis or human immunodeficiency virus (HIV) infection are summarized in Tables 32.5 and 34.17, respectively.

HAZARDS AT HOME AND IN THE COMMUNITY

Exposures at Home

The average American home is a Pandora's box of potentially harmful exposures. Between kitchen, bathroom, garage, and garden, family members may have access to caustics, a variety of aerosols, pesticides, solvents, paint removers, adhesives, and electrical equipment. These types of exposure should be considered when warning about childproofing for toddlers and when evaluating dermatoses and allergic reactions. Exposures at home may also produce illness in ways that come less readily to mind (Table 7.7). Case reports have documented poisoning from inappropriate use of cosmetics and vitamin supplements. Many hobbies can involve exposure to chemicals with fewer protections than workers in industry enjoy. For example, lead poisoning has been documented from ceramics, stained glasswork, and cosmetics; paint strippers containing methylene chloride can produce carbon monoxide poisoning sufficient to aggravate angina and precipitate infarction; and injudicious combinations of cleaning materials can release hazardous fumes. Homes themselves may have hazards. For example, lead-containing paints are a risk to both children and do-it-yourselfers, and formaldehyde-urea foam insulation can release sensitizing fumes. In cases of illness caused by such exposures, physicians need to take a careful history to recognize the cause.

Heating and ventilation systems deserve special mention. Even up-to-date heating systems can produce carbon monoxide poisoning if flues are blocked or inadequate air for combustion is provided. Because symptoms of early carbon monoxide poisoning are nonspecific and mimic those of stress and depression, a high level of suspicion is critical, especially early in the heating season. With the current emphasis on increased insulation and barriers to air infiltration, houses are often poorly ventilated by fresh air. The increasing use of wood, coal, and kerosene heaters may make matters worse. Use of scrap lumber treated with chemical preservatives is an additional hazard.

Leaking roofs and windows can lead to water damage to ceilings and walls. Condensation onto concrete slabs

Table 7.7. Common Hazards at Home

Heating and air conditioning
Water damage and mold
Insulation and lack of ventilation
Vitamins and health foods
Cleaning chemicals
Lead-containing paint
Electric appliances
Water supply
Hobbies
Home repair
Neighborhood pollution sources

under carpet can cause damp conditions as well. Water damage is the major cause of disruption of lead-containing paint and can give rise to significant growth of mold. Recent identification of mold in flood damaged homes as the cause of an epidemic of pulmonary hemorrhage in infants has brought new attention to the danger of inhaled molds.

Office and commercial buildings are also increasingly tight, as heated or cooled air is recycled. Many epidemics of illness caused by chemical or biological agents circulated through the air are being reported. Building-associated illness can be caused by exposure to particulates, chemical fumes from cleaning materials and office equipment, and mold spores and other biological antigens. Because symptoms are often nonspecific, diagnosis may depend on recognizing a temporal pattern or symptoms in coworkers. Evaluation of the ventilation system often reveals inadequacies and in many situations improved ventilation may be all the therapy that is needed.

Exposures from Sources in the Community

Physicians are increasingly being asked for advice relating to concerns about contaminated drinking water and air and the cleanup of toxic wastes. Many communities dependent on groundwater have had their supplies threatened by illegal dumping of chemicals or by leakage from licensed landfills.

The discovery of a chronic source of environmental contamination is an experience few American communities will escape. There is no substitute in such situations for enlisting the assistance of appropriate experts, and physicians in a community may be expected to take the lead in getting help from state and local agencies. Often there is a continuing role for practitioners to play in facilitating the resolution of problems. In many cases, knowledgeable specialists have difficulty in translating what they have to say into language that the lay public can understand. Physicians, who spend their entire days translating medical science into advice for their patients in the office, are well suited to serve in this role. At the same time, community members may need someone who can represent their acute personal concerns to the authorities in a reasoned way. A physician may have to serve as the advocate and critical reviewer of the community, making sure that the statements and positions of all of those involved are supported by factual evidence and calling on independent expertise when appropriate. The Agency for Toxic Substances and Diseases Registries (USPHS) has made a commitment to support physicians in communities affected by environmental contamination with information and assistance. Emergency help is available 24 hours a day at 404-488-4100.

Air Pollution

Patients with respiratory disease are especially concerned about the effects of air pollution. Patients often

Table 7.8. Checklists for Physicians and Others Involved in Hazardous Materials Incidents

What toxic and hazardous substances have been identified?
    What are the concentrations in air, water, and soil?
    What are the known health hazards at these concentrations?
    What are the potential hazards of fire, explosion, or chemical interactions?
How many people have been exposed and how many are likely to become exposed in the near future?
    What groups in the exposed population are likely to be most susceptible to health effects?
    How many exposures are resulting in hospital admissions? Outpatient visits?
    What clinical findings, if any, are being observed?
What technical resources are available on short notice to assist in evaluation and control? Is there a local Hazardous Materials Team?
Is the community adequately handling the casualties?
    What is the capacity of local hospitals, clinics, and physicians to absorb the additional caseload?
    Should hospital disaster plans be mobilized?
    Are intensive care or specialty services adequate or available to the degree needed?
    Are local physicians experienced and knowledgeable about this kind of problem? If not, what is the best way to obtain expert help quickly?
Is this community covered by a repository (such as a tumor registry of population-based research study) that could be used to follow the exposed population in the future?

develop symptoms of respiratory tract irritation during periods of severe pollution, and patients with cardiac or respiratory disease may suffer exacerbations. Prudent advice is in order in such situations. Advice to move to less polluted areas is rarely practical, and such advice should be given only after a great deal of thought about the impact of a move on the patient's entire life. Durable solutions to problems caused by air pollution depend on efforts to limit industrial discharges and, importantly, the emissions of automobiles. Pollution of indoor air in workplaces and in public facilities from cigarette smoking is an equally important challenge to the medical profession and to each community. In recent years, the increase in smoke-free public places has significantly reduced exposure to this form of air pollution. In most states the American Lung Association is leading the struggle for clean air.

Hazardous Materials: Accidents and Disposal

Physicians with no special background in toxicology or public health may be pressed into service in cases of accidental emissions of toxic fumes or accidents involving transport of hazardous materials.

In responding to such emergencies, a practitioner should clarify immediately that the hazard is being contained as effectively as possible, that people not needed at the scene are not being exposed, and that orderly procedures for the care of casualties are being set up. Many communities have developed a coordinated plan for response to hazardous materials incidents. Usually the local emergency response system (fire department or 911 system) will alert a hazardous materials (HAZMAT) team. A checklist is provided in Table 7.8.

General References

Levy BS, Wegman DH, eds. Occupational health: recognizing and preventing work-related disease. 3rd ed. Boston: Little, Brown, 1994.
    The most readable introductory text, not much help as a reference.
McCunney RJ. A practical approach to occupational and environmental medicine. Boston: Little, Brown, 1994.
    Has good material for the part-time occupational physician.
Paul M. Occupational and environmental reproductive hazards. Baltimore: Williams & Wilkins, 1993.
    The best available text about reproductive health and the environment.
Rom WN, ed. Environmental and occupational medicine. Boston: Little, Brown, 1992.
    Textbook that focuses on human exposures in both environmental and occupational settings.
Rosenstock L, Cullen MR. Clinical occupational medicine. Philadelphia: WB Saunders, 1994.
    A good text organized by both organ system and type of hazard.
Sullivan JB, Kreiger GR, eds. Hazardous materials toxicology. Baltimore: Williams & Wilkins, 1992.
    Excellent source for information on specific environmental toxins.
Zenz C. Occupational medicine. Chicago: Year Book Medical Publishers, 1994.
    Especially good for physicians involved in providing occupational health services.

C H A P T E R 8

Primary Care of the Patient with Cancer

LARRY WATERBURY, MD
MICHAEL J. PURTELL, MD

The purpose of this chapter is to examine the role of the general physician in the care of patients who have cancer. Common cancers are discussed in other chapters (breast, Chapter 89; gastrointestinal, Chapter 38; gynecologic, Chapter 95; lung, Chapter 56; prostate, Chapter 49; skin, Chapter 100). The estimated distribution of newly diagnosed cancers and cancer deaths for 1997 is depicted in Figure 8.1. After initial diagnostic evaluation, the location of the primary cancer is unidentified in some patients with metastatic disease. The most common primary cancers that are eventually identified in such patients are cancers of the pancreas, lung, kidney, and colon (8).

GENERAL ASPECTS OF CARE

Communicating the Diagnosis

A patient's primary physician is the one who is most likely to initiate diagnostic evaluation for cancer and to communicate the diagnosis to the patient. During these initial steps, the following elements are important: promptly scheduling tests and notifying the patient of results; communicating clearly (e.g., using the word *cancer* rather than vague terms such as *a growth*); allowing the patient ample time to react to this news; promptly explaining options/recommen-

dations, based on the type and extent of the cancer; checking patient's understanding of and questions about information that has been given; and including family members that the patient selects in all discussions regarding diagnosis, options, and prognosis. Chapter 3 ("The Doctor–Patient Relationship") discusses in detail approaches to communication with patients and their family members.

Initial Referral and Treatment

When possible, one should refer patients to oncologists whom one trusts and knows to be helpful, considerate clinicians. Multimodality treatment regimens involving the combined efforts of surgical, medical, and radiation oncologists may result in a bewildered patient without a physician who accepts the primary responsibility for care. The patient's personal physician should either coordinate care or identify who will be the coordinator for the patient's care and who will be accessible to the patient to answer questions, provide support, and ensure that necessary information is communicated. By receiving up-to-date and complete information about the diagnostic and therapeutic plans and the patient's evolving status, the patient's personal physician may be able to assess the overall picture and, as time goes on, to identify when problems resulting from treatment (e.g., side effects, expense, family disruption, and deteriorating psychological status of patient) outweigh the likely benefits of continued therapy.

Follow-Up Care

Most oncologists welcome participation of the patient's personal physician in continuing care. This is particularly important when treatment is given in an oncology center in a distant city. Some less toxic ambulatory treatment regimens may even be given by the primary physician under the direction of the specialist.

The follow-up of treated patients requires knowledge of the common sites and manifestations of tumor recurrence and the appropriate timing of follow-up examinations and tests, as well as a great deal of sensitivity in recognizing the feelings of the patient. Chapters elsewhere in this book on specific cancers discuss what is known and what is not known about the utility of follow-up assessments. Some patients function better if they are scheduled to be seen less frequently, not to be constantly reminded of the possibility of recurrence. Others require the constant reassurance of a negative examination and normal tests and are more comfortable with frequent follow-up visits. Usually there is room for considerable flexibility in a follow-up plan without jeopardizing the health of the patient.

Whenever a patient with cancer is seen in follow-up, it is important to explain carefully the meaning of symptoms or physical findings and the rationale for tests. If tests will take several days to return, that should

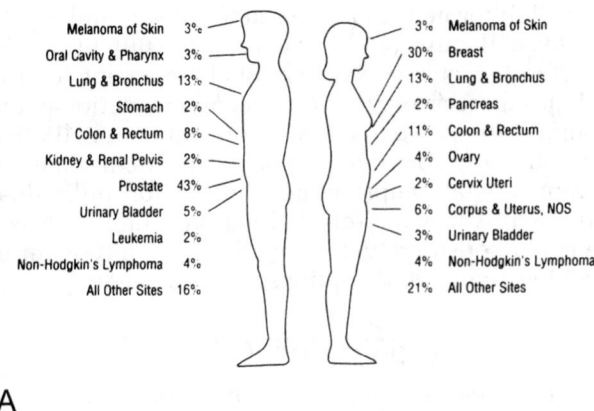

A

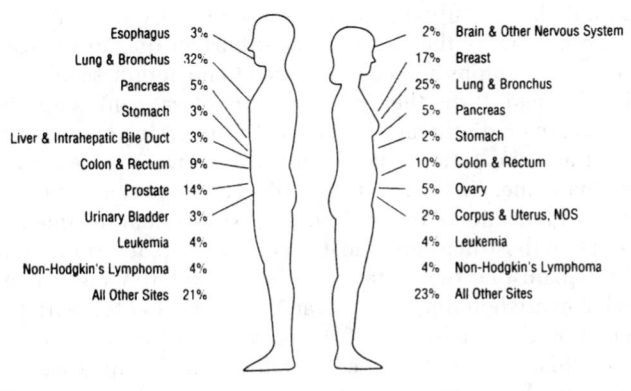

B

Figure 8.1. Estimated new cancer cases **(A)** and estimated cancer deaths **(B)** in 10 leading sites by sex, United States, 1997; excludes basal and squamous cell skin cancer and carcinoma in situ except bladder. *NOS,* Not otherwise specified. (From CA-A Cancer Journal for Clinicians 47:12, 1997.)

be explained and a time for a telephone follow-up arranged.

It is possible that in the future, *tumor markers* that can be measured in the patient's serum—either to screen for cancer or to monitor therapy in patients with disseminated cancer—may be shown to have important utility in patient care. A critical analysis published in 1991 describes potential roles for tumor markers in clinical decision making (2). Although tumor markers can be useful in monitoring the progress of known disease and the response to therapy, these are uses that benefit patients chiefly as part of the care plan of an oncologist or other specialist who is treating them. The routine use of tumor markers to screen for cancer in the asymptomatic patient remains potentially harmful, and there is no current consensus regarding any of the available markers, including the prostate antigen (see discussion in Chapter 49). Generally it is inappropriate to monitor tumor markers routinely as part of the follow-up of patients with cancer who are potentially cured following primary and adjuvant therapy. This

issue has been particularly well studied in patients with breast cancer (1).

The Family's Concerns

The crises attending evaluation for possible cancer and the diagnosis and care for cancer profoundly affect the spouses and families of patients. Common dilemmas for family members include emotional strain, physical demands in caring for the patient, altered roles and lifestyles, finances, and uncertainty about prognosis (9). In addition, there may be questions about the likelihood of cancer occurring in other members of the family. Each of these issues may require consideration by the patient's primary physician (for details see chapters on specific cancers and Chapters 11, "Psychotherapy in Ambulatory Practice," and 19, "Dying, Death, and Bereavement").

Support from the American Cancer Society

The American Cancer Society has chapters in each state and can provide a variety of services to patients and their families. Services vary among states but may include loan of supplies (e.g., hospital beds), transportation to treatment facilities, reduced costs for chemotherapy, respite coverage for caregivers, and a wide range of information about support groups and other help available in the patient's community.

NONOPERABLE CANCERS IN WHICH TREATMENT MAY PROLONG SURVIVAL

Table 8.1 lists a number of nonoperable cancers in which survival may be prolonged by modern treatment regimens; patients with such cancers should be referred to cancer specialists. These patients often benefit from multimodality treatment. Even within this group of cancers, when specialty help is needed, the general physician continues to play an important role, especially if the relationship with the patient or the family has been a lengthy one.

CANCERS UNRESPONSIVE OR POORLY RESPONSIVE TO TREATMENT

Table 8.2 lists a number of cancers less responsive to therapy, where the impact of therapy on survival is unproven or minimal. Diagnosis and initial therapy

Table 8.1.   Some Nonoperable Cancers in Which Treatment Prolongs Survival

Acute leukemia
Hodgkin's disease
Lymphoma
Metastatic testicular cancer
Metastatic ovarian cancer
Small cell carcinoma of the lung
Metastatic breast cancer

Patients with these cancers require specialized treatment, often in centers where multimodality therapy is available.

Table 8.2.   Some Cancers in Which Treatment Provides Palliation in Some Patients (Effects on Survival Unproven or Controversial)

Non–small cell lung cancer (unresectable)
Metastatic large bowel cancer
Metastatic stomach cancer
Metastatic pancreatic cancer
Metastatic malignant melanoma
Metastatic soft tissue sarcomas
Metastatic cervical cancer
Metastatic endometrial cancer
Metastatic hypernephroma
Metastatic prostate cancer (when patient relapses on hormonal therapy)

usually require surgery, but when metastasis is proven, the effect of systemic therapy, radiotherapy, or both is at most palliative (15,16). In such situations, patients often expect their personal physicians to help them select or to actually recommend treatment plans. Several questions come up at this juncture.

Should palliative therapy be recommended? Although it is difficult to generalize, several factors must be considered in attempting to help patients and their families decide whether the patient is likely to benefit from palliative therapy. More than age, the functional status of the patient must be considered in such therapeutic decisions. The infirm, ill, poorly functional patient with widely disseminated and rapidly progressive disease may be more harmed than benefited by the side effects and discomforts of palliative treatment, especially if response rates are small and toxicity of treatment is high. Weight loss before therapy correlates closely with poor response rates in clinical chemotherapy trials in these less responsive cancers (5). Other patients, even if elderly, in good functional status are much more suitable candidates for attempts at palliation. The patient who believes that any chance of response is worth the price of toxicity, and who cannot feel comfortable unless attempting some therapy, should generally be offered treatment.

If some attempt at palliative treatment seems worthwhile, should it be conventional therapy or experimental protocol therapy? Every oncology center has current protocols for the metastatic cancers listed in Table 8.2. Clinical protocols designed to seek improved methods of treatment are important for advances that may improve the outlook and the comfort of future patients. However, experimental therapy may have undesirable consequences for the individual patient. Sometimes, such protocols involve the investigation of treatments with more toxicity than current conventional therapies. They usually require more frequent visits to the physician, as well as more frequent diagnostic tests, because of the necessity to document precisely the objective response. They may therefore also involve increased expense to the patient. The patient's insurance may or may not cover the specific experimental therapy being considered. Patients agreeing to experimental protocol therapy—and their physicians—must

be well informed about the side effects and likely benefits of therapy (12). The helpful consultant should describe the current conventional treatment for the patient's disease and tailor the recommendation to the specific patient. No treatment, conventional palliative chemotherapy or radiotherapy, and experimental therapy are all appropriate choices for individual patients in various clinical situations. Table 8.3 lists the major considerations for patient and physician in selecting among these options.

RADIOTHERAPY

Patient Experience. The patient with cancer often has misconceptions about and limited knowledge of radiotherapy. It is thus important to explain radiotherapy to the patient in terms of the rationale, patient experience, and likely benefits and side effects of this treatment modality. The initial visit usually includes a focused history and physical examination by the radiotherapist. Further diagnostic tests (e.g., radiographs and computerized tomographic scan) may be obtained. If the therapist agrees that treatment is appropriate, the radiotherapy ports may be determined at the first visit and the patient may receive his or her first treatment at that time. The patient is told that skin tattoos may be placed to facilitate the uniformity of subsequent treatments, and that these markings must not be removed. It is important to explain that the therapy machines are bulky and somewhat overwhelming in appearance. Some patients are frightened by the experience; if the referring physician appreciates this, it is useful to contact the radiotherapist and to explain the particular fears of the patient ahead of time. Therapists often give patients and their families a tour of the radiotherapy treatment rooms before starting therapy and spend extra time answering questions about the treatment and its benefits and complications. The patient should be aware that the treatment itself is not painful. The initial consultation is usually time-consuming (several hours), but subsequent treatments are usually scheduled precisely and require only a small amount of time (30 minutes). Treatments are usually given several days a week, and the entire course may take several weeks to complete. The patient usually does not see the radiotherapist at the time of each treatment but is seen by a radiotherapy nurse or technician. The patient therefore needs to know precisely with whom to communicate to address side effects or questions during radiotherapy.

Table 8.3.   Factors Affecting Palliative Treatment Recommendations in Patients with Cancer

The natural history of the untreated cancer
The proven effect of treatment on the natural history
   Likely effects on survival
   Likelihood of lessening morbidity
Toxicity of treatment
Functional status of the patient
Ability of the patient to comprehend the implications of treatment
Psychological state and philosophical position of the patient
Emotional strength and attitudes of immediate family
Financial situation, health coverage status

Table 8.4. Important Side Effects of Radiotherapy

Dermatitis: Less common with newer high-energy machines; avoid sunlight and extreme cold.

Acute radiation pneumonitis: Transient, usually occurring 6–12 wk after treatment; precipitated by corticosteroid withdrawal, concomitant chemotherapy; clinical manifestations include nonproductive cough, dyspnea, fever, leukocytosis with parenchymal infiltrates on radiograph in the area of the radiation ports; may respond to steroid treatment.

Pulmonary fibrosis: Occurs 6–12 months after treatment; not responsive to steroids.

Esophagitis: Usually occurs during treatment; particularly severe when radiotherapy and chemotherapy are administered together.

Nausea, vomiting, and diarrhea: Occur during treatment with most abdominal radiotherapy, usually self-limited.

Enteritis: Rare, more likely with very high-dose treatment; small bowel more sensitive than large bowel and stomach; occurs weeks to years after radiotherapy; manifestations include obstruction, bleeding, perforation; pelvic irradiation (e.g., in the treatment of bladder or prostate cancer) may cause acute *proctitis,* which occasionally becomes chronic, sometimes leading to bleeding or stricture formation.

Pericarditis: Occurs months to years after radiation, usually resolves, occasionally progresses to constrictive pericarditis or tamponade requiring pericardiectomy. There is also an increased incidence of coronary artery disease seen after mediastinal irradiation.

Neurologic side effects: Transverse myelitis, very rare; side effects from CNS irradiation in adults are rare. Lhermitte's sign (the sensation of electric shocks passing down the body when the head is flexed) seen in 10% of patients undergoing mantle irradiation for Hodgkin's disease; after radiotherapy herpes zoster is common.

Hypothyroidism: Common in patients treated for Hodgkin's disease with mantle field; may develop years after treatment.

Sterility: Usually temporary.

Growth retardation in children: Occurs both from direct skeletal effects and from hypopituitarism from CNS irradiation.

Oral and dental side effects: Dry mouth and partial or complete loss of taste or smell are common. Severe dental problems are common after head and neck irradiation because of decrease in saliva formation, increased sensitivity to caries, osteonecrosis.

Cystitis: Occurs during treatment with pelvic irradiation; clinical manifestations include urgency dysuria and hematuria occurring usually during the third and fourth weeks of treatment; usually self-limited and treated symptomatically with fluids and phenazopyridine (Pyridium), 200 mg four times a day; chronic bladder fibrosis is a rare late complication manifested usually by painless hematuria.

See References 3, 4, 6, and 10.

Time Until Symptomatic Response

In addition to the timing and types of side effects that may be experienced, it is important for the patient to know that the response to treatment is often delayed and that sometimes the maximal effect is noted a few weeks after the course of radiotherapy is completed. For example, radiotherapy is useful in the palliation of pain secondary to local bony metastases, but 2 to 3 weeks may elapse before improvement occurs and improvement may not be maximal until a few weeks after treatment is discontinued. Some responses are more rapid, occurring after only a few days of therapy (e.g., relief of superior vena caval obstruction and neurologic deficits from spinal cord obstruction or central nervous system [CNS] metastasis).

An excellent booklet, *Radiation Therapy and You: A Guide to Self-Help During Treatment,* is available free from the National Institutes of Health to patients undergoing radiotherapy (see "General References"). It is helpful to have copies of this booklet available for patients and families to read when radiotherapy is being considered.

Side Effects

Table 8.4 describes important side effects of radiotherapy. The patient will be most concerned by the common side effects that occur during treatment and by those that may remain for a few weeks after treatment is discontinued.

Dermatitis secondary to radiotherapy is less common than it used to be because of the use of the modern high-energy machines. Severe burning requiring specialized treatment is uncommon; however, skin discoloration may occur. The patient should be told that the radiation field should not be exposed to sunlight or extreme cold, and that total but temporary hair loss will usually occur in the areas being radiated and that complete return of hair, after high-dose radiation, may take many months or may not occur.

The most troublesome side effects that occur during radiotherapy are *gastrointestinal.* Patients receiving radiation to the chest or upper back often experience symptoms of radiation esophagitis (odynophagia and sometimes reflux symptoms that may respond to elevation of the head of the bed and to antacids). Severe esophagitis is more likely to occur when radiotherapy has been used in patients who have had prior chemotherapy, especially with such agents as doxorubicin, bleomycin, or *cis*-platinum. *Candida* superinfection of the irritated esophagus is not unusual, especially in patients who are receiving steroids. This usually responds well to treatment with fluconazole (one 50-mg tablet twice a day). Patients should improve with a 1-week course of therapy. Abdominal irradiation can cause diarrhea that may persist to some degree during the entire course of treatment. In addition to replacing fluids and electrolytes, some dietary maneuvers may minimize diarrhea; these are listed in Table 8.5. Nausea and anorexia are the most troublesome side effects of abdominal irradiation and are discussed separately later in this chapter.

Patients who receive radiotherapy to the head or neck are subject to *oral and dental complications.* Before treatment all patients should have a complete dental examination by a dentist experienced in the treatment of patients who have undergone radiotherapy.

Table 8.5. Dietary Maneuvers for Therapy-Induced Diarrhea

Clear liquids (warm or at room temperature)
Avoid fiber (roughage) in the diet
Take smaller amounts of food more often
Avoid fatty foods
Avoid highly spiced foods
Avoid carbonated drinks, beans, cabbage, broccoli, cauliflower, and corn

Damage to the teeth, gums, and bone, plus the xerostomia that results from high-dosage radiotherapy to the oral mucous membranes and salivary glands, may result in severe problems. Many of these can be prevented by appropriate prophylaxis (aggressive treatment of periodontal disease and infected teeth before radiation) and an ongoing program during and after radiotherapy, which should be strictly followed. The use of artificial saliva (Saliva Substitute, Roxane Laboratories) may be helpful for patients with xerostomia.

Corticosteroids and Radiotherapy

The patient's primary care physician may sometimes be involved with the early treatment of CNS metastases or spinal cord compression, using corticosteroids in conjunction with radiotherapy. Multiple regimens are used. A common regimen consists of dexamethasone (Decadron), 4 to 25 mg four times a day, continued until the patient has received several courses of radiotherapy and then slowly tapered over 2 to 3 weeks. Steroids decrease the local edema that occurs in these situations and help protect against radiation-induced edema during the first few days of therapy.

Cumulative Dosage

There is a maximal cumulative dosage of radiotherapy that can safely be given to any one site without the risk of significant permanent tissue damage. This dosage varies for each organ system. If ports do not overlap, definitive full-dose radiotherapy can be given to multiple sites either concomitantly or sequentially. Problems occur when ports are contiguous or overlapping. For example, it is often more beneficial to give palliative total spine irradiation to patients with several isolated spine metastases than to treat only focal symptomatic areas, which may preclude later palliative radiotherapy to symptomatic contiguous areas.

CHEMOTHERAPY

Patients Experience. The chemotherapy experience for the patient is so varied (depending on the disease being treated) that it is hard to give a general description. The medical oncologist giving therapy can best explain to the patient the specifics of treatment, including how it is administered, the frequency of treatment, the hoped-for response, and the side effects. The most common troublesome side effects for the patient are hair loss and nausea and vomiting. The frequency and degree of hair loss vary with the treatment regimen, but it is helpful for the patient to know that hair will regrow once the treatment is discontinued. The treatment of nausea and vomiting is discussed later in this chapter. Table 8.6 lists other acute and chronic side effects of various chemotherapeutic agents. Knowledge of the long-term side effects of various agents is particularly important for the primary physician, who may be responsible for follow-up care of patients with good prognoses after chemotherapy.

An excellent free booklet, *Chemotherapy and You: A Guide to Self-Help During Treatment,* written for patients, is

Table 8.6.   Common Side Effects of Chemotherapy[a]

Hair loss: Alkylating agents, vincristine, vinblastine, adriamycin, mithramycin, daunomycin
Hypercalcemia: Estrogens, antiestrogens (tamoxifen)
Fluid retention: Estrogens, androgens, steroids
Skin darkening: Adriamycin (nails), 5-FU, bleomycin, busulfan, methotrexate[b]
Dermatitis: Methotrexate, alkylating agents, vinblastine, 6-MP, 6-thioguanine, bleomycin (may be delayed)[b]
Marrow depression: Almost all, except vincristine, bleomycin, nitrosoureas may be delayed
Neurologic: cis-platinum (deafness), vincristine, vinblastine, methotrexate, hexamethylmelamine, 5-FU (ataxia), procarbazine, ifosphamide (encephalopathy, seizures), taxol, vinorelbine
Diarrhea: Vinorelbine, 5-FU, leukovorin, camptosar
Gastrointestinal ulcerations: methotrexate, 5-FU, bleomycin (mucocutaneous), adriamycin, leukovorin
Cardiomyopathy: Adriamycin, daunorubicin, mitoxantrone, infusional 5-FU
Pulmonary fibrosis: Bleomycin, alkylating agents, mitomycin-C
Renal damage: cis-platinum, methotrexate, streptozotocin, ifosphamide, nitrosoureas
Red urine: Adriamycin, daunomycin
Hepatic toxicity: Mithramycin, methotrexate, nitrosoureas, cytosine arabinoside, 6-MP
Sexual and gonadal dysfunction: Many drugs and regimens
Secondary neoplasm: Alkylating agents, especially when combined with radiotherapy
Flulike symptoms, malaise: Biologics (IL-2, interferon), gemcitabine
Fever: Bleomycin, biologics
Hypersensitivity reaction: Taxol, etoposide

[a] See Reference 13.

[b] 5-FU, 5-fluorouracil, 6-MP, 6-mercaptopurine.

available through the National Institutes of Health (see "General References"). It is helpful to have this booklet available for patients and families to read when chemotherapy is being considered.

Chemotherapy-Induced Granulocytopenic Fever

The most common side effect of cytotoxic chemotherapy is myelosuppression and the associated risk of systemic infection (14). Granulocytopenia is defined as an absolute neutrophil count of less than 1000 cells/mm^3. However, a significant risk of infection is not incurred until the level falls below 500/mm^3. In particular, the incidence of culture-proven septicemia correlates best with the number of days a patient remains with a neutrophil count below 100/mm^3. The nadir of the white count, and hence the largest risk of serious infection, usually occurs 10 to 14 days after chemotherapy is administered. It is the responsibility of the treating oncologist to monitor the neutrophil counts and instruct patients when to check their temperatures, and when to seek help if a fever or other signs (e.g., malaise, chills, cough) of infection develop. However, there may be circumstances when the patient's primary care physician may be contacted by the patient.

It has been dogma that any granulocytopenic patient is at great risk for Gram-negative bacteremia, especially *Pseudomonas,* and that all febrile neutropenic patients need immediate hospitalization with appropriate empiric antibiotic coverage. For the primary physician, who may not have the patient's latest hemogram and may not have followed the recent course of the patient, this still may be the best guideline. On admission the patient should have blood or urine cultures and a chest radiograph. A history of new symptoms and an examination guided by symptoms, but always including attention to the mouth, skin, and perirectal area, may reveal a source. Unlike unimpaired patients, immunocompromised patients can have a life-threatening septicemia with few or no focal signs or symptoms. Therefore, instead of watching and waiting at the time of admission, one should initiate treatment with broad-spectrum antibiotics such as semisynthetic penicillin and an aminoglycoside or third-generation cephalosporin to which *Pseudomonas* is sensitive. In recent years, the incidence of *Pseudomonas* bacteremia has markedly decreased in these patients; *Escherichia coli* and *Klebsiella pneumoniae* remain the most common infections, and the incidence of Gram-positive infections, especially coagulase-negative staphylococci, has risen, probably because of the increased use of indwelling venous access devices. On occasion, when the patient is not sick and the expected length of neutropenia is short, the experienced oncologist may elect to treat the febrile neutropenic patient as an outpatient.

NAUSEA, VOMITING, AND ANOREXIA

Nausea and vomiting can be the most troublesome side effects of radiotherapy and chemotherapy. In the past, the symptomatic treatment of nausea was only moderately effective, and vomiting was particularly troublesome with therapies containing *cis*-platinum. However, antiemetic regimens combining corticosteroids (dexamethasone, 10 to 20 mg intravenously) with a serotonin blocker (e.g., ondansetron, 10 to 30 mg intravenously) have greatly reduced the incidence of nausea and vomiting in the first 24 hours after therapy with *cis*-platinum and other strongly emetic regimens (7). Lorazepam may have a role in relaxing the anxious patient before chemotherapy, and because of its interference with short-term memory, it may also lessen the chance of a patient developing anticipatory nausea. The nausea of less emetigenic regimens usually can be controlled with a 10- to 20-mg dose of dexamethasone supplemented with prochlorperazine (either 10 mg intravenously or 10 to 20 mg by mouth). Nausea that begins several days after the administration of the chemotherapy and lasts up to a week or more is still a difficult problem to treat, especially after administration of *cis*-platinum. Attempts to treat with a short course of oral dexamethasone (20 mg/day), with prochlorperazine (one or two 10-mg capsules orally or 25-mg suppository every 4 to 6 hours) are only moderately successful. In addition to pharmacologic palliation, the patient with marked nausea will find that it is often helpful to be extremely still, lying down in a quiet room without external stimuli.

A number of *dietary maneuvers* may be helpful to the patient experiencing nausea and vomiting after therapy. The patient who experiences severe nausea and vomiting after therapy should probably drink only clear liquids until the symptoms are decreased. In general, it is more helpful to take smaller portions of food frequently than to take larger meals less often, to take foods that are low in fat, and to avoid overly sweet foods. Mild nausea, especially that experienced before therapy or in anticipation of therapy, may be helped by taking dry toast or crackers in small quantities. It is recommended that patients not lie down just after eating. Some patients find also that it is helpful not to drink liquids with their food (because this may increase their feeling of bloating and subsequent nausea). Many patients become nauseated at the smell of food cooking, and it may be helpful for them to go to another part of the house or to stay out of the house when food is being prepared. Greasy and fried foods seem to be the worst offenders in this regard and are best avoided.

One of the major problems with intensive cancer therapy is *general anorexia* often associated with alterations in taste and smell, which may result in considerable nutritional problems and weight loss (11). Consultation with a dietitian may be extremely helpful in such a situation.

An excellent free booklet, *Eating Hints: Recipes and Tips for Better Nutrition during Cancer Treatment,* is available through the National Institutes of Health (see "General References"). It contains all sorts of dietary advice for patients with cancer, including many recipes.

TERMINAL CARE

The primary physician who has participated in various phases of cancer care and who has an ongoing relationship with the patient and his or her family is often in the best position to help during a patient's terminal illness. The physician who develops some expertise in this regard can find enormous gratification from this role. Chapter 19 deals with many of the issues important in caring for terminally ill patients and their families, including the very important issues of pain control, hospice care, and bereavement. An excellent publication, *Coping with Cancer: A Resource for the Health Professional,* is available free of charge from the National Institutes of Health (see "General References"). In addition to other useful information, it lists organizations and agencies that provide useful services that may aid the physician in providing support for the dying patient.

General References

DeVita VT, Hellman S, Rosenberg SA, eds. Cancer, principles and practice of oncology. 5th ed. Philadelphia: Lippincott-Raven, 1997.
  Exhaustive textbook.
Drugs of choice for cancer chemotherapy. Med Lett 37:25, 1995.
  Useful periodic review of drugs, toxicities, and indications.
Loescher LJ, Welch-McCaffrey D, Leigh SA, et al. Surviving adult cancers. Part I: physiologic effects. Ann Intern Med 111:411, 1989; Welch-McCaffrey D, Hoffman B, Leigh SA, et al. Surviving adult cancers. Part 2: psychosocial implications. Ann Intern Med 111: 517, 1989.

Companion critical review articles that summarize knowledge and knowledge gaps regarding physiologic and psychosocial aspects of long-term survival in treated patients with cancer. Murphy GP, Lawrence W, Lenhard RE, eds. American Cancer Society textbook of clinical oncology. Atlanta: American Cancer Society, 1995.

Provided free by the American Cancer Society. Good source of condensed data about all cancers and their treatment.

Booklets from the National Institutes of Health cited in this chapter are available free of charge from the Office of Cancer Communications, Department of Health and Human Services, NIH, Bethesda, MD 20205, telephone 301-496-4070.

Specific References

1. ASCO Breast Cancer Surveillance Expert Panel. Recommended breast cancer surveillance guidelines. J Clin Oncol 15:2149, 1997.
2. Bates SE. Clinical applications of serum tumor markers. Ann Intern Med 115:623, 1991.
3. Berk L. An overview of radiotherapy trials for the treatment of brain metastases. Oncology 9:1205, 1995.
4. Blayney DW, Longo D. Radiation induced pericarditis. N Engl J Med 306:550, 1982.
5. Dewys WD. Prognostic effect of weight loss prior to chemotherapy in cancer patients. Am J Med 69:491, 1980.
6. Gross NJ. Pulmonary effects of radiation therapy. Ann Intern Med 86:81, 1997.
7. Hainsworth JD, Hesbeth PJ. Single-dose ondansetron for the prevention of cisplatin induced emesis: efficacy results. Semin Oncol 19(Suppl 15):14, 1992.
8. Le Chevalier T, Cvitkovic E, Caille P, et al. Early metastatic cancer of unknown primary origin at presentation: a clinical study of 302 consecutive autopsied patients. Arch Intern Med 148:2035, 1988.
9. Lewis FM. The impact of cancer on the family: a critical analysis of the research literature. In: Patient education and counseling. Limerick: Elsevier Scientific Publishers Ireland, 1986;269.
10. Morgenstern L, Thompson R, Friedman NB. Radiation enteritis. Am J Surg 134:166, 1971.
11. Ottery FD. Supportive nutrition to prevent cachexia and improve quality of life. Semin Oncol 22(Suppl 2):98, 1995.
12. Penman DT. Informed consent for investigational chemotherapy: patients' and physicians' perceptions. J Clin Oncol 2:849, 1984.
13. Perry LC. Toxicity of chemotherapy. Semin Oncol 19(5), 1992.
14. Pizzo PA. Management of fever in patients with cancer and treatment-induced neutropenia. N Engl J Med 328:1323, 1993.
15. Richter MP, Coia LR. Palliative radiation therapy. Semin Oncol 12:375, 1985.
16. Romond EH, Metcalfe MS, MacDonald JS. Palliative chemotherapy and hormonal therapy. Semin Oncol 12:384, 1985.

CHAPTER 9

Selected Special Services: Disability Insurance, Vocational Rehabilitation, and Home Health Services

L. RANDOL BARKER, MD

Maintenance of a patient's overall health often requires efforts beyond those of the physician and the patient. Often, assistance comes from community-based programs to which physicians may refer their patients. Many of these programs provide services for patients with specific types of illness; the roles of such categorical community services are described in the appropriate chapters in this book. Other services are designed to assist patients regardless of their type of illness. This chapter describes three fundamental services of this kind: social security income support programs for disabled people, vocational rehabilitation, and home health services. The purpose of this chapter is to explain eligibility for these services, the nature of the benefits, and the role of physicians in enabling their patients to receive these services. Chapter 7 provides similar information about another noncategorical program, worker's compensation, which is designed to provide coverage for health care costs and income support to people with work-related diseases.

SOCIAL SECURITY PROGRAMS FOR DISABLED PEOPLE

Loss or decrease of a person's ability to earn a living accompanies many illnesses. Beginning with 1954 amendments to the Social Security Act, income support for medically disabled people has been available in the United States. Further modifications since 1954 have led to the program that exists today. Three fundamental benefits are currently available through the Society Security Administration: Disability Insurance (DI), Supplemental Security Income (SSI), and Medicare (health insurance for DI recipients). Medicaid is a federally and state-administered health insurance program that is available automatically in many states for people who receive SSI and for mothers of dependent children whose incomes are below the poverty level. Detailed information about each of these services is available from any local social security office.

Definition of Medical Disability

The Social Security Act defines disability as "inability to engage in any substantial gainful activity by reason of a medically determinable physical or mental impairment that can be expected to result in death or has lasted or can be expected to last for a continuous period of not less than 12 months."

Disability Insurance (Title II)

Eligibility

To be eligible for disability insurance payments, a disabled worker must have paid into the social security program for a minimum period of time before becoming disabled; in addition, there is a requirement for coverage during 5 of the 10 years before the onset of disability. Today, 9 of 10 workers pay the social security tax (FICA). For younger workers (up to age 31), there are modified requirements to meet insured status.

Disabled dependents of a fully insured worker who is retired, disabled, or deceased may be eligible for disability insurance payments in two situations: *a child* who became disabled before age 22 (eligible for disability insurance payments at the time that the child's parent retires, becomes disabled, or dies; payments may begin as early as age 18 and continue as long as the child's disability lasts) and *a widow or widower* who is between 50 and 59 years of age and who did not work under social security but who became medically disabled before or within 7 years of the death of a fully insured spouse.

Benefits

Disability insurance payments go to disabled workers before the age of 65 (after 65, Social Security Retirement Income replaces disability payments) and to eligible children, widows, or widowers as long as they remain disabled. The first monthly disability insurance check is not paid for the first 5 months after the onset of the worker's disability (e.g., a patient who is certified as disabled 6 calendar months after becoming disabled, immediately becomes eligible for a check covering the 1 month in excess of the required 5-month wait). Supplemental Security Income (see below) is often awarded to people who qualify for disability benefits, effective the first day of the month that follows the month in which they apply

for benefits. Income from DI for a disabled worker is the same amount as the retirement income the worker would receive if he or she were 65. The average monthly payment to a disabled worker in 1996 was $704, and to a worker with a wife and dependent children, $1069. In that year, 4.4 million workers and 1.7 million spouses and children were receiving DI benefits.

In addition to income support, disabled people under 65 receive Medicare (Social Security Health Insurance) after they have been eligible for disability benefits for 24 months.

Process of Disability Determination

There are three basic steps in the process of determining medical disability.

First Step. The patient completes a detailed application at a local social security office. The patient must not be gainfully employed at the time of application (*gainful employment* is defined as an activity that yields a monthly income of $500 or more). Most patients initiate disability claims by themselves, but at times a physician or social worker suggests application to a patient who is not aware that his or her condition qualifies as a medical disability.

Second Step. The patient's physician receives a request for medical information and returns this report to the state Disability Determination office. The report sent by the patient's physician should be succinct and precise, and it should provide objective data regarding the condition for which disability is being claimed. It should be divided into the following subheadings: history, physical, laboratory reports, diagnosis, treatment, and response. The information provided should permit claim reviewers to determine both the severity and the duration of the patient's condition. If malingering is suspected, the report should describe the circumstances that raise doubts rather than recording this assessment without supporting information. In this report the physician is not expected to rate the ability of the patient to work. The most helpful guide for completing these medical reports is the booklet *Disability Evaluation Under Social Security* (available free from any social security office or the state Disability Determination office). This manual, which was most recently revised in 1994, contains the criteria for medical disability for most common conditions. These criteria are the basis for most allowances made by disability claim reviewers. Tables 9.1 through 9.6 contain the criteria for several common conditions that may cause medical disability: symptomatic ischemic heart disease, chronic obstructive airway disease, cerebrovascular accident, epilepsy caused by major motor seizures, arthritis of a major weight-bearing joint, and rheumatoid arthritis. Since 1980 the Social Security Administration has paid a small fee to physicians for medical reports for the DI program; a small fee has also been paid for SSI reports since the inception of that program in 1974. Previously, patients were expected to pay for these reports. In some states, doctors also have

Table 9.1. Impairments Qualifying a Person with *Ischemic Heart Disease* for Medical Disability Under Social Security

Ischemic Heart Disease with Chest Discomfort Associated with Myocardial Ischemia

A. Sign- or symptom-limited exercise test demonstrating at least one of the following manifestations at a workload equivalent to 5 METs or less:

1. Horizontal or downsloping depression, in the absence of digitalis glycoside therapy or hypokalemia, of the S-T segment of at least –0.10 millivolts (–1.0 mm) in at least three consecutive complexes that are on a level baseline in any lead (other than aVR) and have a typical ischemic time course of development and resolution (progression of horizontal or downsloping S-T depression with exercise, and persistence of depression of at least –0.10 millivolts for at least 1 minute of recovery); or

2. An upsloping S-T junction depression, in the absence of digitalis glycoside therapy or hypokalemia, in any lead (except aVR) of at least –0.2 millivolts or more for at least 0.08 seconds after the J junction and persisting for at least 1 minute of recovery; or

3. At least 0.1 millivolt (1 mm) S-T elevation above resting baseline during both exercise and 3 minutes or more of recovery in ECG leads with low R and T waves in the leads demonstrating the S-T segment displacement; or

4. Failure to increase systolic pressure by 10 mm Hg, or decrease in systolic pressure below usual clinical resting level (see 4.00C2b); or

5. Documented reversible radionuclide "perfusion" (thallium-201) defect at an exercise level equivalent to 5 METs or less

OR

B. Impaired myocardial function, documented by evidence (as outlined under 4.00C3 or 4.00C4b) of hypokinetic, akinetic, or dyskinetic myocardial free wall or septal wall motion with left-ventricular ejection fraction of 30% or less, and an evaluating program physician, preferably one experienced in the care of patients with cardiovascular disease, has concluded that performance of exercise testing would present a significant risk to the individual, and resulting in marked limitation of physical activity, as demonstrated by fatigue, palpitation, dyspnea, or anginal discomfort on ordinary physical activity, even though the individual is comfortable at rest

OR

C. Coronary artery disease, demonstrated by angiography (obtained independent of Social Security disability evaluation), and an evaluating program physician, preferably one experienced in the care of patients with cardiovascular disease, has concluded that performance of exercise testing would present a significant risk to the individual, with both 1 and 2:

1. Angiographic evidence revealing
   a. 50% or more narrowing of a nonbypassed left main coronary artery
   or
   b. 70% or more narrowing of another nonbypassed coronary artery or
   c. 50% or more narrowing involving a long (greater than 1 cm) segment of a nonbypassed coronary artery or
   d. 50% or more narrowing of at least two nonbypassed coronary arteries
   or
   e. Total obstruction of a bypass graft vessel

2. Resulting in marked limitation of physical activity, as demonstrated by fatigue, palpitation, dyspnea, or anginal discomfort on ordinary physical activity, even though the individual is comfortable at rest.

From Disability Evaluation Under Social Security, 1995. Number codes refer to additional details in this booklet.

MET, Metabolic equivalent.

access to a free teledictation service for dictating their reports.

Third Step. The information provided by the patient and the physician (the disability claim) is re-

viewed at the state Disability Determination office by a team consisting of a disability claims examiner and a physician. If deemed necessary, an independent medical examination is purchased by the Disability Determination office. In keeping with the 1974 Freedom of Information Act, patients may have access to their disability claim files. If an insured worker has an impairment that does not meet the standard criteria for disability but nevertheless prevents the worker from doing his or her usual job, other factors (limitations of age, education, training, work experience) may also be considered by the Disability Determination team in establishing whether he or she is unable to perform any gainful work. However, most findings of disability are based on the standard Social Security Administration criteria.

Appeal Process

If the initial claim of disability has been denied, the claimant may file for reconsideration within 60 days of receiving a denial notice. The case is then reevaluated by a different claim examining team. If the claim is denied at this reconsideration, the claimant has 60 days to file a request for a hearing. Hearings are conducted by administrative law judges. If the claim is again denied, the claimant may make an additional appeal for review by the Appeals Council. After that, the case may be taken to the United States District Court.

A patient's personal physician can be instrumental in ensuring that the patient gets the fullest consideration throughout the Disability Determination process. If the physician thinks that there are aspects of the patient's illness that make it more severe than the criteria indicate, the physician should communicate this information in writing, together with support for this opinion, to the Disability Determination office.

Return to Work

All claims are reviewed for referral to Vocational Rehabilitation (see below) at the time the disability decision is made. In addition, every person with a

Table 9.2. Impairments Qualifying a Person with *Chronic Obstructive Pulmonary Disease* for Medical Disability Under Social Security

Chronic obstructive pulmonary disease from any cause, with the FEV_1 equal to or less than the values specified in this table corresponding to the person's height without shoes. (In cases of marked spinal deformity, see 3.00E.)

Height Without Shoes (cm)	Height Without Shoes (in)	FEV_1 Equal to or Less Than (L, BTPS)
154 or less	60 or less	1.05
155–160	61–63	1.15
161–165	64–65	1.25
166–170	66–67	1.35
171–175	68–69	1.45
176–180	70–71	1.55
181 or more	72 or more	1.65

From Disability Evaluation Under Social Security, 1995.

FEV_1, Forced expiratory volume in 1 second.

Table 9.3. Impairments Qualifying a Person with *Cerebrovascular Accident* for Medical Disability Under Social Security

Central nervous system vascular accident. With one of the following more than 3 months after vascular accident:
A. Sensory or motor aphasia resulting in ineffective speech or communication
B. Significant and persistent disorganization of motor function in two extremities, resulting in sustained disturbance or gross and dexterous movements, or gait and station

From Disability Evaluation Under Social Security, 1995.

Table 9.4. Impairments Qualifying a Person with *Epilepsy Due to Major Motor Seizures* for Medical Disability Under Social Security

Major motor seizures (grand mal or psychomotor), documented by EEG and by detailed description of a typical seizure pattern, including all associated phenomena: occurring more frequently than once a month, in spite of at least 3 months of prescribed treatment.[a] With
A. Daytime episodes (loss of consciousness and convulsive seizures) *or*
B. Nocturnal episodes manifesting residuals that interfere significantly with activity during the day

From Disability Evaluation Under Social Security, 1995.
[a] Adherence to therapy must be objectively confirmed by measurements of drug levels that are in the therapeutic range.

permanent impairment is reevaluated every 7 years, and all other people (i.e., those with impairments that may not be permanent) are reevaluated at least every 3 years to determine whether they are still disabled. Even if the original impairment is judged not to be severe on review, payments are continued for those who have started a vocational rehabilitation program because of improvement in their medical condition; benefits continue until the rehabilitation services are completed or until the person stops receiving these services. The purpose of these processes and the following conditions is to encourage disabled people to return to work:

- Disabled beneficiaries may test their ability to work for 9 months while continuing to receive benefits. After this trial work period, a determination is made about whether the work constitutes substantial gainful activity (defined as an activity that yields a monthly income of $500 or more); if it does, benefits are suspended after an additional 3-month adjustment period.
- If a person who still has a disabling impairment stops work again within 36 months after social security payments have been suspended because of substantial gainful activity, the monthly DI benefits can be resumed, usually without a new application.
- A worker can usually continue to have Medicare coverage for 3 years after his or her DI benefits stop because of return to substantial gainful activity. If a worker starts receiving DI benefits again within 5 years after the DI was stopped, and if the patient was previously entitled to Medicare, that protection resumes immediately.

- Work expenses related to the impairment that are paid for by a disabled person may be deducted from the patient's earnings in determining whether these constitute substantial gainful activity. This is true even if these expenses also apply to needs for daily living (e.g., a wheelchair).
- In addition to disabled workers, workers' children who became disabled before the age of 22 and disabled widows and widowers can also have a trial work period.

Supplemental Security Income

Supplemental Security Income (SSI) is a federal program that was introduced in 1974. It is paid for out of general funds rather than Social Security funds, but it is administered by the same state agencies that administer the Disability Determination program. The application process is similar to that described above for Social Security Disability Insurance. Applications are filed at a local SSA office, and the same criteria are used to evaluate SSI disability claims as are used for DI claims.

Table 9.5. Impairments Qualifying a Person with *Arthritis of a Major Weight-Bearing Joint* for Medical Disability Under Social Security

Arthritis of a major weight-bearing joint (due to any cause) with history of persistent joint pain and stiffness with signs of marked limitation of motion or abnormal motion of the affected joint on current physical examination. With
A. Gross anatomic deformity of hip or knee (e.g., subluxation, contracture, bony or fibrous ankylosis, instability) supported by radiographic evidence of either significant joint space narrowing or significant bony destruction *and* markedly limiting ability to walk or stand *or*
B. Reconstructive surgery or surgical arthrodesis of a major weight-bearing joint and return to full weight-bearing status did not occur, or is not expected to occur, within 12 months of onset

From Disability Evaluation Under Social Security, 1995.

Table 9.6. Impairments Qualifying a Person with *Rheumatoid Arthritis* for Medical Disability Under Social Security

Active rheumatoid arthritis and other inflammatory arthritis. With both A and B
A. History of persistent joint pain, swelling, and tenderness involving multiple major joints (hip, knee, ankle, shoulder, elbow, or wrist/hand) *and* with signs of joint inflammation (swelling and tenderness) on current physical examination despite prescribed therapy for at least 3 months, resulting in significant restriction of function of the affected joints, and clinical activity expected to last at least 12 months
B. Corroboration of diagnosis at some point in time by either
   1. Positive serological test for rheumatoid factor *or*
   2. Antinuclear antibodies *or*
   3. Elevated sedimentation rate *or*
   4. Characteristic histologic changes in biopsy of synovial membrane or subcutaneous nodule (obtained independent of Social Security disability evaluation)

From Disability Evaluation Under Social Security, 1995.

The basic differences between SSI and Social Security benefits are as follows:

- *Eligibility.* SSI is available for two groups of people when they are not insured by social security: those under 65 who are medically disabled and all uninsured people over the age of 65. SSI for people over 65 is similar in purpose to social security retirement income. In addition to these two groups, people who have presumptive disability (claim for total disability being processed) and disabled people who are in the 5-month waiting period for their DI payments to begin may be eligible for SSI. Eligibility in all of these groups is based on need (total resources found to be below a certain defined level) and the absence of gainful employment (defined as earned monthly income of $500 or more).
- There is no waiting period. A person becomes eligible for the first SSI payment the first day of the month after he or she files a disability claim.
- In most states, people approved for SSI are also eligible for Medicaid and other social services provided by their state.
- All people receiving SSI are reviewed once each year to determine whether their income and other resources still make them eligible to receive SSI. Like DI recipients, they are reviewed every 3 or 7 years to establish whether their disability is still present (see above).

The maximal monthly income from SSI in 1997 was $484 for an individual and $726 for a couple. In 1996 there were 6.6 million recipients of SSI, on the basis of disability, blindness, and age (over 65 and without social security).

As described for DI, report of a patient's physician must be received before income support under SSI can be initiated.

VOCATIONAL REHABILITATION

State Vocational Rehabilitation agencies existed before the federal Disability Determination program was created in 1954. In many states, these agencies administer the Disability Determination program in addition to providing vocational rehabilitation services.

Eligibility

To be eligible for Vocational Rehabilitation, a person must have an impairment that interferes with his or her capacity to obtain suitable employment or that is a threat to his or her present career; this does not mean that the person has to meet the criteria for medical disability discussed earlier. The person must have a reasonable chance of being able to engage in a suitable occupation after Vocational Rehabilitation services are provided. A suitable occupation would include being a homemaker provided that Vocational Rehabilitation would enable the person to remain in his or her own home instead of requiring institutional care.

Services

The services provided by Vocational Rehabilitation agencies vary among states. However, they usually include the following:

- *A medical examination.* A complete medical examination is provided to determine the extent of a person's disability.
- *Counseling and guidance.* A trained rehabilitation counselor is assigned to guide each client through the rehabilitation process.
- *Physical aids.* Items such as artificial limbs, braces, hearing aids, eyeglasses, and wheelchairs may be provided if needed.
- *Job training.* Training for the proper job is provided when necessary. This may be given at a vocational school, college or university, or rehabilitation facility, or in the home.
- *Help with transportation expenses.*
- *Equipment and licenses.* Tools, equipment, and licenses necessary for getting started in the right job may be provided.
- *Job placement.* Placement in the right job is an important part of the rehabilitation process. The abilities of each client are carefully matched to job requirements.
- *Follow-up.* The counselor follows up on each placement to make sure that the client's job is suitable.

Physician's Role

As noted earlier, all people applying for social security disability benefits are screened for referral to Vocational Rehabilitation. For those people, the report of the patient's physician (see above) may be used by the Vocational Rehabilitation agency. For people who are not applying for medical disability, the physician is often asked to provide a general medical report for the Vocational Rehabilitation agency. An important role of physicians is to encourage patients to apply for Vocational Rehabilitation and to maintain continued interest in their progress. It has been estimated that every $1000 spent for Vocational Rehabilitation increases by $35,000 the lifetime earnings of those who are rehabilitated.

HOME HEALTH SERVICES

A consequence of illness as distressing to the patient as the loss of the ability to earn an income is the temporary or permanent loss of the ability to remain at home. Most people require acute hospital care one or more times in their adult lives, and a small proportion also require long-term institutional care. The principal objectives of home health services are to minimize the need for admission to acute or long-term care facilities and to decrease length of stay and associated costs in these facilities. Numerous studies show that these objectives are attained when home health services are used appropriately (1).

National Trends

Home health care is the sector of the health care industry that has grown the most in recent years (1). Between 1989 and 1995 the number of home care agencies grew from 11,097 to 18,874, and employment in home care rose 125%, as compared to 25% for the entire health care industry. Although total spending on home health services has grown dramatically, the average annual growth rate in the cost of home health services (the Consumer Price Index) between 1987 and 1994 was 2.0%, substantially lower than the rates for physician services (6.3%) or hospital services (9.3%).

Growth in home health initially accelerated after passage of the Omnibus Reconciliation Acts of 1980 and 1981, which increased funding for home health services by Medicare and Medicaid. Between 1980 and 1995, the number of patients served grew from about 0.9 million to approximately 3.6 million for Medicare and from about 0.4 million to approximately 1.4 million for Medicaid. More recently, cost-effectiveness initiatives from the managed care industry have further promoted home care as an alternative to hospital care.

Range of Services and Providers

Home health services provided include basic care provided by informal caregivers (family members and friends), home food services available at a nominal cost to the patient (Meals-on-Wheels), care provided by physicians or their associates who make home visits, services provided by the personnel of home health agencies, specimen collection and performance of diagnostic procedures such as radiographs and electrocardiograms by clinical laboratories, and delivery/rental by medical suppliers of infusion equipment, medications, and durable medical equipment such as hospital beds. Even when professional help is involved, most of the responsibility for carrying out care is assumed by the patient or a member of the patient's family; as noted in Chapter 1, it is the assumption of responsibility by patients and their families that most distinguishes ambulatory care from institutional care.

Overall coordination of the home care provided by home health agencies is usually provided by a nurse case manager. A substantial proportion of the care is often carried out by home health aides, analogous to nursing aides on hospital wards, under the supervision of the nurse. In recent years, nurse practitioners, enterostomal therapists, and clinical pharmacy consultants have been added to the staffs of many home health agencies, so that more sophisticated care can be provided. In addition to nursing, home care services may include physical, occupational, and speech therapy; nutritional, behavioral, and social work counseling; and mental health services. Home health agencies provide the professional services of *hospice programs* (see Chapter 19) in many communities or may have their own hospice programs. In addition, *maternal and child health programs* have been developed to respond to the needs created by rapid discharge of mothers and newborns.

In recent years, home health agencies and suppliers have added services that require skilled use of equipment traditionally used only in hospitals. These services include the administration of *intravenous therapies,* ranging from short-term normal saline and electrolyte infusions to courses of antibiotics, cancer chemotherapy, cardiac medications, and total parenteral nutrition; and the care of *ventilator-dependent patients* at home. These initiatives have emerged in response to efforts to reduce the length of costly hospitalization and to patients who prefer home care to hospital care for parenteral therapy that may have to be administered for 1 week or more. Day-to-day supervision of the overall care of patients receiving in-home parenteral therapy or ventilator support is usually not provided by the company that supplies and monitors the equipment; therefore, this responsibility is assumed by a nurse case manager who knows the physician's comprehensive plan for the patient and is in close contact with the supplier.

The types of clinical problems most commonly referred to home health agencies are listed in Table 9.7.

Criteria for Third-Party Reimbursement

Any patient or patient's family may purchase services from a home health agency. During the past 20 years, much of the cost of home care has been covered by Medicare, Medicaid, other third-party payers, and managed care organizations. The number and types of services authorized are being more tightly controlled today as part of cost-containment efforts. This has promoted the development of care guidelines and increased focus on instructing patients and family members to carry out care plans.

Of the nearly 19,000 home care agencies and hospices in the United States in 1995, about two-thirds were certified for Medicare reimbursement, and Medicare was the largest payer for home care (approximately 60% of all patients receiving home care). Pa-

Table 9.7. Problems Most Commonly Referred for Home Health Services

Postsurgical wound care (teach or provide dressing changes)
Orthopedic problems (rehabilitation after hospitalization)
Congestive heart failure (monitor for change in status, provide dietary counseling, assess medication compliance)
Diabetes (e.g., supervise insulin technique, provide dietary counseling, teach blood or urine monitoring of glucose, care of the lower extremities)
Hypertension (supervise and reinforce compliance with medication, check blood pressure response in patient's home)
Incurable cancer and AIDS (provide dietary counseling, intravenous therapies, psychological support, and other aspects of hospice care)
Stroke and other incapacitating neurologic problems (provide physical and occupational therapy)
Decubitus and stasis ulcers (teach or provide debridement and dressing changes)
Dementia in an older person living alone (assess environment for health hazards)
Chronic obstructive pulmonary disease (assess home for oxygen therapy, teach energy conservation strategies)

Table 9.8. Criteria for Third-Party Reimbursement for Home Health Services

Medicare[a]

Part A pays for all covered services (skilled nursing, home health aide, social work, physical, occupational, and speech therapy). Care must be provided by a certified home health agency and must be medically necessary. There is no limit to the number of visits, as long as the patient's condition meets criteria for services. The following conditions must be met to qualify for reimbursement:

1. Patient is confined to home.
2. Need for intermittent skilled nursing, physical therapy, or speech therapy. (One of these three services must be needed to qualify for reimbursement for the other services provided by home health agencies, i.e., social work, occupational therapy, home health aide, and nutrition services.)
3. Physician must sign renewal of orders every 60 days.

Medicaid

Coverage for home health services varies by state.

Veterans Administration

Home Care from Hospital-Based Programs

Blue Cross and Other Private Health Insurance

Coverage for home health services varies by plan.

[a] Note that since 1981, Part A Medicare has covered patients even if they have not been recently hospitalized.

tients must meet certain criteria for services to be reimbursed by Medicare and other payers (Table 9.8). Because of the Medicare criterion that the patient must have a medical problem requiring skilled care, payment for the services of a home health aide is often denied after the active problem becomes stable, even when the home health aide's services are important in maintaining the patient's health.

Physician's Role

For most home health services that are reimbursed, the patient's physician must approve and sign orders for all services and revisions of services.

The quality of the communication between physicians and home care providers often determines how much the patient will benefit from home health services. When physicians provide clear and complete initial information and both physicians and home care providers can reach each other easily when needed, patients who would otherwise require in-hospital care can receive excellent care in their homes.

The American Academy of Home Care Physicians (10480 Little Patuxent Parkway, Suite 760, Columbia, MD 21044, telephone 410-730-1623) is an organization of physicians and other home care professionals, founded in the late 1980s, that is dedicated to improving the quality of home care. The organization's newsletter and annual meeting focus on the evaluation of and education about home health care ideas and programs.

General References

Disability evaluation under Social Security. United States Department of Health and Human Services pub. no. (SSA) 05-10089, January 1995.
> Gives criteria for impairments that qualify a person for medical disability under social security (available free from local Social Security Office and State Disability Determination Service).

Rothkopf MM, ed. Standards and practice of homecare therapeutics. 6th ed. Baltimore: Williams & Wilkins, 1997.
> A practical resource for physicians who authorize home care for their patients. Contains separate chapters on each of the sophisticated modes of care now available through home health agencies.

Social Security Administration Office of Program, Policy, and Evaluation and Communications. Understanding SSI. SSA pub. no. 17-008, ICN 443175, May 1996.
> Explains all aspects of SSI. Useful for patients and providers.

Specific Reference

1. Basic statistics about home care 1996. Washington, DC: National Association for Home Care, October 1996.

Psychiatric and Behavioral Problems

CHAPTER 10

Evaluation of Psychosocial Problems

L. RANDOL BARKER, MD
CHESTER W. SCHMIDT, JR, MD

Patients with psychologic and social problems often consult their general physicians, usually complaining of not feeling well in some physical sense. The problems these patients present range from temporary distress to enduring and disabling conditions.

The temporary disturbances that are most often seen by the generalist are anxiety regarding the meaning of a new symptom (e.g., cancer fear), frustrations attending an illness that interrupts valued activities (e.g., recovery phase after myocardial infarction), or dysphoric mood related to recent social stress (e.g., anxiety in the mother of a teenager who has run away from home). Such problems are common in people with excellent previous mental health. These disturbances usually resolve when the interviewing and counseling skills discussed in Chapters 3, 4, and 11 are used in conjunction with management of the patient's medical problem.

Patients with more persistent psychosocial problems are difficult to care for unless one has a knowledge of common psychosocial syndromes and uses a systematic approach to the patient. This chapter and Chapter 11 provide general approaches for the evaluation and treatment of such patients. Later chapters cover the specific psychosocial syndromes seen by generalists.

EPIDEMIOLOGY

The Epidemiologic Catchment Area (ECA) Survey, conducted in 1980 to 1982, identified the frequency of common psychosocial syndromes in a *representative sample of American communities* (4). Table 10.1 lists the four most common disorders in major sex and age subgroups. Approximately 12% of adults reported symptoms of a diagnosable mental disorder during the past 6 months, and 25% had had a mental illness at some time in their lives. Of subjects meeting criteria for disorders other than alcohol or other drug abuse/dependence, approximately 30% had more than one disorder; of those with alcohol or drug abuse/dependence, 45 and 72%, respectively, had coexisting mental disorders (6). These figures probably underrepresent the true prevalence of mental disorders because the study instrument did not identify patients with two common syndromes, adjustment disorder and generalized anxiety disorder. More than half of those with mental illness reported that the only health care providers they saw were generalists, and of these people, the majority had not discussed their mental illness with their health care providers (2).

In American primary care settings, one in three patients has a significant psychosocial problem (3). A World Health Organization (WHO) survey of 14 countries found a similarly high rate of mental disorders in primary care patients; the rates of both occupational and physical disability were higher in patients with mental illness than in those without (5). These findings combined with the ECA community-based data point to the importance of evaluating patients for mental illness.

SYNDROMAL DIAGNOSIS

Accurate diagnosis of a psychosocial problem is essential for prognosis and management. The *Diagnostic and Statistical Manual of Mental Disorders,* fourth edition (DSM-IV), published in 1994 by the American Psychiatric Association, is a particularly useful resource because it provides diagnostic criteria, epidemiologic information, and prognostic profiles for most of the psychosocial syndromes encountered in office practice. DSM-IV criteria are stated wherever relevant in the chapters that follow.

Despite the availability of diagnostic criteria, reaching an accurate psychosocial diagnosis in general medical practice can be difficult. There are several reasons for this:

- When the presenting symptoms are somatic, physical illness must always be considered, even when the patient's presentation suggests a psychosocial problem.
- Psychosocial symptoms or findings are not often specific for one syndrome.
- The necessary information is different from that needed to evaluate a physical symptom; the most salient information is subjective, obtained by inquiring about or observing thoughts, feelings, behaviors, events, and relationships.

After initial information gathering about mental symptoms, it is usually possible to decide which general phenomenon is the dominant problem (e.g., anxiety, depression, somatization, cognitive impair-

Table 10.1.   Four Most Common Psychiatric Disorders by Sex and Age Based on 6-Month Prevalence Rates[a]

Rank	18–24 yr	25–44 yr	45–64 yr	65+ yr	Total
Men					
1	Alcohol abuse/ dependence	Alcohol abuse/ dependence	Alcohol abuse/ dependence	Severe cognitive impairment	Alcohol abuse/ dependence
2	Drug abuse/ dependence	Phobia	Phobia	Phobia	Phobia
3	Phobia	Drug abuse/ dependence	Dysthymia	Alcohol abuse/ dependence	Drug abuse/ dependence
4	Antisocial personality	Antisocial personality	Major depressive episode without grief	Dysthymia	Dysthymia
Women					
1	Phobia	Phobia	Phobia	Phobia	Phobia
2	Drug abuse/ dependence	Major depressive episode without grief	Dysthymia	Severe cognitive impairment	Major depressive episode without grief
3	Major depressive episode without grief	Dysthymia	Major depressive episode without grief	Dysthymia	Dysthymia
4	Alcohol abuse/ dependence	Obsessive– compulsive disorder	Obsessive– compulsive disorder	Major depressive episode without grief	Obsessive– compulsive disorder

From Myers JK, Weissman MM, Tischler GL, et al. Six-month prevalence of psychiatric disorders in three communities. Arch Gen Psychiatry 41:959, 1984.
[a] Dysthymia included. The basis for ranking was the mean 6-month prevalence rates for New Haven, Baltimore, and St. Louis combined.
DIS, Diagnostic Interview Schedule.

ment, or maladaptive behavior). To refine the diagnosis, additional information is needed. For example, consider a patient with a depressed mood. With a systematic approach, the diagnosis of depression may be more accurately formulated as one of the following:

- Adjustment disorder with depressed mood
- Major depression
- Dysthymic disorder (depressive neurosis)
- Depression related to a recently prescribed drug
- Alcoholism presenting as depression

INFORMATION GATHERING

The order in which information is gathered and the particular information gathered vary depending on the style one has developed with previous patients and the diagnosis being considered. With a minimal amount of prompting, many patients volunteer information that would otherwise require systematic questioning. Both the efficiency and the accuracy of the interview are probably enhanced when this occurs. Other interviewing skills useful in eliciting a psychosocial history are described in Chapter 3.

Building on the patient's initial account, one should assess relevant aspects of the social history, the patient's mental status, the patient's personality and coping styles, the chronology of the patient's problem, and the family history of psychosocial problems. With the patient's permission, additional information should be obtained from family members, other physicians, and previous medical records whenever possible. Current medications should be identified because psychologic disturbances can be caused or worsened by a large number of drugs (1). Tables in other chapters list drugs that may cause anxiety (Table 13.1),

depression (Table 15.4), psychotic symptoms (Table 16.2), delirium (Table 17.3), and sexual dysfunction (Table 18.4).

Social and Developmental History

The history should always include a profile of the patient's current life situation (e.g., marital status, family structure, household makeup, educational level, occupation, recreational activities, and substance use). At times, it is also helpful to know the principal patterns and events that have characterized a patient's development from childhood until the present (e.g., family makeup, interactions, conflicts, losses; relationships in school, the armed services, jobs) and to have patients depict their view of the type of person they are and have been. Some of this information is known already to the patient's personal physician, making the assessment of a new psychosocial problem simpler at times. When a psychosocial problem seems likely, the presenting symptom should be reexplored in the context of social interactions (e.g., "Tell me just where you were and who was there the last time you noted the nausea and quivering in your stomach"), and the patient should be asked to describe any recent changes in life situation and to discuss the nature of critical relationships (e.g., with spouse, children, and work associates). If substance abuse or domestic violence, which is often related to substance abuse, is suspected, skillful inquiry is needed to make a diagnosis (see Chapter 21 on alcoholism and domestic violence and Chapter 22 on illicit drugs).

Much psychosocial illness is related to *stressors and maladjustments* that are disclosed by the patient during this inquiry. McWhinney has summarized the social factors most commonly related to psychosocial distress (Table 10.2). The significance of a report of one of these factors becomes clear when it is integrated into the rest of the history (e.g., an interpersonal conflict may be the stressor causing an adjustment disorder or it may be a symptom of alcoholism, depression, or sexual dysfunction).

In addition to providing clues to the diagnosis, the social history usually discloses important assets and liabilities in the patient's life. This information is useful in planning treatment for a psychosocial problem.

Mental Status

When the patient's behavior is the principal problem or when psychologic symptoms are causing a great deal of subjective distress (e.g., marked anxiety or depression) or suggest a major psychiatric disorder (e.g., dementia, schizophrenia, or manic–depressive illness), a brief mental status examination should be performed.

The mental status examination is a systematic assessment of the patient's current mental functioning. The elements of the mental status examination most useful for the general physician include the following:

- *Appearance:* Grooming, attention to dress, motor activity (quiet versus agitated).
- *General level of consciousness:* Alert, sleepy, stuporous, obtunded.

Table 10.2. Common Social Factors Related to Psychologic Symptoms

Loss: (a) Personal loss—loss of a loved one through death or desertion. *(b)* Loss of things—imposed loss of home, cherished possession, or job.
Conflict: (a) Interpersonal—conflict within family, with neighbors, or at work, where hostility is recognized. *(b)* Intrapersonal—role conflict or conflicting demands on the patient (as in a working mother).
Change: (a) Development—where time of life is the major problem (as in adolescence, menopause, or senescence).
(b) Geographic—where a move to an unfamiliar environment is the major problem (as in immigration).[a]
Maladjustment: (a) Interpersonal—problems between people with no overt conflict (as in failure to achieve a satisfactory sexual relationship without hostility between partners). *(b)* Personal—failure to adjust to the environment (home or job) in the absence of the above-mentioned loss, conflict, or change.
Stress: (a) Acute—unexpected event not covered under loss, conflict, or change (for example, the sudden illness of self or of a family member or friend). *(b)* Chronic—long-term situation not included in loss, conflict, or change (e.g., the presence of a handicapped child in the family).
Isolation—not from any recent loss, change, or conflict (as in an elderly widow).
Failure or frustrated expectations—when the patient's goals in life are not fulfilled and when there is no evidence of an intervening event covered by loss, conflict, or change (e.g., failure at school or failure to achieve occupational promotion).

From McWhinney IR. Beyond diagnosis: an approach to the integration of behavioral science and clinical medicine. N Engl J Med 287:384, 1972.
[a] See Table 1.7 (shows developmental challenges at each stage in family life cycle).

- *Orientation:* The patient knows who he or she is, where he or she is, and the date (day, month, and year).
- *Speech:* Ability to use customary syntax. Note slurring, inability to find the right word, pressured speech, flight of ideas, looseness of association, muteness.
- *Memory:* Recent memory, or knowledge of recent events, capacity to remember names of current treating physicians. Remote memory, or ability to give history and present illness in proper historical sequence.
- *Attention and concentration:* Ability to understand and follow questions or instructions.
- *Intelligence:* Can be estimated from level of schooling achieved, vocational history, use of language.
- *Mood:* A pervasive, sustained emotion described by the patient (depressed, euphoric, neutral).
- *Affect:* An observable and immediately expressed emotion (e.g., anger, anxiety, sadness, fear, humor, lability). Note whether display of affect is consistent with the content of speech, thoughts, and behavior.
- *Perceptions:* Presence of hallucinations (i.e., visual, auditory, or somatic perception occurring in the absence of appropriate external stimuli), delusions (i.e., fixed beliefs that are false), paranoid ideas, or persistent phobias (i.e., fears directed toward specific objects or situations).
- *Suicidal thoughts:* Statement or actions that indicate the patient wishes to harm or kill himself or herself.
- *Homicidal or violent thoughts:* Statements or actions that indicate patient wishes to harm or kill others.
- *Judgment:* Capacity to understand one's current situation or to demonstrate appropriate compliance with instructions for care.

Most of the data needed for a brief mental status examination are observable while the patient gives the history. Depending on the cues the patient provides, he or she should be questioned more about his or her mental status and other features of the syndromes suggested by the history. For patients whose mental status suggests focal or global cognitive impairment, a more formal cognitive examination can be administered in a few minutes (see Mini-Mental Status Examination, Table 17.1). For those who describe cardinal symptoms of anxiety, affective, or psychotic disorders, focused interviewing is necessary (see Chapters 13, 15, and 16, respectively).

Personality

Personality is the enduring attitudes and patterns of behavior that typify an individual. Generally a physician becomes acquainted with a patient's personality, particularly the patient's behavior pattern in the face of illness, through caring for that patient during months or years. Some patients exhibit the features of a maladaptive personality, and recognition of this may be helpful in planning the patient's care, as discussed in more detail in Chapter 14.

Coping Responses

Coping responses are behaviors that people assume in adapting to life stresses. There are several common coping responses that should be recognized because patients may use them to avoid confronting a problem for which help is needed. When maladaptive coping is recognized, the physician can often help the patient to disclose the primary problem and to reach a healthier adaptation to it.

Denial is a common response by which a distressing problem is avoided. Denial may be silent (i.e., a patient with bloody stools may withhold this information to avoid confronting the fear of cancer) or it may be voiced openly (e.g., a man who greatly fears sudden death during convalescence from a myocardial infarction may boast of robust health and deny angina or other symptoms he is experiencing).

Rationalization serves the same function as denial. It is a process in which a patient gives plausible explanations for behavior designed to avoid unpleasant realities (e.g., a relapsing alcoholic explains that the demands at work increased so much lately that it was impossible to continue to go to Alcoholics Anonymous meetings).

Regression is reversion to dependent behavior typical of childhood. Regressive behavior is a common response to major illness or other circumstances that threaten a person's autonomy (e.g., a man who is recovering slowly from a hip fracture complains excessively about small problems at home, gets upset when his son cannot continue to visit daily, and expects his wife to order for him when they go out to a restaurant on the weekend).

Projection is a process in which an unpleasant aspect of one's self is ascribed to another person (e.g., a teenager who is angry about limits set by her mother criticizes her older sister for being hostile to their mother).

Displacement is a process in which feelings toward one person are directed toward another (i.e., a researcher who is furious at a colleague who has beaten him to an important finding becomes irritable toward his wife for no apparent reason).

Chronology

Accurate information about the chronology of a psychosocial problem is important for diagnosis, prognosis, and management. Therefore, as the interview is closing, one should ensure that the patient has provided the following essential information: duration of the present episode, the times and circumstances during which the current symptoms have either improved or worsened (if temporal relationships are unclear, it is helpful to have the patient keep a log of symptoms and events for 1 week or more), the patient's optimal level of functioning during the past year (when was it and how long did it last?), and the time and circumstances of any previous episode of similar symptoms or of previous mental illness.

Family History

In the family of a patient with a chronic psychosocial disorder, occurrence in others of the same disorder or other psychiatric problems is common. Information about psychiatric illness in the family may strengthen one's diagnostic hunches and may help the patient to recognize the nature of his or her own problem.

OVERALL FORMULATION OF THE PROBLEM

When the essentials of a patient's psychosocial history have been collected, a useful way to formulate the problem is the five-axis approach recommended by the American Psychiatric Association.

- *Axis I.* Psychosocial syndromes, plus conditions not attributable to a formal mental disorder that are a focus of attention (e.g., psychologic factors affecting medical condition, malingering, uncomplicated bereavement, noncompliance with medical treatment, or academic or occupational problems)
- *Axis II.* Personality disorders or styles and specific developmental disorders
- *Axis III.* General medical conditions
- *Axis IV.* Psychologic and environmental problems (see categories in Table 10.3)
- *Axis V.* Global Assessment of Functioning: current level and highest level for at least a few months during the past year (Table 10.4)

CASE STUDY

Mr. J, a 60-year-old married security guard, underwent coronary artery bypass graft (CABG) surgery in January 1993. His postoperative hospital course was uneventful. Shortly after discharge, he came twice in the same day to the emergency department complaining of severe chest pain and cold upper extremities. Evaluation revealed mild tenderness at the location of his sternotomy scar. The next day he returned, this time describing inability to sleep in addition to the previous symptoms. A thorough evaluation, including an exercise stress test, did not disclose a physical basis for his symptoms.

The patient's wife described regressive behavior since the patient returned home (e.g., he wanted her to bring his meals to him in bed, asked her to pick his clothes for him each day, was having occasional urinary incontinence, and had put her in charge of dispensing all of his medicines). He was not sleeping well and awakened his wife whenever he could not sleep. Additional inquiry and observation revealed a somewhat diminished sense of self-worth and some doubts

Table 10.3. Axis IV: Categories for Psychosocial and Environmental Problems

Problems with primary support group
Problems related to the social environment
Educational problem
Occupational problem
Housing problem
Economic problem
Problems with access to health care services
Problems related to interaction with the legal system/crime
Other psychosocial problem

Reprinted with permission from the DSM-IV. Copyright 1994, American Psychiatric Association.

Table 10.4. Global Assessment of Functioning (GAF) Scale

Consider psychologic, social, and occupational functioning on a hypothetical continuum of mental health–illness. Do not include impairment in functioning caused by physical (or environmental) limitations.

Code	
100	Superior functioning in a wide range of activities, life's problems never seem to get out of hand, is sought out by others because of his or her many positive qualities. No symptoms.
91	
90	Absent or minimal symptoms (e.g., mild anxiety before an exam), good functioning in all areas, interested and involved in a wide range of activities, socially effective, generally satisfied with life, no more than everyday problems or concerns (e.g., an occasional argument with family members).
81	
80	If symptoms are present, they are transient and expectable reactions to psychosocial stressors (e.g., difficulty concentrating after family argument); no more than slight impairment in social, occupational, or school functioning (e.g., temporarily falling behind in schoolwork).
71	
70	Some mild symptoms (e.g., depressed mood and mild insomnia) OR some difficulty in social, occupational, or school functioning (e.g., occasional truancy, or theft within the household), but generally functioning pretty well, has some meaningful interpersonal relationships.
61	
60	Moderate symptoms (e.g., flat affect and circumstantial speech, occasional panic attacks) OR moderate difficulty in social, occupational, or school functioning (e.g., no friends, unable to keep a job).
51	
50	Serious symptoms (e.g., suicidal ideation, severe obsessional rituals, frequent shoplifting) OR any serious impairment in social, occupational, or school functioning (e.g., no friends, unable to keep a job).
41	
40	Some impairment in reality testing or communication (e.g., speech is at times illogical, obscure, or irrelevant) OR major impairment in several areas, such as work or school, family relations, judgment, thinking, or mood (e.g., depressed man avoids friends, neglects family, and is unable to work; child frequently beats up younger children, is defiant at home, and is failing at school).
31	
30	Behavior is considerably influenced by delusions or hallucinations OR serious impairment in communication or judgment (e.g., sometimes incoherent, acts grossly inappropriately, suicidal preoccupation) OR inability to function in almost all areas (e.g., stays in bed all day; no job, home, or friends).
21	
20	Some danger of hurting self or others (e.g., suicide attempts without clear expectation of death, frequently violent, manic excitement) OR occasionally fails to maintain minimal personal hygiene (e.g., smears feces) OR gross impairment in communication (e.g., largely incoherent or mute).
11	
10	Persistent danger of severely hurting self or others (e.g., recurrent violence) OR persistent inability to maintain minimal personal hygiene OR serious suicidal act with clear expectation of death.
1	
0	Inadequate information.

Reprinted with permission from the DSM-IV. Copyright 1994, American Psychiatric Association.

regarding his future. He was worried specifically that he would not return to work, as he had expected to preoperatively, and his calculations suggested that his income would be significantly lower if he applied for social security benefits.

The patient eventually disclosed that he was sure that he had been on the pump too long and that he feared that his incision would break down (this had happened to a friend after CABG).

Mr. J had always seemed to be a self-reliant man. He had worked as a security guard, on medical therapy for his angina, for several years. The CABG was recommended when his angina worsened in November 1992, making it difficult for him to walk the distances required at his job. He had never developed markedly regressive behavior in the past, although he had depended on his wife to make decisions about almost all purchases they made, had never been separated from her for a full day during their long and tranquil marriage, and often referred to her as "Mother." There was no history of significant psychiatric illness in his family.

Based on this story and additional inquiry, the formulation of Mr. J's illness was

- *Axis I.* Adjustment disorder, with depressed mood and physical complaints
- *Axis II.* No personality disorder; history of dependency that made him vulnerable to the behavior he exhibited after CABG
- *Axis III.* (a) Coronary artery disease; (b) status post-coronary artery bypass graft, with good technical result
- *Axis IV.* Economic problems
- *Axis V.* Global Assessment of Functioning (GAF): Current GAF = moderate symptoms and functional impairment (Code 60 in Table 10.4); past year GAF = slight symptoms and functional impairment (Code 80 in Table 10.4)

COMORBIDITY IN THE PATIENT'S FAMILY

Psychosocial problems create substantial stress for the spouse, children, and other people with close ties to the affected patient. This is particularly true of chronic problems such as alcoholism, affective disorders, anxiety disorders, and the somatoform disorders. The impact of the patient's illness on others should always be considered in the evaluation of psychosocial problems. As pointed out in other chapters in this section, there are important ways in which the comorbidity of the family can be alleviated as part of the overall approach to these trying problems. Chapter 3 describes how to conduct a family meeting around a specific problem, and Chapter 11 describes the process for formal family counseling.

ASSESSMENT OF COMPETENCE, DECISION-MAKING CAPACITY, NEED FOR COMMITMENT

The three situations covered here require input by a physician or multiple physicians who know or have examined a patient. A physician assesses the patient's competence and decision-making capacity implicitly at every medical encounter. At times, assessment of these must be done explicitly.

Competence and *incompetence* are legal terms, and

generally their use should be restricted to situations in which a formal determination has been made. Under the law, people are presumed competent to manage their own affairs until a judicial determination has been made. A physician may be called upon to provide evidence to be used in such a determination. Common civil issues that require determination of mental competence include competence to accept or refuse medical care, commitment to hospitals, contesting of wills, and guardianship decisions. In the ambulatory setting, perhaps the most common problem presented by marginally competent patients is unreliable self-care; here, the assistance of a reliable household member or visiting nurse is essential, in addition to the measures needed to obtain a legal decision about competence.

Decision-making capacity is a clinical term referring to the capacity of the patient to make a particular decision. It is also called *clinical competency.* Judgments regarding such capacity are made by clinicians every day, particularly when informed consent is sought for performing medical procedures. Decision-making capacity is said to be present when the patient demonstrates the following:

- Capacity to comprehend information relevant to the decision
- Capacity to deliberate about the choices in accordance with personal values and goals
- Capacity to communicate (verbally or nonverbally) with caregivers

Patients may have the capacity to make one decision (e.g., to assign power of attorney to a relative) but not another (e.g., to decide whether to undergo an experimental surgical procedure), so decision-making capacity must be addressed each time a decision is required. The presence of a psychiatric or neurologic disorder does not necessarily imply incapacity. Although patients who are demented, delirious, delusional, or hallucinating often lack decision-making capacity, they may actually be able to make some decisions themselves. Therefore, they require the same assessment as patients without these disorders or symptoms.

Commitment laws in most states require examination by a physician and do not specify examination by a psychiatrist. Therefore, the patient's primary physician is occasionally required to assist in a commitment determination. A complete psychiatric evaluation, including a complete mental status examination, is necessary to determine whether the patient is dangerous to himself or herself or to others, which is the usual test for commitment.

General References*

American Psychiatric Association. **Diagnostic and Statistical Manual of Mental Disorders.** 4th ed. (DSM-IV). Washington, DC: American Psychiatric Association, 1994.
> Diagnostic criteria and epidemiologic information for all recognized psychiatric disorders.

Cadoret RJ. Chapter 2. In: Cadoret RJ, King LJ, eds. Psychiatry in primary care. St. Louis: CV Mosby, 1983.
> Chapter 2 covers in greater depth the approaches to evaluation by the generalist that are described in this chapter.

Michels R, Marzuk PM. Progress in psychiatry. N Engl J Med 329:552, 628, 1993.
> Two-part extensively referenced review of epidemiology, diagnosis, and management of common mental disorders.

Specific References

1. Drugs that cause psychiatric symptoms. Med Lett 40:21, 1998.
2. Ford DE, Kamerow DB, Thompson JW. Who talks to physicians about mental health and substance abuse problems? J Gen Intern Med 3:363, 1988.
3. Houpt JL, Orleans CS, George LK, et al, eds. The importance of mental health services to general health care. Cambridge, MA: Ballinger, 1979.
4. Myers JK, Weissman MM, Tischler GL, et al. Six-month prevalence of psychiatric disorders in three communities. Arch Gen Psychiatry 41:959, 1984.
5. Ormel J, VonKorff M, Ustun B, et al. Common mental disorders and disability across cultures: results from the WHO collaborative study on psychological problems in general health care. JAMA 272:1741–1748, 1994.
6. Regier DA, Farmer ME, Rae DS, et al. Comorbidity of mental disorders with alcohol and other drug abuse; results from the Epidemiologic Catchment Area (ECA) study. JAMA 264:2511, 1990.

---

*Bold print (general references) and bold numerals (specific references) denote published controlled clinical trials, meta-analyses, or consensus-based recommendations.

CHAPTER 11

Psychotherapy in Ambulatory Practice

ROBERT P. ROCA, MD, MPH
L. RANDOL BARKER, MD

Psychotherapy consists of verbal and behavioral processes that are used for the purpose of relieving symptoms and resolving intrapersonal and interpersonal conflicts. Although many different techniques have been described, there are fundamental principles that are common to all. Generalist physicians have many opportunities to use psychotherapy, both formally and informally.

GENERAL PRINCIPLES
Demoralization

Most candidates for office psychotherapy suffer from demoralization, a painful sense of disappointment and personal inadequacy in the face of life circumstances. By the time such patients acknowledge their distress to the doctor, their usual problem-solving methods have failed and their usual sources of support have been exhausted. Demoralization can usually be formulated as the product of *interactions between environmental stressors and personal vulnerabilities.* Environmental stressors may be remediable (e.g., temporary unemployment) or irremediable (e.g., conjugal bereavement). Personal vulnerabilities may be constitutional (e.g., mental retardation) or learned (e.g., excessive dependency or perfectionism). Particular personal vulnerabilities make individuals susceptible to particular stressors. For example, an exceedingly dependent person may be especially sensitive to the death of a spouse; rigid, controlling parents may be especially distressed by the rebelliousness of their adolescent children.

Psychotherapy may be viewed as an interactive process intended to restore morale. It involves both cognitive and relational tasks. The primary *cognitive task* is to develop a working formulation of patients' difficulties as products of environmental stressors and personal vulnerabilities, to appreciate the personal strengths and resources available to patients for problem solving and amelioration of emotional distress, and to help patients apply these strengths and resources to regain a sense of mastery over life problems. Some strategies useful for these purposes are described in later sections of this chapter ("Psychosocial Treatment Techniques" and "Forms of Counseling").

The *relational task* is to promote in patients what Jerome Frank has called expectant trust (see "General References"). This describes an attitude on the part of patients that their physician cares about them, is competent to help, is confident of their recovery, and is committed to remain available until relief is obtained. Expectant trust is an important element in psychotherapeutic success and is enhanced by several of the techniques described in this chapter. Its effective mobilization also requires an understanding of the concepts of transference and countertransference.

Transference

Patients' expectations of their doctors have complex psychosocial roots. In part, they grow out of patients' experiences with their parents in circumstances of fear, pain, and other forms of distress. As a result of these experiences, patients consciously and unconsciously may come to expect that new people in their lives, particularly caretakers such as physicians, will treat them as their parents did. These expectations are known as transference phenomena: *patients transfer expectations onto their physicians.* When the transferred expectations are positive (positive transference), physicians have at their disposal a powerful resource in their work to help their patients feel better. Positive transference may partly explain placebo responses and must be borne in mind when the effects of new therapeutic interventions are being evaluated.

Not all transference phenomena are positive. Everyone experiences anger, frustration, and other painful emotions in response to the disappointments and deprivations that invariably accompany growing up. These experiences sometimes leave psychologic scars that may contaminate the relationship of the patient with caretakers or authority figures such as physicians. For example, patients who were abandoned by their parents may unconsciously expect that their physician will also abandon them and may therefore cling to the doctor with pathologic dependency. Other sorts of early life experiences may lead to passivity, hostility, compulsiveness, and other maladaptive responses.

Thus negative expectations (negative transference), as well as positive expectations, may be transferred onto physicians and may give rise to maladaptive reactions that complicate the physician–patient relationship and interfere with therapeutic success if not properly managed.

In psychotherapy, transference phenomena are regarded as tools and opportunities as well as potential obstacles. Psychologic distress is often the result of interpersonal problems with family, friends, and associates. Transference phenomena create, in the presence of the psychotherapist, modified but reasonably accurate representations of patients' current and past relationships. As patients, through transference, begin to treat the therapist as a significant person from the past, the therapist gains valuable insight into the roots of patients' interpersonal difficulties and may ultimately use these insights to help patients improve their relationships.

The type and intensity of the transference and the opportunities for its use in treatment vary with the intensity of the therapeutic relationship and the frequency of visits. In short-term counseling, intense therapeutic relationships generally do not develop, and the transference is predominantly positive.

Countertransference

Physicians, like their patients, must endure the trials and tribulations of childhood and adolescence and may thereby develop positive and negative *expectations that are transferred onto other people, including their patients.* These expectations, called countertransference, may compromise the ability of the physician to care for particular patients. For example, the physician son of an abusive alcoholic father may have such a personal emotional stake in promoting the abstinence of his male alcoholic patients that he becomes enraged and ineffective with them when they relapse. It is the responsibility of the physician to be aware of countertransference phenomena and to prevent their intrusion into the doctor–patient relationship, particularly in the context of counseling. The physician may find psychotherapy helpful for this purpose.

PSYCHOSOCIAL TREATMENT TECHNIQUES

Because the simple disclosure of emotional distress and its causes may bring considerable relief to patients, the process of psychosocial evaluation often has therapeutic value in itself. General aspects of evaluation for psychosocial problems are described in Chapter 10. This section describes the principal techniques used in counseling, and the following section describes the forms of planned counseling useful in office practice.

Establishing a Therapeutic Relationship

As noted above (see "Transference"), the therapeutic relationship recapitulates to some extent the parent–child relationship. Several elements are generic to an effective therapeutic relationship. The patient must trust the physician. Trust is promoted by showing interest consistently, accepting sensitive information without being judgmental, taking the patient's concerns seriously, and controlling inappropriate reactions to difficult patients (see Table 3.7). In addition to establishing trust, physicians should ensure that their patients understand how to gain access to them and recognize limits regarding access during ongoing treatment. It is useful to reflect on whether these trust-promoting and condition-setting actions have been accomplished before embarking on counseling.

Identifying and Addressing Information Needs

Misinformation or lack of information causes much emotional distress. Fear of dread illness, misunderstanding of an established condition, or conviction that one's symptoms must be caused by physical illness are common forms of misinformation that patients bring to office visits. Through skillful interviewing, the physician can usually help patients identify and clarify their information needs. The next step is providing information tailored to the patient's needs and confirming that it has been received. Clear explanations of normal physiology, disease processes, treatment regimens, and so on are often overlooked as powerful aids in counseling. Besides imparting knowledge, such explanations draw patients into collaborative relationships with their physicians. Depending on the problem, other counseling techniques may be as important as or more important than this first step, particularly when somatic complaints are caused by a psychosocial problem.

The following interventions are often therapeutic in themselves:

- Identification/clarification regarding *feared or existing physical disorder.* For example,

  The son of a recently deceased diabetic patient thinks he also has diabetes and receives reassurance and advice after a negative workup for diabetes.
  A woman with mitral valve prolapse who has adopted inappropriate activity limitations receives reassurance regarding the benign course of her condition and assurance that she can resume valued activities that she has curtailed. The American Heart Association booklet *Mitral Valve Prolapse* is given to her; it reinforces what her physician has said.

- Identification/clarification regarding a *psychophysiologic basis for somatic symptoms.* For example,

  A man with panic disorder obtains partial relief from an explanation of how hyperventilation leads to central nervous system symptoms.

- Identification/clarification of the *role of a psychosocial stressor in producing symptoms.* For example,

  A man with an adjustment disorder, with anxious mood, recognizes the role of his impending job layoff in precipitating his symptoms; his and his family's fear that he is going crazy is alleviated.

- Identification of a working *diagnosis, the plan, and the likely prognosis.* For example,

A woman with the syndrome of major depression develops some hopefulness when she is told the diagnosis, the plan to use gradually increasing doses of antidepressants, and the likelihood of significant improvement after a few weeks. A man with the syndrome of hypochondriasis is not given the name of his syndrome, but he reaches a truce with his physician after being informed that he will probably continue to have some symptoms but that he can engage in valued activities that he has curtailed.

Eliciting and Responding to Feelings

The discomfort of psychosocial illness is often caused by the feelings the patient is experiencing. The fundamental ways in which one can help the patient deal with feelings are through empathic listening and by allowing the patient to vent feelings in the office.

Empathic Listening

Patients find it reassuring when physicians pay close attention to what they are saying and to the feelings that they are showing. Granting the patient time to reflect, remembering details of the history, responding with appropriate affect to situations described by the patient, and indicating what one has observed or heard about the patient's feelings are actions that demonstrate concern, diminish the isolation that accompanies unexpressed feelings, and enhance the patient's self-esteem. For example,

A man with generalized anxiety disorder feels better after a visit to his physician at which the physician listens attentively, summarizes what the patient has said, and tells him that he understands how distressing it must be to have tension headaches and difficulty concentrating on his work when he is plagued by worries.

Legitimizing Feelings

Patients often feel embarrassed or isolated by their reactions to a situation. One way to help alleviate those feelings is to point out that anyone in the patient's situation might have similar reactions. For example,

A college professor who is confronting surgery for breast cancer describes constant anger since this problem came up; she was preparing to move to another city when she discovered the lump in her breast. She says that it helped when her physician acknowledged the anger and stated, "This anger that upsets you so is very understandable. Anyone in your situation would feel the same way."

Ventilation of Feelings

Patients who do not share strong feelings about past or current experiences usually feel better after releasing their pent-up emotions. An outpouring of emotion can be elicited sometimes by stating that the patient looks tense, angry, or depressed or by commenting that the experience that the patient has just described must have made the patient feel upset. Encouraging patients to express feelings may loosen their defenses just enough to allow the ventilation to take place. For example,

A middle-aged woman with chronic depression (dysthymic disorder) always feels better temporarily when she cries in the presence of her physician about her feelings of guilt caused by the anger she develops toward members of her family in her week-to-week life.

Problem Solving

Demonstrating Respect and Facilitating Choice

When counseling a patient, one should avoid acting as a powerful, all-knowing figure. As noted earlier (under "Demoralization"), patients often attempt to resolve their problems before seeking professional help. Furthermore, they may describe themselves as usually able to handle problems. Inquiring about and acknowledging previous efforts, even when they have been inept or unsuccessful, and supporting any voiced characterization of themselves as problem solvers, can help ready patients for addressing a current problem. The fundamental strategies for facilitated problem solving then become to help the patient recognize assets (e.g., supportive people, enjoyed activities) and to help the patient identify options and make choices that favor resolution of current problems. It is occasionally necessary to be more directive.

Contingency Planning

The life situations that create stress for patients are often manageable even after slight changes. Distressed patients often cannot see a means of making these changes. Once the particular facts of a patient's dilemma are known, the physician and the patient can consider concrete plans for dealing with specific problems that may arise in the days or weeks ahead. In making contingency plans, it is useful to present hypothetical situations and to have the patient decide how to handle them. For example,

A woman who lives alone is distraught because her only child, a grown daughter who recently moved to another city, has hinted that she may not be able to get home for Christmas. The woman's physician encourages her to make another plan for Christmas rather than face the prospect of being alone. She telephones later in the week to say that she still does not know whether her daughter will be able to come for Christmas; however, she has invited several friends to have Christmas dinner (contingency plan) with her and feels much better.

Advice (Persuasion)

The physician is considered by the patient to be an expert and should judiciously exercise that expertise. Concrete recommendations may be helpful for patients who are upset and temporarily unable to use their own coping skills. The physician's advice provides patients with something to hang onto until they can make decisions themselves. For example,

A middle-aged man with major depression who is beginning to improve is tactfully dissuaded from entering a doctoral program that is known to be particularly demanding. (This example makes the point that stressful life changes should be discouraged during recovery from a major depressive illness.)

Advice may also be used in a confrontational manner, forcing patients to face the fact that they are engaging in dangerous or destructive behavior. The shock of the confrontation may pierce their complacency and facilitate behavioral change.

Managing Abnormal Illness Behavior

Abnormal illness behavior is present when the patient's symptoms or impairments or actions (i.e., illness) are disproportionate to detectable disease. Patients with somatoform disorders (see Chapter 12) express their distress mainly in terms of somatic complaints or dreaded conditions; patients with other psychosocial problems also do so at times. The following general strategies are useful in patients whose psychosocial problems present mainly as abnormal illness behavior:

1. *Do not facilitate or reinforce abnormal illness behavior.*
   a. Avoid unnecessary testing.
   b. Avoid unnecessary prescribing.
   c. Avoid unnecessary referral to specialists.
   d. Schedule regular visits (i.e., do not make visits contingent on a new or worsening symptom) and stay within a time frame agreed upon for visits.
2. *Permit the patient to have some symptoms* (do not view elimination of symptoms as an essential goal).
3. *Encourage the patient to talk about his or her life situation instead of about somatic symptoms.*

EXAMPLE

A patient with somatization disorder (see Chapter 12) and an unremarkable recent urinalysis states that she plans to see the urologist who took care of her friend's bladder problem and is persuaded to come for brief weekly visits to her primary physician instead. At the weekly visits, the physician focuses chiefly on the patient's efforts to keep her teenage daughter in school and commends her for any success that she reports in handling these and other domestic problems.

Involving Family, Friends, and Environment

Family members, close friends, and the environment may be valuable resources in the care of patients. When including family members and others in the care of a patient, there is a risk of disclosing confidential information about the patient. The best way to limit this risk is to obtain the patient's permission to speak with others or, when appropriate, to include the patient in meetings with family members (see scheme in Table 3.1 for conducting a family meeting). The following are common interventions that may enhance the usefulness of these meetings.

- *Meeting the family's information needs.* The family and close friends of a patient with a psychosocial problem often suffer much because of the patient's illness. They often have the same kinds information needs as the patient (see above). If they are to understand the patient's feelings and behavior and to handle appropriately their own feelings and behavior toward the patient, these needs must be addressed. For example,

A 70-year-old man who has a major depression tells his physician that his son will probably telephone the physician to ask for information. The son telephones his father's physician and says that he is very concerned. He reports that his father has been angrily criticizing his young grandchildren for all kinds of petty reasons and that this is not the way he used to treat the children. Furthermore, the son is worried that his father must have an ulcer because he leaves the table rubbing his stomach and shaking his head after eating a few bites of each meal. The physician empathizes with the patient's son and explains that the behavior change is typical for a depressed man, that the antidepressant medication that has just been started should lead to some improvement within 2 to 3 weeks, that the history and physical examination did not reveal evidence for anything like an ulcer, and that it is likely that his father will recover entirely within 2 to 4 months. The son voices a mix of relief and tentative hope that things will go the way the physician predicts.

- *Enlisting the family's help.* For some conditions in which the patient demonstrates a failure to make choices favoring improvement, the family may be instrumental in promoting such choices. For example,

The family of an alcoholic patient agrees to participate in a family intervention (see Chapter 21) to get the patient to accept treatment.

- *Facilitating healthy choices regarding the patient's environment.* For example,

The mood of a woman with a long-standing depression (dysthymic disorder) improves after she is encouraged to take a job as a companion and housekeeper for an elderly woman who had a stroke.

Knowing and Using Community Resources

Support groups, recreational or vocational programs, and home health services are among the community resources that may help patients with psychosocial problems. A physician's awareness of and enthusiasm about a community resource can be instrumental in determining its impact on a patient. For example,

The depressed and anxious wife of an alcoholic man experiences marked improvement in her symptoms after she has been active in Al-Anon, a resource suggested by her physician.

An elderly woman joins a geriatric day-care program, which provides supervision and activity for her 5 days a week. This resource, which was suggested by her physician, enables the patient's family to continue to have her live with them and alleviates the patient's feelings of anger and guilt toward family members who felt compelled to check on her frequently during the day.

FORMS OF COUNSELING

The treatment techniques described earlier in this chapter help at times in the care of all patients. Several forms of planned counseling, each of which integrates a number of these treatment techniques, are helpful in the care of selected patients.

Supportive Therapy

The purpose of supportive therapy is to help a patient cope with both ongoing medical problems and stressful life circumstances. Unlike short-term counseling (see next section), the duration of supportive therapy is open ended, and it is often incorporated into the routine management of a chronic disease. Patients should participate in the decision about the frequency of visits and, in so doing, make a contribution at least to that portion of the treatment contract.

EXAMPLE: SUPPORTIVE THERAPY

A physician decides that this form of psychotherapy will be helpful in the long-term treatment of a diabetic patient with a history of poor compliance and multiple family problems. The patient is seen once a month for 20 minutes. The purposes for the sessions are the following:

- To monitor the patient's diabetes
- To enhance compliance
- To review family problems

The verbal exchange between the physician and the patient during the visit consists of a review of the medical regimen and glucose monitoring, check for new symptoms, brief review of what has occurred in the patient's life since the last visit, elicitation and acknowledgment of feelings, and discussion of ways to cope with existing family problems. In this manner, a significant supportive service is provided in the context of management of the patient's chronic disease.

Short-Term Counseling

This form of intervention is especially useful in the treatment of the patient who accepts a psychologic formulation for symptoms and who wants help in resolving a crisis related to those symptoms. The goals of treatment are to strengthen the defenses of the patient and to relieve symptoms without uncovering long-standing intrapsychic conflicts underlying the current problem.

It is usually important at the outset of counseling to establish a *therapeutic contract,* specifying the purpose, length, frequency, and cost of the sessions. These details form the boundaries within which the treatment will take place and may become significant during the course of treatment. Patients often react to the boundaries as part of the transference phenomenon (described above) by objecting to them or by attempting to change or violate them. Although there are exceptions, the boundaries should not be modified because of a change in the relationship between the patient and the physician that arises as a result of transference. The contractual agreements should remain stable throughout the course of treatment.

The exigencies of practice usually require that sessions be brief (15 to 20 minutes) and limited in number (5 to 10). The short-term nature of treatment helps limit the emergence of negative transference reactions and inappropriate dependency. Patients are usually seen individually, although at times couples and families may be treated together (see also "Family Counseling," below). The aim of such short-term treatment is restoration of morale and relief of emotional distress, not personality change. Treatment should focus on problems that are conscious (i.e., readily accessible, not repressed) and current; one should gently divert patients from repeated recitations of past experiences and injuries. The interactive style should be natural and conversational rather than remote and analytical and should be tailored to enhance expectant trust (see above). When appropriate, one should point out that the patient's emotional state is an understandable and valid reaction to difficult life circumstances and then, having validated the feelings of distress, express confidence that they will improve. The physician's role is to facilitate problem solving, usually not to prescribe solutions. To promote problem solving, one should be prepared to help patients identify their strengths and resources, praise their demonstrations of adaptiveness, and help them explore how they might build on their strengths to solve problems. Patients should be encouraged to try options identified in the sessions by means of homework assignments carried out between sessions.

Throughout the course of short-term counseling, it is important to listen for or screen for evidence of a complicating major psychiatric disorder, such as panic disorder, major depression, or alcoholism, because in these conditions psychotherapy may need to be supplemented by pharmacotherapy or other interventions (see Chapters 13, 15, and 21).

EXAMPLE: SHORT-TERM COUNSELING

A 25-year-old woman came for evaluation because of severe leg pain. She had suffered a severe burn injury 1 year before and had experienced leg pain intermittently since then. The physician commented that she appeared tired and tense. At this, she became tearful and said that she and her husband had separated and that, although she felt this was for the best, she was extremely anxious and uncertain that she could manage on her own. She had frightened herself during the previous week by thinking that she might be better off dead.

The history revealed that she was not suicidal and did not meet criteria for major depression or panic disorder. The physician viewed the patient as demoralized and sought to identify the pertinent personal vulnerabilities and environmental stressors. On the basis of a long relationship, the physician knew the patient to be a quiet, self-conscious woman who depended on attractiveness as a source of self-esteem. She was also ambitious and hard working and had enjoyed considerable occupational success. Her major stressor had been the burn injury. She had been spared facial disfigurement but had considerable scarring on her trunk and lower extremities, which she kept covered at all times. Another stressor was the dissolution of her marriage. She regarded this as a positive development, yet she became tearful when discussing it. When the physician pointed this out, she revealed that she was apprehensive about dating again. She felt certain that the scarring from her burns would make her unattractive to men and that she would therefore remain alone, unable to remarry and have children.

The physician responded that her distress was very understandable in view of the problems she had identified, especially her fears of future loneliness. The physician also told her that these fears might be premature and needed to be examined and proposed meeting weekly for five visits, 20 minutes each, to talk about her choices and assumptions. She agreed.

During the next session she complained about her dissolving marriage. After 5 to 10 minutes the physician praised her for having stuck with it as long as she had and for managing to hold a demanding job so successfully at the same time. She then spoke of compliments given her by coworkers, one of whom had always paid special attention to her. She was grateful for this now but insisted that no one would take an interest in her if he knew of her injuries. The physician asked her how she knew this, reiterated the position that her assumptions warranted exploration, and asked how she might comfortably undertake this. She considered some options and over the course of several weeks tried several, initially simply discussing her injury with others to assess people's responses to the news of her injuries and finally allowing some friends to see her scarring. The physician praised her for her courage as she proceeded with these explorations and empathized with her as she dealt with feelings generated by recalling the accident and risking rejection by testing people's responses to her.

By the end of the allotted 5 weeks, she was no longer convinced that the future was hopeless. Although still anxious about the ongoing separation and her potential opportunity to date again, she was no longer feeling overwhelmed and believed herself capable of overcoming her self-consciousness about the injury. The physician acknowledged her progress and offered future support.

Family Counseling

The goals of this form of counseling are to facilitate effective communication among family members, bring to their awareness maladaptive patterns of behavior that may be destructive to one or more members of the family, and have family members change those maladaptive patterns to constructive patterns of behavior. The specific techniques are similar to those used in individual counseling.

EXAMPLE: FAMILY COUNSELING

A couple asked their family physician for help in dealing with their adolescent daughter, who was continually misbehaving at school and home. Evaluation of the problem revealed that the parents had been inconsistent in limit setting for their daughter and the family considered the girl to be the black sheep of the family. Counseling for the whole family was recommended. During the first session the family members had their usual conflict in the presence of the physician: Both parents and the other siblings attacked the daughter, blaming her for all of the family's troubles. The physician interrupted the attack and proposed that this exchange must resemble what goes on at home, indicated that the situation seemed uncomfortable for all who were present, and ventured that they would probably like to do something about it. After everyone concurred with these points, the physician shifted the focus to the develop-

ment of a contract between the parents and their daughter designed to define the rules they expected her to follow and the consequences of violating the rules. The next session was a review of the parents' and daughter's adherence to the contract. The parents reported that the daughter broke the contract by misbehaving, but one of the older siblings pointed out the parents were inconsistent in their application of the agreed-upon limit-setting rules. This revelation confronted the family with the fact that the girl's behavior was a shared responsibility within the family. Over the remaining sessions, the physician continued to encourage the family to establish fair rules to which all could adhere consistently. By focusing on the behavior of the entire family, the pressure on the daughter was relieved, destructive patterns of interacting were interrupted, and new, constructive patterns were introduced.

BEHAVIOR MODIFICATION

The impact of office psychotherapy and the impact of the strategies for managing many medical problems described in this book depend on the elements essential to any change in a patient's behavior: being concerned about one's problem, becoming motivated to make a change, taking action to make a change, and maintaining the change. The conceptual bases for promoting behavior change and skills for facilitating behavior change are described in detail in Chapter 4. Skills and interventions useful for addressing specific conditions are described in most chapters of this book.

General References

Frank J, Frank J. Persuasion and healing. 3rd ed. Baltimore: Johns Hopkins University Press, 1993.
> Presents model of the patient in distress and the components of practical psychotherapy. Commonalities among Western and non-Western societies are described in this monograph.

Frank JD. The influence of patients' and therapists' expectations on the outcome of psychotherapy. Br J Med Psychol 41:349, 1968.
> A classic paper on the effect of expectations on treatment outcome.

Jacobson GF. In: Arieti S, ed. American handbook of psychiatry. 2nd ed. New York: Basic Books, 1974.
> A concise review of the subject of crisis theory and technique.

McDaniel SH, Campbell TL, Seaburn DB, eds. Family-oriented primary care: a manual for medical providers. New York: Springer-Verlag, 1990.
> Helpful for improving one's grounding in theoretical and practical aspects of family involvement in the care of patients with medical and psychosocial problems.

Stuart MR, Lieberman JA. The fifteen-minute hour. Applied psychotherapy for the primary care physician. 2nd ed. New York: Praeger, 1993.
> Provides an overview of rationale for short-term counseling and describes empirically validated techniques for use in a primary care practice.

CHAPTER 12

Somatization

ROBERT P. ROCA, MD, MPH

ILLNESS BEHAVIOR AND SOMATIZATION

People consulting physicians are expected to have discernible pathologic or pathophysiologic abnormalities (i.e., disease) accounting for their symptoms. The magnitude of their complaints and the associated disability are expected to be proportional to the disease diagnosed. They are supposed to pursue and cooperate with medical care and to resume normal social functioning as soon as possible. This sequence of responses is called *normal illness behavior* (18).

Sometimes there is a discrepancy between diagnosable disease and the magnitude and duration of symptoms and disability. Patients may complain of weakness or pain in the absence of objective findings. They may have pseudoseizures. They may visit their physicians repeatedly with fears of having acquired immunodeficiency syndrome (AIDS) despite several negative human immunodeficiency virus (HIV) serologies and normal physical examinations. Such responses are examples of *abnormal illness behavior.*

Patients exhibiting abnormal illness behavior are often manifesting *somatization,* a phenomenon in which unexplained or amplified physical symptoms are linked to psychologic factors or conflicts. Somatization is a feature of many formal psychiatric disorders. Its causes are incompletely understood, but factors promoting somatization can often be discovered in individual cases.

WHY PATIENTS SOMATIZE

Explanations of somatization come from at least four distinct perspectives (17): Somatization may be viewed as a symptom of a disease, a manifestation of personality, a modeled or reinforced behavior, or an understandable product of a patient's life story. Each perspective calls for different observations and illuminates different aspects of the phenomenon of somatization.

Somatization as a Symptom of Disease

Somatization may occur as a symptom of psychiatric disease, particularly major affective disorder, panic disorder, schizophrenia, and dementia.

Unexplained physical symptoms may also be caused by undiagnosed physical disease, even when the symptoms seem to be expressing a psychologic conflict or need. Studies of one subset of somatizing patients—those originally diagnosed as hysterics—have shown that up to 30% may ultimately be found to have medical or neurologic disorders that, in retrospect, explain the presenting hysterical symptoms (14).

Somatization as a Manifestation of Personality

The concept of personality implies enduring attitudes and habitual patterns of response. Personality may be viewed as approximations of ideal prototypes (e.g., histrionic or obsessive–compulsive type), as discussed in Chapter 14, or clusters of individual traits (e.g., dependency, assertiveness). Somatization has been associated with personality viewed both ways. Patients with histrionic and obsessive–compulsive personality types may be predisposed to develop somatization disorder and hypochondriasis, respectively (see below). Furthermore, patients who are highly introspective (i.e., tend to devote diffuse attention to thoughts and feelings about the self) (10) and neurotic (i.e., emotionally unstable, vulnerable to stress, and self-conscious) (8) tend to experience and report unexplained physical symptoms (8).

Somatization as Reinforced Behavior

Somatization may be viewed as behavior modeled or reinforced by the patient's environment (15). This perspective prompts exploration for a history of similar symptoms in the patient or a close contact and encourages a search for evidence of social benefit associated with the patient's current symptoms.

CASE STUDY

A 20-year-old woman was evaluated in the office for back pain. Physical examination was unimpressive, and an exten-

Table 12.1.   Psychiatric Disorders Associated with Somatization

Mental disorders
  Mood disorders, especially major depression
  Anxiety disorders, especially panic disorder
  Schizophrenia
Personality disorders, especially histrionic, dependent, and obsessive–compulsive
Reactive emotional states
  Adjustment disorder with anxiety or depression
  Psychologic factors affecting physical conditions
Somatoform disorders
  Somatization disorder
  Undifferentiated somatoform disorder
  Hypochondriasis
  Conversion disorder
  Somatoform pain disorder
  Body dysmorphic disorder
Disorders with voluntary symptom production
  Factitious disorder with physical symptoms
  Malingering

sive workup was unrevealing. Discussions with the family disclosed that the patient's father was about to lose his disability income and that financial hardship was expected. The timing of the patient's symptoms strongly suggested that she was amplifying symptoms in the hope of becoming eligible for disability and thereby helping ameliorate the family's anticipated financial crisis.

Somatization and the Life Story

Somatization may be viewed as a maladaptive but understandable expression of difficulties originating in early life experiences. Although particular formulations can never be proven, they may help physicians comprehend illness behavior that is otherwise irritating and baffling. For example, patients who suffer parental deprivation and neglect often carry into adulthood potent admixtures of hostility and dependency that may be activated in relationships with physicians. Such patients may develop physical symptoms without diagnosable disease and pursue unrevealing medical evaluations. Often hostile and demanding, they demean the competence and the commitment of their physicians, even as they crave medical attention and insist on even more care. Such behaviors may be seen as expressions of angry disappointment with their earliest caretakers, who did not adequately meet their dependency needs, now displaced onto the physician by means of transference (see Chapter 11). Such a formulation may help the physician respond to such patients less defensively and permit the development of a workable doctor–patient relationship. Other common formulations of this type are discussed elsewhere (1,2).

Reaching a Working Formulation

The development of a working formulation thus requires considering the relative merits of four distinct explanatory points of view in a particular case. There are four fundamental questions: Does the patient have

a mental illness of which somatization is a symptom? Does the patient have personality traits or a personality type associated with somatization? Is the patient's abnormal illness behavior modeled or reinforced by some aspect of the patient's environment? Is this behavior understandable when one considers the patient's unique life history and current predicament? As shown below, the working formulation will often carry specific therapeutic implications.

Somatizing patients often fall into defined diagnostic groups. The psychiatric disorders associated with somatization are listed in Table 12.1. This chapter describes patients in three groups: those with reactive emotional states, those with primary somatizing disorders (see "Somatoform Disorders"), and those in whom symptom production is deliberate. Mood disorders (Chapter 15), anxiety disorders (Chapter 13), schizophrenia (Chapter 16), and personality disorders (Chapter 14) are discussed in detail elsewhere in this book.

REACTIVE EMOTIONAL STATES (DEMORALIZATION)
Adjustment Disorders

Description

Adjustment disorders are reactive emotional states resulting from difficulty in meeting the demands of the environment (24). Patients feel overwhelmed by illness, marital discord, or other problems and become demoralized. Their distress may be expressed in somatic terms, both because somatic complaints legitimize a visit to the doctor and because emotional distress may cause somatic symptoms such as light-headedness, fatigue, nausea, urinary frequency, palpitations, precordial pain, and breathlessness. When such symptoms arise in response to psychosocial problems, a diagnosis of adjustment disorder may be made (see APA criteria, Table 12.2).

Table 12.2.   Diagnostic Criteria for Adjustment Disorder

A. The development of emotional or behavioral symptoms in response to an identifiable stressor(s) occurring within 3 months of the onset of the stressor(s).
B. These symptoms or behaviors are clinically significant as evidenced by either of the following:
  1. Marked distress that is in excess of what would be expected from exposure to the stressor
  2. Significant impairment in social or occupational (academic) functioning
C. The stress-related disturbance does not meet the criteria for any specific Axis I disorder and is not merely an exacerbation of a preexisting Axis I or Axis II disorder.[a]
D. Does not represent bereavement.
E. The symptoms do not persist for more than 6 months after the termination of the stressor (or its consequences).
  Acute: if the symptoms have persisted for less than 6 months
  Chronic: if the symptoms have persisted for 6 months or longer

Reprinted with permission from the DSM-IV. Copyright 1994, American Psychiatric Association.

[a] See Chapter 10 for definition of Axis I and Axis II disorders.

Case Study

A shy 26-year-old parochial school teacher was evaluated for dizziness, abdominal cramps, nausea, excessive urination, and a sensation of fullness in the bladder. When physical examination and laboratory tests revealed no physiologic disturbance, a more detailed history was taken. It showed that his symptoms began shortly after a confrontation with his school principal over his attempt to organize a teacher's union and his criticism of several school policies. In his ensuing anger, he applied for a job that he did not really want. His symptoms prevented him from taking the scheduled examination for the position. (Diagnosis: adjustment disorder, with anxiety and physical symptoms.)

Patients such as this one are often unaware (or only partially aware) of the relationship between their psychologic disturbance and somatic symptoms. As illustrated in the following example, diagnosis may be particularly difficult when the symptoms of psychosocial distress resemble those of a patient's established disease process.

Case Example

A 54-year-old widowed white woman recovering from a myocardial infarction complained to her physician on several occasions of fatigue, breathlessness, and pleuritic-like chest pain unrelated to exertion. Her physical examination and ECG had not changed since discharge from the hospital. Questioning revealed that she was forced to leave her job after her heart attack and was barely able to afford the $40/month needed for medication. She tearfully revealed that although her son had offered to help pay for her medication, her daughter-in-law hinted that they could really not afford to help. This proud and formerly self-sufficient woman, who was initially reluctant to accept any help, was now made to feel like a charity case by her son's wife, and she acknowledged that the periodic symptoms in her chest invariably occurred while she was thinking about her plight. (Diagnosis: adjustment disorder, with mixed emotional features and physical symptoms.)

In this case, emotional distress produced symptoms suggesting cardiac disease. The correct diagnosis was made when the appropriate history was elicited.

Three strategies are important in evaluating patients who may have adjustment disorders:

- *Elicit the relevant history.* Asking the patient open-ended questions such as "How are things at home (or at work)?"often reveals clues about potential sources of psychosocial distress. It is important to allow patients to expand on their personal history. Most patients are grateful for a physician's interest, respect time limits, and with reassurance and encouragement, will go on to solve the precipitating problem themselves. Even before the physician has taken a psychosocial history, patients may provide verbal and nonverbal cues suggesting distress (e.g., saying "Things aren't the way they used to be" or wringing hands and looking away when describing a new somatic symptom; a bizarre description of the symptoms or failure to respond to previous treatment known to work specifically for a somatic disorder) (9). Many patients who are initially reluctant to acknowledge psychosocial distress eventually open up in response to gentle, persistent encouragement from a trusted physician.
- *Rule out major depression.* Patients who attribute their low mood to identifiable psychosocial stressors do not necessarily have an adjustment disorder. Such symptoms as persistently depressed mood, loss of interest in usual activities, poor concentration, reduced energy, diminished appetite, and disturbed sleep suggest a major depressive disorder for which antidepressant medication is usually indicated (see Chapter 15). The presence of an apparent psychosocial precipitant should never deter one from inquiring about these symptoms.
- *Temper the workup.* Patients should be examined, and appropriate laboratory tests should be ordered. However, extensive workups to exclude improbable diagnoses should be undertaken only after careful consideration and after allowing some time to elapse, because such workups may imbed patients in the sick role and prolong their disability.

Management

The identification of a psychosocial basis for patients' somatic complaints is often sufficient to allow them to marshal their own resources for coping (11). When these measures fail, the patient may need goal-focused short-term counseling (see Chapter 11). In selected cases, short-term prescription of anxiolytic or hypnotic medications may be helpful.

There have been only a few reports of the outcome of minor mood disturbances managed by generalists (3,4,11,25). From these studies, the following tentative conclusions can be stated:

- A large proportion of patients get better after just one office visit. Most often, this visit includes empathic listening, a partial physical examination, and reassurance that the patient does not have a serious physical problem.
- Short-term prescribing of drugs for anxiety or insomnia may not increase the proportion of patients who show significant improvement (about two-thirds of patients) when they are reevaluated after 1 month (3). This conclusion derives from a single careful study in which patients with minor mood disturbances were allocated at random to receive brief counseling plus a benzodiazepine drug or just brief counseling.

Several practical considerations regarding longitudinal management are suggested by these findings:

- It is generally prudent to determine the impact of an initial visit on a patient's distress (by brief telephone or office follow-up within a week) before considering a psychotropic drug for an adjustment disorder.
- Some patients (approximately one-third) who seem to have an adjustment disorder do not respond to the strategies described previously. At follow-up visits, such patients should be interviewed systematically to look for evidence of other syndromes, especially panic disorder (see Chapter 13), major depression (see Chapter 15), alcoholism, chemical dependency,

or domestic violence affecting themselves or a member of their household (see Chapters 21 and 22), or one of the somatoform disorders described later in this chapter. For all of these problems, specific treatment in addition to office psychotherapy is indicated.

Psychologic Factors Affecting Medical Condition

Description

Psychologic factors may exacerbate somatic symptoms caused by a concurrent physical disorder. The resulting symptoms are sometimes called *psychophysiologic*. Table 12.3 lists the most common conditions in which such symptoms may occur. When the features listed in Table 12.4 are present, the DSM-IV diagnosis is psychologic factors affecting medical condition.

Most of the conditions listed in Table 12.3 may occur with or without a significant psychologic component. Detailed descriptions of most of these conditions are found elsewhere in this book, as indicated in the table. For a patient's symptoms to be interpreted as psychophysiologic, they should bear a temporal relationship to stressful life situations and should subside when the stressful situation abates.

Conversion symptoms (see below) are differentiated from psychophysiologic symptoms by the absence of a pathophysiologic condition in the former. Psychophysiologic problems are closely related to adjustment disorders, but they are distinguishable from them in that the somatic symptoms are caused by a recognized pathophysiologic condition and the same symptoms may occur in the absence of psychosocial stressors.

This diagnosis is also used when psychologic factors interfere with the treatment of a general medical condition (e.g., when strong denial of illness interferes with adherence to medication regimens).

Management

When initiation or exacerbation of a physical condition is related to environmental stressors, management is the same as that described for adjustment disorder.

SOMATOFORM DISORDERS

As a group, the somatoform disorders are characterized by the occurrence of physical symptoms lacking an organic basis and linked, by positive evidence or strong presumption, to psychologic factors or conflicts. They may be acute or chronic, mild or severely disabling. Because patients with these disorders believe themselves to be physically ill, they are treated primarily by nonpsychiatrists and do not generally accept psychiatric referral. In addition to the management strategies described here, the strategies for managing abnormal illness behavior, described in Chapter 11, are usually helpful.

Somatization Disorder

Description

The best-studied disorder in this group is somatization disorder, formerly known as hysteria or Briquet's syndrome. This is a chronic disorder beginning before age 30 in which the patient seeks treatment for multiple, widely distributed symptoms lacking any known pathologic basis or pathophysiologic mechanism. To

Table 12.3.   Common Conditions in Which Psychophysiologic Symptoms Are Important

Physiologic System	Symptomatic Condition	For Further Information, See Chapter
Cardiovascular	Migraine headache	79
	Vasovagal syndrome (fainting)	81
	Hypertension (usually asymptomatic)	62
	Supraventricular tachycardia	59
	Angina	57
Gastrointestinal	Irritable bowel syndrome	40
	The following symptoms may occur singly or together: anorexia, nausea, vomiting, abdominal cramps, diarrhea, constipation, aerophagia, acid-peptic symptoms	36, 37, 39
Genitourinary	Menstrual disturbance	77
	Difficulties in micturition: frequency (in both sexes), retention (females), hesitancy (in males)	
	Sexual disorders	18
	Dyspareunia	
	Anorgasmia	
	Inhibited sexual excitement	
	Delayed ejaculation, premature ejaculation	
Musculoskeletal	Pain secondary to increased muscle tension: occipital or bitemporal headaches, backaches, myalgia in various muscle groups	65, 79
	Fatigue	
	Tremor	82
	Rheumatoid arthritis	70
Respiratory	Hyperventilation syndrome	13
	Bronchospasm	55
	Dyspnea	54
Skin	Hyperhidrosis	100
	Pruritus	100

Table 12.4.   Diagnostic Criteria for Psychologic Factors Affecting Physical Condition

A. The presence of a general medical condition (coded on Axis III)
B. Psychologic factors adversely affect the general medical condition in one of the following ways:
    1. The factors have influenced the course of the general medical condition as shown by a close temporal association between the psychologic factors and the development or exacerbation of, or delayed recovery from, the general medical condition.
    2. The factors interfere with the treatment of the general medical condition.
    3. The factors constitute additional health risks for the individual.
    4. The factors elicit stress-related physiologic responses that precipitate or exacerbate symptoms of a general medical condition (e.g., chest pain or arrhythmia in a patient with coronary artery disease).

Reprinted with permission from the DSM-IV. Copyright 1994, American Psychiatric Association.

Table 12.5.   Diagnostic Criteria for Somatization Disorder

A. History of many physical complaints beginning before the age of 30, occurring over a period of several years, and resulting in treatment being sought or significant impairment in social or occupational functioning.
B. Each of the following criteria must have been met at some time during the course of the disorder. To count a symptom as significant, it must not be fully explained by a known general medical condition, or the resulting complaints or impairment are in excess of what would be expected from the history, physical examination, or laboratory findings.
    1. Four pain symptoms: A history of pain related to at least four different sites or functions (such as head, abdomen, back, joints, extremities, chest, rectum, during sexual intercourse, during menstruation, or during urination)
    2. Two gastrointestinal symptoms: A history of at least two gastrointestinal symptoms other than pain (such as nausea, diarrhea, bloating, vomiting other than during pregnancy, or intolerance of several different foods)
    3. One sexual symptom: A history of at least one sexual or reproductive symptom other than pain (such as sexual indifference, erectile or ejaculatory dysfunction, irregular menses, excessive menstrual bleeding, vomiting throughout pregnancy)
    4. One pseudoneurologic symptom: A history of at least one symptom or deficit suggesting a neurologic disorder not limited to pain (conversion symptoms such as blindness, double vision, deafness, loss of touch or pain sensation, hallucinations, aphonia, impaired coordination or balance, paralysis or localized weakness, difficulty swallowing, difficulty breathing, urinary retention, seizures; dissociative symptoms such as amnesia, or loss of consciousness other than fainting)

Reprinted with permission from the DSM-IV. Copyright 1994, American Psychiatric Association.

meet APA criteria for this disorder, the patient must have a history of at least eight such symptoms, drawn from the four symptom subgroups listed in Table 12.5: pain symptoms (at least four), gastrointestinal symptoms (two or more), sexual symptoms (at least one), and pseudoneurologic symptoms (at least one). Accurate diagnosis often requires review of old records and careful history taking to determine that a sufficient number of unexplained symptoms have been presented for evaluation and treatment or have caused the patient to take over-the-counter remedies or alter lifestyle. *Seven symptoms are especially useful in screening*: shortness of breath without exertion, dysmenorrhea, burning sensations in sexual organs, difficulty swallowing (lump in throat), amnesia, vomiting, and pain in extremities. The presence of three of these symptoms without adequate physical explanation identifies somatization disorder with a sensitivity of 87% and specificity of 95% (19). Symptoms are often described in dramatic and colorful terms but details tend to be vague and contradictory.

Somatization disorder occurs in 0.2 to 2.0% of women in the general population but is much more common in women seen in clinical settings (16). It is rare in men. Histrionic personality traits may be present. Somatization disorder occurs in 10 to 20% of the female first-degree relatives of women with somatization disorder, whereas antisocial personality disorder and alcoholism are over-represented among their male relatives.

Common complications include substance abuse and iatrogenic illness. One classic study found that women with hysteria undergo more than three times as many operations as control women and lose, by weight, more than three times the mass of organs (5).

The disorder is chronic. In a retrospective study of 49 patients, nearly 70% of women were still symptomatic 15 years after diagnosis (7). However, the mortality of women with somatization disorder is the same as that of normal women (6), and the likelihood of developing another medical or psychiatric disorder explaining the symptoms is only 10% in long-term follow-up (20).

Case Study

A 43-year-old married white woman was referred for psychiatric evaluation by her internist who, noting her presentation with ill-defined symptoms, was requesting help with management. She complained of generalized muscle aching and periodic sensations throughout her body described as what one has when hearing someone scratch his fingers on a blackboard. She also complained of skin lesions on her back and stated that she was hypothyroid and suffered from a chronic urinary tract infection. Her history included tonsillectomy, groin lymph node biopsy (twice), hysterectomy, bladder suspension (twice), rectocele repair, removal of abdominal adhesions, multiple cystoscopies, appendectomy, and removal of a tongue papilloma. The patient stated she had Ménière's disease and episodes of sudden shortness of breath. She also carried a diagnosis of fibrositis, for which she had taken steroids in the past, and restless leg syndrome. She had stopped having sexual intercourse with her husband because of pain that 10 gynecologists could not cure. Her current medicines were Clinoril, Valium, and Bellergal. She mentioned that she had always been ill and that she hated men. Her psychosocial history included marriage to an alcoholic who abused her and a positive family history of suicide. In presenting her symptoms, the patient was extremely vague and interjected facts about her emotional life with an inappropriate laugh. She believed that her symptoms were caused by food allergy. She had stopped eating and at the time of her initial visit to her internist had ingested only distilled water for 4 days. Physical examination and laboratory tests were normal.

Management

Because these patients adhere vigorously to the idea that they are physically ill, they usually do not accept psychiatric referral, and their treatment lies largely in the hands of nonpsychiatrists. Guidelines for management include the following:

- Review all available medical records to determine the range of symptomatic complaints brought to physicians and the adequacy of documented evaluations.
- Respond to physical symptoms by taking a careful history and doing the appropriate physical examination; avoid hospitalization, specialty consultations, and invasive laboratory tests unless objective indications exist (see strategies for managing abnormal illness behavior in Chapter 11).
- Review the four explanatory perspectives (see "Why Patients Somatize") for factors that might be promoting the development of somatization: psychiatric disease (especially major depression), personality disorders (especially histrionic type), behavioral models (e.g., sick family members) or environmental reinforcers (increased attention from parents) supporting the sick role, and aspects of the patient's life story (e.g., poor attention to early childhood dependency needs) that make his or her symptoms (e.g., endless recitation of complaints keeping the patient under very close medical scrutiny) understandable. When possible, address the apparently etiologic factors in the treatment plan (e.g., treat major depression with antidepressants; counsel family members to give attention for healthy behavior but to refrain from rewarding illness behavior).
- Do not expect symptoms to remit entirely, and do not promise the patient cure or complete resolution of symptoms.
- Assure the patient of your continuing availability and schedule regular brief visits so that access to medical attention does not require the development of new symptoms.

- Do not tell the patient that the symptoms are entirely psychologic, but point out that emotional factors worsen physical distress and attempt to direct the patient to discuss life problems. Praise evidence of coping with the demands of daily life despite illness and discomfort.
- Help the family of the patient recognize that despite the abundance and persistence of symptoms, no serious disease has been found, and encourage them to support a strategy that deemphasizes expensive and elaborate diagnostic tests and stresses the maintenance of function in the face of symptoms.

The usefulness of measures such as these in the management of somatization disorder has been demonstrated in a randomized, controlled study (21).

Undifferentiated Somatoform Disorder

This is a residual category designed to accommodate patients who do not fully meet criteria for somatization disorder (see APA criteria, Table 12.6). Symptoms must be present for at least 6 months for the diagnosis to be made. There need be no identifiable precipitant. Although the disorder has not been well studied, it is believed to be much more common than somatization disorder. Its prognosis and clinical course are unknown.

Multisomatoform Disorder

This category does not appear in DSM-IV. It has been proposed as an alternative to "undifferentiated somatoform disorder" for patients with a 2-year history of apparent somatoform symptoms and at least three current somatoform symptoms, reported from a 15-symptom checklist (13). Of 1000 participants in the PRIME-MD (23) study, 82 (8.2%) met criteria for this condition. These patients had significant elevations in disability days and doctor visits as well as impairments in health-related quality of life and were far more likely than patients with other psychiatric conditions to be judged "difficult" by their physicians. Although there are no specific studies of treatment for multisomatiform disorder, it is likely that techniques useful in full-fledged somatization disorder (as described previously) would be helpful in patients with this less broadly symptomatic form of somatization (22).

Table 12.6. Diagnostic Criteria for Undifferentiated Somatoform Disorder

A. One or more physical complaints (e.g., fatigue, loss of appetite, gastrointestinal or urinary complaints)
B. Either 1 or 2;
    1. After appropriate investigation, the symptoms cannot be explained by a known general medical condition or pathophysiologic mechanism (e.g., the effects of injury, medication, drugs, or alcohol).
    2. When there is a related general medical condition, the physical complaints or resulting social or occupational impairment are grossly in excess of what would be expected from the physical findings.
C. The symptoms cause clinically significant distress or impairment in social, occupational, or other important areas of functioning.
D. The duration of the disturbance is at least 6 months.
E. Does not occur exclusively during the course of another disorder (e.g., another somatoform disorder, sexual dysfunction, mood disorder, anxiety disorder, sleep disorder, or psychotic disorder).

Reprinted with permission from the DSM-IV. Copyright 1994, American Psychiatric Association.

Table 12.7.   Diagnostic Criteria for Conversion Disorder

A. One or more symptoms or deficits affecting voluntary motor or sensory function suggesting a neurologic or general medical condition.
B. Psychologic factors are judged to be associated with the symptom or deficit because the initiation or exacerbation of the symptom or deficit is preceded by conflicts or other stressors.
C. The symptom or deficit is not intentionally produced or feigned (as in factitious disorder or malingering).
D. The symptom or deficit cannot, after appropriate investigation, be fully explained by a neurologic or general medical condition, and is not a culturally sanctioned behavior or experience.
E. The symptom or deficit causes clinically significant distress or impairment in social, occupational, or other important areas of functioning; or warrants medical evaluation.
F. The symptom or deficit is not limited to pain or sexual dysfunction, does not occur exclusively during the course of somatization disorder, and is not better accounted for by another mental disorder.

Reprinted with permission from the DSM-IV. Copyright 1994, American Psychiatric Association.

Conversion Disorder

Description

Conversion disorder is a disorder in which an unexplained loss or alteration of body functioning develops in the presence of evidence that the symptoms solve or express a psychologic conflict or need (see APA criteria, Table 12.7). The symptoms often simulate neurologic disease but conform to the patient's notion of body function rather than to the rules of neuroanatomy, and medical evaluation yields no evidence of diagnosable disease. Amnesia, aphonia, blindness, paralysis, numbness, and seizures are among the most common conversion symptoms. The disorder probably occurs more often in women than men and generally begins in adolescence or early adulthood. Patients may have histrionic or dependent personalities and may exhibit remarkable serenity (la belle indifference) in the face of their impairments.

Conversion disorder is unique among DSM-IV somatoform disorders in that the definition not only describes the diagnostic criteria but also proposes psychologic mechanisms as explanations. A mechanism called *secondary* gain is invoked when unexplained symptoms allow the patient to avoid onerous tasks or undesirable duties (see "Somatization as Reinforced Behavior," above).

CASE EXAMPLE

A 15-year-old girl with a history of migraine headache and transient visual field cuts was evaluated for a new visual field cut that had developed without headache over the previous 24 hours. On examination, the visual defect was found to split the macula. At the time of psychiatric interview she revealed that she expected her visual problems to prevent her from obtaining a driver's license when she turned 16. She went on to say that she was afraid to drive, that no other woman in her family drove, and that she would be called upon by everyone to provide transportation. She was referred to a pediatric neurology service, where she received physical therapy and daily psychotherapy. Her field defect resolved.

A second mechanism, *primary gain,* is invoked when conversion symptoms appear to resolve an internal conflict created by a feeling, impulse, or wish that the individual finds frightening or morally unacceptable (see "Somatization and the Life Story," above).

CASE STUDY

A 50-year-old man was admitted to the hospital because of amnesia. He spoke normally and was otherwise neurologically intact, although he could not remember his name or any other details of personal history. After about 24 hours he began speaking freely about anger related to the recent dissolution of his marriage. Particularly upsetting had been news that his boss was dating his wife. Immediately before the development of amnesia he had thought that he might be provoked to violence if he discovered them together. His amnesia completely resolved in 2 days, and he was discharged from the hospital. He briefly participated in outpatient psychotherapy. The working formulation was that the amnesia had served to remove unacceptable violent intentions from his awareness and protect him from acting on them.

Acute conversion symptoms have a good prognosis for recovery, especially if the patient has no other psychiatric disorder.

Management

Guidelines for the treatment of patients with conversion disorder include the following:

- Be certain that the patient has had an adequate medical evaluation because some patients with conversion symptoms have an undiagnosed medical disorder (14).
- Review the various explanatory perspectives for factors that might be promoting the development of conversion symptoms: psychiatric illness (especially major depression), personality disorders (especially dependent and histrionic types), behavioral models (e.g., sick family members) or environmental reinforcers (increased attention from family members) supporting the sick role, and aspects of the patient's life story (e.g., violent feelings toward an abusive alcoholic father) that make the symptoms understandable (e.g., paralysis of the hand when the patient considered violent revenge against his father). When possible, address specific interventions to the etiologic factors identified (e.g., treat major depression with antidepressants; counsel family members to reward healthy behavior instead of illness behavior; refer the angry child of an alcoholic to Al-Anon).
- Emphasize the evidence that no serious disease is present, and express optimism about the prospect of full recovery. Consider physical therapy or some other physical rehabilitative intervention to help the patient save face during recovery.
- Do not bluntly confront the patient with the psychologic origins of the symptoms, but stress that emo-

tional factors may exacerbate such problems. Review the patient's current life circumstances and difficulties, and consider undertaking a course of short-term counseling (see Chapter 11).

Hypochondriasis

Description

This is a chronic disorder in which unrealistic interpretation of physical symptoms leads the patient to fear the presence of a serious illness in the face of repeated reassurances based on adequate medical evaluation (see APA criteria, Table 12.8). Onset is generally in the third decade but may occur later. Both sexes are equally affected. Obsessive–compulsive personality traits are often observed. Anxiety, depression, drug dependence, and iatrogenic disease are common complications. The disorder tends to be chronic, with waxing and waning intensity. Symptomatic exacerbations occur in response to psychosocial stress and to stimuli that provoke bodily preoccupation and fear of disease.

Case Study

A 30-year-old accountant had always been self-conscious about his physical appearance, a concern that he attempted to allay by weight lifting. After his father died of a heart attack he became concerned that he might have heart disease and was fearful about the implication of insignificant chest pains. He also worried about his blood pressure, which was transiently elevated at the time of his yearly physical examinations. His most recent examination revealed insignificant liver enzyme elevations, a finding over which he fretted for weeks. Despite these concerns he rarely missed a day's work. He was not sure that he did not have a serious disease but thought he had best trust his physician.

Patients such as this young man are easy to care for; however, others present more difficult management problems. Often they read whatever they can find and doctor shop. They may lose time from work and, in severe cases, become bedridden.

Management

Because patients with hypochondriasis believe that they are physically ill, they rarely accept psychiatric treatment. Guidelines for management by generalists are similar to those for other chronic somatoform disorders and include the following:

- Respond to physical symptoms by taking a careful history and doing the appropriate physical examination; reassurances cannot be given to the patient if the physical complaints are not investigated. At the same time, avoid hospitalization, specialty consultations, and invasive laboratory tests unless objective indications exist.
- Review the four explanatory perspectives (see "Why Patients Somatize") for factors that might be promoting hypochondriasis: psychiatric illness (especially major depression and anxiety disorders), personality disorder (especially obsessive–compulsive type), behavioral models or environmental reinforcers supporting the sick role (e.g., family members who were excessively concerned about patient's childhood health and lavished attention in response to minor ailments), and aspects of the patient's life story (e.g., religious upbringing with particular emphasis on sexual morality and punishment of sinners) that make the symptoms empathically understandable (e.g., hypochondriacal fear of AIDS in a man with repeatedly negative HIV antibody tests who had a single extramarital encounter 5 years before). When possible, address specific interventions to etiologic factors identified (e.g., treat major depression with antidepressants; counsel family members to give attention for healthy behavior but to refrain from rewarding illness behavior).
- Do not expect symptoms to remit entirely, and do not promise the patient cure or complete resolution of symptoms (see strategies for managing abnormal illness behavior in Chapter 11).
- Assure the patient of your continuing availability and schedule brief visits so that access to medical attention does not depend on the development of new symptoms.
- Do not tell the patient that the symptoms are entirely psychologic, but point out that emotional factors worsen physical distress and attempt to direct the patient to discuss life problems.
- Help the family of the patient recognize that despite the persistence of symptoms, no serious disease has been found, and encourage them to support a strategy deemphasizing expensive and elaborate diagnostic tests and stressing the maintenance of function in the face of symptoms.
- Some patients may accept short-term counseling (see Chapter 11). The development of a relationship characterized by expectant trust is crucial if pa-

Table 12.8.   Diagnostic Criteria for Hypocondriasis

A. Preoccupation with fears of having, or the idea that one has, a serious disease based on the person's misinterpretation of bodily symptoms.

B. The preoccupation persists despite appropriate medical evaluation and reassurance.

C. The belief in A is not of delusional intensity (as in delusional disorder, somatic type) and is not restricted to a circumscribed concern about appearance (as in body dysmorphic disorder).

D. The preoccupation causes clinically significant distress or impairment in social, occupational, or other important areas of functioning.

E. The duraton of the disturbance is at least 6 months.

F. The preoccupation does not occur exclusively during the course of generalized anxiety disorder, obsessive–compulsive disorder, panic disorder, a major depressive episode, separation anxiety, or another somatoform disorder.

Specify with poor insight if, for most of the time during the current episode, the person does not recognize that the concern about having a serious illness is excessive or unreasonable.

Table 12.9. Diagnostic Criteria for Pain Disorder

A. Pain in one or more anatomic sites is the predominant focus of the clinical presentation and is of sufficient severity to warrant clinical attention.
B. The pain causes clinically significant distress or impairment in social, occupational, or other important areas of functioning.
C. Psychologic factors are judged to have an important role in the onset, severity, exacerbation, or maintenance of the pain.
D. The pain is not better accounted for by a mood, anxiety, or psychotic disorder and does not meet criteria for dyspareunia.

Reprinted with permission from the DSM-IV. Copyright 1994, American Psychiatric Association.

tients are to be persuaded that their worries are excessive and that they should participate more fully in life activities. Kellner describes such a short-term treatment approach requiring 10 sessions over 5 months (12).

Pain Disorder

Description

This is a chronic disorder characterized by unexplained or amplified complaints of pain (see APA criteria, Table 12.9). It usually has its onset in the fourth or fifth decades and is associated with marked functional disability. The diagnosis is most useful when psychologic factors can be linked to the onset and maintenance of pain. A typical scenario begins with lower back pain, often developing on the job, initially diagnosed as a sprain. The patient may see his or her general physician and attempt to return to work. Soon thereafter the pain recurs, sometimes after apparent reinjury. Specialty consultations (e.g., orthopedic, neurosurgical) ensue. Conservative treatments (e.g., physical therapy) are ineffective. Surgery may be performed, perhaps with transient benefit, but soon there is a resurgence of symptoms described as worse than ever. After 6 to 12 months of illness the patient is out of work, socially isolated, physically inactive, dependent on narcotic analgesics, angry, and demoralized. He or she may believe that health professionals and family members do not regard the pain as real.

Management

Treatment of somatoform pain disorder is similar to the management of other somatoform disorders:

- Respond to pain complaints with thorough history and physical examination and determine that adequate medical, surgical, and neurologic evaluations have been done, but avoid procedures and hospitalization in the absence of clear indications.
- Review the four explanatory perspectives (see "Why Patients Somatize") for factors that might be promoting unexplained or amplified pain complaints, and design a treatment plan that addresses specific etiologic factors identified: major psychiatric disease (especially major depression and chemical dependency, both of which are common in patients with somatoform pain), personality traits (especially exaggerated dependency), environmental reinforcers (e.g., financial compensation, relief from work responsibility, sympathy of family and friends), and aspects of life history that make the pain complaints empathically understandable (e.g., abusive or negligent parenting leading to a yearning to be cared for in a passive–dependent way, often hidden behind a defiant, pseudoindependent facade).
- Convey optimism that improvement is likely but do not promise cure or complete resolution of symptoms.
- Assure the patient of your continuing availability and schedule regular, brief visits so that access to medical attention does not require exacerbation of symptoms.
- Consider topical treatments and physical therapy because of their intrinsic value, safety, and symbolic value as indicators that the physical reality of the patient's pain is recognized.
- In general, avoid prescribing benzodiazepines and narcotic analgesics and persuade addicted patients to pursue detoxification. In selected patients who are functional on a stable opioid regimen, it is reasonable to maintain the regimen as part of a contractural plan for the management of chronic pain (see Chapter 22 for details).
- Do not tell the patient that the symptoms are entirely psychologic, but stress that emotional factors undoubtedly worsen physical distress, and attempt to direct the patient to discuss life problems, especially interpersonal conflicts and disappointments.
- Enlist the support of the patient's family in an effort to reinforce maintenance of function in the face of symptoms rather than persistence of disability.
- Consider referral to a center specializing in the multidisciplinary care of patients with chronic pain syndromes.

Body Dysmorphic Disorder

Description

Body dysmorphic disorder is a disorder characterized by an excessive or completely unfounded preoccupation with a defect in personal appearance (see APA criteria, Table 12.10). The prevalence of the disorder is unknown, but it may be common. Onset typically occurs between adolescence and age 30. Perceived facial imperfections, such as the shape of the nose or jaw, are the most common sources of concern.

Table 12.10. Diagnostic Criteria for Body Dysmorphic Disorder

A. Preoccupation with an imagined defect in appearance. If a slight physical anomaly is present, the person's concern is markedly excessive.
B. The preoccupation causes clinically significant distress or impairment in social, occupational, or other important areas of functioning.
C. The preoccupation is not better accounted for by another mental disorder (e.g., dissatisfaction with body shape and size in anorexia nervosa).

Reprinted with permission from the DSM-IV. Copyright 1994, American Psychiatric Association.

CASE EXAMPLE

A 60-year-old man entered into psychiatric treatment for chronic depression. He reported long-standing attitudes and patterns of behavior suggesting obsessionality and extreme self-consciousness. He also reported a preoccupation beginning in adolescence with the shape of his jaw. He had undergone elaborate surgical treatment for this but continued to feel that other people were put off by his appearance, a belief contributing to his social discomfort. The examining psychiatrist found nothing remarkable about the appearance of his face. The patient's preoccupation with this perceived defect was partially ameliorated by antidepressant treatment, but he continued to regard himself as misshapen.

Management

Little is known about the treatment and prognosis of the disorder. Some authors believe it should be regarded as a symptom, not as a distinct condition. In general, patients should be discouraged from pursuing surgical solutions, especially when their concerns are entirely unfounded. Otherwise, many of the management guidelines described earlier for other chronic somatoform disorders are applicable. In particular, it is useful to review the four explanatory perspectives for factors promoting the development and maintenance of the symptoms and to treat any specific etiologic factor identified: an associated major psychiatric illness, usually major depression; personality types predisposing to the disorder, especially obsessive–compulsive and avoidant types (see Chapter 14); behavioral models for these concerns (e.g., parents who were dissatisfied with similar physical attributes in themselves); aspects of the life story that make the symptoms empathically understandable (e.g., early experiences with critical parents leading the patient to feel like a freak or alien).

DISORDERS WITH VOLUNTARY SYMPTOM PRODUCTION

The fundamental feature of these disorders is the deliberate simulation of physical symptoms. This characteristic distinguishes these patients from those with chronic somatoform disorders, described above, in whom symptom genesis is not apparently voluntary.

Factitious Disorder with Physical Symptoms

Description

Factitious illness is characterized by the deliberate simulation of physical symptoms for the sole purpose of assuming the role of patient. When this behavior is chronic and leads to multiple hospitalizations, it is known as chronic factitious disorder with physical symptoms (see APA criteria, Table 12.11) or *Münchhausen's syndrome*. When there is deliberate simulation of a psychiatric syndrome, it is designated as factitious disorder with psychologic symptoms.

Patients may report invented symptoms (e.g., severe right lower quadrant abdominal pain) or deliberately produce physical signs by heating thermometers, tying tourniquets around their legs, or ingesting anticoagu-

Table 12.11. Diagnostic Criteria for Factitious Disorder with Physical Symptoms

A. Intentional production or feigning of physical or psychologic signs or symptoms.
B. The motivation for the behavior is to assume the sick role.
C. External incentives for the behavior (such as economic gain, avoiding legal responsibility, or improving physical well-being, as in malingering) are absent.
D. The behavior is not better accounted for by another mental disorder.

Reprinted with permission from the DSM-IV. Copyright 1994, American Psychiatric Association.

lant drugs. The history may be dramatic but vague in medically relevant detail. Onset is usually in early adulthood, often shortly after hospitalization for a bona fide physical illness. Job stability, family life, and other interpersonal relationships suffer profoundly as a result of multiple lengthy hospitalizations.

Management

The main goals of management are to prevent unnecessary hospitalization and to avoid invasive procedures. The management of the hospitalized patient may be facilitated by early psychiatric consultation to assist in diagnosis, determine whether other treatable psychiatric disorders are present, help plan tactful confrontation of the patient with the diagnosis, and attempt to persuade the patient to accept psychiatric hospitalization.

Malingering

Description

Malingering is the deliberate simulation of physical (or psychologic) symptoms to achieve a specific benefit. It is an important and common problem in settings where sickness is rewarded with certain benefits (e.g., avoidance of military service or court appearances; financial compensation for injuries). Malingering may be of three types (see Ford, "General References"):

- Pure malingering, in which there is deliberate deception by the description or production of nonexistent symptoms or signs (rare)
- Partial malingering, which involves the conscious and voluntary exaggeration of symptoms of a real disease
- The deliberate attribution of an actual disability to an injury or accident that did not cause it

The diagnosis of malingering should be suspected whenever symptoms or disability greatly exceeding objective disease are accompanied by obvious social or financial benefit. Other observations suggesting the diagnosis include inconsistency of symptoms (e.g., a blind person detected reading), unusually vague or markedly exaggerated reports of symptoms, and the expression of indignant anger in response to gentle confrontation.

Malingering must be distinguished from factitious disorders, in which the patient has no goal aside from achieving patienthood, and from conversion disorders, in which symptom production is not conscious and intentional.

Management

The goal of management is to persuade malingering patients to give up their symptoms. Patients should gradually and tactfully be made aware that malingering is suspected, and the gratifications associated with the sick role should be removed. Reports of symptoms should be given minimal attention. Because serious psychiatric disorders may underlie apparent malingering, psychiatric consultation should be obtained if possible.

General References*

American Psychiatric Association. **Diagnostic and Statistical Manual of Mental Disorders.** 4th ed. (DSM-IV). Washington, DC: American Psychiatric Association, 1994.
   Recently updated diagnostic criteria and epidemiologic information for all recognized psychiatric disorders.
Ford CV. The somatizing disorders: illness as a way of life. New York: Elsevier, 1983.
   Practical, well-referenced monograph covering all disorders in which somatization is the principal feature.
Kaplan CK, Lipkin M, Gordon GH. Somatization in primary care: patients with unexplained and vexing medical complaints. J Gen Intern Med 3:177, 1988.
   Review article focusing on origins of somatization and on diagnosis and management by the primary care physician.

Specific References

1. Barsky AJ. Patients who amplify bodily sensations. Ann Intern Med 91:63, 1979.
2. Barsky AJ, Klerman GL. Overview: hypochondriasis, bodily complaints, and somatic styles. Am J Psychiatry 140:273, 1983.
3. Catalan J, Bath D, Edmonds G, Ennis J. The effects of non-prescribing of anxiolytics in general practice. I. Controlled evaluation of psychiatric and social outcome. Br J Psychiatry 144:593, 1984.
4. Catalan J, Bath D, Bond A, Martin P. The effects of non-prescribing of anxiolytics in general practice. II. Factors associated with outcome. Br J Psychiatry 144:603, 1984.
5. Cohen ME, Robins E, Purtell JJ, et al. Excessive surgery in hysteria. JAMA 151:977, 1953.
6. Coryell W. Diagnosis-specific mortality. Primary depression and Briquet's syndrome (somatization disorder). Arch Gen Psychiatry 38:939, 1981.
7. Coryell W, Norten SG. Briquet's syndrome (somatization disorder) and primary depression: comparison of background and outcome. Compr Psychiatry 22:249, 1981.
8. Costa PT, McCrae RR. Hypochondriasis, neuroticism, and aging. Am Psychol 40:19, 1985.
9. Drossman DA. The problem patient: evaluation and care of medical patients with psychosocial disturbances. Ann Intern Med 88:366, 1978.
10. Hansell S, Mechanic D. Introspectiveness and adolescent symptom reporting. J Hum Stress 11(Winter):165, 1985.
11. Johnstone A, Goldberg D. Psychiatric screening in general practice. Lancet 1:605, 1976.
12. Kellner R. Psychotherapeutic strategies in hypochondriasis: a clinical study. Am J Psychother 36:146, 1982.
13. Kroenke K, Spitzer RL, deGruy FV, et al. Multisomatiform disorder: an alternative to undifferentiated somatoform disorder for the somatizing patient in primary care. Arch Gen Psychiatry 54:352, 1997.
14. Lazare A. Conversion symptoms. N Engl J Med 305:745, 1983.
15. Lipowski ZJ. Somatization: the concept and its clinical application. Am J Psychiatry 145:1358, 1988.
16. Manu P, Lane TJ, Matthews DA. Screening for somatization disorder in patients with chronic fatigue. Gen Hosp Psychiatry 11:294, 1989.
17. McHugh PR, Slavney PR, eds. The perspectives of psychiatry. Baltimore: Johns Hopkins University Press, 1983.
18. Mechanic D. The concept of illness behavior: culture, situation, and personal disposition. Psychol Med 16:1, 1986.
19. Othmer E, DeSouza C. A screening test in somatization disorder (hysteria). Am J Psychiatry 142:1146, 1985.
20. Perley MJ, Guze SB. Hysteria: the stability and usefulness of clinical criteria. N Engl J Med 266:421, 1962.
21. Smith GR, Monson RA, Ray DC. Psychiatric consultation in somatization disorder: a randomized controlled study. N Engl J Med 314:1407, 1986.
22. Smith GR, Rost K, Kashner TM. A trial of the effect of a standardized psychiatric consultation on health outcomes and costs in somatizing patients. Arch Gen Psychiatry 52:238, 1995.
23. Spitzer RL, Williams JBW, Kroenke K, et al. Utility of a new procedure for diagnosing mental disorders in primary care: the PRIME-MD 1000 study. JAMA 272:1749, 1994.
24. Stoeckle J, Zola IK, Davison GE. The quantity and significance of psychological distress in medical patients. J Chronic Dis 17:959, 1964.
25. Thomas KB. Temporarily dependent patient in general practice. BMJ 1:625, 1974.

---

*Bold print (general references) and bold numerals (specific references) denote published controlled clinical trials, meta-analyses, or consensus-based recommendations.

C H A P T E R   13

Anxiety

ROBERT P. ROCA, MD, MPH

Anxiety is the term applied to a psychophysiologic state characterized by worry (apprehensive expectation), muscle tension, autonomic hyperactivity, and hypervigilance. Anxiety may improve performance in response to danger or challenge and thus may serve an adaptive function. However, when excessive or inappropriate in form or context, it leads to subjective distress and impairment in social and occupational functioning.

NORMAL ILLNESS-RELATED ANXIETY

Patients visiting their physicians or awaiting the results of tests are often anxious. Although such anxiety may be understandable and realistically related to concerns about the meaning of symptoms and consequences of disease, it nonetheless requires recognition and management because it may interfere with medical care. For example, it has been found that survivors of myocardial infarction and their spouses recollected little of the information given to them during in-hospital convalescence, partly as a result of anxiety (56). Such findings highlight the importance of detecting normal illness-related anxiety and treating it skillfully. The following approaches are helpful:

- Assume that patients with new symptoms have concerns about serious illness. It is helpful to ask patients for their ideas about the causes of their symptoms. Often, a relative or friend has had a similar symptom related to a serious disease.
- Avoid comments or jargon that might sensitize or frighten patients (e.g., commenting, while examining a skin lesion, "It's been a long time since I've seen one like that.").

- Prepare the patient for painful procedures with explanations. Assume that any procedure may be frightening to a patient.
- Assume that any patient recovering from serious illness is anxious about the future; determine whether any unnecessary disability in such patients is caused by fear or inadequate education. Hospitalized patients often get incomplete explanations of their illnesses at the time of discharge.

DRUG-RELATED ANXIETY

In evaluating patients with symptoms of anxiety, it is important to identify all medications or substances taken during or just before the onset of symptoms of anxiety. Prescribed drugs, over-the-counter preparations, caffeine, alcohol, and other substances can cause symptoms similar to those found in the primary anxiety disorders described below. Common examples of such compounds are listed in Table 13.1.

When considering the role of caffeine in producing anxiety, it is helpful to know the approximate amount of caffeine in commonly consumed beverages and substances. *Coffee* (cup): brewed 60 to 180 mg, instant 30 to 120 mg, decaffeinated 2 to 5 mg; *tea* (cup): brewed U.S. brands 20 to 90 mg, imported brands 25 to 100 mg; *soft drinks* (6 oz portion): 15 to 23 mg; *dark chocolate* (1 oz): 5 to 35 mg.

Patients who experience prominent anxiety, panic attacks, obsessions, or compulsions in relation to the ingestion of these substances are classified by the American Psychiatric Association (APA) as having a substance-induced anxiety disorder.

ANXIETY DISORDERS

The anxiety disorders described in this chapter are a group of conditions in which anxiety is the predominant symptom. Anxiety causes distress and dysfunction because it is *excessive* (adjustment disorder with anxious mood, generalized anxiety disorder) or *inappropriate in form or context* (phobia, panic disorder, obsessive–compulsive disorder, posttraumatic stress disorder). Anxiety is a component in the presentation of some patients with attention deficit/hyperactivity disorder (Chapter 5), somatoform disorders (Chapter 12), affective disorders (Chapter 15), cognitive impairment (Chapter 17), and substance abuse (Chapters 21 and 22).

Adjustment Disorder with Anxiety

Description

The term *adjustment disorder with anxiety* is used when excessive and maladaptive anxiety occurs in response to a recent, identifiable stressor. This "reactive" anxiety resolves when the stressor remits or when the patient reaches a new level of adaptation or adjustment. APA criteria are listed in Table 13.2.

Table 13.1. Drugs and Other Substances that May Exacerbate (or Produce) Anxiety

Toxic Symptoms
Anticholinergic drugs
Drugs of abuse[a]
  Marijuana and other drugs that alter perception
  Stimulant drugs of abuse
  Inhalants
  Phencyclidine
  Hallucinogens

Sympathomimetic Drugs
Decongestants (found in most over-the-counter cold remedies)
β_2 bronchodilators
Weight-reduction agents

Thyroid Hormone

Xanthine-Containing Drugs, Foods, and Beverages
Bronchodilators with theophylline
Many over-the-counter cold and arthritis remedies
Caffeine (use and discontinuation)[b]

Withdrawal Symptoms
Sedative–hypnotics
Alcohol
Tobacco

[a] See Chapter 22.

[b] See text for approximate amount of caffeine in common beverages.

CASE STUDY

A 55-year-old married man presented to the office because of nonexertional chest pain, dizziness, and breathlessness. He had suffered a heart attack 3 months before but had recovered uneventfully. A recent stress test had shown no signs of coronary insufficiency or serious arrhythmia. His wife reported that the patient had not been himself since leaving the hospital and that "every little thing gets on his nerves." Although he had formerly been "on the go all of the time," he was now afraid to go out of the house. Physical examination now showed no evidence of heart failure, and the electrocardiogram (ECG) was unchanged. The physician reviewed the encouraging results of the ECG and treadmill test, reassured the patient about his symptoms, explained that anxiety is common after myocardial infarction, and asked the patient to enroll in a cardiac rehabilitation program, to telephone in 1 week to report on his symptoms, and to return to the office in 2 weeks for follow-up examination and a review of his progress. The physician also demonstrated some simple relaxation techniques (see below) and gave the patient a small supply of diazepam to be used on an as-needed basis.

Treatment

By definition, an adjustment disorder with anxious mood is expected to remit as the precipitating problems are resolved or a new level of adjustment is reached. Management includes the following steps:

- Advise the patient to moderate or eliminate use of caffeine and other stimulants.
- Consider short-term counseling (see Chapter 11) to meet the patient's informational needs, assist in problem solving, provide encouragement, and restore morale.
- Offer *training in relaxation* and other techniques of self-regulation (see below).

- Consider instituting a short course of *anxiolytic medication*, usually a benzodiazepine (see below).

Generalized Anxiety Disorder

Description

Generalized anxiety disorder is chronic and is characterized by persistent and excessive worry, muscle tension, autonomic hyperactivity, and hypervigilance. APA criteria are listed in Table 13.3.

CASE STUDY

A 63-year-old woman came to her physician complaining of continuous tightness in the chest. She had always been prone to worry and "bad nerves" but had been much more anxious in the year since her husband had died and she had become responsible for managing all aspects of the household. Three of her adult children, one of whom had mental retardation, lived at home, and she continued to prepare their meals and do their laundry. She admitted that she was "scared of everything," generally tense ("Little things make me jump"), and often experienced feelings of shakiness, diaphoresis, and fluttering in the chest, usually in response to contemplating driving by herself or engaging in another feared activity. She did not describe discrete intense panic episodes (see below) or symptoms of major depression (see Chapter 15). Physical examination, electrocardiogram, and exercise stress test were normal. Although she was reluctant to take medications, she agreed to try alprazolam (Xanax) 0.25 mg three times per day. In addition, she agreed to meet with her physician on a monthly basis for 12 months for counseling. During counseling sessions she learned simple relaxation techniques (see below), helped construct a program of systematic desensitization regarding driving, and developed a plan to request that her children participate more consistently in the running of the household. At the end of 1 year she was greatly improved and asked to begin tapering the alprazolam. She was driving regularly to visit friends across town with growing confidence.

Epidemiology and Origins

Generalized anxiety disorder (GAD) occurs in 3 to 5% of general medical outpatients (8,81), often in the

Table 13.2. Diagnostic Criteria for Adjustment Disorder

A. The development of emotional or behavioral symptoms in response to an identifiable stressor(s) occurring within 3 months of the onset of the stressor(s).
B. These symptoms or behaviors are clinically significant as evidenced by either of the following:
   1. Marked distress that is in excess of what would be expected from exposure to the stressor
   2. Significant impairment in social or occupational (academic) functioning
C. The stress-related disturbance does not meet the criteria for any specific Axis I disorder and is not merely an exacerbation of a preexisting Axis I or Axis II disorder.[a]
D. Does not represent bereavement.
E. The symptoms do not persist for more than 6 months after the termination of the stressor (or its consequences).

Acute: if the symptoms have persisted for less than 6 months
Chronic: if the symptoms have persisted for 6 months or longer

Reprinted with permission from the DSM-IV. Copyright 1994, American Psychiatric Association.

[a] See Chapter 10 for definition of Axis I and Axis II disorders.

Table 13.3.   Diagnostic Criteria for Generalized Anxiety Disorder

A. Excessive anxiety and worry (apprehensive expectation), occurring more days than not for at least 6 months, about a number of events or activities (such as work or school performance).
B. The person finds it difficult to control the worry.
C. The anxiety and worry are associated with at least three of the following six symptoms (with at least some symptoms present for more days than not for the past 6 months):
   1. Restlessness or feeling keyed up or on edge
   2. Being easily fatigued
   3. Difficulty concentrating or mind going blank
   4. Irritability
   5. Muscle tension
   6. Sleep disturbance (difficulty falling or staying asleep, or restless unsatisfying sleep)
D. The focus of the anxiety and worry is not confined to features of an Axis I disorder, e.g., the anxiety or worry is not about having a panic attack (as in panic disorder), being embarrassed in public (as in social phobia), being contaminated (as in obsessive-compulsive disorder), being away from home or close relatives (as in separation anxiety disorder), gaining weight (as in anorexia nervosa), or having a serious illness (as in hypochondriasis), and is not part of posttraumatic stress disorder.[a]
E. The anxiety, worry, or physical symptoms cause clinically significant distress or impairment in social, occupational, or other important areas of functioning.
F. Not due to the direct effects of a substance (e.g., drugs of abuse, medication) or a general medical condition (e.g., hyperthyroidism), and does not occur exclusively during a mood disorder, psychotic disorder, or pervasive developmental disorder.

Reprinted with permission from the DSM-IV. Copyright 1994, American Psychiatric Association.
[a] See Chapter 10 for definition of Axis I and Axis II disorders.

guise of a medical disorder (4). Symptoms usually begin in the teens or twenties (2) during times of stress. Although anxiety is generally persistent thereafter, the severity of symptoms fluctuates markedly as life stresses come and go. Major depressive disorder, alcoholism, and other anxiety disorders often complicate the clinical course (2,14).

The causes of generalized anxiety disorder are not fully understood. There is little evidence for a strong genetic contribution (23,76). Anxious mothers (82) and traumatic early life experiences, especially the death of a parent (77), may be predisposing factors, although patients with this disorder do not characterize their childhoods as more difficult than nonanxious people do (42). Events in later life, especially unexpected events perceived as important and negative (13), may also play a role in the emergence of symptoms.

Evaluation and Treatment

A systematic approach to the evaluation and treatment of the patient with GAD includes the following steps:

- Take a medical history and perform a focused physical examination to look for evidence of medical disorders (e.g., hyperthyroidism, pheochromocytoma, hypoglycemia) that may present with symptoms of anxiety.
- Inquire about consumption of alcohol, caffeine-containing beverages, and other drugs (e.g., diet pills), and counsel patient to eliminate ingestion of caffeine and other stimulants and to moderate alcohol consumption.
- Inquire about life stresses and encourage patient to find solutions to problems; anxious patients are often demoralized and benefit from short-term counseling (see Chapter 11) aimed at solving problems and restoring self-esteem.
- Instruct the patient in self-regulation techniques such as *progressive muscle relaxation* (see below) and encourage regular practice.
- Consider a trial of *buspirone* (see below for specific discussion). It is well tolerated and effective in the treatment of generalized anxiety disorder, particularly for the core symptoms of worry and apprehensive expectation, although its onset of action is slower than that of benzodiazepines and it may not be particularly effective in patients with histories of long-term benzodiazepine use. It carries essentially no risk of tolerance or dependency. Effective therapy is continued for at least 6 to 12 months.
- If there are prominent symptoms of hypervigilance (especially sleep disturbance), autonomic hyperactivity, and muscle tension, consider a 1- to 2-month course of *benzodiazepines* to supplement and facilitate short-term counseling (20,68); patients should be allowed to use the medications on an as-needed rather than a standing basis if they prefer. Some patients benefit from long-term occasional use of benzodiazepines at times of unusual stress. Long-term continuous use is controversial, but benzodiazepines appear to retain their anxiolytic potency over time and may therefore continue to be of assistance to patients. Antihistamines may be given in place of benzodiazepines to anxious patients at high risk for drug abuse (see below for discussions of both classes of agents).
- Consider the use of an *antidepressant medication*, particularly trazodone or a tricyclic agent. In a placebo-controlled trial, imipramine, trazodone, and the benzodiazepine diazepam were associated with moderate to marked improvement in approximately 70% of patients, compared with 47% of placebo-treated subjects (68). The antidepressants are more useful for the treatment of worry and apprehension than for the treatment of muscle tension and hypervigilance. They must be taken for several weeks before they become effective, and they carry little risk of tolerance or dependence. Effective therapy is generally continued for 6 months to 1 year.
- No response to treatment or relapse should lead to reassessment of the diagnosis, examination for medical and psychiatric comorbidity (especially major depression), and possible psychiatric referral.

Phobias

Description

As a group, phobias are enduring fears of harmless objects or situations (phobic stimuli), leading patients to avoid contact with them (phobic avoidance). Patients with *specific phobia* fear discrete objects and situations, such as animals, heights, air travel, needles, and visits to the doctor, whereas patients with *social phobia* have specific fears of social humiliation and the scrutiny of others. People with *agoraphobia* fear being alone and being in situations from which escape is difficult (literally, fear of the agora, or marketplace). Although phobic patients generally recognize their fears to be excessive and unreasonable, they nonetheless seek to avoid the phobic stimulus because exposure provokes intense anxiety. The diagnosis of phobia is made only if avoidance of the feared object or situation leads to social or occupational impairment or if the patient experiences great distress as a result of the symptom.

APA criteria for specific phobia and social phobia are listed in Tables 13.4 and 13.5, respectively. Because agoraphobia is usually a complication of panic disorder, it is described in this chapter under "Panic Disorder."

CASE STUDY

A 50-year-old married business executive sought treatment because of an addiction to chlordiazepoxide. In his early twenties he had first become aware of his discomfort in large groups, particularly when he was the focus of attention. He discovered that regular use of chlordiazepoxide improved his general level of comfort, and by age 50 he was using 80 mg/day routinely. He avoided parties whenever possible but was often obliged to make professional presentations before clients and supervisors. In the days preceding a presentation, he would experience great anticipatory anxiety associated with the fear that he would be unable to recall what he wanted to say or that his throat would close up, preventing him from speaking. In response to this fear, he would increase his daily

Table 13.4.   Diagnostic Criteria for Specific Phobia

A. Marked and persistent fear that is excessive or unreasonable, cued by the presence or anticipation of a specific object or situation (e.g., flying, height, animals, receiving an injection, seeing blood).

B. Exposure to the phobic stimulus almost invariably provokes an immediate anxiety response, which may take the form of a situationally bound or situationally predisposed panic attack. Note: In children, the anxiety may be expressed by crying, tantrums, freezing, or clinging.

C. The person recognizes that the fear is excessive or unreasonable. Note: In children, this feature may be absent.

D. The phobic situation is avoided, or else endured with intense anxiety or distress.

E. The avoidance, anxious anticipation, or distress in the feared situations interferes significantly with the person's normal routine, occupational (academic) functioning, or social activities or relationships with others, or there is marked distress about having the phobia.

F. The anxiety, panic attacks, or phobic avoidance associated with the specific object or situation are not better accounted for by another mental disorder, such as obsessive–compulsive disorder (e.g., fear of contamination), posttraumatic stress disorder (e.g., avoidance of stimuli associated with a severe stressor), separation anxiety disorder (e.g., avoidance of school), social phobia (e.g., avoidance of social situations because of fear of embarrassment), panic disorder with agoraphobia, or agoraphobia without history of panic disorder.

Reprinted with permission from the DSM-IV. Copyright 1994, American Psychiatric Association.

Table 13.5.   Diagnostic Criteria for Social Phobia

A. A marked and persistent fear of one or more social or performance situations in which the person is exposed to unfamiliar people or to possible scrutiny by others. The individual fears that he or she will act in a way (or show anxiety symptoms) that will be humiliating or embarrassing. Note: In children, there must be evidence of capacity for social relationships with familiar people and the anxiety must occur in peer settings, not just in interactions with adults.

B. Exposure to the feared social situation almost invariably provokes anxiety, which may take the form of a situationally bound or situationally predisposed panic attack. Note: In children, the anxiety may be expressed by crying, tantrums, freezing, or withdrawal from the social situation.

C. The person recognizes that the fear is excessive or unreasonable. Note: In children, this feature may be absent.

D. The feared social or performance situations are avoided, or else endured with intense anxiety or distress.

E. The avoidance, anxious anticipation, or distress in the feared social or performance situation interferes significantly with the person's normal routine, occupational (academic) functioning, or social activities or relationships with others, or there is marked distress about having the phobia.

F. The fear or avoidance is not due to the direct effects of a substance (e.g., drugs of abuse, medication) or a general medical condition, and is not better accounted for by panic disorder with or without agoraphobia, separation anxiety disorder, body dysmorphic disorder, a pervasive developmental disorder, or schizoid personality disorder.

G. If a general medical condition or other mental disorder is present, the fear in A is unrelated to it; for example, the fear is not of stuttering, trembling (in Parkinson's disease) or exhibiting abnormal eating behavior (in anorexia nervosa or bulimia nervosa).

Reprinted with permission from the DSM-IV. Copyright 1994, American Psychiatric Association.

chlordiazepoxide dosage by 50 to 100%. On the day of the presentation he would take 200 to 300 mg and would perform well. He was dissatisfied with this practice because he now felt depressed and believed that the medication might be playing a role. His diagnosis at the time of evaluation was social phobia and benzodiazepine dependence. A slow chlordiazepoxide taper was undertaken and completed within 6 months. At the same time, he participated actively in a program of in vivo desensitization (see below) involving regular attendance at social activities of graded difficulty and the pursuit of opportunities to give group presentations at work without the assistance of benzodiazepines. His social anxiety declined and his confidence grew as he succeeded in attending parties and giving talks without substantial reliance on medication. Ultimately he continued to use chlordiazepoxide at low dosages before stressful gatherings but no longer had a habit of daily use.

Epidemiology and Origins

Specific phobias are among the most common psychiatric disorders in the community, with 6-month prevalence rates ranging between 5.4 and 13.4% (59). They occur approximately twice as often among women as men and tend to drop in prevalence after age 65. Phobias beginning in childhood often improve with maturity, whereas those beginning in adulthood rarely resolve without treatment. *Social phobia* has a community prevalence of 1 to 2%. It is equally common among men and women and declines in prevalence with increasing age (59).

Between 7 and 8% of general medical outpatients may have phobias (81). In this setting, phobias related to medical procedures (e.g., phlebotomy) may interfere with the delivery of medical care, and phobias related to dread diseases (e.g., cancer, acquired immunodeficiency syndrome [AIDS]) may prevent patients from undergoing examinations that could disclose evidence of the feared illness.

Patients with social phobia may become addicted to alcohol or sedative–hypnotics as a result of self-directed efforts to ameliorate their social anxiety. Furthermore, phobias and phobic anxiety may be risk factors for ischemic heart disease and other forms of cardiovascular morbidity. There is a significant association between measures of phobic anxiety (fears of enclosed spaces, illness, going out alone, heights, and crowds) and the probability of subsequent ischemic cardiac events (39). Such relationships may be mediated by anxiety-related hyperventilation, which has been shown to cause coronary vasospasm and cardiac ischemia (66), or by anxiety-induced arrhythmia (49).

Treatment

Approaches to treating phobic anxiety are based on the notion that this form of anxiety develops as a product of the pairing of an innocuous stimulus with a threatening one. Phobic avoidance emerges and is maintained by the anxiety-preventing consequences of the avoidance. The treatment of phobias has advanced greatly with the development of behavioral therapies aimed at extinguishing phobic anxiety and phobic avoidance. Three commonly used techniques are desensitization, participant modeling, and social skills training.

Systematic desensitization begins with the gradual exposure of the patient to increasingly vivid and anxiety-provoking mental images of the phobic stimulus. As anxiety is generated, the patient induces relaxation by use of a relaxation technique (see below). By exercising a response incompatible with anxiety (i.e., relaxation) in response to the phobic stimulus, the patient gradually extinguishes the phobic anxiety. This treatment occurs over a series of sessions until the patient is comfortable enough to encounter the stimulus in vivo. Related to systematic desensitization is *flooding or implosion,* in which the imagery is presented suddenly rather than gradually.

In vivo desensitization involves the gradual, stepwise exposure of the patient to the feared stimulus in real life. The patient is often initially accompanied by the therapist or a trained family member. Progress from less to more anxiety-producing tasks is accomplished by mastering anxiety at each level. The basis for the technique is that repeated exposure leads to extinction of phobic anxiety.

Participant modeling is a form of in vivo desensitization in which the therapist models the desired interaction with the feared object. This kind of procedure may be useful with severe needle phobics, whose avoidance of needles may be potentially life threaten-ing (e.g., in patients requiring insulin). Therapy involves the following steps (74):

- Education aimed at providing realistic information about the feared object
- Response modeling, in which the therapist handles the feared object
- Joint performance, in which the patient and therapist are both exposed to the phobic stimulus
- Self-directed practice (e.g., inserting a needle into an orange)

Social skills training, especially assertiveness training, is particularly useful in the treatment of social phobics. Its object is to promote the development of comfort in anxiety-provoking social settings (e.g., public speaking or business meetings) by use of modeling and role plays.

Behavioral techniques such as these have been used successfully in treating phobias related to hemodialysis, needles, and return to work after medical illness. They may be carried out by nonphysicians and are usually effective within 15 sessions or less. Among patients treated by these techniques, phobias, hypochondriacal symptoms, and work adjustment often improve within 6 months, and visits to physicians decrease markedly (53,54).

Several pharmacologic agents appear to be effective in the treatment of social phobia. The monoamine oxidase inhibitor phenelzine (48) and the serotonin reuptake inhibitors (SSRIs) sertraline and fluvoxamine (44,80) have particularly strong empirical support for use in this setting. The well-tolerated SSRIs have been shown in placebo-controlled trials to reduce patients' social anxiety scores by 40 to 45%, about double the impact of placebo (44,80).

Panic Disorder

Description

Panic disorder is characterized by recurrent, discrete attacks of intense fear or discomfort associated with somatic and/or psychic symptoms of anxiety. The attacks generally last for a few minutes and are usually unprecipitated, coming out of the blue, even waking the person from sleep at night. People who experience panic attacks often grow uncomfortable being in places from which escape might be difficult or embarrassing or in which help might not be available in the event of a panic attack; this fear and the associated phobic avoidance are called *agoraphobia.*

APA diagnostic criteria for panic disorder without and with agoraphobia are summarized in Table 13.6.

Case Study

A 27-year-old male business executive was referred because of anxiety. He had no psychiatric history, did not abuse drugs or alcohol, and did not consume caffeine excessively. He had recently married and was in the process of buying a house. Immediately before the onset of his symptoms, his father had suffered a nonfatal myocardial infarction. Subsequently, the

Table 13.6. Diagnostic Criteria for Panic Disorder Without and with Agoraphobia

Without Agoraphobia
A. Both 1 and 2:
   1. Recurrent unexpected panic attacks.
   2. At least one of the attacks has been followed by a month or more of (a) persistent concern about having additional attacks, (b) worry about the implications of the attack or its consequences (e.g., losing control, having a heart attack, "going crazy"), or (c) a significant change in behavior related to the attacks.
B. Absence of agoraphobia (defined below).
C. The panic attacks are not due to the direct effects of a substance (e.g., drugs of abuse, medication) or a general medical condition (e.g., hyperthyroidism).
D. The anxiety is not better accounted for by another mental disorder, such as obsessive–compulsive disorder (e.g., fear of contamination), posttraumatic stress disorder (e.g., in response to stimuli associated with a severe stressor), separation anxiety disorder, or social phobia (e.g., fear of embarrassment in social situations).

With Agoraphobia
A. Both 1 and 2:
   1. Recurrent unexpected panic attacks.
   2. At least one of the attacks has been followed by a month or more of (a) persistent concern about having additional attacks, (b) worry about the implications of the attack or its consequences (e.g., losing control, having a heart attack, "going crazy"), or (c) a significant change in behavior related to the attacks.
B. The presence of agoraphobia, that is, anxiety about being in places or situations from which escape might be difficult (or embarrassing) or in which help may not be available in the event of having an unexpected or situationally predisposed panic attack. Agoraphobic fears typically involve characteristic clusters of situations that include being outside the home alone, being in a crowd or standing in a line, being on a bridge, and traveling in a bus, train, or car.
   Note: Consider the diagnosis of specific phobia if limited to one or only a few specific situations, or social phobia if the avoidance is limited to social situations.
C. Agoraphobic situations are avoided (e.g., travel is restricted), or else endured with marked distress or with anxiety about having a panic attack, or require the presence of a companion.
D. The panic attacks are not due to the direct effects of a substance (e.g., drugs of abuse, medication) or a general medical condition (e.g., hyperthyroidism).
E. The anxiety or phobic avoidance is not better accounted for by another mental disorder, such as specific phobia (e.g., avoidance limited to a single situation like elevators), separation anxiety disorder (e.g., avoidance of school), obsessive–compulsive disorder (e.g., fear of contamination), posttraumatic stress disorder (e.g., avoidance of stimuli associated with a severe stressor), or social phobia (e.g., avoidance limited to social situations because of fear of embarrassment).

Reprinted with permission from the DSM-IV. Copyright 1994, American Psychiatric Association.

patient began experiencing frequent episodes of chest pain, dyspnea, and palpitations associated with fear of dying and feelings of panic. Medical workup disclosed no evidence of hyperthyroidism or cardiovascular disease, and he was diagnosed as having panic disorder. He was placed on desipramine and alprazolam and was counseled to eliminate stressors. His panic attacks ceased within a week. He was followed in short-term counseling every 3 weeks, and after 6 months his medications were tapered without symptomatic relapse.

Epidemiology and Origins

Less common than specific phobia and generalized anxiety disorder, panic disorder has a prevalence in the community of 1 to 2% and may be more common in women than in men (71,81). The initial attacks usually occur in the second or third decades, are often vividly recalled, and in approximately 50% of cases, develop during a time of stress (2). Frequently associated psychiatric conditions include major depression, generalized anxiety disorder, agoraphobia (see the next section), and obsessive–compulsive disorder (15–17).

Patients with panic disorder present special differential diagnostic challenges to general physicians and cardiologists. Although panic symptoms are often difficult to distinguish from angina and may lead to unnecessary cardiac catheterization (9), patients with panic disorder have an increased cardiovascular mortality (24), perhaps as a result of hyperventilation-induced coronary vasospasm (66), and may have a very high prevalence of mitral valve prolapse (55), a controversial finding of uncertain significance. In addition, panic symptoms may be simulated by a number of noncardiac medical disorders, including alcohol and sedative–hypnotic drug withdrawal, marijuana use, pheochromocytoma, hyperthyroidism, hypoglycemia, and temporal lobe epilepsy.

Recent studies support the view that panic disorder is *primarily a biological disorder.* Genetic factors have been implicated by family studies demonstrating a 10-fold increase in panic disorder among first-degree relatives of panic probands (63) and a markedly higher concordance rate for panic disorder among monozygotic than among dizygotic twins (76). Furthermore, lactate infusion (34) and hyperventilation (22) may stimulate panic attacks in people with panic disorder, suggesting the existence of specific biological triggers. Finally, pharmacologic treatments may by themselves dramatically reduce the frequency of panic episodes (see below). These observations all suggest an important role for biological factors in the etiology of panic disorder.

There are also *learning* (or *conditioning*) *theories* to explain panic disorder. These propose that panic attacks develop when physical sensations occurring at times of stress are interpreted as signs of grave illness, giving rise to panic. The physical sensations of arousal thus become conditioned phobic stimuli, provoking the panic symptomatology (conditioned response) (7). Conditioning models have been particularly persuasive in accounting for the development and maintenance of agoraphobia (33).

Agoraphobia

Agoraphobia is the most disabling psychiatric complication of panic disorder. The first sign is usually the avoidance of selected settings from which escape would be difficult or embarrassing in the event of a panic attack (e.g., traveling in bus, train, or car; being out of the house alone; standing in the checkout line at a store). With the persistence of panic attacks, the inventory of phobic stimuli expands by generalization, and the patient adopts a variety of behaviors aimed at avoiding contact with a growing number of feared objects and situations (Table 13.7) (18). Ultimately, this fear of having a panic attack (anticipatory anxiety) may become incapacitating, and the patient may become homebound.

Agoraphobia occasionally occurs in the absence of panic attacks (agoraphobia without history of panic disorder in DSM-IV) but this is apparently rare, at least in clinical samples (5). Among patients with panic disorder, those most likely to develop agoraphobia are women who have persistent panic attacks (i.e., no history of clinical remissions), a high degree of interpersonal sensitivity, and a history of anxiety or depression in childhood (5).

Evaluation and Treatment

A systematic approach to the evaluation and treatment of panic disorder includes the following steps:

- Take a history and perform a focused physical examination, looking for evidence of a medical disorder that could simulate panic disorder (e.g., insulin-induced hypoglycemia, temporal lobe seizures, arrhythmias).
- Inquire about the use of caffeine-containing beverages, stimulant drugs, alcohol, marijuana, and other substances associated with panic symptoms during intoxication or withdrawal.
- Inquire about life stresses and encourage the patient to solve problems (see Chapter 11). Although this may not eliminate panic attacks, it will help reduce the levels of generalized anxiety that often develop in patients with panic disorder.
- *Use pharmacologic means* to reduce the frequency and intensity of panic attacks. Serotonin reuptake inhibitors (62), tricyclic antidepressants, and monoamine oxidase (MAO) inhibitors are effective in the prophylaxis of panic attacks (51). In a placebo-controlled trial, there was a 50% or greater decrease from the baseline frequency of panic attacks in approximately 80% of paroxetine-treated patients versus approximately 50% of placebo subjects (62). Benzodiazepines such as the triazolobenzodiazepine

alprazolam (6) are also useful in panic disorder. Because of its rapid onset of action, alprazolam may be started as a single agent at a dosage of 0.25 mg three times a day and increased to 6 mg/day in divided doses. In a large placebo-controlled trial (6), reduction in the frequency of panic attacks and of phobic avoidance became apparent within the first week of therapy; after 4 weeks, 82% of treated versus 43% of placebo patients had improved moderately and 50% versus 28% of placebo subjects were free of panic attacks. If there is concern about the possibility of alprazolam abuse (21), an antidepressant may be used instead as a single agent. The SSRI paroxetine, the tricyclic imipramine, and the MAO inhibitor phenelzine are most often used, although other SSRIs and tricyclics are effective. As a rule, dosages required for prophylaxis of panic attacks approximate those required for antidepressant effect (see Chapter 15). Symptoms may not improve for several weeks and may even intensify at first (44). For these reasons, some physicians combine alprazolam and an antidepressant at the beginning of therapy and taper alprazolam, the more rapidly effective agent, after several weeks. Effective drug treatment is generally continued for at least 6 to 12 months before tapering is attempted. Relapse is common and may indicate the need for chronic therapy.

The conditioned avoidances of agoraphobics may be reduced by behavioral exposure techniques such as those described earlier in this chapter for other phobias.

Patients often gain relief from learning that panic disorder is a common, treatable disease, not a sign of weakness. Education by the physician, supplemented by readily available books written for the lay person (1,36), may help reduce the patient's sense of isolation and embarrassment and provide practical advice about managing panic symptoms.

Obsessive–Compulsive Disorder

Description

The essential features of obsessive–compulsive disorder (OCD) are recurrent, resisted, troubling *thoughts* (e.g., objects are contaminated), and repetitive, purposeful, but senseless *actions* (e.g., washing hands 100 times per day). It is the presence of these obsessions and compulsions that distinguishes OCD from obsessive–compulsive *personality* disorder (see Chapter 14), a personality type characterized by meticulousness, perfectionism, and rigidity. The APA diagnostic criteria for OCD are listed in Table 13.8.

Table 13.7. Frequency of Strategies Adopted by Patients with Agoraphobia to Reduce Anticipatory Anxiety

Strategy	Patients (%)
When out, having a way open for quick return home	91
Being accompanied by husband/wife	85
Sitting near a door in hall, restaurant, etc.	76
Focusing one's mind on something else	63
When out for a walk, taking dog, perambulator, etc.	62
Talking problems over with a friend	62
Talking problems over with one's doctor	62
Being accompanied by a friend	60
Talking "sense to myself" (reassuring oneself)	52
Wearing sunglasses	36

From Burns LE, Thorpe GL. Epidemiology of fears and phobias. J Intern Med Res 5:1, 1977.

CASE STUDY

An 83-year-old widow was referred for evaluation because of disabling fears of contamination. She was a retired mathematics teacher who liked her subject because one and one always equal two; "I like the certainty." A practicing Catholic, she recalled that during adolescence she had once delayed disposing of a sanitary napkin because she had sneezed over it after returning home after Mass and

Table 13.8. Diagnostic Criteria for Obsessive–Compulsive Disorder

A. Either obsessions or compulsions:
Obsessions as defined by 1, 2, 3, and 4:

1. Recurrent and persistent thoughts, impulses, or images that are experienced, at some time during the disturbance, as intrusive and inappropriate, and cause marked anxiety or distress.
2. The thoughts, impulses, or images are not simply excessive worries about real-life problems.
3. The person attempts to ignore or suppress such thoughts or impulses or to neutralize them with some other thought or action.
4. The person recognizes that the obsessional thoughts, impulses, or images are a product of his or her own mind (not imposed from without as in thought insertion).

Compulsions as defined by 1 and 2:

1. Repetitive behaviors (e.g., handwashing, ordering, checking) or mental acts (e.g., praying, counting, repeating words silently) that the person feels driven to perform in response to an obsession, or according to rules that must be applied rigidly.
2. The behaviors or mental acts are aimed at preventing or reducing distress or preventing some dreaded event or situation; however, these behaviors or mental acts either are not connected in a realistic way with what they are designed to neutralize or prevent, or are clearly excessive.

B. At some point during the course of the disorder, the person has recognized that the obsessions or compulsions are excessive or unreasonable. Note: This does not apply to children.
C. The obsessions or compulsions cause marked distress, are time-consuming (take more than an hour a day), or significantly interfere with the person's normal routine, occupational functioning, or usual social activities or relationships with others.
D. If another Axis I disorder is present, the content of the obsessions or compulsions is not restricted to it (e.g., preoccupation with food in the presence of an eating disorder, hair pulling in the presence of trichotillomania, concern with appearance in the presence of body dysmorphic disorder, preoccupation with drugs in the presence of a substance use disorder, preoccupation with having a serious illness in the presence of hypochondriasis, or guilty ruminations in the presence of major depressive disorder).[a]
E. Not due to the direct effects of a substance (e.g., drugs of abuse, medication) or a general medical condition.

Reprinted with permission from the DSM-IV. Copyright 1994, American Psychiatric Association.

[a] See Chapter 10 for definition of Axis I and Axis II disorders.

worried that bits of the communion wafer might have lodged in it. She had received psychiatric treatment several times for obsessive–compulsive symptoms but had recently been doing well until she was forced to change apartments. After the move she became preoccupied with worries about contamination with germs. Especially vexing was deciding when she had adequately washed her hands after defecating; she was consumed by uncertainty about how long she should wash and how she could safely dispose of the towel after drying her hands. Her main fear was that others might be contaminated and become ill as a result of her carelessness. As a result of these ideas, she washed her hands excessively, did not leave her apartment, ate poorly (so she would defecate less), and was unable to engage in normal conversation. Treatment consisted of strict direction to limit hand washing, exhortation about the unreasonableness of her worries, and the use of *fluoxetine*, an antidepressant with specific antiobsessional properties (see below). Within 2 weeks she showed improvement, and by the end of 8 weeks she was able to dispel obsessive ideas effortlessly and felt no compulsion to wash excessively.

Epidemiology and Origins

One to two percent of people in the community (59) and in the general medical clinic (80) meet criteria for OCD. Its prevalence is slightly higher among women and tends to decline with age. Symptoms usually have their onset in adolescence or early adulthood. In one study of patients with OCD (67), the most common obsessions were fear of contamination (55%), of acting aggressively (50%), and of performing unacceptable sexual activities (32%). Somatic obsessions were present in 34% of patients (e.g., a woman who performed breast self-examinations 100 times per day to reassure herself that she had not developed breast cancer [67]), and 36% had obsessive thoughts involving the need for symmetry. The most common compulsions involved checking, cleaning, and counting. In most cases the symptoms were chronic and continuous, with some tendency for symptomatic worsening during times of stress. Associated psychiatric diagnoses included major depression (30%), simple phobia (7%), and panic disorder (5%).

Explanations for OCD have been advanced from several perspectives. Psychoanalytic writers have viewed obsessive–compulsive symptoms as products of reaction formation against unacceptable wishes and impulses, often related to aggression and sexuality. Behavioral theorists and practitioners have stressed the anxiety-reducing effects of compulsive rituals and have proposed that compulsions are maintained precisely because of their positively reinforcing ameliorating effects on conditioned anxiety. The importance of personality traits in the development of OCD is suggested by data showing that preexisting obsessive traits (e.g., meticulousness, perfectionism, indecisiveness) are very common in clinical samples of patients who go on to develop OCD (67) and that people who are obsessional, anxious, or self-conscious may be especially vulnerable to the emergence of OCD in response to life change (58).

Much recent research suggests that OCD has biologic origins. The importance of genetic factors is supported by studies showing high concordance for OCD among monozygotic twins (19) and increased risk for OCD among first-degree relatives of probands with Gilles de la Tourette's syndrome (64). Brain imaging studies demonstrate abnormalities of the left orbital frontal gyri (10) and the caudate nuclei (10,50). Clinical studies linking OCD with head trauma (57) and other neurologic disorders (38) add support to the conception that OCD may be a manifestation of brain disease. Of great theoretical and practical importance is the demonstration that certain antidepressant medications, especially the tricyclic agent clomipramine and agents that inhibit the reuptake of serotonin (e.g., fluoxetine), may dramatically diminish obsessive–compulsive symptoms. The effectiveness of fluoxetine suggests a role for central serotonergic neuronal systems in the pathophysiology of this disorder.

Evaluation and Treatment

A systematic approach to the evaluation and treatment of OCD involves the following steps:

- In the history and physical examination, look for evidence of medical conditions, medications, or dietary practices that may simulate or exacerbate symptoms of anxiety.
- Consider use of *psychosocial treatments*. Most experts recommend the use of cognitive-behavioral therapy as a first-line treatment for every patient willing to participate (52). This suggestion follows from the view that compulsions are maintained by their temporary amelioration of conditioned anxiety. Patients are taught to control their obsessive ruminations by commanding themselves to stop ruminating when obsessive ideas arise (thought stopping), and they are exhorted to resist carrying out their compulsive acts so that they can learn that there are no dire consequences associated with nonexecution of the rituals (response prevention). These techniques are often helpful if patients can be persuaded to practice them.
- Consider use of *antidepressant medications* shown to have specific efficacy in OCD. First-line drugs, all of which are significantly more effective than placebo, include the tricyclic clomipramine and the SSRIs fluvoxamine, fluoxetine, and sertraline (37,75,78). Clomipramine, the first drug approved for use in OCD, is highly sedating and strongly anticholinergic and is usually reserved for patients not responding to the SSRIs. In patients who respond to drugs, the improvement is not sustained if the drug is discontinued. Practical information about antidepressant drugs is found in Chapter 15.
- Consider short-term *problem-solving counseling* (see Chapter 11). Although this may not bring total relief, it is clear that symptomatic exacerbations of this chronic disorder tend to come at times of stress and change, and short-term counseling may help reduce the impact of such influences. On the other hand, insight-oriented, introspective psychotherapies have generally been ineffective in the treatment of OCD.

Posttraumatic Stress Disorder

Description

People who have experienced *severe physical or emotional trauma* may develop a syndrome characterized by intrusive recollections or dreams of the event, avoidance of stimuli provoking memories of the event, and a heightened level of arousal. When such symptoms have been present for less than 3 months, a diagnosis of acute posttraumatic stress disorder (PTSD) is appropriate. When this syndrome has been present for at least 3 months, the diagnosis of chronic PTSD is made. APA criteria are summarized in Table 13.9.

CASE STUDY

A 45-year-old mechanic sustained burns on the arms and thorax when an engine exploded during repair. He had no

Table 13.9. Diagnostic Criteria for Posttraumatic Stress Disorder

A. The person has been exposed to a traumatic event in which both of the following have been present:
  1. The person has experienced, witnessed, or been confronted with an event or events that involve actual or threatened death or serious injury, or a threat to the physical integrity of oneself or others.
  2. The person's response involved intense fear, helplessness, or horror. Note: In children, it may be expressed instead by disorganized or agitated behavior.
B. The traumatic event is persistently reexperienced in at least one of the following ways:
  1. Recurrent and intrusive distressing recollections of the event, including images, thoughts, or perceptions. Note: In young children, repetitive play may occur in which themes or aspects of the trauma are expressed.
  2. Recurrent distressing dreams of the event. Note: In children, there may be frightening dreams without recognized content.
  3. Acting or feeling as if the traumatic event were recurring (includes a sense of reliving the experience, illusions, hallucinations, and dissociative flashback episodes, including those that occur upon awakening or when intoxicated). Note: In young children, trauma-specific reenactment may occur.
  4. Intense psychologic distress at exposure to internal or external cues that symbolize or resemble an aspect of the traumatic event.
  5. Physiologic reactivity upon exposure to internal or external cues that symbolize or resemble an aspect of the traumatic event.
C. Persistent avoidance of stimuli associated with the trauma and numbing of general responsiveness (not present before the trauma), as indicated by at least three of the following:
  1. Efforts to avoid thoughts, feelings, or conversations associated with the trauma
  2. Efforts to avoid activities, places, or people that arouse recollections of the trauma
  3. Inability to recall an important aspect of the trauma
  4. Markedly diminished interest in participation in significant activities
  5. Feeling of detachment or estrangement from others
  6. Restricted range of affect (e.g., unable to have loving feelings)
  7. Sense of a foreshortened future (e.g., does not expect to have a career, marriage, children, or a normal life span)
D. Persistent symptoms of increased arousal (not present before the trauma), as indicated by at least two of the following:
  1. Difficulty falling or staying asleep
  2. Irritability or outbursts of anger
  3. Difficulty concentrating
  4. Hypervigilance
  5. Exaggerated startle response
E. Duration of the disturbance (symptoms in B, C, and D) is more than 1 month.
F. The disturbance causes clinically significant distress or impairment in social, occupational, or other important areas of functioning.

Acute: if duration of symptoms is less than 3 months
Chronic: if duration of symptoms is 3 months or more
With Delayed Onset: onset of symptoms at least 6 months after the stressor

Reprinted with permission from the DSM-IV. Copyright 1994, American Psychiatric Association.

history of psychiatric disorder. His surgical treatment was successful, leaving him with little residual physical disability. However, after discharge he experienced marked sleep disturbance, generalized anxiety, and loss of interest in usual activities. He avoided proximity to fire in any form and could not tolerate listening to reports about fires on the radio. Tricyclic antidepressant treatment aided sleep, improved his mood, and reduced the frequency of his intrusive memories and recurrent dreams, but it did not affect his avoidance behavior. On the anniversary of his injury he would not leave his room because he could not be persuaded that it was safe to do so.

Epidemiology and Origins

The prevalence of PTSD in the community is approximately 1%. Among men, the full syndrome is usually found among Vietnam veterans who were injured in combat; among women, the most common precipitant is physical assault. Individual posttraumatic stress symptoms (particularly nightmares, feelings of jitteriness, and sleep disturbance) are much more common, occurring in approximately 15% of the population. Combat, physical assault, seeing someone hurt or die, and experiencing a serious threat or close call are the most common traumata associated with such symptoms (40).

PTSD generally develops soon after the traumatic event, although onset may be delayed among combat veterans and survivors of burn injury (72). Although symptoms may persist for years after the traumatic event, about half of patients report resolution of symptoms within 6 months (40).

People with PTSD are twice as likely as people without PTSD to have another psychiatric disorder, particularly OCD, dysthymia, substance abuse, bipolar affective disorder, and antisocial personality. There is also an increased risk of PTSD among people with a history of childhood behavioral problems, especially lying, stealing, truancy, vandalism, and school expulsion. Among people with a history of four such behaviors, 6% meet formal criteria for PTSD and 29% report at least one symptom (40).

Explanations of PTSD have been advanced from several perspectives. From the behavioral viewpoint, the posttraumatic symptoms (e.g., hyperarousal, intrusive recollections) are viewed as products of classically conditioned linkages between innocuous stimuli (e.g., a news report about a fire) and the original traumatic event (e.g., painful injury in a fire). The avoidance symptoms are explained in terms of operant conditioning: Avoidance of stimuli reminiscent of the traumatic event is reinforced by its protection of the patient from the symptoms of phobic anxiety (i.e., hyperarousal). Biological theorists have proposed explanations involving changes in central adrenergic autonomic arousal (45) and in cerebral mechanisms regulating sleep cycles (73). Important roles for personality traits and early life experience have been suggested by observations of burn patients and other trauma victims demonstrating relationships between maladaptive personality traits, early life behavioral problems, and poor posttraumatic adjustment (3,40,72).

Treatment

Behavioral, psychotherapeutic, and pharmacologic treatment approaches have all been advocated. *Behavioral treatments* such as desensitization are generally required to help patients overcome the conditioned avoidance of stimuli reminiscent of the traumatic event. Psychotherapy is virtually always needed to assist patients in dealing with anger about the injury, guilt about survival, and similar themes common among people with PTSD.

Antidepressant and anxiolytic medications have been used with variable efficacy. Tricyclic antidepressants and MAO inhibitors may be effective in ameliorating hyperarousal, intrusion, and avoidance symptoms as well as relieving concurrent major depression (25,46). Serotonin-specific reuptake inhibitors such as fluoxetine may be effective in ameliorating "numbing," particularly in noncombat trauma victims (79). Benzodiazepines are sometimes used, but there is no empirical evidence for their effectiveness in this setting, and they are relatively contraindicated in patients at high risk for chemical dependency. Neuroleptic drugs are almost never indicated (27).

TREATMENT OF ANXIETY DISORDERS: GENERAL MEASURES

Specific treatments and results are described above for each specific anxiety disorder. This section describes nonpharmacologic and pharmacologic measures that may be of use in multiple anxiety disorders.

Nonpharmacologic Approaches

A variety of cognitive and behavioral interventions are useful in the treatment of anxiety disorders.

Education and Explanation

Patients with panic attacks, obsessions and compulsions, posttraumatic distress symptoms, and generalized anxiety often feel different, isolated from others, and confused about the nature of their malady. They benefit greatly from learning that they have a diagnosable disorder, that they are not alone in their suffering, and that there are effective treatments. Several popular books can be recommended to patients who are interested in reading about anxiety disorders (1,36).

Self-Regulation Techniques

Many patients benefit from learning specific techniques that reduce motor tension, hyperarousal, and autonomic hyperactivity. These self-regulation techniques include muscle relaxation, diaphragmatic breathing, biofeedback, self-hypnosis, and meditation exercises (32). Interested generalists can develop skills in teaching these techniques to their patients. Alternatively, patients can be referred to behavioral therapists for instruction.

In *progressive muscle relaxation and diaphragmatic breathing* (Table 13.10), patients learn to ameliorate anxiety by sequential contraction and relaxation of muscle groups or by slow inhalation using the diaphragm. With regular practice, patients can apply these techniques in times of distress and achieve considerable relief. Commercially available audiotapes may help guide patients through the procedure (see "General References"), and *The Relaxation Response* (11), written for the layperson, may also be useful.

Table 13.10. Essential Steps in Progressive Muscle Relaxation, Rapid Muscle Relaxation Techniques, and Diaphragmatic Breathing

	Exercise
A. Progressive Muscle Relaxation[a]	
Muscle(s)	
Forehead/scalp	Raise the eyebrows high; hold; feel strain; relax.
Forehead	Scowl or frown; bunch eyebrows with nose upward; relax.
Eyes	Squeeze eyes shut; hold; feel strain in temples; relax.
Mouth	Smile broadly until mouth quivers slightly; relax; press lips tightly inward; hold; relax.
Jaw	Grit teeth gently but firmly; hold; relax; part lips slightly.
Neck/arm/shoulder	Press head back against right hand; relax; repeat exercise with left hand.
Neck/arm/shoulder	Press head forward against right hand placed on forehead; relax; repeat with left hand.
Back/legs/abdomen	Sitting, grip chair sides firmly; raise legs slightly; lift buttocks 1 inch from chair; point toes forward, then backward; relax.
Hands/arm	Make fist; clench tightly; relax.

B. Rapid Relaxation[b]
1. Sit or lie down. The quieter the place, the better.
2. Take a deep breath through your mouth, hold it for 10 seconds, and exhale slowly.
3. Mentally repeat the word "relax" 4 times in a calm manner.
4. Gradually space out repeating "relax" until each repetition takes about 7 seconds.
5. Keep practicing until you achieve the level of relaxation you desire.

C. Diaphragmatic Breathing
While sitting or lying down with a pillow at the small of your back
1. Breathe in slowly and deeply by pushing your stomach out.
2. Say the word "relax" silently to yourself before exhaling.
3. Exhale slowly, letting your stomach come in.
4. Repeat entire procedure 10 times consecutively, with emphasis on slow, deep breaths.
Practice should take place 5 times per day, 10 consecutive diaphragmatic breaths each sitting. Time for mastery is after 1–2 wk of daily practice.

[a] Subject instructed to practice this seated comfortably or reclining.
[b] For immediate relaxation in everyday stressful situation.

In *biofeedback* (28) patients learn to control anxiety with the aid of electromyographic information provided to them in the form of visual or auditory messages. During treatment sessions electrodes are placed in a muscle (e.g., frontalis) or muscle group. Patients then attempt to reduce muscle tension, receive immediate feedback about the effectiveness of their efforts (e.g., a reduction in the amplitude of a tone fed back to them through earphones), and learn to alter their technique to achieve more complete electromyographic (and clinical) relaxation.

Self-hypnosis training often begins with office-based sessions during which the therapist uses a standard hypnotic induction technique and then, for example, asks the patient to notice the warm, tingling feeling starting in the legs and feet and spreading slowly throughout the body. Pleasant, peaceful mental images might be suggested. Patients are taught to induce these states on their own and are advised to practice them regularly, reinforced by periodic office visits for reassessment and further practice. Physicians may develop skills in performing hypnosis by attending seminars such as those sponsored by the Society for Clinical and Experimental Hypnosis.

Meditation techniques (e.g., Zen, yoga, transcendental meditation) have been practiced for centuries but have recently become popular treatments for anxiety because they favorably alter anxiety-related physiologic variables such as respiratory rate, oxygen consumption, and galvanic skin response, a measure of autonomic activity. Meditation techniques that are effective in ameliorating anxiety include or encourage the following elements (12):

- *A mental device.* There should be a constant stimulus such as a sound, word, or phrase repeated silently or audibly, or fixed gazing at an object.
- *Passive attitude.* If distracting thoughts occur during the repetition or gazing, they should be disregarded and attention should be redirected to the chosen stimulus. The patient should not worry about the quality of performance.
- *Decreased muscle tone.* The patient should be in a comfortable position so that minimal muscular work is required.
- *Quiet environment.* An environment with minimal distractions should be chosen. If visual fixation on an object is not used, the patient's eyes should generally be closed.

Pharmacologic Treatments

Patients with anxiety disorders often benefit from pharmacologic treatment. The agents used most often are discussed in this section.

Benzodiazepines

Benzodiazepines are prescribed in ambulatory settings primarily for the treatment of anxiety and insomnia. Adverse side effects include oversedation, ataxia, diminished cognitive function, and rarely, ventilatory depression. The anxiolytic effects of these compounds are believed to result from *enhancement of the activity of γ-aminobutyric acid* (GABA), an inhibitory neurotransmitter hypothesized to play a role in the mediation of anxiety. The use of these agents in the treatment of specific anxiety disorders is described above in the sections describing the disorders. Their use as hypnotic agents is described in Chapter 85.

Pharmacology. Although the effects of the various benzodiazepines on the cognitive and somatic symptoms of anxiety are fundamentally similar, these agents differ in terms of certain clinically important pharmacologic properties. These are described in this section and summarized in Table 13.11.

Route of Administration. All of the anxiolytic benzodiazepines are well absorbed orally, although the rates of absorption vary widely (see below). Diazepam and lorazepam are available for intravenous use; this is rarely required in the ambulatory treatment of anxiety. Lorazepam is very well absorbed after intramuscular administration. If diazepam must be given by this route, the deltoid muscle should be selected as the injection site. The intramuscular absorption of chlordiazepoxide is particularly slow, even after deltoid injection, and intramuscular administration is rarely indicated (35).

Onset of Action. The onset of action after oral dosing depends on the rate of absorption from the gastrointestinal tract. The rate of absorption is governed primarily by intrinsic physicochemical properties of the drugs, including lipid solubility. Diazepam and clorazepate are especially rapidly absorbed and produce prompt sedation, relaxation, and even euphoria, a property associated with abuse liability. Prazepam is slowly absorbed and slow in onset. Other benzodiazepines develop their clinical effects at intermediate rates.

Duration of Action. The duration of action depends primarily on lipid solubility. Agents with higher lipid solubility (e.g., diazepam) are more rapidly redistributed from their sites of action in the central nervous system to peripheral adipose tissue and, therefore, may produce more short-lived clinical effects after single doses than less lipid-soluble drugs (e.g., lorazepam), even those with shorter elimination half-lives. Persistence of drug effect after *multiple* doses depends on elimination half-life.

Rate of Elimination. Elimination half-life is affected by several factors, including lipid solubility. The more highly lipid-soluble drugs are more completely distributed in body fat relative to blood; therefore, these agents have larger volumes of distribution and are less available to the liver for metabolic transformation and elimination. This is especially important in the elderly, who generally have more body fat than younger people and are therefore particularly vulnerable to drug accumulation.

Table 13.11. Usual Dosage and Pharmacokinetics of Anxiolytic Benzodiazepines

Drug (Trade Name), Year Introduced	Onset of Effect After Oral Dose[a]	Available Strengths (mg)	Oral Daily Dosage Range Divided Two or Three Times a Day (mg)	Active Metabolites Present	Elimination Half-Life[b] (hr)
Alprazolam[c] (Xanax), 1981	Intermediate	0.25, 0.5, 1 (scored tablets)	0.75–6	No	8–16
Chlordiazepoxide[c] (Librium; Libritabs), 1960	Intermediate	5, 10, 25 (capsules); 5, 10, 25 (tablets)	15–100	Yes	5–30
Clonazepam[d] (Klonopin), 1990	Intermediate	0.5, 1, 2 (tablets)	1.5–20	Yes	18–50
Clorazepate dipotassium[c] (Tranxene; Tranxene SD), 1972	Rapid	3.75, 7.5, 15 (capsules); 11.25, 22.5 (tablets)	15–60	Yes	36–200
			22.5 (single doses are intended for patients stabilized on 3.75 or 7.5 mg three times a day)	Yes	36–200
Diazepam[c] (Valium), 1961	Rapid	2, 5, 10 (tablets)	4–40	Yes	20–50
Diazepam (Valrelease), 1982	Slow	15 (capsules)	15–30 (single dose is equivalent to 5 mg of Valium three times a day)	Yes	20–50
Halazepam (Paxipam), 1981	Slow to intermediate	20, 40 (tablets)	80–160	Yes	50–100
Lorazepam[c] (Ativan), 1977	Intermediate	0.5, 1, 2 (tablets)	1–6	No	10–20
Oxazepam[c] (Serax), 1963	Slow to intermediate	10, 15, 30 (capsules) 15 (tablets)	30–120 30–120	No	5–10
Prazepam (Centrax), 1977	Slow	5, 10 (capsules)	20–60	Yes	36–200

[a] Drugs with more rapid onset of action are those more rapidly absorbed.

[b] Elimination half-life of lipophilic activity.

[c] Generic available.

[d] Clonazepam is not FDA approved for treatment of anxiety. Approved as an anticonvulsant.

The elimination half-life of a benzodiazepine is also influenced by aspects of its hepatic metabolism. Most of the benzodiazepines are metabolized in the liver by microsomal P-450 oxidative pathways (hydroxylation and N-dealkylation) to compounds that retain some pharmacologic activity. Several of the drugs are transformed to desmethyldiazepam (half-life 50 hours), a metabolite that accounts for all or most of the activity of clorazepate, prazepam, and halazepam. The elimination half-lives of drugs metabolized to this long-lived intermediary compound are long. All benzodiazepines are finally inactivated in the liver by glucuronide conjugation. Certain agents (oxazepam, lorazepam, temazepam) require only conjugation; they do not undergo oxidation and have no active metabolites. The elimination of drugs requiring oxidation may be prolonged by aging, liver disease, and concurrent pharmacotherapy (e.g., cimetidine, oral contraceptives). Conjugation is not affected by these factors. For this reason, oxazepam, lorazepam, and temazepam may be less prone to accumulation with multiple dosing in patients who are elderly, have liver disease, or take multiple medications.

Tolerance, Dependence, and Abuse.   Tolerance is a decline in the effectiveness of a drug at a given dosage with continuing usage. Physical dependence is the development of stereotyped physical signs and symptoms in response to the withdrawal of a substance. Psychological dependence is a subjective craving for a drug, usually accompanied by drug-seeking efforts.

Although tolerance to the hypnotic effects of benzodiazepines usually develops, it is generally believed that tolerance to their anxiolytic effects is less common (61). However, both physical and psychologic dependence may occur, particularly when high dosages are taken for long periods; and drug discontinuation may lead to the development of a withdrawal syndrome. Common withdrawal symptoms include tension, irritability, sleep disturbance, loss of appetite, pain, tremor, paresthesias, photophobia, and hyperacusis (61). Rarely, seizures or delirium may occur (35). In one study (65), minor withdrawal symptoms occurred in 35% of patients with panic disorder who were slowly tapered off alprazolam after 2 months of active treatment; seizures and delirium were not observed. It is important to distinguish between withdrawal (development of new symptoms that resolve with resumption of medication) and rebound (temporary return of original symptoms at greater-than-pretreatment frequency or severity), a common, self-limited postdiscontinuation phenomenon (65,69).

The following measures may be useful in *managing the discontinuation of benzodiazepines* (61):

- Although both the dosage and duration of treatment must be ample in order for patients to experience the benefits of therapy, not all patients require high dosages (e.g., alprazolam 6 mg/day) or long-term treatment (e.g., more than 1 year), both of which make discontinuation more difficult; therefore, dosage and duration of treatment should be minimized.

- Patients should understand that they may experience rebound or withdrawal symptoms after discontinuation and that these do not indicate the need for long-term treatment.
- Patients should be seen weekly and be able to reach the physician by phone between visits so that they feel some control over their level of discomfort.
- Tapering of the drug should occur over 4 to 16 weeks, with 10 to 20% reductions in the daily dosage every week. The rate should be closely tailored to the patient's level of discomfort.
- It may be helpful to switch the patient from a short-acting to a long-acting benzodiazepine (e.g., clonazepam [41]) before beginning the taper; this may reduce fluctuations in medication levels during the day and thereby reduce withdrawal symptoms.
- It is important to watch for emergence of relapse (as opposed to rebound and withdrawal) during the taper and to be prepared to treat this.

Abuse of benzodiazepines is uncommon among patients for whom these agents are prescribed to control anxiety (83). Those who are at high risk of abusing benzodiazepines are patients with concurrent or previous abuse of other drugs such as alcohol, barbiturates, or illicit substances (see Chapter 22). Screening for these problems, as described in Chapter 21, is the best way to avoid prescribing benzodiazepines to potential abusers. Treatment of patients who abuse benzodiazepines is similar to treatment of those with alcoholism and other forms of substance abuse, described in Chapters 21 and 22.

Antidepressants

Tricyclics and MAO inhibitors are useful as antipanic agents and may be effective in ameliorating the psychic symptoms associated with generalized anxiety (43) as well as the intrusive memories associated with posttraumatic stress disorders. Trazodone may be comparably effective in generalized anxiety disorder (65). As reviewed above, several SSRIs have been shown to be effective in panic disorder, OCD, social phobia, generalized anxiety disorder, and possibly PTSD. Detailed guidelines for their use are found in Chapter 15.

Buspirone (Buspar)

Buspirone is the first available azaspirodecanedione. Its overall effectiveness as an anxiolytic is comparable to that of benzodiazepines (31), although it has a slower onset of action and may be more effective in treating the cognitive and interpersonal aspects of anxiety than the somatic elements (30,70). It differs from benzodiazepines in that it has no anticonvulsant or muscle relaxant properties, is nonsedating, does not impair psychomotor function, does not produce euphoria, and does not amplify the effects of alcohol or ameliorate symptoms of alcohol or sedative-hypnotic withdrawal. The most common side effects include nervousness, headache, dizziness, light-headedness, and nausea (60). Tolerance and dependence are not believed to occur, and its abuse liability appears to be low. Its central mechanism of action is unknown; however, it clearly interacts with central serotonergic, GABAergic, and dopaminergic systems differently than do benzodiazepines (26).

Buspirone is well absorbed orally but is subject to a significant first-pass effect in the liver. Although it is largely protein bound in the circulation, it has not been shown to displace phenytoin, digoxin, propranolol, or warfarin from plasma proteins at therapeutic dosages. It undergoes oxidative metabolism in the liver and is excreted by the kidneys; hence liver and kidney disease may slow its metabolism and clearance. Half-life is usually in the range of 2 to 11 hours and may be prolonged in the elderly (29).

Buspirone is available in 5- and 10-mg tablets. The usual starting dosage is 5 mg three times per day. Anxiolytic effects generally require 2 weeks to develop. If there has been only modest response after 2 weeks, the dosage may be increased to 20 mg three times per day; further increases rarely improve its effectiveness. Withdrawal and rebound effects are not believed to occur after discontinuation.

β-Adrenergic Blockers

Propranolol and the other β-blockers may be more effective than benzodiazepines in reducing the autonomic symptoms (e.g., palpitations) that occur in some anxious patients (47). β-Blockers may be particularly helpful prophylactically in acutely anxiety-provoking situations such as public speaking and taking examinations. β-Blockers do not appear to be useful in preventing panic attacks; however, they may be tried in patients who cannot tolerate the drugs of choice for this disorder (i.e., alprazolam, antidepressants). Details regarding the use of β-blocking drugs are found in Chapter 62.

Antihistamines

Antihistamines may be used to control anxiety as alternatives to benzodiazepines. They appear to be safer for patients with chronic obstructive pulmonary disease, in whom benzodiazepines may suppress ventilation, and they are useful in patients who might abuse benzodiazepines. Their major disadvantage is that they are very sedating. Hydroxyzine (Vistaril, Atarax) is most often used for this purpose and may be prescribed at dosages ranging from 10 to 25 mg three times per day.

General References*

American Psychiatric Association. **Diagnostic and Statistical Manual of Mental Disorders.** 4th ed. (DSM-IV). Washington, DC: American Psychiatric Association, 1994.
> Diagnostic criteria and epidemiologic information for all recognized psychiatric disorders.

Shader RI, Greenblatt DJ. Use of benzodiazepines in anxiety disorders. N Engl J Med 328:1398, 1993.
> Excellent recent review.

---

*Bold print (general references) and bold numerals (specific references) denote published controlled clinical trials, meta-analyses, or consensus-based recommendations.

Relaxation Cassettes

A variety of audiocassette programs that provide self-instruction in relaxation techniques are available from Guilford Publications, Inc., 72 Spring St., New York, NY 10003; and New Harbinger Publications, 5674 Shattuck Ave., Oakland, CA 94609.

Specific References

1. Agras MW. Panic: facing fears, phobias, and anxiety. New York: WH Freeman, 1985.
2. Anderson DJ, Noyes R, Crowe RR. A comparison of panic disorder and generalized anxiety disorder. Am J Psychiatry 141:572, 1984.
3. Andreasen NJ, Noyes R, Hartford CE. Factors influencing adjustment of burn patients during hospitalization. Psychosom Med 34:517, 1972.
4. Appenheimer T, Noyes R. Generalized anxiety disorder. Prim Care 14:635, 1987.
5. Aronson TA, Logue CM. On the longitudinal course of panic disorder: developmental history and prediction of phobic complications. Compr Psychiatry 28:344, 1987.
6. **Ballenger JC, Burrows GD, DePont RL, et al. Alprazolam in panic disorder and agoraphobia: results from a multicenter trial. Arch Gen Psychiatry 45:413, 1988.**
7. Barlow DH. Behavioral conception and treatment of panic. Psychopharmacol Bull 22:802, 1986.
8. Barrett JE, Barrett JA, Oxman TE, et al. The prevalence of psychiatric disorders in primary care practice. Arch Gen Psychiatry 45:1100, 1988.
9. Bass C, Cawley R, Wade C, et al. Unexplained breathlessness and psychiatric morbidity in patients with normal and abnormal coronary arteries. Lancet 1:605, 1983.
10. Baxter LR, Phelps ME, Mazziotta JC, et al. Local cerebral glucose metabolic rates in obsessive–compulsive disorder. Arch Gen Psychiatry 44:211, 1987.
11. Benson H. The relaxation response. New York: William Morrow, 1976.
12. Benson H, Beary JF, Carol MP. The relaxation response. Psychiatry 37:37, 1974.
13. Blazer D, Hughes D, George LK. Stressful life events and the onset of a generalized anxiety syndrome. Am J Psychiatry 144:1178, 1987.
14. Brawman-Mintzer O, Lydiard RB. Generalized anxiety disorder: issues in epidemiology. J Clin Psychiatry 57(Suppl 7):3, 1996.
15. Breier A, Charney DS, Heninger GR. Major depression in patients with agoraphobia and panic disorder. Arch Gen Psychiatry 41:1129, 1984.
16. Breier A, Charney DS, Heninger GR. The diagnostic validity of anxiety disorders and their relationship to depressive illness. Am J Psychiatry 142:787, 1985.
17. Breier A, Charney DS, Heninger GR. Agoraphobia with panic attacks. Arch Gen Psychiatry 43:1029, 1986.
18. Burns LE, Thorpe GL. The epidemiology of fears and phobias. J Intern Med Res 5(Suppl 5):1, 1977.
19. Carey G, Gottesman II. Twin and family studies of anxiety, phobic, and obsessive disorders. In: Klein DF, Rabkin JG, eds. Anxiety: new research and changing concepts. New York: Raven Press, 1981;116–136.
20. **Chouinard G, Annable L, Fontaine R, Solyom L. Alprazolam in the treatment of generalized anxiety and panic disorders: a double-blind placebo-controlled study. Psychopharmacology 77:229, 1982.**
21. Ciraulo DA, Sands BF, Shader RI. Critical review of liability for benzodiazepine abuse among alcoholics. Am J Psychiatry 145:1501, 1988.
22. Clark DM, Salkovskis PM, Chalkley AJ. Respiratory control as a treatment for panic attacks. J Behav Ther Exp Psychiatry 16:23, 1985.
23. Cloninger CR, Martin RL, Clayton P, Guze SB. A blind follow-up and family study of anxiety neurosis: preliminary analysis of the St. Louis 500. In: Klein DF, Rabkin J, eds. Anxiety: new research and changing concepts. New York: Raven Press, 1981.

24. Coryell W, Noyes R, Clancy J. Excess mortality in panic disorder: a comparison with primary unipolar depression. Arch Gen Psychiatry 39:701, 1982.

25. Davidson J, Kudler H, Smith R, et al. Treatment of posttraumatic stress disorder with imipramine and placebo. Arch Gen Psychiatry 47:259, 1990.

26. Eison AS, Temple DL. Buspirone: review of its pharmacology and current perspectives on its mechanism of action. Am J Med 80(Suppl 3B):1, 1986.

27. Friedman MJ. Toward a rational pharmacotherapy for posttraumatic stress disorder: an interim report. Am J Psychiatry 145:281, 1988.

28. Gaarder KR, Montgomery PS. Clinical biofeedback: a procedural manual for behavioral medicine. 2nd ed. Baltimore: Williams & Wilkins, 1981.

29. Gammans RE, Mayol FG, Labudde JA. Metabolism and disposition of buspirone. Am J Med 80(Suppl 3B):41, 1986.

30. Goa KL, Ward A. Buspirone: a preliminary review of its pharmacologic properties and therapeutic efficacy as an anxiolytic. Drugs 32:114, 1986.

31. Goldberg HL, Finnerty RJ. The comparative efficacy of buspirone and diazepam in the treatment of anxiety. Am J Psychiatry 136:1184, 1979.

32. Goldberg RJ. Anxiety reduction by self-regulation: theory, practice, and evaluation. Ann Intern Med 96:483, 1982.

33. Goldstein AJ, Chambless DL. A reanalysis of agoraphobia. Behavior Ther 9:47, 1978.

34. Gorman JM, Dillon D, Fyer AJ, et al. The lactate infusion model. Psychopharmacol Bull 21:428, 1985.

35. Greenblatt DJ, Shader RI, Abernethy DR. Current status of benzodiazepines. N Engl J Med 309:354, 1983.

36. Greist JF, Jerreson JW, Marks IM. Anxiety and its treatments: help is available. Washington, DC: American Psychiatric Press, 1986.

37. Greist JH, Jefferson JW, Kobak KA, et al. Efficacy and tolerability of serotonin transport inhibitors in obsessive–compulsive disorder: a meta-analysis. Arch Gen Psychiatry 52:53, 1995.

38. Grimshaw L. Obsessional disorder and neurological illness. J Neurol Neurosurg Psychiatry 27:229, 1964.

39. Haines AP, Imeson JD, Meade TW. Phobic anxiety and ischaemic heart disease. BMJ 295:297, 1987.

40. Helzer JE, Robins LN, McEvoy L. Post-traumatic stress disorder in the general population: findings of the Epidemiologic Catchment Area Survey. N Engl J Med 317:1630, 1987.

41. Herman JB, Rosenbaum JF, Brotman AN. The alprazolam to clonazepam switch for the treatment of panic disorder. J Clin Psychopharmacol 7:175, 1987.

42. Hoehn-Saric R. Characteristics of chronic anxiety patients. In: Klein DF, Rabkin J, eds. Anxiety: new research and changing concepts. New York: Raven Press, 1981.

43. Hoehn-Saric R, McLeod DR, Zimmerli WD. Differential effects of alprazolam and imipramine in generalized anxiety disorder: somatic versus psychic symptoms. J Clin Psychiatry 49:293, 1988.

44. Katzelnick DJ, Kobak KA, Greist JH, et al. Sertraline for social phobia: a double-blind, placebo-controlled crossover study. Am J Psychiatry 152(9):1368, 1995.

45. Kolb LC. A neuropsychological hypothesis explaining post-traumatic stress disorders. Am J Psychiatry 144:989, 1987.

46. Kosten TR, Frank JB, Dan E, et al. Pharmacotherapy for post-traumatic stress disorder using phenelzine or imipramine. J Nerv Ment Dis 179:366, 1991.

47. Lead article: beta-adrenergic blockade and anxiety. Lancet 2:611, 1976.

48. Liebowitz MR, Schneier F, Campeas R, et al. Phenelzine vs atenolol in social phobia. Arch Gen Psychiatry 49:290, 1992.

49. Lown B. Mental stress, arrhythmias, and sudden death. Am J Med 72:177, 1982.

50. Luxenberg JS, Swedo SE, Flament MF, et al. Neuroanatomical abnormalities in obsessive–compulsive disorder detected with quantitative x-ray computed tomography. Am J Psychiatry 145:1089, 1988.

51. Lydiard RB, Ballenger JC. Antidepressants in panic disorder and agoraphobia. J Affect Disord 13:153, 1987.

52. March JS, Frances A, Carpenter D, Kahn D. The Expert Consensus Guideline Series: treatment of obsessive–compulsive disorder. J Clin Psychiatry 58(Suppl 4):1, 1997.

53. Marks I. Fears and phobias. London: Heinemann, 1969.

54. Marks I. Recent results of behavioral treatments of phobias and obsessions. J Intern Med Res 5(Suppl 5):15, 1977.

55. Matuzas W, Al-Sadir J, Uhlenhuth EH, Glass RM. Mitral valve prolapse and thyroid abnormalities in patients with panic attacks. Am J Psychiatry 144:493, 1987.

56. Mayou R, Williamson B, Foster A. Attitudes and advice after myocardial infarction. BMJ 1:1577, 1976.

57. McKeon J, McGuffin P, Robinson P. Obsessive–compulsive neurosis following head injury: a report of four cases. Br J Psychiatry 144:190, 1984.

58. McKeon J, Roa B, Mann A. Life events and personality traits in obsessive–compulsive neurosis. Br J Psychiatry 144:185, 1984.

59. Myers JK, Weissman MM, Tischler GL, et al. Six-month prevalence of psychiatric disorders in three communities. Arch Gen Psychiatry 41:959, 1984.

60. Newton RE, Marunycz JD, Alderdice MT, Napoliello MJ. Review of the side effect profile of buspirone. Am J Med 80(Suppl 3B):17, 1986.

61. Noyes R, Garvey MJ, Cook BL, Perry PJ. Benzodiazepine withdrawal: a review of the evidence. J Clin Psychiatry 49:382, 1988.

62. Oehrberg S, Christiansen PE, Behnke K. Paroxetine in the treatment of panic disorder: a randomized, double-blind, placebo-controlled study. Br J Psychiatry 167:374, 1995.

63. Pauls DL, Slymen P. A family study of panic disorder. Arch Gen Psychiatry 40:1065, 1983.

64. Pauls DL, Towbin KE, Leckman JF, et al. Gilles de la Tourette's syndrome and obsessive–compulsive disorder. Arch Gen Psychiatry 43:1180, 1986.

65. Pecknold JC, Swinson RP, Kuch K, Lewis CP. Alprazolam in panic disorder and agoraphobia: results from a multicenter trial. III. Discontinuation effects. Arch Gen Psychiatry 45:429, 1988.

66. Rasmussen K, Ravnsbaek J, Funch-Jensen P, Bagger JP. Oesophageal spasm in patients with coronary artery spasm. Lancet 1:174, 1986.

67. Rasmussen SA, Tsuang MT. Clinical characteristics and family history in DSM-III obsessive–compulsive disorder. Am J Psychiatry 143:317, 1986.

68. Rickels K, Downing R, Schweizer E, Hassman H. Antidepressants for the treatment of generalized anxiety disorder: a placebo-controlled comparison of imipramine, trazodone and diazepam. Arch Gen Psychiatry 50:884–895, 1993.

69. Rickels K, Fox IL, Greenblatt DJ, et al. Clorazepate and lorazepam: clinical improvement and rebound anxiety. Am J Psychiatry 145:312, 1988.

70. Rickels K, Weisman K, Norstad D. Buspirone and diazepam in anxiety: a controlled study. J Clin Psychiatry 43:81, 1982.

71. Robbins LN, Helzer JE, Weissman MM, et al. Lifetime prevalence of specific psychiatric disorders in three sites. Arch Gen Psychiatry 41:949, 1984.

72. Roca RP, Spence R, Munster A. Post-traumatic adaptation and distress among adult burn survivors. Am J Psychiatry 149:1234, 1992.

73. Ross RJ, Ball WA, Sullivan KA, Caroff SN. Sleep disturbance as the hallmark of posttraumatic stress disorder. Am J Psychiatry 146:697, 1988.

74. Taylor CB, Ferguson JM, Wermuth BM. Simple techniques to treat medical phobias. Postgrad Med J 53:28, 1977.

75. Thoren P, Asberg M, Cronholm B, et al. Clomipramine treatment of obsessive–compulsive disorder: I. A controlled clinical trial. Arch Gen Psychiatry 37:1281, 1980.

76. Torgersen S. Genetic factors in anxiety disorders. Arch Gen Psychiatry 40:1085, 1983.

77. Torgersen S. Childhood and family characteristics in panic and generalized anxiety disorders. Am J Psychiatry 143:630, 1986.

78. Turner SM, Jacob RG, Beidel DC, et al. Fluoxetine treatment of obsessive–compulsive disorder. J Clin Psychopharmacol 5:201, 1985.

79. van der Kolk BA, Dreyfuss K, Michaels M, et al. Fluoxetine in post-traumatic stress disorder. J Clin Psychiatry 55:517, 1994.

80. van Vliet IM, den Boer JA, Westernberg HG. Psychopharmacological treatment of social phobia: a double blind placebo controlled study with fluvoxamine. Psychopharmacology (Berlin) 115:128–134, 1994.

81. Von Korff M, Shapiro S, Burke JD, et al. Anxiety and depression in a primary care clinic. Arch Gen Psychiatry 44:152, 1987.

82. Windheuser HJ. Anxious mothers as models for coping with anxiety. Behav Anal Mod 2:39, 1977.

83. Woods JH, Katz JL, Winger G. Benzodiazepines: use, abuse, and consequences. Pharmacol Rev 44:151, 1992.

C H A P T E R   14

Maladaptive Personalities

ROBERT P. ROCA, MD, MPH

CONCEPT OF PERSONALITY

The enduring attitudes, behaviors, and capacities that distinguish individuals from each other are collectively called personality. Personality has been conceptualized in many ways, two of which are in common use. One approach is to specify *categories of personality* and to classify individuals according to the type they most closely resemble. The ancient Greek topology of personality (phlegmatic, melancholic, sanguine, and choleric) was of this sort, and the American Psychiatric Association uses a similar approach in the classification of personality disorders published in the most recent *Diagnostic and Statistical Manual of Mental Disorders* (DSM-IV) (see below).

Another approach is to view personality as a *mosaic of dimensional traits,* each of which is possessed by individuals in differing degrees (2). Intelligence, as defined by the *intelligence quotient* (IQ), is a model of such a trait. IQ scores are normally distributed in the population and are highly correlated with academic and occupational achievement. People with above-average IQ scores tend to be successful in school and work, whereas those with below-average IQs often have difficulty meeting the demands of daily life independently. Knowledge of a person's position on the dimension of intelligence thus illuminates strengths and vulnerabilities and allows one to predict circumstances that the person might find overwhelming.

CASE STUDY

A 30-year-old man was admitted to the hospital for cellulitis of the feet. His physician discovered that he had only completed the third grade and that he was unable to read, write, or calculate. Further investigation disclosed that he had recently lost his job in a laundromat and that he had been observed walking barefoot in a dumpster looking for items he needed. His physician explained to him, carefully and repeatedly, the relationship between his infection and his behavior. A social worker was called to help him apply for financial assistance and other entitlements.

Dimensions can be converted into categories, albeit with some loss of precision. Mental retardation, for example, is said to be present when the IQ is less than 70. Although this is a useful categorical definition, it is somewhat misleading because the impairment of someone with an IQ of 68 is not substantially more than that of someone with an IQ of 72 who, by definition, would not be considered mentally retarded. Such a case illustrates that thinking in rigidly categorical terms may obscure areas of vulnerability that a dimensional approach might bring to light.

Other personality traits may be described dimensionally, although none has been studied as thoroughly as intelligence. We use dimensional thinking intuitively when we recognize that some people are more meticulous, more gregarious, or more ambitious than others. Psychologists use this approach more technically when they administer standardized tests to describe quantitatively how introverted or neurotic someone is. At some arbitrary point, the meticulous person may be categorized as obsessional or the introverted person as schizoid and thus be said to have a personality disorder; however, it is useful to recognize that certain patients are more meticulous or introverted than others even when they are not categorically obsessional or schizoid. A dimensional view facilitates the recognition of such important personality traits and thus prepares one to take these attributes into account when dealing with patients.

Development of Personality

Personality evolves out of interactions between constitutional, or inborn, factors and the molding influences of the environment. Constitutional factors include capacities, such as intelligence, and aspects of temperament, such as sociability and emotionality, all of which may have neurobiological correlates and genetic determinants (3). The most important environmental influences are interpersonal relationships, usually with parents. Many theories have been offered to account more specifically for personality development, but none has yet proved fully adequate, and none is endorsed in this chapter.

Conceptualization of Personality Disorder

Personality disorders are among the most controversial conditions in psychiatry. There is no doubt that some people have enduring patterns of maladaptive attitudes and behaviors that interfere with their ability to work effectively and to develop and sustain gratifying interpersonal relationships. It is also clear that such people are at increased risk for long-term social impairment and for many major psychiatric illnesses (4,5). The controversy lies in how best to conceptualize and subdivide these disorders. This chapter describes three such conceptualizations.

The dominant approach in the United States—that adopted by the American Psychiatric Association in its most current *Diagnostic and Statistical Manual* (DSM-IV)—is prototypical and categorical. In this scheme, the diagnostic criteria for the personality disorders are lists of attitudes and behaviors (e.g., self-dramatizing, attention seeking) that, in combination, evoke an ideal prototype (e.g., the histrionic personality). Only a person exhibiting the requisite number of such attitudes and behaviors (at least four, in the case of histrionic personality disorder) is said to have the condition. Personality disorder is rare when defined in this way.

Maladaptive personalities can also be conceptualized in terms of quantitative deviations from normal along specific personality dimensions. Many clinically important personality traits may be viewed dimensionally; people may be high or low in obsessionality or dependency or self-importance. Normal endowments of these and other traits are usually considered healthy, whereas excesses are likely to produce special vulnerabilities. For example, excessive obsessionality may lead to great distress in circumstances that require flexibility and emotional spontaneity, and poor self-esteem may predispose one to demoralization in response to criticism from a superior. These examples illustrate that dimensional thinking about personality disturbances calls for consideration of the environmental stresses that expose the vulnerability as well as the trait-based vulnerability itself. Because there are many relevant dimensions, and because most people have at least one trait in excess, a dimensional approach illuminates areas of vulnerability in most patients.

Finally, personality disorders may be viewed as incomplete or atypical expressions of schizophrenia, mood disorders, or other major psychiatric illnesses.

Subtyping of Personality Disorder

As noted above, the American Psychiatric Association adopted a categorical approach to the classification of personality disorders. DSM-IV describes 10 types of personality disorders and groups them into *three clusters:* the dramatic (histrionic, borderline,

narcissistic, and antisocial types), the anxious or fearful (obsessive–compulsive, dependent, and avoidant types), and the odd or eccentric (schizoid, schizotypal, and paranoid types) clusters. In the descriptions of the categorical disorders that follow in this chapter, it is clear that many of the disorders may be viewed as manifestations of extreme positions on dimensions of personality such as emotionality, narcissism, trust, sociability, self-esteem, and assertiveness. It is also seen that the types within each cluster tend to share traits and vulnerabilities and, therefore, implications for management. A few disorders are linked to major psychiatric illnesses. It is important to emphasize that a patient with clinically obvious disturbances involving dimensions of personality may meet criteria for several DSM-IV personality disorders or may meet criteria for none.

Management of Personality Disorders

General Guidelines

Several points are useful to bear in mind when dealing with personality-disordered patients of any subtype:

- Because the maladaptive trait or traits are of long standing and deeply ingrained, it is doubtful that they will change in response to the physician's efforts. The general approach to management is therefore to recognize these sources of vulnerability, take them into account when interacting with the patient, and minimize their adverse impact on the provision of medical care.
- Patients often become angry or depressed when their maladaptive traits are pointed out to them, and either of these responses defeats the physician's purposes. Yet it is often important to call patients' attention to ways in which they are undermining their medical care. When such action is necessary, it is helpful to refer to specific behaviors rather than to aspects of personality and to present one's observations plainly but compassionately and without criticism (e.g., "It is difficult for us to provide you with the care you need when you curse at us and criticize every effort we make. I need to ask you to stop behaving in this way").
- In general, counseling by the general physician, if undertaken at all, is best symptom-focused and short-term (see Chapter 11). For long-term treatment, patients with seriously disturbed personalities should be referred to a mental health professional.

DRAMATIC CLUSTER

Patients with personality disturbances in this cluster tend to occupy extreme positions on the dimensions of emotionality and narcissism. They are intensely emotional, sometimes acting impulsively, aggressively, or self-destructively. They are also self-absorbed, lacking in empathy for others, and extreme (unrealistically high or low) in their self-regard. They tend to be demanding of others, and their relationships are unstable, tempestuous, and exploitive, qualities that may characterize their interactions with physicians and complicate the provision of medical care.

Description of Dramatic Subtypes

Histrionic Personality

The essence of the histrionic type is excessive emotionality, self-dramatization, and attention-seeking. Patients meeting criteria for the categorical disorder are self-centered, unusually eager for approval and praise, overly concerned with physical attractiveness, and often inappropriately sexually seductive or flattering ("Of all the doctors I've had, you are the first to really listen to me"). Their style of speech is dramatic, impressionistic, and factually imprecise, and their expression of emotions is often exaggerated, rapidly shifting, and apparently shallow. They may manifest an unusually warm and sometimes seductive manner with the physician and present to the office with complaints that are dramatically expressed but vague in medically relevant detail. Histrionic patients may be especially inclined to develop somatization disorder (see Chapter 12).

Narcissistic Personality

The narcissistic personality type is characterized by an exaggerated sense of self-importance, intolerance of criticism, and insensitivity to the needs of others. Narcissistic people may exploit others for their own ends, require constant admiration and attention, believe themselves entitled to special treatment, and envy those who are more successful, attractive, intelligent, or otherwise praiseworthy. Such patients are often difficult to care for because they tend to believe that their problems are unique and can be solved only by remarkable physicians. They may challenge the doctor's knowledge, skill, and judgment and expect that their convenience will be the prime consideration in the scheduling of tests and appointments.

Borderline Personality

Extreme instability—in mood, interpersonal relationships, and self-regard—is the essence of the borderline personality, a disorder once alleged to lie on the border of schizophrenia. Recent data more strongly support a link with depressive disorders. Substance abuse, sexual impulsiveness, poor self-esteem, self-mutilation, recurrent (often manipulative) suicidal threats, and brief bouts of intense depression and rage superimposed on chronic feelings of emptiness or boredom characterize the long-term functioning of these patients. A shifting tendency to view other people as all good or all bad and to react to them with extremes of idealization and devaluation creates difficulties in all interpersonal relationships, including those with physicians and other caretakers, who are designated as either good or bad and are pitted against one another (staff splitting).

Antisocial Personality

The antisocial personality type is characterized by a chronic and pervasive pattern of irresponsible and socially unacceptable behavior. Truancy, vandalism, fire setting, lying, and theft in childhood give way to impulsiveness, recklessness, aggressiveness, sexual promiscuity, financial irresponsibility, and outright criminality in adulthood. Often complaining of mistreatment themselves, they shamelessly exploit others in their relationships. In medical settings they may be malingerers (see Chapter 12), consciously feigning disease for obvious gain; in their dealings with medical staff they may be either demanding and abusive or flattering and ingratiating, depending on what they perceive to be most expedient.

Management of Dramatic Subtypes

When dealing with dramatic patients one can expect a show of emotional extremes and a pressure to bestow emotional and material favors as well as medical care. It is helpful to maintain equanimity in the face of the patient's emotional excesses, to avoid defensiveness when challenged, and to give special attention to professional boundaries. Socializing or becoming unusually familiar with histrionic or borderline patients is particularly risky. Because patients with these traits lack empathy and exploit others, it is often necessary to spell out, firmly but nonpunitively, the limits of acceptable behavior with medical staff, nurses, and other members of the health care team; such limit setting is most often needed with narcissistic and antisocial patients.

ANXIOUS OR FEARFUL CLUSTER

Patients with personality disturbances in this cluster tend to be self-doubting, timid, and tense. Lacking confidence in themselves, they may seek to avoid making decisions or taking on responsibility, preferring to have others decide or perform for them; however, they are often dissatisfied with and critical of the efforts of others. They tend to be socially unassertive, submitting to the wishes of others and even avoiding friendship in the first place for fear of ultimate rejection. Levels of generalized anxiety are chronically high.

Description of Anxious Subtypes

Avoidant Personality

The avoidant person craves social contact but avoids it because of intense social discomfort related to expectations of criticism and rejection. These people often complain of loneliness, but are too shy to make the social contacts required to solve the problem unless they are certain of acceptance. Major depression (5) and social phobia commonly occur. Because physicians are generally viewed as accepting of their patients, avoidant people may feel particularly comfortable in the presence of their doctors and may develop symptoms justifying regular visits to alleviate their loneliness.

Dependent Personality

Dependent people lack self-confidence and go to great lengths to ensure the availability of others on whom they can depend for advice and reassurance. Because they feel uneasy and helpless when alone, they may endure abuse and perform unpleasant or demeaning tasks to preserve the dependent relationship. They are exceedingly sensitive to criticism and abandonment. Patients of this type may become quite dependent on their physicians, particularly when other relationships are unsatisfactory, and may use vague, chronic complaints as a means of remaining in close touch, especially in times of stress. Such patients may also become ill before a period of planned unavailability on the part of the physician (e.g., a vacation).

Obsessive–Compulsive Personality

People with obsessive–compulsive personalities are rigid, parsimonious, morally scrupulous, and emotionally constricted. Exceedingly committed to work, they are reluctant to delegate duties, convinced that no one else can do things correctly, yet they are also indecisive and at times are rendered ineffective by perfectionism or preoccupation with trivial details. They tend to describe upsetting emotional experiences in a cool, detached manner (isolation of affect). When ill, they often present their physicians with extremely detailed accounts of their symptoms and request lengthy explanations of their disease and its treatment, including very precise instructions about medication use and likely side effects. They are usually aware of hospital rules and routines and are intolerant of lateness and inefficiency. People with obsessive–compulsive personalities may be especially prone to developing hypochondriasis (see Chapter 12) and obsessive–compulsive disorder, a condition characterized by recurrent, resisted thoughts and repetitive, senseless actions (see Chapter 13).

Passive–Aggressive Personality

Although not listed in DSM-IV, passive–aggressive personality disorder warrants brief mention because of its potential impact on the provision of medical care. Passive–aggressive people do not want to meet the expectations of others but do not want to be held responsible for this decision. Thus they do not say no directly but express hostile resistance in terms of procrastination, intentional inefficiency, and feigned forgetfulness. Usually dependent and lacking in self-confidence, they seek the counsel of others, yet often paradoxically resist following the advice of those whom they consult. In medical settings they insist that they intend to comply with treatment recommendations but then, for example, forget to keep a symptom log required to assess the effectiveness of a new treatment or forget to make it to the laboratory for an important blood test.

Management of Anxious Subtypes

The general guidelines described above are applicable. Because patients with these types of personality traits tend to develop anxious attachment to their physicians, the management of dependency is a central issue. It may be necessary to allow patients to be excessively dependent, within manageable bounds, during times of unusual stress. It may be helpful to give them regular, brief appointments so that they do not need to develop new symptomatic complaints to gain access to attention (see Chapter 12), and it may be useful to advise them to call weekly at a specified time to provide updates on their status; this may preempt emergency calls at less convenient times. Such patients also generally benefit from advance notice about vacations and may appreciate meeting the covering physician ahead of time. Treatment for generalized anxiety disorder, phobias, and major depression may be indicated in selected cases (see Chapters 13 and 15).

ODD OR ECCENTRIC CLUSTER

Patients with disorders in this cluster occupy extreme positions on the dimensions of trust and sociability. They tend to be highly suspicious and to isolate themselves from other people due to anxious mistrust, awkwardness, or indifference.

Description of Eccentric Subtypes

Paranoid Personality

Patients with paranoid personalities tend to perceive threats and insults at every turn. Expecting to be exploited or harmed by others, they hear veiled threats in neutral remarks and readily question the loyalty of friends and the fidelity of spouses. They are guarded, easily slighted, defensive, and unforgiving. Although their suspiciousness does not carry the intensity or conviction of a true delusion, schizophrenia and delusional disorders are overrepresented in their families (3). In medical settings these patients may be reluctant to provide a complete history, especially a social history ("What does this have to do with my medical problem?") and may balk at undergoing laboratory tests ("You doctors are just trying to make money off me").

Schizotypal Personality

Schizotypal people exhibit odd behavior, have peculiar beliefs, and suffer social isolation—as a result of their own social anxiety as well as the impact of their beliefs and behavior on others. Their affect is often constricted, their talk vague and digressive, and their appearance unkempt. They tend to be suspicious and superstitious. People with this disorder are generally severely impaired, often meeting criteria for other personality disorders simultaneously (5). There are family links with schizophrenia (1), and some argue that this disorder should be classified as a variant of schizophrenia rather than a personality disorder (3). Schizotypal patients may be guarded and suspicious in medical settings but may also present to physicians with unusual symptoms (e.g., feelings of electricity in my scalp) and idiosyncratic theories of causation ("Could my neighbors be doing this to me?").

Schizoid Personality

The essential features of the schizoid personality are indifference to the company of others and constricted emotionality. These people are loners who seldom marry, prefer solitary activities, and appear cold and aloof. Despite its name, this disorder does not appear to be closely linked to schizophrenia. Schizoid people tend to shun contact with physicians and may appear very uncomfortable when hospitalization thrusts them into close and constant proximity to others.

Management of Eccentric Subtypes

The general guidelines described above apply here as well. The most important specific principle of management is to work gradually toward the establishment of rapport by meticulous honesty, composure in the face of the patient's suspiciousness and reserve, and a consistent demonstration of sincere concern for the patient's well-being and respect for his or her privacy.

General References*

American Psychiatric Association. **Diagnostic and Statistical Manual of Mental Disorders.** 4th ed. (DSM-IV). Washington, DC: American Psychiatric Association, 1994.
> Diagnostic criteria and epidemiologic information for all recognized psychiatric disorders.

Specific References

1. Kendler KS, Gruenberg AM, Strauss JS. An independent analysis of the Danish adoption study of schizophrenia. II. Arch Gen Psychiatry 38:982, 1981.
2. McHugh PR, Slavney PR. The perspectives of psychiatry. Baltimore: Johns Hopkins University Press, 1983.
3. Rutter M. Temperament, personality, and personality disorder. Br J Psychiatry 150:443, 1987.
4. Rutter M, Quinton D. Parental psychiatric disorder: effects on children. Psychol Med 14:853, 1984.
5. Zimmerman M, Coryell W. DSM-III personality disorder diagnoses in a nonpatient sample. Arch Gen Psychiatry 46:682, 1989.

*Bold print (general references) and bold numerals (specific references) denote published controlled clinical trials, meta-analyses, or consensus-based recommendations.

C H A P T E R 15

Affective Disorders

J. RAYMOND DEPAULO, JR, MD

Clinically significant depressions often go undetected and undiagnosed in the ambulatory medical setting (44). As a consequence, many depressed patients remain untreated for depression but receive costly and misdirected diagnostic procedures and symptomatic therapies (15,37). Undiagnosed depressions exact an even bigger toll on patients and families in the form of severe and persistent functional impairments (25). This chapter outlines the public health consequences of depressive conditions and describes the spectrum of mood disorders that afflict patients. It provides an approach to the treatment of these patients by the generalist.

PUBLIC HEALTH IMPACT OF AFFECTIVE DISORDERS

By any measurement, depressive conditions are major public health problems. In a medical outcome study of community-dwelling people, the *poor functioning uniquely associated with depressive symptoms* was comparable to or worse than that uniquely associated with eight major chronic medical conditions (45). The eight conditions compared to depressive symptoms were current arthritis, current advanced coronary artery disease (recent myocardial infarction), current angina, current back problems, current severe lung problems, current gastrointestinal disorders (ulcers or inflammatory bowel disorders), diabetes, and hypertension. The depressed subjects ranked fourth in impairment in physical functioning, third in impairment in role functioning, second (behind advanced coronary disease) in the number of bed days, and worst of all in social functioning and in their sense of well-being about their current health.

Excess deaths attributed to depression are primarily from suicides. Studies of populations of depressed patients show that 15% eventually die by suicide (12). Suicide is the ninth leading cause of death in the United States. Fifty to 75% of suicides (30,000 per year) occur in people with depressive disorders (3). Among 19- to 24-year-olds in the United States, suicide is the third leading cause of death. In this group, illicit substance abuse is a powerful factor thought to account for the recent increase in adolescent suicide (rates doubled between 1960 and 1980 in white males). In the Old Order Amish population, where there is very little if any drug and alcohol abuse, more than 90% of all suicides between 1880 and 1980 occurred in people with major depression or bipolar disorder (7). It was also observed that these suicides clustered in families with multiple family members with major depression and bipolar disorder.

In recent years, several studies have shown that the *incidence and outcome of other medical disorders are affected adversely by depression.* For example, the incidence of myocardial infarction is increased about fourfold in subjects with a prior episode of major depression (30). The odds of dying in the 18 months following a myocardial infarction are three times greater in patients with concurrent depression than in those without depression (8).

In economic terms, the most recent and systematic study (11) estimated that the annual cost of depressive disorders to the U.S. economy was $44 billion. This is substantially higher than the estimated annual costs of stroke ($18 billion), about the same as the estimated annual cost of coronary artery disease ($44 billion), and just under half of the estimated annual cost of all cancers ($104 billion) (10). Neither this study nor others have considered the costs of depressive conditions related to the increased morbidity and mortality from other medical conditions that may be attributable to depression.

BEREAVEMENT AND ADJUSTMENT DISORDERS

Some mood disturbances are "normal" or even inevitable sequelae of personal, medical, or financial setbacks. It is important to evaluate and help patients in these situations (bereavement and adjustment disorders) because they affect the patient's sense of well-being and the risk of several medical conditions. Bereavement, for example, is associated with increased rates of medical visits, heart attacks, and death in the first year following the loss of a spouse (34). Several medical conditions have been noted to have poor medical outcomes in patients with mild depressions (i.e., adjustment disorders that do not meet criteria for major depressive disorders) (40).

Bereavement or Grief Reactions

Although grief reactions are individual in their content, they share a number of characteristic features. Their intensity tends to reflect the bereaved person's closeness to the deceased. The reaction tends to proceed in phases (24,27), beginning at the time at which the death is made known. The *first phase* is called the numbness or shock phase. Although painful, this first period of about a week is remarkable for the organized or calm way in which many bereaved people appear to go through the societal rituals of mourning, funeral, burial, and the visits with close family and friends. In retrospect, patients describe themselves as confused and not fully appreciating their loss during this first week. A *second phase* emerges with the completion of the structured rituals of mourning, with increasingly intense feelings of sadness, loneliness, and pining for the lost loved one. The most intense feelings of loss come in waves or surges that initially may be as relentless as ocean surges but within several weeks begin to come less frequently. Although the waves diminish in frequency and intensity, they are quite frequent in the first 6 to 12 months. They recur less frequently for years, perhaps for a lifetime, when reminders of the loved one are encountered. As they diminish in frequency, a *third phase* emerges as the person returns to his or her normal daily activities such as work, school, and social activities. Apathy, a diminished sense of organization, a disinterest in doing a job that was previously engaging, and an inability to enjoy things are the characteristic signs of this period. The feelings of apathy and disengagement usually remit slowly and incrementally over many months as they are replaced by a sense of re-engagement in old and new activities. Patients seek or are brought to primary care clinicians during any of the three phases of bereavement. In the early ones, it is usually because of sleeplessness or agitation, which need some intervention such as validating the reasons for distress, reassuring advice for patient and family, instructing family members on how to help, and if necessary, prescribing small amounts of hypnotic or anxiolytic medications. Later, patients may come on their own because they are concerned about their own physical health or persistent problems in functioning at work or at home. It is crucial to remember that in susceptible patients major depression is often precipitated by the loss of a loved one. This often becomes apparent in the third phase of bereavement. (See below for differential diagnostic pointers.) Chapter 19 ("Dying, Death, and Bereavement") contains additional information about the experience of the family members of dying and deceased patients.

Adjustment Disorder with Depressed Mood

Adjustment disorder with depressed mood is a normal or an exaggerated emotional reaction to a loss or stressful life event that has just occurred or is imminent. Table 15.1 shows the APA criteria for the diagnosis of adjustment disorder. The diagnosis of adjustment disorder in terms of the presence of emotional or behavioral symptoms and stressors is usually straightforward. The critical and sometimes difficult part is ruling out Axis I disorders such as major depression and Axis II or personality disorders (see definition of axes in Chapter 10). It is almost axiomatic that patients with any form of depression or with personality disorders would be more likely to overreact or to become functionally impaired in the face of a significant stressor. In fact, major depressive disorders regularly present themselves in the context of an apparent adjustment disorder. At the time of presentation, the patient's distress is often focused on the stressor, and the doctor needs to help the patient adapt to the stressor. This empathic task is distinct from the diagnostic task. If the history does not suggest a coexisting Axis I or II disorder, the appropriate intervention is very similar to the approaches described above for bereaved patients and in Chapter 11 ("Psychotherapy in Ambulatory Practice").

EVALUATION OF PATIENTS WITH DEPRESSIVE SYMPTOMS

Depressed patients who seek medical attention usually do not complain of depressed mood as a primary symptom. If they acknowledge depressed feelings, they usually do so in relation to other complaints, which they see as primary. They usually present to generalists with three types of general complaints: (*a*) a variety of

Table 15.1. Diagnostic Criteria for Adjustment Disorder

A. The development of emotional or behavioral symptoms in response to an identifiable stressor occurring within 3 months of the onset of the stressor.
B. These symptoms or behaviors are clinically significant as evidenced by either of the following:
  1. Marked distress that is in excess of what would be expected from exposure to the stressor
  2. Significant impairment in social or occupational (academic) functioning
C. The stress-related disturbance does not meet the criteria for any specific Axis I disorder and is not merely an exacerbation of a preexisting Axis I or Axis II disorder.[a]
D. Does not represent bereavement.
E. The symptoms do not persist for more than 6 months after the termination of the stressor (or its consequences).

  Acute: if the symptoms have persisted for less than 6 months
  Chronic: if the symptoms have persisted for 6 months or longer

Reprinted with permission from the DSM-IV. Copyright 1994, American Psychiatric Association.
[a] See Chapter 10 for definition of Axis I and Axis II disorders.

somatic symptoms including vegetative symptoms of depression (loss of energy, inability to concentrate, poor sleep, poor appetite, weight loss, decreased motivation or interests) and autonomic anxiety symptoms (tachycardia, chest discomfort, or lightheadedness), (*b*) aches and pains that may have anatomic bases but are out of proportion to what the patient usually experiences (e.g., worsening of migraine headaches, irritable bowel, or back pains) or what is expected (e.g., postsurgical pain that continues to require narcotic analgesics a month after surgery), and (*c*) nervous complaints such as increased tension and feelings of anxiety, often expressed in relation to stressful life circumstances such as marital distress or job difficulty (46,47). The presence of a mood disturbance should not be taken to explain or invalidate all physical complaints because coexistence of psychiatric and medical disorders is the rule rather than the exception.

Even when they are specifically asked about mood, almost half of depressed patients deny depression or sadness as their predominant mood. They describe their predominant mood as apathetic (e.g., "blah"), anxious, or even "numb" (i.e., unable to experience normal emotions including sadness, love, and grief). If the patient does have a mood disturbance and if appropriate inquiries are made, it is likely that several classic features of depression will emerge. Changes in mood (sadness, anger), decreased mental agility and physical energy, pessimistic feelings about the future, and negative self-attitude are features central to depressive disorders. Despite the difficulty inherent in describing these pathologic states, patients should be asked specifically about them as well as about their sleep, appetite, and libido.

The term *atypical depression* refers to major depression or dysthymic states in which hypersomnia, overeating, and lethargy are seen more often than insomnia, anorexia, and psychomotor agitation (39). These patients also seem particularly prone to panic-type anxiety symptoms. Patients with atypical depression have the characteristic depressive changes in self-attitude and vital sense, but describe their mood more as a fatigued feeling than as sadness. The term *atypical* may not be strictly justified because all three of the atypical symptoms are common in depressed patients. However, it does serve to remind clinicians to survey both sides of eating and sleeping behavior. Thus, when asked, "How is your appetite?" a depressed patient may respond, "Good," or "Too good," or "No problem." It is deceptively easy to misinterpret these answers as negative screening responses rather than as clues to depression associated with overeating.

Family members, if available, should be asked to corroborate and augment the information obtained from the patient. With the patient's agreement, the physician also should share with the family the diagnostic assessment, the plans for treatment, and the prognosis because the depressed patient will be hard pressed to remember what is said and will tend to interpret everything too negatively (see "Counseling the Family" later in this chapter).

DYSTHYMIC DISORDER

Dysthymia is a chronic (lasting 2 years or more) depressive state in which the number of depressive symptoms experienced is fewer than what is required for the diagnosis of major depressive disorder (see Tables 15.2 and 15.3 for diagnostic criteria for these two disorders). The dysthymic state is associated with marked impairment in social functioning, especially in close personal relationships. Because the low mood is so persistent, these patients, their family and friends, and their doctors often judge the problem to be an innate part of a chronically unhappy person's disposition, that is, a personality disorder. In reality, the unhappy disposition of dysthymic patients depends to a large degree on treatable depression (23).

Diagnosis

Although each patient's sense of what is normal determines why one patient complains to the doctor and another does not, when depressive symptoms cause suffering or interfere with normal functioning they become a disorder warranting detection and intervention. Even milder forms of depression cause serious functional impairments that are as severe as chronic medical conditions such as ulcerative colitis and rheumatoid arthritis (45).

Presenting or complicating problems associated with depressed mood in dysthymic patients include suicide attempts or self-injurious behavior (usually

Table 15.2. American Psychiatric Association Diagnostic Criteria for Dysthymic Disorder[a]

A. Depressed mood for most of the day, for more days than not, as indicated either by subjective account or observation made by others, for at least 2 years.
B. Presence, while depressed, of at least three of the following:
  1. Low self-esteem or self-confidence, or feelings of inadequacy
  2. Feelings of pessimism, despair, or hopelessness
  3. Generalized loss of interest or pleasure
  4. Social withdrawal
  5. Chronic fatigue or tiredness
  6. Feelings of guilt, brooding about the past
  7. Subjective feelings of irritability or excessive anger
  8. Decreased activity, effectiveness, or productivity
  9. Difficulty in thinking reflected by poor concentration, poor memory, or indecisiveness
C. During the 2-year period of the disturbance, the person has never been without the symptoms in A and B for more than 2 months at a time.
D. No major depressive episode during the first 2 years of the disturbance, that is, not better accounted for by chronic major depressive disorder, or major depressive disorder in partial remission.
E. Has never had a manic episode, or an unequivocal hypomanic episode.
F. Does not occur exclusively during the course of a chronic psychotic disorder, such as schizophrenia or delusional disorder.
G. Not due to the direct effects of a substance (e.g., drugs of abuse, medication) or a general medical condition (e.g., hypothyroidism).

Reprinted with permission from the DSM-IV. Copyright 1994, American Psychiatric Association.
[a] Criteria for children have been omitted from this table.

Table 15.3. American Psychiatric Association Diagnostic Criteria for Major Depressive Episode[a]

A. At least five of the following symptoms have been present during the same 2-week period and represent a change from previous functioning; at least one of the symptoms is either (1) depressed mood or (2) loss of interest or pleasure.
  1. Depressed mood most of the day, nearly every day, as indicated by either subjective report (e.g., feels sad or empty) or observation made by others (e.g., appears tearful)
  2. Marked diminished interest or pleasure in all, or almost all, activities most of the day, nearly every day (as indicated either by subjective account or observation made by others)
  3. Significant weight loss or weight gain when not dieting (e.g., more than 5% of body weight in a month), or decrease or increase in appetite nearly every day
  4. Insomnia or hypersomnia nearly every day
  5. Psychomotor agitation or retardation nearly every day (observable by others, not merely subjective feelings of restlessness or being slowed down)
  6. Fatigue or loss of energy nearly every day
  7. Feelings of worthlessness or excessive or inappropiate guilt (which may be delusional) nearly every day (not merely self-reproach or guilt about being sick)
  8. Diminished ability to think or concentrate, or indecisiveness, nearly every day (either by subjective account or as observed by others)
  9. Recurrent thoughts of death (not just fear of dying), recurrent suicidal ideation without a specific plan, or a suicide attempt or a specific plan for committing suicide
B. The symptoms cause clinically significant distress or impairment in social, occupational, or other important areas of functioning.
C. Not due to the direct effects of a substance (e.g., drugs of abuse, medication) or a general medical condition (e.g., hypothyroidism).
D. Not occurring within 2 months of the loss of a loved one (except if associated with marked functional impairment, morbid preoccupation with worthlessness, suicidal ideation, psychotic symptoms, or psychomotor retardation).

Reprinted with permission from the DSM-IV. Copyright 1994, American Psychiatric Association.
[a] Criteria for children have been omitted from this table.

nonfatal but often requiring heroic medical interventions to prevent a fatal outcome), multiple medical complaints and excessive medical care-seeking behavior or abnormal illness behavior (see Chapter 12 for additional detail), serious diagnosable medical disorders, alcohol and drug abuse (see Chapters 21 and 22), family and marital discord, and job difficulties.

Patients with dysthymic disorder usually have the characteristic sustained changes in self-attitude and vital sense seen with major depression (see below). However, they appear much less prominent, probably because of the chronicity of dysthymia. Hypersomnia, difficulty in getting up, increased appetite and weight gain, and loss of energy and libido are common, as are anxiety symptoms.

Table 15.2 shows the criteria of the APA for making the diagnosis of dysthymic disorder.

Treatment

As studies reveal greater similarities between patients with dysthymia and those with major depression, the treatment of dysthymia increasingly resembles the treatment of major depressive episodes. Several SSRI and tricyclic antidepressants (see below) have been shown to be effective in reducing depressive symptoms (17). In addition, brief psychotherapies are also known to be helpful (see Chapter 11). The major differences in treatment for the two types of depression relate to the increased rate of comorbid problems in behavior, personality, and life problems associated with the more chronic form of depression (dysthymia).

Recognizing that depression plays an important part in their life problems can be helpful for dysthymic patients. However, appreciating the difference between accepting medical regimens to treat mood disorders and making the effort required to overcome maladaptive behavior patterns is equally important.

Prognosis

In contrast to the major affective syndromes, prognosis in dysthymic disorders is more problematic in that they typically continue beyond a 2-year period, and when they will remit cannot be estimated with much confidence. There is a high rate of major depressive episodes, and these dysthymic patients tend to respond well to antidepressants. Poor outcomes are most common in patients with severe social maladjustments and personality disorders (see Chapter 14).

EPIDEMIOLOGY OF MAJOR AFFECTIVE DISORDERS

Mania and major depression are the two syndromes that give the traditional name *manic depressive disorder* to this group of disorders. These disorders are characteristically episodic with complete remissions between episodes. Most patients suffer only recurrent depressive episodes *(the unipolar group),* few suffer only manic episodes (they are grouped with patients with bipolar disorder), and the remainder suffer from both manic and depressive episodes *(the bipolar group).* Based on a national community survey of mental disorders, the Epidemiologic Catchment Area study (see "General References"), it is estimated that 6 to 12% of women and 2 to 5% of men experience at least one major depressive episode during their adult life; it may occur at any age. Only 0.6 to 1.2% of adults develop a bipolar disorder; it is equally common in men and women and the first manic episode usually occurs before age 30.

MAJOR DEPRESSIVE DISORDER

The most common form of clinical depression is major depressive disorder (see Table 15.3 for APA diagnostic criteria). Most depressed people visit a health care facility during the depressive episode but only approximately 30% are diagnosed and given treatment for depression (9,36).

Diagnosis

The *differential diagnosis* of symptoms that suggest major depression varies depending on age, the patient's presenting manifestations, and other associated factors. In *elderly patients* with memory complaints, the differential diagnosis is complex because memory complaints without substantial memory performance problems are common. On the other hand, a modest but reversible dementia can result from the depression alone (so-called pseudodementia; see Chapter 17). In addition, depression and dementia syndromes can be related to underlying neuropathologic disorders, particularly Parkinson's disease and stroke (see Chapters 82 and 83). In *younger patients,* it is important to differentiate major depression from schizophrenia, especially when hallucinations or delusions are part of the presenting picture (see Chapter 16). In younger adults with none of the features of schizophrenia, the differential is between adjustment disorder and major depression in those with recent onset of symptoms, and between adjustment disorder and dysthymia in those with more chronic presentation. Because stressful life events are common precipitating factors of major depressions, their presence is not useful for making or excluding the diagnosis. In patients with panic attacks or obsessive–compulsive symptoms, it is important to remember that both panic disorder and obsessive–compulsive disorder (see descriptions in Chapter 13) may occur in the context of a major depressive syndrome. Depressed patients of all ages should be screened for *chronic alcoholism* (see Chapter 21) and checked for use of *other substances or medications* that can cause or exacerbate symptoms of depression (Table 15.4). Finally, it is important to differentiate unipolar from bipolar depressive states because antidepressants can precipitate manic or mixed manic mood swings in patients with bipolar disorder.

Table 15.4. Drugs and Substances that May Cause or Precipitate Mood Disorder

Depressed States
Alcohol
Amphetamine or cocaine withdrawal
Antihypertensive drugs (clonidine, methyldopa, reserpine,
  β-blockers)
Benzodiazepines
Dapsone
Glucocorticoids
Oral contraceptives
Interferon
Cyclosporin

Hypomanic or Manic States
Antidepressants (all classes)
Bromocriptine
Cyclobenzaprine
Glucocorticoids
Interferon
Cyclosporine
L-Dopa
Metoclopramide
Quinacrine
Stimulant drugs (amphetamine, cocaine, phencyclidine)
Thyroid hormones
Zydovudine

Adapted from Drugs that cause psychiatric symptoms. Med Lett Drugs Ther 35:65, 1993.

A fully developed major depression is characterized by a sustained alteration in mood, self-attitude, and vital sense. The sustained lowering of mood is impervious to environmental influence once the depression becomes severe. Events that are not usually stressful are perceived as overwhelmingly stressful by a depressed patient as the syndrome develops. The *change in self-attitude* is usually manifested in expressions of guilt, inferiority, uselessness, and hopelessness as the mood descends. The *changes in vital sense* (i.e., the subjective assessment of one's physical and mental functioning) include feelings of confusion or poor memory with the inability to concentrate, a lack of energy and easy fatigability, and a sense of ill health, occasionally reaching delusional intensity with the conviction that one is dying of cancer or acquired immunodeficiency syndrome (AIDS) when there is no evidence of these diseases.

Marked psychomotor retardation (i.e., slowed speech and movements), *delusions* with depressive content, and *diurnal mood variation* (worst mood in the morning) occur in a minority of patients but are diagnostically useful when present because they are fairly specific to this disorder.

The specific criteria of the APA for major depressive episode (Table 15.3) require at least five of nine depressive symptoms and related functional impairment for 2 weeks, not caused by the direct effect of a medication or a drug of abuse or of a general medical condition. A patient with a history of an episodic disorder and a fully developed symptom cluster as described is not difficult to diagnose. However, many patients with major depression present with a dominant somatic complaint or with a clear "reason" to be depressed, guilty, or hopeless. In such patients, recognition of a treatable major depression may be delayed. When major depression is strongly suspected, probing inquiry about symptoms from both the patient and those close to the patient usually clarify the diagnosis.

Treatment

Once the diagnosis of major depression is made, treatment consists of explaining the diagnosis to the patient (and family), prescription and monitoring of antidepressant medications, and providing supportive counseling of the patient and family.

Antidepressant Treatment

General Points. For the patient with major depression who is in good physical condition and who is neither overwhelmed with depressive delusions nor suicidal (see "Suicide Prevention," below), antidepressant medication is the appropriate initial treatment. Any antidepressant drug is effective in approximately 70% of patients with major depression, and no antidepressant on the market has been shown to be more effective than the others. Patients who fail to respond to an antidepressant from one class often respond to a drug from a different class. Because depressed patients tolerate side effects (and what they perceive to be side effects) poorly and often stop antidepressants without completing a full 8-week trial of the medication, the selection of the antidepressant to prescribe first has more to do with convenience of administration and side effects than with the probability of a good response. The exception to this rule is the patient who has had a prior good or poor response to a particular antidepressant. The mechanism of therapeutic action of antidepressant drugs is unknown. Although much indirect evidence suggests that they exert their therapeutic effects by enhancing catecholaminergic and serotonergic neurotransmission, their clinical use remains empirical.

Among patients with the syndrome of depression, those with delusions, hallucinations, and profound psychomotor retardation tend to be less responsive to drugs than those without these clinical features. Referral for psychiatric consultation and consideration for electroconvulsive therapy are appropriate for such patients. Among patients with suicidal intent (see "Suicide Prevention," below), antidepressants, especially tricyclics, should be dispensed in small amounts to avoid providing enough drug for a lethal overdose (26).

Characteristics of Available Antidepressants. Characteristics of available antidepressant drugs are listed in Table 15.5. *Tricyclic antidepressants* (TCAs), the oldest class, are listed in two subgroups: secondary and tertiary amines. The monoamine oxidase (MAO) inhibitors are not listed. These drugs, which were the main alternatives to tricyclics before 1990, are uncommonly used today even by psychiatrists specializing in treatment of depression.

There are four *selective serotonin reuptake inhibitors (SSRIs)* on the market in the United States: fluoxetine (Prozac), fluvoxamine (Luvox), paroxetine (Paxil), and sertraline (Zoloft). They are similar in efficacy and side effect profiles. Fluvoxamine is sedating in large doses and, along with paroxetine, is often more sedating than fluoxetine and sertraline.

A newer antidepressant, *nefazodone* (Serzone), is a less sedating relative of the older antidepressant *trazodone* (Desyrel). These agents also inhibit serotonin reuptake but are not as specific as SSRIs. Nefazodone is well tolerated at therapeutic dosages of 300 to 600 mg/day and is a good second-line antidepressant, joining bupropion. Although trazodone is often too sedating for antidepressant use, it is useful in small doses (e.g., 50 mg/night) as a non–habit-forming alternative to benzodiazepine hypnotics for depressed patients.

Bupropion (Wellbutrin) is an antidepressant of the aminoketone class, unrelated to the tricyclic and SSRI antidepressants but related to the phenylethylamines. It inhibits serotonin, norepinephrine, and dopamine reuptake. An uncommon but serious side effect is seizures, which occur in 0.4% of patients treated at dosages up to 450 mg/day. This is only slightly greater than the rate of seizures with tricyclics. At higher dosages originally approved by the FDA (up to 700 mg) bupropion was associated with a higher rate of seizures, thus leading to the recommended 450-mg limit on total daily dosage. For the same reason, the limit for any single dose is 150 mg, and doses should be separated by at least 4 hours. Therefore, most

Table 15.5.   Characteristics of Antidepressant Drugs

Drug	Strengths of Available Oral Preparations (mg)	Low or Starting Dosage Range	Usual Dosage Range	Common Side Effects	Special Considerations
Tricyclics					
Secondary amines					
Nortriptyline[a] (Pamelor, Aventyl, others)	10, 25, 50, 75, 100	25 mg QHS	50–150 mg QHS	Dry mouth, sedation, orthostatis, constipation, weight gain, sexual dysfunction	Titrate to AM trough serum level 90–150 ng/dL
Desipramine[a] (Norpramin, others)	10, 25, 50	25–50 mg QHS	150–250 mg QHS	Same as other tricyclics	Titrate to level >150 ng/dL upper limit unclear–?250 ng/dL
Tertiary amines					
Amitriptyline[a] (Elavil, others)	10, 25, 50, 75, 100	25–50 mg QHS	150–250 mg QHS	Same as other tricyclics, but more severe	Titrate to combined amitriptyline plus nortriptyline level >150 ng/dL upper limit unclear–?250 ng/dL
Doxepin[a] (Sinequan, Adapin, others)	10, 25, 50, 100	25–50 mg HS	150–250 mg QHS	Same as amitriptyline	Titrate to level >125–250 ng/dL
Imipramine (Tofranil, others)	10, 25, 50, 100	25–50 mg HS	150–250 mg QHS	Same as amitriptyline	Titrate to level >180 ng/dL
SSRIs					
Fluoxetine (Prozac)	10, 20	10–20 mg QD	20 mg QD	Insomnia, gastrointestinal discomfort, restlessness, diarrhea, headache, sweating, anxiety, sexual dysfunction	Very long half life; Note: all SSRIs can raise levels of other drugs, including anticonvulsants, tricyclics, theophylline, digoxin, coumadin, some antiarrhythmics, β-blockers, calcium channel blockers, nonsedating antihistamines
Sertraline (Zoloft)	50, 100	25–50 mg QD	100–200 mg QD	Same as fluoxetine but perhaps more gastrointestinal symptoms; less restlessness	
Paroxetine (Paxil)	20, 30	10–20 mg QD	20 mg QD	Same as fluoxetine but less insomnia, sometimes sedation	May be taken at bedtime
Fluvoxamine (Luvox)	50, 100	25–50 mg QD	150–200 mg QD	Similar to sertraline but more sedating	
Others					
Nefazodone (Serzone)	100, 150	37.5–75 mg BID	100–200 mg BID	Nausea, dry mouth, headache, sedation, occasional orthostasis	
Trazodone (Desyrel, others)	50, 150, 300	25–100 mg QHS	300–500 mg QHS	Same as nefazodone but more sedation	Useful in low dose (25–100 mg HS) as relatively safe hypnotic without dependence or cognitive impairment
Bupropion (Wellbutrin)	75, 100	75 mg QD or BID	100–150 mg BID–TID	Insomnia, gastrointestinal upset, more reduction of seizure threshold than others; less sexual dysfunction than other antidepressants	Incompatible with ritonavir; new SR preparation for better BID dosing
Venlafaxine (Effexor)	37.5, 75	37.5–75 BID	100–150 BID	Nausea, insomnia, sedation, sweating, gastrointestinal discomfort	May have more rapid relapse of symptoms with cessation than others, can cause blood pressure increase
Mirtazapine (Remeron)	15, 30	7.5–15 mg QHS	15–45 mg QHS	Sedation, weight gain, dizziness, rarely granulocytopenia	New, currently should be used as third- or fourth-line antidepressant

[a] Generic preparation available.

patients need a two- or three-times-daily dosing schedule to achieve a therapeutic daily dosage of 300 to 450 mg.

Venlafaxine (Effexor) is a newer antidepressant, also of the phenylethylamine class. It is usually given twice daily at total daily dosages of 150 to 300 mg for most patients. Diastolic hypertension occurs in a small fraction of patients, particularly at higher dosages. Monitoring of blood pressure for 2 weeks after any dosage elevation is therefore recommended.

Mirtazapine (Remeron) is a new antidepressant with limited use in the United States. It is associated with significant sedation and has a sufficiently long half-life to allow bedtime dosing. A less common but serious side effect is granulocytopenia. Mirtazapine is currently recommended only for patients who have not responded to other antidepressants.

Alternative Treatments.   A number of nutritional supplements and herbs have been claimed by enthusiasts to be safe and effective for depression. Patients often inquire about them and often state that they would prefer them to the established antidepressants. The reasons vary from the patient who has failed trials with standard antidepressants to the misconception that herbal and nutritional preparations must be safer than the FDA-approved medications for which numerous possible adverse reactions are listed. A recent flurry of articles describe the herb *St. John's wort* as a "natural" antidepressant. In fact, several studies suggest that it has antidepressant properties, but further studies are needed to compare it with established antidepressants (21).

Selection and Dosage Adjustment of Antidepressants.   Because of a favorable side effect profile and their ease of use, the SSRIs have become the drugs of first choice for most depressed patients. Because almost every depressed patient is more prone to or more intolerant of some side effects than others, the selection of the antidepressant to use in a particular instance also depends on the apparent fit between the patient's medical history and an antidepressant's side effect profile. The SSRIs also appear to have a significant advantage over the TCAs in their relative safety in overdose (4,13). Both fluoxetine and the tricyclic nortriptyline have been shown to be safe to use in the first trimester of pregnancy. Although both were associated with a small increase in spontaneous abortions, neither was associated with any increase in fetal abnormalities (28).

Some managed care programs have limited the use of SSRIs because they are more expensive than the tricyclics, which were the antidepressants of first choice before the 1990s. *SSRIs cost $1.50 to $2.00 per day, whereas the oldest tricyclic, imipramine, can cost as little as $0.05 per day.* A policy of limiting access to SSRIs conflicts with data from cost–benefit studies showing that the cost of tests to monitor drug levels, visits, and drug changes in TCA-treated patients more than offset the differences in the cost of the SSRIs (20,32,38).

In the otherwise healthy depressed patient, it is reasonable to initiate antidepressant treatment with 20 mg/day of *fluoxetine* or *paroxetine.* These two SSRIs are administered once a day and require no titration of the daily dosage (35). Studies of these two SSRIs show that most responders do as well on the usual starting dosage of 20 mg/day as on higher dosages (2,42). For patients who are very sensitive to medication side effects, initiating treatment at 10 mg/day and advancing to 20 mg/day after 1 week is a reasonable option.

For patients given *sertraline,* a starting dosage of 25 to 50 mg/day is advisable. The 25-mg dosage can be increased to 50 mg as soon as the patient can tolerate this dosage of medication (usually 1 or 2 days). At the 50-mg daily dosage, some patients need no more upward titration. Therefore, it is advisable to wait 2 weeks before considering the next dosage increase. If the patient appears to be improving rapidly, waiting another 2 weeks is almost always advisable. If there is doubt about the degree of improvement or if none is evident, increasing the dosage by another 25 to 50 mg/day is advisable every 2 weeks until the patient is markedly improved or the dosage has reached 200 mg/day.

Treatment with the tricyclic *nortriptyline,* from the tricyclic group (secondary amines) with fewer side effects, should begin with 25 to 50 mg/day and should be maintained at 50 mg for 2 weeks; if improvement is apparent, no change should be considered for another 2 weeks. If improvement is marginal or absent after the first 2 weeks, a plasma tricyclic level should be obtained. The optimal nortriptyline level is 90 to 150 ng/mL. The process of dosage adjustment to produce an effective result is repeated every 2 weeks until the patient is improved greatly or 4 weeks of optimal treatment has proven fruitless.

Treatment with *imipramine, desipramine, amitriptyline,* and *doxepin* should begin at a dosage of 50 mg/day, increased in 50-mg increments as tolerated to 150 mg/day. A blood level should be measured after 2 weeks at a stable dosage and then dosage adjusted to achieve a therapeutic blood level of 150 ng/mL or greater for all four of these tricyclics (Table 15.5). Starting dosages of TCAs should be reduced by approximately 50% in *older patients* (especially those with medical illnesses). TCA dosage may be increased every 2 to 4 days in young physically healthy patients, but weekly increases are safer for older or infirm patients. Giving the total daily dosage at bedtime is desirable for most patients.

Bupropion can be started at 75 mg on day 1 and increased to 75 mg twice daily on day 2. Thereafter, it can be increased in 75-mg increments up to 150 mg three times a day. The usual therapeutic dosage is 300 to 450 mg/day so that stopping at 150 mg twice daily is warranted until it is clear that this dosage is insufficient (2 to 4 weeks at that dosage without a substantial improvement).

Antidepressant Side Effects.   Patients must be encouraged to tolerate the mild side effects that often occur before the therapeutic effects of antidepressant drugs begin. Many depressed patients tolerate even mild side effects poorly and need frequent reassurance that the treatment is safe and likely to be effective (in 3 to 8 weeks). Apart from the specific warnings regarding drug–drug interactions contained in Table 15.6, no known measures are clinically useful in preventing or alleviating side effects of antidepressant drugs.

The common side effects of *all SSRIs* are transient mild nausea, transient insomnia, and transient nervousness and muscular irritability. All SSRIs have good antianxiety properties when taken for 2 weeks or more at a steady dosage.

All SSRIs cause *sexual dysfunction* in approximately 20% of patients. The most common sexual side effect is orgasmic delay, but decreased interest and, in some, erectile problems may occur. The sexual side effects of tricyclics are at least as prevalent; most often they affect erectile function in men. Bupropion and nefazodone appear to have a lower incidence of sexual side effects.

The most common side effects of the *tricyclics* are anticholinergic: dry mouth, constipation, and less often, delayed micturition, blurred vision, and an anticholinergic delirium. The side effect of greatest concern in TCA-treated patients is orthostatic hypotension. This is particularly problematic in elderly patients and in any patients with unsteady gait or balance problems. In addition, TCAs may produce increased appetite with weight gain, granulocytopenia (rarely), hypomania or mania, slowed cardiac conduction, and cardiac arrhythmias.

Because of the *cardiac side effects,* tricyclics should be given cautiously to patients who have preexisting conduction abnormalities or any unstable cardiac conditions, such as a recent myocardial infarction. However, nortriptyline has been studied in cardiac patients and, if needed, can be safely administered to those with preexisting stable heart disease (43). SSRIs, venlafaxine, and bupropion have few cardiac effects and thus offer greater safety in the cardiac patient.

Bupropion is contraindicated in patients with a seizure disorder. The FDA recommends that the dosage not exceed 150 mg/dose or 450 mg/day to minimize the risk of seizures.

Table 15.6.   Drugs that May Interact with Antidepressants

Antidepressant Drug Class	Interaction
Tricyclic	
Anticholinergic antispasmodics	Enhanced anticholinergic side effects
Anticholinergic antiparkinsonian drugs	Enhanced anticholinergic side effects
Antihypertensive drugs	Enhanced orthostatic hypotension
SSRIs	
TCAs, anxiolytics, hypnotics, neuroleptics	SSRIs block metabolism so blood levels rise; TCA plasma levels may rise two-fold or more
MAO inhibitors	Potentially fatal serotonin syndrome

The major concern associated with the use of *MAO inhibitors* is acute hypertension caused by foods containing the sympathomimetic agent, tyramine, cheeses, wines, beers, broad bean pods, and sympathomimetic drugs. Hypotension, headaches, and nausea are more common adverse reactions.

Drug Kinetics and Interactions. Among the TCAs and SSRIs, fluoxetine has an unusually long half-life (7 days for its active metabolite norfluoxetine). This property can be advantageous when this antidepressant is stopped because it is less often associated with a withdrawal syndrome when discontinued, compared with other SSRIs and venlafaxine. The long half-life increases the time required to achieve washout before change to another antidepressant. It is mandatory to await complete washout when the switch is from an SSRI or venlafaxine to an MAO inhibitor, a distinctly uncommon transition in the primary care setting.

All SSRIs inhibit one or more of the cytochrome P-450 enzymes, but the clinical impact of this property, first reported in 1991, has proved to be modest (6). In patients taking paroxetine, fluoxetine, and sertraline, blood levels of coadministered benzodiazepines, antipsychotics, tricyclic antidepressants, and flecainide-type antiarrhythmic agents may increase. Because of their inhibition of the 3A4 enzyme, nefazodone and fluvoxamine should not be coadministered with the antihistamines astemizole and terfenadine.

Duration of Drug Treatment. In a patient with persistent and significant depressive symptoms, an adequate therapeutic trial usually requires 2 months at a therapeutically effective dosage. After recovery from a first or infrequently recurrent depressive syndrome, the medication that induced the remission should be continued usually for 12 months, the time of highest risk for relapse (22). Most patients with a history of episodes and relapses should be advised to continue their antidepressant for a number of years. The terms *indefinite* and *for the rest of your life* may convey a sense of pessimism to patients who view their depressive symptoms as a personal weakness. In such a circumstance, making the commitment to very long-term treatment often should be an incremental decision, made after comparing 1 and then 2 years of treatment experience with the period before treatment. The use of a lower dosage of the patient's antidepressant for "maintenance" treatment is not recommended; a controlled study of this practice showed that patients taking half of the acute antidepressant dosage had no better outcome than the placebo group (19). After electroconvulsive therapy (see below), maintenance treatment with antidepressants is essential for most patients to reduce the risk of relapse.

Drug Discontinuation. Before discontinuation, whether done electively (in well patients) or necessarily (when an adequate trial of a particular antidepressant has failed), patients should be told that withdrawal symptoms (nausea, dizziness, headache, increased perspiration, and increased salivation) may occur, especially when shorter half-life SSRIs, venlafaxine, or tricyclics are discontinued abruptly. To reduce the risk of withdrawal symptoms, antidepressants that have been given for 2 months or more should be tapered over about 10 days before discontinuation.

Counseling and Psychotherapy

For the first 6 to 8 weeks, the patient with major depression should be seen at least every other week for adjustment of medication and for brief supportive psychotherapy as described in Chapter 11. For patients with major depression, the first priority in supportive counseling is consistent repetition of the answers to three questions most troublesome to depressed patients "What is wrong with me?"; "Is this treatment going to work?" (or this question may be presented as a concern: "I think this pill is making me worse. I want to stop it."); and "What is going to happen to me (e.g., if this doesn't work for me)?" The answers are "You have clinical depression. We don't understand how it is caused but it is not your fault. It is a medical disease. You will get better. We are going to continue to care for you and fight the depression with you until you are better." Answers to these questions and supportive counseling are important for members of the *patient's family* as well (see below).

A second focus of counseling is more directive. *Major life decisions* should be delayed, if at all possible. Job-related and personal relationship changes should be deferred until the patient's ability to maintain a more objective and positive perspective recovers. It is remarkable how many patients resign jobs and separate from spouses based on distorted depressive perceptions about not being able to do their usual work, not being able to feel love for one's spouse, and feeling somehow that "facing this (negative conclusion) reality" will allow them and their loved ones "to move on."

Frank discussion of *suicidal feelings,* plans, and intentions should be a routine part of each visit (see "Suicide Prevention," below). Candid discussion of the level of risk and protective measures available is equally important and may require the participation of a family member or loved one.

The patient should be checked routinely for the *side effects* that are most typical of the patient's antidepressant (see above). This is not only out of medical necessity but because the more depressed the patient, the less tolerant he or she will be of minor adverse drug effects and the more likely to give up on the treatment before it has been given an adequate trial (6 to 8 weeks at a full therapeutic dosage). The support of the doctor in encouraging persistence with drug therapy is crucial.

Office Psychotherapy. Traditional, or "insight-oriented," psychotherapy has been a two-edged sword for depressed patients. On one hand, it engages depressed patients in an empathic consideration of their feelings and concerns. On the other hand, the causal theories behind the practice point in the wrong direction (i.e., toward the patient), and when the depression persists, suggest that the patient rather than the treatment has failed.

The briefer and more present-oriented psychothera-

pies (*cognitive therapy* and *interpersonal therapy*) have moved away from the causal theories that spawned them and can be shown to help patients recover more quickly, especially when used with concurrent antidepressant medication (14). Some of the more common *cognitive distortions* that depressed patients experience and express are listed in Table 15.7. Even one who is not trained in cognitive therapy can help patients by gently challenging negative thoughts such as those listed. A supportively offered challenge can help patients access what they already know and have experienced, both of which usually argue against the most negative and distorted conclusions of the depressed state. *Interpersonal therapy* refers to a focus on the social contexts and consequences of the patient's depression. It includes skills such as identifying and addressing stressors, pointing out assets, and providing alternative choices. These and other skills useful in interpersonal therapy are described in Chapter 11.

Cognitive and interpersonal psychotherapy also can help, in combination with antidepressants, to reduce the risk of relapse during the months following successful treatment (18,19). Even these modes of psychotherapy are not indicated in the most acute depressive states because psychotherapy requires that the patient be able to concentrate, recall, and maintain a level of objectivity and hopefulness.

Referral for Treatment

General physicians should be able to treat most of the patients in whom they diagnose major depression. However, some depressed patients should be referred to a psychiatrist: those in whom the diagnosis is not clear enough to allow confident treatment; those who show no improvement after 8 weeks of treatment with

---

Table 15.7.   Cognitive Distortions in Depression

All-or-nothing thinking: Thinking occurs in black-and-white terms with no recognition of a middle ground. Things are wonderful or awful. One's actions reflect either perfection or total failure.

Overgeneralization: Words such as "always" and "never" may portray a single negative event as a never-ending pattern of defeat.

Selective abstraction: A single negative detail is focused on and ruminated about until it colors everything.

Disqualifying the positive: Positive experiences are often discounted as not relevant, not real, or not deserved.

Arbitrary inferences: It is assumed that things are or will be negative, regardless of the facts.

Magnification or minimization: One's own failures and others' successes are magnified; one's own successes and others' failures are minimized.

Emotional reasoning: Bad feelings are taken as the litmus test of reality.

"Should" statements: Repetitive "I should/should not" or "I must/must not" statements often contribute to depression, resentment, guilt, and hopelessness.

Labeling and mislabeling: Mistakes or shortcomings become sweeping self-condemnations.

Personalization: Depressed people often assume they are the cause of some unfortunate or unpleasant event for which, in actuality, they are not responsible.

Adapted from Burns DD. Feeling good: the new mood therapy. New York: New American Library, 1980.

therapeutic dosages of antidepressant medications (about one in three patients); those who cannot or will not take antidepressant medications; those who are overtly suicidal; and those with delusions, hallucinations, or depressive stupor (i.e., mute and unresponsive). In these patients, hospitalization, more intensive counseling, more aggressive drug therapy, or electroconvulsive therapy (see below) is usually suggested by the psychiatric consultant.

Many patients resist the idea of seeing a psychiatrist. A primary care physician with whom a patient has good rapport can be most persuasive in helping the patient understand why the consultation or referral for treatment is being pursued. Patients need to know that their situation is not hopeless and that referral does not mean that they are being shunned by their personal physician (as many depressed patients fear). Rather, they should understand that additional treatments, with which the psychiatrist has more experience, are available.

Electroconvulsive Therapy

Electroconvulsive therapy (ECT) is an effective and rapid treatment for major depressive disorder. The decision to use ECT should be made by the psychiatrist with the informed consent of the patient and, when available, the informed consent of the patient's family. This treatment was previously given only to hospitalized patients, but outpatient ECT is increasingly available and suitable for medically and behaviorally stable patients. There is some evidence that among patients with clear-cut major depression, those with the more severe symptoms will have a better therapeutic response. The indications for moving quickly to ECT are issues mandating a more rapid response, as in the malnourished, dehydrated, or suicidal patient; the presence of medical illness that makes drug therapy excessively risky; the presence of delusions or overwhelming severity of the depression; and failure of drug therapy. The likelihood of marked benefit from ECT is higher than with antidepressants: approximately 80% in patients with major depression. The benefit is short term, meaning that it lasts for weeks up to 6 months. Thus, for patients with clearly episodic depressions that are severe but infrequent, ECT is an excellent first choice and is certainly not a last resort. The benefit usually requires 6 to 12 treatments given 2 to 3 times per week. The procedure involves anesthetization with a short-acting barbiturate, which is administered before a muscle relaxing agent, usually succinyl choline. The current is administered usually in a unilateral fashion (33), but some patients appear to respond best to bilateral treatments. The general advantage of unilateral electrode placement is that it produces less severe memory impairments.

The *mechanism of action of ECT* is unknown. The therapeutic effect is related to the electrical seizure discharge in a more complex way than previously appreciated. It was formerly believed that the benefit and the seizure were both all-or-none phenomena. It is now known that the seizure is important but that electrode placement and to some degree the amount of electrical energy above that needed for the seizure contribute to the benefit (33). Although there is usually transient memory loss, therapeutic benefit is not linked to the memory disturbance. Although there are other methods of inducing seizures, electric current is easiest to control and, therefore, safest.

Aside from the small risk of brief anesthesia, the *adverse effects* that follow ECT involve primarily memory. Commonly, retention of new and occasionally old memories is mildly defective for weeks to months following a series of ECT treatments. These memory gaps are usually spotty and involve primarily declarative memories (events, things that were heard or read) as opposed to procedural memories (how to perform a task). Typically, the patient in whom this effect becomes clinically apparent (perhaps 40% of treated patients) has trouble recalling names of recent acquaintances, including doctors and nurses, or forgets events that occurred during or just before beginning ECT. Clinically apparent memory defects typically resolve within 2 months. Formal testing reveals mild defects up to 3 months, but none at 6 months after treatment (41).

Depressed patients with brain tumors ordinarily should not receive ECT if there are good alternatives. This concern relates to the possibility that already increased intracranial pressure may be further increased by ECT. Patients with dementias from neuropathologic causes treated with ECT may have temporary worsening of their cognitive impairments, but the effective treatment of depression actually helps overall social functioning. ECT should be avoided, if possible, within 3 months of myocardial infarction, cerebrovascular accident, or perforated viscous repair. Neither anticoagulation therapy nor the presence of a cardiac pacemaker is a hard-and-fast contraindication for ECT.

MANIA

Diagnosis

The manic syndrome, like major depression, is defined by a sustained change in mood, self-attitude, and vital sense. The manic patient's mood may be euphoric or irritable or may alternate between the two. *Self-attitude* is one of overconfidence; when more severe, it is reflected in an inflated sense of power, position, and importance. *Heightened vital sense* is manifested in the patient's sense of quickened and totally accurate thinking. The patient has an overconfident ease in decision making and a sense of heightened perception of sounds, colors, and tastes, and sees only continued supreme well-being in his or her future. The patient manifests dramatically increased energy and a decreased need for sleep. In the speeded up and overconfident state, the patient is observed by his or her family to be very distractible in speech (jumping from topic to topic) and behavior (jumping from one new project to another, completing none). Finally, judgment ranges from poor to catastrophic as patients spend impulsively, including giving away money and personal belongings on the street, and are uncharacteristically disinhibited and provocative in word and deed.

Delusions and hallucinations, when present, are either persecutory or grandiose. Occasionally symptoms thought to be characteristic of schizophrenia (see Chapter 16) occur, leading to the clinical rule that "schizophrenic" symptoms are not in themselves diagnostic but should be judged by the company they keep. In the presence of the characteristic manic syndrome, symptoms thought of as first-rank symptoms of schizophrenia would be considered as part of a mania if they follow the course of the other manic symptoms, remitting as the mood and behavior normalize. The diagnosis of *schizoaffective disorder–manic type* is reserved for patients in whom the psychotic symptoms persist well beyond the manic syndrome so that the patient is psychotic in the absence of the manic symptoms throughout most of the course of the illness. Whether these patients have an unusually severe form of bipolar disorder or a condition more related to schizophrenia is currently unknown. The specific criteria of the APA for mania are shown in Table 15.8.

Initial Treatment

General Principles

Because the disruptive and disinhibited symptoms of mania are more difficult to manage both in medical terms and in dealing with the patient's behavior, manic patients are referred to psychiatrists in most instances. This does not mean that referral occurs in an orderly way, because the patient's acceptance of the need for help is the exception rather than the rule. Thus, a patient's personal physician can be a crucial, or the only,

Table 15.8. American Psychiatric Association Diagnostic Criteria for a Manic Episode

A. A distinct period of abnormally and persistently elevated, expansive, or irritable mood, lasting at least 1 week (or any duration if hospitalization is necessary).
B. During the period of mood disturbance, at least three of the following symptoms have persisted (four if the mood is only irritable) and have been present to a significant degree:
   1. Inflated self-esteem or grandiosity
   2. Decreased need for sleep (e.g., feels rested after only 3 hours of sleep)
   3. More talkative than usual or pressured to keep talking
   4. Flight of ideas or subjective experience that thoughts are racing
   5. Distractibility (i.e., attention too easily drawn to unimportant or irrelevant external stimuli)
   6. Increase in goal-directed activity (either social, at work or school, or sexually) or psychomotor agitation
   7. Excessive involvement in pleasurable activities that have a high potential for painful consequences (e.g., the person engages in unrestrained buying sprees, sexual indiscretions, or foolish business is investments)
C. The mood disturbance is sufficiently severe to cause marked impairment in occupational functioning or in usual social activities or relationships with others, or to necessitate hospitalization to prevent harm to self or others.
D. Not due to the direct effects of a substance (e.g., drugs of abuse, medication) or a general medical condition (e.g., hyperthyroidism).

Reprinted with permission from the DSM-IV. Copyright 1994, American Psychiatric Association.

clinician involved with the manic patient in the initial presentation. Because of an already established relationship with the patient or his or her family, this physician may persuade the patient to take some medication and to accept a referral to a psychiatrist or to a hospital inpatient unit, which is usually required in a full-blown manic syndrome. Basic knowledge about the use of neuroleptic drugs and mood-stabilizing medications, such as lithium and sodium valproate, is therefore important for primary care physicians.

In its milder form (called *hypomania*), the manic syndrome may be successfully treated in an outpatient setting. In the mildest situation, a brief period of hypomania may emerge shortly after a depressed patient has begun an antidepressant medication. These hypomanias may abate on their own in some cases even while the antidepressant is continued. However, this is not a certainty, and rapid escalation to a dangerous mania may also occur. Thus, very close monitoring and careful cessation of antidepressant treatment are appropriate conservative measures for the hypomanic patient. When the symptoms escalate even modestly, antimanic medications are needed promptly. Clinical experience suggests that delay can be disastrous because the syndrome progresses very rapidly and the patient's insight and judgment deteriorate at the same pace. *Neuroleptics* reduce manic symptoms and behavior more rapidly than most mood stabilizers. Thus, they are used alone (see below) or in combination with a mood stabilizer in the early days of treatment.

Winning the cooperation of the acutely manic patient can be very difficult. The euphoric or irritable manic patient often will not accept the notion that his or her behavior is disturbed, much less that it requires inpatient therapy. Explaining the need for medical treatment in a manner that does not inflame the patient and provoke even more disordered behavior is a valuable skill. If possible, consultation with the family about the diagnosis and plan of treatment should be arranged before, not after, confronting the patient with the diagnosis and treatment plan. Despite the uncontrollable behavior of the manic patient, family members may be afraid to support the doctor's resolve to have the patient treated. They may fear being seen by the patient as betraying his or her trust, lest the patient become even more irritable or violent. The clinician's task is to calm the patient and family, persuade the manic patient to accept hospitalization voluntarily if needed, and to resort to civil commitment if necessary.

Although *laws on commitment* vary among states, all states currently have legal provisions to allow the involuntary hospitalization of patients with mental disorders who are clearly dangerous to themselves or others and for whom no less restrictive alternative is appropriate. These difficult processes often require the teamwork of the clinician, the family, and the staff of an emergency room to be successful.

Medication for Severe Mania

Severe acute mania requires treatment initially with *neuroleptics* and later with both mood stabilizers, such as lithium, and neuroleptics. For the first week or two this treatment is usually carried out in the hospital. The generalist's role with such patients many include initial diagnosis, treatment with sufficient medication to get the manic patient to the hospital, and then continued participation in follow-up care.

For acute manic agitation the use of parenteral fluphenazine (Prolixin) or another high-potency neuroleptic is usually effective. Modest doses (5 to 10 mg intramuscularly) calm most patients with little or no depression of blood pressure and little sedation. Older, more sedating phenothiazines such as chlorpromazine (Thorazine) are more difficult to work with because repeated doses are often necessary to break the agitated manic state and these preparations often produce significant orthostatic hypotension. Within 15 to 20 minutes, intramuscular high-potency neuroleptics usually bring about a calming effect that may last for several hours. This period can be used to get the patient admitted to hospital. Even in this short period, however, patients may develop *extrapyramidal side effects* from the high-potency neuroleptics, most often acute dystonic reactions. This condition is alleviated by 50 mg of intramuscular diphenhydramine (Benadryl) or 1 to 2 mg of trihexyphenidate (Cogentin). New neuroleptic agents now available (e.g., Olanzapine) or soon to be available (e.g., Quetiapine, Seroquel) may also prove useful as alternatives to standard neuroleptics in the manic state, especially because they have less propensity for inducing extrapyramidal side effects. This benefit may be particularly salient for affectively ill patients, who are thought to have greater susceptibility to the extrapyramidal effects of neuroleptic drugs, including tardive dyskinesia. These preparations have their own troublesome side effects, which include sedation and orthostatic blood pressure changes.

Maintenance Therapy for Bipolar Disorder

To date, lithium is the only medication for which efficacy has been unequivocally established for preventing relapses in patients with bipolar disorder or mania after acute episodes have remitted (31). Most controlled comparisons of carbamazepine and lithium suggest that they are approximately equivalent in prophylactic efficacy (5). There are as yet no rigorous therapeutic trials comparing lithium with other anticonvulsants that may be useful for maintenance treatment of bipolar disorder. The latter agents include valproate and two newer anticonvulsants, lamotrigine and gabapentin (29). Several other agents, including calcium channel blockers and high-potency benzodiazepines, particularly clonazepam, may also have antimanic utility.

Lithium

Dosage and Schedule. When lithium is the mood stabilizer selected, it is prescribed in divided doses, beginning with 300 to 600 mg on the first day and increasing the dosage in small increments every 3 to 4 days until the therapeutic blood level is achieved. The usual maintenance dosage is 600 to 1800 mg given

Table 15.9. Important Drug Interactions with Lithium

Drugs that May Enhance Lithium Toxicity
Ace inhibitors[b]
Amiloride[a]
Ethacrynic acid[a]
Furosemide[a]
NSAIDs[a]
Spectinamycin[a]
Spironolactone[a]
Tetracycline[a]
Thiazide diuretics[a]
Triamterene[a]

Drugs that May Increase Lithium Excretion
Acetazolamide[c]
Theophylline[c]

Drugs that May Aggravate Lithium Tremor
Caffeine[b]
Neuroleptics[b]
Theophylline[b]
Tricyclic antidepressants[b]
Valproate[b]

[a] Decreased renal excretion.
[b] Mechanism not established.
[c] Increased renal excretion.

in divided doses (two to three times daily with standard preparations and once or twice daily with slow-release preparations). Blood levels, which should be measured 12 hours after a dose (trough levels), should be monitored once or twice per week at first. Even when thoroughly stabilized in a compliant patient, lithium levels should be checked at least six times per year. In addition, because of the possibility of long-term renal effects, maintenance dosage should be aimed at maintaining the lowest therapeutic level (probably 0.6 to 0.9 mEq/L) and not necessarily the level required for acute antimanic activity (0.9 to 1.4 mEq/L). Lithium should be used cautiously with other medications because a number of important drug interactions are associated with its use (Table 15.9).

Side Effects. The adverse effects of lithium can be divided into three groups: early (associated with rapidly rising blood levels), maintenance (associated with stable levels within the therapeutic range), and toxic (usually associated with high lithium levels).

The *early side effects* include nausea and vomiting, diarrhea, mild lassitude, and drowsiness. These effects typically resolve as the serum level stabilizes in the therapeutic range.

The number of possible *side effects from the maintenance dosage* is large enough to warrant a medical review of systems to detect them. The three most important ones are hand tremor, thyroid disturbances, and renal toxicity.

- An accentuated *physiologic (postural) tremor* (see Chapter 82) appears in a large percentage of patients (perhaps 60%) but is rarely severe. A family history of benign essential tremor and of concomitant use of other psychotropic drugs is often associated with more severe tremor.
- In approximately 3% of patients, lithium therapy causes nontoxic *goiter and mild alterations of thy-*

roid function tests (i.e., borderline low thyroxine levels or elevated thyroid-stimulating hormone values). Less often, frank hypothyroidism may occur, usually in patients who had subclinical hypothyroidism before receiving lithium. For these reasons thyroid function should be assessed before lithium treatment is begun.

- Finally, long-term lithium therapy is associated with a *renal concentrating defect* (partial nephrogenic diabetes insipidus due to vasopressin resistance). This abnormality causes symptoms of polyuria and polydipsia in approximately 10% of patients. The concentrating defect predisposes the patient to dehydration and, therefore, to frank lithium intoxication. Polyuric patients must be counseled to maintain good hydration even under circumstances that might inhibit their interest in adequate water intake (including depression) or that would increase water loss (e.g., diarrhea). They should also be instructed to report the onset of polyuria at any time in the course of lithium treatment. A patient's usual daily urine volume and glomerular filtration rate (GFR) should be assessed (see Chapter 47) before lithium is started and yearly thereafter.

The *toxic effects of lithium* occur uncommonly at normal serum levels, but increase in frequency as serum levels exceed 1.5 mEq/L. Premonitory signs are the recurrence of gastrointestinal side effects and worsening of polyuria and hand tremor, lethargy, and clumsiness. Obvious changes in the level of consciousness are reflected in confusion, delirium, stupor, and finally coma. Focal as well as nonlocalizing neurologic signs are often present. Levels above 4.0 mEq/L are potentially fatal; death in coma or due to aspiration pneumonitis can occur. The toxic syndrome is not usually relieved rapidly, even though blood levels can be reduced rapidly. A rather prolonged 10- to 14-day resolution of the mental state is usual. Management of suspected lithium intoxication begins with an emergency measurement of serum lithium level and the discontinuation of lithium when the early signs of the disorder appear. If the clinical or laboratory evaluations suggest the likelihood of the toxic syndrome, hospitalization is mandatory.

The most important treatment strategy for lithium intoxication is prevention. Overingestion and inadequate renal excretion (at times, related to one of the drugs listed in Table 15.8) are the only causes of the disorder.

PROGNOSIS AND LONG-TERM TREATMENT OF AFFECTIVE DISORDERS

Because of the fundamental similarities, the prognoses of unipolar depression and bipolar disorder are discussed together. Before modern treatment, patients with these disorders usually recovered spontaneously within 6 to 18 months. With antidepressants, mood stabilizers such as lithium, and ECT, remissions usually can be achieved much more quickly. However,

even with modern treatment, approximately 20% of patients with severe major depressions may not recover fully in a 2-year period after entering treatment (16). Manic episodes tend to be briefer and are less likely to become chronic; however, some patients with bipolar disorder have chronic depressions or such frequent cycling of their illness that they are never well and may become completely disabled. *Predictors of poor outcome* include severity sufficient to require hospitalization and long duration of major symptoms (1 year) before treatment. It has also been noted that many nonrecovering patients have not been aggressively treated after failure to respond to a trial of antidepressant medications. Although some patients fail to respond to all treatments, clinical experience teaches that most correctly diagnosed patients in whom initial treatment fails will eventually respond to a second, third, or fourth treatment effort.

Relapse. A hallmark of the course of unipolar and bipolar disorders is the tendency to remit and to *relapse.* The frequency of relapse is variable. However, fewer than 20% of major affective syndromes resolve without relapsing at some point. There is a tendency for relapses to become more frequent later in the life of the patient (or later in the course of the illness).

The use of lithium and antidepressants has been shown to be beneficial in preventing recurrent affective episodes (31). Depressive relapses that occur in patients taking lithium or tricyclics are usually less severe and of shorter duration. Lithium is the only treatment demonstrated to reduce the frequency of manic relapses. Other mood stabilizers have been shown to have antimanic activity (see above), but current data are insufficient to establish long-term efficacy of these medications.

Maintenance treatment is usually continued indefinitely in patients with a clearly relapsing disorder. The patient's personal physician can often provide the basic treatment, particularly if that physician is following the patient regularly for chronic medical problems. Brief visits every 2 to 3 months are sufficient when the patient is well. The objectives of these visits are to monitor the mood state, the drug therapy, and the social progress of the patient. Recovery of social ease and full functioning lags several months behind the recovery of mood-related symptoms (25).

The patient and his or her family should be educated about the relapsing and remitting course of the illness, and they should know that relapses will probably be fewer, milder, and of shorter duration with drug therapy. Individual aspects of the patient's illness, particularly the early symptoms of relapse, must be remembered by the patient and the family, and there should be a plan for management of these symptoms when they recur.

COUNSELING THE FAMILY

Family members of patients with serious affective disorders often experience feelings of confusion, hopelessness, guilt, and recrimination toward the patient.

These are not only painful feelings; they impede the family's attempts to support their ill relative. Physicians need to address the family's needs directly through meetings with them. Above all, the family must recognize major affective disorders as diseases and realize that these disorders are not caused by the family, the patient, or even the social predicaments affecting the patient. The family also should know that although the pathophysiology of affective disorders is unknown, empirical treatments are effective and the prognosis for complete recovery from an episode is generally good, although relapses occur frequently. These points usually require some repetition and are best repeated in response to questions that the family should be encouraged to raise in such a meeting or consultation.

The patient education materials provided by the APA and the National Institute of Mental Health and the books by DePaulo and Ablow and by Papolos and Papolos can also be recommended to patients and families (see "General References"). In addition, interested families may gain considerable help from patient and family-member support groups (see sources of information in "General References").

It is equally important to reassure families and patients with dysthymic and transiently demoralized mood states that the patients are not suffering from major mental illness.

Heritability of Depression

Evidence from many studies of concordance comparing identical and nonidentical twins has established a substantial genetic contribution to major affective disorders. No genes have yet been isolated, although linked loci on two chromosomes have been identified that are likely to harbor genes related to bipolar disorder. These modest findings to date support the supposition that there is genetic heterogeneity and that the disease genotype is an ensemble of genes acting in concert to predispose people to these illnesses. It appears that a sibling or offspring of a patient with a major affective disorder has a 10% chance of developing the disorder. However, in some families this risk may be as high as 50%. Counseling patients and their families about the genetic risk should be tailored to the needs and relevant history in each family. The major themes of counseling should be that most cases are genetically influenced, that effective treatment is available, and that treatment is greatly enhanced by early detection of the disorder.

CYCLOTHYMIC DISORDER

An episodic bipolar affective disorder that is sufficiently mild or so brief that the episodes fail to meet the APA criteria for major depression or mania (Tables 15.3 and 15.8) is categorized as a cyclothymic disorder. These patients must be distinguished from patients with the personality traits of emotional lability and self-dramatization, described in Chapter 14, who often report rapid but unsustained mood changes. The family histories of cyclothymic patients are similar to those of patients with bipolar affective disorders. The long-term course is also similar to that of bipolar disorders, and 35% of such patients have been found to experience full-blown manic, hypomanic, or depressive episodes in a 2- to 3-year period of follow-up (1).

SUICIDE PREVENTION

The rate of suicide in most countries is low enough (11 per 100,000 in the United States) that successful prediction of an individual suicide at a given point in time is very unlikely.

Practical strategies in this area are to protect those with high risk in the short term and to reduce the risk in these patients over a longer term. *Risk factors* for successful suicide include depressive disorder (greater severity is associated with greater risk), older age, male gender, alcoholism, living alone, previous suicide attempt, and refusal to accept referral for psychiatric treatment. Retrospective studies of patient groups with major affective disorders in the era before affective drugs were available suggest that approximately 15% of the deaths were caused by suicide. In addition, clinical observations suggest that the risk of suicide increases when improvement begins (or just after a depressed patient is discharged from the hospital) or when the depressive ruminations become frankly delusional convictions. Retrospective studies also suggest that there are fewer suicides in patients treated with ECT or long-term lithium.

The most crucial activities of physicians in preventing suicides are the diagnosis, treatment, and prophylaxis of major depressive episodes. When evaluating any patient with depressed mood, direct and open inquiry should be made regarding suicidal ideas, specific plans, and available means that the patient might be inclined to use. This information, as well as information about the capability and availability of constant family supervision, are essential in determining whether treatment may be attempted safely on an outpatient basis. This evaluation should also be guided by the knowledge that delusional depressed patients have a significantly increased risk of suicide and that patients with prior suicide attempts are more likely than others to attempt it again when depressed. When treating depressed outpatients, it should be recalled that most people who commit suicide with pills have obtained the lethal dose in a single prescription at a recent visit to a physician (26). This could represent as little as a 1- to 2-week supply of a tricyclic antidepressant medication. Thus, small prescriptions and, at times, family supervision of medications are needed. Finally, short-term protection of patients with suicidal intent via hospitalization, including involuntary commitment, is sometimes required.

Most patients who present to emergency facilities after *overdose of pills* do not have major depression, but have adjustment disorders and personality disorders, and they usually do not die by suicide. However, they should be methodically evaluated in the same manner as noted above because many such patients are prone to take overdoses again when stressed. These patients may benefit from brief hospital admissions when social support for them is lacking and suicidal feelings are intense. All should have some outpatient counseling.

General References*

Agency for Health Care Policy and Research. **A clinical practice guideline. Depression in primary care.** U.S. Public Health Service, AHCPR Publication Nos. 93-0550 through 93-0553. Washington, DC: US Department of Health and Human Services, 1993.

> This outstanding two-volume plus two-brochure set contains critically assessed clinical practice guidelines from an expert multidisciplinary primary care panel and is available from the Agency for Health Care Policy and Research, 2101 East Jefferson St., Rockville, MD 20852, at a nominal cost.

Altshuler LL, Cohen L, Szuba MP, et al. Pharmacologic management of psychiatric illness during pregnancy: dilemmas and guidelines. Am J Psychiatry 153:5, 592, 1996.

> A review of the treatment of depressed pregnant women.

American Psychiatric Association. **Diagnostic and Statistical Manual of Mental Disorders.** 4th ed. (DSM-IV). Washington, DC: American Psychiatric Association, 1994.

> Diagnostic criteria and epidemiologic information for all recognized psychiatric disorders.

Boswell EB, Stoudemire A. Major depression in the primary care setting. Am J Med 101:6A, 3S–9S, December 30, 1996.

> An up-to-date review article.

DePaulo JR, Ablow KR. How to cope with depression: a complete guide for you and your family. New York: Fawcett Crest, 1989.

> A book written for patients, families, and general health professionals.

Goodwin FK, Jamison KR. Manic–depressive illness. New York: Oxford University Press, 1990.

> A comprehensive survey of the clinical and scientific literature on bipolar disorders.

Papolos D, Papolos J. Overcoming depression. New York: Harper & Row, 1987.

> An excellent book for patients and families.

Robins LN, Helzer JE, Weissman MM, et al. Lifetime prevalence of specific psychiatric disorders in three sites. Arch Gen Psychiatry 41:949, 1984.

> This is an early report of the national Epidemiologic Catchment Area (ECA) survey of mental disorders.

Shearer SL, Adams GK. Nonpharmacologic aids in the treatment of depression. Am Fam Physician 47:435, 1993.

> This concise article provides excellent practical advice for primary care clinicians in treating depressed patients. It focuses on patient and family education, self-help, and behavioral advice.

Patient Education Pamphlets

The American Psychiatric Association, 1400 K St. NW, Washington, DC 20005: *Facts about Depression, Facts about Manic–Depressive Disorders, Facts about Teen Suicide,* and *Facts about Mental Health of the Elderly.*

The National Institute of Mental Health, 5600 Fishers Lane, Rockville, MD 20857: *Depression: What You Need to Know, Helpful Facts about Depressive Disorders,* and *National Educational Program on Depressive Disorders.*

Sources of Information about Support Groups for Depressed Patients and Their Families

Depression and Related Affective Disorders Association (DRADA), Meyer 3-181, Johns Hopkins Hospital, 600 N. Wolfe St., Baltimore, MD 21287-7381 (telephone 410-955-4647).

---

*Bold print (general references) and bold numerals (specific references) denote published controlled clinical trials, meta-analyses, or consensus-based recommendations.

National Alliance for the Mentally Ill (NAMI), 2101 Wilson Blvd., Suite 302, Arlington, VA 22201 (telephone 800-950-6264).

National Depressive and Manic Depressive Association, 730 N. Franklin St., Suite 501, Chicago, IL 60610 (telephone 800-82-NDMDA or 312-939-2442).

National Mental Health Association (NMHA), National Mental Health Information Center, 1021 Prince St., Alexandria, VA 23314-2971 (telephone 800-969-6642).

Specific References

1. Akiskal HS, Djenderejiian AH, Rosenthal RH, Khani MK. Cyclothymic disorder: validating criteria for inclusion in the bipolar affective group. Am J Psychiatry 134:1227, 1977.
2. Altamura AC, Montgomery SA, Wernicke JF. The evidence for 20 mg a day of fluoxetine as the optimal dose in the treatment of depression. Br J Psychiatry 153:109, 1988.
3. Barraclough B, Bunch J, Nelson B, Sainsbury P. A hundred cases of suicide: clinical aspects. Br J Psychiatry 125:355, 1974.
4. Battersby MW, O'Mahoney JJ, Beckwith AR, Hunt JL. Antidepressant deaths by overdose. Aust N Z J Psychiatry 30:2–223, 1996.
5. Dardennes R, Even C, Bange F, Heim A. Comparison of carbamazepine and lithium in the prophylaxis of bipolar disorders. A meta-analysis. Br J Psychiatry 166:3–378, 1995.
6. DeVane CL. Pharmacokinetics of the newer antidepressants: clinical relevance. Am J Med 6A:97–13S, 1994.
7. Egeland JA, Sussex JN. Suicide and family loading for affective disorders. JAMA 254:915, 1985.
8. Frasure-Smith N, Lesperance F, Talajic M. Depression and 18 month prognosis after myocardial infarction. Circulation 91(4):999, 1995.
9. German PS, Shapiro S, Skinner EA. Mental health of elderly: use of health and mental health services. J Am Geriatr Soc 33(4):246, 1985.
10. Greenberg PE, Stiglin LE, Finkelstein SN, Berndt ER. Depression: a neglected major illness. J Clin Psychiatry 54:419, 1993.
11. Greenberg PE, Stiglin LE, Finkelstein SN, Berndt ER. The economic burden of depression in 1990. J Clin Psychiatry 54:405, 1993.
12. Guze SB, Robins E. Suicide and primary affective disorders. Br J Psychiatry 117:437, 1970.
13. Kapur S, Mieczkowski T, Mann JJ. Antidepressant medications and the relative risk of suicide attempt and suicide. JAMA 268:24, 3441, 1992.
14. Karasu TB. Toward a clinical model of psychotherapy for depression, II: an integrative and selective treatment approach. Am J Psychiatry 147(3):269–278, 1990.
15. Katzelnick DJ, Kobak KA, Greist JH, et al. Effect of primary care treatment of depression on service use by patients with high medical expenditures. Psychiatr Serv 48:1, 59, 1997.
16. Keller, MB, Klerman GL, Lavori PW, et al. Long-term outcome of episodes of major depression. JAMA 252:788, 1984.
17. Kocsis JH, Frances AJ, Voss C, et al. Imipramine for treatment of chronic depression. Arch Gen Psychiatry 29:240, 1973.
18. Kupfer DJ, Frank E. Relapse in recurrent unipolar depression. Am J Psychiatry 144:1, 86, 1987.
19. Kupfer DJ, Frank E, Perel JM, et al. Five-year outcome for maintenance therapies in recurrent depression. Arch Gen Psychiatry 49:10, 769, 1992.
20. Lapierre Y, Bentkover J, Schainbaum S, Manners S. Direct cost of depression: analysis of treatment costs of paroxetine versus imipramine in Canada. Can J Psychiatry 40:7, 370, 1995.
21. Linde K, Ramirez G, Mulrow CD, et al. St. John's wort for depression: an overview and meta-analysis of randomised clinical trials. BMJ 313(7052):253, 1996.
22. Maj M, Veltro F, Pirozzi R, et al. Pattern of recurrence of illness after recovery from an episode of major depression: a prospective study. Am J Psychiatry 149:795, 1992.
23. Markowitz JC, Moran ME, Kocsis JH, Frances AJ. Prevalence and comorbidity of dysthymic disorder among psychiatric outpatients. J Affect Disord 24:63, 1992.
24. McHugh PR. Psychologic illness in medical practice: the concept of disease in psychiatry. Cecil textbook of medicine. Philadelphia: WB Saunders, 1979;15:664.

25. Mintz J, Mintz LI, Arruda MJ, Hwang SS. Treatments of depression and the functional capacity to work. Arch Gen Psychiatry 49:761, 1992.

26. Murphy GE. The physician's responsibility for suicide. I. An error of commission. II. Errors of omission. Ann Intern Med 82:301–305, 1975.

27. Parkes CM. The first year of bereavement. A longitudinal study of the reaction of London widows to the death of their husbands. Psychiatry 33:444, 1970.

28. Pastuszak A, Schick-Boschetto B, Zuber C, et al. Pregnancy outcome following first-trimester exposure to fluoxetine. JAMA 269:17, 2246, 1993.

29. Post RM, Ketter TA, Denicoff K, et al. The place of anticonvulsant therapy in bipolar illness. Psychopharmacology (Berlin) 128:2, 115, 1996.

30. Pratt LA, Ford DE, Crum RM, et al. Depression, psychotropic medication, and risk of myocardial infarction. Circulation 94(12):3123, 1996.

31. Prien RF, Klett CJ, Caffey EM Jr. Lithium carbonate and imipramine in prevention of affective episodes: a comparison in recurrent affective illness. Arch Gen Psychiatry 29:240, 1973.

32. Revicki DA, Brown RE, Keller MB, et al. Cost-effectiveness of newer antidepressants compared with tricyclic antidepressants in managed care settings. J Clin Psychiatry 58:2, 47, 1997.

33. Sackeim HA, Prudic J, Devanand DP, et al. Effects of stimulus intensity and electrode placement on the efficacy and cognitive effects of electroconvulsive therapy. N Engl J Med 328:12, 839, 1993.

34. Schaefer C, Quesenberry CP Jr, Wi S. Mortality following conjugal bereavement and the effects of a shared environment. Am J Epidemiol 141:1142, 1995.

35. Sclar DA, Robison LM, Skaer TL, et al. Antidepressant pharmacotherapy: economic evaluation of fluoxetine, paroxetine and sertraline in a health maintenance organization. J Intl Med Res 23:395, 1995.

36. Shapiro S, Skinner EA, Kramer M, et al. Measuring need for mental health services in a general population. Med Care 23:1033, 1985.

37. Simon GE, VonKorff M, Barlow W. Health care costs of primary care patients with recognized depression. Arch Gen Psychiatry 52:10, 850, 1995.

38. Simon GE, VonKorff M, Heiligenstein JH, et al. Initial antidepressant choice in primary care. Effectiveness and cost of fluoxetine vs. tricyclic antidepressants. JAMA 275:24, 1897, 1996.

39. Sovner D. The clinical characteristics and treatment of atypical depression. J Clin Psychiatry 42:285, 1981.

40. Spitzer RL, Kroenke K, Linzer M, et al. Health-related quality of life in primary care patients with mental disorders. JAMA 274:19, 1511, 1995.

41. Squires LR, Chace PM. Memory functions six to nine months after electroconvulsive therapy. Arch Gen Psychiatry 32:1557, 1975.

42. Tignol J. A double-blind, randomized, fluoxetine-controlled, multicenter study of paroxetine in the treatment of depression. J Clin Psychopharmacol 13(6, Suppl 2):188S, 1993.

43. Veith RC, Raskind MA, Caldwell JH, et al. Cardiovascular effects of tricyclic antidepressants in depressed patients with chronic heart disease. N Engl J Med 306:954, 1982.

44. Wells KB, Hays RD, Burnam MA, et al. Detection of depressive disorder for patients receiving prepaid or fee for service care. JAMA 262:3298, 1989.

45. Wells KB, Stewart A, Hays RD, et al. The functioning and well being of depressed patients: results from the medical outcomes study. JAMA 262:914, 1989.

46. Widmer RB, Cadoret RJ, North CS. Depression in primary care: changes in pattern of patients visits and complaints during subsequent developing depressions. J Fam Pract 9:1017, 1979.

47. Wilson DR, Widmer RB, Cadoret RJ, Judiesch K. Somatic symptoms: a major feature of depression in a family practice. J Affect Disord 5:199, 1983.

CHAPTER 16

Schizophrenia

CHESTER W. SCHMIDT, JR, MD

Schizophrenia is a mental disorder, or group of disorders, for which the etiology is unknown. The American Psychiatric Association lists the essential features of the disorder as the presence of certain psychotic features for a significant length of time (i.e., a 1-month period, with some signs persisting for at least 6 months), characteristic chronic symptoms involving multiple psychologic processes, deterioration from a previous level of functioning, and median age of onset is mid-20s for men and late 20s for women. As noted under "Diagnosis," none of these symptoms is pathognomonic for schizophrenia, and each is seen in other psychotic states.

Familiarity with schizophrenia is important to the generalist for two reasons: In the prodromal stage, the patient often presents first to a general physician, and the interested generalist can provide much of the care for a patient with this lifelong disorder.

EPIDEMIOLOGY

Schizophrenia has been found in all societies throughout the world. The distribution is assumed to be similar through all populations. Epidemiologic studies in Western societies have found the lifetime prevalence of schizophrenia to be slightly less than 1 case per 100 persons. Lifetime incidence rates have been reported to range from 0.6 to 1.9% (7). Studies of incidence and prevalence in Europe using strict and somewhat narrow criteria for schizophrenia have produced case numbers and rates lower than similar studies done in the United States using broader criteria. In 1943, Lemkau et al. (4) determined that 15 to 25% of patients with schizophrenia never enter the hospital. Developments in psychopharmacology over the past three decades and the wide availability of ambulatory treatment resources have expanded the number of patients who never enter the hospital and have greatly reduced the duration of confinement for those who require hospitalization.

Schizophrenia is equally common in males and females. Onset is usually during young adulthood, with the first hospitalization generally occurring between the ages of 25 and 34 years. Most schizophrenic patients are single and are found in lower socioeconomic groups. The proposed reason for the clustering of patients in the lower socioeconomic groups is a downward social drift resulting from deterioration of social and vocational function.

CAUSES

The cause or causes of schizophrenia remain unknown. Numerous constitutional, genetic, neurologic, anatomic, biochemical, nutritional, psychosocial, and psychoanalytical theories have been offered. It is known that people related to schizophrenic patients are at higher risk for the disorder. The increased risk ranges from 3% for second-degree relatives, to 7 to 15% for siblings and children of one schizophrenic parent, to 40% for children of two schizophrenic parents. Concordance rates are 10 to 15% in dizygotic twins and 45% in monozygotic twins. This evidence indicates that there is a genetic factor, but such a factor has yet to be defined. An important clue to the etiology of schizophrenia emerged from studies of the pharmacologic effects of neuroleptic antipsychotic agents on schizophrenia. These antipsychotic agents antagonize dopamine-mediated neurotransmission, leading to the speculation that excessive activity of the dopamine systems may be part of a biochemical defect in schizophrenic patients (8).

NATURAL HISTORY OF SCHIZOPHRENIA

Although the first episode of acute psychosis usually occurs in late adolescence or early adulthood, *prodromal manifestations* of the disease are often present for years before the acute episode. During the prodromal phase, patients gradually withdraw from social relationships into their own inner psychologic world. They become indifferent to their grooming, develop suspicious attitudes about others, and ignore social graces and social rituals. They appear different, peculiar, and sometimes bizarre. Withdrawal often results in a gradual deterioration of scholastic and vocational abilities, although some patients who have achieved substantial social skills (including marriage and family), educational skills (college or graduate level work), and vocational skills (stable and productive work) show little deterioration of their baseline function. The development of these skills may be a function of the age at onset of the disorder: The older the patient is, the more likely it is that he or she will have developed social, educational, and vocational talents. In other patients the deterioration of social and vocational skills may be so striking that the patient seems to have

a changed personality. In many cases of early-onset schizophrenia, the patient has developed only marginal social and vocational skills so that his or her deterioration appears more insidious.

In one study of the prodromal stage of schizophrenia (9), most patients demonstrated some dysphoria (anxiety or depression) in association with social deterioration, and more than half of them developed vague somatic complaints for which they sought help from a generalist physician.

Acute psychotic episodes are marked by the presence of a variety of positive and disorganized symptoms: delusions (content of thought); hallucinations (perception); blunted, flattened, or inappropriate affect; illogical thinking and loosening of associations (form of thought); preoccupation with fantasies and an inner psychologic world (autism); inability to carry out goal-directed behavior because of preoccupation with consequences of alternatives (ambivalence); and stereotyped, bizarre, and sometimes rigid posturing. These episodes are often associated with stressful life events. Before neuroleptics were available, these episodes could last from weeks to years. Currently, most episodes are brought under pharmacologic control within several weeks to 2 months. After treatment, positive and disorganized psychotic symptoms subside and in some cases seem to disappear completely. Most patients then display negative symptoms: affective flattening, reduced speech and thought productivity, anhedonia, and a decrease in motivation. Scholastic and vocational ability may slip further. With each subsequent psychotic episode the patient may slip further and further into a dependent, regressed state in which he or she is unable to function and becomes entirely dependent on family or society. Less than 20% work full-time; the majority are financially supported by welfare programs or federal disability programs. Institutionalization is required in some cases because the patients lose all ability to care for themselves.

Thus, schizophrenia is a lifelong disease consisting of psychotic symptoms that periodically become intense and an arrest or deterioration of social and vocational functioning, probably caused by massive withdrawal of interest in the outside world.

DIAGNOSIS

The diagnosis of schizophrenia, especially during the initial episodes of acute psychosis, is based on clinical judgment and diagnostic criteria that, until recently, were unreliable. No pathognomonic symptoms, signs, or laboratory findings point to the diagnosis. The medical history of the patient does not contribute to the diagnosis and, as discussed above, family history of the disease provides only partial information.

The diagnostic criteria for schizophrenia described in the American Psychiatric Association's *Diagnostic and Statistical Manual of Mental Disorders* (DSM-IV) are an excellent synthesis of several recognized diagnostic formulations (Table 16.1). Diagnosis rests on the findings of the symptoms of psychosis elicited by a

Table 16.1. Diagnostic Criteria for Schizophrenia

A. Characteristic symptoms: Two (or more) of the following, each present for a significant portion of time during a 1-month period (or less if successfully treated):
   1. Delusions
   2. Hallucinations
   3. Disorganized speech (e.g., frequent derailment or incoherence)
   4. Grossly disorganized or catatonic behavior
   5. Negative symptoms, i.e., affective flattening, alogia, or avolition

   (Note: Only one criterion A symptom is required if delusions are bizarre or hallucinations consist of a voice keeping up a running commentary on the person's behavior or thoughts, or two or more voices conversing with each other.)

B. Social/occupational dysfunction: For a significant portion of the time since the onset of the disturbance, one or more major areas of functioning such as work, interpersonal relations, or self-care is markedly below the level achieved before the onset (or when the onset is in childhood or adolescence, failure to achieve expected level of interpersonal, academic, or occupational achievement).

C. Duration: Continuous signs of the disturbance persist for at least 6 months. This 6-month period must include at least 1 month of symptoms (or less if successfully treated) that meet criterion A (i.e., active-phase symptoms), and may include periods of prodromal or residual symptoms. During these prodromal or residual periods, the signs of the disturbance may be manifested by only negative symptoms or two or more symptoms listed in criterion A present in an attenuated form (e.g., odd beliefs, unusual perceptual experiences).

D. Schizoaffective and mood disorder exclusion: Schizoaffective disorder and mood disorder with psychotic features have been ruled out because either 1) no major depressive, manic or mixed episodes have occurred concurrently with the active-phase symptoms, or 2) if mood episodes have occurred during active-phase symptoms, their total duration has been brief relative to the duration of the active and residual periods.

E. Substance/general medical condition exclusion: The disturbance is not due to the direct psychologic effects of a substance (e.g., a drug of abuse, a medication) or a general medical condition.

F. Relationship to a pervasive developmental disorder: If there is a history of autistic disorder or another pervasive developmental disorder, the additional diagnosis of schizophrenia is made only if prominent delusions or hallucinations are also present for at least a month (or less if successfully treated).

Reprinted with permission from the DSM-IV. Copyright 1994, American Psychiatric Association.

mental status examination (see Chapter 10) and a history that documents the prodromal phase.

DIFFERENTIAL DIAGNOSIS

Any kind of psychotic state may resemble acute schizophrenia. However, differences in symptoms permit differentiation and diagnosis. *Delirium, dementia, and amnestic and other cognitive disorders* (see Chapter 17) are marked by disturbances in consciousness (delirium); by disorientation with respect to time, place, and person; and by impairment in intellectual functions (e.g., memory and calculations). In addition, especially in patients under 50, there is usually evidence from the history, physical examination, and laboratory tests of specific organic findings that are etiologically related to the mental condition. *Single psychotic symptoms,* such as persecutory delusions

and auditory hallucinations, may occur de novo in elderly patients as symptoms of dementia or paraphrenia (see Chapter 17). Illicit drugs, especially amphetamine and phencyclidine (see Chapter 22), may mimic the acute phase of schizophrenia. In addition, a number of *prescription drugs* may occasionally produce hallucinations and other manifestations that suggest psychosis (Table 16.2). History of drug usage and absence of the prodromal phase help differentiate these conditions from schizophrenia.

The *psychotic symptoms of major affective episodes* (both mania and depression, see Chapter 15) can also be similar to those seen during acute episodes in the course of schizophrenia. Affective disorders differ from schizophrenia in that psychotic symptoms (e.g., delusions and hallucinations) appear after the development of the affective disturbance (depression or mania). In schizophrenia, marked depression or mania may appear, but the affective disturbance occurs after the onset of the psychotic symptoms. These principles of differential diagnosis are far from perfect, and patients with both types of disorder have been mislabeled. Because of the often poor prognosis associated with schizophrenia, mislabeling has significant consequences such as attitudes toward the patient and the actual treatment provided.

Several *other psychoses* (i.e., schizophreniform disorder, brief reactive psychosis) have symptoms similar to the acute psychotic phase of schizophrenia. How-

Table 16.2. Prescription Drugs that Have Been Reported Occasionally to Cause Hallucinations or Other Manifestations of Psychosis

ACE inhibitors	Fluoxetine (Prozac)
Acyclovir (Zovirax)	Ganciclovir (Cytovene)
Albuterol (Proventil; Ventolin)	Histamine H_2-receptor antagonists
Amantadine (Symmetrel)	Isoniazid (INH, others)
Amiodarone (Cordarone)	Levodopa (Sinemet)
Amphetamine-like drugs	Methyldopa (Aldomet)
Anabolic steroids	Methylphenidate (Ritalin)
Anticonvulsants	Metronidazole (Flagyl)
Antidepressants, tricyclic	Nalidixic acid (NegGram)
Antihistamines	Narcotics
Atropine and anticholinergics	Nonsteroidal anti-inflammatory
Baclofen (Lioresal)	drugs
Benzodiazepines	Pantazocine (Talwin)
β-Adrenergic blockers	Pergolide (Permax)
Bromocriptine (Parlodel)	Phenelzine (Nardil)
Bupropion (Wellbutrin)	Phenylephrine (Neo-Synephrine)
Caffeine	Prazosin (Minipress)
Chloroquine (Aralen)	Procainamide (Pronestyl)
Ciprofloxacin (Cipro)	Procaine penicillin G
Clonidine (Catapres)	Pseudoephedrine
Cocaine	Quinacrine (Atabrine)
Corticosteroids (prednisone,	Quinidine
cortisone, ACTH, other)	Salicylates
Cyclobenzaprine (Flexeril)	Selegiline (Eldepryl)
Cyclosporine (Sandimmune)	Sulfonamides
Deet (Off)	Tamoxifen (Nolvadex)
Digitalis glycosides	Thyroid hormones
Disopyramide (Norpace)	Trazodone (Desyrel)
Disulfiram (Antabuse)	Verapamil
Ethchlorvynol (Placidyl)	Zidovudine (Retrovir)

Adapted from Drugs that cause psychiatric symptoms. Med Lett 35:65, 1993 (includes references to reports).

ever, these psychoses do not include a prodromal phase of withdrawal and deterioration, and patients return to their baseline level of function after recovery from the psychotic episode and do not experience progressive deterioration of function or recurrence of psychotic episodes.

Schizoid personality, described in Chapter 14, is a personality type that is not accompanied by the psychotic features in the diagnosis of schizophrenia (Table 16.1).

TREATMENT AND PROGNOSIS

Neuroleptic Antipsychotic Drugs

The primary treatment of the acute and chronic psychotic manifestations of schizophrenia in ambulatory or hospitalized patients is with the neuroleptic antipsychotic agents (agents that may produce unwanted symptoms that resemble neurologic disease). There are several classes of neuroleptics, with numerous drugs in each class. The common drugs are listed in Table 16.3, together with available strengths and potency equivalents to chlorpromazine.

Although the structures of the various antipsychotics are well known, the pharmacology is not. Dose–

response relationships have not yet been worked out for humans. The drugs produce effects within 1 hour after oral administration and within 10 to 15 minutes after intramuscular injection. They are lipid soluble with a high affinity for cell membranes. The drugs and their metabolites are distributed generally throughout the central nervous system with no local or regional accumulation. Metabolites are partially excreted each day, with significant portions retained in lipid-rich tissues and connective tissues. As these tissues become saturated, the drugs undergo slow turnover. The drugs are detoxified and inactivated mainly through oxidation by hepatic microsomal enzymes, and they are excreted through both the bile and the urine.

There is no evidence that these agents are addicting, although tolerance to some of the side effects (sedation, hypotension, anticholinergic effects, and parkinsonian symptoms) has been reported. The drugs are fairly safe; large amounts must be taken acutely to produce symptoms of stupor or coma.

The mechanisms of action of the antipsychotics are not fully understood. Although it has been speculated that specific antipsychotic activity may result from the dopamine-antagonist action of these agents, the drugs have a variety of effects on many metabolic processes.

Table 16.3. Available Strengths and Equivalent Doses of Commonly Used Neuroleptic Antipsychotic Agents

Generic Name	Trade Name	Available Strengths of Oral Preparations (mg)	Approximate Equivalent Dose (mg)
Phenothiazines			
Aliphatic			
Chlorpromazine[a]	Thorazine	10, 25, 50, 100, 200	100
Triflupromazine	Vesprin	10, 25	30
Piperidines			
Mesoridazine	Serentil	10, 25, 100	50
Piperacetazine	Quide	10, 15	12
Thioridazine[a]	Mellaril	10, 15, 25, 50, 100, 150, 200	95
Piperazines			
Fluphenazine[a,b]	Prolixin, Permitil	1, 2.5, 5, 10	2
Perphenazine[a]	Trilafon	2, 4, 8, 16	10
Trifluoperazine[a]	Stelazine	1, 2, 5, 10	5
Thioxanthenes			
Aliphatic			
Chlorprothixene	Taractan	10, 25, 50, 100	65
Piperazine			
Thiothixene[a]	Navane	1, 2, 5, 10, 25	5
Dibenzazepine			
Loxapine	Loxitane, Daxolin	10, 25, 50	15
Butyrophenone			
Haloperidol[a,c]	Haldol	0.5, 1, 2, 5, 10	2
Indolone			
Molindone	Moban	5, 10, 25	10
New Antipsychotics			
Clozapine	Clozaril	25, 100	50
Risperidone	Risperdal	1, 2, 3, 4	1–2
Olanzapine	Zyprexa	5, 7.5, 10	2–3

[a] Generic available.

[b] Long-acting fluphenazine decanoate or enanthate, for injection, comes in a concentration of 25 mg/mL; also available for injection as fluphenazine hydrochloride, a short-acting preparation.

[c] Haloperidol for injection comes in a concentration of 2 mg/mL.

Treatment of Acute Psychotic Episodes

All of the conventional neuroleptic antipsychotics are equally efficacious for controlling psychotic symptoms associated with schizophrenia. The choice of one drug over another depends on predicted differences in side effects, history of a particular patient's response, and the clinician's familiarity with the agent. The treatment of acute psychotic episodes should begin with the equivalent of 300 to 1000 mg of chlorpromazine (Thorazine) a day, in divided doses (usually three times daily). Only one antipsychotic should be given at a time because administration of more than one agent increases the probability of side effects.

Combativeness, hyperactivity, and agitation are usually controlled within 24 to 48 hours after beginning treatment. If these symptoms are not modified within that period, the dosage should be increased 100 to 200 mg/day, up to the equivalent of 800 to 1000 mg of chlorpromazine. It may be necessary to administer the drugs intramuscularly during the acute phase of agitation if the patient is unable to take oral medication. The butyrophenone haloperidol (Haldol), 2 to 5 mg, is a good choice for intramuscular injection because of its minimal effects on circulatory regulation; an equivalent intramuscular dose of chlorpromazine (25 mg) can also be used, but the likelihood of orthostatic hypotension (occasionally leading to syncope) is greater. For patients who do not respond to an adequate trial (4 to 6 weeks) of at least one antipsychotic, a trial of Clozapine should be considered. Because Clozapine may cause fatal agranulocytosis in 1% of patients, a history of blood dyscrasias and poor compliance are contraindications. Clozapine trial should be at least 3 months at a dosage of 200 to 600 mg/day.

Delusions, hallucinations, associational defects, negativism, and *withdrawal* begin to subside within 1 to 2 weeks after treatment begins. Continued improvement of these symptoms may take place over an additional 4 to 8 weeks. If very high dosages of antipsychotic agents were initially required, the dosage should be reduced to the equivalent of 400 to 600 mg of chlorpromazine as soon as possible. This adjustment in dosage can usually be made 1 to 2 weeks after reaching the peak dosage.

Early Side Effects of Neuroleptics

Antipsychotic drugs with lower potency per milligram, such as chlorpromazine (Table 16.3), produce *sedation,* which may be a useful side effect in treating hyperactive or combative patients but a disadvantage in regressed, withdrawn patients. The *anticholinergic property* of all phenothiazines produces annoying symptoms of dry mouth, stuffy nose, blurred vision, and occasional urinary retention in older patients and (at high dosages) delirium. These side effects often abate or disappear within 2 to 4 weeks. The most worrisome side effect is drug-induced *Parkinson's syndrome.* It occurs with greatest frequency in association with drugs of higher potency per milligram, such

as haloperidol, the piperazine class of phenothiazines, thioxanthene, loxapine, and molindone (Table 16.3). The syndrome usually appears within 5 to 30 days after beginning treatment and includes tremor, rigidity, bradykinesia, fixed facies, drooling, and stooped posture. Because this problem commonly causes patients to discontinue antipsychotic treatment, it should be managed properly. Management consists of reduction of dosage, if possible; change to another drug; or antiparkinsonism medication (for details, see Chapter 82). In most cases reduction of dosage or addition of small amounts of an antiparkinsonism agent controls these side effects. The parkinsonian effects of neuroleptic drugs tend to decrease after 1 or 2 months. Therefore, withdrawal of antiparkinsonism drugs should be attempted after 6 to 12 weeks. Prophylactic treatment of all patients with antiparkinsonism drugs is generally discouraged because of the additional anticholinergic effects of these drugs.

Acute dystonias occur in occasional patients, within 1 to 5 days of initiating any neuroleptic; they are most often seen with haloperidol and the piperazine class of phenothiazines. The symptoms are the sudden onset of severe, tonic contractions of the musculature of the neck (torticollis), the spine, and the heels (opisthotonos); of extraocular muscles (oculogyric crises) of the mouth; and of the tongue. These symptoms remit promptly after parenteral injection of diphenhydramine (Benadryl, 25 to 50 mg intramuscularly) or benztropine (Cogentin, 2 mg intravenously). Neuroleptic treatment can be continued in these patients; an antiparkinsonism agent should be added for about 1 month to protect against recurrent dystonia. *Akathisia* may also occur early in treatment. This side effect is marked by motor restlessness with pacing, fidgeting, and restless legs. It does not resolve with treatment as predictably as the acute dystonias. Treatment is the same as that prescribed for drug-induced Parkinsonism. In a small, controlled trial the lipophilic β-blocker propranolol, in daily doses of 20 to 60 mg, was shown to improve symptoms of akathisia in most patients (5).

A number of *nonneurologic side effects* can result from administration of the antipsychotics. *Cardiovascular toxicity* is usually limited to orthostatic hypotension; this problem is most commonly seen with the aliphatic and piperidine classes of phenothiazines and with chlorprothixene. Frank syncope may occur, rarely, after intramuscular administration of low-potency antipsychotics. Ventricular tachycardia is a rare side effect; there are no baseline characteristics that help one recognize patients at risk for this problem. Reversible *cholestatic jaundice* may occur as an allergic response. *Agranulocytosis* is an exceedingly rare side effect.

The *neuroleptic malignant syndrome* is a rare, and occasionally lethal, idiosyncratic complication. It usually occurs at the onset of treatment, when the dosage is increased, or when a second drug is introduced. Over 24 to 72 hours, the patient develops muscle rigidity and a high temperature (as high as 42°C). Patients with this syndrome should be hospitalized immediately in an intensive care unit because hypoventilation occurs as a consequence of the rigidity of the patient's chest wall muscles.

Because *older schizophrenic patients* are more prone to the development of the common side effects, dosages should be lower for these patients by the equivalent of 100 to 200 mg of chlorpromazine. The very high dosages described for treatment of combativeness and hyperactivity should be avoided in elderly patients.

Long-Term Drug Treatment of Schizophrenia

Interested generalists can assume responsibility for the long-term care of schizophrenic patients. Pharmacotherapy is the principal mode of long-term treatment. Many studies show that 60 to 70% of schizophrenic patients relapse within 1 year if they do not receive medication (3). Most patients require antipsychotics indefinitely, but all patients should be treated for at least 2 years after an acute episode.

The goal of long-term pharmacotherapy is to minimize psychotic symptoms with the lowest dosage of antipsychotic possible. Moderate maintenance dosages appear to be as effective as, and safer than, the larger dosages that have been popular in the United States in recent years (1). For most patients a moderate dosage is the equivalent of 100 to 200 mg of chlorpromazine daily. Patients on this dosage often continue to have psychotic symptoms but do not seem to be disturbed by them (e.g., "I still hear the voices but they don't bother me").

Compliance Problems

Some patients temporarily have difficulty maintaining a regular medication schedule because of psychotic disorganization, negativism, or fear of medication. Inability to comply with the medication regimen may signal the onset of an acute episode. With the first indication of a disruption in medication schedule, the patient should be evaluated, frequency of visits increased to at least once a week, and medication increased if warranted. If the patient remains unable to comply, a long-acting intramuscular agent, fluphenazine decanoate (Prolixin Decanoate, available in doses of 25 mg/mL), 1 to 2 mL every 2 to 4 weeks, should be used. The patient can be returned to an oral medication when symptom control is reestablished. Long-acting intramuscular agents are also useful for new patients for whom no information is available on compliance in aftercare or ambulatory programs.

Nonresponders

Of schizophrenic patients, 5 to 25% do not respond to neuroleptics, and a similar number are intolerant of the side effects. Both groups of patients are candidates for treatment with *clozapine* (Clozaril) (6), a tricyclic dibenzodiazepine. The recommended starting dosage is 25 mg once or twice per day, to be increased 25 mg every other day to 100 mg, then to be increased 50 mg every other day to 300 to 450 mg by 2 weeks. Clozapine is available in 25- and 100-mg tablets. The risk of agranulocytosis is 1 to 2% and requires initial weekly blood monitoring. Because of dose-related incidence of seizures, the dosage should not exceed 600 mg.

Late Side Effects of Neuroleptics

Onset of the early-type side effects, described above, is uncommon in patients taking maintenance dosages of antipsychotics (see above). When an increase in medication is necessary, drug-induced parkinsonism may appear. Patients who experience symptoms of parkinsonism over a long period should try other antipsychotic medications until one is found that does not produce the side effect. As noted above, long-term use of antiparkinsonism medication is to be avoided if possible (see Chapter 82 for further discussion of drug-induced parkinsonism).

Tardive dyskinesia is an extrapyramidal syndrome that occurs in patients after prolonged (months to years) moderate- to high-dosage neuroleptic treatment. The cumulative prevalence is approximately 24%, 27% in women and 22% in men. The prevalence reaches its peak in men at age 50 to 70 years but continues to rise after 70 years in women. Asians have lower prevalence than North Americans, Europeans, and Africans (10). The disorder has been reported in association with long-term treatment with anticonvulsants. Up to 25% of patients treated with neuroleptics who are evaluated for drug-induced tardive dyskinesia are found to have another disorder causing their dyskinesia.

The syndrome of tardive dyskinesia consists of *involuntary or semivoluntary movements* of choreiform, ticlike nature, sometimes associated with a dystonic component that classically involves the tongue, facial, and neck muscles. Early manifestations include fine wormlike movements of the tongue at rest, facial tics, and jaw movements. Later symptoms are buccolingual-masticatory movements, chewing motions, lip smacking, puffing of cheeks, blinking of eyes, and choreoathetoid movements of the extremities. Younger patients often have significant involvement of the extremities and trunk. Although the syndrome is painless, it can be socially embarrassing and can interfere with the patient's ability to feed and care for himself or herself.

The prognosis for remission of tardive dyskinesia is poor, regardless of treatment, and symptoms last for years if not indefinitely. The emphasis of neuroleptic use should therefore be on prevention of tardive dyskinesia, by careful selection of patients for long-term neuroleptic treatment and the use of the lowest possible dosage. At the first sign of the disorder, neuroleptics should be tapered and discontinued if possible. Symptoms gradually diminish or disappear over several months in approximately one-third of patients who can be taken off drugs early.

Because there is no satisfactory treatment for tardive dyskinesia, understanding support by physician and family members is especially important in long-term care of the patient. Antiparkinsonism medications usually worsen the symptoms. One short-term effective treatment is the use of more potent antipsychotics to suppress the symptoms, but this usually requires increasing dosages of the suppressing agent, and subsequent withdrawal of antipsychotics often leads to worsening of the symptoms for a period of time. In case reports, benzodiazepines, pure lecithin, lithium, and sodium valproate have been reported to be useful, but there are no well-delineated guidelines for selecting one of these drugs.

Overall Treatment of the Patient

The schizophrenic patient is sensitive to change or instability in any aspect of his or her life. Whenever possible, one practitioner should provide continuous care so that that practitioner becomes a predictable resource for helping the patient to maintain his or her role in the community. Although few schizophrenic patients work full time (20% or less), they should be referred for vocational rehabilitation (see Chapter 9) or sheltered workshops when requested. Most patients determine their own levels of social activity, and it is fruitless to push them into unwanted activities. The clinician should be available to the patient's family or to foster care providers for periodic review of the patient's progress and expectations. The book *Surviving Schizophrenia* should be recommended to the patient's family (see "General References").

Recreational or social activities are enjoyed by some patients, but many do not care for them. Ideally, residential facilities are available when there is no family for the patient to live with or when the family is a harmful influence. However, in many communities such facilities do not exist. For some patients the clinician and the ambulatory center itself become the sources of the few social contacts that the patient has outside his or her home and inner psychologic world.

Regular office visits should be scheduled. Frequency of visits should be determined on the basis of the current status of the patient, history of the course of the patient's illness, reliability of the patient in taking medication, and the patient's ability to recognize early signs of onset of acute episodes. Office visits need last only 15 to 20 minutes and should include an interim history, a brief mental status examination, a review of the effectiveness of medications and of significant side effects, and provision of support or advice regarding the ways in which the patient is dealing with day-to-day matters. In other words, these office visits may be defined as supportive therapy, as described in Chapter 11.

In addition to individual office visits, *a family management approach* may be useful for patients who are having difficulties with their families (2). The method involves a two-step process:

1. Sessions devoted to educating the patient and family about the nature, course, and treatment of schizophrenia
2. Family sessions aimed at reducing existing family tensions and improving problem-solving skills of the family in coping with causes of stress (see "Family Counseling" in Chapter 11)

Management is enhanced if the clinician has ready access to social services, emergency mental health services, and psychiatric day-care and inpatient services. Social services, especially for financial support (e.g., welfare, food stamps, disability payments), are important in the treatment of schizophrenic patients because of their usual dependent status. Many acute episodes of psychosis are precipitated by threatened or actual withdrawal of welfare and disability payments.

The generalist caring for a schizophrenic patient may need psychiatric consultation for confirmation of the initial diagnosis, decisions regarding hospitalization, or treatment recommendations when symptoms respond poorly to antipsychotics or when side effects are intolerable.

Prognosis of the Treated Patient

Schizophrenia is a lifelong disease that requires an open-ended commitment by the clinician. The patient's life is disrupted by periodic psychosis, sometimes necessitating hospitalization, and by an arrest or deterioration of social function. Some patients are able to work and maintain satisfying interpersonal relationships. Many lead lonely, withdrawn, socially marginal existences. Psychopharmacologic treatment is effective for controlling the symptoms of acute psychosis and suppressing the intensity of psychotic symptoms over long periods. Suppression of psychosis may permit the patient to use his or her intellectual and social talents more effectively in developing and maintaining some role in the community. The new antipsychotics (Table 16.3) are reported to have a positive effect on the deterioration of social function that is so characteristic of schizophrenia.

General References*

American Psychiatric Association. **Diagnostic and Statistical Manual of Mental Disorders.** 4th ed. (DSM-IV). Washington, DC: American Psychiatric Association, 1994.
> Diagnostic criteria and epidemiologic information for all recognized psychiatric disorders.

Bleuler E. Dementia praecox or the group of schizophrenias. New York: International Universities Press, 1950.
> A classic work on schizophrenia.

Drugs for psychiatric disorders. Med Lett 33:43, 1991.
> Concise information on actions and side effects of all currently used antipsychotic drugs.

Practice guidelines for the treatment of patients with schizophrenia. Am J Psychiatry 154(4, Suppl), April 1997.
> A current, thorough review of the comprehensive treatment of schizophrenia, including treatment of neuroleptic-induced side effects.

---

*Bold print (general references) and bold numerals (specific references) denote published controlled clinical trials, meta-analyses, or consensus-based recommendations.

Torrey EF. Surviving schizophrenia: a family manual. New York: Harper & Row, 1995.

> A thorough book that contains invaluable information for families of schizophrenic patients and for physicians.

Specific References

1. Baldessarini RJ, Cohen BM, Teicher MH. Significance of neuroleptic dose and plasma level in the pharmacologic treatment of psychoses. Arch Gen Psychiatry 45:79–91, 1988.
2. Falloon IR, Boyd JL, McGill CW, et al. Family management in the prevention of exacerbation of schizophrenia. N Engl J Med 306:1437, 1982.
3. Hogarty GE, Goldberg SC, Schooler NR, Ulrich RF. Drug and sociotherapy in the aftercare of schizophrenic patients: two-year relapse rates. Arch Gen Psychiatry 31:603, 1974.
4. Lemkau PU, Tietze C, Cooper M. Survey of statistical studies on prevalence and incidence of mental disorder in sample population. Public Health Rep 58:1909, 1943.
5. Lipinski JF, Zubenko GS, Barreira P, et al. Propranolol in the treatment of neuroleptic-induced akathisia (Letter). Lancet 2:685, 1983.
6. Meltzer HY. Treatment of the neuroleptic-nonresponsive schizophrenic patient. Schizophr Bull 18(3):515–542, 1992.
7. Regier DA, Boyd JH, Burke JD, et al. One-month prevalence of mental disorders in the United States. Arch Gen Psychiatry 45:977, 1988.
8. Snyder SH. The dopamine hypothesis of schizophrenia: focus on the dopamine receptor. Am J Psychiatry 133:197, 1976.
9. Van Putten T. Why do schizophrenic patients refuse to take their drugs? Arch Gen Psychiatry 31:67, 1974.
10. Yassa R, Jeste DV. Gender differences in tardive dyskinesia: a critical review of the literature. Schizophr Bull 18(4):701–715, 1992.

C H A P T E R 17

Mental Illness in the Elderly: Principles and Common Problems

PETER V. RABINS, MD, MPH

Although overall rates of mental disorders are similar across the adult age span, the elderly are the least likely to seek help for mental illness. Those who do are most likely to receive treatment from a primary care provider during a routine medical visit (6).

GENERAL PRINCIPLES

Importance of Diagnosis

Making the correct diagnosis is a crucial first step in determining proper treatment. The most common mistakes made in assessing psychiatric symptoms in older patients are ascribing them to normal aging, confusing symptoms with syndromes, and not appreciating the frequent interaction between physical and psychiatric disorders. Asking the appropriate questions and attempting to elicit the classic signs and symptoms should lead to the correct diagnosis even when the presentation is unusual.

Relationship Between Physical and Mental States

Physical and psychiatric illnesses commonly coexist in the elderly. A prudent strategy when facing a patient with both physical and psychiatric complaints is to establish a differential diagnosis for each symptom before assuming that either the physical or the psychiatric disorder is primary. The two types of symptoms may be related in a number of ways.

Mental distress complicating a primary physical illness. Demoralization, anxiety, grief, irritability, and frustration are especially common in older patients with significant physical illness. These feelings usually begin after the onset of the physical illness, vary over time, and respond to the techniques for psychotherapy described in Chapter 11.

Physical complaints as the primary manifestation of psychiatric disorder. Particularly in older patients, focused complaints of physical ill health may be the most prominent or only sign of mental illness, especially depression. Although the physical complaint must be appropriately evaluated, a psychiatric cause should be suspected when the somatic complaint is bizarre, seems to be exaggerated, or has been evaluated without a cause being found, or when the patient has some symptoms of depression.

Psychiatric disorders arising from specific diseases. Cancer of the pancreas, hypothyroidism, and several structural brain diseases (stroke, Parkinson's disease, dementia) are commonly accompanied by a depression. Because the rates of depression are higher in these disorders than in arthritic or orthopedic conditions with similar levels of impairment, it is likely that the medical disorder is the cause of the depression or that the medical and psychiatric disorders share a common etiology. These depressions respond well to antidepressant treatment.

Psychiatric syndromes caused by medication and by substance abuse. Psychiatric syndromes can be precipitated by a variety of medications and by alcohol abuse. Corticosteroids, β-blockers, and other drugs that affect the adrenergic system can induce depressive symptoms. Anticholinergic compounds, dopaminergic agonist compounds, benzodiazepines, and H_2 blockers can induce delirium. Patients with dementia are more vulnerable to developing cognitive side effects from these compounds than are cognitively normal elderly people. Alcoholism, often hard to recognize in elderly patients, can also cause symptoms of depression and anxiety or cognitive defects (see Chapter 21). Abstinence can lead to resolution of the psychiatric symptoms.

Importance of Psychosocial Factors

Psychosocial factors are important to consider in patients of all ages. They become particularly important in the elderly because reduced physical mobility, isolation from family and friends, and financial limitations are more common and can directly interfere with the treatment of medical and psychiatric disorders. For elderly patients with mental illness, referring the patient to a social service agency or enlisting the help of the patient's family may be especially important in ensuring successful treatment and follow-through. Even when dementia is present, psychosocial interventions provide an important avenue for relieving morbidity.

Importance of Cognitive Assessment

Because dementia and delirium are common disorders of the elderly, it is important to be familiar with the assessment of cognitive function. The Mini-Mental

Table 17.1. Mini-Mental Status Examination: Instructions for Administration and Scoring[a]

The Test Takes 5 to 10 Minutes to Administer.

Orientation
1. Ask for year, season, date, day, month. Then ask specifically for parts omitted. One point for each correct. (0–5)
2. Ask in turn for name of state, county, town, hospital or place, floor or street. One point for each correct. (0–5)

Registration
Ask the patient whether you may test his or her memory. Then say the names of three unrelated objects, clearly and slowly, about 1 sec for each. After you have said all three, ask the patient to repeat them. This first repetition determines his or her score (0–3) but keep saying them until he or she can repeat all three up to six trials. If the patient does not eventually learn all three, recall cannot be meaningfully tested.

Attention and Calculation
Ask the patient to begin with 100 and count backward by 7. Stop after five subtractions (93, 86, 79, 72, 65). Score total number of correct answers, one point for each. (0–5)
If the patient cannot or will not perform this task, ask him or her to spell the word *world* backward. The score is the number of letters in correct order, e.g., dlrow = 5, dlrwo = 3. (0–5)

Recall
Ask the patient whether he or she can recall the three words you previously asked him or her to remember. (0–3)

Language
Naming: Show the patient a wrist watch and ask him or her what it is. Repeat for pencil. (0–2)
Repetition: Ask the patient to repeat this phrase after you: "No ifs, ands, or buts." Allow only one trial. (0 or 1)
Three-stage command: "Take a piece of paper in your right hand, fold it in half, and put it on the floor." Give the patient a piece of blank paper and repeat the command. Score 1 point for each part correctly executed. (0–3)
Reading: On a blank piece of paper print the sentence "Close your eyes," in letters large enough for the patient to see clearly. Ask him or her to read it and do what it says. Score 1 point only if the patient actually closes his or her eyes. (0–1)
Writing: Give the patient a blank piece of paper and ask him or her to write a sentence for you. Do not dictate a sentence; it is to be written spontaneously. It must contain a subject and verb and be sensible. Correct grammar and punctuation are not necessary. (0–1)
Copying: On a clean piece of paper, draw intersecting pentagons, each side about 1 inch, and ask him or her to copy it exactly as it is. All 10 angles must be present and 2 must intersect to score 1 point. Tremor and rotation are ignored. (0–1)
Estimate the patient's level of sensorium along a continuum, from alert on the left to coma on the right.

From Folstein MF, Folstein SE, McHugh PR. "Mini-mental state": a practical method for grading the cognitive state of patients for the clinician. J Psychiatr Res 12:189, 1975.

[a]Total possible score is 30 points. Patients with a total of 23 points or less are highly likely to have a cognitive disorder.

Status Examination delineated in Table 17.1 is a reliable, brief, standardized screening tool. It can be useful in following patients over time. It may be normal in initial evaluation of mildly demented patients.

SPECIFIC PSYCHOGERIATRIC DISORDERS

Psychiatric disorders in older patients may present with the classic symptoms described in other chapters of this book. The following pages focus on several syndromes that are particularly important in the elderly.

Depression

Depressive Symptoms

Symptoms of depression and sadness become more common in late life even though the syndrome of major depression is less common in the elderly. This dissociation may be caused by both the criteria used to make diagnoses and intrinsic differences between the young and old. The *Diagnostic and Statistical Manual of Mental Disorders,* 4th edition (DSM-IV), divides mood disorder into several categories (see Chapter 15). The differences among them depend on both symptom clustering and course. The presentation of these disorders in older patients may differ from the presentation in younger patients in several ways.

An adjustment disorder with depressed mood is characterized by sad or low mood that follows, within 3 months, a clearly identifiable stressor or precipitant. In elderly patients stressors such as those listed above ("Importance of Psychosocial Factors") are particularly common. The approaches to office psychotherapy described in Chapter 11 are fully applicable to elderly patients with adjustment disorders.

A dysthymic disorder, conversely, is characterized by the presence of depressive symptoms for more than 2 years. Mood often fluctuates widely but in no discernible pattern. The patient may experience hours, days, or weeks of improved mood, mixed with prolonged periods of unhappiness. In the elderly, a dysthymic disorder should be considered when the patient reports chronic depressive symptoms throughout his or her life and denies the cyclicity and periods of normal mood found in recurrent depressive or bipolar disorder (see Chapter 15). It may require specialty referral because of its chronicity.

Major Depression

The diagnostic criteria of the major affective disorders and their treatment, as described in Chapter 15, are generally applicable to the elderly. Hypochondriacal features, agitation, and suspiciousness or frank paranoia often accompany depression in the elderly and are common sources of diagnostic confusion. A recent study demonstrates that the elderly with major depressive disorder are less likely to report being sad than the young (5). Therefore, denial of sadness does *not* rule out the diagnosis of major depression.

Elderly patients with a hypochondriacal focus usually deny that their mood is sad but focus on physical symptoms for which there is minimal or no evidence of abnormality on physical examination or laboratory assessment. Depressed hypochondriacal patients often have changes in their vital sense ("something is wrong with me") and a negative self-attitude ("I've done something to deserve this or cause this"). Therefore, the patient should be asked specifically about these cardinal features of major depression when hypochondriasis is present.

Because suspiciousness and paranoia are common in depressed elderly patients, other evidence for a major depression should be sought when these symptoms are present. When paranoia and depression coexist, depression is most commonly the primary disorder.

As in younger patients, major depression in the elderly often requires pharmacotherapy or electroconvulsive therapy (ECT). Practical details about these modes of treatment are given in Chapter 15. Tricyclic antidepressants with the most pronounced anticholinergic properties (e.g., amitriptyline and doxepin) should be avoided. The tricyclics with the highest likelihood of causing orthostatic hypotension (e.g., amitriptyline and imipramine) should also be avoided or closely monitored because elderly patients are at higher risk of falls and are more likely to be receiving antihypertensive drugs or other compounds that also can cause orthostasis. Nortriptyline and desipramine are the tricyclic agents that are least likely to cause these side effects. A usual starting dosage in the otherwise healthy elderly person is 10 to 25 mg at bedtime; however, a dosage of 10 mg should be prescribed in the frail elderly or in patients with the potential for medical complications from the drugs. Fluoxetine (Prozac), sertraline (Zoloft), and paroxetine (Paxil) are nontricyclic antidepressants and are usually the agents of first choice for older patients. The long half-life of fluoxetine suggests that it should be used in lower dosages in the elderly than in young patients. Fluoxetine should be started at a dosage of 10 mg in the morning. The maximum dosage is 40 to 60 mg. Sertraline should be started at a dosage of 25 to 50 mg in the morning; 200 mg is the maximum dosage. Paroxetine should be started at a dosage of 10 mg in the morning; 30 mg is the maximum dosage.

ECT is sometimes safer than pharmacotherapy for older patients with cardiac disease. It is equally effective in all age groups (see details regarding ECT, Chapter 15, "Affective Disorders"). Low-dose neuroleptic drugs (see Table 16.3) are indicated when *delusions* complicate depression, especially when the suspiciousness is significantly interfering with the patient's function, is life threatening (e.g., the patient will not eat because he or she believes that the food is poisoned), or causes distress for the patient or those close to him or her.

Depression-Induced Cognitive Impairment

Patients with the onset of depression in late life can present with the belief that they are becoming demented. Some depressed patients perform poorly on routine tests of cognitive function. Previously this condition was called "*pseudodementia,*" but this term has fallen into disfavor because patients with this syndrome perform in the demented range in standardized tests of cognitive function and because up to 50% of these patients eventually develop a progressive dementing illness (2). Nonetheless, recognition of the syndrome is important because both the mood disorder and cognitive function can improve with antidepressant treatment. Depression-induced cognitive impairment should be considered when the onset of cognitive impairment has been subacute (less than 6 months and particularly less than 3 months),when the history of an episode of depression earlier in life is elicited, when a dementia is complicated by hypochondriacal or bizarre delusions (9), when the patient constantly emphasizes his or her cognitive disability (a behavior that is uncommon in Alzheimer's disease), or when a cognitively impaired patient reports early morning awakening, lack of energy, self-blame, or guilt. At times it is difficult to distinguish whether the patient has a primary dementing illness with secondary depression or primary depression with reversible dementia. In such cases a therapeutic trial of an antidepressant (e.g., at least 4 weeks at a therapeutic dosage, as described in Chapter 15) may be the best way to determine which disorder is primary.

Depression Coexisting with Brain Disease

Major depression may complicate primarily organic disorders of the central nervous system. Stroke, Parkinson's disease, and Alzheimer's disease are three common late-life disorders in which major depressive symptoms occur in 20 to 50% of patients (12). The importance of recognizing these as coexisting disorders is that the physical disorder and the psychiatric disorder may both need to be treated if either problem is to improve. For example, depression has been shown to interfere directly with rehabilitation from *stroke.* Thus, the treatment of depression after stroke improves the degree of recovery from the stroke; at the same time, gains from rehabilitation improve the patient's morale and mood (see details in Chapter 83). In *Parkinson's disease,* depressive symptoms and parkinsonian symptoms (e.g., psychomotor retardation) often overlap, and it can be difficult to determine which disorder is causing specific symptoms. In planning treatment, it is best to focus on the depressive or parkinsonian symptoms separately and to treat first the disorder that is causing the worst impairment in function. The treatment of Parkinson's disease is described in Chapter 82. The treatment of depression in patients with *Alzheimer's disease* or multi-infarct dementia can improve cognitive performance, behavior, and mood, although some cognitive impairment will persist.

Paranoia and Suspiciousness

Suspiciousness is more common among the elderly than in younger people. This becomes clinically relevant when the suspiciousness interferes with the patient's life. Several types of disorders can present with suspiciousness.

Suspiciousness as an Isolated Symptom

Some elderly people become more suspicious as they age but have no accompanying signs or symptoms of other mental illness. It is important to determine whether there is a basis for the patient's suspiciousness because financial abuse of the elderly is not uncommon and concerns about the environment being unsafe can

be appropriate. An understandable reaction to difficult circumstances should not be assumed, however, and a review of symptoms that explore other psychiatric conditions is necessary.

Suspiciousness Complicating Depression

As noted above, suspiciousness occurs in some elderly patients with major depression. Depression should be considered primary if the person feels deserving of persecution or punishment or has changes in vital sense and other manifestations of depression (see Chapter 15).

Late-Life Schizophrenia or Paraphrenia

Older patients occasionally develop a syndrome similar to schizophrenia in young people (see Chapter 16). Such patients have *delusions* (fixed, false, idiosyncratic ideas) and *auditory* or *visual hallucinations,* and lack symptoms of depression or cognitive impairment.

The treatment of late-life schizophrenia and paranoia is similar to that for younger patients (see Chapter 16) except that significantly lower dosages of neuroleptic drugs are effective. Although no single neuroleptic is more efficacious than another, those likely to induce orthostatic hypotension, such as chlorpromazine (Thorazine), or with high anticholinergic effects, such as thioridazine (Mellaril), are less desirable, especially if the patient is taking an antidepressant that also has anticholinergic properties. A starting dosage of 0.5 mg of risperidone (Risperdal) two to three times daily or 0.5 to 2 mg daily, or thiothixene (Navane) 1 mg at bedtime (may be increased to 2 mg twice daily) is recommended. Thiothixene is significantly less expensive than risperidone. Of these drugs, risperidone is least likely to cause parkinsonian side effects or orthostasis at low dosages. Because old age is a risk factor for developing tardive dyskinesia, an attempt should be made to discontinue neuroleptic treatment after the patient has stabilized. Chapter 16 describes the use of neuroleptic drugs in detail.

Paranoia and Persecutory Delusions as Symptoms of an Organic Disease

Paranoia can be symptomatic of a focal brain disease (e.g., tumor or stroke), a diffuse brain disease such as Alzheimer's disease (3), a systemic condition such as a metabolic disorder (e.g., hyperthyroidism or hypoparathyroidism), or psychoactive substance abuse. Any patient with a persistent suspicious belief should have a clinical assessment for evidence that supports the presence of one of these causes.

Aging-Associated Cognitive Decline

Some older patients complain of memory loss or slower rate of processing information, or members of their families notice these phenomena, but a history from both the patient and family reveals no social or occupational dysfunction and screening cognitive tests reveal no abnormality. It appears that fewer than 20% of these patients develop a dementia (4). Those unlikely to have a dementia complain of such things as misplacing keys or having more difficulty remembering names or words than they once did; on questioning they acknowledge that names and words often come to them minutes later and that they have not forgotten important engagements or events. Patients who are especially concerned about memory difficulties and report a decline in function in social, personal, or occupational realms should be referred to a neuropsychologist for *formal neuropsychologic evaluation* to better formulate the problem. Careful attention should be given to the medical status of such patients because they could have a subclinical delirium (see below). When no dysfunction is identified and objective testing makes a progressive dementia unlikely, reassurance and an agreement to reassess the patient in 6 months may help relieve the anxiety associated with this condition.

Patient Experience. Formal neuropsychologic testing consists of a several-hour battery of pencil-and-paper tests that examine the following cognitive domains: memory, perception, judgment, and language. A formal report to the referring physician compares the patient's performance with that of age-matched normals. The results either support one in reassuring a patient or can guide referral of the patient for further evaluation.

Dementia

Definition and Epidemiology

Dementia is characterized by a decline in cognitive abilities from a previous level, a decline that is generalized or global and not isolated to one cognitive function such as memory (i.e., amnesia) or language (i.e., aphasia), and the presence of clear consciousness. Dementia can have many etiologies, but fewer than 2% of affected patients have dementia from a reversible etiology.

Moderate to severe dementia affects approximately 5% of people over 65. However, most dementia occurs among the very old; the prevalence is 20% in people 80 and older, and approximately 30% in people over 90. These prevalence rates have been found in numerous European, North American, and Japanese prevalence studies.

Etiologic Evaluation

The assessment of a person with complaints of cognitive decline has three purposes. The first purpose is to identify the probable cause of the dementia, including the identification of treatable disorders. The three most common causes of treatable dementia in elderly patients are medication toxicity, depression, and thyroid disease. In younger patients, acquired immunodeficiency syndrome (AIDS) dementia is now an important cause (see Chapter 34). Commonly used medications that have been associated with global cognitive impairment are the benzodiazepines (most common), H_2 blockers, and anticholinergic drugs. The second purpose of assessment is to identify treatable symptoms and comorbidity in the patient.

Because few patients have a truly reversible dementia, the treatment of medical and behavioral comorbidity is the main focus of both the assessment and the treatment of almost all patients in the ambulatory setting. The third purpose is to identify issues in the caregiver and environment that are amenable to intervention.

The first step in the etiologic evaluation of dementia is *to search for treatable causes,* beginning with the history, physical examination, mental status examination (Table 17.1), and a number of screening tests.

Clinical Characteristics. In considering possible etiologies, it is useful to *determine whether the dementia has the clinical characteristics of subcortical or cortical dementia.* Most treatable dementias present as subcortical dementias. *Subcortical dementias* are characterized by memory loss, apathy, slowness, and movement disorder with intact language (i.e., the patient is able to name objects, repeat a phrase, and follow the three-step command; see Table 17.1) and normal visuospatial function (i.e., the patient is able to copy the diagram on the Mini-Mental Status Examination). Causes of subcortical dementia include hypothyroidism, Parkinson's disease, multiple sclerosis, normal pressure hydrocephalus, the dementia syndrome of depression, and most instances vascular dementia. The *cortical dementias* are characterized by memory loss plus multiple defects in higher cortical functions: *aphasic language* (making paraphasic errors such as substituting a letter, as in *tee* instead of *tie,* or saying an incorrect word, such as *paper* instead of *pencil*), *apraxia* (inability to perform skilled movements such as showing how to drink with a cup on command), or *agnosia* (inability to recognize common objects or sensory stimuli). Alzheimer's disease is the most common cortical dementia, but frontal dementias, Lewy body dementia, and rare dementias such as Creutzfeldt–Jakob disease are included in this category.

Screening Tests. The Agency for Health Care Policy and Research (AHCPR) 1996 Consensus Statement on the differential diagnosis of dementia suggests the following inexpensive screening tests, each targeted at potentially treatable causes, for all patients: complete blood count (CBC), serum electrolyte levels, creatinine clearance, liver function tests, calcium and phosphate concentrations, thyroid-stimulating hormone (TSH), vitamin B_{12} level, and serologic tests for syphilis (1). Imaging of the brain is listed as optional. It is reasonable to obtain a noncontrast computerized tomography (CT) study on all patients with symptoms 2 years or less in duration, onset before age 70, or focal findings on neurologic examination. A CT or magnetic resonance imaging (MRI) scan can identify focal lesions such as a tumor, subdural hematoma, or abscess; demonstrate findings compatible with hydrocephalus; or provide confirmatory evidence for vascular etiology of the dementia. However, it is impossible to diagnose Alzheimer's disease solely by any imaging study. Likewise, overreliance on CT or MRI scan reports of "white matter hyperintensities" has led to an overdiagnosis of vascular dementia. A 1997 consensus statement issued by multiple organizations concurs with the AHCPR recommendations (see "General References").

Alzheimer's disease is diagnosed by inclusion and exclusion criteria. The diagnosis should be made when other specific causes of dementia, including vascular disease, have been excluded, when the condition has been slowly progressive, and when the cognitive disorder includes language impairment, apraxia, or agnosia in addition to memory impairment.

Vascular dementia should be diagnosed when the history suggests distinct episodes of worsening (a stair-step course), when evidence of vascular disease and hypertension are present on examination, and when the neurologic examination reveals asymmetries in reflexes, strength, or sensation.

The *frontal dementias* are a group of slowly progressive diseases that present with pronounced changes in behavior and personality. They are neuropathologically heterogeneous. On CT scanning, they show disproportionate frontal atrophy.

Lewy body dementia presents in a fashion similar to Alzheimer's disease but extrapyramidal symptoms (rigidity and parkinsonian tremor), hallucinations, and delusions are present early in the course. Neuroleptic medications should be avoided, if possible, because they can cause marked worsening of the parkinsonian symptoms.

Management

The management of irreversible dementia can be divided into six aspects:

1. *The assessment process.* This is the first step in management. The diagnosis has often been suspected by the family or patient, but at times abnormal behavior has been misinterpreted as purposefully irritating. As specific a diagnosis as possible should be made and conveyed to the family. The family may ask about long-term prognosis. The average patient with Alzheimer's disease lives 7 to 10 years after early symptoms, but life span while demented can be as long as 20 years. In general, a dementia that has progressed slowly will continue to do so, whereas a history of rapid progression predicts rapid decline. Although the patient has the right to know his or her diagnosis, many lack the ability to realize that they have a deficit. Patients who, when asked, deny that they have any problems with their memory usually do not accept that there is a problem when told directly. Some patients, and most families, experience a measure of relief when it is pointed out that the patient's dementia is a medical problem and not just part of getting older or becoming intentionally stubborn.

The evaluation process should elicit specific *problems in behavior caused by the dementia* (see commonly cited problems, Table 17.2). Difficulty in speaking, dressing, and performing potentially dangerous activities as driving, smoking, and cooking should be inquired about. When present, these problems should be explained as the result of the illness. The family or other caregivers should then try to adapt the environment to the disordered behaviors and should

Table 17.2. Behavior Problems of Patients and Problematic Activities of Daily Living Cited by Families of Demented Patients[a]

Behavior	Percentage of Families Reporting Occurrence	Percentage of Families Reporting Behavior as a Problem
Memory disturbance[b]	100	93
Catastrophic reactions[b,c]	87	89
Demanding/critical behavior	71	73
Night walking	69	59
Hiding things	69	71
Communication difficulties	68	74
Suspiciousness[b]	63	79
Making accusations[b]	60	82
Difficulty eating meals	60	55
Daytime wandering	59	70
Difficulty bathing	53	74
Hallucinations	49	42
Delusions	47	83
Physical violence	47	94
Incontinence[b]	40	86
Difficulty cooking	33	44
Hitting[b]	32	81
Impaired driving	20	73
Smoking	11	67
Inappropriate sexual behavior	2	0

Adapted from Rabins PV, Mace NL, Lucas MJ. The impact of dementia on the family. JAMA 248:333, 1982.

[a]Based on an open-ended interview with the primary caregivers of 55 patients with irreversible dementia.

[b]Cited as most serious problem.

[c]See example in text.

take steps to eliminate dangerous behaviors. Helping caregivers to specifically identify each problem can enable them to institute common-sense solutions they have not otherwise tried. In regard to the patient who continues to drive, the physician should instruct the patient to stop driving rather than asking a family member to do so. Most states require periodic relicensure for older people and some even require physicians to report all patients with dementia. Because these regulations can be helpful, it is important to be aware of them in one's state.

Families needing legal and financial advice should be advised to seek this out early and not wait for a crisis. Guidelines for assessing competence or for obtaining legal guardianship are described in Chapter 10.

2. *Good general medical care.* Congestive heart failure, urinary tract infection, and seemingly minor medical abnormalities can lead to marked deterioration of the demented patient's functioning. Likewise, patients taking drugs that can affect cognition (e.g., cimetidine, β-blockers, benzodiazepines, methyldopa, digoxin, anticholinergics) should be carefully monitored, and all unnecessary medication should be discontinued. A search for superimposed medical illness should be instituted if there is a sudden deterioration in behavior, cognition, or functional ability. Correction of coexisting medical conditions has been shown to improve functioning in demented patients.

3. *Environmental changes, behavioral management, and treatment of depression.* Not sleeping at night,

suspiciousness, easy irritability, and catastrophic reactions (see below) can be more problematic than cognitive impairment. Nonpharmacologic environmental approaches should be tried first. For insomnia these include keeping the person more active in the daytime (day-care centers are a significant help in this regard) and not letting the patient nap during the day. Irritability, suspiciousness, and frustration are usually best managed by eliminating tasks that the patient can no longer do and avoiding situations that frustrate the patient. It is prudent to have the demented patient wear a medical alert bracelet that describes his or her condition.

Neuroleptic (antipsychotic) medications should be used only when other approaches have failed and a specific target symptom (hallucinations, delusions, aggression) is present that presents a danger to the patient or others or is very distressing to the patient. Importantly, these drugs are not indicated for controlling wandering or swearing. The usual dosages for these drugs are listed above (see "Late-Life Schizophrenia or Paraphrenia"). After target symptoms have been controlled for several months, the dosage can often be lowered, and drugs can be discontinued in about one-fourth of patients. Patients taking these drugs must be monitored for two common side effects, orthostatic hypotension and extrapyramidal symptoms (see details in Chapter 16). If only insomnia is a problem, chloral hydrate, 500 to 1000 mg, causes the least paradoxical agitation and the least daytime drowsiness.

Aggressive behavior may be treated with neuroleptic drugs. If these do not control aggressiveness, small dosages of divalproex sodium (Depakote) may be effective. The starting dosage is one 125-mg pill or sprinkles daily, cautiously increased to 250 mg twice daily. Dosage should be adjusted based on clinical response and blood levels. Even at these dosages ataxia may occur and limit its use.

Depression is present in at least 20% of patients with dementia (3). When it has the characteristics of an adjustment disorder or demoralized state (see above), it is best managed with supportive therapy (see Chapter 11). However, major depressions with symptoms of early morning awakening, anorexia, self-blame, worthlessness, nihilistic attitudes, or morbid hypochondriasis also occur. Their treatment is discussed under organic depression, above.

In a *catastrophic reaction,* demented patients with at least partial insight into their disability may become profoundly distressed when brought into a situation in which they are forced to confront their failing aptitudes. Often an overwhelming sense of frustration, fear, anger, or anxiety ensues. These poorly controlled emotions further impair the patient's already limited functional ability, leading to total decompensation of a previously coping patient.

EXAMPLE

A 72-year-old woman with a history of several small strokes experienced moderate forgetfulness and confusion but was generally calm and pleasant. Keeping track of the date with a calendar and making copious notes to herself, she managed to maintain an independent existence at home. At the supermarket checkout counter she could not find her wallet but insisted she had money to pay for her food. The clerk grew impatient, and the patient became increasingly agitated, tearful, and accusatory. When the store manager was called, she picked up grocery items and began throwing them.

These catastrophic reactions can have an adverse impact on both the patient and the patient's family. The explanation of their cause and their prevention through avoidance of provoking circumstances can forestall the need for institutionalization. The use of small dosages of a neuroleptic (see "Late-Life Schizophrenia or Paraphrenia," above) may be beneficial in patients in whom episodes like this recur despite the caregiver's best efforts.

4. *Family support.* Family distress is common. Treating it starts with the assessment and problem-solving approach outlined above. The latter gives families a sense of control and the hope that most problems can be managed despite the irreversibility and probable progression of the underlying disorder. Feelings of guilt, anger, discouragement, and demoralization are common, as are concerns about loss of friends, hobbies, and leisure time; family conflicts; and worry that the principal caregiver will become ill. Allowing families time to express these feelings and concerns and acknowledging that they are common can be helpful. Referring them to support groups can also be helpful. There is evidence from one controlled trial that a combination of counseling that addresses caregivers' needs and support group participation can delay the need for nursing home placement of demented patients, in this study for an average of 329 days (8).

The *Alzheimer's Disease Association* can provide information about nearby resources and has a toll-free telephone number (1-800-621-0379). It is also helpful to recommend a book such as *The 36-Hour Day* (see "General References"), which explains dementia and offers practical advice for dealing with the vexing problems created by a demented family member.

5. *Longitudinal care.* Because the dementing illnesses are progressive (new symptoms appear while old symptoms worsen), expected changes should be described to families. It is also prudent to discuss the possibility of eventual nursing home placement soon after the diagnosis is made. Although most families report that they do not want to place their loved one in a nursing home, it is important to urge them not to promise this unconditionally because medical issues or behavioral problems may develop to the point where placement is necessary. The family's emotional needs may change over time. Here again, a nonjudgmental, listening approach helps family members to feel supported.

6. *Decisions about limiting therapy.* Chapter 6, "Geriatric Medicine," describes the processes whereby patients and their families may plan in advance the limitation of therapy (living wills and other forms of advance directives) and the delegation of decision

making to others. These processes are especially important in planning the care of a demented patient early in the patient's course of dementia.

Drugs for Dementia

Donepezil (Aricept), a cholinesterase inhibitor, has been approved for the treatment of cognitive impairment in patients with Alzheimer's disease. Its effectiveness is modest (about 6 months improvement in some measures of cognitive function on average). The starting dosage is 5 mg at bedtime. If no side effects develop it should be increased to 10 mg at bedtime in 4 to 6 weeks (10). The advantages of donepezil over the previously released cholinesterase inhibitor tacrine (Cognex) are that it has not been associated with hepatic toxicity and can be taken once instead of four times a day.

As discussed above, neuroleptic drugs can be prescribed empirically for delusions, hallucinations, aggression, and agitation. They are 19% more effective than placebo for aggression but few studies support their efficacy for other symptoms (11).

Delirium

Definition and Diagnosis

The essential features of delirium are cognitive impairment, clouding of consciousness, and difficulty sustaining and shifting attention. Delirious patients may appear drowsy or hyperalert (hypervigilant), trail off in the middle of sentences, fail to answer questions or ask that questions be repeated, or appear perplexed. Perceptual disturbances such as illusions (misinterpretations of real external stimuli) or hallucinations are common. Delirium usually has rapid onset, brief duration, and marked fluctuation throughout the day. Delirium is especially common in patients with dementia. Both demented and delirious patients may experience memory impairment, disorientation, hallucinations, delusions, and disturbed thinking. However, the demented patient is alert, whereas the delirious patient is drowsy and waxes and wanes over minutes or hours. The abrupt onset of delirium (within hours or days) differs from dementia, which develops over months or years in most instances.

The presence of cognitive impairment and rapid fluctuation distinguishes delirium from schizophrenia and other psychotic disorders. The hallucinations and delusions associated with delirium are often fleeting and poorly systematized in comparison with those of other psychotic disorders, in which they are sustained and well organized. The electroencephalogram (EEG) in the delirious patient often reveals a generalized slowing of background activity, whereas the EEG is generally normal in schizophrenic and depressed patients.

In some patients, the manifestations of delirium may be so subtle that they are not recognized by an examiner who is unfamiliar with the patient's baseline status. At other times the symptoms suggest depression, dementia, or schizophrenia. The elderly are especially prone

to delirium as a result of medical illness and drug intoxication (7).

The key to accurate diagnosis of delirium is a high index of suspicion in any elderly patient with a history of recent or sudden change in mental status and behavior. The EEG shows diffuse slowing in both delirium and dementia. In delirium, the EEG slowing is often marked, even when the cognitive and behavioral impairment is minor; conversely, severe cognitive impairment and a mildly abnormal EEG are most common in dementia.

Etiologic Evaluation

Delirium can result from a wide range of organic causes that adversely affect the brain metabolism (Table 17.3). Special attention should be given to medications in the elderly because they may produce a delirium at therapeutic dosages. β-Blockers, H_2 blockers, benzodiazepines, and the many compounds with anticholinergic activity are common causes of delirium. Although electrolyte disturbances are the most common metabolic cause of delirium, any disorder of metabolic homeostasis can cause delirium. Withdrawal from alcohol or sedatives is often overlooked in

Table 17.3. Etiologic Classification of Delirium

In a Medical or Surgical Illness (No Focal or Lateralizing Neurologic Signs; Cerebrospinal Fluid Usually Clear)
Metabolic disorders: hepatic stupor, uremia, hypoxia, hypercapnia, hypoglycemia, porphyria, hyponatremia
Congestive heart failure
Pneumonia, septicemia, typhoid fever, other febrile illnesses (especially in elderly)
Hyperthyroidism and hypothyroidism
Postoperative and posttraumatic states

In Neurologic Disease that Causes Focal or Lateralizing Signs or Changes in the Cerebrospinal Fluid
Cerebrovascular disease
Subarachnoid hemorrhage
Hypertensive encephalopathy
Cerebral contusion
Subdural hematoma
Tumor
Abscess
Meningitis
Encephalitis
Status epilepticus (by EEG)
Postconvulsive delirium

The Abstinence States and Exogenous Intoxications (Signs of Other Medical, Surgical and Neurologic Illnesses Absent or Coincidental)
Withdrawal of alcohol (delirium tremens), barbiturates, and nonbarbiturate sedative drugs, following chronic intoxication
Drug intoxication from benzodiazepines, opiates, neuroleptics, antidepressants, antihistamines, H_2 blockers, centrally acting antihypertensives, anticholinergics, digitalis, illicit drugs (see Chapter 22), etc.

Beclouded Dementia
Any dementing or other brain disease in combination with infective fevers, drug reactions, heart failure, or other medical or surgical disease

Adapted from Adams RD. Delirium and other acute confusional states. In: Isselbacher KJ et al, eds. Harrison's principles of internal medicine. 9th ed. New York: McGraw-Hill, 1980.

the elderly as a possible cause of delirium. Multiple causes are suspected and no one specific cause is identified in 30 to 50% of cases. When there is no obvious cause for a patient's apparent delirium, an EEG may be helpful in confirming that delirium is present.

The key to treatment is the identification of the underlying causes when they can be identified. The physical, neurologic, and laboratory examination should focus on causes that are likely in a particular patient. Attention to nutrition, fluid intake, and electrolyte balance is crucial.

The treatment of the behavioral and emotional complications of delirium can become as urgent as the identification of the underlying cause. Frequent reorientation and reassurance, a well-lighted environment, and avoidance of overstimulation are important aspects of treatment. If the agitation, hallucinations, or delusions do not respond to environmental intervention and are overwhelming to the patient or adversely affecting the patient's safety, then a low-dosage neuroleptic given by mouth or intramuscularly (e.g., haloperidol, 0.5 to 1.0 mg every 4 hours) can be ordered.

General References*

Alzheimer's Association telephone number: 800-272-3900; website: http://www.ALZ.ORG.
> A resource for professionals and families.

Blazer DG. Depression in late life. 2nd ed. St. Louis: CV Mosby, 1993.
> Helpful overview of all aspects of this problem.

Cummings JL, Benson DF. Dementia: a clinical approach. Boston: Butterworth-Heinemann, 1992.
> An excellent overview for the clinician.

LaRue A. Aging and neuropsychological assessment. New York: Plenum, 1992.
> A readable introduction to geriatric neuropsychology.

---

*Bold print (general references) and bold numerals (specific references) denote published controlled clinical trials, meta-analyses, or consensus-based recommendations.

Mace NL, Rabins PV. The 36-hour day. New York: Warner, 1991.
> A book that provides detailed practical information for caregiver of persons with dementia. Available in most bookstores for the general public.

Small GW, Rabins PV, Barry PP, et al. **Diagnosis and treatment of Alzheimer disease and related disorders: consensus statement of the American Association for Geriatric Psychiatry, the Alzheimer's Association, and the American Geriatrics Society.** JAMA 278(6):1363–1371, 1997.
> Well-referenced report that addresses all aspects of dementia.

Specific References

1. Agency for Health Care Policy and Research. Recognition and initial assessment of Alzheimer's disease and related dementias. AHCPR Publication No. 97-0702, 1996.
2. Alexopoulos GS, Meyers BS, Young RC, et al. The course of geriatric depression with "reversible dementia": a controlled study. Am J Psychiatry 150:1693–1699, 1993.
3. Burns A, Jacoby R, Levy R. Psychiatric phenomena in Alzheimer's disease: III. Disorders of mood. Br J Psychiatry 157:81, 1990.
4. Caine ED. Amnestic disorders. J Neuropsychiatry 5:6, 1993.
5. Gallo HH, Rabins PV, Lyketsos CG, et al. Depression without sadness: functional outcomes of nondysphoric depression in later life. J Am Geriatr Soc 45:1–9, 1997.
6. Kramer M, German PS, Anthony JC, et al. Patterns of mental disorders among the elderly residents of eastern Baltimore. J Am Geriatr Soc 33:236, 1985.
7. Lipowski ZJ. Delirium in the elderly patient. N Engl J Med 320:578, 1989.
8. Mittelman MS, Ferris SH, Shulman E, et al. A family intervention to delay nursing home placement of patients with Alzheimer disease. JAMA 276(21):1725–1731, 1996.
9. Rabins PV, Merchant A, Nestadt G. Criteria for diagnosing reversible dementia caused by depression: validation by two-year follow-up. Br J Psychiatry 144:488, 1984.
10. Rogers SL, Friedhoff LT. The efficacy and safety of donepezil in patients with Alzheimer's disease: results of a US multicentre, randomized, double-blind, placebo-controlled trial. Dementia 7:293–303, 1996.
11. Schneider LS, Pollock VE, Lyness SA. A meta-analysis of controlled trials of neuroleptic treatment in dementia. J Am Geriatr Soc 28:553, 1990.
12. Starkstein SE, Robinson RG, Price TR. Comparison of patients with and without post-stroke major depression matched for size and location of lesions. Arch Gen Psychiatry 45:247, 1988.

CHAPTER 18

Sexual Disorders

CHESTER W. SCHMIDT, JR, MD

The sexual difficulties described by patients to their physicians are evenly divided into sexual problems that accompany physical illness, those that are secondary to side effects of medication or abuse of drugs, and those that are unrelated to physical problems and are purely psychologic in origin. Typically the psychologically based sexual problems are related to both psychosocial antecedents and current stressful life situations, which are often self-limited. Problems related to medical or psychologic conditions that are reversible or are expected to resolve lend themselves to treatment by counseling techniques that rely heavily on catharsis, reassurance, and education (see Chapter 11, "Psychotherapy in Ambulatory Practice"). Although data documenting results of treatment for these types of problems in the ambulatory setting are limited, clinical experience suggests that the outcome for sexual problems related to reversible conditions is usually good, with improvement rates approaching 75%.

NORMAL SEXUAL RESPONSE CYCLE

To assess these disorders rapidly and accurately, it is helpful to be familiar with the normal sexual response cycle and the major physiologic factors that mediate each phase of the cycle. The human sexual response cycle is divided into four phases.

The *first phase is one of desire* and consists of fantasies and wishes to engage in sexual activity. This response is psychic in origin, but the psychic stimulation is mediated, at least in men, by circulating androgens.

The *second phase is the arousal phase* and consists of a number of physiologic changes plus the subjective sense of sexual pleasure. In both sexes there is an increase in heart rate, an increase in breathing rate, and development of muscular tension throughout the body, most pronounced in the pelvic area and thighs. For both sexes the major physiologic change is the development of vascular congestion in the genital area. For females, the manifestations of vasocongestion are vaginal lubrication and swelling of the external genitalia. In males, vasocongestion leads to erection. Vasocongestion may occur via either of two neurologic pathways. *(a)* A local reflex pathway is initiated by tactile stimulation of the penis or clitoris and mediated by sensory fibers entering the dorsal root ganglia at S2 through S4 and by parasympathetic fibers from these ganglia to the perivesicular, prostatic, and cavernous plexuses; postganglionic fibers from these plexuses go to the blood vessels of the corpora cavernosa. *(b)* A cortical pathway is initiated by psychic stimuli and mediated by parasympathetic and sympathetic fibers that originate at the T12–L1 level of the spinal cord. Each of these pathways promotes rapid inflow and retention of blood in the penis and the vulva.

The presence of these two spinal centers governing erection has important clinical implications. Patients with complete cord transections above the sacral center but below the thoracic center may still be capable of psychogenic erections mediated by impulses descending from higher centers and exiting the cord at T12–L1. With a cord lesion above both spinal centers, psychogenically produced erections are blocked, but the patient may still be capable of reflexogenic erections from direct tactile stimulation of the penis or clitoris even though he or she is unable to experience the sensation.

In addition to neurologic pathways, erection in the male depends on intact arterial blood flow from the right and left internal pudendal arteries.

The *third phase is orgasm.* Subjectively, for both sexes orgasm is a peaking of sexual pleasure accompanied by a sense of release from sexual tension. Physiologically in the male, the most obvious manifestation of orgasm is ejaculation. Ejaculation is mediated by the sympathetic nervous system and consists of two processes: emission, resulting from contraction of the vas deferens, prostate, and seminal vesicles; and actual ejaculation, resulting from rhythmic contraction of the muscles of the pelvic floor and from closure of the internal sphincters of the bladder (preventing retrograde ejaculation). In the female, the rhythmic contractions take place within the musculature of the outer third of the vagina and in the perineal muscles. The subjective component of orgasm is a cortical sensory phenomenon, purely psychic in origin; it can occur without ejaculation or bladder neck closure.

The fourth phase is called resolution, which subjectively is accompanied by a sense of pleasure, warmth, well-being, and relaxation. Physiologically there is a gradual return of heart rate, breathing rate, and muscle tension to the baseline state. Most males are refractory to entering another cycle of sexual activity for some time (minutes in younger men and an hour or longer in middle-aged and older men). Women are not subject to this refractory period and may have multiple orgasms following continued or additional stimulation.

COMMON SEXUAL DISORDERS

The nomenclature and criteria used to classify sexual disorders in this chapter are based on the American Psychiatric Association *Diagnostic and Statistical Manual of Mental Disorders,* 4th edition (DSM-IV). The assessment and management of sexual desire disorders, sexual arousal disorders, orgasmic disorders, sexual pain disorders, and sexual dysfunction caused by general medical conditions are discussed here.

Organic Causes

As is pointed out in the criteria for each of these disorders, the impact of a medical condition should be considered before attributing a disorder solely to psychologic factors. Because sexual functioning involves neural, vascular, and endocrine physiologic mecha-

nisms, as well as cellular receptor activity, many medical conditions and drugs can impair normal function. To make matters more complicated, these pathologic conditions can adversely affect one or more phases of the sexual response cycle (Tables 18.1 to 18.4).

General Characteristics

Frequency

The exact incidence of sexual disorders is unknown. Estimates of lifetime incidence range from a high of 75% in marriages and other long-term relationships to a low of 25%. In a study of patients seen by general internists, 53% of new patients reported sexual dysfunctions or concerns that they would like to discuss with their physician (4). In all likelihood, the higher estimates include concerns about the normalcy of or risks associated with one's sexual behavior, or formal sexual disorders in their milder and more transient forms. Each type of sexual dysfunction can be found in both heterosexual and homosexual individuals and couples. The sex ratio varies for the particular dysfunction. For example, certain orgasm disorders are more common in females. By definition, premature ejaculation is confined to men, and vaginismus is restricted to women.

Age of Onset of Common Sexual Disorders

Psychologic and behavioral antecedents of sexual disorders can sometimes be found in both adolescent and childhood sexual behaviors and fantasies; however, the common age of onset is early adulthood. Onset can occur at any time during adult life, especially for dysfunctions associated with medical conditions or substances/drugs and for those that are situational or transient.

Predisposing Personality Factors

In general, competent and satisfying sexual function is considered to be associated with a healthy and

Table 18.1. Medical Conditions that May Affect Sexual Response in Both Sexes

Organic Factor	Sexual Disorders
Alcoholic neuropathy	Hypoactive arousal, hypoactive orgasm
Angina pectoris or recent myocardial infarction	Hypoactive desire
Any chronic systemic disease	Hypoactive desire, hypoactive arousal
Chronic pain	Hypoactive desire
Degenerative arthritis and disc disease of lumbosacral spine	Hypoactive desire, hypoactive arousal
Diabetes mellitus	Hypoactive arousal, retrograde ejaculation (men)
	Hypoactive orgasm (women)
Endocrine disorders (thyroid deficiency states, Addison's disease, Cushing's disease, hypopituitarism, hyperprolactinemia)	Hypoactive desire, variable effect on arousal
Multiple sclerosis	Hypoactive desire, hypoactive arousal, hypoactive orgasm
Cord lesions	
Low lesion	Hypoactive reflex arousal (psychogenic arousal and reflex ejaculation may be preserved)
High lesion	Hypoactive psychogenic arousal (reflex arousal and ejaculation may be preserved)
Radical pelvic surgery	Hypoactive arousal, hypoactive orgasm
Temporal lobe lesions	Hypoactive or increased desire
Vascular disease	
Large vessel (Leriche syndrome	Hypoactive arousal
Small vessel (pelvic vascular insufficiency)	Hypoactive arousal

Table 18.2.   Medical Conditions that May Affect Sexual Response: Men Only

Organic Factor	Sexual Disorders

Dyspareunia (genital pain during intercourse)
   Disturbed penile anatomy (chordee, Peyrone's disease, traumatic
      fracture, traumatic amputation)
   Penile skin infections
   Prostatic infections
   Testicular disease (orchitis, epididymitis, tumor, trauma)
   Urethral infections (gonorrhea, nonspecific urethral infections)
	Hypoactive desire, hypoactive arousal, and hypoactive orgasm

Hypogonadal androgen-deficient states (Klinefelter's syndrome, testicular agenesis, Kallman's syndrome, testicular tumors, orchitis, hyperprolactinemia, castration)	Hypoactive desire, hypoactive arousal, hypoactive orgasm
Mechanical problems (inguinal hernia, hydrocele)	Hypoactive arousal

Surgical procedures
   Abdominoperineal bowel resection
   Lumbar sympathectomy
   Radical perineal prostatectomy
	
	Hypoactive arousal
	Hypoactive orgasm
	Hypoactive arousal

Table 18.3.   Medical Conditions that May Affect Sexual Response: Women Only

Organic Factor	Sexual Disorders
Complications of Surgery Ovarian approximation to vagina Posthysterectomy scarring Shortened vagina	Hypoactive desire, hypoactive arousal, hypoactive orgasm, and vaginismus may occur with any of the organic factors listed at the left.
Dyspareunia (Painful Intercourse) Agenesis of the vagina Clitoral phymosis Imperforate hymen, rigid hymen, tender hymenal tags Infections of external genitalia: herpes genitalis, labial cysts, furuncles, Bartholin cyst infections Infections of the vagina: herpes genitalis, *Candida albicans, Trichomonas* Injuries due to birth trauma: episiotomy scars, tears, uterine prolapse Irritations of the vagina: chemical dermatitis (douches), atrophic vaginitis, intercourse with insufficient lubrication	
Miscellaneous Pelvis Problems Cystitis, urethritis, urethral prolapse Endometriosis, ectopic pregnancy, pelvic inflammatory disease, ovarian cysts and tumors, pelvic tumors Intrauterine device complications	

adaptive personality development. Therefore, defects in personality structure accompanied by maladaptive personality traits (see Chapter 14) or psychopathology may affect sexual function. However, a study involving 288 patients referred because of a diagnosis of a sexual dysfunction revealed that only 30% of the sample fulfilled criteria for an additional psychiatric disorder (6). Negative attitudes toward sexuality caused by particular experience, internal psychic conflicts, or adherence to rigid cultural values can predispose patients to the development of these dysfunctions.

Course and Severity

The course of sexual dysfunctions varies. Dysfunctions may develop after a period of normal functioning or they may be lifelong. They may be generalized, occurring with all partners, or situational, limited to certain partners. There are differing degrees of impairment, from partial or intermittent to total and unremitting. Usually, early age of onset and total impairment indicate chronicity and predict a poor treatment outcome. Conversely, a history of prior adequate sexual function, situational symptoms, and partial impairment are predictive of a self-limited course and a favorable treatment outcome.

Complications

The major complications are disrupted marital or sexual relationships. In addition, presence of the dysfunction may give rise to a variety of symptoms such as depression, anxiety, guilt, shame, frustration, and anger. These symptoms not only affect the patient but may intrude into most of his or her relationships.

Table 18.4. Common Drugs and Substances That May Affect Sexual Response[a]

Drugs	Sexual Disorders Reported
Alcohol and sedatives (high dose)	Hypoactive desire, hypoactive arousal, delayed orgasm
Amiodarone	Hypoactive desire
Androgens	Increased desire (women)
	Hypoactive or increased desire, and/or hypoactive arousal
Anticonvulsants	
Carbamazepine	Hypoactive arousal
Phenytoin	Hypoactive desire, hypoactive arousal
Antidepressants	
Fluoxetine	Hypoactive desire, hypoactive orgasm
Tricyclics	Hypoactive or increased desire and/or hypoactive arousal
Antihypertensives	
Centrally acting (β-blockers, clonidine, guanabenz, methyldopa, reserpine)	Hypoactive desire, hypoactive arousal, (?) hypoactive orgasm
α-Blockers, hydralazine	Hypoactive arousal
Peripherally acting (guanethidine, guanadrel)	Retrograde ejaculation, hypoactive desire
Antipsychotics	Hypoactive or increased desire, hypoactive arousal, retrograde ejaculation (Merllaril)
Digoxin	Hypoactive desire, hypoactive arousal
Disopyramide	Hypoactive arousal
Disulfiram	Hypoactive arousal, delayed ejaculation
Diuretics	Hypoactive arousal
Estrogens, progesterone	
Men	Hypoactive desire, hypoactive arousal, hypoactive orgasm
Women	Hypoactive desire
H$_2$ blockers (cimetidine, famotidine, ranitidine)	Hypoactive desire, hypoactive arousal
L-Dopa	Increased desire (elderly men)
Lithium	Hypoactive desire, hypoactive arousal
Marijuana (high dose)	Hypoactive arousal (low dose may produce increased desire in men)
Metoclopramide	Hypoactive desire, hypoactive arousal
Narcotics	Hypoactive desire, hypoactive arousal, hypoactive orgasm
Stimulants (high dose) (cocaine, amphetamines)	Hypoactive desire, hypoactive arousal, hypoactive orgasm (low dose may produce increased desire)
Verapamil	Hypoactive arousal

[a]See also drugs that cause sexual dysfunction: an update. Med Lett 34:73, 1992 (contains exhaustive table, with references for each drug listed) and Buffum J. Prescription drugs and sexual function. In: Hall R, ed. Psychiatric medicine, Vol 10, No 2. Orlando, FL: Ryandic Publishing, 1992.

General Approach to the Patient

Because patients often have difficulty initiating discussion about sexual activities and problems, it is important to inquire about sexual orientation and function as part of the primary care of each patient. In a study in a general medicine practice, 90% of patients appreciated being asked about sexual function (4). Table 18.5 outlines interviewing approaches that may be useful in this inquiry. In patients who name a problem, the history of the present problem may be imprecise. Thus, sufficient time should be set aside with the patient to obtain a clear account of the problem. Occasionally, more than one scheduled session may be necessary. The setting for the discussion should be private. For patients whose difficulties involve a partner or a spouse, it is important to have the partner's view of the problem. Sometimes the more functional partner will seek help to gain support for bringing the less functional partner into the evaluation.

The evaluation should be organized to obtain information about the onset and duration of the problem; about factors that make the problem better or worse; about concurrent events such as birth of children, changes in relationships or vocation, or onset of physi-cal or emotional illness; and about use of new medications. It is always important to elicit from patients their ideas about the cause of sexual problems and their expectations of treatment.

Sexual Desire Disorders

Diagnostic Classification

Medical conditions or medications that cause decreased sexual desire should be specifically diagnosed. Predominantly psychogenic disorders have been classified as follows in DSM-IV.

Hypoactive Sexual Desire Disorder (Loss of Libido)

A. Persistently or recurrently deficient (or absent) sexual fantasies and desire for sexual activity. The judgment of deficiency or absence is made by the clinician, taking into account factors that affect sexual functioning, such as age, sex, and the context of the person's life.

B. The disturbance causes marked distress or interpersonal difficulty.

C. Does not occur exclusively during the course of another Axis I disorder (except another sexual dysfunction) and is not caused exclusively by the direct physiologic effects of a substance (e.g., drugs of abuse, medication) or a general medical condition.

Sexual Aversion Disorder

A. Persistent or recurrent extreme aversion to and avoidance of all or almost all genital sexual contact with a sexual partner.

B. The disturbance causes marked distress or interpersonal difficulty.

C. The sexual dysfunction is not caused by another Axis I disorder (except another sexual dysfunction).

Assessment

As seen in Tables 18.1 to 18.4, many medical conditions and drugs have the potential for decreasing sexual desire. In practice, most of these conditions are known to or easily diagnosed by the patient's physician. Only a few conditions may present with the initial complaint of decreased or absent desire.

Congenital or acquired *hypogonadism* may be associated with decreased sexual interest in men (16). Because the testosterone level needed to maintain libido is usually lower than that needed for full stimulation of the prostate and seminal vesicles, the patient should also complain of a decrease or absence of emission when loss of sexual desire is due to hypogonadism. Hypogonadism that occurs before puberty results in eunuchoidism (lack of development of secondary sex characteristics). Similar striking physical findings are not present in patients who acquire hypogonadism after puberty; however, subtle physical changes do occur: decrease in beard growth, tendency to female body habitus, and decrease in size of testes.

An evaluation for hypogonadism should be undertaken in any male with persistent loss of libido (see details in Chapters 74 and 77).

In both sexes, *prolactin-secreting microadenomas* of the pituitary may cause loss of sexual interest. In men this is partly caused by a prolactin-mediated decrease in gonadotropin output, accompanied by a low testosterone level. Hyperprolactinemia causes amenorrhea and galactorrhea in females, but galactorrhea is rare in affected men. Diagnosis can be made in both sexes by measuring serum prolactin levels (normal is less than 15 mg/mL). (See additional details in Chapter 77.)

In both sexes, *alcohol or other substance abuse* can cause decreased sexual desire. Patients who abuse drugs are usually guarded or untruthful about their habits; therefore, persistence and use of collateral interviews are often necessary in diagnosing the primary problem (see Chapters 21 and 22).

Depression is a common cause of loss of sexual desire. Even mild depressive states may result in decreased sexual desire, but in patients with severe depressions, this loss is universally observed. The relationship between loss of sexual desire and the presence of depression may be recognized by noting the patient's mood as well as by obtaining a history of depressive symptoms (see Chapter 15). Life stresses (e.g., loss of a job, death of a family member or of a friend, birth of a new family member, recent illness such as myocardial infarction) are common sources of decreased sexual desire related to depression or anxiety.

In married couples, decreased sexual desire in one or both partners is often the result of *marital strife*. Arguments between partners create anger that eventually

---

Table 18.5.   Suggested Questions Regarding Sexual Practices and Problems

Suggested Opening (Legitimizing Statement)
"Something that I ask each of my patients about is sexual activity. Is that alright with you?"

Suggested Initial Question(s)
(Open-ended question) "Can you tell me about your present sexual activity (practices)?"
or
(Closed, somewhat leading question) "Have you noticed any problem in your ability to have and enjoy sexual relations?"
or
(Closed, but facilitative question) "Do you have any problems or questions related to your current sexual activities?"

Screening Questions for Sexual Dysfunction (Ask for Clarification of any Positive Response)
(Both sexes) "Have you noticed any loss of interest in having sex?"
(Men) "Any problems having an erection?"
(Women) "Any problems with lubrication or swelling of the vagina when you are sexually aroused?"
(Both sexes) "Any problems having an orgasm?"
(Both sexes) "Any pain during intercourse?"

Screening Questions Regarding Sexual Orientation
(Both sexes) "Have you ever had sex with men, women, or both?"
or
(Men) "Do you ever have sex with another man?"
(Women) "Do you ever have sex with another woman?"

Screening Questions for Risk of or History of Sexually Transmitted Disease[a]
(Both sexes) "In the past few years about how many partners have you had for sexual relations?"
(Both sexes) "Have you ever had any kind of infection that you got from having sex?"

Open Question to Obtain Additional Information
"Is there any other information or any other questions about your sexual activities that you would like to discuss with me?"

[a]See list of safe and unsafe sexual practices and instructions for use of a condom (Table 34.2).

interferes with their sexual relationship. Although spouses may be aware of their anger toward each other, they may fail to draw a connection between loss of sexual interest and their mutual differences. Assessment requires a history taken from the couple together and then separately. Review of their current life situation usually elicits the precipitating stresses and highlights the conflicts. The uncovering of extramarital relationships during the assessment requires careful handling. If both partners are aware of the relationship, it can be discussed openly. If the extramarital relationship is revealed to a physician during the individual interviews, the physician should ask what the partner intends to do about the relationship and with the secret information now shared with the physician. The responsibility for telling the other partner should be left to the patient. In some cases the extramarital relationship is a peripheral issue, and airing it could be destructive to an otherwise salvageable relationship.

Certain patients may give a history of *aversion to or avoidance of all forms of genital contact* with a sexual partner, in contrast to a history of gradual or sudden loss of sexual desire. The complaint is often of long standing but may be of recent onset. The aversion may be so severe as to be associated with panic attacks should the patient find him- or herself confronted with a sexual experience.

Finally, decreased or absent sexual desire may be caused by the anxiety and frustration of *repeated sexual failure* associated with one of the other sexual disorders discussed below.

Treatment

Depending on the cause, hypogonadism in men may be treated by surgery, radiotherapy, hormone replacement, or hormone suppression (in the case of hyperprolactinemia). These treatment modalities are discussed in Chapter 77.

In both sexes, if a drug (Table 18.4) is suspected of interfering with sexual desire, it should be discontinued when possible as a diagnostic-therapeutic test. If loss of sexual drive is secondary to alcohol or substance abuse, treatment should be aimed at controlling the abuse (see Chapters 21 and 22).

Patients with coronary artery disease, especially those who have had myocardial infarction, have particular problems associated with sexual function. The treatment of these patients is discussed as part of the overall approach to rehabilitation after infarction in Chapter 58.

Transient hypoactive sexual desire disorders secondary to *psychologic factors* such as stress, anger, or other interpersonal problems can be managed effectively with short-term counseling. When alcoholism, depression, or another psychosocial disorder is the primary problem, specific treatment for that disorder should accompany the counseling. The design of a counseling program should include an agreement between the patient or couple and the physician to meet for a specific number of sessions (usually two to five) for approximately 30 minutes per session.

EXAMPLE

A couple in their mid-twenties presents with a history of recent loss of sexual desire on the husband's part and a decrease in the frequency of their sexual relationships. Assessment reveals a history of mutually satisfying sexual experiences until 1 month ago, when the husband was threatened with a job layoff. Although the husband still has his job, the layoff is still a possibility. The wife reports that the husband has become quiet, sullen, and generally less interested in activities he usually enjoys. They report fighting frequently over small issues. The assessment is that the husband has an adjustment disorder with depressive features (see Chapter 15). During the initial counseling session, the physician suggests that a relationship exists between changes in the husband's behavior and the threatened layoff. The wife indicates that the husband has refused to discuss his concerns because it is unmanly. During the next counseling session, the physician assists the couple in sharing their anguish with each other and developing contingency plans to cope with the potential layoff. As they are drawn into the discussions of planning, the couple's anger with each other subsides and a collaborative relationship is reestablished. The third session is used to review what contingency plans they have made. As an aside, they report that they have resumed their sexual relationship. During the final session the physician reviews the relationship between stress, anger, and the change in sexual functioning; points out that anger subsided when they worked together and that good sex is difficult to experience when they are angry with each other; and encourages them to use what they have learned when stresses arise in the future.

Aversion disorders usually require psychotherapy and treatment of associated panic attacks with low-dosage antidepressant medication (see details regarding panic attacks in Chapter 13).

Patients and their physicians often attempt to treat decreased sexual desire with drugs such as testosterone, alcohol, antianxiety compounds, or stimulants. There is no scientific basis for prescribing drugs for sexual desire disorders, except testosterone for the treatment of confirmed hypogonadism and bromocriptine for treatment of hyperprolactinemia (15), as discussed in Chapter 77.

Sexual Arousal Disorders

Diagnostic Classification

An arousal disorder that is secondary to a medical condition or medication should be diagnosed as a symptom associated with the condition or medication.

Psychogenic disorders have been classified as follows in DSM-IV.

Female Arousal Disorders

A. Persistent or recurrent inability to attain or to maintain until completion of the sexual activity an adequate lubrication–swelling response of sexual excitement.
B. The disturbance causes marked distress or interpersonal difficulty.
C. The sexual dysfunction is not better accounted for by another Axis I disorder (except another sexual dysfunction) and is not caused by the direct physiologic effects of a substance (e.g., drugs of abuse, a medication) or a general medical condition.

Male Erectile Disorder (Impotence)

A. Persistent or recurrent inability to attain or maintain an adequate erection until completion of the sexual activity.
B. The disturbance causes marked distress or interpersonal difficulty.
C. The dysfunction is not better accounted for by another Axis I disorder (other than a sexual dysfunction) and is not caused exclusively by the direct physiologic effects of a substance (e.g., a drug of abuse, a medication).

Assessment

An initial history (including psychosocial evaluation, see Chapter 10) and physical examination will usually lead to a formulation that the problem is either organic (i.e., one of the causes in Tables 18.1 to 18.4) or predominantly psychogenic. The general features in a male patient's history listed in Table 18.6 are helpful in making this important distinction.

Organic Dysfunction. In both sexes, partial or complete failure to begin and maintain genital vasocongestion can be caused by a large number of medical conditions and drugs. Importantly, when sexual desire is intact, a male erectile disorder is unlikely to be caused by a hypogonadal condition because libido is typically diminished in patients with hypogonadal conditions. In younger patients, drugs are the most common cause of erectile disorders (Table 18.4). In older men, new onset of erectile disorders are mostly caused by vascular or neurologic disease (13). The other conditions that may cause sexual arousal disorders (Tables 18.1 to 18.3) usually present with other manifestations before the patient complains of this problem.

In male patients with *diabetes mellitus,* it is estimated that 25 to 60% will eventually develop erectile disorders (5). Because some patients present with erectile disorder as the initial symptom of diabetes, a fasting blood glucose is indicated for any male patient who presents with a chief complaint of erectile disorder that is not caused by an obvious psychosocial stressor or a recently started medication. There is no definitive information at this time about the effect of diabetes on the arousal phase in women; clearly, it can inhibit orgasm in women (11).

Two conditions in women may contribute to arousal disorders: *vaginitis* and *atrophic vaginal changes* secondary to estrogen deficiency (see Chapter 94). Surprisingly, some women do not associate the presence of vaginitis or atrophic changes with the discomfort or pain these conditions can cause when intercourse is attempted. Therefore, the history should include questions to determine whether pain occurs during intercourse, and the physical examination should include a pelvic examination to look for evidence of atrophy (see Chapter 94).

Occlusive vascular disease causing diminished blood flow to the internal pudendal arteries is more likely to affect men than women. Female arousal disorders have been described with large vessel disease (Leriche's syndrome) as well as with medium and small vessel disease. If it is suspected that there is a vascular basis for male erectile disorder, the patient should be offered a referral to a vascular surgeon for evaluation (see Chapter 87). The diagnostic techniques that may be used include angiography of the medium-size vessels of the corpus cavernosa, comparison of penile systolic pressures to limb systolic pressures, Doppler measurement of penile blood flow, and nocturnal penile tumescence studies (NPT) (9).

The *hypogonadal* states that cause hypoactive desire (see above) can also cause arousal disorders (18), and the approach to diagnosis is the same (see Chapter 77).

Psychogenic Dysfunction. If the assessment for an organic cause, which often includes a trial off a potentially offending drug, does not yield a convincing diagnosis, a psychogenic basis should be assumed, and further inquiry followed by appropriate brief counseling (see below) should be used as a diagnostic-therapeutic trial.

Inability to attain and maintain levels of arousal that permit a smooth and trouble-free progression from the beginning of a sexual experience to its completion can be caused by any external or internal psychologic events that interfere with the patient's ability to focus on the physical and psychologic stimuli that maintain the sexual arousal. A dramatic example of an external event is the ringing of a telephone during the sexual experience. An internal psychologic event might be a recurring thought about how one is performing. The history and assessment should be structured to uncover the presence of external events and the specific content of the psychologic events when present. A common finding is a persistent preoccupation and anxiety about performing successfully. This problem may be primary or may occur as a secondary response to the frustration associated with organic dysfunction. Worry about a successful performance becomes more and more absorbing during the course of the sexual experience, so that the psychologic activity crowds out the patient's capacity to focus on the sexual stimuli that

---

Table 18.6.   Clinical Features Differentiating Predominantly Psychogenic from Predominantly Organic Erectile Dysfunction

	Psychogenic	Organic
Onset	Usually abrupt, with temporal relationship to specific stress (e.g., marital difficulties, loss of job, bereavement, fatigue)	Usually insidious decline from previous competency (90–95% of cases)
Course	Selective, intermittent, episodic, transient	Usually persistent, with progressive deterioration
Degree of impairment	Evidence of potential to respond to erotic stimuli and fantasies, with masturbation, other partner	Unable to obtain erection with masturbation, erotic stimuli, other partner
Nocturnal or morning erection	Generally present	Generally absent or reduced in frequency intensity

From Vliet LW, Meyer JK. Erectile dysfunction: progress in evaluation and treatment. Johns Hopkins Med J 151:246, 1982.

maintain the arousal response. When such patients realize they are losing arousal, they try all the harder, shutting off completely their ability to respond to sexual stimuli. Masters and Johnson have called this process *spectatoring* (see "General References"). The term describes a process whereby the patient, through observation of his performance, psychologically takes himself out of the experience. The mental process is guaranteed to result in loss of sexual arousal. Typically this process may begin after one or two failed experiences secondary to external events or stresses. Once the process begins, it becomes internally reinforcing, leading to further worry and further failure. When this process is suspected, the history should focus on the patient's mental experiences during sexual intercourse. Such information is difficult for most patients to describe, and more than a single interview may be required.

Other common causes of psychologically inhibited sexual arousal are *stressful life situations.* Patients who have recently lost a job, lost a relative, are concerned about retirement, or have developed an illness may be unable to clear their minds of their worries during a sexual experience and therefore cannot respond. Similarly, feelings of anger or resentment directed toward the sexual partner can interfere with the ability to become sexually aroused.

If the patient with suspected psychogenic impotence does not respond to brief counseling (see below), then he should be offered referral to a sleep laboratory for *nocturnal penile tumescence (NPT) studies* (9). The diagnostic usefulness of NPT monitoring is based on the assumption that during sleep, the psychologic factors impeding erectile function during wakefulness are no longer operative, allowing a demonstration of the integrity of one's physiologic capacity. Organic deficits, however, would persist during sleep, and therefore interfere with the number and duration of erectile episodes. Research has tended to confirm this assumption, with two exceptions: in certain psychiatric disorders (e.g., endogenous depression) in which rapid eye movement (REM) sleep patterns are also disrupted, and in a few men with organically proven erectile failure who occasionally have an episode of full erection during sleep, such as in patients with lower body spasms caused by spinal cord injury, patients with a vascular steal syndrome, and in a previously unrecognized syndrome of impaired penile tumescence in the presence of sleep apnea, hypoventilation with decreased oxygen saturation, myoclonic jerks, and bradycardia.

Patient Experience. This is similar to the experience for evaluation of sleep disorders (see Chapter 85). The patient is usually scheduled to sleep on three consecutive nights in the sleep laboratory. Parameters monitored include electroencephalography, eye movements (to document the presence of REM sleep), heart rate, blood pressure, changes in penile circumference at the tip (just proximal to the glans) and base using two mercury-filled strain gauges, and an assessment of the degree of penile rigidity during at least one of the erectile episodes. Rigidity is assessed using a specifically designed tonometer that measures the amount of force required to buckle the erect penis. The patient is also briefly awakened to

observe his erection, and asked to evaluate the quality of this erection, and to estimate its sufficiency for intromission. The technician records his estimate of the degree and rigidity of the erection. A photograph of the erect penis is taken, and later reviewed with the patient. This photograph provides visual evidence of normal erectile capacity to the patient with psychogenic dysfunction, it aids in the interpretation of numerical data obtained, and it reveals or confirms the presence of an anatomic deformity interfering with normal erection or intromission.

A do-it-yourself device (the Dacomed Snap-Gauge) for assessing nocturnal erections has been promoted in recent years. Because the role of this potentially cost-saving device has not been validated in careful studies, its place in the evaluation of male erectile disorders is unclear.

If an NPT study indicates an organic disorder (i.e., no or only partial erections occur during sleep), additional evaluation for vascular or neurologic disorders should be carried out. If an NPT study supports a psychogenic erectile disorder, psychiatric referral is warranted.

Treatment for Organic Causes. The method of treatment of organically based sexual arousal disorders in men depends on whether the physiologic impairment is reversible.

If a disease process, such as an infection, has not caused irreversible anatomic or physiologic changes, treatment of the disease is indicated. Similarly, side effects of drugs can be reversed by reduction of dosage or, ideally, discontinuation of the medication. An adequate trial off a drug would be 1 week or more. Testosterone replacement for hypogonadism produces improvement in sexual arousal within a few weeks (see Chapter 77 for details). Whenever one is treating a patient with a reversible organic cause, treatment should be accompanied by encouragement and practical advice, as discussed below.

When a disease process has caused *permanent impairment* of neural, vascular, or anatomic function in males, prosthetic devices that cause erection or pharmacologic measures can be considered, usually in consultation with a urologist.

The most common indication for *penile prosthetic devices* has been in sexually impaired diabetic patients who are otherwise healthy. Counseling of the patient and his spouse or partner is an essential element of a rehabilitative program before and after surgery. Currently, two types of penile prosthetic devices allow the affected male to engage in intercourse. The Small-Carrion (17) prosthesis is a set of semirigid Silastic rods that are placed in the penis, creating a permanent modest erection. The second prosthesis is a hydraulic device (7) that, when implanted, permits voluntary stiffening of the penis. Prosthesis insertion is usually done in an ambulatory surgery unit, followed by meticulous wound care and observation for wound infection. Patients should not resume sexual activity for 6 weeks. Uncommon late complications are erosion of the prosthesis into the urethra and penile pain during intercourse.

Intracavernosal injection of vasodilating substances such as papaverine hydrochloride (smooth muscle relaxant), phenoxybenzamine hydrochloride and phentolamine (β-adrenergic blockers), or prostaglandin E (Alprostadil) has become an important nonsurgical technique for treating organically caused arousal disorder (8); it may also be helpful as adjunctive treatment for men with psychogenic impotence (10). Patients can be taught, with supervision, to inject themselves painlessly with 28-gauge needles. The amount of substance necessary to cause erection may vary from patient to patient and must be determined by the physician (usually a consulting urologist) with a challenge injection, which also serves the function of initiating instruction of the patient. This method of treatment has been more effective for men with neurogenic impotence than for those with vascular or other causes for their impotence. Erection occurs 8 to 10 minutes after injection and lasts 2 to 4 hours, with partial detumescence after ejaculation. Priapism and orthostatic hypotension have been the major untoward effects of treatment with papaverine or β-blockers; penile pain after injection is more common with prostaglandin E. Fibrosis at injection sites leading to deformity of the penis is an uncommon late complication.

Alprostadil (prostaglandin E) can now be administered through a novel transurethral drug delivery system (Medicated Urethral System for Erection, or MUSE). The advantage of this method is substitution of a small pellet inserted via an applicator into the urethra rather than injection into the corpora. Some men experience urethral burning, but adherence to proper techniques of administration will minimize any discomfort. In controlled trials, 65% of men reported successful intercourse with MUSE compared with 19% using a placebo pellet (14).

Yohimbe, an orally administered β-adrenergic blocker, has yielded inconsistent results in men with organic erectile disorder (12) and has been effective in some with psychogenic erectile disorder (10,15). Yohimbe is available as Yohimex (5-mg tablets) and Yocon (5.4-mg tablets), and the usual dosage is one tablet three times a day. Occasional side effects at this dosage are nausea, dizziness, or nervousness. The clinical effect may not be seen until the patient has been on medication for 3 weeks. Considering the relative costs of medication versus psychotherapy, a trial of this drug may be indicated for selected patients.

Sildenafil (Vicra) is a phosphodiesterase inhibitor that can be taken orally and has shown promise in the treatment of male erectile disorders (1). In the context of erotic stimulation, it facilitates the blood flow to the corpus cavernosum. The recommended dose is one 50-mg tablet about 1 hour before sexual activity. In patients with the following conditions, which are associated with increased levels of sildenafil, a 25-mg tablet should be used: age above 65, hepatic impairment, severe renal impairment, and concomitant use of potent cytochrome P4503A4 inhibitors (e.g., erythromycin, ketoconazole). The drug is contraindicated in patients using nitrates because of potentiation of hypotension.

Little is known about the response to treatment in women with disease processes that impair the physiologic capacity for sexual arousal. As in men, side effects of drugs can be eliminated by adjustment of dosage or discontinuation of the drug, and dyspareunia caused by vulvovaginal conditions and atrophic vaginitis can usually be eliminated (see Chapter 94).

Treatment for Psychogenic Causes. The strategy for management of psychologically based sexual arousal disorders in both sexes depends on whether the patient has had the dysfunction for a sustained period or whether the dysfunction has appeared recently and there is a history of competent sexual functioning. As discussed earlier, transient inhibition of sexual excitement is often secondary to stressful life situations or marital discord (adjustment disorders). These clinical situations often respond to brief counseling. The elements of counseling are similar to those described in the previous example of the couple with sexual desire disorders. The role of the therapist is to help the couple recognize the effect of the stress on their relationship as well as the effect of their feelings (often anger) on their ability to relate sexually. Encouragement of collaborative contingency planning for resolving problems reduces anxiety and anger, often helping the couple to return to their baseline level of sexual function. The same principles and steps are applicable to an individual patient.

When spectatoring is a major factor and does not remit after open discussion, referral to a professional skilled in sex therapy usually brings excellent results. A successful form of treatment is one developed by Masters and Johnson that combines cognitive as well as behavioral techniques to replace spectatoring with appropriate sexual focus and behavior.

The following factors favor a *good prognosis* after treatment for psychogenic impotence: history of adequate prior sexual functioning, acute versus insidious onset, short duration of sexual impairment, stable social situation, motivation for treatment, presence of sexual desire, partner willing to participate in treatment, absence of severe marital conflicts, and absence of significant concurrent psychopathy.

Even in patients for whom excellent function can be expected, return to normal sexual arousal can be impaired by worry and hesitation. This is especially true when impaired arousal has been present for more than a few weeks, which is often the case. Such patients should be invited to discuss this situation freely and given permission and encouragement to experiment in one or more ways (e.g., masturbation, erotic pictures or movies, new techniques) in order to test or promote their sexual functions. Of course, such advice should be consistent with the patient's personal beliefs.

Patients who have suffered with a sexual arousal disorder over a long period or have never functioned competently may be given a trial of short-term counseling (see Chapter 11). If the counseling does not result in reasonable improvement, referral for more expert help should be considered.

Orgasm Disorders

Diagnostic Classification

Orgasm disorders caused by medical conditions or medications should be diagnosed as symptoms associated with the responsible conditions or medications

(Tables 18.1 to 18.4). Psychogenic disorders have been classified as follows in DSM-IV.

Female Orgasmic Disorder

A. Persistent or recurrent delay in or absence of orgasm following a normal sexual arousal phase. Women exhibit wide variability in the type and intensity of stimulation that triggers orgasm. The diagnosis of female orgasmic disorder should be based on the clinician's judgment that the woman's orgasmic capacity is less than would be reasonable for her age, sexual experience, and the adequacy of sexual stimulation she receives.
B. The disturbance causes marked distress or interpersonal difficulty.
C. The orgasmic disorder is not better accounted for by another Axis I disorder (except another sexual dysfunction) and is not caused exclusively by the direct physiologic effects of a substance (e.g., a drug of abuse, a medication) or a general medical condition.

Male Orgasmic Disorder

A. Persistent or recurrent delay in or absence of orgasm following a normal sexual excitement phase during sexual activity that the clinician, taking into account the person's age, judges to be adequate in focus, intensity, and duration.
B. The disturbance causes marked distress or interpersonal difficulty.
C. The orgasmic disorder is not better accounted for by another Axis I disorder (except another sexual dysfunction) and is not caused exclusively by the direct physiologic effects of a substance (e.g., a drug of abuse, a medication) or a general medical condition.

Premature Ejaculation

A. Persistent or recurrent ejaculation with minimal sexual stimulation before, upon, or shortly after penetration and before the person wishes it. The clinician must take into account factors that affect duration of the arousal phase, such as age, novelty of the sexual partner or situation, and recent frequency of sexual activity.
B. The disturbance causes marked distress or interpersonal difficulty.
C. The premature ejaculation is not caused exclusively by the direct effects of a substance (e.g., withdrawal from opioids).

Assessment

The orgasmic response is physiologically governed by the autonomic nervous system in both sexes. The organic conditions that effect orgasm are for the most part neurologic disorders, drugs that affect the autonomic system, and surgical or traumatic interruption of the involved neural pathways (Tables 18.1 to 18.4). History taking and physical examination should focus on these possibilities. In women, diabetic autonomic neuropathy is probably the most common organic cause of orgasm disorders (11). Men who are experiencing retrograde ejaculation often state that they have lost their ability to have orgasms. If history reveals that the patient has the subjective sensations of orgasm but has no ejaculate (and the patient is not taking a drug

that can cause retrograde ejaculation; Table 18.4), the patient should have a urologic evaluation of the function of the internal sphincter of the bladder.

Isolated psychogenic anorgasmia in men is a rare disorder associated with severe personality disturbances. Cases can be divided roughly into two personality types: severe obsessive–compulsive character disorder and severe sadomasochistic character disorder.

Premature ejaculation is the most common male orgasmic disorder. There are no known organic causes for premature ejaculation; therefore, the assessment of this dysfunction should focus on psychologic issues. Whereas some men recognize that orgasm regularly occurs too soon for their partner to enjoy intercourse fully, others do not; therefore, both partners should be interviewed in order to make the diagnosis. Typically the couple reports that the male experiences orgasm as he is attempting to penetrate, just after he has penetrated, or within several thrusts after penetration.

Men usually have had the dysfunction since they became sexually active. Although occasionally patients may report the recent onset of premature ejaculation, these men have invariably experienced this disorder for a sustained period in the past. Another variation is the patient who reports good control with a girlfriend but premature ejaculation with his spouse.

The personality structure of the premature ejaculator is often passive–aggressive (see Chapter 14). Evaluation of the relationship usually reveals an ongoing struggle between the couple. The woman is openly angry about some issue (not necessarily the sexual problem), and the man is complacent, content, and puzzled that his partner is upset. Transient episodes of premature ejaculation may be precipitated by marital conflict. Some men who are sufficiently frustrated by the disorder may develop a sexual arousal disorder secondarily.

Psychologically caused orgasm disorder is a common problem in women. Numerous studies estimate that 10% of the female population is anorgasmic to any stimuli and 30 to 50% of all married women are occasionally anorgasmic with intercourse. Assessment should focus on the duration of the problem, a history of sexual functioning, the status of the relationship with the spouse or partner, and the presence of a stressful situation. A history of recent onset, competent past functioning, and identifiable precipitating stresses predicts a good response to treatment. Patients who have been anorgasmic for many years and are seeking help because of a change in their relationship or life situations are more difficult to treat.

Some women complain of anorgasmia, but evaluation reveals that the patient is actually experiencing a sexual arousal disorder. Because treatment may differ for these disorders, clarification of the phase in which the dysfunction is operating may be important.

Treatment

Men. Men rarely experience loss of orgasmic capacity because of organic factors while retaining the capacity for erection. In fact, it is more common for men to lose their potency while retaining the capacity for emission and some of the subjective sensations associated with orgasm. Most of the physical conditions, diseases, and drugs listed in Tables 18.1, 18.2, and 18.4 affect the capacity for erection before orgasmic function is impaired. There may be isolated instances of side effects of drugs in which males report loss of ability to experience orgasm, but retain the capacity for erection. In these instances, it is important to distinguish retrograde ejaculation from anorgasmia. Retrograde ejaculation can occur with some drugs, including thioridazine (Mellaril) and guanethidine (Ismelin), while the other components of orgasm remain intact.

Men with orgasm disorders on a psychogenic basis usually have long-standing personality disorders requiring expert psychotherapy to effect improvement.

There are several *behavioral methods of treatment for premature ejaculation.* The key to helping the premature ejaculator is to teach him to become aware of his progression through the sexual response cycle and then, with his partner, to practice one of two control techniques. Patients without regular partners cannot readily use this behavioral method. The techniques are squeeze technique and stop and go. The squeeze technique requires the partner to place her thumb and first two fingers around the coronal ridge of the penis and press firmly for 10 seconds. The pressure results in a 10 to 25% loss of erection and a decrease in the subjective sense of arousal. The technique teaches the couple a method of control that can be practiced well before the patient reaches high levels of sexual arousal. The stop and go method accomplishes the same thing by discontinuing all forms of stimulation. The patient and his partner alternately stimulate and practice control with these techniques until they are confident of their ability to exercise control. At this point they progress to coitus, interrupting the experience as necessary with the squeeze or stop and go technique. Additional details can be found in Masters and Johnson's *Human Sexual Inadequacy* (see "General References").

Advances in the pharmacologic management of premature ejaculation include the use of Alprostadil (prostaglandin E) by injection or transurethral administration (see above) and selective serotonin reuptake inhibitor (SSRI) antidepressants. Alprostadil maintains erection time, thus prolonging coitus. The SSRI antidepressants (see Chapter 15) have sexual side effects, including delayed orgasm. Dosages for treating premature ejaculation are generally those used for initiating antidepressant therapy.

Women. Apart from managing local vaginal conditions and discontinuing possible causal drugs, there are no organic therapies for this dysfunction in women. Therefore, in female patients with known neuronal damage, including diabetic neuropathy, the goal of therapy should be to help the patients adjust to the permanent loss of their sexual responsiveness.

Transient forms of anorgasmia caused by psychogenic factors are amenable to treatment with coun-seling. A history of previous orgasmic response is a good prognostic indicator. The block in orgasmic response is often due to the process of spectatoring described above. The interfering process is usually secondary to stressful life situations or marital discord. Counseling for married women and women who have a regular sexual partner should include the partner, provided that it is agreeable to the patient. Counseling should be aimed primarily at resolving the dominant problems, which are usually life stresses or interpersonal strife. With the single patient, counseling should be directed at helping the patient suppress or remove the psychologic events (i.e., spectatoring) that are occurring at a critical time, when the patient has reached a high plateau level of excitement and is prepared for orgasmic release. The interfering psychologic events may be removed by having the patient focus to the best of her ability on the physical stimuli that she is experiencing during the excitement phase.

Women with anorgasmia of long duration can be given a trial of counseling. If counseling does not result in substantial improvement, referral for additional evaluation and treatment should be made.

Sexual Pain Disorders

Diagnostic Classification

The diagnosis of psychogenic dyspareunia should be made only after all physical causes have been ruled out (Tables 18.2 and 18.3). The DSM-IV diagnostic criteria for sexual pain disorder are listed below.

Dyspareunia

A. Recurrent or persistent genital pain associated with sexual intercourse in either a male or a female.
B. The disturbance causes marked distress or interpersonal difficulty.
C. The disturbance is not caused exclusively by vaginismus or lack of lubrication, is not better accounted for by another Axis I disorder (except another sexual dysfunction), and is not caused exclusively by the direct physiologic effects of a substance (e.g., a drug of abuse, a medication) or a general medical condition.

Vaginismus. Recurrent or persistent involuntary spasm of the musculature of the outer third of the vagina that interferes with sexual intercourse.

A. The disturbance causes marked distress or interpersonal difficulty.
B. The disturbance is not better accounted for by another Axis I disorder (e.g., somatization disorder) and is not caused exclusively by the direct effects of a general medical condition.

Assessment

The common causes of genital pain during intercourse (dyspareunia) are presented in Tables 18.2 and 18.3. In both sexes, the complaint of discomfort or pain during intercourse requires a careful history, physical examination, and laboratory testing. The most common causes are infections or atrophic vaginitis in women, and urethral or prostatic infection in men. Psychogenic dyspareunia is uncommon, and this diagnosis should be made only after organic causes have been excluded.

Vaginismus is a disorder of women. There are relatively few causes of organic vaginismus, and they are usually secondary to dyspareunia. Diagnosis of functional vaginismus may be made when pelvic examination is attempted and the physician finds it impossible to pass a finger or speculum into the vagina because of contraction of the musculature around the vaginal outlet. Patients may also have a history of inability to be penetrated during coitus because of tightness of the vaginal outlet caused by muscular spasm.

Treatment

The treatment of dyspareunia caused by organic conditions in both men and women is directed at the condition, usually an infection or atrophic vaginitis, causing the pain (see Chapters 27 and 94). Patients with *psychogenic dyspareunia* have many of the features described above for those with psychogenic sexual arousal disorders or orgasm disorders; that is, they report a history of competent sexual function without pain and have current life stress or marital discord. Therefore, the counseling techniques used in the treatment should be similar to those described for the other two disorders. An important strategy in counseling is to allow the patient a face-saving way of giving up the pain without directly confronting him or her with the idea that the pain is of psychogenic origin.

A few patients have psychogenic dyspareunia over a sustained period. Such patients usually have severe underlying psychiatric conditions and require referral for expert evaluation and treatment.

The treatment of organic vaginismus is the same as the treatment of the organic causes of dyspareunia.

The *treatment of functional vaginismus* is based on desensitizing the patient to the experience of penetration. Couples are provided with a series of exercises to be performed in the privacy of their home. Following a relaxing bath, the couple engages in general body touching, excluding the genitals. Next, they repeat general touching but include the genitals, avoiding any touching that is frankly stimulating. At following sessions, they repeat the touching but add the passage of graded-sized dilators, still avoiding stimulating or efforts to attain orgasm. When dilators have reached the size approximating the size of the penis, then the penis can be substituted as a dilator. The same process can be applied by having the woman dilate herself. One problem with the single patient is the possibility that the experience during the sessions at home will not generalize a sexual experience with a partner. Should this occur, treatment may have to be delayed until the patient has a regular partner with whom she has a reasonably good relationship and who can participate in the outlined program.

HOMOSEXUALITY

General Characteristics

The American Psychiatric Association removed homosexuality from its list of mental disorders in 1973. The diagnostic term *Sexual Disorder, Not Otherwise Specified* may be used for patients who experience persistent and marked distress about their sexual orientation.

Thirty years ago, Kinsey et al. (see "General References") estimated that 10% of white American men and 5% of white women were predominantly homosexual. Recent reports from several European and American studies estimate that only 1 to 2% of the male and female population is exclusively homosexual. Estimates of the prevalence of homosexuality in African Americans and of the prevalence of bisexual sexual behaviors in the population have not been published.

Predisposing Factors

Various attempts to relate homosexuality to abnormal pituitary and sex hormone function have been unsuccessful. The evidence to support the contention that homosexuality is genetically determined is scant. Many theories about the cause of homosexuality involving psychosocial predisposition have been proposed. However, no studies have clearly demonstrated psychosocial precipitants.

Course

Most people who accept a homosexual orientation continue that orientation throughout life. Some homosexuals are socially open about their lifestyle; many are covert, largely because of negative attitudes (homophobia) that are common in American communities. Aspects of life as a homosexual that are predictably stressful include the process of discovering one's sexual orientation, disclosure to others (coming out), and the threat of hate crimes.

Complications

In the past, but possibly to a lesser degree at the present time, the principal complication was the social stigma. Bias against homosexuals leads to occupational and other social problems for some, as summarized in Table 18.7. Recently, many American communities have enacted or are considering legislation that explicitly protects homosexuals from job, housing, and other discrimination. On the other hand, some communities, and many fundamentalist religious groups, support legal and moral discrimination against homosexuality. Recently, also, criminal penalties for homosexuality have been eliminated for consenting adults. The principal legal difficulty currently is for people who are promiscuous and who use public facilities for their sexual activities. Homosexuality is entirely compatible with the development of sustained, affectionate, long-term relationships, and there is no evidence that homosexuals are subject to or manifest greater levels of major psychopathology than heterosexuals.

Table 18.7. Influence of Homosexuality on Vocation and Social Life (Results of a Study of 143 Subjects)

	Male Homosexuals % N = 86	Female Homosexuals % N = 57
Social		
No negative influence[a]	51	72
Deprived of family life	35	9
Social contacts limited to other homosexuals	14	19
Ambitions		
No negative influence	68	88
Imposed restrictions on choice of work or advancement	32	12
Job		
No negative influence	84	88
Reprimanded, fired, or asked to resign because of homosexuality	16	12

From Saghir M, Robins E. Male and female homosexuality—a developmental, psychiatric, and sociologic investigation. Baltimore: Williams & Wilkins, 1973.

[a]All negative influences listed are those that subjects felt were specifically a result of being identified as a homosexual.

Assessment and Management

Assessment of patients who express concerns about homosexual fantasies or experiences should focus on the frequency of the experiences, on the patients' decisions to continue with homosexual experiences, and on whether they feel comfortable with those decisions. Patients who ultimately choose a gay lifestyle and are comfortable with that choice do not present problems. However, patients who are anxious or depressed about their homosexual inclinations may need therapy. Adolescents or adults who anxiously report isolated episodes of homosexual experiences or fantasies may need brief supportive counseling (see Chapter 11).

Studies have found that many gay men prefer their personal physician to know of their homosexuality and indicate that they are more satisfied with the care they obtain when their physician is aware of their orientation (3). Studies of lesbians have shown that many are reluctant to disclose their sexual orientation to their physicians because of fear of judgmental attitudes (19).

Male homosexuals require special considerations in their routine medical care. Those who have multiple partners should always be asked about their knowledge of safe sex practices (see Chapter 34) and about symptoms that might be caused by sexually transmitted disease, including human immunodeficiency virus (HIV) infection (see Chapter 34), and they should be screened periodically for type B hepatitis (Chapter 43), syphilis (Chapter 30), and gonorrhea (Chapter 27). Men who practice receptive anal intercourse are subject to both infectious and traumatic anorectal conditions (see Chapter 94).

Most sexually transmitted diseases are uncommon in *lesbian patients,* with the exception of three forms of vaginitis—candidiasis, trichomoniasis, and nonspecific vaginitis—each of which should be considered when a known lesbian patient has a vaginal discharge (see Chapter 93) (19). It is possible that the risk of breast cancer is increased in lesbians. In the absence of adequate information, cancer screening recommendations for lesbians should be those for other women according to age group (see Chapter 2) (19).

SPECIAL CONSIDERATIONS FOR SELECTED AGE GROUPS

Elderly Patients

Aging people do not lose their capacity for sexual function on the basis of the aging process alone. It is important to invite questions regarding sexual function in the general care of older patients because they are often embarrassed to bring up this aspect of their health. Patients who have any of the sexual disorders discussed above should be evaluated in the same manner as one would evaluate a younger patient. The predictable changes associated with aging are slower arousal phase, increased ability to stay at plateau levels of arousal, and in men, a longer refractory period. Women commonly experience dyspareunia as a result of atrophic vaginitis following menopause; management of this treatable problem is described in Chapter 77.

Children

It is unusual for children to complain of sexual difficulties. However, parents occasionally ask their own physicians questions about the developing sexuality of their children. Parents may express concern about the appearance of sexual behavior in children such as mutual exploration of playmates' genitalia or masturbation. The parents can be assured that the behavior is normal and that the behavior should be discouraged in a nonpunitive fashion. Failure to control the behavior may require further evaluation of both the child and the family.

Occasionally, a physician may recognize the presence of *sexual abuse within a family,* either on the basis of physical findings or from information disclosed by a child during a medical visit. If the abuse has been committed by someone outside the family, both the child and parents may require supportive counseling to help them vent their fear and anger about the experience. Discovery of sexual abuse within a family should be fully evaluated. This should be initiated by reporting the problem to the division of protective services of the local department of social services.

Adolescents

Adolescent sexual difficulties (see Chapter 5) may be brought to the attention of the physician by either the adolescent or the adolescent's parents. Adolescents who are sexually active may have questions about their sexual function, birth control, venereal disease, or abortion. In most states, a physician may provide service for sex-related problems to the adolescent with or without the parental consent.

Adolescents may request consultation about *isolated homosexual experiences* or homosexual fantasies. In most cases, the physician's role is to reassure the adolescent that these experiences are normal and not indicative of the development of life-long homosexuality. Adolescents who have developed a homosexual orientation or who are in the process of doing so may be brought to the physician by parents disturbed at the discovery of homosexual activities. In these instances, counseling should be given to the parents to help them accept the adolescent's orientation. Older adolescents (above 17 years) are unlikely to change their orientation. Younger adolescents (below 17 years) have not consolidated their personality development and should be offered referral for psychiatric evaluation and possible treatment.

GENDER IDENTITY DISORDERS

Gender identity disorders are divided into childhood and adult disorders. The essential feature of both groups of disorders is the incongruence between anatomic sex and gender identity.

Predisposing Factors

No known genetic or biochemical predisposing factors have been elucidated. There is some evidence that these disorders may stem from faulty parent–child relationships in situations in which parents have confused sexual identity or have a need to raise a child of one sex in the role of the opposite sex.

Prevalence

These disorders are apparently rare. Male cases are more common than female cases, the reported ratio varying from 8 to 1 to as low as 2 to 1.

Age of Onset

For children, the initial expression of the wish to be in the cross-gender role may take place as early as the fourth birthday. For adults, the manifestations of this disorder usually become apparent in early adulthood, although the adults usually state that they had been aware of wishes to be in the cross-gender role since childhood or adolescence.

Course

The course of the disorder for children is as yet unknown. An undetermined number of affected boys and girls may adopt a homosexual orientation during adolescence or as adults. The course in adults is variable. For some it is chronic and unremitting, with a persistent drive toward attaining surgical reassignment. For others, the intensity of the desire for living and functioning in the cross-gender role waxes and wanes, often associated with current life stress and the appearance of psychiatric symptoms, principally depression. Females who are interested in sexual reassignment are a more homogeneous group than the males, in that they are more likely to have a history of homosexuality and by and large have a more stable course with or without treatment.

Complications

The principal complications are those associated with the desire and attempt to live and function socially and occupationally in the cross-gender role. In addition, there is a moderate degree of associated psychopathology, including episodes of depression and suicide attempts. In rare instances, affected males may attempt to mutilate their genitals.

Assessment

The assessment of these disorders in adults is fairly simple: Most such patients identify themselves as being unhappy with their anatomic sex and interested in a surgical reassignment. No endocrinologic studies are indicated, and physical findings show that the people seeking surgical reassignment are genetically normal men or women. However, the generalist may see rare cases of patients who have a congenital inter-sexed condition and who are confused about their sexual identification.

Treatment

Patients with gender identity disorders should be referred to psychiatrists or to special programs that have the expertise to treat these problems. Gender-disordered patients who are in a cross-gender program and who need continuous administration of cross-gender hormones may be transferred to the generalist. Some physicians may not agree with such treatment, and these patients should select physicians who are comfortable working with it.

THE PARAPHILIAS

The paraphilias is a group of disorders in which sexual interests are directed primarily toward objects other than other human beings, toward sexual acts not usually associated with coitus, or toward coitus performed under bizarre conditions.

The formal diagnosis of each of these conditions includes as criteria that the person has acted on the specific urges or is markedly distressed by them and that the problem has been present for at least 6 months.

Exhibitionism

Exhibitionism is the displaying of the genital organs for the purpose of sexual gratification. This is predominantly a male activity. Orgasmic release is usually achieved through masturbation.

Fetishism

Fetishism is the nearly exclusive displacement of erotic interest in sexual satisfaction to an object or to a body part other than those usually associated with genital sexuality. Common fetish objects are female undergarments (particularly worn or soiled ones), feet, and shoes. Orgasmic release may be achieved by any of the behavior used by adults in sexual activities.

Zoophilia

Zoophilia is the use of animals as a preferred or exclusive method of achieving sexual excitement. The animal may be the object of intercourse or may be trained to excite the human partner sexually by licking or rubbing. The animal is preferred no matter what other forms of sexual outlet are available.

Pedophilia

Pedophilia is a condition in which adults compulsively involve children in their sexual activities. The sexual behavior that results in orgasmic release may be heterosexual or homosexual and includes any behavior used by adults in their sexual activities. In most cases, however, the pedophile is concerned with mutual masturbation or fondling rather than coitus.

Voyeurism

Voyeurism is a deviation in which sexual stimulation and gratification are obtained from looking at the sexual organs of others or from observing their sexual activities. Orgasmic release is usually achieved by masturbating during or just after the period of observation.

Sadism and Masochism

Sadism and masochism are deviations in which sexual arousal and gratification depend on either inflicting pain (sadism) or experiencing it (masochism). There is a broad spectrum of behavior, ranging from the dim awareness of cruelty or suffering as part of the sexual experience to overt behavior, including extreme physical injury and murder. Aspects of sadism and masochism are usually found in the same person, even though one or the other behavior appears dominant.

General Characteristics of the Paraphilias

Predisposing Factors

The cause is unknown. However, history of physical or sexual abuse during childhood appears in a modest number of cases.

Prevalence

The disorders are rare. The sex ratio is predominantly in favor of males, with the exception of sexual sadism and masochism.

Course

The course of these disorders is usually chronic. Peaks of deviant activity may accompany current life stress or be associated with psychiatric symptoms, principally depressive episodes. If the deviant behavior brings the person into conflict with society, the outcome can often include arrest and incarceration. Treatment is difficult because of the egosyntonic nature of the behavior. Anxiety and depression may be associated with the fear of being discovered, arrested, or punished; however, once these dangers have passed, the uncomfortable affect disappears and the person has little motivation for treatment.

Complications

Because these disorders are often associated with other defects in personality development, the capacity for developing long-term, affectionate relationships may be impaired. The possibility of being involved in criminal violations has already been mentioned. In some instances the behavior may bring the person into extremely dangerous situations, resulting in severe injury or death.

Assessment

It is not difficult to diagnose a specific paraphilia once the history is obtained. No specific laboratory tests are indicated. The physical examination is usually normal. Sadistic or masochistic behavior may produce physical injuries. Hypersexuality, including some deviant behavior, has been reported to be associated with temporal lobe epilepsy (2). Thus, in cases in which there is suggestion of a seizure disorder, an electroencephalogram is indicated. Psychiatric disorders, principally depression secondary to loss, may precipitate bursts of deviant behavior in paraphiliacs. Abuse of alcohol or other substances may also increase the behavior.

Stress, anxiety, organic brain syndrome, and mental retardation may lead to episodic deviant behavior, but these episodes are not diagnosed as paraphilia.

Treatment

Psychotherapy or other psychologic treatment designed to control or eliminate paraphiliac behavior is best provided by a psychiatrist. The general physician's role in the care of these patients is in the management of concurrent medical problems. Of major concern are recognition and treatment of venereal disease in patients whose sexual behavior is promiscuous, and the possibility of child abuse in families that have paraphiliac members. Many people who engage in paraphilias were subjected to physical or sexual abuse as children. The pattern is often passed on from generation to generation.

General References*

American Psychiatric Association. **Diagnostic and Statistical Manual of Mental Disorders.** 4th ed. Washington, DC: American Psychiatric Association, 1994.
> Diagnostic criteria and epidemiologic information for all recognized psychiatric disorders.

Crenshaw TL, Goldberg JP. Sexual pharmacology: drugs that affect sexual function. New York: WW Norton, 1996.
> The definitive reference about the effects of drugs on sexual function.

Drugs that cause sexual dysfunction: an update. Med Lett 34:73, 1992.
> Well-referenced brief review. Exhaustive list of drugs and, for each, type of sexual dysfunction that it may cause.

Kinsey AC, Pomeroy WB, Martin CE. Sexual behavior in the human male. Philadelphia: WB Saunders, 1948.
> Long-standing and still widely cited resource (now somewhat outdated).

Krane RJ, Goldstein I, Saenz de Tejada I. Impotence. N Engl J Med 231:1648, 1989.
> Extensively referenced review.

Masters WH, Johnson VE. Human sexual inadequacy. Boston: Little, Brown, 1970.
> The original and still used descriptive work on the behavioral treatment of common sexual disorders.

Meyer K, Schmidt CW, Wise TN, eds. Clinical management of sexual disorders. Baltimore: Williams & Wilkins, 1983.
> Textbook that addresses the evaluation, diagnosis, and treatment of a wide variety of sexual disorders.

The Psychiatric Clinics of North America. Sexuality. Philadelphia: WB Saunders, 1980.
> A concise review.

Segraves RT. Effects of psychotropic drugs on human erection and ejaculation. Arch Gen Psychiatry 46:275, 1989.
> An excellent review of the physiology and receptor chemistry associated with male arousal.

Wagner G, Kaplan HS. The new injection treatment for impotence: medical and psychological aspects. New York: Brunner/Mazel, 1993.
> Detailed book that gives equal weight to physiologic and psychologic aspects of injection treatment for impotence.

---

*Bold print (general references) and bold numerals (specific references) denote published controlled clinical trials, meta-analyses, or consensus-based recommendations.

Specific References

1. Anonymous. SCRIP World Pharmaceutical News. London: PJB Publications, No. 2129, May 17, 1996:24.
2. Blumer D. Changes of sexual behavior related to temporal lobe disorders in man. J Sex Res 6:173, 1970.
3. Dardick L, Grady KE. Openness between gay persons and health professionals. Ann Intern Med 93:115, 1980.
4. Ende J, Rockwell S, Glasgow M. The sexual history in general medicine practice. Arch Intern Med 144:558, 1984.
5. Ellenberg M. Impotence in diabetes: the neurologic factor. Ann Intern Med 75:213, 1971.
6. Fagan P, Schmidt CW, Wise TN, Derogatis R. Sexual dysfunction and dual psychiatric diagnoses. Compr Psychol 29(3):278, 1988.
7. Furlow WL. Surgical treatment of erectile impotence using the inflatable penile prosthesis. Sex Disabil 1:299, 1978.
8. Intracavernous injections for impotence. Med Lett 32:115, 1990.
9. Karacan I. Diagnosis of impotence in diabetes mellitus: an objective and specific method. Ann Intern Med 92:334, 1980.
10. Kiely EA, Williams G, Goldie L. Assessment of the immediate and long-term effects of pharmacologically induced penile erections in the treatment of psychogenic and organic impotence. Br J Urol 59:164, 1987.
11. Kolodny RC. Sexual dysfunction in diabetic females. Diabetes 20:557, 1971.
12. Morales A, Condra MS, Owen JA, et al. Is yohimbine effective in the treatment of organic impotence? Results of a controlled trial. J Urol 137:1168, 1987.
13. Mulligan T, Katz G. Why aged men become impotent. Arch Intern Med 149:1365, 1989.
14. **Padma-Nathan H, et al. Treatment of men with erectile dysfunction with transurethral alprostadil. N Engl J Med 336:1, 1997.**
15. **Reid K, Morales A, Harris C, et al. Double-blind trial of yohimbine in treatment of psychogenic impotence. Lancet 2(8556):421–423, 1987.**
16. Schmidt CW Biochemical treatment of sexual disorders. Psychiatr Clin North Am 3:89, 1980.
17. Small MP. The Small–Carrion penile prosthesis: surgical implant for the management of impotence. Sex Disabil 1:282, 1978.
18. Spark RF, White RA, Connolly PB. Impotence is not always psychogenic: newer insights into hypothalamic–pituitary–gonadal dysfunction. JAMA 243:750, 1980.
19. White J, Levinson W. Primary care of lesbian patients. J Gen Intern Med 8:41, 1993.

C H A P T E R   19

Dying, Death, and Bereavement

LARRY WATERBURY, MD
MICHAEL J. PURTELL, MD

Family physicians traditionally took care of their patients from cradle to death, and then they managed the grief and bereavement of the survivors. This situation has changed dramatically in the last 40 to 50 years, partly because of the mobility of the society and partly because of the increased specialization of physicians. Until 40 or 50 years ago, dying patients stayed at home or returned home from the hospital to be with their family when death was imminent. The physician had a major role in managing the moment of death.

During the second half of the 20th century, interest in the care of dying patients has grown steadily, stimulated in the last decade by the growth of the hospice movement. It is likely that, because of this interest, the general physician again will be able to treat many dying patients in their own homes.

SOCIOPSYCHOLOGIC ISSUES

Fear of Death

Humans are the only creatures known who bury their dead; they have done this since the very dawn of human culture, possibly as far back as 50,000 BC. Before the 11th century AD, life after death was seen as a kind of sleep for an indeterminate period. Death was calmly accepted, without fear. Then the concept of the last judgment began to be taken seriously. An awe and fear of death became manifest in art and culture. The image of purgatory, heaven, and hell, which preoccupied the minds of medieval people, continues to exert its influence on a significant sector of society today.

Although they are aware that death is their ultimate fate, contemporary people are often incapable of facing their own death. The fear of death is intricately linked with facing the finality of one's being and the separation from one's loved ones. Therefore, it is unusual for one to reflect persistently on death unless his or her own life is threatened or unless a close friend or relative is dying.

Fear of Dying

Fear of dying should not be confused with fear of death. Death is the ultimate moment of the cessation of life, and dying is the process whereby that moment is approached. Fear of dying is actually a combination of fear of death and fear of living in dread of death. Whether one is dying at home or in a hospital, one cannot escape the agony of dying. Writings of doctors who attended many deaths at home give vivid descriptions of patients ravaged by pain and disease to such a point that they were often beyond caring and their presence was extraordinarily stressful for their family and friends. On the other hand, dying in a hospital's impersonal environment surrounded by machines and by unfamiliar staff cannot be glamorized either. The technology that has given us the knowledge and equipment to prolong life is greatly responsible for "the medicalization of death" that we see today. The treatment of a dying patient ends with the onset of irreversible coma, and what is left afterward is management of death. Death has been dissected and seen as a phenomenon of several steps: cessation of consciousness, cessation of breathing, and cessation of brain activity, manifested by a flat electroencephalogram. The contemporary fear of dying also involves the dread of a protracted death.

A dying person often continues to hope for a miraculous recovery, but when the hopelessness of the treatment becomes evident, a strange sense of helplessness comes over the patient. Self-blame for not having taken good care of oneself and guilt about one's conduct may cause a patient to view the terminal illness as some kind of punishment. The fear of physical injury and mutilation from drastic treatment, chemotherapy, radiotherapy, or surgical therapy is not to be discounted. Finally, the fear of a crippled existence and of being left alone to die in isolation away from family, friends, and children is present in the back of the mind of many terminally ill patients.

Emotional Reactions in the Face of Death

Terminally ill patients often go through a series of five stages in accepting the reality of their impending death (4). The duration of these stages and the intensity and sequence with which they are experienced are highly variable from one patient to the next. The stages are

1. Shock and denial
2. Anger
3. Bargaining
4. Depression
5. Acceptance

During the first stage, when patients are informed of their diagnosis and poor prognosis, they are usually unable to "hear" it. Some patients may be shocked and surprised temporarily, but a profound sense of disbelief in the physician's pronouncements keeps them calm. They may go from physician to physician to find someone to tell them what they would like to hear—that their condition is not serious. This denial of illness can be best summed up in a phrase: "No, not me." Eventually, all such attempts are deemed to be futile and the patient has to face reality.

During the stage of anger it may be difficult to deal with patients. They complain about their care and, as a result, family, friends, and physicians may avoid them. This rejection further increases their rage. They are likely to ask, "Why me?" They often feel cheated and envious of others. If one does not feel guilty and lose one's self-esteem, he or she is likely, after this period of anger, to move on to the stage of bargaining. On the other hand, if one feels that he or she deserves punishment for past doings as an explanation of one's illness, he or she is likely to become very depressed. From being very mad the patient moves to being very sad.

During the stage of bargaining the dominant theme is "Yes, it is me, but . . ." With the realization of an impending death, patients offer to do things that they did not do before or to live their lives differently in exchange for the prolongation of their life. A number of patients go through a religious experience, and some of them believe that they are "born again." Often at this stage the patient looks comfortable and peaceful, but that sense of well-being is short lived. As the illness advances and suffering is compounded, the patient becomes depressed.

During the stage of depression the reality of impending death sinks even deeper. Patients may have already gone through many real (and imagined) losses by this time, such as loss of a body organ, missing important events in the lives of their family members, or loss of their job or savings. Depression at this stage is not so much compounded by anger as it is colored with resignation. Patients begin to separate from everyone and everything they loved before. At this time they do not want any false hopes. It is a very private and personal time in their lives. They may not want any visitors and may not even say much to their own immediate family members. They want their family's love, affection, and respect but may not be able to give them anything in return. They may exhaust their caregivers by developing regressive behavior patterns, such as failing to accomplish activities of daily living of which they are capable, making many small demands, and becoming incontinent. This stage is very difficult for the family.

Finally, when patients have finished their business—experienced anger and experienced grief—they move to the *stage of acceptance.* If patients have the strong support of their family, they go through all stages to arrive at a final stage of equanimity characterized by tranquillity, in which the patient is neither happy nor sad. At this stage, a patient may simply say "My time is coming close," "It is all right," or "I am ready."

CARE OF A DYING PERSON

Most patients who experience prolonged but predictable dying are patients in the terminal stage of cancer or, currently, acquired immunodeficiency syndrome (AIDS). This discussion focuses on terminal care for such patients, much or all of which can be provided out of hospital. Chapters 8 and 34, respectively, describe the care of patients with cancer and patients with AIDS before the terminal stage.

Throughout the care of a patient with terminal illness, it is important to determine the physical stage of the illness but also the patient's psychologic stage of accepting impending death (see above) and the patient's concerns regarding family or business affairs. Terminally ill patients' needs differ widely, and every effort should be made to provide care that is adapted to these unique needs.

Communication

Communication of Diagnosis, Treatment Plan, and Prognosis

People have different opinions about the need for and importance of communication about the diagnosis, treatment plan, and prognosis of terminally ill patients. A common practice in the past, which still prevails in some societies (9), was to maintain a conspiracy of silence in which the patient's physician in collusion with family members covered up the diagnosis of a terminal illness to "protect" the dying patient from emotional shock. This practice may lead to isolation of the patient from family, friends, and physician. Honesty and sincerity toward the patient usually make dealing with terminal illness more bearable for patient, family members, and physicians and others involved in caring for the patient. Although most patients become temporarily demoralized in the face of this news, they appreciate the truth in the long run. Moreover, it is then easier for their families to relate to them in an open and honest manner. Families participating in a conspiracy of silence have greater emotional difficulties than do families in situations in which truth has prevailed. Occasionally, patients indicate that they do not want to know the unpleasant truth; in that case, one should respect that wish. However, invariably these patients, and those whose physician and family withhold the diagnosis from them, come to know the nature of their illness even if it has not been told directly to them.

Giving and Discussing Bad News. When one is ready to discuss the diagnosis and expected course of the illness with a terminally ill patient, a number of considerations can be helpful. It is important to sit down with the patient and the family in a private place, to avoid lengthy introductions, to be precise and concise but not hurried, and to pay attention to the emotional reactions of the patient and of the family members, responding with silent pauses, followed by verbal acknowledgment of the patient's emotional reactions, rather than providing details about the patient's disease. It is also important not to use euphemisms (e.g., *swelling, tumor,* or *lump*) but to acknowledge the presence of cancer or malignant disease and to pledge to help reduce suffering as much as possible, affirming that one will be involved and supportive to the very end. Most patients do not hear the bad news when it is first delivered and must be told the truth in small doses in the course of several interviews.

Often terminally ill patients receive attention during the early stages of their illness, but that attention wanes as their disease progresses. This occurs largely because of the helplessness that others feel when confronting the patient's plight. The stages of denial, anger, and depression often cause a withdrawal of family, friends, physicians, and other caregivers, and these behaviors establish a vicious cycle; that is, the more the patient is ignored, the more unmanageable and inaccessible the patient becomes. For these reasons, a most important principle of the care of a terminally ill patient is for all parties to maintain a consistency of involvement. The physician should counsel family members in this regard and should plan regular contacts with the patient, either by scheduling office visits or by making visits to the home. These actions can reduce patients' anguish, making it easier for them to express feelings and ask questions. Above all, continued and consistent involvement of physician, family, and other caregivers gives dignity to dying people. The patient continues to feel like a person until the very end.

Advance Directives from the Patient

There is good evidence that patients with terminal illness would welcome early in their clinical course a discussion of the degree and type of support they wish to receive as they become more ill. One study (8) revealed that almost 80% of patients with terminal cancer would not want ventilators or other life support and 50% would want only treatment directed at comfort and pain relief. Ninety percent favored the routine availability of living wills or proxy designation. The majority felt that discussions of these issues should occur early after the diagnosis of a serious illness. Other data suggest that most physicians remain hesitant to initiate discussions of advance directives with patients, especially early in the course of the illness (11). It is important for the physician to help patients and families express their preferences because patients' preferences often are not to have heroic treatment or even continuing supportive care at the end of their terminal illness. These discussions, difficult as they are, spare the patient inappropriate interventions and help maintain dignity during the dying process. Chapter 6 ("Geriatric Medicine: Special Considerations") describes in detail the process of helping patients to delineate advance directives.

The educational organization Choice in Dying provides helpful information regarding living wills and other ways to protect the autonomy of a dying person (200 Varick Street, New York, NY 10014, 212-366-5540).

Communication with the Patient's Family

The emotional problems of the family of the dying person need attention. Family members go through stages of emotional adjustment and have difficulties in accepting the diagnosis and projected course of a terminal illness, just as the patient does. By encouraging open communication between the patient and the family, the physician can make an important contribution in the care of the dying person. Each family member will react differently to the impending death of a person, depending on his or her age, personality, role, and relationship with the patient and the rest of the family. To be effective, the physician must be aware of these factors and allocate time to meet the needs of individual family members. It may be helpful to convene a *family meeting* one or more times to deal with decisions (see the practical approach to this in Chapter 3).

The important advice to family members includes the fact that a dying person has a great need to have access to his or her children and the children have a great need to be close to their dying parent. The physician should encourage these necessary contacts. In addition, the family should be urged to find ways to gratify small needs of the patient. Removing restrictions from food, alcohol, and cigarettes is not only humane but sensible. Considerations such as these are described in an excellent booklet for families, *Taking Time, Support for People with Cancer and the People Who Care About Them* (available free from the National Cancer Institute, Bethesda, MD 20205; phone 1-800-422-6237). It was prepared by patients with terminal cancer and their families to help others deal with many draining and awkward experiences that they will face.

Management of Pain, Anxiety, Depression, Delirium, Dyspnea

Pain

A large number of patients with cancer have significant pain during the terminal stage of their illness. Therefore, a basic principle in the care of these patients is to provide adequate relief of pain. This often requires the administration of narcotics. Because of fear of inducing addiction, patients may receive dosages of narcotics that are too small or too infrequent to relieve pain adequately. In fact, the risk of addiction in this setting is slight; narcotics should be given on schedule (not as needed), including at night, when it is often better to disturb patients for their medication than to wait for pain to waken them.

Another misconception about narcotic use in patients with cancer concerns *tolerance.* Many patients with cancer who take narcotics do not develop tolerance and are able to remain on the same dosage of medication for prolonged periods. When tolerance does occur, it usually manifests itself as a decrease in the duration of analgesia and can be treated by shortening the dose interval or increasing the dosage or both. When the requirement for medication increases, this is often caused by disease progression rather than the development of tolerance. *Physical dependence* (abstinence syndrome occurring at the time of abrupt withdrawal of narcotics) develops within 2 weeks of the initiation of narcotic therapy in most patients.

Important considerations in *selecting medication* for pain are effectiveness, route of administration (e.g., the cachectic patient may have few sites for injections), available forms for oral administration (e.g., some patients may be able to take only liquids easily; liquid morphine is especially useful for such patients), and duration of pain relief. Table 19.1 summarizes practical information about a number of narcotics that are used in controlling pain.

It is often more accurate to *assess the adequacy of pain* relief after a given regimen has been in place for 24 hours. It is best to prevent pain from surfacing by using appropriate dosages and dosing intervals, rather than to gradually increase the dosage until pain is relieved. Thus, narcotics should be prescribed to be taken at a given interval routinely, not only as needed. Appropriate intervals may be as frequent as hourly for oral liquid morphine. In evaluating pain control over time, it is helpful to use a visual analog scale, such as the scale illustrated in Figure 19.1, providing an ongoing record of the effectiveness of pain treatment (7).

Sometimes pain control is inadequate with oral or

Table 19.1. Selected Drugs for Treating Pain

Constituents	Trade Name	Available Preparations	Usual Dose Range[a]	Approximate Equivalent IM Dose of Morphine	Peak Effect (hr)	Duration (hr)	Federal Narcotic Schedule
Moderately Potent							
Codeine phosphate		Tablets, 30, 60, mg	30–120 mg	1–6 mg	2	3–4	II
		Injectable, 10 mg/5 mL					
Codeine–acetaminophen[b]	Tylenol No. 3	Tablets, 30 mg codeine	1–2 tablets	1–2 mg	2	3–4	III
	Tylenol No. 4	Tablets, 60 mg codeine	1 tablet	2 mg	2		
		Elixir, 12 mg codeine/ 5 mL	15–30 mL				
Oxycodone	Roxicodone	Tablets, 5 mg	1–3 tablets	1–5 mg	1	3–4	II
		Liquid, 5 mg/5 mL	5–15 mL	1–5 mg	1	3–4	
	Oxycontin[c]	Controlled-release tablets 10, 20, 40 mg	10–80 mg	2–16 mg	3	12	
Oxycodone aspirin– phenacetin–caffeine	Percodan	Tablets, 5 mg oxycodone	1–3 tablets	1–5 mg	1	3–4	II
Oxycodone acetaminophen	Tylox[d]	Capsules, 5 mg oxycodone	1–2 capsules	1–3 mg	1	3–4	II
	Percocet[b] Roxicet[b]	Tablets, 5 mg oxycodone	1–3 tablets	1–5 mg	1	3–4	
Most Potent							
Morphine sulfate[a]		Injectable, 10 mg/mL	10–30 mg	10–30 mg	0.5	3–4	II
		Constant infusion[e]	1–20 mg/hr	NA	NA	NA	
		Liquid, multiple concentrations	20–200 mg	4–40 mg	1	2–3	
		Tablets 30, 60 mg	30–90 mg	6–20 mg	1	3–4	
	MS Contin[c]	Controlled release 15, 30, 60, 100 mg	30–200 mg	6–40 mg	3	8–12	
	RMS suppos	Suppository, 5, 10, 20, 30 mg	30–90 mg	6–20 mg	1	3–4	
Methadone[f]	Dolophine	Tablets, 5, 10 mg	2.5–20 mg	1–10 mg	2	4–5	II
		Injectable, 10 mg/mL		10 mg			
Meperidine	Demerol	Tablets, 50, 100 mg	50–300 mg	2–10 mg	2	3–4	II
		Syrup, 50 mg/5 mL					
		Injectable, 25, 50, 75, 100 mg/mL	50–150 mg	6–20 mg	1	2–4	
Hydromorphone	Dilaudid	Tablets, 1, 2, 3, 4 mg	2–8 mg	4–10 mg	1	3–4	II
		Suppository, 3 mg					
		Injectable, 1, 2, 3 mg/mL	1–2 mg	10 mg	0.5	3	
Levorphanol[f]	Levo-Dromoran	Tablets, 2 mg	2–4 mg	5–10 mg	2	4–5	II
Fentanyl transdermal patch[e]	Duragesic[c]	Patch 25, 50, 75, 100 µg/hr	50–300 µg/hr	30–360 mg/day	12	48–72	II

[a]Higher doses are needed in patients who develop tolerance. (oral/parenteral ratio = 6 to 1 for one dose, 3 to 1 for multiple doses)

[b]Each tablet contains 300 mg acetaminophen; elixir contains 120 mg (Perocet) or 325 mg (Roxicet) acetaminophen per 5 mL.

[c]Controlled-release treatment may need to be supplemented with short-acting oral narcotics.

[d]Each capsule contains 500 mg acetaminophen.

[e]See text for further details.

[f]The plasma half-life of methadone and levorphanol is long (≥15 hr) and cumulative effects may occur with continual use of these drugs.

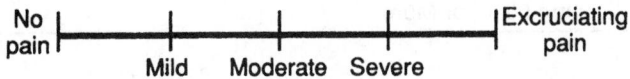

Figure 19.1. Visual analog scale for rating pain severity.

intramuscular medication. *Constant infusion of narcotics* may provide more even and satisfactory pain relief (3). In these instances, morphine or hydromorphone is usually prescribed and the medication is delivered via a small portable pump. The pump allows an infusion of a constant dose plus a periodic bolus programmed to allow the patient to better control the degree of analgesia *(patient-controlled analgesia, or PCA).* The subcutaneous route is far preferable to the intravenous route because of ease of care (family members can be taught how to change the subcutaneous site). Medicare and other third-party payers will pay for constant infusion of narcotics for cancer pain, making this an important option for patients without prescription plans.

An alternative to constant narcotic infusion is *transdermal administration,* using fentanyl patches. The patches provide constant narcotic blood levels (achieved 8 to 12 hours after initial application) for 48 to 72 hours. The patches are expensive (two to four times the cost of equianalgesic doses of oral narcotics), and one usually needs to supplement with as-needed oral narcotics when the patches are initially applied and for breakthrough pain. Blood levels remain constant at the time of changing the patch (usually after 72 hours) because, when the old patch is removed, the skin depot continues to release drug as the new depot accumulates. One should start low and slowly build up the dosage, supplementing with oral analgesics as needed. If a patient is overmedicated, the drug will be in the blood for hours after the patch is removed.

All narcotic analgesics may cause the following *side effects:* sedation, respiratory depression, emesis, suppression of cough, constipation, bladder spasm, or urinary retention. In the terminally ill patient, rarely, there may be a need to reverse narcotic effect because of respiratory depression. When possible one should simply withhold the next dose. If reversal is needed, this can be achieved with small doses of naloxone (0.1 to 0.2 mg intravenously every few minutes) but with the use of naloxone one runs the risk of acute withdrawal and severe pain.

Nausea is an extremely common side effect of narcotic usage in terminally ill patients and should be treated actively. Phenothiazines are usually helpful for narcotic-induced nausea. Prochlorperazine (Compazine, 5 to 10 mg orally or 25 mg by suppository every 4 to 6 hours) causes less sedation and hypotension than chlorpromazine. Haloperidol (0.5 to 2 mg orally or subcutaneously every 6 to 8 hours) is useful for nausea in the agitated patient. Methylprogesterone (Megace) 160 to 800 mg/day can help nausea as well as stimulate appetite. Metoclopramide (Reglan, 10 to 20 mg orally or intramuscularly every 6 hours) is useful if gastric

fullness is a common complaint. Dexamethasone (4 mg every 8 to 24 hours) may also be helpful in the nauseated patient; hyoscyamine (Levsin tabs, 1 or 2 tabs every 4 hours) is useful for controlling secretions.

Constipation is a universal problem in the terminally ill patient who is taking narcotics; it should be treated prophylactically. Bulk laxatives require an adequate intake of food and fluid to be effective and may have little use in the terminally ill patient with poor oral intake. A stool softener alone is rarely effective for narcotic-induced constipation. More useful, sequential strategies are the following:

1. Use daily a preparation that combines a stool softener and a mild stimulant laxative such as dioctyl sodium sulfosuccinate plus casanthranol (Peri-Colace, 1 daily to 2 three times daily) or docusate sodium plus senna (Senokot-S, 1 daily to 4 three times daily).
2. If no success, add bisacodyl (Dulcolax, 5 mg by mouth at bedtime to 15 mg three times daily or milk of magnesia, 30 to 60 mL once or twice daily).
3. If still unsuccessful, add lactulose (Chronulac, 10 g/15 mL, 30 to 45 mL at bedtime or twice a day).
4. If constipation continues, check for *impaction.* If present, with a hard stool, try glycerine suppositories or olive oil retention enemas. If there is no impaction, add bisacodyl suppositories (Dulcolax, 10 mg) or Fleets enema.

A number of adjunctive pharmacologic and non-pharmacologic measures may help the terminally ill patient with pain. Aspirin and other nonsteroidal anti-inflammatory drugs at dosages similar to those used for musculoskeletal pain are often helpful for many types of pain, especially bone pain caused by metastases. Table 19.2 summarizes practical information and indications for other nonnarcotic drugs to control pain. Tricyclic antidepressants may be helpful for neuropathic pain, especially if the pain is associated with insomnia or depression. Corticosteroids are useful for spinal cord compression, brain tumors, and other nerve compression syndromes. They also, at least in the short run, increase appetite, mood, and general sense of well-being. Methylphenidate (Ritalin) may be useful to combat the lethargy of analgesics. Transcutaneous nerve stimulation may be helpful temporarily for localized (particularly neuropathic) pain. A number of psychologic approaches (hypnosis, relaxation training, guided imagery, distraction techniques) are also useful for the cancer patient with pain (see practical approaches described in Chapter 13).

Anxiety

The family's and physician's concern and accessibility may be all that are necessary to relieve the anxiety of the dying patient. Anxiolytic drugs also can be of some help in the management of these patients. Commonly prescribed anxiolytic drugs belong to the benzodiazepine group; their use for the control of anxiety is described in detail in Chapter 13. When insomnia is also a major problem, a benzodiazepine hypnotic can

Table 19.2.   Adjuvant Analgesic Drugs for Adults and Children Weighing 50 kg or More

Class and Drug	Approximate Dosage Range	Administration	Use
Corticosteroids			
Dexamethasone	16–96 mg/day	Oral or intravenous	For pain associated with brain metastases and epidural spinal cord compression
Prednisone	40–80 mg/day	Oral	
Anticonvulsant Agents			
Carbamazepine	200–1600 mg/day	Oral	For neuropathic pain
Gabapentin	900 mg–1 g/day	Oral	
Phenytoin	300–500 mg/day	Oral	
Antidepressant Agents			
Amitriptyline	25–150 mg/day	Oral	For neuropathic pain
Doxepin	25–150 mg/day	Oral	
Imipramine	20–100 mg/day	Oral	
Neuroleptic Agents			
Methotrimeprazine	40–80 mg/day	Intramuscular	For analgesia, for sedation, as antiemetic agent
Antihistamines			
Hydroxyzine	300–450 mg/day	Intramuscular	As adjuvant to opioids for postoperative and other types of pain; for relief of complicating symptoms including anxiety, insomnia, and nausea
Local Anesthetic and Antiarrhythmic Agents			
Lidocaine	5 mg/kg per day[a]	Intravenous or subcutaneous	For neuropathic pain
Mexiletin	450–600 mg/day	Oral	
Tocainide	20 mg/kg per day[a]	Oral	
Psychostimulants			
Dextroamphetamine	5–10 mg/day	Oral	To improve opioid analgesia and decrease sedation
Methylphenidate	10–15 mg/day	Oral	

Adapted from Agency for Health Care Policy and Research (AHCPR). Management of cancer pain: clinical practice guideline, Publication No. 94-0592, 1994.
[a]The dosage give is per kilogram of body weight per day.

be used to induce sleep (see Table 85.8). The sedating antihistamine hydroxyzine (Atarax, Vistaril), 25 to 50 mg by mouth three times daily, may also help patients who have anxiety associated with pain.

Depression

Most patients who go through the depressive stage of dying do not require antidepressant medications, although periodically some may require antianxiety medications. The family's and the physician's support is most therapeutic for this kind of depression. Some patients develop severe depression, particularly after a brief stage of anger, when they conclude that they are being punished for their sins. Loss of self-esteem, guilt feelings, psychomotor retardation, early morning awakening with a diurnal variation in mood, and even suicidal thoughts may appear in this setting. When a number of these and other indicators of a major depression are present, antidepressants may bring relief. There is a detailed discussion of the use of these drugs in Chapter 15.

Delirium

Periodic or persistent delirium (inattentiveness, inaccessibility, inability to recognize loved ones, gross confusion) is very common in the final days or weeks of terminal disease (5). The cause is almost always an identifiable metabolic derangement, infection, excess

analgesic or psychotropic medication, tumor metastasis to the brain, or a combination of these factors. Loss of clear communication as a result of delirium is distressing to the patient's family. Management of easily reversible causes is therefore very important except in the patient whose death is imminent. A list of the principal causes of delirium is found in Chapter 17.

Dyspnea

Dyspnea is a common and distressing symptom for the dying patient. Physical impediments to breathing and psychologic fears and discomfort are often combined when a patient is near death. In this situation, a number of measures can help. If patients have rapidly recurring pleural effusions, a small-diameter tube can be placed in the radiology suite, left in for days to weeks, and managed at home without the discomfort associated with chest tube placement and sclerosis. Positioning the patient upright in bed or in a chair and administering oxygen (if the patient is hypoxic) are useful. Patients may feel better if air is circulated by them from a fan or an open window. If the patient and caretaker can be taught relaxation techniques (see Chapter 13) and calming strategies this can be very useful. Low dosages of opiates (e.g., morphine 2 mg intravenously every 1 to 2 hours as needed) may be helpful for the terminally ill dyspneic patient and when carefully titrated can calm without leading to respiratory depression. The usefulness of nebulized morphine has been examined in a few studies, with mixed results, and more work must be done to determine effectiveness. In using systemic morphine the following points are important:

- The beneficial effect on dyspnea does not usually last as long as the effect on pain and one may have to administer morphine in small doses hourly or by continuous infusion.
- Physician worry about respiratory depression is a major impediment to helping dying patients with dyspnea; most patients, especially if they are not narcotic naive, do not develop significant respiratory depression and, if they do, tolerance to that effect usually develops quickly. Other medications that may be helpful for dyspnea include steroids (for radiation pneumonitis or chemotherapy-induced hypersensitivity lung disease) and phenothiazines (chlorpromazine and promethazine have been shown to decrease dyspnea in patients with chronic lung disease, probably because of their sedative effects, as has Buspirone).

Hospice Care

In many communities, patients and their families can be cared for by their physician in cooperation with a hospice, a program designed to provide terminal care, including relief of pain, to the dying patient and to provide support to the family. Services are delivered either in the patient's home, a hospital, a nursing home, or other hospice facility by a multidisciplinary team under the direction of the physician.

In hospice care, the primary focus changes from curing and caring to simply caring, and the overall goal changes from prolongation of life to the enhancement of the quality of life during the patient's final days. Since the introduction of the hospice movement in the United States and the founding of the first hospice here in 1974, hospice programs have been developed in

most communities, and most third-party payers now provide hospice benefits. *Eligibility criteria* for hospice benefits under Medicare, in accord with 1982 legislation, are the following: The patient must be terminally ill with a life expectancy of 6 months or less, be unable to benefit from further aggressive (curative) therapy, be able to receive most care at home, and have a caregiver (relative or friend) who will assume the responsibility for custodial care of the patient and be the decision maker in the event the patient becomes incompetent to make decisions. Table 19.3 summarizes in detail the processes and services included in Medicare hospice benefits.

The mushrooming of hospice programs may create an erroneous impression that hospice-type care can be provided only in hospices. Comprehensive humanistic treatment for the dying patient and the family can be offered by any physician. Home health agencies can play a pivotal role in this care (see Chapter 9). The essentials for the delivery of hospice-type care at home are physician knowledge and skill in prescribing for symptom relief, physician availability, willingness and ability to work with a multidisciplinary team, and willingness to spend extra time and effort to foresee and alleviate the problems faced by the dying patient and the family.

Dying patients and their families especially appreciate the assurance that the place of care can be changed at appropriate moments from acute medical services to hospice services or to home, and families appreciate the physician's willingness to certify the patient's death at home when the patient has voiced a preference for death at home.

Information on hospice care in the United States is provided by both the National Hospice Organization, 1901 N. Moore Street, Suite 901, Arlington, VA 22209, 703-243-5900, and the Hospice Association of America, 228 7th Street SE, Washington, DC, 202-546-4759.

MANAGEMENT OF GRIEF

If death of a loved one has been unexpected, grief usually begins with an initial stage of shock and disbelief accompanied by a general numbing of all affect. If death has been anticipated, however, this stage is less prominent. There is often a feeling of relief that the dead person's suffering has ended. Soon afterward (within hours to a few days) there is a more demonstrative phase characterized by protest and anguish, often accompanied by tears. These feelings come in waves and may be precipitated by even an indirect reference to the lost person; ordinarily, they do not persist for more than 1 or 2 months. Other symptoms of mourning normally occur throughout the first year after the death of a loved one. During this year, survivors are continuing to grieve while they reorient their lives. As time passes there often is a preoccupation with memories of the lost person. Guilt feelings for not having done enough for the deceased are very common. In some cases, this guilt may be expressed as hostility toward

---

Table 19.3.   Medicare Hospice Benefits

The Medicare hospice benefit is divided into four benefit periods:
   An initial 90-day period
   A subsequent 90-day period
   A subsequent 30-day period
   A subsequent fourth and final extension period of indefinite duration

The beneficiary must be recertified as terminally ill at the beginning of each benefit period. The following covered hospice services are provided as necessary to give palliative treatment for conditions related to the terminal illness: nursing care; services of a medical social worker, physician, counselor (including dietary, pastoral, and other), and home care aide and homemaker; short-term inpatient care (including both respite care and procedures necessary for pain control and acute and chronic system management); medical appliances and supplies, including drugs and biologicals; physical and occupational therapies; and speech-language pathology services. Bereavement service for the family is provided for up to 13 months following the patient's death.

Reprinted with permission from Hospice facts and statistics. Hospice Association of America, 1997 (see "General References").

the physician. Bereaved people often have the experience of seeing the dead person in a crowd or in some other individual fleetingly, which is then followed by the reality of permanent loss. The bereaved person is likely to visit the grave during the first year of loss more frequently than in later years. Sometimes, there is a dramatic change in personality, and the manners and the terminal symptoms of the dying patient are assumed by the bereaved person. This is another way of resolving grief, by attempting to make the lost person a part of the survivor.

Approximately 80% of bereaved people are depressed and have disturbed sleep; 40% have a poor appetite, weight loss, difficulty in concentrating, and general loss of interest in daily life (1). Depression is especially common in spouses in the middle or later years of their lives; about one-third of spouses have symptoms that meet the criteria for the diagnosis of a major depression (see Chapter 15) (2). Although depression may last for many months, 80% of individuals show improvement within 10 weeks. However, two-thirds of bereaved spouses at the end of the first year of bereavement continue to have some symptoms of apathy, aimlessness, and a disinclination to look to the future. Only a small fraction of these survivors develop complicated or atypical mourning.

The management of normal grief during the first year of bereavement should be individualized, depending on the patient's personal, family, and social background. All bereaved people need to be reminded that their grief and its psychophysiologic concomitants are normal. This has to be done with special care, acknowledging the irreparable loss while encouraging them to lead a full life without feeling guilty. Bereavement support groups exist in many communities and are usually known to clergy and social workers. Sharing feelings with others who have lost a loved one may be particularly helpful during this lonely time. A physician's encouragement can be important in helping a grieving person decide to seek such support. When severe emotional reactions become prolonged, pastoral counseling or psychotherapy may be necessary.

Bereaved persons may have new somatic symptoms or amplification of preexisting symptoms. When evaluation reveals no change in physical status, the management strategies suggested for adjustment disorders are appropriate (see Chapter 12). In time, with the completion of their grieving reaction, those patients give up their physical symptoms and again become actively engaged in a new life.

Some bereaved persons may need short-term medication for the relief of insomnia and anxiety. A benzodiazepine hypnotic (see Chapter 85) at bedtime if needed for sleep, or one of the anxiolytic benzodiazepines (see Chapter 13) as needed for anxiety, should be considered for 1 to 2 weeks in the management of normal grief. On the other hand, many patients may be satisfied with an empathetic and supportive physician.

Additional ways in which a physician can be supportive early after a patient's death are to visit the funeral home and to telephone or write to the family, acknowledging one's own sense of loss, supporting the family in what they have done to help in the terminal care of the patient, and inviting contacts at a later time. The latter idea is suggested by a finding that more than half of bereaved spouses report that they had unanswered questions about their spouse's death 1 year later (10).

During the first year of bereavement special attention should be paid to the patient during holidays, anniversaries, or on other important dates. Some symptoms of acute grief are likely to resurface around these times. Supportive therapy at such times usually controls the symptoms.

The physician is in a good position to detect the early signs of pathologic mourning, when a person either shows no signs of grieving or shows the exaggerated features of grieving characterized by excessive or prolonged (longer than a year) social isolation, unmoderated guilt or anger, panic attacks, and physical symptoms without any clear-cut organic etiology. In such cases, consultation with a psychiatrist is appropriate to help remove obstacles that have inhibited the mourner from undergoing a normal grief reaction (6).

General References*

Agency for Health Care Policy and Research (AHCPR). **Management of cancer pain: clinical practice guideline.** U.S. Public Health Service, AHCPR Publication No. 94-0592. Washington, DC: U.S. Department of Health and Human Services, 1994.
> A 200-page document providing critical assessment and practical guidelines. Companion guides for patients and families are also available (free copies available on request by telephone: 1-800-4-CANCER).

Bowlby J. Separation. New York: Basic Books, 1973.
> This is the second volume of Bowlby's classic work on attachment and loss; it deals with the issues of anxiety and anger generated in the anticipation of and in the event of separation from a loved one.

Bowlby J. Loss. New York: Basic Books, 1980.
> This is the third and final volume of Bowlby's work on attachment and loss. This is probably the best book ever written on the subject of bereavement.

Bulkin W, Lukashok MS. Rx for dying: the case of hospice. N Engl J Med 318:376, 1988.
> Editorial review, contains Medicare hospice guidelines and references to literature on the hospice movement in the United States.

Cherny NI, Foley KM, eds. Pain and palliative care. In: Hematology/oncology clinics of North America. Vol. 10. Philadelphia: WB Saunders, 1996.
> Contains excellent reviews of hospice care and management of pain and other symptoms.

Council on Scientific Affairs, American Medical Association. **Good care of the dying patient.** JAMA 276:474, 1996.
> Standards of excellence in supportive care of the terminally ill.

Creagan ET. Psychosocial issues in oncologic practice. Mayo Clin Proc 68:161, 1993.
> Excellent review of many of the practical issues in the care of terminally ill patients and their families.

Kaye P. Symptom control in hospice & palliative care. Essex, CT: Hospice Education Institute, 1989.
> Practical tips used in an English hospice.

---

*Bold print (general references) and bold numerals (specific references) denote published controlled clinical trials, meta-analyses, or consensus-based recommendations.

Kubler-Ross E. On death and dying. New York: Macmillan, 1969.
> A classic work on the subject of death and dying.

Levy MH. Pharmacologic treatment of cancer pain. N Engl J Med 335:1124, 1996.
> Recent, very readable review of the management of cancer pain.

Nelson T. It's your choice, the practical guide to planning a funeral. Glenview, IL: Scott, Foresman, 1982.
> A practical paperback on making funeral plans in the face of impending death.

Zimmerman JM, ed. Hospice: complete care for the terminally ill. 2nd ed. Baltimore: Urban & Schwarzenberg, 1986.
> Well-referenced and practical book that covers all aspects of the hospice approach to terminal care.

Specific References

1. Clayton PJ, Halikas JA, Maurice WL. The bereavement of the widowed. Dis Nerv Syst 32:597, 1971.
2. Clayton PJ, Halikas JA, Maurice WL: The depression of widowhood. Br J Psychiatry 120:71, 1972.
3. Kerr IG, Sone M, DeAngelis C, et al. Continuous narcotic infusion with patient-controlled analgesia for chronic cancer pain in outpatients. Ann Intern Med 108:554, 1988.
4. Kubler-Ross E. On death and dying. New York: Macmillan, 1969:38–137.
5. Massie MJ, Holland J, Glass E. Delirium in terminally ill cancer patients. Am J Psychiatry 140:1048, 1983.
6. Melges FT, DeMaso DR. Grief-resolution therapy: relieving, revising, and revisiting. Am J Psychother 34:51, 1980.
7. Portenoy RK. Pharmacologic management of cancer pain. Semin Oncol 22 (Suppl 2):112,1995.
8. Steinberg MD, Fleishman S, Gitman P, Hotchbiss E. Patient preference for treatment options and advance directives in terminal care (abstract). Am Soc Clin Oncol 7:268, 1988.
9. Thomsen OO, Wulff HR, Martin A, Singer PA. What do gastroenterologists in Europe tell cancer patients? Lancet 341:473, 1993.
10. Tolle SW, Bascom PB, Hickam DH, Benson JA Jr. Communication between physicians and surviving spouses following patient deaths. J Gen Intern Med 1:309, 1986.
11. Wanzev SH, Federman DO, Adelstein ST, et al. The physician's responsibility toward hopelessly ill patients. N Engl J Med 320:844, 1989.

C H A P T E R 20

Tobacco Use and Dependence*

GEORGE E. BIGELOW, PhD
CYNTHIA RAND, PhD

Tobacco use, primarily in the form of chronic cigarette smoking, is the greatest single cause of illness, disability, and death in the United States. Smoking causes an estimated 430,000 deaths annually—nearly 20% of all deaths. The perniciousness of the habit relates largely to a long history of social acceptability and failure by society to recognize and respond to smoking as health-damaging behavior. This has been changing, and continues to change; both society and health professionals are now acting to restrict, proscribe, and treat smoking.

U.S. public policy toward tobacco is in transition at the time of this writing. The FDA has declared its intent to regulate tobacco products as drug-delivery devices for nicotine. State governments are suing the tobacco

*Preparation of this chapter was supported in part by Research Scientist Award K05-DA-00050 from the National Institutes of Health. Carol S. Haines, MD, contributed to this chapter in previous editions.

industry to recover costs of smoking-related illnesses. The tobacco industry has negotiated a proposed settlement with government and health representatives that would substantially limit tobacco marketing and advertising in exchange for limitations on the industry's future financial liability; however, acceptance will require federal legislation, and the outcome remains far from certain. Nevertheless, these events represent important progress in the growing public and professional recognition of the enormous and adverse influence of tobacco use on health.

PREVALENCE OF TOBACCO USE

The decline of smoking prevalence in the United States in recent decades represents an impressive success of public health and prevention efforts. Beginning in 1965 adult smoking prevalence declined by 0.5 to 1.0% per year, from 42% in 1965 to 25% in 1993. Table 20.1 summarizes by demographic characteristics the 1993 data for prevalence of adult cigarette smoking from the National Health Interview Survey. Prevalence is inversely related to education and socioeconomic status, and there are large differences among selected demographic subgroups. Smoking prevalence has been fairly constant in recent years among adults, but has been increasing among adolescents since 1992. Adult smoking prevalence is higher among African Americans than whites, but adolescent prevalence is appreciably lower among African Americans. Other forms of tobacco use occur predominantly in males: pipe and cigar use in approximately 3 and 5%, respectively, and smokeless products (snuff, chewing tobacco) in approximately 6%. However, in some locales and subgroups (e.g., young men in rural or southern areas) the prevalence of smokeless tobacco use may approximate that of smoking.

CAUSES AND RISK FACTORS

The development of tobacco dependence can be viewed as a *pediatric disorder*. Smoking typically begins in the preteen or teenage years; initiation beyond early adulthood is rare. The habit is so widespread that it is not limited to any specific environmental, physiologic, or psychologic circumstances. Social influences (e.g., peer pressures, efforts to display independence and to appear mature and self-confident) are major factors in promoting and sustaining initial smoking experiences. Aversive initial experiences (e.g., coughing, nausea, dysphoria) are described even by people who proceed to chronic dependence. Nicotine is the pharmacologic agent responsible for maintaining tobacco use, but it is the strong learned behavioral habits that make tobacco use truly addictive (33).

Certain risk factors are associated with an increased likelihood of becoming a chronic cigarette smoker. Smoking runs in families. An individual with parents and siblings who smoke is four times as likely to become a smoker as is an individual from a nonsmoking family. The familial association results from both genetic factors (5) and environmental factors. In the past, males were more much likely to smoke than females, but this is no longer the case. There is no distinct personality type that is characteristic of smokers, but on average they tend to be somewhat more extroverted than nonsmokers, to be more adventuresome or risk taking, and to be more likely to deviate from social norms or rules. These latter characteristics may, in adolescence, increase the probability of experimenting with smoking, with a consequent increased risk of chronic dependence. Smoking is also more prevalent in those with other substance use disorders (e.g., 70 to 90% prevalence in alcoholics and other drug abusers). This relationship may reflect similar or overlapping etiologic influences. Smoking may thus serve as a conveniently visible risk factor or marker for those at increased risk of other substance use disorders.

PRIMARY PREVENTION

Primary prevention efforts must be directed to *preadolescents and adolescents.* An important element is changing societal norms about the acceptability of tobacco use. Formal preventive interventions should begin in elementary grades and continue for several years. Effective interventions are not simple fact-based health education, but instead teach specific skills for resisting social pressure and include explicit instructions and rehearsals with peers in vignettes about resisting offers to use cigarettes, alcohol products, and illegal drugs. Children who receive such training have reduced rates of smoking onset (3). As community health leaders, physicians should encourage and support preventive interventions, including bans on to-

Table 20.1. Percentage of Adults (Age ≥18) Who Smoke Cigarettes, United States, 1993

	Men	Women	Total
Race/Ethnicity			
White	27.0	24.0	25.4
African American	32.4	21.0	26.0
Hispanic	28.3	12.7	20.4
Native American	35.9	40.9	38.7
Asian/Pacific	27.4	9.5	18.2
Age (yr)			
18–24	28.8	22.9	25.8
25–44	31.1	27.3	29.2
45–64	29.2	23.0	26.0
65+	13.5	10.5	11.8
Education (yr) (For Ages ≥25 yr Only)			
9–12	42.1	32.3	36.8
12	32.0	26.9	29.2
13–15	28.4	22.1	25.0
16+	14.8	11.9	13.5
Socioeconomic Status			
At or below poverty line	38.1	28.2	32.1
Above poverty line	26.1	21.7	23.8
Total	27.7	22.5	25.0

From Centers for Disease Control. MMWR 43:925–930, 1994.

bacco use in public areas, enforcement of prohibitions on tobacco sales to minors, and restrictions on advertising that glamorizes smoking or appeals to youth.

COURSE OF THE HABIT

The health hazards of smoking are now widely recognized, and the social acceptability of smoking has declined. Consequently, most smokers vacillate between defending and justifying their habit and trying to end it. Most smokers would like to quit, and about half attempt to stop in a given year. Adverse health events and advice from physicians are potent forces in promoting increased cessation efforts by patients. In the United States there are now nearly twice as many former smokers (approximately 97 million) as there are current smokers (approximately 50 million).

Patterns of Quitting and Relapse

Approximately 60 to 80% of smokers who attempt to quit achieve at least a minimal period of abstinence. However, the relapse rate is high, and approximately two-thirds of quitters resume smoking within 3 to 6 months, often within only a few days. Only 15 to 20% of quitters remain cigarette free for 6 months or more. Cessation should not be considered successful until abstinence has been sustained for at least 6 months. The probability of relapse after 6 months of abstinence is small.

Approximately 95% of smoking cessation occurs as the result of smokers' self-directed personal efforts, without formal treatment. Abrupt (so-called cold turkey) cessation is more likely to be successful than is gradual reduction. Most successful quitters require more than one attempt before becoming permanent ex-smokers. Repeated quitting and relapse are characteristic of the normal, successful cessation process. *The risk of relapse is increased* when patients are under emotional stress (e.g., anger, frustration, anxiety, depression), when ex-smokers are exposed to cues associated with prior smoking (e.g., after meals, when consuming alcoholic beverages), and in people whose spouse or friends continue to smoke (31).

HEALTH CONSEQUENCES
Risk of Disease

Although smoking dramatically increases overall population morbidity and mortality, its effects on individual smokers are unpredictable, and some smokers escape major health consequences. Age-adjusted mortality rates for smokers are 70% greater than those for nonsmokers. Life expectancy is significantly shortened by smoking (e.g., 8.1 years less for the 30-year-old two-pack-a-day smoker than for a comparable nonsmoker). Risk is dose related in that it increases with increasing number of cigarettes smoked, with increasing number of years smoking, and with depth of inhalation.

Smoking is associated with increased risk of cancer (especially of the respiratory tract), cardiovascular disease, chronic obstructive pulmonary disease, gastric ulcer, prostate cancer, cervical cancer, and postmenopausal osteoporosis. Smoking by pregnant women reduces fetal growth and birth weight and increases the risk of fetal death; smoking interacts with the use of oral contraceptives by women and increases their risk of myocardial infarction, subarachnoid hemorrhage, and thromboembolic disease.

The *risks of cancer* and chronic pulmonary disease in smokers are 10 times those in nonsmokers. The percentage of oral, throat, and lung cancer deaths attributable to smoking exceeds 80%. The *risk of atherosclerotic cardiovascular disease* is approximately doubled in smokers. The percentage of cardiovascular disease deaths attributable to smoking is 20%. Because of the much greater population prevalence of cardiovascular disease, it is in this area that the greatest overall health benefits of smoking cessation occur.

Benefits of Cessation

The greatest immediate benefit of smoking cessation is the reduction of cardiovascular risk. Within hours of smoking cessation, both carbon monoxide and nicotine, the two cigarette products thought to be primarily responsible for cardiovascular disease, are dissipated from the body, with a consequent reduction in cardiac work requirement concurrent with an increase in oxygenation. There is also prompt reduction in the risk of upper respiratory infection. Slower to accrue is a reduction in the rate of decline of pulmonary function and a reduction in cancer risk; benefits of cessation are measurable in these domains within 3 to 5 years after smoking cessation.

Health benefits of smoking cessation are greater for smokers who quit before the development of symptoms; however, the benefits of cessation also extend to those who have already experienced symptoms of smoking-related disease. For example, individuals who stop smoking after myocardial infarction have improved survival rates compared with those who continue smoking (4). Similarly, there are pulmonary benefits to smoking cessation even late in life (15).

Low-Yield Cigarettes

Because the risks of smoking are dose related, it is tempting to believe that substantial health benefits might be achieved by switching to low-yield cigarettes. This is no longer the case; the variations in currently marketed tobacco yields have little health impact (23,32) and there are negligible correlations between the stated yield values and blood levels of nicotine and its major metabolite, cotinine (1). Biological yield may differ substantially from stated yield because of behavioral variations in the way the cigarettes are smoked. When nominal yields change, smokers tend to change their behavior so as to keep biological delivery unchanged (e.g., by smoking more cigarettes, inhaling more smoke). The primary manufacturing technique for producing current low-yield cigarettes is to place ventilation holes in the sides of the filter to dilute the smoke stream with air. With these low-yield brands it is especially likely that biological delivery will significantly exceed assay delivery because the smoker's fingers tend to block these ventilation holes (25). Smokers should be cautioned that so-called low-yield cigarettes may still have high biological delivery.

Physical Dependence and Craving

Chronic tobacco use produces physical dependence on nicotine. Upon cessation of use, an *abstinence syndrome* typically occurs (16,17). The subjective aspects of the syndrome can be very distressing, and include irritability, restlessness, sleep disturbances, difficulty in concentrating, anxiety, gastrointestinal disturbances, hunger, weight gain, and most important, craving for cigarettes. Most patients feel normal again within approximately 2 weeks of abstinence, except that craving for tobacco may persist for months or years. Nicotine substitution treatment is effective in reducing the abstinence syndrome. The physiologic aspects of the tobacco abstinence syndrome are generally inconsequential, consisting of a slight and gradual decline in heart rate and blood pressure.

Craving for tobacco is an extraordinarily persistent obstacle to sustained abstinence. Many ex-smokers report craving years after cessation. The duration of craving is highly variable, but it should be expected to persist for at least 3 to 6 months, with its frequency and urgency diminishing over that interval. Craving may be a learned phenomenon rather than part of an abstinence syndrome because it is high even in smokers making no attempt to quit or reduce their smoking.

Passive Smoking

Passive smoking—exposure of nonsmokers to air contaminated by the smoking of others—is not only an irritant to many nonsmokers; it has definite adverse health effects. Although the levels of smoke products detected in the blood and urine of passively exposed nonsmokers are low relative to those in smokers, there are significant health risks associated with passive smoking (2,6,10). Passive exposure to the smoke of spouses is associated with impaired pulmonary function, increased lung cancer risk, and increased coronary heart disease risk. Children passively exposed to smoke by parents have increased rates of respiratory infections, slower developmental increases in pulmonary function, and an increased incidence of asthma attacks. Maternal smoking contributes to reduced birth weight, and smokers who stop the habit during pregnancy have significantly heavier babies than do those who continue smoking (30).

Physicians should try to protect nonsmokers from cigarette smoke and should recognize that most ventilation systems simply diffuse and redistribute smoke rather than remove it. Smoking (including employee smoking) should be emphatically prohibited in physicians' offices, and physicians should support similar efforts in all public settings, especially in health care facilities.

RECOGNITION AND DIAGNOSIS

Nicotine dependence is a diagnosable substance use disorder in the American Psychiatric Association's 1994 *Diagnostic and Statistical Manual.* The diagnostic criteria are identical to those for other substance-related disorders (see Chapter 22), reflecting the growing recognition of extensive commonalities among alcoholism, drug abuse, and tobacco dependence.

There is widespread failure of health professionals to recognize and diagnose tobacco dependence and to maintain it on an active problem list. Tobacco use status should be considered at every visit at the office reception point (28). There should be a clear and prominent chart indication to prompt attention at subsequent visits.

Assessment of smoking status is normally via patient self-report. Objective biological indices may become more important as the social acceptability of admitting to smoking declines. Smoking status can be assessed by measuring carbon monoxide concentrations in expired breath. Urine test-strips for nicotine and its metabolites are being developed. The value of objective assessment is indicated by the fact that up to 20 to 30% of self-reported quitters show biological evidence of continuing to smoke.

TREATMENT

Substantial evidence, assistive materials, and pharmacologic modalities, summarized here, are now available for the rational planning of smoking cessation interventions with patients. Detailed office approaches are described in the next section.

Role of the Physician

Concern about health remains the most cited reason smokers quit, and smokers cite physicians as the people most able to influence their decisions to attempt to quit. The physician's optimal role in the treatment of tobacco dependence is to advise and assist all smoking patients to stop. It is a mistake to rely heavily on referral to specialized smoking cessation programs. Results of referral are disappointing when compared with those obtained by devoting equal or less time to brief direct advice.

Brief advice by a physician can significantly increase rates of smoking cessation (26,30); medical economic analyses have shown that smoking cessation advice is as cost-effective as other common interventions, such as treatment of hypercholesterolemia or mild hypertension (8). An increase in smoking cessation rates, from 1 to 3%, can be expected if physicians simply caution each smoker to quit during routine office visits for other problems. Providing a self-help pamphlet with how-to-quit suggestions can yield quit rates of 7 to 12% in general practice. Investing a few more moments to negotiate a quit date can increase the quit rate to 15%. Addition of pharmacologic treatment (see below) will further increase success. Among certain patients advice alone can achieve impressive efficacy. For example, the smoking cessation rate after a first myocardial infarction is as high as 50% for patients given directive smoking cessation advice by their physician, compared with approximately 35% for patients receiving usual care (4). Similarly high rates of cessation are seen in prenatal care settings, where up to 20 to 30% of smokers may quit during a pregnancy (30).

It is important to recognize that the absolute rates of cessation are likely to remain frustratingly low. However, in terms of overall health benefit to a patient population, routine smoking cessation advice from physicians is very worthwhile.

Motivational Communication

The goal of effective doctor–patient communication is to provide advice that maximizes a smoker's motivation and decision to quit. A common error is to rely too much on fact-based health education that implicitly seeks to motivate through fear. Smokers are well aware of the health risks of smoking and do not respond to that information alone. The five actions described in the next section ("Recommended Office Approach") integrate what is known about motivational communication into a practical approach for helping smokers to quit. The approach includes many of the behavioral strategies described in Chapter 4. It focuses on one clear and simple message—"I strongly advise you to quit"—delivered in a manner free of blame or rancor. The advice *should be personally relevant to patients, should describe in a positive way the benefits* to be gained, and *should prescribe a particular course of action.* These three objectives can be attained by pointing out the association between smoking and the specific symptoms, illnesses, or health risks of the individual patient; by pointing out that smoking cessation can prevent, reverse, or stop the progression of disease (whichever is appropriate); and by stating clearly, simply, and directly the course of action to be taken: to stop smoking. A general statement that "Smoking is bad for your health and you can kill yourself if you continue" fails on all three of these points. It is not specifically personal, it describes no benefit, and it is not sufficiently directive. More personalized and directive statements can be more persuasive (e.g., "I strongly advise you to stop smoking; both your coughing and your recurring colds and flus are caused in part by your smoking; I want you to try to quit smoking, and then we should see some improvement").

Patients differ in their readiness and willingness to change their smoking habit. The goal is to move patients along the continuum depicted in Figure 4.1. When patients are ready to attempt cessation the goal should be to agree on a cessation date and provide therapeutic assistance. Patients not yet ready for cessation may become ready in response to repeated nonjudgmental encouragement and motivational advice.

Brochures for Office Use

Self-help smoking cessation brochures can provide useful motivational advice and specific helpful techniques for smokers. A wide variety are available, and these change periodically. Local offices of the American Cancer Society, the American Heart Association, or the American Lung Association should be contacted to obtain copies of their smoking cessation self-help brochures. The National Cancer Institute offers a *Quit for Good Kit* for physicians that includes patient self-help brochures (telephone 1-800-4-CANCER).

Pharmacologic Treatments

There have been substantial changes in recent years in the availability of pharmacologic treatments for tobacco dependence. Nicotine chewing gum and some nicotine transdermal patch products are now available over the counter without prescription. Additional types of nicotine substitution treatment products have been introduced, including a nicotine nasal spray and a nicotine vapor inhaler. Also, bupropion, the first nonnicotine smoking cessation product, has been introduced. Characteristics and 1997 costs of the available products are summarized in Table 20.2. Additional products are under development, including a lozengelike oral transmucosal nicotine. Table 20.3 shows the *costs of smoking and the costs of pharmacologic treatment* with available products.

Mechanism and Indication

Smoking cessation medications are intended to aid patients who are making a serious attempt to stop tobacco use. They will not themselves induce such an attempt. They enhance the success of motivated behavior change efforts; they do not cause or motivate such behavior change directly. Nicotine substitution products suppress the nicotine abstinence syndrome and reduce subjective desire or craving for tobacco. The mechanism of bupropion's efficacy is uncertain, although it also appears to suppress nicotine withdrawal and craving. Medications are to be used in conjunction with a complete cessation of tobacco use. If tobacco use persists beyond the first couple of weeks of treatment, the medication should probably be discontinued until some future renewed effort at total cessation is attempted.

Efficacy

Strong data support the efficacy of all these marketed treatments (11,12,21), but none is clearly superior. All have been shown to increase smoking cessation rates by approximately 50 to 100% over placebo comparison conditions. The absolute rates of smoking cessation depend on many factors: patient motivation and setting, intensity of concurrent behavioral counseling, the definition of cessation, and the time of assessment. Most clinical efficacy trials described in product labeling are conducted in patients sufficiently motivated to volunteer for smoking cessation treatment and in con-

Table 20.2.   Summary of Smoking Cessation Products

Type and Brand Name	Dosage	Package	1997 Retail Cost	Comments
Over-the-Counter Products				
Nicotine gum				
Nicorette	2 mg × 9–24/day	108 pieces	$50	Give special instructions on how to "chew-and-park" the gum.
		48 pieces	$29	
	4 mg × 9–24/day	108 pieces	$56	Emphasize importance of adequate use.
		48 pieces	$32	Target is 9–24 per day for 4–6 weeks, then gradual tapering over 2–4 weeks.
Nicotine patch				
Nicoderm CQ	21 mg/24 hr	14 patches	$50	Target is maintenance for 4–10 weeks, possibly followed by gradual dosage tapering over 2–6 weeks.
		7 patches	$30	
	14 mg/24 hr	7 patches	$30	
	7 mg/24 hr	7 patches	$30	
Nicotrol	15 mg/16 hr	14 patches	$50	
		7 patches	$30	
Prescription Products				
Nicotine patch				
Habitrol	21 mg/24 hr	30 patches	$129	
	14 mg/24 hr	30 patches	$127	
	7 mg/24 hr	30 patches	$120	
Prostep	22 mg/24 hr	7 patches	$40	
	11 mg/24 hr	7 patches	$38	
Nicotine nasal spray				
Nicotrol NS	1 mg × 8–40 mg/day 2 sprays = 1 mg	10 mL at 10 mg/mL	$41	Target is maintenance for 6 or more weeks, possibly followed by gradual tapering of use, up to 12 weeks total. Provides most rapid onset of nicotine effects.
Nicotine vapor inhaler				
Nicotrol inhaler	10 mg/cartridge (delivers 4 mg)	42 cartridges per box	$50	Absorption is via oral mucosa, not lungs. Similar in appearance to a cigarette; may stimulate sensory/manipulation aspects of smoking. 6 to 16 cartridges per day for up to 12 weeks.
Bupropion SR				
Zyban	150 mg 1/day × 3 days then 2/day	60 tablets	$90	Begin 1 week before quit date. No dosage tapering needed. May be combined with nicotine replacement product for greater total effectiveness.

Table 20.3.   Cost of Smoking Versus Cost of Treatment

Annual Cost of Smoking

		Packs Per Day		
		½	1	2
Price per pack[a]	$1	$182	$ 365	$ 730
	$2	$365	$ 730	$1430
	$3	$547	$1095	$2190

Cost of Treatment[b]

Nicotine gum	$230
Nicotine patch	$220
Nicotine nasal spray	$280
Bupropion	$360

[a]Varies by region and taxation.
[b]Estimates based on current retail prices and typical 8-wk treatment course.

junction with individual or group counseling treatment; success is generally defined as 4 weeks of smoking abstinence during active treatment. Under these conditions cessation success rates of 30 to 50% are often achieved in active medication groups, compared with rates of 10 to 30% in placebo groups. Success rates decline to half these values when assessed 6 to 12 months after the end of treatment. Despite variations in the absolute rates of success, the relative efficacy of active pharmacologic treatment over placebo is robust and is preserved across different populations, settings, counseling levels, and follow-up periods.

Nicotine Patch

The nicotine transdermal patch is the treatment of choice at present. This preference relates primarily to its ease of use and relatively good patient compliance. Patches may be worn for either 24 or 16 hours/day. The rationale for 24-hour use is to minimize nicotine withdrawal on waking. The rationale for 16-hour (daytime only) use is to minimize sleep disturbances that may accompany 24-hour use. The most common side effect is skin irritation at the site of patch application. On the basis of a placebo-controlled trial, the nicotine patch has been shown to be effective and safe for use in a wide spectrum of patients with chronic cardiac problems (22). There is no significant medical difference between over-the-counter and prescription products. Table 20.4 outlines the 8-week schedules and basic instructions that are recommended in consensus guidelines. Lower starting dosages are advised for light smokers (15 cigarettes/day or less).

Nicotine Chewing Gum

A potential advantage of nicotine gum is the ability to adjust dosage individually and to schedule use as needed in response to situational variations in nicotine withdrawal and craving. Its major potential disadvantage is the extensive behavioral compliance required for effective use, and the common failure of patients to use enough. Patients must be instructed in proper chewing technique, and must understand that the nicotine is absorbed primarily through the oral mucosa, but very poorly if swallowed. Proper use involves a few chews until a peppery taste or tingling is felt, parking the gum inside the cheek to allow absorption, then repeating at about 1-minute intervals. Nicotine absorption is not rapid, so a regularly timed dosing schedule of 1 gum every 1 to 2 hours is generally more successful than self-selected dosing. Acidic beverages (coffee, juices, soda, and wine) should be avoided before or during gum use because their pH reduces nicotine absorption. The 4-mg dosage form is intended for patients with higher levels of nicotine dependence. Convenient indices of dependence level are number of cigarettes smoked per day (25 or more is considered high dependence) and how soon after waking the first cigarette is smoked (smoking within just a few minutes of waking reflects high dependence).

Nicotine Nasal Spray

The nicotine nasal spray more closely simulates the pharmacokinetics of nicotine delivery via tobacco smoking than do the other nicotine substitution medications. It produces a larger and more rapid increase in blood nicotine levels, although still less than that achieved with smoking. The nasal spray may be especially beneficial to highly dependent smokers, who may need more rapid and more substantial nicotine delivery. The nasal spray's more rapid onset makes as-needed dosing more practical than with gum, but regularly scheduled dosing is still the recommended procedure.

Nicotine Vapor Inhaler

The nicotine vapor inhaler is similar in appearance to a cigarette and may be especially useful to patients who desire the physical manipulation and sensory aspects of smoking. There is no heat or combustion; puffs on the inhaler draw air over an internal nicotine-laden plug. Each puff delivers a very small dose of nicotine vapor (approximately 0.013 mg) to the mouth, where the nicotine is absorbed through the oral mucosa.

Bupropion

Zyban is a sustained-release tablet formulation that contains 150 mg of the antidepressant bupropion. The mechanism of action of bupropion in promoting smoking cessation is unknown, but it probably relates to its inhibition of norepinephrine and dopamine uptake. This is the only marketed nonnicotine smoking cessation medication. It is effective as a sole treatment, but its efficacy can be further enhanced by combination use with a nicotine substitution product. In a controlled trial, in patients who were not depressed, bupropion, 300 mg (150 mg twice daily), yielded a 1-year cessation rate of 23.1% compared with 12.4% in placebo-treated patients [18]. Treatment was initiated 1 week before patients' quit dates and discontinued after 7 weeks. For

Table 20.4.   Schedules and Basic Instructions Recommended for the Use of Nicotine Patches

Dosage and schedule	Treatment of 8 weeks or less has been shown to be as efficacious as longer treatment periods. Based on this finding, the following treatment schedules are suggested as reasonable for most smokers. Clinicians should consult the package insert for other treatment suggestions. Finally, clinicians should consider individualizing treatment based on specific patient characteristics, such as previous experience with the patch, amount smoked, and degree of addictiveness.[a]		
	Brand	**Duration**	**Dosage**
	Nicoderm and Habitrol	4 weeks	21 mg/24 hr
		then 2 weeks	14 mg/24 hr
		then 2 weeks	7 mg/24 hr
	Prostep	4 weeks	22 mg/24 hr
		then 4 weeks	11 mg/24 hr
	Nicotrol[b]	4 weeks	15 mg/16 hr
		then 2 weeks	10 mg/16 hr
		then 2 weeks	5 mg/16 hr
Prescribing instructions	*No smoking* while using the patch. *Location*—At the start of each day, the patient should place a new patch on a relatively hairless location between the neck and waist. *Activities*—No restrictions while using the patch. *Time*—Patches should be applied as soon as patients waken on their quit day.		

From Agency for Health Care Policy and Research. Smoking cessation: clinical practice guideline, no. 18. (USDHHS) AHCPR Publication No. 9600692. Washington, DC: US Government Printing Office, 1996.

[a]These dosage recommendations are based on a review of the published research literature and do not necessarily conform to packet insert information.

[b]Note: The 10-mg and 5-mg patches have been discontinued.

the first 3 days, patients took 150 mg/day, then 150 mg twice daily. All patients received simple smoking cessation counseling.

Bupropion is also marketed as an antidepressant under the brand name Wellbutrin (see Chapter 15); patients should not use the two preparations simultaneously.

Combined Nicotine Substitution Treatments

Some studies suggest that combinations of nicotine substitution products (e.g., patch plus gum) might be more effective than single products (9). Theoretically, such an approach has some merit, but data are at present insufficient to permit firm recommendation.

Chronic Treatment

Current recommendations are for nicotine substitution medications to be used for no more than 2 to 3 months during which they are tapered gradually and discontinued. However, some patients who succeed at stopping smoking continue to use nicotine substitution products for longer periods and may be at risk for smoking relapse if nicotine substitution is stopped. There is no consensus on the appropriate response to this circumstance. However, the health risks of chronic nicotine maintenance are certainly much lower than the risks of smoking.

Potential Medication Interactions

Nicotine substitution treatment typically yields nicotine blood levels well below those achieved during tobacco use. Therefore, potential medication interactions relate primarily to the cessation of tobacco use rather than to the administration of smoking cessation medications. Following tobacco cessation a *dosage decrease* may be required for acetaminophen, adrenergic antagonists (e.g., prazosin or labetalol), caffeine, imipramine, insulin, oxazepam, pentazocine, propranolol or other β-blockers, and theophylline. Following tobacco cessation a *dosage increase* may be required for adrenergic agonists such as isoproterenol or phenylephrine. Bupropion is contraindicated within 14 days of monoamine oxidase (MAO) inhibitor use.

Weight Gain

Weight gain is a common, distressing consequence of smoking cessation. Weight gain results both from dietary changes (increased snacking and selection of high-calorie foods) and from discontinuation of the metabolic effects of nicotine (26,27). Weight gain of patients remaining abstinent for 1 year averages 5 to 15 lb. This magnitude of weight gain is medically insignificant relative to the health benefits of smoking cessation. Unfortunately, the anticipated social, cosmetic, and economic (e.g., wardrobe cost) consequences of weight gain deter some smokers from quitting and contribute to relapse in others. Smoking cessation is most successful if patients accept temporary weight gain rather than struggling against it during the early cessation period. Nicotine substitution treat-

ment (14,20) and bupropion both significantly attenuate weight gain after smoking cessation.

Organized Treatment

Physicians often would like to refer smokers to formal cessation programs. For the small minority of smokers who attend them, organized programs at little or no cost are often available through local voluntary service organizations such as the Lung Association or Heart Association. Commercial programs offer no clear advantages. Most organized programs incorporate standard behavioral principles of self-monitoring, control of environmental cues, and scheduling of rewards. These principles are also well represented in various self-help guides and in the patient education materials packaged with cessation medications.

Relapse Prevention

As with most addictive disorders, the likelihood of relapse after cessation is high. Most relapse occurs within the first few days or weeks of cessation, although patients are at some risk of relapse even after months of abstinence. New quitters face many urges to smoke again. Anticipation and advance planning can prevent relapse. Self-help educational brochures are useful for this purpose. They provide warnings about relapse risk circumstances and suggest coping strategies. In addition, they help patients recognize the normality of "slips" and the importance of continued commitment to cessation. Practical aspects of addressing relapse are described in the next section.

RECOMMENDED OFFICE APPROACH

Most physicians are motivated to counsel smoking cessation for the patient with chronic obstructive pulmonary disease (COPD) or the inpatient recovering from a myocardial infarction (MI). However, too often physicians neglect smoking cessation counseling in routine office care (13,19,29). Patients with smoking-related diseases obviously require strong smoking cessation interventions, but it is the smoking patient who has not yet experienced negative health consequences of smoking who stands to benefit most from smoking cessation. This section describes the primary care smoking cessation practice developed and recommended in a 1996 Clinical Practice Guideline compiled by the Agency for Health Care Policy and Research (AHCPR; see "General References").

Although physicians agree that it is appropriate and important for doctors to counsel patients to stop smoking, they are inconsistent in providing such advice. Reported barriers to counseling include a belief that such advice is ineffectual, the belief that most smoking patients are uninterested in counseling, perceived lack of skills, and time constraints (13,19). However, studies have repeatedly found that brief, directive smoking interventions delivered during routine care are cost-effective, and have the potential for significant public health benefit (see p. 226). A routine office visit for the treatment of eczema, flu, or indigestion can be used successfully to change smoking behavior, in the same way that it may also be used to screen for hypertension. These office-based smoking cessation practices are most effective when the smoking cessation interventions are viewed as essential components of good care. Just as measuring blood pressure at each office visit is now standard practice, so also should smoking status assessment and smoking cessation interventions be systematically integrated into standard office practice (28).

Motivating Smokers to Quit Smoking

Effective motivational counseling for smoking cessation recognizes that smokers cycle through different levels of readiness before attempting smoking cessation (see Fig. 4.1). Many factors can influence a smoker's progress through the stages of a change process. Life events, health symptoms, workplace smoking restrictions, and the price of a pack of cigarettes can all move a smoker closer to cessation. Alternatively, stress, weight gain, family problems, and smoking peers can all act as barriers to change. The strong, directive advice a smoker receives from his or her doctor on the personal importance of quitting smoking is often one of the significant forces that move a smoker closer to quitting. Concern about health is one of the most common reasons smokers cite as a motivation for quitting. Physicians can increase overall motivation for cessation by underscoring the personal *relevance* of quitting for that patient. The *risks* of smoking to both the smoker and his or her family can be highlighted, as well as the *rewards* of quitting, such as better health, saving money, improved vitality, and fewer wrinkles. And finally, because developing sufficient motivation for change may take a smoker months or years, the effort to motivate patients should be *repeated* at every clinical contact. Thus, physicians who consistently and repeatedly use these *4 Rs* and provide smoking patients with advice and encouragement to quit smoking over the course of their medical care are most likely to see success. This *4 R* strategy should be used in conjunction with the actions outlined in Figures 20.2 to 20.6 (Figure 20.1).

Actions: Ask, Advise, Identify, Assist, and Arrange

The AHCPR guidelines were derived from rigorous review of approximately 3000 scientific reports. Those satisfying scientific quality criteria were analyzed us-

ACTION	STRATEGIES FOR IMPLEMENTATION
Relevance	Motivational information given to a patient has the greatest impact if it is relevant to a patient's disease status, family or social situation (e.g., having children in the home), health concerns, age, gender, and other important patient characteristics (e.g., prior quitting experience).
Risks	The clinician should *ask the patient to identify the potential negative consequences of smoking.* The clinician may suggest and highlight those that seem most relevant to the patient. The clinician should emphasize that smoking low-tar/low-nicotine cigarettes or use of other forms of tobacco (e.g., smokeless tobacco, cigars, pipes) will not eliminate these risks. Examples of risks follow. • Acute risks: Shortness of breath, exacerbation of asthma, impotence, infertility, increased serum carbon monoxide. • Long-term risks: Heart attacks and strokes, lung and other cancers (larynx, oral cavity, pharynx, esophagus, pancreas, bladder, cervix, leukemia), chronic obstructive pulmonary diseases (chronic bronchitis and emphysema). • Environmental risks: Increased risk of lung cancer in spouse and children; higher rates of smoking by children of smokers; increased risk for SIDS, asthma, middle ear disease, and respiratory infections in children of smokers.
Rewards	The clinician should *ask the patient to identify the potential benefits of quitting smoking.* The clinician may suggest and highlight those that seem most relevant to the patient. Examples of rewards follow. • Improved health • Improved sense of taste • Improved sense of smell • Cost savings • Improved self-esteem • Better-smelling home, car, and breath • No more worrying about quitting • A good example for children • Healthy babies and children • No worrying about exposing others to smoke • Feeling better physically • Freedom from addiction • Better performance in sports
Repetition	The motivational intervention should be repeated every time an unmotivated patient visits the office setting.

Figure 20.1. The 4 R strategy: Components of clinical interventions to enhance motivation to quit smoking. (From AHCPR, 1996.)

ACTION	STRATEGIES FOR IMPLEMENTATION
Implement an office-wide system that ensures that, for EVERY patient at EVERY office visit, tobacco-use status is queried and documented.*	Expand the vital signs to include tobacco use. • Data collected by health care team. • Implemented using preprinted progress note paper that includes the expanded vital signs, a vital signs stamp, or, for computerized records, includes an item assessing tobacco-use status. VITAL SIGNS Blood Pressure: _____ Pulse: _____ Weight: _____ Temperature: _____ Respiration Rate: _____ Tobacco Use: Current Former Never (circle one) * Alternatives to the vital sign stamp are to place tobacco-use status stickers on all patient charts or to indicate smoking status using computer reminder systems.

Figure 20.2.   ASK: Systematically ask about tobacco use at every visit. (From AHCPR, 1996.)

ACTION	STRATEGIES FOR IMPLEMENTATION
In a clear, strong, and personalized manner, urge every smoker to quit.	Advice should be • Clear: "I think it is important for you to quit smoking now and I will help you." "Cutting down while you are ill is not enough." • Strong: "As your clinician, I need you to know that quitting smoking is the most important thing you can do to protect your current and future health." • Personalized: Tie smoking to current health/illness or the social and economic costs of tobacco use, motivation level/readiness to quit, or the impact of smoking on children and others in the household. Encourage office staff to reinforce the cessation message and support the patient's quit attempt.

Figure 20.3.   ADVISE: Strongly advise all smokers to quit. (From AHCPR, 1996.)

ACTION	STRATEGIES FOR IMPLEMENTATION
Ask every smoker if he or she is willing to make a quit attempt at this time.	• If the patient is willing to make a quit attempt at this time, provide treatment assistance. • If the patient prefers a more intensive treatment or the clinician believes intensive treatment is appropriate, refer to interventions administered by a smoking cessation specialist and follow up with the patient regarding quitting. • If the patient clearly states he/she is not willing to make a quit attempt at this time, provide a motivational intervention.

Figure 20.4.   IDENTIFY: Identify smokers willing to quit and to make a quit attempt. (From AHCPR, 1996.)

ACTION	STRATEGIES FOR IMPLEMENTATION
Help the patient with a quit plan.	Set a quit date. Ideally, the quit date should be within 2 weeks, taking patient preference into account. A patient's preparations for quitting: • Inform family, friends, and coworkers of quitting and request understanding and support. • Remove cigarettes from your environment. Before quitting, avoid smoking in places where you spend a lot of time (e.g., home, car). • Review previous quit attempts. What helped you? What led to relapse? • Anticipate challenges to planned quit attempt, particularly during the critical first few weeks. These include nicotine withdrawal symptoms.
Encourage nicotine replacement therapy except in special circumstances.	Encourage the use of nicotine patch or nicotine gum therapy for smoking cessation.
Give key advice on successful quitting.	Abstinence: Total abstinence is essential. "Not even a single puff after the quit date." Alcohol: Drinking alcohol is highly associated with relapse. Those who stop smoking should review their alcohol use and consider limiting/abstaining from alcohol during the quit process. Other smokers in the household: The presence of other smokers in the household, particularly a spouse, is associated with lower success rates. Patients should consider quitting with their significant others or developing specific plans to stay quit in a household where others still smoke.
Provide supplementary materials.	Sources: Federal agencies, including AHCPR; nonprofit agencies (ACS, ALA, AHA); or local/state health departments. Type: Culturally/racially/educationally/age appropriate for the patient. Location: Readily available in every office.

Figure 20.5.   ASSIST: Assist the patient in quitting. (From AHCPR, 1996.)

ACTION	STRATEGIES FOR IMPLEMENTATION
Schedule follow-up contact, either in person or via telephone.	Timing: Follow-up contact should occur soon after the quit date, preferably during the first week. A second follow-up contact is recommended within the first month. Schedule further follow-up contacts as indicated. Actions during follow-up visit: Congratulate success. If smoking occurred, review circumstances and elicit recommitment to total abstinence. Remind patient that a lapse can be used as a learning experience. Identify problems already encountered and anticipate challenges in the immediate future. Assess medication use and problems. Consider referral to a more intense or specialized program.

Figure 20.6.   ARRANGE: Arrange follow-up contact. (From AHCPR, 1996.)

ing meta-analytic techniques. This permitted the authors to synthesize outcome data from different smoking cessation treatments and to identify effective treatment elements. The resulting guidelines are based on sound scientific evidence, and they recognize the time constraints of practitioners. The AHCPR-recommended practices are *designed to require 3 minutes or less.* They consist of five actions that are described more fully below: ask, advise, identify, assist, and arrange.

Office-based practices should systematically *ask* every patient at every office visit about his or her tobacco use (Fig. 20.2). Clinicians are more likely to intervene with smoking patients when there are office procedures designed to increase the assessment and documentation of smoking status (28). Smoking status should be considered *a vital sign* that is automatically collected, updated, and integrated into the permanent medical record.

The clinician should next *advise* every smoking patients in a strong, direct, personalized manner of the importance of quitting smoking (Fig. 20.3). Even brief (3 minutes or less) advice to quit smoking will increase smoking cessation rates (29).

After advising cessation, the clinician should assess the smoker's motivation and *identify* smokers willing to make a quit attempt and the type of treatment they will accept (Fig. 20.4). For the unmotivated smoker, the physician can attempt to enhance motivation for future cessation.

For patients interested in quitting smoking, the clinician should *assist* in formalizing a quit plan by setting a quit date within 2 weeks (Fig. 20.5). Brief counseling can encourage the patient to inform his or her family of the quit date, remove cigarettes from the environment before quitting, review previous quit attempts to identify aids and barriers, and anticipate challenges, such as withdrawal symptoms. Nicotine replacement therapy (see above) should be encouraged for most patients. Patients should be advised that *total abstinence is essential,* that alcohol should be avoided, and that smoking friends and family members should either join the plan to quit or not smoke around them.

Finally, for patients who have set a quit date, a follow-up contact should be *arranged,* preferably within 2 weeks of the quit date (Fig. 20.6). This contact can be used to reinforce success, troubleshoot problems, monitor nicotine replacement therapy, and refer to more intensive smoking cessation assistance if necessary.

Dealing with Relapse

Risk of relapse is very high for patients who slip and have even one cigarette. Drinking alcohol, socializing with smokers, and high-stress events can all trigger relapse episodes. Patients should be counseled in advance about factors associated with the risk of relapse and reinforced in the continuing challenge of staying abstinent. If relapse occurs it is important to reassure the patient that relapse is not an indicator that they cannot quit smoking, but instead a common event that most former smokers have experienced before successful quitting. A relapse experience is discouraging for a patient, but can provide information on the risks and barriers to be addressed in the next cessation effort. Patients should be encouraged to retry cessation as soon as they are ready, and encouraged to use more intensive interventions (e.g., multisession group programs, longer duration pharmacotherapy) if acceptable.

OTHER FORMS OF TOBACCO USE

This chapter focuses on cigarette smoking because it is the most prevalent form of tobacco use and has the greatest health impact. Other forms of tobacco use—cigars, pipes, snuff, chewing tobacco—also have deleterious health effects (7). Mortality rates associated for these other forms of tobacco use are intermediate between those of cigarette smokers and nonusers of tobacco; for example, the total mortality of cigar or pipe smokers is approximately 15 to 20% higher than that of comparable nonsmokers. Site-specific cancer rates in the oral–nasal cavity are five times as great as in nonusers of tobacco, and there is increased risk of cardiovascular disease. Treatment approaches for these other varieties of tobacco dependence are the same as for cigarette smoking.

PHYSICIANS AND PUBLIC POLICY

The likelihood of success in overcoming addiction to nicotine is increased not only by the personal motivation and willpower of the cigarette smoker, but also by a social and legal environment that encourages nonsmoking, restricts access to tobacco, and reduces the social acceptability of smoking. An increasing body of evidence supports the value of increased taxation on tobacco, restrictive smoking policies, and counter-tobacco advertising in reducing smoking prevalence in a community (10,11,13,17). Just as public policies that ensure clean water and adequate sanitation facilities have made dysentery and cholera rare diseases in this country, emerging public policies designed to restrict and control the use of tobacco may someday make smoking-related diseases rare, rather than the leading cause of preventable death that they are now. Tobacco use is as much a public health risk as the infectious diseases of the past century, and the primary care clinician should be a vocal member of the antitobacco activism within his or her community.

General References*

Agency for Health Care Policy and Research. **Smoking cessation: clinical practice guideline, no. 18. (USDHHS) AHCPR Publication No. 96-0692.** Washington, DC: U.S. Government Printing Office, 1996.
> Clinical practice guideline for smoking cessation. Copies of the full guideline and of a brief "Quick Reference Guide for Primary Care Clinicians" are available by phoning 800-358-9295.

American Psychiatric Association. **Practice guideline for the treatment of patients with nicotine dependence.** Am J Psychiatry 153(Suppl 10):1–31, 1996.
> Discusses psychosocial/behavioral treatments, hypnosis, acupuncture, and a broad range of attempted pharmacotherapies.

Bartecchi CE, MacKenzie TD, Schrier RW. The human costs of tobacco use (first of two parts). N Engl J Med 330:907–912, 1994; and MacKenzie TD, Bartecchi CE, Schrier RW. The human costs of tobacco use (second of two parts). N Engl J Med 330:975–980, 1994.
> Two-part review of the health and economic consequences of tobacco use. Includes a description of the tobacco industry's actions to promote and society's actions to prevent tobacco use.

Benowitz NL. Pharmacologic aspects of cigarette smoking and nicotine addiction. N Engl J Med 319:1318–1330, 1988.
> An excellent overview of the pharmacologic aspects of smoking and nicotine dependence.

Fiore MC, Jorenby DE, Baker TB, et al. Tobacco dependence and the nicotine patch: clinical guidelines for effective use. JAMA 268: 2687–2694, 1992.
> An excellent discussion of smoking cessation treatment incorporating nicotine replacement, primarily with the transdermal patch. Includes specific recommendations for office practice.

Giovino GA, Henningfield JE, Tomar SL, et al. Epidemiology of tobacco use and dependence. Epidemiol Rev 17:48–65, 1995.
> An overview of the historic and current epidemiology of tobacco use and of the tobacco dependence syndrome.

---

*Bold print (general references) and bold numerals (specific references) denote published controlled clinical trials, meta-analyses, or consensus-based recommendations.

Kessler DA, Witt AM, Barnett PS, et al. The Food and Drug Administration's regulation of tobacco products. N Engl J Med 335:988–994, 1996.

>An informative overview of the empirical basis for regulating tobacco products as drug delivery devices for nicotine, including industry manipulation of nicotine and direction of advertising to youth.

National Tobacco Control Organizations

Action on Smoking and Health (ASH), 2013 H Street NW, Washington, DC 20006, http://ash.org.

Americans for Non Smokers Rights (ANR), 2530 San Pablo Avenue, Suite J, Berkeley, CA 94702, http://www.no-smoke.org.

Smokescreen, a free Website that makes powerful "electronic advocacy" easy to use, www.smokescreen.org.

Technical Information Center of the Office on Smoking and Health at the Centers for Disease Control and Prevention (telephone 770-488-5708). Provides free bibliographic assistance for locating articles on any smoking-related issue. It can also provide copies of the annual Surgeon General's Report on Smoking and Health, as well as other publications.

Specific References

1. Benowitz NL, Jacob P. Nicotine and carbon monoxide intake from high- and low-yield cigarettes. Clin Pharmacol Ther 36:265–270, 1984.
2. Brownson RC, Alavanja MCR, Hock ET, et al. Passive smoking and lung cancer in nonsmoking women. Am J Public Health 82:1525–1530, 1992.
3. Bruvold WH. A meta-analysis of adolescent smoking prevention programs. Am J Public Health 83:872–880, 1993.
4. Burling TA, Singleton EG, Bigelow GE, et al. Smoking following myocardial infarction: a critical review of the literature. Health Psychol 3:83–96, 1984.
5. Carmelli D, Swan GE, Robinette D, et al. Genetic influence on smoking: a study of male twins. N Engl J Med 327:829–833, 1992.
6. Chilmonczyk BA, Salmun LM, Megathlin KN, et al. Association between exposure to environmental tobacco smoke and exacerbations of asthma in children. N Engl J Med 328:1665–1669, 1993.
7. Council on Scientific Affairs. Health effects of smokeless tobacco. JAMA 255:1038–1044, 1986.
8. Cummings SR, Rubin SM, Oster G. The cost-effectiveness of counseling smokers to quit. JAMA 261:75–79, 1989.
9. Fagerstrom KO, Schneider NG, Lunell E. Effectiveness of nicotine patch and nicotine gum as individual versus combined treatments for tobacco withdrawal symptoms. Psychopharmacology 111:271–277, 1993.
10. Fielding JE, Phenow KJ. Health effects of involuntary smoking. N Engl J Med 319:1452–1460, 1988.
11. Fiore MC, Smith SS, Jorenby DE, Baker TB. The effectiveness of the nicotine patch for smoking cessation: a meta-analysis. JAMA 271:1940–1947, 1994.
12. Fiscella K, Franks P. Cost-effectiveness of the transdermal nicotine patch as an adjunct to physicians' smoking cessation counseling. JAMA 275:1247–1251, 1996.
13. Frank E, Winkleby MA, Altman DG, et al. Predictors of physicians' smoking cessation advice. JAMA 266:3139–3144, 1991.
14. Gross J, Stitzer ML, Maldonado J. Nicotine replacement: effects on postcessation weight gain. J Consult Clin Psychol 57:87–92, 1989.
15. Higgins MW, Enright PL, Kronmal RA, et al. Smoking and lung function in elderly men and women. JAMA 269:2741–2748, 1993.
16. Hughes JR. Tobacco withdrawal in self-quitters. J Consult Clin Psychol 60:689–697, 1992.
17. Hughes JR, Hatsukami D. Signs and symptoms of tobacco withdrawal. Arch Gen Psychiatry 43:289–294, 1986.
18. Hurt RD, Sachs DPL, Glover ED, et al. A comparison of sustained-release bupropion and placebo for smoking cessation. N Engl J Med 337:1195–1202, 1997.
19. Jaen CR, Stange KC, Nutting PA. Competing demands of primary care: a model for the delivery of clinical preventive services. J Fam Pract 38:166–171, 1994.
20. Jorenby DE, Hatsukami DK, Smith SS, et al. Characterization of tobacco withdrawal symptoms: transdermal nicotine reduces hunger and weight gain. Psychopharmacology 128:130–138, 1996.
21. Jorenby DE, Keehn DS, Fiore MC. Comparative efficacy and tolerability of nicotine replacement therapies. CNS Drugs 3:227–236, 1995.
22. Joseph AM, Norman SM, Ferry LH, et al. The safety of transdermal nicotine as an aid to smoking cessation in patients with cardiac disease. N Engl J Med 335(24):1792–1798, 1996.
23. Kaufman DW, Helmrich SP, Rosenberg L, et al. Nicotine and carbon monoxide content of cigarette smoke and the risk of myocardial infarction in young men. N Engl J Med 308:409–413, 1983.
24. Kozlowski LT, Frecker RC, Khouw V, Pope MA. The misuse of less-hazardous cigarettes and its detection: hole-blocking of ventilated filters. Am J Public Health 70:1202–1203, 1980.
25. Pederson LL. Compliance with physician advice to quit smoking: a review of the literature. Prev Med 11:71–84, 1982.
26. Perkins KA, Epstein LH, Marks BL, et al. The effect of nicotine on energy expenditure during light physical activity. N Engl J Med 320:898–903, 1989.
27. Rigotti NA. Cigarette smoking and body weight. N Engl J Med 320:931–933, 1989.
28. Robinson MD, Laurent SL, Little JM Jr. Including smoking status as a new vital sign: it works. J Fam Pract 40:556–563, 1995.
29. Russell MAH, Wilson C, Taylor C, Baker CD. Effect of general practitioners' advice against smoking. BMJ 2:231–235, 1979.
30. Sexton M, Hebel JR. A clinical trial of change in maternal smoking and its effect on birth weight. JAMA 251:911–915, 1984.
31. Shiffman S. Relapse following smoking cessation: a situational analysis. J Consult Clin Psychol 50:71–86, 1982.
32. Sparrow D, Stefos T, Bosse R, Weiss ST. The relationship of tar content to decline in pulmonary function in cigarette smokers. Am Rev Respir Dis 127:56–58, 1983.
33. Stolerman IP, Jarvis MJ. The scientific case that nicotine is addictive. Psychopharmacology 117:2–10, 1995.

CHAPTER 21

Alcoholism and Associated Problems*

MICHAEL I. FINGERHOOD, MD

Along with cardiovascular disease and cancer, alcoholism ranks among the top three causes of death and disability in the United States. One in three Americans reports that drinking has caused trouble in his or her family (21). The estimated cost of alcoholism to society in 1988 was $85.8 billion (52), with an untold additional cost in the suffering of people who are close to alcoholics. It is also estimated that more than three-fourths of the alcoholics in the United States do not receive treatment for their alcoholism (13). Many of these people have early alcoholism and would be likely to recover successfully if diagnosed and treated.

Until recently, alcoholism was widely regarded as a hopeless condition with a poor prognosis for recovery. Yet alcoholism is one of the most treatable of all medical and psychiatric conditions, with a high long-term success rate when a disease model of alcoholism is used in diagnosis and treatment.

DEFINITION OF ALCOHOLISM

A useful, broad definition of alcoholism is *recurring trouble associated with drinking alcohol.* The trouble may occur in one or more of several domains, including interpersonal (e.g., valued relationships, especially within the family), educational, legal, financial, medical, or occupational. Although there are many exceptions, trouble caused by alcoholism usually occurs in that order of progression, so that one's health and job are last to be overtly affected. The trouble may include the physiologic manifestations of dependence or addiction: *tolerance* (the need for increased amounts of a substance to achieve intoxication or desired effect) and *withdrawal* symptoms. The drinking that is characteristic of alcoholism includes one or more of the following abnormal patterns: inability to control one's use of alcohol (always present), drinking alone, avoiding

---

*L. Randol Barker coauthored this chapter in previous editions of this book.

situations where alcohol is not available, drinking before going to a party, gulping drinks, and continuing to drink alcohol despite occupational, psychosocial, or physical problems caused by drinking.

Consensus Definition

In 1992, a multidisciplinary committee of the National Council on Alcoholism and Drug Dependence and the American Society of Addiction Medicine issued its revised definition of alcoholism: "Alcoholism is a primary, chronic disease with genetic, psychosocial, and environmental factors influencing its development and manifestations. The disease is often progressive and fatal. It is characterized by impaired control over drinking, preoccupation with the drug alcohol despite adverse consequences, and distortions in thinking, most notably denial. Each of these symptoms may be continuous or periodic" (38). Unlike previously issued definitions, this one specifically included denial as a key component of the definition of alcoholism.

Alcoholism is classified by the American Psychiatric Association (APA) under the broad rubric *Substance-Related Use Disorders* (5). In its subclassification for these disorders, the APA has generic criteria for *substance abuse* (abnormal use, with unwanted consequences) and *substance dependence* (more intensive abuse patterns or physiologic manifestations of addiction). The criteria for these two subclassifications are found in Chapter 22. Another widely used term for these disorders is *chemical dependence*. Many people with chemical dependence abuse multiple psychoactive substances (e.g., an alcoholic patient may also abuse cocaine or a benzodiazepine). Chapter 22 describes polydrug abuse and delineates the characteristics of the specific substance use disorders that are common in the United States.

CAUSES

The causes of alcoholism are multifactorial and poorly understood (31,58). A predisposition to alcoholism appears to be inherited by at least half of all alcoholic patients, and there is some evidence that inherited factors are associated with the inability to control use of alcohol (12,17). Social conditioning and enabling behavior by others close to the individual (see "Co-Alcoholism," below) and being a child in a dysfunctional family (see below) are important nongenetic factors. For about 10 to 20% of alcoholic men, another mental disorder (especially antisocial personality disorder, primary abuse of other substances, or an affective disorder) may play a role (51). For alcoholic women, there is evidence that preexisting mental illness, especially a phobic disorder or major depression, may play a role. In addition, for elderly alcoholics whose problem began after the age of 50, the losses and isolation that accompany aging are often associated with the onset of problem drinking. These factors do not account for all alcoholism. They only add credence to the concept that alcoholism is a complex disease and not the result of moral turpitude.

ALCOHOLIC BEVERAGES: CONTENT AND METABOLISM

Alcoholic beverages can be divided into nondistilled (wine and beer) and distilled varieties. The concentration of alcohol (ethanol) in wine ranges from 10 to 22% by volume and is 12 to 14% in most wines. Beer usually contains 4 to 5% alcohol by volume, but beers fermented in the bottle contain a higher percentage of alcohol. The distilled alcoholic beverages—whiskey, brandy, rum, gin, and vodka—contain a higher percentage of alcohol. Alcoholic fermentation ceases when the concentration of alcohol exceeds 15% by volume; therefore, to manufacture more potent beverages, distillation or fortification is necessary. In the United States, the word *proof* is preceded by a number that is double the percentage of alcohol by volume; thus, 90 proof whiskey contains 45% alcohol by volume. One drink of distilled alcohol (1 fluid oz), one glass of wine (4 oz), and one beer (12 oz) contain approximately the same amount of alcohol.

In a 154-pound (70-kg) person, on an empty stomach, one drink of distilled alcohol (usually 1 fluid oz or 30 mL) produces a peak blood alcohol level (BAL) of approximately 25 mg/dL within 30 minutes of ingestion. Approximately 15 mg/dL is metabolized per hour. For example, the alcohol in 120 mL of whiskey would take about 5 to 6 hours to be metabolized. The rate of metabolism is higher—even in the range of 20 to 25 mg/dL per hour—in the alcoholic who drinks heavily each day for many months. To reach a BAL of 300 mg/dL, a 70-kg person generally has to consume 14 to 20 drinks over a few hours.

EPIDEMIOLOGY

Prevalence

In a survey of representative American communities, alcoholism was found to be the most common psychosocial disorder in American men between the ages of 18 and 65 and the fourth most common in American women in the age range 18 to 24 years (40). Alcoholism affects approximately 10% of adult Americans. Among the homeless, this figure runs higher, with some estimates running as high as 45%. Studies of teenage students show that the rates of problem drinking (heavy drinking or drinking to get drunk) exceed the rates of alcoholism in adults, even though the purchase of alcohol by teenagers is illegal (7).

In 1990, yearly consumption of alcohol in the United States was 2.43 gallons of pure alcohol, the equivalent of about 576 twelve-ounce cans of beer, for every person over the age of 15 (52). Per capita alcohol consumption peaks under the age of 50 and declines with increasing age. Because about one-third of the adult population is abstinent, the consumption of alcohol is concentrated in the approximately 94 million drinking Americans. About one-third of that number (30 million) consume approximately 70% of all the alcohol produced. It is this group that uses the health system more often, is most at risk of trauma, and has the recurring problems that constitute alcoholism (73).

Among *general hospital inpatients,* recent studies documented alcoholism in 25% of patients. However, caregivers involved in the treatment of these patients significantly underdiagnosed alcoholism (36,57). Similar percentages have been reported from *emergency departments, clinics, and office practices.* A conservative estimate would be that at least 1 in 10 ambulatory patients has alcoholism or another form of chemical dependence and that at least another 10 or 20% are suffering from a concomitant condition seen in family members that is now called co-alcoholism or codependence (see below). Alcoholism afflicts all ethnic, cultural, and socioeconomic groups, and no single group is immune.

Mortality and Morbidity

Prospective studies show that alcoholic patients have two to four times higher death rates and much higher rates of medical and psychosocial morbidity than do matched controls (34,43). The most common causes of early death in alcoholics are cirrhosis of the liver, cancers of the respiratory and gastrointestinal tracts, accidents, suicide, and ischemic heart disease. Most alcoholics smoke and, in fact, lung cancer is the most common cancer diagnosed in alcoholics (30). During 1995, alcohol-related motor vehicle accidents resulted in 17,274 deaths in the United States (41). Alcohol-related traffic accidents are the leading cause of death for teenagers and young adults. In 1988, 5% of deaths in the United States were alcohol related (52).

Importantly, it has been found that alcoholic men who achieve long-term abstinence do not differ from nonalcoholic men in mortality rate (16). However, relapse was significantly related to mortality.

Use of Health Services

Alcoholics who are untreated for their alcoholism tend to be high users of medical care. Overall, it is estimated that 20% of spending for hospital care and 12% of the total expenditure for adult health care are for problems caused by alcoholism (64). A study representing a variety of hospital types showed that alcoholics constituted a major proportion of the high-cost 13% of patients who consumed as many resources as the low-cost 87% (73). The high-cost group was further characterized by having repeated hospitalizations for the same disease and having a five times higher incidence of unexpected complications of their illnesses than the low-cost group. Other studies show that when alcoholics are successfully treated, their use of health services decreases to that of the general population (29).

NATURAL HISTORY OF ALCOHOLISM

The natural history of alcoholism in men has been delineated in retrospective and prospective studies. In Jellinek's classic retrospective study of recovering alcoholic men (31), the majority of subjects identified multiple phases in the progression of their disease: an initial phase, lasting months to years, in which they used alcohol to relieve tension and developed tolerance to alcohol; a phase in which they experienced blackouts (amnesia for drinking-associated events), increasing preoccupation with getting alcohol, and profound loss of control over use of alcohol; a phase in which there were overt psychologic and behavioral consequences (rationalization, grandiosity, aggressive behavior, remorse, efforts to abstain); and a stage characterized by chronic intoxication and serious deterioration of health and psychosocial functioning. In Vaillant's more recent prospective study (58), this multiphase course of alcoholism characterized three-quarters of men who became alcoholic. Most of the remaining men exhibited abnormal drinking patterns, usually rituals to constrain the uncontrolled drinking that they themselves recognized as abnormal, and had less alcohol-related trouble with family, job, and health. Importantly, in these and other studies of the course of alcoholism it has been found that periodic abstinence or moderation of use is typical. Although anecdotal information suggests that an occasional person with what appears to be alcoholism can return to normal drinking, this is very uncommon and not clinically useful to consider.

MANIFESTATIONS OF ALCOHOLISM

Alcoholism is a protean disease, and it is probably the most common great masquerader today. Table 21.1 lists medical, psychosocial, legal, and other manifestations often associated with alcoholism. Manifestations are ranked in the table according to their strength as diagnostic features, ranging from those that are diagnostic of alcoholism to those that should make one at least consider alcoholism. A number of the most important manifestations of alcoholism are discussed here.

Legal Problems

A history or record of driving while intoxicated (DWI) highly suggests alcoholism. In one study of about 21,000 consecutive people with DWIs (22), approximately 75% of first-time offenders were found to be alcoholic. Of those with two DWI arrests, more than 90% were alcoholic, and of those with three, essentially 100% were alcoholic. A prison record is also strongly suggestive because most prison inmates have a history of alcoholism or other chemical dependence. Child and spouse/partner abuse is also highly associated with alcoholism.

Table 21.1. Medical, Psychiatric, Legal, and Other Findings Suggestive (0 to *) to Highly Suggestive (to ***) or Diagnostic (****) of Alcoholism**

Presenting Complaint and History

**** Drinking problem, recurring[a]	* Depression
*** Blackouts with drinking	* Suicide attempt
*** Spouse/other complains of patient's drinking	* Sexual dysfunction
*** Driving while intoxicated (DWI) record	* Legal problem
*** Prison record	* Noncompliance in treatment
*** Change in alcohol or drug tolerance	* School learning problem
** Frequent requests for mood-changing drugs	* Hypertension
** Gastrointestinal bleeding, especially upper	Headache
** Traumatic injuries, fracture	Palpitations
** Parent, grandparent, or relative alcoholic	Abdominal pain
** Friends alcoholic or other chemical dependence	Amenorrhea
** Family or other violence	Weight loss
** Child abuse or neglect	Vague complaints
** First seizure in an adult	Insomnia
** Job performance problem	Anxiety
* Unexplained syncope	Marital discord
	Financial problem

Alcohol or Other Drug Use History

**** Alcohol use recurring, interfering with health, job, or social functioning[a]	** Other drug misuse or dependence
	* Cigarette smoker
*** Patients says, "I can stop drinking anytime," or the equivalent; or patient gets evasive or angry, or talks glibly during taking of drinking history	
*** Patient states that he or she has consciously stopped drinking completely for any length of time	

Physical Examination

*** Odor of beverage alcohol on breath	* Borderline tachycardia
*** Parotid gland enlargement, bilateral	* Thin extremities in proportion to trunk
*** Spider nevi or angioma	* Splenomegaly
*** Tremulousness, hallucinosis	* Hypertension
** Cigarette stains on fingers	Diaphoresis
** Breath mints odor	Alopecia
** Many scars or tattoos	Abdominal tenderness
** Hepatomegaly	Cerebellar signs (e.g., nystagmus)
** Gynecomastia	
** Small testicles	
** Unexplained bruises, abrasions, or cuts	

Laboratory Abnormalities

**** Blood alcohol level greater than 300 mg/100 mL[a]	** Abnormal liver function tests (especially AST > ALT)
*** Blood alcohol level greater than 100 mg/100 mL without impairment	** Anemia, macrocytic or megaloblastic, microcytic, or mixed
*** High serum ammonia	* Hyperuricemia
*** γ-Glutamyl transpeptidase elevation	* Creatine kinase elevation
** Blood alcohol level positive, any amount	* Hypophosphatemia or hypomagnesemia
** High amylase (nonspecific for pancreas)	Electrolyte imbalance (hyponatremia, hypokalemia)
	Low white blood cell or platelet count
	Hyperlipoproteinemia, type 4 or 5

Diagnosis

**** Hepatitis, alcoholic[a]	** Attempted suicide
*** Pancreatitis, acute or chronic	** Gastritis
*** Cirrhosis	** Refractory hypertension
*** Portal hypertension	** Cerebellar degeneration
*** Wernicke–Korsakoff syndrome	** Peripheral neuropathy
*** Frequent trauma	** Aspiration pneumonia
*** Cold injury	* Gout
*** Nose and throat cancer	* Cardiomyopathy
** Other chemical dependence	* Tuberculosis
** Drownings	* Anxiety
** Burns, especially third degree	* Depression
** Leaves hospital against medical advise	* Marital discord or family problem

[a]Major criteria of the National Council on Alcoholism for the diagnosis of alcoholism (see "General References").

Behavioral, Psychiatric, and Neurologic Problems

Accidents and trauma, including burns, are often associated with alcoholism; in more than half of patients with severe trauma, alcohol or other psychoactive drug use can be detected (54). Among patients with symptoms of chronic mental illness, especially symptoms of depression and anxiety, alcoholism is common. Usually alcoholism is the primary problem in these patients, and treatment of mental symptoms is not successful until the alcoholism is treated.

Alcohol Intoxication

The best known acute consequence of alcoholism is alcohol intoxication, which should usually present no diagnostic problem. Because this condition is so common, diagnostic errors are made when it is forgotten that "drunken" behavior—often with evidence of recent alcohol use—may be caused by a host of conditions, such as infection, metabolic disturbance, neurologic disease, or other drug toxicity. Because alcoholics are especially prone to many disorders that may be manifested as deranged behavior, they should be examined systematically before a diagnosis of simple drunkenness is made.

Alcohol intoxication may be characterized by one or more of the following: relaxation and sedation, euphoria, impaired coordination, loudness, lowered inhibitions, poor memory and judgment, labile mood, slurred speech, nausea, vomiting, and obtundation (Table 21.2). An initial period of excitement and euphoria is often followed by depression and sleep, or possibly coma. The duration and magnitude of the intoxication depend on the amount and the rapidity with which the alcohol was drunk and whether the patient drank on an empty stomach (enhancing the rate of absorption). Tolerance is also a significant factor, as an alcoholic may acquire the (reversible) capacity to increase the rate of alcohol metabolism. Moreover, alcoholics characteristically develop substantial central tolerance, so that they appear fairly sober at blood alcohol levels of 150 mg/dL or more. Most nonalcoholic people become intoxicated at levels between 100 and 200 mg/dL, and some at levels as low as 30 mg/dL. Levels over 400 mg/dL may be lethal, with death usually resulting from depressed respiration or aspiration of vomitus.

Blackouts

Blackouts, amnesia for events that occurred during a period of intoxication, are common. However, 10 to 25% of alcoholics do not have memory blackouts, and some normal drinkers have experienced blackouts after drinking.

Alcohol Idiosyncratic Intoxication

Alcohol idiosyncratic intoxication (pathologic intoxication) is an uncommon syndrome characterized by an extreme, often aggressive or violent reaction to drinking alcohol, which is often followed by amnesia for the episode. The behavior is atypical of the person when not drinking. The duration of this condition is brief (hours), and the person returns to his or her normal state as the blood alcohol level falls. Temporal lobe epilepsy, sedative-hypnotic use, and malingering should be ruled out.

Alcohol Amnestic Disorder (Korsakoff's Psychosis)

Alcohol amnestic disorder is characterized chiefly by short-term memory impairment, associated with some loss of long-term memory, in the absence of clouded consciousness (delirium) or general loss of intellectual abilities (dementia). (For definitions and detailed discussions of delirium and dementia, see Chapter 17.) Patients with less advanced forms of this disorder may be substantially impaired, but they may appear superficially to be normal, particularly because they often attempt to minimize their impairment and to confabulate in order to fill in memory gaps.

The amnestic disorder often follows an episode of *Wernicke's encephalopathy,* a syndrome of global confusion, ataxia, and impaired eye movement, caused by thiamine deficiency, which may occur suddenly or gradually over several days. Parenteral thiamine given during an acute episode of Wernicke's encephalopathy may prevent the amnestic syndrome.

With abstention from alcohol and good nutrition for several months, some patients recover entirely from the alcohol amnestic syndrome. Many remain grossly impaired and require institutional care; of these approximately 20% improve modestly with good long-term institutional support (46).

Table 21.2. Expected Effects According to Blood Alcohol Level for a Person Without Tolerance to Alcohol

Blood Alcohol Level (mg/dL)	Expected Effect	Approximate Location of Physiologic Disturbance
25–50	Relaxation, sedation	
50–100	Coordination impaired; euphoric; loud conversation; apparent reduction of social inhibitions	Cerebral cortex
100–200	Ataxia; depressed fine motor ability, decreased mentation, attention span, and memory; poor judgment; labile mood; beginning of slurred speech	Limbic system and cerebellum
200–300	Marked ataxia and slurred speech, nausea and vomiting, tremor, irritable	Reticular activating system
300–400	Stage 1 anesthesia (unconsciousness), memory lapse	Reticular activating system
>400	Respiratory failure, coma, death	Medulla oblongata

Dementia Associated with Alcoholism

When more generalized intellectual impairment develops after years of heavy drinking, the diagnosis of dementia associated with alcoholism is appropriate. An estimated 70% of actively drinking chronic alcoholics have some cognitive impairments, as measured by psychologic testing. Perhaps 10% of these have dementia that is sufficiently apparent and noticeable without psychologic testing. Because even detoxified alcoholics are likely to show some cognitive impairment for a period after cessation of drinking, this diagnosis should not be made unless dementia persists for at least 1 month after drinking has stopped. Other causes of dementia must be excluded (see Chapter 17).

All alcoholics with any signs of dementia should be treated with high-dosage thiamine (100 mg/day) and multivitamins long term. Some improve over months to years of abstinence.

Other Medical Complications

The various *deficiency states* involved in a diet composed largely of nutritionally empty alcoholic calories (7 calories/g), as well as the *direct toxic actions of alcohol* itself, have been implicated in the pathogenesis of many of the medical consequences of alcoholism. These disorders are legion, spare no body system, and most are related to the quantity and duration of alcohol consumption. Among the more common medical complications of alcoholism are gastritis; fatty liver, hepatitis, or cirrhosis; pancreatitis; cerebellar ataxia; gout; peripheral neuropathy; rhabdomyolysis; hematologic abnormalities (elevated mean corpuscular volume of red blood cells, anemia, thrombocytopenia); hypoglycemia; ketoacidosis; electrolyte abnormalities (hyponatremia, hypokalemia); pulmonary infections suggesting aspiration or impaired defenses (tuberculosis and pneumonia); cancers of the liver, respiratory, and gastrointestinal tract; atrial fibrillation; cardiomyopathy; hypertension; and trauma.

Chronic hypertension is a recognized manifestation of alcoholism. Because it often remits within weeks of discontinuing alcohol, it may be the most common reversible cause of hypertension (see Chapter 62).

Because it is both serious and preventable, the *fetal alcohol syndrome* deserves special mention. It is manifested by morphologic abnormalities, low birth weight, and developmental and cognitive impairment. This syndrome is a consequence of alcohol ingestion during pregnancy. The risk of minor abnormalities (e.g., low birth weight) begins with the consumption of one drink per day; this risk increases with increasingly larger amounts of alcohol consumption. Because of this, it is prudent to advise women not to drink during pregnancy.

Medical Consequences: A Summary View

Nearly all of the medical consequences of alcoholism tend to have certain common characteristics:

- Drinking alcohol causes them.
- A poor diet generally makes most of them worse and makes them occur earlier.
- Harmful habits, such as cigarette smoking and the misuse of other drugs, also tend to compound the medical consequences.
- If the patient continues to consume alcohol, damage involving major organs progresses slowly, but relentlessly, over the course of a few years, often ending in organ failure. The organs affected by alcohol and the rate of decline in function of these organs vary greatly among patients. Severity of damage is loosely correlated with dosage of alcohol; *for one organ, the liver, damage is more common in women at any level of alcohol consumption.*

This progression of organic damage occurs no matter what medical or psychologic intervention the patient receives, as long as drinking continues. If the patient stops drinking, many of the pathophysiologic processes caused by alcohol will reverse rapidly, such as those in the blood and bone marrow (cytopenias), those in the small intestine (malabsorption), hypertension, and fluid and electrolyte imbalance. Other processes do not reverse rapidly with abstinence, but they usually do not progress and often improve over weeks and months. Alcoholic hepatitis, chronic pancreatitis, and cognitive deficits are conditions that tend to improve more gradually.

SCREENING FOR AND DIAGNOSING ALCOHOLISM

Overview

Except when a patient presents with overt behavioral or medical evidence of alcoholism (see diagnostic manifestations in Table 21.1), the diagnosis of alcoholism requires skillful interviewing and careful evaluation of other information. Such an approach is needed for most alcoholics, whose disease is a private problem experienced by them and those who are close to them. In addition to unwanted psychosocial and physiologic consequences of alcoholism, two cardinal features inevitably emerge when one is obtaining information from an alcoholic or others who know him or her: evidence of inability to control the use of alcohol and denial that a significant problem exists.

Loss of Control

Continuous inability to control the use of alcohol is not always present in alcoholics. Indeed, many can go for periods of a few hours (e.g., at a social gathering) to a few months of apparently normal drinking. Therefore, the absence of overt loss of control for a period of time does not rule out alcoholism. In such patients, the loss of control returns eventually. Inability to control one's drinking may be manifested acutely, when the person drinks more than was intended to or is unable to stop drinking and becomes intoxicated; or it may follow a chronic pattern, in which the patient drinks heavily for a few days or most days of each week, often alone, and cannot stop. In addition, some alcoholic patients describe rituals to constrain their intake because of previous trouble with control (e.g., never having a first drink until after dinner). Nonalcoholic people do not describe drinking in these ways, and such information usually indicates that there is a serious problem. Control of alcohol consumption is always an issue for the alcoholic.

Denial

Denial (i.e., the direct or implied message that there is no problem) is present in nearly all actively drinking alcoholics. Denial behavior and responses may be caused by one or more of the following mechanisms: conscious lying (one of the least common mechanisms); classic denial (an adaptive coping response to avoid the shame, lowered self-esteem, and distressing inability to overcome the drinking problem that are experienced by most alcoholics); memory blackout caused by drinking; euphoric recall (the patient remembers only the good times experienced when drinking); the fact that no one points out problems related to drinking; wishful thinking; denial on the part of the family and other close people, including helping professionals; ignorance of what an alcoholic is; toxic effects on information processing and memory; stigma related to the term *alcoholic;* fear of the unknown; and a complex thinking quandary. This last mechanism consists of genuine confusion on the part of the patient; he or she knows that something is wrong but somehow cannot connect it with drinking alcohol (62).

Denial presents in some of the following ways: rationalizations (e.g., "I drink because my work is more than anyone should try to do"), glibness and humor, hostility ("I came to you about my blood pressure and I would appreciate it if we could stay out of my personal life"), comparison of oneself with a "real problem drinker" ("Now see here, I have a lovely family, a job that I enjoy . . . I have nothing in common with those poor guys who have lost it; those are your alcoholics"), reticence to discuss drinking, and the assertions by other physicians or family members that the patient has no problem with alcohol. An alcoholic patient's denial responses are usually the result of years of complex adapting to dependence on alcohol. This helps explain why these responses may seem to be refractory and may cause much frustration during screening/diagnostic interviewing and during efforts to get the patient to accept the diagnosis and agree to treatment (32).

Screening for Alcoholism

Because alcoholism is common and because the evidence for it is usually private information that patients do not volunteer, all patients should be screened for this problem. The goal of screening, and of further inquiry when there are positive responses to screening, is to be confident that one has ruled out alcoholism, has

---

1. Integrate alcohol use inquiry into interview so that it follows inquiry about less sensitive habits.

   Example: "We have talked about your usual diet and your smoking. Can you tell me how you use alcoholic beverages?" (or "How about alcoholic beverages . . .?").

   If the patient says that he/she has never used alcohol and shows no sign of discomfort, inquire about problem use in others (e.g., "Anyone in your family or other close persons who have a drinking problem?"). This helps to identify a risk factor for alcoholism and to identify patients who may suffer because of the alcoholism of another person.[a]

2. **General Questions:** For patients who report present or past use of alcohol, screen for evidence of alcoholism, with a general question such as the following:

   "Has (Did) your use of alcohol caused (cause) any kinds of problems for you?" or "Have you ever been concerned about your drinking?"

3. **CAGE Questions:**[b] If the patient has not disclosed a problem with drinking, use these four focused questions and probe for clarification of positive or ambivalent responses.

   "I'd like to ask you a few more questions about alcohol that I ask all of my patients . . ."

   C "Have you ever felt you ought to CUT DOWN on your drinking (use of _____)?"

   A "Have people ANNOYED you by criticizing your drinking (use of _____)?"

   G "Have you ever felt bad or GUILTY about your drinking (use of _____)?"

   E "Have you ever had a drink first thing in the morning (EYE OPENER) to steady your nerves or get rid of a hangover?" (For other substances: "Have you found that you have to take some _____ most days/some days to feel okay?")

   ---
   [a]See section on "Co-Alcoholism."
   [b]Modifications of questions for substances other than alcohol are shown in parentheses.

Figure 21.1.   A recommended approach to the use of interviewing to screen all patients for alcoholism and problems with alcohol in the family.

detected definite alcoholism, or must continue to consider alcoholism as a possible diagnosis.

There are a number of ways to screen for the cardinal features of alcoholism (27). The approach outlined in Figure 21.1 incorporates the four so-called CAGE questions into the interview (19). In this approach, exploratory inquiry about the use of alcoholic beverages follows inquiries about less sensitive habit information, and the inquiry begins with an open-ended question that prompts patients to respond with more than a simple *yes* or *no* or with a quantitative reply (e.g., "a few beers"). In patients who report any current or recent use of alcohol, discomfort, glibness, voluntary reporting of heavy use, or other information suggesting alcoholism (Table 21.1), including that from the patient's medical history, there is increased likelihood that a problem exists. In the absence of such clues, all patients who report alcohol use should still complete the follow-up questions listed in Figure 21.1 or other questions that focus on similar content.

The approach in Figure 21.1 is designed to uncover specific data that point to the diagnosis of alcoholism. The CAGE questions are derived from the larger Michigan Alcoholism Screening Test (MAST), a standardized instrument that has been used extensively for alcoholism screening (Table 21.3) (27,44). The questions in the MAST may be helpful when one is attempting to uncover occult alcoholism. The questions are best used to gather additional information within the flow of obtaining a history related to drinking, complementing and adding information to positive CAGE answers. The CAGE questions have the advantage of being simple to incorporate into an office interview, being phrased in a nonthreatening way, and focusing on several features that are present in most patients with alcoholism:

- *Inability to control* one's drinking, which leads to cutting back or quitting attempts (C).
- *Domestic problems* caused by one's drinking and that evoke negative responses from other people (A). The phrasing of this question places the blame on the one criticizing, so that a positive response is not self-incriminating.
- *Bad feelings* that one has about drinking-related actions (G). The phrasing of this question allows the patient to blame the drinking and not him- or herself.
- *Physiologic dependence* (E), as denoted by the need to drink to suppress withdrawal symptoms.

Studies of the CAGE questions have shown that they are sensitive (70 to 90% of alcoholics respond positively to one or more of the questions; most have at least two positive responses) and specific (80 to 95% of nonalcoholic people respond negatively to all four

Table 21.3. Michigan Alcoholism Screening Test (MAST)[a]

	Yes	No
0. Do you enjoy having a drink now and then?	0	
1. Do you feel you are a normal drinker? (By normal we mean you drink less than or as much as most other people and you have not gotten into any recurring trouble while drinking.)		2
2. Have you ever awakened the morning after some drinking the night before and found that you could not remember a part of the evening?	2	
3. Does either of your parents, or any other near relative, or your spouse, or any girlfriend or boyfriend ever worry or complain about your drinking?	1	
4. Can you stop drinking without a struggle after one or two drinks?		2
5. Do you feel guilty about your drinking?	1	
6. Do friends or relatives think you are a normal drinker?		2
7. Are you able to stop drinking when you want to?		2
8. Have you ever attended a meeting of Alcoholics Anonymous (AA)?	5	
9. Have you gotten into physical fights when you have been drinking?	1	
10. Has your drinking ever created problems between you and either of your parents, or another relative, your spouse, or any girlfriend or boyfriend?	2	
11. Has any family member of yours ever gone to anyone for help about your drinking?	2	
12. Have you ever lost friends because of your drinking?	2	
13. Have you ever gotten into trouble at work or at school because of drinking?	2	
14. Have you ever lost a job because of drinking?	2	
15. Have you ever neglected your obligations, your school work, your family, or your job for 2 or more days in a row because you were drinking?	2	
16. Do you drink before noon fairly often?	1	
17. Have you ever been told you have liver trouble? Cirrhosis?	2	
18. After heavy drinking have you ever had severe shaking, or heard voices or seen things that really weren't there?	2 (5 DTs)	
19. Have you ever gone to anyone for help about your drinking?	5	
20. Have you ever been in a hospital because of drinking?	5	
21. Have you ever been a patient in a psychiatric hospital or on a psychiatric ward of a general hospital where drinking was part of the problem that resulted in hospitalization?	2	
22. Have you ever been seen at a psychiatric or mental health clinic or gone to any doctor, social worker, or clergy for help with any emotional problem, where drinking was a part of the problem?	2	
23. Have you ever been arrested for drunk driving, driving while intoxicated, or driving under the influence of alcoholic beverages or any other drug? (If YES, How many times? _____)	2 each	
24. Have you ever been arrested, or taken into custody, even for a few hours, because of other drunk behavior, whether due to alcohol or another drug? (If YES, How many times? _____)	2 each	

[a]Interpretation of standard MAST: 0 to 3 points, probable normal drinker; 4 points, borderline score; 5 to 9 points, 80% associated with alcoholism/chemical dependence; ≥10 points, 100% associated with alcoholism. The values assigned to each response are shown.

questions) (27). These test characteristics of the CAGE questions are superior to laboratory tests—γ-glutamyl transpeptidase (GGT), other liver function tests, and mean corpuscular volume (MCV)—that are often measured in patients with alcoholism (8,27). However, abnormalities in these tests may be helpful in supporting persistent inquiry and in confrontation (see below) in the suspected alcoholic.

Screening questions that focus on one common consequence of alcoholism—*trauma*—may be sensitive, especially the question, "Have you ever been injured after drinking?" (54). A positive response to this question, or a history of unexplained repeated trauma or traffic accidents, may be important in patients whose CAGE responses are equivocal or in patients who have few of the social contacts that are implied in the CAGE questions. The latter group includes antisocial younger drinkers, older people, and others who commonly become isolated.

Importantly, the approach in Figure 21.1 does not include direct inquiry about quantity or frequency of alcohol use. Although *quantitative inquiry* may be helpful for identifying an occasional patient who is ready to discuss problems associated with drinking, its disadvantages are that it does not focus on inability to control use or on adverse consequences of drinking, there is no gold standard for the cutoff quantity below or above which one can confidently exclude or diagnose alcoholism (27), and problem drinkers usually underreport the amount and frequency of their drinking (18) and may become guarded in their response to subsequent questions about patterns of use and consequences.

Diagnosis of Alcoholism

The confident diagnosis of alcoholism requires nonjudgmental exploration of any positive information obtained in screening. This may include asking for clarification (e.g., "Can you tell me more about the last time you decided to cut back a bit?" or "Exactly what does she say to annoy you?" or "How do you feel after you take that morning drink on the days that you do take it?"), gentle confrontation ("That must have made you feel pretty bad; sounds like the drinking had a lot to do with it") (49).

At times, a *planned interview with a family member or close friend,* by telephone or in person, may be needed to make a confident diagnosis of alcoholism. This means requesting the patient's permission to discuss his or her drinking with another person; the patient's response to this request may reveal a problem that was denied in response to screening questions (e.g., "No, no, don't talk to her; she'll tell you I overdo it every night, but that's her problem, not mine"). Questions to another person regarding the patient's drinking patterns and consequences of the drinking (asking the same questions contained in the CAGE and MAST instruments; i.e., "Has your husband ever felt he ought to cut down on his drinking?") usually yield abundant evidence for alcoholism when the problem is present. An exception may be the relatives of an elderly alcoholic who have little contact with him or her or have tacitly agreed to ignore or deny a frustrating, seemingly hopeless situation. In this instance, educating the family about the disease concept of alcoholism may be needed before they are willing to describe the patterns and consequences of the patient's drinking.

Through contact initiated by one or more family members, information will be produced that supports the diagnosis of alcoholism. Family members should be encouraged to tell the patient that they have contacted his or her doctor to describe these concerns. The ways in which the family can influence the treatment of the patient and can get help for themselves are described below.

In summary, except for the presence of the diagnostic manifestations of alcoholism (Table 21.1), there is no simple way to diagnose alcoholism. When the problem is not overt, skillful interviewing of the patient and evaluation of multiple pieces of information are needed to make this diagnosis. This process may be accomplished at one or two visits or over weeks to months.

GENERAL PRINCIPLES OF TREATMENT
Definition of Successful Treatment

Alcoholism is a highly treatable disease. Successful treatment depends largely on the skills of those who motivate the alcoholic patient to accept the diagnosis, to undergo detoxification (see below), and to enter and adhere to a long-term treatment process. *Treatment success can be defined as the achievement of abstinence or progressively longer periods of abstinence from alcohol (and other drugs), with improved life functioning for patients and their families.* (A case example is shown in Fig. 21.2.) Using this definition, when treatment is initiated and maintained for about 3 years, at least 70% of alcoholic patients successfully recover from alcoholism (68). This rate of recovery compares favorably with reported rates of spontaneous recovery from alcoholism, which range from 4 to 26%. Factors associated with good and poor outcomes after treatment are summarized below (see "Prognosis with Treatment").

The appropriate terms for describing an alcoholic in recovery are *recovered alcoholic* (a public or polite term) or *recovering alcoholic* (a personal or clinical term). The terms *ex-, reformed, former,* or *cured alcoholic* are inappropriate.

Despite reports that some alcoholics can learn controlled drinking, this goal of treatment has been shown in careful studies to be unrealistic for most alcoholics and should be avoided.

Avoiding a Psychoanalytic Approach

It has been repeatedly shown that treating alcoholics as though their abnormal drinking behavior were secondary to underlying psychopathology is usually unsuccessful and often countertherapeutic. Insight-

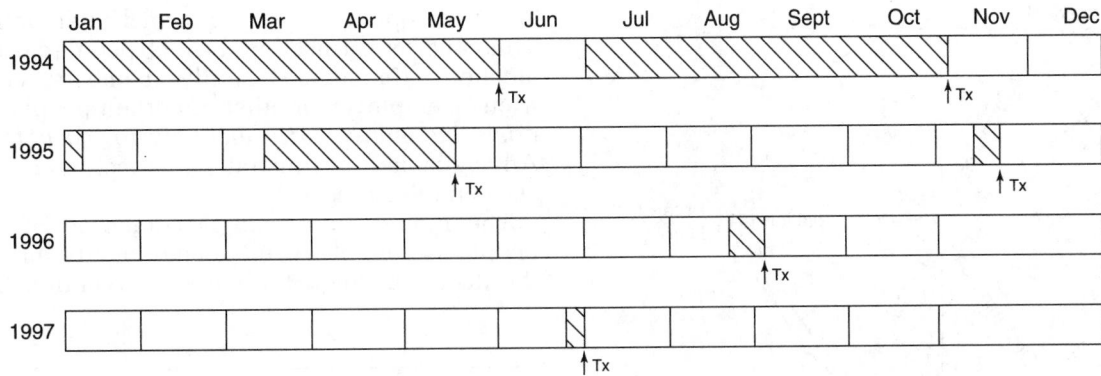

Figure 21.2. Drinking–sober profile of a 53-year-old factory supervisor who had been abusing alcohol for 15 years. The achievement of longer and longer periods of abstinence is typical of the process of recovery from alcoholism. *Hatched areas*, drinking; *clear areas*, abstinence; *Tx*, came in for treatment after having dropped out of treatment.

oriented or in-depth psychotherapy early in the treatment of alcoholism is therefore contraindicated. By contrast, supportive and directive psychotherapy, using the treatment methods outlined below and focused on the alcoholism as a primary disease, is usually effective in helping the alcoholic patient reach a successful recovery.

Breaking Down Denial and Motivating the Patient

Denial (see above) is the major obstacle to having a patient accept the diagnosis of alcoholism and agree to treatment. Three motivational techniques are fundamental in breaking down denial in patients, and in their family members if necessary: confrontation, showing empathy, and offering hope. These techniques are equally important in one-on-one interviews and the other paths to treatment that are described below. *Confrontation* is telling the person what one observes, including that one has diagnosed the disease alcoholism. The patient usually denies the diagnosis and may even get angry. However, with persistent and nonjudgmental confrontation, most patients eventually admit that they have a problem with alcohol. It is important in a confrontation not to argue with the patient but simply to restate the facts.

Statements that convey empathy and offer hope are important in allaying the person's denial, anxiety, anger, and shame. They should be interspersed with confrontational statements. Empathy is conveyed by stating that one recognizes the patient's feelings ("I can see that this is upsetting you") and by conveying concern ("I am very concerned about you"). Offering hope is crucial. The patient must hear, repeatedly, that there is a way out and that there is relief from the misery and bewilderment of the condition. The way out is through abstinence from alcohol and other psychoactive drugs—one day at a time—and regular use of group treatment, which includes self-help groups and group therapy (see below).

Motivation of the patient is an ongoing process. In a model described by Prochaska and DiClemente

(Fig. 21.3), one must first facilitate the patient to move from the state of *precontemplation* to *contemplation*. The patient must seriously be ready for change *(determination), take action* (detoxification and treatment) and, finally, work toward long-term sobriety (*maintenance*). Unfortunately, because alcoholism is a chronic disease, *relapse* is a likely part of the cycle (45).

After a confident diagnosis of alcoholism has been made, the objectives of care are to have the patient accept the diagnosis and agree to treatment. Specific aspects of this process are described here, beginning with one-on-one confrontation of the patient.

One-on-One Confrontation

Using the motivational techniques described above, one can often persuade an alcoholic patient to accept treatment. Several actions are critical in the one-on-one confrontation of the patient:

- Stating the diagnosis
- Explaining the disease model
- Making the model specific to the patient
- Telling about treatment
- Getting the patient (and the family) to accept (support) treatment
- Following through

Figure 21.4 summarizes a recommended approach that includes each of these actions. This approach may be incorporated into the interview at a single visit or into interviews at multiple visits. The term *drinking problem* may be used early in the discussion, before the patient's feelings regarding alcoholism are known. Even in the most denying and uncooperative patient, naming the diagnosis is useful because it plants a seed that is likely to grow, given time and motivation. One must be rather directive in confronting a patient with alcoholism. It is important, however, to include questions that *give the patient some sense of control* during this rather one-sided interaction (see items 3, 5, 7, and 10 in Fig. 21.4). Because most alcoholic patients have negative emotional responses, either overt or private,

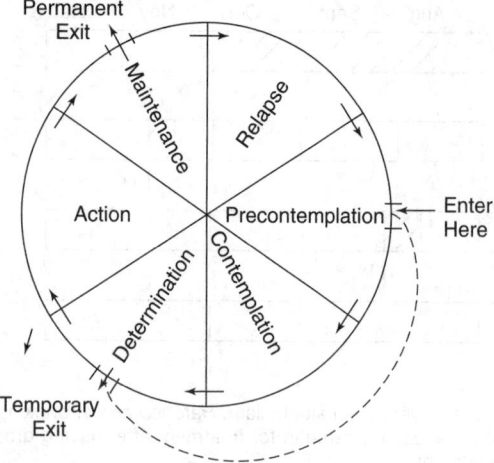

Figure 21.3. A stage model of the process of change. (Adapted from Prochaska JO, DiClemente CC. Transtheoretical therapy: toward a more integrative model of change. Psychother Theory Res Pract 19:276–288, 1982. Reprinted with permission from Miller WR, Jackson KA. Practical psychology for pastors. Englewood Cliffs, NJ: Prentice-Hall, 1985:130.)

to being told their diagnosis, it should be assumed that they will not register much of what one says and that *brevity, repetition, and directness* are essential. Repeated *statements of concern, optimism, and support* for the person are as important as statements of fact about the disease. Such statements help patients while they are hearing a diagnosis that inevitably brings shame, and help convince them that they have a disease for which they are not to blame. To ensure that patients do not conclude that they cannot avoid further drinking because they have a disease, one should tell them that it is their responsibility to seek treatment.

The first goal of treatment is abstinence from alcohol and other psychoactive drugs. However, it is never sufficient simply to tell the patient to stop drinking. Early in treatment, the patient must accept help in the difficult process of recovery. *This help is multidimensional.* In addition to regular follow-up by a supportive physician who believes the patient can recover, the most important elements are a plan for detoxification, Alcoholics Anonymous (AA) or group therapy, and family involvement (see below). Inpatient treatment in a specialized alcoholism treatment facility may be needed. Each of the possible treatment options should be explained to patients and their families. If one is not familiar with these, one should ask an alcoholism counselor to explain them to the patient. If the patient is in a crisis and not enough time is available during the first visit, a return appointment should be scheduled within a few days or the patient should be immediately referred to a reliable treatment program.

Formal Intervention

All too often, alcoholics with concerned families do not respond to efforts to motivate them to accept treatment. In this situation, the family should be told

about the option of using a formal intervention (33). This consists of a meeting at which people closest to the alcoholic (immediate family members, concerned friends, employer, or other important people) *create a crisis that motivates the alcoholic to accept treatment.* An available film illustrates this technique well (see "General References").

The intervention team is composed of as many people as possible who are emotionally important to the alcoholic. Before the actual intervention, this team

---

STATING THE DIAGNOSIS

1. Tell the patient the diagnosis (e.g., "I think that you have the disease alcoholism . . . and I am very concerned about you").

2. Acknowledge the patient's reaction (e.g., "I can see that this is making you pretty uncomfortable . . .").

EXPLAINING THE DISEASE MODEL

3. Ask the patient to tell you his/her idea of what alcoholism is. (Patient usually describes stereotype model of a skidrow alcoholic . . . "and that's not me!". . .)

4. Clarify the patient's model by stating four basic facts:
   a) Alcoholism is a disease ("a disease like other medical diseases . . . for example diabetes").
   b) Like other diseases, alcoholism has an early stage way before what you described.
   c) Like other diseases, alcoholism is not the patient's fault.
   d) Alcoholism can be treated and the chances of recovery are excellent.

MAKING THE MODEL SPECIFIC

5. Ask the patient if he/she knows why you think he/she has alcoholism.

6. Tell the patient the evidence that he/she has alcoholism. (Always restate concern for the patient; if appropriate, stress features of early alcoholism.)

TELLING ABOUT TREATMENT

7. Ask the patient what he/she knows about the treatment of alcoholism.

8. Tell the patient the basic facts about treatment:
   a) Abstinence
   b) Requires the help of other people

GETTING THE PATIENT (AND FAMILY) TO ACCEPT TREATMENT

9. Offer the patient treatment options that you know of (always include a local program that offers detoxification and Alcoholics Anonymous).

10. Get the patient to select a treatment plan and to make contact promptly (e.g., call available detoxification program, call local AA office and let patient speak with AA representative).

11. With the patient's permission, contact his/her spouse or significant person(s) (tell the diagnosis and plan, and initiate plans for family treatment).

FOLLOWING THROUGH

12. Schedule follow-up appointment in 1 or 2 weeks (consider 1 or 2 days if patient has not agreed to make a treatment decision).

Figure 21.4. A recommended approach for one-on-one confrontation of the patient in whom alcoholism has been diagnosed.

meets to talk about the alcoholism, to come together in their thinking, and to agree that their purpose is to show the patient in unmistakable terms that there is a problem and that he or she needs treatment. The process is initiated by having each participant put in writing specific dramatic instances of drinking-related incidents that led to anger, fear, disappointment, sadness, embarrassment, or other distress for the team member. The team then rehearses confronting the alcoholic. Each person learns to begin with an expression of concern for the alcoholic, to describe the disturbing event and how it made that person feel, and to name specific measures they will take if the patient does not agree to treatment (e.g., loss of job, no further visits by grandchildren). As part of a formal intervention, arrangements may be made in advance to have the person admitted for alcoholism treatment. Financing of treatment, packing clothes, arranging for absence from work, and other details must all be worked out by the team ahead of time.

Motivating Through Employee Assistance Programs

Increasingly, employers have recognized the economic and human costs of alcoholism and have developed employee assistance programs to motivate and assist alcoholics into treatment. Employers threaten to terminate employees who have deteriorating job performance due to alcoholism unless they get treatment and remain in treatment. Physicians asked to write work excuses can often work with employee assistance programs to coerce the denying alcoholic to get appropriate treatment for alcoholism. This approach uses the strong motivation to keep a job as leverage for getting treatment and following through to recovery—leverage the physician alone may not have on the patient.

The problem of the impaired professional and the use of measures similar to employee assistance programs are discussed below.

DETOXIFICATION

Approximately 90% of alcoholics can be detoxified from alcohol by outpatient procedures (26,69), leaving approximately 10% that require inpatient treatment for detoxification. With the cost of treatment now a major consideration, the decision between inpatient and outpatient detoxification should be based mostly on medical history and severity of alcohol withdrawal symptoms.

Alcohol Withdrawal Symptoms

The diagnosis of alcohol withdrawal requires a history of recent heavy drinking followed by reduced intake or cessation of use, the absence of other conditions that could cause symptoms mimicking withdrawal, and one or more of the four major manifestations of alcohol withdrawal (tremors, seizures, hallucinosis, and delirium tremens). These occur also in other conditions, ranging from withdrawal from other sedative-hypnotic drugs to meningitis (see list of causes of delirium in Chapter 17, Table 17.5).

Tremulousness usually begins 8 to 12 hours after the patient's last drink and peaks in 24 to 36 hours. *Withdrawal seizures* occur within 8 to 24 hours. Withdrawal seizures may occur independent of other manifestations of alcohol withdrawal. Both seizures and tremulousness can occur before the blood alcohol level has reached zero.

The *alcohol hallucination* is almost never the mythical pink elephant. Rather, it is usually one of moving insects, small animals, or threatening voices. In a series of 50 consecutive patients, 58% of their hallucinations were purely visual, 16% were purely auditory, and 26% were mixed (60). In certain patients these hallucinations may not be all negative; that is, the patient becomes used to them and is no longer frightened. Hallucinations may begin up to several days after the patient stops or markedly reduces alcohol use (usually in the first 48 hours). Typically, alcoholic hallucinosis lasts from minutes to days (usually less than 1 week) but in a very small percentage of patients, hallucinosis may continue for weeks or months and, rarely, as a continuous symptom.

Delirium tremens is a late manifestation of withdrawal, occurring anytime from 48 hours (most common interval) to 14 days (uncommon) after cessation of drinking. It may begin after the patient has shown signs of improvement from the early manifestations of withdrawal. Any of the symptoms of delirium, described in Chapter 17, may signal the onset of delirium tremens.

At least half of ambulatory alcoholic patients who stop drinking develop none of the four major manifestations of withdrawal (69). Additional minor symptoms are common. Anorexia, nausea, and sometimes vomiting are present in varying degrees. Tachycardia, systolic hypertension, and paroxysmal diaphoresis also are common. Generalized weakness may be prominent, and tinnitus, hyperacusis, itching, muscle cramps, and mood and sleep disorders are sometimes experienced. The patient is often hyperalert, startles easily, has difficulty concentrating, and usually craves alcohol or other drugs to quiet symptoms.

Selection of Patients for Inpatient Versus Outpatient Detoxification

There are a number of indications for referring a withdrawing alcoholic patient for *inpatient detoxification* (Table 21.4). Inpatient detoxification provides careful 24-hour monitoring and treatment of withdrawal, evaluation of intercurrent medical problems, and removal of patients from the environment that has facilitated their drinking. If medically stable, patients participate in groups (usually AA) and receive individual counseling.

For mildly symptomatic patients with a stable home environment and supportive family and friends, *outpatient detoxification* supervised at daily visits to a treatment program or physician's office is as effective

Table 21.4.   Indications for Referring a Withdrawing Alcoholic for Inpatient Detoxification

Evidence of hallucinations, severe tachycardia, severe tremor, fever, extreme agitation, or a history of severe withdrawal symptoms
History of seizure disorder
Presence of ataxia, nystagmus, confusion, or ophthalmoplegia, which may be indicative of Wernicke's encephalopathy
Severe nausea and vomiting that would prevent the ingestion of medication
Evidence of acute or chronic liver disease that may alter the metabolism of drugs used in the treatment of withdrawal
Presence of cardiovascular disease such as severe hypertension, ischemic heart disease, or arrhythmia, for which the sympathetic surge of catecholamines during withdrawal poses particular risk
Pregnancy
Presence of associated medical or surgical conditon requiring treatment
Lack of medical or social support system to allow outpatient detoxification

as inpatient detoxification. Patients may contract to attend an AA meeting daily with a friend or family member. For moderately sick patients, the choice of outpatient versus inpatient detoxification should be based on what programs are available. Some outpatient detoxification programs are intensive, requiring patients to spend entire days being monitored, with patients receiving medication as needed and participating in group counseling, but going home to sleep. Other outpatient detoxification programs consist of only brief daily visits.

Using Drugs in Detoxification

A useful *tool for making decisions about pharmacologic treatment in the withdrawing alcoholic* is the Clinical Institute Withdrawal Assessment for Alcohol (CIWA-Ar) (Table 21.5) (56). Pharmacologic therapy is not indicated for a score less than 10. For scores of 10 to 20, clinical judgment should determine the need for pharmacologic treatment. For scores greater than 20, treatment with drugs is indicated and should be administered either on an outpatient or inpatient basis. For scores of 20 to 40, a score can be repeated after administering a dose of medication, and patients without improvement will need more intensive monitoring as inpatients. Notably, pulse and blood pressure are not part of the CIWA scale. Although elevations of blood pressure and pulse do occur in alcohol withdrawal, the other signs and symptoms are more reliable in the assessment of severity of withdrawal. Thus, one should not make a decision about whether to prescribe drugs for alcohol withdrawal based solely on blood pressure and pulse.

Detoxification using orally administered psychoactive drugs appears to be most effective when combined with the nonpharmacologic techniques described in the next section and when treatment is given early. The safest and most effective drugs for this purpose are the benzodiazepine sedative-hypnotics. All of the benzodiazepines are effective. Diazepam (Valium) has an advantage of having a rapid onset of action, long

half-life, and low cost, because it is available in generic form. Its long half-life permits loading on the first day; that is, 5 to 10 mg every 1 to 4 hours until severe symptoms dissipate, which will reduce or perhaps eliminate the need for further dosing on subsequent days. Lorazepam (Ativan) does not require hepatic metabolism and is safer in patients with severe liver disease (i.e., prolonged prothrombin time). Patient response to a dose of benzodiazepine is unpredictable and not necessarily related to the amount of drinking. Ideally, patients should be monitored for response after initial dosing to make an assessment of indicated dosage and dosing interval. Dosing should be titrated to effect. Essential to management is early recognition of withdrawal, early treatment, frequent monitoring, and continual treatment. Given the decision to use sedative drugs in the detoxification process, one can choose low or high dosages (Table 21.6). Low dosages of sedative-hypnotic drugs may be tried first for most patients. The advantage of low-dose treatment is that the patient remains more alert. High dosages of these drugs may be indicated when the low dosage does not suppress or prevent symptoms in the first few hours.

The aim of drug treatment is to alleviate the most bothersome symptoms and signs of withdrawal. Symptom-driven therapy, compared to fixed schedule therapy, has been shown to decrease treatment duration and the amount of benzodiazepine used (48). The drug should be given such that withdrawal symptoms are improved without oversedating the patient. If the patient is being treated as an outpatient, each day's medication should be entrusted to a family member or friend who will be staying with the patient. Most patients need to be medicated for only 24 to 72 hours. The route of administration of benzodiazepines should be by mouth or, if this is not possible, by slow intravenous push (diazepam, lorazepam, or chlordiazepoxide). Other drugs have been used for management of alcohol withdrawal, most notably clonidine and β-blockers. Both of these drugs effectively alleviate the sympathetic markers of withdrawal (hypertension and tachycardia) but do little for the more severe aspects of withdrawal (seizures and hallucinosis). For this reason, if a patient is so symptomatic that the use of drugs is deemed appropriate, a benzodiazepine should be the drug of choice.

For patients in *early delirium tremens* (DTs), a slow intravenous push of diazepam, 10 mg, is the most effective initial treatment. This should be repeated every 30 to 60 minutes as needed to lessen the agitation. At times it may be needed more frequently. After diagnosis and initial therapy, these patients should be admitted to the hospital.

Detoxification Without Drugs

Candidates for nonpharmacologic outpatient detoxification should be ambulatory and, except for their chronic alcoholism and acute withdrawal, should be otherwise free from serious chronic illness or acute problems. The primary aim in nonpharmacologic detoxification is to provide a nonthreatening, positive environment for the patient (Table 21.7). The patient should be kept ambulatory when possible and given a regular diet. Except when asleep or resting comfortably, patient should be encouraged to perform purposeful activities, such as carrying out small duties or attending introductory group education and therapy sessions.

Nonpharmacologic therapy can be just as effective as drug therapy in the detoxification of ambulatory un-

---

Table 21.5. Addiction Research Foundation Clinical Institute Withdrawal Assessment for Alcohol (CIWA-Ar)[a]

Patient _____   Date |__|__|__| Time _____:_____
                                   y   m   d   (24-hour clock, midnight = 00:00)

Pulse or heart rate, taken for one minute:_____   Blood pressure _____/_____

NAUSEA AND VOMITING—Ask "Do you feel sick to your stomach? Have you vomited?" Observation. 0 no nausea and no vomiting 1 mild nausea with no vomiting 2 3 4 intermittent nausea with dry heaves 5 6 7 constant nausea, frequent dry heaves and vomiting	TACTILE DISTURBANCES—Ask "Have you any itching, pins and needles sensations, any burning, any numbness, or do you feel bugs crawling on or under your skin?" Observation. 0 none 1 very mild itching, pins and needles, burning or numbness 2 mild itching, pins and needles, burning or numbness 3 moderate itching, pins and needles, burning or numbness 4 moderately severe hallucinations 5 severe hallucinations 6 extremely severe hallucinations 7 continuous hallucinations
TREMOR—Arms extended and fingers spread apart. Observation. 0 no tremor 1 not visible, but can be felt fingertip to fingertip 2 3 4 moderate, with patient's arms extended 5 6 7 severe, even with arms not extended	AUDITORY DISTURBANCES—Ask "Are you more aware of sounds around you? Are they harsh? Do they frighten you? Are you hearing anything that is disturbing you? Are you hearing things you know are not there?" Observation. 0 not present 1 very mild harshness or ability to frighten 2 mild harshness or ability to frighten 3 moderate harshness or ability to frighten 4 moderately severe hallucinations 5 severe hallucinations 6 extremely severe hallucinations 7 continuous hallucinations
PAROXYSMAL SWEATS—Observation. 0 no sweat visible 1 barely perceptible sweating, palms moist 2 3 4 beads of sweat obvious on forehead 5 6 7 drenching sweats	VISUAL DISTURBANCES—Ask "Does the light appear to be too bright? Is its color different? Does it hurt your eyes? Are you seeing anything that is disturbing to you? Are you seeing things you know are not there?" Observation. 0 not present 1 very mild sensitivity 2 mild sensitivity 3 moderate sensitivity 4 moderately severe hallucinations 5 severe hallucinations 6 extremely severe hallucinations 7 continuous hallucinations
ANXIETY—Ask "Do you feel nervous?" Observation. 0 no anxiety, at ease 1 mildly anxious 2 3 4 moderately anxious, or guarded, so anxiety is inferred 5 6 7 equivalent to acute panic states, as seen in severe delirium or acute schizophrenic reactions	HEADACHE, FULLNESS IN HEAD—Ask "Does your head feel different? Does it feel like there is a band around your head?" Do not rate for dizziness or lightheadedness. Otherwise, rate severity. 0 not present 1 very mild 2 mild 3 moderate 4 moderately severe 5 severe 6 very severe 7 extremely severe
AGITATION—Observation. 0 normal activity 1 somewhat more than normal activity 2 3 4 moderately fidgety and restless 5 6 7 paces back and forth during most of the interview, or constantly thrashes about	ORIENTATION AND CLOUDING OF SENSORIUM—Ask "What day is this? Where are you? Who am I?" 0 oriented and can do serial additions 1 cannot do serial additions or is uncertain about date 2 disoriented for date by no more than 2 calendar days 3 disoriented for date by more than 2 calendar days 4 disoriented for place and/or person

Total CIWA-A Score_____
Rater's Initials_____
Maximum Possible Score 67

Table 21.6.   Characteristics of Benzodiazepines Used Orally in the Treatment of Alcohol Withdrawal

Drug	Onset of Action	Rate of Metabolism	Liver Metabolized	Low Dosage (mg/6 hr)	High Dosage (mg/2–4 hr)
Chlordiazepoxide	Intermediate	Long	Yes	25	100
Diazepam	Fast	Long	Yes	2–5	10–20
Lorazepam	Intermediate	Intermediate	No	0.5	2
Oxazepam	Slow	Short	No	10–15	30

Table 21.7.   Environmental Modification in Treating Alcohol and Other Sedative Withdrawal

Sense	Therapeutic	Countertherapeutic
Visual	Lights on, not bright	Lights off
	Familiar people, pictures, clock, clothes	Marked shadows
Sound	Soft music	Loud or abrupt noises
	Soft conversation	
	Reassurance and reality Orientation by staff	
Touch	Reassuring touch by staff (e.g., taking pulse, hand on shoulder)	Bed clothes High bed Restraints
	Comfortable chair	IVs and tubes
	Low bed	
	Regular clothes	
General	Respect	Hostility, even if subtle
	Positivity, optimism	Negativity or pessimism

Modified from Baum R, Iber FL. Initial treatment of the alcoholic patient. In: Gitlow SE, Peyser HS, eds. Alcoholism: a practical treatment guide, New York: Grune & Stratton, 1980; 73–87.

complicated patients (69). The advantages of nonpharmacologic detoxification without drugs, as compared with traditional detoxification with drugs, are that it can be done largely by nonmedical personnel, it is less expensive, and the patient is more likely to remain alert and, therefore, able to participate in treatment. The only routine medication should be vitamins (50 to 100 mg of thiamine, 1 mg of folate, and a potent multivitamin daily). These vitamins should be continued for the first month or more of recovery.

Many communities have established alcoholism facilities that provide a sheltered, supportive environment to care for alcoholics, using a social model for nondrug detoxification. Patients are screened and evaluated to detect any obvious medical problems before or shortly after being admitted. Should complications arise, backup hospital/medical support is available.

The length of stay varies in each program from 3 days to more than 30 days. Most social setting programs use AA extensively, and many of the larger programs use many of the techniques used in other alcoholism treatment centers. These centers can be either day treatment or residential facilities.

For detoxification at home without the use of drugs, a reliable family member or other person should be present to observe the patient for at least 2 full days. The physician supervising such detoxification should be in touch with the patient or the family member daily during the 2 to 4 days required for detoxification. The following is a checklist for home detoxification:

- The patient should be motivated to do it at home.
- A reliable person should be with or frequently check on the patient.

- There should be access to a telephone to call the physician or counselor two or more times per day for reassurance and to monitor withdrawal.
- There should be no active medical problems requiring aggressive treatment, and no high-dosage chemical dependence to drugs other than alcohol.
- There should be arrangements to see a supervising physician, nurse, or counselor each day.
- The patient should be as active as possible (attend AA, take food and fluid as desired, and take multivitamins daily).
- Involvement in a strong outpatient program should start upon completion of detoxification.

Prevention of Withdrawal Seizures

There is no consensus about whether *phenytoin* (Dilantin) should be included in the detoxification of patients with a history of withdrawal seizures. It has been shown that phenytoin at a dosage of 300 mg/day for 5 days can prevent most withdrawal seizures, even though therapeutic plasma levels of phenytoin are not reached (50). However, in another study, when patients received an intravenous load of phenytoin or placebo within 6 hours of a first alcohol withdrawal seizure, phenytoin provided no benefit in preventing further seizures (3).

There is evidence that a *high-dosage benzodiazepine* regimen for withdrawal can prevent seizures (53). Thus, patients who are significantly symptomatic and receiving sufficient pharmacologic therapy with a benzodiazepine do not require phenytoin. However, only mildly symptomatic patients with a history of a withdrawal seizure should receive prophylactic phenytoin if they are not going to be treated with a benzodiazepine. This recommendation is based on the fact that a seizure may occur without the presence of any other manifestations of alcohol withdrawal (42).

TREATMENT AFTER DETOXIFICATION
Overview

Treatment consists of motivating the patient, initiating a treatment plan, and providing regular follow-up. The clinician who initially motivates an alcoholic to accept treatment may elect not to coordinate the overall treatment but to provide a referral elsewhere. For this important referral, one should select a specialist or a program with demonstrated expertise in helping alcoholics recover. The simplest ways to find such expert help are to call the local National Council on Alcoholism, to ask a colleague who has had experience in referring or treating alcoholics, or to refer the patient to an existing community alcoholism treatment program.

In selecting skilled help, one should look for several characteristics. The effective alcoholism specialist or program tends to be abstinence-oriented; use AA or group therapy as a mainstay of treatment; offer disulfiram to patients; avoid the use of psychoactive drugs in long-term treatment, especially the sedative-hypnotics; refer the spouse to Al-Anon or family therapy; provide close follow-up; and avoid insight-oriented psychotherapy, unless indicated later in the course of recovery. The physician who makes the referral should reinforce participation in the treatment program whenever the patient returns for follow-up.

The importance of being competent in handling alcoholism has been highlighted in legal decisions in recent years in which physicians have lost suits brought by families and patients for failure to diagnose alcoholism, failure to refer alcoholics for treatment, or failure to provide treatment for alcoholism.

Alcoholics Anonymous and Group Therapy

Alcoholics and other chemical-dependent people seem to recover best in group treatment settings. Groups effectively break down the denial process and heal the associated guilt and shame through a combination of identification, nonjudgmental acceptance, confrontation, and support. Every alcoholic should be strongly encouraged to attend AA regularly. Studies show that regular AA attendance is strongly correlated with long-term recovery and improved functioning (28,59). Formal alcoholism group therapy is also successful.

Many patients are reluctant to attend AA or a therapy group. Therefore, when referring a patient, it is important to convey that one is familiar with these programs and has confidence in them. Immediate action, taken while the patient is in the office, may consist of having the patient contact a family member or friend who is active in AA, telephoning the local AA office and letting the patient request a contact to take him or her to a convenient AA meeting, or telephoning an alcoholism treatment program and arranging an intake appointment for the patient.

The best way for physicians to learn about these programs is to attend one or more AA meeting and, if available, open group therapy meetings. To locate such meetings, one should call the local AA office or the local National Council on Alcoholism. The AA process is summarized in Table 21.8.

Psychotherapy

It is commonly thought that all alcoholic patients have a primary and causative underlying psychologic problem. If treatment of this condition is successful, the alcoholism is expected to resolve because it is considered to be chiefly a manifestation of the underlying psychologic problem. Although this approach may seem theoretically valid, this therapeutic strategy rarely works unless there happens to be a coexisting

psychosis. Patients with alcoholism cannot gain insight into aspects of their lives successfully until they have maintained sobriety. Early psychotherapy may impede maintenance of sobriety and trigger relapse. Even in cases with coexisting psychosis, the alcoholism must also be treated. After establishing rapport, therefore, the initial effort in psychotherapy should be to work with the patient toward abstinence and regular participation in group treatment.

Ongoing supportive psychotherapy, by the patient's personal physicians, as described in Chapter 11, is useful for reinforcing the patient's understanding of the disease and the recovery process; for monitoring patient's functioning in important life areas, such as family, job, and interpersonal relations; and for assisting the patient in change and growth.

Discussions with the Spouse or Closest Family Members

As part of the early treatment of an alcoholic patient, the situation should be discussed with the spouse or person closest to the patient. Through such discussions, which should be conducted without breaking the patient's confidentiality, one can ensure that the family agrees with the goal of abstinence; explore the spouse's own drinking pattern; discern any special problems occurring in any of the close family members, including the children; educate the spouse about the enabling process; refer the spouse to Al-Anon, teenage children to Alateen, or some other available family resource; and schedule a follow-up visit after the spouse has attended several Al-Anon meetings. *If the family does not change and grow, usually through regular attendance at Al-Anon meetings, it will be more difficult for the patient to recover.* Family treatment and the Al-Anon process are described below (see "Co-Alcoholism").

Disulfiram (Antabuse)

Although controlled studies have not shown unequivocally that it increases duration of sobriety (4,72), the use of disulfiram to prevent drinking should be considered for some patients. Patients must be in active recovery, including AA and individual or group therapy. Disulfiram should not be used as the focus of treatment, but as an adjunct. The risks of prescribing disulfiram have probably been overemphasized. Disulfiram is available, as Antabuse, in the form of scored tablets containing 250 or 500 mg.

Disulfiram–Alcohol Interaction

Alcohol is initially oxidized by the hepatic enzyme alcohol dehydrogenase to acetaldehyde, and disulfiram inhibits acetaldehyde oxidation by interfering with aldehyde dehydrogenase. This effect may persist for up to 2 weeks after cessation of disulfiram. The symptoms of the alcohol–disulfiram reaction are related to *elevated acetaldehyde;* they are usually proportional to the amounts of disulfiram and alcohol ingested. Some people have typical symptoms after

Table 21.8. The Process of Alcoholics Anonymous

AA was founded in 1935 by two chronic alcoholics, one a stockbroker and one a physician.

Meetings

AA meetings are held frequently in all communities in the United States and in most other countries. Meetings are either open or closed (most are open and most welcome nonalcoholics interested in treating alcoholism). A published directory of meetings, places, times, and information by telephone are available from each local chapter of AA. By contacting AA, an alcoholic can almost always arrange to be taken to a meeting in his or her community, often on the day he or she makes the request. Many AA members attend meetings several times a week. Some attend at least one meeting per day. Lifelong activity in AA is the basis for maintaining health for many recovering alcoholics.

Meetings are usually 1 hour in length. Most are held in the evening, although there are many daytime meetings as well. Meetings begin with a recitation by one member of the Twelve Steps and the Twelve Traditions and are devoted to examination and interpretation of these, as illustrated in personal experiences described by a number of members. One member of the group chairs the meeting and calls on speakers. Speakers introduce themselves by their first names (e.g., "I'm Joe—I'm an alcoholic"). Meetings end with group recitation of the Lord's Prayer or the Serenity Prayer "God grant me the Serenity to accept the things I cannot change, Courage to change the things I can, and Wisdom to know the difference."

AA on the surface can sometimes look insubstantial and unsophisticated, often turning off newcomers. Often the spiritual overtones of the program are rejected. However, the program is *profound and life changing.* Without an administrative structure, owning no property, and having no dues or fees, it continues to grow because it works and meets human need.

Publications

AA provides printed educational aids in the form of pamphlets (available at meetings) and "the Big Book" (*Alcoholics Anonymous,* a collection of personal stories that illustrate vividly the ways that lives are damaged by alcoholism and the AA path to recovery). One can obtain this book or other literature at meetings, at the local AA office, or by writing AA World Services, Box 459, Grand Central Station, New York, NY 10017.

The 12 Steps and the 12 Traditions

The 12 Steps

1. We admitted we were powerless over alcohol, that our lives had become unmanageable.
2. Came to believe that a power greater than ourselves could restore us to sanity.
3. Made a decision to turn our will and our lives over to the care of God *as we understood Him.*
4. Made a searching and fearless moral inventory of ourselves.
5. Admitted to God, to ourselves, and to another human being the exact nature of our wrongs.
6. Were entirely ready to have God remove all these defects of character.
7. Humbly asked Him to remove our shortcomings.
8. Made a list of all persons we had harmed, and became willing to make amends to them all.
9. Made direct amends to such people wherever possible, except when to do so would injure them or others.
10. Continued to take personal inventory, and when we were wrong promptly admitted it.
11. Sought through prayer and meditation to improve our conscious contact with God, *as we understood Him,* praying only for knowledge of His will for us and the power to carry that out.
12. Having had a spiritual awakening as the result of the Steps, we tried to carry this message to alcoholics, and to practice these principles in all our affairs (note: for this step, Altman substitutes "others" for the word "alcoholics").

Boiled down, these steps mean, simply:
a. Admission of alcoholism.
b. Personality analysis and catharsis.
c. Adjustment of personal relations.
d. Dependence on some higher power.
e. Working with other alcoholics.

The 12 Traditions

1. Our common welfare should come first; personal recovery depends upon AA unity.
2. For our group purpose there is but one ultimate authority—a loving God as He may express Himself in our group conscience. Our leaders are but trusted servants; they do not govern.
3. The only requirement for AA membership is a desire to stop drinking.
4. Each group should be autonomous except in matters affecting other groups or AA as a whole.
5. Each group has but one primary purpose—to carry out its message to the alcoholic who still suffers.
6. An AA group ought never endorse, finance, or lend the AA name to any related facility or outside enterprise, lest problems of money, property, and prestige divert us from our primary purpose.
7. Every AA group ought to be fully self-supporting, declining outside contributions.
8. Alcoholics Anonymous should remain forever nonprofessional, but our service centers may employ special workers.
9. AA, as such, ought never to be organized; but we may create service boards or committees directly responsible to those they serve.
10. Alcoholics Anonymous has no opinion on outside issues; hence the AA name ought never be drawn into public controversy.
11. Our public relations policy is based on attraction rather than promotion; we need always maintain personal anonymity at the level of press, radio, and films.
12. Anonymity is the spiritual foundation of our Traditions, ever reminding us to place principles before personalities.

drinking as little as 7 mL of alcohol (about half of a drink). A very small percentage of patients seem to be able to drink despite taking disulfiram with no significant symptoms. In these latter patients, the dosage can be increased up to 500 mg/day, but only if the patient seems motivated to abstinence.

The common symptoms of the alcohol–disulfiram reaction usually begin within 10 minutes of drinking and include flushing, throbbing in the head and neck, headaches, anxiety, general discomfort, sweating, and respiratory difficulty. The reaction typically lasts between 30 minutes and several hours. Less often, nausea, vomiting, hypotension, thirst, chest pain, palpitation, dyspnea, hyperventilation, tachycardia, syncope, weakness, blurred vision, and confusion can occur.

Office Prescribing of Disulfiram

Patients who are motivated to succeed in recovery and who have experienced relapse or dread the likelihood of relapse are candidates for disulfiram. Table 21.9 summarizes a practical plan that can be used in office practice. This supervised approach is similar in its demands on patients and physicians to the initiation and management of long-term treatment. A detailed patient education guide accompanies packages of Antabuse. Patients should carry an identification card that identifies them as taking disulfiram.

Advantages of Disulfiram

Disulfiram has several advantages: Because the drug is taken daily, it is a constant reminder that one cannot drink safely; it provides evidence of compliance in the treatment program; it is compatible with other forms of treatment of alcoholism; and it can also provide family and employer with reassurance that as long as it is taken daily, the alcoholic cannot get drunk. Patients should consider four additional advantages: The decision not to drink has to be made only once a day; because of this, patients tend not to worry about whether they can drink; not worrying or thinking about drinking saves considerable energy; and this makes recovery easier.

Side Effects and Contraindications

Disulfiram at recommended dosages is well tolerated by most patients. Some patients complain of drowsiness, fatigability, headaches, a garliclike or metallic aftertaste, and breath odor and acneform eruptions. To avoid the problem with drowsiness, the disulfiram can be taken at bedtime. The other side effects usually subside within a few days or weeks with continued

Table 21.9. The Suggested Approach to Supervised Use of Disulfiram

1. Satisfy the following indications: the patient is willing to take medication several times a week under supervision, the patient can recall making the decision to take the first drink of a relapse, and the patient is actively involved in an organized outpatient treatment program.
2. Rule out contraindications and ask yourself the following question: "Can this patient survive a disulfiram–alcohol reaction?"
3. Ensure sober state before the initiation of treatment.
4. Be sure patient and spouse know how to avoid hidden alcohol in foods, OTC medications, toiletries, etc.
5. Have the patient read, discuss, and sign a consent form before initiating treatment.
6. Begin with a dosage of one tablet (250 mg) daily.
7. *Keep the medication bottle in the office* and have the patient come in three times a week to be dispensed two (or three) doses by the office staff. After 1 month, decrease the visits to twice a week and increase the number of pills dispensed accordingly. After another month, go to weekly visits and continue these for the duration of disulfiram treatment. See the patient at least monthly and repeat laboratory testing every 3 months.
8. If the patient misses more than one or two appointments in a row, have the office staff contact the people on the consent form, and stop administering the medication.

therapy. More rarely, confusion (particularly in the elderly), optic neuritis, polyneuritis, and peripheral neuritis may occur.

Contraindications for the use of disulfiram include a history of hypertension, diabetes, emphysema, seizures, significant liver or renal disease, coronary artery disease, hypothyroidism, pregnancy, or a history of drinking while taking disulfiram. If alcohol-related liver disease is present, prescribing of disulfiram should be delayed until the levels of serum aspartate aminotransferase (AST) and serum alanine aminotransferase (ALT), two serum markers of liver disease, are less than three times the normal range. Disulfiram may impair the metabolism and *potentiate the effects of caffeine, warfarin, and phenytoin,* and it may interact additively to *potentiate the neurologic side effects of isoniazid* (ataxia, psychosis). It should be used with caution in conjunction with these drugs or with the following other classes of drugs: β- or α-adrenergic antagonists, vasodilators, sympathomimetic amines, monoamine oxidase inhibitors, tricyclic antidepressants, and neuroleptics. Most cough syrups no longer contain alcohol, but an alcoholic patient should avoid medications such as cough syrups and foods (salad dressings) that name alcohol as an ingredient.

Naltrexone

Naltrexone (Revia) is a second drug that is potentially useful as an adjunct to a formal treatment program for individuals with alcohol dependence. Unlike disulfiram, patients do not get sick if they drink while taking naltrexone. Naltrexone has been shown to *reduce alcohol craving* and as a result may be particularly useful in preventing relapse in motivated patients (61). However, the numbers of patients in most studies have been small and there is little long-term data. Most published studies look at the impact of naltrexone on drinkers for less than 6 months.

Naltrexone is an opiate antagonist and therefore it cannot be prescribed to patients on opiate analgesics. Furthermore, patients maintained on naltrexone will not obtain pain relief if prescribed an opiate. The notion of using naltrexone for alcohol dependence was based on laboratory studies that showed that rats increased alcohol intake after administration of small doses of opiates.

Naltrexone is well tolerated, with nausea as its main side effect. To avoid nausea, patients should be prescribed 25 mg (half tablet) a day for 2 days and 50 mg/day thereafter. Naltrexone can be used in combination with disulfiram. Although there is no clear evidence of hepatotoxicity, the makers of naltrexone advise monitoring of liver function tests (initially at monthly intervals and then less frequently). If naltrexone is tolerated and is successful in aiding abstinence, the recommended initial course of treatment is 3 months. Naltrexone does not cause physical dependence and can be stopped at any time without withdrawal symptoms. If a patient is going to have elective surgery, naltrexone should be stopped at least 72 hours beforehand to allow the use of opiate analgesia.

A decision to stop naltrexone or disulfiram is best made jointly by the physician, the spouse or other close person, the AA sponsor, and the patient. It should be based on the strength of the person's recovery. Important guidelines in this decision are active AA or group therapy participation, coping with crises without recourse to drinking, improved family relationships, dissolution of denial, social ease (diminution in social anxiety), growth in self-esteem, and prolonged abstinence.

Psychoactive Drugs

Although many alcoholics have symptoms such as anxiety, insomnia, and tremors that might be helped by sedatives, in actuality these drugs usually interfere with successful recovery. Anxiolytic drugs may have a role in acute detoxification (see above), and major tranquilizers, antidepressants, and lithium have usefulness in treating, respectively, the schizophrenic, the severe protracted depressive, and the manic–depressive alcoholic (as long as these patients are being treated concomitantly for alcoholism). Apart from these situations, psychoactive drugs should not be prescribed for alcoholics. There are many reasons for this: all sedatives are cross-tolerant with alcohol and thus have a built-in escalation factor; combining sedatives with alcohol is often dangerously synergistic; inability to control consumption, a cardinal feature of alcoholism, occurs with prescribed sedative drugs; memory blackouts may also occur with other sedatives and minor tranquilizers; patients may alter the prescription to obtain excess quantities of these drugs; prescribing these drugs reinforces psychoactive substance use as a coping mechanism and impairs development of the patient's own coping mechanisms; and the drugs interfere with learning to relate to others in a healthy manner. Bissell (10) said: "I do think we need to give our patients a substitute for alcohol, but I don't think that substitute can be another sedative. I think it has to be our concern, our time, our caring, and ourselves."

Follow-Up: Prevention and Management of Relapse

Next to dealing with denial and motivating the patient, follow-up is the most difficult part of treatment. One reason is that when an alcoholic recovers there may be an early honeymoon period during which the patient feels and looks so good that one is lulled into believing that regular follow-up is unnecessary. However, because it takes about 2 to 3 years of appropriate treatment before recovery can be secure, regular follow-up is indicated.

During the first 6 weeks after stopping drinking, patients need much support and direction, for this is the time when they are most likely to relapse. Therefore, at least weekly patient contacts are indicated for this time, with a gradually decreasing frequency thereafter. Some of these contacts may be by telephone.

Other *high-risk times for relapse* include special days and occasions such as vacations, holidays, business trips, birthdays, anniversaries, or crises such as separation, divorce, death of a close person, or illness in the family. Other relapse danger times are when a patient stops taking disulfiram or stops attending AA or group therapy meetings.

"Dry drunks" are often part of the natural history of recovery. This is the name given by recovering alcoholics to the negative emotions and behaviors reminiscent of those that occurred when the patient was drinking. Dry drunks may last from a few hours to several weeks or even months. Treatment is by recognition, education, and alteration of the diet and other current life habits. Dry drunks are often associated with eating poorly. Regular well-balanced meals should be recommended, and caffeine intake, including coffee, tea, colas, and chocolate, should be markedly decreased or discontinued. Increased attendance at AA or group therapy meetings at this time is very important. Moderation in the patient's work and recreational activities and rest should be advised.

The *relapse process generally begins long before the person drinks.* This process often progresses in the following sequence: reactivation of denial, progressive isolation and defensiveness, building a crisis to justify symptom progression, immobilization, confusion and overreaction, depression, loss of control over behavior, recognition of loss of control, option reduction, and debilitation, which ends in drinking, using other drugs, or some other debilitating condition (25).

Although it should not be telegraphed to the patient, relapse is part of the natural history of successful recovery for most alcoholics (25), and one should not become discouraged if it happens (Fig. 21.3 illustrates the long-term course of a typical recovering alcoholic). Instead, one should immediately recruit the patient back into treatment using the same motivational techniques used initially. Relapse is a time for both patient and therapist to learn about their mistakes and to correct them by strengthening treatment.

INPATIENT REHABILITATION

Although controlled studies differ over the advantage of inpatient rehabilitation over outpatient treatment, inpatient rehabilitation for 2 to 6 weeks may be especially helpful for selected patients (35,63). It is always planned for in advance when a formal intervention is used (see above). Other indications for inpatient rehabilitation are strong denial, especially if it persists in outpatient treatment; unsuccessful or too slow recovery despite adequate outpatient treatment; weak or unavailable support systems; danger to self or others; severe medical, psychiatric, or other problems related to the alcoholism; and patient's desire for inpatient treatment.

Although treatment goals among inpatient rehabilitation programs vary, some of the major goals include breaking down denial, educating about alcoholism/chemical dependence, providing an introduction to group treatment (self-help groups and group therapy), becoming aware of feelings and beginning to learn to handle them, learning how to ask for help, learning how to communicate directly and honestly, learning how to enjoy life while abstinent, beginning family restoration, and developing a specific, appropriate, and structured long-term recovery program.

PROGNOSIS WITH TREATMENT

A number of factors, described here, are associated with a good or poor prognosis for recovery. Even factors traditionally thought to be major barriers to treatment success—a skid row lifestyle or being an unattached young adult—do not always preclude successful recovery (7,20).

Factors Associated with a Good Prognosis

The first of these factors is *clinician commitment and patient motivation*. Most patients are only marginally motivated to get well. They can be characterized as being quite ambivalent: A part of them wants to get well, and another part of them wants to continue drinking and stay sick (patients usually do not know what is wrong with them because no one has told them of the diagnosis in an effective way). Such patients have a good chance of getting into recovery if their physician is committed to the treatment of the patient's alcoholism and consistently uses the motivational techniques described previously.

The *presence of a crisis situation* is also a positive prognostic factor if the crisis is used as a motivational tool. The crisis may be the threat of a job loss, family separation or divorce, a DWI charge, a health-related crisis, an organized formal intervention (see above), or some other dramatic event. A physician actually precipitates a crisis whenever the confrontation approach described previously (Fig. 21.4) is used. As in that approach, it is critical to act promptly if a situational crisis is to be used effectively to motivate the patient to accept treatment. If exploitation of this crisis does not work, at least a seed has been planted that may eventually yield results.

A third factor associated with a good prognosis is *appropriate treatment for at least 2 years*. Patients whose alcoholism began before age 25 usually require at least 3 years of treatment. Many alcoholics who begin treatment either believe they can do it on their own or return to drinking and drop out of treatment. To recover effectively, most alcoholics need to be with people who are themselves recovering successfully. This favorable environment is found most easily in self-help groups such as AA and in group therapy. Thus, when the patient shows any indication of dropping out of treatment, it is important to promptly persuade against this.

The prognosis is also better *if family, job, health, and cognitive function are intact*. The status of family, job, health, and cognitive function usually correlates with how far along the alcoholism has advanced. Thus, making a diagnosis early in the course of the alcohol-ism generally portends a better prognosis because each of these aspects of the patient's life tends to be more intact early in the illness. Also, in early illness the patient's and family members' denial systems and other defense systems tend not to be as strong.

If one or more members of the patient's family is receiving treatment for co-alcoholism (see below), the patient generally has a better prognosis.

Additional factors that increase the likelihood of long-term success are prompt recognition and intervention when relapse occurs (see above) and the acceptance by patient and physician of a threefold recovery model that views alcoholism as a physical, mental, and spiritual illness (65,66).

Factors Associated with a Poor Prognosis

If the patient has *no perceived threat of loss* from continued drinking, the prognosis for recovery is generally worse.

A second factor that may worsen the prognosis is one of the *following forms of inappropriate treatment*: disulfiram alone, psychoanalytically oriented psychotherapy in the first year of alcoholism treatment, controlled drinking treatment, use of sedatives in long-term management, inpatient or outpatient treatment that does not treat alcoholism as a primary illness, and treatment that is too short in duration.

Although many patients who have a continued self-destructive bent do not tend to recover, some do. Often, intensive inpatient alcoholism treatment for 2 months or longer can be helpful in such patients. However, economic restraints most often limit this option.

Cognitive impairment or psychosis often makes treatment difficult. However, the presence of these factors alone does not preclude a full attempt at treatment. With abstinence there is often surprising improvement over time.

Acceptance of a *derelict subculture status* by the patient makes the prognosis virtually hopeless. However, it can be helpful to screen for a potentially reversible derelict status by looking at prior career and duration of dereliction (20). For example, a person who up until 2 years ago was in a productive profession or trade and is now on skid row has potential for recovery. By contrast, a skid row person who has had no constructive activities for many years generally has little chance for reaching a successful long-term recovery.

If patients have *powerful enablers* (see "Co-Alcoholism," below) to deny, cover up, and protect them from the consequences of drinking or drug using, it is less likely that they will make a successful recovery.

SPECIAL POPULATIONS
Alcoholism in the Elderly

It is estimated that alcoholism is present in 3 to 4 million Americans over the age of 60, with prevalence estimates of 2 to 10% (11). Most elderly alcoholics have not been diagnosed, and even fewer are in treatment.

This is true despite the fact that the elderly alcoholic is more likely to have seen a physician recently than a younger alcoholic.

The diagnosis of alcoholism can be more difficult in the elderly because they are less likely to face job loss, legal problems, marital problems, or fear of premature death. However, any change in functional status can be an important clue. The CAGE questionnaire, discussed previously, has been validated in the elderly using a cohort of 323 elderly patients in an outpatient medical practice of an urban university teaching hospital. The sensitivity and specificity for a score of ≥ 1 was 86% and 78%, respectively, and 70% and 91% for a score of ≥ 2. In this population, scores of 2, 3, and 4 yielded positive predictive values of 79, 82, and 94%, respectively (15). The CAGE may not be effective in detecting elderly binge drinkers who are at high risk of falling (2). As an adjunct, a geriatric version of the MAST has been developed (Table 21.10).

Elderly patients with alcoholism tend to fall into two groups: *early onset and late onset.* Two-thirds of patients fall into the early onset group. These are patients who have had ongoing alcoholism but may have avoided some of the usual sequelae. They are often hidden functional alcoholics who, as they lose mobility or cognitive abilities, become unable to function normally and become unhidden. The late onset patients are likely to have had a recent stressor (i.e., loss of spouse, retirement, or a new impairment in activities of daily life). Occasionally, late onset alcoholism occurs in a previous teetotaler (6). Compared with younger patients with alcoholism, the elderly are more likely to be separated, divorced, or widowed and are more likely to live alone.

The elderly are more sensitive to the acute effects of alcohol, with amplification of preexisting deficits. Dysphoria predominates over euphoria. In addition, there is more likely to be interaction with prescribed drugs.

It is estimated that only 15% of alcoholics over the age of 60 are receiving adequate treatment (11). Once a patient is confronted and agrees to treatment, there are some aspects of treatment specific to the elderly.

The elderly patient who experiences significant alcohol withdrawal is best monitored in an inpatient setting. For patients with mild withdrawal, treated at home, family or friends should stay with them for at least the first week of abstinence. In addition, home health care, if available, should be considered.

Table 21.10. Michigan Alcohol Screening Test—Geriatric Version (MAST-G)[a]

		Yes	No
1. After drinking have you ever noticed an increase in your heart rate or beating in your chest?	1.	(1)	(0)
2. When talking with others, do you ever underestimate how much you actually drink?	2.		
3. Does alcohol make you sleepy so that you often fall asleep in your chair?	3.		
4. After a few drinks, have you sometimes not eaten or been able to skip a meal because you didn't feel hungry?	4.		
5. Does having a few drinks help decrease your shakiness or tremors?	5.		
6. Does alcohol sometimes make it hard for you to remember parts of the day or night?	6.		
7. Do you have rules for yourself that you won't drink before a certain time of the day?	7.		
8. Have you lost interest in hobbies or activities you used to enjoy?	8.		
9. When you wake up in the morning, do you ever have trouble remembering part of the night before?	9.		
10. Does having a drink help you sleep?	10.		
11. Do you hide your alcohol bottles from family members?	11.		
12. After a social gathering, have you ever felt embarrassed because you drank too much?	12.		
13. Have you ever been concerned that drinking might be harmful to your health?	13.		
14. Do you like to end an evening with a night cap?	14.		
15. Did you find your drinking increased after someone close to you died?	15.		
16. In general, would you prefer to have a few drinks at home rather than go out to social events?	16.		
17. Are you drinking more now than in the past?	17.		
18. Do you usually take a drink to relax or calm your nerves?	18.		
19. Do you drink to take your mind off your problems?	19.		
20. Have you ever increased your drinking after experiencing a loss in your life?	20.		
21. Do you sometimes drive when you have had too much to drink?	21.		
22. Has a doctor or nurse ever said they were worried or concerned about your drinking?	22.		
23. Have you ever made rules to manage your drinking?	23.		
24. When you feel lonely, does having a drink help?	24.		

Copyright by The Regents of the University of Michigan, 1991.

For further information, contact Frederic Blow, PhD, at University of Michigan Alcohol Research Center, 400 E. Eisenhower Pkwy, Suite A, Ann Arbor, MI 48104, 313-998-7952.

[a]Scoring: 5 or more "yes" responses indicative of alcohol problem.

Once the patient is medically stable, treatment toward continued abstinence should be initiated. Treatment must be specifically tailored for the elderly. Because of decreased mobility and an inability to drive, patients may find AA meetings more difficult to reach. Meetings during the day must be found for the elderly afraid to go out at night. The elderly tend to be more comfortable in smaller groups. These can often be found in meetings that run in a senior center. The senior center can also be a source of activities to fill the new void of free time formerly spent drinking.

As the elderly are often on many medications and more likely to have other chronic medical illnesses, disulfiram should generally be avoided. Many elderly alcoholics would benefit from a 30-day stay at an inpatient treatment center. Some centers have recovery programs specifically for the elderly alcoholic. Access to this type of treatment is usually related to insurance and cost.

Alcoholism in Women

Alcoholism is more likely to go unrecognized in women than in men (24,71), yet suicide, trauma, and liver disease are more common in female alcoholics than in male alcoholics. An additional concern is the pregnancy-related complication of fetal alcohol syndrome, mentioned previously. Alcoholism decreases a woman's average life expectancy by 15 years (47).

Women tend to drink more subtly and covertly. Partly, this is related to society considering drinking in public, especially in a tavern or bar, less acceptable in women than in men. Thus, women often drink at home. Women who are unmarried, divorced, or unemployed drink more. Alcoholic women are also more likely to have alcoholic spouses.

The techniques discussed previously should be used to screen, diagnose, and confront women with alcoholism. There are some particular obstacles to treatment. Women are more likely to need provision of child care while they are in treatment. In addition, alcoholic women tend to have less spouse support than do alcoholic men. There are treatment programs aimed specifically toward women, including AA, which has women-only meetings. Alcoholic women, who make up only approximately 30% of AA, should generally seek other women to be their sponsors.

The Impaired Physician or Other Professional

The prevalence among physicians of alcoholism and other chemical dependence is probably similar to that for the general population (37). Each year, a substantial number of physicians are lost to the profession because of chemical dependence or other treatable illnesses, and many more practice despite being seriously troubled or impaired. In recent years, numerous professional organizations have implemented such programs, including organizations of physicians, nurses, dentists, pharmacists, psychologists, social workers, lawyers, and others.

Definitions

Impaired professionals may be further defined as those who are troubled by personal difficulties to the extent that they cannot offer reasonable patient care, effectively help others through interpersonal skills, or maintain skills by continuing education, or they demonstrate a definite decline from their prior level of functioning, even if they are currently performing adequately. Impairment may be further characterized by denial and ambivalence on the part of the physician, the family, and the community, all of whom may ignore the problem until it is too late. Intervention with appropriate treatment as soon as alcoholism is recognized is a major goal of the impaired physician movement.

Recognition and Management

The manifestations, symptoms, or signs of impairment from alcoholism and other chemical dependence among professionals are the same as those seen in nonprofessionals.

When one is concerned about impairment in a colleague, it is advisable to contact one or more close associates of that colleague to confirm the impairment. Likely reasons for the impairment may be uncovered in this discreet inquiry; often alcoholism or other chemical dependence is the underlying problem. Persuasion of an impaired physician to accept the existence of a problem and to agree to rehabilitation can be attempted by a concerned colleague, an approach similar to that for other people with alcoholism (Fig. 21.4). Such efforts are likely to be met with intense denial. A second approach is to use the state's physician rehabilitation committee. Each state medical society has a committee and maintains telephone access for confidential reporting of impaired physicians. Subcommittees undertake verification of the problem, followed by confrontation of the troubled physician, similar to the formal intervention technique described above. The goal of this process is to rehabilitate the physician, usually through intensive treatment in a residential facility (55).

Recently, the Association of Program Directors in Internal Medicine issued a position paper regarding alcohol and other chemical dependence among resident physicians. Recommendations included keeping residents well informed regarding program policy related to substance abuse, a clearly defined process for (self) referral, and how to help a colleague suspected of substance abuse (1).

BRIEF INTERVENTION FOR NONDEPENDENT DRINKERS

Brief interventions are time-limited sessions provided by primary care providers that focus on *reducing alcohol use in the nondependent drinker.* Many targeted people may be in the early stages of alcoholism, having not yet lost control of their drinking. Brief interventions have been found to be effective in reducing alcohol consumption (or achieving treatment referral) of problem drinkers (9,23,70).

Brief intervention is a process of assessing alcohol use, giving feedback, contracting and goal setting, arriving at a strategy for behavior modification, and providing a plan for follow-up. There must be an emphasis on personal responsibility for change and clear advice to change. Therapeutic empathy describes the recommended counseling style. Typically, the goal of brief intervention is not abstinence. Therefore, patients must receive follow-up to determine whether they are not just problem drinkers but are indeed alcoholics.

The approach to brief intervention parallels the approach previously mentioned in confronting the patient with alcoholism. *Six essential elements* should be included: *(a)* feedback of personal risk (patient-focused review of the evidence for existing or potential risk related to drinking), *(b)* emphasis on personal responsibility for change (empowering the patient to take control of the decision for change), *(c)* clear advice for change ("Based on all we have discussed, you need to make a change"), *(d)* offering a menu of alternative options ("Here's some ways you can make a change"), *(e)* therapeutic empathy as an innate part of the intervention ("I know this may be difficult"), and *(f)* enhancement of patient self-efficacy ("This is not hopeless; with change, things will get better for you"). Chapter 4 describes in detail the concepts that underlie these behavior modification techniques.

The brief intervention procedures used in studies vary, but none involve more than six contacts. No outside referrals are made, but written materials are often helpful. Typical follow-up sessions are usually 15 minutes. Studies show reduction of alcohol consumption in problem drinkers by 10 to 35% at 1-year follow-up. Some studies show an impact on drinking with just one interventional session. This further illustrates the importance of addressing alcohol use in all patients, even those who are not alcoholic, because problem drinking, independent of alcohol dependence, plays an enormous role in contributing to trauma, especially automobile accidents.

CO-ALCOHOLISM (CODEPENDENCE)

Co-alcoholism can be defined as ill health or maladaptive, problematic, or dysfunctional behavior that is associated with living with, working with, treating, or otherwise being close to a person with alcoholism. Co-alcoholism is a specific example of the more general phenomenon codependence (i.e., suffering or dysfunction associated with or caused by focusing on the needs or behaviors of others) (67). The long-term sequelae of one type of codependence—growing up in a family dominated by alcoholism or by other unhealthy or dysfunctional abnormal patterns—is described below ("Adult Children of Dysfunctional Families").

Co-alcoholism affects not only individuals and families, but also helping professionals, communities, businesses, other institutions, and even whole societies. Its signs and symptoms range from passive acceptance and absence of overt problems to the following range of manifestations:

In People Close to an Alcoholic

- Behaviors that protect the alcoholic (enabling)
- Behavioral or psychologic symptoms, such as anxiety disorders, depression, insomnia, hyperactivity, aggression, anorexia nervosa, bulimia, and suicidal gestures
- Functional or psychosomatic illness
- Family violence or neglect
- Alcoholism or another chemical dependence

In Helping Professionals

- Failure to diagnose alcoholism
- Failure to treat alcoholism as a primary illness
- Treating the alcoholic with sedatives or tranquilizers
- Treating the co-alcoholic with sedatives or tranquilizers

As noted earlier, some of these co-alcoholic behaviors have been the basis for a number of successful lawsuits against physicians in recent years.

In Society at Large

- Not confronting relatives, friends, and colleagues who are inappropriately intoxicated or are chronically abusing alcohol or drugs
- Placing a positive social value on those who drink
- Stigmatizing those who are alcoholics or those who do not drink

Co-Alcoholism in the Individual

The following is a *typical case history of co-alcoholism in an individual.*

A 38-year-old white, married woman presented with recurring episodes of upper abdominal pain of about 4 years' duration. During that time she had been evaluated by two internists and had been hospitalized once. After extensive evaluations, the working diagnosis was functional abdominal pain. She was treated with antispasmodics and sedatives but there was no substantial improvement. The pain occurred almost every day. On a follow-up visit 6 months later, the patient said that a friend had suggested that she attend the self-help group Al-Anon because her husband's drinking had been bothering her for at least 5 years. The patient reported that after she attended 12 Al-Anon meetings over 3 months, her abdominal pain gradually abated. On follow-up 2 years later, she had continued to attend Al-Anon and the symptoms had not recurred. In the meantime, the patient's husband had continued to drink.

This case study illustrates a common manifestation of co-alcoholism: a psychosomatic illness that resolved after the patient recognized an alcohol problem in the family and attended Al-Anon regularly.

Recognition and Treatment of the Co-Alcoholic Patient

When a patient has unexplained somatic or psychologic symptoms, it is helpful to ask whether the patient has ever been concerned about the drinking (or drug use) of anyone close to him or her. If the answer is *yes,* the patient should be asked to describe the problem. If the patient is vague or doubtful, one can administer some or all of the questions in the *Family Drinking Survey* shown in Table 21.11. One can also ask the possible co-alcoholic to answer CAGE questions (Fig. 21.1) or the questions on the MAST (Table 21.3) as though the questions were addressed to, and answered honestly by, the potentially alcoholic person to whom he or she is close (39). A positive score on one of these is a strong indication of co-alcoholism.

Initially, the psychologic and behavioral adjustments of the co-alcoholic are normal responses to an abnormal situation. However, these adaptive responses eventually lead to the person becoming dysfunctional.

Co-alcoholism, like alcoholism, is chronic, progressive, and characterized by denial, ill health, or maladaptive behavior, and by a lack of knowledge about alcoholism.

The major strategies in treating a patient with co-alcoholism are remarkably similar to those for treating the alcoholic:

- Have the patient accept the fact that he or she is a co-alcoholic.
- Motivate the patient to get help (occasionally by using a coercive intervention, such as the formal intervention described above).

Table 21.11. Family Drinking Survey

	Yes	No
1. Does someone in your family undergo personality changes when he or she drinks to excess?		
2. Do you feel that drinking is more important to this person than you are?		
3. Do you feel sorry for yourself and frequently indulge in self-pity because of what you feel alcohol is doing to your family?		
4. Has some family member's excessive drinking ruined special occasions?		
5. Do you find yourself covering up for the consequences of someone else's drinking?		
6. Have you ever felt guilty, apologetic, or responsible for the drinking of a member of your family?		
7. Does one of your family member's use of alcohol cause fights and arguments?		
8. Have you ever tried to fight the drinker by joining in the drinking?		
9. Do the drinking habits of some family members make you feel depressed or angry?		
10. Is your family having financial difficulties because of drinking?		
11. Did you ever feel like you had an unhappy home life because of the drinking of some members of your family?		
12. Have you ever tried to control the drinker's behavior by hiding the car keys, pouring liquor down the drain, etc.?		
13. Do you find yourself distracted from your responsibilities because of this person's drinking?		
14. Do you often worry about a family member's drinking?		
15. Are holidays more of a nightmare than a celebration because of a family member's drinking behavior?		
16. Are most of your drinking family member's friends heavy drinkers?		
17. Do you find it necessary to lie to employers, relatives, or friends in order to hide your spouse's drinking?		
18. Do you find yourself responding differently to members of your family when they are using alcohol?		
19. Have you ever been embarrassed or felt the need to apologize for the drinker's actions?		
20. Does some family member's use of alcohol make you fear for your own safety or the safety of other members of your family?		
21. Have you ever thought that one of your family members had a drinking problem?		
22. Have you ever lost sleep because of a family member's drinking?		
23. Have you ever encouraged one of your family members to stop or cut down on his or her drinking?		
24. Have you ever threatened to leave home or to leave a family member because of his or her drinking?		
25. Did a family member ever make promises that he or she did not keep because of drinking?		
26. Did you ever wish that you could talk to someone who could understand and help the alcohol-related problems of a family member?		
27. Have you ever felt sick, cried, or had a "knot" in your stomach after worring about a family member's drinking?		
28. Has a family member ever failed to remember what occurred during a drinking period?		
29. Does your family member avoid social situations where alcoholic beverages will *not* be served?		
30. Does your family member have periods of remorse after drinking occasions and apologize for his or her behavior?		
31. Please write any symptoms or medical or nervous problems that you have experienced since you have known your heavy drinker. (Write on back if more space is needed.)		

If you answer "Yes" to any two of the above questions, there is a good possibility that someone in your family has a drinking problem.

If you answer "Yes" to four or more of the above questions, there is a definite indication that someone in your family *does* have a drinking problem.

These survey questions are modified or adapted from validated survey instruments such as the Children of Alcoholics Screening Test (CAST) and the Howard Family Questionnaire, and from the Family Alcohol Quiz from Al-Anon.

- Refer the patient to Al-Anon or Alateen (As is true of AA referrals, enthusiasm for and a good understanding of the Al-Anon process on the part of the referring physician are critical to successful referral. The Al-Anon process is described in Table 21.12).
- Provide supportive psychotherapy at follow-up visits (see description of techniques, Chapter 11) and refer the patient or the family for additional therapy, especially group therapy for codependents or adult children of dysfunctional families (see below).
- Assist in the process of getting the alcoholics who are

the source of the problem into treatment. (This is not the responsibility of the co-alcoholic, however.)

Co-Alcoholism in the Helping Professions

Co-alcoholism includes behavior on the part of professionals that enables alcoholics to remain enmeshed in their disease, as noted above. Enabling behavior often coexists with otherwise excellent clinical skills. The *Professional Enablers Screening Test* (Table 21.13) is useful for identifying the various ways in which

Table 21.12.   The Al-Anon Process

Al-Anon began in the 1940s as an AA auxiliary and initially called itself AA Family Groups. In 1952, the wives of the two founders of AA established Al-Anon.

Al-Anon is a fellowship of family members of alcoholics who meet together to share their experiences, strengths, and hopes so that they can achieve health and serenity. The organization is modeled after AA and uses the 12 Steps of AA (see Table 21.8) as its principles for individual recovery. Its focus is not on the alcoholic but on the family members; thus, it powerfully frees families from their dependence on the alcoholic.

Al-Anon meetings are all open to the public and often meet at the same time and location as AA meetings. In most communities, Al-Anon has a telephone listing where meeting information, help, and literature can be obtained. Where there is no local Al-Anon office, the AA office can provide Al-Anon information.

Al-Anon meetings generally last 1 hour and follow the format of AA meetings (see Table 21.8), but they are usually smaller and discussion of topics is often freer than in AA.

Al-Anon is the sponsor of Ala-Teen and Ala-Tots, which are organizations for teenage and young children of alcoholics, respectively. These groups follow the Al-Anon discussion format and in general are not open to the nonalcoholic public, but helping professionals are usually welcome if they request to attend ahead of time. In the last several years in some areas, Al-Anon members have begun groups for adult children of alcoholics. These groups offer help to adults who may no longer live with an alcoholic family member, but whose life continues to be adversely affected by the legacy of growing up in an alcoholic home. These are especially powerful, and many patients with this background can be profoundly helped.

Al-Anon publishes a number of pamphlets that are available at meetings for families. *Al-Anon Faces Alcoholism,* Al-Anon's "Big Book," describes the family's plight with alcoholism through a variety of stories that graphically describe how families become sick in response to the alcoholic. Its other major book, *Living with an Alcoholic,* offers practical suggestions for recovery.

More information can be obtained by writing Al-Anon Family Group Headquarters, Box 182, Madison Square Station, New York, NY 10010.

Table 21.13.   Professional Enablers Screening Test[a]

Please check your answer to each question. For medically oriented questions, please check the space to which you would subscribe, even though you may not be a physician.

	Yes	No
1. Do you sometimes avoid raising sensitive issues related to drinking because it might offend your patient, or make him or her angry or feel bad?	(2)	
2. Do you generally treat the heavy-drinking person's problems without focusing most of the treatment on the drinking behavior?	(5)	
3. Do you avoid confronting your heavy-drinking patient when there is good evidence that he or she has misinformed you about his or her drinking?	(2)	
4. Do you generally suggest to your alcoholic patients that they cut down on their drinking?	(3)	
5. Do you believe what your heavy-drinking patient tells you about his or her drinking without using other sources such as a spouse, employer, screening test, blood alcohol test, or other laboratory test?	(5)	
6. Do you generally prescribe a sedative or minor tranquilizer for the nervous conditions or sleep problems of your alcoholic patients?	(5)	
7. Do you refer most of your alcoholic patients to attend Alcoholics Anonymous meetings regularly?		(5)
8. Do you refer many of your alcoholic patients to an alcoholism therapy group?		(3)
9. Do you prescribe disulfiram (Antabuse) to many of your alcoholic patients?		(3)
10. When your alcoholic patient has a minor crisis requiring hospitalization, do you routinely hospitalize him or her in a community hospital general ward?	(5)	
11. Do you refer most of the spouses of family members of your alcoholic patients to attend Al-Anon meetings regularly?		(5)
12. Do you subscribe to the theory that most alcoholics have an underlying psychologic disorder that is the major cause of the alcoholism?	(5)	
13. Do you believe that most alcoholics will not respond positively to treatment for their alcoholism?	(5)	

[a]Numbers in parentheses are the scores recommended for the corresponding responses. A score of 0 to 3 points indicates a probable nonenabler, 4 to 6 points may indicate a possible enabler, 7 points or more indicates a probable enabler.

enabling may occur in the context of medical practice. Societal norms (including one's own approach to the use of alcohol or other drugs), plus nonawareness of modern approaches to diagnosis, motivation, and treatment of the alcoholic, are probably the major reasons for co-alcoholism in helping professionals. Several steps are recommended for the professional who wishes to cease being an enabler:

- Update one's knowledge of alcoholism.
- Attend a number of AA and Al-Anon meetings.
- In one's own practice, try using skills such as those described in this chapter. The best cure for co-alcoholism in the physician is success in getting a number of alcoholics and their families into the recovery process.

DOMESTIC VIOLENCE

Domestic violence is present in all demographic and socioeconomic strata. It is especially prevalent in women whose partners abuse alcohol or other drugs and in women who themselves abuse substances. It is estimated that 75% of wives of alcoholics have been threatened and 45% have been assaulted by their alcoholic partners. *Domestic violence has been defined* by the American Medical Association as an ongoing debilitating experience of physical, psychologic, or sexual abuse in the home, associated with increased isolation from the outside world and limited personal freedom and accessibility to resources (see "General References").

In the United States, it is estimated that 2 million women per year are victims of domestic violence and more than 12 million will be abused some time during their lives. Most of these women never seek help from health care providers for the consequences of domestic violence. However, studies demonstrate a relationship between domestic violence and medical and psychiatric illness.

Brief screening for domestic violence should be incorporated into the medical interview of all women. Because some women may not initially recognize themselves as victims of domestic violence, questioning should be specific (Table 21.14). The issue should

Table 21.14.   A Recommended Approach to the Use of Interviewing to Screen Patients for Domestic Violence

Integrating domestic violence inquiry into interview as part of social history:

"Because abuse and violence have unfortunately become a common part of a woman's life, I ask all my patients about it routinely."

We all occasionally fight at home. What happens when you and your partner disagree?

Have you ever been treated badly or threatened by your partner?

Has your partner ever prevented you from leaving the house, seeing friends, getting a job, or continuing your education?

Does your partner ever force you to have sex or force you to engage in sex that is uncomfortable to you?

(if appropriate) You mentioned your partner drinks (uses drugs). How does he act when he is drinking (using drugs)?

Table 21.15.   Clinical Signs and Symptoms Suggestive of Domestic Violence

Alcohol or drug abuse
Anxiety
Atypical chest pain
Change in appetite
Chronic headaches
Chronic pain of unclear etiology
Depressed mood
Difficulty concentrating
Dizziness
Fatigue
Frequent evidence of minor trauma
Frequent requests for pain medications or tranquilizers
Frequent visits with vague somatic complaints
Gastrointestinal upset, diarrhea, or dyspepsia
Insomnia
Palpitations
Panic attacks
Paresthesias
Pelvic pain
Suicide attempts or gestures

be dealt with sensitively, validating the difficulty most women have in discussing the issue. The patient may be reluctant to disclose information because of shame, humiliation, low self-esteem, or fear of retaliation by the perpetrator. Some women may also believe that they deserve the abuse and do not deserve help or may feel that they need to protect their partner, who is their only source of affection and support. There may also be a belief on the part of the victim that the medical provider will not understand the problem or will not believe her.

In addition to screening, certain patient problems should alert one to the possibility of domestic violence (Table 21.15). Problems may range from direct evidence of physical trauma (contusions, abrasions, and broken bones) to nonspecific complaints of fatigue and difficulty concentrating. The screening information and medical history related to domestic violence must be well documented in the medical record because they provide evidence that may be used in a legal case. The record should include detailed descriptions of any injuries and, if possible, photographs of injuries sustained.

Once evidence of abuse is obtained, one must validate the seriousness of the situation to the patient. This must occur even if the patient is not yet ready to leave the abusive spouse. In addition, the immediate safety of the woman should be assessed. Unfortunately, the level of severity of past violence may not be a predictor of the severity of future violence. If safety is in question, the woman (and her children) should be advised to stay with family or friends, or at a shelter that specializes in caring for abused women and their families. Medical attention may also be needed for abused children in the household.

Often, the patient resists taking action. One should continue to show concern and work to motivate the patient toward change. Once the patient has agreed to take action, community resources must be accessed. These resources, which may differ by community can provide support, safety, and advocacy. The *National Domestic Violence Hotline* (1-800-799-SAFE) is a 24-hour service that helps women find a safe place to stay in their communities. At times, psychiatric or substance abuse referral may also be appropriate.

ADULT CHILDREN OF DYSFUNCTIONAL FAMILIES

In recent years, it has been recognized that many adults in our society grew up in families made dysfunctional by alcoholism or other abnormal behaviors that dominated life at home. The term *adult children of alcoholics* (ACOA) is widely used for those whose childhood was affected by alcoholism or other chemical dependence in one or both parents.

A dysfunctional family tends not to support the psychologic and spiritual growth of each of its members. Trying to be real (i.e., expressing oneself through one's actual feelings and thoughts) in such a family is generally so painful that the child develops a mask, which can be called a false self or codependent self. Living through this false self is survival-oriented but not fulfilling. From becoming entrenched in living this way, such people come to think that that is all there is to life. When they become adults and leave their family of origin, they generally continue in this stance, unhappy and unfulfilled. Many develop alcoholism or other chemical dependence.

Because the ACOA concept has been widely publicized in the lay media, many affected people recognize their situation and seek help from programs in their communities. However, some present their problems in medical visits.

Among the many adult problems that derive from these childhood roles are difficulty in showing feelings and developing intimate relationships, high tolerance for inappropriate behavior in others, difficulty getting one's own needs met, being either very responsible (helping others, never saying no) or irresponsible, and seeking approval of others. Many people with these patterns enter the helping professions. Although supportive psychotherapy (see Chapter 11) can be helpful, these people tend to have recurring problems unless they enter a full recovery program (65,67).

The major process in a full recovery program includes identifying and experientially working through one's psychologic and spiritual wounding, much of it from one's family of origin. Like recovery from alcoholism and other chemical dependence, a major treatment modality for the adult child syndrome is long-term group therapy in a group that is specific for this condition. Such group therapy has become more widely available in recent years. Also important to full recovery is participation in self-help programs, including Al-Anon groups (described above), ACOA groups (available in many communities, often in association with Al-Anon), or Co-Dependents Anonymous groups (not specific to alcoholism, available in many communities). Individual counseling, keeping a journal or diary, educational experiences, and intensive residential treatment may also be helpful for some people (14,65,67).

General References*

Alcoholics Anonymous. The story of how many thousands of men and women have recovered from alcoholism ("The Big Book"). 3rd ed. New York: Alcoholics Anonymous World Services, 1976.
> The nature of alcoholism and the recovery process using AA are illustrated in a large number of personal stories.

American Medical Association. **Diagnostic and treatment guidelines on domestic violence.** Chicago: American Medical Association, 1992.
> An excellent brief monograph written for clinicians.

Barnes HN, Aronson MD, Delbanco TL, eds. Alcoholism: a guide for the primary care physician. New York: Springer-Verlag, 1987.
> An excellent guide for clinicians caring for patients with alcoholism.

Bean MH. Alcoholics Anonymous. I. Principles and methods. Psychiatr Ann 5:5, 1975.
> A psychiatrist's lucid account of the AA process, based on her personal visits to 40 different AA groups.

Bean MH, Zinberg NE, eds. Dynamic approaches to the understanding and treatment of alcoholism. New York: Free Press, 1981.
> Detailed description of the denial process and other psychodynamic aspects of the alcoholic's behavior.

Drews T. Getting them sober: a guide for those who live with an alcoholic. Plainfield, NJ: Haven Books, 1980.
> Widely available paperback for families of alcoholics; quick reading. Advice regarding numerous practical issues.

The Enablers and *The Intervention* (films). Minneapolis: Johnson Institute, 1978.
> Two of the best films ever made on alcoholism. The technique of formal intervention is shown.

Gorski TT, Miller M. Staying sober: a guide for relapse prevention. Independence, MO: Independence Press, 1986.
> A book that describes in detail the relapse process and how to deal with it. For recovering alcoholic patients.

Gravitz H, Bowden J. Recovery guide for adult children of alcoholics. New York: Simon & Schuster, 1986.
> For therapists and laypeople, a practical and readable map of recovery.

Jellinek EM. The disease concept of alcoholism. New Haven: College and University Press, 1960.
> Landmark monograph reviewing the history of the disease concept.

O'Connor PG, Schottenfeld RS. Patients with alcohol problems. N Engl J Med 338(9):592–602, 1998.
> Well-referenced update on the full spectrum of problems associated with alcohol, focusing on the needs of the generalists.

Rogers RL, McMillin CS, eds. Don't help: a positive guide to working with the alcoholic. New York: Bantam, 1989.
> Practical account of techniques for group or individual counseling that, in conjunction with AA, are often effective in long-term treatment of alcoholism.

Turner RC, Lichstein PR, Peden JG Jr, et al. Alcohol withdrawal syndromes: a review of pathophysiology, clinical presentation, and treatment. J Gen Intern Med 4(5):432, 1989.

Vaillant G. The natural history of alcoholism. Cambridge, MA: Harvard University Press, 1983.
> Detailed monograph, much of it based on the author's longitudinal studies.

Whitfield CL. Healing the child within: discovery and recovery for adult children of dysfunctional families. Pompano Beach, FL: Health Communications, 1987.
> A clinical introduction to the problems of adult children of alcoholics and other dysfunctional families and to successful recovery from these problems.

Whitfield CL. A gift to myself: a personal notebook and guide for healing my child within. Deerfield Beach, FL: Health Communications, 1990.
> A detailed description of the recovery process for adult children of dysfunctional families.

---

*Bold print (general references) and bold numerals (specific references) denote published controlled clinical trials, meta-analyses, or consensus-based recommendations.

Specific References

1. Aach RD, Girard DE, Humphrey H, et al. Alcohol and other substance abuse and impairment among physicians in residency training. Ann Intern Med 116:245, 1992.
2. Adams WL, Barry KL, Fleming MF. Screening for problem drinking in older primary care patients. JAMA 276:1964, 1996.
3. Alldredge BK, Lowenstein DH, Simon RP. Placebo-controlled trial of intravenous diphenylhydantoin for short-term treatment of alcohol withdrawal seizures. Am J Med 87:645, 1989.
4. American College of Physicians. Disulfiram treatment of alcoholism. Ann Intern Med 111:943, 1989.
5. American Psychiatric Association. Diagnostic and statistical manual of mental disorders. 4th ed. (DSM-IV). Washington, DC: American Psychiatric Association, 1994.
6. Atkinson RM, Tolson RL, Turner JA. Late versus early onset problem drinking in older men. Alcohol Clin Exp Res 14:574, 1990.
7. Bean-Bayog M. The adolescent drinker. In: Barnes HN, Aronson MD, Delbanco T, eds. Alcoholism: a guide for the primary care physician. New York: Springer-Verlag, 1987.
8. Beresford TP, Blow FC, Hill E, et al. Comparison of CAGE questionnaire and computer-assisted laboratory profiles in screening for covert alcoholism. Lancet 336:482, 1990.
9. Bien TH, Miller WR, Tonigan JS. Brief interventions for alcohol problems: a review. Addiction 88:315, 1993.
10. Bissell LC. The treatment of alcoholism: what do we do about long-term sedatives? Ann N Y Acad Sci 252:396, 1975.
11. Bloom PL. Alcoholism after sixty. Am Fam Physician 28:111, 1983.
12. Blum K, Noble EP, Sheridan PJ, et al. Allelic association of human dopamine D2 receptor gene in alcoholism. JAMA 263:2055, 1990.
13. Bowen OR, Sammons JH. The alcohol-abusing patient: a challenge to the profession. JAMA 260(15):2267, 1988.
14. Brown S. Treating adult children of alcoholics: a developmental perspective. New York: Wiley, 1988.
15. Buchsbaum DG, Buchanan RG, Welsh J, et al. Screening for drinking disorders in the elderly using the CAGE questionnaire. J Am Geriatr Soc 40:662, 1992.
16. Bullock KD, Reed RJ, Grant I. Reduced mortality risk in alcoholics who achieve long-term abstinence. JAMA 267:668, 1992.
17. Conneally PM. Association between the D_2 dopamine receptor gene and alcoholism: a continuing controversy. Arch Gen Psychiatry 48:664, 1991.
18. Cyr MG, Wartman SA. The effectiveness of routine screening questions in the detection of alcoholism. JAMA 259(1):51, 1988.
19. Ewing JA. Detecting alcoholism: the CAGE questionnaire. JAMA 252:1905, 1984.
20. Fagan RW, Mauss AL. Social margin and social reentry: an evaluation of a rehabilitation program for skid row alcoholics. J Stud Alcohol 47(5):413, 1986.
21. Fein R. Alcohol in America: the price we pay. Newport Beach, CA: Care Institute, 1984;10.
22. Fine E. Philadelphia DWI study. U S J Alcohol Drug Abuse 19(March), 1983.
23. Fleming MF, Barry KL, Manwell LB, et al. Brief physician advice for problem alcohol drinkers: a randomized controlled trial in community-based primary care practices. JAMA 277:1039, 1997.
24. Gore-Gearhart J, Beebe DK, Milhorn HT, et al. Alcoholism in women. Am Fam Physician 44:907, 1991.
25. Gorski TT. Relapse prevention planning: a new recovery tool. Alcohol Health Res World 6:11, 1986.
26. Hayashida M, Alterman AI, McLellan T, et al. Comparative effectiveness and costs of inpatient and outpatient detoxification of patients with mild-to-moderate alcohol withdrawal syndrome. N Engl J Med 320:358, 1989.
27. Hays JT, Spickard WA Jr. Alcoholism: early diagnosis and intervention. J Gen Intern Med 2:420, 1987.
28. Hoffman NG, Harrison PA, Belille CA. Alcoholics Anonymous after treatment: attendance and abstinence. Int J Addict 18:311, 1983.
29. Holder HD, Blose JO. The reduction of health care costs associated with alcoholism treatment: a 14-year longitudinal study. J Stud Alcohol 53:293, 1992.
30. Hurt RD, Offord KP, Croghan IT, et al. Mortality following inpatient addictions treatment. Role of tobacco use in a community-based cohort. JAMA 275:1097, 1996.
31. Jellinek EM. Phases of alcohol addiction. Q J Stud Alcohol 13(4):673, 1952.
32. Johnson B, Clark W. Alcoholism: a challenging physician–patient encounter. J Gen Intern Med 4:445, 1989.
33. Johnson VE, ed. I'll quit tomorrow. New York: Harper & Row, 1980.
34. Klatsky AL, Armstrong MA, Friedman GD. Alcohol and mortality. Ann Intern Med 117:646, 1992.
35. Miller WR, Hester RK. Inpatient alcoholism treatment: who benefits? Am Psychol 41(7):794, 1986.
36. Moore RD, Bone LR, Geller G, et al. Prevalence, detection and treatment of alcoholism in hospitalized patients. JAMA 261:403, 1989.
37. Moore RD, Mead L, Pearson TA. Youthful precursors of alcohol abuse in physicians. Am J Med 88:332, 1990.
38. Morse RM, Flavin DK. The definition of alcoholism. JAMA 268:1012, 1992.
39. Morse RM, Swanson WM. Spouse response to a self-administered alcoholism screening test. J Stud Alcohol 36:400, 1975.
40. Myers JK, Weissman MM, Tischler GL, et al. Six-month prevalence of psychiatric disorders in three communities. Arch Gen Psychiatry 4:959, 1984.
41. National Highway Traffic Safety Administration. Traffic safety facts, 1995: alcohol. Washington, DC: US Department of Transportation, National Highway Traffic Safety Administration, National Center for Statistics and Analysis, Research and Development, 1996.
42. Ng SK, Hauser WA, Brust JC, et al. Alcohol consumption and withdrawal in new-onset seizures. N Engl J Med 319:666, 1988.
43. Pell S, D'Alonzo CA. A five-year mortality study of alcoholics. J Occup Med 15:120, 1973.
44. Powers JS, Spickard A. Michigan Alcoholism Screening Test to diagnose early alcoholism in a general practice. South Med J 77:852, 1984.
45. Prochaska JO, DiClemente CC. Toward a comprehensive model of change. In: Miller WR, Heather N, eds. Treating addictive behaviors: process of change. New York: Plenum, 1986.
46. Reuler JB, Girard DE, Cooney TG. Wernicke's encephalopathy. N Engl J Med 312:1035, 1985.
47. Roman PM. Biological features of women's alcohol use: a review. Public Health Rep 103:628, 1988.
48. Saitz R, Mayo-Smith MF, Roberts MS, et al. Individualized treatment for alcohol withdrawal. A randomized double-blind controlled trial. JAMA 272:519, 1994.
49. Samet JH, Rollnick S, Barnes H. Beyond CAGE: a brief clinical approach after detection of substance abuse. Arch Intern Med 156:2287, 1996.
50. Sampliner R, Iber F. Diphenylhydantoin control of alcohol withdrawal seizures. JAMA 230:1430, 1974.
51. Schuckit MA. The clinical implications of primary diagnostic groups among alcoholics. Arch Gen Psychiatry 42:1043, 1985.
52. Secretary of Health and Human Services. Eighth special report to the U.S. Congress on alcohol and health. Washington, DC: US Department of Health and Human Services, September 1993.
53. Sellers EM, Naranjo CA, Harrison M, et al. Diazepam loading: simplified treatment of alcohol withdrawal. Clin Pharmacol Ther 822, December 1983.
54. Skinner HA, Holt S, Schuller R, et al. Identification of alcohol abuse using laboratory tests and a history of trauma. Ann Intern Med 101:847, 1984.
55. Spickard WA Jr. The impaired physician. In: Barnes HN, Aronson MD, Delbanco TL, eds. Alcoholism: a guide for the primary care physician. New York: Springer-Verlag, 1987.
56. Sullivan JT, Sykora K, Schneiderman J, et al. Assessment of alcohol withdrawal: the revised clinical institute withdrawal assessment for alcohol scale (CIWA-Ar). Br J Addict 84:1353, 1989.
57. Umbricht-Schnecter A, Santora P, Moore RD: Alcohol abuse: comparison of two methods for assessing its prevalence and associated morbidity in hospitalized patients. Am J Med 91:110, 1991.

58. Vaillant GE, ed. The natural history of alcoholism, revisited. Cambridge, MA: Harvard University Press, 1996.
59. Vaillant G, Clark W, Cyrus C, et al. Prospective study of alcoholism treatment: eight-year follow-up. Am J Med 75:455, 1983.
60. Victor M, Hope JM. The phenomenon of auditory hallucinations in chronic alcoholism. J Nerv Ment Dis 126:451, 1958.
61. Volpicelli JR, Alterman AI, Hayashida M, O'Brien CP. Naltrexone in the treatment of alcohol dependence. Arch Gen Psychiatry 49:876, 1992.
62. Wallace J. Alcoholism from the inside out: a phenomenological analysis. In: Estes NJ, Heinemann ME, eds. Alcoholism: development, consequences, and interventions. St Louis: CV Mosby, 1977.
63. Walsh DC, Hingson RW, Merrigan DM, et al. A randomized trial of treatment options for alcohol abusing workers. N Engl J Med 325:775, 1991.
64. West LJ, Maxwell DS, Noble EP, Solomon DH. Alcoholism. Ann Intern Med 100:405, 1984.
65. Whitfield CL. Advances in alcoholism and chemical dependence. Am J Med 85:465, 1988.
66. Whitfield CL. Alcoholism, attachments and spirituality: stress management and serenity during recovery. Baltimore: Perrin and Thegell, 1984.
67. Whitfield CL, ed. Healing the child within: discovery and recovery for adult children of dysfunctional families. Deerfield Beach, FL: Health Communications, 1987.
68. Whitfield CL. Outpatient management of alcoholism. Psychiatr Ann 12:447, 1982.
69. Whitfield CL, Thompson G, Lamb A, et al. Detoxification of 1,024 alcoholics without psychoactive drugs. JAMA 239:1409, 1978; and letter response, 241:2597, 1979.
70. Wilk AI, Jensen NM, Havighurst TC. Meta-analysis of randomized control trials addressing brief interventions in heavy alcohol drinkers. J Gen Intern Med 12:274, 1997.
71. Wilsnack SC, Wilsnack RW. Epidemiology of women's drinking. J Subst Abuse Treat 3:133, 1991.
72. Wright C, Moore RD. Disulfiram treatment of alcoholism. Am J Med 88:647, 1990.
73. Zook CJ, Moore FD. High-cost users of medical care. N Engl J Med 302:996, 1980.

C H A P T E R 22

Illicit and Therapeutic Use of Drugs with Abuse Liability*

MICHAEL I. FINGERHOOD, MD

DEFINITIONS

Drugs with abuse liability modify mood, feeling, thinking, and perception. Many are commonly pre-

*John T. Sullivan contributed to this chapter in the fourth edition.

scribed and are useful therapeutic agents. The use and abuse of such substances date back thousands of years. Plant alkaloids, alcohol, and an ever-increasing array of newly synthesized chemicals have also been used in illicit endeavors. Patterns of use and the social acceptance of use of these agents have differed from time to time and from place to place. Successive generations of the same society have held discordant views about which substance to use, at what age, in what amount, and under which circumstances (e.g., attitudes regarding alcohol use in the preprohibition and postprohibition eras in the United States). Neighboring cultures have also differed about the sanctioned use of psychoactive substances. In 20th-century Western society, there are two forms of fairly innocuous use of illicit substances, experimental and social-recreational use, and two defined patterns of abnormal use, substance abuse and substance dependence.

Experimental Use

The experimental use of illicit substances is sporadic; the initial trial and experience usually are associated with youthful rites of passage. These experiments usually have little impact on mental health. They are potentially dangerous because of possible dosage errors, because unsterile methods of exposure may occur, because of behaviors that may endanger the user or other people, and because some people may find the drug experience extraordinarily rewarding, leading to repeated use. Incorrect labeling of such drugs (a common problem) increases the risk of these untoward consequences. Experimentation is common but decreasing compared with prior surveys. A 1992 national high school survey (23) revealed that 48% of all respondents had engaged in an experimental trial of an illicit drug (primarily marijuana) and 90% had tried alcohol on at least one occasion.

Social-Recreational Use

The social and recreational use of illicit substances suggests that they have been used repetitively but that control has been exerted over the dosage and the time of use. The risks of unintended overdosage, improper exposure, and mislabeling are increased by the frequency of use. Recreational use often is not psychologically disabling even though adverse consequences may occur. Adequate social and behavioral function is maintained. Most American use of alcohol and marijuana conforms to this pattern of social-recreational use.

Abuse and Dependence

The 1994 revision of the *Diagnostic and Statistical Manual of the American Psychiatric Association* (DSM-IV) delineates two diagnostic categories for the substance-related disorders (1). The diagnostic criteria are the same for all psychoactive substances, including alcohol.

The DSM-IV Criteria for Substance Abuse

A. A maladaptive pattern of substance use leading to clinically significant impairment or distress, as manifested by *one or more of the following* occurring at any time during the same 12-month period:
1. Recurrent substance use resulting in a failure to fulfill major role obligations at work, school, or home (e.g., repeated absences or poor work performance related to substance use; substance-related absences, suspensions, or expulsions from school; neglect of children or household)
2. Recurrent substance use in situations in which it is physically hazardous (e.g., driving an automobile or operating a machine when impaired by substance use)
3. Recurrent substance-related legal problems (e.g., arrests for substance-related disorderly conduct)
4. Continued substance use despite having persistent or recurrent social or interpersonal problems caused or exacerbated by the effects of the substance (e.g., arguments with spouse about consequences of intoxication, physical fights)
B. Has never met the criteria for substance dependence for this class of substance

The DSM-IV Criteria for Substance Dependence

A maladaptive pattern of substance use, leading to clinically significant impairment or distress, as manifested by *three or more of the following* occurring at any time in the same 12-month period:
1. Tolerance, as defined by either of the following:
   a. Need for markedly increased amounts of the substance to achieve intoxication or desired effect
   b. Markedly diminished effect with continued use of the same amount of the substance
2. Withdrawal, as manifested by either of the following:
   a. The characteristic withdrawal syndrome for substance (refer to the criteria sets for withdrawal from the specific substances)
   b. The same (or closely related) substance is taken to relieve or avoid withdrawal symptoms
3. The substance is often taken in larger amounts or over a longer period than was intended.
4. There is a persistent desire or unsuccessful efforts to cut down or control substance use.
5. A great deal of time is spent in activities necessary to obtain the substance (e.g., visiting multiple doctors or driving long distances), use the substance (e.g., chain smoking), or recover from its effects.
6. Important social, occupational, or recreational activities are given up or reduced because of substance use.
7. Continued substance use despite knowledge of having had a persistent or recurrent physical or psychologic problem that was likely to have been caused or exacerbated by the substance (e.g., current cocaine use despite recognition of cocaine-induced depression, or continued drinking despite recognition that an ulcer was made worse by alcohol consumption).

An important difference between DSM-IV and the third edition is that the diagnosis of psychoactive substance dependence no longer requires the presence of tolerance or a withdrawal syndrome. The diagnosis of dependence may now be made solely on the basis of impairment in psychosocial functioning.

Polydrug Abuse

Polydrug use, abuse, and dependence are extremely common. For example, more than 80% of alcoholics are cigarette smokers. Many younger alcoholics also abuse cocaine. Heroin and cocaine addicts often abuse alcohol. Alcoholics are at greater risk of abusing benzodiazepines (compared to non–drug abusing populations). People in methadone maintenance programs often abuse cocaine, benzodiazepines, and alcohol, and more than 90% are cigarette smokers. Use of speedballs (heroin and cocaine) is common. Use of a particular drug can be a function of price and availability, as illustrated by geographic differences in the patterns of drug abuse. Sometimes a drug interaction is desired (e.g., anxiolytic effects of alcohol counteract anxiogenic effects of cocaine). Mixed dependencies are often seen in detoxification units and are preferably treated on an inpatient basis. In general, people who find one drug of abuse particularly rewarding are likely to find other drugs of abuse also to be rewarding.

Classification by Pharmacologic Effect

Later sections of this chapter describe the manifestations and the principles of management for selected substances of abuse common in the United States today (Chapters 20 and 21 describe tobacco and alcohol abuse/dependence, respectively). A list of all drugs that have abuse potential would be extremely long. However, it is possible to group the various substances into broad classes, the members of which share common characteristics and are readily distinguishable from other classes (Table 22.1). Psychoactive substances may thus be generally classified as depressants, opioids, stimulants, and drugs that alter perception (including hallucinogens).

SOCIAL AND EPIDEMIOLOGIC ASPECTS

Social Aspects

Drug abuse has been a dominant public health concern for the past 20 years. Quite apart from toxic effects that may represent specific health threats to the individual abuser (discussed at greater length below under each substance), there are major societal consequences. The loss of impulse control directly associated with drug abuse, especially that caused by depressant intoxication (primarily alcohol), is clearly recognized as conducive to acts of violence (assault, rape, murder, and suicide). Impaired judgments and performance secondary to intoxication

Table 22.1.   Categories of Psychoactive Drugs

CNS Depressants
Alcohol
Sedative-hypnotics
  Barbiturates
  Nonbarbiturate sedative-hypnotics
  Meprobamate (Equanil or Miltown)
  Benzodiazepines
  Glutethimide (Doriden), methaqualone (Quaalude)
Inhalants
  Nitrous oxide, toluene, volatile hydrocarbons

Opioids
Morphine, hydromorphone (Dilaudid), heroin, meperidine (Demerol), codeine, methadone

Stimulants
Cocaine, amphetamine, methylphenidate (Ritalin), MDMA, phenmetrazine (Preludin), caffeine, nicotine, arecoline

Drugs that Alter Perception (Including Hallucinogens)
Marijuana, LSD, dimethyltryptamine tryptamine (DMT), psilocybin, PCP, belladonna alkaloids (atropine, scopolamine)

are associated with greatly increased rates of vehicular and workplace accidents and trauma, as well as impaired work performance and attendant economic loss.

Finally, not as a result of pharmacologic effects, but as an unintended byproduct of illicit status, substances of abuse are closely linked to crime (3). Illegal status puts a premium on the cost of satisfying addiction and provides a high economic stimulus to hook and supply consumers. Tens of billions of dollars annually in property crime and robberies are committed by addicts to pay the hugely inflated price of their addiction. Thousands of homicides annually are linked to drug abuse, many by dealers to acquire and police their turf. Many more billions of dollars are spent in the criminal justice system in the apprehension, trial, and imprisonment of addicts and dealers. More than 80% of people in prison in the United States have committed drug-related crimes.

Prevalence Trends

Although there is no question that drug abuse continues to be one of the most serious problems faced by public health and law enforcement authorities, survey data suggest that the use of some illicit substances has been declining modestly in important segments of the population. Nevertheless, in 1996 there were an estimated 2.1 million users of cocaine and 600,000 heroin-dependent people in the United States. Since 1975, a national survey of high school seniors and young adults has been conducted by the University of Michigan Institute for Social Research (23). The principal measure of use frequency is the 30-day prevalence, meaning the percentage of respondents who admit to use of a particular drug at least one time during the past 30 days. Table 22.2 summarizes these data for selected drugs; the table also summarizes the 30-day prevalence of daily use of these drugs by high school seniors. Trends from these survey data indicate that use by high school seniors of marijuana, stimulants, tranquilizers, nitrites, sedatives, and most hallucinogens has continued to decline annually since 1980. The prevalence of cocaine use, which had increased from 1.9% in 1975 to a high of 6.7% in 1985, declined to 1.9% in 1992. Alcohol use peaked at 72% in 1980 and declined to 57.1% in 1992, with a dramatic decline from a 34.7% daily use recorded in 1988 to a 3.7% daily use for the last 30 days in 1992. Less than 2% of respondents reported using lysergic acid diethylamide (LSD) or inhalants with any regularity. A notable finding of the survey is that the decline in use of most drugs has been accompanied by *changes in attitudes.* An increasing number of high school seniors have endorsed the belief that drug use is harmful. The number who say they disapprove of drug use has also increased. These findings suggest that drug education efforts and media representations of the adverse consequences of drug use are effective.

A disturbing note that augurs poorly for a continued decline in high school senior use is the finding that among 8th graders (surveyed in 1992), there is a pattern of drug use and experimentation that would predict a rise in use by the time these students complete high school (31).

In addition, there is an upward trend for emergency room visits related to heroin, with 76,000 such visits in 1995. This increase is postulated to be related to the increasing purity of heroin sold on the street.

Drug use and abuse are not evenly distributed throughout various segments of society. The incidence and prevalence of regular use and abuse are greater among inner-city populations characterized by low levels of employment and educational achievement. Minorities are overrepresented in this population. These groups have not shown as great a decline in drug use as the more middle-class populations have.

Table 22.2. Prevalence of Use of Selected Drugs Reported by High School Students, Class of 1992 (Shows Percentage of Respondents)

Drugs	Used One or More Times Last 30 Days	Used Daily for the Last 30 Days
Marijuana/hashish	14.0	2.2
Inhalants	2.7	0.3
LSD	1.9	0.0
PCP	0.4	0.1
Cocaine	1.9	0.1
Heroin	0.2	0.0
Other opiates	1.5	0.1
Stimulants	3.7	0.2
Sedatives	1.4	0.0
Tranquilizers	1.3	0.1
Alcohol	57.1	3.7
Cigarettes	28.4	19.1

Adapted from Johnson LD, O'Mallay PM, Backman JG. Drug use, drinking, and smoking: national survey results from high school, college, and young adult populations. Rockville, MD: US Department of Health and Human Services, Public Health Services, Alcohol, Drug Abuse, and Mental Health Association, 1992.

Special Populations

Among adolescents in whom drug use problems are severe enough to present for detoxification, polydrug abuse is almost invariable. Median age of first use of primary drug of abuse was 15, and median age for admission for detoxification was 17, in a study conducted in Baltimore (14). Drug use included alcohol (94%), cannabis (84%), cocaine (65%), heroin (43%), phencyclidine (PCP) (37%), inhalant (36%), barbiturates (34%), and amphetamines (32%). Physical dependence was reliably seen only with heroin. PCP use was more common among Caucasians and heroin use was more common among African Americans. Most came from unstable family backgrounds.

The *elderly* are not at high risk for illicit drug use. Addiction to illicit drugs tends to wane over the years in those who survive beyond their fifties or sixties. Most drug problems in the elderly occur with alcohol, tobacco, and prescription drugs (opioids for analgesia and benzodiazepines for insomnia). Occasionally, elderly people are seen in methadone programs, where they tend to do well.

Women are at lower risk of drug abuse than men but still make up about a third of the treatment population. They also are more likely than men to abuse illicit drugs by smoking or snorting rather than injecting. Particular problems include prostitution and consequent high rates of sexually transmitted diseases, as well as pregnancy, child care problems, and single-parent status. Access to and acceptance of prenatal care improve pregnancy outcome (perinatal morbidity and mortality). Alcohol is the most teratogenic of the drugs of abuse. Longer-term effects for other drugs are less certain. Neonatal opioid withdrawal is common and usually is easily treated.

Psychiatric disorders are more common among substance abusers than in the population as a whole. These both precede onset of substance abuse and result from substance abuse. Consequences of substance abuse also mimic psychiatric disorders. For example, patients with anxiety disorders may self-medicate with alcohol or benzodiazepines. Withdrawal from these substances produces anxiety regardless of whether the patient has an anxiety disorder. Stimulants acutely produce psychotic reactions, and depression is seen during withdrawal. Substance abusers are often given personality disorder diagnoses (especially the antisocial type). A low mood state (hypophoria) is common among substance abusers (see Gold and Slaby in "General References" for a review of psychiatric disorders associated with substance abuse).

CAUSES

Predisposing Factors

Drug abuse as defined above is merely an operational definition. The causes are clearly complex. Some of the factors involved are listed below.

- *Pharmacologic.* Certain drugs, classes of drugs, and routes of administration are consistently reported to be rewarding or reinforcing.

- *Genetic.* Certain individuals appear to be biologically predisposed to the rewarding effects of drugs of abuse and to the acquisition of drug dependence. This is most well recognized for alcohol and tobacco but is increasingly being recognized for other drugs of abuse.
- *Learning and behavior.* Repeated use of drugs (rewarding stimulus) elicits various conditioned responses and behaviors that perpetuate drug use.
- *Personality and psychiatric disorder.* People who have difficulty in deferring gratification seem to be predisposed to drug abuse. Those with mood or anxiety disorders may find that certain drugs of abuse normalize these states.
- *Social, environmental, and cultural.* Different societies have different attitudes and customs regarding use of psychoactive substances (e.g., French attitude toward wine). People who have few other rewarding activities (e.g., gainful employment) may be predisposed toward drug abuse as a rewarding activity.

These causes do not speak to possible legal consequences or to therapeutic maneuvers. Four models, described here, have been proposed to encompass these concerns. The models, although distinct, are not mutually exclusive, and most people fit into more than one model, illustrating the complexity of their disease.

Etiologic Models

Moral Failure Model

This view attributes substance abuse to a failure by parents or parental surrogates (e.g., religious training, schools, movies, television, records loosely grouped as society) to inculcate values and to the absence of an ongoing morality that would prevent the use and abuse of drugs. From a public health viewpoint the model has utility. When applied to the person already dependent on drugs and with a long criminal record, it is not useful unless there is some religious conversion experience or complete acceptance of a 12-step program (e.g., Alcoholics Anonymous or Narcotics Anonymous).

Legal Model

Proponents define behavior as aberrant only when specific acts violate existing law and then recommend existing legal remedies such as trial, fines, and imprisonment to deal with these infractions. This view tends to underestimate the impairment related to drug dependence, and therefore the "rationality" of the behavior. It also tends to counter the disease or illness concept of addiction.

Disease Model

The disease model hypothesizes a host susceptibility to drugs of abuse that is lifelong, progressive, and incapable of modification and hence can be coped with only by total abstinence. It takes as its substrate only those meeting the definitions of substance abuse or dependence (see above) and does not concern itself with social or experimental use. The disease model partially encompasses research advances in psychopharmacology.

The disease model was originally proposed to counter adverse societal attitudes and judgmental views toward alcohol and drug abuse. This model also offers a nonstigmatizing explanation of substance abuse to organizations such as Alcoholics Anonymous and Narcotics Anonymous. These organizations have helped unleash a vast movement for self-improvement that has helped a significant number of abusers. The disease model is the paradigm for the proponents of *methadone maintenance,* developed in the 1960s. Chronic narcotic abuse was seen as a biological modification of the brain that required supplementation by a narcotic substitute that does not lead to significant dysfunction.

Psychosocial Model

The psychosocial model sees chemical dependency as the inadvertent effect of repeated self-medication by a vulnerable population intent on relieving overwhelming anxiety or psychic pain attendant on loss, hopelessness, boredom, depression, and fear. Drugs of abuse are potent and effective, albeit short-term, chemical alleviators of these symptoms. Vulnerability in this model is not a function of genetic constitution (although this may define an enhanced susceptibility) but of membership in at-risk populations who, because of youthful immaturity, socioeconomic disability, and the lack of responsible familial or peer support systems, have not developed the same repertoire of behaviors that the greater part of society uses to cope with adversity. This model has the virtue of defining an at-risk population from among the young, the dropouts, and the socially and economically disadvantaged that best fits the majority of abusers in our current epidemic. The model helps explain the potential for endemic abuse by people who, although they may be socially and economically advantaged, may also turn to repetitive self-medication in the face of losses or situational anxiety, demoralization, or physical pain. The psychosocial model avoids a simplistic expectation of cure by mere detoxification or by enforced abstinence if release back into the same environment is contemplated without remediation of the conditions of vulnerability. The model also relies on support systems and self-help as a condition of remission.

TOLERANCE AND PHYSICAL DEPENDENCE

Most drugs of abuse share the capacity to induce tolerance. *Tolerance* is defined as the phenomenon whereby with repeated use an increased amount of drug is required to produce a given effect. Alternatively, the same amount of drug produces a lesser effect with repeated administration. The time required for the induction of tolerance ranges from days after repeated intravenous or intramuscular administration of opioids, to weeks or months after repeated oral administration of opioids, barbiturates, alcohol, and other sedatives.

Physical dependence is defined as the phenomenon

whereby abrupt cessation of a drug results in withdrawal symptoms and signs (the abstinence state). Withdrawal symptoms and signs are often the opposite of the biological effects exerted by the drug in question (Table 22.3).

Physical dependence is not synonymous with addiction. People who are prescribed benzodiazepines may exhibit physical dependence (sometimes called therapeutic dependence) but not fulfill criteria for substance dependence (see DSM-IV criteria above). Similarly, many people exhibit a withdrawal syndrome for caffeine but also do not fulfill criteria for substance dependence.

COMPLICATIONS OF INJECTING DRUGS

Cutaneous complications in chronic injecting drug users include needle marks or scars, usually in the antecubital fossae of both arms, on the forearms and wrists, or on the backs of the hands. The presence of old abscess scars and of bluish phlebitis scars from past injections also indicates chronic use. Long-time users are usually forced to seek new injection sites as old sites become unusable because of scarring, and they may exhibit fresh needle marks on the legs and neck.

Skin and soft tissue infections are extremely common and account for 57% of hospital admissions for injecting drug users (17). The prerequisites for infection include damage or irritation to tissues and colonization with an organism that causes infection. The various drugs of abuse are not equally irritating. Repetitive trauma from repeated injections contributes to the infectious process. *Staphylococcus aureus* is the most common pathogen (staphylococcal colonization is universal among injecting drug users). Streptococci (groups A and G) are the next most common pathogens. However, almost every common pathogen (as well as some uncommon ones) are seen. The types of infec-

tions include cellulitis, abscess, multiple chronic ulcerations, necrotizing fasciitis, pyomyositis, septic phlebitis, and infected aneurysms (17). Regional lymphangitis and lymphadenitis are common with all of these conditions. More unusual infections introduced at the site of injection include wound botulism, candidiasis, and tetanus.

When needles are shared, there is a high risk of acquiring *hepatitis.* Seroprevalence surveys among injecting drug users reveal positive hepatitis C serology in up to 86% (9). Many have chronically elevated transaminase activity, although the natural history of hepatitis C in this population is not yet well described. Hepatitis B virus is also common among injecting drug users with carrier (antigen positive) rates of 4% and previous infection (antibody positive) rates ranging from 30 (9) to 94% (27). People who have been infected with hepatitis B virus are at risk for infection with hepatitis D virus (delta virus). Hepatitis B vaccine should be given to seronegative injecting drug users. Chapters 32 ("Immunization to Prevent Infectious Disease") and 43 ("Diseases of the Liver") describe hepatitis vaccines and hepatitis in detail.

Approximately 30% of recent cases of acquired immunodeficiency syndrome (AIDS) in the United States and 50% in Europe relate to injecting drug use (7). Prevalence of *human immunodeficiency virus (HIV) infection* among populations of United States injecting drug users ranges from less than 10% in Los Angeles to 56% in New York City and San Juan (24). Rapid spread among this population has also occurred in Thailand, Brazil, and India so that large numbers of AIDS cases will be seen in these countries in the future. Injecting drug users are the main sources of heterosexual, and subsequent perinatal, transmission of HIV. Compared with homosexuals who are HIV positive, injecting drug users who are HIV positive are more likely to have morbidity related to bacterial infections

Table 22.3.   Characteristics of Dependence on Drugs of Abuse

Drug	Physiologic Effect	Withdrawal Symptoms and Signs (1 to 7 days After Last Dose)	
Opioids	Pupillary constriction Analgesia Constipation Respiratory depression	Pupillary dilation Myalgia Diarrhea Stimulation of respiratory centers ("yawning") Rhinorrhea Gooseflesh Nausea and vomiting Restlessness	
Alcohol, barbiturate, benzodiazepines	Induction of sleep (hypnosis) Sedation Alcohol usually decreases but may increase seizure activity (other sedatives decrease seizure activity)	Insomnia Nausea Tremulousness Anxiety Irritability Autonomic hyperactivity (sweats, tachycardia, hypertension) Delirium Seizures Death (alcohol and barbiturates)	Minor symptoms Onset 24–72 hr after last dose Duration 72–96 hr after last dose Major symptoms Onset 72 hr to 1 wk after last dose Duration up to 2 wk after last dose
Cocaine	Pupillary dilation Tachycardia Hypertension	Bradycardia Hyperphagia Fatigue Hypersomnolence	

(endocarditis, pneumonia, and abscesses). In general, studies have found that modest behavior change among injecting drug users has occurred as a result of concern about AIDS. This relates mostly to risk reduction rather than to elimination (smoking or snorting rather than injecting drugs). Multiple simultaneous interventions appear to be needed. These include access to drug abuse treatment (including methadone), education, counseling, social support, and needle and syringe exchange/availability (15). Despite these interventions, a proportion (especially those with antisocial personality) do not significantly change their behavior. Chapter 34 describes HIV infection in detail.

Endocarditis, usually caused by bacteria at injection sites, most often affects the tricuspid valve. *S. aureus* is the most common causative organism. Mitral and aortic valves are not uncommonly involved and are more likely to be affected if there is preexisting pathology. Streptococci (enterococcus, viridans, and β-hemolytic) are next most common and are more likely to affect left-sided valves. Other organisms include Gram-negatives *(Pseudomonas)* and fungi *(Candida).* Polymicrobial and culture-negative endocarditis also occur. Diagnosis is usually not difficult. Prognosis is related to size of vegetations and to complications such as heart failure and embolic events. Treatment should be in a controlled inpatient setting. Chapter 31 describes the posthospital management of endocarditis.

Skeletal infections account for a significant number of admissions of injecting drug abusers (7). Osteomyelitis and septic arthritis occur, mainly by hematogenous but occasionally from contiguous spread. The lumbar spine, sternoarticular structures, and the pelvis and its articular structures are commonly involved. Synovial joints (most commonly the knee) and occasionally the appendicular skeleton can be involved. The most common organisms are aerobic Gram-negative bacilli (mostly *Pseudomonas aeruginosa).* Tuberculosis and fungal infections are also encountered. Gonococcal arthritis is commonly seen among drug-abusing women who prostitute. Chapter 31 describes the ambulatory aspects of diagnosis and management of osteomyelitis.

Pulmonary complications, other than septic emboli, are mostly related to obtundation and drug intoxication with consequent aspiration pneumonia (or pulmonary edema from opiates), lung abscess, and empyema. Microembolization, talc granulomas, pulmonary fibrosis, and uncommonly, pulmonary hypertension are sometimes seen. Pneumothorax may occur as a complication of attempted injection in the neck.

Defects in host defense mechanisms (independent of HIV-induced problems) are present in injecting drug users. Cell-mediated immunity is depressed, but the mechanisms involved are not clearly understood. Other factors such as malnutrition and concurrent alcohol abuse complicate the study of this problem. Humoral immune response is not diminished. There are polyclonal increases in immunoglobulin, probably related to repeated antigenic exposure, that result in elevated total protein levels. Thrombocytopenia commonly occurs as a result of circulating immune complexes reacting with platelets. Up to 25% of drug users have a biological false-positive serologic test result for syphilis. Usually, the positive titer is 1:4 or less and the more specific fluorescent treponemal antibody (FTA) test is negative.

SELECTED DRUGS OF ABUSE
Sedative-Hypnotics and Benzodiazepines
Usual Effects and Therapeutic Use

Sedatives cause intoxication similar to that seen with alcohol. Sufficient amounts are often taken to produce a depression of cortical function and to relax social and personal inhibitions. A high, or a state in which mood is elevated and anxiety is reduced, is described in abusers. Normal individuals and those with anxiety disorders do not usually find these effects pleasurable or reinforcing. Because of their safety profile, benzodiazepines have become the only sedative-hypnotics prescribed for anxiolytic or sedating purposes. The proper prescribing of benzodiazepines for this purpose is discussed in Chapter 13. This class of medicine should be avoided in all patients with a history of substance abuse. Phenobarbital should be the only prescribed barbiturate, with its indication being for seizure prevention. Shorter-acting barbiturates are contained in migraine medicines such as fiorinal. These medications have a high abuse potential and should be avoided.

Acute Adverse Effects

Overdose may lead to slurred speech, impaired judgment, and unsteady gait. Even greater overdose may lead to stupor, coma, respiratory depression, vasomotor collapse, and death. Benzodiazepines (compared with barbiturates) cause less loss of motor coordination and almost never cause death when taken alone in large doses (unless given rapidly intravenously, e.g., midazolam or diazepam). However, the combination of alcohol and benzodiazepines can be lethal.

Chronic Adverse Effects

Almost no organ toxicity is associated with chronic administration of these drugs. From this standpoint they are safer than alcohol. Patients should receive prescriptions for sedatives with a clear plan and clear instructions. If prescribed for insomnia, benzodiazepines should be prescribed for short-term treatment (52). Otherwise, if patients use the medications on a regular basis, they will induce tolerance and increase the dosage. Such escalation of the dosage is especially common in those with histories of drug or alcohol abuse, particularly patients who are on methadone maintenance. After chronic use, an abstinence syndrome often occurs (Table 22.3).

Currently, the most commonly abused sedatives are alprazolam (Xanax), clonazepam (Clonopin), and diazepam (Valium). Escalating drug use may go undetected until confusion, irritability, slurred speech, or ataxia are recognized as signs of sedative intoxication. Physical examination may include ecchymoses from injuries sustained during an intoxicated state. Sedative-hypnotics can also produce anterograde amnesia. This is mostly dosage-related and has been most often described with triazolam (Halcion), midazolam (Versed), and diazepam (Valium). Physical dependence on benzodiazepines and the potential for major withdrawal symptoms may occur in as little as 2 months if dosages substantially above therapeutic levels are used. From a clinical point of view, most patients who abuse and have significant physical dependence on benzodiazepines abuse other drugs concurrently. It has been well established that withdrawal symptoms occur (8,36,51) in patients taking therapeutic dosages daily for 6 months or more. In the latter cases, the risk of withdrawal can be reduced by simply tapering the dosage. Although chronic use may create the risk of withdrawal symptoms, there is evidence that patients may use benzodiazepines on a chronic basis without developing tolerance to the anxiolytic effects of the medication (4,52).

Treatment

Nonbenzodiazepine sedative overdose is a life-threatening occurrence that should be treated in an emergency department. Because of physical dependence (detailed above), patients who use excessive dosages of sedative drugs are at risk of serious withdrawal reactions (including life-threatening seizures). Chapter 13 ("Anxiety") delineates guidelines for the withdrawal of benzodiazepines in the patient who has developed physical dependence. Outpatient treatment for therapeutic dependence can often be managed by tapering the prescribed benzodiazepine or switching to a benzodiazepine with a longer half-life and tapering it over several weeks (43). Onset time of withdrawal symptoms (Table 22.3) is inversely related to the half-life of the benzodiazepine of use. Inpatient treatment is often required for high-dose abuse and is best managed using phenobarbital, which has a long half-life (80 to 100 hours) and provides the pharmacokinetic umbrella to cover the patient for withdrawal symptoms (44).

Opioid (Narcotic) Analgesics

Opioids are commonly prescribed drugs and play an essential role in the care of patients. It has been widely observed that the fear of causing opioid addiction has led physicians to undermedicate in the management of acute pain (2). This is a common, legitimate criticism of physicians. Less commonly, there has been a tendency in treating patients with chronic pain to continue the use of opioid analgesics when the development of tolerance has rendered them less effective or even countertherapeutic. Patients who have been taking opioid analgesics for long periods may experience little pain relief and may, in fact, confuse incipient

withdrawal toward the end of a dosing interval with the onset of pain (34). An understanding of the tolerance induction, physical dependence, and addiction can ensure more rational prescribing patterns.

The opiate-dependent patient is not generally seen in office practice seeking treatment for drug dependence, although a review of medical histories given by patients entering methadone maintenance programs indicates that they often receive treatment for a range of other medical problems. Patients often appear in office practice settings attempting to obtain prescription drugs when they experience difficulty in obtaining heroin (diacetylmorphine). Morphine, hydromorphone (Dilaudid), and meperidine (Demerol) are the drugs most preferred by addicts, but they will readily use the whole range of less potent opioid and nonopioid analgesics if preferred drugs are unavailable. The term *opioid* refers both to drugs derived from opium (opiates) and to synthetic drugs with similar actions. If analgesics are difficult to obtain, opioid addicts temporarily use virtually any depressant drug. Alcohol, barbiturates, nonbarbiturate sedative-hypnotics, the benzodiazepines, and promethazine hydrochloride (Phenergan) are often abused by patients maintained on methadone because of their tendency to potentiate the effects of methadone.

Usual Effects and Therapeutic Use

Opiates are the prototype for managing pain in patients. To prevent abuse, they should be prescribed on a fixed schedule. For a comparison of the different opioids, see Chapter 19, Table 19.1.

Used for short intervals after an acute pain syndrome, opioids are safe and effective. Abuse liability increases with potency. Heroin, the most commonly abused illicit opioid, is usually injected intravenously but can also be injected subcutaneously (skin-popping), smoked, or sniffed (snorting). Heroin crosses the blood–brain barrier more effectively than other opioids. The effects after use consist of a brief and intense period of euphoria followed by several hours of a pleasant dreamy state in which the user may slowly nod as if falling asleep. Areas of pain feel numbed. The skin may itch (because of histamine release), which leads to characteristic scratching. Other effects include increased talkativeness (soapboxing) and sometimes increased activity and conjunctival suffusion (red eye). Stomach turning and vomiting (pleasant sick) occur. Physiologic effects include miosis and respiratory depression.

Acute Adverse Effects

Opioid overdose is characterized by depressed consciousness and respiration. Pulmonary edema, a common complication of opioid overdose, contributes to hypoxia and may cause death, even while the needle is still in the vein. Some opioids, such as propoxyphene (Darvon) and meperidine, cause convulsions at high dosages. The latter has a proconvulsive metabolite (normeperidine) that accumulates in patients with renal failure and often causes seizures.

Chronic Adverse Effects

The adverse effects of chronic heroin abuse result from use of dirty needles (see "Complications of Injecting Drugs," above), the adulterants mixed with the heroin, and the associated lifestyle (poor nutrition, lack of health care, and criminal activity) rather than from the drug itself. Heroin is usually mixed with milk sugar (lactose) and quinine under nonsterile conditions. Other more dangerous adulterants may also be included to mask the dilution of the heroin. Heroin nephropathy, a focal glomerulosclerosis, is predominantly reported in African Americans. Its precise cause is unclear, but it is thought to be related to an adulterant.

An analog of meperidine, 1-methyl-4-phenyl-1,2,5,6-tetrahydropyridine (MPTP), which is a commercially available compound, has been used intravenously by drug abusers as a form of synthetic heroin. Some MPTP users have developed a severe form of *parkinsonism*. Others who have not developed parkinsonism have evidence of nigrostriatal dopamine depletion.

Analgesic nephropathy is associated with combination products that include codeine, caffeine, aspirin, and phenacetin. Large dosages over many years are required to produce this complication. Reinforcing effects resulting in repeated dosing probably relate to the codeine and caffeine in the products.

Tolerance (defined above) to heroin develops quickly and can be demonstrated to some degree after only a few days of administration of the drug. The degree of tolerance and the consequent severity of withdrawal symptoms depend primarily on dosage levels and the frequency and duration of use. However, the severity of a patient's addiction to heroin is as much a function of psychologic and social factors as it is a simple consequence of tolerance or of withdrawal symptoms.

Opioid withdrawal is characterized by anxiety, nausea, yawning, diarrhea, sweating, rhinorrhea, dilated pupils, and piloerection (gooseflesh). In the advanced stages of withdrawal, the patient experiences vomiting and muscle spasms that often appear as jerky kicking movements of the legs. Although the untreated addict experiences significant anxiety and discomfort during withdrawal, the process itself presents no serious medical risks. Opioid addicts tend to confuse anxiety with the early symptoms of withdrawal, so the diagnosis of withdrawal should be made on the basis of observable signs rather than solely on subjective reports of anxiety and nausea.

Treatment

Opioid overdose must be treated in an emergency room. Emergency treatment requires cardiorespiratory monitoring and support. The opioid antagonist naloxone (Narcan) is safe and effective in countering the central nervous system (CNS) depression caused by opioid overdose, but may precipitate withdrawal. The initial dose is 0.4 mg intravenously. This may need to be repeated because naloxone has a shorter duration of action than most opioid agonists.

Any patient who has been abusing heroin or other opioids and is willing to accept help should be referred for treatment. Few addicts voluntarily seek treatment before being faced with the destructive consequences of their drug use.

Detoxification may be accomplished using clonidine hydrochloride in conjunction with other pharmacologic aids (dicyclomine for abdominal cramps and ibuprofen for bone pain) to provide symptomatic treatment of withdrawal symptoms. Clonidine is more effective in suppressing signs than in relieving symptoms of withdrawal (21). Clonidine is dosed at 0.1 mg every 6 hours for the first day, followed by 0.1 mg every 8 hours the second day, and 0.1 mg every 12 hours on the third day. Dosages are held for systolic blood pressure less than 100. Transdermal clonidine (TTS-2 patch) may be an effective adjunct in outpatient treatment. However, it has a delayed onset of action because it does not cross the dermis for at least 24 hours after placement. However, the patch lasts 7 days and assists in alleviating any protracted withdrawal symptoms. It can be prescribed only if blood pressure allows.

Detoxification may also be accomplished by *substituting methadone for the opioid previously used* by the patient and then gradually reducing the dosage over time, usually longer than a week. The initial dose should be sufficient to suppress withdrawal symptoms without causing sedation. Methadone detoxification is normally done on an ambulatory basis by specially licensed drug treatment programs. *Buprenorphine* (22) may be preferable to methadone because of superior safety and possibly a lesser physical dependence potential. It is illegal for a care provider to prescribe an opiate for the treatment of opiate withdrawal. As with detoxification from any substance, the patient should be engaged in a program of outpatient chemical dependency counseling during and after detoxification (see sections on detoxification and rehabilitation, below).

The efficacy of the treatment of opiate withdrawal in the primary care setting is not well studied, but success is likely to be low. In addition, clonidine has street value and has its own abuse potential. In the primary care setting, the clonidine patch is probably the safest modality to use for opiate withdrawal and ideally the patch should be placed in the office.

Inhalants: Solvent Abuse

The inhalation of solvents is a form of substance abuse that is most commonly found among children and adolescents. Because solvents are easily obtainable and inexpensive, they are likely to be preferred by people who lack the money or other resources needed to obtain more desirable drugs. A partial list of specific substances subject to this type of abuse includes gasoline, ignition spray, airplane glue, paint thinner, spray paint, lighter fluid, nail polish remover, cleaning fluid, and shoe polish. Toluene and other similar chemicals are the psychoactive substances. Inhalation is typically accomplished by saturating a rag with the substance and holding it directly over the face or placing it in a bag that is then placed over the nose and the mouth.

Usual Effects

The effects of solvents are immediate and of short duration, usually dissipating in a few hours or less (depending on the dosage). Acute intoxication is similar to alcohol intoxication except for the shorter duration.

Acute Adverse Effects

A hangover, with symptoms of headache and nausea, that is similar but perhaps milder than the hangover produced by alcohol has been observed. Some users experience apparent delirium characterized by tactile hallucinations, spatial distortions, and body image distortions. Sudden sniffing deaths have been described when inhalants were used during strenuous activity or under conditions in which blood oxygen is reduced. Such deaths apparently occur as a result of cardiac arrhythmias. Other deaths have been caused by suffocation when the user loses consciousness with the bag containing the solvent covering the nose and mouth.

Chronic Adverse Effects

The effects of solvents on the CNS, liver, kidneys, and bone marrow are not well understood. Cerebellar damage (which is partially reversible with abstinence) and peripheral neuropathy occur with long-term use. Numerous studies have demonstrated organ damage from long-term exposure to low concentrations of industrial solvents, but it is less clear to what extent these findings can be generalized to the short-term, high-concentration exposures experienced by inhalant abusers.

There is evidence that tolerance develops with chronic solvent abuse, but withdrawal symptoms and signs are uncommon, probably because the concentration of the substance in neurons is not sustained.

Treatment

Because the acute effects of solvents are usually of short duration, abusers rarely present for medical treatment. On rare occasions a patient may be brought in for treatment of a solvent-induced delirium. Chronic solvent abuse requires the same type of intense counseling and rehabilitative intervention indicated for other forms of self-destructive substance abuse (see below).

Cocaine and Other Stimulants

Cocaine, the amphetamines, methylphenidate, and phenmetrazine are the most commonly abused stimulant drugs. (Nicotine is discussed in Chapter 20.)

Cocaine is used in several forms. The route for cocaine intake depends on the form used. As the natural water-soluble powder, cocaine hydrochloride,

it is either sniffed (snorted) and absorbed through the nasal mucosa or injected intravenously. Forms of cocaine that can be smoked (using a water pipe or in cigarette form) are produced by extracting or freeing the cocaine alkaloid from the hydrochloride salt. When ether is used as the reagent in this process, the resulting product is referred to as freebase. When baking soda and water are used as reagents, the resulting product is crack, so named because of the crackling sound that is produced when the drug is smoked. Although they may differ in appearance and concentration, freebase and crack are pharmacologically the same.

Cocaine use appears in variable patterns. In the early stages, sessions of cocaine use typically last 2 to 4 hours, with intervals of days or weeks between sessions. Some users are able to maintain this pattern of use without progressing further. However, many users follow a pattern of rapidly escalating use in which both the length of sessions and the rate of consumption increase; users of freebase and crack may be more likely to succumb to this pattern than are users who snort cocaine powder.

Chronic abusers typically engage in runs, or periods of intensive cocaine use that can last anywhere from a few hours to several days. A run is terminated when the user runs out of cocaine or money or is too physically exhausted to continue. A run may be followed by a crash that lasts 1 or 2 days. During the crash, the user may experience some or all of the following: depression, hypersomnia, hyperphagia, fatigue, anxiety, irritability, and craving for cocaine.

Amphetamines are swallowed or injected intravenously. Two nonamphetamine stimulants, *methylphenidate* (Ritalin) and *phenmetrazine* (Preludin), which can mimic the effects of naturally occurring stimulants such as cocaine, are taken orally or intravenously.

Abusers of stimulants develop some tolerance to the euphoric effects of the drugs but may become more sensitive to other effects such as irritability, restlessness, hypervigilance, and paranoia. Users report that in any given session of cocaine use the duration and intensity of the euphoric effect seem to recede with successive doses, a phenomenon called chasing the dragon's tail.

Usual Effects and Therapeutic Use

CNS stimulants produce euphoria, increased confidence and energy, increased heart rate and blood pressure, dilated pupils, constriction of peripheral blood vessels, and increased body temperature. Effects are caused by sympathetic stimulation centrally and peripherally. Other acute effects include freezing (i.e., parkinsonian signs and symptoms). Aphonia and dysphonia are not uncommon. The duration and intensity of effect depend on the dosage and the route of administration. Single oral doses of amphetamines produce effects lasting 2 to 4 hours. The effects of cocaine, when sniffed, are rapid in onset but short in duration. Smoking freebase or crack produces an intense, short-duration effect (i.e., peak effect in 2 to 3 minutes, duration about 10 minutes) because smoking is an extremely efficient method of drug administration. Intravenous dosing produces similar (or greater) intensity and longer duration of effects.

Its capacity to produce euphoria gives cocaine a high abuse potential. In animals, cocaine produces certain reinforcing responses that exceed those of other drugs of abuse. The administration of cocaine in humans is associated with an increased desire for more cocaine (i.e., the presence of the drug itself in the body increases desire for cocaine). Users often delay entry into treatment until they are physically and emotionally exhausted or are faced with serious financial, legal, or medical problems.

Amphetamines, as stimulants, gained a resurgence as agents used in weight loss programs. *Phentermine* and *fenfluramine* in combination had been shown to be effective in causing weight loss. However, fenfluramine has since been removed from the market because of the discovery of its causing cardiac vascular damage (see Chapter 76, "Obesity").

Acute Adverse Effects

Very large doses of all of the stimulants may cause hyperpyrexia, arrhythmias, hypertension, and coronary and cerebral artery vasospasm, leading to myocardial infarction, stroke, convulsion, cardiovascular collapse, and death (50). Large doses of cocaine may also cause respiratory depression with a fatal outcome.

Chronic Adverse Effects

The chronic abuser of cocaine, amphetamines, and other long-acting stimulants is typically hyperactive, jittery, and irritable while using, and depressed, exhausted, or lethargic afterward. Often, previously stable people may develop unexplained financial problems or uncharacteristic overnight disappearances. With chronic heavy use there is usually a history of sleep disturbance and weight loss. The patient may be emotionally labile, and periods of irritability, depression, and fatigue may alternate with periods of elation and enthusiasm (mania). Physical examination may reveal needle marks; rhinitis; teeth worn from bruxism (grinding of teeth); ulcers on the lips, tongue, or nose; tremor; flushing; cardiac arrhythmias; and excessive sweating. Although cocaine may initially enhance sexual functioning, chronic use often interferes with sexual performance. Extremely heavy users may exhibit rapid, repetitious, and ritualistic body movements.

A *reversible organic delusional disorder* that resembles paranoid schizophrenia is occasionally seen. This syndrome may occur in normal subjects with no previous psychiatric history (16). Subjects who have taken higher dosages of a stimulant (e.g., 10 mg of dextroamphetamine every hour) have developed the disorder within 24 hours, as have high-dose cocaine (39) and methylphenidate (35) users. Cases of persistent psychotic disorders have been reported. Intravenous Ritalin abusers almost uniformly develop talc lung because talc is a filler in the Ritalin tablet.

Treatment

No data at present distinguish stimulant-abusing patients who should be hospitalized from those who may succeed as outpatients. Clearly, patients who present a risk of suicide should be hospitalized, as should patients who are unable to maintain abstinence long enough to begin a program of outpatient treatment. Although virtually all patients experience a moderate mood disturbance after a session of cocaine use, only a small percentage become suicidal. Only a minority of cocaine abusers use the drug on a daily basis for more than 1 or 2 days. In most cases, sessions of continuous cocaine use do not exceed 12 hours, and episodes of use are often separated by periods of abstinence lasting several days or more. Abstinence may occur because the user is unable to obtain more cocaine, is too exhausted to continue using, or is making an attempt to stop or control use. In many instances these periods of abstinence last several days or more, long enough for the patient to recover from the fatigue and hypophoria that normally follow use. Motivated patients with appropriate external supports can be engaged in outpatient treatment during such breaks in cocaine use. Treatment preferably involves daily counseling sessions during the first few weeks of abstinence. Necessary external supports include stable employment, a drug-free home environment, and active involvement in Narcotics Anonymous. For such patients, hospitalization should probably be considered only after an initial attempt at outpatient treatment has failed. No specific pharmacologic treatment is indicated for cocaine withdrawal because symptoms are mild. Currently, no drugs have been convincingly demonstrated to be efficacious in maintaining abstinence. A variety of drugs, including fluoxetine, desipramine, and ondansetron, have been studied for their effects in reducing the reinforcing responses to cocaine in humans (42). To date, none has become clinically useful.

Marijuana/Hashish

Marijuana consists of the dried leaves of the *Cannabis sativa* plant, which are usually smoked in pipes or cigarettes (joints). *Hashish* is a concentrated resin of cannabis and contains approximately 5 to 10 times the concentration of the principal psychoactive ingredient—9-tetrahydrocannabinol (THC)—as does *marijuana*. The discussion that follows applies to both marijuana and hashish. Cannabis can also be added to foods such as brownies, but when it is eaten, effects appear less rapidly and are less under control of the user.

Usual Effects and Therapeutic Use

The effects of marijuana from usual smoked doses last from 3 to 6 hours. The more common effects are elation, a high, an increased tendency to laughter and silliness, tachycardia, reddening of the eyes, and a later stage of relaxation. At higher dosages these effects are enhanced; the user may misjudge the effects of time, and perception of sound, color, and other sensations may be distorted or sharpened. Short-term memory and logical thinking are impaired, as is the ability to drive a car or perform other complex tasks (20,28). Additive effects occur with alcohol or other CNS depressants. Dosages three to five times higher than those producing relaxation and mild euphoria can result in effects similar to those of LSD and other hallucinogenic substances (depersonalization, auditory and visual hallucinations). Thus, some of the usual effects of marijuana that might be enjoyable to the experienced user can be frightening to the inexperienced user. The setting is also important in determining the effects of the drug. When smoked in a pleasant and familiar setting, marijuana is less likely to produce a negative response than when used in unfamiliar or threatening surroundings.

Cannabis has effects that are *potentially useful for therapeutic purposes* (e.g., decreased intraocular pressure, antiemetic properties). However, other currently approved drugs are of similar or superior efficacy for these indications and have fewer side effects. Accordingly, there are no strong pharmacologic indications for the introduction of cannabis as a therapeutic agent. The principal psychoactive substance in cannabis is marketed in oral preparations. Dronabinol (Marinol) is a schedule II drug in the United States and nabilone is available in Canada. Both are indicated for use as appetite stimulants.

Acute Adverse Effects

Considering the large number of regular users in the United States, it is clear that adverse reactions to marijuana requiring medical treatment are rare. The most common adverse response is an *acute anxiety reaction* that is similar to the panic attacks described in Chapter 13. It is different in that it includes paranoid ideation, and the usual effects of the drug in exaggerated form, which are not typically features of panic attacks. These reactions are most likely to occur in novice users or in users who unexpectedly receive a much larger than usual dose. Most reactions last only the few hours it takes for the effects of the drug to wear off. Some patients experience persistent anxiety for several days after the initial panic subsides. It has been estimated that three intense panic reactions occur per 100,000 exposures (33).

There have also been reports of *delirium* induced by marijuana. A dysphoric reaction characterized by disorientation, catatonialike immobility, acute panic, and heavy sedation has also been reported. These conditions tend to remit within 2 to 4 hours as the effects of the marijuana diminish.

Reports of *enduring psychotic reactions* after heavy marijuana use have appeared, largely in countries where marijuana is used at much higher dosages than in the United States. Reports of confirmed psychotic reactions to marijuana in this country are rare.

Chronic Adverse Effects

There is substantial evidence that marijuana at dosage levels associated with common social usage results in loss of energy and drive, impaired memory, and apathy. This is sometimes called the *amotivational syndrome.*

Smoking marijuana, even a few cigarettes daily for only a few weeks, adversely affects *pulmonary function* (46). Heavy cannabis users tend to be heavy tobacco smokers. The tar content of cannabis smoke is 50% higher than that of tobacco. Accordingly, users have chronic bronchitis and other respiratory diseases. It has also been reported that marijuana smoke contains 70% more carcinogens than does tobacco smoke (32). Although there is reason for concern, there are no data yet that demonstrate an association of neoplasia with marijuana. There have been conflicting findings concerning possible adverse effects of marijuana on the immune system. Some studies report changes in immunologic responsiveness, but the clinical implications of these changes are currently unknown. There is evidence that marijuana reduces testosterone levels in men, although the average level for users remains within normal limits (25).

Animal studies involving very high dosages of THC have yielded evidence of *teratogenicity.* There are no reports of a higher level of birth defects among children born to mothers who were regular users of marijuana during pregnancy. Several studies (11,12,18) suggest that more subtle effects, such as neurologic abnormalities and reductions in birth weight and height, may be associated with maternal use of marijuana.

Tolerance and Withdrawal. Regular use induces moderate tolerance. High dosages followed by sudden cessation produces a mild withdrawal syndrome in both animals and humans. In one study (33), volunteers who smoked an average of five marijuana cigarettes a day for 64 days exhibited restlessness, sleep disturbance, loss of appetite, and irritability when they stopped using marijuana. Because most social use is not regular and of high dosage, neither tolerance nor physical dependence is a major issue.

Treatment

Because they must be closely observed and may take several hours to recover, patients with *panic reactions* are best managed in a setting such as a drug abuse program, mental health center, or emergency department where continuing observation and supportive contact can be provided (45). Generally, these patients require simple reassurance and an explanation that they are experiencing a drug reaction that will dissipate as the drug is eliminated from their bodies.

Delusional or delirious patients should be seen in an emergency department because they present more complicated management problems and may require sedation or hospitalization. Furthermore, other causes of delirium should be ruled out. Restraints should be used only when absolutely necessary for the safety of the patient or others. Drugs should also not be used unless the patient is extremely agitated and difficult to control.

Treatment for chronic use should involve the support necessary for abstinence: a drug-free environment, active participation in 12-step meetings of Alcoholics Anonymous or Narcotics Anonymous, and in some circumstances group counseling.

Phencyclidine (PCP)

Phencyclidine is a *barbituratelike anesthetic* and derivative of ketamine. However, PCP exhibits selective action as an anesthetic, appearing to depress sensory tracts—including proprioception, pain, touch, and temperature—to a greater degree than it depresses cortical function. The resultant state of sensory deprivation and relative cortical wakefulness makes for a peculiar sense of detachment, disembodiment, and weightlessness (26). These sensations are intensely pleasurable for some, whereas for others they induce intense anxiety and even panic. PCP was developed as an anesthetic but was abandoned for this purpose when it was found to cause disturbing side effects. It continues to be used by veterinarians as an animal tranquilizer or immobilizing agent. Pure PCP is a white powder that dissolves in water. It is usually sprinkled on marijuana, dried parsley flakes, or other organic material and smoked. Less often, it is obtained in powder or tablet form and ingested or sniffed (snorting). Street names for the drug vary considerably from region to region, but it is most commonly known as angel dust, flakes, crystal, greens, hog, or sheets.

Usual Effects

The effects of PCP are dose related, although both intraindividual and interindividual responses vary. People who take PCP in the low dosages normally associated with street use may experience exhilaration, euphoria, inebriation, tranquilization, and perceptual disturbances. Some unpleasant effects commonly reported include disorientation, hallucinations, anxiety, paranoia, hyperexcitability, and irritability. At usual street dosages, most users reach peak intoxication in 5 to 30 minutes and remain high for 4 to 6 hours. It may take 24 hours or more before the user feels completely normal again.

Acute Adverse Effects

Even at low dosages, PCP is capable of occasionally causing severe reactions that may precipitate *extreme agitation and acts of violence* toward the user and to others. With higher dosages users are more likely to exhibit delirium, which may include hallucinations.

There is a difference between the delirium that is seen in acute PCP toxicity and what has been called *PCP psychosis,* a disorder closely resembling schizophrenia that develops after acute intoxication and persists for 24 hours or more. Such psychoses may develop out of the original intoxication or may occur days after the intoxication has cleared.

Ataxia, nystagmus, slurred speech, and ptosis are common features of acute PCP toxicity. Very high dosages of PCP, which are normally the result of oral ingestion rather than smoking, can result in coma, severe respiratory depression, seizures, and death.

Chronic Adverse Effects

Chronic use of PCP may produce persistent changes in personal habits (hygiene or dress), problems with memory or speech, sleep disturbances, mood changes (depression, irritability), paranoid or frankly delusional thinking, and unusual excitability or lethargy. Little is known about long-term physical effects.

Treatment

Consistent correlation has been found between the patient's initial level of consciousness and the time course of improvement. Patients with delirium clear in 3 to 8 hours, patients who remain stuporous or comatose for 1 to 4 hours clear in 5 to 62 hours, and patients whose stupor or coma lasts 6 or more hours clear in 75 to over 200 hours. Therefore, patients who are delirious at presentation can be treated in an emergency department and do not require hospitalization. Repeated mental status examinations should be performed to ensure that the patient is in a state of clear consciousness for at least 4 hours before discharge. Members of the family should be cautioned that the patient should stay in the company of family members or reliable friends for several days. Patients can have the onset of severe depression or a PCP psychosis for several days after the acute effects of the drug have subsided. Patients who remain comatose or stuporous for more than 2 hours or who develop a PCP psychosis require hospitalization. PCP abuse usually occurs in the setting of polysubstance abuse and long-term treatment should include traditional 12-step meetings.

Lysergic Acid Diethylamide (LSD)

Lysergic acid diethylamide is the prototype of a number of alkaloid substances of high potency that predictably cause *hallucinations.* Others include psilocybin, dimethyltryptamine (DMT), and mescaline. All are classified as hallucinogens and are CNS depressants at higher dosages. LSD (acid) is sold illicitly in the form of powder, tablets, or capsules. Sugar cubes, small squares of gelatin (window pane), or paper (blotter acid) that have been impregnated with the drug are also available. LSD is usually ingested orally and its effects appear within 30 to 40 minutes, reaching a peak at about 90 minutes, with physiologic effects gone by 6 hours but subjective effects persisting for 8 to 12 hours.

Usual Effects

LSD usually produces some combination of the following subjective effects: depersonalization, altered time perception, labile mood, perceptual distortions (usually visual), body image distortion, and feelings of increased insight. Physiologic effects include slight rises in blood pressure and heart rate, fever, lack of coordination, dilated pupils, increased salivation and lacrimation, hyperreflexia, and occasionally vomiting.

Acute Adverse Effects

Inexperienced users may have an *acute panic reaction* that occurs because the normal effects of the drug are unfamiliar or unexpected. In more severe reactions, users of LSD may experience *hallucinations* (usually visual) and *delusions* that may persist beyond the time when the drug is circulating in the blood.

Flashbacks, spontaneous recurrences of the original LSD experience, have been estimated to occur in 1 of every 20 users (from days to years later). They are more likely to occur in chronic users (and can occur following the use of any hallucinogenic drug, including marijuana). There have also been reports of *prolonged psychotic reactions* after the use of LSD, although these are rare.

Patients with acute LSD toxicity can be differentiated from those with PCP toxicity or schizophrenia in several ways. LSD causes dilation of the pupils, which is absent in PCP toxicity and schizophrenia. PCP toxicity usually is characterized by clouding of consciousness, and the patient often exhibits ataxia, nystagmus, and ptosis, which are not features of LSD toxicity or of schizophrenia.

Chronic Adverse Effects

Some degree of tolerance develops with repeated use of LSD, but no withdrawal syndrome has been observed.

Treatment

Adverse reactions to LSD usually remit in 8 to 24 hours, and hospitalization is usually unnecessary. However, the patient should be observed until symptoms clear. Referral to an emergency room or to a drug abuse program that can provide this type of support will usually be necessary. The same supportive measures described earlier for the treatment of adverse reactions to marijuana are appropriate. Extremely agitated patients should be given diazepam (Valium), 20 mg orally or intramuscularly, before being sent to a treatment center.

Anabolic Androgenic Steroids

These drugs are used to enhance athletic performance. They are derivatives of testosterone and promote growth of skeletal muscle and may increase lean body mass. Use is widespread but data are limited. One study demonstrated that 6.6% of male high school seniors had used anabolic steroids (6). A telephone survey in 1988 suggested that there were one million users in the United States (49). They are mostly used in cycles of weeks or months. Stacking (use of more than one preparation) and pyramiding (dosages gradually increased and then tapered) are common patterns of administration. Dosages used are much greater than those administered for therapeutic purposes.

Usual Effects and Therapeutic Use

Acute experimental administration of testosterone to people with histories of drug abuse reveals that testosterone at both therapeutic and supratherapeutic dosages cannot be distinguished from placebo under double-blind conditions. The same subjects can reliably detect and report euphoria from small dosages of morphine (10). Total body weight increases in less than a week, partly because of salt and water retention and also because of a true increase in lean body mass. No studies have shown an increase in strength in nonathletes. Some studies show an increase in strength in trained weight lifters.

Recent studies of anabolic androgenic steroids show them to be of therapeutic benefit in people with weight loss related to HIV infection. Both oxandrolone, an oral synthetic anabolic steroid, and testosterone are prescribed *for involuntary weight loss* and wasting related to medical illness. In these settings they are safe to prescribe, with low abuse potential.

Chronic Adverse Effects

Although it is not clear that there are any acute adverse effects, there clearly are chronic adverse effects if these drugs are taken in excess. These include decreases in sperm count and reversible decreases in size of testes, masculinization in women (e.g., hoarse voice and clitoral hypertrophy), premature fusion of epiphyses in adolescents, decreased glucose tolerance, an unfavorable lipid profile (increased low-density lipoprotein, decreased high-density lipoprotein), acne, alopecia, hirsuteness, peliosis hepatis, and complications of injecting drug use (see above). There is a tenuous link with malignancy and case reports of myocardial infarction and other vascular events. The best documented psychological effect is an increase in aggression. Some users apparently fulfill DSM-IV criteria for psychoactive substance abuse and dependence as defined at the beginning of this chapter (5). More systematic studies are needed. Users have lower rates of tobacco consumption and higher rates of alcohol consumption than the population at large.

Atropinic Drugs

Belladonna derivatives such as atropine (the alkaloid produced by deadly nightshade [*Atropa belladonna*] and also by jimsonweed [*Datura stramonium*]) and scopolamine are acetylcholine antagonists that at high dosages produce hallucinations, delirium, and varying states of excitement, insomnia, or amnesia. These effects may be followed by CNS depression and coma. The undesired pharmacologic effects of these drugs—dryness of the mouth, blurred vision, anhidrosis, and tachycardia—limit their appeal as psychoactive agents. Thus, the rare instances of abuse are mostly by teenagers experimenting with jimsonweed in rural areas or, in the past, by use of over-the-counter soporifics that contained scopolamine until it was banned by the FDA some years ago. Treatment of toxic overdose is a medical emergency requiring gastric lavage and ingestion of activated charcoal to limit intestinal absorption, maintenance of vital signs, administration of physostigmine, and lowering of body temperature.

Arecoline (Betel/Areca Nuts)

Arecoline is a *parasympathomimetic alkaloid somewhat similar in structure to nicotine.* It is used for its psychoactive effects by about a billion people, mostly in Southeast Asia and the Indian subcontinent. It is the world's fourth most popular psychoactive drug (after caffeine, alcohol, and nicotine). It is a cholinergic drug because it exerts effects similar to acetylcholine including sweating, salivation and increases in other body secretions, and increase in bladder tone, and can decrease elevated body temperature. At low dosages it produces general arousal and is usually classified as a stimulant (47). Effects are generally a mixture of arousal and depression according to dosage and individual responsiveness to cholinergic agents. The nuts have a bitter taste and produce reddened saliva and stained teeth, and chronic use commonly leads to grinding of the teeth and cancer of the oral cavity. They are usually chewed with lime to enhance absorption. Treatment of arecoline poisoning consists of administration of atropine and cardiorespiratory support.

PHARMACOLOGIC APPROACHES TO TREATMENT OF DRUG ABUSE

Detoxification

With the exception of opioid-addicted patients who enter methadone maintenance treatment, rehabilitation usually begins with detoxification. This is the process or set of procedures involved in readjusting the patient to a lower or absent tissue level of the substance of abuse. Where they are available, the specific pharmacologic approaches to detoxification have been described above under descriptions of individual drugs of abuse.

Detoxification is the first and easiest task for the recovering addict. Patients tend to attach too much significance to the task of physiological withdrawal and too little significance to the behavioral changes that are required to prevent relapse (see "Rehabilitation," below).

With proper support, many chemically dependent patients can be detoxified on an *outpatient* basis. Such patients should be seen on a daily basis throughout the detoxification and should be participating concurrently in an intensive program of counseling and education. Medications should be administered on a daily basis so that the patient has only the dosages needed between visits. Clearly many patients do not have the social support and accessibility to appropriate programs for this to occur. The other conditions needed for successful outpatient detoxification are described in detail in Chapter 21, "Alcoholism."

In general, *inpatient* detoxification is necessary when the patient is unable to discontinue use of illicit substances despite appropriate medication and psychologic support; the patient has concurrent medical problems that require hospitalization or significant medical problems that would be exacerbated by detoxification (e.g., symptomatic coronary artery disease); the patient has developed an extremely high tolerance and has a history of major withdrawal symptoms such as seizures and delirium tremens; the patient presents a clear risk of suicide or, because of chronic intoxication and impaired judgment, is a danger to self or others; and the patient is dependent on multiple drugs.

For most patients, it is not physical dependence that presents the major obstacle to recovery. Rather, it is the propensity to relapse, and the factors that influence this, that determine the success of the patient's efforts to become drug free.

Methadone Maintenance

Methadone maintenance is the most widely used chemotherapeutic approach to the treatment of opioid addiction. Methadone is *a long half-life opioid* that is taken orally in a single daily dose. Methadone is substituted for the opioid previously used by the patient, at a dosage that prevents withdrawal but causes less sedation or intoxication. The starting dose is usually 30 mg. The methadone dosage is gradually increased, thereby increasing the patient's tolerance for all opioids to a level where the user is less able to experience a significant effect, even from large dosages of illicit narcotics. Although this methadone blockade can be overridden by a sufficiently large dose of another narcotic, the payoff for doing so is small in relation to the cost. Patients taking methadone are partially tolerant to its euphoric–sedative effects and are thus able to function normally in home and work settings.

Numerous studies have shown methadone maintenance to be a cost-effective approach in treating opioid addiction (38). Meta-analyses of various clinical trials demonstrate that methadone in well-run clinics is superior to placebo with similar psychosocial supports (in terms of retention in treatment and reduction of heroin use). Nevertheless, a randomized, controlled trial of methadone versus nonmethadone treatment has not been conducted. Methadone maintenance produces substantial reductions in crime and increases economic productivity of patients in treatment. It has also taken on a new significance because of its potential for reducing the spread of AIDS.

Contingency management treatment has been most often applied to methadone maintenance programs. Attempts are made to change behavior by manipulating consequences. Rewards or punishments are provided as incentives for desirable behavior. For example, take-home privileges are linked to the provision of clean urine tests.

Although demonstrably cost-effective, methadone treatment has *several limitations.* As with other forms of chemical dependency treatment, there is a high turnover and rate of relapse. Patients are required to take methadone under observation at a clinic at least three times a week, and this requirement sometimes conflicts with work and family commitments. Although methadone is effective in suppressing the use of opioids, it has no such effect on alcohol or other drugs, and many methadone-maintained patients develop problems with other substances. Methadone-maintained patients become both physically and psychologically dependent on the drug, and many experience considerable difficulty in making the transition from methadone to abstinence. Some treatment professionals believe that opioid addicts have a biochemical abnormality that is corrected by methadone so that it may be necessary for them to remain on methadone for life. No scientific evidence supports this view at this time. However, it is likely that genetic studies will reveal a biological predisposition to opioid use, as has been demonstrated with alcohol and tobacco. Some patients who make appropriate changes in lifestyle and develop good social and emotional support systems are able to detoxify successfully from methadone.

Newer pharmacologic treatments have been introduced in the last few years. These include *L-acetylmethadone* (LAAM) and *buprenorphine*. LAAM has a longer half-life than methadone and can be given three times weekly, thus decreasing the need for take-home medication and decreasing the possibility of diversion. Buprenorphine, not yet approved for oral use in the United States, is a partial opioid agonist that has a superior safety profile to both methadone and LAAM (with significantly lower chance of respiratory depression). It is as effective as methadone in treating opiate addiction (22). It also may produce less physical dependence. It is therefore likely to become the drug of choice for maintenance opioid treatment.

Naltrexone

Naltrexone is an orally administered *opioid receptor antagonist* that is highly effective in blocking the effects of opioids. It is a long-acting drug that can effectively block the effects of opioids when administered three times a week. Because naltrexone causes an acute withdrawal reaction, candidates for naltrexone treatment must first be detoxified from the opioid to which they are addicted. Unlike methadone, which works by increasing the patient's tolerance for opioids, naltrexone competes with opioids at the receptor site. Another important difference is that naltrexone is not addicting, and patients can discontinue use without difficulty. The major disadvantage of naltrexone is that few patients are willing to use the drug and stay on it for an appropriate length of time. Its effectiveness is thus limited to highly motivated patients or patients who can be required to take the drug. Like methadone, naltrexone is not effective in blocking the use of other substances of abuse. A patch preparation of naltrexone is under development.

The pharmacologic equivalents of methadone and naltrexone have not been developed for other drugs such as cocaine.

REHABILITATION

All forms of drug abuse optimally require both acute and long-term intervention. Acute interventions (see above) include the management of overdose, toxicity, and withdrawal under medical supervision (if this is indicated). However, when the immediate physical consequences of drug abuse have been successfully treated, there remains a need to identify and treat, if possible, any underlying conditions that motivated drug misuse in the first place. Many drug abusers have significant problems of psychologic and social adjustment and may benefit from counseling and rehabilitation over extended periods. As described below, the general physician's major role in dealing with long-term rehabilitation is to motivate patients to cease drug abuse and to enter and continue in rehabilitation programs.

Effective rehabilitation programs stress the development of practical social and vocational skills, and the avoidance of social environments conducive to drug use. In recent years, there has been an increasing recognition that families may actually enable drug abuse by one or more members. Family therapy has been used successfully with opiate addicts (41) and appears to be the treatment of choice with drug-abusing teenagers who are still living with their parents.

Because many drug abusers have important deficits in education and vocational preparation, lack basic social and recreational skills, and are handicapped by problems of poor impulse control and low self-esteem, the process of rehabilitation often takes considerable time. Learning disabilities are also common among this population (37). As with alcoholism, relapse is common and recurrent treatment episodes are often required.

There is evidence that existing treatment modalities shorten the course of substance abuse disorders and reduce the amount of injury to both the individual and the community. There is evidence that treatment reduces the economic costs that result from drug abuse and that these cost reductions substantially exceed the actual cost of providing care (38). However, it must also be acknowledged that definitive treatment methods that result in lasting abstinence from drugs in a significant proportion of patients do not currently exist.

Principal Types of Rehabilitation Programs

Residential Treatment Programs

Two types of residential treatment programs are commonly encountered in the United States.

Therapeutic communities typically require patients to commit themselves to 6 months or more of treatment. Patients are subjected to an intense, aggressively confrontational form of group therapy that is intended to facilitate change by stripping away antisocial, drug-oriented beliefs and values and replacing them with socially adaptive beliefs and values. Therapeutic communities tend to have high dropout rates in the first few weeks of treatment because many patients are not willing to make the commitment required by this form of treatment. Patients who remain for the duration of treatment, however, often achieve an enduring drug-free adjustment.

A more common form of residential treatment is the *intermediate-term residential program*. These programs are typically 4 weeks in duration and were originally designed to treat alcoholism. Over the last two decades, they have evolved into chemical dependence programs that accept patients with a wide range of substance abuse problems. Intermediate-term residential programs use a more traditional group therapy approach that is less aggressive than the approach used by therapeutic communities. They also place a strong emphasis on education. In most facilities, patients attend lectures and films designed to increase their understanding of the disease of chemical dependency and the nature of the recovery process. Traditionally, intermediate-term residential programs have been viewed as the treatment of choice for chemical dependency, but in recent years they have come under pressure from a variety of groups concerned about the rising cost of health care benefits. Residential treatment is considerably more expensive than outpatient care, and comparisons of the two approaches for one form of drug abuse—alcoholism—show little difference in outcome for comparable patients (29). There are few data for other drugs of abuse. In response to the demand for more cost-effective treatment approaches, intermediate-term residential facilities now offer flexible lengths of stay rather than admitting all patients for the same 28- or 30-day program.

Intensive Outpatient Treatment Programs

Demands for more cost-effective forms of treatment have led to a greater emphasis on the use of outpatient approaches. Intensive outpatient programs offer a combination of education and group counseling similar to that found in the intermediate-term residential programs, but they provide treatment in the evenings so patients do not have to be absent from home or work. Intensive outpatient programs have patients attend treatment sessions four to six times a week and offer 12 to 20 hours of therapeutic activities each week for 4 to 6 weeks or longer. Traditional individual psychotherapy (rather than counseling) has not proved particularly effective in treating drug dependence.

Self-Help Groups

Self-help groups such as *Alcoholics Anonymous* (AA) and *Narcotics Anonymous* (NA) provide another valuable resource for people seeking help for a substance abuse problem. These 12-step programs provide a clearly defined sequence of steps that the addict must take to recover. They also provide immediate access to the emotional support and encouragement of others who have successfully coped with similar problems. AA and NA both maintain hotlines that are listed in the telephone directories of every major community in the United States and Canada. The NA process is identical to the process of AA, which is described in Chapter 21, Table 21.8. Most drug-free treatment programs incorporate the tenets of NA into their approach and encourage patients to get actively involved with a 12-step program.

Nar-anon provides support for members of the addict's family using 12 steps modeled on the 12 steps of Al-Anon (see Chapter 21, Table 21.12). Even if the patient refuses to accept treatment or try self-help groups, family members (who may be codependents) can be referred to Nar-anon. Codependents may experience a wide range of physical and emotional stresses as a result of another family member's addiction. Codependents often experience guilt, shame, loss of self-esteem, diminished self-confidence, and social isolation. They often believe that they are in some way to blame for the substance abuser's problems, a belief that is often fostered by the substance abuser, who is more than happy to shift responsibility to others. Codependents often engage in enabling behaviors— actions that are intended to help the substance abuser but only shield the substance abuser from the consequences of his or her behavior and therefore delay serious efforts at recovery. Codependents often resort to a variety of strategies intended to control or prevent access to drugs by the substance abuser. Such efforts are usually unsuccessful. Recovery usually occurs when the substance abuser feels the need for change and is willing to accept full responsibility for making change occur. Substance abusers who recover are motivated to change in large part by the unpleasant and painful consequences of their drug use. Nar-anon helps family members recognize and discontinue enabling behaviors and helps them cope with the physical and emotional stresses that result from living with a substance abuser.

Common Obstacles to Recovery

Many patients, particularly those in the early stages of addiction, have difficulty accepting the requirement of total abstinence. Although they might not admit it, many patients enter treatment with the unstated agenda of gaining control of their drug use rather than stopping it. They are reluctant to give up the pleasurable effects of drugs or they doubt their ability to cope with emotional distress without the relief afforded by drugs. They secretly hope to learn how to enjoy the benefits of drugs while avoiding the problems that have accompanied their drug use in the past. This is part of the process of denial. Other patients enter treatment believing that they have a problem with one type of drug but not with others. Cocaine addicts, for example, often think that they do not have a problem with alcohol or marijuana and see no reason to give up the use of those drugs. Experience has shown, however, that *continued use of nonproblem drugs tends to predispose patients to relapse with their problem drug.* Furthermore, patients who continue to use other drugs are less likely to make the changes in lifestyle that are important in maintaining recovery over the longer term.

One of the most important tasks for the patient in early recovery is to sever ties with drug users and to develop new relationships with nonusers or, at least, with nonabusers. The relationships with other abusers tend to be superficial and based mainly on the shared activity of getting high. In addition to forming new relationships, the recovering addict must learn to form a new type of relationship, one that involves a level of trust, honesty, and intimacy that may seem alien to some. Such relationships are fundamental to recovery because they are the primary source of support for the addict struggling with the physical and emotional demands of recovery. During their addiction, most addicts learn to use drugs as a quick and effective, though ultimately destructive, method of dealing with physical or emotional distress. In recovery, the addict must learn other strategies to cope with distress.

The active abuse of drugs during adolescence and early adulthood seems to interfere with the development of basic social skills. In addition, addicts are often hampered by diminished self-esteem and self-confidence and by the expectation that they will be rejected by society. Meeting people for the first time and attempting to initiate new relationships generate anxiety for most people under the best circumstances. When normal social anxiety is compounded by the social and emotional deficits that characterize most addicts in early recovery, the task of forming new relationships can become so intimidating that it may be avoided altogether. The recovering addict who feels lonely or isolated is tempted to resume contact with old friends who are still using drugs.

Another important lifestyle change has to do with the use of leisure time. Drug use is, among other things, a recreational activity. Getting and using drugs provides a daily routine that fills time and provides stimulation and challenge. For some addicts, the enjoyment of certain aspects of the drug-oriented lifestyle is as important as the reinforcing effects of drug use in maintaining drug involvement. For other users, being high makes it possible to tolerate what would otherwise be a tedious daily routine. It is important for the addict in early recovery to identify new activities that will provide a reasonable amount of stimulation and satisfaction. Boredom greatly increases the risk of relapse, and the recovering addict who fails to find employment that is in some way rewarding or to develop satisfying leisure activities is in danger of relapse.

Self-help groups (see above) are an invaluable resource for people in early recovery. In addition to providing emotional support and guidance, they are the best available forum for meeting nonusers and developing new friendships. They also sponsor social and recreational activities and provide opportunities for addicts in early recovery to learn new ways of managing leisure time from people who are further along in recovery.

In summary, recovery from chemical dependency requires a multitude of changes in beliefs, relationships, and lifestyle. Some of the required changes are difficult to accomplish, and the need for them is not immediately apparent to many addicts. In early episodes of treatment, most addicts make some of the needed changes but not enough to avoid relapse over the long term. As a result, *relapse rates* among patients successfully completing treatment run as high as 80% in the year after treatment. Of course, results highly depend on how the population is selected. Socially stable, higher socioeconomic groups have a better prognosis. With successive treatment episodes, however, one can hope to see a changing pattern in which periods of abstinence grow longer and periods of active drug use grow shorter. Perhaps it is best to view relapse as an indication that the patient has so far failed to make all of the necessary changes needed to support an enduring recovery. Instead of regarding relapse as an indication that the patient's case is hopeless, the patient's physician can encourage the patient to identify the reasons for the current relapse and to make changes that will help the patient avoid a recurrence. The approach should not be very different from that of other chronic diseases such as hypertension or diabetes, in which complete cure is uncommon.

Urine Testing

Urine testing to establish drug abuse seems a tempting and objective means of cutting through the problems of denial, unreliable histories, and the less than clear-cut signs and symptoms presented to arrive at a diagnosis. In the general physician's office, however, testing for drug abuse can prove problematic. The patient already knows whether he or she is abusing drugs. The question is whether the patient is willing to share that information with the family or physician.

The testing requires *informed voluntary consent* of any person 18 years of age or older, except in true emergencies. Faced with this requirement, laboratory testing yields no more information than the patient is willing to provide by history. Testing at the request of an employer or school authority, in particular, is fraught with ethical questions. Nevertheless, many employers now require drug testing (which is legal). This often provides evidence of illicit drug use that the patient is not willing to share.

There are problems of *sensitivity and specificity* in using urine screening tests to identify drug abusers. False negative results occur (because of deception in collection and insensitive testing), false positive results are reported (because of innocent confounding substances or doubts about the source of the specimen, the chain of command, and the normal frequency of testing error), and most significantly, problems of interpretation of results are seen. Experimental, social, and recreational use of illicit substances is so widely practiced that a positive test by no means establishes abuse or dependency. It also does not provide evidence of intoxication or impairment. Furthermore, prescribed drug use such as a benzodiazepine for anxiety or codeine for pain leads to positive urine tests. Codeine (like heroin) is detected as morphine in the urine.

The testing of minors under the age of 18, which theoretically can be authorized by parents and legal guardians regardless of the wishes of the patient, raises issues of patient trust, ethics, and legality if contested. Possible drug use can be explored most productively in the context of the total family relationship, without the referring physician appearing to have to take sides.

In most instances, testing (like ongoing therapy) should probably be performed by the consulting specialist or treatment program. Avoiding urine testing in the primary care setting also helps facilitate the doctor–patient relationship. It is hoped that people who relapse will be open and honest and will be more likely to show up for medical visits if they do not have to worry about urine testing.

THE GENERAL PHYSICIAN'S ROLE

Addressing Drug Abuse

Since the 1920s, with the exception of small numbers of psychiatrists and substance abuse specialists from other disciplines, physicians in the United States have been reluctant to become involved in problems of substance abuse and dependence. This is understandable because, beginning with the passage of the Harrison Narcotic Act in 1914, laws did not permit maintenance prescribing. From 1920 to 1940, some physicians, nurses, and pharmacists who persisted in regarding narcotic addiction as a medical problem and in prescribing or dispensing narcotics in violation of the Harrison Act were prosecuted and imprisoned. This campaign led to avoidance of the problems of addiction by physicians and other health care providers. Physicians are still reluctant to become involved in problems with addiction because of a lack of knowledge of how to deal with these patients, their own attitudes toward substance abuse, and the understandable response to the difficult behaviors these patients often exhibit.

In recent years, substance abuse (including alcohol and nicotine abuse) has been recognized as the major cause of much of the morbidity seen in medical practice (30)—usually a mix of physical, mental, and social consequences—and the responsibility of physicians to care for the patient with substance abuse has been emphasized. In light of the complexity of long-term rehabilitation of the patient with substance abuse, the major role of the physician is recognition of the problem, motivation of the patient to accept treatment, referral to a treatment program, ongoing care for the patient's other medical problems, and, importantly, continued motivation to remain in recovery from previous substance abuse.

Discovery of a substance abuse problem starts with a suspicion of the diagnosis if signs, symptoms, and elements of the history suggest the possibility, even in the most unlikely subjects. People from all walks of life abuse drugs. The stereotype of the drug abuser is of a young, antisocial male of unkempt appearance who uses drugs for their euphoric effect. Although this is often the case, the abuse of illicit drugs such as marijuana and cocaine also occurs commonly among middle- and upper-class Americans, and the misuse and abuse of prescription analgesics and anxiolytics by people who are in the mainstream of American society have been recognized for many years. Patients with chronic anxiety, insomnia, or pain are at risk of abusing medications used to treat those conditions. In some instances, escalated use (and sometimes abuse) develops not because the patient is primarily seeking drug-induced euphoria or intoxication but because the tolerance that develops during continued use leads the patient to increase the dosage to inappropriate levels. Elderly patients are at particular risk because they are more likely to be given medications. Changes in the pharmacokinetics of drugs secondary to the aging process also make the elderly more vulnerable to normally prescribed dosages (48) (see Chapter 6). Furthermore, they often have less recourse to nonpharmacologic alternatives in coping with pain, psychologic distress, or insomnia.

Advice on history taking includes the following: Do not use the label *addict,* ask questions about drug use in the context of general medical history, develop a nonjudgmental approach, use direct questions, learn to recognize qualified answers, be persistent and friendly, and do not discuss rationalizations. It is often helpful to obtain information from a family member or close friend, with the patient's consent.

Interviewing techniques helpful in screening for alcoholism and motivating the alcoholic to accept treatment are described in Chapter 21. Techniques such as the CAGE questionnaire, as shown in Figure 21.1, can be adapted to screen patients for the abuse of other drugs and substances. Another questionnaire, known as the *Drug Abuse Screening Test* (DAST) is shown in Table 22.4 (40). A score greater than 4 indicates a significant substance abuse problem. The diagnostic accuracy of this instrument has been established (13).

Prescribing Controlled Drugs

Prescription drug abuse can be best avoided by careful and thoughtful prescribing of medications. Office-based physicians prescribe large amounts of controlled drugs. A summary description of the various *schedules under the Controlled Substances Act* is shown in Table 22.5. Refills of schedule II drugs and more than five refills in 6 months for schedule III or IV drugs is a violation of federal law. When prescribing these drugs, it is important to realize that chronic pain, anxiety, and insomnia usually cannot be treated with controlled drugs on a long-term basis without inducing some tolerance and physiologic dependence.

Table 22.4. Drug Abuse Screening Test (DAST-20)

Name: _____   Date: _____

The following questions concern information about your potential involvement with drugs *not including alcoholic beverages* during the past 12 months. Carefully read each statement and decide if your answer is 'Yes' or 'No.' Then, circle the appropriate response beside the question.

In the statements 'drug abuse' refers to (1) the use of prescribed or over-the-counter drugs in excess of the directions and (2) any nonmedical use of drugs. The various classes of drugs may include: cannabis (e.g., marijuana, hash), solvents, tranquilizers (e.g., Valium), barbiturates, cocaine, stimulants (e.g., speed), hallucinogens (e.g., LSD), or narcotics (e.g., heroin). Remember that the questions *do not* include alcoholic beverages.

Please answer every question. If you have difficulty with a statement, then choose the response that is mostly right.

These questions refer to the past 12 months.

Circle Your Response

1. Have you used drugs other than those required for medical reasons?	Yes	No
2. Have you abused prescription drugs?	Yes	No
3. Do you abuse more than one drug at a time?	Yes	No
4. Can you get through the week without using drugs?	Yes	No
5. Are you always able to stop using drugs when you want to?	Yes	No
6. Have you had 'blackouts' or 'flashbacks' as a result of drug use?	Yes	No
7. Do you ever feel bad or guilty about your drug use?	Yes	No
8. Does your spouse (or parents) ever complain about your involvement with drugs?	Yes	No
9. Has drug abuse created problems between you and your spouse or your parents?	Yes	No
10. Have you lost friends because of your use of drugs?	Yes	No
11. Have you neglected your family because of your use of drugs?	Yes	No
12. Have you been in trouble at work because of drug abuse?	Yes	No
13. Have you lost a job because of drug abuse?	Yes	No
14. Have you gotten into fights when under the influence of drugs?	Yes	No
15. Have you engaged in illegal activities in order to obtain drugs?	Yes	No
16. Have you been arrested for possession of illegal drugs?	Yes	No
17. Have you ever experienced withdrawal symptoms (felt sick) when you stopped taking drugs?	Yes	No
18. Have you had medical problems as a result of your drug use (e.g., memory loss, hepatitis, convulsions, bleeding, etc.)?	Yes	No
19. Have you gone to anyone for help for a drug problem?	Yes	No
20. Have you been involved in a treatment program specifically related to drug use?	Yes	No

Practitioners must be vigilant to avoid being "duped," acquiescing to patient demands by prescribing inappropriately. To avoid possible abuse, medications with abuse liability should be prescribed on a fixed schedule. This strategy improves control of symptoms, minimizes the development of symptoms (rather than reacting to symptoms after they occur), and avoids patient focus on immediate relief. Medications should be prescribed for short periods during treatment of acute problems. Patients should be seen for reassessment at frequent intervals and telephone refills should be avoided.

There is a definite risk of *theft of prescription blanks* or *alteration of a prescription.* All prescription pads should be safeguarded and, ideally, marked "not for scheduled drugs." Prescription blanks for scheduled drugs should be kept locked separately. Prescriptions should be written clearly, and the number of pills to be dispensed and the number of refills should be written out (not just a number). If no refills are to be given, "no refill" should be noted. All prescribing of scheduled drugs should be documented clearly in the chart.

Practitioners should be suspicious of patients who lose prescriptions or medications; obtain prescriptions from multiple practitioners; run out of medication before the time that would be expected; demand one specific drug as the only one that will work; have a sudden deterioration in work, school, or relationships; have a history of substance abuse; have a history of violent behavior; and have slurred speech or unexplained cognitive impairment. Prescribing practices that may be illegal, dangerous, or inappropriate, or indicate drug abuse, are listed in Table 22.6.

Two classes of controlled drugs, *benzodiazepines and narcotics,* are the most commonly abused prescription drugs (19). Long-term use of these drugs is sometimes appropriate (see Chapter 13, "Anxiety," and "Chronic Pain Management," below). However, intermittent use is required to avoid physical dependence. Nonpharmacologic modalities should always be used to increase the interval between doses, decrease the required dosage, and permit intermittent use of these drugs if possible.

Nonscheduled drugs with abuse liability include muscle relaxants, clonidine, and antiemetics. Clonidine, prescribed for hypertension, commonly finds its way onto the streets, where it is sold to opiate addicts to alleviate opiate withdrawal. Muscle relaxants are abused commonly as sleeping pills.

Chronic Pain Management

Chronic pain of nonmalignant origin is not a single entity. It has a variety of causes and contributing factors. It may fit best the syndromal formulation of somatoform pain (see details in Chapter 12). Treatment may vary from behavioral and physical therapy approaches to medications, including opioids. Pain is

Table 22.5.   Controlled Substances Act

The Controlled Substances Act (Title II of the Federal Comprehensive Drug Abuse Prevention and Control Act of 1970) is designed to improve regulation of the manufacturing, distribution, and dispensing of controlled substances by providing a "closed" system for legitimate handlers of these drugs. If not specifically exempted, every person who manufactures, distributes, *prescribes,* administers, or dispenses any controlled substance must register annually with the Attorney General. Accurate records of drugs purchased, distributed, and dispensed must be maintained and kept on file for two years by all persons who regularly dispense and charge for controlled substances in the course of their practice.

Each drug or substance subject to control is assigned to one of five schedules depending upon the potential for abuse, medical usefulness, and degree of dependence if abused. The five schedules and the drugs included in them follow:

Schedule I: Drugs and other substances having a high potential for abuse and no current accepted medical usefulness. Included are certain opium derivatives (e.g., *heroin*), some synthetic opioids (e.g., α-methylfentanyl), and hallucinogens (e.g., LSD).

Schedule II: Drugs having a high potential for abuse and accepted medical usefulness; abuse leads to severe psychologic or physical dependence. In general, drugs in this schedule were previously controlled under the Narcotic Acts (e.g., opium and derivatives, other *opioids, cocaine*). Stimulants, such as amphetamine and related compounds, and the short-acting *barbiturates* also are in this schedule.

Schedule III: Drugs having less abuse potential and accepted medical usefulness; abuse leads to moderate dependence. Included in this schedule are certain stimulants and depressants (e.g., barbiturates not included in other schedules), as well as preparations containing *limited quantities of certain opioid drugs.*

Schedule IV: Drugs having a low abuse potential, accepted medical usefulness, and limited dependence. Included in this schedule are certain depressants not in another schedule (e.g., chloral hydrate, phenobarbital, the *benzodiazepines*).

Schedule V: Drugs, including a few *over-the-counter preparations,* having a low abuse potential, accepted medical usefulness, and limited dependence. Mixtures containing limited quantities of opioids with nonopioid drugs are included in this schedule.

From Drug evaluations. 6th ed. Chicago: American Medical Association, 1986.

one of the most common reasons patients consult a physician, yet it is often inadequately treated. There is much controversy over the long-term use of opioids for nonmalignant pain. Opioids can clearly be of benefit in some patients with chronic pain who have not responded to other pharmacologic therapies, including nonsteroidal anti-inflammatory drugs (NSAIDs), and have no history of substance abuse. Success or benefit should be measured by improvement in quality of life, as measured by greater ability to perform activities of daily life. Side effects such as respiratory depression and sedation tend to be rare in patients with chronic pain and should not prevent the proper prescribing of opioids.

Evaluation of a patient with chronic pain should include the following: a pain history with specific details of the impact of pain on the patient; using a 10-point pain scale (1 = minimal pain and 10 = severe pain), an assessment of pain in a typical day (worst score, best score, average score, and response of pain score to pharmacologic and nonpharmacologic interventions); a directed physical examination; a review of previous diagnostic studies; a review of previous interventions; an alcohol and drug history; and an assess-

ment of coexisting diseases or conditions. Treatment should be based on the findings in this evaluation and the presenting cause of pain.

Nonpharmacologic therapies, including acupuncture, acupressure, exercise, hydrotherapy, biofeedback, relaxation techniques, massage, and physical therapy, should all be considered and prescribed, if appropriate, as adjuncts to the management of chronic pain. They provide an opportunity for patients to be active in their approach to overcoming chronic pain. Psychosocial stress and mood have an impact on pain perception and the ability to cope with pain. Patients should not lose their "identity" to their diagnosis of chronic pain, and these nonpharmacologic modalities often contribute to a better sense of well-being.

The relationship between pain and depression is complex because many patients with depression have a history of chronic pain and vice versa. Depression does lower pain tolerance and increase analgesic requirements. There have been a variety of trials using tricyclic antidepressants as adjuncts for pain control. In addition, when given at bedtime, they enable sleep, which may have a positive impact on pain during the day. Pain improvement may occur at lower than therapeutic blood levels. Nortriptyline at a dosage of 10 or 25 mg at bedtime is a usual starting point, with gradual increase of dosage depending on effect. Other antidepressants have also been found to be useful as pain management adjuncts, with paroxetine (Paxil) deserving particular mention. Details regarding antidepressants are found in Chapter 15.

Other drugs to be considered as adjuncts for pain management following a trial of nortriptyline or paroxetine include the *anticonvulsants* phenytoin and carbamazepine and the *topical analgesic cream capsaicin.* The anticonvulsants are particularly effective for chronic pain of neuropathic origin. They are dosed

Table 22.6.   Generally Inappropriate Prescribing Practices

Combinations of scheduled drugs
Two prescriptions for the same scheduled drug filled on the same or consecutive days
Prescriptions for lethal dosages over a few days
Continuous prescription of scheduled drugs for long durations (some exceptions)
Regular prescriptions of "preferred" drugs of abuse (e.g., Desoxyn, Dilaudid, Demerol, Dexedrine, Preludin)
A crescendo prescribing pattern of progression to multiple scheduled drugs
Prescribing for two or more members of a family the same drug or combination of scheduled drugs
Prescriptions that contain refills for schedule II drugs
Writing for more than five refills in 6 months for schedule III or IV drugs
Two scheduled drugs for the same purpose
Regularity and sheer volume of prescriptions for scheduled drugs
Prescribing scheduled drugs to known drug abusers
Prescribing scheduled drugs to family members
Prescription of scheduled drugs from two or more practitioners simultaneously
Prescriptions that lead to purchases of scheduled drugs far exceeding dispensing records

Adapted from Hollister AS. Patterns of scheduled drug prescribing abuse by Tennessee physicians. Subst Abuse 11:69, 1990.

at the usual anticonvulsant dosages and require blood monitoring (see Chapter 80). Side effects often limit their usage. Capsaicin, a topical substance P inhibitor, is available without prescription and is often useful as an adjunct for treatment of postherpetic neuralgia, arthritis, diabetic neuropathy, and reflex sympathetic dystrophy.

If a *trial of opioids* is deemed appropriate, the provider should ensure that the patient is informed of the risks and benefits of opioid use. Most patients should have already been tried on a course of NSAIDs. The provider may choose to continue an NSAID while initiating opioid therapy. Specific conditions under which opioids will be prescribed should be agreed upon (i.e., strict adherence with directions, no telephone refills, and patient responsibility for the prescription and all pills). Only one provider should be responsible for all prescriptions related to chronic pain. A written agreement specifying these conditions may be useful. See additional pointers above ("Prescribing Controlled Drugs").

In general, *long-acting opioids* should be used for chronic pain because they reduce the need for frequent dosing, have reduced abuse liability, and alleviate pain while preventing the re-emergence of pain. Both morphine and oxycodone are available as long-acting, twice-a-day preparations for the treatment of pain. Fentanyl is available in patch formulation that lasts for 3 days. The fentanyl patch should be prescribed only to patients who are already opioid experienced. Details regarding opioid analgesics are found in Table 19.1.

Review of treatment efficacy should be an ongoing process. Patients should keep a pain diary with a record of daily activity and pain scores during a typical day. Monthly follow-up visits should include a review of the pain diary, an assessment of functional status, efficacy of analgesia, drug side effects, quality of life, and any sign of medication misuse. All of this information should be documented in the patient chart on each visit.

General References*

Aronoff GM, ed. Evaluation and treatment of chronic pain. Baltimore: Williams & Wilkins, 1992.
> An in-depth guide to providing care to patients with chronic pain.

Benzodiazepine dependence, toxicity and abuse. A Task Force Report of the American Psychiatric Association. Washington, DC: American Psychiatric Association, 1990.

Brecher EM, ed. Licit and illicit drugs. Boston: Little, Brown, 1972.
> Although dated, still an excellent overview of the history of drug abuse in the United States.

Gawin FH, Ellinwood EH Jr. Cocaine and other stimulants. N Engl J Med 318(18):1173, 1988.
> Review covering epidemiology, pathophysiology, and treatment for the stimulants discussed in this chapter.

---

*Bold print (general references) and bold numerals (specific references) denote published controlled clinical trials, meta-analyses, or consensus-based recommendations.

Gold MS, Slaby AE, eds. Dual diagnosis in substance abuse. New York: Marcel Dekker, 1991.
> Recent review of psychiatric disorders and substance abuse.

Hollister LE. Health aspects of cannabis. Pharmacol Rev 38:1, 1986.
> Excellent review of cannabis.

Levine DP, Sobel JD, eds. Infections in intravenous drug abusers. New York: Oxford University Press, 1991.
> A comprehensive review of infectious diseases in drug abusers.

Marlatt AG, Gordon JR, eds. Relapse prevention. New York: Guilford Press, 1985.
> An excellent review of literature on relapse and relapse prevention.

McLellan AT, Luborsky L, O'Brien CP, et al. Is treatment for substance abuse effective? JAMA 247(10):1423, 1982.
> Evidence from multiple programs that current rehabilitation approaches are effective.

Mendelson JH, Mello NK. Management of cocaine abuse and dependence. N Engl J Med 334:965, 1996.

Sullivan JT, Sellers EM. Treating alcohol, barbiturate and benzodiazepine withdrawal. Ration Drug Ther 20:1, 1986.
> Covers pharmacologic treatment of CNS depressant withdrawal.

US Department of Health and Human Services. Drug abuse and drug abuse research. The Third Triennial Report to Congress. Rockville, MD: DHHS, 1991.
> A summary of recent advances in the epidemiology, health implications, prevention, and treatment of drug abuse in the United States.

Specific References

1. American Psychiatric Association. Diagnostic and statistical manual of mental disorders. 4th ed. (DSM-IV). Washington, DC: American Psychiatric Association, 1994.
2. Angell M. The quality of mercy. N Engl J Med 306:98, 1982.
3. Ball JC, Nurco DN. Criminality during the life course of heroin addiction. In: Problems of drug dependence 1983. Rockville, MD: Department of Health and Human Services, 1984.
4. Benzodiazepine dependence, toxicity, and abuse. The Task Force Report of the American Psychiatric Association. Washington, DC: American Psychiatric Association, 1990.
5. Brower KJ, Blow FC, Young JP, Hill EM. Symptoms and correlates of anabolic-androgenic steroid dependence. Br J Addict 86:759, 1991.
6. Buckley WE, Yesalis CE, Friedl KE, Anderson WA. Estimated prevalence of anabolic steroid use among male high school seniors. JAMA 26:3441, 1988.
7. DesJarlais DC, Friedman SR. AIDS prevention programs for injecting drug users. In: Wormser GP, ed. AIDS and other manifestations of HIV infection. New York: Raven Press, 1992.
8. Dysken MW, Chan CH. Diazepam withdrawal psychosis: a case report. Am J Psychiatry 134:573, 1977.
9. Fingerhood MI, Jasinski DR, Sullivan JT. Prevalence of hepatitis C in a chemical dependence population. Arch Intern Med 153:2025, 1993.
10. Fingerhood MI, Sullivan JT, Testa MP, Jasinski DR. Abuse liability of testosterone. J Psychopharmacol 11:59, 1997.
11. Finnegan LP. Pulmonary problems encountered by the infant of the drug-dependent mother. Clin Chest Med 1:311, 1980.
12. Fried PA. Marijuana use by pregnant women: neurobehavioral effects in neonates. Drug Alcohol Depend 6:415, 1980.
13. Gavin D, Ross H, Skinner H. Diagnostic accuracy of the drug abuse screening test. Br J Addict 84:301, 1989.
14. Golden A, Sullivan JT, Kwiterovich P, Jasinski DR. Patterns of drug abuse among adolescents presenting for detoxification. Abstract presented at AMERSA National Conference, 1990.
15. Gostin LO, Lazzarini Z, Jones S, Flaherty K. Prevention of HIV/AIDS and other blood-borne diseases among injection drug users. A national survey on the regulation of syringes and needles. JAMA 277:53, 1997.
16. Griffith JD, Cavanaugh JH, Oates JA. Psychosis induced by the administration of d-amphetamine to human volunteers. In: Efron DH, ed. Psychotomimetic drugs. New York: Raven, 1970.

17. Hasan SB, Albu E, Gerst PH. Infectious complications in IV drug abusers. Infect Surg 52:398, 1988.

18. Hingson R, Alpert JJ, Day N, et al. Effects of maternal drinking and marijuana use on fetal growth and development. J Pediatr 70:539, 1982.

19. Hollister AS. Patterns of scheduled drug prescribing abuse by Tennessee physicians. Subst Abuse 11:69, 1990.

20. Hollister LE. Health aspects of cannabis. Pharmacol Rev 38:1, 1986.

21. Jasinski DR, Johnson RE, Kocher TR. Clonidine in morphine withdrawal: differential effects on signs and symptoms. Arch Gen Psychiatry 42:1063, 1985.

22. Johnson RE, Jaffe JH, Fudala PJ. A controlled trial of buprenorphine treatment for opioid dependence. JAMA 267:2750, 1992.

23. Johnston LD, O'Malley PM, Bachman JG. Drug use, drinking, and smoking: national survey results from high school, college, and young adults populations. Rockville, MD: United States Department of Health and Human Services, Public Health Service, Alcohol, Drug Abuse, and Mental Health Administration, 1992.

24. Khabbaz RF, Onorato IM, Cannon RO, et al. Seroprevalence of HTLV-I and HTLV-II among intravenous drug users and persons in clinics for sexually transmitted diseases. N Engl J Med 326:375, 1992.

25. Kolodny RC, Lessin PJ, Toro G, et al. Depression of plasma testosterone with acute marijuana administration. In: Braude MC, Szara S, eds. Pharmacology of marijuana. New York: Raven, 1976.

26. Luisada PV. Phencyclidine. In: Lowinson JH, Ruiz P, eds. Substance abuse: clinical problems and perspectives. Baltimore: Williams & Wilkins, 1981.

27. Machnick MG, Horchang HL, Peteman RR. Liver disease associated with intravenous drug abuse. In: Levine DP, Sobel JD, eds. Infections in intravenous drug abusers. New York: Oxford University Press, 1991.

28. Melges FT, Tinklenberg JR, Hollister LE, Gillespie HK. Temporal disintegration and depersonalization during marijuana intoxication. Arch Gen Psychiatry 23:204, 1970.

29. Miller WR, Hester RK. Inpatient alcoholism treatment: who benefits? Am Psychol 41:794, 1986.

30. Moore RD, Bone LR, Geller G, et al. Prevalence, detection, and treatment of alcoholism in hospitalized patients. JAMA 261:403, 1989.

31. National Institute on Drug Abuse. Statistical series G, trend data through January-June 1992. Washington, DC: US Government Printing Office, 1992.

32. Novotny M, Lee ML, Bartle KD. A possible chemical basis for the higher mutagenicity of marijuana smoke as compared to tobacco smoke. Experientia 32:280, 1976.

33. Nowlan R, Cohen S. Tolerance to marijuana: heart rate and subjective high. Clin Pharmacol Ther 22:550, 1977.

34. O'Brien CP, Weisbrot MM. Behavioral and psychological components of pain management. In: Brown RM, Pinkert TM, Ludford JP, eds. Contemporary research in pain and analgesia. Washington, DC: US Government Printing Office, 1983.

35. Parran TV, Jasinski DR. Intravenous Ritalin abuse: prescription drug abuse. Arch Intern Med 151:781, 1990.

36. Pevnick JS, Jasinski DR, Haertzen CA. Abrupt withdrawal from therapeutically administered diazepam. Arch Gen Psychiatry 35:995, 1978.

37. Rhodes SS, Jasinski DR. Learning disabilities in alcohol dependent adults: a preliminary study. J Learn Disabil 25:551, 1990.

38. Rufener BL, Rachal JV, Cruze AM. Management effectiveness measures for NIDA drug abuse treatment programs. Vol. 1, Rockville, MD: US Department of Health, Education and Welfare, 1984.

39. Schuckit MA, ed. Drug and alcohol abuse. New York: Plenum, 1989.

40. Skinner HA. The drug abuse screening test. Addict Behav 7:363, 1982.

41. Stanton MD, Todd TC. The family therapy of drug abuse and addiction. New York: Guilford, 1982.

42. Sullivan JT, Jasinski DR, Preston KL, et al. Cocaine blocking effects of ondansetron. Proceedings of the 53rd annual scientific meeting, The Committee on Problems of Drug Dependence, NIDA Res Monogr 119:466, 1992.

43. Sullivan JT, Sellers EM. Detoxification for triazolam physical dependence. J Clin Psychopharmacol 12:124, 1992.

44. Sullivan JT, Sellers EM. Treating alcohol, barbiturate and benzodiazepine withdrawal. Ration Drug Ther 20:1, 1986.

45. Talbott JA. Emergency management of marijuana psychosis. In: Bourne PC, ed. Acute drug abuse emergencies. New York: Academic Press, 1976.

46. Tashkin DP, Shapiro BJ, Lee YE, Harper CE. Subacute effects of heavy marijuana smoking on pulmonary function in healthy men. N Engl J Med 294:125, 1976.

47. Taylor P. Cholinergic agonists. In: Goodman-Gilman A, Rall TW, Nies AS, Taylor P, eds. The pharmacologic basis of therapeutics. New York: Pergamon, 1990.

48. Thompson TL, Moran ML, Nies AS. Psychotropic drug use in the elderly. N Engl J Med 308:134, 1983.

49. US Olympic Committee. Sportsmediscope 1:7, 1988.

50. Wetli CV, Wright RK. Death caused by recreational cocaine use. JAMA 241:2519, 1979.

51. Winokur A, Rickels K, Greenblatt DJ, et al. Withdrawal reaction from long-term, low-dosage administration of diazepam. Arch Gen Psychiatry 35:101, 1980.

52. Woods JH, Katz JL, Winger G. Use and abuse of benzodiazepines: issues relevant to prescribing. JAMA 260:3476, 1988.

SECTION

3

Allergy and Infectious Diseases

C H A P T E R   23

Allergy and Related Conditions

MARTIN D. VALENTINE, MD

Allergy is a state of increased immunologic reactivity resulting from the synthesis of immunoglobulin E (IgE) antibodies after exposure to foreign immunogenic protein. Subsequent allergen–IgE antibody interaction stimulates release of chemical mediators that cause the symptoms of allergy. Although allergic symptoms are undesirable, the allergen–antibody–mediator sequence may have originally evolved as a host defense mechanism.

Many Americans have acute and chronic conditions generally considered to be allergic in origin. Approximately 9% of all office visits to physicians are for one of these conditions (5). Most visits are for conditions that are known to be mediated by antibodies of the IgE class or for conditions that resemble IgE-mediated allergy. Because the symptoms in these patients result from the release or formation of a limited number of chemical mediators, effective pharmacologic treatment may be similar whether or not allergy in the true sense is involved.

It is believed that the ability to synthesize large amounts of IgE with specificity for certain antigens may be inherited. The risk of developing an allergy for a child if one parent is allergic is one chance in three, increasing to two in three if both parents are allergic.

This chapter is concerned with IgE-mediated allergy and similar conditions (with the exception of asthma, which is discussed in Chapter 55). Other immunopathologic conditions that are not IgE mediated (drug-induced hepatitis, autoimmune hemolytic anemia, contact dermatitis) are discussed elsewhere in this book.

PATHOPHYSIOLOGY

Antibody

Acute allergic reactions are mediated by IgE antibodies. Never present in large amounts, IgE concentration in serum is greatest between puberty and young adulthood. As indicated in Figure 23.1, IgE binds to surface receptors on tissue mast cells and blood basophils. The release of histamine and other chemical mediators from these cells is initiated by the bridging of a pair of IgE molecules on cell surface receptors by an antigen molecule of appropriate specificity.

Allergens

Allergens that have clinical relevance are usually proteins with a molecular weight between 10,000 and 40,000 Da. Low-molecular-weight substances such as penicillin can be allergenic if they can combine as haptens with host proteins.

Mediators

The release or formation of biologically significant chemical mediators is a prerequisite to the development of allergic symptoms. In general, mediators initiate smooth muscle contraction, and alter vascular tone and permeability. *Histamine,* released from mast cells and basophils, causes pruritus, flushing, nasal stuffiness, conjunctival injection, bronchoconstriction, uterine contraction, increased permeability of venules, and hypotension. *Anaphylatoxin,* a substance formed during complement activation, induces histamine release. *Cytokines* (interferons, interleukins, growth and various other factors that modulate cell growth and secretory processes) also play roles in the clinical expression of allergies. *Bradykinin* and similar polypeptides with potent vasodepressor activity may be responsible in part for the shock of anaphylaxis. *Leukotriene* D_4 (LTD_4) is a 5-lipoxygenase metabolite of arachidonic acid with bronchoconstrictor and vasodilator activity. It and *prostaglandin* D_2 (PGD_2) have been found in the nasal secretions of patients with allergic rhinitis challenged intranasally with allergen.

PHYSIOLOGIC BASIS FOR TREATMENT

Pharmacologic

Drugs can favorably influence the outcome of an allergic condition by acting at various sites in the sequence of the allergic reaction (Table 23.1). Although no drug prevents antigen–antibody interaction, disodium cromoglycate (Cromolyn, Intal), nedocromil

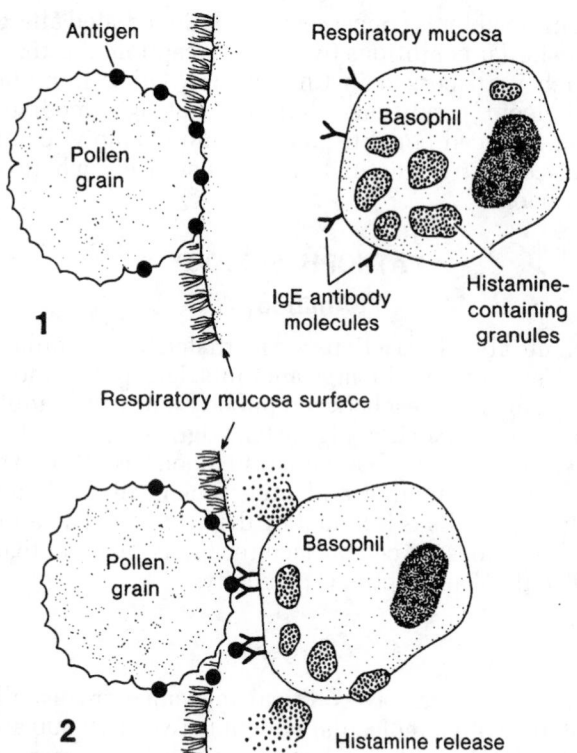

Figure 23.1. Steps in the IgE-mediated response of respiratory mucosa to pollen antigen. *Step 1,* pollen grains containing antigen reach nasal mucosa containing mast cells and basophils with IgE antibodies to antigen. *Step 2,* antigen bridges adjacent IgE molecules, initiating histamine release.

(Tilade), and ketotifen (Zaditen) prevent mediator release after this interaction has occurred. Zileuton (Zyflo) inhibits 5-lipoxygenase, montelukast (Singulair), and zafirlukast (Accolate) blocks LTD_4 receptors. The formation or release of some mediators is modulated by variation in cellular and tissue levels of cyclic adenosine monophosphate (cAMP), which acts as a second messenger for certain energy-requiring metabolic steps. β-Adrenergic agonists appear to inhibit mediator release and relax bronchial smooth muscle by increasing cAMP. The methylxanthines, such as theophylline, produce similar effects by preventing enzymatic breakdown of cAMP. Conventional (H_1) antihistamines inhibit histamine effects by competing with histamine for H_1 receptor sites. The usefulness of antihistamines is limited by their inability to compete successfully with high tissue concentrations of histamine adjacent to its cellular sites of origin, and also because nearly all antihistamines are central nervous system (CNS) depressants. Corticosteroids have antiinflammatory and topical vasoconstrictor effects and inhibit histamine release from basophils but not from mast cells.

Immunologic

Immunization of humans with extracts of pollens has been shown to result in the appearance in serum of blocking antibody (immunoglobulin G), suppression of specific IgE production, and a reduction in the sensitivity of mediator-containing cells to antigen challenge.

ALLERGIC RHINITIS AND SIMILAR NASAL CONDITIONS

Epidemiology and Natural History

The prevalence of allergic rhinitis in the United States varies from region to region, depending on the amount and type of airborne allergens present. Onset of symptoms is most common between the ages of 10 and 20. The prevalence is approximately 10% in the age group 16 to 64 and may be as high as 20 to 25% in young adults (5).

During the 10 years after onset, about one-third of young adults get better, and almost half get worse. Some have a permanent remission of symptoms; in the longitudinal study of the Tecumseh population, typical allergic rhinitis remitted entirely in 8% of subjects during a 4-year interval (1). The severity of symptoms tends to decrease in most subjects after age 40. Therefore, it is important to consider other causes for apparent allergic rhinitis that begins after age 40. Whereas it is generally thought that asthma develops in many people with allergic rhinitis, in fact only about 10% develop both conditions.

Causes of Noninfectious Rhinitis

Noninfectious rhinitis refers to conditions in which there is usually no purulent discharge from the nose; purulent discharge is typical of nasal and paranasal infections such as viral upper respiratory infection and acute and chronic sinusitis (see Chapter 28). Grossly

Table 23.1. Site of Action of "Antiallergic" Drugs

Drug	Action Site	Mode of Action
Cromolyn, Nedocromil	Mast cell, polymorphonuclear leukocytes	Inhibits mediator release
Adrenergics		
α	Postcapillary venules, arterioles	Vasoconstriction
β_2	Mast cell, basophil	Inhibits mediator release (increases cAMP)
Methylxanthines	Mast cell, basophil	Inhibits mediator release (increases cAMP)
	Bronchial muscle	Relaxes bronchial muscle
H_1 antihistamines	H_1-receptor blockade	Competitive inhibition
H_2 antihistamines	H_2-receptor blockade	
Corticosteroids	Basophils	Inhibits mediator release
	Neutrophils	Prostaglandin inhibition
	Lymphocytes	IgE synthesis inhibition
Zafirlukast, other LTD_4 blockers	LTD_4-receptor blockade	Competitive inhibition
Zileuton, other enzyme inhibitors	5-Lipoxygenase inhibitors	Enzyme inhibition

Table 23.2. Miscellaneous Nonallergic Causes of Noninfectious Rhinitis

Rhinitis Medicamentosa
Sympatholytic antihypertensive medication:
  α-Blockers
  β-Blockers
  Guanethidine
  Methyldopa
  Reserpine
Aspirin sensitivity (other NSAIDs also)
Topical decongestant abuse (rebound rhinitis)

Endocrine
Hypothyroidism
Pregnancy
Oral contraceptives

Anatomic
Nasal polyp
Deviated nasal septum
Nasal tumor

Vasomotor Rhinitis

purulent secretions occasionally occur in noninfectious rhinitis; microscopically, large numbers of eosinophils are seen. Subjects with noninfectious rhinitis may belong to one of three categories: typical seasonal allergy, perennial (year-round) allergy, and miscellaneous nonallergic causes for nasal symptoms. The latter are listed in Table 23.2 and are described below. The classification of an individual patient depends chiefly on information obtained in the history. Some patients may have elements of more than one of these conditions.

History

Symptoms of Noninfectious Rhinitis. The symptoms that trouble patients most are obstruction of nasal airflow, dry mouth (from mouth breathing), nasal discharge (usually clear), itching of the nose and the soft palate, and sneezing. In addition, cough and discharge, itching, and puffiness of the eyes may occur, and there may be periodic loss of smell and taste. Occasionally, acute sinusitis (see Chapter 28) or serous otitis media (see Chapter 96) may occur as complications. Although these symptoms are not incapacitating, they may interfere significantly with the patient's usual activities and may lead to minor mood disturbance (see Chapter 12) in susceptible people. As shown in Figure 23.2, there is considerable day-to-day variability in the severity of symptoms in patients with typical seasonal allergy. Furthermore, the symptoms may vary substantially from year to year.

In nasal allergy caused by *seasonally prevalent allergens,* symptoms recur each year at approximately the same time. Pollen counts are higher in the morning, and outdoor symptoms are apt to be worse at that time. In *nonseasonal allergy,* symptoms may be induced by exposure to allergens (e.g., animal dander) any time during the day. In *vasomotor rhinitis* (see below), obstructive symptoms are prominent and, in contrast

to allergic rhinitis, irritative symptoms (sneezing and itching) are usually not pronounced.

Allergic Causes of Nasal Symptoms. *Environmental exposures.* In seasonal allergy (hay fever), the specific source of the patient's trouble can often be identified in a carefully taken history. Skin testing and in vitro immunologic tests can be used to provide definitive evidence; these measures are appropriate when the incrimination of a specific allergen, such as dog dander, will assist in environmental treatment or when immunotherapy is being considered (see below). In patients with year-round allergic symptoms, differentiation from nonallergic rhinitis may be more difficult. Indirect evidence for an allergic cause of nasal symptoms includes other manifestations of atopy and a history of typical allergic rhinitis in one or both parents. The absence of blood or nasal eosinophilia (25% eosinophils in Giemsa-stained nasal smear) mitigates against an allergic etiology.

Pollen. To a certain extent, even a limited knowledge of local pollen-releasing flora will assist one in history taking. The general rule is that plants capable of causing nasal allergy produce copious quantities of pollen in inconspicuous, unattractive flowers that depend on wind for pollination. Therefore, pollen from attractive, pleasantly scented flowers, such as roses, is not allergenic because these flowers depend on insects for pollination. So-called rose fever is usually caused by allergy to grass pollen, which is prevalent when roses are in bloom; the pleasant scent of the rose simply aggravates the patient already irritated by the allergic reaction initiated by grass pollen. In sections of the country where the seasons are well demarcated, tree pollens are found in early spring, followed in late spring by grass pollen (Table 23.3). Late summer produces ragweed pollen in the East and Midwest and cedar pollen in other sections. Mold spores are also prevalent in the fall, but snow during the winter usually prevents further dissemination of spores.

House dust, a mongrel material of uncertain heritage, can be more of a problem during the heating season in northern climes because all heating systems, but particularly forced air systems, tend to disperse dust particles. Among important components of urban dust are fragments of cockroach exoskeleton and excreta; the house dust mite, a nonparasitic organism that exists on human skin scales after they are shed; and aerosolized fragments of the saliva and skin of mammalian pets. Animal hair per se, comprising primarily insoluble collagen, is allergenic only by virtue of its burden of dander (shed skin). Symptoms caused by animal allergens may be more pronounced in pollen seasons in pollen-sensitive patients and in circumstances when patients and their pets spend more time indoors (e.g., during winter).

Nonallergic Causes of Nasal Symptoms. As noted above, a number of other conditions may cause symptoms of chronic nasal obstruction. Most of these can be diagnosed or excluded on the basis of the history and physical examination.

Rhinitis medicamentosa refers to symptoms pro-

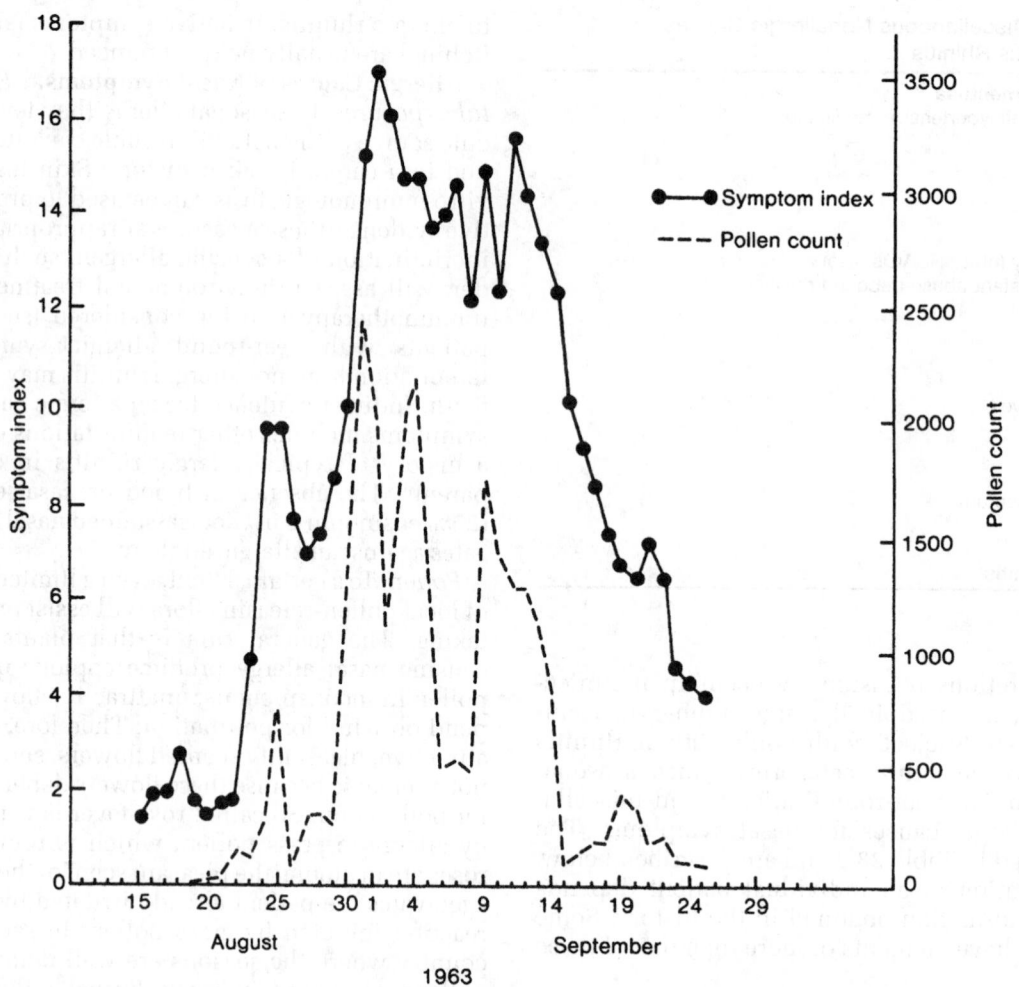

Figure 23.2.   Day-to-day variation in self-reported symptoms during the pollen season in an untreated patient with allergy to ragweed pollen.

Table 23.3.   Seasonal Occurrence of Pollens in Selected Regions

Pacific Northwest	*North Central*	*Northeast*
Trees: Apr–May	Trees: Mar–May	Trees: Apr–May
Grasses: Apr–Oct	Grasses: May–Aug	Grasses: May–July
Weeds: June–Sept	Ragweed: Aug–Sept	Ragweed: Mid-Aug–Sept
North California	Other weeds: June–Sept	Other weeds: May–Sept
Trees: Feb–May	*Midwest*	*Mid-Atlantic*
Grasses: Apr–Sept	Trees: Mar–May	Trees: Mar–May
Sagebrush: July–Oct	Grasses: May–July	Grasses: May–June
Other weeds: Mar–Oct	Ragweed: Aug–Oct	Ragweed: Mid-Aug–Sept
South California	Other weeds: July–Oct	Other weeds: May–Sept
Trees: Feb–June	*South Central*	*Southeast*
Grasses: Apr–Oct	Mountain cedar: Dec–Feb	Trees: Feb–May
Sagebrush: July–Oct	Other trees: Feb–Apr	Grasses: May–Oct
Other weeds: June–Oct	Grasses: Feb–Aug	Ragweed: Aug–Oct
	Ragweed: Aug–Oct	Other weeds: May–Oct
	Other weeds: June–Oct	

duced by the administration of several *sympatholytic drugs* (Table 23.2) or *aspirin* (and other nonsteroidal anti-inflammatory drugs [NSAIDs]), and to symptoms associated with abuse of topical decongestants. People susceptible to aspirin-induced symptoms develop profuse rhinorrhea, conjunctival suffusion, and severe bronchospasm minutes to hours after ingestion of aspirin or another NSAID; they may also develop an anaphylactoid reaction (see below). The aspirin rhinitis–bronchospasm reaction, if not fatal, is self-limited and probably does not exist in a subacute or chronic form. Abuse of topical decongestants, associated with frequent use, leads, after 1 to 2 weeks, to tolerance and then to rebound engorgement of submucosal blood vessels as the vasoconstrictive effect of the medication fades. The diagnosis of rhinitis medicamentosa can be made most efficiently by discontinuing the suspected drug. Symptoms usually remit within 1 to 5 days. The persistence of symptoms after a drug has been stopped suggests allergic or vasomotor rhinitis. Symptoms of topical decongestant abuse may persist for more than a week; the management of this problem is described below.

The nasal symptoms, chiefly obstructive, that may accompany *pregnancy,* oral *contraceptive use,* and *hypothyroidism* are most readily recognized because of their temporal association with one of these conditions and their remission when the inciting condition is no longer present.

The recognition of *anatomic causes* for chronic nasal symptoms depends chiefly on the physical examination (see below). An uncommon problem such as a tumor may be suspected if there are new and progressive symptoms, especially in older patients. Polyps or deviated nasal septum may produce chronic obstructive symptoms that are difficult to separate from perennial allergy or vasomotor rhinitis. In patients with the combination of aspirin-induced bronchospasm and nasal symptoms (see below), polyps are common. When one of these anatomic causes is suspected, the patient should be referred to an otolaryngologist.

In more than half of the patients with chronic, nonseasonal nasal symptoms, the clinical evidence does not support the diagnosis of perennial allergy or one of the miscellaneous causes just described. These patients are thought to have the poorly understood condition known as *vasomotor rhinitis* (VMR) (9). As is true of allergic rhinitis, symptoms of VMR are also thought to be provoked by environmental stimuli. The pathophysiology of this condition seems to involve inappropriate heightened reactivity of the nasal membranes to a variety of stimuli. Typically the patient awakes in the morning without symptoms but develops nasal congestion, with or without discharge, and sneezing shortly after getting out of bed; moreover, exposure to a cold bedroom or bathroom, particularly to cold bathroom tiles, is often identified by the patient as an inciting stimulus. Pleasant scents (in perfumes or household products such as soaps and detergents), cooking odors, products of combustion, and emotional stress may all precipitate symptoms. Management of VMR is described below.

Physical Examination

Allergic and vasomotor rhinitis, with or without conjunctivitis, usually presents with swollen nasal membranes and enlarged turbinates that are often described as pale or blue. The usual healthy pink appearance is absent. It may be difficult to differentiate edematous membranes or turbinates from nasal polyps; the appearance of pearly glistening globules, resembling peeled green grapes, in the nasal cavity suggests polyps and requires the opinion of an oto-

laryngologist. Polyps usually arise from stalks originating in the ethmoid sinuses. They are often visible on speculum examination; at times, they may fill the nasal cavity.

Management of Allergic Rhinitis

Table 23.4 outlines the management of seasonal or perennial allergic rhinitis.

Avoidance and Environmental Control

The treatment of choice is removal of a suspected allergen from the environment or removal of the patient from the allergenic environment. If this is not possible, other environmental manipulations may be carried out. Because the allergic patient is rarely affected by only one allergen, general control of the environment with respect to removal of as many irritants as possible is often beneficial, even though the irritants play only a contributory role. Thus, the allergic patient benefits from avoiding smoke in the environment, although smoke is not usually regarded as an antigen-containing substance. *Animal-sensitive* patients benefit by removing the animal from the home or attempting to reduce direct contact with it. Improvement of symptoms after pet-ectomy is gradual because of persistence of allergen in the environment, even for several months; thorough vacuum cleaning and washing of all fabrics and surfaces, if feasible, hasten the elimination of allergens. If it is questionable whether a pet is actually producing allergic symptoms, it is appropriate to send the patient, not the pet, for a short stay away from home. If the symptoms improve when the patient is away from home but come back at home, this is presumptive evidence of the presence of allergens in

Table 23.4.   Management of Allergic Rhinitis

Avoidance and Environmental Control
Control dust
Isolate furred animals
Obtain machine-washable polyester pillows
Seal mattress in zippered cover
Close windows, use air conditioning
Adjust humidity to 30–40% in winter
Filter air
    Electrostatic
    HEPA

Pharmacologic Treatment[a]
Antihistamine alone (for discharge, sneezing, itchy eyes)
Decongestant alone (for obstruction)
Antihistamine–decongestant combination
Topical anticholinergic (Ipratropium) for watery rhinorrhea
Topical antihistamine (Azelastine)
Topical disodium cromoglycate (cromolyn)
Topical corticosteroid
Systemic corticosteroid

Immunotherapy
Rational choice of allergens
    History
    Skin testing
Adequate dosage essential

[a]See details in Tables 23.5 to 23.7.

the home, usually from an animal or an unsuspected source of mold or related fungal growth, such as a contaminated humidifier reservoir or dust mites.

The *quality of the air in closed environments* can have a significant impact on symptoms. Regulation of the relative humidity is useful; it should be maintained between 35 and 40% during the winter. Humidifier reservoirs must be kept clean. Reduction of humidity in warm, humid summer weather may also be beneficial, although this is less critical unless the degree of humidity is such that it supports visible mold growth. Air conditioning and dehumidifiers are thus often necessary where the relative humidity is always high. Any heating, humidifying, or air-cooling device that depends on the delivery of forced air must have an effective air filter. Several types of filtration media and devices are available. Homes with forced warm air heating systems may have an oil-fired heater, but more often have a heat pump or gas-fired burner. Regardless of the type of fuel, the usual plastic or fiberglass mesh filter, changed monthly if the homeowner remembers, is nothing more than a mechanical filter (much like a window screen to prevent insects, birds, and other large creatures from invading the home.) The most sophisticated device, formerly called an electrostatic filter, is now known as an electronic air cleaner. It is expensive and requires professional installation. It is the most efficient furnace filter, but perhaps not a great deal better than a number of passive filters, which incorporate either chemically treated cellulose or plastic mesh that acquires an electrostatic charge from the flow of air. Electronic and electrostatic filters depend on electrostatic precipitation of particulate matter as it is drawn through a charged field by a blower. Another type depends on the trapping of particulate matter in a specially treated cellulose high-efficiency particulate air (HEPA) filter. Maintenance of the electrostatic filtration device requires replacement or periodic cleaning (usually by washing) of the particle-trapping device. With a HEPA filter, accessory filters may need to be replaced on a regular basis. These prefilters are necessary for trapping larger particles that would otherwise impair the efficiency of the unit. In addition to air-filtering devices, the following are desirable: floors that are bare or carpeted with washable rugs, windows that are curtained with washable curtains rather than dust-catching Venetian blinds, bedrooms furnished with washable materials and containing a minimum of dust-catching books and bric-a-brac, and use of pillows of washable polyester and mattresses encased in zippered plastic covers.

Drug Therapy

Symptomatic drug treatment of allergic rhinitis is empiric and usually involves striking a satisfactory balance between the beneficial effects of the drug and the undesirable side effects. The goal of therapy is reduction of symptoms to a level that enables the patient to function normally because complete elimination of symptoms is usually impossible (Fig. 23.3). Antihistamines are the mainstays of empiric therapy. Sympathomimetic decongestants, cromolyn, topical or systemic corticosteroids, and topical ophthalmic agents may be added to antihistamines depending on the patient's needs.

Antihistamines. In many patients, an antihistamine alone may provide adequate relief most of the time. This is particularly true when irritative symptoms (sneezing, itching, discharge) are the major problems. Many antihistamines are available. The older agents produce some sedation and drying of the mucous membranes, and their efficacy in suppressing nasal symptoms generally parallels the degree of these two side effects. As indicated in Table 23.5, there are several classes of antihistamines from which to choose in the treatment of allergic rhinitis. Individual patients may respond more readily to a given class, but within classes, differences in efficacy tend to be slight. Once an effective class has been found for a patient, preference within the class is determined by the relative absence of side effects. Because there is an enormous cost difference between generic and brand-name antihistamines, once a patient has found an effective product, he or she should be encouraged to try an equivalent generic drug. Subtle manufacturing differences between clinically equivalent products may make a particular one more suitable for a given patient. A useful procedure is to choose one drug from each class as a starting point, beginning with the drugs listed first in each class in Table 23.5. At first it is better to avoid sustained-release preparations; they may be used later for convenience once the right drug is found.

As shown in Table 23.5, antihistamines are available in a variety of strengths and forms; some are available without prescription. All have their onset of action in 10 to 30 minutes. Sustained-released preparations may need to be taken every 8 hours for continuous effect. Antihistamines appear to be more effective if dosing is begun in anticipation of symptoms (i.e., before exposure to animals or before the beginning of the grass or ragweed pollen season).

To obviate sedation, some patients omit daytime doses and use a sustained-release preparation at bedtime to help ensure a good night's sleep and to adequately control the irritative symptoms that are so common upon awakening in the morning. Terfenadine and astemizole have little or no sedative or anticholinergic effects. Cardiac arrhythmia secondary to a delay in the myocardial conduction system has been associated, rarely, with terfenadine or astemizole when taken in excess of the recommended dosage or as an overdose, or when one of these drugs has been taken concomitantly with erythromycin, clarithromycin (Biaxin), ketoconazole (Nizoral), or itraconazole (Sporanox). Because of this association, the widely prescribed form of terfenadine, Seldane, was taken off the market in 1998. Astemizole should not be prescribed because of an unnecessary risk/benefit ratio and because safer alternatives exist. To date, rhythm disturbances have not been observed with the recently released fexofenadine (Allegra, or terfenadine carboxylate), or loratadine (Claritin). Loratadine is chemically related to azatadine (Optimine) and cyproheptadine (Periactin), but does not seem to cause dry mouth or seda-

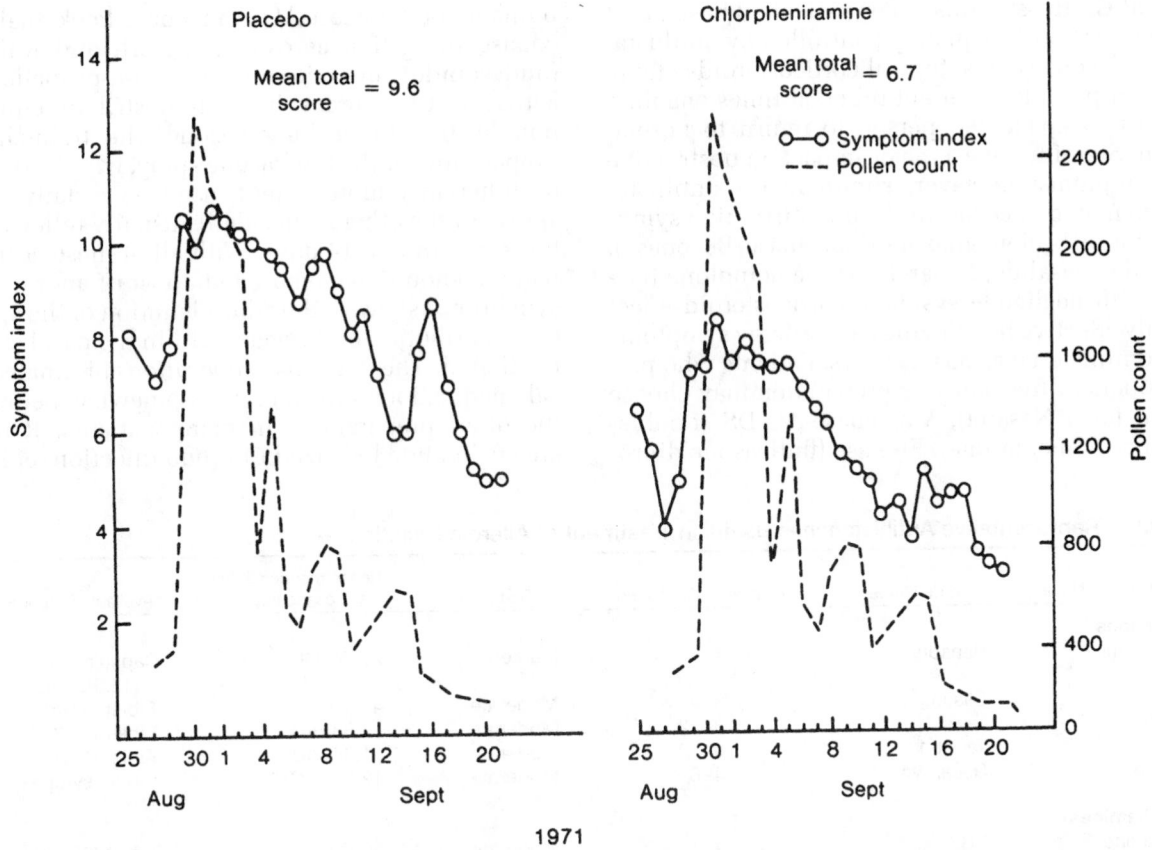

Figure 23.3. Symptom level in patients with allergic rhinitis taking antihistamines. These two sets of data compare the response of carefully matched groups of ragweed-allergic patients either to placebo or to an antihistamine (chlorpheniramine) during the ragweed pollen season. It can be seen that the antihistamine reduces but does not eliminate symptoms (the symptoms recorded by patients were sneezing, stuffy nose, runny nose, red itchy eyes, and cough). (Adapted from Valentine MD, Norman PS, Lichtenstein LM. Evaluation of an antihistamine in ragweed hay fever. In: McMahon FG, ed. Evaluation of gastrointestinal, pulmonary, anti-inflammatory, and immunological agents. Mount Kisco, NY: Futura, 1974.)

tion when taken in the usual dosage of 10 mg once daily. Astelin (azelastine) is a novel antihistamine preparation, delivered in a small dose by nasal spray. Its use is sometimes associated with nasal drying and unpleasant taste as it drains from the nasal cavity posteriorly.

Sympathomimetic Decongestants. Sympathomimetic decongestants may add significantly to the beneficial effects of antihistamines. They may be particularly effective in patients who have pronounced obstructive symptoms caused by nasal mucosal edema; presumably decongestants work by vasoconstriction, which decreases the blood flow to nasal mucosa. A second beneficial property of these agents is that they have a stimulatory effect on the CNS, which may counteract antihistamine-induced sedation. Table 23.6 summarizes practical information about a number of commonly prescribed *antihistamine–decongestant combinations* (may require written prescription). Extendryl and Atrohist Plus incorporate the anticholinergic agent methscopolamine for additional drying effects and are usually never necessary.

Sympathomimetic decongestants are also available alone in over-the-counter oral preparations and in topical drops and sprays (see Table 28.1). These forms may be useful in patients with allergic rhinitis whose most troublesome symptom is nasal obstruction or in those who cannot tolerate antihistamines. Decongestant treatment without antihistamine is the treatment of choice in patients with acute sinusitis and serous otitis media, two conditions that may complicate any allergic or nonallergic process producing congestion of the nasal mucosa.

In therapeutic dosages, oral sympathomimetic decongestants may occasionally cause tachycardia and blood pressure elevation (4). Therefore, it is important to determine the patient's blood pressure response before prescribing a sympathomimetic for prolonged use; this can be done within 1 to 3 hours of administration of the drug. Patients with allergic rhinitis should be strongly warned against the routine use of nasal decongestant sprays or drops because this may lead to rhinitis medicamentosa (see above). Perhaps the best advice for the patient who cannot part with a decongestant spray is to use it only at times when symptom relief is crucial—for example, at bedtime if nasal obstruction makes it difficult to get to sleep (and when the stimulatory effects of oral sympathomimetic decongestants may interfere with sleeping).

Topical Corticosteroids. For patients whose nasal symptoms are not adequately controlled by antihistamines or decongestants, topical corticosteroids (Table 23.7) often provide excellent relief, at times enabling an almost incapacited person to return to normal function. Steroids have a major impact on obstructive nasal symptoms; however, simultaneous antihistamine use may be needed to suppress irritative symptoms. Esters of beclomethasone (Vancenase, Beconase), flunisolide (Nasalide, Nasarel), or triamcinolone (Nasacort) with negligible systemic corticosteroid effect are highly effective in relieving nasal allergy symptoms when administered as nasal sprays. Patients who prefer a propellant-free aqueous preparation may choose Nasalide (also Nasarel), Vancenase-AQ-DS (double-strength beclomethasone), Flonase (fluticasone dipropionate), or Nasacort-AQ. Vancenase Pockethaler, Beconase inhalation aerosol, Nasacort, and Rhinocort (budesonide) are micronized, Freon-propelled, dry aerosols. Two sprays in each nostril of either the double-strength beclomethasone, the triamcinolone preparation, or the fluticasone spray, which are said to be inherently more potent, used once daily, or two sprays of the others twice daily, usually relieve symptoms within 7 to 14 days. With all of these agents the patient should be instructed to sniff more or less synchronously with the administration of the spray so that distribution of the agent within the nasal cavity is facilitated. The *aqueous preparations* of inhaled topical medications are tolerated somewhat better than the other preparations in many patients. Rare side effects include localized *Candida* infection, epistaxis,

Table 23.5.   Representative Antihistamines Useful in Treatment of Allergic Rhinitis

Class and Generic Name	Trade Name	Duration of Action (hr)	Sedation	Recommended Adult Dosage (mg)	Available Preparations (mg)
Ethanolamines					
Diphenhydramine[a,b]	Benadryl	4–6	Marked	25–50 QID	Capsule (25, 50), elixir (12.5/5 mL)
Carbinoxamine[c]	Clistin	3–4	Moderate	4 QID	Tablet, elixir
Clemastine	Tavist	8–12	Moderate	2.68 BID	Tablet (2.68)
	Tavist-1[b]	8–12	Moderate	1.34 BID	Tablet (1.34)
Doxylamine	Decapryn	4–6	Moderate	12.5–25 QID	Tablet, syrup
Ethylenediamines					
Tripelennamine[a,c]	PBZ	4–6	Moderate	50 QID	Tablet (25, 50), elixir (37.5/5 mL)
Alkylamines					
Chlorpheniramine[a–c]	Chlor-Trimeton	4–6	Mild	4 QID	Tablet (4), syrup (2/5 mL)
Dexchlorpheniramine[c]	Polaramine	4–6	Mild	2 QID	Tablet (2), syrup (2/5 mL)
Brompheniramine[a–c]	Dimetane	4–6	Mild	4 QID	Tablet (4), elixir (2/5 mL)
Triprolidine[a,b]	Actidil	8–12	Mild	2.5 BID	Tablet (2.5), syrup (1.25/5 mL)
Phenothiazines					
Promethazine[a]	Phenergan	4–6	Moderate	12.5–25 QID	Tablet (12.5, 25, 50), syrup (2.5/5 mL)
Trimeprazine[a,c]	Temaril	4–6	Moderate	2.5–7.5 QID	Capsule (2.5), syrup (2.5/5 mL)
Piperidines					
Azatadine	Optimine	8–12	Moderate	1–2 BID	Tablet
Cyproheptadine[d]	Periactin	4–6	Marked	4 QID	Tablet (4), syrup (2/5 mL)
Butyrophenone					
Fexofenadine	Allegra	8–12	Little or none	60 BID	Tablet (60)
Miscellaneous					
Loratidine	Claritin	12–24	Little or none	10 daily	Tablet (10) (available as a liquid)
Astemizole	Hismanal	Up to several weeks	Little or none	10 daily on empty stomach	Tablet (10)
Piperazine					
Cetirizine	Zyrtec	18–24	Moderate	5–10 mg HS	Tabs (5, 10 mg) elixir 5/5 mL
Hydroxyzine[a,d]	Atarax, Vistaril	6–12	Moderate	10–25 BID, TID	Capsule (10, 25, 50, 100), suspension (10/5 mL)

[a]Generic available.

[b]Over-the-counter drug.

[c]Sustained-release preparation available.

[d]More useful in urticaria and pruritus.

mucosal ulceration, and nasal septal perforation. Patients must be told to expect gradual improvement, over the course of days, in contrast to the immediate response to be expected from a topical vasoconstrictor. Dexamethasone as a nasal aerosol has also been available for some time but is rarely indicated because of the increased risk of adrenal gland suppression that is present with this high-potency preparation, when used in maximal dosage. Both flunisolide and beclomethasone have been used safely for prolonged periods. All nasal aerosols occasionally cause transient, mild, local irritation.

Patients who are using intranasal corticosteroids occasionally report symptoms of an intercurrent *infec-*

tious rhinitis. Although the manufacturers advise patients to notify their physicians in this instance, there is no evidence for a need to discontinue the topical spray. Topical steroids may also be continued while sinusitis is being treated with a decongestant or antibiotic.

Systemic corticosteroids are occasionally justified in treating seasonal allergy. For example, in a patient who usually requires topical steroids for obstructive symptoms, a 3- or 4-day course of prednisone (20 mg/day) may be needed to relieve nasal obstruction sufficiently so that the aerosol can effectively reach the nasal mucosa. Only rarely should a longer course of steroids (2 to 3 weeks) be used to treat allergic rhinitis. The

Table 23.6.   Representative Antihistamine–Decongestant Combinations Useful in Treating Allergic Rhinitis

Trade Name	Contents	mg/unit	Form Available	Usual Adult Dosage
Deconamine-SR	Chlorpheniramine	8	TDC[a]	1 q12hr
	Pseudoephedrine	120		
Ornade	Chlorpheniramine	12	TDC ("spansule")	1 q12hr
	Phenylpropanolamine	75		
Naldecon	Chlorpheniramine	5	Timed-release tablet	1 q8–12hr
	Phenyltoloxamine	15		
	Phenylephrine	10		
	Phenylpropanolamine	40		
Nolamine	Chlorpheniramine	4	Timed-release tablet	1 q8–12hr
	Phenindamine	24		
	Phenylpropanolamine	50		
Fedahist	Chlorpheniramine	8	"Timecaps"	1 q12hr
	Pseudoephedrine	120		
	Chlorpheniramine	10	"Gyrocaps"	1 q12hr
	Pseudoephedrine	65		
Dimetapp	Brompheniramine	12	Extentab	1 q12hr
	Phenylpropanolamine	75		
Bromfed	Brompheniramine	12	TDC	1 q12hr
	Pseudoephedrine	120		
Bromfed-PD	Brompheniramine	6	TDC	1 q12hr
	Pseudoephedrine	60		
Atrohist Plus	Chlorpheniramine	8	Timed-release tablet	1 q12hr
	Phenylephrine	25		
	Phenylpropanolamine	50		
	Hyoscyamine	0.19		
	Atropine SO$_4$	0.04		
	Scopolamine HBr	0.01		
Actifed	Triprolidine	2.5	Tablet or capsule	1 TID
	Pseudoephedrine	60		
Claritin-D	Loratadine	5	Timed-release tablet	1 BID
	Pseudoephedrine	120		
Claritin-D-24 hr	Loratadine	10	Timed-release tablet	1 qAM
	Pseudoephedrine	240		
Trinalin	Azatadine	1	Timed-release tablet	1 q12hr
	Pseudoephedrine	120		
Drixoral	*d*-Brompheniramine	6	Timed-release tablet	1 q12hr
	Pseudoephedrine	120		
Extendryl	Chlorpheniramine	8	TDC	1 q12hr
	Phenylephrine	20		
	Methscopolamine	2.5	TDC	1 q12hr
Extendryl Jr	(Half the strength of Extendryl)			
Extendryl Chewable	Chlorpheniramine	2	Chewable tablet	1 q4–6hr
	Phenylephrine	10		
	Methscopolamine	1.25		
Rondec-T	Carbinoxamine	4	Tablet	1 TID
	Pseudoephedrine	60		
Rondec-TR	Carbinoxamine	8	Timed-release tablet	1 BID
	Pseudoephedrine	120		
Tavist-D	Clemastine	1	Tablet	1 BID
	Phenylpropanolamine	75		

[a]Timed disintegration capsule.

Table 23.7.   Forms and Dosage of Topical Steroids for Allergic Rhinitis

Trade Name	Drug	Form	Dispenser	Dosage
Beconase-AQ	Beclomethasone	Aqueous solution	Manual pump, metered dose	Two sprays in each nostril BID
Beconase Inhalation Aerosol	Beclomethasone	Micronized powder	Freon-propelled	Two puffs in each nostril BID
Vancenase-AQ-DS	Beclomethasone	Aqueous solution	Manual pump, metered dose	Two sprays in each nostril QD
Vancenase Pockethaler	Beclomethasone	Micronized powder	Freon-propelled	Two puffs in each nostril BID
Nasalide, Nasarel	Flunisolide	Aqueous solution	Manual pump, metered dose	Two sprays in each nostril BID
Nasacort	Triamcinolone	Micronized powder	Freon-propelled	Two puffs in each nostril QD
Nasacort-AQ	Triamcinolone	Aqueous suspension	Manual pump	Two sprays in each nostril QD
Tri-nasal	Triamcinolone	Aqueous suspension	Manual pump	Two sprays in each nostril QD
Rhinocort	Budesonide	Micronized powder	Freon-propelled	Two sprays in each nostril QD
Flonase	Fluticasone	Aqueous solution	Manual pump	Two sprays in each nostril QD
Decadron Turbinaire	Dexamethasone	Micronized powder	Freon-propelled	Two puffs in each nostril BID–TID

prednisone can usually be tapered rapidly during the last few days of treatment (see further discussion of steroid use in Chapter 74). Although parenteral, depot steroid injections are convenient, they are generally not indicated because oral prednisone permits greater dosing flexibility and, possibly, less risk of adrenal gland suppression.

Cromolyn Sodium.   A nasal aerosol is available of cromolyn sodium (Nasalcrom), an agent that inhibits mediator release in the mast cells of the nasal mucosa. Aerosolized cromolyn must be administered approximately every 4 hours by metered dose to each nostril to prevent symptoms. Mild side effects (chiefly nasal irritation) are common, but they are transient and well tolerated. The disadvantages of this drug are high cost to the patient and the frequent dosing schedule. However, for selected patients with unequivocal seasonal allergic symptoms, a trial of cromolyn may be worthwhile because of the absence of antihistamine sedation. In animal-sensitive patients, a trial of cromolyn before exposure is worthwhile; if effective, the drug should be continued every 4 hours during the period of exposure. In 1997, Nasalcrom was approved for over-the-counter (OTC) sales.

Ipratropium.   *Ipratropium* (Atrovent), an anticholinergic agent, is available as 0.03% and 0.06% nasal sprays for allergic rhinitis when watery rhinorrhea is a problem.

Management of Eye Symptoms.   Often, the nasal symptoms of allergic rhinitis are controlled by one of the drugs mentioned above, but the eye symptoms persist. In this situation any of the various OTC topical preparations containing α-adrenergic agents such as Vasocon, Naphcon, or Opcon may be effective; two drops should be instilled three to four times daily. Prefrin is an OTC compound of antipyrine, phenylephrine, and pyrilamine, which may be used as an alternative. Several preparations are available in the "A" form, denoting inclusion of antihistamine. For the patient who is seriously impaired by conjunctival symptoms despite topical vasoconstrictors, either of two weak topical steroids (HMS Liquifilm or FML Liquifilm) may be tried for brief periods; however, an ophthalmologist should be consulted, at least by telephone, first. Prolonged use of ophthalmic steroids should be avoided unless the patient has periodic slitlamp examinations by an ophthalmologist, because of the danger of herpetic keratitis. Compounds often called "mast cell stabilizers"—substances that inhibit release of histamine from mast cell granules—such as ophthalmic cromolyn (Crolom, formerly Opticrom), tromethamine (Alomide), and Patanol, are sometimes effective alternatives to ocular steroids. Livostin (levocabastine), an antihistamine for ophthalmic use, is also effective in allergic conjunctivitis.

Other preparations for the control of allergic eye symptoms have been introduced in recent years. One is Acular, a preparation of the NSAID diclofenac (Voltaren) for ophthalmic use. Because drugs applied to the conjunctival sac are significantly absorbed, Acular would be contraindicated in NSAID-sensitive patients (see below). An ophthalmic form of nedocromil solution, not yet available for general use, has been found to be at least as effective as topical cromolyn in allergic conjunctivitis. Nedocromil is a quinolone whose properties resemble those of cromolyn.

Any *contact lens wearer* should consult an ophthalmologist before using any eye drop. The preservative *benzalkonium chloride,* itself a potential sensitizer, can be adsorbed by many contact lenses. One complication of contact lens use, giant papillary conjunctivitis, is often treated with topical cromolyn.

Referral to an Allergist

Patients who do not respond to the measures outlined above should be referred to an allergist for evaluation to confirm the diagnosis of allergic rhinitis or to disclose any other cause for nasal symptoms and to determine whether the patient may be a candidate for immunotherapy.

The immunologic tests done by an allergist are primarily scratch or intracutaneous tests using solutions of suspected offending allergens. These skin tests are more sensitive, although no more specific, than the in vitro radioallergosorbent test (RAST), in which the patient's serum level of allergen-specific IgE antibody is measured. Moreover, the skin test is far less expensive than the RAST; therefore, the latter should be reserved for instances when the skin is not suitable for testing (e.g., in patients with dermatographism or generalized atopic dermatitis) or when skin reactivity seems to be equivocal when compared with negative and positive controls.

Immunotherapy with sufficient dosages of appropriate allergens has been shown to reduce symptoms in 95% of patients with seasonal allergic rhinitis caused by ragweed or grass pollens (Fig. 23.4); however, nearly one-third of patients seem to benefit from a placebo (2). Although there are few controlled studies of animal dander immunotherapy, some allergists try this mode of therapy in selected animal-hypersensitive patients when manipulation of the environment and pharmacologic control are ineffective. House dust mites (*Dermatophagoides* species), commensal occupants of human habitats, are important sources of airborne allergen in some areas. Control is difficult and no practical miticide is available at present. Mite extract is also available for diagnosis and immunotherapy.

Because allergic rhinitis is often present in multiple family members, parents may question their physicians about the value of immunotherapy for their affected children. Immunotherapy is rarely indicated

in early childhood. Although it may yield apparently good results in the prepubertal child, it should be borne in mind that puberty may also be accompanied by a diminution in symptoms of allergic rhinitis. Therefore, immunotherapy is indicated chiefly in the postpubertal patient.

Immunotherapy is often arbitrarily recommended for 2 to 3 years. Initially, the patient is given frequent injections of the selected allergen extract in progressively higher dosages until a maintenance dosage is achieved, after which booster injections are given approximately once or twice per month for the duration of immunotherapy. After 2 or 3 years, a decision must be made whether to continue treatment or to stop it and watch for recurrence of symptoms. Some patients who respond well to several years of immunotherapy may continue to enjoy reduced symptoms even after immunotherapy is stopped. Allergen preparations modified with formalin (allergoid) or glutaraldehyde are awaiting FDA approval; this sort of chemical modification allows less frequent dosing and a somewhat reduced risk of systemic reactions to therapy.

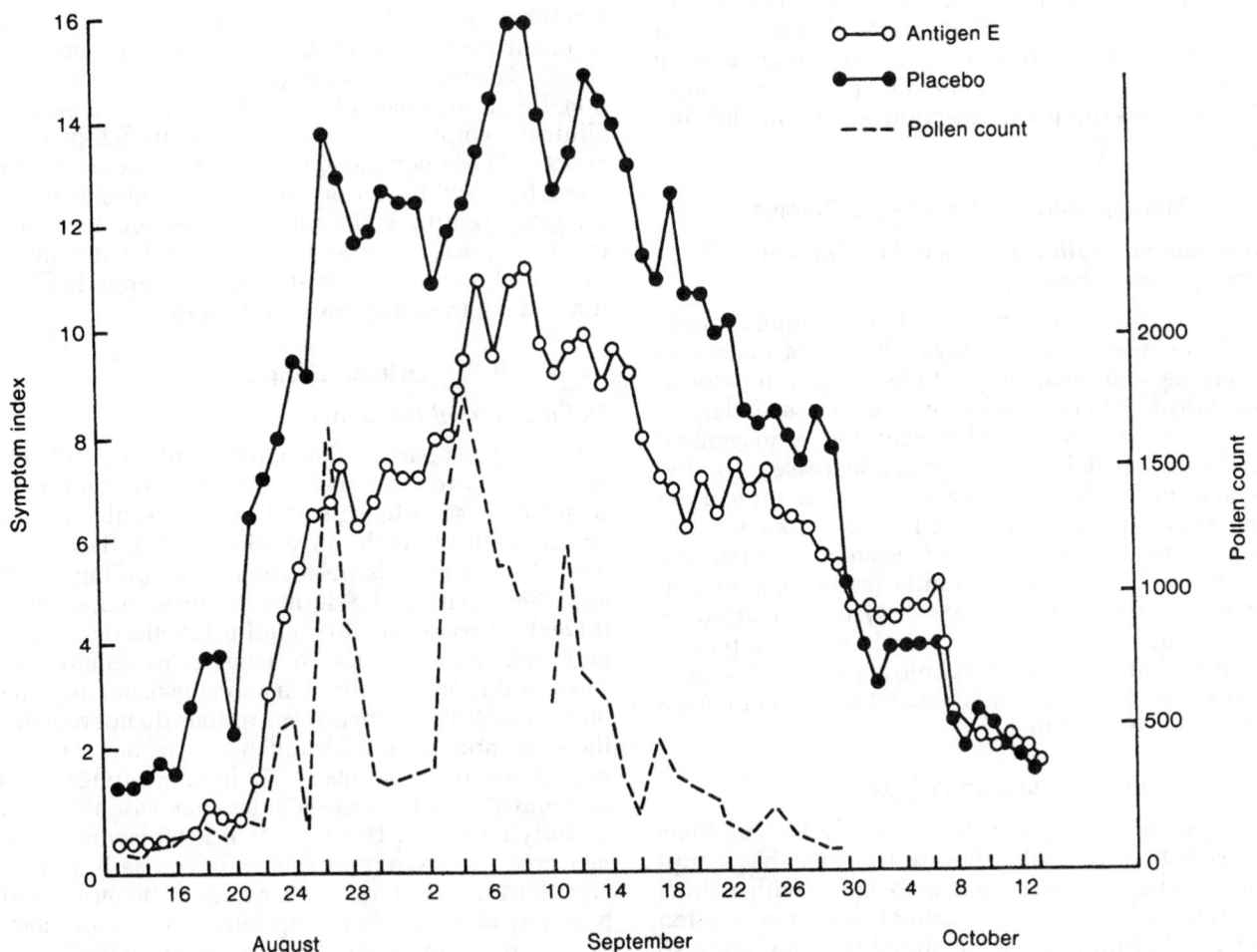

Figure 23.4. Daily symptom scores of patients immunized with a ragweed antigen (Antigen E), compared with matched patients "immunized" with a placebo. (From Lichtenstein LM, Norman PS, Winkenwerder WL. A single year of immunotherapy for ragweed hay fever: immunologic and clinical studies. Ann Intern Med 75:663, 1971.)

The patient's general physician may at times be asked to administer maintenance subcutaneous allergen injections. Three types of untoward reactions may occur after allergen injections:

- *An immediate local reaction,* characterized by formation of a wheal and flare at the site within 15 to 30 minutes of injection. An eruption that is as large as a half dollar is an indication not to increase the dosage of allergen in the subsequent injection. This type of reaction may result from inadvertent administration of the dose too superficially.
- *A delayed local reaction,* which begins 2 to 4 hours after the injection of allergen and reaches a peak at 18 to 24 hours. This is most commonly seen when dust and mold spore antigens are included in the extract and may be caused by nonallergens present in the raw material used to make the extract. This type of delayed, large local skin reaction may prevent an increase in the dosage of allergen because of local discomfort.
- *A generalized or constitutional reaction.* This may be immediate or delayed, but usually occurs within 30 minutes of treatment; therefore, patients are required to wait for 30 minutes after each injection before leaving the doctor's office. Many allergists advise their more sensitive patients to carry an emergency epinephrine self-treatment kit (Epi-Pen, Center Laboratories) for use if a reaction occurs after leaving the office.

Management of Nonallergic Rhinitis

Management of Rhinitis Caused by Topical Decongestant Abuse

Rhinitis medicamentosa of the rebound variety should be suspected whenever there is a history of worsening symptoms of nasal obstruction in association with more than a week of regular (i.e., several times daily) use of a topical decongestant. Management consists of explaining the probable reason for the problem to the patient, discontinuing the topical decongestant, and prescribing a 1- to 2-week course of corticosteroid in aerosol form (see above), which will relieve the symptoms of rhinitis medicamentosa. In very severe cases, several days of systemic corticosteroids should precede topical steroid use. The patient usually has an underlying chronic nasal condition, and appropriate management is needed when that condition has been identified.

Management of Intranasal Polyps

Polyps (see description above) may cause symptoms of obstruction to nasal airflow or they may be asymptomatic. They may be seen in association with asthma precipitated by aspirin (see below), and there is often associated chronic or acute sinusitis. They are also often seen in patients with cystic fibrosis. The treatment of symptomatic polyps consists of topical corticosteroids (see above) or polypectomy. When polyps

are suspected, the patient should be referred to an otolaryngologist to confirm the diagnosis and to plan appropriate management.

Management of Vasomotor Rhinitis

This nonallergic condition (9) shows little or no response to antihistamines, but symptoms may diminish when the patient is treated with oral decongestants alone. Symptoms may also respond to intranasal corticosteroids (see above), which can be prescribed for use during troublesome exacerbations. The most important consideration in management for patients with vasomotor rhinitis is ensuring that they understand the chronicity of their condition, the limited symptomatic treatment available, and the importance of avoiding irritants in their environment and of not abusing topical decongestants.

GENERALIZED ALLERGIC AND ALLERGIC-LIKE REACTIONS

Two categories of generalized reactions may be seen in ambulatory settings: urticaria/angioedema (usually not life threatening) and anaphylaxis/anaphylactoid reactions (often life threatening). The underlying mechanisms for these generalized reactions are either classic IgE-mediated allergy or one of a number of nonallergic processes in which mediator release and clinical symptoms resemble those in IgE-mediated allergy. These generalized reactions may be precipitated by a wide variety of foreign substances and physical stimuli. At the end of this section, the following five specific causes of generalized reactions are discussed: penicillin, *Hymenoptera* venom, foods, iodinated contrast materials, and aspirin.

Urticaria/Angioedema

Definition and Incidence

Urticaria and angioedema differ pathologically only with respect to the microscopic depth of the process, which consists primarily of the extravascular accumulation of fluid, with no evidence of inflammation. Raised erythematous areas of edema involving only the superficial part of the dermis are urticarial eruptions (hives), whereas edema extending into the deep dermis and subcutaneous tissue constitutes angioedema. These eruptions usually itch and may occur anywhere on the body. True urticarial eruptions do not remain in the same area of skin for much longer than 24 hours; persistence of eruptions for 72 hours or longer in the same area of skin suggests cutaneous vasculitis as an underlying cause. During a typical episode of acute urticaria, evanescent eruptions may arise in different areas for 1 day or more. Urticaria ceases being acute and becomes chronic after eruptions have continued to appear, recur, or persist for 6 weeks or longer.

Urticaria is particularly common in prepubertal females but occurs at some time in approximately one-fifth of the population.

Causes and Evaluation

A number of causes are recognized for urticaria/angioedema (Table 23.8). Both urticaria and angioedema may occur alone or together in each of the conditions listed in the table; the exception to this rule is the rare syndrome, hereditary angioedema, in which angioedema alone occurs.

The definite (or most likely) cause of acute urticaria can often be determined by a history of an exposure preceding the onset of symptoms. The onset of acute urticaria/angioedema may occur from minutes to hours after the exposure to an inciting substance. (Additional discussion of reactions to selected common substances is found in a later section of this chapter.)

A number of urticaria/angioedema states are initiated by *physical stimuli*. The most common is *dermatographism*, a linear wheal with flare that occurs at the site of brisk stroking with a firm object; the eruption fades within 30 minutes. Several less common conditions are induced by physical stimuli: *pressure urticaria/angioedema*, which is characterized by local swelling, sometimes painful, that occurs immediately or within 4 to 6 hours after constant pressure has been applied (e.g., by tight garments); exposure to low temperatures *(cold urticaria)*; exposure to sunlight or intense artificial light *(solar urticaria)*; so-called *cholinergic urticaria* (because it can be reproduced locally in affected subjects by the injection of cholinergic agents), which develops after an increase in core body temperature caused by a hot bath, exercise, or fever; and urticaria developing shortly after the local application of heat *(heat urticaria)*.

It is particularly important to consider *hereditary*

angioedema (HAE), a rare but potentially life-threatening condition, in any patient with isolated episodes of angioedema, particularly if there is a history of other family members with angioedema. Onset of symptoms usually occurs before age 20. Typically, the patient does not describe itching. Local trauma may precipitate peripheral attacks. Visceral attacks may occur spontaneously, characterized by abdominal pain. Life-threatening oral or laryngeal edema may occur during any attack. HAE is associated with deficiency of the inhibitor of the first complement component, C1, but does not seem to be triggered by an immune process except in the acquired form of the disease. The diagnosis is suggested by a low level of serum C4 and a normal C3 level. Patients with these findings should be referred to an allergist for definitive evaluation, which involves a functional assay for the inhibitor. An acquired form of C1 inhibitor deficiency has recently been recognized in which the pathophysiology involves consumption of the inhibitor through chronic activation of C1 by circulating immune complexes, the entire syndrome being secondary to lymphoproliferative or other malignant disorders. In both the inherited and the acquired forms, the diagnosis must be confirmed immunologically. Another cause of low values of C4 in urticaria is cutaneous vasculitis; this is usually accompanied by an elevated erythrocyte sedimentation rate.

It is often difficult to determine the cause of chronic urticaria. The diagnostic workup may include complete blood counts with differential, sedimentation rate, urinalysis, stool examination for ova and parasites, and tests for hepatitis antigen (see Chapter 43), cytomegalovirus antibody, heterophil antibody (Monospot test, see Chapter 53), cold agglutinins, cryoglobulins, and C3, C4, or antinuclear antibody. Despite screening tests for underlying conditions, in more than 70% of patients with chronic urticaria no cause is found (so-called idiopathic urticaria).

Management

Many patients with minor episodes of urticaria/angioedema simply tolerate it or learn by trial and error how to eliminate the causative factors. Others seek help from their physicians.

The intense itching of acute urticaria usually responds promptly to the subcutaneous administration of epinephrine (for adults, 0.2 to 0.3 mL of a 1:1000 solution of aqueous epinephrine, repeated after 15 minutes if necessary). An antihistamine such as diphenhydramine (50 mg) or chlorpheniramine (4 mg) should be given orally at the same time. If the parenteral route is used, the initial dosage should be reduced 50% to avoid marked sedation.

Additional antihistamines are helpful in preventing prolonged symptoms from urticaria. Hydroxyzine (Vistaril or Atarax) appears to be the most effective for controlling itching (6), particularly in chronic urticaria. A low dosage (10 mg every 8 hours) should be tried initially, as the usual dosage (25 mg every 8 hours)

Table 23.8.   Causes of Urticaria/Angioedema

Acute (Episode Lasting 6 Weeks or Less)
Allergy (IgE-mediated)
    Foods, drugs, insect stings
Infection
    Virus (mononucleosis, hepatitis)
    Bacterial (β-hemolytic streptococcus)
Idiosyncrasy
    NSAID
    Iodinated contrast material
Physical agents
    Dermatographism
    Heat
        Generalized ("cholinergic")
        Localized
    Cold
    Solar
    Pressure
Idiopathic

Chronic or Recurring
Hereditary angioneurotic edema
Hepatitis
Parasitic infestation
Neoplasm (especially Hodgkin's lymphoma)
Collagen-vascular disease
    Systemic lupus erythematosus
    Polyarteritis
Idiopathic

is much more likely to cause significant sedation. Cetirizine (Zyrtec, a metabolite of hydroxyzine) may be effective in a dosage of 10 mg at bedtime. If hydroxyzine or cetirizine is ineffective, cyproheptadine (Periactin) may be tried, beginning with 2 mg every 12 hours and increasing to a maximum of 4 mg four times daily. The addition of an H_2 antagonist (cimetidine or ranitidine) may enhance the effectiveness of conventional (H_1) antihistamines in the management of urticaria. Ephedrine, 25 mg every 4 to 6 hours, may be added to H_1 plus H_2 regimens with some additional beneficial effect resulting from the α-, β_1-, and β_2-adrenergic effects of this compound.

These measures are useful in most of the allergic and nonallergic urticaria/angioedema states. There are exceptions, however. *Cold urticaria* seems to respond best to cyproheptadine (Periactin), 4 mg every 6 hours. *Pressure urticaria,* when severe enough to require treatment, usually does not respond to antihistamines and may require a short course of corticosteroids. *Solar urticaria* should be managed with a combination of topical sunscreens and hydroxyzine. *Attacks of HAE* may be prevented by long-term treatment with a non-virilizing androgen derivative (8). This form of treatment should usually be planned in conjunction with a consulting allergist. Life-threatening acute attacks of HAE require hospitalization for observation in an intensive care unit. If C4 levels are less than 50% of normal, any surgical procedure proposed for such patients should not be attempted without pretreatment because of the risk of precipitating local attacks through trauma. Stanozolol (Winstrol), 4 mg four times a day for 3 days given preoperatively, appears to have sufficient effect to prevent HAE attacks in the intraoperative and postoperative periods.

Avoidance. When there is a clear indication that certain conditions promote urticaria, it is important to avoid reexposure because more severe reactions may result. Acute generalized urticaria/angioedema after exposure to a foreign substance signifies that there is a risk of a life-threatening reaction (see below) on reexposure. In addition, in patients with a history of solar, cold, or cholinergic urticaria, there is a small risk of vascular collapse on subsequent exposure. These disquieting facts should be made known to affected subjects and their families in order to emphasize the importance of avoiding exposure, of obtaining immediate medical attention if recurrent exposure occurs, and of administering emergency treatment if there is a severe reaction (anaphylaxis; see next section).

Anaphylaxis/Anaphylactoid Reactions

Definition

Life-threatening acute generalized reactions are not uncommon in ambulatory practice. Table 23.9 lists substances that have been documented as causes of such reactions; other important causes are insect stings and ingested foods (see below).

Anaphylaxis is an immune response to an agent to which a person has become hypersensitive by prior exposure. A variety of symptoms may occur. Initially, there may be a diffuse erythema of the skin followed by a sense of warmth and then generalized urticaria. Severe and rapidly progressive respiratory distress caused by bronchospasm or angioedema involving the larynx may follow. Gastrointestinal symptoms may include vomiting, abdominal cramps, and diarrhea (occasionally bloody). Vascular collapse, with or without other symptoms, can occur (anaphylactic shock). Reactions clinically indistinguishable from anaphylaxis can also occur when no allergic basis can be established for the reaction (idiopathic anaphylaxis or anaphylactoid reaction).

Management

The recommendations of the National Institutes of Health Task Force on Allergy for the initial management of anaphylaxis and anaphylactoid reactions are summarized in Table 23.10. Because bronchospasm, hypotension, and other hazardous manifestations can recur over a number of hours, the patient should either be hospitalized or kept under close observation during the 12 to 24 hours after anaphylaxis.

Avoidance of the offending substance is, of course, critical in patients with a history of anaphylaxis. The self-treatment kit described below under "Hymenoptera Venom Allergy" should be prescribed for patients who are at risk of recurrent accidental exposures.

Penicillin Allergy

Penicillin allergy is a common concern in ambulatory practice, where short courses of penicillin or one of the semisynthetic penicillins are often prescribed. The physician may be confronted with either of two problems.

The most common problem is the patient who needs penicillin and gives a history of penicillin allergy. For the infections treated in ambulatory practice, there is almost always a suitable alternative to a penicillin (throughout this book, the appropriate alternative is named wherever a penicillin is recommended). The most prudent strategy is to select an alternative drug whenever there is a possibility of prior penicillin allergy, even though this will lead to some unnecessary substitution, because almost half of patients giving a history of penicillin allergy do not in fact show allergic reactions when rechallenged with penicillin (10). In an ambulatory patient who has been labeled allergic to penicillin on the basis of an atypical allergic reaction, genuine penicillin allergy can be confirmed or excluded by skin testing, ideally using both major and minor determinant penicillin antigens (10); this may be particularly desirable in young adults who may be denied access to penicillin throughout their lives on the basis of unsubstantiated penicillin allergy. When such patients are seen in ambulatory practice, the best plan is to select alternatives to penicillin when antibiotics are needed and to refer them to an allergist for administration and interpretation of these critical skin tests. At present, the major determinant is available

Table 23.9. Causes of Anaphylaxis or Anaphylactoid Reactions[a]

Route of Administration[b]	Agent
Injection	Heterologous antisera
	Snake venom, rabies, diphtheria, antilymphocyte serum, antitumor antibody, clostridia
	Heterologous culture media of vaccines
	Flu, measles
	Antibiotics
	β-Lactam: penicillin, semisynthetic penicillins, cephalosporins
	Others: tetracyclines, aminoglycosides, chloramphenicol, amphotericin B, vancomycin, polymyxin, bacitracin
	Other drugs
	Protamine
	Venoms
	Hymenoptera
	Other: deer fly (*Chrysops discalis*), kissing bug (*Reduviidae*), snake, other insects, Gila monster
	Blood products
	Red blood cells
	Plasma factors: IgA, δ-globulin, clotting factors
	Hormones
	Insulins, ACTH, methylprednisolone,[c] progesterone[c]
	Enzymes
	Chymotrypsin, chymopapain, trypsin, penicillinase, L-asparaginase, streptokinase
	Allergen extracts
	Diagnostic
	Therapeutic
	Miscellaneous
	Dextran, dialyzer hypersensitivity
	Generalized anesthesia induction
	Thiobarbiturates, myorelaxants
Ingestants	Foods
	Nuts, berries, beans, legumes, seafood, many others
	Drugs
	Others
	Bee pollen tablets
Inhalant	Penicillin, cromolyn
	Polymerized corn starch powder
	Psyllium
Topical	Skin: antibiotics, certain physical stimuli, *p*-phenylenediamine, latex rubber
	Intravaginal: sperm and seminal products, latex condom
	Ophthalmic: fluorescein dye
	Rectal: latex tubing used for barium enema
Physical stimuli	Exercise, cholinergic, cold
Unknown	Idiopathic anaphylaxis, systemic mastocytosis
Miscellaneous	Echinococcus cyst

From Shatz GS. Anaphylaxis. In Korenblat PE, Wedner HJ, eds. Allergy theory and practice. 2nd ed. Philadelphia: WB Saunders, 1992.

IgA, Immunoglobulin A; *ACTH*, adrenocorticotropic hormone.

[a]Incomplete list.

[b]Certain antigens may have more than one route of administration.

[c]Immunologic mechanism possible but not proved.

commercially as Pre-Pen from the Schwarz Pharmaceutical Company. The minor determinant mixture is not available yet; until it is available, testing should be carried out with Pre-Pen and penicillin G at a concentration of 10,000 units/mL. This will detect 90% of penicillin-allergic patients.

Approximately half of patients with confirmed penicillin allergy also have positive skin tests to cephalosporins (10). Therefore, cephalosporin antibiotics should not be given to persons allergic to penicillin, and vice versa.

Less commonly, the physician in ambulatory practice will have to manage a first reaction to penicillin. Table 23.11 shows the approximate incidence of each of three types of allergic reactions (immediate, accelerated, and late) following either parenteral or oral administration of penicillin. The management of the more common late reactions (usually nonurticarial morbilliform rashes) is reassurance and a short course of an antihistamine if itching is a problem. The acute management of accelerated and immediate reactions is described in the preceding sections on urticaria and anaphylaxis. Long-term management requires ensuring that the patient and the immediate family know that all forms of penicillin and the related cephalosporin antibiotics should be avoided.

Ampicillin Rash

Ampicillin (and amoxicillin) commonly causes a *nonallergic maculopapular rash* that is not pruritic. The rash appears 48 to 72 hours after starting ampicillin. It occurs in approximately 9% of all patients given ampicillin and as many as 50% of patients with mononucleosis for whom ampicillin has been prescribed (5). The risk of developing this type of rash is also higher in patients with lymphatic leukemia and

Table 23.10. Treatment of Anaphylaxis or Anaphylactoid Reaction

When applicable, place tourniquet above site of injection or sting to obstruct venous return or stop the administration of the causative agent. Remove tourniquet temporarily every 10–15 minutes.

Place patient in recumbent position and elevate lower extremities.

Administer aqueous epinephrine 1:1000, 0.3–0.5 mL subcutaneously or intramuscularly (or if necessary 0.1 in 10 mL saline solution given intravenously over several minutes) and repeat as necessary.

When applicable, inject aqueous epinephrine 1:1000, 0.1–0.3 mL at the site of the injection.

Establish and maintain airway, first with oral airway. If necessary, use endotracheal tube.

Give oxygen as needed.

Monitor vital signs frequently.

If patient is not responding, give diphenhydramine hydrochloride (Benadryl), 50 mg intravenously over 3 minutes (maximum, 200 mg/kg in 24 hours).

If blood pressure cannot be obtained, give normal saline intravenously and maintain blood pressure with norepinephrine bitartrate (Levophed), 1 or 2 ampules (32 µg/min) in 500 mL of 5% glucose in water. Titrate to maintain blood pressure.

If severe asthma without shock give aminophylline, 500 mg intravenously over 10–20 minutes.

While corticosteroids will not be helpful for the acute anaphylaxis, they may prevent protracted anaphylaxis.

Modified from Asthma and the other allergic diseases, NIAID Task Force.

hyperuricemia and in those taking allopurinol. Rechallenge with ampicillin at a later time often causes no recurrence of the rash or other adverse reactions; therefore, a well-documented history of this kind of ampicillin rash is not a contraindication to subsequent ampicillin (or other penicillin) treatment.

Hymenoptera Venom Allergy

Stings by yellowjackets, hornets, honeybees, and wasps result in generalized allergic reactions of varying severity in approximately 0.4% of the population (5).

IgE-mediated hypersensitivity to these insect venoms may be confirmed by skin testings with suitable dilutions of available venoms; this is most appropriately done by an allergist. Because victims, unless already familiar with the distinguishing features of the various Hymenoptera, are often unable to tell bees from yellowjackets, hornets, or wasps, skin testing with individual venoms is particularly important. After a generalized allergic reaction to an insect sting has been treated (see above), the physician should immediately initiate a plan to protect the patient's future health. Avoidance of recurrent exposure is critical. Wearing shoes at all times is the single most important safeguard to the patient. However, because of the likelihood of reexposure, despite the patient's best efforts, the patient (and ideally a companion whenever the patient is outdoors) should know both the early signs of a generalized reaction and how to administer emergency treatment. An emergency self-treatment kit containing a syringe preloaded with epinephrine should be prescribed. An example is the Ana-Kit (Bayer), which contains a calibrated syringe that allows subcutaneous

administration of two measured doses (0.3 mL each) of epinephrine, two chewable 4 mg tablets of chlorpheniramine, two sterile swabs, a tourniquet, and instructions. The Epi-Pen and Epi-Pen Jr. kits (Center Laboratories) provide a single 0.3- or 0.15-mg dose of epinephrine, respectively, in an automatic injector, which some patients may prefer. It is prudent for general physicians to be familiar with one of these kits, to keep one in the office, and to review its use with any susceptible patient.

Any adult patient with sensitivity to one of these venoms confirmed by skin testing who has had a history of a potentially life-threatening reaction has a greater than 50% chance of a similar reaction if stung again and should therefore be offered immunotherapy with the venoms to which he or she is reactive. Such treatment is analogous to that described above for seasonal allergy; it reduces the likelihood of a future severe reaction to less than 5%. Once immunotherapy is instituted for insect venom hypersensitivity, it must be maintained through the use of booster injections at 4- to 6-week intervals for a minimum of 5 years. Children through age 16 whose systemic reactions have been confined to the skin (urticaria or angioedema) have a 10 to 20% risk of future systemic reactions of similar or milder type, and a minuscule risk of a more severe reaction. Therefore, in this group of patients, immunotherapy may be offered but may be of small benefit (11).

Even patients who do not have life-threatening generalized reactions (i.e., those who have urticaria/angioedema or other cutaneous symptoms) may be at increased risk of a more severe reaction on reexposure; therefore, such patients also should be referred to an allergist for skin testing and for a careful explanation of the available methods of protection (immunotherapy or an emergency self-treatment kit). Patients whose reactions have been toxic but local (confined to an area contiguous to the site of the sting) are not considered candidates for immunotherapy, even if the reaction is large.

Food Allergy

The gastrointestinal tract is sufficiently permeable to antigens found in food that some people experience one or more manifestations of allergy after the ingestion of a food to which they have become sensitive. Clinically apparent food allergy is much more common in young children than in adolescents or adults. In adults, food allergy usually manifests as urticaria/angioedema or anaphylaxis minutes to hours after ingestion of food. In children (particularly those sensitive to cow's milk), rhinitis, eczema, asthma, and colic may also occur. The most common causes of food allergy are listed in Table 23.12. Allergy to shellfish has nothing to do with susceptibility to the nonimmunologic reactions to iodinated contrast materials seen after administration of these materials (see below).

Evidence of sensitization to foods can be detected by *skin testing*. However, it has been established that only

50 to 60% of subjects with positive skin puncture tests have a reaction on double-blind food challenge. Conversely, virtually no patients with negative skin tests have been found to have positive responses to placebo-controlled, double-blind challenge. Thus, although the puncture test is useful for screening, the placebo-controlled, double-blind food challenge is the definitive test for establishing the diagnosis of food allergy. A blind challenge should not be carried out when an anaphylactic reaction is thought to be caused by a particular food because of the potential danger of the reaction.

There is no good evidence for non–antibody-mediated food hypersensitivity, although some practitioners believe that a variety of unorthodox techniques can substantiate antibody-independent food sensitivity. Various symptoms, including hyperactivity, depression, difficulty in concentration, and memory loss, have been blamed on food allergy. Evidence to support such notions consists of uncontrolled observations by physicians who strongly believe in the existence of such entities.

The management of food allergy is avoidance and, in selected instances, prescription of and education about self-treatment kits (see above). Although no evidence exists that food sensitivity can be neutralized by injections of tiny concentrations of food extracts or by the sublingual administration of drops of food extract, at least one experimental immunotherapy protocol attempting to reduce anaphylactic sensitivity to peanuts is in progress in the United States, with promising preliminary results.

Reactions to Iodinated Contrast Materials

Patients receiving intravenous iodinated contrast materials may develop one of three reactions that resemble allergic reactions. Neither IgE-mediated allergy nor other immunologic mechanisms have been found to explain these reactions, although complement activation may be shown in vitro. The three types of reaction are

- *Rash.* Onset of urticaria/angioedema, usually accompanied by generalized itching.
- *Anaphylactoid.* Cough, dyspnea, wheezing, syncope, with or without urticaria/angioedema.
- *Vasomotor.* An exaggerated response to dye injection, with more than the usual amount of flushing

and nausea, often accompanied by a sensation of numbness and tingling of the extremities and transient hypotension of a mild degree.

It has been estimated that there is a 1 to 2% risk of developing one of these reactions in the general population and an approximately 35% risk in patients with a history of a reaction (5). At present, there is no method such as a skin test or a small trial dose to prospectively identify the patient at risk. There is no evidence that a history of allergy to iodides or seafood predisposes a patient to a reaction to contrast media.

Management of the acute reaction is similar to that described for generalized allergic reactions. The patient should be carefully educated about the risk of recurrence, and repeated studies with iodinated contrast materials should be avoided whenever possible. In the event that a patient with a history of a reaction (either urticaria/angioedema or anaphylactoid) must undergo a later study, the following regimen should be followed: prednisone, 50 mg, by mouth 13, 7, and 1 hour before the procedure; diphenhydramine, 50 mg, and ephedrine, 25 mg, by mouth 1 hour before the procedure. This regimen reduces but does not entirely eliminate the risk of a subsequent reaction (3).Use of newer (and costlier) nonionic contrast agents is said to reduce reaction risk significantly (12).

Reactions to Aspirin and Other NSAIDs

Aspirin (acetylsalicylic acid) and other NSAIDs can produce urticaria/angioedema, an anaphylactoid reaction, or mild to severe asthma (usually in association with rhinorrhea, described above) in susceptible subjects. These reactions usually occur in patients with a history of some type of allergy. It has been estimated that the respiratory tract manifestations of aspirin sensitivity may develop in up to 10% of asthmatic patients (5); the problem is particularly common in patients with both bronchial asthma and nasal polyps.

IgE-mediated allergy to aspirin has not been demonstrated. Further evidence against an allergic basis is the fact that affected patients, when tested, show similar reactions to other NSAIDs (see description of these drugs in Chapter 70) not related antigenically to aspirin. The yellow food-coloring dye tartrazine (used in some foods, beverages, and medications) may also elicit urticaria in NSAID-sensitive patients.

The first generalized or respiratory tract reaction to

Table 23.11. Estimated Incidence of Allergic Reactions to Penicillin[a]

Type of Reaction	Manifestations	Time of Occurrence after First Dose of Penicillin	Percentage of Treated Patients Showing Reaction
Late reactions	Skin rash	≥72 hr	1.4
Accelerated reactions	Urticaria	1–72 hr	0.3
Immediate reactions	Generalized urticaria	2–30 min	0.3
	Anaphylaxis	2–30 min	0.04
	Anaphylactic deaths[b]		0.001

[a]Modified from Asthma and the other allergic diseases, NIAID Task Force Report. NIH pub. no. 79-387, May 1979.

Results are based on 70 to 80 million therapeutic courses of penicillin or semisynthetic penicillin or cephalosporin given per annum in the United States.

[b]From 400 to 800 deaths per year in the United States.

Table 23.12. Foods that Most Often Cause Allergic Reactions

Most Common
Seafood
Eggs
Nuts
Seeds

Others
Milk
Chocolate
Grains (barley, rice, wheat)
Fruits (citrus, melons, bananas, strawberries)
Vegetables (tomatoes, celery, spinach, corn, potatoes, soybeans)

Table 23.13. Aspirin Preparations and Some Commonly Purchased Aspirin-Containing Products

Alka-Seltzer[a]	Excedrin[a]
Anacin[a]	Fiorinal
Anahist	Goody's Headache Powders[a]
Arthritis Pain Formula[a]	Measurin
Ascodeen-30	Midol[a]
Ascriptin[a]	Momentum Muscular Backache Formula[a]
Aspergum[a]	Pabirin
Bayer Aspirin[a]	Panalgesic[a]
Bufferin[a]	Percodan
Cama Inlay-Tabs[a]	Persistin
Cirin	Phenaphen
Congesprin[a]	Quiet World Analgesic/Sleeping Aid[a]
Cope	Rhinex
Coricidin[a]	St. Joseph Cold Tablets for Children[a]
Darvon Compound	Sine-Off Tablets, Aspirin Formula[a]
Dristan[a]	Stanback[a]
Duradyne DHC Tablets	Stero-Darvon
Duragesic Tablets	Supac
Easprin	Synalgos
Ecotrin[a]	Triaminicin[a]
Empirin	Vanquish[a]
Emprazil	Viro-Med[a]
Equagesic	4-Way Cold Tablets[a]

[a]Over-the-counter.

aspirin or another NSAID usually occurs in adulthood, most typically a number of years after the onset of asthma (7). Symptoms may occur immediately after ingestion of aspirin or another NSAID or a number of hours later. Because of this delay, the role of aspirin or another NSAID may be overlooked by the patient; therefore, any patient with an unexplained generalized reaction or the onset or exacerbation of the respiratory tract symptoms described above should be questioned about the use of aspirin or one of the other NSAIDs.

The management of the generalized reactions in these patients is the same as that described for urticaria/angioedema and for anaphylaxis. Management of acute respiratory tract symptoms is similar to that described for allergic/nonallergic rhinitis and that described in Chapter 55 for acute asthma. Avoidance of NSAIDs and of products containing aspirin (Table

23.13) is essential after the diagnosis has been established. Affected patients should be explicitly instructed to use only acetaminophen (Tylenol or a generic) when they need a mild analgesic or antipyretic. An oral desensitization regimen using aspirin has been reported to lessen chronic nasal and sinus symptoms in some aspirin-sensitive patients. This regimen should be regarded as experimental and should not be undertaken in the ambulatory patient or in the hospitalized patient without expert consultation.

General References

deShazo RL, Smith DL, eds. Primer on allergic and immunologic diseases. 3rd ed. JAMA 268(20):2785–2996, 1992.
> Intended as a survey, aimed primarily at physicians early in their training.

Kaplan AP, ed. Allergy. 2nd ed. Philadelphia: WB Saunders, 1997.
> Authoritative and current text, especially accessible to the nonallergist.

Middleton E Jr, Reed CE, Ellis EF, eds. Allergy: principles and practice. St. Louis: CV Mosby, 1983.
> A two-volume compendium with chapters by many authorities. It is worthwhile to read on a given topic both in this and in Samter (see below), as the viewpoints are often complementary.

Samter MD, ed. Immunological diseases. 5th ed. Boston: Little, Brown, 1995.
> Authoritative, fact-filled text, with a little more emphasis on basics.

Specific References

1. Broder I, Higgins MW, Mathews KP, Keller JB. Epidemiology of asthma and allergic rhinitis in a total community, Tecumseh, Michigan. J Allergy Clin Immunol 54:100, 1974.
2. Graft DG, Valentine MD. Immunotherapy. In: Kaplan AP, ed. Allergy. New York: Churchill Livingstone, 1985.
3. Greenberger PA, Patterson R, Radin RC. Two pretreatment regimens for high-risk patients receiving radiographic contrast media. J Allergy Clin Immunol 74:540, 1984.
4. Horowitz JD, Howes LG, Christophidis N, et al. Hypertensive responses induced by phenylpropanolamine in anorectic and decongestant preparations. Lancet 1:60, 1980.
5. NIAID Task Force Report. Asthma and the other allergic diseases. NIH publication no. 79-387, May 1979.
6. Rhoades RB, Leifer KN, Cohan R, Wittig HJ. Suppression of histamine-induced pruritus by three antihistamine drugs. J Allergy Clin Immunol 55:180, 1975.
7. Samter M, Beers RF Jr. Intolerance to aspirin. Clinical studies and consideration of its pathogenesis. Ann Intern Med 68:975, 1968.
8. Sheffer AL, Fearon DT, Austen KF. Hereditary angioedema: a decade of management with stanozolol. J Allergy Clin Immunol 80:855, 1987.
9. Stewart TW Jr. Vasomotor rhinitis: neglected cause of nasal congestion. Postgrad Med 67:171, 1980.
10. Sullivan TJ, Wedner HJ, Shatz GS, et al. Skin testing to detect penicillin allergy. J Allergy Clin Immunol 68:171–180, 1981.
11. Valentine MD. Anaphylaxis and stinging insect hypersensitivity. JAMA 268:2830, 1992.
12. Wolf GL, Mishkin MM, Roux SG, et al. Comparison of rates of adverse drug reactions: ionic contrast agents, ionic agents combined with steroids, and nonionic agents. Invest Radiol 26:404, 1991.

C H A P T E R   24

Undifferentiated Acute Febrile Illness

NATHANIEL F. PIERCE, MD

Acute febrile illnesses are common and have many possible causes, ranging in significance from trivial to life threatening. For those that require treatment, accurate diagnosis is needed to guide the choice of therapy. In most instances, fever is accompanied by localizing complaints or physical findings that suggest specific diagnoses and guide decisions about diagnostic studies or treatment. Thus, for example, fever plus flank pain suggests the diagnosis of urinary tract infection, indicates the need for a urinalysis, and is likely to require antibiotic therapy.

A more difficult problem is posed, however, when fever occurs as an isolated complaint or is accompanied only by nonspecific constitutional symptoms, such as chills, malaise, anorexia, or modest weight loss. Although such acute undifferentiated febrile illnesses may raise the fear of serious illness for both patient and physician, most are benign and resolve spontaneously in 2 weeks or less, without a specific diagnosis being made. In very few instances do undifferentiated febrile illnesses persist and remain unexplained despite continued careful observation of the patient and the performance of routine diagnostic laboratory tests. Only when fever has lasted at least 3 weeks in such patients should it be designated fever of unknown origin (FUO). Patients with FUO require more extensive diagnostic evaluation, sometimes in the hospital.

This chapter describes a rational approach to the diagnosis and management of acute undifferentiated febrile episodes, emphasizing a balance between cautious observation and active investigation.

NORMAL TEMPERATURE RANGE

In most healthy people, the normal oral temperature varies between 96.5°F (35.8°C) and 99°F (37.2°C), the lowest value occurring between 2 and 4 AM, and the highest between 6 and 10 PM. In very hot weather, a person's temperature may be 0.5° to 1°F (0.3° to 0.6°C) higher than normal. Vigorous exercise, such as marathon running, also causes the temperature to rise temporarily.

ETIOLOGIC CONSIDERATIONS

Infections

Infection is the most common cause of acute undifferentiated fever; however, other causes are possible. Most episodes of undifferentiated fever caused by infection are self-limited, eventuate in complete recovery without treatment, and are likely to be caused by a virus. The viral agents that cause these episodes are rarely identified, and attempts to identify causative viruses are not usually warranted.

For certain infections that begin as undifferentiated fever, diagnostic signs or symptoms develop after one or several days. These include a number of common benign conditions, as well as uncommon conditions, some of which require prompt diagnosis and treatment. Most common among these are viral infections such as infectious mononucleosis (see Chapter 53), viral hepatitis (see Chapter 43), varicella (chickenpox), rubeola (measles), rubella (German measles), and recent human immunodeficiency virus (HIV) infection (see Chapter 34); rickettsial infections, such as Rocky Mountain spotted fever and Q fever; Lyme disease, a spirochetal infection transmitted by deer ticks (see Chapter 30); a variety of localized bacterial infections, such as those involving the pleura, biliary tract, retroperitoneum, urinary tract, liver, and spleen; and several bacteremic infections, especially acute bacterial endocarditis and *Salmonella* bacteremia. If there has been recent travel to certain developing countries (see Chapter 33), the list of etiologic considerations should include malaria, dengue fever, scrub typhus, and leptospirosis, and the possibility of viral hepatitis and *Salmonella* bacteremia is increased. Table 24.1 summarizes salient features of important infections that may present with acute undifferentiated fever and that are not discussed elsewhere in this text.

Drugs

A small portion of acute undifferentiated febrile episodes in ambulatory patients is caused by hypersensitivity to drugs. Almost any drug can cause fever, but digitalis preparations and insulins almost never do. Those most often responsible are listed in Table 24.2. Fever may begin promptly after starting the drug or may be delayed by several weeks; however, a drug taken regularly for 3 months or longer is unlikely to cause

Table 24.1.   Some Acute Nonbacterial Infections for Which Undifferentiated Fever May Be the First Manifestation

Infection	Transmission	Incubation Period (days)	Clinical Features
Chickenpox (varicella)	Person-to-person via respiratory secretions and direct contact; highly contagious	10–21	Malaise and fever precede or occur simultaneously with rash. Rash develops in crops as pruritic maculopapules evolving in hours to vesicles and in days to dried scabs. All stages of rash are seen in the same skin area.
German measles (rubella)	Person-to-person via respiratory secretions and direct contact; highly contagious	14–21	1- to 7-day prodrome of malaise, headache, fever, mild conjunctivitis followed by maculopapular (occasionally confluent) rash that begins on forehead and spreads to trunk and extremities.
Leptospirosis (*Leptospira interrogans*)	Reservoir: wild and domestic animals. Contact of the skin, especially if abraded, or of mucous membranes, with water, moist soil, or vegetation contaminated with urine of infected animals, as in swimming or accidental or occupational immersion	4–19	Fever with sudden onset, headache, chills, severe myalgia (calves and thighs), and conjunctival suffusion. Other manifestations that may be present are diphasic fever, meningitis, rash (palate, exanthem), hemolytic anemia, hemorrhage into skin and mucous membranes, hepatorenal failure, jaundice, mental confusion/depression, and pulmonary involvement with or without hemoptysis. Specific treatment: penicillins, cephalosporins, erythromycin.
Measles (rubeola)	Person-to-person via respiratory secretions	9–11	3- to 4-day prodrome with fever, malaise, hacking cough, rhinitis, subsiding 1–2 days after onset of maculopapular rash spreading from face to neck to trunk, to feet (by third day).
Q fever (*Rickettsia burnetii*)	Spread by airborne rickettsiae in dust contaminated by infected animals (cattle, sheep, goats) or by direct contact with infected animals or their tissue	14–26	Headache, chills, fever, anorexia, myalgias lasting 3 days to 2 weeks. Cough with rales after a few days, persisting after fever remits. Treated with tetracycline or chloramphenicol.
Rocky Mountain spotted fever (*Rickettsia rickettsii*)	Bite of infected tick or contamination with tick tissues or feces	3–14	Abrupt onset of severe headache, chills, myalgia, fever. Rash (second to fourth day of fever) initially *macules* on wrists, ankles, palms, soles, extending in 6–12 hours to buttocks, trunk, face; becomes *maculopapular* by day 2–3 and *petechial* by about day 4, progressing to ecchymoses. Rash may be missed on dark skin. Early treatment with chloramphenicol or tetracycline is life-saving.

Table 24.2.   Drugs that Often Cause Fever Due to Hypersensitivity

Allopurinol	Nifedipine
Amphotericin B	Nitrofurantoin
Antihistamines	*p*-Aminosalicylic acid
Atropine	Penicillamine
Barbiturates	Penicillins
Bleomycin	Phenolphthalein[b]
Captopril	Phenytoin
Cephalosporins	Procainamide
Clofibrate	Propylthiouracil
Ethambutol	Pyrazinamide
Heparin	Quinidine
Hydralazine	Salicylates[c]
Ibuprofen	Streptomycin
Iodides[a]	Sulindac
Isoniazid	Sulfonamides
Methyldopa	

[a] Including intravenous contrast media.
[b] Found in many nonprescription laxatives.
[c] When toxic levels occur.

fever. Drug fever may be low grade or may exceed 104°F (40°C). Chills are uncommon with drug fever, but their presence does not exclude this diagnosis. Urticaria, maculopapular skin rash, and eosinophilia occur in many cases. Rarely, hypersensitivity to commonly prescribed drugs may begin with fever, followed by the syndrome of *serum sickness* (rash, lymphadenopathy, arthritis, nephritis, edema); these drugs include barbiturates, methyldopa, penicillin, phenytoin, and sulfonamides. A lupuslike syndrome characterized by fever, arthralgias, and positive antinuclear antibody (ANA) titers may follow the initiation of hydralazine or procainamide. When a drug is the cause of a patient's fever, its removal is usually followed by defervescence in 1 to 2 days; however, fever may last up to 2 to 3 weeks if the drug is eliminated slowly (e.g., iodides). Readministration of the suspected drug usually causes fever within a few hours, thus confirming its causative role. This confirmatory test should be considered only if the drug is expected to be important for future therapy and the original febrile episode was not associated with organ damage.

An ambulatory patient may have *drug-induced fever caused by mechanisms other than hypersensitivity*, most of them rare. Temperature elevation caused by altered thermoregulation can occur because of direct effect on the central nervous system (amphetamines, cocaine, phenothiazines); decreased heat loss caused by diminished sweating, especially in the presence of high ambient temperature (drugs with anticholinergic activity); or hypermetabolism (monamine oxidase inhibitors, excessive thyroid hormone, cimetidine). Fever caused by the pharmacologic action of a drug may be seen in the Herxheimer reaction that follows antimicrobial treatment of syphilis or Lyme disease (see details in Chapter 30) and in association with chemotherapy that causes rapid destruction of tumor cells. Administration-related fever may occur after any intravenous infusion of a drug because of either contamination with bacterial pyrogens or phlebitis. In addition, repeated intramuscular injections at the same site can cause a sterile abscess that releases endogenous pyrogens.

Other Causes

Other acute processes that may cause undifferentiated fever include vascular occlusive or inflammatory events such as deep vein thrombophlebitis, minor pulmonary emboli, and asymptomatic myocardial infarction. Similarly, fever may be the only manifestation of acute hemolytic episodes, as occur in acute autoimmune hemolytic anemia or hemolytic anemia caused by glucose-6-phosphate dehydrogenase (G6PD) deficiency. Recent immunization with certain vaccines (see Chapter 32) may also cause fever. Leukopenia caused by medications such as ACE inhibitors, carbamazepine, ticlopidine, and antithyroid agents may present with undifferentiated fever.

High-Risk Patients

In patients with certain preexisting conditions, serious infections play an increased role in causing acute undifferentiated fever.

Patients with lymphomas or HIV infection and those receiving therapeutic dosages of corticosteroids (more than 20 mg/day of hydrocortisone or an equivalent dosage of another corticosteroid), especially if combined with other immunosuppressive agents, are at increased risk of developing primary or reactivation tuberculosis or other mycobacterial infections, acquiring or reactivating certain fungal infections (e.g., cryptococcosis, histoplasmosis, and coccidioidomycosis), reactivating certain viral infections (e.g., herpes zoster or cytomegalovirus infections), or developing infections caused by *Pneumocystis carinii* or *Toxoplasma*; the approach to these problems in patients with HIV infection is described in detail in Chapter 34.

Patients with established rheumatic valvular disease, certain types of congenital heart disease (e.g., ventricular septal defect, patent ductus arteriosus, or coarctation of the aorta), or prosthetic heart valves or vascular grafts are at increased risk of bacterial endocarditis (acute or subacute) or other endovascular infection.

Patients with multiple myeloma, surgical splenectomy, or autosplenectomy caused by sickle cell disease are at increased risk of serious spontaneous bacter-

emia, especially that caused by *Streptococcus pneumoniae, Haemophilus influenzae, Neisseria meningitidis,* or *Salmonella.* Patients with granulocytopenia (fewer than 1000 granulocytes/mm^3) are at increased risk of being bacteremic when febrile (see "Ambulatory Approach to Management" in Chapter 8).

Patients with advanced hepatic cirrhosis, especially when it is accompanied by ascites, may develop spontaneous bacterial peritonitis, often without localizing signs or symptoms. And patients who administer illicit drugs to themselves intravenously are at risk of developing bacterial sepsis, HIV infection, and hepatitis B or C because of nonsterile technique.

In other patients, especially elderly people, alcoholics, and those with diabetes mellitus, the usual signs and symptoms of some acute bacterial infections may be diminished or absent. Fever may be the only manifestation of pneumonia, empyema, or localized intra-abdominal infection in such patients, and the febrile response to these infections may be less than usually seen in younger nondiabetic or nonalcoholic patients.

Fever Lasting More Than 3 Weeks

The major causes of unexplained fever lasting more than 3 weeks differ appreciably from those described above. The most common causes are *(a)* chronic infections, especially tuberculosis, subacute bacterial endocarditis, chronic osteomyelitis, cytomegalovirus infections, occult intra-abdominal abscesses, urinary tract infections, and HIV infection; *(b)* collagen-vascular or rheumatic diseases, especially systemic lupus erythematosus, temporal arteritis, rheumatic fever, and rheumatoid arthritis; *(c)* certain neoplasms, especially lymphoma, acute leukemia, hypernephroma, hepatoma, pancreatic carcinoma, carcinoma of the lung, and malignancies involving bone; and *(d)* miscellaneous disorders such as granulomatous hepatitis, hyperthyroidism, drug fever, inflammatory bowel disease, sarcoidosis, thyroiditis, and recurrent pulmonary emboli.

Early diagnosis of these disorders is sometimes possible, especially when localizing symptoms or signs, or known risk factors, are present. Otherwise, these diagnoses are usually considered only when fever has been unexplained for at least 3 weeks despite preliminary diagnostic studies.

DIAGNOSTIC APPROACH
General Objectives

There are two general objectives in managing patients with acute undifferentiated fever: early diagnosis in the few instances of serious illness that require specific treatment, and the avoidance of unnecessary and expensive diagnostic studies and of blind therapy for the majority of patients whose course will prove benign and self-limited. The key to achieving these objectives is sequential evaluation, as summarized in Table 24.3 and described below.

Table 24.3. Acute Undifferentiated Febrile Illness: Summary of Sequential Evaluation Process

Evaluation Process	Comment
Initial Evaluation	
1. History, physical examination; if negative and not seriously ill, observe 7–10 days; *frequent phone contact*	Spontaneous defervescence common, benign illness common
2. More thorough evaluation of high-risk patients,[a] including laboratory studies	Increased risk that fever is caused by serious illness, usually infection
3. If seriously ill: more extensive laboratory studies; may need hospitalization and treatment	
Repeat Evaluations (at Weekly Intervals)	
1. Carefully repeated history and physical examination, expanded laboratory evaluation	Thorough reevaluation often detects cause of fever
2. Discontinue recent drugs, document fever	
After 3 Weeks	
1. Begin evaluation for true FUO, may include hospitalization	Spontaneous defervescence uncommon, fever usually caused by serious illness with substantial risk of mortality

[a]See text.

Initial Evaluation

The initial evaluation of most patients with an acute undifferentiated febrile illness requires about 15 minutes. A febrile illness is present if an oral temperature exceeding 99.5°F (37.6°C) is found on examination or by history. The evaluation of such patients should aim to detect signs, symptoms, or historical information that will identify the most likely reasons for the fever. A history of similar symptoms among others at home or at work suggests an infectious process. Fever with no other signs or symptoms in a patient recently started on a new drug, especially one known to cause fever (Table 24.2), suggests drug fever. If no localizing signs or symptoms are found and the patient does not seem seriously ill, no further evaluation is needed. The patient should be reassured and instructed to keep a record of morning and evening temperatures at home. A telephone call should be scheduled after 1 or 2 days as a simple means of following the course of the illness, detecting new complaints, and providing reassurance. If undifferentiated fever persists for 7 to 10 days, the patient should return for a thorough reevaluation.

Exceptions to this pattern of management are patients whose *constitutional symptoms are severe,* who have underlying conditions that predispose to serious infections or mask their manifestations (see above), who have been recently hospitalized or have undergone invasive diagnostic studies, or who describe fever of at least 2 weeks' duration when first seen. The initial evaluation of such patients should be expanded to include a thorough history and physical examination, as described below under "Reevaluation," and the following laboratory studies: chest radiograph with posteroanterior (PA) and lateral views, complete blood count (CBC) with differential, erythrocyte sedimentation rate, liver function tests, at least two blood cultures (aerobic and anaerobic), urinalysis, and quantitative urine culture if the urinalysis reveals pyuria or bacteriuria. Positive findings should be used to guide further studies or treatment. Patients with severe constitutional symptoms may require hospitalization and prompt antimicrobial therapy for possible bacteremia, especially if underlying conditions predisposing to bacteremia are present or hematologic findings suggestive of bacteremia are found (e.g., Döhle bodies or vacuoles in granulocytes, an increased erythrocyte sedimentation rate, or increased numbers of band-forms with an elevated or depressed total white blood cell count). If not hospitalized, such patients should be reevaluated daily by telephone or at an office visit until severe symptoms subside or the cause of fever is determined.

Reevaluation

Patients with unexplained fever that has lasted 1 week or more after the initial evaluation should be thoroughly reevaluated.

The *history* should be reviewed, including recent travel (especially to areas of poor sanitation; see Chapter 33, "Medical Advice for the International Traveler"), contact with people with infectious or febrile illnesses (especially hepatitis, mononucleosis, or HIV infection), drug use (including recently prescribed drugs, over-the-counter medications, and illicit drugs), alcohol abuse, homosexual activity, intravenous drug abuse, and familial disorders associated with fever or infection. The medical and surgical history should be explored. The review of systems should be repeated to detect any new complaints or subtle complaints missed at the initial evaluation. Seemingly trivial symptoms, such as vague abdominal discomfort, may prove of great value in localizing the cause of fever.

The *physical examination* should be meticulously reperformed. As with the history, subtle findings may prove invaluable. Essential procedures that are sometimes ignored, but should be included, are funduscopic examination (after dilating the pupils, if necessary); examination for a tender or enlarged temporal artery; search for a new or changing heart murmur; detection of an enlarged or tender thyroid gland; search for pericardial, pleural, or hepatic friction rubs; search for hepatomegaly or splenomegaly; detection of subtle abdominal or hepatic tenderness; examination of the rectum and prostate; pelvic examination; thorough search for lymphadenopathy including epitrochlear nodes; and examination of skin and mucous membranes (including conjunctivae) for petechiae and of nail beds for splinter hemorrhages.

Laboratory studies should also be initiated. A CBC, differential white blood cell count, and urinalysis should be performed. Additional studies should include a chest radiograph (PA and lateral views), erythrocyte sedimentation rate, serum alkaline phosphatase, serum aminotransferases, and a test for occult fecal blood. At least two blood cultures (each cultured aerobically and anaerobically) should be obtained. The urine should be cultured if pyuria or bacteriuria is observed. An intermediate-strength purified protein derivative (PPD) skin test should be applied unless there is a documented history of a positive PPD or of tuberculosis (see details for placing and interpreting PPD in Chapter 29). If there has been travel within 6 months to an area where malaria is endemic, appropriate blood smears should be examined (see other considerations related to fever after travel to developing countries in Chapter 33). Any medications started during the previous 2 months should be discontinued or, if that is not possible, replaced by chemically unrelated substitutes. This is especially important for the drugs listed in Table 24.2.

Patients whose fever remains unexplained after re-evaluation should chart their temperature at least twice daily for another full week. If unexplained fever persists, the history and physical examination should again be reviewed. Additional laboratory studies should include skin tests for cutaneous anergy (if intermediate PPD was negative), an electrocardiogram, serum calcium determination, serum titers of antistreptolysin O, rheumatoid factor, antinuclear antibody, HIV antibody, and a Monospot test. The CBC, differential white blood cell count, and urinalysis should be repeated.

If fever is still unexplained, temperature should be charted again for a full week. Documentation of temperature recordings by an independent observer is important to rule out *factitious fever.* Patients remaining febrile for at least 3 weeks after initial evaluation and lacking a recognized cause or provisional diagnosis despite the approach described above should be studied more extensively, usually in the hospital.

MANAGEMENT OF FEVER

Fever is not usually harmful, and *antipyretic therapy* is not often needed. Moreover, such treatment may confuse the clinical picture by altering the temperature pattern. In certain circumstances, however, control of fever is desirable. These include patients with severely compromised cardiac function in whom fever-associated tachycardia further stresses the heart and patients, such as alcoholics or those with dementia,

who develop increasing confusion or delirium when febrile. *Aspirin* is usually effective as an antipyretic but may cause an uncomfortable diaphoresis or precipitate shaking chills. These side effects can be minimized by giving 0.3 to 0.6 g aspirin regularly at 3- to 4-hour intervals. *Acetaminophen,* in similar dosage, may be used in patients who are allergic to aspirin, in patients with hemorrhagic diatheses, or in patients with a history of gastrointestinal bleeding or with poor tolerance of aspirin. Acetaminophen is preferred in teenage or younger children when there is a possibility that fever is caused by influenza or varicella infection; use of aspirin during these infections has been linked to the occurrence of Reye's syndrome.

Antimicrobial drugs have no place in the treatment of patients with acute undifferentiated fever, except in those who appear dangerously ill or who have seriously compromised defenses against infection. The premature use of antibiotics serves only to confuse interpretation of the patient's clinical course, add unnecessary expense, and risk the addition of drug toxicity to the patient's complaints. In most instances, antibiotics should be withheld until a diagnosis for which they are indicated is made.

The *daily activities* of febrile patients need not be severely restricted but should be moderated to provide additional rest, light meals, and the avoidance of strenuous or tiring tasks.

General References

Benenson AS, ed. Control of communicable diseases in man. 16th ed. Washington, DC: American Public Health Association, 1995.
> Periodically updated resource with systematically presented information on all communicable diseases.

Esposito AL, Gleckman RA. A diagnostic approach to the adult with fever of unknown origin. Arch Intern Med 139:575, 1979.
> This article includes initial evaluation of patients with acute undifferentiated fever as well as those with true fever of unknown origin.

Knockaert DC, Varmesti LJ, Bobbabis HJ. Recurrent or episodic fever of unknown origin: review of 45 cases and survey of the literature. Medicine 72:184, 1993.
> A review of episodic FUO, an entity more likely to be associated with uncommon diseases.

Larson EB, Featherstone HJ, Petersdorf RG. Fever of undetermined origin: diagnosis and follow-up of 105 cases, 1970–1980. Medicine 61:269, 1982.
> A follow-up of Petersdorf's original study on fever of unknown origin, documenting the changing diagnostic composition of this syndrome.

Lipsky BA, Hirschmann JV. Drug fever. JAMA 245:851, 1981.
> A concise review of the problem of drug fever, with typical clinical examples and guidelines for management.

MacKowick PA, LeMaistre F. Drug fever: a critical appraisal of conventional concepts. Ann Intern Med 106:728, 1987.
> A review of 148 episodes, with a valuable description of clinical features and causative agents.

Mellors JW, Horwitz RI, Harvey MR, Horwitz SM. A simple index to identify occult bacterial infection in adults with acute unexplained fever. Arch Intern Med 147:666, 1987.
> A valuable report on clinical and hematologic features that help to identify patients with acute unexplained fever caused by occult bacterial infection.

Petersdorf RG, Beeson PB. Fever of unexplained origin: report on 100 cases. Medicine 40:1, 1961.
> The classic study of fever of unknown origin.

CHAPTER 25

Bacterial Infections of the Skin

NATHANIEL F. PIERCE, MD

Most skin infections are trivial and can be managed at home without medical assistance. Each year, however, approximately 5% of the population develops a skin infection that requires medical attention. The severity of these infections depends on the virulence of the infecting organisms and the state of host defenses. The most common infecting organisms are *Streptococcus pyogenes* and *Staphylococcus aureus*. In otherwise healthy people these often cause only modest morbidity and respond rapidly to appropriate treatment. They can, however, cause serious infections, especially in diabetic patients, patients with impaired blood supply to or impaired lymphatic or venous drainage of the infected site, or patients with defects in leukocytic or immunologic defense mechanisms. Serious infection is also more likely when other bacteria, or combinations of bacteria, are involved, as occurs in bites or contaminated wounds.

SUPERFICIAL INFECTIONS CAUSED BY S. pyogenes AND S. aureus

Impetigo, ecthyma, and erysipelas are superficial infections usually caused by group A hemolytic strep-

tococci *(S. pyogenes)* and *S. aureus*. These infections arise from breaks in the skin that are often so minor they are unnoticed.

Impetigo

Impetigo occurs mostly among preschool children, especially in warm humid climates or when personal hygiene is poor. Under these conditions, the disease is highly contagious and outbreaks may occur. Older children and adults are only occasionally affected.

Impetigo *begins as a pruritic, focal, superficial eruption of small 1- to 2-mm vesicles,* often on the face near the nares, chin, or lower extremities. There is usually no history of trauma. In several days the vesicles change to pustules that break, become crusted, and have an erythematous base. Regional lymphadenopathy is common, but there are no constitutional symptoms. The process may spread because of scratching. Healing occurs without scarring. Impetigo may recur if personal hygiene is not improved.

A bullous form of impetigo is caused by *S. aureus.* It can cause epidemics among newborns, but occurs only sporadically among children; adult cases are uncommon. The process begins as a macular erythematous rash. The characteristic thin-walled, fluid-filled, superficial bullae appear within 1 to 3 days, range from 1 to several centimeters in diameter, and usually involve exposed areas of the body. These rupture, desquamation occurs, and healing without scarring follows in about 7 days. In its most dramatic form, this process causes the scalded skin syndrome, a disease of small children in which there is extensive superficial desquamation.

Ecthyma

Ecthyma occurs under the same conditions of poor hygiene that promote impetigo. It is characterized by 3- to 10-mm *discrete ulcerating lesions with an adherent necrotic crust and surrounding erythema;* a small amount of pus often underlies the crust. The ulcer is sufficiently deep to cause permanent scarring. Lesions are most common on the anterior tibial surface at sites of minor trauma or insect bites. Untreated, the lesions tend to spread distally and there may be associated lymphadenopathy; systemic symptoms, however, are lacking. Cultures of pus may yield both *S. pyogenes* and *S. aureus.* There is evidence that *S. aureus* may cause a majority of cases (3). Lesions with a similar appearance may result from bacteremia with *Pseudomonas aeruginosa.*

Erysipelas

Erysipelas involves progressive, often rapid spread of infection through superficial layers of skin and lymphatics. It may occur after a minor wound in normal skin but is more likely when prior injury or disease has impaired the lymphatic or venous drainage of the skin or left extensive scarring, as, for example, in a patient with chronic venous insufficiency of the lower extremities or with a radical mastectomy. Most episodes of erysipelas are caused by *S. pyogenes*. A few are caused by *S. aureus* or other agents, such as *Pasteurella multocida* or *Erysipelothrix rhusiopathiae* (see Table 25.4), and these cannot always be distinguished clinically.

Erysipelas is characterized by a *rapidly spreading area of marked erythema with warmth, local pain, an elevated sharp margin between involved and uninvolved skin, and firm edema that gives the skin a typical "orange peel"* appearance. There may be seropurulent drainage at the inoculation site, but fluctuation and dermal necrosis are lacking. Erythema often extends centrally along superficial draining lymphatics; regional lymph nodes are often enlarged and tender. Systemic toxicity, chills, and fever are common. If it is untreated, metastatic infection may occur, and there is appreciable mortality. Facial infections are especially dangerous because of possible intracranial spread via draining lymphatics or veins. Extensive involvement of the trunk also carries an increased risk of death.

Management

Bacterial cultures of the lesions of impetigo, bullous impetigo, and ecthyma are not usually helpful. Impetigo and ecthyma may reveal mixed cultures of *S. pyogenes* and *S. aureus,* or either agent alone, whereas lesions of bullous impetigo are often sterile. Blood cultures should be obtained when erysipelas is extensive or associated with marked systemic toxicity (e.g., temperature greater than 102°F [39°C], shaking chills, severe malaise). Attempts to isolate an organism by culturing sterile saline that has been injected and

Table 25.1. Antibiotic Selection for Superficial and Pustular Skin Infections

Infection	Antibiotic[a]	Route
Superficial Infections		
Impetigo	Mupirocin	Topical
	Dicloxacillin[b]	Oral
	Cephalexin[b]	Oral
	Erythromycin	Oral
Ecthyma	As for impetigo	
Erysipelas		
Mild	Penicillin V	Oral
	Erythromycin	Oral
Severe	Penicillin G	Intravenous
Pustular Infections		
Folliculitis	None	
Furunculosis, boils	Dicloxacillin[b]	Oral
	Cephalexin[b]	Oral
	Erythromycin	Oral
Bullous impetigo	As for furunculosis	Oral
Carbuncle	As for furunculosis	Oral
	Nafcillin	Intravenous
	Vancomycin	Intravenous
Cellulitis	As for carbuncle	

[a]Give a single antibiotic. Choices are in order of preference and include alternatives for patients allergic to penicillin. See the text for duration of therapy and adjunctive treatment. Dosage recommendations are in Table 25.2.
[b]Other penicillinase-resistant oral β-lactams may also be given.

Table 25.2. Antibiotic Dosage and Schedule for Skin Infections Caused by *S. pyogenes* and *S. aureus* in Adults[a]

Antibiotic	Dosage
Ambulatory Treatment	
Mild infection	
Mupirocin	2% ointment 2 times/day
Dicloxacillin	250 mg PO 3 times/day
Cephalexin	500 mg PO 4 times/day
Erythromycin	250–500 mg PO 3 times/day
Penicillin V	500 mg PO 3 times/day
Parenteral Treatment	
Severe infection	
Penicillin G	600,000–2,000,000 units IV q6hr
Nafcillin	1.0–1.5 g IV q4hr
Vancomycin	0.25–0.5 g IV q6hr

[a]Selection of antibiotics for specific infections is described in the text and summarized in Table 25.1. The duration of therapy is described in the text.

withdrawn at the edge of the lesion through a fine needle have a low yield, but may be helpful when usual treatment is ineffective (3). If there is seropurulent drainage at the site of inoculation, this should be cultured. Placing the culture swab in a transport medium, such as Carey–Blair medium, preserves the specimen until it reaches the diagnostic laboratory.

Antimicrobial therapy is required for all of these infections (Tables 25.1 and 25.2). To eradicate group A streptococci, antibiotic treatment should be given for 10 days, even though marked improvement may occur earlier.

Impetigo and ecthyma are treated similarly. Topical mupirocin is preferred, except for lesions of the scalp or mouth (2). Dicloxacillin, cephalexin, and other penicillinase-resistant β-lactams are effective oral antimicrobials. Erythromycin is also effective where *S. aureus* are sensitive to it. Adjunctive therapy includes careful daily soaking of lesions to remove crusted debris using warm water with an iodophor (a soap that releases iodine in a nontoxic, nonstaining form, e.g., Betadine skin cleanser) or with a soap that contains hexachlorophene (e.g., pHisoHex). Prevention depends primarily on improved personal hygiene; the most important preventive measure is careful frequent skin cleansing with soap and water.

Treatment of *bullous impetigo* should be directed at penicillin-resistant staphylococci. Oral dicloxacillin and cephalexin are effective; erythromycin is an alternative where *S. aureus* are sensitive to it.

Minor episodes of *erysipelas* may be treated with oral penicillin V or erythromycin. Application of moist heat to the affected area appears to hasten clearing of the infection. Serious episodes are those with marked systemic toxicity, extensive lesions, facial lesions, or those occurring in compromised hosts (e.g., diabetic patients). Such patients usually require hospitalization and treatment with penicillin G intravenously (Tables 25.1 and 25.2). Special attention should also be paid to patients with atherosclerotic peripheral vascular disease who have infections of their lower extremities. In such patients, the affected leg should be rested and elevated; sustained pressure on any part of the leg or foot should be avoided.

Patients with preexisting damage to the veins or lymphatics of an extremity may experience repeated episodes of erysipelas that cause further damage. Patients who have numerous recurrent infections should receive continuous antibiotic prophylaxis with penicillin V (250 mg twice daily), benzathine penicillin (600,000 units intramuscularly monthly), or erythromycin (250 mg twice daily). Reduction of chronic edema by fitted pressure stockings or by diuretics helps reduce susceptibility to this infection.

Superficial skin infections respond rapidly to appropriate therapy. Systemic toxicity and erythema associated with erysipelas usually abate within 3 or 4 days, and discrete skin lesions show marked healing within 10 days. During this period, activity should be restricted in accord with the extent of morbidity. Minor lesions require no restrictions. Patients with any form of impetigo should avoid contact with infants and small children until lesions heal.

Complications

Streptococcal skin infections do not cause rheumatic fever, but may cause *acute glomerulonephritis* if the streptococcal strain is nephritogenic. Nephritis is not prevented by antibiotic therapy. The average latency period between initial symptoms of a streptococcal skin infection and the onset of glomerulonephritis is 2 weeks. If a nephritogenic strain is known to be in the community, initial and 14-day follow-up evaluation should include a urinalysis. Most patients who develop poststreptococcal glomerulonephritis are asymptomatic, but in some, glomerulonephritis is first suggested by gross hematuria, acute hypertension, or signs of salt and water retention, such as dependent edema or congestive heart failure.

Bacteremia with metastatic infection may complicate neglected or severe episodes of erysipelas. Metastatic infection should be considered in patients with severe disease who respond poorly to treatment or develop findings suggestive of distant localized infection. Possible metastatic infections include meningitis, endocarditis, septic arthritis, infection of preexisting pleural effusions or ascites, or solid organ abscesses (e.g., in the liver or spleen).

PUSTULAR INFECTIONS CAUSED BY *S. aureus*

These include folliculitis, furunculosis, hydradenitis suppurativa, and carbuncles. They represent increasingly severe effects of the infection of hair follicles, sebaceous glands, or sweat glands by *S. aureus,* the result being inflammation and abscess formation.

Folliculitis

Folliculitis involves minor inflammation of individual hair follicles, often with formation of small superficial pustules. There is little pain or surrounding erythema. In some people, lesions may recur for months or even years. A common area of involvement is the bearded part of the face, in which minor trauma from shaving may be a contributing factor.

Furunculosis

Deeper infection of follicles or cutaneous glands leads to formation of pustular furuncles (boils are large furuncles). These range in diameter from about 5 mm to 2 to 3 cm and occur most commonly on hairy areas exposed to friction, trauma, or maceration (e.g., the buttocks, neck, face, axillae, groin, forearms, thighs, and upper back). Furunculosis may also complicate the acne of adolescence. Furuncles begin with pruritus, local tenderness, and erythema, followed by swelling and marked local pain. As pus forms in the center of the lesion, the overlying skin becomes thin, the lesion becomes elevated, pain increases, and spontaneous drainage of pus ultimately occurs, usually with prompt relief of pain and rapid healing. Furunculosis may be recurrent in some people, especially diabetic patients and chronic nasal carriers of *S. aureus.*

Hydradenitis Suppurativa

Hydradenitis suppurativa is caused by obstruction of apocrine sweat glands, usually in the axilla, perineum, or groin. The process is chronic, perpetuated in part by the scars, abscesses, and sinus tracts that develop in the involved skin.

Carbuncles

A carbuncle is a coalescent mass of deeply infected follicles or sebaceous glands with multiple interconnecting sinus tracts and cutaneous openings that drain pus ineffectively. Carbuncles usually occur in the thick skin on the back of the neck or the upper back. Once formed, the lesions steadily worsen, with increasing pain, erythema, swelling, purulent drainage, and lateral enlargement; they vary in diameter from 3 to 10 cm or larger. Fever and systemic toxicity are common. Carbuncles occur with increased frequency in diabetics and may recur in the damaged area of skin.

Management

Bacterial cultures of typical pustular lesions are usually unnecessary because virtually all are caused by *S. aureus* and most isolates prove resistant to penicillin G.

Minimal lesions, such as *folliculitis,* require little therapy. Careful, twice-daily cleansing with a mild soap, preferably one containing hexachlorophene, and avoidance of minor trauma and irritants, such as cosmetics or abrasive soaps, are usually sufficient.

Furuncles should be managed initially by gentle application of warm moist heat (either as moist compresses or baths) for about 30 minutes four times a day, and by immobilizing the affected area (e.g., splinting of digits, instructing the patient to avoid pressing on the furuncle). Lesions less than 1 cm in diameter often drain spontaneously after 1 to 3 days and require no further treatment. Larger lesions, painful lesions, or lesions that do not drain spontaneously should be *drained surgically when they are fluctuant.* This can be done in the office by making a single incision into the abscess with a scalpel, after first infiltrating the incision line with 0.5 or 1.0% lidocaine for local anesthesia. Lifting the anesthetized skin with a towel clip when the incision is made helps avoid pain caused by downward pressure from the scalpel. Packing with iodoform gauze for 1 or 2 days may be needed to control oozing of serosanguinous discharge after surgical drainage. Antimicrobial therapy is required only for extensive lesions such as multiple furuncles, carbuncles, or lesions associated with marked surrounding inflammation, or in diabetic patients. In such cases oral dicloxacillin or erythromycin (Tables 25.1 and 25.2) should be given until signs of inflammation completely subside, which may take 2 weeks or longer; when antibiotics are given, indurated furuncles often resolve without becoming fluctuant.

Carbuncles may require extensive surgical drainage, which can usually be done in an outpatient facility. Patients with severe systemic toxicity, such as diabetic patients with carbuncles, require hospital admission and parenteral therapy with a penicillinase-resistant penicillin; vancomycin is an effective alternative for those allergic to penicillin.

Recurrent furunculosis may prove a frustrating problem. Management of individual episodes is as described above, but other steps should also be taken to eliminate colonization with staphylococci. The anterior nares should be cultured. Patients whose nasal cultures contain *S. aureus* should be treated by application of mupirocin ointment to the anterior nares twice daily for 5 days (5). Alternatively, bacitracin ointment may be applied three or four times daily for 14 days. Prolonged therapy with bacitracin ointment may be needed if cultures become positive upon cessation of treatment. During topical treatment, bacterial contamination of skin should be meticulously controlled by having the patient bathe and shampoo three times daily with a hexachlorophene soap and by changing underclothing and bed and bath linens daily.

Recurrent furunculosis may occur in certain *disorders that impair host defenses.* Tests for diabetes mellitus should be made; if positive, control of blood glucose may prove beneficial (see Chapter 72). Defects in polymorphonuclear leukocyte function are a rare cause of recurrent furunculosis but should be considered in patients who show an increased incidence or severity of infections caused by staphylococci. Gram-negative bacteria and fungi may be cultured from the furuncles of such patients. If an unusual problem, such as a leukocyte defect, is suspected, the patient should be referred to a medical center with the capability to investigate such disorders.

Hydradenitis suppurativa is a difficult problem that requires prolonged, often lifelong treatment by multiple methods. These include selective surgical drainage of abscesses; elimination of irritants, such as tight clothing, antiperspirants, and shaving of the axillae; careful frequent cleansing of skin with antiseptic agents; local application of heat; intermittent or long-term systemic antibiotic therapy; and, in some cases, local irradiation or excisional surgery. Management of such patients is best done by physicians especially skilled in the treatment of skin disorders. (See additional discussion in Chapter 100, "Common Problems of the Skin.")

Complications

Staphylococcal skin infections may spread to other sites. This is especially true in patients with extensive inflammation and systemic toxicity, such as those with carbuncles, in whom bacteremia is common. Even an innocent appearing furuncle may, however, cause metastatic infection, especially in patients with a focus of increased susceptibility, such as a ventricular septal defect, an artificial heart valve, or an arthritic joint. Patients at risk of bacteremia who have such susceptible foci or whose systemic complaints (fever, focal pain) persist despite antibiotic treatment should be carefully examined for possible metastatic infection.

CELLULITIS AND WOUND INFECTIONS

Any break in the skin may become infected. This includes not only obvious trauma, such as lacerations, burns, abrasions, and animal or human bites, but also minor injuries such as scratches and insect bites. The features of the resultant infection vary widely and depend on the nature of the wound, the type of infecting organism, and the defensive responses of the infected person. In many instances, early appropriate management given on an ambulatory basis is sufficient. In others, recognition of serious infection and prompt hospitalization for vigorous medical or surgical treatment are of prime importance. Table 25.3 describes findings that require hospitalization or surgical intervention. Table 25.4 lists organisms that may cause life-threatening forms of cellulitis.

Cellulitis Caused by *S. pyogenes* and *S. aureus*

Acute cellulitis is a spreading infection of skin and subcutaneous tissues. The involved area, which en-

Table 25.3. Wound Infections: Findings that Necessitate Hospitalization or Surgical Intervention

Finding	Comment
Extensive cellulitis or erysipelas with systemic toxicity	Needs parenteral antibiotics, close observation
Diminished arterial pulse in cool, swollen, pale, infected extremity	Possible fasciitis, a surgical emergency
Cellulitis with cutaneous necrosis or subcutaneous gas	Needs parenteral antibiotics and possible surgical drainage/debridement
Closed space infection of the hand	Needs surgical drainage

Table 25.4. Causes of Life-Threatening Bacterial Cellulitis

Cause	Important Features
Gram-negative enteric bacilli, especially *Escherichia coli*	Occur in fecally contaminated wounds; gas may be present; surgical drainage required for gas or pus
Mixed anaerobic and enteric aerobic bacteria	Occur in fecally contaminated wounds; gas may be present; symptoms may progress rapidly and may include exquisite pain; surgical drainage required
Bacillus anthracis	Causes anthrax when minor wound is inoculated by spore-contaminated animal products (animal hides and hair, especially from goats); local chancrelike lesion develops followed by systemic toxicity
E. rhusiopathiae	Erysipelaslike lesion with central clearing; due to wound contamination with fish or meat products; treated with penicillin V or tetracycline
P. multocida	Erysipelaslike lesion that follows a dog or cat scratch or bite; treated with penicillin V or tetracycline
Marine vibrios	Necrotizing cellulitis after minor wound is contaminated by sea water or contact with shellfish
Aeromonas hydrophila	Wound contaminated by fresh water swimming

larges steadily, is painful, tender, and intensely erythematous. Chills and fever are common and bacteremia may occur. The lesion differs from erysipelas in that its margin is not as sharply demarcated, nor is it elevated. There may be purulent or serous drainage at the inoculation site; in severe cases, patches of involved skin may become necrotic.

The most common causes of acute cellulitis are *S. pyogenes* and *S. aureus*. Finding Gram-positive cocci in drainage from the wound is presumptive evidence that they are causative. Infection by these agents may progress rapidly, especially when it involves an area of chronic edema. Lower extremity infection in patients with peripheral arterial insufficiency may cause tissue necrosis and secondary infection.

Management of cellulitis should include culture of any wound drainage (as described for erysipelas) and prompt antibiotic therapy. In mild cases, treatment may be given on an ambulatory basis. The treatment should be effective for infections by penicillin-resistant staphylococci, as well as penicillin-sensitive streptococci. Oral dicloxacillin or cephalexin is adequate for infections caused by either type of organism; erythromycin is a suitable alternative for patients who are allergic to penicillin (Tables 25.1 and 25.2). Local application of moist heat is a useful adjunct to antibiotic treatment; care should be taken, however, to avoid causing burns, especially in patients with impaired sensitivity to pain. Improvement is usually apparent in

3 or 4 days; during this period, patients should rest the involved area (with elevation when the cellulitis involves an extremity) and be told to report promptly any worsening of the infection or of constitutional symptoms. Severe infections require hospitalization and parenteral treatment with a penicillinase-resistant β-lactam, such as nafcillin, or vancomycin. This includes patients with extensive lesions, lesions of the face, or serious toxicity.

Secondarily Infected Ulcers

Cutaneous ulcers are caused by a wide variety of conditions, including peripheral vascular disease, arterial insufficiency, pressure sores, and neurologic disorders. Management of the ulcer is generally aimed at the underlying cause and seeks to improve blood flow, reduce edema, and avoid pressure and trauma (see Chapter 88); control of secondary infection is also important. Superficial colonization with a variety of bacteria is unavoidable and without consequence; however, infection that is deeper or laterally invasive prevents healing and may interfere with other treatments, such as skin grafting. Infection is best controlled by repeated careful cleaning and local debridement. Systemic antibiotics should be used only when all other methods fail to control surrounding infection. The choice of antibiotic should be based on cultures of the wound or its purulent drainage. Local antibacterials are sometimes helpful. Those effective against a broad spectrum of bacterial agents include polymyxin–bacitracin–neomycin ointment and topical nitrofurazone (Furacin ointment); these should be applied three times daily until healing occurs or it is apparent that they are ineffective. Soaking with 3% acetic acid three to four times daily is helpful in controlling bacterial growth in ulcers colonized with *Pseudomonas aeruginosa*.

Cutaneous Diphtheria

Cutaneous ulcers or other skin lesions may become secondarily infected with *Corynebacterium diphtheriae,* causing cutaneous diphtheria. Although the cutaneous lesion may appear benign, myocarditis or neuropathy develops in approximately 3% of cases. Outbreaks have occurred in the northwest and southern parts of the United States, primarily among Native Americans or urban indigents. The presence of cutaneous diphtheria in a community should increase suspicion that skin wounds may harbor this agent. The diagnosis should be suspected when existing wounds develop a *gray-yellow or gray-brown covering membrane* and surrounding erythema (1). Typically, the membrane can be easily removed to reveal a clean base. Other minor skin lesions may also become infected. Typical organisms can be seen in methylene blue stains of smears from the wound and confirmed by culture on Loeffler's or tellurite agar. Presumptive cases should be reported to public health officials and treated with equine diphtheria antitoxin (20,000 to 40,000 units intramuscularly or intravenously after testing for hypersensitivity to horse serum) and either erythromycin (1.5 g/day, orally) or procaine penicillin (1.2 million units/day, intramuscularly) for 7 to 10 days.

Bites

Bite wounds become infected with the oral, salivary, or dental flora of the biting person or animal and may cause serious local or systemic infections. Initial management before signs of infection appear is of primary importance in preventing certain infections. Appropriate prophylaxis for tetanus is required for all bite wounds (see Chapter 32).

Human bites are contaminated with a complex variety of aerobic and anaerobic oral bacteria. Without treatment, a severe necrotizing cellulitis often results. Minor lesions that break the skin should be washed thoroughly and treated with a combination of dicloxacillin (250 mg three times a day) and ampicillin (500 mg three times a day) given orally, each for 7 days. Oral clindamycin (150 to 300 mg three times a day) is appropriate for patients who are allergic to penicillin. Antibiotics should be continued for 7 to 10 days. More severe wounds, including wounds of the hands and knuckles, require meticulous debridement and possible tendon repairs. These should be referred for surgical management.

Dog bites carry the risk of local soft tissue infection with various organisms, including *P. multocida*, and raise concern about rabies. Minor abrasions, shallow punctures, or superficial lacerations require no therapy for local infection other than thorough cleansing with soap and water. Puncture wounds should be irrigated vigorously with sterile saline injected through a 20-gauge needle. More extensive or deeper bites require surgical management for debridement and, in some cases, primary closure. Ampicillin (500 mg by mouth three times a day for 7 days) and dicloxacillin (250 mg by mouth three times a day for 7 days) should be given for bites of the hands or face. The same treatment is appropriate for patients who have signs of soft tissue infection when first seen. Patients with hand infection require surgical management and intensive antibiotic therapy.

Rabies precautions should be taken with all dog bites, including bites by domestic pets, even though the risk of rabies from domestic pets—especially when biting was provoked—is very small (4). The dog should be quarantined for 10 days. If the dog's owner cannot be identified, the local health department should be called to take charge of the dog. If its owner is known, it may be observed at its home. If it remains well, there is no risk of rabies. If the dog develops neurologic symptoms or dies, its brain should be examined immediately; prophylaxis is required if evidence of rabies is found. If the dog escapes after biting, and especially if the bite was unprovoked, rabies prophylaxis with human rabies immune globulin and human diploid cell rabies vaccine is indicated (see Chapter 32).

Bites by other domestic animals (e.g., cats) should be managed in the same way as dog bites. Bites by some wild animals carry a greater risk of rabies and are treated similarly, except that rabies prophylaxis is usually required (unless the animal's brain can be examined). Wild animals with the greatest risk of carrying rabies are raccoons, skunks, foxes, coyotes, and bats. The risk of rabies with rodent bites, including squirrel bites, is very small; the local health department should be consulted regarding the need for rabies prophylaxis after a rodent bite.

Guidance on the use of rabies prophylaxis, management of the biting animal, and the risk of rabies among various animal species should be sought from local or state health authorities.

Puncture Wounds

Most puncture wounds involve the feet or hands and may introduce infecting bacteria that cannot be removed by washing or debridement. In all instances, patients should receive appropriate prophylaxis for tetanus (see Chapter 32). *Low-risk wounds* (i.e., those not likely to be contaminated by soil or fecal material and in which the wound site is healthy, well-vascularized tissue) need only be thoroughly washed and observed for several days for signs of developing infection. Should infection develop, any wound drainage should be cultured and treatment begun with dicloxacillin (250 mg three times daily) or erythromycin (250 to 500 mg three times daily) for presumptive staphylococcal or streptococcal infection; the wound site should also be soaked in warm soapy water for 30 minutes at least four times a day. *Higher-risk wounds* (i.e., those likely to be contaminated with fecal material, soil, or foreign debris, or occurring in a diabetic person or in an extremity with an inadequate blood supply) should be treated from the outset with a broad-spectrum antibiotic (in adults, ciprofloxacin 750 mg every 12 hours or another quinolone; in children under 15 years, one of the antibiotics above), and the wound site should be rested and treated with warm soaks as above. The patient should promptly report any evidence of inflammation, swelling, or persisting pain. If purulent drainage develops, this should be cultured. Antibiotic management should be altered if bacteria resistant to the current treatment are isolated. If pus develops, surgical drainage is usually required.

Felon

A felon is an infection of the pulp of the distal phalanx of a finger, usually following a recognized local wound. Abscess formation and tissue necrosis are common, and bony or articular involvement may occur. If the felon is neglected or inadequately treated, severe damage, including loss of function, may occur. The most common causative agents are *S. aureus* and *S. pyogenes,* although Gram-negative bacilli may also be recovered. Treatment involves surgical drainage by a physician who is familiar with the procedure. Concurrent antibiotic therapy should be guided by Gram's stain and culture of infected material.

Paronychia

A paronychia is an infection, often chronic or recurrent, that involves tissue immediately adjacent to a fingernail or toenail. The affected tissue is warm, tensely swollen, erythematous, and painful. When infection is chronic, the nail may become ridged or discolored and may be lost. Paronychia occur most often in people who bite their nails excessively or whose hands are frequently in water (e.g., dishwashers or mothers of infants). Diabetic patients also have an increased risk of this infection. *Candida* species appear to play an etiologic role, although a variety of bacteria are also usually present. Management involves keeping hands as dry as possible (e.g., using waterproof gloves for dishwashing) and applying an anticandidal medication (e.g., nystatin cream) or a broad-spectrum antifungal (clotrimazole or miconazole cream) two times a day for several weeks. When localized swelling does not respond to these measures, drainage may be helpful. This can be done by sliding an 18-gauge needle, bevel down, along the nail into the involved area. Lifting the skin from the nail with the needle usually achieves drainage and relief of pain.

The major cause of paronychia of the toe (usually a great toe) is an ingrown toenail. Diagnosis and management of this problem are described in Chapter 102.

Intertriginous Infections

Approaches to diagnosis of infections involving moist intertriginous areas (toe webs, axillae, groin area) are described in Chapter 100.

General References*

McDonough JJ, Stern PJ, Alexander JW. Management of animal and human bites and resulting human infections. Curr Clin Top Infect Dis 3:11, 1987.
> A thorough review of the subject.

Sapico FL, Witte JL, Canawati HN, et al. The infected foot of the diabetic patient: quantitative microbiology and analysis of clinical features. Rev Infect Dis 6(Suppl 1):S171, 1984.
> A careful study of infected foot ulcers showing that anaerobes outnumbered aerobes, the most common being *Bacteroides* species, anaerobic streptococci, and *Clostridium* species.

Schachner L, Taplin D, Scott GB, Morrison M. A therapeutic update of superficial skin infections. Pediatr Clin North Am 30:397, 1983.
> An excellent review.

Witkowski JA, Parish LL. Bacterial skin infections. Management of common streptococcal and staphylococcal lesions. Postgrad Med 72:166, 1982.
> A practical review of the features and treatment of these infections, with excellent photographs of typical infections.

Specific References

1. Belsey MA, Sinclair M, Roder MR, LeBlanc DR. *Corynebacterium diphtheriae* skin infections in Alabama and Louisiana: a factor in the epidemiology of diphtheria. N Engl J Med 280:135, 1969.
2. Dagan R, Bar-David Y. Double-blind study comparing erythromycin and mupirocin for treatment of impetigo in children: implications for a high prevalence of erythromycin-resistant *Staphylococcus aureus* strains. Antimicrob Agents Chemother 36:287, 1992.
3. Hook EW, Hooton TM, Horton CA, et al. Microbiologic evaluation of cutaneous cellulitis in adults. Arch Intern Med 146:297, 1986.
4. Rabies prevention: United States. MMWR 38:205, 1989.
5. Scully BE, Briones F, Gu J, Neu HC. Mupirocin treatment of nasal staphylococcal colonization. Arch Intern Med 152:353, 1992.

---

*Bold print (general references) and bold numerals (specific references) denote published controlled clinical trials, meta-analyses, or consensus-based recommendations.

C H A P T E R   26

Acute Gastroenteritis and Associated Conditions

RICHARD G. BENNETT, MD

Acute symptoms of gastroenteritis may follow the ingestion of a wide variety of infectious and chemical agents. Ingestion may occur because of direct person-to-person contact or, more commonly, via contaminated food or water. In addition, the ability of viral enteropathogens to spread by air transmission has recently been established (6). With several important exceptions, the acute illnesses caused by these agents are characterized by diarrhea, with or without other gastrointestinal symptoms (nausea, vomiting, abdominal pain) or systemic symptoms and signs (anorexia, fever, malaise, orthostatic hypotension, neurologic deficits).

Diarrhea is defined as an increase in the number or volume of bowel movements, which are usually fluid (see Chapter 39). The diarrhea of gastroenteritis usually begins abruptly, sometimes preceded by systemic symptoms, and the hour of onset can typically be documented by the patient. With few exceptions, the illness is self-limited and terminates within 1 to 5 days.

Tables 26.1 (infectious agents) and 26.2 (chemical agents) summarize the etiologic agents, pathophysiology, clinical and epidemiologic features, and principles of diagnosis and treatment for conditions that may occur in the United States.

EPIDEMIOLOGY

Incidence and Distribution

The incidence of the conditions listed in Tables 26.1 and 26.2 varies from year to year; and the true incidence is never known because a large proportion of cases are not reported to physicians or health authorities. Of 2423 reported outbreaks investigated by the United States Centers for Disease Control and Prevention (CDC) between 1988 and 1992, the *cause* was established for only 1001 (41%). This reflects the current limitations in diagnostic capabilities, particularly for identifying the viral pathogens thought likely to cause many outbreaks. Based on annual surveillance by the CDC, it is known that the greatest number of reported foodborne outbreaks are caused by *Salmonella* spp., followed by *Clostridium botulinum, Staphylococcus aureus,* and *Clostridium perfringens.* The relative numbers of outbreaks do not necessarily correlate with the number of people affected by a specific enteropathogen. Table 26.3 summarizes for the period 1988 through 1992 the number of outbreaks, cases, and deaths resulting from the eight most commonly identified bacteria in investigations of foodborne outbreaks, as well as the average number of cases per outbreak and overall case-fatality rates. The magnitude of disease related to enterohemorrhagic *Escherichia coli* (i.e., strains such as *E. coli* O157:H7 that produce a potent cytotoxin known as verotoxin, or Shiga-like toxin) may have stabilized since this organism was first identified as a human pathogen in 1982. *E. coli* O157:H7 came to national attention during the first 2 months of 1993, when 500 cases were reported from the western United States resulting from a large outbreak related to contaminated hamburger meat eaten at fast-food restaurants (11). Further large-scale outbreaks have not been reported, perhaps as most fast-food restaurants now always cook hamburgers until well done. A recent report showed that *E. coli* O157:H7 was isolated most commonly from visibly bloody stool specimens that yielded a bacterial enteropathogen (37). Although the most common pathogen isolated in waterborne outbreaks is *Giardia,* a large outbreak related to *Cryptosporidium* resulted in 1993 from contamination of the public water supply in Milwaukee, Wisconsin.

Outbreaks unrelated to contaminated food or water and resulting from viral enteropathogens occur most often within institutional settings (e.g., day-care centers and nursing homes) and during the winter.

Studies of outbreaks of *viral gastroenteritis* in adults have shown that the symptoms it produces overlap with the symptoms produced by several common bacterial pathogens (Table 26.4). A viral cause is more likely when secondary cases develop in a household or institution, a pattern that suggests person-to-person spread rather than one-time exposure to a common food.

Sources and Modes of Transmission

The *sources and modes of transmission* of the etiologic agents causing foodborne illness are summarized

Table 26.1.   Characteristics of Acute Illness Caused by Ingestion of Infectious Agents

Agent	Pathogenesis	Usual Clinical Features	Frequency in USA	Usual Pattern[a]
Bacteria				
Bacillus cereus (28)	Enterotoxin produced in food or in intestine	Vomiting if preformed toxin in food; diarrhea; rhabdomyolysis and liver failure reported	Increasing	CSO
Campylobacter jejuni (3,36)	Invasion of large and small intestine	Fever, abdominal pain, diarrhea	Common	S, CSO
Clostridium botulinum	Neurotoxin produced in food	Vomiting, diarrhea, symmetric motor paralysis, cranial nerve and respiratory paralysis, death	Uncommon	CSO
Clostridium difficile (13)	Cytotoxin and enterotoxin produced in large intestine secondary to overgrowth	Fever, abdominal pain, diarrhea (rarely bloody) in a patient currently or recently on antibiotics; relapse of up to 20%	Common in hospitalized or recently hospitalized patients	S
Clostridium perfringens	Enterotoxin released during sporulation in large intestine	Diarrhea, occasionally vomiting	Common	CSO
Escherichia coli (25)				
Enterotoxigenic	Enterotoxin produced in small intestine	Voluminous watery diarrhea without fever (traveler's diarrhea)	Common (travelers)	CSO, S
Invasive	Invasion of large intestinal mucosa	Fever, diarrhea (often bloody)	Rare	CSO, S
Adherent (7,42)	Adheres tightly to small bowel mucosa	Acute diarrhea, which may be prolonged	Unknown, probably uncommon	S
Hemorrhagic (40) (e.g., *E. coli* 0157:H7)	Verotoxin produced in large bowel	Hemorrhagic colitis, may be followed by hemolytic uremic syndrome or thrombotic thrombocytopenic purpura	Common	CSO
Listeria monocytogenes (10)	Colonization	Fever, vomiting, abdominal pain, sepsis	Uncommon	CSO
Salmonella (many species)	Invasion of small and large intestine	Fever and diarrhea	Common	CSO
Salmonella typhi	Invasion of small intestine mucosa, systemic dissemination	Protracted illness: fever, malaise, headache, constipation more often than diarrhea, splenomegaly, occasionally intestinal perforation	Uncommon	S
Shigella sp.	Invasion of large intestine	Fever, diarrhea (often bloody)	Common	S
Staphylococcus aureus (20)	Enterotoxin produced in food	Vomiting dominates, diarrhea	Very common	CSO
Streptococcus group A	Invasion of upper respiratory tract	Streptococcal pharyngitis syndrome (see Chapter 28)	Uncommon (by this mode of transmission)	CSO
Vibrio cholerae (32)	Enterotoxin produced in small intestine	Voluminous watery diarrhea without fever	Rare	CSO, S
Vibrio parahaemolyticus	Probably both invasion and enterotoxin production; exact mechanism unknown	Diarrhea, abdominal cramps	Uncommon	CSO, S
Vibrio vulnificus (24)	Mechanism unknown	Fever, abdominal pain, diarrhea; septicemia "metastatic" cutaneous lesions	Uncommon	S
Yersinia enterocolitica (8)	Invasion of small and large intestine	Fever, abdominal pain, may suggest appendicitis, diarrhea	Uncommon	CSO, S
Viruses				
Norwalk (23)	Invasion of small intestine	Vomiting and diarrhea	Common	CSO
Rotavirus (19,23)	Invasion of small intestine	Severe gastroenteritis in young children, mild in adults	Common	S
Protozoa and Helminths				
Entamoeba histolytica (18)	Invasion of large intestine	Diarrhea, often chronic and bloody	Uncommon (travelers)	CSO, S
Giardia lamblia (39)	Colonization and occasional invasion of small intestine	Diarrhea, flatulence with foul-smelling stools	Uncommon (travelers)	CSO, S
Trichinella spiralis	(a) Encysted trichinae mature, mate, reproduce in small intestine; (b) larvae penetrate intestine, migrate to muscles where they cause inflammation and become encysted	Diarrhea, puffy eyes, muscle aching, fever, occasionally severe heart failure; eosinophilia typical	Uncommon	CSO, S
Cryptosporidium (9)	Colonization	Diarrhea, acute in children and healthy adults; chronic in HIV-infected patients	Common in patients with AIDS	S
Cyclospora (38)	Colonization	Diarrhea, cramping, heartburn, low-grade fever	Uncommon; more common in patients with AIDS	CSO, S

[a]CSO, common source outbreak; S, sporadic.

[b]Anal–oral transmission may occur in homosexual men.

Epidemiologic Features				
Source (Reservoir)	Transmission to Humans	Incubation Period	Diagnosis	Specific Therapy
Soil	Foodborne	2–16 hr	Culture suspected food	None
Animal feces	Foodborne or waterborne[b]	24–48 hr	Culture stool, blood	Erythromycin (see text)
Animal feces, soil	Foodborne (canned, low pH, anaerobic)	12–36 hr	Culture food, identify toxin in food, blood, stool	Polyvalent antitoxin
Ubiquitous, especially in health care environments (spores)	Probably not necessary but may occur in hospitals[b]	2–10 days after beginning antibiotics (rarely up to 6 weeks after antibiotics stopped)	Identify toxin in stool	Metronidazole or vanco-mycin (see text)
Human feces, animal feces, soil	Foodborne (meats)	12–24 hr	Culture suspected food	None
Human feces	Foodborne	24–48 hr	Culture stool, identify en-terotoxin production by bacteria	None
Human feces	Foodborne (cheeses)	24–48 hr	Culture stool	Same as *Shigella* (see text)
Human feces	Probably foodborne	24–48 hr	Culture stool, small bowel	Antibiotics to which or-ganism is sensitive
Animal feces	Foodborne	24–48 hr	Culture stool (see text)	None
Dairy cattle	Foodborne	18 hr–21 days	Stool culture; serum antilis-terolysin O	Ampicillin or trimethoprim-sulfamethoxazole
Animal feces; eggs	Foodborne (many foods, see text), person-to-person[b]	12–48 hr	Culture stool	Ampicillin or Chloram-phenicol, in selected cases only (see text)
Human feces	Person-to-person, food-borne[b]	4 days–3 weeks	Culture blood, stool, anti-bacterial antibodies	Chloramphenicol
Human feces	Person-to-person[b]	12–48 hr	Culture stool	Fluoroquinolone (see text)
Human skin, nares, mouth	Foodborne (many foods, see text)	2–8 hr	Culture food, and food handlers	None
Human pharynx, skin lesions	Foodborne	1–3 days	Culture throat, food, skin lesions of food handlers	Penicillin (see Chapter 28)
Human feces	Waterborne and foodborne	12 hr–5 days	Culture stools, antibacterial and antitoxin antibody	Tetracycline
Sea water	Foodborne (various types of seafood from estuary and sea water)	15–24 hr	Culture stool	None
Sea water	Foodborne (various types of seafood from estuary and sea water)	24 hr–2 days	Culture stool	Antibiotics for Gram-negative sepsis; tetracycline
Animal feces	Foodborne, person-to-person	Probably 3–7 days	Culture stool	Doxycycline or trimethoprim-sulfamethoxazole
Human feces	Foodborne and waterborne, person-to-person (sec-ondary cases)	1–3 days	Rise in antiviral antibody	None
Human feces	Person-to-person (secondary cases)	1–3 days	Virus antigen in stool Rise in antiviral antibody	None
Human feces	Foodborne and waterborne, person-to-person[b]	Few days to months	Examine stool for tropho-zoites	Metronidazole (see text)
Human feces	Waterborne, person-to-person[b]	1–4 weeks	Examine stool for tropho-zoites	Metronidazole (see text)
Animal muscle (swine, many wild animals)	Foodborne	2–28 days	Skin tests, antibody, muscle biopsy	Mebendazole and steroids (see text)
Fresh water; human and animal feces	Waterborne; person-to-person	?2–7 days	Examine stool for tropho-zoites	Evolving
Fresh water (resistant to chlorination)	Waterborne; person-to-per-son?; animal-to-person?	12 hr–11 days	Examine stool for oocysts	Trimethoprim-sulfamethoxazole

Table 26.2.   Characteristics of Acute Illness Caused by Ingestion of Chemical Agents

Agent	Pathogenesis	Clinical Features	Frequency in USA	Pattern[a]
Seafood				
Ciguatera fish poisoning	Toxins from algae concentrated in fish, particularly predatory fish; toxins affect human cell sodium channels	Vomiting, diarrhea, paresthesias (warmth, extremities), metallic taste, blurred vision, sharp pains in extremities, respiratory paralysis	Uncommon (Florida)	CSO, S
Domoic acid (41) (amnesic shellfish poisoning)	Neuroexcitatory amino acid produced by phytoplankton and concentrated by mussels	Vomiting, cramps, headache, neurologic symptoms, antero-grade amnesia, seizures, coma, death	Rare (surveillance for domoic acid in Canada)	CSO, S
Scrombroid fish poisoning	Histamine intoxication	Histamine reaction (flushing, headache, dizziness, burning of mouth and throat; urticaria, pruritus, and bronchospasm)	Uncommon (frozen and fresh fish can be affected)	CSO, S
Paralytic shellfish poisoning	Multiple neurotoxins (saxitoxins) causing motor paralysis	Paresthesias (warmth, extremities), floating sensation, dysphonia, dysphagia, weakness, and respiratory paralysis	Uncommon (surveillance for toxins in shellfish in United States)	CSO, S
Mushrooms				
Muscarine	Muscarinic cholinergic response	Colicky abdominal pain, nausea, vomiting, diarrhea, salivation, miosis, blurred vision, brady-cardia, hypotension	Uncommon	CSO, S
Phalloidin (and other toxins)	Diverse cytotoxin effects, multi-systemic	*Stage 1:* Nausea, abdominal pain, vomiting, bloody diarrhea, marked weakness, hypotension (shock) *Stage 2:* Clinical improvement (day 2 or 3) *Stage 3:* Severe hepatic failure, delirium, frequent fatal outcome		CSO, S
Miscellaneous				
Heavy metals (antimony, cadmium, copper, iron, tin, zinc)	Upper gastrointestinal irritation	Metallic taste to food, nausea, vomiting, or diarrhea	Uncommon	CSO, S
Monosodium glutamate (MSG)	Idiopathic reaction	Burning sensation in chest, neck, abdomen, extremities	Common	S

Data from Gossalin RE, Hodge HC, Smith RP, Gleason MN. Clinical toxicology of commercial products. 5th ed. Baltimore: Williams & Wilkins, 1984; and Morris JG. Natural toxins associated with fish and shellfish. In: Blaser MJ, Smith PD, Randin JI, et al, eds. Infections of the gastrointestinal tract. New York: Raven, 1995.
[a]*CSO,* Common source outbreak; *S,* sporadic.

in Tables 26.1 and 26.2. The features of four of the most well-recognized etiologic agents illustrate the diverse ways that foodborne disease is acquired:

- Humans whose skin or nasal mucosa is colonized are almost always the source of *S. aureus.* Contamination of food with small numbers of staphylococci is undoubtedly very common. Staphylococcal food poisoning occurs when contaminated foods are allowed to stand long enough for organisms to multiply and produce enterotoxin. The principal foods in which this occurs are those high in protein (ham, pork, beef, poultry, either cooked or in salads, and cream-filled cakes and pastries) and those with a high salt or sugar content (ham, salads, and custards) (20).
- Animals are the source of the *Salmonella* serotypes that cause most human disease; only *Salmonella typhi* and *Salmonella paratyphi* are carried by humans. Transmission from animal to humans occurs chiefly by fecal contamination of equipment and personnel involved in the packaging and preparing of food, most commonly poultry and meats. Foodborne outbreaks of salmonellosis have also been recognized, increasingly related to use of under-

cooked eggs (26). Although eggs with visible shell cracks should always be considered suspect, those with intact shells can also be infected (e.g., from a salmonella abscess in the ovary of a hen). Only hard-cooked eggs and pasteurized eggs are absolutely safe; raw egg dishes (e.g., homemade salad dressings, eggnog, ice cream), and undercooked eggs (e.g., scrambled and soft-cooked eggs), should be avoided, particularly by immunocompromised and elderly people (31).

- *Clostridium perfringens* is a ubiquitous organism found in human and animal feces and in soil. Meats are the most frequently contaminated foods; transmission of enough organisms to produce illness occurs typically with inadequately heated or re-heated meats (spores may survive at normal cooking temperatures and then germinate and multiply while foods are being held at warm temperatures or being rewarmed at temperatures that do not inhibit bacterial growth).
- *Enterohemorrhagic E. coli* are found in the intestines of healthy livestock and can contaminate the surface of whole meat products during slaughter and processing. Ground meats pose the highest risk because

Epidemiologic Features				
Source	Transmission to Humans	Incubation Period	Diagnosis	Specific Therapy
Food chain of bottom-dwelling and predatory fish caught in Florida, Hawaii (red snapper, barracuda)	Foodborne	1–6 hr	Clinical and epidemiologic features	Mannitol infusion, atropine for bradycardia, hypotension symptoms may last days to months
Mussels and clams contaminated with domoic acid	Foodborne	Minutes to 48 hr	Clinical and epidemiologic features	Supportive care
Bacteria acting on fish flesh (tuna, mackerel, bonito, skipjack, mahi mahi)	Foodborne ("Peppery" taste of affected fish reported)	Minutes to 1 hr	Clinical and epidemiologic features; elevated urine histamine level	None or antihistamines in severe cases
Toxic dinoflagellates concentrated in filter-feeding bivalves (mussels, clams, oysters, scallops)	Foodborne	<30 min	Clinical and epidemiologic features	None (lasts few hours–few days)
Amanita muscaria	Foodborne	Few minutes–few hours	Clinical and epidemiologic features	Atropine 0.1–0.5 mg SC or IV
Amanita phalloides and other *Amanita* species	Foodborne	6–15 hr	Clinical and epidemiologic features	None
Containers made of alloy that includes a heavy metal	Foodborne (food prepared in, stored in, or eaten from a container from which heavy metal leached)	5 min–8 hr	Clinical and epidemiologic features	None
Foods prepared with large amounts of MSG	Foodborne (Chinese restaurant foods)	3 min–2 hr	Clinical and epidemiologic features	None

surface contamination is distributed throughout the product, and ingestion of raw or undercooked contaminated ground meat can lead to infection that can result in bloody diarrhea and hemolytic uremic syndrome. The mortality among patients with the latter syndrome can be high. The risk of illness is minimized by cooking ground red meat until it is no longer pink or until juices run clear (internal temperature 155°F).

Most episodes of foodborne illness follow the *ingestion of normally safe foods that have been rendered unsafe by one or more of the following factors:* failure to refrigerate foods properly or to heat foods thoroughly, preparing foods a day or more before they are served, allowing foods to remain at warm temperatures, failure to reheat or cook foods at temperatures that kill vegetative bacteria, incorporating raw (contaminated) ingredients into foods that receive no further cooking, failure to clean and disinfect kitchen or processing plant equipment, and contamination by infected food handlers who practice poor personal hygiene. Unfortunately, as the complexity of the international food distribution system increases, unanticipated outbreaks will continue to occur. For example, a recent outbreak of salmonellosis in Finland and the United States was traced to alfalfa sprouts grown from seeds supplied by a Dutch shipper (29).

A small minority of foodborne illnesses are caused by the ingestion of *foods that are always unsafe* because of the presence of toxins that cannot be rendered innocuous by cooking or other means (e.g., ciguatoxin, scombrotoxin, *Amanita* toxins, paralytic shellfish toxin, mushroom toxin, and heavy metals) (15,21).

The *place* of ingestion of the etiologic agent is usually the patient's home or a restaurant and, less commonly, a social gathering or an institutional eating place.

Populations at Risk

For many of the conditions listed in Tables 26.1 and 26.2, *people are at risk at all ages,* and a single episode may not confer protective immunity against a later episode. Although most cases of acute diarrheal episodes occur in children, older adults are at increased risk from dying from gastrointestinal illnesses. Of 28,538 diarrhea-related deaths in the United States between 1979 and 1987, 78% occurred in adults 55 or more years old versus 11% in children less than 5 years old (27). A particularly high rate of diarrheal illness

Table 26.3. Selected Bacterial Foodborne Outbreaks, Cases, Average Number of Cases per Outbreak, Deaths, and Case-Fatality Rate, 1988–1992

Bacteria	Outbreaks	Cases	Cases/Outbreak	Deaths	Case-Fatality Rates (per 1,000)
Bacillus cereus	21	433	21	0	0.0
Campylobacter spp.	27	732	27	2	2.7
C. botulinum	60	133	2	11	82.7
C. perfringens	40	3,801	95	1	0.3
E. coli	11	244	22	0	0.0
Salmonella spp.	549	21,177	39	38	1.8
Shigella spp.	25	4,788	192	0	0.0
S. aureus	50	1,678	34	0	0.0

Data adapted from CDC Surveillance Summaries. MMWR SS-5:45, 1996.

Table 26.4. Comparison of Symptoms of Viral Bacterial Gastroenteritis in Adults

Symptom	Percentage with Symptom				
	Viral Gastroenteritis		Bacterial Gastroenteritis		
	Rotavirus[a]	Norwalk Agent[b]	*Salmonella*[b]	*Shigella*[b]	*S. aureus*
Nausea	2	85	50	45	62
Vomiting	9	84	23	39	86
Abdominal cramps	26	62	78	60	86
Diarrhea	33	44	73	100	67
Fever	5	32	49	72	10
Headache	NR[c]	37	33	6	8

[a]From Wenman WM, Hinde D, Felthman S, Gurwith M. Rotavirus infection in adults. Results of a prospective family study. N Engl J Med 301:303, 1979.
[b]From Adler JL, Zicki R. Winter vomiting disease. J Infect Dis 119:668, 1969.
[c]*NR,* Not reported.

also occurs in people of all ages who travel to developing countries (see Chapter 33).

In the early 1980s, a wide spectrum of intestinal infections was recognized in homosexual and bisexual men and labeled the *gay bowel syndrome* (see also Chapter 92). At the time, these cases were ascribed to a combination of asymptomatic carriage of one or more enteric pathogens and unsafe sexual practices (e.g., oral–genital and genital–anal contact between subjects, exposure to multiple sexual partners). However, many of these reported cases were no doubt related to unrecognized human immunodeficiency virus (HIV) infection because HIV had not been identified at the time the term *gay bowel syndrome* was coined. Now, the diagnosis of HIV infection must be considered in patients with unusual diarrheal syndromes because HIV-infected patients are at increased risk for bacterial infections of the gastrointestinal tract (e.g., salmonellosis, shigellosis), as well as bacterial infections in general. Protracted diarrhea can herald the progression of HIV infection, and a number of enteropathogens can cause not only acute illness but also prolonged symptoms of diarrhea in patients with advanced HIV disease. *Cryptosporidium* infection, usually a benign self-limited diarrheal illness in children and healthy adults, may cause a prolonged and life-threatening illness (9). *Isospora belli,* usually not thought of as a diarrheal pathogen, may also cause diarrheal illness in these patients. Diarrheal illnesses caused by *Campylobacter jejuni,* which are usually short illnesses in normal hosts, may be prolonged in HIV-infected pa-

tients. (See Chapter 34 for additional discussion of infection in HIV-infected patients.)

PATHOGENESIS

As indicated in Tables 26.1 and 26.2, the majority of the etiologic agents produce symptoms caused by either inflammation of the gastrointestinal tract or physiologic events related to one or more toxins.

The common bacterial diarrheal syndromes can be separated into invasive and enterotoxigenic syndromes (Table 26.5) (39,42), and this becomes important when antibiotic treatment is considered. In *invasive disease,* the etiologic agent is found in the intestinal mucosa, and the diarrhea results from destruction of the cells of the mucosa, which often is caused by the inflammation. This usually occurs in the large bowel and produces systemic symptoms (particularly fever), local symptoms (tenesmus, abdominal discomfort), and frequent small amounts of stool that contain pus cells and often blood. Shigellosis is the prototype of this syndrome. In *enterotoxigenic diarrhea,* the organisms do not invade tissue but colonize and multiply on the small bowel mucosal surface; during this process they produce enterotoxins, which act as chemical mediators and cause net secretion of fluid and electrolytes by the small bowel. Little tissue damage is produced, and inflammation of the mucosa is minimal. Symptoms consist of watery diarrhea (which may be voluminous), accompanied by minimal systemic signs, unless dehydration becomes significant. The prototypes of this syndrome are diarrheas caused by *Vibrio cholerae* and by enterotoxigenic *E. coli* (25,32).

Unfortunately, not all enteric diseases caused by bacteria fit into this simple dichotomy. *Enteroadherent strains* of *E. coli* have been characterized that neither invade mucosal cells nor produce enterotoxins, but they tightly adhere to the mucosal surface and produce diarrhea, presumably by interfering with normal absorptive processes. These strains produce diarrhea primarily in small children and many belong to the classic enteropathogenic serotypes (7,42). In addition, *Clostridium difficile, a cause of antibiotic-associated diarrhea* and pseudomembranous colitis, produces two toxins: an enterotoxin (toxin A), which causes secretion of fluid into the gut lumen, and a potent cytotoxin (toxin B), which damages the gut epithelium and leads to inflammation.

PATIENT EVALUATION

Historical Information

In addition to a history of the specific symptoms, the most useful information is as follows:

- A history of *food eaten* within the past 48 hours, particularly noting any deviation from the patient's usual pattern, such as eating an unusual food (e.g., a special fish), eating at a restaurant, or attending a picnic or potluck dinner.
- A history of a *similar illness in others* (family members or members of a group who ate with the patient). This is helpful in suggesting a common source outbreak.
- The probable *incubation period.* This may be helpful in suggesting the most likely cause of a patient's illness (Tables 26.1 and 26.2). For example, the onset of symptoms immediately after ingestion always indicates chemical food poisoning, onset of symptoms within a few hours of eating strongly suggests staphylococcal food poisoning, onset within 24 to 48 hours suggests *Salmonella* infection, and onset of symptoms 1 week or more after exposure suggests a less common problem such as *giardiasis.*

- A *history of taking antimicrobials.* Overall, no etiologic agent can be identified in approximately 80% of these patients. A history of taking clindamycin, ampicillin, or a cephalosporin currently or within the last 2 weeks, usually during hospitalization, supports the diagnosis of antibiotic-associated diarrhea caused by *C. difficile.* This agent causes syndromes that range from enterotoxigenic diarrhea to an invasive disease (see above), and rarely (0.5% of cases) it causes the syndrome of pseudomembranous colitis (14).
- A history of *neurologic symptoms* after ingestion of canned foods should always suggest botulism or one of the other sources of neurotoxins (all rare) listed in Table 26.2.
- A history revealing *risk factors for HIV infection* (see Chapter 34) and chronic diarrhea should suggest the possibility of *Cryptosporidium* (9,22), *Isospora,* or *Salmonella* infection.

Physical Examination

The physical examination is usually of minimal help in establishing a cause. Fever or significant abdominal tenderness in association with diarrhea suggests an invasive organism as the etiologic agent. Poor skin turgor and postural hypotension suggest significant salt and water deficits (uncommon in adults with diarrhea in the United States). Rare conditions in which the physical findings may be helpful are *botulism* and other neurotoxic forms of food poisoning, and *trichinosis* (Tables 26.1 and 26.2).

Laboratory Studies

In most outpatients with acute gastrointestinal illness, no laboratory studies are indicated (4) unless a common source outbreak is suspected. In such cases,

Table 26.5. Characteristics Distinguishing Invasive and Enterotoxigenic Diarrhea

Feature	Invasive Diarrhea	Enterotoxigenic Diarrhea
History	Fever, abdominal pain, tenesmus, may have blood in stool	Watery diarrhea with little or no fever or other systemic symptoms
Physical examination	Fever, abdominal tenderness; proctoscopy may be indicated	May be signs of salt and water depletion
Laboratory studies	Stool culture (may be diagnostic) Fecal leukocytes in large numbers[a] White blood cell count may be elevated	Stool culture usually negative unless special culture techniques available No or few fecal leukocytes White count usually normal, but may be elevated
Therapy	Oral fluids and electrolytes (usually only small quantities needed)	Oral fluids and electrolytes Bismuth subsalicylate, other symptomatic medications as needed[c]
Course	Antimicrobials often indicated[b] Improvements in 1–2 days, particularly if appropriate antimicrobials used	Antimicrobials not indicated Duration of 1–2 days usually; may last up to 5 days

[a]Use a drop of methylene blue stain with liquid stool.
[b]See text for recommendations for specific bacterial pathogens.
[c]See text for details.

special cultures and tests for toxins in stools and in food, primarily for epidemiologic purposes, should be obtained.

In patients evaluated in the emergency room or in patients with a combination of diarrhea for more than 24 hours, fever, and blood in the stool or significant volume depletion, the following laboratory studies are indicated (4,33):

- *Stool culture for Salmonella, Shigella, Campylobacter, and Yersinia.* Unfortunately, enterotoxigenic *E. coli,* invasive *E. coli, Vibrio* spp., and most viral agents cannot be identified in routine laboratory workups because of the special techniques required.
- *Stool examination for fecal leukocytes.* The test is done by mixing a small bit of stool with methylene blue stain on a microscope slide, and placing a coverslip over the mixture. After 2 or 3 minutes, the preparation is examined under the *high dry objective* for the presence of leukocytes. More than 10 leukocytes per high-powered field is indicative of an invasive pathogen.
- *A white blood cell count.* An elevated count or number of immature polymorphonuclear leukocytes supports the diagnosis of invasive diarrheal disease.

In suspected cases, the laboratory should be asked to culture the stool for *E. coli* that cause hemorrhagic colitis or to examine the stool microscopically for *Giardia lamblia, Entamoeba histolytica,* or *Cryptosporidium* (Table 26.1). For optimal identification of trophozoites of the latter organisms, fresh stools should be examined immediately by an experienced observer. For the diagnosis of giardiasis, stools may need to be examined repeatedly. *E. histolytica* trophozoites are best identified from the mucus taken from the base of ulcerations seen at proctoscopy.

When needed to make clinical decisions, additional laboratory tests can be ordered for some conditions (Tables 26.1 and 26.2). Particularly for hospitalized patients with diarrhea and those with postantibiotic diarrhea, tests for *C. difficile* toxins must be specifically ordered because clinical laboratories typically do not culture stool for *C. difficile.* Until recently, the toxins produced by the bacterium were detected in stool specimens with tissue culture assays (requires 48 to 72 hours); immunoassays (latex agglutination tests or enzyme immunoassays) now make possible same-day results. (Also see Chapter 39 for a discussion of the laboratory evaluation of patients with chronic diarrhea.) For hospitalized patients with new diarrhea, ordering a *C. difficile* test alone is the most cost-effective approach, and stool cultures and ova and parasite examinations are usually unrevealing (35).

MANAGEMENT

In all patients with acute diarrhea, symptomatic treatment is of primary importance. In addition, some patients may require specific therapy (i.e., antibiotics), usually indicated on the basis of the history and physical examination. Most episodes of acute diarrhea are self-limited, lasting 1 to 2 days, but occasionally symptoms last 5 to 10 days. Resolution of illness is thought to be caused by the local secretory immune response of the gastrointestinal tract.

Symptomatic Treatment

Fluid Therapy

With the exception of giardiasis, amebiasis, *C. difficile* colitis, and the more severe cases of shigellosis and salmonellosis, practically all acute diarrheal disease seen commonly in the United States can be treated with only symptomatic therapy, the mainstay of which is the replacement of fluids and electrolytes lost in the stool. Because in most patients the disease is mild and the amount of stool is small, replacement is simple. Young, healthy patients should be encouraged to drink a lot of fluids, to avoid spicy foods, and otherwise to eat what they like. Foods with complex carbohydrates (e.g., cereals, rice, toast), but not foods with concentrated simple sugars (most sweet foods), may facilitate fluid reabsorption at the brush border of the intestinal mucosa and help to limit duration of diarrhea (5).

In patients who have a *very large loss of stool,* those who experience weakness and a feeling of being washed out (with or without signs of volume depletion), and older adults (who are at increased risk for hypoperfusion of vital organs with even moderate dehydration because of silent atherosclerosis), replacement should consist of fluids containing electrolytes and glucose. Oral glucose–electrolyte or carbohydrate–electrolyte replacement solutions (e.g., Pedialyte, Rehydralyte, and Ceralyte), and packets containing premeasured salts and sugars that must be dissolved in water (e.g., Orlyte and Oral Rehydration Salts) are available commercially (5,17). These products have been developed primarily for treating children but are adequate for adults. Most have sodium concentrations of 50 to 75 mEq/L and substitute citrate for bicarbonate. A less complete replacement fluid can be made using one pint (500 mL) water, ½ teaspoon table salt (NaCl), and four rounded teaspoons of table sugar (sucrose).

Because of their sugar and salt contents, *none of the following beverages is satisfactory for fluid replacement* in patients whose diarrhea is causing moderate to severe fluid loss: nondietetic soft drinks (hyperosmolar sugar solution), dietetic soft drinks (inadequate amount of simple sugars needed to facilitate intestinal fluid reabsorption), and sports drinks such as Gatorade that are designed to replace the hypotonic fluids lost with perspiration (inadequate amount of salts for replacement of intestinal fluid losses).

Patients should be instructed to replace estimated diarrheal fluid losses roughly on a 1:1 basis. Typically, 1 to 2 L should be drunk in the first 1 to 2 hours after diarrhea commences, and an additional 1 to 2 L a day until symptoms resolve. Hydration is judged adequate if dilute urine is passed every 3 to 4 hours.

Patients experiencing *severe diarrhea or vomiting* that precludes easy replacement with oral replacement fluids and those who have evidence of moderate to severe salt and water depletion should receive initial intravenous fluid replacement with Ringer's lactate or its equivalent. This can be accomplished in ambulatory settings, in the patient's home (see Chapter 9), or in the hospital depending on the availability of resources and the severity and duration of the patient's illness.

Other Symptomatic Measures

Several types of medications are commonly used to treat diarrhea symptomatically. *Diphenoxylate with atropine* (Lomotil) and *loperamide* (Imodium or generic, nonprescription) are agents that cause a decrease in intestinal motility and stool frequency; they may be useful to the patient at times when frequent defecation would be embarrassing. These drugs do not alter the natural course of the disease and are potentially harmful if invasive pathogens such as *Shigella* are causing the diarrhea. These medications should be avoided in frail elderly patients (particularly those recently discharged from the hospital) and those in nursing homes (in whom *C. difficile* infections are common) because toxic megacolon can be precipitated by the use of antiperistaltic drugs.

Kaolin and pectin mixtures (Kaopectate or generic, nonprescription) add to the bulk of the stool, and thus the stools become less watery; actual fluid loss, however, is not affected by these agents. *Bismuth subsalicylate* (Pepto-Bismol or generic, nonprescription) has been demonstrated to decrease the volume of stools in patients with diarrhea caused by enterotoxigenic organisms and to be safe in a variety of diarrheal illnesses (2). This compound has antibacterial activity as well. It may be taken in either liquid or tablet form. The dosage is two tablets or 30 mL every half to 1 hour, as needed, up to a maximum of eight doses per 24 hours. Patients should be advised that this compound can cause black stools regularly and sometimes a blackened tongue.

In patients with *protracted vomiting,* which may occur with staphylococcal food poisoning, the antiemetic drug prochlorperazine (Compazine) may be helpful, given as a 25-mg rectal suppository two or three times daily to healthy adults, and at lower dosages for the elderly.

Specific Treatment

In patients in whom *shigellosis* is strongly suspected or from whom the organism has been cultured in the stool, appropriate antibiotic treatment should be given because this will shorten the illness from 3 to 7 days to 1 to 2 days. A fluoroquinolone antibiotic (e.g., ciprofloxacin 500 mg or norfloxacin 400 mg, twice daily) for 3 days is the current drug of choice (34). An alternative therapy is trimethoprim-sulfamethoxazole, one double-strength tablet every 12 hours for 5 days (16).

If *Salmonella* is isolated from diarrheal stool, patients should not be given antibiotics unless there is evidence of systemic disease, such as high fever or other symptoms or signs of systemic infection. It has been found that routine treatment of *Salmonella* gastroenteritis with antibiotics leads to a prolongation of the carrier state in some people (1). Even without antibiotic treatment, patients may excrete *Salmonella* in the stool for several weeks to months after their acute illness has terminated. If there is systemic disease or if the patient is immunocompromised, the same antibiotics listed above for shigellosis should be prescribed, but the duration of therapy should be 3 to 7 days. Alternatively, chloramphenicol 500 mg four times a day for 3 to 7 days can be prescribed.

Patients infected with *Campylobacter* may benefit from antibiotic therapy, but controlled studies indicate primarily an effect on excretion of the organism rather than a clinical effect. Erythromycin, 500 mg four times a day for 5 days, seems to be the best regimen; most strains are also sensitive to similar dosages of tetracyclines, but resistance to the quinolones is now being reported (34).

In patients who develop *significant diarrhea related to antibiotics,* ideally the antibiotic should be stopped, and another substituted only if antibiotic therapy must be continued. *C. difficile* causes approximately 20% of antibiotic-associated diarrhea in hospitalized patients, but is almost always responsible for severe cases of antibiotic-associated diarrhea accompanied by fever and abdominal pain (pseudomembranous colitis). The diarrhea usually begins during antibiotic treatment or within 2 weeks of stopping antibiotics; occasionally it begins weeks to months later (14). If *C. difficile* is strongly suspected, bismuth subsalicylate (see above) often helps, particularly in patients with mild to moderate diarrhea without significant systemic symptoms. Metronidazole (Flagyl), 250 mg by mouth four times a day for 5 days, shortens the illness in most patients and is indicated when severe diarrhea and other symptoms occur (e.g., low-grade fever and mild abdominal pain). For the 20% of patients with relapsing infection (13) or for those with severe diarrhea and systemic manifestations of illness such as high fever, abdominal pain, or elevated blood leukocyte count indicative of pseudomembranous colitis, the much more expensive antibiotic vancomycin should be given in an oral dosage of 250 to 500 mg four times daily for 7 to 14 days (30).

There is no evidence that antibiotics are useful in patients with *hemorrhagic colitis* caused by *E. coli.* However, antibiotics are definitely useful in the treatment of traveler's disease, most of which is caused by enterotoxigenic *E. coli* (see Chapter 33).

Patients with *giardiasis* and *amebiasis* require appropriate antimicrobial therapy. For giardiasis, the drug of choice is metronidazole (Flagyl), 250 mg three times a day for 5 days. (Quinacrine hydrochloride, an earlier recommended treatment, is no longer available in the United States.) For moderate to severe amebic dysentery, metronidazole should be administered, 750 mg three times a day for 10 days, followed by iodoquinol (Yodoxin; previously diiodohydroxyquin), 650 mg three times a day for 3 weeks, to eradicate the cyst forms (18).

Trichinosis is treated with mebendazole 300 mg

three times daily for 3 days, then 500 mg three times daily for 10 days. High dosages of prednisone (e.g., 40 to 60 mg/day) should be given simultaneously, if symptoms are pronounced, for 3 to 5 days and then tapered.

Patients with *suspected botulism* should be hospitalized in an intensive care unit immediately and should be given polyvalent antitoxin, which must be obtained through the local health department.

Patients with mushroom poisoning caused by *Amanita muscaria* should be treated with atropine and hospitalized (Table 26.2).

Chapter 34 describes the selection of antimicrobial therapy for the diarrheal illnesses associated with HIV infection; for one of these, cryptosporidiosis, no antibiotic therapy has been shown to be effective, but partial response with octreotide 50 mg subcutaneously every 8 hours for 48 hours has been reported.

Patient's Role in Therapy

Acute gastroenteritis, like the common cold, is often diagnosed and handled by the patient without contacting a physician. In some instances, patients contact their physician by telephone, and a working diagnosis and plan of therapy can be established without an office visit. This is particularly true for healthy patients with typical symptoms of staphylococcal food poisoning. In all situations, whether the patient is examined or not, it should be stressed that care of gastroenteritis requires taking of sufficient fluids, at times supplemented by an oral electrolyte solution (see above) and by oral antibiotics if prescribed. Patients should be advised to contact their physician if diarrhea becomes worse or if they develop fever or protracted vomiting. A follow-up visit is not needed unless symptoms persist beyond 2 to 3 days or unless stool cultures have been taken and reveal that antibiotic therapy is indicated. Limitation of activity should be dictated by how the patient feels and by proximity of toilet facilities.

Course of Illness

The dehydrated patient feels almost immediate improvement when adequate oral replacement fluids are given. When the patient is given antimicrobial therapy for an invasive pathogen, diarrhea and fever should decrease notably within 24 to 36 hours.

An *atypical course* occasionally occurs after initial diagnosis and treatment. Any patient may develop an increase in diarrhea after being initially seen, which could result in unanticipated significant dehydration. An increase in severity of symptoms could also occur if the patient develops antibiotic-associated enterocolitis. The occasional patient with antibiotic-resistant *Shigella* may not respond to initial therapy, indicating the need for an alternative drug. The enteric fever syndrome caused by *S. typhi* (typhoid fever), some other *Salmonella* species, and some *Yersinia* species typically begins with constipation, fever, headache,

and abdominal pain, but diarrhea may develop. The progressive course and abdominal tenderness (at times suggesting acute appendicitis) are features that suggest these causes and the need for both stool and blood cultures (8). An initial episode of *ulcerative colitis* (bloody diarrhea) or an initial episode of *Crohn's disease* (pain with nonbloody, intermittent diarrhea that does not remit) could be misdiagnosed as shigellosis. With inflammatory bowel diseases, fluids or antibiotic therapy would not lead to resolution of symptoms.

Rarely, a patient's diarrheal symptoms may persist for more than a week. In this case, the patient should return for further evaluation, particularly repeated stool examinations, which may be necessary to confirm the diagnosis of protozoal infections.

PREVENTION

Primary Prevention

Primary prevention of the diseases discussed above can theoretically be accomplished by the following measures:

- Reducing the agent's presence in the environment
- Increasing resistance of the host (by immunization or prophylactic antibiotics)
- Using environmental measures that block the transmission of the agent

Regulations governing sewage treatment, water purification, and food processing, packing, and preparation provide the principal protective barriers to foodborne disease *outside the home.* Unfortunately, this is often inadequate, as evidenced by the observation that as many as 50% of poultry carcasses sold commercially in supermarkets are contaminated with *Salmonella* or *Campylobacter.*

In the home, almost all forms of foodborne disease can be prevented if several measures are followed routinely (Table 26.6). *Many people do not realize that some of the food they prepare each day is contami-*

Table 26.6.   Measures to Prevent Foodborne Disease in the Home

Refrigerate all foods that are capable of supporting microbial growth (perishable foods).

Avoid keeping perishable food for long periods, even in the refrigerator.

Cook all foods at sufficiently high temperatures before serving, and follow the same procedure when foods are reheated.

Avoid preparing perishable foods a day or more before they are to be served.

Avoid allowing foods to stand at warm temperatures for several hours before being served.

Avoid incorporating raw (contaminated) ingredients into foods that receive no further cooking.

Clean kitchen equipment thoroughly after it has been in contact with perishable foods.

Avoid using utensils that may contain toxic metals.

Avoid foods that are unsafe no matter how they are processed (see text).

nated *before cooking* and that proper cooking and storing, not absence of contamination, is the way in which most food is rendered safe to eat. Whenever food known to be contaminated is eaten raw, the risk of foodborne disease is present. This is particularly important with respect to shellfish, which concentrate microbial organisms from the waters in which they are grown.

Despite routine testing of water by public health authorities for contamination by enteric pathogens, the number of cases of illness related to consumption of *raw seafood* continues to increase. Illnesses arise from bacteria such as *Shigella* and *Vibrio,* particularly *Vibrio vulnificus,* viruses such as hepatitis A and Norwalk, and unusual parasites in sushi (24). Some experts suggest that the risks associated with eating raw seafood are now unacceptable (12,21), and people at risk for gastrointestinal infections should be instructed to avoid eating uncooked seafood.

Secondary Prevention

After an outbreak of an acute enteric illness, appropriate measures should be taken to prevent additional cases.

In the household, any foods suspected of transmitting illness should be thrown away. (In the event that an epidemiologic investigation is warranted, a sample should be submitted to the local health department.) An error in storage or cooking of the suspected food is often evident; the patient's physician should point out this error and, most important, review the standard precautions listed in Table 26.6 to prevent repeated episodes of foodborne illness. When a member of a household has an enteric infection that is transmissible from person to person (Table 26.1), this person should be instructed to wash his or her hands frequently, especially before preparing food for others. *Food-service employees* should not work until the symptoms of infectious gastroenteritis resolve. Those with shigellosis or salmonellosis should not work until two consecutive stool cultures obtained not less than 24 hours apart (and not less than 48 hours after discontinuation of antibiotics if antibiotics were given) are negative.

When *exposure outside* the home is suspected by the physician, the problem should be reported immediately to the local health department; it is the responsibility of the health department to undertake an epidemiologic investigation to protect others. Each year, investigations of 400 to 500 outbreaks of foodborne illness are reported to the CDC, and many lead to measures that interrupt potentially widespread outbreaks of diseases, some of them particularly hazardous, such as botulism.

Prophylaxis for Travelers to the Developing World

The problem of diarrheal illness and other problems related to travel are discussed in Chapter 33.

General References*

Benenson A, ed. Control of communicable diseases in man. 16th ed. Washington, DC: American Public Health Association, 1995.
A concise summary of epidemiology, management, and prevention of communicable diseases.

Blacklow NR, Greenberg HB. Viral gastroenteritis. N Engl J Med 325:252, 1991.
A useful review.

Blaser MJ, Smith PD, Ravdin JI, et al, eds. Infections of the gastrointestinal tract. New York: Raven Press, 1995.
Comprehensive textbook.

Centers for Disease Control and Prevention. Waterborne disease outbreaks, 1986–1988, and foodborne disease outbreaks, 5-year summary, 1983–1987. In: CDC Surveillance Summaries 39(SS-1), 1990.
Summarizes methods for CDC surveillance and patterns in the United States for the 1980s.

Centers for Disease Control and Prevention. Surveillance for foodborne-disease outbreaks, United States, 1988–1992. In: CDC Surveillance Summaries 45(SS-5), 1996.
Most recent summary from CDC of surveillance and patterns of foodborne disease in the United States.

Gorbach SL. Bacterial diarrhoea and its treatment. Lancet 2:1378, 1987.
Useful review article.

Hedberg CW, Osterholm MT. Outbreaks of food-borne and waterborne viral gastroenteritis. Clin Microbiol Rev 6:199, 1993.
Useful review article.

Kapikian AZ. Viral gastroenteritis. JAMA 269:627, 1993.
Useful review article.

The Medical Letter on Drugs and Therapeutics. Drugs for parasitic infections. Med Lett Drugs Ther 34:17, 1992.
Periodically updated source of current recommendations for treatment.

Park SI, Giannella RA. Approach to the adult patient with acute diarrhea. In: Giannella RA, ed. Gastroenterol Clin North Am 22:483, 1993.
Useful review article.

Todd E. Foodborne illness. Epidemiology of foodborne illness: North America. Lancet 336:788, 1990.
Useful review article.

Specific References

1. Aserkoff B, Bennett JV. Effect of antibiotic therapy in acute salmonellosis on the fecal excretion of salmonellae. N Engl J Med 281:636, 1969.
2. Bierer D. Bismuth subsalicylate: its history, chemistry, and safety. Rev Infect Dis 12(S1):S3, 1990.
3. Blaser MJ, Wells JG, Feldman RA, et al. Campylobacter enteritis in the United States. Ann Intern Med 98:360, 1983.
4. Carmeli Y, Samore M, Shoshany O, et al. Utility of clinical symptoms versus laboratory tests for evaluation of acute gastroenteritis. Dig Dis Sci 41:1749, 1996.
5. Carpenter CCJ, Greenough WB, Pierce NF. Oral-rehydration therapy: the role of polymeric substrates. N Engl J Med 319:1346, 1988.
6. Caul EO. Small round structural viruses: airborne transmission and hospital control. Lancet 343:1240, 1994.
7. Clausen CR, Christie DL. Chronic diarrhea in infants caused by adherent enteropathic *Escherichia coli.* J Pediatr 100:358, 1982.
8. Cover TL, Aber RC. *Yersinia enterocolitica.* N Engl J Med 321:16, 1989.
9. Current WL, Reese NC, Ernst JV, et al. Human cryptosporidiosis in immunocompetent and immunodeficient persons. N Engl J Med 308:1252, 1983.

*Bold print (general references) and bold numerals (specific references) denote published controlled clinical trials, meta-analyses, or consensus-based recommendations.

10. Dalton CB, Austin CC, Sobel J, et al. An outbreak of gastroenteritis and fever due to *Listeria monocytogenes* in milk. N Engl J Med 336:100, 1997.
11. Davis M, Osaki C, Gordon D, et al. Update: multistate outbreak of *Escherichia coli* O157:H7 infection from hamburgers: Western United States, 1992–1993. MMWR 42:258, 1993.
12. DuPont HL. Consumption of raw shellfish: is the risk now unacceptable? N Engl J Med 314:707, 1986.
13. Fekety R, McFarland LV, Surawicz CM, et al. Recurrent *C. difficile* diarrhea: characteristics of and risk factors for patients enrolled in a prospective, randomized double-blinded trial. Clin Infect Dis 24:324, 1997.
14. Fekety R, Shah AB. Diagnosis and treatment of *Clostridium difficile* colitis. JAMA 269:71, 1993.
15. Gosselin RE, Hodge HC, Smith RP, Gleason MN. Clinical toxicology of commercial products. 4th ed. Baltimore: Williams & Wilkins, 1976.
16. Gotuzzo E, Oberhelman RA, Maguina C, et al. Comparison of single-dose treatment with norfloxacin and standard 5-day treatment with trimethoprim-sulfamethoxazole for acute shigellosis in adults. Antimicrob Agents Chemother 33:1101, 1989.
17. Greenough WB, Maung U K. Oral rehydration therapy. In: Field M, ed. Current topics in gastroenterology: diarrheal diseases. New York: Elsevier, 1991;485.
18. Guerrant RL. The global problem of amebiasis: current status, research needs, and opportunities for progress. Amebiasis: introduction, current status, and research questions. Rev Infect Dis 8(2):218, 1986.
19. Ho M, Glass RI, Pinsky PF, Anderson LJ. Rotavirus as a cause of diarrheal morbidity and mortality in the United States. J Infect Dis 158:1112, 1988.
20. Holmberg SD, Blake PA. Staphylococcal food poisoning in the United States: new facts and old misconceptions. JAMA 251:487, 1984.
21. Hughes JM, Merson MH. Current concepts: fish and shellfish poisoning. N Engl J Med 295:1117, 1976.
22. Janoff EN, Reller LB. *Cryptosporidium* species, a protean protozoan. J Clin Microbiol 25:967, 1988.
23. Kapikian AZ, Chanock RM. Viral gastroenteritis. In: Evans AS, ed. Viral infections of humans. 3rd ed. New York: Plenum, 1989.
24. Klontz KC, Lieb S, Schreiber M, et al. Syndromes of *Vibrio vulnificus* infections: clinical and epidemiologic features in Florida cases, 1981–1987. Ann Intern Med 109:318, 1988.
25. Levine M. *Escherichia coli* that cause diarrhea: enterotoxigenic, enteropathogenic, enteroinvasive, enterohemorrhagic, and enteroadherent. J Infect Dis 155:377, 1987.
26. Levine WC, Smart JF, Archer DL, et al. Foodborne disease outbreaks in nursing homes, 1975 through 1987. JAMA 266:2105, 1991.
27. Lew JF, Glass RI, Gangarosa RE, et al. Diarrheal deaths in the United States, 1979 through 1987. JAMA 265:3280, 1991.
28. Mahler H, Pasi A, Kramer JM, et al. Fulminant liver failure in association with the emetic toxin of *Bacillus cereus*. N Engl J Med 336:1142, 1997.
29. Mahon BE, Pönkä A, Hall WN, et al. An international outbreak of *Salmonella* infections caused by alfalfa sprouts grown from contaminated seeds. J Infect Dis 175:876, 1997.
30. The Medical Letter on Drugs and Therapeutics. Treatment of *Clostridium difficile* diarrhea. Med Lett Drugs Ther 31:94, 1991.
31. Mishu B, Griffin PM, Tauxe RV, et al. *Salmonella enteritidis* gastroenteritis transmitted by intact chicken eggs. Ann Intern Med 115:190, 1991.
32. Ouchterlony O, Holmgren J, eds. Cholera and related diarrheas. 43rd Nobel Symposium. Basel: Karger, 1980.
33. Riley LW. The epidemiologic, clinical, and microbiological features of hemorrhagic colitis. Annu Rev Microbiol 41:383, 1987.
34. Sack RB, Rahman M, Yunus M, Khan EH. Antimicrobial resistance in organisms causing diarrheal disease. Clin Infect Dis 24:S102, 1997.
35. Siegel DL, Edelstein PH, Nachamkin I. Inappropriate testing for diarrheal diseases in the hospital. JAMA 263:979, 1990.
36. Skirrow MB. *Campylobacter*. Lancet 336:921, 1990.
37. Slutsker L, Ries AA, Greene KD, et al. *Escherichia coli* O157: H7 diarrhea in the United States: clinical and epidemiologic features. Ann Intern Med 126:505, 1997.
38. Soave R. *Cyclospora*: an overview. Clin Infect Dis 23:429, 1997.
39. Stevens DP. Host–pathogen biology. Rev Infect Dis 4:851, 1982.
40. Su C, Brandt LJ. *Escherichia coli* O157:H7 infection in humans. Ann Intern Med 123:698, 1995.
41. Teitelbaum JS, Zatorre RJ, Carpenter S, et al. Neurologic sequelae of domoic acid intoxication due to the ingestion of contaminated mussels. N Engl J Med 322:1781, 1990.
42. Vial PA, Robins-Browne R, Lior H, et al. Characterization of enteroadherent-aggregative *Escherichia coli*, a putative agent of diarrheal disease. J Infect Dis 158:70, 1988.

C H A P T E R   27

Genitourinary Infections

PATRICK A. MURPHY, MD

Urinary tract infection (UTI) is one of the most common disorders seen in primary care. Most of these infections respond well to therapy, but complicated urinary infections can cause significant morbidity and mortality. This chapter provides a practical approach to the diagnosis, evaluation, management, and follow-up of patients with urinary tract infections. Some sexually transmitted diseases (syphilis, Chapter 30; and human immunodeficiency virus [HIV] infection, Chapter 34) and vulvovaginal infections (Chapter 94) may be confused with UTIs, and are discussed elsewhere in this book.

GENERAL CONSIDERATIONS

Gram-negative, aerobic bacteria cause 90 to 95% of urinary tract infections in all age groups, with *Esche-*

richia coli accounting for approximately 80% of community-acquired infections in women and 30 to 50% of nosocomial urinary tract infections in men and women (28). There are more than 100 serotypes of *E. coli*, but only 8 of these commonly cause infection. *Enterobacter, Klebsiella, Proteus* species, and *Pseudomonas* are especially important as causes of nosocomial UTIs or of infection in people with structurally abnormal urinary tracts. Gram-positive bacteria cause 5 to 10% of UTIs; *Staphylococcus saprophyticus* is common in young women in the ambulatory setting (18), and the enterococcus in nosocomial UTIs in patients of either sex. Viruses, mycobacteria, fungi, and parasites rarely cause UTIs. Fungi are most often seen in urine from patients who were recently in hospital and were or still are catheterized. Diabetes mellitus fosters fungal infection of the urine, as does failure to empty the bladder completely.

In women, the major cause of UTI is invasion of the urinary tract by bacteria that have ascended the urethra from the introitus. Women who are prone to infection have colonization of the vaginal introitus with the same serotypes of *E. coli* found in the fecal flora. Risk factors for acute UTIs in women include a history of a recent UTI, increased sexual activity, use of a diaphragm and a spermicide, and failure to void after intercourse (12). There is little evidence to support the commonly held views that the direction of wiping after bowel movements, the use of oral contraceptives, or tampons play a role in the pathogenesis of UTIs in women (9).

Infection of the bladder and kidneys *in men* is unlikely unless there is a structural abnormality of the urinary tract. The much lower incidence of UTI in men has been attributed to the long male urethra, the absence of colonization by bacteria near the meatus, and an antibacterial factor—prostatic antibacterial factor—that is present in the prostatic fluid and is markedly diminished in some men with recurrent prostatic infection. UTIs occur in some male homosexuals who have no abnormalities of the urinary tract (3) and in some men who are not circumcised (30).

The bladder has unique *intrinsic defenses* against infection. The washout of bacteria by periodic voiding is probably one important defense mechanism. The bladder mucosa also removes surface organisms, perhaps by phagocytosis, the secretion of mucus, surface antibody production, or all of these. This defense mechanism is severely limited if residual urine is regularly present after voiding (5).

Host factors play an important role in the pathogenesis of UTIs (29). UTIs occur more often and persistently in both men and women who have structural abnormalities of the urinary tract (e.g., an obstruction) or who have been catheterized or instrumented. Vesicoureteral reflux (the retrograde flow of urine from the bladder to the ureters) may be associated with ascending infection but is not necessarily causal. Infection in women occurs more often in pregnancy (4 to 6% incidence), especially if they also have sickle cell trait (10 to 15% incidence). Diabetes mellitus does not increase the risk of developing a UTI unless there is an associated disorder of bladder emptying or unless the patient has been instrumented. However, once a UTI has developed in a diabetic patient, it may be more virulent.

GENERAL DIAGNOSTIC EVALUATION

The diagnosis of urinary tract infection is suggested by the history and physical examination (see below) and confirmed by examination of the urine. Sometimes, radiographs and instrumentation of the urinary tract are necessary ancillary procedures.

The Patient with Irritative Symptoms: Diagnostic Approach

In young adults, UTIs are characterized by symptoms of bladder irritation such as frequency of micturition and dysuria. There may be urgency of micturition, and if a toilet is not immediately available, there may be minor leakage of urine or even complete incontinence. The urine is commonly cloudy and smells offensive. Suprapubic pressure or pain is commonly described. In a severe infection, there may be hematuria. If so, blood is evenly mixed throughout the volume of urine.

Approximately 30% of women with no fever and with no more symptoms than the above prove to have *pyelonephritis* when subjected to detailed examination (8). Clinical evidence of pyelonephritis would be high fever above 38.5°C, pain in the loin, chills and rigors, and evidence of frank sepsis such as tachypnea and hypotension. It is axiomatic that any woman with a UTI and a positive blood culture has pyelonephritis.

In women usually, but not exclusively, between the ages of 15 and 50, *vaginal infections and sexually transmitted diseases (STDs) may mimic UTIs* (17). A pelvic examination should be performed if the history is suggestive of vulvovaginitis from candidiasis, trichomoniasis, or other infections that may account for the bladder irritative symptoms (see Chapter 94). Chlamydial or gonococcal urethritis should also be considered in sexually active women (see Chapter 94). Both of these infections are most probable in women with many sexual partners but both are found in 2 to 4% of married women presenting for routine antenatal care (6). Chlamydial cervicitis is characterized by mucopurulent cervical discharge with endocervical edema. Gonococcal infection typically causes a purulent discharge from the cervix. Both infections are best detected by an endocervical culture.

In children under the age of 5, UTI may present in atypical ways such as bed wetting, fever, vomiting, or inconsolable crying. Older children generally have the same symptoms as adults. Aged people, especially if demented or psychotic, may have very few symptoms referable to the urinary tract. They commonly experience delirium, fever, urinary incontinence, or even sepsis of unknown cause. Thus, at the extremes of life it is unwise to rely on urinary symptoms.

UTI in pregnancy, known to older obstetricians as pyelitis of pregnancy, is a highly dangerous condition. The diagnosis is difficult because there may be few bladder symptoms. Instead, the patient commonly has intractable vomiting in the second or third trimester, elevated blood pressure with superimposed preeclampsia or eclampsia, renal failure, sepsis, or premature labor. UTI in pregnant women usually takes the form of pyelonephritis because the ureters are dilated and atonic and ascending infection is facilitated. Most cases of frank pyelitis of pregnancy are preceded by asymptomatic bacteriuria, and there is a great opportunity for preventive medicine (see later).

Urine Examination

The urinalysis is the most important initial study in the evaluation of the patient suspected of having a UTI because a negative urinalysis makes a UTI unlikely and because a urinalysis may aid in the localization of an infection within the urinary tract.

Collection

Collection of a *clean-caught* midstream urine specimen can be difficult, especially for women. The superiority of this procedure for reducing contamination compared with routine midstream urine collection has not been demonstrated (19). Therefore, culturing a simple midstream urine specimen voided into a sterile container should be sufficient for most outpatients of both sexes. The midstream collecting procedure may be impossible in women who are very obese or who have other disabilities. In this instance, urine must be obtained by bladder catheterization.

Catheterization of the urinary bladder is accomplished by using a No. 14 catheter inserted through the urethra into the bladder and removed when the specimen has been obtained. This requires careful preparation and cleansing of the urethra with an aseptic solution such as Betadine. Even with this precaution, a single straight catheterization has a 1% risk of inducing a new infection in ambulatory patients (39).

Urinalysis

If the urine specimen cannot be processed by the laboratory within 10 to 15 minutes after collection, it must be refrigerated until it reaches the laboratory.

The *uncentrifuged specimen* can be examined microscopically under a coverslip with use of the *oil immersion lens.* The finding of bacteria by this method has a 90% correlation with the subsequent culture of more than 1 million bacteria/mL of urine. The number of white cells in the uncentrifuged urine can be roughly quantitated microscopically *in a counting chamber by the use of the low-power lens.* In women, the finding of more than 7 white cells/mm^3 is abnormal (although not specific for infection). The finding of 7 or fewer white cells/mm^3 suggests that infection is not present (32). In men, the finding of any number of white cells should be considered abnormal.

Centrifuged urine is more convenient in some ways than is unspun urine. White cell casts are more easily seen in centrifuged urine; they are important because they are proof positive of pyelonephritis. Red cells, white cells, and bacteria are all concentrated and more easily detected. Small numbers of white cells seen in centrifuged urine are unreliable, and pyuria should not be considered significant unless there are more than *10 white cells/high-powered field* (HPF).

As a practical matter, microscopic examination of the urine for bacteria is difficult or impossible in most doctors' offices. Because in many cases there is little doubt about the diagnosis, it is reasonable to either treat the patient empirically (e.g., first or recurrent uncomplicated infections in women) or use the *urine dipstick* as a rapid diagnostic aid. There may be abnormalities in tests for pH, protein, or blood, but these are nonspecific. The abnormalities specifically correlated with infection are found with the dipstick-based *nitrite test* and the *test for leukocyte esterase.* Nitrite is generated by the reductive activity of bacteria on urinary nitrate. Leukocyte esterase reflects the presence of white cells in the urine. If both of these are positive, then UTI is present more than 90% of the time (14,24). Not all bacteria reduce nitrate, and not all UTIs are associated with a sufficient number of white cells in the urine to yield a positive esterase test (e.g., sensitivity of test is 100% for 50 WBC/HPF or more but approximately 40% for 6 to 12 WBC/HPF). An important cause of a false-negative nitrate test is the ingestion of large amounts of vitamin C. If the patient is symptomatic but the dipstick is negative, one should try direct demonstration of bacteriuria by microscopy or culture before deciding that infection is not present.

Culture

Many women know perfectly well that they have a UTI and merely need a prescription with instructions to recontact the office if symptoms persist. Culture of the urine in such patients is *costly ($60 to $80) and inconvenient* and rarely affects one's decision because the patient is better before the answer is known. On the other hand, a urine culture should always be obtained before therapy in patients who have recently been hospitalized or who are seriously ill and febrile. Infections in pregnant women are so serious that urine should always be cultured. Infections in young men are sufficiently unusual that a culture should also be obtained. In other patients, clinical judgment should dictate whether a culture is done.

If a urine culture is performed, the specimen should be refrigerated during transport to the laboratory. Most patients with symptomatic UTIs have at least 10^5 bacteria/mL of urine. However, some people develop symptoms of cystitis in the presence of 10^3 or even 10^2 organisms/mL of urine (33). If such patients are not treated, they tend to return with more severe symptoms and higher bacterial counts in the urine (35).

In patients whose urine is sent for culture, the species of bacteria isolated is also important. *Multiple species suggest contamination,* except in chronically catheterized patients or in special circumstances such as a vesicocolic fistula. Even small numbers of definite pathogens such as *E. coli* or *Klebsiella* should be regarded as suspicious. Conversely, large numbers of skin flora such as *Staphylococcus epidermidis* or *diphtheroids* can usually be ignored. Anaerobic bacteria virtually never cause UTI and if they are repeatedly present it suggests a communication with the bowel. The presence of fungi, usually *Candida,* is seldom correlated with symptoms or signs of UTI and in most cases is inconsequential.

Culture of urine specimens can be difficult in remote parts of the country. Commercially available kits allow one to dip a coated slide into fresh urine, drain, and incubate. Colonies develop directly on the slide and the counts correlate well with those obtained by quantitative plate cultures (21).

Culture-Negative Urine. If the patient has symptoms of cystitis with or without pyuria but the urine does not contain visible or cultured bacteria, the most likely explanation is that the patient has urethritis, prostatitis, or vaginitis. However, adenovirus can cause symptomatic cystitis, and chemical cystitis can be caused by several chemotherapeutic agents. In patients with culture-negative pyuria, tuberculosis of the kidney, bladder stone, bladder tumor, and interstitial cystitis (see below) should be considered.

Localizing the Site of Infection

Several techniques may characterize a UTI as either confined to the bladder or involving the kidneys. However, in most cases it is unnecessary to try to decide whether the patient has cystitis, pyelonephritis, or prostatitis. Many patients with pyelonephritis respond to standard 3-day treatment regimens described below (31).

The simplest indication that a patient has pyelonephritis or prostatitis that requires prolonged treatment is that the UTI relapses after a standard 3-day course of antibiotics that would be expected to clear a simple bladder infection. *Relapse* means that all the infectious episodes are caused by the same organism as defined not only by species, but also by any other available characteristics such as antibiotic sensitivity or serotype. Relapsing episodes are not necessarily caused by pyelonephritis: They may be caused by persistent colonization of the introitus and multiple episodes of ascending infection. Most cases of recurrent UTI are managed by prolonged courses of antibiotics, as discussed in the treatment section below.

In pyelonephritis, the bacteria in the urine are usually coated with antibody. This can be detected using fluorescent goat anti–human immunoglobulin. In cystitis, bacteria in the urine are generally free of antibody. This test is not absolutely reliable: Antibody-coated bacteria may be found in prostatitis, and antibody-negative bacteria may be obtained from some cases of pyelonephritis. For this reason, the test is of limited clinical value and should rarely be performed (27).

Other techniques are cumbersome because they require urethral or ureteral catheterization. The gold standard for localization of upper tract infection is

Table 27.1. Indications for Evaluating Patients with Urinary Tract Infections with Ultrasonography

Acute pyelonephritis in male patients
Acute pyelonephritis in women with persistent high fevers or leukocytosis after 2 or 3 days of antimicrobial treatment
Renal colic (see Chapter 47)
Palpable bladder or renal mass
Urea-splitting organism, usually *Proteus* spp.
Frequently recurrent urinary tract infections in women (more than three or four per year)
Failure to eradicate infection with appropriate therapy

bilateral ureteral catheterization with separate collection of the urine from each kidney. There is a less complicated bladder washout technique that detects pyelonephritis but gives no information about the side of the infection. Radiographic abnormalities such as renal cortical scars are not present in most cases of pyelonephritis. Localization of the UTI is so seldom needed in clinical practice that patients who require it should be referred to a urologist.

Imaging

Uncomplicated UTIs that respond to treatment do not require additional workup. However, some clinical situations warrant investigation for anatomic abnormalities (Table 27.1). In office practice, an intravenous pyelogram (IVP) is no longer the most appropriate way to evaluate renal anatomy. *Sonography* is quicker and less dangerous to renal function. It will detect kidney size, cortical scars, stones, and hydronephrosis. If sonography is normal, IVP is unlikely to add more information (10). Sonography is particularly useful for detecting and estimating the volume of residual urine in patients who cannot empty the bladder.

Computerized tomography (CT) scanning is most useful for the detection of perinephric abscess and as a prelude to operations on the kidneys. *Voiding cystourethrography* is another test that should be delegated to the urologist.

MANAGEMENT OF SYMPTOMATIC URINARY INFECTIONS IN WOMEN

First Infection, Occasional Infection, or Uncomplicated Infection

Most women with UTIs experience only one or occasional uncomplicated infections. The diagnosis of a UTI can be confirmed by urinalysis and urine culture; as discussed above, a therapeutic trial is usually sufficient and is more convenient and far less costly for the patient. Although an uncomplicated infection may clear spontaneously in time, treatment with antibiotics dramatically shortens the symptomatic period and should be given. Forcing fluids, historically a common practice, is discouraged once antibiotic therapy has been initiated because it may actually dilute significantly the concentration of antimicrobial in the urine.

Antibiotic treatment (Table 27.2). Uncomplicated urinary tract infections should usually be treated with

an *antibiotic* for 3 days. Three days of treatment gives the same cure rates as the traditional 7- to 10-day courses and there is little superinfection with *Candida*, a common occurrence with the longer course. One-dose therapy was popular a number of years ago, but the cure rates are less than those attainable with 3 days of therapy (25).

For patients who are not pregnant, a wide range of drugs can be used. Probably the best available therapy is trimethoprim–sulfamethoxazole. This produces little in the way of allergy, kills most Gram-negative rods, tends to sterilize the vaginal introitus, and is inexpensive. Overall, the cure rate is 90 to 95% (22). Patients allergic to sulfonamides can be treated with a quinoline, a tetracycline or nitrofurantoin.

β-*Lactams* such as ampicillin and cephalosporins are less effective than the four drugs mentioned above. However, in pregnant women there is no reasonable alternative to β-lactams because of the risk of harm to the fetus. Therefore, a somewhat increased risk of recurrent urinary infection must be accepted. In the rare pregnant woman with a serious penicillin allergy, one could consider an aminoglycoside, but there is a risk of fetal deafness.

Any of the above treatments generally sterilizes the urine and produces total relief of symptoms in 24 hours or less. In very symptomatic patients, one could add the bladder analgesic *phenazopyridine* (Pyridium) 200 mg three times a day for 1 day or more. This drug, which requires a prescription, usually alleviates annoying symptoms, especially dysuria and urgency, within hours after the first dose. The patient should be told that phenazopyridine will cause the urine to become dark orange.

If the patient remains asymptomatic after treatment, she may be regarded as cured without the need for any additional follow-up.

Table 27.2. Antimicrobial Agents for Uncomplicated Urinary Tract Infections (3-Day Therapy)

Agent	Dosage
First Choice (Effective and Inexpensive)	
Trimethoprim–sulfamethoxazole[a] (Bactrim, Septra, generic)	1 DS q12hr
Second Choice (Effective)	
A Quinolone[b]	
Ciprofloxacin (Cipro)	250 or 500 mg q12hr
Norfloxacin (Noroxin)	400 mg q12hr
Ofloxacin (Floxin)	200 mg q12hr
Tetracycline[a]	500 mg q12hr
Doxycycline[a]	100 mg q12hr
Third Choice (Effective For Cystitis But Not For Pyelonephritis)	
Nitrofurantoin (Furadantin)	50 or 100 mg q12hr
Fourth Choice (Less Effective But Can Be Used During Pregnancy)	
β-Lactams (e.g., amoxicillin, cephalexin)	250–500 mg q8hr

[a]Three-day course costs less than $5.
[b]Three-day course costs $15–$20.

Table 27.3. Points to Consider in Educating Women Who Have Had an Uncomplicated Infection

Infections are often recurrent. However, the following measures may decrease the recurrence rate:

Avoid a full bladder. This is an especially important reminder during travel.
High fluid intake (1 L in 2–3 hr) may eradicate an infection that has just become symptomatic.
Irritation to the urethra, as occurs with sexual intercourse, is associated with the movement of bacteria into the bladder. Voiding after intercourse, therefore, helps to prevent recurrent infection.
Diaphragm use is associated with development of urinary tract infection.

Infections in the absence of structural urologic disorder are rarely, if ever, associated with the development of chronic renal failure.
Prompt recognition and treatment will help to control symptoms.
Even if recurrent infections are frequent, there is much that can be done to control symptoms.

Points to stress to women after a UTI episode are summarized in Table 27.3. The behaviors that most often help prevent recurrent UTI are emptying the bladder after sexual intercourse and avoiding a full bladder. If a woman is using a diaphragm for contraception, a change in contraceptive method could be considered (see Chapter 93 for details regarding contraceptive methods).

Management of Recurrent Infection

Most women with recurrent UTIs have *reinfection* (rather than *relapse,* discussed below). Although the infections are symptomatic and occasionally may be associated with pyelonephritis, recurrent reinfections in women with structurally normal urinary tracts rarely, if ever, lead to chronic renal failure (11).

The approach to women with anatomically normal urinary tracts and the syndrome of reinfection has been vastly improved by the understanding of the pathogenesis of UTI in women. In the past, women were often treated with a variety of painful manipulations such as urethral dilation, urethral incision, transurethral resection of the bladder neck, installation of a variety of intravesical agents, and other inappropriate and ineffective maneuvers. Instead, each episode of bacterial infection should be treated as outlined above in the section on first infections. If there are three or four or more recurrences in a year, the urinary tract should be evaluated for anatomic abnormalities (see above). Patients with structural problems should be referred to the appropriate specialist (urologist or gynecologist). If the urinary tract is normal, prophylactic antimicrobials should be considered.

Prophylactic Antimicrobials

A number of studies have confirmed the efficacy of prophylaxis in reducing the frequency of UTIs in women, and prophylactic therapy has dramatically improved the lives of many women with multiple UTIs (40). The agents that have been used are effective when given as a single small dose at bedtime. A dose taken only after sexual intercourse is also effective in patients whose recurrent UTIs are associated with sexual activity. Patient acceptance is good, and side effects are uncommon.

Many agents have been shown to be effective prophylactically, but nitrofurantoin (Furadantin), a 50-mg tablet at bedtime, trimethoprim–sulfamethoxazole 40/200 mg (half a tablet of regular strength Bactrim, Septra, or generic at bedtime), and cephalexin (Keflex or generic), a 250-mg capsule at bedtime, are used most commonly and are recommended. In some patients, the antibiotic may be effective when given for 3 days of the week. Prophylactic therapy should be continued for 6 months. If there are still frequent recurrences after the cessation of prophylaxis, prophylaxis for a longer period (e.g., a year) should be tried.

Estrogens

In elderly women, the vaginal cells lose glycogen, lactobacilli vanish from the vaginal flora, and the introitus becomes colonized with Gram-negative rods. A controlled trial has demonstrated that the frequency of recurrent UTIs in elderly women can be greatly reduced (from an average incidence of 5.9 to 0.5 episodes per year) by the use of intravaginal estrogen creams (26). Treated patients used intravaginal cream containing 0.5 mg of estriol on the following schedule: nightly for 2 weeks, then twice weekly for 8 months. Presumably, systemic estrogens would have the same effect, and might be preferred for their cardiac effects.

CLINICAL SYNDROMES THAT MIMIC URINARY TRACT INFECTIONS IN WOMEN

There are two syndromes in women that mimic classic UTI. The urethral syndrome is common, and interstitial cystitis is rare.

Urethral Syndrome (Dysuria–Pyuria Syndrome)

The urethral syndrome is characterized by bladder irritation, frequency, urgency, and dysuria without significant (greater than 10^5) bacterial colonies per milliliter on culture. *Dysuria–pyuria syndrome* may be the better term because *dysuria is invariable and most patients have pyuria* (more than 8 white blood cells/mm^3 of clean uncentrifuged urine). Studies show that many women with the syndrome have bacterial infection with low bacterial colony counts (36). These patients respond to the standard therapy for uncomplicated UTI described above.

Sexually Transmitted Infections

The urethral syndrome can also be caused by any of several sexually transmitted infections. *Chlamydia, gonorrhea,* and *herpes simplex* are the most common causes. Other agents such as *Mycoplasma hominis* and *Ureaplasma urealyticum* may be found, but their significance is uncertain.

Any woman who has the acute onset of *dysuria and*

has urine that is apparently sterile may have one of these infections. Correct diagnosis and therapy are somewhat demanding and require facilities that may not be present in most doctor's offices. The patient should have a pelvic examination to check for the signs of common STDs, and the appropriate specimens should be obtained for culture and other examinations (see Chapter 94).

The important *features to look for during pelvic examinations* are herpetic vesicles for herpes simplex, mucopurulent cervical discharge for chlamydia, and frankly purulent cervical discharge and sometimes urethral discharge for gonorrhea. Evidence of other sexually transmitted infections should be noted because they may require separate treatment. Diagnosis may be confirmed by Tzanck test or culture for herpes simplex; enzyme-linked immunosorbent assay (ELISA), fluorescent antibody, or endocervical culture for chlamydia; and endocervical culture for gonorrhea. Tests based on the PCR reaction are becoming available for all three organisms and offer much greater sensitivity. There is even a PCR test for chlamydia that can be done on urine.

Sexually transmitted infections should be treated according to Centers for Disease Control and Prevention (CDC) guidelines, which are updated annually. As of 1996, *ceftriaxone* 250 mg intramuscularly was the standard therapy for gonorrhea; it also eliminates incubating syphilis. *Doxycycline* 100 mg twice daily for 7 days is given also, for chlamydial infection, even if the patient appears to have gonorrhea. Alternatively, both gonorrhea and chlamydia can be treated with *ofloxacin* 400 mg twice daily for 7 days. If the patient clearly does not have gonorrhea, chlamydial infection can be treated with *azithromycin* 1 g orally as a single dose or doxycycline 100 mg twice daily for 7 to 10 days. Severe primary herpes simplex infections should be treated with acyclovir or famciclovir (see details in Chapter 94).

If the patient has not been sexually active ever or for years, then the dysuria/pyuria syndrome is occasionally caused by a viral infection. Adenovirus is the most common cause (20).

Unidentified Etiology

Of women who have the urethral syndrome, 5 to 10% do not have a demonstrable infectious agent even when special culture methods are used; most often these patients do not have pyuria. The cause of the syndrome in these instances is unknown. In this group, treatment with reassurance, sitz baths, and the urinary tract analgesic phenazopyridine (Pyridium), 200 mg three times a day for 5 to 10 days, will provide some relief. The patient should be informed that this medication causes the urine to appear orange. If symptoms persist, referral to a urologist is indicated for cystoscopic evaluation.

Measures to be recommended to patients with this syndrome should be identical to those outlined above for UTI (Table 27.3) or, if there is vaginitis or an STD present, as outlined in Chapter 94.

Interstitial Cystitis

Interstitial cystitis is an occasionally seen disorder affecting middle-aged women, which early in its course may be confused with the urethral syndrome. Interstitial cystitis causes symptoms of suprapubic discomfort, especially when the bladder is full, and symptoms are relieved by voiding. The patient may experience progressive loss of bladder volume and increasing urinary frequency, and eventually may have to void four to six times per hour throughout the night. The urinalysis is often normal, but hematuria may be present. The urine is sterile. This disease is difficult to diagnose. If it is suspected on the basis of the history, referral to a urologist is indicated. The urologist performs cystoscopy and often a biopsy of the bladder to establish the diagnosis (usually a normal-appearing mucosa with a very small vesical capacity is identified; tissue histology may show changes consistent with the diagnosis; mucosal hemorrhage may appear with bladder filling). Also, a cystoscopic evaluation permits the urologist to exclude other causes of the symptoms (e.g., bladder tumor). No definitive therapy has yet been developed for treatment of this condition.

Vaginitis and Cervicitis

For detailed discussion of these conditions, see Chapter 94.

SYMPTOMATIC UTIs IN MEN

Bacterial Cystitis

Bacterial cystitis in men is similar in presentation to that in the female patient and is diagnosed by the same method, but a urine culture should always be obtained. A UTI in a man suggests the presence of an underlying structural problem or the presence of bacterial prostatitis. In the last edition of this book, it was stated that the initial evaluation should always include a prostate examination. However, because young men who are either homosexual or uncircumcised can develop UTIs in the absence of a structural abnormality, some easing of this standard is reasonable in men from either of these groups (3,30). If a workup is initiated, sonography is preferable to IVP as a screening tool.

A small number of young boys develop UTI in the apparent absence of a structural abnormality. Most turn out to have a congenital abnormality such as urethral valves. Young men with UTIs most often have stone or hydronephrosis. Older men generally have prostatic enlargement or stones.

Bacterial cystitis in men should always be treated for a minimum of 7 to 10 days (see daily dosages and schedules for antibiotics, Table 27.2). Structural problems are so common that short courses are ineffective. Even if no structural anomaly is found, men should be carefully followed up because many of the infections will relapse. Many men with relapse-type recurrences have bacterial prostatitis; therefore, a follow-up visit 4 to 6 weeks after the initial infection should be arranged to reculture the urine and, if it is positive, to consider treatment for chronic prostatitis (see below).

Prostatitis

Prostatitis is classified as bacterial prostatitis (acute and chronic), nonbacterial prostatitis (prostatosis), or the much less common prostatic infections caused by a virus, a parasite, tuberculosis, a fungus, or nonspecific granulomatous changes.

Acute Bacterial Prostatitis

Acute bacterial prostatitis is characterized often by the abrupt onset of fever, chills, low back pain, and perineal pain with irritative urinary tract symptoms, although on some occasions systemic symptoms are not pronounced. Perineal discomfort may be worsened by defecation. In addition, the patient may have initial, terminal, or occasionally total hematuria (see Chapter 45). Rectal examination usually discloses a tender, swollen, and boggy prostate. The urine and the expressed prostatic secretions contain leukocytes, and culture often grows the responsible bacterial pathogen, which most commonly is *E. coli* in older men and *Chlamydia* or *N. gonorrhoeae* in younger men.

When the diagnosis is made, the patient may require hospitalization, although if systemic symptoms are minimal, ambulatory therapy is appropriate. Most antibiotics do not achieve high concentrations in prostatic fluid. The best initial choice for younger patients is *ofloxacin* (400 mg twice daily), which penetrates the prostate well and covers the common etiologic organisms. If quinolones cannot be used, then a number of other antibiotics may be tried. *Trimethoprim–sulfamethoxazole* does penetrate prostatic epithelium and is an alternative for treating *E. coli*. Penicillins and cephalosporins do not achieve effective concentrations in the prostate and are not useful. Because of the overriding effects of local antibiotic concentration, antibiotics such as *erythromycin,* which would not normally be used to treat *E. coli,* may also prove effective. Therapy with antimicrobials for acute prostatitis should be continued for 2 weeks. Dosages and schedules are listed in Table 27.2.

Bed rest and sitz baths for 20 to 30 minutes two or three times a day may provide comfort. Occasionally, prostatitis results in acute urinary retention, which requires hospitalization and urgent urologic consultation. The palpable irregularity of the prostate gland after acute infection may persist for several months. The acute infection is readily controlled but recurrences may occur, especially in older patients.

Chronic Bacterial Prostatitis

The organisms that cause chronic bacterial prostatitis most often are Gram-negative bacilli, *E. coli* being the most common organism, followed by *Enterococcus, Proteus,* and *Klebsiella*. Most patients with chronic bacterial prostatitis have mild irritative symptoms (frequency, urgency, and dysuria), and occasionally there is a urethral discharge. Fever is absent.

Patients may also have painless hematuria or painful ejaculation with hematospermia. On rectal examination the prostate gland feels somewhat irregular and may be mildly tender, although the examination is often unremarkable.

Obstructive symptoms are rare. Most often the patients have intermittent symptomatic episodes that have been controlled with short courses of antibiotics. Unfortunately, however, recurrent infection is common because of persistence of bacteria within the urinary tract. Chronic prostatitis may also be a reservoir for acute symptomatic cystitis, pyelonephritis, or epididymitis. Therefore, a prolonged course of therapy is indicated when chronic prostatitis is diagnosed clinically. If the infectious organism is sensitive, *ciprofloxacin 250 mg twice daily for 2 weeks* has been shown to be effective in eradicating infection in over 60% of patients with chronic prostatitis (7).

If all efforts to eradicate infection fail, symptoms usually can be controlled with *suppressive therapy* using a low-dose *trimethoprim–sulfamethoxazole,* one-half tablet of regular strength (Bactrim, Septra, or generic) nightly, indefinitely. The only way to effect a cure is by radical prostatectomy, but the morbidity of this procedure precludes its use for benign disease. Repeated prostatic massage has not been shown to be effective. Patients with refractory chronic bacterial prostatitis should be evaluated by a urologist.

Nonbacterial Prostatitis (Prostatosis)

Some patients have all of the symptoms and signs of chronic bacterial infection of the prostate, but no organism can be demonstrated. They have nonbacterial prostatitis (prostatosis), which is the most common form of prostatic inflammation. These patients have mild perineal pain and irritative symptoms on urination with *cells in the urine sediment, but negative urine cultures.* Culture of the secretions and urine by special techniques occasionally reveals infectious agents such as *Mycoplasma, Gardnerella vaginalis, U. urealyticum,* or *Chlamydia* species; however, the significance of these findings is unknown. Most patients with this condition cannot be cured; nevertheless, treatment with an antimicrobial such as ciprofloxacin or ofloxacin at the dosage and schedule described above for acute prostatitis may control symptoms. An antispasmodic agent such as oxybutynin (Ditropan), 5 mg two to three times a day, may be tried. Therapeutic prostatic massage has not been shown to be of value.

If there is no response to therapy, the patient should be referred to a urologist to exclude conditions such as interstitial cystitis and in situ bladder cancer. Both conditions require cystoscopic examination for confirmation.

Prostatodynia

Patients with a syndrome called prostatodynia have symptoms suggesting prostatic inflammation but have no evidence of inflammation on physical examination, have *no white blood cells in the urine or expressed prostatic secretions, and have sterile urine cultures.* There is some evidence that the syndrome may be caused by a neurologic disorder and that muscle relaxants or α-sympathetic blocking agents such as phenoxybenzamine (Dibenzyline) are effective in treating it. If this syndrome is suspected, urologic consultation is suggested to confirm the diagnosis, to rule out interstitial cystitis and bladder cancer, and to initiate therapy.

Epididymitis

Organisms reach the epididymis through the lumen of the vas deferens from infected urine, the posterior urethra, or the seminal vesicles. Epididymitis is manifested as an abrupt swelling of the epididymis that spreads rapidly, presenting often as a generalized inflammation of the entire hemiscrotum and making the differentiation from an acute orchitis impossible. Often, fever, chills, and irritative bladder symptoms are also present. The differential diagnosis includes torsion of the testicle, acute orchitis, and tumor of the testicle with hemorrhage or hydrocele. *Several observations help differentiate torsion from epididymitis:* Torsion occurs in young boys and epididymitis occurs after puberty, the urinalysis is normal in torsion but usually shows pyuria in epididymitis, and elevation of the scrotum often relieves the pain of epididymitis but intensifies the discomfort in torsion. If there is any doubt about the distinction between epididymitis and testicular torsion, a urologist's opinion should be obtained at once.

Epididymitis may be distinguished from orchitis only in its early stages. However, the presence of a urethral discharge or pyuria suggests epididymitis. A *tumor* of the testis is usually identified by its hardness and insensitivity to pressure. A *hydrocele* is usually easy to identify because it is painless and transilluminates light.

Most cases of epididymitis in young men are caused by *Chlamydia trachomatis* infection. Gonorrhea causes less than 5% of such cases. At any age, UTI with Gram-negative rods can spread to the epididymis; most such patients are over 50. Mumps is reviving as an occasional cause of epididymo-orchitis in patients whose vaccine immunity has waned. Rarely, chronic epididymal infection is caused by tuberculous or fungal disease of the urinary tract. In some instances no infectious agent can be identified. Once the diagnosis of epididymitis is made on clinical grounds, it should be treated while the etiologic organism is being confirmed by culture of the urine.

Presumed chlamydial infection should be treated with doxycycline, azithromycin, or ofloxacin (see daily dosages in Table 27.4), and bacterial pathogens should be treated as usual (Table 27.2). *Treatment should be continued for 14 days.* Gonorrhea should be treated with ceftriaxone plus doxycycline for possible chlamydia coinfection, or with ofloxacin (Table 27.4).

Bed rest, scrotal support, and sitz baths may minimize symptoms while the infection is responding to treatment. The patient should be informed that indu-

Table 27.4. Management of Urethritis in Men

Treatments for gonococcal urethritis and nongonococcal urethritis simultaneously:

Ceftriaxone (Rocephin) 250 mg intramuscularly as single dose
plus
Doxycycline 100 mg twice a day for 7 days *or* 1 g azithromycin by mouth
OR
Ofloxacin 300 mg q12hr for 7 days
Report to local health department. They will follow up and treat sexual partners.
Men who appear to have gonorrhea should be treated for both.

Treatments for nongonococcal urethritis:

Doxycycline 100 mg q12hr for 7 days
OR
Ofloxacin 300 mg q12hr for 7 days
OR
Azithromycin 1 g orally (single dose)

1998 Guidelines for treatment of sexually transmitted diseases. MMWR 47(RR-1), 1998.

ration and edema in the region of the epididymis may persist for as long as 6 to 8 weeks.

The *older patient* with acute epididymitis should always have a urine culture and should be evaluated for obstruction at the bladder outlet (see Chapter 49) as soon as the acute symptoms are controlled. On rare occasions, continued pain from chronic epididymitis may occur; if it does, a urologist should be consulted because an epididymectomy may be required.

Urethritis

Urethritis is an acute inflammation of the urethra that may be classified as gonococcal or nongonococcal (13).

Nongonococcal urethritis is more common, and the most common cause for it is *C. trachomatis.* Symptoms of urethritis in the male patient include a discharge from the urethra, dysuria, and a sensation of itching at the distal end of the penis. There is no associated fever. Nearly 25% of men with a *Chlamydia* infection have no symptoms (34). Culture for *C. trachomatis* is expensive and is not recommended for routine clinical use; however, commercial laboratories increasingly have available low-cost, rapid, and accurate methods of detecting *Chlamydia* in urogenital swab specimens. These methods, as they become more widely available, will help accurately diagnose *Chlamydia* urethritis.

Diagnosis of *gonococcal urethritis* depends on the examination and culture of the urethral discharge. Material from the male urethra is best obtained using a sterile calcium alginate swab (Calgiswab, Type 1). The Calgiswab is much smaller than the usual cotton swab and for this reason is less irritating to the patient. Approximately 10% of men with gonorrhea are asymptomatic, and swabbing the urethra for a culture of *N. gonorrhoeae* is appropriate whenever there is a history of exposure.

Swartz et al. (37) point out the usefulness of counting the white blood cells after staining the discharge with Gram's stain. A Calgiswab is passed into the urethra, then rolled over a 1- to 2-cm area on a slide, which is stained by Gram's stain. Gonococcal urethritis is almost always associated with more than 50 WBC/HPF compared with less than 2 in normal men and a count of 4 to 50/HPF in patients with nongonococcal urethritis. Gonococcal urethritis is diagnosed by the presence on Gram's stain of extracellular or intracellular Gram-negative diplococci.

Management

The management of STDs is continually changing. A full-scale update from CDC was issued in 1998 (Table 27.4). If a person appears to have gonorrhea, he or she should be treated not only for gonorrhea but also for chlamydia. The gold standard is one intramuscular dose of ceftriaxone plus 7 days of doxycycline to deal with chlamydia. An attractive but expensive alternative is to use ceftriaxone plus a single large dose of azithromycin by mouth, which has been shown to eradicate chlamydia. Alternatively, both diseases can be treated with 5 days of ofloxacin by mouth. Many clinics use ciprofloxacin instead. Intramuscular spectinomycin is a treatment useful only for gonorrhea, which might be indicated occasionally.

In nongonococcal urethritis, the discharge continues for a longer period and is more mucoid, and the smear, as noted above, has fewer white blood cells and no stainable bacteria. Treatment with doxycycline 100 mg twice a day for 7 days is usually effective but recurrences may occur. Alternatives are a quinolone for 5 days, or a single large dose of azithromycin.

Because all forms of urethritis must be assumed to be sexually transmitted, the patient's *partner or partners* should be treated with a regimen appropriate for the urethritis and the patient should use a condom until all of the infections have been eradicated.

When patients continue to have recurrences of nongonococcal urethritis or have persistent symptoms unresponsive to antimicrobial agents, they should have bacteriologic studies to evaluate the possibility of a chronic bacterial prostatitis (see above), and they should also undergo urologic investigation for evaluation of possible urethral stricture, foreign bodies, or other intraurethral lesions. A few cases of doxycycline-resistant nongonococcal urethritis are caused by *Ureaplasma* infection (38).

Gonorrhea in women is discussed in Chapter 94.

PERSISTENT UTI IN MEN AND WOMEN

As noted above, treatment in the male or female patient of infection in a normal urinary tract with an appropriate antimicrobial should result in the sterilization of the urine within 72 hours. By this time, symptoms should have abated, or at least markedly diminished. If symptoms continue, a persistent infection may be present, and the urine culture should be repeated. If the urine culture is still positive despite antibiotic therapy, further investigation is required. Modern antibiotics are so effective and the concentra-

tions achieved in urine are so high that persistent infection is unusual.

The possibilities to be considered are that the patient is not taking the antibiotic or has taken it but vomited subsequently; the organism is totally resistant (unusual but seen with certain pseudomonads and enterococci); the patient's renal function is so poor (e.g., creatinine above 3 mg/dL) that little antibiotic reaches the urine; the antibiotic does not work at the current urinary pH; there is a gross structural anomaly such as a vesicocolic fistula or a leaking pyonephrosis or a nidus of sequestered bacteria such as a staghorn calculus, as described in Chapter 47; or the organism is not a bacterium at all, but a fungus. Once one has decided which of the above applies, the indicated treatment is usually obvious.

RECURRENT INFECTION, RELAPSE TYPE, IN MEN AND WOMEN

Recurrent infection with the same organism is called relapse infection and implies the persistence of bacteria in tissue within the urinary tract. Relapse infection is similar to persistent infection except that in relapse the urine has been shown to be sterile while the patient is on or has completed antimicrobial therapy, whereas sterility is never demonstrated with persistent infection. Relapse occurs most often within 6 weeks of completion of a course of antimicrobial therapy. An underlying structural problem is often present in both men and women with this condition. In women, relapse is much less common than reinfection but is difficult to document because most infections are a result of *E. coli*, which has many serotypes that cannot be differentiated by routine bacteriologic laboratory techniques. Therefore, recurrent UTI caused by *E. coli* may be either relapse (same serotype) or reinfection (different serotype). On the other hand, relapse of infection with organisms other than *E. coli* may be diagnosed by routine bacteriologic culture. In women, if recurrent infection with *E. coli* occurs four times in a 12-month period or if relapse infection with other species occurs, evaluation as outlined under "Persistent UTI in Men and Women" to exclude the possibility of structural abnormality is appropriate. If a structural abnormality is identified, it should be corrected if possible.

If a woman or man has a structural or functional abnormality of the urinary tract that cannot be corrected, sterilization of the urinary tract usually is not possible. In a patient who has had recurrent infections because of urine stasis caused by an atonic bladder, *intermittent straight catheterization* by the patient or a trained member of the family may help to prevent recurrent infections (see "Urinary Incontinence" in Chapter 6). In patients with other abnormalities, *suppressive therapy* (see regimens for prophylaxis of recurrent cystitis above) may decrease the frequency of symptomatic exacerbations or episodes of sepsis. Relapsing infection may occur in *patients with no evidence of a structural abnormality*. In women, that usually means that the patient has chronic pyelonephritis. In men, the most common cause is chronic bacterial prostatitis. Chronic pyelonephritis is generally treated with a 6-week course of an appropriate antibiotic, on several occasions if necessary. Some patients may eventually respond to prolonged antibiotic courses of 6 months or more. These prolonged courses are generally indicated only in young patients where there is some hope of cure.

If the patient has chronic bacteriuria that cannot be eradicated, there is good evidence that the ingestion of large quantities of cranberry juice will reduce the number of symptomatic episodes (2).

INFECTION IN CATHETERIZED PATIENTS

In the ambulatory setting, one often sees patients who were catheterized while acutely ill in the hospital, developed infection, and now have bacteriuria, even though the catheter has been removed. In general, these patients should be treated based on antibiotic sensitivities, because otherwise they will probably develop symptomatic episodes of cystitis or pyelonephritis. The usual course of antibiotic is 10 days, and because recurrence is common, a test of cure urine culture should be done.

ACUTE PYELONEPHRITIS IN MEN AND WOMEN

Pyelonephritis is a bacterial infection of the kidney that most often results from ascending infection. It is suggested by flank pain, fever, and often, abdominal pain in addition to symptoms of bladder irritation. Bacterial infection of the kidney may also be present without any of these signs or symptoms or with only bladder irritation (8). The urinalysis will show changes as outlined above, but only the presence of *white blood cell casts* is diagnostic of pyelonephritis.

Clinically apparent acute pyelonephritis *in men* suggests the presence of a structural problem predisposing to infection and is an indication for immediate hospitalization, parenteral antimicrobial therapy, a sonogram, and possibly other urologic investigations. If an abscess is seen or suspected, a CT scan is indicated because abscesses usually need surgical drainage.

In *women,* an underlying structural problem is much less likely to be present. Therefore, the decision for hospitalization and evaluation requires careful consideration. The patient can be treated at home if she does not have complicating medical illnesses, is not severely ill, does not exhibit sepsis, is reliable, can take antimicrobials by mouth, and if access to the physician is guaranteed should symptoms worsen (28). If a patient is treated at home, follow-up in 24 to 48 hours by telephone is necessary. If there has not been significant improvement during that time, the possibility of an undrained infection (e.g., caused by obstruction or abscess) should be considered and prompt hospitalization should be arranged for parenteral antibiotics, sonography, and emergency urologic consultation.

The initial treatment for the patient treated at home can be a 10- to 14-day course of any of the antimicrobial agents listed in Table 27.2, with an appropriate adjustment based on the results of the urine culture and on sensitivity testing. Forcing fluid (once an antimicrobial has been started) is unnecessary and may theoretically be detrimental because the concentration of antimicrobials in the urine and in the renal tissue may be diluted. However, intake should be adequate to replace fluid losses, including the additional fluid lost by fever or by vomiting.

If the acute episode of pyelonephritis promptly resolves, follow-up in 3 to 4 weeks is appropriate. At that time, the urine culture should be sterile. If the urine is not sterile and if the organism is the same one that caused the clinical attack of pyelonephritis, the patient is a candidate for a prolonged course of antibiotic therapy (6 weeks).

ASYMPTOMATIC BACTERIURIA IN MEN AND WOMEN

Not Associated with Pregnancy

Asymptomatic bacteriuria is more common in women and increases in both sexes with advancing age. Among people aged 20 to 50, bacteriuria is present in 0.5% of men and less than 5% of women. In contrast, 3% of men and 20% of women aged 65 to 70 have positive urine cultures. After age 80, 22% of men and 23 to 50% of women have bacteriuria (15).

In addition to advancing age, asymptomatic bacteriuria is also associated with indwelling urinary catheters, urinary incontinence, multiple medical illnesses, impairment of functional status, and impairment of mental status.

Several population studies report an unexplained increase in mortality in elderly patients with asymptomatic bacteriuria (4). This increase in mortality appears to be secondary to concomitant illnesses rather than a direct consequence of the bacteriuria, and treatment of the bacteria does not affect mortality (1). It is not known how often nonpregnant patients with asymptomatic bacteriuria develop symptomatic infections. Treatment with antibiotic therapy is often unsuccessful in eradicating infection and may be associated with the development of more resistant infections (23). Therefore, screening for or treatment of asymptomatic bacteriuria in nonpregnant adult women of any age is not recommended.

Associated with Pregnancy

Asymptomatic bacteriuria in pregnancy is common, affecting up to 6% of women in the first trimester. Recognition of this fact is important because eradication of bacteriuria reduces the high incidence of symptomatic UTI that subsequently occurs during pregnancy and may increase the risk of premature birth (16). The drugs used are β-lactams, which are known to be associated with a higher rate of recurrent infection than quinolones or trimethoprim–sulfamethoxazole. Good follow-up is therefore essential.

General Reference*

Stamm WER, Hooten TM. Management of urinary tract infections in adults. N Engl J Med 329:1328, 1993.

    Well-referenced review article that stresses recent advances and emphasizes cost-effective strategies for treating UTI.

Specific References

1. Abrityn E, Mossey J, Barlin JA, et al. Does asymptomatic bacteriuria predict mortality, and does antimicrobial treatment reduce mortality in elderly ambulatory women? Ann Intern Med 120:827, 1994.

2. Avorn J, Moname M, Gurivitz JH, et al. Reduction of bacteriuria and pyuria after ingestion of cranberry juice. JAMA 271:751, 1994.

3. Barnes RC, Daijuker R, Reddy RE, Stamm WE. Urinary tract infection in sexually active homosexual men. Lancet 2:171, 1986.

4. Boscia JA, Alnityn E. Pyuria and asymptomatic bacteriuria in elderly women. Ann Intern Med 110:404, 1989.

5. Brettman LR. Pathogenesis of urinary tract infections: host susceptibility and bacterial virulence factors. Urology 33(3):9, 1988.

6. Cates W Jr. Epidemiology and control of sexually transmitted diseases: strategic evaluation. Infect Dis Clin North Am 1:1, 1987.

7. Childs SJ, Goldstein EJC. Ciprofloxacin as treatment for genitourinary tract infection. J Urol 141:1, 1989.

8. Fairley KF, Carson NE, Gutch RC, et al. Site of infection in acute urinary tract infection in general practice. Lancet 2:615, 1971.

9. Fihn SD. Behavioral aspects of urinary tract infection. Urology 33(4):16, 1994.

10. Filly R. Ultrasonography. In: Friedland GW, Filly R, Goris ML, et al, eds. Uroradiology: an integrated approach. New York: Churchill Livingstone, 1983.

11. Freedman LR. Natural history of urinary tract infection in adults. Kidney Int 8:S96, 1975.

12. Hooton TM, Hillier S, Johnson C, et al. *Escherichia coli* bacteriuria and contraceptive method. JAMA 265:64, 1991.

13. Jacobs NF, Kraus SJ. Gonococcal and nongonococcal urethritis in men. Ann Intern Med 82:7, 1975.

14. James GP, Paul KL, Fuller JB. Urinary nitrite and urinary tract infection. Am J Clin Pathol 70:671, 1978.

15. Kaye D. Urinary tract infections in the elderly. Bull N Y Acad Med 57(2):209, 1980.

16. Kincaid-Smith P. Bacteriuria in pregnancy. Lancet 1:395, 1965.

17. Komaroff AL. Acute dysuria in women. N Engl J Med 310:368, 1984.

18. Latham RH, Running K, Stamm WE. Urinary tract infections in young women caused by Staphylococcus saprophyticus. JAMA 250:3063, 1983.

19. Leisure MK, Dudley SM, Donowitz LG. Does a clean catch urine sample reduce bacterial contamination? N Engl J Med 328:289, 1993.

20. Manalo D, Mufson MA, Zoller IM, Manded VM. Adenovirus infection in acute hemorrhagic cystitis: a study in 25 children. Am J Dis Child 121:281, 1971.

21. Margileth AM, Pedreira FA, Hirschman GH, et al. Urinary tract bacterial infections. Pediatr Clin North Am 23:71, 1976.

22. McCue JD. Urinary tract infection and dysuria. Cost conscious evaluation and antibiotic therapy. Postgrad Med 80:133, 1986.

23. Nicolle LE, Mayhew WJ, Bryan C. Prospective randomized comparison of therapy and no therapy for asymptomatic bacteruria in elderly institutionalized women. Am J Med 83:27, 1987.

24. Pfolles M, Ringenberg B, Rames L, et al. The usefulness of screening tests for pyuria in combination with culture in the diagnosis of urinary tract infection. Diagn Microb Infect Dis 6:207, 1987.

25. Phillnick JT, Bracikowski SP. Single dose antibiotic treatment for uncomplicated urinary tract infections. Less for less? Arch Intern Med 145:1672, 1985.

26. Raz R, Stamm WE. A controlled trial of intravaginal estriol in post-menopausal women with recurrent urinary tract infections. N Engl J Med 329:753, 1993.

27. Rumans LW, Vosti KL. The relationship of antibody-coated bacteria to clinical syndromes. Arch Intern Med 138:1077, 1978.

28. Safrin S, Siegel D, Black D. Pyelonephritis in adult women: inpatient versus outpatient therapy. Am J Med 85:793, 1988.

29. Sobel JD, Kaye D. Urinary tract infections. In: Mandell GL, Douglas RG, Bennett JR, eds. Principles and practice of infectious diseases. 3rd ed. New York: Churchill Livingstone, 1990.

30. Spach DH, Stapleton AE, Stamm WE. Lack of circumcision increases the risk of urinary tract infection in young men. JAMA 267:679, 1992.

31. Stamey TA: Recurrent urinary tract infections in female patients. Rev Infect Dis 9(Suppl 2):S195, 1987.

32. Stamm WE. Measurement of pyuria and its relationship to bacteriuria. Am J Med 75(Suppl 1B):53, 1983.

33. Stamm WE, Counts GW, Running KR, et al. Diagnosis of coliform infection in acutely dysuric women. N Engl J Med 307:463, 1982.

34. Stamm WE, Koutsky LA, Benedett JK, et al. Chlamydia trachomatis urethral infection in men. Ann Intern Med 100:47, 1984.

35. Stamm WE, Running K, McKwitt M, et al. Treatment of the acute urethral syndrome. N Engl J Med 304:956, 1987.

36. Stamm WE, Wagner KF, Ansel RL, et al. Causes of the acute urethral syndrome in women. N Engl J Med 303:409, 1980.

37. Swartz SL, Kraus SJ, Hermann KL, et al. Diagnosis and etiology of nongonorrhea urethritis. J Infect Dis 138:445, 1978.

38. Taylor-Robinson D, Furr PM. Clinical antibiotic resistance to *Ureaplasma urealyticum*. Pediatr Infect Dis 5(Suppl):5335, 1986.

39. Turck M, Goffe B, Petersdorf RG. The urethral catheters and urinary tract infections. J Urol 88:834, 1962.

40. Vosti K. Recurrent urinary tract infection: prevention by prophylactic antibiotics after sexual intercourse. JAMA 231:934, 1975.

---

*Bold print (general references) and bold numerals (specific references) denote published controlled trials, meta-analyses, or consensus-based recommendations.

C H A P T E R 28

Respiratory Tract Infections

FREDERICK T. KOSTER, MD
L. RANDOL BARKER, MD

UPPER RESPIRATORY INFECTIONS

Magnitude of the Problem

Upper respiratory infections (URIs) are the most common acute illnesses in the United States and in the industrialized world. These infections are the most common causes of absences from school or work. Most URIs are self-diagnosed and self-treated and do not come to the attention of a physician (Americans spend $1 billion annually for over-the-counter medications for the relief of upper respiratory symptoms).

Common Cold

The common cold is a mild, self-limited syndrome caused usually by viral infection of the upper respiratory tract mucosa and characterized by one or more of the following symptoms: nasal discharge and obstruction, sneezing, sore throat, cough, and hoarseness.

Epidemiology and Transmission

The common cold syndrome is caused by a variety of viruses that are clinically indistinguishable from each other, yet have distinct seasonal peaks for unknown reasons. *Rhinoviruses* are the etiologic agent in 25 to 30% of colds, with seasonal peaks in early fall and mid- to late spring. *Coronaviruses* account for another 10 to 15% of annual colds, with a seasonal peak in midwin-

ter. *Influenza, parainfluenza, respiratory syncytial viruses, and adenovirus* are etiologic agents for another 10 to 15%, although this group more commonly has the typical influenza syndrome (see below). Bacteria associated with pharyngitis (see below) can also cause some of the common cold symptoms.

The incidence of the common cold syndrome decreases with age. On the average, adults have two to four colds per year; children have six to eight (42). Because person-to-person spread of colds occurs mainly in the home and at school, schoolchildren usually serve as carriers for introducing colds into the family. Thus, mothers tend to have higher secondary attack rates than do fathers.

Transmission of rhinovirus is most efficient by direct physical contact (28). Frequent, unconscious touching of virus-contaminated nasal mucosa contaminates the subject's hands. Infectious material can survive on the hand for as long as 4 hours (1), during which time hand-to-hand contact with susceptible subjects transmits the virus. Exposure to susceptible subjects across even short distances of air is an inefficient method of transmission of rhinoviruses, although aerosol transmission of particles effectively transmits some viruses (e.g., Coxsackie, influenza, and adenovirus). Thus transmission of colds is probably uncommon in offices, theaters, buses, and so on if nose-to-hand-to-hand-to-nose contact is avoided.

Clinical Characteristics

The correct diagnosis of the common cold is readily made by the patient. After an incubation period of 48 to 72 hours, the syndrome begins with mild malaise, rhinorrhea, sneezing, scratchy throat, and variable loss of taste and smell. These symptoms increase to maximal severity on the second to fourth day. Viral excretion and communicability are maximal during the period of severest symptoms. Fever is usually not present but, if present, rarely exceeds 1°F (0.5°C) elevation. Cough and hoarseness may begin later, and their severity and duration are increased in cigarette smokers. Conversely, neither cigarette smoking nor exposure to cold appears to increase the attack rate of colds. Colds usually last 1 week but in one-quarter of cases last up to 2 weeks.

Identification of the causative virus by clinical observation is not possible, nor is it necessary for management. The primary challenge for the physician is to identify the patients with complicating secondary bacterial sinusitis (see below) and otitis media (see Chapter 96), for whom antimicrobials may be beneficial. The use of radiographs, pneumatic otoscopy, and throat culture is discussed in sections on sinusitis (below), otitis (Chapter 96), and pharyngitis (below), respectively.

Treatment

Patients with typical URI syndromes can be assessed and managed appropriately by a telephone contact (35). Specific antiviral therapy for the uncomplicated common cold is not available, but symptomatic treatment is appropriate. Aspirin and acetaminophen relieve fever, headache, and myalgias, but increase nasal secretions, possibly by decreasing the neutralizing antibody response (25). Naproxen (and presumably other nonsteroidal anti-inflammatory drugs [NSAIDs]) relieves the headache, myalgias, and cough without altering viral shedding or antibody response (65). Bed rest is not necessary to facilitate recovery. Steam inhalation did not alleviate nasal symptoms (20), but sipping hot chicken soup (the only soup studied) increases the clearance of nasal mucus (59). Recovery from hoarseness, caused by inflammation and edema of the vocal cords, may be accelerated by voice rest. Zinc lozenges taken every 2 hours may accelerate recovery of all symptoms but may also cause nausea and bad taste (46).

Nasal congestion is best relieved by *topical decongestants;* sprays rather than drops are preferred for ease of administration (Table 28.1). Patients should be cautioned against using drops or sprays for more than 5 days to avoid the rebound effect, defined as an increase in nasal congestion when decongestant medication is discontinued. In contrast to orally administered decongestants (when used in excess of recommended dosages), there has been no blood pressure–elevating effect reported with topical decongestants. (See additional discussion of topical decongestants in Chapter 23.) Topical ipratropium spray (0.06%) relieves rhinorrhea and sneezing but may cause blood-tinged mucus and nasal dryness (31).

The *oral decongestants* phenylpropanolamine and pseudoephedrine (Sudafed, 30 mg over-the-counter or 60 mg by prescription; also available as Sudafed S.A., a sustained-action preparation containing 120 mg of pseudoephedrine, taken every 12 hours) are somewhat helpful. When prescribed in the recommended dosages, these drugs do not cause blood pressure to increase in treated hypertensive patients (41).

The *combination of decongestant and antihistamine,* helpful in allergic rhinitis (see Chapter 23), offers less consistent relief of common cold symptoms (see Table 23.7) (63,64).

There is no evidence that any *expectorant* is effective in URIs, and it is more rational and far less expensive to use the other ingredients contained in combination cough remedies individually in appropriate dosages. (See discussion of cough suppressants below.)

Antimicrobials are useless in the uncomplicated cold.

Patient Education

Because transmission of colds occurs chiefly by physical contact, it is reasonable to counsel patients and those around them that transmission can be minimized by handwashing, reduced finger-to-nose contact, and reduced exposure to the cold sufferer. Physicians should be particularly vigilant to avoid contact with the patient's secretions and should wash their hands carefully after examining the infected patient. Although physicians with common colds may examine patients if they wash their hands and avoid sneezing on the patient, physicians with the flu syndrome should avoid patient contact (see below).

Viral URIs may be complicated by superimposed bacterial sinusitis, otitis media, or pneumonitis. Therefore, patients should be advised to notify their physician of any symptoms (see below) suggesting one of these syndromes, each of which may require antimicrobial treatment.

Prevention

Prophylactic and therapeutic properties of large doses of *vitamin C* have been examined in a number of trials, and no consistent beneficial effect has been found (10). In the studies suggesting a benefit, the placebo effect could not be excluded because subjects could identify the vitamin C capsule by taste. In dosages above 4 g/day, vitamin C may cause diarrhea and has the potential of precipitating urate, oxalate,

Table 28.1. Over the-Counter Cold Medications[a]

	Generic Name	Trade Name	Effectiveness	Side Effects
Antihistamines	Chlorpheniramine	75 products listed in PDR	Reduces sneezing, nasal mucus, symptom score	Drowsiness
	Diphenhydramine HCl	Benadryl	No difference from placebo	Drowsiness
	Triprolidine	Actifed	No difference from placebo	No
	Astemizole	Hismanol	Seasonal allergic rhinitis	Weight gain
Decongestants	Pseudoephedrine/ phenylephrine spray	89 products listed in PDR	Reduces congestion, sneezing	Tachycardia, palpitations, elevated diastolic BP, fatigue, dizziness, bladder outlet obstruction
	Oxymetazoline spray	Dristan, Afrin	Improved symptom score	Rebound nasal congestion
Expectorants	Guaifenesin	64 products listed in PDR	Marginal reduction sputum quantity, not in cough frequency	No
Combinations	Decongestant/antihistamine	Many[b]	Reduces congestion, post-nasal drip, rhinorrhea	Dry mouth, insomnia, nervousness

[a]See package insert for dosage and schedule information.
[b]See Chapter 23, Table 23.6.

and cystine stones in susceptible people. Other uncommon effects include diminishing the anticoagulant effect of warfarin and confusing urine glucose tests, causing a false-negative glucose oxidase (Dextrostix, Tes-tape), a false-negative urine nitrate test, or a false-positive copper reduction test (Clinitest tablets).

Vaccine development is complicated by the great antigenic diversity of respiratory viruses, including more than 100 serotypes of rhinoviruses and 47 serotypes of adenoviruses.

Flu Syndrome

Flu presents as the abrupt onset of malaise, myalgia, headache, and fever. Coryza and sore throat are also present. Illness is severe for 3 to 14 days, and convalescence lasts for 1 to 4 weeks. As many as 85% of cases of flu syndrome may be caused by the influenza virus during an epidemic (3). Other viruses, especially parainfluenza, respiratory syncytial, and adenovirus, produce the same clinical syndrome and may coinfect patients with influenza (27).

Epidemiology

Epidemic spread of the influenza virus is caused by the appearance of new antigenic variations of the virus in nonimmune populations. Antigenic variations occur almost annually in influenza serotype A, whereas variation occurs much less frequently in influenza B. Major variation is called *antigenic shift* and results in pandemic spread of a new strain, almost always type A, throughout regions of the world where there is little natural immunity. The most recent pandemics were in the winters of 1957 to 1958, 1968 to 1969, and 1977 to 1978, and they varied considerably in severity. Between pandemics, minor antigenic variations occur frequently, resulting in nearly annual epidemics dur-

ing the winter. Such interpandemic spread, although less dramatic, occurs frequently and therefore accounts for greater cumulative morbidity and mortality than pandemic spread. In some years there are no influenza epidemics. In recent years, however, epidemic influenza has occurred regularly and has influenced death rates (Fig. 28.1). Although it is often impossible clinically to separate infections caused by type A or B, influenza A is responsible for greater excess mortality than type B.

Influenza virus appears to be transmitted by virus-containing small particle aerosols dispersed by sneezing, coughing, or talking. The incubation period is 18 to 72 hours. Viral shedding persists for 5 to 10 days, but virus is present in high titer in secretions for only 48 hours after the onset of clinical illness. In the community, person-to-person transmission is rapid, with spread initially among children, then adults. In local epidemics the incidence of cases reaches a peak in 2 to 3 weeks and persists for only 5 to 6 weeks.

Clinical Characteristics

Uncomplicated influenza, type A or B, has an abrupt onset of systemic symptoms including fever, chills, headache, myalgias, and malaise. The fever, which may rise to 106°F (41°C) in some cases, typically lasts 3 days, although often it persists for 5 to 7 days. Headache and myalgias involving the back, arms, legs, and, occasionally, the eyes are the predominant symptoms, persisting as long as the fever. Respiratory symptoms, such as nonproductive cough, nasal discharge, hoarseness, and sore throat, appear as systemic symptoms wane. Cough and weakness usually subside after 2 weeks but may persist for a longer time.

Physical findings include general toxicity, flushed face, hot skin, watery red eyes, clear nasal discharge, tender cervical lymph nodes, and occasionally, local-

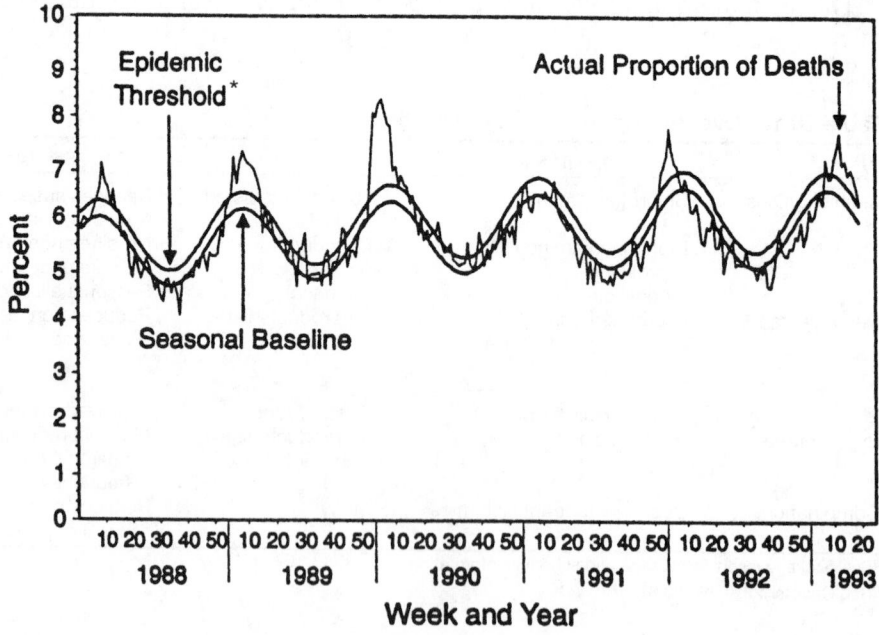

Figure 28.1. Weekly pneumonia and influenza mortality as a proportion of all deaths for 121 cities, United States, January 1, 1988, through May 15, 1993. *The epidemic threshold is 1.645 standard deviations above the seasonal baseline calculated using a periodic regression model applied to observed percentages since 1983. This baseline was calculated using a robust regression procedure.

ized rales in the chest. The white cell count and differential count usually demonstrate mild neutropenia and relative lymphocytosis, caused by absolute granulocytopenia.

Treatment

Amantadine (Symmetrel) and its derivative *rimantadine* (Flumadine) are available for treatment of type A influenza infections. These drugs attenuate clinical disease in all patients with influenza A by reducing the fever by 50% and by shortening the duration of illness by 1 or 2 days; these benefits are seen only if the drug is administered within 24 to 48 hours of onset of illness. Both drugs are available in 100-mg tablets. Side effects, which include insomnia, nervousness, dizziness, and difficulty in concentrating, occur in approximately 7% of adults taking amantadine. These side effects appear a few hours after the first dose, tend to diminish after repeated doses, and disappear upon discontinuation of the drug. Rimantadine rarely causes these side effects. The cost of a therapeutic course (200 mg once a day or 100 mg twice a day for 7 days) is approximately $5 for amantadine and $20 for rimantadine, in contrast to the more costly prophylactic course (12,47) described in Chapter 32. In frail elderly patients and in patients with an elevated creatinine concentration, only 100 mg should be given daily. Treatment with amantadine or rimantadine should be seriously considered for patients at high risk of morbidity and mortality who develop an influenzalike illness in a community where the state or local health department has reported influenza A. Groups at high risk include

- Unvaccinated children and adults with chronic diseases including pulmonary, cardiovascular, metabolic, neuromuscular, or immunodeficiency diseases
- Adults whose activities are vital to community function, including selected hospital personnel
- Patients with life-threatening primary influenza pneumonia, although the efficacy of amantadine in such patients has not been demonstrated

Supportive measures are important for symptomatic relief. Bed rest and adequate fluid intake should be advised. Aspirin, 600 to 900 mg every 3 to 4 hours, or acetaminophen in children or if aspirin is contraindicated, reduces headache, fever, and myalgia. Sponging with tepid water is effective in lowering high fever, whereas sponging with isopropyl alcohol only increases the patient's discomfort. Relief of nasal discharge may be obtained by agents discussed in the section above on the common cold. Relief of cough with cough suppressants is discussed in the section below on acute bronchitis.

Complications

Patients should be advised that dyspnea, hemoptysis, wheezing, purulent sputum, fever persisting more than 7 days, and rarely, dark urine, severe muscle pain, and tenderness herald complications that demand prompt medical attention and usually hospitalization.

Pulmonary complications exhibit a continuous spectrum of severity, from mild airway hyperreactivity without pulmonary infiltrates to segmental influenza pneumonia or secondary bacterial pneumonia to fulminant bilateral influenza pneumonia with the acute respiratory distress syndrome (ARDS).

Airway hyperreactivity may occur after some (30) but not all influenza infections (62) and after other viral respiratory infections (21). It appears to be caused by destruction of epithelial cells secondary to viral invasion and may result from heightened sensitization of afferent cholinergic irritant receptors in the respiratory mucosa. Exposure to inhaled irritants induces a vagally mediated increase in airway resistance, manifested clinically by bronchospasm, coughing, or both; cough may also be caused by direct stimulation of cholinergic irritant receptors because these are the receptors that mediate the cough reflex (for additional details, see Chapter 54). Patients with asthma or chronic bronchitis have even greater bronchoconstrictor responses because of their underlying bronchial smooth muscle hyperreactivity. Airway hyperreactivity can be demonstrated for 3 to 8 weeks after influenza and other viral infections, and occasionally it may last for 4 to 6 months, even in nonatopic patients.

The relationship between airway hyperreactivity and persistent symptoms after influenza is not entirely clear; however, it is likely that nonproductive cough, wheezing, and dyspnea on exertion are related to airway hyperreactivity. These postflu symptoms seem to be particularly common in urban areas during periods of high air pollution. Chest roentgenograms are clear. Both cough and wheezing, following an otherwise uncomplicated flulike infection, may be treated with a trial of an aerosolized bronchodilator (see Chapter 55) as needed and at bedtime. Patients troubled particularly by nighttime cough will obtain additional relief with 15 to 30 mg of codeine at bedtime.

During influenza epidemics, there is a twofold to threefold increase in the incidence of pneumonia (3). The incidence of *postinfluenzal bronchitis and pneumonia* varies with age: low in patients below age 50 and very high in patients over age 70. Mortality from pneumonia during influenza epidemics clearly increases for those with chronic pulmonary disease and congestive heart failure.

Primary influenza viral pneumonia is a rare complication occurring predominantly among people with cardiovascular disease but occasionally in healthy young adults. After several days of typical influenzal symptoms, fever, cough, and dyspnea rapidly progress to cyanosis and delirium, often developing into ARDS. Immediate hospitalization and intensive care are required, but mortality remains high.

Milder influenza pneumonia may be restricted to a single lobe. Patients have persistent fever, cough and dyspnea, localized rales, and normal white blood cell count, and they subsequently experience a benign course.

Secondary bacterial pneumonia and bronchitis complicate up to 10% of cases of influenza A, depending on age group and chronic pulmonary or cardiac disease. Pneumonitic complications of influenza B are less common but are becoming increasingly recognized (2). The presentation is typically biphasic: The initial influenzal illness is followed by several days of clinical improvement, and then there is an exacerbation of fever with production of purulent or bloody sputum. The predominant bacterial pathogen is *Streptococcus pneumoniae,* but *Haemophilus influenzae* and *Staphylococcus aureus* are also common; the last mentioned has a mortality rate of approximately 50% in this setting. The diagnosis and management of pneumonia are discussed below.

Nonpulmonary complications of influenza are unusual. *Myositis,* with thigh pain and inability to walk, occurs occasionally in children and adolescents. Severe myositis with myoglobinuria and acute renal failure has been observed in adults after both influenza A and B. Guillain–Barré syndrome, encephalitis, and transverse myelitis are *neurologic complications* associated rarely with influenza A and, very rarely, B infection, but no firm causal relationship has been established. *Reye's syndrome,* on the other hand, is a rare but severe complication of influenza, usually type B, presenting as a change in mental status and progressing to coma and hepatic failure. The mean age of attack is 6 years and the incidence has fallen markedly in recent years. The syndrome is rare in adults and, unlike the situation in children, there is no known relationship between aspirin and the syndrome in adults. With the exception of mild myositis, all of the nonpulmonary complications of influenza require hospitalization for differential diagnosis and management.

Prevention

The use of influenza vaccine and amantadine prophylaxis in ambulatory practice is discussed in Chapter 32.

Pharyngitis

Etiologic Agents

Sore throat is the fourth most common symptom seen in medical practice. The most important task in the evaluation of pharyngitis is to identify and treat group A streptococcal infections in adults, especially those with a history of rheumatic fever, and to recognize less common causes of pharyngitis associated with more serious systemic illness.

Pharyngitis in the adult is caused by a variety of bacterial and viral pathogens, with no one pathogen predominating (34). Common pathogens, each accounting for 10 to 15% of cases, include β-hemolytic *streptococci* groups A and G, *Mycoplasma pneumoniae,* and TWAR strain of *Chlamydia pneumoniae.* Less common pathogens include *Corynebacterium haemolyticum, Neisseria gonorrhoeae, respiratory syncytial virus, influenza types A and B, parainfluenza, herpes simplex virus, adenovirus,* and *Epstein–Barr virus.* No pathogens are found in at least one-third of cases.

Accompanying signs and symptoms may suggest the cause in some cases. *C. haemolyticum* is characterized by exudative pharyngitis, a scarlatiniform rash, fever, and adenopathy (44). Infectious mononucleosis (see Chapter 53) is characterized by the clinical triad of sore throat, fever, and lymphadenopathy with or without mild tenderness; it can be distinguished with certainty from streptococcal infection on clinical grounds only when hepatosplenomegaly and a maculopapular skin rash (similar to a drug eruption or rubella) are present. Palatal petechiae may be seen in mononucleosis but may also occur with rubella and streptococcal pharyngitis. Pharyngoconjunctival fever, caused by several adenovirus strains, is usually accompanied by influenzalike symptoms and can be distinguished by concurrent conjunctivitis in one-third of cases and a history of swimming pool exposure 1 week before onset. Herpes simplex, Coxsackie virus A, herpangina, and aphthous stomatitis are distinguished by the presence of mucosal vesicles or ulcers (see additional details in Chapter 101). Bacterial epiglottis and peritonsillar abscess may present with a sore throat as the initial primary symptom, but are distinguished by accompanying symptoms (see below).

Bacterial Pharyngitis: Diagnosis, Management, and Course

The most common treatable bacterial pathogens are *group A streptococci, C. haemolyticum,* and *M. pneumoniae.* It has been common practice to treat presumptive bacterial pharyngitis in adults with erythromycin, 500 mg orally twice daily for 10 days, because this regimen covers all three of the common pathogens. This practice may not be wise because of the rising resistance of group A streptococci to erythromycin (60) and the infrequent occurrence of the other two pathogens.

Group A Streptococcal Pharyngitis. Occurring most commonly in the winter and spring, the incubation period for group A streptococcal pharyngitis is 2 to 4 days, followed by the abrupt onset of sore throat, malaise, fever, and headache (61). All of the features of the classic syndrome, including fever, tender tonsillar lymph nodes (at angle of jaw), and creamy white exudate on the tonsils, occur in less than 10% of cases of streptococcal pharyngitis (38), and each of these features may occur in other types of pharyngitis. Importantly, *cough, hoarseness, and rhinorrhea are not usually present in the patient with strep throat.* The distinctive scarlatiniform rash *(scarlet fever)* is characterized by a diffuse red blush appearing on the trunk early in the disease, spreading centrifugally, blanching with pressure, and acquiring a sandpaper texture; 1 week later the skin desquamates, particularly over the palms and soles. This rash is seen not only in group A strep infection but also in toxic shock syndrome and Kawasaki's syndrome; the rash of *C. hemolyticum* is localized to the trunk and does not desquamate.

Because clinical findings are nonspecific, the diagnosis of streptococcal pharyngitis requires a *throat culture.* Currently, many physicians prefer to send throat swabs in transport media to commercial laboratories. Inexpensive office throat culture kits are available and have a high sensitivity (approximately 95%). To avoid false-negative results, correct swabbing and plating techniques must be followed. The tonsillar tissue and posterior pharynx are swabbed vigorously enough to induce a gag reflex; the swab is then rubbed on about one-sixth of a blood agar plate and subsequently streaked with a sterile wire loop. The agar is stabbed several times with the loop to enable recognition of subsurface hemolysis. A bacitracin disc is applied and the plate incubated at 37°C for 18 to 24 hours. With a little practice, one can readily recognize β-hemolytic colonies, estimate the number, and recognize the inhibition of their growth by the bacitracin disc if they belong to group A. Rapid diagnosis using Gram's stain of pharyngeal swab material yields variable results even with skilled observers, and is thus not recommended. Rapid diagnosis using kits to detect streptococcal antigen in throat swab specimens has improved; specificity is adequate, but sensitivity remains less than that of a correctly performed throat culture. If a strep antigen test is used, negative assays must be followed by a standard throat culture. There is no evidence at this time that current strep antigen tests substantially reduce the number of throat cultures performed (9).

In deciding whether to culture or treat a patient for strep throat, the results of a study conducted in multiple primary care settings are helpful (38). In this study, patients complaining of sore throat could be separated into three groups according to clinical features and the results of throat cultures:

- A group with tonsillar exudate, tender anterior cervical adenopathy, and temperature greater than 100°F: 2% of all pharyngitis patients had this constellation of findings, and of these 42.1% had positive strep cultures.
- A group with tonsillar exudate or tender adenopathy or a temperature greater than 100°F: 61% had one of these findings, and of these 13.5% had positive cultures.
- A group with none of the three clinical findings: 37% were in this category, and of these 3.4% had positive cultures.

Based on this study, it would be reasonable to treat patients from the first group with antibiotics before knowing the result of the throat culture, to culture patients from the second group but defer antibiotics until the culture result is known, and to neither culture nor treat patients in the third group. An exception to these guidelines is that all patients with a sore throat who have a history of rheumatic fever should be cultured whether or not the above clinical features are present (7). Although some positive cultures represent asymptomatic carriage, it is best to assume that all positive cultures are significant in these patients and to treat accordingly.

In three types of patients besides those having characteristics of the first group above, antibiotic treatment for streptococcal pharyngitis should be started routinely before throat culture results are known: patients with a history of rheumatic fever not currently taking prophylaxis, young patients with a strong family history of rheumatic fever, and all new cases of pharyngitis in an explosive epidemic of streptococcal disease in semiclosed populations such as groups of military personnel or students living in dormitory settings. (Local health authorities should be notified immediately in this situation.)

Symptomatic *family contacts* of patients with streptococcal pharyngitis should have cultures made and should be treated if the cultures are positive. Routine culture of asymptomatic family members is not indicated.

In adults over the age of 15 without a history of acute rheumatic fever (ARF), first attacks of ARF are rare. Therefore the *principal goals of treatment for streptococcal pharyngitis in adults* are the amelioration of symptoms, the prevention of local suppurative complications, and the prevention of spread. Because early therapy (in the first 2 days) is required for symptomatic relief, most physicians do not wait for culture results in patients with severe pharyngitis. In untreated patients, fever, malaise, and sore throat are self-limited, abating in 3 to 5 days; early treatment may reduce modestly the duration and severity of these symptoms. In patients being treated to prevent recurrence of ARF, therapy within 7 days of onset of pharyngitis is sufficient (see "Rheumatic Fever," below).

The *preferred therapy* for streptococcal pharyngitis is parenteral benzathine penicillin, 1.2 million units given once, because it obviates noncompliance and is the only treatment proven to prevent rheumatic fever. If oral therapy is given, the recommended regimen is penicillin V, 250 mg three times a day for 10 days (36). For patients allergic to penicillin, erythromycin, 250 mg every 6 hours for 10 days, or another macrolide is recommended. A number of oral cephalosporins (10-day courses) and azithromycin (500 mg first day and 250 mg for 4 days) have clinical and bacteriologic cure rates superior to penicillin VK (55,66). It is not yet clear that the increased cost of the extended-spectrum antibiotics is balanced by decreased costs of fewer repeat treatments for clinical failures and increased compliance. (See practical information about antimicrobials below, Table 28.7.) Posttreatment cultures should be performed only if there is a history of rheumatic fever in the patient or in a household contact.

Gonococcal Pharyngitis. Gonococcal pharyngitis should be considered in patients who complain of sore throat in association with urethritis or vaginitis; it occurs alone without genital symptoms in less than 5% and must be diagnosed by throat culture. Special culture techniques should be used to detect gonorrhea in specimens from patients practicing orogenital sex. Gram's stain of direct pharyngeal smear is insensitive and nonspecific. Calcium alginate swabs should be used because ordinary cotton swabs contain fatty acids inhibitory to gonococcal growth. The swab should be immediately plated on a modified Thayer–Martin medium that is incorporated in a number of inexpensive kits for office culture. For throat cultures, however, *N. gonorrhoeae* must be distinguished from *Neisseria meningitidis* and *Neisseria lactamica* by carbohydrate fermentation and serology; therefore, cultures should be sent to state or regional laboratories. Effective treatment, based on the 1989 recommendations of the Centers for Disease Control and Prevention (CDC), is either ceftriaxone, 250 mg as a single intramuscular injection, or erythromycin, 500 mg by mouth four times a day for 7 days. The former, newer regimen is highly effective, is comfortable for the patient, and obviates compliance and drug resistance problems. Ampicillin and spectinomycin should not be used because they are associated with unacceptable failure rates in the treatment of pharyngeal gonorrhea. A follow-up culture 7 days after completion of therapy should be done as a test of cure. Cotreatment for presumed chlamydial infection should be given (doxycycline 100 mg twice daily for 7 days).

Chapters 27 and 94 discuss in detail sexually transmitted infections in men and women, respectively.

Diphtheria. This diagnosis should be suspected when there is a *grayish membrane* in the anterior nares or on the tonsils, uvula, or pharynx. (Infectious mononucleosis and strep throat display a creamy white exudate and do not involve the uvula.) Treatment must begin before bacteriologic confirmation and requires hospitalization for strict isolation, bed rest, close observation, antitoxin, and erythromycin or penicillin for 14 days. Management of contacts is discussed in Chapter 32.

Other Bacteria. Throat cultures often grow pneumococci, staphylococci, groups B and C streptococci, and various Gram-negative enterobacteria. These species, which colonize the pharynx, have only rarely been shown to be etiologic agents in pharyngitis, and patients who harbor them should not be treated with antimicrobial agents.

Vincent's Angina. Vincent's angina is an anaerobic infection of the pharynx characterized by fever, tender lymphadenitis, a large grayish-brown pseudomembrane in the pharynx, and very foul odor. It is a complication of acute necrotizing ulcerative gingivitis, which is described in Chapter 101. Hospitalization for antimicrobial treatment with penicillin or tetracycline is the appropriate management plan.

Rheumatic Fever

Acute rheumatic fever (7) is a clinical syndrome of nonsuppurative inflammatory lesions of the heart, joints, and central nervous system (CNS), following a group A streptococcal pharyngeal infection. Incidence of ARF has been declining in the United States over the past 40 years, but its importance is suggested by recent outbreaks during the last 10 years in the United States, as well as continued endemicity in developing countries, where it accounts for up to 40% of all cardiovascular disease.

Although most cases occur in children aged 6 to 15 years, the attack rate of ARF after untreated exudative pharyngitis in military recruit camp has been as high as 3%. One-third of ARF cases follow asymptomatic streptococcal infection, but almost all cases are associated with a rise in serum antistreptolysin O (ASO). The latent period between clinical streptococcal pharyngitis and onset of ARF is a mean of 19 days, with a range of 1 to 5 weeks.

Diagnosis uses the Jones criteria: two major criteria (carditis, polyarthritis, chorea, subcutaneous nodules, and erythema marginatum), or one major criterion and two minor criteria (fever, arthralgia, heart block, elevated acute-phase reactants including granulocytosis, erythrocyte sedimentation rate, and C-reactive protein). Evidence of recent streptococcal infection must be obtained, either by positive throat culture, strep antigen test, or elevated or rising antistreptococcal antibodies. Within 2 months of onset, 80% of patients with ARF have an ASO titer greater than 200 Todd units/mL, and 95% of patients have at least one elevated titer among the battery of three tests (ASO, anti-DNAse B, and antihyaluronidase). The Streptozyme slide test is insufficiently standardized at this time to be useful.

Carditis is usually associated with a murmur of mitral or aortic regurgitation caused by valvulitis. Echocardiographic signs of valvular disease without audible murmur are not diagnostic. *Polyarthritis* is typically the earliest and most prominent symptom, usually in the knees, ankles, elbows, and wrists. Arthritis lasts 1 to 4 months, typically migrating from joint to joint, residing in each joint for 1 to 2 weeks. It responds dramatically to salicylate therapy. *Chorea,* a less common phenomenon, is an involuntary movement disorder of the trunk or limbs that disappears in sleep and is often associated with weakness and emotional lability. Chorea may occur as an isolated sign of ARF and must be differentiated from other neurologic diseases. Rare major criteria are *erythema marginatum,* a transient, expanding pink rash with serpiginous margins and pale centers, and *subcutaneous nodules,* firm, painless nodules up to 2 cm in diameter found over tendons and bones.

Precise Jones criteria are required to diagnose ARF because overdiagnosis results in unnecessary anguish and future antibiotic prophylaxis. The criteria may be relaxed when the patient has had a previous episode of ARF. Isolated chorea and indolent carditis still present difficult diagnostic challenges.

Treatment for ARF should be initiated only after the diagnosis is certain, with the assistance of an infectious disease or cardiology consultation if there is uncertainty about the diagnosis. Treatment involves bed rest, analgesics, salicylates, and corticosteroids, depending on symptom severity. Corticosteroids should be tapered to avoid rebound signs.

Continuous prophylaxis against recurrent ARF is indicated in young patients, patients at high risk of streptococcal infection (parents of young children, schoolteachers, medical and military personnel, and those in crowded living conditions), and those with ARF within the previous 5 years. Continuous prophylaxis may be provided through any of the following regimens.

- Benzathine penicillin G, 1.2 million units intramuscularly every 4 weeks (the regimen of choice).
- Penicillin V, 125 to 250 mg by mouth twice a day.
- Sulfadiazine is no longer available in the United States.
- Prophylaxis may be discontinued in adults who did not have prior carditis, at age 18 or 5 years after the last attack, whichever is longer (6).

Chronic or Relapsing Sore Throat

Some patients describe a sore throat of several weeks' duration at their first visit. Others have either a prolonged course after an illness that began as a typical acute pharyngitis syndrome or frequent recurrence of sore throats. The conditions that may cause prolonged or recurrent pharyngitis are listed in Table 28.2. Most are discussed in more detail elsewhere in the book, as indicated in the table.

Chronic tonsillitis or *recurrent pharyngitis* may be alleviated in some patients by tonsillectomy. Chronic tonsillitis is a clinical diagnosis made in patients with recurrent sore throats (several in the same year), very large tonsils, and chronically enlarged, periodically tender lymph nodes. Tonsillectomy to alleviate chronic tonsillitis continues to be controversial (54). β-Lactamase–producing organisms in the pharynx, including *S. aureus, Haemophilus* species, *Bacteroides* species, and *Branhamella catarrhalis,* can inactivate penicillin and protect mucosal streptococci; these conditions may underlie some cases of chronic tonsillitis. For recurrent pharyngitis and tonsillitis caused by group A streptococci and aerobic and anaerobic penicillin-resistant pathogens, eradication of streptococci and elimination of recurrent tonsillitis have been

Table 28.2.   Causes of Chronic or Relapsing Sore Throat

Primary Site of Pain	Condition	See for Details
Pharynx	Chronic tonsillitis	
	Smoking (especially marijuana)	Chapters 20, 22
	Postnasal drip	Chapter 54
	Infectious mononucleosis	Chapter 53
	Chronic fatigue syndrome	Chapter 53
	Agranulocytosis	
	Acute leukemia	
	Pemphigus	
Not the pharynx	Septic thyroiditis	Chapter 73
	Subacute thyroiditis	
	Angina (radiating to neck)	Chapter 57
	Esophageal reflux	Chapter 35
	Psychogenic	Chapter 12

achieved in some patients with clindamycin, 300 mg every 8 hours, or amoxicillin–clavulanic acid (Augmentin), 500 mg every 8 hours for 7 days.

Acute Sinusitis

The sinuses are air-filled bony cavities that produce and drain up to 2 pints of mucus every day. This self-cleaning occurs by movement of the mucus, propelled by cilia, through the ostia; the ostia are located behind the several bony plates (turbinates) that one can see on inspection of the lateral surface of each nasal passage. Acute sinusitis is a bacterial infection of one or more paranasal sinuses, which occurs when the normal drainage is impaired by blockage of one or more ostia. Acute sinusitis complicates approximately 0.5% of viral URIs, which commonly cause obstruction of the ostia (29). Sinusitis may also be a complication of noninfectious rhinitis (see Chapter 23), polyps, foreign bodies, swimming and diving, immune deficiency, or anatomic nasal obstruction of sinus drainage. Up to 10% of cases of acute sinusitis are an extension of dental abscess. Nursing home or homebound patients with nasogastric tubes occasionally have occult sinusitis as a cause of persistent fever.

Diagnosis

The pain of sinusitis is caused by periosteal reaction secondary to purulent inflammation behind an obstructed ostium. The pain is dull in the early stages but becomes throbbing in later stages. Coughing, dependency, and percussion over the involved sinus exacerbate the pain. Percussion of the teeth is often painful in maxillary sinusitis. The facial pain associated with the noninfectious causes of nasal congestion (see Chapter 23) may resemble the early pain of acute sinusitis, but it is less localized and does not become progressively worse. Other causes of facial pain to be distinguished from sinusitis are dental abscess (see Chapter 101), migraine, cluster headache, and trigeminal neuralgia (see Chapter 79).

In addition to pain and tenderness, the patient's report of a colored nasal discharge, observation of purulent mucus draining from the ostia after noseblowing, and poor response to nasal decongestants are findings that support the diagnosis of sinusitis (76).

Nontender edema of the eyelids, seen predominantly in children, may occur with uncomplicated ethmoid and maxillary sinusitis. Acute sinusitis may present without pain as in subacute sinusitis (see below), usually in the guise of a cold persisting for more than 2 weeks and accompanied by cough caused by postnasal drip, purulent nasal discharge persisting throughout the day, and headache.

Examination should include the pharynx, nose, ears, and teeth. Transillumination of the sinuses can be attempted (75), but it is unreliable without experience.

Radiologic examination of the sinuses is unnecessary in patients with typical signs and symptoms. It is

Figure 28.2. Acute infectious maxillary sinusitis. Waters view shows complete opacity of the right maxillary sinus caused by thickening of the lining mucosa or fluid accumulation. The mucoperiosteal line is preserved. The left maxillary sinus is normal in appearance.

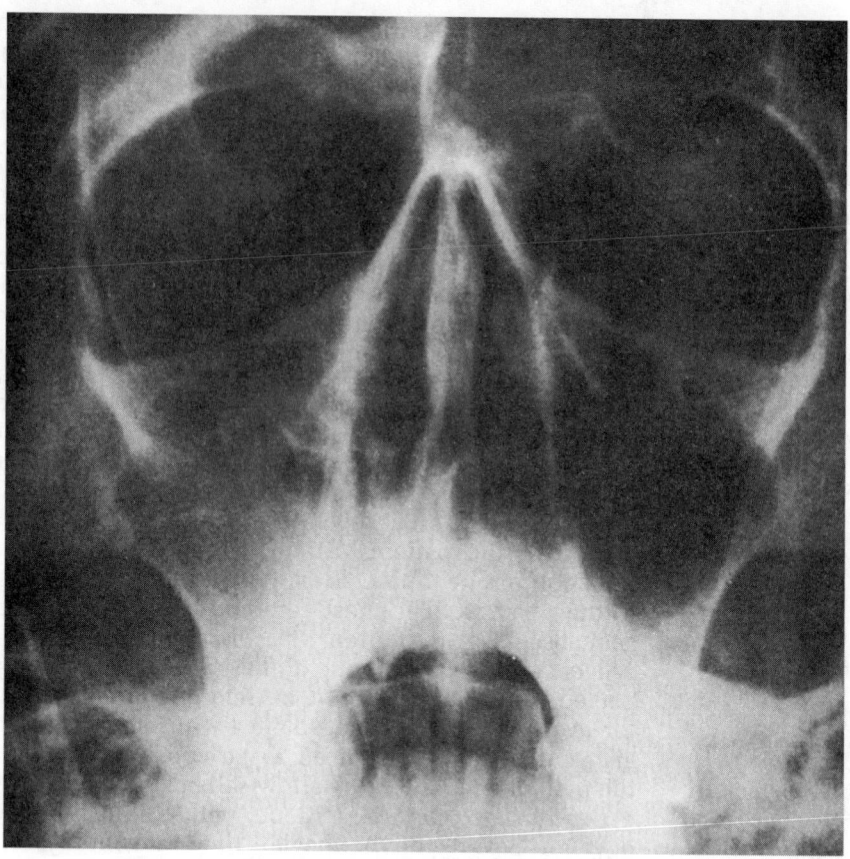

most helpful in the diagnostic workup of headache and in patients who do not respond to therapy or who are toxic and require accurate diagnosis early. Figure 28.2 shows the typical radiologic changes seen in acute maxillary sinusitis. Computerized tomography (CT) is highly sensitive but lacks specificity (75).

Acute sinusitis can be treated without culture. Nasopharyngeal swabs are usually contaminated with normal flora and are of no use. *S. pneumoniae* and unencapsulated *H. influenzae* are the bacterial agents formed by antral puncture in 60% of acute purulent sinusitis and probably in most acute exacerbations of chronic sinusitis. Anaerobes, *Streptococcus pyogenes, Neisseria catarrhalis,* β-hemolytic streptococci, *M. pneumoniae, C. pneumoniae,* and Gram-negative aerobes each cause a small percentage of infections. *S. aureus* causes less than 5% and tends to be associated with pansinusitis and general toxicity.

Management and Course

The combination of topical decongestants and antibiotics was not superior to decongestants alone in a large community-based clinical trial that compared amoxicillin with placebo (71). This trial, with a placebo arm, differs from a clinical trial, without a placebo arm, that showed similar response patterns when the same regimen was taken for 3 instead of 10 days (the regimen was trimethoprim–sulfamethoxazole [TMP/SMX] one double-strength [DS] tablet

twice a day) (73). There may be a subset of patients with sinusitis for whom antibiotics will accelerate recovery, but at present there are not obvious characteristics that identify this subset.

Improvement in sinus drainage is important. A decongestant spray, such as Neo-Synephrine 0.25 or 0.5%, or oxymetazoline 0.05%, is administered as an initial spray to decrease congestion in the membranes of the anterior nares, followed 5 to 10 minutes later by a second spray delivered deeper to the middle meatus. This is repeated every 4 to 8 hours for 2 to 4 days, followed by oral decongestants (see details on the common cold, above) for an additional 2 weeks. Pain relief is important, and codeine may be required. Patients who plan to fly, especially in nonpressurized aircraft, should take an oral decongestant before takeoff, supplemented with topical decongestant spray every 4 hours.

Resolution of facial pain, headache, and fever is expected within several days. If no response occurs by this time, the diagnosis should be confirmed by radiography using a single Waters view (occipitomeatal view) (74), and referral to an otolaryngologist for antral puncture or endoscopic drainage may be advisable. Toxic patients, especially those with frontoethmoid sinusitis, should be referred at initial presentation for hospitalization, drainage, culture, and definitive parenteral antibiotics. Patients whose symptoms worsen during the first 48 hours of vigorous ambulatory therapy should be referred. Patients with severe facial pain benefit from early antral puncture for pain relief.

Complications of acute sinusitis are unusual. They should be regarded as medical emergencies because they represent direct extension of infection to adjacent orbits, bone, blood vessels, and CNS. Nontender periorbital edema indicates restriction of orbital venous outflow through congested ethmoid veins, is not associated with decreased visual acuity, and is appropriately managed with vigorous medical therapy. However, *tender periorbital swelling,* associated with proptosis and chemosis, represents orbital cellulitis and requires immediate referral to an otolaryngologist. Subsequent progression of cellulitis to subperiosteal or orbital abscess, associated with ophthalmoplegia and loss of vision, requires emergency surgical drainage. Osteomyelitis is most often a complication of frontal sinusitis. Cavernous sinus thrombosis should be suspected in the patient with signs of orbital complications plus extreme toxicity. Intracranial extension is rare but life threatening, presenting most commonly as meningitis. Abscesses in the brain and epidural and subdural spaces present more insidiously. Frontal lobe abscess may present as mild headache, low-grade fever, malaise, and personality change. In poorly controlled diabetics and immunocompromised hosts, *rhinocerebral mucormycosis* begins in the nose and maxillary sinuses and may be recognized by a black eschar on the nasal turbinates.

Chronic Sinusitis

When the symptoms of acute sinusitis, especially pain and fever, subside with therapy, purulent nasal discharge may continue. Despite persistence of radiologic changes, this stage usually resolves after an additional 2 to 3 weeks of conservative management with oral decongestants.

The term *chronic sinusitis* is used when symptoms persist *more than 3 months,* usually in a relapsing pattern following short-term therapy and improvement. Chronic sinusitis results from obstruction to sinus drainage and the loss of normal ciliated epithelial lining of the sinus cavity, leading to a low-grade infection by anaerobic and aerobic bacteria. Acute exacerbations may occur, caused primarily by the organisms that most commonly cause acute sinusitis (*H. influenzae* and *S. pneumoniae*). Chronic sinusitis may complicate certain systemic diseases, such as sarcoidosis, Wegener's granulomatosis, IgA deficiency, human immunodeficiency virus (HIV) infection, and allergic rhinitis with asthma. In extensive disease, bilateral occlusion of the ostiomeatal complex and severe mucosal thickening by CT correlate with asthma and peripheral eosinophilia (52).

Diagnosis and Management

The working diagnosis of chronic sinusitis can be made on the basis of features in the history and physical examination. Persistent purulent nasal discharge and postnasal drip with associated cough, despite adequate medical therapy, are the primary features of chronic sinusitis. Facial pain and tenderness are minimal or absent. Because CT scanning is more sensitive and more specific than plain radiographs, consultants often prefer the former when they choose to make diagnostic or treatment decisions on the basis of radiologic examination.

Oral penicillin V or amoxicillin for 1 month is the most appropriate *antimicrobial regimen;* amoxicillin–clavulanate or clindamycin are appropriate alternatives (see dosages and schedules in Table 28.7). For patients whose main symptom is chronic cough, a 1- or 2-week trial of an antihistamine–decongestant preparation provides symptom relief and may be all that is needed in up to one-third of patients (57). *Topical corticosteroids,* in dosages similar to those used for allergic rhinitis (see Chapter 23), may also lead to resolution of symptoms in chronic sinusitis. For patients whose syndrome does not resolve with one or more of these empirical treatments, referral to an otolaryngologist for consideration of *surgical drainage* is recommended.

Pharyngeal Abscess

Occasionally, after several days of symptoms of a URI, the patient develops a complicating infection of one of the closed compartments adjacent to the pharynx. The most common of these pharyngeal abscesses are peritonsillar abscess and retropharyngeal abscess. When one of these conditions is suspected, the patient should be referred immediately for evaluation and management by an otolaryngologist. Other conditions to consider when the patient is unable to swallow saliva because of pain are listed in Table 28.3.

Peritonsillar Abscess

Patients with peritonsillar abscess develop severe odynophagia; they are not only unable to take liquids, but also may be unable to swallow their own saliva, resulting in early dehydration. The voice acquires a muffled quality, and trismus may be present. Fever, malaise, and systemic toxicity are typical. Dramatic relief may occur if the abscess drains spontaneously before the patient seeks medical attention. On physical examination, there is a swelling of the anterior tonsillar pillar at its superior pole. The involved tonsil itself may or may not be enlarged, but it is displaced medially. This condition is almost always unilateral.

Table 28.3. Differential Diagnosis of Severe Throat Pain, Odynophagia, and Inability to Swallow Saliva

Peritonsillar abscess	Toxic epidermal necrolysis
Retropharyngeal abscess	Stevens–Johnson syndrome
Vincent's angina	Botulism
Diphtheria	Tetanus
Pharyngeal zoster	Gastrointestinal reflux
Epiglottitis	

Retropharyngeal Abscess

The symptoms of this condition are similar to those of peritonsillar abscess. In addition, there may be respiratory embarrassment if the process extends inferiorly toward the larynx. Trismus is uncommon. On examination, a swelling in the posterior oropharynx is readily seen. Lateral soft tissue radiographs of the neck may disclose expansion of the soft tissue density in the posterior pharyngeal space.

Management

Unless the airway or swallowing is compromised, needle aspiration and outpatient treatment with oral penicillin are effective (32). This can be performed by an otolaryngologist, oral surgeon, or experienced emergency room physician. Half of the cases of peritonsillar abscess are caused by group A *S. pyogenes.* Although some cultures grow penicillin-resistant organisms, there is no different in cure rate between those receiving penicillin and those receiving broader-spectrum agents. The acute failure rate of needle aspiration is 6%; incision and drainage is appropriate for acute failures. Non–group A strep peritonsillar abscesses recur in 10% of cases; abscess tonsillectomy may be required for repeated recurrences (32).

Epiglottitis

Acute epiglottitis is a life-threatening but curable condition. The epiglottis serves as a valve that closes over the proximal portion of the trachea during swallowing to prevent aspiration. When the epiglottis becomes inflamed, the resultant edema causes it to curl posteriorly and inferiorly, thereby reducing the glottic aperture. Inspiration, which draws the epiglottis down, further reduces the effective airway.

Epiglottitis is a rare complication of URIs. Since the introduction of the *H. influenzae* B vaccine, the incidence in children has decreased and now the incidence in adults is higher than in children (22).

The diagnosis of epiglottitis should be suspected in patients with a sore throat, odynophagia, and muffled voice, all of short duration. Only one-half of patients are febrile and show evidence of pharyngitis, and only one in three patients has cervical adenopathy. Sitting erect, complaint of dyspnea, and stridor noted in inspiration are indications of airway obstruction. Soft tissue radiographs of the neck may show edema of the epiglottis and narrowing of the aperture. The diagnosis is confirmed by indirect laryngoscopy, which reveals marked edema of the epiglottis and supraglottic tissue; this procedure must be performed only in circumstances in which emergency intubation could be carried out because it may induce (rarely in adults) additional obstruction.

Management requires admission for observation; patients with signs of airway obstruction noted above should be admitted to an intensive care unit, where close observation and emergency tracheotomy are possible (22). The remainder of the patients can be managed conservatively in a general ward with antibiotic treatment of the most common organisms, including *S. aureus, H. influenzae, S. pneumoniae,* and *S. pyogenes.* Topical or systemic corticosteroids do not prevent airway obstruction.

Telephone Assessment and Self-Care for URI

Most physicians welcome the opportunity to assess URI symptoms initially by telephone. The telephone assessment should accomplish the following:

- Differentiate between infectious and allergic problems
- Among the patients with acute infections, distinguish those with possible bacterial infections or superinfections who should be examined to determine whether antibiotics should be prescribed
- Identify those who may have complications of a URI that require office evaluation
  - The following symptoms and signs should be sought: symptoms lasting more than 3 weeks; fever lasting more than 1 week, or associated with delirium; purulent nasal discharge with sinus pain; purulent sputum, chest pain, dyspnea, or hemoptysis; ear pain or discharge; sore throat and a history of rheumatic fever; the combination of cough and fever over 102°F (39°C) or fever for more than 4 days; hoarseness for more than 1 month; pleuritic chest pain; marked odynophagia; and the combination of dysphagia, stridor, and difficulty in breathing.
- For patients not needing an office visit, provide simple instructions for self-care based on the measures described earlier

Increasing numbers of patients consult self-care algorithms. The book *Take Care of Yourself* by Vickery and Fries (see "General References") is one of the most widely distributed collections of algorithms. In one evaluation (5), strict adherence to the algorithms for colds, influenza, cough, and sore throat would have increased the number of patient visits to a physician. Thus, this standard set of instructions exhibited sensitivity, missing few people who need to be examined, yet lacked specificity and led to unnecessary visits. This study points to the need to search for symptom complexes that better identify patients likely to be helped by a visit to a physician.

LOWER RESPIRATORY INFECTIONS

The cardinal manifestation of lower respiratory tract infection is cough, usually accompanied by auscultatory evidence of lower tract inflammation (rhonchi, rales, wheezes, signs of consolidation). Bronchitis and pneumonia are the major infectious syndromes of the lower respiratory tract in adults. The differential diagnosis of lower respiratory tract infections can be facilitated by the information found in Table 28.4, which summarizes by time course and etiologic agent the common and less common bronchitis and pneumonia syndromes.

Table 28.4. Differential Diagnosis of Cough Caused by Infectious Agents

Acute (<2 Weeks)
Acute bronchitis/URI
    Common: respiratory viruses, influenza A and B, respiratory
        syncytial virus
    Uncommon: *S. pneumoniae, H. influenzae, M. pneumoniae,*
        C. pneumoniae, L. pneumophilia, M. catarrhalis
Pneumonia (see also Table 28.5)
    Common: *S. pneumonia, H. influenzae, M. pneumoniae,*
        C. pneumoniae
    Uncommon: influenza, respiratory syncytial virus, *L. pneumophila,*
        M. catarrhalis plague, varicella, tuberculosis
    Note: person-to-person transmission: tuberculosis, influenza,
        plague, varicella
Acute pulmonary edema caused by hantavirus

Persistent (>2 Weeks)[a]
Repeated aspiration
    Glottic dysfunction (old age, sedation)
    Esophageal dysfunction, obstruction
Tuberculosis
    Pulmonary/pleural
    Laryngeal (normal chest radiograph)
Fungal pneumonias
    Histoplasmosis
    Coccoidioidomycosis
    Blastomycosis
Postinfectious bronchospasm

[a]See Chapter 54 for noninfectious causes.

Acute Bronchitis

Clinical Characteristics

Acute bronchitis is an inflammatory condition of the tracheobronchial tree that results from respiratory infections with common cold viruses, influenza, adenovirus, *M. pneumoniae, C. pneumoniae, B. catarrhalis,* and rarely, *Bordetella pertussis.* The role of secondary bacterial invasion by *S. pneumoniae* and *H. influenzae* is unclear. The illness is characterized by cough, with or without sputum production, persisting longer than expected (usually 1 to 2 weeks) after the onset of an acute URI.

Rhinovirus and coronavirus, by virtue of their high prevalence, are common etiologic agents for mild bronchitis of short duration and without fever. Influenza, adenovirus, and *M. pneumoniae* cause a more severe bronchitis associated with fever and burning substernal pain. Mucoid sputum production develops in half of all cases and is not helpful in distinguishing etiologic agents. Frequency and duration of cough are increased in cigarette smokers.

Patients with a cough as the predominant or only respiratory symptom may have pneumonia, bronchitis, or one of a variety of noninfectious conditions associated with persistent cough. Diagnostic efforts should be directed at identifying patients with pneumonia and with noninfectious causes of cough, leaving acute bronchitis as a diagnosis of exclusion.

The diagnosis of pneumonia is discussed below. In approaching the patient who has a persistent cough without apparent infectious cause, it is helpful to consider what is known about the anatomy and physi-

ology of the cough reflex (see Chapter 54). Airborne irritants, especially smog containing sulfur dioxide, and allergens cause bronchitic symptoms. Repeated small aspiration of oral and upper airway secretions, especially in the elderly and in the alcoholic patient with incompetent glottic function, is also associated with nighttime cough.

Bacterial cultures of sputum should not be performed because a contribution of colonizing bacteria to acute bronchitis has not been demonstrated and sputum is readily contaminated by nasopharyngeal flora. Culture techniques for viral agents and *M. pneumoniae* are not widely available. *M. pneumoniae* may be implicated if the patient is a young adult, cases of persistent cough or interstitial pneumonitis are occurring in family contacts, and the case occurs in the summer or early fall. The diagnosis can be confirmed by a fourfold or greater rise in specific complement fixation titer between acute and convalescent serum.

The prevalence of *pertussis* is increasing among adults; rates exceeding 20% of adults with a cough persisting 2 weeks or more have been reported in urban areas (51,78). Adults serve as a reservoir of infection for nonimmune children. Pertussis is characterized by initial nonspecific symptoms of malaise and rhinorrhea followed by 1 to 14 weeks of *severe paroxysms* of repetitive coughs without inspiration. The paroxysm is terminated by an inspiratory whoop. The clinical symptoms are attenuated in previously immunized adults and children. Because of the nonspecific nature of the symptoms, the duration of cough of 2 weeks is used as the threshold to initiate investigation of sporadic cases, and 1 week is used during an outbreak. Culture, using a *nasopharyngeal swab,* on special media for *Bordetella* is the standard diagnostic assay but is uncommonly positive, particularly after antibiotics or later in the course of illness. Direct immune fluorescent staining of organisms on smear of nasopharyngeal secretions is useful in outbreak investigations. Diagnosis by a single positive antibody test in acute serum is increasingly used to detect sporadic cases (51,78).

Treatment

Treatment of cough, not accompanied by systemic symptoms such as fever, myalgias, malaise, and chest pain, is only symptomatic. Cough suppression is occasionally achieved by dextromethorphan but usually requires simple codeine sulfate, 15 to 30 mg every 4 to 6 hours (especially at bedtime). Antihistamines should be avoided, and oral fluid intake encouraged, to prevent inspissated secretions.

Smokers with acute bronchitis should be strongly encouraged to stop smoking at least for the duration of the acute illness. Smokers with a history of chronic cough before their bronchitis may be more motivated to discontinue smoking permanently in the face of the acute illness. In 50% of those who discontinue smoking, the chronic cough resolves completely within 1 month. Behavioral approaches to smoking cessation are described in Chapter 20.

Randomized controlled trials with the highest methodologic rigor studying antibiotic efficacy in acute bronchitis conclude that antibiotic treatment has no role in this illness (24,53). A cough with purulent sputum, accompanied by systemic symptoms and a clear chest radiograph, occasionally responds to antibiotics that target common encapsulated bacteria, but these examples are uncommon. Sputum color is not necessarily an accurate indicator of purulence. *If pertussis is suspected,* appropriate diagnostic studies (see above) should be performed rather than using presumptive therapy with antibiotics, unless the patient is located in an epidemic. Treatment for pertussis is a 14-day course of either erythromycin 40 to 50 mg/kg per day (maximum 2 g/day) divided in two doses; TMP/SMX is an alternative for patients allergic to erythromycin.

Some patients persist with a hacking, productive cough, perhaps caused by a cycle of coughing and bronchial irritation. If no other evidence of active infection or bronchospasm is present, these patients may be treated with aerosolized beclomethasone (70). (See practical information about available preparations in Chapter 55.) Dramatic reduction in cough will be seen in 48 to 72 hours if the patient has airway reactivity responsive to inhaled steroids.

Acute Exacerbations of Chronic Bronchitis

Clinical Characteristics

Respiratory infections contribute to the episodic worsening of cough and increased sputum production in the patient with chronic obstructive pulmonary disease (COPD), and they are the most common identifiable causes of death in these patients. Evidence that infections in adulthood play an independent role in the deterioration of pulmonary function is lacking, however (68).

The most important indicator of intercurrent infection is the patient's report of a change in color, consistency, and amount of sputum. Patients who consistently produce purulent sputum most of the time may notice increasing cough, dyspnea, and fatigue. Systemic toxicity with fever and chills is generally absent unless pneumonia is present.

The role of bacteria in acute exacerbations of chronic bronchitis is difficult to assess. The bronchial secretions of patients with chronic bronchitis contain pneumococci, unencapsulated *Haemophilus* species, and normal pharyngeal flora, which persist through asymptomatic intervals. The development of purulent sputum is not correlated with the presence of one or more specific bacterial species. These bacteria appear de novo during acute exacerbations in only a small percentage of uncolonized patients. Similarly, the acquisition of a new serotype of either pneumococci or encapsulated *Haemophilus* species is usually not followed by a clinical exacerbation. In summary, a primary role for these bacteria in the pathogenesis of clinical exacerbations remains unclear, and performing Gram's stain and a culture of the sputum during acute exacerbations will not provide useful information.

Viruses (influenza, parainfluenza, respiratory syncytial, rhinovirus, and coronavirus) may cause up to 50% of acute infectious exacerbations. *M. pneumoniae* may be the agent in up to 10% of episodes.

Treatment

Acute exacerbations of chronic bronchitis should always be managed with more vigorous applications of routine therapy for chronic symptoms. Clearance of secretions should be promoted with postural drainage and therapeutic dosages of bronchodilators (see Chapter 55). Cough suppressants and sedatives should be avoided. Smokers should be strongly counseled to discontinue smoking at least until their acute symptoms have resolved. As noted above, chronic cough will resolve completely within 1 month in half of all patients who are motivated by an acute illness to discontinue smoking permanently.

Antimicrobial prophylaxis is commonly used in the management of chronic bronchitis, but the efficacy of this practice has not been demonstrated convincingly (68). Many studies suggest that continuous prophylaxis with tetracycline at low dosages reduces the frequency of exacerbations during the winter months. However, the conclusions of most studies do not stand up to rigorous analysis. In addition, there is considerable concern that widespread use of prophylactic antibiotics without clear effectiveness may promote emergence and dissemination of antibiotic-resistant strains in the community.

Efficacy of short-term antibiotic therapy given for acute exacerbations has been evaluated in a meta-analysis of randomized trials (58). A small but consistent beneficial effect of antibiotic treatment was found to be significant, especially for the patients with low baseline peak flow rates (58). For the individual patient, efficacy may be best estimated on the patient's reported response to antibiotics during previous exacerbations. A reasonable approach is to provide reliable patients who have three or more acute exacerbations per year with a prescription for a 7- to 10-day course of one of the following: tetracycline, 250 mg two to four times daily; amoxicillin, 250 to 500 mg three times daily; or TMP/SMX, two tablets twice daily. The patient is instructed to begin the antibiotic within 24 hours of the first sign of a "chest cold" because early initiation of therapy may be more effective in alleviating symptoms and preventing time lost from work (68). Oral penicillin V and chloramphenicol are inappropriate alternatives because penicillin is not effective against the *Haemophilus* species and there are many safer alternatives to chloramphenicol.

Some patients managed at home for acute exacerbations do not improve by any criteria or deteriorate after self-initiated therapy. These patients should be asked to keep in touch by telephone during the acute episode so that symptoms indicating pneumonia are detected earlier.

Pneumonia

More than 3 million episodes of pneumonia occur annually in the United States, responsible for more than 30 million days of disability requiring bed rest, and 600,000 hospitalizations. With influenza, pneumonia ranks fifth among all diseases as a cause of death and first among infectious diseases, and its mortality rate has been rising during the last two decades (56).

Definition

Pneumonia is a lower respiratory tract infection accompanied by systemic and respiratory tract symptoms and evidence of consolidation on chest radiograph.

Distinction from Bronchitis. Bronchitis and pneumonia represent a continuum of lower respiratory infection. Aspirated pathogens, including bacteria, fungi, and viruses, invade the bronchial epithelium and alveoli. The extent of involvement of adjacent lung parenchyma determines whether there is an infiltrate on chest roentgenogram. The alveolar inflammation spreads like a grass fire, and the advancing edge of edema and leukocyte infiltration are not radiologically apparent. Patients seen early and those with emphysema and reduced parenchyma may fail to show any infiltrate or may show a patchy infiltrate on their chest film despite the presence of considerable inflammation. Thus, the clinical distinction between acute bronchitis and acute pneumonia is often an arbitrary radiologic distinction. Early management and the decision for hospitalization must focus on the overall condition of the patient in terms of signs and symptoms of systemic toxicity as well as of localized pulmonary infection.

Pneumonia Syndromes and Causes

Important clues for the etiologic diagnosis of pneumonia may be obtained from a knowledge of seasonal, environmental, and occupational predilections of the different agents that cause pneumonias (Table 28.5).

Bacterial pneumonias make up the majority of all adult pneumonias, and the largest fraction of these are caused by *S. pneumoniae* (4,14,49,67). Pneumococcal pneumonia may occur in a previously healthy adult, or after a URI, usually with the abrupt onset of shaking chills, fever, pleuritic chest pain, and cough productive of purulent or rusty sputum. Bacterial pneumonias are commonly preceded by a viral prodrome of headache, myalgias, and malaise. In the setting of compromised pulmonary clearance of secretions (depressed consciousness, morbid obesity, abdominal surgery, chronic bronchitis, congestive heart failure, and alcoholism) that predisposes to pneumococcal and other bacterial pneumonias (37), onset of clinical symptoms may be more insidious. Other types of bacterial pneumonias are more common in different clinical settings: *staphylococcal* and *H. influenzae* after influenza A or B; *Haemophilus, Klebsiella,* and anaerobic pneumonias in *alcoholics;* and anaerobic and *Gram-negative pneumonias* in *recently hospitalized patients.* In the elderly, particularly those in nursing homes, *S. pneumoniae* continues to be the most common cause of pneumonia, but Gram-negative aerobes, nontypable strains of *H. influenzae,* and mixed pneumococcal–Gram-negative anaerobes are common causes. *Group B streptococci, M. catarrhalis,* and *Legionella pneumophila* are also occasional causes of pneumonia in the elderly. *M. catarrhalis* is particularly common in patients with chronic obstructive lung disease.

The so-called *atypical pneumonia syndrome,* most common in patients under age 40, is distinguished by a prodrome of headache and myalgia preceding the onset of respiratory symptoms. Respiratory pathogens commonly causing "atypical pneumonia" include *M. pneumoniae, L. pneumophila, C. pneumoniae* (TWAR strain), a number of viruses (influenza A and B, respiratory syncytial virus, parainfluenza, adenovirus), *Chlamydia psittaci, Coxiella burnetii* (Q fever), *Coccidioides immitis,* and *Pneumocystis carinii.* Nonetheless, all of these pathogens may present as a pneumonitis that clinically is indistinguishable from pneumococcal pneumonia (4,67), rendering the designation "atypical pneumonia" of little use clinically.

Complications of M. pneumoniae are more common in severely ill patients, and fulminant infection can occur irrespective of age or host status (11). Complications include sinusitis, otitis media, myringitis (diagnostic if bullae are seen), erythema multiform or erythema nodosum, intravascular hemolysis, meningoencephalitis, toxic psychosis, myocarditis, and pericarditis. Persistent hacking cough, lasting as long as 6 weeks despite therapy, is common and requires symptomatic relief with codeine (see Chapter 54). Relapse of the primary disease occurs in up to 10% of cases, usually 2 to 3 weeks after the initial illness, and is probably related to the fact that mycoplasma persists in bronchial epithelium for up to 14 weeks.

Pneumonia caused by C. pneumoniae is characterized by fever, cough, and sore throat, and it often presents as a biphasic illness, with severe pharyngitis and laryngitis in the first phase (26).

Legionnaire's disease (Legionella pneumophila and other species) can often be distinguished by accompanying signs such as diarrhea, headache, relative bradycardia, abdominal pain, liver enzyme elevations, and hematuria, but these signs can also accompany pneumonia caused by viruses or mycoplasma (14). Signs of encephalopathy (confusion, delirium, stupor) are not uncommon in Legionnaire's disease.

Because 50% of first opportunistic infections in acquired immunodeficiency syndrome (AIDS) are episodes of *P. carinii* pneumonia (PCP) and it has become a common cause of community-acquired pneumonia in urban settings (46), this diagnosis should be entertained if the onset of fever, cough, and dyspnea is insidious over 1 to 4 weeks and the immune status of the host is unknown (see details in Chapter 34).

Hantavirus pulmonary syndrome (HPS) is a rare pneumonitis with a high mortality rate (13), now recognized throughout the United States and western Canada (39). Following 1 to 7 days of nonspecific viral

Table 28.5. Clues to the Presumptive Diagnosis and Treatment of Acute Pneumonia[a]

Organisms	Seasonal Incidence	Incubation Period (Days)	Epidemiologic Setting	Clinical Clues	Antibiotics[c]
Common Bacteria					
S. pneumoniae	All year		Elderly; smokers; cardiopulmonary disease, alcoholism	None[b]	Erythromycin (mild cases only), penicillin (when dx known), cephalosporins, trimethoprim–sulfamethoxazole, some quinolones (see text), not tetracycline
H. influenzae	All year		Same	None[b]	Amoxicillin, amoxicillin–clavulanate, trimethoprim–sulfamethoxazole, quinolones, azithromycin, clarithromycin
M. catarrhalis	All year		COPD	None	Erythromycin (not amoxicillin), trimethoprim–sulfamethoxazole; quinolones
L. pneumophila	All year; Summer outbreaks	2–10	Construction sites; air-cooling apparatus	Diarrhea[b]; Fever >40°C	Erythromycin (not β-lactams), quinolones
C. pneumoniae (TWAR)	All year	Not known	Young adults, person-to-person	Diarrhea[b]; Pharyngitis; Laryngitis	Erythromycin (not β-lactams)
Anaerobes	All year	1–5	Aspiration	Consolidation in dependent lobe	Amoxicillin–clavulanate, clindamycin, penicillin VK
Gram-negative aerobes	All year	1–5	Aspiration, alcoholism, elderly, recent hospitalization with antibiotics, institutionalization	Delirium; sepsis	Clindamycin (usually needs IV antibiotics)
Uncommon Bacteria (<1% Incidence)					
Psittacosis	All year	6–15	Exposure to birds, especially parrots, turkeys, pigeons (20% have no bird exposure)		Erythromycin; doxycycline
Q fever	All year	14–28	Contact with sheep, goats, cattle, especially at parturition		Doxycycline; quinolones
Tularemia (pulmonary)	All year	2–4	Handling infected rodents, rabbits		Doxycycline
Plague (pneumonia)	Spring to fall	2–4	Handling infected rodents, humans, cats	Delirium, sepsis, bubo	Gentamicin; doxycycline
Other Pathogens					
M. pneumoniae	Summer to fall	14–28	Multiple members of household ill, often at 3- to 4-week intervals	Pharyngitis, laryngitis, bullous myringitis, dry hacking cough persisting >1 week	Erythromycin, tetracycline, doxycycline, quinolones
Respiratory syncytial virus	Spring	2–8	Contact with bronchiolitis in children, nosocomial spread		—
Influenza A and B	Winter, spring	1–3	Accompany school absenteeism	Severe headache, myalgias	Amantadine, rimantidine (influenza A only)
Parainfluenza 1, 2, 3	All year	3–8	Croup in household	Conjunctivitis	—
Adenovirus	Winter	4–5	Closed populations	Conjunctivitis	—
Hantavirus	All year	8–21	Close contact with deer mice	Severe myalgias, pulmonary edema	Ribavirin (in clinical trial only)
P. carinii	All year	Unknown	HIV risk group		Trimethoprim–sulfamethoxazole

[a]Tuberculosis and some fungal pneumonias may be indistinguishable from acute pneumonia (symptoms <7 days).

[b]No difference in prodromal symptoms and respiratory tract symptoms among these four pathogens.

[c]See practical information regarding available strengths, dosage, side effects in Table 28.7. See text for duration of antimicrobial treatment.

prodrome of fever, myalgias, chills, and headache, the respiratory phase is heralded by dry cough and dyspnea, with rapid onset of pulmonary edema caused by a capillary leak syndrome. The most lethal complication is cardiogenic shock. Laboratory clues to HPS include thrombocytopenia, atypical lymphocytosis, and transaminasemia in every case, and the frequent occurrence of acidosis, mild coagulcpathy, and proteinuria. Any patient from a rural area with potential rodent exposure in whom HPS is clinically suspected should be hospitalized where immediate access to intensive care is possible.

Evaluation

Physical Examination. The physical examination does not usually distinguish between bacterial and atypical pneumonia syndromes. Crepitant rales that do not clear with cough are suggestive of pneumonia of either type. Signs of consolidation (increased tactile fremitus, dullness to percussion, bronchial breath sounds, and egophony) are more common in bacterial pneumonia. In early stages of pneumonia, the examination may be normal, despite an infiltrate on radiograph. On the other hand, rales and rhonchi may indicate pneumonia before the appearance of an infiltrate.

Laboratory Examination. Every patient suspected of having pneumonia should have a chest radiograph, pulse oximetry to measure O_2 saturation of hemoglobin, peripheral blood white cell count and differential count, and two blood cultures before initiating antibiotics (77). A white cell count over 15,000 is usually associated with bacterial pneumonia. Although the radiograph is essential for the firm diagnosis of pneumonia, a normal radiograph does not necessarily rule out pneumonia and radiograph patterns are not specific in terms of the cause (4,14). In one study (69) in which diagnosis was attempted by six radiologists from the blinded chest film alone, mycoplasmal pneumonia was incorrectly identified as bacterial in a significant proportion of patients.

A sputum Gram's stain is occasionally helpful in directing initial therapy, but discordant results between Gram's stain and culture in pneumococcal pneumonia, and the lack of diagnostic data from many other common respiratory pathogens including *Legionella, mycoplasma,* and *chlamydia,* render the Gram's stain of limited utility. In pneumonia caused by *staphylococci, Hemophilus species,* and *Enterobacteriaceae,* the Gram's stain of the sputum usually contains large numbers of Gram-positive cocci in clusters, small Gram-negative coccobacillary, and Gram-negative rods, respectively. The rapid Gram's stain technique requires only 1 to 2 minutes: heat fixation; 5 seconds crystal violet, water rinse; 5 seconds Gram's iodine, water rinse; decolorization of the thin part of the smear with 4 to 5 drops of 95% alcohol, water rinse; 5 seconds safranine, water rinse; blot dry. The sputum sample is probably of lower respiratory tract origin if there are fewer than 10 squamous epithelial cells and more than 25 polymorphonuclear leukocytes/high dry

(×100) field, except in leukopenic patients. The appearance of columnar ciliated epithelial cells ensures lower tract origin.

Sputum cultures have limited utility in the management of ambulatory pneumonias because sputum samples are often contaminated by oral pneumococci, and cultures are usually negative if any prior antibiotic therapy has been administered (67,77).

Serologic Diagnosis. Few pathogens can be diagnosed by serologic study of the acute serum specimen; exceptions include many but not all cases of pertussis and all cases of hantavirus infection (39). During an apparent community outbreak of a respiratory illness caused by unculturable agents, it is helpful to the public health authorities when practitioners collect and save acute and convalescent serum for later study at reference laboratories. Guided by epidemiologic clues (Table 28.5), measurement of acute and convalescent titers for antibodies to *M. pneumoniae, Q fever, psittacosis, influenza, Legionella species, tularemia, C. immitis,* and *Histoplasma capsulatum* is available at most state diagnostic laboratories and many commercial laboratories.

The presence of serum *cold agglutinins* is often used as a rapid diagnostic test for mycoplasmal pneumonia but has several drawbacks, including the requirement of delivery to the laboratory at 37°C, insensitivity to detect true positive mycoplasmal infection, and lack of specificity caused by positive cold agglutinins among cases of pneumococcal and adenoviral pneumonia.

Management: Decision About Hospitalization

Because an etiologic diagnosis of pneumonia would require many different tests, and as many as 50% of cases cannot be defined despite extensive state-of-the-art diagnostic techniques (4), treatment decisions focus on the antibiotic selection and the need for hospitalization. The desire to avoid unnecessary hospitalization has led to studies defining low-risk patients with community-acquired pneumonia (17,18).

A meta-analysis of pneumonia outcomes revealed 11 prognostic factors associated with increased mortality: altered mental status, male gender, absence of pleuritic chest pain, hypothermia, systolic hypotension, tachypnea, diabetes mellitus, neoplastic disease, leukopenia, and multilobar pulmonary infiltrates (17). A survey of practitioners making decisions on hospitalizations indicated that hypoxemia, inability to maintain oral intake, and lack of patient home care support were nearly universal and appropriate criteria for admission (19). Their estimation of the patient's risk of death based on examination and comorbidity usually overestimated the risk of death, resulting in excessive use of hospitalization (19). The large *Pneumonia Patient Outcome Research Team* (PORT) study, which used the experience of more than 14,000 patients with community-acquired pneumonia (18), established that *when the answers to all of the following three questions are "no",* the patient is in the lowest of five risk classes (group I) with a 30-day mortality rate of 0.1 to 0.4% (18):

- Is the patient older than 50 years?
- Is one or more of the following coexisting conditions present: neoplastic (except skin cancer), cerebrovascular, renal, liver disease or congestive heart failure?
- Is one or more of the following abnormalities on physical examination present: altered mental status, pulse above 125/minute, respiratory rate above 30/minute, systolic blood pressure below 90 mm Hg, temperature below 35°C or above 40°C?

If the answers to any of the three questions was "yes," further risk assessment was determined by a point scoring system including the additional characteristics listed in Table 28.6, each of which was independently associated with increased morbidity. The study found that classification in risk groups I, II (70 points or less), or III (71 to 90 points) predicted the safety of ambulatory management as the initial approach to a patient with pneumonia (18). These PORT-derived indicators of risk can be used as general guidelines until prospective studies provide even more precise rules, but clinical judgment must always supersede any rules (15,72). Additional unusual complications such as concomitant meningitis or septic arthritis, hemoptysis, prior splenectomy, and need for respiratory isolation of potential tuberculosis or pneumonic plague must be considered.

Failure to respond to initial therapy for reasons such as the following may dictate the need for hospital admission: impaired host defenses, pulmonary embolism, airway obstruction, continued aspiration, noncompliance, vomiting medications, empyema, dental abscess, antibiotic/resistance.

Management: Ambulatory

Choice of Antimicrobial Therapy (Table 28.7). In view of the large array of efficacious antibiotics and the difficulty in arriving at a definitive etiologic diagnosis for most cases of pneumonia, a wide variety of empiric regimens have been recommended in textbooks and journals, reflecting regional and experiential biases of the authors. Empiric regimens must necessarily use broad-spectrum antibiotics, and some experts believe that their use will enhance the dissemination of broadly resistant respiratory pathogens.

The American Thoracic Society (ATS) has issued the following consensus guidelines for the initial treatment of immunocompetent adults with community-acquired pneumonia (CAP) (50); these guidelines are reasonable and practical but require further study to show that adherence improves outcome (16). The guidelines placed ambulatory patients in two groups.

First group: For ambulatory patients with no comorbidity and less than 60 years of age, a macrolide is recommended as first-line therapy. Erythromycin, 500 mg three to four times daily, and the newer macrolides clarithromycin and azithromycin provide coverage for pneumococcal, chlamydial, Legionella, and mycoplasmal infections. The newer macrolides, which are expensive, are not associated with the frequent abdominal pain caused by erythromycin, and provide better coverage for Haemophilus species. Because of the latter feature, the ATS guideline recommends the newer macrolides for the treatment of CAP in smokers. Azithromycin has the advantage of once-daily dosing. Erythromycin and clarithromycin, but not azithromycin, can raise blood theophylline levels, occasionally into the toxic range, and dosages of the latter drug should be monitored and adjusted. In addition, erythromycin and clarithromycin have been associated, rarely, with an increased risk of lovastatin-induced rhabdomyolysis and an increased risk of terfenadine-induced arrhythmia. Alternatives to the macrolides are those fluoroquinolones (lexofloxacin, gresafloxacin, or trovafloxacin), which are efficacious for treating S. pneumoniae, M. pneumoniae, Chlamydia trachomatis, Legionella, M. catarrhalis, and Gram-negative aerobes.

Second group: For ambulatory patients with either COPD, a comorbid illness (see those listed in Table 28.6), or age over 60, who are at greater risk for infection with Gram-negative aerobes, Haemophilus species, and pneumococcus, the guidelines suggest a second-generation cephalosporin (e.g., cefaclor available in generic form) or a combination agent (TMP/SMX or β-lactam/β-lactamase inhibitor). The ATS guideline makes the addition of a macrolide optional, depending on the epidemiologic and clinical history suggesting Legionella or another "atypical pneumonia" agent. Although the prevalence of antibiotic-resistant pneu-

Table 28.6. Point Scoring System for Step 2 of the Prediction Rule for Assignment to Risk Classes II (≥70 Points), III (71–90 Points), IV, and V

Characteristic	Points Assigned[a]
Demographic factor	
Age	
Men	Age (yr)
Women	Age (yr) − 10
Nursing home resident	+10
Coexisting illness	
Neoplastic disease	+30
Liver diseae	+20
Congestive heart failure	+10
Cerebrovascular disease	+10
Renal disease	+10
Physical examination findings	
Altered mental status	+20
Respiratory rate ≥30/min	+20
Systolic blood pressure <90 mm Hg	+20
Temperature <35°C or ≥40°C	+15
Pulse ≥125/min	+10
Laboratory and radiographic findings	
Arterial pH <7.35	+30
Blood urea nitrogen ≥30 mg/dL (11 mmol/L)	+20
Sodium <130 mmol/L	+20
Glucose ≥250 mg/dL (14 mmol/L)	+10
Hematocrit <30%	+10
Partial pressure of arterial oxygen <60 mm Hg	+10
Pleural effusion	+10

Adapted from Fine MJ, Auble TE, Yealy DM, et al. A prediction rule to identify low-risk patients with community-acquired pneumonia. N Engl J Med 336:243–250, 1997.

[a]A total point score for a given patient is obtained by summing the patient's age in years (age minus 10 for women) and the points for each applicable characteristic.

Table 28.7.   Oral Antimicrobial Drugs Used in Ambulatory Treatment of Respiratory Infections

Drug[a] (Trade Name)	Available Strengths (mg)	Usual Adult Dosage and Schedule[c]	Common Side Effects	Drug and Food Interactions and Instructions
Penicillin V	250, 500	250–500 mg TID–QID	Diarrhea, nausea, vomiting, vaginitis, skin	Rash with infections mononucleosis or concomitant allopurinol, false-positive Clinitest (use Clinistix or Tes-tape)
Amoxicillin	250, 500	250–500 mg TID–QID		
Amoxicillin–clavulanate (Augmentin)[b]	250, 500	250–500 mg q8hr		
Erythromycin	250, 500	250–500 mg TID–QID	Nausea, vomiting, abdominal pain, diarrhea (less with azithromycin and clarithromycin)	False elevation of aminotransferase, raises serum theophylline and terfenadine levels, potentiates warfarin and glucocorticoids, increases risk of lovastatin-induced rhabdomyolysis
Azithromycin[b] (Zithromax)	250	500 mg loading dose 250 mg daily 1 hr before eating for 4 days		
Clarithromycin[b] (Biaxin)	250, 500	500 mg BID		
Tetracycline	250, 500	250–500 mg TID–QID	Skin photosensitivity, nausea, vomiting, heartburn, diarrhea, mucosal candidiasis	Food, milk, antacids, iron interfere with absorption
Doxycycline	100	100 mg BID		
Trimethoprim (T) plus sulfamethoxazole (S) (TMP/SMX)	80 T/400 S (single-strength) 160 T/800 S (double-strength)	2 single-strength or 1 double-strength BID	Skin rash, gastrointestinal upset, elevates serum creatinine	Prolongs half-life of warfarin, phenytoin, and oral hypoglycemics
Clindamycin	150, 300	150–450 mg TID–QID	C. difficile–induced diarrhea	To avoid possible esophageal irritation, take with a full glass of water
Cefuroxime axetil[b] (Ceftin)	125, 250, 500	250–500 mg BID	Nausea, vomiting, diarrhea	Absorption enhanced with food, false-positive Clinitest
Cefaclor	250	250–500 mg q8hr		
Loracarbef (Lorabid)	200, 400	200–400 mg q12hr		
Ciprofloxacin[b] (Cipro)	250, 500, 750	500 mg BID	Nausea, diarrhea, vomiting, restlessness	Prolongs half-life of theophylline; antacids interfere with absorption; CNS side effects increased with caffeine
Levofloxacin (Levofloxin)	500	500 mg QD		
Ofloxacin[b] (Floxin)	400	400 mg BID		

[a]No trade name is listed for those available in generic preparations.
[b]Courses of these cost more than $50.
[c]See text for duration of antimicrobial treatment.

mococci is increasing (8), there is not yet evidence that empiric regimens for pneumonia should be revised to account for resistance patterns (41). Furthermore, a prospective cohort study recently showed that the outcomes of patients greater than 60 or having one comorbidity did not differ significantly when those given only a macrolide antibiotic were compared with those given an ATS-recommended regimen (23). Most macrolide-treated patients received erythromycin, at a cost that was one-tenth the cost of most of the ATS-recommended agents.

The widespread availability of *home intravenous antibiotic services* makes it feasible to avoid or shorten hospitalization yet provide the advantages of intravenous antibiotics for patients deemed stable yet unable to tolerate oral antibiotics.

Duration of Antimicrobial Treatment.   Duration of therapy for community-acquired pneumonia is not well defined. Considerations such as the presence of coexisting illness and the severity of illness at the onset of antibiotic therapy must be taken into account. The ATS guidelines suggest that bacterial infections, such as *S. pneumoniae* pneumonia, should be treated

for approximately 7 to 10 days, whereas cases of *M. pneumoniae* and *C. pneumoniae* may need longer therapy ranging from 10 to 14 days. For most infections, a 5-day course of azithromycin is adequate therapy because of its prolonged biological half-life. *Legionella pneumophila* should be treated for 21 days.

Follow-Up.   The patient should be advised to keep in close contact by telephone, maintain good hydration with oral fluids, use aspirin or acetaminophen to control fever and headache, and avoid cough suppressants and cigarettes. A telephone contact with the patient 24 hours after the initial visit provides a check on antibiotic compliance and side effects and on the status of symptoms; also it reassures the acutely ill patient that he or she has access to the physician should the condition worsen or fail to improve.

A follow-up visit to the office 3 to 4 days later will help assess response to therapy. Symptoms of pneumococcal pneumonia in the uncompromised host abate dramatically within 48 to 72 hours of initiation of therapy, and somewhat longer with other pathogens and compromised host defenses (50). If substantial clinical response to the initial antibiotic therapy has not occurred in this time, the patient must be reevaluated. Possible reasons for clinical failure include poor compliance with the antibiotic regimen, resistance of the etiologic organism to the empiric antibiotics, unusual pathogens such as tuberculosis, viral or fungal pneumonia, or a noninfectious cause such as pulmonary embolus or carcinoma (50). In any case, hospitalization is usually required to determine the cause of therapeutic failure.

Complete resolution of symptoms caused by an episode of pneumonia may not occur for 30 days or more after diagnosis (43). This includes cough, fatigue, dyspnea, and sputum production but not pleuritic chest pain.

Following clinical resolution of the pneumonia, a chest radiograph is recommended to exclude persistent radiographic abnormalities suggestive of endobronchial obstruction, particularly in smokers and patients over the age of 40. The rate of radiographic resolution depends on age and multilobar involvement; follow-up at 2 weeks is appropriate for the young adult with one lobe involvement, whereas the elderly with multilobar disease should be followed at 8 weeks (45).

Pneumonia in HIV-Infected Patients

HIV-infected patients are more susceptible to infection with a wide variety of pulmonary pathogens. PCP presents with the insidious onset of fever, nonproductive cough, and exertional shortness of breath (33). Findings on the chest examination may or may not reveal rales. Examination may reveal other evidence of immunosuppression such as oral thrush, hairy leukoplakia, or cutaneous lesions of Kaposi sarcoma. The chest radiograph usually reveals a diffuse interstitial infiltrate, although diffuse or focal airspace consolidation can be caused by PCP. Several antimicrobial agents are effective in treating PCP, and patients with mild PCP can be treated in the ambulatory setting. A systematic approach to the HIV-infected patient is described in Chapter 34.

Prevention of Pneumonia

Polyvalent pneumococcal vaccine and influenza vaccines are discussed in detail in Chapter 32. No special precautions need to be taken to isolate the ambulatory patient with pneumonia. Household contacts of these patients need no special surveillance, with the exceptions of pneumonic disease caused by tuberculosis (see Chapter 29), tularemia, plague, and meningococci.

Pleurodynia

Pleurodynia is an uncommon acute illness caused by members of the Coxsackie virus family. It occurs in summer and early fall. The presenting symptoms may suggest the onset of pneumonia: abrupt onset of *severe paroxysmal pain of the thorax or abdomen,* worse with cough or breathing. Other manifestations of pleurodynia include fever, headache, cough, and anorexia.

The physical examination is often normal except that the patient splints to avoid pain, which is commonly felt in the lower rib cage or under the sternum. The chest radiograph is usually normal. Most patients recover within 3 days to 1 week. Rare complications are orchitis, pericarditis, and aseptic meningitis.

General References*

Benenson AS, ed. Control of communicable diseases in man. 15th ed. Washington, DC: American Public Health Association, 1995.
> A concise summary of causes, prevention, and management of communicable diseases.

Mandell GL, Bennett JE, Dolin R, eds. Principles and practice of infectious diseases. 4th ed. New York: Churchill Livingstone, 1995.
> The standard textbook of infectious diseases.

Vickery DM, Fries JF. Take care of yourself: a consumer's guide to medical care. 4th ed. Reading, MA: Addison-Wesley, 1990.
> Simple algorithms for self-care of common medical problems.

Specific References

1. Ansari SA, Springthorpe VS, Sattar JA, et al. Potential role of hands in the spread of respiratory viral infections: studies with human parainfluenza virus 3 and rhinovirus 14. J Clin Microbiol 29:2115–2119, 1991.
2. Baine WB, Luby JP, Martin SW. Severe illness with influenza B. Am J Med 68:181, 1980.
3. Barker WH, Mullooly JP. Pneumonia and influenza deaths during epidemics: implications for prevention. Arch Intern Med 142:85, 1982.
4. **Bartlett JG, Mundy LM. Community-acquired pneumonia. N Engl J Med 333:1618–1624, 1995.**
5. Berg AO, LoGerfo JP. Potential effect of self-care algorithms on the number of physician visits. N Engl J Med 300:535, 1979.
6. Berrios X, del Campo E, Guzman P, Bisno AL. Discontinuing rheumatic fever prophylaxis in selected adolescents and young adults. Ann Intern Med 118:401, 1993.
7. Bisno AL. Group A streptococcal infections and acute rheumatic fever. N Engl J Med 325:783, 1991.
8. **Breiman RF, Butler JC, Tenover FC, et al. Emergence of drug-resistant pneumococcal infections in the United States. JAMA 271:1831–1835, 1994.**
9. Burke P, Bain J, Lowes A, Athersuch R. Rational decisions in managing sore throat. BMJ 296:1646, 1988.
10. **Chalmers TC. Effects of ascorbic acid on the common cold: an evaluation of the evidence. Am J Med 58:532, 1975.**
11. Chan ED, Welsh CH. Fulminant *Mycoplasma pneumoniae* pneumonia. West J Med 162:133–142, 1995.
12. **Delker LL, Moser RH, Nelson JD, et al. Amantadine: does it have a role in the prevention and treatment of influenza? A National Institutes of Health Consensus Development Conference. Ann Intern Med 92:256, 1980.**
13. Duchin J, Koster FT, Peters CJ, et al. Hantavirus pulmonary syndrome: a new illness in the southwestern United States. N Engl J Med 330:949–955, 1994.
14. Fang GD, Fine M, Orleff J, et al. New and emerging etiologies for community-acquired pneumonia with implications for therapy. Medicine 19:307, 1990.
15. Farr BM. Prognosis and decisions in pneumonia. N Engl J Med 336:288–289, 1997.
16. **Fein AM, Neiderman MS. Guidelines for the initial management of community-acquired pneumonia: savory recipe or cookbook for disaster? Am J Respir Crit Care Med 152:1149–1153, 1995.**
17. Fine MJ, Smith MA, Carson CA, et al. Prognosis and outcomes of patients with community-acquired pneumonia. JAMA 275:134–141, 1996.

---

*Bold print (general references) and bold numerals (specific references) denote published controlled clinical trials, meta-analyses, or consensus-based recommendations.

18. Fine MJ, Auble TE, Yealy DM, et al. A prediction rule to identify low-risk patients with community-acquired pneumonia. N Engl J Med 336:243–250, 1997.

19. Fine MJ, Hough LJ, Medsger AR, et al. The hospital admission decision for patients with community-acquired pneumonia: results from the Pneumonia Patient Outcomes Research Team Cohort Study. Arch Intern Med 157:36–44, 1997.

20. Forstall GJ, Macknin ML, Yen-Lieberman BR, Medendrop SV. Effect of inhaling heated vapor on symptoms of the common cold. JAMA 271:1109–1111, 1994.

21. Fraenkel DK, Bardin PG, Sanderson G, et al. Lower airways inflammation during rhinovirus colds in normal and in asthmatic subjects. Am J Respir Crit Care Med 151:879–886, 1995.

22. Frantz TD, Rasgon BM, Quesenberry CP Jr. Acute epiglottis in adults: analysis of 129 cases. JAMA 272:1358–1360, 1994.

23. Gleason PP, Kapoor WN, Stone RA, et al. Medical outcomes and antimicrobial costs with the use of the American Thoracic Society guidelines for outpatients with community-acquired pneumonia. JAMA 278(1):32–39, 1997.

24. Gonzales R, Sande M. What will it take to stop physicians from prescribing antibiotics in acute bronchitis? Lancet 345:665–666, 1995.

25. Graham NMH, Burrell CJ, Douglas RM, et al. Adverse effects of aspirin, acetaminophen, and ibuprofen on immune function, viral shedding, and clinical status in rhinovirus-infected volunteers. J Infect Dis 162:1277–1282, 1990.

26. Grayston JT. Infections caused by Chlamydia pneumoniae strain TWAR. J Infect Dis 15:757, 1992.

27. Gross PA, Rodstein M, LaMontagne JR, et al. Epidemiology of acute respiratory illness during an influenza outbreak in a nursing home. Arch Intern Med 148:559, 1988.

28. Gwaltney JM Jr, Moskalski PB, Hendley JO. Hand to hand transmission of rhinovirus colds. Ann Intern Med 88:463, 1978.

29. Gwaltney JM Jr, Phillips CD, Miller RD, et al. Computed tomographic study of the common cold. N Engl J Med 330:25–30, 1994.

30. Hall WJ, Douglas RG Jr. Pulmonary function during and after common respiratory infections. Annu Rev Med 31:233, 1980.

31. Hayden FG, et al. Effectiveness and safety of intranasal ipratropium bromide in common colds: a randomized, double-blind, placebo-controlled trial. Ann Intern Med 125:89–97, 1996.

32. Herzon FS. Peritonsillar abscess: incidence, current management practices, and a proposal for treatment guidelines. Laryngoscope 105(Suppl 74):1–17, 1995.

33. Hopewell PC. Pneumocystis carinii pneumonia: diagnosis. J Infect Dis 157:1115, 1988.

34. Huovinen P, et al. Pharyngitis in adults: the presence and coexistence of viruses and bacterial organisms. Ann Intern Med 110:612, 1989.

35. Jepson S, Holbrook JH, Hale D, Lyon J. Management of upper respiratory tract infections by telephone. West J Med 160:529–533, 1994.

36. Klein JO. Management of streptococcal pharyngitis. Pediatr Infect Dis J 13:572–575, 1994.

37. Koivula I, Sten M, Makela PH. Risk factors for pneumonia in the elderly. Am J Med 96:313–320, 1994.

38. Komaroff AL, Pass TM, Aronson MD, et al. The prediction of streptococcal pharyngitis in adults. J Gen Intern Med 1:1, 1986.

39. Koster FT, Jenison S. Hantavirus infections. In: Blacklow N, Bartlett JG, Gorbachs S, eds. Infectious diseases. 4th ed. Philadelphia: WB Saunders, 1997.

40. Kroenke K, Omori DM, Simmons JO, et al. The safety of phenylpropanolamine in patients with stable hypertension. Ann Intern Med 111:1043, 1989.

41. Lonks JR, Medeiros AA. The growing threat of antibiotic-resistant Streptococcus pneumoniae. Med Clin North Am 79:523–535, 1995.

42. Lorber B. The common cold. J Gen Intern Med 11:229–236, 1996.

43. Metlay JP, Fine MJ, Schulz R, et al. Measuring symptomatic and functional recovery in patients with community-acquired pneumonia. J Gen Intern Med 12:423–430, 1997.

44. Miller RA, Brancato F, Holmes KK. Corynebacterium hemolyticum as a cause of pharyngitis and scarlatiniform rash in young adults. Ann Intern Med 105:867, 1986.

45. Mittl RL Jr, Schwab RJ, Duchin JS, et al. Radiographic resolution of community-acquired pneumonia. Am J Respir Crit Care Med 149:630–635, 1994.

46. Mossad SB et al. Zinc gluconate lozenges for treating the common cold: a randomized, placebo-controlled study. Ann Intern Med 125:81–88, 1996.

47. Mostow SR. Prevention, management and control of influenza: role of amantadine. Am J Med 82(Suppl 6A):35, 1987.

48. Mundy LM, Auwaerter PG, Oldach D, et al. Community-acquired pneumonia: impact of immune status. Am J Respir Crit Care Med 152:1309–1315, 1995.

49. Musher DM. Infections caused by Streptococcus pneumoniae: clinical spectrum, pathogenesis, immunity, and treatment. Clin Infect Dis 14:801, 1992.

50. Neiderman MS, Bass JB, Campbell GD, et al. Guidelines for the initial management of adults with community-acquired pneumonia: diagnosis, assessment of severity, and initial antimicrobial therapy. Am Rev Respir Dis 148:1418–1426, 1993.

51. Nennig ME, Shinefield HR, Edwards KM, et al. Prevalence and incidence of adult pertussis in an urban population. JAMA 275:1672–1674, 1996.

52. Newman LJ, Platts-Mills TAE, Phillips CD, et al. Chronic sinusitis: relationship of computed tomographic findings to allergy, asthma and eosinophilia. JAMA 271:363–367, 1994.

53. Orr PH, Scherer K, Macdonald A, Moffatt MEK. Randomized placebo-controlled trials of antibiotics for acute bronchitis: a critical review of the literature. J Fam Pract 36:507–512, 1993.

54. Paradise JL, Bluestone CD, Bachman RZ, et al. Efficacy of tonsillectomy for recurrent throat infection in severely affected children: results of parallel randomized and non-randomized clinical trials. N Engl J Med 310:674–683, 1984.

55. Pichichero ME. Cephalosporins are superior to penicillin for treatment of streptococcal tonsillopharyngitis: is the difference worth it? Pediatr Infect Dis J 12:268–274, 1993.

56. Pinner RW, Teutsch SM, Simonsen L, et al. Trends in infectious disease mortality in the United States. JAMA 275:189–193, 1996.

57. Pratter MR, Bartter T, Akers S, et al. An algorithmic approach to chronic cough. Ann Intern Med 119:977, 1993.

58. Saint S, Bent S, Vittinghoff E, Grady D. Antibiotics in chronic obstructive pulmonary disease exacerbations: a meta-analysis. JAMA 273:957–960, 1995.

59. Sakethoo K, Januszkiewicz A, Sackner MA. Effects of drinking hot water and chicken soup on nasal mucus velocity and nasal airflow resistance. Chest 74:408, 1978.

60. Seppala H, Nissinen A, Jarvinen H, et al. Resistance to erythromycin in group A streptococci. N Engl J Med 326:339–340, 1991.

61. Shulman ST. Streptococcal pharyngitis: diagnostic considerations. Pediatr Infect Dis J 13:567–571, 1994.

62. Skoner DP, Doyle WJ, Seroky J, Fireman P. Lower airway responses to influenza A virus in healthy allergic and nonallergic subjects. Am J Respir Crit Care Med 154:661–664, 1996.

63. Simons FER, Simons KJ. The pharmacology and use of H_1-receptor-antagonist drugs. N Engl J Med 330:1663–1670, 1994.

64. Smith MBH, Feldman W. Over-the-counter medications. A critical review of clinical trials between 1950 and 1991. JAMA 269:2258, 1993.

65. Sperber SJ, Hendley JO, Hayden FG, et al. Effects of naproxen on experimental rhinovirus colds: a randomized, double-blind, controlled trial. Ann Intern Med 117:37–41, 1992.

66. Still JG. Management of pediatric patients with group A beta-hemolytic Streptococcus pharyngitis: treatment options. Pediatr Infect Dis J 14:S57–61, 1995.

67. Sue DY. Community-acquired pneumonia in adults. West J Med 161:383–389, 1994.

68. Tager I, Spiezer FE. Role of infection in chronic bronchitis. N Engl J Med 292:563, 1975.

69. Tew J, Colenoff L, Berlin BS. Bacterial or nonbacterial pneumonia: accuracy of radiographic diagnosis. Radiology 124:607, 1977.

70. Thompson AB, Muellen MB. Aerosolized beclomethasone in chronic bronchitis. Am Rev Respir Dis 146:389, 1992.
71. van Buchem FL, Knottnerus JA, Schrijnemaekers VJJ, Peeters MF. Primary-care–based randomised placebo-controlled trial of antibiotic treatment in acute maxillary sinusitis. Lancet 349:683–687, 1997.
72. Weingarten SR, Reidinger MS, Hobson P, et al. Evaluation of a pneumonia practice guideline in an interventional trial. Am J Respir Crit Care Med 153:1110–1115, 1996.
73. Williams JW Jr, Holleman DR Jr, Samsa GP, Simel DL. Randomized controlled trial of 3 vs. 10 days of trimethoprim/sulfamethoxazole for acute maxillary sinusitis. JAMA 273:1015–1021, 1995.
74. Williams JW Jr, Roberts L, Distell B, Simel DL. Diagnosing sinusitis by x-ray: comparing a single Waters view to 4-view paranasal sinus radiographs. J Gen Intern Med 7:481–485, 1992.
75. Williams JW Jr, Simel DL. Does this patient have sinusitis? Diagnosing acute sinusitis by history and physical examination. JAMA 270:1242–1246, 1993.
76. Williams JW Jr, Simel DL, Roberts L, Samsa GP. Clinical evaluation for sinusitis: making the diagnosis by history and physical examination. Ann Intern Med 117:705, 1992.
77. Woodhead MA, Arrowsmith J, Chamberlain-Webber R, et al. The value of routine microbial investigation in community-acquired pneumonia. Respir Med 85:313–317, 1991.
78. Wright SW, Edwards KM, Decker MD, Zeidin MH. Pertussis infection in adults with persistent cough. JAMA 273:1044–1046, 1995.

C H A P T E R 29

Tuberculosis in the Ambulatory Patient

PATRICK A. MURPHY, MD

EPIDEMIOLOGY

Incidence Trends

At the time of writing this chapter in the previous edition, the United States was experiencing an actual increase in tuberculosis incidence. The cause was the human immunodeficiency virus (HIV) epidemic, which had created large numbers of susceptible hosts. In addition, the number of cases of tuberculosis (TB) caused by bacilli resistant to most or all standard antituberculous drugs rapidly increased. These multiple drug–resistant (MDR) bacilli were highly lethal for patients with HIV infection, and it was feared that they would also produce untreatable infections in the normal population. Because of these problems, there has been a resurgence of interest in the disease, changes in medical and hospital practices, and intense follow-up of diagnosed cases by public health officers.

All this activity has paid off, and the current situation looks better (8). In 1995, there were 22,813 new cases of TB in the United States, almost back to the 1985 level of 22,201. Furthermore, 36% of all the cases occurred in people born in other countries, and of those, two-thirds were born in Haiti, Mexico, India,

China, Vietnam, or the Philippines. It seems likely that most of such cases were acquired abroad and imported. The number of cases in United States natives fell 10% between 1994 and 1995, whereas the incidence in immigrants rose 5%. More than half of all imported tuberculosis presents within 5 years of entry into the United States. MDR tuberculosis is still virtually 100% lethal in the HIV-infected person; however, the incidence of MDR tuberculosis nationwide has decreased slightly.

This improvement in the national picture can be attributed to many causes. Skin testing for tuberculosis has come back as a diagnostic procedure and is mandatory for health care workers. Patients discovered by this method are promptly given isoniazid preventive therapy. Clinical suspicion for tuberculosis by doctors has escalated, and tuberculosis is being considered as a possible cause of almost any chest illness, and almost any abnormal chest radiograph. Microbiologic methods for diagnosis have improved: PCR allows diagnosis of tuberculosis from the sputum, and metabolic inhibition tests allow early detection of drug-resistant bacilli. Four-drug therapy for tuberculosis has virtually replaced the old two- and three-drug regimens, and therapy is commonly enforced by directly observing the patient take his or her medicines. Finally, hospitals, clinics, and prisons have refined their ventilating systems to reduce airborne transmission of tuberculosis. These changes in practice are discussed below.

HIV and Tuberculosis

It is estimated that a normal adult newly infected with TB has approximately a 5% chance of developing clinical illness in the first 5 years after infection, and a total lifetime risk of approximately 10%. The other 90% of normal people infected with TB have a positive skin test but never develop clinical illness. In contrast are people who are tuberculin positive as a result of a long-standing infection who then acquire HIV infection. Such people have an annual incidence of clinical disease of 8 to 10%, and essentially a 100% lifetime incidence (14). Even more devastating are the consequences of being HIV positive and then becoming infected with TB. Because HIV seropositivity is often unknown to or concealed by the HIV-infected person, precise estimates of annual risk in this situation are not available. However, there are enough epidemics of severe primary TB among HIV-infected people exposed to an index case of tuberculosis to make it clear that the risk must be considerably higher than the 8 to 10% quoted above for the situation in which TB is acquired first. The annual risk is almost certainly over 50% and may approach 100% (10).

There are two other reasons why HIV infection amplifies TB rates. The first is based on the intensity of exposure needed to become infected. Tuberculosis is acquired by inhaling dried droplet nuclei, which typically contain one to three organisms. A normal person usually must inhale several hundred such nuclei be-

fore one of them successfully establishes a caseous focus. Most cases of TB in normal people follow long-standing, intense exposure to an infected person living in the same house or working in daily close contact. By contrast, a person infected with HIV acquires tuberculosis after inhaling an average of less than 10 infected nuclei, meaning that HIV-infected people often acquire TB after casual contact with an infected person. The other reason why HIV infection amplifies TB rates is that the clinical disease is often severe, and many bacilli are coughed out. Each case of TB in an HIV-infected person is therefore more infectious for other people than is the average case of TB in an immunocompetent person (10).

No matter how immunosuppressed one is, one cannot develop tuberculous infection unless one is exposed to the organism. HIV infection acquired by a young male homosexual in Iowa is highly unlikely to be complicated by TB because there is little chance that he will ever be exposed to a case of pulmonary TB.

Reactivation and Primary Tuberculosis

There are now two distinct epidemiologic profiles of clinical TB. Most sporadic symptomatic cases still arise as reactivation disease in a patient who was infected many years ago and was never treated or was inadequately treated. When the patient becomes old or develops an immunosuppressive illness, the disease reactivates. Such patients are infectious for others, and TB cases can develop in people closely exposed to them. The response to primary tuberculous infection depends on the kind of person infected. Children are highly susceptible to TB and tend to have clinical symptoms shortly after primary infection. Primary infection in an adult usually causes no symptoms, but the newly infected person becomes tuberculin positive (17). As discussed above, primary TB in an HIV-infected person tends to be severe and progressive (10).

Causes

The cause of TB in an immunologically normal person residing in the United States is almost always *Mycobacterium tuberculosis.* Atypical mycobacteria, such as *Mycobacterium kansasii* and *Mycobacterium avium-intracellulare,* and certain fungi, such as *Cryptococcus neoformans* and *Histoplasma capsulatum,* may produce disease indistinguishable from TB and should be considered in the differential diagnosis. All these diseases are more common and more severe in the immunosuppressed. In foreign countries bovine bacilli can be important.

Drug Resistance

In populations who have never been treated with antituberculous drugs, primary resistance of tubercle bacilli to most drugs occurs at a low level (approximately 1 to 3%). Because the mechanisms of resistance are different for every drug, primary resistance to multiple drugs is uncommon. However, during the past 50 years many inner-city patients have been placed on antituberculous drugs without close supervision. Such patients are likely to take drugs singly, because of real or perceived side effects from multiple drugs, and to discontinue therapy entirely after symptoms improve. Not only do the bacilli in these patients become resistant to many antituberculous drugs, but these resistant organisms may infect other people. In such cases, the TB is "primary" because the infected person has a new infection. Nonetheless, the tubercle bacilli may be resistant to one or more of the standard antituberculous drugs. In 1965, before the HIV epidemic, children in Brooklyn with TB had isoniazid-resistant organisms 15% of the time (17).

The HIV epidemic has amplified the problem of drug-resistant tubercle bacilli that already existed in large cities. It is now not uncommon for tubercle bacilli to be resistant to all three standard antituberculous drugs: isoniazid (INH), rifampin (RIF), and ethambutol (EMB). Some strains have been resistant to all known antituberculous drugs. Such MDR strains are disastrous for the HIV-infected person because the disease cannot be controlled and they die of it rapidly. MDR strains are also a major public health hazard for immunocompetent people who are exposed to intense concentrations of infectious droplet nuclei. There is no reason to believe that these organisms are any more virulent than average, and presumably a normal person infected with such strains would have a 10% lifetime risk of developing clinical disease.

DIAGNOSIS

History

When symptomatic, TB almost always presents with signs and symptoms of weeks to months duration. Almost the only time it presents as acute disease is in rare cases of acute meningitis or tuberculous pneumonia. The history should be directed toward both defining the symptom complex and determining possible exposure to known sources of disease.

Because TB has multiple presentations, one should be suspicious about anyone with chronic unexplained symptoms. Weight loss (documented over a defined period), fever (particularly in the late evenings), night sweats (to be differentiated from environmentally induced sweats), decreased appetite, and the loss of a sense of well-being are the most important nonspecific symptoms. Persistent cough (usually with sputum production), hemoptysis, and pleuritic chest pain are more specific findings suggestive of pulmonary involvement.

It is important to know whether the patient has previously had TB, has previously been skin tested for TB (if so, when and what the results were), and when the patient has had previous chest films (and where they can be obtained).

Possibly significant history also includes any family member or close friend with known TB, any person in school or at work with known disease, and any recent history of travel to a country where TB is common.

Because extrapulmonary TB may occur in any organ (e.g., pleura, lymph nodes, endometrium, kidneys, ureters, bones and joints, skin, meninges, small intestine, and peritoneum) or as a disseminated (miliary) form, symptoms and signs in any organ must raise the consideration of TB.

Physical Examination

The physical examination may be entirely negative, even with obvious evidence of pulmonary disease on the chest radiograph. The following positive findings, when present, may be of considerable help in suggesting the diagnosis: rales localized to the upper posterior chest or auscultatory evidence of pulmonary cavitation (bronchovesicular breathing and whispered pectoriloquy), evidence of pleural effusion, supraclavicular and infraclavicular retraction, lymphadenopathy, evidence of weight loss, and fever. Although rare in the United States, large, matted, nontender cervical lymph nodes (at times with draining sinuses) are almost diagnostic of scrofula, a form of tuberculous adenitis (which may also be caused by atypical mycobacteria) seen primarily in children.

Tuberculin Skin Tests

The standardized skin test for evidence of tuberculous infection uses 5 units of Tween-stabilized intermediate strength purified protein derivative (PPD), which is injected intradermally on the volar skin of the forearm. The use of control tests with "anergy panel" antigens has been abandoned. The PPD test requires intradermal injection, which is a highly skilled procedure. Tine tests and automated methods of introducing antigen into the skin such as the Heaf gun can be used in population surveys. Positive results elicited with these methods should be confirmed with the standard PPD. The PPD reaction should be read at 48 hours. A practical method for determining the diameter of the indurated area is the *ballpoint pen method:* a line is drawn from a point 1 to 2 cm away from the margin of a positive reaction; when the pen tip reaches the margin of the indurated area, definite resistance is felt; this is repeated on the opposite side, and the diameter of the indurated reaction is measured.

The diameter required for a positive test varies according to circumstances.

A: Cases in which more than 5 mm is regarded as positive
   People with HIV infection
   People with recent close contact with a case of pulmonary tuberculosis
   People with fibrotic changes on their chest radiograph suggestive of healed tuberculosis
B: Cases in which more than 10 mm is regarded as positive

In general, those with chronic illnesses known to predispose to tuberculosis, or those from areas with a high incidence of TB
People with silicosis, malnutrition, or diabetes
People on renal dialysis, corticosteroids, or chemotherapy for cancer
Children less than 4 years of age
People born in high-prevalence areas
The poor
People from prisons, nursing homes, and other group residences
C: Cases in which more than 15 mm is regarded as positive
People generally healthy and not exposed to TB

A *PPD conversion* requires an increase of 10 mm within 2 years for patients under 35 years of age. In patients over 35 years, the requirement is an increase of 15 mm within 2 years. Note that a change from 8 to 12 mm is *not* a PPD conversion, and a change from 10 to 20 mm would not be a conversion for a healthy person over 35 years. These guidelines have replaced the old uniform 10-mm standard because they generate fewer false-positive PPD conversions (7). They are not foolproof and should be applied with common sense. In particular, it has been suggested that even 2 mm induration may be significant in an HIV-infected patient (13).

The tuberculin skin test is an excellent way of diagnosing recent tuberculous infection in children or young adults. Such people are rarely tuberculin positive in the absence of recently acquired tuberculous infection. The test is also useful for investigating family members or health care personnel who have had known exposure to patients with infectious TB. Because it is not specific or sensitive enough to guide a clinical decision, the tuberculin test is less useful for the evaluation of patients with nonspecific symptoms that may be caused by TB. In some populations of elderly patients, up to 50% may be tuberculin positive as a result of long-standing infection that is inactive and has nothing to do with the present illness. Fully 20% of patients who do have active clinical TB are PPD negative. When one adds in other clinical variables such as tumors, steroid therapy, radiation therapy, and organ transplants, a negative PPD test is often uninterpretable. Also, a negative PPD test may be harmful if it is used to rule out the diagnosis of TB in a patient whose clinical state may be caused by active disease.

A *person with a known positive tuberculin skin test should not have it repeated.* In such patients, there is a risk of producing a very strong positive reaction characterized by tender induration, axillary adenopathy, temperature elevation, and sloughing of the epidermis after a week. When a patient develops this complication, it should be treated with a sterile gauze dressing impregnated with a topical steroid, such as 0.1% triamcinolone.

The Centers for Disease Control and Prevention (CDC) recommends that *previous BCG vaccination* be disregarded when interpreting the response to a PPD (2). The reason is that most BCG vaccines do not appear to convert to a positive PPD. On the other hand, necrotic tuberculin reactions are particularly common in people who were vaccinated with BCG in childhood and become health care workers who must be PPD tested every 6 or 12 months. If the vaccination was 20 to 30 years earlier, the first tuberculin test is commonly negative. However, if repeated testing is done, the immunologic memory revives and the reaction becomes progressively more intense. Not only does this raise unwarranted fears of tuberculous infection, but the reactions are very painful. The CDC regulations do not cover this situation; however, it is prudent not to do more than one tuberculin test in anyone previously vaccinated with BCG.

M. tuberculosis shares antigens with related mycobacteria, so a positive skin test is not specific. However, most cross-reactions are less than 10 mm in diameter. Skin testing with specific atypical mycobacterial antigens should not be done: The antigens are not available for general use and the results are difficult to interpret.

The *booster phenomenon* may interfere with the interpretation of the tuberculin test (20). Patients with a remote tuberculous or atypical mycobacterial infection who have become skin-test negative may, upon repeat annual skin testing, develop a positive response because of the boosting effect of the repeated test. This boosting effect can be detected by administering a second tuberculin test 1 week after the first test in patients who initially have a negative response. If the second response is positive, these patients can be said to have had past infection but are not considered to have a recently acquired infection. The booster phenomenon is important in elderly people, in whom it is common, and in people such as hospital employees who may be skin tested frequently.

Current practice in hospitals is that all employees not known to be PPD positive are tested on entry. If they are PPD negative on entry and have contact with patients, they are retested annually, or more often if the hospital is in an area where TB is common.

Laboratory Evaluation

Chest Radiograph

Both posteroanterior (PA) and lateral views should be obtained. If the standard radiograph is normal but the patient has strong clinical evidence for TB, an apical lordotic view or a computerized tomography (CT) scan of the chest should also be obtained. The radiologic findings typical of TB (e.g., apical scarring, hilar adenopathy with peripheral infiltrate, upper lobe cavitation, miliary infiltrate) are not specific; however, a negative chest film rules out pulmonary TB (with the rare exception of early miliary disease), making the chest film a very sensitive test.

Cultures and Smears of Sputum

Sputum, for smear and culture, should be obtained at least three times. A *positive sputum smear* highly suggests TB (not absolutely diagnostic because of the possibility of atypical infection or of contamination), and a *positive culture is diagnostic.* If sputum is difficult to obtain, one can obtain assisted sputum after the patient has inhaled hypertonic saline aerosol. This procedure is obviously dangerous to personnel and should be done only in a special room with proper precautions for infection control. If clinical features suggest infection outside the lung, then smears and cultures of other body fluids such as urine and cerebrospinal fluid (CSF) are appropriate.

Cultures usually become positive within 3 or 4 weeks. Any tubercle bacillus isolated from a patient should be tested for sensitivity to standard drugs, because it may be necessary to change treatment if the organism shows resistance. The state health laboratory will be glad to do this if necessary. In parts of the world with very limited funds, it may be necessary to confine drug susceptibility tests to tubercle bacilli from patients who have failed standard therapy.

Miscellaneous Laboratory Tests

In patients with active TB, the hematocrit value may be normal or low. The anemia caused by TB is normochromic and normocytic, the so-called anemia of chronic disease (see Chapter 50). The white blood cell count and differential count are usually normal; occasionally a monocytosis is seen in patients with severe disease. The urine should be tested routinely; if sterile pyuria is found, it is suggestive of renal TB and cultures should be sent.

Tests of liver function such as serum aminotransferases, alkaline phosphatase, and bilirubin may be helpful if disseminated disease or liver involvement is suspected. Also, these values provide baselines in case the patient develops hepatitis caused by antituberculous drugs. Other procedures, such as thoracentesis, lumbar puncture, and liver biopsy, are indicated only when specific organ involvement is suspected.

Presumptive Diagnosis

The presumptive diagnosis of active TB can be made when any of the following is found:

- A typical chest radiograph
- A positive sputum smear
- A biopsy showing caseating granulomas with or without acid-fast organisms
- A recent change (within 1 year) of the tuberculin skin test from negative to positive, associated with other characteristic systemic symptoms or signs

The diagnosis of active TB is confirmed by a positive culture from any body fluid or biopsy specimen. All patients with a presumptive or confirmed diagnosis of TB must be reported promptly to the appropriate local health department.

Diagnosis of Tuberculosis in HIV-Infected Patients

In 1993, pulmonary TB in an HIV-positive patient was designated as an *acquired immunodeficiency syndrome (AIDS)-defining condition* (see Chapter 34).

When clinical TB appears before the development of other AIDS-indicator conditions, presentation occurs in a typical fashion, with pulmonary disease predominantly in the apices and often with cavitation. Fever, sweats, cough, anorexia, and wasting are common complaints. When TB appears after AIDS is already established, many patients have progressive primary disease, with extensive lower lobe involvement, no cavitation, and hilar adenopathy (10). Extrapulmonary TB is more common in patients with AIDS and involves lymph nodes, liver, brain, meninges, bone marrow, adrenals, and the genitourinary tract. Aspiration or biopsy of the suspected site of infection should be performed for acid-fast stain and culture. When acid-fast bacilli (AFB) are found in one of these specimens, treatment for *M. tuberculosis* should be initiated while awaiting culture results, even though *M. avium-intracellulare* is more common.

MANAGEMENT AND COURSE

Treatment

When TB is diagnosed in association with systemic signs or symptoms, the patient should be treated for active disease. Patients with positive tuberculin reactions as the only manifestation of disease are more difficult to treat (see "Isoniazid Prophylaxis," below).

Isolation

Any patient with symptomatic TB should be hospitalized at once in respiratory isolation in a negative-pressure room. Isolation must be instituted as soon as the diagnosis is made or even strongly suspected. One can never prevent a patient walking into an emergency room and exposing a doctor, two or three nurses, a clerk, a radiology technician, and other patients to the risk of TB. But an undiagnosed patient who stays on a medical ward for 2 weeks may easily expose 200 people. Isolation should be maintained until the patient is clearly noninfectious (see below).

In some communities, no hospital has the required isolation rooms and MDR tubercle bacilli are uncommon or unknown. In these circumstances, a patient who has a home can be started on treatment and sent home. The logic is that everyone in the home has already been exposed. The patient is instructed not to leave the house for 2 weeks, and not to allow any previously unexposed visitors for the same period. Therapy in the home should be directly observed (see below), and the patient allowed to leave the house or have visitors only when clearly improving. It should be noted that this exception to the guidelines does not apply to patients who are homeless or are unlikely to follow directions because of alcoholism or drug addiction. It also does not apply in communities where MDR tuberculosis is common.

Drug Therapy for Tuberculosis

The imperatives of the MDR tuberculosis situation have resulted in a *standard four-drug protocol* for treating tuberculosis (6). There is little room for individual variation, and attempts to use nonstandard methods usually result in telephone calls from the local health department. The pressure is in favor of *rendering the patient noninfectious in the shortest possible time.* That way, fewer nurses are required to supervise the therapy.

The current standard initial regimen is as follows:

- *Isoniazid* (INH) 300 mg/day (available strengths: 100 and 300 mg)
- *Rifampin* (RIF) 600 mg/day (available strength 600 mg)
- *Ethambutol* (EMB) 15 mg/kg per day, commonly 1200 mg/day (available strengths 100 and 400 mg)
- *Pyrazinamide* (PZA) 2000 mg/day (available strength 500 mg)

These drugs are given for 2 months, and then the EMB and PZA are discontinued. INH and RIF are continued for another 4 months, making *6 months of treatment in all.* When the cultures become available, sensitivities should be checked. If the bacilli are susceptible to all four drugs and if directly observed therapy (see below) is used, more than 98% of cases of tuberculosis are permanently cured (9,11).

The enthusiasm for four-drug supervised therapy should not obscure the fact that this regimen is not appropriate for everyone. It is possible to cure TB with two or three drugs, but it takes longer. Patients should receive special consideration if they cannot take all the components of the standard regimen.

Drug Toxicity

Patients may develop a number of toxicities from antituberculous medications (Table 29.1).

- *Isoniazid* (15,16). Hepatic toxicity is the most common adverse reaction; it occurs at a biochemical level in approximately 20% of patients who take the drug, and the incidence of toxicity increases with age and

Table 29.1. Drugs for the Treatment of Mycobacterial Disease in Adults[a]

Commonly Used Agents	Available Strengths of Oral Tablets or Capsules (mg)	Dosage		Most Common Side Effects	Tests for Side Effects	Drug Interactions[b]
		Total Once Daily Dose	Twice Weekly Dosage			
Isoniazid[c]	100, 300	5–10 mg/kg up to 300 mg PO or IM	15 mg/kg PO up to 900 mg	Peripheral neuritis, hepatitis, hypersensitivity	Aminotransferases (not as a routine)	Carbamazepine: increased toxicity, both drugs Disulfiram: psychosis, ataxia Phenytoin: toxicity increased
Rifampin	150, 300	10 mg/kg up to 600 mg PO	10 mg/kg up to 600 mg PO	Hepatitis, febrile reaction, purpura (rare)	Aminotransferases (not as a routine)	May reduce the effect of the following drugs due to increased hepatic metabolism: oral contraceptives, quinidine, corticosteroids, anticoagulants, disopyramide, diazepam, barbiturates, methadone, digitoxin, digoxin, oral hypoglycemics; *p*-aminosalicylic acid may interfere with absorption of rifampin
Streptomycin		15–20 mg/kg up to 1 g IM	25–30 mg/kg up to 1 g IM	Eighth nerve damage, nephrotoxicity	Vestibular function, audiograms; blood urea nitrogen and creatinine	Neuromuscular blocking agents; may be potentiated to cause prolonged paralysis
Pyrazinamide	500	15–30 mg/kg up to 2 g PO	50–70 mg/kg up to 4 g	Hyperuricemia, hepatotoxicity	Uric acid, aminotransferases	
Ethambutol	100, 400	15–25 mg/kg PO	50 mg/kg PO up to 2.5 g	Optic neuritis (reversible with discontinuation of drug; very rare at 15 mg/kg), skin rash	Red-green color discrimination and visual acuity,[d] difficult to test in a child under 3 years	

[a]Adapted from American Thoracic Society. Treatment of tuberculosis and tuberculosis infection in adults and children. Am Rev Respir Dis 134:355, 1986; and MMWR 42:2, 1993.

[b]Reference should be made to current literature, particularly on rifampin, because it induces hepatic microenzymes and therefore interacts with many drugs.

[c]With pyridoxine 25 mg/day for poorly nourished or pregnant patients, to prevent peripheral neuropathy.

[d]Initial examination should be done at start of treatment.

with excessive alcohol intake. Pregnant women are at increased risk of INH toxicity. Laboratory evidence of mild injury to the liver is not in itself a reason to stop the drug, however, because in most subjects, the aminotransferase level returns to normal while the drug is being continued. If the patient develops jaundice or develops fever with elevated liver enzymes, the drug should be stopped. The liver injury is usually reversible and will heal without further therapy. However, in some patients (elderly men and particularly those with chronic alcohol-related liver disease), the liver injury may be severe and sometimes fatal. INH liver toxicity most often occurs early in therapy, so that the first 2 to 3 months are the most critical in the detection of adverse drug reactions. Specific guidelines for monitoring for INH hepatitis are contained in the section on prevention (below). Sensory peripheral neuropathy is an uncommon complication of INH therapy that occurs only in patients on an inadequate diet; it can be prevented by taking 25 mg of pyridoxine every day.

- *Ethambutol.* The most serious side effect of EMB is *optic neuritis,* resulting in decrease of visual acuity and in inability to distinguish the color green. This problem was seen frequently when the drug was given in a dose of 25 mg/kg. It is extremely uncommon at the current recommended daily dose of 15 mg/kg.

- *Rifampin.* Serious allergic complications of RIF therapy, including thrombocytopenia manifested by purpura, petechiae, and hematuria, acute renal failure, and a flu syndrome, occur in approximately 1% of patients and necessitate cessation of therapy. There is a modest increase in hepatic toxicity that may be additive to INH toxicity, so patients taking both drugs should be supervised closely. Patients should be warned that RIF will result in an orange-red color in secretions such as urine and saliva and may irreversibly stain contact lenses. Rifampin accelerates the metabolism of other drugs (Table 29.1) and may necessitate an increase in the dosage of these drugs. Interaction with HIV protease inhibitors is a major problem and requires expert advice.

Special Situations

Pregnant women are difficult to treat because of the need to consider the effects of prescribed drugs on the fetus. The standard recommendation, for areas where MDR tuberculosis is uncommon, is a three-drug regimen of INH, RIF, and EMB. There is worldwide experience with this regimen and it is generally regarded as safe. Pyrazinamide is a category C drug that could be added if necessary; streptomycin (STR) is category D and its use is discouraged. For other antituberculosis drugs one should seek expert advice.

Patients with *renal failure* are difficult to treat because both EMB and PZA are excreted largely by the kidneys. If renal function is only moderately reduced, this situation can be dealt with by dosage reduction However, if the patient is on hemodialysis, the calculations become a nightmare. Because the toxicity of

EMB is blindness and that of PZA is severe hepatitis, errors are serious. Both rifampin and isoniazid can be given in full dosage to people with no renal function. INH plus RIF given together for 9 months cures all forms of TB. It seems better to accept the longer treatment. If there is a real possibility of MDR TB, and a four-drug regimen is necessary, INH, RIF, PZA, and STR might be the safest. The hepatotoxicity of PZA is generally reversible, and although ototoxicity of STR is irreversible, the blood level of STR can be measured.

Patients who have HIV infection but are infected with drug-sensitive tubercle bacilli have a good prognosis for cure of the TB. It is usual to treat for 9 months rather than 6, and to be meticulous about follow-up.

Drug Resistance. If the bacilli prove to be resistant to either INH or RIF, treatment should be modified to a three- or four-drug regimen in which the bacilli are susceptible to all components. Such a regimen should be continued for at least 12 months, and perhaps 18 months in a case of extensive disease. If the bacilli are resistant to both INH and RIF, the organism is by definition a multi–drug resistant one. The patient should be referred for treatment to an expert, either in a university or in the state health department. What the expert will do is keep the patient in isolation as long as bacilli are found on sputum culture. All available secondary antibiotics will be tried against the organism. A selection will be made from possibilities such as capreomycin and clofazimine. Regimens of six or seven drugs are not uncommon. If the response to the best available therapy remains poor, the addition of γ-interferon infusions can be tried (18). If the patient is HIV infected, the outlook is probably hopeless, but there are occasional survivors (12). Details about longitudinal management of patients with drug resistant TB are found below ("Course in Treated Patients").

Additional Therapy

The patient may have symptoms that require special management (e.g., high fever and toxicity for which corticosteroids may be helpful, or a pleural effusion that needs draining). The patient should be encouraged to eat an adequate diet. If the patient is eating poorly, pyridoxine (25 mg/day) should be taken with INH to prevent peripheral neuropathy. Pyridoxine should also be taken routinely by pregnant patients and by patients with other diseases that may cause peripheral neuropathy (e.g., alcoholism, diabetes, end-stage renal disease).

Course in Treated Patients

Follow-Up Schedule

Physicians in the United States are rarely expected or allowed to supervise the treatment of a patient with TB. Directly observed therapy is so clearly superior for most patients that only completely reliable patients should be treated in a physician's office. Health departments will supervise therapy, test contacts, and provide prophylactic INH if necessary, provide free drugs, and perform sputum cultures and radiographs as tests of cure (9). It is hard to compete with that, and it has actually been shown that both death rates and recurrence rates are higher for patients treated by physicians (1). However, in rural areas of the United States or in other countries, the physician may have to supervise therapy for TB.

After treatment has been initiated, the patient should be seen or contacted at least once a month, chiefly to ensure drug compliance and to monitor for drug side effects. Sputum cultures should be obtained monthly for the first 3 months. At 3 months and between 6 months and 1 year, chest radiographs should be obtained. *Sputum culture should be negative after 3 months of therapy,* although occasionally nonculturable acid-fast organisms are seen on smear for longer periods. A test-of-cure culture should be done on all patients at 5 or 6 months. Resolution of pulmonary infiltrates is often slow; the former practice of monthly chest radiographs is therefore not warranted. Chest radiographs are most helpful in excluding progression of disease and in documenting the patient's status when TB is cured.

If the patient has sensitive bacilli and follows a recommended and supervised regimen for the prescribed time, then relapse is so rare that postcure follow-up is not strictly necessary. If the patient has a chronic disease, such as HIV, TB follow-up can be integrated with that of the chronic disease.

Usual Response

Patients with active TB who comply with therapy have an excellent prognosis. Exceptions are patients with organisms resistant to the usual antituberculous drugs or patients who develop adverse effects from the antituberculous therapy. The patient should show some symptomatic improvement within 1 week of being started on antituberculous therapy. Improvement is usually indicated by an increased sense of well-being, an increase in appetite, and a decrease in cough, fever, and night sweats; temperature should be normal within 14 days of initiating treatment. Most patients are back to their usual state of health in 1 to 2 months.

The improvement is caused by the prompt antibacterial effects of the drugs, which lead to a decrease in the inflammatory response of the host. After 2 or 3 weeks of therapy, the patient who is improving clinically (decreased cough, absence of fever, improved appetite) can be considered *noninfectious.* If the patient is known to be infected with an MDR organism, three sputa must be negative on smear before the patient can be released from isolation.

Respiratory Isolation for Ambulatory Patients

Health care workers who are the first points of contact in facilities serving patients at risk for TB should be trained to ask questions to detect patients who should be isolated because of signs or symptoms suggestive of TB. Even clerks can ask questions about chronic respiratory symptoms, and alert the doctor or nurse. Patients with signs or symptoms suggestive of TB should be evaluated promptly to minimize the time spent in ambulatory care areas. TB precautions should be applied while the diagnostic evaluation is being conducted.

TB precautions in the ambulatory care setting consist of placing the patient in a separate waiting area apart from other patients and not in open waiting areas, ideally in a room meeting TB isolation requirements, and giving the patient a surgical mask and instruction to keep it on. Patients should also be given tissues and instructed to cover their mouths and noses when coughing or sneezing, if they must remove their mask to facilitate respiratory clearance.

Ventilation in ambulatory care areas serving patients at high risk for TB should be designed and maintained to reduce the risk of TB transmission. General use (e.g., waiting rooms) and special areas (e.g., treatment or TB isolation rooms in ambulatory areas) should be ventilated in the same manner as described for similar inpatient areas. Enhanced general ventilation or the use of air disinfection techniques, such as in-room recirculation of air through high-efficiency particulate air (HEPA) filters or ultraviolet irradiation of the upper room air, may be useful. Ambulatory care settings in which patients with TB are frequently seen should have a negative-pressure room.

In general, *patients suspected or confirmed to have active TB should be considered infectious* if cough is present, they are undergoing cough-inducing procedures, sputum AFB smears are positive, or they are not receiving chemotherapy, have just started chemotherapy, or have a poor clinical or bacteriologic response to chemotherapy. A person with drug-susceptible TB who is on adequate chemotherapy and has had a significant clinical and bacteriologic response to therapy (reduction in cough, resolution of fever, and progressively decreasing quantity of bacilli on smear) is probably no longer infectious.

Patients with active TB who need to be seen in a clinic should have appointments scheduled to avoid exposing HIV-infected or otherwise severely immunocompromised patients. This could be accomplished by setting aside certain times of the day for appointments for these patients or having them seen in areas where immunocompromised patients are not treated.

Patients with infectious TB should have at least two negative sputum smears for AFB before being placed in indoor environments that are especially conducive to transmission, such as shelters for the homeless, or in settings where highly susceptible people, such as those with HIV infection, will be exposed (3).

Drug Resistance

The treatment of patients with drug-resistant tubercle bacilli has become common in certain U.S. cities such as New York and Miami. In other cities, drug resistance to even one antibiotic occurs less than 3% of the time, and MDR strains have rarely been observed. However, the population is so mobile that a patient who has acquired infection in one city may present for treatment in another.

Because MDR strains do not constitute the majority of strains in any city, it is customary to start treatment in all patients with a standard regimen. Exceptionally, the patient may give a clear history of exposure to a known case of MDR TB or come from an epidemic situation where an MDR organism is known to be responsible. In these cases, the patient can be started at once on the best available regimen.

Patients infected with MDR strains may show a delayed clinical response during the first few weeks of therapy. Because the laboratory may take 8 to 10 weeks to provide sensitivity data on the original isolates, it may be difficult to detect this problem early. Newer tests based on firefly luciferase assays may permit detection of drug-resistant tubercle bacilli in as little as 8 hours, but such assays are not yet commercially available.

The cardinal rules for management of proved or suspected MDR tuberculosis are as follows: Never add one drug to a failing regimen (5); refer the patient to the TB section of the local health department before any changes in regimen are tried; and keep the patient in respiratory isolation until he or she is demonstrably cured. Control of MDR infection with chemotherapy is difficult. Treatment may require empiric regimens containing up to six drugs and lasting 18 to 36 months; at times resectional surgery may be required (see review by Iseman, "General References"). If a patient has MDR TB complicating HIV infection, the patient usually dies despite taking all available antituberculous drugs.

Patient's Role in Therapy

In most of the world, TB treatment is initiated and conducted entirely in the ambulatory setting. The patient's role in the successful treatment of TB, daily self-administration of drugs for a period of 6 or 9 months and return for regular follow-up visits, is crucial. Because poor compliance accounts for most therapeutic failures in the treatment of TB, the most important function of monthly visits is the assessment, reinforcement, and documentation of compliance.

The patient should be advised about the communicable nature of TB, which is particularly important until one has been on therapy for at least 2 weeks. During those first 2 weeks, patients should avoid intimate contact with others and should cough into tissue, which then should be incinerated or disposed of in closed plastic bags. After 2 weeks, most patients can be considered noncontagious, and activities can be dictated solely by their sense of well-being.

Directly Observed Therapy

Directly observed therapy (DOT) is a response to the present epidemic of uncontrolled drug-resistant TB in some U.S. cities. The preferred DOT regimen is a *four-drug, 6-month regimen.* All drugs are given twice per week, either on Monday–Thursday or Tuesday–Friday. In general, the doses of drugs are increased over those given daily, but for each drug, there is a maximum dose, which is given in Table 29.1. The patient must go to a treatment center and swallow the medication while a nurse is watching. In cities, it may be possible to have nurses take TB therapy into schools, factories, or prisons where large numbers of patients are congregated. Disabled patients can receive supervised therapy in their homes. The regimen is modified as necessary by the results of sensitivity tests on the patient's tubercle bacilli. Patients who do not keep appointments are pursued into their homes by health department personnel and, if necessary, by the police. Some cities have laws that permit the incarceration of uncooperative infectious tuberculous patients, and in extreme cases they are applied. There is no doubt that supervised therapy is effective (9). On the other hand, this approach is an affront to human dignity and it is not always feasible. Vast numbers of uneducated and even illiterate patients have been treated successfully by traditional methods; most societies simply do not have funds to pay for supervisors; and in rural areas, patients would have to make long journeys to be treated. The problem is that lack of compliance is difficult to predict (see Chapter 4); even such traditional indicators as alcoholism, drug addiction, and psychosis correlate significantly but poorly (19).

PREVENTION OF TUBERCULOSIS
Case Detection Among Known Contacts

An integral part of initiation of care in any patient with active TB in the United States is case reporting to the local health authority and investigation of contacts. This entails tuberculin testing of all household and intimate nonhousehold contacts and retesting of nonreactors in 3 months. Reactors are examined by chest radiograph and, if free of active disease, are given chemoprophylaxis with INH (see below). With the exception of evaluating family members, this type of investigation is usually difficult for a physician to carry out alone and should be done by the local city or county health department. Such departments have trained personnel who are available to visit homes and workplaces to detect cases in contacts.

Tuberculin Testing in Prevention

Ideally, the tuberculin skin test status of all people should be determined at some time in their early adult life (see description of technique for skin testing above). In almost all school-age children, screening for tuberculin positivity is coordinated with school health programs. In adult populations, a number of factors such as urban residence, the presence of chronic disease, a history of residence in underdeveloped countries, and health care occupation increase the importance of periodic tuberculin testing. This is particularly true for people for whom INH would be recommended if the PPD was positive.

Because of the increased risk of contact with unrecognized cases of TB, physicians and hospital personnel who work with populations that have an increased prevalence of TB have an increased chance of acquiring infection. Both for personal protection and because of the risk of transmitting TB to patients, these physicians and other health workers should have annual tuberculin testing and should take INH chemoprophylaxis if they convert from negative to positive.

Isoniazid Prophylaxis

INH prophylaxis (300 mg/day for 6 to 12 months) has been shown to prevent 55 to 90% of expected new cases of active TB among special groups of people at high risk (3,4). Because of the small but real risk of INH-induced hepatitis, however, the recommendations for the use of INH have changed somewhat in recent years. At present, INH prophylaxis is recommended for people in the following groups:

- Close contacts of active infectious cases, especially young children and HIV-infected people, regardless of PPD status
- People with recent skin test conversion (not those with booster responses)
- People with positive skin tests and an abnormal chest radiograph suggestive of old TB (i.e., apical scarring, calcified hilar lymph node)
- People with a history of old TB who have never been given antibacterial treatment
- People with positive skin tests who will be given corticosteroid or immunosuppressive therapy, who have silicosis, who have a history of a gastrectomy, or who have conditions such as Hodgkin's disease or HIV infection, which reduces T-cell activity
- People with a positive skin test only, who are under the age of 35 years

Twelve months is recommended for patients with HIV infection and other forms of immunosuppression. Other infected patients should receive a minimum of 6 continuous months of therapy. It is recommended that children receive 9 months of therapy. For patients at especially high risk of TB whose compliance is questionable, supervised preventive therapy may be indicated. When resources do not permit supervised daily therapy, INH may be given under supervision twice weekly at the dosage of 15 mg/kg.

The guidelines recommended by the American Thoracic Society for *monitoring patients taking INH* are the following (3):

- Patients receiving preventive therapy, or responsible adults in households with children on preventive therapy, should be questioned carefully at monthly intervals for symptoms consistent with those of liver damage or of other toxic effects (i.e., unexplained anorexia, nausea, or vomiting of more than 3 days' duration, fatigue or weakness of more than 3 days' duration, and new and persistent paresthesias of the hands and feet) and for signs consistent with those of liver damage or of other toxic effects (i.e., persistent dark urine, icterus, rash, and elevated temperature of more than 3 days' duration without explanation).

- No more than a 1-month supply of INH should be dispensed at any visit. If signs and symptoms of toxicity appear, INH should be stopped immediately and the patient should be reevaluated. INH preventive therapy should not be prescribed if monthly monitoring cannot be accomplished. The reason for these recommendations is that an analysis of 20 fatal cases of hepatitis caused by prophylactic INH treatment showed that only one occurred in a patient seen every month. The great majority of the fatalities occurred in patients handed a year's supply of INH and never seen again (16).

Monitoring by routine laboratory tests (e.g., aminotransferases, serum bilirubin, and alkaline phosphatase) is not always useful in predicting hepatic disease in INH recipients and therefore is not recommended routinely. However, in evaluating signs and symptoms such tests are mandatory. Preventive therapy should be reinstituted only if biochemical studies are normal and signs and symptoms are absent.

Because it has been recognized that monthly monitoring may fail to detect an occasional patient with severe hepatitis, monthly measurement of aminotransferase levels is recommended for patients who are in the groups at the highest risk of developing INH hepatitis: those over 35 years of age, daily drinkers, patients concomitantly taking other potentially hepatotoxic drugs, and patients with a history of liver disease. This would detect the transient aminotransferase elevation that occurs in approximately 20% of subjects taking INH; a cutoff level, such as a level three or five times normal, is recommended as the criterion for discontinuing INH.

General References*

Barnes PF, Barrows SA. Tuberculosis in the 1990s. Ann Intern Med 119(5):400, 1993.
    Well-referenced review of literature on TB published since 1987.
Iseman MD. Treatment of multidrug-resistant tuberculosis. N Engl J Med 329:784, 1993.
    Practical approaches to MDR as of 1993.

Specific References

1. Alwood K, Keruly J, Moore-Rice K, et al. Effectiveness of supervised intermittent therapy for tuberculosis in HIV infected patients. AIDS 8:1103–1108, 1994.
2. Advisory Council for Elimination of Tuberculosis and Advisory Committee on Immunization Practices (ACIP). The role of BCG vaccine in the prevention and control of tuberculosis in the United States. MMWR 45(RR-4):1–18, 1996.
3. American Thoracic Society. Control of tuberculosis in the United States. Am Rev Respir Dis 146:1623, 1992.
4. Centers for Disease Control and Prevention. The use of preventive therapy for tuberculous infection in the United States. MMWR 39:9, 1990.
5. Centers for Disease Control and Prevention. National action plan to combat multidrug resistant tuberculosis. MMWR 41:56, 1992.

---

*Bold print (general references) and bold numerals (specific references) denote published controlled clinical trials, meta-analyses, or consensus-based recommendations.

6. Centers for Disease Control and Prevention. Initial therapy for tuberculosis in the era of multidrug resistance. MMWR 42(RR7):1, 1993.

7. Centers for Disease Control and Prevention. Federal Register 59, #208, p. 54273, 1994.

8. Centers for Disease Control. Tuberculosis morbidity: United States, 1995. MMWR 45:365, 1996.

9. Chaulk CP, Moore-Rice K, Rizzo R, et al. Eleven years of community-based directly observed therapy for tuberculosis. JAMA 274:945, 1995.

10. Daley CL, Small RM, Schechter GF, et al. An outbreak of tuberculosis with accelerated progression among persons infected with human immunodeficiency virus: an analysis using restriction fragment length polymorphisms. N Engl J Med 326:231, 1992.

11. Dutt AK, Moers D, Stead WW. Short-course chemotherapy for extrapulmonary tuberculosis. Nine years' experience. Ann Intern Med 104:7, 1986.

12. Friedan TR, Sherman LF, Maw KL, et al. A multi-institutional outbreak of highly drug resistant tuberculosis. JAMA 286:1229, 1996.

13. Graham NMH, Nelson KE, Solomon L, et al. Prevalence of tuberculin positivity and skin test anergy in HIV-1 seropositive and seronegative intravenous drug users. JAMA 267:369, 1992.

14. Hopewell PC. Impact of human immune deficiency virus infection on the epidemiology, clinical features, management and control of tuberculosis. Clin Infect Dis 15:540, 1992.

15. Kopanoff DE, Snider DE, Caras CJ. Isoniazid related hepatitis. Am Rev Respir Dis 117:991, 1978.

16. Moulding TS, Redeker AG, Kanel GC. Twenty isoniazid associated deaths in one state. Am Rev Respir Dis 140:700, 1989.

17. Reider HL, Cauther GM, Comstock GW, Snyder DE. Epidemiology of tuberculosis in the United States. Epidemiol Rev 11:79, 1989.

18. Road I, Hacham R, Leeds N, et al. Use of adjunctive treatment with interferon gamma in an immunocompromised patient who had refractory multidrug resistant tuberculosis of the brain. Clin Infect Dis 22:572, 1996.

19. Sumartojo E. When tuberculosis treatment fails: a social behavioral account of patient adherence. Am Rev Respir Dis 147:1311, 1993.

20. Thompson NJ, Glassroth JL, Snider DE Jr, Farer LS. The booster phenomenon in serial tuberculin testing. Am Rev Respir Dis 119:587, 1979.

C H A P T E R 30

Selected Spirochetal Infections: Syphilis and Lyme Disease*

JOHN A. FLYNN, MD
ANNE MARIE ROMPALO, MD, ScM

This chapter describes two spirochetal infections, syphilis (caused by *Treponema pallidum*) and Lyme disease (caused by *Borrelia burgdorferi*), each of which has acute and chronic manifestations.

SYPHILIS

Epidemiology

Syphilis has been a major public health concern since the late 15th and early 16th centuries, when an epidemic of syphilis swept through Europe with higher associated morbidity and mortality than is currently seen with the disease. It is estimated that in the early 1900s, 10% of the adult American population had syphilis (4). Consequently, recognition of this complex disease and its varied manifestations was an essential component of medical education. In the 1990s, the disease is far less common.

Following the introduction of penicillin in the 1940s, primary and secondary syphilis declined, reaching a nadir of 6392 cases in 1956 (15). The prevalence of syphilis gradually increased until the mid-1980s, when rates suddenly began to increase by 10 to 15% per year. This increase coincided with an epidemic of crack cocaine use and was accompanied by a demographic shift in the portion of the population most affected, from homosexually active men to het-

---

*Edward W. Hootz, III, MD, contributed to this chapter in the fourth edition.

erosexual men and women (25,46). It has been suggested that in addition to cocaine-related prostitution, diminution in funds available for efforts to control non–human immunodeficiency virus (HIV), sexually transmitted diseases (STDs) may have contributed to the dramatic change in syphilis rates in the late 1980s. The epidemic increase of the 1980s appears to have peaked in 1990, when 50,233 cases of primary and secondary syphilis were reported (15,25).

The recent epidemic of syphilis has also disproportionately affected racial minorities (25). In 1991, primary and secondary syphilis rates were 2.4 and 1.6 per 100,000 among white, non-Hispanic males and females, respectively, whereas comparable rates for African Americans were 141 and 108 per 100,000. Recent increases in syphilis rates for women have also contributed to a more than 15-fold rise in reported cases of congenital syphilis between 1985 and 1991 (15,60).

Stages of the Disease

The acquired form of the disease has different stages (Table 30.1): primary, secondary, early and late latent, and tertiary or late syphilis. The clinical manifestations of the primary and secondary stages may be subtle and often overlap. Only one-third of untreated patients develop tertiary manifestations.

Primary Syphilis

Primary syphilis is characterized by the development of a *chancre* at the site of intimate sexual contact (genitals, anus, mouth, breast, and occasionally elsewhere). It appears 10 to 90 days (average 21 days) after infection by *T. pallidum,* the etiologic organism. It usually starts as a single painless papule that varies in size from a few millimeters to a few centimeters in diameter and progresses to a highly infectious, painless ulcer with indurated edges. Multiple lesions occur in approximately 30% of cases. There is associated painless regional and generalized lymphadenopathy. If secondary infection of the chancre occurs, the lesions may become painful. Major considerations in the differential diagnosis of a genital ulcer are summarized in Table 30.2. The herpes simplex virus remains the most common cause of chancrelike genital ulcers, but chancroid should be considered in the differential diagnosis of genital ulcers in certain geographic areas of the United States where it continues to be reported. Definitive diagnosis is made by microscopic examination of exudate expressed from the ulcer (see "Direct Microscopic Examination"). Serologic tests for syphilis (STS) are usually reactive (see "Serology for Diagnosis and Follow-Up").

Surveillance of the sexual contacts of newly diagnosed patients with infectious (primary or secondary) syphilis has shown active infection in about one-third to one-half of those who had such contact in the month preceding the patient's diagnosis (47).

Secondary Syphilis

If untreated during the primary stage, approximately 50% of patients develop secondary syphilis 6 weeks to 6 months after initial contact, and the other half

Table 30.1. Outline of the Clinical Stages of Syphilis

Stage	Characteristic Findings	Usual Onset after Exposure	Duration of Stage in Untreated Patients	Dark Field
Primary	Chancre—may be absent or not visible (e.g., in vagina or mouth)	10–90 days (average 21 days)	2–6 weeks	+ (Chancre, lymph nodes)
Secondary	Rash, condyloma latum, lymphadenopathy	6 weeks to 6 months	2–6 weeks; recurrences in 25% over 4 years	+ (Especially moist lesions)
Latent			May be lifelong because only ⅓ of untreated patients develop tertiary syphilis	Negative
Early	None	<1 year after infection		
Late	None	>1 year after infection		
Late (tertiary)				
Benign	Gumma	2–10 years	Indolent	Negative
Cardiovascular	Aorta aneurysm Aortic insufficiency Coronary artery disease, especially of the ostia	10–30 years	Progressive; may be fatal	Aorta may be +
Neurosyphilis		2–35 years	Progressive; may be fatal	Brain may be +
Asymptomatic	None			
Acute syphilitic meningitis	Headache, cranial nerve lesions, papilledema	6 weeks to 2 years	Not applicable	
Meningovascular	Signs of infection depend on area involved	2–10 years		
Paresis	Minor personality change to frank psychosis	15–35 years		
Tabes dorsalis	Signs of posterior column degeneration	5–30 years		

Table 30.2. Differential Diagnosis of a Genital Sore

Primary Syphilis (Chancre)
Incubation period 10–90 days (average, 21 days)
Usually painless (in absence of secondary infection)
Not vesicular
Usually single indurated ulcer but multiple lesions are seen in
  30% of cases
Spirochete on dark-field examination
Nontender inguinal adenopathy

Herpes Simplex
Incubation period 24–48 hours
Usually painful
Vesicular
Usually multiple ulcers
Multinucleated giant cells on Giemsa stain plus virus on culture
Tender inguinal adenopathy

Chancroid
Multiple soft superficial erosions
Painful
Nontender adenopathy. *Haemophilus ducreyi* on Gram's stain of
  dried smear (small Gram-negative bacillus)

Granuloma Inguinale
Soft, occasionally raised, granulating lesions in inguinal area
Donovan bodies on smear (histiocytes with intracytoplasmic
  encapsulated Gram-negative bacilli)

Other Considerations
Trauma, carcinoma, scabies, lichen planus, psoriasis, fixed drug
  eruption (especially phenolphthalein), fungus infection, folliculitis

advance into a latent stage of disease. When the secondary stage begins, the chancre is still present in 15 to 20% of cases. The most characteristic finding is a nonpruritic rash that is usually maculopapular, but not vesicular or bullous. It can involve all areas of the skin, especially the trunk, palms, and soles. Scalp and eyelash involvement of hair follicles may lead to alopecia. Mucous patches (gray oral patches on an erythematous base) are particularly infectious. Condylomata lata are flat, wartlike lesions usually found in moist intertriginous regions such as the genital or anal area. They are also highly infectious. They must be distinguished from the more common verrucous, fleshy genital wart (condyloma acuminatum, see Chapter 94). Dark-field or direct fluorescent antibody for *T. pallidum* (DFA-TP) examination of moist skin lesions of the condyloma latum should be positive. In as many as one-half of the patients, skin lesions may not occur or may not be detected.

Constitutional symptoms such as fever, headache, malaise, and generalized lymphadenopathy are common. Other systemic manifestations occur in 1 to 2% of cases and include hepatitis, immune complex nephropathy, and aseptic meningitis. Serologic tests for syphilis are reactive in virtually 100% of patients at this stage (see "Serology for Diagnosis and Follow-Up").

Untreated, the clinical manifestations of secondary syphilis last for 2 to 6 weeks and may recur in approximately 25% of patients at some time during the first 4 years after infection; 90% of all relapses occur within a year. Although recurrences are usually identical to initial episodes, condyloma lata may be more common in the recurrent episode than in the initial episode. The major considerations in differential diagnosis are drug reactions, psoriasis, and pityriasis rosea (see descriptions of these conditions, Chapter 100).

Latent Syphilis

As the name implies, latent syphilis is the period after infection with *T. pallidum* in which there are no clinical manifestations. In the United States, the division between early and late latent infection has been set at 1 year because recurrent secondary manifestations rarely occur after more than 1 year. Because sexual transmission occurs only through direct lesion contact, a person who has sexual contact with a partner with latent syphilis more than 1 year before diagnosis is unlikely to be infected; this is therefore a useful demarcation for reporting purposes.

The majority of patients with latent disease come to diagnosis through routine serologic testing (see "Serology for Diagnosis and Follow-Up"). Detection early in this stage is important not only for epidemiologic purposes but also to prevent further complications in the one-third of untreated patients who go on to develop late manifestations of syphilis.

Tertiary (Late) Syphilis

Tertiary or late disease is divided into three principal forms: late benign (gummatous) syphilis, cardiovascular syphilis, and late neurosyphilis. Since the advent of penicillin therapy, all forms of tertiary syphilis have become uncommon, although there is conjecture that they are more common in HIV-positive patients (see "HIV Infection and Syphilis," below). In addition, the late manifestations have become milder and more subtle (27).

Late benign syphilis is characterized by the development of a gumma, a granulomatous lesion that may grow to several centimeters in size. The gumma is thought to be a hypersensitivity reaction because viable organisms are rarely seen. Gummas usually occur within 2 to 10 years of infection, most commonly on the skin (ulcerative or nodular–ulcerative), in bone, or in the liver, and are especially destructive when in the brain, liver, or heart. Diagnosis is made on the basis of typical pathologic findings and of dramatic healing of visible gummas after treatment.

Cardiovascular syphilis, which is very uncommon today, was reported in 13.6% of untreated men and 7.6% of untreated women 5 to 30 years after acquisition of the disease. However, recent reports of probable syphilitic aortitis confirm previous studies that revealed unsuspected tertiary syphilis in a significant number of patients autopsied in areas where the prevalence of syphilis was thought to be low (61). Syphilitic aortitis occurs when *T. pallidum* destroys the elastic tissue of the media of the aorta and produces an endarteritis of the vasa vasorum. Clinical manifestations include aneurysm of the ascending aorta and progressive dilation of the aortic ring, resulting in aortic insufficiency and heart failure. When the coronary ostia are involved, angina pectoris may result. Linear calcification of the ascending aorta is a common radiologic finding in syphilitic aortitis; it may precede clinical symptoms and signs of aortic involvement.

Neurosyphilis

Asymptomatic neurosyphilis is defined by the occurrence of a reactive Venereal Disease Research Laboratory (VDRL) test for syphilis, a lymphocytic pleocytosis, or an elevated protein concentration test in the cerebrospinal fluid (CSF) of a syphilis patient who has no neurologic or psychiatric signs or symptoms and no other illnesses to explain the findings. The prevalence of asymptomatic neurosyphilis varies according to disease stage. Laboratory-detected abnormalities in CSF are most common in patients with secondary syphilis and become less common with increasing duration of infection (25). The diagnosis of asymptomatic neurosyphilis and its significance are subjects of controversy (11,34). The following facts are important to know: First, dissemination of *T. pallidum* to the central nervous system is very common at all stages, even primary syphilis, and *T. pallidum* may be demonstrable in the spinal fluid of patients without other CSF abnormalities. Second, studies performed in the preantibiotic era indicated that the intensity of CSF abnormalities in patients with asymptomatic neurosyphilis correlate with the likelihood of developing clinically apparent neurosyphilis (21). Third, in the preantibiotic era only about 10% of patients developed clinical neurosyphilis. Fourth, with the widespread use of intramuscular penicillin, even at dosages that did not produce spirocheticidal levels in the central nervous system, the incidence of clinical neurosyphilis fell to nearly zero. Consequently, the regimens recommended for the routine treatment of primary, secondary, and early latent syphilis have not been substantially altered in the most recent guidelines of the U.S. Centers for Disease Control and Prevention (CDC) (51). However, interest in this issue is ongoing because patients infected with HIV seem to develop neurosyphilis more often despite treatment with intramuscular or intravenous penicillin, possibly because of their immunocompromised state (18,24). HIV-infected patients with neuropsychiatric manifestations can present difficult diagnostic problems because of limitations in the diagnostic tests for neurosyphilis (see below) and the lack of specific markers for both syphilitic and HIV infection of the central nervous system. Diagnosing asymptomatic neurosyphilis and defining its natural history in HIV-infected patients are even more difficult (24). However, because of concerns about the sufficiency of current treatment schedules, this issue is receiving considerable attention (see "HIV Infection and Syphilis," below).

Symptomatic neurosyphilis, which is also uncommon, occurred in 9.4% of men and 5% of women with untreated syphilis in the Oslo study of the natural history of untreated syphilis (see "General References"). The risk of developing symptomatic neuro-syphilis after a primary infection is greater in whites than in blacks. Symptomatic neurosyphilis is divided into various types depending on the site of major involvement.

- *Syphilitic meningitis.* Although many patients with secondary and early latent syphilis complain of mild photophobia, headache, or meningismus, a small percentage develop a severe syphilitic meningitis. This syndrome is characterized by severe headache, meningismus, seizures, and cranial nerve signs, including papilledema or involvement of the 3rd, 6th, 7th, and 8th nerves. CSF examination usually reveals increased numbers of mononuclear cells, elevated protein concentration, and reactive CSF VDRL tests. The clinical and laboratory manifestations of syphilitic meningitis usually resolve with treatment (3,25).
- *Meningovascular syphilis* usually occurs within 2 to 10 years after untreated primary infection. Common manifestations include headache, irritability, and personality changes. Vasculitis involving small end arteries results in focal neurologic signs. The severity of the patient's disability depends on the extent and location of the accompanying cerebrovascular inflammation and occlusion.
- *Tabes dorsalis* usually occurs 5 to 30 years after infection. It is characterized by symptoms and signs of posterior column degeneration (ataxia, areflexia, broad-based gait, incontinence, impotence, abdominal pain crises, and paresthesias or lightning pains in the extremities). Characteristic findings also include trophic joint changes (Charcot's joints), the Argyll–Robertson pupil (small, irregular pupil that accommodates but does not react to light), and optic atrophy (in approximately 10% of patients).
- *The syndrome of general paresis* usually occurs 15 to 35 years after infection. It is caused by destruction of the parenchyma of the cerebral cortex. It consists of personality changes, irritability, poor judgment, insomnia, and memory loss. The progressive dementia in these patients may be characterized by periodic euphoria and delusions of grandeur.

A diagnosis of neurosyphilis is based on spinal fluid findings: elevated protein concentration, an increased number of mononuclear cells, and a reactive serologic test for syphilis (see "Serology for Diagnosis and Follow-Up"). Although there is little doubt that reactive CSF VDRL tests indicate neurosyphilis, many patients with central nervous system (CNS) syphilis have only elevated cell counts or protein concentrations as CSF manifestations of infection. In such patients, and particularly those with concomitant HIV infection, efforts should be made to rule out other CNS infections. The role of the CSF fluorescent treponemal antibody absorption (FTA-ABS) test in neurosyphilis diagnosis is controversial. Most studies agree that a nonreactive CSF FTA-ABS is useful for ruling out neurosyphilis, but the significance of a reactive CSF FTA-ABS without other CSF abnormalities is unclear (11,12,25,29).

Serology for Diagnosis and Follow-Up

Direct Microscopic Examination

As syphilis decreased in prevalence, both the availability of dark-field microscopy and the competency of those performing it declined. Some reference laboratories now perform direct fluorescent microscopy using specific antisera (DFA-TP) to identify the organism. Large medical centers with special STD clinics and larger health departments ordinarily provide reliable testing. One should call ahead to ensure that a working microscope and a knowledgeable reader are available. To obtain material, one should abrade the lesion gently with gauze so as to produce a nonbloody, serous exudate; after wiping the surface, squeeze the lesion between gloved thumb and forefinger; collect the exudate in a capillary tube or on a microscope slide; and give it to someone who knows how to do the test. Microscopic examination should be performed on three consecutive slides in highly suspect patients before syphilis is definitively ruled out. This is especially true if antibiotic ointments have been used. Dark-field examination should not be done on material obtained from oral lesions because of the potential for confusion with *Treponema macrodentium,* a common mouth inhabitant. The DFA-TP test is more specific and can be performed on oral smears.

Serologic Tests in Diagnosis

Serologic tests are of two basic types: nontreponemal and treponemal. Nontreponemal tests detect reagin, a nonspecific antibody to cardiolipin, a normal component of many tissues. Wassermann in 1906 was the first to use this reaction to detect patients with syphilis. Since then about 100 different forms of the original Wassermann test have been developed. Of the five flocculation tests in common use today, the VDRL and the rapid plasma reagin (RPR) tests are most commonly used.

The treponemal tests include the FTA-ABS and the microhemagglutination test for *T. pallidum* (MHA-TP or HATTS). Both tests detect specific antibodies to *T. pallidum.* Figure 30.1 shows the pattern of reactivity of various serologic tests during the course of untreated syphilis.

The sensitivity (the percentage of syphilitic patients with a reactive test) varies at each stage of the disease and for different tests (Table 30.3). The RPR is slightly more sensitive than the VDRL; the FTA-ABS tests and hemagglutination procedures are more sensitive than the VDRL and RPR. The range of values for sensitivity is accounted for by differences in case definition in different studies. Where case definition is more rigorous (e.g., using a positive dark-field or DFA-TP to ensure the diagnosis of primary syphilis rather than simply clinical criteria), the sensitivity is higher.

STS specificity (the percentage of nonsyphilitic patients with a negative test) is also shown in Table 30.3. There are two major reasons for the variance in specificity given for each test. First, study populations differ in the proportion of patients with conditions

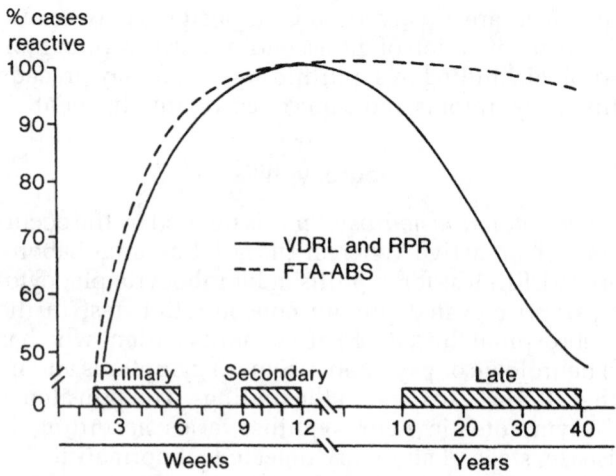

Figure 30.1. Serology of untreated syphilis. (Adapted from Wallace AL, Norins LC. Syphilis serology today. Prog Clin Pathol 2:198, 1969.)

that cause false-positive test results. For example, studies of the specificity of the VDRL or the FTA-ABS in a group of nuns or other healthy volunteer populations have revealed very few false positives. On the other hand, studies in STD clinic populations, facilities serving drug addicts, or arthritis clinic populations with many patients with systemic lupus have yielded higher rates of false positives and consequently lower estimates of specificity. Second, test performance can vary in different laboratories, with devastating effects on both the specificity and sensitivity of vulnerable tests such as the FTA-ABS (12). Table 30.3 gives consensus sensitivity and specificity figures for serologic tests done on serum from patients in an STD clinic population and performed at the CDC Reference Laboratory (32). As with any other test, one must determine how applicable they are to tests done in one's patient population and at one's reference laboratory. Most of the discussion of treponemal tests is confined to the FTA-ABS test, which is used more extensively than the MHA-TP.

When a nontreponemal test is reactive and the FTA-ABS or the hemagglutination test is consistently nonreactive, the patient is considered to have a *biological false-positive* test result. Acute biological false-positive VDRL and RPR tests are defined as those lasting less than 6 months. Historically, they have been reported in patients with viral and bacterial pneumonia, hepatitis, pregnancy, mononucleosis, measles, and malaria, and after smallpox vaccination. Chronic false-positive nontreponemal test reactions (those lasting more than 6 months) occur in diseases of disordered immunity, such as systemic lupus erythematosus, rheumatoid arthritis, and Waldenström's macroglobulinemia, as well as in chronic liver disease, and in intravenous drug addicts, elderly patients (approximately 1% of people over 70 and 10% of people over 80), and occasional patients on a hereditary basis. Biological false-positive VDRL or RPR titers are usually

1:8 or lower but occasionally can be higher, especially in hereditary cases. A false-positive nontreponemal test result should not be dismissed but should be used as a clue to the diagnosis of the conditions listed above. However, in as many as 50% of cases, no explanation can be found and the patient remains symptom free. Whatever the case, a patient should be informed of his or her test status in order to prevent inappropriate labeling and treatment for syphilis.

When properly performed, the FTA-ABS tests have a specificity of 98%. A positive FTA-ABS test is essentially a true positive in patients with related treponemal conditions such as yaws, pinta, and bejel. These must be considered in evaluation of patients from regions where those diseases are endemic, such as parts of Africa and Central and South America. False-positive reactions occur in patients with lupus erythematosus, rheumatoid arthritis, chronic liver disease, and some infections, and in other patients for unexplained reasons. Because small errors in laboratory technique can affect the results of the FTA-ABS tests more than the results of the nontreponemal tests, the FTA-ABS should be performed only when nontreponemal tests are reactive (12). Exception should be made when either primary or tertiary syphilis is highly suspect and the nontreponemal test is negative, there are neurologic or psychiatric signs suggestive of tabes or paresis, or signs of aortic insufficiency and aneurysm of the ascending aorta are present. In these situations, the treponemal test may occasionally be the only reactive test (Table 30.3).

In diagnosing latent syphilis, a single reactive nontreponemal test, even if confirmed by a treponemal test result, should not be relied on as the only datum, especially if there is no other reason to suspect syphilis. The test should be repeated to ensure that blood specimens were not mixed up. The clinical, psychologic, and social implications of this diagnosis are too serious to rely on a single datum.

The sensitivity of the CSF VDRL for the detection of neurosyphilis ranges from 10 to 89%. It is highest for meningitis, meningovascular, and paretic forms and lowest for asymptomatic neurosyphilis and tabes dorsalis. Although it is virtually 100% specific for neurosyphilis, instances of false-positive CSF VDRL have been reported after traumatic lumbar puncture and in a case of meningeal tumor. The CSF VDRL, with all of its limitations, remains the test of choice in the workup for neurosyphilis in selected patients (11).

Serologic Tests in Screening

A nontreponemal serologic test for syphilis should be used as a screening test in patients who are sexually active with multiple partners or who are at increased risk for acquisition of syphilis (5). Patients who are being screened for or who are found to have another STD should also have a screening STS. In most office settings, an STS should be done routinely on a sexually active patient's first visit. In subsequent visits, a repeated STS should be done only in patients deemed to have been at risk for acquiring a new infection during the interval.

Pattern of Serologic Tests after Treatment

The nontreponemal test has been reported to revert to nonreactive in more than 85% of patients adequately treated for primary or secondary syphilis over time (Fig. 30.2). A common misconception is that the FTA-ABS always remains reactive for life, even following adequate syphilis therapy. In a recent study, approximately 10% of primary syphilis patients had become FTA-ABS nonreactive 12 months after penicillin therapy (48). The tendency to lose FTA-ABS reactivity after therapy also appears to be more pronounced in patients with HIV infection (20,47). The FTA-ABS should be repeated once, 12 months after syphilis is diagnosed and treated. If it remains reactive, it should not be repeated. In later serologic testing of patients who have had syphilis, the nontreponemal test titer becomes the most useful tool (see "Follow-Up") (49,50). In patients treated for early latent syphilis, nontreponemal tests become nonreactive within 5 years of treatment in approximately 75%, whereas only about 25% of patients with treated late latent syphilis are seronegative in 5 years (16). Many middle-aged and older people with a titer of 1:4 or lower reactivity in the nontreponemal test fall into the category of adequately treated serofast syphilis; differentiation from late latent syphilis can sometimes be made through careful history.

Table 30.3. Sensitivity and Specificity of Serologic Tests for Syphilis[a] at Different Stages

Stage of Syphilis	VDRL[b]		RPR[b]		FTA-ABS[b]		MHA-TP[b]	
	Sens.	Spec.	Sens.	Spec.	Sens.	Spec.	Sens.	Spec.
Primary	80% (59–87)	98% (80–99)	86% (81–100)	98% (80–99)	98% (93–100)	98% (84–99)	82% (64–90)	99% (98–100)
Secondary	100 (99–100)	98	100 (99–100)	98	100 (99–100)	98	100 (96–100)	99
Latent	96 (73–100)	98	99	98	100 (96–100)	98	100 (96–100)	99
Tertiary (late)	71	98	73	98	96	98	94	99

[a]The consensus figures for the sensitivity and specificity are for tests done in the CDC Reference Laboratory (15) on samples derived from a well-run STD clinic. The figures in parentheses demonstrate the variability in published reports. Responsible factors include study of populations with different prevalences of syphilis and other confounding illnesses, variable performance by the laboratory, and different clinical criteria for the diagnosis of syphilis.
[b]See text for fuller discussion of these tests.

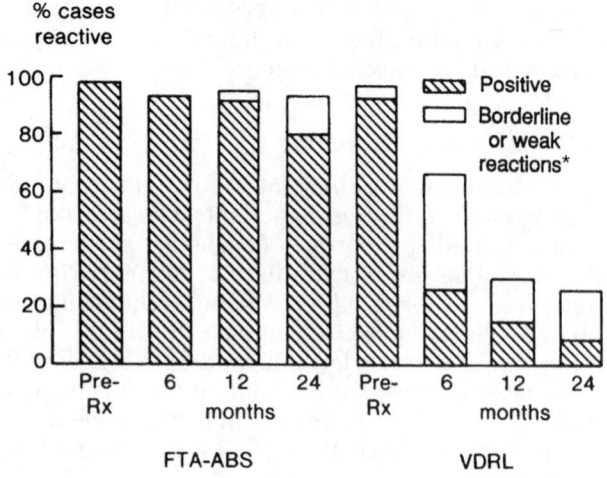

% cases reactive

Positive
Borderline or weak reactions*

FTA-ABS   VDRL

Figure 30.2. Serologic reactivity of 80 patients treated for dark-field positive primary or secondary syphilis and observed for 2 years, with use of FTA-ABS and VDRL tests. *These reactions are now classified as nonreactive. (Adapted from Schroeter AL et al. Treatment for early syphilis and reactivity of serologic tests. JAMA 221:471, 1972.)

Treatment

Regimens

The treatment of choice for *primary, secondary, and early latent syphilis,* as well as for known contacts of a patient with infectious syphilis, is 2.4 million units of benzathine penicillin G (LA Bicillin) intramuscularly (51). An alternative for patients allergic to penicillin is oral doxycycline 100 mg twice a day for 2 weeks, or tetracycline 500 mg orally four times a day for 2 weeks. In penicillin-allergic patients who cannot tolerate tetracycline or doxycycline, ceftriaxone (1 g intramuscularly daily for 8 to 10 days) may be used; however, published experience with this regimen is meager. Follow-up is essential with any regimen, but it is especially important when alternatives to penicillin are used. The regimen of single-dose ceftriaxone (250 mg intramuscularly), but not of quinolones or spectinomycin, for the therapy of gonorrhea is effective against incubating syphilis acquired simultaneously (26,50).

The treatment of choice for *late latent syphilis, gummas, and cardiovascular syphilis* is 2.4 million units of benzathine penicillin G intramuscularly (LA Bicillin) weekly for 3 weeks (7.2 million units total). For patients who are allergic to penicillin, alternative drugs can be used; however, the CDC suggests that a CSF examination be done first to exclude neurosyphilis because it may not respond to benzathine penicillin or an alternative regimen. It is best to validate a history of penicillin allergy by careful history and, when possible, by skin testing, using the major and minor penicillin determinants if available (see Chapter 23). Alternative regimens are tetracycline (500 mg orally four times a day for 4 weeks) or doxycycline (100 mg orally twice daily for 4 weeks). Erythromycin is no longer advocated because of the lack of studies demonstrating efficacy in late latent and late syphilis as

well as concerns about the association of congenital syphilis with treatment failure. It is also worth noting that some would treat cardiovascular syphilis with the regimen for neurosyphilis, which follows.

In patients who have *confirmed neurosyphilis,* a stage in which benzathine penicillin treatment failures have been documented (19), therapy should consist of 18 to 24 million units of intravenous aqueous crystalline penicillin G daily (3 to 4 million units every 4 hours) for 10 to 14 days. When outpatient compliance can be ensured, an alternative regimen is procaine penicillin G 2.4 million units intramuscularly once daily plus probenecid 500 mg by mouth four times a day for 10 to 14 days. As noted above, a history of penicillin allergy should be evaluated, and in the occasional patients in whom it is confirmed, consultation with an infectious disease expert is desirable to select the best alternative treatment.

Effectiveness

The effectiveness of treatment, usually as measured by nontreponemal test serologic response, varies depending on the stage of syphilis treated. In one study of patients with *primary and secondary syphilis,* retreatment was required in 5% of patients after the usual dosages of benzathine penicillin G, and in 10% of patients after the usual dosages of tetracycline (49). In a recent study of 103 HIV-positive and 444 HIV-negative patients with primary, secondary, and early latent syphilis, 24% were classified as serologic treatment failures at 3 months, 17% at 6 months, and 14% at 12 months. Among HIV-negative patients, serologic treatment failure was more common in early latent stage, but among HIV-positive patients failure rates were similar for all stages. Of note, only one clinical treatment failure during the 1-year follow-up period was detected in an HIV-infected patient. This failure was evidenced by a new palmar–plantar rash accompanied by a fourfold titer increase. The criterion for serologic treatment failure in this study was failure of the RPR titer to decrease fourfold or become nonreactive within 3, 6, 9, and 12 months after therapy (47).

The effectiveness of treatment in patients with *latent syphilis* is difficult to assess because of the absence of any markers to follow. However, in one follow-up study, all 469 patients with late latent syphilis treated at various centers at the recommended dosages of penicillin were symptom free 12 years later (28).

The effectiveness of treatment of *cardiovascular syphilis* has been debated. Most investigators believe that treatment may arrest the disease but not reverse it. Because of the weakening of the media of the aorta, aneurysms may continue to enlarge even after adequate treatment.

The results of treatment for *neurosyphilis* vary directly with the extent of the disease and inversely with its duration. Thus, treatment often reverses the signs and symptoms of acute meningovascular syphilis and stabilizes tabes dorsalis, but is less effective in reversing the signs of general paresis, especially if given late in its course (65). In addition to the reversal of clinical signs, the return of any CSF reactivity to normal is an index of effective therapy. If the initial CSF examination reveals a pleocytosis, the lumbar puncture should be repeated every 6 months until the cell count is normal. If the examination shows no improvement in 6 months or is not normal by 2 years, retreatment is probably indicated.

Jarisch–Herxheimer Reaction

The Jarisch–Herxheimer reaction is an acute febrile reaction accompanied by headache, myalgia, and other symptoms that may occur within the first 24 hours after any therapy for syphilis (30,41). It may be caused by lysis of *T. pallidum;* however, the pathogenesis of this reaction is poorly understood. The reaction resolves after several hours. The Jarisch–Herxheimer reaction is common among patients with early syphilis. When it occurs during treatment of secondary syphilis, skin lesions may become more prominent. Because the Jarisch–Herxheimer reaction is common, patients should be told that the reaction usually is mild and lasts only a few hours and that it can be treated with mild analgesics. Uncommonly, the reaction may be severe and consist of high fever, chills, headache, muscle and joint pains, sore throat, and transient hypotension. It may produce significant exacerbation of neurologic signs in a small percentage of patients treated for neurosyphilis. For this reason, corticosteroid therapy has been used both before and after treatment, but its efficacy is not established (30). The Jarisch–Herxheimer reaction may induce early labor or cause fetal distress among *pregnant women* and they should be counseled to contact their obstetricians in light of this possible reaction. However, therapy of pregnant women should not be withheld or delayed over this concern.

Practical Approach to the Patient

Sexually active patients in whom syphilis is a consideration usually present to their physicians because of a sore or rash, referral as a known contact of a patient with syphilis, worry about a recent sexual liaison, or a positive serologic test in routine premarital, blood donor, or health screening. The diagnosis of syphilis must be made carefully because it can have a major impact on the relationships of patients with their contacts and on how they view themselves. Furthermore, all sexually active women with reactive nontreponemal serologic tests should have a pelvic examination before syphilis staging is considered complete. A systematic approach to diagnosis and management is outlined here.

Evaluation

The history should include a description of any sore or rash, determination of a previous history of STD (especially syphilis), review of the results of previous serologic tests for syphilis, an inquiry into the patient's sexual practices to guide the physical examination, and information about recent partners and their disease status.

The *physical examination* should include a careful search for typical lesions in all areas of sexual contact. Special care should be taken in examining the anogenital area and the mouth. Other features to look for include regional and generalized lymphadenopathy, enlarged liver, and neurologic, psychiatric, and cardiovascular signs when late disease is a concern.

Laboratory data should include direct microscopy of the exudate from any suspicious lesions and serologic testing for syphilis (see "Serology for Diagnosis and Follow-Up"). CSF examination is mandatory in patients with psychiatric or neurologic signs or symptoms. The CDC recommends that all patients with latent syphilis should be evaluated clinically for evidence of tertiary disease (e.g., aortitis, neurosyphilis, gumma, and iritis). Patients with neurologic or ophthalmic signs or symptoms, evidence of active tertiary syphilis, treatment failure, or HIV infection with late latent syphilis or syphilis of unknown duration should have a prompt lumbar puncture to exclude neurosyphilis. In asymptomatic patients, CSF examination may be performed if dictated by circumstances and patient preferences, but it is reasonable to administer the recommended regimen and follow symptoms and serologic response without performing lumbar puncture (11,21,64).

In patients who were treated for syphilis with heavy metals before the penicillin era, the question sometimes arises about the need for further treatment. Most experts do not recommend retreating such patients if there are no suspicious signs or symptoms and there is no history of exposure to infectious syphilis in the interim.

Special difficulty is presented by *patients who are pregnant* and who are found to have an abnormal serologic result when a routine STS is performed either at their initial visit or, in areas of high prevalence, when it is repeated during the third trimester and at delivery. Because pregnancy has been reported to be a cause of a biological false-positive nontreponemal test, the treponemal test is an essential confirmatory test. If the treponemal test is nonreactive and there is no clinical evidence of syphilis, nontreponemal and treponemal tests should be repeated monthly for 3 months. If the treponemal tests remain negative, this can be considered to be a biological false-positive reaction. If there is clinical or serologic confirmation of syphilis, the staging and therapy are similar to those for nonpregnant patients. The only difference in therapy is that in penicillin-allergic patients, tetracycline and doxycycline are contraindicated. Current CDC treatment guidelines suggest that pregnant patients who give a history of penicillin allergy should be skin tested for penicillin with major and minor determinants and, if positive, desensitized (see Chapter 23). Because women treated in the second half of pregnancy are at high risk for premature labor or fetal distress if their treatment precipitates a Jarisch–Herxheimer reaction (see above), treatment should be coordinated with the obstetrician and these women should be advised to seek obstetric attention after treatment if they notice any contractions or decrease in fetal movements. Nontreponemal tests should be repeated in the third trimester and at delivery. Serologic titers may be checked at monthly intervals to determine therapeutic response in women at high risk for reinfection or in high syphilis prevalence areas. All infants born to women with reactive serologic tests for syphilis should have a thorough physical examination looking for evidence of congenital syphilis. A quantitative nontreponemal serologic test for syphilis should be performed on the infant's serum. Pathologic examination of the placenta or umbilical cord using specific fluorescent antitreponemal antibody staining is also recommended (51).

Management

The management plan is contingent on making the appropriate diagnosis. The diagnosis rests on positive results of direct microscopy or on the combination of a reactive nontreponemal and treponemal test. When the diagnosis is made, the disease should be staged appropriately, as outlined above.

The most common errors in the diagnosis of syphilis are failing to take proper note of an abnormal serology and missing the diagnosis entirely, or noting the serologic change but inadequately staging the disease (e.g., "positive VDRL, treat with penicillin"). Treatment of syphilis at a given stage is indicated, not treatment of a reactive VDRL. Appropriate antibiotic regimens are listed above for each stage of syphilis.

Follow-Up. In following up with the patient, the nontreponemal test titer remains the most useful index of the effectiveness of treatment. A high titer is more likely to occur in early syphilis or in active late disease. A nontreponemal test should be performed every 3 to 6 months for a year to see if the patient has a fourfold or greater fall in titer (e.g., a 1:32 titer that falls to 1:2). Failure of nontreponemal test titers to decline fourfold by 6 months after therapy for primary or secondary syphilis identifies patients at risk for treatment failure. These patients should be reevaluated, if originally HIV negative, for HIV infection. They should have additional clinical and serologic follow-up; if follow-up cannot be ensured, they should be re-treated. Some experts recommend CSF examination (34). Patients with latent syphilis should have quantitative nontreponemal serologic tests repeated at 6, 12, and 24 months after initial therapy. If titers increase fourfold, if an initially high titer of 1:32 or more fails to decline at least fourfold within 12 to 24 months, or if the patient develops signs or symptoms attributable to syphilis, the patient should be evaluated for neurosyphilis and re-treated appropriately (51). The same nontreponemal test should be used on all serial specimens because of the differences in their sensitivity: The RPR titer will often be at least one dilution higher than a VDRL done on the same specimen.

Patients who have a *fourfold or greater rise in titer* during follow-up should be considered to be reinfected and should be staged and treated accordingly. In patients with very low titers (e.g., 1:1), as is usually the case in the late latent stage, there is no practical way of assessing the adequacy of therapy.

Contact Tracing. In most jurisdictions, physicians are obligated by law to report the patient's name and the stage of the disease to the health department, both for statistical purposes and for contact tracing by specially trained investigators. Because of rapport with the patient, a physician may choose to coordinate contact tracing. In this era of freer discussion of human sexuality, this poses less of a problem; however, the physician may encounter a patient who does not wish to be straightforward with partners about outside liaisons. This presents a conflict between patient confidentiality and the binding legal requirement to report the patient. Health department investigators make every effort to keep the patient's name from being divulged; however, when a spouse is involved, this may be impossible without resorting to deception, which is not recommended. When the patient balks at informing a spouse or steady partner, it must be impressed upon the patient that the relationship may well benefit from frank and honest discussion of the situation. In any case, not to do so would put the partner at risk and this cannot be condoned.

All identified contacts of patients with infectious syphilis should be thoroughly evaluated for signs of syphilis. When the contact has signs of syphilis, the disease should be staged and treated accordingly and their contacts should be located. Even if there are no signs or serologic evidence of active disease, contacts of patients with primary, secondary, or early latent syphilis should receive prompt treatment for primary syphilis without waiting for clinical manifestations or serologic test results (22). Contacts of patients with late latent or tertiary syphilis should have serologic testing performed but need not be treated if tests are nonreactive.

Education. Education should focus on prevention. If patients have sexual relations with multiple partners, they should be counseled about the risk this entails for contracting syphilis and other STDs. When a patient is treated for infectious syphilis, the patient should be told to abstain from sex until the sore or rash disappears or for at least 1 week, whichever is longer. If a patient plans to continue to be promiscuous, he or she should be cautioned to use a condom as a protection against STD transmission and acquisition. To be effective, condoms must be used during foreplay, be properly worn, and remain intact (13); detailed instructions for condom use are summarized in Table 34.2. Condoms cannot prevent infection if lesions are outside of the area covered. Contraceptive vaginal creams and jellies may provide partial prophylaxis as well. Nonetheless, patients who continue to be promiscuous should have checkups for gonorrhea, HIV, and syphilis whenever they suspect they may have acquired one of these diseases or on a 6-month or yearly basis.

HIV INFECTION AND SYPHILIS

The biological, clinical, psychologic, social, political, and economic consequences of HIV infection are as far reaching as those that were associated with syphilis from the 15th to the mid-20th century. Studies in Africa and the United States show that patients who have had syphilis are at increased risk of being infected with HIV. This results in part from common exposure, through prostitution and intravenous drug use (46), but also because of the facilitation of HIV transmission through genital ulcerations. Safer sexual behavior that decreases the risk of infection with one disease also decreases the risk for the other.

Because of the strong association of these two diseases, patients suspected of having syphilis should be encouraged to be tested simultaneously for HIV infection (44). Although most patients infected with HIV have normal serologic and clinical responses to *T. pallidum,* immunocompromised patients may develop altered seroreactivity, and possibly even altered clinical manifestations of syphilis. When clinical findings suggest that syphilis is present but serologic tests for syphilis are nonreactive or confusing, it may be helpful to perform such alternative tests as biopsy of a lesion, dark-field examination, or direct fluorescent antibody staining of lesion material. There is some evidence that HIV-infected patients are more prone to develop clinical neurosyphilis and to fail to respond to standard treatment for syphilis. This issue is under intense study. At present, standard treatment for syphilis (see above) is still recommended for HIV-infected patients, but VDRL tests at 2-, 3-, 6-, 9-, and 12-month intervals for HIV-infected patients with primary or secondary syphilis are recommended to search for evidence of treatment failure (stable or rising titer) (24). HIV-infected patients with latent syphilis should be evaluated clinically and serologically at 6, 12, 18, and 24 months after therapy. If at any time clinical symptoms develop or nontreponemal titers rise fourfold, a CSF examination should be performed and treatment administered accordingly. Patients in whom treatment has failed should be re-treated in conjunction with an infectious disease consultant. Chapter 34 provides a comprehensive account of the ambulatory care of the HIV-infected patient.

LYME DISEASE

Epidemiology

Since the original clinical description in 1977 of Lyme disease, which is caused by the spirochete *Borrelia burgdorferi,* this condition has become the most common arthropodborne illness in the United States (7). This previously unidentified spirochete was originally isolated from the *Ixodes damini* (also called *Ixodes scapularis*) tick in the northeast United States (6). Subsequently, other forms of *Ixodes* ticks have been found to carry this infection throughout Europe and Asia. In addition to the transmitting tick vector, there must be one or two other animal reservoirs that allow growth of the borrelia. In the United States, the white-footed mouse and the white-tailed deer are the preferred hosts for this very small tick, which is no larger than 2 by 3 mm in its adult form. Through horizontal transmission among these reservoirs, ticks become infected. In endemic areas it has been estimated that up to 50% of ticks may be infected (37). Lyme disease occurs when the infected tick feeds on a susceptible person and transmits the spirochete to that person. By best estimates the probability of acquiring Lyme disease from a single tick bite in an endemic area is 1 to 3% (10). The disease incidence is greatest in the mid-spring through late fall. This correlates with periods of increased tick populations as well as increased outdoor activity of people in endemic areas.

Surveillance of this nationally notifiable disease has been conducted for the past 15 years. The following diagnostic criteria for this surveillance were established in 1990 (63):

- Erythema migrans, or
- At least one late manifestation (defined below) and laboratory confirmation of infection

The highest number of cases are reported in the northeastern, north-central, and mid-Atlantic regions. In 1995, 11,603 cases of Lyme disease were reported in 43 states and the District of Columbia, with an overall incidence rate of 4.4 per 100,000 population. Connecticut (45.6), Rhode Island (34.9), New York (21.9), and New Jersey (21.1) reported the highest rates that year (8). There is no increased risk based on gender. People with significant outdoor exposure in endemic areas have increased risk; however, many cases have occurred where there has not been significant outdoor exposure.

Clinical Manifestations

Different staging systems have been used for Lyme disease. Originally the illness was divided into three sequential stages, with the development of characteristic cutaneous lesions called stage 1. These lesions were previously called erythema chronicum migrans but now are called simply *erythema migrans* (EM). This stage is followed within several weeks to months by multisystemic manifestations of predominantly cardiac and neurologic involvement (stage 2) and then months to years later by the development of arthritis (stage 3). With further clinical observation it has been appreciated that many patients with Lyme disease may not have this characteristic progression of symptoms. Patients may develop EM and no further symptoms in the absence of antibiotic therapy. Others may present with one of the later manifestations of the infection without any history of EM. Most recently, this staging has been modified to divide Lyme disease into early and late infectious complications. *Early infection* includes the localized cutaneous symptoms as well as the symptoms of disseminated disease that can develop within weeks to months of onset of infection. *Late infection* refers to the rheumatic, neurologic, and cutaneous symptoms that develop months to years after the original infection.

Early Manifestations

The early manifestations of Lyme disease occur within weeks to months after the initial infection. Unusual manifestations include uveitis, optic neuritis, hepatitis, osteomyelitis, myositis, and pneumonitis. The more common manifestations are described here.

Localized Infection. Following a tick bite, an incubation period of several days to a month may elapse before the *pathognomonic skin lesion, erythema migrans (EM), forms at the site of the bite.* The common sites are the axillae, groin, and waistline. This lesion starts as an erythematous macule or papule with an outer border and clearing center that expands up to 15 cm in a circumferential manner over several days. The border is sharply demarcated, warm to touch, and nontender. Only one-third of patients are aware of an original tick bite at the time of these symptoms. If untreated, this lesion resolves spontaneously within several weeks. If appropriate antibiotic therapy is initiated, the rash resolves in days. This rash is the single best clinical marker for this condition and occurs in up to 90% of cases (17).

Disseminated Disease. The localized cutaneous infection is often accompanied by *hematogenous dissemination* within the first month. This is typically heralded with a flulike illness that can cause myalgias, arthralgias, fatigue, and a low-grade fever. Generalized lymphadenopathy may also develop. Even without antibiotics, these signs and symptoms resolve in 4 to 6 weeks (57).

Neurologic Manifestations. Up to 20% of untreated patients develop neurologic involvement within 4 to 8 weeks from the resolution of EM in the form of meningitis, cranial neuropathy, or radiculoneuropathy (45). Meningitis is the most common neurologic feature. This presents with fever, meningismus, photophobia, and headache. There is a mild lymphocytic pleocytosis (100 to 500 cells) of the CSF with an elevated protein level (23). The most common cranial neuropathy is a peripheral seventh nerve palsy. This often is unilateral but can be bilateral in up to one-fourth of the cases (9). Most cases resolve within 1 month regardless of treatment. Peripheral radiculoneuropathies occur less often and may involve the motor or sensory nerve fibers alone or together in an asymmetric pattern.

Cardiac Manifestations. Carditis can occur in up to 8% of patients with untreated Lyme disease, typically within 3 months of developing EM. A baseline electrocardiogram should be obtained in patients with the new diagnosis of Lyme disease. The most common finding when a patient has or develops carditis is first-degree atrioventricular (AV) block, but complete heart block requiring temporary pacemaker placement may occur (39). Cardiomyopathy and asymptomatic electrocardiographic changes may also occur. All cardiac involvement usually resolves within 8 weeks and complete heart block usually recedes within 1 week of development, making permanent pacemaker placement unnecessary.

Musculoskeletal Manifestations. More than half of the patients develop migratory arthralgias, myalgias, and bone pain. A self-limited monarticular or oligoarticular arthritis may develop, primarily in the large joints and most often in the knee. Polyarthritis is distinctly unusual.

Dermatologic Manifestations. Multiple disseminated secondary annular lesions may develop in half of the untreated patients (56). These lesions are smaller than the initial lesion and resolve with appropriate antibiotic therapy.

Late Manifestations

The late manifestations of Lyme disease occur many months to years after the initial infection.

Late Musculoskeletal Manifestations. A migratory oligoarthritis may develop in up to 60% of patients with untreated disease (59). They will often experience recurrent attacks of oligoarthritis, most commonly in the knee, that may persist for several weeks to months before resolving. There may be large synovial effusions that can be quite inflammatory (up to 100,000 WBC/mm^3). Even in untreated patients, the arthritis usually resolves. A minority of patients go on to develop a chronic arthritis, even after extensive antibiotic therapy with apparent eradication of all spirochetes. In these cases, an immune response may play a major role based on the presence of certain HLA specificity (DR4 and DR2) as well as the existence of an antibody response to certain outer surface proteins of the spirochete (OspA and OspB) (31,58).

Late Neurologic Manifestations. The most common neurologic manifestation of late Lyme disease is a chronic encephalopathy that can occur years after the initial infection (33). Patients experience memory impairment and mood changes. In addition, a polyradiculopathy may develop in those with encephalopathy. This results primarily in sensory symptoms in the form of paresthesia or radicular pain of the extremities. Motor involvement is unusual. Partial improvement in these symptoms may occur in half of the patients treated with antibiotics, but the natural history appears to be that of a chronic progressive course. All forms of chronic neurologic involvement are believed to be rare, occurring in less than 5% of people with untreated Lyme disease.

Late Dermatologic Manifestations. A late cutaneous manifestation that has been seen primarily in untreated patients infected with Lyme disease in Europe is *acrodermatitis chronica atrophicans* (1). This is a red to blue nodular plaque that develops most commonly on the upper extremities (dorsal aspect of the hand, elbow) and lower extremities (extensor surface of the foot and ankle). In time the involved skin becomes atrophic or sclerotic. There have been cases in which *B. burgdorferi* was cultured from these lesions.

Diagnosis

The diagnosis of Lyme disease should be based primarily on the presence of characteristic clinical findings, response to appropriate antibiotic therapy, and exposure to an endemic area (54). The clinical presentation of erythema migrans rash is so distinctive that any patient presenting with this requires treatment for early Lyme disease. In patients with other associated findings (e.g., facial nerve palsy, complete heart block) and no history of rash, their risk of exposure must be considered. If it is high, serologic testing should be performed.

With the exception of tissue samples from the involved skin lesions in patients with erythema migrans, it is extremely difficult to culture *B. burgdorferi* from any site in infected patients (36). Because this technique is difficult and the skin lesion is pathognomonic, attempts at culturing skin biopsy sites are not usually advised.

The other forms of diagnostic testing involve primarily determining whether there has been an *immune response* to the spirochete, using an enzyme-linked immunosorbent assay (ELISA) to detect IgM and IgG antibodies to *B. burgdorferi*. In patients infected with Lyme disease it takes several weeks before an IgM response can be detected. This may not occur at all in the presence of early antibiotic use. After 4 to 6 weeks, the IgG antibody response should develop in untreated patients. False-positive results have been noted in a number of situations, including viral infections, rheumatoid arthritis, and other autoimmune diseases, as well as in healthy people living in endemic areas (36). Thus, these studies do not have sufficient sensitivity or specificity to be used for screening in the absence of appropriate clinical and environmental findings to fully make or exclude the diagnosis of Lyme disease (2).

Immunoblotting with the Western blot technique is being used to distinguish equivocal and false-positive from true-positive results from ELISA testing (43). DNA detection with polymerase chain reaction (PCR) methods is fraught with technical difficulties that prevent its wide-scale clinical use. The newest promising technique, using recombinant antigens of *B. burgdorferi* in serologic testing, is currently being evaluated for clinical use (38).

Treatment

Lyme disease in all stages should respond with clinical improvement to appropriate antibiotic therapy. It is important to recognize and treat early Lyme disease to prevent the development of later manifestations of the disease. A Jarisch–Herxheimer reaction (described above) has been documented in some patients following treatment. Because early treatment often blunts the immune response, reinfection can occur.

Early Manifestations

EM can be successfully treated with oral doxycycline in adults or amoxicillin in pregnant or lactating women (Table 30.4). In people who are allergic to these medications, oral cefuroxime is the most effective alternative (40). Although erythromycin has been demonstrated to be successful against EM, it is less effective in the treatment of disseminated disease. In most cases the EM rash resolves within days of initiating therapy and 10 days of antibiotic therapy is usually sufficient.

Patients with isolated facial palsy, minor cardiac abnormalities (e.g., first-degree AV block), or disseminated annular lesions at the time of diagnosis should be treated with a 30-day oral regimen (42). If the patient

Table 30.4.   Antibiotic Therapy for Treating Lyme Disease

Oral Therapy for *Localized Disease* (Erythema Migrans)		
Doxycycline	100 mg BID	10 days
	OR	
Cefuroxime	250 mg BID	10 days

Pregnant or Lactating Women		
Amoxicillin	500 mg TID	10 days

Oral Therapy for *Early Disseminated Disease* (First-Degree AV Block, Facial Palsy, Disseminated Annular Lesions)		
Doxycycline	100 mg BID	30 days
	OR	
Cefuroxime	250 mg BID	30 days

Intravenous Therapy for *Early Disseminated Disease* (Complete AV Block, Meningitis, Neuritis)		
Ceftriaxone	2 g QD	30 days
	OR	
Cefotaxime	3 g q12hr	30 days

Oral Therapy for *Late Disease* (Arthritis)		
Doxycycline	100 mg BID	30 days
	OR	
Cefuroxime	250 mg BID	30 days

Intravenous Therapy for *Late Disease* (Persistent Arthritis, Late Neurologic Diseases)		
Ceftriaxone	2 g QD	30 days
	OR	
Cefotaxime	3 g q12hr	30 days

has complete AV block, meningitis, or neuritis, he or she should be given intravenous therapy for 30 days (55). Ceftriaxone is preferred over penicillin because the dosing schedule allows home antibiotic therapy. Patients with significant cardiac involvement may require monitoring and a temporary pacemaker.

Late Manifestations

Late manifestations of Lyme disease require longer courses of antibiotics (Table 30.4). Lyme arthritis should be treated with a 30-day course of oral antibiotics. If the patient does not respond, a 15- to 30-day course of intravenous ceftriaxone should be given (14). A small percentage of patients may develop a postinfectious immune response with persistent arthritis despite extensive antibiotics. Patients with late neurologic manifestations should be treated initially with a 30-day course of intravenous ceftriaxone (55).

Prevention

The risk of being infected by *B. burgdorferi* from a tick bite depends on several variables. This includes the percentage of infectivity of ticks in the endemic area, the number of tick bites received, and the amount of time that the tick is attached. If tick feeding is less than 48 hours, the risk of transmitting infection is remarkably low. However, this risk increases substantially with more than 3 days' exposure to the tick or if the tick becomes engorged.

Several studies have examined the efficacy and cost-effectiveness of *antibiotic prophylaxis following a tick bite*. One study recommended that if the risk of infection following the bite is greater than 3.6% (35), then antibiotic prophylaxis should be given for anyone known to have been bitten by a tick. In two separate placebo-controlled trials, the risk of becoming infected in an endemic area (less than 1.5%) was no greater that the risk of developing side effects from the antibiotic treatment (10,52). Until further data are available, it is difficult to recommend prophylactic therapy for tick bites in endemic areas. However, if a tick from an endemic area has been in place for more than 72 hours or is engorged, it is reasonable to prescribe prophylactic therapy for early Lyme disease with a 10-day course of doxycycline.

Recent preliminary results have been published from a large clinical trial of a *killed vaccine* containing recombinant *Borrelia burgdorferi* outer surface lipoprotein-A (L-OspA) (53). Vaccination requires two injections 1 month apart and sometimes a third booster injection 1 year later. In subjects 15 to 59 years old, efficacy, defined as a percent of expected cases prevented during two "LD seasons," was 82% after two doses and 100% after the third dose. In individuals over the age 60, efficacy rates are only 75% with three injections. To date, the frequency of adverse events has been similar in the vaccine in the placebo group.

The best preventive measure is to educate patients carefully about limiting exposure to infected ticks. They should wear long pants tucked into their socks when walking in such areas. In addition, they should carefully inspect their skin after outdoor activities to allow for rapid detection and removal of ticks.

General References*

Syphilis

Clark EG, Danbolt N. The Oslo study of the natural course of untreated syphilis. Med Clin North Am 48:613, 1964.
   Long-term study of the natural history of syphilis in 1404 subjects.
Holmes KK, Mardh PA, Sparling PF, Weisner P, eds. Sexually transmitted diseases. New York: McGraw-Hill, 1990.
   Detailed accounts of syphilis and other STDs by leading experts.
Hook EW III, Marra CM. Acquired syphilis in adults. N Engl J Med 326:1060, 1992.
   Recent review.
Jones JH. Bad blood. New York: Free Press, 1981.
   A popular account of the Tuskegee study of untreated syphilis in African-American male subjects.
Rosebury T. Microbes and morals. New York: Vebany Press, 1971.
   Fascinating account of the history of sexually transmitted disease.

Lyme Disease

Rahn DW, Malawista SE. **Lyme disease: recommendations for diagnosis and treatment.** Ann Intern Med 144:472, 1991.
Steere AC. Lyme disease. N Engl J Med 321:586, 1989.
   General review of all aspects of Lyme disease by the person who first described and has extensively studied the disease.

Specific References

1. Asbrink E, Hovmark A. Early and late cutaneous manifestations of Ixodes-borne borreliosis (erythema migrans borreliosis, Lyme Borreliosis). Ann N Y Acad Sci 539:4–15, 1988.

2. Bakken LL, Case KL, Callister SM, et al. Performance of 45 laboratories participating in a proficiency testing program for Lyme disease serology. JAMA 268:891, 1992.
3. Balkany TJ, Dans PE. Reversible sudden deafness in early acquired syphilis. Arch Otolaryngol 104:66, 1978.
4. Brandt AM. No magic bullet: a social history of venereal disease in the United States since 1880. New York: Oxford University Press, 1987.
5. Brown ST, Zaidi A, Larsen SA, Reynolds GH. Serological response to syphilis treatment. JAMA 253:1296, 1985.
6. Burgdorfer W, Barbour AG, Hayes SF, et al. Lyme disease: a tickborne spirochetosis? Science 216:1317–1319, 1982.
7. Centers for Disease Control and Prevention. Lyme disease: United States 1991–1992. MMWR 42:345–350, 1993.
8. Centers for Disease Control and Prevention. Lyme disease: United States, 1995. MMWR 45:23, 1996.
9. Clark JR, Carlson RD, Sasaki CT, et al. Facial paralysis in Lyme disease. Laryngoscope 95:1341–1345, 1985.
10. Costello CM, Steer AC, Pinkerton RE, et al. Prospective study of tick bites in an endemic area for Lyme disease. J Infect Dis 150:489–496, 1984.
11. Dans PE, Cafferly I, Oller SE, Johnson RT. Inappropriate use of the cerebrospinal fluid venereal disease research laboratory (CSF-VDRL) test to exclude neurosyphilis. Correspondence. Ann Intern Med 104:86, 724, 1986.
12. Dans PE, Judson FN, Larsen SA, Lantz MA. The FTA-ABS test. A diagnostic help or hindrance? South Med J 70:312, 1977.
13. Darrow WW. Condom use and use-effectiveness in high-risk populations. Sex Transm Dis 16:43, 1989.
14. Dattwyler RJ, Halperin JJ, Volkman DJ, Luft BJ. Treatment of late Lyme borreliosis: randomised comparison of ceftriaxone and penicillin. Lancet 1:1191, 1988.
15. Division of STD/HIV Prevention. Sexually transmitted disease surveillance, 1991. U.S. Department of Health and Human Services, Public Health Service. Atlanta: Centers for Disease Control and Prevention, July 1992.
16. Fiumara NJ. Serologic responses to treatment of 128 patients with late latent syphilis. J Am Vener Dis Assoc 6:243, 1979.
17. Gerber MA, Bell GJ, Burke GS, et al. Lyme disease in children in southeast Connecticut. N Engl J Med 335:17, 1997.
18. Gordon SM, Eaton ME, George R, et al. The response of symptomatic neurosyphilis to high-dose intravenous penicillin G in patients with human immunodeficiency virus infection. N Engl J Med 331:1469, 1994.
19. Greene BM, Miller NR, Bynum TE. Failure of penicillin G benzathine in the treatment of neurosyphilis. Arch Intern Med 140:1117, 1980.
20. Haas JS, Bolan G, Larsen SA, et al. Sensitivity of treponemal tests for detecting prior treated syphilis during human immunodeficiency virus infection. J Infect Dis 162:862, 1990.
21. Hahn RD, Cutler JC, Curtis AC, et al. Penicillin treatment of asymptomatic central nervous system syphilis. I. Probability of progression to symptomatic neurosyphilis. Arch Dermatol 74:355, 1956.
22. Hart G. Epidemiologic treatment for syphilis and gonorrhea. Sex Transm Dis 7:149, 1980.
23. Henriksson A, Link H, Cruz M, Stiernstedt G. Immunoglobulin abnormalities in cerebrospinal fluid and blood over the course of lymphocytic meningoradiculitis (Bannworth's syndrome). Ann Neurol 20:337, 1986.
24. Hook EW. Syphilis and HIV infection. J Infect Dis 160(3):530, 1989.
25. Hook EW III, Marra CM. Acquired syphilis in adults. N Engl J Med 326:1060, 1992.
26. Hook EW III, Roddy RE, Handsfield HH. Ceftriaxone therapy for incubating and early syphilis. J Infect Dis 158:881, 1988.
27. Hooshmand H, Escobar MR, Kopf SW. Neurosyphilis, a study of 241 patients. JAMA 219:726, 1972.
28. Idsoe O, Guthe T, Willcox RR. Penicillin in the treatment of syphilis. The experience of three decades. Bull WHO 474(Suppl):1, 1972.
29. Jaffe HW, Kabins SA. Examination of cerebrospinal fluid in patients with syphilis. Rev Infect Dis 4(Suppl):S842, 1982.

---

*Bold print (general references) and bold numerals (specific references) denote published controlled clinical trials, meta-analyses, or consensus-based recommendations.

30. Kalish RA, Leong JM, Steere AC. Association of treatment resistant chronic Lyme arthritis with HLA-DR4 and antibody reactivity to OspA and OspB of Borrelia. Infect Immun 61(7): 2774, 1993.

31. Larsen SA, Hunter EF, McGrew BE. Syphilis. In: Wentworth B, Judson FN, eds. Laboratory methods for the diagnosis of sexually transmitted diseases. Washington, DC: American Public Health Association, 1984.

32. Logigian EL, Kaplan RF, Steere AC. Neurologic manifestations of Lyme disease. N Engl J Med 323:1438, 1990.

33. Lukehart SA, Hook EW, Baker-Zander SA, et al. Invasion of the central nervous system by *Treponema pallidum*: implications for diagnosis and treatment. Ann Intern Med 110:855, 1988.

34. Magid D, Schwartz B, Craft J, et al. Prevention of Lyme disease after tick bites: a cost effectiveness analysis. N Engl J Med 327:534–541, 1992.

35. Magnarelli LA. Current status of laboratory diagnosis for Lyme disease. Am J Med 98:4A-10S–4A-14S, 1995.

36. Magnarelli LA, Anderson JF. Ticks and biting insects infected with the etiologic agent of Lyme disease, *Borrelia burgdorferi*. J Clin Microbiol 26:1482–1486, 1988.

37. Magnarelli LA, Anderson JF, Fikrig E, et al. Use of recombinant antigens of *Borrelia burgdorferi* in serologic tests for diagnosis of Lyme borreliosis. J Clin Microbiol 34:237–240, 1996.

38. McAlister HF, Klementowicz PT, Andrews C, et al. Lyme carditis: an important cause of reversible heart block. Ann Intern Med 110:339–345, 1989.

39. Nadelman RB, Luger SW, Frank E, et al. Comparison of cefuroxime axetil and doxycycline in the treatment of early Lyme disease. Ann Intern Med 117:273, 1992.

40. Putkonen T, Salo OP, Mustakallio KK. Febrile Herxheimer reaction in different phases of primary and secondary syphilis. Br J Vener Dis 42:181, 1966.

41. Rahn DW, Malawista SE. Lyme disease: recommendations for diagnosis and treatment. Ann Intern Med 114:472, 1991.

42. Recommendations for test performance and interpretation from the Second National Conference on Serologic Diagnosis of Lyme Disease. MMWR 44(31):August 11, 1995.

43. Recommendations for diagnosing and treating syphilis in HIV-infected patients. MMWR 37:39, 1988.

44. Reik L, Steere AC, Bartenhagen NH, et al. Neurologic abnormalities of Lyme disease. Medicine (Baltimore) 58:281, 1979.

45. Rolfs RT, Goldberg M, Sharrar RG. Risk factors for syphilis and cocaine use and prostitution. Am J Public Health 80:853, 1990.

46. Rolfs RT, Joesoef R, Hendershot EF, et al. Treatment of early syphilis in HIV-infected and uninfected persons: a randomized trial of enhanced therapy that included examination of cerebrospinal fluid. N Engl J Med 337:307, 1997.

47. Romanowski B, Sutherland R, Fich GH, et al. Serologic response to treatment of infectious syphilis. Ann Intern Med 114:1005, 1991.

48. Schroeter AL, Lucas JB, Price EV, Falcone VH. Treatment for early syphilis and reactivity of serologic tests. JAMA 221:471, 1972.

49. Schroeter AL, Turner RH, Lucas JB, Brown WJ. Therapy for incubating syphilis. Effectiveness of gonorrhea treatment. JAMA 218:711, 1971.

50. Sexually transmitted disease 1997 treatment guidelines. Centers for Disease Control and Prevention. In press.

51. Shapiro ED, Gerber MA, Holabird NB, et al. A controlled trial of antimicrobial prophylaxis for Lyme disease after deer tick bites. N Engl J Med 327:1769, 1992.

52. Shrestha M, Grodzicki RL, Steere AC. Diagnosing early Lyme disease. Am J Med 78:235, 1985.

53. Sigal LH, Adler-Klein D, Bryant G, et al. Multicenter efficacy trail of a recombinant *Borrelia burgdorferi* (Bb) outer surface protein A (OspA) vaccine for prevention of Lyme disease (LD). Arthritis Rheum 40:5173, 1997.

54. Skoldenberg B, Stiernstedt G, Karlsson M, et al. Treatment of Lyme borreliosis with emphasis on neurological disease. Ann N Y Acad Sci 539:317–323, 1988.

55. Steere AC, Bartenhagen NC, Craft JE, et al. The early clinical manifestations of Lyme disease. Ann Intern Med 99:76–82, 1983.

56. Steere AC, Bartenhagen NH, Craft JE, et al. The early clinical manifestations of Lyme disease. Am J Med 78:235, 1985.

57. Steere AC, Dwyer E, Winchester R. Association of chronic Lyme arthritis with HLA-DR2 and HLA-DR4 alleles. N Engl J Med 323:219–223, 1990.

58. Steere AC, Schoen RT, Taylor E. The clinical evolution of Lyme arthritis. Ann Intern Med 107:725–731, 1987.

59. Syphilis and congenital syphilis: United States, 1985–1988. MMWR 37:32, 1987.

60. Tertiary syphilis deaths: South Florida. MMWR 36:29, 1987.

61. The Jarisch–Herxheimer reaction. Lancet 1:340, 1977.

62. Weber K, Schierz G, Wilske B, et al. Reinfection with erythema migrans disease. Infection 14:32, 1986.

63. Wharton MC, Chorba TL, Vogt RL, et al. Case definitions for public health surveillance, MMWR 39(RR-13):19–21, 1990.

64. Wiesel J, Rose DN, Silver AL, et al. Lumbar puncture in asymptomatic late syphilis. An analysis of the benefits and risks. Arch Intern Med 145:465, 1985.

65. Wilner G, Brody JA. Prognosis of general paresis after treatment. Lancet 2:1370, 1968.

C H A P T E R   31

Ambulatory Care for Selected Infections Including Osteomyelitis, Lung Abscess, and Endocarditis

JOHN G. BARTLETT, MD

Usually, the three types of infections reviewed in detail in this chapter are managed initially with intravenous antibiotics administered in the hospital. Patients with these infections are often seen first in an office setting, and the long courses of antibiotics used to treat them are then completed after discharge from the hospital. These infections involve diverse bacteria and different anatomic sites but share the propensity for relapse caused by persistent bacteria at the infected site. This explains the requirement for prolonged courses of antimicrobial treatment. Antibiotics may be administered by two different routes out of hospital: the oral route, to complete a course initiated parenterally during hospitalization, and the intravenous route, using the same regimen provided for inpatients and used by home health agencies (see details in Chapter 9 and in review cited in "General References").

EXPANDING ROLE OF ORAL ANTIBIOTICS

In the past, there was reluctance to prescribe oral antibiotics to be taken at home for most serious infections; however, this approach is gaining acceptance because of a number of studies indicating efficacy (1,9,10,16,22,24). The advantages of home use of oral agents are patient convenience, the notable reduction in cost, and a reduction in nosocomial infections. These and other considerations are summarized in Table 31.1. Average charges for hospital care that includes intravenous antibiotics are about $1,000/day, whereas for intravenous antibiotics given at home the average charge is $300 to $400/day and for oral agents the cost is $1 to $6/day. The issue of patient convenience is obvious. With regard to nosocomial infections, the cost in terms of morbidity, mortality, and hospital charge is substantial. In 1992, it was estimated that nosocomial infections accounted for 19,000 deaths (0.9% of hospitalized patients) and were a contributing factor in the death of 58,000 (2.7%) patients; the extension in hospital stay averaged 4 days for those with nosocomial infections, at an average cost of $2100 (7). Of particular concern in recent years has been nosocomial acquisition of tuberculosis (especially the multiply resistant strains); *Clostridium difficile*–associated colitis, which is now recognized largely as a nosocomial complication; and Legionnaires' disease. Hospitals also remain the major source of problem pathogens such as *Pseudomonas aeruginosa,* multiply resistant Gram-negative bacilli, methicillin-resistant *Staphylococcus aureus,* and vancomycin-resistant *Enterococcus.*

Some types of infectious diseases have traditionally been treated with parenteral antibiotics but may sometimes be treated with oral agents: *P. aeruginosa* urinary tract infections (including bacterial prostatitis), pulmonary infections in patients with cystic fibrosis, some forms of osteomyelitis, tricuspid valve endocarditis caused by *S. aureus* in intravenous drug abusers, fever in the patient with neutropenia (see Chapter 8), some cases of pyelonephritis, most cases of pneumonia (see Chapter 28), and select fungal infections that traditionally have required amphotericin B.

Newer Antimicrobial Agents

Much of the progress in this area has resulted from the development of oral antimicrobial agents in four classes that have an expanded spectrum of activity: cephalosporins, fluoroquinolones, β-lactam–β-lactamase inhibitor combinations, and the triazole antifungal agents. Among the *cephalosporins* and *carbecephams,* the agents with an expanded spectrum of activity for oral administration include cefaclor, cefuroxime axetil, cefprozil, cefpodoxime, loracarbef, and cefixime. All of these agents are active against most strains of Enterobacteriaceae; activity against major Gram-positive cocci is variable, and none of these agents is active against *P. aeruginosa,* enterococci, or methicillin-resistant *S. aureus.* In general, these agents are advocated for respiratory tract infections, skin and soft tissue infections, and urinary tract infections. The *fluoroquinolones* include norfloxacin, ciprofloxacin, ofloxacin, enoxacin, lomefloxacin, levofloxacin, sparfloxacin, grepafloxacin, and trovafloxacin. There are

Table 31.1.   Advantages and Disadvantages of Home Treatment with Oral Antimicrobial Agents

Advantages
Cost reduction[a]
   Hospital costs (IV antibiotics) $1100/d
   Home care (IV antibiotics) $320/d
   Home care (oral antibiotics) $6/d
Patient convenience
Reduced nosocomial infections
Demonstrated efficacy

Disadvantages
Bioavailability
Need for supportive care or monitoring
Compliance
Possible legal liability
Selected infections that require parenteral agents
Serious side effects that require immediate care

[a]Costs based on 1993 average total charge for Johns Hopkins Hospital for inpatients, industry average charge for home care, and average wholesale charge for many oral antibiotics.

slight differences among these agents in bioavailability, spectrum of activity, pharmacology, and side effects. In general, ciprofloxacin is favored for infections involving *P. aeruginosa;* levofloxacin and sparfloxacin are preferred for infections in which *Streptococcus pneumoniae* is an established or suspected pathogen. *S. aureus* strains are developing resistance to the fluoroquinolones, and resistance to one implies resistance to the entire group. The only available oral β-*lactam*–β-*lactamase* inhibitor is amoxicillin plus clavulanate (Augmentin), which has the spectrum of amoxicillin plus organisms that are penicillin resistant because of β-lactamase production: *S. aureus,* many Gram-negative bacilli, *Haemophilus influenzae,* and many anaerobes.

For oral treatment of serious anaerobic infections, either of two older drugs, metronidazole and clindamycin, is usually an option.

Newer Antifungal Agents

The triazoles include ketoconazole, fluconazole, and itraconazole. These drugs are now supplanting amphotericin B for many fungal infections. All three are effective against most strains of *Candida albicans* and may be used for mucocutaneous candidiasis, but use for parenchymal and systemic *Candida* infections is limited. Fluconazole has established efficacy for cryptococcosis. Itraconazole now appears to be the preferred agent for most cases of histoplasmosis, blastomycosis, and paracoccidioidomycosis and for many cases of coccidioidomycosis and aspergillosis.

Risks and Burdens of Home Treatment

The use of oral agents in the home setting for infections traditionally treated with intravenous antibiotics in the hospital is not without some risks and burdens. Supportive care requiring some hospital resources for very sick patients is an example. Although monitoring of drug levels is rarely an issue with oral

agents, compliance is always a concern, and physicians have been notoriously unable to predict which patients will take their medications (see Chapter 4 for details). In many communities, this issue is now addressed for tuberculosis by direct observation of pill taking, although here the circumstances are somewhat different because antituberculous drugs can be given twice weekly and the need is justified on the basis of public health concerns. Selected pathogens are difficult or impossible to treat with currently available oral agents. These include the fluoroquinolone-resistant strains of *P. aeruginosa,* most infections involving methicillin-resistant *S. aureus,* and cytomegalovirus. An additional concern about outpatient management is the fact that patients are not under direct observation, so emergency care is not immediately available for serious side effects. The major example is IgE-mediated hypersensitivity caused by β-lactam agents, which occurs with the frequency of about 1:2,500 to 1:25,000 courses of penicillin G. Finally, there may be concern about legal liability when the use of oral antibiotics is not considered the standard of care, even if efficacy and safety seem well established. Because many third-party payers now mandate home care for stable patients who require long-term antibiotics, the latter concern is unlikely to deter expanded home treatment.

OSTEOMYELITIS

Definition

Osteomyelitis is an infection of bone. There are *four major categories:* osteomyelitis following hematogenous spread of infection, osteomyelitis secondary to a contiguous focus of infection, infection of prosthetic joints, and osteomyelitis associated with vascular insufficiency. These four categories differ according to patient age, bones involved, predisposing conditions, usual bacterial pathogens, and presentation (Table 31.2). Osteomyelitis is also classified as *acute or chronic:* acute osteomyelitis indicates newly recognized bone infection; chronic osteomyelitis indicates prior infection or clinical symptoms exceeding 10 days (16).

Clinical Presentation and Bacteriology

Hematogenous

Hematogenous osteomyelitis is classically described as a disease of *children,* usually under 16 years of age, which is usually caused by *S. aureus* (16). The tendency for this infection to occur during active growth reflects the enhanced susceptibility of the vascular network of the metaphysis, especially of the femur or tibia. About one-third of patients have a history of preceding nonpenetrating trauma in the area that is subsequently involved. The infection begins in the metaphyseal sinusoidal veins; it is contained by the epiphyseal growth plate and tends to spread laterally, with perforation of the cortex and lifting of the loose periosteum.

Hematogenous osteomyelitis of the long bones in

Table 31.2.   Types of Osteomyelitis

	Hematogenous	Secondary to Contiguous Infection	Complications of Vascular Insufficiency
Approximate proportion of all cases	20%	50%	30%
Most common age groups	1–16 yr >50 yr	Any age	>50 yr
Bones involved	Long bones (children) Vertebrae (adults)	Hip, femur, tibia, digits	Feet
Predisposing causes	Trauma Bacteremia	Surgery Soft tissue infection	Diabetes mellitus Vascular insufficiency
Usual bacteria	*S. aureus* Gram-negative bacilli	Often polymicrobial: Gram-negative bacilli, *S. aureus*	Usually polymicrobial: Gram-negative bacilli, anaerobes, streptococci, *S. aureus*
Presentation			
Initial episode	Fever, local pain swelling, tenderness, limited movement	Fever, local pain swelling, tenderness, limited movement	Ulceration drainage ± pain
Recurrent episode	Sinus drainage ± pain	Sinus drainage ± pain	Drainage ± pain

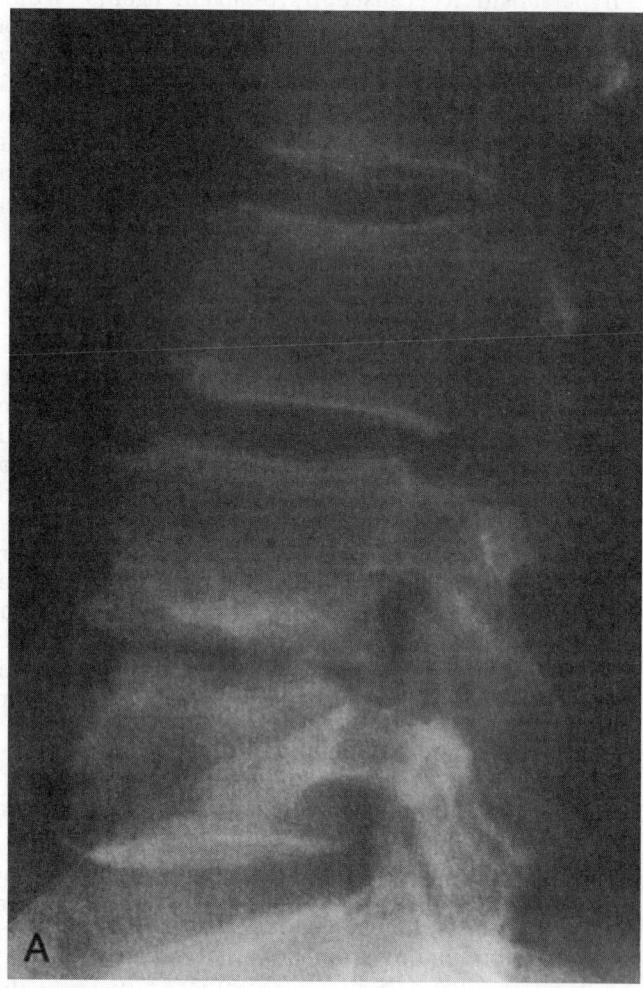

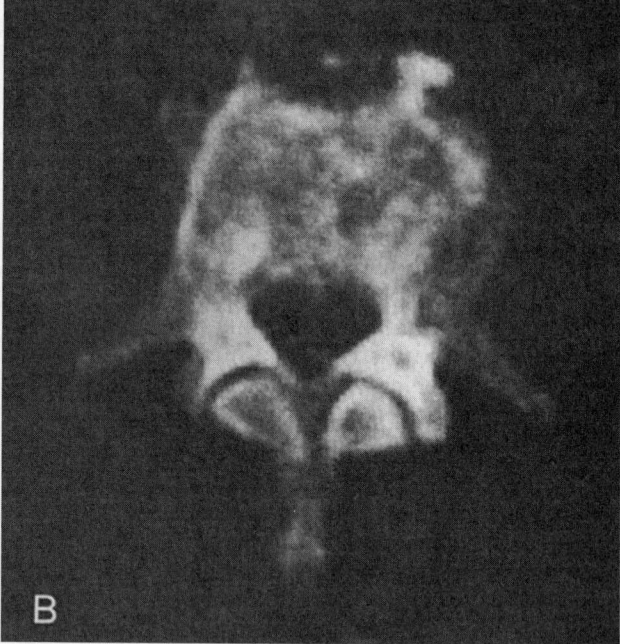

Figure 31.1.   A. L3–4 staphylococcal osteomyelitis of 3 months' duration, with disc narrowing and sclerosis seen on plain film. **B.** Computerized tomographic scan in same patient showing small soft tissue abscess and minimal bone destruction. Hazy bone outline. (From Post MJD, ed. Computed tomography of the spine. Baltimore: Williams & Wilkins, 1984;740.)

adults is rare, different in presentation, and bacteriologically distinct. In these patients, the growth cartilage has been resorbed so the subarticular space is more vulnerable, and the periosteum is firmly attached so that subperiosteal abscess formation is uncommon. The most common form of hematogenous osteomyelitis in adults involves the vertebrae (Fig. 31.1) and the most common pathogens are Gram-negative bacilli and

S. aureus. The initial site of infection is the richly vascularized bone adjacent to cartilage; there is subsequent involvement of adjacent bone plates and of the intervertebral disc. The infection may extend longitudinally to involve adjacent vertebrae, anteriorly to produce a paraspinal abscess, or posteriorly to form an epidural abscess.

Acute hematogenous osteomyelitis usually presents with precipitous onset of pain, swelling, chills, and fever. With vertebral osteomyelitis, there is fever with back pain, stiffness, and often point tenderness over the infected vertebra. Many patients have a more subacute presentation, with vague symptoms of 1 to 2 months' duration before presentation, with few constitutional complaints. One well-described variant is Brodie's abscess (also called a cold abscess): subacute staphylococcal osteomyelitis located in the metaphysis of a long bone, which presents with local pain and fever. Patients with recurrent or chronic osteomyelitis often simply note increased or persistent drainage and pain after an episode involving the same anatomic location.

Contiguous Infection

Osteomyelitis secondary to contiguous foci of infection accounts for at least half of all cases. The most common precipitating factor is previous surgery, usually involving the lower extremities, such as open reduction of fractures of the femur or tibia. Next in frequency is a soft tissue infection involving the digits of the hands or feet. These infections usually become apparent within 1 month of a precipitating event, although many patients have chronic or recurrent infections that occur intermittently for years or decades.

Prosthetic Joint Infections

Infections that complicate prosthetic joints are classified as acute infection (within 12 weeks of surgery) or chronic (within 3 to 24 months of surgery) (16). There may be later infections resulting from transient bacteremia in a fashion analogous to the pathogenesis of endocarditis, with the joint serving as a susceptible nidus. The presentation of an infected prosthesis is a painful, unstable joint, often with little or no fever and nonspecific radiographic findings. The diagnosis is best established with semiquantitative culture of an aspirate from the joint space or bone–cement interface. *Staphylococcus epidermidis* accounts for 75% of cases; next in frequency are *S. aureus,* streptococci, *Peptococcus magnus,* enteric Gram-negative bacilli, and *Candida* spp.

Vascular Insufficiency

Osteomyelitis associated with vascular insufficiency is most common in patients with diabetes mellitus or severe atherosclerosis (6,11). The most common sites of infection are the toes or small bones of the feet, usually with overlying soft tissue infections (Fig. 31.2). These infections are often detected with the routine radiographs performed to evaluate chronic draining sinuses or skin ulcers that are so common in the patients at risk. Probing that demonstrates extension of ulcers to bone is essentially diagnostic of osteomyelitis, and this finding supersedes all scanning techniques in terms of specificity (6,11). Both the

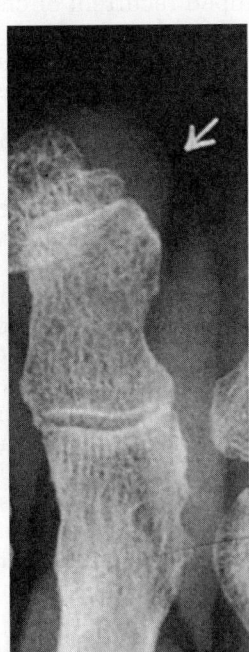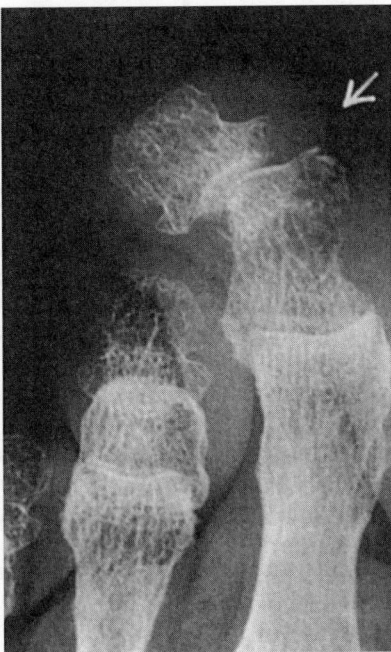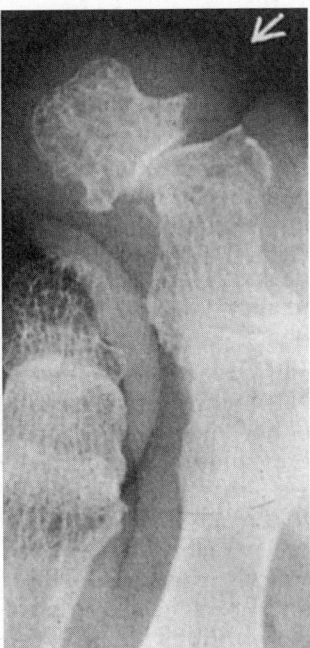

Figure 31.2.   Arrows indicate, from left to right, infected soft corn, sinus tract, and osteomyelitis in the distal interphalangeal joint. As destruction increases, the joint becomes dislocated. (From Gamble FO, Yale I. Clinical foot roenterology. Baltimore: Williams & Wilkins, 1966.)

adjacent soft tissue infection and the osteomyelitis usually involve a *polymicrobial flora* that may include anaerobic bacteria, coliforms, pseudomonads, streptococci, and *S. aureus.*

Laboratory Evaluation

Diagnostic studies include radiographs, radionuclide studies, computerized tomography (CT), or magnetic resonance imaging (MRI) to demonstrate typical bone changes and cultures to identify the etiologic organism.

The earliest changes on plain radiographs are lytic lesions; other findings may include soft tissue swelling, periosteal reaction, cortical irregularity, demineralization, and sequestrum formation. However, typical changes are not visible on plain films until 30 to 50% of the bone has been resorbed, and this usually requires 10 to 14 days. In a patient with a normal plain film but clinical findings suggesting osteomyelitis, a technetium bone scan or a [111]indium leukocyte scan can be helpful. Both of these tests are sensitive in early osteomyelitis (70 to 90%), but they lack specificity (50 to 75%) (16,18,25). The bone scan uses [99]technetium as a marker bound to diphosphonate that concentrates in bone because of incorporation at sites of osteoblastic activity. Abnormal studies may occur when there is increased blood flow associated with soft tissue infections or with osteoblastic activity caused by other processes, such as degenerative joint disease. Most authorities regard ^{99}Tc as the preferred scintigraphic method (18,30). Computerized tomography and magnetic resonance imaging are also useful in showing osteomyelitis. CT scans are particularly useful in guiding needle biopsy or percutaneous aspirations. MRI is particularly sensitive and may show osteomyelitis before changes are evident by scintigraphy (16). Prosthetic material that is ferromagnetic is a contraindication to MRI, but most materials now used in orthopedic surgery do not interfere with MRI.

Because antimicrobial treatment, often prolonged, is the mainstay of management, accurate bacteriologic data are helpful for making the diagnosis and planning treatment. The list of possible organisms is long, and sensitivity patterns for these organisms show considerable variation, making empirical selection of antimicrobials hazardous. These considerations may justify an aggressive attempt to identify the responsible organism. Conclusive bacteriologic studies require isolation of the pathogen from the bone or blood cultures.

Under ideal circumstances, an orthopedist should perform a *needle aspiration* over the involved bone, either blindly or, preferably, under CT guidance (13). If subperiosteal pus is obtained, surgical drainage is mandatory. If no pus is obtained, the needle is inserted into bone to obtain a specimen. The diagnostic yield with a needle aspirate of bone is approximately 60%, and for a surgical biopsy it is approximately 90% (16). Cultures from draining sinus tracts tend to show poor correlation with cultures obtained directly from bone

(20). Needle aspirate specimens should be submitted for Gram's stain and for culture of aerobic and anaerobic bacteria. Care must be exercised in the interpretation of culture results, even of bone aspirates, because these are often contaminated, especially if the specimen is obtained by traversing soft tissue infections (29). Organisms recovered in low concentrations, especially those growing only in the broth culture, must be viewed with skepticism. Common skin contaminants include *S. epidermidis,* diphtheroids, and Propionibacterium. These organisms tend to cause osteomyelitis only in the presence of prosthetic devices. Gram's stain of exudate or tissue aspirate should verify the culture results and represents an important correlate in determining the etiologic organism. The semiquantitative results of cultures are an important and often overlooked component of interpreting culture results, especially when the organisms detected are common contaminants.

Treatment

General Principles

Immobilization was commonly advocated in the treatment of osteomyelitis in the preantibiotic era. However, it appears to be less important at present, and most authorities conclude that strict immobilization is unnecessary.

Antimicrobial Treatment: Acute Osteomyelitis

For newly diagnosed or acute osteomyelitis, the standard recommendation has been a 3- to 6-week course of parenteral antibiotics (3,27,31). This recommendation is based on several studies that note that patients often developed recurrent or chronic disease when treatment was less than 21 days. The standard regimen for acute staphylococcal osteomyelitis in adults is a penicillinase-resistant penicillin such as nafcillin, given intravenously at a dosage of 1.5 to 2 g every 6 hours. Alternative parenteral regimens are cefazolin (1.0 to 1.5 g every 8 hours), vancomycin (1 g every 12 hours), or clindamycin (600 mg every 8 hours) (16). In stable patients, these regimens can be initiated in the hospital and completed at home.

To decrease cost, length of hospitalization, and patient discomfort, a *modified regimen,* consisting of a short course of parenteral antibiotics followed by a prolonged course of oral agents, has been developed (5,10,16,17,19,24). The intravenous antibiotic is given for at least 3 days, or until the patient is afebrile, or for an arbitrarily defined period such as 1 to 2 weeks. An alternative oral agent selected by in vitro sensitivity tests is then taken by mouth, usually at home, to complete a total 3- to 6-week course, usually 4 weeks. The drugs recommended for oral administration are clindamycin (300 mg every 6 hours), an oral antistaphylococcal penicillin such as dicloxacillin or cephalexin (500 mg every 6 hours), or a fluoroquinolone. It should be noted that the importance of bactericidal activity and the relative merits of drugs for bone penetration as factors in drug selection are debated issues that remain unresolved.

Antimicrobial Treatment: Chronic Osteomyelitis

Therapeutic guidelines are less precise for chronic osteomyelitis. Because necrotic bone may serve as a nidus for sequestered bacteria, surgical excision of dead tissue and adequate debridement are often essential components of treatment. Antibiotic selection should be based on bacteriologic diagnosis using deep aspirates or, preferably, cultures obtained from bone. The daily dosage, route of administration, and duration of treatment are somewhat arbitrary, but most authorities recommend prolonged courses. The initial treatment may be parenteral antibiotics for 1 to 3 months in the hospital or in the home, followed by oral agents for several months (31). An alternative approach is the use, from the outset of treatment, of oral agents to which the patient's infecting organism is sensitive for extended periods, such as 6 months or longer (5,10,16,17,19,21,24). Fluoroquinolones such as ofloxacin or ciprofloxacin alone or in combination with clindamycin or metronidazole have established efficacy for osteomyelitis with a mixed anaerobic–coliform flora (10). Oral cephalosporins may also be used for infections involving Gram-negative bacilli; metronidazole by mouth is preferred for oral treatment of deep infections involving anaerobes, although clindamycin and amoxicillin–clavulanate (Augmentin) are probably effective as well. Various authors have used a variety of dosages of these antibiotics. Guidelines should be sought in published reports or the most current editions of manuals on the use of antibiotics for specific infections.

Late Complications

The major complication of osteomyelitis is recurrence that may happen months, years, or decades after the initial event. The patient should be warned of this potential complication. The clinical features of recurrences are fever, draining sinuses, local pain, elevated sedimentation rate, and the typical changes noted on radiographs or scans as summarized above. Chronic osteomyelitis may be complicated by secondary amyloidosis, although it has become extremely rare since the advent of antibiotics. Another complication is epidermoid carcinoma arising in a draining sinus of osteomyelitis, which occurs in 0.2 to 1.5% of cases, with a mean delay of 34 years (32).

Patients with orthopedic devices such as prosthetic joints are at risk for infection after transient bacteremia. However, unlike the situation with endocarditis, there are no guidelines from authoritative sources to direct preventive treatment. It is reasonable to administer prophylactic antibiotics for the procedures that are considered a risk by the American Heart Association for patients susceptible to endocarditis (see Chapter 86, Table 86.13). However, the major pathogens for infected orthopedic devices are *S. aureus, S. epider-*

midis, and to a lesser extent, *Streptococcus,* whereas endocarditis prophylaxis is directed primarily against *Streptococcus.* For the former organisms, some recommend prophylaxis with an oral cephalosporin or clindamycin: one dose 1 hour before dental work in patients with periodontal disease or potential dental infection and two subsequent doses (26). However, the American Academy of Oral Medicine has deferred issuing a formal standard for antibiotic prophylaxis in patients with orthopedic prostheses.

LUNG ABSCESS

Definition

Lung abscess refers to pulmonary suppuration with parenchymal necrosis caused by bacterial infection. The lesions are traditionally classified on the basis of clinical and bacteriologic observations. Lung abscesses are considered *acute or chronic* depending on the duration of symptoms at the time of initial presentation, with the usual dividing line being 4 to 6 weeks. Clinically, lung abscesses are often grouped as *putrid* lung abscess, in reference to the foul odor of sputum that is regarded as diagnostic of anaerobic infection, or *nonspecific* lung abscess, indicating that aerobic sputum cultures have not grown out a pathogen. Anaerobic bacteria are the presumed pathogens in these cases also. Lung abscesses may also be classified clinically as primary or secondary, depending on predisposing conditions. *Primary* lung abscesses are those that occur in patients who are prone to aspiration or in previously healthy patients. *Secondary* abscesses are complications of a local lesion such as a pulmonary malignancy or of a systemic disease that compromises immunologic defenses. Approximately 80% of lung abscesses are primary; 60% are putrid, and 40% are nonspecific (probably mostly anaerobic) (2). Patients with lung abscess often present in the ambulatory care setting because of the chronicity of these infections. Most patients are hospitalized for diagnostic studies and initial treatment with intravenous antibiotics. The hospital course is usually followed by prolonged courses of antibiotics and follow-up chest radiographs.

Clinical Presentation and Bacteriology

Many bacteria are potential pulmonary pathogens, but few organisms are likely to cause parenchymal necrosis. The most common pathogens are anaerobic bacteria that make up the normal flora of the gingival crevice and are aspirated during periods of altered consciousness. The usual pathogens in such cases are *Prevotella* spp., *Bacteroides* spp., anaerobic streptococci, and *Fusobacterium nucleatum* (2). The most common aerobic bacteria that cause suppurative pulmonary infections are *S. aureus* and *Klebsiella pneumoniae;* less common causal pathogens are *Streptococcus pyogenes, S. pneumoniae, H. influenzae, P. aeruginosa, Legionella, Nocardia,* and enteric Gram-negative bacilli other than *K. pneumoniae.* It is important to exclude other etiologic agents such as mycobacteria and fungi that may cause chronic abscesses requiring an entirely different antimicrobial regimen. Tuberculosis should be suspected in any patient with a lung abscess, especially patients with a cough for 1 month to 1 year, nonputrid sputum, and typical clinical features of night sweats and weight loss.

Patients with anaerobic lung abscesses usually have indolent complaints that last for weeks or even months. Common symptoms include fever, malaise, cough, and sputum production. Pleuritic pain and hemoptysis are common and may persuade a chronically ill patient to seek medical attention. Chills are occasionally noted, but true rigors are rare. The common observation of anemia and weight loss reflects the chronicity of many of these infections. The sputum is usually purulent, and putrid odor is noted in approximately 60% of bacteriologically confirmed anaerobic lung abscesses. The usual sites of involvement are the anatomic segments of the lung where aspiration is most likely to occur by gravitational flow in the recumbent position. These are the superior segments of the lower lobes and the posterior segments of the upper lobes. Less common abscess sites are the basilar segments of the lower lobes, which are dependent in the upright or semi-upright position.

Lung abscesses caused by aerobic bacteria are usually found in specific clinical settings. Staphylococcal pulmonary infections with abscess formation are particularly common in young children and in adults with influenza or hospital-acquired pneumonia. *Klebsiella* is often suspected as a cause of lung abscess in alcoholic patients, but even in these patients anaerobic organisms are far more common. The immunologically compromised patient may have pulmonary suppuration caused by a variety of bacterial and nonbacterial organisms, but anaerobes appear to be distinctly unusual in this population.

Laboratory Examination

The initial evaluations in patients with the symptoms of lung abscess are those recommended for patients with suspected pulmonary infections in general. These include a chest radiograph, a complete blood count, blood cultures, and an examination of expectorated sputum. Gram's stain of respiratory secretions typically shows a mixed or polymicrobial flora. The lung abscess generally is readily apparent with the chest radiograph (Fig. 31.3), although other causes of a pulmonary cavity must be considered in the differential diagnosis. Alternative considerations include a cavitating neoplasm, cavitating pulmonary infarction, tuberculosis, fungal infection, an infected pulmonary cyst or bulla, and a loculated empyema (i.e., pleural space infection) with an air–fluid level caused by a bronchopleural fistula, gas-producing organisms, or Wegener's granulomatosis.

When a cavitary lesion appears to be caused by bacterial infection, there is controversy about the approach to identifying the likely pathogen. Sputum should be examined using Gram's stain and Ziehl–Nielson stain to determine from the outset whether an anaerobic pathogen or *Mycobacterium tuberculosis* is the likely cause of the abscess.

Expectorated sputum is easily obtained from most patients, and standard cultures usually show a predominance of an aerobic organism when it is the etiologic pathogen. The problem with these specimens is that they are inappropriate for anaerobic culture, and the results with aerobic cultures are often misleading because of contamination by bacteria that reside in the upper airway.

Bronchoscopy is generally not useful for microbiological studies except for mycobacterial and nonbacterial pathogens; an exception is when specimens are obtained with a specialized double catheter and are cultured quantitatively for aerobes and anaerobes.

Antimicrobial Treatment

Antimicrobials are the mainstay of treatment for lung abscess (Table 31.3). The best-studied regimens are those for anaerobic lung abscesses because these account for most cases. Nevertheless, there is considerable controversy regarding the selection of agents and the duration of treatment.

Anaerobic Infections

With regard to drug selection, the initial antimicrobial recommended by most authorities is *clindamycin,* which is active against most anaerobic bacteria. In approximately 25% of patients, anaerobic organisms resistant to penicillin are present, and nearly all of these organisms are highly sensitive to clindamycin. Not surprisingly, comparative trials showed that clindamycin was superior to penicillin in terms of the primary response rates and the duration of fever after the institution of treatment (15), two factors that may allow earlier hospital discharge. The initial treatment is usually given parenterally (600 mg intravenously every 8 hours) until the patient is afebrile and there is subjective improvement. This generally requires 3 to 7 days but may be considerably longer in patients with very large lung abscesses, patients with prolonged symptoms before treatment, and patients with pleural complications (primary empyema). The major alternative antibiotics are amoxicillin–clavulanate (875 mg orally twice daily) or penicillin (10 million units intravenously daily) plus metronidazole (500 to 750 mg twice daily).

Aerobic Infections

Guidelines for antimicrobial selection are less precise for lung abscesses involving other organisms. In these cases, the antibiotic is selected on the basis of in vitro sensitivity tests. Abscesses involving *S. aureus* or Gram-negative bacilli are regarded as more serious infections, and intravenous antibiotics should be given for a more prolonged period; in selected stable patients, the intravenous regimen can be completed at home.

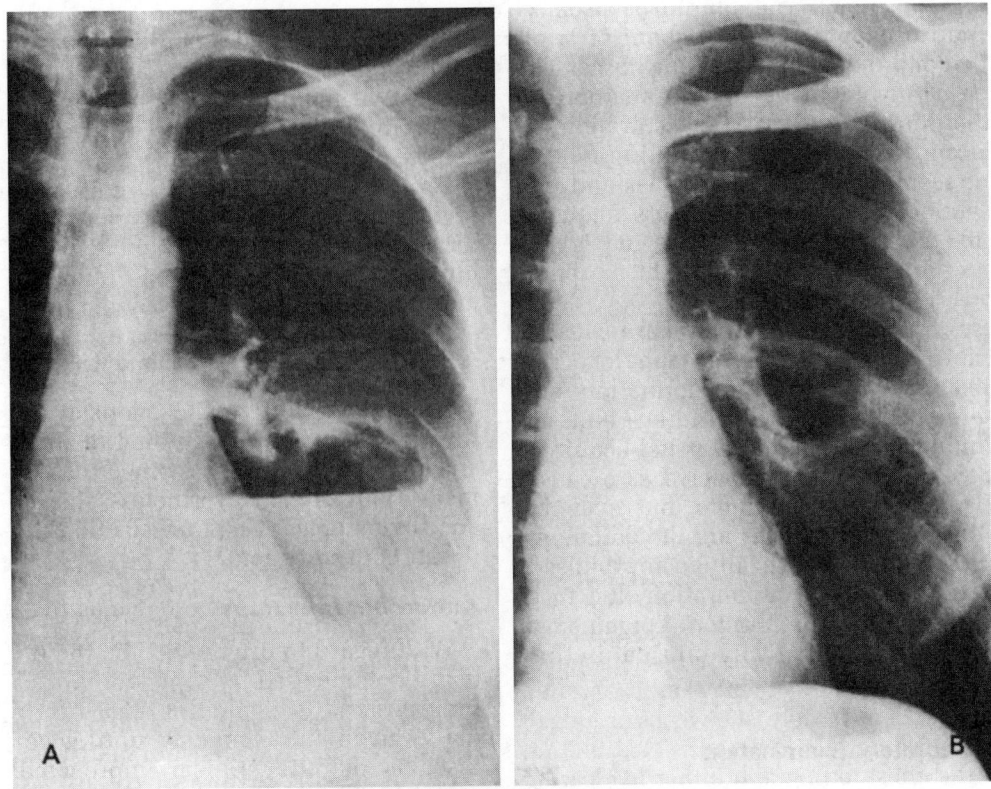

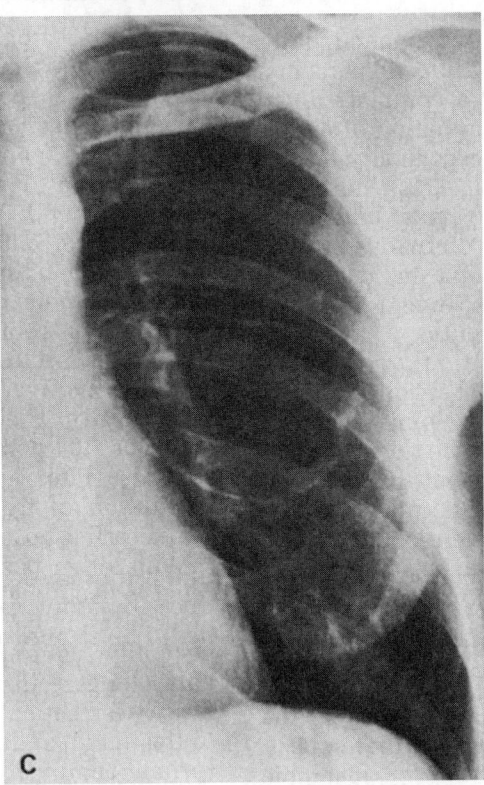

Figure 31.3. Putrid lung abscess. **A.** July 6, 1976. The patient developed fever and coughed up foul sputum after an epileptic attack. The huge cavity with an air–fluid level in the left lower lobe suggests a pyopneumothorax. However, the irregularity of the cavity wall indicates that it lies within the lung rather than in the pleura. **B.** August 3, 1976. On antibiotic therapy, the cavity has become much smaller and there is no longer an air–fluid level. **C.** September 20, 1976. Although the patient is clinically well, the cavity has increased in size. Its wall is thin and smooth, and there are infiltrations in the lung around the cavity. The ballooning of the cavity was noted after an attack of asthma. The increase in size was caused entirely by air trapping because of the bronchospasm and does not indicate reactivation of the infection. (From Rabin CB, Baron MG. Radiology of the chest. 2nd ed. Baltimore: Williams & Wilkins, 1980;340.)

Table 31.3. Antimicrobial Regimens for Primary Lung Abscess

Intravenous[a]	Oral[a]	Comments
Aqueous penicillin G 5–10 million units/day	Penicillin G or V 500–750 mg four times a day *or* Amoxicillin 500 mg four times a day *or*	Regarded as standard *Advantages:* Inexpensive and well tolerated *Disadvantages:* Approximately 20% fail to respond and additional patients have delayed response
	Amoxicillin–clavulanate 250–500 mg every 8 hours[b] *or*	*Advantage:* Coverage for organisms that produce β-lactamase *Disadvantage:* Expensive
Clindamycin 600 mg every 6–8 hours	Clindamycin 300 mg four times a day	*Advantage:* Opitmal response rates *Disadvantages:* Expensive; side effects include 10–20% with diarrhea and occasional patients with pseudomembranous colitis

[a]Intravenous treatment until patient is afebrile and clinically improved; oral treatment is given either to complete an arbitrary total course of 3 to 6 weeks of treatment or until chest radiographs show clearance or a small, stable residual lesion.

[b]Both strengths listed are for amoxicillin; both contain 125 mg of clavulanate.

Duration of Treatment

Rigorous studies to determine the optimal duration of antimicrobial treatment for lung abscesses have not been done. The duration of treatment is arbitrary, but most authorities recommend at least 6 weeks or longer depending on results of serial radiographs. Antibiotics are given until the chest radiograph either is clear or shows only a small stable residual lesion (Fig. 31.3). These recommendations are based on experiences in which patients have had relapses despite treatment for at least 1 month; in these patients the infiltrate was still resolving when drugs were discontinued, and the patients were subsequently readmitted for recurrent abscesses in the same pulmonary segment. The usual oral regimen with clindamycin is 300 mg four times daily.

Regardless of the total duration of treatment, adequate follow-up is necessary to ensure resolution with serial radiographs. These should be obtained at 2- to 3-week intervals, or earlier if there is clinical deterioration. Most patients with lung abscess treated with antibiotics improve clinically before there is demonstrable improvement in the chest radiograph; cavities gradually close, but 20 to 30% persist beyond 6 weeks, and the roentgenographic criteria for cure as defined above may require several months (14).

Inadequate Response to Treatment

Failure to show progressive improvement, especially if accompanied by clinical symptoms, necessitates a change in medical therapy, bronchoscopy (to rule out obstruction), or on rare occasions, surgery. The major indications for surgery are an abscess that is totally refractory to antibiotic treatment, life-threatening or persistent hemorrhage, and abscesses occurring in association with an obstructed bronchus (12).

ENDOCARDITIS

Definition

Endocarditis refers to infections involving heart valves, usually caused by bacteria, but occasionally caused by other microbes such as *Rickettsia* or fungi. There is a spectrum of clinical findings, but patients with the subacute form of the disease may have symptoms that are notably vague and nonspecific. The principal criteria for making the diagnosis are documented fever, heart murmur, and positive blood cultures. A unique feature of the disease is that most patients have continuous bacteremia so that blood cultures are positive in 95% of patients, regardless of the temporal relationship between blood samplings and temperature profile. All patients with endocarditis should be hospitalized for complete diagnostic evaluation, supportive care, and initiation of treatment with antibiotics, given intravenously. This discussion addresses the management of these patients in the ambulatory care setting following hospitalization.

Treatment

Antimicrobial Treatment out of Hospital

Antibiotics are selected for patients with endocarditis according to in vitro sensitivity tests, with emphasis on bactericidal activity. Most patients are treated with specific regimens according to guidelines from authoritative sources. The standard of treatment has traditionally been 4 to 6 weeks of intravenous antibiotics. Many authorities now endorse a 2-week regimen of penicillin and streptomycin for infections caused by penicillin-sensitive strains of *Streptococcus viridans* and *Streptococcus bovis* (4), and most recommend prolonged courses for patients with prosthetic valve endocarditis (28). When intravenous antibiotics are planned for several weeks, part of the parenteral course can be administered at home to expedite hospital discharge.

Abbreviated courses of intravenous or oral antibiotics have been suggested for staphylococcal tricuspid valve endocarditis as a complication of intravenous drug abuse (9,23). The advantages of this plan are that it is substantially less expensive, it reduces the problem of venous access, and it appears to be highly effective. The *oral regimen* studied most extensively is ciprofloxacin (750 mg twice daily) plus rifampin

(300 mg twice daily), but *S. aureus* is showing escalating rates of resistance to all fluoroquinolones, so use should be restricted to cases showing good bactericidal activity in vitro. Alternatively, initial treatment may be with intravenous agents such as nafcillin (2 g every 4 hours) with or without gentamycin (1 mg/kg every 8 hours) for 2 weeks, followed by oral administration of ciprofloxacin or cephalexin (500 mg every 6 hours) (8). The duration of treatment should be 4 weeks.

Patients with *prosthetic valve endocarditis* have infections that have proved particularly difficult to cure without intervening surgery. Nevertheless, intravenous antibiotics are given with the aim of avoiding re-operation; this is a realistic goal with antibiotic-sensitive organisms. The most common pathogen in these cases is *S. epidermidis,* which is treated for at least 6 weeks with intravenous drugs selected on the basis of in vitro sensitivity tests. The usual regimen is a penicillinase-resistant penicillin (nafcillin or oxacillin, 2 g every 4 hours) or vancomycin (30 mg/kg daily) for at least 6 weeks combined with gentamycin (1 mg/kg every 8 hours) for the first 2 weeks (4). For methicillin-resistant strains the regimen is vancomycin and rifampin (300 mg orally every 12 hours) for at least 6 weeks and gentamycin for 2 weeks. Many authorities recommend prolonged courses of oral antibiotics after the initial intravenous regimen, such as dicloxacillin or cephalexin in a divided dose of 2 g/day. Because these patients are often stable, it is reasonable to complete a course of dicloxacillin or cephalexin combined with rifampin, 600 to 900 mg/day, out of hospital. This oral regimen is continued for arbitrarily defined periods that range from several weeks to 6 months or longer (28). Because *rifampin reduces the effect of warfarin,* which is part of the medical regimen of patients with prosthetic valves, patients taking rifampin typically need an increase in their warfarin dosage.

Long-Term Follow-Up and Prognosis

Patients with endocarditis treated medically or surgically should be followed carefully after discontinuation of antibiotics. Major *complications* during this recovery phase include congestive heart failure, relapse, mycotic aneurysms, and recurrences involving new organisms.

Blood cultures are commonly recommended after discontinuation of antibiotic treatment, usually 2 to 3 days later. Patients who have had an inadequate course of therapy usually relapse within this time frame. Patients most likely to relapse are those with prosthetic valve endocarditis and endocarditis involving organisms resistant to antibiotics. The presence of positive blood cultures without a clearly identifiable portal of entry in the recovery phase is presumptive evidence of relapse. The usual recommendation is another course of antibiotics or surgery for a refractory infection. The choice between these two approaches is made on the basis of the extent of the initial treatment course, underlying valve disease, and the in vitro sensitivity of the organism, with particular attention to bactericidal activity. The patient should also be warned

of the possibility of relapse and should be instructed to monitor temperature, especially in the evening, when elevations are most likely to be noted.

Cardiac function should be followed carefully during and after antibiotic treatment for endocarditis. Valve replacement is a rather common practice during active infection, especially in the 6 to 20% of patients who satisfy certain, often somewhat arbitrary criteria. It should be noted, however, that the mortality rate of surgery performed during active infection is substantially higher than surgery performed on an elective basis. When possible, valve replacement should be conducted 6 weeks or longer after antibiotics have been discontinued. The major indication is congestive heart failure that proves difficult to control with medical management.

Mycotic aneurysms may become apparent at any time during the course of endocarditis, but most become clinically apparent several months or even years after treatment. These lesions usually occur at arterial bifurcations and have been reported in up to 15% of cases. The vessels most often involved are intracranial; next in frequency are chest and abdominal arteries. The diagnostic evaluation usually consists of computed tomography, when the central nervous system is involved, and arteriography for lesions suspected there or in other locations. Surgical correction is almost always indicated.

Anticoagulation is usually avoided during active endocarditis because of the danger of bleeding from unrecognized aneurysms or from embolic infarctions. However, in patients who are receiving anticoagulants for prosthetic valves, anticoagulation should be continued in the absence of a bleeding complication.

It must be remembered that any patient with endocarditis is at risk for another infection. These patients should be warned about this potential complication with endoscopy, surgery, and dental procedures. It is good practice to supply all patients who are at risk for endocarditis with the wallet-sized card provided by the American Heart Association that contains recommendations for *antibiotic prophylaxis* with various procedures (see Chapter 86, Table 86.13). This serves the dual role of emphasizing the importance of prophylaxis to the patient and ensuring that specific guidelines will be available to health professionals who may be performing procedures on the patient that can cause bacteremia.

General References*

Gilbert DN, Dworkin RJ, Raber SR, Leggett JE. Outpatient parenteral antimicrobial-drug therapy. N Engl J Med 12:829, 1997.
    Detailed review of available infusion systems and of medical information related to parenteral administration of antibiotics to outpatients.

Osteomyelitis

Lew DP, Waldvogel FA. Osteomyelitis. N Engl J Med 336:999, 1997.
Waldvogel FA, Medoff G, Swartz M. Osteomyelitis: a review of clinical features, therapeutic considerations and unusual aspects. I, II, and III. N Engl J Med 282:198, 260, 316, 1970.

*Bold print (general references) and bold numerals (specific references) denote published controlled clinical trials, meta-analyses, or consensus-based recommendations.

Waldvogel FA, Vasey H. Osteomyelitis: the past decade. N Engl J Med 303:360, 1980.

   Thorough, well-references reviews, updated periodically.

Lung Abscess

Bartlett JG. Anaerobic bacterial infections of the lung and pleural space. Clin Infect Dis 16:S248, 1993.

Gopalakrishna KV, Lerner PI. Primary lung abscess. Cleve Clin Q 42:3, 1975.

Perlman LV, Lerner E, D'sops N. Classification and analysis of 97 cases of lung abscess. Am Rev Respir Dis 99:390, 1969.

Endocarditis

Bayliss R, Clark C, Oakley CM, et al. The microbiology and pathogenesis of infective endocarditis. Br Heart J 50:513, 1983.

Bayliss R, Clark C, Oakley CM, et al. The teeth and infective endocarditis. Br Heart J 50:506, 1983.

Watanakununakorn C, Burkert T. Infective endocarditis in a large community teaching hospital. Medicine 72:90, 1993.

Specific References

1. Austrian R, Winston AL. The efficacy of penicillin V (phenoxymethylpenicillin) in the treatment of mild and of moderately severe pneumococcal pneumonia. Am J Med Sci 232:624, 1956.
2. Bartlett JG. Anaerobic bacterial infections of the lung. Chest 91:901, 1987.
3. Bell S. Further observations on the value of oral penicillins in chronic staphylococcal osteomyelitis. Med J Aust 2:591, 1976.
4. Bisno AL, Dismukes WE, Durak DT, et al. Antimicrobial treatment of infective endocarditis due to viridans streptococci, enterococci, and staphylococci. JAMA 261:1471, 1989.
5. Black J, Hunt TL, Godley PJ, Matthew E. Oral antimicrobial therapy for adults with osteomyelitis or septic arthritis. J Infect Dis 155:968, 1987.
6. Caputo GM, Cavanagh PR, Ulbrecht JS, et al. Assessment and management of foot disease in patients with diabetes. N Engl J Med 331:854, 1994.
7. Centers for Disease Control and Prevention. Public focus: surveillance, prevention and control of nosocomial infections. MMWR 41:783, 1992.
8. Chambers HF, Miller RT, Newman MD. Right-sided *Staphylococcus aureus* endocarditis in intravenous drug abusers: two-week combination therapy. Ann Intern Med 109:619, 1988.
9. Dworkin RJ, Sande MA, Lee BL, Chamgers HF. Treatment of right-sided *Staphylococcus aureus* endocarditis in intravenous drug users with ciprofloxacin and rifampin. Lancet 2:1071, 1989.
10. Gentry LO, Rodriguez-Gomez G. Ofloxacin versus parenteral therapy for chronic osteomyelitis. Antimicrob Agents Chemother 35:538, 1991.
11. Grayson ML, Gibbons GW, Balogy K, et al. Probing to bone in infected pedal ulcers: a clinical sign of underlying osteomyelitis in diabetic patient. JAMA 273:721, 1995.
12. Hagan JL, Hardy JD. Lung abscess revisited. A survey of 184 cases. Am Surg 197:755, 1983.

13. Howard CB, Einhorn M, Dagan R, et al. Fine-needle bone biopsy to diagnose osteomyelitis. J Bone Joint Surg BR 76:311, 1994.
14. Landay MJ, Christensen EE, Bynum LJ, Goodman C. Anaerobic pleural and pulmonary infection. AJR 134:233, 1980.
15. Levinson ME, Mangura CT, Lorber B, et al. Clindamycin compared with penicillin for the treatment of anaerobic lung abscess. Ann Intern Med 98:466, 1983.
16. Lew DP, Waldvogel FA. Osteomyelitis. N Engl J Med 336:999, 1997.
17. Lew DP, Waldvogel FA. Quinolones and osteomyelitis: state of the art. Drugs 49(Suppl 2):100, 1995.
18. Littenberg B, Mushlin AL. Technetium bone scanning in the diagnosis of osteomyelitis: a meta-analysis of test performance. J Gen Intern Med 7:158, 1992.
19. MacGregor RR, Graziani AL. Oral administration of antibiotics: a rational alternative to the parenteral route. Clin Infect Dis 24:457, 1997.
20. Mackowiak POA, Jones SR, Smith JW. Diagnostic value of sinus-tract cultures in chronic osteomyelitis. JAMA 239:2772, 1978.
21. Mader JT, Norden C, Nelson JD, et al. Evaluation of new anti-infective drugs for the treatment of osteomyelitis in adults: Infectious Diseases Society of American and the Food and Drug Administration. Clin Infect Dis 15(Suppl 1):S155, 1992.
22. Malik IA, Abbas Z, Karim M. Randomized comparison of oral ofloxacin alone with combination of parenteral antibiotics in neutropenic febrile patients. Lancet 339:1092, 1992.
23. Munoz P, Berenguer J, Rodriques-Zreixems M, et al. Ciprofloxacin and infective endocarditis. Infect Dis Clin Pract 2:119, 1993.
24. Nelson JD. A critical review of the role of oral antibiotics in the management of hematogenous osteomyelitis. In: Remington RS, Swartz MN, eds. Clinical topics in infectious diseases. Vol. 4. New York: McGraw-Hill, 1996;64–74.
25. Newman LG, Waller J, Palestro CJ, et al. Unsuspected osteomyelitis in diabetic foot ulcers. Diagnosis and monitoring by leukocyte scanning with indium In 111 oxyquinoline. JAMA 266:1246, 1991.
26. Norden CW. Antibiotic prophylaxis in orthopedic surgery. Rev Infect Dis 13:S842, 1991.
27. Norden C, Nelson JD, Mader JT, Calandra GB. Evaluation of new anti-infective drugs for the treatment of infections of prosthetic hip joints: Infectious Diseases Society of America and the Food and Drug Administration. Clin Infect Dis 15(Suppl 2):S177, 1992.
28. Sande MA, Scheld WM. Combination antibiotic therapy of bacterial endocarditis. Ann Intern Med 92:390, 1980.
29. Sugarman B, Hawes S, Musher DM, et al. Osteomyelitis beneath pressure sores. Arch Intern Med 143:683, 1983.
30. Tumeh SS, Tohmeh AG. Nuclear medicine techniques in septic arthritis and osteomyelitis. Rheum Dis Clin North Am 17:559, 1991.
31. Wagner DK, Collier BC, Rytel MW. Long-term intravenous antibiotic therapy in chronic osteomyelitis. Arch Intern Med 145:1073, 1985.
32. West WF, Kelly P, Martin WJ. Chronic osteomyelitis. I. Factors affecting the results of treatment in 186 patients. JAMA 213: 1837, 1970.

CHAPTER 32

Immunization to Prevent Infectious Disease*

WILLIAM H. BARKER, MD

Protection against infectious diseases can be conferred by active immunization with vaccines and by passive immunization with immune globulin (IG) preparations. Additional vaccines will become available in the next few years, and additional information will be generated to improve our understanding of the mechanisms of immune response to vaccines. Therefore, it can be expected that recommendations appropriate today will be revised in the future. This chapter describes vaccines and IG preparations available in the United States, focusing on several questions commonly considered in practice: Who should receive specific immunization? When should they receive it? and What are the common side effects or adverse

reactions? Chapter 33 provides similar information on immunization for travelers to developing countries.

PATIENT ASSESSMENT

History

A history of immunizations should be obtained from all patients. In young adults, this information may be readily available, but in older persons it is often hard to obtain. Patients may or may not keep personal records that are of use. People who have served in the military will have received routinely recommended immunizations as well as several additional vaccines not generally administered to the general population. People who often travel abroad should have this information recorded on their International Vaccination Card. Immunization history is particularly important in determining whether to give tetanus toxoid or antitoxin after an injury, whether diphtheria should be seriously considered in the diagnosis of acute pharyngitis (see Chapter 28), and what immunizations are needed by patients who plan to travel outside the United States (see Chapter 33).

A history of allergic reactions or other untoward reactions to vaccines or their components should always be excluded before giving an immunization. Most modern vaccines are highly purified, and allergic reactions after their use are rare. However, a history of a severe adverse reaction to a vaccine is a contraindication to its further use. Anyone with a history of severe allergic reactions after eating eggs should not receive vaccines made in eggs (e.g., influenza and yellow fever vaccines). Viral vaccines prepared in tissue culture often contain small amounts of antibiotics (especially neomycin) to which some patients may be allergic. For patients with previous allergic reactions to any vaccine, the contents of each vaccine should be determined from the package insert before administration. Some patients may experience unusually severe toxic inflammatory reactions to bacterial vaccines such as typhoid and cholera vaccines.

Immunization with live virus vaccines is generally contraindicated in patients with known *immunodeficiency syndromes* or recent treatment with *immunosuppressive drugs*. Patients known to be infected with the human immunodeficiency virus (HIV) may be at increased risk when receiving live vaccines, although adverse effects have been documented infrequently. *Pregnant women*, in whom a vaccine virus might pose a risk to the fetus, should generally not be given live vaccines. In addition to ascertaining by history that a woman of childbearing age is not pregnant, it is important to counsel the patient to use contraceptive practices to prevent pregnancy for 3 months after immunization with a live vaccine (see Chapter 93, "Birth Control"). The risk of unavoidable and imminent exposure of a nonimmune pregnant woman to certain viruses, notably polioviruses and yellow fever virus, may justify use of the corresponding live vaccines. Prophylactic use of IG and the various hyperimmune globulin preparations is considered safe in pregnancy.

*Louis F. Fries, MD, and Neal A. Halsey, MD, contributed to this chapter in previous editions.

Recent administration of IG preparations requires that the use of some live virus vaccines be postponed because passively acquired immunity may interfere with the active response to the vaccine (24). IG preparations should not be administered earlier than 2 weeks after live virus vaccine so that the vaccine virus can stimulate an active immune response. Yellow fever and oral polio vaccines are exceptions because interference does not occur. These vaccines can be given without regard to IG administration.

Minor illness (e.g., upper respiratory infection with or without a low-grade fever) is not a contraindication to necessary immunization. A patient with moderate or *severe acute illness* should generally not be immunized until after the illness has resolved, both because vaccine side effects might add to the patient's morbidity and because the effectiveness of the vaccination may be diminished.

Physical and Laboratory Evaluation

When immunization is contemplated, physical examination and laboratory testing usually add little to the assessment of the patient. Pregnancy or an acute illness (see above) may be confirmed on examination if the history suggests one of these; and findings suggestive of an immunodeficiency syndrome should be pursued with appropriate clinical laboratory studies.

Serologic tests are useful in deciding whether to immunize adults in selected situations. When considering the use of hyperimmune globulin preparations or hepatitis B vaccine for protection against hepatitis B, the demonstration of preexisting antibody to hepatitis B makes additional protection superfluous. The decision regarding screening for antibodies before vaccination should be based on the estimated prevalence of markers for hepatitis B infections in the population from which the patient comes and the cost of serologic testing (see below). Similarly, when considering the use of rubella vaccine in a woman of childbearing age, the presence of antibodies to rubella virus obviates the need for vaccination.

IMMUNIZATION PROCEDURES

The package insert for a vaccine always includes information about dosage, route, site of administration, interval between immunizations, common and uncommon side effects, contraindications, potential trace contaminants that may cause hypersensitivity reactions, and appropriate storage conditions for the vaccine.

Simultaneous Vaccine Administration

Many widely used vaccines can be given simultaneously. The Advisory Committee on Immunization Practices (ACIP) of the Centers for Disease Control and Prevention list the following guidelines for simultaneous vaccine administration. Inactivated vaccines can be administered simultaneously at separate sites or at the same site with combination preparations. Tetanus and diphtheria toxoids (Td) are most effectively given together as a combined vaccine. However, when vaccines commonly associated with side effects are given together, the side effects may be accentuated and consideration should be given to vaccinating on separate occasions. An inactivated vaccine and a live, attenuated virus vaccine can be administered simultaneously at separate sites. Some live virus vaccines are routinely given together. Measles, mumps, and rubella (MMR) vaccines constitute a combined live virus vaccine that can be given to any age group.

Patients should be informed of the risks and benefits associated with any vaccine in understandable lay terms. The range of common side effects and appropriate symptomatic therapies should be explained. Because of the rare possibility of anaphylactic reactions, patients receiving any immunization should be observed for about 15 minutes. Finally, patients should be clearly informed of the name of the immunizations they have received and be encouraged to keep a written record of them. Official immunization cards are available in every state for this purpose.

Physicians and health care providers are required to maintain permanent records of immunization and to report certain adverse effects after immunization with the usual childhood vaccines to the U. S. Department of Health and Human Services (4). These recording requirements are summarized in the FDA Drug Bulletin (6). Similar record keeping for all immunizations in childhood and adulthood is prudent.

CURRENT RECOMMENDATIONS FOR VACCINES AND IMMUNE GLOBULINS

Table 32.1 summarizes the major and commonly used vaccines and IG preparations available in the United States. The following sections provide practical information on selected infectious diseases for which immune protection of adults is most likely to be undertaken in ambulatory practice.

INFORMATION FOR PATIENTS ABOUT VACCINATION SCHEDULES

Table 32.2, furnished by the National Coalition for Adult Immunization (NCAI), provides a quick reference that can be provided to adults so that they are aware of appropriate scheduling of recommended vaccines. Chapter 5 ("Adolescent Patients") provides similar information for adolescents. A *new strategy for ensuring vaccination of adolescents* recommends routine preventive care visits to health care providers for patients 11 to 12 years of age to vaccinate adolescents who have not been previously vaccinated with varicella virus vaccine, hepatitis B vaccine, or the second dose of MMR vaccine; to provide a booster dose of tetanus and diphtheria toxoids; to administer other vaccines that may be recommended for certain adolescents; and to provide other recommended preventive services (23).

Table 32.1. Characteristics and Administration of Commonly Used Vaccines and Immune Globulin Preparations (See Details in Text)

Vaccine or Immune Globulin (Ref)	Type of Preparation	Population to Be Immunized[a]	Usual Age and Immunization Schedule[b]	Common Adverse Reactions[c]
Diphtheria toxoid (12)	Toxoid	All	Childhood; series of 3 primary injections (day 0, 1 mo, 6–12 mo) with boosters every 10 yr[d]	Local pain and swelling
Tetanus toxoid (12)	Toxoid	All	Childhood; series of 3 IM injections (day 0, 1 mo, 6–12 mo) with boosters every 10 yr[d]	Local pain and swelling
Tetanus immune globulin (TIG) (12)	High-titered human immune globulin	Unimmunized person with wound	Single IM injection (250 units)	Not significant
Acellular pertussis vaccine (13)	Fractionated killed bacteria and toxoid	All children	2, 4, 6 mo, 15–18 mo, and 4–6 yr	Mild fever, fretfulness
Measles vaccine (19)	Live, attenuated virus[a]	All children	12–15 mo and 4–6 yr or 11–12 yr	Fever, rash
Rubella vaccine (19)	Live, attenuated virus[a]	All children and unimmunized women	12–15 mo and 4–6 yr or 11–12 yr, women through childbearing age with measles vaccine as MMR	Arthralgias, fever
Mumps vaccine (19)	Live, attenuated virus[a]	All children and young adults without history of mumps	12–15 mo and 4–6 yr or 11–12 yr with measles vaccine as MMR	Not significant
Polio vaccine, oral (OPV) Parenteral (IPV)	Live, attenuated virus; Killed virus	All; All	Ages 2, 4 mo, 12–18 mo, and 4–6 yr; Children or adults (preferred for adults); primary series of 3 doses	Rare paralytic disease; Not significant
Polio, IPV and OPV (20)		All	IPV at 2 and 4 mo; OPV at 12–18 mo and 4–6 yr	Not significant
Haemophilus influenzae type B	Conjugated purified polysaccharide	All children, high-risk adults (asplenic)	Children, some adults; series of 3 injections beginning at 2 mo	Not significant
Hepatitis B vaccine (15)	Recombinant proteins from yeast	All (eventually)	Childhood, selected adults; 3 injections (0 time, 1 mo, 6 mo in adults; birth, 1–2 mo, third dose at 6–12 mo in children)	Not significant
Hepatitis B immune globulin (15)	High-titered human γ-globulin	Persons exposed to hepatitis B	0.06 mL/kg at time of exposure and again 1 mo later	Not significant
Hepatitis A vaccine (14)	Killed virus	Selected children and adults with high risk of exposure, travelers to Hepatitis A endemic lands	Initial dose followed by booster dose 6–12 mo later	Local soreness
Influenza vaccine (16)	Killed virus (whole virus and "split virus" preparations) preparations of virus change yearly	Persons at high risk, elderly, or chronically ill	Adults: single injection (whole virus) repeated yearly; Children under 12: split virus preparation, 2 doses	Fever, local tenderness
Immune globulin (IG)	Pooled human γ-globulin	Persons exposed to hepatitis A and B or measles	Usually adults; Hepatitis A: 0.02 mL/kg, once; Hepatitis B: 0.06 mL/kg, twice; Measles: 0.25 mL/kg, once	Pain
Meningococcal vaccine (18)	Purified polysaccharide (serogroups A, C, Y, W135)	Only during epidemic disease; those at high risk	All ages; young adult military; Single injection	Erythema at injection site
Rabies vaccine (21)	Killed virus	Persons bitten by possibly rabid animal or at high risk of exposure; Unimmunized persons	Any age; postexposure: 5 doses of vaccine IM (days 1, 3, 7, 14, 28); Any age; preexposure: 3 doses of vaccine IM (days 0, 7, 21 or 28)	Pain, rare neurologic reactions, urticaria
Rabies immune globulin (HRIG) (21)	High-titered human γ-globulin	Unimmunized persons with suspicious animal bite	Any age; single injection, up to ½ unfiltrated into wound	Not significant
Pneumococcal vaccine (17)	Polyvalent purified polysaccharide (23 serotypes)	Persons with asplenia, or chronic illness, elderly	Any age (>2 yr); single injection, booster after ≥5 years (high-risk only) (see text)	Erythema at injection site
Bacillus Calmette–Guérin vaccine (BCG) (1)	Live, attenuated bacteria	Newborns in developing countries and persons with high risk of developing multiple drug-resistant tuberculosis	Infants and children; single injection, intradermal	Prolonged granuloma or ulcer at injection site, lymphadenitis
Varicella vaccine (22)	Live, attenuated virus	All children, susceptible persons ≥13 yr (especially if in contact with immunosuppressed persons)	Children 11–12 yr: single dose at 12–18 mo (if susceptible); Persons ≥13 yr: 2 doses 4–8 weeks apart	Erythema soreness at injection site
Varicella zoster immune globulin (VZIG) (22)	High-titered human δ-globulin	Immunocompromised people without history of varicella who are exposed to varicella	125 units/10 kg once, within 96 hr of exposure	Not significant

[a]Populations cited represent general ambulatory patients. Certain subsets (HIV-infected, other immunocompromised persons) may benefit from specifically tailored immunization programs (see Chapter 34).
[b]All injections are intramuscular unless otherwise specified. Schedules given are for adults unless the vaccine is used solely in pediatric age group.
[c]Reactions listed are most common and/or serious. This listing is *not* exhaustive. Allergic hypersensitivity is possible with almost any vaccine, but is rare.
[d]Boosters of diphtheria and tetanus are particularly important for those traveling to underdeveloped countries. Diphtheria and tetanus vaccines should be given in combined (Td) preparation. (See also Table 32.4).
[e]Given as the combination mumps, measles, and rubella vaccine (MMR). (See additional details about measles vaccine in Tables 32.5 and 32.6)

Table 32-2. Information About Immunization Schedules that Can Be Provided to Adults

Infection Prevented	Timing of Immunizations			
ADULT				
Hepatitis A (Hep A) for those at risk[a]	Two doses are recommended for long-term protection.			
	First dose		Second dose 6 to 12 months later	
Hepatitis B (Hep B) for those at risk[a]	First dose	Second dose 1 month later	Third dose 5 months after second dose	
Measles, mumps, rubella (MMR)	One dose is recommended for adults born in 1957 or later if not previously immunized. (Second dose may be required in some work or school settings.)			
Tetanus, diphtheria (Td) if initial series not given during childhood	First dose	Second dose 1 month later	Third dose 6 months after second dose	Booster shot every 10 years
Varicella (chickenpox)	Two doses are recommended for those 13 and older who have not had chickenpox.			
	First dose		Second dose 1 to 2 months later	
OLDER ADULTS AND THOSE WITH CHRONIC ILLNESSES				
Influenza (flu)	Given yearly in the fall to people age 65 or older. Also recommended for people younger than 65 who have medical problems such as heart disease, lung disease, and other conditions, and for others who work or live with high-risk individuals.[a]			
Pneumonia (pneumococcal only)	Usually given once at age 65 or older. A repeat dose 5 years later may be given to those at highest risk.[a] Also recommended for people younger than 65 who have chronic illnesses such as those listed for influenza, and also those with kidney disorders and sickle cell anemia.[a] Can be given at any time during the year.			

Modified from the National Coalition for Adult Immunization.
[a]Consult your doctor to determine your level of risk.

DELIVERY SYSTEMS AND CME

Underutilization and missed opportunities to provide indicated vaccination among adults enrolled in medical practices have been repeatedly documented, particularly among minority groups (26). A variety of simple techniques for improving vaccination delivery, including reminder mailings, standing orders, staff nurse roles, and tracking systems, have been shown to be effective in both private office and clinic settings (8). Continuing medical education on such techniques as well as updates on developments in adult vaccination may be accessed from the Association of Teachers of Preventive Medicine (202-463-0550) and the NCAI (301-656-0003).

PROTECTION AGAINST SELECTED INFECTIONS

Diphtheria

Fewer than five cases of diphtheria are reported each year in the United States (12). People who have never received diphtheria toxoid should be immunized and diphtheria toxoid should be given as booster doses with tetanus toxoid (Td) whenever tetanus toxoid is indicated.

For unimmunized school-aged children and adults, *adult type* (Td) tetanus and diphtheria toxoids are used. This preparation contains only approximately 25% of the diphtheria toxoid contained in the pediatric DTP (diphtheria and tetanus toxoids and pertussis vaccine) and no pertussis antigen to minimize the risk of local reactions in sensitized adults. Primary immunization in these age groups consists of an initial dose, a 1 month dose, and a third dose at 6 to 12 months. A Td booster is recommended every 10 years to ensure protection. In adults, there is a 25 to 50% incidence of local soreness, swelling, and itching after Td injections; fever occurs in less than 10% and urticaria in approximately 2% of individuals. Serious reactions (swelling of the whole arm, or anaphylaxis) occur rarely (12).

For asymptomatic unimmunized contacts of patients with diphtheria, management includes prophylactic antibiotics (600,000 units of benzathine penicillin intramuscularly or a 7-day course of erythromycin, 250 mg four times daily), primary vaccination as outlined above, and daily surveillance for 7 days for clinical evidence of diphtheria (see Chapter 28).

Tetanus

Approximately 50 cases of tetanus are reported each year in the United States. Although natural immunity to tetanus has been found in some adult populations, everyone should be regarded as susceptible unless actively immunized. Most cases in the United States occur in people over age 60, primarily in those who were never immunized. Tetanus usually occurs after penetrating wounds from accidents and animal bites (see Chapter 25). The incubation period is 4 to 21 days with an average of 10 days.

In those who have received a primary series of three doses of toxoid at any time in their life, an injection of adsorbed toxoid once every 10 years is sufficient to boost antitoxin titers to protective levels. The need for booster doses of combined diphtheria–tetanus toxoids (Td) in people with wounds depends on the number of previous doses of tetanus toxoid received and the type of wound (Table 32.3). Only alum-adsorbed toxoids should be used. Fluid toxoids are still available in the United States, but these preparations are less immunogenic than alum-adsorbed preparations (12).

Patients who require *tetanus immune globulin* (TIG) because they have not been adequately immunized (Table 32.3) should be given 250 units intramuscularly. This preparation is made from human serum, and therefore hypersensitivity reactions do not occur. Patients who require TIG should at the same time (but at a different site) be given their first dose of toxoid, followed by repeated doses of toxoid 1 month and 6 to 12 months later.

Hepatitis A

Hepatitis A is primarily transmitted by the fecal–oral route and constitutes a significant risk for people living in settings with potentially poor food, water, or personal hygiene and with high endemic rates of hepatitis A.

Two inactivated hepatitis A vaccines (Havrix, Smith Kline Beecham, and Vaqta, Merck) were licensed for use in the United States in the early 1990s. These vaccines are highly immunogenic and have shown more than 90% effectiveness in preventing clinical disease in field experiences. Long-term duration of immunity has not been tested, given the relative recency of development of these vaccines.

Vaccines should replace immune globulin for preexposure prophylaxis against hepatitis A. However, vaccines have little to offer patients exposed to active hepatitis A because of the relatively short incubation period. Exposed persons should receive passive protection with pooled human *IG,* optimally within 2 weeks of exposure. The usual dose is 0.02 mL/kg intramuscularly.

Active immunization with hepatitis A vaccine is recommended for international travelers to regions

Table 32.3. Summary Guide to Tetanus Prophylaxis in Routine Wound Management (United States)

History of Adsorbed Tetanus Toxoid Doses	Clean, Minor Wounds		All Other Wounds[a]	
	Td[b]	TIG[c]	Td[b]	TIG[c]
Uncertain or <3	Yes	No	Yes	Yes
≥3[d]	No[e]	No	No[f]	No

From MMWR 40(RR-10):1, 1991.

[a]Such as, but not limited to, wounds contaminated with dirt, feces, and saliva; puncture wounds; avulsions; and wounds resulting from missiles, crushing, burns, and frostbite.

[b]Td, tetanus and diphtheria toxoids, adsorbed (for adult use). For children <7 years old, DTP (DT, if pertussis vaccine is contraindicated) is preferred to tetanus toxoid alone. For persons ≥7 years old, Td is preferred to tetanus toxoid alone.

[c]*TIG,* Tetanus immune globulin.

[d]If only three doses of fluid toxoid have been received, a fourth dose of toxoid, preferably an adsorbed toxoid, should be given.

[e]Yes, >10 years since last dose.

[f]Yes, >5 years since last dose. (More frequent boosters are not needed and can accentuate side effects.)

with poor sanitation and endemic hepatitis, children living in communities with known high endemic rate of hepatitis A, homosexually active men, users of illicit injectable drugs, people working closely with nonhuman primates, and patients who receive clotting factor replacement concentrates (14).

Vaccine should be administered intramuscularly in the deltoid muscle, generally in a two-dose schedule, with the second dose given at 6 to 12 months; the dosage of vaccine antigen varies by patient age and by specific product. Side effects include soreness and redness at injection site, usually within 3 days, and occasional headache. Serious adverse events have not been observed.

Hepatitis B

The timing and patterns of appearance of antigens and antibodies after hepatitis B infection are illustrated in Chapter 43, Figure 43.1. Although IG in large doses (two doses of 0.06 mL/kg intramuscularly 4 weeks apart) may be useful in preventing hepatitis B, a *hyperimmune globulin preparation* (hepatitis B immune globulin [HBIG]) is preferred and is approximately 75% effective in preventing hepatitis in patients known to have direct exposure to hepatitis B virus (25). When HBIG is given at the same time as hepatitis B vaccine (see below), protection is enhanced. Exposed patients who already have antibody to the hepatitis B surface antigen (anti-HB$_s$) do not require prophylaxis.

Recombinant HB$_s$Ag vaccines (Recombivax HB, Merck; Engerix-B, Smith Kline Beecham) made in yeast have replaced plasma-derived vaccines in the United States. Recombinant vaccines are similar to the plasma-derived products in immunogenicity and efficacy (approximately 90%). The vaccines are given intramuscularly at 0, 1 to 2, and 4 to 6 months. Recommended doses vary according to age; patients who are immunocompromised or who are receiving hemodialysis should be given larger doses as specified in package inserts. The preferred vaccination site is the arm because suboptimal antibody responses have occurred when the vaccine was injected into the buttock. Soreness and redness may occur at the injection site and anaphylaxis has been documented, but this is rare. Booster doses are not routinely recommended at present; however, after 5 to 8 years, 30 to 60% of vaccine responders experience decline in antibody titers to less than 10 mIU/mL. Subclinical infections have been shown to occur in vaccinated persons, but protection against developing the chronic carrier state after the completed immunization schedule has been shown to persist for at least 9 years. The few instances of chronic carrier state developing several years after an active antibody response have occurred in immunocompromised individuals, primarily people with HIV infection.

Table 32.4 summarizes the current recommendations of the ACIP for *postexposure prophylaxis* for infants born to mothers with acute or chronic hepatitis

Table 32.4.   Recommended Prophylaxis After Perinatal, Sexual, or Household Exposure to Hepatitis B Virus

Type of Exposure	Type of Infection in Contact	Type of Prophylaxis
Perinatal	Acute or chronic	Vaccination + HBIG[a]
Sexual	Acute	HBIG[b] + Vaccination
	Chronic	Vaccination
Household contact	Chronic	Vaccination
	Acute	
	No exposure	None
	Known exposure	HBIG[b] ± vaccination
	Infant (<12 months)	Vaccination
		HBIG[a] if not vaccinated

From CDC 1997.
[a]0.5 mL.
[b]0.06 mL/kg.

B infection, sexual contacts and household contacts of persons with hepatitis B infections. Table 32.5 summarizes recommendations for postexposure prophylaxis for people who have had percutaneous, ocular, or mucous membrane exposure to blood from patients with known or suspected acute or chronic hepatitis B infections.

The American Academy of Pediatrics and the ACIP have recommended that *all infants* routinely receive hepatitis B vaccine, and routine vaccination of adolescents is encouraged when resources are available. Hepatitis B vaccine is also recommended for others who are at increased risk of exposure: health care professionals exposed frequently to blood or blood products (e.g., laboratory and blood bank personnel, operating room staff, surgeons, dentists, endoscopists, pathologists, staff in oncology, and dialysis units and emergency room staff), homosexually active men, family members or sexual partners of chronic HB$_s$Ag carriers, prostitutes, patients who frequently receive transfusions of blood or blood products, patients in hemodialysis units, inmates and staff of institutions for the mentally retarded, inmates of long-term correctional institutions, users of illicit injectable drugs, selected international travelers (see Chapter 33), people from countries with high endemic rates of HBV infection, and members of a family that adopt HB$_s$Ag-positive children. The vaccine is not routinely recommended for individuals who come in contact with HB$_s$Ag carriers at work or school. Screening for antibodies to hepatitis B virus before immunization is cost-effective only in populations in which the prevalence of such antibodies is high (e.g., intravenous drug abusers). Vaccination of individuals who have anti-HB$_s$ from previous infection does not result in increased adverse effects (15).

People at high risk of repeated exposure to blood or blood products should consider *testing for anti-HB$_s$* 1 to 3 months after the third dose of vaccine to ensure that they have responded (Tables 32.4 and 32.5). Testing at intervals of 1 year or more after vaccination may not accurately determine whether some people have responded to the vaccine (see above). The need for booster doses for adults who receive a primary series in infancy remains to be assessed.

Hepatitis C and Non–A, Non–B Hepatitis

There is no IG preparation known to be protective against the multiple agents of non–A, non–B hepatitis, which are now the most common cause of posttransfusion hepatitis. Most non–A, non–B infection is caused by hepatitis C. All blood donors are now screened for hepatitis C (10).

Hepatitis in ambulatory patients is discussed in Chapter 43.

Influenza

Inactivated virus vaccines have been available for the prevention of influenza for many years. Earlier vaccines often led to fever and malaise, but current preparations are highly purified and side effects in carefully controlled placebo studies are essentially limited to soreness at the site of the injection. Specifically, there is no evidence of increased frequency of flulike upper respiratory illness after vaccination (11). Patients with egg allergy should not receive influenza vaccination. Whole and split virus vaccines are available; either may be used in adults. The vaccine recommended each year is polyvalent, which contains antigens from the type A and B strains that are expected to prevail during that season. The efficacy of the vaccine depends on the closeness in matching between the vaccine strains and the viruses circulating that year. Influenza vaccine has had consistently high (70 to 80%) protective efficacy against acute influenza among healthy young adults in most years. Although somewhat less protective against acute upper respiratory tract influenza in older patients, influenza vaccine is generally 50 to 70% protective against life-threatening pneumonia and other cardiovascular complications in this vulnerable age group (7). A protective antibody response occurs within 2 to 3 weeks of vaccination.

Annual immunization with the current year's vaccine beginning in October, before influenza season, is recommended for those in whom influenza causes the highest morbidity and mortality. This includes all individuals over age 65 and patients of any age with significant heart, lung, metabolic, immunocompromising disease, or chronic debilitating conditions. The vaccine is also recommended for those involved in critical jobs in which absenteeism may be detrimental (e.g., firemen, policemen, selected hospital personnel). Consideration should also be given to vaccinating close contacts or caregivers interacting with the above groups and to children or teenagers receiving chronic aspirin therapy because they are at risk of Reye's syndrome. Trivial intercurrent illnesses, such as mild upper respiratory tract infections, should not be viewed as contraindications to timely influenza immunization of high-risk individuals. Medicare now reimburses physicians for influenza vaccination of patients over 65 (16).

Amantadine prophylaxis. During confirmed local outbreaks of influenza A, the antiviral drug amantadine (Symmetrel) or its derivative rimantadine (Flumadine) can be used prophylactically as well as therapeutically (see Chapter 28 for a discussion of therapeutic use). Amantadine prevents clinical disease caused by influenza A (but not type B) viruses in 70 to 90% of subjects. The prophylactic use of this drug during a local influenza A outbreak is recommended for the same high-risk patient, patient contact, and critical occupation groups as listed above under influenza vaccination.

Amantadine or rimantadine, 200 mg, should be given once daily during the local outbreak. Because of the increased risk of side effects, people over 70 should be given only 100 mg/day and frail elderly persons should receive only 50 mg/day (available in liquid form). If influenza vaccine is given, amantadine can be given simultaneously and then stopped after 2 weeks when protective antibodies will have developed. Patients should be warned of transient central nervous system side effects, which occur during the first few days in 5 to 10% of subjects: insomnia, light-headednesss, nervousness, drowsiness, and difficulty in concentration. These side effects are less common in people taking rimantadine (5).

Influenza in ambulatory patients is discussed in Chapter 28.

Pneumococcal Disease

Purified polyvalent polysaccharide vaccine is available for the prevention of disease caused by *S. pneumoniae*. Protective efficacy is estimated to be in the range of 50 to 80% against bacteremic illness with the pneumococcal serotypes in the vaccine that has been manufactured since 1983 (23 serotypes that are responsible for 80 to 90% of invasive of pneumococcal disease in the United States, including the 6 serotypes responsible for most penicillin-resistant pneumococcal disease). The vaccine is given as a single 0.5-mL dose, administered intramuscularly or subcutaneously, and it produces few untoward effects. It may be administered simultaneously with influenza vaccine, prefer-

ably in the opposite arm, without diminishing antibody response. It is recommended for all people 65 or older and for people 2 to 64 years of age with immunocompromising disease, chronic cardiac or pulmonary disease, diabetes, alcoholism, or functional (e.g., sickle cell disease) or anatomic asplenia.

Revaccination at 5-year intervals is now recommended for the following two groups: people less than 65 years of age at high risk (e.g., immunocompromised persons, because they have relatively rapid decline in antibody titer) and people 65 years of age or older who received their initial dose before they were 65 years of age. Physicians may administer a booster dose to those initially vaccinated after age 65, with no increased risk of side effects, although such boosters are not recommended by the ACIP (17).

Pneumococcal pneumonia in ambulatory practice is discussed in Chapter 28.

Measles

Measles is a moderately severe illness in most people and has been associated with an overall case fatality rate of 3:1,000 in recent years. Case fatality rates are higher in young infants and adults than in school-aged children. Since 1963, inactivated and subsequently live, attenuated measles vaccines have been available. From the 1960s, when measles vaccination of children was introduced generally in the United States, the number of cases reported annually fell from more than 400,000 to less than 1,500. However, from 1989 to 1991, more than 55,000 cases were reported, with 11,000 hospitalizations and 130 deaths (2). Although most cases in recent years have occurred in unvaccinated preschool children, measles continues to cause disease in adolescents and adults, especially in schools and other group settings. Recent data show that a single dose of measles vaccine does not confer lifelong immunity in a small proportion of people. In response to these problems, a *two-dose vaccine schedule*, preferably provided as MMR (see below), is now recommended with initial dose at 12 to 15 months of age and second dose at 4 to 6 years of age (Table 32.6). Measles vaccine is associated with transient fever (103°F or greater) or rash 7 to 12 days after vaccination in

Table 32.5. Recommendations for Hepatitis B Prophylaxis After Percutaneous or Permucosal Exposure

Exposed Person	Treatment When Source is Found to Be:		
	HB$_s$Ag Positive	HB$_s$Ag Negative	Source Not Tested or Unknown
Unvaccinated	HBIG × 1[a] and initiate HB vaccine[b]	Initiate HB vaccine[b]	Initiate HB vaccine[b]
Previously vaccinated			
Known responder	No treatment	No treatment	No treatment
Known nonresponder	HBIG × 2 *or* HBIG × 1 and initiate revaccination	No treatment	If high-risk source, treat as if HB$_s$Ag positive
Response unknown	Test exposed for anti-HB$_s$ 1. If inadequate,[c] HBIG × 1 plus HB vaccine 2. If adequate, no treatment	No treatment	Test exposed for anti-HB$_s$ 1. If inadequate,[c] initiate revaccination 2. If adequate, no treatment

From CDC 1997.

[a]HBIG dose, 0.06 mL/kg IM.

[b]Adult dose, product specific.

[c]Adequate anti-HB$_s$ is ≥10 mIU/mL by radioimmunoassay or positive by electroimmunoassay.

Table 32.6. Current Recommendations for Measles Vaccination

	Criteria for Adequate Protection
Routine childhood schedule, U.S. Most areas	Two doses,[a,b] first dose at 12–15 months second dose at 4–6 years (entry to kindergarten or first grade)[c]
High-risk areas[d]	Two doses,[a,b] first dose at 12 months second dose at 4–6 years (entry to kindergarten or first grade)[c]
Colleges and other educational institutions after high school	Documentation of receipt of two doses of measles vaccine after the first birthday[b] or other evidence of measles immunity[e]
Medical personnel beginning employment	Documentation of receipt of two doses of measles vaccine after the first birthday[b] or other evidence of measles immunity[e]

From CDC 1997.

[a]Both doses should preferably be given as combined measles, mumps, rubella (MMR) vaccine.

[b]No less than 1 month apart. If no documentation of any dose of vaccine, first dose of vaccine should be given at the time of school entry or employment and second dose no less than 1 month later.

[c]Some areas may elect to administer the second dose at an older age or to multiple age groups.

[d]A county with more than five cases among preschool-aged children during each of at least 5 years, a county with a recent outbreak among unvaccinated preschool-aged children, or a county with a large inner-city urban population. These recommendations may be applied to an entire county or to identified risk areas within a county.

[e]Prior physician-diagnosed measles disease, laboratory evidence of measles immunity, or birth before 1957.

approximately 5% of vaccines. Guidelines for *control of measles outbreaks* in preschool-aged children, in institutions (e.g., day centers, schools, colleges), and in medical facilities are provided in Table 32.7. Special attention should be directed toward ensuring immunity in all health care providers and providing measles vaccine to adolescents and young adults.

Unimmunized household contacts of persons with measles, especially infants born to nonimmune women, should be given IG 0.25 mL/kg (up to 15 mL maximum). Immunocompromised children and adults exposed to measles should receive 0.5 mL/kg (maximum dose 15 mL) of IG (19).

Mumps

From 1967 to 1995, the number of cases of mumps reported annually in the United States fell from more than 100,000 to less than 1,000 because of the widespread use of mumps vaccine in children.

Live, attenuated mumps virus vaccine, preferably given as MMR (see below) is recommended routinely for children and for unvaccinated young adults with no history of physician-diagnosed mumps; most people born before 1957 can be considered immune. Because the mumps virus can cause severe illness in adults (orchitis, meningitis, or pancreatitis), there is good reason to provide protection to young adults who may

be susceptible. Outbreaks of mumps have been reported among college and university students, and this group merits special attention. A single dose of mumps vaccine, alone or in MMR, yields durable protection in approximately 90% of recipients (19).

Rubella

Since 1970, live, attenuated rubella virus vaccine has been administered routinely to children 1 year of age and older. The major rationale for use of this vaccine is prevention of the spread of rubella virus to pregnant women and thus reduction of the incidence of the congenital rubella syndrome. From 1972 to 1996, the number of cases of rubella reported annually in the United States fell from more than 56,000 to less than 200. Reported cases of congenital rubella syndrome remained constant at 50 to 60 from 1970 to 1980, then fell dramatically to 13 in 1983 and 1 in 1988. In 1990 and 1991, a resurgence of rubella was observed with more than 40 cases of documented congenital rubella syndrome reported in the United States.

Anyone working in a medical facility who does not have documentation of past rubella vaccination or serologic evidence of immunity should be vaccinated against rubella. Adults, and especially nonpregnant adolescent girls and women in the childbearing age group, should be offered rubella vaccine if they have not received vaccine or are not known to have serologic evidence of immunity. Serologic testing before vaccination is unnecessary because prior immunity does not increase the risks of vaccination. Vaccinated women should be cautioned against becoming pregnant (see Chapter 93, "Birth Control") for the 3 months after receiving rubella vaccine because of the theoretical possibility of fetal damage. However, no cases of congenital abnormalities have been observed in more than 300 susceptible women who received rubella vaccine just before or during pregnancy, and the theoretical risk is less than 1% (19). Approximately 25% of postpubertal women receiving rubella vaccine experience arthralgias in the first 1 to 3 weeks after immunization. Frank arthritis is much less common and all symptoms are usually mild and transient.

MMR Vaccine

In most cases, MMR is the vaccine of choice when any of its components is indicated, although the three vaccines are available separately. *A two-dose schedule is now highly recommended for all children.* The first dose of MMR should be administered at 12 to 15 months of age; the second dose is now recommended at 4 to 6 years, before school entry, but may be given at 11 to 12 years of age. The measles component is associated with the occurrence of fever or mild rash within 7 to 12 days after injection. MMR or its component vaccines should not be given to pregnant women. Anaphylaxis or other serious systematic adverse reactions are rare with MMR or any of the three individual component vaccines.

Most adults born before 1957 are assumed to be immune to mumps, measles, and rubella. *Adults born in 1957 or later* who do not have a medical contraindication should receive at least one dose of MMR vaccine unless they have documentation of vaccination with at least one dose of measles–rubella–and–mumps-containing vaccine or other acceptable evidence of immunity to these three diseases: laboratory evidence of immunity or physician documented diagnosis of the disease. Serosurveys document a lack of identifiable antibody to measles, mumps, or rubella among 15 to 20% of young adult Americans (9). Adolescents and college students who have no documentation of live measles, rubella, or mumps vaccinations or other acceptable evidence of immunity are recommended to receive a two-dose course of MMR vaccine, with the second dose administered no sooner than 1 month after the initial dose. Students with medical contraindications to vaccination with MMR and any of its component vaccines should be given a letter of explanation to present to the health officials of their educational institution (19).

Meningococcal Disease

Meningococcal disease is a serious, potentially fatal infection that usually occurs sporadically, with highest incidence in infants and relatively rare occurrence among the general population but may occur in epidemics within defined communities. A quadrivalent meningococcal polysaccharide vaccine (Menomune, Connaught) is available and recommended for use in mass vaccination campaigns to control epidemics of type C meningococcal disease, but it is not for general public use. When an epidemic is identified by public health officials, vaccination of persons in the affected community consists of a single 0.5 mL subcutaneous injection (18).

Polio

Wild poliovirus and new onset poliomyelitis have been eradicated from the Western Hemisphere, and global eradication is anticipated within several years. Vaccine-associated paralytic polio (VAPP) among primary vaccines with oral polio vaccine (OPV) or their household contacts remains a rare but real risk in the United States, where 125 cases occurred between 1980 and 1994—approximately 1 case per 750,000 first doses of OPV. Revised ACIP recommendations issued in 1997 conclude that the following three polio vaccine options offer equal protection against polio but favor the adoption of the first option because of greater protection against VAPP: sequential administration of two doses of inactivated polio vaccine (IPV) at 2 and 4 months of age followed by OPV at 12 to 18 months and 4 to 6 years of age, a full series of OPV, and a full series of IPV.

Polio vaccination for adults in the United States is recommended for travelers to remaining polio endemic parts of the world, unvaccinated adults whose children will be receiving OPV, and laboratory workers who handle specimens that may contain polioviruses.

The recommended schedule for *unvaccinated adults* consists of two doses of IPV injected at 4- and 8-week intervals and a third dose at 6 to 12 months. For adults at increased risk of exposure to wild poliovirus (travelers, laboratory workers) who have previously completed a primary OPV or IPV series, a single dose of OPV or IPV may be administered (20).

Rabies

Indigenously acquired human rabies is rare in the United States. In 1992, only one human case was reported. Theoretically, all clinical cases of rabies are preventable if protective treatment is given promptly after exposure. The incubation period is usually 2 to 8 weeks, but it may be as short as 10 days or as long as 1 year or more.

Since 1982, inactivated rabies virus vaccine produced in human diploid cells has been in use in the United States. It causes fewer and milder reactions than the older duck embryo-derived vaccine. Formulations for intramuscular or intradermal injection are

Table 32.7. Recommendations for Measles Outbreak Control[a]

Outbreaks in preschool-aged children	Lower age for vaccination to as low as 6 months of age in outbreak area if cases are occurring in children <1 year of age[b]
Outbreaks in institutions (day-care centers, K–12th grades, colleges, and other institutions)	Revaccination of all students and their siblings and of school personnel born in or after 1957 who do not have documentation of immunity to measles[c]
Outbreaks in medical facilities	Revaccination of all medical workers born in or after 1957 who have direct patient contact and who do not have proof of immunity to measles[c]
	Susceptible personnel who have been exposed should be relieved from direct patient contact from the 5th to 21st day after exposure (regardless of whether they received measles vaccine or IG) or if they become ill for 7 days after they develop rash

From CDC 1997.

[a]Mass revaccination of entire populations is not necessary. Revaccination should be limited to populations at risk, such as students attending institutions where cases occur.

[b]Children initially vaccinated before the first birthday should be revaccinated at 15 months of age. A second dose should be administered at the time of school entry or according to local policy.

[c]Documentation of physician-diagnosed measles disease, serological evidence of immunity to measles, or documentation of receipt of two doses of measles vaccine on or after the first birthday.

available, as is a hyperimmune globulin derived from human sera (HRIG).

For *postexposure prophylaxis* following an animal bite (see Chapter 25), the recommended treatment schedule is as follows: on day 1, simultaneous administration of HRIG (20 IU/kg, up to half infiltrated into the wound and the remainder intramuscularly), and the first dose of vaccine, also given intramuscularly; additional vaccine doses are given on days 3, 7, 14, and 28. The effectiveness of this regimen, followed exactly, in protecting humans from rabies has been well established. Adverse reactions (urticaria, anaphylaxis, transient headache, and fever) occur in less than 0.5% of persons receiving this vaccine (3,21).

For *preexposure prophylaxis*, people working in areas where rabies is enzootic or in occupations where potential for rabies exposure is high (e.g., veterinarians) should be vaccinated before exposure. In this situation, the appropriate formulation may be given intradermally in 0.1-mL doses or intramuscularly in 1.0-mL doses on days 0, 7, and 21 or 28 with booster doses every 2 years (see Chapter 33 for details regarding frequency of vaccine for those living in high-risk areas). Preexposure immunization does not eliminate the need for postexposure prophylaxis, but it obviates the need for HRIG and decreases the number of vaccine doses required to two (days 0 and 3).

Tuberculosis

Efforts to control tuberculosis in the United States are based on early identification and treatment of active disease and on isoniazid prophylaxis of the contacts of tuberculous patients and other groups at increased risk (see Chapter 29). Because most new TB cases are reactivation of disease in older individuals and because efficacy has been questioned in the past, indications for immunization with Bacillus Calmette–Guérin (BCG) vaccine in the United States have been limited. However, the recent spread of multiple drug–resistant tuberculosis (MDR-TB), unresponsive to isoniazid and rifampin, as well as recent meta-analyses indicating up to 80% BCG effectiveness in protecting children against serious forms of TB have prompted reconsideration of the potential use of BCG in the United States (1).

At present, BCG should be considered for the following two groups:

- Infants and children who have a negative tuberculin skin test and *(a)* who have repeated exposure to persistently untreated or unsuccessfully treated, sputum-positive pulmonary tuberculosis and cannot be separated from the presence of the infectious patient or reliably receive isoniazid, or *(b)* who have repeated exposure to active disease caused by MDR-TB organisms and cannot be separated from the infectious patient
- Health care workers who have negative tuberculin skin tests and work in settings with recurrent transmission of MDR-TB

BCG is a live, attenuated vaccine derived from *Mycobacterium bovis*. The Tice strain (Organon, Inc.) is the only BCG vaccine licensed in the United States. It is administered percutaneously through multiple punctures in the upper arm, with doses differing by age of recipient. A small ulcerating postule typically occurs at the vaccination site several weeks after receiving the vaccine.

BCG vaccine is contraindicated in people receiving immunosuppressive therapy or who have immunocompromising conditions, including HIV infection.

Varicella

Varicella (chickenpox) is a highly contagious, generally self-limited disease of childhood caused by varicella zoster virus. In 1965, approximately 20% of children 11 to 12 years old remained susceptible (i.e., had no history of varicella). Although varicella occurs infrequently among adolescents and adults, it is more severe among these groups and among immunocompromised people in all age groups. Complications include pneumonia, encephalitis, and occasionally death.

In 1995, a live, attenuated varicella virus vaccine (Varivax, Merck) was licensed for use in people 12 months of age or older in the United States. Although primarily intended for children, the vaccine is recommended for everyone 12 years of age or older, particularly those who are susceptible (those with negative or unknown history of varicella) and who have close occupational (health care workers) or household contact with immunocompromised people or others at high risk of serious complications. Because 70 to 90% of adults without a reliable history of varicella are actually immune, serologic testing before vaccination is likely to be cost-effective in these subjects (22). Varicella vaccine should not be given to anyone with primary or acquired immunodeficiency, including HIV.

Vaccination of healthy adolescents and adults consists of two 0.5-mL doses administered subcutaneously at 4- and 8-week intervals. Adverse effects have been limited to pain and redness at the injection site (22).

Postexposure prophylaxis. Varicella zoster immune globulin (VZIG), available from American Red Cross distribution centers, is indicated for immunocompromised adolescents and adults who are susceptible to varicella (i.e., have negative history for chickenpox and no history of receiving varicella vaccine) and have been exposed to an active varicella case. It is effective in preventing or suppressing varicella if given within 96 hours of exposure. Healthy adults and pregnant women who are susceptible to varicella (see above) are at increased risk of varicella complications and may also be given VZIG for postexposure prophylaxis at their physician's discretion. Recommended prophylactic dosage of VZIG is 125 units/10 kg (22 lb), administered intramuscularly. The major adverse reaction is discomfort at the injection site; anaphylactic shock is rare (22).

General References*

ACP Task Force on Adult Immunization and Infectious Diseases Society of America. Guide for adult immunization. 3rd ed. Philadelphia: American College of Physicians, 1994.
> Contains all standard recommendations in a single source with critical discussions of efficacy, indications, administration, and adverse effects of vaccines and immune globulin preparations and new section on practice strategies for maximizing vaccine delivery.

Benenson AS, ed. Control of communicable diseases in man. 16th ed. Washington, DC: American Public Health Association, 1995.
> A concise summary of epidemiology and management of virtually all communicable diseases, updated at 5-year intervals.

Fedson DS. Adult immunization: summary of the National Vaccine Advisory Committee report. JAMA 272:1133–1137, 1994.

Gardner P, Schaffner W. Current concepts: immunization of adults. N Engl J Med 328(17):1252, 1993.
> Concise review article of all major vaccines for adults.

Gardner P, Eickhoff T, Poland GA, et al. Adult immunization. Ann Intern Med 124:35–40, 1996.
> Concise review of two vaccines licensed since 1993 review: hepatitis A and varicella.

Recommendations of the Advisory Committee on Immunization Practices (ACIP). Use of vaccines and immune globulins in persons with altered immunocompetence. MMWR 42(RR-4):1–18, 1993.

Recommendations of the Advisory Committee on Immunization Practices (ACIP). Vaccine side effects, adverse reactions, contraindications and precautions. MMWR 45(RR-12):1–35, 1996.
> Summary of extensive literature review conducted by Institute of Medicine.

Specific References

1. Advisory Council for Elimination of Tuberculosis and Advisory Committee on Immunization Practices (ACIP). The role of BCG vaccine in the prevention and control of tuberculosis in the United States. MMWR 45(RR-4):1–18, 1996.
2. Atkinson WL, Orenstein WA, Krugman S. The resurgence of measles in the United States, 1989–1991. Annu Rev Med 43:451–463, 1992.
3. Bernard KW, Roberts MA, et al. Human diploid cell rabies vaccine: effectiveness of immunization with small intradermal or subcutaneous doses. JAMA 247:1138, 1982.
4. Chen RT, Rastogi SC, Mullen JR, et al. The vaccine adverse event reporting system (VAERS). Vaccine 12:542–550, 1994.
5. Douglas RG Jr. Drug therapy: prophylaxis and treatment of influenza. N Engl J Med 322:443, 1990.
6. Food and Drug Administration. New reporting requirements for vaccine adverse events. FDA Drug Bull 18(2):16, 1988.
7. Gross PA, Hermogenes AW, Sacks HS, et al. The efficacy of influenza vaccine in elderly persons. A meta-analysis and review of the literature. Ann Intern Med 123:518–527, 1995.
8. Gyorkos W, Tannenbaum TN, Abrahamowicz M, et al. Evaluation of the effectiveness of immunization delivery methods. Can J Public Health 85(Suppl):S14–S30, 1994.
9. Kelly PW, Petrucelli BP, Stehr-Green P, et al. The susceptibility of young adult Americans to vaccine preventable infections. JAMA 266:2724–2729, 1991.
10. Lemon SM, Thomas DL. Vaccines to prevent viral hepatitis. N Engl J Med 336:196–204, 1997.
11. Margolis KL, Nichol KL, Poland GA, Pluskar RE. Frequency of adverse reactions to influenza vaccine in the elderly. JAMA 264:1139–1146, 1990.
12. Recommendations of the Advisory Committee on Immunization Practices (ACIP). Diphtheria, tetanus, and pertussis: recommendations for vaccine use and other preventive measures. MMWR 40(RR-10):1–28, 1991.
13. Recommendations of the Advisory Committee on Immunization Practices (ACIP). Pertussis vaccination. Use of acellular pertussis vaccines among infants and young children. MMWR 46(RR-7):1–29, 1997.
14. Recommendations of the Advisory Committee on Immunization Practices (ACIP). Prevention of hepatitis A through active or passive immunization. MMWR 45(RR-15):1–30, 1996.
15. Recommendations of the Advisory Committee on Immunization Practices (ACIP). Hepatitis B virus infection: a comprehensive immunization strategy to eliminate transmission in the United States. MMWR (in press).
16. Recommendations of the Advisory Committee on Immunization Practices (ACIP). Prevention and control of influenza. MMWR 46(RR-9):1–25, 1997. (Note: Update for each year issued by ACIP.)
17. Recommendations of the Advisory Committee on Immunization Practices (ACIP). Prevention of pneumococcal disease. MMWR 46(RR-8):1–24, 1997.
18. Recommendations of the Advisory Committee on Immunization Practices (ACIP). Control and prevention of meningococcal disease and control and prevention of serogroup C meningococcal disease: evaluation and management of suspected outbreaks. MMWR 46(RR-5):1–21, 1997.
19. Recommendations of the Advisory Committee on Immunization Practices (ACIP). Measles, mumps, and rubella: vaccine use and strategies for measles, rubella, and congenital rubella syndrome elimination and mumps control. MMWR 1997 (in press).
20. Recommendations of the Advisory Committee on Immunization Practices (ACIP). Poliomyelitis prevention in the United States: introduction of a sequential vaccination schedule of inactivated poliovirus vaccination followed by oral poliovirus vaccine. MMWR 46(RR-3):1–25, 1997.
21. Recommendations of Immunization Practices Advisory Committee (ACIP). Rabies prevention: United States 1991. MMWR 40(RR-3):1–19, 1991.
22. Recommendations of the Advisory Committee on Immunization Practices (ACIP). Prevention of varicella. MMWR 45(RR-11):1–36, 1996.
23. Recommendations of the Advisory Committee on Immunization Practices (ACIP), the American Academy of Pediatrics, the American Academy of Family Physicians, and the American Medical Association. Immunization of adolescents. MMWR 45(RR-13):1–16, 1996.
24. Siber GR, Werner BG, Halsey NA, et al. Interference of immune globulin with measles and rubella immunization. J Pediatr 122(2):204, 1993.
25. Stevens CE, Taylor PE, Tong MJ, et al. Yeast-recombinant hepatitis B vaccine. Efficacy with hepatitis B immune globulin in prevention of perinatal hepatitis B virus transmission. JAMA 257(19):2612, 1987.
26. Williams WW, Hickson MA, Kane MA, et al. Immunization policies and vaccine coverage among adults. The risk for missed opportunities. Ann Intern Med 108(4):616, 1988.

*Bold print (general references) and bold numerals (specific references) denote published controlled clinical trials, meta-analyses, or consensus-based recommendations.

C H A P T E R   33

Medical Advice for the International Traveler

STEPHEN D. SEARS, MD, MPH
DAVID A. SACK, MD

SCOPE OF THE PROBLEM

International travel is increasing in popularity. Americans are visiting exotic locales on adventure travel tours and trekking to increasingly remote regions of the world. It is estimated that 25 to 40 million Americans travel by air to foreign countries each year. This does not include the many who take boats, cruises, or cars to Canada and Mexico. Of these millions, it is estimated that 3 to 5 million journey to developing areas of the world where infectious diseases that are uncommon in developed countries are encountered. Malaria, schistosomiasis, yellow fever, polio, typhoid fever, and amebiasis are just a few of the diseases that are more prevalent in tropical developing countries. Many travelers make little or no provision for the prevention of illness while traveling. This is unfortunate because the overall attack rate for several infectious diseases is much higher in international travelers than it is in comparable populations that remain at home. This fact is well illustrated by the results of a study of Swiss travelers that found that three-quarters had at least one symptom of infectious illness while traveling; of the 16,500 travelers surveyed in this study, more than 30% had at least one episode of a diarrheal illness (21). In a follow-up study, not only were travelers found to have illnesses while traveling, but almost one-third became ill within a month of returning home (22). Another study of 2000 travelers returning to the United Kingdom found that 43% became ill during or shortly after their journeys (17) and, in a recent review, 75% of travelers did not take sufficient basic precautions against infection (15).

The previously cited studies offer a small glimpse into the medical problems of travelers. Even so, there is no reliable measurement of the amount or severity of disease encountered by the traveler. Only a portion of the most dramatic cases of illness in travelers, such as malaria, Lassa fever, or African trypanosomiasis, are ever reported to public health authorities. At present, there is no mechanism for obtaining accurate surveillance data on the incidence or prevalence of illness in American travelers, nor are there data on significant risk factors for acquiring infectious diseases. This lack of data hampers scientific investigation of interventional strategies in travelers. Even so, significant progress has been made in the prevention of malaria, traveler's diarrhea, and diseases for which immunizations exist.

Factors such as the low cost of air travel and expectations of safe water, safe food, and unrestricted access to swimming place large numbers of Americans at risk of contracting diseases in the tropics and presenting to their physicians at home; for example, a college student on a safari in Kenya can be bitten by an Anopheles mosquito carrying sporozoites of *Plasmodium falciparum* and 2 weeks later be back at college when the fever and chills begin.

To prevent unnecessary illness, it is imperative that travelers undertake appropriate *pretrip health planning*. When approached by a person about to embark upon an international journey, it is important to ascertain several key aspects of the proposed trip. Where are you going? Where will you stay? What is the purpose of your trip? Where will you be eating? In restaurants or in private homes? Is sex with other travelers or local residents likely? With this information, one can categorize the types and magnitude of risk. A businessperson staying for a short time in a first-class hotel in a large city in a developing country has different risks than does a college student who will be living in villages in several developing countries. Most travelers fit somewhere between these two extremes and a travel consultation must be individualized to fit the traveler's lifestyle, itinerary, medical history, use of medications, allergies, and previous immunizations.

Sources for current recommendations. Immunizations, malaria prevention, food and water safety, diarrhea, schistosomiasis, and a number of general health hazards are topics that should be discussed with the traveler. Two useful resources that are updated yearly provide practical information on these issues: *Health Information for International Travel,* published by the United States Public Health Service (available from the Centers for Disease Control and Prevention, Atlanta, GA 30333) and *Vaccination Certificate Requirements for International Travel and Health Advice to Travelers,* published by the World Health Organization (available from WHO Publication Center, 49 Sheridan Ave., Albany, NY 12210). Other valuable resources include the International Association for Medical Assistance to Travelers (IAMAT, 417 Center

St., Lewistown, NY 14092), which provides information on tropical diseases as well as a list of English-speaking physicians overseas, and the Centers for Disease Control and Prevention (CDC) Traveler's Information Hotline (404-332-4559; will fax current information on all regions).

In addition, online resources now available include the CDC Home Travel Information Page (http://www.cdc.gov/Travel/Travel.html/) and World Health Organization Home Page (http://www.who.ch/). Another useful site is the U.S. State Department Travel Warnings and Consular Information sheets (http://www.stolaf.edu/network/travel-advisories.html).

IMMUNIZATIONS

Vaccines are now available against a number of the major viral and bacterial diseases encountered in developing areas. For patients traveling to these areas, it is necessary to administer travel-specific vaccines and to update primary vaccines (Table 33.1). Immunizations can be broadly separated into those that are legally required and those that are recommended. *Legally required vaccinations* are public health measures that certain countries demand before entry, to benefit the country as a whole, whereas *recommended immunizations* are designed to benefit only the patient.

Table 33.1. Vaccines and Immune Globulin for International Travel

Vaccine/Immune Globulin	Patient Age	Route[a]	Dose	Booster	Comments
Yellow fever	>9 mo	SC	0.5 mL	0.5 mL q10yr	May be required.
Cholera	6 mo–4 yr	SC or IM	0.2 mL	0.2 mL q6mo	May be required.
	5–10 yr		0.3 mL	0.3 mL q6mo	Limited efficacy.
	>10 yr		0.5 mL	0.5 mL q6mo	
Typhoid parenteral	<10 yr	SC	0.25 mL	0.25 mL q3yr	Local reactions common.
	>10 yr		0.50 mL	0.5 mL q3yr	
Typhoid oral (TY21a)	>1 yr	Oral	1 dose QOD × 4	Repeat series q5yr	Keep refrigerated, avoid antibiotics.
Typhoid parenteral (ViCPS)	≥2 yr	IM	0.5 mL	2 yr	Well tolerated.
Poliomyelitis					
OPV	All ages	Oral	3 doses	1 dose pretravel	IPV is preferable for adults.
IPV	All ages	SC	3 doses	1 dose q10yr	
Japanese encephalitis	<3 yr	SC	0.5 mL	1 dose at 1 and 4 yr	Just licensed by the FDA.
	>3 yr		1.0 mL		
Hepatitis A					
Havrix	2–17 yr	IM	0.5 mL × 2	6–12 mo then 10 yr	
	>17 yr	IM	1 mL × 2	6–12 mo then 10 yr	
Vaqta	2–17 yr	IM	0.5 mL × 2	6–12 mo then 10 yr	
	>17 yr	IM	1 mL × 2	6–12 mo then 10 yr	
Immune globulin (short term <3 mo)	<23 kg	IM	0.5 mL	—	Immune globulin is used for prophylaxis of hepatitis A; consider screening for anti-HAV in frequent travelers.
	23–45 kg		1.0 mL	—	
	>45 kg		2.0 mL	—	
Tetanus–diphtheria	>7 yr	IM	3 doses	1 dose q10yr	Always use combined vaccine.
Meningitis A, C, Y, W135	>2 yr	IM	0.5 mL	Unclear	For specific areas of travel.
Rabies	All ages	IM	1.0 mL (3 doses)	1 dose q2yr	Still requires postexposure treatment.
		ID	0.1 mL (3 doses)	1 dose q2yr	
Hepatitis B	All ages	IM	1.0 mL (3 doses)	Unclear	Protection lasts 5–7 yr.

[a]*SC,* Subcutaneous; *IM,* intramuscular; *ID,* intradermal.

No vaccines are legally required to enter or return to the United States. However, many countries have strict entry requirements, and travelers who arrive without proper vaccination certificates may be denied entry, quarantined, or possibly vaccinated at the point of entry. Therefore, it is important to determine what vaccines are required before beginning a journey.

Currently, the only legally required vaccination is for yellow fever, and each country has its own requirements. In the past, smallpox and cholera vaccinations were required by many countries, but in 1980 the World Health Organization declared the global eradication of smallpox, and on January 1, 1982, smallpox was deleted from the list of diseases subject to regulation. Although cholera vaccination is not endorsed by the World Health Organization for entry into any country, some local authorities may still require proof of cholera vaccination, especially if the traveler is arriving from endemic areas.

Yellow Fever

Yellow fever, once almost controlled, has made a dramatic resurgence (18). Yellow fever vaccine, containing a live, attenuated strain of the yellow fever virus, is one of the most important and effective vaccines. It is required by some countries before travelers are allowed entrance, particularly when areas to be visited are endemic for yellow fever and when travelers have recently left a country endemic for yellow fever. If yellow fever exists in the country of destination, the traveler should be vaccinated regard-

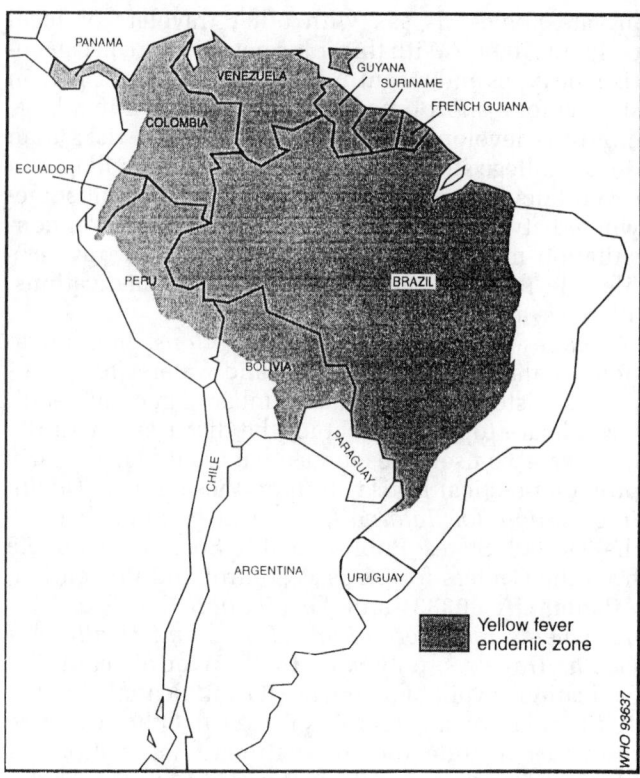

Figure 33.2. Yellow fever endemic zone in the Americas. (From Health Information International Travel, 1996. US Department of Health and Human Services.)

less of the regulations of the country (Figs. 33.1 and 33.2). The vaccine is nontoxic and induces long-lasting immunity. Reactions, which are generally mild, occur in 1 to 5% of patients. These include mild headache, myalgia, low-grade fever, or other minor symptoms 5 to 10 days after inoculation. Because yellow fever vaccine is a live, attenuated virus, it could pose a risk to pregnant women, although teratogenicity has not been encountered. Pregnant women who must travel to areas endemic for yellow fever should be vaccinated. It is presumed that the unknown but small risk to the fetus is less than the risk to the mother. If at all possible, the trip should be postponed until after delivery. The vaccine is contraindicated in immunocompromised patients, including patients with acquired immunodeficiency syndrome (AIDS) with CD4 counts below 200. Because the vaccine strain is grown in chick embryo culture, it should not be given to travelers with known hypersensitivity to eggs. Yellow fever immunization is also discouraged in children less than 9 months of age because of neurotoxicity in infants. Yellow fever vaccine is available only through official yellow fever vaccine centers; locations of these centers can be obtained by calling the local health department. The dose of vaccine is 0.5 mL subcutaneously, and it must be given within 1 hour of reconstitution. The vaccine should be stored at 5°C until it is reconstituted. The vaccine gives solid immunity for at least 10 years. If it is contraindicated for a traveler to receive yellow fever

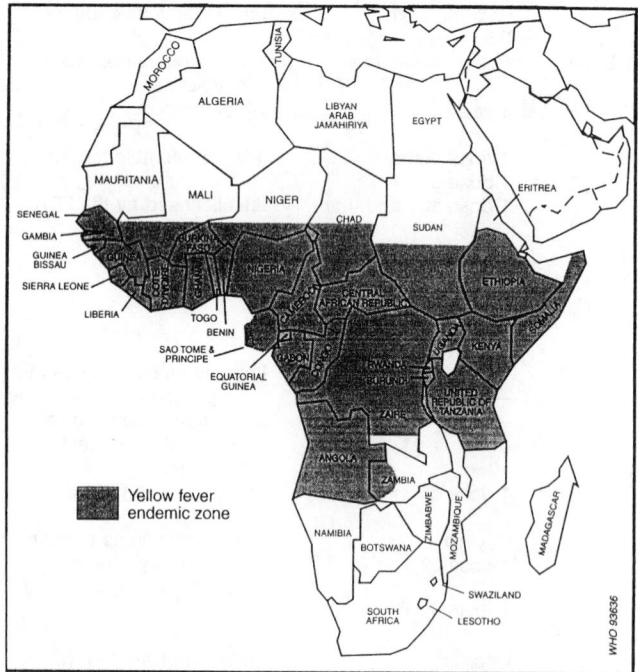

Figure 33.1. Yellow fever endemic zone in Africa. (From Health Information International Travel, 1996. US Department of Health and Human Services.)

vaccine for any of the above reasons, a detailed letter explaining the contraindications should be provided to the traveler.

Cholera

Since January 1991, more than a million cases of cholera have occurred in South and Central America, and cholera occurs in nearly all developing countries. In addition, a new cholera epidemic erupted in India in 1992 with a non-01 vibrio cholerae strain and has spread rapidly (14). Even so, the risk to travelers remains low, especially for those who use caution in food and water acquisition. In 1973, the World Health Assembly recommended discontinuing required vaccination against cholera. By 1992, all countries had officially discontinued this requirement, but a few in Africa still have unofficial requirements at certain border crossings for travelers coming from areas endemic for cholera. Thus, there is still some possibility of difficulty at borders unless a certificate of vaccination is obtained. Unless the vaccine is legally required, the killed whole cell injectable vaccine is discouraged because the vaccine causes excessive local inflammation and is not warranted considering the low risk. Travelers in countries outside the United States may wish to take one of the new safe *oral cholera vaccines* if they travel to high-risk areas. The oral killed whole cell B subunit vaccine is given as a two-dose series and provides protection for about 3 years, whereas the oral live cholera vaccine CVD103-HgR is given as a single dose. Neither is available yet in the United States, but they are becoming increasingly available in Europe and other countries. For travelers following usual tourist routes and using standard precautions in countries endemic for cholera, the estimated attack rate is less than 1 per 100,000 returning travelers, but recent studies in Japanese travelers suggest that the rate of cholera infection may be much higher than previously assumed (24). Furthermore, the estimated rates are likely to be significantly underestimated because many cholera episodes may be not be distinguished from other episodes of traveler's diarrhea, and being treated overseas, they may not be reported to the CDC. Nonetheless, rather than recommend immunization routinely, one should emphatically instruct travelers to areas endemic for cholera not to eat uncooked vegetables, to use caution with undercooked seafood, and always to drink boiled water or bottled beverages.

Typhoid Fever

Typhoid fever remains a danger for high-risk travelers; more than 60% of the cases reported in the United States occur after international travel. Areas with the greatest risk are parts of South America and the Indian subcontinent, although the risk is present in almost all developing countries (3). *Salmonella typhi* is transmitted by the ingestion of fecally contaminated food and water; typhoid vaccination, although not legally required, is recommended for travelers who are likely to stray off the usual tourist route, stay in small villages, and eat local food. With the increasing prevalence of antimicrobial resistance to *S. typhi,* vaccination takes on even greater significance.

Three vaccines currently are licensed for protection against typhoid fever: a live, attenuated oral vaccine (Ty21a), a newly licensed capsular polysaccharide parenteral vaccine (ViCPS, Typhim Vi), and the older heat phenol inactivated parenteral vaccine. The efficacy of these vaccines is 60 to 70% depending on the degree of subsequent exposure. Ty21a is a mutant of *S. typhi* that produces enough endotoxin to be immunogenic and nonpathogenic and has limited replication. Ty21a is taken as four separate doses over 7 days; it must be refrigerated and is well tolerated, although abdominal cramps sometimes occur with the vaccine. Antibiotics should not be taken during the week that the oral vaccine is being administered. Typhim Vi is composed of purified Vi (Virulence) antigen, the capsular polysaccharide produced by *S. typhi.* Primary vaccination with ViCPS consists of one 0.5-mL (25-µg) dose given intramuscularly. The vaccine is discouraged for children under 2 years of age because of poor immunogenicity at this age. The heat phenol inactivated parenteral vaccine should always be used without the paratyphoid component. The parenteral vaccine often causes pain at the injection site, fever, headache, and malaise for 1 to 3 days. If the traveler has never been vaccinated, the primary sequence is two inoculations 1 month apart (see Table 33.1 for dosages). The parenteral inactivated vaccine causes significantly more adverse events and is not more effective than either ViCPS or Ty21a. Therefore, either oral Ty21a or ViCPS is generally preferred.

Polio

Paralytic poliomyelitis has been eradicated from the Americas (2). In developing countries outside the Americas, polio rates are falling but travelers should still be protected. Travelers who have previously completed a primary series with either the Sabin (oral, live) or Salk (parental, inactivated) vaccine should have a booster dose if they have not previously received a booster as an adult. A history of at least three doses of oral polio vaccine (OPV, Sabin) or four doses of inactivated polio vaccine (IPV, Salk) with IPV boosters each 5 years until age 18 is evidence of adequate primary immunization. Such fully immunized people need only one dose of polio vaccine before traveling to high-risk areas. If a traveler is only partially immunized, the primary series should be completed.

Adults who require a primary series should receive IPV. Recently, a new inactivated polio vaccine of enhanced potency has been released (eIPV). IPV is preferred in adults because the risk of OPV-associated paralysis is somewhat higher in adults than in children. If children are not already vaccinated, they should receive a primary series. If an unimmunized adult traveler does not have time to complete a primary IPV series before departure, a single dose of OPV may offer reasonable protection. On return, primary immunization with IPV should be completed. Live (OPV) vaccine should not be given routinely to women known to be pregnant, although teratogenicity has not been shown. If the risk of polio is significant and the pregnant woman is unimmunized, primary vaccination with IPV would be prudent. Because OPV is a live virus, immunocompromised patients and their families should not receive OPV; instead they should be immunized with IPV. Table 33.1 summarizes information regarding dosages for polio vaccines.

Tetanus and Diphtheria

Tetanus occurs worldwide but is slightly more common in the tropics. Many adult travelers may not be protected against tetanus (10). Thus, tetanus immunization should be kept up to date in travelers. Boosters must be given every 10 years regardless of age. Travelers, if they injure themselves, are less likely to seek medical help, so adequate pretravel immunization becomes more important. *Diphtheria* is endemic in many developing countries and is currently epidemic in the countries of the former USSR and most cases occur in unimmunized or partially immunized people. Therefore, routine immunization with tetanus–diphtheria (Td) rather than with tetanus toxoid alone should be given. For primary immunization, patients older than 7 years should receive three doses of Td. (Before age 7, the primary immunizing agent is the diphtheria–pertussis–tetanus combination [DPT].) The first doses are 1 to 2 months apart and the third 6 to 12 months later. Local reactions may occur within 12 to 48 hours after vaccination. Severe local reactions can occur in adults if the booster is given within a short time of the previous vaccine. The only contraindication to Td is a history of hypersensitivity reactions after immunization.

Hepatitis A

Hepatitis A (HA) continues to be an important risk for travelers to many areas of the developing world and is the most common vaccine-preventable disease of travelers. Although the risk is less for people who travel on ordinary tourist routes and stay for short periods, it may be considerable for those who bypass the tourist routes and stay for extended periods. HA illness may be asymptomatic but can also be severe, with jaundice and significant morbidity. Protection against HA is strongly recommended for international travelers to developing areas (13). Although immune globulin provides passive protection against HA for a few months and is safe and effective, HA vaccine (active immunization) is generally preferred for most travelers. Two vaccines are licensed, Havrix (SKF) and Vaqta (Merck), and both prevent approximately 90% of expected HA infections. Travelers to HA-endemic areas should ideally receive the first dose of vaccine at least 1 month before travel. Recent evidence suggests that vaccine is protective even when given immediately before a trip,

even though protective antibodies may not be measurable. Immune globulin is less expensive and is still a reasonable choice for travelers making only one trip who need limited (up to 3 months) HA protection. For travelers leaving immediately, administering both immune globulin and HA vaccine is both safe and effective. The recommended schedules for both Havrix and Vaqta include a primary immunization for all patients and a booster in 6 to 12 months for patients 2 to 18 years of age. A booster for subjects over 18 ensures optimal long-term protection. The dosage of immune globulin may be based on weight, but for adults injection of 2 mL for stays of less than 3 months is adequate in practice. The vaccines are well tolerated and adverse events are rare. The only side effect of immune globulin is muscle soreness at the injection site. Immune globulins for intramuscular injection prepared in the United States carry no risk of transmission of human immunodeficiency virus (HIV) or other infectious agents, but those produced in developing countries should not be used. Pregnancy is not a contraindication to immune globulin. Screening for anti–hepatitis A virus in frequent travelers should also be considered (see details in Chapter 43).

Hepatitis B

Hepatitis B vaccination is now recommended for all infants and adolescents. Although the risk of hepatitis B is generally low for the routine traveler, this may be an opportunity to provide this important vaccine. Health care workers who are likely to have contact with blood or secretions from patients in areas endemic for hepatitis B should receive hepatitis B vaccine. Travelers who will live for more than 6 months in countries with a high prevalence of hepatitis B antigenemia should also be strongly considered for vaccination. The prevalence of hepatitis B virus carriers is 5 to 15% in sub-Saharan Africa and Southeast Asia, including China and Indonesia, and 1 to 5% in North Africa, South Central Asia, and Southern Europe. Because hepatitis B can be transmitted through sexual contact, travelers should be counseled appropriately when going to endemic areas. Vaccination or hepatitis B immune globulin (HBIG) prophylaxis may be appropriate for people who are likely to have sexual contacts. Primary adult vaccination consists of three intramuscular doses of 1 mL of vaccine. The first two doses are given 1 month apart and the third dose should be given 6 months later. This is often difficult in travelers, and accelerated vaccine schedules have been defined and may be useful for travelers with high exposure risks (see additional details in Chapters 32 and 43).

Rabies

Rabies remains uncontrolled in many areas of the developing world, but the risk to travelers is low. Rabies transmission occurs when the rabies virus is introduced into open cuts or wounds, usually through the bite of an infected animal, so counseling on avoidance of animal bites and avoiding street dogs is essential. *Preexposure rabies prophylaxis,* which consists of three inoculations of human diploid cell killed virus vaccine (1 mL intramuscularly on days 0, 7, and 21 or 28) is appropriate for long-term travelers who will live in endemic areas. People who anticipate animal exposure, such as veterinarians, animal handlers, and laboratory workers, should also be vaccinated and should also receive a booster dose of vaccine (1 mL) every 2 years. Children are especially at risk because of the increased likelihood of contact with stray dogs. The human diploid cell vaccine (HDCV) is more immunogenic and causes fewer reactions than the old duck embryo vaccine. Occasional local reactions and rare systemic reactions such as headaches, myalgias, and dizziness may occur. Vaccine from animal brain tissue is still being used in some developing countries, so if travelers require rabies vaccine, they should be sure to obtain the HDCV.

The HDCV may also be administered to travelers by the intradermal route (0.1 mL on days 0, 7, and 21 or 28) if the three-dose series is completed 30 days or more before departure. Intradermal rabies vaccine is as immunogenic as intramuscular vaccine, but because the dose is one-tenth of the intramuscular dose, it is less costly. The HDCV should not be administered by the intradermal route when chloroquine or mefloquine, which may interfere with the immune response to the HDCV, is being used.

Pregnancy is not a contraindication to preexposure prophylaxis. If the previously vaccinated traveler is exposed to rabies, he or she should still seek medical help for *postexposure immunization* described in Chapter 32. Any animal bite should be thoroughly cleansed with soap and water to help reduce the risk of rabies.

Tuberculosis

Tuberculosis continues to be a worldwide health problem, but the risk to the short-term traveler is small. Mycobacterium tuberculosis is primarily a respiratory pathogen contracted by inhaling droplet nuclei, but unpasteurized milk products can also spread the disease. Travelers who will be spending extended periods in tuberculosis endemic areas should have a tuberculin skin test before departure. Calmette–Guérin bacillus (BCG) vaccine use is controversial and most U.S. experts do not recommend it. Periodic skin tests in long-term travelers are recommended to detect subclinical infections.

Measles, Mumps, Rubella, Influenza

In most developing and developed countries other than the United States, measles, mumps, and rubella remain uncontrolled. Therefore, children should receive routine immunizations against these diseases before travel. Adolescents and adults who have neither had these diseases nor been immunized against them are at risk of becoming infected while traveling. People

born after 1957 should have a booster dose of vaccine if they have not already received it. Rubella vaccine is indicated for females of child-bearing age without serologic evidence of prior rubella infection.

Certain travelers may benefit from pretrip vaccination with influenza and pneumococcal vaccine. Influenza causes morbidity and mortality throughout the world and poses risk to unvaccinated travelers. Increasing penicillin resistance in pneumococci throughout the world is of concern. The same criteria for selecting candidates for influenza and pneumococcal vaccine in the United States should be used.

Chapter 32 contains details regarding dosages and schedules for these vaccines.

Japanese Encephalitis

Japanese encephalitis (JE) is a mosquitoborne viral encephalitis that occurs in epidemics in much of Asia, including China, and endemically in the tropical areas of Southeast Asia. The risk to short-term travelers and those who confine their travel to urban centers is low. People at greatest risk are those living for prolonged periods in endemic or epidemic areas (Fig. 33.3). A vaccine to protect against JE is in the United States. The vaccine (JE-VAX, Japanese encephalitis vaccine, inactivated) distributed by Connaught Laboratories, should be considered for patients planning long-term residence in endemic areas and for travelers visiting rural

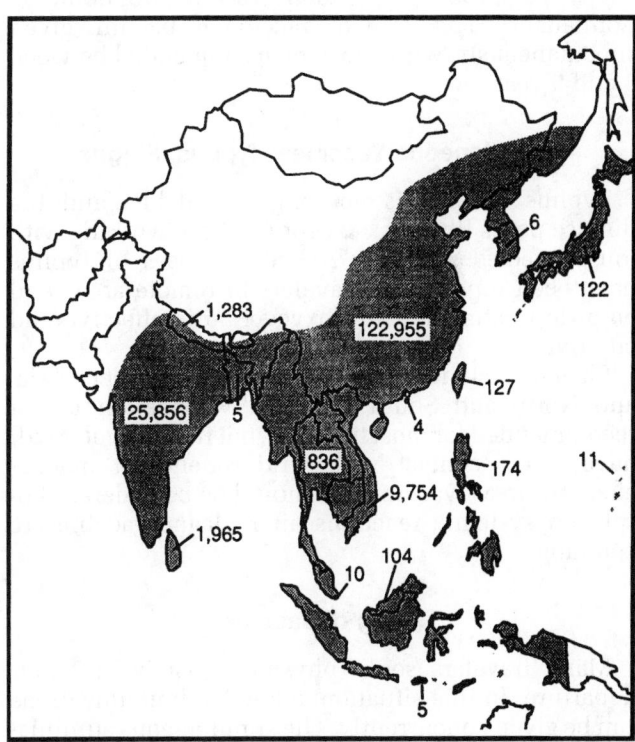

Figure 33.3. Reported Japanese encephalitis cases by endemic countries and regions of Southeast Asia where viral transmission is proven or suspected, 1986–1990. (From Tsai TF. Japanese encephalitis vaccines. In: Plotkin SA, Mortimer E, eds. Vaccines. 2nd ed. Philadelphia: WB Saunders, 1994.)

farming areas or sleeping in unscreened rooms in endemic or epidemic areas. It is especially recommended for people staying more than 1 month in an endemic country. JE vaccine is associated with a 10 to 20% rate of side effects, including fever, headache, myalgias, and malaise. Serious allergic reactions have also been documented, but the vaccine is overall immunogenic, efficacious, and safe and has been used to vaccinate millions of people. The primary series consists of three subcutaneous injections at weekly intervals, with boosters at 1 and 4 years, and the series should be completed at least 3 weeks before departure.

Meningococcal Meningitis

Meningococcal meningitis occurs throughout the developing world, often in devastating epidemics. Although cases in American travelers are rare, vaccine may be indicated in travelers going to countries with high rates of infection. Areas where pretravel immunization has been recommended include New Delhi, Northern India, and Nepal; the meningitis belt of Sahel (sub-Saharan Africa), including the dry inland regions of west African countries; Saudi Arabia after outbreaks in pilgrims returning from Mecca; and East Africa, including Burundi, Kenya, Tanzania, Mozambique, and Zambia. Although meningococcal meningitis epidemics have occurred in Latin America, the prevalent type has been B, a serotype not covered by the vaccine. The vaccine available for use in the United States is the A, C, Y W-135 Quadrivalent vaccine (Menomune, Connaught). The dose of vaccine is 0.5 mL given subcutaneously, with boosters recommended between 3 and 5 years.

Miscellaneous Vaccines: Typhus, Plague

Typhus vaccine is no longer available, and the disease poses little risk except for those working with louse-infected refugees. Anecdotal cases of typhus have been reported in travelers to remote areas and empiric treatment with doxycycline is effective and curative.

Plague exists in certain rural areas in Africa, Asia, and North and South America. Vaccination is not recommended for most travelers, but if the traveler will have direct contact with wild rodents in plague-enzootic areas, vaccination should be considered. Local and systemic reactions after plague vaccine are common.

Timing of Vaccines

Many travelers see a physician just before their departure. In this situation, all active immunizations can be given concurrently. The simultaneous administration of injectable cholera and yellow fever vaccine may rarely be associated with lower than expected antibody levels to both vaccines. The clinical relevance of this is unknown because injectable cholera vaccine is almost never given. Simultaneous administration of

multiple vaccines produces good antibody responses to all the antigens. However, when it is possible, multiple vaccinations should be spread out over time, and all should be completed by 1 week before arrival in a developing country to decrease the likelihood of reactions and to ensure that adequate antibody levels have been attained (7). When vaccines are administered concurrently, they should be given with separate syringes at different body sites. Killed vaccines can be given at the same time as immune globulin. With certain live, attenuated vaccines (especially measles, mumps, rubella), passively acquired antibody may interfere with replication of the vaccine virus and poses the possibility of decreasing the efficacy of the vaccine. Therefore, if possible, live virus vaccines should be given at least 14 days before the administration of immune globulin and probably 3 months after administration. Immune globulin does not interfere with yellow fever or oral polio vaccines, both of which are live.

MALARIA PROPHYLAXIS

Malaria is a potentially fatal parasitic disease caused by infection of red blood cells with *Plasmodium* species. It is usually transmitted by *Anopheles mosquitoes* but can be acquired from transfused blood and intravenous drug use. Malaria tends to be more severe in immunologically virgin travelers than in residents of endemic areas. The disease is characterized by high fevers, chills, sweats, myalgias, and headache with no obvious focal signs or symptoms of infection. Malaria exists worldwide. The risk of contracting malaria varies from country to country and from season to season depending on local conditions such as rainfall, altitude, and mosquito density. Because malaria is almost totally preventable in travelers, there should be no deaths in travelers caused by malaria. Each year, however, American travelers still die because of inadequate protection against malaria. Prevention of malaria requires a twofold approach: minimizing mosquito contact and taking appropriate prophylactic medicine (16).

To avoid mosquito exposure, travelers should sleep in screened rooms and under mosquito nets. Anopheles mosquitoes feed predominantly from dusk to dawn. Therefore, travelers who must be out during this time should try to cover the body with clothing and use insect repellent on exposed areas. Long-sleeved shirts, long-legged trousers, and occasionally a face net should be worn if at all possible. Mosquito repellent containing N, N-diethylmetatoluamide (DEET) (20 to 40%) should be applied to exposed skin. Use of 100% DEET is not recommended and can be toxic for children. Outdoor nighttime activity should be avoided whenever possible.

Even with appropriate mosquito protection, travelers may get bitten by malarious mosquitoes. It is therefore necessary to take an appropriate *chemoprophylactic* drug (Table 33.2) when traveling to a malarious area. Malaria chemoprophylaxis should preferably

Table 33.2.   Drugs Used in the Prophylaxis of Malaria[a]

Drugs	Adult Dosage	Pediatric Dosage
Chloroquine phosphate (Aralen)	500 mg salt orally, once/wk	5 mg/kg base (8.3 mg/kg salt) orally, once/wk, up to a maximal dose of 300 mg base
Hydroxychloroquine sulfate (Plaquenil)	400 mg salt orally, once/wk	5 mg/kg base (6.5 mg/kg salt) orally, once/wk, up to a maximal adult dose of 310 mg base
Mefloquine	228 mg base (250 mg salt) orally, once/wk	15–19 kg: ¼ tablet/wk 20–30 kg: ½ tablet/wk 31–45 kg: ¾ tablet/wk >45 kg: 1 tablet/wk
Doxycycline	100 mg orally, once/day	>8 yr of age: 2 mg/kg of body weight orally/day, up to adult dose of 100 mg/day
Proguanil (not available in United States)	200 mg orally, once/day in combination with weekly chloroquine	<2 yr: 500 mg/day 2–6 yr: 100 mg/day 7–10 yr: 150 mg/day >10 yr: 200 mg/day
Primaquine	15 mg base (26.3 mg salt) daily, once/day for 14 days	0.3 mg/kg base (0.5 mg/kg salt) orally once/day for 14 days
For presumptive therapy: pyrimethamine–sulfadoxine (Fansidar)	3 tablets (75 mg pyrimethamine and 1500 mg sulfadoxine orally as a single dose)	5–10 kg: ½ tablet 11–20 kg: 1 tablet 21–30 kg: 1.5 tablets 31–45 kg: 2 tablets >45 kg: 3 tablets

[a]See text for indications according to geographic region and *Plasmodium* species.

begin 1 to 2 weeks before travel and should continue for 4 weeks after leaving the malarious areas. Before deciding on a chemoprophylactic regimen, it is important to obtain recent information regarding country-specific malaria risk. The CDC maintains up-to-date information that is available by calling 404-332-4555. Regardless of the chemoprophylaxis used, it is still possible to contract malaria. Symptoms of malaria can develop as early as 1 week after initial exposure and as late as several months after departure from a malarious area.

In selecting the appropriate chemoprophylactic agents, several factors must be taken into consideration (25). The most important consideration is whether the traveler will be at risk of acquiring chloroquine-resistant *Plasmodium falciparum* (CRPF) malaria (see below).

For travel to malarious areas where CRPF has not been reported or is at a very low level (e.g., Central America), once weekly *chloroquine phosphate,* 500 mg of the phosphate salt (300 mg base), should be taken. Chloroquine is usually well tolerated, but a few people may experience mild side effects, including itching, nausea, and disorientation. Side effects can be minimized by taking the drug with meals or in divided twice-weekly doses. As an alternative, the related compound *hydroxychloroquine* may be better tolerated. Amodiaquine, another related compound (not available in the United States), should not be used because of associated hepatotoxicity and marrow depression. When chloroquine is used for prolonged periods at high dosages, as in the therapy of rheumatoid arthritis, it may be associated with a severe retinopathy. This serious side effect is extremely rare when chloroquine is used at the low dosages for malaria chemoprophylaxis. The risk of retinopathy appears to increase after a cumulative dosage of 100 g of base, and periodic retinal examinations should be considered in patients who have taken this much chloroquine. Chloroquine is

safe in pregnant and lactating women and should be recommended to pregnant women traveling to malaria endemic zones.

Most malaria endemic areas now have strains of *P. falciparum* that are resistant to chloroquine, and travelers to these areas (Fig. 33.4) are at risk of contracting chloroquine-resistant malaria if chloroquine alone is used for chemoprophylaxis. For these areas, once-per-week *mefloquine* (250 mg) is recommended. In two areas, eastern Thailand and rural Cambodia, mefloquine resistance has been reported. Minor side effects reported with mefloquine include dizziness and gastrointestinal disturbances that tend to be transient and self-limited. Mefloquine has occasionally been associated with asymptomatic bradycardia and a prolonged QT interval and should be used with caution, if at all, by travelers who take β-blockers, quinidine, calcium channel blockers, or other cardiac drugs that alter conduction. Mefloquine should also be used with caution, if at all, in travelers with a seizure disorder or underlying psychosis. Mefloquine is safe in the second and third trimesters of pregnancy. There is insufficient information regarding its safety in the first trimester. Mefloquine prophylaxis should begin 1 week before travel to malarious areas and it should be continued weekly for 4 weeks after leaving such areas.

There are a number of *alternative chemoprophylactic regimens for CRPF.* For travelers who are unable to take mefloquine or those traveling to areas where mefloquine resistance has been reported, daily doxycycline is an acceptable regimen. Prophylaxis with doxycycline (100 mg) should begin 1 to 2 days before, during, and for 4 weeks after traveling to the malarious area. Travelers who use doxycycline must be alert to potential side effects, including sun sensitivity and gastrointestinal tract intolerance. Proguanil (Paludrine) has been used both alone and in combination with other antimalarials, but it is

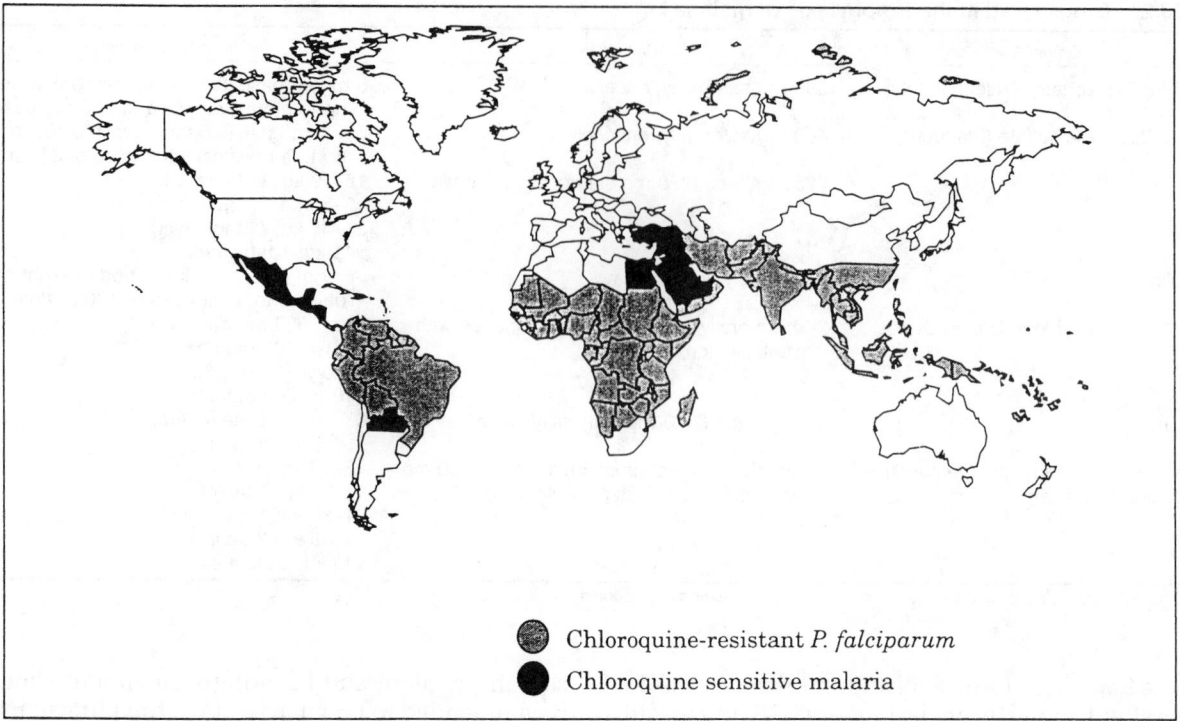

Chloroquine-resistant *P. falciparum*

Chloroquine sensitive malaria

Figure 33.4.   Distribution of malaria and chloroquine-resistant *Plasmodium falciparum,* 1996. (From Health Information International Travel, 1996. US Department of Health and Human Services.)

not available in the United States. Daily proguanil (200 mg) in combination with chloroquine may be useful in East Africa, but has not been as effective in Thailand and Papua New Guinea.

Travelers who decide to take chloroquine alone or chloroquine and proguanil should take with them a treatment supply of pyrimethamine–sulfadoxine (Fansidar). These travelers are at risk of acquiring CRPF and should be advised to take the Fansidar promptly if they have a febrile illness and cannot obtain medical care promptly (Table 33.2). Mefloquine should not be used for self-treatment because of the likelihood of dosage-dependent side effects.

Routine malaria prophylaxis with chloroquine or mefloquine does not prevent delayed attacks of malaria from *Plasmodium vivax* or *Plasmodium ovale* because these species have an extraerythrocytic chronic liver phase not eradicated by these two agents. *Primaquine* is an 8-aminoquinolone drug that is effective against the chronic liver forms of vivax and ovale malaria. For travelers with minimal mosquito exposure and short stays in endemic areas, primaquine is not routinely indicated. However, primaquine prophylaxis should be considered in travelers who have had extended stays in areas endemic for either *P. vivax* or *P. ovale* malaria and who have had significant mosquito exposure. Primaquine, 15 mg of base daily for 14 days, is usually given during the last 2 weeks of chloroquine chemoprophylaxis. Primaquine can cause hemolysis in people with glucose 6-phosphate deficiency (G6PD), and it has several other potential side effects, such as

headache, nausea, vomiting, and gastrointestinal distress. Before treatment with this drug, the patient's G6PD status should be determined.

FOOD AND WATER

Food and water are the most common vehicles for the introduction of infectious agents into the body. It is best for the traveler to the developing world to consider any uncooked food and any product containing unpasteurized milk as possibly contaminated and therefore not safe to consume. Meats can harbor pathogens such as *Trichinella spiralis* and *Taenia solium* and *Taenia saginata*. Raw or undercooked freshwater fish and crustaceans can transmit liver flukes and tapeworms. Even after foods have been cooked, it is imperative that food be properly stored. Food held at ambient temperatures is a medium in which bacterial pathogens can multiply rapidly. Creamy desserts are often vehicles for *Salmonella* and staphylococcal food poisoning and should be avoided in areas with poor refrigeration (see clinical description in Chapter 26). Fruits that can be peeled are safe as long as they are peeled by the consumer just before eating. The traveler should be wary of cheese products made from unpasteurized milk as possible sources of *Brucella* and other enteric pathogens. Salads should be avoided because lettuce and leafy vegetables are difficult to clean properly and often harbor infectious parasite eggs, cysts, and bacteria.

Although water may be safe in hotels in large cities,

only water that has been adequately boiled or chlorinated should be considered safe to drink. If the traveler is uncertain about the purity of the water, it should be boiled. Routine chlorination may not kill all parasites. In areas where purified water is not available or where hygiene and sanitation are poor, travelers are advised to drink only the following beverages: those that use boiled water, such as hot tea or coffee; canned or bottled carbonated beverages, including carbonated bottled water and soft drinks; and beer or wine.

Boiling is by far the most reliable method of making water safe to drink. If the water contains sediment or floating matter, it should be strained with a cloth before boiling or chemical treatment. The water should be boiled vigorously for at least 10 minutes to kill cysts, viruses, and bacteria, then allowed to cool to room temperature. If boiling is not possible, water can be *chemically disinfected* with tincture of iodine or tetraglycine hydroperiodide tablets. The purification tablets can be purchased from a pharmacy or a sporting goods store. The traveler should follow the manufacturer's instructions. If the water is cloudy, the number of tablets should be doubled. If the water is extremely cold, it should be allowed to warm up before the tablets are added. Tincture of iodine should be used as follows:

Per Quart or Liter of Water	Timing
Clean water, 5 drops	Let sit 30 minutes
Cloudy or cold water, 10 drops	Let sit several hours

Water may also be adequately purified by the use of small portable *water filters* that are available in sporting goods stores. These remove all waterborne parasitic and bacterial agents and some remove viruses. The water can be consumed immediately after treatment.

It should be remembered that where water may be contaminated, ice (as well as containers for drinking) should also be considered contaminated. If at all possible, boiled or bottled water should be used for making ice, rinsing drinking vessels, and brushing teeth. If boiled or bottled water is unavailable, the hot water tap can be used as a last resort. Although many infectious agents do not grow at these temperatures, hot tap water is by no means completely safe.

DIARRHEA

Diarrhea is the most common illness among travelers to developing countries, affecting from 30 to 60%; thus, it affects the enjoyment of the trip for many people. Most cases do not pose a serious health threat; however, some episodes are severe and may lead to dehydration. Cases occur when fecally contaminated food or water is ingested, so the precautions mentioned above for food and water should be followed. Even with good personal hygiene and avoidance of suspect food and water, the attack rate for traveler's diarrhea remains high. Approximately 75% of episodes are caused by bacterial agents, with more than 50% caused by enterotoxigenic *Escherichia coli.* Because the causative agents can be assumed to be bacterial three-fourths of the time,

several strategies to prevent bacterial diarrhea or to treat it early have been studied (5).

Prophylaxis

In January 1985, a consensus conference on traveler's diarrhea held at the National Institutes of Health recommended against the use of routine prophylactic antimicrobials. The potential risk of adverse reactions to the prophylactic agent was thought to outweigh the benefits. Although routine prophylaxis was not thought to be appropriate, it was also concluded that some travelers may wish to consult with their physician and may elect to use prophylactic antimicrobial agents for travel under special circumstances, once the risks and benefits are clearly understood (4). The antimicrobials that have been used in this way include ciprofloxacin (250 or 500 mg/day), norfloxacin (400 mg/day), doxycycline (100 mg/day with meals), and trimethoprim–sulfamethoxazole (one double-strength tablet daily) (6), continued for 2 days after departure from a developing country. If prophylaxis is used, it should be limited to less than 3 weeks, and the quinolones listed are preferred in most cases because of the excellent coverage for the enteric pathogens, with consequent high efficacy rates (prevents more than 95% of expected illness) and low rate of adverse reactions. If doxycycline is being used for another indication (e.g., malaria prophylaxis or acne), additional antidiarrheal prophylaxis is not needed; because of possible photosensitivity, people taking doxycycline should wear hats and garments that prevent sun exposure.

Pepto-Bismol, a nonprescription product containing bismuth subsalicylate, can also prevent approximately 65% of diarrhea episodes; the dosage is two tablets four times a day with meals. Pepto-Bismol turns the tongue and stools black; it may cause tinnitus.

Examples of travelers who would benefit from prophylaxis are those with preexisting medical conditions (e.g., cardiovascular disease) that would place the person at great risk if diarrhea and even mild dehydration develop. Prophylaxis is also sometimes appropriate for people who will be at high risk for a very limited time (e.g., volunteers in a refugee camp for less than 3 weeks).

Treatment

Most cases of diarrhea are self-limited and may require only rest and replacement of fluids and salts. This can best be accomplished with oral rehydration solution (ORS) (e.g., CeraLyte, Cera Products, Inc., Columbia, Maryland), but certain home-available fluids (e.g., juices, soups) can also be used. Especially when diarrhea is severe, ORS should be used because it contains a complete formulation to replace the needed electrolytes in the appropriate concentrations. The traveler should drink a volume of ORS to approximate the volume of diarrhea losses, although an exact balance of intake and output is not necessary. If no commercial ORS is available, a similar solution can be made by adding one-half teaspoon salt, one-half teaspoon baking soda, and 4 tablespoons sugar to 1 pint (500 mL) water. (If baking soda is not available, 1 teaspoon salt should be used.) The electrolyte concentrations of fluids for sweat replacement (e.g., Gatorade) are not equivalent to ORS. Any ORS remaining after 24 hours should be discarded because there is a chance of bacterial contamination.

Early antimicrobial treatment with ciprofloxacin (250 or 500 mg twice daily), norfloxacin (400 mg twice daily), doxycycline (100 twice daily), or trimethoprim–sulfamethoxazole (one double-strength tablet twice daily) will shorten the episode caused by susceptible strains of bacteria. Generally the drug should be started soon after diarrhea begins and continued for 3 days, although a single dose of ciprofloxacin (500 mg) has been shown to be effective (19). If the illness is thought to be *shigellosis* on the basis of signs and symptoms (blood in the stool, fever, and severe cramps), one of the quinolones for 5 days is the regimen of first choice; the second choice would be trimethoprim–sulfamethoxazole for 5 days. Most shigellae are resistant to tetracyclines and sulfa, however.

Antimotility drugs such as diphenoxylate/atropine (Lomotil) and loperamide (Imodium) may provide temporary relief when diarrhea is especially inconvenient, such as during an 8-hour country bus trip, or other emergent situations. There continues to be concern that dysentery can be prolonged if antimotility drugs are used and these agents should be used with care (if at all) with fever or dysentery because of potential clinical deterioration with an invasive bacterial pathogen. They have been used together with antimicrobial agents such as the quinolones to provide more rapid relief than might occur with the antimicrobial alone; however, the improvement is marginal. If loperamide (no prescription needed), which does not

cause atropinelike side effects, is used, the dose is two 2-mg tablets after each voluminous, watery stool.

Bismuth subsalicylate (Pepto-Bismol) is also helpful, although large amounts are needed to significantly reduce diarrhea. The dosage is 30 mL liquid (or two tablets) every half hour to 1 hour, up to eight doses in 24 hours. Precautions with this drug include complications caused by the salicylates it contains and by the fact that it binds tetracyclines.

Kaopectate, Enterovioform, and Streptotriad are not efficacious and should not be used.

The choices among the modalities described above should be based on the patient's symptoms. Fluid replacement should be encouraged for any episode of diarrhea but is all that is necessary in mild cases. For diarrhea of moderate severity (two to three unformed stools per day, no fever, no symptoms of frank dysentery, i.e., severe crampy pain or bloody stools), nonspecific symptomatic therapy may be all that is needed. Either bismuth subsalicylate or loperamide is useful. Antimicrobial agents should be used only for moderately severe to severe illness (more than four unformed stools per day, mild fever, dysentery).

For diarrhea that is very severe, is associated with repeated vomiting, or does not improve after several days, the traveler should be advised to consult a physician rather than attempt self-treatment. A doctor should also be consulted if there is blood in the stool; there is a fever higher than 101°F, especially if accompanied by shaking chills; or antimicrobial therapy does not provide rapid improvement.

Finally, in preparation for possible diarrhea, the traveler should be reminded that *toilet tissue* is difficult to find in many developing countries and that it is prudent to take a supply.

Additional information regarding the pathogenesis, epidemiology, and treatment of diarrheal illnesses is contained in Chapter 26.

Figure 33.5. Geographic distribution of *S. mansoni* and *S. intercalatum*. (From Warren KS, Mahmoud AAF, eds. Tropical and geographical medicine. New York: McGraw-Hill, 1990.)

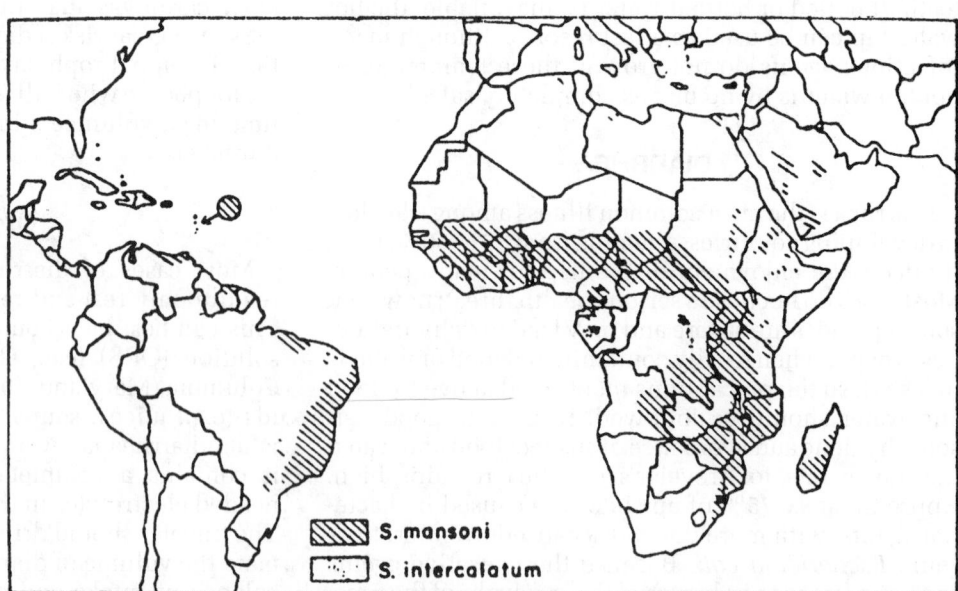

S. mansoni

S. intercalatum

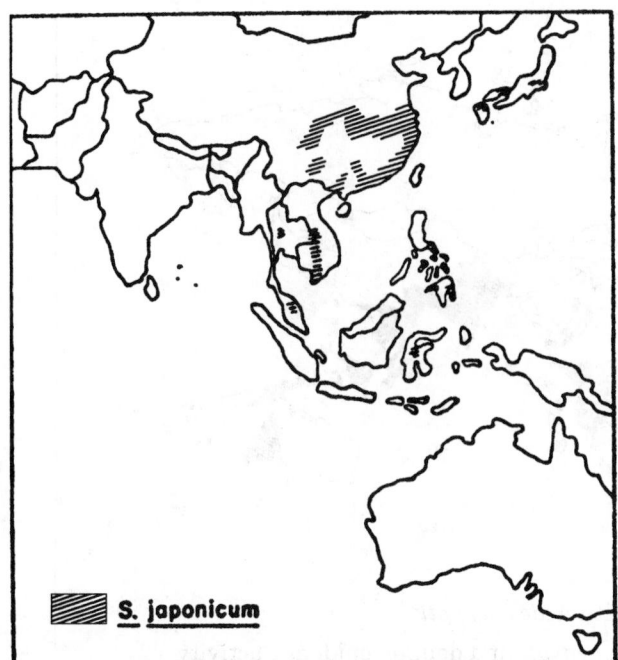

Figure 33.6. Geographic distribution of *S. japonicum.* On the mainland of Indochina, *S. mekongi* is probably the predominant species. (From Warren KS, Mahmoud AAF, eds. Tropical and geographical medicine. New York: McGraw-Hill, 1990.)

SCHISTOSOMIASIS

Schistosomiasis is one of the world's major public health problems. Three predominant species exist *(Schistosoma mansoni, Schistosoma japonicum, Schistosoma haematobium)* and are found worldwide (Figs. 33.5 through 33.7). Although few travelers are aware of schistosomiasis, it is a common disease in much of the developing world (12). After infection, the disease may lie dormant until it causes problems later in life. People contract schistosomiasis by wading or swimming in fresh or estuary water that harbors the snail vector of this trematode parasite. The cercariae (larval stage) can penetrate the skin and pass into the bloodstream without causing any symptoms at the time. Symptoms that may occur with schistosomiasis depend on the stage of the infection. Sometimes, there may be a rash at the site where the cercariae invaded, but this is uncommon. About 4 or 5 weeks after infection, an episode of fever, cough, and general malaise may occur. Still later (6 months to several years), more severe complications may occur, usually related to liver or urinary tract disease.

In recent years, severe cases of schistosomiasis have occurred in Americans after river rafting in Ethiopia and after swimming in fresh water in Kenya. Although treatment has improved with the advent of praziquantel, it is better to advise travelers to avoid fresh water contact in endemic areas and thereby prevent disease acquisition. For a returning traveler who has been exposed to fresh water in a schistosome-endemic area, screening tests including a complete blood count and

specific serology may be useful. This is particularly important in a patient with unexplained systemic symptoms. Eosinophilia in the peripheral blood may be present during the initial stages of the parasitic infection, although it is not a constant finding in late chronic infections. Positive serology indicates likely exposure, especially in the nonimmune traveler. If serology is positive, a further laboratory evaluation including urinalysis and stool examination for ova should be undertaken, recognizing that the acute syndrome described above may occur before there is detectable egg excretion. Proven or strongly suspected acute schistosomal infection requires treatment with *praziquantel* (Biltricide), which is effective in early schistosomal infection. This drug is supplied in 600-mg tablets, scored so that they can be broken into four 150-mg units. Treatment is accomplished in 1 day by giving a single dose of 40 mg/kg for *S. mansoni* or *S. haematobium* and three doses (20 mg/kg each) 4 to 6 hours apart for *S. japonicum.*

DENGUE

In recent years the incidence of dengue fever has increased dramatically in most of the countries in the Caribbean (Fig. 33.8). Dengue fever is a mosquitoborne viral illness transmitted by *Aedes aegypti* mosquitoes. It occurs in parts of tropical Asia, Africa, and the Pacific. Dengue fever is characterized by sudden onset of high fevers, severe frontal headaches, joint and muscle pains, and a general feeling of malaise. In addition, many patients have nausea, vomiting, and a rash that typically appears 3 to 5 days after the onset of fever. The rash may spread from the trunk to the arms,

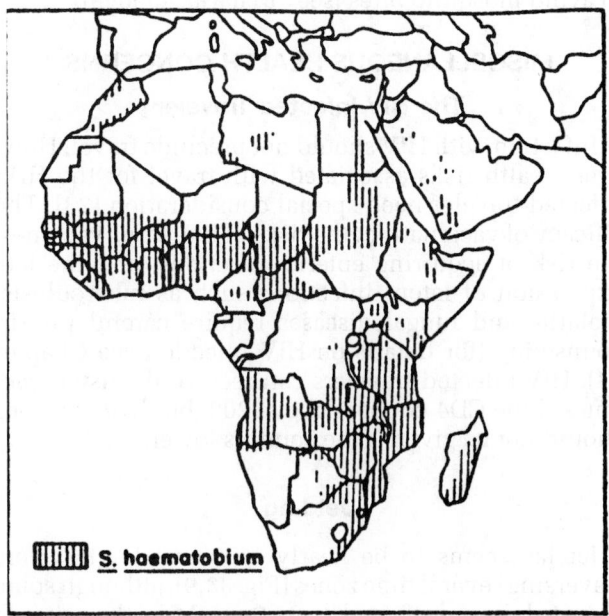

Figure 33.7. Geographic distribution of *S. haematobium.* (From Warren KS, Mahmoud AAF, eds. Tropical and geographical medicine. New York: McGraw-Hill, 1990.)

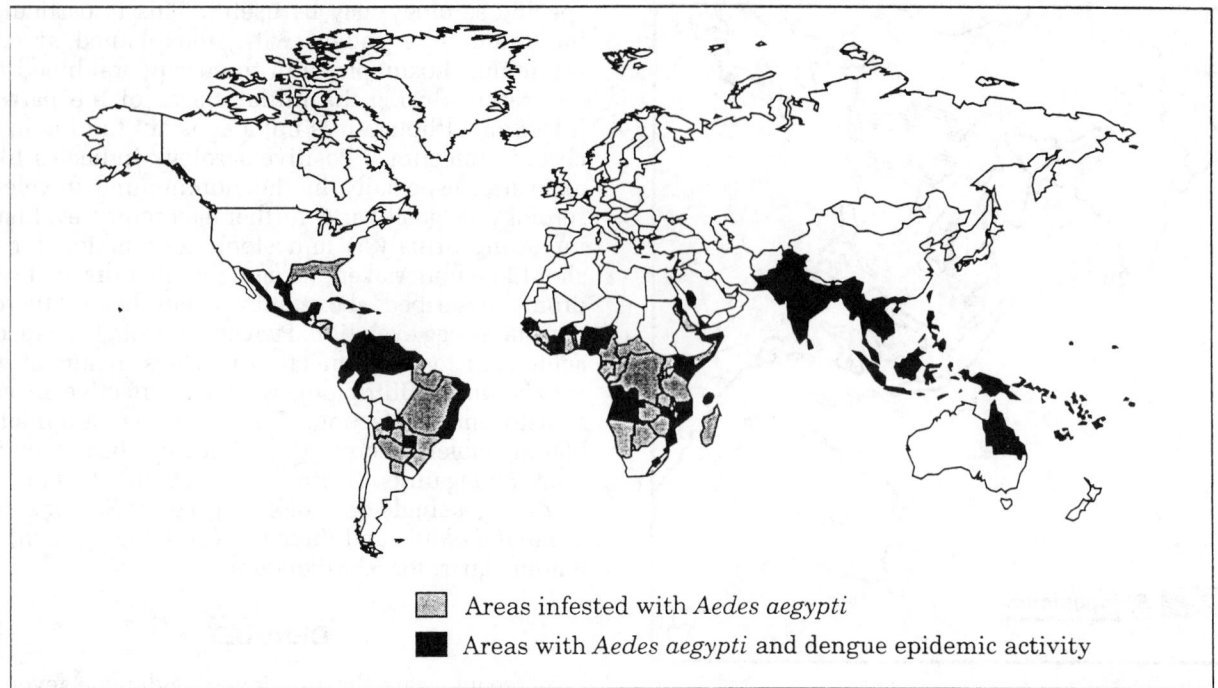

Figure 33.8. World distribution of dengue, 1996. (From Health Information International Travel, 1996. US Department of Health and Human Services.)

legs, and face and, generally, is benign and self-limited, although prolonged convalescence is often seen. Most dengue is subclinical or nonspecific in presentation but it may also present as a severe and fatal hemorrhagic disease called dengue hemorrhagic fever. Currently, there is no specific treatment for dengue and vaccines are not available. Travelers to areas where dengue is endemic therefore need to take precautions to avoid mosquito bites (see "Malaria," above).

MISCELLANEOUS HEALTH CONCERNS

The HIV-Infected Traveler

Infection with HIV should not preclude travel. However, health risks associated with travel for the HIV-infected traveler need special consideration (23). The efficacy of vaccination, the risks of live virus vaccines, the risk of acquiring enteric infections, and the late expression of latent infections such as tuberculosis, malaria, and fungal diseases require careful pretrip counseling (for details on HIV infection see Chapter 34). HIV-infected travelers can receive the usual vaccines if the CD4 count is above 200, but live vaccines should not be given if the count is lower.

Jet Lag

Jet lag seems to be nearly universal for travelers traversing several time zones (Fig. 33.9), although some seem to be more affected than others. More than simple travel fatigue, jet lag occurs when the body's physiologic clock has not yet adjusted to the new time zone. Symptoms include sleepiness during the daytime,

lying awake and hungry at night, and often a feeling that one's thinking processes are not quite normal. Several days to a week are usually needed to recover completely from jet lag.

Although time is the only cure, a *few suggestions* seem to help. Patients should be advised to avoid overeating and excess alcohol ingestion during air travel and to keep a light snack handy for middle-of-the-night hunger. Also, they should be advised to try to schedule a day of rest after passing six or more time zones before proceeding with their business or vacation. Taking a mild sleeping medication before bed for 2 or 3 days may also help them get back on schedule (see also Chapter 85, "Sleep Disorders"). *Melatonin,* a hormone produced in the pineal gland that is a potent modulator of circadian rhythms, has been investigated as a prophylactic agent for jet lag. It appears that use of melatonin improves the symptoms of jet lag in most travelers when taken as 3 to 6 mg 30 minutes before bedtime (local time) for the first 5 days after arrival. (Melatonin preparations are available without prescription.) For short-term use such as for jet lag, it appears safe.

Accidents

The major cause of serious morbidity and leading cause of mortality in travelers to the developing world is accidents, especially involving motor vehicles (9). Other major accidents include drowning, electric shocks, and trauma associated with dangerous sports (hang gliding, whitewater rafting). Injury prevention strategies should be part of routine travel advice.

Defensive driving is a must. In developing areas, roads are generally not as well built as in developed areas, and road hazards are common. Compounding the problems of accidental trauma is the usual lack of a developed emergency medicine infrastructure. Many countries have no formal emergency transport system, and hospital supplies are often lacking. Blood is often not available or not carefully screened, and quality control is not available. For serious trauma, it is often best to arrange transport to a medical facility in or operated by a developed nation.

Injectable Medications and Blood Transfusions

Travelers should be advised to avoid, if possible, receiving any injectable medication or blood transfusions when traveling in the developing world. Both hepatitis B and HIV can be readily transmitted by this route because needles and syringes may not always be sterilized properly. In addition, blood in most developing countries is not routinely screened for HIV (and may also not be screened for hepatitis B).

Motion Sickness

Travelers with a history of motion or sea sickness can attempt to avoid these symptoms by taking one of the antihistamines useful for this problem or ginger root derivatives. In a recent study of whale watchers in the North Sea, meclizine, cyclizine, dimenhydrinate, and ginger root were found to have equivalent efficacy (20). Further details are found in Chapter 81.

Swimming and Bathing

Swimming in contaminated water may result in eye, ear, skin, and some intestinal infections. Wading, washing, and swimming should be avoided in water that is likely to be infested with the snail hosts of schistosomiasis (see above) or with human sewage or with animal urine that may contain *Leptospira*. Generally, only chlorinated pools should be considered safe places to swim in developing countries. Ocean beaches may be safe, if not contaminated by sewage, but bathers should be advised to wear light shoes to protect against exposure to coral and other contact hazards.

Insects

The bites, stings, and contact of some insects cause unpleasant reactions. Many insects, such as mosquitoes, can bite and transmit disease without the traveler being aware of the bite. Insect repellents, protective clothing, and mosquito netting, which prevent the bite of insects, are the best prevention for some communicable diseases, particularly malaria (see above). Travelers therefore should take a supply of insect repellent cream, lotion, or spray.

Sunburn

Sunburn is a particular hazard in tropical and high-glare environments. Sunshades, sunscreens (see Chapter 100), broad-brimmed hats, and protective clothing are important preventive measures. Many sunscreen lotions must be reapplied after bathing or heavy perspiration. For maximal protection, travelers should apply all sunscreen products before going outside. A small percentage of people who take the antibiotic tetracycline (including doxycycline) may develop an exaggerated burn after exposure to the sun; this may be important if this antibiotic is being taken daily for diarrhea prevention.

High Altitude

High altitudes can be a problem for people with preexisting heart or lung disease, and portable oxy-

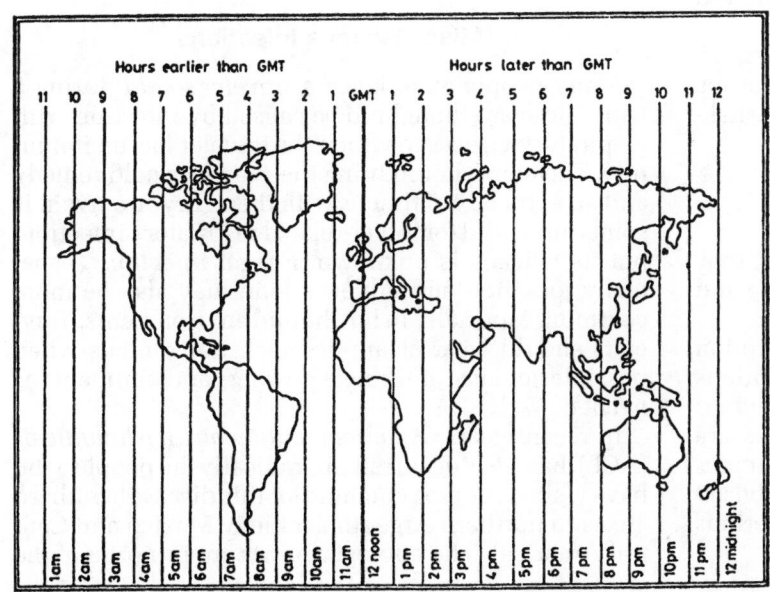

Figure 33.9. Time zones (jet lag typically occurs when five or more zones are crossed). *GMT,* Greenwich meridian time. (From Walker E, Williams G, Raeside F, Calvert L. ABC of healthy travel. 4th ed. London: BMJ Publishing Group, 1997.)

gen may be advisable for these situations. Rapid exposure to altitudes more than 8000 feet above sea level can cause serious medical problems. The incidence and severity of mountain sickness are related to the altitude, rate of ascent, and prior acclimatization. Initial symptoms include dizziness, headache, extreme fatigue, chilliness, nausea, and vomiting. More severe symptoms may also occur, most commonly difficulty in concentrating, extreme shortness of breath, and more severe headache. In most people, symptoms are mild and clear within 24 to 48 hours. If symptoms persist or are severe, a return to lower altitude may be required. Administration of oxygen generally relieves acute symptoms. Preventive measures include adequate rest before travel, avoidance of alcohol and tobacco, and decreased physical activity at high altitude.

The carbonic anhydrase inhibitor acetazolamide (Diamox) has been shown to reduce the time needed for acclimatization to high altitudes. It is prescribed at a dosage of 125 to 250 mg three times a day beginning 1 day before ascent and continued for 2 to 3 days after ascent. Two other drugs, dexamethasone and nifedipine, have also been studied in high-altitude illness and may be useful in patients already ill. Although acetazolamide is considered the drug of choice for the prevention of high-altitude sickness, the definitive treatment consists of moving to a lower altitude as soon as possible (11). Acetazolamide should not be used by sulfa-allergic people.

Snakes and Scorpions

Poisonous snakes live in many developing countries, although most travelers will never see them unless they visit a zoo. If travelers will be walking through brush or jungle, or will be walking at night, they should wear good-quality leather boots that go above the ankle. Not all snake bites are poisonous and not all poisonous snake bites are fatal, but immediate treatment by a physician is essential. If possible, the traveler should bring the snake for identification.

Scorpion bites are painful but seldom dangerous, except possibly to infants. Exposure to bites can be avoided by sleeping under mosquito netting and shaking clothing and shoes before putting them on.

Medicines

If travelers are taking prescribed medications, they should obtain an adequate supply before leaving and keep all medications in their luggage.

Many medications are sold without prescription overseas. However, the traveler should be cautious about purchasing medicines. Although medicines made by recognized pharmaceutical companies are generally of high quality, the quality of other medicines may not be guaranteed. The traveler should be advised not to self-medicate, as many medicines have serious side effects.

Pregnant Women and Children

Some medications used commonly in travelers should not be given to pregnant women, in particular doxycycline (impairs tooth development in the infant) and Fansidar (see "Malaria," above) (1). Travel late in pregnancy may precipitate labor. In fact, many airlines do not allow air travel during the final month.

Immunizations recommended for children are, in general, the same as those recommended for adults (Table 33.1), except that yellow fever vaccine is not usually required under 1 year of age. Routine baby shots are even more important for children traveling to developing countries because diphtheria, whooping cough, polio, and measles are common. The dosages of medicines have to be adjusted for children. This is especially important for malaria medications. Because children may be restless on long airline trips, some parents are tempted to sedate their children. This is discouraged, however, because children may react adversely to sedatives.

Sexually Transmitted Diseases

Casual sex in travelers may be more common than previously recognized (8). The risk of contracting sexually transmitted diseases is high in some parts of the world. Very importantly, HIV infection has become a global health problem. In addition to the risk of HIV infection, sexually transmitted pathogens such as penicillinase-producing *Neisseria gonorrhoeae* are becoming increasingly common. Likewise, less common pathogens such as chancroid and lymphogranuloma venereum and hepatitis B are more common in certain areas. To reduce the risk of sexually transmitted infections, travelers need to be discriminating in sexual relations and avoid multiple partners, anonymous partners, prostitutes, and people who have had multiple sexual partners. If a traveler chooses to have sexual relations, condoms should always be used during intercourse.

Miscellaneous Infections

Many people experience a *traveler's cold* during a trip. These are thought to be caused by infection with respiratory viruses to which the traveler has no immunity. Travelers should bring their favorite cold remedy and an extra box of tissues with them. Erythromycin is sometimes used for travel-related respiratory infection, but its efficacy is unknown. *Fungal infections,* especially jock itch and athlete's foot, may also be more common, especially in hot, humid environments. Travelers should wear clean, dry socks, or sandals when possible, and use antifungal powders and ointments as needed.

In recent years, *American cutaneous leishmaniasis* (ACL) has also occurred sporadically in people who have visited the area endemic for this disease (southern Texas to northern Argentina, chiefly Mexico and Central America). The etiologic agents are protozoa of the

Leishmania species, which are inoculated by female sandflies that inhabit forested lowlands. The skin lesion of ACL evolves over weeks to months from a papule to a nodule to an ulcer with raised indurated borders that eventually heals with a scar. Diagnosis requires identification of organisms in skin scrapings or biopsied tissue. Using insect repellent and wearing long sleeves and trousers are usually effective in preventing sandfly bites.

Long-Term Travelers

Recommendations for long-term travelers are generally the same regarding food and water, immunizations, malaria prophylaxis, and so on; however, a few issues may require increased emphasis and the need for certain interventions may increase. For example, the reasons for immunizing short-term travelers against hepatitis B, typhoid, meningitis, or Japanese encephalitis may not be compelling, but the benefit for a long-term traveler will be greater because the duration of time at risk is greater. Hence, the need for complete immunizations for endemic diseases of the area should be stressed. With recommendations for universal hepatitis B protection for infants, the importance of this vaccine for young travelers living overseas should be stressed. Furthermore, travelers may be willing to avoid fresh garden salads for short times, but long-term residents may choose to grow their own garden or find safe vegetables.

The commonly used antimalarials (chloroquine, mefloquine, and Paludrine) can all be used safely for several years if indicated; therefore, long duration of stay is not a contraindication for these drugs, although the cost of long-term usage must be discussed when choosing an antimalarial.

If the traveler hires people to work in the house, these employees should be screened medically before starting work. The examination should include a chest radiograph to rule out active tuberculosis and stool analysis to rule out fecal parasites and *S. typhi.*

Medical Emergencies

If the traveler becomes seriously ill or injured while traveling, the U.S. consulate can provide advice on where to go for help.

INTERNATIONAL TRAVELER'S HEALTH KIT

The following is a suggested first aid and health kit that represents the minimal necessary equipment for the traveler to the developing world (supply can be obtained from various travel catalogs and suppliers):

- International Immunization Card with documentation of vaccines received
- Appropriate medication for malaria prophylaxis
- Mosquito repellent
- Water purification tablets or tincture of iodine, or water filters

- Oral rehydration salt packets (available in the United States from CERA Products, Columbia, Maryland, 410-997-2334 and Jianas Brothers, Kansas City, Missouri, 816-421-2880)
- Antimicrobial medication for treatment or prevention of diarrhea as arranged with the traveler's physician
- Imodium or Lomotil, if indicated
- Sunscreen
- Adhesive bandages (for blisters)
- A spare pair of glasses or at least the lens prescription
- Any prescription medication the traveler takes regularly
- The traveler's favorite cold remedy
- Fever thermometer
- Aspirin or acetaminophen (paracetamol in most other countries)
- Astringent or antiseptic
- Antifungal powder
- Toilet paper

POSTTRAVEL SCREENING

Most people who acquire viral, bacterial, or parasitic infections in developing countries become ill within 6 weeks after returning, but certain infectious diseases, such as malaria and schistosomiasis, may not manifest themselves until later. The traveler should be advised to seek medical help for any unexplained symptoms during the 12 months after the end of a trip. When an unexplained late illness occurs, it is necessary to identify all of the developing countries that the traveler visited to know which infectious disease risks he or she encountered.

For travelers who stay for long periods in the developing world, it is prudent to provide routine screening on arrival home. This should include a complete blood count, liver function tests, tuberculosis skin test, stool examination for occult blood, urinalysis, and stool examination for ova and parasites. If these tests all are normal, the traveler has probably not acquired a serious unrecognized infectious disease, but posttrip surveillance for another 6 months is still warranted.

General References*

Advice for travelers. Med Lett 38:17, 1996.
    Up-to-date summary.
Barnett ED, Chen R. Children and international travel: immunizations. Pediatric Infect Dis J 14:982–992, 1995.
    A good review of the issues unique to the pediatric traveler.
Blair JE. Protecting travelers against infections: immunizations and other preventive strategies. Postgrad Med 100(6):159–172, 1996.
    Up-to-date summary.
Gardner P, ed. Health issues of international travelers. Infectious Diseases Clinics of North America. Philadelphia: WB Saunders, 1992.
    Comprehensive review of travel medicine.

---

*Bold print (general references) and bold numerals (specific references) denote published controlled clinical trials, meta-analyses, or consensus-based recommendations.

Health Information for International Travel. Supplement to Morbidity and Mortality Weekly Report, DHHS publ no. (CDC) 92-8280, Atlanta, Centers for Disease Control and Prevention.

   A practical manual, updated yearly, available free of charge.

Jong EC, McMillan R. The travel and tropical medicine manual. 2nd ed. Philadelphia: WB Saunders, 1995.

   A relevant manual written for the clinician that contains a list of travel clinics.

Mathews DS, Pust RE, Cordes DH, et al. Prevention and treatment of travel-related illness. Am Fam Physician 44:1343, 1991.

   Practical information.

Patterson JE, Patterson TF, Biafj BM, et al. Assuring safe travel for today's elderly. Geriatrics 44:44, 1989.

   Good review of age-related health risks.

Schroeder D, ed. Staying healthy in Asia, Africa, and Latin America. 3rd ed. Stanford, CA: Volunteers in Asia Press, 1993.

   A handbook that contains the nuts and bolts of health maintenance for traveling in the developing regions of the world.

Specific References

1. Barry M, Bia F. Pregnancy and travel. JAMA 261:728, 1989.
2. CDC 1992 Update. Eradication of paralytic poliomyelitis in the Americas. MMWR 41:681, 1992.
3. CDC Recommendations and Reports. Typhoid immunization: recommendations of the Advisory Committee on Immunization Practices (ACIP). MMWR 43:1–7, 1994.
4. Consensus Conference. Traveler's diarrhea. JAMA 253:2700, 1985.
5. DuPont HL, Ericsson CD. Prevention and treatment of traveler's diarrhea. N Engl J Med 328:1821, 1993.
6. Ericsson CD, Johnson PC, DuPont HC, et al. Ciprofloxacin or trimethoprim–sulfamethoxazole as initial therapy for travelers diarrhea. Ann Intern Med 106:216, 1987.
7. Falvo C, Horowitz H. Adverse reactions associated with simultaneous administration of multiple vaccines to travelers. J Gen Intern Med 9:255–260, 1994.
8. Gagneux OP, Blockliger CU, Tanner M, Hatz CF. Malaria and casual sex: what travelers know and how they behave. J Travel Med 3:14–21, 1996.
9. Hargarten SW, Barker TD, Guptill K, et al. Overseas fatalities of United States citizen travelers: an analysis of deaths related to international travel. Ann Emerg Med 20:622, 1991.
10. Hilton E, Singer C, Kozarsky P, et al. Status of immunity to

tetanus, measles, mumps, rubella, and polio among U.S. travelers. Ann Intern Med 115:32, 1991.
11. Honigman B, Theis MK, Koziol-McLain J, et al. Acute mountain sickness in a general tourist population at moderate altitudes. Ann Intern Med 118:587–592, 1993.
12. Jelinek T, Nothdurft H, Loscher T. Schistosomiasis in travelers and expatriates. J Travel Med 3:160–164, 1996.
13. Lemon SM, Thomas DL. Vaccines to prevent viral hepatitis. N Engl J Med 336:196–204, 1997.
14. Mahon BE, Mintz ED, Greene KD, et al. Reported cholera in the United States 1992–1994: a reflection of global changes in cholera epidemiology. JAMA 276:307–312, 1996.
15. Packham CJ. A survey of notified travel-associated infections: implications for travel health advice. JL Pub Hlth Med 17:217–222, 1995.
15a. Petrie K, Dawson AG, Thompson L, Brook R. A double-blind trial of melatonin as a treatment for jet lag in international cabin crew. Biological Psychiatry 33(7):526–530, 1993.
16. Rangel-Frausto MS, Edmond MD. Malaria: protection of the international traveler. Infect Control Hosp Epidemiol 14:155–160, 1993.
17. Reid D, Dewar RD, Fallon RJ, et al. Infection and travel: the experience of package tourists and other travelers. J Infect 2:65, 1980.
18. Robertson SE, Hull BP, Tomori O, et al. Yellow fever: a decade of reemergence. JAMA 276:1157–1162, 1996.
19. Salam I, Katelams P, Leigh-Smith S, Farthing MJG. Randomized trial of single-dose ciprofloxacin for traveler's diarrhea. Lancet 44:1537–1539, 1994.
20. Schmid R, Schick T, Steffen R, et al. Comparison of seven commonly used agents for prophylaxis of sea sickness. J Travel Med 1:203–206, 1994.
21. Steffen R, van der Linde F, Gyr K, Schar M. Epidemiology of diarrhea in travelers. JAMA 249:1176, 1983.
22. Steffen R, Rickenbach M, Wilhelm U, et al. Health problems after travel to developing countries. J Infect Dis 156:84, 1987.
23. Wilson ME, VonReyn CF, Fineberg MD, et al. Infections in HIV-infected travelers: risks and prevention. Ann Intern Med 114:582, 1991.
24. Wittlinger F, Steffen R, Watanabe H, et al. Risk of cholera among western and Japanese travelers. J Travel Med 2:154–158, 1995.
25. Wyler DJ. Malaria chemoprophylaxis for the traveler. N Engl J Med 329:31–37, 1993.

C H A P T E R 34

Ambulatory Care for the HIV-Infected Patient

JANET HORN, MD
LORI FANTRY, MD, MPH

Since the last edition of this book, the prognosis for patients with human immunodeficiency virus (HIV) in the United States has greatly improved. For example, in 1996, for the first time since the beginning of the epidemic, the number of deaths related to HIV/AIDS (acquired immunodeficiency syndrome) decreased by 48% in New York City. In addition, AIDS is no longer the leading cause of death in 25- to 44-year-old adults. Many HIV-infected people have increased longevity and better quality of life because of advances in the prevention and treatment of opportunistic infections (OIs). In addition, in many areas of the country, funding for the care of HIV-infected patients has greatly increased and thus improved the lives of these patients. Finally, newly developed antiviral agents have radically altered the course of HIV disease. These changes have made the care of HIV-infected patient more rewarding yet more complex.

GENERAL CONSIDERATIONS

Causes

The human immunodeficiency virus or HIV-1, originally called human lymphotropic virus type III (HTLV-III), was isolated and found to be the etiologic agent of AIDS in 1983. Other related human retroviruses include HIV-2, HTLV-I, and HTLV-II. HIV-2, found primarily in West Africa, has also been associated with AIDS but has a more prolonged incubation period (22). HTLV-1 has been associated with tropical spastic paraparesis and T-cell leukemia/lymphoma, and HTLV-II has not yet been associated definitively with any human disease.

HIV is a member of the *lentivirus subfamily of human retroviruses*. These viruses code for an enzyme known as reverse transcriptase, which permits transcription of viral RNA into proviral DNA and subsequent integration into the host's cellular genome, leading to a persistent and latent infection. The retroviruses are associated with diseases of long incubation period, involvement with the hematopoietic and central nervous systems, and immune suppression.

Epidemiology

The Centers for Disease Control and Prevention (CDC) estimates that almost 1 million Americans are infected with HIV. Because HIV seropositivity is not a reportable condition, these figures are derived from numerous sources regarding high-risk behaviors and the numbers of people who engage in these behaviors and, in fact, the most recent estimates of infection are lower than previous estimates. As of October 1995, 501,310 cases of AIDS had been reported to the CDC (4). The major distribution characteristics of the AIDS epidemic in adults in the United States are as follows.

AIDS has been diagnosed in all 50 states. The case incidence is especially high in large cities in the states with high incidence rates (i.e., California, Texas, New York, New Jersey, Maryland, Florida, Georgia, and the District of Columbia). The region of the country with the most rapidly growing proportion of the population with AIDS is the South.

AIDS occurs in adults who belong to the major risk groups for HIV infection: homosexual and bisexual men, intravenous drug users (IDUs) of both sexes, prostitutes, hemophiliacs, and infants of women in high-risk groups. Rarely are the risk factors for acquisition of HIV infection unknown.

In the late 1980s, the proportion of AIDS diagnoses in homosexual and bisexual men began to decline while that in IDUs increased, as evidenced by an increase in the proportion of patients with AIDS who report injecting drug use (IDU): from 17% during 1981 to 1987 to 27% reported from 1993 to 1995. Heterosexual transmission, the major mode of transmission in developing countries, has also become increasingly important in the United States and Europe.

AIDS onset is most common in the age range 20 to 50 years, with the peak incidence between 30 and 39 years. Primary HIV infection precedes AIDS by about 10 years (see below), meaning that a substantial proportion of infection occurs in adolescents and young adults.

The proportion of AIDS cases who are women has increased from 8% during 1981 to 1987 to 18% from 1993 to 1995. Women account for 63% of all cases transmitted by heterosexual contact.

Of the cases reported from 1993 to 1995, 38% occurred in African Americans and 18% occurred in Hispanics. In contrast, of the cases reported from 1981 to 1987, 25% occurred in African Americans and 14% occurred in Hispanics.

Transmission and Prevention of Transmission

HIV-1 occurs in highest concentrations in blood and semen. It also occurs in lower concentrations in cervical and vaginal secretions, saliva, tears, breast milk, and amniotic fluid. HIV transmission is most commonly through blood and semen, but vaginal secretions and breast milk also have been implicated in the transmission process.

Sexual Transmission

HIV infection can be transmitted during sexual intercourse between men and between men and women. *The following patterns, practices, and situations carry the greatest risk of infection:*

- Unprotected receptive anal intercourse, especially if the mucosal lining has been torn, which may happen with penile insertion itself but is more likely to happen with such sexual practices as fisting.
- Unprotected receptive vaginal intercourse, especially during menses.
- Unprotected vaginal or rectal intercourse when either partner has genital ulceration (e.g., due to primary syphilis, chancroid, or genital herpes). Genital ulcers can act as conduits for infected blood from or for infected semen, blood, or vaginal secretions into the person with the ulcer.

The prevention of sexual transmission of HIV requires that sexually active people choose sexual practices that eliminate the high-risk situations listed above, as well as other lower-risk practices including all unprotected insertive anal and vaginal intercourse and oral–genital contact. In the care of every patient who is sexually active and in public education messages, the fundamentals of safe, possibly safe, and definitely unsafe sex should be clearly communicated (Table 34.1). Specific instructions for the most effective use of condoms (Table 34.2) are particularly important.

Transmission Through Transfusion of Blood and Blood Products

HIV can be transmitted only by whole blood, blood cellular components, plasma, and clotting factors. No other blood products (e.g., immune globulin preparations, albumin, plasma protein fraction, hepatitis B vaccine) have been implicated.

The risk of acquiring HIV through a blood transfusion is now infinitesimally small. The estimated risk of HIV infection is 1:153,000 per unit of blood transfused (13). This low risk has been achieved by blood

Table 34.1.   Safe Sex Guidelines

Safe Sex Practices
Massage
Hugging
Mutual masturbation
Social kissing (dry)
Body-to-body rubbing
Voyeurism, exhibitionism, fantasy

Possibly Safe Sex Practices
French kissing (wet)
Anal intercourse **with condom**[a]
Vaginal intercourse **with condom**[a]
Limiting the number of partners with whom one has sex

Unsafe Sex Practices
Semen, vaginal fluid, menstrual blood, or urine in mouth or in contact with the skin where there is an open cut or sore
Anal intercourse **without condom**[a]
Vaginal intercourse **without condom**[a]
Rimming (oral–anal contact)
Fisting (possible percutaneous inoculation with blood from trauma caused by inserting fist into anus)
Having sex when either partner has an open genital sore

[a]See instructions for condom users in Table 34.2.

Table 34.2   Instructions for Condom Users

Use a condom every time you have intercourse.
Always put the condom on the penis before intercourse begins.
Put the condom on when the penis is erect.
Do not pull the condom tightly against the tip of the penis. Leave a small empty space—about 1 or 2 cm—at the end of the condom to hold semen. Some condoms have a nipple tip that will hold semen.
Unroll the condom all the way to the bottom of the penis.
If the condom breaks during intercourse, withdraw the penis immediately and put on a new condom.
After ejaculation withdraw the penis while it is still erect. Hold onto the rim of the condom as you withdraw so that the condom does not slip off.
Use a new condom each time you have intercourse. Throw used condoms away.
If a lubricant is desired, use water-based lubricants such as contraceptive jelly. Lubricants made with petroleum jelly may damage condoms. Do not use saliva because it may contain virus.
Store condoms in a cool, dry place if possible.
Condoms that are sticky or brittle or otherwise damaged should not be used.

Adapted from Population Reports XIV, No. 3, 1986.

donor education programs (to eliminate donors who belong to high-risk groups), uniform blood product screening since April 1985, HIV-inactivating treatment of clotting-factor concentrates, the use of autologous blood transfusions for elective surgery, and efforts to avoid all nonessential transfusions.

Needle Transmission

Needle transmission explains the large proportion of patients with AIDS in the United States in whom the only identified risk factor is the sharing of needles for intravenous drug injection. HIV-infected patients in this group pose a threat to both needle partners and sexual partners. In developing countries, this mode of transmission may also occur because of reuse of improperly cleaned needles and syringes for the injections of medicines.

Definitive interruption of transmission by this mode requires that the user discontinue the practice as part of a recovery program (see Chapter 22, "Use and Abuse of Illicit Drugs and Substances"). The interruption of transmission by those who continue intravenous drug use requires that they avoid needle sharing. Syringe and needle exchange programs have been shown to decrease needle sharing and to decrease spread of HIV infection. Therefore, drug treatment centers often serve the dual purpose of drug treatment and prevention of HIV transmission. Community-based outreach workers have also been successful in reaching IDUs. It is unknown whether cleansing needles with bleach before reuse is effective in preventing infection. Protective behaviors have been difficult to promote in this subset of people who engage in a variety of high-risk behaviors.

Perinatal Transmission

Although several modes may account for perinatal transmission from an HIV-infected woman to her infant, most infants acquire their infection at or near the time of delivery because of inoculation or ingestion of maternal blood. Intrauterine transmission by cord blood is less common and transmission postnatally through breastfeeding is rare (20). It is estimated that 7 to 39% of infants born to HIV-infected mothers become infected, with the highest rates occurring in infants born to mothers with high viral loads, late-stage disease, early fetal membrane rupture, and placental inflammation. Prevention of perinatal transmission requires primary prevention through safer sex practices and secondary prevention through HIV testing and subsequent counseling of HIV-infected women about the risks of pregnancy. In addition, zidovudine (AZT) monotherapy has been shown to prevent approximately two-thirds of predicted transmission of HIV to the fetus.

Casual Contact and the Risk of HIV Transmission

Casual transmission of HIV does not occur. Thus, household contacts of HIV-infected patients who are not sexual partners are not at risk during ordinary circumstances. Although the virus has been isolated in urine and saliva, there have been no documented cases of transmission through kissing or through exposure to urine, stool, or saliva. However, it is generally recommended that the same precautions taken to prevent transmission of hepatitis B in the household setting be observed by HIV-infected people (see Chapter 43). Precautions for avoiding transmission to health care workers and caretakers are described at the end of this chapter.

Pathogenesis of Disease in HIV-Infected Patients

HIV causes illness by impairing important components of the patient's immune system, making the patient susceptible to a wide variety of infections. This virus also causes illness by its direct effect on other body systems, especially the nervous system (27).

HIV preferentially infects human *T lymphocytes of the helper/inducer subset* (also called *T4 or CD4 cells*), resulting in both quantitative and qualitative defects in helper-cell function. Because helper T lymphocytes are crucial in cell-mediated immunity, HIV infection impairs this type of immunity, making the patient susceptible to a number of opportunistic infections. Uninfected people usually have more than 800 CD4 cells/mm^3 of blood, whereas HIV-infected patients with opportunistic infections usually have less than 200 CD4 cells/mm^3. Thus, monitoring the CD4 cell count has become useful for predicting the degree of suppression of a patient's cell-mediated immunity, guiding the differential diagnosis of new symptoms, and deciding when to initiate antiretroviral treatment and prophylaxis for opportunistic infection (see below).

Other abnormalities of immune function are also found in HIV-infected people. HIV can infect and impair the function of macrophages and monocytes as well as CD4 lymphocytes. HIV infection may also result in B-lymphocyte activation and nonspecific hypergammaglobulinemia, which may impair de novo antibody response to some antigens; this may place the patient at increased risk for infection with encapsulated bacteria. In addition, some studies suggest that HIV infection may cause derangements in polymorphonuclear neutrophil phagocytosis and intracellular killing.

Although most of the illnesses in patients with HIV infection are caused by impaired resistance to infection, a number of clinical manifestations are direct consequences of HIV infection or the immune response to HIV infection. There is good evidence that the virus plays an etiologic role in some neurologic syndromes. The virus may directly affect the nervous system both centrally and peripherally, causing HIV meningitis, dementia, and peripheral neuropathy. In addition, the virus, or in some cases the immune response to the virus, causes disease in the gastrointestinal tract, heart, lungs, and possibly the kidneys.

Natural History and Prognosis in HIV Infection

A longitudinal study of gay men in San Francisco showed that the mean length of time from seroconversion to AIDS, using the definition of AIDS before 1993, was 10 years. The time from infection to symptoms, however, varied considerably from person to person and probably reflects variations in individuals' immune systems and the infectivity of different strains of the virus. Expanded use of antiretroviral therapy, prophylaxis against opportunistic infections, and treatment of AIDS-associated conditions results in delayed progression and longer life expectancies for HIV-infected people. An overview of the natural history of HIV infection, based on CD4 counts and viral load, is shown in Figure 34.1. Because the virus may remain clinically silent with no demonstrable signs of immunodeficiency or symptoms for many years (23), asymptomatic patients play a major role in transmitting the virus.

Initial infection with HIV may be asymptomatic or may manifest itself as a mild to severe flulike illness 2 to 6 weeks after exposure. During the period of initial infection, blood virus levels are high, HIV is widely disseminated, and there is a transient decrease in circulating CD4 cells. The symptoms are nonspecific and may include fever, myalgia, malaise, headache, pharyngitis, anorexia, and nausea; often patients do not seek medical attention and the acute infection remains undiagnosed. There is an immune response to HIV between 1 week and 3 months after infection, and antibodies are detectable 6 to 24 weeks after the initial exposure. The early immune response is associated with a dramatic decrease in viremia, but viral replication is never completely curtailed, particularly in lymphoid tissue.

Prognosis. The marker of disease progression that is most familiar to clinicians and has served the test of time is the CD4 lymphocyte count. The absolute number and percentage of CD4 lymphocytes gives the clinician an indication of the degree of immunosuppression and hence can be used to determine what types of associated conditions the patient is susceptible to and give an estimate of life expectancy. The absolute number of

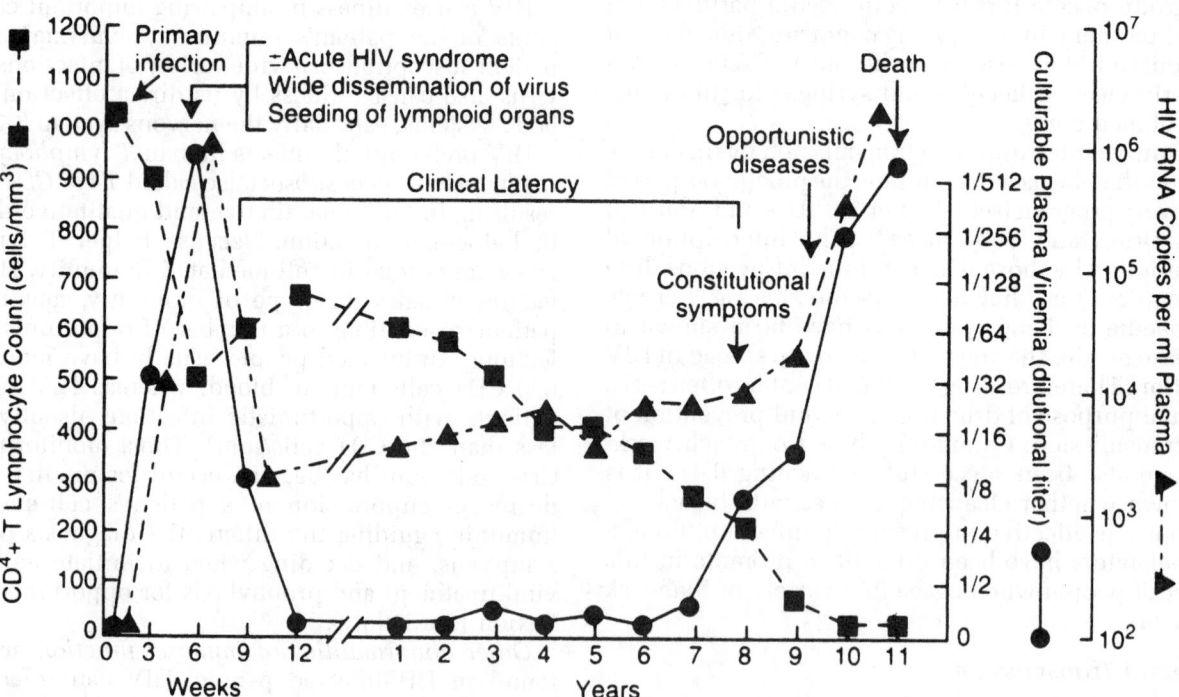

Figure 34.1. Natural history of HIV infection, based on CD4 counts and viral load. (From Fauci AS, et al. Ann Intern Med 124:654, 1996.)

Table 34.3 Equivalence for Absolute Numbers of CD4 Cells and CD4 Percentages

CD4 Cells (per mm³)	CD4 Cell Percentage of Total Lymphocytes
>500	>29
200–500	14–29
<200	<14

Adapted from Centers for Disease Control and Prevention. 1993 revised classification system for HIV infection and expanded surveillance case definition for AIDS among adolescents and adults. MMWR 41(RR-17), 1992.

CD4 cells is subject to more variability because of normal biological fluctuations in total lymphocyte counts. Table 34.3 shows equivalences for absolute counts and percentages of CD4 lymphocytes. Within a year of seroconversion, CD4 cell counts usually drop 200 to 300/mm³ from the normal range of 800 to 1200. This decline is followed by an increase to near baseline and then a slow decline of less than 100 cells per year (Fig. 34.1). People with CD4 cell counts greater than 500 are usually asymptomatic and have virtually no risk of developing an AIDS-indicator condition, except for tuberculosis (TB), cervical cancer, recurrent bacterial pneumonias, or superficial Kaposi's sarcoma (KS), within 18 months. In contrast, those with CD4 cell counts of 100 or less are often symptomatic and have a 60% chance of developing an AIDS-indicator disease (excluding TB, cervical cancer, and recurrent bacterial pneumonias) within 18 months.

A second prognostic indicator of disease progression that has recently come into widespread use is *HIV viral load* (measured as circulating HIV RNA) (30). Recent studies show that viral load is an even better marker of disease progression than CD4 lymphocyte counts and when used with CD4 cell counts is the best indicator of disease progression. A change in viral load usually occurs before a change in CD4 lymphocyte count, so changes in therapy can be made sooner if viral load is used. Nevertheless, changes in viral load should be interpreted with caution because there is wide intrapatient variation and serial changes are significant only when they are greater than 50% (.3 log). Plasma HIV RNA varies from nondetectable, which is currently less than 400 copies/mL with most commercially available assays, to greater than 1 million copies/mL. Immediately after infection, plasma viral load begins to rise and peaks at greater than 100,000 copies/mL. It then declines and plateaus in about 150 days to a steady state called the viral set point. The viral set point remains constant for months to years and is an excellent indicator of risk for disease progression. Viral load again rises just before the development of opportunistic diseases and reaches its highest value with end-stage disease.

The usefulness of the combined baseline CD4 and HIV RNA counts in prognosis was reported in 1997 and is summarized in Figure 34.2. The cohort of patients was enrolled in the mid-1980s, meaning that the findings in Figure 34.2 represent the natural history of HIV infection before the introduction of current disease-modifying therapy.

Guidelines for the use of CD4 count and viral load in clinical decision making are found below (Tables 34.8 and 34.14 through 34.16).

Classification System for HIV Infection and Case Definition for AIDS

Since January 1993, the CDC has used a revised HIV classification system that emphasizes the importance of the CD4 (T lymphocyte) count (Table 34.4). This replaced the previous classification system published by the CDC in 1986, based exclusively on clinical disease criteria. Patients are now classified according to three categories of CD4 cell counts:

1. More than 500/mm³
2. 200 to 499/mm³
3. Less than 200/mm³

They are also classified according to three clinical categories:

A. Asymptomatic, acute HIV, or persistent generalized lymphadenopathy
B. Symptomatic, not (A) or (C) conditions
C. AIDS-indicator conditions

Once a person meets criteria for symptomatic HIV or AIDS, that person remains in the same category or advances to a more advanced stage despite interventions that may eliminate symptoms or increase CD4 cell counts. Patients in categories 3 or C meet the case definition of AIDS.

Symptomatic disease in category B includes any condition attributable to immunodeficiency from HIV infection or complicated by HIV infection (except those in categories A and C). Examples of these conditions include bacillary angiomatosis; oropharyngeal candidiasis; vulvovaginal candidiasis that is persistent, frequent, or poorly responsive to therapy; cervical dysplasia (moderate or severe) or cervical carcinoma in situ; constitutional symptoms such as fever (38.5°C or higher) or diarrhea lasting more than 1 month; oral hairy leukoplakia; herpes zoster of more than one dermatome or recurring at least once; idiopathic thrombocytopenic purpura; listeriosis; pelvic inflammatory disease; and peripheral neuropathy.

The CDC has also expanded the list of *AIDS-indicator conditions* (Table 34.5). In addition to the 23 clinical conditions originally used to define AIDS, pulmonary tuberculosis, recurrent pneumonia (at least two episodes per year), and invasive cervical cancer are now AIDS-indicator diseases.

There is substantial intralaboratory and interlaboratory variation in CD4 counts, which are derived from three other measures: the total white cells, the percentage of lymphocytes, and the percentage of lymphocytes that are CD4 cells. Because of this variability in CD4 counts, it is recommended that clinical decisions be

Figure 34.2. Kaplan–Meier curves showing AIDS-free survival by HIV-1 RNA category among groups with different baseline CD4 lymphocyte counts. The five categories of HIV-1 RNA were the following: I, 500 copies/mL or less; II, 501 to 3,000 copies/mL; III, 3,001 to 10,000 copies/mL; IV, 10,001 to 30,000 copies/mL; and V, more than 30,000 copies/mL. Numbers in parentheses are the sample sizes of the groups at baseline. Groups that were too small to provide estimates were omitted. (From Mellors JW, Munoz A, Giorgi JV, et al. Plasma viral load and CD4+ lymphocytes as prognostic markers of HIV-1 infection. Ann Intern Med 126:946–954, 1997.)

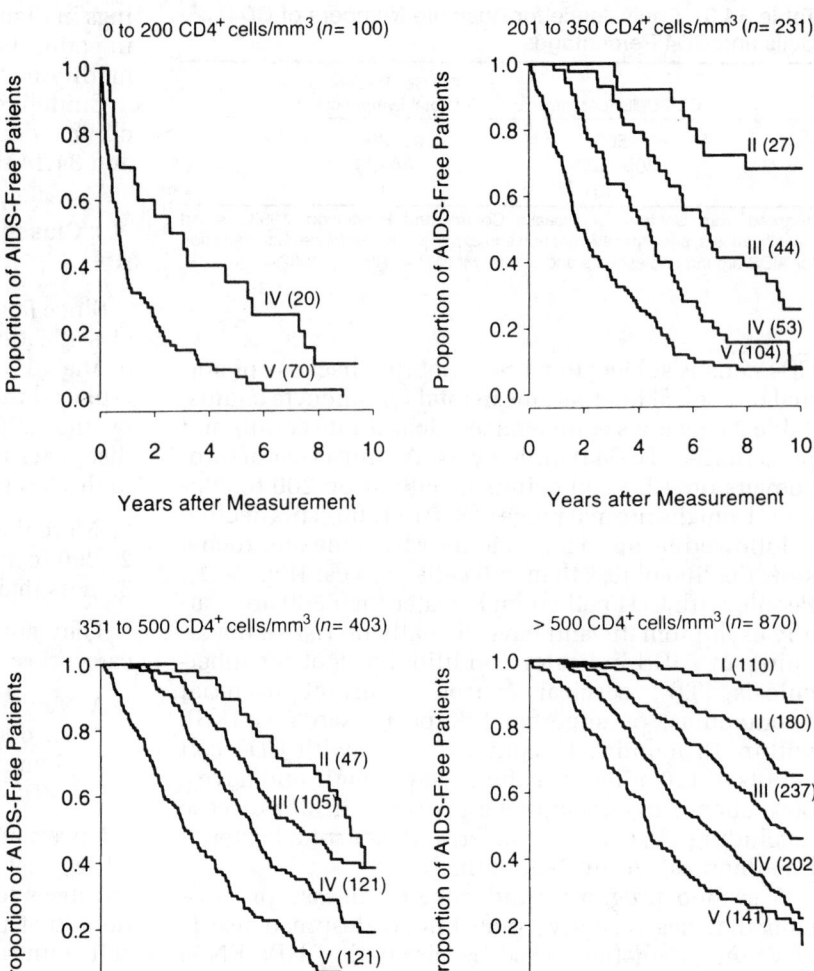

Table 34.4. HIV Classification System

CD4+ T-Cell Categories	Clinical Categories		
	(A) Asymptomatic Acute (Primary) HIV or PGL[a]	(B) Symptomatic, Not (A) or (C) Conditions	(C) AIDS-Indicator Conditions[b]
(1) ≥500/mm³	A1	B1	C1
(2) 200–499/mm³	A2	B2	C2
(3) <200/mm³ (AIDS indicator T-cell count[b])	A3	B3	C3

[a]PGL, Persistent generalized lymphadenopathy.

[b]Row 3 and Column C (shaded) illustrate the expanded AIDS surveillance case definition. Patients with AIDS-indicator conditions (Category C, see Table 34.5) as well as those with CD4+ T-lymphocyte counts less than 200/mm³ (Categories A3 or B3) became reportable as AIDS cases in the U.S. and Territories, effective January 1, 1993.

based on at least two CD4 counts that fall within the range that determines that decision (e.g., decision to initiate *Pneumocystis carinii* pneumonia prophylaxis because the CD4 count is less than 200/mm³).

SEROLOGIC DIAGNOSIS AND ASSOCIATED COUNSELING

Serologic Tests

Antibody to HIV usually appears 6 to 12 weeks after infection but may take as long as 6 months to appear. However, the body's immune response to HIV does not lead to elimination of the virus from host tissues. As described above, a persistent carrier (and persistent seropositive) state follows infection with this type of virus. The diagnosis of HIV infection is based on detection of *anti-HIV antibodies* by the enzyme-linked immunosorbent assay (ELISA), confirmed by the more specific Western blot (WB) method. In the WB method, several individual HIV proteins are transferred onto nitrocellulose paper and reacted against the patient's serum and known positive and negative sera; HIV antibody is detected by an anti–human immunoglobulin antibody coated with an enzyme that, in the presence of substrate, produces a colored band. A positive WB test (the presence two of three colored bands representing p24, gp41, and gp120 or gp160) indicates that the patient has been infected with HIV (6).

ELISA tests are reported as positive or negative. WB tests are reported as positive, negative, or indeterminate. The routine processing of a specimen that is positive on initial ELISA testing always includes rerun of the ELISA, to confirm the result, followed by the WB test. Turnaround time from obtaining the patient's initial specimen to reporting of the WB result is about 1 week in most laboratories.

The currently used ELISA tests have a sensitivity greater than 99% and a specificity of 99.5%. False-positive ELISA tests (ELISA positive, WB negative) may occur when nonspecific serologic reactions are present in patients who have other types of immunologic abnormalities or who have had multiple transfusions or multiple pregnancies. False-positives are most common in patients from groups at low risk of acquiring HIV infection. False-negative ELISA results may occur in recently infected patients who have not made an antibody response.

Patients whose WB tests are reported as indeterminate are those whose sera yield only one of the necessary positive color bands. In most cases, the person is not infected with HIV, especially if the person is at low risk. However, this result may signify that a person is in the process of primary infection and will eventually convert to WB positive. For this reason, the patient should be tested again; if the result remains indeterminate, testing should be repeated in 3 to 6 months. If the WB pattern remains indeterminate for 6 months—in the absence of any known risk factors or clinical findings to suggest HIV infection—the test may be considered negative. Patients who have risk factors or findings compatible with HIV-induced disease should have continued evaluation.

In 1996, the FDA licensed the *first home HIV test kits.* These systems require the purchaser to pierce his or her skin with the lancet supplied in the kit, place a few drops of blood on a filter paper test card, and then send the sample to a central laboratory. Routine testing with ELISA and, if necessary, Western blot is then performed. Sensitivity and specificity are comparable to routine testing on serum. Counseling is provided over the telephone. The FDA has also approved an oral specimen collection device as well as a urine HIV test.

Indications for Serologic Testing

HIV testing and counseling are indicated both to prevent further transmission of disease and to allow people already infected to be identified so that they can seek appropriate medical care. It is especially important now that we have potent drugs to halt the progression of HIV and prevent infection in newborns. Mandatory testing is performed in the military, many prison populations, and the Job Corps and on all donors of blood, semen, and organs.

According to the CDC, voluntary testing should be performed in all patients who have sexually transmitted diseases, are current or former IDUs, are hemophiliacs, have active tuberculosis, have received blood transfusions or blood products between 1978 and 1985, are prostitutes, are from developing countries with high rates of HIV infection, have regular sexual partners with risk factors or known to be HIV-infected, have signs or symptoms suggestive of HIV infection, consider themselves at risk for HIV infection or request testing, and are exposed to blood or other at-risk body fluids (including health care workers who perform invasive procedures); all pregnant women should also have voluntary testing performed.

Some authorities also recommend that all patients between the ages of 15 and 54 admitted to a hospital with an AIDS diagnosis rate of 1 or more per 1000 discharges be tested for HIV infection (7). This is based on the findings that many hospitalized HIV-infected patients present with conditions other than those directly related to HIV infection.

Pretest and Posttest Counseling

The most important aspect of HIV testing is pretest and posttest counseling. Because of the ominous meaning of HIV infection, it is important to ensure privacy and to allow sufficient time to respond to the

Table 34.5. AIDS-Indicator Conditions in HIV-Infected Persons

Candidiasis
  Bronchi
  Trachea
  Esophagus
  Lungs
Cervical cancer, invasive
Coccidioidomycosis, disseminated or extrapulmonary
Cryptococcosis, extrapulmonary
Cryptosporidiosis, extrapulmonary
Cytomegalovirus disease (other than liver, spleen, or nodes)
Encephalopathy, HIV-related (dementia)
Herpes simplex
  Chronic ulcer >1 month's duration
  Bronchitis
  Pneumonitis
  Esophagitis
Histoplasmosis, disseminated or extrapulmonary
HIV wasting syndrome (>10% weight loss and either chronic weakness and fever or chronic diarrhea, ≥30 days)
Isosporiasis, intestinal of >1 month's duration
Kaposi's sarcoma
Lymphoma
  Burkitt's
  Immunoblastic
  Primary of the brain
Mycobacterium
  M. avium complex, disseminated or extrapulmonary
  M. kansasii, disseminated or extrapulmonary
  M. tuberculosis, pulmonary or extrapulmonary
  Other species, disseminated or extrapulmonary
P. carinii pneumonia
Pneumonia, two or more episodes within a year
Progressive multifocal leukoencephalopathy
Salmonella septicemia, recurrent
Toxoplasmosis, brain

Adapted from Centers for Disease Control and Prevention. 1993 revised classification system for HIV infection and expanded surveillance case definition for AIDS among adolescents and adults. MMWR 41 (No. RR-17): 1992.

Table 34.6. HIV Pretest and Posttest Counseling: Points for Discussion

Pretest Counseling

Meaning of positive test:
 Positive test means HIV infection
 Positive test does NOT mean AIDS[a]
 Positive test means patient is an HIV carrier
Confidentiality of test results and medical information
Availability of anonymous and confidential counseling and testing sites
Potential adverse psychosocial consequences if information becomes known, e.g., possible adverse effects on employment, housing, insurance status
Sources of additional AIDS/HIV-related information[b]
Means for reducing risk of HIV transmission or exposure (depends on patient's current or likely high-risk behaviors)
 "Safe sex" practices (see Tables 34.1 and 34.2)
 Sterilization of intravenous drug equipment
 Treatment for drug addiction
 Discontinuation of sharing intravenous needles

Posttest Counseling

Interpretation of HIV antibody test results
Information about long-term chances of developing symptoms
Planning for medical follow-up
Referral to psychosocial support services
Reinforcement of recommendations for prevention of HIV transmission/exposure
Discussion of notification of sexual partners or needle-sharing partners
Reproductive issues in women

[a]Most people with a positive test will develop AIDS. Length of time from infection to development of AIDS is variable but averages 10 years.
[b]A single source for information is the National AIDS Information Clearing House, P.O. Box 6003, Rockville, MD 20850 (800-458-5231).

patient's feelings and questions. Many settings require the patient's written informed consent as part of pretest counseling. Recommended points of discussion during counseling are shown in Table 34.6. Information about behaviors associated with the risk of acquiring HIV infection is important in both stages of counseling. Details have been published regarding counseling of patients infected with HTLV-I and HTLV-II also (8).

Information about available printed materials useful in posttest counseling and about regional programs for HIV-infected patients can be obtained by contacting the National AIDS Information Clearing House (P.O. Box 6003, Rockville, MD 20850; telephone 800-458-5231).

EARLY EVALUATION AND TREATMENT OF THE HIV-INFECTED PATIENT

Baseline History, Physical Examination, and Laboratory Studies

The apparently asymptomatic patient with HIV infection requires an initial evaluation and ongoing psychosocial support and medical assessment. This section describes important manifestations to be sought in initial and subsequent evaluations of HIV-positive patients and prophylactic guidelines, as established by the U.S. Public Health Service in

collaboration with the Infectious Diseases Society of America (10). Descriptions of symptomatic manifestations are found under "The Symptomatic HIV-Infected Patient."

Some patients, when initially infected with HIV, may have a mild to severe mononucleosislike illness lasting 1 to 2 weeks. Symptoms include fevers, diaphoresis, malaise, myalgias, arthralgias, pharyngitis, retro-orbital headaches, and in some patients, lymphadenopathy (31). When asked specifically, at least half of all HIV-positive patients reveal a *history of an illness with these features of acute HIV infection.* Less common manifestations of acute HIV infection include polyneuropathy, brachial neuritis, and odynophagia with esophageal ulcers. The incubation period (time from exposure to onset of illness) for the acute syndromes may range from 5 days to 3 months, usually 2 to 4 weeks. Some observations suggest that patients who experience symptoms associated with seroconversion have a worse prognosis.

In addition to the HIV-oriented review of systems summarized in Table 34.7, seropositive patients should be asked about a history of sexually transmitted diseases, tuberculosis or a positive purified protein derivative (PPD) test, exposure to or history of hepatitis B, immunosuppressive therapy (e.g., an asthmatic patient who intermittently requires corticosteroids), and previous immunizations including pneumococcal and hepatitis B vaccines. Important information to obtain in the social history includes current sexual practices (type and number of sexual partners), types of contraception used, and past or present intravenous drug use.

The *baseline physical examination* should include all organ systems, with special emphasis on the oral cavity, skin, lymph nodes, and in women, the reproductive system. Physical manifestations in these organ systems are particularly important because diseases may be found that are potentially treatable (i.e., seborrheic dermatitis) or that carry prognostic significance (i.e., oral candidiasis).

The baseline laboratory evaluation should establish a database that will be useful for identifying already-present abnormalities and for comparison when abnormalities are identified at a later time in the care of the

Table 34.7. HIV-Oriented Review of Symptoms

General: Weight loss, fever, night sweats
Skin: New rashes, pigmented lesions, itching
Lymphoid system: Asymmetric or rapidly growing lymph nodes
HEENT: Change in vision, unusual headaches, congestion or running nose, oral lesions
Respiratory: Cough, shortness of breath, decrease in exercise tolerance
Gastrointestinal: Pain or difficulty in swallowing, nausea or vomiting, diarrhea, painful defecation
Neuropsychiatric: Difficulty thinking, depression, change in personality, numbness or tingling, muscle weakness, loss of sensation

patient. This database should include a complete blood count (CBC) (including a differential and platelet count), hepatitis B surface antigen and antibody, syphilis serology, *Toxoplasma* antibody, HIV viral load, and CD4 lymphocyte count. Many experts recommend repeating the HIV viral load in 2 to 4 weeks to establish a more certain baseline. Baseline serologic tests for antibody to cytomegalovirus (CMV) are not generally useful because of the high prevalence of positive tests in the normal population. Unless the patient has a history of a positive PPD skin test or tuberculosis, the patient should have a PPD. A chest radiograph should be performed in all patients who have a positive PPD (5 mm or more induration), or have respiratory symptoms or a history of respiratory disease.

Many patients who complain of no symptoms at baseline will have one or more abnormalities found on physical examination or laboratory evaluation, most commonly generalized lymphadenopathy (see definition below), reduced CD4 count, elevated HIV viral load, or mild suppression of the elements of the bone marrow (23). If a history of constitutional symptoms (weight loss, fevers, night sweats) is elicited, this should be evaluated further, as discussed in the next section. Findings in the oral cavity that may not cause symptoms but suggest some degree of immunodeficiency include oral hairy leukoplakia or early *Candida* infection (see descriptions below). A finding of an isolated low platelet count may be indicative of immune thrombocytopenic purpura, which may also be predictive of progression of disease. Laboratory abnormalities (e.g., hypochromic anemia) should be evaluated in the same manner as in a non–HIV-infected patient.

Health Maintenance: Monitoring Schedules, Immunizations, and OI Prophylaxis

Table 34.8A outlines the recommended monitoring schedule for HIV-infected patients *according to CD4 cell count.* Table 34.8B and this section address immunizations and OI prophylaxis to prevent first episodes of preventable diseases. Later sections address the treatment of OIs ("The Sympomatic HIV-Infected Patient") and the schedule for viral load monitoring and the initiation and long-term use of antiretroviral drugs ("Antiretroviral Treatment").

Prevention of First Episodes of Opportunistic Infections

Immunizations. Preventive care for HIV-infected patients should include various vaccinations (Table 34.8B).

Because pneumococcal pneumonia is the leading cause of bacterial pneumonia in HIV-infected patients, *pneumococcal vaccine* is recommended for all HIV-infected patients. It should be given early in the course of HIV infection or, if given in later stage disease, after the patient has been started on appropriate antiviral therapy. Although the pneumococcal vaccine is less immunogenic in HIV-infected than in HIV-negative patients, it has been shown to stimulate antibody levels sufficient to provide protection, especially in patients with early asymptomatic disease. The use of *influenza vaccination* is more controversial because there are no data documenting higher case rates or mortality among HIV-infected patients and a recent analysis suggests that it may not be cost-effective (28,29).

Hepatitis B vaccine should be given in hepatitis B surface antigen and antibody-negative patients who have continued risk factors for hepatitis B because of the increased risk for chronic hepatitis in HIV-infected patients.

Although data on the efficacy of *other killed or inactivated vaccines* is not available, it is still recommended that routine vaccines such as tetanus be given to HIV-infected patients.

Live, attenuated vaccines such as polio, typhoid, yellow fever, and vaccinia should not be given. Measles vaccine, however, has been shown to be safe in HIV-infected children and can be given according to the recommendations for HIV-negative people.

For details regarding dosages and schedules of immunizations, see Chapter 32.

Antimicrobial Prophylaxis. Table 34.8B delineates recommendations for antimicrobial prophylaxis for infections caused by *Pneumocystis carinii, Mycobacterium avium,* and *Toxoplasma gondii.* These indications for prophylaxis are guided largely by CD4 counts and not symptomatic infection. Recommended prophylaxis regimens for other OIs, initiated *after episodes of symptomatic infection,* are found below ("The Symptomatic HIV-Infected Patient").

Pneumocystis carinii pneumonia (PCP) prophylaxis should be initiated when the CD4 cell count is less than

Table 34.8A. Health Maintenance in the HIV-Infected Patient: Monitoring Timing and Frequency Based on CD4 Count

CD4 Cell Count (per mm³)	>600	500–600	200–499	100–200	<100
CD4 cell count	6 mo	3 mo	3 mo	3 mo	3 mo
HIV viral load	6 mo	3 mo	3 mo	3 mo	3 mo
Syphilis serology	12 mo	12 mo	12 mo	12 mo	12 mo
Hepatitis B serology	Once	Once	Once	Once	Once
Tuberculosis screening[a]	12 mo	12 mo	12 mo	12 mo	12 mo
Pap smear	6–12 mo	6–12 mo	6–12 mo	6–12 mo	6–12 mo
Ophthalmologic examination (CMV)	No	No	No	No	6 mos

[a]When positive do not repeat.

Table 34.8B. Health Maintenance in the HIV-Infected Patient: Immunizations and Antimicrobials Treatment to Prevent First Episodes of Disease Caused by Opportunistic Infections

Category 1: Strongly Recommended as Standard of Care			
Pathogen	Indication[a]	First Choice	Alternatives
Pneumocystis carinii	CD4 <200 or oropharyngeal candidiasis or unexplained fever >2 weeks	TMP/SMX, 1 DS QD, 1SS QD or 1 DS 3 times per week	Dapsone 50 mg BID or 100 mg QD Dapsone 50 mg QD + pyrimethamine 50 mg QWK + leucovorin 25 mg QWK Dapsone 200 mg + pyrimethamine 75 mg + leucovorin 25 mg QWK Aerosol pentamidine 300 mg via Respirgard II nebulizer every month
Mycobacterium tuberculosis	PPD reaction ≥5 mm or prior PPD result without treatment or contact with active case of tuberculosis	Isoniazid 300 mg + pyridoxine 50 mg QD × 12 months or isoniazid 900 mg + pyridoxine 50 mg BIW × 12 months	Rifampin 600 mg QD × 12 months
Isoniazid-resistant	Same with exposure to INH resistant TB	Rifampin 600 mg QD × 12 months	Rifabutin 300 mg QD × 12 months
Multidrug resistant	Same with exposure to MDR TB	Expert consultation	
Toxoplasma gondii	IgG antibody to Toxoplasma and CD4+ count <100 mm^3	TMP/SMX, 1 DS PO QD	TMP/SMX 1 SS PO QD Dapsone 50 mg PO QD *plus* pyrimethamine 50 mg PO QWK *plus* leucovorin 25 mg PO QWK
Mycobacterium avium complex	CD4+ count <50 mm^3	Clarithromycin, 500 mg PO BID or Azithromycin, 1200 mg PO QWK	Rifabutin, 300 mg PO QD Azithromycin 1200 mg PO QD plus rifabutin 300 mg PO QD
Streptococcus pneumoniae	All patients ≥2 years old	Pneumococcal vaccine, 0.5 mL × 1 and revaccinate ≥5 years after first dose	IV or IM immunoglobulin
Varicella virus	Significant exposure to chickenpox or shingles for patients with no history of either condition or, if available, negative antibody titer	Varicella zoster immune globulin (VZIG), 5 vials (1.25 mL each) IM, given ≤96 hr after exposure, ideally within 48 hr	Acyclovir 800 mg PO 5/day
Category 2: Generally Recommended			
Pathogen	Indication	First Choice	Alternatives
Hepatitis B	All susceptible (anti-HBc-negative) patients	Energix B, 20 µg IM × 3 or Recombivax HB, 10 µg IM × 3	None
Influenza A	All patients (annually, before influenza season)	Whole or split virus, 0.5 mL IM/yr	Rimantadine, 100 mg PO BID or amantadine, 100 mg PO BID

Modified from Johns Hopkins HIV Report, September 1997; excerpted from MMWR 46 (RR-12):1–46, 1997.

[a]*Note:* Lowest CD4 count a patient has reached is used to determine need for prophylaxis, even for patients responding to antiretroviral therapy.

200 or if the patient already has had PCP or now has oral candidiasis or unexplained fever for more than two weeks (5,10). Doses and regimens for the oral agents effective for prophylaxis are shown in Table 34.8B. Aerosolized pentamidine (300 mg every 4 weeks administered over 20 to 25 minutes with a jet nebulizer) is an alternative to the oral regimens. Oral TMP/SMX is the preferred agent because it has been shown to be most efficacious and it also has the added benefit of being inexpensive (less than $50 for a year of treatment) (5,16).

The most common *side effects with TMP/SMX prophylaxis,* in descending order of frequency, include rash, pruritus, nausea and vomiting, fever, anemia, neutropenia, and elevated liver function tests. These side effects often occur within the first month of starting therapy, but some, especially cutaneous reactions and fever, may occur even years after initiation of therapy. Complete blood cell counts should be monitored within the first 4 weeks of starting therapy and at

least every 3 months thereafter. Liver function tests, BUN, and serum creatinine should also be monitored at least every 3 months. These side effects occasionally necessitate discontinuation of therapy. Often, however, TMP/SMX can be reintroduced, especially when given in gradually increasing doses using the liquid formulation.

If life-threatening reactions occur, such as Stevens–Johnson syndrome, or the patient is unwilling to restart TMP/SMX because of prior side effects, dapsone or aerosolized pentamidine can be substituted. The major toxicities of dapsone are rash and cytopenias. The side effects of aerosolized pentamidine include cough and bronchospasm, most often seen in smokers or in patients with preexisting asthma. Pretreatment with a metered-dose bronchodilator often prevents this problem. In addition, because of the risk of aerosolization of a mycobacterial infection not previously suspected, use of aerosolized pentamidine should be used only in specially designated areas and in patients proven not to have active TB. Trials are ongoing to study *atovaquone* and the other agents for PCP prophylaxis.

All HIV-infected patients with *positive tuberculin tests,* regardless of age, should be treated prophylactically with isoniazid 300 mg for at least 12 months. If the patient is known to have been exposed to a strain that is resistant to isoniazid but sensitive to rifampin, rifampin should be used as preventive therapy (see details in Chapter 29).

Patients with antibodies to *Toxoplasma gondii* and CD4 cell counts less than 100 cells/mm^3 should be given TMP/SMX (one double-strength per day) for prophylaxis (10). Dapsone and pyrimethamine are acceptable alternatives if TMP/SMX is not tolerated. Folinic acid is also given, with the regimen at 25 mg/week to prevent bone marrow toxicity associated with pyrimethamine.

Prophylaxis is recommended against *Mycobacterium avium complex* (MAC) when CD4 cell counts are less than 50 cells/mm^3 (10). Effective regimens include azithromycin 1200 mg once a week, clarithromycin 500 mg twice daily, or rifabutin 300 mg daily. Azithromycin and clarithromycin are more efficacious than rifabutin, and azithromycin has the added advantage of once-weekly dosing.

Oral ganciclovir has been shown to prevent *CMV retinitis* in patients with low CD4 cell counts but because of toxicity and difficulty defining which patients are at risk, CMV prophylaxis is not recommended (10). Screening every 6 months for CMV retinitis is recommended for patients with CD4 cell counts less than 75 cells/mm^3.

With the advent of new antiviral agents that can raise CD4 cell counts for prolonged periods (see below), there has been debate about whether prophylactic agents need to be continued when the CD4 cell count rises above the value used as the threshold for prophylaxis. Currently, it is recommended that prophylaxis be instituted and maintained based on the lowest CD4 cell count recorded even when CD4 counts rise after initiation of effective antiviral agents.

Coexisting Medical Problems

HIV-positive patients are as likely as HIV-negative patients to have common acute or chronic diseases. The two groups should be approached in the same way in addressing these problems and in addressing indicated preventive care (see Chapter 2).

Many HIV-infected patients describe minor problems, such as fatigue, night sweats, mild chronic diarrhea, pruritus, and low-grade temperature elevation, for which specific infectious causes cannot be identified. Many of these problems probably are manifestations of chronic HIV infection. In addition, for some patients a focus on somatic concerns is the way in which they present their mental distress (see Chapter 12 for a detailed discussion of somatization). When an identifiable opportunistic infection has been excluded (see below) and there is no evidence of a conventional infection, simple palliative measures should be recommended (e.g., increased rest, the use of acetaminophen or aspirin as needed, skin lubricants). Patients should be encouraged to discuss their mental distress at the same time that they are queried and advised about physical symptoms.

Psychosocial and Ethical Aspects

Dealing with the psychosocial issues accompanying the diagnosis of asymptomatic HIV infection is usually much more difficult than the medical management. Patients who have learned that they have a fatal disease that may have been acquired sexually and is stigmatizing for a variety of reasons usually feel extremely isolated and despondent. Because patients' emotional responses may impair the ability to process information, it is important to check their comprehension of the facts, to be prepared to reiterate points covered in the posttest counseling session (Table 34.6), and to respond to the feelings and questions that these points will evoke. The patient must understand how the virus is and is not transmitted, the usual course of the disease, and available therapeutic interventions.

The HIV-infected patient has an intense need for hope and support. In addition to ensuring the patient of one's ongoing support and using counseling techniques that are helpful for a patient in crisis (see Chapter 11), it is appropriate to offer psychologic or psychiatric consultation after the diagnosis of HIV positivity. Among the major psychosocial consequences of this diagnosis are the uncovering of homosexuality in men whose gay orientation has been confidential; the threatened loss of family, social, and occupational relationships; an increase in the release of irresponsible promiscuity in antisocial people (especially IDUs); and a greatly increased risk of suicide. These problems particularly require expert counseling.

HIV-positive patients should be assured of confidentiality about their condition but at the same time be instructed to inform others who may have been infected by them. Although asymptomatic HIV infection is not reportable in most jurisdictions, the patient's physician may have a responsibility to inform others who may be infected if the patient will not do so. This raises the difficult conflict between the patient's right to confidentiality and the rights of other people to protect their health. Laws governing physicians' actions and obligations and ethical aspects of caring for an HIV-infected patient are discussed further in a later section ("Public Health and Legal Responsibilities of the Physician").

THE SYMPTOMATIC HIV-INFECTED PATIENT

General Principles

The most important aspect of the primary care of the symptomatic HIV-infected patient is knowing the patient well. Many newly diagnosed HIV-positive patients are young and have been previously healthy;

symptoms and illness are often new to them. They may either overreact to each symptom or deny symptoms entirely. Good rapport with patients is thus essential for having them disclose information and for distinguishing the significance of new symptoms.

Guidelines for monitoring objective findings and making treatment decisions are described in this section and under "Antiretroviral Treatment." The section below, "Overall Principles of Treatment," summarizes critical points. Sources for the most current recommendations are named in "General References."

The *CD4 lymphocyte count* is the most useful marker for guiding treatment decisions in the care of HIV-infected patients (Table 34.8). For deciding on early and long-term treatment with antiretroviral drugs, the *viral load,* in addition to the CD4 count, should be used (see Table 34.8 and "Antiretroviral Treatment," below). It is generally thought that the CD4 count is an indicator of the patient's current immunologic and clinical status and that the viral load indicates future progression. When a patient's CD4 count is between 200 and 500, new symptoms should lead to a careful search for an opportunistic infection; when a patient's CD4 count is less than 200, new symptoms are likely to be due to an opportunistic infection; and when a patient's CD4 count is greater than 500 cells/mm³, new symptoms are more likely to be due to non–HIV-associated conditions.

Common OIs and other manifestations of HIV infection are described in this section, by symptoms and by organ systems involved.

In the 1990s, the four most common AIDS-indicator conditions are three OIs (PCP, MAC, and *esophageal candidiasis*) *and the HIV wasting syndrome.* Tables 34.9 and 34.10 summarize the principal features, diagnostic approaches, and acute and maintenance antimicrobial treatments for the OIs of HIV-infected patients (19). Practical details regarding antiretroviral treatment are found below.

The less severe opportunistic infections of HIV-infected patients can be diagnosed and treated in ambulatory settings. Only severely ill patients need hospitalization. For acute problems diagnosed in the hospital, completion of the course of antimicrobial treatment and maintenance antimicrobial treatment can usually be accomplished after discharge from the hospital (see "Duration and Location of Treatment for Opportunistic Infections," below).

Constitutional Manifestations and Lymphadenopathy

Fatigue is probably the most common symptom described by HIV-infected people. When fatigue is present without associated objective findings, a psychological basis for this symptom should be considered (see below).

Fevers, night sweats, or weight loss may be the presenting manifestations of one of the opportunistic infections described below or of a malignancy, or they may be due to HIV infection itself. When one or more of these symptoms are present, a careful evaluation for a treatable problem is mandatory. Some constitutional symptoms (e.g., fever above 38°C or diarrhea lasting longer than 1 month) categorize the patient as having symptomatic HIV infection (Table 34.4), which in some states is reportable (see above).

The laboratory evaluation of fever, chills, or night sweats should include a CBC with differential, liver function tests, chest radiograph, serum cryptococcal antigen test, blood and urine cultures, and sputum cultures if sputum is available. If the history, physical examination, and these screening laboratory data do not reveal an explanation for fever, a more extensive workup should be performed. Considerations should be given to blood, bone marrow, and stool cultures for MAC, and to specialized imaging techniques (computerized tomography [CT] or gallium scans) to look for an occult infection. MAC is now the most common mycobacterial species isolated from AIDS patients. Infection with this organism, which may be suppressed but not cured, typically causes systemic symptoms as well as wasting and persistent diarrhea. This species of *Mycobacterium* is not communicable.

Lymphadenopathy is always a troublesome finding because it may represent reaction to HIV, infection with another agent, or a malignancy. Prospective studies of a large cohort of homosexual men show approximately a 30% frequency of persistent generalized lymphadenopathy—defined as nodes 1 cm or greater in diameter in two or more noncontiguous extrainguinal sites—during the first 6 months after diagnosis of HIV positivity (23). Nodes most often enlarged are anterior and posterior cervical, axillary, submental, and femoral nodes; preauricular and epitrochlear nodes are rarely enlarged. Patients with generalized lymphadenopathy often have one or more other abnormalities in the history, physical examination, or laboratory evaluation, but no single abnormality coexists predictably with adenopathy. Lymphadenopathy per se has not been found to be predictive of the patient's future experience (25).

Young, sexually active patients with HIV infection are at risk for other diseases causing diffuse adenopathy, such as secondary syphilis, hepatitis B, toxoplasmosis, and infectious mononucleosis. These can usually be diagnosed or excluded by using specific serologic studies and referring to the baseline results of such studies (see baseline evaluation of asymptomatic patients, above). If a patient's lymphadenopathy is most pronounced in the inguinal region, with or without an active genital lesion or a history of a lesion, other sexually transmitted diseases such as chancroid or lymphogranuloma venereum should be considered. If lymphadenopathy is localized in one area, progressively enlarging, associated with constitutional symptoms, or of a different texture (very firm or irregular), biopsy should be considered to exclude malignancy. With the increasing and successful use of antimicrobial agents as prophylaxis against opportunistic infections, lymphoma more often may be a presenting illness in

Table 34.9. Principal Features of Common Opportunistic Infections In HIV-Infected Patients

Organ System/Organism	Mode of Transmission/ Isolation Procedures	Major Clinical Features	Definitive Diagnosis: Method/Source	Antimicrobial Agents[a]
Respiratory System				
P. carinii[b,c]	Endogenous Patient not contagious No isolation	Dry cough, mild SOB, subacute presentation, may have no findings on P.E.	Cytologic stain: bronchial lavage or lung tissue	1. TMP/SMX or 2. Pentamidine or 3. Dapsone/TMP or 4. Atovaquone (mild cases) or 5. Clindamycin/primaquine
M. tuberculosis[b,d]	Aerosolized droplets Human-to-human Respiratory isolation	Productive cough, SOB, fever usually with findings on P.E.	Smear or culture: bronchial lavage	Isoniazid, rifampin, ethambutol, and pyrazinamide
Neurologic System				
C. neoformans[b,c] (meningitis)	Cat exposure Patient not contagious No isolation	Headache, fever, change in mental status; often no findings on P.E.	Positive India ink or cryptococcal antigen or culture: CSF	1. Amphotericin B ± (flucytosine) or 2. Fluconazole
T. gondii[b,c] (cerebritis or abscess)	Not human-to-human Patient not contagious No isolation	Headache, seizures, focal neurologic deficit, ± fever	1. Head CT with contrast 2. A single specimen for toxoplasma serology not helpful 3. Definitive dx: brain biopsy 4. Dx often made by response to empiric Rx	1. Pyramethamine and sulfadiazine and folinic acid or 2. Clindamycin as alternative to sulfa drugs
Herpes simplex or varicella-zoster (encephalitis)	Human-to-human Wound and skin precautions if peripheral lesions present	Headache, seizures, change in mental status, ± fever	1. Head CT, cerebritis or WNL 2. LP, pleocytosis 3. EEG, focal temporal slowing 4. Brain biopsy, culture: definitive 5. Empiric Rx often tried	Acyclovir
Progressive multifocal leukoencephalopathy[b] (JC virus)	? mode of transmission No isolation	Change in mental status	1. Head CT with contrast or MRI: distinctive pattern 2. Brain biopsy, definitive	None
Oral Cavity and Gastrointestinal System				
Thrush (C. albicans)[c]	Endogenous No isolation	White plaques in mouth	Potassium hydroxide microscopy or culture: Scraping of plaque	1. Nystatin or 2. Clotrimazole or 3. Ketaconazol or 4. Fluconazole or 5. Itraconazole
Candida esophagitis[b,c]	Same as above	Dysphagia/odynophagia ± thrush	Biopsy of esophagus for pathology	1. Fluconazole or 2. Ketaconazole or 3. Itraconazole or 4. Amphotericin B
Herpes simplex esophagitis[b,c]	Human-to-human transmission Contact of mucous membrane/open skin wound with lesion Wound and skin precautions if peripheral lesions present	Dysphagia/odynophagia ± oral mucocutaneous HSV infections	1. Biopsy of esophagus for pathology, culture 2. May be assumed with definite oral herpes and esophageal symptoms	1. Acyclovir or 2. Famciclovir or 3. Valacyclovir
Cytomegalovirus[b,c] esophagitis/ ileocolitis	Human-to-human Sexual, intravenous, vertical, breast milk, ? other No isolation (? pregnant caretakers)	Esophagitis: same as above Ileocolitis: cramping abdominal pain ± fever ± diarrhea	Biopsy of site for pathology, culture	1. Ganciclovir or 2. Foscarnet

Table 34.9—continued.   Principal Features of Common Opportunistic Infections In HIV-Infected Patients

Organ System/Organism	Mode of Transmission/Isolation Procedures	Major Clinical Features	Definitive Diagnosis: Method/Source	Antimicrobial Agents[a]
Oral Cavity and Gastrointestinal System—cont'd				
Salmonella sp.[c]	Fecal–oral transmission Enteric precautions	Diarrhea, fever, systemic toxicity	Stool culture	1. TMP/SMX or 2. Fluoroquinolones
Cryptosporidium[b]	Not human-to-human No isolation	Chronic, profuse diarrhea	1. Stool O & P exam 2. Biopsy	?
I. belli	Not human-to-human No isolation	Chronic, profuse diarrhea	1. Stool O & P exam 2. Biopsy	TMP/SMX
Other Organ Systems				
Skin				
Mucocutaneous herpes simplex virus[c,e]	Human-to-human Contact of mucous membrane or open skin with active lesion Skin and wound precautions until lesion crusted	Classic vesicular lesion and distribution	Smear (Tzanck prep) or culture	1. Acyclovir or 2. Famciclovir or 3. Valacyclovir
Varicella-zoster (shingles)	Same as HSV	Same as HSV in dermatomal distribution	Same as above: Only culture differentiates from HSV	1. Acyclovir or 2. Famciclovir or 3. Valacyclovir
Eye				
Cytomegalovirus[b,c] (retinitis)	Same as for cytomegalovirus under GI above	Asymptomatic, or loss of vision	1. Ophthalmologist-diagnosed classic retinal lesion 2. Positive CMV urine or blood cultures	1. Ganciclovir or 2. Foscarnet 3. Cidofovir 4. Ganciclovir implants
Disseminated Infections				
M. avium complex[b,c]	Not human-to-human No isolation	Wasting syndrome, diarrhea/abd pain, FUO	1. Blood cultures 2. Stool cultures 3. Tissue biopsy (bone marrow, liver, colon)	1. Clarithromycin/ethambutol or 2. Fluroquinolones or azithromycin or rifabutin
Histoplasmosis[b,c]	Not human-to-human No isolation	Nonspecific: FUO, weight loss Pulmonary Sx	1. Bone marrow biopsy and culture 2. Blood culture 3. Biopsy of lymph node, liver, lungs	1. Amphotericin B or 2. Itraconazole (maintenance itraconazole)
Coccidioidomycosis[b,c]	Not human-to-human No isolation	Same as above plus CNS: meningoencephalitis cutaneous: nodules, ulcers	1. Sputum/tissue pathology 2. Cultures: Bone marrow, blood, lymph node, liver, urine 3. ± Serology	1. Fluconazole or 2. Amphotericin B

HSV, Herpes simplex virus; SOB, shortness of breath; P.E., physical examination; WNL, within normal limits; LP, lymphocyte predominant; FUO, fever of unknown origin; O & P, ova and parasite.

[a]For details regarding treatment, see Table 34.10 and text section entitled "Duration and Location of Treatment."
[b]AIDS-defining illness (see Table 34.5).
[c]Requires maintenance after initial treatment.
[d]See Chapter 29 for details.
[e]Maintenance should be considered.

Table 34.10. Practical Information About Antimicrobial Agents Used for the Treatment of the Opportunistic Infections Listed in Table 34.9

Antimicrobial Agent	Organisms and Syndromes	Dosage/Schedule/Route	Duration/Maintenance	Common Adverse Effects	Drug Interactions	Dosage Change with Renal/Hepatic Failure	Available Strengths, Preparations
Antifungal							
Nystatin	*Candida* spp.: Thrush	Suspension 100,000 units TID PO	2 wk ± maintenance or PRN	1. Transient nausea, vomiting (N and V) 2. Unpleasant taste	None	None	100,000 units per 5 mL suspension
Amphotericin B oral suspension	Same as nystatin	100 mg QID	2 wk	1. Rash 2. Nausea/vomiting	None	None	100 mg/mL in 24-mL bottles
Clotrimazole	Same as nystatin	Troches 10 mg five times/day PO	1–2 wk ± maintenance or PRN	1. Nausea	None	None	10 mg/troche
Fluconazole	*Candida* spp.: Thrush Esophagitis Cryptococcus Meningitis	100 mg/day PO (200 mg first day) 100 mg/day PO 400 mg/day PO	2 wk 2 wk 6–10 wk after prior therapy with amphotericin B, maintenance of 200 mg/day	1. GI side effects 2. Headache 3. ↑ LFTs	1. Warfarin: potentiated 2. Phenytoin: increased levels 3. Hypoglycemics: increased levels	↓ with renal failure	Tablets: 50, 100, 200 mg Suspension: 10 mg/mL
Ketoconazole	*Candida*: Thrush Esophagitis	200 mg/day PO 200–400 mg/day PO	2 wk Maintenance Rx	1. N and V 2. Mild ↑ LFTs 3. Severe hepatitis (1/15,000) 4. Adrenal insufficiency	1. H$_2$ blockers, antacids: prevent absorption of ketoconazole 2. Warfarin: anticoagulant effect enhanced 3. Hypoglycemics: severe ↓ glucose 4. Rifampin: causes ↓ levels of ketoconazole 5. Phenytoin: may alter concentration of either	Renal: none Precaution with hepatic failure	200-mg capsule
	Histoplasmosis	200–400 mg/day PO	Maintenance only				
	Coccidioidomycosis	200–400 mg/day PO	2 wk				
Itraconazole	*Candida* spp.: Thrush Esophagitis	200 mg QD		1. Gastrointestinal 2. Headache	Decreased levels with rifampin, rifabutin, phenytoin, midazolam, cyclosporine, oral hypoglycemics, digoxin, H$_2$ blockers, omeprazole, antacids, sulcrafate, and ddl. Do not use with terfenadine, astemizole, and cisapride. Increased levels of ribabutin, phenytoin, midazolam, cyclosporine, hypoglycemics, and digoxin.	None	100-mg capsules, 10 mg/mL in 150 mL bottles Oral solution: 10 mg/mL
	Histoplasmosis	300 mg QD 200 mg QD	3 days chronic				

Table 34.10—continued. Practical Information About Antimicrobial Agents Used for the Treatment of the Opportunistic Infections Listed in Table 34.9

Antimicrobial Agent	Organisms and Syndromes	Dosage/Schedule/Route	Duration/Maintenance	Common Adverse Effects	Drug Interactions	Dosage Change with Renal/Hepatic Failure	Available Strengths, Preparations
Antifungal—cont'd Amphotericin B[a]	*Aspergillosis* spp.: Pneumonia	1.0–1.4 mg/kg/day IV	Total dosage 30–40 mg/kg	1. ↓ renal function 2. Anemia, thrombocytonia (leukopenia—rare) 3. Reactions assoc. with infusion: fever, chills, H/A 4. Thrombophlebitis 5. Anaphylaxis, hepatotoxicity—rare	May cause additive nephrotoxicity with aminoglycosides	When creatinine >3.5, ↓ daily dose by ½ or use same dose QOD	100 mg per vial
	Candida: Thrush Esophagitis	0.3–0.5 mg/kg day IV	1. Up to 500 mg total				
	Other organs	0.6–1.0 mg/kg day IV	2. 1.5–2.0 g total				
	C. neoformans: Meningitis	0.5–1.0 mg/kg day IV	To total of 1.0 g, then maintenance of at least 100 mg/wk				
	Histoplasmosis Disseminated	0.5–1.0 mg/kg day IV	Total = 2.0–2.5 g				
	Coccidioidomycosis Disseminated	0.5–1.0 mg/kg day IV	Total = 2.0–2.5 g				
5-Flucytosine (usage limited due to bone marrow suppression)	*Cryptococcus* meningitis (synergistic with amphotericin)	50–150 mg/kg/day in four divided doses PO (IV available on request) can reduce amphotericin dosage	Only to be used with amphotericin × 6 weeks	1. N and V, diarrhea 2. Bone marrow suppression 3. Hepatotoxicity	Avoid when using other marrow-suppressive drugs	1. ↓ in renal failure 2. Caution in hepatic failure	Capsules: 250, 500 mg
Antiprotozoan Trimethoprim (TMP)/sulfamethoxazole (SMX)	*P. carinii* pneumonia	5 mg/kg TMP component IV q8hr or equivalent (2 DS tabs QUID) PO 1 DS daily or 1 SS daily or 1 DS 3×/wk	21 days Maintenance	1. Nausea, vomiting 2. Rash; drug fever 3. Hematologic: bone marrow ↓ 4. Reversible renal impairment	1. ? potentiation of warfarin phenytoin 2. Avoid when using other drugs	1. Renal; use cautiously	DS tablets: 160 mg TMP component, 800 mg SMX component
Dapsone-TMP	*P. carinii* pneumonia	100 mg PO dapsone q day; TMP 15 mg/kg/day	Maintenance	Same as TMP/SMX	Same as TMP/SMX	Same as TMP/SMX	100-mg tablet (dapsone)

Drug	Indication	Dose	Duration	Toxicity	Interactions	Dose in renal failure	How supplied
Pentamidine	P. carinii pneumonia	4 mg/kg/day IV slowly (IM causes sterile abscesses)	21 days	1. Rapid infusion: tachycardia, orthostatic hypotension 2. Renal insufficiency 3. Hypo/hyperglycemia 4. Bone marrow ↓	None	No guidelines available	300 mg (for IV use)
		300 mg aerosolized qmo	Maintenance	Bronchospasm		None	
Clindamycin + primaquine	P. carinii pneumonia	600 mg IV q6hr or 300–450 mg PO q6hr 15 mg base PO QD	21 days				
Atovaquone	P. carinii pneumonia	750 mg PO BID	21 days	Rash, nausea, diarrhea			Liquid
Trimetrexate (with folinic acid)	P. carinii	45 mg/m²	21 days	1. Bone marrow suppression 2. Increase LFTs 3. Headache 4. Nausea	Avoid other bone marrow toxic agents	Decrease	25-mg vials
Pyrimethamine	T. gondii cerebritis/abscess (used in conjunction with sulfadiazine or clindamycin)	100–200 mg loading dose → 75–100 mg/day PO (must supplement with folinic acid → 10–50 mg/day)	≥6 wk	1. Hematologic: ↓ bone marrow (↓ WBC, ↓ platelets, megaloblastic anemia)	Avoid other bone marrow toxic drugs	No guidelines available	25-mg tablet
Sulfadiazine	T. gondii (with pyrimethamine, folinic acid)	25–50 g/day PO 6–8 g/day in 4 divided doses PO 2–4 g/day in 4 divided doses	Maintenance ≥6 wk Maintenance	Same as TMP/SMX	Same as TMP/SMX	Same as TMP/SMX	500-mg tablet
Clindamycin	T. gondii (alternative to sulfadiazine)	900–1200 mg q6–8hr IV 300–450 mg q6–8hr PO	≥6 wk Maintenance	1. Nausea, vomiting, diarrhea 2. Pseudomembranous colitis 3. Mild elevation of aminotransferases 4. Hypersensitivity	1. Enhanced action of curarelike drugs 2. Worsened colitis	1. None 2. Avoid with hepatic dysfunction	Capsules: 75, 150, 300 mg
Antiviral Acyclovir	Herpes simplex infections: Esophagitis Encephalitis	5 mg/kg IV q8hr 10 mg/kg IV q8hr Mucocut: 200–400 mg BID–TID PO	7–10 days or until lesions crusted or gone Maintenance	1. Nausea, vomiting, lightheadedness 2. Renal insufficiency with rapid infusion 3. Neurotoxicity 4. Hematologic unusual	1. Possible additive nephrotoxicity with aminoglycosides	1. ↓ with renal failure	200 mg capsule
	Varicella-zoster infections: Shingles	10 mg/kg IV q8hr or 600–800 mg 5 × day PO	7–10 days or until lesions crusted				
	Encephalitis	10 mg/kg IV q8hr					

Table 34.10—*continued.* Practical Information About Antimicrobial Agents Used for the Treatment of the Opportunistic Infections Listed in Table 34.9

Antimicrobial Agent	Organisms and Syndromes	Dosage/Schedule/ Route	Duration/Maintenance	Common Adverse Effects	Drug Interactions	Dosage Change with Renal/Hepatic Failure	Available Strengths, Preparations
Antiviral							
Ganciclovir	Cytomegalovirus infection: Retinitis Colitis Other disseminated	5 mg/kg IV q12hr induction then 5 mg/kg IV QD	2–3 wk Maintenance (dose not clearly est.)	1. Neutropenia, thrombocytopenia 2. Neurotoxicity—confusion 3. GI—nausea, vomiting		↓ with renal failure	
Ganciclovir implants	CMV retinitis		Permanent	Retinal detachment	None	No change	
Ganciclovir oral	CMV infection	1 g TID	Permanent	Bone marrow suppression	Avoid other bone marrow toxic agents	Decrease	250-mg capsules
Foscarnet	CMV infection	60 mg/kg IV q8hr 90 mg/kg IV QD	14–21 days Maintenance	Renal failure 1. Genital ulcerations 2. Hypocalcemia hypophosphatemia hypokalemia hypomagnesemia	1. Renal toxicity with other nephrotoxic drugs 2. ↑ Risk of hypocalcemia with pentamidine	↓ or D/C with renal failure	
Valacyclovir	Varicella-zoster Herpes simplex	1 g TID 1 g BID	7–10 days 7–10 days	1. Headache 2. Nausea	None	Decrease	500 mg
Famciclovir	Varicella-zoster	500 mg TID	7–10 days		None	Decrease	Tablets: 125, 250, 500 mg
Cidofovir	CMV	5 mg/kg/wk 5 mg every other wk	2 wk Maintenance	1. Neutropenia 2. Proteinuria	Avoid other nephrotoxic agents	Decrease	375 mg in 5-mL vial

[a]Dosage based on cumulative, not daily dose. *DS*, double strength; *SS*, single strength.

these patients. Chapter 53 provides additional details regarding the causes of lymphadenopathy and the indications for a lymph node biopsy.

Respiratory Tract Manifestations

The lung is the organ most often involved in HIV-related opportunistic infections. In approximately 60% of patients with AIDS, the diagnosis of AIDS is made on the basis of PCP, and an additional 20% of patients experience at least one episode in the course of their disease (15). Despite the frequency of this pathogen as the etiologic agent for pneumonia in patients with AIDS, other opportunistic and conventional agents such as *Streptococcus pneumoniae* (pneumococcus) may cause pneumonia, either as the sole agent or simultaneously. For this reason, a systematic diagnostic approach to lower respiratory tract symptoms is very important in HIV-infected patients with pneumonia. Moreover, as chemoprophylaxis for *Pneumocystis* becomes more widely used for patients with HIV infection, other causes for respiratory infection will probably become more prevalent.

P. carinii *Pneumonia*

Symptoms of PCP are similar to those of other pneumonias, but the symptoms may be less acute in onset. Common complaints include fever, night sweats, dyspnea, and nonproductive cough. The duration of respiratory symptoms is usually 1 to 3 weeks, although the systemic symptoms may have been present for several months. Because many of these patients have been previously healthy, their clinical presentation may be subtle. For example, it is common for a patient with PCP to have had no more than a mild dry cough and a modest decrease in exercise tolerance. Either thrush or hairy leukoplakia (see below) may be present, or may have occurred in the past, as an indicator of immunosuppression. The physical examination is often not specific. Fever, tachycardia, and tachypnea may be present and, if so, indicate more severe disease. Auscultation of the chest is often unremarkable, and the chest radiograph may be normal (15).

Diagnostic evaluation. HIV-infected patients with only a history of respiratory symptoms should undergo a stepwise laboratory evaluation that is designed to diagnose or rule out PCP and other pulmonary infections. In patients with abnormal chest radiographs, the pattern of infiltrates is helpful in determining the next step. The timing of onset of symptoms is also helpful. A lobar infiltrate on radiograph and a history of acute onset of symptoms is most consistent with a community-acquired pneumonia, either typical (e.g., pneumococcal) or atypical (e.g., mycoplasmal). A lobar infiltrate in the presence of subacute or chronic symptoms is more consistent with mycobacterial or fungal disease. A diffuse interstitial pattern is the most common presenting pattern on chest radiograph in patients with PCP who have not taken prophylactic medicine; some have only focal infiltrates, however, and up to

10% initially have normal chest radiographs. Recent studies show that with the increased use of PCP prophylaxis, patterns other than the typical diffuse interstitial pattern are becoming more common. Because PCP is so common in HIV-infected patients, a normal radiograph in the presence of even minimal lower respiratory tract symptoms should be followed by screening tests such as pulse oximetry (including check for desaturation with walking), pulmonary function tests, or gallium lung scanning.

In the presence of any objective findings of pulmonary infection (radiographic infiltrates, hypoxia, abnormal diffusing capacity, or pulmonary uptake of gallium), one should attempt to make a specific diagnosis by *inducing the production of sputum;* this is done in settings that are equipped to have the patient inhale an aerosol of hypertonic saline, produced by an ultrasonic nebulizer. *P. carinii* is diagnosed by microscopic examination of sputum; there is no technique for culturing this organism. Examination of induced sputum for *P. carinii* has a sensitivity of approximately 80% in selected patients, although its negative predictive value is low (15). Therefore, if a specific diagnosis is not made on induced sputum, the patient should undergo fiberoptic bronchoscopy with *bronchoalveolar lavage.* Sputum can also be stained and cultured for mycobacteria, fungi, and viruses. Patients with no diagnosis even after bronchoalveolar lavage should have *transbronchial biopsy.* Hospital admission for open-lung biopsy may be indicated in selected cases; however, an open-lung biopsy is seldom necessary. When PCP is suspected, antimicrobial treatment can be initiated because this will not alter the chance of identifying the organism, even in specimens obtained after a week of treatment. Often the patient's response to anti-PCP therapy supports the diagnosis of PCP. Particularly in patients who already have had an AIDS-indicator condition (Table 34.5), and in whom the definitive diagnosis of PCP is not mandatory, the response to therapy may obviate an invasive diagnostic procedure.

Details of treatment for PCP are summarized in Tables 34.9 and 34.10. The first-line agent for the treatment of PCP is TMP/SMX. If the patient is allergic to or unable to tolerate TMP/SMX, dapsone-TMP, trimethotrexate, pentamidine isethionate, or clindamycin with primaquine may be used. Each of these agents may cause serious adverse reactions in 25 to 50% of patients treated for 2 weeks or more. *Atovaquone,* an anti-PCP agent with fewer side effects, is also available but is recommended only for mild PCP because it has been shown to be less efficacious than other agents in more severe disease (17).

Symptomatic improvement often occurs within 24 to 48 hours, but it may be slower in some patients. The chest radiograph usually reverts to normal within 2 weeks of initiating treatment. Patients should not be considered to have failed treatment until at least 5 to 7 days of therapy without improvement have elapsed. At this time, discontinuation of the initial therapy and substitution of an alternative drug is warranted.

Patients who require a change in drug because of toxicity usually do well, whereas those who require a change because of treatment failure often do poorly. Of patients with first episodes of PCP, 70 to 80% recover. Higher mortality rates are seen in patients who are sick enough to require hospital admission and who have, or develop in the hospital, severe hypoxemia, elevated lactate dehydrogenase levels, and severe lung damage (1). The use of *corticosteroids* has been shown to be effective in patients with severe PCP, defined as P_{O_2} of 70 or less (24). However, before instituting corticosteroids, it is best to have a definite diagnosis of PCP to avoid possible permissive effects of corticosteroids on another opportunistic infection.

Secondary Prevention for PCP. Recurrences of PCP are common after successful therapy; 50 to 60% of patients who survive 1 year from an initial episode relapse without preventive therapy. PCP prophylaxis, described above, should be instituted after the acute episode.

Tuberculosis

Mycobacterial infections are well-recognized complications of immunosuppression. The incidence of *Mycobacterium tuberculosis,* which is highly communicable, is increasing in patients with AIDS, and TB may be the presenting illness in some HIV-infected patients. To reflect this, the 1993 CDC case definition for AIDS added pulmonary TB in an HIV-infected person as an AIDS-indicator condition (Table 34.5). Chapter 29 ("Tuberculosis in the Ambulatory Patient") discusses the approach to prophylaxis and treatment of TB in HIV-infected patients, including patients infected with multidrug-resistant strains of *M. tuberculosis.*

Other Respiratory Tract Infections

If the chest radiograph of an HIV-infected patient shows a lobar infiltrate, sputum should be obtained and processed for a Gram's stain and routine culture, mycobacterial and fungal stains and culture, and diagnostic tests (immunofluorescent staining of sputum and serologic tests) for *Legionella* and *Mycoplasma* as described in Chapter 28. Treatment should be based on guidelines for treatment of community-acquired pneumonia, described in Chapter 28, unless or until a specific pathogen is identified.

HIV-infected patients may also have a *simple bronchitis* or *sinusitis* presenting with cough and a negative chest radiograph. Although it would be reasonable to treat for one of these entities if the patient is not acutely ill, PCP should be suspected if the patient does not respond.

Neurologic Manifestations

The nervous system is often involved in patients with HIV infection. More than 10% of patients with AIDS have an initial AIDS-indicator neurologic disease (Table 34.5), and more than two-thirds are found to have neurologic involvement at autopsy (21). Involve-ment of the nervous system may be categorized as disease secondary to HIV infection itself or disease secondary to opportunistic pathogens or neoplasms. Manifestations may be caused by diseases of the central nervous system (CNS) or the peripheral nervous system, as shown in Table 34.11. Tables 34.9 and 34.10 summarize features and treatment of the principal opportunistic CNS infections of patients with AIDS.

Global CNS Disorders Caused by HIV

In a small proportion of patients, *acute HIV CNS infection* may occur, manifested as a focal or diffuse encephalitis or aseptic meningitis; there may be associated cranial neuropathies, myelopathy, or peripheral neuropathy. Several of these manifestations may occur simultaneously. Typically, these acute CNS manifestations resolve within 1 to 4 weeks.

In later stages of HIV infection, many patients develop the AIDS dementia complex, a disorder characterized by cognitive, motor, and behavioral dysfunctions. Dementia is the most common CNS complication of AIDS, found eventually in up to 65% of patients. This disorder is included in the CDC case definition of AIDS (Table 34.5). Diagnostic features include positive HIV serology, history of cognitive/behavioral changes (especially impaired concentration and attention, apathy, and memory loss), and associated neurologic findings including hyperreflexia, hypertonia, signs of myelopathy (spastic paraparesis or ataxia), and frontal release signs. In early stages of HIV infection of the CNS, the mental status and neurologic examinations

Table 34.11.   Neurologic Syndromes in HIV-Infected Patients

Diffuse Brain Disease
Encephalitis (toxoplasmosis, CMV)
AIDS dementia complex

Meningitis
Aseptic (acute HIV infection)
Cryptococcal
Tuberculous
Lymphomatous

Focal Brain Disease
Toxoplasmosis
Primary CNS lymphoma
Progressive multifocal leukoencephalopathy (JC virus)
Tuberculoma
Cryptococcoma
Herpes simplex/varicella-zoster virus encephalitis

Peripheral Neuropathies/Radiculopathies/Myelopathies
Neuropathies/radiculopathies
   Mononeuritides (brachial plexopathy)
   Guillain–Barré syndrome
   Sensorimotor polyneuropathy
   CMV polyradiculopathy
   Varicella-zoster (may involve multiple dermatomes)
Myelopathies
   Transverse myelitis (varicella-zoster virus, cytomegalovirus, lymphoma)
   HIV vacuolar myelopathy

can be completely normal. Cerebrospinal fluid findings are nonspecific: normal or slightly elevated protein concentration, normal glucose concentration, a slight mononuclear pleocytosis, negative cryptococcal antigen, and nonreactive VDRL test. CT scan or magnetic resonance imaging (MRI) of the brain may show atrophy with changes in white matter.

Before making a working diagnosis of AIDS dementia, it is important to exclude metabolic or toxic encephalopathies, opportunistic infections, neoplasms, and neurosyphilis. The Mini-Mental Status Examination is helpful for identifying most significant cognitive abnormalities in a brief office interview (see Chapter 17, Table 17.1). In a patient whose Mini-Mental Examination is normal, neuropsychologic testing may be useful in assessing suspected early AIDS dementia and in following the course of the disease; this may be especially important in assessing patients whose work requires a high level of cognitive function. Characteristic abnormalities include difficulty with complex sequencing, impairment of fine and rapid motor movements, and slowed verbal fluency. In rare instances, brain biopsy may be indicated to exclude other metabolic, neoplastic, or infectious causes. There are reports of improved cognitive function after several weeks of zidovudine (AZT) (1000 to 1200 mg/day) and protease inhibitor therapy.

Opportunistic CNS Infections

Opportunistic infections of the CNS occur in many HIV-infected patients. *Cryptococcus neoformans* is the most common pathogen causing meningitis in AIDS patients; this meningitis usually presents as a nonfulminant process. Focal CNS disease is most often caused by *Toxoplasma gondii,* although primary CNS lymphoma, tuberculoma, or cryptococcoma may present in the same way. *Progressive multifocal leukoencephalopathy* (PML) may also present as a focal CNS disease. This is a progressive demyelinating disorder caused by reactivation of a papovavirus in immunosuppressed patients, including those with AIDS. It presents as a subacute disease, progressing over several weeks, with focal neurologic deficits without alteration of consciousness until its terminal stages. Currently, only experimental protocols are available for treatment of this condition.

The clinical presentation of opportunistic CNS infections in patients with HIV may be subtle. Headache and fever are the most common presenting symptoms of CNS infections, although fever may not be present. Focal neurologic findings and meningismus are found in fewer than half of patients with CNS infection. Therefore, a high index of suspicion must be maintained in any HIV-positive patient with a low CD4 count with new onset of severe headache, a change in a usual headache pattern, or persistent headache. Because sinusitis may present with fever and a headache and is common in HIV-infected patients, this diagnosis should be considered as well.

Laboratory evaluation. Because the physical examination usually is not diagnostic, a thorough laboratory evaluation is important in any patient with new neurologic symptoms. The evaluation should begin with plain and contrast-enhanced CT scan of the head to exclude mass lesions. The presence of a ring-enhancing lesion is fairly characteristic for toxoplasmosis, although lymphoma and other causes cannot be excluded. Because toxoplasmosis is the most common cause of such a lesion and because definitive diagnosis requires a brain biopsy, it is reasonable to begin empirical treatment for toxoplasma on the basis of the CT scan. If after 10 to 14 days of therapy the patient has not clinically improved or the CT scan shows no improvement, further diagnostic measures should be considered.

Unless the CT scan shows a mass lesion that might lead to herniation, *lumbar puncture* should also be performed in evaluating new CNS symptoms. Cerebrospinal fluid (CSF) should be evaluated for opening pressure, cell count, protein and glucose concentrations (with a simultaneous serum glucose), Gram's stain, India ink preparation, culture for bacteria, mycobacterial and fungal stains and cultures, cryptococcal antigen, and a VDRL test. Cryptococcal meningitis may be present even with few or no cells in the CSF; in most cases, cryptococcal antigen is present in both the CSF and the serum. A working diagnosis of neurosyphilis should be considered in the presence of a positive serum VDRL, CSF pleocytosis, and negative cultures and stains for other organisms, even if the CSF VDRL is negative.

If the CT scan, CSF examination and culture, and serologic studies do not reveal a cause for the patient's symptoms, an MRI scan should be obtained. Once opportunistic infections and neoplasms are excluded, especially in a patient in whom mental status changes are pronounced, the AIDS dementia complex should be the working diagnosis.

Peripheral Neuropathy

Peripheral neuropathies may occur at all stages of HIV infection, including demyelinating neuropathies such as the Guillain–Barré syndrome in early HIV infection, painful sensory neuropathy of the feet, and infectious radiculopathies caused by varicella-zoster virus or CMV. Chapter 84 ("Peripheral Neuropathy") provides additional information about these syndromes in HIV-infected patients.

Psychiatric Manifestations

Psychiatric disorders may predate the acquisition of HIV infection in some patients, and treatment of patients with a preexisting psychiatric illness and HIV infection may be extremely challenging. Virtually all HIV-infected patients go through a stressful experience upon learning that they are infected (see above). In the months to years that follow diagnosis of HIV infection, these patients may require supportive counseling and the assistance of professional social workers and social service agencies to deal with psychosocial problems. Some patients develop major psychiatric disorders, symptoms of which may be difficult to distinguish from the symptoms of organic CNS disease or drug toxicity (26). For example, apathy and mental slowing are often prominent in the presentation of major depression in HIV-infected patients, and paranoid thoughts or other symptoms of functional psychosis may accompany symptoms that suggest delirium or cognitive impairment. When organic causes have been excluded or when there is a strong possibility that both organic and functional CNS syndromes coexist in a patient, psychotropic medications should be prescribed.

For major depression, which is more common in HIV-infected persons than in the general population, antidepressant treatment is usually effective. Either a tricyclic antidepressant with minimal anticholinergic effects (nortriptyline or desipramine) or a nontricyclic antidepressant should be selected because these patients seem to be prone to the anticholinergic effects of the tricyclics (including delirium). The usual dosages of all antidepressants are appropriate in patients who are in the early stages of HIV infection. The dosages should be lower than the usual recommended dosages in patients who are in the late stages and these patients seem to be more sensitive to all of the effects of antidepressants. (See Chapter 15, "Affective Disorders," for practical information about antidepressants.) Early experience suggests that psychostimulant drugs (e.g., methylphenidate and dextroamphetamine) may be particularly helpful in alleviating the apathy in depressed HIV-infected patients (26). Advice regarding the use of these drugs should be sought from a psychiatrist who has used them to treat depression.

For patients who develop *psychotic symptoms,* the high-potency neuroleptic haloperidol is recommended, as it has few anticholinergic side effects. Psychotic symptoms in HIV-infected patients respond to rather low dosages of haloperidol (e.g., 1 to 5 mg one to three times a day). Details regarding the use of neuroleptic drugs are found in Chapter 16, "Schizophrenia."

Oral Cavity and Gastrointestinal Manifestations

The oral and gastrointestinal manifestations of HIV infection may be caused by opportunistic pathogens or, in the case of some patients with diarrhea, by nonopportunistic pathogens. Tables 34.9 and 34.10 summarize the features and treatment of the opportunistic oral and gastrointestinal infections most common in HIV-infected patients.

Oral Lesions

Oral lesions are common in HIV-positive patients, and they are often the first symptoms of immunodeficiency. The most common oral problem is *thrush, or candidiasis,* which occurs most typically as a whitish coating of the oral mucosa or tongue (see Chapter 101, Fig. 101.6). Five to 10% of patients develop thrush within the first 6 months of known seropositivity, and

it occurs in one-third to one-half of patients at some point in their disease. Other manifestations of oral *Candida* infection are angular cheilosis and erythema without coating. The topical regimens listed in Table 34.10 usually control symptoms of thrush; if they fail, systemic ketoconazole or fluconazole usually work.

The many other oral manifestations of HIV infections include oral hairy leukoplakia Kaposi's sarcoma (KS), mass lesions secondary to neoplasms and opportunistic infections, and difficult-to-control periodontal disease. *Oral hairy leukoplakia* (OHL) is particularly important to recognize because, like herpes zoster infection (shingles) and thrush, it is a manifestation of immunodeficiency. It presents as symptomless hypopigmented shaggy lesions, histologically showing hyperparakeratosis of the mucosa, on the lateral aspects of the tongue. It may be confused with thrush, from which it may be distinguished by scraping the lesion and examining the scrapings microscopically after application of potassium hydroxide (see technique, Chapter 100). The absence of typical fungal forms generally excludes thrush. A distinct *HIV gingivitis* that may lead to severe periodontitis and occasionally acute necrotizing gingivitis may occur despite good oral hygiene. Management of periodontal disease may include topical treatment (e.g., povidone-iodine or chlorhexidine) or systemic antibiotics. Management of these problems requires coordination of care with a dentist. *Oral Kaposi's sarcoma* appears as bluish, black, or red flat lesions, usually on the hard palate. Biopsy of suspicious lesions establishes the diagnosis.

Tracheitis and Esophagitis

Tracheitis and esophagitis should be considered when the patient complains of odynophagia, dysphagia, or retrosternal chest pain. The most common cause of esophagitis in HIV-infected patients is *Candida albicans;* most patients have oral thrush concomitant with or preceding esophagitis. Candida infection distal to the oral cavity constitutes an AIDS-indicator condition (Table 34.5). Esophagitis may also be caused by herpes simplex virus or CMV. Rarely, KS, primary lymphoma, and esophageal squamous cell carcinoma have been found as the cause of esophageal symptoms. In a patient with thrush and severe odynophagia, the clinical diagnosis of *Candida* esophagitis can be made. Odynophagia without thrush should be evaluated with endoscopy or a barium swallow. Definitive diagnosis of symptoms of tracheitis or esophagitis requires endoscopic biopsy of the involved portion of the airway or esophagus.

Gastric and Hepatobiliary Diseases

The stomach is the most common gastrointestinal location for visceral Kaposi's sarcoma; lesions are commonly found by endoscopy in patients with cutaneous KS. Gastric lymphomas may also be found.

Acalculous cholecystitis occurs occasionally in HIV-infected patients and usually is secondary to *Cryptosporidium* or *Microsporidium.*

Parenchymal hepatic disease is also common in HIV-infected patients. They commonly have elevated concentrations of serum alkaline phosphatase and serum aminotransferases. The underlying pathology includes, most often, fatty infiltration, portal inflammation, and noncaseating granulomas. Serologic evidence of past hepatitis B infection is almost universal. Often, liver abnormalities are caused by an already-diagnosed disseminated infection. When this is not likely, liver biopsy is appropriate especially because chronic active hepatitis secondary to hepatitis B and C is treatable with α-interferon. MAC is the most common opportunistic pathogen isolated. KS is also found commonly.

Diarrhea

Diarrhea occurs in approximately 50% of patients during the course of HIV infection; when careful evaluation does not yield a cause (about one-third of the time), diarrhea can be ascribed to HIV infection (18).

Large volume diarrhea, indicative of small bowel disease, often with associated crampy abdominal pain and weight loss, is common. The opportunistic and conventional enteric pathogens that may cause small bowel disease include *Isospora belli, Microsporidia* and *Cryptosporidium,* CMV, MAC, *Giardia lamblia, Salmonella, Shigella,* and *Campylobacter.* Multiple stool specimens for culture and microscopic examination for ova and parasites are necessary to diagnose each of these entities. Some entities, such as CMV and MAC, require more invasive procedures such as small or large bowel biopsy for diagnosis. HIV itself may be associated with abnormal small bowel mucosa. Chapter 26 contains details regarding the diagnosis and management of gastroenteritis caused by conventional pathogens.

It has been pointed out that the rate of control of chronic diarrhea (approximately 75% of patients) is no better, but more costly, when an extensive investigation is conducted than when the initial approach is limited to stool cultures, specific treatment when a pathogen is identified, and diphenoxylate hydrochloride or imodium for symptom control if no treatable pathogen is identified. When this strategy is followed, more extensive evaluation would be reserved for patients (approximately 25%) whose stool frequency is still abnormal after 1 month (18).

Diarrhea indicative of colorectal disease is also common in HIV-infected patients. This presents as frequent small-volume stools, tenesmus, and proctalgia. Laboratory examination and culture of stool specimens are helpful for establishing a diagnosis, and in some cases sigmoidoscopy or colonoscopy with biopsy may be used.

In patients who practice receptive anal intercourse, *perianal herpetic ulcerations* may account for proctalgia and tenesmus, as may a number of other sexually transmitted infections (e.g., syphilis, gonorrhea, chlamydia).

HIV Wasting Syndrome

The diagnosis of *HIV wasting syndrome,* an AIDS-indicator condition (Table 34.5), is made in patients with the combination of pronounced weight loss (10% or more from baseline) plus either chronic diarrhea (at least two loose stools per day for 30 days or more) or chronic weakness and fever (intermittent or constant for 30 days or more) in the absence of other opportunistic infection or malignancy that could explain the findings. To date, no efficacious treatment for this syndrome has been confirmed. Optimal use of antiretroviral drugs and of therapy for lesions of the oral cavity and esophagus, in conjunction with good nutrition, is important. Clinical trials are in progress to evaluate the reported benefits of anabolic steroids in some patients.

Cutaneous Manifestations

A wide variety of skin lesions may occur in HIV-positive patients (12). Probably the best known is *Kaposi's sarcoma,* which occurs more often in homosexual men than in patients from other risk groups. KS is thought to arise from lymphatic endothelial cells. It presents as painless, violaceous papules, usually 0.5 to 2 cm in diameter, often multiple, occurring most commonly on the face, on the extremities, and in the oral cavity. The lesions are bluish in light-skinned patients and may appear nearly black in dark-skinned patients. KS requires a biopsy for definitive diagnosis. This is especially important because it is an AIDS-indicator condition (Table 34.5). KS may also involve the lungs, oral cavity, and the gastrointestinal tract.

Seborrheic dermatitis and exacerbations of *psoriasis* are also commonly seen in HIV-infected patients. Diagnosis and management of these two conditions are described in Chapter 100 ("Common Problems of the Skin").

A number of the *invasive opportunistic infections* of HIV-infected patients, such as cryptococcosis, atypical mycobacterial infection, and histoplasmosis, may present with cutaneous lesions that are rather insignificant in appearance. In the presence of symptoms of systemic disease, one should be highly suspicious and consider biopsy of new skin lesions.

Mucocutaneous herpes simplex virus infection, described in Chapter 100, is another syndrome often seen in HIV-infected patients, and if persistent for more than a month, it is also an AIDS-indicator condition. *Shingles,* or reactivation of latent varicella-zoster infection, is also common in HIV-infected patients and may involve multiple dermatomes. Diagnosis is based on a cytologic examination of the vesicle fluid (the Tzanck smear), viral cultures, or PCR (see details in Chapter 100). The mucocutaneous erosions caused by these viruses also predispose the patient to local and disseminated bacterial superinfection.

Diagnosis and treatment for herpes virus infections are summarized in Tables 34.9 and 34.10. The treatment of KS may vary from expectant observation to a variety of antineoplastic regimens. The consultation of an oncologist should be obtained in deciding on the management of this tumor.

Other Organ Systems

Other organ systems are involved in HIV-infected patients, although not as often as those mentioned above.

The predominant *ophthalmologic* disease is CMV retinitis, which may be completely asymptomatic but, if left untreated, progresses to blindness. CMV retinitis occurs in approximately 20% of patients with AIDS. Routine funduscopic examination is crucial, especially in patients with proven CMV disease in the past and in patients with CD4 counts less than $75/mm^3$. Diagnosis is confirmed by an ophthalmologist because the lesions, which are hemorrhagic and exudative, are specific for this entity.

Hematologic disease is usually secondary to involvement of the bone marrow by one of the opportunistic infections, such as TB, MAC, or histoplasmosis, or secondary to adverse effects of medications used to treat these patients, especially AZT (see below) and TMP/SMX. Bone marrow aspirate and biopsy are often indicated to ascertain the cause of the abnormality.

Both reversible and irreversible *renal abnormalities* are encountered in patients with HIV infection. Although some of these abnormalities may be caused by HIV infection, many result from identifiable causes, especially drug toxicity.

The diagnostic approach to *cardiac disease* in HIV-infected patients should also focus on identifiable causes other than HIV infection. A distinct HIV cardiomyopathy has been described. One common cardiac disease is the infective endocarditis seen in IDUs, which is unrelated to their HIV infection.

With the increase in the numbers of HIV-infected women, involvement of the *reproductive tract* has been recognized. Women with HIV infection often have chronic vulvovaginal candidiasis or herpes, unresponsive to therapy, as the first manifestation of underlying immunodeficiency. Immunosuppressed women may also be at more risk for the progression to malignancy of cervical papillomavirus infection, and such patients should be followed with Papanicolaou smears every 6 to 12 months (see Chapter 95 for technique).

Duration and Location of Treatment for Opportunistic Infections

Duration of therapy is an important consideration for the opportunistic agents that cause AIDS-defining infections. For each specific treatment shown in Table 34.10, the recommended length of treatment is listed. In the absence of a fully functional immune system, most opportunistic infections are never completely cured despite apparently successful therapy; therefore, for many of these infections some form of *maintenance therapy* is recommended as prophylaxis against recurrent infection (also called secondary prophylaxis or suppressive therapy). This is especially true of PCP, cryptococcal meningitis, cerebral toxoplasmosis, thrush, esophageal candidiasis, mucocutaneous herpetic infections, and CMV retinitis. Maintenance (prophylactic) regimens for these infections are also shown in Table 34.10.

Because of the need for prolonged therapy, *home administration of intravenous antibiotics and fluids* is used with increasing frequency. Home treatment often follows a brief hospital admission when the patient is evaluated, specific treatment is initiated, and a Hickman catheter is placed for long-term use. The catheter is placed, under sterile conditions in an operating room, in the subclavian vein; it requires twice-daily flushing with heparin. Even medications as difficult to administer as amphotericin B and intravenous pentamidine are now being given in the patient's home by nurses trained to monitor the patient during drug infusion. In patients with chronic intractable diarrhea, intermittent home intravenous fluid replacement may be needed, and patients with reversible causes of weight loss can receive total parenteral nutrition at home. Chapter 9 provides details regarding referral of patients for home health services.

ANTIRETROVIRAL TREATMENT

Since the last edition of this book, several developments have appreciably altered the approach to and monitoring of antiretroviral therapy (2). These include the development and increasing use of the measurement of a patient's viral load to monitor progression of disease and response to treatment; the development of many new antiretroviral drugs, including those with a different mechanism of inhibiting viral replication, the protease inhibitors (PIs) (14); and a better understanding of the mechanisms of viral resistance to antiretroviral drugs, which has led to more rational approach to therapy. These advances have accounted for dramatic improvement in prognosis, such as a 50% reduction in progression to AIDS or death in zidovudine-treated patients whose regimen was modified as outlined below and over 90% success in attaining undetectable HIV RNA with PI-containing regimens versus no such results in matched patients on regimens that do not contain a PI (14).

For the above reasons, the goals of anti-HIV therapy have also changed, and now include, in addition to suppression of viral replication, the possibility of viral eradication.

Viral Load

As noted above, combined baseline viral load and CD4 counts give the most useful information about prognosis without treatment (Fig. 34.2). The viral load has been shown to be a better indicator of disease progression than the CD4 count, and thus a better guide to the need to initiate or change antiretroviral therapy. In multiple longitudinal studies, subjects in the quartile with the lowest viral load (less than 500 HIV RNA copies per mL of plasma) had the lowest risk of progression to AIDS and death; those in the quartile with the highest viral load (30,000 to 50,000 HIV RNA copies per mL) were at the greatest risk of progression (2). Like the CD4 count, the viral load may fluctuate, depending on multiple factors, and thus should be measured several times 2 to 4 weeks apart wherever it is being used to make a treatment decision. In the view of most experts, any viral load greater than 10,000 should be regarded as unacceptable and some even consider anything above detectable unacceptable.

Antiretroviral Drugs

Tables 34.12A–C and 34.13 summarize practical information about available antiretroviral drugs. In recent years, two new classes of antiretroviral agents have been added to the original *nucleoside reverse transcriptase inhibitors* (NRTIs), of which zidovudine (AZT, ZDV) was the first. These include the *nonnucleoside reverse transcriptase inhibitors* (NNRTIs), which have the same mechanism of action but a different structure, and the *protease inhibitors* (PIs), which

Table 34.12A. Characteristics of Nucleoside Reverse Transcriptase Inhibitors (NRTIs)

Generic Name Trade Name	Zidovudine (AZT, ZDV) Retrovir	Didanosine (ddl) Videx	Zalcitabine (ddC) HIVID	Stavudine (d4T) Zerit	Lamivudine (3TC) Epivir
Form	100, 300 mg caps, IV, vials, combination pill with lamivudine (Combivir)	25, 50, 100, 150 mg tabs Buffered powder packets: 100, 167, 250 mg Liquid: 20 mg ddl/ mL Mylanta DS	0.375, 0.75 mg tabs	15, 20, 30, 40 mg caps	150 mg tabs, combination pill with AZT (Combivir) Oral solution: 10 mg/mL
Dosing recommendations	200 mg TID or 300 mg BID	Tablets >60 kg: 200 mg BID <60 kg: 125 mg BID	0.75 mg TID[a]	>60 kg: 40 mg BID[a] <60 kg: 30 mg BID	150 mg BID[a] <50 kg: 2 mg/kg BID
Oral bioavailability	60%	Tablet: 40% Powder: 30%	85%	86%	86%
Serum half-life	1.1 hours	1.6 hours	1.2 hours	1.0 hour	3–6 hours
Intracellular half-life	3 hours	25–40 hours	3 hours	3.5 hours	12 hours
Elimination	Metabolized to AZT Glucuronide (GAZT) Renal excretion of GAZT	Renal excretion—50%	Renal excretion—70%	Renal excretion—50%	Renal excretion unchanged
Major toxicity	Bone marrow suppression: anemia or neutropenia Subjective complaints: GI intolerance, headache, insomnia, asthenia	Pancreatitis, peripheral neuropathy, nausea, diarrhea	Peripheral neuropathy, stomatitis	Peripheral neuropathy	(Minimal toxicity)

From Johns Hopkins HIV Report, December, 1997.
[a]Adjust for renal failure.

Table 34.12B. Nonnucleoside Reverse Transcriptase Inhibitors (NNRTIs)

Generic Name Trade Name	Nevirapine Viramune	Delavirdine Rescriptor
Form	200 mg tabs	100 mg tabs
Dosing recommendations	200 mg PO QD × 14 days, then 200 mg PO BID	400 mg PO TID (four 100 mg tabs in ≥3 oz water to produce slurry)
Oral bioavailability	>90%	85%
Serum half-life	25–30 hours	5.8 hours
Elimination	Metabolized by cytochrome P-450; 80% excreted in urine (glucuronidated metabolites, <5% unchanged), 10% in feces	Metabolized by cytochrome P-450; 51% excreted in urine (<5% unchanged), 44% in feces
Drug interactions	Induces cytochrome P-450 enzymes The following drugs have suspected interactions that require careful monitoring if coadministered with nevirapine: rifampin, rifabutin, oral contraceptives, midazolam, triazolam, and protease inhibitors	Inhibits cytochrome P-450 enzymes Contraindicated drugs: terfenadine, astemizole, ergot derivatives, amphetamines, anticonvulsants (phenytoin, carbamazepine, phenobarbital), triazolam, midazolam, cisapride, rifabutin, and rifampin Antacids and didanosine: separate administration by ≥1 hr
Major toxicity	Rash, hepatitis	Rash, headaches

From Johns Hopkins HIV Report, December, 1997.

Table 34.12C.   Characteristics of Protease Inhibitors

Generic Name Trade Name	Indinavir Crixivan	Ritonavir Norvir	Saquinavir Fortovase	Nelfinavir Viracept
Form	200, 400 mg caps	100 mg caps 600 mg/7.5 mL PO solution	200 mg caps	250 mg tablets 50 mg/g oral powder
Dosing recommendations	800 mg q8hr Take 1 hr before or 2 hr after meals; may take with skim milk or low fat meal	600 mg q12hr[a] Take with food if possible	1200 mg TID Take with large meal	750 mg TID Take with food (meal or light snack)
Oral bioavailability	65%	(Not determined)	~ 12%,	20–80%
Serum half-life	1.5–2 hours	3–5 hours	1–2 hours	3.5–5 hours
Route of metabolism	P-450 cytochrome 3A4	P-450 cytochrome 3A4, >2D6	P-450 cytochrome 3A4	P-450 cytochrome 3A4
Storage	Room temperature	Refrigerate; single dose may be at room temperature for 12 hr	Room temperature	Room temperature
Adverse effects	Nephrolithiasis GI intolerance, nausea Lab: Increase indirect bilirubinemia (inconsequential), transaminase elevation Misc: Headache, asthenia, blurred vision, dizziness, rash, metallic taste, thrombocytopenia	GI intolerance, nausea, vomiting, diarrhea Paresthesia—circumoral and extremities Asthenia Taste perversion Lab: triglycerides increase ≥200%, transaminase elevation, elevated CPK and uric acid	GI intolerance, nausea, and diarrhea Headache Transaminase elevation	Diarrhea Transaminase elevation
Drug interactions	Inhibits cytochrome P-450 (less than ritonavir) Not recommended for concurrent use: rifampin, terfenadine, astemizole, cisapride, triazolam, midazolam, ergot alkaloids Indinavir levels increased by: ketoconazole,[b] delavirdine Indinavir levels reduced by rifampin, rifabutin, nevirapine, grapefruit juice Didanosine: reduces indinavir absorption unless taken >2 hr apart	Inhibits cytochrome P-450 (potent inhibitor) Ritonavir increases levels of multiple drugs that are not recommended for concurrent use[c] Didanosine: reduced absorption of both drugs: take ≥2 hr apart Ritonavir decreases levels of ethinyl estradiol, theophylline, sulfamethoxazole, and zidovudine Ritonavir increases levels of clarithromycin and desipramine	Inhibits cytochrome P-450 Saquinavir levels increased by: ritonavir, ketoconazole, grapefruit juice, nelfinavir, delavirdine Saquinavir levels reduced by: rifampin, rifabutin, and (?) phenobarbital, phenytoin, dexamethasone and carbamazepine, and nevirapine Not recommended for concurrent use: terfenadine, astemizole, cisapride, ergot alkaloids	Inhibits cytochrome P-450 (less than ritonavir) Nelfinavir levels reduced by rifampin, rifabutin Not recommended for concurrent use: rifampin, triazolam, midazolam, ergot alkaloids, terfenadine, astemizole, cisapride Nelfinavir decreases levels of ethinyl estradiol and norethindrone Nelfinavir increases levels of rifabutin, saquinavir, and indinavir

From Johns Hopkins HIV Report, December, 1997.

[a]Dose escalation for Ritonavir: day 1–2: 300 mg BID; day 3–5: 400 mg BID; day 6–13: 500 mg BID; day 14: 600 mg BID. Combination treatment regimen with Saquinavir (400–600 mg PO BID) plus Ritonavir (400–600 mg PO BID).

[b]Decrease indinavir to 600 mg q8hr.

[c]Drugs contraindicated for concurrent use with Ritonavir: amiodarone (Cardarone), astemizole (Hismanal), bepridil (Vascar), bupropion (Wellbutin), cisapride (Propulsid), clorazepate (Tranxene), clozapine (Clozaril), diazepam (Valium); ecainide (Enkaid), estazolam (ProSom), flecainide (Tambocor), flurazepam (Dalmane), meperidine (Demerol), midazolam (Versed), piroxicam (Feldene), propoxyphene (Darvon), propafenone (Rythmol), quinidine, terfenadine (Seldane), triazolam (Halcion), zolpidem (Ambien), and ergot alkoloids.

act at a different locus in the process of viral replication than NRTIs or NNRTIs (14). In addition to the adverse effects listed in Table 34.12C, the PIs have been associated with the development of diabetes mellitus.

The development of agents that act at different loci in the viral replication cycle has led to the application of principles used with other infectious agents to prevent resistance and promote eradication, such as the principles applied in the treatment of tuberculosis. The hallmark of these principles is the use of several agents simultaneously (combination therapy). Thus, monotherapy, or the use of a single agent, such as AZT, is no longer considered appropriate.

Although the full extent to which the PIs have expanded the efficacy of antiretroviral treatment is still unknown, multiple clinical trials have shown that PI-containing regimens dramatically increase CD4 counts, decrease viral load, delay clinical progression, and prolong life (14). However, the duration of the efficacious effects is unknown, with recent studies showing secondary failure in as early as 6 months. Consensus recommendations for antiretroviral treatment were extensively revised during 1997 in light of the availability of PIs.

Recommendations

Current treatment recommendations always include at least three agents, usually two NRTIs and a PI. Depending on the circumstances, appropriate combinations may consist of two NRTIs and an NNRTI or two PIs and two NRTIs. Consensus recommendations current in early 1998 are summarized in Tables 34.14 through 34.16. These tables address the following four questions: when to start antiretroviral treatment, what to start with, when to change therapy, and what to change to.

Because so many agents are available currently, there are many ongoing trials to determine which particular combinations are most efficacious for lowering the viral load. With several agents being used simultaneously, there is a high likelihood of side effects and drug–drug interactions. Because of the exceedingly rapid pace at which these new drugs and the related clinical trial data are being released, primary care physicians should consult sources of timely updates (see "General References") and infectious disease consultants. This is analogous to the relationship between primary care physicians and oncologists in the care of patients with a neoplastic disease.

Drug Resistance

It is now understood that the short duration of the antiviral response (decreased viral load and increased CD4 in some patients) is caused by the virus's ability to mutate to avoid the effects of antiretroviral drugs. The problem of drug resistance is not unique to HIV. It has complicated the treatment of other infectious agents, such as *M. tuberculosis,* other bacteria (*Pseudomonas* species, *Neisseria gonorrhea*), and other viruses (e.g., CMV and herpes simplex virus). With increasing knowledge of the resistance mechanisms of HIV, strategies to forestall or prevent the emergence of resistance are being developed, particularly the combined use of agents with different mechanisms of action on viral replication (Tables 34.15 and 34.16).

When resistance develops to some of the antiretroviral agents, it may also develop simultaneously to another drug that has never been used. Thus, knowledge of the *cross-resistance patterns* of various antiretroviral agents is important in changing therapy. It is now known that the development of resistance to the protease inhibitors is closely related to the amount of drug in the patient's body and thus the patient's compliance in taking the prescribed dosage at the appropriate time (see Table 34.12C). Taking these drugs at a reduced dosage or only occasionally results in a level of drug at which selection for drug-resistant variants occurs.

OVERALL PRINCIPLES OF TREATMENT

The following overall principles for treatment are derived from the *1996 Consensus Statement of the International AIDS Society* (2). They apply to patients who have not been on any agents previously, as well as those who have previously been treated.

- The viral load and CD4 count are both used to monitor the patient's response to therapy (see recommended intervals in Table 34.8A); however, the viral

Table 34.13. Dosage Modifications for Combinations of Nonnucleoside Reverse Transcriptase Inhibitors and Protease Inhibitors

	Modification of Coadministered Drug					
Initial Drug	Nevirapine	Delavirdine	Indinavir	Saquinavir	Ritonavir	Nelfinavir
Neveripine	—	No data	1000 mg TID	Avoid	No change	No change
Delavirdine	No data	—	600 mg TID	No change	No change	No data
Indinavir	No change	No change	—	Avoid	No data	500 mg TID
Saquinavir	Avoid	No data	Avoid	—	400 mg BID	No change
Ritonavir	No change	No change	No data	400 mg BID	—	250 mg TID
Nelfinavir	No change	No data	600 mg TID	No change	No change	—

Table 34.14. Antiretroviral Therapy: When to Start

Clinical Category	CD4+ T Cell Count and HIV RNA	Recommendation
Symptomatic (AIDS, thrush, unexplained fever)	All	Treat.
Asymptomatic	CD4+ T Cells <500/mm³ *or* HIV RNA >10,000 (bDNA) *or* >20,000 (RT-PCR)	Treatment should be offered. Strength of recommendation is based on prognosis for disease-free survival and willingness of the patient to accept therapy.[a]
Asymptomatic	CD4+ T Cells >500/mm³ *and* HIV RNA <10,000 (bDNA) *or* <20,000 (RT-PCR)	Some experts would delay therapy and observe; however, some experts would treat.

Developed by the Panel on Clinical Practices for Treatment of HIV Infection convened by the Department of Health and Human Services (DHHS) and the Henry J. Kaiser Foundation (final version was released November 4, 1997; reproduced from Johns Hopkins HIV Report, December 1997.

[a]Some experts would observe patients with CD4+ T cell counts between 350–500/mm³ and HIV RNA levels <10,000 (bDNA) or <20,000 (RT-PCR).

Table 34.15. Antiretroviral Therapy: What to Start With

Preferred Combination Regimens: Strong evidence of clinical benefit and sustained suppression of plasma viral load:
One choice each from Column A and Column B. Drugs are listed randomly, not in priority order.

Column A (PIs)	Column B (NRTIs)
Indinavir	ZDV + ddI
Nelfinavir	d4T + ddI
Ritonavir	ZDV + ddC
Saquinavir	ZDV + 3TC
	d4T + 3TC

Alternative: Less likely to provide sustained virus suppression:
1 NNRTI (Nevirapine) + 2 NRTIs (Column B above)
Saquinavir (hard gel capsule) + 2 NRTIs (Column B above)
Not generally recommended: Clinical benefit demonstrated but initial virus suppression is not sustained in most patients:
2 NRTIs (Column B)
Not recommended: Evidence against use, virologically undesirable, or overlapping toxicity:
All monotherapies, d4T + ZDV, ddC + ddI, ddC + d4T, ddC + 3TC

Developed by the Panel on Clinical Practices for Treatment of HIV Infection convened by the Department of Health and Human Services (DHHS) and the Henry J. Kaiser Foundation (final version was released November 4, 1997; reproduced from Johns Hopkins HIV Report, December 1997.

load is more sensitive and should generally be used to decide on the institution or alteration of antiretroviral therapy.

- The CD4 count indicates the degree of immunosuppression and should be used to determine when to begin prophylaxis for opportunistic infections (see Table 34.8B).
- Decisions regarding therapy should *never* be based on a single measurement of the viral load or CD4 count. A repeat measurement should be obtained to confirm the initial measurement.
- The goal of antiretroviral therapy is undetectable viral load. Repeatedly measured viral loads greater than 20,000 are unacceptable and warrant initiation or alteration of therapy.
- Monotherapy with PIs, NNRTIs, and lamivudine is never acceptable because resistance develops rapidly. Other agents (e.g., didanosine) can be used alone in special circumstances but are not nearly as efficacious as when used in combination. AZT monotherapy in the HIV-infected pregnant woman, to reduce the risk of vertical transmission of the virus, is an exception to this principle.
- Because patient compliance in taking the PIs is crucial to avoid resistance, both verbal and written patient instructions about dosages and intervals are mandatory.
- Therapy should be initiated with three medications, preferably two NRTIs and one PI (e.g., AZT, 3TC, and indinavir).
- The viral load should be monitored at least 2 to 4 weeks after the initiation of or change in antiretroviral therapy, and then at 3 months to assess continued efficacy. Thereafter, viral load and CD4 should be monitored every 3 to 6 months (see also Table 34.8A). A 0.5 log decrease in viral load is regarded as significant.
- Therapy should definitely be altered if there is failure to obtain a 0.5 log decrease in viral load confirmed by

two measurements. At any viral load above detectable, it may be wise to alter therapy because it is now known that viral resistance occurs rapidly and this therapy will ultimately fail. Transient increase in viral load, which resolves after about 1 month, may follow immunizations or intercurrent acute illnesses.

- If therapy is to be altered, two agents should be changed, not just a single agent.

PROBLEMS UNIQUE TO SPECIFIC PATIENT POPULATIONS

Injecting Drug Users

Injecting drug users (IDUs) have difficult medical and social problems, even in the absence of HIV disease. Hospital admission for complications related to drug use, including endocarditis, thrombophlebitis, and cellulitis, is common. In some cases, the intravenous drug user uses multiple substances, including alcohol with its related medical complications. Thus, when an intravenous drug user is infected with HIV, the care becomes even more challenging. Although infection must always be considered in such patients when they have signs of an acute illness (tremors, tachycardia, fever, prostration, changes in sensorium), they should also be evaluated for drug toxicity or withdrawal.

Lack of intravenous access is a common and frustrating problem in these patients. Often, placement of a central line expedites therapy and prevents much of the frustration experienced in looking for peripheral vascular access. Unfortunately, a central line also provides active drug users with a site for injecting themselves, while being treated in the hospital or at home.

In addition to their medical problems, drug abusers also present many behavioral problems. Often noncompliant with medication and manipulative, and at times callous about the risks they pose to others, these patients require much patience and expertise. Effective treatment for their substance abuse is critical to having them follow appropriate care for their HIV infection.

Information regarding prevention of needle transmission of HIV is described above. Treatment of substance abuse is described in Chapter 22 ("Illicit and Therapeutic Use of Drugs with Abuse Liability").

Women

HIV-infected women generally fall into one of two categories, based on age. A minority are older female patients who have acquired their infection through transfusion of blood products and who have an underlying medical condition. Most are younger patients who have histories of intravenous drug use or multiple sexual partners from an early age; thus they are at risk not only for other diseases transmitted by needle sharing and sexual promiscuity, but also for unplanned pregnancy. Because the diagnosis of HIV seropositivity may come as a surprise, these young women often deny the diagnosis and do not return for medical follow-up.

Women capable of childbearing should be counseled about the risk of transmission of HIV infection to their newborn should they become pregnant; the risk of transmission to the fetus is currently estimated as 7 to 40%. Barrier contraception (condom use by the partner) is of paramount importance to prevent not only pregnancy but also transmission of HIV (for details, see "Sexual Transmission," above).

It is now known that treatment with zidovudine (AZT) during pregnancy reduces the risk of transmission of HIV to the fetus by about two-thirds and thus should be prescribed to pregnant HIV-infected women (3,20). Most pregnant women also merit more aggressive treatment (see above) despite the lack of studies to evaluate the safety of most antiretroviral drugs in pregnancy, especially during the first trimester (see Bartlett in "General References").

SPECIAL CONSIDERATIONS

Social and Economic Issues

As noted above, under "Early Evaluation and Treatment of the HIV-Infected Patient," the diagnosis of HIV seropositivity or AIDS can be devastating to the patient. Patients with AIDS are faced not only with coping with a fatal disease, which is sexually transmissible, but also with the social stigma attached to the disease. These patients must confront the need to inform their sexual partners (for the partners' own protection) and the risk of losing close friends. They must face the risk of employment, housing, or insurance discrimination. Women must face the effect of this disease on their childbearing future, as well as the effect on children they are already rearing. Because many people who are seropositive are in dire financial straits before their illness, the disease may create an unbearable financial burden. In addition to the medical complications of AIDS, these social and economic problems will come to the attention of the patient's physician, who must repeatedly present unpleasant facts to the patient and help the patient come to terms with them.

The patient's financial stress may be ameliorated somewhat by the fact that AIDS (and some HIV-related illnesses that do not meet diagnostic criteria for AIDS) qualifies a patient for Social Security Disability. This means that the patient receives Social Security income immediately but must wait 24 months before receiving Medicare health insurance. A patient who meets the needs criteria for Supplemental Security Income (SSI) can obtain health insurance through Medicaid immediately (see Chapter 9 for further information). In 1997, the 1-year retail cost of each of the protease inhibitors ranged from $6000 to $8000, giving an idea of the size of the health care cost of AIDS, even for the ambulatory patient.

A newer and rather unusual problem has arisen since the advent of the newer antiretroviral agents, especially the PIs, and the more widespread use of combination therapy: that of patients having unexpected restored health after years of considering themselves to be terminally ill. This has raised many psychologic and practical issues, including making plans for a future never expected, returning to work after being on disability, and the guilt of surviving when so many early in the epidemic did not.

In addressing the social aspects of the patient's

Table 34.16.   Antiretroviral Therapy: When to Change and What to Change to

When to Change Therapy

The goal of therapy is a viral burden of <500 copies/mL at 4–6 months after starting a new regimen. The probability of achieving this goal can be crudely predicted at 1–2 months, at which time there should be a decrease in viral burden of at least one log (10-fold). The decision to change therapy is confounded by prior drug exposures, toxicities, and a lack of substitute regimens with acceptable tolerance, established efficacy or probability of adherence. In some instances, because of limited options, it is preferred to continue a regimen that incompletely suppresses the virus.

What to Change to[a]

Prior Regimen	New Regimen (Not Listed in Priority Order)
2 NRTIs +	2 new NRTIs +
Nelfinavir	Ritonavir *or* Indinavir *or* Saquinavir + Ritonavir *or* NNRTI[b] + Ritonavir *or* NNRTI[b] + Indinavir[c]
Ritonavir	Saquinavir + Ritonavir[c] *or* Nelfinavir + +NNRTI[b] *or* Nelfinavir + Saquinavir
Indinavir	Saquinavir + Ritonavir *or* Nelfinavir + NNRTI[b] *or* Nelfinavir + Saquinavir
Saquinavir	Ritonavir *or* Ritonavir + Saquinavir *or* NNRTI[b] + Indinavir
2 NRTIs + Nevirapine	2 new NRTIs + a protease inhibitor
2 NRTIs	2 new NRTIs + a protease inhibitor
	2 new NRTIs + Ritonavir + Saquinavir
	1 new NRTI + a protease inhibitor + an NNRTI
	2 protease inhibitors + an NNRTI[b]
1 NRTI	2 new NRTIs + a protease inhibitor
	2 new NRTIs + NNRTI[b]
	1 new NRTI + NNRTI[b] + a protease inhibitor

Developed by the Panel on Clinical Practices for Treatment of HIV Infection convened by the Department of Health and Human Services (DHHS) and the Henry J. Kaiser Foundation (final version was released November 4, 1997; reproduced from Johns Hopkins HIV Report, December 1997.

[a]These suggested alternative regimens have not been proven to be clinically effective.

[b]Of the two available NNRTIs, clinical trials support a preference for nevirapine over delavirdine based on results of viral load assays. These two agents have opposite effects on CYP 450 pathway and this must be considered in combining these drugs with other agents.

[c]There are some clinical trials with viral burden data to support this recommendation.

disease, the *patient's right to privacy and confidentiality* should be ensured at the outset, and patients should be asked to specify the people to whom they plan to disclose the nature of their illness. Intensive psychologic counseling is of paramount importance in helping AIDS patients cope with these decisions and the many changes in their lives caused by their disease. A team approach to the management of all aspects of AIDS is crucial. In addition to the physician's input, the supportive counseling of a social worker and help from community-based support groups and health department AIDS services should be enlisted.

Death and Dying

Because AIDS is in many a fatal disease, dealing with the issues of death and dying is extremely important. It is probably not appropriate to begin such discussions when a patient first learns of seropositivity, other than to answer questions about the prognosis frankly. It should be emphasized that HIV infection has a long latency period (Fig. 34.1) and that it is not known that all HIV-positive people will develop AIDS. In these circumstances, hope is extremely powerful in maintaining the patient's psychologic and physical well-being.

The more appropriate time to explore the issues of death and dying is when the patient develops signs and symptoms related to progressive immunodeficiency. Open discussions should be initiated about financial planning and about advance directives regarding resuscitation and other aspects of care when one may not be competent. These discussions should take place early in the course of AIDS while the patient is still fully competent. Again, the team approach is important here because the patient needs as much support as possible. Issues of death, dying, and bereavement are discussed in further detail in Chapter 19, and Chapter 6 describes legal considerations in specifying and documenting advance directives.

Public Health and Legal Responsibilities of the Physician

No disease in recent times has emphasized to a greater extent the confrontation between the defense of individual privacy and the protection of public health. Clearly, this remains a major challenge to health care professionals dealing with HIV infection. The physician's primary responsibility is to the patient. The unique trust inherent in the physician–patient relationship allows the physician to guide the patient to protect those who may be at risk because of intimate exposure. The physician has the responsibility of emphasizing to the patient, on multiple occasions if necessary, the importance of informing sexual or needle-sharing partners of seropositivity. Guidelines governing the physician's responsibility when the patient refuses to inform others are included in many state laws, and advice regarding these guidelines should be sought from public health authorities in one's state. Many states now have confidential programs for sexual partner notification.

Physicians are required by law to report all newly diagnosed cases of AIDS, using confidential morbidity report forms. Some states now require reporting of most symptomatic HIV-associated diseases.

Information and Support for Household Members

People who live with or care for HIV-infected patients at home have special needs.

First, they need clear information about the transmission of HIV infection, about both the safety of nonintimate contact with the patient and the risks and precautions related to intimate contact. Household caretakers should be advised to follow the precautions recommended to health care workers for the care of all patients, the so-called universal precautions described in the next section. Guidelines for social interaction in the household should be based on information described above ("Transmission and Prevention of Transmission").

Second, people close to patients with HIV infection and AIDS invariably have a variety of intense emotional reactions and must also confront distressing social implications of the patient's illness. Thus, taking the time to share information and, more important, to respond to the questions and feelings of the patient's caretakers is a critical part of caring for patients with HIV and AIDS.

Precautions for Health Care Workers

The possibility of transmission of HIV to health care workers and caretakers in the patient's household has been of concern since the identification of HIV as the cause of AIDS. The cumulative results of several studies of health care workers have shown that health care workers are at an extremely low but finite risk of occupational infection with the virus (11). The predominant occupational risk for infection is through accidental needlestick exposure; however, the risk of infection after an exposure to HIV-infected blood through a needlestick is less than 0.5% (9).

It has been shown that accidental infection is preventable by conscientious use of the *universal precautions* summarized in Table 34.17. The word "univer-

---

Table 34.17. Health Care Workers' Universal Precautions that Should Be Used in the Care of *All* Patients

Wear gloves for touching blood and body fluids, mucous membranes, or nonintact skin of the patient.
Wash hands immediately before and after patient care.
Wear gown, mask, and goggles if aerosolization or splattering of blood or body fluids is likely.
Handle sharp instruments with great care and discard them immediately in containers designed for this purpose. Used venipuncture needles MUST NOT be recapped.
Clean blood spills promptly with disinfectant such as 1:10 dilution of bleach.
Refrain from direct patient care if you have exudative skin lesions.

Table 34.18.   Medical Management of HIV Infection: Postexposure Prophylaxis for Health Care Workers

Provisional Public Health Service recommendations for chemophrophylaxis after occupational exposure to HIV, by type of exposure and source material, 1996

Type of Exposure	Source Material	Antiretroviral Prophylaxis[a]	Antiretroviral Regimen[b] (Recommended Duration: 4 weeks)
Percutaneous	Blood[c]	Recommend	ZDV plus 3TC plus IDV
	Highest risk		
	Increased risk	Recommend	ZDV plus 3TC ± IDV
	No increased risk	Offer	ZDV plus 3TC
	Fluid containing visible blood, other potentially infectious fluid or tissue	Offer	ZDV plus 3TC
	Other body fluid (e.g., urine)	Not offered	
Mucous membrane	Blood	Offer	ZDV plus 3TC ± IDV
	Fluid containing visible blood, other potentially infectious fluid[d] or tissue	Offer	ZDV ± 3TC
	Other body fluid (e.g., urine)	Not offered	
Skin, increased risk	Blood	Offer	ZDV plus 3TC ± IDV
	Fluid containing visible blood, or other potentially infectious fluid[d] or tissue	Offer	ZDV ± 3TC
	Other body fluid (e.g., urine)	Not offered	

From Bartlett J. Medical management of HIV infection. Baltimore: Port City Press, 1997.

[a]Recommend postexposure prophylaxis (PEP); *offer* indicates offering PEP; *not offer,* PEP should not be offered.

[b]ZDV (200 mg PO TID or 300 mg PO BID); 3TC (lamivudine, 150 mg PO BID). *IND,* indinavir (800 mg PO TID).

[c]Highest risk: large volume inoculum and high HIV titer specimen.

[d]Includes semen, vaginal secretions, cerebrospinal, synovial, pleural, peritoneal, pericardial, and amniotic fluid (note that all seroconversions have involved blood or bloody body fluid or viral cultures in labs).

sal" refers to the fact that these precautions should be followed in the direct care of all patients and in handling the body fluids of all patients (9).

If a health care worker has a percutaneous injury (needlestick or cut), or contact of mucous membrane (eye or mouth) or skin with blood, tissues, or other body fluids, the source patient should be assessed clinically and, if consent is obtained, that patient should be tested for HIV infection (11). As soon as possible after exposure, the exposed worker should be counseled and, if consent is obtained, tested for HIV infection. If the source patient is HIV negative and has no clinical indicators of or risk factors for HIV infection, no further follow-up of the exposed worker is necessary. If the source patient's HIV status cannot be determined or the patient is HIV infected, the exposed worker should be retested periodically (6 weeks, 12 weeks, and 6 months after exposure) for 6 months and told to seek medical care for any acute illnesses that occur during this period. The Public Health Service now recommends *postexposure prophylaxis* (PEP) for occupational exposures to HIV in certain situations (Table 34.18). Prophylaxis is recommended for exposures associated with the highest risk for HIV transmission, offered for those exposures with a lower but nonnegligible risk, and unjustified for exposures with a negligible risk. PEP should be initiated within 1 to 2 hours after exposure; although animal studies suggest that PEP is not effective when begun later than 36 hours after exposure, it should still be considered after 1 to 2 weeks after exposure because of the beneficial effects of early treatment of acute HIV infection. The optimal duration of therapy is unknown, but 4 weeks is suggested. Because of the higher risk of transmission of hepatitis B virus (HBV), a person with a needlestick injury

should also be evaluated and treated appropriately for possible HBV (see details in Chapter 32).

General References*

American Medical Association web site. http://www.ama-assn.org/special/hiv/hivhome.html.
> Offers continuing medical education on HIV care and access to the National Library of Medicine's AIDS line.
> (Other web site with HIV information: http://www.thebody.com/learning.html)

Bartlett J. Medical management of HIV infection. Baltimore: Port City Press, 1997.
> Practical manual, especially regarding details about antimicrobial drugs, updated every 1 to 2 years. Interim updates at Johns Hopkins AIDS Service Web Site http://www.hopkins-aids.edu.

Bartlett JB, Finkbeiner AK. The guide to living with HIV infection. 2nd ed. Baltimore: Johns Hopkins University Press, 1993.
> An invaluable practical resource for caretakers and family members.

Centers for Disease Control and Prevention. **United States Public Health Service/Infectious Disease Society of America guidelines for the prevention of opportunistic infections in persons infected with human immunodeficiency virus: a summary.** MMWR 46(RR-12):1–46, 1997.
> The most recent summary of guidelines for OI prophylaxis.

Cotton DJ, ed. AIDS clinical care. Massachusetts Medical Society, Waltham.
> Excellent monthly review of issues related to HIV care including a feature topic, case history, and review of recent journal articles.

Sande MA, Volberding PA, eds. The medical management of AIDS. 5th ed. Philadelphia: WB Saunders, 1997.
> Practical information on all aspects of HIV infection.

For federally approved treatment guidelines and information, the

---

*Bold print (general references) and bold numerals (specific references) denote published controlled clinical trials, meta-analyses, or consensus-based recommendations.

HIV/AIDS Treatment Information Service may be called: 800-448-0440 (TDD/Deaf access, 800-243-7012) Monday through Friday, 9 AM to 7 PM EST, fax 301-738-6616, P.O. Box 6303, Rockville, MD 20849-6303.

Specific References

1. Brenner M, Ognibene FP, Lack EE, et al. Objective clinical and histological prognostic factors for patients with *Pneumocystis carinii* pneumonia and acquired immunodeficiency syndrome. Am Rev Respir Dis 136:1199, 1987.

2. Carpenter CJ, Fischl MA, Hammer SM, et al. Consensus statement. Antiretroviral therapy for HIV infection in 1996. Recommendations of an international panel. JAMA 276:146, 1996.

3. Centers for Disease Control and Prevention. Zidovudine for the prevention of HIV transmission from mother to infant. MMWR 43:285, 1994.

4. Centers for Disease Control and Prevention. First 500,000 AIDS cases, United States, 1995. MMWR 44, 1995.

5. Centers for Disease Control and Prevention. Recommendations for prophylaxis against *Pneumocystis carinii:* Guidelines for prophylaxis against *Pneumocystis carinii* pneumonia for adults and adolescent persons infected with human immunodeficiency virus. U.S. Public Health Service Task Force on antipneumocytis prophylaxis for patients with human immunodeficiency virus infection. MMWR 4138(RR-4):1, 5, 1989.

6. Centers for Disease Control and Prevention. Interpretation and use of the Western blot assay for serodiagnosis of human immunodeficiency virus type I infections. JAMA 262(24):3395, 1989.

7. Centers for Disease Control and Prevention. Public Health Service guidelines for counseling and antibody testing to prevent HIV infection and AIDS. MMWR 36:509, 1987.

8. Centers for Disease Control and Prevention. Recommendations for counseling persons infected with human T-lymphotropic virus, types I and II. Recommendations on prophylaxis and therapy for disseminated *Mycobacterium avium* complex for adults and adolescents infected with HIV. MMWR 42, 1993.

9. Centers for Disease Control and Prevention. Recommendations for prevention of HIV transmission in health care settings. MMWR 36(Suppl 2):1S, 1987.

10. Centers for Disease Control and Prevention. United States Public Health Service/Infectious Disease Society of America guidelines for the prevention of opportunistic infections in person infected with human immunodeficiency virus: a summary. MMWR 46(RR-12):1–46, 1997.

11. Centers for Disease Control and Prevention. Update: Provisional Public Health Service recommendations for chemoprophylaxis after occupational exposure to HIV. MMWR 45(22):468–472, 1996.

12. Coopman SA, Johnson RA, Platt R, Stern RS. Cutaneous disease and drug reactions in HIV infection. N Engl J Med 328:1670, 1993.

13. Cummings PD, Wallace EL, Schorr JB. Exposure of patients to human immunodeficiency virus through the transfusion of blood components that test antibody-negative. N Engl J Med 321:941, 1989.

14. Deeks SG, Smith M, Holodniy M, et al. HIV-1 protease inhibitors. A review for clinicians. JAMA 277:145, 1997.

15. Hopewell PC. Diagnosis of *Pneumocystis carinii* pneumonia. Medical management of AIDS. Infect Dis Clin North Am 2(2):409, 1988.

16. Hughes WT, Kuhn S, Chaudhary S, et al. Successful chemoprophylaxis for *Pneumocystis carinii* pneumonitis. N Engl J Med 297:1419, 1977.

17. Hughes WT, Leoung G, Kramer F, et al. Comparison of atovaquone with TMP–SMX to treat *Pneumocystis carinii* pneumonitis in patients with AIDS. N Engl J Med 328:1521, 1993.

18. Johanson JF, Sonnenberg A. Efficient management of diarrhea in the acquired immunodeficiency syndrome (AIDS). Ann Intern Med 112:942, 1990.

19. Kaslow RA, Phair JP, Friedman HB, et al. Infection with the human immunodeficiency virus: clinical manifestations and their relationship to immune deficiency. Ann Intern Med 107:474, 1987.

20. Landesman SH, Kalish LA, Burns DN, et al. Obstetrical factors and the transmission of human immunodeficiency virus type 1 from mother to child. N Engl J Med 334:1617, 1996.

21. Levy RM, Bredesen DE, Rosenblum ML. Neurological manifestations of the acquired immunodeficiency syndrome (AIDS): experience of UCSF and review of the literature. J Neurosurg 62:75, 1985.

22. Markowitz DM. Infection with the human immunodeficiency virus type 2. Ann Intern Med 118:211, 1993.

23. Moss AR, Bachetti P. Natural history of HIV infection. AIDS 39(2):55, 1989.

24. Montaner JSG, Lawson LM, Levitt N, et al. Corticosteroids prevent early deterioration in patients with moderately severe *Pneumocystis carinii* pneumonia and the acquired immunodeficiency syndrome (AIDS). Ann Intern Med 113:14, 1990.

25. Osmond P, Chaisson RE, Moss AR, et al. Lymphadenopathy in asymptomatic patients seropositive for HIV. N Engl J Med 317:246, 1987.

26. Ostrow D, Grant I, Atkinson H. Assessment and management of the AIDS patient with neuropsychiatric disturbances. J Clin Psychiatry 49(Suppl 5):14, 1988.

27. Panteleo G, Graziosi C, Fauci AS. The immunopathogenesis of human immunodeficiency virus infection. N Engl J Med 328:327, 1993.

28. Poland GA, Love KR, Hughes CE. Routine immunization of the HIV-positive asymptomatic patient. J Gen Intern Med 5:147, 1990.

29. Rose DN, Schechter CB, Sacks HS. Influenza and pneumococcal vaccination of HIV-infected patients: a policy analysis. Am J Med 94:160, 1993.

30. Saag MS, Holodniy M, Kurtizkes DR, et al. HIV viral markers in clinical practice. Nature Med 2:625, 1996.

31. Schacker T, Collier AC, Hughes J, et al. Clinical and epidemiological features of primary HIV infection. Ann Intern Med 125:257, 1996.

SECTION

4

Gastrointestinal Problems

CHAPTER 35

Disorders of the Esophagus: Dysphagia, Noncardiac Chest Pain, and Gastroesophageal Reflux

PHILIP O. KATZ, MD

PHYSIOLOGY OF SWALLOWING

Normal swallowing requires the coordination of the skeletal muscles of the pharynx, the cricopharyngeus muscle (the upper esophageal sphincter), and the proximal third of the esophagus, with the smooth muscle of the distal body of the esophagus and the lower esophageal sphincter. Thus, the initiation of swallowing is voluntary, but involuntary processes subsequently propel the swallowed bolus through the esophagus into the stomach. The following sequence of events occurs during normal swallowing: relaxation of the upper esophageal sphincter to permit entry of the bolus into the esophagus, closure of the sphincter to prevent esophageal or pharyngeal regurgitation and aspiration, propulsion of the bolus distally by esophageal peristalsis, relaxation of the lower esophageal sphincter (LES) to allow easy entrance of the bolus into the stomach, and prompt closure of the LES to prevent reflux of gastric contents.

DYSPHAGIA

Dysphagia, difficulty in swallowing, may result from a disturbance of any of the anatomic structures or of the physiologic events involved in normal swallowing. It is an extremely specific symptom and should never be dismissed as an emotional problem or symptom of globus hystericus (discussed later in this chapter). The patient often says that food sticks in his or her chest, often pinpointing the precise area. Occasionally, dysphagia may be accompanied by pain on swallowing, *odynophagia,* but the two symptoms are distinct and may occur independently. Two types of dysphagia exist: oropharyngeal dysphagia (the inability to initiate the act of swallowing) and esophageal dysphagia (difficulty in transporting material down the esophagus).

Clinical Evaluation

History

Because of the complexity of the swallowing mechanism, the causes of dysphagia are varied. Certain aspects of the history are helpful in elucidating the underlying disorder. Difficulty in swallowing solids strongly suggests an anatomic obstruction such as carcinoma, stricture, or esophageal ring, whereas difficulty in swallowing solids and liquids suggests a motility disturbance such as achalasia, scleroderma, or diffuse esophageal spasm.

The history may also be useful in identifying the region of abnormal function as either oropharyngeal or esophageal. Symptoms suggestive of *oropharyngeal dysphagia* include difficulty in initiating a swallow, regurgitation of liquid through the nose, aspiration with swallowing, and an inability to propel a bolus of food into the esophagus. Patients with *esophageal dysphagia* complain of retrosternal fullness after swallowing and of the feeling that food is stuck at a certain point in the esophagus, often relieved by regurgitation. Esophageal dysphagia is most commonly caused by structural abnormalities (ring, stricture, or tumor) but may be caused by reflux esophagitis or a primary motility disorder. Several common causes of dysphagia are listed in Table 35.1.

Mild weight loss may be described by patients with any type of chronic dysphagia, the result of a voluntary decrease in intake of food that often accompanies their symptoms. More severe weight loss with anorexia suggests carcinoma or achalasia.

Special Studies

To delineate the cause of dysphagia, one or more of the following procedures should be used: radiologic studies, esophagoscopy, and esophageal motility studies. The workup can establish a diagnosis in 95% of cases. Consultation with a gastroenterologist is recommended for most patients with dysphagia, both for evaluation of the clinical problem and for the performance of esophagoscopy and motility studies.

Radiology. The initial study in most patients with dysphagia should be a *barium swallow,* a procedure that can identify motility disturbances and anatomic deformities. A barium swallow is also the easiest procedure for the patient to tolerate (it takes only 15 to 20 minutes and is associated with essentially no discomfort). As with all radiologic studies, the radiologist should be told which disorders are most suspected. Without this communication, the radiologist may perform a routine barium swallow looking only for carci-

Table 35.1. Types of Dysphagia

Symptoms	Causes
Oropharyngeal	
Nasal regurgitation, cough, aspiration with swallowing, difficulty initiating swallow	Central nervous system: Cerebrovascular accident, Parkinson disease, brainstem tumors
	Muscle: Myasthenia, polymyositis, thyroid disease, systemic lupus erythematosus
	Structural: Web, Zenker diverticulum, extrinsic compression
Esophageal	
Dysphagia for solids	Carcinoma, stricture
Continuous	
Intermittent	Ring, diverticulum, esophagitis
Dysphagia for solids and liquids	Motility disorder, severe narrowing from tumor, stricture, esophagitis

noma, stricture, or reflux. Special techniques must be applied to identify esophageal rings and diverticula. Careful fluoroscopic control is required to evaluate motility. In addition, to observe the rapid activity of pharyngeal contractions and to detect abnormal esophageal contractions, the barium swallow should be recorded on videotape or cine film if oropharyngeal dysphagia is suspected. A marshmallow or other solid bolus should be added if esophageal dysphagia is suspected. This will help localize the site of the obstruction. A double contrast study (carbon dioxide pellets are added to the barium meal to distend the esophagus) should be performed to identify mucosal abnormalities associated with gastroesophageal reflux. In this way, barium studies often can detect both organic and functional abnormalities that have led to dysphagia. However, a negative study does not exclude either anatomic (e.g., reflux esophagitis, small ulcers, or early cancer) or motor disorders of the esophagus, and a positive study seldom permits a specific diagnosis to be made; therefore, a barium swallow is almost always followed by endoscopy or esophageal manometry.

Endoscopy. *Esophagoscopy* is an essential part of the evaluation of dysphagia. Because the barium swallow may miss some lesions, endoscopy should be performed in all patients with persistent dysphagia, particularly in those with persistent difficulty in swallowing solid food. Esophagoscopy is complementary to the radiographic examination. The procedure is well tolerated and can be performed on an ambulatory basis even in the elderly. When a lesion is detected by radiography, endoscopy provides the most direct approach to establish the nature of the lesion, whether inflammatory or neoplastic. Biopsies and brushings for cytologic evaluation can be obtained under visual guidance. Furthermore, the instrument may disrupt esophageal webs or rings that are causing the dysphagia and thus may be both a diagnostic and a therapeutic tool. Inability to pass the endoscope through the esophagus into the stomach confirms an anatomical cause of the dysphagia and rules out a primary motor disturbance (e.g., achalasia). The patient's experience

with upper gastrointestinal endoscopy is described in Chapter 38.

Recording of Esophageal Motility. *Esophageal manometry* is the best procedure for the evaluation of esophageal motor function (Table 35.2). This study measures the strength, function, and coordination of the upper and lower esophageal sphincters, and the body of the esophagus in response to a swallow. The procedure is well tolerated, takes only about 30 minutes, and involves the passage of a narrow catheter through the nose or the mouth into the stomach. Recordings are made of the amplitude and coordination of contractions within the pharynx and esophagus. Various motility abnormalities can be diagnosed by use of this technique. Esophageal manometry should be performed in all patients for whom a structural cause for the dysphagia cannot be found.

Specific Causes of Dysphagia

Carcinoma of the Esophagus

Cancer of the esophagus should always be suspected as the cause of dysphagia in patients over the age of 40. The incidence of esophageal carcinoma in the United States is approximately 9300 cases per year. Men, especially African-American men, are more likely to develop squamous cell esophageal cancer than are women. Predisposing factors include cigarette smoking, heavy alcohol use, lye strictures, achalasia, and, for adenocarcinoma, Barrett's mucosa. For unknown reasons, there is an increased incidence of esophageal carcinoma in South Carolina, Washington, DC, and Alaska (19).

In the majority of cases, esophageal cancer is of the squamous cell type. These tumors are most common in the middle to distal third of the esophagus. Adenocarcinoma is more likely to be seen when the normal squamous cells of the esophagogastric junction are destroyed by reflux and replaced by columnar cells (Barrett's mucosa). Carcinoma of the cardia of the stomach may extend into the lower esophagus and obstruct the esophageal lumen. Adenocarcinoma of the gastric cardia and gastroesophageal junction is rising in incidence.

Diagnosis. The diagnosis of esophageal cancer is generally made only after symptoms have developed, by which time the lesion is already advanced, with involvement of regional lymph nodes. In patients with predisposing conditions, such as Barrett's mucosa, earlier detection of the cancer may be achieved by regular endoscopic surveillance every 1 to 2 years with cytologic brushings of the entire esophagus. Most patients present with dysphagia for solid food for several months that progresses to dysphagia for solids and liquids, usually with progressive weight loss. Odynophagia (pain on swallowing) may accompany the dysphagia. Occult blood loss is common but hematemesis is unusual.

The diagnostic workup in all patients includes a barium swallow and upper endoscopy. If the radiograph is negative, the endoscopic examination may still reveal mucosal lesions. When the tumor is already defined by radiograph, endoscopy is necessary to establish a histologic diagnosis, which is important in deciding whether surgery or radiation therapy is indicated. Multiple biopsies and directed brush cytologies obtained via the endoscope provide a positive tissue diagnosis in more than 95% of cases of esophageal cancer. However, radiologic evaluation remains important because it provides useful information about the degree of esophageal obstruction, the length of the tumor, and the appearance of the fundus of the stomach. With the combined use of these two techniques, cancer of the esophagus can be differentiated from other esophageal lesions, such as peptic stricture of the esophagus, achalasia, severe esophagitis, and esophageal varices.

After the diagnosis is confirmed, a computed tomographic (CT) scan of the chest should be considered to evaluate the possibility of extraesophageal extension, but it is most useful to rule out hepatic metastases. Endoscopic ultrasound is being used with increased frequency for staging. Its efficacy is not yet established. Regardless of the staging procedure, more than 50% of patients with tumor apparently confined to the esophagus have extensive, incurable disease at operation.

Therapy. Therapy for esophageal cancer is generally *surgery* (5) or *radiation*. The choice between these two forms of therapy depends on the cell type and the location of the neoplasm. Adenocarcinoma is less radiosensitive, usually occurs in the distal third of the esophagus, and therefore is better suited for a surgical approach. Squamous cell carcinoma is radiosensitive, and numerous studies suggest that radiation of lesions in the distal and middle thirds of the esophagus is as effective as is surgery (see Chapter 8 for a discussion of radiotherapy in the treatment of cancer). Surgical resection is more extensive and less well tolerated in more proximal tumors. Combination radiotherapy and resection have been reported to improve survival, but more experience with this approach is needed. With either approach, the prognosis is poor: 75% of patients die within 1 year of diagnosis, and 90% die by 5 years.

Patients with adenocarcinoma detected during regular screening of Barrett's mucosa may have a better prognosis. Preoperative chemotherapy has met with recent success and should be considered before surgery, even in patients with resectable cancer.

Palliation (maintenance of an open esophagus so that the patient can swallow food and saliva) should be the major aim of therapy if the tumor is not resectable. Dilation of the lumen with mercury-weighted rubber dilators, guidewire-assisted polyvinyl dilators, or various balloon dilators may all achieve successful palliation. Treatment with thermal coagulating dilators or laser therapy occasionally may be helpful. Esophageal prostheses have been used in palliation, particularly with tracheoesophageal fistulas. Chemotherapy or surgical palliation should also be considered in selected cases. Unfortunately, no well-designed clinical trials that compare different modalities have been done, so the choice of palliation must be individualized after consultation with a surgeon, an oncologist, and a gastroenterologist.

Achalasia

Achalasia is characterized by the complete absence of esophageal peristalsis and failure of LES relaxation. The condition occurs in all age groups, with a peak incidence in the fourth and fifth decades. The incidence of this disorder is approximately 1 in 100,000 population per year. Men and women are equally susceptible to the disease. Patients present most commonly with progressive dysphagia for both solids and liquids and, often, with regurgitation of ingested material. Pulmonary symptoms such as nocturnal coughing and even aspiration pneumonia may be the initial mode of presentation. Occasionally, substernal chest pain is associated with the dysphagia.

Pathogenesis. The pathogenesis of achalasia is unknown. Several studies have described abnormalities in the myenteric ganglion cells in the distal esophagus (LES zone), in the body of the esophagus, and in the vagal nucleus and its peripheral fibers. However, these

Table 35.2. Esophageal Motility Disorders

Disorder	Manometry: Esophageal Body	Manometry: Lower Esophageal Sphincter	Primary Symptoms
Primary			
Achalasia	Absent peristalsis, low amplitude	High pressure, normal, incomplete relaxation (may be normal early in the disease)	Dysphagia, regurgitation, chest pain
Diffuse esophageal spasm	Simultaneous contractions mixed with normal peristalsis	Normal pressure, ⅓ with incomplete relaxation	Chest pain, dysphagia
Nutcracker esophagus	High amplitude, normal peristalsis	Normal pressure	Chest pain
Hypertensive LES	Normal amplitude	High pressure, normal relaxation	Chest pain
Nonspecific motility disorder	Nontransmitted, low amplitude with normal peristalsis	Normal pressure	Dysphagia, chest pain
Secondary			
Reflux esophagitis	Low amplitude, poor peristalsis	Low pressure	Heartburn, dysphagia
Scleroderma	Aperistalsis (smooth muscle), low amplitude	Low to absent pressure	Dysphagia, heartburn
Polymyositis	Proximal muscle disorder (low amplitude, disordered peristalsis)	Normal pressure	Regurgitation, oropharyngeal dysphagia

findings have not been consistent. Pharmacologic studies have further supported the concept of denervation of the esophagus. There is an exaggerated response of the LES and the body of the esophagus to cholinergic stimulation and to the hormone gastrin, consistent with the concept of denervation hypersensitivity. The cause of the neuropathic injury is unknown.

Diagnosis.   The routine chest radiograph often suggests the diagnosis. The normal gastric air bubble is absent, and an air–fluid level in the dilated esophagus is sometimes seen behind the heart. With a very dilated and tortuous esophagus, the mediastinum appears widened. The typical features on barium esophagogram (Fig. 35.1) include smooth, tapered narrowing of the distal end of the esophagus that fails to open properly; retention of barium and secretions in the more proximal esophagus; and absence of peristalsis. The distal narrowing is often described as a bird beak or pen quill deformity. The patient must be examined while upright to demonstrate the height of the retained barium-filled column.

Esophageal manometry has demonstrated three distinct abnormalities in patients with achalasia: absence of peristalsis of the smooth muscle of the esophagus, failure of the LES to relax after a swallow, and elevated LES pressure. If possible, manometry should be done in every patient with the disease to confirm the diagnosis. In achalasia, the basal LES pressure usually is elevated, at times to very high levels, and the degree of relaxation is incomplete, generally less than 50%. Thus, there is a constant high-pressure zone that impedes the passage of the esophageal contents. Peristalsis is also absent, further impairing the propulsion of the bolus distally. Manometry may demonstrate high-amplitude, simultaneous, repetitive contractions that are not peristaltic. These patients are classified by some as having vigorous achalasia and often have severe chest pain (1).

Patients who present early in the course of disease with mild symptoms and minimal esophageal dilation may, at manometry, appear to have normal LES relaxation (because of a manometric artifact) and normal sphincter pressure and yet have true achalasia. In such cases, technetium-labeled food studies with the patient in the upright position should be performed to confirm delayed emptying and the abnormal LES (9).

Differential Diagnosis.   Achalasia must be differentiated from other disorders that lead to obstruction of the passage of food into the stomach. *Esophageal strictures,* both peptic and neoplastic, and *carcinomas at the esophagogastric (EG) junction* may result in symptoms and even in a radiographic and manometric picture similar to that of achalasia (17). Thus, all such patients should be evaluated with endoscopy. Failure to pass the endoscope into the stomach indicates an anatomic obstruction. *Scleroderma,* with its associated esophageal motility disturbance, may result in dysphagia with diminished peristalsis seen on the radiograph. If stricture has not occurred, the patient will demonstrate a wide-open sphincter through which barium passes easily. By the time patients with esophageal scleroderma develop stricture and dilation of the esophagus that may mimic achalasia, they usually have

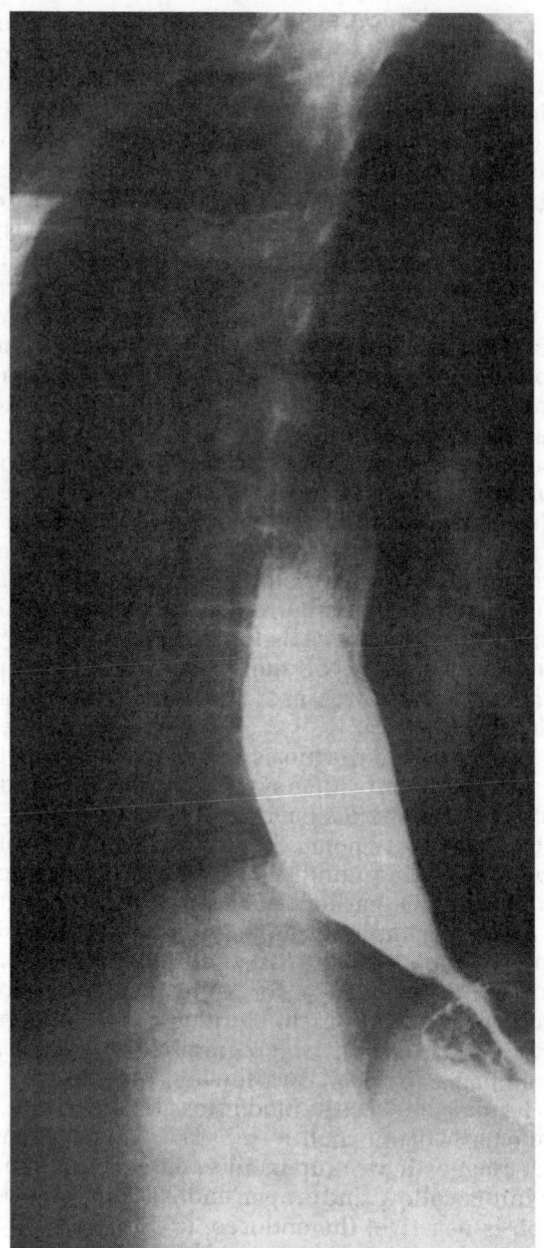

Figure 35.1.   Barium swallow in a patient with achalasia. The esophagus is dilated and the tapered distal segment never opens normally. Under fluoroscopy, no peristalsis is seen, but simultaneous contractions are noted.

other obvious stigmata of scleroderma (particularly tight skin of the face and hands or Raynaud's phenomenon). Furthermore, on esophageal manometry the LES pressure in scleroderma is low rather than high, as it is in achalasia, but, as in achalasia, the disorder of motility is confined to the smooth muscle portion (distal two-thirds) of the esophagus, with a normally functioning proximal segment. In patients from South America, *Chagas' disease* may result in a megaesophagus and present with manometric patterns identical to that of achalasia. Patients with *idiopathic intestinal pseudoobstruction* have a manometric pattern similar to that of achalasia (15); esophageal manometry may be used to help confirm the diagnosis.

Therapy. Two types of definitive therapy exist for achalasia: pneumatic dilation and surgery. Both forms of therapy are aimed at reducing the pressure gradient between the esophagus and the stomach, thus decreasing the severity of the dysphagia. The aperistalsis and impaired sphincter relaxation persist after therapy. *Pneumatic dilation,* an outpatient procedure, is performed by a trained gastroenterologist. The esophagus is aspirated completely before the dilation. After premedication with analgesics and sedatives, a balloon dilator is passed into the stomach. The dilator is a weighted tube, the distal portion of which includes an inflatable balloon. Under fluoroscopic guidance, the balloon portion is positioned across the LES. It is then inflated for 10 to 30 seconds, causing a forceful disruption of the LES muscle. The dilator is then removed and can be expected to be blood streaked. The patient usually experiences chest pain during the procedure. The major risk of the procedure is esophageal perforation, which occurs in up to 5% of dilations. Satisfactory results (long-term improvement in dysphagia, weight gain, and decrease in retention of barium) can be expected in approximately 85% of cases. In successful cases, there is immediate relief of symptoms. The patient is observed for 4 to 6 hours and discharged. Dilation can be repeated if symptoms of dysphagia recur or worsen, but most patients have only minimal symptoms for many years after therapy. Repeat esophageal manometry is not necessary if symptoms have been relieved.

Surgical therapy involves a transection of the circular muscle of the LES zone to the level of the mucosa, the Heller myotomy. This surgical approach provides results similar to those after pneumatic dilation, with a success rate of 80 to 85%. The procedure may cause significant reflux esophagitis in 10 to 25% of patients. As a result of this complication, some advocate combining a fundoplication with the myotomy. Until re-cently, the procedure required a thoracotomy, but it can now be performed by either a laparoscopic or thoracoscopic approach. These minimally invasive techniques have made myotomy a better tolerated procedure with shorter hospitalizations, but because pneumatic dilation can be performed on outpatients, it is usually the procedure of choice. Surgery is reserved for failure of repeated dilations to provide symptomatic relief, esophageal perforation secondary to pneumatic dilation, inability to perform dilation because of the shape of the esophagus or the presence of a large epiphrenic diverticulum, and inability to exclude carcinoma.

Medical therapy with nitrates, calcium channel blockers (Table 35.3), and even mercury bougienage may offer transient improvement in some patients. Pharmacologic therapy should be reserved for patients in whom pneumatic dilation or myotomy is contraindicated or for patients with very mild disease.

Recently, botulinum toxin, injected into the LES via endoscopy, has been studied as a treatment of achalasia (12). A decrease in LES pressure and improved esophageal emptying are seen immediately after injection. An initial success rate of 70 to 80% has been reported on the first injection, with most patients relapsing (and requiring repeat treatment) in 6 months to 1 year. This procedure can be performed by a trained endoscopist and has no more risk than esophagoscopy alone. The therapy should be considered for patients in whom surgery has high risk and in whom the risk of perforation with pneumatic dilation is also high.

Complications. Many studies suggest that patients with achalasia are at increased risk of esophageal cancer. The incidence of this complication ranges from 6 to 29% in various series (11). Cancer in patients with achalasia should not be confused with cancer of the esophagogastric junction presenting with an achalasia-like picture. The cancer that develops in patients with

Table 35.3. Therapy for Spastic Esophageal Motility Disorders Associated with Chest Pain

Treatment Modality	Dose	Mode of Administration	Major Complications
Reassurance			
Nitrates[a]			
Nitroglycerin	0.4 mg SL	Usually before meals and PRN	Headache
Isosorbide[a]	10–30 mg PO	30 min before meals	
Anticholinergics			
Dicyclomine (Bentyl)	10–20 mg	4 times a day	Dry mouth, blurred vision
Sedatives/antidepressants			
Diazepam (Valium)	2–5 mg	4 times a day	Drowsiness
Trazodone (Desyrel)	50–100 mg	4 times a day	Drowsiness, impotence
Doxepin (Sinequan)[a]	50 mg	At bedtime	Drowsiness
Calcium channel blockers[a]			
Nifedipine (Procardia)	10–30 mg	4 times a day	Dizziness, nausea, dyspepsia
Diltiazem (Cardizem)	90 mg	4 times a day	Headache, edema, nausea
Smooth muscle relaxants[a]			
Hydralazine[a]	20–50 mg	3 times a day	Headache, lupuslike syndrome
Static dilation	50 French	Repeat as needed	None
Pneumatic dilation[b]			Perforation (3–5%)
Esophagomyotomy[c]			Thoracotomy required; gastroesophageal reflux (20%)

[a]Orthostatic hypotension is a common complication of this class of drugs.
[b]May be indicated if dysphagia is a prominent symptom.
[c]Rarely indicated (intractability).

primary achalasia usually occurs many years after the diagnosis of achalasia has been established, is of the squamous cell type, and generally occurs in the midportion of the esophagus. There is no evidence that successful therapy of achalasia prevents the development of cancer. Thus, patients with achalasia probably should be considered for periodic endoscopy with esophageal cytology every 3 to 5 years after diagnosis, although no definitive studies have been done to support this recommendation.

Diffuse Esophageal Spasm

Clinical Presentation. Symptomatic diffuse esophageal spasm (DES) (14) is a disorder characterized by intermittent nonperistaltic (simultaneous) esophageal contractions that result in dysphagia and substernal chest pain. The disorder is seen equally in both sexes and at all ages (although it appears to be rare in children). The dysphagia is intermittent and is experienced for both solids and liquids. The pain is also intermittent and may be provoked by certain foods, particularly hot and cold beverages. At other times, the pain occurs spontaneously and may even awaken the patient at night. The pain is highly variable in quality and is sometimes described as knifelike or as dull and crushing; it may radiate to the neck, back, or arms. It may be brief or last for hours. Because of its location, radiation, and crushing quality, it is often confused with the pain of ischemic heart disease. When no cardiac disease is found, many of these patients are believed to have a psychogenic disturbance. Thus, this condition is often undiagnosed and is easily confused with other conditions.

Diagnosis. The procedures for the diagnosis of this condition include radiographic studies and esophageal manometry. A carefully performed *barium swallow,* or *videoesophagogram,* may demonstrate nonperistaltic, spontaneous, and simultaneous contractions (tertiary waves) of the body of the esophagus. However, these abnormal contractions are often encountered during routine barium swallow, especially in the elderly, and by themselves do not make a diagnosis of esophageal spasm without the appropriate clinical history. Furthermore, because DES is an intermittent condition, the barium swallow may be normal or too insensitive to detect the motility disturbance. Because the barium study is not specific, it should be done only on patients with dysphagia. Patients with suspected DES should have *esophageal motility studies* to confirm the diagnosis, even if they have had a barium swallow. Provocative agents (e.g., edrophonium) can be used during the motility studies to identify more clearly patients who experience chest pain associated with abnormal esophageal contractions (described later in this chapter) (8).

Therapy. Therapy for DES and other motility disorders that cause chest pain is discussed in greater detail later in this chapter and is listed in Table 35.3.

Other Primary Motility Disorders

In addition to achalasia and DES, three distinct primary motility abnormalities of the esophagus have been described that are associated rarely with dysphagia. The *nutcracker esophagus* and the *hypertensive lower esophageal sphincter* (excessively high LES pressures with normal esophageal peristalsis) are two abnormalities associated primarily with chest pain and, rarely, with dysphagia; they are discussed later in this chapter. Some patients with dysphagia referred for esophageal motility testing demonstrate contractions in the distal esophagus with amplitude of smooth muscle contraction below 30 mm Hg in more than 30% of swallows. This is called *ineffective esophageal motility* because contractions of this low amplitude are incapable of effective propagation of a bolus. This abnormality is seen commonly with gastroesophageal reflux, and rarely it may be seen with dysphagia alone.

Secondary Motility Disorders

Chronic reflux esophagitis (discussed later) may cause scarring of the distal esophagus, which can result in decreased force of esophageal contractions and/or ineffective esophageal motility, either of which can lead to dysphagia. There is ample evidence that acute acid reflux does not induce esophageal spasm, but chronic reflux may cause symptoms and motility abnormalities that are radiographically similar. Treatment is aggressive antireflux therapy. Improvement in dysphagia and contraction abnormalities is variable, but the pain of chronic reflux usually diminishes with treatment.

Abnormalities of esophageal contractions associated with dysphagia may be seen in patients with hyperthyroidism or hypothyroidism, amyloidosis, and myotonic dystrophy. Diabetes mellitus has been associated with multiple radiographic and manometric abnormalities, but patients are seldom symptomatic. Collagen vascular disease, particularly scleroderma, may affect the esophagus as well. Chronic idiopathic intestinal pseudoobstruction may produce manometric abnormalities indistinguishable from those of achalasia. Many authorities have used esophageal manometry to help make this diagnosis. Use of the term *presbyesophagus* should be abandoned. Aging itself does not produce significant alteration of esophageal motility.

Scleroderma of the Esophagus

The esophagus is involved in up to 80% of patients with scleroderma. At times the esophageal symptoms are the presenting complaints that lead to the diagnosis. Indeed, the esophagus may demonstrate the characteristic abnormalities even before skin changes occur. The main symptoms of esophageal scleroderma are heartburn and dysphagia. The cause for these symptoms can be readily appreciated by examining the changes in esophageal motility. In esophageal scleroderma, the LES pressure is very low, resulting in free gastroesophageal reflux. In addition, the peristaltic waves initially are of reduced amplitude, progressing later to complete aperistalsis in the smooth muscle portion of the esophagus, sparing the skeletal muscle portion. Because peristalsis is impaired, the refluxed acid remains in the esophagus for an abnormally long time, perhaps accounting for the common development of an esophageal stricture in this disorder. Thus, the dysphagia may be caused by the primary motor abnormality or may signify the development of a peptic stricture.

The pathogenesis of scleroderma is unknown. In the esophagus, the disorder is not simply secondary to replacement of muscle fibers with collagen because the motility dysfunction can be demonstrated in the absence of histopathologic changes. Several studies have suggested a neural defect rather than a primary myogenic disorder.

Scleroderma is a chronically progressive disease for which no specific treatment exists. Therapy of esophageal manifestations is directed at symptomatic relief and prevention of strictures.

Patients with scleroderma, whether they have dysphagia or heartburn, should be referred to a gastroenterologist for evaluation of esophageal motility and to rule out reflux esophagitis and stricture formation. If reflux is present, the patient should be treated with intensive antireflux therapy (Table 35.4) to try to prevent stricture formation. Strictures should be dilated by bougienage, followed by long-term medical therapy with proton pump inhibitors. In general, patients with scleroderma require a high dosage of an H_2 antagonist or a proton pump inhibitor (Table 35.4) for

treatment of esophagitis. Antireflux surgery should be avoided because the motility disorder may lead to significant dysphagia after fundoplication.

Esophageal Webs and Rings. Dysphagia for solid foods may be caused by esophageal webs or rings. An *esophageal web* is a mucosal structure that protrudes into the lumen, most commonly in the proximal esophagus. The association of iron deficiency anemia with a proximal esophageal web constitutes the *Plummer–Vinson syndrome. Esophageal rings* are located in the distal esophagus and may be either mucosal or muscular; rings can be demonstrated in up to 10% of the population but rarely cause symptoms.

The ring that occurs just above the gastroesophageal junction is called *Schatzki's ring.* The origin of these lesions is unclear, but they are probably acquired. They are often found in asymptomatic individuals. There is some evidence that gastroesophageal reflux is associated with the development of Schatzki's ring.

Symptoms arise when the ring narrows the esophageal lumen to less than 13 mm in diameter and are rare if the lumen is more than 20 mm in diameter. A typical presenting symptom of a patient with an esophageal ring is intermittent dysphagia for solid foods. The

Table 35.4.   Treatment of Gastroesophageal Reflux

Intervention	Specific Change	Mechanism of Improvement
Phase I		
Elevate head of bed (6- to 8-inch blocks)		Decreased acid contact time
Avoid drugs that decrease LES pressure	Theophylline, nitrates, calcium channel blockers, benzodiazepines	Avoids decrease of lower sphincter pressure
Avoid irritants	Citrus, coffee	Avoids direct mucosal damage
Stop smoking		Removes inhibition of H_2 blockers, increases lower sphincter pressure
Avoid eating before sleep	3 hours	Avoids gastric distension
Antacids	As needed	Decreases gastric acid
Alginic acid (Gaviscon)	As needed	Barrier protectant
H_2 antagonists (OTC)	As needed	Decreases gastric acid
Phase II		
H_2 antagonists[a]		
Cimetidine (Tagamet)	400 mg BID (nonerosive symptomatic disease)	Decreases acid secretion
	800 mg BID (erosive esophagitis)	
Ranitidine (Zantac)	150 mg BID (nonerosive symptomatic disease)	
	150 mg QID (erosive esophagitis)	
Famotidine (Pepcid)	20 mg BID (nonerosive symptomatic disease)	
	40 mg BID (erosive esophagitis)	
Nizatidine (Axid)	150 mg BID (all forms of reflux disease)	
Cisapride	10 mg QID	Both cisapride and metoclopramide increase LES pressure, increase esophageal clearance, and accelerate gastric emptying
Metoclopramide (Reglan)	5–10 mg QID	
Sucralfate (Carafate)	1 g QID	Mucosal protection (not FDA approved for treatment of reflux)
Proton pump inhibition		
Lansoprazole (Prevacid)	30 mg/day (AM)	
	15 mg/day (AM) maintenance	
Omeprazole (Prilosec)	20 mg/day (AM)	Decreases acid secretion
Phase III		
Surgery	Nissen fundoplication	Creates intra-abdominal esophagus and increased lower sphincter pressure
	Belsey Mark IV repair	
	Hill procedure	

[a]Nocturnal H_2 antagonists are insufficient antireflux therapy.

patient may point to the area of the ring. At times a bolus of food may become impacted; the patient then regurgitates and then may be able to resume eating without further difficulty. The intermittency of the dysphagia, the chronicity of the condition, and the difficulty in making the diagnosis unless specifically suspected often result in misdiagnosis and inappropriate therapy.

The diagnosis of esophageal ring is best made by barium swallow with a barium-coated marshmallow. The lower esophageal ring is best detected when the lower segment of the esophagus is distended, as it is during a Valsalva maneuver. Endoscopy is sometimes helpful to differentiate rings from annular strictures secondary to either reflux esophagitis or carcinoma. Cervical webs are often missed on conventional radiography but may be detected with cine studies. The webs usually are detected on the anterior surface of the esophagus, and lateral and oblique films are needed to demonstrate these lesions. Endoscopy often fails to visualize cervical webs and may disrupt the lesion during blind passage of the instrument into the esophagus. The endoscope may reveal an esophageal ring during air sufflation of the distal esophagus.

If the webs are associated with iron deficiency, treatment of the anemia causes rapid regression of the web. Otherwise, therapy involves mechanical disruption of the ring or web as well as reassurance, along with the recommendation to chew food well and slowly. Bougienage with a large-caliber dilator often disrupts the lower esophageal ring with complete relief of the dysphagia. The procedure causes transient discomfort but much less pain than does pneumatic dilation. It is ordinarily done by a gastroenterologist in his or her office. Rarely, symptoms may persist after bougienage, and pneumatic dilation or even surgery may be necessary.

Globus Hystericus

Globus hystericus is a diagnosis often made in patients with dysphagia who have no demonstrable organic disease. However, this condition does not produce dysphagia and should not be used to explain away the symptom of dysphagia. Patients with globus describe the sensation of a lump in the throat, but they do not actually have difficulty swallowing. At times, these symptoms may be more pronounced with eating. However, when specifically questioned, patients deny dysphagia or food sticking or being held up in this region and they state that the symptom is present even when they are not eating. The pathogenesis of this condition is unknown, but hypertonicity of the upper esophageal sphincter, as a primary disorder or as a consequence of esophageal reflux, has been suggested. Gastroesophageal reflux should be ruled out (see below) before a psychologic disturbance (see Chapter 12) is diagnosed. Reassurance and an explanation of the problem form the basis for treatment. Mild sedation may be helpful. The significance of this disorder is mainly its differentiation from other conditions that produce true dysphagia.

ESOPHAGEAL CHEST PAIN

Chest pain is a common and difficult diagnostic challenge. It is now well accepted that esophageal disease can be implicated as a cause of recurrent anginal chest pain. The prevalence of esophageal chest pain is unknown. However, 10 to 30% of first cardiac catheterizations done to evaluate chest pain are normal. At least 50% of patients with normal coronary catheterizations have identifiable esophageal abnormalities; 50% of patients with normal coronary arteries continue to be disabled by chest pain, despite being told that they do not have heart disease (13). These patients still receive cardiac drugs, continue to have approximately two physician visits a year for chest pain, and are hospitalized about once a year for continuing evaluation, at significant cost.

Etiology and Pathogenesis

Esophageal chest pain has been attributed to stimulation of esophageal chemoreceptors by acid reflux or of mechanoreceptors by smooth muscle spasm or esophageal distension. Cold or hot liquids may cause severe chest pain, suggesting that there may also be alteration in temperature receptors in the esophagus. Transient myoischemia may be a cause of pain in patients with spastic motility disorders. Such patients have an increased frequency of psychiatric disorders and have personality profiles similar to those of patients with the irritable bowel syndrome (Chapter 40), suggesting that chronic stress may play a role in the pathogenesis of chest pain. Panic disorder has been diagnosed in up to one-third of patients with chest pain and normal coronary angiograms (7).

Two major abnormalities have been associated with esophageal chest pain: esophageal motility disorders and gastroesophageal reflux disease (GERD).

Recent studies using ambulatory pH monitoring have demonstrated gastroesophageal reflux in approximately 45% of patients with unexplained chest pain. The typical symptom of gastroesophageal reflux—heartburn—is seen in about half of patients with GERD-related chest pain. Approximately 30% of patients with esophageal chest pain have a demonstrable motility disorder, and of this group, the most common disorder is the *nutcracker esophagus* (hypertensive esophagus, supersqueezer). This manometric abnormality is characterized by normal peristaltic contractions in the distal esophagus with contraction amplitude greater than 2 standard deviations above normal (less than 180 mm Hg) associated with chest pain (Table 35.2). Many of these patients have prolonged duration of contractions as well. *Diffuse esophageal spasm* (DES) (see above) is the motility disorder usually considered the principal cause of esophageal chest pain; however, studies have found it to be uncommon, representing less than 10% of esophageal motility abnormalities in patients with noncardiac chest pain (4). Other disorders, such as an *isolated elevated LES pressure* (hypertensive LES) and *achalasia,* are rarely associated with noncardiac chest pain. A large number of patients (approximately 35%) have contraction abnormalities that do not fit into one of the four categories defined here. These patients are grouped under the general category of *nonspecific esophageal motility disorders* (NEMDs).

Evaluation requires consultation with a gastroenterologist. Few patients have spontaneous chest pain during stationary esophageal motility testing (even if esophageal motility is abnormal) but have their typical chest pain reproduced when the esophagus is stimulated with intravenous edrophonium (Tensilon). This cholinergic agonist reproduces chest pain accompanied by high-amplitude esophageal contractions in 20 to 30% of patients with chest pain and normal coronary arteries. Edrophonium does not cause narrowing of the coronary arteries, nor does it cause chest pain in normal subjects or in patients with irritable bowel syndrome. A positive test indicates that the chest pain is of esophageal origin.

Diagnosis

Unfortunately, the history is not reliable in differentiating esophageal from cardiac pain or in differentiating the various esophageal causes of chest pain. Location, exertional onset, and radiation do not distinguish the two entities. Heartburn, dysphagia, or odynophagia suggests an esophageal etiology, but overlap does exist. Pain lasting longer than 1 hour is more likely to be esophageal but is occasionally seen with cardiac disease. Therapeutic trials with antacids or nitrates do not distinguish between the two diseases. Intraesophageal acid perfusion can cause pain and ST-T wave changes indistinguishable from coronary artery disease, so cardiac disease must be ruled out before the esophagus can be implicated. A musculoskeletal etiology should be sought by careful examination of the chest wall and the costochondral joints. Peptic ulcer disease should be excluded by history, and if biliary tract disease is suspected, it should be excluded by ultrasound. Endoscopy is normal in 80 to 90% of cases and should not be routine (3). If heartburn is present, consideration should be given to a short (3- to 4-week) therapeutic trial of antireflux therapy. If this trial is unsuccessful, the patient should be referred, if possible, to a gastroenterologist who has equipment to perform 24-hour ambulatory esophageal pH monitoring. With this latter method, the frequency of reflux can be assessed, episodes of pain can be correlated with episodes of reflux, and esophageal pH can be monitored during exercise. If this study is negative, esophageal manometry with provocative testing with edrophonium should be performed. Using this systematic approach, an esophageal etiology can be established in more than 60% of patients with noncardiac chest pain.

Treatment

If gastroesophageal reflux is diagnosed, treatment should proceed in a stepwise fashion as outlined later in this chapter, although most patients require higher dosages of H_2 antagonists or proton pump inhibitors for pain relief. Treatment of patients who have only positive provocative tests is more difficult and controversial (Table 35.3). Reassurance should be given to all patients, specifically indicating that the esophagus is the cause of their pain and that the heart is normal. Many experience a decrease in pain with this single intervention. Patients with spastic disorders or with nutcracker esophagus may respond to a nitrate or a calcium channel blocker. Hydralazine may be tried in patients with symptomatic esophageal spasm if nitrates or calcium blockers are not successful. Trazodone HCl (Desyrel), an antidepressant, has been used successfully to relieve chest pain in these patients and is particularly useful in patients with other symptoms suggestive of depression. Recently, imipramine (50 mg at bedtime) has been shown to lower the frequency of esophageal chest pain (2). This dosage, lower than that used to treat depression, is suspected to have a visceral analgesic effect on smooth muscle. Tranquilizers and anticholinergics have been used successfully in some patients. Patients with symptoms unresponsive to these measures may respond to biofeedback or to other psychologic interventions. Rarely surgery with a long esophageal myotomy is required in patients with severe pain in whom pharmacologic therapy has failed. Many patients with esophageal chest pain, whatever the cause, continue to have intermittent symptoms despite therapeutic intervention.

GASTROESOPHAGEAL REFLUX

Gastroesophageal reflux disease (GERD) is common in the United States. Approximately 10% of Americans experience daily heartburn and up to 33% have symptoms monthly. Most patients complain of burning substernal pain that radiates upward, often aggravated by meals and by lying down and relieved by sitting up. Approximately 10% of people have chest pain, consistent with angina pectoris, as the sole manifestation of reflux. An unknown number of people have hoarseness, cough, or wheezing as manifestations of GERD. In most cases the diagnosis and treatment of GERD can be managed successfully by the primary care provider; however, 10 to 15% of patients develop complications and require referral to a gastroenterologist.

Etiology and Pathogenesis

The etiology of GERD is unknown. Several defects contribute to the development and progression of the disease. By far the most significant is an abnormality of the antireflux barrier: the lower esophageal sphincter (LES). Two major abnormalities of the LES are associated with an increased frequency of reflux: *a low basal LES pressure* and *transient LES relaxation* unassociated with a swallow. The latter abnormality is the most common cause of an episode of reflux. Abnormal esophageal epithelial resistance (increased permeability to hydrogen ions), abnormalities of gastric emptying, gastric distension, and the nature of the gastric refluxate (acid, pepsin, and bile) all contribute to the development of GERD.

Diagnosis

Several diagnostic tests are readily available to establish the clinical diagnosis. No single test provides complete information about the cause and consequences of reflux, so careful selection among the available modalities is required. In patients with mild heartburn, a therapeutic trial of phase I therapy, including antacids or H_2-receptor antagonists in over-the-counter (OTC) doses, is an effective diagnostic approach. If successful, no further workup may be needed. Patients with dysphagia and chest pain who have other atypical symptoms or who fail to respond to phase I measures should have a diagnosis established by one of the tests described below.

A *barium swallow* is the simplest, least expensive procedure used to diagnose GERD. A double-contrast study should always be performed to evaluate for mucosal irregularities associated with esophagitis. Several points are important in interpreting the barium study. Hiatal hernia is present in 40 to 60% of the general population. Mild free reflux may be seen in 30% of normal individuals. These findings, together or alone, should not be used to make a diagnosis of reflux disease. The presence of mucosal irregularities, stricture, or esophageal ulcer suggests a high likelihood (85 to 95%) that GERD is present. A normal barium swallow may be seen in 40 to 60% of patients with symptomatic GERD and does not rule out significant disease. It is most useful as a screening study to rule out complications and to evaluate patients with dysphagia; otherwise, endoscopy is the procedure of choice.

Endoscopy (esophagoscopy) is the best study for the diagnosis and evaluation of reflux esophagitis or of other complications of GERD such as stricture or Barrett's epithelium. If esophagitis is present at endoscopy, the diagnosis of GERD is established with 95% certainty, and no further workup is required. If a stricture is encountered, it should be biopsied to rule out carcinoma (dilation may be done at the same sitting in some patients). If Barrett's mucosa is observed, biopsies can be taken to confirm the diagnosis and to rule out dysplasia or in situ carcinoma.

The diagnosis of GERD is established in most patients by the combination of history and endoscopy. However, if the diagnosis is still in doubt, 24-hour *ambulatory pH monitoring* should be performed. (Endoscopy may be normal in 40% of patients in whom reflux is subsequently verified by prolonged intraesophageal pH monitoring.) The test is performed by placing a 2-mm flexible antimony probe transnasally 5 cm above the LES. The probe is connected to a recording box similar to a Holter monitor and worn about the waist. The patient can then be observed at home eating a normal diet. Ambulatory monitoring is extremely useful in patients with noncardiac chest pain, in patients with chronic pulmonary or otolaryngologic symptoms suggestive of reflux, or in patients with typical symptoms when a diagnosis is elusive. Probes may be placed at multiple levels in the esophagus to evaluate patients with atypical symptoms. All patients who are being considered for surgery should have pH monitoring to confirm the diagnosis before the operation. The study is extremely reproducible and is currently the most sensitive and specific diagnostic test for the presence of abnormal acid reflux.

A suggested approach to the diagnosis of GERD is outlined in Figure 35.2.

Treatment

Treatment is divided into phases (Table 35.4). *Phase I therapy* is aimed predominantly at modification of lifestyle. This includes elevating the head of the bed on 6- to 8-inch blocks or using a wedge designed to be placed in the bed under the shoulders and upper back. The patient should avoid sleeping on more pillows because this might actually increase abdominal pressure and contribute to more reflux. Certain foods (e.g., coffee, citrus juice, and spices) are direct esophageal irritants and should be avoided. The patient should be instructed not to lie down after a meal because this promotes greater reflux. Avoidance of food 3 hours before going to bed has also been shown to decrease episodes of reflux. Drugs that decrease LES pressure (e.g., calcium channel blockers, nitrates, sedatives, and theophylline) should be avoided. Antacids and OTC H_2 antagonists are part of phase I therapy and should be used as needed to relieve daytime symptoms. Phase I therapy alone is successful for approximately 25% of patients with symptoms. If symptomatic improvement is not seen in 2 to 3 weeks, prescription therapy should be started.

Phase II therapy is primarily pharmacologic and is aimed at decreasing gastric acid secretion (H_2 antagonists or proton pump inhibitors), augmenting LES pressure, and improving esophageal clearance with prokinetic agents (metoclopramide or cisapride) or enhancing mucosal protection (sucralfate). H_2 antagonists and prokinetic agents have similar healing rates when compared to placebo in acute studies, although the largest and most consistent experience is with H_2 antagonists. Treatment should be begun with an H_2 antagonist in twice-daily dosage or with a prokinetic agent and should be continued for 8 to 12 weeks. Average acute healing rates are approximately 50% with this regimen. If symptoms do not resolve, the physician has three choices: A second drug can be added, higher-dosage H_2 blockers can be tried for an additional 8 to 12 weeks, or a proton pump inhibitor can be started. Current data suggest that a proton pump inhibitor is the most successful and least costly of the three options. Healing rates for both omeprazole and lansoprazole are 80 to 90% at 8 weeks. Omeprazole has recently received FDA approval for initial treatment of gastroesophageal reflux. Using this agent as first-line therapy is extremely effective but costly.

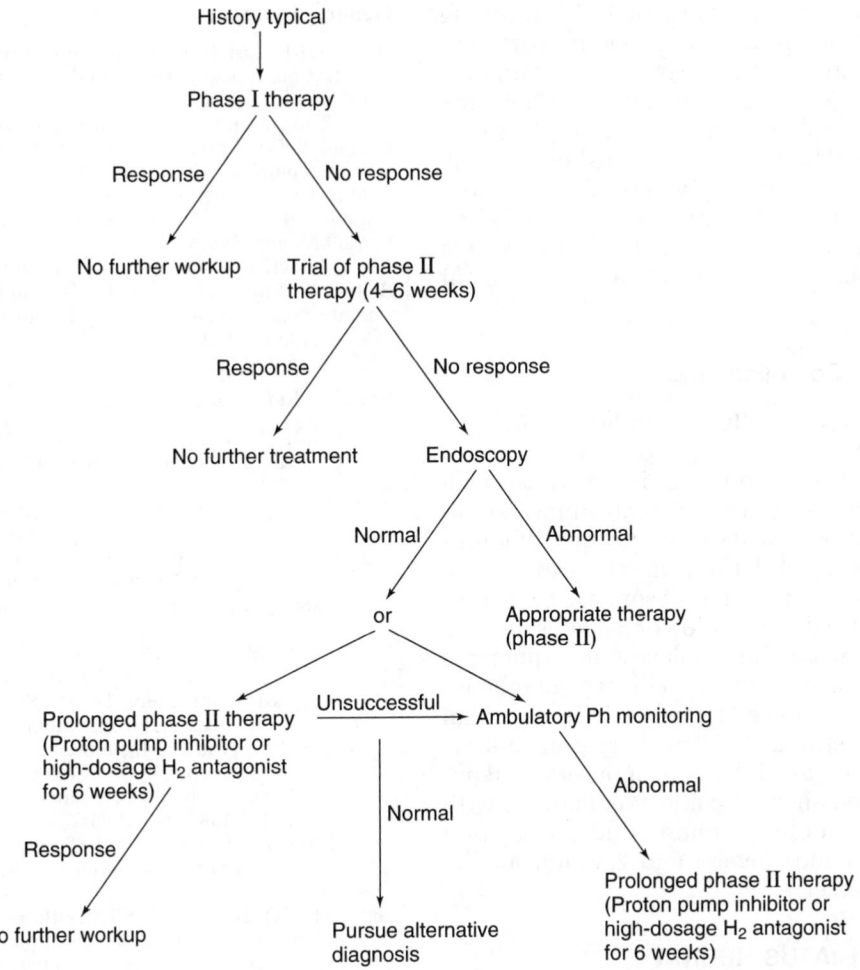

Figure 35.2. Approach to patients with gastroesophageal reflux.

Long-Term Treatment

It is now clear that GERD is a chronic disease. Symptomatic and endoscopic relapse of esophagitis is seen in up to 80% of patients initially treated successfully. Therefore, most patients require some form of long-term therapy (6,18), which must be individualized. H_2-receptor antagonists at full dosage are approved for maintenance treatment and are effective in maintaining symptomatic and endoscopic remission in 40 to 60% of patients. Cisapride has shown similar results in clinical trials but is not approved by the FDA for this treatment. The proton pump inhibitors omeprazole and lansoprazole give the best symptomatic relief and are the most effective agents in maintaining remission of esophagitis (approximately 80% of patients, on daily therapy) (8). Patients with erosive esophagitis or Barrett's esophagus usually require proton pump inhibitors to maintain symptomatic remission, whereas patients with nonerosive esophagitis can often be maintained with H_2-receptor antagonists or prokinetic agents. However, continuous treatment with proton pump inhibitors for 5 years or longer is safe and no special monitoring, including measurement of serum gastrin, is necessary (10).

Surgery (phase III) is indicated in 5 to 10% of patients with reflux disease. Indications are strictures unresponsive to medical therapy, hemorrhage secondary to erosive esophagitis, esophageal ulcers unresponsive to medical therapy, aspiration pneumonia secondary to reflux, reflux-induced hoarseness, and symptoms refractory to medical management. Barrett's esophagus is considered by some authorities to be an indication for surgery. However, most would attempt to treat such patients with aggressive medical therapy before surgery because there is no indication that surgery alters the risk of esophageal cancer. Before surgery all patients should have esophageal manometry to evaluate LES pressure and esophageal peristalsis. Then ambulatory pH monitoring must be done to confirm the diagnosis of abnormal acid exposure before surgery. Operations incorporating a fundoplication around the distal esophagus provide symptomatic improvement in approximately 90% of patients. This operation can now be done laparoscopically with success equal to that of the open procedure. In experienced hands, hospitalization is reduced to 1 to 2 days, with a marked decrease in pain and an earlier return to normal activity. Simple repair of hiatus hernia, if present, has not been as effective, nor have the benefits been as long lasting. Fundoplication provides an effective barrier to reflux. Several variations of the operation are available, and local surgical expertise generally dictates the specific operation that is performed. Complications include dysphagia, which is usually transient, and the gas-bloat syndrome from inability to belch. Antireflux surgery for patients with scleroderma should be avoided at all costs, as it may markedly exacerbate dysphagia. Vagotomy is not indicated in the treatment of GERD.

Complications

The complications of reflux include hemorrhage, ulcerations, stricture formation, and development of Barrett's mucosa (16). Esophagitis is the cause of 5 to 10% of all cases of upper gastrointestinal hemorrhage. Peptic ulcers and strictures must be differentiated from malignancy and from ingestion of caustic substances. The presence of a midesophageal ulcer or stricture should raise the suspicion of Barrett's mucosa (columnar-type mucosa that replaces the squamous mucosa of the tubular esophagus). This type of mucosa contains several different cell types, including parietal cells capable of secreting acid. Of further significance is that this mucosa is a metaplastic response to inflammation and is a premalignant condition. Patients with Barrett's mucosa should therefore undergo regular endoscopic surveillance (every 1 to 2 years) for the development of cancer.

HIATUS HERNIA

Herniation of a part of the stomach through the diaphragm through the normal esophageal hiatus into the thorax is called a hiatus hernia. The defect is common, but the precise prevalence is very much influenced by the zeal of the radiologist during the performance of an upper gastrointestinal series. Estimates of prevalence therefore range from 30 to 60% overall. The defect is twice as common in women as in men and is extremely common in elderly people, affecting perhaps 70 to 80% of the population who are older than age 60. Many physicians still erroneously correlate hiatus hernia with reflux esophagitis, but certainly a hernia may exist without producing symptomatic reflux, and reflux may occur without hernia. If a patient has clear-cut reflux esophagitis, the treatment should not be influenced by the presence of a hiatus hernia. If a patient who does not have reflux is inadvertently discovered to have a hiatus hernia, no treatment is indicated. (In the past, needless surgery was done to reduce a hiatus hernia in patients whose symptoms were not clearly attributable to the defect.)

A *paraesophageal hernia,* the hernia of part of the stomach through the diaphragm adjacent to the gastroesophageal junction, is potentially dangerous because about one-third of the time the hernia incarcerates and produces acute obstruction, a surgical emergency.

General References*

De Vault KR, Castell DO. Guidelines for the diagnosis and treatment of gastroesophageal reflux disease. Arch Intern Med 155:2165, 1995.
    The guidelines of the American College of Gastroenterology.
Maton PN. Omeprazole. N Engl J Med 324:965, 1991.
    A comprehensive review.
Mattox HE III, Richter JE. Prolonged ambulatory esophageal pH monitoring in the evaluation of gastroesophageal reflux disease. Am J Med 89:345, 1990.
    A review of current indications for this evolving technology.
Richter JE, Bradley LA, Castell DO. Esophageal chest pain: current controversies in pathogenesis, diagnosis and therapy. Ann Intern Med 110:66, 1989.
    A comprehensive review of the subject.

Specific References

1. Bondi JL, Goodwin DH, Garrett JM. Vigorous achalasia: its clinical interpretation and significance. Am J Gastroenterol 58:145, 1972.
2. Cannon RO, Quyyumi AA, Mincemoyer R, et al. Imipramine in patients with chest pain despite normal coronary angiograms. N Engl J Med 330:1411, 1994.
3. Cherian P, Smith LF, Bardhan KD, et al. Esophageal tests in the evaluation of non-cardiac chest pain. Dis Esophagus 8:129, 1995.
4. Dalton CB, Castell DO, Hewson EG, et al. Diffuse esophageal spasm. A rare motility disorder not characterized by high-amplitude contractions. Dig Dis Sci 36:1025, 1991.
5. Ellis FH Jr. Treatment of carcinoma of the esophagus or cardia. Mayo Clin Proc 64:945, 1989.
6. Howden CS, Castell DO, Cohen S, et al. The rationale for continuous maintenance treatment of reflux esophagitis. Arch Intern Med 155:1465, 1995.
7. Katon W, Hall ML, Russo J. Chest pain: relationship of psychiatric illness to coronary arteriographic results. Am J Med 84:1, 1988.
8. Katz PO, Dalton CB, Richter JE, et al. Esophageal testing of patients with non-cardiac chest pain or dysphagia. Results of three years experience with 1161 patients. Ann Intern Med 106:593, 1987.
9. Katz PO, Richter JE, Cowan R, Castell DO. Apparent complete lower esophageal sphincter relaxation in achalasia. Gastroenterology 90:978, 1986.
10. Klinkenberg-Knol EC, Festen HPM, Jansen JBMJ, et al. Long-term treatment with omeprazole for refractory reflux esophagitis. Ann Intern Med 121:161, 1994.
11. Meijssen MAC, Tilanus HW, van Blankenstein M, et al. Achalasia complicated by oesophageal squamous cell carcinoma. A prospective study in 195 patients. Gut 33:155, 1992.
12. Pasricha PJ, Rai R, Ravich WJ, et al. Botulinum toxin for achalasia: long-term outcome and predictors of response. Gastroenterology 110:1410, 1996.
13. Richter JE, Bradley LA, Castell DO. Esophageal chest pain: current controversies in pathogenesis, diagnosis and therapy. Ann Intern Med 110:66, 1989.
14. Richter JE, Castell DO. Diffuse esophageal spasm: a reappraisal. Ann Intern Med 100:242, 1984.
15. Schuffler MD, Pope CE II. Esophageal motor function in idiopathic intestinal pseudoobstruction. Gastroenterology 70:677, 1976.
16. Spechler SJ, Goyal RK. Barrett's esophagus. N Engl J Med 315:362, 1986.
17. Tucker HJ, Snape WJ Jr, Cohen S. Achalasia secondary to carcinoma: manometric and clinical features. Ann Intern Med 89:315, 1978.
18. Vigneri S, Termini R, Leandro G, et al. A comparison of five maintenance therapies for reflux esophagitis. N Engl J Med 333:1106, 1995.
19. Yakshe PN, Fleischer DE. Neoplasms of the esophagus. In: Castell DO, ed. The esophagus. Boston: Little, Brown, 1992.

*Bold print (general references) and bold numerals (specific references) denote published controlled clinical trials, meta-analyses, or consensus-based recommendations.

C H A P T E R 36

Abdominal Pain

MARVIN M. SCHUSTER, MD

Abdominal pain is one of the most common presenting complaints of ambulatory patients. Many patients complain of having chronic pain that is constant or recurrent, and in this population it is important to consider functional as well as organic causes for the symptom. Acute abdominal pain (onset within 24 hours before the patient seeks help) almost always reflects an organic process. In any case, whether chronic or acute, abdominal pain resulting from an organic cause is more often a symptom of gastrointestinal (GI) disease than of nongastrointestinal disease.

The caregiver's response to the patient with abdominal pain is influenced by its rapidity of onset, its apparent severity, its location, and accompanying signs and symptoms (e.g., fever, GI bleeding, diarrhea) that may suggest a specific process. Although there is no information about the relative frequency of the various causes of abdominal pain, experience suggests that, most often, *acute pain* is self-limited (abates within hours) and the pain is usually attributed (without proof) to viral gastroenteritis or dietary indiscretion. *Chronic pain,* if associated with an organic process, is most often caused by peptic, gallbladder, or diverticular disease, chronic relapsing pancreatitis (primarily in alcoholics), or carcinoma (most commonly pancreatic or colonic). The symptoms and signs that accompany these processes are discussed in a general way in this chapter and more specifically in the chapters devoted to these conditions. Chronic pain that is not associated with a demonstrable organic process is most often caused by the irritable bowel syndrome (see Chapter 40).

The significance of pain is determined by two major factors: the characteristics of the pain and the characteristics of the patient. The significance of pain to the patient depends on its severity and frequency, the degree to which it interferes with daily life or sleep patterns, and its meaning (both implied and symbolic). Even severe pain can be tolerated for brief periods if it appears infrequently, whereas less severe pain may be less tolerable if it interrupts important activities or disturbs sleep. Pain that has no anticipated end is generally less well tolerated than pain that, even though intense, has a predictable span. The threshold of pain tolerance varies considerably from one individual to another, because of both neurologic and psychologic factors. When pain suggests to the patient a serious underlying disorder, such as cancer, this concern itself may decrease tolerance for pain. Also, pain that is primarily organic may be reinforced by the secondary psychosocial gains it provides.

Elderly patients with abdominal pain require special attention (3). Even serious underlying conditions may be manifested by minimal subjective complaints and objective signs. For example, the diagnosis of appendicitis and of ruptured appendix is easily missed because pain may not be severe and fever and leukocytosis may be minimal or absent. Therefore, careful follow-up of abdominal pain in the elderly warrants repeated abdominal and rectal examinations and serial determinations of temperature and laboratory tests (e.g., white blood cell and differential counts).

Management of any type of pain can be significantly improved by consideration of certain general principles. For example, reassurance that pain can be relieved by medication or surgery can significantly raise the threshold of tolerance. On the other hand, the existence of severe pain sensitizes patients to additional, less intense pain (e.g., lumbar puncture or venipuncture), and the patient's overreaction to the second pain should not be taken to imply that the primary pain is psychogenic. Another common misconception is that alleviation of pain by placebo implies psychogenic origin; in fact, organic pain may be more readily relieved by placebo than is psychogenic pain. A post hoc rationalization that accounts for this phenomenon views the patient with organic pain as a person who wants desperately to get rid of the pain, whereas the person with psychogenic pain may be unwilling to give it up because of secondary gain.

TYPES OF ABDOMINAL PAIN

A few general concepts concerning abdominal pain are reviewed here because understanding them can be helpful diagnostically. Pain involving the digestive system can be visceral, parietal, referred, neurogenic, or psychogenic. Pain caused by metabolic disease is ordinarily visceral or neurogenic.

Visceral Pain

Visceral pain can result from spasm or stretching of the muscle wall of a hollow viscus, from distension of the capsule of a solid organ such as the liver, or from inflammation and ischemia of a visceral structure. Tenderness associated with visceral pain (sometimes including rebound tenderness) is often felt directly over the part of the digestive system that is involved, although (except for the terminal ileum) small bowel tenderness is usually not well localized. Abdominal viscera are insensitive to cutting, tearing, crushing, and burning.

Parietal Pain

The parietal peritoneum, mesentery, and posterior peritoneal covering are sensitive to forces similar to those that affect the viscera, but the omentum and anterior abdominal wall are less sensitive. Parietal tenderness is more localized than visceral tenderness, and rebound tenderness is experienced over the involved area. Parietal pain that is the result of generalized inflammation (peritonitis) encompasses a large area of the peritoneum. A rigid abdomen, associated with pain, usually means that the inflammation is severe.

Referred Pain

Both visceral and parietal pain may be referred to a remote site along shared nerve pathways (dermatomes). Gallbladder pain, for example, typically radiates to the infrascapular area, and right diaphragmatic pain to the right shoulder. Esophageal pain can be confused with the pain of myocardial ischemia because the sites to which the pain radiates may be identical (e.g., the neck and left arm). The more severe the visceral pain, the more likely it is to be referred to the back, as with esophageal spasm or with cholecystitis. The skin overlying the dermatome to which the pain is referred may be hypersensitive. Deep palpation of the primary site of the painful organ may intensify the pain, not only locally, but at its referred site, whereas the reverse is not true; deep palpation over the referred site does not usually enhance pain over the primary site.

Abdominal Pain Caused by Metabolic Disease

Metabolic disease may produce intestinal pain by a direct effect on the alimentary tract (e.g., when intestinal spasm is induced by porphyria, lead poisoning, or familial Mediterranean fever). In hereditary angioneurotic edema, C1 esterase deficiency may produce intestinal swelling, which can result in pain as a result of partial obstruction or intestinal spasm. On the other hand, metabolic disorders may secondarily produce GI pain; for example, hyperparathyroidism may produce a painful peptic ulcer or pancreatitis. Hyperlipidemia also may cause pancreatitis but may be associated with abdominal pain in the absence of pancreatic disease.

Neurogenic Pain

Neurogenic abdominal pain (causalgia) is experienced by the patient as a burning sensation along the route of distribution of the nerve and is sometimes associated with hyperesthesia. Usually the spinal root is involved by herpes zoster, carcinoma, or arthritis, but peripheral neuropathies caused by operative trauma or diabetes mellitus may also produce neurogenic abdominal pain. There is no relationship of neurogenic pain to digestive function (e.g., eating or defecating).

Psychogenic Pain

Psychogenic pain may represent a conversion reaction that results in the perception of pain when no organic dysfunction exists, or it may result from psychophysiologic reactions characterized by pathologic or physiologic responses to psychologic stress (see Chapter 12). For example, emotional stress can lead to painful intestinal spasm in patients with irritable bowel syndrome (Chapter 40). This spasm is a measurable physiologic event. Similarly, stress may lead to peptic symptoms as a result of gastric hypersecretion, which also can be quantitated. Pain or tenderness that represents a conversion reaction (emotions converted into somatic complaints) may disappear during periods of distraction. Such pain may be inconsistent and incompatible with known neuroanatomy and neurophysiology.

HISTORICAL CLUES TO DIAGNOSIS

Although the successful diagnosis of conditions that present with abdominal pain depends on meticulous pursuit of leads that are provided by history and physical examination, familiarity with standard questions and examination techniques assists in ensuring completeness. A history of previous episodes of pain, medications taken (e.g., nonsteroidal anti-inflammatory drugs [NSAIDs] or warfarin), and the existence of a chronic disease (e.g., diabetes mellitus or diverticulosis) is important. Questions relating to local features include the nature and quality of pain; its location, radiation, intensity, timing, duration, and course; and the factors that precipitate, aggravate, and alleviate it. Associated symptoms and signs include tenderness, fever and chills, anorexia, nausea and vomiting, diarrhea and constipation, obstruction, borborygmus, rectal bleeding, passing of mucus, jaundice, and genitourinary symptoms. Although aggravation of pain by emotional tension is seen with functional disorders such as irritable bowel syndrome, the pain of many organic disorders can also be accentuated by stress.

Rapidity of Onset of Pain

The temporal development of abdominal pain is an important factor that guides the physician in evaluation. In particular, pain that develops abruptly or within minutes and becomes rapidly severe is very ominous (Table 36.1).

In addition, situations in which a silent period follows the initial symptoms are notoriously deceptive problems. For example, a perforated viscus or an intestinal infarction may be characterized by resolu-

Table 36.1. Causes of Acute Abdominal Pain According to Rapidity of Onset

Intestinal Causes	Extraintestinal Causes
Abrupt Onset (Instantaneous)	
Perforated ulcer	Ruptured or dissecting aneurysm
Ruptured abscess or hematoma	
Intestinal infarct	Ruptured ectopic pregnancy
Ruptured esophagus	Pneumothorax
	Myocardial infarct
	Pulmonary infarct
Rapid Onset (Minutes)	
Perforated viscus	Ureteral colic
Strangulated viscus	Renal colic
Volvulus	Ectopic pregnancy
Pancreatitis	Splenic infarct
Biliary colic	
Mesenteric infarct	
Diverticulitis	
Penetrating peptic ulcer	
High intestinal obstruction	
Appendicitis (gradual onset more common)	
Gradual Onset (Hours)	
Appendicitis	Cystitis
Strangulated hernia	Pyelitis
Low small intestinal obstruction	Salpingitis
Cholecystitis	Prostatitis
Pancreatitis	Threatened abortion
Gastritis	Urinary retention
Peptic ulcer	Pneumonitis
Colonic diverticulitis	
Meckel diverticulitis	
Crohn's disease	
Ulcerative colitis	
Mesenteric lymphadenitis	
Abscess	
Intestinal infarct	
Mesenteric cyst	

Adapted from Ridge JA, Way LW. Abdominal pain. In: Sleisenger MH, Fordtran JS, eds. Gastrointestinal disease, 5th ed. Philadelphia: WB Saunders, 1993;156.

tion of the intense initial pain hours after perforation or infarction first occurs and by a recurrence of pain several hours later when peritonitis and volume depletion are well established.

Almost always, therefore, if the patient complains of an abrupt onset of severe abdominal pain on the day that he or she visits the physician, even if the pain has resolved and the abdominal examination is unrevealing, a complete blood count, urinalysis, chest radiograph, plain and upright films of the abdomen, and close surveillance over several hours are imperative.

When the onset of pain is more gradual, many more causes are possible, and considerable judgment is necessary in determining the urgency and direction of the evaluation. The caregiver must be guided by the patient's history, the nature and location of the pain, and the examination. In all cases, follow-up examination is warranted. Newly experienced abdominal pain, even if it is felt to be innocuous, should never be dismissed without follow-up (at least by telephone) within a few days so that any important new symptoms are not missed. It is best for the physician to initiate this follow-up because it obviates the need for the patient to decide whether a change in symptoms is important enough to trouble the physician.

Nature and Location of Pain

Esophageal pain is generally described as pressing, constricting, or burning (Tables 36.2 and 36.3). It is usually located in the substernal area and, when severe, radiates through to the back. The location of the pain is a good clue to the location of the underlying disease. Although pain from the lower esophageal region may be referred higher, lesions high in the esophagus do not refer to the lower part of the esophagus (see also Chapter 35).

Gastric pain is usually experienced in the subxiphoid area or the left upper quadrant. Although gastritis is perceived as a true pain (often burning or cramping in quality), the distress caused by both duodenal and gastric ulceration is experienced as a gnawing discomfort or as a hunger sensation rather than as pain. The discomfort caused by peptic ulcer is often precipitated by fasting and is relieved by eating. Thus, pain of peptic ulcer usually awakens the patient between 1 and 3 AM. In contrast, pain of gastritis may be aggravated by eating or relieved only momentarily and then subsequently intensified over 10 to 15 minutes. A change from ulcer distress to a burning, boring, or knifelike pain (especially when there is radiation through to the back) is an indication of a complication of ulcer: penetration. Pain that is precipitated by meals also suggests gastric outlet obstruction (often caused by pyloric channel ulcer) or high intestinal obstruction (see also Chapter 37).

Duodenal pain is felt also in the epigastric area or slightly to the right of it, and it may radiate through to

Table 36.2. Nature and Location of Gastrointestinal Pain

Organ Involved	Nature of Pain	Location of Pain
Esophagus	Burning, constricting	Upper lesions: high substernal
		Lower lesions: low sternal or referred upward
		Severe: back
Stomach	Gnawing discomfort, sensation of hunger	Epigastric Left upper quadrant
Duodenum	Gnawing discomfort, sensation of hunger	Epigastric
Small intestine	Aching, cramping, bloating, sharp	Diffuse Periumbilical Terminal ileum: right lower quadrant
Colon	Aching, cramping, bloating, sharp	Lower abdomen Sigmoid: left lower quadrant Rectum: midline and sacrum
Pancreas	Excruciating, constant	Upper abdomen radiating to back
Gallbladder	Severe, later dull ache	Right upper quadrant Radiates to right scapula or interscapular area
Liver	Ache, occasionally sharp	Right lower rib cage Right upper quadrant if liver is enlarged

Table 36.3. Differential Diagnosis of Abdominal Pain Caused by Gastrointestinal Disorders

	A. Character, Location, Production or Relief		
Disorder	Character	Location	Produced or Relieved by
Peptic ulcer	Gnawing hunger discomfort, occasionally burning, gastric (within minutes after meals), duodenal (usually several hours after meals)	Subxiphoid, may radiate to back	Produced by empty stomach, relieved by food, antacids, or H_2-receptor blockers
Penetrating ulcer	Severe boring contrast pain	Subxiphoid radiating to back	May awaken patient in early morning hours, may be relieved by antacids or H_2-receptor blockers
Perforated ulcer	Abrupt, severe pain followed within 6 hr by deceptive refractory period with diminishing of pain	Initially epigastric, then right lower quadrant (right gutter)	Initial pain spontaneous, peritonitis aggravated by movement
Small bowel obstruction	Crampy severe pain with partial obstruction, constant pain develops with complete obstruction or strangulation	Generalized periumbilical or localized over strangulation	Relieved by intubation decompression
Large bowel obstruction	Crampy pain initially, constant pain with subsequent distension or strangulation, onset less sudden than upper intestinal obstruction	May be localized or generalized	Occasionally relieved by intubation decompression
Intestinal infarct	Severe, excruciating, abrupt onset	Generalized	Relieved only by surgery
Intussusception	Sudden onset severe crampy pain	Periumbilical	Temporary relief may occur with emesis
Appendicitis	Initially colic then continuous with varying intensity	Initial colic in periumbilical area, subsequently continuous in right lower quadrant, occasional testicular radiation	Aggravated by extension of right leg
Pancreatitis	Severe constant pain	Epigastric, radiation to back or lower abdomen	Often initiated by alcoholic binge or eating after binge, by common duct obstruction, penetrating ulcer, or blunt trauma
Cholecystitis	Constant, severe pain preceding nausea and vomiting; subsidence of pain followed by aching	Right upper quadrant radiating to infrascapular region	Precipitated by heavy meal and aggravated by deep inspiration
Biliary colic	Crampy, severe pain	Epigastric, radiating to right upper quadrant and subscapular region	Precipitated by heavy meal within 1–3 hr
Diverticulitis	Crampy or continuous pain	Left lower quadrant, may radiate to back	Relieved by anticholinergics and antibiotics
Crohn's disease	Crampy with partial obstruction and continuous pain with inflammatory mass	Periumbilical or right lower quadrant, may radiate to back	May be precipitated by milk; relieved by defecation or intubation decompression
Ulcerative colitis	Crampy pain usually, may be constant with toxic dilation	Often left lower quadrant or any area of colon, generalized with toxic megacolon or perforation	Precipitated by emotional stress or infection; toxic megacolon by opiates or enemas; relieved temporarily by defecation

	B. Abnormal Physical Findings, Associated Signs, and Laboratory Features		
Disorder	Abnormal Physical Findings	Associated Signs and Symptoms	Laboratory Features
Peptic ulcer	Subxiphoid tenderness	Nausea, vomiting, retrosternal burning; weight gain with duodenal ulcer; weight stable or loss with gastric ulcer	Endoscopic or radiographic demonstration of ulcer, possible occult blood in stool or melena, and iron deficiency anemia
Penetrating ulcer	Marked subxiphoid tenderness	Writhing, clutching abdomen	Amylase may be elevated
Perforated ulcer	Initially rigid with rebound, during refractory stage tenderness disappears to return later, absence of liver dullness with intraperitoneal air	Patient lies rigidly still, pale, perspiring; emesis may be present	Upright film shows free air under diaphragm, leukocytosis
Small bowel obstruction	Borborygmus, high-pitched sound with rushes initially; later quiet abdomen; tenderness may be mild or rebound tenderness may be present	Emesis (may be feculent with lower obstruction), obstipation, may be weak with shocklike appearance	Plain film of abdomen showing air–fluid levels may show stepladder pattern

Table 36.3—*continued.*   Differential Diagnosis of Abdominal Pain Caused by Gastrointestinal Disorders

| | B. Abnormal Physical Findings, Associated Signs, and Laboratory Features | | |
Disorder	Abnormal Physical Findings	Associated Signs and Symptoms	Laboratory Features
Large bowel obstruction	Initially hyperperistalsis with high-pitched rushes, subsequently distension and decrease in bowel signs	Nausea but less vomiting than with high obstruction, obstipation, or marked constipation	Large bowel distension with air-fluid levels and no air demonstrated distal to obstruction
Intestinal infarct	Quiet bowel sounds, tenderness present but not commensurate with pain, later rebound tenderness	Shock, bloody diarrhea, melena, vomiting; history of intestinal angina	Leukocytosis, hemoconcentration; bloody fluid on paracentesis; plain film of abdomen may reveal normal gas pattern or no gas pattern due to fluid-filled loops
Intussusception	Tender mass in abdomen, high-pitched peristaltic rushes	Initially normal stool after onset, then blood, mucus, and constipation; vomiting is late; fever after strangulation	Barium enema demonstrates coiled spring appearance of invagination; with ileocecal intussusception, small bowel loop is in colon
Appendicitis	Localized rebound tenderness, hyperesthesia over area	Initially diarrhea, then constipation; nausea and vomiting may be present; fever, tachycardia; rectal tenderness in right perirectal area	Leukocytosis
Pancreatitis	Marked epigastric tenderness, guarding and upper abdominal distension; the pain of chronic pancreatic disease may be less pronounced	Emesis almost invariable, fever, with hemorrhagic pancreatitis purple color in flank or periumbilical region; emesis is less common in patients with chronic pancreatic disease	Marked leukocytosis, hyperamylasemia; serum calcium depression on days 2 to 4, toxic psychosis on days 2 to 4; radiograph may show calcification, localized ileus, or colon cutoff sign; upper gastrointestinal series demonstrates pancreatic enlargement and spicules in C loop of duodenum; may have left pleural effusion
Cholecystitis	Tenderness over gallbladder area, especially on deep inspiration; Murphy sign may be positive	More common in obese women 40 years or older after pregnancy; high incidence among some American Indian populations	Leukocytosis; plain film may show calcified stone; oral cholecystogram nonvisualized during attacks, TcHIDA nonvisualized; cholangiograms may show radiopaque stones
Biliary colic	As above	As above; jaundice may be present	Radiopaque stones may be seen on plain film; nonvisualization on cholecystogram during colic; subsequently may show radiolucent stones; IV cholangiogram may show dilated duct; bilirubin, alkaline phosphatase increase; may have hyperamylasemia
Diverticulitis	Guarding and tenderness in left lower quadrant	Constipation, fever, tachycardia; rectal tenderness on left; may have urinary frequency or dysuria from periocolonic involvement	Leukocytosis, barium enema shows diverticula but may not visualize during acute episode, may show partial obstruction
Crohn's disease	Tender mass in right lower quadrant, borborygmus	Nausea, vomiting, diarrhea, fever; may have perirectal fistula; tender mass in right rectal area, occasional clubbing	Anemia, elevated sedimentation rate; small bowel series shows cobblestone appearance or string sign
Ulcerative colitis	Tender over involved area, distended especially over transverse colon with toxic megacolon	Frequent passing of small amounts of bloody liquid stool; tenesmus with rectal involvement; fever, tachycardia, arthralgia, erythema nodosa; proctoscopy reveals bleeding and friability	Anemia; elevated sedimentation rate; barium enema demonstrates ulcerations, shortening, effacement of colon

Modified from Handbook of Differential Diagnosis, vol 2, part 1: The abdomen. Nutley, NJ: Rocom Press, 1974.

the back. When an ulcer is perforated, the pain appears abruptly in the epigastric region and later settles into the right lower quadrant as gastric contents are spilled into the right gutter.

Small intestinal pain is generally diffuse and poorly localized. It is experienced in the periumbilical area and, when severe, radiates through to the back. Pain deriving from the terminal ileum may be localized to the right lower quadrant. Uncommonly it may radiate down the leg. Small intestinal pain is generally crampy, sharp, or aching. *Bloating, distension,* and *dull ache* are terms that often are associated with prolonged mechanical obstruction or reflex ileus, whereas more acute forms may be manifested by sharp, steady pain. Associated fever and chills suggest inflammatory bowel disease.

Colonic pain is better localized, often to the lower abdomen. *Sigmoid pain* is felt in the left lower quadrant, and *rectal pain* is often described by the patient as being located over the rectum, usually in the midline. Gas pocketed in the splenic flexure of the colon (seen most commonly in patients with the irritable bowel syndrome) produces left upper quadrant or left chest pain that may be confused with the pain of myocardial ischemia. Temporary relief is obtained by passing gas (see also Chapter 40). Colonic pain generally is crampy or of an aching quality unless perforation occurs, and then it is often severe and constant. Associated fever and chills suggest diverticulitis, diverticular abscess, or ulcerative colitis.

Pancreatic pain is excruciating and constant and usually located in the upper abdomen with radiation through to the back, but it may be felt in almost any area of the abdomen. Chronic pancreatic pain (caused by inflammation, pseudocyst, or carcinoma) is similar in nature and location to acute pancreatic pain but may be less severe. Pancreatitis is almost invariably associated with vomiting. If vomiting is not present, other diagnoses, such as pancreatic carcinoma, should be considered.

Appendicitis often begins as diffuse abdominal pain that intensifies over hours as it settles in the right lower quadrant. The pain of appendicitis is often aggravated by extension of the right leg.

Gallbladder pain generally begins in the right upper quadrant or epigastrium and radiates to the interscapular area or to the right infrascapular area. It is excruciatingly severe, may be aggravated by deep inspiration, and is replaced by a dull, aching sensation that persists for hours after the severe pain subsides. Tenderness can often be elicited by deep palpation under the rib in the area of the gallbladder, especially during deep inspiration. Gallbladder pain often appears several hours after a heavy dinner.

Associated fever and chills suggest ascending cholangitis (see also Chapter 90).

Hepatic pain localizes over the liver, and a tender liver can be demonstrated by palpating the edge during deep inspiration or by fist percussion over the lower right rib cage anteriorly (or over the right upper quadrant if the liver is enlarged).

Genitourinary pain (e.g., renal colic) is discussed in Chapters 27 and 47.

PHYSICAL EXAMINATION

The patient's general appearance provides clues about the severity, the duration, and often the cause of the underlying condition. The cold, sweat, and pallor of shock along with the marble skin (superficial vessels seen over blanched skin) indicating vasoconstriction are signs of significant hemorrhage. Tachycardia and perspiration are seen in both shock and sepsis, but the skin in shock is cold and clammy, whereas in sepsis it is warm and moist. Signs of sepsis suggest bacterial enteritis, inflammatory bowel disease, intra-abdominal abscess, cholangitis, pancreatitis, peritonitis, or pyelonephritis.

The position assumed by the patient may be characteristic of a particular disorder. A position of truncal flexure often typifies patients with pancreatitis, whereas patients with gallbladder colic tend to pace or writhe about and appear restless in their unsuccessful attempt to find a comfortable position. This is in sharp contrast to the immobile position assumed by patients with peritonitis, who attempt to avoid even the slightest jarring movement.

Inspection of the abdomen is facilitated by using incident lighting to visualize abdominal asymmetry and to outline masses and pulsations. In thin patients with partial obstruction, peristaltic intestinal movement may be seen through the abdominal wall, and churning peristalsis may coincide with reports of crampy abdominal pain. Flank discoloration *(Gray–Turner sign)* or periumbilical discoloration *(Cullen sign)* results from retroperitoneal or intraperitoneal hemorrhage dissecting into the subcutaneous tissues and may indicate hemorrhagic pancreatitis. A strangulated hernia may protrude visibly from ventral defects, from the inguinal area, or into the scrotum, where peristaltic contractions may occasionally be appreciated. Patients with subphrenic abscess or gallbladder disease may have inspiratory pain that results in splinting and avoidance of deep inspiration.

Auscultation should always be performed before palpation so that abdominal sounds may be evaluated before they are altered by palpation. At times borborygmus is audible without the stethoscope. Specifically, one should search for hyperperistaltic or hypoperistaltic sounds, for the high tinkles of obstruction, and for bruits suggesting vascular distortion from aneurysms, compression of blood vessels, or invasion of blood vessels (as in invasion of the splenic artery in advanced pancreatic carcinoma). Although a silent abdomen implies reflex ileus, bowel sounds may also be quiet or significantly diminished late in the course of mechanical obstruction. Whenever obstruction (especially gastric outlet obstruction) is considered, an attempt should be made to elicit a succussion splash. This is done by placing the stethoscope over the area (e.g., the stomach) and shaking the patient gently but abruptly. A sloshing sound indicates the presence of air and fluid. This finding in the stomach 3 hours or more after eating or drinking indicates delayed gastric emptying or, rarely, marked hypersecretion.

Gentle percussion should precede palpation and is an excellent means for detecting rebound tenderness, masses, and tympany (either generalized or localized) over an area of ileus or obstruction. Because air rises to the area between the liver and the abdominal wall, absence of liver dullness with the patient in a recumbent position is an important finding indicating the presence of free air in the abdominal cavity.

Before *palpation,* it is wise to ask the patient to point to the site of maximum pain. Gentle palpation should at first avoid that site to minimize the chances that muscle guarding will interfere with the examination. The patient should be lying perfectly supine with knees flexed to facilitate relaxation of abdominal muscles. Guarding may be localized over specific lesions (often inflammatory), or there may be marked rigidity if pain is severe, as in perforation or penetration. Subxiphoid tenderness suggests an active ulcer. Tenderness over the liver, especially when the liver edge is brought down against the examining finger by deep inspiration, suggests inflammation in this organ. With gallbladder disease, tenderness is localized to the region of the gallbladder, and with cystic or common duct obstruction, a distended viscus can sometimes be felt as well. Right lower quadrant tenderness is found with appendicitis as well as with Crohn's disease involving the ileum or the ileocecal area. A left lower quadrant tender sigmoid cord is felt most commonly with irritable bowel syndrome but can also indicate diverticular disease. A distinct tender mass in the right lower quadrant suggests inflammation (usually Crohn's disease) extending beyond the bowel; a similar finding in the left lower quadrant suggests diverticulitis. Boardlike rigidity indicates an intra-abdominal catastrophe such as perforation or infarction. Pulsatile masses should be differentiated from laterally expansile masses because the former can represent a mass overlying an artery, whereas the latter implies aneurysmal dilation. When localized perforation has occurred, rebound tenderness may be localized over the area. Hyperesthesia may exist over the segmental distribution of the spinal nerve that innervates the particular area of the viscus. This finding is detected by gently rubbing the fingers over the skin of the involved dermatome.

Rectal examination can be extremely helpful in localizing areas of tenderness as well as in palpating masses through the rectum. Periappendiceal abscesses can sometimes be identified in this manner, as can a perforated diverticulum. On digital examination the finger should complete a circle that includes the entire perirectal area.

Genital and pelvic examination, like the rectal examination, should be performed in all patients with abdominal pain because it can detect hernias as well as genitourinary and other pelvic problems.

If analgesic drugs have been administered, it is useful to reexamine the patient after pain has been relieved to identify masses or localized tenderness that may have been obscured by guarding and rigidity.

LABORATORY TESTS

A complete blood count, urinalysis, and test for occult blood in the stool are required in every person with serious acute abdominal pain, as are a chest radiograph and plain and upright films of the abdomen. Other laboratory tests should be ordered as indicated by the specific findings.

A low hematocrit value or hemoglobin concentration can call attention to intraperitoneal or retroperitoneal bleeding, whereas hemoconcentration raises consideration of mesenteric vascular occlusion. High white blood cell count and high erythrocyte sedimentation rate suggest inflammation or infection. Blood in the urine points to kidney disease as a possible source of pain, and white cells point to infection.

The presence of occult blood in the stool reinforces concern about the GI tract as a source of painful symptoms and may be an early sign of vascular ischemia or intussusception, or a sign of more common lesions such as peptic ulcer, polyp, or inflammatory bowel disease.

RADIOLOGY

Plain and upright films of the abdomen are helpful in delineating gas patterns, which may demonstrate displacement of intestine by intra-abdominal masses or may show localized loops of ileus such as one sees with *pancreatitis* or *pyelonephritis*. Air is distributed more widely in the small bowel in *reflex ileus* and in *intestinal obstruction*. In the latter the typical stepladder pattern is often encountered, with slight separation of the loops caused by edema of the wall of the small bowel; an upright film demonstrates air–fluid levels in the dilated loops. Absence of air distal to a specific point suggests *obstruction* at that point. *Volvulus* can be diagnosed on the plain film, which demonstrates a sausage-shaped air-filled or air- and fluid-filled viscus coming to an apex. In gastric volvulus the greater curvature is seen above the lesser curve, and a double air–fluid level is a classic finding, one level being in the lesser curvature of the fundus and the other in the antrum (because of the inverted U-shaped stomach under these conditions). Free air under the diaphragm on the upright film indicates a *perforated viscus* unless the patient has had recent surgery (at which time air was introduced) or has *pneumatosis cystoides intestinalis,* in which case a large amount of air may appear subdiaphragmatically from ruptured pseudocysts. The important clue to pneumatosis cystoides intestinalis is the presence of free air in the absence of signs or symptoms of perforation or peritonitis. Radiopaque gallbladder or kidney stones or pancreatic calcification seen on plain film may help corroborate a suspected diagnosis or point attention toward one of these organs.

Contrast studies have been largely replaced by endoscopic procedures in the evaluation of patients with abdominal pain. Endoscopy is both more sensitive and more specific than contrast radiology of the bowel, although it is considerably more expensive. An *upper GI series* (see Patient Experience, Chapter 37) is useful if extrinsic compression on the stomach or duodenum or partial gastric outlet obstruction are suspected at endoscopy. *Barium enema* (see Patient Experience, Chapter 38) can be useful in demonstrating a low site of obstruction and reducing an intussusception. A barium enema should always be preceded by digital examination of the rectum and by proctoscopy to be certain that the rectum is normal (e.g., that there is no rectal carcinoma). When pain is thought to result from gallbladder disease (see Chapter 90) and opaque stones are not visible on plain abdominal film, ultrasonography is an excellent means of demonstrating stones in the gallbladder but is not reliable in detecting ductal stones. An *oral cholecystogram* may demonstrate radiolucent stones; if the gallbladder is not visualized with reinforced dosage, a diseased gallbladder is likely. A *TcHIDA or PipHIDA radioisotopic study* may demonstrate obstruction of the common or cystic duct. This technique requires injection of isotope and serial views for 1 hour. (A sonogram is usually performed beforehand to localize the gallbladder.)

Ultrasonography is also useful in showing pancreatic edema or pseudocysts, evaluating a suspected abdominal aortic aneurysm, and evaluating a patient who is difficult to examine for an intra-abdominal mass; this technique has the advantage of avoiding irradiation. Sonography is often unsatisfactory in obese patients and in those with metal abdominal sutures because adipose tissue and metal reflect sound.

Computed tomography (CT) is a sensitive means of demonstrating masses, infarcted tissue, and cysts but is expensive and exposes the patient to radiation.

Magnetic resonance imaging (MRI) is not used as an initial imaging study of the abdomen but is used selectively to define mass lesions, especially in the liver, kidneys, or adrenal glands, and vascular abnormalities, such as hemangiomata or renal or hepatic vein thrombosis. It is considerably more expensive than a CT scan. HASTE MRI, a new technique (1,2), can demonstrate viscera without movement artifact. It is also effective in showing flowing fluids and therefore can demonstrate partial or complete vascular occlusion.

Table 36.4 compares the ultrasound, CT, and MRI techniques and the patient experience during the performance of these procedures.

Selective mesenteric angiography should be performed in patients suspected of having mesenteric vascular ischemia (particularly in elderly patients with postprandial abdominal pain) or mesenteric vascular occlusion (e.g., in women taking contraceptive medication). This is particularly helpful in older patients because normal arteriographic findings rule out mesenteric vascular disease; on the other hand, occlusion of even two of the three major aortic branches (celiac, superior mesenteric, and inferior mesenteric arteries) may occur without symptoms of mesenteric vascular disease. It may be prudent to hospitalize the patient for this procedure. The patient experience is similar to that described for renal arteriography (see Chapter 62).

ENDOSCOPY

Upper GI endoscopy (esophagoscopy, gastroscopy, duodenoscopy) requires referral to a gastroenterologist. It should be considered the ambulatory procedure of choice to diagnose upper GI disease and to obtain a biopsy for diagnosis (e.g., when cancer is suspected). Endoscopy should be performed promptly when abdominal pain is associated with upper GI bleeding (see Chapter 38), but these patients should be hospitalized. The patient's experience during the procedure is described in Chapter 38.

Proctoscopy should be performed in any patient with abdominal pain and rectal bleeding or a change in bowel habits or in any patient in whom inflammatory bowel disease (proctitis, ulcerative colitis, Crohn's disease) is suspected. Moreover, anal lesions such as hemorrhoids and fissures are best demonstrated by proctoscopy. The procedure routinely should precede roentgenographic examination of the lower bowel because the barium enema does not visualize the lower rectum.

For *proctosigmoidoscopy,* whether prior preparation

Table 36.4.   Ultrasound, Computed Tomographic (CT) Scanning, and Magnetic Resonance Imaging (MRI): Comparison of the Technique and the Patient Experience

Characteristic	Ultrasound	CT	MRI
Basis of tissue attenuation	Tissue elasticity, acoustic impedance	Electron density; linear attenuation coefficient	Nuclear resonance
Radiation dose or toxic effect	None known at diagnostic energy levels	8–10 R (skin exposure)	None known
Morphologic detail	Good	Excellent	Excellent
Contrast medium useful	No	Iodinated intravascular and oral agents; diatrizoate meglumine (Gastrografin)	No (in abdomen)
Time for examination	½–1 hr	½–1 hr	1 hr
Operator skill	Substantial	Minimal	Minimal
Ease of interpretation	Complex, many artifacts	Straightforward	Moderately straightforward
Preparation	Nothing by mouth after midnight (for pelvis, three glasses of water 1 hr before study and do not void)	Evacuate barium from recent gastrointestinal studies (or wait 1 wk)	None
Cooperation	Lie still, supine, be able to hold breath	Lie still, supine, be able to hold breath	Lie still, supine, breathe quietly

Adapted from Ferrucci JT Jr. Body ultrasonography (first of two parts). N Engl J Med 300:538, 1979.

is appropriate depends on the suspected pathology. If *proctosigmoidoscopy* is performed to detect or biopsy a mass lesion, a laxative is used the day before and a cleansing enema is given on the morning of the procedure. On the other hand, mucosal lesions (e.g., inflammatory bowel disease) are best demonstrated without preparation (other than a natural bowel movement the morning of the procedure). Most enema preparations tend to produce some mucosal edema that may obscure mucosal lesions. Proctosigmoidoscopy is not painful, but an uncomfortable sensation is produced by the distension of the rectosigmoid region by the instrument used and by air.

Fiberoptic sigmoidoscopy can generally be performed if a laxative is administered the day before the procedure and if an enema is given on the morning of the procedure. Many general physicians have been trained to perform this procedure, but in the absence of such training referral to a gastroenterologist is appropriate. The patient's experience during the procedure is described in Chapter 36.

Colonoscopy, like upper endoscopy, requires referral to a gastroenterologist. It should be considered in patients with abdominal pain who have occult rectal bleeding (see Chapter 38), in those with suspected diffuse colonic inflammatory disease (ulcerative colitis, Crohn's disease) or suspected ischemic colitis, and in patients with polypoid lesions on barium enema who require biopsy or, often, resection of the lesion. Colonoscopy cannot be performed within a day or two of a barium radiograph of the lower or upper GI tract. The patient's experience during the procedure is described in Chapter 38.

In addition to concerns about facts relating to endoscopy, many patients have specific apprehensions and misconceptions that can be managed appropriately only if the patient is encouraged to express them. The most common questions concern the indication for the procedure, its anticipated benefits, and technical details about the procedure itself, including prior preparation, side effects, and risks. Much of the patient's anxiety can be allayed if the referring physician can answer these questions appropriately. The physician may find it helpful to emphasize that the fiberoptic instruments can be passed with little discomfort and that photographs can be taken for detailed study, as well as brushings for cytology and biopsy for histology.

TREATMENT

The treatment of patients with abdominal pain depends on the severity of the pain, its rapidity of onset, and the nature of the underlying condition, if known. Severe pain with an abrupt or rapid onset often reflects a GI disorder that will require surgical intervention (Table 36.1). Hospitalization and consultation with a surgeon should be requested immediately in almost all cases. Less severe pain (pain that does not prevent the patient from ambulating, talking normally, thinking coherently, and so on) should not be treated aggressively with analgesic drugs until an attempt has been made to establish a diagnosis because the pain often abates spontaneously within minutes or hours and does not recur. In such circumstances, no further evaluation is indicated. If the pain recurs or persists and the cause is not obvious, the screening tests described in this chapter should be done. If these tests do not provide a diagnosis, referral to a gastroenterologist is indicated.

As a general rule, analgesic drugs may be prescribed to patients with persistent pain, but opiates should be avoided if possible because they may aggravate the underlying condition. (For example, morphine may aggravate pancreatitis by producing duodenal and ampullary spasm, thus enhancing pancreatic duct obstruction, and opiates or anticholinergics may produce toxic megacolon in patients with active ulcerative colitis. Furthermore, there is a risk of narcotic addiction in any patient whose pain is likely to be of prolonged duration.)

General References

Ferrucci JT Jr. Body ultrasonography (first of two parts). N Engl J Med 300:538, 1979.
> Good review of the clinical uses of sonography, with useful comparison of computerized tomographic scanning.

Glasgow RE, Mulvihill SJ. Abdominal pain, including the acute abdomen. In: Feldman M, Scharschmidt BF, Sleisenger HH, eds. Sleisenger and Fordtran's gastrointestinal and liver disease, 6th ed. Philadelphia: WB Saunders, 1997;1:80.

Handbook of differential diagnosis, vol. 2., part I, The abdomen. Nutley, NJ: Rocom Press, 1974.
> Excellent illustrations by M. F. Netter and good tables.

Nathan L, Huddleston JH. Acute abdominal pain in pregnancy. Ob Gyn Clin North Am 33:55, 1995.

Pearigen PD. Unusual causes of abdominal pain. Emerg Med Clin North Am 14(3):593, 1996.

Specific References

1. Beall D, Regan F. MRI of bowel obstruction using the Haste sequence. J Comput Assist Tomogr 20:823, 1996.
2. Regan F, Fradkin J, Khazan R. Choledocholithiasis evaluation with magnetic resonance imaging. Am J Radiol 167:1441, 1996.
3. Sanson TG, O'Keefe KP. Evaluation of abdominal pain in the elderly. Emerg Med Clin North Am 14(3):615, 1996.

C H A P T E R 37

Peptic Ulcer Disease

PHILIP O. KATZ, MD

EPIDEMIOLOGY: NATURAL HISTORY

Peptic ulcer disease is a common clinical problem. It is estimated to have a lifetime incidence of 5 to 10%. Between 1 and 2% of the population has an ulcer at any time and approximately 200,000 to 400,000 new cases are seen in the United States each year. The rate of hospital admissions for uncomplicated duodenal ulcer has decreased significantly in the last 35 years, but the incidence of gastric ulcer and complications of ulcer disease—bleeding and perforation—have not diminished, suggesting that the treatment of peptic disease has become primarily an ambulatory function. Duodenal ulcer is twice as common in men than in women and 1.5 times as common as gastric ulcer. The peak incidence for duodenal ulcer is in the fifth decade in men and in the sixth decade and older in women. Gastric ulcer is slightly more common in men than in women, and in both sexes, it is more common in the elderly.

Ulcers are usually less than 1 cm in diameter, although giant ulcers (larger than 2.5 cm) occasionally occur. Duodenal ulcers are almost always located in the duodenal bulb or immediately postbulbar, within 3 cm of the pyloric duodenal junction. Ulcers distal to the duodenal bulb should raise the suspicion of the Zollinger–Ellison syndrome (discussed later in this chapter) or Crohn's disease of the duodenum. Gastric ulcers are most commonly located on the lesser curvature, at the junction of the body and antrum of the stomach. There is no risk of cancer in a duodenal ulcer, but 1 to 3% of gastric ulcers occur in carcinomas.

Untreated duodenal ulcer disease can be chronic. Estimates are that 60 to 80% of patients have a recurrence within 1 year of diagnosis if curative therapy is not given. Many recurrences are asymptomatic. Recurrences decrease over 10 to 20 years, but symptomatic duodenal ulcer is often seen in the elderly. The recurrence rate of gastric ulcers has not been studied as extensively but appears to be lower. Both duodenal and gastric ulcers tend to recur in the same place as the index ulcer. Long-term studies suggest that bleeding or perforation occurs at a rate of 1 to 3% a year, with a lifetime incidence of approximately 20%, if the ulcer is not adequately treated. Recurrent hemorrhage occurs in approximately 50% of patients who have had a prior bleed. A few studies suggest that the complication rate may be reduced by maintenance therapy (2) and can be eliminated if the bacterium *Helicobacter pylori* is eradicated (see below). The major risk of death from ulcer disease is on the first presentation (3).

RISK FACTORS

Certain factors are associated with an increased risk of developing peptic ulcer disease (Table 37.1). Genetic factors appear to play an important role. Men are more prone to both duodenal and gastric ulcers than are women. Duodenal ulcer is three times more common in first-degree relatives of a patient with a duodenal ulcer than in the general population. Furthermore, certain genetic markers, such as pepsinogen I, HLAB5, and red blood cell acetylcholinesterase, can identify groups at increased risk. With the aid of such markers, peptic ulcer disease has been shown to be genetically heterogeneous. In certain families there appears to be an autosomal dominant mode of inheritance, whereas in others no discernible pattern is found.

The role of *stress* in the pathogenesis of peptic ulcer disease is well recognized but difficult to quantitate. Nevertheless, it is clear that threats to the psychologic or physical well-being of some people appear to predispose them to the symptoms of peptic ulcer. Why some people react to stress by developing ulcer symptoms and others by developing another disease (e.g., asthma or hypertension) is unknown (see Chapter 12 for a discussion of psychosomatic illness).

Cigarette smoking has been repeatedly demonstrated to be associated with an increased frequency of duodenal ulcer disease, with frequencies ranging between 33 and 100% above those found among nonsmokers (19). In addition, there is evidence that cigarette smoking may delay the healing of both gastric and duodenal ulcers and increase the frequency of their recurrence

Table 37.1.   Diagnostic Tests for *Helicobacter pylori*

Method	Specimen	Cautions	Sensitivity (%)	Specificity (%)	Comments
For Patients Who Do Not Require Endoscopy					
Serology test (in office)	Serum or whole blood	Lipidemia	90–95	90	Performed in 5–20 min; detects IgG (elevated in patients with *H. pylori*).
Multiwell ELISA (in laboratory)	Serum	Recent antibiotics make interpretation of a single sample difficult; 1–5% of patients do not produce detectable antibody	90–95	90	Decrease in paired antibody titers can be assessed. Patients with rapid antibody decrease are cured. Persistent antibody after therapy is common and may slowly decrease (12–18 mo), which may represent cure or continued infection.
Urea breath test	Breath sample	Antibiotics and PPIs can cause false-negative results; should be done 4 weeks or more after last antibacterial therapy; not affected by H_2-receptor antagonists	95	95	Urease of *H. pylori* generates labeled CO_2 from breakdown of ingested urea. Breath sample taken 20–40 min after fasting. Patient ingests isotope in liquid (^{13}C) or capsule (^{14}C).
For Patients Undergoing Endoscopy and Biopsy					
Rapid urease test	1–2 mucosal biopsies	Same as for breath test: do not take samples from ulcers or lesions	90	98	Simple biopsy test: Urease of *H. pylori* generates ammonia and causes pH change. One-step test, no reagents, result in 1–24 hr. Least expensive method of endoscopic diagnosis.
Histology	2 mucosal biopsies	Still regarded by many as the gold standard for *H. pylori* detection	95	98	Simple and very accurate: Specimen can be reexamined in equivocal cases. Provides a permanent record. Special stains occasionally necessary to detect organism.
Culture of biopsy	1–2 mucosal biopsies	3–6 days on moist, brain–heart blood agar in *Campy pac* or 10% CO_2, 37°C	80	100	Provides antibiotic sensitivity information (if necessary).

ELISA, Enzyme-linked immunosorbent assay.

(21). There is no epidemiologic evidence that alcohol is ulcerogenic, although it is a known cause of acute gastritis. Coffee, both caffeinated and decaffeinated, is a mild stimulant of gastric acid secretion. Symptoms may be exacerbated by coffee, but a definite causal relationship with ulcer disease has not been demonstrated.

Certain disease states have been associated with an increased risk of peptic ulcer disease. Evidence of such associations must be carefully evaluated in light of the high prevalence of ulcer disease in the general population and the frequent use of ulcerogenic drugs. However, there is good evidence linking duodenal (but not gastric) ulcer disease with chronic obstructive pulmonary disease, alcoholic cirrhosis, chronic renal failure, and hyperparathyroidism.

Conditions that lead to increased gastric acid secretion also predispose to ulcer disease. The Zollinger–Ellison syndrome, or gastrinoma (discussed later in this chapter), is the best example of such a condition.

Extensive small bowel resection may also lead to hyperplasia of antral gastrin-containing cells and result in ulcer disease. Retained antrum after gastric surgery is yet another example of a situation in which uninhibited acid production is associated with recurrent ulcerations.

Many drugs are reputed to be ulcerogenic, although the evidence is not well established for most of them. Aspirin is one drug that causes gastric and duodenal ulcers. Experimentally, aspirin disrupts the gastric mucosa both physiologically and anatomically, leading to ulcer formation. The risk of gastric ulcer increases sixfold when patients use more than three aspirin a day (1). Aspirin use also increases the risk of bleeding from peptic lesions (see Chapter 51). Enteric coated or buffered aspirin has no advantage over regular aspirin with respect to these untoward effects. Alcohol used concomitantly with aspirin increases the risk for ulcer bleeding.

There is good evidence that all nonsteroidal anti-inflammatory drugs (NSAIDs) can cause gastric and duodenal ulcers. The greatest risk of NSAID-induced gastric or duodenal bleeding appears to be in women over 60 years of age (12), in patients with a history of ulcers, and in patients who are taking corticosteroids concurrently. Prospective and retrospective studies have concluded that chronic use of corticosteroids by patients who are not taking NSAIDs does not increase the risk of peptic ulcer disease or its complications (5).

It is now well accepted that *Helicobacter pylori* infection is the most common and important risk factor for duodenal ulcer. The risk of gastric ulcer is probably multifactorial, although many gastric ulcers are associated with *H. pylori* and the decreased recurrence of gastric ulcer after eradication of infection suggests that *H. pylori* is a risk factor.

PATHOPHYSIOLOGY

Duodenal Ulcer

Duodenal ulcer disease has always been viewed as the result of an imbalance between the normal duodenal defense mechanisms and the amount of acid delivered to the duodenum from the stomach. Multiple abnormalities have been identified that result in this imbalance: increased parietal cell mass, increased capacity of parietal cells to secrete acid, increased vagal drive to secrete acid, defective inhibition of gastrin release and of gastric secretion after gastric acidification or after a meal (these first four abnormalities result in a considerably increased acid production compared with normal), abnormally rapid gastric emptying, and altered duodenal defense mechanisms, including bicarbonate secretion, mucus production, vascular integrity, and endogenous prostaglandin production. It is now clear that these imbalances are caused by hypersecretory states, ingestion of NSAIDs, and, most important, *H. pylori* infection.

Helicobacter pylori

H. pylori is a Gram-negative spiral organism found exclusively in gastric epithelium (20). It may be seen in the duodenal bulb in regions where there is gastric metaplasia. The organism is found in 10% of healthy people under 30 and in approximately 60% of healthy people over 60. The rate of infection is higher in lower socioeconomic areas and developing countries. The organism is probably spread by person-to-person contact.

H. pylori is the etiologic agent for chronic nonerosive antral gastritis, is present in the stomach in more than 90% of patients with a duodenal ulcer, and is the most common cause of that disease (20). It is estimated that 15 to 20% of infected patients will develop an ulcer in their lifetime. Other diseases associated with *H. pylori* infection are the rare B-cell mucosa-associated lymphoid tissue (MALT) lymphoma and gastric adenocarcinoma.

Eradication of the organism appears to result in accelerated duodenal ulcer healing (14) and significantly decrease ulcer recurrence 1 and 2 years after treatment (14,16). The rate of reinfection is unknown but appears to be less than 1% up to 5 years after treatment. Eradication of *H. pylori* also reduces recurrent bleeding in patients who have bled.

Gastric Ulcer

The pathogenesis of gastric ulceration is unclear. It is generally believed that the basic defect in gastric ulcer formation is the disruption of the gastric mucosal barrier. It has been shown that this barrier can be broken by such irritants as bile, alcohol, and aspirin. These experimental observations help explain the epidemiologic data associating alcohol with acute gastritis, and aspirin with gastric ulcers and erosions. Furthermore, in patients with gastric ulcers, radiologic and manometric studies have suggested that there is an increased duodenal gastric reflux. This reflux of bile across an incompetent pyloric sphincter results in the disruption of the mucosal barrier. Once the barrier is broken, hydrogen ion may diffuse back into the gastric cells, leading to ulceration via local histamine release, vasodilation, and tissue damage. Thus, according to this concept, gastric ulcer formation requires injury to the gastric mucosal barrier and the presence of some, but not necessarily an excessive amount of, acid. *H. pylori* infection has been associated with gastric ulcer disease in a majority of patients and the presence of gastritis may make the mucosa more susceptible to injury.

DIAGNOSIS

History

The most common symptom of peptic ulcer disease is epigastric distress—vague discomfort or a feeling of gnawing hunger—usually in the midline. If actual pain occurs, it is typically aching or burning.

Classically, the distress of duodenal ulcer occurs 1 to 3 hours after a meal and may awaken the patient from sleep, usually between 1 and 2 AM; it is relieved within minutes by food, antacids, or vomiting. Pain is minimal before breakfast. In patients with gastric ulcers, the history is more variable. In some, a similar distress–food–relief pattern exists, whereas in others there is no relationship with food. Occasionally, the distress is actually exacerbated by food.

Other less common symptoms of ulcer disease include nausea, vomiting, and dyspepsia. However, in some patients with ulcers, one or more of these symptoms may occur in the absence of typical ulcer pain. Weight loss occurs in up to 50% of patients with a benign gastric ulcer and is therefore not a helpful feature in distinguishing a benign from a malignant ulcer. Patients with duodenal ulcer often gain weight because they eat more in an attempt to control their pain.

The history may also suggest certain complications. Pyloric obstruction presents first with early satiety and then with persistent vomiting, often of undigested food. A change in the quality of the pain or radiation of the pain to the back or shoulder suggests penetration of the ulcer. A history of melena suggests bleeding. Occasionally, one of these complications is the first clinical manifestation of peptic ulceration.

Physical Examination

The physical examination may provide supportive, although nonspecific, information. Localized epigastric tenderness is common. The presence of a succussion splash 4 hours or more postprandially is evidence of gastric outlet obstruction. Rectal examination should be included in the initial physical examination to obtain a stool specimen for testing for occult blood.

Radiologic Studies

Confirmation of the presence of peptic ulcer disease can be made with barium studies or endoscopy. The barium study has been used less and less over the years because it is less accurate than endoscopy and because endoscopy allows biopsy of the mucosa for *H. pylori.*

Patient Experience. The patient should be told that the upper gastrointestinal series requires a series of radiographs to be taken after he or she swallows a bolus of mint-flavored barium, that peristalsis is monitored fluoroscopically during the procedure, and that to coat as much of the stomach and duodenum as possible, the patient will be prone. The entire procedure takes approximately 20 to 25 minutes. Double (air) contrast studies, done after swallowing barium and a tablet that releases carbon dioxide into the stomach, do not alter this experience.

Duodenal Ulcer

The radiographic diagnosis of duodenal ulcer disease depends on the detection of an ulcer crater. Overall, the sensitivity of radiographic studies in detection of duodenal ulcer is 40 to 80%, with the greatest sensitivity achieved with double-contrast radiographs. Ulcers less than 0.5 cm in diameter are often missed radiographically. Ulcers larger than 2.5 cm are classified as giant duodenal ulcers. Duodenal ulcers do not carry the risk of malignancy that gastric ulcers do, so follow-up radiographs to confirm healing generally are not needed. In patients with chronic ulcer disease with severe deformity of the bulb, radiographic distinction between old scarring with deformity and new active ulcerations is often difficult. Comparison with previous films and correlation with the clinical state are needed in these cases.

Gastric Ulcer

A well-performed double-contrast radiographic study can detect approximately 65 to 80% of gastric ulcers seen at endoscopy; of greater importance is the differentiation of benign from malignant ulcers. In evaluating a gastric ulcer, the radiologist generally describes it as benign, malignant, or indeterminate. As many as 10% of gastric ulcers may be classified in this last category. Although the radiographic impression of a benign or malignant ulcer is generally very accurate, discrepancies still occur. The prevalence of malignancy in an ulcer diagnosed radiographically as benign ranges from 3 to 7%, with higher frequencies when indeterminate lesions are included, although air contrast techniques may decrease this error rate. Furthermore, barium studies may miss benign lesions, particularly when multiple ulcers are present. Even carefully performed radiography misses up to 20% of ulcers seen by endoscopy. Thus, although a barium study is often the initial procedure of choice for gastric ulcers, it must be recognized that its sensitivity is less than that of endoscopy and that it is associated occasionally with erroneous results.

Endoscopy

Experienced endoscopists diagnose up to 95% of gastroduodenal ulcers (the ulcer ultimately is proved by a second endoscopy, surgery, or radiography) (8). When both ulcers and erosions (duodenitis) are considered as diagnostic criteria, the sensitivity of radiography in the detection of both duodenal and gastric lesions is 54%, compared with 90% for endoscopy. The question of the primary diagnostic procedure of choice for the diagnosis of ulcers remains to be settled. Clearly, the decision must be based on the clinical presentation as well as the overall condition of the patient. Guidelines for endoscopy in peptic ulcer disease can only be suggested. In patients with typical symptoms of duodenal ulcer, a diagnosis can be strongly suggested by response to a therapeutic trial of medical therapy. Patients with long-standing abdominal pain refractory to medical treatment, recurrent symptoms after curative therapy, or negative radiographs should undergo endoscopy. Other indications for endoscopy include suspected outlet obstruction, active or suspected gastrointestinal bleeding, the need to evaluate equivocal or indeterminate findings on upper gastrointestinal series, and the need to confirm the presence or absence of *H. pylori.* There is a higher diagnostic yield of endoscopy in patients over the age of 65 (11). No follow-up endoscopic evaluation of an uncomplicated duodenal ulcer is required because the risk for malignancy is nil.

Another controversial issue is the indication for endoscopy when a gastric ulcer is diagnosed by radiograph. The argument for endoscopy in all patients with gastric ulcer is that 3 to 7% of radiographically benign ulcers are later found to be malignant, and it is known that malignant ulcers sometimes appear to have healed when follow-up radiographs are taken. The argument against routine endoscopy is that most endoscopies only confirm the radiographic impression, so the patient incurs unnecessary discomfort, risk, and cost. Unfortunately, no data are available to help, nor are any likely to be forthcoming because of the large number of patients required to do a conclusive study. It is the position of the American Society for Gastrointestinal Endoscopy (4) that all patients with gastric ulcers that appear benign should have endoscopy with biopsy at some point in the therapy (after 8 weeks of therapy, for example). It is reasonable to do early endoscopy in all patients with ulcers that are not clearly radiographically benign or that are large (more than 2.5 cm). Biopsies can be obtained at that point and all parties can be reassured. The ulcers should then be followed until they have healed, as confirmed by endoscopy. For a review of patient experience, see Chapter 38.

Gastric Analysis

Gastric secretory studies have enhanced the understanding of the pathophysiology of ulcer disease but are of limited clinical usefulness. Although many patients with duodenal ulcer disease can be shown to hypersecrete acid, more than half of such patients actually have normal levels of acid production. Furthermore, the presence of hypersecretion does not predict the development of ulcer disease in an individual patient. Dyspepsia with a negative radiograph is not an indication for gastric analysis.

In patients with gastric ulcers, gastric analysis is not helpful. No reliable criteria exist to differentiate benign from malignant gastric ulcers.

The main indications for gastric analysis are for preoperative evaluation of patients with suspected Zollinger–Ellison syndrome or in postgastrectomy patients with recurrent ulcer disease. However, gastric analysis is not useful as an indicator of the type of surgery needed; more acid production does not necessarily require more gastric resection (18).

Serum Gastrin Measurements

Measurements of the level of gastrin in the blood are readily available and are useful in the evaluation of selected patients with peptic ulcer disease. The fasting basal serum gastrin level is usually normal (less than 150 pg/mL) in patients with duodenal and gastric ulcer disease but is elevated, often to very high levels (usually 1000 pg/mL or more), in patients with the Zollinger–Ellison syndrome. Therefore, fasting gastrin determinations are useful in screening for this condition. In patients with frequently recurrent ulcers and in patients refractory to conventional therapy—features suggestive of the syndrome—two or three fasting serum gastrin determinations should be made to rule out this condition because the levels may fluctuate. Also, in all patients undergoing elective ulcer surgery, a preoperative gastrin level should be measured to rule out Zollinger–Ellison syndrome. (Hypergastrinemia is discussed later in this chapter.)

Diagnosis of *H. pylori*

Several diagnostic tests are available for the detection of *H. pylori* infection (5–7,10,12) (Table 37.1). The gold standard is *histologic testing* (9), using at least two biopsies obtained endoscopically from different parts of the antrum to ensure that the infection is not missed. This method has a sensitivity and specificity of 85 to

100%. It is time-consuming, requires analysis by an experienced pathologist, and is expensive. *H. pylori* is identified in the mucosa with the use of hematoxylin and eosin, Warthin–Starry, or Giemsa stains. The sensitivity for cultures (essentially done for research only) is usually 50 to 95%, but the specificity approaches 100%.

For patients undergoing endoscopy, one of the most cost-effective tests is the rapid *urease (CLO) test*. In this commercially available test, the biopsy is placed in a gel-containing urea, phenol red, and a bacteriostatic agent. *H. pylori* causes a color change from yellow to red if the test is positive. This test is approximately 95% sensitive and 95% specific.

Several noninvasive tests are available for use in the office (13). One of these is a fingerstick serologic test for the detection of immunoglobulin G (IgG) antibody. The method is approximately 90% sensitive and specific. A decline in IgG concentration correlates well with eradication of *H. pylori* 12 to 24 months after treatment (7).

Another noninvasive test, recently released, is the *urea breath test*. It entails giving the patient ^{13}C-labeled urea by mouth and then measuring the patient's breath for the labeled bicarbonate, which is generated when *H. pylori* splits the urea. This test is 96% sensitive and 98% specific. The ^{13}C test is read by a mass spectrometer, so it must be sent out of the office for reading. This is a reliable, noninvasive test for evaluation of eradication of the organism (6).

Summary

If endoscopy is planned, a rapid urease test is the diagnostic procedure of choice for *H. pylori*. If a patient with a duodenal (or gastric) ulcer has a negative rapid urease test, a serologic test should be performed to rule out a false-negative result. This is more cost-effective (and accurate) than histologic examination or culture (10,15). Follow-up, if necessary, should include the urea breath test. If endoscopy is not necessary, diagnosis can be made by serology unless there is a history of infection.

MEDICAL THERAPY

The treatment of peptic ulcer disease involves two issues: healing of the ulcer and prevention of its recurrence. Both can be accomplished with successful eradication of *H. pylori,* if present. Acute treatment also includes relief of pain with pharmacologic agents. Rarely, a patient is refractory to medical treatment or has complications and requires surgery.

Nonpharmacologic Therapy

There is no evidence that dietary modification affects the course of peptic ulcer disease. Frequent feedings, bland diets, increased milk consumption, and decreased consumption of spices and fruit juices have never been demonstrated to affect healing. Although alcohol and caffeine increase acid secretion, no evidence exists that discontinuing either of these substances enhances healing, and it is reasonable to allow patients to continue to consume them in moderation. Dietary restrictions should be limited to substances that cause symptoms; otherwise, patients should be allowed to eat as they wish.

The most important nonpharmacologic intervention is to discontinue cigarette smoking (see Chapter 20) (19,21). Cigarette smoking both increases the risk and delays the healing of duodenal ulcers. Impaired healing of duodenal ulcers in smokers compared with nonsmokers has been repeatedly demonstrated in controlled trials with H_2 antagonists. The impact of smoking is more dramatic when recurrence of ulcers is examined. Nonsmokers who are not prescribed maintenance therapy and do not have *H. pylori* eradicated have a yearly recurrence rate of approximately 20% (equal to smokers treated with maintenance therapy) compared with a recurrence rate of approximately 70% in nontreated smokers in whom the organism is not eradicated (21). Smoking may predispose patients to perforation and bleeding. The effect of smoking on gastric ulceration appears to be similar to that on duodenal ulceration, although it has not been studied as extensively. If *H. pylori* is eradicated, duodenal ulcers do not appear to recur even if smoking is continued. Nevertheless, it seems prudent to recommend smoking cessation in these patients.

Aspirin and other NSAIDs are well-known risk factors for gastric erosions and ulcers. There is a trend toward an increased risk of duodenal ulcers and erosions as well. All such agents should be discontinued, if possible, when a patient has a peptic ulcer.

Duodenal Ulcer

Pharmacologic Therapy

Patients with a proven diagnosis of duodenal (or gastric) ulcer associated with *H. pylori* infection should receive treatment aimed at eradication of *H. pylori* and appropriate pharmacologic therapy to decrease duode-

nal ulcer pain. Appropriate treatment results in healing of 85 to 95% of duodenal ulcers and reduction of duodenal ulcer recurrence to less than 1% per year. There are several important treatment principles: Therapy with a single antibiotic is not effective, no single regimen has proven effective for all patients, and substitution of an antibiotic of the same class for a recommended antibiotic (e.g., ampicillin for amoxicillin or doxycycline for tetracycline) results in a dramatic decrease in healing rates. Each regimen discussed in this section should be evaluated based on efficacy, antimicrobial resistance, side effects, compliance, cost, and previous treatment.

Several regimens have received FDA approval (23) (see Table 37.2): Dual therapy with omeprazole (20 mg twice a day) and clarithromycin (500 mg three times a day) given for 14 days is a well-tolerated regimen with an eradication rate of 75 to 85%. Omeprazole (20 mg/day) should be continued for 2 additional weeks. Ranitidine, bismuth citrate (RBC, 400 mg three times a day) given for 4 weeks plus clarithromycin (500 mg three times a day) for 2 weeks has an eradication rate of 80 to 85%. Triple therapy with bismuth subsalicylate (2 tablets four times a day), metronidazole (250 mg four times a day), and tetracycline (500 mg four times a day) taken for 14 days, prepared as a blister pack for each day's dosage, has recently been approved for treatment by the FDA and has an eradication rate above 90%. Combined treatment with a single daily dose of an H_2-receptor antagonist for 6 weeks is part of the approved regimen. Many experts substitute omeprazole (20 mg daily) for 4 weeks instead of the H_2-receptor antagonist. Compliance is key with the regimen. More than 60% of the doses must be completed to ensure optimal eradication rates. Side effects have been variable with this regimen, ranging from 10 to 30%, and may be reduced by the addition of omeprazole. The blister pack should greatly improve compliance. Patients who are intolerant of tetracycline can be given amoxicillin (500 mg four times a day) in its place. The

Table 37.2. Drugs Approved for Treatment of Peptic Ulcer Disease

Drug	Available Strengths	Initial Dose[a,b]	Principal Side Effects
Cimetidine (Tagamet)[c]	200 mg 300 mg 400 mg 800 mg	400 mg BID 800 mg at bedtime	Gynecomastia, confusion, impotence, blood dyscrasia, drug interaction
Ranitidine (Zantac)	150 mg 300 mg	150 mg BID 300 mg at bedtime	Gynecomastia, impotence, hepatitis (rare)
Famotidine (Pepcid)[c]	20 mg 40 mg	20 mg BID 40 mg at bedtime	Headache, decreased libido, depression, mild increase in aminotransferase
Nizatidine (Axid)	150 mg 300 mg	150 mg BID[d] 300 mg at bedtime	Sweating, urticaria (<1%), somnolence, elevated liver enzymes
Sucralfate (Carafate)[c]	1 g	1 g QID[d] 2 g BID	Constipation
Omeprazole (Prilosec)	20 mg	20 mg QD (AM)	Nausea, headache
Lansoprazole	15 mg	15 mg QD[d]	

[a]Duodenal ulcer, 4–6 weeks.
[b]Gastric ulcer, 8–12 weeks (document healing).
[c]Available in liquid suspension.
[d]Not approved for gastric ulcer by the FDA.

regimen that appears to have become favored, especially by gastroenterologists, is called *proton pump inhibitor (PPI)-based triple therapy.* Although it has not been approved by the FDA, eradication rates of up to 95% have been reported with 7 to 14 days of treatment with omeprazole (20 mg twice a day), metronidazole (500 mg twice a day), and clarithromycin (500 mg twice a day). To ensure an optimal response, treatment for at least 10 days appears appropriate. Amoxicillin (1000 mg twice a day) may be substituted for metronidazole with similar healing rates. It is likely that no further treatment beyond 14 days is required for treatment of duodenal ulcer when PPI-based triple therapy is used. It appears that the PPI lansoprazole (30 mg twice a day) may be substituted for omeprazole.

No individual regimen should be relied on exclusively. The choice must be individualized and based on compliance, cost, resistance, and efficacy. Current estimates are that metronidazole resistance rates are approximately 11% and clarithromycin resistance rates are approximately 5%. Amoxicillin and tetracycline resistance are uncommon. It is hoped that future treatment will be simpler and equally effective.

If *H. pylori* is successfully eradicated, maintenance therapy should not be needed. If symptoms recur after seemingly successful treatment, the patient should be tested for the presence of the organism (urea breath test or repeat endoscopy, depending on availability and cost). If *H. pylori* is present, it is probably not reinfection but incomplete treatment, and another course of treatment should be prescribed. If *H. pylori* is not found, evaluation for another cause of symptoms should be pursued.

In the case of *H. pylori*–negative duodenal ulcer (probably caused by NSAIDs), traditional treatment with H$_2$-receptor antagonists, sucralfate, or PPIs in recommended doses should be given (Table 37.3). Maintenance therapy should be considered only if severe gastrointestinal bleeding was associated with a duodenal ulcer. This can be accomplished with one-half the daily dose of whatever drug was given for acute healing.

Gastric Ulcer

In general, the same drugs available to treat duodenal ulcers are effective in the treatment of gastric ulcer. If *H. pylori* is present (and it should be sought), it should be eradicated, regardless of whether NSAIDs are thought to be implicated.

In general, healing must be documented, preferably by endoscopy. No dietary restriction affects healing, and hospitalization (in the absence of complications) is unnecessary. NSAIDs, including aspirin, should be discontinued. Smoking cessation should be strongly recommended. Maintenance therapy should be prescribed according to the guidelines for duodenal ulcer.

The prevention and treatment of gastropathy, associated with NSAIDs, are discussed in Chapter 70.

SURGICAL THERAPY

Surgery is effective therapy for the relief of ulcer symptoms and for the prevention of ulcer recurrence. With current therapy, surgery is almost never necessary except in emergencies. Although certain postoperative problems are common, most patients feel significantly better after surgery.

Indications

The indications for ulcer surgery are perforation, uncontrolled hemorrhage, gastric outlet obstruction, and rarely, intractability.

Before any elective surgery, some preoperative assessment should be made to rule out Zollinger–Ellison syndrome, hypercalcemia, and persistent *H. pylori* infection.

Types of Operations

Various operations are available for the treatment of ulcer disease. The physician should discuss with the surgeon the various alternatives and reach an agreement about which operation may be best suited

Table 37.3. Therapeutic Options for Eradication of *H. pylori*

Regimen	Drugs	Dosage	Duration
Dual therapy	Omeprazole	40 mg QD	2 wk
	Clarithromycin	500 mg TID	
	or		
	RBC	400 mg BID	4 wk
	Clarithromycin	500 mg TID	2 wk
Bismuth-based triple therapy	Bismuth subsalicylate	2 tablets QID	2 wk
	Metronidazole	250 mg QID	
	Tetracycline or	500 mg QID	
	amoxicillin	500 mg QID	
PPI-based triple therapy	Metronidazole or	500 mg BID	10–14 days
	amoxicillin	1000 mg BID	
	Omeprazole	20 mg BID	
PPI plus two antibiotics	Clarithromycin	500 mg BID	
Quadruple therapy	Bismuth-based triple therapy plus omeprazole	Triple therapy plus omeprazole 20 mg daily	14 days

RBC, Ranitidine and Bismuth Citrate.

for the individual patient. Of course, the final decision is generally made in the operating room after the surgeon has evaluated the gastroduodenal area. The patient should also be educated about the rationale for the planned surgical approach and the expected outcome.

Duodenal Ulcer

Three major operations are currently used for duodenal ulcer: *vagotomy with pyloroplasty, vagotomy with antrectomy,* and *parietal cell (or highly selective) vagotomy.* The first two procedures involve a selective vagotomy (gastric vagal fibers only) plus a drainage procedure to facilitate gastric emptying postoperatively. The third procedure involves cutting vagal fibers to the body (acid-secreting cells) of the stomach, preserving antral innervation, and eliminating the need for a drainage procedure. Vagotomy with pyloroplasty has the lowest mortality, shortest operation time, and a recurrence rate of 6 to 8%. Vagotomy with antrectomy is technically more difficult and may predispose patients to more postoperative morbidity (because an anastomosis to the remaining stomach is required) but has the lowest recurrence rate (less than 2%) (17). Postoperative complications (Table 37.4) are significantly more common with either procedure than with parietal cell vagotomy. A parietal cell vagotomy has a recurrence rate of 10% at 10 years (17), approximately four to five times that of vagotomy with antrectomy. Long-term complications (of dumping syndrome and diarrhea) are less than 60% those of vagotomy with antrectomy. In the hands of experienced surgeons a parietal cell vagotomy is the operation of choice. The higher recurrence rate (which can be managed medically in 80%) is an acceptable tradeoff for the decreased complication rate.

Gastric Ulcer

For gastric ulcers the type of surgery is less certain because understanding of the condition is less clear. In contrast to duodenal ulcer disease, a vagotomy may not be indicated in all patients with a gastric ulcer who undergo surgery. However, in patients who have evidence of concomitant duodenal ulcer disease (approximately 10 to 40% of patients with gastric ulcers) and in patients who have pyloric ulcers, which generally behave as duodenal ulcers, a vagotomy is clearly indicated. If the ulcer is within the antrum, an antrectomy or hemigastrectomy that includes the ulcer is often the preferred operation. When the ulcer cannot be included in the gastric resection, a full-thickness biopsy of the ulcer should be taken for frozen section to rule out malignancy. The recurrence rate for gastric ulcers after these types of operation is very low (1 to 2%).

After antrectomy or hemigastrectomy, the stomach may be anastomosed to the duodenum (Bilroth I anastomosis) or to the jejunum (Bilroth II). The type of anastomosis is determined by the surgeon based on the degree of duodenal deformity and on technical considerations.

Postgastrectomy Syndromes

Many problems develop after gastrectomy (Table 37.4). In 10% of patients, postgastrectomy complications are severe. Many of these conditions result from the altered physiology created by the surgery.

ZOLLINGER–ELLISON SYNDROME

The Zollinger–Ellison syndrome dramatically represents the relationship between gastrin, acid secretion, and ulcer formation. The syndrome results from a *non-β islet cell tumor* of the pancreas that autonomously secretes gastrin and is therefore called a *gastrinoma.* In most cases, multiple tumors are present, most commonly found in the head of the pancreas. These tumors vary considerably in size from several millimeters, often undetectable at surgery, to huge masses that may even be palpable through the abdominal wall. Approximately two-thirds of gastrinomas are malignant in their biologic behavior and histologic appearance; they can metastasize and be a cause of death, although generally they are slow growing.

With the introduction of readily available measurement of gastrin, the appreciation of the clinical features of Zollinger–Ellison syndrome has changed. The original description of the syndrome focused on the virulent nature of the ulcer diathesis and on the atypical location for the ulcers. It is now recognized, however, that 75% of ulcers in patients with Zollinger–Ellison syndrome occur in the duodenal bulb and appear as routine single duodenal ulcers. However, the finding of postbulbar and jejunal ulcerations should alert the physician to the possibility of the syndrome. More than one-fourth of patients undergo ulcer surgery before the diagnosis of the syndrome, which is usually made only when anastomotic ulcers develop. Diarrhea is another common symptom, occurring in more than one-third of patients, and may precede the formation of ulcers by several years; however, 7% of patients have diarrhea and never develop an ulcer. (The diarrhea is caused principally by the increased secretion of gastric acid, which, when it enters the duodenum, lowers the pH of the normally alkaline duodenal fluid and thereby interferes with absorption of water and electrolytes.)

Diagnosis

The diagnosis of Zollinger–Ellison syndrome should be considered under the following conditions: failure of medical therapy, giant ulcer, multiple ulcers, postbulbar or jejunal ulcers, anastomotic ulcer, ulcer disease in association with diarrhea (but not diarrhea secondary to drugs), and radiographic or secretory evidence of gastric hypersecretion.

The diagnosis of Zollinger–Ellison syndrome is usually based on the fasting serum gastrin concentration, normally less than 150 pg/mL. Elevations greater than 1000 pg/mL in association with the typical clinical picture are nearly diagnostic of a gastrinoma. How-

Table 37.4. Postgastrectomy Syndromes

Syndrome	Clinical Features	Pathophysiology	Diagnosis and Treatment
Early			
Stomal dysfunction	Vomiting, gastric retention	Edema, inflammation, hypokalemia	Electrolyte repletion, time, no suction
Duodenal stump dehiscence	Pain, fever, signs of abscess, sepsis, death	Bilroth II anastomosis: tension and poor closure, adjacent pancreatitis, excessive inflammation in area of surgery	Reoperation
Afferent loop syndrome	Pain, vomiting bile without food, may occur acutely or chronically	Bilroth II anastomosis: afferent loop too long, kinked, twisted, herniated, etc; loop fills, then empties	Reoperation
Vagotomy complications			
Transient dysphagia	Dysphagia	Lower esophageal sphincter dysfunction	Usually transient, disappears in 1–2 wk
Diarrhea	Diarrhea transient or slight, 20–40% of patients; troublesome, 5%; occurs mainly with selective vagotomy and drainage procedure	Most common after truncal vagotomy; appears to be related to increased output of dihydroxy bile salts, the cause of which is uncertain	Cholestyramine, Amphojel
Late or Persistent			
Dumping syndrome	Early phase: with or shortly after meals—nausea, abdominal fullness or pain, cramping, palpations, dizziness, sweating	Distension of gastric pouch and upper jejunum from rapid emptying; peripheral intravascular volume depletion from rapid entry of fluid into jejunum due to osmotic changes in jejunum; vasomotor symptoms related to release of vasoactive substances into circulation, such as serotonin and bradykinin	Small frequent meals, high protein, low carbohydrate, small volume of liquids only
	Late phase: symptoms of hypoglycemia	Early hyperglycemia → insulin production → late hypoglycemia	
Gastric cancer	Increased incidence of 3–5% in gastric stump 15–20 yr after surgery	Possibly related to chronic gastritis developing after gastrectomy	Endoscopy for diagnosis, surgical resection
Diarrhea	Chronic diarrhea	Rapid gastric emptying, lactose intolerance unmasked by vagotomy, malabsorption, Z–E syndrome, bile acid output increased, bacterial overgrowth	Lactose-free diet; if no response, malabsorption workup (Chapter 39)
Stomal or recurrent ulcer	Recurrent ulcer symptoms; hemorrhage in approximately 50%	Hyperacidity caused by inadequate resection, incomplete vagotomy, retained antrum, unrecognized Z–E syndrome (gastrinoma)	Endoscopy; H_2 antagonists, (successful in 80%), reoperation
Anemia	Iron deficiency	Chronic blood loss; impaired iron absorption	Repletion of deficient nutrient
	Nutritional anemia	Defective vitamin B_{12} absorption because of decreased intrinsic factor production (resection and gastritis); possible blind loop bacterial overgrowth; folate deficiency	
Osteomalacia	Bone pain	Diminished calcium intake, poor vitamin D absorption; duodenal bypass	

Z–E, Zollinger–Ellison.

ever, in patients with mild elevations of the serum gastrin concentration (between 150 and 300 pg/mL) and in postoperative patients, differentiation between Zollinger–Ellison syndrome and other causes for hypergastrinemia is important. Consultation with a gastroenterologist is advisable. Other conditions that may lead to hypergastrinemia include retained antrum, G-cell hyperplasia, postvagotomy plus pyloroplasty, small portion of the population with routine duodenal ulcer disease, and pernicious anemia. Also, H_2-receptor blockers cause a slight increase in the serum gastrin concentration, so these drugs should be stopped 12 hours before blood is drawn for the measurement. Proton pump inhibitors may cause elevation of serum gastrin for weeks to months after being stopped.

Differentiation of these disorders from the Zollinger–Ellison syndrome requires the use of provocative tests, the secretin and calcium infusion tests, generally performed by a gastroenterologist. The *secretin test* is preferred because it is more reliable and is safer. In both tests, the response of the serum gastrin level to the infusion of a stimulating substance is monitored. In the secretin test, the serum gastrin level rises, usually within the first half hour after the injection of secretin in patients with Zollinger–Ellison syndrome, whereas in all other disorders the gastrin level falls or is unchanged.

In the *calcium infusion test,* serum gastrin determinations are made immediately before and then repeatedly for 4 hours after the intravenous administration of calcium. In all conditions, the gastrin level increases. However, in the Zollinger–Ellison syndrome, the response is exaggerated with a rise more than 50% over basal levels.

Gastric analysis may provide further supportive data. Marked hypersecretion is found in both the basal state and after pentagastrin stimulation. Because the stomach is being influenced by an autonomous tumor, further stimulation with exogenous pentagastrin provides little additional stimulation to secretion. Thus, the basal acid output (BAO) to maximal acid output (MAO) ratio is 0.6 or greater in this syndrome. However, there is considerable overlap with normal values, so the gastric secretory data alone cannot be used to make the diagnosis.

Various attempts have been made to localize the gastrinoma in the hope that excision of an isolated tumor would be curative. Unfortunately, such efforts have been unsuccessful because multiple tumors are often present, small lesions are undetectable by surgical inspection of the pancreas, and these tumors often have metastasized by the time surgical exploration is performed [18]. The use of selective pancreatic venography with measurements of gastrin levels from each venous site may provide an improved method to localize the gastrinoma.

Therapy

Because the tumor mass is rarely localized and therefore rarely curable by local resection, therapy is directed at the end organ. Total gastrectomy historically has been the procedure of choice. Although little evidence exists to suggest that gastrectomy alters the biologic behavior of the gastrinoma, it does prevent the consequences of the hypersecretion of acid. In the past, patients died from this condition most often because of the virulent nature of the ulcer diathesis, including frequent recurrences, diarrhea, and even malabsorption, as well as multiple operations. Complete removal of the end organ prevents these complications. In some patients a parietal cell vagotomy may be an alternative to gastrectomy.

In recent years it has become clear that medical therapy is successful in controlling the ulcer disease and the diarrhea and that surgery is most often unnec-essary. The H^+–K^+–ATPase inhibitors omeprazole and lansoprazole are also extremely successful in controlling acid secretion in these patients, although high doses are often required. Long-term treatment with these agents is approved and is safe.

NONULCER DYSPEPSIA

Dyspepsia is a symptom of persistent epigastric discomfort, occasionally related to meals and sometimes associated with nausea, belching, or bloating [20,21]. It is estimated to be present in 7% of the United States population, most of whom rarely seek medical treatment. When patients with dyspepsia are evaluated with endoscopy, only 20 to 25% have demonstrable peptic ulcer disease or gastric cancer. Nonulcer dyspepsia presents a diagnostic and therapeutic dilemma.

If large groups of patients with nonulcer dyspepsia are evaluated, four major diseases are found to be associated: irritable bowel syndrome (IBS), cholelithiasis, gastroesophageal reflux, and chronic pancreatic disease. In IBS (see Chapter 40) the dyspepsia is associated with diffuse abdominal pain and altered bowel habits. Patients with gastroesophageal reflux disease have associated heartburn. Chronic pancreatic disease is less common but is usually associated with more severe pain and steatorrhea. The most difficult diagnostic dilemma, because of the high prevalence of gallstones in the general population, is distinguishing patients with symptomatic gallstones from patients with dyspepsia and asymptomatic (incidental) gallstones (see Chapter 90). It is now well established that patients with dyspepsia do not respond to cholecystectomy unless they have had an identifiable attack of acute cholecystitis or a history of biliary colic. The absence of either should suggest that gallstones are not the cause of dyspepsia.

Patients without one of these identifiable conditions are said to have *essential dyspepsia.* The etiology of this condition is unknown. A small subset of patients has been described with delayed gastric emptying of solids; however, correlation of improvement of symptoms with treatment has been poor. Approximately 50% of patients have *H. pylori* gastritis (see previous discussion). Again, symptomatic response to treatment for this infection has been inconsistent. It is clear that patients with essential dyspepsia do not have increased basal acid secretion, nor has a definite association with stress been documented.

The approach to the patient can be difficult. The yield of diagnostic procedures is low and, particularly with cholelithiasis, may be confusing. Response to empiric therapy with H_2 blockers has been disappointing and may be misleading and lead to inappropriate long-term therapy.

Until more controlled trials are available, patients younger than 40 years with a short history and no evidence of organic disease by physical examination and appropriate laboratory tests may be treated with reassurance, some modification of their diet, and avoidance of caffeine, alcohol, and tobacco. Drugs with a low incidence of side effects—such as H_2 blockers, sucralfate, and antacids—may be used, if necessary, in short courses of 3 to 4 weeks. If no response occurs in 4 weeks and no evidence of reflux disease or IBS is present, endoscopy should be performed. If endoscopy is negative, the other diagnoses should be pursued. Patients over age 60 are candidates for early investigation (within 1 to 2 weeks), particularly if symptoms are severe and have occurred for the first time. In this group the diagnostic yield for endoscopy is 60% (8,22). Patients who are not responsive to these measures are often treated for *H. pylori* infection (Table 37.3) if these organisms are demonstrated on gastric biopsy. Response is variable, and such treatment is not yet supported by appropriately designed trials.

The long-term prognosis is good with or without treatment in patients in whom endoscopy is negative.

GASTRITIS

Gastritis—inflammation of the stomach mucosa—is a nonspecific diagnosis that is made by endoscopic biopsy. It may be variably associated with dyspepsia, although a cause-and-effect relationship has not been documented. Several types of gastritis are seen in clinical practice.

Acute erosive, or *hemorrhagic, gastritis* is seen most commonly in seriously ill hospitalized patients; in patients taking NSAIDs, including aspirin; after heavy alcohol ingestion; and rarely in patients prescribed potassium chloride or iron supplements. Symptoms are variable but usually include nausea or vomiting and gastrointestinal bleeding that requires hospitalization.

Nonerosive or *chronic antral gastritis* is a histologic entity commonly seen in the general population, particularly the elderly. It is now well accepted that this condition is caused by *H. pylori* infection. However, it is unclear whether the histologic (or endoscopic) entity of gastritis is associated with symptomatic disease. There has been no demonstrated correlation between eradication of *H. pylori,* histologic resolution of gastritis, and relief of dyspepsia, bloating, abdominal pain, gas, and so on. In practice, patients with these syndromes should be treated as having nonulcer dyspepsia. Symptomatic treatment of patients with nonerosive gastritis is the same as it is for patients with nonulcer dyspepsia.

General References*

Feldman M, Scharschmidt F, Sleisenger MH, eds. Sleisenger and Fordtran's gastrointestinal and liver disease: pathophysiology,

---

*Bold print (general references) and bold numerals (specific references) denote published controlled clinical trials, meta-analyses, or consensus-based recommendations.

diagnosis, management, 6th ed. Philadelphia: WB Saunders, 1997. The standard text.

Specific References

1. Aspirin Myocardial Infarction Study Research Group. A randomized, controlled trial of aspirin in persons recovered from myocardial infarction. JAMA 243:661, 1980.
2. Bardhan KD, Hinchliffe RFC, Bose K. Low dose maintenance treatment with cimetidine in duodenal ulcer: intermediate term results. Postgrad Med J 62:347, 1986.
3. Bonnevie O. Survival in peptic ulcer. Gastroenterology 75:1055, 1978.
4. Committee on Endoscopic Utilization. Appropriate use of gastrointestinal endoscopy. Manchester, MA: American Society for Gastrointestinal Endoscopy, June 6, 1986.
5. Conn HO, Poynard T. Corticosteroid therapy does not induce peptic ulcer. J Intern Med 236:619, 1994.
6. Cutler AF, Havstad S, Ma CK, et al. Accuracy of invasive and noninvasive tests to diagnose *Helicobacter pylori* infection. Gastroenterology 109:136, 1995.
7. Cutler AF, Prasad VM. Long-term follow-up of *Helicobacter pylori* serology after successful eradication. Am J Gastroenterol 91:85, 1996.
8. Dooley CP, Larson AW, Stace NH, et al. Double contrast barium meal and upper gastrointestinal endoscopy. A comparative study. Ann Intern Med 101:538, 1984.
9. Faigel DO, Furth EE, Childs M, et al. Histological predictors of active *Helicobacter pylori* infection. Dig Dis Sci 41:937, 1996.
10. Fallone CA, Mitchell A, Paterson WG. Determination of the test performance of less costly methods of *Helicobacter pylori* infection. Clin Invest Med 18:177, 1995.
11. Fjosne U, Kleveland PM, Waldum H, et al. The clinical benefit of routine upper gastrointestinal endoscopy. A comparative study. Scand J Gastroenterol 21:433, 1986.
12. Fries JF, Miller SR, Spitz PW, et al. Toward an epidemiology of gastropathy associated with nonsteroidal antiinflammatory drug use. Gastroenterology 96:647, 1989.
13. Graham DY, Evans DJ, Peacock J, et al. Comparison of rapid serological tests (FlexSure HP and QuickVue) with conventional ELISA for detection of *Helicobacter pylori* infection. Am J Gastroenterol 91:942, 1996.
14. Graham DY, Lew GM, Evans DG, et al. Effect of triple therapy (antibiotics plus bismuth) on duodenal ulcer healing. A randomized controlled trial. Ann Intern Med 115:266, 1991.
15. Greenberg PD, Koch J, Cello JP. Clinical utility and cost effectiveness of *Helicobacter pylori* testing for patients with duodenal and gastric ulcers. Am J Gastroenterol 91:228, 1996.
16. Hentschel E, Brandstätter G, Dragosics B, et al. Effect of ranitidine and amoxicillin plus metronidazole on the eradication of *Helicobacter pylori* and the recurrence of duodenal ulcer. N Engl J Med 328:308, 1993.
17. Jordan PH, Thornby J. Should it be parietal cell vagotomy or selective vagotomy–antrectomy for treatment of duodenal ulcer. A progress report. Ann Surg 205:572, 1987.
18. McCarthy D. The place of surgery in the Zollinger–Ellison syndrome. N Engl J Med 302:1344, 1980.
19. McCarthy DM. Smoking and ulcers: time to quit (editorial). N Engl J Med 311:726, 1984.
20. National Institutes of Health. *Helicobacter pylori* in peptic ulcer disease. JAMA 272:65, 1994.
21. Sontag S, Graham DY, Belsito A, et al. Cimetidine, cigarette smoking, and recurrence of duodenal ulcer. N Engl J Med 311:689, 1984.
22. Talley NJ, Phillips SF. Nonulcer dyspepsia: potential causes and pathophysiology. Ann Intern Med 108:865, 1988.
23. Walsh JH, Peterson WL. The treatment of *Helicobacter pylori* infection in the management of peptic ulcer disease. N Engl J Med 334:984, 1995.

C H A P T E R   38

Gastrointestinal Bleeding

LAWRENCE J. CHESKIN, MD

The presence of blood in the stool or the upper gastrointestinal (GI) tract is always a significant finding that requires thorough investigation. GI bleeding may present as occult blood, melena (black stool) or intermittent hematochezia (the passage of overtly bloody stool), or hematemesis. Massive hemorrhage requires immediate hospitalization and often emergency diagnostic procedures. (The vomiting of blood, also, almost always dictates immediate hospitalization.) Otherwise, the evaluation of GI bleeding can often be performed in an ambulatory setting. Table 38.1 shows the common conditions associated with GI bleeding.

TESTS FOR DETECTION OF BLOOD IN STOOL

In normal subjects, the hemoglobin concentration of the stool is less than 2 mg hemoglobin per gram of stool, as measured by tagged red cell assay. The most commonly used test for fecal occult blood is the *modified guaiac slide test (Hemoccult)*. This test depends on the peroxidase activity of hemoglobin and reflects the concentration of hemoglobin in the stool. In mass screening programs, 1 to 16% of subjects have positive test results. Of these, 2 to 17% prove to have cancer (2 to 14% early stage cancer) (2) and 9 to 36% have adenomatous polyps. The rest have other causes of bleeding (e.g., gastritis or peptic ulcer), or no detectable source. The test is more specific than it is sensitive; one study predicted that testing stool for occult blood in asymptomatic people over age 45 as the primary screening method would fail to detect half of the cases of colorectal cancer (1). Because colonic cancers and polyps may bleed intermittently, sensitivity is improved when multiple stool specimens are evaluated. Left-sided lesions are detected more often than right-sided ones. In asymptomatic patients with a positive slide test who have carcinoma, more than 80% have early lesions limited to the bowel. Thus, a positive test for occult blood in the stool requires further investigation and may favorably influence the patient's prognosis.

Laxatives increase the numbers of both true-positive and false-positive results of the Hemoccult test (probably by an irritant effect on the normal colonic mucosa and on colonic lesions such as cancer). For this reason, some screening programs recommend a high-bulk diet for several days before the stool is tested in the hope of maximizing the discovery of occult lesions. False-negative results are more likely in patients taking large doses of vitamin C. Positive tests without clinical significance may result variably from hemoglobin or from peroxidase-rich foods (rare red meat and uncooked vegetables such as broccoli, turnips, and cauliflower), and from iron compounds. Salicylates and other nonsteroidal anti-inflammatory agents may cause occult GI bleeding, either because of a direct irritant effect on the stomach or duodenum or because of unmasking of an underlying lesion. Rehydration of the fecal material also increases the false-positive rate and is not recommended.

The optimal number and timing of the collection of stool samples have not been determined. The object is to detect bleeding from lesions that are known to bleed sporadically. To enhance compliance, convenience for the patient is also important. The usual recommendation is to obtain two different samples from three different stools over 3 days every year in patients over 40 years of age (see Chapter 2) (2). Patients should avoid raw red meat, large doses of vitamin C and aspirin, and other nonsteroidal anti-inflammatory agents for 3 days before and during the period of testing. The stool slides can be stored up to 6 days if necessary without a decrease in the sensitivity of the test.

EVALUATION OF PATIENTS WITH GASTROINTESTINAL BLEEDING

Choosing Appropriate Tests

The history and physical examination direct the sequence of the various tests used to investigate GI bleeding. The patient's age, medical history, and social history; the nature of associated symptoms; and the severity of bleeding are all important factors. For example, patients with peptic symptoms or with risk factors such as the use of nonsteroidal anti-inflammatory medications (see Chapter 37) require an initial evaluation of their esophagus, stomach, and duodenum, whereas patients with a change in bowel habits require an initial evaluation of their colon and rectum. In general, patients under the age of 50 are less likely to have a colonic lesion than are patients 50 or older. Peptic disease and benign rectal lesions are more evenly distributed in adults of all ages.

In asymptomatic patients with occult fecal blood or

Table 38.1.   Common Causes of Gastrointestinal Bleeding

Occult Bleeding
Gastritis, especially caused by nonsteroidal anti-inflammatory
   agents or ethanol
Peptic ulcer disease
Colonic polyps
Colonic cancer
Gastric cancer
Esophagitis

Melena
Peptic ulcer disease
Hemorrhagic gastritis
Gastric carcinoma

Hematochezia
Diverticulosis
Angiodysplasia
Rectal outlet disorders (hemorrhoids, cryptitis, fissures)
Inflammatory bowel disease
Colonic polyps
Colonic cancer

Hematemesis
Peptic ulcer disease
Esophageal varices
Mallory–Weiss tear
Hemorrhagic gastritis
Gastric cancer

in patients with hematochezia but with no other symptoms, the lower bowel should generally be investigated first. In patients with hematemesis or melena but with no other symptoms, the upper GI tract should be investigated first. One reasonable approach to the evaluation of lower and upper GI bleeding is described in the next two sections of this chapter.

Lower Gastrointestinal Tract

For patients presenting with hematochezia, flexible or (less commonly) rigid proctosigmoidoscopy is usually the first test done to evaluate the lower bowel. If inconclusive, it should be followed by an *air-contrast barium enema* or a *colonoscopy*. Barium enema is slightly less costly than *flexible sigmoidoscopy;* colonoscopy is approximately four times as costly (six times, if performed with polypectomy). In patients over the age of 40 or 50, colonoscopy should be performed as the initial test.

The finding of hemorrhoids, polyps, or even a rectal cancer on flexible sigmoidoscopy does not obviate examination of the rest of the colon. However, in patients under 50, if the pattern of bleeding is consistent with rectal disease (see Chapter 92) and a rectal lesion is seen during proctosigmoidoscopy, colonoscopy is not always necessary. Also, diverticulosis (see Chapter 41), found on barium enema, should not be considered the cause of intermittent mild hematochezia until colonoscopy has failed to provide another explanation.

For patients with occult fecal blood and no localizing symptoms, a colonoscopy or a flexible sigmoidoscopy plus a barium enema is the minimum recommended workup (2).

Proctosigmoidoscopy

Anorectal lesions are poorly visualized by barium enema. Cryptitis, bleeding hemorrhoids, fissures, and proctitis can be seen only by rigid or flexible proctoscopy. Even rectal polyps or cancer are much better revealed by proctoscopy than by a barium enema. The preparation of the patient for this procedure and the patient's experience during the procedure are described in Chapter 36.

Flexible sigmoidoscopy is used to evaluate the rectum and descending colon. It is better tolerated and identifies more proximal lesions than does rigid proctosigmoidoscopy. It is most useful in screening asymptomatic patients for colorectal adenoma or carcinoma (18). It is not recommended for evaluating patients with GI bleeding because colonoscopy is still required to exclude more proximal colonic lesions.

Barium Enema

The *barium enema* is a valuable test in the detection of colonic lesions. Even in patients with suspected anorectal disease, a colonoscopy or barium enema is indicated to rule out other lesions, particularly in patients at high risk for polyps and cancer. The barium enema may also detect diverticula, inflammatory bowel disease, strictures, extraluminal masses, or intramural filling defects from endometriosis or metastatic tumor.

The double (air) contrast barium technique is preferred in the search for a colonic source of bleeding. This technique has the advantage over the conventional single-contrast barium enema in providing much better detail of the mucosa. Early changes of inflammatory bowel disease can also be detected by this technique, although not with as high a sensitivity as colonoscopy. However, because of the risk of perforation, the double-contrast barium enema should not be performed in patients suspected of having an obstructing lesion or acute diverticulitis.

Patient Experience. The patient's colon must be cleaned before the study can be performed satisfactorily. A reasonable regimen is the ingestion of 2 to 3 L of liquids and a low-residue diet (see Table 39.2, Chapter 39) the day before the examination and administration of a laxative, such as 2 to 4 tablespoons of milk of magnesia at night; on the morning of the examination, a sodium phosphate (Fleet) enema is self-administered. This preparation is effective in approximately 90% of patients. Patients who are chronically constipated may need 2 days of preparation. The preparation often causes cramping and urgency but is important to the examination and should be encouraged.

The patient should be told that the barium will be introduced into the rectum through a lubricated plastic enema tip while the patient lies on his or her left side on a hard table. Often a balloon is then inflated around the tip to seal the rectal ampulla. The patient is then told to lie supine while the barium is allowed to flow in, intermittently, under fluoroscopic observation. Often, the patient experiences cramping during this process. After the colon is filled, several films are taken, with the patient in various positions. The barium is then evacuated. The films are developed and an additional film is taken after evacuation. The entire procedure takes 45 to 60 minutes.

The air-contrast barium enema differs from the standard technique in that a smaller amount of very dense barium is introduced, followed by insufflation of air. All patients experience cramping during this procedure (usually more than is experienced during the standard barium enema), and atropine may be given to inhibit cramping. The patient is flatulent for several hours after the procedure.

Colonoscopy

Colonoscopy is indicated in patients with GI bleeding of suspected colonic origin, either as the initial test or as a follow-up examination when proctosigmoidoscopy and barium enema have not provided an unequivocal diagnosis. Most gastroenterologists perform colonoscopy instead of a barium enema plus flexible sigmoidoscopy because of its higher positive predictive value in the evaluation of rectal bleeding (9). Also, in patients with polyps, colonoscopy provides a way to remove the polyps without major surgery. An experienced endoscopist can reach the cecum in more than 90% of cases. The complications from the procedure are mainly perforation and hemorrhage; the overall complication rate for diagnostic colonoscopy is 0.3 to 0.4%, with a mortality rate of 0.02%. If polypectomy is performed, the morbidity rate increases to 1 to 2%, but the mortality rate remains the same.

The sensitivity of colonoscopy in experienced hands is much higher than that of even an air-contrast barium enema (see previous discussion): Only 2% of polyps are not diagnosed. In a study of anemic patients with occult bleeding, colonoscopy revealed polyps (greater than 5 mm in diameter) or cancer in 15% of patients with negative barium enema examinations and, in patients with rectal bleeding, 34% had a significant lesion (including 11% with cancer) when the barium enema was reported as negative or simply as showing diverticulosis (17).

Patient Experience. Preparation for colonoscopy usually includes a liquid diet for 2 or 3 days and laxatives and enemas (prescribed by the consultant gastroenterologist). An alternative preparation is to drink 4 L of a nonabsorbed isosmolar salt solution the night before the procedure (Golytely or Colyte). Elderly patients may have difficulty ingesting this amount of fluid, in which case the standard laxative preparation (see the previous section, "Barium Enema") may be preferable. Just before the procedure, the patient is sedated intravenously (usually with meperidine plus diazepam or midazolam). During the procedure, the patient may experience discomfort when the bowel is distended with air for inspection and as the colonoscope is maneuvered through the bowel lumen. There is no additional discomfort when a biopsy or polypectomy is performed. The duration of the procedure is variable, depending on the tortuosity of the colon, the presence of disease, and the skill of the endoscopist, but the average is 30 to 60 minutes. Someone must be available to accompany the patient home after the procedure because of possible lingering sedation. In patients who are at

risk of endocarditis (see Chapter 60), antibiotic prophylaxis must be given by the endoscopist before and after the procedure (see Table 86.12).

Upper Gastrointestinal Tract

The sequence of tests performed in evaluating the upper GI tract depends on the severity of the bleeding and the suspected diagnosis. *Upper endoscopy,* or *esophagogastroduodenoscopy (EGD),* has become the procedure of choice for most patients with upper GI bleeding. An *upper GI series* is sometimes done first in patients with suspected peptic disease or carcinoma when the bleeding is chronic or occult. On the other hand, if an inflammatory process is suspected (esophagitis or gastritis), endoscopy should be done because contrast radiography is less sensitive in detecting mucosal lesions that are not severe. Also, in acutely bleeding patients, *endoscopy* is indicated because actively bleeding lesions can often be treated at the time of the procedure, by endoscopic sclerotherapy in the case of bleeding esophageal varices or by electrocautery in the case of bleeding ulcers or angiodysplasias. If an upper GI series has been performed first and is negative or reveals a gastric ulcer (Chapter 37) or a tumor, endoscopy should be the next routine procedure. Upper GI series and upper endoscopy have approximately the same cost. If the upper and lower GI tracts have been evaluated in a patient with GI bleeding and the studies have been negative, a *small bowel series* should be considered to investigate the possibility of Crohn's disease and other disorders that affect mainly the small intestine.

Radiologic Studies

The *upper GI series* is helpful in the detection of mass lesions in the esophagus and stomach and in identifying gastric and duodenal ulcerations, although it does not allow mucosal biopsy for *Helicobacter pylori.* It is well tolerated and inexpensive. The patient's experience during the performance of an upper GI series is described in Chapter 37.

The conventional *small bowel series* is very poor at detecting small lesions of the intestine (e.g., cancer or leiomyoma). Disorders such as Crohn's disease or lymphoma are more likely to be revealed by radiograph (although a definitive diagnosis can be made only by biopsy). These sources of bleeding are uncommon and should be suspected only when the more common conditions (peptic ulcer disease, colonic polyps) have been excluded. The patient should be warned that the small bowel series requires spending 1 to 5 hours in the radiology department, during which time films are taken every 30 minutes.

Endoscopy

Upper endoscopy is the most widely used means of investigating GI blood loss. This technique not only is more sensitive than radiography but also provides a direct means of obtaining specimens for histologic examination. Because of its greater sensitivity, endoscopy is indicated even if barium studies have been negative in the evaluation of a suspected upper GI source of bleeding.

Patient Experience. Upper endoscopy is an outpatient procedure that usually takes less than 15 minutes. The patient fasts overnight before the procedure. Just before the procedure, the patient is sedated with intravenous medication (meperidine plus diazepam or midazolam) and the throat is anesthetized with a topical anesthetic. Some gagging is common during passage of the endoscope into the esophagus. Under direct vision, mucosal biopsies and cytologic brushings can be obtained from suspicious lesions for histologic confirmation. Biopsies are completely painless. Complications include perforation and bleeding but are extremely uncommon. Newer, smaller-caliber endoscopes have greatly improved patient tolerance of the procedure. After the procedure, because of the sedation, someone must be available to drive the patient home. The patient typically has a sore throat for several hours.

SELECTED LESIONS THAT BLEED

The most common cause of upper GI bleeding—peptic disease—is discussed in Chapter 37. Several common causes of lower GI bleeding are discussed in other chapters: benign anorectal disorders (Chapter 92), inflammatory bowel disease (Chapter 39), and diverticulosis (Chapter 41).

Colonic Polyps

Colonic polyps or colonic cancer should be suspected in any patient over 40 years of age who has GI bleeding or a change in bowel habits. Bleeding may be occult or may occur as intermittent hematochezia. The patient is often totally asymptomatic but may complain of a change in bowel habits, abdominal pain, or passing mucus through the rectum. It is believed that all cancers of the colon (except those associated with ulcerative colitis; see Chapter 39) arise from these benign epithelial tumors, although only a small percentage of premalignant polyps grow into invasive cancers. It has been estimated that it takes a minimum of 5 years for an early polyp to become an invasive cancer. Thus, the removal of polyps before they become malignant has the potential to prevent the occurrence of colonic cancer in predisposed individuals. Although polyps are most common in the rectosigmoid region, they may be found anywhere in the colon. The detection of a polyp on proctoscopy or barium enema is an indication for referral to a gastroenterologist.

The risk of polyps becoming malignant is related to their histologic type and size. *Hyperplastic polyps* make up 10 to 30% of all colorectal polyps. They tend to be small (less than 0.5 cm) and located in the distal colon or rectum, and they probably have no malignant potential. *Villous and tubular adenomas* make up almost two-thirds of all colorectal polyps, are found in 25% of people by age 50 (and in 50% by age 80), and carry a definite risk of malignant transformation that

increases as they increase in size. The risk that a villous adenoma over 2 cm is cancerous is more than 50% (Table 38.2) (15). Fortunately, if the cancer remains confined to the mucosa of the polyp *(carcinoma in situ)*, colonoscopic polypectomy is curative. Once the cancer has infiltrated the stalk of the polyp, surgery is indicated. Because the cancerous change in the polyp may be focal, single biopsies of a polyp are not sufficient to exclude the presence of a malignancy; the entire polyp must be excised.

Once an adenomatous or villous polyp has been detected, surveillance for additional polyps is indicated. In 30% of patients, more than one polyp is present at the time of initial investigation and the risk of recurrence rises with the number and size of polyps that are initially discovered. Subsequent development of new polyps occurs in at least 10% of patients. The patient should continue to be tested yearly for occult blood in the stool. The finding of a single positive test is an indication for a repeated evaluation. Even when the stools are negative for blood, periodic evaluation of the colon is still recommended. Colonoscopy, or air-contrast barium enema plus flexible sigmoidoscopy, should be repeated every 3 years. If a follow-up examination reveals no further polyps, the screening interval may be increased to once every 5 years.

Multiple polyposis syndromes are rare inherited abnormalities that are significant for their malignant potential. *Familial polyposis, Gardner's syndrome,* and *Turcot syndrome* all are associated with multiple adenomatous polyps of the colon (Fig. 38.1) and therefore carry a high risk of the development of carcinoma. Gardner's syndrome includes osteomas and soft tissue tumors, and Turcot syndrome includes tumors of the central nervous system. Familial polyposis and Gardner's syndrome are inherited as an autosomal dominant defect, Turcot syndrome as an autosomal recessive. The diagnosis of a polyposis syndrome is usually made when the patient is in his or her twenties, with cancer developing in virtually all patients by some 20 years later. There is considerable controversy about the therapy for these conditions. Colonic resection is indicated, but its extent and timing are not uniformly agreed on. Ideally, when rectal polyps are present, a proctocolectomy should be performed to eliminate the risk of cancer. However, because the patients are generally asymptomatic and young, the prospect of an ileostomy (see Chapter 42) is often overwhelming to them. Newer operations involving ileorectal pull-through procedures are now available, and results are encouraging (see Chapter 42). Consultation with a

Table 38.2. Polyps: Relationship of Size, Histologic Type, and Risk of Carcinoma

Histologic Type	% That Are Cancerous		
	Under 1 cm	1–2 cm	More than 2 cm
Tubular adenoma	1.0	10.2	34.7
Intermediate type	3.9	7.4	45.8
Villous adenoma	9.5	10.3	52.9

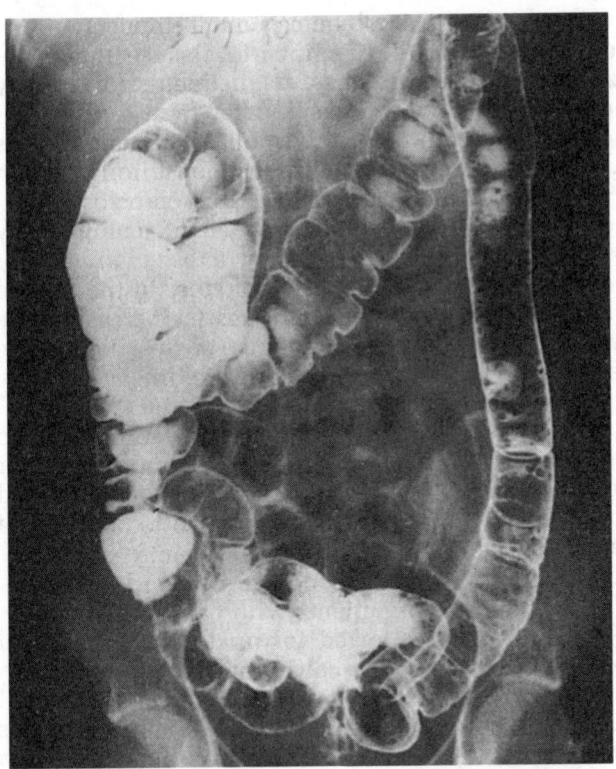

Figure 38.1. Double (air) contrast barium enema performed in a patient with familial polyposis. With this technique, numerous polyps of varying sizes may be seen throughout the colon.

gastroenterologist and a gastrointestinal surgeon is recommended as soon as the diagnosis is made.

Colonic polyposis syndromes should be distinguished from conditions associated with juvenile polyps or hamartomas that are of low malignant potential. The *Peutz–Jeghers syndrome* consists of multiple hamartomas, predominantly of the small intestine, associated with buccal and cutaneous pigmentation. Although the malignant potential of the hamartomas is low, duodenal and ovarian carcinomas have been reported in 2 to 5% of patients. Rarely, juvenile polyps may occur throughout the GI tract. In the absence of associated extracolonic manifestations, this syndrome is called *generalized juvenile polyposis;* when accompanied by alopecia, nail bed changes, hyperpigmentation, and malabsorption, it is called the *Cronkhite–Canada* syndrome.

Colorectal Cancer

Epidemiology and Etiology

Cancers of the colon and rectum account for 14% of all cancers and are the second leading cause of cancer death overall in the United States. There is approximately a 5% lifetime chance of developing a colorectal cancer.

Colorectal cancer occurs with increasing frequency in older age groups, with two-thirds occurring in people over 65 years of age. Geographic differences in the mortality rates due to this neoplasm suggest an etiologic role for dietary and environmental factors. In particular, a high-fat, low-fiber diet appears to be associated with an increased risk of colorectal cancer. For unclear reasons, the proportion of cancers in the right side of the colon has increased in recent years, with a commensurate drop in the proportion of rectosigmoid lesions (6). Currently, about half of colorectal cancers are within reach of the flexible sigmoidoscope. The remaining half are proximal to the splenic flexure and accessible only with a colonoscope. The three main predisposing conditions for colorectal cancer are colonic polyps, familial polyposis (see previous discussion), and ulcerative colitis (see Chapter 39). The presence of these conditions dictates the need for a strict colonoscopic surveillance program in patients with these conditions and at times even prophylactic surgery to prevent the development of cancer. (See Chapter 39 for the risk of cancer in ulcerative colitis.) Although it is accepted that a family history of colorectal cancer predisposes one to polyps and colorectal cancer, there is some evidence that the risk does not rise significantly above that of the general population unless more than one first-degree relative has had colorectal cancer (7).

Screening Tests

Because of the high incidence of colon cancer and its precursor, the colonic polyp, screening tests should be performed routinely in all patients over 50 years old. A number of large, randomized trials show that annual or biennial fecal occult blood testing decreases the 8- to 15-year cumulative mortality from colorectal cancer by 16 to 33%, compared with no screening (8,10,12,13). The most comprehensive screening program would involve periodic colonoscopy, but its cost and complications make this perhaps less desirable for patients who are at average risk. One reasonable compromise between cost and efficacy is the guidelines offered by the American Cancer Society, which are that two specimens from three consecutive stools should be tested for occult blood annually by use of the guaiac-card test. These cards are convenient for the patient because they can be mailed to the physician's office without a significant loss in sensitivity.

In addition, a yearly rectal examination should be performed in the average-risk patient 50 and over. Proctosigmoidoscopy, preferably by use of a flexible sigmoidoscope, should also be performed to ensure a normal rectal and rectosigmoid area. Subsequently, flexible sigmoidoscopy can be performed every 5 years in the asymptomatic patient who has negative tests for fecal occult blood. A retrospective case-control study published in 1992 of patients 45 years of age and older who had been followed for 17 years revealed that screening sigmoidoscopy reduced deaths from colon cancer by nearly 60% (18).

Diagnosis

History. The chromosomal changes that accompany the progression of normal colonic mucosa to adenoma to carcinoma have been elucidated (11).

There may soon be a means to detect people who are at increased risk of developing colorectal cancer so that surveillance can be focused on them. Unfortunately, most patients with adenocarcinoma of the colon are diagnosed only after symptoms have developed. Fewer than 10% are asymptomatic at time of diagnosis, and it is in this group that the highest chance for cure exists. The major presenting symptoms are abdominal pain (25 to 75%) and a change in bowel habits (20 to 50%), either constipation or diarrhea. Abdominal pain is least common in patients with cancer of the rectum, where even large lesions can be accommodated without producing symptoms. Gross blood in the stool is another common complaint, occurring in 75% of patients with rectal cancer and 30 to 40% of patients with colonic cancer above the rectum. Unfortunately, this hematochezia is often mistakenly attributed to hemorrhoids. Presentation with anemia or with weight loss is also common.

Physical Examination.   The findings on physical examination vary according to the location and extent of the lesion. The primary tumor may be palpable as an abdominal mass, particularly in cancer of the right colon, where lesions can remain asymptomatic for long periods. Metastatic disease may be suggested by the presence of a large, hard, nodular liver; ascites; peripheral adenopathy; or the palpation of a mass in the cul-de-sac on rectal examination. Signs of anemia may be present, particularly in lesions of the cecum and ascending colon that may bleed occultly for months or even years before the diagnosis is made. Most patients have a positive test result for occult blood sometime during their course of illness.

Barium Enema.   The diagnosis of colon cancer is sometimes made by barium enema. Findings may include a polypoid mass, stenosis (either as a stricture or with an "apple-core" appearance), distortion of the mucosa, and localized rigidity of the bowel wall. At times, distortion or fixation of adjacent structures may be seen. The development of a gastrocolic fistula, best seen on barium enema, is also suggestive of a primary colonic neoplasm.

It has traditionally been said that the accuracy of the barium enema for the diagnosis of colon cancer is excellent, except at opposite ends of the large bowel. The cecum is often difficult to evaluate because of the inability to cleanse the region completely and, at times, to distinguish a prominent ileocecal valve or sphincter from a mass. The rectum is also difficult to visualize optimally because often it is obscured by the balloon through which the barium is administered. Thus, proctoscopy or flexible sigmoidoscopy is usually recommended in addition to a barium enema in patients suspected of having a colorectal carcinoma. However, a recent study found no difference in sensitivity of the barium enema in detecting cancer in the right colon or the left colorectum (17).

Endoscopy.   The role of endoscopy in the diagnosis of colorectal cancer continues to increase. Some polypoid lesions, even if large or sessile, can be removed via the colonoscope, avoiding surgery in many cases. In addition, colonoscopy has an important role in the evaluation for other colonic lesions. The prevalence of coexistent polyps in patients with colon cancer is high, ranging from 10 to 30%. These residual polyps may develop later into carcinoma, accounting for the incidence of a second colon cancer in 5 to 10% of patients with cancer of the colon who have been followed for up to 25 years (15). In addition, synchronous colon carcinomas occur in 3 to 5% of patients. Thus, colonoscopy is helpful in ensuring that the rest of the colon is free of neoplastic lesions. Optimally, colonoscopy should be performed preoperatively; otherwise, it should be done within the first year postoperatively. In a very large recent survey in Indiana, the sensitivity of colonoscopy for the detection of colorectal carcinoma was 95%, whereas that of barium enema was 83% (17). Also noteworthy is that there is a significant miss rate for colonoscopy. For precursor polyps, colonoscopy failed to detect 27% of lesions 0.5 cm or smaller, and 6% of lesions 1 cm or larger (16).

Carcinoembryonic Antigen

Carcinoembryonic antigen (CEA) is a normal fetal antigen found in the blood of many patients with colorectal carcinoma (from 30% of patients with local disease to 83% of patients with metastatic disease). It is also commonly found in the blood of patients with other malignancies, in cigarette smokers, or with a variety of benign conditions, including peptic ulcer, pancreatitis, diverticulitis, and inflammatory bowel disease. Therefore, the CEA titer is not a useful screening test for the presence of colorectal cancer.

Although its efficacy and cost-effectiveness for this purpose have been questioned (14), the assay may be helpful in the postoperative treatment of patients who have elevated blood CEA levels at the time of diagnosis. Persistently elevated CEA levels postoperatively suggest metastatic disease; falling levels that then rise on follow-up evaluation suggest the reemergence of the malignancy, usually at a remote site.

Therapy

Surgery is the most effective therapy for most cases of colon carcinoma. Inoperable tumors (including metastatic tumors) respond 20 to 40% of the time to 5-fluorouracil plus other chemotherapeutic agents, preferably prescribed by or with the advice of an oncologist. However, there is no clear effect of such therapy on survival. Operable tumors at an advanced stage (Table 38.3) should be treated with the same drugs, and in such cases, there is some survival benefit.

Anal cancers should be treated, if possible, in specialized centers with radiation and chemotherapy and then, if possible, should be surgically removed.

Preoperative Evaluation

Before surgery, most patients should undergo evaluation for metastatic disease. Liver function tests should be performed routinely, as well as computerized tomography (CT) or ultrasound of the liver. In patients with bowel obstruction or bleeding, surgery may still be needed as palliation, despite the presence of liver metastases. In patients asymptomatic from their bowel

Table 38.3.   Colon Carcinoma

Classification[a]	Staging and 5-Year Survival	
	Microscopic Findings	5-Year Survival (%)
A	Disease limited to mucosa	95
B	Tumor extends to serosa	60–70
C	Tumor extends to serosa and nodes involved	<40
D	Distant metastases	<5

[a]Modification of the Dukes classification.

lesions, the presence of multiple hepatic metastases should deter surgical intervention (single hepatic metastases are often resectable). However, abnormal liver function tests alone should not be considered absolute evidence of metastatic disease. A histologic diagnosis should be made, if possible. Needle liver biopsy is a simple way to obtain tissue and may be guided by ultrasound or CT. A preoperative CEA level should also be determined as a baseline.

For patients requiring an ostomy, preoperative evaluation by an enterostomal therapist is helpful, not only to discuss with the patient problems and concerns about the ostomy, but also to mark the proper location of the ostomy preoperatively (see Chapter 42).

Prognosis

The prognosis of colorectal carcinoma is based on several variables. The major variable is the extent of the tumor, in terms of its invasion through the bowel wall and of its lymph node involvement (Table 38.3). Vessel invasion and the degree of differentiation of the tumor histologically also affect survival. The pathologist's interpretation of the resected specimen is much more meaningful than the surgeon's estimation of curability.

Follow-up Care

Most patients undergoing resection for colorectal cancer do well in the early postoperative period. Diarrhea may be present early but is usually transient and easily controlled with antidiarrheal medication. The patient with a colostomy needs continued follow-up care by the surgeon and the enterostomal therapist to ensure proper functioning and handling of the ostomy (see Chapter 42).

The long-term follow-up is aimed at detection of recurrence or spread of the cancer and at continued surveillance for new colonic lesions. Most commonly, metastases occur in adjacent nodes, with eventual spread to the liver. Physical examinations, liver function tests, and CEA levels are usually done every 2 to 6 months for 3 to 5 years. Abdominal CT scans must be obtained to assess a confirmed rise in CEA levels or liver function tests, but whether long-term outcome is improved is unclear, despite earlier detection of recurrent tumor.

To evaluate for synchronous colonic lesions, colonoscopy should be performed within the first 6 to 12 months postoperatively if it has not already been done preoperatively. If no lesions are found, colonoscopy should be repeated 3 years later. The interval may then be increased to once every 5 years if no recurrence or adenomatous polyps are detected. Yearly evaluation for occult fecal blood loss should also be performed,

with three to six Hemoccult cards. If any of these are positive, colonoscopy should be repeated.

Arteriovenous Malformations of the Colon

Arteriovenous malformations of the colon are a common source of GI bleeding (3,4), most often in the elderly and in patients with chronic renal failure. A variety of terms have been used to describe these abnormalities, including *angiodysplasia, hemangioma,* and *vascular ectasia.* The etiology of the disorder is unknown. Although the lesions may occur throughout the GI tract, they appear most commonly in the mucosa of the cecum and ascending colon, where multiple lesions are often found, ranging in size from 1 mm to more than 1 cm. An association of angiodysplasia of the colon with aortic stenosis has been observed repeatedly (3).

The prevalence of angiodysplasias and the frequency with which they cause bleeding are uncertain. With increasing use of endoscopy and selective angiography, the disorder is being recognized more often. In one study of patients over the age of 60 without a history of GI bleeding, submucosal vascular ectasis was detected in 53% and mucosal lesions in 27% (3). Angiodysplasias may be the most common cause of bleeding from the right colon, and they and diverticula are the most common causes of major lower intestinal bleeding in the elderly (19).

These lesions, when they bleed, often produce hematochezia. The bleeding is sometimes brisk and may be massive, but occult blood loss may also occur, and seems to be an increasingly common presentation of this disorder (5). Bleeding often stops spontaneously but commonly recurs. The lesions cannot be detected by barium enema, are not recognizable from the serosal surface by the surgeon, and are often overlooked by the pathologist. The diagnosis is best made by selective arteriography (by which a malformation can be visualized even when the bleeding has stopped) or by colonoscopy. However, like diverticula, the mere presence of angiodysplasias does not incriminate them as the source of bleeding, and other potential sources should be sought. Lesions that have bled should be excised, preferably by surgical resection of the involved segment of colon. However, colonoscopic cauterization of discrete mucosal lesions can be performed by an experienced gastroenterologist.

Physicians should be aware of this disorder, especially in elderly patients with GI bleeding in whom initial evaluation is unrevealing, but the diagnosis is made only after consultation with a gastroenterologist or radiologist.

General References*

American College of Physicians. Suggested technique for fecal occult blood testing and interpretation in colorectal cancer screening. Ann Intern Med 126:808, 1997.
   The formal position of the ACP.

*Bold print (general references) and bold numerals (specific references) denote published controlled clinical trials, meta-analyses, or consensus-based recommendations.

Potter GD, Sellin JH. Lower gastrointestinal bleeding. Gastroenterol Clin North Am 17(2):341, 1988.

Ransohoff DF, Lang CA. Sigmoidoscopic screening in the 1990s. JAMA 269:1278, 1993.

Ransohoff DF, Lang CA. Screening for colorectal cancer with the fecal occult blood test: a background paper. Ann Intern Med 126:811, 1997.
> The supporting data for the ACP position (see American College of Physicians, 1997).

Winauer SJ, Fletcher RH, Miller L, et al. Colorectal cancer screening: clinical guidelines and rationale. Gastroenterology 112:594, 1997.
> Consensus guidelines endorsed by the American Gastroenterological Association, the American Cancer Society, the American College of Gastroenterology, the American Society for Gastrointestinal Endoscopy, and others.

Specific References

1. Allison JE, Feldman R, Tekawa IS. Hemoccult screening in detecting colorectal neoplasm: sensitivity, specificity, and predictive value. Long term follow-up in a large group practice setting. Ann Intern Med 112:328, 1990.
2. American College of Physicians. Suggested technique for fecal occult blood testing and interpretation in colorectal cancer screening. Ann Intern Med 126:808, 1997.
3. Boley SJ, Sammartano R, Adams A, et al. Nature and etiology of vascular ectasias of the colon. Gastroenterology 72:650, 1977.
4. Cheung PS, Wong SK, Boey J, et al. Frank rectal bleeding: a prospective study of causes in patients over the age of 40. Postgrad Med J 64:364, 1988.
5. Coppell MS, Gupta A. Changing epidemiology of GI angiodysplasia with increasing recognition of clinically milder cases. Am J Gastroenterol 87:201, 1992.
6. Devesa SS, Chow WH. Variation in colorectal cancer incidence in the United States by subsite of origin. Cancer 71:3819, 1993.
7. Grossman S, Milos ML. Colonoscopic screening of persons with suspected risk factors for colon cancer. I. Family history. Gastroenterology 94:395, 1988.
8. Hardcastle JD, Chamberlain JO, Robinson MH, et al. Randomized controlled trial of fecal-occult-blood screening for colorectal cancer. Lancet 348:1472, 1996.
9. Irvine EJ, O'Connor J, Frost RA, et al. Prospective comparison of double contrast barium enema plus flexible sigmoidoscopy v. colonoscopy in rectal bleeding. Gut 29:1188, 1988.
10. Kewenter J, Brevinge H, Engaras B, et al. Results of screening, rescreening, and follow-up in a prospective, randomized study for detection of colorectal cancer by fecal occult blood testing. Results for 68,308 subjects. Scand J Gastroenterol 29:468, 1994.
11. Kinzler KW, Nilber TMC, Vogelstein B, et al. Identification of a gene located at chromosome 5q21 that is mutated in colorectal cancers. Science 251(4999):1366, 1991.
12. Kronborg O, Fenger C, Olsen J, et al. Randomized study of screening for colorectal cancer with faecal-occult-blood test. Lancet 348:1467, 1996.
13. Mandel JS, Bond JH, Church TR, et al. Reducing mortality from colorectal cancer by screening for fecal occult blood. N Engl J Med 328:1365, 1993.
14. Moertel CG, Fleming TR, Macdonald JS, et al. An evaluation of the CEA test for monitoring patients with resected colon cancer. JAMA 270:943, 1993.
15. Muto T, Bussey HJ, Morson BL. The evolution of cancer of the colon and rectum. Cancer 36:2251, 1975.
16. Rex DK, Cutler CS, Lemmel GT, et al. Colonoscopic miss rates of adenomas determined by back-to-back colonoscopies. Gastroenterology 112:24, 1997.
17. Rex DK, Rahmani EY, Haseman JH, et al. Relative sensitivity of colonoscopy and barium enema for detection of colorectal cancer in clinical practice. Gastroenterology 112:17, 1997.
18. Selby J-V, Friedman GD, Quesenberry CP Jr, et al. A case-control study of screening sigmoidoscopy and mortality from colorectal cancer. N Engl J Med 326:653, 1992.
19. Tedesco F, Wayne J, Raskin J, et al. Colonoscopic evaluation of rectal bleeding: a study of 304 patients. Ann Intern Med 89:907, 1978.

CHAPTER 39

Constipation and Diarrhea

LAWRENCE J. CHESKIN, MD

CONSTIPATION

Definition

Constipation is often defined as the infrequent, difficult passage of stool. However, it may mean different things to different people: that the stools are too infrequent, too difficult to expel, too hard, or too small, or that there is a sensation of incomplete evacuation. Of these, frequency of bowel movements is the most readily measured. Several studies have identified a wide variation in the frequency of bowel movements among normal subjects of both sexes and of all ages, ranging from three per day to three per week. Therefore, someone who has fewer than three bowel movements per week is constipated, by definition. On the other hand, a change in frequency of movements from, say, two per day to three per week may also signify constipation. However, it is probably not necessary to do a workup or to treat people merely because they report fewer than three bowel movements per week. Even one movement per week is acceptable if it does not represent a recent change in bowel frequency and is not associated with symptoms such as pain on defecation or bloating. Constipation is among the most prevalent gastrointestinal (GI) complaints, accounting for more than 2.5 million physician visits in the United States annually, and more than half a billion dollars in sales of laxatives.

Almost always, constipation is caused by a delay in transit within the colon or by a pelvic outlet delay (see also Chapter 40). A wide variety of conditions may affect colonic transit (Table 39.1). There may be structural abnormalities that obstruct the passage of intraluminal contents, or there may be conditions that alter colonic motility. Evaluation of patients with constipation must therefore include consideration of a wide variety of possible etiologies. Although it is difficult to be precise about the relative frequencies of these

Table 39.1.   Various Causes of Constipation

Idiopathic Causes (Possible Mechanisms)
Dietary factors: low residue
Motility disturbances: colonic inertia or spasm (irritable bowel
   syndrome)
Sedentary living

Structural Abnormalities
Anorectal disorders: fissures, thrombosed hemorrhoids
Strictures
Tumors

Endocrine/Metabolic Causes
Hypercalcemia
Hypokalemia
Hypothyroidism
Pregnancy

Neurogenic Causes
Cerebrovascular events
Hirschsprung's disease
Parkinson's disease
Spinal cord tumors
Trauma

Smooth Muscle/Connective Tissue Disorders
Amyloidosis
Scleroderma

Drugs
Antacids: aluminum- and calcium-containing compounds
Anticholinergics
Antidepressants
Calcium channel blockers (especially verapamil)
Cholestyramine
Narcotics
Sympathomimetics: pseudoephedrine

Psychogenic Causes (Especially Depression)

etiologies, chronic constipation (months or longer) is most commonly caused by a motility disorder (as in sedentary people eating a low-fiber diet or in patients with the irritable bowel syndrome), the use of constipating drugs, local anorectal problems (fissures, hemorrhoids, and tumors), and pelvic outlet delay.

Evaluation

History

The history provides the most useful information about the etiology of constipation. It may reveal a gross misconception about normal bowel habits or a neurotic preoccupation with bowel function. Reassurance that there is a broad range of normal bowel frequency may be all the treatment that is needed in many cases of self-defined constipation. It is important to determine whether there is a history or suggestion of a systemic process (e.g., hypothyroidism, hyperparathyroidism, or scleroderma), a neurologic disorder (e.g., cerebrovascular disease or Parkinson's disease), or the taking of drugs (e.g., anticholinergics, calcium channel blockers, opiates, or antidepressants), all of which are known to impair colonic motility. Most systemic or neurologic diseases are almost certain to affect organs outside the GI tract so that, in addition to constipation, patients

have symptoms that reflect extraintestinal dysfunction. On the other hand, even local processes (e.g., strictures or tumors) often produce other GI symptoms in addition to constipation, such as abdominal pain or rectal bleeding. Thus, rectal bleeding should always be thoroughly evaluated (see Chapter 38) even though in constipated patients it often is caused by perianal disease (fissures, hemorrhoids). Abdominal pain with constipation is also a prominent feature of the irritable bowel syndrome (see Chapter 40). Most patients with idiopathic diet-related or drug-induced constipation are otherwise asymptomatic, although a complaint of a bloated sensation is common if constipation is prolonged.

Physical Examination

The physical examination should be focused on the identification of underlying causes of constipation. The general examination is rarely helpful unless an abdominal mass is detected. Rectal examination is often helpful because it can identify fissures and hemorrhoids as well as anal stenosis or stricture secondary to surgery or inflammation. The anal sphincter is normally closed. A gaping anal opening or asymmetry of the anal opening may indicate a neurologic disorder (spinal cord trauma, peripheral neuropathy) that impairs sphincteric function. After inspection, a careful digital examination should be performed to evaluate the strength of the anal sphincters, the presence of masses, the consistency of the stool, and the presence of any painful or tender areas. The stool should also be tested for occult blood.

Endoscopy

Flexible sigmoidoscopy should be performed routinely in newly constipated patients in whom the cause is not obvious. Because it is important to exclude carcinoma in older patients (over 50) with new onset constipation, even if the sigmoidoscopy reveals an apparently benign cause of constipation, the remainder of the colon should be visualized with a barium enema (see "Radiographic Studies"). However, most gastroenterologists recommend that a colonoscopy be performed in older patients instead of a flexible sigmoidoscopy and a barium enema. In such patients anoscopy may be needed to search properly for hemorrhoids or fissures (see Chapter 92). Flexible sigmoidoscopy can be performed in the office with the patient in the knee–chest position on a routine examining table, or in the left lateral position. Sigmoidoscopy should be performed to the highest level possible, with limitations imposed by the patient's tolerance of the procedure, the presence of stool, and the length of the instrument (a flexible sigmoidoscope is usually 60 cm in length and can often be passed to the splenic flexure). Even a good air-contrast barium enema is not a substitute for endoscopy because subtle mucosal abnormalities cannot be detected, and the most distal 15 to 20 cm of the colon are difficult to evaluate radiographically. The patient's experience during flexible sigmoidoscopy is described in Chapter 36.

Inflamed *hemorrhoids* and *fissures* found during anoscopy or flexible sigmoidoscopy may be secondary to constipation, but may also cause pain on defecation, and thus may promote constipation. These lesions are also common causes of bleeding in the chronically constipated patient. A spotty or diffuse brown pigmentation of the mucosa, *melanosis coli,* is indicative of *chronic laxative abuse,* particularly of the anthraquinone family (e.g., cascara, senna, and aloe). A mass lesion, such as a *carcinoma* or *polyp,* may also be identified by flexible sigmoidoscopy or colonoscopy.

A *rectal biopsy* may diagnose amyloidosis, ulcerative colitis, or Crohn's disease, and a deeper, suction biopsy of a rectal valve may diagnose Hirschsprung's disease. Biopsies of the rectal mucosa can be taken safely below the peritoneal reflection (approximately 12 cm proximal to the anus in men, 8 cm in women). Punch biopsies can be performed by any physician who has had appropriate training and experience. Suction biopsies should be performed only by a surgeon or gastroenterologist. Rectal biopsy should be painless unless a tender, inflamed lesion is biopsied; if it is done properly, the risk of bleeding and perforation, the major complications, is low.

Radiographic Studies

Radiographic examination is helpful primarily in the detection of obstructing lesions. A colonoscopy or a barium enema should be performed in all adult patients who complain of constipation of recent onset (within the preceding 6 months). The costs of radiographic and endoscopic procedures are compared in Chapter 38. The plain film of the abdomen may occasionally diagnose an obstructing carcinoma before a barium study has been done. The presence of a megacolon or a volvulus, of either the sigmoid or the cecum, also may be easily diagnosed by a plain film. The more recent the onset of constipation, the more likely it is that the colonoscopy or the barium enema (see "Patient Experience," Chapter 38) will yield positive results. Obstructing neoplasms and strictures can be identified by barium studies. Sometimes, patients with Hirschsprung's disease reach adolescence or adulthood without the diagnosis having been made. A narrowed rectal segment on a radiograph is a clue to the diagnosis. The radiologist may also comment on the motility of the colon, particularly if there is significant spasm or if haustral markings are absent, as seen in patients who use laxatives habitually or who have an atonic megacolon. Repeated endoscopic or barium studies are rarely helpful unless some aspect of the history or physical examination suggests a new development.

Other Studies

Colonic motility tests and *transit studies* are additional procedures that may provide insight into the pathophysiology of constipation. These studies are generally available only in specialized centers. They should be performed in the few patients who are severely impaired by constipation and who are refractory to conventional therapy.

Colonic motility studies are performed by placing catheters to monitor intracolonic pressures in the rectal and sigmoid regions. The study can identify various patterns of colonic activity in patients with constipation. In some, high-amplitude phasic contractions are seen spontaneously, as well as in response to stimulation. This type of segmental activity is sometimes associated with pain and is believed to cause constipation by impeding the distal flow of luminal contents. In other patients, an atonic pattern is found, characterized by a decreased response to stimulation and a loss of resistance to distension (5).

Colonic transit time can be measured by plotting the expulsion of radiopaque markers (Sitzmarks, commercially available) after daily ingestion of a capsule containing 24 markers. Once a steady state is reached, the number of markers entering the GI tract must equal the number being excreted, and the transit time in hours is equal to the number of markers still in the colon on plain film (7). Moreover, the distribution of these markers may have a relationship to the underlying motility disturbance. The retention of markers only in the rectum suggests a failure of expulsion, whereas retention throughout the colon suggests generalized colonic inertia.

Treatment

The treatment for constipation should, if possible, be based on correction of the underlying abnormality; for example, if there is a systemic disease that can be treated (e.g., hypothyroidism) or a constipating drug that can be stopped. The use of laxatives as a reflex response to complaints of constipation should be discouraged. Successful therapy must include discussion with the patient about the broad limits of normal bowel function and the patient's own concepts of normal bowel activity.

Bowel Retraining

Bowel retraining is an important initial aspect of therapy for patients whose constipation does not have an identifiable and remediable cause. The patient should be encouraged to have a regular daily routine with time set aside for having a bowel movement, preferably within 5 to 10 minutes after a meal, to take advantage of the strong stimulus of the gastrocolic reflex. This behavior modification program allows the patient to become more aware of and responsive to the normal urges to defecate. Patients should be advised always to respond to such urges. In severely constipated patients, a bowel retraining program may be initiated, with enemas or suppositories used to enhance bowel activity at the desired time. For enemas, lukewarm tap water should be used because all other solutions may be irritating if used repetitively. The enema should also be done soon after eating a meal to take advantage of the gastrocolic reflex. For suppositories, bisacodyl (Dulcolax) should be used, again just after eating; however, they should not be used for more than a few days because they may eventually be irritating. Glycerin suppositories are commonly used but not very effective.

Diet

Diet is an important factor in bowel function. There is epidemiologic evidence that greater amounts of crude dietary fiber are associated with a lesser prevalence of constipation as well as of other GI disorders, including diverticular disease and colorectal cancer. The mechanism for the effect on constipation is unclear. Studies in normal volunteers show that when fiber is added to the diet, stool weight increases but the effect on whole gut transit time varies. Some studies show a speeding of transit when baseline transit is slow but no change or slowing when the baseline transit is rapid (4,9). Several mechanisms may account for these observations: Fiber may act as a bulk-forming agent, fiber may increase the concentration of fecal bile salts (which have a pronounced cathartic effect), and fiber, metabolized by colonic bacteria to nonabsorbable volatile fatty acids, may act as an osmotic cathartic. The low-fiber diet generally consumed in the United States, along with other variables such as sedentary lifestyle, may account for the large number of patients who complain of constipation. As an initial step in treatment, the patient should be advised to follow a diet rich in fiber. As listed in Table 39.2, a variety of foods are high in fiber. As a practical matter, it may be reasonable to add a commercial fiber preparation to a high-fiber diet. Maintaining an adequate intake of fluids, particularly difficult in some older patients with constipation, can be helpful in maintaining proper stool water content.

Laxatives

Despite numerous warnings, laxatives are still popular in the treatment of constipation. The presence of 700 or more commercially available laxatives and enema preparations attests to the widespread use of these agents. The mechanism of action for most laxatives is poorly understood, and the potential for toxicity is often underestimated (Table 39.3). Few data are available for comparison among the various laxatives, and the decision to use a particular laxative often is determined by individual preference rather than by objective evidence of efficacy or safety.

There are a number of different mechanisms by which a laxative effect may be achieved. *Bulk-forming agents* are natural or synthetic polysaccharides or cellulose derivatives that exert their laxative effect primarily by absorbing water and increasing fecal mass. Psyllium seed and bran are examples of such laxatives. In addition to their hydrophilic properties, these agents are metabolized by colonic bacteria, resulting in accumulation of osmotically active metabolites. These laxatives are effective in increasing the frequency and in softening the consistency of stool. There have been isolated reports of obstruction secondary to hydrophilic agents in patients with esophageal

Table 39.2.   Fiber Content of Various Foods

Type of Food	Dietary Fiber per Average Serving (g)
Vegetables	
Beans (navy, lima, kidney, baked)	8.5–10.0
Beans (string)	2.0
Broccoli	3.2
Brussels sprouts	2.3
Cabbage	2.0
Carrots	2.0
Celery	1.0
Corn	2.6
Corn on the cob	5.9
Lettuce	1.0
Potato (baked with skin)	3.0
Potato (french fried)	1.6
Peas (canned)	6.0
Rice	0.8
Fruit	
Apple with peel	2.0
Apple juice	0.0
Banana	1.5
Grapefruit (fresh)	0.6
Orange	2.0
Peach	2.0
Raspberries	4.6
Strawberries	1.6
Bread	
Whole wheat	1.3
White, rye, French	0.7
Cereal	
All-Bran (100%)	8.4
Corn flakes	2.6
Wheaties	2.6
Other Foods	
Meats: chicken, liver, fish, lamb	0.0
Cheese, milk, yogurt	0.0

or small bowel strictures. In most cases, however, this type of laxative is highly effective and the potential for adverse effects appears to be low. However, in patients with an atonic form of constipation, particularly with megacolon, these agents are often ineffective and produce an uncomfortable sensation of bloating and gaseousness at high dosages. Bloating is common in all patients when they begin to take bulk agents, but it is generally transient and can be minimized by increasing the dosage gradually over a period of weeks. A recent meta-analysis found that laxatives and fiber increased the frequency of bowel movements by a mean of 1.4 times per week (12). Fiber and bulk laxatives also reduced constipation-related abdominal pain.

Dioctyl sodium sulfosuccinate (Colace) is often labeled as a *stool softener* or a wetting agent. It works by lowering surface tension, allowing water to enter the stool more easily. It is generally well tolerated.

The *saline laxatives* are magnesium or sodium salts (e.g., milk of magnesia and sodium phosphate), which are poorly absorbed and therefore act as hyperosmolar solutions. They may also stimulate the release of cholecystokinin, a hormone that stimulates colonic motility. Complications include hypermagnesemia in

Table 39.3.   Laxatives

Classification and Active Ingredient	Examples	Dosage	Average Onset of Action	Potential Adverse Effects
Bulk				
Psyllium seed	Konsyl	1 tsp to 2 tbsp/day	12–24 hr or more	Increased gas and bloating sensation; bowel obstruction if stricture present
	Effer-Syllium			
	Perdiem (with senna)			
Plus dextrose	Metamucil			
Bran		4+ tbsp/day		
Calcium polycarbophil	FiberCon	4–8 tablets/day		
Emollient (Softeners)				
Dioctyl sodium (or calcium) sulfosuccinate (docusate sodium)	Colace, Peri-Colace (with casanthranol) Surfak	1–3 caps/day	24–48 hr	
Stimulant				
Phenolphthalein	Ex-Lax	1–2 tablets (100–200 mg)	6–8 hr	Dermatitis; electrolyte imbalance, melanosis coli
Bisacodyl	Dulcolax	2–3 tabs (10–15 mg)	6–12 hr	
Senna	Senokot, Perdiem (with psyllium)	1–4 tsp or 2–4 tabs	6–12 hr	
Cascara (casanthranol)	Peri-Colase (with dioctyl sodium)	1–2 tabs	8–12 hr	
CO_2	Ceo-two suppositories	1–2	10–30 min	
Osmotic				
Ricinoleic acid	Castor oil	1–2 tsp		Electrolyte imbalance
Lactulose[a]	Cephulac, Chronulac	1–2 tbsp/day	24–48 hr	Excessive gas production
Magnesium salts	Milk of Magnesia, magnesium citrate	2–4 tbsp	3–6 hr or less	Hypermagnesemia, hypocalcemia, hyperphosphatemia in chronic renal failure
Sodium salts	Phospho-Soda	2 tbsp in ½ glass of water	2–6 hr	
	Fleet enema (sodium phosphate)	120 mL	2–5 min	Dehydration; hypocalcemia; hyperphosphatemia in chronic renal failure

[a]Requires a prescription.

patients with renal failure and hypocalcemia from phosphate overdoses.

Stimulant laxatives, such as anthraquinone derivatives (senna, aloe, cascara) and diphenylmethane compounds (phenolphthalein, bisacodyl), exert their effects primarily by altering electrolyte transport by the intestinal mucosa and thereby increasing intestinal motor activity. The effect of these agents is claimed to be more specific on the colon. Phenolphthalein, an ingredient found in many over-the-counter preparations, has been associated with severe allergic dermatitis and the Stevens–Johnson syndrome. The chronic use of the anthraquinone derivatives has been reported to induce damage to the myenteric plexus, and thus may eventually impair bowel motility. Agents such as these that affect electrolyte transport may result in significant hypokalemia, factitious diarrhea, protein-losing enteropathy, and salt overload. Although these agents are undoubtedly effective, their chronic use may lead to significant side effects, and they should be avoided when possible.

Castor oil, previously thought to be a stimulant laxative, is now understood to exert its cathartic effect by alteration of intestinal fluid and electrolyte secretion. Ricinoleic acid, the active ingredient of castor oil,

has effects on the small and large intestine similar to those of bile acids: It inhibits absorption of sodium and glucose and stimulates fluid and electrolyte secretion by increasing cellular cyclic adenosine monophosphate (cAMP) and by inhibiting sodium–potassium adenosine triphosphatase (ATPase). This increase in intraluminal fluid content may then secondarily affect intestinal motility. Its use is not recommended because of the potential for fluid–electrolyte disturbances.

Lactulose (Cephulac or Chronulac syrup) is a semi-synthetic disaccharide that is not metabolized by intestinal enzymes. As a result, water and electrolytes are retained within the intestinal lumen by the osmotic effect of this undigested sugar. In addition, this agent is converted by colonic bacteria to organic acids, which may further alter electrolyte transport and/or affect colonic motility. Lactulose is commonly used in patients with hepatic encephalopathy (see Chapter 43). It has also been shown to be an effective laxative in patients with chronic constipation. There is little current information on the relative merits of lactulose and bulk laxatives except that lactulose is expensive and requires 24 to 48 hours to achieve its effect.

Surgery is rarely necessary in the treatment of constipated patients. However, it is required for resection of an obstructing lesion, and myectomy may be needed for treatment of Hirschsprung's disease. Various procedures have been recommended for patients with megacolon who suffer from recurrent volvulus, ranging from simple tacking down of the loose mesentery to resection of bowel. Finally, in severe cases of intractable constipation, extensive surgery has been advocated, varying from resection of redundant sigmoid loops to subtotal colectomy with ileal proctostomy. The exact role and precise indication for this type of surgery remain to be more clearly defined. A recent study suggests that subtotal colectomy is effective and well tolerated in patients with severe atonic constipation (6).

General Recommendations

Therapy of constipation should always be directed first at identifying and treating any underlying disorder (Table 39.1). If the constipation is drug induced, the drug should be discontinued (if possible) or an alternative that is less constipating should be substituted. Otherwise, fiber and fluids should be added to the diet, and if necessary, a bulk laxative should be prescribed. When constipation is idiopathic, caused by an irreversible underlying disorder (e.g., diabetes mellitus), or secondary to a necessary drug, dietary changes and some form of laxative therapy may be necessary.

In practically all patients with constipation, a high-fiber diet or a bulk laxative is helpful. The amount of dietary fiber or bulk laxative that is needed varies from patient to patient and must be determined individually. Because the only significant side effect from this form of therapy is excessive gas and a bloated sensation, the dosage can be gradually increased until either the constipation is resolved or the side effects become too uncomfortable. For most patients, this form of therapy is successful and appears to be very safe on a chronic, defined (i.e., not as needed) basis. No other laxatives are needed.

However, in patients with partial bowel obstruction (as recognized on radiograph) or in those with an atonic form of constipation (e.g., institutional megacolon), the high fiber–bulk laxative approach is not usually effective. A patient with constipation caused by partial obstruction usually must be treated surgically. A patient with an atonic colon may need a stimulant laxative. Senna compounds, bisacodyl (either as a tablet or as a suppository), or enemas are most effective in such cases. Combinations of a stimulant laxative with a bulk agent (e.g., Perdiem) or with a softener (e.g., Peri-Colace) are reasonable and effective forms of therapy. Bulk agents alone in such cases simply distend the already distended bowel further without improving bowel function.

Special consideration must be given to the bedridden or chair-bound patient. In such patients, use of laxatives may result in incontinence because the patient may not be able to recognize or respond quickly enough to the sudden urge to defecate. In these circumstances, bulk agents are useful to keep the stool soft, but suppositories or enemas should also be used (simple tap water enemas are usually sufficient; also see Table 39.3), with the patient already positioned on the commode. In this fashion, the embarrassment and soilage of fecal incontinence can be avoided, and fecal impactions can be prevented. Enemas or suppositories may be used regularly (daily to every third day) to prevent fecal impactions and overflow diarrhea and incontinence.

A pamphlet for patients, titled *What Is Constipation?*, is sponsored by the National Institute of Arthritis, Diabetes, Digestive and Kidney Diseases. (This pamphlet may be ordered [and then duplicated] from Clearinghouse, 1555 Wilson Boulevard, Suite 600, Rosslyn, VA 22209-2461.)

DIARRHEA

Diarrhea is a troublesome problem that almost everyone has experienced. In infants and children, diarrhea can rapidly lead to death if untreated. The frail elderly also are at increased risk, when they become volume depleted, of strokes or of other major ischemic events. In most adult cases, the diarrheal illness begins abruptly, lasts only a day or two, and resolves without serious sequelae (see Chapter 26). Only occasionally does the illness continue for more than a week or do symptoms recur after the initial attack. The task facing the clinician is to identify the few patients with a significant underlying disorder who may require a specific therapeutic approach.

Definition

Patients complaining of diarrhea generally have an increase in the frequency and fluid volume of the bowel movement. Stool weight is the best objective measurement of diarrhea, with mean weights in the United States ranging normally between 100 and 200 g/day. In the patient with chronic diarrhea, objective documentation of daily fecal output is sometimes necessary (see below). Most patients with significant diarrhea produce more than 250 g of stool per day. A subset of patients with diarrhea present with the frequent passage of small volumes of liquid stool. Patients with inflammatory conditions or space-occupying lesions of the rectum may present in this fashion. Patients with the irritable bowel syndrome have stool volumes either within or slightly above the normal range. Patients with secretory forms of diarrhea, or small bowel disorders with malabsorption, often pass very large volumes of stool, in the range of 500 to 1000 g/day or more.

Pathophysiology

There are four basic mechanisms of diarrhea: osmotic load within the intestine, resulting in retention of water within the lumen; excessive secretion of electrolytes and water into the intestinal lumen; exudation of protein and fluid from the intestinal mucosa; and altered intestinal motility, resulting in rapid transit through the colon.

Osmotic diarrhea occurs when poorly absorbed material retains fluid within the intestinal lumen. This mechanism operates in patients with malabsorption or with lactose intolerance, in which undigested sugars accumulate within the intestinal lumen and exert a considerable osmotic load. Magnesium-containing laxatives and some magnesium-containing antacids (e.g., Maalox) probably produce diarrhea through a similar mechanism.

Secretory diarrhea occurs when the intestinal mucosa secretes increased amounts of water and electrolytes under the stimulation of a variety of substances. Cholera is the prototype, but a number of other enterotoxin-producing organisms (e.g., enterotoxigenic *Escherichia coli*) produce diarrhea in the same way (see Chapter 26). Other substances that induce secretory diarrhea include bile acids and long chain fatty acids (e.g., after ileal resection or in Crohn's disease or a malabsorption syndrome), certain GI hormones, and anthraquinone laxatives. Many of these stimulating agents have been shown to increase intracellular cAMP and to inhibit sodium potassium ATPase. The increase in cAMP leads to increased secretion.

Exudative diarrhea results from the outpouring of protein, blood, or mucus from an inflamed or ulcerated mucosa. Ulcerative colitis, Crohn's disease, invasive infections (see Chapter 26), and infiltrative disorders such as Whipple's disease and lymphoma are examples of this mechanism.

Motility disorders may lead to diarrhea, although the exact correlation between the abnormal motility and the diarrhea is not completely understood. The irritable bowel syndrome (see Chapter 40) is generally believed to be a motor disorder that causes abdominal pain and altered bowel habits, with diarrhea predominating in many patients. Diabetes mellitus may also lead to diarrhea caused by neurogenic dysfunction. Other conditions, such as scleroderma, can lead to stasis of the bowel with resultant bacterial overgrowth, steatorrhea, and diarrhea.

It is not always possible to identify one particular mechanism to account for diarrhea in a given patient; sometimes more than one mechanism is operative. However, an appreciation of pathophysiology enables the physician to understand the clinical features of a diarrheal illness better and to select appropriate therapy.

Evaluation of Acute Diarrhea

Acute diarrhea caused by infectious agents and by ingested toxins is discussed in greater detail in Chapter 26. Most patients who present to the physician with a sudden onset of diarrhea have a benign, self-limited illness. These patients do not require extensive evaluation and can be simply reassured. However, a small percentage of such patients have a significant underlying illness for which specific therapy is needed.

If diarrhea persists for more than 72 hours or if there is gross blood in the stool, an evaluation is indicated. In any case, the patient should always be evaluated before

medicine is prescribed because in certain situations, even nonspecific antidiarrheal therapy may be harmful. In particular, it has been shown that opiate-containing antidiarrheal drugs such as Lomotil or Imodium may prolong the course of acute infectious diarrhea by hindering the natural mechanism of clearing the body of the organism (3).

History

The history reveals whether the illness is acute or chronic and also provides clues to the underlying cause. The sudden onset of loose, watery stool is most commonly caused by an infectious process, and much less often by ingestion of drugs or poisons. Infectious diarrhea is likely to affect more than one person. Often, no specific bacterial agent is identified and the syndrome is assumed to be a viral gastroenteritis. Bacteria may cause diarrhea by a direct effect on the bowel or by elaboration of a toxin that produces intestinal dysfunction. Toxin-induced diarrhea, often associated with vomiting, begins within 6 hours of ingestion of contaminated food, whereas bacteria-induced diarrhea does not begin for 12 to 24 hours. Bloody diarrhea should never be ascribed to viral or toxin-mediated diarrhea; it is more likely to be caused by bacterial infection *(Shigella, Campylobacter, Yersinia, Salmonella,* invasive *E. coli),* ulcerative colitis, or ischemic bowel disease. Information about recent travel should include not only trips out of the country but also camping or fishing trips. *Giardiasis,* for example, may be carried by beavers, which contaminate water supplies and cause both epidemic outbreaks and individual cases of acute diarrhea among campers and hikers. Recent use of drugs is a common cause of new-onset diarrhea (Table 39.4) that may not be readily recognized by the physician or the patient. Some antihypertensives (e.g., methyldopa, hydralazine, reserpine, and guanethidine), magnesium-containing antacids, broad-spectrum antimicrobials, and quinidine are commonly used drugs that can lead to diarrhea (see below).

A number of intestinal disorders associated with *human immunodeficiency virus* (HIV) cause diarrhea, so appropriate questions should be asked to identify patients who are at risk of having HIV infection (see Chapter 34). Patients with CD4 counts below 50/mm^3 or viral burdens greater than 70,000 copies/mL are at particular risk of acquiring acute and chronic parasitic and bacterial infections such as *Microsporidium, Cyclospora, Isospora belli, Mycobacterium avium intracellulare,* and *Campylobacter jejuni.*

Physical Examination

The physical examination in acute diarrhea is generally unremarkable. The patient's state of hydration should be estimated because it is an important measure of the severity of the diarrhea and of the need for hospitalization. Abdominal examination may reveal mild diffuse tenderness. The bowel sounds are clearly active or hyperactive. Rectal examination is essential because diarrhea may be the initial manifestation of obstructing rectal carcinoma; furthermore, in the geri-

Table 39.4.   Common Drugs that May Induce Diarrhea

Antibiotics[a]
Clindamycin
Ampicillin
Cephalosporins

Antacids
Magnesium-containing

Antihypertensive Agents
Guanethidine
Hydralazine
Methyldopa
Propranolol
Reserpine

Cardiovascular Agents
Digitalis
Quinidine

Antimetabolites
Colchicine

Alcohol

Nutritional Supplements
Hyperosmolar solutions (enteral feedings)

Potent Diuretics
Furosemide
Ethacrynic acid
Bumetanide

[a]All antibiotics can induce diarrhea.

atric population, fecal impactions may result in overflow diarrhea, and constipating agents may be mistakenly recommended.

Stool Examination

If diarrhea has continued for more than 3 to 4 days, the stool should be examined for the presence of blood, fecal leukocytes, and enteric pathogens. Blood in the stool suggests mucosal disruption and is not a feature of osmotic, secretory, or motor diarrhea. Inflammatory conditions such as ulcerative colitis and pseudomembranous colitis (see Chapter 26), as well as *Shigella* and invasive strains of *E. coli*, often cause bloody diarrhea.

Fecal leukocytes are best seen by microscopic examination of the liquid portion of the stool after staining with methylene blue or Gram's stain (see Chapter 26, where the technique is described). They are not seen in infectious processes that do not invade the mucosa such as viral enteritis, in toxin-mediated diarrhea such as cholera, or in infection with noninvasive *E. coli* (see Chapter 26). *Salmonella, Shigella, Amoeba,* and *Campylobacter,* which are invasive organisms, typically lead to exudation of fecal leukocytes, as does chronic inflammatory bowel disease. In these conditions, in which the mucosal barrier is broken, the course of the diarrheal illness is unpredictable and may even become life-threatening. The absence of fecal leukocytes or blood is therefore very reassuring and, in these cases, the disease is usually transient.

Stool cultures for bacterial pathogens should be

obtained in all patients who have fecal leukocytes. Specific isolation techniques are needed to diagnose *Yersinia* and *Campylobacter,* common causes of acute diarrhea, and should be requested. Acute infectious diarrhea secondary to *Salmonella* or *Shigella* or other invasive organisms is impossible to differentiate from acute inflammatory bowel disease, especially without a stool culture. In the absence of fecal leukocytes, stool cultures are generally negative and are not routinely recommended. Gram's stain of the stool for bacteria is not helpful except in cases of suspected staphylococcal enterocolitis or gonococcal proctitis.

Examination of the stool for parasites such as *Entamoeba histolytica* and *Giardia lamblia* is important if diarrhea persists more than a few days, even in the absence of a history of travel, because the organism may be passed by contact with a carrier. Microscopic examination of the inflammatory exudate of a patient with acute amebic colitis almost always demonstrates motile trophozoites, but only if the slide is prewarmed (e.g., over a light bulb) and then examined immediately. Slides sent to a laboratory for processing are unlikely to reveal amebae. Rectal biopsy may identify the organisms in the exudate. Serologic tests for amebae can be useful but do not distinguish recent from distant infection. Measuring acute and convalescent titers is more specific for recent infection, but gives the diagnosis only in retrospect. *Giardia* can be detected on examination of fresh stool in only approximately 50% of patients. Duodenal aspiration or biopsy is more sensitive in diagnosing giardiasis.

Endoscopy

Flexible sigmoidoscopy is important in patients with acute diarrhea associated with fecal leukocytes or bloody diarrhea if the cause is not obvious. The examination should be performed without a prior enema because enemas may alter the appearance of the mucosa and reduce the chance of detecting intestinal pathogens such as amebae. The marginal diagnostic return in examining the entire colon is quite small, so flexible sigmoidoscopy is preferable to colonoscopy in evaluation of acute diarrheal illness.

Many acute diarrheal illnesses produce a similar abnormal but nonspecific mucosal appearance on sigmoidoscopy. However, certain findings suggest specific diseases. In viral enteritis, giardiasis, toxin-mediated diarrhea, drug-induced diarrhea, and other conditions not accompanied by fecal leukocytes or blood loss, the sigmoidoscopy is normal. In *ulcerative colitis* the rectal mucosa is involved in at least 95% of cases, and the mucosa is uniformly abnormal with bleeding and a granular, friable appearance. *Crohn's disease* uncommonly affects the rectum, but is often apparent in the sigmoid or more proximal portions of the colon. It may appear as discrete aphthoid ulcers or patches of grossly abnormal mucosa with normal intervening tissue. *Amebiasis* occasionally produces flask-shaped ulcers that may be single or multiple, with normal intervening mucosa; more often, however, it produces a pattern very similar to ulcerative colitis. In *shigellosis,* multiple small superficial ulcers may be seen, but the appearance may also be indistinguishable from that of ulcerative colitis. *Pseudomembranous colitis* is identified by the presence of numerous raised yellow plaques covering an inflamed mucosa. Occasionally a carcinoma or large villous adenoma may be detected by sigmoidoscopy. Sigmoidoscopy also provides an opportune time to obtain samples of stool and exudate for culture and microscopic examination. The patient's experience with sigmoidoscopy is described in Chapter 36.

Radiographic Studies

Radiography is of limited use in the evaluation of acute diarrhea and may, in fact, be confusing. In patients suspected of having inflammatory bowel disease or ischemic colitis, plain films of the abdomen may demonstrate an irregular appearance of the bowel wall secondary to mucosal edema, often described as thumbprinting. In the gravely ill patient with fulminant colitis, the radiograph may confirm the presence of toxic megacolon. In most cases of acute diarrhea, a plain film is not needed. Barium studies during the acute phase of the diarrhea are likewise not needed and in certain conditions may even be hazardous, as in patients with severe colitis or ischemic bowel disease. Similarly, a small bowel series during acute viral enteritis may be frighteningly abnormal, resembling sprue, and yet may rapidly return to normal after resolution of the acute illness.

Evaluation of Chronic Diarrhea

The approach to patients with either acute diarrhea that lasts longer than 3 to 4 days or chronic diarrhea (lasting longer than 3 weeks) is very much the same. Although the physician may be reassured by knowing that the majority of such patients do not suffer from any serious progressive or disabling disease, the patient requires a specific diagnosis and effective therapy. The differential diagnosis is so varied, and the available tests are so numerous, that the diagnostic workup of chronic diarrhea poses a difficult problem. The following discussion provides a practical approach to this problem.

History

The history is often helpful in differentiating organic from functional diarrhea (as in irritable bowel syndrome; see Chapter 40). If organic diarrhea is suspected, it is important to determine whether the pathogenic mechanism is osmotic, secretory, motor, or exudative (see above).

In patients with so-called *functional diarrhea,* the history of diarrhea often dates back many months or years, although occasionally it can be traced to a specific acute diarrheal illness. Despite the chronicity, no sequelae, such as weight loss, anemia, or hypoalbuminemia, have occurred. The patient typically complains of several watery, at times explosive bowel movements early in the morning, and then no subsequent movements the rest of the day. Nocturnal bowel

movements are rare. The total stool output is usually small, however—often less than 200 g/day and rarely, if ever, more than 500 g/day. Mucus often is present. There is no blood in the stool unless secondary conditions, such as anal fissures, have developed. Postprandial pain is a feature of irritable bowel syndrome (see Chapter 40), but is absent in many patients. The condition often waxes and wanes in severity, and stress often exacerbates the symptoms.

The most common cause of chronic secretory diarrhea is *laxative abuse.* It should be suspected in apparently healthy patients with large-volume diarrhea, especially if they have *melanosis coli* on sigmoidoscopic examination (see above). Although such patients may have emotional problems with which the physician must deal (see Chapter 12), often the abuse simply reflects a misconception about normal bowel movement frequency and an attempt to adhere to that standard.

In patients with organic disease, the history may indicate the part of the intestinal tract that is involved. The passage of a large volume of frothy, malodorous stool without blood suggests small bowel diarrhea, often secondary to malabsorption. The frequent passage of small volumes of poorly formed, bloody stools suggests inflammatory, exudative disorders of the colon such as ulcerative colitis. The presence of recognizable fat droplets (oil) suggests malabsorption, often secondary to pancreatic insufficiency. (Floating stools and undigested food in the stools are not always helpful observations because they may be seen in both organic and functional diarrheal states.) The association of diarrhea with the ingestion of certain dietary products (milk, fruit, hyperosmolar solutions, and sorbitol-containing gum or candy) may not be recognized by the patient unless he or she is specifically asked. A detailed drug history is also important because many drugs may cause diarrhea (Table 39.4).

Other symptoms may help the physician to arrive at a specific diagnosis. *Arthritis* and *arthralgias* may suggest the presence of one of several uncommon bowel diseases, such as inflammatory bowel disease and Whipple's disease; conversely, diarrhea may be an important feature of Reiter's syndrome (see Chapter 71). *Weight loss,* in the absence of anorexia, should suggest malabsorption, hyperthyroidism, or a malignant tumor. *Abdominal pain* may reflect the irritable bowel syndrome (see Chapter 40), in which case it is generally in the left lower quadrant or the suprapubic region; or a disease of the small bowel (e.g., Crohn's disease), in which case it is often periumbilical or in the right lower quadrant; or a gastrinoma (Zollinger–Ellison syndrome), in which case peptic ulcers are responsible for upper abdominal pain.

Physical Examination

The physical examination may reveal additional information about the etiology of the diarrhea. Patients with malabsorption may have evidence of weight loss, peripheral neuropathy (secondary to vitamin B deficiency), and carpopedal spasm (secondary to hypocalcemia). Erythema nodosum and pyoderma gangrenosum are seen in some cases of inflammatory bowel disease. Hyperpigmentation is a feature of Whipple's disease and Addison's disease. Diabetic diarrhea is often associated with other evidence of autonomic dysfunction, such as postural hypotension. Nondeforming arthritis is a feature of Whipple's disease and of inflammatory bowel disease. Hepatosplenomegaly and lymphadenopathy suggest lymphoma or Whipple's disease. The abdominal examination may reveal an arterial bruit or an aortic aneurysm, which suggests ischemic bowel disease. A rectal examination may disclose perianal disease (e.g., abscesses or fistulas, secondary to Crohn's disease), a rectal tumor, or a fecal impaction.

Endoscopy

Flexible sigmoidoscopy may be performed during the initial visit without a prior cleansing enema. Examination and biopsy of the rectosigmoid mucosa may suggest specific etiologies (ulcerative colitis, Crohn's disease, amebiasis, pseudomembranous colitis, Whipple's disease, or amyloidosis). Even a grossly normal-appearing mucosa is worth biopsying because collagenous or microscopic colitides, for example, may be present in patients with chronic watery diarrhea. The finding of melanosis coli (spotty or diffuse brownish mucosal pigmentation) in a patient complaining of diarrhea indicates laxative abuse. At the time of sigmoidoscopy, stool specimens are obtained for microscopic evaluation and culture. Gonococcal proctitis appears similar to ulcerative proctitis (see below) and requires direct plating on a warm special culture medium (Thayer–Martin) with prompt incubation. Routine stool cultures should be taken as well. The stool should be examined for leukocytes, blood, fat (Sudan stain), and parasites (see Chapter 26).

After this initial evaluation, the etiology of the chronic diarrhea in most patients is either evident or strongly suspected. It is usually possible to distinguish functional from organic diarrhea, detect evidence of inflammatory or infiltrative disease, suspect the presence of malabsorption, characterize the diarrhea as small bowel or large bowel, and even suggest the underlying pathophysiology. Further evaluation is then dictated by the results of this initial workup.

Laboratory Studies

Laboratory studies should be selected to support the clinical impression, but rarely are able to make or exclude a specific diagnosis. For example, the erythrocyte sedimentation rate (ESR) may be elevated in a variety of inflammatory diseases that cause diarrhea, but a normal ESR does not exclude inflammatory bowel disease or a connective tissue disorder.

Radiologic Studies

A plain film of the abdomen may reveal pancreatic calcifications (indicative of chronic pancreatitis), a dilated small bowel, or an abnormal bowel contour (as in inflammatory bowel disease or lymphoma).

In the patient over 40 years old with chronic or recurrent diarrhea, a *barium enema* or *colonoscopy* is indicated during the initial evaluation. In younger patients, such studies are unlikely to be useful unless a specific disorder is suspected. The presence of blood in the stool, at any age, is a clear indication for a colonoscopy or barium enema, regardless of the presence of hemorrhoids or fissures. Neoplastic and inflammatory conditions may be diagnosed in this way, and ulcerative colitis and Crohn's disease of the colon can be differentiated in most cases. When inflammatory bowel disease is suspected, during the barium enema an attempt should be made to reflux contrast material into the terminal ileum to rule out Crohn's disease of the ileum.

The timing of the barium enema is important. Barium interferes with the collection of stool for measurement of volume and fat and with the detection of parasites. A barium enema should be delayed for 1 week after a rectal biopsy to prevent colonic perforation. The patient's experience with the barium enema is discussed in Chapter 38.

A *small bowel series* (see Chapter 38 for a discussion of the patient's experience with this procedure) is helpful in distinguishing mucosal disease (celiac sprue), inflammatory conditions (Crohn's disease), and infiltrative processes (Whipple's disease or amyloidosis). In addition, a small bowel series is indicated in postsurgical patients to clarify the anatomy (e.g., a blind loop or fistulas) and to detect localized areas of dilation and stasis.

Other Studies

A *quantitative 72-hour stool collection,* although regarded as unpleasant by both the patient and laboratory personnel, is a very informative test. It should be used early in the evaluation of patients in whom the initial routine workup does not suggest a diagnosis. The test can be performed in the ambulatory setting by having the patient collect all stool in a preweighed container supplied by the clinical laboratory. The test should be performed before barium studies or other invasive tests. The normal stool is less than 250 g/day (or less than 250 mL/day). Most patients with irritable bowel syndrome or other functional forms of chronic diarrhea have stool weights and volumes within this range. A stool volume of more than 1000 mL/day suggests a secretory diarrhea or malabsorption.

Fecal fat should also be measured during this collection. Normally less than 7% of ingested fat is secreted in the stool per day (4 to 7 g on an average American diet containing 60 to 100 g of fat). Although less reliable, a qualitative test for stool fat by Sudan stain can be useful as a rapid screening test for steatorrhea. The presence of steatorrhea dictates a different approach to the remainder of the workup (see below). In the absence of excessive fat excretion or evidence of an exudative process (e.g., inflammatory bowel disease), high-volume diarrhea suggests a secretory process. The *osmolality* and *electrolyte concentration* of the specimen can also be measured. In osmotic diarrhea, the measured fecal osmolality is more than twice the sum of the concentration of fecal sodium and potassium because of the presence of unmeasured osmotically active substances. In secretory diarrhea, the calculated and measured osmolality are nearly the same.

In patients suspected of having a secretory diarrhea, further evaluation generally requires hospitalization and consultation with a gastroenterologist. In secretory diarrhea, having the patient ingest nothing by mouth for 48 hours does not alter the volume of diarrhea, whereas in osmotic diarrhea the stool volume significantly decreases. Causes of chronic secretory diarrhea include hormone-secreting tumors and surreptitious laxative abuse. Evaluation of such patients often requires availability of various hormone assays.

Evaluation of Malabsorption

When the quantitative or qualitative fecal fat demonstrates steatorrhea, the evaluation of the diarrhea should be focused on the cause of malabsorption. Malabsorption can result from small intestinal disease, pancreatic disease, hepatobiliary disease, or gastric disease. A series of diagnostic studies is used initially to define the organ involved and then to diagnose the specific disease. Consultation with a gastroenterologist is generally recommended to help perform and analyze these various tests.

The D-xylose test measures the absorptive capacity of the proximal small bowel and is useful in distinguishing malabsorption from maldigestion (pancreatic enzyme deficiency). D-xylose does not require the pancreatic stage of digestion to be absorbed by an intact small intestinal mucosa. After absorption it enters the blood and is excreted in the urine. The test is performed in the same manner as an oral glucose tolerance test and can be performed in the ambulatory setting by most clinical laboratories. A 25-g oral dose of xylose is given, and the patient's urine is collected over the next 5 hours. A blood sample is collected 1 hour after ingestion. In disorders of the intestinal mucosa (e.g., celiac disease and Whipple's disease), xylose is poorly absorbed and low levels are found in the serum and urine. Uncommonly, massive bacterial overgrowth may also produce an abnormal D-xylose test that reverts to normal with antibiotic treatment. Because an abnormal xylose test suggests mucosal disease, a *small bowel biopsy* should be performed next. Dehydration, renal insufficiency, third spacing of fluid, vomiting, and hypothyroidism may spuriously decrease urine (but not serum) levels of D-xylose.

If the xylose test is normal, maldigestion, usually caused by *pancreatic insufficiency,* is the most likely cause of steatorrhea. In chronic pancreatitis, pancreatic calcifications may be seen on an abdominal plain film, and diabetes mellitus is sometimes present. Pancreatic insufficiency can be confirmed by measuring pancreatic secretions or by measuring intraluminal contents after a test meal. These older tests involve intubation of the duodenum, with collection of intraluminal contents. Newer methods do not require intubation but simply entail urine collection, as in the Bentiromide

test, which uses a nonabsorbable synthetic peptide that is cleaved by pancreatic enzymes, then becomes absorbable and is measured when it is excreted in the urine. Often, however, if a presumptive diagnosis of pancreatic insufficiency is made, the patient is treated empirically with pancreatic enzymes (e.g., Viokase, three to six tablets with meals, or Pancrease, two to three tablets with meals). If the diagnosis is correct, symptoms are moderately improved, but not entirely eliminated. Diagnostic and therapeutic decisions should be made in consultation with a gastroenterologist.

Endoscopic biopsy of the small intestine is often useful in the detection of various disorders that may cause malabsorption and/or diarrhea. Disorders that may be diagnosed by small bowel biopsy include sprue, Whipple's disease, intestinal lymphoma, amyloidosis, lymphangiectasia, and eosinophilic gastroenteritis. Giardiasis can also be diagnosed by examination of the intestinal mucosa and the intestinal mucus or fluid.

Disorders of the terminal ileum (Crohn's disease, ileal resection) may also lead to diarrhea and malabsorption. Evaluation may include a *Schilling test* or a *bile salt breath test.* The Schilling test measures vitamin B_{12} absorption, which is abnormal in disorders of the terminal ileum, the site of B_{12} absorption. Absorption is impaired despite the presence of intrinsic factor (see Chapter 50) or the administration of antibiotics.

Similarly, the bile salt breath test measures bile acid absorption, which is also abnormal in disorders of the terminal ileum, the site of bile salt absorption. The patient is given orally a radiolabeled (^{14}C) bile salt. In the presence of terminal ileal disease, the bile salt is malabsorbed and excess acid reaches the colon, where bacteria deconjugate it and release $^{14}CO_2$, which diffuses across the colon and is excreted in the breath. Therefore, in ileal disease, the level of $^{14}CO_2$ in the patient's expired air is abnormally high. The same abnormality can be seen when there is bacterial overgrowth in the small bowel, so that the bile acid is deconjugated and metabolized there instead of in the colon. Bile acid malabsorption caused by bacterial overgrowth is reversed when the patient is given antibiotics. Both the Schilling test and the bile salt breath test are performed by nuclear medicine specialists.

Specific Causes of Chronic Diarrhea

Lactose Intolerance

Lactose is by far the most commonly malabsorbed carbohydrate (see Chapter 40). Lactose intolerance results from a deficiency or total absence of the enzyme lactase in the brush border of the intestinal mucosa, which causes maldigestion and therefore malabsorption of lactose. The unabsorbed carbohydrate exerts an osmotic effect that draws water into the intestinal lumen. In the colon, the lactose is metabolized by bacteria to organic acid, CO_2, and hydrogen. The acid contributes to the diarrhea by both an osmotic effect and an irritant effect on the colonic mucosa. Thus, the unabsorbed carbohydrate, if present in sufficient quantities (the critical amount varies widely), may cause diarrhea, gaseousness, bloating, and abdominal cramps.

Lactose intolerance may be present either as an inherited condition, "lactase nonpersistence" after childhood, or one that is acquired because of damage to the intestinal epithelium (e.g., caused by infectious enteritis or sprue). Even in patients with a genetic disorder, the onset of the disease is unpredictable and may not occur until adult life. The secondary cases are usually, but not always, reversible if the underlying disease is successfully treated. The severity of the clinical symptoms is highly variable.

In some patients even small amounts of lactose produce severe symptoms, whereas in others large quantities may be consumed with no or only minimal symptoms. Isolated lactase deficiency is most common in African Americans (70 to 100% prevalence) and in Asians (more than 90%) but may also be found in 12% of the white population in the United States (2). The condition is more pronounced in certain clinical settings: when superimposed on another diarrheal disorder, most commonly irritable bowel syndrome; after gastric surgery, which permits rapid delivery of lactose to the small bowel; and when a patient consumes extra amounts of milk as part of (misguided) therapy for ulcer disease.

The diagnosis of lactose intolerance is suggested by the history and the response to a lactose-free diet. However, nearly a third of patients with symptomatic lactose intolerance may not have made the correlation between the dietary intake and the resulting symptoms because a wide variety of foods, ranging from bread to instant coffee, contain lactose (see Chapter 40, Table 40.2).

Ordinarily, a 3-week trial of a diet that is free of milk and milk products is a satisfactory therapeutic trial to test the diagnosis of lactose intolerance. Other tests are indicated only in equivocal cases or when the patient's nutritional status would be compromised by eliminating milk products unnecessarily.

Specific tests for the diagnosis of *lactose intolerance* include the lactose tolerance test and the *hydrogen breath test*. The lactose tolerance test measures changes in the concentration of serum glucose at 1 and 2 hours after ingestion of 50 g of lactose. A rise in glucose of 20 mg/100 mL above fasting is normal. The test has approximately a 30% false-positive rate, and its validity depends on a variety of factors besides simply the presence of the lactase enzyme. The hydrogen breath test is easier to perform and is more accurate. Unabsorbed lactose is fermented by colonic bacteria, and the resultant hydrogen is absorbed and expired in the breath. In normal subjects, after a lactose load, there is only a trace amount of hydrogen in the expired air, whereas in lactose-deficient patients substantial levels are recorded. This test is widely available; it is usually performed by a nuclear medicine specialist or in a gastrointestinal laboratory and requires 2 to 4 hours of the patient's time.

Fecal Impaction

Although it is the result of chronic constipation, fecal impaction (12) commonly causes diarrhea. The adults most at risk for impaction are elderly sedentary people, often bedridden. The feces are usually impacted in the rectum or in the rectosigmoid region but occasionally may extend high up into the colon (rarely, even to the cecum). The leaking of colonic fluid around the impaction, resulting in the passage of frequent, small-volume, watery bowel movements, accounts for the diarrhea. Other symptoms are common but are usually nonspecific: a sense of fullness in the rectum, vague lower abdominal pain, nausea, and headache. On physical examination, the firm stool is palpable in the left lower quadrant of the abdomen, which is best examined bimanually (a finger of one hand in the rectum and the other hand on the abdomen). The impaction is best removed manually if it is low enough, or through the sigmoidoscope if it is not. Repeated enemas (e.g., a Fleet enema; Table 39.3) may be helpful once some of the very hard stool is removed. Complications of impaction include recurrent urinary tract infection (because of compression of the ureters, more common in women), urinary incontinence, intestinal obstruction, perforation of the colon, and local ulceration (stercoral ulcer). Prevention of fecal impaction is an important goal in the sedentary elderly and is best done by increasing dietary fiber, adding a bulk laxative (Table 39.3) if necessary, and urging that at least 2 quarts of liquid be ingested each day, in addition to that consumed in the course of meals. Patients should also be sure to obey promptly the urge to defecate.

Ulcerative Colitis

Ulcerative colitis is a chronic inflammatory disorder of the colonic and rectal mucosa; its cause is unknown. It is recommended that patients with this condition be followed by their personal physician in consultation with a gastroenterologist. The disorder may affect patients of any age, with a peak incidence in the third decade and a second peak in the seventh decade.

The clinical picture of ulcerative colitis is highly variable. The disorder may be limited to the rectum (ulcerative proctitis) or may involve the entire colon. Symptoms may range from occasional rectal bleeding, even without diarrhea, to profuse purulent and bloody diarrhea. The severity of the initial presentation and the extent of the disease at the time of the initial attack have been shown to be useful predictors of the eventual course of the disease. Most patients (approximately 60%) have mild disease, that is, fewer than four bowel movements a day without fever, weight loss, or hypoalbuminemia. The vast majority of these patients have colitis limited to the rectosigmoid region or descending colon. Approximately 10 to 15% of patients with ulcerative colitis develop severe pancolitis with accompanying deterioration in their general health. Another 25% have moderate disease with more troublesome diarrhea, often containing blood, accompanied by crampy lower abdominal pain. Patients with moderate or severe disease may also have systemic symptoms of fever, fatigue, and weight loss. The clinical course is characterized by periodic exacerbations that generally respond well to adjustments in medical therapy. The smallest group of patients with ulcerative colitis consists of those with severe disease. This group includes the 1% of patients who present initially with fulminant colitis. In patients with severe colitis, symptoms may suddenly worsen, with profuse diarrhea, rectal bleeding, and high fevers. Plain films of the abdomen may demonstrate a dilated bowel (toxic megacolon). Mortality is high in this group of patients.

Because there is no specific test for, or histopathology of, ulcerative colitis, the diagnosis depends on the constellation of symptoms, the appropriate endoscopic and histologic appearance of the colonic mucosa, the exclusion of other inflammatory conditions, and the natural history of the disorder. Patients with acute presentations, depending on the circumstances, must be differentiated from patients with bacterial diarrheas (see Chapter 26), amebiasis, Crohn's disease (see below), and ischemic colitis (*ischemic colitis* presents with acute abdominal pain and the passage of bloody stool; this is a disease of middle-aged or older people who usually have evidence of generalized atherosclerosis).

Treatment. *Medical therapy* for ulcerative colitis is determined by the severity of the attack. (The use of antidiarrheal drugs in patients with chronic diarrhea is discussed later in this chapter.) Mild attacks may respond to sulfasalazine (Azulfidine), whereas moderate or severe attacks require treatment with oral or intravenous steroids. Steroids are very useful for acute exacerbations but are not helpful in preventing relapses. Conversely, sulfasalazine is of limited value in the treatment of acute attacks but has been shown to reduce the frequency of exacerbations and may allow reduction of the dosage of steroids. A minority of patients with ulcerative colitis need continuous steroid therapy. Other drugs, such as cytotoxic agents, require further evaluation before they can be recommended. 5-Aminosalicylic acid (Mesalamine or olsalazine, by enema or suppository, or Asacol, orally in a sustained-release tablet) may be used in patients intolerant to sulfasalazine (11), preferably in consultation with a gastroenterologist.

It has been discovered that nicotine alleviates symptoms in patients with ulcerative colitis (10), but whether it should be recommended treatment remains to be clarified.

Surgery in ulcerative colitis is curative, and patients should be counseled early in their course about the role of surgery in the treatment of this disorder. Patients should be informed about the indications for surgery and the types of operations that are available. Early attention to this issue enables the patient to accept an operation more readily if it is needed. Surgery for ulcerative colitis involves a proctocolectomy with an ileostomy to which a stomal appliance is attached to ensure continence (see Chapter 42). Construction of a continent ileostomy (Kock pouch) avoids the need for a stomal appliance, but the procedure is technically difficult and often requires revision. Another alternative is construction of an internal pouch from a loop of small bowel anastomosed to the anus (Park's procedure). These last two procedures are most successful in motivated young patients undergoing elective colectomy.

Cancer of the Colon. The risk of colorectal cancer is increased 5 to 10 times in patients with ulcerative colitis. The major risk factors are duration of disease (risk increases significantly after 8 to 10 years of disease), extent of colonic involvement (pancolitis carries the highest risk, whereas the risk in patients with ulcerative proctitis is similar to that of the general population), and age of onset of disease (patients under the age of 25 at the time of onset have the highest risk, independent of the extent of disease). The cancer may be found anywhere in the colon, although most commonly it is within the rectum or rectosigmoid. It may be multicentric and does not arise in adenomatous polyps. It is important that the patient know about the risk of cancer because it may influence a decision to undergo colectomy. After they have had the disease for 8 to 10 years, high-risk patients should have yearly evaluations of the colon by colonoscopy. Because dysplastic changes of the colonic mucosa have been identified as precancerous and have been shown to correlate closely with the development of cancer elsewhere in the colon, serial colonic and rectal biopsies should be obtained during this yearly colonoscopy in high-risk patients.

Crohn's Disease

Crohn's disease, or *regional enteritis,* is a chronic inflammatory condition of unknown cause involving all layers of the intestine, as opposed to just the mucosa in ulcerative colitis. The condition most commonly affects the terminal ileum, but any area from the esophagus to the anus can be involved. The onset of the disease most commonly is in adolescence and young adulthood. The incidence of Crohn's disease has been rising in recent years, particularly Crohn's disease of the colon.

Presentation. Crohn's disease may be localized initially to the small bowel, involve small bowel and colon, or be confined to the colon only. The inflammatory process often remains confined to the initial site of involvement unless surgery is performed. Recurrence is the rule after surgery, and the condition may then involve additional segments of bowel. Spontaneous progression of the disease tends to be in a proximal (orad) direction. As the inflammatory process persists, the bowel wall becomes thickened and stenotic, leading to bowel obstruction. Fistula formation is characteristic and may involve any contiguous structure. As a result, abscess formation and infection may complicate the clinical course. Diarrhea, abdominal pain, and weight loss are the most common symptoms. Unlike in ulcerative colitis, rectal bleeding is not a prominent feature unless the colon is the major site of involvement.

The *differential diagnosis* includes disorders of both

the small and large bowel. Occasionally the patient presents with fever and acute right lower quadrant pain resembling acute appendicitis. When there is terminal ileal involvement, Crohn's disease must be distinguished from lymphoma and tuberculosis. Colonic involvement may suggest ulcerative colitis, ischemic colitis, or carcinoma. Involvement of the distal small bowel and the right colon, the presence of characteristic skip areas, stricturing of the bowel, perianal disease, and fistula formation are helpful diagnostic features that suggest Crohn's disease.

Treatment. *Medical therapy* for Crohn's disease is similar to that for ulcerative colitis, depending heavily on corticosteroids and sulfasalazine. These agents may be effective in treating the recurrent attacks that characterize Crohn's disease, but neither agent has been shown to be effective in preventing relapses. In addition, sulfasalazine has not been shown to be useful in disease limited to the small bowel. Metronidazole (Flagyl) seems to be effective for perianal fistulas. Immunosuppressants, such as 6-mercaptopurine and azathioprine (Imuran), have produced variable results, and their use in this condition is controversial.

Surgery is sometimes necessary in Crohn's disease for resection of fibrotic obstructing lesions, drainage of abscesses, and resection of complicated fistulas. Occasionally the disease is refractory to medical therapy, and the diseased bowel must be resected. It must be recognized that surgery is not intended to be curative, so removal of normal bowel to achieve wide, disease-free margins is not indicated. In the rare patient whose disease is extensive and unresponsive to medical and surgical intervention or in whom a short bowel syndrome has developed secondary to the disease and to repeated surgery, long-term home parenteral hyperalimentation can be beneficial in providing good nutritional support and ameliorating symptoms.

Course. Despite its chronicity and tendency for recurrence, Crohn's disease takes a highly variable course. Prolonged asymptomatic periods occur, even after years of disease activity and multiple operations. There is a poor correlation between the clinical severity and the radiologic appearance of the disease, so follow-up radiographs are not indicated unless there is a suspicion of a new development in the disease (e.g., a fistula). The risk of colorectal carcinoma is elevated significantly only in Crohn's disease involving the colon, and even then probably not to the same degree as in ulcerative colitis. Mortality from the disease is low, but morbidity is high. Because the natural history is so variable, the physician should approach the patient with Crohn's disease in a positive and hopeful fashion, yet be aware of the potential for significant morbidity. All patients should be followed in close consultation with a gastroenterologist.

Drug-Induced Diarrhea

A variety of commonly used medications may cause diarrhea (Table 39.4). The diarrhea may be a direct result of the pharmacologic activity of the drug (e.g., magnesium-containing antacids or colchicine), or the mechanism for the induction of diarrhea may be unknown (e.g., hydralazine or propranolol). The diarrhea

may also signify drug toxicity (e.g., digitalis). Certain drugs have repeatedly been associated with diarrhea (antibiotics, antacids, quinidine, digitalis, alcohol), whereas in other cases (hydralazine, propranolol) the relationship is rare and not well defined.

Diarrhea associated with antibiotics may range from a mild increase in the frequency and volume of stools to a toxic, life-threatening condition. Diarrhea may develop during the course of antibiotic therapy, after parenteral or oral use, but may also occur up to months after discontinuation of the drugs. The antibiotics most commonly associated with diarrhea are ampicillin, tetracycline, clindamycin, and the cephalosporins.

In the more severe forms of antibiotic-associated diarrhea, the diarrhea is bloody and is accompanied by abdominal cramps and fever. Endoscopy may reveal pseudomembranes, which appear as raised yellowish plaques on edematous, friable mucosa. Histologically these pseudomembranes are collections of fibrin, mucin, and leukocytes. *Pseudomembranous colitis* is caused by proliferation of *Clostridium difficile* and the elaboration of its toxin. This organism accounts for the vast majority of cases of pseudomembranous colitis and for 20 to 30% of antibiotic-associated diarrhea in general. The toxin elaborated by *C. difficile* can be assayed in stool. The organism can also be cultured but is difficult to grow. Because culture is less sensitive than the toxin titer and does not correlate as well with symptoms, it is not recommended.

Therapy involves discontinuation of the antibiotics and, in cases of pseudomembranous colitis, administration of metronidazole (Flagyl), 500 mg four times a day for 7 days (see Chapter 26). This antimicrobial is effective against clostridial organisms, and the response is fairly rapid. Relapses after discontinuation of metronidazole are not uncommon. In such cases, a second course should be administered. Vancomycin, a much more expensive drug (approximately 100 times the cost of metronidazole), can be prescribed (125 to 500 mg four times a day for 7 days) for cases repeatedly resistant or relapsing after metronidazole. Oral cholestyramine has also been used effectively to bind the toxin. Antidiarrheal medications are contraindicated because they may actually prolong the duration of the disease. It is probably unnecessary to treat patients who are found to have *C. difficile* toxin-positive stools, as is common in nursing homes, unless there are accompanying symptoms or an outbreak is in progress. Symptomatic patients can be treated with bismuth subsalicylate (Pepto-Bismol), 30 mL or 2 tablets every 4 hours, while awaiting the assay of the toxin.

Postsurgical Diarrhea

A variety of surgical procedures may result in diarrhea. Predictably, *extensive small bowel resections* (e.g., for mesenteric vascular occlusions) result in severe diarrhea and steatorrhea (short bowel syndrome). Management of such patients requires careful attention to nutritional factors and often requires narcotics for control of the diarrhea. Long-term home hyperalimentation has allowed patients to overcome the severe malabsorption that would accompany massive small bowel resection.

Resection of the ileum is less well tolerated than resection of the jejunum because the ileum serves as the only site for absorption of bile acids. When the ileal resection is limited (less than 100 cm), the total bile acid pool remains sufficient to prevent significant steatorrhea. However, there is still an excessive loading of bile acids into the colon, where they stimulate mucosal secretion and result in diarrhea. Therapy for this form of diarrhea is aimed at binding the fecal bile acids with an agent such as cholestyramine. The dosage is 4 g given before meals and at bedtime. When ileal resection is more extensive (more than 100 cm), the total bile acid pool becomes diminished below the critical level needed for proper digestion and absorption of fat, and steatorrhea develops. The use of cholestyramine in this situation further depletes the bile acid pool and worsens the steatorrhea and diarrhea. Therefore, dietary fat should be supplied in the form of medium-chain triglycerides, which do not require bile acids for absorption. Commercial preparations are available (e.g., Portagen), and consultation with a nutritionist as well as a gastroenterologist is recommended.

Diarrhea may also follow *gastric surgery* with vagotomy. At times the vagotomy causes diarrhea by altering intestinal motility and, for unclear reasons, by increasing the concentration of fecal bile acids. Therapy with cholestyramine has been successful in this postvagotomy syndrome. Gastric surgery may also unmask latent lactase deficiency or, rarely, latent celiac disease. The blind loop syndrome with resultant bacterial overgrowth, dumping syndrome, inadvertent gastroileal anastomosis, and gastrocolic fistula are all complications that may result in diarrhea in patients after gastrectomy (see Chapter 37).

Diarrhea occurs rarely after routine cholecystectomy, associated with an increased concentration of fecal bile acids. Therapy with cholestyramine is effective. Subtotal colectomy, with an ileal–rectal anastomosis (e.g., for multiple polyposis), often results in diarrhea that is usually easily controlled by antidiarrheal medication and diminishes with time. Segmental colonic resection usually does not result in diarrhea because of the large functional reserve of the normal colon.

Symptomatic Antidiarrheal Therapy

Diarrhea is merely a symptom, and therapy, if possible, should be directed at the primary underlying process. However, a wide variety of agents are available for symptomatic control of diarrhea. The efficacy of these agents is highly variable and the mechanism of action of many is poorly understood. Symptomatic treatment should be avoided in patients with acute infectious diarrhea (except at minimal dosages to prevent marked discomfort) because early suppression of bowel movements in these conditions prolongs the diarrhea.

Hydrophilic bulk-forming agents, such as psyllium (Metamucil, Konsyl), have been shown to improve the consistency of ileostomy and colostomy effluent (see Chapter 42; see preparation and dosages in Table 39.3). These agents, which paradoxically are also used in treating constipation, are particularly useful in patients with irritable bowel syndrome (Chapter 40).

Another group of antidiarrheal medications consists of those classified as *absorbents* on the premise that these agents absorb factors within the intestinal lumen that cause diarrhea. Medications of this group include kaolin and pectin (Kaopectate), bismuth salts (Pepto-Bismol), aluminum hydroxide (Amphojel), and cholestyramine (Questran). Most are available over the counter, but their value is not well established. However, Pepto-Bismol has been shown to be effective in controlling the symptoms of traveler's diarrhea (see Chapter 26). Cholestyramine is effective in treating bile acid–induced diarrhea, as occurs in patients after ileal resection, vagotomy, or cholecystectomy. This drug also may bind other compounds, such as digoxin and warfarin, and thereby decrease their absorption.

Opioid derivatives are probably the most effective antidiarrheal medications. Opiate drugs delay the transit of intraluminal contents through the small and large intestines. A central effect is also likely. In patients with extensive small bowel resection, codeine may be the only effective form of therapy. The synthetic agents diphenoxylate-atropine (Lomotil) and loperamide (Imodium) are also effective and generally are well tolerated. The atropine in Lomotil contributes little to its antidiarrheal effect and may cause significant toxicity. Imodium has the theoretical advantages of a more favorable ratio of GI effects to central nervous system effects and a longer duration of action. An over-the-counter formulation is now available. Imodium has the practical disadvantage of being expensive. The development of megacolon, prolongation of symptoms, and worsening of pseudomembranous colitis have all been linked to the injudicious use of these agents in patients with bacterial diarrhea. The potential risk for abuse is theoretically less for Imodium.

Another group of drugs that is under investigation is classified as antisecretory. Some of these drugs inhibit the synthesis of prostaglandins, which increase intestinal secretion by stimulating adenylate cyclase activity within intestinal cells. (Adenylate cyclase is the enzyme that catalyzes the formation of cAMP, the concentration of which influences certain transport systems in cell membranes). Other drugs of this class inhibit adenylate cyclase directly. For example, indomethacin inhibits prostaglandin synthesis and has been shown experimentally to inhibit the effect of enterotoxin. Propranolol, an inhibitor of adenylate cyclase, suppresses bile acid–induced fluid accumulation in intestinal loops. Certain diuretics, such as ethacrynic acid, which act on electrolyte transport, have also been shown to be effective enterotoxin antagonists. Endorphinlike peptides are also under study as antidiarrheal agents. Investigation into their mechanism of action may lead to the development of new effective forms of therapy against diarrhea. Recently, a somatostatin analog (octreotide) has been made available for the treatment of GI endocrine tumors (e.g., VIP-oma, gastrinoma, carcinoid). It is not recommended for use in other forms of diarrhea.

Because there are few data to allow an objective comparison of the various antidiarrheal medications, the choice of drug must be based on efficacy, safety, and cost. For acute, self-limited illnesses, drugs such as kaolin-pectate and bismuth salts are often tried by patients, even before a physician is consulted. For such patients, diphenoxylate–atropine (Lomotil) or loperamide (Imodium) is highly effective. Patients should be instructed to use medication after a diarrheal movement, not to exceed 8 tablets/day. Loperamide may provide longer diarrhea-free intervals with fewer side effects (8). Oral rehydration therapy (see Chapters 26 and 33 for details on products) is important, especially with voluminous diarrhea in the frail elderly, and in children. Both glucose-based and rice-based electrolyte solutions are available for rehydration (1). It should be recognized that commercial rehydration solutions designed for athletes (e.g., Gatorade) have inadequate concentrations of electrolytes and therefore are not satisfactory in the treatment of diarrhea.

For patients with chronic diarrhea, the choice of medication is based on the severity and cause of the diarrhea. In patients with the diarrhea-predominant form of the irritable bowel syndrome (Chapter 40), hydrophilic agents may be useful. The dosage should be titrated to the desired bowel habits, with dosages ranging from 1 teaspoon to 2 tablespoons/day mixed in 8 ounces of juice or water per dose. In patients with diarrhea from other causes, diphenoxylate–atropine or loperamide should be tried. These medications can be given in divided doses throughout the day. Diarrhea can also be prevented by taking one or two tablets before engaging in an event associated with diarrhea (e.g., meals or examinations).

In more severe cases of diarrhea, narcotics are necessary. Tincture of opium is convenient because it can easily be titrated (by the drop) to control diarrhea at the lowest possible dosage. A recommended starting dosage is six drops every 4 to 6 hours, to be adjusted by one or two drops per dose depending on the patient's response. Codeine, at a dose of 15 to 30 mg, may also be used with the same dosage schedule.

General References*

Cranston D, McWhinnie D, Collin J. Dietary fibre and gastrointestinal disease. Br J Surg 75:508, 1988.
> A review of the relationship of fiber to constipation, diverticular disease, and colorectal cancer.

Gerding DN. Disease associated with *Clostridium difficile* infection. Ann Intern Med 110:255, 1989.
> A good review of the clinical spectrum from asymptomatic carriers to fulminant disease.

Sawer MK, Gehlbach SH. Bacterial disease of the colon. Prim Care 15:125, 1988.
> A good review. Emphasizes selection of patients with self-limited disease and discusses oral rehydration as primary treatment in these patients.

Simon D. Pharmacotherapy of gastrointestinal tract infections in patients with AIDS. Pract Gastroenterol 17(3):9, 1993.

Specific References

1. Aver ME, Snyder JD. Oral therapy for acute diarrhea: the underused simple solution. N Engl J Med 323:891, 1990.
2. Bourlioux P, Pouchart P. Nutritional and health properties of yogurt. World Rev Nutr Diet 56:217, 1988.
3. Dupont HL, Hornick RB. Adverse effects of Lomotil therapy in shigellosis. JAMA 226:1525, 1973.
4. Harvey RF, Pomare EW, Heaton KW. Effects of increased dietary fibre on intestinal transit. Lancet 1:1278, 1983.
5. Kaufman N, Schuster MM. Colonic motility studies differentiate three types of constipation. Gastroenterology 76:1166, 1979.
6. Lubowsky CZ, Chen FC, Kennedy ML, et al. Results of colectomy for severe slow transit constipation. Dis Colon Rectum 39:23–29, 1996.
7. Metcalf AM, Phillips SF, Zinsmeister AR, et al. Simplified assessment of segmental colonic transit. Gastroenterology 92:40, 1987.
8. Palmer KR, Corbett CL, Holdsworth CD. Double blind cross-over study comparing loperamide, codeine, and diphenoxylate in the treatment of chronic diarrhea. Gastroenterology 79:1272, 1980.
9. Payler DK, Pomare EWJ, Heaton KW, et al. The effect of wheat bran on intestinal transit. Gut 16:209, 1975.
10. **Pullan RD, Rhodes J, Garresh S, et al. Transdermal nicotine for active ulcerative colitis. N Engl J Med 330:811, 1994.**
11. **Sutherland LR, May GR, Shaffer EA. Sulfasalazine revisited: a meta-analysis of 5-aminosalicylic acid in the treatment of ulcerative colitis. Ann Intern Med 118:540, 1993.**
12. Tramonte SM, Brand MB, Mulrow CD, et al. The treatment of chronic constipation in adults. J Gen Intern Med 12:15–24, 1997.

*Bold print (general references) and bold numerals (specific references) denote published controlled clinical trials, meta-analyses, or consensus-based recommendations.

C H A P T E R 40

Irritable Bowel Syndrome

MARVIN M. SCHUSTER, MD

DEFINITION AND EPIDEMIOLOGY

Irritable bowel syndrome (IBS) is the most common gastrointestinal condition encountered in medical practice (5,9,10). The syndrome is diagnosed on the basis of abdominal pain, altered bowel habits, and the absence of detectable organic disease. A related condition, painless (or nervous) diarrhea, should be considered either as a separate entity, or at best a variant of IBS, because it affects patients with different personality profiles, is more directly and immediately related to emotional stress, and has a different course and prognosis. Symptoms of IBS generally appear during late teenage years or in the early twenties and more commonly afflict women than men, the disorder having a female to male predominance of 2:1. The symptoms rarely appear for the first time after the age of 50, so this diagnosis should be made extremely reluctantly in the older patient who has had a recent onset of symptoms. There is some question about whether recurrent abdominal pain of childhood is a form of IBS or leads to IBS in later life.

There are many other terms by which irritable bowel syndrome is known. These include *mucus colitis, nervous colitis, spastic colon, nervous colon, irritated colon,* and *unstable colon.* The term *colitis* is especially inappropriate because no inflammation is present and because it is frightening to the patient, who easily confuses it with ulcerative colitis. This misconception imposes unnecessary stress on pa-

tients whose condition is readily aggravated by stress. The term *irritable bowel syndrome* is more appropriate than other terms because it refers to general gastrointestinal irritability, indicating that areas other than the colon may be involved, and it also emphasizes that this is a syndrome, not a specific disease.

PATHOPHYSIOLOGY

The signs and symptoms of irritable bowel syndrome appear to be related predominantly to exaggeration of normal intestinal motility patterns. In normal subjects the dominant type of motor activity is segmenting contractions, which tend to retard the forward movement of intraluminal contents. This impeding activity represents approximately 90% or more of the wave types recorded in normal individuals. When this type of activity is excessive, constipation ensues. In diarrheal states this activity is markedly diminished or abolished and is replaced by infrequent mass propulsive movements (which may occur five or six times a day during episodes of diarrhea). The symptoms of IBS (abdominal pain, constipation, diarrhea) are related to excessively strong, spastic contractions either of the segmenting (impeding) or propulsive type. The motility pattern of IBS has been described as the paradoxical motility of constipation and diarrhea, but the paradox is a spurious one if these basic principles are understood.

Ambulatory recordings reveal high-amplitude progressive contractions (HAPCs) (2) that sweep down the colon six to eight times per 24 hours in normal subjects. HAPCs are associated with meals and defecation. They are seen less than once per 24 hours in constipation-predominant IBS, and their decreased frequency is another reason (in addition to hypersegmentation) for constipation in IBS.

Motility can be influenced by a number of factors, such as meals, emotionally stressful situations, anxiety, and various drugs (e.g., opiates). In IBS, exacerbation of symptoms by meals (i.e., pain, distension, and occasional diarrhea) is thought to be related to an exaggeration of the normal biphasic postprandial response: the gastroileocolic response, which consists of an early neurogenic (reflex) component during the first 15 to 30 minutes postprandially, and hormonally stimulated contractions that appear after 40 minutes. The hormonal phase may be initiated by gastrointestinal hormones released during feeding. For example, cholecystokinin, which is released as food enters the duodenum, can reproduce postprandial symptoms in some patients with IBS, and these symptoms are associated with increased motility. Whether this or other hormones of this type are clinically important is unknown.

Recent studies point to heightened visceral sensory perception as an additional factor in the pathophysiology of IBS (1,6,7).

DIAGNOSIS

History

Most patients with IBS come to medical attention after their symptoms have been present for months or years. Major complaints are those of pain and altered bowel habits. Which of these two components is emphasized depends on which is the more disturbing to the patient. This, in turn, is determined by the intensity of each symptom, by the patient's reaction to it, and by the disruptive effects of the symptom on the patient's function and activities. For example, some patients are less bothered by abdominal pain, which can be hidden from others, but are perturbed by urgent diarrhea, which interferes with their job or social functions. The pattern of symptoms varies considerably from person to person but remains fairly consistent for a given patient, with changes occurring predominantly in intensity or frequency of occurrence. Typically, symptoms are intermittent, with symptom-free periods lasting days, weeks, or rarely, months. Some patients have symptoms every day.

Pain

The quality of pain may be described by one patient as crampy, by another as sharp or burning. For most, the pain is relieved temporarily by a bowel movement. One of the most important features that differentiates functional from organic pain is that the pain does not awaken the patient from sleep. It is important that the question concerning this feature be carefully phrased because there is an important distinction between awakening with pain and being awakened by pain. Patients with IBS who are depressed have early-morning awakening and, after awakening, experience pain, but close questioning can reveal that the patient was not awakened by the pain. The location of pain may vary from person to person but is fairly consistent for a given person. Pain may be localized to any quadrant, although it is more common in the lower abdomen than anywhere else and in the left lower quadrant more often than in the right. Although the pain usually does not radiate, some patients describe transmission into the lower back or down the legs. The distribution of the pain is generally over a wide enough area that the patient, when asked to point to the location of the pain, does so with the flat of his or her hand rather than with a finger, and often makes a circular motion covering a broad area. More often than not, the onset of pain does not appear to correlate with any known precipitating stressful event; instead, periods of illness may correlate with general periods of stress over months or years. It is important to determine what life experiences or interpersonal relationships constitute stress for a particular person so that this history can be taken into account when establishing a treatment program.

Altered Bowel Habits

The altered pattern of defecation in patients with IBS may consist of constipation, diarrhea, or, more commonly, alternating constipation and diarrhea, with one of the two predominating. (Chapter 39 discusses these symptoms in detail.) As with pain, the altered pattern of defecation, though variable from person to person, is fairly consistent for a given patient, changing only in periodicity and intensity.

Not infrequently the major disordered bowel function occurs in the morning, with the first stool being normal in consistency, followed in rapid succession by increasingly loose stools, sometimes associated with flatulence and sometimes precipitated by meals. The bowel movements are accompanied by a great deal of urgency and are preceded by cramps that are relieved by defecation. Formed stools are often compressed and of narrow pencil-sized diameter because of the molding effect of rectosigmoid spasm. In other instances spasm of the colon results in the passage of scybalous, dehydrated stools described by the patient as hard pellets. Mucus may cover the stools or be passed separately. Stools may mistakenly be called diarrheal when they consist of frequently passed small quantities of soft fragments that are narrow in caliber. Explosive defecation may result from evacuation of gas along with the stool. Fecal incontinence (usually slight staining), which occurs in approximately 20% of patients with IBS, may result from the repetitive reflex relaxations that occur in association with repetitive spastic distal colonic contractions.

Painless Diarrhea. Patients who have diarrhea but do not have abdominal pain generally are thought to have a disorder that is different from IBS, although sometimes painless diarrhea is classified as a variant of the irritable bowel syndrome. Compared with those of patients with IBS, their symptoms are more directly related to a stressful event, follow more immediately upon that stress, and respond more readily and dramatically to alleviation of stress. Also, the prognosis is generally better than it is in classic IBS.

Relationship of Symptoms to Meals

Some patients with IBS experience exacerbation of their symptoms postprandially. They appear to be a special subset of patients. Some patients report intolerance of specific foods, most commonly milk and milk products, caffeine, fried foods, and red wine.

Gas

Intestinal gas derives from swallowing of air, bacterial breakdown of poorly digested foods, or diminished absorption of gas (which may occur during the rapid transit that accompanies diarrhea). Aerophagia is aggravated by frequent swallowing while chewing gum and during nervous states and is induced by a dry throat or by the excessive intake of carbonated beverages, including beer. Increased gas production follows eating of legumes (e.g., beans) that contain stachyose and raffinose, substances that can be digested only by colonic flora, resulting in release of large amounts of hydrogen in the colon. If patients have milk intolerance because of lactase deficiency, undigested lactose enters the colon, where it is broken down by colonic bacteria, also resulting in gaseous distension.

Although gaseous distension is a common complaint, actual measurements demonstrate that patients with IBS have no more gas than do normal subjects. Instead, they have a decreased tolerance to distension from normal amounts of gas, a factor that may be related to hypermotility of their bowel and to the lowered threshold for distension-induced spasm. Because gas tends to rise, it usually forms pockets under the splenic flexure, which is the highest portion of the colon in the upright position. This entrapment of air is further facilitated by distal rectosigmoid spasm that impedes its passage. The *splenic flexure syndrome* that ensues is experienced as chest pain, which may mimic the pain of myocardial ischemia. A similar *hepatic flexure syndrome* can accompany gas trapped on the right side and may mimic the pain of cholecystitis. Relief often occurs with passage of gas.

Studies in which air has been instilled into the small bowel demonstrate that patients with IBS tend to reflux gas more readily into the stomach than do normal subjects, which may explain their complaint of increased belching. This complaint also seems to result from abnormal intestinal motility.

Upper Gastrointestinal Symptoms

One-fourth to one-half of patients with IBS complain of dyspeptic symptoms such as heartburn, indigestion, pain, and nausea (but rarely vomiting). These upper gastrointestinal symptoms reinforce the concept that the motor abnormality is not restricted to the colon alone.

Significance of Weight Loss and Bleeding

IBS per se is not associated with either weight loss or gastrointestinal bleeding, and the appearance of either of these two symptoms in patients with IBS should alert the physician to another disorder. However, significant depression accompanying IBS may explain substantial weight loss, just as anal fissures or hemorrhoids resulting from the altered bowel habits of the syndrome may explain bright red rectal bleeding. Nevertheless, either of these two symptoms warrants a meticulous search for other disorders, including cancer. A sudden change in symptom pattern after many years also warrants a search for a new disorder.

Psychologic Factors

Seventy percent of patients with IBS have abnormal scores on psychologic testing (Table 40.1). The psychologic disturbances that most commonly accompany IBS are somatoform disorder, anxiety, depression, and cancerophobia. Of these, anxiety is the most readily detected and perhaps the easiest to treat by pharmacologic means, psychologic approaches, or environmental manipulation. Depression is generally masked and is commonly overlooked by patient and physician alike (see Chapter 15). This is in part because somatization, a common manifestation of depression, results in a focus on complaints that may misdirect the physician's attention from underlying psychologic factors. Depression should be suspected in patients who appear preoccupied or sad or who by their report or the report of family members have lost interest in matters that formerly interested them. Studies show a high frequency of reported physical and, particularly, sexual abuse among patients with IBS (3). It is important to solicit this information and to deal with it therapeutically (see Chapter 18).

Community studies comparing people with IBS who do not seek medical attention with those who do demonstrate that patients who seek medical attention have more psychologic distress than those who do not (11). Cancerophobia may be suggested when the patient compares his or her symptoms with those of a relative or friend who has had cancer. In addition to determining whether the patient has an unwarranted and excessive fear of cancer, an attempt should be made to elicit from the patient and other informants any other fears or concerns that the patient has with respect to him- or herself and the illness.

Physical Examination

Except for an anxious demeanor, patients with IBS usually look remarkably healthy, and physical examination is correspondingly normal, with the common exception of mildly increased tympany to percussion over one or more areas of the colon and a tender, cordlike sigmoid palpable in the left lower quadrant. A palpable sigmoid itself is not an unusual finding, even in normal people, because firm stool may be present in this area, but tenderness is significant. Tenderness may

Table 40.1. Psychologic Features of Irritable Bowel Syndrome

Psychopathology	Diagnostic Features	Treatment
Depression	Sad, tearful, hopeless, fatigue, loss of interest, early morning awakening	Antidepressant medication, environmental manipulation
Anxiety	Symptoms increased by stress	Relaxation training, environmental manipulation, coping techniques
Gratification from illness behavior	Symptoms often interfere with work or socializing	Treat as a physical deformity, encourage maximal activity, discourage talking to others about illness, recognize chronic nature of disorder
Cancer phobia	Patient or family reports fear; patient describes similarity of his or her symptoms with those of a known cancer victim	Adequate early workup, then limit further investigation; discuss openly with patient

After Whitehead WE, Schuster MM. Psychological management of irritable bowel syndrome. Pract Gastroenterol 3:32, 1979.

Table 40.2.   Lactose-Free Diet[a]

Type of Food	Food Allowed	Food to Be Avoided
Milk and milk products	Nutramigen and soya bean milk used in place of milk, nondairy "milk" that does not contain lactose, Lactaid milk	All milk of any species and all products containing milk as skim, dried, evaporated, condensed yogurt, cheese,[b] ice cream, malted milk, sherbets
Meat, fish, fowl	Plain beef, chicken, fish, turkey, veal, pork, ham, liver, or other organ meats	*Creamed* or *breaded* meat, fish, or fowl; sausage products such as weiners, liver sausage; cold cuts that contain milk
Eggs	All	None
Vegetables	All	Creamed, breaded, or buttered vegetables, any vegetables to which lactose has been added during processing
Potatoes and substitutes	White potatoes, sweet potatoes, yams, macaroni, noodles, rice, spaghetti	Any creamed, breaded, or buttered potatoes or starch and instant potatoes if lactose has been added during processing
Breads and cereals	Any that do not contain milk or milk products	Prepared mixes such as muffins, biscuits, waffles, pancakes, dry cereals with added skim milk powder; instant cream of wheat and other instant hot cereals (read labels carefully)
Fats	Margarines that do not contain milk or milk products, salad dressings that do not contain milk or milk products, bacon, salad oils, shortening	Margarines and dressings containing milk or milk products; butter, cream cheese
Soups	All except those listed under foods excluded	Cream soups, chowders, commercially prepared soups that contain lactose
Desserts	Water and fruit ices; Jello, angel food cake; home-made cakes, pies, cookies made without milk from acceptable ingredients; ice cream made with non-dairy mix	Commercial cakes and cookies and mixes; custard, puddings, ice cream made with milk; any containing chocolate
Fruits	All fresh, canned, or frozen that are not processed with lactose	Any canned or frozen that are processed with lactose
Miscellaneous	Nuts and nut butter, unbuttered popcorn, olives, pure sugar candy, jelly or marmalade, sugar, Karo, chewing gum	Gravy, white sauce, coffee, powdered drink, caramels, molasses, molasses candies, most instant coffee (Folger's instant coffee and Tang are lactose free)

[a]In all instances labels should be carefully read and any product that contains milk, lactose, dry milk solids, or curds should be omitted. Also avoid whey and sugar substitutes with lactose. For milk products use Coffee-mate, soy milk baby formulas, or Lactaid milk.

[b]Swiss, Jarlsberg, Edam, and sharp cheddar are the only cheeses allowed.

be present in other areas also, particularly in the right lower quadrant, where a squishy cecum may be palpated.

Digital rectal examination is usually unremarkable but may reveal excessive tenderness. Proctoscopic examination should demonstrate no structural abnormality but often does reveal rectal and rectosigmoid spasm and excessive tenderness that precludes advance beyond 12 or 13 cm. At times excessive mucus is encountered.

In patients with symptoms of IBS, the physician should look for signs of hyperthyroidism, masses, adenopathy, and partial intestinal obstruction, as well as for abdominal bruits, which might signal ischemic intestinal angina in the elderly.

Laboratory Tests

Basic laboratory tests should be carried out to demonstrate the absence of anemia; a normal white blood cell count and sedimentation rate; the absence of blood, ova, and parasites on three stool examinations; a negative flexible sigmoidoscopy; and (when symptoms are severe enough or prolonged enough to warrant the study) a barium enema negative except for spastic contractions. Effacement of haustra may be seen in the barium enema if there has been prolonged laxative abuse (see Chapter 39). Occasionally a small bowel series is necessary to rule out Crohn's disease, especially when diarrhea predominates or when there is associated weight loss. Painful splenic flexure symptoms sometimes require studies to rule out coronary artery disease (see Chapter 57).

The basic principle in the selection and timing of laboratory tests is to perform as early as possible the tests that are necessary to convince both the physician and the patient that organic disease has been ruled out. It is generally imprudent to postpone some tests for a later date or to repeat tests continually because this behavior arouses the suspicion that the diagnosis is uncertain, that the disease might be progressive, or that a new and more dire problem such as cancer or colitis may be developing.

Differential Diagnosis

Many symptoms of IBS are nonspecific and can be produced by other disorders. A careful travel history should be obtained to assess the likelihood of *bacterial infection* or *parasitic infestation,* including giardiasis and amebiasis.

Because patients with *lactose intolerance* often do not associate their symptoms with milk, the failure to find a direct relationship between milk intake and diarrhea should not dissuade the physician from testing for milk tolerance. Lactose intolerance is best ruled out by a therapeutic trial on a lactose-free diet (see the sample lactose-free diet in Table 40.2) for 3 weeks, eliminating all milk and milk products, including butter, cottage cheese, yogurt, and soft cheeses. Aged cheeses, such as Swiss and Jarlsberg, are permissible because most of the lactose in them has been eliminated. Yogurt contains little lactose and may be reintroduced later as tolerated. Acidophilus milk (cultured with *Lactobacillus acidophilus*), contrary to popular misconception, contains the same amount of lactose as regular milk. However, the amount of lactose in milk can be virtually eliminated by adding 12 drops of lactase (Lactaid, obtained over the counter) to a quart of milk, which is then permitted to remain overnight in the refrigerator; this procedure reduces, but does not eliminate entirely, the symptoms of lactose intolerance (8). Lactaid milk, available commercially, is 70% lactose free and is tolerated in small quantities (added to cereal or coffee, for example) by most lactose-intolerant patients. Also, Lactaid tablets or Lactrase capsules taken just before ingestion of milk products reduce the lactose load substantially. Otherwise, nondairy (lactose-free) substitutes such as Coffee-mate, Cremora, or Mocha Mix may be used. Margarine may be substituted for butter. If all symptoms disappear on a lactose-free diet, then the diagnosis is lactose intolerance. Partial improvement implies that, in addition to IBS, the patient has lactose intolerance and that some of the symptoms (usually those of gaseous bloating and diarrhea) are caused by the intolerance. The therapeutic dietary trial is more useful than a lactose tolerance test, which simply tests the patient's response to a given amount of lactose in a single dose at a particular time (see also Chapter 39).

Among the other disorders that can mimic symptoms of diarrhea-predominant IBS are hyperthyroidism, nontropical sprue, carcinoid, Zollinger–Ellison syndrome, medullary carcinoma of the thyroid, diabetic autonomic neuropathy, Addison's disease, Whipple's disease, and human immunodeficiency virus (HIV)-associated diarrhea (see Chapter 34). Constipation-predominant IBS may be mimicked by hypothyroidism, hyperparathyroidism, diverticular disease, intestinal obstruction, and colon cancer. Suspicion of any of these disorders justifies the appropriate tests to rule them out. Further evaluation of patients with atypical symptoms of IBS should be done in consultation with a gastroenterologist.

NATURAL HISTORY

There is evidence that approximately 15% of the general adult population have the IBS but have not sought medical attention for it (12). Patients who seek medical attention have more psychopathology than those who do not and may give a false impression of an increased incidence of psychopathology in IBS. Approximately one-fourth of patients who seek medical treatment for IBS ultimately have a permanent remission. It is unclear whether this represents the natural course of the disease or a response to early treatment of mild disease. The patient who is referred for gastroen-

terologic consultation often has correspondingly more severe and chronic symptoms and generally experiences a more prolonged course.

Although there is little information concerning patients with IBS who present to the primary care physician, it has been shown that the course of patients seen by gastroenterologists follows a fairly consistent pattern that is characteristic for the given individual. In fact, the pattern is so consistent that any significant change should be accepted as a warning of a new superimposed problem warranting further investigation.

THERAPY

General Principles

Because the underlying etiology of IBS is unknown, treatment is symptomatic and relies on education, reassurance, diet, supportive and behavioral therapy, and pharmacotherapy aimed at both the underlying motor disorder and its psychologic concomitants. Successful management requires an interest in the patient and the disorder, an understanding on the part of both patient and physician of what is known about IBS, and above all, a recognition of the chronic nature of the disorder, which implies acceptance of a prolonged cooperative therapeutic endeavor.

Education and Reassurance

Treatment begins with the first interview and physical examination, which should be designed to begin to establish a relationship of mutual interest and confidence and should be thorough enough to demonstrate to the patient that the physician has taken the complaints seriously and is performing all necessary maneuvers to rule out organic causes. At the same time, attention to the details of all contributing factors, including diet, emotional reactions, interpersonal relationships, social interactions, and the patient's fears and concerns, provides ample evidence to the patient that these are important factors with which he or she must deal. The worst mistake that a physician can make is to downplay the symptoms on the grounds that they exist only in the patient's mind. This is incorrect physiologically and therapeutically; a definite motor disorder exists and can be demonstrated by both myoelectric and motility recordings.

It is important to take the time to explain to the patient the present understanding of the disordered motility and the factors influencing it to emphasize that although the disorder is chronic, it can be managed by appropriate cooperation between patient and physician. The demonstrated ability of the physician to predict the course promotes confidence. Furthermore, if the patient knows what to anticipate and understands that treatment can be expected to ameliorate rather than eliminate the disorder, he or she is better prepared to face recurrence, which otherwise might be disappointing and frightening. Labeling and understanding the abnormal motor activity can be reassuring to the patient and may provide him or her with the patience required to wait for gradual improvement. At the same time, the positive implications of the diagnosis should be underscored, emphasizing that IBS, although often persistent, does not lead to cancer, colitis, or ileitis and does not alter life expectancy.

Diet

Even when the patient keeps a meticulous daily log relating onset of symptoms to life events (including activities, interpersonal relations, and food intake), it is often difficult to make direct associations with any degree of specificity. It is best to explain to patients who have postprandial distress that although some foods may be bothersome, it is usually the act of eating (rather than a specific food) that aggravates the symptoms. Because a lactose-free diet can provide dramatic relief for patients who are lactose intolerant, it is worthwhile trying such a diet in every patient. (Patients who improve on a 3-week lactose-free trial may then add small amounts of lactose-containing foods until symptoms appear. This will establish the level of lactose that can be tolerated by that person.) Otherwise, the most that can be said about food intolerance is that some people react badly to coffee, carbonated beverages, and spicy sauces, although no convincing evidence exists in this regard. Therefore, patients may wish to abstain from these foods for a period, noting whether symptoms recur on at least two occasions when each substance is reintroduced. Any food that is definitely associated with precipitation of symptoms should obviously be avoided, but one should be careful not to create a dietary cripple.

Some patients with constipation-predominant IBS derive benefit from a diet that includes a large amount of *bran.* This can be administered as 2 tablespoons of Miller's unprocessed bran three times daily. Bran can be obtained from a health food store. Because it looks and tastes like sawdust, it can be camouflaged in cereal, baked in cookies, or taken with a beverage. Studies of diverticular disease show that the effect of bran on transit and motility appears to be specific and is not common to all fibers (4). Therefore lettuce, celery, and fruits may not produce similar results. Bran has been shown to increase the size of stool and the frequency of its passage. Patients should be warned that flatulence might increase some when bran is first administered but that it diminishes by the end of 3 weeks in 80% of patients. However, 15 or 20% of people find these side effects intolerable even after 3 weeks. Dosage should be titrated for each patient, weighing the beneficial effects against the annoying side effects.

Drugs

The *hydrophilic colloids* (bulk agents such as Metamucil, Konsyl, or L.A. Formula, containing psyllium seed) may be especially useful in patients who have alternating constipation and diarrhea. Because of their hydrophilic qualities, they tend to bind water and therefore decrease the fluidity of diarrheal stools, while preventing excess dehydration in constipated patients. Initially, 1 to 2 tablespoons of hydrophilic powder are prescribed in conjunction with a meal two to three times a day, and the dosage is gradually diminished to once a day (adjusting to the patient's response). It is better to prescribe the agent before or after a meal rather than at bedtime, so that it becomes mixed with the meal as it traverses the gastrointestinal tract. When taken at night the medication can result in the passage of rock-hard stool followed by a gelatinous mass. Patients who are thin should take the bulk agent after meals because it tends to suppress appetite, whereas obese patients may derive benefit from taking it before meals, thus achieving satiation without high caloric intake. Although there are ample theoretical grounds for prescribing antispasmodic medication, clinical experience with spasmolytic agents is disappointing. Nevertheless, some patients improve with *antispasmodic drugs,* particularly those whose symptoms are induced by meals and those who complain of tenesmus. Well-controlled studies are needed to determine whether anticholinergic medication has more than a placebo effect. When used for those whose symptoms are related to meals, anticholinergics should be prescribed 30 to 45 minutes before meals so that the major benefit of the drug is available at the time of anticipated symptoms. Patients with tenesmus should take the drug on a regular basis, timing the dose so that it is given as close as possible to 1 hour before anticipated symptoms. There is no evidence that one anticholinergic is better than another, but it seems logical to use drugs that have the highest ratio of antispasmodic to antisecretory effect, so that a large dosage can be administered to suppress spasm without producing undesirable side effects such as dry mouth. Mebeverine, a spasmolytic agent with little or no antisecretory effect, is available in most countries outside the United States and is prescribed in dosages of 100 to 200 mg four times a day (½ hour before meals if symptoms are meal related). In the United States dicyclomine hydrochloride (Bentyl) is given in dosages of 20 to 40 mg four times a day, as tolerated. The major side effects are tachycardia and orthostatic hypotension. Thus, baseline and follow-up recordings of pulse rate and blood pressure with the patient seated and standing are important. Dicyclomine should be prescribed in small quantities to elderly people who are susceptible to orthostatic changes; for example, 10-mg doses can be given on a divided basis, gradually increasing to reach the desired effect as tolerated. If improvement ensues, long-term medication for months or years is warranted. Tolerance usually does not develop, but change to a different anticholinergic may be helpful if benefit decreases. A therapeutic trial should be carried out for at least 3 weeks to test the efficacy of the drug.

Significant diarrhea may respond to *diphenoxylate–atropine* (Lomotil), 1 to 2 tablets every 6 hours while diarrhea persists, or to *loperamide* (Imodium), which has a longer duration of action and may be given in 1 to 2 tablets every 8 hours. Care should be taken to discontinue medication as soon as the diarrhea is controlled to avoid inducing constipation, especially in patients who are prone to having alternating diarrhea and constipation. Patients who have strongly diarrhea-predominant IBS and who do not respond to these medications may benefit from *codeine,* 30 to 60 mg every 6 hours, especially if pain is disabling. Because of its potentially addicting qualities, codeine should be prescribed with caution, although addiction is rare when codeine is taken for diarrhea. This is partially because intestinal tolerance to the drug does not develop. The same dosage that controls diarrhea at one stage continues to control it subsequently, and escalating dosages are not required as they are in patients who have developed central nervous system addiction.

Analgesic medication should be avoided if possible and, when needed, should be prescribed in the mildest form and lowest dosage possible. However, aspirin and acetaminophen are rarely effective. Pentazocine (Talwin), 50 to 100 mg, can be given every 6 hours as needed for severe pain, but the number of tablets taken should be monitored. Morphine generally should be avoided, especially when constipation exists, because it tends to aggravate spasm.

Gas Control

Most medications designed to alleviate gaseous distension have proved to be disappointing. However, simethicone (Mylicon), 2 to 4 tablets with meals, or activated charcoal, 4 tablets with meals and at bedtime, can be prescribed as a therapeutic trial. Phazyme 95 or 125, 1 to 2 tablets with meals and at bedtime, or similar enzymes such as Ilozyme, Pancrease, Viokase, or Cotazym can also be tried, although their efficacy has not been documented.

Psychologic Management

Psychologic management begins with the recognition of depression, anxiety, and somatization of affect (Table 40.1). Symptoms of IBS often are anxiety provoking and perpetuated by social reinforcement (secondary gain). Psychologic evaluation and management usually can be effectively performed by the interested physician without the need for psychiatric referral. The condition itself is not an indication for psychiatric consultation. Referral should be reserved for patients who would need expert psychotherapy whether or not they have IBS.

Psychologic management is dictated by answers to the following questions:

- Is there evidence of anxiety, and are the symptoms aggravated by stress? If so, what are the specific stresses? Stress-induced anxiety can be handled by avoiding or modifying situational factors and by teaching relaxation techniques (using audiotapes). Occasionally, mild tranquilizing agents are indicated (see Chapter 13).

- Is the patient depressed? As with anxiety, attempts should be made to determine specific depressing situations, especially to determine whether simple maneuvers can alter them. If not, the patient sometimes can learn new ways of handling situations that cannot be avoided. Tricyclic antidepressants (see Chapter 15) may prove helpful in depression.

- Does gratification from illness behavior (see Chapter 12) reinforce the illness? Evidence that this is so derives from the history that the illness keeps the patient from job-related or social discomfort and stress. The spouse, family, or friends respond sympathetically to the patient's symptoms, providing further reinforcement. The patient's motivation is generally unconscious, and it is a strategic error to accuse a patient of trying to derive benefit from the illness. Treatment is designed to reduce the amount of gratification that illness behavior evokes. The patient is asked not to discuss his or her illness with family members, but instead to reserve complaints for the physician. In return, family members are instructed to help the patient by discouraging excessive discussion of his or her illness and by avoiding overly sympathetic responses. The patient is instructed to view the illness as a physical disability that may be overcome by pushing performance to maximal capacity.

- What misconceptions does the patient have about the illness? The answer to this question can be obtained from questions directed to the patient as well as to his or her family members, who may provide information that the patient is reluctant to give. A rational explanation of the patient's disorder is necessary, but the physician should also listen attentively to the patient's fears (of cancer, for example) and should deal with them as well. Patience is required because these issues may need to be worked through repetitively. A steady, supportive approach is most desirable, as well as a clear demonstration that the physician is acquainted with and sensitive to the patient and his or her disorder and needs. Regular (although not necessarily frequent) follow-up visits supply reassurance to the patient, whereas as-needed visits are often viewed as abandonment or as an indication of impotence on the part of a physician who feels incapable of providing further help. Furthermore, as-needed visits lend themselves to greater abuse by the patient who is seeking secondary gains.

PROGNOSIS

Whether treatment alters the prognosis or simply affects the patient's ability to accept or deal with his or her symptoms has not been established. It is difficult to determine the impact of a specific form of treatment on the natural course of IBS for a number of reasons. First, each patient is different: Some have milder symptoms, some more severe; some have frequent recurrences, some infrequent. Second, patients with painless diarrhea are included in some studies and excluded from others. The prognosis for this group is better than that of patients with pain, and the number of such patients included in any given study markedly influences the results of a particular treatment program. Third, the more serious the associated psychologic factors, the more prolonged the course of IBS, no matter what the underlying precipitating factors and presentation. Fourth, physicians are different in their training, interest, background, and approaches. Fifth, various treatment programs have been fashionable from time to time and none has undergone systematic, long-term evaluation in a manner that provides useful scientific data. All of these factors underscore the need for organized, individualized, multifaceted management by a physician who is interested, educated, skillful, and compassionate.

General References

Lynn RB, Friedman LS. Irritable bowel syndrome. N Engl J Med 329:1940, 1993.
> An authoritative review.

Olden KW, Schuster MM. Irritable bowel syndrome. In: Feldman M, Scharschmidt F, Sleisinger MH, eds. Sleisinger and Fordtran's gastrointestinal and liver disease, 6th ed. Philadelphia: WB Saunders, 1997;1536.
> A comprehensive review of pathophysiology, clinical features, and treatment of IBS.

Read NW, ed. Irritable bowel syndrome. London: Grune & Stratton, 1985.
> An authoritative anthology by international experts on specific aspects of IBS and its management.

Thompson WG. The irritable gut. Baltimore: University Park Press, 1979.
> A delightfully written overview of functional disorders of the gut, including irritable bowel syndrome.

Whitehead WE, Schuster MM, eds. Gastrointestinal disorders: behavioral and physiological basis for treatment. Orlando, FL: Academic Press, 1985;155.

Specific References

1. Accarino A, Azpiroz F, Malagelada JR. Selective dysfunction of mechanosensitive intestinal afferents in irritable bowel syndrome. Gastroenterology 108:636, 1995.
2. Crowell MD, Bassotti G, Cheskin LJ, et al. Prolonged ambulatory monitoring of high amplitude propagated contractions from the colon. Am J Physiol 261:G-263, 1991.
3. Drossman DA, Laserman J, Nachman G, et al. Sexual and physical abuse in women with functional and organic gastrointestinal disorders. Ann Intern Med 113:828, 1990.
4. Eastwood MA, Smith AN, Brydon WG, Pritchard J. Comparison of bran, ispaghula and lactulose on colon function in diverticular disease. Gut 19:1144, 1978.
5. Harvey RF, Salih SY, Read AE. Organic and functional disorders in 2000 gastroenterology outpatients. Lancet 1:632, 1983.
6. Mayer EA, Gebhart GF. Basic and clinical aspects of visceral hyperalgesia. Gastroenterology 107:271, 1994.
7. Mayer EA, Raybould HE. Role of visceral afferent mechanisms in functional bowel disorders. Gastroenterology 99:1688, 1990.
8. Reasoner J, Maculan TP, Rand AG, Thayer WR. Clinical studies with low-lactose milk. Am J Clin Nutr 34:54, 1981.
9. Sircus W, Eastwood MA. Frequency of functional gastrointestinal disorders. Lancet 2:613, 1977.
10. Talley WJ, Zinsmeister AR, Von Dyke C, Melton LJ. Epidemiology of colonic symptoms and irritable bowel syndrome. Gastroenterology 101:927, 1991.
11. Whitehead WE, Bosmajian L, Zonderman AB, et al. Symptoms of psychologic distress associated with irritable bowel syndrome. Comparison of community and medical clinic samples. Gastroenterology 95:709, 1988.
12. Whitehead WE, Winget C, Fedoravicius A, et al. Learned illness behavior in patients with irritable bowel syndrome and peptic ulcer. Dig Dis Sci 27:202, 1982.

C H A P T E R   41

Diverticular Disease of the Colon

LAWRENCE J. CHESKIN, MD

DEFINITIONS

The terminology for conditions subsumed under the phrase *diverticular disease* is widely misunderstood. The phrase refers to a variety of clinical states that may differ in etiology and prognosis. The nomenclature of diverticular disease of the colon is listed in Table 41.1. As can be seen from this classification, *diverticulosis* is simply the presence of colonic diverticula, without presuming that there are accompanying signs and symptoms. *Symptomatic diverticular disease* is diverticulosis associated with pain or altered bowel habits in the absence of evidence of diverticular inflammation. *Diverticulitis* is inflammation of one or more diverticula, generally implying perforation of a diverticulum, and is almost always symptomatic. The *prediverticular state* is characterized by the radiographic, pathologic, and often clinical features of diverticulosis without the formation of diverticula. The distinction between these entities is more than semantic, as the pathophysiology and natural history of each of these conditions probably vary.

EPIDEMIOLOGY AND PATHOGENESIS

The prevalence of diverticular disease in Western countries is strongly correlated with advancing age: Approximately 20% of men and women over 40, 50%

Table 41.1.   Nomenclature of Diverticular Disease of the Colon

Diverticulosis (presence of multiple diverticula)
    Asymptomatic
    Symptomatic (pain, altered bowel habits)
    Complicated by hemorrhage
Diverticulitis (necrotizing inflammation in one or more diverticula)
    With microperforation (local inflammation)
    With macroperforation, manifested by abscess, fistula, peritonitis, obstruction, or hemorrhage
Prediverticular state: muscular thickening and shortening of colonic wall without recognizable diverticula

over 60, and as many as 66% over age 85 have diverticulosis of the colon. These figures reflect a striking rise in the frequency of the condition over the last 70 years (5% of people over 60 were affected in the early years of this century), coincident with the advent of milling, which removes two-thirds of the fiber content of flour. In addition, it is known that vegetarians have a much lower prevalence of diverticular disease than nonvegetarians. In animals, a lifelong low-fiber diet is associated with the formation of diverticula, whereas a high-fiber diet is not. This evidence has led to the hypothesis that a low-fiber diet increases intraluminal pressure and that the increased pressure leads to herniation of the mucosa through weakened or porous parts of the colonic muscle. In support of this hypothesis is the demonstration in some cases of diverticular disease of higher resting pressures in the colon and of exaggerated contractile activity in response to meals and cholinergic stimulation (3). Thus, both a low-fiber diet and disordered colonic motility have been implicated in the pathogenesis of diverticulosis.

Another aspect in the pathogenesis of this condition is the weakness in the colonic wall through which the mucosa herniates to form the diverticulum. The site of herniation occurs at areas of least resistance, most often at points of penetration of intramural vessels through the circular muscle layer. The association of colonic diverticula with scleroderma and with Marfan's and Ehlers–Danlos syndromes suggests that loss of muscle mass or defects in collagen may be important factors. Changes in collagen synthesis are known to occur with aging and may explain the increased prevalence of diverticular disease in elderly people. Thus, the formation of diverticula may also involve a degenerative process of the colonic muscle with a change in tensile strength of the wall of the colon.

ASYMPTOMATIC DIVERTICULOSIS

A substantial majority of patients with diverticulosis detected on barium enema are entirely asymptomatic. The diverticula may be localized to the sigmoid colon or may involve the entire colon diffusely. The sigmoid colon is almost always involved (95% of the time), and sigmoid diverticula account for 75% of all colonic diverticula. It is believed that this predilection is explained by the narrow caliber of the sigmoid colon, resulting in higher intraluminal pressures and hence a greater risk of herniation. The more distal the position in the colon, the higher the prevalence of diverticula. However, rectal diverticula rarely occur.

The natural history of diverticulosis is variable. A large majority of patients never present clinically, either because their diverticulosis is asymptomatic or because the symptoms are not severe enough to cause them to seek medical attention. Symptomatic diverticular disease presents either as painful diverticular disease (75%) or as diverticulitis or hemorrhage (25%). In most cases, diverticula precede the onset of symptoms by several years. In a minority of cases, however, typical symptoms precede anatomic disease (the prediverticular state).

Although a diet high in fiber may be beneficial in preventing the development of diverticula, there is little evidence that therapy for asymptomatic diverticulosis is of any value in preventing or even delaying the occurrence of symptomatic diverticular disease or of such complications as diverticulitis or hemorrhage. Maintenance of regular bowel habits without the use of laxatives is probably the best advice for asymptomatic patients. It is also prudent to alert them to the manifestations of symptomatic diverticular disease and to urge them to seek medical care promptly should such symptoms develop.

PAINFUL DIVERTICULAR DISEASE

Diagnosis

Diverticular disease may at times become symptomatic. When the predominant symptoms are abdominal pain and an alteration in bowel habits, the cause is usually painful diverticular disease. The hallmark of this disease is abdominal pain without evidence of an inflammatory process. The pain may be colicky or steady, is generally in the left lower quadrant, and is usually made worse by meals (presumably because of gastrocolic reflex) and at least partially relieved by having a bowel movement or by passing flatus. Bowel habits, usually during the painful episodes, become irregular in 46 to 63% of cases, with development of constipation, diarrhea, or both in an alternating fashion. Constipation is more common than the other alterations in bowel habit. These attacks are usually episodic rather than continuous. Symptoms may also include nausea, heartburn, and flatulence.

Physical examination may reveal tenderness, at times significant, in the left lower quadrant of the abdomen. A tender sigmoid loop, which feels like a sausage, may be palpable, but there is no other palpable mass and the entire abdominal examination is often unremarkable. The stool should be negative for occult blood, but rectal bleeding may be found because of coincidental rectal outlet disorders such as fissures or hemorrhoids. The presence of fever, leukocytosis, or peritoneal signs points toward the more serious diagnosis of diverticulitis.

Proctosigmoidoscopy, if performed during an attack, shows a normal colonic mucosa. However, considerable pain and spasm may be caused by the procedure.

The *barium enema* (see Chapter 38) is important both for the diagnosis of diverticulosis and for excluding other reasons for symptoms. Spasm may be a feature of diverticular disease, but fistulas or a mass suggests diverticulitis, carcinoma, or Crohn's disease. Particularly in elderly patients, in whom the prevalence of diverticulosis is so high, it is important not to assume that the patient's symptoms have been explained once diverticula are found; carcinoma, for example, may be the real cause.

Therapy

The therapy for symptomatic diverticular disease is based on the assumption that low-fiber diets and increased colonic pressure are important pathogenetic factors. Diets high in fiber (see Chapter 39, Table 39.2) are prescribed and have been shown to be effective in improving bowel transit and relieving symptoms. Commercial preparations of hydrophilic colloids made from vegetable fiber are available and convenient but are more expensive than dietary sources (see Chapter 39, Table 39.3). Thus, patients should be instructed about high-fiber diets and, if necessary, should be given fiber supplements at a dosage of 4 to 10 g (1 tablespoon one to three times a day in a glass of water or juice). Artificial fiber products in tablet form are also available (Fiberall, Fibercon).

In addition to dietary maneuvers, anticholinergic drugs or antispasmodic drugs may be helpful for the relief of abdominal pain. Although these agents are not of proven value for this condition, some patients do respond. Dicyclomine (Bentyl), at a dosage of 10 to 20 mg before meals and at bedtime, or hyoscyamine (e.g., Levsin) 0.125 to 0.25 mg every 4 hours as needed may be helpful. Other more potent anticholinergics may produce adverse side effects and may aggravate the constipation.

The patient should be told that the course of the disease is unpredictable and that attacks will probably be experienced at irregular intervals (months to years) for the rest of his or her life. There is no benefit in continuing to take medication for the condition between attacks, but maintenance of a high-fiber diet is prudent.

DIVERTICULITIS

Diverticulitis results from perforation of one or more diverticula, usually in the sigmoid colon. Perforation may result from persistently high colonic pressures or from an inflammatory process that weakens the wall of the diverticulum. The perforation may be grossly evident, with fistulization and abscess formation, or it may be only microscopic and well confined. Diverticulitis increases in incidence with age and with duration of the underlying diverticulosis, and is more common in patients with the largest number of diverticula. Fistulas may form to the bladder, vagina (especially after hysterectomy), small bowel, or skin (5). The long-term risk of developing diverticulitis among patients with diverticulosis is 10 to 25% but probably is much lower in asymptomatic diverticulosis.

Diagnosis

The cardinal symptoms of acute diverticulitis are abdominal pain and fever. In classic cases, the pain is severe, abrupt in onset, and persistent, worsening with time and localizing to the left lower quadrant. The pain is often accompanied by anorexia, nausea, and vomiting. Altered bowel habits, especially constipation, are common. Urinary tract symptoms and purulent vaginal discharge may occur because of fistula formation or because of inflammation of contiguous structures.

Abdominal tenderness and fever are found on physical examination. Localized peritonitis may be noted by the marked direct and rebound tenderness over the involved area, generally most pronounced in the left lower quadrant. The abdomen is often distended and tympanitic to percussion and the bowel sounds diminished. A mass may be felt at the site of inflammation in the left lower quadrant or on pelvic or rectal examination. Rectal bleeding occurs in approximately 25% of patients and is usually occult.

Leukocytosis is almost always present. Pyuria and/or hematuria may be found when there is involvement of the bladder or ureter.

It must be appreciated that the presentation of acute diverticulitis may be muted in the elderly patient. A high degree of suspicion is required in this population because there may be no fever, no leukocytosis, and minimal abdominal pain.

The *differential diagnosis* includes painful diverticular disease, carcinoma of the colon, and inflammatory or ischemic bowel disease. The presence of peritonitis, fever, and leukocytosis rules out simple symptomatic diverticular disease. The other conditions are distinguished from diverticulitis by their clinical course and by barium enema or endoscopy.

The *diagnosis* of acute diverticulitis is made largely on clinical grounds, but some tests may be useful in confirming the clinical impression. Plain abdominal radiographs (flat and upright or decubitus) may show signs of ileus and the location of the inflammatory mass, or air in the bladder in some cases of colovesical fistula. Plain films are also important in detecting free air caused by perforation, a surgical emergency. A limited flexible sigmoidoscopy is indicated in many cases when the diagnosis is in doubt, both to rule out other processes in the left colon and to see whether there are indeed diverticula in the sigmoid colon. Once their presence is verified, the procedure is terminated to avoid worsening or causing perforation. Weeks later, after successful medical therapy, it is safe to complete the examination of the rest of the colon, by either colonoscopy or barium enema. This is not so much to make the diagnosis of diverticulitis as to exclude other conditions, such as carcinoma or Crohn's disease. Abdominal computerized tomography (CT) may be very helpful in visualizing diverticular abscesses in the pericolonic tissues and has largely supplanted other radiographic and endoscopic modalities as an adjunct to the clinical diagnosis of diverticulitis (4).

Therapy

Most patients with diverticulitis should be hospitalized, placed on bowel and bed rest, and given analgesics, intravenous hydration, and antimicrobial drugs (such as clindamycin and gentamicin, or cefotetan to treat both aerobic and anaerobic infection). Selected patients, with mild tenderness and low-grade fever, may be treated on an ambulatory basis with oral broad-spectrum antibiotics (e.g., trimethoprim/sulfamethoxazole double-strength twice daily plus metronidazole 500 mg every 6 hours for 10 days to 2 weeks).

Although more than 75% of patients respond to conservative medical management, it is wise to obtain surgical consultation early in the hospital course to facilitate operative intervention should it prove necessary. The patient's condition usually improves markedly in 3 to 10 days if medical therapy is successful. For patients who respond to conservative management, a recurrence rate of 25%, mostly in the first 5 years, can be expected.

Failure to resolve the acute inflammatory process, recurrent attacks of diverticulitis, and obstructive stricture formation are indications for surgical intervention (1). It seems reasonable that patients be placed on a high-fiber diet after recovery from an acute episode of diverticulitis.

DIVERTICULAR BLEEDING

Diverticular disease is the most common cause of gross lower gastrointestinal bleeding in adults, followed closely by bleeding from angiodysplasias. Both diverticulosis and angiodysplasias are common in the older population, and both are commonly found in the proximal colon. Diverticular bleeds, in contrast to diverticulitis, occur in the right colon in two-thirds of cases (even though diverticula are more common in the left colon). The average age of patients with diverticular bleeding is approximately 70. Bleeding is the presenting manifestation of diverticular disease in 16% of patients. The exact cause of diverticular bleeding is uncertain. Diverticulitis is rarely, if ever, associated with gross bleeding. There is no evidence that dietary therapy reduces the risk of hemorrhage. Most instances of bleeding occur in patients who are otherwise asymptomatic.

Massive hemorrhage is a common mode of presentation for diverticular bleeding, although in many cases the bleeding is occult and chronic. It should be appreciated that massive lower gastrointestinal bleeding in a patient known to have diverticula is not necessarily diverticular in origin. In 30% of cases, colonoscopy detects a second lesion (e.g., cancer or angiodysplasia) (2). Occult bleeding also should be ascribed to diverticulosis only after other causes have been excluded by a thorough evaluation (see Chapter 38).

Patients with diverticular hemorrhage require hospitalization for hemodynamic stabilization, diagnosis, and therapy. Approximately 70% of patients stop bleeding spontaneously. The recurrence rate is 20 to 25% and increases with each subsequent episode of bleeding.

General References

Almy T, Howell D. Diverticular disease of the colon. N Engl J Med 302:324, 1980.
>   A good review of pathophysiology and classification of diverticular disease. Well referenced.

Deckmann RC, Cheskin LJ. Diverticular disease in the elderly. J Am Geriatr Soc 40:986, 1993.
>   A general review with emphasis on presentation in the elderly.

Specific References

1. Levien DH, Mazier WP, Surrell JA, Raiman PJ. Safe resection for diverticular disease of the colon. Dis Colon Rectum 32:30, 1989.
2. Tedesco F, Waye J, Raskin J, et al. Colonoscopic evaluation of rectal bleeding: a study of 304 patients. Ann Intern Med 89:907, 1978.
3. Trotman IF, Misiewicz WP. Sigmoid motility in diverticular disease and the irritable bowel syndrome. Gut 29:218, 1988.
4. Welch CE. Computerized tomography scans for all patients with diverticulitis. Am J Surg 155:366, 1988.
5. Woods RJ, Lavery IC, Fazio VW, et al. Internal fistulas in diverticular disease. Dis Colon Rectum 31:591, 1988.

C H A P T E R 42

Care of Patients with Colostomy or Ileostomy

MARVIN M. SCHUSTER, MD

Ostomies are openings of a portion of the gastrointestinal tract—usually the ileum or the colon—that have been surgically diverted to the abdominal wall. It is estimated that there are more than 1 million ostomates (the preferred term for people with ostomies) in North America. Unfortunately, the amount of time devoted in medical school curricula and postgraduate training to the care of ostomies is not commensurate with these numbers, so few physicians have the necessary background to be appropriately helpful to the ostomate. This is particularly unfortunate in light of the fact that the partial or total colectomy that results in an ileostomy or colostomy often cures the underlying condition, leaving a healthy patient who is capable of normal function, assuming that he or she receives appropriate preoperative preparation and postoperative ostomy care.

Ninety percent of *ileostomies* are performed for ulcerative colitis. Less often, other conditions, such as Crohn's disease of the colon or familial polyposis, require this operation. Most of the patients are young, 75% or more being between 20 and 45 years of age.

In contrast, *colostomies* are usually performed for cancer of the rectum and, less often, for diverticulitis or for neurologic impairment or gunshot wounds that have led to incontinence. Both children and young adults with congenital disorders, such as imperforate anus, may have colostomies, but 80% of patients who have colostomy surgery are over the age of 50.

Appropriate management of the stoma begins before surgery and continues for a short period after successful surgery and for a longer period when old problems persist or new ones arise.

PREOPERATIVE CARE

Ostomy management should begin as soon as ostomy surgery is seriously considered. For preparation of the patient to be most effective, family members should be included because the approach is best tailored to meet the needs of the patient and the family. Preparation should include a brief description of the surgery, emphasizing the benefits to be derived, and of the stoma, stressing the fact that the stoma itself need not interfere with any aspect of future life except for vigorous body contact sports. Emphasis is placed on the fact that modern developments in appliances permit normal functioning and that there is no way that anyone will be able to tell that the clad patient has an ostomy. After these introductory comments, the patient and family should be given an opportunity to voice their concerns and to ask questions, both during this first discussion and later, when the initial shock has worn off.

Many resources are available during the preoperative stage: the informed physician or surgeon, specially trained stoma nurses or enterostomal therapists (most of whom are nurses who have had specialized training at one of the schools of enterostomal therapy), and members of the visiting committee of the local chapter of the United Ostomy Association. The latter are usually lay ostomates trained as members of the visiting committee, who are specifically selected whenever possible to match the patient in age and sex (and often in socioeconomic status), so that the patient can identify readily with the visitor. The benefits to be derived from the visiting team cannot be overemphasized; even the most comforting professionals cannot be as reassuring to the patient as some kindred soul who has undergone similar surgery, has adjusted to it, and is leading a healthy, productive, and joyful life.

Pamphlets available through the local ostomy chapters can promote the patient's acceptance of the procedure, provide an optimistic projection for the future, and educate the patient in the use of ostomy appliances and colostomy irrigation. In addition, videotapes on preoperative preparation are available; they are particularly useful when viewed by the patient after the first discussion of the topic because they not only depict healthy ostomates who discuss their initial and subsequent adjustment but also provide basic anatomic information and information concerning appliances. Such information allays fears and misconceptions and provides the basis for logical questions.

What to Tell the Patient About Conventional Ileostomy

Conventional ileostomies require that the patient continuously wear a pouch, which is applied to the body using a skin barrier (a waferlike adhesive) to provide a watertight seal. In this manner the intestinal contents (a better term than *stool* or *waste material*) discharge into the pouch, which can be emptied into the toilet simply by unclipping the end of the pouch four or five times a day. The contents are liquid and usually odorless. The pouch is flat and cannot be detected through the clothing or even in a bathing suit. The seal is tight enough so that people can swim, dive, dance, and participate in sports such as skiing or baseball. Modern materials are so effective that the pouch can be worn for a week at a time without being removed.

What to Tell the Patient About a Kock or Internal Pouch

The Kock or internal pouch (sometimes called continent ileostomy) consists of several loops of small intestine sutured to each other and opened so that they form a reservoir pouch (artificial rectum) within the abdomen. This reservoir is connected to the abdominal wall with a short segment of ileum and opens into the abdominal wall much as a conventional ileostomy does, except that it can be placed much lower on the abdomen because it will not require an external pouch if it performs well. Between the pouch and the short ileal conduit, a nipple valve is constructed by inverting the ileum into the pouch in such a manner that it prevents leakage and therefore provides continence. To evacuate the contents of the pouch, the patient inserts a Silastic catheter into it through the ileostomy and the nipple valve. The ileal contents then drain through the catheter into the toilet bowl. Although frequent drainage is necessary initially, eventually most patients drain three or four times a day. Because it does not require an external appliance, the stoma can be placed near the groin, permitting the wearing of brief attire, such as a bikini.

This type of surgery is not recommended for patients who have Crohn's disease involving the ileum. Moreover, one-third of the operations are initially unsuccessful in providing total continence and therefore require revision and, in some instances, more than one revision. These factors must be taken into consideration when deciding the appropriate form of surgery for the specific patient, especially when patients with conventional ileostomies ask about the advisability of converting their conventional, well-functioning ileostomy to the continent ileostomy. This operation is also not appropriate for people who have neurologic disorders that impair manual dexterity and interfere with insertion of the Silastic catheter. For these reasons the Kock procedure has been largely replaced by the endorectal pull-through operation (see the next section).

What to Tell the Patient About Sphincter-Saving Operations

The operation that has largely replaced the Kock pouch as a continent procedure is the *endorectal pull-through with ileal pouch* (1). Like the Kock procedure, the endorectal pull-through involves the construction of a reservoir pouch formed by suturing several adjacent loops of small bowel to each other and opening up the contiguous walls to form a reservoir. The distal (efferent) limb is then brought through the rectal stump, which has been denuded of its mucosa, and the distal ileum is sutured to the distal rectal wall from inside. The denuded rectum then adheres to the serosal surface of the efferent ileal limb. Thus, the anal sphincters are spared and nerve damage from anterior dissection is avoided. This approach can be used when rectal involvement from ulcerative colitis is not so severe that it prevents lifting the mucosa off the submucosal surface and removing it. Generally this procedure is contraindicated in Crohn's disease because of the risk of local inflammation around the intestinal surface and anastomosis and because of the danger of fistula formation. When successful, this sphincter-forming surgery can preserve continence. The construction of an adequate reservoir and the appropriate placement of the efferent limb are technically difficult. Therefore, this procedure should be performed only by surgeons who have had substantial experience with the operation.

The *ileoanal anastomosis,* an increasingly popular procedure, differs from the endorectal pull-through in that, in the former procedure, the ileal pouch is attached directly to the anus.

What to Tell the Patient About Colostomy

There are basically four different types of colostomies: the *dry colostomy*, the *wet colostomy*, the *loop colostomy*, and the *continent colostomy* using a magnetic cap. Most permanent colostomies are dry sigmoid colostomies, which result from rectal resection, usually for cancer of the rectum. Because only the rectum has been removed, the usual stool consistency is not altered. This is an important feature because it means that patients who have frequent and erratic bowel habits, as in the irritable bowel syndrome, will continue to have these bowel habits and therefore will have unpredictable evacuation. They will probably have to wear an appliance. Patients who have more regular bowel habits can often develop controlled evacuations by use of irrigation (enemas) that they initially administer daily for proper control and later, in most instances, every 2 days. Some colostomates simply wear a small adhesive bandage or gauze pad, although most prefer to wear a small appliance (stoma cap) to protect them against incontinence during those few days a year when they develop the same episodes of diarrhea that affect the general population. Patients who have irritable bowel syndrome (see Chapter 40) or nervous diarrhea when they are stressed will continue to have similar symptoms after surgery and therefore may not achieve continence during intervals between irrigations.

The wet colostomy refers to loose stool that occurs when a colostomy is situated proximal to the splenic flexure. This type of colostomy usually is performed as a temporary bypass and is generally less desirable because evacuations are more frequent and cannot be controlled by irrigation, and because the contents are malodorous because of colonic bacterial action. A permanent ileostomy is generally preferable to a permanent wet colostomy. The wet colostomy requires an appliance large enough to contain the colonic evacuations.

Loop colostomies and double-barrel colostomies are performed as (usually temporary) diverting procedures in the proximal colon. The loop is brought over a glass or plastic rod, and the resultant irregular oblong shape may make a watertight appliance fit difficult.

Informed consent for colostomy requires that the patient be made aware of possible postoperative impotence. If impotence does occur, psychologic adjustment to it is improved with preoperative counseling. Impotence is uncommon among ileostomates, but some degree of sexual impairment occurs in 80% of colostomates, 50% of whom are totally impotent after surgery. This is due to the wide resection that is necessary for rectal cancer surgery, the major indication for a colostomy, as well as the advanced age of the colostomate compared to the ileostomate. Patients may be reassured that sexual counseling is available if problems arise and that many couples find alternative satisfactory means of sexual gratification. It is appropriate to offer men the possibility of penile prostheses or intracavernosal or transurethral delivery of a vasodilating drug to produce potency (see Chapter 18). Obviously these concerns are less significant for the female ostomate, who does not experience impaired performance, although impaired gratification may still be an important factor.

POSTOPERATIVE MANAGEMENT

Only late postoperative problems are discussed here because the early problems will be managed in the hospital. Four major categories of problems are psychologic adjustment, sexual adjustment, appliance management, and local and physiologic problems. Again, all can be minimized by appropriate preoperative preparation and counseling of the patient and the patient's family by an informed physician working with the appropriate members of the health care team.

Psychologic Adjustment

A concerted effort should be made postoperatively by the medical team, the family, and particularly the spouse to restore self-esteem and foster independence. During the early postoperative months, men tend to depend on their wives for nursing care, but women seem to prefer help from other women (daughters, mothers, sisters) rather than from husbands. This is explained by the fact that wives express more concern about being physically unacceptable to the husband than vice versa. On the other hand, one-fifth of wives have been reported to react by vomiting, fainting, or showing frank expressions of disgust when first exposed to their husband's stoma. This obviously engenders a sense of rejection, degradation, and loss of self-esteem. All too often little consideration is given by the physician to the possibility of such exaggerated responses or to their consequences. Attendance at meetings of local ostomy chapters is a good way to prepare the family during the postoperative period. Formal psychotherapy may be needed when depression is severe, when suicidal inclinations appear prominent, or when behavior is bizarre.

Sexual Adjustment

When debilitating illnesses, such as inflammatory bowel disease, have led to decreased libido and impaired sexual function, ileostomy may lead to improved postoperative sexual function and more satisfactory sexual relations. This is less often true when colostomies, performed with proctectomy and radical pelvic dissection, lead to neurologic impairment of potency. Even in these circumstances psychologic factors may play a major role, as demonstrated by a survey that reported that all men who had had extramarital affairs before surgery terminated these relationships postoperatively, feeling that only their wives would accept them (2). Also, cessation of relationships involving a female colostomate was invariably initiated by the female and was never reported to be a result of rejection by the husband.

In general, impaired sexual relationships may result from neurologic impairment, depression with loss of libido, inhibitions caused by a sense of humiliation and embarrassment, or in some unfortunate instances, rejection by the spouse. An awareness of these possibilities will prepare the physician to assist with preventive or corrective measures. Frank discussions with the male patient may in some instances indicate the advisability of urologic referral for treatment of impotence (see Chapter 18).

Appliance Management

Modern improvements have impressively decreased the number of problems that are directly attributable to the appliance.

Skin Problems

Skin breakdown, a problem that used to plague 50% of ileostomates, is now uncommon because of effective skin barriers that have replaced the old cement adhesives. Hypersensitivity to adhesives or to the pouch can be diagnosed when the contour of skin reaction conforms to that of the adhesive or the pouch. If hypersensitivity is suspected, a patch test using the arm or trunk distant from the stoma may confirm the suspicion. Skin problems are more common among ileostomates than colostomates because ileostomy effluent contains digestive enzymes. Skin that has been excoriated by ileal leakage should be treated with a cortisone spray, such as Kenalog, and an antifungal powder, such as Mycostatin, neither of which interferes with adherence of the appliance. Patients with more serious skin problems should be referred to gastroenterologists and to enterostomal therapists experienced with ostomy care. Skin complications for proximal colostomies may be similar to those of ileostomies.

Odor

Odor problems are more commonly encountered by colostomates than ileostomates because of putrefactive bacteria present in the colon. Some bacterial colonization of the ileum takes place after colectomy, but odor problems occur only occasionally in 50% of ileostomates and more often in about a third. Sudden increase in gas and odor may signify partial intestinal obstruction. Dietary factors such as oils, fat-soluble vitamins, eggs, and onions may be associated with offensive odors and may be diagnosed by careful dietary history or by use of elimination diets. Odors may also be caused by malabsorption resulting from small bowel disease or resection. A number of deodorants are available that can be placed into the pouch (Nilodor, Banish, Aspirin, and Ostoban powder), and oral bismuth subcarbonate also may be helpful.

Leakage

Under ordinary circumstances, leakage is rarely seen with new appliances, but it may become a problem if pregnancy or postoperative weight gain (as, for example, when a patient has been emaciated from inflammatory bowel disease) changes body contour, requiring refitting of the appliance. The stoma may shrink during the first 6 to 8 weeks after surgery, and good follow-up care is vital for at least the first postoperative year. Minimal bleeding at the stoma may occur occasionally and is no cause for alarm. A soft, wet cloth should be used to clean the stoma because dry materials may stick to the surface and cause bleeding. Skin excoriation can occur as a result of perspiration under the pouch, particularly in hot weather. This can be prevented by wearing a cover over the pouch and powdering the skin liberally.

Equipment Update

Stoma nurses and enterostomal therapists are usually familiar with state-of-the-art supplies and equipment. Such products include the following:

- Durahesive flexible wafer (Sur-Fit Natur) allows removal and replacement of the pouch without disturbing the skin barrier, helps avoid discomfort and skin irritation, and allows easy repositioning for supine bedside drainage without removal of the pouch.

- Stomahesive paste and Stomahesive protective powder can be used to fill in skin irregularities around the stoma.
- The Guardian two-piece system has the only drainable pouch with replaceable filters.
- First Choice drainable pouch with convex barrier is a one-piece unit that provides excellent skin protection for flush, recessed, or retracted stomas.
- I LE-SORB absorbent gel packets placed in the pouch transform diarrheal water into a gel, which keeps the contents of the pouch away from the stoma.
- Closed-pouch styles and closed minipouches are interchangeable with the two-piece units for patients who have colostomies.
- Stoma caps provide a convenient stomal covering for discharge that is controlled by irrigation. The caps contain carbon cloth filter to absorb the odorous components of flatus.

Local and Physiologic Complications

Ileostomates are much more likely to experience complications of this type than are colostomates, and most of these complications appear within the first year after surgery. Obstruction caused by volvulus, herniation, or adhesions is the most common problem, whereas prolapse, retraction, and fistula formation are seen less often. These problems usually require consultation with a surgeon or gastroenterologist and often need surgical correction. Crampy abdominal pains, abdominal distension, vomiting, and excessive diarrheal discharge suggest the presence of obstruction. Gastroenteritis may mimic some of these symptoms but persists only for several days.

Because of the absence of normal colonic absorptive function, ileostomates may be susceptible to dehydration or electrolyte imbalance (particularly salt depletion), especially in hot weather because of sweating and increased incidence of infectious diarrhea. For this reason ileostomates should be encouraged to increase water and salt intake during the summer unless there are medical contraindications. Antidiarrheal agents such as deodorized tincture of opium, Lomotil, or Imodium may be needed during these periods and also should be available during travel to countries where traveler's diarrhea may be a problem (see Chapter 33).

With these minimal precautions, neither ileostomy nor colostomy imposes any dietary restrictions, except that ileostomates should avoid excessive quantities of peanuts or fibrous foods such as bean sprouts (see Chapter 39, Table 39.2 for the fiber content of various foods), which have been reported to be associated with obstruction. Taken in moderation, however, these foods usually present no problem.

Effects of Small-Bowel Resection or Colectomy on Handling of Medications

For the most part colectomy does not influence drug absorption because most drugs are absorbed in the small bowel. A major exception is sulfasalazine (Azulfidine), one of the drugs most commonly used for inflammatory bowel disease. The inactive form of this drug is broken down by colonic bacteria into an active constituent that is reabsorbed into the bloodstream and secreted in connective tissue of the gut. Colectomy obviously can seriously impair this process. On the other hand, because sulfasalazine is most effective for colonic involvement in inflammatory bowel disease, it is not often required after colectomy.

When resection of parts of the small bowel is performed for the treatment of inflammatory bowel disease, the patient is left with decreased absorptive surface and often intestinal hurry. This rapid transit may lead to poor absorption of medication and foodstuffs. Particularly, enteric and sustained-release preparations should be avoided under these circumstances. Patients with short bowel syndrome are especially prone to have problems and may benefit from medications prescribed in liquid rather than tablet form because liquid is more rapidly absorbed.

Residual inflammatory disease and bacterial overgrowth in the terminal ileum of ostomy patients may result in poor absorption of vitamin B_{12} and the need for vitamin B_{12} replacement.

Colostomy Irrigation

Although a few colostomates (having distal colostomy) find that they can have controlled bowel movements by careful dietary manipulations, the vast majority use irrigation to control evacuation. This simply involves the instillation of 1 L of warm tap water through the colostomy. The replacement of the old irrigating catheter with the blunt cone (which is placed against the stoma to prevent backflow) has virtually eliminated the problems of perforation. Although tepid water is preferred to avoid cramping, some patients find cold water more effective. It is normal for patients to have an initial evacuation followed within ½ hour by further excretion; for this reason the patient should be advised to continue wearing the irrigation sleeve (long pouch) with the end closed for ½ hour after irrigation. Cramps experienced during the irrigation may be caused by rapid instillation of water or air distension of the bowel resulting from failure to expel the air from the irrigating tip or from obstruction. Constipation and diarrhea should be handled in the same way as in patients who have intact colons (see Chapter 39), relying on dietary manipulations as much as possible (prunes and bran for constipation and hard cheeses and rice for diarrhea).

General References

Beart RW Jr. Sphincter saving operations for chronic ulcerative colitis. Adv Surg 23:195, 1990.

Schuster MM, Bengel JR. Ileostomy and colostomy management. In: Spittell J Jr, ed. Clinical medicine, vol 10. New York: Harper & Row, 1982;1–19.

 A comprehensive review directed primarily at physicians.

Sparberg M. Ileostomy care. Springfield, IL: Charles C Thomas, 1971.

Walter FC. Modern stoma care. New York: Churchill Livingstone, 1976.

The preceding two references are useful texts for both physicians and patients.

White CA, Hunt JC. Psychological factors in postoperative adjustment to stoma surgery. Ann R Coll Surg Engl 79:3, 1997.

Specific References

1. Coran AG, Sarahan TM, Dent TL, et al. The endorectal pull-through for the management of ulcerative colitis in children and adults. Ann Surg 197:99, 1983.
2. Dyk RB, Sutherland AM. Adaptation of spouse and other family members to the ostomy patients. Cancer 9:123, 1956.

C H A P T E R   43

Diseases of the Liver

ESTEBAN MEZEY, MD

HEPATITIS

Hepatitis is an inflammatory condition that may be localized in the liver or may be part of a generalized systemic process. Acute hepatitis is usually a self-limited disease. The principal causes of acute hepatitis are viruses, drugs, and alcohol. Chronic hepatitis is unresolved hepatitis that has persisted for longer than 6 months. Cirrhosis is often the principal consequence of chronic hepatitis.

Acute Hepatitis

Viral Hepatitis

Viral hepatitis is a systemic infection whose principal manifestations are hepatic. The four types of viral hepatitis that are well-defined, separate entities are designated type A, B, C, and E. Delta hepatitis (hepatitis D virus) is infection by a defective viruslike particle that is dependent on persisting or concomitant infection with type B virus.

The characteristic features of type A, B, C, and E hepatitis are shown in Table 43.1. *Type A hepatitis,* previously known as infectious hepatitis, is more common than the other types. It is usually transmitted by the fecal–oral route and has a particularly high incidence wherever people come in close contact

Table 43.1. Comparison of Selected Characteristics of Various Types of Viral Hepatitis

Characteristic	Type A	Type B	Type C	Type E
Hepatitis A antibody	Appearance of or increase in titer	Absent or no change in titer	Absent or no change in titer	Absent or no change in titer
Hepatitis B surface antigen	Absent	Present in early stage of illness	Absent	Absent
Hepatitis C antibody	Absent	Absent	Appears 10–20 weeks after infection	Absent
Incubation period	15–50 days	50–160 days	15–160 days	35–40 days
Route of infection	Oral and parenteral	Usually parenteral, also oral or sexual	Usually parenteral, also oral or sexual	Oral
Age preference	Children	Any age	Any age	15–40 years
Seasonal incidence	Autumn–winter, epidemic outbreaks	All year	All year	Epidemic outbreaks
Severity	Usually mild	Often severe	Often mild	Mild, severe in pregnancy
Mortality	0.1%	0.1–1.0%	0.1%	0.5% (20% in pregnancy)
Prophylactic value of γ-globulin	Good	Good with hyperimmune hepatitis B globulin	Unclear	Unclear
Hepatitis vaccine	90–100% efficacy	90% efficacy		

under poor hygienic conditions. A number of epidemics have been described after fecal contamination of the water or food supply. Ingestion of contaminated shellfish has been associated with sporadic cases as well as with epidemics.

Type B hepatitis, previously called serum hepatitis, is usually transmitted by the parenteral route from blood, blood products, or contaminated needles. It is also commonly transmitted by sexual contact and from the mother to the fetus. *Delta hepatitis* is transmitted by the same routes as type B hepatitis (24). Its incubation period ranges from 3 to 13 weeks. Infection with delta agent may become manifest as a biphasic pattern of hepatitis when there is simultaneous infection with hepatitis B virus, or as a clinical exacerbation of hepatitis in patients who are carriers of hepatitis B virus with or without chronic liver disease. Delta hepatitis has been implicated in cases of fulminant hepatitis and in worsening of chronic liver disease with more rapid progression to cirrhosis. However, the incidence of delta hepatitis is unknown.

Hepatitis C accounts for most cases of hepatitis acquired by blood transfusion. In the United States, 19% of cases of hepatitis C are acquired by blood transfusion, 28% by parenteral use of illicit drugs, 6% by sexual or household exposure to people who have had hepatitis or multiple partners, and less than 4% by occupational exposure to infected blood. The source of the remaining 43% of cases is unknown (3). Ear piercing in men and intranasal cocaine use have been found to be more common in blood donors infected with hepatitis C virus than in noninfected donors (7).

Hepatitis E is a common cause of hepatitis epidemics in developing countries, but it can also occur sporadically in developed countries. The virus is transmitted by the fecal–oral route, usually by ingestion of contaminated water. It is associated with a high mortality in pregnant women (22).

Hepatitis G is a single-stranded RNA virus that has a genomic sequence similar to hepatitis C virus. It is present in 1.8% of blood donors and often is found in the blood of patients with hepatitis C infection. In a few cases hepatitis G is the only virus identified in patients

with hepatitis, and in most of these cases the hepatitis is mild. However, definitive proof is lacking to implicate hepatitis G virus as a causative agent of hepatitis.

Clinical Presentation. The clinical symptoms of the various types of hepatitis are similar. However, in contrast to the other types of viral hepatitis, acute viral hepatitis C is usually a mild illness that is very likely to persist and develop into chronic hepatitis. Most cases of hepatitis are anicteric, patients have a few nonspecific symptoms such as fatigue and nausea, and the disease is often misdiagnosed as a flulike illness. The correct diagnosis, if suspected, is made by demonstrating bilirubin in the urine and an increase in serum aminotransferases. In icteric disease the symptoms that usually precede jaundice are anorexia, fatigue, abdominal discomfort, and nausea. Erythematous skin rashes, urticaria, arthralgias, and low-grade fever may also appear. These initial symptoms are followed within 10 days by the appearance of dark urine, often pruritus, and jaundice. It is at this stage that most patients seek medical attention. On physical examination a tender palpable liver is found in approximately 70% of the patients. Posterior cervical lymphadenopathy and splenomegaly may also be present. Jaundice usually increases in intensity in the first few days and then begins to decrease, disappearing completely by 2 to 8 weeks after onset.

Laboratory Features. A mild degree of transient anemia, granulocytopenia, lymphocytosis with the appearance of atypical lymphocytes, and mild hemolytic anemia, with an increase in the reticulocyte count, are commonly found in patients with viral hepatitis. Both direct (conjugated) and total fraction of serum bilirubin rise; the height reached by the total bilirubin is an indication of the severity of the disease. However, total serum bilirubin levels higher than 30 mg/dL are almost invariably caused by complicating hemolysis. The serum aminotransferases generally rise before the onset of detectable jaundice, may reach levels as high as several thousand units, and may remain elevated for several weeks. The height reached by the aminotransferases in the serum provides only a rough estimate of the degree of hepatocellular injury and is of no prognostic value. However, a rapid fall in aminotransferases from a high peak value to normal in less than 1 week may be an indication of fulminant hepatitis with massive necrosis and collapse of liver parenchyma. The serum alkaline phosphatase usually rises in the early, cholestatic phase of hepatitis, remains elevated throughout the illness, and is often the last serum enzyme to return to normal levels after clinical recovery. The concentration of serum albumin is normal in acute hepatitis. Serum γ-globulins often are transiently elevated. The prothrombin time is usually normal and, if prolonged, is usually responsive to the administration of vitamin K. Prolongation of the prothrombin time with no response to vitamin K administration suggests severe hepatitis; if the prolongation increases, it is indicative of fulminant hepatitis. Vitamin K, 10 to 15 mg, is usually given by the subcutaneous route; when it is given intravenously, the rate of administration should be no faster than 1 mg/minute to avoid an anaphylactoid response.

Immunologic Features.   A marked advance in the diagnosis of hepatitis occurred with the discovery in 1964 of an antigenic substance in the blood that was later documented to be associated only with type B hepatitis. This antigen, initially named Australian antigen because it was first detected in the serum of an Australian aborigine, is now designated hepatitis B surface antigen (HB$_s$Ag). In 1973 the hepatitis A antigen was discovered, and the determination of serum antibodies to this antigen began to be used for the identification of type A hepatitis. Delta virus, which is associated with HB$_s$Ag, was discovered in 1977. In 1989 an antibody to hepatitis C was developed as a diagnostic test for the identification of parenterally transmitted non-A, non-B hepatitis (17). The hepatitis C RNA test became available soon thereafter. Various serologic tests have been used for the detection of hepatitis E virus in epidemiologic studies, but no standard test is currently available.

In acute *type A hepatitis,* fecal excretion of hepatitis A antigen (HA Ag) can be demonstrated a few days before the increase in serum aminotransferases, rising to a peak during maximal serum aminotransferase elevation, and then falling as jaundice appears. Antibody to hepatitis (anti-HA, predominantly IgM) appears in the serum as HA Ag disappears from the stool and rises rapidly to high levels. Afterward, antibody titers (predominantly IgG) remain detectable for at least 10 years, indicative of immunity against reinfection. Because hepatitis A infection is very common, many healthy people have detectable anti-HA in the serum. The prevalence of positive anti-HA is approximately 30% in the United States and as high as 90% in certain areas of Latin America and Asia (32). Hence, identification of an acute episode of hepatitis as type A requires a high titer of anti-HA of the IgM class or the appearance of or a rise in anti-HA titer in the serum collected during the convalescent stage compared with the acute stage of hepatitis.

The *hepatitis B virus* by electron microscopy appears as a double-shelled 42-nm spherical particle, originally called the Dane particle. The outer shell of this particle is HB$_s$Ag, and the inner core contains an antigen that has been designated the hepatitis B core antigen (HB$_c$Ag). The inner core also contains double-stranded DNA and DNA polymerase activity. In acute type B viral hepatitis, HB$_s$Ag first appears in the blood 1 to 2 weeks before and usually disappears by 2 months after the onset of clinical symptoms (Fig. 43.1). Antibody to hepatitis B core antigen (anti-HB$_c$) appears in the serum at the onset of clinical symptoms, reaches a peak soon after the maximal level of serum aminotransferase is reached, and then falls gradually, becoming undetectable 1 to 2 years after the infection. Antibody to the hepatitis B surface antigen (anti-HB$_s$) usually appears during the convalescence, when HB$_s$Ag is no longer detectable, and then persists for many years. The presence of HB$_s$Ag or IgM anti-HB$_c$ or a rise in anti-HB$_s$ titer during the acute illness is evidence that the hepatitis is caused by the hepatitis B virus (16). Persistence of HB$_s$Ag in the serum beyond 3 months after the infection suggests that the patient has become a chronic carrier of the hepatitis B virus (25). High titers of anti-HB$_c$, but absent anti-HB$_s$, are usually found in association with HB$_s$Ag in the carrier state. The presence of anti-HB$_s$ indicates that the patient has had a prior infection with type B hepatitis and now is immune to reinfection. In 1972 a new antigen called e antigen was discovered in HB$_s$Ag-positive sera. The e antigen (HB$_e$Ag), although associated only with type B hepatitis, is immunologically distinct from HB$_s$Ag and HB$_c$Ag. HB$_e$Ag appears transiently in the serum during the early phase of acute type B hepatitis. In chronic carriers of HB$_s$Ag, the presence of HB$_e$Ag is a marker of active virus replication and correlates with infectivity of the carrier (11). Some studies suggest that the presence of HB$_e$Ag in the chronic carrier is an indicator of progression of acute hepatitis B to chronic hepatitis or cirrhosis.

Hepatitis delta virus (HDV) is a defective viruslike particle that is composed of a small RNA genome

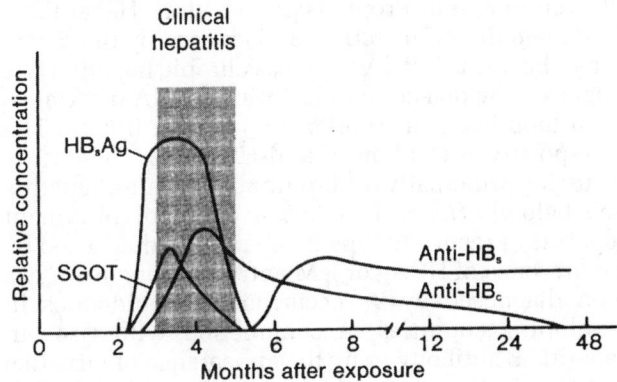

Figure 43.1. Pattern of appearance of hepatitis B surface antigen (HB$_s$Ag) and antibodies to hepatitis B surface antigen (anti-HB$_s$) and to hepatitis B core antigen (anti-HB$_c$) in acute hepatitis B infection. SGOT is now called aspartate aminotransferase (AST). (From Mezey E. Specific liver diseases. In: Halsted JA, Halsted CH, eds. The laboratory in clinical medicine. 2nd ed. Philadelphia: WB Saunders, 1981.)

surrounded by delta antigen (HDAg) and a coat of HB_sAg. Acute hepatitis delta infection (24) is associated with a brief rise in delta antigen (HDAg) that lasts approximately 10 days followed by the appearance of delta antibody (anti-HD). Initially the antibody is of IgM type, lasting 10 to 20 days, followed by the appearance of IgG anti-HD. A characteristic of hepatitis delta infection is a lowering of HB_sAg titers; probably hepatitis D virus requires hepatitis B virus for its replication.

Hepatitis C is caused by a single-stranded RNA virus. There are at least five major genotypes of the hepatitis C virus, which have different geographic distribution and influence on the clinical course of the disease and its response to therapy (6). Hepatitis C virus RNA (HCV RNA) is detectable within 10 days of infection and persists during the development of acute and chronic hepatitis. Anti-HC becomes detectable 12 to 15 weeks after infection. In most cases it persists in the blood regardless of the outcome of the disease (3).

Hepatitis E is caused by a 27- to 34-nm nonenveloped RNA single-stranded polyadenylated virus. A variety of immunoassays have been developed for the diagnosis of hepatitis E, and these assays have been used in clinical and epidemiologic studies of various epidemics in different parts of the world. A hepatitis E RNA test has also been used in some of these studies (22).

At present the practical usefulness of the immunologic markers for hepatitis is as follows: *Hepatitis A infection* is confirmed by the demonstration of a rise in anti-HA titer in the serum collected during convalescence as compared with the acute stage of hepatitis, or preferably, during the acute illness, by the presence of anti-HA of the IgM class. *Infection with hepatitis B* is usually confirmed by the presence of HB_sAg, but if the antigen is absent and it is clinically indicated, the diagnosis can be confirmed by demonstrating IgM anti-HB_c. The determination of anti-HB_s is useful to find out whether a person is immune to hepatitis B or whether that person is a candidate for prophylaxis, a subject that is discussed later in this chapter (see "Prevention and Prophylaxis of Viral Hepatitis"). *Acute hepatitis C infection* is diagnosed by the detection of hepatitis C RNA, whereas chronic hepatitis C is diagnosed by detection of hepatitis C RNA or by anti-HC 6 months or more after the onset of illness. The false-positive detection of anti-HC is less than 10%, occurring principally in chronic autoimmune hepatitis (see below). *Hepatitis D,* as a cause of fulminant hepatitis or recurrent type B hepatitis, is diagnosed by the presence of HDAg or IgM anti-HD. *Hepatitis E* has been diagnosed by its occurrence in epidemics in developing countries in conjunction with rises in hepatitis E antibody or by the appearance of viruslike particles in the stool, which have been identified to date only in the course of epidemiologic investigations.

Management. Acute viral hepatitis usually resolves completely in 1 to 3 months. There is no specific therapy. Bed rest is indicated initially in the symptomatic patient because it often alleviates the symptoms, although there is no evidence that it changes the overall course of the illness (23). As the patient's symptoms improve, a gradual increase in activity is allowed as tolerated by the patient. Intake of a normal-calorie, high-protein diet should be encouraged, although it is often difficult for the patient to eat because of nausea and anorexia. However, these symptoms are usually minimal in the morning, so the patient should be encouraged to eat a large breakfast. Strict isolation of the patient to his or her own room and bathroom is often impractical and probably unnecessary. General hygienic measures, such as washing the hands after contact with the patient and careful handling of stool and blood samples, are mandatory (see "Prevention and Prophylaxis of Viral Hepatitis").

Hospitalization is indicated in patients in whom the diagnosis is uncertain and in those who have severe symptoms of nausea and vomiting, changes in mental status, or a prothrombin time that is prolonged more than 4 seconds above the control value. In addition, it is advisable to admit to the hospital patients who do not have somebody at home who can observe and help them.

Nausea can be controlled with oral Benadryl, 25 mg three times a day, or by Compazine, 10 mg two to four times a day, without danger of central nervous system depression. Acetaminophen, 500 mg four times a day, can be safely given for abdominal discomfort (the risk of hepatotoxicity is at much higher dosages). No sedatives should be given because they may precipitate hepatic encephalopathy. Corticosteroids are of no value in the treatment of acute viral hepatitis.

Patients should be followed at intervals varying from 1 to 3 weeks and should not be discharged from ambulatory care or returned to full activity until all symptoms have disappeared and all laboratory tests have returned to normal. Patients are advised not to ingest alcoholic beverages until 1 month after all laboratory tests have returned to normal.

In patients with hepatitis B, HB_sAg should be measured after 6 months. If HB_sAG is still detectable at that time, the patient should be managed in consultation with a hepatologist.

Liver Biopsy.   Liver biopsies are indicated only if the diagnosis is uncertain or if the clinical course of the disease is prolonged beyond 6 months. A specialist in liver disease should be consulted to evaluate the patient and to perform the liver biopsy.

In patients who do not require hospitalization for another reason, liver biopsies today can be performed as outpatient procedures in a hospital. The patient should be demonstrated to have a history of normal hemostasis, a prothrombin time less than 4 seconds above control, and a platelet count greater than 80,000/ mm^3. A liver biopsy is contraindicated if there is an infiltrate in the right lower lung or a right-sided pleural effusion, absent hepatic dullness to percussion, suspected liver hemangioma or abscess, massive ascites, extrahepatic obstruction, or severe anemia (hemoglobin less than 10 g/dL).

Patient Experience. After application of local anesthesia, the liver biopsy is performed by the intercostal right subcutaneous route using suction with a needle 1.6 mm in diameter. It entails minimal risk when done by a skilled operator. The most common complication is pleuritic pain lasting a few hours after the biopsy, which is noted in approximately 5% of the cases. The most serious complications are bleeding and bile peritonitis, which occur in less than 1% of cases. The incidence of mortality from liver biopsy is 0.2%. After the procedure, patients are observed for approximately 6 hours and, if no complications have occurred, are sent home accompanied by a friend or relative.

Prognosis. Most patients with acute viral hepatitis recover from their illness without any sequelae. The mortality rate from all types of hepatitis is less than 0.1%. The principal cause of death is the development of fulminant hepatitis, which is more common in type B hepatitis. Fulminant hepatitis usually overcomes the patient within 10 days of the onset of the symptoms of hepatitis. Older patients and patients with other medical illnesses, such as diabetes mellitus, are more likely to have a prolonged course and higher mortality. Type E hepatitis, transmitted by the fecal–oral route, results in a high mortality in pregnant women. Indications of a poor prognosis are changes in mental status, a nonpalpable liver that is also small on hepatic scan, a liver that decreases rapidly in size, or a prothrombin time that is prolonged more than 4 seconds above normal.

Chronic hepatitis occurs in approximately 85% of patients with hepatitis C, and 15 to 20% of those patients eventually develop cirrhosis. Chronic hepatitis and cirrhosis occur in 3 to 5% of patients with type B hepatitis. Chronic hepatitis and cirrhosis do not occur after type A or type E hepatitis. These complications should be suspected in patients who continue to have clinical and laboratory evidence of liver disease 6 months after the onset of acute hepatitis (13). Most patients clear the HB_sAg from their serum within 3 months of the onset of the illness. Approximately 10% of patients with type B hepatitis become chronic carriers of HB_sAg. Chronic carriers of HB_sAg with abnormal levels of serum aminotransferases should be evaluated for the development of chronic active hepatitis by liver biopsy. An increased incidence of hepatocellular carcinoma has been found in carriers of HB_sAg and hepatitis C RNA.

Differential Diagnosis. A number of other viruses have been reported to cause hepatitis. *Cytomegalic inclusion infection,* usually clinically inapparent in the adult, can present with manifestations of hepatitis in patients being administered immunosuppressive therapy, in those who have diseases characterized by immunosuppression (see Chapter 34), or after blood transfusions in healthy subjects; the diagnosis can be made promptly, if necessary, by examination of biopsy specimens for intranuclear inclusions and detection of the virus in tissue with specific antibodies. Alternatively, the diagnosis can be made by showing a rise of specific IgM antibody to the virus or by culture of the urine. *Mononucleosis* (caused by the Epstein–Barr virus, EBV) is often associated with hepatocellular dysfunction with mild transient jaundice in 5 to 10% of patients. It is diagnosed by the presence in the serum of a heterophil antibody that is not absorbed by guinea pig kidney or by a positive mononucleosis spot test. Demonstration of IgM EBV antibodies specific for EB virus confirms the diagnosis (see Chapter 53).

Hepatitis caused by *leptospirosis* should be suspected in patients who have been in close contact with rodents or with food, water, soil, or other material contaminated with the urine of rodents; the diagnosis is established by recovery of leptospiras in culture of the blood or by a rise in antibodies in the course of the disease. *Drug-induced hepatitis* (see below) presents with clinical features that are indistinguishable from viral hepatitis, and a history of drug intake is a most important clue in suspecting the diagnosis. *Alcoholic hepatitis* (see below) usually develops after recent heavy alcohol ingestion; the serum aminotransferases are rarely elevated more than 10 times above normal and the elevation is primarily in the serum aspartate aminotransferase (AST). In patients with marked cholestasis, as evidenced by persistent elevation of the bilirubin, high serum alkaline phosphatase, and pruritus in association with persistent dark urine and light stools, the diagnosis of *extrahepatic biliary obstruction* should be entertained. An abnormal sonogram may provide a clue to extrahepatic obstruction if the biliary ducts are found to be dilated, and the patient should then be referred to a specialist in liver diseases for further evaluation.

Prevention and Prophylaxis of Viral Hepatitis. General hygienic measures, such as washing the hands after contact with the patient, are the most effective means of preventing the spread of hepatitis from patients to others. The patient's dishes and eating utensils can be shared by other people only if cleaned by heating above 120°C for 15 to 20 minutes in a dishwasher after the patient has used them. Assignment of the patient to a separate bathroom is ideal but often impractical. The viruses can be present in feces, blood, and other body fluids of the patients. The handling of all of these materials should be done with care. Because the virus appears in the stool during the prodromal period of hepatitis, the precautions mentioned should be taken routinely in environments where there is a high risk of development of hepatitis, such as in institutions for the mentally retarded.

The screening of blood for HB_sAg and anti-hepatitis C before transfusion has markedly decreased the risk of posttransfusion infection by hepatitis B and hepatitis C viruses to 1 in 63,000 and 1 in 100,000 units transfused, respectively (26). Other sources of type B and C that can easily be controlled are contaminated needles, pins used to test sensation, and dental and surgical instruments. All used needles or pins should be discarded in specially labeled bottles containing 40% formalin, which is known to inactivate the hepatitis viruses. The preferred method for cleaning surgical and dental instruments is by heat sterilization. The risk that most health care workers who are HB$_s$Ag positive pose to their patients is minimal if high standards of hygiene are maintained. The exceptions are dentists and surgeons (15), who often develop cuts on their hands while operating. Dentists are urged to wear gloves regardless of whether they are HB$_s$Ag positive to protect themselves and their patients. Patients who have had hepatitis B or hepatitis C and have recovered (clinically and serologically) may be infectious for many years and therefore should not be allowed to donate blood. Spouses of patients with hepatitis B should receive hepatitis B vaccine. Unvaccinated sexual partners of patients who have recovered from hepatitis B may be at risk. Sexual partners of patients in monogamous relationships with chronic hepatitis C have less than a 2% risk of infection.

Standard immune serum globulin (ISG) is known to prevent the clinical manifestations of hepatitis A in 80 to 90% of persons when administered within 2 weeks after exposure. However, it does not prevent subclinical infection. The recommended dosage of standard ISG is 0.02 mL/kg. *Hepatitis A vaccine* is indicated for close personal contacts of patients with known hepatitis A, inmates of institutions during an epidemic of hepatitis A, and travelers to areas where hepatitis is endemic. It is not indicated for casual acquaintances or coworkers of the patient or for people who are known to have anti-HA antibody in their serum. To obtain immediate and long-term protection in people recently exposed to hepatitis A, the vaccine is combined with the administration of ISG. The hepatitis A vaccine results in the development of protective anti-HA antibody 2 weeks after its administration, a protection that lasts approximately 6 months, at which time a booster dose is given to extend the protection for up to 10 years. The vaccination (Havrix or Vagta) is given as an injection of 0.5 mL to children and adolescents aged 2 to 17 years and as a 1-mL injection to adults (19).

The role of standard ISG in the prevention of type B hepatitis is uncertain. *Hepatitis B immune globulin* (containing a high titer of anti-HB$_s$) prevents approximately 75% of cases of type B hepatitis (if given immediately after exposure) in people who have been stuck with needles contaminated by HB$_s$Ag-positive patients, in sexual partners of HB$_s$Ag-positive patients, in newborns of HB$_s$Ag-positive mothers, and in the staff of dialysis units (27). It is not indicated for casual or work contacts of patients with type B hepatitis or for patients who have been demonstrated to have anti-HB$_s$. Testing for anti-HB$_s$ should be done routinely before administration of hepatitis B immune globulin, provided that the results of the tests can be obtained within 1 week of exposure to the virus.

Chapter 32 contains details regarding indications, dosages, and schedules for primary prevention of hepatitis B with *hepatitis B vaccine,* postexposure prophylaxis for adults and newborn infants exposed to people who have active hepatitis B or are known HB$_s$Ag carriers, and postexposure prophylaxis for adults exposed to people whose HB$_s$Ag status is unknown.

There have been insufficient studies to know whether the incidence of posttransfusion hepatitis C or hepatitis E is decreased by the administration of standard ISG. No vaccines are currently available for the prevention of hepatitis C or hepatitis E.

Drug-Induced Hepatitis

The liver is the principal organ concerned with drug metabolism; hence, it is not surprising that it is also a principal target for drug toxicity. Every drug has the potential for producing hepatocellular damage. Drug-induced hepatitis results from either direct hepatotoxicity or an idiosyncratic reaction (host hypersensitivity). Hepatotoxic reactions caused by direct toxins such as carbon tetrachloride and inorganic phosphorus are dose dependent and reproducible with a brief interval after exposure to the drug. Idiosyncratic reactions are the more common response to drugs. Characteristically, they are not dose dependent, occur in only a small number of people who are exposed, and are preceded by a sensitizing period of 1 to 4 weeks of exposure or a history of exposure. Drug reactions may be cholestatic, simulate viral hepatitis, or combine features of both processes.

Cholestatic Reactions. Cholestasis is caused by a direct dose-related effect of the administration of anabolic steroids and oral contraceptives. Cholestasis occurs in 1 to 2% of patients receiving anabolic steroids but occurs less often after the ingestion of oral contraceptive drugs. Jaundice and pruritus are prominent symptoms. The elevated serum bilirubin is composed principally of the direct conjugated fraction. Serum alkaline phosphatase and cholesterol are elevated, whereas serum aminotransferases are normal or only slightly elevated. Cholestasis disappears soon after withdrawal of the offending drug.

A much larger number of drugs cause cholestasis through *hypersensitivity.* Examples are phenothiazine derivatives such as chlorpromazine, antibiotics such as erythromycin, antithyroid drugs such as propylthiouracil and methimazole, hypoglycemic agents such as tolbutamide and chlorpropamide, immunosuppressant drugs such as azathioprine, and cytotoxic drugs such as chlorambucil. Common clinical features of these drug reactions are fever, right upper quadrant abdominal pain, pruritus, skin rash, and eosinophilia. Serum aminotransferases are moderately elevated (less than 10 times above normal). The clinical and laboratory abnormalities usually subside between 2 and 4 weeks after discontinuation of the drug, although on occasion cholestasis persists for months to years. Severe pruritus is treated with cholestyramine (Questran) given in a dosage of 4 g three times a day before meals. Relief of pruritus is obtained in 4 to 7 days after starting this medication. Patients with cholestasis should be hospitalized whenever the jaundice persists unchanged or increases 2 to 4 weeks after discontinuation of the drug to investigate the possibility of other causes of cholestasis (see Chapter 90).

Hepatocellular Reactions. Most agents that produce direct hepatocellular damage are toxins rather than drugs. *Acetaminophen,* however, is a drug that produces hepatic necrosis in all people if ingested in a large dose (greater than 10 g), usually in a suicide attempt. Alcoholics and patients taking drugs such as phenobarbital, which are inducers of microsomal enzymes, are at risk of developing hepatic necrosis after the ingestion of lower doses of acetaminophen. Shortly after ingestion the patient develops nausea and vomiting, but evidence of hepatocellular damage often does not become apparent until 48 hours later, when serum aminotransferases rise and the prothrombin time becomes prolonged. The patient's condition then deteriorates; jaundice appears and central nervous system depression may occur. The mortality rate of patients who took an overdose of acetaminophen was found to be 3.5% in one large study (5). Thus, patients who are known to have or are suspected of having ingested toxic amounts of acetaminophen should be hospitalized.

Idiosyncratic hepatocellular reactions have been reported after the administration of a number of drugs, the most common of which are isoniazid, α-methyldopa, nitrofurantoin, ketoconazole, phenylbutazone, and halothane. Asymptomatic increases in serum aminotransferases, which subside despite continued administration of the drug, have been reported in 5 to 10% of patients taking isoniazid or α-methyldopa (33). Because of the often transient nature of the serum aminotransferase elevations, there is no need to monitor this test in asymptomatic patients. However, the development of symptoms of fatigue and anorexia or of nausea and general malaise is an indication for the determination of serum aminotransferases; if aminotransferase activity is increased, the drug should be discontinued immediately because this often heralds the onset of severe hepatocellular damage. In some cases rifampin, an occasional cause of hepatotoxicity itself, potentiates the hepatotoxic effects of isoniazid. The incidence of acute hepatitis in patients taking these drugs is 0.1 to 0.3%. Women and older patients are more likely to be affected. The onset of the reaction is between 1 and 10 weeks after the start of therapy. The symptoms, laboratory tests, and findings on liver biopsy are indistinguishable from those of viral hepatitis (see above), so serologic tests to rule out viral hepatitis are often obtained. The hepatitis usually resolves within a few weeks after the drug is discontinued. However, a mortality rate as high as 12% has been reported for severe hepatitis caused by isoniazid. Moreover, chronic active liver disease can develop if the drug responsible for the hepatitis is continued. Administration of corticosteroids is not indicated in drug-induced hepatitis.

Alcoholic Hepatitis

This condition is seen most often after prolonged heavy alcohol intake. Women are more susceptible to alcoholic liver disease than men, and it usually does not develop in men who drink less than 40 g ethanol/day or in women who drink less than 20 g ethanol/day (equivalent to 4 and 2 ounces [120 and 60 mL] of 86

proof whiskey, respectively). Many of the presenting clinical characteristics of patients with alcoholic hepatitis (e.g., anorexia, significant fatigue, jaundice, and tender hepatomegaly) are indistinguishable from those of viral hepatitis. However, patients with alcoholic hepatitis are more likely to have fever and leukocytosis. The elevation of the serum aminotransferases is rarely 10 times above normal, and often there is a prolongation of the prothrombin time. The elevation of AST is characteristically greater than that of alanine aminotransferase (ALT). Patients with alcoholic hepatitis and jaundice should be admitted to the hospital and have a definite diagnosis established by liver biopsy, if not contraindicated by abnormal hemostatic function. Liver biopsy differentiates alcoholic hepatitis from drug-induced hepatitis and viral hepatitis and gives an indication of any underlying chronic liver disease. The illness is often more severe than in patients with viral hepatitis, and decompensation with hepatic encephalopathy and death can occur. Approximately one-third of patients with alcoholic hepatitis have been shown to progress to cirrhosis, often within 6 months (20). However, if patients can abstain from further drinking of alcohol (see Chapter 21), approximately one-third recover completely, both clinically and histologically, usually within a month.

Chronic Hepatitis

Chronic hepatitis is inflammation of the liver detected by abnormal liver tests or abnormal liver histology that has persisted for longer than 6 months. The spectrum of chronic hepatitis varies from a benign reversible process to an unrelenting process that often progresses to cirrhosis. Liver biopsy is essential both for the diagnosis and to establish the severity of the disease and the need for treatment. The liver histology is graded semiquantitatively according to the degree of necrosis and inflammation and the degree of fibrosis to indicate whether there is minimal, mild, moderate, or severe activity, or whether there is cirrhosis (9).

The principal causes of chronic hepatitis are infection with hepatitis viruses, both type B and type C, autoimmune (formerly called lupoid hepatitis), and drugs such as isoniazid, α-methyldopa, and nitrofurantoin. In addition, *Wilson's disease,* α₁-antitrypsin deficiency, and *primary biliary cirrhosis* may present with clinical and histologic features of chronic hepatitis.

The onset of chronic hepatitis is usually insidious. The patient may be asymptomatic and liver disease may be detected by aminotransferase elevations done on routine testing, or there may be symptoms of general malaise, fatigue, abdominal discomfort, anorexia, and jaundice. In about a third of the patients, the disease evolves from a clinically overt episode of acute hepatitis. Physical examination in patients with chronic hepatitis often reveals hepatomegaly and, sometimes, when the disease is more advanced, splenomegaly, spider angiomas, palmar erythema, and gynecomastia. Elevations of serum aminotransferases may be the only laboratory abnormality, but elevations of bilirubin and globulins are also common. Decreases in serum albumin and prolongation of the prothrombin time reflect loss of hepatocellular function and a poor prognosis. Older male patients are more likely to have HB_sAg in the serum and to present with an acute onset of illness. Patients with chronic hepatitis caused by hepatitis C virus may have arthralgias, vasculitis, palpable purpura, and peripheral neuropathy caused by *type II cryoglobulinemia*. Characteristically these patients have false-negative test results for anti–hepatitis C and undetectable hepatitis C RNA because these factors are concentrated in the cryoprecipitates (1).

Patients with *autoimmune hepatitis* are more likely to be women and to present with acne, amenorrhea, arthralgia and arthritis, pleurisy, or intermittent fever (8). In addition, they may have associated thyroiditis, Sjögren's syndrome, ulcerative colitis, glomerulonephritis, or hemolytic anemia. Laboratory tests on these patients show evidence of immunologic hyperactivity: Serum γ-globulin is often markedly elevated, and there is elevation in the titers of antinuclear antibodies and smooth muscle antibodies. A small subgroup of patients with chronic autoimmune hepatitis have normal titers of antinuclear antibodies, but have elevated liver–kidney microsomal (anti-LKM) antibodies. In addition, antimitochondrial antibodies are found in 15% of these patients.

The diagnosis of *Wilson's disease* (which affects approximately 1 in 1 million people) should be considered in all patients, particularly those under 25 years of age, who have clinical and laboratory features of otherwise unexplained chronic hepatitis (30). Wilson's disease is discussed in more detail in the section on cirrhosis. The diagnosis of chronic hepatitis caused by α_1-*antitrypsin deficiency* (which affects 1 in 1000 people) is suggested by the finding of an absent or low α_1-globulin on serum protein electrophoresis (10). The diagnosis is established by demonstrating a low value of α_1-antitrypsin in the serum by quantitative measurement and by protease inhibitor (Pi) typing (10). The common allele is PiM, whereas liver disease occurs in approximately 20% of people who are homozygous for the allele PiZ. Liver biopsy reveals periodic acid-fast Schiff (PAS)–positive cytoplasmic inclusions that are resistant to diastase in both homozygous and heterozygous patients for the allele PiZ. There is no known medical therapy for this deficiency, which is transmitted by codominant inheritance. The diagnostic characteristics of *primary biliary cirrhosis* are discussed in the section on cirrhosis later in this chapter. The diagnosis of *drug-induced chronic hepatitis* (see "Drug-Induced Hepatitis") depends on a careful history and the demonstration of improvement of the patient after discontinuation of drugs that are known to produce this illness. In most cases, chronic active hepatitis caused by drugs reverts to normal after discontinuation of the offending drug (33).

The clinical course of patients with chronic active hepatitis is variable. Patients can be asymptomatic for a long time, have periods of intermittent worsening and remission, or have a progressive course to cirrhosis and death if untreated (29). Delta hepatitis is associated with clinical exacerbation of chronic hepatitis B and more rapid progression to cirrhosis (24).

Therapy. *Corticosteroids* have been shown to be beneficial in symptomatic patients with chronic autoimmune hepatitis. Clinical, biochemical, and histologic improvement and even remission have been observed, and mortality rates have been reduced after therapy with corticosteroids (29). Prednisone or prednisolone, 40 to 60 mg, is given initially to suppress the activity of the disease and then is tapered slowly, usually over 1 to 3 months, to a maintenance dosage of 10 to 20 mg. Symptomatic improvement followed by a fall in serum aminotransferases occurs in the first few weeks. Treatment with corticosteroids is decreased to the smallest dosage possible to maintain normal or minimal elevations of the serum aminotransferases. Discontinuation of the corticosteroid therapy often results in a relapse. Azathioprine at an initial dosage of 100 mg a day in combination with prednisone is often effective in maintaining a remission (8). Asymptomatic patients with chronic hepatitis are usually treated only if they have persistent elevations of serum aminotransferases and histologic evidence of at least a mild grade of activity and evidence of early fibrosis. Administration of corticosteroids to patients with chronic viral hepatitis is contraindicated because it appears to favor replication of hepatitis viruses, resulting in a higher morbidity and mortality (18).

Interferon-α therapy is effective in eliminating evidence of viral replication (HB_eAg) and in normalizing serum aminotransferase in more than one-third of patients with type B hepatitis (14). Higher dosages and prolonged administration of interferon-α result in improvement in 15 to 25% of patients with chronic delta hepatitis (13). Interferon-α therapy normalizes serum aminotransferases in half of patients with type C hepatitis, but the relapse rate within 6 months of completion of therapy is 51% (13). Hence, the rate of sustained response is only 15 to 25%. The response rate was improved in some pilot studies when interferon-α was combined with ribavirin. Decisions about the use of interferon should be made in consultation with a hepatologist.

No specific therapy exists for type E hepatitis.

UNEXPLAINED ELEVATIONS OF LIVER ENZYMES IN THE SERUM

Elevations of serum aminotransferases and alkaline phosphatase are occasionally found in normal subjects or in patients not suspected of having liver disease. In such a situation the abnormality should first be confirmed by repeated testing. Next, it is important to remember that elevated serum aminotransferases and alkaline phosphatase do not necessarily originate from the liver. For example, elevated serum aminotransferases can be caused by injury to the heart and striated muscle; if the source of the serum aminotransferases is muscle, the more specific creatine kinase will also be elevated. An isolated increase of serum alkaline phosphatase can originate from liver or bone. The hepatic origin of alkaline phosphatase can be confirmed by demonstration of an elevated 5'-nucleotidase, which, unlike alkaline phosphatase, is present only in the liver and the epithelium of the bile ducts. By contrast, an elevated serum alkaline phosphatase accompanied by a normal serum 5'-nucleotidase is almost invariably caused by bone disease; a common cause of such an occurrence is a recent bone fracture. Any persistent elevation of serum aminotransferases for longer than 6 months that remains unexplained is an indication for liver biopsy to rule out chronic hepatitis. A persistent elevation of serum alkaline phosphatase in the absence of an elevated serum bilirubin can occur in patients with fatty liver, which is common in diabetic and obese patients or can be the result of space-occupying lesions, such as granulomas or metastatic carcinoma. A computerized tomographic (CT) scan with contrast of the liver is recommended in these cases to rule out metastatic carcinoma, but a liver biopsy is indicated only if the CT scan shows a space-occupying lesion or if there is clinical suspicion of diseases such as tuberculosis and sarcoidosis that may result in hepatic granulomas.

ALCOHOLIC FATTY LIVER

Alcoholic fatty liver is caused by alterations of lipid metabolism caused by alcohol and therefore occurs in all persons who ingest alcohol in excessive amounts. It is manifested mainly by a feeling of abdominal fullness caused by hepatomegaly and mild elevation of the serum aminotransferases (rarely more than two times above normal). On occasion marked fatty infiltration is associated with symptoms of malaise, weakness, anorexia, tender hepatomegaly, and even jaundice. These symptomatic patients require further evaluation, occasionally including liver biopsy, to distinguish fatty liver from alcoholic hepatitis and cirrhosis. The treatment of fatty liver consists of abstinence from alcohol. With abstinence the abnormal accumulation of fat disappears within 4 to 6 weeks. As the patient improves, the liver decreases in size and becomes nontender. Serum bilirubin and aminotransferases promptly return to normal. Recurrent episodes of symptomatic fatty liver are common after heavy alcohol ingestion, but there is no evidence that this lesion itself leads to cirrhosis.

NONALCOHOLIC STEATOHEPATITIS

Fatty liver is a common finding in nonalcoholic obese patients and in patients with type 2 diabetes (28). Fatty liver is present in 80 to 90% of morbidly obese patients. Most of the patients are asymptomatic and liver disease is discovered by finding elevated serum aminotransferases. The principal symptoms when present are fatigue and right upper abdominal discomfort. Hepatomegaly is a finding in 90% of the patients, but splenomegaly is rare. If the diagnosis is in doubt, it can be confirmed by ultrasonography. Weight reduc-

tion by intake of a calorie-restricted low-fat diet often results in a decrease in fatty infiltration, improvement of symptoms, a decrease in liver size, a fall in serum triglycerides, and sometimes in a fall in serum aminotransferases. Fatty liver with evidence of inflammation and fibrosis (steatohepatitis) can have a slow progression toward cirrhosis.

CIRRHOSIS

Cirrhosis is a chronic diffuse liver disease characterized by widespread hepatic fibrosis and nodule formation. The fibrosis is the result of extensive destruction of liver cells, and the nodularity represents regeneration. For clinical purposes cirrhosis can be classified into the following major categories: alcoholic, viral (hepatitis B and C), cardiac, and biliary cirrhosis; Wilson's disease; hemochromatosis; and schistosomiasis. The two major morphologic types of cirrhosis are *micronodular,* which is characterized by regular small nodules, and *macronodular,* in which there is extensive scarring of the liver and the presence of irregular nodules of various sizes (31). Alcoholic cirrhosis is characteristically micronodular, whereas cirrhosis caused by chronic viral hepatitis is characteristically macronodular. On occasion cirrhosis of the alcoholic is of the macronodular type; this is more common in chronic alcoholics who no longer drink alcohol. The onset of cirrhosis is usually insidious and is associated with nonspecific symptoms such as fatigue, anorexia, weight loss, nausea, and abdominal discomfort. As the disease progresses, signs of hepatocellular failure become prominent: jaundice, edema, ascites, electrolyte abnormalities, bleeding tendencies, spider angiomas, palmar erythema, gynecomastia, impotence, and loss of axillary and pubic hair. Hepatomegaly and portal hypertension resulting in splenomegaly and a venous collateral circulation are common. The most severe complications of cirrhosis are hepatic encephalopathy, bleeding from esophageal varices, and infection. Patients with alcoholic cirrhosis often have recurring episodes of hepatocellular failure, precipitated by superimposed alcoholic hepatitis and fatty infiltration induced by alcohol ingestion. Clinical improvement often occurs after abstinence from alcohol and after bed rest and optimal nutrition. By contrast, patients with macronodular cirrhosis are more likely to present insidiously with evidence of portal hypertension. When hepatocellular failure occurs in these patients, it is usually a terminal event because it is the result of excessive fibrosis and reduced hepatic parenchymal mass rather than of reversible lesions such as necrosis and fatty infiltration found in alcoholic cirrhosis. Rapid deterioration of patients with cirrhosis should raise the suspicion of a complicating *hepatocellular carcinoma.* Common laboratory findings in patients with cirrhosis include anemia, a normal or slightly decreased white blood cell count, and moderate thrombocytopenia. The most common abnormal liver tests are hyperbilirubinemia, a depressed serum albumin, elevated serum globulins, and a prolonged prothrombin time.

Differential Diagnosis

The diagnostic characteristics of some of the other types of cirrhosis are as follows:

- *Cardiac cirrhosis* develops only after prolonged and severe cardiac failure, usually caused by valvular disease, particularly in patients with tricuspid incompetence or constrictive pericarditis. Jaundice, hepatomegaly, and ascites are prominent features, but the diagnosis can be established with certainty only by liver biopsy. Treatment of cardiac failure—for example, of constrictive pericarditis by pericardiectomy—results in improvement of liver function.

- *Primary biliary cirrhosis* (21) is a chronic disease of unknown cause that is characterized by progressive intrahepatic cholestasis and is most often seen in middle-aged women. The principal manifestations are jaundice with pruritus, hepatomegaly, hypercholesterolemia with the formation of xanthoma and xanthelasma, and steatorrhea caused by the decreased delivery of bile acids to the intestine. Antimitochondrial antibodies are found in 95% of these patients, and their presence is virtually diagnostic. Liver biopsy in the early stages reveals injury to the septal and large intralobular bile ducts with surrounding accumulation of inflammatory plasma cells and lymphocytes and with granuloma formation. In the end stages of the disease, cirrhosis develops that is nearly indistinguishable from other causes of nonalcoholic cirrhosis. Treatment with ursodeoxycholic acid (Actigall) has been found to reduce serum bilirubin and aminotransferases and delay clinical progression of the disease, although it does not affect histologic progression (21).

- *Wilson's disease* is a rare disorder of copper metabolism that is inherited as an autosomal recessive disorder (30). Its symptoms result from hepatic and neurologic dysfunction. In children the principal symptoms are caused by liver involvement, whereas in adults neurologic symptoms tend to predominate. The diagnosis should be suspected in all children or young adults who develop cirrhosis because treatment with copper-chelating agents can arrest the disease and alleviate all symptoms. A characteristic finding that is virtually diagnostic is the presence of Kayser–Fleischer rings, which are greenish-brown rings found on the posterior surface and in the periphery of the cornea. Because these rings cannot often be seen by the naked eye, it is important to refer all suspected patients to the ophthalmologist for slitlamp examination of the cornea. Serum ceruloplasmin, the copper-binding protein, is reduced in most but not all cases. Histologic examination of a liver biopsy is not diagnostic. However, quantitative determination of copper with a finding of more than 250 mg/g of dry liver weight or the urinary excretion of more than 50 mg/24 hours is diagnostic. Hospitalization is not required for treatment of Wilson's disease with d-penicillamine, a chelating agent with considerable toxicity, best administered by a hepatologist.

- *Hemochromatosis* is an inherited disorder of iron metabolism, resulting in excessive body iron; it is characterized principally by cirrhosis, diabetes mellitus, and grayish pigmentation of the skin. Other symptoms are cardiac failure and arrhythmias, peripheral neuritis, arthritis, and testicular atrophy. The iron overload appears to be caused by an increased absorption of dietary iron, and the mode of inheritance is autosomal recessive. The disease usually appears in people over 40 years of age and develops earlier in men, probably because of the menstrual loss of iron in women. The diagnosis is made by demonstrating a high serum iron (greater than 150 mg/dL), a high saturation of iron-binding protein (greater than 50%), and increased serum ferritin, usually in a patient with a family history of the disease (4). Therapy consists of removal of excess iron by repeated phlebotomy (1 to 2 units weekly).

- *Hepatic schistosomiasis* may occur in people from tropical areas who have been infected by schistosome cercariae while swimming or walking in infested water. The liver disease is caused by the deposition of ova of *Schistosoma mansoni* in the portal areas, with the development of an inflammatory reaction, often with granuloma formation and periportal fibrosis. Jaundice is uncommon in these patients on presentation. The most common laboratory abnormalities are increases in serum alkaline phosphatase and mild elevations of serum bilirubin and aminotransferases. The diagnosis of active infection is made by demonstrating mobile *Schistosoma* ova on fresh examination of rectal biopsy, and the diagnosis of liver involvement is made by showing the presence of ova capsules on liver biopsy.

Management

The treatment of uncomplicated cirrhosis consists of voluntary restriction of activity if the patient has weakness and fatigue, a diet high in protein but low in salt, and abstinence from alcohol (see Chapter 21). This regimen almost invariably results in improvement of hepatocellular function in patients with alcoholic cirrhosis and occasionally in patients with nonalcoholic cirrhosis. Tranquilizers and sedatives should be avoided. Infection and gastrointestinal bleeding, which in addition to alcohol ingestion are common precipitating factors of decompensation, should be searched for and treated. Vitamin K, 15 mg subcutaneously, may improve prolongation of the prothrombin time. Multivitamins and folic acid, 1 mg/day, may be given if the patient's dietary intake appears to be inadequate or if there is evidence of vitamin deficiencies. Potassium deficiency is common and may contribute to the precipitation of hepatic encephalopathy, but its extent is difficult to assess because serum potassium concentration is a poor reflection of the total body potassium. However, when serum potassium falls below 3.5 mEq/L, the deficit often can be replaced by giving 30 mL of 10% potassium chloride orally two or three times a day, if tolerated, or K-dur tablets 20 mEq, two or three times daily.

Fluid retention is treated with sodium restriction (500 mg of sodium chloride per day) and diuretics. The induced diuresis should be slow and should result in a loss of no more than 2.27 kg (5 lb) of weight per week because of the danger of precipitating electrolyte depletion and hypokalemia. Diuresis can be initiated by spironolactone, 100 mg a day, and the dosage can be increased gradually to 200 mg/day to obtain a diuresis. A loop diuretic (e.g., furosemide) is added to the regimen gradually if diuresis is inadequate. The dosage of the diuretics is decreased or the diuretics discontinued if the patient develops hyponatremia or impaired renal function. Patients with ascites that is unresponsive to sodium restriction and high dosages of diuretics should be referred to a hepatologist for management by either therapeutic paracentesis or transjugular intrahepatic portasystemic stent–shunt (TIPS). The development of acute hepatic encephalopathy manifested by asterixis or changes in mental status is an indication that the patient should be hospitalized for evaluation and treatment. Acute and chronic gastrointestinal bleeding is also an indication for hospitalization.

Protein can be restricted in stable cirrhotic patients to 45 g/day without development of a negative nitrogen balance as long as a minimum of 400 g of carbohydrate is ingested a day. A change from animal protein to a vegetable protein diet may also improve hepatic encephalopathy. The exact mechanism whereby vegetable protein is better tolerated is unknown. However, vegetable protein contains smaller amounts of ammonia, methionine, and aromatic acids and also results in alterations of small intestinal and colonic bacterial flora so that the excretion of fecal nitrogen is increased (12). Lactulose is a nonabsorbable synthetic disaccharide that reduces blood ammonia and improves encephalopathy in more than 80% of patients when administered in dosages of 20 to 30 g (30 to 45 mL) three to four times a day. Lactulose usually is effective only when it also increases the frequency of bowel movements. Other than producing mild abdominal cramps and flatulence, lactulose is devoid of side effects. The mechanism of its action is not well defined, but its effectiveness is related to its ability to trap nitrogen in the stool and decrease ammonia production. Some of the decrease in ammonia production may be caused by a decrease in contact time of the stool with colonic bacteria. The beneficial effects of a vegetable protein diet and lactulose on hepatic encephalopathy are additive. Chronic hepatic encephalopathy can be treated with protein restriction and lactulose on an ambulatory basis. Patients with decompensated cirrhosis who are not responding to therapy should be considered for liver transplantation and should be referred to a hepatologist for evaluation.

General References*

Alter MJ, Mast EE. The epidemiology of viral hepatitis in the United States. Gastroenterol Clin North Am 23:437–455, 1994.

---

*Bold print (general references) and bold numerals (specific references) denote published controlled clinical trials, meta-analyses, or consensus-based recommendations.

Update on the epidemiology of all forms of viral hepatitis.

Maddrey WC, Sorrell MF. Transplantation of the liver. 2nd ed. Norwalk, CT: Appleton & Lange, 1995.

Mezey E. Fatty liver. In: Schiff ER, Sorrell MF, Maddrey WC, eds. Schiff's diseases of the liver. 8th ed. Philadelphia: JB Lippincott, 1998.
Discusses various causes, clinical presentation, and management of fatty liver.

Okuda K. Hepatocellular carcinoma: recent progress. Hepatology 15:948, 1992.

Zakim D, Boyer TD. Hepatology. A textbook of liver disease. 3rd ed. Philadelphia: WB Saunders, 1996.
A comprehensive textbook of liver disease.

Zimmerman HJ. Update on hepatotoxicity due to classes of drugs in common clinical use: non-steroidal drugs, anti-inflammatory drugs, antibiotics, antihypertensives, and cardiac and psychotropic agents. Semin Liver Dis 10:322, 1990.
A comprehensive source of information on drug hepatotoxicity.

Specific References

1. Agnello, V, Chung RT, Kaplan LM. A role for hepatitis C virus in type II cryoglobulinemia. N Engl J Med 327:1490, 1992.
2. Alter MJ. Epidemiology of hepatitis C in the West. Semin Liver Dis 15:5, 1995.
3. Alter MJ, Margolis HS, Krawczynski K, et al. The natural history of community-acquired hepatitis C in the United States. N Engl J Med 327:1899, 1992.
4. Bassett ML, Halliday JW, Ferris RA, Powell LW. Diagnosis of hemochromatosis in young subjects: predictive accuracy of biochemical screening tests. Gastroenterology 87:628, 1984.
5. Black M. Acetaminophen hepatotoxicity. Annu Rev Med 35:577, 1984.
6. Bukh J, Miller RH, Purcell RH. Genetic heterogeneity of hepatitis C virus: quasispecies and genotypes. Semin Liver Dis 15:41–63, 1995.
7. Conry-Cantinela C, VanRaden M, Gibble J, et al. Routes of infection, viremia, and liver disease in blood donors found to have hepatitis C infection. N Engl J Med 334:1691, 1996.
8. Czaja AJ. Autoimmune liver disease. In: Zakim D, Boyer TD. Hepatology. A textbook of liver disease. 3rd ed. Philadelphia: WB Saunders, 1996; 1259.
9. Desmet VJ, Gerber M, Hoofnagle JH, et al. Classification of chronic hepatitis: diagnosis, grading, and staging. Hepatology 19:1513, 1994.
10. Fagerhol MK, Laurell CB. The polymorphism of pre-albumins and α_1-antitrypsin in human sera. Clin Chim Acta 16:199, 1967.
11. Grady GF and the U.S. National Heart and Lung Institute Collaborative Study Group. Relation of e antigen to infectivity of HB_sAg-positive inoculations among medical personnel. Lancet 2:492, 1976.
12. Greenberger NJ, Carley J, Schenker S, et al. Effect of vegetable and animal protein diets in chronic hepatic encephalopathy. Am J Dig Dis 22:845, 1977.
13. Hoofnagle JH, DiBisceglie AM. Drug therapy: the treatment of chronic viral hepatitis. N Engl J Med 336:347, 1997.
14. Hoofnagle JH, Shafritz DA, Popper H. Chronic type B hepatitis and the healthy HB_sAg carrier state. Hepatology 7:758, 1987.
15. The Incident Investigation Teams and Others. Transmission of hepatitis B to patients from four infected surgeons without hepatitis Be antigen. N Engl J Med 336:178, 1997.
16. Krugman S, Overby LR, Mushahwar IK, et al. Viral hepatitis, type B. Studies on natural history and prevention re-examined. N Engl J Med 300:101, 1979.
17. Kuo G, Choo Q-L, Alter HJ, et al. An assay for circulating antibodies to a major etiologic virus of human non-A, non-B hepatitis. Science 244:362, 1989.
18. Lam KC, Lai CL, Trepo C, Wu PC. Deleterious effect of prednisolone in HB_sAg-positive chronic active hepatitis. N Engl J Med 304:380, 1981.
19. Lemon SM, Thomas DL. Vaccines to prevent viral hepatitis. N Engl J Med 336:196, 1997.
20. Mezey E. Treatment of alcoholic liver disease. Semin Liver Dis 13:210, 1993.

21. O'Donohue J, Williams R. Primary biliary cirrhosis. QJM 89:5, 1996.

22. Purcell RH. Hepatitis viruses: changing patterns of human disease. Proc Natl Acad Sci U S A 91:2401, 1994.

23. Repsher LH, Freebern RK. Effects of early and vigorous exercise on recovery from infectious hepatitis. N Engl J Med 281:1393, 1969.

24. Rizzetto M, Verme G, Gerin JL, Purcell RH. Hepatitis delta virus disease. Prog Liver Dis 8:417, 1986.

25. Sampliner RE, Hamilton FA, Iseri OA, et al. The liver histology and frequency of clearance of the hepatitis B surface antigen (HB$_s$Ag) in chronic carriers. Am J Med Sci 277:17, 1979.

26. Schreiber GB, Busch MP, Kleinman SH, Korelitz JJ. The risk of transfusion-transmitted viral infections. The Retrovirus Epidemiology Donor Study. N Engl J Med 334:1685, 1996.

27. Seeff LB, Koff RS. Passive and active immunoprophylaxis of hepatitis B. Gastroenterology 86:958, 1984.

28. Sheth SG, Gordon FD, Chopra S. Nonalcoholic steatohepatitis. Ann Intern Med 126:137, 1997.

29. Soloway RD, Summerskill WHJ, Baggenstoss AH, et al. Clinical, biochemical, and histological remission of severe chronic active liver disease: a controlled study of treatments and early prognosis. Gastroenterology 63:820, 1972.

30. Sternlieb I, Scheinberg IH. Chronic hepatitis as a first manifestation of Wilson's disease. Ann Intern Med 76:59, 1972.

31. Summerskill WHJ, Davidson CS, Dible JH, et al. Cirrhosis of the liver. A study of alcoholic and non-alcoholic patients in Boston and London. N Engl J Med 262:1, 1969.

32. Szmuness W, Dienstag JC, Purcell RH, et al. Distribution of antibody to hepatitis A antigen in urban adult populations. N Engl J Med 295:755, 1976.

33. Zimmerman HJ, Maddrey WC. Toxic and drug-induced hepatitis. In: Schiff L, Schiff ER, eds. Diseases of the liver. 7th ed. Philadelphia: JB Lippincott, 1993; 1:707.

Renal and Urologic Problems

SECTION 5

Renal and Urologic Problems

C H A P T E R   44

Proteinuria

EDWARD S. KRAUS, MD

Normally less than 150 mg of protein per 24 hours is present in urine, although values may be as high as 300 mg/24 hours in adolescents. Sixty percent of this urinary protein is plasma protein (two-thirds of it is albumin) that has been filtered by glomeruli and only partially reabsorbed by renal tubules. The remaining 40% is synthesized and secreted into the urine by the renal tubules as well as by the more distal portions of the urogenital tract.

Increased urinary protein excretion (proteinuria) may be caused by renal disease, either glomerular dysfunction that allows more protein to be filtered or changes in the renal tubules so that there is decreased reabsorption of filtered proteins. Alternatively, increased urinary protein excretion may reflect increased metabolic generation of protein. Proteinuria is often encountered when all individuals are screened (2 to 5% prevalence). In most instances proteinuria is simply an abnormal laboratory finding in an asymptomatic patient with no significant impact on his or her present or future health. Approximately 1% of those who have proteinuria when screened have renal or systemic disease with significant physiologic sequelae. Currently, screening for proteinuria is not recommended for the general population (16), but it should be performed in selected groups at risk for renal disease (see "Office Assessment of Patients with Proteinuria"). This chapter discusses the methods of detection of protein in the urine and describes an approach to the evaluation and treatment of patients with proteinuria.

METHODS FOR DETECTING PROTEINURIA

Office screening for proteinuria is easily accomplished by several accessible and inexpensive semiquantitative methods described in detail in this chapter. Most methods are sensitive (dipstick detects 20 to 30 of albumin per deciliter; sulfosalicylic acid and heat and acetic acid, 5 to 10 mg of protein per deciliter), so positive results may be obtained when testing concentrated urine, even though 24-hour urinary protein excretion is normal. With all of these methods, false-positive and false-negative results may occur (Table 44.1).

Dipstick

A dipstick is the most practical and easiest test for semiquantitation of urinary proteins. When moistened with urine, the stick becomes yellow when protein is absent. As protein concentration increases, interference with the dye–buffer combination results in an increasingly green color. Although simple and inexpensive, the technique has several limitations. Because the color reaction is pH dependent, false-positive reactions may be observed if the urine is alkaline (pH greater than 7.5). This error can be avoided by adding a drop of strong acid (e.g., 1 N HCl) before testing to ensure that the pH in the urine is less than 7.0. Also, the dipstick method is sensitive primarily to albumin. Therefore, globulins or parts of globulins (heavy or light chains, Bence Jones protein) may be missed. Because of these limitations, an alternative method of screening for proteinuria should be available in the physician's office. Either of the methods described in this section is satisfactory.

Sulfosalicylic Acid

Another easy and inexpensive semiquantitative test for proteinuria is protein precipitation with a 3 to 10% solution of sulfosalicylic acid (SSA). SSA is available from some pharmacies or from hospital laboratories. SSA is used most often to detect globulins or light chains because the dipstick is insensitive to these proteins. However, false-positive test results occur if the urine is already turbid. In this situation the urine must be filtered before it is tested. False-positive results also occur when the test is done within 3 days of the administration of iodinated radiographic contrast media or after the administration of some drugs (Table 44.1). In addition, the SSA test detects proteins of prostatic and vaginal origin. These contaminants can be avoided by not palpating the prostate before collecting urine from men and by obtaining a clean voided urine specimen from women, which should show no or only a few vaginal cells microscopically.

Heat and Acetic Acid

Heat and acetic acid is more time-consuming and is recommended as a second method of urine protein

Table 44.1.   Urinary Constituents that Alter the Results of Protein Screening Tests

Urinary Constituents	Dipstick	Sulfosalicyclic Acid	Heat and Acetic Acid
Radiographic contrast media	No effect	False positive	False positive
Drugs and drug metabolites[a]	No effect	False positive	False positive
Bence Jones protein	False negative	No effect	False negative[b]
Highly alkaline urine	False positive	False negative	False negative
Urine turbidity	No effect	False positive	False positive
Vaginal or prostatic secretion	No effect	False positive	False positive

Modified from Bradley M, Schumann GB, Ward PCJ. Examination of urine. In: Henry JB, ed. Todd–Sanford–Davidsohn clincial diagnosis and management by laboratory methods. 16th ed. Philadelphia: WB Saunders, 1979.

[a]Tolbutamide, tolmetin, chlorpromazine, sulfisoxazole, and high dosages of cephalosporins and penicillin.

[b]Precipitated protein may disappear rapidly and be missed with continued heating.

testing only when SSA is not available. Glacial acetic acid may be purchased at a photography store and must be diluted for accurate results. The diluted solution, 1 volume of glacial acetic acid to 2 volumes of water, may be stored and used as necessary. The test is performed by heating the top of a test tube containing approximately 10 mL of urine. After the top of the urine begins to boil rapidly, three or four drops of the diluted acetic acid are added. Reheating to boiling causes a white precipitate to form if protein (either globulin or albumin) is present in the urine specimen. False-positive results occur if the specimen is contaminated with prostatic or vaginal secretions or in the presence of certain drugs or radiographic contrast media (Table 44.1). Furthermore, the rapid boiling may mask the visualization of a transient precipitation of Bence Jones protein.

OFFICE ASSESSMENT OF PATIENTS WITH PROTEINURIA

Patients may present for evaluation of proteinuria that has been discovered during evaluation for school, military service, employment, or insurance. If these patients are otherwise healthy, a screening test for proteinuria should be repeated two or three times in the office before further workup is performed. Transient nonrecurrent mild proteinuria may be seen in association with changes in systemic hemodynamics caused by the stress of fever, exercise, exposure to cold, or decompensated congestive heart failure, and thus may not reflect a progressive renal disease.

Historically, chronic proteinuria should be suspected if the patient acknowledges reports of abnormal urinalysis performed as part of previous screening examinations. Patients also may be aware of prior renal or urologic problems but may not associate them with proteinuria. Therefore, a detailed urologic history should be obtained, including history of infection or stones, prior radiologic evaluations, and family history of renal insufficiency. Because drugs such as gold, penicillamine, captopril, and nonsteroidal anti-inflammatory agents can cause proteinuria, medications should be reviewed thoroughly. Proteinuria may represent only one facet of a systemic illness, suggested by dermatologic, rheumatologic, infectious, and cardiovascular review of systems. The date of onset of

edema, nocturia, or hypertension may help determine the duration of a disease associated with proteinuria. Occasionally, the patient may have noticed a foaming of urine upon voiding if proteinuria has been massive.

Physical examination should be reviewed for the presence of signs that may be associated with the cause of renal disease (e.g., diabetic retinopathy, abdominal masses suggestive of polycystic kidneys, or rashes, murmurs, or arthropathy indicative of systemic illness) or that may result from renal disease (e.g., edema) or both (e.g., hypertension).

If screening examinations reveal proteinuria, further laboratory evaluation should include several studies. First, a microscopic urinalysis should be performed. The presence of other abnormalities, such as hematuria, casts, or inflammatory cells, suggests specific patterns of renal disease of which proteinuria may be just a part. Second, serum creatinine concentration or creatinine clearance should be measured to identify whether renal filtration function is impaired (see Chapter 48). Third, proteinuria should be quantitated by either examining a 24-hour urine sample or determining the protein/creatinine ratio in a single voided sample. This will help classify the disorder (see next section) and assist in the development of the differential diagnosis.

24-Hour Urine Collection for Protein

A clean container without preservatives, usually a gallon jug, is given to the patient with instructions about the collection process. The 24-hour collection is best done on a day when the patient will be using one toilet, and it is helpful for the patient to place a note on the toilet on the day of collection as a reminder to collect all required specimens. On the day of collection, the first voided morning specimen is discarded, and then all urine in the next 24 hours, including the next morning's first voided specimen, is collected in the container. Once the urine is collected, it is not critical when protein determination is done. When delays in analysis are prolonged, however, bacterial growth can falsely raise protein concentrations. Therefore, it is advisable to refrigerate the urine until it is brought to the laboratory if the specimen is not brought in on the day the collection is completed. Alternatively, where refrigeration is not possible, 1 to 2 g of boric acid should be added to the container. Other preservatives (e.g., strong acids, thymol) must be avoided because they will interfere with the protein assay.

Quantitation of urine protein is a precise measurement in a well-controlled laboratory, and any value greater than 200 mg/day is considered abnormal. Proteinuria is classified as nonnephrotic if the excretion is between 200 and 3500 mg in 24 hours and is classified as nephrotic (definitely indicative of glomerular disease) when the excretion is greater than 3500 mg in 24 hours, regardless of the presence or absence of other manifestations of the nephrotic syndrome (low serum albumin, edema, high serum cholesterol). The simultaneous measurement of urinary creatinine is helpful as an index of the adequacy of collection. Most patients who are not wasted and are of average body mass produce between 800 and 1500 mg of creatinine per day (21 to 26 mg/kg per day in adult men, 16 to 22 mg/kg per day in adult women).

Protein/Creatinine Ratio

An excellent correlation exists between 24-hour urinary protein excretion and the protein/creatinine concentration ratio (milligrams per deciliter of protein ÷ milligrams per deciliter of creatinine), determined in a random sample of urine obtained during normal daytime activity (1). A ratio of greater than 0.2 is considered abnormal. A ratio greater than 3.5 represents nephrotic range proteinuria. The ratio may overestimate 24-hour urinary protein excretion in certain circumstances, most notably when urine is collected from diabetic patients after strenuous exercise and from patients whose daily urinary creatinine excretion is considerably less than 1 g, such as frail adults. Conversely, determination of this ratio from a first morning urine specimen may underestimate daily urinary protein losses (see "Orthostatic Proteinuria"). The urinary protein/creatinine ratio is especially useful when a 24-hour collection is difficult to obtain or when there is doubt about the completeness of the sample.

NONNEPHROTIC PROTEINURIA

A variety of primary renal and systemic diseases may be associated with nonnephrotic range proteinuria. Also, most, if not all, patients with nephrotic range proteinuria may at some time have had nonnephrotic range protein excretion. Evaluation is best defined by considering patients who have normal physical examinations and laboratory profiles (isolated proteinuria) separately from patients with other stigmata of disease, such as active urinary sediment or hypertension (nonisolated proteinuria).

Isolated Proteinuria in Apparently Healthy Patients

If the initial evaluation is negative except for the presence of isolated proteinuria, the proteinuria may

be further classified as persistent (25 to 30% of patients) or intermittent (70 to 75% of patients) (13). The physician can determine which pattern is present by obtaining five or six specimens for semiquantitative analysis over several months. Also, the 24-hour urine protein excretion is almost always less than 1 g in patients with isolated proteinuria. If the total protein excretion is greater than 2 g/24 hours, the chance of significant occult kidney disease is high, and further investigation for nonisolated proteinuria should be considered.

Intermittent Proteinuria

A study of patients with intermittent isolated proteinuria screened by dipstick (protein in fewer than 80% of specimens) revealed definite abnormalities by light microscopy in the renal tissue of approximately 60% of patients, and approximately 40% had a normal or nearly normal biopsy (10). The significance of these findings is unclear, however, in light of another study that retrospectively analyzed the prognostic significance of proteinuria in male college students and found no excess mortality 37 to 45 years later. Morbidity was not studied (7). More recently, the Framingham study reported that overall mortality and cardiovascular mortality rates in men were slightly but significantly increased (approximately threefold) in association with proteinuria, in some cases intermittent (2).

In any case, patients who are found to have asymptomatic intermittent proteinuria and who have no evidence of systemic or renal disease can be given an optimistic prognosis. It is unnecessary to perform a kidney biopsy in these patients, but it would be prudent to follow them yearly with measurement of urine protein excretion, a urinalysis, and determination of serum creatinine. Should deterioration in renal function, significant increase in protein excretion or new abnormalities occur, reassessment and possibly a renal biopsy are necessary.

Persistent Proteinuria

Patients with protein in more than 80% of urine specimens screened by dipstick are defined as having persistent isolated proteinuria. The disorder may be further classified by evaluating the effect of posture. *Orthostatic persistent proteinuria* is present when the patient is in the upright position only. *Constant persistent proteinuria* is not influenced by the position of the patient.

Orthostatic Proteinuria. A simple method of determining the presence of this phenomenon is to have the patient collect two urine specimens. The patient rests quietly for 2 hours and then voids just before retiring in the evening to ensure an empty bladder on assuming the recumbent posture. The patient then does not get out of bed for 8 hours. Upon arising he or she voids completely into a container labeled *recumbent urine (Specimen 1).* The patient then stays up but is not vigorously active and collects all subsequent urine over the next 8 hours. This specimen is labeled *ambu-*

latory urine (Specimen 2). The protein concentrations in the urine specimens are then compared. This protocol may be simplified if the patient does not drink during the night. In the morning after overnight fluid deprivation, two or more urine specimens are collected consecutively. The first specimen is marked recumbent and should be collected immediately upon arising. The following specimens, collected after the patient is up, active, and ambulating normally for 8 hours, should be labeled *ambulatory*. A semiquantitative test (dipstick or SSA) and a measurement of urine concentration to confirm antidiuresis are performed on each sample (13). In patients with orthostatic proteinuria the recumbent protein excretion is negligible, whereas proteinuria is found when the patient assumes the upright posture.

A renal biopsy is not necessary in the evaluation of a patient with this problem; however, when biopsies have been done as part of a research protocol, minor abnormalities have been defined in approximately one-half of the patients and the others have had a biopsy that appeared normal on light microscopy (studies using electron or immunofluorescent microscopy have not been done) (13). However, it would be prudent to follow the patient by measuring urinary protein excretion and serum creatinine on a yearly basis even after the proteinuria has cleared.

If orthostatic persistent proteinuria is documented, the prognosis seems to be excellent. Military recruits with this problem have been followed for 20 years (15). None developed renal failure, and approximately 80% were no longer proteinuric. Not all patients who were free of protein in the urine at 10-year follow-up remained protein free after 20 years, although none of those patients showed significant deterioration in renal function. Also, a small number of patients reevaluated 42 to 50 years after the establishment of the diagnosis of postural proteinuria manifested good health (14).

Constant Proteinuria. In most patients with constant proteinuria, diverse morphologic changes are identified in kidney biopsy specimens. Few long-term studies of these patients have been made, but their course is likely to be indolent. Renal failure develops very rarely, although most patients develop abnormal urine sediment and 50% develop hypertension (5). It is not necessary to perform renal biopsy when there are no other findings, but yearly reevaluation is appropriate and should include blood pressure measurement, urinalysis, and determination of 24-hour protein excretion and serum creatinine and creatinine clearance. If proteinuria exceeds 2 g/day, additional evaluation including sonogram or intravenous pyelogram and collagen vascular screens may be appropriate.

Nonisolated Proteinuria

If an abnormality related to proteinuria is discovered during initial evaluation (e.g., hypertension, hematuria, casts in the urine, or renal failure), further investigation may be necessary. The direction and extent of the investigation depend on the nature of the abnormality. Renal biopsy may be indicated, especially if there is hematuria, red blood cell casts, mild renal failure, or evidence of systemic disease (e.g., systemic lupus erythematosus [SLE]). Table 44.2 lists some additional investigations that may be indicated to evaluate abnormalities associated with proteinuria. A telephone consultation with a nephrologist may be helpful in determining the need for further evaluation.

Microalbuminuria

In diabetic patients, small increases in urinary albumin excretion (below the detectability limits for usual laboratory screening methods) have been associated with an increased likelihood (up to 9 times greater incidence) of developing diabetic nephropathy, retinopathy, and cardiovascular complications, even if patients are normotensive (11). Small clinical studies further indicate that use of antihypertensive agents (particularly angiotensin-converting enzyme [ACE] inhibitors) (8,9), low-protein diets, and perhaps very tight glucose control may slow the rate of development of these complications (see Chapter 72). In a study by Lewis et al. (8), captopril dosed 25 mg three times a day slowed the rate of decline in creatinine clearance by almost 50%. Meta-analysis of studies published investigating the effect of antihypertensive therapy on renal function in diabetic patients further supports the unique protective role of ACE inhibitors in this population (3).

Consensus statements (see "General References") have been published recently encouraging that both patients with insulin-dependent diabetes for more than 5 to 10 years and non–insulin-dependent diabetic

Table 44.2. Selected Investigations that May Be Appropriate in the Diagnosis of Proteinuria that Is Not Isolated or Is Nephrotic

Antineutrophil cytoplasmic antibody (ANCA) if vasculitis is suspected
Antinuclear antibody if SLE is suspected
Antistreptolysin (ASO) titer if there is a possibility of poststreptococcal glomerulonephritis
Complement (C_3, C_4) if glomerulonephritis is suspected
Complete blood count to provide a baseline evaluation for subsequent use and to provide a clue to a systemic illness (such as leukemia)
Erythrocyte sedimentation rate if collagen vascular disease is suspected
Fasting blood sugar to consider the possibility of diabetes mellitus
Hepatitis B surface antigen, hepatitis C antibodies by second- or third-generation ELISA, if hepatitis-associated vasculitis may be present
Intravenous pyelogram to provide evidence for structural renal disease (e.g., papillary necrosis)
RPR with history or risk factors for sexually transmitted disease
Serum albumin if nephrotic range proteinuria is present
Serum electrolytes (Na^+, K^+, Cl^-, HCO_3^-, Ca^{2+}, PO_4^{2-}) to provide a screen for abnormalities subsequent to renal disease
Serum and urine protein electrophoresis and immunofixation electrophoresis if multiple myeloma is suspected
Uric acid to screen for urate-related renal disease
Urine culture if pyuria is present
Radiograph of chest to provide evidence for systemic disease (e.g., sarcoidosis)

Table 44.3.   Cause of Nephrotic Syndrome in Adults

Most Common
Diabetes mellitus
Idiopathic membranous glomerulopathy
Idiopathic lipoid nephrosis (including minimal change disease, mesangial proliferative glomerulonephritis, focal segmental glomerulosclerosis)

Less Common
Proliferative glomerulonephritis (crescentic glomerulonephritis)
Membranoproliferative glomerulonephritis
Collagen vascular disease
Amyloidosis

An extensive list of potential causes of nephrotic syndrome can be found in Glassock RJ, Adler SG, Ward HJ, Cohen AH. Primary glomerular disease. In: Brenner BM, Rector FC, eds. The kidney. 4th ed. Philadelphia: WB Saunders, 1991;1213.

patients less than 70 years of age be screened annually for the presence of microalbuminuria. Although semi-quantitative dipstick assays exist for the detection of microalbuminuria, quantitative assays performed by a laboratory are still preferred. Microalbuminuria is defined by excretion of 30 to 300 mg albumin in a timed 24-hour urine collection or an albumin/creatinine ratio greater than or equal to 30 mg/g in a spot urine sample. An abnormal result should be rechecked 2 or 3 times over several months. If microalbuminuria is found repeatedly and subsequently does not improve with tighter glycemic control, ACE inhibitor therapy should be considered. Stabilization or up to a 30 to 50% fall of urinary albumin excretion over the ensuing 3 to 6 months would indicate response to this intervention. Patients should be monitored for a rise in serum creatinine or the development of hyperkalemia during the first few weeks after initiation of ACE inhibitor therapy.

NEPHROTIC PROTEINURIA

When a 24-hour protein quantitation reveals more than 3.5 g of protein or when the protein/creatinine ratio is greater than 3.5, nephrotic range proteinuria is established by definition and is indicative of glomerular disease. Once nephrotic range proteinuria has been identified, consultation with a nephrologist is appropriate to help decide the extent of the workup, as well as to provide suggestions for treatment (4). There are many causes of nephrotic syndrome, but few conditions are seen with significant frequency in a general medical practice (Table 44.3). Clinical and laboratory assessments for systemic illness should be performed first in an effort to establish the etiology of the nephrotic syndrome (e.g., detection of Bence Jones proteinuria or collagen vascular screens for SLE). Table 44.2 lists some of the laboratory evaluations that may be helpful in determining the cause of renal disease. When nephrotic range proteinuria develops in a patient who has been diabetic for more than 10 years, the renal lesion is almost always diabetic glomerulosclerosis, particularly if the patient also has diabetic microaneurysms in the retina. In this setting, a renal biopsy is usually unnecessary. On the other hand, a biopsy usually is necessary to diagnose a specific primary renal disease if a diagnosis cannot be made by other tests (e.g., detection of Bence Jones proteinuria or rectal biopsy for amyloid), or it may be needed to guide therapy or to help determine prognosis (e.g., SLE).

Renal Biopsy

Patient Experience. Renal biopsy requires hospitalization for 24 to 48 hours. Generally, in patients without renal failure and normal hemostasis, percutaneous biopsy is performed under local anesthesia with fluoroscopic or sonographic guidance. This technique permits the nephrologist to sample the lower portion of the kidney, thus avoiding the hilar vessels and the renal collecting system. With percutaneous biopsy the patient usually experiences minimal discomfort and is able to be out of bed in 12 hours.

The biopsy core is approximately 1 mm in diameter and approximately 10 to 20 mm in length. Usually two such tissue cores are obtained. The risk associated with percutaneous renal biopsy is small if it is performed by an experienced physician.

Microscopic hematuria is almost inevitable, and usually there is a small hematoma at the biopsy site on the surface of the kidney. However, it is usually of no clinical consequence. Gross hematuria occurs in 5 to 10% of patients, but less than 5% of this group require a transfusion to replace blood loss. Fewer than 1 in 1000 patients require nephrectomy because of continued massive bleeding, and death from biopsy is rare. A renal arteriovenous fistula may develop after biopsy, but it usually closes spontaneously. Rarely this complication may require treatment if bleeding continues or if hypertension develops (6). Even more rarely, there may be perforation of another viscus.

When percutaneous biopsy is not feasible (e.g., because of obesity, an ectopic location, or small size of the kidney), open or laparoscopic biopsy can be obtained; some surgeons perform this procedure under local anesthesia in selected patients.

Regardless of the technique of obtaining the biopsy, the evaluation of tissue by a pathologist experienced in preparation and interpretation of renal biopsy material includes light, immunofluorescent, and electron microscopy.

The physician who has referred to a nephrologist a patient in whom a renal biopsy has been performed should expect communication of the following: the probable diagnosis, based on all aspects of the microscopic assessment; whether specific therapy for the condition is indicated; and what prognostic judgment can be made.

TREATMENT OF PATIENTS WITH PROTEINURIA

Nonnephrotic proteinuria requires no special treatment in itself. Patient care is directed at diagnosis, education, surveillance, and treatment of any underlying disease. However, if the proteinuria is believed to be caused by a drug, it should be discontinued. Proteinuria from drugs may take several months to resolve, but occasionally it is permanent.

Some patients with nephrotic range proteinuria are asymptomatic and require no therapy unless the results of the renal biopsy dictate that treatment be given. When either edema or hypoalbuminemia is present, special therapy may be indicated. In the absence of renal failure, albumin synthesis is either increased or normal in patients with the nephrotic syndrome. Until recently, treatment included provision of a high-protein diet (2 to 3 g of protein per kilogram of dry weight, that is, estimated or actual weight before edema developed). Currently, mild to moderate protein restriction rather than protein supplementation is advised. In addition, judicious use of ACE inhibitors and nonsteroidal anti-inflammatory agents (there should be surveillance for hyperkalemia and acute renal failure) has been associated with a decrease in proteinuria and perhaps stabilization of renal function and improvement of protein and lipid metabolism (12). Appropriate standards for protein intake and pharmacologic intervention in this setting remain controversial and are a subject of intense research.

In the presence of edema, salt restriction to a tolerable level such as a no-added-salt diet (approximately 2 to 3 g of Na; see Chapter 62, Table 62.12) is appropriate. If the edema is more severe and unresponsive to sodium chloride restriction, cautious use of a loop diuretic (furosemide, torsemide, or bumetanide) may be necessary. An attempt should not be made to rid the patient entirely of edema, which could risk contraction of the circulating volume with serious consequences. Potassium-sparing diuretics (spironolactone, triamterene, or amiloride) may be added if renal failure is absent or metolazone or thiazides may be added if loop diuretics have not been entirely adequate. In many instances the patient can establish the correct diuretic dosage schedule by keeping a diary of weights and drug intake. If acceptable control is still not achieved, consultation with a nephrologist is appropriate.

Numerous extrarenal complications are associated with nephrotic syndrome. These include alterations in cellular immunity leading to increased infections, hyperlipidemia, and changes in calcium and bone metabolism. Nephrotic syndrome can be associated with a hypercoagulable state with thrombosis of the renal veins as well as of other vessels. Clues to the development of this complication include pulmonary embolism, sudden deterioration in renal function, significant increase in the level of proteinuria, or the development of hematuria. Suspicion of this complication requires hospitalization of the patient for urgent evaluation. Patients with nephrotic syndrome (especially those with membranous glomerulonephritis) should be counseled about risk factors for deep venous thrombosis, such as long periods of immobilization.

Prediction of the course and selection of specific therapy in patients with nephrotic range proteinuria depend on the pathologic pattern that is identified in the biopsy. Patients with nephrotic range proteinuria need regularly scheduled office visits at 1- to 4-month intervals. Usually this follow-up is done by the primary physician and the patient sees the nephrologist only once a year. The office visit provides an opportunity to review the patient's symptoms and to perform a limited physical examination (which, at a minimum, should include weight, volume assessment, and blood pressure) as well as to evaluate the 24-hour urine protein excretion, or a protein/creatinine ratio, the renal function (creatinine or creatinine clearance), and the serum electrolytes if diuretics are being used. Less often, an assessment of the serum albumin may be necessary.

General References*

Bennett PH, Haffner S, Kasiske BL, et al. Screening and management of microalbuminuria in patients with diabetes mellitus: recommendations to the Scientific Advisory Board of the National Kidney Foundation from an ad hoc committee of the Council on Diabetes Mellitus of the National Kidney Foundation. Am J Kid Dis 25:107, 1995.
> Consensus statement enumerating evidence-based clinical practice guidelines for evaluation and management of proteinuria.

Glassock RJ. Focus on proteinuria. Am J Nephrol 10(Suppl 1):88, 1990.
> Review of the pharmacologic basis for intervention of proteinuria.

Lafayette RA, Perrone RD, Levey AS. Laboratory evaluation of renal function. In: Schrier RW, Gottschalk CW, eds. Diseases of the kidney. 6th ed. Boston: Little, Brown, 1997.
> Excellent summary of the physiologic basis and evaluation of proteinuria.

Specific References

1. Ginsberg JM, Chang BS, Matarese RA, Garella S. Use of single voided urine samples to estimate quantitative proteinuria. N Engl J Med 309:1543, 1983.
2. Kannel WB, Stampfer MJ, Castelli WP, Verter J. The prognostic significance of the proteinuria: Framingham study. Am Heart J 108:1347, 1984.
3. Kasiske BL, Kalil RSN, Ma JZ, et al. Effect of antihypertensive therapy on the kidney in patients with diabetes: a meta-regression analysis. Ann Intern Med 118:129, 1993.
4. Kassirer JP. Is renal biopsy necessary for optimal management of the idiopathic nephrotic syndrome? Kidney Int 24:561, 1983.
5. King SE: Diastolic hypertension and chronic proteinuria. Am J Cardiol 9:669, 1962.
6. Leiter E, Gribetz D, Cohen S. Arteriovenous fistula after percutaneous needle biopsy: surgical repair with preservation of renal function. N Engl J Med 287:971, 1972.
7. Levitt JI. The prognostic significance of proteinuria in young college students. Ann Intern Med 66:685, 1967.
8. Lewis EJ, Hunsicker LG, Bain RP, et al. The effect of angiotensin-converting enzyme inhibition on diabetic nephropathy. N Engl J Med 329:1456, 1993.
9. Mathiesen ER, Hommel E, Parving HH. Efficacy of captopril in postponing nephropathy in normotensive insulin dependent diabetic patients with microalbuminuria. BMJ 303:81, 1991.
10. Muth RG. Asymptomatic mild intermittent proteinuria. A percutaneous renal biopsy study. Arch Intern Med 115:569, 1965.
11. Nelson RG, Knowler WC, Pettitt DJ, et al. Assessment of risk of overt nephropathy in diabetic patients from albumin excretion in untimed urine samples. Arch Intern Med 151:1761, 1991.
12. Praga M, Hernandez E, Montoyo C, et al. Long-term beneficial effects of angiotensin-converting enzyme inhibition in patients with nephrotic proteinuria. Am J Kidney Dis 20:240, 1992.
13. Robinson RR. Isolated proteinuria in asymptomatic patients. Kidney Int 18:395, 1980.
14. Rytand DA, Spreiter S. Prognosis in postural (orthostatic)

---

*Bold print (general references) and bold numerals (specific references) denote published controlled clinical trials, meta-analyses, or consensus-based recommendations.

proteinuria. Forty- to fifty-year follow-up of six patients after diagnosis by Thomas Addis. N Engl J Med 305:618, 1981.

15. Springberg PD, Garrett LE, Thompson AL Jr, et al. Fixed reproducible orthostatic proteinuria: results of a 20-year follow-up study. Ann Intern Med 97:516, 1982.

16. Woolhandler S, Pels RJ, Bor DH, et al. Dipstick urinalysis screening of asymptomatic adults for urinary tract disorders. I. Hematuria and proteinuria. JAMA 262:1215, 1989.

C H A P T E R   45

Hematuria

DAVID A. SPECTOR, MD

Normal individuals excrete up to 2 million red blood cells (RBCs) into the urine daily. This rate extrapolates to one to three RBCs per high-power microscopic field (HPF) using standard urinalysis techniques. The finding of greater numbers of RBCs/HPF constitutes abnormal hematuria, although the exact level separating normal from abnormal is arbitrary. Benzidine- or orthotolidine-impregnated, hemoglobin-sensitive dipsticks, widely used as screening tests for hemoglobinuria (usually caused by lysis of RBCs in the urine and therefore an indication of hematuria), are less sensitive than microscopy but are usually positive in urine containing more than three RBCs/HPF. The rate at which RBCs lyse depends on the concentration of the urine in which they are found and the duration of time they are exposed. Usually some lysis occurs within a few minutes, especially when the urine is dilute. There are certain limits to the use of hemoglobin-sensitive dipsticks (Table 45.1).

Microscopic hematuria may or may not indicate serious genitourinary tract disease (2,8,13). The symptoms, signs, and laboratory findings associated with hematuria and the clinical setting in which it occurs help considerably in predicting the seriousness of the finding. For example, gross hematuria or hematuria associated with proteinuria or pyuria is highly predictive of a significant disease. Conversely, asymptomatic microhematuria in a young adult has little predictive value.

PSEUDOHEMATURIA

A large number of substances can impart a color to urine that may be mistaken for hematuria (19). *Exogenous sources* of some of these substances are listed in Table 45.2. *Endogenous substances* capable of producing a reddish hue include porphyrins, myoglobin, and hemoglobin. Myoglobin and hemoglobin also cause positive reactions in tests for RBCs (e.g., Labstix or Multistix). Therefore, when the urine dipstick is positive and the microscopy is negative for RBCs, myoglobinuria or hemoglobinuria should be suspected. Both are serious findings and warrant further evaluation. Myoglobinuria indicates substantial muscle disease or injury and hemoglobinuria indicates significant hematuria (with lysis of RBCs) or hemolysis. However, the dipstick reaction may not detect hemoglobin (or RBCs) or myoglobin when these substances are present if there is heavy hypochlorite (bleach, chlorine) or peroxidase (from bacteria) contamination of the urine specimen or its container. A false-negative dipstick test may also occur when formaldehyde (e.g., present as a breakdown product of Mandelamine) or large amounts of vitamin C are in the urine because both substances decrease the sensitivity of the test reagent.

INNOCENT HEMATURIA

Microscopic hematuria is often identified after a genitourinary tract examination such as a pelvic or prostate examination, cystoscopy or bladder catheterization, or biopsy of prostate, bladder, or kidney. Occasionally, gross hematuria may be seen in this setting. Gross or microscopic hematuria is also sometimes present after vigorous exercise such as swimming, lacrosse, boxing, football, or running. This finding is most common in long-distance runners, and in one study, 18% of athletes were found to have hematuria after the completion of a marathon (17). Hematuria in all such settings subsides in 24 to 48 hours. It does not signify underlying genitourinary disease when it resolves quickly and does not recur spontaneously. In exercisers (especially runners), proteinuria or cast formation sometimes accompanies the hematuria, and the red cells have been found to be dysmorphic, suggesting that the bleeding site is the glomerulus.

HEMATURIA WITH PYURIA

If a patient is found to have hematuria associated with pyuria (with or without irritative symptoms such as frequency, urgency, or dysuria), an infectious cause is most likely and bacterial cultures should be obtained. If a specific organism is identified, appropriate antimicrobial therapy should be given (see Chapter 27). After treatment, the patient should be followed care-

Table 45.1. Limits of Dipstick Method for Detection of Blood in the Urine

Reasons for a Positive Test
Hematuria greater than approximately 5–10 RBCs/HPF
Hematuria with lysis of RBCs
    From hypotonic urine (specific gravity <1.008)
    From highly alkaline urine (pH >6.5)
Hemoglobinuria from intravascular hemolysis
Myoglobinuria from muscle injury
False-positive reactions
    From hypochlorite (bleach) contamination of container
    From peroxidase (from heavy growth of bacteria)

Reasons for a False-Negative Test
Vitamin C: Ingestion of large amounts of vitamin C (>200 mg/day) results in diminished oxidation potential of the test material. The dipstick test may miss trace quantities of blood, although usually there is a quantitative decrease in the estimate of blood (such as 3+ to 2+). (This is of concern only if RBCs are observed but the dipstick test is negative.)
Formaldehyde: Ingestion of bacterial suppressant agents (such as Mandelamine or Hiprex) that produce formaldehyde in acid urine or contamination of the container with formaldehyde diminish the oxidizing potential of the reagent strips. This results in a quantitative estimate error or, if hematuria is minimal, false-negative results.

fully (including the performance of a urinalysis) for 4 to 6 weeks to ensure that the hematuria has been eradicated and does not recur. If irritative symptoms suggesting infection have been present and the routine culture is sterile, a *sexually transmitted disease* (especially *Chlamydia* infection or gonorrhea), a viral infection, or tuberculosis (now a rare cause of hematuria) should be suspected. *Chlamydia trachomatis infection* (see Chapters 27 and 94), especially, may be manifested by hematuria and pyuria with minimal irritative symptoms. When a sexually transmitted infection is suspected but cannot be proved, a therapeutic trial of an antimicrobial drug may be given (see Chapters 27 and 94). *Viral cystitis* is a fairly common infection of young women. It has a short-lived (2 to 3 days) natural course, and it is nonrecurrent. Suspicion of *tuberculosis of the urinary tract* requires several weeks to confirm by culture (an acid-fast stain of the urine is not a reliable indicator because of the regular presence of acid-fast material from smegma bacilli). Because noninfectious disorders of the bladder (including malignancies) may also present with irritative symptoms (see Chapter 49), one should ensure that those symptoms, especially in patients over age 50, have abated and it is probably prudent to see that the patient's urinalysis is normal on two or three occasions in the following 4 to 6 weeks.

HEMATURIA WITH PROTEINURIA, RED BLOOD CELLS CASTS, OR DYSMORPHIC RED BLOOD CELLS

Hematuria associated with proteinuria reflects either glomerulonephritis or interstitial nephritis. When proteinuria is greater than 3.5 g/24 hours (i.e., nephrotic range) or red cell casts are present, the diagnosis is probably glomerulonephritis (see Chapter 44). The

morphologic appearance on microscopy of the RBCs may help differentiate glomerular from nonglomerular bleeding (4). This observation takes advantage of the deformation of the cytoplasmic content of RBCs after their passage into Bowman space. If more than 80% of at least 100 (counted) red cells appear dysmorphic (abnormal size, shape, and cytoplasmic staining) using Wright's stain (or phase contrast microscopy, if available) of urinary sediment, glomerular bleeding is very likely. In particular, acanthocytes (ringform RBCs with vesicle-shaped protrusions), when present, almost always indicate glomerular disease (10). If glomerulonephritis is suspected, estimation of glomerular filtration rate and quantitative 24-hour urine protein is indicated. Also, a thorough evaluation for a possible cause should be conducted. Chapter 44 (Table 44.2) suggests an approach. Although any form of glomerulonephritis may be present, IgA nephropathy (Berger's disease) (7) and Alport's syndrome (hereditary nephritis, often associated with deafness) are especially likely in situations in which the hematuria has been an incidental finding. Both of these diseases are characterized by recurrent episodes of hematuria (microscopic or gross), fluctuating proteinuria, and a variable course. A nephrologist should be consulted when these or other forms of glomerulonephritis are suspected. Often the nephrologist will perform a renal biopsy (see Chapter 44) to establish the diagnosis, estimate the prognosis, and determine treatment.

ASYMPTOMATIC ISOLATED MICROHEMATURIA

The prevalence of isolated microscopic hematuria is high. In one study, 13% of adult men and postmenopausal women were found to have asymptomatic hematuria (14). On the other hand, studies that have used more stringent definitions of hematuria in a variety of populations demonstrate a 2 to 5% prevalence of microscopic hematuria (Table 45.3).

Table 45.2. Exogenous Substances that May Cause Pseudohematuria[a]

Medications

Analgesics	Phenacetin, phenazopyridine (e.g., Pyridium)
Antimicrobials	Nitrofurantoin, rifampin, sulfonamides
Antimalarials	Chloroquine, primaquine
Laxatives	Anthraquinones: cascara, senna, danthron (e.g., Modane or Dorbane)
Anticancer agents	Doxorubicin, daunorubicin
Others	Deferoxamine (an iron-chelating agent), levodopa, phenothiazines, methyldopa (rare)

Vegetable Dyes
Anthocyanins: beets, blackberries
Paprika
Rhubarb
Fuscin (a reddish dye used in topical agents)

Others

Antiseptics	Mercurochrome, phenols, cresols, povidone-iodine (Betadine)

Urate crystals (in acid urine)

[a]Some of these agents cause hemoglobinuria.

Table 45.3.   Distribution (%) of Selected Urologic Findings in Asymptomatic Patients with Microhematuria

	Ref. 11 (HMO Urology Referrals)	Ref. 9 (246 pts., Urology Referral)	Ref. 8 (636 Young Israeli Men[a])	Ref. 14 (781 pts., Rochester MN Population[a])	Ref. 2 (177 Women, Urology Referral)	Ref. 12 (192 Men >50 Yr Screened for Hematuria)
Neoplasia	8.5	9.3	0.2	1.0	0	8.3
Other Disorders						
Renal calculi	3.4	0	0.6	3.3	1.6	8.9
Ureteral calculi	0.6	1.0	0	0.9	0.6	
Nephritis/renal insufficiency	1.2	2.0	0.1	14.4	0	1.0
Benign prostatic hypertrophy	16.5	8.0	0	37.7	—	47.4
Urinary tract infection	4.3	2.0	0	0.5	b	2.6
Urethrotrigonitis/ prostatitis	37.7	18.0	0.1	1.8	32.6	—
Any Finding[c]	88.3	47.6	d	62.5	63.0	84.9

[a]Complete urologic workup not performed on all patients.

[b]Women with urinary tract infection excluded from study.

[c]Includes those listed above in addition to other findings that may or may not have been related to the hematuria. These include hydronephrosis, renal cysts, polycystic kidney disease, vesicoureteral reflux, interstitial and radiation cystitis, diverticula, ureteropelvic junction obstruction, ureterocele, cystocele, neurogenic bladder, atrophic vagina, scarred kidney, cystitis cystica, polyps, papillary necrosis, calcified renal mass, and trabeculated bladder. Some patients in all series had more than one disorder.

[d]Unable to determine from data.

Causes of Asymptomatic Hematuria

In all series, no specific diagnosis was made for many patients, in part because patient evaluations were usually incomplete. For example, most series did not include a renal biopsy, which may have revealed glomerular or interstitial disease (5,18). The importance of this omission is borne out by one study in which 51 of 65 adult patients with hematuria with minimal or no proteinuria and with a negative urologic workup had a specific diagnosis established only after the performance of a renal biopsy (5).

In addition, most series did not include quantitation of 24-hour urine calcium and uric acid. Hypercalciuria (more than 300 mg/24 hours) or hyperuricosuria (more than 750 mg/24 hours in women; more than 800 mg/24 hours in men) has been shown to be a cause of hematuria (presumably as a result of irritation of the tubules by microcrystals), and it has been shown that thiazide therapy (which reduces calciuria) or allopurinol stops the bleeding (1).

In general, neoplasia is more common in series derived from an older population of patients referred to urologists, and it is rare in series of nonreferred young individuals. Conversely, unsuspected renal biopsy findings are often found in younger patients, although in one study, 40% of renal biopsies were abnormal even in patients in their seventh decade (18). As in patients with combined hematuria and proteinuria, the most likely biopsy findings in patients with asymptomatic hematuria are IgA nephritis, followed by Alport's disease and thin basement membrane disease (18).

EVALUATION OF PATIENTS WITH HEMATURIA

Pseudohematuria and drug-induced hematuria (Table 45.4) should be ruled out. The evaluation then depends on associated symptoms, on whether the bleeding is gross or microscopic, and on the results of the complete urinalysis (see above). Localization of the site of the bleeding in the genitourinary tract is the first priority. The associated symptoms and the history of temporal events often provide a diagnostic clue. For example, colicky flank pain suggests that the hematuria is emanating from the ureter, whereas dysuria and frequency suggest that the bleeding is from the bladder. All patients should be asked about the temporal relationship of the hematuria to exercise and to ingestion of medications or food. The urinalysis is helpful also if findings suggest glomerular disease or infection (see above). In some studies, the seriousness of the underlying lesion is proportional to the number of RBCs/HPF, with patients with gross hematuria especially at risk of serious or life-threatening illness (11).

A history and physical examination should be performed to evaluate the patient for clues to illnesses with which hematuria is associated (e.g., a nodular prostate suggestive of prostate cancer or cutaneous or other abnormalities suggestive of a collagen vascular disease). When the history and physical examination plus selected laboratory tests (e.g., urine culture) and treatment (e.g., antimicrobial agents) do not support a working diagnosis, certain laboratory data should be obtained. This evaluation should include a complete blood count, an estimate of glomerular function (e.g., serum creatinine), a sickle cell preparation (if the patient is African American), a 24-hour urine specimen for determination of the concentration of calcium and uric acid (see above), and an intravenous pyelogram with tomography (if the creatinine concentration is not significantly elevated and the patient has no history of dye allergy). In patients suspected of having a bleeding disorder, a platelet count and the measurement of the

Table 45.4.   Examples of Drugs Causing Hematuria

Antimicrobials
Penicillin analogs[a]
Cephalosporin analogs[a]
Sulfa analogs[a]
Polymycin[a]
Rifampin[a]

Analgesics and Anti-Inflammatory Agents
Aspirin[b]
Phenacetin[b]
Aminosalicylic acid[b]
Nonsteroidal anti-inflammatory agents[a]

Diuretics
Furosemide[a]
Ethacrynic acid[a]
Thiazides[a]

Anticoagulants
Warfarin (Coumadin)[c]

Other
Cyclophosphamide[d]
    Ifosfamide (Isex, an antineoplastic agent)[d]
    Danazol[d]

[a]Infrequent bleeding caused by interstitial nephritis, usually occurring within days to weeks of taking drugs; usually reversible.

[b]Infrequent bleeding caused by medullary/papillary necrosis, usually following many months or years of combination analgesic preparations; partially reversible.

[c]An underlying cause of hematuria is often found and a workup should be considered (6).

[d]Bleeding caused by hemorrhagic cystitis in 10–20% of patients; dose-related and usually reversible.

prothrombin, partial thromboplastin, and bleeding times should be done. If an underlying bleeding diathesis is identified, the search for a pathologic process in the genitourinary tract should continue because one is usually identified (see Chapter 51). In older patients (more than 40 to 50 years old), two or three fresh morning urine specimens should be evaluated by a cytology laboratory for the presence of tumor cells. The sensitivity of cytology in this setting is 30% when an upper tract tumor is present and 50 to 90% when a bladder tumor is present. (The higher rates of detection are in situations in which a higher grade of cancer is present.)

When neoplasia is a consideration (patients over 40 to 50 years of age or those who are younger but have a risk factor for bladder cancer [see below]), a urologist should be consulted and the patient should undergo cystoscopy (see Chapter 49) (3). Risk factors for bladder cancer include a heavy occupational exposure (e.g., to aromatic amines, dyes, benzidine, and paint ingredients [see Chapter 7]), prolonged daily use of analgesics (phenacetin, acetaminophen, and aspirin combinations have been reported to be associated with genitourinary cancer), or heavy smoking. When neoplasia is a strong consideration, the urologist might also suggest the evaluation of the patient by computerized tomographic (CT) scanning, magnetic resonance imaging, or renal angiography.

When neoplasia is not strongly considered and persistent hematuria is present or recurrent, the patient should be referred to a nephrologist for consideration of the performance of a renal biopsy (see Chapter 44).

When no etiologic basis for microscopic hematuria is initially found, follow-up evaluations should be performed. Although in some patients microhematuria is transient and benign, in other patients with persistent hematuria, genitourinary neoplasms or calculi are discovered 1 to 3 years after the onset of hematuria (15,16).

Gross Hematuria

When gross hematuria is present, the evaluation should initially proceed in the same manner as in the patient with microscopic hematuria, but there are several caveats. Blood clots in the urine suggest that bleeding is from the bladder. However, clots may occasionally result from upper tract bleeding, and in

Table 45.5.   Diagnosis Established in 1000 Cases of Gross Hematuria

Diagnosis	% Patients	
Kidney	**15.2**	
Tumor		3.5
Pyelonephritis		3.0
Calculus		2.7
Trauma		2.0
Hydronephrosis		1.5
Polycystic disease		0.6
Chronic glomerulonephritis		0.6
Other		1.3
Ureter	**6.5**	
Calculus		5.3
Tumor		0.7
Other		0.5
Bladder	**39.5**	
Cystitis		22.0
Tumor		14.9
Calculus		1.2
Other		1.4
Prostate	**23.6**	
Benign hyperplasia		12.5
Chronic prostatitis		9.0
Carcinoma		2.1
Urethra	**4.3**	
Stricture		1.7
Calculus		1.3
Gonorrhea		0.4
Tumor		0.3
Other		0.6
Other Causes	**2.4**	
Urinary tuberculosis		0.7
Other infections		1.2
Hemophilia		0.2
Uremic syndrome		0.1
Thrombocytopenia		0.1
Dicumarol poisoning		0.1
"Essential" Hematuria	**8.5**	
Total	**100.0**	

Adapted from Lee LW, Davis E. Gross urinary hemorrhage: a symptom, not a disease. JAMA 153:782, 1953. This study remains among the largest published series to date.

that situation ureteral colic is likely to occur. Another caution is important when gross hematuria develops: Plasma protein may be lost into the urine (and detected by qualitative or quantitative testing) in large quantities, yet not reflect a glomerular disease. However, the concentration of urinary protein rarely exceeds a daily excretion of 1 g when it occurs from gross bleeding. The *three-glass test* is sometimes useful in determining the site of gross bleeding. This test is performed by having the patient void into containers in a sequence: The initial 10 mL of urine represents the urethral specimen, the *middle portion* of urine voided is nondiagnostic of a specific location, and blood in the *terminal portion* (the last few drops of urine) suggests that the site is likely to be the prostate, bladder neck, or proximal urethra. Blood present in all three specimens is not specific for the site of origin.

In patients with persistent gross hematuria, a urologist should always be consulted promptly, as the most opportune time to identify the site is when the bleeding is active.

The surveillance of a patient found to have gross hematuria depends on the cause (Table 45.5). If no cause is found, close surveillance (every 6 months for several years) is indicated because some of these patients have a serious underlying disorder, such as a tumor or glomerulonephritis. This surveillance should include reviewing the history, performing a physical examination, obtaining a urinalysis and determining the urea nitrogen and creatinine concentrations, and in situations in which a tumor is considered, obtaining a urine specimen for cytologic examination and referring the patient to a urologist for a cystoscopic examination.

HEMATOSPERMIA

The presence of blood in the ejaculate of men is an alarming but usually innocuous symptom. This problem occurs most often in men over 40, and most often the episodes recur over several weeks or months. When it occurs in an otherwise asymptomatic man who has a normal physical examination (including rectal examination of the prostate and seminal vesicles) and a normal urinalysis, the patient should be reassured that it is innocuous and that no further workup is necessary. If there is any abnormality, further evaluation for benign prostatic hypertrophy or cancer of the prostate, seminal vesicles, bladder, or urethra should be considered and a urologist should be consulted.

General References

Abarbonel J, Benet AE, Lask D, Kimche D. Sports hematuria. J Urol, 143:887, 1990.

Fogazzi GB, Ponticelli C. Microscopic hematuria diagnosis and management. Nephron 72:125, 1996.

Leary FJ, Aguilo JJ. Clinical significance of hematospermia. Mayo Clin Proc 49:815, 1974.

Sutton JM. Evaluation of hematuria in adults. JAMA 263:2475, 1990.

Specific References

1. Andres A, Praga M, Bello I, et al. Hematuria due to hypercalciuria and hyperuricosuria in adult patients. Kidney Int 36:96, 1989.
2. Bard RH. The significance of asymptomatic microhematuria in women and its economic implications. Arch Intern Med 148:2629, 1988.
3. Carter WC III, Rous SN. Gross hematuria in 110 adult urologic hospital patients. Urology 18:342, 1981.
4. Chang BS. Red cell morphology as a diagnostic aid in hematuria. JAMA 252:1747, 1984.
5. Copley JB, Hasbargen JA. Idiopathic hematuria. A prospective evaluation. Arch Intern Med 147:434, 1987.
6. Cuttino JT Jr, Clark RL, Feaster SH, Zwicke DL. The evaluation of gross hematuria in anticoagulated patients: efficacy of IV urography and cystoscopy. AJR Am J Roentgenol 149:527, 1987.
7. D'Amico G. Clinical features and natural history in adults with IgA nephropathy. Am J Kidney Dis 12:353, 1988.
8. Froom P, Ribak J, Benbassat J. Significance of microhematuria in young adults. BMJ 288:20, 1984.
9. Golin AL, Howard RS. Asymptomatic microscopic hematuria. J Urol 124:389, 1980.
10. Köhler H, Wandel E, Brunck B. Acanthocyturia: a characteristic marker for glomerular bleeding. Kidney Int 40:115, 1991.
11. Mariani AJ, Mariani MC, Macchioni C, et al. The significance of adult hematuria: 1000 hematuria evaluations including a risk–benefit and cost-effectiveness analysis. J Urol 141:350, 1989.
12. Messing EM, Young TB, Hunt VB, et al. Home screening for hematuria: results of a multi-clinic study. J Urol 148:289, 1992.
13. Mohr DN, Offord KP, Melton LJ III. Isolated asymptomatic microhematuria. J Gen Intern Med 2:318, 1987.
14. Mohr DN, Offord KP, Owen RA, Melton J III. Asymptomatic microhematuria and urologic disease. A population-based study. JAMA 256:224, 1986.
15. Murakami S, Igarashi T, Hara S, et al. Strategies for asymptomatic microscopic hematuria: a prospective study of 1,034 patients. J Urol 144:99, 1990.
16. Nieuwhof C, Doorenbos C, Grave W, et al. A prospective study of the natural history of idiopathic non-proteinuric hematuria. Kidney Int 49:222, 1996.
17. Siegel AJ, Hennikens CH, Solomon HS, Von Boeckel B. Exercise-related hematuria. Findings in a group of marathon runners. JAMA 241:391, 1987.
18. Topham PS, Harper SJ, Furness PN, et al. Glomerular disease as a cause of isolated microscopic haematuria. QJM 87:329, 1994.
19. Young DS, Pestoner LC, Gibberman V. Effects of drugs on clinical laboratory tests. Clin Chem 21:1D, 1975.

C H A P T E R   46

Hypokalemia

KEVIN A. ROSSITER, MD

Hypokalemia, serum potassium concentration less than 3.5 mEq/L, is uncommon and occurs in less than 1% of the population of normal, healthy people. However, hypokalemia is common in ambulatory practice, and often reflects the presence of disease or the consequence of drug therapy in that setting. Although the occurrence of hypokalemia is sometimes ignored and the consequences are often thought to be trivial, the role of hypokalemia in medical disorders, including hypertension and cardiovascular and cerebrovascular disease, is important. Hypokalemia may also be life threatening, especially when severe, but may also predispose to death even when mild. Loss of potassium through the gastrointestinal tract or the kidneys accounts for most cases of hypokalemia seen in ambulatory practice, with less common causes occasionally encountered. The physiology of potassium homeostasis, the clinical consequences of potassium depletion, an approach to the differential diagnosis, and the management of hypokalemia are reviewed.

PHYSIOLOGIC BACKGROUND

The serum potassium concentration depends on the total body potassium content and the distribution of potassium between the intracellular and extracellular spaces (32). Total body potassium, normally about 50 mEq/kg, is determined by the external balance between the intake and excretion of potassium. In health, excretion matches intake and total body potassium remains

essentially constant (Fig. 46.1). The internal balance or distribution of potassium between the intracellular and extracellular spaces may vary even in the absence of changes in the external balance of potassium (32).

External Potassium Balance

The average intake of potassium is approximately 1 mEq/kg per day or 60 to 100 mEq/day (36). Normally, about 90% is absorbed and excreted in the urine, with the remainder being eliminated in the stool (Fig. 46.1). However, the gastrointestinal tract losses can increase substantially. In diarrheal states, large amounts of potassium may be lost acutely in the stool. With progressive chronic renal failure, on the other hand, the amount of potassium eliminated by the colon increases substantially through adaptation to preserve normal serum potassium until very severe renal failure is encountered. Only trivial amounts of potassium are lost through the skin (less than 5 mEq/day) unless sweating becomes profuse.

That hypokalemia is so uncommon in normal healthy adults is testimony to the abundance of potassium in the diet of most people and the body's ability to conserve potassium when the potassium is limited. By adjusting the rate of urinary potassium excretion in proportion to intake, the kidney acts as the major regulator of potassium balance. Because potassium is freely filtered by the glomerulus and is nearly completely reabsorbed in the proximal parts of the nephron, urinary potassium excretion is largely a function of distal tubular secretion. Factors affecting the rate of potassium secretion (and excretion) include (Fig. 46.2) the serum potassium concentration, the luminal flow rate, distal sodium and chloride delivery, the plasma aldosterone concentration, distal transepithelial voltage, acid–base balance, antidiuretic hormone concentration, and dietary potassium intake (9). Any factor that increases the urinary flow rate, distal sodium delivery, or aldosterone secretion; decreases distal chloride delivery; or causes metabolic alkalosis will stimulate potassium secretion and predispose to the development of potassium depletion. Urinary potassium excretion can be reduced dramatically to a minimum of 5 to 25 mEq/day. Although dietary deficiency of potassium may facilitate other causes of hypokalemia (e.g., diuretic induced), hypokalemia caused by diet alone is rare in otherwise normal patients unless intake is severely limited for prolonged periods. Therefore, when hypokalemia is encountered, there is almost always some significant factor or disease that must be investigated.

Internal Potassium Balance

Nearly all of the body potassium is located intracellularly, with only the smallest portion in the extracellular space. This distribution is maintained by membrane-bound Na-K-ATPase preserving a ratio of intracellular to extracellular potassium concentration of approximately 30:1 (32). Indeed, less than 2% of total body potassium (50 to 60 mEq) resides in the

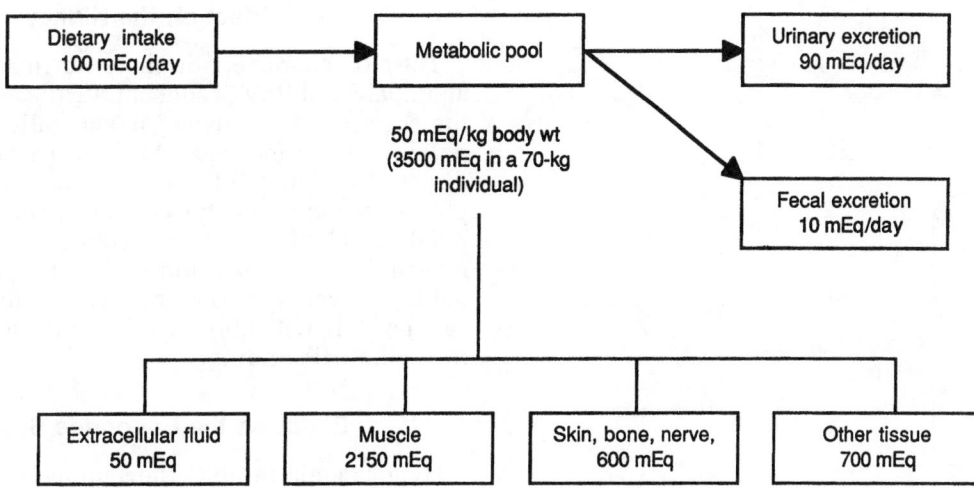

Figure 46.1. Balance of potassium. (Adapted from Kliger AS, Hayslett JP. Disorders of potassium. In: Brenner BM, Stein JH, eds. Acid–base and potassium homeostasis. New York: Churchill Livingstone, 1978.)

extracellular space (Fig. 46.1). Therefore, small transcellular potassium shifts can significantly affect the serum potassium concentration, even in the absence of changes in total body potassium. Factors known to stimulate cellular potassium uptake and thereby predispose to hypokalemia include β_2-adrenergic stimulation, insulin, alkalosis, anabolism, and aldosterone.

The ebb and flow of transcellular potassium shifts are frequent. Potassium is not lost proportionally from the extracellular and intracellular spaces, so it is not surprising that the serum potassium does not always accurately reflect total body stores. The least amount of potassium is in the plasma (the smallest subset of the extracellular fluid) and it is by sampling the blood of that tiny compartment that the assessment of hypokalemia is made. Nevertheless, in the absence of major alterations in internal potassium balance, there is a roughly linear inverse relationship between the decrement in the serum potassium concentration and the magnitude of the potassium deficit. The serum potassium falls approximately 0.3 mEq/L for each 100 mEq of potassium depletion (32). This relationship is valid for deficits up to approximately 500 mEq. With larger deficits, the serum potassium falls less for every 100 mEq of potassium lost. What is impressive and misleading to the clinician is how much potassium can be lost, how large a potassium deficit there might be, and how well preserved the serum potassium often is. In fact, many clinicians dismiss small decrements in potassium as mild. However, because of the flux of potassium across the membranes, these "mild" changes often reveal major deficits.

CONSEQUENCES OF POTASSIUM DEPLETION

Hypokalemia is often detected in a set of electrolytes in an asymptomatic individual. Almost as often, the symptoms of the problems that have led to potassium depletion are prominent, such as vomiting or diarrhea. However, severe but "asymptomatic" potassium depletion may occasionally have serious consequences

(Table 46.1) (36). Many of these desperate consequences are the result of changes in cell membrane potential that affect the function of the neurovascular and cardiovascular systems.

Effect on Neurovascular and Cardiovascular Systems

Of greatest concern is the effect of hypokalemia on the *heart*. Although some claim that severe potassium depletion can cause myocardial necrosis in rare cases, changes in potassium balance can clearly affect cardiac conduction and rhythm. During hypokalemia, characteristic pathologic electrocardiographic changes may be seen (Fig. 46.3). Hypokalemia has also long been known to predispose patients to digitalis intoxication manifested by a variety of rhythm disturbances. Whether mild to moderate hypokalemia per se is a cause of dangerous ventricular ectopy is a matter of controversy (26), certainly hypokalemia is arrhythmogenic in certain patients, such as those with underlying heart disease (4).

Both *smooth and skeletal muscle function* may be altered by potassium depletion. Severe hypokalemia can cause gastrointestinal tract dysmotility, resulting in ileus. Proximal muscle weakness can progress to paralysis. The respiratory muscles may be involved, resulting in respiratory failure. Hypokalemia may also predispose to rhabdomyolysis, at least in part by interfering with exercise-induced vasodilation. On the other hand, postural hypotension and a decrease in systemic vascular resistance have been reported in potassium-depleted patients. Rarely, tetany may be seen even in the absence of changes in pH or serum calcium.

Effect on Blood Pressure

Although hypokalemia is often considered a complication of therapy for hypertension, increasing evidence implicates a stronger role for potassium in the patho-

Luminal
• Flow rate
• Na⁺conc.
• Electrical potential difference (voltage)
• Cl⁻conc.

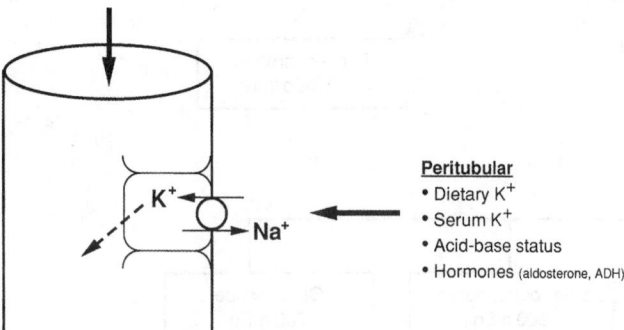

Peritubular
• Dietary K⁺
• Serum K⁺
• Acid-base status
• Hormones (aldosterone, ADH)

Figure 46.2. Factors influencing potassium secretion by the distal tubule. (Modified from Giebisch G. Physiology of potassium metabolism. In: Whelton A, Walker WG, eds. Potassium in cardiovascular and renal medicine. New York: Marcel Dekker, 1986.)

physiology and evolution of hypertension and other cardiovascular and cerebrovascular diseases. Various epidemiologic data show a relationship between hypokalemia and hypertension. Many populations throughout the world who consume a low-potassium diet have been found to have some of the highest prevalence of hypertension and cardiovascular disease (10,18). Large studies also show that a person's blood pressure is partly potassium dependent (13,21). Even when the sodium intake is low, the risk of hypertension has been found to increase as the amount of potassium consumed in the diet decreases, independent of the sodium intake (8). Potassium supplementation in some hypertensive patients is modestly hypotensive in its effect (30,34). Finally, quite separate from the effect on hypertension, potassium supplementation has been shown to reduce the risk of cerebrovascular disease and stroke (12,16).

The mechanisms for the effect of potassium supplementation or high-potassium diet on blood pressure are unclear. Nevertheless, these increasingly important observations suggest that simple strategies may have an enormous impact and offer the opportunity for a simple intervention to lower a patient's likelihood of developing hypertension (1,3,29). Studies show that supplementation of a diet with 48 to 120 mEq/day has the effect of lowering blood pressure (30,34). Increasing dietary potassium also had an effect on hypertension (5,12). Therefore, although hypokalemia is often a complication of therapy for hypertension, the implications of low dietary potassium and the need for supplemental potassium are far broader. The correction of hypokalemia by dietary means or pharmacologic supplementation enhances the treatment of hypertension with minimal risk and expense (39).

Effect on the Kidney

The most characteristic alteration in renal function is an impaired ability to concentrate the urine. However, the severity of the defect is generally mild and the polyuria sometimes seen may be caused in large part by direct stimulation of thirst. With prolonged severe potassium depletion, the glomerular filtration rate and renal blood flow may be reduced. This is usually reversible with potassium repletion. Rarely, acute renal injury can occur. Progressive chronic renal failure can develop, with chronic tubulointerstitial disease as the pathologic finding.

Effect on the Endocrine System

Hypokalemia inhibits the synthesis of aldosterone, increases plasma renin activity, and decreases insulin secretion as well as insulin action. The latter effect may worsen the patient's control of diabetes mellitus. Renal ammonia production, directly stimulated by hypokale-

Table 46.1.   Clinical Sequelae of Hypokalemia

Cardiovascular
Predisposition to digitalis intoxication
Abnormal electrocardiogram
Ventricular ectopic rhythms
Cardiac necrosis
Increased blood pressure

Neuromuscular
Gastrointestinal
  Constipation
  Ileus
Skeletal muscle
  Weakness, cramps
  Tetany
  Paralysis (including respiratory)
  Rhabdomyolysis

Renal
Decreased renal blood flow
Decreased glomerular filtration rate
Renal hypertrophy
Pathologic alterations (interstitial nephritis)
Predisposition to urinary tract infection

Fluid and Electrolyte
Polyuria and polydipsia
  Renal concentrating defect
  Stimulation of thirst center
  ADH release (?)
Increased renal ammonia production
  Predisposition to hepatic coma
  Altered urinary acidification
Renal chloride wasting
Metabolic alkalosis
Sodium retention
Hyponatremia (with or without concomitant diuretic therapy)

Endocrine
Decrease in aldosterone
Increase in renin
Altered prostaglandin metabolism
Decrease in insulin secretion (carbohydrate intolerance)

Modified from Tannen RL. Potassium disorders. In: Kokko JP, Tannen RL, eds. Fluids and electrolytes. Philadelphia: WB Saunders, 1986.

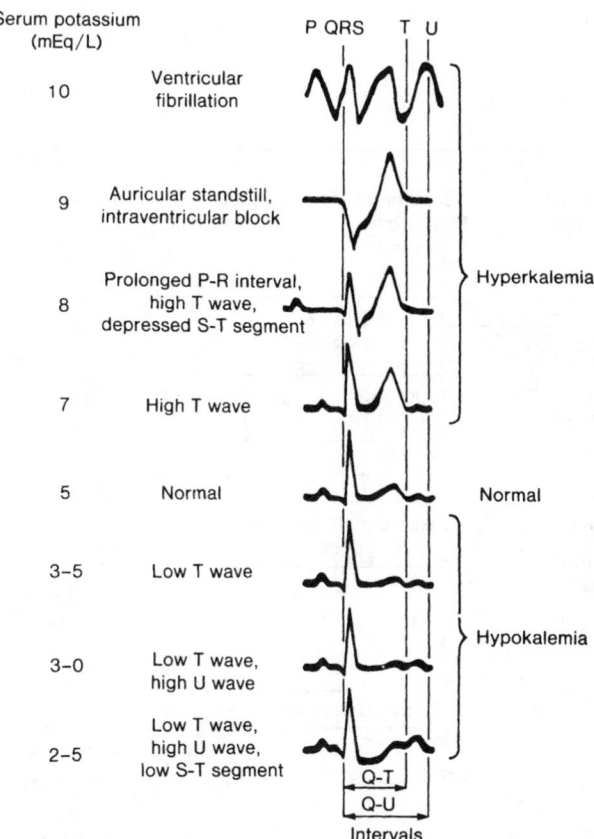

Figure 46.3. Electrocardiogram in assessment of potassium. (Adapted from Burch GE, Winsor T. A primer of electrocardiography. 6th ed. Philadelphia: Lea & Febiger, 1972;128.)

mia, may precipitate or aggravate hepatic encephalopathy in patients with severe liver failure.

DIFFERENTIAL DIAGNOSIS AND MANAGEMENT

Three fundamental mechanisms that reflect the balance of potassium homeostasis, alone or in combination, may lead to hypokalemia: transcellular shift of potassium into cells, reduced potassium intake, and excessive potassium loss.

History and Physical Examination

The history obtained from the hypokalemic patient should focus specifically on diet, medications (especially diuretics, laxatives, and β_2-adrenergic agonists), vomiting, diarrhea, urine output, hypertension, diabetes mellitus, and family history. The patient's medical records should be reviewed for previous potassium measures. If one is found, it will help date the onset of the problem and any temporally related event (e.g., β-adrenergic therapy or new-onset hypertension). This may provide a clue to the diagnosis. The physical examination should include a careful assessment of volume status, including measurement of blood pressure in the supine and upright positions and edema.

Laboratory data should always include glucose, serum blood urea nitrogen, and creatinine. At this point, the etiology of hypokalemia may be obvious, and if the patient responds to therapy as expected, further evaluation may be unnecessary.

Basic Laboratory Assessment

If the cause of hypokalemia remains unclear, the following approach is recommended (Fig. 46.4) (25). First, determine whether there is any reason to suspect an extracellular to intracellular shift of potassium. If not, the patient is most likely to be potassium depleted. In this case, the next step is to determine where the potassium was lost: Was it via a renal or extrarenal route? This often can be achieved by measuring the urinary potassium. If renal potassium excretion is high (greater than 20 mEq/L on a spot urine specimen or greater than 20 mEq in a 24-hour collection) despite hypokalemia, excessive renal potassium losses are, at least in part, responsible for potassium depletion. On the other hand, if renal potassium excretion is appropriately low, this suggests an extrarenal loss of potassium, with appropriate renal conservation. However, in many cases the simple evaluation of isolated urine potassium values is insufficient for a variety of reasons. The transtubular potassium gradient (TTKG) may be used to assist the evaluation (see "Transtubular Potassium Gradient," below).

As shown in Figure 46.4, further studies depend on whether potassium has been lost through a renal or extrarenal route. The acid–base status and blood pressure provide useful clues.

Magnesium depletion and potassium depletion often go hand in hand and magnesium depletion can cause renal potassium wasting. Hypomagnesemia is a common finding in up to 40% of hypokalemic patients. Although the mechanism is incompletely understood, enhanced aldosterone secretion is believed to play a role. Hypomagnesemia (of any cause) can cause hypokalemia as a result of fecal as well as urinary losses. Serum magnesium therefore should be measured during the evaluation of any refractory hypokalemic patient.

Transtubular Potassium Gradient

The urine potassium concentration may be misleading or simply inadequate when examined by itself because of factors other than potassium homeostasis. The urine potassium concentration may reflect neither potassium secretion nor aldosterone activity in the tubule. Rather, the potassium concentration may be influenced by the water flux in the collecting duct during the final steps of forming urine. The movement of water occurs after the major sites that affect potassium content in the urine. The concept of the TTKG (37,38) was developed to provide a noninvasive assessment and index of potassium secretory processes of the kidney.

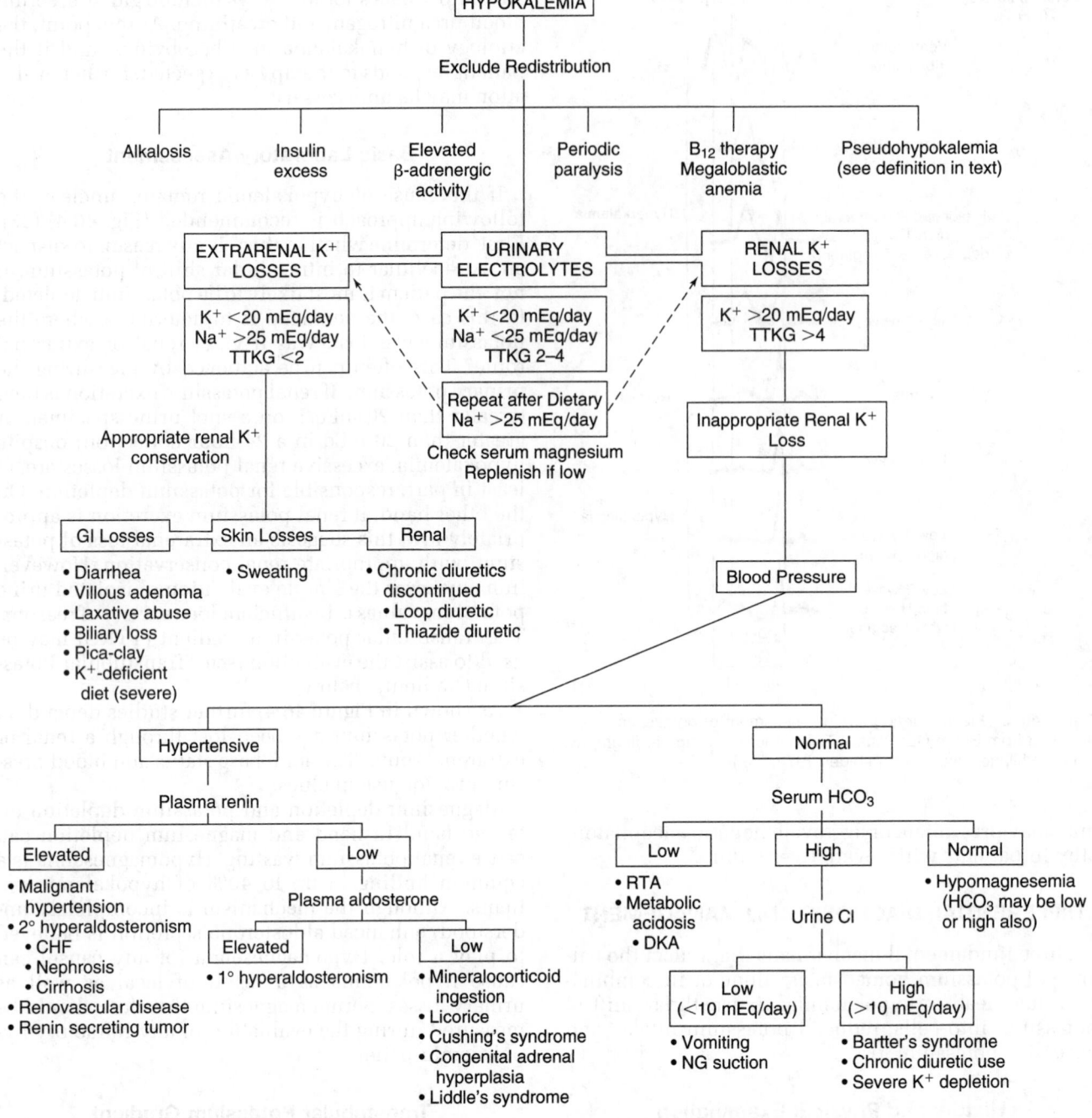

Figure 46.4. Diagnostic approach to hypokalemia. (Modified from Narins RG, Jones ER, Stom MC, et al. Diagnostic strategies in disorders of fluid, electrolyte and acid–base homeostasis. Am J Med 72:496, 1982.)

The TTKG is calculated as follows:

$$TTKG = [K]_{urine}/[K]_{plasma} \div U_{osm}/P_{osm} \quad (46.1)$$

where [K] equals the urine or plasma potassium concentration, and U_{osm} and P_{osm} represent urine and plasma osmolality, respectively. All are obtained in random specimens drawn simultaneously.

This innovative, easy-to-use calculation rooted in physiologic principles has many applications and wide versatility to assist in the evaluation of potassium

disorders (7,14). The expected normal value during hypokalemia caused by extrarenal potassium losses is less than 2. Any deviation from this value when hypokalemia is present reveals that the kidney is contributing in some way to a disorder of potassium homeostasis (Table 46.2).

The following observations and assumptions are necessary: The region of the nephron responsible for final tubular secretion and reabsorption of potassium is the distal convoluted tubule and the cortical collecting duct; the peritubular fluid bathing that section of the nephron has approximately the same potassium concentration as plasma; the potassium concentration in the urine flowing through that section of the nephron reflects the final secretion or reabsorption of potassium (depending in large part but not exclusively on aldosterone); the urine flowing beyond that section of the nephron will be modified further depending on the amount of water removed or added as the urine courses through the medulla (the amount of water removed changes the potassium concentration independently of the forces acting directly on potassium excretion); the amount of water removed can be assessed by measuring the urine osmolality and comparing it with the plasma osmolality; and the urine potassium (when corrected for that water loss) compared with the plasma potassium reflects the net balance of forces acting on potassium in the kidney.

Figure 46.5 illustrates the effect of water reabsorption on the urine potassium concentration and the role of the TTKG.

In certain clinical circumstances, the interpretation of the TTKG requires special consideration. Although it is still reliable, the TTKG must take into account the presence of drugs that block the action of aldosterone or potassium-sparing diuretics; low urinary concentration of sodium (less than 25 mEq), which would independently reduce the secretion of potassium; preexisting severe hypokalemia, which diminishes the normal potassium secretory response to aldosterone; water diuresis, because antidiuretic hormone (ADH) is necessary for normal potassium secretion (the urine osmolality $[U_{osm}]$ must be greater than or equal to the plasma osmolality $[P_{osm}]$); intrinsic renal disease such as interstitial nephritis; diabetes mellitus that is poorly controlled, or diabetic ketoacidosis, which blunts the normal response to aldosterone; extracellular fluid volume contraction and edematous conditions (e.g., heart failure, cirrhosis, or nephrosis), both of which alter urinary osmolality through avid sodium reabsorption and low urea excretion; and diuretics, which may cause an underestimation of potassium secretion if the urine flow rate and volume are large.

Measuring Potassium

The terms *serum potassium* and *plasma potassium* have been used in this discussion. *Plasma potassium* measured from unclotted blood is the most reliable means to assay potassium. However, in clinical practice, potassium is nearly always measured in serum. Blood allowed to clot, as when *serum* is analyzed ("red-top tubes"), usually releases a small amount of potassium. Therefore, serum potassium is likely to be slightly higher than plasma potassium, the true value in the blood. Usually, the difference is very small. However, this can be a problem with hyperkalemia. Occasionally, when the clinician is concerned that the serum potassium level is falsely high, as in marked thrombocytosis, a plasma potassium ("green-top tube") can be obtained to accurately reflect the true blood concentration.

Gastrointestinal Losses Resulting in Potassium Deficiency

Diarrhea

Potassium and bicarbonate are normally present in the stool in high concentrations. When diarrhea is significant, hypokalemia may result. This often is associated with a non–anion gap hyperchloremic metabolic acidosis (caused by the loss of bicarbonate). Occasionally, hypokalemia may be a clue to the presence of a villous adenoma of the colon or surreptitious laxative abuse. Diarrheal states in general are often associated with clinical contraction of the extracellular fluid volume, detected on physical examination by weight loss, low jugular venous pressure, poor skin turgor, tachycardia, and orthostatic hypotension. Urinary potassium excretion should be low when potassium deficiency results from intestinal losses because in this setting the kidney conserves potassium maximally. However, this is true only when the volume status of the patient is maintained. When diarrhea is severe and volume contraction develops, secondary hyperaldosteronism occurs as a protective strategy to preserve salt balance.

Table 46.2. Transtubular Potassium Gradient (TTKG)

Clinical Issue	Hypokalemia		Hyperkalemia	
TTKG	<2	>4	<6	>10
Cause	Extrarenal K⁺ loss with renal conservation of K⁺ Diarrhea Post diuretic use Skin loss	Inappropriate renal K⁺ loss or wasting Current diuretic use Bartter's syndrome Cushing's syndrome RTA I, II Licorice use Normal or excess aldosterone action 1° or 2° hyperaldosteronism Vomiting Malignant hypertension	Failure of kidney to excrete K⁺ appropriately Renal failure (acute or chronic) Interstitial nephritis Aldosterone decreased Hypoaldosteronism Addison's disease RTA Type IV	Exogenous K⁺ with appropriate renal response Excess K⁺ oral or IV Normal aldosterone response Rhabdomyolysis Metabolic acidosis β-Adrenergic blockade

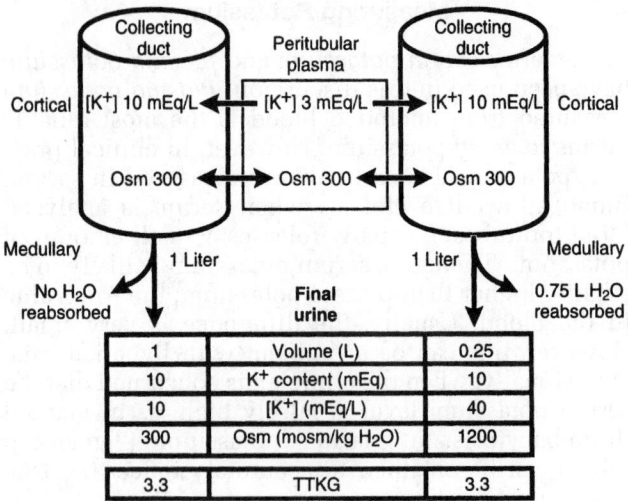

Figure 46.5. The transtubular potassium gradient (TTKG): the role of water reabsorption, urine potassium concentration, and TTKG. (Modified from Halperin ML, Goldstein MB. Fluid, electrolyte and acid–base emergencies. New York: WB Saunders, 1988.)

Potassium losses are accelerated in the urine paradoxically.

Loss of Gastric Fluid

Hypokalemia is well known to accompany vomiting or gastric drainage. Yet, although gastric fluid is rich in hydrochloric acid, it contains only small amounts of potassium (approximately 5 to 10 mEq/L). The major route of potassium loss in this setting is the urine (31). The loss of gastric chloride induces metabolic alkalosis, chloride deficiency, extracellular volume depletion, and secondary hyperaldosteronism. The increased filtered load and increased distal delivery of bicarbonate, decreased distal delivery of chloride, and high levels of aldosterone all act together to stimulate secretion of potassium. The urine will have high concentrations of potassium but very low concentrations of chloride. Under these circumstances, correction of potassium depletion and metabolic alkalosis requires provision of adequate amounts of chloride, potassium, and sodium. Potassium administered with anions other than chloride is not retained but is excreted in the urine (15).

Diuretics

Diuretics that act proximally to potassium secretory sites accelerate potassium excretion by increasing the amount of sodium and water delivered to the distal nephron while simultaneously stimulating the release of aldosterone. Loop diuretics (furosemide, bumetanide, torsemide), thiazides, and chlorthalidone are diuretics that act in this way and may cause hypokalemia. The serum potassium concentration usually reaches a nadir within 7 days after beginning therapy (22). The degree of potassium depletion depends on the concurrent sodium intake. Furthermore, some diuretics cause more severe hypokalemia than others (22): At standard dosages, thiazide and thiazidelike diuretics induce an average fall in the serum potassium concentration of approximately 0.6 mEq/L, and up to 50% of patients develop a serum potassium less than 3.5 mEq/L; furosemide causes less potassium depletion, with an average fall in potassium concentration of only 0.3 mEq/L. The use of multiple kaliuretic diuretics acting at different nephron sites (e.g., furosemide and thiazide) is likely to cause significant hypokalemia (24).

Patients who take diuretics (whether they are edematous or not) often risk becoming potassium depleted, although the exact number of patients at risk varies. Less than 7% (22) to 50% (2) of patients on diuretics may develop hypokalemia. This discrepancy suggests that drug therapy, risk factors, and associated problems may vary. Levels below 3.0 mEq/L suggest one or two situations: *excessive sodium intake* that increases the amount of sodium and water delivered to the distal nephron, which in turn accelerates potassium secretion, or *an unrecognized potassium-wasting state* such as primary or secondary hyperaldosteronism (35). Both should be considered when significant hypokalemia develops after the introduction of potassium-wasting diuretics, particularly if the potassium level before treatment was low.

Metabolic alkalosis often accompanies hypokalemia in patients taking diuretics. Many potassium-wasting diuretics stimulate renal hydrogen ion secretion. Contraction of the extracellular volume may also help maintain the rise in serum bicarbonate concentration. Metabolic alkalosis develops along with chloride deficiency, and can be corrected only by a chloride-containing salt (15).

Monitoring Potassium in Patients Receiving Diuretics

Before administration of diuretics, the serum potassium (as well as the other electrolytes, blood urea nitrogen, and serum creatinine) should be measured. If it is normal, serum potassium should be measured approximately 1 and 4 weeks after the initiation of, or increase in, the dosage of a diuretic. Most patients who develop hypokalemia will have done so within the first week. Subsequently, semiannual assessment is probably adequate in nonedematous, stable, well-nourished patients unless other indications arise. Edematous patients have major underlying diseases and those with heart failure are often treated with digitalis, so the risk of serious consequences of hypokalemia is greater. Therefore, monitoring should be more frequent in these patients.

Prevention and Therapy of Diuretic-Induced Hypokalemia

Whether mild diuretic-induced hypokalemia is dangerous remains controversial (26). When a diuretic is indicated, the physician should use simple measures that can minimize the risk of hypokalemia. These include using the lowest effective dosage of a diuretic agent and prescribing a moderate restriction of dietary salt. (An identical restricted diet may be prescribed as 75 to 100 mEq sodium per day or 2 to 2.5 g sodium or 4 to 6 g sodium chloride; see Table 62.12. These calculations are derived from the facts that 1 g sodium chloride equals 17 mEq sodium and 1 g sodium equals 43 mEq sodium.) Increased dietary potassium should also be suggested because it is easy for a patient to accomplish, cost-effective, and may be associated with other benefits such as lower blood pressure and decreased stroke risk (see above), hypertension, and other cerebrovascular diseases.

Even with preventive measures, approximately 30% of diuretic-treated patients become hypokalemic in the range of 3.0 to 3.5 mEq/L (17). Normalization of serum potassium is always indicated. The management of diuretic-induced hypokalemia should be emphasized and individualized (11) for all patients, but especially for those listed in Table 46.3 (35).

When the diuretic must be continued and normalization of the serum potassium must be restored, the decision must be made whether to use potassium supplements or potassium-sparing diuretics (see Table 62.14). Although a variety of potassium supplements are available (Table 46.4), only *potassium chloride* corrects diuretic-induced hypokalemia associated with metabolic alkalosis (15). Salt substitutes are composed mostly of potassium chloride (approximately 50 to 65 mmol/teaspoon) and are a cheap and effective alternative. However, diuretic-induced hypokalemia may seem to be refractory even to large doses of potassium chloride because the renal clearance of potassium remains high during continued diuretic therapy (6,27). In one study, potassium chloride at dosages up to 96 mmol/day normalized the serum potassium in only 8 of 16 hypertensive patients with diuretic-induced hypokalemia (27). However, understanding the balance of intake and output is essential. If the physician does not prescribe, or the patient does not take, enough potassium supplement to exceed the losses, the serum potassium will never normalize.

Potassium-sparing diuretics (including spironolactone, triamterene, and amiloride) may offer several advantages (17) such as reducing urinary potassium losses, minimizing the development of metabolic alkalosis by reducing acid excretion (spironolactone), and limiting renal magnesium wasting. In one study con-

Table 46.3.   Indications for Potassium Maintenance Therapy

Digitalis therapy
Predisposition to hepatic coma
Serum potassium <3.0 mEq/L
Development of glucose intolerance
Underlying cardiac disease
Symptoms attributable to hypokalemia

Taken with permission from Tannen RL. Diuretic induced hypokalemia. Kidney Int 28:988, 1985.

Table 46.4.   Commonly Available Potassium Chloride Supplements

Product	Amount
Extended-release tablets	
Micro-K Extentabs, Slow K, Klor-Con 8	8 mEq
K-Dur, K-Norm, K-Tab, Ten-K, Micro-K 10 Extentabs, Klor-Con 10	10 mEq
K-Dur	20 mEq
Powders for solution (flavored)[a]	
K-Lor (also 15 mEq), Kato, Klor-Con Klor-Con 125 (25 mEq)	20 mEq/packet
Suspension (no taste)	
Micro-K LS	20 mEq/packet
Efflorescent granules or tablets (flavored)[a]	
Klorvess, Klor-Con/EF (25 mEq)	20 mEq
Solutions (flavored)[a]	
Klorvess 10%, Rum-K 15%	20–30 mEq/15 mL

[a]Taste generally improved by chilling.

version from hydrochlorothiazide (with or without potassium supplements) to hydrochlorothiazide plus amiloride or hydrochlorothiazide plus triamterene without potassium supplements increased the serum potassium by approximately 0.5 to 0.7 mEq/L and brought it into the midnormal range (28).

The *major risk* of attempts to raise the serum potassium is overshoot hyperkalemia. To avoid this, all patients beginning therapy with potassium supplements or potassium-sparing agents should be assessed for risk factors for hyperkalemia. These include renal insufficiency (obvious elevations of serum creatinine greater than 1.2 mg/dL), diabetes mellitus, age 75 or older, and the ingestion of other agents known to interfere with potassium homeostasis (e.g., converting-enzyme inhibitors, nonsteroidal anti-inflammatory drugs, cyclosporine, and heparin). Approximately a 50% reduction in glomerular filtration rate may occur between the age of 20 to 80 years in many people (see Chapter 48), whereas the serum creatinine is still in the normal range. In this setting there may be a loss of the ability of the kidney to readily maintain potassium balance. Therefore, all patients beginning therapy to raise the serum potassium level should have their serum potassium measured after 1 and 4 weeks and then at least every 6 to 12 months, if not more often as indicated. If a hypokalemic patient is found to have renal insufficiency or other risk factors for hyperkalemia, potassium supplements and potassium-sparing diuretics are generally contraindicated.

Assessment of 24-hour urinary potassium excretion along with serum potassium helps in predicting how best to supplement (or restrict) the patient. For example, if the patient is taking 40 mEq of potassium supplementation a day, has a 24-hour urinary excretion of 80 mEq a day of potassium, and has a plasma potassium of 3.0 mEq/L, then more supplements (dietary or pharmacologic) are indicated. Even in the patient with normal renal function, potassium supplements and potassium-sparing diuretics generally should not be given together or along with other drugs that interfere with potassium homeostasis.

Less Common Causes of Hypokalemia

The approach to diagnosing these problems is based on the history, physical examination, urinary electrolyte levels, acid–base status, and occasionally the measurement of plasma renin activity and aldosterone levels.

Deficient Potassium Intake

Potassium is widely distributed in many foods, especially fruits, raw vegetables, many types of fish, beef, and pork (Table 46.5). Therefore, inadequate potassium intake is an unusual cause of hypokalemia except in some high-risk situations (dietary fads, pica, alcoholism, cachexia). Insufficient dietary potassium during anabolic states as cells take up potassium, as when malnourished patients are fed and with treatment for megaloblastic anemia (33), may lead to hypokalemia. In such patients, the urinary potassium excretion is less than 10 to 20 mEq/day while they are hypokalemic unless there is a compounding problem. Dietary deficiency of potassium, particularly in the elderly, may also exacerbate diuretic-induced hypokalemia.

Excessive Urinary Potassium Losses (Renal Potassium Wasting)

The differential diagnosis in this setting is complex, but it can be simplified by assessing the acid–base status and blood pressure of the patient (Fig. 46.4) (25).

When hypokalemia secondary to renal potassium wasting is accompanied by an elevated blood pressure, renin (angiotensin) or mineralocorticoid (or glucocorticoid) excess is suggested. Several causes must be considered (Table 46.6). The evaluation of such a patient is complex. However, certain basic diagnoses may be made in an office. Referral to a center experienced in the evaluation of these syndromes may still be necessary.

Unless the cause is readily apparent (e.g., a patient with essential hypertension treated with diuretics), the first step in the evaluation of renal potassium wasting in a hypertensive patient is the determination of plasma renin activity (Fig. 46.4). If the renin is elevated, this suggests primary renin excess, as may be caused by renovascular, accelerated, malignant hypertension (see Chapter 62), or rarely a renin-producing tumor. On the other hand, if the renin level is low, the plasma renin activity should be remeasured along with the plasma aldosterone level. If both levels are low, the presence of excessive amounts of endogenous or exogenous steroids, other than aldosterone, is likely: Licorice, chewing tobacco, carbenoxolone, and steroid-containing nasal sprays are rare exogenous causes of this syndrome. Finally, if the renin level is low but the simultaneous aldosterone level is high, primary aldosteronism is strongly suggested. The sensitivity and specificity of this screening test may be increased by determining the aldosterone/renin ratio 2 hours after administration of 25 mg of captopril. In primary aldosteronism, the ratio remains high but is suppressed in patients with essential hypertension (19,20).

Primary Hyperaldosteronism. Most patients with primary aldosteronism are asymptomatic (40). Clinical

Table 46.5.   Some Common Potassium-Rich Foods

Food Source	Average Portion	Potassium (mEq)	Sodium (mEq)
Vegetables			
Artichoke	1 large	22.0	3.7
Beans			
Cooked dried	½ cup	10.7	—
Lima	⅝ cup	10.8	—
Brussels sprouts	7 medium	7	—
Corn	1 ear	5.0	—
Potato			
White	1 boiled	7.3	—
Sweet	1 boiled	7.7	—
Tomato			
Fresh	1 medium	9.4	—
Canned	½ cup	5.6	3.3
Squash, winter	½ cup boiled	11.9	—
Meats			
Hamburger	1 patty	9.8	1.7
Rib roast	2 slices	11.2	2.5
Fish, haddock	1 medium fillet	8.0	7.7
Clams	4 large	6.0	1.7
Oysters	6 medium	3.1	3.1
Fruits			
Apple	1 medium	2.8	—
Applesauce	⅓ cup	1.7	—
Apricots	3 medium	7.2	—
Avocado	½ pitted	15.5	—
Banana	1 6-inch	9.5	—
Cantaloupe	¼ medium	6.4	—
Dates	10 pitted	16.6	—
Fruit cocktail	½ cup	4.3	—
Grapefruit	½ medium	3.5	—
Melon	¼ small	6.4	—
Orange	1 small	7.7	—
Peach	1 medium	5.2	—
Pear	1 medium	6.7	—
Plum	2 medium	7.7	—
Prunes, dried	10 medium	17.8	—
Raisins	1 tablespoon	2.0	—
Strawberries	10 large	4.2	—
Watermelon	1 slice	15.4	—
Juice			
Grapefruit	1 cup	10.4	—
Orange	1 cup	12.4	—
Pineapple	1 cup	9.2	—
Prune	1 cup	15.0	—
Tomato	1 cup	13.7	20.9
Vegetable	1 cup	14.1	21.7
Nuts			
Peanuts, roasted	1 tablespoon	2.0	—
Peanut butter	2 tablespoon	2.0	—
Mixed nuts	3.5 oz	2.0	—
Milk			
Buttermilk	9 oz	8.0	14
Skim milk	8 oz	8.5	6
Whole milk	8 oz	9.0	5

manifestations, when present, in addition to hypertension, are related to potassium depletion and occur only when such depletion is severe. These include weakness, paralysis, tetany, arrhythmias, polyuria, and polydipsia. Edema is less common than would be expected because of adaptive factors that diminish sodium retention. Patients with primary aldosteronism usually have hypokalemia, but as many as 25% have serum potassium levels above 3.5 mEq/L. However, many of these patients manifest hypokalemia if challenged with potassium-wasting diuretics or with large intakes of sodium chloride (200 mmol/day, approximately 4 to 5 g of sodium or 10 to 12 g sodium chloride). Both of these interventions result in increased delivery of sodium and water to the distal nephron, where, under the influence of excessive aldosterone, sodium is reabsorbed and potassium and hydrogen ions are secreted. Hypokalemia and metabolic alkalosis ensue. Indeed, the development of severe hypokalemia after the initiation of thiazide therapy is sometimes a clue to a hypermineralocorticoid state. On the other hand, a serum potassium greater than 4.0 mEq/L in a patient on a high-sodium diet (documented by a 24-hour urinary sodium excretion of approximately 200 mEq/day) virtually excludes the diagnosis (40).

When the combination of hypokalemia, suppressed plasma renin activity, and elevated aldosterone levels appears likely, localization procedures (computerized tomography [CT] or magnetic resonance imaging [MRI]) should be undertaken by the consultant to distinguish adenomas from bilateral adrenal hyperplasia. The treatment of adenomas has primarily been surgical and excision has often led to the cure of hypertension and hypokalemia. If bilateral hyperplasia is found, surgery is not indicated because it is seldom curative. A trial of spironolactone is useful in almost all patients. Large doses (up to 400 mg daily) are sometimes necessary and the full effects may not be seen for several weeks. Failure of spironolactone to normalize the blood pressure while normalizing hypokalemia strongly suggests that, regardless of the presence or absence of an adenoma to explain the aldosterone excess, surgery would probably not resolve the hypertension. Although spironolactone has been the mainstay of medical therapy for primary aldosteronism, amiloride (up to 40 mg/day) is also effective and may be the drug of choice for patients intolerant of spironolactone (40).

Normotensive Renal Potassium Wasting. When renal potassium wasting is discovered in a normotensive patient, the acid–base status should be evaluated (Fig. 46.4). If metabolic acidosis is present, renal tubular acidosis or diabetic ketoacidosis (although this is usually apparent by findings other than renal potassium wasting) is suggested. If metabolic alkalosis is present, the urinary chloride provides an important clue to the underlying process. If the urinary chloride concentration is low, the likely cause is upper gastrointestinal fluid loss. If the urinary chloride is high, causes may include the coincident use of diuretics during the time of the sampling, but other causes are possible, such as Bartter's syndrome. It should be emphasized that diuretic abuse and self-induced vomiting are common concealed causes of hypokalemia and metabolic alkalosis.

Urinary electrolyte evaluation with respect to diuretics is often frustrating. The half-life of the various diuretics must be considered. Most loop diuretics, with the exception of torsemide, have fairly short half-lives despite the common perception that they are long acting. Therefore, excess urine chloride may be seen during the period of active or recent drug use with apparently paradoxical low urine chloride after the drug has left the urine.

Bartter's Syndrome. Bartter's syndrome presents with hypokalemic metabolic alkalosis, excessive urinary potassium losses, and normal blood pressure, without edema. Plasma renin activity and aldosterone levels are significantly elevated. This presentation is mimicked by diuretic abuse and surreptitious vomiting, from which Bartter's syndrome must be differentiated. A urine screening test for surreptitious use of diuretics should be done. Also urinary chloride is elevated in Bartter's syndrome and decreased in surreptitious vomiting, both of which may present with hypokalemic metabolic alkalosis. Hypokalemia is usually refractory to potassium supplementation but may be ameliorated by administration of prostaglandin synthesis inhibitors (e.g., nonsteroidal antiinflammatory drugs [NSAIDs]) or amiloride 5 to 10 mg/day (28).

Transient Disorders of Internal Potassium Balance

β_2-Adrenergic agonists lower the serum potassium concentration by stimulating cellular potassium uptake. A reduction in serum potassium is commonly

Table 46.6. Causes of Hypertension with Associated Renal Potassium Wasting

Hyperreninemic Forms
Renovascular
Renin tumor
Malignant or accelerated essential hypertension

Hyporeninemic Steroid-Dependent Forms
Mineralocorticoid
  Exogenous
    Licorice, desoxycorticosterone, fludrocortisone, chewing tobacco, carbenoxolone
  Endogenous
    Adrenal adenoma
    Adrenal glomerulose hyperplasia
    Enzyme deficiency: 17-OHase; 11-OHase
    Liddle's syndrome
Glucocorticoid
  Endogenous
    Cushing's syndrome, pituitary, ectopic ACTH, adrenal cortical
  Exogenous

Taken with permission from Narins RG, Jones ER, Stom MC, et al. Diagnostic strategies in disorders of fluid, electrolyte and acid–base homeostasis. Am J Med 72:496, 1982.

seen when β_2-adrenergic agonists (administered via any route) are used in the treatment of asthma or premature labor. Although the decrease in serum potassium is usually mild, significant hypokalemia can occur, which usually resolves within hours after the drug is discontinued. Similarly, *high levels of endogenous catecholamines* released during stress may explain transient reductions in serum potassium (that resolve with or without potassium supplementation) sometimes seen during acute hospital admissions (23), delirium tremens, and acute myocardial infarction (33).

Metabolic and respiratory alkalosis are associated with small shifts of potassium from the extracellular to the intracellular space. This may sensitize the patient to digitalis, even in the absence of total body potassium depletion.

Insulin stimulates cellular potassium uptake in liver and skeletal muscle, independent of its effects on glucose transport. This dose-dependent action forms the basis for using insulin in the treatment of severe hyperkalemia. When insulin is used to correct hyperglycemia and the initial serum potassium is normal, hypokalemia may ensue.

Hypokalemic periodic paralysis is a rare familial disorder characterized by spontaneous episodes of paralysis that may be precipitated by a variety of stimuli, including insulin, glucose, and a high-carbohydrate meal. A similar syndrome may also be seen in hyperthyroidism, especially in Asian men. Although a profound fall in the serum potassium is regularly demonstrated during paralysis, urinary potassium excretion decreases dramatically, signifying an intracellular shift of potassium. In the thyrotoxic form, β-blocking agents may be effective in preventing attacks.

Vitamin B_{12}, when administered in the therapy of megaloblastic anemia, may cause large intracellular shifts of potassium as metabolic activity is increased in hematopoietic cells. Provision of adequate quantities of potassium and careful monitoring prevent this complication.

Finally, other rare causes of transient hypokalemia have been reported. *Pseudohypokalemia* caused by metabolically active cells incorporating potassium after a specimen of blood has been drawn and left at room temperature has occurred in leukemias. Hypothermia can lower plasma potassium to 3.0 mEq/L or less because of potassium uptake into cells. Rare cases of barium salt poisoning caused by contamination of table salt and blockade of potassium channels inhibiting potassium exit from cells have been reported.

General References*

Greenberg A, et al. Primer on kidney diseases. New York: Academic Press, 1994.

Halperin ML, Goldstein MB. Fluid, electrolyte, and acid–base physiology. Philadelphia: WB Saunders, 1994.
> Thorough text on this subject covering basic science to clinical medicine.

---

*Bold print (general references) and bold numerals (specific references) denote published controlled clinical trials, meta-analyses, or consensus-based recommendations.

Narins RG. Clinical disorders of fluid and electrolyte metabolism. New York: McGraw-Hill, 1994.
> The "gold standard" in the field of fluid and electrolytes.

Weiner ID, Wingo CS. Hypokalemia: consequences, causes, and correction. J Am Soc Nephrology 8(7):1179, 1997.

Specific References

1. Appel LJ, Moore TJ, Obarzanek E, et al. A clinical trial of the effects of dietary patterns on blood pressure. DASH Collaborative Research Group. N Engl J Med 336(16):1117, 1997.
2. Bloomfield RL, Wilson DJ, Buckalew VM. The incidence of diuretic-induced hypokalemia in two distinct clinic settings. J Clin Hypertens 2:331, 1986.
3. Brancati FL, Appel LJ, Seidler AJ, et al. Effect of potassium supplementation on blood pressure in African Americans on a low-potassium diet. A randomized, double-blind, placebo-controlled trial. Arch Intern Med 156(1):61, 1996.
4. Caralis PV, Materson BJ, Perez-Stable E. Potassium and diuretic-induced ventricular arrhythmias in ambulatory hypertensive patients. Miner Electrolyte Metab 10:148, 1984.
5. Chalmers JMT, Morgan T, Doyle A, et al. Australian National Health and Medical Research Council Dietary Salt Study in Mild Hypertension. J Hypertens 4(6):S629, 1986.
6. Down PF, Polak A, Rao R. Fate of potassium supplements in six outpatients receiving long-term diuretics for edematous disease. Lancet 2:721, 1972.
7. Ethier JH, Kamel KS, Magner PO, et al. The transtubular potassium concentration in patients with hypokalemia and hyperkalemia. Am J Kidney Dis 15(4):309, 1990.
8. Frisancho AR, Leonard WR, Bollettino LA. Blood pressure in blacks and whites and its relationship to dietary sodium and potassium intake. J Chronic Dis 37(7):515, 1984.
9. Giebish G. Physiology of potassium metabolism. In: Whelton PK, Whelton A, Walker GW, eds. Potassium in cardiovascular and renal medicine. New York: Marcel Dekker, 1986.
10. Grim CE, Luft FC, Miller JZ, et al. Racial differences in blood pressure in Evans County, GA: relationships to sodium and potassium intake in plasma renin activity. J Chronic Dis 33:87, 1980.
11. Harrington JT, Isner JM, Kassirer JP. Our national obsession with potassium. Am J Med 73:155, 1982.
12. Iimura O, Kijima T, Kikuchi K, et al. Studies on the hypotensive effect of high potassium intake in patients with essential hypertension. Clin Sci 61:77s, 1981.
13. INTERSALT Research Group. INTERSALT: an international cooperative study on electrolytes and blood pressure. BMJ 297:319, 1988.
14. Kamel KS, Quaggins S, Scheich A, et al. Disorders of potassium homeostasis: and approach based on pathophysiology. Am J Kidney Dis 24(4):597, 1994.
15. Kassirer JP, Berkman PM, Lawrenz DR, et al. The critical role of chloride in the correction of hypokalemic alkalosis in man. Am J Med 38:172, 1965.
16. Khaw KT, Barrett-Conner E. Dietary potassium in stroke-associated mortality: a 12-year prospective population study. N Engl J Med 316:235, 1987.
17. Krishna GG, Shulman MD, Narins RG. Clinical use of the potassium-sparing diuretics. Semin Nephrol 8:354, 1988.
18. Langford HG. Dietary potassium and hypertension: epidemiological data. Ann Intern Med 98(Suppl):770, 1983.
19. Laragh JH, Brenner BM. Hypertension: pathophysiology, diagnosis, and management. New York: Raven Press, 1990.
20. Lyons DF, Kem DC, Brown RD, et al. Single dose captopril as a diagnostic test for primary aldosteronism. J Clin Endocrinol Metab 57:892, 1988.
21. McCarron DA, Morris CD, Henry HJ, et al. Blood pressure and nutrient intake in the United States. Science 224:1392, 1984.
22. Morgan DB, Davidson C. Hypokalemia and diuretics: an analysis of publications. BMJ 280:905, 1980.
23. Morgan DB, Young RM. Acute transient hypokalemia: new interpretation of a common event. Lancet 2:751, 1982.
24. Nader PC, Thompson JR, Alpern RJ. Complications of diuretic use. Semin Nephrol 8:365, 1988.

25. Narins RG, Jones ER, Stom MC, et al. Diagnostic strategies in disorders of fluid, electrolyte and acid–base homeostasis. Am J Med 72:496, 1982.
26. Papademetriou V. Diuretics, hypokalemia, and cardiac arrhythmias: a critical analysis. Am Heart J 111:1217, 1986.
27. Papademetriou V, Burris J, Kukich S, et al. Effectiveness of potassium chloride or triamterene in thiazide hypokalemia. Arch Intern Med 145:1986, 1985.
28. Ridgeway NA, Ginn DR, Alley K. Outpatient conversion of treatment to potassium-sparing diuretics. Am J Med 80:785, 1986.
29. Siani A, Strazzulo P, Giacco A, et al. Increasing the dietary potassium intake reduces the need for antihypertensive medication. Ann Intern Med 115:753, 1991.
30. Siani A, Strazzulo P, Russo L, et al. Controlled trial of long term oral potassium supplements in patients with mild hypertension. BMJ 294:1453, 1987.
31. Stein JH. Hypokalemia: common and uncommon causes. Hosp Pract 23:55, 1988.
32. Sterns RH, Cox M, Feig PU. Internal potassium balance and the control of the plasma potassium concentration. Medicine 60:339, 1981.
33. Sterns RH, Spital A. Disorder of internal potassium balance. Semin Nephrol 7:206, 1987.
34. Svetkey LP, Yarger WE, Feussner JR, et al. Double-blind, placebo-controlled trial of potassium chloride in the treatment of mild hypertension. Hypertension 9(5):444, 1987.
35. Tannen RL. Diuretic-induced hypokalemia. Kidney Int 28:988, 1985.
36. Tannen RL. Potassium disorders. In: Kokko JP, Tannen RL, eds. Fluids and electrolytes. Philadelphia: WB Saunders, 1986.
37. West ML, Bendz O, Chen CB, et al. Development of a test to evaluate the transtubular potassium gradient in the cortical collecting duct in vivo. Miner Electrolyte Metab 12:226, 1986.
38. West ML, Marsden PA, Richardson RM, et al. New clinical approach to evaluate disorders of potassium excretion. Miner Electrolyte Metab 12:234, 1986.
39. Whelton PK, Jiang H, Cutler JA, et al. Effects of oral potassium on blood pressure: metaanalysis of randomized controlled clinical trials. JAMA 277(20):1624, 1997.
40. Young WF, Klee GG. Primary aldosteronism: diagnostic evaluation. Endocrinol Metab Clin North Am 17:367, 1988.

CHAPTER 47

Urinary Stones

DAVID A. SPECTOR, MD

Urinary stones are common in the United States. Although urologic intervention or nephrologic consultation may occasionally be required, most patients with stones can be evaluated, treated, and followed by the primary care physician. This chapter reviews the various manifestations of stone disease, the types of urinary stones, the evaluation of patients with stones, the acute and chronic treatment of patients with urinary stones, and when to obtain consultation for these patients.

PRESENTATION OF URINARY STONE DISEASE

Physicians will encounter urinary stone disease in patients with acute colic, persistent or recurrent urinary tract infection, isolated hematuria, no symptoms but a stone discovered incidentally on a radiograph taken for other purposes, or a history of stones.

Acute Colic

Presentation

Most patients with urinary stones at some time have an acute episode of colic. The stone, if obstructing, causes ureteral spasm, resulting in severe intermittent pain. The location of the pain depends on the location of the stone in the ureter but is most often felt in the flank; then, as the stone moves distally, pain radiates in a characteristic pattern around the groin and into the testicles in the male or into the labia majora in the female. Nausea, vomiting, and other gastrointestinal symptoms that often suggest a primary gastrointestinal problem may be associated with pain. Examination reveals an uncomfortable, restless patient. There may be costovertebral tenderness as well as deep tenderness in the abdomen. More important, no signs of peritoneal irritation are present (guarding, rebound, or rigidity). Fever is not present unless urinary tract infection has developed in the obstructed urinary tract.

Urinalysis almost always demonstrates microscopic (or gross) hematuria. The presence of pyuria is important because chronic bacterial infection may be associated with the development of urinary stones; however, pyuria may be absent even if infection is present during complete ureteral obstruction.

Diagnosis and Management

The aims of management of colic should be relief of discomfort, surveillance for infection, and determination of whether stones will pass spontaneously or will require surgical removal. The *abdominal radiograph* is useful in monitoring the site and progression of the stone. Approximately 90% of renal stones are radiodense and can be seen on a good quality radiograph. The size and position of the stone help determine the likely course of the episode of colic and the urgency of intervention. In general, stones that are smaller than 5 mm pass spontaneously, those between 5 and 10 mm have a 50% chance of passing spontaneously, and those larger than 10 mm usually require surgical removal. The common sites where stones become lodged are in the renal calyx, in the ureteropelvic junction, in the ureter at the pelvic brim where the ureter begins to pass over the iliac vessels, in the lower third of the ureter, and at the ureterovesical junction. If there is doubt about whether calcification seen on the plain film is within the urinary tract, an oblique view may help. It is also important to review old abdominal films taken for any reason to see whether a stone was present at that time.

An *intravenous pyelogram* (IVP) or HASTE magnetic resonance imaging (MRI), if available, should also be obtained as soon as possible in the patient with colic because it will help establish the diagnosis, especially in patients with radiolucent stones, and it will provide certain important information that will aid in management. Occasionally, a patient who has acute ureteral colic will have a history of allergy to radiologic dye. In this instance, *an ultrasonic study, or HASTE MRI (if available), of the collecting system of the kidney may*

help in determining the presence of obstruction or a solitary kidney. Alternatively, a urologist could be consulted for consideration of either an *antegrade pyelogram* (i.e., via a catheter passed percutaneously into the renal pelvis) or a *retrograde pyelogram*. These methods are safe for patients with a history of allergy to IVP dye.

Occasionally a patient with a history strongly suggestive of renal colic may have another cause for the pain. A dissection of the aorta, acute back strain or lumbar disc disease, the passage of blood clots in the ureters (as in sickle cell disease or renal infarct), and malingering should be considered. A malingerer is often difficult to identify at first, but usually gives a classic history of acute renal colic and may also relate a history of allergy to IVP dye. Often these patients have blood (obtained from a fingerstick or oral injury) in the urine specimen they give for analysis. (For further information, see Chapter 12.)

Several factors help one decide whether to hospitalize a patient with renal colic, to obtain urgent urologic consultation, or to treat the patient at home. First, the patient with nausea and vomiting cannot be ensured of an adequate fluid intake or adequate oral analgesia and should be admitted to a hospital. Second, fever suggests infection proximal to an obstructing stone, and urgent urologic consultation should be obtained. Third, if an IVP reveals a nonfunctioning kidney (completely obstructed ureter), a partially obstructed ureter from a solitary kidney, or urine extravasation, urgent urologic consultation should be obtained. Fourth, if the stone is larger than 10 mm, spontaneous passage is very unlikely and urologic consultation should be obtained. Of all stones that become symptomatic, 80% are ureteral, and 85 to 90% of these pass spontaneously. Thus, only 10 to 15% of ureteral stones require interventional treatment (3).

Most patients can be treated at home. Forced hydration of 2 to 3 L of fluid every 24 hours is necessary to maintain a good urinary flow and to help in moving the stone. When the patient is voiding, all of the urine voided during the period of intermittent colic should be collected and strained through an old stocking, a fine knit screen, or a filter paper so that the passed stone may be saved and analyzed. It is important to prescribe analgesic medication such as oxycodone (generic, 5 mg, 1 to 3 tablets) or Tylox, which contains oxycodone and acetaminophen (1 to 3 capsules orally every 3 to 4 hours) to control the discomfort. A phenothiazine (e.g., Phenergan, 25 mg) given with the narcotic provides additional relief by controlling any associated nausea. Some prostaglandin synthesis inhibitors such as indomethacin (Indocin or generic, 50 mg three to four times per day), ketorolac (Toradol, 10 mg every 4 to 6 hours orally; also may be given as 30 mg intravenously or intramuscularly every 6 hours), or diclofenac (Voltaren, 50 mg orally two to three times daily) may give effective analgesia in renal colic. This effect may result from reductions in ureteric wall muscle tension, reduced renal pelvic pressure caused by decreased glomerular filtration rate, and a reduction of ureteral edema. Indomethacin may be tried in combination with traditional analgesics when symptoms of colic are prolonged. The patient should be hospitalized if fever, uncontrolled pain, or vomiting develops. If symptoms of colic are intermittent and well controlled at home, the patient should be followed with a weekly radiograph of the abdomen to determine the progression of the stone. If by 6 weeks the stone has not passed, it is unlikely that spontaneous passage will occur and urologic consultation should be obtained. For occupational or social reasons, some patients want to consider surgical removal of the stone earlier and therefore ask their physicians to request urologic consultation sooner.

Stones that pass from the ureter into the bladder generally pass with ease through the urethra. In the event of a bladder outlet obstruction, a stone may be retained in the bladder *(bladder stone),* where it may grow and in time become an infection stone (see "Struvite Stones," below).

Patient Requiring Urologic Referral.   When a patient is referred to a urologist for *stone removal,* there are several options. Lower ureteral stones may be removed using a basket that is inserted through a cystoscope or ureteroscope. This procedure is similar to cystoscopic examination but requires general or spinal anesthesia and hospitalization (see Chapter 49 for patient experience). This procedure has a success rate greater than 95% and a low rate of complications. Until the early 1980s, stones located more proximally required removal by open ureterolithotomy, open pyelolithotomy, or in the case of a staghorn calculus, nephrolithotomy. However, in recent years two new techniques, *percutaneous nephrostolithotomy* (PCNL) and *extracorporeal shock wave lithotripsy* (ESWL), have supplanted traditional open stone removal operations. Both techniques give results similar to operative stone removal but are associated with less convalescent time and less morbidity.

PCNL requires that the patient be sedated and an IVP be performed to localize the kidney and the stone. Under fluoroscopy, a percutaneous nephrostomy tube is placed near the posterior axillary line. Subsequently, the tract is dilated and various nephroscopes, buckets, and forceps are used to extract the calculi. For struvite (triple phosphate, or "infection") calculi (see "Struvite Stones," below), *hemiacidrin (Renacidin) irrigation* is sometimes useful to dissolve residual stones. Antegrade radiographs are performed to confirm stone removal and ureteral patency. Successful removal occurs in more than 95% of renal stones and 88% of ureteral stones. On the other hand, PCNL is associated with a significant incidence of complications including hemorrhage (5 to 12%), AV fistulae (0.6%), perforation/extravasation (5 to 26%), and fever or sepsis (3 to 11%) (15). Typically, a 2- to 3-day hospitalization is needed for a patient to undergo PCNL.

The number of centers providing ESWL has multiplied rapidly in recent years. ESWL sometimes requires that the patient have anesthesia (usually spinal), but most often it is performed with just intravenous

sedation, after which the stone is located by ultrasound or fluoroscopically. A shock wave, generated by an electrode similar to a spark plug, is focused by the lithotripter for a precise impact on the stone (Fig. 47.1). When the shock wave encounters materials (calculus) with different acoustic properties from surrounding tissue, a tensile force is produced that shatters that material. This treatment takes an average of 30 to 45 minutes. ESWL usually is done in outpatient settings. Following ESWL, fragments of stone generally pass in the urine for a few days and usually cause mild

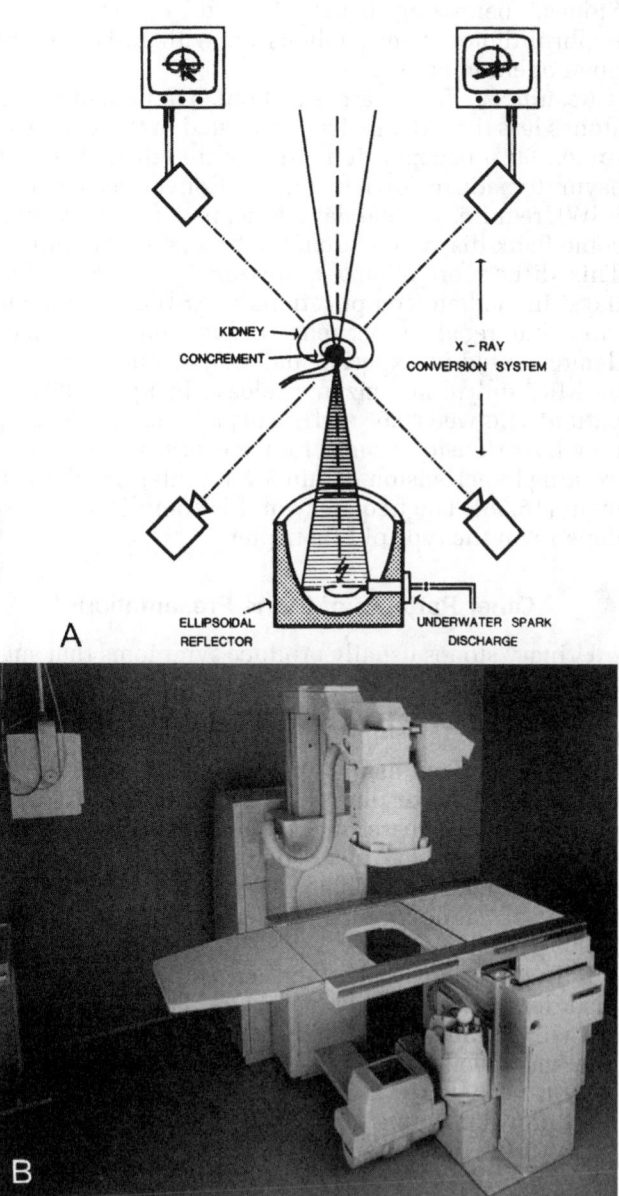

Figure 47.1.   **A.** Schematic drawing of the technical arrangement of a modern lithotripter. (From Chaussey C, Schmidt E, Jocham D. Non-surgical treatment of renal calculi with shock waves. In: Roth RA, Finlayson BF, eds. Clinical management of urolithiasis. Baltimore: Williams & Wilkins, 1993.) **B.** Photograph of a modern lithotripter. (Courtesy of Domier Medical Systems, Inc, Kennesaw, GA.)

colic. Retreatment is needed in a few patients, and macroscopic hematuria occurs transiently in most.

The selection of treatment modalities for a given patient depends in part on the characteristics of the stone being treated and in part on local resources and expertise. Where all modalities are available, ESWL used alone is the treatment of choice in 70% of patients. Patients suitable for treatment using ESWL are those with single or multiple renal stones less than 20 mm in diameter, some smaller staghorn stones (those in which the pelvis is not dilated), and some stones located in the upper third of the ureter. Larger calculi, most staghorn calculi, and calculi composed of cystine (see "Cystine Stones," below) are usually treated by percutaneous nephrolithotomy in combination with ESWL, or by open operation alone.

Results of ESWL are excellent. Of patients with stones less than 10 mm in size located in the kidney or ureter, 90% become stone free or are left with small, asymptomatic residual fragments. Convalescence from ESWL requires several days. Most patients experience some flank discomfort from the trauma to the kidney. This discomfort often requires analgesics for a few days. Immediate complications of ESWL are uncommon, but renal or perirenal tissue injury has been demonstrated in experimental studies and suggested by MRI and tissue enzyme release in up to 85% of patients. Between 0.65 and 8% of patients may develop new hypertension or experience exacerbation of preexisting hypertension within 3 years after ESWL treatment (16,28). The frequency of this complication may depend on the type of lithotripter.

Other Patterns of Stone Presentation

Urinary stones usually produce symptoms that suggest acute colic, at least at some time in their course. When stones are discovered in patients who do not have colic, these patients demand the same evaluation and management (see "Diagnostic Workup of Patients with Urinary Stone Disease," below) as do patients who have passed a stone associated with colic.

Table 47.1. Classification of Stone-Forming Patients by Type of Stone Passed

Type of Stone	Coe Series (1431 Patients)	Other Series Combined (1870 Patients)
Calcium oxalate (with or without phosphate)	69[a]	63.2[a]
Calcium phosphate	2	7.4
Calcium and uric acid	10	
Uric acid	2	5.4
Cystine	1	2.5
Struvite	7	21.5
Unknown	10	

From Coe FL. Nephrolithiasis: pathogenesis and treatment. Chicago: Year Book Medical Publishers, 1988.
[a]All values expressed as percentages of patients in each category.

Table 47.2. Metabolic and Clinical Disorders in 989 Calcium Oxalate Stone Formers

Disorders	No. of Patients (%) Men	Women
Systemic Disease		
Primary hyperparathyroidism[a]	26 (4)	24 (10)
Sarcoid	6 (1)	1 (1)
Cushing's syndrome	5 (1)	1 (0.4)
Paget's disease	1 (0.1)	4 (2)
Renal tubular acidosis, type I	7 (1)	4 (2)
Enteric hyperoxaluria[b]	39 (5)	13 (5)
No Systemic Disease		
Idiopathic (hereditary) hypercalciuria	213 (29)	121 (49)
Hyperuricosuria	126 (17)	9 (4)
Both disorders	120 (16)	22 (9)
No metabolic disorders[c]	186 (26)	52 (11)
Total	**729**	**249**

From Coe FL. Nephrolithiasis: pathogenesis and treatment. Chicago: Year Book Medical Publishers, 1988.
[a]Seventeen additional patients had primary hyperparathyroidism; either their stones were admixed with uric acid, struvite, or cystine; they had stones with no calcium; or their stone type was unknown.
[b]Includes primary hyperoxaluria (three patients) and hyperoxaluria as a consequence of intestinal bypass for obesity.
[c]Urinary citrate data not available. Hypocitraturia has been found alone or in combination with other disorders in 19% of hypercalciurias.

TYPES OF STONES AND THEIR CAUSES

There are four main types of urinary calculi: calcium oxalate or phosphate, uric acid, struvite–triple phosphate (magnesium ammonium phosphate), and cystine. Calcium stones are by far the most common. Table 47.1 shows the classification of stone-forming patients by the type of stone passed.

It is important to be familiar with the metabolic disorders these patients may have. This understanding will be helpful in planning a diagnostic evaluation and specific therapy (see the diagnosis and treatment sections later in this chapter). This is particularly true in the evaluation of the patient with the most common stone type: calcium.

Calcium Stones

Table 47.2 shows the metabolic and clinical disorders in calcium stone formers. This table shows that in almost 80% of patients who have had a calcium stone, the cause is known. In addition to the common disorders shown in the table, other metabolic disorders, such as hypocitraturia, may promote urinary calcium salt precipitation. Hypocitraturia is present as the sole metabolic abnormality in 10% (22) and as one of two or three abnormalities in 19% (25) of calcium stone formers. Urine pH, which affects the prevalence of many types of stones (see "Urinalysis," below), has little influence on the formation of calcium oxalate stones, but calcium phosphate stones are promoted with a pH greater than 6. The approach to these disorders is discussed later in this chapter.

Uric Acid Stones

Uric acid stones are caused by the high insolubility of undissociated uric acid (pK of 5.7, i.e., 50% of uric acid is undissociated at pH 5.7, 90% is undissociated at pH 4.7). Three factors are associated with uric acid stone formation: hyperuricosuria, highly acid urine, and low urinary volume. The lifetime incidence of uric acid stones in the general population is very low (Table 47.3). On the other hand, uric acid stones are very prevalent in patients who have gout, asymptomatic hyperuricemia, and hyperuricosuria, and probably in patients with a history of gout and no hyperuricemia. Many patients have passed uric acid stones long before a gouty attack has occurred. It is known that many patients with gout produce an abnormally high fraction of their daily acid load as titratable acid rather than as ammonium and therefore have an unusually low average urinary pH. Furthermore, patients with chronic diarrhea or patients with excessive fluid loss from the skin may have highly concentrated urine, which predisposes them to the formation of uric acid calculi. Patients who have myeloproliferative disease and those who have solid tumors that are undergoing lysis may have excessive uric acid excretion, which may be associated with uric acid stones and tubular plugs of urate. Patients with gout also have more calcium stones than people in the general population (29). The association may result from crystallization of uric acid, which then forms a nidus for calcium deposition.

Struvite Stones (Infection Stones)

It is generally believed that infection stones form primarily as a consequence of the hydrolysis of urea and the production of ammonium by the bacterial enzyme urease. The production of ammonia leads to a highly alkaline urine, which promotes the precipitation of magnesium, ammonium, and phosphate. These are the components of the infection-induced or struvite stone. Most urea-splitting organisms are *Proteus* species; however, *Pseudomonas, Klebsiella, Staphylococ-*

Table 47.3. Prevalence of Uric Stones in Various Populations

Population	Lifetime Incidence (%)
General population	0.01
Patients with gout	22
Hyperuricosuria in primary gout[a]	
<300 mg/24 hr	11
300–699 mg/24 hr	21
700–1100 mg/24 hr	35
>1100 mg/24 hr	50
Hyperuricemia in men[b]	
7–8 mg/dL	12.7
8–9 mg/dL	22
>9 mg/dL	40

[a]From Yu T-F, Gutman AB. Uric acid nephrolithiasis in gout. Ann Intern Med 67:1133, 1967.

[b]From Hall AP, Barry PE, Dawber TR, McNamara PM. Epidemiology of gout and hyperuricemia. Am J Med 42:27, 1967.

Table 47.4. Urinary Cystine Excretion

Normal individuals	<100 mg
Heterozygotes for cystinuria	150–300 mg
Homozygotes for cystinuria	>600 mg

cus, and some *Escherichia coli* strains are capable of producing urease. Struvite stones do not form de novo but almost always are a complication of another primary stone disease in which infection has become superimposed, and they are especially likely to grow into staghorn calculi (large stones that cannot pass the ureteropelvic junction and that form a cast of all or a portion of the pelvicaliceal system).

Cystine Stones

Cystine stones are rare and usually are seen in young patients because the onset is usually in childhood. The stone forms because of crystallization of cystine when the urine is supersaturated with this substance, which occurs when there is an inherited defect in renal tubular resorption of filtered cystine. This is a particularly virulent form of stone disease and may be associated with staghorn calculi. In addition to cystinuria, there is usually urinary loss of other basic amino acids, including ornithine, lysine, and arginine. The disorder is an inherited autosomal recessive trait, although some heterozygous patients have excess cystine excretion, as is shown in Table 47.4. Cystine is much less soluble in acid urine than it is in alkaline urine; therefore, cystine stones generally form when urine is acid and cystine excretion is greater than 400 mg/24 hours.

NATURAL HISTORY OF URINARY STONE DISEASE

Urinary calculus disease is a chronic illness. Once a stone has formed there is a tendency for recurrence, and management should be tailored to the stone activity, the type of stone, and any associated metabolic abnormality.

Stone activity—the number of stones formed and the change in size of existing stones—is an important, although at times difficult, determination. It requires a yearly review of stones passed and removed, as well as an evaluation by abdominal radiograph of the increase in size of known stones or the appearance of new stones. The activity of urinary calculi depends on a number of factors: stone type, associated metabolic abnormality, treatment received (both specific and nonspecific), and age. Therefore, precise rates of recurrence cannot be given with real accuracy.

Nevertheless, two studies provide useful and corroborative information regarding the recurrence rate after passing a first urinary stone. In one retrospective study of 515 patients followed after a single (first) stone and no medications to prevent a recurrence, there was a 50% recurrence rate at approximately 9 years and about a 75% recurrence rate by 25 years (23). These data are presented as a graph in Figure 47.2. Another study of patients who passed their first calcium stone showed a recurrence in half of the patients by 5 years and in two-thirds by 9 years (2).

Therefore, it is suggested that evaluation for associated metabolic abnormalities be undertaken in every patient who has formed a new stone because recurrence is likely, the basic assessment is noninvasive and inexpensive, and a workup may uncover an especially virulent or important systemic disease or metabolic defect responsible for stone formation.

DIAGNOSTIC WORKUP OF PATIENTS WITH URINARY STONE DISEASE

Evaluation of patients with stone disease can be accomplished entirely in an ambulatory setting. This evaluation depends on a directed history and physical examination, stone analysis if available, and certain laboratory measurements. The extent of the evaluation of patients passing a first stone is somewhat controversial. Some suggest an abbreviated evaluation because not all patients have recurrent stones and because all treatment modalities have potential side effects; others, citing the likelihood of eventual recurrence, fully evaluate patients after the first stone passage (see Coe et al., 1992, in "General References"). A U.S. National Institutes of Health (NIH) consensus development conference on the prevention and treatment of kidney stones (see "General References") suggests a minimum workup of first stone formers. The approach outlined in this section is a reasonable and commonly used method of evaluating patients who have had a urinary calculus.

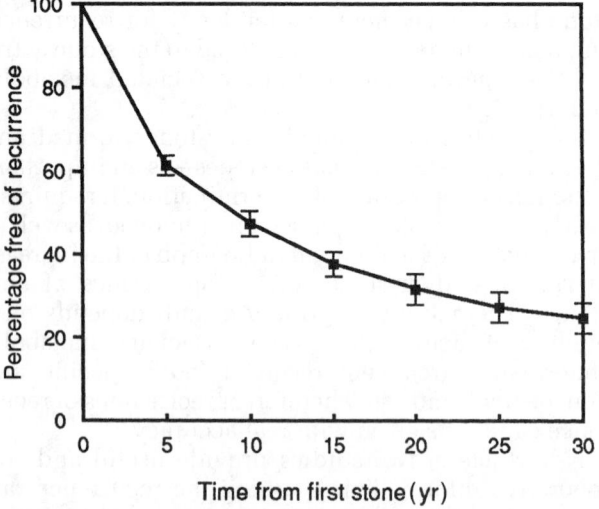

Figure 47.2. Life-table calculation of the time course of recurrence after a first renal stone in 515 patients. (Reproduced with permission from Sutherland JW, Parks JH, Coe FL. Recurrence after a single renal stone in a community practice. Miner Electrolyte Metab 11:267, 1985.)

History

A history is important in determining the activity of stone disease as well as in providing clues to the nature of the stone. The number of passed stones, the frequency of attacks of colic or hematuria, and the history of infection should be obtained. Previous abdominal radiographs and, most important, chemical analysis of prior stones should be obtained, if possible. *Family history* may provide a clue to cystine stones, uric acid stones (gout), and many calcium stones (e.g., those associated with idiopathic hypercalciuria). *Dietary history* may reveal excessive intake of sodium, animal protein, purine, or oxalate (see "Types of Stones and Their Causes," below). High-protein meat diets are associated with production of metabolic acids (which leech bone and cause hypercalciuria), increased urine excretion of urate, and decreased excretion of urinary citrate, all of which may predispose to the development of stone disease. The approximate daily *fluid intake* is also an important part of the history. Some people may ingest as little as 500 to 700 mL/day and thus have concentrated urine most of the day. *Medication history* is important. For example, aspirin at high dosages (more than 5 g/day) and probenecid are associated with increased uric acid excretion and may cause a predisposition to uric acid calculi. On the other hand, use of the xanthene oxidase inhibitor allopurinol has led to development of xanthene stones. Use of calcium-containing antacids (e.g., Camalox, Bisodol, Titralac, Tempo, or Tums) as well as vitamins A and D and loop diuretics (e.g. furosemide) may be associated with hypercalciuria and calcium stone formation. Acetazolamide (Diamox) may be associated with development of chronically alkaline urine and a higher incidence of calculi made of calcium phosphate. Vitamin C at high dosages may cause hyperoxaluria. Triamterene and its metabolites (10) and Acyclovir and Indinavir (11) have been found as the nidus in urinary calculi (or as the only constituent). Moreover, certain medications, such as thiazides or allopurinol, decrease calcium and uric acid excretion, respectively, whereas loop diuretics, conversely, promote hypercalciuria and interfere with results of testing in a patient who is being evaluated for renal stone disease. *Occupational history* is important because environmental temperature (and therefore fluid losses) and accessibility to fluids are factors that influence stone formation by promoting decreased output of highly concentrated urine.

Physical Examination

Physical examination (when there is no colic) occasionally gives clues to specific problems. For example, band keratopathy (stippled calcification of the perimeter of the cornea, which may require a slitlamp for visualization) may be seen in hyperparathyroidism, or there may be signs of sarcoidosis, hyperthyroidism, inflammatory bowel disease, neoplasia, or gouty arthritis. Most often, however, the examination is normal.

Urinalysis

The urinalysis provides a simple assessment that may give specific direction to the determination of the cause of the urinary calculus. It is important that the urinalysis be complete, including the determination of pH. The pH is usually acid in patients with a uric acid or a cystine stone and is invariably alkaline in patients with struvite stones. Also, the pH may suggest the presence of renal tubular acidosis: The first voided morning urine is usually acid, so finding a urine pH above 6.0 in this specimen suggests the possibility of renal tubular acidosis. The microscopic analysis may show hematuria (although this is often absent in the intercritical period), crystals, or evidence of infection. Crystals of cystine have the appearance of a benzene ring and are highly suggestive of cystinuria. Other crystals are more variable and are not diagnostic but may give a clue to the stone composition in patients with lithiasis (see photographs in Coe et al., 1992, ["General References"] for typical examples).

Stone Analysis

If a stone is available, it should be analyzed because the stone type determines the approach to evaluation and treatment. Stones can be analyzed inexpensively at commercial laboratories and may be mailed without preservative for this purpose.

Laboratory Assessment

A laboratory analysis is important even in patients in whom a stone is available for analysis (Table 47.5). This evaluation is necessary because it is increasingly recognized that many patients have more than one metabolic disorder that predisposes them to stone formation. For example, struvite stones often start as some other primary stone type, most often calcium; patients with a calcium oxalate stone may have hypercalciuria, hyperuricosuria, or hypocitraturia. Patients usually comply with the testing necessary for proper evaluation of a metabolic disorder if they understand the ease with which it can be accomplished, the substantial rate of recurrent calculi, and the effectiveness of specific therapy for different metabolic problems (see "Preventive Treatment of Urinary Calculus Disease," below). Furthermore, the 24-hour urine volume and sodium content provide objective guides to when the most basic interventions, such as increasing fluid intake (if urinary volume is low) or decreasing salt intake (if sodium excretion is high), are useful (see "General Measures," below).

Laboratory assessment of patients who have formed urinary calculi is simple and noninvasive and can be performed easily in the office. It is important that this initial evaluation be accomplished without modifying the patient's diet or habits so that an underlying process associated with urinary calculus disease is not masked. The reasons for obtaining most studies listed

Table 47.5. Laboratory Assessment of Patients with Urinary Calculi[a]

Measurement	Day of Testing	
	1	2
24-Hour urinary volume	√	√
24-Hour urinary calcium[b]	√	√
24-Hour urinary uric acid[c]		√
24-Hour urinary creatinine	√	√
24-Hour urinary oxalate	√	√
24-Hour urinary citrate	√	√
24-Hour urinary sodium	√	√
Urinalysis	√	
Urine cystine screen (cyanide–nitroprusside test)	√	
Urine culture (if pyuria)	√	
Urine pH (taken on first voided morning specimen collected under mineral oil)	√	
Serum calcium	√	√
Serum phosphorus	√	
Serum uric acid	√	
Serum chloride	√	
Serum bicarbonate	√	
Serum creatinine	√	
Serum urea nitrogen	√	

[a]During evaluation patients should follow their usual diet and life habits.

[b]The 24-hour urine container should contain 15 mL concentrated HCl (with warning to avoid contact).

[c]The 24-hour urine container should contain a few crystals of thymol to retard bacterial overgrowth.

in Table 47.5 are self-evident. Urinary creatinine is measured to monitor the completeness of collections and to estimate glomerular filtration rate. Urinary sodium (reflecting dietary intake) is measured because increased urinary sodium excretion promotes hypercalciuria. Serum calcium should be repeated at least once and ionized calcium determined, if possible, because the latter is a more accurate index of hypercalcemia. Urinary citrate should be measured in patients with calcium stones. Citrate combines with calcium to form a soluble complex, thus reducing the availability of calcium for crystallizing with oxalate or phosphate, and also directly inhibits crystallization of these substances.

An *IVP*, if not done previously as part of the evaluation of an episode of acute colic, should be done in an attempt to search for underlying structural disease (e.g., anatomic abnormality of the lower tract or medullary sponge kidney).

In addition to the laboratory assessment outlined in Table 47.5, *parathyroid hormone* should be measured if hypercalcemia (see Chapter 74) or hypophosphatemia is present, or if stone analysis indicates that the stone is made up of calcium phosphate. Finally, urinary oxalate should be measured when hyperoxaluria is suspected (Table 47.6). It is not done routinely because hyperoxaluria is uncommon and the analysis cannot be done reliably by all laboratories.

Hypercalciuria

Although calcium excretion varies somewhat with intake of calcium and of protein, generally the upper limits of calcium excretion for patients eating

Table 47.6. Situations in Which Hyperoxaluria May Be Expected

Hereditary overproduction (usually virulent stone disease with frequent recurrences and nephrocalcinosis, often occurring before age 12 years)
Methoxyflurane anesthesia (immediately after)
Ethylene glycol ingestion (immediately after)
Chronic inflammatory bowel disease affecting the ileum, ileal resection, or small bowel bypass
Cellulose phosphate ingestion (during entire period of ingestion)
Oxalate gluttony (tea, spinach, rhubarb)

a normal diet are 250 mg/24 hours for women and 300 mg/24 hours for men. Patients with *hypercalciuria without hypercalcemia* deserve special attention because they are seen commonly and because of the variable pathogenesis of their stones. Table 47.7 lists the causes of hypercalciuria that may not be associated with hypercalcemia.

Most patients have idiopathic hypercalciuria from either a *renal leak* (renal hypercalciuria, 5% of stone formers) or *excessive gastrointestinal absorption* of calcium (absorptive hypercalciuria). In the latter, which is far more common, there is excess gastrointestinal absorption (and then excretion) of calcium after the ingestion of calcium. The differentiation of renal from absorptive hypercalciuria requires the use of an *oral calcium tolerance test* (18), which is not routinely recommended in a general medical office practice but should be performed by a nephrologist or urologist specializing in stone disease. However, it is important to be aware that some patients with absorptive hypercalciuria may have normal calcium excretion if they inadvertently restrict their calcium intake on the day of the urine collection. Therefore, it is advantageous to ensure that the patient is continuing a usual diet for a few days before and during the metabolic evaluation.

PREVENTIVE TREATMENT OF URINARY CALCULUS DISEASE

General Measures

Patients who have formed even a single stone should be educated about the nature of urinary calculi, their natural history, the importance of regular surveillance, and the effectiveness of therapy. Increasing fluid intake and eliminating dietary excesses or deficiencies will probably control calcium stone formation in many patients, although controlled studies providing proof of efficacy of dietary interventions are not available (21).

The decision to use specific therapy (especially pharmacologic therapy) must be made on an individual basis. The rate of stone recurrence for a large population of patients may not apply to an individual patient. It is prudent to use only general and dietetic therapeutic measures if the patient has passed only a single stone and has no evidence of urinary stones on radiograph. However, for recurrent stone formers or patients with radiographic evidence of stones, more specific measures should be used (see below).

Diet

Diet can play a role in most conditions in which stones form. Because obtaining a detailed diet history is often impractical in the office, it is usually helpful to have a dietitian or nutritionist evaluate the patient, both to determine dietary excesses or deficiencies and to begin to plan dietary therapy, depending on the results of the evaluation for metabolic abnormalities. Specific diet restriction is discussed under the various stone types later in this chapter.

Fluid Intake

A low urine volume, reflecting low fluid intake, is common in many stone formers. Regardless of the type of stone that has been formed, a patient should maintain a high intake of fluids to ensure a urinary output of 3 to 4 L/day. This high urinary output prevents supersaturation, and the high flow rate may wash out small crystalline formations before they produce any obstructive or irritative symptoms.

Patients who have had several urinary stones are likely to continue to do so. Such patients should be prescribed a high fluid intake throughout the day and night (20). This can be accomplished by having the patient drink 3 L through the day and then take one or two glasses of water before retiring. This should result in a nocturnal diuresis necessitating voiding 3 to 4 hours later, at which time a further ingestion of one or two glasses of water will continue the diuresis until morning. Although annoying to the patient, once the habit is formed it is a small nuisance compared with subsequent stone formation. Continuing to encourage patients is critical to the success of the treatment program.

Avoidance of Dehydration

Patients should be counseled to avoid dehydration and, consequently, concentrated urine when participating in sports and during travel or work.

Table 47.7. Causes of Hypercalciuria that May Not Be Associated with Hypercalcemia

Idiopathic hypercalciuria
Administration of loop diuretics (furosemide, ethacrynic acid, or bumetanide)
Excessive salt ingestion
Exogenous adrenal corticosteroids
Cushing's syndrome
Paget's disease of bone
Immobilization
Progressive bone disease
Malignant tumors
Hyperthyroidism
Sarcoidosis
Renal tubular acidosis
Other causes of metabolic acidosis
Medullary sponge kidney
Severe phosphate deprivation

Specific Therapy for Calcium Stone Formers

Calcium is present in most urinary calculi, and hypercalciuria is the most common disorder uncovered during the evaluation of patients with urinary calculus disease. In addition to the general measures described earlier in this chapter, there are several specific therapies.

Dietary Measures

Because dietary calcium restriction usually results in a fall in urinary calcium excretion, it has been advocated for patients with calcium stones and hypercalciuria. However, no controlled studies have confirmed the efficacy of this measure. In fact, in two large analyses, dietary calcium was found to be *inversely* related to the risk of developing renal calculi, with a 46% reduction of risk in men and a 35% reduction of risk in women ingesting the highest versus the lowest quintile dietary calcium (6,7). Although the mechanism whereby higher dietary calcium might protect against stones is uncertain, it is known that greater calcium binding of gut oxalate results in decreased oxalate absorption and reduction of urinary oxalate excretion. Therefore, apart from its likely increase in urinary stones, dietary calcium restriction may actually cause significant additional effects, such as reduced bone mineral density and negative calcium balance. Thus, dietary calcium restriction is no longer recommended as a general policy in treating calcium stones. On the other hand, supplemental calcium (e.g., calcium carbonate tablets) has been shown to be a risk factor for renal calculi and should be avoided in patients with renal stones (6,7).

A number of authorities suggest limiting animal protein intake to 1 g/kg daily in patients with renal calculi. In addition to increasing calcium excretion, dietary animal protein intake increases excretion of uric acid and lowers urinary citrate excretion (probably because of acid production consequent to animal protein catabolism). These latter two changes predispose to formation of calcium stones. Recent reports demonstrate a direct relationship between animal protein intake and calcium stone formation (6,7). However, no controlled or prospective trials have reported on the impact of protein restriction on renal calculi formation.

Similar circumstantial data suggest that high dietary potassium intake and prevention of hypokalemia may independently reduce the risk of calcium stones. Thus, potassium bicarbonate, but not sodium bicarbonate, reduces calcium excretion (13), and potassium deprivation increases calcium excretion (14). Furthermore, a higher dietary potassium intake was associated with a 50% reduction in the risk of calcium stones (6). It seems sensible, then, to avoid hypokalemia and, when indicated, to provide alkali (citrate) as the potassium salt (see "Potassium Citrate," below). Finally, because dietary sodium chloride enhances calciuria, all patients with calcium stones should have modest restriction of dietary salt.

Thiazide Diuretics

Thiazide administration has been shown to result in a fall in urinary calcium excretion by as much as 50 to 60% within a day or two. Thiazides are an ideal theoretical choice (if hypokalemia is avoided) in the treatment of renal hypercalciuria, but thiazides also seem to be effective in absorptive hypercalciurias and even in patients with calcium stones associated with normal calcium excretion. Many studies attest to a 60 to 90% efficacy of a thiazide in reducing the frequency of calcium stones in all types of stone formers. Although there are serious methodologic concerns about some of these studies (4), two prospective trials demonstrate at least a 50% reduction in stone relapse in patients taking thiazide (9,12) and most experts consider thiazide the drug of choice in hypercalciurics. However, because of their tendency to raise serum calcium, thiazides should be avoided in patients already hypercalcemic (e.g., those with hyperparathyroidism or sarcoidosis).

Any thiazide diuretic may be used, but trichlormethiazide (2 to 4 mg) or hydrochlorothiazide (25 to 50 mg) twice daily, or chlorthalidone (25 to 50 mg) once daily are most commonly prescribed. The exact dosage of thiazide to be used for the prevention of urinary calculi is uncertain. The incidence of side effects was nearly 35% in one early study (27) using a 50-mg dose of hydrochlorothiazide of twice a day, the regimen that usually resulted in maximal hypocalciuria. Most side effects were seen soon after initiation of the drug. Intolerance of thiazides can be limited to less than 10% of patients by gradually increasing the dosage, and reducing the dosage if side effects develop. Although thiazides elevate the plasma uric acid level (see Chapter 69), this is not detrimental to patients with urate stones. Chapter 46 provides a discussion of the management of the hypokalemic complications of thiazides. If a potassium-sparing diuretic is used, amiloride, 5 to 10 mg daily, is the drug of choice. Also, a preparation containing amiloride and hydrochlorothiazide (e.g., Moduretic) may be used. Triamterene should not be given because of the association of this agent with the formation of urinary calculi (see "History," above). The best choice for prevention or treatment of thiazide-induced hypokalemia is the addition of oral potassium citrate (see the next section). This provides both potassium and base. The latter increases urinary citrate, which is reduced as a consequence of thiazide therapy (17). Citrate therapy has also been useful in hypercalciuric patients who continue to form stones despite thiazide therapy, presumably by increasing urinary citrate concentration (see the next section) (19).

Potassium Citrate

Potassium citrate (e.g., Polycitra-K, Urocit-K) is useful in many metabolic conditions associated with renal stones. Potassium citrate is prescribed at a dosage of 0.5 to 2 mEq/kg per day in two to four doses daily. Its usefulness results from the alkalinizing effect on the urine (for calcium stones associated with renal tubular acidosis, hyperuricosuria, and diarrheal syndromes, and for uric acid and cystine stones); an increase in urinary citrate, a natural inhibitor of stone formation (for calcium stones associated with hypocitraturia); and a mild reduction in calciuria. In a placebo-controlled prospective randomized trial, 30 to 60 mEq potassium citrate daily reduced stone events by 90% compared with placebo and to pretreatment rates in hypocitraturic calcium stone formers (1).

The goals of treatment are to provide enough base to increase urinary pH to 6.0 and 7.0 and to restore normal urinary citrate excretion (more than 320 mg/day and as close as possible to the normal mean of 640 mg/day). Twenty-four-hour urinary citrate or urinary pH measurement should be obtained to determine the adequacy of the initial dosage. Once an acceptable level is achieved it should be confirmed every 6 to 12 months.

Orthophosphate (Inorganic Phosphate)

The administration of inorganic phosphate (e.g., K-Phos) has been shown to reduce urinary calcium and the formation of calcium stones, in part by complexing gut calcium and thereby decreasing absorption, and in part by increasing urine inhibitors of stone formation. Although some trials suggest that orthophosphate reduces renal calculi (24), others do not, and no controlled trial is available. Because of the large doses required and the high incidence of gastrointestinal side effects, this therapy is discouraged for patients without consultation from a nephrologist.

Cellulose Phosphate

Taken with meals, this ion-exchange resin (Calcibind) binds calcium so it is not absorbed. Early trials suggest that this agent might be useful in hyperabsorptive hypercalciuria, but the only controlled trial did not show efficacy (4). Because the incidence of significant side effects including osteoporosis may be high, cellulose phosphate is not recommended without consultation with a nephrologist.

Patients with Calcium or Uric Acid Stones Who Are Found to Have Hyperuricosuria

Patients with calcium stones who have hyperuricosuria or those who have mixed calcium and uric acid stones should be treated as if they had pure uric acid stones.

If purine gluttony is present, hyperuricosuria can be modified by dietary restriction of purine-rich food, such as liver, kidney, and fish roe. However, gluttony is not often the problem, and other means are necessary.

Uric acid stone formation can be significantly modified by *increasing the urinary pH;* increasing the pH of the urine from 4.5 to 5.5 or 6.5 increases uric acid dissociation from 15 to 40% and 80%, respectively. Alkalinization can be accomplished by the administration of sodium bicarbonate several times a day. However, because sodium bicarbonate often causes gas and gastrointestinal discomfort, citrate salts (e.g., Polycitra-K solution containing 2 mEq of base per milliliter) are more palatable and therefore preferable. Most patients require 10 mL three times a day, but the dosage should be adjusted as necessary based on the results of regular urine pH testing. The metabolism of citrate results in the generation of bicarbonate. During the initial week of treatment and periodically thereafter, the patient should be taught to measure the urinary pH several times a day to ensure proper alkalinization (urine pH greater than 6.5).

Should these agents not be effective in controlling recurrence of uric acid stones, if the urine pH cannot be kept above 6.5, or if uric acid excretion is above 650 mg, *allopurinol* (which decreases uric acid production) may be used and effectively reduces stone recurrence. Allopurinol (Zyloprim, available in 100- and 300-mg tablets) should be initiated at a dosage of 100 mg once a day and raised to a level that controls uric acid excretion to below 500 or 600 mg/24 hours (doses greater than 300 mg are divided in two daily doses). Complications from allopurinol are usually minor (minor skin rash, drug fever, or precipitation of an acute gouty attack); the drug should be discontinued when a skin rash or fever occurs because diffuse fatal systemic vasculitis has been reported. The use of allopurinol is especially important as a preventive measure in patients who have excess uric acid excretion because of a myeloproliferative disease or in anticipation of tumor lysis.

Hyperoxaluria

In patients with hyperoxaluria, the aim is lower oxalate excretion (normal excretion is less than 45 mg/day). Treatment depends to some extent on the cause of hyperoxaluria. Reduction of foods with high oxalate content (spinach, rhubarb, chard, nuts, cocoa, and chocolate) helps in many cases of mild hyperoxalemia. The most common setting of severe hyperoxaluria and oxalate stones is in patients with malabsorption, especially in cases of ileal resection. In such circumstances, gut calcium, which ordinarily precipitates with oxalate, binds instead to fats, allowing oxalate to be readily absorbed. Treatment in such circumstances may be complicated and might include reducing dietary oxalate and fat, supplementing calcium and magnesium, prescribing cholestyramine resin to bind oxalate, administering potassium citrate, and recommending high fluid intake. Nephrology consultation for help in managing this complex problem is appropriate.

Cystinuria

Stone formers with cystinuria generally have particularly virulent disease and are best treated in consultation with a nephrologist. Generally it is necessary to raise urinary pH in a manner similar to the method used in patients with uric acid stones (see "Uric Acid Stones," above) and, if stone activity continues, to use d-penicillamine or tiopronin (fewer side effects), which form complexes with cystine and prevent its precipitation.

Struvite or Infection Stones

Infection stones are particularly virulent. Untreated patients with infected staghorn calculi often develop sepsis and require urgent nephrectomy. In addition, when the disease is bilateral, there is an associated 25% mortality rate in 5 years (26). In view of this morbidity and with the recent advance in techniques for controlling infection stones, early urologic referral is suggested. The goal of surgery in such patients is to remove the stone totally. This may be done by a variety of approaches. The mortality for these procedures in skilled hands is less than 1%. Application of hypothermia combined with a technique permitting the kidney to be bivalved has permitted great success in total stone removal with preservation of renal function. However, there is still a high recurrence rate. Also, percutaneous nephrostolithotomy may be used for smaller stones. This procedure usually requires that the stone be broken up by a shock wave probe (ultrasonic lithotripsy) (see "Patient Requiring Urologic Referral," above). In another treatment the stone may be perfused and dissolved by an acid solution—hemiacidrin (Renacidin)—using a percutaneous catheter placed antegrade into the pelvis of the kidney (8).

In addition to the surgical treatment of stone disease, medical therapy is an important adjunct. Associated metabolic abnormalities should be sought and treated. Specific antimicrobial therapy is necessary in conjunction with surgery, and where stones cannot be removed surgically, suppressive therapy with antimicrobials may decrease the incidence of septicemia. The use of oral agents that prevent infecting bacteria from splitting urea (urease inhibitors) has been shown to decrease recurrence of some struvite stones by preventing the formation of highly alkaline urine caused by the ammonium produced by urea-splitting organisms. Acetohydroxamic acid (Lithostat) may be used as an adjunct to antimicrobial therapy and surgery in patients with struvite stones. Acetohydroxamic acid, 250 mg, three to four times a day or a total dosage of 10 to 15 mg/kg per day (but never more than 1.5 g/day) should be used only when the patient is infected with urea-splitting organisms, as evidenced by a high urinary pH. Because of its teratogenic effects, it is contraindicated in women who are pregnant. Also it is not effective in the presence of moderate renal failure (i.e., creatinine 2.5 mg/dL or higher or creatinine clearance 20 mL/minute). Side effects occur in nearly 30% of patients and some are serious, such as thrombophlebitis and hemolysis. Experience with the drug is still limited, and consultation with a urologist is appropriate before prescribing it.

Urinary Calculi in Patients Without an Identifiable Metabolic Disorder

Approximately 10 to 15% of stone formers found after evaluation not to have a metabolic disorder may respond to thiazides or allopurinol, as outlined earlier (5).

General References*

Coe FL, Favus MJ, Pak CYC, et al. Kidney stones: medical and surgical management. Philadelphia: Lippincott-Raven, 1996.
> A multiauthored textbook that covers all aspects of stone disease.

Coe FL, Parks JH, Asplin JR. The pathogenesis and treatment of kidney stones. N Engl J Med 327:1141, 1992.
> This review covers medical aspects of urinary stone disease and provides an extensive documentation of the literature.

National Institutes of Health. Consensus Development Conference on Prevention and Treatment of Kidney Stones. J Urol 141:705, 1989.
> A useful consensus statement.

Preminger GM. Is there a need for medical evaluation and treatment of nephrolithiasis in the "age of lithotripsy?" Semin Urol 12:51, 1994.
> Reviews classification, evaluation, and treatment of urinary calculi.

Specific References

1. Barcelo P, Wuhl O, Servitge E, et al. Randomized double-blind study of potassium citrate in idiopathic hypocitraturia calcium nephrolithiasis. J Urol 150:1761, 1993.
2. Blacklock NJ. The pattern of urolithiasis in the Royal Navy. In: Hodgkinson A, Nordin BE, eds. Renal Stone Symposium. London: Churchill, 1969;33–47.
3. Chaussy CG, Fuchs GJ. Current state and future developments of noninvasive treatment of human urinary stones with extracorporeal shock wave lithotripsy. J Urol 141:782, 1989.
4. Churchill DN. Medical treatment to prevent recurrent calcium urolithiasis. A guide to critical appraisal. Miner Electrolyte Metab 13:294, 1987.
5. Coe FL. Treated and untreated recurrent calcium nephrolithiasis in patients with idiopathic hypercalciuria, hyperuricosuria, or no metabolic disorder. Ann Intern Med 87:404, 1977.
6. Curhan GC, Willett WC, Rimm ER, Stempfer MJ. A prospective study of dietary calcium and other nutrients and the risk of symptomatic kidney stones. N Engl J Med 328:833, 1993.
7. Curhan GC, Willett WC, Speizer FE, et al. Comparison of dietary calcium with supplemental calcium and other nutrients as factors affecting the risk for kidney stones in women. Ann Intern Med 126:497, 1997.
8. Dretler SP, Pfister RC, Newhouse JH. Renal stone dissolution via percutaneous nephrostomy. N Engl J Med 300:341, 1979.
9. Ettinger B, Citron JT, Livermore B, et al. Chlorthalidone reduces calcium oxalate calculous recurrence but magnesium hydroxide does not. J Urol 139:679, 1988.
10. Ettinger B, Oldroyd NO, Surgel F. Triamterene nephrolithiasis. JAMA 244:2443, 1980.
11. Kopp JB, Miller KD, Mican JAM, et al. Crystalluria and urinary tract abnormalities associated with Indinavir. Ann Intern Med 127:119, 1991.
12. Laerum E, Larsen S. Thiazide prophylaxis of urolithiasis: a double-blind study in general practice. Acta Med Scand 215:383, 1984.
13. Lemann J Jr, Gray RW, Pleuss JA. Potassium bicarbonate, but not sodium bicarbonate, reduces urinary calcium excretion and improves calcium balance in healthy men. Kidney Int 35:688, 1989.
14. Lemann J Jr, Pleuss JA, Gray RW, Hoffman RG. Potassium administration reduces and potassium deprivation increases urinary calcium excretion in healthy adults. Kidney Int 39:973, 1991.
15. Lingeman JE. Lithotripsy and surgery. Semin Nephrol 16:487, 1996.
16. Lingeman JE, Woods J, Toth PD, et al. The role of lithotripsy and its side effects. J Urol 141:793, 1989.
17. Nicor MJ, Peterson R, Sakhaee K, et al. Use of potassium citrate as potassium supplement during thiazide therapy of calcium nephrolithiasis. J Urol 131:430, 1984.

*Bold print (general references) and bold numerals (specific references) denote published controlled clinical trials, meta-analyses, or consensus-based recommendations.

18. Pak CYV, Kaplan RA, Bone H, et al. A simple test for the diagnosis of absorptive, resorptive and renal hypercalciurias. N Engl J Med 292:497, 1975.
19. Pak CYC, Peterson R, Sakhaee K, et al. Correction of hypocitraturia and prevention of stone formation by combined thiazide and potassium citrate therapy in thiazide-unresponsive hypercalciuric nephrolithiasis. Am J Med 79:284, 1985.
20. Pak CY, Sakhaee K, Crowther C, Krinkley L. Evidence justifying a high fluid intake in treatment of nephrolithiasis. Ann Intern Med 93:36, 1980.
21. Parivar F, Low RK, Stoller ML. The influence of diet on urinary stone disease. J Urol 155:432, 1996.
22. Preminger GM. The metabolic evaluation of patients with recurrent nephrolithiasis. A review of comprehensive and simplified approaches. J Urol 141:760, 1989.
23. Sutherland JW, Parks JH, Coe FL. Recurrence after a single renal stone in a community practice. Miner Electrolyte Metab 11:267, 1985.
24. Thomas WC Jr. Use of phosphates in patients with calcareous renal calculi. Kidney Int 13:390, 1978.
25. Wilson DM. Clinical and laboratory approaches for evaluation of nephrolithiasis. J Urol 141:780, 1989.
26. Wojewski A, Zajaczkowski T. The treatment of bilateral staghorn calculi of the kidneys. Int Urol Nephrol 5:249, 1974.
27. Yendt ER. Medical management of calcium stones. In: Roth RA, Finlayson B, eds. Stones: clinical management of urolithiasis. Baltimore: Williams & Wilkins, 1983;187–209.
28. Yokoyama M, Shoji F, Yanagizawa R, et al. Blood pressure changes following extracorporeal shock wave lithotripsy for urolithiasis. J Urol 147:553, 1992.
29. Yu T-F, Gutman AB. Uric acid nephrolithiasis in gout. Predisposing factors. Ann Intern Med 67:1133, 1967.

CHAPTER 48

Chronic Renal Insufficiency

GARY R. BRIEFEL, MD

Renal insufficiency, either presenting as a primary renal event or complicating another illness, is a common clinical problem. The understanding of the reasons why patients who have renal insufficiency progress to renal failure has increased, and the ability to modify the natural history has improved. Because patients with beginning stages of renal insufficiency are first discovered by the primary care provider, it is important to be familiar with the initial phases of the evaluation and management.

The healthy kidney performs a wide variety of functions that contribute to the maintenance of the internal environment of the body. In addition to its role in maintaining the balance of water and electrolytes, the kidney has important endocrine and metabolic functions. It produces hormones responsible for normal bone formation (1,25-dihydroxyvitamin D_3), red blood cell production (erythropoietin), and blood pressure control (renin, prostaglandins). The kidney is responsible for degrading a number of polypeptide hormones, including parathyroid hormone, insulin, gastrin, and prolactin. Also, the kidney serves as a major excretory route for many toxic metabolic wastes and a wide variety of drugs or their breakdown products.

In parallel with the progressive destruction of renal mass that occurs with many chronic kidney diseases, patients pass through a sequence of clinical stages before reaching *end-stage renal disease* (ESRD, the point when dialysis is required). The divisions between these stages are somewhat arbitrary and may vary between patients; nevertheless, these distinctions are useful in predicting the kinds of abnormalities that are to be expected for any given degree of renal dysfunction. Frequent reference to the glomerular filtration rate (GFR) throughout this chapter should not be interpreted to mean that the precise value of this measurement must be known in order to manage the patient. Before end-stage renal disease the blood urea nitrogen (BUN) and serum creatinine concentrations are often within the normal range, despite a fall of the GFR to as low as 50 mL/minute. Signs and symptoms, if present during this stage, are usually attributable to the underlying disease (e.g., diabetes mellitus, hypertension). As renal function declines further (GFR 20 to 50 mL/minute), the BUN and serum creatinine levels become noticeably increased and some metabolic abnormalities appear (e.g., metabolic acidosis, carbohydrate intolerance, and reduced synthesis of 1,25-dihydroxyvitamin D_3). Also at this point, the kidney's ability to respond to acute changes in body fluid and electrolyte composition is reduced. In this stage of renal insufficiency, although the BUN and serum creatinine concentration are increased (azotemia), symptoms attributable to the retention of nitrogenous wastes are absent. However, the patient may begin to experience symptoms related to anemia (fatigue), loss of urine-concentrating ability (polyuria), or volume expansion (dyspnea or edema). When the GFR falls below 20 mL/minute (serum creatinine concentration usually greater than 5 mg/dL), the patient enters the stage of renal failure. This stage is associated with a further reduction in the ability of the kidney to maintain homeostasis and is characterized by multiple biochemical abnormalities (e.g., hypocalcemia, hyperphosphatemia, and metabolic acidosis) and fluid overload. The term *uremia* is used to describe the entire set of signs, symptoms, and metabolic disturbances that occur in advanced kidney failure (GFR less than 10 mL/minute, serum creatinine concentration usually greater than 8 mg/dL) and that may affect virtually all organ systems. Examples of some uremic manifestations include nausea, vomiting, anorexia (gastrointestinal tract), lassitude, reversal of the sleep cycle (nervous system), heart failure, hypertension (cardiovascular system), pruritus (skin), and infertility (endocrine system).

EPIDEMIOLOGY OF CHRONIC RENAL INSUFFICIENCY

There is excellent information on the epidemiology of patients who require renal replacement therapy (dialysis or renal transplantation) and enter the ESRD Program (the Medicare-funded program that provides coverage for virtually all patients in the United States needing dialysis). These data are collected and analyzed by the federally funded United States Renal Disease System (USRDS) (41). At the end of 1993, more than 217,000 patients were being treated for ESRD under the Medicare program in the United States with either dialysis or kidney transplantation. That is, 1 of every 1264 residents of the United States is being treated for ESRD. Since 1972, the year Medicare coverage was extended to patients with chronic renal failure who needed dialysis, the incidence of end-stage renal failure in patients who enter dialysis and transplant programs has increased from 71/million per year to more than 214/million per year in 1992 (41). In actual numbers, 57,000 new patients entered the ESRD Program in 1993 and this figure has been increasing yearly by almost 9%. The incidence of ESRD requiring dialysis has been noted to be 30 to 40% higher in men than in women and to peak between the ages of 65 and 74 years. The rate has also been estimated to be from three to four times greater in nonwhites than in whites, because of either higher prevalence of hypertension or a greater end-organ sensitivity to the effect of hypertension in nonwhites (Fig. 48.1).

The reported distribution of patients entering the End-Stage Renal Disease Program by primary diagnosis is as follows: diabetic nephropathy, 35.7%; primary hypertensive disease, 29.1%; glomerulonephritis, 11.7%; interstitial nephritis, 2.9%; cystic kidney disease, 2.9%; collagen vascular disease, 2.1%; obstructive nephrology, 1.9%; acquired immunodeficiency syndrome (AIDS) related, 0.5%; miscellaneous/unknown, 11% (41). Although patients with AIDS-related renal diseases are a small fraction of the total, the incidence rate has doubled between 1990 and 1992 from 0.67 to 1.4 new patients/million.

CLASSIFICATION

Kidney diseases are often classified according to whether they produce acute or chronic renal failure. *Acute renal failure* (ARF) is defined as a deterioration of glomerular filtration that occurs over days or weeks, whereas the course of *chronic renal failure* often runs from months to years. Many diseases that cause ARF are reversible, and recovery is often complete (e.g.,

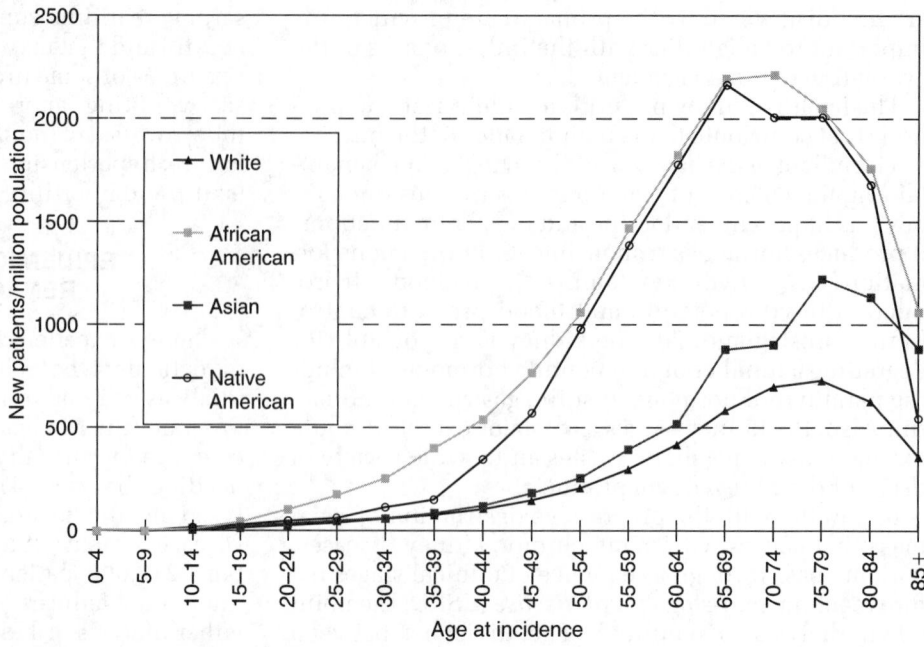

Figure 48.1. Incidence of treated end-stage renal disease by race and age. Rates are per million population. Includes Medicare patients only. (Modified from Agodoa LYC, Held PJ, Port FK, eds. US Renal Data System, USRDS 1996 annual data report. Bethesda, MD: National Institute of Diabetes, and Digestive and Kidney Diseases, 1996.)

aminoglycoside nephrotoxicity). ARF is not commonly encountered in the ambulatory setting, but may be seen with obstruction, drug nephrotoxicity (angiotensin-converting enzyme [ACE] inhibitors), or rapidly progressive glomerulonephritis. Recovery from diseases that produce chronic renal failure is less common. It should be emphasized that some illnesses that produce ARF may not be entirely reversible and can progress to end-stage renal disease (e.g., Goodpasture's syndrome and acute cortical necrosis). Conversely, some chronic forms of renal disease can improve spontaneously or with therapy and may never progress to the point of requiring dialysis treatments (e.g., membranous glomerulopathy or the nephropathy of systemic lupus erythematosus).

The causes of kidney failure may be further subdivided into those with prerenal, renal, or postrenal components. *Prerenal azotemia* is caused by factors that produce a decrease in renal perfusion. Diminished perfusion may result from anatomic lesions such as might occur with renal artery stenosis, but more commonly it is related to decreased cardiac output (heart failure), vasodilation (septic shock), or volume depletion (vomiting or excessive diuretic use). Prerenal azotemia caused by volume depletion, for example, may often be superimposed on existing chronic renal failure from other causes. *Postrenal azotemia* is caused by obstructing lesions that occur distal to the kidney parenchyma involving the renal pelvis, ureters, bladder, or urethra. Common examples of such lesions include prostatic enlargement, nephrolithiasis, and retroperitoneal cancers.

Most diseases that cause chronic renal failure directly involve the kidney parenchyma and are classified according to the anatomic region that is primarily affected (Table 48.1). *Glomerular lesions* can be caused by proliferation of endothelial or mesangial cells (e.g.,

postinfectious glomerulonephritis), thickening of the basement membrane (e.g., membranous glomerulopathy, diabetic nephropathy), glomerulosclerosis (e.g., focal sclerosis), or combinations of the three (e.g., membranoproliferative glomerulonephritis). Any of the diseases that cause glomerular lesions, if sustained, can lead to what is called chronic glomerulonephritis. Clinically, glomerular diseases are often associated with hypertension, edema, renal insufficiency, hematuria, and proteinuria.

Diseases that affect primarily the tubulointerstitial areas of the kidney are characterized morphologically by interstitial inflammation, fibrosis, and tubular atrophy. In the past these lesions were often equated with bacterial infections of the kidney (pyelonephritis), but most are caused by toxins (e.g., analgesics, heavy metals), metabolic derangements (e.g., hyperuricemia, hypercalcemia), or immunologic disorders (e.g., methicillin-induced interstitial nephritis). The glomeruli are only secondarily involved in the tubulointerstitial diseases. *Polycystic and medullary cystic kidney diseases* are a subgroup of the tubulointerstitial nephropathies and are characterized histologically by the presence of a multitude of thin-walled cysts derived from tubular epithelium. Patients with interstitial forms of kidney disease are not usually hypertensive or edematous, and they often produce large volumes of urine with high sodium contents. Typically, nonnephrotic range proteinuria (less than 3 g/day), sterile pyuria, and hyperchloremic metabolic acidosis are present.

Lesions of the renal vessels may be located in the main renal arteries (e.g., atherosclerosis, fibromuscular dysplasia), medium-sized arteries or arterioles (e.g., polyarteritis nodosa, scleroderma), or the renal veins (e.g., renal vein thrombosis). Renal insufficiency is a result of a reduction in blood flow to the glomeruli.

Involvement of the renal vessels is often a part of a systemic illness that also affects vessels in other areas of the body. The clinical features of the renal vasculitides are very similar to those of glomerulonephritis except that nephrotic range proteinuria (more than 3 g/day) is uncommon.

A number of renal diseases can variably affect one or more of the kidney's anatomic regions. For instance, renal involvement in *multiple myeloma* may take the form of a diffuse thickening of the glomerular basement membrane (light-chain nephropathy), or more often it causes a tubulointerstitial nephropathy. *Systemic lupus erythematosus* is another example of a disease that can produce either glomerular or tubulointerstitial damage.

Renal diseases can be further subclassified according to whether they are congenital, part of a systemic disorder, primary to the kidney, or the result of injury. The congenital or hereditary diseases most often encountered are polycystic kidney disease and Alport's

Table 48.1. Classification of Kidney Diseases that May Result in Chronic Renal Failure

Prerenal Diseases
Renal artery stenosis S
Hepatorenal syndrome S

Renal Parenchymal Diseases
Glomerular diseases
  Membranous glomerulonephritis (GN) I
  Membranoproliferative GN I
  Focal glomerulosclerosis I
  HIV nephropathy S
  Rapidly progressive GN I
  Goodpasture's syndrome I, S
  Lupus nephritis I, S
  IgA nephropathy I
  Alport's syndrome (hereditary nephritis) H, S
  Diabetic glomerulosclerosis M, S
Tubulointerstitial diseases
  Drug-induced interstitial nephritis N*
  Chronic pyelonephritis with reflux
  Analgesic nephropathy N
  Radiation nephritis N
  Polycystic kidney disease H, S
  Sickle cell nephropathy S
  Heavy metal nephropathy N
  Gouty nephropathy M, S
  Medullary cystic disease H
Vascular diseases
  Thrombotic thrombocytopenic purpura S
  Hemolytic-uremic syndrome S
  Scleroderma kidney S
  Hypertensive nephropathy S
  Vasculitis I,S
  Wegener's granulomatosis I, S
Miscellaneous
  Myeloma kidney N, S
  Amyloidosis S

Postrenal Diseases
Nephrolithiases
Bilateral ureteral obstruction
Bladder outlet obstruction

H, Hereditary; *I*, immunologically mediated; *M*, metabolic; *N*, nephrotoxic; *S*, part of a systemic disorder.
[a]See Table 48.3.

form of hereditary nephritis. Diabetes mellitus and hypertension are the two most common systemic disorders producing chronic renal failure, and one or other of these diseases is listed for approximately 62% of the patients entering dialysis programs. Immunologic injury to the kidney can be in the form of glomerular immune complex deposition, as in systemic lupus erythematosus, or antiglomerular basement membrane antibody disease, best exemplified by Goodpasture's syndrome. Most immunologically mediated diseases affect predominantly the vessels or glomeruli, but they can also damage the tubulointerstitial areas, as in a drug-induced interstitial nephritis (e.g., methicillin). Drugs (e.g., phenacetin) or toxins (e.g., heavy metals) most often produce damage to the interstitium. Metabolic disorders (e.g., diabetes mellitus, oxalosis) can result in damage to any region of the kidney.

PATHOPHYSIOLOGY OF UREMIA

The course of many chronic kidney diseases is characterized by the progressive loss of functioning nephrons. The kidney undergoes a number of adaptive changes that allow most patients with chronic renal failure to have few signs or symptoms until 80% of the original number of nephrons have been lost.

Once a certain level of renal impairment has been reached, further deterioration seems to be inevitable, even when the original insult is transient and when other causes of additional damage have been excluded. An example of this phenomenon is the course of renal disease after ureteral reimplantation in patients with vesicoureteral reflux and mild renal insufficiency. Even in the absence of continuing reflux or infection, some of these patients will, in time, develop proteinuria and progressive renal insufficiency. Renal biopsies in these patients reveal glomerulosclerosis.

The mechanism that has been postulated to explain the progressive nature of renal disease is related to the adaptive response to injury (8). According to this hypothesis, after a reduction in nephron mass, renal vasodilation occurs and leads to hyperperfusion of the remaining glomeruli. These changes are considered to be adaptive because they result in increased glomerular filtration rates. However, experiments show that this state of *glomerular hypertension,* if sustained, can in itself be harmful (Fig. 48.2). Glomeruli of nephrons exposed to prolonged hyperperfusion begin to leak protein, become sclerotic, and eventually are destroyed. Recent theories implicate toxicity from the filtered proteins, perhaps mediated by release of cytokines or other inflammatory products, as an important mechanism of renal parenchymal damage. As more and more nephrons are lost, the stimulus for hyperperfusion of the residual nephrons is increased and the process becomes self-perpetuating. There is evidence that many diseases that produce limited kidney damage (e.g., patchy cortical necrosis, analgesic nephropathy, radiation nephritis) may progress to end-stage disease by this mechanism.

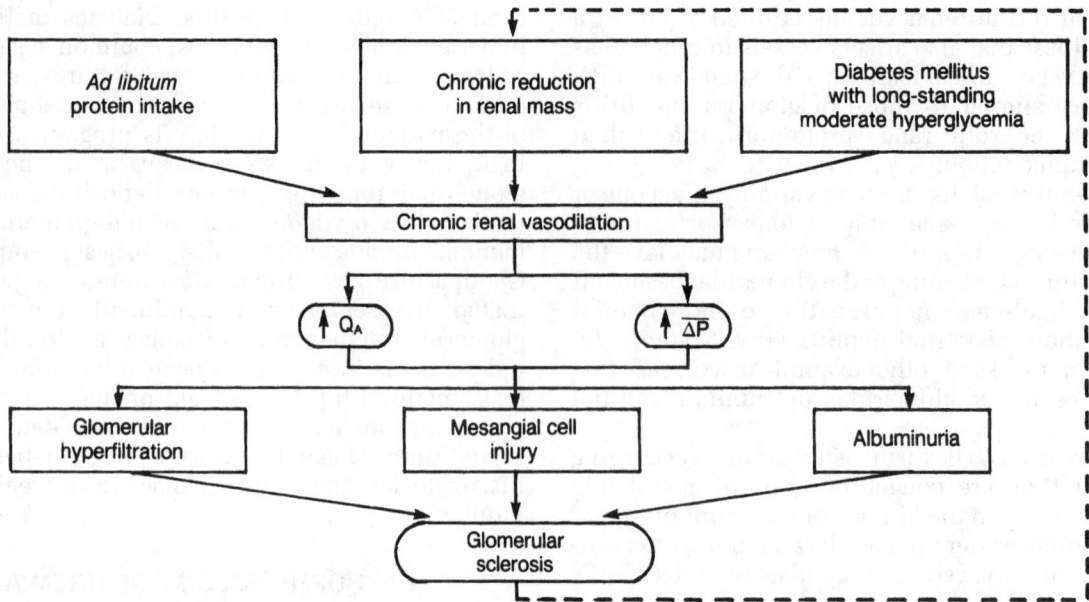

Figure 48.2. Proposed sequence of events whereby a chronic reduction in kidney mass and the consequent increase in glomerular pressures and flows lead to progressive renal damage. Q_A, Blood flow; ΔP, transcapillary hydraulic pressure. (Redrawn from Brenner BM, Meyer TW, Hostetter TH. Dietary protein intake and the progressive nature of kidney disease: the role of hemodynamically mediated glomerular injury in the pathogenesis of progressive glomerular sclerosis, aging, renal ablation, and intrinsic renal disease. N Engl J Med 307:652, 1982.)

The ability of the impaired kidney to maintain the concentrations of individual components of the body's fluids within normal limits is variable. The concentrations of substances that are simply filtered and neither secreted nor resorbed by the tubule, such as urea, begin to rise early in the course of renal impairment (GFR 50% of normal). In contrast, the serum concentration of phosphorus, which is under the influence of parathyroid hormone (PTH), is kept within the normal range until more than 80% of renal function is lost. This is because in renal failure increased PTH activity progressively reduces the amount of phosphorus resorbed by the tubule (normally 80% of filtered phosphorus is resorbed) in parallel with the reduction in renal mass. Once the GFR falls below 20% of normal, this mechanism can no longer keep pace, and the serum phosphorus level begins to rise. Other solutes, such as sodium and potassium, are even better regulated, and their concentrations are maintained within the normal range until the GFR is less than 5 mL/minute.

Eventually the reserve capacity of the kidney is overwhelmed and a number of signs, symptoms, and metabolic abnormalities appear that are characteristic of uremia (Table 48.2). Uremia is a complex syndrome that results from the failure of the kidney to fulfill its excretory, endocrine, and metabolic functions. In the patient with end-stage renal disease, virtually every organ system is affected to some degree. The mechanisms for only some of the abnormalities that appear in uremia are well understood. Efforts to explain the metabolic consequences of renal failure by the retention of toxic wastes are only partially satisfying. Because urea is easily measured, it is the putative toxin that has been most thoroughly examined. Other nitrogenous waste products (e.g., ammonia, guanidinosuccinic acid), middle molecules (polypeptides of intermediate molecular weight), and a variety of organic and inorganic compounds have been implicated in the pathogenesis of uremia. Each of these toxins, individually or together, potentially could interfere with a specific cellular metabolic function and give rise to a manifestation of uremia.

Not all manifestations of uremia can be attributed to the retention of metabolic waste products. Many well-described endocrine and metabolic derangements are of equal significance in the pathogenesis of uremia. A deficiency of certain hormones results when the failing kidney is no longer able to produce them in adequate quantities (e.g., erythropoietin, 1,25-dihydroxyvitamin D_3). Other hormones normally degraded or metabolized by the kidney may be present in excess (e.g., PTH, insulin, prolactin). Alternatively, the damaged kidney may elaborate an excess of hormone (e.g., renin). Hormone levels or activity may also be altered as a consequence of abnormal protein binding (e.g., thyroid hormone), peripheral resistance (e.g., insulin, parathyroid hormone), or loss of feedback control (e.g., luteinizing hormone).

DIAGNOSIS OF CHRONIC RENAL INSUFFICIENCY

Presentation

Kidney disease can most easily be recognized when it is associated with clearly defined clinical symptoms such as urinary tract obstruction or laboratory findings such as proteinuria or hematuria. The recognition of one of these abnormalities is helpful in focusing the ensuing diagnostic evaluation. Often, the presence of renal disease is discovered during the evaluation of a systemic disease of which renal dysfunction is only a part (e.g., diabetes mellitus, hypertension).

Because of the remarkable reserve and adaptive capabilities of the kidney, symptoms of uremia do not appear until glomerular filtration is reduced to 10 to 15% of normal. Therefore, unless clearly overt signs of renal involvement are present (e.g., gross hematuria), many patients progress to advanced renal failure asymptomatically. In other patients, whose renal insufficiency is detected early in its course by routine blood tests, specific findings on history and physical examination may also be absent. Special laboratory testing in these patients often permits establishment of a definitive diagnosis. The complete evaluation may vary from brief evaluation in the patient with advanced renal failure and markedly shrunken kidneys to extensive evaluation in the patient who may have potentially

Table 48.2. Major Physiologic and Clinical Abnormalities of Uremia

Fluid and Electrolyte Abnormalities
Volume expansion
Hyperkalemia
Hypocalcemia
Hyperphosphatemia
Metabolic acidosis

Endocrine–Metabolic Abnormalities
Vitamin D deficiency
Hyperparathyroidism
Carbohydrate intolerance
Impotence and infertility
Hypertriglyceridemia

Hematologic–Immunologic Abnormalities
Impaired platelet function
Abnormal T- and B-cell function
Anemia

Cardiovascular Abnormalities
Hypertension
Accelerated atherosclerosis
Pericarditis

Dermatologic Abnormalities
Pruritus
Increased pigmentation
Acne

Gastrointestinal Abnormalities
Nausea and vomiting
Anorexia
Pancreatitis

Neuromuscular Abnormalities
Peripheral neuropathy
Seizures
Coma
Asterixis
Myoclonus

reversible disease of recent onset. Most of the evaluation can be performed on an ambulatory basis.

History and Physical Examination

Findings in the history and physical examination can provide useful information that helps establish the nature of the kidney disease, estimate its duration, and determine its effect on the patient. One of the major goals in evaluating the patient with recently identified renal failure is to distinguish patients with primary, acquired kidney diseases from those whose renal failure is caused by familial, congenital, or systemic illnesses.

First the family history should be reviewed for the presence of polycystic kidney disease, Alport's syndrome, medullary sponge kidney, hypertension, diabetes mellitus, or renal failure. The presence of a hereditary form of renal disease in the family should help establish the etiology of the patient's kidney problem. Next, the patient's medical history should be reviewed carefully, with a particular emphasis on discovering the presence of a systemic illness that can cause renal failure (e.g., hypertension, diabetes mellitus, collagen vascular disorders). Patients with AIDS may develop a nephropathy that presents with nephrotic syndrome and often progresses to renal failure (34). In the absence of symptoms related to a systemic illness, one needs to question the patient about symptoms associated with abnormalities of the urinary tract. Dysuria, frequency, renal colic, hesitancy, or urinary incontinence point to an abnormality of the lower urinary tract as the cause of the patient's renal dysfunction.

In addition to the symptoms that may prove useful in establishing a diagnosis, several symptoms (e.g., nausea, vomiting, fatigue, nocturia, itching, restless leg) are nonspecific. These "uremic" symptoms are present in most patients with advanced renal failure.

Because symptoms of renal failure often do not appear until late in the course of renal failure, it is sometimes difficult to pinpoint the time of onset of the disease. Important clues can occasionally be found when records of past physical examinations performed for work, insurance, or military purposes are reviewed.

Because drugs may either be the cause of renal dysfunction (e.g., heroin, analgesics, nonsteroidal anti-inflammatory drugs [NSAIDs], aminoglycosides) or aggravate preexisting renal insufficiency (e.g., diuretics) (Table 48.3), there should be a complete inventory of past and current drug use.

The physical examination should be focused on a search for signs of systemic illnesses and for genitourinary structural abnormalities. These might include high blood pressure, hypertensive or diabetic retinopathy, vascular bruits, vasculitic skin rashes, gouty tophi, or ocular abnormalities (e.g., band keratopathy of hypercalcemia). Enlarged kidneys to palpation may be found in patients with polycystic disease or hydronephrosis. A pelvic or rectal examination should be performed to evaluate causes of lower urinary tract

Table 48.3.   Some Commonly Used Drugs that May Adversely Affect Renal Function

Antibiotics
Aminoglycosides (ATN)
Penicillins (IN)
Tetracyclines (increased azotemia and acidosis)

Analgesics
Aspirin (PN and reduction in RBF)
Phenacetin (PN and IN)
Nonsteroidal analgesics (IN, nephrotic syndrome, and reduced RBF)

Diuretics
Thiazides (volume depletion and IN)
Loop agents (volume depletion and IN)

Miscellaneous
Radiocontrast materials (ATN)
Methysergide (retroperitoneal fibrosis causing obstructive uropathy)
Penicillamine (NS)
Gold (NS)
H_2-receptor antagonists (interfere with secretion of creatinine and produce false elevations of the serum creatinine concentration)
ACE inhibitors (precipitate renal failure in patients with renovascular disease)

ATN, Acute tubular necrosis; *IN,* interstitial nephritis; *NS,* nephrotic syndrome; *PN,* papillary necrosis; *RBF,* renal blood flow.

obstruction, such as prostatic or cervical cancer. When obstruction or flaccid neurogenic bladder is suspected, the bladder should be catheterized or evaluated by sonography after the patient voids to measure residual volume (see Chapter 6 for technique). A residual volume that is larger than approximately 200 to 300 mL should raise concern for bladder outlet obstruction (see Chapter 49) or neuropathic bladder (most commonly seen in diabetic patients). Signs of heart failure, pericarditis, or neuropathy are most often related to the stage of renal failure and are not helpful in establishing etiology.

Laboratory Investigation

Laboratory testing of patients with chronic renal insufficiency establishes the severity and etiology of the kidney disease, as well as determines the presence of complicating abnormalities.

Diagnostically, the *urinalysis* can often provide important information. Red blood cells (RBCs), particularly when associated with RBC casts, are most indicative of a glomerular or vascular lesion. In the presence of isolated hematuria, the presence of dysmorphic RBCs in the urinalysis can suggest an upper urinary tract source. White blood cells, with or without casts, are found in the interstitial nephropathies. Hyaline or granular casts are not indicative of a specific pathologic process.

The *urine dipstick* is only a rough guide to the amount of proteinuria (see Chapter 44). Most dipsticks are designed to detect only albumin and may therefore miss the presence of other proteins, such as light chains. The dipstick measures only the concentration of protein, so the reading must be interpreted in conjunction with the urine specific gravity. When

quantification of proteinuria is desired, a 24-hour urine specimen should be obtained and can also be used to calculate the creatinine clearance (see below). Alternatively, the protein/creatinine ratio may be determined in a specimen of urine as described in Chapter 44. The finding of nephrotic range proteinuria (more than 3 g/day) usually indicates a glomerular lesion, whereas lesser amounts are seen in some glomerular or vascular disorders and in most interstitial forms of nephritis (see Chapter 44). In patients over the age of 40 with unexplained renal insufficiency, regardless of the amount of urinary protein detected by dipstick, a serum and urine electrophoresis should be obtained to exclude the possibility of multiple myeloma.

Selected tests should be ordered when an *immunologically mediated disease* is suspected, such as in a patient with vasculitis or an unexplained nephritic picture (RBC casts, nephrotic proteinuria). For example, measurement of the serum complement levels (C3 and C4) and screening for the presence of antistreptococcal antibodies, antinuclear antibodies, rheumatoid factor, and cryoglobulins may be of value when collagen vascular disease or poststreptococcal glomerulonephritis is suspected. Measurement of antineutrophil cytoplasmic antibodies (ANCAs) is useful in diagnosing cases of systemic vasculitis, including Wegener's granulomatosis and polyarteritis nodosa. Hepatitis B surface antigen (see Chapter 43) can be demonstrated in the blood of some patients with membranous glomerulopathy and in some forms of vasculitic renal disease. Hepatitis C infections are associated with mixed cryoglobulinemia and membranoproliferative glomerulonephritis. Hepatitis B and C antigens and antibodies should also be assayed in any patient being referred for dialysis or transplantation because precautions to prevent the spread of hepatitis must be taken if the patient is a potential carrier. A test for human immunodeficiency virus (HIV) antibodies (see Chapter 34) should be performed in patients with nephrotic syndrome or renal failure who are at risk for

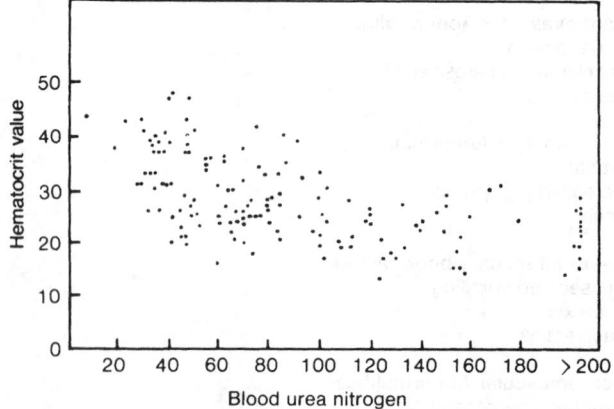

Figure 48.3.   Relationship of blood urea nitrogen concentration to the hematocrit value in patients with chronic renal failure. (From Erslev AJ. Erythrocyte function of the kidney. In: Wesson LG, ed. Physiology of the human kidney. New York: Grune & Stratton, 1969; 521.)

HIV infection. In general, a nephrologist should be consulted to help guide this workup.

The *severity of anemia* (see Chapter 50) roughly parallels the BUN, as shown in Figure 48.3. The absence of anemia in patients with renal insufficiency should suggest either recent onset, the presence of polycystic kidney disease, or hydronephrosis. Both polycystic kidney disease and hydronephrosis can be associated with normal or elevated hematocrit values. The peripheral blood smear should be examined carefully for abnormalities associated with diseases that can produce renal failure. Rouleaux formation may be present in multiple myeloma, and leukopenia may be associated with collagen vascular diseases. A microangiopathic hemolytic anemia can be seen in patients with thrombotic thrombocytopenic purpura, the hemolytic–uremic syndrome, postpartum renal failure, accelerated hypertension, or scleroderma.

Measurements of the concentration of blood glucose, serum electrolytes (Na, K, Cl, HCO_3, Ca, PO_4), and uric acid are helpful in monitoring the patient. Hypercalcemia may suggest a tumor or hyperparathyroidism. The uric acid level is usually elevated in patients with renal insufficiency, but a level greater than 12 mg/dL may indicate the presence of primary hyperuricemia or of a myeloproliferative disorder.

Some *measure of overall kidney function* is needed to determine the degree of impairment, monitor the progression of disease, assess the effects of therapy, and adjust the dosage of drugs that are excreted by the kidney. The GFR is the standard means of expressing the level of renal function. In clinical practice, the GFR may be estimated from the serum creatinine concentration, the endogenous creatinine clearance, or formulas that incorporate the patient's serum creatinine level, age, and weight.

The normal GFR is approximately 100 to 140 mL/minute in men and 85 to 115 mL/minute in women. A gradual deterioration of GFR with age occurs, even in the absence of overt renal disease, in 70% of individuals (29,38). The following equation may be used for estimating the expected creatinine clearance in healthy men.

$$GFR \text{ (mL/minute)} = 133 - 0.64 \times Age \text{ (years)}$$
$$(48.1)$$

The clearance for women aged 50 or greater is approximately 5 to 10 mL/minute less than for men. Thus, at age 70, for example, an individual without renal disease may have lost 30% of his or her previous GFR.

The serum creatinine concentration is a better indicator of renal function than is the level of BUN because the latter is affected by such nonrenal factors as volume status, diet, intestinal bleeding, liver function, and protein catabolism. The general relationship between the serum creatinine concentration and the GFR is shown in Figure 48.4. When trying to determine the extent of renal impairment, it is important to remember that the value of serum creatinine concentration for any level of GFR varies among individuals. This is because the relationship between

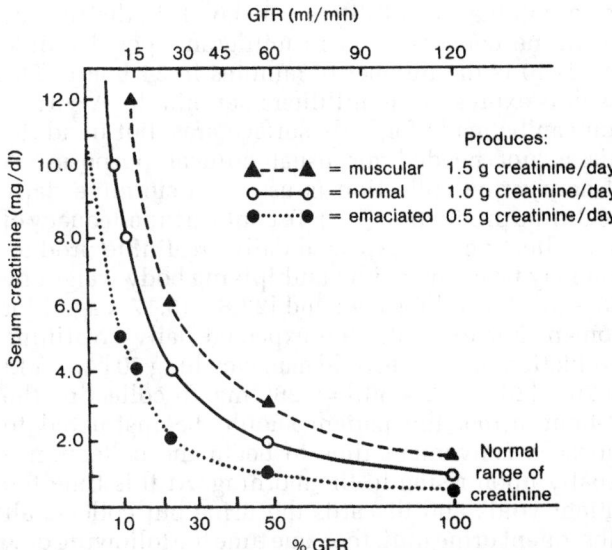

Figure 48.4. Relationship of the serum creatinine concentration to glomerular filtration rate in patients with different muscle mass.

the serum creatinine concentration and the GFR is significantly influenced by nonrenal factors such as the patient's muscle mass and age. Creatinine is produced by muscle, and its production rate directly parallels the muscle mass. The amount of creatinine produced per day also falls with age. As can be seen in Figure 48.4, a small or elderly patient may have a doubling of the serum creatinine concentration, from 0.8 to 1.6 mg/dL, and still have a level within the "normal" range. Also, a young muscular patient who produces 1.5 g of creatinine per day will have a GFR of 30 mL/minute when his or her serum creatinine concentration is 5 mg/dL, whereas an elderly, frail patient who produces only 0.5 g of creatinine per day will have a creatinine clearance of only 10 mL/minute at the same level of serum creatinine. Therefore, although an elevated serum creatinine almost always reflects abnormal renal function, a creatinine concentration in the "normal" range does not mean that GFR is normal, particularly if there is other evidence for the presence of renal disease. Once the factors affecting the level of serum creatinine concentration are understood, the physician should have a clinically useful measure of overall renal function.

Because of the difficulties in estimating the level of renal function from the serum creatinine concentration alone, alternative methods for estimating the GFR are available. These methods are generally used when adjusting dosages of drugs that are excreted by the kidney or when assessing renal function in elderly or small patients.

The endogenous creatinine clearance is a reasonable approximation of GFR in patients with normal or modestly reduced function but overestimates the GFR in advanced renal failure. The formula used for calculating clearance is UV/P divided by 1440, where U is the urine creatinine in milligrams per deciliter, V is urine volume in milliliters per day, P is the plasma creatinine concentration in milligrams per deciliter, and 1440 is the number of minutes in 24 hours. The result is expressed in milliliters per minute. A correction can be made for body surface area, but in adults this is not needed for usual clinical purposes. A 24-hour urine collection is used to determine daily creatinine production (UV). To confirm the adequacy of this collection, the expected daily creatinine production may be estimated by multiplying body weight by [28 − (0.2 × age)] for men and [23.8 − (0.17 × age)] for women. For example, the expected daily creatinine production in a 50-year-old man weighing 70 kg would be 70 × [28 − (0.2 × 50)] = 1260 mg. In collecting the 24-hour urine, the patient should be instructed to choose a convenient time to begin the collection—usually upon rising in the morning. At this time the patient voids and discards the urine but collects all subsequent urine until the same time the following day, when the patient again voids and adds that specimen to the collection. The blood sample for measurement of creatinine is generally obtained at the end of the collection period but may be drawn at any time during the collection. The estimation of the GFR by measuring creatinine clearance is often inaccurate, mainly because of collection errors. Although radionuclide measurements of GFR that do not require urine collection are available, there is rarely a need for such accuracy in office practice and these tests are reserved largely for research purposes.

An alternative to calculating the creatinine clearance that avoids the difficulties entailed in collecting urine samples and can be performed in the office is based on a formula that takes into account the patient's body weight and age:

$$(140 - \text{Age}) \times \text{Body weight in kg} \div \atop 72 \text{ (Serum creatinine concentration)} \qquad (48.2)$$

(The value should be multiplied by 0.85 in the case of a small woman.) It should be recognized that the value of GFR determined by the preceding formula or measured by creatinine clearance may vary significantly from the more accurate determination of GFR by inulin clearance. For clinical purposes, however, these differences are generally considered insignificant.

When monitoring the course of kidney disease, it should be recalled that the serum creatinine concentration increases in a nonlinear fashion as renal function declines (Fig. 48.4). In the early stages of renal insufficiency, when the GFR falls by 50%, the absolute increase in the serum creatinine concentration is small. Therefore, most of the loss of functioning nephrons occurs at levels of serum creatinine that would be considered only modestly elevated. Once the GFR is reduced to 20 to 30% of normal, the curve expressing the relationship between serum creatinine and GFR rises steeply. Absolute changes in the serum creatinine concentration when there is end-stage renal disease are therefore less significant, when related to losses of GFR, than those seen in early renal insufficiency.

Alternative methods of *monitoring the progression of renal disease* have been devised to overcome the limitations of using the serum creatinine concentration alone and because measuring sequential creatinine clearances is often impractical or improperly done. A plot of the reciprocal of the serum creatinine concentration ($[\text{Cr}]^{-1}$) versus time (Fig. 48.5) produces a function that parallels the rate of decline in GFR. In many but not all patients, the plot is linear, with the slope reflecting the rate of progression and the horizontal axis intercept the estimated time of end-stage renal failure. It has been suggested that the slope is constant for an individual and that any deviation reflects the effects of therapy or the presence of a superimposed process. One should be aware of the limitations to this method for monitoring renal function. Comparisons of

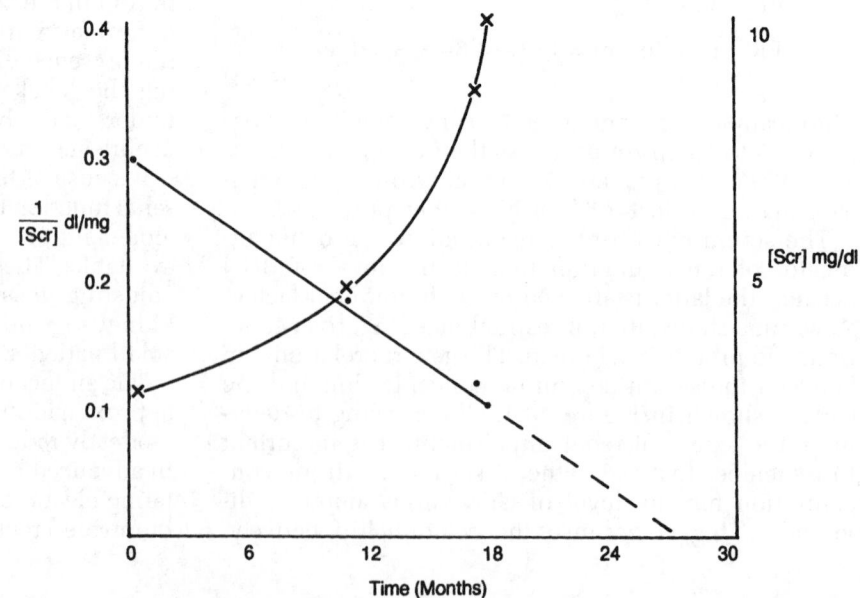

Figure 48.5. Relationship between the serum creatinine concentration ([Scr]) and the reciprocal of serum creatinine concentration (1/[Scr]) over time in a patient during an 18-month period. The linear relationship between the reciprocal of serum creatinine concentration over time suggests that nephrons are being lost at a constant rate. This kind of plot can also be used to monitor the course of renal failure. By extending the line derived from observed data it is possible to make a rough estimate *(dashed line)* of when dialysis will be necessary. [Scr] indicated by line with x marks, 1/[Scr] indicated by solid line.

$[Cr]^{-1}$ versus GFR measured with radioisotope techniques have disclosed discordances in up to 45% of cases (42). For example, the slope of $[Cr]^{-1}$ may overestimate or underestimate the rate of change of GFR using the radioisotope techniques. In some cases the slope of the $[Cr]^{-1}$ remained stable while true GFR declined or vice versa. These discrepancies are caused in part by changes in creatinine metabolism that occur in patients with renal failure. Therefore, mathematical formulations may be useful, but must be interpreted only in conjunction with the remainder of the clinical and laboratory information. It is also important to understand that changes in GFR (reflected by an increasing serum creatinine concentration or a falling creatinine clearance) are not necessarily related to permanent changes in intrinsic kidney function and may be caused by other factors (see "Treating Reversible Causes of Deterioration of Renal Function," below).

Renal Imaging Techniques

Anatomic and functional evaluation of the kidney can be obtained through a variety of tests, not all of which need be performed on any individual patient. Renal imaging techniques in chronic renal failure should be used to establish renal size, detect remediable lesions, and determine etiology.

Renal sonography is a reliable means of estimating kidney size and usually detects the presence of significant hydronephrosis. Because of the risk of radiocontrast dye toxicity in patients with renal impairment (see below), the sonogram should be used in place of the intravenous pyelogram (IVP) as the initial imaging technique in most instances. Median kidney length as measured by sonography is 11.2 cm on the left and 10.9 cm on the right. Renal size is slightly less in women than men and decreases with age in both sexes (11). An abdominal radiograph including kidneys, ureters, and bladder (KUB), with tomograms if necessary, is the simplest and least expensive test for estimating renal size but does not detect the presence of hydronephrosis. Normal kidney length as measured by radiograph is approximately 12 to 13 cm, or roughly the same as three to four lumbar vertebrae and discs. The kidneys appear longer when measured by radiograph because of a projection effect. Small kidneys by either technique usually indicate advanced chronic renal disease. However, normal or large kidneys may be seen in chronic renal failure (e.g., diabetes mellitus, amyloidosis).

Hydronephrosis caused by obstruction should be ruled out in every patient with chronic renal insufficiency. If the screening sonogram reveals the presence of hydronephrosis, a urologist should be consulted. Subsequent evaluation of the obstructed kidney by the urologist may include an IVP, a retrograde pyelogram, a computerized tomographic (CT) scan, or a sonographically guided percutaneous antegrade pyelogram. These evaluations are selected to localize the precise site of the obstruction and to identify its nature. The choice of the procedure depends on the preference of the urologist. However, an added advantage of the antegrade pyelogram technique is that it allows simultaneous placement of a percutaneous nephrostomy

Table 48.4.   Clinical Presentations of Atheromatous Renal Disease

Acute renal failure following reduction in blood pressure (particularly with ACE inhibitors)
Progressive azotemia in a patient with known renovascular disease
Azotemia associated with new-onset hypertension or a change in severity of hypertension
Unexplained azotemia in an elderly patient with peripheral vascular disease
Progressive renal failure with evidence of cholesterol embolization

Adapted from Jacobson HR. Ischemic renal disease: an overlooked entity? Kidney Int 1988;34:729.

tube for drainage. Occasional cases of nondilated hydronephrosis occur, so further evaluation is indicated, even when the sonogram is normal, when the suspicion of obstruction is high (e.g., a patient with a history of renal colic or intra-abdominal malignancy). HASTE magnetic resonance imaging (MRI) can be used to distinguish between acute and chronic obstruction (36).

The *IVP* is most useful in determining the etiology of renal failure in diseases that produce gross anatomic abnormalities such as chronic pyelonephritis, nephrolithiasis, or obstruction from papillary necrosis. Although the cysts in patients with polycystic kidney disease are detected by IVPs, renal ultrasound is a better screening technique. The IVP is not useful in patients with parenchymal disorders that are not associated with gross anatomic defects. The IVP is of value only when the creatinine concentration is relatively low (e.g., less than 2.0 to 2.5 g/dL); and when used in patients with renal insufficiency, IVP-associated dehydration could injure the kidney and could be avoided (see below).

CT scans, commonly believed to be useful in evaluating a patient with renal failure, should not be routinely used in the evaluation of patients with chronic renal disease. Their usefulness is limited, and a nephrologist should be consulted before ordering a CT scan.

Nuclear medicine imaging techniques, useful in the evaluation of patients with hypertension caused by unilateral renal artery stenosis, have been found to be less reliable in detecting bilateral renovascular disease (RVD). Bilateral atheromatous RVD, an often overlooked cause of renal failure (16), is more difficult to diagnose with radionuclide studies because the standard renal scan relies on asymmetric blood flow as a diagnostic criterion. When blood flow to both kidneys is reduced, it is difficult to distinguish bilateral renal artery stenosis from parenchymal diseases. Captopril renography, which depends on captopril-induced hemodynamic alterations (and is helpful in diagnosing unilateral renal artery stenosis in the absence of significant renal failure), may be of value and should be tried in patients with renal insufficiency and suspected bilateral RVD (Table 48.4), but unfortunately it often is not diagnostic (15). Doppler or duplex ultrasonography has been used as a screening tool for diagnosing bilateral renal artery stenosis, but they do not provide anatomic detail and are operator dependent. Because none of the noninvasive tests is of proven efficacy in diagnosing patients with presumed bilateral RVD, an arteriogram should be obtained when the index of suspicion is high and when a therapeutic decision (e.g., balloon dilation) would be made based on the results. Magnetic resonance or CO_2 angiography and intravenous digital subtraction angiography have been suggested as lower-risk methods of imaging the renal arteries; as technology improves they may replace the current imaging methods (23), but they are not yet available. For now, the use of intra-arterial digital subtraction rather than conventional arteriography is recommended because the risks of dye-induced ARF or atheroembolic disease appears to be reduced, probably because of the lesser amount of dye given and the use of smaller catheters. Given the complex decisions encountered when evaluating patients with suspected ischemic renal artery disease, a vascular surgeon and a nephrologist should be consulted before the arteriogram is ordered. The most difficult decisions arise in patients with probable diabetic nephropathy, who often have significant peripheral vascular disease. The decision to perform angiography is usually based on the clinical judgment that the course deviates from what is generally seen in diabetics, or when the vascular component seems prominent (severe hypertension, claudication, bruits). Because these patients often have multiple sites of atheromatous involvement, additional radiologic information beyond the renal arteries (views of the splenic or mesenteric arteries) may be required.

The incidence of *radiocontrast-induced ARF* seems highest in patients with renal insufficiency (serum creatinine concentration greater than 2 mg/dL), diabetic patients, or the elderly. However, some argue that the only significant risk factor is preexisting renal disease. Although incidence rates of ARF as high as 50% have been reported, most of these cases have been clinically insignificant and reversible. More recent reviews of ARF in high-risk patients have found lower rates of ARF (9 to 16%), and it has been suggested that a greater awareness of the role of pretest and posttest hydration may be proving to be of benefit (32). The use of low osmotic radiocontrast agents (sodium meglumine ioxaglate, iohexol) appears to reduce, but does not eliminate, the occurrence of postangiography ARF in patients with preexisting renal insufficiency (24). The benefits of giving mannitol infusions prophylactically are still unsettled. In summary, the presence of renal insufficiency should not be considered an absolute contraindication to the performance of intravascular dye studies, particularly when the needed information cannot be obtained by alternative means. Because the decline in renal function from radiocontrast materials appears to be particularly preventable by avoiding volume depletion, patients should be instructed to maintain salt (6 to 8 g/day) and fluid intake (1 to 2 L/day) both before and after the examination. Low osmotic radiocontrast agents should be used in patients who have preexisting renal insufficiency.

Renal Biopsy

Once the baseline data have been accumulated, a nephrologist should be consulted, at least by telephone, to help interpret the information and to decide whether a renal biopsy is indicated. The renal biopsy provides histologic information and for many disease entities is the most specific diagnostic test available. The biopsy should be considered when the diagnosis is uncertain, to estimate prognosis, to help demonstrate renal involvement of a systemic illness, and to help make therapeutic decisions. Most renal biopsies can be performed percutaneously using local anesthesia. Although overnight observation in the hospital is still common, some nephrologists perform renal biopsies in ambulatory surgery settings with 6- to 8-hour monitoring (see Chapter 44). If the kidneys are very small or if renal failure is advanced, a biopsy is usually not done.

MONITORING THE PATIENT WITH RENAL INSUFFICIENCY

The interval between visits is determined by the stage of renal insufficiency, the rate of progression, and the presence of complicating disorders. Early in the course, patients should have office visits scheduled every 4 to 6 months for monitoring of their symptoms, signs (e.g., weight, blood pressure, edema), and laboratory data (e.g., serum creatinine concentration, BUN, electrolytes, complete blood counts, urinalysis, and possibly creatinine clearance). As renal failure progresses, visits must be spaced more closely, usually at 1-month intervals until dialysis becomes necessary. Once the GFR falls below 10 mL/minute, clinical decisions are based more on the presence of symptoms or specific electrolyte abnormalities, such as hyperkalemia or acidosis, than on further changes in the serum creatinine concentration or creatinine clearance. Drug dosages should be reviewed at each visit and adjusted according to the degree of renal dysfunction (see "Drug Use in Renal Insufficiency," below).

COURSE AND PROGNOSIS

The underlying renal disease largely determines prognosis. Many renal diseases have characteristic rates of progression. For example, patients with polycystic kidney disease typically have very indolent courses and some never progress to end-stage renal failure. More aggressive courses, with advanced renal failure developing within months to a year, are more likely to occur in patients with diseases such as rapidly progressive glomerulonephritis, systemic sclerosis, or malignant hypertension. However, most renal diseases fall into an intermediate group, with end-stage renal failure developing within 1 to 5 years after the initial diagnosis.

Therapy

Goals

The goals of therapy fall into four major categories. The first is to treat the underlying renal disease, if possible (e.g., corticosteroids or chlorambucil for membranous nephropathy). The second is to slow the progression of renal deterioration by modifying the known or suspected factors that aggravate the primary process (e.g., treatment of hypertension, glomerular hyperperfusion) and to avoid factors that may aggravate existing renal failure (e.g., avoiding NSAIDs). The third goal is to treat the specific complications of renal disease (e.g., acidosis), as they occur, and to prevent the long-term complications of uremia before they can become fully established (e.g., secondary hyperparathyroidism). Finally, the patient should be referred to a dialysis and transplantation center well before the need for renal replacement therapy (see "Dialysis and Transplant," below).

Specific Treatments

Once a diagnosis is established, a nephrologist should be consulted to determine whether effective therapy is available for the patient's renal disease. In general, the earlier in the course a treatment is started, the more likely it is to be successful in halting or reversing the disease. When the patient's renal disease is advanced or the effectiveness of the treatment is not well established, it is often advisable to forgo potentially toxic therapies, as the hazards often outweigh the benefits.

Many immunologically mediated renal diseases (e.g., membranous nephropathy, Wegener's disease, Goodpasture's syndrome, lupus nephritis) may respond to treatment with corticosteroids, cytotoxic agents, or plasmapheresis. For others (e.g., IgA nephropathy), there is no proven effective therapy. Patients with immunologically mediated renal diseases who require therapy should be under the care of a rheumatologist or nephrologist.

When the renal disease is associated with a metabolic disorder such as occurs in diabetes mellitus, it is reasonable to treat the underlying abnormality (e.g., hyperglycemia). Treatment directed at metabolic control may slow the course of renal deterioration but is not likely to result in significant reversal of established disease. In fact, the cause-and-effect relationship between hyperuricemia and renal failure in patients with gout is debatable (43).

When a drug (e.g., methicillin, indomethacin) or other toxic substances (e.g., heavy metal) is identified as the cause of renal failure, the offending agent should be withheld or avoided. A trial of corticosteroids may be given to patients with drug-induced interstitial nephritis, but this treatment is still controversial and the decision should be made in conjunction with a nephrologist.

Vascular lesions in the kidney caused by malignant hypertension may resolve slowly and usually only partially with control of blood pressure. In some patients this correlates with significant improvement in the GFR. Patients with renal failure secondary to bilateral RVD may have significant improvement in their renal function after successful angioplasty or bypass surgery, particularly if intervention occurs before renal insufficiency becomes too far advanced (serum creatinine below 4 mg/dL).

Obstructing lesions of the urinary tract may require surgical excision (e.g., benign prostatic hypertrophy) or urinary diversion (e.g., retroperitoneal fibrosis) to preserve or improve renal function. Other patients can be managed more conservatively (e.g., intermittent straight catheterization of the bladder) if the lesion is not amenable to surgical therapy (e.g., flaccid neurogenic bladder).

Nonspecific Treatments

There are important treatment options that can reduce the rate of renal deterioration by as much as one-half, even when no specific therapies can be directed at the primary renal disorder. The first involves the use of protein-restricted diets to retard the progression of renal disease in order to delay or even obviate dialysis (7,31). The GFR in healthy animals and humans varies directly with protein intake. Dietary protein restriction has been shown in animal experiments, using various models of partial renal injury, to reduce the degree of compensatory hypertrophy (see "Pathophysiology of Uremia," above) and to forestall the development of glomerular sclerosis, proteinuria, and progressive renal failure. Dietary treatments have been extensively studied in humans as well (Fig. 48.6). The other intervention shown to protect the kidney is treatment of hypertension that is commonly found in renal diseases of all types. Most of the studies that investigated diet therapy and control of blood pressure divided the patient populations into those with and without diabetes. Therefore, the following discussion separates the interventions by patient population.

Despite several small studies that seemed to confirm the benefits of dietary protein restriction in humans, questions remained about the value of diet therapy in the treatment of chronic renal failure in people. Some, but not all, of these questions have been resolved by the recently completed Modification of Diet in Renal Disease (MDRD) Study (21). Patients with mild to moderate renal insufficiency (GFR 25 to 55 mL/minute) were randomized to either a usual (1.3 g/kg daily) or low protein (0.58 g/kg daily) intake. Patients with more advanced renal insufficiency (GFR 13 to 24 mL/minute) were randomized to low protein (0.58 g/kg daily) or very low protein intake (0.28 g/kg daily) with supplemental keto-amino acids. Both groups were further randomized into a usual (mean arterial pressure [MAP] = 107 mm Hg) or low blood pressure (MAP = 92 mm Hg) group. ACE inhibitors were used in a significant proportion of both groups. Using an intention-to-treat analysis, despite achieving dietary and blood pressure goals, there were no significant differences between the interventions on the rate of decline of GFR (measured by radioisotope techniques), the time until dialysis was required, or mortality. Although the mean protein intake between the groups were different, there was considerable variation and overlap between patients. When the data from the group with advanced renal failure were reanalyzed, correlating actual achieved dietary protein intake with GFR (controlling for other factors known to influence the rate of decline in GFR), it was concluded that within the range of protein intakes between 0.5 and 1.0 g/kg daily, a lower

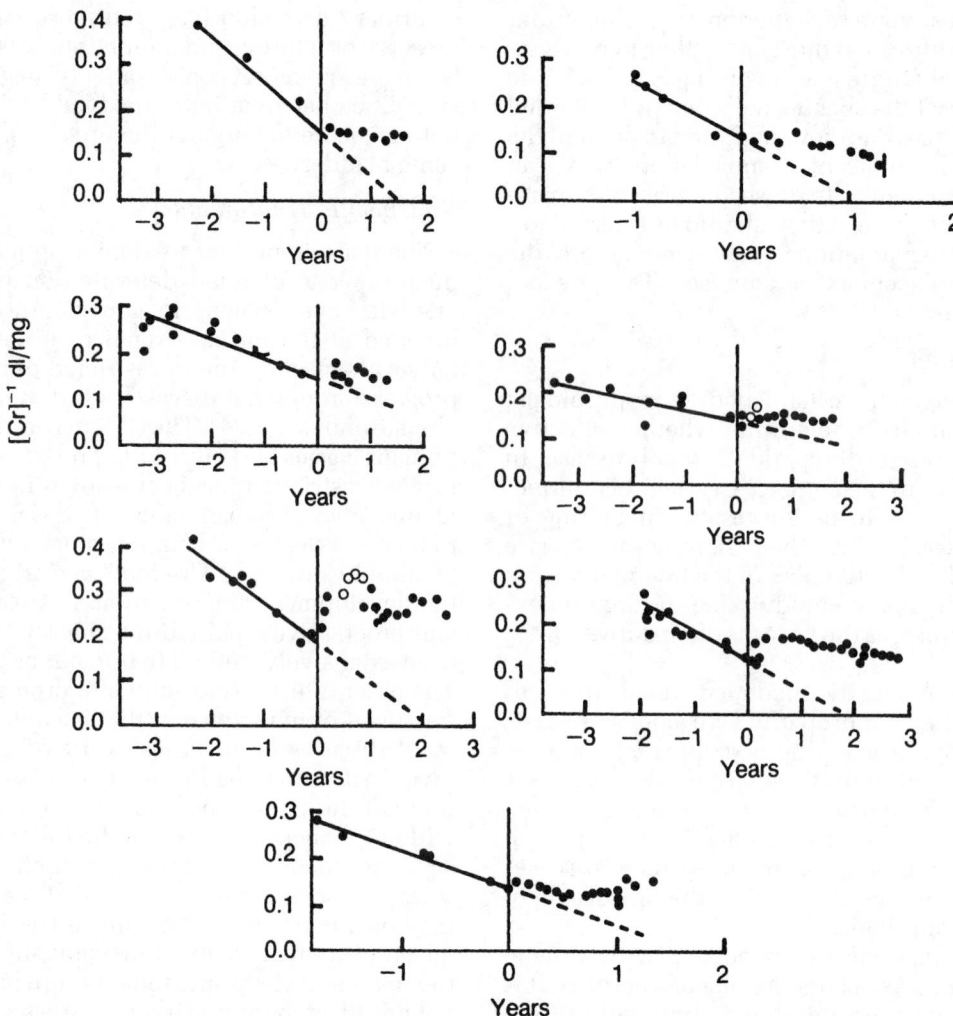

Figure 48.6. Data showing how the rate of progression of renal failure, as determined by a plot of the reciprocal of the serum creatinine concentration over time, in seven patients, was affected by the institution at time 0 of a low-phosphorus, low-protein diet. A decrease in the slope reflects stabilization of renal func- tion. The dashed line indicates the projected course. (Data redrawn from Mitch WM, Walser M, Steinman TI, et al. Effect of a keto acid–amino acid supplement to a restricted diet on the progression of chronic renal failure. N Engl J Med 311:623, 1984.)

protein intake was associated with a slower rate of decline in GFR (25).

Based on current literature, an NIH Consensus Conference (40) made the following recommendations for nutritional management of nondiabetic patients with renal insufficiency. There is insufficient evidence to warrant protein restriction in patients whose GFR is greater than 25 mL/minute, who therefore should be maintained on a normal protein intake of more than 0.8 g/kg daily. A diet restricted in protein (0.6 g/kg daily) should be prescribed for patients with GFR below 25 mL/minute, with the understanding that good dietary counseling be available and that there be careful monitoring for signs of malnutrition (weight loss, serum albumin below 4.0 g/dL, transferrin below 200 mg/dL). Given the remaining controversy over dietary restriction in patients with renal failure, consultation with a nephrologist should be obtained before embarking on such therapy.

Hypertension, present in many patients with renal insufficiency, may also aggravate preexisting kidney failure. Of the 1795 patients with renal insufficiency admitted to the baseline period of the MDRD study, 83% were hypertensive. The factors that correlated with the prevalence of hypertension included older age, lower GFR, the presence of glomerular diseases, high body mass index (BMI), male sex, and African-American race. The presence of hypertension, in the MDRD study, predicted a greater probability of progressive renal insufficiency with a faster rate of decline. That long-term control of hypertension slows the progression of renal insufficiency seems to be beyond debate (see Chapter 62), but a number of important clinical questions remain unresolved. One important question is what levels of blood pressure should be targeted. Few studies have addressed the issue of whether renal function is better preserved by lowering blood pressure below the usual target of

140/90 mm Hg. In addition to varying the protein intake, patients in the MDRD study were randomized into usual and aggressive antihypertensive therapies. Patients in the aggressively treated group (MAP target 92 mm Hg) whose GFRs were between 25 and 55 mL/minute had a more rapid decline in renal function during the first 4 months than the usual care group (MAP target 107 mm Hg) but a more gradual decline thereafter. It was postulated that the initial rapid decline was hemodynamically mediated and did not reflect actual kidney damage. The beneficial effect of aggressive blood pressure control was greatest in patients with proteinuria (above 1 g/day). These findings have led to the recommendation that the target blood pressure should be 130/80 to 85 mm Hg for patients with chronic renal insufficiency without proteinuria, but blood pressure in patients with renal insufficiency associated with proteinuria of greater than 1 g should be lowered to levels near 125/75 mm Hg. Currently, the recommendations for treating hypertension in African Americans, who seem to be more susceptible to the damaging effects of high blood pressure, are not different from those for other populations. This may change once the results of the African-American Study of Kidney Disease and Hypertension study become available.

A second important question is whether certain antihypertensive regimens offer advantages over others. That is, do some antihypertensive medications have effects beyond the consequences of lowering of blood pressure? ACE inhibitors have the theoretical advantage of reducing intraglomerular pressures and proteinuria in addition to reducing systemic blood pressures. Calcium channel blockers may have specific local protective effects on the renal vasculature or glomerular basement membrane that could be advantageous beyond their systemic effects on hypertension. Some, but not all, studies comparing the use of various ACE inhibitors with other antihypertensive medications in humans with nondiabetic renal failure show that ACE inhibitors offer a particular advantage in slowing the progression of renal insufficiency (18,30,44). Although definitive data are lacking, the general recommendations for treating hypertension in patients with renal insufficiency are to use an ACE inhibitor unless renal artery stenosis is suspected or the patient has hyperkalemia (serum potassium above 5.0 mEq/L). The serum potassium and creatinine levels should be checked at 1 to 2 weeks and periodically thereafter. A small rise in creatinine (below 0.5 mg/dL) or potassium (below 0.5 mEq/L) may occur but does not necessarily mean that therapy should stop. Whether angiotensin II receptor antagonists (losartan) are as effective in protecting the kidney as ACE inhibitors remains to be shown. Calcium channel blockers seem to be an adequate alternative to ACE inhibitors when the latter cannot be used or there are other reasons for choosing a calcium channel blocker (44). Whether there are differences between the types of calcium channel blockers in terms of renal protective effect is still unclear.

Therapy directed at correcting volume overload in patients with mild to moderate renal insufficiency is similar to that of patients with normal renal function and hypertension. A salt-restricted diet (e.g., 2 g/day) may be attempted as a first step. Loop diuretics such as furosemide, bumetanide, or torsemide can be added when salt restriction is insufficient or when nondiuretic drugs (e.g., hydralazine, captopril) lead to secondary salt retention. Thiazides are generally avoided in patients with GFRs below 30 mL/minute because they often lose their diuretic effect. Potassium-sparing diuretics (spironolactone, triamterene, amiloride) should not be used in patients with significant renal impairment because of the increased risk of developing hyperkalemia. In patients who have refractory edema or advanced renal failure with severe salt retention, it may be necessary to use large doses of diuretic (furosemide 400 mg, bumetanide 10 mg, or torsemide 200 mg) or to use a combination of loop diuretic and thiazide (metolazone 2.5 to 5 mg) (37). Patients need to have their weight and chemistries closely monitored when using combination diuretic therapy as some patients experience exaggerated responses.

There is often a fine line between effective blood pressure control and hypotension when potent diuretics and antihypertensives are being used; therefore, careful monitoring of blood pressure (both supine and upright) and of serum creatinine concentration are necessary. With the use of potent drugs such as minoxidil (for detailed discussions of these drugs see Chapter 62), bilateral nephrectomy (which results in the requirement for dialysis) for the treatment of refractory cases of hypertension can generally be avoided. Long-term control of hypertension may also be important in reducing the risk of atherosclerosis in patients on dialysis.

Treating Reversible Causes of Deterioration of Renal Function

Before any change in serum creatinine concentration is attributed to the natural progression of the underlying renal disease, several alternative possibilities should be considered (Table 48.5).

Extracellular volume depletion is probably the most common cause for a fall in GFR. It may be related to an intercurrent illness associated with anorexia, fever, gastrointestinal losses of sodium and water, excessive salt restriction, or diuretic use. The usual clinical signs

Table 48.5. Causes of Renal Functional Deterioration

Volume depletion (salt and water depletion)
Congestive heart failure
Drug nephrotoxicity
Ureteral or urethral obstruction
Orthostatic hypotension
Microcrystal deposition (e.g., acute severe hyperuricemia)
Hyperphosphatemia–hypercalcemia
Hypertension
Radiocontrast materials (oral and parenteral)
Glomerular hyperperfusion

of volume depletion (e.g., low jugular venous pressure, orthostatic hypotension, tachycardia, decreased skin turgor, and weight loss) may be absent, and a therapeutic trial of salt (6 to 8 g/day) administration may be required to establish the diagnosis. Weight loss between office visits is usually the most important diagnostic clue to the presence of volume depletion. The urinary sodium concentration or urine osmolality, usually helpful in establishing the diagnosis of volume depletion in oliguric patients, is of little value in the patient with chronic renal failure because concentrating and salt-conserving ability in these patients is often impaired.

Patients with decompensated congestive heart failure may also have superimposed prerenal azotemia. Optimal treatment of heart failure may improve renal function in these patients (see Chapter 61).

Drugs given for treatment of various other disorders can be related to worsening of renal function (Table 48.3). A careful review of both prescribed and over-the-counter medications is therefore necessary when assessing unexpected changes in kidney function. Of the drugs prescribed in the ambulatory setting, diuretics and NSAIDs are probably the most common offenders. Diuretics can aggravate preexisting renal failure by inducing intravascular volume depletion, and less commonly by producing an interstitial nephritis. Careful monitoring of the blood pressure, weight, BUN, and serum creatinine concentration will help detect early signs of prerenal azotemia in patients receiving diuretics. Withholding diuretic therapy for several days usually allows intravascular volume and GFR to return to baseline values.

NSAIDs use can result in a deterioration in kidney function, either by causing a reversible redistribution of renal blood flow or by producing an interstitial nephritis. NSAIDs are most likely to reduce GFR in patients with prerenal states, such as volume depletion, congestive heart failure (CHF), or nephrosis. At this time it cannot be said that one nonsteroidal compound is safer to use in the patient with renal insufficiency than another. It is therefore best to avoid them altogether once the GFR is less than 50 mL/minute.

There are numerous reports of reversible renal dysfunction when ACE inhibitors have been administered to patients with bilateral renovascular disease or renal artery stenosis of a solitary kidney. The former group should be considered for further diagnostic evaluation of their vascular disease.

Obstruction, because of its reversibility, should always be considered in patients with a fall in the GFR. This is particularly true in elderly men predisposed to prostatic hypertrophy or in diabetic patients who may have autonomic neuropathy affecting bladder emptying. Drugs that reduce bladder tone (e.g., antidepressants, antispasmodics, and antiparkinsonian drugs with anticholinergic properties) should always be considered as causes of urinary retention. If obstruction is a possibility, the patient should have a measurement of postvoid residual volume (see Chapter 6 for technique).

Orthostatic hypotension, caused by drugs or autonomic neuropathy, can cause a worsening of renal failure. Drugs and other causes of this problem are summarized in Chapter 81. Orthostatic hypotension should be managed by adjusting or stopping the drugs or prescribing practical measures summarized in Chapter 81.

Microcrystal deposition in the kidney has been suggested as a cause of progressive deterioration in patients with azotemia. Serum uric acid concentrations are often elevated in patients with renal insufficiency. However, there is no evidence that reducing the serum uric acid concentration will prevent further deterioration when the original kidney disease was not caused by tophaceous gout. Allopurinol is not used, therefore, unless it is needed to control symptomatic gout.

Calcium phosphate deposits have been found in the parenchyma of end-stage kidneys regardless of the original disease process. It has been postulated that these deposits have some role in the progression of renal disease. Although dietary phosphorus restriction appears to help reduce the rate of deterioration of renal function in both animal and human kidney failure, the mechanism by which this occurs is still unclear. Nevertheless, many nephrologists currently recommend that patients reduce phosphorus intake to 800 mg (see below) once GFR falls below 30 mL/minute.

Dietary Management

The major goals of dietary management in the patient with chronic renal insufficiency are to optimize intravascular volume, correct electrolyte abnormalities, relieve uremic symptoms, and prevent or slow the progression of kidney disease (Table 48.6). The dietary and general treatment of nephrotic syndrome, occasionally a component of chronic renal failure, is discussed in Chapter 44.

The *volume of the intravascular space* is directly related to salt balance, which is in turn regulated by the kidney. As renal function declines, the ability of the kidney to maintain salt balance in response to changes in sodium intake becomes limited, especially when the changes occur abruptly. The intravascular volume may be depleted if the intake of salt is reduced (e.g.,

Table 48.6. Dietary Management of Renal Failure[a]

Therapy	Goals
Salt: 4–6 g/day	Maintain intravascular volume
Fluid: 1–3 L/day	Avoid dehydration
Potassium: If [K] >5.5 mEq/L, restrict intake to 2–2.4 g/day	Prevent hyperkalemia
Protein: Restrict intake to 0.55–0.6 g/kg per day (50% rich in essential amino acids)	Relieve uremic symptoms Retard progression of renal failure
Calories: 35–45 kcal/kg per day	Maintain nutrition
Calcium: 1–1.5 g/day	Maintain [Ca] = 9–10 mg/dL
Vitamins: multivitamin + folate	Replace vitamins lacking in protein-restricted diet
Phosphorus: Restrict intake to 800 mg/day	Prevent secondary hyperparathyroidism

[a]A dietician should be consulted to teach the patient how to achieve these intakes.

Table 48.7.   Diuretics in Renal Failure

Drug	Available Strengths (mg)	Dosage	Route of Excretion	Comments
Thiazides (Hydrochlorothiazide)	25, 50	12.5–50 mg/day	Renal	May induce volume depletion and hyperuricemia. Loses effectiveness if GFR <30 mL/min but may be used in combination with loop diuretics in advanced renal failure.
Metolazone (Zaroxolyn)	2.5, 5, 10	5–20 mg/day	Renal	May induce volume depletion and hyperuricemia. Effective when GFR >10 mL/min.
Furosemide (Lasix)	20, 40, 80	20–400 mg/day	Renal	May induce volume depletion and hyperuricemia. Effective when GFR >5 mL/min. May produce ototoxicity and rarely interstitial nephritis. May increase nephrotoxicity of antibiotics.
Bumetanide (Bumex)	0.5, 1, 2	1–10 mg/day	Renal	May induce volume depletion and hyperuricemia. Side effects include ototoxicity and muscle pains and may also increase the risk of antibiotic nephrotoxicity.
Torsemide (Demadex)	5, 10, 20, 100	5–100 mg/day	Hepatic/renal	Longer half-life than other loop diuretics.
Ethacrynic acid (Edecrin)		Avoid	Hepatic	Usually avoided in renal failure because the risk of ototoxicity is significantly higher than with furosemide or bumetanide.
Spironolactone (Aldactone) Triamterene (Dyrenium) Amiloride (Moduretic)		Avoid	Hepatic	Avoid when GFR <50 mL/min due to the risk of inducing serious hyperkalemia.

excessive salt restriction, anorexia) or if there are losses of salt (e.g., vomiting, diarrhea, diuretics). A reduction in intravascular volume can lead to a further increase in the SUN and to serum creatinine concentrations above the baseline values (prerenal azotemia). Conversely, the intravascular volume will increase if the intake of salt is suddenly augmented (dietary indiscretion), and the patient can develop hypertension, edema, or heart failure.

Most patients with chronic renal insufficiency maintain sodium balance on a salt intake of 4 to 6 g. Patients with CHF or hypertension may need further limitation of salt intake (2 g of salt), whereas the rare patient with severe salt-wasting nephropathy may require salt supplements to prevent volume depletion. Most of these latter patients have some form of interstitial renal disease.

Salt intake should be adjusted to maintain intravascular volume at the level that maximizes the GFR for any given degree of renal failure. Assessing the state of the intravascular volume can be aided by obtaining serial body weights (rapid changes in weight are usually caused by fluid gains or losses), performing a physical examination (e.g., orthostatic change of pulse and blood pressure, jugular venous pressure, skin turgor, edema), and measuring changes in the SUN and serum creatinine concentrations (increases in the level of SUN are proportionately greater than that of the serum creatinine concentration in states of volume depletion). It is often useful to establish an ideal weight. This is the weight at which the patient has optimal renal function without overt signs of volume overload. For some patients, those with CHF or nephrotic syndrome, for example, a small amount of edema is acceptable because worsening of azotemia

may develop when further diuresis is attempted. Whenever there is a significant change in the GFR, the intravascular volume and the ideal weight should be reevaluated.

When the GFR falls as a result of volume depletion, it is necessary to restore the intravascular volume. This can be accomplished either by adding salt to the diet or by prescribing sodium chloride (600 mg four times a day) or sodium bicarbonate tablets (600 mg four times a day) until the patient's weight and GFR return to baseline values. If oral replacement is not practical (e.g., persistent vomiting), the patient should be hospitalized for intravenous therapy.

If volume overload develops or persists despite salt restriction, diuretics can be used to increase salt excretion (Table 48.7). Because the thiazide diuretics, with the exception of metolazone (Zaroxolyn), lose their effectiveness when the GFR falls below 30 mL/minute, it is often necessary to use a loop diuretic, such as furosemide (Lasix), torsemide (Demadex), or bumetanide (Bumex). Another loop diuretic, ethacrynic acid (Edecrin), has been associated with an unacceptable level of ototoxicity and should not be used in patients with renal insufficiency. The potassium-sparing diuretics spironolactone (Aldactone), triamterene (Dyrenium), and amiloride (Moduretic) are also best avoided without consultation from a nephrologist in patients with significant renal failure because of the risk of inducing serious hyperkalemia.

Potassium restriction is usually unnecessary until the late stages of renal failure (GFR less than 15 mL/minute), except in the small number of patients with the syndrome of hyporeninemic hypoaldosteronism (see below), but careful monitoring of serum potassium levels is indicated nonetheless. If hyperkalemia develops, potassium restriction to between 2 and 2.4 g/day (40 to 50 mEq) is necessary. A dietitian should be consulted to help plan a potassium-restricted diet. Foods with high potassium contents include dairy products, many greens, beans, potatoes, tomatoes, bananas, dates, prunes, raisins, and citrus fruits. Patients who are on sodium-restricted diets must also be informed that many salt substitutes are unacceptable because they are often composed of potassium salts.

The association of hyperkalemia and hyperchloremic metabolic acidosis in patients with mild to moderate renal insufficiency (GFR greater than 25 mL/minute) should lead one to consider the presence of the hyporenin hypoaldosterone syndrome (33). This syndrome occurs most often in azotemic patients with hypertension, diabetes mellitus, or interstitial nephritis. This disorder probably has many causes, but it is caused in part by a suppression of the renin–aldosterone axis. The diagnosis is usually made on clinical grounds, after excluding other reasons for hyperkalemia (e.g., high potassium intake or drugs that reduce the renal excretion of potassium), but it can be more firmly established by the demonstration of a low plasma renin concentration that fails to rise after stimulating the patient with furosemide (Lasix, 40 mg orally) and upright posture for 2 hours. The patient should also have no evidence of glucocorticoid deficiency (random cortisol concentration of 15 to 25 mg/mL; see also Chapter 74). Because, in the absence of aldosterone, potassium excretion by the kidney depends on an adequate urine flow rate (1.5 to 2 L/day), patients with this syndrome are at risk for developing severe hyperkalemia during periods of salt restriction or volume depletion. Normotensive patients may be treated with a mineralocorticoid (fluorohydrocortisone [Florinef], 0.1-mg tablets, ½ to 1 tablet/day). Alternatively, if hypertension is present or develops after the administration of the mineralocorticoid, the patient may be treated with a combination of furosemide (Lasix, 40 to 80 mg twice a day) plus sodium bicarbonate (600 mg four times a day). The furosemide is used to promote a good urine flow rate, whereas the sodium bicarbonate helps prevent salt depletion and also is of use in correcting the associated metabolic acidosis. The goal of therapy is to keep the serum potassium concentration within the normal range. Because therapy is often complicated, these cases are best managed with the help of a nephrologist or endocrinologist.

Although diluting and concentrating abilities are impaired in renal failure, most patients can ingest 1 to 3 L of fluid a day without developing hyponatremia. If hyponatremia occurs, fluids should be limited to less than 1.5 L a day to prevent water intoxication.

Protein-restricted diets, in addition to their use in reducing the rate of decline in kidney function, are indicated for patients with advanced renal failure (GFR less than 15 mL/minute) who develop nausea, vomiting, or other symptoms attributable to uremia. Because many end products of protein metabolism have been implicated in the causation of the uremic syndrome, therapy consists of reducing protein intake to approximately 0.6 g per kilogram of body weight per day (approximately 40 g of protein per day in a 70-kg patient). Normal protein intake in the United States exceeds 70 g/day. Half of the protein intake should be in the form of meats, fish, eggs, or milk because these foods are rich in essential amino acids. For the patient on a protein-restricted diet to maintain adequate nutritional balance, total caloric intake must be adjusted to provide 35 to 45 kcal/kg/day. This can be accomplished by increasing the intake of fats and carbohydrates.

Because protein-restricted diets are often deficient in vitamins, calcium, and phosphorus, patients should receive a daily vitamin supplement and 1 to 1.5 g of elemental calcium per day (a single 600-mg calcium carbonate tablet provides 250 mg of elemental calcium). The reduction in dietary phosphorus is desirable (see below), so phosphorus supplements are not given.

If symptoms such as nausea and vomiting related to uremia persist or the creatinine clearance falls below 5 mL/minute, the patient should be started on dialysis. Further restriction of protein intake is possible but should be attempted only for limited periods and under the direct supervision of a nephrologist. With the present availability of dialysis, little is to be gained by trying to maintain a very symptomatic patient on a highly restricted diet. Proper planning for patients with progressive renal disease should prevent referral of debilitated, malnourished, and neuropathic patients to a dialysis center (see "Symptomatic Therapy of Advanced Renal Failure," below).

Considering the complexity of such diets and the need for individualization of salt, mineral, protein, and potassium intake, consultation with a dietitian or a nephrologist proficient in prescribing renal diets is suggested. Constant encouragement and supervision of dietary therapy are needed. The success of dietary treatment often depends on the involvement of family members as well as an enthusiastic dietitian.

Calcium and Phosphorus

Renal osteodystrophy is a general term that encompasses osteitis fibrosa, osteomalacia, and a variety of other bone lesions that occur in patients with kidney failure. The pathophysiologic factors that lead to osteodystrophy originate in the early stages of renal failure, although clinical manifestations generally do not develop until the patient is on dialysis.

The pathophysiology of renal osteodystrophy is complex but can be briefly summarized as follows: PTH hypersecretion occurs in response to an absolute or relative deficiency of the active form of vitamin D (see below). The relative deficiency of vitamin D, in turn, leads to diminished calcium absorption, skeletal resistance to the effects of PTH, and resetting of the set point of PTH secretion in response to calcium.

The increased rate of PTH secretion is successful at keeping serum calcium and phosphorus levels within the normal range until the GFR is less than 30 mL/minute. In more advanced renal failure, hypocalcemia and hyperphosphatemia develop. Hyperphosphatemia further blunts the calcemic response to PTH and diminishes vitamin D secretion. The most important consequence of prolonged secondary hyperparathyroidism is the development of bone disease (osteitis fibrosa cystica).

Osteomalacia, in renal insufficiency, is caused partly by the failure of the diseased kidney to convert 25-hydroxyvitamin D_3 to its more active form, 1,25-dihydroxyvitamin D_3. The active form of vitamin D is necessary for normal bone mineralization. Serum levels of vitamin D can be in the normal range in patients with renal failure, but with GFRs above 30 mL/minute such levels may still represent a relative deficiency of the vitamin because elevated levels of vitamin D would be expected because of the low calcium concentrations in renal failure. Absolute deficiencies of vitamin D are found once the GFR falls below 30 mL/minute. Abnormal collagen synthesis, the titration of bone buffers, and the accumulation of aluminum in the bone matrix have also been implicated in the pathogenesis of osteomalacia.

Patients with renal insufficiency should have periodic measurements of calcium, phosphorus, magnesium, and alkaline phosphatase. Levels of PTH, when measured by the carboxyl-terminal assay, will be uniformly high because the kidney is responsible for the elimination of that fragment. Therefore, determination of PTH levels, when necessary, should be by an assay that measures the intact or amino-terminal hormone. Bone radiographs or biopsies are not routinely obtained in the patient not yet on dialysis, unless the patient has symptomatic bone disease.

The clinical features of deranged calcium and phosphorus metabolism, including bone pain, fractures, and proximal myopathy, are not often seen until after the patient is on dialysis. However, it is generally acknowledged that preventing parathyroid hyperplasia is easier than reversing it once established. Therefore, therapy to correct these abnormalities should begin during the early stages of renal failure (Table 48.8).

Based on a knowledge of calcium, phosphorus, and

vitamin D alterations in early renal insufficiency, it is possible to outline a plan of therapy directed at reducing the incidence and severity of osteodystrophy in late renal insufficiency. The goals of therapy are to limit the rise in PTH secretion that usually accompanies renal failure and to prevent the development of osteomalacia. These goals can be achieved by maintaining a positive calcium balance, providing vitamin D, and reducing phosphorus intake.

Because calcium absorption is diminished in patients with renal insufficiency, the first step in treatment is to ensure an adequate intake of calcium. This is particularly important if the patient is on a protein-restricted diet that often contains only 300 to 400 mg of calcium (normal calcium intake is 800 to 1000 mg/day). Supplements in the form of calcium carbonate (generic), 600 mg four times per day, will provide 1000 mg of elemental calcium per day. Calcium lactate (generic, 300 mg, in two tablets four times a day) can be substituted if the carbonate is not tolerated because of constipation or bloating.

It has been shown in a prospective, controlled trial that low dosages of orally administered vitamin D (Rocaltrol) given to patients with GFRs between 60 and 20 mL/minute can reverse some of the biochemical and histologic evidence of osteodystrophy (3). If, after consultation with a nephrologist, it is decided to treat early, one should start at the lowest dosage of the vitamin D preparation selected and raise the dosage every 4 weeks until the serum calcium is in the upper range of normal. It appears, from experience, that most patients with renal insufficiency cannot tolerate a Rocaltrol dosage greater than 0.5 g/day without developing hypercalcemia. Hypercalcemia may be associated with increases in the serum creatinine concentration, which should be reversible once the dosage of vitamin D is reduced and calcium levels return to the normal range. Therefore, because of the frequency of hypercalcemia and its potential effects on renal function, it is crucial that serum calcium levels be monitored weekly, after a change in dosage, until the serum calcium concentration stabilizes, and monthly thereafter. There does not appear to be any value to monitoring the levels of vitamin D metabolites during therapy. In general, one expects to see a fall in the levels of alkaline phosphatase and PTH, but as yet there are no treatment guidelines based on these values.

Vitamin D therapy should not be initiated when serum calcium or phosphorus levels are greater than 10.5 and 6 mg/dL, respectively, because of the possibility of inducing metastatic calcification or renal dysfunction. If the serum phosphorus level is elevated, as is common in patients whose GFR is below 30 mL/minute, it is necessary to first reduce the level of phosphorus to normal before starting vitamin D therapy.

The serum phosphorus concentration may rise after institution of vitamin D therapy because both calcium and phosphorus absorption are increased. If dietary phosphate restriction (approximately 800 mg/day) is not sufficient to maintain serum phosphorus levels

Table 48.8. Steps in the Management of Calcium and Phosphorus Balance in Patients with Renal Failure

Therapy	Goals
GFR 50–30 mL/min	
Calcium supplements (1–1.5 g/day)	Maintain serum calcium concentration at 9–10 mg/dL
Vitamin D (Rocaltrol 0.25–0.5 μg/day, available in 0.25-μg tablets)	Maintain serum calcium concentration at 9–10 mg/dL
GFR <30 mL/min	
Restrict phosphorus intake (800 mg/day)	Maintain serum phosphorus concentration at 4.0–6.0 mg/dL
Phosphorus-binding antacids (calcium carbonate, aluminum carbonate, or aluminum hydroxide taken with meals)	Maintain serum phosphorus concentration at 4.0–6.0 mg/dL

within the normal range, phosphate binders must be used (see below).

The form of vitamin D used is important because preparations (e.g., vitamin D_2 or D_3) that require final activation by the kidney have proved to be ineffective at the usual dosages. The most commonly used vitamin D preparations that do not require renal activation are 1,25-dihydroxyvitamin D_3 (Rocaltrol) and dihydrotachysterol (DHT). When given orally, both Rocaltrol (0.25 to 1.0 µg/day) and DHT (0.125 to 0.5 mg/day) are effective in improving calcium absorption and raising serum calcium levels in azotemic patients. Studies comparing the effectiveness of DHT and Rocaltrol have not been performed, although the latter, because it is the native hormone, has possible advantages. Both can produce hypercalcemia, but because of its shorter half-life the hypercalcemia induced by 1,25-dihydroxyvitamin D_3 tends to be of shorter duration.

Restriction of *dietary phosphorus* to approximately 800 mg/day (normal intake is 1 to 1.8 g/day) should be initiated when the serum phosphorus level first becomes elevated. This degree of phosphorus restriction can be achieved by restricting the intake of protein to 60 g/day (foods such as eggs, meat, and fish contain 15 mg of phosphorus per gram of protein) and dairy products (20 to 30 mg/g). Despite restriction of phosphorus intake, the serum phosphorus level often becomes elevated when the GFR falls below 30 mL/minute. At this juncture it is necessary to start treatment with phosphate binders. Calcium-containing compounds such as calcium carbonate and calcium acetate, which bind phosphate in the intestine and thereby reduce phosphate absorption, have supplanted the use of oral antacids containing aluminum hydroxide (Alternagel or Amphojel) or aluminum carbonate (Basaljel). This is because it has been demonstrated that aluminum from the antacids is absorbed and can accumulate in the brain and bones of patients with renal failure. This aluminum accumulation has been implicated in the pathogenesis of the dialysis dementia syndrome (myoclonus, seizures, and dementia), anemia (see Chapter 50), and a particular form of osteomalacia (characterized by the appearance of aluminum in the mineralization front of bone studied histochemically) that develop in some patients with end-stage renal failure. Nephrologists now recommend the addition of aluminum-containing compounds only in re-

Table 48.9. Drugs Whose Bioavailability Is Altered by Phosphate Binders

Decreased
Digoxin
Oral anticoagulants
Tetracycline
Anticholinergics
Aspirin
Chlorpromazine

Increased
Penicillin
Pseudoephedrine

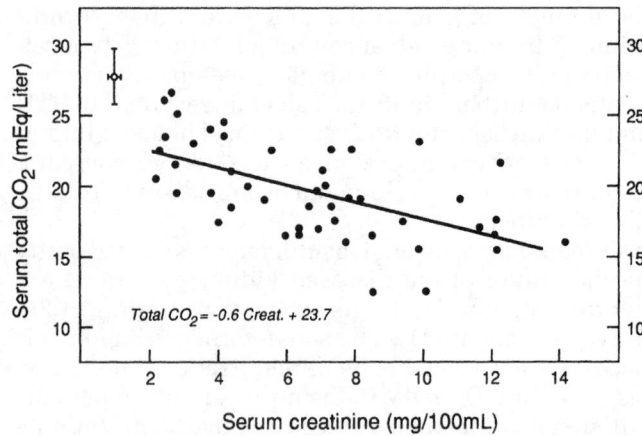

Figure 48.7. Relationship between the serum bicarbonate and serum creatinine concentrations in patients with chronic renal insufficiency. (From Widmer B et al. The influence of graded degrees of chronic renal failure. Arch Intern Med 139:1099, 1979.)

fractory cases of hyperphosphatemia. Other medications (Table 48.9) should not be given simultaneously with phosphate binders because their absorption may be increased or decreased. Furthermore, calcium citrate and aluminum-containing binders should not be given simultaneously because citrate increases the absorption of aluminum. The initial dosage of antacid should be 1 or 2 tablets or capsules given with meals; the dosage should be increased (at 2-week intervals) until the serum phosphorus concentration is reduced to between 4 and 6 mg/dL. Serum phosphorus concentration should be monitored every 1 to 2 months to avoid the syndrome of phosphate depletion (low serum phosphorus), which may result in muscle weakness, osteomalacia, and fractures.

Acidosis

A mild hyperchloremic (normal anion gap) metabolic acidosis develops commonly in patients with early renal insufficiency (Fig. 48.7). This occurs because the decrease in the production of ammonia by the failing kidney results in the inability of the kidney to excrete metabolically produced acids (sulfates and phosphates). The hypochloremic (with an abnormal anion gap) acidosis commonly associated with renal failure does not generally appear until the GFR has fallen below 20 mL/minute.

Chronic metabolic acidosis contributes to the long-term complications of patients who have renal failure by decreasing bone mineralization and suppressing protein synthesis. The goal of treating the acidosis is to maintain a serum bicarbonate level above 20 mEq/L. If protein restriction (see "Dietary Management," above), which reduces exogenous acid load, is insufficient to restore buffering capacity, base in the form of sodium citrate liquid (1 mL liquid = 1 mEq bicarbonate) can be given. Dosages of 30 to 60 mEq/day of base, given in divided doses, are generally sufficient to maintain acid–base balance. Sodium bicarbonate (600 mg =

14 mEq base) can also be used but is less well tolerated than citrate because of gastrointestinal complaints such as belching and bloating. Finally, $CaCO_3$ that is given as a calcium supplement and phosphate binder may also be effective in correcting the acidosis.

Anemia

A normochromic, normocytic anemia develops in patients with chronic renal failure, and its severity is proportional to the degree of renal insufficiency (Fig. 48.3). The hematocrit value generally falls to between 15 and 25% in a patient with advanced renal failure. The anemia of renal failure results mainly from decreased erythropoietin production. Other causes of anemia (e.g., iron deficiency) must also be considered.

All patients should be placed on a multivitamin regimen that includes folate to replace the vitamins lacking in the restrictive diets. Blood transfusion, when necessary, should not be withheld for fear of sensitizing a potential transplant recipient. Patients who have received multiple blood transfusions have higher rates of retention of functioning transplanted kidneys than do those who have not received transfusions. Iron deficiency is almost universal in patients on hemodialysis but may also occur in the predialysis patient, particularly if multiple blood samples have been taken or if there is bleeding. Iron deficiency is best diagnosed in patients with chronic renal failure by measuring the level of serum ferritin. The serum iron and iron-binding capacity are often low in patients with renal failure, but a transferrin saturation less than 15% should suggest the possibility of iron deficiency. The values of serum ferritin that are associated with normal iron stores are higher in patients with renal failure than in those without kidney disease. Therefore, the laboratory should be consulted to interpret serum ferritin levels properly in the uremic patient. The treatment of iron deficiency is the same in azotemic patients as it is in any other patient (see Chapter 50).

Patients whose hematocrit levels fall below 30% or who have symptoms related to anemia can be treated with recombinant human erythropoietin (Epogen, Procrit) given at dosages of 50 to 100 units/kg subcutaneously, two to three times per week (13,28). The higher dosages are associated with a more rapid response, but unless there is some urgency to correct the anemia, starting at the lower dosages is recommended. Most patients become asymptomatic when the hematocrit level is between 30 and 35%, but patients who have severe coronary disease may need further correction. Even patients who are not iron deficient but are taking erythropoietin should be given ferrous sulfate 300 mg and 1 mg of folic acid daily because iron and vitamin stores can be depleted rapidly. Blood pressure with this treatment may become more difficult to control in some patients, and it is therefore recommended that blood pressure measurements be taken on a weekly basis until the hematocrit level stabilizes (usually 6 to 8 weeks).

DRUG USE IN RENAL INSUFFICIENCY

The incidence of adverse drug effects is increased in patients with renal failure, a fact that is attributable largely to the alterations in pharmacokinetics that occur as renal function declines. Adverse drug effects in these patients can be divided into those that are caused by abnormal drug metabolism (e.g., increased incidence of digitalis toxicity) and those that are caused by an effect on renal function that is part of the anticipated pharmacologic action of the drug (e.g., reduction in GFR with diuretics or NSAIDs) (6). In renal failure, drug bioavailability, volume of distribution, and protein binding may be abnormal; however, the most significant derangement is the prolongation of half-life of many drugs or their metabolites. Therefore, it is necessary to have a basic understanding of how a drug's administration should be modified when renal failure is present.

Because even over-the-counter preparations (aspirin, ibuprofen, magnesium-containing antacids) have the potential for causing toxicity, patients should be reminded to telephone their physician before using nonprescription drugs. Whenever possible, drugs that require no modification of dosage or that do not affect kidney function adversely should be substituted for those with a greater potential for inducing toxicity. The avoidance of drugs with marginal efficacy will help reduce the frequency of adverse effects.

A complete review of drug usage in renal failure may be found in *Drug Prescribing in Renal Failure,* published by the American College of Physicians (1). Guidelines are provided in this section for the drugs most commonly prescribed in ambulatory practice (Tables 48.10 and 48.11).

Before initiating therapy with a drug that requires dosage modification in renal failure, it is necessary to have an accurate estimation of GFR. Predicting the GFR from the serum creatinine level alone is not recommended; rather, one should either measure the creatinine clearance directly or use one of the formulas for estimating GFR (see Equations 48.1 and 48.2 above).

Depending on what modifications are required for a particular drug, an appropriate loading and maintenance dosage can be chosen. A loading dose must be given whenever rapid achievement of therapeutic drug levels is desired. Maintenance dosages are adjusted either by lengthening the interval between administrations or by reducing the size of each dose. The use of nomograms or tables does not guarantee that adverse drug effects will not occur. The monitoring of serum drug levels is therefore often helpful, particularly when using drugs with low toxic/therapeutic ratios. Finally, the list of drugs should be reviewed periodically and the patient questioned specifically about side effects.

Antimicrobials

When renal impairment is not advanced (GFR above 50 mL/minute), no change is necessary for most commonly used antimicrobials in the dosages used in

Table 48.10.   Some Commonly Used Drugs that Require Dosage Reduction in Renal Failure (GFR <50 mL/min)

Cardiovascular Drugs
Digoxin (Lanoxin)
Nadolol (Corgard)
Atenolol (Tenormin)
Procainamide (Pronestyl)
Disopyramide (Norpace)

Antihypertensive Drugs
Captopril (Capoten)
Clonidine (Catapres)
Guanethidine (Ismelin)

H$_2$-Receptor Antagonists
Cimetidine (Tagamet)
Ranitidine (Zantac)

Hypoglycemic Drugs
Insulin
Acetohexamide
Chlorpropamide

Drugs Used in the Treatment of Gout
Allopurinol (Zyloprim)

Antibiotics
Most penicillins
Some cephalosporins
Quinolones

ambulatory practice (e.g., penicillins, cephalosporins, erythromycin, metronidazole, chloramphenicol, quinolones). However, the administration of tetracyclines, with the exception of doxycycline, is discouraged in the patient with impaired renal function because these drugs tend to increase the urea nitrogen concentration and could increase symptoms of uremia. Below a GFR of 50 mL/minute, many antibiotics require dosage modification and it is therefore important to check the pharmacokinetics of the drug.

When treating urinary tract infections in patients with GFRs below 50 mL/minute, urinary antiseptic drugs such as nitrofurantoin (Macrodantin) or nalidixic acid (NegGram) should not be used because they are ineffective and there is an increased risk of systemic toxicity associated with the retention of metabolites. Antimicrobials such as ampicillin, fluoroquinolones, and the cephalosporins that are secreted by the renal tubular cells achieve a high urine concentration, even when the GFR is very low. They are effective in the therapy of urinary tract infections in patients with advanced renal failure. Trimethoprim–sulfamethoxazole is also effective in patients with impaired renal function. The dosage of ciprofloxacin/ofloxacin should be reduced by 50% when the GFR falls below 30 mL/minute.

Analgesics

The dosages of acetaminophen, codeine, oxycodone (Tylox), and pentazocine (Talwin) require no modification in renal failure. Furthermore, none of these

drugs adversely affects kidney function in patients with chronic renal insufficiency. There is some epidemiologic evidence that the regular, heavy use of acetaminophen is associated with an increased risk of renal damage. The use of meperidine (Demerol) for more than two to three doses is hazardous because of the accumulation of its metabolites, which may induce seizures.

The use of NSAIDs, including aspirin, is generally not recommended in patients with renal insufficiency because they predictably result in a 25 to 50% decrease in GFR (9). The effects of NSAIDs on GFR result from changes in renal blood flow consequent to inhibition of renal prostaglandin synthesis and are greatest in patients who have diminished effective circulatory volume (patient on diuretics or with CHF). The reduction in GFR is generally reversible once the NSAID is discontinued, but the return to baseline may take up to 1 month. It is unclear whether the reduction in GFR associated with NSAIDs results in any permanent harm to the kidney.

There are several possible approaches to the patient with renal insufficiency for whom it is believed important to use an NSAID. Sulindac (Clinoril) appears not to affect renal prostaglandin synthesis to the same extent as the other NSAIDs and is generally considered to produce lesser effects on GFR in patients with mild renal insufficiency (12). The nonacetylated salicylates are only weak inhibitors of prostaglandin synthesis and theoretically should not affect renal function. Currently, however, there are no data on the safety of

Table 48.11.   Some Commonly Used Drugs that Should Be Avoided in Patients with Renal Failure (GFR <30 mL/min)

Antimicrobials
Cephaloridine (Loridine)
Tetracyclines
Nitrofurantoin (Macrodantin)
Nalidixic acid (NeGram)

Analgesics
Aspirin
NSAIDs (e.g., Motrin, Nalfon)
Meperidine (Demerol)

Diuretics
Potassium-sparing diuretics (Aldactone, Moduretic, Dyrenium)
Ethacrynic acid (Edecrin)
Thiazides (e.g., Diuril)

Antacids
Magnesium-containing antacids (e.g., Maalox, Mylanta)

Hypoglycemic Drugs
Acetohexamide (Dymelor)
Chlorpropamide (Diabinase)
Metformin (Glucophage)

Drugs Used in the Treatment of Gout
Phenylbutazone (Butazolidin)
Sulfinpyrazone (Anturane)
Probenecid (Benemid)

nonacetylated salicylates in patients with renal insufficiency. In any event, when NSAIDs are given to patients with renal failure, it is necessary to monitor kidney function carefully and it is probably prudent to discontinue their use if more than a minimal change in renal function is seen.

Patients with renal insufficiency are predisposed to developing salt retention, hyponatremia, and hyperkalemia when given NSAIDs. Hyperkalemia is more common when NSAIDs are given in conjunction with potassium-sparing diuretics or ACE inhibitors. Finally, there have been numerous case reports of patients with previously normal renal function developing ARF with nephrotic syndrome, as an idiosyncratic reaction, after having been given NSAIDs. When examined by biopsy, these patients generally are found to have an interstitial form of nephritis.

Antiviral agents including acyclovir, ganciclovir, amantadine, and zidovudine (AZT) all require dosage modification when GFR falls below 50 mL/minute.

Sedatives, Hypnotics, and Tranquilizers

In the patient with renal failure, no alteration in dosage is necessary for the benzodiazepines (e.g., Valium, Librium, Dalmane), neuroleptics (e.g., Haldol or Thorazine), and tricyclic antidepressants (e.g., Pamelor) because all are metabolized chiefly by the liver. The metabolism of serotonin reuptake inhibitors such as fluoxetine (Prozac) and sertraline (Zoloft) is unclear. The phenothiazines and tricyclics must be used with caution because they have significant anticholinergic properties and, accordingly, may cause urinary retention. All psychoactive drugs are capable of causing excessive sedation in patients with advanced renal failure. Lithium, which is renally excreted, should be used with great caution once the GFR falls below 50 mL/minute. Levels must be monitored frequently (for details see Chapter 15).

Antacids, H₂-Receptor Antagonists, and Proton Pump Inhibitors

Many commonly prescribed or over-the-counter antacids contain magnesium compounds as a major constituent, and magnesium toxicity may occur when the GFR falls below 30 mL/minute. Therefore, the patient should be instructed to use antacids that are based on aluminum (as opposed to magnesium). Because, with prolonged ingestion, significant amounts of aluminum are absorbed and accumulate in the tissues of patients with renal failure, they should be prescribed only for periods less than 1 month. Sucralfate, although containing aluminum, may be used because the compound is minimally absorbed compared with other aluminum-containing compounds.

The dosage of the H₂-receptor antagonists cimetidine, ranitidine, and famotidine must be reduced 50% as the creatinine clearance falls below 30 mL/minute.

All can cause an increase in serum creatinine levels, probably because of inhibition of the tubular secretion of creatinine.

There are no significant dosage alterations for the hydrogen pump blockers such as omeprazole (Prilosec).

Cardiovascular Drugs

Both the loading and maintenance dosages of digoxin must be reduced once the GFR falls below 50 mL/minute. The loading dosage of digoxin should be reduced by 75% and the maintenance dosage by 50% once the GFR falls below 50 mL/minute. Despite the use of nomograms (2) and the monitoring of drug levels, digoxin toxicity remains a problem in the uremic patient. Therefore, whenever feasible, other treatments for heart failure should be tried before resorting to digoxin.

A large variety of β-blocking agents are now available and each has slightly different pharmacologic or pharmacokinetic properties. The most important consideration in patients with renal failure is the route of excretion. The dosages of propranolol (Inderal), metoprolol (Lopressor), labetalol (Normodyne), and penbutolol (Levatol), which are all metabolized by the liver, are unchanged even in advanced renal failure. Atenolol (Tenormin), nadolol (Corgard), pindolol (Visken), carteolol (Cartrol), timolol (Blocadren), and the metabolites of acebutolol (Sectral) are excreted largely by the kidney and require dosage reduction. All β-blocking agents should be used with caution in patients with impaired renal function because they reduce cardiac output and may thereby aggravate azotemia.

The dosage interval should be increased twofold to fourfold to avoid toxicity when giving procainamide (Pronestyl) and disopyramide (Norpace) in patients with renal failure. Monitoring blood levels of the drug and, in the case of procainamide, its active metabolite (N-acetylprocainamide) is important in guiding therapy. Once the GFR falls below 10 mL/minute, the dosages of flecainide, encainide, and tocainide should be halved. Quinidine and amiodarone do not require dosage modification, even in advanced renal failure.

The use of antihypertensive drugs in patients with renal failure is discussed in Chapter 62.

Hypoglycemic Agents

The half-life of insulin is prolonged in renal failure, so attention to dosage is required in the diabetic patient with developing renal insufficiency to avoid hypoglycemia. The oral hypoglycemic agents acetohexamide and chlorpropamide have active metabolites that accumulate in renal failure and may produce prolonged hypoglycemia. Therefore, non–insulin-dependent diabetic patients taking oral hypoglycemic agents should switch to tolbutamide (Orinase), glipizide (Glucotrol), or glyburide (Micronase, Diabeta) once the GFR falls below 50 mL/minute.

The use of metformin (Glucophage) is discouraged in the presence of even modest degrees of renal insufficiency because the incidence of lactic acidosis increases as GFR declines.

Anticonvulsants

The dosage of phenytoin (Dilantin) is essentially unchanged in renal failure because an increased volume of distribution and a shortened half-life are offset by reduced protein binding. Because the unbound fraction of phenytoin is increased, the therapeutic and toxic effects of Dilantin occur at lower measured total serum levels in patients with renal failure than they do in patients without renal insufficiency (Fig. 48.8).

Drugs Used in the Treatment of Gout

Colchicine may be used for the prophylactic treatment of symptomatic gout in usual dosages (0.6 to 1.2 mg/day). The incidence of colchicine myopathy appears to be increased in patients with kidney impairment, and when it is prescribed the patient should be monitored closely for this complication by measuring creatinine phosphokinase concentration and muscle strength. The dosage of allopurinol must be reduced to 200 mg/day in patients with GFRs below 50 mL/minute and to 100 mg/day when the GFR is below 30 mL/minute. The uricosuric agents probenecid (Benemid) and sulfinpyrazone (Anturane) are ineffective when

the GFR falls below 50 mL/minute and should therefore not be used. Indomethacin (Indocin) is almost entirely metabolized by the liver, so it does not accumulate in patients with even advanced renal failure. However, patients who receive indomethacin for the treatment of acute gout must have their SUN and serum creatinine concentrations monitored carefully because indomethacin can cause a transient worsening of renal function.

CHRONIC RENAL INSUFFICIENCY AND COEXISTING DISORDERS

Nonrenal diseases often occur in patients with uremia. In some, such as patients with systemic lupus erythematosus or diabetes mellitus, the renal disease is part of a generalized illness that affects many other organ systems. Others may have diseases unrelated to the kidneys, such as coronary artery disease, chronic obstructive pulmonary disease, or malignancy. The coexistence of multiple disorders often complicates management. For example, angina in patients with coronary artery disease may be aggravated by the anemia of chronic renal failure.

Diabetes Mellitus

Up to 30 to 40% of patients with Type 1 and 10% of those with Type 2 (the incidence is higher in African Americans, Hispanics, and Native Americans) develop chronic renal failure, and patients with diabetes mellitus account for about one-third of many dialysis populations, with the majority having Type 2. The pathophysiology of diabetic nephropathy is complex and involves genetic, metabolic, and hemodynamic factors. It is becoming increasingly important for the generalist to recognize and treat these patients because efforts to prevent the development of advanced renal failure must take place early, usually before the patient is referred to the nephrologist.

Proteinuria, detected by a urine dipstick, is the earliest clinical manifestation of diabetic nephropathy and is seen 10 to 15 years after the onset of Type 1 diabetes mellitus and sooner in patients with Type 2. By this time, pathologic changes of diabetic glomerulosclerosis are well established, and the ability to change the course of disease is reduced. More subtle degrees of proteinuria, so-called microalbuminuria (30 to 300 mg in 24 hours), predicts the development of diabetic nephropathy and identifies a subpopulation of patients who need more aggressive therapy, including tight glucose and blood pressure control. Without specific interventions, a high proportion of patients with Type 1 and Type 2 who have microalbuminuria develop renal insufficiency.

The Council on Diabetes Mellitus of the National Kidney Foundation has published guidelines for the screening and treatment of diabetic patients with microalbuminuria (5). Screening for microalbuminuria should be performed annually for all diabetics between the ages of 12 and 70. Although timed urine collections are more accurate and preferable, mea-

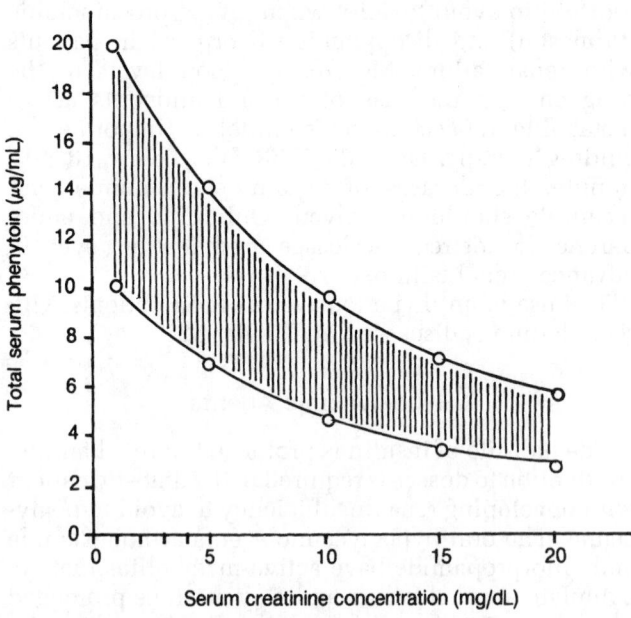

Figure 48.8. Range of total serum phenytoin concentrations in patients with varying degrees of renal failure that provide therapeutic levels of free drug. (Redrawn from Reidenberg NM, Affirme M. Influence of disease on binding of drugs to plasma proteins. Ann N Y Acad Sci 226:115, 1973.)

surement of a morning spot urine for albumin and creatinine, using a specific assay to detect microalbuminuria, is a more practical alternative. Microalbuminuria is present if the albumin excretion rate is between 30 to 300 mg/24 hours or the albumin/creatinine ratio is between 30 to 300 mg/g on two occasions in a 3-month period. Urine protein may be falsely elevated if the patient is performing strenuous exercise, has a febrile illness or urinary tract infection, or is in heart failure.

Short-term studies of patients with early diabetes showed that tight glycemic control can reverse some of the abnormalities, such as hyperfiltration, thought to be important in the development of diabetic nephropathy. The Diabetes Control and Complications Trial (DCCT) (10) showed that the development of microalbuminuria could be forestalled and that the amount of established albuminuria could be reduced when intensive therapy with multiple-dose insulin or an insulin pump was coupled with frequent glucose monitoring in patients with Type 1 diabetes. Although similar data are lacking for populations of patients with early Type 2 diabetes, it makes sense to attempt better glucose control in these patients.

Hypertension is often present in diabetic patients, particularly if they have evidence of nephropathy. A number of studies in both Type 1 and Type 2 diabetes demonstrate that the speed of renal deterioration is correlated with the degree of hypertension and that reducing the blood pressure to normal levels slows the rate. Animal studies and short-term human studies suggest that ACE inhibitors and perhaps calcium channel blockers may provide additional protective effects beyond those afforded by the lowering of blood pressure. These impressions have been confirmed in large-scale, randomized studies (27). Most nephrologists would now recommend the use of an ACE inhibitor as first-line antihypertensive therapy in diabetic patients with nephropathy. Although hyperkalemia and renal insufficiency (in patients with bilateral renal artery stenosis) are uncommon complications of ACE inhibitor therapy, the serum potassium and creatinine levels should be checked approximately 1 week after starting treatment. Competitive inhibitors to angiotensin receptors, such as losartan, may eventually be alternatives to ACE inhibitors, but currently there is insufficient information to make recommendations about their role in the treatment of diabetic nephropathy. In at least one study, the nondihydropyridine calcium channel blockers, verapamil and diltiazem, were as effective as lisinopril in reducing protein excretion and the rate of decline in GFR in patients with Type 2, renal insufficiency, and proteinuria (4). Regardless of what antihypertensive agent is used, it is important to maintain good control of the blood pressure (130/85 mm Hg or lower).

The renoprotective effect of ACE inhibitors appears to extend to normotensive patients with either Type 1 or Type 2 diabetes (22,35). Therefore, the consensus is to treat all diabetic patients who have microalbuminuria or macroalbuminuria, regardless of blood pressure, with ACE inhibitors unless contraindicated.

As in nondiabetic patients, the value of a low-protein diet in retarding the progression of renal damage in diabetic populations remains controversial. If attempted, it is important to refer the patient to a dietitian who is familiar with the prescription of the diets and who will work with the patient over time to help with compliance.

Renal disease may reduce the requirement for insulin, an effect related at least in part to decreased hormone degradation in the renal tubules as nephrons are progressively lost. Some oral hypoglycemic agents, notably chlorpropamide and acetohexamide, also have prolonged half-lives in uremic patients. As a consequence of these pharmacologic abnormalities, the first overt manifestation of renal disease in some diabetic patients is the occurrence of hypoglycemia. Therefore, the dosage of insulin or oral hypoglycemic drugs should be assessed regularly in the patient with renal impairment.

Diabetes per se is not a contraindication to dialysis or transplantation, although the course of diabetic patients is more complicated than that of patients with isolated renal failure. The form of therapy best suited for these patients with end-stage renal failure is uncertain. Hemodialysis, peritoneal dialysis, and transplantation have their proponents. Diabetic patients should be reminded that dialysis and transplantation are supportive therapies for renal dysfunction and will not improve their diabetes. It should also be remembered that the course of dialysis or transplants in these patients is less favorable than that of patients with renal failure without diabetes (see "Dialysis and Transplantation" later in this chapter). The microvasculopathy that destroys the kidney also affects the retinal and peripheral vessels. Because blindness and peripheral vascular disease are important causes of morbidity and mortality in the dialysis and transplant population, it is critical for these patients to have appropriate attention to their eyes (see Chapter 72) and feet (see Chapter 102) (14).

Heart Disease

Patients with congestive heart failure or angina often require more frequent monitoring as renal function declines. Diuretics may lose their effectiveness, or as anemia worsens patients with ischemic heart disease may become more symptomatic. In this situation transfusions are necessary if there has been an inadequate response to antianginal therapy, although erythropoietin may be useful in improving the anemia.

Patients with renal failure have been noted to have an accelerated rate of atherogenesis. This may be explained by the presence of hypertension, glucose intolerance, hypertriglyceridemia, and reduced levels of high-density lipoproteins in this group of patients.

Human Immunodeficiency Virus Infection

A *chronic,* progressive nephropathy characterized by proteinuria and renal failure can be seen in patients with AIDS. Most of these patients have a history of intravenous drug abuse, but AIDS nephropathy has also been found in homosexuals and children. The prognosis of these patients is grim and many die of infections, complications, or inanition before they reach the point of needing dialysis. Uncontrolled studies report a beneficial effect of steroids on the course of HIV nephropathy (39), but treatment remains frustrating. Only a small percentage of the patients who start on a dialysis program live more than 6 months (34), although recent reports suggests a more optimistic prognosis (19). The experience is somewhat better for patients who are HIV positive but have unrelated renal failure.

Malignancy

Renal failure as a result of hypercalcemia, sepsis, or drug nephrotoxicity is not an uncommon occurrence in patients dying with a malignancy. In many of these patients it would be inappropriate to prolong their lives by initiating dialysis. However, patients with multiple myeloma or other neoplasms who may have a long survival might benefit from dialysis. Therefore, dialyzing patients with neoplastic diseases should be recommended only after careful discussion with the patient, the family, an oncologist, and a nephrologist.

Pregnancy and Renal Insufficiency

The presence of even mild renal insufficiency has important ramifications for the health of the mother and baby. The frequency of hypertensive complications is increased and proteinuria is exacerbated in women with renal disease who become pregnant. Aside from the increased incidence of hypertension, women who have antepartum serum creatinine levels 1.4 mg/dL or below do not generally experience a worsening of renal function during the pregnancy. The renal outcome for women with initial serum creatinine levels greater than 1.4 mg/dL is not as good, with almost half experiencing a decline of renal function during pregnancy that persists in many (20). Prematurity and low birth weight are much more common in babies born to women with renal insufficiency, but fetal survival is greater than 90% in most series when women get appropriate prenatal attention and high-quality neonatal intensive care is available.

SYMPTOMATIC THERAPY OF ADVANCED RENAL FAILURE

Patients with advanced renal failure (GFR less than 10 mL/minute) invariably develop a variety of uremic symptoms. Gastrointestinal disturbances such as nausea, anorexia, and vomiting are common. Treatment involves further restriction of protein (see "Dietary Management," above) or antiemetics (e.g., Compazine). Itching is often a bothersome problem of unknown etiology. Reduction of serum phosphorus to normal levels and the use of skin lubricants (see Chapter 100) and antihistamines (e.g., Benadryl, 25 to

50 mg four times/day) are all worth 1- to 3-week trial periods. Ultraviolet light therapy may also be helpful, but this requires consultation with a dermatologist performing this form of therapy. Fatigue, heart failure, and angina may be caused by worsening anemia or volume overload and should respond to erythropoietin or diuretics. Neuromuscular symptoms, such as myoclonus, restless legs, and disturbed sleep, are signs of advanced uremia and should serve as warnings that more severe abnormalities (e.g., seizures, coma) may soon develop.

Although the patient and physician should try to minimize the symptoms of uremia with conservative therapy (with protein-restricted diets) and delay the time when dialysis treatment becomes necessary, there is a point when this effort becomes counterproductive. The persistence of uremic symptoms despite the best conservative medical management is an indication for dialysis regardless of the SUN or serum creatinine concentration.

There are no absolute laboratory criteria defining the time at which dialysis should be initiated, but most patients in whom dialysis is started have serum creatinine concentrations of approximately 8 to 10 mg/dL. Many nephrologists believe that diabetics develop uremic symptoms at lower levels of BUN and creatinine concentrations than do nondiabetics. Delay in starting dialysis can lead to patients developing severe peripheral neuropathy, malnutrition, or pericarditis from which complete recovery might not be possible. A low serum albumin (less than 4.0 g/dL), reflecting malnutrition, has been shown to be a strong predictor for increased mortality in both dialysis and predialysis populations. As patients become uremic, there is a tendency for them to spontaneously decrease their food intake, which predisposes them to malnutrition. Most nephrologists would consider any sign of malnutrition, such as weight loss or low serum albumin (not attributable to other causes), to be an indication to start dialysis (17).

DIALYSIS AND TRANSPLANTATION

In 1992, more than 160,000 patients were being maintained on dialysis in the United States. Most facilities provide hemodialysis, peritoneal dialysis, and transplantation (or referral to a transplant center) for patients with end-stage renal failure (Table 48.12). Either form of dialysis therapy can be performed at a center or at the patient's home. Some patients choose dialysis as a permanent form of treatment, whereas others undergo dialysis temporarily until they receive a kidney transplant. Although dialysis does not correct all of the metabolic abnormalities of chronic renal failure, it has enabled thousands of patients to lead productive lives.

Hemodialysis

The hemodialysis procedure involves circulating the patient's blood through a machine that corrects elec-

Table 48.12. Treatments for End-Stage Renal Failure

Hemodialysis
Home
Hospital based
Satellite or self-care (e.g., those not situated in a hospital)

Peritoneal Dialysis
Continuous ambulatory peritoneal dialysis
Continuous cyclic peritoneal dialysis
Intermittent peritoneal dialysis

Renal Transplantation
Living donor transplant
Cadaveric transplant

trolyte abnormalities and can remove excess fluid and toxic metabolic wastes. In the case of slowly progressive renal failure, provisions for dialysis should be made months in advance of need. The goal of dialysis therapy is to maintain health at a level consistent with a normal lifestyle. Therefore, it is not advisable to wait for signs and symptoms of far-advanced uremia (e.g., pericarditis, seizures, coma, or bleeding) to appear before initiating dialysis. The patient should be referred to a nephrologist associated with a dialysis center when the creatinine clearance approaches 25 mL/minute. In this way the patient may be familiarized with the various forms of therapy offered at that facility and become acquainted with the staff.

Before starting dialysis, it is necessary to provide vascular access to allow for the repeated venipunctures required for this form of therapy. It is important that the access be placed well before the patient needs dialysis treatments; otherwise, it is necessary to use temporary access techniques (central vein or femoral vein cannulation), which are associated with both short-term (pneumothorax, infection) and long-term complications (subclavian vein stenosis or thrombosis). The preferred access is the arteriovenous fistula, which is usually created at the wrist of the nondominant arm. The creation of a fistula can be performed, in most instances, under local anesthesia and often in an outpatient surgical unit. Because a 2- to 3-month maturation period is often necessary before the fistula can be used, arrangements for the creation of the fistula should be made early, and always before the GFR falls to less than 10 to 15 mL/minute. If the patient's vessels are inadequate to support the creation of an arteriovenous fistula, an alternative would be to insert a synthetic (Dacron, Gore-Tex) graft under the skin of the forearm. The synthetic graft can generally be used within 3 weeks of placement. The most common complications after placement of a fistula or graft are clotting and infection.

Hemodialysis is performed in most centers three times a week, and each session lasts about 3 to 4 hours. Except for needle insertion, the procedure is not painful, but some patients do experience muscle cramps, headaches, or nausea during or just after dialysis. Hospital-based dialysis should be reserved for patients who require intensive monitoring. Home dialysis is encouraged for patients with good home situations who have willing and able partners. Home dialysis patients have the advantage of more flexible schedules and a greater sense of control than do hospital-based patients and, therefore, have the greatest chance of maintaining their previous lifestyle. The remainder of the patients can be treated at outpatient dialysis centers.

As a group, hemodialysis patients have an 80% survival rate for the first year, and at 5 years the survival rate falls to approximately 55%. The development of long-term complications of chronic renal failure, including progressive neuropathy, osteodystrophy, cardiovascular disease, and an array of endocrine disturbances, reflects the fact that dialysis does not correct all of the metabolic disturbances of uremia.

Peritoneal Dialysis

Peritoneal dialysis procedures involve the instillation of dialysis fluid through a catheter into the abdominal cavity. Fluid and toxic solutes are transferred across the mesenteric capillary bed into the dialysis fluid, which is then removed through the catheter. Recent improvements in the techniques of peritoneal dialysis have increased its popularity among patients. In the past, peritoneal dialysis required 12 to 16 hours of being connected to an automatic cycling machine, two to three times a week (*intermittent peritoneal dialysis [IPD]*). Even then, its simplicity and freedom from hemodynamic complications made this form of therapy attractive, particularly to the elderly or to those with heart disease. Currently, *continuous ambulatory peritoneal dialysis (CAPD)* has nearly replaced the older machine-based therapy. In this technique the patient constantly carries 2 L of dialysis solution in the abdomen (26). The fluid is exchanged four times a day, every day. However, because fluid movement is determined by gravity, and no machine is necessary, the patient is able to perform dialysis at home, at work, or virtually anywhere. This degree of freedom is one of the most attractive aspects of CAPD. Its other attributes, at least theoretically, are the greater removal of higher-molecular-weight substances than that provided by hemodialysis, and the continuous nature of the dialysis that eliminates the large swings in the concentration of electrolytes and creatinine that occur with the more intermittent forms of therapy. Also, the abdominal catheter for CAPD can be placed at the time of the first dialysis and does not require a maturation period. The major difficulty associated with peritoneal dialysis is the development of peritonitis. The incidence in the typical patient is about one infection every 12 to 24 months, but these infections generally respond to antimicrobials and continued peritoneal dialysis; often treatment of peritonitis does not require hospitalization. However, the peritoneal dialysis catheter may need periodic replacement.

Continuous cyclic peritoneal dialysis (CCPD) is a variant of peritoneal dialysis in which the patient is connected to an automated cycling device that performs the exchanges while the patient is sleeping, further reducing the impact of dialysis on the patient's daytime schedule.

Comparative survival statistics between hemodialysis and peritoneal dialysis are difficult to interpret because of significant population selection biases. Whether hemodialysis or peritoneal dialysis is used depends on the center to which the patient is referred and on patient preference. At most dialysis facilities the patient has a choice and may change dialysis modes if the outcome of one is unsatisfactory.

Renal Transplantation

Of all available therapies, a successful renal transplant provides for the most complete correction of the uremic syndrome. Innovations in antirejection therapy, such as the use of the potent immunosuppressant drugs cyclosporine, tacrolimus, mycophenolate mofetil, or monoclonal antibodies (OKT3), have improved the rate of graft survival.

The success of renal transplantation depends on the antigenic similarity between donor and recipient. Except in the cases of identical twins (in which rejection does not occur), the best results are found in living related donor, HLA-identical transplants. In this instance, kidney survival is greater than 90% at 2 years. More commonly performed are two HLA-matched sibling-to-sibling or parent-to-child organ transplants, with a success rate of 92% at 1 year and 87% at 2 years (Fig. 48.9). Patient survival for non–HLA-identical living related donor transplants is greater than 90% at both the 1- and 2-year intervals. Most patients do not have the possibility of having living related donors (less than 25% of patients are able to receive living related donor transplants) and must await a cadaveric transplant, which, despite the best tissue typing, has a significantly lower success rate of 83% at 1 year and 77% at 2 years. Patient survival rates for cadaveric transplants are 90% at 1 year and 88% at 2 years. Comparison of survival statistics between cadaveric transplants and dialysis patients is complicated because of selection bias. Transplant recipients tend to be younger, have better myocardial function, and have fewer coexisting illnesses than their dialysis counterparts. If these factors are taken into account, no significant difference in the survival rate can be found between patients receiving cadaveric kidney transplants and those being treated by dialysis.

Patients with uncomplicated renal transplants usually require a 4- to 7-day hospitalization. After transplantation (except for those performed between identical twins), the patient requires lifelong immunosuppression, usually with a combination of cyclosporine (Sandimmune) or tacrolimus (Prograf), prednisone, and azathioprine (Imuran) or mycophenolate mofetil (Cell Cept). The patient must understand that there is always the risk of rejection and the possibility of graft failure, with a return to dialysis. Although there is no doubt that a successfully functioning transplant restores health better than any other therapy, patients on immunosuppressive therapy have considerable risks from corticosteroids and immunosuppression, such as obesity, diabetes, cataracts, osteoporosis, serious infections, and malignancies.

The primary physician can be of great value in advising which forms of therapy might coincide best with the patient's expectations. Often, patients have a better understanding of their choices if they visit a dialysis or transplant unit and talk with patients or staff. The decision to suggest a renal transplant is most clear-cut in adolescents or young adults who wish to pursue an active, vigorous life, have a job, and have

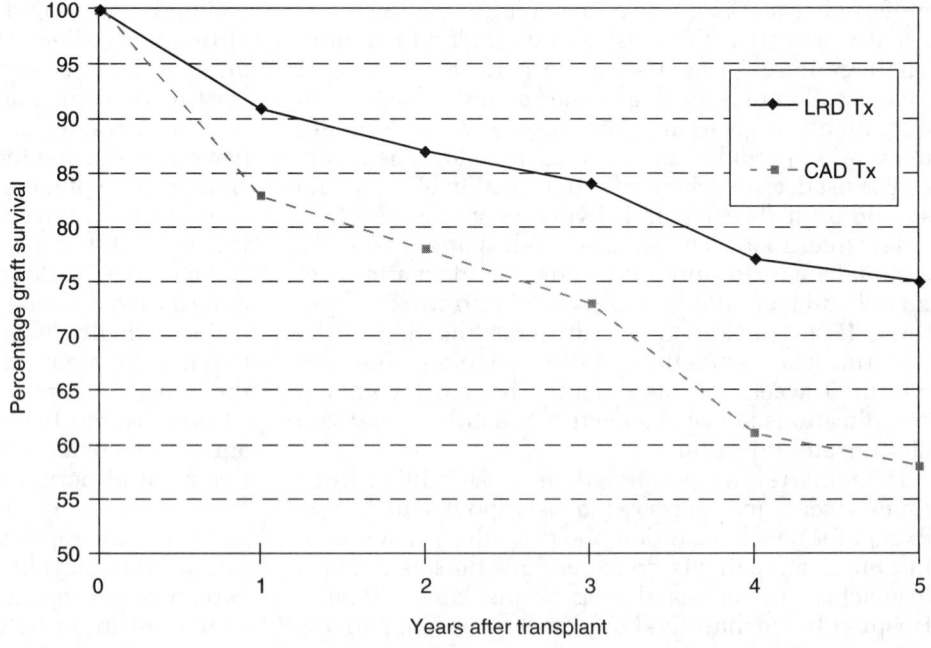

Figure 48.9. Two-year kidney graft survival according to donor source in patients treated with cyclosporine. (Modified from Agodoa LYC, Held PJ, Port FK, eds. US Renal Data System, USRDS 1996 annual data report. Bethesda, MD: National Institute of Diabetes, and Digestive and Kidney Diseases, 1996.)

intact sexual functions. This is particularly so if a well-matched living donor is available. Elderly patients or those with extensive multisystem disease may not be able to tolerate the rigors of transplantation. For others, a period of dialysis and assessment of the patient's adjustment to this therapy often help in determining whether to continue dialysis or consider transplantation. The patient who adjusts well to dialysis can often be fully rehabilitated and can maintain a job as efficiently as the patient with a successful renal transplant. At present it appears that quality of life is the most important criterion determining which form of therapy is selected because survival appears to be similar in patients undergoing either cadaveric transplantation or dialysis.

The personal financial impact of chronic renal failure and the cost of hemodialysis and transplantation, which initially were prohibitively expensive, has been minimized for patients and their families by the extension of the Medicare program to patients under the age of 65 with end-stage renal failure. Nevertheless, patients often have to leave their jobs because of chronic illness or because of the time requirements of therapy.

Despite advances in dialysis and transplantation in recent years, the best hope for patients with chronic renal diseases lies in prevention and appropriate therapy in the early stages of renal insufficiency. These objectives must be accomplished by the patient's primary physician.

General References*

Brenner BM, Rector FC, eds. The kidney. 5th ed. Philadelphia: WB Saunders, 1996.
    Useful general nephrology text.
Felsefeld AJ. Considerations for the treatment of secondary hyperparathyroidism in renal failure. J Am Soc Neprol 8:993, 1997.
    Review of pathophysiology and treatment of renal bone disease.
Garella S. Uremic acidosis. Contrib Nephrol 69:39, 1989.
    Review of the causes, clinical consequences, and treatment of uremic acidosis.
Hood VL, Gennari FJ. End stage renal disease. Measures to prevent it or slow its progression. Postgrad Med 100:163, 1996.
    Review of the therapies directed at slowing the course of progressive renal failure.
Materson BJ, Preston RA. Prevention of diabetic nephropathy. Hosp Pract 32:129, 1997.
    Current review on the effects of intensive therapy on the outcome of long-term complications of Type 1 diabetes.
Remuzzi G, Ruggenenti P, Benigni A. Understanding the nature of renal disease progression. Kidney Int 51:2, 1997.
    Latest theories explaining the mechanisms that lead to progressive renal failure.

Specific References

1. American College of Physicians. Drug prescribing in renal failure. Dosing guidelines for adults. 3rd ed. Publication DRF 90. Philadelphia: American College of Physicians, 1994.
2. Aronson JK. Clinical pharmacokinetics of cardiac glycosides in patients with renal dysfunction. Clin Pharmacokinet 8:155, 1983.
3. Baker LRI, Louise Abrams SM, Roe C, et al. 1,25(OH) 2 D 3 administration in moderate renal failure: a prospective double blind trial. Kidney Int 35:661, 1989.
4. Bakris GL, Copley JB, Vicknair N, et al. Calcium channel blockers versus other antihypertensive therapies on progression of Type II associated nephropathy. Kidney Int 50:1641, 1996.
5. Bennett PH, Haffner S, Kasiske BL, et al. Screening and management of microalbuminuria in patients with diabetes mellitus: recommendations to the Scientific Advisory Board of the National Kidney Foundation from an ad hoc committee of the Council on Diabetes Mellitus of the National Kidney Foundation. Am J Kidney Dis 25:107–112, 1995.
6. Bennett WM, Plamp C, Porter GA. Drug related syndromes in clinical nephrology. Ann Intern Med 87:582, 1977.
7. Bergstrom J. Discovery and rediscovery of low protein diets. Clin Nephrol 21:29, 1984.
8. Brenner BM, Meyer TW, Hostetter TH. Dietary protein intake and the progressive nature of kidney disease: the role of hemodynamically mediated glomerular injury in the pathogenesis of progressive glomerular sclerosis, aging, renal ablation, and intrinsic renal disease. N Engl J Med 307:652, 1982.
9. Clive DM, Stoff JS. Renal syndromes associated with nonsteroidal antiinflammatory drugs. N Engl J Med 310:563, 1984.
10. The Diabetes Control and Complications Research Group. The effect of intensive treatment of diabetes on the development and progression of long-term complications in insulin-dependent diabetes mellitus. N Engl J Med 329:977, 1993.
11. Emanian SA, Nielsen BN, Pederson JF, Ytte L. Kidney dimensions at sonography: correlation with age, sex, and habitus in 665 adult volunteers. AJR Am J Roentgenol 160:83, 1993.
12. Eriksson L, Strufelt G, Thysell H, et al. Effects of sulindac and naproxen on prostaglandin secretion in patients with impaired renal function and rheumatoid arthritis. Am J Med 89:313, 1990.
13. Eschbach JW, Egrie JC, Dowing MR, et al. Correction of the anemia of end-stage renal disease with recombinant human erythropoietin. Results of a combined phase I and II clinical trial. N Engl J Med 316:73, 1987.
14. Friedman EA, L'Esperance JR, eds. Clinical management of diabetes mellitus. In: The diabetic–renal–retinal syndrome. New York: Grune & Stratton, 1980.
15. Geyskes GG, Dei HY, Puylaert CB, et al. Renovascular hypertension identified by captopril-induced changes in the renogram. Hypertension 9:451, 1987.
16. Greco BA, Breyer JA. Atherosclerotic ischemic renal disease. Am J Kidney Dis 29:167, 1997.
17. Hakim RM, Lazarus JM. Initiation of dialysis. J Am Soc Nephrol 6:1319, 1995.
18. Hannedouche T, Landais P, Goldfarb B, et al. Randomized controlled trial of enalapril and beta blockers in non-diabetic chronic renal failure. BMJ 309:833, 1994.
19. Ifudu O, Mayers JD, Mathew JJ, et al. Uremia therapy with end-stage renal disease and human immunodeficiency virus infection: has the outcome changed in the 1990s? Am J Kidney Dis 29:549, 1997.
20. Jones DC, Hayslett JP. Outcome of pregnancy in women with moderate or severe renal insufficiency. N Engl J Med 335:226, 1996.
21. Klahr S, Levey AS, Beck GJ, et al. The effects of dietary protein restriction and blood-pressure control on the progression of chronic renal disease. N Engl J Med 330,877, 1994.
22. Laffel LM, McGill JB, Gans DJ, et al. The beneficial effect of angiotensin-converting enzyme inhibition with captopril in diabetic nephropathy in normotensive Type I patients with microalbuminuria. Am J Med 99:497, 1995.
23. Laissy JP, Benyounes M, Limot O, et al. Screening of renal artery stenosis: assessment with magnetic resonance angiography at 1.0 T. Magn Reson Imaging 14:1033, 1996.
24. Lautin EM, Freeman NJ, Schoenfeld AH, et al. Radiocontrast-associated renal dysfunction: a comparison of lower-osmolality and conventional high-osmolality contrast media. AJR Am J Roentgenol 157:59, 1991.

*Bold print (general references) and bold numerals (specific references) denote published controlled clinical trials, meta-analyses, or consensus-based recommendations.

25. Levey AS, Adler S, Caggiula AW, et al. Effects of dietary protein restriction on the progression of advanced renal disease in the Modification of Diet in Renal Disease Study. Am J Kidney Dis 27:652, 1996.

26. Levey AS, Harrington JT. Continuous peritoneal dialysis for chronic renal failure. Medicine 61:330, 1982.

27. Lewis EJ, Hunsicker LG, Bain RP, et al. The effect of angiotensin-converting enzyme inhibition on diabetic nephropathy. N Engl J Med 329:1456, 1993.

28. Lim VS, DeGowin RL, Zavala D, et al. Recombinant human erythropoietin treatment in pre-dialysis patients. A double-blind placebo controlled trial. Ann Intern Med 110:108, 1989.

29. Lindeman RD, Tobin J, Shock NW. Longitudinal studies on the rate of decline in renal function with age. J Am Geriatr Soc 33:278, 1985.

30. Maschio M, Alberti D, Janin G, et al. Effect of angiotensin converting enzyme inhibitor benazepril in the progression of renal insufficiency. N Engl J Med 334:939, 1996.

31. Maschio G, Oldrizzi L, Tessitore N, et al. Effects of dietary protein and phosphorus restriction on the progression of early renal failure. Kidney Int 22:371, 1982.

32. Parfrey PS, Griffitch SM, Steinman TI, et al. Contrast material–induced renal failure in patients with diabetes mellitus, renal insufficiency or both. A prospective controlled study. N Engl J Med 320:1, 1989.

33. Phelps KR, Lieberman RL, Oh MS, Carroll HJ. Pathophysiology of the syndrome of hyporeninemic hypoaldosteronism. Metabolism 29:186, 1980.

34. Rao TKS, Friedman EA, Nicastri AD. The types of renal disease in the acquired immunodeficiency syndrome. N Engl J Med 316:1062, 1987.

35. Ravid M, Savin H, Jutrin I, et al. Long-term stabilizing effect of angiotensin-converting enzyme inhibition on plasma creatinine and on proteinuria in normotensive type II diabetic patients. Ann Intern Med 118:577, 1993.

36. Regan F, Petronis J, Bohlman M, et al. Perirenal MR high signal: a new and sensitive indicator of acute ureteric obstruction. Clin Radiol 52:445, 1997.

37. Rose BJ. Diuretics. Kidney Int 39:336, 1991.

38. Rowe JW, Andres R, Tobin JD, et al. Age-adjusted standards for creatinine clearance. Ann Intern Med 84:567, 1976.

39. Smith MC, Austen JL, Carey JT, et al. Prednisone improves renal function and proteinuria in human immunodeficiency virus-associated nephropathy. Am J Med 101:41, 1996.

40. Striker G. Report on a workshop to develop management recommendations for the prevention of progression in chronic renal disease. J Am Soc Nephrol 5:1537, 1995.

41. US Renal Data System, Agodoa LYC, Held PJ, Port FK, eds. USRDS 1996 annual data report. Bethesda, MD: National Institutes of Health, National Institute of Diabetes and Digestive and Kidney Diseases, April 1996.

42. Walser M, Drew DH, LaFrance ND. Reciprocal creatinine slopes often give erroneous estimates of progression of chronic renal failure. Kidney Int 36(Suppl 27):S-81, 1989.

43. Yu T-F, Berger L, Dorph DJ, Smith H. Renal function in gout. Factors influencing the renal hemodynamics. Am J Med 67:766, 1979.

44. Zucchelli P, Zuccla A, Borghi M, et al. Long-term comparison between captopril and nifedipine in the progression of renal insufficiency. Kidney Int 42:452, 1992.

C H A P T E R   49

Bladder Outlet Obstruction

RAY E. STUTZMAN, MD

The bladder, bladder outlet, prostate, and urethra may be affected by a wide variety of conditions that result in symptoms of urinary obstruction or bladder irritability. These disorders are common, especially in older men.

Benign prostatic hyperplasia (BPH) is the most common cause of bladder outlet obstruction in men over 50 years of age. Autopsy studies show that 50 to 60% of men over 50 have significant enlargement of the prostate caused by BPH, and the prevalence increases with age. A number of other conditions may also cause symptoms of bladder outlet obstruction in the male: urethral stricture, carcinoma of the prostate, neurogenic bladder, bladder calculus, prostatitis, bladder neck contracture, and carcinoma of the bladder. Functional obstruction, seen in both women and men, may result from chronic bladder distension, debilitating disease, psychogenic retention, or medications.

HISTORY

Bladder outlet obstruction is characterized by symptoms of urinary hesitancy, diminished force and caliber of the stream, and postvoid dribbling. The symptoms of urinary frequency, urgency, and nocturia result from a diminished functional bladder capacity, bladder muscle hypertrophy, and often bladder instability. The hypertrophy results in increased intravesical pressure during voiding, thereby providing compensation for the obstruction. In time, however, the bladder will decompensate, and this may lead to residual urine, infection, hematuria, hydronephrosis, and renal failure.

Patients with *urethral stricture* usually have a history of urethral trauma, instrumentation (most commonly indwelling Foley catheter), or urethritis and, in association with symptoms of bladder outlet obstruction, may notice a split stream. *Carcinoma of the prostate* may present with obstructive symptoms that are often of a shorter duration than those seen in patients with BPH, in whom symptoms of outlet obstruction usually progress over several years. Recent onset of back or bone pain, anorexia, or weight loss suggests malignancy. *Neurogenic bladder* should be suspected when other symptoms of neurologic disease are present, when disorders of bowel or sexual function coexist with bladder outlet obstruction, or when a systemic disease that causes neurologic bladder dysfunction (e.g., diabetes mellitus or spinal cord injury) exists.

A review of current and recently used medications (Table 49.1) is mandatory in the evaluation of the patient with symptoms of bladder outlet obstruction (21). Anticholinergic agents, antispasmodic and antiparkinsonian drugs, as well as many antidepressant drugs depress bladder muscle contractility; sympathomimetic agents (e.g., ephedrine and other decongestants found in over-the-counter cold remedies), β-blocking agents, and levodopa increase bladder outlet resistance. Diuresis (e.g., from a diuretic, glucosuria, or a large, brisk fluid intake) may overstretch a partially decompensated detrusor muscle and cause acute urinary retention.

It is important to distinguish *outlet obstructive bladder symptoms* (hesitancy, decreased stream, postvoid dribbling) from *irritative bladder symptoms* (frequency, urgency, nocturia). Although anatomic or functional obstruction may produce both types of symptoms, irritative symptoms are seen with cystitis, prostatitis, bladder stones, and bladder carcinoma.

Table 49.1. Selected Pharmacologic Agents with Known Influence on Bladder Function

Drugs that Increase Bladder Tone and Contractility
Bethanechol (Urecholine)

Drugs that Decrease Bladder Contractility
Anticholinergic drugs (e.g., Pro-Banthine, Donnatal, Ditropan)
Antihistamines
Calcium antagonists (verapamil, nifedipine, diltiazem)
Prostaglandin inhibitors (e.g., ibuprofen)
Tricyclic antidepressants (e.g., imipramine, nortriptyline)
$β_2$-Adrenergic antagonists (e.g., terbutoline)

Drugs that Increase Bladder Outlet Resistance
Adrenergic agonists (e.g., ephedrine, Sudafed, Ornade)
Antiparkinsonian drugs (e.g., levodopa, Sinemet)
β-Adrenergic antagonists (e.g., propranolol)
Estrogens

Drugs that Decrease Outlet Resistance
Antispasticity drugs (e.g., diazepam, Baclofen)
α-Adrenergic antagonists (e.g., doxazosin, prazosin, phenoxybenzamine, terazosin)

Drugs that Increase Urinary Volume
Diuretics

Finally, the differentiation of polyuria from urinary frequency, and nocturia from enuresis (involuntary bedwetting) can be made by appropriate questioning.

The American Urological Association (AUA) Measurement Committee has developed a symptom assessment tool (Table 49.2) for patients with prostatism (24). This prostate symptom score is based on the answer to seven questions concerning urinary symptoms. Each question allows the patient to choose one out of five answers scaled to indicate increasing severity of the particular symptom. The answers are assigned points from 0 to 5. The total score can therefore range from 0 to 35 (asymptomatic to very symptomatic). There is an additional single question to assess the quality of life. The answer to this question ranges from "delighted" to "terrible," or 0 to 6. The International Consensus Committee (ICC), under the patronage of the World Health Organization (WHO), has agreed to use the symptom index for BPH. The ICC strongly recommends that all physicians who counsel patients with symptoms of prostatism use these measures not only during the initial interview but also during and after treatment in order to monitor response.

PHYSICAL EXAMINATION

The physical examination of the patient with symptoms of bladder outlet obstruction should be carefully focused, with special emphasis on the urinary tract.

The *abdominal examination* may reveal several findings: a distended bladder from retention, renal tenderness (infection or hydronephrosis) or a renal mass (hydronephrosis, neoplasm, or cystic disease), and inguinal hernia from straining at urination when outlet obstruction is present. In the male patient, the *examination of the penis* may reveal phimosis or urethral meatal stenosis that could cause partial obstruction. The examination of the epididymides may show evidence of acute or chronic infection, which may be a complication of bladder outlet obstruction and concomitant prostatitis. A brief *neurologic examination,* particularly of the anal sphincter tone, genital and perineal sensation, and motor, sensory, and reflex activity of the lower extremities, may disclose abnormalities that suggest a neurogenic bladder as the cause of the patient's symptoms.

A careful *rectal examination* of the prostate is important in evaluating the patient with suspected BPH or prostatic carcinoma. Although there are certain limits, rectal palpation permits examination of the lateral lobes of the prostate and the posterior lobe, adjacent to the apex. The anterior lobe cannot be felt, and rarely is the median lobe palpable unless it is markedly enlarged. BPH most commonly involves the lateral and median lobes; moreover, the size of the prostate gland as estimated by rectal examination is not directly related to the degree of urinary obstruction.

The most important information obtained from the rectal examination is the *consistency of the prostate gland.* The patient may be examined when he is in the

Table 49.2. International Prostate Symptom Score (I-PSS)[a]

	Not at All	Less Than 1 Time in 5	Less Than Half the Time	About Half the Time	More Than Half the Time	Almost Always	Your Score
Incomplete emptying: Over the past month, how often have you had a sensation of not emptying your bladder completely after you finished urinating?	0	1	2	3	4	5	
Frequency: Over the past month, how often have you had to urinate again less than 2 hours after you finished urinating?	0	1	2	3	4	5	
Intermittency: Over the past month, how often have you found you stopped and started again several times when you urinated?	0	1	2	3	4	5	
Urgency: Over the past month, how often have you found it difficult to postpone urination?	0	1	2	3	4	5	
Weak stream: Over the past month, how often have you had a weak urinary stream?	0	1	2	3	4	5	
Straining: Over the past month, how often have you had to push or strain to begin urination?	0	1	2	3	4	5	
	None	1 time	2 times	3 times	4 times	5 or more times	
Nocturia: Over the past month how many times did you most typically get up to urinate from the time you went to bed at night until the time you got up in the morning?	0	1	2	3	4	5	
						Total I-PSS Score =	

Quality of Life

	Delighted	Pleased	Mostly Satisfied	Mixed (About Equally Satisfied and Dissatisfied)	Mostly Dissatisfied	Unhappy	Terrible
If you were to spend the rest of your life with your urinary condition just the way it is now, how would you feel about that?	0	1	2	3	4	5	6

[a]From International Consensus Committee under patronage of the World Health Organization (R. 20). Handy cards containing this information are currently available at no cost from Merck and Co., Inc., 215-652-7300.

decubitus, knee–chest, or standing–bending position. The patient should void as fully as possible before the examination because a full bladder may distort the size of the prostate. The patient should be told that he may feel the urge to void when the prostate is examined. To prevent anal sphincter spasm, appropriate time should be used to explain the procedure to the patient. Using ample lubricant, the physician should dilate the anal sphincter slowly and gently by gradually inserting the finger through the anus and asking the patient to bear down slightly. This examination permits the determination of shape, size, and consistency of the prostate; the presence of tenderness; any other rectal masses; and the adequacy of anal sphincter tone.

The normal prostate is palpable 2 to 5 cm from the anal verge through the anterior rectal wall. The examining finger can normally reach over the top (base) of the prostate, as well as over each lateral border. A median sulcus is appreciated in the midline. The palpable prostate can be compared in size, configuration, and consistency with the tip of the nose.

BPH often results not only in obliteration of the median sulcus but also in a failure of the examining finger to reach the base of the gland. The consistency of the gland in BPH is smooth and rubbery, similar to the thenar eminence of the hand. The gland is not tender unless prostatitis is present. BPH may be characterized by symmetric or asymmetric enlargement and can be nodular. The clinical differentiation between carcinoma and asymmetric or nodular BPH is usually based on the degree of induration or hardness of the gland.

Classically, prostatic carcinoma is characterized by a rock-hard nodule or mass involving one or both posterior lobes. The zygomatic arch of the face has a similar consistency to that of prostatic carcinoma. However, not all hard nodules are found on biopsy to be cancer, nor are all cancerous nodules hard. Granulomatous prostatitis, prostatic calculi, spheroids of BPH, or nodularity resulting from transurethral prostatic resection may present as prostatic nodules and induration. Only 30 to 40% of prostatic nodules biopsied as suspicious for carcinoma are positive on histologic examination.

If prostatic carcinoma is suspected, it is important to determine the extent of the local lesion—single nodule, diffuse involvement, or extension outside the capsule—and to refer the patient to a urologist.

PRELIMINARY LABORATORY ASSESSMENT

If the patient is thought to have bladder outlet obstruction caused by BPH, the need and urgency for urologic consultation must be determined. A urinalysis and the determination of the urinary flow rate (see below), the performance of a urine culture (if pyuria is present), and measurement of serum creatinine or, sometimes, the measurement of the postvoid residual volume (see below) provide the data that will aid in making this decision. The measurement of *prostate-specific antigen* (PSA) should be obtained in patients suspected of having carcinoma.

PSA and Screening for Prostate Cancer

Prostate-specific antigen (PSA) is an enzyme synthesized only by prostatic epithelial cells. The ejaculate contains a high concentration of PSA. However, PSA is not specific for prostate carcinoma. Elevated serum PSA levels may be found in prostate carcinoma, glandular hyperplasia associated with BPH, acute bacterial prostatitis, prostate abscess, prostatic infarction, and manipulation of the prostate (e.g., cystourethroscopy, needle biopsy of the prostate, or transurethral resection of the prostate [TURP]). Ejaculation within 48 hours may elevate the PSA. Digital rectal examination and transrectal ultrasound do not appear to alter significantly the level of serum PSA. In 70% of men, PSA is less that 2 ng/mL. It is estimated that 40 to 50% of men with prostate carcinoma have a PSA greater than 10 ng/mL, whereas less than 5% of patients with BPH have such levels. When the physician elects to screen for asymptomatic prostate cancer in a man, the serum PSA determination is not adequate but should be used in conjunction with a digital rectal examination. There remains controversy concerning the routine screening of men for asymptomatic prostate cancer. A popular position that has been widely publicized in the lay and medical literature is the recommendation that all men between the ages of 50 and 75 years who also have at least a 10-year life expectancy should have a yearly PSA and digital rectal examination (9). On the other hand, there is no evidence yet that the early detection of asymptomatic prostatic cancers has changed survival, and indeed, it may lead to significant mental and physical morbidity (e.g., from anxiety, or from morbidity related to surgery or radiation) (7,12). Therefore, screening for prostate cancer remains controversial. The general physician should always discuss the risks and benefits of an evaluation aimed at the early detection of prostate cancer with patients who might be considered candidates for screening. Ongoing studies on the course of prostate cancer with and without treatment in the future will guide clinicians concerning this consideration. Men who have a family history of prostate cancer are at increased risk and should be screened yearly, starting at age 40. African Americans also have an increased risk of developing prostate cancer and should be screened regularly. In both of these instances, the patient should understand the implications and subsequent diagnostic and therapeutic considerations of finding a biopsy positive for cancer. PSA density (PSAD), a quotient of serum PSA and prostate volume determined by ultrasonography performed by a urologist or ultrasonographer, may be useful in distinguishing BPH from prostate cancer in the patient with a history or physical examination that raises concern about cancer. The rate of change in PSA levels may be a sensitive and specific early clinical marker for the development of prostate cancer (8). A serial increase of 0.75 ng or more in the level of PSA over base levels, drawn at 6- to 12-month intervals, is strongly suggestive of prostatic carcinoma despite normal digital rectal examinations. An increase in volume of the prostate in BPH occurs more slowly, so PSA does not rise rapidly in that condition. If a significant increase in levels occurs, transrectal ultrasound and prostate biopsy (both done by the consulting urologist or sonographer) should be considered. PSA exists in both a bound and a free form. Patients with prostate cancer often have less free or unbound PSA, usually less than 10%; on the other hand, patients with BPH usually have greater than 25% free PSA.

Patient Experience. Needle biopsy of the prostate is usually done in a urologist's office or in an ultrasound suite. Prostate biopsy currently is most commonly done in conjunction with transrectal ultrasound (TRUS) (see below). No anesthesia or sedation is required and the patient can eat and drink normally on the day of the procedure. Aspirin should be stopped for a week and anticoagulants should be stopped until the anticoagulant effect has gone to avoid an increased risk of bleeding. A prophylactic antimicrobial (usually a fluoroquinolone) is given the evening before and the morning of the procedure. The procedure usually takes 20 to 30 minutes and the patient feels no more discomfort than with a typical rectal examination. The ultrasound probe, which is slightly larger than the index finger, is introduced into the rectum, allowing the prostate gland to be visualized. Usually a total of 10 to 12 needle core specimens are obtained from suspicious as well as normal areas. The biopsy apparatus has a spring-loaded gun mechanism and the operator informs the patient that a loud noise will be heard when it is fired. The patient usually remains under surveillance for 30 to 60 minutes to be sure that the procedure was accomplished without incident. Most men notice slight blood in their urine or stool for a day or two. Bloody semen may be experienced for several ejaculations. The patient is informed that these findings are common and of no concern unless they persist.

Most important, serum PSA concentration is the most reliable marker for response to treatment in prostate carcinoma. Serum PSA values should be negligible within 3 to 4 weeks following a radical prostatectomy. The failure of this to occur is an indication of residual disease. Elevated PSA levels also drop after primary radiation therapy but never reach zero. Regardless of the treatment, a rising PSA level means progression of the disease.

URODYNAMIC ASSESSMENT

Urodynamic evaluation of the urinary tract includes urinary flow rate (uroflowmetry), cystometry, and pressure flow studies. *Uroflowmetry* should be done by the general physician because it is easy to perform, is noninvasive, and may provide valuable information about the degree of obstruction and thereby guide the initiation of treatment. *Urinary flow rate* may be assessed by measuring the volume of urine voided during a 5-second period (4). Normal males have 5-second volumes exceeding 75 mL, whereas men with urinary obstruction have flows less than 50 mL in 5 seconds. *Cystometry* performed by a urologist is indicated in patients with clinical suspicion of voiding dysfunction unrelated to bladder outlet obstruction, primarily patients with urgency, frequency, or a suggestion of a neurologic disorder. There is no evidence that routine cystometry is of value in the management of urinary outlet obstruction secondary to BPH.

If the patient does not have hematuria, urinary tract infection, or renal failure and if the diagnosis of BPH is likely, further evaluation depends on whether the patient is a candidate for surgery (Table 49.3). If there is no indication for surgery, then no further evaluation is necessary at this juncture.

UROLOGIC INVESTIGATION

When surgery is a consideration and a patient is referred to a urologist, several further assessments often are made.

Imaging

Intravenous urography once was used routinely in the evaluation of men with bladder outlet obstructive symptoms, but because it is invasive and has some side effects, this is no longer true. It now is limited, for the most part, to an evaluation of a patient with hematuria.

Table 49.3. Indications for Surgery in Patients with BPH and Bladder Outlet Obstruction

Urinary retention
Intractable symptoms caused by obstruction
Recurrent or persistent urinary tract infection
Recurrent prostatic bleeding
Significant postvoid residual urine
Changes of the kidneys, ureters, or bladder caused by prostatic obstruction
Abnormally low urinary flow rate
Bladder calculi

If an intravenous urogram is believed to be necessary (e.g., to evaluate a patient with hematuria), the physician should determine that the serum creatinine concentration is less than 1.8 mg/dL. If the patient gives a history of a previous reaction, even if mild or moderate in severity, there is approximately a 35% chance of a recurrent reaction. However, nonionic contrast agents may be used with a much lower risk. A decision to perform a study in this instance must be made on an individual basis and in consultation with a radiologist and urologist. *Ultrasonography* of the urinary tract, a simple, noninvasive technique, appears to provide more useful information and is used more commonly. It is the procedure of first choice to evaluate the upper urinary tract for the presence of hydronephrosis, stones, renal masses, and anomalies. Ultrasonography is useful to quantitate the postvoid residual urine, identify bladder calculi, and estimate the size of the prostate. *Transrectal ultrasonography* (TRUS), because it can clearly visualize the prostate, is in common use. This procedure is useful when evaluating a patient with an abnormal prostate on rectal examination or an elevated PSA. It is usually ordered by a urologist and usually is done in combination with a prostate biopsy. The size of the prostate gland can be calculated and abnormal areas within the gland can be delineated; cancer, for example, is usually hypoechoic. If cancer is suspected or known, TRUS assists in staging (i.e., extensive local disease or invasion of the seminal vesicles). TRUS is used for localization in performing needle biopsy of the prostate. A *renal scan* may be used to evaluate renal blood flow or delayed excretion suggestive of obstruction. A *retrograde ureteropyelogram* done in conjunction with cystoscopy by a urologist (see below) provides visualization of the ureters, renal pelvis, and calyces. The contrast media used during this procedure is rarely absorbed and can be used safely in patients with contrast media allergy (e.g., from an intravenous pyelogram). If the history suggests a urethral stricture (see above), a *retrograde urethrogram* may be performed. This procedure requires instillation of contrast material into the urethra with appropriate radiographs. Anesthesia is not needed during this procedure, and only minimal discomfort is experienced during injection into the urethra.

Instrumentation

A general physician or a urologist gains considerable information in the evaluation of a patient with symptoms of bladder outlet obstruction by performing several invasive procedures. Because these procedures may be associated with the development of infection, they should not be done casually.

Bladder Catheterization for Postvoid Volume

Inserting a urethral catheter immediately after a patient has voided will determine the amount of residual urine (more than 100 mL is abnormal), as well as help determine whether there is a urethral stricture (see also Chapter 6). There is a risk of urosepsis if infection is present; also, hematuria or urinary retention may result from the instrumentation. *Ultrasound* of the lower abdomen and pelvis accurately estimates postvoid residual urine without an invasive procedure such as catheterization. In fact, when available, ultrasound has virtually replaced catheterization in the determination of the postvoid residual volume. Simple to use, accurate, portable ultrasound units are available and are useful for the general physician to purchase. If a neurogenic bladder is suspected, the patient should be referred to a urologist for a consultation and the performance of a cystometrogram and possibly a cystourethroscopy.

Cystometrogram

A cystometrogram is easily performed by a urologist in the office. The procedure is similar to a catheterization for residual urine. After the catheter is placed, a sterile solution is used to fill the bladder and to record and classify the detrusor response to the increasing volume.

Cystourethroscopy

Cystourethroscopy is a procedure that permits visualization of the entire urethra, the prostate, and the bladder.

Patient Experience. Cystourethroscopy usually is done in a urologist's office or in an outpatient clinic using topical anesthesia without premedication. A lighted rigid or flexible instrument, typically 6 mm in diameter, is used. The patient often perceives a feeling of suprapubic pressure as the bladder is being filled with the irrigating fluid, but the degree of discomfort is usually slight. The examination takes just a few minutes. However, if a retrograde ureteropyelogram is performed, another 15 minutes may be required. After cystoscopy, patients often experience dysuria. The patient should have been advised about this and informed that it may be relieved by voiding while sitting in a bathtub filled with warm water or by taking phenazopyridine (Pyridium), 100 mg three times a day for 1 or 2 days. Hematuria after cystoscopy is also common and may persist for 2 or 3 days. The patient should be informed of this possibility, reassured that it is not uncommon, and advised to force fluids (2 to 3 L/day). Infection in the urinary tract occurs only rarely after cystoscopy. Occasionally, acute urinary retention results from edema of the prostate subsequent to instrumentation. If this complication occurs, the insertion of an indwelling catheter and possibly hospitalization are necessary. An uncommon long-term complication of cystoscopy is urethral stricture. The use of smaller instruments and new flexible cystoscopes decreases the incidence of this complication.

The urologist learns a great deal from the cystoscopic examination. The entire urethra is seen. The size of the prostate, the degree of occlusion, trabeculation in the bladder, the presence of a bladder stone, and diverticula are all directly visualized. This information is most important in helping the urologist determine the need for and the type of surgery.

TREATMENT OF BLADDER OUTLET OBSTRUCTION
Benign Prostatic Hyperplasia

For more than 50 years the traditional operative approaches for BPH have been TURP and open prostatectomy. Questions have been raised about the morbidity and mortality of these procedures (17). Several simpler and less invasive surgical therapies have been developed or are being investigated. In addition, a number of nonsurgical treatments are being used. These surgical and nonsurgical options are discussed below.

A theoretical alternative to any treatment, particularly in a patient with acute or chronic urinary retention, is to remain on long-term indwelling catheterization or to have clean intermittent catheterization. Suprapubic cystostomy, used extensively in the past, is rarely needed today because of the improvement in urethral catheters and the widespread use of intermittent catheterization. Occasionally suprapubic catheterization is used acutely, and in this situation, the fistula heals quickly after the catheter is removed, provided any outlet obstruction has been removed. Long-term catheterization of any sort is associated with recurrent urinary tract infections and urosepsis; therefore, other options for treating a patient with bladder outlet obstruction should always be considered first. Finally, bethanechol (Urecholine), a cholinergic agent commonly prescribed in the past for an adynamic bladder without outlet obstruction, is rarely used today because of the cardiovascular and gastrointestinal side effects and the availability and ease of intermittent catheterization.

Surgical Management of BPH

Transurethral Resection of the Prostate. TURP is still the most commonly used procedure in the surgical treatment of BPH; more than 90% of prostatectomies for benign disease are performed this way but this percentage seems to be decreasing as new techniques and nonsurgical therapies are advancing. It requires hospitalization for 1 to 2 days, although occasionally it is done as an outpatient procedure; general or spinal anesthesia is used.

Complications have been minimized by the use of smaller, more efficient instruments, by improved lighting, and by isotonic irrigating fluids. Nevertheless, bleeding, infection, and plasma hypoosmolality (from absorption of irrigation fluid) may occur. Long-term complications of TURP include urethral stricture, bladder neck contracture, and incontinence (15).

A common consequence of TURP is *retrograde ejaculation,* a situation characterized by the ejaculation of semen into the bladder rather than externally through the urethra. This phenomenon occurs because the bladder neck is opened as part of the TURP and cannot subsequently contract, as is necessary to produce antegrade ejaculation. Retrograde ejaculation results in sterility but does not usually affect orgasm. This consequence should be discussed with sexually active patients and their partners before prostatectomy.

TURP should not produce organic erectile impotence; however, psychogenic impotence may follow this and other genitourinary surgery. The management of psychogenic impotence is described in Chapter 18.

Most patients can resume normal physical and sexual activity in approximately 4 weeks following TURP. However, complete healing of the prostatic fossa usually takes 2 to 3 months, and during this period a urinalysis may reveal white and red blood cells.

Open Prostatectomy. Open prostatectomy requires a slightly longer hospitalization and recovery period. This approach is used when, in addition to having a large prostate, the patient has a bladder condition that can be repaired at the same time (e.g., bladder diverticulum or bladder stone). Organic erectile impotence occurs occasionally, especially when the perineal approach has been used. If this complication occurs, an evaluation should be performed before attributing the impotence to the surgery and presuming it to be irreversible.

It is important for a patient undergoing any form of prostatectomy for BPH to understand that the entire prostate gland is not removed. Because of the presence of residual prostate tissue, these patients have a risk equal to that of the general population of developing prostatic carcinoma. Prostate cancer screening should be used by the physician in men electing such screening (see above), even though they have had any form of prostatectomy. Because residual prostatic tissue remains, recurrent symptoms or complications from prostatic hypertrophy may develop later. The frequency of recurrence depends primarily on the extent of the initial surgery and is highly variable.

Transurethral Incision of the Prostate and Bladder Neck. Transurethral incision of the prostate (TUIP) is gaining increasing favor and replacing TURP in selected cases. The indication for incision of the prostate is the same as it is for TURP, except that it may be used in younger men and in patients whose prostate gland seems of nearly normal size in rectal examination, usually considered to be less than 30 g by urologists. Incision is performed primarily through the muscle of the bladder neck and through the prostate adenoma to the level of the verumontanum. Usually two incisions are made. In comparing TUIP with TURP, there are fewer complications with TUIP and the postoperative flow rates and relief of symptoms are comparable with either procedure. There are no significant differences in subjective prostate-related symptoms or uroflowmetry in the two groups. However, there is a higher incidence of bladder neck contracture after TURP. The additional advantages of TUIP are that the patient's postoperative stay is shorter, there is a shorter operative time and decreased perioperative morbidity, and some procedures have been performed using only local anesthesia. Finally, the incidence of retrograde ejaculation is less with TUIP. The major disadvantage of TUIP is the potential for missing major localized prostate cancer; therefore, some urologists advocate either a biopsy of the prostate or at least one loop incision (similar to that done in TURP) for tissue at the time of the TUIP.

Other Procedures to Relieve Bladder Neck Obstruction. *Balloon dilation* has been performed recently. However, objective evaluation of the procedure shows little benefit over urethral instrumentation or watchful waiting.

A permanently implanted *urethral stent* made of various materials from stainless steel to a biodegradable substance has been used with varying results. The placement of a urethral stent is limited, therefore, primarily to high-risk patients who have suffered urinary retention and are poor operative risks. The advantages of the stent are that there is no significant intraoperative or postoperative hemorrhage and no need for an indwelling urethral catheter, the procedure can usually be done under local anesthesia, and the patient most often does not require hospitalization. Stent dislodgement, urinary infection, and stones forming on the stent all have been reported. In selected cases it is considered as an alternative to chronic indwelling catheter or intermittent clean catheterization.

Transurethral microwave hyperthermia (TUMT) is an FDA-approved outpatient procedure that seems to improve the patient's symptoms objectively and subjectively without causing significant tissue damage (2). The temperature of the prostate is raised to approximately 45° to 55°C. Findings after hyperthermia of the prostate show that there is a definite improvement, on the order of 50%, in the obstructive symptoms. These procedures are well tolerated with only a few transient and usually mild adverse effects. Histologic analysis of material obtained following hyperthermia shows significant tissue reaction and evidence of widespread cell death of prostate tissue. On the other hand, TRUS measurement of the size of the gland has failed to demonstrate any overall reduction in the volume of the prostate during follow-up.

Laser Treatment of the Prostate. The use of lasers may be an alternative to TURP. The laser is in direct contact with the prostatic urethra and results in incision and vaporization of prostatic tissue. Studies of laser prostatectomy suggest that acute or delayed complications typical of TURP are seen. Laser prostatectomy may be performed as an outpatient procedure, with similar benefits to TURP, transurethral vaporization of the prostate (TVP), and transurethral needle ablation (TUNA).

Transurethral Vaporization of the Prostate. Transurethral vaporization appears to be providing results comparable to those of TURP. A more powerful electrical current in the resectoscope loop results in vaporization of tissue with minimal bleeding. There is also a wedge loop that can provide vaporization, as well as removal of prostatic tissue. This results in less bleeding, shorter catheterization, and shorter hospital stay. Some of these procedures can now be done on an outpatient basis, with removal of the catheter within 24 to 48 hours. Another advantage of the TVP is that most of the equipment necessary for this procedure is available in most operating rooms and hospitals; expensive equipment, as is necessary in laser therapy, is not needed.

Transurethral Needle Ablation (TUNA). TUNA is a newer technique involving the insertion of a needle transurethrally into the prostate, causing tissue necrosis by radio frequency. This procedure can be done on an outpatient basis under local anesthesia, usually with an indwelling catheter for 1 to 2 days. Although still new and not widely available, this procedure is very promising because of its simplicity, decrease in morbidity, and successful outcome.

Nonsurgical Treatment of BPH

Nonsurgical therapy for BPH currently relies on two different pharmacologic approaches:

- Eliminating the dynamic component of the bladder outlet obstruction through the use of β-adrenergic antagonists (e.g., terazosin, doxazosin)
- Producing a state of androgen deprivation with luteinizing hormone-releasing hormone (LHRH) antagonists, antiandrogens, or 5α-reductase inhibitors (e.g., finasteride)

The rationale for α-antagonists in BPH is based on the fact that smooth muscle makes up a significant component of the human prostate. In fact, the prostate is composed primarily of glandular epithelium, smooth muscle, and connective tissue. Several α-blockers have been used; doxazosin and terazosin, selective long-acting α1-adrenergic blockers, have been most extensively studied (13,14). The typical dosage of terazosin (e.g., Hytrin, available in 1-, 2-, 5-, and 10-mg tablets) is 2 to 10 mg/day in one or two daily doses. The blood pressure must be monitored and the drug should be started at a dosage of 1 mg at bedtime (to minimize the hypotensive effect) and increased in 3 to 7 days if no response has occurred. Doxazosin (e.g., Cardura, available in 1-, 2-, 4-, and 8-mg tablets) is taken as 2 to 8 mg/day in a single dose. If the patient is taking other antihypertensive agents, closer monitoring of the blood pressure is needed. Generally, dosage adjustment can be made weekly. In patients who initially have low blood pressure, α-blockers are probably best avoided. In selected patients with minimal to moderate outlet symptoms, the results of treatment with α-blockers have been excellent, with a measured increase in urinary flow rate, decrease in some of the irritative voiding symptoms, and minimal side effects. α-Blockers are effective in both larger and smaller glands.

Hormonal therapy (androgen deprivation) including castration has long been known to decrease the size of the prostate when BPH is present. However, the side effects of both medical or surgical castration precluded such therapy except in elderly symptomatic patients who were considered to be too high a risk for surgical intervention or for the administration of an anesthetic. The development of a 5α-reductase inhibitor, *finasteride* (Proscar), has significantly altered the management options for patients with BPH (22). *Finasteride* produces a profound fall in serum and intraprostatic dihydrotestosterone (DHT) levels without lowering testosterone levels. It possesses no androgenic, antiandrogenic, or steroid hormone-related properties. In approximately 30% of patients over 6 months it causes a 30% reduction in prostate volume. To date there have been no clinically significant adverse effects and no significant changes in other hormone parameters. Patients who take finasteride have approximately a 50% drop in their pretreatment PSA level. The dosage of finasteride (Proscar) is 5 mg orally every day in a single dose. It must be given for at least 6 months for the trial to be considered adequate. If a patient stops finasteride, the prostate size will return to pretreatment levels and the bladder outlet obstructive symptoms will recur. If the patient does benefit from finasteride, the drug should be continued indefinitely. The administration of finasteride does not preclude surgical treatment if the patient alters his decision to take the drug for any reason or fails to respond to the medication after 6 months. Finasteride is most effective in glands that are larger on examination, usually considered to be more than 40 g by urologists (5); glands that are very large (more than 70 g) are usually so large that the examiner cannot reach the base (upper portion) with the examining finger, assuming the bladder is not distended.

Finasteride, terazosin, or both have been compared with placebo in men with BPH (14a). Terazosin was effective in this study but fenasteride was not and the combination was no more effective than terazosin alone. However, in an accompanying editorial, Walsh (19a) points out that BPH is a heterogenous disorder and that the Lepor study did not control for prostate gland size as had been done in the earlier fenasteride study (22). Walsh suggests, as indicated above, that fenasteride be used only when the gland is large, whereas α-antagonists can be used with large and small glands.

Estrogens are thought to play a considerable causative or permissive role in BPH; estrogen deprivation, therefore, may represent a useful treatment in BPH. Aromatase inhibitors have attracted attention for use in the treatment of several estrogen-dependent clinical disorders. These agents are still under investigation and cannot be recommended yet.

Currently, there are many alternatives in the management of acute urinary retention and significant bladder outlet obstruction from BPH. All alternatives must be considered and thoroughly discussed with the patient in consultation with the urologist.

In summary, most patients with mild or moderate symptoms of bladder outlet obstruction should be reassured and can be followed by watchful waiting. If they do have significant bothersome symptoms, the initial therapy would be α-blockers. If the prostate is large this can also be combined with finasteride if adequate response is not achieved with α-blockers alone. In patients who have acute urinary retention following an operative procedure or from medication, an α-blocker is appropriate to give them a trial at voiding; also, these patients can be taught intermittent self-catheterization to see whether they will have returned to their prior voiding pattern. In patients requiring invasive procedures, still the most accepted method is a TURP, but some of the newer modalities, such as transurethral vaporization of the prostate and transurethral needle ablation of the prostate, may be suggested by the consulting urologist.

Urethral Stricture

A urethral stricture may be treated with urethral dilation, transurethral incision of the stricture, or open urethral surgery. The method selected depends on the length and location of the stricture, the patient's overall health, and the urologist's experience.

PROSTATIC CARCINOMA

Prostatic carcinoma is the most commonly diagnosed cancer among American men and may present with bladder outlet obstruction, although this is a far less common cause than with BPH. The most common physical finding leading to the diagnosis of adenocarcinoma of the prostate is a prostatic nodule or induration discovered on a routine rectal examination of the prostate or an elevated PSA. Either finding should lead to a urologic consultation and a biopsy of the prostate. Approximately 30 to 40% of prostatic nodules or induration in the prostate are adenocarcinomas. The prevalence of unsuspected or incidental carcinoma of the prostate found at TURP ranges from 4% in the fourth decade to 80% in the ninth decade of life. The prevalence at autopsy is even higher because many cancers begin in the outer periphery of the prostate gland and are missed by incomplete transurethral resection.

The therapy of prostatic carcinoma is somewhat controversial but may be approached on the basis of the stage of disease classified by the Whitmore–Jewett system (10) (Table 49.4). This is usually established clinically by digital rectal examination, PSA levels, and a bone scan. TRUS may be helpful in the assessment of local disease and in estimating the volume of neoplasm. This is usually done in conjunction with the biopsy of the prostate (see above). Magnetic resonance imaging (MRI) or computerized tomography (CT) scan is usually not indicated.

The tissue obtained by biopsy (see above) is described using the *Gleason Scoring System* for adenocarcinoma of the prostate. This system divides the cancer into five histologic grades, with Gleason pattern

1 being well differentiated and Gleason pattern 5 being poorly differentiated. The cancer patterns are scored based on the predominant histologic grade seen at two sites. The most differentiated cancer (and those with the best prognosis) would be scored as grade 1 + 1, or a Gleason score of 2. The most poorly differentiated cancers would be scored as grade 5 + 5, or a Gleason score of 10. This information assists the urologist in planning the management options. In addition, the urologist stages the patient with adenocarcinoma of the prostate.

Most urologists, pathologists, and oncologists have now adopted the TNM staging classification for prostate carcinoma (18). Table 49.5 compares the TNM classification with the Whitmore–Jewett staging system. Significant in this classification is T1c, a tumor identified by needle biopsy performed because of an elevated PSA, but with a normal rectal examination. Regional lymph nodes are assessed by N, and the distant metastases are assessed by M.

If the neoplasm is limited to the prostate (no evidence of local spread or metastatic disease) and the patient is under 75 years of age, has an anticipated 10-year survival, and has no contraindicating medical diseases, he is a candidate for a curative treatment. Radiation therapy and radical prostatectomy are primary considerations. Radical prostatectomy appears to provide slightly less morbidity and longer survival (16). In the hands of a urologist experienced in this type of surgery, the complications are minimal and less than 2% of patients develop incontinence. A modification of the traditional radical prostatectomy permits the removal of all cancerous tissue, yet spares the pelvic nerves that control erection; there is preservation of preexisting potency in up to 70% of younger patients (19).

Stage A (T1, N0 M0) prostatic carcinoma is disease unsuspected on rectal examination of the prostate, but discovered at the time of prostatectomy, usually TURP, for obstructive symptoms thought to be secondary to benign hyperplasia. If carcinoma is reported, the percentage or volume of neoplasm to the total amount of tissue removed and the histologic grade of the neoplasm should be noted. This information will aid in the management and determination of prognosis of the patient. Stage A is further subdivided into stage A1 (T1a) disease, well-differentiated carcinoma in less than 5% of resected tissue. All other incidentally discovered carcinomas are stage A2 (T1b) and are considered potentially more aggressive. The urologist initiates a metastatic evaluation with a nuclear bone scan. PSA should be measured if not already done and always before treatment and, because it is of great value in following a patient, after treatment.

If there is no evidence of local or distant metastatic disease, the management in stage T1a disease is controversial. In a younger patient (less than age 65 years) with T1a disease who is at a higher risk for recurrence because of his expected longevity, radical prostatectomy is recommended. For the older patient (over 65 years), observation is often recommended. The patient with T1b disease is at considerable risk for

Table 49.4.   Staging of Prostatic Carcinoma

Stage	Description
A	Clinically undetectable; found on pathologic examination after prostatectomy
A1	Focal and well differentiated
A2	Diffuse (>5%) or poorly differentiated
B	Limited to prostate on rectal examination
B1	Solitary nodule; <1.5 cm; one lobe
B2	One whole lobe or both lobes
C	Locally extending outside of prostatic capsule or into seminal vesicles
D	Metastatic disease
D1	Pelvic lymph node metastases
D2	Distant metastases, usually bone

Table 49.5.   TNM Classification and Whitmore–Jewett Staging System

TNM	Description	Whitmore–Jewett	Description
T1a	Nonpalpable, with 5% or less of resected tissue with cancer (TURP or open prostatectomy)	A1	Same as TNM
T1b	Nonpalpable, with greater than 5% of resected tissue with cancer (TURP or open prostatectomy)	A2	Same as TNM
T1c	Nonpalpable, but serum PSA is elevated	0[a]	Same as TNM
T2a	Palpable, half of 1 lobe or less	B1N	Palpable nodule, less than 1 lobe
T2b	Palpable, greater than half of 1 lobe but not both lobes	B1	Palpable, less than 1 lobe
T2c	Palpable, involves both lobes	B2	Palpable, 1 entire lobe or more
T3a	Palpable, unilateral capsular penetration	C1	Palpable, outside capsule, not into seminal vesicles
T3b	Palpable, bilateral extracapsular extension	C2	Same as TNM
T3c	Palpable, invasion of seminal vesicles	C3	Same as TNM
T4	Tumor is fixed or invades adjacent structures (i.e., bladder neck, sphincter, rectum, pelvic wall)	C4	Same as TNM
N	Regional lymph node metastases	D1	Same as TNM
M	Distant metastases (i.e., bone)	D2	

Modified from Partin AW, Yoo S, Carter HB, et al. The use of prostate-specific antigen, clinical stage and Gleason score to predict pathological stage in men with localized prostate cancer. J Urol 150:110, 1993.

[a]Not defined in original Whitmore–Jewett classification.

developing metastases, and radical prostatectomy is recommended.

The management of patients with T1c, biopsy done because of an elevated PSA, is also controversial. Management options include watchful waiting, radical prostatectomy, and radiation therapy. The age of the patient, the grade of the tumor, and the estimated volume of the cancer, such as number of positive biopsy cores, must be considered in recommending management.

Stage B (T2, N0 M0) carcinoma is defined as disease limited to the prostate gland that is detected clinically either as a nodule or as diffuse hardness with no extension or fixation. If the neoplasm is limited to the prostate and the patient is under 75 years of age, has an anticipated 10-year survival, and has no contraindicating medical diseases, he is a candidate for curative radical prostatectomy or definitive radiation therapy.

Local extensive prostatic cancer, *stage C (T3 and T4, N0 M0),* is usually treated by definitive radiotherapy. The decision to treat a patient with prostate cancer with radiotherapy also requires a risk–benefit discussion by the urologist, oncologist, or radiotherapist. Although radiotherapy is generally well tolerated, there is some risk for the subsequent development of symptomatic chronic proctitis, usually manifest by bleeding and tenesmus, impotence, and chronic cystitis usually associated with bleeding. The prevalence of these complications is variable and depends in part on the dosage of radiotherapy and the size of the delivery port. The age and general health of the patient are major considerations in determining management options. If significant bladder outlet obstruction is present, the patient may also need a TURP; this combination of treatment results in an increased risk of urinary incontinence.

Studies show that the obturator and iliac nodes are usually the first sites of metastases, and these structures are positive in 5 to 50% of patients with prostatic cancers. Unfortunately, current imaging techniques, including CT and MRI, are not reliable in detecting early lymph node metastases and are not routinely indicated in the preoperative evaluation of a patient with prostate cancer. A PSA level greater than 20 mg is suggestive of nodal metastases but does not preclude surgical therapy or radiation therapy.

Metastatic, or stage D (M+), prostatic cancer is best managed by hormonal therapy (i.e., androgen deprivation) via surgical (castration) or pharmacologic methods. Studies show that hormonal therapy initiated at the time of diagnosis does not prolong survival but may delay the onset of symptomatic metastases compared with hormonal therapy initiated only in response to symptoms (e.g., bone pain). Diethylstilbestrol (3 mg/day) and orchiectomy give similar results, producing an 85 to 90% partial symptomatic response rate in previously untreated patients. The duration of response is 18 months on average (3,6), although prolonged remissions have been documented. There is no advantage of combining orchiectomy and estrogen therapy. Generally, estrogen therapy, which causes salt and water retention, should be avoided in patients who also have an edema-forming illness (e.g., severe congestive heart failure or nephrotic syndrome) not controlled by diuretics. Diethylstilbestrol is no longer commonly used. LHRH analogs (leuprolide, goserelin) are expensive (approximately $500 per monthly injection, covered by Medicare); they have proven to be just as effective as surgical castration (23). These analogs in combination with potent antiandrogens (flutamide, bicalutamide) provide total androgen blockage. However, data do not indicate that the total androgen blockage provides long-term survival any better than either chemical or surgical castration alone. An antiandrogen is recommended, however, in patients initially starting on LHRH agonists, as these initially cause a rise in the testosterone and then it drops after approximately 3 to 4 weeks. The antiandrogen is usually given for only 3 to 6 weeks.

The physician should be aware of the effects of androgen ablation, either by chemical or surgical castration. Patients after several years may experience osteopenia and osteoporosis, anemia, loss of libido, hot flashes (as experienced in some women following menopause), and some loss of well-being and masculine prowess.

There has been no major contribution to the treatment of metastatic prostate cancer since the landmark observation of Huggins and Hodges (11) regarding the efficacy of androgen ablative therapy. A number of investigational trials have used cytotoxic chemotherapy in all stages of prostatic carcinoma, but no method is as effective as androgen deprivation. Cytotoxic chemotherapy also is only partially effective in patients who fail hormonal therapy or who have extensive metastatic disease. Tumor necrosis factor and suramin are still under investigation but may provide a response in 20 to 30% of patients in early trials. Gene therapy and vaccines are under investigation and initial results appear encouraging.

Much of the controversy in the diagnosis and treatment of prostatic cancer results from the inability to assess accurately the influence of prostatic cancer on longevity (1,20). Many patients with low-grade and low-stage disease should be treated by watchful waiting, particularly those over 75. A more aggressive approach should be taken in patients who are young (30 to 60). It is estimated that a significant number of young patients with prostate cancer have a genetic basis for their disease and their family members should be screened and followed closely. It is currently typical to offer aggressive treatment, primarily radical prostatectomy, to younger men with prostate cancer in the belief that it is a more aggressive form. Radiation therapy is recommended primarily in patients 70 and older with locally confined disease or in younger patients with T3 disease (stage C) who are not considered surgical candidates.

Controversy remains in the use of adjuvant hormonal therapy in the treatment of prostate cancer. For patients who are surgical candidates, there are no data to support the use of hormonal therapy before surgery. In selected patients, especially those with T3 disease (stage C), radiation therapy should be considered.

Cryotherapy or freezing of the prostate for cancer is still experimental. It is not recommended currently in the primary treatment of prostate cancer.

However, because prostatic cancer occurs in older men who often have coexisting diseases that influence longevity and because the natural history of the disease is not well understood, there is great variability in survival among men with prostate cancer. The best estimates for survival with various stages of prostatic cancer with the treatments discussed above are listed in Table 49.6.

URINARY INCONTINENCE

Urinary incontinence is a common problem of the elderly and of younger women. It may be a manifestation of urinary outlet obstruction. The evaluation of incontinence is described in Chapter 6. In general, younger patients with incontinence are best referred to a urologist or gynecologist for evaluation and definitive treatment, which is usually surgical when the problem

Table 49.6. Survival with Appropriately Managed Prostatic Carcinoma Using Both the Whitmore–Jewett and the TNM Systems

Stages		% Men Surviving with Prostate Cancer at Various Stages Who Receive Treatment	
	5 yr	10 yr	15 yr
A1 T1	Normal life expectancy		
A2	50–80	40–70	15–35
B T2	50–90	40–70	15–40
C T3	15–70	5–60	0–30
D M+	5–30	3–10	0–3

is pure stress incontinence. Elderly patients with urinary incontinence are usually treated by the general physician or geriatrician; their treatment is described extensively in Chapter 6, "Geriatric Medicine: Special Considerations."

General References*

Blasko JC, Lange PH. Prostate cancer: the therapeutic challenge of locally advanced disease. N Engl J Med 337:340, 1997.
Chodak GW. Screening for prostate cancer in 1993: is it appropriate, or not? Semin Urol 11:47, 1993.
Fitzpatrick JM, ed. Société Internationale d'Urologie reports: nonsurgical treatment of BPH. New York: Churchill Livingstone, 1992.
Osterling JE. Benign prostate hyperplasia. Medical and minimally invasive treatment options. N Engl J Med 332:99, 1995.
   A thorough review of therapeutic possibilities in managing men with symptomatic BPH.
Resnick MI, Kursh E, eds. Current therapy in genitourinary surgery. 2nd ed. St Louis: CV Mosby, 1992.
Rittmaster RS. Finasteride. N Engl J Med 330:120, 1994.
   A good review of this drug in the treatment of BPH.
Special issue: medical management of prostatic disease. J Androl 12:234, 1991. Special issue: prostate carcinoma. J Urol 147:784, 1992.
Walsh PC. Benign prostate hyperplasia. In: Walsh PC, Retik AB, Stamey TA, Vaughan ED Jr, eds. Campbell's urology. 7th ed. Philadelphia: WB Saunders, 1998.

Specific References

1. Adolfsson J, Carstensen J. Natural course of clinically localized prostate adenocarcinoma in men less than 70 years old. J Urol 146:96, 1991.
2. Baert L, Ameye F, Pike MC, et al. Transurethral hyperthermia for BPH patients with retention. J Urol 147:1558, 1992.
3. Bailar JC, Byar DP. Estrogen treatment for cancer of the prostate: early results with three doses of diethylstilbestrol and placebo. Cancer 26:257, 1970.
4. Bloom DA, Foster WD, McLeod DG, et al. Cost-effective uroflowmetry in men. J Urol 133:421, 1985.
5. Boyle P, Gould AL, Roehrborn CG. Prostate volume predicts outcome of treatment of benign prostate hyperplasia with finasteride: meta-analysis of randomized clinical trials. Urology 48:398, 1996.
6. Byar DP. The Veterans Administration cooperative urologic research group's studies of cancer of the prostate. Cancer 32:1126, 1973.
7. Carr TW. Natural history of prostate cancer. Lancet 341:91, 1993.
8. Carter HB, Pearson JD, Metter EJ, et al. Longitudinal evaluation of prostate-specific antigen levels in men with and without prostate disease. JAMA 267:2215, 1992.

*Bold print (general references) and bold numerals (specific references) denote published controlled clinical trials, meta-analyses, or consensus-based recommendations.

9. Cupp MR, Oesterling JE. Prostate-specific antigen, digital rectal examination, and transrectal ultrasonography: their roles in diagnosing early prostate cancer. Mayo Clin Proc 68:297, 1993.

10. Garnick MB, Fair WR. Prostate cancer: emerging concepts. Ann Intern Med 125:118, 1996.

11. Huggins C, Stevens RE, Hodges, CV. Studies on prostatic cancer: II. The effects of castration on advance carcinoma of the prostate gland. Arch Surg 43:209, 1941.

12. Kramer BS, Brown ML, Prorock PC, et al. Prostate cancer screening: what we know and what we need to know. Ann Intern Med 119:914, 1993.

13. Lepor H, Meretyk S, Knapp-Maloney G. The safety, efficacy and compliance of terazosin therapy for benign prostatic hyperplasia. J Urol 147:1554, 1992.

14. Lepor H, Kaplan SA, Klimberg I, et al. Doxazosin for benign prostatic hyperplasia: long-term efficacy and safety in hypertensive and normotensive patients. J Urol 157:525, 1997.

14a. Lepor H, Willingford WO, Barry MJ, et al. N Engl J Med 335:533, 1996.

15. Mebust WK, Holtgrewe HL, Cockett ATK, Peters PC. Transurethral prostatectomy: immediate and postoperative complications. A cooperative study of 13 participating institutions evaluating 3885 patients. J Urol 141:243, 1989.

16. Partin AW, Steinberg GD, Pitcock RV, et al. Use of nuclear morphometry, Gleason histologic scoring, clinical stage, and age to predict disease-free survival among patients with prostate cancer. Cancer 70:161, 1992.

17. Roos NP, Wennberg JE, Malenka DJ, et al. Mortality and reoperation after open and transurethral resection of the prostate for benign prostatic hyperplasia. N Engl J Med 320:1120, 1989.

18. Schroder FH, Hermanek P, Denis L, et al. TMN classification of prostate cancer. Prostate 4:129, 1992.

19. Walsh PC, Lepor H, Eggleston JC. Radical prostatectomy with preservation of sexual function: anatomical and pathological considerations. Prostate 4:473, 1983.

19a. Walsh P. Treatment of benign prostate hyperplasia. N Engl J Med 335:586, 1996.

20. Wason J, Fleming C, Bruskewitz R, et al, for The Prostate Patient Outcome Research Team. The treatment of localized prostate cancer: what are we doing, what should we know, and what should we be doing? Semin Urol 11:23, 1993.

21. Wein AJ: Drug treatment of voiding dysfunction, Parts I–II. AUA Update Ser 7:14, 1988.

22. The Finasteride Study Group. The effect of finasteride in men with benign prostatic hyperplasia. N Engl J Med 327:1185, 1992.

23. The Leuprolide Study Group. Leuprolide versus diethylstilbestrol for metastatic prostate cancer. N Engl J Med 311:1281, 1984.

24. The Measurement Committee of the American Urological Association. The AUA symptoms index for benign prostatic hyperplasia. J Urol 148:1549, 1992.

Hematologic Problems

CHAPTER 50

Anemia

LARRY WATERBURY, MD

GENERAL CONSIDERATIONS

Anemia, a reduction of the proportion of red cells or of hemoglobin in the blood, is a condition, like hypoxia or jaundice, that always reflects a primary underlying disease. Although sometimes symptoms (e.g., shortness of breath on exertion) or signs (e.g., pallor) are associated with anemia, the diagnosis of the condition depends essentially on one or more laboratory measurements, such as the hematocrit value (the amount of red cells in a volume of blood) or the hemoglobin concentration. In general, anemia is defined in a man as a condition in which the hematocrit value is less than 42% or the hemoglobin concentration is less than 14 g/100 mL and in a woman as a hematocrit value less than 37% or a hemoglobin concentration less than 12 g/100 mL. When anemia is diagnosed, other measurements (see "Approach to Evaluation of Anemia," below) are important in establishing the cause of the process and selecting appropriate therapy.

Most routine complete blood counts (CBCs) obtained in clinical practice in this country are determined by automated counting methods (Table 50.1). The CBC usually reports the hemoglobin (Hb) concentration, hematocrit (Hct) value, red blood cell count (RBC), white cell count, mean corpuscular volume (MCV), mean corpuscular hemoglobin (MCH), and mean corpuscular hemoglobin concentration (MCHC). One commonly used automated system (Coulter) measures the hemoglobin, RBC, and MCV, and from these variables calculates the hematocrit value, MCH, and MCHC. With the use of the automated counters, the indices (MCH, MCHC, MCV), especially the MCV, are precise, accurate measurements that can be used in approaching the diagnostic workup of anemia. The calculated Hct value is slightly lower than that obtained by centrifugation (packed cells trap plasma, distorting the ratio of red cells to plasma). The red cell distribution width (RDW) calculated by most automated systems is a measure of variation in size. It is often increased in many anemias (e.g., moderate to severe iron deficiency, megaloblastic anemias, many hemolytic anemias, anemias associated with reticulocytosis).

APPROACH TO EVALUATION OF ANEMIA

The routine database that should be obtained on every anemic patient includes the hematocrit value, hemoglobin concentration, MCV, MCHC, and reticulocyte count (Table 50.2). A smear of the peripheral blood should be obtained by fingerstick or from unanticoagulated blood on the tip of a venipuncture needle. (Anticoagulants may distort the morphology of the blood cells.) The smear may be stained in the physician's office or be transported to an outside laboratory to be stained and interpreted. On the basis of all of these data and a complete history and physical examination, the physician can progress a long way toward an etiologic diagnosis of the anemia. Three questions should be asked:

What is the MCV? With the use of the automated counters, the MCV is a direct measurement of red cell size. The normal range varies with individual laboratories but is approximately 82 to 98 fL. Actually, it is helpful to use a broader normal range of 80 to 100 fL to classify the anemia as microcytic (MCV less than 80 fL), normocytic (MCV 80 to 100 fL), or macrocytic (MCV greater than 100 fL). Microcytic and macrocytic anemias have very limited differential diagnoses, so by simply noting the MCV the diagnostic approach can be easily focused when the anemia is microcytic or macrocytic.

What is the basic mechanism of the anemia? There are only three ways patients become anemic: decreased effective production of red cells by bone marrow, bleeding, or hemolysis. The most helpful laboratory measurement in defining the mechanism of anemia is the reticulocyte count. The reticulocyte count is used to assess the appropriateness of the response of the bone marrow to anemia. The normal reticulocyte count

Table 50.1.   Representative Normal Values (Coulter S)

	Men	Women
Hemoglobin, g/dL of blood	14–18	12–16
Hematocrit value, %	42–54	37–47
MCV, fL	82–98	82–98
MCH, pg	27–32	27–32
MCHC, g/dL of red blood cells	31.5–36	31.5–36

is approximately 1%, representing the 1% of new cells that are released into the circulation from the bone marrow daily (the ordinary red cell life span being approximately 100 days). Under the stimulus of erythropoietin, in the anemic patient the bone marrow should be able to triple acutely its output of new cells; when anemia is chronic and severe, the bone marrow may be able to increase its output of cells to 8 to 10 times normal. This increased bone marrow activity is reflected in an appropriately elevated reticulocyte count. The reticulocyte count must be adjusted for the level of anemia to obtain a value known as the reticulocyte index (Table 50.3), a more accurate reflection of erythropoiesis. In patients with bleeding or hemolysis the reticulocyte index should be at least 3%, whereas in patients with anemia caused by decreased production of red cells the reticulocyte index is less than 3%, and often less than 1.5%.

In addition to the reticulocyte index, serial hematocrit values over a few days or weeks may provide clues to the mechanism of the anemia. Total shutdown of production in the marrow in the absence of bleeding or hemolysis results in a fall in the hematocrit value of only 3 or 4 percentage points/week. If the value has fallen more rapidly, bleeding or hemolysis must have taken place. Anemia with an appropriate reticulocyte response in the absence of bleeding usually means hemolysis.

Does the patient have another problem that is commonly associated with anemia? Table 50.4 lists anemias commonly associated with various clinical characteristics and diseases. For this purpose race and sex are also taken into consideration. Women are iron deficient more often than are men, and African-American patients are more likely than are whites to have hemoglobinopathies or glucose-6-phosphate dehydrogenase deficiency.

In summary, the initial database should enable the physician to classify the anemia on the basis of the MCV, categorize the basic mechanism of the anemia, and consider possible causes based on the patient's problem list. This initial assessment should then suggest the appropriate further diagnostic workup.

ANEMIA WITH A LOW MCV

Table 50.5 lists the anemias commonly associated with a low MCV. For the most part the diagnosis rests between iron deficiency anemia and thalassemia. Occasionally the anemia of chronic inflammation and, even more rarely, sideroblastic anemia are microcytic, although more often they are normocytic or, in the case of sideroblastic anemia, macrocytic.

Iron Deficiency Anemia

Although dietary iron deficiency does occur in the infant and during the rapid growth phase of adolescence, in the United States iron deficiency generally occurs only as a result of bleeding. Iron deficiency from menstruation and from pregnancy is extremely common in women; however, iron deficiency in a man or in a postmenopausal woman should be considered to be caused by gastrointestinal bleeding until proven otherwise.

Diagnosis

The history and physical examination may yield information that suggests the presence of iron deficiency (11). Such information includes a history of multiple pregnancies in a woman; strange dietary habits such as the eating of ice, starch, or clay (pica); any history of gastrointestinal bleeding; and physical findings of a sore tongue, brittle and ridged fingernails, spoon nails, or cheilosis. The physical findings are seen only in patients with long-standing and severe iron deficiency.

Most of the body's iron is incorporated in hemoglobin, but approximately one-third of it is stored in reticuloendothelial sites, primarily in the spleen, liver, and bone marrow. In patients with slow continued bleeding, the reticuloendothelial iron stores supply the requirement of the bone marrow for iron until the stores are depleted. It is at this point that iron deficiency anemia begins to develop. In iron deficiency, cell size (MCV) correlates with the degree of anemia, so very mild iron deficiency anemia may be associated with normal-sized cells (see "Mild Iron Deficiency," below, and Table 50.6 (14). The MCV progressively decreases as the anemia becomes more severe, but the MCHC usually remains normal until the hematocrit value falls below 30%. As the anemia becomes more marked, the red cells also become progressively more distorted (poikilocytosis). Table 50.6 illustrates the relationship between the hematocrit value, the MCV, and the degree of red cell distortion (poikilocytosis) seen in iron deficiency anemia of varying degrees of severity.

Often the diagnosis of iron deficiency is obvious after the initial history, physical examination, and standard laboratory evaluation. If not, a number of other tests may be useful; the *reticulocyte index* is inappropriately low for the degree of anemia. The *serum iron concentration (SI)* is low but is usually low also in patients with acute and chronic inflammation and malignancy. Furthermore, an acute infectious process such as pneumococcal pneumonia will cause an immediate drop in the serum iron even though the patient is not iron deficient. Classically, the *total iron-binding capacity*

Table 50.2.   Routine Database for Anemic Patients

Hematocrit value
Hemoglobin concentration
MCV
MCHC
Reticulocytic count (and calculation of reticulocytic index)
Evaluation of a peripheral blood smear (fingerstick)

Table 50.3.   Reticulocyte Index

$$\text{Reticulocyte index} = \text{Reticulocyte count} \times \frac{\text{Patient Hct}}{\text{Normal Hct}}$$

Example: reticulocyte count 6%, hematocrit 15%

$$\text{Reticulocyte index} = 6\% \times \frac{15\%}{45\%} = 2\%$$

(TIBC) is elevated. It is a measure of serum transferrin, the iron transport protein that supplies bone marrow red blood cell precursors with iron. However, many iron-deficient patients have a normal TIBC, and it may be low in cases of chronic inflammation or malignancy regardless of whether or not iron deficiency is present. The *bone marrow iron stain* is the most definitive way to prove a diagnosis of iron deficiency because iron stores are depleted when iron deficiency anemia is present and are normal or elevated in patients with microcytic anemia from other causes.

Serum ferritin may be helpful in the assessment of body iron stores (18). Ferritin is a water-soluble complex of iron and a binding protein, apoferritin. The serum ferritin concentration reflects the status of the reticuloendothelial stores and, in general, is a more specific test than the serum iron and iron-binding capacity in the diagnosis of iron deficiency. A low serum ferritin concentration almost always reflects iron deficiency. A very high serum ferritin concentration usually signifies iron overload, as in the patient who has received multiple transfusions. However, in many clinical situations, the serum ferritin may be spuriously normal or even elevated in the presence of iron deficiency anemia (Table 50.7). In these situations it may be difficult to make a definitive diagnosis of iron deficiency without a bone marrow iron stain. (Although response to a so-called therapeutic trial of iron may allow a presumptive diagnosis of iron deficiency, in general it is inappropriate to subject people to an expensive and uncomfortable evaluation of their gastrointestinal tract without the definitive information provided by marrow iron stain.)

Treatment

After institution of oral iron therapy, the reticulocyte response is maximal at around 7 to 10 days. The hematocrit value begins to rise after approximately 1 week, and in the uncomplicated case a normal hematocrit value is reached in a few weeks. However, it takes many months of therapy for patients to replete their iron stores. Iron absorption is variable and unpredictable. Even under optimal conditions only a fraction of ingested iron is absorbed. In the menstruating woman with iron deficiency anemia, treatment for a year may be necessary; in the man with iron deficiency anemia, treatment for 6 months is often indicated. Iron deficiency is common in menstruating women, especially in those with heavy menstrual periods and a history of multiple pregnancies. Some may require constant iron therapy to maintain a normal hematocrit value. Standard treatment with oral iron consists of 1 tablet of iron (e.g., ferrous sulfate, 300 mg, which contains 60 mg of elemental iron) three times daily on an empty stomach (1 hour before meals). If it is difficult for patients to take

Table 50.4.   Anemias Associated with Various Clinical Settings

Female
Iron deficiency

African Americans
G6PD deficiency, hemoglobinopathies, thalassemia

Mediterranean Origin
G6PD deficiency, thalassemia

Far East Origin
Hemoglobinopathies, thalassemia

Viral Infections
Immune hemolysis
Decreased production

Bacterial Infection
Anemia of inflammation
Microangiopathic hemolysis
Oxidative hemolysis (G6PD deficiency)
Other hemolytic mechanisms

Malignancy
Iron deficiency caused by bleeding from a colon cancer
Microangiopathic hemolysis
Immune hemolysis
Decreased production

Alcoholic Liver Disease
Bleeding
Hypersplenism
Folate deficiency
Decreased production
Sideroblastic anemia
Iron deficiency
Hemolysis

Hyperthyroidism or Hypothyroidism
Decreased production
Pernicious anemia
Iron deficiency

Renal Failure
Decreased production
Hemolysis
Bleeding

Aortic Valve Replacement
Microangiopathic hemolysis

Malignant Hypertension
Microangiopathic hemolysis

Rheumatoid Syndromes
Anemia of inflammation
Iron deficiency
Immune hemolysis

Collagen Vascular Disease
Immune hemolysis
Anemia of inflammation

Drugs
α-Methyldopa: Immune hemolysis
Quinine/quinidine: Immune hemolysis
Penicillin: Immune hemolysis (rare)
Butazolidin/chloramphenicol: Dose-related marrow depression; idiosyncratic aplastic anemia
Gold: Aplastic anemia
Antituberculosis drugs: Sideroblastic anemia
Phenytoin: Megaloblastic anemia (folate); pure red cell aplasia
Sulfa/sulfones: G6PD hemolysis
Methotrexate: Megaloblastosis
Amphotericin, cis-platinum, zidovudine: Production defect

the noontime dose, it is reasonable to omit it. There are numerous preparations of iron other than ferrous sulfate, but there is usually no justification for recommending any of them unless a reduction in the dosage of elemental iron is required (see "Side Effects," below). Generally, time-release capsules and enteric coated preparations are to be avoided. They are costly and absorption is variable. Oral iron should be taken between meals, separate from H_2 blockers, antacids, and omeprazole. Preparations containing iron, including ferrous sulfate, can be obtained without prescription.

Side Effects. Approximately 15% of patients have gastrointestinal side effects from oral iron, most commonly constipation, but nausea, abdominal cramping, and diarrhea are also seen. When such side effects develop, the practitioner may elect to administer iron only once a day or may instruct the patient to take iron with meals instead of on an empty stomach (but not with tea or antacids). Taking iron with food decreases iron absorption by approximately 50%, but absorption is still sufficient to replenish the body's iron if treatment is continued long enough. If symptoms still continue after these alterations in dosage and schedule, it is helpful to decrease the individual dosage of oral iron. If the dosage is decreased to less than 40 mg of elemental iron, symptoms often abate. This can be done by using pediatric liquid preparations, which are usually well tolerated. If these adjustments in the dosage and schedule of oral iron administration are made, parenteral iron is rarely indicated. However, parenteral therapy is indicated in patients with small and large bowel inflammation, rapid gastrointestinal transit, or malabsorption, and when the patient has severe iron deficiency and noncompliance has been repetitively proven. Iron dextran is the most commonly used form of parenteral iron and is usually given in 2.0-mL (100-mg) doses intramuscularly or intravenously. If the intravenous route is chosen, it must be given no more rapidly than 1.0 mL/minute. Guidelines for the dosage of parenteral iron are provided in the *Physicians' Desk Reference* but may be calculated grossly by age and hemoglobin concentration (Table 50.8). A test dose of 0.5 mL is administered an hour before the first therapeutic dose to ensure that the patient is not allergic to the preparation. Injections may be given daily until the calculated required dosage has been administered. Side effects from parenteral iron include pain and rash at the injection site, arthralgias, staining of the skin, fever, and rare anaphylactoid reactions.

Thalassemia

In the normal adult three hemoglobins are present in mature red cells: A, the major component, and two minor components, A_2 and F (fetal). Each hemoglobin molecule consists of four heme groups and four globin chains; the globin chains in each molecule are of two different types. All three hemoglobins have two -globin chains but differ in the second set (β, δ, γ) of globin chains (Table 50.9).

Thalassemia is an inherited defect in globin chain production. Anemia is caused by a combination of decreased hemoglobin production and, usually, mild hemolysis. β-Thalassemia (29) is seen in the United States primarily in African-American patients, patients from Southeast Asia, or those of Mediterranean (Greek and Italian) origin. The genetics of α-thalassemia are complicated, and the disorder appears to have a wider racial distribution than does β-thalassemia, but it is especially common in African Americans (27). Most patients are heterozygous and are clinically asymptomatic but may have microcytosis. The diagnosis is important because the entity is often confused with iron deficiency anemia, resulting in lifelong repetitive workups for gastrointestinal bleeding and inappropriate treatment with iron. Microcytosis in African-American patients is more likely caused by α-thalassemia than by iron deficiency.

Diagnosis

Table 50.10 lists the typical database for the patient with heterozygous α- or β-thalassemia. The combination of a low MCV and only a very mild anemia should alert the physician to the diagnosis because in iron deficiency the degree of microcytosis parallels the severity of the anemia (Table 50.6).

Table 50.5. Causes of Anemia with Low MCV

Iron deficiency
Thalassemia
Anemia of chronic inflammation (occasionally)
Sideroblastic anemia (congenital, rare)
Some hemoglobinopathies (e.g., HbE)
Aluminum toxicity

Table 50.6. Representative Datebase at Various Stages in the Slow Development of Severe Iron Deficiency Anemia[a]

Hct (%)	42	42	35	27	19
MCV (82–98 fL)	92	88	82	75	68
MCHC (32–36 g/dL)	33	33	33	31	29
SI (65–175 µg/dL)	70	60	35	20	20
TIBC (250–375 µg/dL)	300	300	300	400	450
Serum ferritin (10–200 µg/mL)	60	30	5	3	1
Peripheral smear	Normal	Normal	Normal	1 + poikilocytosis 1 + hypochromia	4 + poikilocytosis 4 + hypochromia
Bone marrow iron stores	Present	Absent	Absent	Absent	Absent

Hct, Hematocrit value; *MCV*, mean corpuscular volume; *MCHC*, mean corpuscular hemoglobin concentration; *SI*, serum iron; *TIBC*, total iron-binding capacity.
[a]Numbers in parentheses are the range of normal values.

Table 50.7.   Inappropriately Normal or Elevated Serum Ferritin Levels

Acute liver disease
Cirrhosis
Hodgkin's disease
Acute leukemias
Solid tumors (occasionally)
Fever
Acute inflammation
Renal dialysis patients
After taking oral iron for 2–3 weeks or after recent treatment with
    parenteral iron

Table 50.8.   Representative Total Body Iron Deficits (mg) at Various Body Weights and Hemoglobin Concentrations

Patient Weight (lb)	Iron Deficit at Various Hemoglobin Levels			
	4 g/dL	6 g/dL	8 g/dL	10 g/dL
100	2250	1750	1400	1000
120	2650	2100	1650	1150
140	3050	2500	1950	1350
160	3550	2850	2200	1550
180	3950	3200	2500	1750

In the forms of β-thalassemia most commonly seen in the United States, there is a decreased production of β chains with a compensatory increase in the production of δ chains, resulting in a decreased production of hemoglobin A and an increased production of hemoglobin A_2. This increase can be assessed by electrophoresis of the hemoglobin and is a definitive diagnostic test for β-thalassemia. Less commonly, in this country, increases in hemoglobin F may be seen in patients with β-thalassemia.

The α-thalassemias are more difficult to diagnose because a decreased production of α chains will affect the relative concentrations of all of the normal adult hemoglobins. A definitive diagnosis of one of the α-thalassemia syndromes may be difficult and may require family studies or techniques available primarily in research laboratories. However, the diagnosis of presumptive α-thalassemia in the setting of an appropriate database (hematologic values consistent with the diagnosis in the absence of iron deficiency and of β-thalassemia) is reasonable even in the absence of laboratory confirmation.

Patient Education

It is important to explain to patients with heterozygous thalassemia that the clinical features of their condition mimic iron deficiency. The patient should be put on guard against repetitive diagnostic workups for iron deficiency. The physician should emphasize the benign nature of the illness and that the anemia, being mild, usually does not cause any symptoms. The patient should be cautioned against taking oral iron because thalassemic patients actually have an increase in iron stores. Genetic counseling is important; a couple, both heterozygous for β-thalassemia, has a 25% chance of having a child with homozygous β-thalassemia. Furthermore, the genes for thalassemia and those

for hemoglobin S and C are alleles. Hemoglobin S–β-thalassemia is a clinically significant disease.

Miscellaneous

The anemia of chronic disease and the anemia of malignancy may be associated with a low MCV (although the MCV is usually normal). These entities are discussed under "Anemias with Normal Mean Corpuscular Volume and an Inappropriately Low Reticulocyte Index" later in this chapter. Sideroblastic anemias (characterized by increased iron stores and ringed sideroblasts in the bone marrow) are occasionally microcytic, and some hemoglobinopathies are associated with a low MCV (hemoglobin E). The former are best treated in consultation with a hematologist; the latter are seen primarily in Southeast Asians. Aluminum toxicity, sometimes seen in dialyzed patients with chronic renal failure, sometimes causes a further reduction in red cell mass, with microcytosis (21).

ANEMIA WITH A HIGH MCV

An MCV greater than 100 fL is abnormal and an attempt should be made to explain the abnormality. Table 50.11 lists conditions associated with an elevated MCV (13). For the most part, the diseases associated with an elevated MCV are liver disease, the megaloblastic anemias (including drug-induced megaloblastosis), and the refractory anemias with hypercellular bone marrows (myelodysplasias). Occasionally an elevated MCV measured by the automatic counter is spurious, caused by red cell antibodies or marked rouleaux formation in patients with a very high erythrocyte sedimentation rate. Because young red cells are large, patients with a marked reticulocytosis may have an elevated MCV.

Liver Disease

Chronic hepatocellular and obstructive liver disease results in loading of cholesterol in the lipid portion of

Table 50.9.   Globin Chain Composition of Normal Adult Hemoglobins

		Percentage of Total in Normal Adults
Hgb A	$\alpha_2\beta_2$	97
Hgb A_2	$\alpha_2\delta_2$	2
Hgb F	$\alpha_2\gamma_2$	1

Table 50.10.   Heterozygous Thalassemia: Typical Database

Hct	37%
HCV	69 fL
MCH	20 pg
MCHC	32 g/dL
Reticulocyte count	2.5%
Red blood cell morphology	Microcytosis, poikilocytosis, stippling
Ferritin	Normal or increased

Abbreviations are as in Table 50.6.

Table 50.11. Differential Diagnosis of MCV Greater Than 100 fL

Spurious
Reticulocytosis (marked)
Liver disease
Alcoholism
Myelodysplastic syndromes
Myelophthisis
Drugs
Megaloblastic anemias
Normal variant

the red cell membrane so that the cell increases in size. Thus, the MCV is often elevated but is usually not greater than 115 fL (Table 50.16). On smears, cells appear to be round and centrally targeted, without significant variation in shape. This morphologic abnormality is not a cause of anemia. However, patients with liver disease often have other reasons to be anemic (bleeding, hemolysis, folic acid deficiency). The severe alcoholic often has an elevated MCV even in the absence of overt liver disease or marked megaloblastosis (10). Presumably the elevated MCV results from periodic episodes of alcoholic liver disease, folic acid deficiency, or both. Because of poor diet, the alcoholic often becomes folic acid depleted. In addition, alcohol interferes with folic acid metabolism.

Megaloblastic Anemia

A megaloblast is a larger than normal hematopoietic precursor with a nucleus that contains characteristic granular chromatin, the result of abnormal DNA synthesis (23). Table 50.12 lists the various etiologies of megaloblastic anemia related to vitamin B_{12} (cobalamin) or folic acid deficiency (essential cofactors in DNA synthesis). The body's stores of B_{12} are such that a diet without B_{12} (one in which animal protein is completely excluded) would not result in megaloblastosis due to B_{12} deficiency for several years; therefore, dietary B_{12} deficiency is extremely rare. By far, the most common etiology of B_{12} deficiency is pernicious anemia, an acquired autoimmune defect of the gastric mucosa resulting in deficient formation of intrinsic factor, which binds ingested B_{12} and allows its absorption in the terminal ileum. Patients with pernicious anemia are usually elderly and often complain of sore mouth, indigestion, and constipation or diarrhea. Neurologic problems, including peripheral neuropathy, dorsal column dysfunction (loss of vibratory and position sense in the lower extremities), and changes in affect, are common. If the deficiency is not corrected, lateral column dysfunction (weakness and spasticity) also occurs. The anemia develops so slowly that patients often have very low hematocrit values and yet remarkably good cardiovascular compensation for their anemia. Such patients usually have an expanded total blood volume and are prone to develop heart failure if given transfusions. B_{12} deficiency from other causes (Table 50.12) is less common. Patients who have had total gastrectomy or ileal resection or who have

ileal disease (Crohn's disease, tropical sprue) are likely to develop B_{12} deficiency and should receive prophylactic B_{12}. B_{12} deficiency after partial gastrectomy is much less common. There is evidence that B_{12} malabsorption may occur and lead to neuropsychiatric sequelae secondary to vitamin B_{12} deficiency, despite normal hematologic values and normal Schilling tests (discussed later in this chapter). In such cases vitamin B_{12} levels are usually low, although often not as low as those seen in pernicious anemia. Diagnosis may require more sensitive (and more expensive) tests of B_{12} metabolism such as measurement of serum or urine methylmalonic acid and serum homocysteine (24). The mechanism of B_{12} deficiency in such patients is unclear, although it may be caused, at least in some patients, by an inability to absorb food-bound B_{12}, even though they secrete normal amounts of intrinsic factor (4). Patients who are suspected of having such problems should be referred to a hematologist or a neurologist for further evaluation. A therapeutic trial of vitamin B_{12} is often recommended.

In contrast to vitamin B_{12}, the body's stores of folic acid are depleted rapidly when patients eat a diet deficient in folate. (The main sources of folate in the diet are leafy vegetables, fruits, nuts, and liver.) Therefore, folic acid deficiency is most often dietary. For example, pregnant women have an increased need for folate and without prenatal supplementation may develop folate deficiency, as may patients whose dietary intake is severely restricted because of chronic disease or multiple surgical procedures. Intestinal malabsorption due to any cause is also a common cause of folate deficiency. Finally, a number of drugs may be associated with folate deficiency: Phenytoin (Dilantin) interferes with folate absorption, alcohol interferes with folate utilization, and methotrexate and trimethoprim–sulfamethoxazole (Bactrim, Septra) interfere with folate metabolism. Also, some chemotherapeutic agents used

Table 50.12. Causes of Megaloblastosis Due to Vitamin B_{12} and Folic Acid Deficiency

B_{12}
Pernicious anemia (acquired and congenital)
Gastrectomy
Ileal resection
Crohn's disease and tropical sprue
Fish tapeworm infestation
Blind loop syndrome
Nutritional deficiency (vegan diet, rare)
Familial selective malabsorption (Imerslund's syndrome)

Folic Acid
Dietary (old age, alcoholism, chronic disease)
Malabsorption (sprue)
Hemodialysis
Severe exfoliative skin disease (e.g., psoriasis)
Drugs
   Interference with absorption or use (phenytoin, alcohol)
   Dihydrofolate reductase inhibitors (methotrexate, trimethoprim)
Increased requirements
   Pregnancy
   Infancy
   Hemolysis (e.g., sickle cell anemia)

Table 50.13. B$_{12}$ and Folate Concentrations

Serum B$_{12}$ Concentration
Spuriously low in some patients with folate deficiency
Spuriously low in some pregnant patients
May be spuriously low in patients taking large daily doses of vitamin C
May be low in strict vegetarians
May be elevated for weeks after one injection of B$_{12}$
Increased in myeloproliferative syndromes

RBC Folate Concentration
Reflects chronic folate deficiency
Falsely low in some patients with B$_{12}$ deficiency
Falsely high in patients with reticulocytosis

Serum Folate Concentration
A measure of recent dietary intake of folate
May be low, normal, or elevated in B$_{12}$ deficiency

in the treatment of cancer and to induce immunosuppression in patients with a variety of disorders (e.g., psoriasis, systemic lupus) cause megaloblastosis (e.g., hydroxyurea, cytosine arabinoside, methotrexate, azathioprine) by inhibiting DNA synthesis.

Diagnosis

The morphology of the peripheral blood and bone marrow is the same in patients with folic acid and B$_{12}$ deficiencies (23). With a severe megaloblastic anemia the MCV often is significantly elevated. An MCV of greater than 120 fL is almost always caused by a megaloblastic anemia. The red cells in the peripheral blood are characterized by marked variation in size and shape. The common cell is a macroovalocyte (large egg-shaped cell). One may also see Howell–Jolly bodies (nuclear fragments), Pappenheimer bodies (iron granules), and nucleated red blood cells. The nuclei of the neutrophils are often hypersegmented, and commonly there is a neutropenia and thrombocytopenia. The bone marrow is typically markedly cellular, revealing characteristic megaloblastic changes of all cell lines. The bone marrow iron stain usually reveals increased numbers of iron-containing nucleated red cells (sideroblasts).

Folic Acid and B$_{12}$ Assay. Classically, in B$_{12}$ deficiency the serum B$_{12}$ level is quite low (less than 100 pg/mL) and the serum folate level is high. Spuriously normal B$_{12}$ levels may occasionally be seen in B$_{12}$ deficiency (see above), and spuriously low levels may be seen without B$_{12}$ deficiency in some patients with folic acid deficiency (Table 50.13). The serum folate assay has little clinical usefulness in the workup of megaloblastic anemia secondary to folic acid deficiency. The red cell folate concentration does reflect chronic folate deficiency, although it may be falsely low in some patients with B$_{12}$ deficiency (Table 50.13).

The Schilling Test. The Schilling test is a measure of B$_{12}$ absorption and requires the measurement of total radioactivity excreted during a 24-hour period after the ingestion of radioactive B$_{12}$. This test is useful primarily in cases in which the data are confusing or in patients already treated with B$_{12}$, when the serum

levels are no longer helpful. The Schilling test requires a cooperative patient who can collect a 24-hour urine sample. The test includes the following steps: After voiding, the patient takes 0.5 µCi of ^{60}Co or ^{57}Co cyanocobalamin by mouth. A 24-hour urine collection is initiated; at 2 hours, 1 mg of B$_{12}$ is given by injection (the flushing dose) and the percentage of the radioactive B$_{12}$ excreted in 24 hours is determined. Normally 7% or more of the dose is excreted in 24 hours. Incomplete collection results in a spuriously low Schilling test and a false diagnosis of B$_{12}$ malabsorption. In addition, if there is severe megaloblastic anemia, there are changes in the gastrointestinal mucosa that affect B$_{12}$ absorption. For example, the Schilling test may be abnormal in folic acid deficiency because of the effect of folate deficiency on the intestinal mucosa, until the megaloblastic process is treated for a week or two (Table 50.14).

Table 50.15 outlines a stepwise approach to the use of the laboratory in differentiating between folic acid and B$_{12}$ deficiency in a patient with a megaloblastic anemia.

After a diagnosis of vitamin B$_{12}$ deficiency is established and treatment is initiated (see below), there is no need for periodic determination of serum vitamin B$_{12}$.

Other Laboratory Features. Megaloblastic anemias are essentially hemolytic in that there is marked destruction of abnormally formed cells within the marrow (ineffective erythropoiesis), which often results in indirect hyperbilirubinemia and an elevated level of serum lactate dehydrogenase. The serum iron concentration is usually elevated, and the reticulocyte index is inappropriately low.

Gastric achlorhydria is present in pernicious anemia, and antibodies to gastric mucosal cells and to intrinsic factor are often present, as are other autoantibodies, especially antithyroid and antiadrenal antibodies. The most useful of these tests is the assay of anti–intrinsic factor antibody in serum, which is reasonably specific for pernicious anemia and is present in approximately 70% of cases. Anti–intrinsic factor antibody assay may be helpful in the occasional patient with megaloblastic anemia of uncertain etiology. There is an increased prevalence of thyroid disease (hypothyroidism, hyperthyroidism, and euthyroid goiter) in patients with pernicious anemia.

Treatment

The usual treatment for B$_{12}$ deficiency is monthly intramuscular administration of 1000 µg of B$_{12}$ for the

Table 50.14. Causes, Other Than Pernicious Anemia, of a Positive Schilling Test

Incomplete urine collection
Renal failure
Some patients with megaloblastic anemia before treatment
Gastric antibodies to intrinsic factor
Defective intrinsic factor
Drugs (alcohol, colchicine, neomycin, cholestyramine)
Pancreatic insufficiency
Partial gastrectomy

Table 50.15.   Differentiating Between Folate and B_{12} Megaloblastosis

Etiology by History	RBC Folate	Serum B_{12}	Interpretation	Further Testing
Suggests folate	↓	Normal or ↑	Folate deficiency	None
Suggests folate	↓	Slightly ↓	Folate deficiency	Recheck B_{12} after folate treatment for 1 week
Suggests B_{12}	Normal or ↑	↓	B_{12} deficiency	None
Suggests B_{12}		↓	B_{12} deficiency	May confirm with Schilling test
	(serum folate usually ↑)			
All other combinations → Schilling test				

Table 50.16.   Laboratory Features in Three Conditions Associated with an Elevated MCV

	Liver Disease	Megaloblastic Anemia	Myelodysplastic Syndrome
MCV	Usually <115 fL	Often >115 fL	Usually <115 fL
White blood cell count (WBCs)	Variable	Often decreased	Often decreased
Platelet count	Variable	Often decreased	Often decreased
Red blood cell (RBC) morphology	Target cells, no poikilocytosis	Marked anisocytosis and poikilocytosis, macro-ovalocytes	Marked anisocytosis and poikilocytosis, may mimic megaloblastic anemia
Nucleated RBCs	Not common	Common	Common
WBC morphology	Normal	Hypersegmented nuclei of neutrophils	May have abnormal mononuclear cells, no nuclear hypersegmentation of neutrophils
Platelet morphology	Normal	Normal	May be large and degranulated
RBC folate	Depends on diet	Decreased in folate deficiency, normal or slightly decreased in B_{12} deficiency	Normal or elevated
Serum B_{12}	Normal	Decreased in B_{12} deficiency, may be slightly decreased in folate deficiency	Normal or elevated

rest of the patient's life. Many physicians treat patients daily while they are in the hospital, particularly if they have neurologic signs; however, there is little evidence that this practice is more efficacious than just starting patients on maintenance monthly B_{12} injections.

One to five mg of folic acid daily is adequate treatment for patients with folic acid deficiency. Treatment should be given at least until a normal hematocrit level is reached and should be continued if the patient is not eating an adequate diet or if the underlying cause persists (e.g., malabsorption). Patients with a chronic hemolytic state, such as those with sickle cell anemia, patients on hemodialysis (folic acid is dialyzable), and pregnant patients, should receive prophylactic treatment. Whether patients are hospitalized depends on the severity of their symptoms and signs, the severity of the anemia, and in the case of folate deficiency, the nature of the underlying disease.

With appropriate treatment of megaloblastic anemia, there is a rapid reticulocytosis, which reaches a peak at approximately 7 to 10 days; the hematocrit value begins to rise in approximately 1 week, and in uncomplicated cases it rises at a rate of 4 to 5 percentage points/week. The leukopenia and thrombocytopenia respond dramatically, and white blood cell and platelet counts may return to normal in a day or two. There is a variable response of the neurologic complications of B_{12} deficiency. Megaloblastic madness usually abates dramatically. Dorsal column problems and peripheral neuropathies usually improve, but more slowly. Lateral spinal tract signs are usually refractory to treatment.

Myelodysplasic Syndromes

These syndromes are acquired disorders of bone marrow stem cells, seen usually in elderly patients, that at presentation may mimic a megaloblastic anemia (17). However, the morphologic features of the bone marrow, and usually the peripheral smear, are different (Table 50.16). White cell and platelet morphology may be abnormal, the serum B_{12} and folic acid levels are high, and the patients do not respond to folic acid or B_{12}. In the bone marrow, ringed sideroblasts (red cell precursors containing granules of iron that form a ring around the nuclei) are common, as are megaloblastoid changes. Approximately 25% of patients develop acute nonlymphocytic leukemia, usually within a year but sometimes only after several years.

ANEMIAS WITH NORMAL MCV AND APPROPRIATE RETICULOCYTE INDEX (HEMOLYSIS AND BLEEDING)

Anemias caused by bleeding and hemolysis are associated with an appropriate bone marrow response manifested by an appropriate reticulocyte index (Table 50.3). The MCV is usually normal; however, if the reticulocyte count is high, the MCV may be slightly elevated. The diagnosis of hemolysis is suggested by an anemia with a reticulocyte index of at least 3% in the absence of overt bleeding. Bleeding is far more common than hemolysis, and bleeding in certain body sites (e.g., retroperitoneal bleeding in patients taking anticoagulants or bleeding into the site of a hip fracture) may be associated with a marked drop in hematocrit value and a high reticulocyte count, without external evidence of blood loss. Furthermore, the correction of anemias that are caused by decreased bone marrow production may also give a database that mimics hemolysis (e.g., patients with an appropriate reticulocyte response after being treated with iron, folic acid, or B_{12}, or after alcohol withdrawal).

Approach to Hemolysis

It is appropriate to attempt to prove that hemolysis is occurring before obtaining diagnostic tests in a search for specific etiologies. The diagnostic approach to hemolysis varies depending on whether hemolysis is primarily intravascular or extravascular.

Intravascular Hemolysis

Table 50.17 lists hemolytic mechanisms associated with intravascular destruction of red cells. Almost all of them require that the patient be hospitalized and that, if possible, diagnostic testing and treatment be planned in consultation with a hematologist. In intravascular hemolysis red cell lysis occurs within the vascular space, resulting in hemoglobinemia. The plasma becomes visibly red or brown (methemoglobinemia) at a low concentration of hemoglobin (approximately 30 mg/100 mL). Free hemoglobin initially binds to haptoglobin (a binding protein produced in the liver). Once haptoglobin is saturated, free hemoglobin passes through the glomerulus and hemoglobinuria occurs. Some of the hemoglobin in the renal tubules is absorbed by the renal tubular cells, which slough into the urine several days later and stain positively for iron (urine hemosiderin). The latter test, therefore, is helpful in documenting the presence of intravascular hemolysis several days after it has occurred. Table 50.18 suggests an appropriate database when hemolysis is suspected in the clinical states associated with intravascular hemolysis.

Extravascular Hemolysis

Most hemolysis occurs extravascularly within cells of the reticuloendothelial system. A diagnosis of extravascular hemolysis is more difficult to prove than that of intravascular hemolysis. There is no hemoglobinemia, hemoglobinuria, or hemosiderinuria. Haptoglobin is only partially saturated because there is only a slight leakage of free hemoglobin into the circulation.

Table 50.17. Clinical States Associated with Intravascular Hemolysis

Acute hemolytic transfusion reactions
Severe and extensive burns
Physical trauma (e.g., march hemoglobinuria)
Severe microangiopathic hemolysis (e.g., aortic valve prosthesis)
G6PD deficiency
Paroxysmal nocturnal hemoglobinuria

Table 50.18. Appropriate Database when Intravascular Hemolysis Is Suspected

Observation of the color of the serum/plasma
Observation of the color of the urine
Measurement of free plasma hemoglobin
Heme pigment test of the urine if there are no red cells in the urine sediment
Measurement of serum haptoglobin
Iron stain of urine sediment for hemosiderin several days after a presumed hemolytic event

There may be indirect hyperbilirubinemia, but this is an extremely insensitive sign of hemolysis. There is an increase in fecal and urine urobilinogen, but this is difficult to quantitate. Other tests of hemolysis, such as red cell survival, are difficult, and the results are not known for several days. The physician often must be satisfied with only a presumptive diagnosis of extravascular hemolysis. Therefore, when extravascular hemolysis is suspected, it may be appropriate to obtain tests diagnostic of specific disease states based on a knowledge of the patient's other problems and on the baseline database (Table 50.19).

Information from the Peripheral Smear

In hemolytic states the peripheral smear often reveals only evidence of the response of the bone marrow to hemolysis (large polychromatophilic or finely stippled red cells). It is a common misconception that one always sees fragmented red cells on smear (seen only in microangiopathic hemolytic anemias). However, the smear may give further clues about the specific etiology of the hemolysis, as indicated below.

Spherocytes.   Spherocytes are seen in small numbers in many hemolytic states. When present in large numbers they suggest either hereditary spherocytosis, autoimmune hemolysis, or one of the hemoglobin C hemoglobinopathies.

Elliptocytes.   In large numbers these suggest a diagnosis of hereditary elliptocytosis.

Fragmented Cells (Schistocytes).   Sharply pointed fragmented cells (helmet cells, spiculated cells, triangle cells) are seen in microangiopathic states (see below).

Spiculated Cells.   Sometimes spiculated cells are seen in patients with severe liver disease and hemolysis (usually in a terminal stage of liver disease). Spiculated cells are also one type of schistocyte found in the blood of patients with microangiopathic hemolysis.

Bite Cells (Blister Cells).   Bite cells are sometimes seen in patients with oxidative hemolysis (e.g., glucose-6-phosphate dehydrogenase deficiency). In bite cells, all of the hemoglobin appears to be pushed to one side of the cell.

Poikilocytosis and the Hemoglobinopathies.   In patients with sickle cell disease and in the various other sickle cell syndromes, the peripheral smear is often diagnostic (see below).

Table 50.19. Most Common Causes of Extravascular Hemolysis

Autoimmune hemolysis
Delayed hemolytic transfusion reactions
Hemoglobinopathies
Hereditary spherocytic and nonspherocytic anemias
Hypersplenism
Hemolysis with liver disease

Hemolysis with a Positive Coombs' Test

Once hemolysis is suspected, the diagnostic testing should be guided by the patient's problem list (9,28). Because of the relatively common occurrence of immune hemolysis and the important therapeutic implications of such a diagnosis, it is desirable to obtain a Coombs' test at this stage in the workup.

Positive Direct Coombs' Test

The direct Coombs' test is done by mixing the patient's cells with Coombs' antiserum containing antibody to IgG and to complement. If the test is positive, the physician should first ascertain from the laboratory personnel that the positive result is attributable to antibody and/or complement on the red cell surface. If this is the case, it is important to determine whether the antibody is an alloantibody or an autoantibody.

Alloantibodies are antibodies induced by prior transfusion or, in a woman, by placental transfer of fetal red cells. The antibodies are directed against specific minor red cell antigens, and it is important to identify them in case future transfusions are necessary. Ordinarily the antibody is present primarily in the patient's plasma and is identified by an antibody screen (indirect Coombs' test). However, a direct Coombs' test would also be positive because of the presence of alloantibodies if the patient had been recently transfused with cells that were still circulating and sensitized by the antibody.

In a patient with hemolysis, if there has not been a recent transfusion, a positive direct Coombs' test generally implies the presence of an autoantibody. In this situation the antibody may be present in the serum as well as on the surface of the red cells. Table 50.20 describes the differences between alloantibodies and autoantibodies. Autoantibodies are classified as either warm antibodies or cold antibodies. Warm antibodies are usually IgG and cannot be identified by direct agglutination of red cells, but require a Coombs' test. Cold antibodies, however, are usually IgM, cause direct agglutination of red cells in the cold, and result in a positive Coombs' test because of fixation of complement to the red cell, which is identified by nonspecific Coombs' antiserum.

Hemolysis Caused by Warm Antibodies

Table 50.21 lists the conditions commonly associated with autoimmune hemolysis resulting from a warm antibody. Patients may develop such antibodies secondary to the use of certain drugs or to one of a number of conditions, including infections (particularly viral), collagen vascular disease (systemic lupus erythematosus [SLE]), lymphoproliferative diseases, and other malignancies. The classic example of a drug that induces a positive Coombs' test is α-methyldopa (Aldomet) (30). A positive Coombs' test is not usually observed unless the patient has been taking large doses of Aldomet for a long period; in such circumstances a positive Coombs' test is not uncommon, but hemolysis is rare.

Autoimmune hemolysis is a relatively infrequent condition; sometimes it precedes the development of SLE or lymphoma. Patients usually have anemia, which may be severe. On physical examination the spleen is slightly enlarged in 50% of patients, and mild jaundice and fever are not uncommon. The peripheral smear shows marked polychromatophilia, spherocytosis, and often but not always, an elevated reticulocyte index. Autoimmune hemolysis that is temporary, such as that caused by drug administration or viral infections, usually requires no treatment (although if a drug is implicated, it should be discontinued). The process gradually remits over 2 to 4 weeks. Patients receiving methyldopa who do not have hemolysis but are found, incidentally, to have a positive Coombs' test, need not discontinue use of the drug. Patients with chronic primary autoimmune hemolysis should be referred to a hematologist, who usually prescribes corticosteroids, which are usually effective if first given at a reasonably high dosage and slowly tapered as the anemia improves. Occasionally, splenectomy is required for refractory cases. In patients with secondary chronic

Table 50.20. Comparison of Alloantibody and Autoantibody

	Alloantibody	Autoantibody
Direct Coombs' test	Often negative; may be positive if sensitized foreign red cells are still circulating	Positive
Indirect Coombs' test	Positive	Positive or negative
Antibody screen (panel)	Specificity is seen	Panagglutination, no specificity seen

Table 50.21. Autoimmune Hemolysis Caused by a Warm Antibody: Differential Diagnosis

Idiopathic
Secondary
  Infection (particularly viral)
  Drugs
    α-Methyldopa
    Penicillin
    Quinine/quinidine
  Collagen vascular disease (systemic lupus erythematosus)
  Lymphoproliferative disorders
  Miscellaneous (e.g., thyroid disease, malignancy)

Table 50.22. Hemolysis with Fragmented Red Cells on Peripheral Smear: Differential Diagnosis

Aortic value prosthesis
Arteritis (e.g., malignant hypertension, polyarteritis)
Disseminated intravascular coagulation
Thrombotic thrombocytopenic purpura
Hemolytic–uremic syndrome
Malignancy
Giant hemangiomas
Renal transplant rejection
Eclampsia

autoimmune hemolysis, treatment of the underlying disease is the most important therapy. Autoimmune hemolysis may sometimes present as a fulminant life-threatening anemia, sometimes associated with reticulocytopenia. In such cases patients should be hospitalized immediately and transfused despite the incompatible cross-match.

Cold Agglutinin Hemolysis

The most common etiology of autoimmune hemolysis caused by a cold antibody is a viral illness or *Mycoplasma* pneumonia (19). Severe hemolysis is rare. Chronic idiopathic cold agglutinin hemolysis or cold agglutinin hemolysis secondary to a lymphoproliferative disease is often more refractory to treatment with steroids and splenectomy than is the case with warm antibody hemolysis. Transfusion therapy may be a problem in such cases because the antibody is a panagglutinin and reacts with all blood types; therefore, a compatible cross-match may be impossible to obtain. Ordinarily, the IgM antibody in cold agglutinin hemolysis is not significantly hemolytic, and transfusions with warmed washed red cells may be attempted when absolutely necessary (20).

Hemolysis with Fragmented Red Cells on Peripheral Smear

Table 50.22 lists the conditions associated with hemolysis and the presence of fragmented red cells on peripheral smear. The peripheral blood contains sharply pointed poikilocytes (schistocytes). Such cells are characteristic and are clearly differentiated from abnormally shaped red cells seen in other conditions (3). The hemolysis may be severe and in such cases is usually intravascular, resulting in hemoglobinemia, hemoglobinuria, haptoglobin saturation, and subsequently, hemosiderinuria (see above). Red cell fragmentation may occur after insertion of a prosthetic aortic valve. Rarely this may be associated with clinically significant hemolysis. More often, red cell fragmentation is caused by arteriolar lesions (e.g., fibrin, inflammation) that cause damage to red cells as they pass through the damaged vessel. When fragmented red cells are accompanied by thrombocytopenia, one should consider the possibility of disseminated intravascular coagulation (see Chapter 51) and of throm-

botic thrombocytopenic purpura. This latter syndrome is often accompanied by fever and neurologic deficits, which characteristically fluctuate. Patients suspected of having this condition should be hospitalized immediately and treated in consultation with a hematologist. The hemolytic–uremic syndrome is a related (perhaps identical) syndrome, more common in children, characterized by the prominence of renal failure over other organ dysfunction.

Hemolysis with Enlarged Spleen (Hypersplenism)

Not all large spleens cause cytopenias, and the degree of cytopenia does not necessarily correlate with the size of the spleen (12). Thrombocytopenia and leukopenia are more common than is anemia. Splenomegaly, from almost any cause, may result in hypersplenism, but the syndrome is seen most often in patients who have chronic liver disease and congestive splenomegaly. Splenomegaly is sometimes seen in patients with hemolysis from other mechanisms, such as autoimmune hemolysis or hereditary spherocytosis. Rarely, splenectomy is necessary because of severe cytopenias resulting from hypersplenism. Occasional patients with Felty's syndrome (see Chapter 70) are benefited by splenectomy, as are some patients with chronic leukemia or lymphoma.

Glucose-6-Phosphate Dehydrogenase Deficiency

Glucose-6-phosphate dehydrogenase (G6PD) deficiency (2) is seen primarily in African-American patients in the United States. Inheritance is sex linked. Ten percent of African-American males are affected (hemizygotes), as are 20% of African-American females (heterozygotes). In the affected African-American patients, hemolysis caused by G6PD deficiency is an acute intravascular hemolytic event usually precipitated by infection or an oxidant drug. Drugs known to precipitate hemolysis include sulfonamides, nitrofurantoin, and primaquine. Caucasian-type G6PD deficiency is seen primarily in patients from Mediterranean countries and usually is more severe than the African type, sometimes causing chronic, persisting, partially compensated hemolysis.

Diagnosis after a hemolytic event may be difficult, especially in the female heterozygotes. Screening tests for G6PD deficiency may be normal at this time, and even the affected hemizygote African-American male may have a normal screening test for several weeks after hemolysis (young cells contain more G6PD activity). Occasionally a characteristic cell (bite cell) is seen in the peripheral blood during a hemolytic event.

Although the frequency of the genetic defect is high, the incidence of severe hemolysis with provocation (infection, drugs) is low. Ordinarily routine screening before treatment with a known oxidant drug (e.g., sulfonamide) is not recommended. Affected patients should be given a list of drugs to avoid (2), including over-the-counter medications such as phenacetin.

Sickle Cell Disorders

Approximately 8% of the African-American population in the United States carry the sickle cell gene (1). The gene is also present to much less an extent in Greeks, Italians, Arabians, and people from India. Hemoglobin S results from a mutation in the β-globin chain in hemoglobin that, when oxygen tension is reduced, causes the formation of rigid elongated tactoids that distort red cell shape and increase red cell rigidity. The clumping together of sickled cells leads to tissue ischemia and infarction. A number of common inherited disorders involving hemoglobin S are listed in this section.

Sickle Cell Trait

Most people who are heterozygous for hemoglobin S (sickle cell trait) are completely well and are not anemic. The peripheral smear appears normal, although sickling is seen if the blood is deoxygenated. Hemoglobin electrophoresis reveals approximately 40% hemoglobin S and 60% hemoglobin A, whereas hemoglobins A_2 and F are present in normal concentration.

Most patients with sickle trait lead a normal life. However, rare clinical events attributable to the presence of sickle cell hemoglobin do occur. For example, splenic infarction at high altitudes (above 10,000 feet) has been reported. (Oxygen pressures in commercial aircraft are high enough that people with sickle cell trait may fly safely.) Occasionally, infarctions occur in more vital organs during vigorous exercise. All people with sickle cell trait have renal tubular dysfunction resulting in hyposthenuria; on occasion severe hematuria may occur from hypertonicity in the renal medulla, resulting in sickling and leading to ischemia and tubular infarction. People with sickle cell trait have a higher incidence of renal infections, especially during pregnancy.

It is important to identify patients with sickle cell trait so that they may be given genetic counseling. A couple, both heterozygous for hemoglobin S, should be informed that they have a 25% chance of having a child with sickle cell anemia. Prenatal diagnosis of sickle cell anemia by amniocentesis is now possible.

Sickle Cell Anemia (Hemoglobin SS)

Sickle cell anemia exists in approximately 0.15% of the African-American population (1,7,31). The disease is usually severe, resulting in significant morbidity as well as shortened life expectancy. One of the most disturbing clinical features of the illness is the occurrence of painful (thrombotic) crises: recurrent episodes of severe pain, usually in the limbs and the abdomen, caused by sickling-induced ischemia. Patients have a lifelong, often severe anemia, with hematocrit values that range from the high teens to the low thirties (average is mid-twenties). The primary mechanism of the anemia is extravascular hemolysis, so that there is a chronic reticulocytosis and a chronic indirect hyperbilirubinemia. The patients usually have a leukocytosis, the white cell count rising occasionally as high as

30,000 to 40,000 cells/mL during a painful crisis. A mild thrombocytosis is also common. The peripheral smear shows markedly distorted red cells, including characteristically sickled cells. Upon electrophoresis, only hemoglobin S with a variable amount of hemoglobin F (no hemoglobin A) is detected.

The multiple and repetitive episodes of organ ischemia caused by sickling result in a host of abnormalities. The bones characteristically appear abnormal on radiograph, revealing old infarctions that mimic the changes of osteomyelitis. The medullary spaces are usually widened by the marked compensatory expansion of bone marrow. The spine often takes on a distorted appearance, and aseptic necrosis of the femoral (and, rarely, humeral) head is common, sometimes requiring joint replacement. Puberty is often delayed. Splenomegaly usually disappears by age 8 because of repeated infarctions of the spleen. An adult with sickle cell anemia is essentially autosplenectomized. This lack of splenic function contributes to the propensity for infections, related especially to a decreased ability to resist pneumococcal infections. Gallstones (pigment stones) are common, and sicklers do develop cholecystitis, which may be extremely difficult to differentiate clinically from a syndrome of intrahepatic cholestasis secondary to sickling in the hepatic sinusoids. There is some hazard to surgery, but patients with recurrent abdominal pain consistent with cholecystitis, who have gallstones, should probably have elective cholecystectomy (see Chapter 90). Pregnancy in women with SS disease is complicated by an increased risk of pyelonephritis, pulmonary infarction, antepartum hemorrhage, prematurity, and fetal death. With time, patients develop cardiomegaly and chronic myocardial disease related to repetitive microinfarctions of the heart. Murmurs are common and may suggest rheumatic or congenital heart disease. Patients with sickle cell anemia develop venous thromboses and pulmonary embolism. They also develop thromboses in situ in the lungs, followed, after many years, by chronic scarring and fibrosis. Pulmonary thrombosis/embolism may lead to pulmonary hypertension and heart failure. Cerebral vascular accidents are common, including infarction and intracerebral and subarachnoid hemorrhage. Seizures are common as well. Up to 75% of patients with sickle cell anemia develop leg ulcerations that may be chronic and extremely difficult to heal. Patients with sickle cell anemia are prone to serious retinopathy, which rarely may lead to blindness because of plugging of small retinal capillaries and subsequent neovascularization. It is important for these patients to be examined yearly by an ophthalmologist because some of the problems can be prevented by photocoagulation of abnormal new retinal vessels (22).

SC Disease

The genes that code for hemoglobin S and hemoglobin C are alleles. The C hemoglobin mutation is common in African Americans (approximately 2% prevalence), and patients doubly heterozygous for S and C constitute approximately 0.15% of that population. The syndrome is similar to that of SS disease but is usually somewhat more mild. In contrast to sickle cell anemia, the spleen is palpable in 50% of adult patients.

S–β-Thalassemia

Patients doubly heterozygous for hemoglobin S and β-thalassemia trait have a syndrome similar to sickle cell anemia but usually more mild. Characteristically the MCV is low. The spleen may be palpable, and the hemoglobin electrophoresis reveals 70 to 80% hemoglobin S and smaller amounts of hemoglobin A and F (the reverse of the pattern in sickle cell trait).

Treatment

Painful Thrombotic Crises. Painful crises are often severe and may last for a few hours to several days and occasionally for several weeks. They may be associated with high fever and neutrophilia, which makes it difficult but important to differentiate crises from infection. No specific therapy exists. The patient is usually treated with narcotics and hydration. Because patients can become addicted to narcotics because of the repetitive episodes of severe pain, it is important to limit strictly the amount of narcotics given them in ambulatory practice. When pain is severe and persistent, hospitalization is indicated.

Infection. As mentioned, patients with sickle cell anemia are prone to infections, especially with the pneumococcus. Patients with sickle cell anemia should receive pneumococcal vaccine (see Chapter 32) and should be encouraged to seek medical help at the first evidence of infection or fever.

Hemolytic and Aplastic Crises. Acceleration of hemolysis is unusual. If hematocrit values drop significantly below baseline, it is probably because of decreased marrow production, associated with infection. Such episodes are much more common in children. If they occur, hospitalization and transfusion are often necessary. Patients with chronic severe hemolysis have an increased requirement for folic acid, and folic acid deficiency may occur, resulting in reticulocytopenia and more severe anemia. Therefore, daily folic acid therapy (1 mg) is reasonable for all patients with sickle cell anemia.

Thromboembolization. When patients with sickle cell disease develop deep vein thrombosis or pulmonary embolism, they should be treated with anticoagulants, as would any patient with such problems (see Chapter 52). However, venography should be avoided because of the danger of developing leg ulcers in any patient with SS hemoglobin whose lower extremities are traumatized. It is often difficult to distinguish pulmonary thrombotic/embolic problems from pneumonia. The *acute chest syndrome,* an episode characterized by chest pain, shortness of breath, and cough—often with fever and a pulmonary infiltrate—is common in patients with sickle cell anemia and usually warrants hospitalization to evaluate the diagnostic possibilities and institute appropriate treatment.

Leg Ulcers. Leg ulcers are often large and are particularly refractory to treatment. Skin grafting is usually only temporarily helpful and often does not seem to be worth the time and discomfort involved. It is important to keep the ulcers clean, to elevate the legs frequently, and to use surgical stockings and elastic wraps (see Chapter 88).

Hematuria. Patients with sickle cell trait, sickle cell anemia, SC disease, and sickle cell thalassemia all are prone to bouts of severe hematuria related to sickling and to medullary ischemia precipitated by the hypertonicity of the renal medulla. Bleeding can occur for days or even weeks. Maintenance of a high urine flow is important to prevent clots from causing obstruction, and usually the hematuria stops spontaneously.

Priapism. Priapism is common in SS and SC disease and often results in permanent impotence once it has resolved. If urologic intervention is to be attempted, it must be done within a few hours of the onset of the priapism. It is often only temporarily helpful. Once impotence has occurred, penile protheses are often helpful (see Chapter 18).

Preventive Treatment with Hydroxyurea. A large controlled study has demonstrated that treatment with hydroxyurea does decrease the incidence of painful crises in some patients with sickle cell anemia (8). The mechanism may be partly (but not completely) caused by increased intracellular levels of hemoglobin F. The benefit is modest in most patients and a therapeutic trial requires close monitoring by a hematologist. The long-term side effects of hydroxyurea must be weighed carefully before a patient is placed on therapy (8).

Recommendations for Preventive Care

Patients with sickle cell disorders have a lifelong chronic illness and require frequent and recurrent use of the health care system. The patient needs one general physician who is familiar with him or her. The availability of emergency care 24 hours a day is also exceedingly important.

Infection. There should be rapid evaluation of fever, chills, or other signs of infection. The patient should be immunized with the pneumococcal vaccine (see Chapter 32). Because heart murmurs and cardiomegaly are common, it is often difficult to know whether a patient with sickle cell anemia has valvular heart disease. If any doubt exists, it is reasonable to prescribe prophylactic antibiotics before dental procedures (see Chapter 86).

Narcotic Abuse. As mentioned earlier in this chapter, analgesics should be given at dosages sufficient to relieve pain during a thrombotic crisis. However, the use of narcotics on an ambulatory basis should be avoided if possible because addiction can occur. Easy access to the primary physician should help to obviate giving patients a supply of narcotics to take in case of pain.

Folic Acid. It is generally recommended that patients receive 1 mg of folic acid daily.

Ophthamologic Examination. Patients should see an ophthalmologist yearly.

Incentive Spirometry. There is evidence that incentive spirometry may decrease pulmonary complications in patients with pain crises.

Transfusions. In general, transfusions should be avoided because of the dangers of iron overload, sensitization to minor red cell antigens, infection, and other hazards of transfusion. Exchange transfusion (supervised by a hematologist) may help interrupt a prolonged pain crisis and is indicated in severe, life-threatening acute chest syndrome (see above), and hypertransfusion is useful in preventing recurrent neurologic vascular events.

Hydroxyurea. Patients with frequent, severe, life-altering painful crises should be referred to a hematologist for consideration for therapy with hydroxyurea.

ANEMIAS WITH NORMAL MCV AND AN INAPPROPRIATELY LOW RETICULOCYTE INDEX

Mild normocytic anemias without appropriate reticulocyte responses are among the most common problems seen in clinical practice. Before considering possible etiologies and embarking on a diagnostic workup, it is important to be sure that the hematocrit value/hemoglobin concentration is reproducibly low. Moreover, the normal values for the laboratory should be known. For example, in some laboratories a hematocrit value of 35% in a woman is normal. One should also consider the variation in normal values related to age, sex, pregnancy, and other factors. Finally, one should be sure that volume overload is not the etiology. Volume shifts may result in swings in hematocrit value of 6 or 8 percentage points. Table 50.23 lists the differential diagnosis of a normocytic anemia with an inappropriately low reticulocyte count.

Anemia of Renal Failure

Patients with uremia are anemic primarily because of decreased production of erythropoietin (15). The red cell morphology on smear is usually normal, but occasionally spiculated cells (burr cells) may be seen. An occasional patient may have a microangiopathic peripheral smear. There may be a mild thrombocytopenia, and the nuclei of the neutrophils may be hypersegmented even in the absence of folic acid deficiency. The hematocrit value depends on the degree of renal failure (see Fig. 48.3, Chapter 48). Significant anemia is unusual if the creatinine is less than 2 mg/100 mL. The hematocrit value seen in patients with renal failure on dialysis is extremely variable (from the low teens, requiring transfusion, up to the mid-thirties). Recombinant human erythropoietin is helpful for the treatment of anemia of renal failure. Responses can be dramatic, and although the preparation is expensive, side effects are few (e.g., hypertension in some patients) (16). Patients in renal failure may also be anemic because of iron deficiency (secondary to blood loss) or because of folate deficiency (because folic acid is dialyzable). Some patients with glomerulonephritis or arteritis may have a microangiopathic hemolytic anemia.

Anemia of Chronic Disease

Any chronic inflammatory disease (e.g., rheumatoid arthritis) or malignant neoplastic disease may cause mild to moderate anemia, unrelated to blood loss or hemolysis (5,6,26). (If the hematocrit value is less than 25%, another explanation should be sought.) Red cell morphology is usually normal but occasionally the MCV may be less than 80 fL, requiring differentiation of the process from other causes of a microcytic anemia (see above). The serum iron and the total iron-binding capacity are low; the percentage of saturation may be just as low as it is in iron deficiency (less than 10%). The serum ferritin is normal or elevated, and bone marrow iron stores are normal or increased.

In addition to chronic infections, an acute infection or inflammation will cause a decrease in serum iron, reticulocytopenia, and bone marrow red cell production. If present for 1 week or more, therefore, an acute inflammatory process may result in a fall in the hematocrit value of several percentage points.

Mild Early Iron Deficiency

Although severe iron deficiency results in microcytic anemia (see above), in the early stages mild iron deficiency may result in anemia with a normal peripheral smear and a normal MCV. Diagnosis can usually be made by measurement of serum ferritin or by a bone marrow iron stain. In addition, a patient with severe iron deficiency, when it accompanies a macrocytic anemia such as a megaloblastic anemia (as in an alcoholic patient with iron deficiency and folic acid deficiency) may have a severe anemia that is normocytic. The reticulocyte count is inappropriately low until (in the alcoholic patient) alcohol is withdrawn and iron and folate are administered.

Anemia in the Elderly

Old age per se is not an explanation for a significant normocytic anemia (25). Hematocrit values in healthy patients in their seventies are only slightly lower than they are in the normal adult range (Table 50.1). However, it is in elderly patients that frustrating, mild, unexplained, normocytic anemias occur. In such pa-

Table 50.23.   Anemia with a Normal MCV and Low Reticulocyte Index: Differential Diagnosis

Renal failure
Anemia of chronic disease (inflammatory disease and malignancy)
Anemia of hypoendocrine states (hypothyroidism, etc.)
Mild (early) iron deficiency
Combined iron deficiency and megaloblastic anemia
Drug-induced marrow depression
Primary bone marrow disorders
Bone marrow infiltration (myelophthisis)
Bleeding or hemolysis plus one of the above

tients the following possible explanations should be considered: fluid overload, blood loss from phlebotomy if the patient has been hospitalized recently, and any recent inflammatory disease (viral or bacterial infection, inflammatory joint problem) that may depress bone marrow production and, if present for several days, may result in a drop in hematocrit value. If none of these explanations seems appropriate and there is no reason to suspect an underlying problem, it is reasonable simply to follow the hematocrit value without further diagnostic workup. If it is known that the onset of the anemia is recent (e.g., if there is a record of a normal hematocrit value 3 months previously), other efforts should be made to explain it. For example, the possibility of occult gastrointestinal bleeding with early iron deficiency or the anemia of chronic disease or malignancy should be entertained.

General References

Charache S, Johnson CS, eds. Sickle cell disease. Hematol Clin North Am 10:1221–1407, 1996.

Waterbury L. Hematology. 4th ed. Baltimore, MD: Williams & Wilkins, 1996.

Williams WJ, Beutler E, Erslev AJ, Lichtman MA, eds. Hematology. 5th ed. New York: McGraw-Hill, 1995.

Specific References

1. Abramson H, Bertles JF, Wethers DL, eds. Sickle cell disease. St Louis: Mosby, 1973.
2. Beutler E. Glucose-6-phosphate dehydrogenase deficiency. N Engl J Med 324:169, 1991.
3. Brain MC. Microangiopathic hemolytic anemia. N Engl J Med 281:833, 1969.
4. Carmel R, Sinow RM, Siegel ME, Samloff IM. Food cobalamin malabsorption occurs frequently in patients with unexplained low serum cobalamin levels. Arch Intern Med 148:1715, 1988.
5. Cartwright GE. The anemia of chronic disorders. Semin Hematol 3:351, 1966.
6. Cash JM, Sears DA. The anemia of chronic disease: spectrum of associated diseases in a series of unselected hospitalized patients. Am J Med 87:638, 1989.
7. Charache S. Treatment of sickle cell anemia. Annu Rev Med 32:195, 1981.
8. Charache S, Barton FB, Moore RD. Hydroxyurea and sickle cell anemia. Clinical utility of a myelosuppressive "switching" agent. The Multicenter Study of Hydroxyurea in Sickle Cell Anemia. Medicine 75:300, 1996.
9. Collins PW, Newland AC. Treatment modalities of autoimmune blood disorders. Semin Hematol 29:64, 1992.
10. Colman N, Herbert J. Hematologic complications of alcoholism: overview. Semin Hematol 17:164, 1980.
11. Cook JD. Clinical evaluation of iron deficiency. Semin Hematol 19:6, 1982.
12. Dameshek W. Hypersplenism. Bull N Y Acad Med 31:113, 1955.
13. Davidson RJL, Hamilton PJ. High mean red cell volume: its incidence and significance in routine hematology. J Clin Pathol 31:493, 1978.
14. England JM, Ward S, Down MC. Microcytosis, anisocytosis and the red cell indices in iron deficiency. Br J Haematol 34:589, 1976.
15. Erslev AJ. Management of anemia of chronic renal failure. Clin Nephrol 2:174, 1974.
16. Eschbach JW, Eqrie JC, Downing MR, et al. Correction of the anemia of end-stage renal disease with recombinant human erythropoietin. Results of a combined phase I and II clinical trial. N Engl J Med 316:73, 1987.
17. Ganser A, Haelyer D. Clinical course of myelodysplastic syndromes. Hematol Oncol Clin North Am 6:607, 1992.
18. Halliday JW, Powell LW. Serum ferritin and isoferritins in clinical medicine. Prog Hematol 11:229, 1979.
19. Jacobson LB, Longstreth GF, Edgington TS. Clinical and immunologic features of transient cold agglutinin hemolytic anemia. Am J Med 54:514, 1973.
20. Jefferies LC. Transfusion therapy in autoimmune hemolytic anemias. Hematol Clin North Am 8:1087, 1994.
21. Kaiser L, Schwartz KA. Aluminum induced anemia. Am J Kidney Dis 5:348, 1985.
22. King W, Nadel AJ. Ophthalmologic complications in hemoglobinopathies. Hematol Oncol Clin North Am 5:535, 1991.
23. Lindenbaum J. Status of laboratory testing in the diagnosis of megaloblastic anemia. Blood 61:624, 1983.
24. Lindenbaum J, Healton EB, Savage DG, et al. Neuropsychiatric disorders caused by cobalamin deficiency in the absence of anemia or macrocytosis. N Engl J Med 318:1720, 1988.
25. Lipschitz DA, Udupa KB, Milton KY, Thompson CO. Effects of age on hematopoiesis in man. Blood 63:502, 1984.
26. Means R, Krantz SB. Progress in understanding the pathogenesis of the anemia of chronic disease. Blood 80:1639, 1992.
27. Pierce HI, Kurachi S, Sofroniadou K, Stamatoyamopoulos G. Frequencies of thalassemia in American blacks. Blood 49:981, 1977.
28. Pirofsky G. Clinical aspects of autoimmune hemolytic anemia. Semin Hematol 13:251, 1976.
29. Rawley PT. The diagnosis of β-thalassemia trait: a review. Am J Hematol 1:129, 1976.
30. Salama A, Mueller-Eckhardt C. Immune-mediated blood cell dyscrasias related to drugs. Semin Hematol 29:54, 1992.
31. Vichinsky EP. Comprehensive care in sickle cell disease: its impact on morbidity and mortality. Semin Hematol 28:220, 1991.

C H A P T E R 51

Disorders of Hemostasis

PHILIP D. ZIEVE, MD

In a healthy person a number of different processes interact to ensure that blood is maintained in a fluid state until the integrity of a blood vessel wall is compromised; at that point, a plug is rapidly formed to prevent exsanguination. Three major systems are involved in this regard: the vasculature itself, the blood platelets, and the coagulation system.

EVALUATION OF PATIENTS

The history is the most important aid in determining whether a patient has a hemorrhagic diathesis (4). Patients with congenital disorders of hemostasis or acquired disorders of long standing almost certainly have had unexpectedly excessive bleeding in response to minor trauma or to surgery. The clinician should ask specifically whether the patient has required transfusion after an operative procedure or a seemingly minor trauma.

Bleeding caused by injury to the vasculature is overwhelmingly more common than bleeding caused by defective hemostasis. Therefore, patients with gastrointestinal or genitourinary hemorrhage, for example, are more likely to have a lesion (e.g., a peptic ulcer, carcinoma, diverticulum, or tumor of the kidney or of the bladder that has bled) than a disorder of hemostasis. Similarly, nose bleeds, bleeding gums, or excessive menstrual flow probably reflect local (usually benign) problems. Furthermore, even if patients have hemostatic dysfunction, they are likely to bleed from local lesions, the propensity to bleed of which has been accentuated by the hemostatic abnormality.

Specific disorders of hemostasis may be suspected strongly on the basis of the patient's history and because of characteristic findings on physical examination (Fig. 51.1; see below), but in almost all instances laboratory tests are required before a specific diagnosis can be made. Screening tests, procedures that are extremely sensitive to alterations in hemostasis, are ordinarily relied on first in a patient with a suspected hemorrhagic diathesis (Table 51.1). If any of these tests is abnormal or if it is strongly suspected that a disorder of hemostasis exists, even if the tests are not abnormal, more specific tests are indicated; these are best performed in consultation with a hematologist.

DISORDERS OF BLOOD VESSELS

Vascular disease is diagnosed uncommonly as a cause of a hemorrhagic diathesis, in part because, except for trauma, disorders of the vasculature that result in untoward bleeding are rare (3) and in part because there is no reliable screening test to detect generalized vascular dysfunction. The primary hemor-

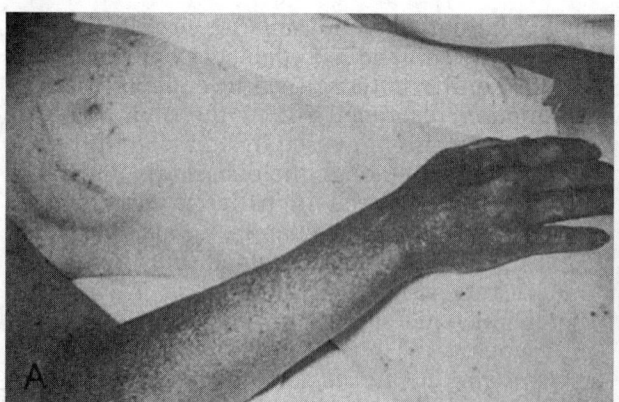
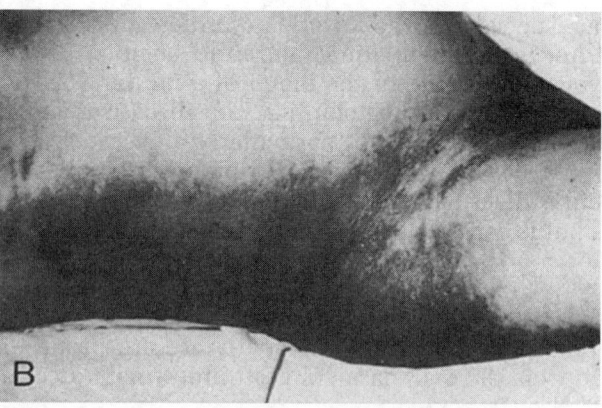

Figure 51.1. Bleeding caused by thrombocytopenia compared with bleeding caused by abnormal coagulation. **A.** Immune thrombocytopenic purpura with typical petechial lesion. **B.** Hemophilia A with extensive purpuric bleeding. (From Zieve PD, Levin J. Disorders of hemostasis. Philadelphia: WB Saunders, 1976.)

Table 51.1. Laboratory Evaluation of Hemostatic Function

System	Screening Tests	Specific Tests
Blood vessels	None	Depends on suspected underlying disorder (see text)
Platelets Quantitative	Scanning of a stained smear of the peripheral blood	Platelet count
Qualitative	Bleeding time	Platelet aggregation
Coagulation	Partial thromboplastin time, prothrombin time, thrombin time	Factor assays

rhagic manifestation of vascular disease is purpura, a confluent purplish discoloration of the skin caused by extravasation of blood from cutaneous and subcutaneous blood vessels. Although patients with an abnormal vasculature may occasionally experience bleeding from large blood vessels, most commonly they bleed into the skin or mucous membranes. Because purpura is a common response to minor trauma, it cannot in itself be taken as evidence of an underlying hemorrhagic diathesis.

Cutaneous Lesions

Unexplained bruises, especially on the lower extremities, are common and usually are not associated with an underlying disease process. A history of easy bruisability therefore is unlikely, in itself, to lead to a diagnosis of a disorder of hemostasis. Similarly, *senile purpura,* which occurs characteristically on the dorsum of the hand and the extensor surfaces of the forearms, does not represent a generalized hemorrhagic diathesis but results from the loss of connective tissue support to intracutaneous blood vessels, which then are easily traumatized and bleed within the substance of the skin. Identical lesions are seen sometimes in patients with Cushing's syndrome or in patients who have received corticosteroid therapy.

Allergic purpura (Henoch–Schönlein purpura) (6,20) is a hypersensitivity reaction to an antigenic stimulus that usually cannot be identified (although sometimes a drug or a bacterial infection can be incriminated as a provocative agent). Characteristically, patients develop a symmetric petechial rash, which is most prominent on the extremities. The lesions are slightly raised, distinguishing them from the petechiae of thrombocytopenia. No hemostatic dysfunction is associated with this condition; the cutaneous manifestations of the disorder are part of a widespread small-vessel vasculitis, the manifestations of which also may include arthralgias (sometimes with evidence of joint effusions), fever, malaise, abdominal pain, gastrointestinal bleeding, and renal disease caused by a focal glomerulonephritis that occasionally may progress to chronic renal failure. There is no specific treatment for this condition; although if the patient is taking a drug that is suspected to be a sensitizing agent, it should be discontinued. Most patients recover spontaneously within 3 or 4 weeks, but sometimes signs and symptoms of the disease continue or recur for up to a year. Patients should be reassured while they are symptomatic that unless they have evidence of progressive renal disease, they will ultimately recover.

Autoerythrocyte sensitization (25) is a disorder characterized by apparently spontaneous painful ecchymoses, usually on the lower extremities and anterior trunk. The disorder is named as it is because of a belief at one time that it arose as the result of a hypersensitivity response to the patients' red cells or red cell stroma, and in fact the lesions can sometimes be produced by injection of autologous red cells into the skin of these patients. It has become apparent, however, that virtually all patients with the disorder, most of whom are women, are severely psychoneurotic and in some instances frankly psychotic; many people believe now that the lesions are self-inflicted.

Cryoglobulinemia (14,15) as a primary abnormality or as a special feature of an underlying disease such as dysproteinemia (see "Dysproteinemia" later in this chapter), lymphoma, or collagen vascular disease may also cause purpuric bleeding, especially on the lower extremities. The cryoglobulins may be isolated monoclonal proteins or may be immune complexes of monoclonal IgG or IgM and polyclonal IgG, or of mixed polyclonal immunoglobulins. There is often an associated glomerulonephritis and, in the patient with immune complex formation, sometimes evidence of hepatitis B infection (14).

The diagnosis of cryoglobulinemia may be made by placing a sample of the patient's serum in a refrigerator overnight and then inspecting the serum to see whether a white gel or precipitate has formed that disappears when the specimen is warmed. The blood for this test should be drawn in a warm syringe, and then it should be allowed to clot and retract in a 37°C water bath. Primary cryoglobulinemia is poorly responsive to treatment; secondary cryoglobulinemia may respond to treatment of the underlying disease.

Hyperglobulinemic purpura of Waldenström (18) is a rare, poorly defined condition characterized by purpura, especially of the lower extremities, an elevated erythrocyte sedimentation rate, mild anemia, and a polyclonal increase in the blood of a mixture of IgG and anti-IgG immunoglobulins. The disease is more common in women and, particularly after the age of 40, may be associated with an underlying collagen vascular disorder. The primary condition is untreatable but is generally benign.

Patients with other small-vessel vasculitides sometimes also present with petechialike lesions and systemic disease (e.g., renal or pulmonary disease) typically much more severe than it is in patients with allergic purpura. These conditions are sometimes associated with antineurophilic cytoplasmic antibodies (ANCA). Such patients are best managed in consultation with a rheumatologist.

Mucocutaneous Lesions

Some patients with vascular disease are prone to bleeding from the oral, nasal, or gastrointestinal mucosa, as well as from the skin. Such patients may present to their physicians not only with cutaneous hemorrhage but with bleeding gums, epistaxis, hematemesis, or melena.

Amyloidosis

Mucocutaneous bleeding may be a symptom of amyloidosis because of the deposition of amyloid within the walls of blood vessels (13,19). Periorbital bleeding and bleeding in skin folds are especially common. The skin in the areas of hemorrhage sometimes appears thickened because of palpable amyloid deposits within it. Patients suspected of having this disorder should have skin biopsies with appropriate staining as well as serum and urine electrophoresis in an attempt to make a specific diagnosis.

Dysproteinemia

Myeloma or macroglobulinemia may be associated with untoward bleeding, either because of increased viscosity of the blood or because the coating of blood vessels and platelets with the abnormal protein interferes with normal hemostatic function (23). Abnormal coagulation is also common in patients with these disorders. Patients suspected of having dysproteinemia should have samples of their serum and urine examined by electrophoresis in an attempt to demonstrate a monoclonal protein. If the diagnosis of dysproteinemia seems likely on the basis of this test and the clinical presentation, consultation with a hematologist or oncologist is appropriate.

Vitamin C Deficiency

There are three situations in which symptomatic vitamin C deficiency (scurvy) might be seen in this country: in chronic alcoholics, food faddists, and chronically ill or debilitated patients (17). Because humans, unlike most animals, are unable to synthesize vitamin C, they depend on exogenous sources such as fruits or leafy vegetables. People who cannot or will not eat an adequate diet of foods that contain the vitamin are subject to the manifestations of scurvy. The signs and symptoms of scurvy are attributable largely to the formation of defective connective tissue, because of the human body's absolute dependence on vitamin C for the synthesis of normal collagen. Mucocutaneous bleeding is common in patients with vitamin C deficiency who characteristically have large ecchymoses on their extremities, bleeding gums, and, very suggestive of this disorder, perifollicular hemorrhages that appear commonly on the lower extremities and anterior trunk. Sometimes patients with vitamin C deficiency develop hemarthroses similar to those seen in patients with severe coagulation disorders. All manifestations of scurvy are readily reversed by administration of vitamin C, so that although the disorder is uncommon it should be considered in patients with compatible signs and symptoms. Vitamin C deficiency can be confirmed by assay of the blood, but this is usually unnecessary because if the diagnosis is suspected, a therapeutic trial of vitamin C (250 mg once a day) is innocuous.

Hereditary Hemorrhagic Telangiectasia

Hereditary hemorrhagic telangiectasia is an inherited abnormality of blood vessels (an autosomal dominant condition) in which there is dilation of abnormally thin-walled venules and capillaries (24). The dilations result in characteristic telangiectases, which are small, flat, red, or purple lesions that blanch on pressure. They occur throughout the body but can be seen externally most commonly on the lips, tongue, hand, and mucous membranes of the nose. Lesions of larger blood vessels also occur in this disease, most commonly pulmonary arteriovenous fistulas, which develop in up to one-third of patients and may cause high-output heart failure. Vascular malformations of the liver or the brain also may occur. The mucocutaneous lesions may bleed excessively when traumatized. Recurrent epistaxis is the most common symptom of patients with the disorder, but the most troublesome problem is recurrent gastrointestinal bleeding, which is notoriously difficult to manage. Accessible lesions can ordinarily be treated by local compression. No pharmacologic agent will alter the course of the condition, but symptoms are variable; many patients experience little difficulty during the course of their life.

DISORDERS OF PLATELETS

Platelets provide a cellular defense against the loss of blood from traumatized vessels, especially where blood flow is relatively rapid, as it is on the arterial side of the circulation and in the left heart. Platelets are particularly effective in sealing leaks from small arterioles and capillaries; when platelets are abnormal, either quantitatively or qualitatively, these vessels bleed most prominently. The platelet plug is initiated by the exposure of platelets to subendothelial collagen, which is exposed by injury to the vascular intima. The absorption of a protein, von Willebrand factor (VWF; see below), to specific receptor sites on the platelet surface is important in the mediation of this process. Thereafter, aggregating agents such as thrombin and adenosine diphosphate cause the accretion of platelets at that site, eventually forming an adhesive plug that within minutes prevents the further flow of blood. Eventually the plug is replaced by fibrin laid down by the activation of the coagulation mechanism, which occurs simultaneously with the initiation of platelet plug formation.

Thrombocytopenia is one of the most common acquired disorders of hemostasis. The normal platelet count is between 150,000 and 400,000/mm^3, but the platelet count ordinarily must be reduced to below 50,000/mm^3 before untoward bleeding is observed, and even then bleeding usually does not occur unless the patient is traumatized. So-called spontaneous bleeding is unlikely unless the platelet count is reduced to below 20,000/mm^3. The characteristic lesion of thrombocytopenia is the petechia, a small purpuric hemorrhage occurring on the skin or mucous membranes, especially at sites of elevated capillary pressure, such as the lower extremities, the forearm after inflation of a blood pressure cuff, or the face after prolonged crying or coughing. In fact, if capillary pressure is raised high enough, or if capillaries are damaged after sunburn, for example, petechiae may be seen in otherwise normal people. Although cutaneous bleeding may be the first clue to the diagnosis of thrombocytopenia, morbidity from the disorder is more likely to result from gastrointestinal or genitourinary hemorrhage. As previously mentioned, if bleeding from these sites occurs, the patient should be examined at an appropriate time to determine whether an organic lesion, such as a carcinoma of the colon or of the kidney, has bled in association with defective hemostasis. The most feared complication of thrombocytopenia is intracerebral bleeding that, although it occurs infrequently, is still one of the major causes of death in patients with the disorder.

Evaluation of the Thrombocytopenic Patient

The best screening test for the evaluation of the numbers of platelets in the blood is observation of a stained smear of the peripheral blood. With relatively little experience it is easy to determine whether the platelet count is unusually low or high. In unanticoagulated blood (e.g., from a fingerstick), at least one clump of platelets should be seen, on the average, in every oil immersion field. In anticoagulated blood, one platelet should be seen for every 10 to 20 red cells. If a quantitative abnormality is suspected, a precise platelet count can be obtained. The bleeding time is not useful as a screening test for detecting quantitative abnormalities of platelets or for predicting which patients are likely to bleed excessively when traumatized (26). However, despite its limitations, the bleeding time is still used commonly to evaluate qualitative abnormalities of platelet function, described later in this chapter.

Patients with an immune thrombocytopenia (see below) characteristically have increased amounts of γ-globulin adsorbed to their platelets. Serologic tests to detect these proteins are widely available but have proved to be nonspecific and therefore of little value in establishing a precise diagnosis.

In ambulatory practice, in most patients encountered with platelet counts lower than normal, the precise pathophysiology of thrombocytopenia is not clear.

Many patients are found to have thrombocytopenia during the course of routine hematologic studies performed to obtain baseline data, or as part of an evaluation of an apparently unrelated condition. If the platelet count is more than 50,000/mm^3 in such circumstances, and the history, physical examination, and other hematologic evaluations do not suggest that an underlying disease is present that urgently requires diagnosis and treatment, it is probably justifiable simply to follow the patient with serial platelet counts (performed monthly until it is determined how stable the counts are). If the counts do not decrease further and if no other evidence of a disease process emerges, there is no need to stress the patient with further diagnostic procedures.

Symptomatic thrombocytopenia caused by decreased production of platelets is usually observed in conjunction with processes such as aplastic anemia, leukemia, disseminated tuberculosis, or metastatic carcinoma that affect other hematologic cell lines. In contrast, severe thrombocytopenia caused by increased destruction of platelets does not necessarily indicate the presence of a disease process that is affecting parts or systems of the body other than the blood platelets or their precursors. To be reasonably certain about the pathophysiology of thrombocytopenia, however, it is sometimes necessary to perform an aspiration of the bone marrow and to evaluate the numbers of megakaryocytes and the appearance of the other blood-cell precursors. Patients who have thrombocytopenia because of diseases involving the bone marrow, except in cases of megaloblastic anemia, have reduced numbers of megakaryocytes; if the underlying disease process is severe, it is likely that abnormalities of production of, or qualitative changes in, other cell lines also will be noted. On the other hand, if the patient is thrombocytopenic because of increased destruction of platelets, the numbers of megakaryocytes will be increased and the marrow will otherwise appear normal (although increased erythroid activity might be seen in those patients who are bleeding). If it is decided that a bone marrow aspirate is indicated because of thrombocytopenia with a hemorrhagic diathesis or because of a suspicion of a generalized underlying disease affecting the bone marrow, referral to a consultant in hematology is warranted. Depending on the nature of the underlying disease, it would then be appropriate for the hematologist to initiate and maintain therapy, or to refer the patient back to the primary physician. Recently it has been proposed (1,11) that bone marrow aspirate need not be done routinely in patients with isolated thrombocytopenia (thought to be immune mediated) except for patients who are over 60 (myelodysplastic syndromes are more common in this group) or unless splenectomy is being considered (see below).

Decreased Production of Platelets

Decreased production of platelets is a common mechanism for thrombocytopenia in ambulatory patients (Table 51.2). Apparent suppression of thrombopoiesis is often associated with viral infections such as benign upper respiratory infections, infectious mononucleosis, and childhood exanthems. In most cases, bone marrow aspirates show megakaryocytes in normal or reduced numbers, although they sometimes

Table 51.2. Thrombocytopenia Caused by Decreased Production of Platelets

Generalized Disorders of Hematopoiesis
Aplastic anemia[a]
Invasive procedures: leukemia, metastatic carcinoma, disseminated infection (e.g., tuberculosis)[a]
Folate or vitamin B_{12} deficiency
Drugs: cytotoxic agents, choloramphenicol, alcohol[b]

Specific Disorders of Thrombopoiesis
Certain infections (usually viral)[b]
Certain drugs (in most cases, cause and effect have not been demonstrated)[b]

[a]Not discussed in the text of this chapter.
[b]Processes most likely to be seen in ambulatory practice.

appear morphologically abnormal. At other times, increased numbers of megakaryocytes are seen, suggestive of a destructive process (perhaps immunologic) to which the marrow has responded with increased production of platelets. In general, patients with benign *viral infections* are not likely to have severe thrombocytopenia and so are not at major risk of bleeding. The process ordinarily dissipates as the infection resolves.

Certain drugs predictably produce thrombocytopenia by affecting thrombopoiesis. Among these, cytotoxic agents are unlikely to be administered by the general internist. Although thiazide diuretics have been reported to produce mild to moderate thrombocytopenia commonly, a clear-cut cause-and-effect relationship has not been demonstrated unequivocally. In the reported studies platelet counts have fallen several weeks after the beginning of therapy, sometimes associated with morphologically abnormal megakaryocytes. Rarely, however, thiazides have been clearly implicated in immunologically induced destructive thrombocytopenia (see "Increased Destruction of Platelets"). Thiazide diuretics also are a common cause of allergic purpura (see above), but patients with this condition have normal platelet counts.

A large number of drugs have been implicated, on occasion, in the production of thrombocytopenia by the suppression of thrombopoiesis. Therefore, if patients are symptomatic from thrombocytopenia or have counts below 50,000/mm^3 and the cause of thrombocytopenia is unknown, it would be reasonable to discontinue administration of all drugs that are not considered absolutely essential.

Management

Clearly, if the cause of the decreased platelet production can be removed (e.g., discontinuing administration of an offending drug), that should be done. If there is no evidence of mucous membrane or internal bleeding, treatment of the thrombocytopenia itself usually is unnecessary. Bleeding patients should be hospitalized for platelet transfusions. Also, some patients with chronic diseases of the bone marrow, such as myelodysplasia or aplastic anemia, may require periodic platelet transfusions. Such patients should be followed by a hematologist or an oncologist as well as by a primary physician.

Increased Destruction of Platelets

Destruction of platelets as a cause of thrombocytopenia is infrequently seen in ambulatory practice but, when seen, is most likely to have an immunologic basis (Table 51.3). *Autoimmune thrombocytopenia* (1,9,11), the most common antibody-induced disorder associated with a low platelet count, is a diagnosis made in a practitioner's office by exclusion. Such patients characteristically present with petechial bleeding. Physical examination reveals no other evidence of disease; in particular, the spleen usually is not palpable. Bone marrow aspirates appear normal except for increased numbers of megakaryocytes. An acute disease, often preceded by benign viral infection, is seen more commonly in children and, by definition, lasts less than 6 months. The chronic illness (often still called ITP, idiopathic thrombocytopenic purpura) lasts longer than 6 months and is seen more often in women than men (ratio of 3 or 4 to 1). It sometimes is associated with an underlying lymphoproliferative disorder, a collagen vascular disease, especially systemic lupus erythematosus, and more rarely, autoimmune hemolytic anemia. There is an increased incidence of immune thrombocytopenia in association with human immunodeficiency virus (HIV) infection (17,22) (see Chapter 34). Autoimmune thrombocytopenia has been shown to be caused by an antibody adsorbed to the surface of circulating platelets that results in their premature destruction by the reticuloendothelial system. It has been demonstrated that the disorder is characterized by ineffective production of platelets as well (12).

Many drugs (16) have been associated with thrombocytopenia on an immunologic basis. Heparin is the drug most commonly implicated (see Chapter 52). Many other drugs (e.g., quinine, quinidine, and digoxin) have been implicated rarely. If a patient presents to the practitioner with severe thrombocytopenia caused by increased destruction of circulating platelets, it is important to ask what drugs the patient is

Table 51.3. Thrombocytopenia Caused by Increased Destruction of Platelets

Immunologic
Autoimmune[a]
  Primary
  Secondary to an underlying disease (e.g., systemic lupus, lymphoma, viral infections such as EB or HIV infection)
Isoimmune
  Neonatal
  Posttransfusion[b]
Drug induced
  Quinidine
  Quinine
  Gold
  Heroin

Nonimmunologic
Infections[b]
Drug induced: alcohol[a]
Mechanical injury[b]

[a]Processes most likely to be seen in ambulatory practice.
[b]Not discussed in the test.

taking and to consider stopping them if there is any question that the drugs are involved in the process. Occasionally, patients with rheumatoid arthritis treated with gold salts develop thrombocytopenia that has an immunologic basis; in fact, this process appears to be much more common than the generalized suppression of hematopoiesis occasionally associated with the administration of gold. In addition, several cases have been reported in which heroin addicts have thrombocytopenia of an immune type, apparently produced by heroin (or an adulterant used with it).

It is not unusual for *alcoholics* to develop thrombocytopenia, usually to a moderate degree, after a binge. Alcohol appears to damage platelet membranes, causing their premature destruction, and to inhibit compensatory increase in platelet production by marrow megakaryocytes. Once the binge is over, the platelet count returns to normal (or transiently higher than normal) in 4 to 5 days. Alcoholics of long standing who have developed cirrhosis of the liver and portal hypertension may have chronic thrombocytopenia because of increased sequestration of platelets in their spleens.

Management

An American Society of Hematology Practice Guidelines Panel has recently made recommendations about the treatment of isolated immune thrombocytopenia (1,11). The panel found that there was no experimental evidence on which recommendations could be based, so they resorted to achieving a consensus among experts. The recommendations that follow are not precisely those of the panel but are consistent with its views: If the platelet count is less than 20,000/mm^3, treatment should be instituted immediately with the equivalent of 60 to 100 mg (1 mg/kg of body weight) of prednisone, even if the patient is asymptomatic or has only a few petechiae. Patients with mucous membrane or internal bleeding should be hospitalized; patients with severe internal bleeding should receive intravenous γ-globulin in the hospital as well; such bleeding will not occur (caused by thrombocytopenia) if the platelet count is 50,000/mm^3 or greater. In general, the risk of major bleeding appears greater in elderly patients (5,16).

Most patients with platelet counts of 20,000 to 30,000/mm^3 or less because of chronic immune thrombocytopenia ultimately require splenectomy.

Treatment of immune thrombocytopenia in patients with HIV infection is the same as it is for patients who do not have HIV infection (28).

Although approximately 70% of patients respond within days to corticosteroids with a rise in platelet count sufficient to maintain adequate hemostasis, most relapse as the dosage is tapered. (A reasonable schedule is to reduce the dosage by 10 mg/day each week to half the initial dosage and then by 5 mg/day each week). If patients do not respond to corticosteroids initially, if mucous membrane or internal bleeding recurs, or if the platelet count falls below 30,000/mm^3 as the dosage of corticosteroids is tapered, splenectomy is indicated. Adequate platelet counts (greater than 50,000/

mm^3) are maintained in approximately 80% of splenectomized patients.

Decisions about treatment for patients with refractory thrombocytopenia (persistent after splenectomy) should be made, if possible, with the help of a hematologist.

Increased Sequestration of Platelets

Patients with large spleens often have thrombocytopenia because of redistribution of platelets within a larger splenic pool, most commonly because of congestive splenomegaly associated with portal hypertension. Splenectomy reverses thrombocytopenia but should be considered only if there is a clear-cut hemorrhagic diathesis and if the underlying disease responsible for the enlarged spleen permits an operation to be performed.

Increased Use of Platelets

Patients with disseminated intravascular coagulation (7) characteristically have thrombocytopenia, almost always in association with multiple defects in coagulation. Such patients often present acutely ill because of the underlying disease that has incited the hemostatic disorder. For example, in patients with various complications of pregnancy, with disseminated carcinoma, or in some patients with septicemia, hemostatic mechanisms have been activated because of exposure of the circulating blood to thromboplastic material. The hemorrhagic diathesis is manifest most commonly by widespread bruising, petechiae, and mucous membrane bleeding, occasionally, but not often, associated clinically with evidence of venous or arterial thrombosis. In addition to thrombocytopenia, patients have disordered coagulation, which can be identified by measuring the prothrombin time, the partial thromboplastin time, and the concentration of fibrinogen in the plasma, and by the demonstration of increased titers of fibrinogen and fibrin degradation products in the plasma or serum. These products are formed by the lysis of fibrinogen and fibrin by plasmin, the major proteolytic enzyme of the blood. Patients who are strongly suspected of having disseminated intravascular coagulation or in whom the diagnosis has been made should be hospitalized for further treatment and to identify and treat the underlying disease.

Qualitative Disorders of Platelets

A number of inherited abnormalities of platelets have been identified that result in impaired hemostasis even though platelet counts are often within normal limits (2). In general the hemorrhagic diathesis associated with these conditions is milder than it is in patients with severe thrombocytopenia. Practitioners are unlikely to see these patients, but if patients have unexplained bleeding, such as purpura, epistaxis, or menorrhagia, with apparently normal coagulation and normal or slightly reduced platelet counts, it is reasonable to perform a bleeding time (see below), which is often abnormal in patients with qualitatively abnormal platelets. Similar abnormalities may be acquired in patients with various disease states (10), most commonly uremia; in fact, patients with chronic renal failure who have a tendency to bleed often improve after hemodialysis. Perhaps the most common acquired qualitative disorder of blood platelets occurs after the ingestion of aspirin, which often prolongs the bleeding time and irreversibly interferes with platelet aggregation and the release of certain intracellular platelet constituents. Although untoward bleeding is unusual in patients who have taken aspirin, the drug may intensify a preexisting tendency to bleed. Other nonsteroidal anti-inflammatory drugs (NSAIDs) also may impair platelet function but, compared to aspirin, the effect is even less predictable and is more quickly reversible when the drug is stopped.

Patient Experience. The bleeding time should be performed using a commercially available, spring-loaded, disposable device (Simplate) that makes a small incision in the forearm. The examiner should puncture the skin with the disposable lancet. A blood pressure cuff should be inflated to 40 mm Hg above the elbow during the test. The time between the instant the puncture is made and the point at which blood from the wound can no longer be adsorbed onto a piece of filter paper is the bleeding time (normally 2 to 9 minutes). The patient should be warned of the very transient sharp pain that will be experienced when the wound is made and of the small scar, usually inapparent, that may form when the wound heals.

Thrombocytosis

Platelet counts above 400,000, unless associated with a myeloproliferative disorder such as polycythemia vera, myeloid metaplasia, or chronic granulocytic leukemia, are not in themselves associated with an increased risk of morbidity from excessive bleeding or clotting. However, they may signify the presence of an underlying disease that requires attention. If on a routine evaluation, a large number of platelets are on the patient's peripheral blood smear, a platelet count should be obtained. If thrombocytosis exists, the most common causes are *inflammatory disease* and *solid tumor malignancies*. However, because a large number of conditions have at least on occasion been associated with an elevated platelet count, there is no reason to perform more than the usual comprehensive history and physical examination and any laboratory tests suggested by these examinations in an attempt to explain the thrombocytosis.

Patients with myeloproliferative disorders, if they have thrombocytosis, usually have large distorted platelets on smear and other hematologic abnormalities typical of the particular disease. Many of those patients also have splenomegaly. The treatment of thrombocytosis associated with myeloproliferative disease should be planned in consultation with a hematologist.

COAGULATION DISORDERS

The generation of a solid fibrin clot from circulating soluble fibrinogen is the body's major defense against the loss of blood from the vasculature, especially from blood vessels larger than the capillary, arteriole, and venule. Coagulation (8) is initiated by the exposure of proteins to thromboplastic substances (tissue factor) when blood vessels are injured. Thereafter, a series of enzymatic reactions occurs that results in the conversion of fibrinogen by the proteolytic enzyme thrombin to fibrin. The best screening tests to detect abnormalities of clotting are the partial thromboplastin time (PTT) and the prothrombin time (PT). Both of these tests are reliably performed by hematology laboratories. The PTT and the PT measure different phases of the early parts of the coagulation process (8), but both measure the later phase of the process—the conversion of prothrombin to thrombin and the subsequent conversion of fibrinogen to fibrin. The clotting time is an insensitive test and should not be relied on as a screening procedure to detect abnormalities in this system.

There are enzymatic mechanisms that oppose coagulation and prevent unwarranted widespread clotting of the blood when a blood vessel is injured. A number of cases have been reported of patients with an increased tendency to thrombosis and low levels of activity of one of the various protease inhibitors that normally circulate in the blood and regulate coagulation (see Chapter 52). *The fibrinolytic system* generates the proteolytic enzyme plasmin, which adsorbs to the clots and results in their ultimate dissolution. Bleeding as the result of increased endogenous fibrinolytic activity is essentially unheard of. Fibrinolytic therapy is commonly used in the treatment of various thrombotic diseases (e.g., acute myocardial infarction) but such therapy requires hospitalization.

Patients who have a deficiency of one or more of the coagulation proteins are more likely to have extensive soft tissue bleeding or major hemorrhage in response to trauma than are patients with disorders of the vasculature or of blood platelets (petechiae, discussed earlier in this chapter, are never a sign of abnormal coagulation). Hereditary disorders of coagulation are rare. They are ordinarily readily diagnosed because of the history of lifelong bleeding and, in the case of hemophilia, because of a history of characteristic hemorrhage into joints and soft tissues. Patients who have a severe hemorrhagic diathesis because of a hereditary abnormality of clotting almost always have markedly low levels of the deficient coagulation protein. Therefore, screening tests such as the partial thromboplastin time are almost always abnormal and provide clues to the presence of the disorder. It is unlikely that the practitioner will encounter such patients because most of them are diagnosed in childhood and are treated by hematologists thereafter. However, if such a patient is encountered who is suspected of having a hereditary disorder of coagulation but who has not previously been diag-

Table 51.4. Advice to Give Patients with a Disorder of Hemostasis

Take only medicine prescribed by your physician. Do not take aspirin or cold remedies. You may take Tylenol instead of aspirin for pain, colds, etc.

Do not drink any alcoholic beverage.

Avoid any activity that might expose you unnecessarily to trauma (e.g., contact sports)

Wear a bracelet (prescribed by the physician) identifying you as a "bleeder" and giving the name of your disorder.

Call your physician:
    If you experience any abnormal bleeding (including excessive menstrual bleeding)
    Before you visit your dentist
    Before seeing any other physician
    If you are hospitalized for any reason without your physician's knowledge

nosed, referral to an appropriate center would be warranted.

von Willebrand's disease (27) is an inherited abnormality of hemostasis (autosomal dominant) in which there is a reduction in the concentration or structure of a protein, the von Willebrand factor (VWF), which ordinarily binds to platelets and mediates their adhesion to subendothelial collagen in the course of platelet plug formation (see above). Normally VWF forms a complex with antihemophilic globulin (factor VIII:C), the protein that is deficient in the blood of patients with classic hemophilia, so that patients with von Willebrand's disease often have reduced levels of factor VIII. The qualitative disorder of platelets is reflected in a prolonged bleeding time and decreased platelet adhesiveness. The platelets of these patients characteristically do not aggregate in vitro, as normal platelets do, when exposed to the obsolete antibiotic ristocetin. The course of the disease as well as the extent of the laboratory abnormalities vary from one patient to another, but in general the hemorrhagic diathesis is milder than it is in hemophilia A. Patients bleed most commonly from their gastrointestinal tract; it is not unusual that symptoms of the disease are not apparent until the patient is an adult. The bleeding time and partial thromboplastin time are useful screening tests, but any patient suspected of having the disorder should have plasma factor VIII assayed as well. The diagnosis and treatment of patients with von Willebrand's disease require the ongoing participation of a hematologist.

Acquired disorders of coagulation are more common than are congenital ones. By their nature they are more likely to be associated with multiple defects in hemostasis, such as those seen in patients with disseminated intravascular coagulation (discussed earlier in this chapter) or in patients taking anticoagulant drugs (see Chapter 52). The diagnosis and management of these problems are discussed in those sections.

ADVICE TO PATIENTS WHO HAVE A DISORDER OF HEMOSTASIS

Table 51.4 lists some rules to give patients who have hemostatic dysfunction (see Chapter 52, Table 52.2). It is also important that the patient know the name of his or her disease and its clinical manifestations.

General References*

Colman RW, Hirsh J, Marder VJ, Salzman EW, eds. Hemostasis and thrombosis: basic principles and clinical practice. 3rd ed. Philadelphia: JB Lippincott, 1994.
    An authoritative, exhaustively referenced text.

Jennette JC, Falk RJ. Small-vessel vasculitis. N Engl J Med 337:1512, 1997.

Ratnoff OD, Forbes CD, eds. Disorders of hemostasis. New York: Grune & Stratton, *1996*.
    A well-edited review.

Specific References

1. The American Society of Hematology ITP Practice Guideline Panel. Diagnosis and treatment of idiopathic thrombocytopenic purpura: recommendations of the American Society of Hematology. Ann Intern Med 126:319, 1997.
2. Bellucci S, Tobelem G, Caen JP. Inherited platelet disorders. In: Brown EB, ed. Progress in hematology. New York: Grune & Stratton, 1983;13:223.
3. Bick RL. Vascular disorders associated with thrombohemorrhagic phenomena. Semin Thromb Hemost 5(3):167, 1979.
4. Collier BS, Schneiderman P. Clinical evaluation of hemorrhagic disorders: the bleeding history and differential diagnosis of purpura. In: Hoffman R, Benz EJ Jr, Shattil SJ, et al, eds. Hematology. Basic principles and practice. New York: Churchill Livingstone, 1991;1252.
5. Cortelazzo S, Finazzi M, Molteni A, et al. High risk of severe bleeding in aged patients with chronic idiopathic thrombocytopenic purpura. Blood 77:31, 1991.
6. Cream JJ, Gumpel JM, Peachey RDG. Schönlein–Henoch purpura in the adult. A study of 77 adults with anaphylactoid or Schönlein–Henoch purpura. Q J Med 39:461, 1970.
7. Deykin D. The clinical challenge of disseminated intravascular coagulation. N Engl J Med 283:686, 1970.
8. Furie B, Furie BC. Molecular and cellular biology of blood coagulation. N Engl J Med 326:800, 1992.
9. George JN, El-Harake MA, Raskob GE. Chronic idiopathic thrombocytopenic purpura. N Engl J Med 331:1207, 1994.
10. George JN, Shattil SJ. The clinical importance of acquired abnormalities of platelet function. N Engl J Med 324:27, 1991.
11. George JN, Woolf SH, Raskob GE, et al. Review: idiopathic thrombocytopenic purpura: a practice guideline developed by explicit methods for the American Society of Hematology. Blood 88:3, 1996.
12. Gernsheimer T, Stratton J, Ballem PJ, Slichter SJ. Mechanisms of response to treatment in autoimmune thrombocytopenic purpura. N Engl J Med 320:974, 1989.
13. Glenner GG. Amyloid deposits and amyloidosis. N Engl J Med 302:1283, 1333, 1980.
14. Gorevic PD, Kassab HJ, Levo Y, et al. Mixed cryoglobulinemia: clinical aspects and long-term follow-up of 40 patients. Am J Med 69:287, 1980.
15. Grey HM, Kohler PF. Cryoimmunoglobulins. Semin Hematol 10:87, 1973.
16. Guthrie TH Jr, Brannan DP, Prisant LM. Idiopathic thrombocytopenic purpura in the older adult patient. Am J Med Sci 296:17, 1988.

---

*Bold print (general references) and bold numerals (specific references) denote published controlled clinical trials, meta-analyses, or consensus-based recommendations.

17. Hodges RE, Hood J, Canham JE, et al. Clinical manifestations of ascorbic acid deficiency in man. Am J Clin Nutr 24:432, 1971.

18. Kyle RA, Gleich GJ, Bayrid ED, Vaughn JH. Benign hypergammaglobulinemic purpura of Waldenström. Medicine 50:113, 1971.

19. Kyle RA, Greipp RR. Amyloidosis (AL): clinical and laboratory features in 229 cases. Mayo Clin Proc 58:665, 1983.

20. Martinez-Taboada VM, Blanco R, Garcia-Fuentes M, Rodriguez-Valverde V. Clinical features and outcome of 95 patients with hypersensitivity vasculitis. Am J Med 102:186, 1997.

21. Miescher PA. Drug-induced thrombocytopenia. Semin Hematol 10:311, 1973.

22. Morris L, Distenfeld A, Amorosi E, Karpatkin S. Autoimmune thrombocytopenic purpura in homosexual men. Ann Intern Med 96:714, 1982.

23. Perkins HA, MacKenzie MR, Fudenberg HH. Hemostatic defects in dysproteinemias. Blood 35:695, 1970.

24. Perry WH. Clinical spectrum of hereditary hemorrhagic telangiectases (Osler–Weber–Rendu disease). Am J Med 82:989, 1987.

25. Ratnoff OD. The psychogenic purpuras: a review of autoerythrocyte sensitization, autosensitization to DNA, hysterical and factitial bleeding, and the religious stigmata. Semin Hematol 17:192, 1980.

26. Rodgers RPC, Levin J. A critical reappraisal of the bleeding time. Semin Thromb Hemost 16:1, 1990.

27. Ruggeri ZM, Zimmerman TS. von Willebrand factor and von Willebrand disease. Blood 70:895, 1987.

28. Walsh C, Krigel R, Lennette E, Karpatkin S. Thrombocytopenia in homosexual patients. Prognosis, response to therapy, and prevalence of antibody to the retrovirus associated with acquired immunodeficiency syndrome. Ann Intern Med 103:542, 1985.

C H A P T E R   52

Thromboembolic Disease

PHILIP D. ZIEVE, MD
LARRY WATERBURY, MD

Patients with acute vascular occlusions, whether they be venous or arterial, almost always require hospitalization for initial diagnosis and treatment. The responsibility of the clinician in the office is to recognize the problem, to arrange for hospitalization in an appropriate facility, and ultimately to manage the patient after discharge from the hospital.

VENOUS THROMBOEMBOLISM

Risk Factors

Most patients who present to the physician with venous occlusion have formed clots in the veins of the lower extremities. The primary pathologic process is stasis of blood (e.g., as might be seen in people who are chronically ill, obese, or for other reasons lead sedentary lives or who have sustained trauma to their lower limbs). *Upper extremity deep vein thrombosis* in ambulatory patients is uncommon but in general is associated with similar risk factors and the same complications as is lower extremity thrombosis and warrants the same diagnostic and therapeutic considerations (59).

There is an association between the use of *oral contraceptive agents* and venous thromboembolism (an increased risk historically of 5- to 10-fold). The risk exists only during the time the contraceptive is being used but does not increase with duration of use (70). Because oral contraceptives currently contain considerably less estrogen than they once did, the risk appears to have diminished substantially. Postmenopausal hormonal replacement is not associated with a risk of thromboembolic disease.

Occasionally, an underlying *malignancy,* not always apparent, is associated with venous (or arterial) thromboembolic disease (23,58,62). Also occasionally, an *inherited deficiency of a naturally occurring anticoagulant* (e.g., *protein C,* an inhibitor of activated coagulation factors V and VIII [9]; *protein S,* a cofactor in reactions that involve protein C [9,17]; or *anti-*

thrombin III, an inhibitor of thrombin as well as of several other activated coagulation factors [11]) is implicated in the genesis of recurrent thrombosis. *Resistance to activated protein C* is the most common inherited abnormality in patients with deep vein thrombosis (68); the resistance is due to a mutation in the factor V molecule, so-called *factor V Leiden* (65). Also, rarely, an inherited or acquired abnormality of fibrinogen (a *dysfibrinogenemia*), revealed usually by a prolonged thrombin time (see Chapter 51) or of fibrinolysis, may be associated with thromboembolic disease. Evaluation of abnormalities of coagulation that might cause hyperthrombotic states are done reliably only by specialized laboratories.

Antibodies to phospholipid or, more precisely, to protein-phospholipid complexes, may potentiate venous and arterial thromboses (51). Some of these antibodies are identified by their ability to prolong various phospholipid-dependent coagulation tests— most often the recalcified plasma clotting time and the activated partial thromboplastin time. These times are prolonged in normal plasma mixed with the plasma of affected patients. Such antibodies were first recognized in patients with systemic lupus erythematosus (SLE) and are called *lupus anticoagulants.* Other antiphospholipid antibodies are directed against cardiolipin and are detected by immunoassay. Concordance is limited between lupus anticoagulants and anticardiolipin antibodies. Antiphospholipid antibodies are present in about one-third of patients with SLE, often in patients with other diseases of connective tissue and uncommonly in the rest of the population. The incidence of thrombotic events is highest in patients with SLE (in whom it also may be associated with thrombocytopenia and spontaneous abortion). In other people, the risk is not well defined, but in one large retrospective study, the risk was five times that in a control group, when the antibody titers were high (22). Currently, it seems prudent to test for antiphospholipid antibodies in all patients with SLE who have a thrombotic event or who are contemplating pregnancy and in other patients who experience thrombotic events without associated risk factors. The antibodies characteristically persist for months, or sometimes years, and may recur. When patients with antiphospholipid antibodies develop venous or arterial thromboses, they should be anticoagulated (see below).

Hyperhomocystinemia, a risk factor for arterial thrombosis, appears to predispose patients to venous thrombosis as well; in one study, 10% of patients with deep venous thrombosis had elevated plasma levels of homocysteine (26).

Patients without apparent risk factors who experience recurrent thromboses or patients who have a positive family history who experience one thromboembolic event should be evaluated for an inherited or acquired abnormality of coagulation, preferably in consultation with a hematologist. Assays of coagulation factors or of their inhibitors should be done by an experienced laboratory at least 2 months after an acute event and after anticoagulation has been discontinued.

Phospholipid antibody titers or homocysteine levels can be measured any time.

Presentation and Evaluation

Superficial thrombophlebitis is readily recognized as inflammation of a visible tender, often palpably thrombosed, vein. There is no risk of embolism from such clots, unless the deep veins are also involved. In one study, superficial thrombophlebitis was much more likely to be associated with deep vein thrombosis (DVT) if the superficial veins were not varicose (6) (see Chapter 88). Otherwise, treatment does not require administration of anticoagulant drugs (see below) and is confined to nonsteroidal anti-inflammatory drugs, elevation of the extremity, local moist heat, and if there is concomitant infection, antibiotics. However, many believe that patients with phlebitis of the entire superficial saphenous vein to the groin should be anticoagulated. If DVT is suspected in a patient with superficial phlebitis, ultrasonography (see below) should be performed.

Signs and symptoms of pulmonary embolism (see Chapter 54) may be the sole manifestation of venous thrombosis in the deep veins of the lower extremities. More commonly, patients present with swelling, pain, and tenderness of the affected extremity, although swelling alone may be the presenting symptom. In any case, the prevention of pulmonary embolism is the primary reason why diagnosis and treatment of venous thrombosis are urgent. On the basis of history and physical examination alone, however, it is difficult to distinguish DVT from other processes. At least half of the time other diagnoses (especially musculoskeletal injury) prove to be responsible for these signs and symptoms (37). Therefore, patients suspected of having thrombosis of the deep veins or of having had pulmonary embolism without clinical evidence of peripheral thrombosis must undergo specific diagnostic studies so that appropriate therapy for venous thromboembolism may be instituted. The test of reference is contrast venography. If characteristic filling defects are seen in radiographs of the veins after injection of contrast material, the diagnosis is established. However, because of the relative difficulty, discomfort, and occasional side effects (see below) of the procedure, noninvasive tests have largely replaced venography in the diagnosis of DVT.

Patient Experience. Contrast venography is performed after injection of the contrast medium into a dorsal vein of the foot. The patient should be warned that the procedure sometimes is associated with unpleasant burning or cramping in the lower extremity while the dye is being injected (especially in patients with phlebitis). Venography itself may cause thrombosis; the incidence of superficial and deep vein thrombosis, proved by repeated venography, is approximately 2% (7,46).

One of two noninvasive tests is commonly used in the diagnosis of DVT: *impedance plethysmography* (IPG) (33,34,38) and *Doppler ultrasonography* (74). Both depend on the skill of the technician who performs the test, and the sensitivity and specificity of the tests should be established by every vascular laboratory. Both tests are more sensitive in detecting thrombosis in deep veins of the thigh but are insensitive in detecting thrombosis in deep veins of the calf. However, calf vein thrombi are unlikely to embolize unless they first propagate into the thigh (53,57). Because of limitations in the specificity of IPG (e.g., false-positive tests are common in patients with right-sided heart failure or with conditions that cause external venous compression), ultrasonography has become the preferred test. The sensitivity of IPG has been questioned as well (1). Doppler ultrasonography (74) (so-called duplex ultrasonography) combines ultrasonography with Doppler technology to provide visualization of the venous channels and a measurement of the flow of blood through them. During the performance of the test, an external probe is applied to the thigh and the failure of the vein underlying the probe to collapse is a sensitive and specific sign of thrombosis. The cost of a Doppler ultrasonogram is two to three times the cost of IPG and is approximately the cost of a venogram.

A model has been developed to establish the pretest probability of DVT and to estimate the predictive value of the noninvasive tests (73) (Table 52.1). By use of the pretest probability a sensible diagnostic therapeutic approach to patients with suspected DVT has been suggested (Table 52.2). Even though the approach cannot be considered definitive until larger scale prospective studies have been done, it does provide some direction on the basis of objective data, rather than on unsubstantiated clinical impression, as has often been

Table 52.1. A Model for Predicting Pretest Probability (PTP) for Deep Vein Thrombosis

Major Points
Active cancer (including treatment within previous 6 months)
Recent immobility for more than 3 days, whatever the cause
  (e.g., bed rest, paralysis, plaster cast)
Major surgery within 4 weeks
Tenderness along the distribution of the deep venous system
Measurable swelling of the thigh and calf
Calf swelling alone >3 cm on symptomless side (measured 10 cm
  below tibial tuberosity)
At least 2 first-degree relatives with a history of DVT

Minor Points
Recent trauma (within 60 days) to the symptomatic leg
Pitting edema (symptomatic leg only)
Dilated superficial veins (nonvaricose, in symptomatic leg only)
Hospitalization within 6 months
Erythema of symptomatic leg

Probability of DVT
High
  ≥3 major points and no alternative diagnosis
  ≥2 major points, ≥2 minor points and no alternative diagnosis
Low
  1 major point, ≥2 minor points and an alternative diagnosis
  1 major point, ≥1 minor point and no alternative diagnosis
  0 major points, ≥3 minor points and an alternative diagnosis
  0 major points, ≥2 minor points and no alternative diagnosis
Moderate
  All other combinations

Modified from Wells PS, Hirsh J, Anderson DR, et al. Accuracy of clinical assessment of deep-vein thrombosis. Lancet 345:1326, 1995.

Table 52.2. Predictive Value of Ultrasonography (US)

	Normal	Abnormal
Low PTP	DVT ruled out	Venography (treat for DVT if abnormal)
Moderate PTP	Repeat US in 1 week (treat for DVT if abnormal)	Treat for DVT
High PTP	Venography (treat for DVT if abnormal)	Treat for DVT

Modified from Wells PS, Hirsh J, Anderson DR, et al. Accuracy of clinical assessment of deep-vein thrombosis. Lancet 345:1326, 1995.
PTP, Pretest probability (see Table 52.1).

the case. On the basis of the model, patients with low pretest probability and normal ultrasonography (nearly half the study group) can be considered not to have a DVT.

Patients with *calf vein thrombosis* alone need not be given anticoagulant drugs (see below); they can be treated in the same way as are patients with superficial thrombophlebitis. If ultrasonography (or IPG) is unavailable, however, patients with venographically demonstrable calf vein thrombosis should be anticoagulated because there is no easy way, on follow-up, to detect propagation of the clot (40).

Once a definite diagnosis of DVT is made, the patient must be hospitalized for treatment (the probable approval of low-molecular-weight heparin for the treatment of DVT will modify this dictum—see below).

Patient Experience. IPG is performed by inflating a pneumatic cuff at the midthigh to occlude venous return and then rapidly deflating it. The changes in blood volume are measured by changes in electrical resistance detected by a pair of electrodes attached to the cuff. No discomfort is associated with this procedure, other than the mild transient sensation of increased pressure during the few seconds of inflation.

Doppler ultrasonography takes about 10 minutes to perform and is painless; the patient lies quietly while transducers are placed on the thigh; during the test, a probe is applied with gentle pressure over the vein being evaluated.

If patients have signs and symptoms of *pulmonary embolism* (see Chapter 54), the first diagnostic procedure should be a *ventilation/perfusion scan of their lungs.* If the scan is negative or is read as low probability and the patient has signs and symptoms of venous occlusion of the lower extremities, further diagnostic studies should be done (see above) to establish that diagnosis. If the lung scan is interpreted as indeterminate or high probability, the patient should be hospitalized—in the first instance for pulmonary angiography and in the second for treatment. In many instances, however, the clinician will elect to admit the patient to the hospital on the basis of the clinical presentation and then obtain all necessary diagnostic procedures.

Treatment

The most important therapy for patients with DVT in the lower extremities is anticoagulation, instituted to prevent extension of the clot. The larger the clot, the more likely it is to break off and become an embolus. Anticoagulation is usually instituted in the hospital with heparin, which is administered for 5 to 10 days, the approximate time for clots to become adherent to the vessel wall. Heparin is used because its onset of action is immediate, compared with coumarin compounds, the other major class of anticoagulant drugs.

Warfarin

Warfarin is the coumarin commonly used in the anticoagulation of ambulatory patients. Coumadin is the brand name product that is commonly prescribed; other products, including generic products, are reliable but are not interchangeable because of variation in bioavailability. Ordinarily, patients who have been hospitalized for diagnosis and initial treatment of venous thromboembolic disease are given warfarin while heparin is being administered so that by the time that drug is discontinued, the full effect of the coumarin has become established. Coumarins interfere with the synthesis of vitamin K–dependent clotting factors (factors II, VII, IX, and X) by the liver. Their effect is not fully realized until they have been given for approximately 5 days. The administration of warfarin usually is initiated in dosages of 10 mg/day (1-, 2-, 2.5-, 4-, 5-, 7.5-, and 10-mg tablets are available) and then adjusted, depending on the therapeutic response, which is monitored by use of the prothrombin time, a reproducible, dependable test performed reliably by most clinical laboratories.

There is an internationally accepted uniform system for reporting the prothrombin time (42). The system dictates that all results be related to those obtained by use of a standardized thromboplastin, the critical reagent used in the performance of the test. The relationship is expressed as an *International Normalized Ratio (INR)*, and laboratories doing prothrombin times should report their results in terms of the INR. (The INR is the ratio of the patient's prothrombin time to the normal standard prothrombin time of the testing laboratory, raised by an exponent, the International Sensitivity Index [ISI], supplied by the manufacturer of the thromboplastin.) Because there is still some question about the reliability of the ISI provided by a given manufacturer, however, it is best, if possible, to have sequential prothrombin times done by the same laboratory or, if a different laboratory is to be used, to have prothrombin times done on the same plasma by both laboratories to establish the appropriate standards of comparison.

In most circumstances, the goal of anticoagulant therapy with warfarin is to maintain the INR between 2.0 and 3.0 because it is within this range that a reasonable therapeutic effect is achieved and the risk of untoward bleeding is small. The ratio of the patient's prothrombin time to that of the control will vary, depending on the ISI of the thromboplastin that is used. These recommendations result in significantly lower prothrombin times than have been thought appropriate in the past. During the first several weeks of administration of warfarin, the prothrombin time should be measured at least every few days until it is determined

that the proper dosage schedule has been achieved. Thereafter it is appropriate to measure the anticoagulant response monthly. At the same time it is prudent to examine the patient's urine and stool for occult blood and to assess the hematocrit value or hemoglobin concentration.

During the course of anticoagulation with coumarin compounds, patients should be instructed to avoid predictable trauma such as might be expected from playing contact sports or from working in an environment associated with a high risk of injury. Intramuscular injections should not be given to the anticoagulated patient; subcutaneous injections, done properly, are safe. Venipunctures are also safe, but the wound should be compressed for 10 to 15 minutes after the needle is withdrawn. Arterial punctures are contraindicated as outpatient procedures, for which prolonged compression and observation of the puncture site are impractical.

Factors Affecting Response. Ordinarily, patients taking a given dose of warfarin maintain a consistent hypoprothrombinemic response, once a steady state is reached. However, a number of factors might alter the patient's responsiveness to warfarin after a period of stability (Table 52.3). Sometimes, the amount of vitamin K ingested in the patient's diet might be altered drastically, increasing the potency of warfarin if less vitamin K is ingested and decreasing it if considerably more is ingested. Significantly decreased ingestion of vitamin K is almost always associated with a markedly decreased intake of food (e.g., in patients who are anorexic because of illness or who have instituted severe dietary restrictions in an attempt to lose weight). The effect of reduction in intake of vitamin K is most pronounced in those patients who are concomitantly receiving antibiotics, which inhibit the synthesis of vitamin K by normal flora of the intestinal tract. Because the vitamin K–dependent clotting factors are synthesized in the liver and because coumarins are metabolized by the liver, patients who develop inter-

Table 52.3. Some Factors that May Affect a Patient's Response to Warfarin

Enhanced Response	Reduced Response
Vitamin K deficiency	Barbiturates
Liver disease	Carbamazepine (Tegretol)
Drugs	Chlordiazepoxide (Librium)
Anabolic steroids	Cholestyramine
Amiodarone	Griseofulvin
Cimetidine[a]	Nafcillin
Clofibrate	Rifampin
Cotrimoxazole (e.g., Bactrim)	Sucralfate
Erythromycin	Spironolactone
Isoniazid	Foods[b]
Metronidazole (Flagyl)	Avocado
Miconazole	Fish
Phenylbutazone	Broccoli
Piroxicam (Feldene)	Spinach
Propranolol	Cabbage
Sulfinpyrazone	Kale
	Cauliflower

[a]The effect of other H_2 blockers is uncertain.
[b]Rich in vitamin K.

current hepatic illness (e.g., hepatitis) should be watched carefully for enhanced effective anticoagulation. In such a circumstance, it would be wise to measure prothrombin times more frequently but it would not be necessary to discontinue warfarin unless bleeding ensued or the prothrombin time became significantly prolonged over the baseline therapeutic control.

One of the major problems in dealing with a patient taking coumarin anticoagulants is the possibility of *drug interaction.* A number of pharmacologic agents potentiate the anticoagulant effect of coumarins, and a few inhibit it. (See Table 52.3, which lists the drugs for which good supporting evidence is available; other possible interactions for which the evidence is less strong are listed on p. 233S in Reference 30.) One should be cautious, however, when initiating any new forms of therapy or discontinuing old ones in a patient who is receiving coumarin anticoagulants. Prothrombin times should be checked more frequently for several weeks to ensure that the pharmacologic response to coumarin has not been altered. In general, the likelihood of a potentiated response is much higher than that of an inhibitory one, so there is greater risk of an increased susceptibility to bleeding than of an inhibition of anticoagulation. One should also be careful about the use of drugs such as aspirin that have an effect on hemostasis that might be enhanced by warfarin or that may produce bleeding by injuring the gastric mucosa. Other nonsteroidal anti-inflammatory drugs (see Chapter 70) also have at least a potential for compromising hemostasis (few data are available) and should be used cautiously.

Complications. By far the major complication experienced by patients taking coumarin anticoagulants is hemorrhage (44,50). In general the risk of hemorrhage is increased by the intensity of treatment and by the presence of comorbid conditions (e.g., hepatic or renal disease) (18,44). The risk appears greatest within the first month of initiation of treatment. Elderly patients, who are likely to be sicker, to have a greater propensity to fall, to have lesions that are prone to bleed, and to be taking multiple medications, are probably at greater risk. Minor episodes (e.g., small bruises and bleeding gums after brushing of the teeth) are relatively common but ordinarily do not require a change in the dose schedule of the anticoagulant. Occult rectal bleeding, minor bleeding from hemorrhoids, microscopic hematuria, and menorrhagia are encountered in less than 10% of patients. When bleeding of this kind is observed, every attempt must be made to establish the site of bleeding by the use of appropriate diagnostic studies (41). If prothrombin times have been maintained within the therapeutic range, the rapidity and extent of bleeding will dictate whether the anticoagulant drug should be discontinued, at least temporarily. Major genitourinary or gastrointestinal bleeding sufficient to lower the hematocrit value or hemoglobin concentration, or bleeding of any degree in the central nervous system, dictates prompt discontinuation of the anticoagulant and immediate hospitalization for further diagnosis and treatment. It is prudent to administer 25 mg of vitamin K 1 (AquaMEPHYTON) intravenously at a rate no greater than 5 mg/minute while arranging for hospitalization. (The prothrombin time will begin to shorten in 4 to 6 hours and, in most patients, will be in a safe range in 12 to 24 hours.) Bleeding is often associated with an independent organic process (e.g., a peptic ulcer, a carcinoma of the colon or a genitourinary abnormality); bleeding of this kind is likely to occur even when the prothrombin time is in the therapeutic range (12,40).

There is a major risk in the use of coumarin compounds in *pregnant patients* (24,48). Major hemorrhagic complications occur in the fetus as well as teratogenic effects unrelated to the anticoagulant action. Therefore it is recommended that pregnancy be avoided in women who are being treated with coumarin drugs because a normal infant can be expected only about two-thirds of the time. The risk of heparin in pregnancy is less clear cut; an increased incidence of fetal wastage has been reported (24) but also has been disputed; in any case, if anticoagulation is necessary, heparin is clearly safer than coumarins (see below) (21,48).

Advice for management of patients who are taking a coumarin compound and who are to undergo a surgical procedure is provided in Chapter 86.

Rarely, patients given a coumarin anticoagulant will develop *hemorrhagic infarcts* in their skin (often in women's breasts) within 10 days, with eventual sloughing of necrotic tissue. This complication is much more likely in people with protein C or protein S deficiency (see above). Under such circumstances, the drug ordinarily is stopped immediately (although it is unclear whether it is necessary to do so).

Table 52.4 provides useful information for patients at the onset of anticoagulation or at the time that the patient is discharged from the hospital. Selection of pa-

Table 52.4. Advice to Be Given to Patients Taking a Coumarin Anticoagulant

Take only medicines prescribed by your doctor. Do not take mineral oil, laxatives, aspirin (or any product such as a cold remedy that contains aspirin), or any other proprietary anti-inflammatory agents or any multivitamin preparation that contains vitamin K. You may take acetaminophen (e.g., Tylenol) instead of aspirin for pain.

Take your coumarin at the same time each day.

Avoid wide variation in the kinds and amounts of food you eat, especially fish, broccoli, spinach, cabbage, kale, or cauliflower.

Do not drink more than 1 or 2 glasses of beer or wine or the equivalent of more than 1 ounce (1 "shot") of whiskey/day.

Avoid any activity that might expose you unnecessarily to trauma—for example, contact sports.

Call your doctor immediately:

If you experience any abnormal bleeding.

Before you visit the dentist.

Before seeing any other physician.

If you cannot keep your scheduled appointment.

Before leaving on a trip.

If you are hospitalized, for any reason, without your doctor knowing about it.

tients who can follow these rules will diminish considerably the incidence of hemorrhagic complications in patients taking anticoagulant drugs (see also Chapter 51, Table 51.5).

Heparin

Because heparin must be administered parenterally, it is not commonly prescribed to outpatients. If, however, because of unacceptable side effects unrelated to its anticoagulant activity, a coumarin could not be used, subcutaneous heparin has sometimes been required after hospitalization. It has typically been administered every 12 hours in doses designed to maintain the partial thromboplastin time (PTT, like the prothrombin time, a reliable, easily obtained test) at 1.5 to 2 times control (35). Once a dosage regimen is established by this technique (usually in the range of 15,000 to 17,500 units twice a day), it probably is unnecessary to measure the PTT again unless the patient develops bleeding or recurrent thrombosis. It has been demonstrated that prevention of recurrent thromboembolism is comparable to that achieved by the use of warfarin (35). So-called low-dose heparin (5,000 units twice a day) is inadequate treatment for patients with established thrombosis (36).

Low-Molecular-Weight Heparin and Heparinoids. In recent years, a number of *low-molecular-weight heparins* that appear to have significant advantages over conventional standard (unfractionated) heparin have been developed. The new preparations have greater bioavailability, a more predictable dose response, and a longer half-life than the standard product (32). These differences permit the administration of a fixed dose of heparin subcutaneously once or twice a day and eliminate the need to monitor the patient's PTT. A number of clinical trials (39,43,49) and meta-analyses (47,66) have concluded that the efficacy and safety of low-molecular-weight heparin are at least as good as that of standard heparin. Currently, three low-molecular-weight heparins are licensed in the United States: enoxaparin (Lovenox), dalteparin (Fragmin), and ardeparin (Normiflo). They are approved for prophylaxis but not for treatment of DVT. In the near future it is likely that these and other low-molecular-weight heparins will be approved for treatment and that additional preparations will be licensed. At that time, it should be possible to treat uncomplicated patients (e.g., with no evidence of pulmonary embolism, no increased risk of bleeding) on an ambulatory basis (as in hospitalized patients, for 5 days, until the effect of warfarin, started on day 1 or 2, is optimal).

Danaparoid (Orgaran) has recently been approved for prophylaxis of DVT (13). It is a mixture of low-molecular-weight sulfated glycosaminoglycans from which the heparin has been removed. Its effects on coagulation are similar, but slightly different, than those of heparin. Sufficiently large trials comparing danaparoid with low-molecular-weight heparin have not yet been reported to assess relative risks and benefits precisely.

Heparin-Induced Thrombocytopenia. Unfractionated, standard heparin (see above) causes antibody-mediated thrombocytopenia in up to 3% of patients to whom it is administered (72). The risk increases with duration of therapy; the first cases are usually observed after 5 to 7 days of treatment. (A mild transient drop in platelet count early in the course of therapy is more common and is of no significance.) Many of these thrombocytopenic patients develop concomitant venous or arterial thrombosis (71). Therefore, platelet counts, hematocrit values, and fecal occult blood should be measured every 2 to 3 days in patients administered heparin. Platelet counts under 40,000 to 50,000/mm^3, thrombocytopenic bleeding, or thrombosis associated with a platelet count that has fallen below 150,000/mm^3 dictate that the heparin be discontinued and that an alternative form of therapy for thromboembolic disease be sought. Heparinized ambulatory patients who exhibit untoward bleeding or clotting should be hospitalized, and a platelet count should be done as part of their evaluation.

The risk of thrombocytopenia appears to be much less with the use of low-molecular-weight heparin or heparinoids (see above) than with the use of standard heparin, although few direct comparisons have been done (72). Nevertheless, low-molecular-weight heparin or a heparinoid should not be substituted for standard heparin if thrombocytopenia occurs.

The administration of warfarin early in the course of treatment with heparin (see above) has probably attenuated the risk of heparin-induced thrombocytopenia and thrombosis.

Other Complications. Prolonged use of unfractionated heparin (4 months or more) in dosages exceeding 10,000 units/day has been reported to cause *osteoporosis;* spontaneous spinal and rib fractures have been observed. The risk of this complication developing is unknown, nor is it known whether low-molecular-weight heparin ever causes osteoporosis; until more data are accumulated, treatment with heparin for longer than 3 months is at least relatively contraindicated.

Both standard heparin (especially the bovine preparation) and low-molecular-weight heparin also commonly cause *reversible elevation* of *aminotransferase activity,* without other evidence of hepatic dysfunction (15). No pathologic correlation with this reaction has been identified, so if it occurs, heparin may continue to be administered.

Finally, both standard and low-molecular-weight heparin predictably suppress aldosterone production and induce hyperkalemia in 7 to 8% of treated patients (54). The risk is especially great in patients prone to hyperkalemia for other reasons (e.g., diabetic mellitus, chronic renal disease); in such patients, potassium levels should be measured every 3 to 4 days (54).

Aspirin

A meta-analysis has concluded that aspirin is of some use in reducing the incidence of DVT and, especially, pulmonary emboli in immobilized patients (2,5). There is no justification for prescribing aspirin as a treatment of venous thrombosis.

Course

It has been standard practice for many years to continue anticoagulation for at least 3 months in patients with DVT (10). It is likely that patients who have developed DVT in response to a transient risk (e.g., surgery, trauma) may not need anticoagulation for longer than 4 to 6 weeks (14,55). However, a randomized prospective study suggests that patients without apparent risks should be treated for 6 months after a first episode of venous thromboembolism (64). Patients with persistent risk (e.g., cancer, recurrent thromboembolic disease, or abnormalities of hemostasis that predispose them to thrombosis—see above), should be treated indefinitely (14,63).

Patients should be advised to avoid prolonged sitting or standing in one position, should be encouraged to elevate their legs for two to three periods of 30 minutes each day, and to wear elastic stockings to promote venous return. Although the effectiveness of these maneuvers has not been established, there is little or no risk associated with any of them, and they may be of some value.

When a decision is made to discontinue anticoagulation therapy, it may be terminated abruptly without fear of an increased risk of early recurrence of venous thrombosis; the so-called rebound phenomenon has never been demonstrated.

Recurrent DVT may be difficult to diagnose (45); it is not a common problem in appropriately managed patients—see above. Many patients who have had a documented acute DVT develop recurrent pain and swelling of the same extremity. Even contrast venography may be equivocal in such patients because of persistent occlusion of a vein by a previous clot. In such circumstances, Doppler ultrasonography is probably the most reliable test, if it (or IPG) has been demonstrated to have become normal after treatment of an acute thrombotic event; normalization occurs in 70% of patients by 3 months and in 90% by 9 months (33). If ultrasonography (or IPG) has not become normal and if a contrast venogram is not interpretable, or if recurrent thrombosis has been definitively diagnosed, anticoagulation for a year is probably reasonable.

Postphlebitic Syndrome

Some patients, after repeated attacks of thrombosis of the veins of the lower extremities, develop chronic changes in those veins with loss of competence of the valves and hemorrhage of small tributary veins leading to chronic edema and discoloration of the legs and ankles (8,68). Sometimes painful stasis ulcers that make it difficult for the patient to move about also develop. The treatment of this postphlebitic syndrome is the promotion of venous return from the lower extremities by the use of support stockings during the day and by elevation of the lower extremities for several hours each day. In those patients who have developed ulcers, bed rest with persistent elevation of the extremity above the level of the heart is recommended and, if necessary, administration of appropriate antibiotics. On such a regimen, the ulcers usually heal, although they may recur if the patients are not careful to continue to follow prescribed conservative therapy (see Chapter 88). Signs and symptoms of chronic venous insufficiency are often manifest in patients with no history or evidence of DVT (16).

ARTERIAL THROMBOEMBOLISM (SEE ALSO CHAPTERS 59, 83, AND 87)

Unlike clots that form in the venous circulation, arterial thrombosis is primarily initiated by platelet plug formation, begun by the adherence of ambient platelets to altered surfaces in arterial vessels. The major risk factor, by far, is *atherosclerosis;* but, rarely, underlying *malignancy,* an *antiphospholipid antibody,* or *hyperhomocystinemia* may be associated with an increased propensity to arterial thrombosis (see above). Symptoms and signs of thromboembolism appear more abruptly than those of venous occlusion and commonly are associated with necrosis of tissue that had been fed by the now obstructed vessel. Heparin and coumarin anticoagulants, both experimentally and clinically, are of little use in preventing the formation of such clots or in preventing their propagation. (There is, however, compelling evidence that warfarin anticoagulation decreases considerably the risk of arterial emboli in patients with chronic atrial fibrillation [see Chapter 59]. Warfarin is also prescribed commonly for patients with dilated cardiomyopathy [see Chapter 61].) There is a great deal of interest, therefore, in the use of drugs that interfere with platelet plug formation and that might be useful in the prophylaxis of arterial thromboembolism. Although a number of agents have been tested and others are being actively evaluated, of the currently approved drugs, only aspirin and ticlopidine (see below), have been shown to be efficacious. Dipyridamole (Persantine), a commonly prescribed drug, has never been shown clearly to be useful (19).

Aspirin

Aspirin interferes with platelet function and therefore inhibits platelet plug formation. It interferes with the formation of a potent aggregating and vasoconstricting substance, thromboxane A 2, formed in platelets by the metabolism of prostaglandins. Aspirin inhibits the rate-limiting enzyme in this reaction, cyclo-oxygenase; as a result, the aggregation of platelets by collagen or connective tissue is inhibited and the release of substances, which themselves stimulate platelet aggregation, is impaired.

Aspirin inhibits not only prostaglandin synthesis in platelets but also the formation by vascular endothelium of prostacyclin, a potent inhibitor of platelet aggregation. Although there is not precise information on the proper dosage of aspirin to be administered to achieve an optimal effect (presumably at the point where there is maximum inhibition of thromboxane A 2 synthesis and minimum inhibition of prostacyclin synthesis) (20), there is no evidence that aspirin at any dosage is thrombogenic.

Unless aspirin is administered to patients with an underlying hemostatic disorder (including the administration of an anticoagulant drug; see above), a hemorrhagic diathesis is unusual. However, aspirin does have a toxic effect on the mucosa of the gastrointestinal tract that may result in bleeding or may increase the likelihood of hemorrhage from preexistent peptic ulcerations (61).

A number of studies have been performed to assess the efficacy of aspirin for *secondary prevention* of thromboembolic events in patients with a history of cardiovascular and cerebrovascular disease. A meta-analysis (a statistical evaluation of the sum of all published interpretable trials) of 70,000 patients with a history of arterial vascular disease or of a condition that predisposes patients to vascular disease reported that allocation to antiplatelet treatment (essentially aspirin) reduced overall vascular events by approximately 25% and reduced death from vascular events by 18% (2,3). There was no significant difference between patients with cardiovascular disease and those with cerebrovascular disease, and no significant difference in effect between 75 and 325 mg/day of aspirin. A study of 333 men with stable angina, a subset of the large Physicians' Health Study, reported that 325 mg of aspirin every other day did not affect the frequency of chest pain but did reduce risk of a first myocardial infarction by 87% during the 5 years of the study (60).

It is reasonable to recommend aspirin, 75 to 100 mg/day, to patients with transient ischemic attacks (TIAs), unstable angina, stable angina, myocardial infarction, thrombotic stroke, or peripheral arterial disease (28,75). There is little risk of major hemorrhagic side effects at these dosages (325 mg/day, in fact, increases the risk only slightly) (31,61).

It has become a routine in most centers to administer aspirin (325 to 975 mg/day), usually with dipyridamole (105 mg three times a day), indefinitely to patients who have undergone coronary artery bypass surgery. A meta-analysis has supported the use of antiplatelet agents in this regard (27) and, indeed, in a wide variety of patients in whom maintenance of vascular patency is important (e.g., after angioplasty or after a procedure to establish vascular access for hemodialysis) (2,4). It is unlikely that dipyridamole is important to this regimen (see above).

There have also been three studies of aspirin in the *primary prevention* of atherosclerotic disease (given prophylactically to apparently healthy people) (52,56,67). The combined studies showed a one-third reduction in the number of nonfatal myocardial infarctions (29) but no reduction in overall mortality from vascular disease. A later expanded meta-analysis of studies of 30,000 healthy people who were at apparently low risk of atherosclerotic disease showed minimal benefit of antiplatelet therapy (again, primarily aspirin) in protecting against vascular events, including death from vascular disease (2,3). There is therefore no compelling reason to prescribe aspirin as a prophylactic agent to such people.

Ticlopidine

Ticlopidine inhibits the aggregation of platelets by adenosine diphosphate (ADP). A multicenter study showed ticlopidine to be approximately 20% more effective than aspirin in preventing death from any cause and in preventing fatal and nonfatal major strokes in a population of men and women who had recently experienced TIAs or minor strokes (25). However, the incidence of side effects, especially diarrhea, was considerably greater than with aspirin, and severe reversible neutropenia occurred in approximately 1% of patients. The value of the drug in patients with coronary artery disease is unknown. The recommended dosage is 250 mg twice a day, resulting in a cost more than 100 times that of aspirin. Therefore, ticlopidine, marketed as Ticlid, should be prescribed only for patients at risk for major stroke who cannot take aspirin. If prescribed, the manufacturer recommends the patient's white blood cell count and differential count be measured every 2 weeks for 3 months.

General References*

American College of Chest Physicians Conference on Antithrombotic Therapy. Chest 108:225S, 1995.
> A consensus on the use of antithrombotic therapy using evidence-based criteria.

Thomas DP, Roberts HR. Hypercoagulability in venous and arterial thrombosis. Ann Intern Med 126:638, 1997.
> Concise review of the subject.

Ginsberg JS. Management of venous thromboembolism. N Engl J Med 335:1816, 1996.
> Concise well-referenced review with sensible recommendations.

Specific References

1. Anderson DR, Lensing AWA, Wells PS, et al. Limitations of impedance plethysmography in the diagnosis of clinically suspected deep-vein thrombosis. Ann Intern Med 118:25, 1993.
2. Antiplatelet trialists' collaboration. Collaborative overview of randomized trials of antiplatelet therapy.
3. I. Prevention of death, myocardial infarction, and stroke by prolonged antiplatelet therapy in various categories of patients. BMJ 308:81, 1994.
4. II. Maintenance of vascular graft or arterial patency by antiplatelet therapy. BMJ 308:159, 1994.
5. III. Reduction in venous thrombosis and pulmonary embolism by antiplatelet prophylaxis among surgical and medical patients. BMJ 308:235, 1994.
6. Bergquist D, Jaroszewski H. Deep vein thrombosis in patients with superficial thrombophlebitis of the leg. BMJ 292:658, 1986.
7. Bettmann MA, Robbins A, Braun SD, et al. Contrast venography of the leg: diagnostic efficacy, tolerance, and complication rates with ionic and nonionic contrast media. Radiology 165:113, 1987.

---

*Bold print (general references) and bold numerals (specific references) denote published controlled clinical trials, meta-analyses, or consensus-based recommendations.

8. Beyth RJ, Cohen AM, Landefeld S. Long-term outcomes of deep-vein thrombosis. Arch Intern Med 155:1031, 1995.

9. Clouse LH, Comp PC. The regulation of hemostasis: the protein C system. N Engl J Med 314:1298, 1986.

10. Coon WW, Willis PW III. Recurrence of venous thromboembolism. Surgery 73:823, 1973.

11. Cosgriff TM, Bishop DT, Hershgold EJ, et al. Familial antithrombin III deficiency: its natural history, genetics, diagnosis and treatment. Medicine (Baltimore) 62:209, 1983.

12. Culclasure TF, Bray VJ, Hasbargen JA. The significance of hematuria in the anticoagulated patient. Arch Intern Med 154:649, 1994.

13. De Valk HW, Banga JD, Wester JW, et al. Comparing subcutaneous danaparoid with intravenous unfractionated heparin for the treatment of venous thromboembolism. A randomized controlled trial. Ann Intern Med 123:1, 1995.

14. Duiguid DL. Oral anticoagulant therapy for venous thromboembolism. N Engl J Med 336:433, 1997.

15. Dukes GE, Sanders SW, Russo J, et al. Transaminase elevations in patients receiving bovine or porcine heparin. Ann Intern Med 100:646, 1984.

16. Editorial. Post-thrombotic venous disorders. Lancet 1:1488, 1985.

17. Engesser L, Brockmans AW, Briet E, et al. Hereditary protein S deficiency: clinical manifestations. Ann Intern Med 106:677, 1987.

18. Fihn SD, McDonell M, Martin D, et al. Risk factors for complications of chronic anticoagulation. A multicenter study. Ann Intern Med 118:511, 1993.

19. Fitzgerald GA. Dipyridamole. N Engl J Med 316:1247, 1987.

20. Fitzgerald GA, Oates JA, Hawiger J, et al. Endogenous biosynthesis of prostacyclin and thromboxane and platelet function during chronic administration of aspirin in man. J Clin Invest 71:676, 1983.

21. Ginsberg JS, Hirsh J, Turner DC, et al. Risk to the fetus of anticoagulant therapy during pregnancy. Thromb Haemostas 61:197, 1989.

22. Ginsberg KS, Liang MH, Newcomer L, et al. Anticardiolipin antibodies and the risk for ischemic stroke and venous thrombosis. Ann Intern Med 117:997, 1992.

23. Goldberg RJ, Serreff M, Gore JM, et al. Occult malignant neoplasm in patients with deep venous thrombosis. Arch Intern Med 147:251, 1987.

24. Hall JG, Pauli RM, Wilson KM. Maternal and fetal sequelae of anticoagulation during pregnancy. Am J Med 68:122, 1980.

25. Hass WK, Easton JD, Adams HP Jr, et al. A randomized trial comparing ticlopidine hydrochloride with aspirin for the prevention of stroke in high risk patients. N Engl J Med 321:501, 1989.

26. den Heijer M, Koster T, Blom HJ, et al. Hyperhomocysteinemia as a risk factor for deep-vein thrombosis. N Engl J Med 334:759, 1996.

27. Henderson WG, Goldman S, Copeland JG, et al. Antiplatelet or anticoagulant therapy after coronary artery bypass surgery. A meta-analysis of clinical trials. Ann Intern Med 111:743, 1989.

28. Hennekens CH, Buring JE, Sandercock P, et al. Aspirin and other antiplatelet agents in the secondary and primary prevention of cardiovascular disease. Circulation 80:749, 1989.

29. Hennekens CH, Peto R, Hutchison GB, Doll R. An overview of the British and American aspirin studies (Letter). N Engl J Med 318:923, 1988.

30. Hirsh J, Dalen JE, Deykin D. Oral anticoagulants. Mechanism of action, clinical effectiveness, and optimal therapeutic range. Chest 108:231S, 1995.

31. Hirsh J, Dalen JE, Fuster V, et al. Aspirin and other platelet-active drugs. The relationship among dose, effectiveness, and side effects. Chest 108:247S, 1995.

32. Hirsh J, Levine MN. Low molecular weight heparin. Blood 79:1, 1992.

33. Huisman MV, Büller HR, ten Cate JW, et al. Utility of impedance plethysmography in the diagnosis of recurrent deep-vein thrombosis. Arch Intern Med 148:681, 1988.

34. Huisman MV, Büller HR, ten Cate JW, et al. Management of clinically suspected acute venous thrombosis in outpatients with serial impedance plethysmography in a community hospital setting. Arch Intern Med 149:511, 1989.

35. Hull R, Delmore T, Carter C, et al. Adjusted subcutaneous heparin versus warfarin sodium in the long-term treatment of venous thrombosis. N Engl J Med 306:189, 1982.

36. Hull R, Delmore T, Genton E, et al. Warfarin sodium versus low-dose heparin in the long term treatment of venous thrombosis. N Engl J Med 301:855, 1979.

37. Hull R, Hirsh J. Advances and controversies in the diagnosis, prevention, and treatment of venous thromboembolism. In: Brown BE, ed. Progress in hematology. New York: Grune & Stratton, 1981;12:73.

38. Hull RD, Hirsh J, Carter CJ, et al. Diagnostic efficacy of impedance plethysmography for clinically suspected deep-vein thrombosis. Ann Intern Med 102:21, 1985.

39. Hull RD, Raskob GE, Rosenbloom D, et al. Treatment of proximal vein thrombosis with subcutaneous low-molecular-weight heparin vs intravenous heparin. Arch Intern Med 157:289, 1997.

40. Hyers TM, Hull RD, Wey JG. Antithrombotic therapy for venous thromboembolic disease. Chest 108:335S, 1995.

41. Jaffin BW, Bliss CM, Lamont JT. Significance of occult gastrointestinal bleeding during anticoagulation therapy. Am J Med 83:269, 1987.

42. Koepke JA, Triplett DA. Standardization of the prothrombin time—finally. Arch Pathol Lab Med 109:800, 1985.

43. Koopman MM, Prandoni P, Piovella F, et al. Treatment of venous thrombosis with intravenous unfractionated heparin administered in the hospital as compared with subcutaneous low-molecular-weight heparin administered at home. N Engl J Med 334:682, 1996.

44. Landefeld CS, Beyth RJ. Anticoagulant-related bleeding: clinical epidemiology, prediction, and prevention. Am J Med 95:315, 1993.

45. Leclerc JR, Jay RM, Hull RD, Hirsh J. Recurrent leg symptoms following deep vein thrombosis. A diagnostic challenge. Arch Intern Med 145:1867, 1985.

46. Lensing AWA, Prandoni P, Büller HR, et al. Lower extremity venography with Iohexol: results and complications. Radiology 177:503, 1990.

47. Lensing AWA, Prins MH, Davidson BL, Hirsh J. Treatment of deep venous thrombosis with low-molecular weight heparins. A meta-analysis. Arch Intern Med 155:601, 1995.

48. Letsky EA, de Swiet M. Thromboembolism in pregnancy and its management. Br J Haematol 57:543, 1984.

49. Levine M, Gent M, Hirsh J. A comparison of low-molecular-weight heparin administered primarily at home with unfractionated heparin administered in the hospital for proximal deep-vein thrombosis. N Engl J Med 334:677, 1996.

50. Levine MN, Raskob G, Landefeld S, Hirsh J. Hemorrhagic complications of anticoagulant treatment. Chest 108:276S, 1995.

51. Love PE, Santoro SA. Antiphospholipid antibodies: anticardiolipin and the lupus anticoagulant in systemic lupus erythematosus (SLE) and in non-SLE disorders. Prevalence and clinical significance. Ann Intern Med 112:682, 1990.

52. Manson JE, Stampfer MJ, Coldity GA, et al. A prospective study of aspirin use and primary prevention of cardiovascular disease in women. JAMA 266:521, 1991.

53. Moser KM, LeMoine JR. Is embolic risk conditioned by location of deep venous thrombosis? Ann Intern Med 94:439, 1981.

54. Oster JR, Singer I, Fishman LM. Heparin-induced aldosterone suppression in hyperkalemia. Am J Med 98:575, 1995.

55. Petitti DB, Strom BL, Melmon KL. Duration of warfarin anticoagulant therapy and the probabilities of recurrent thromboembolism and hemorrhage. Am J Med 81:255, 1986.

56. Peto R, Gray R, Collins R. Randomized trial of prophylactic daily aspirin in British male doctors. BMJ 296:313, 1988.

57. Philbrick JT, Becker DM. Calf deep venous thrombosis. A wolf in sheep's clothing. Arch Intern Med 148:2131, 1988.

58. Prandoni P, Lensing AWA, Büller HR. Deep-vein thrombosis and the incidence of subsequent symptomatic cancer. N Engl J Med 327:1128, 1992.

59. Prandoni P, Polistena P, Bernardi E, et al. Upper extremity deep

vein thrombosis. Risk factors, diagnosis, and complications. Arch Intern Med 157:57, 1997.

60. Ridker PM, Manson JE, Gaziano JM, et al. Low-dose aspirin therapy for chronic stable angina. A randomized placebo-controlled clinical trial. Ann Intern Med 114:835, 1991.

61. Roderick PJ, Wilkes HC, Meade TW. The gastrointestinal toxicity of aspirin: an overview of randomized controlled trials. Br J Clin Pharmacol 35:219, 1993.

62. Sack GH, Levin J, Bell WR. Trousseau's syndrome and other manifestations of chronic disseminated coagulopathy in patients with neoplasms: clinical, pathophysiologic, and therapeutic features. Medicine (Baltimore) 56:1, 1977.

63. Schulman S, Granqvist S, Holmström M, et al. The duration of oral anticoagulant therapy after a second episode of venous thromboembolism. N Engl J Med 336:393, 1997.

64. Schulman S, Rhedin A-S, Lindmarker P, et al. A comparison of six weeks with six months of oral anticoagulant therapy after a first episode of venous thromboembolism. N Engl J Med 332:1661, 1995.

65. Simoni P, Prandoni P, Lensing AWA, et al. The risk of recurrent venous thromboembolism in patients with an arg$^{506}\rightarrow$ gln mutation in the gene for factor V (factor V Leiden). N Engl J Med 336:399, 1997.

66. Siragusa S, Cosmi B, Piovella F, et al. Low-molecular-weight heparins and unfractionated heparin in the treatment of patients with acute venous thrombo-embolism: results of a meta-analysis. Am J Med 100:269, 1996.

67. The Steering Committee of the Physicians' Health Study Research Group. Final report on the aspirin component of the ongoing physicians' health study. N Engl J Med 321:129, 1989.

68. Strandness DE, Langlois Y, Cramer M, et al. Long term sequelae of acute venous thrombosis. JAMA 250:1289, 1983.

69. Svensson PJ, Dahlbäck B. Resistance to activated protein C as a basis for venous thrombosis? N Engl J Med 330:517, 1994.

70. Vessey M, Mant D, Smith A, Yeates D. Oral contraceptives and venous thromboembolism: findings in a large prospective study. BMJ 292:526, 1986.

71. Warkentin TE, Kelton JG. A 14-year study of heparin-induced thrombocytopenia. Am J Med 101:502, 1996.

72. Warkentin TE, Levine MN, Hirsh J, et al. Heparin-induced thrombocytopenia in patients treated with low-molecular-weight heparin or unfractionated heparin. N Engl J Med 332:1330, 1995.

73. Wells PS, Hirsh J, Anderson DR, et al. Accuracy of clinical assessment of deep-vein thrombosis. Lancet 345:1326, 1995.

74. White RH, McGahan JP, Daschbach MM, Hartling RP. Diagnosis of deep-vein thrombosis using duplex ultrasound. Ann Intern Med 111:297, 1989.

75. Willard JE, Lange RA, Hillis LD. The use of aspirin in ischemic heart disease. N Engl J Med 327:175, 1992.

C H A P T E R 53

Selected Illnesses Affecting Lymphocytes: Mononucleosis, Chronic Lymphocytic Leukemia, and the Undiagnosed Patient with Lymphadenopathy

LARRY WATERBURY, MD
PHILIP D. ZIEVE, MD

This chapter reviews two well-defined conditions that affect lymphatic organs and lymphocytes—the mononucleosis syndrome and chronic lymphocytic leukemia—and two other common conditions that are less well defined: the undiagnosed patient with lymphadenopathy and the chronic fatigue syndrome.

INFECTIOUS MONONUCLEOSIS

Several infections are caused by herpes viruses, including infectious mononucleosis (Epstein–Barr virus [EBV]), cytomegalovirus (CMV) infections, herpes simplex infections (see Chapters 94 and 100), and varicella–zoster infections (see Chapter 100).

Epidemiology and Pathogenesis

The EBV is the cause of infectious mononucleosis (5), an acute febrile illness that affects primarily teenagers and young adults (the age group between 15 and 25 years). Infection with the virus is extremely common; for example, more than 50% of college students of both sexes have antibodies to it, and each year 12% of college students who do not have antibodies to EBV develop them (most of them in the course of clinical mononucleosis) (17). Because of the ubiquity of exposure early in life, infectious mononucleosis is rare in people over the age of 30 and, when it does occur, may present atypically (see below). The virus seems to be spread by oral contact, first infecting the throat; then B lymphocytes generate a T-cell response that results in atypical lymphocytosis, which is a hallmark of the disease.

Signs and Symptoms

Clinical illness usually begins after a 1- to 2-month incubation period. Classically, patients have pharyngitis, lymphadenopathy, splenomegaly, and marked atypical lymphocytosis. Table 53.1 lists the relative frequency of the characteristic signs and symptoms associated with the illness. Pharyngitis occasionally can be extremely severe and is often accompanied by an exudate, which may be foul smelling. Rarely, it may be so severe that it leads to respiratory obstruction. Of the few patients who do not have pharyngitis (especially children), most simply have a nonspecific febrile illness associated with malaise. Other patients have mild jaundice and a syndrome that mimics infectious hepatitis. Posterior cervical adenopathy is characteristic of almost all patients, and there is often generalized lymph node enlargement as well; approximately 60% have an enlarged spleen. Some patients may experience a protracted course with nonspecific symptoms, slight to moderately tender lymphadenopathy, and splenomegaly that persist for weeks. Most patients are significantly improved by the end of 3 weeks.

Patients usually present to the physician at the end of the first week of a nonspecific illness characterized by malaise and perhaps by anorexia, mild headache, and fever (up to 104°F). Adenopathy, splenomegaly, and pharyngitis usually appear at about this time and slowly resolve over the following weeks. However, as noted below, the classic laboratory features of the disease may not be present until the second or third week of the clinical illness. Patients over 40 years of age tend to have more prolonged fever and less adenopathy than do young adults (8).

Laboratory Features

The hematocrit value is usually normal, although occasionally mild hemolysis and, rarely, a severe au-

toimmune hemolytic anemia are seen. The peripheral white cell count is usually elevated, reaching its height during the second and third weeks of the clinical illness. Early in the course there may be a severe absolute neutropenia, and occasionally the absolute neutrophil count is less than 500/μL. The differential count of the white cells is characterized by an absolute lymphocytosis with large numbers (more than 10% of the total white cell population) of atypical lymphocytes (large lobulated or indented nuclei and vacuolated or bluish cytoplasm). The platelet count is normal to slightly decreased in most patients; severe thrombocytopenia may occur rarely. Slight increases in the activity of hepatic enzymes are common but never reach the height seen in viral hepatitis; however, older patients tend to have more marked hepatic dysfunction, and in this group jaundice is common (8).

Serologic Features

Diagnosis is based on the presence of typical clinical features and characteristic serologic tests. A number of different EBV antibodies have been identified (5). They are summarized in Table 53.2. *Immunoglobulin M antibody to viral capsid antigen* (IgM anti-VCA) appears within 1 to 6 weeks after onset of infection and disappears within 3 to 6 months; a rising titer during the first few weeks of clinical illness is the most useful and generally the most easily available serologic evidence of recent primary infection. *Antibodies to the early antigen (EA) complex of EBV of the diffuse (D) type* (known as anti-D antibodies) also appear early in primary infection and disappear by 2 to 3 months, but anti-D antibody testing is much less available than IgM anti-VCA testing. *Heterophil antibodies* are elevated in most patients; the highest titers are reached during the first week of clinical illness. Differential absorption studies are needed to identify the presence of those heterophil antibodies that are specific for infectious mononucleosis (the antibodies are absorbed by bovine red cells but not by guinea pig kidney). A number of rapid macroagglutination slide tests are commercially available (14). Most use horse red cells (e.g., the Mono-Test), which are more sensitive than sheep red cells in the detection of heterophil antibodies. Some kits use differential absorption techniques as well. In general, the slide kits are sensitive to the detection of heterophil antibodies but also may yield positive results in other conditions associated with such antibodies (serum sickness, viral hepatitis, CMV infections, other viral illnesses, leukemia).

Table 53.1. Signs and Symptoms of Infectious Mononucleosis

Common Symptoms	%	Common Signs	%	Less Common Signs and Symptoms	%
Malaise	100	Adenopathy	100	Jaundice	10
Sore throat	85	Fever	90	Arthralgia	5
Warmth, chilliness	70	Pharyngitis	85	Skin rash	5
Anorexia	70	Splenomegaly	60	Diarrhea	5
Headache	50	Bradycardia	40	Photophobia	5
Cough	40	Periorbital edema	25		
Myalgia	25	Palatal enanthem	25		

Table 53.2. Serologic Evidence of Epstein–Barr Virus Infection

IgM antibody to viral capsid antigen (IgM anti-VCA). Appears early in primary infection and disappears within 3 to 6 months.

IgG antibody to viral capsid antigen (IgG anti-VCA). Appears slightly later than IgM anti-VCA and remains detectable for life.

Antibodies to the early antigen (EA) complex of EBV of the diffuse (D) type (anti-D). Anti-D antibodies appear early in primary infection and disappear by 2 to 3 months.

Antibodies to EB nuclear antigen (anti-EBNA). Anti-EBNA appears very late (months) after primary infection and is detectable for life.

From Evans AS et al. Seroepidemiologic studies of infectious mononucleosis with EB virus. N Engl J Med 279:1121, 1968.

In patients with classic symptoms of infectious mononucleosis, a positive mononucleosis slide test is sufficient serologic confirmation for the diagnosis for clinical purposes. Some 5 to 10% of patients with clinical infectious mononucleosis and serologic evidence of recent primary EBV infection are heterophil antibody negative. Another 5 to 10% of patients with clinical features of infectious mononucleosis have another illness (e.g., CMV infection, toxoplasmosis).

Complications

Severe complications of infectious mononucleosis are rare but do occur (4). They include neurologic problems (encephalitis, meningitis, peripheral neuropathy, Guillain–Barré syndrome), bacterial superinfection, and splenic rupture. The latter has accounted for a number of deaths, especially because the diagnosis is easily missed. The diagnosis should be suspected if there is a recent history of sudden, brief, sharp abdominal pain. Occasional deaths have been seen also with severe pharyngitis and airway obstruction. All of these complications are even more rare when the mononucleosis syndrome is caused by an infectious agent other than the EBV (see below). The pharyngitis in infectious mononucleosis may closely resemble that of exudative streptococcal pharyngitis, and all patients should have throat cultures to rule out bacterial infection.

Treatment

No specific treatment exists for infectious mononucleosis, and all that is usually necessary is patient education and supportive care. There is no evidence that prolonged bed rest is helpful. It is reasonable for patients to avoid strenuous activities until they feel strong enough to participate. Contact sports should be avoided if the spleen is tender or significantly enlarged. Because splenomegaly may persist for months, however, it seems unreasonable to avoid such sports until the spleen is no longer palpable. Although contacts do occasionally develop infectious mononucleosis, there is no evidence that the disease is highly infectious and patients should not be rigidly restricted from interpersonal contacts. (However, the patient continues to shed the virus for several months after onset of the illness. Close personal exposure during this period only occasionally results in transmission of the disease.)

Surgery is indicated for splenic rupture (16). Corticosteroids are usually reserved for patients with severe pharyngitis and impending airway obstruction; in this situation they are usually dramatically effective. Ordinarily a high dosage (40 to 60 mg of prednisone daily) is given initially, with rapid tapering of treatment by 1 week to 10 days.

Other Causes of the Mononucleosis Syndrome

Cytomegalovirus Infection

Although CMV infections may cause devastating clinical illness in the newborn (in utero) and in the immunocompromised host, infection in the noncompromised adult causes a clinical syndrome essentially indistinguishable from infectious mononucleosis except that exudative pharyngitis is unusual in CMV infection. Unlike exposure to EBV, which has occurred in most adults in the United States by age 25, primary CMV infections usually occur at an older age, making CMV mononucleosis the most common cause of the mononucleosis syndrome in patients over 25 to 30 years of age. Up to 50% of people over the age of 40 have antibodies to CMV, although most do not have a history of infection. Diagnosis usually depends on the demonstration of at least a fourfold rise in CMV complement-fixing antibodies over 4 to 6 weeks. When available, the demonstration of IgM antibodies to CMV antigens or the demonstration of cytolytic antibodies to CMV antigens is more useful in proving recent primary infection (Table 53.3).

Table 53.3. Causes Other Than EBV for the Mononucleosis Syndrome: Serologic Diagnosis of Recent Infection

CMV	Fourfold to eightfold rise in complement fixation titer.
	Elevated IgM or cytolytic antibodies to CMV antigen, if available, are more helpful.
Toxoplasmosis	Dye test (DT) or immunofluorescent antibody (IFA) titers of >1:1000 plus an IgM-IFA titer of >1:64.
Hepatitis A	Elevated titer of IgM antibody to hepatitis A antigen (IgM anti-HAAg). (See Chapter 42.)
Hepatitis B	Elevated hepatitis B surface antigen (HBsAg). Chronic carrier state identification will require follow-up measurement of HBsAg, HBeAg, and lack of rise of anti-HBs. (See Chapter 42.)
Rubella	The hemagglutination inhibition antibody (HIA) titer is the most widely used. The antibody is first detected after onset of the rash, and the titer rises rapidly for 1 to 2 weeks thereafter. If one does not catch this rise with acute and convalescent sera, the titer usually remains high for several months, so a single high titer is not meaningful. However, a low titer (<1:16) 2 weeks after the rash is strongly against the diagnosis.
HIV infection	Serologic evidence of infection may follow by weeks signs and symptoms of the mononucleosis syndrome.

Toxoplasmosis

Acute toxoplasmosis may also cause a clinical syndrome that resembles infectious mononucleosis, but pharyngitis does not occur and splenomegaly and lymphadenopathy are usually not as prominent. Diagnosis usually depends on a constellation of serologic findings indicative of recent primary infection (Table 53.3).

Other Infections

Other infections may mimic infectious mononucleosis. These include hepatitis A, hepatitis B, hepatitis C, rubella, adenovirus infection, and acute human immunodeficiency virus (HIV) infection. Sometimes an etiologic agent cannot be identified even after extensive serologic testing. Table 53.4 suggests a stepwise plan for the serologic evaluation of patients with the mononucleosis syndrome. Seronegative patients need further evaluation only if symptoms persist for more than a week or two, or if symptoms intensify or if worrisome adenopathy persists (see "The Undiagnosed Patient with Lymphadenopathy," below).

The Chronic Fatigue Syndrome

Since 1985, there has been an epidemic in the United States, predominantly in young women, of an illness characterized universally by debilitating fatigue and by a host of other symptoms (sore throat, tender lymph nodes, myalgia, joint pain, headaches, malaise, impaired memory or concentration), many of them suggestive of EBV infection. Initially people who complained of these symptoms were thought to have chronic mononucleosis because of the demonstration of antibodies to EBV in their blood. It soon became evident, however, that antibody titers to a number of viruses (CMV, herpes simplex, measles) were elevated in the blood of these patients, casting doubt on the role of EBV as an etiologic agent of the illness. Therefore, the illness was renamed the chronic fatigue syndrome, and criteria were formulated for its diagnosis (6). It has become obvious that the prevalence of psychiatric illness (e.g., depression, somatoform disorder, anxiety) is increased considerably in patients with the syndrome, so that it is tempting to think that all of the symptoms reflect underlying psychopathology. Recent studies failed to identify differences between controls and cases in a host of tests of immunologic function (12), and to date, no infectious cause has been identified. Affected patients are likely to remain symptomatic indefinitely; they need the understanding and support of their families and their physicians and specific attention to psychiatric problems when they are manifest (see Chapters 12, 13, and 15). The likelihood of patients returning to totally normal function is low. Poor prognostic features include older age, more chronic illness, the presence of comorbid psychiatric disease, and a persistent belief by the patient that the illness has a physical cause (9). Psychiatric intervention, especially cognitive therapy, may be helpful (2,18).

CHRONIC LYMPHOCYTIC LEUKEMIA

Clinical Features

Chronic lymphocytic leukemia (CLL) is the most common type of leukemia in the United States. It is primarily a disease of older men (19) in that two-thirds of patients are 60 or older and two to three times as many men are afflicted as are women. A mild tendency for the disease to segregate in families suggests that genetic factors may play a role in its acquisition (1).

Many patients are asymptomatic when diagnosed (see below), but complaints of malaise and increased fatigability are common. Ultimately most patients develop generalized lymphadenopathy and splenomegaly.

A persistent absolute lymphocytosis (greater than 10,000 μL for 3 months or longer) is the hallmark of the disease; lymphocyte counts as high as 200,000 to 300,000/μL may be seen occasionally. Other tests (bone marrow aspiration, lymph node biopsy) are ordinarily not necessary to establish the diagnosis.

As the disease progresses, hypogammaglobulinemia, anemia, granulocytopenia, and thrombocytopenia may develop. Autoimmune disorders (autoimmune hemolytic anemia and thrombocytopenia and pure red cell aplasia) develop in 10 to 15% of patients.

Treatment and Course

The survival of patients with CLL correlates best with the stage of their disease at diagnosis (3,13). For

---

Table 53.4. Stepwise Serologic Testing in the Diagnosis of the Cause of the Mononucleosis Syndrome

1. Typical clinical features with a positive heterophil slide test. This essentially establishes a diagnosis of infectious mononucleosis, usually caused by EBV. *Recommendation:* No further testing is needed.
2. Typical clinical features with a negative heterophil slide test at the time the patient first presents to the physician. *Recommendation:* Draw acute serum samples (save frozen in two containers) for pertinent serologic testing for EBV, toxoplasmosis, CMV, hepatitis A, hepatitis B, and rubella (see Table 53.3). Repeat heterophil slide test during the third week of clinical illness. If positive, no further testing is necessary. If negative, repeat EBV serology (at least 2 weeks after acute sample) and send with one of the acute serologic samples for EBV IgM anti-VCA testing (and anti-D testing if available). If the EBV serologies are diagnostic of recent infection, no further testing is necessary.
3. Typical clinical features, negative slide test at week 3 of clinical illness, and negative EBV serology (IgM anti-VCA or anti-D). *Recommendation:* Draw convalescent sera for testing for toxoplasmosis, CMV, hepatitis A, hepatitis B, and rubella and send with acute sera for appropriate serologic testing (see Table 53.3). Consider HIV infection in patients at risk.
4. Typical or atypical clinical features with negative serologies for all of the above. Consider other causes (e.g., leukemia, lymphoproliferative disease, granulomatous disease, collagen vascular disease). *Recommendation:* Consider lymph node biopsy and other tests (e.g., bone marrow aspiration and biopsy).

example, asymptomatic patients with only an absolute lymphocytosis have an essentially normal life expectancy. Patients with lymphadenopathy alone have a median survival of 6 to 8 years, and patients with significant anemia or thrombocytopenia have a median survival of 2 to 3 years.

There is no good evidence that treatment influences survival, but it can be helpful in decreasing the severity of signs and symptoms in the later stages of the disease. Thus, stable, asymptomatic patients with or without lymphadenopathy or splenomegaly do not require treatment. On the other hand, patients with marked constitutional symptoms (weight loss, severe malaise) or with symptomatic anemia or thrombocytopenia should be treated. For years standard treatment of CLL included alkylating agents (e.g., chlorambucil) and prednisone. Recent studies suggest that treatment of CLL with the purine analogue fludarabine results in a higher rate of remission (especially complete remission) and in more prolonged remissions than does treatment with alkylating agents (15). Aggressive treatment (including bone marrow and stem cell transplant) of early stage disease in younger patients with CLL is undergoing active investigation. Patients with autoimmune hemolysis and thrombocytopenia require more aggressive treatment with corticosteroids, and splenectomy is sometimes necessary in severely anemic or thrombocytopenic patients who are unresponsive to corticosteroids. A hematologist or medical oncologist should be consulted at the time of diagnosis of CLL and should be involved in the care of patients who require treatment.

Differential Diagnosis

A number of neoplastic conditions other than CLL may be associated with a chronic lymphocytosis: macroglobulinemia, B- and T-cell lymphomas, hairy cell leukemia, prolymphocytic leukemia, and adult T-cell leukemia. The morphology of the cells or other manifestations of the disease usually lead to the correct diagnosis. These conditions should be managed in close consultation with an oncologist.

A syndrome has been recognized (11), most often in older people, characterized by a clonal proliferation of large granular T lymphocytes (up to 10,000/mm^3) and, usually, chronic neutropenia. Anemia (rarely, red cell aplasia) and thrombocytopenia are uncommon. Lymphocytic infiltration of the bone marrow and spleen (with splenomegaly) is characteristic; lymph node involvement is rare. Some patients have coexistent seropositive rheumatoid arthritis; most patients, with or without arthritis, have serologic abnormalities (e.g., in addition to increased titers of rheumatoid factor, antinuclear antibodies, polyclonal hypergammaglobulinemia, and circulating immune complexes). The major morbidity from the disease is caused by recurrent bacterial infections; otherwise, most patients require no treatment and their mortality rate is low.

THE UNDIAGNOSED PATIENT WITH LYMPHADENOPATHY: WHEN TO RECOMMEND LYMPH NODE BIOPSY

Lymphadenopathy is a common physical finding that is associated with multiple disease processes (10). The decision about when to biopsy an enlarged lymph node is difficult (7). The problem arises most often in younger patients. Older patients with localized lymphadenopathy unexplained by infection or inflammation should be assumed to have cancer until proven otherwise, and the biopsy decision, therefore, is usually an easy one. However, lymphadenopathy in children and in young adults is usually caused by inflammation, and biopsy is usually not diagnostic. The clinician is often concerned in such circumstances about the possible harm from a delay in the diagnosis of a malignancy (Hodgkin's disease or non-Hodgkin's lymphoma most commonly) or a granulomatous condition (e.g., tuberculosis, sarcoid) for which specific treatment is indicated. However, harm can result from unnecessary biopsy. For the patient, there is both psychologic and physical discomfort from the procedure, and most important, there can be uncertainty about the interpretation of the biopsy of a reactive node. The histology of reactive nodes, especially those encountered in the mononucleosis syndrome, can be difficult to interpret. Reed–Sternberg cells (ordinarily pathognomonic of Hodgkin's disease) can be seen in the nodes of patients with infectious mononucleosis, and reactive nodes can sometimes look like and be interpreted as diagnostic of Hodgkin's disease or of non-Hodgkin's lymphoma. Because of these problems, biopsy of a lymph node should be avoided in a patient with the mononucleosis syndrome if possible. However, because patients with systemic lymphoma, Hodgkin's disease, miliary tuberculosis, and so on may have symptoms suggestive of the infectious mononucleosis syndrome (e.g., fever, anorexia, weight loss, malaise), one of the main reasons to pursue, by serologic studies (see above), a specific cause for the syndrome is to attempt to make a diagnosis without having to do a biopsy.

If a specific diagnosis cannot be made on the basis of serologic studies, few criteria can be relied on to decide whether a biopsy is indicated. However, one helpful retrospective study reported that in the age range of 9 to 25 years, three variables were important in determining whether a lymph node biopsy might be diagnostic of an illness requiring specific treatment (20): the size of the node to be tested by biopsy, the presence or absence of ear–nose–throat symptoms, and the presence or absence of an abnormality on chest radiograph. Nodes greater than 2 cm in diameter were more likely to contain important histologic information than were smaller nodes. An abnormal chest radiograph (adenopathy, infiltrate) in a patient with peripheral adenopathy correlated with useful biopsy information. Patients with cervical lymphadenopathy but without any ear–nose–throat symptoms were more likely to have a diagnostic lymph node biopsy. Table 53.5 summarizes

Table 53.5.   When to Recommend Lymph Node Biopsy in the Teenager and Young Adult

Features Against Early Biopsy

Mononucleosis syndrome, especially when proven serologically.

Ear–nose–throat symptoms (earache, sore throat, coryza tonsillar or dental infection).

Lymph nodes less than 2 cm in diameter.

Normal chest radiograph especially when associated with one of the above.

Features for Early Biopsy

Systemic illness with atypical features of the mononucleosis syndrome and without serologic proof of a cause of the mononucleosis syndrome (see Table 53.4).

Lymph nodes greater than 2 cm in diameter and an abnormal chest radiograph, absence of ear–nose–throat symptoms, or no proof of a typical mononucleosis syndrome.

Localized supraclavicular lymphadenopathy. This may be seen in the mononucleosis syndrome but in its absence is suggestive of mediastinal (right supraclavicular) or abdominal (left supraclavicular) granulomatous or neoplastic disease.

some of the features that can be used, especially in the young patient, to help determine the advisability and timing of a lymph node biopsy.

General References*

Betts RF. Infectious mononucleosis syndromes. In: Beutler E, Lichtman MA, Coller BS, Kipps TJ, eds. Williams hematology. 5th ed. New York: McGraw-Hill, 1995;997.

Dighiero G, Travade P, Chevret S. B-cell chronic lymphocytic leukemia: present states and future directions. Blood 78:1901, 1991.

Kipps TJ. Chronic lymphocytic leukemia and related diseases. In: Beutler E, Coller BS, Kipps TJ, eds. Hematology. 5th ed. New York: McGraw-Hill, 1995;1017.

Specific References

1. Conley CL, Misiti J, Laster AJ. Genetic factors predisposing to chronic lymphocytic leukemia. Medicine (Baltimore) 59:323, 1980.

2. Deale A, Chalder T, Marks I, Wessely S. Cognitive behavior therapy for chronic fatigue syndrome: a randomized controlled trial. Am J Psych 154:408, 1997.

3. Dighiero G, Travade P, Chevret S, et al. B-cell chronic lymphocytic leukemia: present status and future directions. Blood 78:1901, 1991.

4. Dorman JM, Glick TH, Shannon DC, et al. Complications of infectious mononucleosis. Am J Dis Child 128:239, 1974.

5. Evans AS, Niederman JC, McCollum RW. Seroepidemiologic studies of infectious mononucleosis with EB virus. N Engl J Med 279:1121, 1968.

6. Fukuda K, Straus SE, Hickie I. The chronic fatigue syndrome: a comprehensive approach to its definition and study. Ann Intern Med 121:953, 1994.

7. Greenfield S, Jordan MC. The clinical investigation of lymphadenopathy in primary care practice. JAMA 240:1388, 1978.

8. Horwitz CA, Henle W, Henle G, et al. Infectious mononucleosis in patients aged 40 to 72 years: report of 27 cases, including 3 without heterophil-antibody responses. Medicine (Baltimore) 62:256, 1983.

9. Joyce J, Hotopf M, Wessely S. The prognosis of chronic fatigue and chronic fatigue syndrome: a systematic review. QJM 90:223, 1997.

10. Libman H: Generalized lymphadenopathy. J Gen Intern Med 2:48, 1987.

11. Loughran TP, Starkebaum G. Large granular lymphocyte leukemia. Report of 38 cases and review of the literature. Medicine (Baltimore) 66:397, 1987.

12. Mawle AC, Nisenbaum R, Dobbins JG, et al. Immune responses associated with chronic fatigue syndrome: a case-control study. J Infect Dis 175:136, 1997.

13. Rai KR, Han T. Prognostic factors and clinical staging in chronic lymphocytic leukemia. Hematol Oncol Clin North Am 4:447, 1990.

14. Rippey JH, Bowman HE. Infectious mononucleosis test performance on CAP survey specimens. Am J Clin Pathol 72:363, 1979.

15. Rozman C, Montserrat E. Chronic lymphocytic leukemia. N Engl J Med 333:1052, 1995.

16. Rutkow IM: Rupture of the spleen in infectious mononucleosis. Arch Surg 113:718, 1978.

17. Sawyer RN, Evans AS, Niederman JC, McCollum RN. Prospective studies of a group of Yale University freshmen. I. Occurrence of infectious mononucleosis. J Infect Dis 123:263, 1971.

18. Sharpe M, Hawkins K, Simkin S, et al. Cognitive behaviour therapy for the chronic fatigue syndrome: a randomized controlled trial. BMJ 312:22, 1996.

19. Skinnider LF, Tan L, Schmidt J, Armitage G. Chronic lymphocytic leukemia. A review of 745 cases and assessment of clinical staging. Cancer (Philadelphia) 50:2951, 1982.

20. Slap GB, Brooks SJ, Schwartz JS. When to perform biopsies of enlarged peripheral lymph nodes in young patients. JAMA 252:1321, 1984.

*Bold print (general references) and bold numerals (specific references) denote published controlled clinical trials, meta-analyses, or consensus-based recommendations.

Pulmonary Problems

C H A P T E R 54

Common Pulmonary Problems: Cough, Hemoptysis, Dyspnea, Chest Pain, and Abnormal Chest X-Ray*

PETER WHITE, JR, MD
STEVE N. GEORAS, MD

Patients who develop acute respiratory problems usually present with symptoms that result in the rapid diagnosis and treatment of the underlying disorder. On the other hand, chronic diseases of the lung that cause slowly progressive symptoms may go undetected unless incidentally discovered as part of a general medical evaluation. This chapter discusses common pulmonary problems with which the general physician is often confronted: cough, hemoptysis, dyspnea, noncardiac chest pain, and the abnormal chest x-ray.

COUGH

Cough is an important defense mechanism that clears the airways of both secretions and inhaled

particles (18). Although it is often associated with other respiratory symptoms, cough may be the symptom that prompts a patient to seek medical advice. A cough is composed of three phases: a deep inspiration, closure of the glottis accompanied by a rapid increase in intrathoracic pressure, and a final opening of the glottis with an explosive release of pressure.

Mucosal neural receptors that initiate a *cough reflex* are located throughout the nasopharynx, ears, larynx, trachea, and bronchi down to the level of the terminal bronchioles. Stimulation of these receptors in the nasopharynx may cause sneezing, whereas stimulation of tracheal and bronchial receptors may also cause bronchospasm. After activation of the receptors, impulses are conducted along afferent pathways in the ninth and tenth cranial nerves to the cough center in the medulla. The reflex is complete through efferent pathways that cause forceful contraction of the diaphragm and other expiratory muscles. Although many different stimuli activate these receptors, all essentially initiate cough by some form of mechanical or chemical irritation. Additional factors, such as acute inflammation of the airways, may disrupt the bronchial mucosa, increase its permeability, and expose the receptors. The accompanying increases in respiratory secretions will lead to cough. Environmental pollutants, such as cigarette smoke, can directly stimulate the receptors without necessarily provoking an inflammatory reaction. Finally, although stimulation of irritant receptors may cause reflex bronchoconstriction, the bronchospasm itself, through reflex pathways, induces cough.

Acute Cough Syndromes

Table 54.1 shows the causes of cough. Generally, acute coughs are self-limited and caused by viral *upper respiratory infections* (18). In contrast, cough that is triggered by mild bronchospasm may persist for weeks to months after a viral upper respiratory tract infection (see below). Usually viral infections, atypical pneumonias, and *Pneumocystis carinii* pneumonia are associated with nonproductive coughs, and bacterial infections are associated with significant sputum production. Younger patients tend to have a more productive cough associated with *pneumonia,* whereas older individuals, especially those with chronic obstructive pulmonary disease (COPD), may retain secretions because of impaired ability to clear them. When a productive cough follows a typical viral syndrome, it may signal the development of a superimposed bacterial bronchitis or pneumonia. High concentrations of air pollutants, such as insoluble gases (e.g., ozone, SO_3, or NO2), which are not irritating to the upper airway, can cause either a dry or a productive cough secondary to chemical irritation.

Chronic Cough Syndromes

A persistent cough (generally lasting more than 3 weeks) is often more bothersome than the acute cough

---

*Philip L. Smith, E. James Britt, and Peter B. Terry contributed to this chapter in previous editions.

Table 54.1.   Causes of Cough

Causes	Examples
Common Causes	
Acute	
Inflammation	Tracheitis, bronchitis, pneumonia
Irritation	Environmental pollutants
Bronchospasm	Infection
Chronic	
Inflammation	Bronchitis, pollution, cigarettes, bronchiectasis, aspirated foreign body, chronic pneumonia (tuberculous and nontuberculous mycobacterial infection, *Pneumocystis pneumonia* in AIDS)
Irritation	Cigarettes, cancer, postnasal drip
Bronchospasm	Asthma, heart failure
Less Common Causes	
Drug-induced	Angiotensin-converting enzyme inhibitor, β-blockers (oral or ophthalmic)
Irritation	Esophageal reflux, chronic aspiration, auditory canal stimulation (cerumen, hair), aortic aneurysm
Inflammation	Sarcoid, alveolitis, bronchiolitis obliterans organizing pneumonia (BOOP)

syndrome described above. The most common cause of chronic coughing is *cigarette smoking* (18). The so-called smokers cough, a manifestation of *chronic bronchitis,* is generally described as hacking, worse in the morning, and may be described as productive or dry, as sputum is often ignored by cigarette smokers. The number of cigarettes smoked bears little relationship to the development of cough except when more than three packs of cigarettes are smoked daily. By definition, patients with chronic bronchitis have productive coughs that may interfere with their sleep. Perhaps because they inhale more deeply, smokers of marijuana may complain of a persistent cough after smoking only one to two cigarettes daily. Patients with central *bronchogenic and mediastinal tumors* often present with cough, whereas patients with metastatic tumors or peripheral lung cancers that arise outside the airways or beyond irritant receptors seldom do. In nonsmokers, the most common cause of chronic cough is *postnasal drip,* resulting from chronic sinusitis or allergic rhinitis (18,27). It is important to recognize that *bronchospasm* in smokers, as well as nonsmokers, can be associated with a chronic dry cough. Cough may be the only manifestation of mild *asthma* (cough variant asthma) and need not be associated with dyspnea, wheezing, or changes in baseline pulmonary function (7). A dry, hacking cough associated with dyspnea is common in patients in *heart failure* (see Chapter 61). Similarly cough may precede the complaint of dyspnea in patients with pulmonary emboli or bronchiolitis obliterans organizing pneumonia (BOOP) (a patchy pneumonia, probably immunologic, often idiopathic, that often responds to treatment with corticosteroids). *Chronic pulmonary infections,* such as tuberculosis or nontuberculous mycobacterial pneumonia in immunocompetent patients, and *Pneumocystis carinii* pneumonia in patients with acquired immunodeficiency syndrome (AIDS), commonly cause coughing. A chronic nonproductive cough occurs in up to 2% of patients taking an *angiotensin-converting enzyme inhibitor* and remits shortly after the drug is discontinued (3).

There are numerous less common causes of chronic cough. *Reflux esophagitis* may present with only minimal gastrointestinal (GI) symptoms and a significant, nagging cough, and occasionally, hoarseness (see Chapter 35). A nocturnal cough that is precipitated or increased by lying flat makes this diagnosis more suspect. A chronic cough may be caused by a process that stimulates the neural receptors in the pleura and pericardium (18). Even *impacted cerumen* in the external auditory canal can elicit a chronic cough. If the history and physical examination are unrevealing, it is often tempting to attribute chronic cough to a psychogenic cause; however, this is a rare cause of coughing, most often reported in children (19). Characteristically, psychogenic cough is nonproductive, subsides during sleep, and is related to emotional stress.

Evaluation

The acute and chronic cough syndromes are evaluated in similar ways. Usually a history and physical examination yield a presumptive diagnosis. Information should be obtained about the development, duration, character and precipitants of the cough, environmental or occupational exposure, smoking history, and any history of asthma or COPD. A history of constant swallowing or of throat clearing is associated with postnasal drip, even though the patient may deny many other symptoms associated with sinusitis.

Although the physical examination seldom provides a specific diagnosis, it may provide important clues. Careful examination of the ears, nose, throat, and lungs may yield relevant clues to a diagnosis. Cobblestoning in the posterior oropharynx represents lymphoid hyperplasia and is commonly seen in patients with chronic sinusitis. Examination of the chest may reveal rhonchi caused by the loose secretions that result from acute or chronic infection. A localized wheeze suggests a bronchogenic tumor, whereas wheezing at end expiration suggests active bronchospasm. Finally, the physical examination allows the quality and severity of the cough to be observed. A harsh cough associated with loose secretions is characteristic of tracheobronchitis resulting from viral upper respiratory infection. When little or no coughing occurs in the course of the visit, the patient should be asked to cough to determine whether the cough is productive or is associated with wheezing. This is also useful because some patients refuse to admit to expectoration of sputum and often unconsciously swallow their secretions.

If a diagnosis is not obvious after a history and physical examination, a chest x-ray is indicated. It may reveal a tumor, a pneumonia, or another chronic inflammatory process involving the lung parenchyma. The x-ray also may demonstrate atelectasis associated with a bronchogenic tumor or an aspirated foreign body. Patients with coughing from viral and bacterial tracheobronchitis, asthma, or cigarette smoking usually have a normal or unremarkable chest x-ray. In patients with a normal x-ray, spirometry can be used to look for obstructive airways disease. However, a normal spirogram does not necessarily exclude the diagnosis (see Chapter 55). When the chest x-ray is normal, bronchoscopy seldom provides additional useful information (18). Although a proximal bronchogenic tumor can be hidden on a chest x-ray by the mediastinal shadows, patients with these tumors often have associated hemoptysis (see below) (38). If the history, physical examination, chest x-ray, and spirogram are unrevealing and if the patient's cough persists after stopping new medicines and angiotensin-converting enzyme inhibitors and β-blockers (including eye drops), referral to a subspecialist may be appropriate. Additional tests would include methacholine challenge (asthma), high-resolution chest computerized tomography (CT) scan (bronchiectasis, interstitial lung disease), sinus x-ray or CT (chronic sinusitis), cine esophagram or 24-hour pH probe (gastroesophageal reflux), and rarely, bronchoscopy (endobronchial tumor or aspirated foreign body) or cardiac evaluation (heart failure, aortic dissection, or aneurysm). A diagnostic algorithm for evaluating chronic cough has been published (18).

Therapy

The specific therapy of the various acute inflammatory and irritating processes likely to cause coughing is discussed in detail in individual chapters dealing with these topics.

In general, viral tracheobronchitis requires only symptomatic therapy because coughing usually subsides spontaneously in 2 to 4 weeks. Patients with persistent coughing and a history or physical examination compatible with bronchospasm may benefit from bronchodilators. Treatment should begin with an inhaled β$_2$-sympathomimetic agonist. A detailed therapeutic approach to the pharmacologic treatment of bronchospasm is presented in Chapter 55.

Cessation of cigarette smoking and avoidance of a polluted environment may be the most important aspects of the therapy of both acute and chronic cough. In one study of 200 patients with a chronic cough, 50% had relief within 1 month of cessation of cigarette smoking, and eventually 77% of these patients had complete resolution of their cough (37). Thus, the patient who continues to smoke and to complain of cough is particularly frustrating because it is often difficult to convey that smoking as few as one or two cigarettes a day causes airway irritation and inflammation.

Removal of impacted cerumen in the auditory canal provides immediate relief (see Chapter 96). The treatment of postnasal drip and reflux esophagitis are discussed in Chapters 28 and 35, respectively. Approximately one-fourth of patients with chronic cough referred for subspecialty evaluation had more than one cause (18). Thus, if specific therapy does not eliminate the cause, additional testing and treatment should be pursued.

After specific therapy has been initiated, the use of *antitussives* should be considered. Despite the enormous demands made for antitussives, there are few situations in which these preparations are absolutely necessary. Moreover, the expectoration of sputum is a major goal in the therapy of patients with chronic obstructive airways disease. Therefore, when antitussives are needed in patients with productive coughs, it is usually better to attempt cough reduction (not total suppression), primarily to allow patients to sleep and to avoid posttussive syncope or stress incontinence or exacerbating strained chest wall or abdominal muscles. In the United States, several hundred cough and decongestant preparations, usually sold as combination products, are available. Many of these preparations combine so-called expectorants with antitussives and should be avoided because, insofar as they have an effect, they work at cross purposes. In one of the few published prospective double-blind studies of patients with cough associated with the common cold, dexbrompheniramine, an antihistamine (contained, for example, in Cheracol and Drixoral), and pseudoephedrine, a vasoconstrictor, reduced symptoms compared with placebo (9). Another randomized study of 97 patients with cough secondary to upper respiratory tract infections found no difference between guaifenesin alone versus guaifenesin plus codeine or guaifenesin plus dextromethorphan in reducing coughing (8).

Antitussives act on the cough reflex either by anesthetizing the peripheral irritant receptors or by increasing the threshold of the cough center. The two most effective nonnarcotic antitussives are *dextromethorphan* and *benzonatate* (Table 54.2). Dextromethorphan is chemically derived from the opiates; however, it is classified as nonnarcotic because at prescribed dosages it has no sedative or analgesic effects and therefore has little potential for abuse. It is available over the counter in a variety of preparations (e.g., Dimetane DX). Dextromethorphan suppresses cough centrally. Occasionally, the drug causes nausea, dizziness, or vertigo; and overdosage of more than 200 mg may lead to central

Table 54.2. Nonnarcotic Antitussives

Drug	Brand Name	Usual Dose	Site of Action	Comment
Dextromethorphan	Many preparations	15–30 mg four times a day	Central	Considered most effective central agent
Benzonatate	Tessalon	100–200 mg four times a day	Peripheral	Considered most effective peripheral agent

nervous system (CNS) depression. Benzonatate is a peripherally acting anesthetic similar to tetracaine. Rarely, it causes headaches, dizziness, and nausea or GI upset. The drug should not be chewed or sucked because this will result in an unpleasant taste and prolonged oral pharyngeal anesthesia. Overdosage has been associated with CNS stimulation and tremors, which may lead to seizures followed by profound CNS depression. It is reasonable to treat patients initially with dextromethorphan and, if intolerable cough persists, to substitute benzonatate.

If nonnarcotic antitussives are ineffective, *codeine* can be tried. Many clinicians prescribe codeine preferentially to patients with persistent cough because it is a more potent cough suppressant than the nonnarcotic agents. Codeine is effective in dosages of 15 to 30 mg administered every 3 to 6 hours. The common side effects—nausea, vomiting, constipation, dry mouth, and sedation—are usually not experienced at these lower dosages.

HEMOPTYSIS

Hemoptysis is defined as the expectoration of blood from below the vocal cords. It can range from flecks of blood in sputum to the coughing of large amounts (more than 1 L) of blood. Distinguishing between hemoptysis and hematemesis can be difficult. Blood from the lungs is usually bright red and frothy, has an alkaline pH, and is usually mixed with sputum containing macrophages and white blood cells. Often, patients with hemoptysis complain of a tickling or irritation in their chest. On the other hand, hematemesis is characterized by blood that is darker brown, has an acid pH, and is mixed with food particles. Sometimes blood from a lesion in the sinuses or in the upper airway will be aspirated and later expectorated, making it appear that the bleeding occurred in the lower respiratory tract. A careful history and physical examination must be performed to avoid inappropriate evaluation or treatment. The patient should be instructed to collect and save the bloody sputum so that the hemoptysis can be quantified. Nevertheless, a history of hemoptysis should not be ignored if a patient cannot produce a specimen on command because the symptoms can be intermittent. The various pulmonary causes of hemoptysis are summarized in Table 54.3.

In the typical ambulatory practice, blood streaking of the sputum is caused by *chronic bronchitis* 50 to 60% of the time, and by *lung cancer* 10 to 20% of the time; but the likelihood of a particular diagnosis depends on the patient population (e.g., smokers versus nonsmokers) (6,33). *Bronchiectasis* in the industrial world is less common today because of mass screening for tuberculosis, childhood vaccinations for measles and whooping cough, and antibiotic treatment of serious respiratory infections. *Active cavitary tuberculosis* is also a less common cause of hemoptysis than it once was, but residual upper lobe bronchiectasis, the result of old tuberculosis infection, is still seen. *Bronchogenic carcinoma* (see Chapter 56) presents with

Table 54.3. Pulmonary Causes of Hemoptysis

Causes	Examples
Common	
Inflammation	Bronchitis, bronchiectasis (including cystic fibrosis), tuberculosis, pneumonia, lung abscess
Neoplasm	Lung cancer
Less Common	
Inflammation	Goodpasture's syndrome, idiopathic pulmonary hemosiderosis, Wegener's granulomatosis, SLE, systemic necrotizing vasculitis
Infection	Parasitic, preexisting cavitary disease with mycetoma (old Tb or fibrocystic sarcoidosis), broncholithiasis
Neoplasm	Bronchial carcinoid, endobronchial metastasis
Vascular disease	Pulmonary embolus with infarction, arteriovenous malformation, aortic aneurysm, mitral stenosis, tricuspid endocarditis, pulmonary hypertension
Iatrogenic cause	Bronchoscopy, transthoracic lung biopsy, transtracheal oxygen catheter, pulmonary artery catheterization
Drugs	Anticoagulation, aspirin, crack cocaine, solvents, penicillamine
Chest trauma	

hemoptysis at two stages: blood-streaked sputum may be a brief manifestation of a small irritative mucosal lesion. This symptom may resolve only to be replaced later by major hemoptysis from a large endobronchial tumor that is friable or necrotic or is eroding central vessels. Approximately 10% of patients with lung cancer have hemoptysis at presentation, and approximately 60% of patients experience hemoptysis at some time during their disease (30). Usually blood from a *necrotizing pneumonia* or a *lung abscess* is mixed with pus, and the sputum appears red-brown or red-green. Hemoptysis from *pulmonary emboli,* a manifestation of pulmonary infarction, is assumed to be rare due to the lung's dual blood supply. However, in patients with significant heart or lung disease, pulmonary infarction occurs in approximately 20% of patients with pulmonary emboli (25). In one study, approximately 30% of patients with documented pulmonary emboli complicated by pulmonary infarction had hemoptysis (2). Even with the advent of fiberoptic bronchoscopy, the cause of hemoptysis remains undiagnosed 8 to 15% of the time (1,4). The 5-year survival rate for patients with cryptogenic hemoptysis (hemoptysis with normal chest x-ray and a negative bronchoscopy) is very good (85 to 95%) (4).

Less common causes of hemoptysis are also listed in Table 54.3, but this ranking reflects to some extent the location of a practice. For example, mycetomas and parasitic infections that cause hemoptysis are much more common in areas of the country where those problems are endemic. Hemoptysis is common in *bronchial carcinoids* by virtue of their endobronchial location and marked vascularity. Hemoptysis caused by *pulmonary metastasis* from a solid tumor is rare. Its presence raises the possibility of endobronchial metastases, which are most common in patients with breast, colon, and kidney cancer, and those with malignant melanoma. Patients with *mitral stenosis* and pulmonary vascular congestion are prone to hemoptysis with any source of lung irritation. Although certainly less common today, this valvular abnormality is often silent and the history of rheumatic fever forgotten. Patients taking the *anticoagulants* warfarin or heparin may develop hemoptysis. Whether this symptom is a clue to a specific bronchial lesion is unclear, insofar as no substantial experience with this problem has yet been published. Any inflammation of the airways in a patient taking anticoagulants may be complicated by hemoptysis. Occasionally, *blunt chest trauma* produces hemoptysis in an otherwise healthy individual.

Evaluation

The diagnostic evaluation of hemoptysis is aimed at determining the cause, localizing the site, and quantifying the amount of bleeding. The history and physical examination are directed at uncovering clues to the causes outlined in Table 54.3. An attempt should be made to quantitate the amount of hemoptysis by history and by collection of expectorated blood. Massive hemoptysis, generally defined as greater than 600 mL of blood during a 24-hour period, represents a medical emergency, and survival of the patient depends on rapid diagnosis and treatment (4).

During the physical examination, extrathoracic sources of bleeding from the nasal passages, sinuses, and pharynx should be sought. Physical findings may be helpful. Digital clubbing may be seen in non–small cell lung cancer, lung abscess, or bronchiectasis. Scattered ecchymoses, multiple petechiae, or GI bleeding suggests a coagulopathy, and telangiectasias of the skin, lips, or buccal mucosa is consistent with hereditary hemorrhagic telangiectasis (or Osler Weber Rendu syndrome). Ulceration and crusting of the nasal septum may represent upper airway involvement of Wegener's granulomatosis. The significance of unilateral wheezing or crackles must be interpreted with caution because these sounds may be produced by aspirated blood or secretions rather than by endobronchial tumor.

A chest x-ray is essential because acute inflammatory diseases, such as active tuberculosis, pneumonia, and lung abscess, will produce obvious radiographic abnormalities. Typically lung cancers associated with hemoptysis are centrally located squamous cell carcinomas, and approximately half are cavitary. However, localization of the bleeding source is often precluded by bilateral aspiration of blood or by the presence of bilateral pulmonary disease. Patients with bronchitis often have normal chest x-rays, and the findings on plain film of focal bronchiectasis may be nonspecific. If the bronchiectasis is a result of old tuberculosis, however, apical scarring may suggest the diagnosis; otherwise, there may be increased or crowded lung markings, thickened dilated bronchi, multiple cystic cavities (1 to 3 mm in diameter), or infiltrates due to recurrent infection. The chest CT scan is more sensitive than the chest x-ray in detecting bronchiectasis and is generally sufficient to make the diagnosis. Differentiating bronchitis from bronchiectasis by history and chest x-ray is sometimes difficult. This distinction may not be critical, however, because the acute medical management of bronchitis and bronchiectasis in patients with hemoptysis is the same.

When the chest x-ray is normal or nonlocalizing, endobronchial malignancy is the principal diagnosis to exclude, although bronchitis is the most likely diagnosis. Individuals under 40 years old, including smokers, with hemoptysis that has lasted less than 1 week are unlikely to have cancer (32). In such patients, observation is a reasonable initial approach.

Persistent or recurrent hemoptysis mandates a thorough evaluation that includes bronchoscopy. Patients with normal chest x-rays who are at increased risk for lung cancer (over 40 years old, greater than 20-pack-year cigarette smoker) should undergo bronchoscopy. Still, only 5% of these patients will have lung cancer discovered at bronchoscopy (see Chapter 56) (26,28). Sputum cytology may provide the diagnosis in as many as half of these patients (5,29), but bronchoscopy is generally still required to locate the site of malignancy (lung versus upper aerodigestive tract) and to plan for therapy (28). The role of chest CT scan in patients with hemoptysis and normal chest x-rays has not been determined, but most clinicians view bronchoscopy and chest CT scans as complementary (16).

Therapy

Patients with bronchitis or bronchiectasis can usually be treated on an ambulatory basis with antimicrobial drugs, such as amoxicillin, doxycycline, or TMP/SMX for 10 to 14 days. Blood streaking of the sputum usually resolves within 2 to 3 days, but a full course of antibiotic therapy should be completed. Blood irritates the tracheobronchial tree and triggers constant cough, which by itself is traumatic. Mild cough suppression may help (see above), but heavy sedation is undesirable. The patient must maintain the ability to expectorate blood as it accumulates. No clinical criteria or radiographic signs predict massive hemoptysis, and the quantity of hemoptysis does not necessarily indicate the seriousness of the patient's underlying disease. Thus, given the tendency for rebleeding and the often unpredictable clinical course of hemoptysis, a low threshold for hospitalization is warranted.

DYSPNEA

Breathing is an unconscious act that usually occurs effortlessly; yet even normal people become aware of their breathing during deep sighs or during moderate to severe exercise. Dyspnea, the abnormal, uncomfortable sensation of breathlessness, is difficult to define because patients often cannot accurately perceive or quantitate the feeling. Similar to an individual's threshold for the recognition of pain, the complaint of dyspnea depends on both the individual's limit for discomfort and the specific circumstances that provoke shortness of breath. Thus, dyspnea must be defined in terms of what is abnormal for a particular individual in the context of his or her level of fitness and of the amount of activity that is associated with breathlessness. Some patients become dyspneic with relatively small measurable alterations in ventilation, whereas others (e.g., patients who are hyperventilating with Kussmaul's breathing) may not complain of dyspnea. Fortunately, a reasonable correlation exists between the degree of dyspnea and objective measurements of physiologic dysfunction.

Often, the actual complaint of dyspnea may not be expressed as such, and it may vary depending on the type of precipitating illness as well as on whether it developed abruptly or over a longer period. Thus, asthmatic patients may complain of acute shortness of breath, tightness in the chest, or an inability to exhale, whereas patients with acute pulmonary embolism may state that their breath has suddenly "been taken away," and they cannot get enough air even though they ventilate easily. In contrast, patients with emphysema who have modified their lifestyles may dismiss the sensation of breathlessness as part of their advancing age. (23)

Normal Ventilation

No single mechanism is responsible for dyspnea. Because dyspnea is the result of a variety of diverse influences acting alone or together, a brief discussion of the control of ventilation may help the practicing physician understand the complexity of dyspnea and the reason why this sensation often does not immediately respond to correction of obvious physiologic abnormalities. Normally, ventilation is coupled to the individual's metabolic demands as reflected in the oxygen consumption and carbon dioxide elimination necessary to meet a given level of activity. These needs are sensed by peripheral (carotid and aortic bodies) and central (medullary) chemical chemoreceptors that respond to the O_2, CO_2, and pH of blood and cerebrospinal fluid. The acute stimulation of these receptors provokes changes in minute ventilation. In addition, the control and regulation of the rate and pattern of breathing are influenced by the reflex effects of activation of neural receptors that lie in the lung parenchyma, airways, blood vessels, respiratory muscles, and chest wall. For example, receptors in the chest wall and diaphragm will respond to increased stiffness (decreased compliance) in the lung that occurs with fluid accumulation or with interstitial fibrosis. In addition, interstitial edema may activate C fibers located in the alveolar interstitium and may reflexly cause dyspnea in patients with pulmonary edema. Other receptors located in the airway epithelium cause rapid shallow breathing, coughing, and bronchospasm when irritating substances are inhaled. Finally, the CNS alone can cause large alterations in breathing that lead to hyperventilation in association with anxiety attacks (see

Chapter 13). This discussion should help in understanding, for example, why the correction of arterial hypoxemia alone in a patient with an asthmatic attack usually does not relieve the sensation of breathlessness. In this situation, dyspnea results from the complex interaction of both chemical and neural stimuli to breathe, coupled with an inividual's response to these signals. Therefore correction of only one of these problems is not sufficient to abolish dyspnea.

Evaluation

The causes of dyspnea are diverse and include essentially all diseases that result in significant functional impairment of either the respiratory system (gas exchange and pulmonary mechanics) or the cardiovascular system (circulatory and cardiac function) as well as any hematologic abnormality that impairs oxygen delivery. Table 54.4 summarizes the general disease categories likely to cause abnormal breathlessness.

In ambulatory practice, the major causes of dyspnea are obstructive airways disease and arteriosclerotic and hypertensive heart disease, either alone or in combination. The prevalence of symptomatic lung disease in a specific geographic region or socioeconomic group is further modified by the prevalence of cigarette use, urban pollution, and occupational exposure to inhaled toxic substances. The clinical circumstances and sequence of events in which dyspnea occurs will aid in its evaluation.

One of the first steps in evaluating a patient who complains of dyspnea is deciding whether the symptoms reflect an acute or a chronic event because the more serious causes of dyspnea tend to present abruptly. In general, dyspnea of sudden onset is easier to evaluate, but the workup must proceed quickly to determine whether the patient should be admitted to the hospital for more intensive evaluation and therapy. On the other hand, the evaluation of chronic dyspnea can usually be accomplished more slowly in an ambulatory setting.

Acute Dyspnea

The history, physical examination, and chest x-ray form the focal point of the evaluation of a patient with acute dyspnea. In a young patient, the medical history and physical examination alone often suggest the presumptive diagnosis. When necessary, additional distinction of primary cardiac from pulmonary disorders will be aided by the chest x-ray, spirogram, and electrocardiogram (ECG).

Acute tracheobronchitis should be considered in the middle-age smoker with cough, dyspnea, and purulent sputum in association with a clear chest x-ray. When wheezing and rhonchi are present, the term *asthmatic bronchitis* is often used. *Spontaneous pneumothorax* (see below) presents with sudden sharp chest pain and dyspnea. A small but significant pneumothorax on chest x-ray can easily be missed, and diagnostic accuracy will be improved with an expiratory film. Previously undiagnosed *interstitial*

Table 54.4. Causes of Dyspnea

	Acute	Chronic
Common		
Pulmonary		
Obstructive airways disease	Asthma, bronchitis	Asthma, COPD
Restrictive lung disease	Pneumothorax	Diffuse interstitial lung disease, pleural effusion
Inflammatory	Pneumonia	
Vascular	Pulmonary embolism	
Cardiac	CHF (angina equivalent)	CHF (cardiomyopathy)
Other	Psychogenic	Chronic anemia, obesity
Less Common		
Pulmonary		
Upper airway obstruction	Epiglottitis, foreign body aspiration	Goiter
Restrictive lung disease		Diaphragm paralyses, neuromuscular disease, kyphoscoliosis, pulmonary metastases (lymphangitic)
Vascular		Pulmonary hypertension (thromboembolic, idiopathic), hepatopulmonary syndrome (cirrhosis)
Cardiac		CHF (pericardial disease)
Other	CO intoxication, acute blood loss or hemolysis, thyroid disease	

lung disease, bullous lung disease, and *cystic fibrosis* may also present with spontaneous *pneumothoraces.* In these cases, the chest film should demonstrate characteristic abnormalities.

Acute dyspnea in association with fever, cough, and purulent sputum with localized infiltrates suggests *pneumonia,* usually bacterial (see Chapter 28). Diffuse infiltrates and nonproductive cough suggest atypical pneumonia (see Chapter 28).

The patient with acute dyspnea and known *heart failure* has usual cardiac symptoms and signs, including paroxysmal nocturnal dyspnea, crackles, cardiomegaly, and a symmetric interstitial pattern with or without pleural effusions. *Psychogenic dyspnea,* or the hyperventilation syndrome, has a rapid onset and is usually found in conjunction with anxiety disorders (see Chapter 13). This syndrome should be considered in young patients in whom dyspnea is unrelated to exertion and is associated with somatic complaints and excessive fearfulness (31).

Less common but important causes of acute dyspnea include acute *foreign body aspiration,* usually evident from the history of aspiration and a physical examination that demonstrates decreased breath sounds over the part of the lung supplied by the occluded bronchus. During the heating season or in certain industrial settings, *carbon monoxide intoxication* should be considered as a cause of headaches and dyspnea. Diagnosis requires a high degree of suspicion and awareness of the problem. Confirmation requires measurement of carboxyhemoglobin with a cooximeter. The partial pressure of oxygen measured in the arterial blood gas sample will remain normal.

Pulmonary Embolism

Pulmonary embolism (PE) is a major life-threatening cause of acute dyspnea, but the diagnosis can be difficult. Its evaluation requires a systematic approach with a logical sequence of diagnostic testing because approximately 75% of patients presenting with suspected deep venous thrombosis (DVT) or PE do not have these conditions (14).

The incidence of PE is high in patients with chronic obstructive lung disease or congestive heart failure and in those with risk factors for venous thromboembolism (e.g., active cancer, prolonged immobilization, or a strong family history of DVT) (14). In a multicenter study, 60% of patients with PE were men, and of the women under age 45 who had PE, 75% were found to be using oral contraceptives (see Chapter 93). In this same study, the most common symptoms present at the time of diagnosis were dyspnea and chest pain, which were found in more than 80% of patients. Hemoptysis, cough, and apprehension were seen less often (2). The physical examination is usually not helpful in the diagnosis, especially because many of the patients have underlying respiratory and cardiovascular diseases that may themselves produce abnormal physical findings: tachycardia, tachypnea, and an accentuated second pulmonic heart sound.

Most laboratory tests are not useful in the diagnosis of PE (34). Chest x-rays are often abnormal, but the findings are nonspecific (localized infiltrates, atelectasis, an elevated hemidiaphragm, or a pleural effusion). The arterial gas tensions are also often abnormal (reduced Pao_2 and $Paco_2$) but are not helpful diagnostically, in part because of considerable variation and in part because of the high prevalence of cardiopulmonary diseases that alter both the Pao_2 and $Paco_2$.

The most useful procedure in the screening of patients for PE is a ventilation/perfusion ($\dot{V}/\dot{Q}$) scan of the lungs. Whether the patient is hospitalized before having the scan depends on the severity of the presentation.

Patient Experience. Little discomfort is associated with a lung scan. The patient should be instructed that he or she will inhale a mixture of oxygen and xenon for 3 to 4 minutes, followed by a venous injection of radioactive-labeled technetium. Several different projections are then recorded on a scanner while the patient is lying on a table.

The V̇/Q̇ scan is a highly sensitive test, but it can be nonspecific depending on the configuration, location, and number of perfusion defects seen. There are well-established criteria for interpreting the results of V̇/Q̇ scans. In general, the greater the perfusion defects without corresponding ventilation defects, the "higher probability" the scan. If the V̇/Q̇ scan is normal, the diagnosis of an acute PE is excluded. Conversely, a high probability scan is associated with an 85 to 90% chance of PE. Unfortunately, only 10 to 15% of patients will have a high probability scan, and less than 5% will be normal. Most patients will have an intermediate probability (or nondiagnostic) V̇/Q̇ scan and require further testing to confirm or exclude the diagnosis. It is worth remembering that a "low-probability" scan does not exclude the diagnosis of PE. In particular, if there is a high clinical suspicion, up to 40% of patients with low-probability V̇/Q̇ scans will have documented PE on pulmonary angiography (35).

In patients with nondiagnostic V̇/Q̇ scans, abnormal compression ultrasonography (or impedance plethysmography) may detect a proximal DVT and confirm the need for anticoagulation (17). Approximately 10% of these patients will have a DVT detected by initial testing and should be hospitalized for initiation of anticoagulant therapy (see Chapter 52). Because ultrasonography does not detect calf-vein thromboses, some patients with an initially negative test are at risk for propagating a thrombus and suffering a PE. This occurs 2 to 15% of the time, depending on risk factors for DVT. If there is adequate cardiopulmonary reserve, serial noninvasive testing (e.g., at days 5 and 10) is a reasonable strategy (11). Alternatively, if clinical suspicion for PE is high or there is limited cardiorespiratory reserve, pulmonary angiography may be warranted. Spiral CT scans are being increasingly used to test for PE noninvasively (13). Enthusiasm for this mode is tempered by the limited experience to date, and the poor visibility of thrombi outside of large vessels.

The resolution of PE varies and can occur as early as 1 to 2 weeks in patients who have had small emboli. With larger emboli and in patients with underlying cardiopulmonary disease, there may be angiographic evidence of emboli that persists for 2 or 3 months (10). If chest pain occurs after discharge, a subsequent lung scan (and perhaps, depending on the results, angiography) is necessary to determine whether embolization has recurred.

Evaluation of Chronic or Progressive Dyspnea

In contrast to acute dyspnea, chronic dyspnea is usually more difficult to diagnose and often requires more extensive diagnostic procedures; therefore the evaluation should proceed in a logical sequence to avoid expensive and invasive laboratory testing. Because shortness of breath is appropriate to certain levels of activity depending on the fitness of the individual, the physician must decide whether the patient's symptoms are abnormal and over what period they have developed. Many patients with chronic cardiopulmonary disease or chronic anemia adapt to the insidious onset of dyspnea by subconsciously changing daily habits and avoiding physical activity. The degree of dyspnea should be determined by comparing the patient's abilities to perform work with an appropriate peer group and with his or her baseline performance. Thus, the complaint of dyspnea in a 35-year-old who normally runs 5 miles and now becomes short of breath after running only 2 miles should not be ignored.

The most useful initial test is the chest x-ray, which is often abnormal and therefore directs subsequent evaluation. Patients with *COPD* associated with emphysema have hyperinflation, decreased lung markings, and often evidence of bullous formation (see Chapter 55). Large *pleural effusions, lung cancer,* or *heart disease* associated with dyspnea results in obvious changes in the chest roentgenogram with evidence of fluid occupying at least half of one hemithorax, large mass lesions, or cardiomegaly, respectively. *Interstitial lung disease* that has led to fibrosis is revealed by chest x-ray, although the precise cause often requires intensive investigation (see below). *Unilateral hemidiaphragm paralysis* results in obvious asymmetry in lung expansion. Patients with this condition often describe orthopnea secondary to difficulty with diaphragmatic excursion in the recumbent position.

Patients with dyspnea and a normal or nonspecific chest x-ray represent a challenging group to diagnose. An approach for doing the workup in these patients is shown in Table 54.5. Most of these patients have obstructive lung disease (23). A spirogram is useful to

Table 54.5. Workup of Chronic Dyspnea When the Initial Workup (e.g., Chest X-Ray, Spirometry) is Unrevealing

Disease Suspected	Test
Pulmonary	
Obstructive airways disease	Home peak flow monitoring, bronchoprovocation
Interstitial lung disease	Helium lung volumes, diffusing capacity, high-resolution chest CT scan
Respiratory muscle weakness	Helium lung volumes, diffusing capacity, inspiratory/expiratory pressures
Pulmonary hypertension (thromboembolic, idiopathic)	V̇/Q̇ scan, echocardiography, pulmonary angiography
Unclear	Helium lung volumes, diffusing capacity
Cardiac	
Coronary artery disease	ECG/MUGA: rest ± exercise
Cardiomyopathy	Echocardiogram
Other	
Thyroid disease	Thyroid function tests
Anemia	Hemoglobin concentration or hematocrit value
Mixed cardiac/respiratory disease	Cardiopulmonary exercise testing
Deconditioning	Cardiopulmonary exercise testing
Anxiety/hyperventilation	Cardiopulmonary exercise testing

screen for occult lung disease because a normal spirogram nearly excludes significant parenchymal disease. Although patients with exercise-induced asthma may have a normal spirogram during symptom-free periods, more commonly there is evidence of slight reduction in the baseline forced expiratory volume as a percentage of forced vital capacity. Home peak flow monitoring may confirm the diagnosis in these patients. Additional specialized procedures that aid in the diagnosis of exercise-induced asthma are discussed in Chapter 55. One study reported 72 patients referred for evaluation of chronic dyspnea not diagnosed by history, physical examination, chest x-ray, or spirometry. The two most common diagnoses were asthma/reactive airway diseases (approximately 17%) and hyperventilation syndrome (approximately 20%), but there was a wide spectrum of underlying diseases in the remaining cases. Notably, 20% of patients remained undiagnosed despite extensive evaluation (12).

In general, *obesity* is not associated with dyspnea unless body weight is markedly increased (50 to 100% or more or 100 pounds or more over ideal weight). *Primary pulmonary hypertension* may be associated with subtle dilation of the pulmonary arteries on chest x-ray and is most commonly seen in young asthenic women. *Upper airway obstruction* due to *goiter,* for example, often is not apparent on a routine posteroanterior and lateral chest x-ray. Anemia does not usually cause dyspnea unless it has developed acutely (blood loss or hemolysis) or unless it is relatively severe (e.g., hematocrit values of 20% or less). Some patients with advanced *hepatic cirrhosis* complain of severe dyspnea, especially worse when upright ("platypnea"). These patients experience excess shunting of blood through abnormal vascular channels in the lung (the *"hepatopulmonary syndrome"*) (20).

In patients in whom the diagnosis is uncertain, laboratory testing should include a hemoglobin determination or hematocrit value to determine whether the patient is severely anemic or polycythemic, and thyroid function studies if there are symptoms of thyroid dysfunction (e.g., unexplained weight gain, fatigue).

1. *Complete pulmonary function tests.* In addition to baseline spirometry (see Chapter 55), other pulmonary function tests include the measurement of *total lung capacity* and *functional residual capacity,* which quantitate the degree of hyperinflation or restriction. Categorization of a disorder as obstructive or restrictive will direct the physician to a narrowed list of causes. *The diffusing capacity* measures the amount of alveolar capillary surface area available for gas exchange. Thus, the diffusing capacity is reduced in patients with PE and other vascular occlusive diseases as well as in patients with emphysema. In contrast, an elevated diffusing capacity is found in conditions that elevate the pulmonary blood volume—for example, erythrocytosis, early congestive heart failure, or obesity. These additional tests should be considered only if spirometry is abnormal. Measurement of inspiratory and expiratory pressures helps characterize neuromuscular problems. *Flow-volume loops* help identify upper airway sources of obstruction. The experience of the patient during the performance of these tests is described in Chapter 55.

2. *Cardiovascular testing.* The use of specialized non-invasive cardiovascular evaluation, including *echocardiograms* and *gated heartpool nuclear scanning* to assess right and left ventricular function or the presence of valvular heart disease is discussed in Chapters 60 and 61.

3. *Exercise testing.* If a patient is dyspneic on exertion and baseline testing of cardiopulmonary function, as described above, is normal or only mildly abnormal, exercise testing should be considered.

In general, two types of exercise tests are available. The first is a standard *cardiac stress test,* during which the patient is exercised and observed for the development of chest pain and for electrocardiographic or radionuclide ischemic changes (see Chapter 57). The second type of exercise testing is a *cardiopulmonary stress test* in which cardiac function, pulmonary gas exchange, ventilation, and physical fitness are quantitated at specific work loads. The two types of tests are similar, but the patient should be told that the cardiopulmonary test requires continuous exercise while breathing into a mouthpiece, and measurement of oxygenation is made either by an oximeter or by means of an indwelling arterial line. Such complicated cardiopulmonary stress testing is justified and useful to determine whether dyspnea is due to cardiac disease; pulmonary disease, including exercise-induced asthma or occult pulmonary vascular disease; deconditioning; or combinations of the above. This type of testing is particularly useful in evaluating patients for disability compensation because static pulmonary function and noninvasive cardiac testing may not accurately predict the functional state of a given patient during actual working conditions. The referring physician can usually determine presumptively the most likely cause for dyspnea and can make the appropriate referral for the specific exercise test. In large hospital centers with combined cardiopulmonary laboratories, simultaneous consultation and exercise testing by cardiologists and pulmonologists may be available.

This approach to the evaluation of dyspnea will almost always answer the questions necessary for diagnosis of the underlying condition and for establishment of a therapeutic regimen.

Therapy

Treatment of dyspnea is primarily aimed at therapy of the underlying cardiac, pulmonary, or hematologic disorders that cause abnormal breathlessness. In certain patients with underlying irreversible lung disease, specific measures that improve respiratory muscle function may alleviate symptomatic dyspnea. Training programs that increase both muscle strength and endurance are available in selected pulmonary rehabilitation centers and have resulted in decreased shortness of breath in some patients. Because anxiety and depression are commonly associated with the development of chronic cardiopulmonary disorders associated with dyspnea, appropriate anxiolytics or antidepressants may be useful (see Chapter 13). In patients with pulmonary disease, buspirone (20 to 30 mg/day) may be an effective anxiolytic and does not impair respiratory drive. Selective serotonin reuptake inhibitors (SSRIs) may be particularly useful in patients with panic attacks (31). Low-dose narcotics (e.g., morphine sulfate) can be extremely useful as a palliative therapy for patients with end-stage COPD or lung cancer, but should be used with caution because they can impair ventilatory drive.

NONCARDIAC CHEST PAIN

Chest pain is a particularly frightening symptom because of the widespread knowledge and concern about heart disease; however, nonspecific musculoskeletal pain is more common than angina, especially in younger patients (less than 40 years old). Most patients with chest pain can be evaluated and treated in an ambulatory setting; a few patients require referral to a specialist. The common noncardiac cause of chest pain is discussed in this section, which should be read in conjunction with Chapter 57.

Afferent neural impulses responsible for thoracic pain are carried by the sympathetic chain, vagus, and phrenic nerves. Visceral structures, which include the lung, diaphragm, heart, and esophagus, all lie within the thoracic cage and have overlapping innervation. Chest pain arising from these different organs often have similar referral patterns; therefore, irritation of the diaphragmatic pleura, diaphragm, or pericardium from either thoracic or abdominal disease causes chest pain that radiates to the shoulder. In addition, patients may have difficulty localizing pain from the deeper anatomic structures within the chest, whereas diseases involving the superficial structures, muscles, and ribs are more easily localized. Because there is no sensory innervation of the lung parenchyma, alveolar or interstitial disease does not cause chest pain unless the pulmonary vasculature, bronchi, or pleura are involved. Recent studies have found that enhanced visceral (esophageal) pain perception underlies many cases of unexplained anginalike chest pain (15).

Table 54.6 lists causes of chest pain.

Musculoskeletal pain is common in young individuals who increase their exercise abruptly (including patients who acutely hyperventilate as part of an anxiety state; see Chapter 13). A history of unusual exertion with increased breathing plus tenderness of intercostal muscles usually suffices to make this diagnosis.

Pain caused by *tracheitis* or *tracheobronchitis* is a distinctive substernal burning sensation that is precipitated by coughing and is most often associated with viral respiratory infections. This is in contrast to the sharp, stabbing, pleuritic chest pain experienced with pneumonia. The latter is clearly localized to the

Table 54.6.   Causes of Chest Pain

Causes	Examples
Common	
Chest wall	Nonspecific musculoskeletal, costochondritis, Tietze's syndrome
Cardiac	Angina
Pulmonary	Tracheitis, pleurodynia, pneumonia
Gastrointestinal	Esophageal reflux/spasm
Neurologic	Cervical spine disease (radicular)
Less Common	
Chest wall	Herpes zoster, thoracic outlet syndrome, fractured rib, tumor
Cardiac	Dissecting aortic aneurysm, pericarditis
Pulmonary	Pneumothorax, pulmonary hypertension, pulmonary infarction
Gastrointestinal	Peptic ulcer disease, abdominal infection/peritonitis

chest wall and arises from stretching the inflamed parietal pleura during breathing or coughing. *Pleurodynia* (or epidemic myalgia), characterized by fever, headache, and sudden onset of intense lower-thoracic pleuritic pain, is usually due to Coxsackie B viruses.

Other causes of chest pain include *costochondritis* (Tietze's syndrome), which is an anterior localized pain associated with tenderness over one or more costochondral junctions; *herpes zoster,* which commonly causes unilateral aching or itching, limited to one dermatome, which may precede by several days the eruption of vesicles; *rib fracture or bone metastases,* which are more chronic and pleuritic in nature; and *cervical spine disease* with referred pain to the chest (see Chapter 64). Acute stabbing chest pain can occur with a *spontaneous pneumothorax,* which occurs primarily in young men or in older patients with obstructive pulmonary disease. Often, a small (less than 20%) pneumothorax is not accompanied by significant dyspnea in otherwise healthy individuals. Pleuritic chest pain associated with *PE* results from infarction of parenchymal lung tissue with irritation of the parietal pleura and is almost always associated with dyspnea; and in most patients, the chest x-ray will show an infiltrate. The pain associated with *pulmonary hypertension* is heavy and aching and often similar to that of cardiac ischemia (see Chapter 57). *GI disorders,* such as reflux esophagitis or gastric or duodenal ulcer, are usually distinguished from cardiopulmonary chest pain by their association with eating and by their relief by antacids (Chapters 35 and 37).

Evaluation

Many common causes of noncardiac chest pain can be diagnosed by a thorough history and physical examination. Because discrete anatomic structures must be involved to cause noncardiac chest pain, the physical examination is more useful in the diagnosis of noncardiac chest pain than in the diagnosis of dyspnea and hemoptysis. Inspection of the chest wall may reveal the characteristic unilateral eruption of herpes zoster along a dermatome. Light palpation over the chest wall elicits pain and crepitus from fractured ribs. Mild pressure over the costochondral junctions anteriorly reproduces the pain of Tietze's syndrome. (In general, cardiac pain is not worsened by pressure over the chest wall.) In pneumonia or pulmonary infarction a distinct friction rub can be heard directly over the specific area of chest pain. With pericardial involvement a friction rub that varies with respiration or with the cardiac cycle is usually present. A thorough abdominal examination is important because diseases involving the abdominal visceral organs can cause referred chest pain that is indistinguishable from that produced by involvement of the thoracic structures. Often, laboratory studies and a chest x-ray will not be necessary for the diagnosis of these common causes of chest pain.

Therapy

The treatment of chest pain requires therapy of the underlying disease process, as well as analgesic drugs for the pain itself. Tracheal irritation is limited to the duration of the viral illness but can be treated by cough suppression and bronchodilators (see "Cough," above). Tietze's syndrome is treated with standard anti-inflammatory agents and heat. Although the pain of herpes zoster is often severe, it may be controlled with mild narcotics such as codeine, 30 to 60 mg every 4 to 6 hours. The chest pain experienced in pulmonary hypertension often does not respond to treatment with nonnarcotic analgesics, and narcotics may be required if the hypertension does not improve with treatment.

Pleuritic pain in patients with pneumonia or PE responds to specific therapy of the inflammatory process. Nevertheless, narcotics may be needed to reduce splinting of the chest wall and thereby to prevent atelectasis. Codeine (60 mg every 4 hours) is usually adequate therapy.

THE ABNORMAL CHEST X-RAY

A chest x-ray must always be compared with prior films because an abnormality that has been stable in size for more than 2 years is almost certainly benign and may not require further evaluation. Also, depending on the appearance of the abnormality and the patient's age, the most appropriate plan may be observation with serial chest x-ray.

Specific Patterns Indicative of an Abnormal Chest X-Ray

This section reviews common abnormalities that indicate the presence of pulmonary disease that requires further evaluation.

Air Bronchogram

Normally, bronchi beyond the mainstem division cannot be seen; however, when the alveoli surrounding a bronchus are devoid of air because of consolidation, or less commonly, collapse, an air bron-

chogram (Fig. 54.1) can be seen. The presence of an air bronchogram indicates an alveolar filling process and is most commonly seen in pneumonia and pulmonary edema (cardiogenic and noncardiogenic). However, an air bronchogram is not present in every consolidated lung because bronchi may fill with secretions or exudate. Therefore its absence is less significant than its presence.

Silhouette Sign

The obliteration on a chest x-ray of the margin of a normally opaque structure in the chest by an abnormal pulmonary density is called the silhouette sign. If the physician has knowledge of thoracic anatomy and of spatial relations, the silhouette sign can be used to localize abnormalities within the lung parenchyma. Edges of organs that are in contact with parenchymal infiltrates will be obliterated because the normal air interface is eliminated. On the other hand, intrathoracic lesions that are not anatomically contiguous will not interfere with the outlines of nearby structures. For example, obliteration of the cardiac border, an anterior structure, localizes an abnormality to the right middle lobe or the lingular segment of the left upper lobe (Fig. 54.2). In contrast, an infiltrate that overlaps but does not obliterate the cardiac border is posterior and represents a lower lobe lesion. Lower lobe abnormalities obliterate diaphragmatic borders and on the lateral chest x-ray are seen as an increased density over the vertebrae (spine sign). Obliteration of the left border of the aortic knob, a posterior structure, occurs with lesions in the apical posterior segment of the left upper lobe whereas obliteration of the ascending aorta, an anterior structure, occurs with lesions in the anterior segment of the right upper lobe.

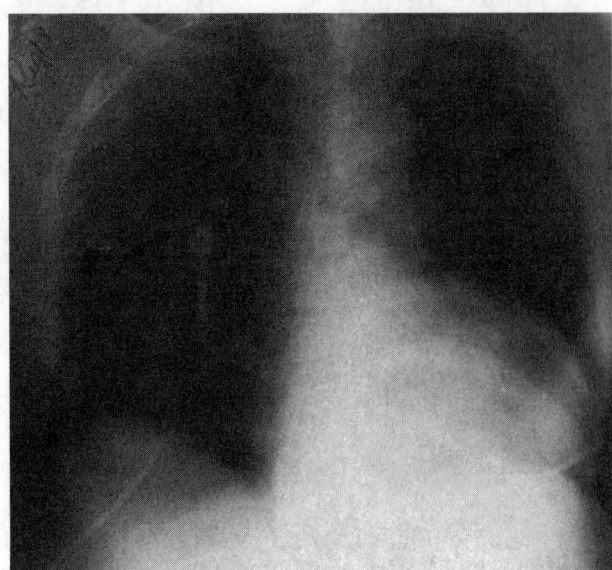

Figure 54.1. Air bronchogram. The patient had fever and sputum production; the initial x-ray demonstrates a branching air bronchogram seen behind the heart on the left, which is consistent with a lower-lobe infiltrate.

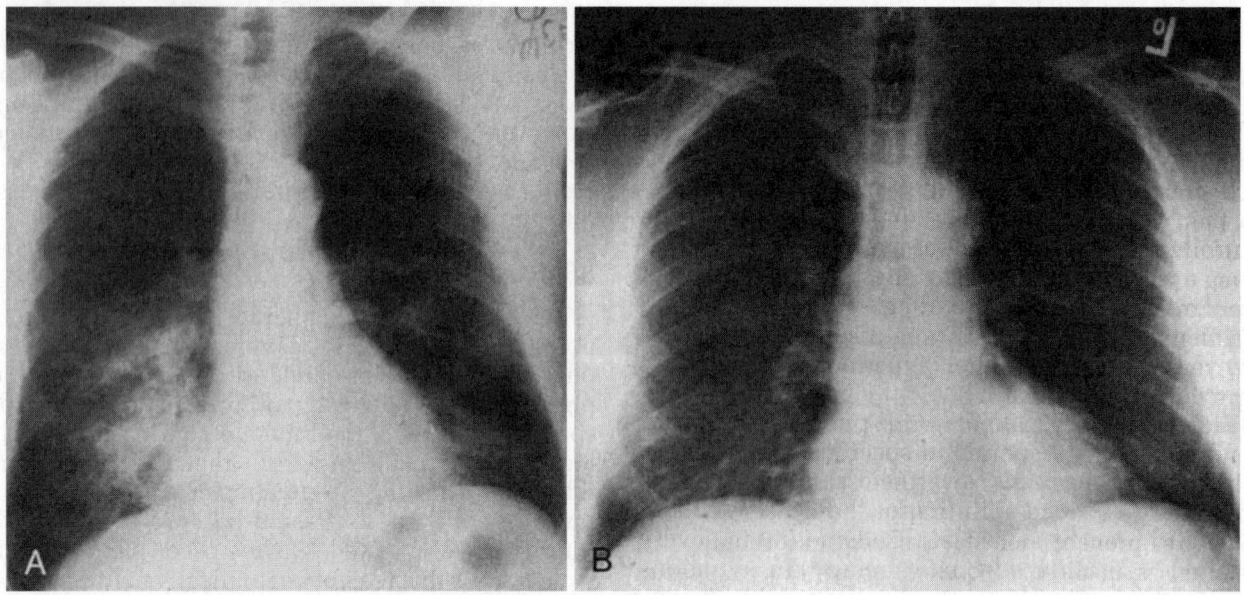

Figure 54.2. Silhouette sign. In this figure, a middle lobe infiltrate obscures the border of the heart **(A).** A previous x-ray is shown for comparison **(B).**

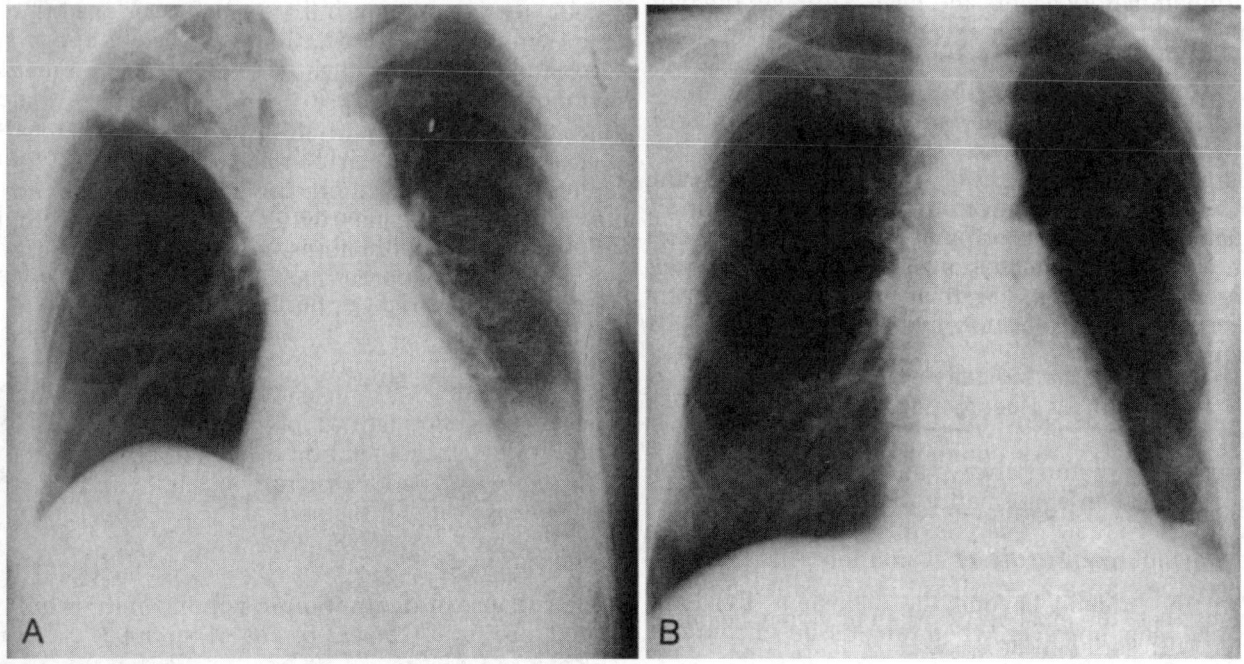

Figure 54.3. Collapse. This demonstrates collapse of the right upper lobe and partial collapse of the left lower lobe in a patient complaining of cough and increased sputum **(A).** The middle lobe fissure is displaced upward and there is blunting of the left hemidi-

aphragm. Note that there is no air bronchogram in either collapsed segment. Aggressive physical therapy was initiated, and within 24 hours, there is resolution of the collapse on the right and almost complete resolution on the left **(B).**

Collapse

The collapse (Fig. 54.3) or diminution in volume of the whole lung, a lobe, or a segment of one of the lobes can be an important clue to the presence of asymptomatic pulmonary disease, such as bronchogenic carcinoma, or it may be the cause of a symptom, such as dyspnea in an asthmatic patient with mucous plugging. The primary mechanisms that cause pulmonary

collapse are *bronchial obstruction* from either an intrinsic bronchial mass or an extrinsic or intrinsic stenosis of the bronchus, *compression of the lung* from a large pleural effusion or from a pneumothorax, *peripheral bronchial plugging* with subsequent pulmonary collapse, and *contraction of the lung* secondary to chronic inflammatory disease. The signs of collapse are related to anatomic landmarks within the lung and are manifested by displacement of the fissure in the lung, loss of aeration within the pulmonary parenchyma, and crowding of the vascular and bronchial lung markings. Other signs that suggest collapse reflect the secondary effects of loss of lung volume such as elevation of the diaphragm, shift of the mediastinal structures toward the collapsed area, diminution of the size of a hemithorax, compensatory hyperinflation, hilar displacement, and tracheal deviation. These latter signs are much more difficult to interpret in patients with underlying lung disease, in whom many of these signs may exist in the absence of collapse.

Septal Markings

Normally, lung markings reflect vascular patterns within the pulmonary parenchyma and are rarely due to the bronchi or the lymphatics. Three types of linear shadows represent septal markings within the lung: *Kerley A lines,* thin nonbranching lines several inches long radiating from the hilum that appear to cross blood vessels; *Kerley B lines* (Fig. 54.4), up to 1 inch in length, found at the lateral lung bases, on the posteroanterior film or in the retrosternal clear space on the lateral film, radiating from the pleura; and *Kerley C lines,* fine interlacing structures throughout the lung parenchyma

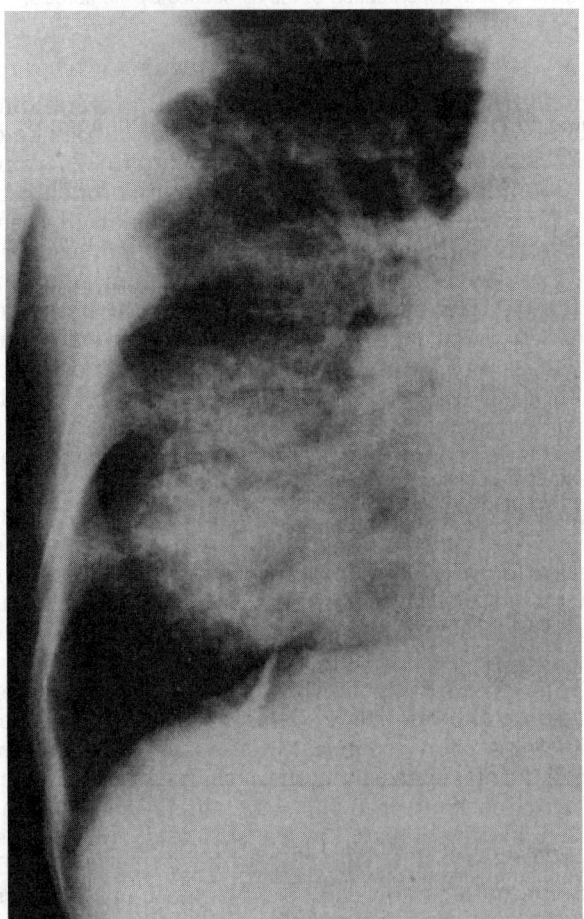

Figure 54.4. Kerley B lines. A close view of the right lower lung in a patient with congestive heart failure demonstrates horizontal linear lines that run to the edge of the lung.

that produce a spiderweb appearance. The fine linear or reticular pattern represented by Kerley's lines are specific for interstitial lung disease. The most common cause of these lines is interstitial edema caused by congestive heart failure.

Common Problems in Patients with Abnormal Chest X-Rays

In this section, three general categories are discussed in which the chest x-ray provides the basis for diagnosis and further evaluation. A general approach is outlined, including the initial evaluation that should be completed by the physician before referral to a pulmonary specialist or a thoracic surgeon. Often, this diagnostic evaluation can be completed in an ambulatory setting.

Infiltrates

Infiltrates represent alveolar or interstitial lung disease and seldom show borders except at pleural surfaces. They may be radiographically separated into diffuse and focal infiltrates. *Diffuse* implies bilateral generalized involvement, if not of the entire lungs, then at least most of both lung fields. *Focal* implies discrete lesions that may or may not be bilateral but that have intervening normal lung tissue between the localized lesions.

Alveolar. *Alveolar infiltrates* (Fig. 54.5A) can be recognized by their fluffy margins, their coalescence into rosette formations, their occasional butterfly configuration involving hilar and central lung zones, and the presence of air bronchograms or air alveolograms.

Although there are numerous causes of diffuse interstitial pulmonary disease, there are a few causes of diffuse alveolar lung disease. Therefore the distinction between an alveolar and an interstitial process is important. Unfortunately, it is not always possible to distinguish between the two entities and there may be a combination of both. Moreover, a disorder that begins as an interstitial process can often merge into an alveolar process, such as interstitial edema in early congestive heart failure progressing to florid pulmonary edema.

The causes of *diffuse alveolar pulmonary disease* of the lung are shown in Table 54.7. The three most common causes are *infection, edema,* and *hemorrhage,* and they are characterized by rapid progression and regression. In contrast, diffuse interstitial disease develops more slowly. Therefore the time course for the development of pulmonary symptoms and roentgenographic abnormalities is an important aspect in the differential diagnosis of diffuse lung disease.

Interstitial. An *interstitial pattern* may be primarily linear (reticular) or may consist of multiple, discrete, noncoalescent round nodules, 1 to 5 mm in diameter (Fig. 54.5B). Although there can be a summation effect, these small nodular densities retain a distinct identity in comparison to the larger, fluffier infiltrates characteristic of alveolar disease. In certain disease processes, such as tuberculosis, histoplasmosis, or healed viral pneumonia, these nodules may

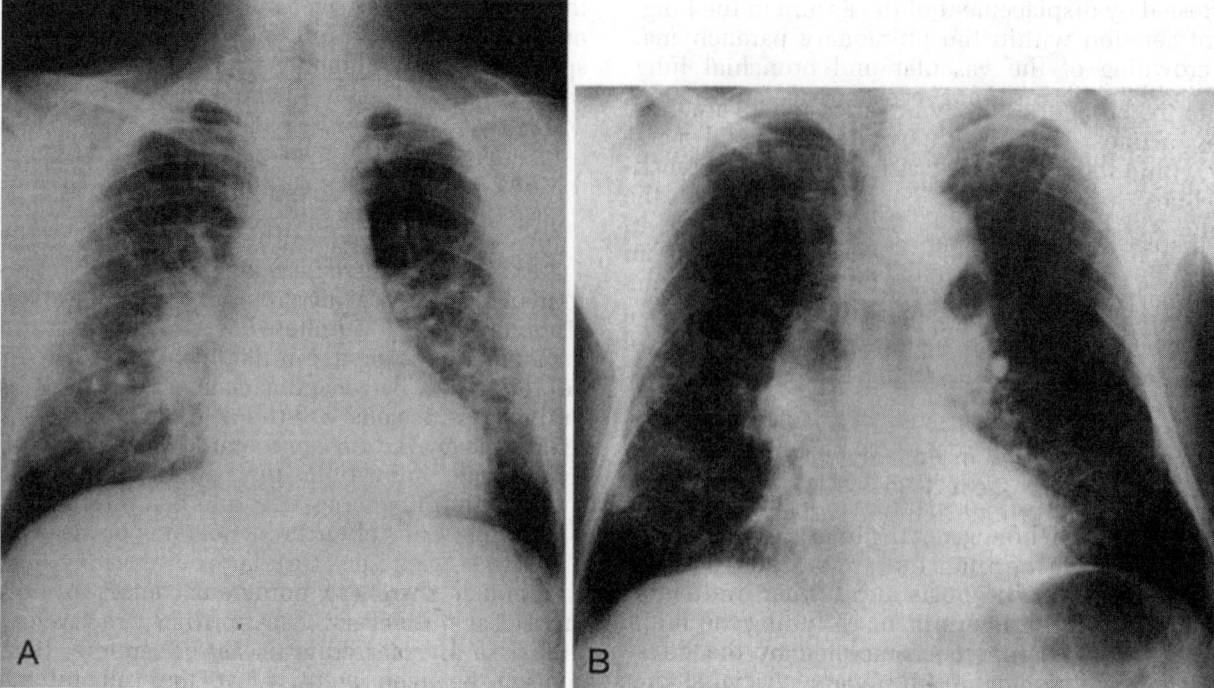

Figure 54.5. **A.** Alveolar patterns. This patient has progressive dyspnea after inhaling fumes from an automobile accident. Compared to **B,** little air is visible in the infiltrate because fluid is filling the alveoli. **B.** Interstitial pattern. This demonstrates bilateral interstitial infiltrates in a patient with progressive dyspnea and with fibrosis on biopsy. Compared to **A,** there is a lacy reticular appearance with accentuation of the air spaces by the fibrosis.

Table 54.7.   Causes of Diffuse Alveolar Pulmonary Disease

Disorder	Common	Uncommon
Infection (pus)	Pneumonia	
Edema (fluid)	Cardiac and non-cardiac	
	Pulmonary edema	
Hemorrhage (blood)		Anticoagulation, trauma, hemoptysis, Goodpasture's syndrome, idiopathic pulmonary hemosiderosis
Cells		Bronchoalveolar cell cancer, lymphoma, sarcoidosis, eosinophilic granuloma, pulmonary eosinophilic disorders
Foreign material		Lipoid pneumonia
Protein		Alveolar proteinosis

calcify and thus appear more dense. *Honeycombing* is seen in advanced interstitial lung disease and represents end-stage irreversible scarring with thickened or dilated airways. It can be identified on a chest x-ray as round or oval irregular air spaces that have a reasonably uniform diameter of 1 to 10 mm and are arranged in weblike bunches, thus giving the impression of a honeycomb. Honeycombing is seen in a variety of fibrosing lung diseases, including idiopathic pulmonary fibrosis, sarcoidosis, asbestosis, chronic hyper-

sensitivity pneumonitis, and eosinophilic granuloma. Bilateral interstitial infiltrates in the lower lung fields are a commonly seen radiographic pattern. The most common diagnoses with this pattern are bronchiectasis, chronic aspiration, collagen vascular diseases, asbestosis, sarcoidosis, or idiopathic pulmonary fibrosis. Localized interstitial processes often represent residues of prior pulmonary infections. If new, they may represent acute processes such as mycoplasma pneumonia or lymphangitic spread of carcinoma.

Although interstitial lung disease can be idiopathic, this is a diagnosis of exclusion; and the primary goal in the evaluation is to determine whether a treatable disease is present (Table 54.8). The initial medical history, physical examination, and laboratory testing should be oriented toward evaluating the patient for the presence of sarcoidosis, pulmonary involvement associated with collagen vascular disease, granulomatous lung infection (mycobacterium, fungus), or pneumoconiosis secondary to occupational exposure (see Chapter 7). Additional testing often includes complete pulmonary function testing (spirometry, lung volumes, diffusing capacity, room air arterial blood gas measurement), formal cardiopulmonary exercise testing, chest CT, and fiberoptic bronchoscopy with lavage and transbronchial lung biopsy. The transbronchial lung biopsy is often useful in diagnosing and guiding therapy in patients with sarcoidosis, lymphangitic spread of tumor, infectious disease, collagen vascular pulmonary diseases, and idiopathic pulmonary fibrosis. If the tissue obtained with transbronchial biopsy is inadequate for diagnosis, consultation with a thoracic surgeon for a surgical lung biopsy (video assisted thoracoscopy or open lung biopsy) may be indicated.

Slowly Resolving or Recurrent Infiltrates. *Endobronchial tumor* must be considered in patients who have a slowly resolving pneumonia. Most patients with community-acquired pneumonia respond rapidly to antibiotic therapy, and their chest x-ray will return to baseline over 2 to 4 weeks (see Chapter 28). In one study, radiographic resolution of pneumonia was inversely related to age and was delayed in smokers, patients with multilobar infiltrates, and in hospitalized patients (24). Patients with chronic obstructive lung disease (see Chapter 55) who have difficulty mobilizing their bronchial secretions and patients with superimposed congestive heart failure or with necrotizing or multilobar pneumonia may have pulmonary infiltrates that persist for 4 to 5 months. If a patient shows symptomatic improvement and slow but progressive roentgenographic clearing, observation is warranted. If roentgenographic abnormalities persist and the patient fails to show clinical improvement or if the pulmonary infiltrate is found in an asymptomatic individual, further evaluation to exclude lung cancer is warranted (see Chapter 56). In contrast to an older patient, a younger patient with recurrent sinopulmonary infections should be suspected of having an abnormal host defense such as cystic fibrosis or an immunoglobulin deficiency state, which may escape detection until adolescence or early adulthood. In addition, an undiagnosed immunodeficiency such as AIDS should be considered if a patient with a presumed community acquired pneumonia fails to respond to appropriate antibiotics (see Chapter 34).

Older patients with *recurrent pneumonias* should also be evaluated for the possibility of lung cancer (36). In evaluating patients with recurrent pneumonia, it is essential to review previous chest x-rays to document the anatomic location and the characteristics of the recurrent pulmonary infiltrate. In general, if a pneumonia recurs in multiple lobes or in pulmonary segments that are unrelated anatomically, bronchogenic carcinoma is unlikely. For example, a recurrent pneumonia that initially involves the right upper lobe and subsequently the right lower lobe is unlikely to be the result of a single endobronchial tumor. In addition to the anatomic location, the time during which recurrent pneumonias have occurred should be considered. If the interval is more than 2 years, malignancy is unlikely.

Apical. Often, roentgenographic patterns that range from increased pulmonary markings or minor scarring to cystic or cavitary disease in the upper lobes will be interpreted by a radiologist as showing old granulomatous disease or active tuberculous infection. The evaluation of these patients includes questioning about previous tuberculous lung disease (including the type and duration of antituberculous therapy) and an assessment of the reactivity of the tuberculin skin test. Comparison with prior chest x-rays is useful because the activity of an infiltrate cannot be determined from an isolated chest x-ray. If old chest x-rays demonstrate that no change has occurred, further evaluation may be unnecessary. The evaluation and treatment of patients with tuberculosis are discussed in Chapter 29.

Superior sulcus tumors, usually squamous cell carcinomas, arise in the extreme apex of the lung and may be difficult to distinguish from pleural thickening or old granulomatous disease. Later in the disease course, x-rays may reveal erosion of adjacent ribs or vertebrae by the tumor (see Chapter 56).

Pleural Effusion

Small amounts of free fluid within the pleural space will obliterate the costophrenic or costocardiac angles. Because the density of pleural fluid is greater than the density of the lung, a subpulmonic collection will laterally displace the crest of the diaphragm (Fig. 54.6A). An increased density between the stomach gas bubble and pulmonary tissue may also indicate the presence of fluid within the pleural space. The diagnosis of a large pleural effusion is not difficult because fluid within the pleural space on an upright chest x-ray will form a concave density across the chest cavity; decubitus x-rays will demonstrate free

Table 54.8.   Causes of Diffuse Interstitial Pulmonary Disease

Disorder	Common	Uncommon
Known Causes		
Cardiovascular	Early heart failure	
Infection	Atypical and viral pneumonia, *Pneumocystis* infection	Miliary tuberculosis, fungal pneumonia
Collagen vascular disease		Scleroderma, rheumatoid arthritis, systemic lupus erythematosus
Occupational (*Pneumoconiosis*)		Asbestosis, silicosis, coal miner's pneumoconiosis
Hypersensitivity and drug reactions		Hypersensitivity pneumonitis, nitrofurantoin, cytotoxic drugs
Physical agents		Radiation
Neoplastic		Lymphoma, lymphangitic spread of tumor
Unknown Causes		
	Sarcoidosis	Idiopathic pulmonary fibrosis, eosinophilic granuloma, lymphocytic interstitial pneumonitis

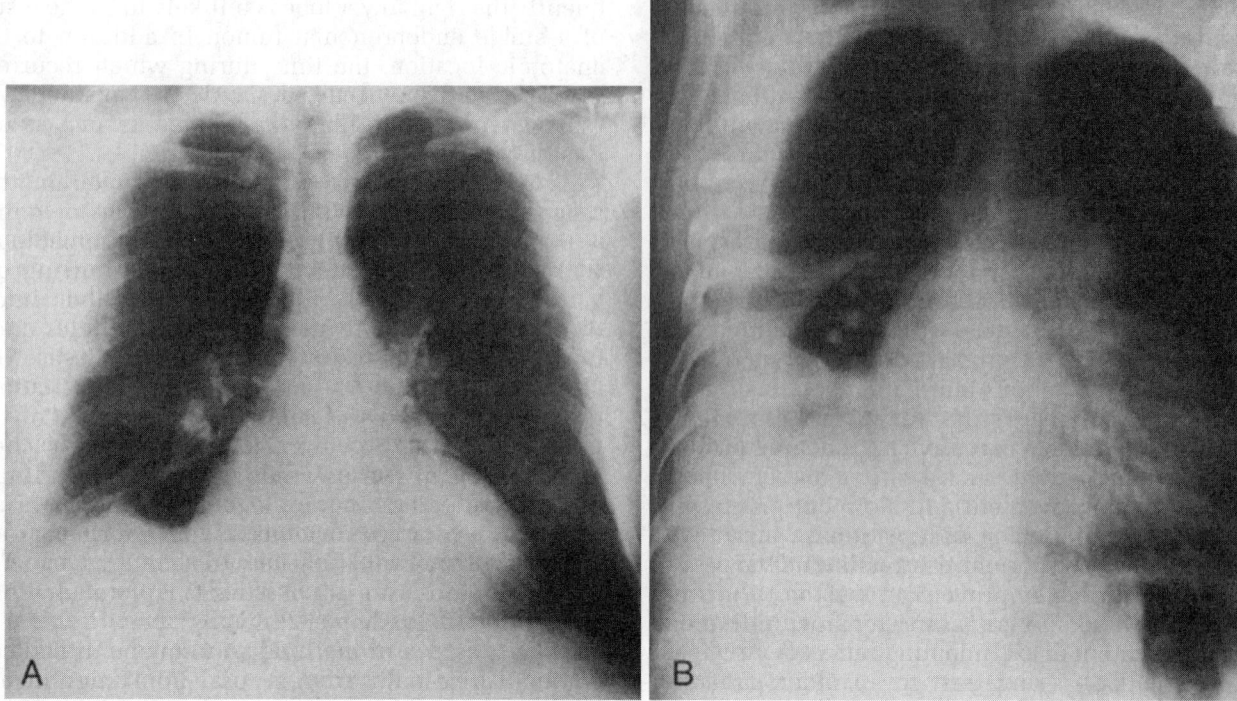

Figure 54.6. Subpulmonic effusion. The diaphragm appears to be elevated on the right **(A).** This represents subpulmonic fluid; when the patient is placed in the right lateral decubitus position **(B),** fluid layers on the right and tracks in the minor fissure and along the apex and the diaphragm.

flowing pleural fluid in the dependent hemithorax (Fig. 54.6B). If the patient is recumbent, the pleural fluid will layer over the entire hemithorax, causing the lung to appear opaque.

In general, when pleural effusion is seen on a chest x-ray, a sample should be obtained for analysis. The obvious exception is a patient who develops acute pulmonary edema associated with a rapidly developing pleural effusion that resolves with therapy for congestive heart failure (see Chapter 61). The causes of pleural effusion are listed in Table 54.9. A diagnostic thoracentesis to determine the cause of the effusion can generally be done when the thickness of the fluid between the inner border of the rib and lung is more than 1 cm on a lateral decubitus x-ray. The fluid should be sent for white blood cell and differential count, total protein concentration, lactate dehydrogenase (LDH) concentration, glucose concentration, Gram's stain, cultures (aerobic and anaerobic bacteria, mycobacterium, fungus), and cytopathology (if malignancy is suspected). Most pleural effusions are clear and straw colored, and deviations from this norm this may be diagnostically helpful. For example, a bloody effusion suggests tumor, and less commonly, PE with infarction, tuberculosis, or trauma; a lime-green effusion suggests tuberculosis; a white milky effusion suggests a chylous exudate; and a viscous fluid with feculent odor strongly suggests an anaerobic empyema.

It is important to classify pleural effusion as either transudative or exudative. *Transudates,* caused by in-creased hydrostatic pressure or decreased plasma oncotic pressure have low protein and LDH concentration and are generally due to congestive heart failure, cirrhosis with ascites, or nephrotic syndrome. They do not require further diagnostic evaluation, and treatment is directed at the underlying cause. *Exudates,* due to increased protein permeability of the pleural blood vessels, are generally caused by inflammation or tumor infiltration. Exudates are defined by one of the following criteria: *(a)* pleural fluid protein concentration that is greater than 50% of the concentration of serum protein, *(b)* pleural fluid LDH concentration that is greater than 60% of the concentration of serum LDH, or *(c)* pleural fluid LDH concentration that is greater than 67% of the upper limit of normal serum LDH (22). Pleural effusions with protein concentrations greater than 3 g/100 mL are nearly always exudates. A cell count and pleural fluid cytologic study should be performed because the presence of polymorphonuclear leukocytes in pleural fluid suggests acute inflammation and infection, whereas more than 50% lymphocytes suggests tuberculosis or malignancy. The presence of more than 5% pleural mesothelial cells makes the diagnosis of tuberculosis unlikely. Low pleural fluid glucose concentration (less than 50 mg/dL) occurs in infections (parapneumonic, tuberculosis), rheumatoid arthritis, and occasionally malignancy. If a pleural effusion is bloody or appears infected, the patient should be hospitalized for further diagnostic studies and therapy (e.g., pleural biopsy, chest tube drainage).

Pneumothorax

There are three major types of pneumothorax: spontaneous, iatrogenic, and traumatic. Of these, the general physician is most commonly faced with a spontaneous pneumothorax either in a young healthy individual or in an older patient with underlying pulmonary disease. In the former, a subpleural apical bleb ruptures into the pleural space, causing varying amounts of air to collect. Patients with spontaneous pneumothoraces tend to be tall, thin young male smokers (21). These patients generally are at rest when they first experience symptoms. In the older patient, emphysema with concomitant bullous disease is commonly associated with a pneumothorax (Fig. 54.7). The abrupt onset of pleuritic chest pain or dyspnea is characteristic. Pneumothoraces are diagnosed by demonstrating a visceral pleural line on the chest x-ray.

After the diagnosis of pneumothorax is made, the patient may need observation (ambulatory or inpatient) or insertion of a chest tube. Needle aspiration to expand the lung is discouraged because further laceration can occur. In general, patients with underlying lung disease should be hospitalized and may require a chest tube because of their limited pulmonary reserve. On the other hand, a healthy patient with a small pneumothorax (less than 15%) who is not in distress may remain at home and be followed by serial chest x-rays. The rate of reabsorption is slow; assuming approximately 1.25% of the volume is reabsorbed per day (21), a 15% pneumothorax will take approximately 12 days to reabsorb spontaneously.

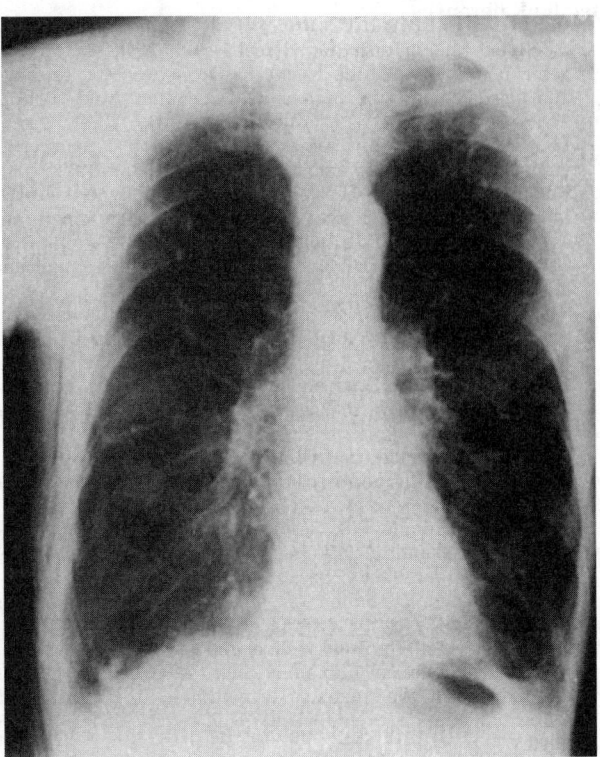

Figure 54.7. Pneumothorax. If the x-ray is not carefully examined, the pneumothorax in the right lower lung can easily be missed. Note the widespread bullae throughout the lung.

Solitary Nodule

A solitary nodule is a radiologic finding that always requires evaluation. A detailed discussion of the problem is to be found in Chapter 56.

Table 54.9.   Causes of Pleural Effusion

Effusion	Effusion	Effusion
Transudate	CHF Cirrhosis, nephrosis	Pericardial disease Myedema, peritoneal dialysis
Exudate		
Malignancy	Metastatic disease (solid tumors)	Lymphoma, mesothelioma
Infection	Bacterial (parapneumonia) and empyema), tuberculosis	Atypical pneumonias, fungal, viral, parasites (amebiasis, paragonimiasis)
Trauma Gastrointestinal	Hemothorax	Chylothorax Pancreatitis, esophageal rupture, subphrenic abscess
Collagen vascular disease		Systemic lupus erythematosus, rheumatoid arthritis
Miscellaneous		Pulmonary infarction, benign asbestos effusion, drug hypersensitivity, postmyocardial infarction syndrome, uremia, trapped lung, lymphatic abnormalities

General References*

Felson B, Weinstein AS, Spitz HB. Principles of chest roentgenology. Philadelphia: WB Saunders, 1965.
> A programmed text on the fundamentals of reading a chest x-ray.

George RB, Light RW, Matthay MA, Matthay RA. Chest medicine. Essentials of pulmonary and critical care medicine. 3rd ed. Baltimore: Williams & Wilkins, 1995.
> Concise complete general textbook of pulmonary medicine.

Irwin RS, Curley FJ. The treatment of cough. A comprehensive review. Chest 99:1477, 1991.
> A thorough review by a leader in the field.

Jones NL, Campbell EJ. Clinical exercise testing. 2nd ed. Philadelphia: WB Saunders, 1982.
> The standard text on this subject.

Reed JC. Chest radiology. Plain film patterns and differential diagnoses. 4th ed. St. Louis: Mosby-Year Book, 1997.
> A thorough textbook that gives a discussion and comprehensive differential diagnosis of common radiographic patterns of chest disease.

Tapson VF, Fulkerson WJ, Saltzman HA. Venous thromboembolism. Clin Chest Med 16(2):229–387, 1995.
> Up-to-date monograph on epidemiology, pathophysiology, diagnosis, and treatment.

*Bold print (general references) and bold numerals (specific references) denote published controlled clinical trials, meta-analyses, or consensus-based recommendations.

Specific References

1. Adelman M, Haponik EF, Bleecker ER, Britt EJ. Cryptogenic hemoptysis: clinical features, bronchoscopic findings, and natural history in 67 patients. Ann Intern Med 102:829, 1985.

2. Bell WR, Simon TL, DeMets DL. The clinical features of submassive pulmonary emboli. Am J Med 62:355, 1977.

3. Bucknall CE, Neilly JB, Carter R, et al. Bronchial hyperreactivity in patients who cough after receiving angiotensin converting enzyme inhibitors. BMJ 296:86–88, 1988.

4. Cahill BC, Ingbar DH. Massive hemoptysis: assessment and management. Clin Chest Med 15:147, 1994.

5. Clee MD, Sinclair DJM. Assessment of factors influencing the result of sputum cytology in bronchial carcinoma. Thorax 36:143, 1981.

6. Corey R, Hla KM. Major and massive hemoptysis: reassessment of conservative management. Am J Med Sci 294:301–309, 1987.

7. Corrao WM, Braman SS, Irwin RS. Chronic cough as the sole presenting manifestation of bronchial asthma. N Engl J Med 300:633, 1977.

8. Croughan-Minihane MS, Petiti DB, Rodnick JE, Eliaser G. Clinical trial examining the effectiveness of three cough syrups. J Am Board Fam Pract 6:109, 1993.

9. Curley FJ, Irwin RS, Pratter MR, et al. Cough and the common cold. Am Rev Respir Dis 138:305, 1988.

10. Dalen JE, Banas JS Jr, Brooks HL, et al. Resolution rate of acute pulmonary embolism in man. N Engl J Med 280:1194, 1969.

11. Dalen J. When can treatment be withheld in patients with suspected pulmonary embolism? Arch Intern Med 153:1415, 1993.

12. DePaso WJ, Winterbauer RH, Lusk JA, et al. Chronic dyspnea unexplained by history, physical examination, chest roentgenogram, and spirometry: analysis of a seven-year experience. Chest 100:1293, 1991.

13. Gefter W, Hatabu H, Holland GA, et al. Pulmonary thromboembolism: recent developments in diagnosis with CT and MR imaging. Radiology 197:561, 1995.

14. Ginsberg JS. Management of venous thromboembolism. N Engl J Med 335:1816, 1996.

15. Goyal RK. Changing focus on unexplained esophageal chest pain. Ann Intern Med 124:1008, 1996.

16. Haponik EF, Britt EJ, Smith PL, et al. Computer chest tomography in the evaluation of hemoptysis. Chest 91:80, 1987.

17. Hull RD, Raskob G, Ginsberg JS, et al. A noninvasive strategy for the treatment of patients with suspected pulmonary embolism. Arch Intern Med 154:289, 1994.

18. Irwin RS, Curley FJ, French CL. Chronic cough: the spectrum and frequency of causes, key components of the diagnostic evaluation, and outcome of specific therapy. Am Rev Respir Dis 141:640, 1990.

19. Kravitz H, Gomberg RM, Burnstine RC, et al. Psychogenic cough tic in children and adolescents. Clin Pediatr 8:580, 1969.

20. Lange P, Stoller J. The hepatopulmonary syndrome. Ann Intern Med 122:521, 1995.

21. Light RW. Management of spontaneous pneumothorax. Am Rev Respir Dis 148:245–248, 1993.

22. Light RW, MacGregor I, Luchsinger PC, Ball WF. Pleural effusions: the diagnostic separation of transudates and exudates. Ann Intern Med 77:507, 1972.

23. Mahler DA, Horowitz MB. Clinical evaluation of exertional dyspnea. Clin Chest Med 15:259, 1994.

24. Mittl RL Jr, Schwab RJ, Duchin JS, et al. Radiographic resolution of community-acquired pneumonia. Am J Respir Crit Care Med 149:630–635, 1994.

25. Moser KM. Pulmonary embolism. In: Murray JF, Nadel JA, eds. Respiratory medicine. 2nd ed. Philadelphia: WB Saunders, 1994.

26. O'Neil KM, et al. Hemoptysis indications for bronchoscopy. Arch Intern Med 151:171, 1991.

27. Poe RH, Harder RV, Israel RH, Kallay MC. Chronic persistent cough. Experience in diagnosis and outcome using an anatomic diagnostic protocol. Chest 95:723, 1989.

28. Poe RH, et al. Utility of FOB in patients with hemoptysis and normal CXR. Br J Dis Chest 81:186, 1987.

29. Savage PJ, Donovan WN, Dellinger RP. Sputum cytology in the management of patients with lung cancer. South Med J 77:840–842, 1984.

30. Shields TW, Ritts RE. Bronchial carcinoma. Springfield, IL: Charles C. Thomas, 1974.

31. Smoller JW, Pollock MH, Otto MW, et al. Panic anxiety, dyspnea, and respiratory disease. Am J Respir Crit Care Med 154:6, 1996.

32. Snider GL. When not to use the bronchoscopy for hemoptysis. Chest 76:1, 1979.

33. Soll B, Selecky PA, Chang R, et al. The use of the fiberoptic bronchoscope in the evaluation of hemoptysis. AARD 15:165, 1978.

34. Szucs MM Jr, Brooks HL, Grossman W, et al. Diagnostic sensitivity of laboratory findings in acute pulmonary embolism. Ann Intern Med 74:161, 1971.

35. The PIOPED Investigators. Value of the ventilation/perfusion scan in acute pulmonary embolism. Results of the prospective investigation of pulmonary embolism diagnosis (PIOPED). JAMA 263:2753, 1990.

36. Winterbauer RH, Bedon GA, Ball WC Jr. Recurrent pneumonia. Predisposing illness and clinical patterns in 158 patients. Ann Intern Med 70:689, 1969.

37. Wynder EL, Kaufman PL, Lesser RL. A short-term follow-up study on ex-cigarette smokers. Am Rev Respir Dis 96:645, 1967.

38. Zavala DC. Diagnostic fiberoptic bronchoscopy: techniques and results of biopsy in 600 patients. Chest 68:12, 1975.

C H A P T E R   55

Obstructive Airways Diseases: Asthma and Chronic Obstructive Pulmonary Disease

ROBERT A. WISE, MD
MARK C. LIU, MD

Obstructive lung diseases are the most common forms of chronic pulmonary disease encountered in ambulatory practice. The most common causes of chronic obstructive lung diseases are *asthma, chronic bronchitis,* and *emphysema.* Less common disorders that lead to chronic obstructive lung disease include bronchiectasis, chronic forms of bronchiolitis, and cystic fibrosis. These disorders have different clinical presentations, causes, pathophysiologies, and prognoses, but all share the same physiologic abnormality—chronic airflow limitation (9).

EPIDEMIOLOGY

Obstructive airways diseases are increasing in prevalence and severity throughout the world. Over the past decade, the prevalence of emphysema and chronic bronchitis in the United States increased by 40%, whereas the prevalence of asthma increased by 20%. Approximately 2.0 million people in the United States have emphysema; 12.6 million have chronic bronchi-

tis; and 10.3 million have asthma. Each year, more than 80,000 deaths are attributed to chronic bronchitis and emphysema, the fourth leading cause of death; 5,000 deaths are caused by asthma, with increasing mortality mainly in women and in inner-city minorities (4). The direct health care costs for chronic bronchitis, emphysema, and asthma are about $3 billion each (4). Between 1979 and 1993, the age-adjusted mortality from chronic obstructive lung disease increased 47%, which is particularly notable because the other five leading causes of death showed a 30% reduction in mortality during this interval (35).

PATHOPHYSIOLOGIC ABNORMALITIES IN OBSTRUCTIVE LUNG DISEASE

The diagnosis, severity, clinical course, and response to treatment can best be established by objective tests of lung function. How these disorders lead to chronic airflow limitation, and how this limitation is measured in the ambulatory patient, are discussed below.

Forced Expiratory Spirometry

Obstructive lung diseases cause the lung to empty slowly during a forced expiratory maneuver. Normal people can forcefully expel all of the air that can leave their lungs (the vital capacity) within 4 to 6 seconds. People with established obstructive lung disease may continue to expire during a forced expiratory maneuver for 10 to 20 seconds or more.

Forced Expiratory Vital Capacity: FVC and FEV_1

The forced expiratory vital capacity (FVC) test is used to diagnose and follow the course of obstructive lung diseases. The test is performed by having the patient blow forcefully into a device that records the volume of air leaving the lungs as a function of time. The record of the maneuver is called a *spirogram,* and the test itself is called forced *expiratory spirometry.* Devices that record the spirogram may either measure flow directly (a pneumotachometer) and calculate volume electronically, or measure volume directly (a spirometer). Many such devices are commercially available and are accurate and reliable, but it is important to ascertain that the devices meet established standards that are promulgated for either screening or diagnostic purposes (8–10,99). More common than inaccurate equipment is the inability of the technician to elicit maximum effort, cooperation, and coordination from the test subject. A good spirometry technician has been likened to a combination of a bully with a cheerleader in obtaining maximal efforts (93). Attention to detail in calibrating the equipment and in measuring the test, experienced judgment in determining which maneuvers represent the subject's true lung function, sensitivity to the test subject, and enthusiastic supportive coaching are important qualities in a successful spirometry technician (6). Excellent texts

Table 55.1.   Indications for Spirometry

Establish diagnosis of obstructive lung disease.
Establish prognosis of obstructive lung disease.
Evaluate acute bronchodilator response.
Evaluate response to treatment.
Measure physiologic impairment for disability rating.
Evaluate thoracic and nonthoracic surgical risk.

Table 55.2.   Criteria for Good Spirometry Session

At least three technically acceptable maneuvers
  Rapid start of expiration
  Continuous effort without hesitation or coughing
  Prolonged effort until plateau (at least 6 seconds)
At least two reproducible maneuvers
  FEV_1 and FVC within 5% or 200 mL of highest value

are available on spirometry testing in the ambulatory setting (51). Anyone caring for patients with obstructive lung diseases should have ready access to spirometry. General indications for spirometry are listed in Table 55.1.

The *forced expiratory maneuver* is performed by having the patient take a maximal inspiration and then forcefully blow all of the air into the spirometer. A technically satisfactory maneuver is one that has a rapid onset, has a smooth contour without hesitation or coughing, and is prolonged until airflow ceases, with a minimum duration of 6 seconds. The test is repeated until three technically satisfactory maneuvers are obtained, two of which give reproducible measurements. Reproducible measurements are defined as being within 5% of each other or within 200 mL, whichever is greater (Table 55.2).

Many measures can be derived from the forced expiratory spirogram, but the most useful are the total amount of air leaving the lung, the FVC; the amount of air leaving the lung in the first second, the FEV_1; and the percentage of total air that leaves the lung in the first second, the FEV_1/FVC ratio or FEV_1%. The volume measures are expressed as absolute values adjusted to reflect the volume of gas at body temperature with 100% humidity (BTPS). The FEV_1 and FVC are compared to predicted values based on age, gender, race, and height from a healthy reference population, usually as a percent of predicted (7). Airflow limitation is said to exist when the FEV_1% is reduced below the value found in 95% of healthy nonsmokers (Table 55.3) (40). The severity of airflow obstruction is determined by the reduction in FEV_1. Because diseases of airflow limitation also cause increased trapping of gas in the lung at the end of a forced expiration, FVC commonly is reduced as well. This should not, however, be confused with disorders that are associated with small lungs, the *restrictive lung diseases* (see Chapter 54). Despite the low FVC, the maximum gas volume of the lung—the *total lung capacity (TLC)* (see below)—is usually increased in patients with obstructive disease. Typically, restrictive lung diseases cause an increase in FEV_1/FVC ratio

in combination with a reduced FVC (Table 55.4 and Fig. 55.1).

The degree to which airflow limitation can be reversed rapidly can be measured by performing spirometry before and after treatment with an inhaled bronchodilator. Normally, the increase in FEV_1 is less than 12% of the baseline value; and the increase in FVC, less than 15%. Although this test is helpful in determining the potential for improvement when there is a rapid response to inhaled bronchodilators, many patients without a rapid response show improvement after several weeks or months of treatment with bronchodilators or anti-inflammatory agents.

Patient Experience. Forced expiratory spirometry can be safely and accurately performed on people with normal lung function as well as those with advanced lung disease, even those who are critically ill. After a nose clip is attached, the patient inspires deeply and then forcefully expires for about 6 seconds. Because of the high intrathoracic pressures generated, patients occasionally experience light-headedness during the maneuver. This can be minimized by having the patient sit during the test. Some patients experience soreness of the chest wall or abdomen for a day or two after the test, although analgesics are rarely needed.

Flow-Volume Loops

Forced expiratory airflow is high during the initial part of expiration and gradually falls to zero throughout the course of the maneuver. The forced expiratory maneuver then can be plotted as flow in relation to volume. If this is also done during a forced inspiration, the resultant display is called a flow-volume loop. Flow-volume loops can be readily calculated and displayed with small computers attached to flow or volume measuring devices. The flow-volume loop does

Table 55.3.   Predicted Normal and Lower Limits of Normal FEV_1/FVC Ratio for 68″ Tall Person

Age (Years)	Men		Women	
	Predicted (%)	Lower Limit Normal (%)	Predicted (%)	Lower Limit Normal (%)
20	85.0	76.7	86.7	77.6
30	83.5	75.2	84.1	75.1
40	82.0	73.7	81.6	72.6
50	80.4	72.2	79.1	70.0
60	78.9	70.6	76.6	67.5
70	77.4	69.1	74.1	65.0
80	75.9	67.6	71.5	62.5

Adapted from Crapo RO, Morris AH, Gardner RM. Reference spirometric values using techniques and equipment that meet ATS recommendations. Am Rev Respir Dis 123:659, 1981.

Table 55.4.   Interpretation of Spirometry

Ventilatory Defect	FEV_1	FVC	FEV_1/FVC
Obstructive	Decreased	Normal or decreased	Decreased
Restrictive	Decreased	Decreased	Normal or increased

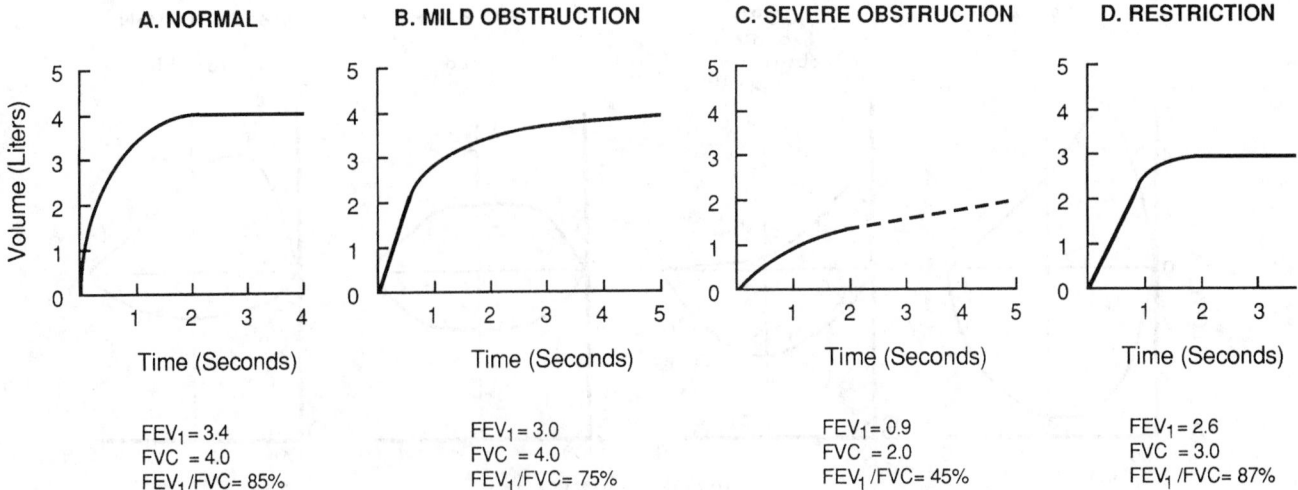

Figure 55.1. Spirographic tracings of forced expiration. Exhaled volume is plotted against time. The forced vital capacity (FVC) is represented by the total volume expired. One-second forced expiratory volume (FEV$_1$) is the volume of air expired during the first second. **A.** Normal spirogram. **B.** Spirogram from a patient with mild obstructive airways disease. **C.** Spirogram from a patient with severe obstructive defect. If the spirogram were incorrectly terminated after 2 seconds, the FVC would be artificially reduced (see text). When it is performed correctly (dotted lines), it is obvious that there is airway obstruction and that there is no restrictive disease. **D.** Spirogram showing restrictive pulmonary disease (FEV$_1$/FVC is normal but FVC is reduced).

not give information about the presence of obstructive airway disease that is not present in the traditional volume-time tracing of the spirogram, and does not allow the easy hand-measurement of the FEV$_1$ that can be done with the traditional mechanically linked spirometer tracing. The flow-volume loop is useful to detect upper airway disorders that affect the early portions of the forced expiration or that impede forced inspiration, such as laryngeal tumors, tracheal stenosis, or vocal cord paralysis (67) (Fig. 55.2). Because these disorders of the upper airway may mimic the dyspnea and wheezing of obstructive lung diseases and because they are potentially curable, the flow-volume loop can provide important information when the diagnosis is uncertain.

Other Lung Function Tests

Ordinarily, tests of lung function other than spirometry are not feasible to implement in the clinic or office setting, and they require referral to a pulmonary function laboratory. They are mainly helpful in the initial evaluation of patients with lung disease.

Measurement of lung volume by *helium dilution, nitrogen washout,* or *body plethysmography* are helpful tests to establish the diagnosis of obstructive lung disease. The total lung capacity is usually increased (hyperinflation), as is the residual volume (air trapping) in both emphysema and acute asthma. In contrast, restrictive disorders such as sarcoidosis, asbestosis, or interstitial pulmonary fibrosis cause reductions in lung volume. Because helium dilution and nitrogen washout measure lung volume only in units of lung that are well ventilated, they tend to underestimate the true lung volume in people with emphysematous

bullae or acute asthma with air trapping. Body plethysmography, which measures compressible gas volume in the chest, is more accurate in these conditions but, because of the expense and technical difficulty of this measurement, is often unavailable. In most circumstances, the dilution or washout methods provide sufficient accuracy to distinguish obstructive lung diseases from restrictive lung diseases.

Patient Experience (Lung Volume Measurements). With the helium dilution and nitrogen washout methods, the patient quietly breathes either a mixture of helium and oxygen or pure oxygen for 5 to 7 minutes. Because these tests require complete collections of expired gas, the patient must be able to form a tight seal around a mouthpiece. After the resident gas in the lung is measured (functional residual capacity, FRC), the patient must perform two or three slow vital capacity maneuvers for calculation of the subdivisions of lung volume.

With the body plethysmography method, the patient sits in a tightly sealed box, about the size of a telephone booth, and breathes through a mouthpiece. At intervals, the technician closes a shutter on the mouthpiece and instructs the subject to perform a panting maneuver against the closed mouthpiece. The test is safe and painless, although about 1 in 10 people either find the box too confining or are unable to coordinate the panting maneuver. After the resident compressible gas in the lung is measured (thoracic gas volume, TGV), the patient performs several slow vital capacity maneuvers.

Measurement of the *carbon monoxide diffusing capacity (Dco)* by the single-breath method is widely available in pulmonary function laboratories. This test measures the effective area of the alveolar–capillary

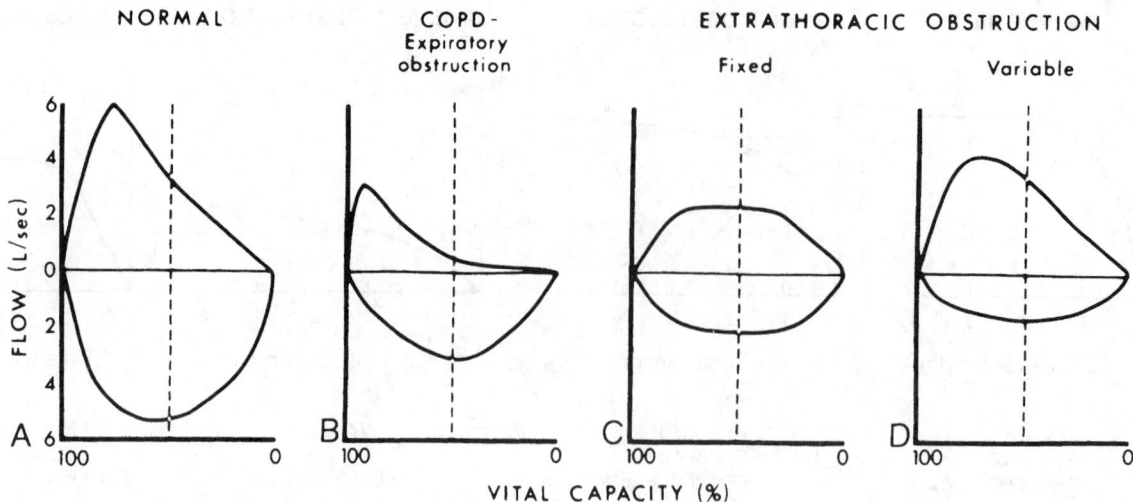

Figure 55.2. Flow-volume curves (loops) of maximal forced expiration (upper) and maximal inspiration (lower). Expiratory and inspiratory flow is plotted against lung volume expressed as a percentage of vital capacity. The dotted line can be used to compare flow rates at 50% of the vital capacity, where inspiratory flow rates normally exceed expiratory flow rates. **A.** Normal flow-volume curves. **B.** Flow-volume curves illustrating expiratory airflow obstruction showing decreased flow rates at all points in lung volume throughout maximal expiration. **C.** Fixed extrathoracic airway obstruction (cancer or stenosis of the larynx) produces a pat- tern where there is a decrease and flattening of both inspiratory and expiratory flow-volume curves. Inspiratory flow rate at 50% of the vital capacity is equal to similar expiratory flow rate. **D.** Variable extrathoracic obstruction (vocal cord paralysis) produces a pattern where there is a decrease and flattening of maximal inspiratory flow-volume curves. Inspiratory flow rates at 50% of the vital capacity are less than similar expiratory flow. (Modified from Hyatt RE, Black LF. The flow-volume curve: a current perspective. Am Rev Respir Dis 107:191, 1973.)

membrane available for gas transfer. Because of the destruction of alveolar septa, the Dco is reduced in emphysema. The magnitude of reduction in Dco is well correlated with the anatomic severity of emphysema, as well as the amount of emphysema found in high-resolution computerized tomographic scans of the chest (23).

Because the Dco is also reduced in diseases that affect the interstitium of the lung (e.g., pulmonary fibrosis and sarcoidosis) and diseases that affect the pulmonary blood vessels (e.g., pulmonary emboli and primary pulmonary hypertension), a reduction in Dco must be evaluated in the context of other lung function tests and clinical findings. Because the Dco is often elevated in asthma, however, it helps determine the degree of reversibility of lung function that can be expected. When the diffusing capacity is below 50 to 60% of the predicted value, about half of the individuals with obstructive lung disease have oxygen desaturation with exercise and may benefit from supplemental oxygen (107). When the Dco exceeds 60% of predicted, oxygen desaturation with exercise is uncommon.

Patient Experience (Diffusing Capacity). The patient takes in a full vital capacity breath of gas containing a small concentration of carbon monoxide and holds his or her breath for 10 seconds. The maneuver is conducted two or three times to obtain reproducible measurements. The amount of carbon monoxide taken up does not cause appreciable increases in carboxyhemoglobin, and the test can be safely performed on patients who are anemic or who have coronary artery disease.

The expired alveolar air is analyzed to determine the rate of uptake of carbon monoxide. Because it requires a 10-second breath-hold and about 1 L of vital capacity to collect an alveolar gas sample effectively, those who are severely dyspneic, who are unable to hold their breath because of problems with cooperation or comprehension, or who have less than 1 L of vital capacity usually cannot perform this maneuver.

Mechanisms of Airflow Limitation

Because the common finding of this group of diseases is a reduction in forced expiratory airflow, it is important to understand the mechanism by which this reduction occurs. During forceful expiration, the pleural pressure rises around both the alveoli and the conducting airways. The pressure in the alveoli is slightly higher than the pleural pressure because the lung has elastic properties that tend to compress the alveolar gas, similar to an inflated latex balloon. This pressure difference between the alveoli and the pleural space is called the *elastic recoil pressure* and is equal to the distending pressure that prevents collapse of the alveolus. During expiration, the pressure near the alveoli is close to alveolar pressure, but falls along the length of the airways because of the airway resistance. As pleural pressure is increased, the expiratory flow increases and the pressure drop along the airway becomes greater. When the pressure in the airway falls below a critical level with respect to the surrounding pleural pressure, the condition of flow limitation occurs. Under the condition of flow limitation, further increases in pleural pressure do not increase airflow. The precise mechanism by which flow limitation occurs is not fully understood, but it has been hypothesized that there is development of a narrowing at a site in the airway that acts like a nozzle or a fluttering of the airway that creates turbulence.

Although it is not understood exactly what occurs at the site of flow limitation in the airway, the general pathophysiologic processes that lead to reduced flows during forced expiration are understood (Table 55.5). Everyone has flow limitation during a forced expiration, but people with obstructive airways diseases demonstrate flow limitation with less effort and at lower airflow. The three lung abnormalities that reduce flow during forced expiration are decreased lung recoil pressure, increased resistance of the airways, and increased tendency of airways to collapse. Decreased lung recoil pressure causes a lower distending pressure between the airway and the surrounding pleural pressure, thereby promoting the tendency of the airways to narrow. Increased resistance of the airways, particularly in the periphery of the lung, causes increased pressure drops along the airways during expiration, promoting the tendency of the airways to narrow. Increased airway collapsibility caused by bronchial smooth muscle constriction, inflammatory products encroaching upon the airway lumen, or decreased tethering of the airway by the alveolar septa also causes airways to collapse more easily.

In general, one can attribute the airflow limitation in *emphysema* to the decreased elastic recoil of the lung; the airflow limitation in *chronic bronchitis* to the increased peripheral airway resistance; and the airflow limitation in *asthma* to the increased tendency of airways to collapse. Although all of these disorders are classified as *obstructive lung diseases,* it must be emphasized that physical obstruction of the airways is not the only mechanism causing reduced forced expiratory flow.

ASTHMA

Definition

Asthma is a disorder characterized symptomatically by cough, chest tightness, shortness of breath, and wheezing associated with limitation of airflow (see above). The symptoms may be acute and episodic or may wax and wane over long periods. One or more of the symptoms may be dominant, but usually all are present. The airflow obstruction is variable and usually, although not always, returns to the normal range

Table 55.5.   Mechanisms of Airflow Limitation

Mechanism	Disease	Anatomic Correlate
Decreased elastic recoil	Emphysema	Destruction of alveolar septa
Increased airway resistance	Chronic bronchitis	Peribronchial fibrosis, mucous gland hyperplasia
Increased airway collapsibility	Asthma	Smooth muscle hyperplasia, submucosal inflammation, mucous plugging of small airways

between exacerbations. Between episodes, most asthmatics are symptom free, but they are susceptible to attacks of wheezing, cough, and chest tightness when exposed to various "triggers." Commonly reported triggers for asthma attacks are shown in Table 55.6. Inflammation of the airways and bronchial hyperreactivity are nearly universally found in asthmatics (66).

About 1 in 20 residents of the United States has asthma, and it is even more common in other developed countries. About half of the asthmatics in the United States have onset of the disease during childhood. In the prepubertal age group, the disease is more common in males, whereas the reverse is true for adults. About half of the children with asthma will have spontaneous resolution of their disease by young adulthood. After the third decade, there is an increasing prevalence of asthma with advancing age.

Allergy to common aeroallergens is present in most childhood asthmatics, and chronic allergic exposure is considered to be a potential underlying cause in the development of childhood asthma as well as an exacerbating trigger. In the older population, specific allergies are not as tightly linked to the presence of asthma, although those with allergies are more likely to have asthma than those without allergies (29).

Pathophysiology

Airways Reactivity

Asthma is a disorder characterized by recurrent bronchospasm induced by either specific allergic stimuli or nonspecific irritant or physicochemical stimuli. This increased tendency to have bronchospasm is synonymously called bronchial reactivity, airways reactivity, bronchial hyperreactivity, or bronchial hyperresponsiveness. This characteristic is defined by exaggerated declines in lung function after inhalation challenge with nonspecific bronchoconstrictor agents such as methacholine or histamine, with physical agents such as cold dry air ventilation or exercise-induced hyperpnea, or with specific allergic agents such as inhaled allergens.

Virtually all asthmatics with active disease display airways reactivity, and the degree of reactivity roughly correlates with the severity of asthma. About one in eight individuals without clinical asthma also shows laboratory evidence of airways reactivity. Most smokers with mild chronic obstructive lung disease without clinical evidence of asthma have airways reactivity. Therefore laboratory evidence of airways reactivity is not by itself diagnostic of asthma. However, testing for airways reactivity is useful when a negative result can rule out the diagnosis of asthma: the person with chronic persistent cough (see Chapter 54), episodic unexplained dyspnea (see Chapter 54), or occupationally associated respiratory symptoms. Although the testing procedure for airway reactivity is not complex, it is not performed on a regular basis except in specialty clinics and therefore usually requires referral to a pulmonary function laboratory.

Table 55.6.   Common Triggers for Asthma

Exercise	Viral respiratory infections
Cold Air	Strong odors/irritants
Seasonal aeroallergens	Cigarette smoke
Ragweed pollen	Perfume
Tree pollen	Detergents
Grass pollen	Oxidant air polluntants
Indoor aeroallergens	
Dust mite feces	
Cockroaches	
Warm-blooded pets	
Mold spores	

Patient Experience (Airway Reactivity Testing). The testing procedure is safe if the baseline level of lung function is no more than mildly impaired. The patient should not use oral theophylline for 24 hours before the test, or inhaled bronchodilators for 12 hours before. All prescribed oral or inhaled corticosteroids or other anti-inflammatory drugs should be continued. The patient breathes increasing concentrations of methacholine or histamine, either through repeated vital capacity breaths or through quiet tidal breathing. After each concentration, spirometry is performed. When the FEV$_1$ falls by 20% or more or the highest concentration is reached, the test is terminated and the bronchoconstriction is reversed with an inhaled bronchodilator. When conducted in a supervised setting, the test is safe, although many people with reactive airways experience coughing or chest tightness.

Specific airway inhalation challenge with antigen is rarely necessary for clinical purposes unless it is absolutely necessary to document whether a specific agent exacerbates asthma, such as a work-related exposure where employment decisions must be made. However, the response to specific antigen challenges do give insight into the pathogenesis of chronic asthma. After inhalation of an antigen of sufficient dose, acute bronchoconstriction lasts for 20 to 60 minutes, the *early-phase reaction.* Untreated, this early bronchospasm resolves within 1 to 2 hours, although it may be reversed with inhaled bronchodilators. Approximately 4 to 24 hours later, however, bronchospasm recurs in about half of allergic people. It is generally thought that the early-phase reaction is due to bronchial smooth muscle constriction but that the *late-phase* reaction is the consequence of inflammatory cells and their products in the airways.

Exercise-induced bronchospasm is present in 50 to 90% of asthmatics. Following cessation of vigorous exercise, normal individuals show a small amount of bronchodilation. In contrast, susceptible asthmatics develop bronchoconstriction 5 to 20 minutes after stopping exercise. Similar responses can be elicited by breathing cold, dry air. Postulated causes for exercise-induced bronchoconstriction include increases in the osmolality of the airway fluid lining layer because of drying of the airways causing release of inflammatory mediators; direct response of the airways to cooling during exercise hyperpnea; or vascular engorgement of the bronchial mucosa. Exercise-induced bronchospasm can be effectively prevented by pretreatment

with either an inhaled β2-adrenergic agonist or cromolyn (see below).

Patient Experience (Exercise Bronchoprovocation). The patient should not use any theophylline for 24 hours before testing, or any inhaled bronchodilator, cromolyn, or nedocromil for 12 hours before testing. The patient exercises on a bicycle ergometer or treadmill to tolerance. After stopping exercise, spirometry is performed several times for the following 30 minutes. If bronchospasm occurs, it is reversed with an inhaled bronchodilator.

Airway Inflammation

The mechanisms that cause nonspecific airways reactivity are not entirely understood; however, it is now recognized that airway inflammation is linked to the presence of airways reactivity. Even mild asymptomatic asthmatics show submucosal infiltration with neutrophils, eosinophils, monocytes, T lymphocytes, and mast cells; edema; vascular engorgement; subepithelial collagen and fibronectin deposition; and epithelial desquamation (115). Patients with more severe asthma show hyperplasia of smooth muscle, mucous gland hypertrophy, thickening of the subepithelial basement membrane, and widespread mucous plugging of the small airways.

Numerous theories explaining how airway inflammation leads to airways reactivity have been advanced. It is likely that asthma is the common expression of several mechanisms or that one mechanism is predominant in some situations but not others. Whatever the mechanism, there is strong evidence that treatment of the underlying airway inflammation can reduce airways reactivity and improve asthma symptoms (19).

Pathophysiology of the Acute Asthmatic Attack

The acute asthmatic attack may occur suddenly as a consequence of exposure to an allergic or irritant substance producing severe bronchospasm in an individual with previously well-controlled asthma and normal lung function. More commonly, the attack occurs after many days of progressive reductions in lung function, increasing lability of lung function, progressive exertional dyspnea and cough, and increasing requirements for symptomatic use of inhaled bronchodilators (86).

During the acute attack, bronchospasm, mucosal edema, and mucous plugging lead to narrowing and closure of small peripheral airways. This causes an increase in resistance to inspiratory and expiratory airflow and, more important, trapping of air. The patient must breathe at high volume to keep the airways open. The consequences of this hyperinflation are increased work of breathing, impaired mechanical advantage of the shortened respiratory muscles and of the flattened diaphragm, pulmonary hypertension, and markedly negative inspiratory swings in pleural pressure to initiate airflow. If the attack is severe or prolonged, respiratory muscle fatigue can occur with consequent hypoventilation, carbon dioxide retention, hypoxemia, respiratory failure, and death (94). Arterial blood gas tensions in nonsevere asthma attacks usually show hypocapnia from hyperventilation. A normal arterial carbon dioxide tension may indicate either resolution of the attack or impending respiratory failure, and must therefore be correlated with other clinical features (90). Ventilation–perfusion mismatch accounts for the hypoxemia that accompanies an asthma attack; however, treatment with β-adrenergic bronchodilators usually worsens ventilation–perfusion matching, causing transient worsening hypoxemia as the asthma attack improves. Resolution of the attack is often preceded by the expectoration of copious secretions with small mucous plugs. As the attack resolves, dyspnea and chest tightness disappear before wheezing resolves, whereas abnormalities of lung function can persist for many days or weeks.

Clinical Presentations

Clinical presentations of asthma differ with regard to chronicity and to inciting factors. There is broad overlap between these categories of asthma, and they should not necessarily be considered to have differing underlying mechanisms.

Extrinsic asthma is a condition in which the worsening of the asthma can be clearly associated with exposure to a specific allergen (Table 55.6). The most common perennial allergens associated with worsening of asthma include molds (particularly *Alternaria*), house dust mites, cockroaches, cat dander, and dog dander. The most common seasonal allergens include ragweed (autumn), tree pollen (spring), and grass pollens (summer). Diagnosis of a specific allergen triggering asthma requires a clear history of worsening asthma after exposure, improvement of the asthma when the allergen is removed, and positive wheal and flare reaction to the offending agent on allergy skin testing. Clear association of asthma with a specific allergen is important because control of the environmental exposure or specific immunotherapy can be time-consuming, expensive, or impractical. When an aeroallergen is clearly associated with asthma symptoms, immunotherapy with weekly allergy injections may lead to mild, although transient, improvement in the disease (41).

Intrinsic asthma is a condition in which there is no clear association with specific allergen exposure. This form of asthma is more common in adults than in children and typically causes perennial symptoms. Acute episodes may be triggered by viral illnesses, but often no specific provocative stimulus can be found. In about half of the cases, the asthma persists or worsens throughout life, leading to incompletely reversible abnormalities of pulmonary function. When this is associated with chronic cough and sputum production, it is often called *chronic asthmatic bronchitis* and may be difficult to distinguish from smoking-related chronic obstructive lung disease. The cause of this form of asthma is unclear. Many patients show some traits of allergic tendencies with elevation of serum IgE levels and sputum eosinophilia, but allergy skin testing is usually negative. In some cases, it appears that the onset of the disease followed a severe lower respiratory tract viral infection, whereas in others it may be associated with long-term exposure to specific allergens or respiratory irritants (31,130).

Occupational asthma (see Chapter 7) is a condition in which a specific occupational exposure leads to cough, wheezing, and chest tightness. If exposure to the offending antigen persists, a chronic asthmatic condition with sensitivity to nonspecific agents may occur. If exposure to the sensitizing agent is stopped soon enough, symptoms and nonspecific airway reactivity often resolve, although it may take up to 2 years. Because the prognosis for remission is better in those who cease exposure early, the treating physician needs to diagnose occupational asthma early and to initiate steps to avoid continued exposure (36). Common substances that may cause occupational asthma are shown in Table 55.7.

Reactive airways dysfunction syndrome (RADS) is a disorder that follows an intense short-term exposure to

Table 55.7. Occupational Exposures Causing Asthma

Agent	Specific Examples	Occupation
Birds	Pigeons, chickens	Pigeon breeders, poultry workers
Chemicals	Hexachlorophene, formalin, ethylene diamine, metabisulfite	Hospital workers, photographers, food preparation workers, water purification workers
Crustaceans	Crabs, shrimp	Food processing workers
Drugs	Antibiotics, sulfa derivatives	Workers in pharmaceutical industry, agricultural feed mixing
Enzymes	B. subtilis, trypsin, papain	Detergent handlers, pharmaceutical industry workers
Epoxy resins	Anhydride compounds	Workers in manufacturing, auto body repair
Laboratory animals	Rats, mice, rabbits, guinea pigs	Laboratory workers, veterinarians
Metals	Platinum, nickle, chromium, cobalt, vanadium	Workers in metal plating, leather tanning, hard metal industry
Plants	Grain dust, flour	Grain handlers, bakers, millers
Plastics and rubber	TDI (toluene di-isocyanate), DDI (diphenylmethane di-isocyanate), Azodicarbonamide	Polyurethane plastic, paint, varnish, and rubber workers
Soldering fluxes	Colophony, aminoethylethanolamine	Electronics, aluminum fabrication workers
Vegetable products	Gum acacia	Printing workers
Wood dust	Cedar, redwood	Carpenters, construction workers, woodmill workers

Adapted from Chan-Yeung M. Occupational asthma. Chest 98:148S–161S, 1990.

a toxic, nonallergenic substance such as sulfuric acid, nitric acid, chlorine, or hydrochloric acid fumes. After the exposure—often the result of an industrial accident or fire—and resolution of the resultant acute lung injury, the individual is left with chronic airways reactivity to nonspecific physicochemical agents such as tobacco smoke or cold air. The disorder may resolve after several months but often leads to chronic airways reactivity (3,25).

Exercise-induced bronchospasm is present in most asthmatics, although some children and young adults may experience asthma only after exercise. This syndrome may be confused with exertional dyspnea or angina, although careful questioning will reveal that the dyspnea occurs after a 5- to 20-minute symptom-free interval after the cessation of sustained activity. Exercise-induced bronchospasm is thought to be caused by the airway cooling and drying effect of exercise hyperpnea and is therefore worse with outdoor exercise in cold weather (87). Exercise in a warm, humid environment such as an indoor swimming pool is often well tolerated. The symptoms can be prevented by inhalation of a β-agonist bronchodilator or sodium cromolyn (see below) about 20 minutes before exercise.

Triad asthma (Sampter's syndrome) is a syndrome of nasal polyps, asthma, and aspirin sensitivity. One of three asthmatics with nasal polyps has aspirin sensitivity, in comparison to 1 in 15 asthmatics without nasal polyps. These individuals often have severe chronic asthma and occasionally experience systemic anaphylactic reactions to aspirin or aspirinlike compounds (132), including nonsteroidal anti-inflammatory drugs (NSAIDs). Even asthmatics who are aware that they are sensitive to aspirin, which occurs in 10% of asthmatics, may be inadvertently using compounded drugs that contain aspirin. (See Chapter 23 for a list of common medicines that contain aspirin.) The mechanism by which this occurs is thought to involve blockade of cyclooxygenase–derived prostaglandins and the induction of lipoxygenase-derived leukotrienes from inflammatory cells. Surgical removal of the nasal polyps may make the asthma better, but the polyps often recur and require long-term topical or systemic corticosteroid treatment. If aspirin is required for treatment of another condition, rapid desensitization can be performed, but daily maintenance doses of aspirin are required to sustain the effect. Aspirin-sensitive asthma is an indication for the use of leukotriene antagonists or inhibitors such as zafirlukast or zileuton.

Cough-variant asthma is a condition in which wheezing, dyspnea, and chest tightness are minimal symptoms, but chronic cough is the major complaint. Approximately 30% of patients with chronic persistent cough of more than 8 weeks' duration have airways reactivity and respond to treatment with bronchodilators or corticosteroids (70).

Allergic bronchopulmonary aspergillosis (ABPA) is an uncommon form of asthma that is difficult to treat and can lead to chronic respiratory failure. The disorder is caused by local allergic reaction to non-invasive *Aspergillus* or to other fungal species colonizing the airway. *Aspergillus fumigatus,* a ubiquitous saprophyte, is the most common organism, but other fungi can cause the same syndrome (74). The chronic inflammatory condition leads to dilation and bronchiectasis of the central airways, recurrent mucous plugging and segmental atelectasis, and eventually fibrotic destruction of lung parenchyma. Criteria for the diagnosis of ABPA include recurrent atelectasis and pulmonary infiltrates; blood and sputum eosinophilia; immediate skin test reactivity to *Aspergillus;* serum precipitins to *Aspergillus;* elevated serum IgE; specific IgG and IgE antibodies to *Aspergillus* by RAST or ELISA testing (see below); and proximal bronchiectasis on chest computerized tomography (59).

Inhaled or systemic antifungal therapy is not helpful in eradicating the offending agent. The usual treatment consists of systemic corticosteroids with starting dosages of 0.5 to 1.0 mg/kg per day of prednisone or equivalent. At least 6 months of therapy are usually required, but many patients are never able to tolerate permanent steroid cessation. Early diagnosis and treatment are necessary to prevent the progressive bronchiectasis and lung fibrosis that can occur. The effectiveness of therapy is monitored with serum IgE levels and chest x-rays. Because ABPA is found in approximately 10% of cystic fibrosis patients, the physician should consider screening for cystic fibrosis with sweat chloride concentrations or genetic analysis in patients with ABPA.

Intractable asthma is defined as dyspnea, wheezing, and frequent exacerbations despite maximum therapy with bronchodilators and inhaled and systemic corticosteroids (83). When symptoms are intractable, the possibility should be considered that a condition that mimics asthma (see below) is present. Other circumstances that may contribute to intractable asthma include an occult persistent exposure to an allergen or irritant at home or at work, use of β-blockers either systemically or as eye drops, use of aspirin or related drugs, exposure to dietary chemicals such as sulfites, hypothyroidism or hyperthyroidism, gastroesophageal reflux, sinusitis, bronchopulmonary aspergillosis, and mucocutaneous fungal infection. However, the most likely cause of intractable asthma is nonadherence to prescribed treatment, a behavior that is often underestimated (76,116).

Wheezing conditions not from asthma may be confused by the patient or physician with asthma, often as an intractable case. Such conditions include congestive heart failure, mitral stenosis, cystic fibrosis, immotile cilia syndrome, immunoglobulin deficiency, laryngeal tumors, vocal cord paralysis, laryngospasm, airway foreign body, hypereosinophilic syndromes, endobronchial sarcoidosis, bronchiolitis obliterans, Churg–Strauss vasculitis, multiple pulmonary emboli, reaction to angiotensin-converting enzyme inhibitors, and in underdeveloped countries, pertussis and diphtheria.

Evaluation of Chronic Asthma

Medical History and Clinical Interview

A thorough medical history is essential for establishing the diagnosis of asthma and for guiding treatment. The following factors should be evaluated: duration, frequency, and severity of attacks; seasonal variation of disease; specific trigger factors; occupational and recreational exposures; home conditions; other allergic conditions; and medication use and adherence.

Asthmatics describe their episodic shortness of breath differently than do patients with other forms of lung disease or heart failure (49). Asthmatics use terms such as *chest tightness* and *wheeziness* rather than *air hunger, suffocation,* or *rapid breathing.* Asthmatics often say the site of obstruction is in their neck. They report more difficulty with inspiration than expiration in contrast to patients with emphysema, who cannot distinguish inspiratory from expiratory distress (58).

Asthma should not be considered well controlled if there is more than occasional requirement for symptomatic use of inhaled bronchodilators or if there is nocturnal awakening with symptoms. The presence of nocturnal symptoms is such a characteristic feature of asthma that the absence of this history should stimulate the investigation of other causes of episodic wheezing and chest tightness. Although pollen seasons and common aeroallergens vary geographically, asthma that is worse in the early fall suggests ragweed allergy; worse in the summer, grass pollen allergy; and worse in the spring, tree pollen allergy. Specific asthma triggers (Table 55.6) should be elicited. Because the symptoms of asthma may follow an allergic exposure by 2 to 24 hours, elicitation of such exposures requires careful questioning or the maintenance of a prospective asthma diary recording exposures, symptoms, and peak flow. Occupational exposures may be obvious (Table 55.7) but can also occur from operations in an adjacent work space or via ventilation systems. Strong evidence of an occupational trigger exposure is the absence of symptoms on weekends and during vacations. Occasionally it is necessary to have a work-site inspection performed by an expert in occupational medicine (see Chapter 7). Recreational activities may involve exposures similar to those in the workplace such as toluene di-isocyanate (TDI) in those who use polyurethane paint or varnish, molds in those who engage in water sports or boating, or seminal fluid allergy in those who have coitus (122).

In cases in which it is unclear whether the home exposure is important, the patient should be questioned about whether the asthma worsened upon moving to a new home and whether it improves during periods away from home. Perennial allergen and irritant exposures at home contribute to the chronic airway inflammation that causes asthma, particularly in children (130). House dust mites feed on desquamated human skin and produce allergenic feces that are easily respirable. Dust mites thrive in a humid, warm environment, particularly in feather pillows, comforters, carpets, upholstered furniture, and mattresses. Cockroaches and their excreta are highly allergenic. Pets, particularly cats and dogs, secrete antigen in their saliva that may persist in the home environment many years after the pets are no longer present. Frequent vacuuming, while useful in eliminating home allergens, also disperses antigen into the air for several hours. Smokers in the home also disperse irritant side stream smoke that worsens asthma. Humidifiers or other causes of high ambient humidity promote the growth of molds as well as of dust mites. Urea-formaldehyde foam insulation can cause low-level irritant exposure that is a potential aggravator of asthma. Newly varnished floors or furniture can give off isocyanate fumes that worsen asthma.

Knowledge of associated allergic conditions is helpful. Histories of allergic rhinitis, eczema, and urticaria can assist in determining specific asthma triggers and would support more specific therapies directed toward those allergens. Chronic allergic or infectious sinusitis can exacerbate asthma, and symptoms or sinus pain or drainage should be elicited.

Gastroesophageal reflux, often asymptomatic, may trigger nocturnal asthma either through reflex distension and irritation of the esophagus or through aspiration of gastric contents into the larynx and lower airways (33). *Tartrazine* (yellow dye #5) is found in yellow or orange foods, particularly powdered orange juice substitutes. Although tartrazine was once thought to be a common cause of asthma in aspirin-sensitive individuals, it is now considered that true tartrazine sensitivity is exceedingly rare. *Sulfites,* present in dried fruits, wines, processed potatoes, seafood, and salad greens, can cause acute asthma attacks. The mechanism is thought to be from production of sulfur dioxide. In rare cases, large doses of *monosodium glutamate,* found in oriental cooking or snack foods, can bring on asthma. It should not be assumed that asthmatics do not smoke *cigarettes.* In some urban populations, as many as 40% of asthmatics are cigarette smokers. Air pollution, particularly respirable particulates, ozone, SO_2, and NO_2 have been implicated as an exacerbating factor in asthma during atmospheric inversions in the summer (1,11,121).

Only approximately 50% of asthmatics adhere to their prescribed drug regimen, often without admitting this to the treating physician. Adherence worsens as the drug program becomes more complex, and there is less adherence with drugs that prevent but do not relieve symptoms (24). It is important to elicit in a friendly and supportive manner whether the patient is actually following the prescribed program. This can be aided by questions such as, "How often do you have difficulty taking your medications on a routine basis?" or "What problems have you had in taking your medicines?" Barriers to adherence (see Chapter 4) include failure to accept or understand the benefit and purpose of medication and environmental controls, the high cost of drugs and supplies, frequent dosing of multiple drugs, side effects of treatment, and disorganized, stressful living conditions. These elements need to be explored and modified when possible.

Physical Examination

The physical examination of the patient with asthma should be directed toward confirming the diagnosis, estimating the severity of disease, evaluating related conditions, and ruling out other disorders that mimic asthma.

During an *acute asthmatic attack,* the patient appears frightened and fatigued. The respiratory pattern is deep and slow with a prolonged expiratory phase, but may progress to rapid shallow breathing with expiratory grunting that heralds the onset of respiratory failure. Speech is telegraphic or absent. Coughing is ineffective. The chest appears hyperinflated, with reduced tidal expansion compared to the strong respiratory efforts. The sternomastoid muscles are contracted with each inspiration during severe episodes. Hyperinflation of the lungs causes the lower lateral rib cage to move inward with each inspiratory contraction of the flattened diaphragm rather than outward as normally occurs. Tachycardia is present, with weakening of the pulse during inspiration. An inspiratory fall in systolic blood pressure *(pulsus paradoxus)* of more than 15 mm Hg is present in severe attacks but may disappear with the onset of respiratory failure (123). The chest has diffuse polyphonic expiratory wheezes, but in the most severe attacks may be silent. Inspiratory wheezing suggests the presence of upper airway obstruction, whereas localized or monophonic wheezing suggests mechanical bronchial obstruction from tumor or foreign body. Absent breath sounds in one hemithorax with wheezing in the other should raise the possibility of *pneumothorax*—a potentially lethal complication.

In chronic asymptomatic asthma, the examination of the chest may be entirely normal, although the presence of mild airflow obstruction can be determined by listening for wheezes during a forced expiration. However, this finding is neither sensitive nor specific for asthma. Associated allergic rhinitis causes the nasal mucosa to be pale and edematous. Nasal polyps appear as tan-gray mucoid lesions that obstruct the nasal aperture.

Examination should be directed at disorders that may mimic asthma. Listening over the neck during forced inspiration or with the arm extended over the head can bring out inspiratory stridor with upper airway obstruction. Findings of congestive heart disease such as chest crackles, cardiomegaly, or mitral murmurs should be carefully evaluated. High-pitched monophonic localized inspiratory squeaks suggest the presence of bronchiolitis.

Laboratory Testing

Spirometry (see above) should be performed in all asthmatics in the asymptomatic phase and periodically during the course of therapy to establish a baseline measure and to monitor therapy. Persistent abnormali-

ties of pulmonary function, which form the basis for recurrent attacks of asthma, are present in the asymptomatic phase (89). The chest x-ray is usually normal in asymptomatic asthma but shows hyperinflation during acute attacks. Allergic bronchopulmonary aspergillosis shows characteristic central bronchiectasis and signs of mucoid impaction. During severe acute asthma attacks, pneumothorax or pneumonia may require specific treatment. Peripheral blood eosinophilia is common in asthma and roughly correlates with the severity of disease (45). Microscopic examination of unstained sputum can distinguish eosinophils from neutrophils when there is purulence, guiding the need for corticosteroids versus antibiotics (52). Other features characteristic of asthmatic sputum are *Charcot–Leyden crystals,* which are spear-shaped crystals of lysophospholipase derived from eosinophil granules; *Curschmann spirals,* which are mucous casts of small airways; and Creola bodies, which are clumps of *desquamated ciliated epithelial cells.*

Skin testing for specific allergens is helpful to diagnose specific allergies, particularly when environmental control procedures are costly or difficult, such as changing occupations or residences or eliminating a beloved pet. However, positive allergy skin tests do not indicate the presence of allergy to a particular substance unless there is a compatible history. *Radioallergosorbent tests* (RASTs) measure allergen-specific IgE in the blood and may be substituted for skin testing, but they are often more expensive. *Total serum IgE* is elevated in asthma but is useful mainly for diagnosis and monitoring of allergic bronchopulmonary aspergillosis (see above). *Methacholine challenge* is helpful when the diagnosis of asthma is uncertain. A normal methacholine challenge in a symptomatic person virtually eliminates the diagnosis of asthma, although some asthmatics have normal methacholine challenge tests during remission. *Flow-volume loops* and *nasopharyngoscopy* are useful tests to determine whether vocal cord dysfunction is mimicking asthma (39,50).

Treatment

The goals of the treatment of asthma are to keep the patient symptom free day and night, with full activity levels, normal lung function, absent side effects, and satisfaction with the process of care. For most patients who can adhere to a comprehensive asthma management plan (76), these are realistically attainable goals.

Treatment in the ambulatory setting has four major components: monitoring of symptoms and lung function, control of environmental triggers, education of the patient and family, and drug therapy (Table 55.8).

Table 55.8. Components of Asthma Treatment

Monitor symptoms and lung function.
Control adverse environmental exposures.
Educate patient and family.
Administer drug therapy.

Home Monitoring of Lung Function

Monitoring lung function with objective tests is important in asthmatics who have to use symptomatic bronchodilator treatments more than once or twice per week. Inexpensive, reliable peak flow monitors are commercially available. Recording peak flow gives an indication of the maximal benefit that can be expected from treatment, can forecast the worsening of asthma before severe symptoms develop, allows objective identification of harmful environmental or occupational exposures, and facilitates telephone contact between the patient and medical caregivers. A practical regimen is to record the peak flow daily in the morning. If it is less than 80% of the patient's personal best level, additional recordings during the day are warranted. The determination of a patient's personal best level can be obtained during a 2- or 3-week period of intensive asthma treatment and should be periodically updated. The patient should establish a new personal best peak flow when he or she puts a new peak flow meter into use. Asthma diaries are helpful in recording patterns of peak flow variation, symptoms, and use of symptomatic bronchodilators (Fig. 55.3).

Control of Environmental Triggers and Complicating Conditions

Environmental controls for asthma include the identification and removal of nonspecific irritants and the reduction of exposure to specific allergens. Smoking should be discouraged, and *smoking cessation* may require repeated strong personalized messages, referral to smoking cessation group programs, and nicotine replacement therapy (see Chapter 20). Household members should also be discouraged from smoking or to confine smoking to parts of the house not occupied by the asthmatic patient.

Gastroesophageal reflux may worsen asthma, particularly at night. Small, frequent feedings; elevation of the bed; and antacids, histamine-2 receptor blockers, or proton pump blockers may be prescribed (see Chapter 35) (125). In some cases of severe steroid-dependent asthma, surgical treatment of reflux is remarkably effective (79). *Allergic or infectious sinusitis* should be aggressively treated with antibiotics, intranasal steroids, intranasal cromolyn, or surgical procedures (17,61).

Common specific perennial *allergen sources* include house dust mite, cockroaches, molds, and pets. *House dust mites* can be controlled by maintaining a low relative humidity, removing carpeting and stuffed furniture from the bedroom, and covering mattresses and pillows with impermeable covers. Asthmatics should avoid vacuuming or entering a freshly vacuumed area for 1 to 2 hours or should wear a protective facemask. High efficiency vacuum cleaners are available but are of unproven value. Bedding should be washed weekly in hot water (above 130°F) to eliminate dust mites. *Fur-bearing animals* shed allergenic dander, saliva, and urine, and they should be eliminated from the household if they exacerbate asthma. If the patient or family is unwilling to part with the pet, other partially effective measures include washing the pet frequently, excluding the pet from the asthmatic's bedroom, and blocking forced hot air vents in the asthmatic's bedroom (44). *Cockroach infestation* is a particularly important cause of asthma in inner cities (72) and can be controlled with insecticides. The preferred methods of cockroach control are boric acid powder, poison baits, and traps. *Insecticide sprays,* particularly cholinesterase inhibitors, can cause severe asthma exacerbations by themselves. *Molds* can be controlled in the home by the use of dehumidifiers and by providing adequate ventilation in the kitchen and bathroom. Indoor air cleaning devices using high-efficiency filters or electrostatic filters can diminish suspended particles of tobacco smoke and mold spores, but they have not been found to improve asthma symptoms in controlled studies. Therefore, they are not recommended for routine use and do not substitute for other methods of environmental control. Room or house humidifiers should be avoided because they can increase concentrations of mold spores and house dust mites.

During specific pollen allergy seasons or high air pollution days, asthmatics should stay indoors at midday when the pollen concentration and air quality are worst. Outdoor exercise during high air pollution periods should be avoided because high levels of ventilation increase the damaging effect of air pollutants. Closing doors and windows and using a recirculating air conditioner are appropriate preventive measures.

Exposure to occupational allergens ideally should be controlled by ventilation changes in the workplace, but often personal respiratory protection or even job reassignment are required to control this exposure. Sources of nonspecific respiratory irritants should be avoided. These include unvented gas, kerosene, or wood burning stoves and heaters. In highly sensitive individuals, aerosol sprays and perfumed cosmetics may worsen asthma and should be eliminated.

Drugs that worsen asthma such as aspirin and other NSAIDs and β-adrenergic blockers should be avoided or should be monitored closely if no alternatives are possible. Many patent medications for upper respiratory infections, sinusitis, gastroenteritis, musculoskeletal pain, or menstrual pain contain aspirin, which can worsen asthma in susceptible unaware individuals, and the use of such drugs should be avoided. β-Adrenergic blockers may inadvertently be used as eye drops for treatment of glaucoma, with the potential for severe asthma exacerbation.

Annual influenza vaccination is recommended for asthmatics of all ages because the infection can precipitate severe and prolonged exacerbations of asthma.

Education of the Asthmatic

Education of the patient is an important obligation of the physician (108). Excellent materials are available from volunteer and government agencies to assist in this process. The specific aims of the education should be to recognize the signs and symptoms of asthma, to use the peak flow meter correctly, to take medication

ASTHMA SYMPTOM AND PEAK FLOW DIARY

___My predicted peak flow
___My personal best peak flow
___My Green (OK) Zone (80-100% of personal best)
___My Yellow (Caution) Zone (50-80% of personal best)
___My Red (Danger) Zone (below 50% of personal best)

Date	a.m.	p.m.	a.m.	p.m.	a.m.	p.m.	a.m.	p.m.	a.m.	p.m.	a.m.	p.m.	a.m.	p.m.
Peak flow reading														
No asthma symptoms														
Mild asthma symptoms														
Moderate asthma symptoms														
Serious asthma symptoms														
Medicine used to stop														
Urgent visit to the doctor														

1. Take your peak flow reading every morning (a.m.) when you wake up and every night (p.m.) at bedtime. Try to take your peak flow readings at the same time each day. If you take an inhaled beta$_2$-agonist medicine, take your peak flow reading *before* taking that medicine. Write down the highest reading of three tries in the box that says peak flow reading.
2. Look at the box in the upper left of this sheet to see whether your number is in the green, yellow, or red zone.
3. In the space below the date and time, put an "X" in the box that matches the symptoms you have when you record your peak flow reading.
4. Look at your asthma control plan for what to do when your number is in one of the zones and you have asthma symptoms.
5. Put an "X" in the box beside "medicine use" if you took *extra* asthma medicine to stop your symptoms.
6. If you made any visit to your doctor's office, emergency room, or hospital for treatment of an asthma episode, put an "X" in the box marked "urgent visit." Tell your doctor if you went to the emergency room or hospital.

No symptoms = No symptoms (wheeze, cough, chest tightness, or shortness of breath) even with normal physical activity.
Mild symptoms = Symptoms during physical activity, but not at rest. It does not keep you from sleeping or being active.
Moderate symptoms = Symptoms while at rest; symptoms may keep you from sleeping or being active.
Serious symptoms = Serious symptoms at rest (wheeze may be absent); symptoms cause problems walking or talking; muscles in neck or between ribs are pulled in when breathing.

Figure 55.3. Asthma symptom and peak flow diary.

properly, to establish and follow treatment plans for exacerbations, to avoid and control asthma triggers, and to make appropriate use of urgent medical care. Important specific topics are listed in Table 55.9.

Asthmatic patients need to be instructed in the proper use of *metered-dose inhalers* (MDIs) used to deliver inhaled medications. Patients should be observed using their inhaler during office visits and proper technique should be repeatedly taught because some studies have shown that 40% of asthmatics do not use their inhalers properly. Proper technique (Table 55.10) involves the following steps: gently shaking the MDI; holding it 2 inches away from the open mouth; triggering the device at the onset of inspiration from normal end-tidal lung volume; inhaling slowly to total lung capacity over 5 seconds; holding the breath at total lung capacity for 5 to 10 seconds; and exhaling slowly (100). For patients who cannot perform this maneuver properly despite training and practice, the effectiveness of the MDI can be enhanced by use of a spacer or reservoir device. Some drugs are available in single- or multiple-dose dry powder inhalers or breath-triggered MDIs; these devices are breath-activated and are effective for people with poor coordination; however, they require good inspiratory flows to work properly. In the uncommon cases where use of an MDI is not effective, small electrically powered nebulizers can deliver bronchodilators. However, use of nebulizers is limited by their lack of portability, their expense, and the need for meticulous cleaning and preparation of solutions. Rinsing the mouth after inhalation of drugs effectively

Table 55.9. Components of Asthma Education

Description of asthma
What asthma medicines do
Community resources for asthma patients and their families
Correct use of metered dose inhaler and nebulizer
How to use a peak flow meter
How to record an asthma diary
Warning signs of asthma attacks
Asthma trigger control plan
Steps to manage an asthma attack
School, work, and exercise activity plans

Table 55.10. Proper Use of Metered-Dose Inhaler (MDI)

Action	Reason for Action
Shake MDI gently.	Disperses drug evenly with vehicle. Check that canister is full.
Hold the MDI 2 fingerbreadths from the widely opened mouth.	The larger droplets will rain out in the air rather than impact in the mouth. This prevents mouth and throat irritation with some vehicles, and thrush with inhaled corticosteroids.
Breathe normally and pause at quiet end-expiration.	Inhaling from a low lung volume allows greater peripheral penetration of the drug.
Actuate the MDI at the onset of inspiration and slowly inhale over 4–6 seconds.	Slow inspiratory flow rates enhance deposition of particles in the peripheral airways and reduce turbulence and impaction in the upper airway.
Hold the breath for 5–10 seconds at total lung capacity.	Small respirable particles will be allowed to settle in the smaller airways during the breath-hold.
Exhale slowly.	Slow expiration reduces exhalation of drug from the lung.

Adapted from Newhouse MT, Dolovitch MB. Control of asthma by aerosols. N Engl J Med 315:870, 1986.

Table 55.11. Self-Management of Acute Exacerbations

Monitor peak flow and symptoms.
Use inhaled β-adrenergic agonist every 20 minutes for three doses, then every 3–4 hours for 6–12 hours as needed.
Contact physician or visit emergency department if there is incomplete response to initial treatment and peak flow is 50–70% of baseline.
Go to emergency department if poor response to initial therapy, or if peak flow is <50% of baseline.

reduces local oropharyngeal side effects and minimizes systemic absorption.

Each asthmatic should have a well-understood action plan for treatment of exacerbations, and should also understand signs of worsening asthma and what action should be taken. Such a plan should be based on the patient's history of severity of exacerbations, access to health care, and reliability. A typical action plan is shown in Table 55.11.

Drug Treatment for Asthma

Drugs should be used in the treatment of asthma in a stepped approach to normalize activity levels and lung function and to minimize exacerbations (Table 55.12). Once control of asthma is achieved, the program can be slowly tapered to maintain the lowest necessary drug dosage (20,88). It is important to distinguish between drugs that are used for short-term relief of symptoms and drugs that are used for long-term control of the underlying disease. Failure of the patient to understand this distinction often leads to underuse of anti-inflammatory agents and to overreliance on inhaled bronchodilators, with consequent failure to meet the goals of asthma care.

For *mild asthma,* inhaled selective β_2-agonists should be prescribed. Use should be confined to the minimum number of inhalations needed to control symptoms. Table 55.13 lists several selective β_2-agonists available in MDIs. The choice of which β_2-agonist to use should be made initially on the basis of the subjective reaction of the patient and cost because little else distinguishes most of the agents available by prescription in the United States. Nonprescription asthma inhalers should be avoided because many contain epinephrine, which has potentially serious cardiovascular side effects from its α- and β_1-adrenergic properties. Because selective β-agonists are so effective in relieving symptoms of bronchospasm, but without treating the underlying airway inflammation, they have the potential for permitting patients to increase exposure to harmful agents and to delay more definitive treatment. There remains controversy whether the regular use of short-acting β-agonists can lead to worsening of asthma, so it is prudent to limit their use to symptomatic relief (135).

Long-acting selective β-agonists may lead to the development of tolerance to their protective effect against nonspecific bronchial challenge, while the acute bronchodilating effects of these drugs are unchanged (38). The typical MDI contains 200 to 300 inhalations, and therefore should last about 3 to

Table 55.12.   Stepwise Approach to Asthma Care

	Symptoms	Lung Function	Quick Relief Drugs	Long-Term Control Drugs
Step 1 Mild intermittent	Symptoms less than twice weekly Brief exacerbations Nocturnal symptoms less than two times per month	FEV$_1$ or PEFR 80% predicted	Short-acting inhaled β-agonists Use of β-agonist more than twice weekly may indicate need to start control treatment	None needed
Step 2 Mild persistent	Symptoms more than twice weekly but not daily Limitation of activity during exacerbations Nocturnal symptoms more than two times per month	FEV$_1$ or PEFR 80% predicted	Short-acting inhaled β-agonists Use of β-agonist more than once daily may indicate need to increase control treatment	Low-dose inhaled corticosteroid, or cromolyn, or nedocromil, or sustained-release theophylline
Step 3 Moderate persistent	Daily symptoms Daily use of short-acting bronchodilator Nocturnal symptoms more than once weekly	FEV$_1$ or PEFR 60 to 80% predicted	Short-acting inhaled β-agonists Use of β-agonist more than once daily may indicate need to increase control treatment	Medium-dose inhaled corticosteroid, or low-dose inhaled corticosteroid with long-acting bronchodilator (e.g., salmeterol or theophylline)
Step 4 Severe persistent	Continual symptoms Limited physical activity Frequent exacerbations Frequent nocturnal symptoms	FEV$_1$ or PEFR 60% predicted	Short-acting inhaled β-agonists Use of β-agonist more than once daily may indicate need to increase control treatment	High-dose inhaled corticosteroid and long-acting bronchodilator (e.g., salmeterol or theophylline) or oral corticosteroid as needed to treat and prevent exacerbations

Principles of Stepwise Care of Asthma

Gain control of asthma as quickly as possible, then decrease treatment to the least medication necessary to maintain control.
A short course of oral corticosteroids may be needed at any step to gain control of asthma or treat exacerbations.
Review treatment at 1- to 6-month intervals for possible stepwise reduction in treatment.
If control is not maintained, review patient inhaler technique, adherence, and control of environmental irritants, allergens, or adverse drug response (e.g., aspirin, β-blockers).

Adapted from National Heart, Lung, and Blood Institute. Expert Panel Report II: Guidelines for the Diagnosis and Management of Asthma (see "General References," Consensus Statements and Guidelines for Management of Asthma and COPD).

Table 55.13. β-Sympathomimetic Agonists

Generic Name	Trade Name	β₂ Selectivity	Onset of Action (min)	Inhalation Peak Effect (min)	Duration of Effect (hr)	Dosage Form
Isoetharine	Bronkosol Bronkometer	$\beta_2 >$ β_1	5	5–15	2–3	Metered-dose inhaler, 340 µg/puff Nebulized solution, 1%
Metaproterenol	Alupent	$\beta_2 >>>$ β_1	1–5	30–60	2–5	Metered-dose inhaler, 650 µg/puff Nebulized solution, 5%
Terbutaline	Brethine Bricanyl Brethaire	$\beta_2 >>>$ β_1	1–5	30–60	2–5	Metered-dose inhaler, 200 µg/puff Injection, 1 mg/mL
Bitolterol	Tornalate	$\beta_2 >>>$ β_1	3–5	30–60	4–8	Metered-dose inhaler, 370 µg/puff
Pirbuterol	Maxair	$\beta_2 >>>$ β_1	5	30–60	4–5	Metered-dose inhaler, 200 µg/puff
Albuterol	Proventil Ventolin	$\beta_2 >>>>$ β_1	5–15	60–90	3–6	Metered-dose inhaler, 90 µg/puff Nebulized solution 0.5%
Salmeterol	Serevent	$\beta_2 >>>>>\beta_1$	10–20	180	12+	Metered-dose inhaler, 25 µg/puff

4 weeks or longer. More common use of bronchodilator MDIs usually indicates the need for more intensive anti-inflammatory therapy. In general, however, modern selective β-agonists are safe and effective drugs, and they should not be withheld from the symptomatic asthmatic. The most common side effects are tremor and cardiac arrhythmias. An often neglected side effect of chronic use of β-agonists is hypokalemia (apparently caused by an intracellular shift of potassium), which can be corrected with supplemental potassium (see Chapter 46). Long-acting β-agonists such as salmeterol that have a slower onset of action and longer duration of retention are used for long-term control of symptoms and should be avoided for symptomatic control. The use of such agents for short-term relief of symptoms may lead to excessive adrenergic stimulation. Therefore agents in this class should be prescribed in conjunction with a shorter-acting agent to be used for acute relief of symptoms.

If the need for inhaled bronchodilators exceeds three to four uses daily (excluding prophylactic use for exercise), an inhaled anti-inflammatory agent should usually be prescribed. *Inhaled nonsteroidal antiallergy drugs* include cromolyn (Intal-2 metered sprays four times a day) and nedocromil (Tilade-2 metered sprays two to four times a day). These agents diminish airways reactivity over several weeks and have virtually no side effects. They also may be used to inhibit exercise-induced bronchospasm. Their use is limited, however, by the lack of availability of the high-concentration preparations that have been shown to be most effective, the recommended frequency of dosing, and the high cost of these drugs. In selected cases, it is an acceptable alternative to prescribe a long-acting bronchodilator, such as inhaled salmeterol, or oral long-acting theophylline. In mild persistent asthma, particularly those who exhibit aspirin sensitivity, leukotriene inhibitors and antagonists, may also be used (see above).

Inhaled corticosteroids are important anti-inflammatory agents. They reduce airway inflammation and airway reactivity (71). Because of their poor absorption and rapid metabolism, systemic steroid effects are minimal. Most of the side effects are caused by local effects such as oral candidiasis, which can be

avoided by use of a spacer/reservoir device or by rinsing the mouth with water after each use. Although biochemical evidence of chemical adrenal suppression and increased bone metabolism is found with high-dose inhalation (more than 1200 µg/day) of these agents, clinically noteworthy systemic toxicity is rarely observed. However, reports of increased prevalence of glaucoma in older people receiving large doses of inhaled steroids and decreased growth in children receiving moderate to large doses of inhaled steroids emphasize the importance of using the smallest effective dose (57). Inhaled corticosteroids available in the United States include beclomethasone, budesonide, flunisolide, fluticasone, and triamcinolone. All are approximately equivalent in efficacy and side effects, although some have more convenient dosages and delivery devices. The drug is usually started at a dosage that is adequate to control asthma symptoms and is decreased to the lowest effective dosage (20). The effect of a change in dosage of inhaled corticosteroids may take 3 to 4 weeks to ascertain. Table 55.14 shows the equivalence of available formulations of inhaled corticosteroids.

If inhaled corticosteroids do not control symptoms and optimize lung function, consideration should be given to adding a second long-acting drug, such as an oral or inhaled long-acting β-agonist or a long-acting oral theophylline preparation, to control asthma. These drugs are particularly helpful when the main symptoms occur at night. A long-acting *theophylline* preparation may be given at a dosage of 400 to 1200 mg/day in one or two daily doses. Theophylline should be started at a low dosage that is increased at weekly or longer intervals with monitoring of blood levels to titrate to a serum theophylline level of 10 to 15 µg/mL (117). Theophylline is a mild bronchodilator and also has a modest anti-inflammatory effect (140). Side effects of theophylline include anorexia, nausea, gastroesophageal reflux, anxiety, and palpitations. Serious toxic effects at serum levels above 20 µg/mL include seizures and atrial and ventricular tachyarrhythmias. Because theophylline is metabolized by the liver, there are interactions with numerous other drugs. Erythromycin, ciprofloxacin and

Table 55.14. Approximate Comparative Daily Dosages for Inhaled Corticosteroids in Adults

Drug	Low Dose	Medium Dose	High Dose
Beclomethasone	168–504 µg	504–840 µg	>840 µg
42 µg/puff	4–12 puffs	12–20 puffs	>20 puffs
84 µg/puff	2–6 puffs	6–10 puffs	>10 puffs
Budesonide Turbuhaler	200–400 µg	400–600 µg	>600 µg
200 µg/dose	1–2 inhalations	2–3 inhalations	>3 inhalations
Flunisolide	500–1000 µg	1000–2000 µg	>2000 µg
250 µg/puff	2–4 puffs	4–8 puffs	>8 puffs
Fluticasone	88–264 µg	264–660 µg	>660 µg
44 µg/puff	2–6 puffs		
110 µg/puff		2–6 puffs	>6 puffs
220 µg/puff			>3 puffs
Triamcinolone	400–1000 µg	1000–2000 µg	>2000 µg
100 µg/puff	4–10 puffs	10–20 puffs	>20 puffs

Adapted from National Heart, Lung, and Blood Institute. Expert Panel Report II: Guidelines for the Diagnosis and Management of Asthma (see "General References," Consensus Statements and Guidelines for Management of Asthma and COPD).

other quinolones, and cimetidine decrease theophylline metabolism and elevate serum levels. Cigarette smoking and hyperthyroidism are associated with increased metabolism and decreased theophylline levels. Congestive heart failure and hepatic insufficiency require a reduction in dosage.

An oral, long acting β-agonist, albuterol (4-mg tablets), may be given twice daily. Maximal dosages of oral β-adrenergic agonists are often limited by tremor and a sensation of nervousness, and therefore should be titrated upward starting at one-half to one-quarter the maximum recommended dosage. Tolerance to this side effect occurs over several weeks, whereas the bronchodilator action is retained. The availability of *inhaled long-acting β-agonists* such as salmeterol has supplanted the use of oral agents except in circumstances where cost, compliance, or patient preference dictate their use. The role of the new class of antileukotriene drugs (62), leukotriene receptor blockers (zafirlukast—Accolate, 20 mg twice a day) and 5-lipoxygenase inhibitors (zileuton—Zyflo, 600 mg four times a day), is unclear. Antileukotriene drugs are probably most effective for the patient with mild or moderate asthma, for the patient with aspirin sensitivity, and for the patient who cannot use higher dosages of inhaled corticosteroids (104).

Inhaled anticholinergic drugs (e.g., ipratropium bromide) are safe and effective bronchodilators in asthma, and they add some marginal benefit when added to β2-adrenergic agonists (64).

When these measures are ineffective in controlling asthma or when previously stable asthma is punctuated by an exacerbation, oral corticosteroids should be used. These may be prescribed as a 5- to 14-day course starting at 30 to 60 mg/day of prednisone or equivalent prednisolone and either stopping abruptly or tapering gradually. In more difficult cases, tapering of the steroids may take several months or require chronic treatment with daily or every-other-day prednisone. In dosages above 20 mg/day for long periods, serious complications, including diabetes mellitus, posterior subcapsular cataracts, osteoporosis with compression fractures, and hypothalamic–pituitary–adrenal axis suppression, are common. Because of the serious side effects of chronic steroid use, vigorous efforts should be made to optimize adherence with environmental controls and maximum inhalational drug therapy in these patients. Other disorders that mimic asthma should be investigated. If long-term steroids are necessary, tuberculin skin testing should be performed, although the benefit of isoniazid prophylaxis compared with monitoring with chest x-rays in this setting is controversial (120). In those receiving long-term therapy, particularly postmenopausal women, prophylaxis of corticosteroid-induced osteoporosis with alendronate (Fosamax) should be considered.

For asthmatic patients who cannot taper steroids, several options may be considered, although none is well established at present. These include methotrexate, cyclosporine, troleandomycin, oral gold salts, hydroxychloroquine, and intravenous immunoglobulin infusions (32,133). In the future, monoclonal antibodies to IgE, or methods of controlling IgE production at the level of the T-helper cell may be forthcoming. If gastroesophageal reflux and associated asthma exacerbations can be documented by esophageal pH probe recording and manometrics, medical (or, in refractory cases, surgical) treatment of the reflux should be considered (79) (see Chapter 35). Initiation of these treatments should be undertaken by someone familiar with the treatment of steroid-dependent asthmatics because many such patients can be successfully tapered with consistent comprehensive care.

Emergency Treatment of the Acute Asthmatic Attack

When asthma fails to respond to home management (Table 55.12), the patient should be instructed to receive emergency treatment in a hospital emergency department or a similarly equipped facility. Both patients and physicians should understand that untreated severe asthma can be fatal and should recognize the individual at risk (131) (Table 55.15). Treatment should be initiated with nebulized treatments of selective β-adrenergic agonists given as three treatments in the first 60 to 90 minutes (Table 55.16). MDI administration of four to eight inhalations using a reservoir device is as effective as nebulizer therapy, and may be used when a nebulizer is not readily available (68).

Supplemental oxygen should be given to patients who are hypoxemic or to those in whom arterial oxygen saturation is unknown. Because bronchodilators initially can worsen ventilation–perfusion matching, oxygen saturation may fall during the early phases of treatment even as lung function is improving. Peak flow measurement or spirometry should be performed on admission and after each nebulizer treatment to determine response. Arterial blood gases should be checked in patients who appear severely ill to determine whether hypercapnia is present and whether mechanical ventilation might be required. A chest x-ray should be performed in patients in whom the possibility of pneumonia, pulmonary edema, or pneumothorax is suspected. Serum theophylline levels should be measured in patients taking theophylline to guide possible therapy with this drug.

If the initial treatment is unsuccessful, one should consider initiating systemic corticosteroids at a dosage of 60 to 125 mg prednisolone intravenously every 6 hours (81). Hourly treatments with nebulized bronchodilators should be continued, and the response measured. If there is no response to nebulized bronchodilators over the first 2 to 3 hours, subcutaneous epinephrine 0.2 to 0.4 mg or terbutaline 0.25 mg may be administered (16). In patients with peak flow less than 50% of baseline, intravenous theophylline may be beneficial in improving lung function and preventing hospital admission, starting with an infusion of 0.6 mg/kg lean body weight (118,144). The infusion rate should be 0.3 mg/kg for patients with hepatic disease or for those taking drugs that diminish aminophylline metabolism. In patients not previously taking theophylline, a loading dose of 5 to 6 mg/kg should be given. In those who have been taking theophylline, the dosage should be guided by serum levels, with no more than a 3 mg/kg loading dose. Intravenous fluids should be given for dehydration, but excessive administration of intravenous fluids may worsen the asthma by promoting airway mucosal edema.

After the initial treatment, if the patient shows deterioration with peak flow to FEV_1 less than 25% of baseline, develops altered sensorium, has an arterial oxygen tension less than 60 mm Hg on supplemental oxygen, or has arterial carbon dioxide tension greater than 40 mm Hg, the patient should be transferred to an intensive care facility for further treatment, monitoring, and possible intubation and mechanical ventilation.

In most circumstances, the response to the first 4 hours of therapy should determine whether the patient needs to be admitted to the hospital. Considerations that favor hospitalization include peak flow less than 40% of baseline, continued severe symptoms, a recent history of failed emergency treatment, a history of respiratory failure, and inadequate home support or access to medications.

Management of the Pregnant Asthmatic

Pregnancy has an unpredictable effect on asthma— about one-third of patients experience no change in symptoms, one-third improve, and one-third get worse. Poorly controlled asthma poses an increased risk of prematurity, intrauterine growth retardation, and perinatal morbidity. Prolonged or severe asthmatic attacks with hypoxemia or acid–base disturbances pose significant risks to the fetus, which has borderline oxygenation. Thus, prompt and aggressive management of acute asthmatic episodes should take precedence over concerns that the medications used to manage asthma may pose theoretical risks to the fetus.

In pregnant women, during an acute asthmatic attack, initial treatment should include supplemental oxygen to maintain an oxygen saturation of greater than 95% to prevent fetal hypoxemia. Epinephrine should be avoided if possible because of its tendency to reduce placental blood flow. Fetal monitoring should also be instituted in all but mild asthma attacks.

In general, management of pregnant and nonpregnant asthmatics is the same. Control of symptoms should be attempted with minimal use of medications, but no special attempt to discontinue medications is indicated.

β_2-Adrenergic agents and theophylline are smooth muscle relaxants and may therefore inhibit uterine contractions during labor. They have been used for decades and are generally safe for the fetus. Epinephrine causes vasoconstriction because of its α-adrenergic properties and may diminish placental and fetal blood flow. The most commonly used systemic corticosteroids, prednisone and prednisolone, cross the placenta poorly, so steroid production by the fetus is unaffected. Adrenal steroid suppression in the mother, however, may require administration of supplemental corticosteroids during the stresses of labor and delivery. Long-term use of oral steroids in other conditions has been associated with lower birth weight infants, so it is prudent to maximize inhaled forms of therapy before instituting long-term oral ste-

Table 55.16. Dosages of Inhaled β-Adrenergic Agonists in Acute Asthma Exacerbations in Adults

Drug	Dose (Nebulized in 3–5 mL Sterile Saline Solution)
Albuterol	2.5 mg (0.5 mL of 0.5% solution)
Metaproterenol	15 mg (0.3 mL of 5% solution)
Isoetharine	5 mg (0.5 mL of 1% solution)

Table 55.15. Risk Factors for Fatal Asthma

Previous episode of mechanical ventilation for asthma
Hospitalization for asthma in previous year
Steroid-dependent asthma
Nonadherence to medical treatment
Overuse of inhaled β-adrenergic agonists
Recent steroid taper or abrupt withdrawal
Lack of objective measures of asthma severity
Psychiatric disorder
Inner-city residence, poverty

roids. The benefits of inhaled steroids and cromolyn outweigh any potential risk to the pregnant asthmatic or her fetus. As a general rule, it is prudent to rely on drugs that have a long record of safe experience in pregnant asthmatics (see "General References," Management of Asthma During Pregnancy).

Course and Prognosis

Asthma that begins at an early age generally improves, and rates of prolonged remission have been reported from 30 to 70% (105). The severity of asthma correlates with the remission rate, so children with mild disease are likely to remit, whereas those with severe disease often continue to be symptomatic. Some childhood asthmatics experience a remission but then have a recurrence of asthma in adulthood. Such patients tend to develop disease that is persistent and severe.

Patients who first develop asthma as adults often develop irreversible airway obstruction. Additional risk factors such as cigarette smoking, environmental exposures, and infection may influence the progression of asthma to chronic obstructive pulmonary disease (COPD) (see below).

Death from asthma or one of its complications is uncommon, with overall death rates in the United States of about 1 per 100,000 population. Considering disease prevalence (approximately 10 million asthmatics in the United States), this is a low mortality rate. However, asthma mortality increased 31% between 1980 and 1990, with the greatest burden of death sustained by inner-city African-American males (97). The cause for this disturbing trend is unknown, but the increased incidence of and mortality from asthma in the United States are representative of similar trends around the world. Some of these changes in mortality rate may be the result of improved recognition and reporting, increased rates in the elderly because more individuals are living to old age, or changes in environmental factors such as air pollution or allergen exposure. Inadequate recognition of disease severity and access to medical care may also be important factors. Of great concern is the possibility that these changing trends are the result of inappropriate management, particularly the widespread use of inhaled β_2-agonists, whose overuse has been identified as a risk factor for fatal or near-fatal asthma attacks. This possible association emphasizes the need to manage asthma comprehensively and to limit reliance on the use of bronchodilators alone.

CHRONIC OBSTRUCTIVE PULMONARY DISEASE

Definition

Many attempts to define COPD have been made, leading to some confusion about terminology. The American Thoracic Society definition follows: Chronic obstructive pulmonary disease (COPD) is a disorder characterized by abnormal tests of expiratory flow that do not change markedly over periods of several months' observation. The qualification is intended to distinguish COPD from asthma. The airflow obstruction may be structural or functional. Specific causes of airflow obstruction such as localized disease of the upper airways, bronchiectasis, and cystic fibrosis are excluded. Bronchial hyperreactivity may be present with COPD as measured by an improvement in airflow following the inhalation of β-adrenergic agents or worsening after inhalation of methacholine or histamine (9).

COPD may further be subclassified into emphysema and chronic bronchitis.

Emphysema is defined by morphologic criteria as abnormal dilation of the terminal airspaces of the lung with destruction of alveolar septa in the absence of interstitial fibrosis (98). Whereas a formal diagnosis of emphysema requires gross anatomic inspection of the lung, a clinical diagnosis can be reasonably based on a compatible history, physical examination, pulmonary function tests, and radiographic studies. *Panacinar emphysema* is a condition in which all of the airspaces in an acinus are equally dilated. Typically, the bases of the lung are more involved than the apices. This is the usual finding in α_1-antitrypsin deficiency and in some elderly nonsmoking individuals. *Centroacinar emphysema* describes the condition in which the respiratory bronchiole at the proximal end of the acinus is more dilated than other portions of the acinus. Commonly, the apices of the lung are more involved in this disorder, which occurs predominantly in cigarette smokers. Peripheral airways disease is commonly associated with centroacinar emphysema, manifested by inflammation, fibrosis, and tortuousity of the terminal and respiratory bronchioles. The physiologic abnormality is the consequence of both the emphysema and the small airway narrowing and fibrosis.

Chronic bronchitis is a condition of chronic cough and sputum production that excludes other specific disorders such as bronchiectasis, tuberculosis, or cystic fibrosis. The formal epidemiologic definition of this disorder is the presence of cough and sputum production for the majority of days of the week for at least 3 months of the year for at least 2 years in a row. However, nearly everyone with chronic bronchitis has cough and sputum production on a perennial basis. Chronic bronchitis is common in cigarette smokers and is often incorrectly perceived by the patient to be a normal smoker's cough. The morbid anatomy of chronic bronchitis shows hyperplasia and hypertrophy of the mucous glands of the large central airways with central mucous plugging, variable degrees of smooth muscle hyperplasia, and airway wall thickening and inflammation (69). Chronic bronchitis can occur in the absence of major physiologic abnormalities, and the extent that it contributes to mortality and morbidity in COPD is controversial. In patients with advanced COPD, mortality is best predicted by the postbronchodilator FEV_1, with no additional information provided by the presence of sputum production (14). Some epidemiologic studies of people with less severe disease have shown some excess mortality associated with cough and phlegm, but the magnitude is not large (110). Approximately 50% of those with abnormal lung function report cough and phlegm, and the magnitude of the physiologic abnormality is worse in those who report more severe cough and phlegm. However, individual smokers with chronic bronchitis can develop severe airflow limitation without emphysema. These individuals are often classified as having *chronic obstructive bronchitis* or, when there is more prominent reversible airflow obstruction, *chronic asthmatic bronchitis.*

Natural History

COPD is a chronic disease that has its origins in early adulthood, or possibly even childhood, but does not produce symptoms or impairment of activity until it is far advanced, usually in late middle-age or in the elderly. The normal aging process causes slowly progressive degeneration of lung function after young adulthood, so a normal person loses approximately 20% of vital capacity and approximately 25% of FEV_1 between the ages of 25 and 75. The average decline in FEV_1 is about 30 mL/year, with some acceleration after the age of 65. These changes are the result of loss of elastic recoil in the lung from the degradation of elastin fibers, similar to the changes that occur in the skin that cause wrinkles. In most cigarette smokers, the rate of decline of FEV_1 is normal or only moderately increased. In susceptible smokers, however, there is an accelerated degeneration of lung function, 80 to 150 mL/year loss of FEV_1 (54,55,139). Over the course of several decades, this leads to progressive breathlessness and, if unchecked, to disability, respiratory failure, and death. It has been suggested that children who have serious respiratory ailments or exposure to respiratory toxins such as passive cigarette smoke will be at increased risk for development of COPD because of impaired lung function as young adults, and consequently less reserve capacity (Fig. 55.4).

Because of the reserve capacity of the lungs, the early stages of COPD do not cause any limitation of activity. When the FEV_1 reaches approximately 50% of predicted, there is ventilatory limitation of exercise capacity, but this is often ignored or attributed to deconditioning; and heavy exercise is progressively curtailed. Respiratory infections may cause severe and prolonged symptoms in this phase of the disease, often causing the patient to seek medical care. When the FEV_1 reaches approximately 30 to 35% of predicted (about 1.2 L in a man and 1.0 L in a woman), symptoms prevent normal execution of daily living and work activities, and about half of the afflicted individuals stop working. With continued decline in the FEV_1, chronic hypoxemia, hypercapnia, and cor pulmonale develop. Viral infections, mucous plugging, or respiratory irritants—including exposure to air pollutants—can precipitate episodes of acute respiratory failure, leading to hospitalization, mechanical ventilation, or death. More than half of the patients with COPD compatible with emphysema die within 10 years after

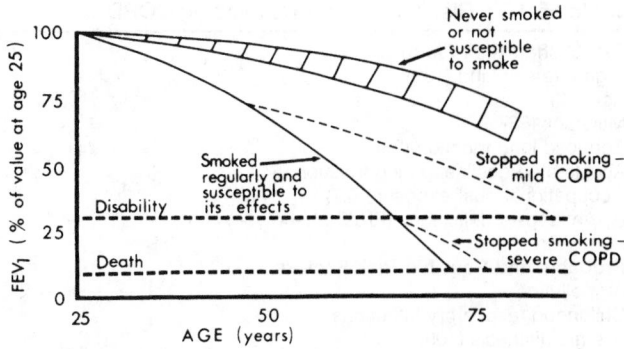

Figure 55.4. Effect of risk factors from smoking on the loss of lung function (FEV_1). The upper curves are derived from subjects who do not smoke or are not susceptible to the effects of smoking. They lose lung function gradually throughout adult life (15 to 30 mL/year). Lower curves show accelerated loss of lung function in subjects who are susceptible to the effects of cigarette smoke. At age 65 there is respiratory disability because FEV_1 has decreased to 25 to 30% of predicted (1 to 1.2 L), and further functional deterioration will eventually cause death because of complications of respiratory insufficiency. If that subject stops smoking, life may be prolonged but a respiratory death will still eventually result. If intervention is initiated earlier in life (40 to 50 years) when there is mild COPD, accelerated loss of lung function is reversible and a respiratory death will be avoided. Although this figure illustrates theoretical loss of FEV_1 for an adult cigarette smoker, susceptible smokers will lose lung function at different rates, thereby becoming disabled at different ages. (Modified from Fletcher C, Peto R. The natural history of chronic airflow obstruction. BMJ 1:1645,1977.)

initial diagnosis, whereas approximately 15% of those with chronic asthmatic bronchitis die in the first decade after diagnosis (27). The prognosis for the individual patient has not improved over the last 30 years.

Cigarette smoking is a major risk factor for development of COPD. Both observational studies and clinical trials have shown that cessation of smoking earlier in the course of disease can slow the rate of degeneration of lung function to the normal or near-normal range (15,145). When the disease is far advanced, however, degeneration of lung function may continue irrespective of smoking cessation (12).

Pathogenesis

It is impossible to predict which individuals are susceptible to COPD. However, several risk factors have been identified that increase an individual's risk for developing COPD (30,63) (Table 55.17).

Among these risk factors, *cigarette smoking* is the most prominent and potentially the most amenable to change. The mechanism by which cigarettes lead to COPD is thought to be mediated by proinflammatory components of cigarette smoke such as the hydrocarbon compound *acrolein.* Fourfold to fivefold increases in the numbers of activated neutrophils are present in the terminal air spaces and the peribronchial regions in smokers. These cells produce elastase that destroys the elastin elements in the alveolar walls and induces emphysema in animal models. Normally, the small

Table 55.17.   Risk Factors for Developing COPD

Established Risk Factors
Cigarette smoking (139)
Age (63)
Male sex (63)
Reduced lung function (28)
Accelerated decline in lung function (54)
Occupational dust exposure (22)
α_1-Antitrypsin deficiency (Pi-ZZ phenotype) (42)

Probable and Possible Risk Factors
Air pollution
Childhood respiratory infections
Allergic diathesis (105)
Airways reactivity (105)
Low socioeconomic status (139)
Poor nutrition
ABO blood type (139)
ABH nonsecretor status
Family members with COPD (139)

Adapted from Burrows B. Airways obstructive diseases: pathogenetic mechanisms and natural histories of the disorders. Med Clin North Am 74:547, 1990; and from Higgins M. Risk factors associated with chronic obstructive lung disease. Ann N Y Acad Sci 624:7, 1991.

amount of neutrophil elastase is inactivated by anti-elastases present in serum and lung liquid lining layer, α_1-antitrypsin being present in the largest quantities. Alveolar macrophages, when activated by constituents of cigarette smoke, secrete neutrophil chemotactic factors and promote neutrophil degranulation. *Cathepsin B,* a protease produced by human alveolar macrophages, induces emphysema in animal models and is found in 10-fold excess in the lungs of cigarette smokers. The serum antiproteases that are present in the lung are inactivated by oxidative free radicals that are produced by activated neutrophils and alveolar macrophages and that are present in cigarette smoke (127,128). The balance between free protease activity within the alveolus and alveolar duct and local antiprotease activity is thought to determine the rate of destruction of the lung parenchyma (56). In some smokers, even when the levels of antiprotease activity are normal, there may be a reduction in the rate of inactivation of the damaging enzymes.

α_1-*Antitrypsin* deficiency is an uncommon genetic disorder (found in about 1 in 2500 Caucasians of European descent) in which the circulating levels of antiproteases are less than 10% of normal. Normal α_1-antitrypsin activity is produced by the allele Pi-M (protease inhibitor M), for which approximately 90% of the population are homozygous. Pi-S is an allele with intermediate antiprotease activity, and Pi-Z is an allele with marked reduction in antiprotease activity. More than 75 minor alleles of the Pi gene have been identified, although most are rare and are uncommonly associated with disease (42). Individuals who are homozygous for the Pi-Z phenotype are at the greatest risk for developing premature emphysema. Such individuals account for approximately 1 to 2% of cases of emphysema. The Pi-Z phenotype is the result of a single DNA base substitution causing an amino acid substitution that prevents secretion of the material from liver cells (42). Serum levels are less than 15% of normal, despite hepatic intracellular accumulation of

the enzyme inhibitor. In addition, the Pi-Z inhibitor has a slower reaction rate in neutralizing proteases, so what is secreted is less effective. Most studies have shown little if any increased risk for emphysema in people with intermediate levels of α_1-antitrypsin—the Pi-MS, Pi-MZ, and Pi-SZ phenotypes—suggesting that there is a threshold level of antiprotease activity for development of premature emphysema in deficient patients. Although affected people present for medical care with severe emphysema in the third and fourth decades, many people with α_1-antitrypsin deficiency have normal or only mildly abnormal lung function if they do not smoke (124).

Occupational exposure to a number of mineral and organic dusts has been implicated in the development of COPD (22). In most of these circumstances, however, the offending agents are additive or synergistic with the effects of cigarette smoking, and it is uncommon to find occupationally related COPD in the absence of cigarette smoking. The mechanism is presumed to be the result of nonspecific irritation or activation of alveolar macrophages, enhancing lower respiratory inflammation. Although far-advanced silicosis and asbestosis may be associated with airflow obstruction, the predominant lesion in these disorders is fibrosis with localized compensatory emphysema and honeycombing leading to restrictive ventilatory defects. Occupational exposure to sensitizing agents found in grain, wood, and cotton dust, and polyurethane compounds not only may cause asthma but may lead to fixed airflow obstruction with chronic asthmatic bronchitis if the exposure is prolonged.

Nonspecific airway reactivity occurs in approximately 70% of people with COPD, even those with mild abnormalities and minimal symptoms, and is more common in women than in men (73). However, the interpretation of this finding is controversial. One school of thought, the so-called Dutch hypothesis, holds that this is a constitutional state that predisposes the individual to develop accelerated degeneration of pulmonary function when exposed to cigarette smoke or to other environmental agents (126). The alternative viewpoint is that airways reactivity is a marker for inflammatory or geometric changes that have already occurred, and therefore is the result of the disease process, not the cause.

The magnitude of airway reactivity correlates with the rate of decline of lung function (105) as well as with markers of inflammation (114). Whereas inflammatory mediators or airway wall thickening may contribute to increased tendency for airways to narrow, it is also possible that destruction of alveolar septal attachments and thickening of airway walls, which are the result of smoking-induced inflammation and early emphysema, lead to the increased tendency of the airways to constrict (47). This hypothesis is supported by the findings that airway reactivity is inversely correlated with baseline lung function in smokers (105), does not disappear with smoking cessation (114), and is induced in animals with emphysema caused by proteolytic enzymes.

Abnormal lung function during early adulthood is a

predictor of accelerated degeneration in lung function, a phenomenon known as the *horse race effect* (28). Presumably, those with lower lung function have already experienced some degeneration in lung function. Even individuals within the normal range of lung function who show lower spirometric indices have increased mortality from lung disease and other causes.

Aging is normally associated with changes in lung function, including reduction in vital capacity and FEV_1, and increases in residual volume and functional residual capacity. Physiologically, all of these changes can be attributed to a reduction in the elastic recoil of the lung that accompanies the aging process. The mechanism for these changes is unknown but is presumed to be the cumulative effect of endogenous and exogenous factors that degrade the elastin in the lung, and the balance of processes that repair or prevent this damage. Emphysema of the panacinar type, which is similar to that occurring with α_1-antitrypsin deficiency, is found in some elderly nonsmoking individuals, particularly women. Development of emphysema in smokers may reflect either the additive effects of toxic exposure that accelerate the normal aging of the lung or interference with the processes that inhibit such degeneration. Most of the increased mortality from COPD over the last two decades has been confined to individuals over the age of 65, raising the possibility that the disease is being unmasked as mortality from heart disease, stroke, and infectious diseases is declining.

COPD is more common among the poor and poorly educated. Although cigarette smoking is more common in lower socioeconomic groups, the indigent have worse lung function even when adjusted for smoking status. Race is not thought to be a component; some evidence suggests that African Americans are less susceptible to COPD than Caucasians (137). Factors that may contribute include crowded living conditions with exposure to frequent viral respiratory infections, indoor air pollutants from heating or cooking devices in poorly ventilated homes, poor nutrition, exposure to passive cigarette smoke, inadequate access to medical care for childhood respiratory infections, or increased exposure to respiratory irritants and toxins in the workplace. Although COPD mortality rates are highest in Caucasian men, women and African Americans have shown disproportionate increases in COPD mortality over the past decade, likely reflecting changing smoking patterns over the past 30 years.

The evidence that high levels of air *pollution* are important in the genesis of COPD is suggestive, but not definitive (65). In animal models, high levels of NO_2 and ozone can induce emphysema independently and can potentiate protease-induced emphysema, suggesting that oxidant air pollutants inhibit lung protective mechanisms. There is convincing evidence that acid aerosols contribute to transient worsening of COPD symptoms and contribute to periodic increases in hospitalizations for respiratory exacerbations (11,21).

Whereas allergic tendencies are strongly associated with the presence of asthma and symptoms of cough and wheeze in nonsmokers, the effect of atopy on respiratory symptoms and on decline in lung function in smokers is less clear. In part, this may be because of the tendency of adolescents and young adults with highly reactive airways to avoid cigarette smoking. Some evidence suggests that allergies or nonspecific elevation of serum IgE levels contribute to the development of fixed airway obstruction in smokers (105).

Evaluation of the Patient with COPD

History

COPD must be considered a diagnostic possibility in all individuals who smoke, even in the absence of respiratory symptoms. The physician should inquire about smoking habits in every patient encounter. Specific questioning about the age of onset, average number of packs per day, and number and duration of quit attempts should be elicited. Often patients report being nonsmokers to the physician when they have only recently quit smoking. Other respiratory symptoms such as cough, phlegm, and exertional dyspnea should be quantified. Morning sputum production is often erroneously considered to be normal by smokers. Shortness of breath can be detected by asking whether the individual has trouble keeping up with peers doing routine activities such as walking, sports, or work activities. More advanced dyspnea is roughly quantified by distance walked or flights of stairs walked before stopping. Sleep disturbances are a common and often overlooked symptom of COPD and may impair quality of life more than exertional dyspnea.

Physical Examination

Although historical and physical findings of COPD may confirm the diagnosis when they are present, they are usually apparent with advanced disease (see below for spirometric guidelines). The absence of these findings is not sensitive enough to exclude the diagnosis in the person at risk (18) (Table 55.18). COPD is often overlooked from clinical findings alone. In one large autopsy series, only one in eight cases of emphysema was diagnosed clinically.

In advanced COPD, general physical findings include those caused by hyperinflation: increase in resting chest anteroposterior diameter, flattening of the angle of the clavicle and trapezius, widening of the xiphocostal angle, and increase in the intercostal spaces. With inspiration there is diminished movement of the rib cage and increased movement of the abdominal wall. The patient has hypertrophied and well-defined abdominal and sternomastoid muscles, but diminished muscle mass in the thighs and legs. The characteristic seated posture is leaning forward with both hands on the knees to fix the shoulders, permitting more effective use of the accessory cervical muscles. Pursed-lip breathing and prolonged time of expiration are spontaneously adopted to diminish the energy expenditure of breathing. The fingers often show tobacco staining. Clubbing of the nails is rare and suggests the presence of bronchiectasis or bronchogenic carcinoma. Chest percussion shows increased reso-

Table 55.18. Sensitivity and Specificity of History and Physical Findings for Diagnosis of Moderate COPD

Historical Items			
Historical Finding	Cutoff	Sensitivity (%)	Specificity (%)
Age	≥75 years	13	99
Previous diagnosis of COPD	Yes vs. no	80	74
Smoking history	≥70 pack-years	40	95
Dyspnea severity (5-point scale)	≥4	60	75
Phlegm	2 oz or more in AM when present	20	95
Theophylline use	Yes vs. no	60	71
Steroid use	Yes vs. no	40	87
Inhaler use	Yes vs. no	27	94
Home oxygen	Yes vs. no	20	96

Physical Examination Items			
Physical Finding	Cutoff	Sensitivity (%)	Specificity (%)
Initial impression[a]	Yes vs. no	25	95
Diaphragm excursion	<2 cm TLC vs. RV	12	98
Chest percussion	Increased Resonance	32	94
Cardiac dullness	Decreased area	16	99
Blow out a match	≤10 cm	53	88
Wheeze	Yes vs. no	9	100
Reduced breath sounds	Yes vs. no	65	96
Forced expiratory time	>10 seconds	12	99
Cardiac point of maximum Impulse	Abdominal	27	98
Final overall opinion	Yes vs. no	51	93

Adapted from Badgett RG, Tanaka DJ, Hunt DK, et al. Can moderate chronic obstructive pulmonary disease be diagnosed by historical and physical findings alone? Am J Med 94:188, 1993.
[a]Based on general inspection.

nance and low diaphragms that move poorly with full inspiration and expiration. Auscultation shows diminished transmission of breath sounds over areas of emphysema and is the most reliable physical finding indicative of chronic airflow limitation. Early inspiratory crackles indicate opening of closed airways and are common in COPD, whereas late and pan-inspiratory crackles are more common with interstitial lung diseases (113). Wheezing may be elicited in most COPD patients by forced expiration, but the presence of wheezing during quiet breathing is more common with reversible bronchospasm.

In far advanced disease with *cor pulmonale,* elevated right atrial pressures cause neck vein distension, peripheral edema, and hepatomegaly. The pulmonary hypertension and distension of the right ventricle cause a pronounced cardiac impulse in the epigastrium. Tricuspid regurgitation from dilation of the right ventricle and pulmonary hypertension causes a systolic murmur over the epigastrium that increases with inspiration. In contrast to other forms of pulmonary hypertension, a ventricular heave and increased intensity of the second heart sound are not usually appreciated because of the interposed emphysematous lung.

Additional Studies

The ability to blow out a paper match from more than 10 cm away with an open mouth is a rudimentary lung

function test that is helpful when abnormal, but it is not sensitive (129). Another simple bedside lung function test is to measure the forced expiratory time with a stethoscope over the trachea during a forced vital capacity maneuver. However, it is not accurate enough in practice to screen for airflow limitation (75).

The *chest x-ray* is abnormal only in advanced disease. Signs of COPD include hyperinflation with flattening of the diaphragm, increased retrosternal airspace on the lateral view, narrow cardiac silhouette, paucity and tapering of peripheral blood vessels, and bullae (119). In some smokers with COPD, particularly those with bronchitic symptoms, there may be small rounded opacities or increased linear markings that represent thickened airway walls.

High-resolution computerized tomography of the chest is becoming the standard for evaluation of emphysema in the absence of an anatomic diagnosis. In practice, however, this study is rarely necessary because less expensive tests of lung function—spirometry and the diffusing capacity—are usually adequate to distinguish asthma from emphysema and to follow the course of the disease and the response to treatment.

Spirometry (see above) should be performed initially and during routine visits, as well as during exacerbations of disease (53). As a general rule, FEV_1 measurements greater than 2 L indicate mild obstruction; 1 to 2 L, moderate obstruction; and less than 1 L, severe obstruction. Peak flow monitoring, useful in asthma, may be misleading in COPD, because the peak flow can be well maintained despite worsening disease.

Sensitive tests, such as the *single-breath nitrogen washout test* (see above), measure the function of the small airways. Such tests are abnormal in most smokers and do not predict who will develop symptomatic COPD. Therefore, they are not routinely recommended. In smokers, forced expiratory spirometry is effective in screening for COPD. With serial measures of spirometry, it is possible to identify individuals who are demonstrating accelerated declines in lung function before symptoms intervene. Of spirometric indices, a FEV_1/FVC ratio below 70% predicts future decline in lung function (28).

Bronchodilator testing can reveal reversible bronchospasm, and the postbronchodilator measure of FEV_1 is the best overall predictor of life expectancy in COPD. Failure to respond rapidly to a single dose of an inhaled bronchodilator does not indicate that lung function will not improve with more long-term treatment. About one in five patients who do not demonstrate a rapid bronchodilator response will show improvement in lung function after several weeks of treatment with bronchodilators or corticosteroids (48). Abnormal methacholine reactivity is common in COPD but does not usually provide sufficient information to warrant its routine use.

The *carbon monoxide diffusing capacity test* (see above) is helpful in distinguishing emphysema from asthma. Cigarette smokers without emphysema have mild reductions in diffusing capacity because of the accumulation of carbon monoxide in the blood, which is only partially reversible with smoking cessation. A diffusing capacity below 70% of the predicted value is present with emphysema but may also be found with interstitial fibrosis and pulmonary vascular diseases. In chronic asthmatic bronchitis, the diffusing capacity tends to be preserved (77).

Measurements of lung volume (see above) help distinguish obstructive lung diseases from restrictive lung diseases, and they are particularly helpful during the initial assessment or when it is unclear whether an interstitial process is present such as that caused by occupational exposure to silica or asbestos. Measurements of airway resistance and lung compliance are often abnormal in COPD but do not add useful clinical information in most circumstances.

Exercise testing is indicated in individuals who demonstrate reduction in diffusing capacity below 50 to 60% of predicted and who are not hypoxemic at rest, if supplemental oxygen is being considered for improving exercise capacity. Exercise testing should be performed in a monitored facility. Measurement of oxygen saturation with a pulse oximeter usually suffices to determine whether oxygen should be prescribed. More complex and invasive exercise testing with measurement of arterial blood gas tensions, oxygen consumption, and ventilation are used for evaluation for disability (see Chapter 9), or if the cause for dyspnea is unclear.

Hypoxemia occurs in COPD as a consequence of ventilation–perfusion mismatching. In those with advanced disease, particularly obese individuals, hypoventilation and hypercapnia also promote hypoxemia. With exercise, particularly at higher altitude, hypoxemia can worsen because of impairment of diffusion of oxygen across the alveolar–capillary membrane. Measurement of arterial oxygen tension at rest should be done for patients who have moderately advanced disease, with FEV_1 below about 1.5 L, because this group is at risk to have chronic hypoxemia and to develop cor pulmonale. At higher altitudes, hypoxemia develops with less severe pulmonary involvement, and oxygen tensions should be measured more frequently. When the FEV_1 falls below 1.0 L, chronic hypercapnia becomes more common, often in the patients with the least dyspnea.

Other blood tests are indicated only as needed for the general care of the patient. An elevated hematocrit value is uncommon in COPD in comparison with similar levels of hypoxemia at altitude, but when it does occur, it should alert the clinician to the possible presence of chronic hypoxemia. Hypokalemia and hypomagnesemia are common as a consequence of β-adrenergic agonists in conjunction with diuretics and, if severe, may contribute to respiratory muscle failure (80).

Screening evaluation for *severe α_1-antitrypsin deficiency* can be done with serum protein electrophoresis to see if there is a marked decrease in the α_1-globulin level, although intermediate deficiencies require direct measurements of protease inhibitor levels. This need not be done routinely unless there is a strong family history of premature emphysema or of α_1-antitrypsin deficiency, the chest x-ray suggests panacinar emphysema, or the patient has severe COPD at a relatively young age.

Cystic fibrosis may present in adulthood with chronic cough and phlegm associated with chronic airflow limitation. It should be suspected if there is radiographic evidence of bronchiectasis; a family history of cystic fibrosis or severe chronic childhood lung disease; if the patient has allergic bronchopulmonary aspergillosis; or if sputum cultures persistently grow mucoid colonies of Pseudomonas. Elevations of chloride in sweat iontophoresis samples confirm the diagnosis, but genetic testing is available in reference laboratories to define polymorphisms of the CFTR gene.

The *electrocardiogram* in COPD shows a vertical or indeterminate heart axis and low voltage. Enlarged P waves, right axis deviation, or right ventricular hypertrophy is present with cor pulmonale. Echocardiography can confirm right ventricular dilation and tricuspid valve insufficiency. If available, *Doppler studies* of tricuspid retrograde flow can be used to estimate pulmonary artery pressures. Transesophageal echocardiography (see Chapter 60) gives better views, but the more invasive nature of the procedure limits its application; and if there is severe hyperinflation, the study is often technically inadequate. In most circumstances echocardiography should be reserved for patients in whom there is a question of associated left ventricular dysfunction or of valve disease.

Sputum examination by Gram's stain or wet preparation during exacerbations can help determine whether there is a predominance of neutrophils or eosinophils, guiding the choice between corticosteroids and antibiotics. Culture of the sputum is unnecessary unless pneumonia is present or unusual or resistant organisms are suspected. Most exacerbations are thought to be provoked by viral infections, and when bacterial superinfection occurs, it is usually with common pathogens such as *Streptococcus pneumoniae, Haemophilus influenzae,* or *Moraxella (Branhamella) catarrhalis* (96).

Management

The components of care in COPD consist of education about the disease, prevention of disease progression, treatment of complications, drug treatment to maximize lung function, and rehabilitation to optimize activity levels.

Education is important so that the patient can develop an understanding of what COPD is, how it is caused, and what possible courses the disorder may take. The patient should be given realistic expectations about the long-term progressive course of the disease, tempered by the understanding that temporary worsenings are treatable. The patient should try to achieve maximum social and physical functioning and to make use of whatever family, social, and medical support is available. Simple measures such as the availability of special parking areas for the disabled, wheelchairs and motorized carts in shopping malls and airports, portable oxygen, and oxygen supplementation during air travel are not always known by patients with advanced COPD, who may unnecessarily confine themselves to home and become socially isolated. Local volunteer health associations commonly sponsor groups in which these issues are discussed, and they often provide instructional materials. Patients and their families should understand that the dyspnea that occurs with exertion is not harmful to the lung and that with appropriate pacing of activities, a certain level of dyspnea is actually desirable to achieve and maintain physical conditioning. Inquiries about sexual functioning should not be avoided. Education of the patient's bed partner about proper techniques and the use of prophylactic bronchodilators and oxygen can establish more normal sexual functioning, even with severe disease. Advance directives regarding intensive or long-term medical care should be discussed with patients and their families, and the physician should encourage this communication. Both physician and patient should understand that episodes of acute respiratory failure in COPD that require mechanical ventilation are often successfully treated, but that the long-term survival is poor, although unpredictable, in those who have incapacitating dyspnea, cor pulmonale, or poor nutrition (92).

Prevention of disease progression and complications
is one of the most important goals of treatment. By the time most patients present with advanced disease, they have discontinued smoking, although a sizable minority have not. Many with mild or moderate disease continue to smoke, unaware of their illness and the potential for arresting its progression by smoking cessation. The practical approaches to smoking cessation are discussed in Chapter 20. In the patient with lung disease, the physician should deliver a strong personalized smoking cessation message that emphasizes the definite and progressive nature of the disease, the likelihood of early disability with continued smoking, and the potential for arresting the disease when smoking is stopped. Referral to a smoking group program and use of nicotine gum or skin patch replacement therapy are advised.

Exposure to respiratory irritants should be avoided in the workplace as well as the home, and if the disease is complicated by allergy or overlaps with allergic asthma, environmental control measures should be instituted. Smoking of marijuana and cocaine may cause airway irritation, and although there is little evidence that they contribute to airway reactivity or to development of COPD, their use should be discouraged.

Pneumococcal vaccination (see Chapter 32) is recommended, although it is not uniformly successful in older patients with chronic obstructive lung disease. In those who have severe nutritional compromise or who are using corticosteroids, vaccination every 6 years can increase antibody levels. *Influenza vaccination* annually (see Chapter 32) or amantadine/rimantadine prophylaxis for unimmunized individuals during an influenza epidemic can prevent or attenuate this potentially fatal infection.

Patients with α_1-antitrypsin deficiency are candidates for intravenous replacement therapy with protease inhibitors, although the long-term benefits of this treatment are not yet established (5).

Treatment of Complications

Tracheobronchial infections are common in COPD, heralded by a change in the quantity, viscosity, or color of sputum. Although most infections are initiated by viruses, bacterial contamination or superinfection of the lower respiratory tract is common. Broad-spectrum and inexpensive antibiotics such as tetracycline, erythromycin, amoxicillin, or trimethoprim–sulfamethoxazole can shorten the duration of these symptoms, although there is little evidence that long-term use of antibiotics will halt the progression of disease (13,96). When the patient is intolerant of first-line antibiotics or when there is a evidence of resistant organisms, cephalosporin, amoxicillin–clavulanate, or quinolone antibiotics should be prescribed. Care should be taken to monitor for theophylline toxicity if erythromycin or quinolones are prescribed since these drugs inhibit hepatic metabolism of theophylline.

Chronic hypoxemia causes pulmonary hypertension and cor pulmonale, a condition associated with poor survival if untreated. Oxygen therapy prolongs survival and improves physical and psychologic functioning in hypoxemic patients with COPD (82,103). When indicated (Table 55.19), oxygen can be administered with a nasal cannula. Oxygen concentrators, compressed oxygen tanks, and liquid oxygen storage reservoirs are all suitable for home use (106,111). Portable liquid oxygen systems and small compressed oxygen tanks with demand valves allow mobility out of the home and should be used whenever possible. Oxygen should be prescribed at the lowest level necessary to maintain an arterial oxygen saturation at or above 90%, usually 1 to 4 L/minute for a minimum duration of 18 hours/day. The patient should understand that oxygen is used to prevent cardiac complications, and not as a symptomatic treatment for dyspnea. Reservoir or demand-valve oxygen delivery systems conserve oxygen use, prolonging ambulatory oxygen systems. Transtracheal oxygen catheters are used for the occasional patient who requires high oxygen concentrations or who cannot tolerate a nasal cannula (134).

If desaturation occurs with exercise, increased flows of oxygen during activity can improve exercise tolerance and enhance the ability to engage in an exercise conditioning program. *Nocturnal hypoxemia* in COPD is common and often unsuspected. The role for screening for nocturnal oxygen desaturation and the treatment for it are not well established. Nonetheless, it is prudent to test for nocturnal hypoxemia (in a sleep center or a hospital) in individuals who have erythrocytosis, unexplained peripheral edema without waking abnormalities of blood gases, or daytime hypersomnolence. Oxygen treatment for nocturnal hypoxemia improves sleep quality as well as daytime activity levels.

When *pulmonary hypertension* and *cor pulmonale* are present, treatment consists of continuous oxygen to overcome hypoxemia and diuretics to control peripheral edema. Digitalis is not useful unless there is concomitant left ventricular disease or atrial tachyarrhythmias. Calcium channel blockers can vasodilate the pulmonary circulation, but they often worsen hypoxemia and their benefit is not established. Almitrine, not available in the United States, improves arterial oxygen tension through improved ventilation–perfusion matching but does not reduce pulmonary artery pressure (141). Phlebotomy can be used to maintain a hematocrit value less than 50%, although persistent erythrocytosis suggests inadequate oxygen supplementation or another cause (37).

Supraventricular tachyarrhythmias are common in patients with COPD, as a consequence of right atrial enlargement, increased endogenous adrenergic tone,

hypoxemia, and drug treatment—particularly theophylline. Treatment is similar to that in nonpulmonary patients (see Chapter 59). However, the presence of COPD should not prevent evaluation for treatable causes of arrhythmias such as pulmonary embolism, hyperthyroidism, or valvular heart disease, which may be difficult to diagnose in these patients.

Control of *mucus hypersecretion* with the use of expectorants is not of proven benefit in improving lung function, although some patients report improvement in symptoms (112). Iodinated glycerol has been removed from the U.S. market because of the frequency of adverse effects, particularly thyroid disease.

Hypercapnia may actually be an adaptive response to obstructive lung disease by decreasing the work of breathing, preventing respiratory muscle fatigue, and allowing a diminished sensation of dyspnea. Respiratory stimulants may therefore be detrimental over long periods. Bronchospasm (see below), obesity (see Chapter 76), and sleep apnea (see Chapter 85) are reversible conditions that can contribute to hypercapnia and therefore should be evaluated and treated. Sedatives with potential for respiratory depression should be avoided.

Malnutrition is present in 50% of patients with advanced COPD, usually when the FEV_1 is less than 35% of predicted. This is the consequence of increased metabolic demands as well as of insufficient caloric intake. Body weight less than 90% of ideal is associated with increased mortality and decreased exercise capacity in patients with otherwise similar lung function (142,143). The physician should monitor body weight in COPD patients and prescribe caloric supplementation as needed.

Drug Therapy to Maximize Lung Function

Bronchodilators and anti-inflammatory agents are used in COPD to reverse bronchospasm and to prevent bronchoconstriction in response to provocative agents. Small amounts of bronchoconstriction and air trapping can cause marked deterioration in symptoms, and conversely, small amounts of bronchodilation can cause considerable improvement in functional capacity. The use of anti-inflammatory agents to alter the course of the disease is not yet established.

Drug treatment should use the minimum number of agents and the least frequent dosing schedule possible, starting with the agents having the greatest benefit and least toxicity. The recommended stepped treatment approach is to start with anticholinergic agents, then β-adrenergic agents, followed by theophylline and corticosteroids (53). Response to treatment is judged by symptomatic improvement as well as by spirometry.

Ipratropium bromide (Atrovent) is an inhaled anticholinergic drug that causes 4 to 8 hours of bronchodilation through inhibition of vagal stimulation of the airways. It appears to be particularly effective in patients with chronic asthmatic bronchitis, and it does not lead to tolerance, making it the first-choice bronchodilator for COPD patients. The dosage is started at two MDI inhalations three times daily, and

Table 55.19. Indications for Continuous Oxygen Therapy

Arterial oxygen tension ≤55 mm Hg or sat O_2 ≤88% while in usual state of health

Arterial oxygen tension ≤60 mm Hg or sat O_2 ≤89% with evidence of chronic hypoxemia such as erythrocytosis, ankle edema, venous engorgement, electrocardiographic p-pulmonale, or psychologic impairment can be increased to six inhalations four times daily. Systemic side effects are uncommon. Local side effects include mouth irritation and cough, which can be diminished by good inhaler technique or by use of a spacer (60) (see above). Although ipratropium provides sustained benefit in patients with moderate disease, it does not inhibit progression of the disease if smoking is continued (15).

β-Adrenergic agonists are used at dosages comparable to those used in asthma (see above). Although there is concern that self-medication with these agents is overused in asthmatics, the dosages used in COPD are often less than are needed to achieve adequate bronchodilation (53). The dosages of inhaled selective β-agonists should be increased before oral agents are prescribed so that tremor and hypokalemia are minimized. For nocturnal symptoms, inhaled long-acting agents such as salmeterol are useful. Spacer devices, breath-actuated MDIs, and dry-powder inhalers of β-adrenergic agonists are useful for those who cannot coordinate the use of conventional MDIs (see above).

Theophylline is best taken in a long-acting preparation once or twice daily. Although it is possible to monitor blood levels, there is only a rough correlation between side effects and serum levels. The use of theophylline in COPD has diminished in recent years, but it is still an effective second-line drug (78). As with asthma, this drug is most useful for the prevention of nocturnal symptoms. Although the bronchodilating effects of theophylline are moderate compared with inhaled drugs, it has other pharmacologic actions that improve the well-being of the COPD patient, including improvement in diaphragm function, prevention of respiratory muscle fatigue, increased ventilatory drive, potentiation of catecholamine function, prevention of microvascular permeability, increased mucociliary clearance, prevention of late-phase antigen responses, inhibition of mast cell histamine release, and suppression of leukocyte activation (109). Clinical trials showing improvement in functional status beyond that gained from the effects of bronchodilation are consistent with improvement in respiratory muscle function (95,144).

Oral corticosteroids are widely used in COPD for treatment of exacerbations (2). Among chronic symptomatic patients, some 10 to 20% show substantial short-term improvement, defined as 25% or greater increase in FEV_1. In general, the patients studied have had far-advanced disease and have not differed from other COPD patients except in their steroid response (91). Some have suggested that long-term low-dose oral steroids may slow the progression of the disease, but the evidence is not strong in comparison to the well-defined side effects of such treatment. If patients have an inadequate response to inhaled bronchodilators and theophylline, it is reasonable to try a short-term trial of oral corticosteroids with monitoring of lung function. If there is no improvement in lung function after a 2- to 4-week trial of corticosteroids, they should be discontinued. If there is a response to initial treatment, the dosage should be tapered slowly to achieve the least dosage compatible with relief of symptoms. In steroid-responsive individuals, the use of inhaled corticosteroids may allow lower oral dosages to be used.

Inhaled corticosteroids (see above) by themselves are beneficial in a minority of COPD patients, although the benefit is less than with oral corticosteroids. Furthermore, some patients who respond to oral corticosteroids do not respond to inhaled agents. Although inhaled steroids do inhibit inflammation in COPD, they do not reduce airway reactivity as they do in asthma (136). Inhaled corticosteroids may decrease the progression of airflow limitation, but the benefit is mainly in nonsmokers or those with asthmatic bronchitis (46).

Pulmonary Rehabilitation

Lacking the capacity to restore damaged lung parenchyma, efforts should be made to optimize activity levels through rehabilitation programs. The content of such programs varies widely but includes some or all of the following elements: education about COPD and its treatment, support group discussions, pacing and energy conservation training for daily activities, aerobic exercise conditioning, upper-extremity exercises, respiratory muscle training, and pursed-lip and diaphragm breathing exercises. Generally, these programs have demonstrated improved exercise endurance and sense of well-being without changes in lung function, although not all individuals benefit and it is unclear which components of these programs are most important (34,102). If a coordinated rehabilitation program is not accessible, many of these elements can be provided individually to ambulatory patients. For example, a regular daily walk for 15 to 30 minutes at a pace that induces mild to moderate dyspnea can be safely prescribed for most patients with COPD. Support groups for patients and families are widely available through volunteer agencies.

Surgery

Surgical resection of bullae is rarely indicated for treatment of COPD. An individual with a single large bulla that occupies more than one-third of the hemithorax with preserved carbon monoxide diffusing capacity is likely to do best after bullectomy (101). Unilateral and bilateral lung transplantation is successful in some patients with severe emphysema, but the indications are not established and the procedure is limited by expense, risk, and lack of donor organs (84,85,138). Lung volume reduction surgery (43), where lung tissue is removed surgically, leads to increased elasticity of the remaining lung, and may improve the contour and function of the diaphragm. The operative mortality from the procedure is ranges from 4 to 14%; the duration of benefit is unknown; and selection criteria for this operation are not well defined; therefore, although promising, lung volume reduction surgery should be approached as an experimental procedure (26) (see Fein et al., "General References").

The perioperative management of patients with COPD is discussed in Chapter 86.

Prognosis (See also "Natural History," above)

In general, the prognosis of patients with chronic airways obstruction can be estimated from the FEV_1. One study showed that in moderate obstruction, when FEV_1 was greater than 1.25 L, the 5-year survival of patients was only slightly decreased from that of matched controls. If FEV_1 was between 0.75 and 1.25 L, 5-year survival decreased to approximately 66% of expected, and if less than 0.75 L, to 33% of expected (27). Cardiac disease, resting tachycardia, hypercapnia, and hypoxemia pose additional risks to survival, whereas a significant response to bronchodilator therapy (greater than 10% improvement in FEV_1) is associated with improved survival. Serial tests of lung function at 6- to 12-month intervals help identify patients with accelerated rates of decline.

General References*

Asthma

Clark TJH, Godfrey S, Lee TH, eds. Asthma. 3rd ed. New York: Chapman & Hall Medical, 1992.
> An authoritative text on asthma etiology, diagnosis, and treatment.

Kaliner AB, Barnes PJ, Persson CGA. Asthma: its pathology and treatment. Vol 49. (In series Lung biology in health and disease, edited by Claude Lenfant.) New York: Marcel Dekker, 1991.
> Contains good discussions of the cellular basis of asthma.

Szefler SJ, Leung DYM, eds. Severe asthma: pathogenesis and clinical management. Vol 86. (In series Lung biology in health and disease, edited by Claude Lenfant.) New York: Marcel Dekker, 1996.
> Excellent reference for treatment of steroid-dependent asthma. Good treatment of drug adherence issues.

Chronic Obstructive Pulmonary Disease

Cherniack NS, ed. Chronic obstructive pulmonary disease. Philadelphia: WB Saunders, 1991.
> A multi-authored text with authoritative reviews of all aspects of chronic obstructive pulmonary disease.

Consensus Statements and Guidelines for Management of Asthma and COPD

Agency for Health Care Policy and Research. **Smoking cessation clinical practice guideline.** JAMA 275:1270, 1996.

American Thoracic Society. **Standards for the diagnosis and care of patients with chronic obstructive pulmonary disease.** Am J Respir Crit Care Med 152(5 Pt 2):S77, 1995.

Beveridge RC, Grunfeld AF, Hodder RV, Verbeek PR. **Guidelines for the emergency management of asthma in adults.** CAEP/CTS Asthma Advisory Committee. Canadian Association of Emergency Physicians and the Canadian Thoracic Society. Can Med Assoc J 155(1):25, 1996.

Chan-Yeung M. **Assessment of asthma in the workplace.** ACCP consensus statement. Chest 108:1084, 1995.

Fein AM, Branman SS, Casaburi R, et al. **Lung volume reduction surgery. Official statement of the American Thoracic Society.** Am J Respir Crit Care Med 154:1151, 1996.

Joint Task Force on Practice Parameters. **Practice parameters for the diagnosis and treatment of asthma.** Joint Task Force on Practice Parameters, representing the American Academy of Allergy Asthma and Immunology, the American College of Allergy,

Asthma and Immunology, and the Joint Council of Allergy, Asthma and Immunology. J Allergy Clin Immunol 96(5 Pt 2):707, 1995.

McDonald CF, Burdon JG. **Asthma in pregnancy and lactation. A position paper for the Thoracic Society of Australia and New Zealand.** Med J Aust 165:485, 1996.

National Asthma Education and Prevention Program Expert Panel Report II. **Guidelines for the Diagnosis and Management of Asthma.** HHS publication 97-451. Bethesda, MD: The National Heart, Lung and Blood Institute, 1997 (http://www.nhlbi.nih.gov/nhlbi/nhlbi.htm).

National Asthma Education and Prevention Program Working Group. **Considerations for Diagnosing and Managing Asthma in the Elderly.** NIH publication 96-3662. Bethesda MD: The National Heart, Lung and Blood Institute, 1996 (http://www.nhlbi.nih.gov/nhlbi/nhlbi.htm).

National Asthma Education Program Working Group. **Management of asthma during pregnancy.** NIH publication 93-3279A. Bethesda, MD: The National Heart, Lung and Blood Institute, 1992. (http://www.nhlbi.nih.gov/nhlbi/nhlbi.htm).

North of England Asthma Guideline Development Group. **North of England evidence based guidelines development project: summary version of evidence based guideline for the primary care management in adults.** BMJ 312(7033):762, 1996.

Siafakas NM, Vermeire P, Pride NB, et al. **Optimal assessment and management of chronic obstructive pulmonary disease (COPD).** The European Respiratory Society Task Force. Eur Respir J 8:1398, 1995.

Specific References

1. Abbey DE, Petersen F, Mills PK, Beeson WL. Long-term ambient concentrations of total suspended particulates, ozone, and sulfur dioxide and respiratory symptoms in a nonsmoking population. Arch Environ Health 48:33, 1992.
2. Albert RK, Martin TR, Lewis SW. Controlled clinical trial of methylprednisolone in patients with chronic bronchitis and acute respiratory insufficiency. Ann Intern Med 92:753, 1980.
3. Alberts WM, do Pico GA. Reactive airways dysfunction syndrome. Chest 109:1618, 1996.
4. American Lung Association. Lung disease data, 1993. New York: American Lung Association, 1993.
5. **American Thoracic Society. Guidelines for the approach to the patient with severe hereditary alpha-1-antitrypsin deficiency. Am Rev Respir Dis 140:1494, 1989.**
6. American Thoracic Society. Pulmonary function laboratory personnel qualifications. Am Rev Respir Dis 134:623, 1986.
7. American Thoracic Society. Lung function testing: selection of reference values and interpretative strategies. Am Rev Respir Dis 144:1202, 1991.
8. American Thoracic Society. Standardization of spirometry— 1987 update. Am Rev Respir Dis 136:1285, 1987.
9. American Thoracic Society. Standards for the diagnosis and care of patients with chronic obstructive pulmonary disease (COPD) and asthma. Am Rev Respir Dis 136:225, 1987.
10. American Thoracic Society. Standardization of spirometry, 1994 update. Am J Respir Crit Care Med 152:1107, 1995.
11. American Thoracic Society. Health effects of outdoor air pollution. Am J Respir Crit Care Med 153:3, 1996.
12. Anthonisen NR. Chronic obstructive pulmonary disease. Can Med Assoc J 138:503, 1988.
13. **Anthonisen NR, Manfreda J, Warren CWP, et al. Antibiotic therapy in exacerbations of chronic obstructive pulmonary disease. Ann Intern Med 106:196, 1987.**
14. Anthonisen NR, Wright EC, Hodgkin JE, IPPB Trial Group. Prognosis in obstructive pulmonary disease. Am Rev Respir Dis 133:14, 1986.
15. **Anthonisen NR, Connett JE, Kiley JP, et al. Effects of smoking intervention and the use of an inhaled anticholinergic bronchodilator on the rate of decline of FEV_1; The Lung Health Study. JAMA 272:1497, 1994.**
16. **Appel D, Karpel JP, Sherman M. Epinephrine improves expiratory flow rates in patients with asthma who do not respond to inhaled metaproterenol sulfate. J Allergy Clin Immunol 84:90, 1989.**

---

*Bold print (general references) and bold numerals (specific references) denote published controlled clinical trials, meta-analyses, or consensus-based recommendations.

17. Aubier M, Levy J, Clerici C, et al. Different effects of nasal and bronchial glucocorticosteroid administration on bronchial hyperresponsiveness in patients with allergic rhinitis. Am Rev Respir Dis 146:122, 1992.

18. Badgett RG, Tanaka DJ, Hunt DK, et al. Can moderate chronic obstructive pulmonary disease be diagnosed by historical and physical findings alone? Am J Med 94:188, 1993.

19. Barnes PJ. A new approach to the treatment of asthma. N Engl J Med 321:1517, 1989.

20. Barnes PJ. Inhaled glucocorticoids for asthma. N Engl J Med 332:868, 1995.

21. Bates DV, Sizto R. The Ontario Air Pollution Study: identification of the causative agent. Environ Health Perspect 79:69, 1989.

22. Becklake MR. Occupational exposures: evidence for a causal association with chronic obstructive pulmonary disease. Am Rev Respir Dis 140(3 Pt 2):S85, 1989.

23. Bergin C, Muller N, Nichols DM, et al. The diagnosis of emphysema; a computed tomographic-pathologic correlation. Am Rev Respir Dis 133:541, 1986.

24. Birkhead G, Attaway NJ, Strunk RC, et al. Investigation of a cluster of deaths of adolescents from asthma: evidence implicating inadequate treatment and poor patient adherence with medications. J Allergy Clin Immunol 84(4 Pt 1):484, 1989.

25. Boulet LP. Increases in airway responsiveness following acute exposure to respiratory irritants. Reactive airway dysfunction syndrome or occupational asthma? Chest 94:476, 1988.

26. Brenner M, Yusen R, McKenna R Jr, et al. Lung volume reduction surgery for emphysema. Chest 110:205, 1996.

27. Burrows B, Bloom JW, Trayer GA, Cline MG. The course and prognosis of different forms of chronic airways obstruction in a sample from the general population. N Engl J Med 317:1309, 1987.

28. Burrows B, Knudson RJ, Camilli AE, et al. The horse-racing effect and predicting decline in forced expiratory volume in one second from screening spirometry. Am Rev Respir Dis 135:788, 1987.

29. Burrows B, Martinez FD, Halonen M, et al. Association of asthma with serum IgE levels and skin-test reactivity to allergens. N Engl J Med 320:271, 1989.

30. Burrows B. Airways obstructive diseases: pathogenetic mechanisms and natural histories of the disorders. Med Clin North Am 74:547, 1990.

31. Busse WW, Lemanske RF Jr, Dick EC. The relationship of viral respiratory infections and asthma. Chest 101(6 Suppl):385S, 1992.

32. Busse WW, McGill K, Jarjour NN. Current management of asthma patients with corticosteroid resistance. Am J Respir Crit Care Med 154(2 Pt 2):S70, 1996.

33. Castell DO. Asthma and gastroesophageal reflux. Chest 96:2, 1989.

34. Celli BR. Pulmonary rehabilitation in patients with COPD. Am J Respir Crit Care Med 152:861, 1995.

35. Center for Disease Control and Prevention. Mortality patterns—United States, 1993. MMWR 45:161–164, 1996.

36. Chan-Yeung M. Occupational asthma. Chest 98:148S, 1990.

37. Chetty KG, Brown SE, Light RW. Improved exercise tolerance of the polycythemic lung patient following phlebotomy. Am J Med 74:415, 1983.

38. Cheung D, Timmers MC, Zwinderman AH, et al. Long-term effects of a long-acting beta 2-adrenoceptor agonist, salmeterol, on airway hyperresponsiveness in patients with mild asthma. N Engl J Med 327:1198, 1992.

39. Corren J, Newman KB. Vocal cord dysfunction mimicking bronchial asthma. Postgrad Med 92:153, 1992.

40. Crapo RO, Morris AH, Gardner RM. Reference spirometric values using techniques and equipment that meet ATS recommendations. Am Rev Respir Dis 123:659, 1981.

41. Creticos PS, Reed CE, Norman PS, et al. Ragweed immunotherapy in adult asthma. N Engl J Med 334:501, 1996.

42. Crystal RG, Brantly ML, Hubbard RC, et al. The alpha-1-antitrypsin gene and its mutations: clinical consequences and strategies for therapy. Chest 95:196, 1989.

43. Davies L, Calverley PM. Lung volume reduction surgery in chronic obstructive pulmonary disease. Thorax 51(Suppl 2):S29, 1996.

44. de Blay F, Chapman MD, Platts-Mills TA, et al. Airborne cat allergen (Fel d I). Environmental control with the cat in situ. Am Rev Respir Dis 143:1334, 1991.

45. Djukanovic R, Roche WR, Wilson JW, et al. State of the art: mucosal inflammation in asthma. Am Rev Respir Dis 142:434, 1990.

46. Dompeling E, van-Schayck CP, van-Grunsven PM, et al. Slowing the deterioration of asthma and chronic obstructive pulmonary disease observed during bronchodilator therapy by adding inhaled corticosteroids. A 4-year prospective study. Ann Intern Med 118:770, 1993.

47. Drazen JM, Hirschman C, Macklem PT, et al. Mechanics of bronchoconstriction influenced by inflammation. In: Holgate ST, ed. The role of inflammatory processes in airway hyperresponsiveness. Boston: Blackwell, 1989.

48. Eaton ML, Green BA, Church MS, et al. Efficacy of theophylline in irreversible airflow obstruction. Ann Intern Med 92:758, 1980.

49. Elliott MW, Adams L, Cockcroft A, et al. The language of breathlessness. Use of verbal descriptors by patients with cardiopulmonary disease. Am Rev Respir Dis 144:826, 1991.

50. Elshami AA, Tino G. Coexistent asthma and functional upper airway obstruction. Case reports and review of the literature. Chest 110(5):1358, 1996.

51. Enright PL, Hyatt RE. Office spirometry: a practical guide of the selection and use of spirometers. Philadelphia: Lea & Febiger, 1987.

52. Epstein RL. Constituents of sputum; a simple method. Ann Intern Med 77:259, 1972.

53. Ferguson GT, Cherniack RM. Current concepts: management of chronic obstructive pulmonary disease. N Engl J Med 328:1017, 1993.

54. Fletcher C, Peto C, Tinker C, Speizer FE. The natural history of chronic bronchitis and emphysema. New York: Oxford University Press, 1976.

55. Fletcher C, Peto R. The natural history of chronic airflow obstruction. BMJ 1:1645, 1977.

56. Fujita J, Nelson NL, Daughton DM, et al. Evaluation of elastase and antielastase balance in patients with chronic bronchitis and pulmonary emphysema. Am Rev Respir Dis 142:57, 1990.

57. Garbe E, LeLorier J, Boivin JF, Suissa S. Inhaled and nasal glucocorticoids and the risks of ocular hypertension or open-angle glaucoma. JAMA 277:722, 1997.

58. Govindaraj M. What is the cause of dyspnea in asthma and emphysema? Ann Allergy 59:63, 1987.

59. Greenberger PA. Allergic bronchopulmonary aspergillosis and funguses. Clin Chest Med 9:599, 1988.

60. Gross NJ. The influence of anticholinergic agents on treatment for bronchitis and emphysema. Am J Med 91:11S, 1991.

61. Grossman J. One airway, one disease. Chest 111(2 Suppl):11S, 1997.

62. Hay DW. Pharmacology of leukotriene receptor antagonists. More than inhibitors of bronchoconstriction. Chest 111(2 Suppl):35S, 1997.

63. Higgins M. Risk factors associated with chronic obstructive lung disease. Ann N Y Acad Sci 624:7, 1991.

64. Higgins RM, Stradling JB, Lane DJ. Should ipratropium bromide be added to beta-agonists in treatment of acute severe asthma? Chest 94:718, 1988.

65. Hodgkin JE, Abbey DE, Euler GL, Magie AR. COPD prevalence in nonsmokers in high and low photochemical air pollution areas. Chest 86:830, 1984.

66. Horwitz RJ, Busse WW. Inflammation and asthma. Clin Chest Med 16:583, 1995.

67. Hyatt RE, Black LF. The flow-volume curve: a current perspective. Am Rev Respir Dis 107:191, 1973.

68. Idris AH, McDermott MF, Raucci JC, et al. Emergency department treatment of severe asthma. Metered-dose inhaler plus holding chamber is equivalent in effectiveness to nebulizer. Chest 103:665, 1993.

69. Jeffrey PK. Morphology of the airway wall in asthma and in chronic obstructive pulmonary disease. Am Rev Respir Dis 143:1152, 1991.

70. Johnson D, Osborn LM. Cough variant asthma: a review of the clinical literature. J Asthma 28:85, 1991.

71. Juniper EF, Kline PA, Vanzieleghem MA, et al. Effect of long-term treatment with an inhaled corticosteroid (budesonide) on airway hyperresponsiveness and clinical asthma in nonsteroid-dependent asthmatics. Am Rev Respir Dis 142: 832, 1990.

72. Kang BC, Johnson J, Veres-Thorner C. Atopic profile of inner-city asthma with comparative analysis on the cockroach-sensitive and ragweed-sensitive subgroups. J Allergy Clin Immunol 92:802, 1993.

73. Kanner RE, Connett JE, Altose MD, et al. Gender difference in airway hyperresponsiveness in smokers with mild COPD. The Lung Health Study. Am J Respir Crit Care Med 150:956, 1994.

74. Kauffman HF, Tomee JF, van der Werf TS, et al. Review of fungus-induced asthmatic reactions. Am J Respir Crit Care Med 151:2109, 1995.

75. Kern DG, Patel S. Auscultated forced expiratory time as a clinical and epidemiologic test of airway obstruction. Chest 100:636, 1991.

76. Kinsman RA, Dirks JF, Pahlem NW. Noncompliance to prescribed-as-needed medication use in asthma: usage patterns and patient characteristics. J Psychosom Res 24:97, 1980.

77. Knudson RJ, Kaltenborn WT, Burrows B. Single breath carbon monoxide transfer factor in different forms of chronic airflow obstruction in a general population sample. Thorax 45:514, 1990.

78. Lam A, Newhouse MT. Management of asthma and chronic airflow limitation. Are methylxanthines obsolete? Chest 98: 44, 1990.

79. Larrain A, Carrasco E, Galleguillos F, et al. Medical and surgical treatment of nonallergic asthma associated with gastroesophageal reflux. Chest 99:1330, 1991.

80. Lipworth BJ, McDevitt DG, Struthers AD. Prior treatment with diuretic augments the hypokalemic and electrocardiographic effects of inhaled albuterol. Am J Med 86:653, 1989.

81. Littenberg B, Gluck EH. A controlled trial of methylprednisolone in the emergency treatment of acute asthma. N Engl J Med 314:150, 1986.

82. Long term domiciliary oxygen therapy in chronic hypoxic cor pulmonale complicating chronic bronchitis and emphysema: report of the Medical Research Council Working Party. Lancet 1:681, 1981.

83. Luskin AT. Recalcitrant asthma: an allergist's approach. Allergy Proc 11:281, 1990.

84. Lynch JP, Trulock EP. Lung transplantation in chronic airflow limitation. Med Clin North Am 80:657, 1996.

85. Mal H, Andreassian B, Pamela F, et al. Unilateral lung transplantation in end-stage pulmonary emphysema. Am Rev Respir Dis 140:797, 1989.

86. McFadden ER Jr. Exertional dyspnea and cough as preludes to acute attacks of bronchial asthma. N Engl J Med 292:555, 1975.

87. McFadden ER Jr. Heat and water exchange in human airways. Am Rev Respir Dis 146(5 Pt 2):S8, 1992.

88. McFadden ER Jr, Gilbert IA. Medical progress: asthma. N Engl J Med 327:1928, 1993.

89. McFadden ER Jr, Kiser R, DeGroot WJ. Acute bronchial asthma: relations between clinical and physiologic manifestations. N Engl J Med 288:221, 1973.

90. McFadden ER Jr, Lyons HA. Arterial blood gas tensions in asthma. N Engl J Med 278:1027, 1968.

91. Mendella LA, Manfreda J, Warren CPW, et al. Steroid response in stable chronic obstructive pulmonary disease. Ann Intern Med 96:17, 1982.

92. Menzies R, Gibbons W, Goldberg P. Determinants of weaning and survival among patients with COPD who require mechanical ventilation for acute respiratory failure. Chest 95: 398, 1989.

93. Miller A. Pulmonary function tests in clinical and occupational lung disease. New York: Grune & Stratton, 1986.

94. Molfino NA, Nannini LJ, Martelli AN, Slutsky AS. Respiratory arrest in near-fatal asthma. N Engl J Med 324:285, 1991.

95. Murciano D, Auclair MH, Pariente R, Aubier M. A randomized, controlled trial of theophylline in patients with severe chronic obstructive pulmonary disease. N Engl J Med 320: 1521, 1989.

96. Murphy TF, Sethi S. Bacterial infections in chronic obstructive pulmonary disease. Am Rev Respir Dis 146:1067, 1992.

97. National Asthma Education Program. Executive Summary. Guidelines for the Diagnosis and Management of Asthma. NIH Publication No. PHS 91-3042A. Bethesda, MD: US Department of Health and Human Services, 1991.

98. National Heart, Lung, and Blood Institute, Division of Lung Diseases. Workshop report: the definition of emphysema. Am Rev Respir Dis 132:182, 1985.

99. Nelson SB, Gardner RM, Crapo RO, Jensen RL. Performance evaluation of contemporary spirometers. Chest 97:288, 1990.

100. Newhouse MT, Dolovitch MB. Control of asthma by aerosols. N Engl J Med 315:870, 1986.

101. Nickoladze GD. Functional results of surgery for bullous emphysema. Chest 101:119, 1992.

102. Niederman MS, Clemente PH, Fein AM, et al. Benefits of a multidisciplinary pulmonary rehabilitation program; improvements are independent of lung function. Chest 99:798, 1991.

103. Nocturnal oxygen therapy trial group. Continuous or nocturnal oxygen therapy in hypoxemic chronic obstructive lung disease: a clinical trial. Ann Intern Med 93:391, 1980.

104. O'Byrne PM. Leukotrienes in the pathogenesis of asthma. Chest 111(2 Suppl):27S, 1997.

105. O'Conner GT, Sparrow D, Weiss S. The role of allergy and nonspecific airway hyperresponsiveness in the pathogenesis of chronic obstructive pulmonary disease. State of the art review. Am Rev Respir Dis 140:225, 1989.

106. O'Donohue WJ Jr. Home oxygen therapy. Med Clin North Am 80:611, 1996.

107. Owens GR, Rogers RM, Pennock BE, Levin D. The diffusing capacity as a predictor of arterial oxygen desaturation during exercise in patients with chronic obstructive pulmonary disease. N Engl J Med 310(19):1218, 1984.

108. Parker S, Mellins RB, Soga D. Asthma education: a national strategy. Am Rev Respir Dis 140:848, 1989.

109. Pauwels RA. New aspects of the therapeutic potential of theophylline in asthma. J Allergy Clin Immunol 83(2 Pt 2):548, 1989.

110. Peto R, Speizer FE, Cochrane AL, et al. The relevance in adults of air-flow obstruction, but not of mucus hypersecretion, to mortality from chronic lung disease: results from 20 years of prospective observation. Am Rev Respir Dis 128:491, 1983.

111. Petty TL. Home oxygen therapy. Mayo Clin Proc 62:841, 1987.

112. Petty TL. The National Mucolytic Study. Results of a randomized, double-blind, placebo-controlled study of iodinated glycerol in chronic obstructive bronchitis. Chest 97:75, 1990.

113. Piirila P, Sovijarvi AR, Kaisla T, et al. Crackles in patients with fibrosing alveolitis, bronchiectasis, COPD, and heart failure. Chest 99:1076, 1991.

114. Pride NB. Bronchial hyperreactivity in smokers. Eur Respir J 1:485, 1988.

115. Pueringer RJ, Hunninghake GW. Inflammation and airway reactivity in asthma. Am J Med 92(6A):32S, 1992.

116. Rand CS, Wise RA. Measuring adherence to asthma medication regimens. Am J Respir Crit Care Med 149(2 Pt 2):S69, 1994.

117. Rogers RM, Owens GR, Pennock BE. The pendulum swings again: toward a rational use of theophylline. Chest 87:280, 1985.

118. Rossing TH, Fanta CH, Goldstein DH, et al. Emergency therapy of asthma: comparison of the acute effects of parenteral and inhaled sympathomimetics and infused aminophylline. Am Rev Respir Dis 122:365, 1980.

119. Sanders C. The radiographic diagnosis of emphysema. Radiol Clin North Am 30:1019, 1991.

120. Schatz M, Patterson R, Kloner R, Falk J. The prevalence of tuberculosis and positive tuberculin skin tests in a steroid-treated asthmatic population. Ann Intern Med 84:261, 1976.

121. Schwartz J, Slater D, Larson TV, et al. Particulate air pollution and hospital emergency room visits for asthma in Seattle. Am Rev Respir Dis 147:826, 1993.

122. Shah A, Sircar M. Postcoital asthma and rhinitis. Chest 100:1039, 1991.

123. Shim C, Williams MH Jr. Pulsus paradoxus in asthma. Lancet 1:530, 1973.

124. Silverman EK, Province MA, Rao DC, et al. A family study of the variability of pulmonary function in α_1-antitrypsin deficiency: quantitative phenotypes. Am Rev Respir Dis 142:1015, 1990.

125. Simpson WG. Gastroesophageal reflux disease and asthma. Diagnosis and management. Arch Intern Med 155:798, 1995.

126. Sluiter HJ, Keeter GH, de Monchy JG, et al. The Dutch hypothesis (chronic non-specific lung disease) revisited. Eur Respir J 4:479, 1991.

127. Snider GL. Chronic obstructive pulmonary disease: risk factors, pathophysiology and pathogenesis. Annu Rev Med 40:411, 1989.

128. Snider GL, Lucey EC, Stone PJ. Pitfalls in antiprotease therapy of emphysema. Am J Respir Crit Care Med 150(6 Pt 2):S131, 1994.

129. Snider TH, Stevens JP, Wilner FM, Lewis BM. Simple bedside test of respiratory function. JAMA 170:1631, 1959.

130. Sporik R, Holgate ST, Platts-Mills TA, Cogswell JJ. Exposure to house-dust mite allergen (Der p I) and the development of asthma in childhood. A prospective study. N Engl J Med 323:502, 1990.

131. Strunk RC. Identification of the fatality-prone subject with asthma. J Allergy Clin Immunol 83:477, 1989.

132. Szczeklik A. Aspirin-induced asthma: pathogenesis and clinical presentation. Allergy Proc 13(4):163, 1992.

133. Szefler SJ. Anti-inflammatory drugs in the treatment of allergic disease. Med Clin North Am 76:953, 1992.

134. Tarpy SP, Celli BR. Long-term oxygen therapy. N Engl J Med 333:710, 1995.

135. Taylor DR, Sears MR, Cockcroft DW. The beta-agonist controversy. Med Clin North Am 80:719, 1996.

136. Thompson AB, Mueller MB, Heires AJ, et al. Aerosolized beclomethasone in chronic bronchitis: improved pulmonary function and diminished airway inflammation. Am Rev Respir Dis 148:389, 1992.

137. Tockman MS, Khoury MJ, Cohen BH. The epidemiology of COPD. In: Chronic obstructive pulmonary disease, lung biology in health and disease. 2nd ed. New York: Marcel Dekker, 1985;28:43.

138. Trulock EP. Lung transplantation: state of the art. Am J Respir Crit Care Med 155:789, 1997.

139. U.S. Surgeon General. The Health Consequences of Smoking: Chronic Obstructive Lung Disease. DHHS Publication No. 84-50205. Washington, DC: US Government Printing Office, 1984.

140. Weinberger M, Hendeles L. Theophylline in asthma. N Engl J Med 23;334:1380, 1996.

141. Weitzenblum E, Schrijen F, Apprill M, et al. One year treatment with almitrine improves hypoxaemia but does not increase pulmonary artery pressure in COPD patients. Eur Respir J 4:1215, 1991.

142. Wilson DO, Rogers RM, Hoffman RM. Nutrition and chronic lung disease. Am Rev Respir Dis 132:1347, 1985.

143. Wilson DO, Rogers RM, Wright EC, Anthonisen NR. Body weight in chronic obstructive pulmonary disease. Am Rev Respir Dis 139:1435, 1989.

144. Wrenn K, Slovis CM, Murphy F, Greenberg RS. Aminophylline therapy for acute bronchospastic disease in the emergency room. Ann Intern Med 115:241, 1991.

145. Xu X, Dockery DW, Ware JH, et al. Effects of cigarette smoking on rate of loss of pulmonary function in adults: a longitudinal assessment. Am Rev Respir Dis 146:1345, 1992.

CHAPTER 56

Lung Cancer*

LINDA F. BARR, MD

EPIDEMIOLOGY

Lung cancer is the leading cause of visceral cancer and of cancer-related death in the United States. More than 170,000 cases of lung cancer were diagnosed in 1995 with an estimated 157,400 deaths (18). Of these cancers, 80 to 90% are caused by tobacco smoke, most importantly from cigarettes, but also from pipes and cigars. Indeed, the increasing death rates from lung cancer in the past 50 years lag 20 years behind a parallel rise in cigarette smoking. The lifetime lung cancer mortality for the general population is approximately 10% for smokers and 1% for nonsmokers (3).

For smokers, the major determinant of risk of lung cancer is the number of cigarettes smoked per day, not the amount of tar in each cigarette. The relative risk rises from 5.5 for those who smoke 1 to 10 cigarettes a day, to 14.2 for 20 cigarettes a day, and to 20.4 for 21 to 30 cigarettes a day. Lung cancer rates decrease when smoking is stopped, and approach those of people who

*Philip L. Smith contributed to this chapter in a previous edition.

have never smoked by 10 years after cessation; for former heavy smokers, some risk remains (19). The U.S. Environmental Protection Agency has recognized also that the inhalation of smoke from others' cigarettes (passive smoking) may also lead to a slightly increased risk of lung cancer.

Other exposures that increase the risk for lung cancer and examples of relevant occupations are listed in Table 56.1 (45). It is especially important to identify people with an asbestos exposure. Not only do these individuals have an increased incidence of mesothelioma, but they also have a sixfold greater risk of developing lung cancer than the general population; and those exposed people who smoke are 60 times more likely to develop bronchogenic carcinoma than are nonsmoking, nonexposed people (39).

The risk of exposure to *radon* as another pulmonary carcinogen has received a great deal of public attention. Radon is a naturally produced radioactive gas that is found universally in the soil and air. The contribution of radon exposure to excess lung cancer in uranium and other underground miners (including those who mine iron, zinc, tin, and fluorspar) is well established. Of unproven but theoretical concern is the exposure to radon from contaminated soil beneath some homes. It is estimated that such exposure may be responsible for about 10,000 lung cancer deaths annually. Because of uncertainty in the risk estimates, it has been suggested that corrective measures should be taken for individual homes when tests (commercially available) show that

the exposure rate approaches that found in mines. Whether such measures are effective in reducing the risk of lung cancer is unknown. The interaction between risks of lung cancer from radon exposure and from cigarette smoking is unclear (26).

It is important to consider two other groups with increased risk of bronchogenic carcinoma. First, those with previous lung cancers or with other tobacco-associated cancers are at markedly increased risk of developing a second cancer of the respiratory or upper digestive tract (discussed later). Second, some studies suggest that genetic predisposition may influence the risk of lung cancer, albeit only slightly (40).

SCREENING

The diagnosis of lung cancer is generally made in the last quarter of the tumor's life cycle, usually after metastases have occurred and essentially have determined the outcome of therapy (46). This observation underlies the dismal survival of patients with the disease: For all stages combined, 5-year survival for patients with non–small cell lung cancer is 14% and for those with small cell lung cancer is 6% (18). Thus, there is much interest in detecting lung cancers at an earlier, curable stage. Unfortunately, a large multicenter study showed that screening heavy cigarette smokers with yearly chest x-rays and sputum cytology, although improving the detection of cancer and increasing the chances that the tumor could be resected, still did not lead to a significant reduction in mortality (17).

There are presently no similar studies to address the impact of screening for early lung cancer detection in other groups with increased risk. Thus, although routine screening using chest roentgenography and sputum cytology (see below) would not be recommended for cigarette smokers, no recommendations can be made regarding any other single risk group, nor can the impact of such screening on those with multiple risk factors be gauged at this time. The failure of the chest x-ray as a screening tool likely relates to its relative insensitivity: A tumor diameter of 1 cm is the usual size first detected on the chest x-ray, and approximately 30 cell doublings are required to reach this size (32). Although sensitive molecular techniques such as the polymerase chain reaction allow the detection of genetic abnormalities arising from very few expectorated cells in the patient's sputum, it is as yet unclear which abnormalities need to be screened and how this information can be used clinically.

HISTOLOGY

Lung cancer is classified broadly into two major groups—*non–small cell lung cancer* and *small cell lung cancer*—both of which are associated with cigarette smoking. Non–small cell lung cancer is comprised of *squamous cell, large cell,* and *adenocarcinomas.* The approximate distribution of types of lung cancer among patients with different smoking histories

Table 56.1. Occupational Agents Associated with Lung Cancer

Agent	Occupational Examples
Arsenic	Copper smelting, pesticide manufacturing, manufacture of "pressure-treated" wood
Asbestos	*Historically:* production, shipfitters; *currently:* maintenance and construction workers exposed to asbestos insulation, mechanics exposed to asbestos brake linings
Beryllium	Mining, refining, manufacture of ceramics, electronic and aerospace equipment
Bis(chloromethyl)ether	Production, construction
Cadmium	Electroplating, manufacture of plastics and alloys, pigments, battery electrodes
Chromium, hexavalent	Manufacturing of pigments, stainless steel, plating
Mustard gas	Production, warfare
Nickel	Manufacturing of stainless steel, nonferrous alloys, batteries, and electroplating
Polycyclic aromatic compounds	Aluminum production, coal gasification, coke production, soot, and iron and steel founding
Radon	Mining
Vinyl chloride	Production of polyvinyl chloride
Probable Carcinogens	
Acrylonitrile	Manufacture of acrylic fiber for textiles, pipes
Diesel exhaust	Mining, trucking, construction
Formaldehyde	Manufacture, biology
Silica	Mining, masonry, concrete, pottery

Based on classifications of the International Agency for Research on Cancer and the National Institute of Occupational Safety and Health.

is listed in Table 56.2 (5). Five percent of lung cancer is made up of rarer tumors including carcinoids, sarcomas, and mesotheliomas.

The incidence of bronchioloalveolar carcinoma has doubled over the past 20 years, and in one study, this tumor constituted 15% of all lung cancers (5). The reason for this increase is unclear. Patients with this cancer tend to be younger, are more likely to be female, and are less likely to be smokers than those with other lung cancers. The treatment of bronchioloalveolar carcinoma is similar to that of non–small cell carcinoma, and the prognosis varies, depending on the histologic subtype and stage of disease. (6).

HISTORY

The symptoms of lung cancer may be categorized as those caused by mass effect of the tumor in the airway, those caused by impingement of the tumor on extrapulmonary mediastinal structures, those of paraneoplastic syndromes, and those of distant metastases.

Pulmonary Symptoms

Of patients with lung cancer, 90% have symptoms at the time of diagnosis, and most of these symptoms are respiratory. These include cough, dyspnea, chest pain, hemoptysis, and symptoms related to postobstructive pneumonia. Cough occurs in almost all patients during the course of lung cancer. Cough and sputum are nonspecific symptoms in smokers, but the appearance of a chronic cough, with or without expectoration, in an older smoker should raise a suspicion of lung cancer (47).

The incidence of hemoptysis as a presenting complaint of lung cancer ranges in the literature from 6 to 51% (21), generally manifest as blood-streaked sputum rather than as massive hemoptysis. Assuming that there is no other explanation that can be diagnosed by history, physical examination, and a routine chest x-ray, the issue with these patients is whether to proceed with an investigation into the cause of the hemoptysis (see Chapter 54). Factors that favor a bronchoscopic investigation into the cause of mild

hemoptysis are patient age greater than 40 years, an abnormal chest x-ray, a history of hemoptysis of more than 1 week, a history of tobacco smoking, a chronic cough, or the presence of anemia or weight loss. Lung cancer is found at bronchoscopy in one-third of patients with hemoptysis with one or more of these risk factors (44). Whether bronchoscopy is indicated in the absence of these other factors is unclear. With rare exceptions, a negative bronchoscopy is reliable for excluding cancer in patients with hemoptysis and negative radiologic studies (1).

Chest pain is reported by approximately half of patients with lung cancer on presentation, usually as an intermittent dull ache on the side of the tumor. The cause of this pain is unclear, and if the tumor appears otherwise resectable, this symptom should not preclude surgery. A more severe pain may indicate metastatic disease to the parietal pleura or to a bone and may necessitate a bone scan. Shoulder pain, sometimes mistaken for arthritis, may be caused by a Pancoast (superior sulcus) tumor (see below) or may be caused by a tumor involving the diaphragm.

Extrapulmonary Thoracic Symptoms

Extrapulmonary symptoms caused by intrathoracic extrapulmonary extension include superior vena cava syndrome, Pancoast tumor syndrome, Horner's syndrome, dysphagia, hoarseness, and cardiac disease. Patients with such symptoms should be rapidly evaluated for definitive diagnosis and treatment. The *superior vena caval (SVC) syndrome* consists of edema and rubor of the upper trunk and face, sometimes with syncope. It is caused by obstruction of the superior vena cava by involvement of the mediastinum with tumor. The chest x-ray usually shows a right upper lobe mass, a widened mediastinum, and in 25% of cases, a right pleural effusion.

The *Pancoast syndrome* is caused by a tumor that is located at the pulmonary apex and that involves adjacent structures such as the chest wall, lymphatics, ribs, vertebrae, vessels, and nerves. The tumor may cause shoulder pain; arm pain and paresthesia, usually in the ulnar distribution, indicate encroachment of the brachial plexus.

Horner's syndrome is due to tumor invasion of the sympathetic trunk and consists of miosis, ptosis, enophthalmos, facial flushing, and anhidrosis on the affected side.

Hoarseness may be caused by involvement of the trachea with tumor or by vocal cord paralysis caused by entrapment of the recurrent laryngeal nerve by a mediastinal mass. This symptom should be evaluated with a flow-volume loop or laryngoscopy. *Wheezing,* although usually caused by small airways obstruction, may also be produced by upper airway or bronchial obstruction by an intrinsic or extrinsic mass. Therefore, upper airway involvement should be ruled out in all wheezing patients by auscultation over the neck, with emergent evaluation (flow-volume measurement or laryngoscopy) when indicated.

Table 56.2. Histologic Type of Lung Cancer by Smoking Habits

Type	Never Smoked (%)	Pipe/ Cigar (%)	Current Cigarette Smoker (%)	Ex-Cigarette Smoker (%)
Non–small cell carcinoma				
Squamous cell		33.3	45.9	15.5
Adenocarcinoma	30.0	20.0	8.5	25.2
Large cell	10.0	13.3	13.0	9.7
Bronchioloalveolar	50.0	33.3	9.8	26.2
Small cell carcinoma			15.4	2.0
Other types	10.0		7.4	21.4
No. of patients	10	15	377	103

Modified from Auerbach O, Garfinckel L. The changing pattern of lung carcinoma. Cancer 68:1973, 1991.

Extrathoracic Symptoms

Anorexia, cachexia, weight loss, and fever are common in patients with lung cancer, particularly as the disease advances. Extrathoracic metastatic disease is found at autopsy in most patients with non–small cell lung cancer and in almost all patients with small cell lung cancer. Metastases may be seen in any organ. Common metastatic sites for lung cancer include the pleura, bone, brain, liver, and adrenal glands. In addition, small cell lung cancer frequently invades the bone marrow, leading to hematologic abnormalities.

Paraneoplastic Syndromes

Paraneoplastic syndromes are common in patients with lung cancer. It is important to recognize that the symptoms of the paraneoplastic syndrome may precede the other symptoms of lung cancer; manifestations of these syndromes may mimic metastatic disease and mislead treatment decisions; and these symptoms generally improve with successful treatment of the underlying malignancy.

Endocrine syndromes may be seen in 10 to 15% of patients. The most common is *hypercalcemia* secondary to a parathyroid hormone–like substance, usually caused by a non–small cell carcinoma. The syndromes of *inappropriate antidiuretic hormone release* and of *ectopic adrenocorticotropic hormone (ACTH) secretion* are less common and more likely to be seen in patients with small cell lung cancer then in those with non–small cell cancer. Increased levels of these ectopic hormones can be found in the blood of many more patients with small cell lung cancer than the few percent that manifest these syndromes. The *ectopic ACTH syndrome* is characterized by mild hypertension, hyperglycemia, hypokalemia, and alkalosis, generally without the other manifestations of Cushing's syndrome.

Clubbing and hypertrophic pulmonary osteoarthropathy are common in, although not limited to, patients with lung cancer. Clubbing is seen in one-third of patients with lung cancer. Hypertrophic pulmonary osteoarthropathy with pain, swelling and tenderness, and positive bone scan of affected bones may be seen in as many as 10% of these patients, and lung cancer is the underlying cause in more than 80% of adult cases of this osteoarthropathy.

Neurologic paraneoplastic processes are rare but dramatic and may be the presenting symptoms of small cell lung cancer (36). In the *Eaton–Lambert syndrome,* proximal muscle weakness and paresthesias may mimic myasthenia gravis from which it can be distinguished by electromyography. The diagnosis of other neurologic paraneoplastic syndromes including peripheral neuropathies, subacute cerebellar degeneration, cortical degeneration, polymyositis, and intestinal dysmotility may be facilitated by the measurement of type I antineuronal nuclear antibody (ANNA-1) (36), which is available, however, only in a few specialized centers.

Patients with lung cancer also may demonstrate an increased tendency to clot, manifest either as typical or atypical *(Trousseau's syndrome)* venous or arterial thromboembolic disease (see Chapter 52).

PHYSICAL EXAMINATION

The physical examination is usually unrevealing in lung cancer. Occasionally, the pulmonary examination reveals local wheezing from bronchial obstruction or evidence of pleural effusion. In addition, a general physical examination may show evidence of metastasis or of a paraneoplastic syndrome, and it is also important for establishing the physiologic ability of the patient to undergo therapy. The patient should be evaluated for supraclavicular adenopathy, the most common site of peripheral lymph node metastasis because a positive needle aspiration cytology from this area is a less invasive means of both diagnosis and of establishing unresectability.

DIAGNOSTIC PROCEDURES

Chest X-Ray

A review of old chest x-rays can demonstrate the rapidity of disease onset and may aid in prognostication. A mass with a doubling time of less than 2 weeks or greater than 450 days is unlikely to be malignant. For a more extensive discussion of radiologic characteristics helpful in differentiating benign from malignant pulmonary lesions, see the section "Solitary Pulmonary Nodule."

Certain chest x-ray patterns are suggestive of particular types of lung cancer. Squamous cell and small cell carcinomas tend to be centrally located, and adenocarcinomas and large cell carcinomas tend to arise peripherally. The centrally located tumor is more likely to present with symptoms of obstruction: atelectasis, pneumonia, and dyspnea. Small cell lung cancer may demonstrate only hilar adenopathy with no visible primary tumor on the initial chest x-ray. Squamous cell carcinoma is the most likely bronchogenic carcinoma to cavitate, although even this tumor cavitates uncommonly. Bronchioloalveolar cell carcinoma also usually presents peripherally and tends be multifocal. This cancer has a variety of radiologic manifestations and may appear as a single mass or as multiple nodules, or it may imitate a pneumonia.

Computerized Tomographic Scanning and Magnetic Resonance Imaging of the Chest

A computerized tomographic (CT) scan of the chest is useful in determining the anatomic extent of the lung cancer and in guiding diagnostic and therapeutic procedures. CT scanning is now done routinely in the evaluation of patients with suspected lung cancer. CT may demonstrate additional lesions that are unseen on chest x-ray. Furthermore, CT may aid in characterizing the size, shape, and composition of these lesions. For example, CT is better than the chest x-ray in determining calcification of a solitary pulmonary nodule; a densely calcified nodule is more likely to be benign (42).

Also, CT may demonstrate fat in a nodule, highly suggestive of a hamartoma. In addition, the presence and size of mediastinal or hilar lymph nodes can be evaluated by CT. Nodes greater than 1 cm in diameter have a 60% chance of representing metastatic disease (29), and if a surgical cure is contemplated, sampling by transbronchial needle aspiration, mediastinoscopy, or mediastinotomy is required (see below). Finally, extending CT cuts down through the upper abdomen may demonstrate hepatic or adrenal metastases, although these radiographic findings will require biopsy if therapy would be influenced by the histology of these lesions. Magnetic resonance imaging (MRI) is not as informative as CT scanning for evaluating pulmonary parenchymal disease, nor is it helpful for evaluating mediastinal nodes. Spiral CT or MRI are useful in specific cases—for example, in the evaluation of the possibility of vascular invasion by tumor.

Sputum Cytology

The frequency of diagnosis of lung cancer from cytology submitted from spontaneously expectorated sputum depends on the cell type and the location of the tumor (30). Squamous cell tumors shed cells into the airways, and cytologies are positive approximately 80% of the time. However, patients with a peripheral adenocarcinoma have positive cytologies less than 5% of the time. Regardless, the completion of the diagnostic evaluation should not be delayed in situations in which sputum cytologic examination is not readily available. Patients should be instructed to produce a forceful cough. Three early morning specimens should be collected in a tightly fitting container, and if they cannot be submitted to the laboratory within 2 to 3 hours of collection, a fixative should be added and the specimens can be pooled and submitted together. Saccomanno's solution, which contains alcohol and Carbowax, is one of the best fixatives; it can be prepared by the laboratory and stored by the physician for later use. More than three samples does not increase the likelihood of a positive diagnosis of cancer. If the patient is not producing sputum, induction by the inhalation of an aerosolized solution of saline can be helpful. The patient inhales normal saline or a balanced salt solution (Hanks' BSS) that is aerosolized by an ultrasonic nebulizer (DeVilbiss 3583). In general, sputum induction is not a routine office procedure and should be done by experienced personnel. In addition to the sputum collected immediately after induction, good material is produced on the following morning. The addition of chest vibration or percussion does not improve the yield from sputum cytology. In cases in which there is obstruction of the bronchus as evidenced by the physical examination or the chest x-ray, it is reasonable to start collecting sputum after therapy, including antibiotics and perhaps bronchodilators, which may reestablish airway patency and allow sputum to be produced.

Bronchoscopy

Bronchoscopy is useful for both the diagnosis and staging of bronchogenic carcinoma (4). Bronchoscopy is important to search for a second, synchronous malignancy and to evaluate vocal cord function. A fixed vocal cord would suggest involvement of the recurrent laryngeal nerve in the mediastinum. Furthermore, the bronchoscope visualizes the proximal extent of the tumor because distance from the carina determines surgical resectability (although newer techniques—so-called tracheal "sleeve" resections—do sometimes allow resection of tumors close to the carina). Multiple diagnostic procedures may be done through the bronchoscope: transbronchial biopsy using forceps, brushing for cytology, and bronchoalveolar lavage. In addition, *transbronchial needle aspiration* (TBNA) allows sampling of hilar, subcarinal, and other mediastinal lymph nodes. Fiberoptic bronchoscopy is an outpatient procedure and can be done comfortably using mild sedation, a short-acting narcotic (fentanyl), a drying agent (usually atropine), and topical lidocaine. Occasional circumstances dictate preoperative endotracheal intubation or the use of a rigid bronchoscope, both of which are done with general anesthesia.

The diagnostic yield of bronchoscopy is 60 to 80% for tumors greater than 2 cm in diameter and 20 to 40% for those less than 2 cm, and is higher for visualized masses in the central airways. Necrotic tumors, submucosal carcinoma, and large tumors that displace feeding bronchi may be more of a diagnostic challenge and may require more than one bronchoscopic procedure to obtain diagnostic material. Many peripheral tumors are accessible by bronchoscope using fluoroscopically guided needles, brushes, and biopsy forceps. However, masses that are smaller than 2 cm or in the outer third of the lung are usually better approached by percutaneous transthoracic needle aspiration.

Although generally a safe and well-tolerated procedure, potential complications of bronchoscopy include pulmonary hemorrhage, pneumothorax, laryngospasm or bronchospasm, and transient cardiac arrhythmias. Patients with primary or secondary coagulation disorders, thrombocytopenia, uremia, pulmonary hypertension, or the superior vena cava syndrome are at an increased risk for bleeding. Pneumothorax complicates approximately 5% of transbronchial forceps biopsies, and less than 1% of transbronchial needle aspiration procedures, although only half of these patients require a chest tube. Transient atrial and ventricular arrhythmias occur in approximately 5% of elderly bronchoscopy patients and may be related to transient hypoxemia. However, death is rare and almost always is associated with a transbronchial biopsy that has caused significant bleeding.

The interval between a myocardial infarction and safe performance of fiberoptic bronchoscopy is unknown and must be established on an individual basis, balancing the goals of the procedure and the therapeutic implication of results. Approximately 16% of patients have a low-grade fever after bronchoscopy, but the incidence of pneumonia is low. Although the incidence of bacteremia during bronchoscopy is less than 2%, some advocate prophylactic antibiotics for patients at risk for bacterial endocarditis (20).

Patient Experience. Bronchoscopy may be performed on an ambulatory basis by a pulmonologist or a thoracic surgeon. The patient is told to fast (including liquids) 12 hours before bronchoscopy (although generally medicines may be taken with a sip of water) and not to eat for approximately 4 hours after its completion when the effects of topical anesthesia wear off. The only discomfort the patient will experience is coughing caused by irritation of the trachea and main bronchi, which is treated with topical lidocaine. There is usually no pain associated with this procedure.

In the unusual situation in which sputum cytology demonstrates malignancy but the chest x-ray and chest CT do not localize a suspicious area ("occult carcinoma"), a long bronchoscopic procedure is undertaken under general anesthesia, in which a meticulous upper airway evaluation is followed by sequential sampling of each pulmonary segment. Positive findings mandate a confirmatory procedure in which repeat sampling is done of subsegments corresponding to the positive material. The yield of this procedure is 13 to 35%, and up to 15% of these patients have multicentric carcinomas. New metachronous primary lung cancer develops in these patients at the rate of 5% per year. Almost all of these patients are heavy smokers and have increased surgical morbidity and mortality; thus lung-sparing surgery or photodynamic therapies may be indicated (12).

Percutaneous Transthoracic Needle Aspiration

CT-directed percutaneous transthoracic needle aspiration (PTNA) of the lung is most useful when a mass or a nodule is located peripherally near the pleura or in the apex of the lung. It is especially helpful in the diagnosis of metastatic carcinoma because these tumors arise outside of the airway and are difficult to diagnose by bronchoscopy, particularly when they are less than 2 cm in size. It may also be preferred when infection is in the differential diagnosis because the interpretation of the significance of an infectious agent obtained by bronchoscopy is complicated by the passage of the scope through the nonsterile nasopharynx or oropharynx. PTNA is performed by either a radiologist or pulmonologist with fluoroscopic or CT guidance. The technique and experience of the operator and of the cytopathologist are of paramount importance in the success of the procedure, and the yield is increased with a repeat procedure. However, the false-negative rate for any fluoroscopically guided procedure is significant. Thus, nondiagnostic or nonspecific findings require follow-up, the nature of which is determined by the adequacy of the sample and the clinical scenario. PTNA is an outpatient procedure, done with local anesthetic, and requires a cooperative patient (23).

Contraindications to the procedure include large blebs or blood vessels that are in the direct path of the needle, a patient with an uncontrollable cough, in which case general anesthesia may be necessary, and contralateral pneumonectomy, in which case the production of a pneumothorax would be devastating. In addition, patients with pulmonary hypertension have an increased risk of bleeding.

Patient Experience. The patient will feel a mild pressure with the introduction of the needle. Otherwise, there is no significant pain. Potential complications include a 5% risk of bleeding (usually of minimal amount), and a 10 to 15% risk of pneumothorax (only one-half of these require chest tube insertion). Most patients can resume normal activity within 24 hours.

Mediastinoscopy, Mediastinotomy, and Thoracoscopy

Mediastinoscopy and mediastinotomy are indicated when radiographically enlarged mediastinal lymph nodes cannot be adequately sampled by use of less invasive techniques (TBNA or PTNA; see above). Lymph nodes accessible to cervical mediastinoscopy are those in the pretracheal area from the thoracic inlet to 1 cm beyond the carina bilaterally. Those anterior to the aortic arch and in the aortic–pulmonary window (usually associated with a left upper lobe carcinoma) are not accessible to the cervical mediastinoscope and require anterior mediastinotomy. Potential complications include wound infection, injury to major vascular structures, and recurrent laryngeal nerve paralysis (28). These procedures are done by thoracic surgeons and require general anesthesia and hospitalization.

A biopsy done through a thoracoscope may be better tolerated than one done during a limited thoracotomy, and thoracoscopy may also be helpful, in selected cases, in the removal of peripheral lung masses (31), and in diagnosing the cause of pleural effusions. This procedure can be done under general anesthesia or in the sedated patient with local anesthetic. The procedure involves inducing a controlled pneumothorax, then examining the visceral and parietal pleuras with either a rigid or fiberoptic endoscope. Some techniques require the insertion of instruments through additional incision(s). The patient generally has 2 to 3 days of hospital observation after thoracoscopy. The incidence of complications is similar to that of the closed procedures (7).

STAGING

The staging of the patient with lung cancer has two goals: to determine the anatomic extent of the tumor and to determine the physiologic capacity of the patient to undergo therapy.

For non–small cell lung cancer, the anatomic extent of the tumor is defined by the TNM classification system, where T = tumor size, N = nodal involvement, and M = distant metastases. The TNM categories are then grouped into four stages with therapeutic and prognostic implications (Tables 56.3 and 56.4, and Fig. 56.1)

Small cell lung cancer is classified by a two-stage system. In limited stage disease, the cancer is confined to the hemithorax and the regional lymph nodes (including mediastinal, ipsilateral hilar, and supraclavicular nodes), which essentially delineate the extent of disease that can be contained within a tolerable radiation port. Extensive stage disease is that which lies outside these boundaries.

For all lung cancer patients, staging includes a chest CT with cuts down through the liver and adrenals, a complete blood count with a differential count, an alkaline phosphatase level, serum electrolytes including serum calcium, and coagulation studies. The goal of the staging of small cell lung cancer is to determine whether the disease is limited or extensive because the former is treated with radiation and chemotherapy (and, in rare cases, with surgery), and the latter with chemotherapy alone. Thus, the staging of small cell lung cancer, as determined by the oncologist, may include cranial and abdominal CT scans, bone scans, symptom-directed x-rays, and possibly a bone marrow examination because these areas are commonly involved with this tumor. For non–small cell lung cancer, additional staging recommendations are controversial.

Brain and bone scans have traditionally been recommended only for appropriate symptoms or signs (41). However, the absence of neurologic symptoms and signs does not reliably exclude brain metastases, and one group advocates cranial CT in the initial staging of all patients with non–small cell lung cancer (16). Finally, any patient with bronchogenic carcinoma, who has symptoms not clearly attributable to the tumor should have further evaluation to rule out a synchronous malignancy.

TREATMENT

Non–Small Cell Lung Cancer

The most important prognostic criterion for non–small cell lung cancer is the TNM classification because it defines resectable, and thus most of the potentially curable, disease. Surgery is the standard treatment for those without clinical evidence of mediastinal or metastatic disease and is an option for selected patients with tumor involvement of the mediastinum or chest wall. Surgical resection results in a 5-year survival of 50 and 30% for patients with clinical Stage I and Stage II non–small cell lung cancer, respectively (Fig. 56.1). Surgical resection is appropriate for selected patients with Stage IIIA disease. Five-year survival in this group is 15% by presurgical staging, but

---

Table 56.3.   Staging of Lung Cancer—TNM Definitions

Primary Tumor (T)

TX	Primary tumor cannot be assessed, or tumor proven by presence of malignant cells in sputum or bronchial washings but not visualized by imaging or bronchoscopy
TO	No evidence of primary tumor
Tis	Carcinoma in situ
T1	Tumor 3 cm or less in greatest dimension, surrounded by lung or visceral pleura, without bronchoscopic evidence of invasion more proximal than lobar bronchus (i.e., not in main bronchus)[a]
T2	Tumor with any of the following features of size or extent:
	More than 3 cm in greatest dimension
	Involves main bronchus, 2 cm or more distal to the carina
	Invades the visceral pleura
	Associated with atelectasis or obstructive pneumonitis that extends to the hilar region but does not involve the entire lung
T3	Tumor of any size that directly invades any of the following: chest wall (including superior sulcus tumors), diaphragm, mediastinal pleura, or pericardium; tumor in the main bronchus less than 2 cm distal to the carina but without involvement of the carina; or associated atelectasis or obstructive pneumonitis of the entire lung
T4	Tumor of any size that invades any of the following: mediastinum, heart, great vessels, trachea, esophagus, vertebral body, or carina; or tumor with a malignant pleural effusion[b] or pericardial effusion, or satellite nodule(s) within the primary bearing lobe

Lymph Node (N)

NX	Regional lymph nodes cannot be assessed
NO	No regional lymph node metastasis
N1	Metastasis in ipsilateral peribronchial or ipsilateral hilar lymph nodes, including direct extension
N2	Metastasis in ipsilateral mediastinal or subcarinal lymph node(s)
N3	Metastasis in contralateral mediastinal, contralateral hilar, ipsilateral or contralateral scalene, or supraclavicular lymph node(s)

Distant Metastasis (M)

MX	Presence of distant metastasis cannot be assessed
MO	No distant metastasis
M1	Distant metastasis[c]

From Reference 33.

[a]The uncommon superficial tumor of any size with its invasive component limited to the bronchial wall, which may extend proximal to the main bronchus, is also classified as T1.

[b]Most pleural effusions associated with lung cancer are caused by tumor. However, there are a few patients in whom multiple cytologic examinations or pleural fluid are negative for cancer. In these cases, the fluid is nonbloody and is not an exudate. When these elements and clinical judgment dictate that the effusion is not related to the tumor, the effusion should be excluded as a staging element and the patient should be staged T1, T2, or T3. Pericardial effusion is classifed according to the same rules.

[c]Tumor nodule(s) in the ipsilateral lung nonprimary tumor–bearing lobe are classified as M1.

Table 56.4.   Staging of Lung Cancer—New International Revised Stage Grouping

Stage 0	Tis
Stage IA	T1, N0, M0
Stage IB	T2, N0, M0
Stage IIA	T1, N1, M0
Stage IIB	T2, N1, M0
	T3, N0, M0
Stage IIIA	T1-3, N2, M0
	T3, N1, M0
Stage IIIB	T4, Any N, M0
	Any T, N3, M0
Stage IV	Any T, Any N, M1

From Reference 33.

it is considerably better for those defined by surgical staging. However, these outcomes contrast with those of patients who cannot be surgically resected, those with Stage IIIB cancer (for whom 5-year survival is 5%), and those with Stage IV (metastatic) cancer for whom 5-year survival is rare.

Unfortunately, only a small proportion of patients have surgically resectable disease. Recently, therapy for locally advanced non–small cell lung cancer (Stages IIIA and IIIB) has undergone change. Combined modality therapy using various combinations of chemotherapy, radiation therapy, and surgery has been shown to improve survival for this group of patients (14). Although these benefits are modest to date, promising new chemotherapeutic agents are on the horizon, and primary care physicians should encourage their patients to participate in approved prospective clinical trials at local medical centers.

Surgical Considerations

Patients with non–small cell lung tumors that appear anatomically localized after staging evaluation are considered surgical candidates if the risks of the thoracotomy, and of the removal of functional lung tissue are considered medically reasonable. The prediction of residual lung function following resection is based on pulmonary function studies. If x-rays show a patchy distribution of baseline lung disease, a nuclear perfusion study may be needed to determine the contribution of the proposed lung resection to the total lung function; and the predicted postoperative FEV_1 is calculated from this fraction. All patients should be evaluated as potential candidates for both pneumonectomy and lobectomy in case operative findings dictate that the former will be necessary for cure. A pneumonectomy is feasible if the preoperative FEV_1 is 2 L or more or 80% predicted, if the maximum voluntary ventilation is 50% or more than predicted, or if the maximal oxygen consumption on exercise testing is more than 20 mL/kg per minute. Alternatively, a lobectomy or pneumonectomy is feasible if the predicted postoperative FEV_1 is 0.8 L or more or 40% of predicted. For borderline cases, or when the degree of dyspnea or disability is greater than the FEV_1 would predict, a DL_{CO} 40% or more of predicted or a change of oxygen saturation of 2% or less with exercise suggests that a patient is operable (see Chapter 55 for a description of pulmo-

nary function tests). Patients who do not meet these criteria or those who have hypoxemia or hypercarbia on baseline arterial blood gas have a high risk for respiratory complications after thoracotomy. Additional considerations such as cardiovascular status, other comorbid disease, and the informed patient's wishes need to be considered in the surgical decision (15).

Possible postoperative pulmonary complications of patients undergoing thoracotomy include the need for prolonged mechanical ventilatory support or the development of bronchospasm, atelectasis, and pneumonia. Several prophylactic measures decrease the risk for these complications in patients with chronic obstructive lung disease. Preoperative measures include the sustained cessation of smoking, use of inhaled bronchodilators and theophylline, treatment of pulmonary infection with antibiotics, and treatment of increased secretions with measures such as chest physiotherapy and postural drainage. Finally, all patients need to be taught how to use the incentive spirometer.

Thoracotomy results in a temporary decrease in vital capacity of 30% (in part due to pain and atelectasis), as well as increased upper airway bacterial load. Thus, important postoperative measures include using adequate but not excessive pain control, encouraging the patient to cough frequently and to use the incentive spirometer, and providing early ambulation. Normal activities can be resumed within several weeks of surgery, depending on the pulmonary reserve. Follow-up at least every 3 to 4 months for the first few years after resection, and at least yearly thereafter, is often advised to detect metastasis or local recurrence and second primary malignancies (the latter discussed later) but probably has no influence on overall survival.

Radiotherapy

Definitive radiotherapy is not as effective a therapy as surgery, but it offers a potential for cure or for prolonged survival when surgery is not an option. Although compromised lung function may limit the ability to deliver radiation, definitive radiotherapy may cure 15 to 20% of patients with Stages I and II disease who have contraindications to surgery (22). As discussed earlier, radiotherapy has a role as part of a multimodal therapy for Stage IIIA and IIIB disease.

The complications of external radiation include pneumonitis, pulmonary fibrosis, and dysphagia from transient esophagitis. The rate of these complications depends on the time and dosage of radiation delivery and the volume of normal tissue exposed. However, complication rates have fallen in recent years as techniques have improved. Minimizing pulmonary risk in a patient with underlying lung disease requires individualization of radiation protocols by the radiation oncologist (see Chapter 8), taking into account the extent of the pulmonary disease and the anatomy of the tumor.

Palliative Therapies

For patients who are not candidates for other therapies, local symptom palliation may be accomplished

Figure 56.1. Cumulative survival of non–small cell lung cancer patients according to clinical **(A)** and surgical–pathologic **(B)** stage. (Roman numerals refer to stages [see Table 56.3]. Operative deaths excluded [1975–1982 collected series].) (From Mountain CF. Lung cancer staging classification. Clin Chest Med 14:43, 1993.)

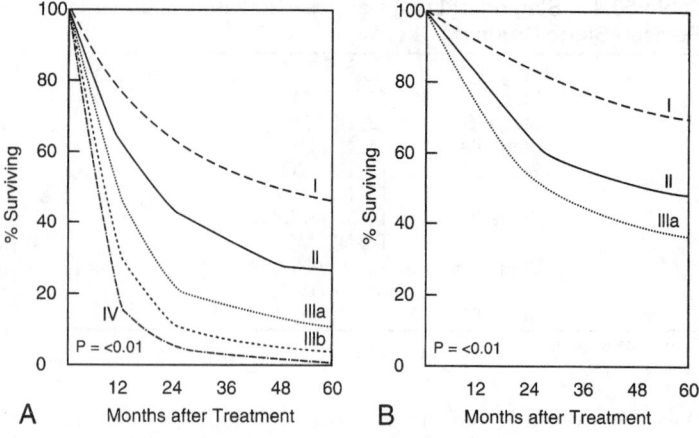

by palliative external beam radiation therapy. Palliative radiotherapy is delivered over shorter intervals and in lower dosages than those used for definitive therapy, and it relieves hemoptysis, SVC syndrome, and dyspnea in 60 to 80% of patients. However, it is rare for vocal cord paralysis to respond. Although less than 20% of non–small cell lung cancer patients with atelectasis respond to radiotherapy, 57% of those with small cell lung cancer reexpand collapsed lobes or lungs (43).

Laser therapy, brachytherapy, and the bronchoscopic placement of prosthetic stents are other options for the symptomatic relief of major airway obstruction These procedures may require hospitalization and need to be performed by physicians familiar with their use. The neodymium-yttrium-aluminum-garnet (YAG) laser is useful for debulking endobronchial obstructing lesions. Symptomatic relief is immediate and dramatic but may last only 1 to 3 months in two-thirds of patients because of tumor regrowth. Thus repeated procedures may be required, with increasing procedure-related mortality. Endoscopically placed brachytherapy with [192]iridium is used to reduce either endobronchial or extraluminal compressing masses. This therapy relieves symptoms more rapidly than external radiation, although not as rapidly as laser therapy, and has a longer duration of response with fewer complications compared with laser. Brachytherapy also does not cause the regional pneumonitis that limits the use of external radiation. The risks of brachytherapy and laser therapy are bronchial perforation and hemorrhage with asphyxiation. In addition, local edema with critical airway occlusion can complicate laser therapy, and fistulas may form after brachytherapy. The roles of laser or brachytherapy as definitive therapies for bronchogenic carcinoma remain to be defined (10,12).

Small Cell Lung Cancer

Almost all patients with small cell lung cancer have either clinically evident or subclinical metastases at presentation. Therefore surgery or local radiation is unlikely to be effective. Chemotherapy is the standard treatment. It increases survival for most patients with both extensive and limited disease and has the potential for cure of a few patients with limited disease. The standard chemotherapeutic protocol uses a combination of two to three agents given every 3 to 4 weeks for six to eight courses. Some protocols add thoracic and/or cranial irradiation. The major toxicity of the chemotherapeutic agents used for small cell lung cancer is myelosuppression (see Chapter 8 for other common adverse effects of chemotherapy). Table 56.5 shows the influence of combination chemotherapy on survival of patients with small cell lung cancer. For the elderly (70 years or older) or those with severe cardiopulmonary or renal disease or decreased performance status, aggressive chemotherapy may not be appropriate because of a decreased ability to tolerate its associated side effects. However, oral etoposide or a related agent as a single chemotherapeutic agent has acceptable toxicity in these patients, results in response rates of 65 to 80%, and has been shown to increase survival to a median of 9 to 11 months (9). Newer drugs, in development, may prove to be less toxic, but in all cases, quality of life should be discussed with the patient before a final choice of medication is made. Chemotherapy for lung cancer may be given to ambulatory patients and is best administered by an oncologist.

Five-year survivors of small cell lung cancer therapy face a high rate of recurrent small cell cancer, second primary cancers (see below), and an increase in the incidence of leukemia and of myelodysplastic syndromes. Patients who receive cranial irradiation have a 20% incidence of central nervous system toxicity, which may not appear for several years (2), although reduction of dosage in recent years may attenuate this risk.

Follow-Up of Patients Surviving Lung Cancer

Patients who have had a lung cancer have a significant risk of a second primary cancer. In one large study of patients with resected Stage I non–small cell lung cancer, one-third had second synchronous or metachronous cancers discovered over 10 years of follow-up, of which one-third were second primary lung cancers (27). How these patients should be followed has yet to be defined. A yearly chest x-ray, in addition to close attention to standard recommendations for early detection of (extrapulmonary) cancers, such as yearly history and physical examination, monitoring for occult fecal blood, and routine mammography, would be advisable. The role for chemoprophylaxis with retinoids, beta-carotene, alpha-tocopherol, or other agents to reduce the risk of new bronchogenic carcinoma in those with previous cancers of the aerodigestive tract remains under investigation (see Reference 35).

PLEURAL EFFUSIONS

Patients with bronchogenic carcinoma and effusion usually have dyspnea and cough, although one-quarter are asymptomatic of the effusion. In contrast, most patients with malignant mesothelioma and effusion have chest pain. In one-third of patients with carcinomatous pleurisy, the effusions are bilateral, and three-quarters of patients have moderate to large pleural effusions. Indeed, the absence of a mediastinal shift in the setting of a large effusion is highly suggestive of a tumor either fixing the mediastinum, obstructing a main bronchus, or simulating an effusion in the pleural space. There are two categories of pleural effusion in the setting of lung cancer: carcinomatous involvement of the pleura (malignant effusion) and what has been termed *paramalignant* effusion in which the pleura is not involved with tumor. Malignant effusion is usually exudative, is usually serosanguinous but may be bloody, and may have a lymphocytosis, a low pH, and a low glucose concentration. The paramalignant effusion may be either exudative or transudative and may be due to mediastinal carcinoma obstructing lymph drainage or secondary to postobstructive pneumonia or atelectasis (38). The patient with a malignant effusion is not surgically curable, and most patients die within 6 months of diagnosis. However, those with paramalignant effusions may be candidates for surgery, generally as part of a combined modality therapy. Thus, the

cause of pleural effusion needs to be established in patients with otherwise curable bronchogenic carcinoma, as well as for those with nonresectable carcinoma to help direct palliative therapy.

Thoracentesis, with cytologic evaluation of fluid, provides diagnoses in more than two-thirds of cases of malignant effusions, with the yield improved by repeating the procedure, as well as by blind pleural biopsy. Potential complications of either of these procedures include pneumothorax (5 to 10%), bleeding (approximately 1%), and parietal pleural seeding (1 to 2%). Unfortunately, for 10 to 20% of patients with malignant effusions, these studies are nondiagnostic (37). Both thoracentesis and pleural biopsy are routinely done in an ambulatory setting, the latter only by pulmonologists or thoracic surgeons.

A more sensitive examination for pleural disease in the patient with suspected malignant effusion is thoracoscopy (described earlier). Thoracoscopically directed pleural biopsy correctly identifies malignancy in 97% of affected patients.

Patient Experience. For thoracentesis and pleural biopsy, patients are administered a local anesthetic before the insertion of a needle into the pleural space. The patient feels the prick of the small needle when the anesthetic is injected and feels usually some pain when the actual thoracentesis is performed. If a significant pneumothorax occurs, shortness of breath will be experienced.

For diagnostic thoracoscopy, a short-acting sedative (e.g., Versed) and a short-acting opiate (fentanyl) are injected intravenously. Then a small incision is made under local anesthesia and an endoscope is passed into the pleural space. Patients feel primarily pressure during the performance of the procedure.

Both thoracentesis and thoracoscopic evaluation of the pleura take approximately 30 minutes to perform.

The treatment of pleural effusions in the setting of lung cancer depends on the cause. Palliative systemic chemotherapy is the main option for patients with small cell lung cancer and is one option in patients with unresectable non–small cell cancer. Otherwise, various palliative procedures have been tried.

Those patients with effusions secondary to mediastinal lymphatic obstruction may be candidates for external radiotherapy. Effusions secondary to postobstructive processes may be amenable to external radiotherapy or to laser therapy, brachytherapy, or placement of a prosthetic stent, all procedures directed at reestablishing bronchial patency.

Malignant effusions, which usually recur after they are drained, may be treated with repeated thoracentesis. However, the most common approach to the malignant effusion is pleurodesis of the pleural space. In general, the optimal candidate for this procedure is one who has already demonstrated symptom relief with thoracentesis, has a prognosis of greater than a few months, and has an effusion that is not acidotic (pleural fluid pH less than 7.30 is associated with a poor response to pleurodesis). For pleurodesis, the pleural space is drained as completely as possible with a chest

Table 56.5. Influence of Therapy on Survival of Patients with Small Cell Lung Cancer

Era	Survival	
	Limited Disease	Extensive Disease
Prechemotherapy		
Supportive care (median)	3 mo	1.5 mo
Surgery (5 yr)	<1%	
Radiotherapy (5 yr)	1–3%	
Chemotherapy		
Single agent (median)[a]	6 mo	4 mo
Combination		
Median	10–14 mo	7–11 mo
5 yr	2–8%	0–1%
Combination with chest irradiation		
Median	12–16 mo	7–11 mo
5 yr	6–12%	0–1%

From Ihde DC. Chemotherapy of lung cancer. N Engl J Med 327:1434, 1992.
[a]Some recent results suggest that longer median survival may be possible in selected patients.

tube in the hospital or with a pig-tailed catheter (inserted under radiologic guidance, as an outpatient procedure), and a sclerosing agent (e.g., doxycycline or bleomycin) is instilled into the pleural space. The sclerosing agent may need to be reinstilled after a few days if the first treatment is ineffective. This procedure is helpful in three-quarters of selected patients. Pre-medication for pleurodesis includes additional nar-cotic and simultaneous intrapleural instillation of lidocaine to decrease the pleural pain associated with this procedure. The patient generally requires narcot-ics while the chest tube is in. Surgical pleural abrasion or pleurectomy has a higher morbidity and mortality than closed pleurodesis, but may be useful for selected patients (38).

SOLITARY PULMONARY NODULE

A solitary pulmonary nodule (SPN) is defined as a single focal spherical density in the pulmonary paren-chyma that is not associated with any other parenchy-mal process or with adenopathy. Its diameter is vari-ously designated in the literature as up to 3 to 4 cm. One-half of these lesions are malignant, either primary pulmonary cancers or metastases from an extrapulmo-nary source. Surgical resection is possible in 80% of those with an SPN, and the 5-year survival rate is 40%. These figures are significantly better than those for lung cancer as a group. The nonmalignant lesions are due to a diverse group of processes, including granulomatous processes (e.g., tuberculosis or fungal diseases), ham-artomas, bronchial adenomas, organizing pneumonia, pulmonary infarcts, and arteriovenous malformations (25). The management of the SPN for an individual patient is based on a risk–benefit analysis including the probability that the nodule is malignant, the risks of the contemplated diagnostic and therapeutic procedures, the accuracy of biopsy techniques, the risk that a delay in therapy will affect outcome, and finally, the in-formed patient's preference.

There are three possible strategies for managing a patient with an SPN. The first is to do no further follow-up. The second is to refer the patient for an immediate invasive study for diagnosis or treatment. The third is to observe the SPN carefully over time ("watchful waiting") for any signs that would move the patient to one of the other management strategies. The answers to four questions will allow the physician to determine the most appropriate management for the individual patient.

Question 1: Is the visualized lesion really a solitary pulmonary nodule? It has been estimated that 10 to 20% of lesions interpreted as possible SPNs on the initial chest x-ray are not actual SPNs (24). In these cases, what appeared to be a pulmonary nodule may actually be an extraparenchymal process (e.g., bone, vascular, or chest wall lesions), or alternatively, the pulmonary nodule may not be a solitary process (i.e., additional disease is present). Other radiologic studies, including a review of old films and CT scans, may be helpful.

Question 2: What is the age and stability of the nodule? Comparison of the current studies with prior x-rays is needed to answer this question. The doubling time for a pulmonary malignancy ranges from 20 to 400 days. Thus, the lack of growth of a SPN for several years is sufficient evidence of benign disease.

Question 3: What are the characteristics of the patient that increase the risk for malignancy? The establishment of smoking status (or other toxic expo-sure as outlined in Table 46.1) is one cornerstone of this investigation. The second is the patient's age: The prevalence of malignancy in SPNs is 1% in patients less than 35 years old, but increases rapidly with years above this age (13). Furthermore, the history of a malignancy mandates a more aggressive approach be-cause in 80% of these patients, the SPN will prove to be either a primary or metastatic malignancy (34). It is important that an SPN in a patient with a known extrapulmonary primary tumor be biopsied because these nodules are more likely to be a new primary tumor of the lung than to be a metastasis (8).

Question 4: What are the risk characteristics of the nodule? The most important of these is the growth rate, as previously discussed. Second, although calcifica-tion may be seen in malignant disease, certain patterns of calcification favor a benign diagnosis. A dense central nidus and a diffuse or a laminated pattern of calcification are reliable signs of healed granuloma. A popcorn pattern of calcification suggests a hamartoma. However, an eccentric nidus of calcification is uninfor-mative and may be due to a cancer engulfing a prior calcified lesion. CT densitometry is more sensitive than chest x-ray for demonstrating calcification (42). Other characteristics, including nodule size (a diam-eter of greater than 3 cm is more likely malignant) and shape (an irregular lesion with poorly defined or spiculated borders is suggestive of malignancy), may be helpful in the context of the other factors discussed.

To answer these questions, the workup of the SPN includes first obtaining the necessary films to verify the presence of an SPN, then examining all prior x-rays, and finally, obtaining a chest CT to confirm the pres-ence of disease, demonstrate associated disease, exam-ine the characteristics of the nodule (including size, shape, and the presence of calcification, fat, fluid and vessels), and evaluate the diagnostic approach. Using these data, a risk analysis may be formulated based on the determinations as outlined above. It is important to discuss this analysis with the patient to establish the goals and plans at this point. For some patients, the benign nature of the process may be assured after some or all of these steps; and these patients will not require further evaluation. For other patients, a choice will need to be made about whether to proceed to an immediate diagnostic or treatment procedure, or whether to watch and wait.

The diagnostic techniques for obtaining a biopsy of an SPN include (a) fluoroscopically directed trans-bronchial biopsy (TBBx) or transbronchial needle as-piration (TBNA), done through a fiberoptic broncho-scope; (b) fluoroscopically directed percutaneous transthoracic needle aspiration (PTNA); *(c)* thoracoscopic biopsy; or *(d)* thoracotomy. These procedures have been discussed earlier. The diagnostic yield of TBBx is 30 to 70%, and of PTNA is 70 to 90% (11,25). Nonneoplastic causes of peripheral nodules (especially certain infections) may be diagnosed by TBBx or PTNA. However, the specter of false-negative results from biopsies obtained by both of these techniques mandates that nonspecific findings be followed by either another procedure or by watchful waiting. The choice of the initial diagnostic technique and of the follow-up management is best determined by a pulmonologist in consultation with the patient.

Based on the discussion above, the watchful waiting strategy would be appropriate management, for example, for a patient less than 35 years old with no risk factors and with a small well-defined nodule; a patient with a nodule of less than 2.5 cm that has been unchanged in size for 2 years by prior chest x-rays; a patient with few risks who has had negative diagnostic studies; or a patient for whom the risk of the diagnostic and therapeutic procedures outweigh the risks of watchful waiting. Given the range of tumor doubling times, it is unlikely that the delay inherent in this strategy would result in a significant decrease in survival for the patient with a pulmonary nodule that is malignant (13). A scheme for monitoring serial x-rays might be to obtain repeat films every 3 to 4 months for 1 year, then every 6 months for 1 year, then to repeat at yearly intervals thereafter. The total number of years to follow a nodule depends on the suspicion of malignancy based on the above criteria. For patients for whom the level of suspicion is low, serial studies for 2 years are adequate. For the patient for whom the level of suspicion for malignancy is high, a 5-year follow-up is necessary to encompass the unusually slow-growing carcinoma (usually an adenocarcinoma).

General References*

Demetri G, Elias A, Gershenson D, et al. NCCN small-cell lung cancer practice guidelines. Oncology 10(Suppl):179, 1996.

Ettinger DS, Cox JD, Ginsberg RJ, et al. NCCN non-small-cell lung cancer practice guidelines. Oncology 10(Suppl):81, 1996.

Ginsberg RJ, Vokes EE, Raben A. Non-small cell lung cancer. In: DeVita VT Jr, Hellman S, Rosenberg SA, eds. Cancer: principles and practice of oncology. 5th ed. Philadelphia: Lippincott-Raven, 1997;858.

Ihde DC, Glatstein E, Pass HI. Small cell lung cancer. In: DeVita VT Jr, Hellman S, Rosenberg SA, eds. Cancer: principles and practice of oncology. 5th ed. Philadelphia: Lippincott-Raven, 1997;911.

Pass HI, Mitchell JB, Johnson DH, Turrisi AT, eds. Lung cancer. Philadelphia: Lippincott-Raven, 1996.

Specific References

1. Adelman M, Haponik EF, Britt EF, Bleeker ER. Cryptogenic hemoptysis: clinical features, bronchoscopic findings, and natural history of 67 patients. Ann Intern Med 102:829, 1985.
2. Albain KS, Crowley JJ, Livingston RB, et al. Long-term survival and toxicity in small cell lung cancer: expanded Southwest Oncology Group experience. Chest 99:1425, 1991.
3. Ames BN, Magaw R, Gold LS. Ranking possible carcinogenic hazards. Science 236:271, 1987.
4. Arroliga AC, Matthay RA. The role of bronchoscopy in lung cancer. Clin Chest Med 14:87, 1993.
5. Auerbach O, Garfinckel L. The changing pattern of lung carcinoma. Cancer 68:1973, 1991.
6. Barkley JE, Green MR. Bronchioloalveolar carcinoma (Review). J Clin Oncol 14:2377, 1996.
7. Boutin C, Viallat JR, Cargnino P, Farisse P. Thoracoscopy in malignant pleural effusions. Am Rev Respir Dis 124:588, 1981.
8. Cahan WG. Multiple primary cancers of the lung, esophagus and other sites. Cancer 40:1954, 1977.
9. Carney DN, Grogan L, Smit EF, et al. Single-agent oral etoposide for elderly small cell lung cancer patients. Semin Oncol 17(Suppl 2):49, 1990.
10. Chin HW, Anderson W McD. Intraluminal brachytherapy for endobronchial carcinoma. Pulmonary and critical care update. A Program of the American College of Chest Physicians. 8(19), 1993.
11. Cortese DA. Solitary pulmonary nodule: observe, operate, or what? (Editorial). Chest 81:662, 1982.
12. Cortese DA, Edell ES. Role of phototherapy, laser therapy, brachytherapy, and prosthetic stents in the management of lung cancer. Clin Chest Med 14:149, 1993.
13. Cummings SR, Lillington GA, Richard RJ, et al. Managing solitary pulmonary nodules. The choice of strategy is a "close call." Am Rev Respir Dis 134:453, 1986.
14. Dillman RO, Herndon J, Seagren SL, et al. Improved survival in Stage III non-small-cell lung cancer: Seven-year follow-up of Cancer and Leukemia Group B(CALGB) 8433 trial. J Natl Cancer Instit 88:1210, 1996.
15. Dunn WF, Scanlon PD. Preoperative pulmonary function testing for patients with lung cancer. Mayo Clin Proc 68:371, 1993.
16. Ferrigno D, Buccheri G. Cranial computed tomography as a part of the initial staging procedures for patients with non-small-cell lung cancer. Chest 106:1025, 1994.
17. Frost JK, Ball WC Jr, Levin ML, et al. Early lung cancer detection: Results of the initial (prevalence) radiologic and cytologic screening in the Johns Hopkins study. Am Rev Respir Dis 130:549, 1984.
18. Fry WA, Menck HR, Winchester DP. The National Cancer Data Base report on lung cancer. Cancer 77:1947, 1996.
19. Garfinckel L, Silverberg E. Lung cancer and smoking trends in the United States over the past 25 years. CA 41:137, 1991.
20. Haponik EF, Kvale P, Wang KP. Bronchoscopy and related procedures. 2nd ed. In: Fishman AP, ed. Pulmonary disease and disorders. New York: McGraw-Hill, 1988;437.
21. Hyde L, Hyde CI. Clinical manifestations of lung cancer. Chest 65:299, 1974.
22. Ihde DC, Minna JD. Non-small cell cancer. I. Biology, diagnosis and staging. Curr Probl Cancer 15:61, 1991.
23. Khouri NF, Stitik FP, Erozan YS, et al. Transthoracic needle aspiration biopsy of benign and malignant lung lesions. AJR 144:281, 1985.
24. Khouri NF, Meziane MA, Zerhouni EA, et al. The solitary pulmonary nodule. Assessment, diagnosis and management. Chest 91:128, 1987.
25. Lillington GA, Caskey CI. Evaluation and management of solitary and multiple pulmonary nodules. Clin Chest Med 14:111, 1993.
26. Lubin JH, Boice JD. Lung cancer risk from residential radon: meta-analysis of eight epidemiologic studies. J Natl Cancer Instit 89:49, 1997.
27. Martini N, Bains MS, Burt ME, et al. Incidence of local recurrence and second primary tumors in resected stage I lung cancer. J Thorac Cardiovasc Surg 109:120, 1995.
28. McElvein RB. Procedures in the evaluation of chest disease. Clin Chest Med 13:1, 1992.
29. McLoud T, Bourgouin P, Greenberg R, et al. Bronchogenic carcinoma: analysis of staging in the mediastinum with CT by correlative node mapping and sampling. Radiology 182:319, 1992.
30. Mehta AC, Marty JJ, Lee FYW. Sputum cytology. Clin Chest Med 14:69, 1993.

---

*Bold print (general references) and bold numerals (specific references) denote published controlled clinical trials, meta-analyses, or consensus-based recommendations.

31. Miller DL, Allen MS, Deschamps C, et al. Video-assisted thoracic surgical procedure: management of a solitary pulmonary nodule. Mayo Clin Proc 64:462, 1992.

32. Mizuno T, Masoka A, Ichimura H, et al. Comparison of actual survivorship after treatment with survivorship predicted by actual tumor volume doubling time from tumor diameter at first observation. Cancer 53:2716, 1984.

33. Mountain CF. Revisions in the international system for staging lung cancer. Chest 111:1710–1717, 1997.

34. Neifeld JP, Michaelis LL, Doppman JL. Suspected pulmonary metastases: correlation of chest x-ray, whole lung tomography, and operative findings. Cancer 39:383, 1977.

35. Omenn GS, Goodman GE, Thornquist MD, et al. Effects of a combination of beta-carotene and vitamin A on lung cancer and cardiovascular disease. N Engl J Med 334:1150, 1996.

36. Patel AM, Davila DG, Peters SG. Paraneoplastic syndromes associated with lung cancer. Mayo Clin Proc 68:278, 1993.

37. Poe RH, Israel RH, Utell MJ, et al. Sensitivity, specificity and predictive values of closed pleural biopsy. Arch Intern Med 144:325, 1984.

38. Sahn SA. Malignant pleural effusions. Clin Chest Med 6:113, 1985.

39. Selikoff IJ, Hammond EC. Asbestos and smoking. JAMA 242:458, 1979.

40. Sellers TA, Potter JD, Bailey-Wilson JE, et al. Lung cancer detection and prevention: evidence for an interaction between smoking and genetic predisposition. Cancer Res 52(Suppl):2694S, 1992.

41. Shepherd FA. Screening, diagnosis, and staging of lung cancer. Curr Opin Oncol 5:310, 1993.

42. Siegelman SS, Zerhouni EA, Leo FP, et al. CT of the solitary pulmonary nodule. AJR 135:1, 1980.

43. Slawson R, Scott R. Radiation therapy in bronchogenic carcinoma. Radiology 132:175, 1979.

44. Snider GL. When not to use the bronchoscope for hemoptysis (Editorial). Chest 76:1, 1979.

45. Steenland K, Loomis D, Shy C, Simonsen N. Review of occupational lung carcinogens. Am J Ind Med 29:474, 1996.

46. Weiss W. Lung cancer: diagnosis and preoperative evaluation. J Respir Dis 1:345, 1984.

47. Weiss W, Seidman H, Boucot K. The Philadelphia Pulmonary Neoplasm Research Project: symptoms in occult lung cancer. Chest 73:57, 1978.

Cardiovascular Problems

CHAPTER 57

Angina Pectoris

NISHA CHANDRA STROBOS, MD

Chest pain is one of the most common complaints of patients in an ambulatory practice. The major early objective in the diagnosis of such patients is the separation of noncardiac from cardiac pain. Chapters 35 and 54 describe the various causes of noncardiac pain and their distinguishing characteristics. This chapter describes the diagnosis and treatment of the most common cause of cardiac pain: transient myocardial ischemia—angina pectoris. Chapter 58 describes the posthospital medical care and rehabilitation of patients who have had a myocardial infarction.

Ischemic heart disease caused by atherosclerosis is one of the most common ailments in the Western world; in the United States it remains the leading nontraumatic cause of disability and death, even though, because of increased public awareness and health education, the mortality from ischemic heart disease has declined more than 20% in the last 25 years. However, it is now the leading cause of death in American women, ahead of death from cancer (see below).

Patients with chest pain often seek medical attention. It is essential that physicians know how to respond to such patients in order to make appropriate diagnostic and therapeutic decisions. In the approach to the patient with chest pain, a detailed history and physical examination must not be replaced by sophisticated noninvasive or invasive cardiovascular procedures. A detailed history and physical examination permit the physician to tailor these studies to meet more specifically the needs of the patient, thereby increasing the efficiency of these often expensive procedures.

PATHOPHYSIOLOGY

Angina is caused by a mismatch between myocardial oxygen supply and demand. Normally, the myocardium produces most of its energy by means of aerobic metabolism. Oxygen demands are a function of the amount of work that cardiac muscle is called upon to perform. That work, in turn, is a function of the heart rate, the systolic blood pressure, the duration of systole, the tension of the walls of the left ventricle, and the contractility of the myocardium. Tension (T), described by the Laplace relationship ($T = P \times r \div 2h$), is directly proportional to the ventricular blood pressure (P) and volume (r = radius of the ventricular cavity) and is inversely proportional to the thickness (h) of the ventricular wall. Contractility essentially is the amount of work that the myocardium can do under a given load and, in the normal heart, is influenced primarily by the peripheral vascular tone (generated by the sympathetic nervous system) and by the intracellular and extracellular electrolyte concentration of cardiac muscle. These relationships, which affect the heart's ability to do work, are also important in the pathophysiology of heart failure (see Chapter 61).

In practical terms, these concepts reveal why the heart is more prone to ischemia when its rate is increased (e.g., by exertion or emotional stress), when left ventricular tension is increased (e.g., by increased blood pressure or by ventricular dilation), or when myocardial contractility is increased (e.g., by the sympathetic discharge that accompanies exertion or emotional stress). An increased demand for myocardial oxygen is met by an increase in coronary blood flow. This flow occurs primarily during diastole (because during systole the coronary arteries are squeezed and deliver much less blood to the myocardium) and is determined by two major factors: coronary perfusion pressure and coronary vascular resistance. However, there is little change in total coronary flow over a wide range of coronary perfusion pressures because of flow autoregulation. Hence, changes in coronary blood flow occur primarily as a result of changes in coronary vascular resistance. Coronary vascular resistance, in turn, is determined by the degree of collateralization and the patency of the coronary blood vessels; when the vessels are narrowed by spasm or by an atherosclerotic plaque, coronary resistance increases and oxygen demands may not be satisfied. With exercise, coronary blood flow may need to increase as much as four to five times above resting levels.

Recent studies highlight the importance of the coronary endothelium in patients with coronary artery disease (60). The endothelium serves several purposes, including the maintenance of a nonthrombogenic surface and inhibition of vascular smooth muscle growth and inflammatory activity. In addition, a vasorelaxant compound produced by the endothelium, called *endothelium-derived relaxing factor* (EDRF), has been shown to be critical for normal vasoreactive function, vascular smooth muscle relaxation, and consequently vascular dilation. EDRF, now identified as nitric oxide, is produced by healthy endothelium in response to vasodilators such as bradykinin, acetylcholine, serotonin, and substance P. Patients with hyperlipidemia and documented coronary artery disease have been shown to have impaired coronary vasoreactivity, which can improve dramatically following treatment with lipid-lowering agents (76). In fact, endothelial function and vasoreactivity have been shown to be impaired even before significant atherosclerosis has become angiographically apparent.

Most patients with angina have fixed atherosclerotic lesions of 70% or more in at least one major coronary vessel. The classical teaching has been that obstructive coronary lesions that are not hemodynamically significant at rest become symptomatic (flow limiting) only in response to an increase in myocardial oxygen demand. However, it has been demonstrated that changes in coronary vasomotor tone, rather than changes in myocardial oxygen demand, can often result in ischemia in patients with stable angina (60). This phenomenon, vasospasm (see below), is probably also related to disordered endothelial function and may be one of the triggers for atherosclerotic plaque rupture and the subsequent development of an unstable coronary syndrome.

If the myocardium receives insufficient blood to satisfy its metabolic demands, the resultant ischemia usually results in pain, arrhythmia, or left ventricular dysfunction. When ischemic, the heart is also much more susceptible to arrhythmias, which can, in themselves, produce symptoms. Transient myocardial ischemia causes transient chest pain, or angina pectoris; prolonged ischemia often causes myocardial infarction. The character of the pain is the same in both situations. Ischemia can occur without the development of chest pain—a condition called silent ischemia, discussed elsewhere in this chapter. The treatment of ischemia is directed at reducing myocardial oxygen demand and increasing coronary blood flow.

RISK FACTORS

Both genetic and environmental factors influence the development of atherosclerotic heart disease. Research has been targeted at defining the role of these factors in the premature development of cardiovascular disease. The recognition of risk factors is especially important because they may be modified to prevent disease. In this regard, it is noteworthy that the Lipid Research Primary Prevention Trial has conclusively shown that a reduction in plasma cholesterol lowers the incidence of coronary artery disease (42). The West of Scotland study demonstrated that such reductions of cholesterol in asymptomatic patients significantly reduce mortality from coronary artery disease (CAD) (71). A pamphlet titled *Risk Factors and Coronary Disease: A Statement for Physicians* is available from the American Heart Association; it summarizes the various risk factors that have been identified and makes recommendations for dealing with them (Table 57.1). It can be obtained in bulk by calling or writing the local chapter of the Heart Association.

It is difficult to assign a specific risk to a particular factor because often the risk is proportionate to the degree of exposure (e.g., the number of cigarettes smoked a day or the concentration of cholesterol in the blood) and because the various factors interact in a complicated way to compound the risk of disease in a given patient. However, it is imperative to attenuate the

Table 57.1. Risk Factors for Coronary Artery Disease

Factor	Comment	Documentation
Blood pressure (Chapter 62)	Risk is directly proportionate to increase of systolic or diastolic blood pressure.	Excellent
Blood lipids (Chapter 75)	Risk is directly proportionate to increase in concentration of total cholesterol and low-density lipoprotein (LDL) and inversely proportionate to concentration of high-density lipoprotein (HDL).	Excellent
Diabetes mellitus (Chapter 72)	Risk is 2 times control in diabetic men, 3 times control in diabetic women.	Excellent
Cigarette smoking (Chapter 20)	Proportionate to number of cigarettes smoked per day (3 times control at a pack or more per day).	Excellent
Oral contraceptives (Chapter 93)	Risk is much greater in women over age 35, and when higher dosages of estrogen are taken (see Chapter 93).	Excellent
Personality type	A competitive, driving person (so-called type A personality) is more prone to coronary artery disease.	Good
Sedentary living	People who do not exercise regularly may have a greater risk of myocardial infarction than do those who exercise regularly.	Fair
Diet[a] (Chapter 75)	High lipid content of diet may potentiate coronary artery disease.	Good in humans Excellent in animals

[a]Alcohol and caffeine, although claimed by some in the past to be independent risk factors, have not been established to be so. However, obesity, by increasing the severity of hypertension, hyperlipidemia, and diabetes mellitus, may have an important influence on the development of coronary artery disease.

risk associated with all modifiable factors. The importance of abstinence from tobacco (both active and passive smoking exposure) and control of blood pressure and plasma lipids in all patients with CAD cannot be overemphasized. Recent studies confirm that coronary lesions can actually regress if stringent lipid control is achieved (57). This is particularly important in diabetic patients, who are at high risk for recurrent ischemic events (see Chapter 72).

Although it is not a risk factor per se, recent myocardial infarction is a powerful predictor of new angina; almost 50% of patients with no history of angina develop typical angina in the first year after myocardial infarction.

DIAGNOSIS
History

Onset of Ischemic Pain

Many patients with ischemic cardiac pain can document the circumstances of their first pain. This is not as true in patients with pain of neuromuscular or gastrointestinal origin unless trauma or some catastrophe such as a bowel perforation has occurred. The ability of the patient to describe the first experience with chest pain is extremely useful, therefore, in differential diagnosis.

Character and Location of the Ischemic Pain

The discomfort of myocardial ischemia can be variously described; many do not describe it as a pain, so it is often more effective to ask the patient to describe the discomfort. Some describe it as squeezing, crushing, burning, or smothering, whereas others describe it as a shortness of breath or simply a feeling of heaviness. Some patients may use a Levine's sign, a fist held firmly against the chest, to describe the discomfort. A sharp pain is unlikely to be of cardiac origin, but the patient should be asked to characterize it further, if possible, because "sharp" to some patients means severe rather than knifelike or piercing. Ischemic pain begins and ends gradually, is usually steady in character, but occasionally may wax and wane.

Typically, the discomfort is midline and substernal; it often radiates to the shoulder, arm, hand, or fingers, usually to the left. Radiation down the inside of the arm into the fingers supplied by the ulnar nerve is classic. Pain may radiate also into the neck, the lower jaw, or the intrascapular region. Occasionally, the patient may have pain only in a referred location and experience no chest discomfort at all. The atypical pain may be such that the patient consults a dentist because pain in the lower jaw that is due to myocardial ischemia is ascribed to a toothache. In addition, the pain of myocardial ischemia is diffuse and cannot be easily localized. Rarely is the patient able to point with one finger to the location of the pain; when pain can be localized in this way, it is likely to be noncardiac in origin (see Chapter 54). The elderly, especially the frail elderly, are especially likely to experience atypical pain (or dyspnea instead of pain) with respect to character and location.

Initiation of Ischemic Pain

The single most important diagnostic feature of the discomfort of myocardial ischemia is its often predictable relationship to exertion, emotional stress, or other situations that may either increase myocardial oxygen demand or decrease myocardial oxygen supply. The cause of atypical pain, pain in an unusual location or of an unusual character, may be clarified by this relationship. Pain that is experienced at rest, if it is caused by cardiac ischemia, suggests unstable angina (see below), variant angina (see below), or myocardial infarction.

Anxiety and mental stress are an important and often overlooked provoking factor in many patients. Myocardial oxygen demand may be increased by anxiety to an extent and duration greater than that produced by exercise, resulting in prolonged pain. Recent data demonstrate that mental stress more than doubles the risk of myocardial ischemia in the hour following the stressful episode (34). This is important in understanding environmental factors in a patient with angina.

Angina is more likely to occur during cold or windy weather because of increased peripheral vascular resistance and consequently increased myocardial work, and perhaps because of cold-activated reflexes that produce a decrease in coronary flow. In some patients a specific diurnal pain pattern may be evident with angina, occurring only with an early daily activity such as an early morning shower or a walk from a car to a place of work. It is important to recognize this pattern because it has specific therapeutic implications. Sometimes ischemic discomfort follows a heavy meal, perhaps because of the shunting of blood to abdominal viscera and because of increased sympathetic tone.

Nocturnal angina may be a consequence or manifestation of left ventricular failure or may represent unstable angina (see below). Similarly, patients who describe breathlessness and chest pain with exertion may have angina as a consequence of transient left ventricular failure.

An increase in carboxyhemoglobin level is an important although seldom recognized cause of angina in some people with specific environmental exposures. Commonly, this may occur through exposure to high carbon monoxide (CO) levels in heavy traffic or through inhalation of CO in tobacco smoke. Studies confirm that patients with stable angina may have pain at much lower work loads than usual if exposed to levels of CO that are commonly encountered in congested city traffic or in traffic tunnels (3).

Relief of Ischemic Pain

Because angina is caused by a discrepancy between oxygen supply and demand, relief of pain is achieved by increasing coronary blood flow or decreasing oxygen demand. Cessation of effort or relief of anxiety decreases oxygen demand, and angina begins to disappear within minutes thereafter. So-called walk-through angina is uncommon. Most people must stop or at least slow the activity responsible for precipitating the pain before it is relieved. A history of relief of pain by sublingual nitroglycerin is also useful. However, the patient must be told that the use of nitroglycerin in this way is a diagnostic trial and that the prescription of nitroglycerin does not necessarily mean coronary artery disease. The physician and the patient both need to know that the relief of chest pain by nitroglycerin is not specific for myocardial ischemia. For example, the pain of esophageal spasm is commonly relieved by nitroglycerin (see Chapter 35). A placebo effect may relieve chest discomfort from other causes as well.

Duration of Ischemic Pain

Angina pectoris responds promptly to measures directed at reducing myocardial oxygen demand (cessation of effort usually) or possibly at increasing coronary blood flow. Pain is usually relieved within 5 minutes; if it persists beyond 20 minutes, a myocardial infarction is likely and the patient should be hospitalized.

Physical Examination

The examination should be done with particular attention to uncovering circumstantial evidence that would support a diagnosis of cardiovascular disease: high blood pressure, evidence of abnormal lipid metabolism such as xanthomas (see Chapter 75), funduscopic changes reflecting long-standing hypertension or diabetes mellitus, or evidence of peripheral vascular disease (see Chapter 87). Such physical findings sug-

gest ischemic heart disease, although none is pathognomonic; in many patients the physical examination is entirely normal. Physical findings (e.g., S_4, paradoxic splitting of S_2, or a murmur of mitral insufficiency; see Chapter 60) may be present transiently during an episode of chest pain. The blood pressure should also be recorded if the patient is examined while he or she is experiencing chest pain; transient hypertension during an ischemic attack is common. Hypotension detected during myocardial ischemia is an ominous sign and probably indicates global ischemia produced by left main coronary artery disease or severe three-vessel disease. This is important to recognize because early arteriography and bypass surgery should be considered in such patients.

Electrocardiogram

A 12-lead standard electrocardiogram (ECG) should be obtained as soon as possible in any patient with suspected ischemic cardiac pain.

The most reliable ECG sign of chronic ischemic heart disease is a Q wave, recorded by the leads of the ECG that are measuring electrical activity of a part of the myocardium that has been previously infarcted (Fig. 57.1A). Nonspecific ST–T wave changes, abnormalities of conduction (except for left bundle branch block, LBBB; see below), and arrhythmias do not help establish the diagnosis of myocardial ischemia. ST depression with a flat or downsloping ST segment, however, is indicative of subendocardial ischemia (Fig. 57.1B). It is seldom present in the resting ECGs of patients with

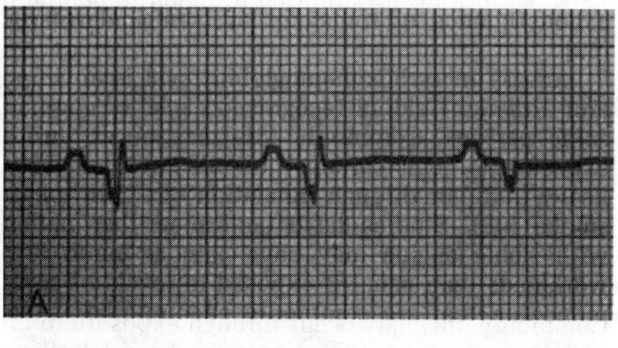

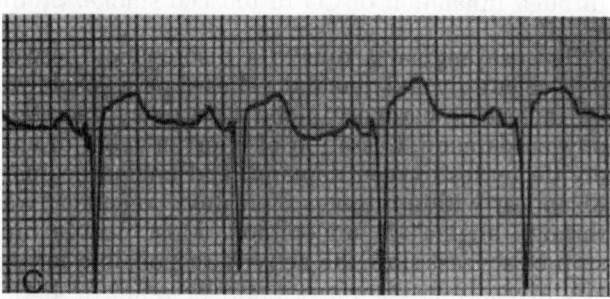

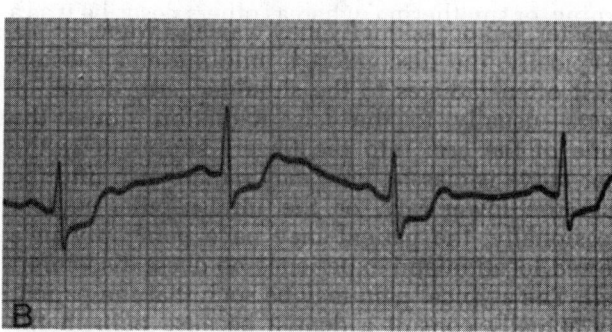

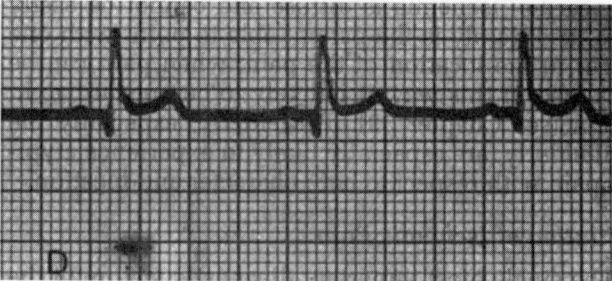

Figure 57.1. Electrocardiographic strips of patients with suspected ischemic heart disease. **A.** Q waves suggestive of chronic myocardial disease. **B.** ST depression developing after exertion.

C. ST elevation during coronary artery spasm (vagrant angina).
D. Early repolarization (a normal variant).

ischemic heart disease unless they are experiencing angina at the time the tracing is being recorded. On the other hand, these transient ischemic changes are seen commonly when a patient with ischemic heart disease is exercised to a point at which chest pain develops. Such ECG changes, appearing with exercise or pain and resolving with rest or with the resolution of pain, strongly indicate myocardial ischemia. Therefore, the necessity of repeating the ECG at rest or after the chest pain has been resolved cannot be overemphasized. ST elevation at rest (Fig. 57.1C) during an episode of chest pain suggests variant angina (see below) or myocardial infarction and allows localization of the diseased coronary artery. T-wave inversion in an ECG taken at rest is a nonspecific finding but can also be seen after infarction or as a specific transient finding in a patient experiencing angina. Thus, ECG changes noted during episodes of chest pain not only confirm the diagnosis of myocardial ischemia but also indicate to some degree the extent and location of the ischemic myocardium. As a general rule, the more widespread the changes the more myocardium is involved.

Listed below are some important general guidelines for use of the ECG in evaluating chest pain. It is important to caution that some exceptions to these guidelines do exist.

A large proportion of all patients with known coronary artery disease have a normal resting ECG, if the ECG is done at a time when the patient is not experiencing chest pain and if the patient has not had a previous myocardial infarction. Therefore, the finding of a normal resting ECG in such a patient is not good evidence against the diagnosis of coronary artery disease.

Patients with a normal resting ECG often have ischemic ECG changes during episodes of angina. Also, such patients usually have a positive exercise stress test (see below). The absence of changes in such circumstances suggests that ECG "silent" areas of the heart (the apex, the posterolateral wall) are ischemic or that the pain may not be caused by ischemia.

A patient with a baseline abnormal resting ECG caused by previous infarction, left ventricular hypertrophy, bundle branch block, and so on may develop only minor ECG changes during an attack of angina, making confirmation of the diagnosis difficult. However, a careful review of the ECG in such patients may unmask subtle findings (e.g., pseudonormalization of downsloping ST waves and of inverted T waves in V_4–V_6 in patients with LBBB that strongly suggest ischemia.

An abnormal resting ECG, in the absence of other evidence, does not justify a diagnosis of ischemia or coronary artery disease. Although there is a high degree of statistical correlation between an abnormal ECG and coronary artery disease, most people in whom this correlation exists have other evidence of coronary artery disease, such as clinically documented infarction, typical angina pectoris, or arteriographically proven disease. When a patient has a negative cardiac history, a normal cardiovascular examination, and an abnormal ECG, it is likely that the ECG abnormalities

are caused by some form of cardiac abnormality other than coronary artery disease or that there is no cardiac disease. The QRS abnormalities of infarction are conduction abnormalities that may have many other causes. Thus, a pattern suggesting old infarction can be seen in patients without coronary artery disease and may be caused by healed myocarditis, an infiltrative disease such as amyloidosis or sarcoidosis, or Wolff–Parkinson–White syndrome (see Chapter 59). Similarly, ST-segment elevation suggesting acute infarction may be seen in the resting ECG of healthy people with so-called early repolarization. This pattern (Fig. 57.1D) is found most often in young adult men, usually in the midleft chest leads but also in right chest leads and limb leads. The ST elevation may reach 4 mm, but there is no ST depression in reciprocal leads and the ST elevation usually normalizes during exercise. The presence of nonspecific ST–T abnormalities in an otherwise well person should not be regarded as evidence of heart disease in the absence of other confirmatory findings. Nonspecific ST–T abnormalities per se are rarely diagnostic of anything and that is why they are called nonspecific.

There is a high degree of correlation between LBBB and organic heart disease (see Chapter 59), especially coronary artery disease. Right bundle branch block (RBBB), on the other hand, especially in younger patients, is seen commonly in the absence of other cardiac abnormalities. It is presumed that RBBB in the absence of other evidence of cardiac disease is congenital; in many instances it is a totally benign finding.

Stress Tests

Standard Exercise Electrocardiography

The exercise stress test not only is a means of establishing the diagnosis of myocardial ischemia, but can also be used to assess the efficacy of antianginal therapy and the extent of myocardium at risk, to identify patients likely to have more severe coronary artery disease, and to assess serially the degree of conditioning or exercise capacity in patients of all age groups.

The rationale behind exercise stress testing is that as the work performed by the patient increases, cardiac work is increased. This increase in work results in an increase in myocardial oxygen utilization, which demands an increase in coronary blood flow. If narrowed or obstructed coronary arteries prevent the required increase in coronary blood flow, ischemia may occur and be manifest as chest pain or ECG changes (22).

Various techniques have been devised, but the most commonly used and best standardized ones require the patient to be monitored with a 12-lead ECG while walking on a treadmill at work loads that can be progressively increased by increasing the speed and inclination of the device. A bicycle ergometer (with hand pedals) may be substituted for a treadmill, permitting the patient to exercise with his or her arms instead of legs. This is particularly useful in patients who cannot use the treadmill because of claudication, arthritis, or amputation, and in the evaluation of patients who have chest pain predominantly or exclusively with work that involves the arms and shoulders.

The stress test should be performed in a facility that has equipment and staff trained to deal with arrhythmias and other cardiac emergencies. With properly selected patients and an appropriately equipped laboratory and a trained staff, an exercise stress test is a safe procedure with reported mortality rates of approximately 0.01%.

Ordinarily a patient exercises until a predetermined heart rate is attained. This is usually 90% of the maximal heart rate predicted on the basis of the patient's age (see Table 58.7, Chapter 58). This goal can be modified according to the preexercise evaluation of the patient, keeping in mind the needs of the patient and the physician. For example, in a young person in whom there is a low probability of ischemic heart disease, attempting to reach the maximal heart rate or exercising the patient to the point of exhaustion is reasonable and adds to the sensitivity of the study. A negative study under such circumstances is strong evidence against myocardial ischemia. On the other hand, in an older patient a negative study (no chest pain and no ischemic ECG changes) may be clinically meaningful at a lesser work load if the work load approximates that patient's normal daily activity.

Criteria

The electrocardiographic criterion for a positive stress test is generally considered to be downsloping or horizontal ST depression of more than 1 mm (Fig. 57.1B). Correlation of significant angiographic (usually defined as 50% luminal narrowing of at least one major coronary vessel) and electrocardiographic results shows a 65% sensitivity of the test (9). This means that only 65% of patients with documented significant coronary artery disease have an abnormal exercise ECG and 35% have a false-negative result. However, the specificity of the exercise ECG is 90%, which means that 90% of people without coronary artery disease have a normal exercise ECG and 10% have a false-positive response. If stricter criteria for a positive stress test are used, such as 2 mm ST depression for the diagnosis of ischemia, the sensitivity decreases and the specificity increases. It is important to note that with more extensive coronary disease (e.g., severe three-vessel or left main disease), false-negative studies are rare (9).

False-positive stress tests are often encountered in patients taking various medications (e.g., digitalis or phenothiazines), in women, and in patients with left ventricular hypertrophy or mitral valve prolapse (79). In such patients or in patients with baseline ST-segment abnormality or conduction defects such as LBBB and RBBB or other conduction system disorders (e.g., Wolff–Parkinson–White syndrome), the sensitivity of the exercise stress test can be enhanced by concurrent radioisotopic or echocardiographic imaging and is commonly used.

Occasionally, especially in patients after transmural myocardial infarction, ST-segment elevation may be noted during exercise. Studies show that this finding in itself does not indicate ischemia but rather relates to the size of the underlying infarct and probably suggests left ventricular dysfunction. ST elevation in leads without Q waves, however, does indicate ischemia.

In evaluating the results of exercise stress testing, it is important to keep in mind Bayes' theorem: The predictive accuracy (number of subjects with true positive tests divided by the number of positive tests) of any diagnostic test is directly related to the sensitivity of the test (the percentage of patients with the disease in whom the test is positive), the specificity of the test (the percentage of patients without the disease in whom the test is negative), and the prevalence of the disease in the population studied (8,55) (see Chapter 1). This relationship exists whenever the specificity of any test is less than 100%. In populations that have a high prevalence of disease, the predictive accuracy is very high even when sensitivity and specificity are low. Conversely, the predictive accuracy is very low in groups of patients with a low prevalence of disease even when the procedure has high specificity and high sensitivity. Therefore the predictive accuracy of an exercise stress test depends on the characteristics of the population studied. In men with classic angina pectoris or previous myocardial infarction, a positive exercise stress test accurately predicts the presence of occlusive coronary artery disease approximately 85% of the time (78).

Occasionally, an otherwise asymptomatic patient is found to have a positive exercise test (when performed, for example, before the patient's initiating an exercise program). In such patients, a false-positive result must be ruled out and the diagnosis confirmed, if necessary, by stress-thallium testing. The MRFIT study (47) showed that such asymptomatic people have a significantly higher incidence of cardiac events over 7 years than patients who do not have a positive stress test. Aggressive modification of risk factors and antianginal therapy may effectively improve outcome in such patients. Hence, if the diagnosis of ischemia is confirmed, even in the asymptomatic patient, antianginal therapy is warranted.

Indications for Exercise Stress Testing

In general, exercise stress testing is used for diagnostic or prognostic purposes or to assess the effectiveness of therapy.

To clarify the cause of chest pain. This is probably the most common reason for recommending an exercise stress test in an ambulatory population. In some practices, exercise stress tests are recommended for many patients to provide reassurance that chest pain is not caused by cardiac ischemia. In such cases, factors influencing sensitivity, specificity, and predictive accuracy of the test must be kept in mind.

To assess prognosis in patients with known ischemic heart disease and after myocardial infarction. A positive stress test after minimal exertion, hypotension with exercise, or extensive sustained ST depression in several ECG leads probably indicates severe three-vessel disease or left main coronary artery disease (9). Studies from the prethrombolytic era suggested that a positive submaximal stress test in patients after myocardial infarction identified a high-risk population (see Chapter 58) and recommended that such patients be considered for coronary arteriography. The 1996 American Heart Association–American College of Cardiology Guidelines support symptom-limited treadmill testing at 3 weeks after myocardial infarction (2).

Serial stress tests, at 18-month intervals, can also be used to follow patients with stable angina. A deterioration in performance (angina or ischemic changes on the ECG at a lower work load) strongly suggests worsening coronary artery disease. Occasionally, the physiologic significance of an anatomic lesion (e.g., 30 to 50% left anterior descending coronary artery stenosis) noted at coronary arteriography may be questionable. In such a patient, a positive stress test in the appropriate ECG leads (i.e., V_1 to V_4 in this example) or a reperfusion defect on a thallium scan (see below) would clearly define the hemodynamic significance of the anatomic lesion.

To ascertain the effects of medical or surgical (revascularization) management of coronary artery disease, particularly when baseline studies have been performed. The exercise stress test documents objectively whether a patient has improved and, if so, to what extent. The documentation of improvement with a stress test is often reassuring to the patient and in many instances necessary before an employer will allow a patient to return to work (especially if physical labor is required). On the other hand, patients with worsening coronary artery disease can also be identified, and in such patients more aggressive evaluation, such as coronary arteriography, may be indicated.

Some physicians believe that an exercise stress test is advisable in an apparently healthy middle-age or elderly person who wishes to undertake a new physically stressful activity. For example, a preliminary exercise stress test is considered an appropriate part of the evaluation of a person who wishes to join an exercise program or to begin mountain climbing or running, especially if that person has previously led a largely sedentary life or has coronary risk factors; the caveats regarding predictive accuracy should be recalled when interpreting stress tests in such patients. Table 58.5 (Chapter 58) lists the metabolic equivalents (METs) of a number of common activities. Stress test data reported in terms of METs achieved before symptoms appear are useful in counseling the patient regarding safe levels of exercise and activity.

To document the response of a patient with a cardiac arrhythmia to exercise and to document the response of the arrhythmia to therapy (see Chapter 59). This is particularly useful in patients in whom the history suggests an exercise-induced arrhythmia. A decrease in ventricular ectopy with exercise in a patient with known ventricular arrhythmias is often a favorable prognostic sign.

Contraindications to Exercise Stress Testing

There are a number of contraindications to stress testing. The recent onset of unstable angina pectoris after a period of stabilization or an acute myocardial infarction is a relative contraindication to exercise stress testing. Most of these patients should not be subjected to maximal exercise stress tests. However, modified submaximal stress tests can be performed with a reasonable degree of safety in selected patients as early as day 4 or 5 after myocardial infarction. The information thus obtained may be invaluable for making recommendations about physical activity and further therapy.

Uncontrolled hypertension is a relative contraindication and depends on the level of blood pressure and the degree of end organ impairment.

Exercise stress testing should not be performed in patients with severe uncontrolled congestive heart failure because of the risk of acute pulmonary edema, hypotension caused by low cardiac output, and serious arrhythmias.

Significant ventricular arrhythmias are a relative contraindication to exercise stress testing. However, it may be difficult to know before the test whether a given ventricular arrhythmia is significant because patients with frequent multifocal premature ventricular contractions may show a decrease or an increase in ectopic activity when stressed. If ventricular ectopy increases with exercise, the test should be terminated.

Suspected severe valvular disease, particularly obstructive valvular disease such as mitral stenosis, aortic stenosis, or subvalvular aortic outflow obstruction, may impose serious risks to patients who are exercised. This is because the heart may be unable to increase cardiac output in response to an increased demand. In such patients the usual increase in blood pressure with exercise significantly increases ventricular afterload and thus reduces perfusion. Again, however, modified stress tests can probably be performed with a reasonable degree of safety in appropriately selected patients.

Exercise stress testing should be performed with caution in a variety of other conditions. Exercise testing is contraindicated in patients with myocarditis, acute pericarditis, severe pulmonary hypertension, recent pulmonary embolism, atrial fibrillation with an uncontrolled ventricular response, intercurrent acute systemic illness, or significant infection. Patients with a high degree of atrioventricular (AV) block should be exercised cautiously because they may not be able to increase their heart rate appropriately. Patients with severe chronic pulmonary disease, such as increased bronchospasm, increased hypoxemia, or cardiac arrhythmias, may have difficulty when exercised. However, exercise stress tests in such patients, with concomitant pulmonary function studies and blood gas analyses, can provide useful information (see Chapter 55).

Neurologic or orthopaedic disease may make it difficult for the patient to participate in an exercise stress test. Modifications of stress testing, by use of a bicycle ergometer, for example, can sometimes circumvent these problems.

Patient Experience. The patient spends 1 to 1.5 hours at the stress test laboratory and should not eat for at least 2 hours before the test; the preceding meal should be light and should not contain butter, cream, coffee, tea, or alcohol; comfortable clothes and shoes should be worn. The patient should be told which regular medicines should be taken on the day of the test (if not told at the time the appointment was made, the patient should be instructed to telephone the stress test laboratory to inquire about medications several days in advance). Before testing, ECG leads are applied to the chest and a blood pressure cuff is applied to one arm. The test consists of walking on a treadmill; the speed and the slope of the treadmill are increased during the test. Alternatively, the test may consist of pedaling on a bicycle ergometer. The patient is asked to exercise to a point where discomfort is experienced; if chest pain, shortness of breath, claudication, or light-headedness are experienced, the test is terminated. The degree of exercise is consistent with the age and physical condition of the patient. The duration of the test is determined by the time it takes to reach an age-predicted maximal heart rate (usually no more than 10 to 15 minutes).

If radioisotope scanning is included in the stress test (see below), the patient receives an intravenous injection containing [201]thallium at the time of maximal exercise and undergoes cardiac scanning immediately after exercise and again 3 hours later. If technetium sestamibi is used, the second scan may be after 24 hours. If an echocardiogram is included in the stress test, the patient has a baseline two-dimensional echocardiogram recorded and a repeat echocardiogram at peak exercise and in recovery.

Radioisotope Imaging

In an effort to improve the sensitivity and specificity of stress testing, especially in patients with baseline ST–T abnormalities, various imaging testing modalities have been developed. They evaluate myocardial function or flow. Pharmacologic testing has also been used in patients unable to exercise (e.g., patients with severe arthritis or peripheral vascular disease) or with limited exercise ability (patients with severe lung disease). Pharmacologic testing is often coupled with an imaging modality to improve the sensitivity and specificity of the test. Commonly used imaging modalities include radioisotope imaging with [201]thallium or [99]technetium-based agents such as ^{99m}Tc-sestamibi, 2D echocardiography, and position emission tomography.

[201]*Thallium* is the isotope most often used for assessing regional myocardial blood flow, either by planar imaging or by single-photo emission computerized tomography (SPECT), a slightly more sensitive, and more expensive, technique (43). The rationale for using thallium is based on its ability to substitute biologically for ionic potassium. It is very efficiently extracted by healthy myocardial cells and uptake is proportionate to regional perfusion. Low-energy emissions permit recording of the myocardial pattern of radioactivity. Areas of infarcted or ischemic myocardium have no or diminished uptake and hence show reduced or absent activity, so-called cold spots. The perfusion defects seen in transiently ischemic myocardium disappear or fill in as the ischemic episode resolves (i.e., during the reperfusion scan).

[201]Thallium scans are commonly performed as part of an exercise stress test or in conjunction with the intravenous administration of adenosine, dipyridamole, or dobutamine (pharmacologic stress testing; see below). The cost is almost three times the cost of the standard test. Thallium is injected intravenously at the time of peak exercise (or at the time of peak infusion during a pharmacologic stress test), and scintigraphic images obtained shortly thereafter depict regional myocardial perfusion at the time of peak stress. Scintigraphic images taken 3 hours later show redistribution of isotope; a filling in of a cold spot defined on the stress images is likely to indicate transient ischemia. On the other hand, a persisting cold spot, or one with only partial redistribution, is likely to be caused by infarction.

Thallium scanning with exercise stress testing is at least as sensitive and is more specific for detection of occlusive coronary artery disease than ECG exercise stress testing (remembering that predictive accuracy depends on the population under investigation; see above) (8). A normal maximal stress–thallium study rules out significant coronary artery occlusions with 90% confidence. Recent studies indicate that a reinjection of a small dose of thallium at the time of redistribution imaging (i.e., 3 hours) further increases the sensitivity of the test (23). It is not reasonable, however, to recommend that all patients undergoing exercise testing should incur the additional expense of a thallium scan. The use of thallium with exercise stress testing is of particular value in conditions that render ECG interpretation difficult or impossible (e.g., diffuse ST–T changes, bundle branch block). It has been shown to be particularly useful in patients after transmural myocardial infarction (30).

Besides its value in evaluating selected patients for exercise-related ischemia, [201]thallium scanning is also useful for detecting evidence of a recent or remote myocardial infarction (e.g., in patients with nonspecific ECG changes and a history of a clinical event too remote to be evaluated by measurement of cardiac enzymes) and for identifying viable myocardium in an area of previous infarction. A resting defect on a [201]thallium scan is more sensitive than an ECG Q wave for identifying an old infarction. Thallium studies can also be used to localize and identify the ischemia-producing blood vessel in patients with known coronary artery disease. This allows a more focused planning of future therapeutic strategies.

[99m]*Technetium sestamibi,* a radioactive tracer, can also be used to assess myocardial perfusion.

^{99m}Tc-teboroxime is an alternative agent that can be used, and others are likely to be made available in the near future. The shorter half-life of ^{99m}technetium (6 hours) compared to ^{201}thallium (73 hours) allows administration of a larger tracer dose and provides better imaging. It is particularly useful in large, obese patients or in patients with breast attenuation on ^{201}thallium imaging. Because of its washout characteristics, two separate injections are commonly made: with stress and during rest imaging.

Position emission tomography (PET) studies usually use oxygen-15 (half-life 2 minutes), nitrogen-13 (half-life 10 minutes), carbon-11 (half-life 20 minutes), or fluorine-18 (half-life 110 minutes) as the tracer and require a local or on-site cyclotron for tracer production. Rubidium-82 (half-life 75 seconds) does not require a cyclotron and can be used to assess myocardial perfusion along with nitrogen-13 and oxygen-15 water. PET scanning is usually used during pharmacologic vasodilation and qualitative or semiquantitative changes in rubidium-82 estimated myocardial flow are calculated. PET scanning using F-18 fluorodeoxyglucose as a marker for glucose utilization and tissue viability is particularly useful in evaluating regional wall viability in patients with CAD and LV dysfunction. Because of the associated expense, few centers are capable of performing PET imaging on a routine clinical basis.

Radioisotope imaging with stress MUGA (gated blood pool) scans can also be used to assess ischemia. The cost is almost twice that of a standard exercise stress test. The rationale for this test is based on the fact that myocardium that becomes ischemic during graded exercise develops regional wall motion abnormalities that can be detected by sequential image analyses. The patient exercises on a semirecumbent bicycle, a posture that is comfortable for sustained exercise for many people. The test may be useful in patients whose stress–thallium study is equivocal or if exercise-induced left ventricular dysfunction is suspected.

Pharmacologic Stress Testing

Patients who are unable to exercise because of physical limitations can be evaluated after intravenous administration of dipyridamole, adenosine, or dobutamine in conjunction with an imaging modality. Dipyridamole and adenosine dilate the normal coronary arteries, thus creating an intracoronary steal syndrome with reduced blood flow to areas of myocardium supplied by vessels with fixed stenosis. Because of its ultrashort duration of action, adenosine is preferred to dipyridamole in this test. Dobutamine at high dosages (20 to 40 µg/kg per minute) increases the heart rate, blood pressure, and myocardial contractility, and thereby increases myocardial oxygen demand.

Mild side effects (nausea, flushing, headaches) are common with all three of these agents and occur in 25 to 80% of patients. Both dipyridamole and adenosine (but not dobutamine) can produce severe bronchospasm and hence must be used with great caution in patients so predisposed. Adenosine can also cause transient heart block.

The sensitivity and specificity of pharmacologic stress testing with dipyridamole or adenosine approximates that of stress–thallium imaging (70). However, the sensitivity of dobutamine stress electrocardiography is considerably less than that of stress–thallium imaging (44), and the test should not be performed if another modality is available.

Stress Echocardiography

Occasionally *two-dimensional echocardiography* (2D echo) is used instead of radioisotope scanning (19,65). The cost is approximately the same. In such cases a baseline 2D echo is obtained before exercise and again at peak exercise. Wall motion changes are evaluated. This test is called a stress echo; it has no clear-cut advantage over radioisotopic imaging except that there is no exposure to radioactivity.

Pharmacologic stress echocardiography (e.g., using dobutamine) is a technique developed to evaluate patients who cannot exercise. The results and safety of the procedure are comparable to those of a routine exercise stress test (19,45,69) and much better than those of dobutamine stress electrocardiography (see above) (21).

Ambulatory Electrocardiography

The ambulatory ECG (Holter monitor) may also be useful in detecting myocardial ischemia, especially in patients suspected of having variant angina. However, it is not a good tool for screening patients to make the diagnosis of coronary artery disease. In patients with coronary artery disease who are symptomatic during ambulatory ECG monitoring, ST-segment elevation or depression can be observed during episodes of pain and at other times as well (silent ischemia; see below). In patients with silent ischemia the ambulatory ECG is particularly useful in quantitating the degree and frequency of ischemia and in assessing the efficacy of therapy.

Ultrafast CT Scanning

Studies in the 1970s demonstrated that coronary calcification (detected by cardiac fluoroscopy) was useful in identifying patients with angiographically significant CAD (at least 70% stenosis) (6). The concept of using coronary calcification as a marker of CAD has been revisited in the 1990s; the degree of coronary calcification is calculated and scored by ultrafast CT scanning. This inexpensive screening tool ($350 to $375 per test) may be useful in middle-age patients with atypical chest pain. Although the sensitivity and specificity of this diagnostic tool are not significantly better than those of treadmill testing alone, its negative predictive value is high (11).

Coronary Arteriography

Figure 57.2 shows diagrammatically the coronary arteries and their branches as they appear on coronary arteriography. This technique provides direct information about the presence of coronary artery disease and defines the distribution and severity of obstructive coronary lesions. Coronary arteriography is usually performed in conjunction with detailed intracardiac hemodynamic monitoring and a left ventriculogram. The addition of the latter two procedures allows for the detailed evaluation of valvular lesions and overall left ventricular function. Coronary angiography has greatly expanded our understanding of the prognosis of coronary artery disease and it has become a major tool for decision making in the individual patient. Postmyocardial infarction studies in the 1970s identified that coronary anatomy predicted recurrent ischemia, but not mortality. Also, the degree of vascular occlusion was not predictive of future ischemic events (73).

Indications

Our expanding clinical experience and the changing spectrum of therapeutic options make it difficult to define firm guidelines for the use of coronary arteriography. Certain indications for coronary arteriography are generally accepted. However, some physicians believe that coronary arteriography should be performed in all (or almost all) patients with angina or myocardial infarction—especially those who are less than 50 years of age—and others believe that it should be used only as a last resort.

The referring physician should know the morbidity and mortality of the procedure. Ideally, each laboratory should systematically and periodically analyze its performance.

The principal indications for coronary arteriography are as follows.

To determine the suitability for revascularization of patients who have failed maximal medical therapy (see below). This indication is clear-cut because revascu-larization offers an excellent chance for clinical improvement.

To detect left main or severe three-vessel coronary artery disease. Patients with these lesions can often be identified on the basis of the history or stress test performance (see above). In addition, patients who are post-MI, with a positive early submaximal exercise stress test or clinical evidence of ischemia, are a high-risk population and should undergo early arteriography. Demonstration of left main or severe three-vessel disease in such patients is an indication for early coronary bypass surgery. Also, because patients with a subendocardial infarction are at high risk for further ischemic events, early coronary arteriography may be useful in this population. Although it has not been shown to alter 1-year mortality, there is a decreased rehospitalization rate and a decreased need for anti-ischemic medication in patients who have revascularization procedures as the result of the demonstration of major occlusive lesions by angiography (4). Angiography is done in up to 60% of patients postinfarction, but probably no more than 30 to 35% warrant the procedure (63).

To permit decisions concerning management in young patients with coronary artery disease who want to continue an active or stressful lifestyle. Ideal recommendations regarding therapy and prognosis can be made only with knowledge of coronary anatomy. This is particularly true if exercise stress testing or radioisotope imaging suggests that there is a large amount of myocardium at risk for infarction.

To evaluate patients with chest pain suggestive of angina in whom the diagnosis remains unclear despite other tests (e.g., thallium imaging) *and in whom it is important to know whether coronary artery disease exists* (e.g., airplane pilots). This becomes particularly important in patients with atypical chest pain and a

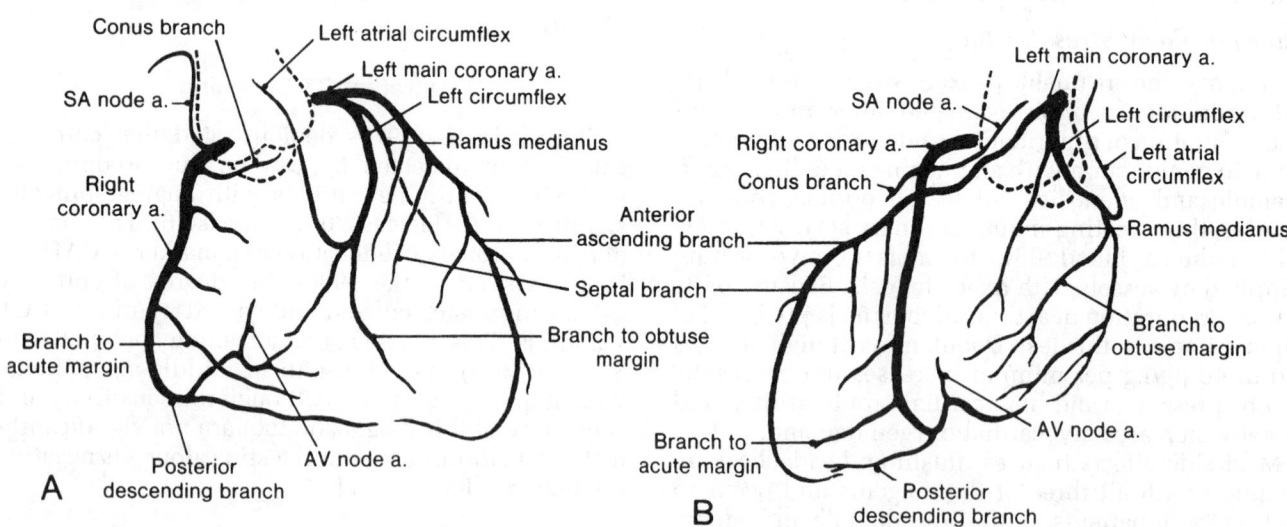

Figure 57.2. Anatomic representation of the coronary arteries. These vessels are represented as they would be seen on the angiogram. No attempt to convey the third dimension has been made. Careful study of the changes in position of the various branches with rotation of the heart is essential to intelligent interpretation of arteriograms. **A.** Anteroposterior. **B.** Lateral. (From Abrams HL, Adams DF. The coronary arteriogram. First of two parts. Structural and functional aspects. N Engl J Med 281:1276, 1969.)

fear of death or of a heart attack. In such patients, the knowledge that the coronary arteries are anatomically normal may be essential to prevent the patient from becoming a "cardiac cripple."

Inherent in the recommendation for coronary arteriography is the assumption that the patient is a potential candidate for coronary revascularization. If the patient's general medical condition or other medical problems preclude revascularization or if the patient refuses to consider revascularization regardless of catheterization results, arteriography is ill-advised.

Technique and Patient Experience. Usually the patient is hospitalized the morning of the catheterization. The procedure is not painful and the patient remains awake throughout the study. One hour before the procedure, the patient is given a sedative, usually diazepam (Valium), 10 mg orally. What happens next depends on the technique used. There are two commonly used techniques; both are performed under fluoroscopic control.

By the Sones technique, an incision is made, under local anesthesia, over the right brachial artery, and the catheter is threaded through a small incision into the artery and then via the subclavian and brachiocephalic arteries into the aorta near the coronary sinuses. By the Judkins technique, a special catheter is inserted percutaneously into the femoral artery and then threaded up the aorta to the coronary sinuses. The tip of the catheter is moved into the right or left sinus; contrast medium is injected; and then, under direct fluoroscopic visualization, the orifices of the right and left coronary arteries are injected sequentially with contrast medium. The patient is asked to hold his or her breath during the few seconds of the injection. The catheter used in the Judkins technique is designed to enter easily either the right or left artery, so that after one arterial system is visualized adequately, the catheter must be withdrawn and the complementary catheter inserted.

After the coronary circulation has been visualized, ventricular pressures are measured and dye is injected directly into the left ventricular cavity to observe ventricular contraction. During ventriculography, aneurysms and valvular lesions, such as mitral regurgitation, can also be assessed. (Another special catheter is introduced in the Judkins technique for this phase of the study.) Ejection fraction (the ratio of stroke volume to end-diastolic volume) is measured, then the catheter is withdrawn, and (if the Sones technique has been used) the incisions are sutured.

During this procedure the patient feels slightly woozy from the sedation; there is no pain except for a sensation of hot flushing when the dye is injected and pressure on the groin as the catheter is held in place. The patient is usually discharged from the hospital the same day. (See also *Heart Catheterization,* an illustrated brochure published for patients by the American Heart Association.) Recently, the technique of angiography and PTCA via the radial artery has been shown to be effective and is gaining increasing popularity, especially as an outpatient procedure (40).

Complications

The major complications of coronary arteriography are myocardial infarction, stroke, and death. Other complications include false aneurysms, arterial thrombosis, bleeding, transient impairment of renal function, allergy to contrast material (see Chapter 23), arrhythmias, and hypotension.

The risks of complications after coronary arteriography are related to the experience of the laboratory performing the studies and to the types of patients being studied. Risks tend to be lower in young, otherwise healthy patients and higher in older patients with poor left ventricular function, particularly those with associated peripheral vascular disease. The incidence of side effects, especially impairment of renal function, is also higher in diabetic patients or patients with dehydration or prior therapy with other nephrotoxic agents. Risks are lower in established laboratories doing a large number of procedures, and the low risk is related to the experience and proficiency of the team performing the study.

Interpretation

If there is 70% or more obstruction of a coronary artery, a significant impairment of coronary blood flow, even at rest, may be expected. A 50% narrowing may produce no significant decrease in flow at rest but may produce serious physiologic impairment when there is an increase in myocardial oxygen demand. Sometimes the consulting cardiologist uses the combined results of stress testing or thallium–stress testing and arteriography to determine whether a given coronary occlusion may be significant enough to consider revascularization. For example, marked anterior ST depression and chest pain and an anterior thallium reperfusion defect during an exercise stress test may indicate that there is a severe decrease in flow through a left anterior descending coronary artery even when the arteriogram demonstrates a lesion that obstructs 50% or less of the lumen.

PROGNOSIS

Mortality

The crude annual mortality rate after the onset of angina in persons without known infarction was reported in the 1970s at approximately 5% (39). Recent data suggest that 2-year mortality is approximately 1.3% (75). In contrast, the crude first-year mortality rate remains between 10 and 30% for patients with unstable angina (see below), 8 to 10% for patients surviving 30 days after myocardial infarction, and 5 to 10% for patients with stable angina of 2.5 years' duration (4,14,35,36).

Stress testing (see above) helps detect patients with angina who have good or poor prognoses and complements the predictive value of arteriography. Patients with typical symptoms of ischemia who have positive exercise stress tests have an annual incidence of subsequent events and mortality that is higher than that of patients who have negative stress tests (25). Symptomatic patients with equivocal tests have intermediate risks. The prognosis is worse when ST depression is more downsloping, when the ST depression occurs earlier during exercise, when the degree to which the ST segments are depressed increases, when the ST depression persists longer after termination of exercise, or if left ventricular function is reduced. This information may be helpful in selecting patients for further studies such as coronary arteriography.

The two most important determinants of mortality in patients with coronary artery disease are the location and extent of coronary artery occlusion and the left ventricular ejection fraction (13). Coronary arteriography identifies with considerable precision the subsets of patients with poor or good prognoses, regardless of clinical manifestations of their coronary artery disease. Data from the Coronary Artery Surgery Study (CASS) registry of more than 14,000 patients indicate that the annual mortality rate for patients with one-vessel disease is 2%, for two-vessel disease 4%, for three-vessel disease 8% (46), and for left main disease 27 to 37% (15). In patients with reduced left ventricular ejection fraction (ejection fraction 35 to 40%), these figures are considerably worse (53).

In terms of assessing the effect of therapy, the Veterans Administration study demonstrated significantly better survival with surgery than with medical therapy in patients with left main coronary artery disease, and in patients with three-vessel disease and impaired left ventricular function (72). The European Cooperative Coronary Surgical Study Group data support these findings but also show a benefit for surgery (over medical therapy) in patients with 75% lesions in two vessels, one of which is the proximal left anterior descending (27). The CASS randomized study compared medical and surgical therapy in patients with mild angina and found no significant difference in 5-year survival among patients with one-, two-, or three-vessel disease with normal left ventricular function (16).

Chapter 58 provides additional information about prognosis for subsets of patients with unstable angina or recent myocardial infarction.

Morbidity

Although angina may spontaneously remit after it has been present for a long interval (as a consequence of myocardial infarction or collateral circulation), the usual course is one of periodic symptoms and, for many patients, progressive disease (gradually worsening angina, unstable angina, myocardial infarction, congestive heart failure, arrhythmias, or sudden death) (36). A recent European study followed 3000 patients for 2 years. During this period, 28.2% underwent coronary artery bypass grafting (CABG), 7.5% underwent PTCA, and 1.6% underwent both procedures. A total of 3.6% definite coronary events (sudden coronary death, fatal myocardial infarction, nonfatal myocardial infarction) occurred, of which more than one-third were in those

undergoing revascularization; 1.3% patients died of cardiac causes in 2 years of follow-up (75).

The impact of angina on a patient's functional capacity depends on the nature of his or her usual activities and the status of the disease. As described below, pharmacologic and nonpharmacologic measures can have an important impact on changing these limitations of activity, even though such measures usually have no impact on the overall mortality. Many patients with angina can continue to engage in most if not all of their usual activities after therapy. (Table 9.1, Chapter 9, lists the criteria that qualify a person with ischemic heart disease for Social Security benefits.)

TREATMENT OF ANGINA PECTORIS

A useful booklet, *Living with Angina,* can be obtained from the local chapter of the American Heart Association. It will help the patient better understand his or her illness and the rationale behind its treatment.

General Therapeutic Considerations

In evaluating and treating patients with angina, it is of paramount importance to identify and treat underlying contributing factors.

Hypertension is often present in patients with angina. There is a linear relationship between left ventricular work and myocardial oxygen demand. Left ventricular systolic pressure increases in response to an increase in peripheral vascular resistance. Both systolic and diastolic hypertension can increase myocardial oxygen demand. An attempt should always be made to reduce resting blood pressure to normal in patients with chronic hypertension, including those with isolated systolic hypertension. This can be of crucial importance in reducing the frequency and severity of angina pectoris in the hypertensive patient. β-Blockers and selected calcium channel blockers (see Chapter 62) are excellent choices in such patients because they have other antianginal properties and may also control hypertension without diuretics in some patients. Agents such as hydralazine and minoxidil that cause a reflex tachycardia may be less desirable.

It is important to achieve a maximal level of pulmonary compensation in patients with *angina and coexisting lung disease* (see Chapter 55). Chronic hypoxemia and acidosis and the increased work of breathing in patients with pulmonary disease increase myocardial oxygen demand or decrease myocardial oxygen delivery, or both. β-Selective bronchodilators are less likely to accelerate the heart rate and are often useful in such patients.

Abstinence from tobacco products is essential because nicotine in tobacco can cause coronary vasoconstriction. In heavy smokers without clinical lung disease, a decrease in smoking may also decrease susceptibility to angina. Various techniques that are used to achieve this goal are described in Chapter 20. Similarly, passive tobacco smoke should be avoided.

Carbon monoxide exposure in heavy traffic should also be avoided in patients whose angina is precipitated in this setting.

The possibility of *hyperthyroidism* (see Chapter 73) in patients with angina should never be overlooked, particularly in older patients or in patients with increasing angina. Often, particularly in the older patient, other obvious signs of hyperthyroidism may not be present. For example, hyperthyroidism may be manifest only by an increased frequency or severity of angina, an increase in heart rate in people with atrial fibrillation, or increasing heart failure.

Anemia also requires serious consideration, particularly when the hemoglobin concentration falls below 7 g/dL. This is the point at which cardiac output must increase to maintain peripheral oxygen delivery at rest.

Heart failure (see Chapter 61) in patients with angina should always be treated. The real possibility that latent heart failure exists in patients with unstable angina (see below) or nocturnal angina should be considered. Diuretics or the use of vasodilators or digitalis may be effective in such patients and may reduce the frequency and severity of angina or eliminate angina altogether. The calcium channel blocker amlodipine has little negative inotropic effect and may be useful in such patients because it reduces preload and afterload, helps decrease left ventricular end-diastolic pressure, lowers peripheral vascular resistance, and thus improves left ventricular function.

Lipids and Diet

Recently, the reasons for the decrease in mortality from heart disease from 1980 to 1990 were analyzed (see Chapter 75). More than 50% of the decline in mortality could be attributed to primary and secondary risk factor reductions (38). Strikingly, more than 70% of the decline in mortality occurred in patients with known CAD. These observations are further supported by the West of Scotland trial, which demonstrated a significant mortality reduction with treatment of hyperlipidemia in asymptomatic people, with the greatest benefit being in patients with other risk factors for CAD (71). The value of secondary prevention has been definitively established by two recent trials, the 4S study and the CARE trial; both demonstrated a significant reduction in mortality when LDL was lowered to approximately 100 to 120 mg/dL (66,67). Other trials also have clearly demonstrated coronary artery lesion regression with vigorous, sustained normalization of elevated cholesterol to a low-density lipoprotein cholesterol level of less than 120 mg/dL (10). Recent data suggest also that lowering of LDL is associated with normalization of disordered endothelial function (see above).

Patients with CAD and hyperlipidemia should be encouraged to follow the AHA Step I and, if needed, Step II diet (see Chapter 75). If LDL remains above 140 mg/dL in patients with known CAD, the National Cholesterol Education Program recommendations call for the initiation of lipid-lowering pharmacologic therapy to achieve an LDL of 100 mg/dL or less (28) (see Chapter 75).

Alcohol

Alcohol is an acute pressor agent and may be responsible for as many as 10% of all cases of hypertension (61). However, moderate drinking (1 to 3 drinks per day) is clearly accompanied by an increase in HDL cholesterol (41). This effect may be related to antioxidants and flavonoids, found more often in red wine. The extent to which the increase in blood pressure associated with heavy drinking mitigates the beneficial effect on HDL remains to be determined. In an editorial, Victor and Hansen comment, "In the absence of alcohol related illness, therefore, a drink or two a day still seems safe and advisable from a cardiovascular standpoint" (77).

Antioxidants

Although antioxidants may be important in inhibiting atherosclerosis, clinical trials with antioxidants such as vitamin E have not yet shown a conclusive long-term benefit (48).

Fish Oil

Epidemiologic studies in the early 1990s suggested that eating fish conferred protection against CAD. However, in 1995, after studying 44,895 male health professionals, Ascherio et al. reported no beneficial effect of increasing fish intake from 1 to 2 servings per week to 5 to 6 per week (5).

Physical Conditioning

Physical conditioning can also improve the exercise tolerance and psychologic well-being of patients with stable angina. For interested patients, referral to a physician-supervised exercise program is the best plan. In recent years, most large communities have developed such programs for patients with coronary artery disease. Chapter 58 describes the physiologic basis of physical conditioning and describes a supervised exercise program for cardiac patients. The booklet, *Exercise Testing and Training of Individuals with Heart Disease or at High Risk for Its Development: A Handbook for Physicians,* available from the American Heart Association, provides additional information on this subject.

In addition to recommending exercise programs for selected patients, patients with angina should be counseled about physical activities that may increase their symptoms. Physicians should specifically discuss with patients (and their partners) the safety of sexual intercourse, a subject that people are often reluctant to broach. The level of sexual activity and the degree of physical exertion recommended ideally should be based on the results of an exercise stress test. The energy requirements for a broad range of activities are summarized in Table 58.5 (Chapter 58).

Medical Treatment

The basic objective in treating patients with angina pectoris is to relieve or prevent pain by improving the relationship between myocardial oxygen demand and supply. This objective can be attained by increasing coronary blood flow or by decreasing myocardial oxygen demand. Angina that occurs with exercise is usually caused by an increase in myocardial oxygen demand that cannot be met because of fixed arterial obstruction. A decrease in or cessation of the work that produced angina usually results in a prompt reduction in myocardial oxygen demand. Thus, rest or a decrease in the level of activity may relieve angina in 1 to 2 minutes. When anxiety is a contributing or provoking factor, it may take longer for myocardial work to decrease and the episode of angina may be prolonged.

The major advance in the medical management of angina has been the demonstration that long-acting nitrates, β-blocking agents, and calcium channel blockers can decrease the frequency of anginal attacks and can increase the exercise tolerance and work capacity of many people with angina. In general, the duration or intensity of exercise before angina is doubled when these drugs are used optimally. Table 57.2 lists practical information about the drugs used most often in the treatment of angina.

Nitrates

Traditionally, nitroglycerin and related compounds have been the mainstay of treatment of patients with angina pectoris. Initially these agents were thought to increase coronary blood flow by producing coronary artery dilation. Although nitrates may increase coronary blood flow in patients with spasm or may increase collateral flow to obstructed vessels, evidence suggests strongly that the mechanism of action of nitrates in most patients is not an increase in blood flow but a decrease in myocardial oxygen demand and peripheral vascular resistance. These compounds produce dilation of the venous circulation, which reduces venous return and decreases ventricular volume. The decrease in ventricular volume improves the efficiency of the heart and decreases wall tension. These effects ultimately reduce myocardial oxygen demand. Nitrates also produce arterial dilation to a lesser degree, and thereby reduce the resistance to ventricular ejection. This effect further decreases myocardial oxygen demand by reducing left ventricular work. Thus, the beneficial antianginal effect of nitrates is caused primarily by peripheral vasodilation.

Sublingual nitroglycerin is still the drug of choice for the relief and prevention of discrete episodes of angina pectoris in most patients. The initial dose should be small (0.4 mg) to minimize unpleasant side effects (flushing, headache, light-headedness) in patients in whom higher dosages may be unnecessary. Patients should be taught that it is important that their pain be relieved as soon as possible and they should be instructed to take nitroglycerin whenever such symptoms appear. Use of nitroglycerin in this way may do more than simply prevent ischemic pain. Angina often produces some anxiety, which may increase heart rate, left ventricular contractility, and hence myocardial oxygen demand. Thus, ischemia may be increased and the severity and the duration of pain may be prolonged. In addition, some patients, during periods of ischemia, develop serious arrhythmias, hypotension, or incipient heart failure, which may be aborted by the prompt administration of nitroglycerin. If pain is not relieved by 2 to 3 tablets of nitroglycerin (the patient should wait for 3 minutes between doses), or if the use of nitroglycerin increases suddenly and dramatically, the patient should be instructed to call his or her physician or to go to an emergency facility immediately because of the danger of impending myocardial infarction. Because nitroglycerin may lose potency on storage, patients should be advised not to keep tablets longer than 3 to 4 months after opening the bottle, and if pain is not relieved and usual side effects are also not experienced, the problem may be caused by a change in the drug rather than a change in cardiac status. Prophylactic use of nitroglycerin is of particular value in patients who have angina in response to specific and reproducible stress despite other therapies. For example, the patient who develops angina after walking from a car to a place of work can be taught to take nitroglycerin after the car is parked, to wait a few minutes, and then to walk to work, thereby preventing pain altogether. The use of prophylactic nitroglycerin before sexual intercourse may also prevent angina and may alleviate the anxiety that is naturally associated with sexual activity when angina is anticipated.

It is important to teach the patient to use sublingual nitroglycerin correctly. The patient should cease the activity that has caused angina, take sublingual nitroglycerin, and sit down to avoid the possible untoward effects of hypotension (increased in the standing position). When initiating treatment with sublingual nitroglycerin, it is advisable to administer the first dose in the office so that the patient can experience the side effects and receive reassurance from a physician or nurse that this is an expected response. Patients who start taking nitroglycerin at home may otherwise become so frightened by side effects that they may delay taking it or avoid its use altogether. The most common side effects are flushing and headache; both may diminish with increasing usage of the drug. A nitroglycerin lingual spray has been developed that is designed to deliver 0.4 mg of nitroglycerin sublingually with each compression of the nebulizer. Some patients find this preparation more acceptable and reliable than the tablet.

Long-acting nitrates. As shown in Table 57.2, long-acting nitrates are available in a variety of preparations. Careful studies confirm the clinical efficacy of both

Table 57.2.   Selected Drugs Used in the Treatment of Angina[a]

Class	Brand Name	Available Strengths	Usual Starting Dosage	Usual Maximum Dosage	Onset	Duration
Nitrates						
Nitroglycerin (sublingual)[b]	Nitrostat and others	0.15-, 0.30-, 0.40-, 0.60-mg tablets, sublingual	1 tablet (0.4 mg) at time of, or in anticipation of, pain	2-3 tablets at time of pain	30 sec	3-5 min
Topical Ointment[c]	Nitro-Bid, Nitrol	2% ointment	½ inch every 4-6 hr as needed	4-5 inches q3-4hr	30-60 min	3-6 hr
Patch[c]	Transderm Nitro, Nitro-Dur, and Nitrodisc	2.5-, 5-, 10-, 15-mg/24 hr rated release (0.1, 0.2, etc., mg/hr)	5 mg	2-3 patches that deliver 15 mg/24 hr	30 min	24 hr
Long-Acting						
Erythrityl[b] tetranitrate	Cardilate	5-, 10-, 15-mg tablets, oral or sublingual; 10-mg tablets, chewable	5 mg sublingually in anticipation of pain or 10 mg orally or chewed three times a day	100 mg/day in divided doses	5 min (sublingual and chewed)	4 hr
Isosorbide[b] dinitrate	Isordil, Sorbitrate, and others	5-, 10-, 20-mg tablets, oral; 40-mg tablets or capsules, oral	10 mg BID or TID	60-80 mg BID or TID	15-30 min	4-6 hr
Isosorbide mononitrate	Ismo	20 mg	20 mg BID given 7 hr apart	40 mg BID given 7 hr apart	60 min	5 hr after 2nd dose
β-Adrenergic Blockers[b]						
Propranolol[b]	Inderal	10-, 20-, 40-, 80-mg tablets, oral	10-20 mg three or four times a day	320 mg a day in divided doses	1-1.5 hr	4-6 hr
Nadolol	Corgard	40-, 80-, 120-mg tablets, oral	40 mg once a day	240 mg	1-2 hr	24 hr
Atenolol	Tenormin	50-, 100-mg tablets, oral	50 mg once a day	100-150 mg	1-2 hr	24 hr
Metoprolol	Lopressor	50-, 100-mg	100 mg in two divided doses; in older persons, 25 mg BID	200 mg BID	1-2 hr	24 hr
Calcium Channel Blockers						
Nifedipine	Procardia	10-mg capsule	10 mg three or four times a day; 10 mg at time of pain if sublingual	40 mg q6hr	20-30 min	8 hr
Nifedipine, extended release	Procardia XL	30, 60, 90 mg	30 mg QD (for converting pts from TID to XL, add up mg dose, e.g., 30 mg TID = 90 mg XL)	90 mg QD	1-2 hr	>24 hr
Verapamil	Calan, Isoptin	80-, 120-mg tablets	80 mg three or four times a day	120 mg QID	30-45 min	6-8 hr
Verapamil SR	Isoptin SE, Calan SR	120, 180, 240 mg	120-180 mg QD	240 mg BID	1-2 hr	24 hr
Diltiazem	Cardizem	30-, 60-mg tablets	30 mg four times a day	60 mg q6hr	30-45 min	6-8 hr
Diltiazem CD	Cardizem CD	180, 240, 300 mg	180-240 mg QD	360 mg QD	1-2 hr	24 hr
Nicardipine	Cardene	20-, 30-mg capsules	20 mg three times a day	40 mg TID	30-120 min	8 hr
Amlodipine	Norvasc	2.5, 5, 10 mg	5 mg QD, increase dosage after 3-5 days, small or elderly pts start 2.5 mg QD	10 mg QD	Several hours	24 hr

[a]Other drugs, other dosages of the drugs listed, and combinations of different drugs are marketed. The drugs and dosages shown are the ones most often used.
[b]Generic available. Table 59.3 provides information on the pharmacology of all six of the currently available β-blockers.
[c]The brand name of these preparations is followed by a number (5, 10, 15, 20). It is important to know whether that number refers to milligrams per 24 hours (Transderm-Nitro or Nitrodisc) or to square centimeters of the patch (Nitro-Dur). Nitro-Dur contains 4 mg/cm of patch, reported now as release/hr.

nitroglycerin ointment and isosorbide tablets (20,74). Their effects last from 4 to 6 hours after administration. Patients restudied an average of 6 months after beginning isosorbide tablets maintained the same increase in exercise tolerance (20). The dosage of nitrate needed to improve symptoms may be high; fortunately, available preparations permit a great deal of flexibility in dosage, as shown in Table 57.2.

In selecting among available preparations, the major considerations should be the known efficacy, convenience, and cost of a particular nitrate for the patient. Using these criteria, isosorbide is probably the best choice for ambulatory patients. The disadvantages of nitroglycerin ointment are that it is messy to apply, it is difficult to apply similar amounts evenly each time, and irritation of the skin may occur after prolonged use. Its major advantage is that it can be removed promptly if a patient develops a significant side effect (e.g., severe hypotension) shortly after application.

A *nitrate patch* for once-a-day use also is available. It provides controlled release of 0.2, 0.4, or 0.6 mg/hour of nitroglycerin through a semipermeable membrane applied to the skin by means of an adhesive tape. It has two advantages compared with nitroglycerin ointment: It is not messy to use and it delivers a standardized dose. However, constant serum levels of nitrate predispose to the development of tolerance. A tachyphylactic effect has been conclusively demonstrated in patients with heart failure treated with the nitroglycerin patch (1,68), and a similar effect occurs in patients with angina treated with frequent oral doses (e.g., every 4 hours) of nitrates. It appears that a 12- to 14-hour nitrate-free interval is needed for the drug to exercise its maximal effect. Therefore, patients who develop increasing angina while using the patch may benefit from being changed to an oral nitrate regimen or from having the patch removed at night (24). A mononitrate preparation (e.g., isosorbide mononitrate, or Ismo) has the advantage of twice-a-day oral dosing (commonly 20 mg, 7 hours apart) and has not been shown to produce tachyphylaxis (7).

The side effects of all long-acting nitrates are similar to those produced by sublingual nitrates. Many patients have already experienced the headache produced by sublingual nitroglycerin before being treated with a long-acting preparation.

Because of persistent headache, some patients are unable to take long-acting nitrates, although in most patients this is not a problem. Because nitrates can produce orthostatic hypotension and occasionally syncope, it is very important to check a patient's orthostatic blood pressure response before and after initiating treatment with or increasing the dosage of a long-acting nitrate. Two relative contraindications to long-acting nitrates are a history of migraine or cluster headache and demonstrated orthostatic hypotension before initiation of treatment.

β-Blocking Agents

A number of β-blockers are currently available in the United States. These agents vary in their cardioselec-

tivity, metabolism, and to some degree, side effects (see below and Chapters 59 and 62).

In many respects β blockade is an ideal approach to the treatment of angina. It decreases heart rate, contractility, and in many patients systemic blood pressure. These effects alone or in combination significantly reduce myocardial oxygen consumption and thus prevent the frequency or severity of angina in most patients.

An added benefit for patients with ischemic heart disease is that β blockade often effectively prevents arrhythmias (see Chapter 59). It may decrease or eliminate premature ventricular contractions (PVCs), and the ventricular rate in patients with atrial fibrillation may also be decreased. Furthermore, when PVCs are frequent, the number of hemodynamically effective ventricular contractions is diminished, which decreases coronary as well as peripheral perfusion. In patients who are in atrial fibrillation, decreasing the ventricular response improves left ventricular dynamics by decreasing heart rate, increasing diastolic filling period, and decreasing myocardial oxygen consumption.

The dosage of a β-blocker can be rapidly increased over hours or days until the desired effect is obtained. The heart rate is a useful guide to treatment; sinus bradycardia at a rate at rest between 50 and 60 beats/minute is a reasonable goal. However, the ideal dosage is one that not only results in mild sinus bradycardia at rest but also blocks an increase in heart rate with exercise. The dosage necessary to produce this effect and that necessary to relieve angina pectoris may vary considerably.

Because β-agents decrease myocardial contractility, they must be used cautiously in patients with heart failure. If failure increases (sometimes expressed first as decreased exercise tolerance), reducing the dosage of the β-blocker or adding a vasodilator may improve cardiac compensation and at the same time reduce the severity or frequency of anginal attacks (see Chapter 61).

Extreme caution must be exercised when using any β-blocker in patients with second- or third-degree block (see Chapter 59) because life-threatening bradycardia can be precipitated in such patients.

The nonselective β-blockers (propranolol, nadolol, pindolol, timolol) are contraindicated in patients with intrinsic asthma. A history of allergic asthma or bronchospasm during pulmonary infections should therefore be sought in all patients for whom β-blockers are being considered. Furthermore, patients with chronic obstructive lung disease may develop increased bronchospasm from β-blockers even if they have no history of allergic or intrinsic asthma; therefore, in such patients a selective β-blocker with minimal β$_2$-blocking effects should be used. Metoprolol and atenolol are both cardioselective and can often be safely used in such patients and in patients with peripheral arterial disease, particularly Raynaud's disease, in whom nonselective β-blockers may exacerbate symptoms. However, even these agents have β$_2$-blocking effects at moderate and high dosages and should be used cautiously in these situations.

Although impotence occurs in 1% or less of the susceptible population, it is perhaps the major reason that the use of β-blockers is limited in middle-age men. It can sometimes be overcome by prescribing a β-blocker with poor lipid solubility and thus less penetration of the nervous system (e.g., atenolol instead of propranolol). Atenolol also is less likely to cause depression or to alter sleep patterns, occasional side effects of other β-blockers.

Several of the newer β-blockers can be administered once or twice a day, a feature that significantly promotes patient compliance. Because some β-blockers are excreted entirely by the kidneys, the interval between doses should be increased in patients with renal insufficiency who are taking those preparations (see Table 59.3).

Calcium Channel Blockers

Calcium channel blockers have added a new dimension to the treatment of angina. These drugs reduce the influx of calcium into the slow channels of the myocardium and smooth muscle (see Chapter 59) and thereby cause several important hemodynamic effects: dilation of coronary arteries and prevention of coronary vasospasm and production of systemic vasodilation, thus effectively reducing preload and afterload. They have been shown to be effective in the treatment of both stable and unstable angina and are also effective antihypertensive agents (29,50). A number of calcium channel blockers are currently available in the United States (Table 57.2). Although many are effective in the treatment of hypertension (see Chapter 62), only six currently are approved for use in patients with angina (nifedipine, nicardipine, amlodipine, verapamil, diltiazem, and bepridil).

Nifedipine is the one most often prescribed for patients with angina. It is a potent coronary and systemic vasodilator. The common side effects of nifedipine are dizziness, flushing, headache, nausea, diarrhea, and, because of systemic vasodilation, peripheral edema. The major adverse effect is severe hypotension, which, in association with a reflex tachycardia, can actually intensify myocardial ischemia in an occasional patient. All side effects can usually be controlled by a reduction in dosage of the drug. Nifedipine and other calcium channel blockers should be used cautiously in patients taking digoxin because excretion of digoxin may be inhibited and digitalis toxicity may be induced. At higher dosages in patients with reduced left ventricular function, negative inotropy may be observed with nifedipine. It is also an effective antihypertensive, especially in older patients. A recent meta-analysis (59) suggests that short-acting calcium blockers, when used to treat hypertension, may worsen mortality. This effect is probably restricted to the short-acting forms of nifedipine, and is not seen with the longer-acting daily preparation. The once-a-day preparation is less likely to be associated with hypotension and peripheral edema. The delivery system of this preparation is such that the tablet is excreted in the stools. To avoid alarm, patients should be warned of this phenomenon.

Nicardipine is structurally similar to nifedipine but is much less likely to cause hypotension or left ventricular dysfunction. Thus, it is particularly useful in patients with angina and modest heart failure or in those with borderline blood pressure.

Amlodipine also has been shown to be an effective antianginal and antihypertensive agent. Its safety and efficacy in patients with significant left ventricular dysfunction (51,52) make it a particularly attractive anti-ischemic agent. An added advantage is its once-a-day dosing and the infrequent incidence of side effects. It has few if any effects on the AV node. Reflex tachycardia following administration is also unusual.

Verapamil is most often prescribed for the treatment of hypertension or arrhythmias but it too is an effective antianginal agent. However, it has a more potent negative inotropic effect than other calcium channel blockers and significantly retards AV conduction. Therefore it should not be used in patients with compromised left ventricular function or with sinus bradycardia, sick sinus syndrome, or AV block (see Chapter 59). In these situations, amlodipine or nicardipine are safer choices. Verapamil might reasonably be prescribed and be particularly beneficial in a patient with a supraventricular arrhythmia who also has angina.

Diltiazem also significantly retards AV conduction, but it has less of a negative inotropic effect than does verapamil and, in contrast to nifedipine, is unlikely to cause hypotension or other side effects (e.g., flushing, headache, edema). It is available as a twice-a-day or a once-a-day preparation.

Bepridil, although approved for treatment of patients with stable angina, is not often used because of its tendency to cause prolongation of the QT interval. It should be prescribed only for patients who are not helped by other forms of treatment.

Caution must be exercised when treating older patients with calcium blockers, especially if used in conjunction with a β-blocker or other agents that slow AV conduction (e.g., digitalis) or if used in patients with preexisting conduction system disease. In such patients, significant heart block and bradycardia can be precipitated but usually resolve after stopping administration of the calcium blocker or after the administration of calcium intravenously. This effect, although most commonly seen with verapamil and diltiazem, may occur with other calcium blockers, but not with amlodipine.

Initiating and Adjusting Long-Acting Drugs for Angina

The choice of an antianginal regimen should be made after evaluation of the patient's age, angina frequency, lifestyle, and possible mechanism of angina. In addition, the patient's financial resources should be considered because many of the newer agents, although effective, are expensive and not available as generic substitutes. In patients with stable angina, either a nitrate preparation or a β-blocker can be tried initially (Table 57.2). If the patient does not improve, the dosage can be increased weekly until a response is achieved. If the type of treatment selected initially fails to help at a maximally tolerated dosage, another agent can be added or substituted. Because nitrates and β-blockers decrease myocardial oxygen demand by different mechanisms, the concomitant use of the two types of therapy is reasonable.

A number of relative contraindications to long-acting nitrates and β-blockers have been mentioned above; these contraindications are important in selecting the initial treatment in some patients.

A good argument can be made for administering a β-blocker to most patients with angina, especially younger patients desirous of an active lifestyle, unless there is a specific contraindication. If a β-blocker is effective in reducing or eliminating angina pectoris, additional preparations may be unnecessary. In patients on maximally tolerated β blockade who continue to have pain, addition of a long-acting nitrate preparation or a calcium channel blocker may bring symptoms under better control.

Because of the possible risk of precipitating worsening angina when a β-blocker is abruptly discontinued and because of indirect evidence for a similar problem when long-acting nitrates are abruptly discontinued, these drugs should be tapered over several days when they are being stopped. (However, if a patient is taking a β-blocker and a calcium blocker, the former can be rapidly withdrawn with no ill effect [32].) All patients should be warned about this problem so that they do not casually stop and start these drugs; a corollary to this is the importance of explaining that these drugs are being prescribed chiefly to prevent symptoms, so that patients whose symptoms remit do not conclude that they can try stopping medication themselves.

In general, β-blockers are prescribed first to patients with predictable angina (chest pain reproducible after a given effort) who are likely to have fixed obstruction of their coronary arteries, unless there is a specific contraindication such as chronic obstructive lung disease. A calcium channel blocker is prescribed to patients who have variable chest pain, in whom coronary artery spasm (see "Variant Angina," below) may be playing a role, or to those intolerant of β-blockers.

Because patients who fail to improve after maximal medical management for angina pectoris are considered candidates for coronary arteriography and possible revascularization, it is important to define maximal medical therapy. In practical terms, administration of a β-blocker in increasing doses until side effects preclude further increase, in conjunction with a dose of long-acting nitrates increased to the point where side effects begin to become intolerable, together with maximal dosages of calcium channel blockers, would be considered to constitute maximal medical management in most patients. If a β-blocker and a calcium channel blocker are used together, the dosage of both may have to be lower than if either is used alone because of an additive adverse effect on blood pressure

and, depending on the agents used (see above), left ventricular function. Similarly, if a nitrate and nifedipine are used together, severe hypotension is more likely and the dosages may have to be reduced. If side effects limit the addition of the third drug, the combination of a β-blocker and calcium channel blocker is likely to be more effective than a β-blocker and a long-acting nitrate.

Role of Anticoagulants and Drugs that Interfere with Platelet Plug Formation

Despite their occasional use, there are no data to support the use of anticoagulants or dipyridamole in patients with angina. The role of aspirin in the treatment of patients with atherosclerotic heart disease is discussed in Chapter 52. In essence, aspirin 325 mg/day is extremely beneficial to patients with stable or unstable angina and after myocardial infarction (36,62).

Percutaneous Transluminal Coronary Angioplasty

Percutaneous transluminal coronary angioplasty (PTCA) is an important option for the treatment of coronary artery disease that cannot be controlled by the administration of drugs. This technique has the ability to restore nearly normal coronary flow in diseased native coronary arteries, without the cost and morbidity of bypass surgery. It involves the compression of a critical coronary lesion against the wall of the affected coronary artery by means of an inflatable balloon mounted on a special catheter. Patients are identified as candidates for PTCA after cardiac catheterization has clearly delineated coronary anatomy and after it has been determined that bypass surgery would otherwise be indicated. PTCA was initially used to treat patients with single-vessel, proximal, discrete, noncalcific coronary lesions. However, in skilled hands, three-vessel coronary lesions can be successfully dilated also. Although there are no absolute contraindications to the procedure, patients with arterial dissection or eccentric and long stenotic lesions are poor candidates and have a higher risk of complications and restenosis with PTCA. These patients are best treated with surgery.

Patients who are appropriate candidates for PTCA undergo the procedure either immediately after cardiac catheterization or at a later time, depending on the clinical situation and the needs of the particular patient. The catheter is usually introduced through a femoral artery under local anesthesia. A brachial approach can also be used but requires a cutdown. The coronary orifice is reached with a preshaped guiding catheter through which the balloon catheter with the balloon decompressed is inserted. The balloon is positioned halfway across the lesion, and translesional pressure gradients are measured. (Most significant coronary lesions cause a significant pressure drop across the lesion.) Under fluoroscopic control, the balloon is inflated with increasing pressures until there is no more indentation of the balloon or until the previously recorded pressure gradient is essentially abolished and dye injections through the guiding catheter show normal flow and a sufficiently patent coronary artery. Steerable catheters have been designed and have significantly widened the spectrum of lesions that can be successfully treated by PTCA. The dilation results in an actual intimal tear and occasionally a coronary dissection may occur. Therefore a cardiac surgical team is ordinarily on standby during the procedure. Barring complications, the patient's experience during PTCA and the time of the procedure are the same as they are for coronary angiography (see above). The incidence of major side effects (including dissection, myocardial infarction, and sudden death) is related to the skill and experience of the operator and can be as low as 2 to 4%. Overall, the procedure is successful 80 to 90% of the time. After successful angioplasty, patients are prescribed aspirin indefinitely. Patients taking ticlopidine can develop leukopenia, so blood counts should be checked at 2-week intervals (see Chapter 52).

The major limitation of PTCA is restenosis. The usual restenosis rate after PTCA is 30%, but the rate can be as high as 40 to 50% for certain left anterior descending coronary lesions. Most restenoses occur within the first 6 months and can be successfully treated a second time by PTCA (49). A lack of symptoms after 6 to 8 months usually indicates a favorable long-term prognosis. The use of intracoronary stents into the coronary artery at the site of dilation has dramatically reduced the incidence of restenosis. In addition, in patients with unstable coronary syndromes, the intravenous use of a IIb/IIIa platelet glycoprotein blocking agent for 24 to 36 hours after a PTCA or stent placement has further reduced restenosis rates (26) but that approach is still experimental. (Glycoprotein IIb/IIIa is the receptor to which platelet aggregating agents bind and is therefore essential to platelet plug formation.)

PTCA with or without stent placement is an especially attractive therapeutic option in younger patients (40 to 50 years of age) in whom coronary bypass grafts, given the current state of the art, could be expected to remain patent for only 10 to 12 years. Also, the comparative cost and morbidity of PTCA versus bypass surgery make the former more attractive if the therapeutic benefit is likely to be the same. Patients can usually be discharged on the second hospital day and can often return to gainful employment 1 week after PTCA, compared with 3 to 6 months after bypass surgery. After PTCA, it is advisable to have patients undergo a stress test within a few weeks. The results are useful in gauging the patient's ability to return to work.

In an effort to reduce restenosis and achieve better patency, a technique called atherectomy has been developed. During this procedure, the atherosclerotic plaque is actually shaved away through a specially designed catheter. In skilled hands, the technique is as effective as PTCA, and in a controlled trial, the two techniques appear to have comparable long-term results (17). However, the procedure is not widely available.

Surgical Management

Coronary artery bypass surgery is one of the most common surgical procedures performed in this country today. It is accepted generally that patients with incapacitating angina pectoris who have good left ventricular function and who have failed maximal medical therapy should be considered as candidates for coronary arteriography and subsequent surgery. It has been demonstrated that patients with left main coronary artery disease or its equivalent benefit symptomatically and have increased longevity after surgical intervention designed to increase coronary blood flow (72). Recommendations and results regarding surgery for patients with other lesions are discussed above.

The two surgical methods used today consist of saphenous vein bypass graft or implantation of an internal mammary artery into the native coronary artery circulation. Some surgeons also use gastric arterial conduits in patients undergoing repeat surgical procedures. The technique used is often based on the surgeon's preference and experience. A well-illustrated brochure, *Coronary Artery Bypass Surgery*, that explains the procedure and the patient's experience is available from the local chapter of the American Heart Association.

Patients with good left ventricular function have a 1 to 2% mortality rate from surgery and less than 5% of patients develop evidence of myocardial infarction during the perioperative period. Perioperative infarction is more likely to occur in older patients and in patients with severe disease distal to a proximal obstruction. Another major complication of bypass surgery is stroke, the mechanism of which may relate to hypoperfusion of a watershed bed or embolization during aortic cross-clamping. The risk of perioperative stroke is highest in patients above the age of 70 years and can be as high as 5 to 10%.

Approximately 60% of properly selected patients initially have complete (or nearly complete) relief of angina pectoris, and another 20% have a significant decrease in angina (37). There is a demonstrable increase in exercise tolerance after surgery in approximately 60 to 80% of such patients.

Historically, up to 50% of patients have developed recurrent angina within 5 years of bypass surgery. The diagnosis of recurrent angina should be confirmed by exercise stress testing. Initial treatment is the same as it is for patients who have not had bypass surgery: nitrates, β-blockers, or calcium channel blockers. Patients who prove to be unresponsive to medical treatment should undergo coronary angiography in an effort to delineate new lesions that could be amenable to percutaneous angioplasty or repeat bypass surgery. In an attempt to prevent formation of such lesions, it is now common practice to administer aspirin to patients after bypass surgery (see Chapter 52) and to treat hyperlipidemia aggressively (see Chapter 75).

The *postpericardiotomy syndrome* develops in approximately 30% of patients after bypass surgery, usually within 2 to 4 weeks (but sometimes as early as a few days or as late as 6 months after the operation). The syndrome is characterized by fever, pleuritic chest pain, and often pleural and pericardial effusions. Large effusions may require drainage, but most patients respond to diuretics and a nonsteroidal anti-inflammatory agent (e.g., indomethacin, 25 to 50 mg three times a day for 1 to 2 weeks). Patients who are refractory to such treatment usually respond to prednisone, initially 60 mg a day for 2 to 3 days with tapering of the dosage over 7 to 10 days. It has been suggested that graft occlusion is more likely in patients with postbypass pericarditis. Constrictive pericarditis is a late rare complication of the postpericardiotomy syndrome; when it occurs, pericardial stripping is often necessary.

Dysesthesia, swelling, and itching are common in the leg from which the vein was harvested and can persist for several months. The swelling usually responds to the use of support hose or elevation of the legs periodically during the day. If the itching is severe and there is no evidence of local infection, topical corticosteroid ointments are often effective.

Bypass surgery has been shown to prolong life in several patient subsets (see above). In addition, 60% of patients who either were working just before bypass surgery or discontinued work because of cardiac symptoms return to work after surgery. Early ambulation is advisable and the role of cardiac rehabilitation, as early as 6 to 8 weeks postoperatively, cannot be overemphasized (see detailed discussion in Chapter 58).

The BARI study compared revascularization in diabetic patients with CABG versus PTCA, and demonstrated the superiority of CABG in this particular subset of patients (12). Randomized studies comparing PTCA and CABG have been difficult to perform because many physicians exhibit a bias toward selecting patients with three-vessel disease. However, randomized trials and meta-analyses show comparable mortality and infarction rates at 3 years (56). Approximately 18% of patients who have had PTCA require CABG within 1 year; after a year the need for an additional procedure falls dramatically (56).

In recent years, bypass surgery in patients over 75 years of age has become increasingly common. Changing demographics, the improved care of elderly patients with coronary artery disease, and improved anesthesia techniques have prompted this change in practice. However, perioperative complications in such patients are often much higher than in those less than 70 years of age, and recuperation is slow. The decision to operate on such patients must take this higher morbidity into consideration and be driven primarily by a failure of maximal medical therapy. The benefit of CABG in reducing mortality in patients older than 70 years is not yet clear.

UNSTABLE ANGINA

Unstable angina is a term used to describe pain caused by cardiac ischemia that is becoming more intense, occurs more frequently (often provoked by diminishing effort, perhaps even at rest), and is relieved less readily by nitroglycerin. The syndrome has also been called crescendo angina and preinfarction angina. Sometimes unstable angina develops in a patient with previously stable, reasonably controlled angina; at other times, it develops in a patient with recent onset of ischemic symptoms. During the episode, the ECG shows ST elevation or depression or T-wave inversion that reverts to normal when the pain has abated. Because of the increased risks of myocardial infarction and sudden death and because of the need for aggressive medical therapy, patients with unstable angina should be hospitalized. Aggressive medical treatment with heparin, β-blockers, calcium channel blockers, and intravenous nitroglycerin is usually implemented. The TIMI III trial demonstrated that patients with unstable angina derived no benefit from thrombolytic therapy or routine early catheterization (64). Intravenous platelet glycoprotein IIb/IIIa inhibitors (see above) are being tested in patients with unstable angina, and appear to be promising (18). Coronary arteriography is indicated in patients in whom pain is not controlled by medical therapy, however, to determine their suitability for coronary bypass surgery or PTCA (see above).

The prognosis of these patients after hospital discharge is described in Chapter 58.

VARIANT ANGINA

Variant angina (Prinzmetal's angina) is, in a sense, unstable in that it occurs usually at rest but, unlike typical angina, does not occur on exertion or in response to emotional stress. Attacks of pain are experienced often at the same time each day, often awakening the patient early in the morning. During the attacks, there is ST-segment elevation that reverts to baseline when the attack is over; in about one-third of the patients there are also transient AV blocks or arrhythmias (including ventricular tachycardia or fibrillation). Unlike unstable angina, pain is usually promptly relieved by sublingual nitroglycerin.

Coronary artery spasm often plays a major role in the pathogenesis of variant angina. Two groups of patients have been identified. By far the larger group (85% of patients) have fixed, often proximal obstruction of a major coronary artery; angina in this group often is associated with spasm of the artery near the site of obstruction. The variant syndrome in this group of patients commonly follows months or years of stable typical angina pectoris or follows a myocardial infarction.

The smaller group with variant angina (15% of patients) have normal coronary arteries but have spasm of one of the arteries, thereby reducing blood supply to the myocardium, resulting in ischemic pain. These patients are usually younger and are predominantly women. There is usually no history of typical angina or myocardial infarction in these patients, and rarely a history of a systemic arteritis syndrome may be obtained. The ST elevation observed during the anginal attack is a manifestation of coronary artery spasm. It can often be confirmed by arteriography, either by the spontaneous occurrence of arterial spasm and chest pain during the procedure or by induction of arterial spasm by the administration of ergonovine. It is important to perform arteriography in such patients because those with normal coronary arteries are obviously not candidates for bypass surgery or PTCA and most respond favorably to treatment with calcium channel blockers, the drugs of choice in such patients. If used without calcium channel blockers, β-blockers may potentiate coronary artery spasm because of unopposed α-adrenergic vasoconstriction. However, a double-blind study of patients with rest angina showed that β-blockers, when added to nifedipine and nitrates, significantly reduced the number of episodes of angina in treated patients as compared with a control group treated with nifedipine and nitrates alone (32).

ANGINA WITH NORMAL CORONARY ARTERIES

Several investigators have reported large series of patients with typical angina, angiographically normal coronary arteries, and no obvious myocardial abnormality (54). Such patients may have ischemic exercise ECG responses. There are several possible causes for this condition. Accumulating evidence implicates coronary spasm (see above) in many patients; therefore it is important during angiography to confirm the diagnosis, if possible, by infusing ergonovine. The symptoms may also be caused by abnormal coronary reserve (e.g., in patients with hypertension, aortic stenosis and regurgitation, and hypertropic cardiomyopathy). Abnormalities of platelet function, small vessel disease, and mitral valve prolapse have been found in some patients. The prognosis of such patients is generally favorable (58), with survival being comparable to age- and sex-matched controls with normal coronaries. In the treatment of such patients, nitrates, calcium channel blockers, and β-blockers are often effective.

Angina and myocardial infarction, probably caused by coronary vasospasm, have also been reported in otherwise healthy patients who use cocaine. Coronary vasospasm usually occurs acutely after ingestion or inhalation of cocaine, but can also be observed up to an hour after use as a result of vasoactive byproducts of cocaine metabolism. Prolonged episodes of angina in such patients usually respond well to treatment with calcium channel blockers because concurrent hypertension is common.

SILENT ISCHEMIA

Many episodes of myocardial ischemia are painless. Such silent ischemia may be detected either during exercise treadmill testing (ETT) or by continuous ECG monitoring. Asymptomatic ischemic ST-segment changes on ECG monitoring are common in patients with coronary artery disease and have been correlated with transient abnormalities in myocardial perfusion and function.

Many ambulatory patients with stable angina experience asymptomatic episodes of ischemia that often occur at low heart rates during activities of everyday life, without an apparent significant increase in myocardial oxygen demand; such episodes may even be precipitated by mental stress. Studies in patients with unstable angina or in the early postinfarction phase have identified silent ischemia to be a powerful predictor of poor outcome (31,33). Patients with unstable angina who also have silent ischemia have a significantly greater frequency of bypass surgery, angioplasty, or recurrent symptomatic angina than patients without silent ischemia (33). In high-risk patients after myocardial infarction (e.g., patients with ejection fractions below 40%) silent ischemia detected on predischarge ECG monitoring has been shown to be the single most powerful predictor of poor outcome (31). The presence of silent ischemia within the first 3 days of myocardial infarction has also been shown to be associated with a greater frequency of recurrent ischemic events. Although several studies have identified silent ischemia to be a poor prognostic factor for patients with coronary artery disease (31), it is unknown whether treatment in such patients conclusively affects prognosis favorably.

CORONARY ARTERY DISEASE IN WOMEN

A large body of data suggests that women with coronary artery disease have different outcomes than men (79). Coronary artery disease in women was previously seen predominantly in postmenopausal women, but it has now become increasingly common in premenopausal women as well. Coronary artery disease is now the leading cause of death in women in the United States. This change may relate to the high prevalence of smoking and hyperlipidemia in younger women. Risk factors for coronary artery disease include a positive family history of coronary artery disease, diabetes mellitus, tobacco use, hypertension, hyperlipidemia, and possibly (especially in younger women who smoke) oral contraceptives.

The accurate diagnosis of coronary artery disease in women is harder to establish because symptoms are often atypical and false-positive stress tests are more common. Hence, stress–thallium testing is often necessary. However, the sensitivity of this test is reduced because of the occurrence of breast tissue attenuation in some patients. Unlike in men, stress MUGAs have a low specificity and sensitivity in women because 50% of normal women do not have substantial increases in left ventricular ejection fraction with exercise. Therefore coronary fluoroscopy is possibly the most useful test to screen for coronary artery disease in women because the presence of calcium in the coronary vessels (on fluoroscopy or on ultrafast CT; see above) is highly predictive of significant coronary artery disease. Women are also more likely to have atypical angina pain, and variant angina is also common in women. Thus, physicians must be suspicious of and be alert to atypical presentations in even young women with risk factors for coronary artery disease. The treatment of angina in women is the same as that described above.

In terms of outcome, women are more likely than men to have non–Q-wave myocardial infarction. However, they have a substantially higher postinfarction mortality that is independent of age. They also have worse outcomes after cardiac catheterization, PTCA, or coronary artery bypass surgery. The reason for these differences in outcome is unknown and is the focus of active ongoing research.

General References*

Gersh BJ, Braunwald E, Rutherford JD. Chronic coronary artery disease. In: Braunwald E, ed. Heart disease. A textbook of cardiovascular medicine. 5th ed. Philadelphia: WB Saunders, 1997;1289.
    A complete discussion of the diagnosis and management of angina pectoris.
Maddahi J. Myocardial perfusion imaging for the detection and evaluation of coronary artery disease. In: Skorton DJ, ed. Marcus cardiac imaging. A companion to Braunwald's heart disease. 2nd ed. Philadelphia: WB Saunders, 1996;971.

Specific References

1. Abrams J. Interval therapy to avoid nitrate tolerance: paradise regained? Am J Cardiol 64:931, 1989.
2. ACC/AHA Guidelines for the Management of Patients with Acute Myocardial Infarction. A report of the American College of Cardiology/American Heart Association Task Force on Practice Guidelines (Committee on Management of Acute Myocardial Infarction). J Am Coll Cardiol 28:1328, 1996.
3. Alldred EN, Bleecker ER, Chaitman BR, et al. Short-term effects of carbon monoxide exposure on the exercise performance of subjects with coronary artery disease. N Engl J Med 321:1426, 1989.
4. Anderson HV, Cannon CP, Stone PH, et al. One-year results of the thrombolysis in myocardial infarction (TIMI) IIIB clinical trial. A randomized comparison of tissue-type plasminogen activator versus placebo and early invasive versus early conservative strategies in unstable angina and non-Q wave myocardial infarction. J Am Coll Cardiol 26:1643, 1995.
5. Ascherio A, Rimm EB, Stampfer MJ, et al. Dietary intake of marine n-3 fatty acids, fish intake, and the risk of coronary disease among men. N Engl J Med 332:977, 1995.
6. Bartel AG, Chen JTT, Peter RH, et al. The significance of coronary calcification detected by fluoroscopy: a report of 360 patients. Circulation 49:1247, 1974.
7. Belder MA, Schneeweiss A, Camm AJ. Evaluation of the efficacy and duration of action of isosorbide mononitrate in angina pectoris. Am J Cardiol 65:6, 1990.
8. Beller GA, Gibson RS. Sensitivity, specificity, and prognostic significance of noninvasive testing for occult or known coronary disease. Prog Cardiovasc Dis 29:241, 1987.
9. Bogaty P, Dagenais GR, Cantin B, et al. Prognosis in patients with a strongly positive exercise electrocardiogram. Am J Cardiol 64:1284, 1989.
10. Brown G, Albers JJ, Fisher LD, et al. Regression of coronary artery disease as a result of intensive lipid lowering therapy in men with high level of apolipoprotein B. N Engl J Med 323:1289, 1990.
11. Budhoff MJ, Georgiou D, Brody A, et al. Ultrafast computed tomography as a diagnostic modality in the detection of coronary artery disease: a multicenter study. Circulation 93:898, 1996.
12. Bypass Angioplasty Revascularization Investigation (BARI) Investigators. Comparison of coronary bypass surgery with angioplasty in patients with multivessel disease. N Engl J Med 335:217, 1996.
13. Califf RM, Mark DB, Harrell FE, et al. Importance of clinical measures of ischemia in the prognosis of patients with documented coronary artery disease. J Am Coll Cardiol 11:20, 1988.
14. Califf RM, White HD, Van de Werf F, et al. One-year results from the Global Utilization of Streptokinase and TPA for Occluded Coronary Arteries (GUSTO-I) Trial. Circulation 94:1233, 1996.
15. Caracciolo EA, Davis KB, Sopko G, et al. Comparison of surgical and medical group survival in patients with left main coronary artery disease. Long-term CASS experience. Circulation 91:2325, 1995.
16. CASS Principal Investigators and Their Associates. Coronary artery surgery study (CASS): a randomized trial of coronary artery bypass surgery. Circulation 68:939, 1983.
17. CAVEAT Investigators, United States and Europe. The coronary angioplasty versus excisional atherectomy trial preliminary results. Circulation 86:(Suppl)I-374, 1992.
18. Coller BS, Anderson KM, Weisman HF. The anti–GPIIb-IIIa agents: fundamental and clinical aspects. Haemostasis 26 (Suppl 4):285, 1996.
19. Dagianti A, Penco M, Agati L, et al. Stress echocardiography: comparison of exercise, dipyridamole and dobutamine in detecting and predicting the extent of coronary artery disease. J Am Coll Cardiol 26:18, 1995.
20. Danahy DT, Aronow WS. Hemodynamics and antianginal effects of high-dose oral isosorbide dinitrate after chronic use. Circulation 56:205, 1977.
21. Daoud EG, Pitt A, Armstrong WF. Electrocardiographic response during dobutamine stress echocardiography. Am Heart J 129:672, 1995.
22. Detrano R, Gianrossi R, Mulvihill D, et al. Exercise-induced ST segment depression in the diagnosis of multivessel coronary disease: a meta analysis. J Am Coll Cardiol 14:1501, 1989.
23. Dilsizian V, Smeltzer WR, Freedman NMT, et al. Thallium reinjection after stress-redistribution imaging: does 24-hour delayed imaging after reinjection enhance detection of viable myocardium? Circulation 83:1247, 1991.
24. Elkayam U. Tolerance to organic nitrates: evidence, mechanisms, clinical relevance, and strategies for prevention. Ann Intern Med 114:667, 1991.
25. Ellstad MH, Wan MKC. Predictive implications of stress testing: follow-up of 2700 subjects after maximum treadmill stress testing. Circulation 51:363, 1975.
26. EPIC Investigators. Use of a monoclonal antibody directed against the platelet glycoprotein IIb/IIIa receptor in high-risk coronary angioplasty. N Engl J Med 330:956, 1994.
27. European Coronary Surgery Study Group. Prospective randomised study of coronary artery bypass surgery in stable angina pectoris: second interim report. Lancet 2:491, 1980.
28. Expert Panel on Detection, Evaluation, and Treatment of High Blood Cholesterol in Adults. Summary of the second report of the National Cholesterol Education Program (NCEP) Expert Panel on Detection, Evaluation, and Treatment of High Blood Cholesterol in Adults (Adult Treatment Panel II). JAMA 269:3015, 1993.
29. Gerstenblith G, Ouyang P, Achuff SC, et al. Nifedipine in unstable angina. A double-blind randomized trial. N Engl J Med 306:885, 1982.
30. Gibson RS, Watson DD, Craddock GB, et al. Prediction of cardiac events after uncomplicated myocardial infarction; a prospective study comparing predischarge exercise thallium-201 scintigraphy and coronary angiography. Circulation 68:321, 1983.
31. Gottlieb SO, Gottlieb SH, Achuff SC, et al. Silent ischemia on Holter monitoring predicts mortality in high-risk postinfarction patients. JAMA 259:1030, 1988.

*Bold print (general references) and bold numerals (specific references) denote published controlled clinical trials, meta-analyses, or consensus-based recommendations.

32. Gottlieb SO, Weisfeldt ML, Ouyang P, et al. Propranolol for unstable angina in the era of calcium antagonists: a double blind randomized trial. Circulation 70 (Suppl 2):48, 1984.

33. Gottlieb SO, Weisfeldt ML, Ouyang P, et al. Silent ischemia as a marker for early unfavorable outcomes in patients with unstable angina. N Engl J Med 314:1214, 1986.

34. Gullette ECD, Blumenthal JA, Babyak M, et al. Effects of mental stress on myocardial ischemia during daily life. JAMA 277:1521, 1997.

35. GUSTO Investigators. An international randomized trial comparing four thrombolytic strategies for acute myocardial infarction. N Engl J Med 329:673, 1993.

36. Hennekens CH, Buring JE, Sandercock P, et al. Aspirin and other antiplatelet agents in the secondary and primary prevention of cardiovascular disease. Circulation 80:749, 1989.

37. Hultgren HN, Peduzzi P, Detre K, et al. The 5 year effect of bypass surgery on relief of angina and exercise performance. Circulation 72(Suppl 5):79, 1985.

38. Hunink MGM, Goldman L, Tosteson ANA, et al. The recent decline in mortality from coronary heart disease, 1980–1990. The effect of secular trends in risk factors and treatment. JAMA 277:535, 1997.

39. Kannel WB, Feinleib M. Natural history of angina pectoris in the Framingham study: prognosis and survival. Am J Cardiol 29:154, 1972.

40. Kimeneij F, Laarman GJ, Odekerken D, et al. A randomized comparison of percutaneous transluminal coronary angioplasty by the radial, brachial and femoral approaches: The Access Study. J Am Coll Cardiol 29:1269, 1997.

41. Langer RD, Criqui MH, Reed DM. Lipoproteins and blood pressure as biological pathways for effect of moderate alcohol consumption on coronary heart disease. Circulation 85:910, 1992.

42. Lipid Research Clinics Program. The lipid research clinics coronary primary prevention trial results. II. The relationship of reduction in incidence of coronary heart disease to cholesterol lowering. JAMA 251:365, 1984.

43. Maddahi J: Myocardial perfusion imaging for the detection and evaluation of coronary artery disease. In: Skorton DJ, ed. Marcus cardiac imaging. A companion to Braunwald's heart disease. 2nd ed. Philadelphia: WB Saunders, 1996;971.

44. Mairesse GH, Marwick TH, Vanoverschelde J-LJ. How accurate is dobutamine stress echocardiography for detection of coronary artery disease? Comparison with two-dimensional echocardiography and technetium-99m methoxyl isobutyl isonitrile (MIBI) perfusion scintigraphy. J Am Coll Cardiol 24:920, 1994.

45. Mertes H, Saivada SG, Ryan T, et al. Symptoms, effects, and complications associated with dobutamine stress echocardiography: experience in 1118 patients. Circulation 88:15, 1993.

46. Mock MB, Ringqvist I, Fisher LD, et al. Survival of medically treated patients in the Coronary Artery Surgery Study (CASS) registry. Circulation 66:562, 1982.

47. Multiple Risk Factor Intervention Trial Research Group. Baseline rest electrocardiographic abnormalities, antihypertensive treatment, and mortality in the Multiple Risk Factor Intervention Trial. Am J Cardiol 55:1, 1985.

48. National Cholesterol Education Program. Second report of the expert panel on detection, evaluation, and treatment of high blood cholesterol in adults (Adult Treatment Panel II). Circulation 89:1329, 1994.

49. O'Keefe JH, Rutherford BD, McConohay DR, et al. Multivessel coronary angioplasty from 1980 to 1989: procedural results and long-term outcome. J Am Coll Cardiol 16:1097, 1990.

50. Packer M. Combined beta-adrenergic and calcium-entry blockade in angina pectoris. N Engl J Med 320:709, 1989.

51. Packer M, Nicod P, Khandheria BR, et al. Randomized, multicenter, double-blind, placebo-controlled evaluation of amlodipine inpatients with mild-to-moderate heart failure. J Am Coll Cardiol 17:274A, 1991.

52. Packer M, O'Connor CM, Ghali JK, et al. Effect of amlodipine on morbidity and mortality in severe chronic heart failure. N Engl J Med 335:1107, 1996.

53. Passamani E, Davis KB, Gillespie MJ, et al. A randomized trial of coronary artery bypass surgery. Survival of patients with a low ejection fraction. N Engl J Med 312:1665, 1985.

54. Pasternak RC, Thibault GT, Savoia M, et al. Chest pain with angiographically insignificant coronary arterial obstruction. Clinical presentation and long-term follow-up. Am J Med 68:813, 1980.

55. Patterson RE, Horowitz SF. Importance of epidemiology and biostatistics in deciding clinical strategies for using diagnostic tests: a simplified approach using examples from coronary artery disease. J Am Coll Cardiol 13:1653, 1989.

56. Pocock SJ, Henderson RA, Rickards AF, et al. Meta-analysis of randomized trials comparing angioplasty with bypass surgery. Lancet 346:1184, 1995.

57. Post Coronary Artery Bypass Graft Trial Investigators. The effect of aggressive lowering of low-density lipoprotein cholesterol levels and low-dose anticoagulation on obstructive changes in saphenous-vein coronary-artery bypass grafts. N Engl J Med 336:153, 1997.

58. Proudfit WL, Bruschke AVG, Sones FM. Clinical course of patients with normal or slightly or moderately abnormal coronary arteriograms: 10 year follow-up of 571 patients. Circulation 62:712, 1980.

59. Psaty BM, Smith NL, Siscovick DS, et al. Health outcomes associated with antihypertensive therapies used as first-line agents. A systematic review and meta-analysis. JAMA 277:739, 1997.

60. Quyyumi AA, Cannon RO, Panza JA. Endothelial dysfunction in patients with chest pain and normal coronary arteries. Circulation 86:1864, 1992.

61. Randin D, Vollenweider P, Tappy L, et al. Suppression of alcohol-induced hypertension by dexamethasone. N Engl J Med 332:1733, 1995.

62. Ridker PM, Manson JE, Gaziano JM, et al. Low-dose aspirin therapy for chronic stable angina. A randomized clinical trial. Ann Intern Med 114:835, 1991.

63. Rogers WJ, Bowlby LJ, Chandra NC, et al. Treatment of myocardial infarction in the United States (1990 to 1993). Observations from the National Registry of Myocardial Infarction. Circulation 90:2103, 1994.

64. Role of thrombolytic therapy and/or catheterization. The results of TIMI-III. Proceedings of the 65th American Heart Association Sessions. New Orleans, November 1992.

65. Ryan T, Vasey CG, Presti CF, et al. Exercise echocardiography: detection of coronary artery disease in patients with normal left ventricular wall motion at rest. J Am Coll Cardiol 11:993, 1988.

66. Sacks FM, Pfeffer MA, Moye LA, et al. The effect of pravastatin on coronary events after myocardial infarction in patients with average cholesterol levels. Cholesterol and Recurrent Events Trial Investigators. N Engl J Med 335:1001, 1996.

67. Scandinavian Simvastatin Survival Study Group. Baseline serum cholesterol and treatment effect in the Scandinavian Simvastatin Survival Study (4S). Lancet 345:1274, 1995.

68. Schaer DF, Buff IA, Katz RJ. Sustained antianginal efficacy of transdermal nitroglycerin patches using an overnight 10-hour nitrate-free interval. Am J Cardiol 61:46, 1988.

69. Secknus MA, Marwick TH. Evolution of dobutamine echocardiography protocol and indications: safety and side effects in 3,011 studies over 5 years. J Am Coll Cardiol 29:1234, 1997.

70. Shaw LJ, Eagle KA, Gersh BJ, Miller DD. Meta-analysis of intravenous dipyridamole–thallium-201 imaging (1985 to 1994) and dobutamine echocardiography (1991 to 1994) for risk stratification before vascular surgery. J Am Coll Cardiol 27:787, 1996.

71. Shepherd J, Cobbe SM, Ford I, et al. Prevention of coronary heart disease with pravastatin in men with hypercholesterolemia. West of Scotland Coronary Prevention Study Group. N Engl J Med 333:1301, 1995.

72. Takaro T, Hultgren HW, Lipton MJ, et al. The V.A. cooperative randomized study of surgery for coronary arterial occlusive disease. II. Subgroup with significant left main lesions. Circulation 54(Suppl 3):107, 1976.

73. Taylor GJ, Humphries JO, Mellits ED, et al. Predictors of clinical course, coronary anatomy and left ventricular function after

recovery from acute myocardial infarction. Circulation 62:960, 1980.

74. Thadani U, Fung HL, Darke AC, Parker JO. Oral isosorbide dinitrate in angina pectoris: comparison of duration of action and dose–response relation during acute and sustained therapy. Am J Cardiol 49:411, 1982.

75. Thompson SG, Kienast J, Pyke SDM, et al. Hemostatic factors and the risk of myocardial infarction or sudden death in patients with angina pectoris. N Engl J Med 332:635, 1995.

76. Treasure CB, Klein L, Weintraub WS, et al. Beneficial effects of cholesterol-lowering therapy on the coronary endothelium in patients with coronary artery disease. N Engl J Med 332:481, 1995.

77. Victor RG, Hansen J. Alcohol and blood pressure: a drink a day. N Engl J Med 332:1782, 1995.

78. Weiner DA, Ryan TJ, McCabe CH, et al. Exercise stress testing. Correlations among history of angina, ST-segment response and prevalence of coronary-artery disease in the coronary surgery study (CASS). N Engl J Med 301:230, 1979.

79. Wenger NK. Coronary heart disease in women: clinical syndromes, prognosis, and diagnostic testing. Cardiovasc Clin 19:173, 1989.

C H A P T E R 58

Postmyocardial Infarction Care, Cardiac Rehabilitation, and Physical Conditioning

PETER V. VAITKEVICIUS, MD
KERRY J. STEWART, EDD

EPIDEMIOLOGY OF MYOCARDIAL INFARCTION

Overview

Cardiovascular disease remains the major cause of mortality in the United States. In 1994, coronary artery disease (CAD), hypertension, and stroke accounted for more than 950,000 deaths, or 42% of all deaths (34). About half of these deaths were caused by myocardial infarction (MI). Nearly three-quarters of all deaths from CAD occur outside the hospital. From 1984 to 1994, the crude death rate from all forms of cardiovascular disease declined by 22.4% and the death rate from MI declined by 28.6%. This reduction is the result of changes in risk factor detection, hospital and ambulatory care of patients, and lifestyle. The absolute number of deaths from cardiovascular disease actually increased in 1993, primarily because of the rise in the total population of older people. In both older and younger patients, some mortality after MI could probably be prevented with more consistent use of interventions known to benefit patients after MI, the focus of this chapter (18,31,32,50,84).

Patients who survive an acute MI are two to nine times more likely to suffer recurring illness or death from CAD. There are approximately 7 million survivors of MI in the United States at any given time (5). Two of every three MI survivors do not make a complete recovery but still have a good long-term prognosis. The longitudinal care of the patient who has survived an MI is usually the responsibility of the patient's personal physician.

Demographic Subgroups

Five percent of MIs occur in patients less than 40 years of age, and 45% of people who have MIs are under age 65. Strikingly, approximately 85% of deaths from MI occur in patients over 65 (34).

It is estimated that in the United States, 1 man in 5 will have an MI before age 60 and that one in 10 to 15 men in this age group will die prematurely of atherosclerotic heart disease. These risks are two to three times lower in age-matched women under the age of 65; they are only slightly lower in women over 65 (34,40,68). Death rates from CAD are highest among African-American men and women. In 1993, age-adjusted death rates per 100,000 population were 139.3 for African-American men versus 133.0 for white men (4.7% higher) and 85.7 for African-American women versus 63.8 for white women (34.3% higher).

Data from the Cardiovascular Health Study show that the *prevalence of MI* in older men (i.e., the history of having had MI) ranges from 18% for ages 65 to 69 to 30% for ages 80 to 84 (34). The prevalence of MI in women ranges from 9.5% for ages 65 to 69 to 17.9% for ages 85 and greater. These findings appear to be related to the higher incidence and prevalence of CAD throughout the adult years in men.

For *patients hospitalized with an acute MI,* women, particularly African-American women, have higher case mortality than men both during hospitalization and in the 48 months after discharge (77). The higher mortality in women admitted for acute MI has been found in all age groups irrespective of type of treatment (8).

PROGNOSIS OF PATIENTS DISCHARGED FROM CORONARY CARE UNITS

Patients discharged after hospitalization in a coronary care unit (CCU) may be divided into three broad categories: those who have had a confirmed MI, those who have had unstable angina, and those who have had cardiac arrest without a confirmed MI. Patients in each of these categories have differing prognoses.

Survivors of Myocardial Infarction

Mortality

The in-hospital mortality for acute MI is now less than 10%. The overall first-year mortality for hospital survivors of an MI is approximately 5 to 10%. Thereafter, the annual mortality remains between 3 and 5% for the next 15 years. These figures are the same for patients surviving *transmural MIs* or *subendocardial MIs* (SEMIs), despite the apparent smaller infarct size, less occlusion of the infarct-related artery, and better overall left ventricular ejection fraction (LVEF) after SEMI. This seeming paradox may be related to the greater persistence of jeopardized myocardium following SEMI (27). Most of the deaths in the first year occur during the 3 months after discharge, and they occur chiefly in patients with one or more of the high-risk characteristics listed in Table 58.1.

The *classification of acute MI developed by Killip* according to the presence and severity of congestive heart failure (CHF) on admission to the hospital is one of the most useful prognostic indices. Class I patients have no evidence of CHF on admission, class II patients have mild CHF, class III patients present with pulmonary edema, and class IV patients have cardiogenic

---

Table 58.1. Characteristics Associated with Increased Mortality After Discharge of Patients Who Have Had MI

Admission Characteristics
History of a previous MI
CHF (chest x-ray or Killip classification)
History of hypertension
Extent of LV ischemia (radionuclide scintigraphy, cardiac enzymes)

Characteristics at Discharge
Early (within 10 days) post-MI angina, with transient ST–T changes[a]
Ejection fraction ≤40% (radionuclide ventriculography, arteriography)
Complex ventricular arrhythmia[b] (Holter monitor)
Left main proximal, left anterior descending, or three-vessel CAD (arteriography)
Positive limited early post-MI ECG stress test (within 2–3 weeks after MI)
Ventricular aneurysm developing in acute stage of MI

Characteristics Following Discharge
ECG abnormalities, especially ischemic ST-segment depression, ≥1 month after MI
Decreased heart rate variability
Cigarette smoking

[a]Mortality risk highest when ECG shows ischemia at a distance (i.e., transient ischemic ST changes in myocardial location that is different from the location of the patient's MI).
[b]Multifocal premature ventricular contractions (PVCs), runs of two or more sequential ectopic ventricular beats, or PVCs with R on T pattern.

shock. Figure 58.1 shows the strikingly different survival rates among patients in these four classes (60). Recently, there has been improvement in survival rates in each of the Killip classes, but the classification remains a valid index of morbidity and mortality after MI.

The clinical factors predictive of an increased mortality after hospital discharge are listed in Table 58.1. Patients with the greatest risk of mortality during the first year following an MI have one or more of the following: a previous MI; development of early (within 10 days) post-MI angina accompanied by transient ST-segment or T-wave changes; an ejection fraction of 40% or less; late hospital phase (predischarge) complex ventricular arrhythmia; proximal left main, left anterior descending, or three-vessel coronary artery disease; a positive stress test at low work load within a few weeks after MI; presence of ischemic ST changes on resting electrocardiogram (ECG) taken 1 month or longer after MI; and lack of heart rate variability (the amount of heart rate fluctuation around the mean heart rate) (80). Left ventricular (LV) aneurysm developing within 2 days of the acute MI also brings a high risk of death during the first year, independent of LV function (47). In addition to these cardiac complications, post-MI depression is strongly associated with post-MI mortality (22).

In patients who are clinically stable 1 to 6 months after hospitalization for an acute MI or unstable angina, the presence of ischemic ST-segment depression in the resting ECG is the strongest predictor of morbidity and mortality over the ensuing 3 years. Posthospitalization stress testing is predictive of future coronary events in stable patients only when ischemia (1 mm or larger ST-segment depression on exercise ECG) or a reversible perfusion defect (on thallium exercise test) is present at a low work load (5 metabolic equivalents [METs] or less) or when there is evidence of exercise-induced LV dysfunction (LV cavity dilation and/or increased thallium uptake by the lung during exercise) (49). Each of these high-risk subsets has made up less than 3% of study populations.

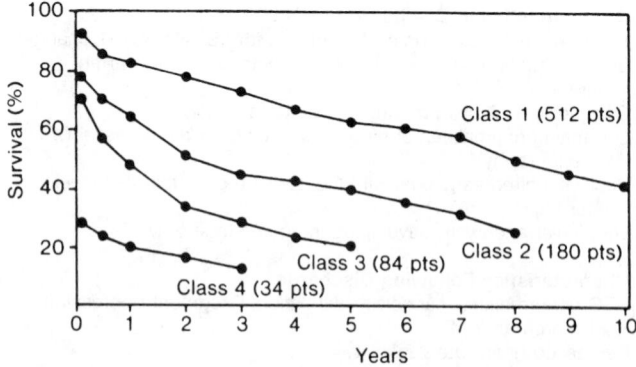

Figure 58.1. Survival after acute MI based on Killip classification (810 patients admitted to the Duke Medical Center Coronary Care Unit from 1967 to 1978). (From Rosati RA, Harris PJ. Acute myocardial infarction. In: Fries J, Ehrlich GE, eds. Prognosis: contemporary outcomes of disease. Bowie, MD: Charles Press, 1981;275–279.)

Morbidity

Studies conducted in the 1970s showed that postinfarction angina occurs during the year after an MI in approximately 75% of patients who had angina before their MI and in approximately 50% of those who did not have it before their MI (82). In patients who are free of angina or other cardiac symptoms in the hospital, a predischarge exercise stress test may be performed safely. Patients who can exercise to 5 to 6 METs or to 70 to 80% of the age-predicted maximal heart rate without an abnormal ECG or blood pressure response have a 1-year mortality of 1 to 2% (44). Exercise testing increases the ability to predict whether a patient will develop angina. Angina during the years after an MI occurs in 86% of patients with positive stress tests (96% of patients with both a positive early post-MI stress test and a previous history of angina) and in 36% of those with negative stress tests (only in 26% of patients with both a negative stress test and no previous history of angina) (82). In addition, patients with a post-MI symptom limited stress test showing early ischemic ST-segment changes (1 mm or more exercise-induced ST-segment depression) or limited work capacity (5 METs or less) have two or more times the risk of recurrent MI and of death over the ensuing year (75). As described below ("Risk Stratification Before Hospital Discharge"), patients with abnormal predischarge stress tests are often catheterized to decide on the advisability of revascularization.

Postinfarction medical complications other than angina include CHF, life-threatening arrhythmias and sudden death, intracavity thrombi with stroke and systemic emboli, and post-MI syndrome (Dressler's syndrome).

The psychologic and social sequelae during the year after an MI depend on both the severity of the patient's MI and the patient's premorbid psychosocial situation. After an MI, 10 to 20% of patients are unable to return to their former occupational and recreational activities. Fortunately, the remaining 80 to 90% of patients are able to do so within 2 to 6 months. Persistent denial, anxiety, depression, and dependency after an MI are associated with a decrease in the rate of return to work and usual social activities, regardless of the patient's physiologic status. Major depression occurs in 15 to 20% of patients and there is evidence that it is associated with a three- to fourfold increased cardiovascular mortality at 6 months (6,22).

Patients with Unstable Angina

Unstable angina is defined as pain caused by cardiac ischemia that is occurring more frequently, is being provoked by less effort, is occurring at rest, or is being relieved less readily by nitroglycerin. Other characteristics are described in Chapter 57.

Patients discharged from the CCU with the diagnosis of unstable angina have 1-year morbidity and mortality rates that may exceed those of patients discharged with the diagnosis of a completed MI. Studies show that the resting ECG and the response to exercise stress testing are especially helpful in predicting future events in patients who are clinically stable after admission for unstable angina (49). The lack of ischemic ST-segment changes during exercise testing helps to identify patients at lower risk (79).

In an individual patient with unstable angina, a more precise prognosis can be given by defining the coronary anatomy by *catheterization.* In studies of patients with unstable angina, coronary catheterization has shown that left main coronary artery disease is more common in patients discharged with the diagnosis of unstable angina than in those discharged with the diagnosis of a completed MI (15 versus 5%, respectively). Another 10% have diffuse coronary artery disease, 10% have normal coronary arteries and are presumed to have coronary artery spasm or small vessel disease as the cause of their chest pain, and the remaining 65% are equally divided among single, double, and triple coronary vessel disease (55). This information is clinically important because of the demonstrated superiority of surgical over medical treatment of left main coronary artery disease. The prognoses associated with each of the above patterns and the management of unstable angina are described in Chapter 57.

Survivors of Cardiac Arrest Who Have Not Had a Myocardial Infarction

The first-year mortality rate of survivors of out-of-hospital cardiac arrest who have not had an MI is approximately three times the mortality rate of survivors of out-of-hospital cardiac arrest who subsequently are shown to have completed an MI. In a study of more than 200 survivors of out-of-hospital cardiac arrest followed for over 4 years, the rate of recurrence of ventricular fibrillation or sudden death in patients without an acute MI was 31%, compared with 5% for out-of-hospital survivors of cardiac arrest who subsequently evolved ECG changes of acute MI. The median time to recurrent circulatory arrest was 20 weeks. More than 70% of the episodes of ventricular fibrillation were unexpected, occurred during sleep or during the usual activities of daily living (64).

Because the survivors of ventricular fibrillation not associated with an MI are a highly unstable group of patients, they require aggressive and highly individualized treatment. The multiplicity of recent advances in electrophysiology, antiarrhythmics, automatic implantable defibrillators, and the many innovative surgical approaches to medically intractable but symptomatic ventricular dysrhythmias dictate prompt referral of such high-risk patients to a consulting cardiologist.

RISK STRATIFICATION BEFORE HOSPITAL DISCHARGE

In 1997, the American College of Physicians (ACP) published the recommendations for in-hospital risk stratification of MI patients that are summarized in Figures 58.2 and 58.3 (see "General References"). This three-phase scheme delineates decision making that is supported by outcome data from clinical trials. It was

published to guide the care of MI patients before they are discharged from the hospital. It draws on a mix of *baseline characteristics and findings from continuous reevaluation of the patient.* Depending on clinical findings, a patient may have undergone thrombolysis, revascularization, or neither in the acute and nonacute phase of risk stratification. In the *predischarge evaluation,* patients at intermediate or low risk (60 to 70% of MI patients) should have assessment of their LV function and noninvasive stress testing. Often, those patients can be discharged after stays as short as 4 to 5 days. The postdischarge prognosis of MI patients and their appropriate management depends on the predischarge evaluation, postdischarge reevaluations, and the rehabilitation and medical approaches described in this chapter.

REHABILITATION AND MANAGEMENT AFTER MYOCARDIAL INFARCTION

Most patients discharged after MI can expect to return to most of their usual activities within 6 weeks to 4 months. For a smaller number of patients, complications of their MI make this outcome impossible. In either situation, an organized plan for care should be followed (Table 58.2). This plan should include the education of the patient and the patient's family. Because of shorter hospital stays, much of the patient education previously included in inpatient cardiac rehabilitation is now conducted in outpatient programs.

Patient Education

Most hospitals initiate education about MI when the patient is clinically stable. The educational program is often the responsibility of a cardiac rehabilitation professional. Patient education should cover the nature of coronary heart disease, cardiac symptoms, cardiac drugs, modification of major risk factors (reducing smoking, hypertension, and hyperlipidemia; promoting exercise), and guidelines for resumption of physical activities (including sexual activity) and return to work. It should be emphasized that MI is a manifestation of a disease process that has been going on for many years. Many patients attribute their MI to what they were doing at the moment it actually occurred. Patients must understand that the MI would have occurred regardless of what they were doing that particular day and that the likelihood of a recurrence may best be diminished by following prescribed medical therapy and making lifestyle changes. These matters may be discussed in a general sense, usually in a group setting.

Individualized information should be provided in a *predischarge conference* at which the patient and the patient's family members are encouraged to ask questions. The conference should include review of any adverse prognostic features identified before discharge (Table 58.1); the medications prescribed at discharge; discussion of specific plans for cardiac rehabilitation, diet, and smoking modification; a chance for ventilation about emotional stress-laden issues; and realistic

Figure 58.2. Flow diagram of risk stratification after myocardial infarction. *CCU,* Coronary care unit; *CHF,* congestive heart failure; *LBBB,* left bundle branch block; *MI,* myocardial infarction; *PTCA,* percutaneous transluminal coronary angioplasty; *ST,* ST segment. (From Clinical Guidelines Parts I and II. Guidelines for risk stratification after myocardial infarction [American College of Physicians]. Ann Intern Med 126:556, 561, 1997.)

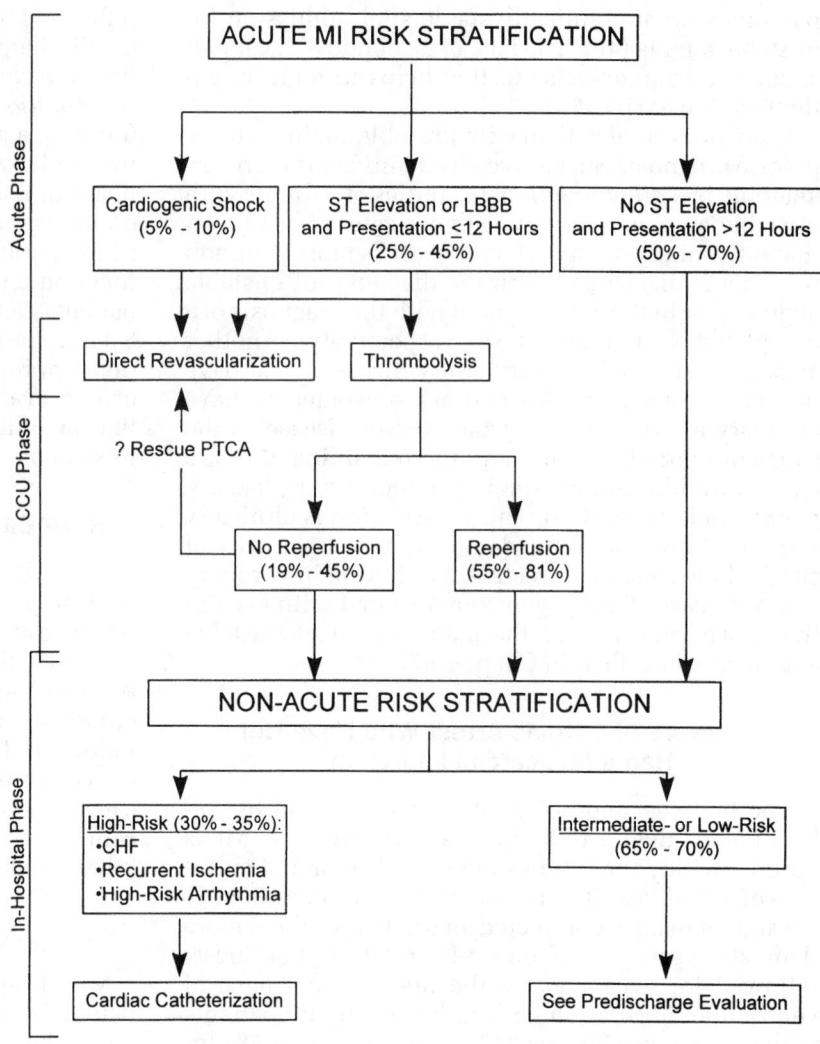

appraisal of expectations of return to work. Because of the high frequency of postinfarction angina, it is especially important to describe this symptom to patients who have never had it and to point out to all patients that it may occur with the increased activity recommended for the coming weeks. Every patient should be given sublingual nitroglycerin, and the correct use of this drug should be reviewed.

Because patients may not retain the information they hear in the hospital, it is important to provide this information in writing and to assess and reinforce patient understanding of it after discharge. The patient education booklet *After a Heart Attack* (available without charge from local chapters of the American Heart Association) gives a useful general account of the disease process, prognosis, coronary risk factors, and rehabilitation process.

Many hospitals have developed *group classes for survivors of MIs and their spouses.* Typically, patients and their spouses are invited to participate in a number of weekly meetings during the first or second month after discharge. Sessions are usually led by a cardiac rehabilitation professional such as a nurse, social

worker, or cardiologist, with the objective of having participants raise questions about the recovery period to provide mutual support by sharing experiences with each other. Additional resources available in many communities are patient-run heart clubs and supervised physical conditioning programs (see "Physical Conditioning," below). The American Association of Cardiovascular and Pulmonary Rehabilitation (7611 Elmwood Ave., Suite 201, Middleton, WI 33562; telephone 608-831-6989; http://www.aacvpr.org) publishes a national directory of cardiac rehabilitation programs and is a good source of professional and patient materials including *Guidelines for Cardiac Rehabilitation* (see "General References"). There are also several nationally distributed newsletters for patients with coronary artery disease (e.g., *The Coronary Club Bulletin,* 9500 Euclid Ave., Cleveland, OH 44195; telephone 216-444-3690). In recent years, the *world wide web* has offered a wealth of patient information dealing with heart disease prevention and rehabilitation. Some examples include Johns Hopkins Bayview Medical Center (http://www.jhbmc.jhu.edu/cardiology/cardiology.html), the American Heart Association (http://www.amhrt.org), Heart Information Network (http://www.heartinfo.org), and Franklin Institute (http://www.fi.edu/biosci/heart.html). Patients can also be directed to support groups such as The Mended Hearts (http://www.mendedhearts.org). Many of these sites provide links to other sources of patient information, support, and online newsletters.

Postdischarge Appointments

In general, each patient who has had an MI should be encouraged to telephone his or her physician at least once during the first week at home, to discuss any questions that arise, and an office visit should be scheduled within 2 to 3 weeks. Before this visit, it is important to review the patient's hospital summary to determine whether adverse prognostic features were present (Table 58.1) and to identify the medications prescribed at discharge. The visit should be divided between an assessment of the patient's progress in rehabilitation (physical activity level, diet and smoking modifications, emotional status, understanding of the overall plan of care, expectation about return to work) and an assessment of the patient's medical status (manifestations of ischemia and heart failure, blood pressure status, and review of current medica-

tions). Two or more additional office visits, similar to the first visit, should be scheduled during the 3 months after an MI, and the patient should be encouraged to telephone at any time about symptoms or questions.

Risk Stratification at 3 to 6 Weeks

About 3 to 6 weeks after MI, a *maximal exercise stress test* should be considered, as this can provide helpful therapeutic and prognostic information regarding the patient's disease. Table 58.3 summarizes the criteria and recommendations of the American College of Physicians, based on stratification into low-risk and moderate-risk findings in this stress test. The stress test is also used to assess functional capacity and is very helpful in guiding the return to work. About 3 months, an ECG should be obtained; this will be the patient's new baseline ECG.

Activity Schedule

Table 58.4 contains a practical summary (for use by the patient) of symptom recognition and a schedule of progressive physical activities for the first 2 months after MI. Table 58.5 lists a broad array of activities corresponding to the recommended energy levels dur-

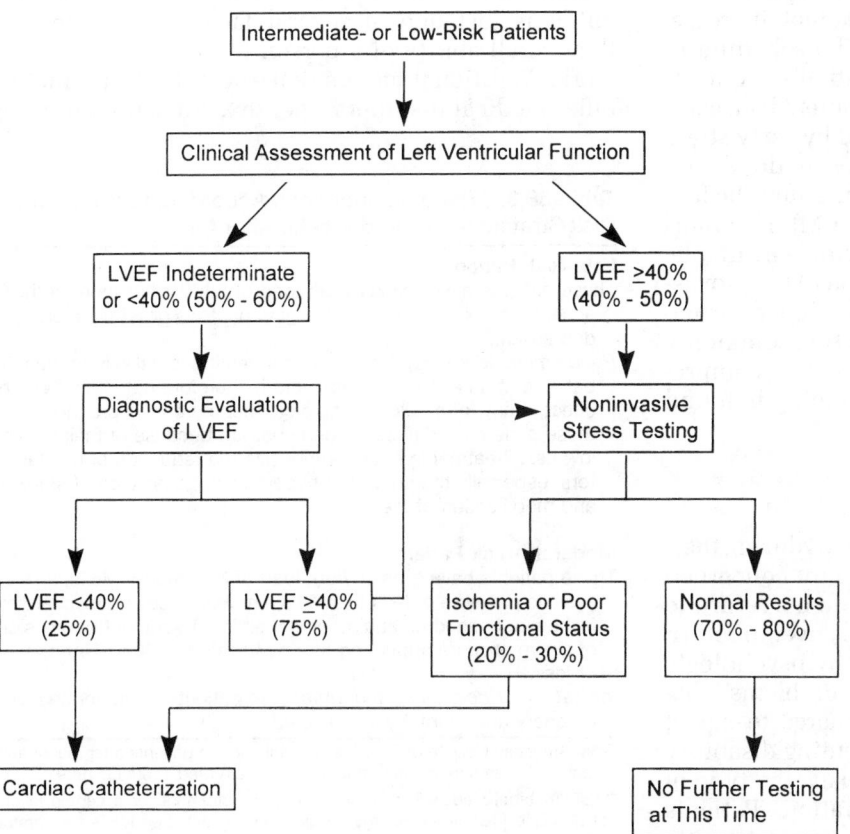

Figure 58.3. Flow diagram for predischarge risk stratification after myocardial infarction. *LVEF,* Left ventricular ejection fraction. (From Clinical Guidelines Parts I and II. Guidelines for risk stratification after myocardial infarction [American College of Physicians]. Ann Intern Med 126:556, 561, 1997.)

Table 58.2. Plan of Care for MI Survivors After Hospital Discharge

Patient Education (Objectives for all Patients)[a]
Understands disease process (damage to the heart that heals in a few months, leaves a scar)
Understands likely prognosis
Understands and follows progressive activity schedule[b]
Understands approximate timetable for return to work[b]
Understands importance of controlling major risk factors (smoking, hypercholesterolemia, hypertension) and takes action to control them
Knows how to recognize principal cardiac symptoms (angina, tachycardia, heart failure, hypotension) and understands how to use sublingual nitroglycerin
Participates in group classes after discharge[c]
Gets answers to questions specific to his or her lifestyle

Medical Management
All patients
    Review in-hospital course for prognosis characteristics (see Table 58.1) and for medications prescribed at discharge
    Assess and reinforce above patient education
    Check periodically for complications of infarction (see Table 58.6)
    Check for behavior–psychiatric complications
    Check ECG 2–3 months after discharge
Selected patients
    β-Blocker, ACE inhibitor, calcium antagonist, or aspirin treatment[d]
    Referral for physical conditioning[d]

[a]Essential to include the patient's spouse in all aspects of education.
[b]Serial exercise stress tests may be used to plan progressive activity (see text).
[c]If programs are available in the community.
[d]See text for details.

ing and after the recuperation period. Resumption of activities with different energy requirements should be gradual; in particular, the duration of certain activities should be brief at first, with gradual increase, according to how the patient feels. The schedule in Table 58.4 can be given to most patients. A more aggressive plan can be tailored for the patient if an early physical conditioning program, guided by early stress testing, is available. Similarly, stress test–guided conditioning can also be planned for patients after the first 1 to 2 weeks of convalescence from an MI. Programs that enroll patients soon after MI are widely available. In addition to the American Association of Cardiovascular and Pulmonary Rehabilitation mentioned earlier, affiliates of the American Heart Association commonly maintain lists of local exercise programs. A comprehensive discussion of exercise conditioning is found below (see "Physical Conditioning").

Return to Work

Because most patients have their first MI during their active working years, they are commonly concerned about returning to work. Patients who do not return to work within 6 months of MI are unlikely ever to return to work (62), and this is often caused by psychologic not physical factors (see "Psychologic Problems," below). Telling the patient, soon after discharge, to expect to return to work is important in preventing disability caused by psychologic factors. Obviously, the type of work is also an important consideration. Patients whose occupations involve mental stress and hectic

schedules should be advised to return to work on a part-time basis at first, leaving plenty of time for rest and relaxation. For patients whose work involves significant physical exertion, the timing of return to work can be based on the information in Tables 58.4 and 58.5 and guided by the results of exercise stress testing and monitored responses during a supervised rehabilitation program. From Table 58.5, it is evident that most occupations require an energy level of 6 METs or less. Occupational activities classified as heavy work, such as digging ditches, require energy expenditure of 7 METs or more. Certain activities may produce an increased work load on the heart because of psychologic stress (e.g., driving a vehicle) or because they entail significant isometric exercise (e.g., carpentry, plumbing, shoveling, operating pneumatic tools, or carrying objects heavier than 30 lb).

Patients with MIs complicated by poorly controlled angina, CHF, or arrhythmias should be evaluated in conjunction with a consulting cardiologist (see "Medical Complications," below) before a plan for returning to work and other activities is recommended. Some of these patients qualify for *permanent medical disability* (see criteria for disability caused by coronary artery disease, Chapter 9, Table 9.1) or for job retraining through vocational rehabilitation. The *fundamental difference between impairment and disability* caused by coronary artery disease was underscored in the report of the 1989 Bethesda Conference on Insurability and Employability of the Patient with Ischemic Heart Disease (12). Impairment is a medically defined disorder and is an important component of disability, but it is just one of several factors that determine the overall ability of a person to perform meaningful work. Additional factors that affect disability include other medical disorders, age, sex, education, training,

Table 58.3. Recommendations According to Stress Test Risk Stratification 3 to 6 Weeks After MI

Low-Risk Patients
These patients have a peak work load of 5 METs[a] or more in the absence of exercise-induced angina pectoris or ST-segment depression.
Recommendations: Further diagnostic testing is unlikely to identify patients at an even lower risk, and is therefore not indicated. The effect, if any, of medical or surgical therapy on the prognosis of these patients is difficult to demonstrate because of their very low risk. Treatment should emphasize the reduction of risk factors, especially the control of hypertension, cessation of smoking, and modification of diet.

Moderate-Risk Patients
These patients have a peak work load of less than 5 METs, a peak systolic pressure of less than 110 mm Hg, or severe myocardial ischemia, defined as angina or ischemic ST-segment depression of 2 mm or more appearing at a heart rate of 130 to 140 bpm or less.
Indication for coronary arteriography: In patients at moderate risk, coronary arteriography is indicated.

From American College of Physicians. Evaluation of patients after recent acute myocardial infarction (position paper). Ann Intern Med 110:485, 1989.
[a]MET (metabolic equivalent) is the energy requirement for a certain level of activity. One MET is the energy requirement at rest. See METs for common activities in Table 58.5.

Table 58.4.   Activity Schedule and Symptom Recognition for Patients Convalescing from MI[a]

General Points

All activities, including sitting and lying down, require energy. The amount of energy required to perform a specific activity is expressed as METs. One MET is your resting energy requirement. As activities become more strenuous, the amount of energy required (METs) also increases, as does the work load imposed on your heart.

The schedule recommended in this program is based on the number of METs needed for various activities. Some specific recommendations are given for each of the first 3 months following your return to home. Table 58.5 gives the energy requirements for a wide variety of additional activities. If the table omits your favorite activities, ask your doctor about them.

Warnings: Generally the following activities impose an added strain on your heart and should be avoided, especially during the first 3 months after a heart attack:

Taking very hot or cold showers or baths
Holding your breath while exercising, lifting, or straining
Working in a bent or stooped position or with arms held above your head
Doing work that requires continuous tensing of your muscles
Working or exercising during very hot, cold, humid, or windy weather (in bad weather, plan your regular exercise at a nearby shopping mall)
Working or exercising during the first hour after a meal or after consuming alcohol
Consuming excessive amounts of alcohol (e.g., more than 1–2 ounces of whiskey, 2–3 beers, 1–2 glasses of wine per day)
Walking or exercising on a hill or an inclined surface
Engaging in any activity that creates emotional stress or worry for you

Recommended Activity Schedule[b]

First Month (1–3 METs)

From discharge to 1 week

Regular exercise: Walk 5 minutes at a leisurely pace once a day on a level surface.

Some specific advice: This week, primarily get used to being at home. Occupy yourself with sit-down activities such as watching television, playing cards, sewing, painting, or sketching. Avoid lifting objects heavier than 5 lb or doing activities that require reaching above your head. You may go up and down the stairs. However, take your time and limit the number of times you need to climb them. Do all of the things you were doing in the hospital. Get up and get dressed each day. You may be surprised at how tired and weak you feel. This is natural. Be sure to take rest periods when you need them, particularly after meals and before you exercise or climb the stairs.

Week 2

Regular exercise: Walk 5 minutes at a leisurely pace twice a day.

Some specific advise: Continue all of your previous activities and add others, such as taking rides in the car (however, no driving yet), cooking a meal, washing clothes in a machine (have someone else remove them), making your bed, attending a relaxing movie, going out to dinner, going shopping with your family (let others lift things from the shelves to the basket and carry the groceries), shooting pool, playing shuffleboard, throwing a softball underhand, playing a piano or organ.

Weeks 3 and 4

Regular exercise: Advance gradually to walking 10 minutes at a leisurely pace twice a day.

Some specific advice: Continue your previous activities and others, such as going to church, sweeping floors, polishing furniture, driving the car (beginning with short drives, avoiding heavy traffic).

Second Month (3–5 METs)

Regular physical exercise: Progressively increase leisurely walking from 15 minutes once a day at a slightly faster pace to 30 minutes once or twice a day.

Some specific advice: Table 58.5 lists the approximate energy requirements of each activity. You may gradually increase your activities by adding additional activities and spending more time at them; consult Table 58.5 for activities requiring 5 METs or less (or more).

Recognizing Heart Symptoms

Your heart will give you warning signs if it is not ready for increased activity. Here are some guidelines to use:

Pulse: Locate your pulse and count the number of times it beats for 15 seconds and multiply that number by 4. This is your heart rate for 1 minute. Take your pulse before you begin your walk or any new activity and at the end of the activity. Contact your doctor before resuming exercise if

There is an increase of 20 heartbeats or more per minute in postexercise pulse over preexercise pulse
Your heart rate exceeds 120/min[c]
You detect abnormal heart action: pulse becoming irregular, fluttering or jumping in chest or throat, very slow pulse rate, sudden burst of rapid heartbeats

Chest pain: Contact your doctor before resuming exercise if you experience pain or pressure in the chest, arm, or throat precipitated by exercise or following exercise. Remember to take your nitroglycerine and rest if you do experience pain.

Dizziness: Contact your doctor before resuming exercise if you become dizzy, light-headed, or faint during exercise.

Breathing difficulty: Contact your doctor before resuming exercise if you become short of breath during or after a new exercise, or if you awaken from sleep short of breath.

[a]Information in Table 58.5 should be given to patients who receive the instructions in this table.
[b]Pace of these activities may be scaled up or down by results of early post-MI stress test when available.
[c]These figures may be markedly modified by results of early stress test or medication.

and psychosocial support. The main points in the report state that most MI patients can return to work; prognosis can be estimated by clinical examination and noninvasive studies that evaluate LV function (echocardiogram), myocardial jeopardy (thallium–stress test), and electrical instability (Holter); cardiac catheterization is not routinely required; special assessment may be needed for jobs requiring sudden or sustained high effort or heat exposure (e.g., firefighters) or for those in which sudden disability may endanger others (e.g., airline pilots); a trial period of progressively increasing part-time work may be necessary

Table 58.5.   Energy Requirements of Certain Activities

Activity Level	Self-Care or Home	Occupational	Recreational	Physical Conditioning
Very light (≤3 METs)	Washing, shaving, dressing Desk work, writing, washing dishes Driving car[a]	Sitting (clerical, assembling) Standing (store clerk, bartender) Driving truck[a] Crane operator[a]	Shuffleboard Horseshoes Bait casting Billiards Archery[a] Golf (cart)	Walking (level, at 2 mph) Stationary bike (very low resistance) Very light calisthenics
Light to moderate (3–5 METs)	Cleaning windows Raking leaves Weeding Power lawn mowing Waxing floors (slowly) Painting Carrying objects 15–30 lb[b]	Stocking shelves (light objects)[b] Light welding Light carpentry[b] Machine assembly Auto repair Paper hanging[b]	Dancing Golf (walking) Sailing Horseback riding Volleyball Tennis (doubles) Sexual intercourse[a] (see details in the text)	Walking (3–4 mph) Level bicycling (6–8 mph) Light calisthenics
Moderate (5–7 METs)	Easy digging in garden Level hand lawn mowing Climbing stairs (slowly) Carrying objects 30–60 lb[b]	Carpentry (exterior home building)[b] Shoveling dirt[b] Pneumatic tools[b]	Badminton (competitive) Tennis (singles) Snow skiing (downhill) Light backpacking Basketball Football Skating (ice and roller) Horseback riding (gallop)	Swimming (breast stroke)
Heavy (7–9 METs)	Sawing wood[b] Heavy shoveling[b] Climbing stairs (moderate speed) Carrying objects 60–90 lb[b]	Tending furnace[b] Digging ditches[b] Pick and shovel[b]	Canoeing[b] Mountain climbing[b] Fencing Paddleball Touch football	Jogging (5 mph) Swimming (crawl stroke) Rowing machine Heavy calisthenics Bicycling (12 mph)
Very heavy (9 METs)	Carrying loads upstairs[b] Carrying objects 90 lb or more Climbing stairs (quickly) Shoveling heavy snow[b] Shoveling for 10 min (16 lb)	Lumber jack[b] Heavy laborer[b]	Handball Squash Ski touring over hills[b] Vigorous basketball	Running (6 mph) Bicycling (13 mph or steep hill) Rope jumping

From Haskell WL. Design and implementation of cardiac conditioning programs. In: Hellerstein HK, ed. Rehabilitation of the coronary patient. New York: John Wiley & Sons, 1978; 203.

[a]May cause added psychologic stress that will increase load on the heart.

[b]May produce disproportionate myocardial demands because of use of arms or isometric exercise. See further discussion regarding isometric (resistive) exercise in physical conditioning section of this chapter.

for smooth transition from total disability to full-time work; and maximal functional capacity should be evaluated as soon as stability is present, usually 3 to 5 weeks after uncomplicated MI, 7 weeks after coronary bypass surgery, and 1 week after coronary angioplasty.

Although cardiac rehabilitation, including education, counseling, and behavioral intervention has many benefits, it has not been shown to alter the rates of return to work. This was the conclusion of the 1995 *Cardiac Rehabilitation Guidelines* of the Agency for Health Care Policy and Research (see "General References"). The expert panel reported that although education and counseling may improve a patient's potential for return to work, many other factors play a role in return to work, including willingness of the employer to rehire the patient, the patient's level of job satisfaction, economic incentives, and perceived stress of the job.

Sexual Activity

It is safe for patients who are symptom free during usual activities of daily living to resume sexual intercourse within 4 to 6 weeks of their MI. Available data

suggest that the energy requirement approximates 3 METs during foreplay and afterplay and 5 METs at climax (35). These are equivalent to the oxygen demands of a brisk walk around the block or climbing one flight of stairs. In a study of patients after MI, coitus accounted for less than 1% of sudden deaths. These usually occurred during extramarital affairs in which the men were considerably older than their companions and often were inebriated at the time of intercourse (78).

When counseling patients about resumption of sexual activity, one should *give specific advice* and encourage questions. The pamphlet *Sex and Heart Disease,* available from the American Heart Association, is a helpful adjunct to counseling. Frequency of sexual intercourse can be similar to the frequency before the patient's MI. Sexual foreplay without completion of intercourse can be recommended to patients who wish to resume sex cautiously. In general, sexual activity can be resumed in the position that was most gratifying before the MI; however, patients should avoid positions in which they support their weight on their arms because this requires sustained isometric type of work (see "Physical Conditioning," below) and may put extra stress on the heart. Sexual activity should be engaged in when both partners are relaxed. It is best to abstain from intercourse for 2 or 3 hours after eating a large meal because eating increases the work of the heart.

Inability to return to a previous pattern of sexual activity may be caused by angina (precipitated by intercourse), new medications, or psychologic stress associated with the recent MI. If an otherwise stable patient develops angina during intercourse, sublingual nitroglycerin can be taken just before sexual activity. The evaluation and management of drug-induced and psychologic sexual dysfunction, both of which may occur after MI, are discussed in Chapter 18.

Psychologic Problems

It is normal for patients to experience *symptoms of anxiety and depression* during the first few weeks after discharge from the hospital. Some of these symptoms are caused by misconceptions about the nature and prognosis of MI, and they respond to clarification of the facts. Most patients do well when encouraged to express their concerns and reassured that their response is normal. A small supply of a minor tranquilizer (see Chapter 13) or a short-acting hypnotic (see Chapter 85) can be prescribed to be used if needed. As noted earlier (under "Patient Education"), participation in group classes and group exercise programs can also help patients adjust to changes in their lives after MI.

Another common psychologic complication of MI is an *inappropriate fear of physical activity of any kind* (i.e., the so-called "cardiac cripple"). Early participation in supervised physical activity including the treadmill test and exercise conditioning have been shown to enhance the patient's self-confidence and ability to perform physical tasks (20). Having the spouse observe the early treadmill test establishes confidence in the spouse that his or her partner is not a cardiac cripple. In some medical centers, spouses are offered an opportunity to walk on the treadmill as well. This serves to establish a reference point for estimating ability to engage in activity. Engaging in a wide range of activities in the months after an MI is important because self-confidence is task specific (19,20). Most cardiac exercise programs (see below) emphasize activities using the legs, such as walking and jogging. Although this increases self-confidence in tasks requiring leg work, it does little for arm self-confidence. To increase arm self-confidence, patients must practice arm exercises as well (19,29). This is especially important for patients who plan to return to work that requires upper body and arm efforts.

Another common problem is *denial of illness persisting beyond the first few days in the hospital.* The behavior associated with persistent denial may create substantial risks. This is especially true of patients who are extremely competitive and are used to controlling most of the circumstances of their lives (2). They are typically determined to return to work as soon as possible and will refuse cardiac rehabilitation on the basis that they can do it better on their own. This

behavior arouses anxiety, fear, and concern in the spouse and family and may lead to significant marital conflict. An open discussion with patient and spouse, with each acknowledging the other's concerns, can often lead to resolution of these conflicts and more appropriate behavior from each partner.

At times it is useful to teach patients to use *various forms of feedback* to guide their activities. Specifically, patients are taught to use a target heart rate based on an exercise stress test; to observe themselves and how they feel, with the basic instruction to rest if fatigue or any cardiac symptoms occur during exercise, and to call the physician if symptoms persist after using nitroglycerin; and to view the spouse as a source of feedback. In most cases, the spouse's observation of how the patient looks is remarkably accurate. If a wife says her husband looks tired or does not look right, she is probably right (and vice versa). By having the patient agree to consider these comments as well meaning, the patient will usually comply with the spouse's advice. Thereafter, the number of reminding behaviors from the spouse is reduced progressively, and the rehabilitation process can proceed with greater enthusiasm from both partners. With more difficult patients or when there is preexisting marital strife, the consultation of a psychiatrist or psychologist may be helpful in managing adjustment problems.

Some patients have *severe psychologic and behavioral problems after MI* that may interfere with their rehabilitation. The most common problem is *persistent depression,* which may have characteristics of a major or minor depressive illness or may present as an adjustment disorder characterized by anxiety, depression, somatization, or a mixture of these responses (65). The diagnosis and management of these problems are discussed in Chapters 12 ("Somatization"), 13 ("Anxiety"), and 15 ("Depression").

Major depression, which is often underdiagnosed in the post-MI period, has a prevalence of 15 to 20% and is an independent risk factor for mortality at 6 months (6,22). These findings highlight the importance of recognizing symptoms of depression and offering patients appropriate treatment, which should include a program of cardiac rehabilitation (15). A study in which depressive symptoms were present in 20% of patients following a major coronary event showed that symptoms resolved in two-thirds of these patients following a program of cardiac rehabilitation (48). Although there have been no clinical trials of their efficacy in the post-MI period, the selective serotonin uptake inhibitors (SSRIs) have an excellent safety profile in cardiac patients and would be appropriate for the treatment of patients with major depression after MI. These drugs are described in detail in Chapter 15.

Studies show that the basic components of *coronary-prone behavior* (type A behavior) are time urgency and free-floating hostility. Long working hours, sustained drive, reasonable competitiveness, and enthusiasm do not appear to constitute coronary-prone behavior. In some patients, the basic components of type A behavior can be modified. Such modification has been associated with significant decrease in morbidity and mortality (23).

Medical Prophylaxis

Overview

There is evidence that medical prophylaxis with β-blocking agents and aspirin reduces the risk of morbidity and mortality after MI. For certain subgroups of patients, long-term treatment with angiotensin-converting enzyme (ACE) inhibitors also improves prognosis. Despite the widespread use of calcium channel blockers after MI, there is no evidence that treated patients benefit. The evidence for current recommendations regarding each of these classes of drugs is thoroughly reviewed by Hennekens et al. ("General References").

β-Blockers

The benefits of β-blocker prophylaxis are modest in low-risk patients (25). Therefore, when there are contraindications for initiating a β-blocker or when a patient develops significant side effects, prophylactic treatment may not be beneficial in low-risk patients. The benefits from β-blockers are related to their mechanism of action. Generally, their benefit is not related to cardioselectivity or membrane stabilization, or intrinsic sympathomimetic activity. The benefits are seen in all ages and in all types of MIs, although older patients (60 years and older) and patients with complicated MIs (compromised LV function and ventricular arrhythmias) seem to show greater benefits than do low-risk patients, as defined in Table 58.3. When initiated early in the course of an infarction (within 6 hours), β-blocker may limit or reduce infarct size. Later in the postinfarct time period, the mechanism for a reduction in mortality is the prevention of reinfarction and the antiarrhythmic property of β-blockers. The *overall magnitude of benefit* from the use of β-blockers seems to be about a one-third reduction in first-year mortality (from approximately 6 to 4% when all randomized patients are considered) and about the same magnitude of reduction in reinfarction during the first post-MI year; these benefits may extend beyond 1 year in some subgroups. *Contraindications* to the use of β-blockers include asthma, bradycardia, and insulin-treated diabetes mellitus. Although CHF is commonly considered a contraindication to the use of β-blockers, an improvement in survival and reduction in expected coronary events have been found even with a history of CHF, as long as the CHF is clinically compensated when β-blocker therapy is initiated (7). Even in patients with severe, uncompensated CHF there is significant improvement in morbidity and mortality associated with the addition of a β-blocker to a baseline regimen of digoxin, diuretics, and ACE inhibitors (39). The *recommended dosage* of a β-blocker is the amount required to produce attenuation of heart rate and blood pressure response to exercise without producing side effects (25). The characteristics of the available β-blocking drugs are summarized in Chapter 62, Table 62.11.

The issue of *duration of β-blocker therapy* is of great practical relevance in the clinical management of post-MI patients because of the their potential side effects (e.g., depression, easy fatigability, cold extremities, and aggravation of hypercholesterolemia). The benefits of the long-term use of β-blockers are still debated (81). Several long-term studies examining their benefit postinfarction support a duration for their use of 2 to 3 years after an acute MI. After this time, the survival benefits are less certain. It is reasonable to conclude that if a patient is tolerating the therapy without the described side effects, β-blocker use should be continued for 2 to 3 years post-MI and longer if not demonstrated to have adverse long-term effects in future studies.

Antiplatelet Therapy

Multiple randomized trials of antiplatelet therapy for secondary prevention of vascular disease show that prolonged treatment with aspirin has no effect on nonvascular mortality but reduces vascular *mortality* by approximately 15% and nonfatal vascular *events* (stroke or MI) by approximately 30% in patients with preexisting cardiac or cerebral vascular diseases (1). Post-MI benefits are similar to those in patients following stroke and transient ischemic attack (TIA). *In absolute terms,* the benefits of antiplatelet therapy accrued to about 40 per 1000 treated patients during the first month of treatment following an acute MI, and to about 40 per 1000 patients with a history of MI who were treated for 3 years. There is no difference in the degree of protection afforded by aspirin alone at a dosage of 325 mg/day and that afforded by higher aspirin dosages or other antiplatelet agents. Aspirin, 100 mg/day, has also been shown to improve coronary artery bypass graft patency at 4 months (90% of grafts patent versus 68% in the placebo group) (42) and to decrease significantly the frequency of restenosis after percutaneous transluminal coronary angioplasty (PTCA) (76) and thrombolysis (58). In patients who are allergic to aspirin, ticlopidine (250 mg twice a day) or sulfinpyrazone (400 mg twice a day) may be considered. These drugs are not as well studied as aspirin, they are more expensive, and the adverse effects can be more pronounced. For additional details regarding antiplatelet agents, see Chapter 52.

ACE Inhibitors

In the *acute management of MI,* it is now routine to consider all patients for treatment with ACE inhibitors, in addition to aspirin and β-blockers. The purpose for the use of these agents postinfarction is to prevent LV remodeling and recurrent ischemic events. After an infarction, *long-term ACE inhibitor treatment* should be offered to all patients with clinical symptoms of heart failure, a reduction in ejection fraction even if asymptomatic, or significant wall motion abnormalities with or without a reduction in ejection fraction. Data to guide recommendations about the duration of therapy are not yet available. It is reasonable to recommend their indefinite use if significant side effects (hypertension, hyperkalemia, decrease in renal function, or persistent cough) are absent.

In *chronic ischemic congestive cardiomyopathy,* the long-term use of the ACE inhibitors is associated with significant improvement in morbidity and mortality irrespective of severity and symptoms of failure. A large placebo-controlled study showed that patients with recent MI and LV dysfunction (ejection fraction of 40% or less by radionuclide ventriculography) who were randomized to captopril experienced a modest reduction in cardiovascular and overall mortality, progression to severe heart failure, and recurrent MI during 3 years of treatment (54). The *absolute incidence* of all cardiovascular events was reduced from approximately 40% in the placebo group to approximately 32% in the treatment group. Another large study showed that asymptomatic patients with LVEF of 35% or less who were randomized to enalapril also experienced a reduction in mortality or progression to heart failure during 3 years of treatment (67). The benefits accrued chiefly to patients with the lowest ejection fractions (28% or less). In these patients, the respective 3-year absolute incidences in placebo and treatment groups were as follows: death (all causes), 21 versus 18%; death or hospitalization for CHF, 33 versus 25%; and development of symptomatic CHF, 39 versus 23%. In asymptomatic patients with reduced ejection fractions, ACE inhibitors should be started at low dosages (e.g., enalapril 2.5 mg/day; captopril 6.25 mg three times daily) with gradual increases (e.g., enalapril up to 10 mg/day; captopril up to 25 or 50 mg three times daily) guided by blood pressure response and renal function. Characteristics of ACE inhibitors are summarized in Chapter 62.

Calcium Channel Blockers

The role of calcium channel blockers (CCBs) for both the acute management and secondary prevention of MI is limited. Short-acting nifedipine (and perhaps other dihydropyridine CCBs) is contraindicated because it was found to increase CAD mortality in multiple secondary prevention trials (26). Despite evidence from subgroup analysis that some patients benefited from short-term post-MI treatment with diltiazem, the large Multicenter Diltiazem Postinfarction Trial also showed marked increase in morbidity in some subgroups (28,30,51). Overall, CCBs have not been demonstrated to significantly improve mortality in MI survivors and should be limited to patients with symptomatic ischemia on β-blockers who are not candidates for revascularization as an additional antianginal, patients who do not tolerate β-blocker therapy, and the control of specific cardiac rhythms (see Chapter 59, "Arrhythmias").

Smoking, Hyperlipidemia, Hypertension, and Exercise

Smoking

Post-MI morbidity and mortality are significantly reduced in patients who discontinue smoking (83). Smokers who have survived an MI are usually motivated to stop; practical ways to assist them, including the prescription of nicotine substitution products, are described in Chapter 20.

Lipid-Lowering Diet and Drugs

The Framingham Study showed that the positive association of cholesterol level, particularly low-density lipoprotein (LDL) cholesterol level, with coronary disease mortality persists until age 80 (38). In the past, this finding was the basis for routinely advising all MI survivors to follow a low-fat diet. More recently, controlled trials show that cholesterol-lowering drugs reverse or delay progression of atherosclerotic plaques (4,53), reduce the incidence of coronary artery events in apparently healthy hypercholesterolemic men (41,43), and improve the prognosis in MI survivors (56,61,63). In the large 4S trial of secondary prevention, men and women 35 to 70 years, with cholesterol in the range 213 to 309 mg/100 mL despite 8-week trial of diet, were randomized to simvastatin 20 to 40 mg daily or placebo (56). Simvastatin subjects had the following *6-year absolute benefits* when compared with placebo subjects: survival, 91.3 versus 87.6%; one or more CAD events, 19 versus 28%; and risk of undergoing myocardial revascularization procedures, 11.3 versus 17.2%. The mean changes in total cholesterol, LDL cholesterol, and HDL cholesterol in the treatment group were −25, −35, and +8%, respectively. In 1994, an expert panel of the National Cholesterol Education Program recommended treatment to attain a target LDL level of 100 mg/100 mL post-MI (see "General References"). A definitive clinical trial using this target level has not yet been conducted, but the 4S study and the more recent pravastatin trial in post-MI patients with total cholesterol levels below 240 mg/100 mL and LDL levels 115 to 174 mg/100 mL both provide indirect support for the 1994 recommendation (56,63).

As pointed out in the recent ACP risk stratification report ("General References"), lipid levels measured within 24 to 48 hours of an MI are accurate and can guide post-MI secondary prevention decisions. Detailed information regarding cholesterol and atherosclerotic disease is found in Chapter 75.

Hypertension

There have been no critical assessments of the treatment of post-MI hypertension. Because of the J-curve finding described in Chapter 62 ("Hypertension"), it is prudent to control this risk factor but to avoid overtreatment (i.e., to a resting diastolic BP below 80 mm Hg).

Exercise

The role of formal exercise programs in rehabilitation after MI is described in detail below ("Physical Conditioning").

Medical Complications

Table 58.6 lists the principal medical complications of MI, the procedures that may be useful in diagnosing or evaluating them, and potential therapies. As noted above ("Risk Stratification Before Hospital

Table 58.6.   Medical Complications of MI

Complications	Diagnostic Procedures for Selected Patients[a]	Management Approaches
Angina or other evidence of reversible ischemia	ECG stress testing, radionuclide stress testing, Holter monitor for silent ischemia, coronary arteriography	Standard antianginal therapy (see Chapter 57), coronary artery bypass or PTCA for selected patients, physical conditioning
CHF	Radionuclide ventriculography or echocardiography (ejection fraction, segmental dysfunction, rupture, ventricular aneurysm)	Afterload reduction, diuretics, inotropics, ?β-blockers, ?anticoagulants (see Chapter 61 for treatment of heart failure); surgery in a few selected patients
Arrhythmias	Holter monitor; ECG stress testing, electrophysiological study in selected patients	β-Blockers, other antiarrhythmics (see Chapter 59); surgery or implanted defibrillator in selected patients
Post-MI syndrome (Dressler's)	Echocardiography (pericardial effusion)	Aspirin or other anti-inflammatory agents (see text)
Systemic emboli	Echocardiography (intracardiac thrombus)	Anticoagulant therapy (see Chapter 52); surgery in selected patients

[a]Should be coordinated and interpreted by consulting cardiologist.

Discharge"), complications identified early are addressed very aggressively before or shortly after discharge. For example, 56% of patients in the National Registry of Myocardial Infarction were catheterized in 1990–1994 (32). In general, the use of sophisticated and costly procedures to evaluate the complications listed in Table 58.6 should be coordinated by a consulting cardiologist.

Postinfarction Angina

As pointed out in the discussion of prognosis above, angina is common in survivors of MI. The evaluation and medical management of angina are described in detail in Chapter 57. Because protection of the heart from transient ischemia may be especially important during recovery from an MI, it is advisable to prescribe β-blockers in most patients (see above) and to undertake aggressive evaluation and management of patients who develop angina within the first 3 months after MI. Because of the poor prognosis associated with angina that occurs very early after an MI, patients with this problem following hospital discharge should be referred to a cardiologist for consideration of coronary catheterization and possible coronary revascularization.

Postinfarction Symptomatic Congestive Heart Failure

Postinfarction symptomatic CHF usually develops before discharge from the hospital. Currently, most patients have their LVEF measured as part of their evaluation before discharge, so that those at increased risk of developing symptomatic CHF after discharge are known. As noted above, it has been shown that ACE inhibitors delay deterioration in functional capacity and improve survival in patients with CHF after MI (37,54). The use of ACE inhibitors and other agents for CHF is described in detail in Chapter 61. Selected patients with persistent CHF may have segmental or global LV dysfunction, or mitral regurgitation, that may improve after cardiac surgery.

Postinfarction Arrhythmias

A substantial proportion of MI survivors have *complex ventricular arrhythmias* (see criteria in Table 58.1)

on 24-hour ambulatory ECG monitoring after the first week of hospitalization. Controlled trials do not show that the suppression of ventricular ectopy with drug therapy improves mortality. The Cardiac Arrhythmia Suppression Trial (CAST) revealed that the use of type I antiarrhythmic agents (encainide and flecainide) in such patients was associated with about three times the sudden death rate of the use of placebo (16). In addition, the use of antiarrhythmic agents in the posthospital treatment of patients with the *combination of complex ventricular arrhythmias and low ejection fractions* documented at the end of their stay in the hospital remains controversial. Early trials using type I drugs did not establish efficacy (45); however, recently reported trials using the type III drug amiodarone suggest a significant reduction in arrhythmias and arrhythmia-related deaths in this high-risk subset of patients (57,59). Recently published trials evaluating the benefits of implantable defibrillators in specific high-risk populations have supported prior beliefs that defibrillators prolong life when compared with antiarrhythmic drugs (49a,75a). Unfortunately, specific recommendations regarding the use of defibrillators in post-MI patients are currently lacking, but ongoing studies are likely to identify patient subgroups who can benefit from a defibrillator (24,51a). Details regarding all options for the management of symptomatic arrhythmias are discussed in detail in Chapter 59.

Postmyocardial Infarction (Dressler's) Syndrome

It is estimated that 3 to 4% of patients develop this complication, usually within 1 to 8 weeks after an MI. The syndrome is characterized by the pain of pericarditis (substernal pain relieved by leaning forward and increased with inspiration), presence of a friction rub, a pericardial effusion (which can best be demonstrated by echocardiography), malaise, fever, leukocytosis, and often a unilateral or bilateral pleural effusion. The principal considerations in the differential diagnosis are pulmonary embolism and recurrence or extension of the recent MI.

A patient with suspected Dressler's syndrome should be considered for hospitalization. A possible recurrent MI should be addressed by monitoring, serial ECGs, and cardiac enzymes. Evaluation for pulmonary embolization requires a ventilation–perfusion lung scan or pulmonary angiography. If these tests do not show an explanation for the patient's symptoms, the clinical diagnosis of Dressler's syndrome can be made with reasonable assurance. Echocardiographic evidence of a pericardial effusion and an elevated erythrocyte sedimentation rate may also be present.

Dressler's syndrome usually responds to salicylates or indomethacin; in patients who do not respond to these drugs, prednisone gives prompt relief of symptoms. However, the use of steroids within 4 weeks of an MI may alter postinfarction healing and may increase the risk of myocardial rupture. The use of steroids should therefore be limited to patients who are more than 4 weeks postinfarction. Once the diagnosis is secure and symptoms are controlled, the patient can be discharged. The anti-inflammatory drug chosen in the hospital should be administered for a few weeks after discharge. Prednisone should be tapered according to the schedule described in Chapter 74. Patients who have recurrent symptoms when anti-inflammatory treatment is discontinued should resume treatment for another month or longer.

Arterial Embolization

Arterial embolization occurs following hospitalization in 5 to 10% of MI survivors. The emboli seem to originate from mural thrombi that are typically seen in the LV apex adjacent to akinetic or dyskinetic wall segments. Approximately 30 to 40% of hearts with akinetic or dyskinetic LV apices show mural thrombi on the echocardiogram. Because of these facts, anticoagulation (see Chapter 52) in patients with mural thrombi is widely practiced, although the impact and appropriate duration of anticoagulation have not been assessed in a prospective trial. However, most cardiologists anticoagulate MI survivors with mural thrombi for 3 to 6 months. One retrospective study showed that in patients with severe CHF (Class III–IV NYHA with LVEF below 20%), warfarin therapy over 6 months decreases the incidence of stroke from 3.3 to 0.6% (21). Patients with atrial fibrillation or a history of embolic events should also be considered for systemic anticoagulation with warfarin.

Shoulder–Hand Syndrome (Reflex Sympathetic Dystrophy)

Shoulder–hand syndrome, characterized by pain and stiffness of the shoulder and pain and swelling of the hand, may occur during the first 1 to 2 months after an MI. It usually affects the left side. This syndrome rarely occurs when patients are mobilized early after an MI. Management of the shoulder–hand syndrome is described in Chapter 83 ("Cerebrovascular Disease").

Referral for Cardiology Consultation

Selected MI survivors may benefit from coronary angioplasty or cardiac surgery, by having their symptoms reduced or their prognosis improved. Patients in the following groups should be referred promptly to a cardiologist to ensure optimal medical therapy and to obtain an opinion about the advisability and the timing of invasive procedures:

- Patients with *uncontrolled angina* refractory to medical therapy, with a markedly positive exercise stress test at low work load or with evidence of LV dysfunction during exercise (e.g., increased lung uptake of thallium during exercise)
- Patients with a *ventricular aneurysm*
- Patients with *CHF refractory to medical therapy* (ACE inhibitors, digitalis, and diuretics)
- Patients with *structural complications* such as ventricular septal defect (suggested by holosystolic murmur and thrill at the left sternal border), papillary muscle rupture (suggested by refractory CHF and holosystolic apical murmur), segmental akinesis, or ventricular aneurysm
- Patients with *electrical instability* (e.g., symptomatic bradycardia, high-grade atrioventricular [AV] blocks, ventricular tachycardia, or other arrhythmias)

Noncardiac Surgery

Noncardiac surgery carries a very high risk during the first 3 to 6 months after an MI (see Chapter 86 for details).

Home Care for Acute Myocardial Infarction

A 1971 controlled trial in Great Britain showed that for patients with uncomplicated acute MIs the outcome is similar whether the patient is cared for in the home or in an intensive care unit (46). Because hospital care is the norm for an acute MI in the United States, it is unlikely that home care will gain significant acceptance. However, management at home may be appropriate for an occasional patient who has a stable acute MI and objects to hospitalization, who is demented and would predictably become very disoriented and agitated in a CCU, or who consults a physician several days after the onset of symptoms of infarction. The scheme for rehabilitation after MI described in this chapter can be adapted to these situations.

MANAGEMENT OF UNSTABLE ANGINA AFTER DISCHARGE FROM HOSPITAL

Of patients admitted to a hospital with unstable angina but without MI, 15 to 30% continue to have pain despite vigorous medical management. Patients in this group have an estimated 25% 1-year mortality rate. Therefore, most are evaluated and referred for coronary angioplasty or coronary artery bypass surgery. These interventions relieve or eliminate symptoms in most cases and improve survival for those with left main coronary artery disease, three-vessel disease, and two-vessel disease with LV dysfunction.

To date, the rehabilitation of the medically managed patient with unstable angina has not been studied as systematically as the rehabilitation of the patient after

MI. These patients should receive education similar to that recommended for patients after MI regarding the nature of coronary artery disease, the recognition of symptoms, and the control of risk factors (see above). Because these patients do not have an ischemic injury that may take 2 or more months to heal, they often return to their usual activities more rapidly than patients who have had an MI. This is true particularly if their angina is well controlled and a stress test shows good effort tolerance (9 METs or more) and minimal or no changes caused by ischemia or LV dysfunction.

Additional information regarding the management of unstable angina is found in Chapter 57.

PHYSICAL CONDITIONING

Regular exercise, with the goal of attaining the physiologic adaptation known as the *conditioning effect,* is safe and beneficial for most patients after MI, just as it is for healthy people and patients with most chronic diseases. The basic principles of exercise training are applicable to people with and without heart disease. *Low-intensity exercise* that does not produce a conditioning effect may be associated with health benefits (see below).

Cardiovascular principles related to exercise are described here; important principles regarding the musculoskeletal system are described in Chapter 67.

Muscular and Cardiovascular Effects

The body responds and adapts to the kind and amount of physical demands placed on it. The response is *specific,* meaning that the greatest changes are observed only in the areas on which demands are placed. For exercise to bring about an improvement in physical fitness, it must *overload* the muscles or organ system involved in the exercise. To overload is to exercise at a greater intensity than the intensity to which one is accustomed. The overload must be applied gradually, in stages, for maximal effectiveness and safety. This is known as progressive resistance. *Threshold of training* is the amount of exercise that must be done to produce fitness improvements. The factors that must be considered when establishing a plan for physical conditioning are as follows.

Type of Activity

As stated, the effects of exercise are specific to the type of activity engaged in and the body function it addresses. Thus, if the objective is to improve cardiovascular endurance, exercise that increases heart rate and peripheral oxygen consumption is required. If the objective is to improve strength, exercise with increasing amounts of resistance is required. There is little carryover of the effects of an exercise from one component of fitness to another.

Activities for cardiovascular fitness entail rhythmic repetitive movements of large muscle groups against small resistance. Such activities are of low intensity and can be performed for a long time. They include walking, jogging, swimming, cycling, rowing, jumping rope, skating, running, and cross-country skiing. These activities increase the demand for oxygen and the muscles adapt by enhanced extraction of oxygen, which is the reason they are called *aerobic* activities. They are also called dynamic activities.

Sustained, slow-movement activity often involving small muscle groups against high resistance is known as *static activity or resistive exercise.* Examples are weight lifting, pushups, situps, isometrics, carrying heavy packages, and hand grips. Most activities requiring lifting and straining, such as shoveling, have a large static component. In such activities there is increased peripheral vascular resistance, with subsequent increase in blood pressure but little increase in heart rate or cardiac output. Such exercises do not bring about enhancement in oxygen extraction, so they are generally not aerobic. There are inadequate data to suggest that brief episodes of moderate resistive exercise are dangerous. In fact, studies show that cardiac patients who were required to carry or lift weights or to perform isometric exercise after MI had fewer ischemic electrocardiographic changes and arrhythmias during resistive exercise than during aerobic exercises (13,74). Gradual involvement in activities such as weight lifting may therefore be beneficial and desirable, especially in patients whose jobs require static efforts.

Intensity

Exercise intensity is set at a level that requires more effort than normal activity. This level is usually set at *70% of predicted maximal oxygen uptake,* a level that is attained when the heart rate reaches approximately 80% of the age-predicted maximal rate. Optimal conditioning occurs when a person sustains this rate during an aerobic activity. Table 58.7 lists *target heart rates* for healthy people in various age groups. Lower levels of aerobic exercise also produce a partial conditioning effect. Exercise prescription for patients with heart disease are discussed later in this chapter.

Duration

Exercise must be performed for a sufficient amount of time to be effective. Duration can be varied in several ways: Increase repetitions while maintaining the same rate, such as in weight training; increase the distance covered at the same rate, such as in walking or jogging; reduce the number of rest periods between different exercises; or reduce the rest time during a rest period.

Table 58.7. Target Heart Rates for Healthy People, by Age (Approximately 80% Maximal Predicted Heart Rate)

Age (yr)	Heart Rate (beats/min)
20–29	170
30–39	160
40–49	150
50–59	140
60–69	130

From Parmley JF Jr, Blair S, Gazes PC, et al., eds. Proceedings of the National Workshop on Exercise in the Prevention, Evaluation, and Treatment of Heart Disease. J South Carolina Med Assoc 65 (Suppl 1):Dec, 1969.

Studies in exercise physiology suggest that the total work done during an exercise session (i.e., duration × intensity) may be more important in eliciting improvements than intensity or duration alone. Therefore, a long, low-intensity workout may be equivalent to a short, high-intensity workout if the total work is the same. A long, low-intensity workout (e.g., long period of sustained walking) may be more suitable for beginners and for middle-aged or older patients because it would reduce the risk of injury. For cardiovascular fitness (using the heart rates listed in Table 58.7), duration should be *at least 20 minutes at the target heart rate.*

Frequency

This factor refers to the number of times per week exercise is to be done. Exercise must be performed regularly, and for most types of exercise three to five times per week is desirable. However, two to three times per week is probably more sensible for the beginner because many musculoskeletal injuries occur at the start of a program from overuse. This can increase to three to five times per week as adaptation takes place.

The principal hemodynamic adaptation to aerobic exercise in patients with heart disease takes place in the peripheral vascular and muscular systems. Trained muscles can extract more oxygen from a given blood flow and there is a better distribution of the cardiac output. Heart rate and blood pressure are lower at rest and at a given submaximal work load. As a result, the patient can do more work with less cardiac effort (i.e., less myocardial oxygen demand). This is extremely beneficial to cardiac patients who have limited blood supply through the coronary arteries. Angina may occur at the same threshold, that is, the same double product (heart rate × systolic blood pressure), but this threshold is reached at a higher level of body work or MET level. METs are used to rate the energy requirement of different physical activities, as indicated by the amount of oxygen extracted during those activities. One MET is 3.5 mL O_2/kg body weight per minute and is equivalent to oxygen requirement at rest; 2 METs are twice the resting requirements, and so on. (See Table 58.5 for the METs required for a broad range of activities.) The higher the MET level attained during exercise testing, the more fit the patient is considered to be. In patients with coronary artery disease, the increase in angina-free exercise capacity achieved with regular exercise is similar to that achieved with medications such as β-blockers and nitrates. In healthy people who practice aerobic exercise there are also changes in the heart itself, including increase in diastolic volume, increase in ejection fraction at rest and to a greater extent during exercise, and enhancement of contractility. Few studies show any of this central effect in cardiac patients. However, there is evidence that cardiac patients may achieve these changes if they train hard and long enough (17). Improvement in coronary collateral circulation or myocardial perfusion has been demonstrated in patients who participate in regular physical exercise and adhere to a low-fat diet (66).

However, the independent effect of exercise on CAD progression is not yet known.

Hormonal and Metabolic Effects

In addition to the effect of training on the cardiovascular and muscular systems, aerobic exercise is associated with beneficial changes in a number of other systems; there is increased vagal tone, lowering of catecholamines, decrease in serum triglycerides, increase in the ratio of high- to low-density lipoprotein, reduction in adipose tissue, slowing of loss of bone mass, augmentation in plasma fibrinolytic activity, and enhanced endogenous opiate activity (may add to sense of well-being). A comprehensive review (Peterson, "General References") distinguishes exercise (planned, structural, repetitive physical activity that leads to physical conditioning) from all other physical activity, and summarizes benefits and risks that accompany both and the specific instructions that can be given to patients.

Conditioning in Healthy People

Healthy people can develop their own physical conditioning programs, using a self-instruction program (10,85). The objective of conditioning programs is to reach an exercise level at which the body achieves 70% of maximal predicted oxygen uptake, a level that is attained when the heart rate reaches approximately 80% of the maximal predicted rate (Table 58.7). As stated previously, optimal conditioning in healthy people occurs with aerobic activity at the target heart rate for 20 minutes, at least three times per week. Lower levels of aerobic exercise also produce a partial conditioning effect in healthy people.

Selected people should consult their physicians before beginning a conditioning program. In general, people over the age of 35 and those with major risk factors for atherosclerosis should have a physical examination and a resting ECG. Exercise stress tests should be considered for people in a number of categories, as summarized in Table 58.8. Nondiagnostic fitness tests for apparently healthy people are usually available at health clubs, YMCAs, wellness centers, and community colleges. The charge varies from $50 to $100. When supervised and interpreted by qualified allied health professionals, these tests can provide the basis for the exercise prescription. Fees are usually nominal and are included in the overall package for exercise sessions.

Low-Intensity Exercise

The conditioning guidelines outlined above refer to exercise that is structured and planned and has the goal of improving cardiovascular fitness in addition to improving health. Physical activity at a lower intensity or duration, or activity that is not structured (e.g., recreational games, gardening, walking, stair climbing), may produce health benefits without actually

Table 58.8. People for Whom Stress Testing Should Be Considered When Beginning Exercise Programs

Status	Test or Training Mode
Healthy, under 35 yr	No special test
Healthy, over 35 yr	Stress test[a]
Coronary prone, all ages	Stress test
Coronary stricken, all ages	Stress test

[a]Tests performed by paramedical personnel to assess baseline exercise capacity.

increasing cardiovascular fitness. For example, in one study (14) there was a dose–response relationship of exercise intensity to increased maximal oxygen uptake (fitness). However, after 6 months, increases in HDL cholesterol occurred in all exercisers whether their exercise intensity was low, moderate, or high. For some patients, the advice to increase physical activity to any level may bring some benefit compared with no activity at all. In a study from the Cooper Clinic in Dallas, Texas (3), there was a decrease in all-cause mortality after 8 years even among people with low to moderate fitness levels compared with the least fit group.

Ideally, patients should be encouraged to exercise sufficiently to improve fitness and health. However, because long-term compliance with a prescribed exercise program is difficult, patients should be encouraged to increase activity in any form. During recent years, several reports from health and government organizations and agencies have recommended regular moderate-intensity physical activity as an option for people who get little or no exercise. A 1995 *NIH Consensus Statement on Physical Activity and Cardiovascular Health* (see "General References") recommends that children and adults alike should set a goal of accumulating at least 30 minutes of moderate-intensity physical activity on most, and preferably all days of the week. The consensus panel concluded that this level of activity confers significant health benefits. Furthermore, people who currently meet these daily standards may derive additional health benefits by becoming more active or including more vigorous activity. Another report, the *1996 Surgeon General's Report on Physical Activity and Health* (see "General References"), addressed the question of whether cardiorespiratory fitness gains are similar when physical activity occurs in several short sessions (e.g., 10 minutes) and when the same total amount and intensity of activity occurs in one longer session (e.g., 30 minutes). The reported concluded, based on expert opinion, that although the health benefits of brief intermittent activity have not yet been demonstrated, it is reasonable to expect them to be similar to those of continuous activity. Moreover, for people who are unable to set aside 30 minutes for physical activity, shorter episodes are clearly better than none. The 1995 document *Physical Activity and Public Health: A Recommendation from the Centers for Disease Control and Prevention and the American College of Sports Medicine* (see

"General References") provides similar recommendations about the need for increased physical activity for cardiovascular health, and further states that two other components of fitness—flexibility and muscular strength—should not be overlooked. The report advises that people who maintain or improve their strength and flexibility may be better able to perform daily activities, less likely to develop back pain, and better able to avoid disability, especially as they advance into older age.

Physical Conditioning in Patients After Myocardial Infarction

Although the focus of this section is on exercise training, the recently published *Cardiac Rehabilitation Clinical Practice Guidelines* (see "General References") from the Agency for Health Care Policy and Research defined the scientific basis for recommendations for multifactorial cardiac rehabilitation services that include medical evaluation, prescribed exercise, cardiac risk factor modification, and education, counseling, and behavioral interventions. The key beneficial health outcomes resulting from multifactorial cardiac rehabilitation are a reduction in mortality, reduction in the number of cardiac events, improvements in symptoms, increased exercise tolerance, improvements in blood lipids, increased smoking cessation, and improved psychosocial outcomes. Provision of these services is physician-directed. They are implemented by a variety of health care professionals. Unfortunately, despite the scientific evidence demonstrating the benefits of cardiac rehabilitation, the report points out that only 11 to 20% of the several millions of patients with coronary heart disease participate in cardiac rehabilitation programs.

Benefits of Conditioning

Cardiac patients who exercise regularly and have become conditioned show better control of angina and enhancement of physical working capacity.

Because of the peripheral cardiovascular adaptations described earlier, angina pectoris occurs at higher exercise levels. This increased anginal threshold allows the patient to do more work, and at any given level of work the patient feels more comfortable because the work represents a lower percentage of a now higher maximal capacity. Similar benefits for patients with LV dysfunction and chronic heart failure have also been demonstrated (9,73). *Rating of perceived exertion* (RPE) is a scale that measures how hard any given level of work feels (Table 58.9). The RPE is administered during exercise testing. The patient is asked to rate the work at each stage of the test. After conditioning, the RPE is lower at any given stage and is associated with a lower heart rate and blood pressure (33). RPE is also a useful way to prescribe exercise. This approach focuses on how the patient actually feels and correlates closely with the target heart rate and desired MET level. For most cardiac patients, a prescription at 13 to

14 ("somewhat hard" to "hard") on the RPE scale is both safe and effective for cardiovascular conditioning.

The *effect of exercise training on longevity in patients after MI* has been established. Meta-analysis of the combined results of 10 randomized clinical trials demonstrates a 25% reduction in cardiovascular mortality, although not in nonfatal reinfarction for patients in rehabilitation programs (52). Benefits of exercise conditioning on the psychometric profile are not firmly established (see Greenland and Chu in "General References").

Risks of Conditioning

With proper selection, supervision, monitoring, and precautions, physical conditioning for cardiac patients has proved to be remarkably safe. Cumulative data from more than 1.5 million person-hours of exercise, done predominantly 3 months after MI, show that the risks of ventricular fibrillation, acute MI, and death are 1 in 10,000 to 1 in 32,000, 1 in 253,000, and 1 in 100,000 to 1 in 212,000 person-hours of exercise, respectively (11). There is no comparable large series on exercise conditioning earlier than 3 months after MI. In the authors' experience with exercise programs beginning an average of 10 days after hospital discharge, there have been few complications during exercise over a 15-year period. These patients exercise three times a week, for an average of 6 to 8 weeks, at a conditioning heart rate of approximately 80% of what they safely achieved on a post-MI stress test, usually performed before hospital discharge.

Cardiovascular Medications and Conditioning

Many patients who enroll in exercise programs are taking one or more medications. Many of these medications alter the cardiovascular response to exercise. Patients enrolled in a conditioning program should always be stress tested (see below) while taking their regular medications, and the effects of their drugs must be considered in interpreting test results. For example, β-blockers attenuate the heart rate response to exercise. Thus, heart rate is not useful as an endpoint for

Table 58.9. Rate of Perceived Exertion (RPE) Scale

6
7 Very, very light
8
9 Very light
10
11 Fairly light
12
13 Somewhat hard
14
15 Hard
16
17 Very hard
18
19 Very, very hard
20

From Borg G. Subjective effort in relation to physical performance and working capacity. In: Pick HL, ed. Psychology: from research to practice. New York: Plenum, 1978;333.

Table 58.10. Effect of Various Classes of Medications on Hemodynamic Status During Exercise

Drug	Peak Heart Rate	Peak Systolic Blood Pressure
Antihypertensives		
ACE inhibitors	=	↓
Hydralazine	↑	↓
Minoxidil	↑	↓
Clonidine	↓	↓
Guanethidine	↓	↓↓
Methyldopa	↓	↓
Prazosin	↑	↓
Nitrates	↑	↓
Antiarrhythmics	=	↓
β-Blockers	↓	↓
Digitalis[a]	=	↑
Calcium blockers		
Nifedipine	↑	↓
Diltiazem	=	↓
Verapamil	↓	↓

Modified from Powles ACP. The effect of drugs on the cardiovascular response to exercise. Med Sci Sports Exerc 13:252, 1981.

↓, decreased; ↑, increased; =, no discernible effect.

[a]Patients with CHF.

stress testing or as a parameter for the patient to monitor during exercise conditioning. In a patient on a β-blocker, symptoms, ECG changes, fatigue, and RPE (Table 58.9) are used as endpoints during stress testing. These parameters are also useful for establishing the exercise prescription in patients on certain medications. Table 58.10 summarizes the *effects of a number of commonly prescribed cardiac drugs on the hemodynamic response to exercise.*

Patients taking a variety of drugs have been evaluated and have participated safely in physical conditioning programs. There is some controversy regarding the effect of β-blockers on the response to training. It has been suggested that β-blockers may attenuate the beneficial effects of training. A clinical trial (69) to establish whether a β-blocker (propranolol) or a calcium channel blocker (diltiazem) limits exercise capacity and training effect shows that neither drug interfered with muscle strength. After starting propranolol, maximal aerobic capacity was reduced by 20%, whereas a 20% increase in aerobic capacity from this reduced level occurred with training while subjects continued to use the drug. Thus, although a training effect can be achieved while using a β-blocker, its use may limit the full benefit of exercise training as measured by maximal aerobic capacity. On the other hand, for patients who are limited by ischemia, the use of a β-blocker may allow the patient to achieve work loads that may not otherwise be attained without anti-ischemic medication.

Referral for Conditioning

The decision to refer a patient for physical conditioning after MI depends on the patient's clinical status, motivation, and the availability of well-supervised and staffed programs designed for such patients. Medically supervised programs, offering ECG monitoring and the immediate availability of emergency care, often accept patients within 1 to 2 weeks of hospital discharge. If such a program is not available, cautious guidelines such as those shown in Table 58.4 are appropriate. After 2 months, when no supervised program is available, patients with uncomplicated MI can be advised to increase their exercise levels gradually, using the results of a stress test to establish target heart rates or RPE.

Before beginning a conditioning program, the patient should have an ECG stress test (see Chapter 57 for a description of the patient's experience), the results of which are used in planning the exercise program. In general, the conditioning target heart rate is 70 to 85% of the maximal heart rate safely achieved on the stress test. Figure 58.4 shows the results of such a stress

test, performed 3 weeks after an MI in a patient who was evaluated just before enrollment in a supervised exercise program.

Contraindications

A patient should not be enrolled in or should discontinue a conditioning program if the following problems are present: poorly controlled angina, severe dyspnea at low work loads, moderate to severe uncontrolled hypertension at rest (diastolic above 110 mm Hg), complex arrhythmias (Table 58.1), atrial fibrillation with a rapid ventricular response, second- or third-degree heart block, significant valvular or congenital heart disease, significant orthopedic or pulmonary limitations, chronic alcoholism, or recent acute physical or mental illness.

```
PATIENT: J T   ID#: 00 00 00    DATE:  6 / 6 / 81
REFERRING PHYSICIAN: CCU


********************************PATIENT DATA*****************************


AGE: 34    SEX: MALE    HGT: 68    WGT: 162   INDICATION: EARLY S/P MI
PRESENT SYMPTOMS: NONE
CCU ADMISSION DATE:   5 / 12 / 81     DX: INFERIOR MI
PRIOR EST:  4 / 14 / 75      RESULTS: NEGATIVE EXERCISE STRESS TEST
MEDS: NITROPASTE
RISK FACTORS: SMOKING FAMILY HX


***********************PRE-EXERCISE SCREENING***********************


SUPINE: HR: 62  BP: 114 / 78      STANDING: HR: 66  BP: 112 / 80
RESTING EKG:AXIS/PATTERNS:    INFERIOR MI
RESTING EKG:RHYTHM:           NORMAL SINUS RHYTHM
POST-HYPERVENTILATION:        NO SIGNIFICANT CHANGES


****************************EXERCISE RESULTS*************************


REASON FOR STOPPING TEST: TARGET HEART RATE ATTAINED
EXERCISE PROTOCOL: MODIFIED NAUGHTON      TOTAL TIME: 14 MIN, 30 SEC
PEAK SPEED: 3 MPH  ELEVATION: 10 % GRADE    METS:  7    NYHA CLASS: 1
PHYSIOLOGICAL DATA: PREDICTED MAX HR:  186    90% MAX HR:  167
PEAK HR:  132        THIS WAS ADEQUATE FOR THE WORK PERFORMED
PEAK BP:  150/120    THIS WAS ADEQUATE FOR THE WORK PERFORMED
THE RATE-PRESSURE PRODUCT WAS:  19800

     EXERCISE EKG:ST-T CHANGES:
THERE WERE NO SIGNIFICANT CHANGES NOTED.

     EXERCISE EKG:RHYTHM:
THERE WERE NO ARRHYTHMIAS NOTED.

     SYMPTOMS:
THERE WERE NO SYMPTOMS REPORTED.

     CONCLUSIONS:
1.   ADEQUATE, NEGATIVE EARLY POST MI STRESS TEST.
2.   ACCELERATED DIASTOLIC BLOOD PRESSURE RESPONSE TO EXERCISE.
     RECOMMENDATIONS:
A.   MAY START MONITORED EXERCISE PROGRAM.
B.   CONSIDER BETA BLOCKADE IN VIEW OF #2 ABOVE.
```

Figure 58.4A. Example of a formal report of an exercise stress test useful for planning rehabilitation, conducted 3 weeks after myocardial infarction.

	Bruce		Protocol Mod. Naughton				
Stage	Treadmill	Mets	Treadmill	Mets	BP	HR	Comments
1	1.7/0*	2	2/0	2	140/100	87	NO SYMPTOMS; NO EKG CHANGES
2	1.7/10	5	2/3.5	3	145/105	92	NO SYMPTOMS; NO EKG CHANGES
3	2.5/12	7	2/7	4	140/115	98	NO SYMPTOMS; NO EKG CHANGES
4	3.4/14	10	2/10.5	5	140/110	108	NO SYMPTOMS; NO EKG CHANGES
5	4.2/16	13	2/14	6	150/120	128	NO SYMPTOMS; NO EKG CHANGES
6			3/10	7	145/95	132	FATIGUE; NO EKG CHANGES
7			3/12.5	8			
8			3/15	9			
9			3/17.5	10			
10							

*Miles per hr/percent elevation

			Recovery	
Min	BP	HR	Comments	
0	145/95	132	NO SYMPTOMS; NO EKG CHANGES	
2	114/85	94	NO SYMPTOMS; NO EKG CHANGES	
4	112/80	88	NO SYMPTOMS; NO EKG CHANGES	
6	112/84	75	NO SYMPTOMS; NO EKG CHANGES	
8	112/84	78	NO SYMPTOMS; NO EKG CHANGES	
10	110/82	84	NO SYMPTOMS; NO EKG CHANGES	

Figure 58.4B. Data from stress test.

Exercise Programs

Exercise sessions should be supervised by personnel trained in exercise physiology and cardiopulmonary resuscitation, with immediate availability of monitoring and resuscitative equipment. Programs that accept patients soon after MI should have equipment for continuous ECG monitoring. Sessions are usually held *three times a week on nonconsecutive days.* The total duration of an average session is about 45 minutes. The pattern for a workout is illustrated in Figure 58.5. During the stimulus phase, the patient exercises at an intensity that elicits a heart rate or RPE (see above) that falls within the prescribed target zone. Figure 58.6 shows recommendations for exercise intensity based on heart rate response during an exercise stress test. Exercising near the 70% level, for 20 to 30 minutes,

promotes fitness, and beginners should be instructed to maintain intensity near this level. Experienced exercisers can advance to the 85% level if a more intense workout is desired. The stimulus, or period at the target heart rate, is preceded by 5 to 10 minutes of warmup and is followed by 5 to 10 minutes of cool-down (Fig. 58.5). Warmup and cool-down should include stretching and range-of-motion calisthenic exercises (see Chapter 67, Fig. 67.18). *Warmup* provides for gradual acceleration of the heart and circulation; it is beneficial to joints and muscles and helps prevent musculoskeletal injuries. *Cool-down* provides for gradual deceleration of the cardiovascular system and prevents pooling of blood in the muscles when exercise stops abruptly. Pooling can lead to a precipitous drop in venous return and, consequently, postexercise hypotension.

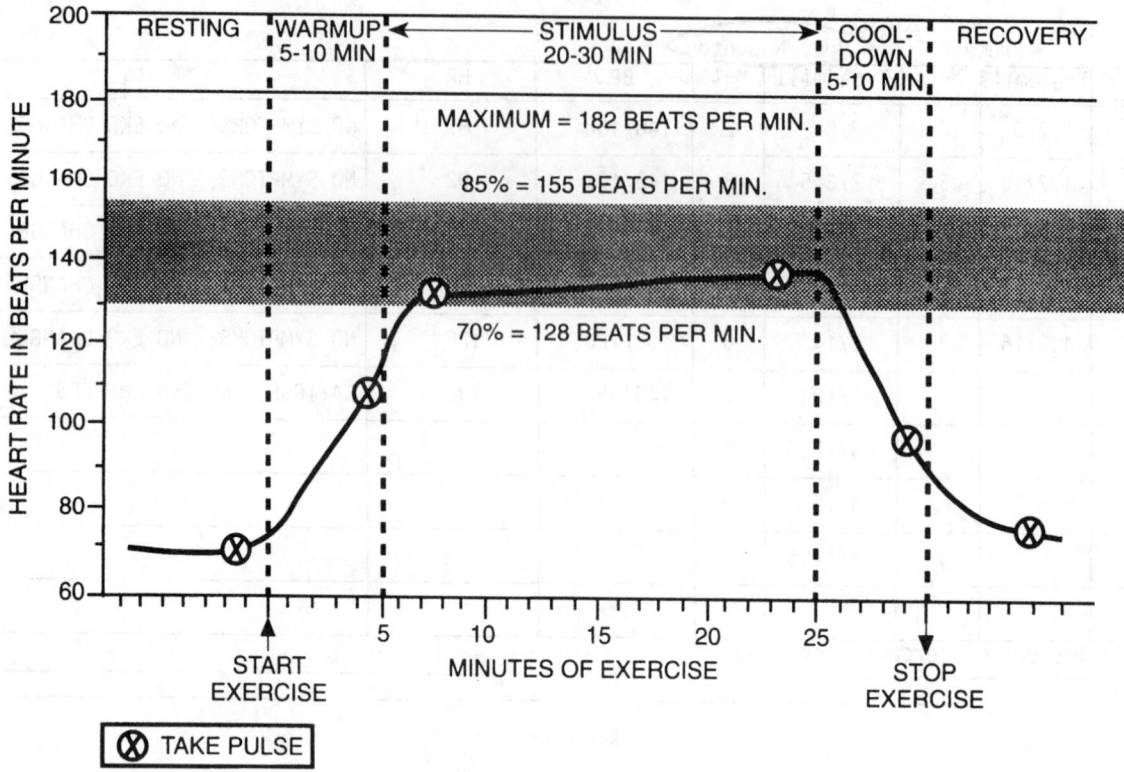

Figure 58.5. The exercise training pattern.

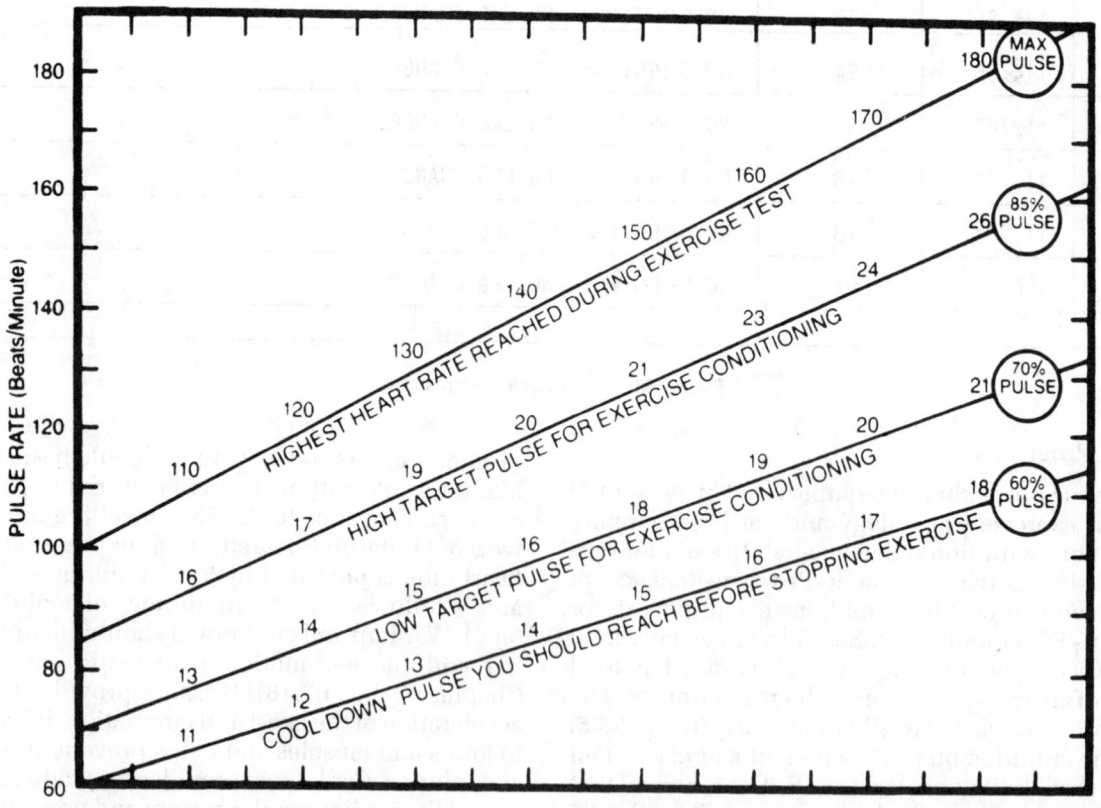

Figure 58.6. Target pulse rates for 10-second counts that should be measured the first 10 seconds after exercise. (To convert the count to beats per minute, multiply by 6.) To determine a patient's target pulse rate range, identify the highest rate safely achieved during the most recent exercise test on the top line (*maximum pulse line*), then locate the corresponding 10-second counts on the 85 and 70% lines directly below. These two values represent the limits of target rate range for exercise conditioning. (From Haskell WL. Design and implementation of cardiac conditioning programs. In: Wenger NK, Hellerstein HK, eds. Rehabilitation of the coronary patient. New York: Wiley, 1978;209.)

As discussed earlier, *training is specific to the muscles used in a particular exercise.* Therefore a training session should consist of a variety of activities designed to provide a well-rounded workout. Exercises for both the legs and arms can be incorporated into the session. Aerobic training of the legs can be achieved through bicycling, walking, jogging, and aerobic dance. The arms can be trained with shoulder wheels, rowing machines, and arm ergometers. Swimming, cross-country ski machines, and combination arm–leg cycles are excellent for exercising both lower and upper extremities at the same time.

For selected cardiac patients, *circuit weight training* can be used to improve both aerobic capacity and upper- and lower-body strength (36). Three-year experience with this type of training indicates increased muscle strength and self-efficacy, enhanced compliance with the exercise program, and no cardiac or orthopedic complications (70). In circuit weight training, the patient uses machines, each of which stresses a different muscle group, and moves from weight machine to weight machine, performing for 30 seconds at 40% of maximal capacity, with 30 seconds of rest between each exercise, for a total of 20 minutes. This type of exercise combines elements of dynamic and static forms of exercise. Established exercise guidelines recommend that patients selected for this type of exercise should be preconditioned in a traditional program of walking and jogging for at least 3 months and achieve at least 6 METs on a treadmill test without symptoms or ischemic ECG changes. However, more recent studies demonstrate the safety and efficacy of weight training incorporated into cardiac rehabilitation as soon as 4 weeks after acute MI in selected patients (71,72). An extensive review of the use of weight training in coronary artery disease and hypertension can be found elsewhere (see Stewart in "General References").

Termination of Supervised Training

Criteria for terminating supervised exercise training and transfer to nonsupervised maintenance programs are not clearly established. ECG monitoring for 6 to 8 weeks, and longer, during early exercise programs is generally recommended. Clinical stability and functional capacity above 7 to 8 METs (Table 58.5) are generally accepted exit criteria.

After a few months of supervised exercise, repeated stress testing is useful for measuring the change in physical working capacity and for adjusting more accurately the optimal exercise training intensity.

Long-Term Maintenance of Physical Conditioning

Long-term compliance with formal exercise programs is often poor. It is necessary to exercise regularly at the proper intensity, frequency, and duration if physical fitness is to be maintained. Measurable deterioration in the conditioning effect occurs after missing only a few weeks. The time required to retrieve lost ground seems to be directly related to the length of time without exercise and the degree of physical fitness achieved before cessation of exercise. Exercise must become a part of a person's weekly routine, not something that is done only sporadically or only during the recovery from MI.

General References*

1996 Surgeon General's Report on Physical Activity and Health (S/N 017-023-00196-5). U.S. Department of Health and Human Services, Centers for Disease Control and Prevention, National Center for Chronic Disease Prevention and Health Promotion, The President's Council on Physical Fitness and Sports.

Significant reviews and summaries promoting the benefits of lifestyle changes.

American Association of Cardiovascular and Pulmonary Rehabilitation. **Guidelines for cardiac rehabilitation programs.** Champaign, IL, Human Kinetics, 1991.

Provides criteria for patient selection and exercise training.

Clinical Guideline Parts I and II. Guidelines for risk stratification after myocardial infarction (American College of Physicians). Ann Intern Med 126:556, 561, 1997.

Guidelines based on critical assessment of 280 published articles. Excellent explanation of the evidence base for rational and cost-effective predischarge care of MI patients.

Expert Panel on Detection, Evaluation, and Treatment of High Blood Cholesterol in Adults. **National Cholesterol in Education Program: second report of the Expert Panel on Detection, Evaluation, and Treatment of High Blood Cholesterol in Adults (Adult Treatment Panel II).** Circulation 89:1329–1445, 1994.

Detailed review of evidence plus explicit guidelines for controlling lipid levels in patients with and without CAD.

Greenland P, Chu JS. **Efficacy of cardiac rehabilitation services with emphasis on patients after myocardial infarction.** Ann Intern Med 109:650, 1988.

Review paper.

Hennekens CH, Albert CM, Goldfried SL, et al. **Adjunctive drug therapy of acute myocardial infarction: evidence from clinical trials.** N Engl J Med 335:1660–1667, 1996.

Critical review of all clinical trials of the use of ACE inhibitors, nitrates, CCBs, antiarrhythmic agents, magnesium in patients with MI.

Peterson DM. **Exercise and physical activity in the adult population: a general internist's perspective.** J Gen Intern Med 8:149, 1993.

Review of benefits and risks of physical activity. Contains specific instructions for patients for whom the primary physician recommends exercise.

Physical activity and cardiovascular health. NIH Consensus Statement 13(3):1–33, Dec. 18–20, 1995.

Expert panel reviews data suggesting physical activity as a major focus for prevention.

Physical activity and public health: a recommendation from the Centers for Disease Control and Prevention and the American College of Sports Medicine. JAMA 273:4, 1995.

Summary statements by organizations heading effort to promote increasing physical activity as a means of prevention.

Stewart KJ. **Weight training in coronary artery disease and hypertension.** Prog Cardiovasc Dis 35(2):159, 1992.

Review article.

Wenger NK, Froelicher ES, Smith LK, et al. **Cardiac rehabilitation clinical guideline no. 17.** Rockville, MD: U.S. Department of Health and Human Services, Public Health Service, Agency for Health Care Policy and Research and National Heart, Lung, and Blood Institute. AHCPR Pub. No. 96-0673, October 1995.

Written by leaders in the field of cardiac rehabilitation and based on critical review of published research.

Books for Laypeople on Exercise and Conditioning

American College of Sports Medicine. ACSM fitness book. Champaign, IL: Human Kinetics, 1992.

Iknoian T. Fitness walking. Champaign, IL: Human Kinetics, 1995.

Sharkey BJ. Fitness and health. 4th ed. Champaign, IL: Human Kinetics, 1997.

---

*Bold print (general references) and bold numerals (specific references) denote published controlled clinical trials, meta-analyses, or consensus-based recommendations.

Specific References

1. Antiplatelet Trialists' Collaboration. Collaborative overview of randomized trials of antiplatelet therapy. I. Prevention of death, myocardial infarction, and stroke by prolonged antiplatelet therapy in various categories of patients. BMJ 308:81, 1994.
2. Baile WF, Engel BT. A behavioral strategy for promoting treatment compliance following myocardial infarction. Psychosom Med 40:412, 1978.
3. Blair SN, Kohn HW, Paffenbarger RS Jr, et al. Physical fitness and all-cause mortality: a prospective study of healthy men and women. JAMA 262:2395, 1989.
4. Blakenhorn DH, Nessim SA, Johnson RL, et al. Beneficial effects of combined cholesterol-niacin therapy on coronary atherosclerosis and coronary venous bypass grafts. JAMA 257:3233, 1987.
5. Braunwald E. Treatment of the patient after myocardial infarction. N Engl J Med 302:290, 1980.
6. Carney RM, Rich MW, Tevelde A, et al. Major depressive disorders in coronary artery disease. Am J Cardiol 60:1273, 1987.
7. Chadda K, Goldstein S, Byington R, et al. Effect of propranolol after acute myocardial infarction. Circulation 73:503, 1986.
8. Chandra NC, Rogers WJ, Tiefenbrunn WJ, et al. The National Registry of Myocardial Infarction Registry Investigators. J Am Coll Cardiol 21:237A, 1993.
9. Coats AJS, Adampoulos S, Meyer TC, et al. Effects of physical training in chronic heart failure. Lancet 335:63, 1990.
10. Cooper KH, ed. The new aerobics. New York: Bantam Books, 1970.
11. Council on Scientific Affairs, American Medical Association. Physician-supervised exercise programs in rehabilitation of patients with coronary heart disease. JAMA 245:1463, 1981.
12. DeBusk RF. Report of the twentieth Bethesda Conference. Insurability and employability of the patient with ischemic heart disease. 38th Annual Scientific Session. Anaheim, CA: American College of Cardiology, March 1989.
13. DeBusk RF, Valdez R, Houston N, Haskell W. Cardiovascular responses to dynamic and status efforts soon after myocardial infarction. Circulation 58:368, 1978.
14. Duncan JJ, Gordon NF, Scott CB. Women walking for health and fitness. How much is enough? JAMA 266:3295, 1991.
15. Duryee R. The efficacy of inpatient education after myocardial infarction. Heart Lung 21:217, 1992.
16. Echt DS, Liebson PR, Mitchell LB, et al. Mortality and morbidity in patients receiving encainide, flecainide, or placebo: The Cardiac Arrhythmia Suppression Trial. N Engl J Med 324:781, 1991.
17. Ehsani AA, Heath GH, Hagberg JM, et al. Effects of 12 months of intense exercise training on ischemic ST-depression in patients with coronary artery disease. Circulation 64:1116, 1981.
18. Ellerbeck EF, Jencks SF, Radford MJ, et al. Quality of care for Medicare patients with acute myocardial infarction: a four-state pilot study from the cooperative cardiovascular project. JAMA 273:1509–1514, 1995.
19. Ewart CK, Stewart KJ, Kelemen MH, et al. Self-efficacy mediates strength gains during circuit weight training in men with coronary artery disease. Med Sci Sports Exerc 18(5):531, 1986.
20. Ewart CK, Taylor CB, Reese LB, DeBusk RF. Effects of early postmyocardial infarction exercise testing on self-perception and subsequent physical activity. Am J Cardiol 51:1076, 1983.
21. Falk RH, Pollak A, Tandon PK, et al. The effect of warfarin on prevalence of stroke in patients with severe heart failure (Abstract). J Am Coll Cardiol 21:218A, 1993.
22. Frasure-Smith N, Lesperance F, Talajic M. Depression following myocardial infarction. Impact on 6-month survival. JAMA 270:1819, 1993.
23. Friedman M. Diagnosis and treatment of type A behavior as a medical disorder. Prim Cardiol 15:68, 1989,
24. Friedman PL, Stevenson WG. Unsustained ventricular tachycardia: to treat or not to treat. N Engl J Med 335:1984–1985, 1996.
25. Furberg CD, Friedwald WT, Eberlein KA. Proceedings of the workshop on the implications of recent beta-blocker trials for postmyocardial infarction patients. Circulation 67:1, 1983.
26. Furberg CD, Psaty BM, Meyer JV. Nifedipine: dose-related increase in mortality in patients with coronary heart disease. Circulation 92(5):1326–1330, 1995.
27. Gibson RS, Beller GA, Gheorghiade M, et al. The prevalence and clinical significance of residual myocardial ischemia two weeks after uncomplicated non–Q wave infarction: a prospective natural history study. Circulation 73:1186, 1986.
28. Gibson RS, Boden WE, Theroux P, and Diltiazem Reinfarction Study Group. Diltiazem and reinfarction in patients with non–Q wave myocardial infarction. Results of a double blind, randomized multi-center trial. N Engl J Med 315:423, 1986.
29. Gillilan RE, Chopra AK, Kelemen MH, et al. Prediction of compliance to target heart rate during walk-job exercise in cardiac patients by a self-efficacy scale. Med Sci Sports Exerc 16:115, 1984.
30. Goldstein RE, Boccuzzi S, Eruess D, et al. Effects of diltiazem on occurrence of heart failure after myocardial infarction (Abstract). Circulation 80(Suppl):II-50, 1989.
31. Grines C, Demaria A. Optimal utilization of thrombolytic therapy for acute myocardial infarction: concepts and controversies. J Am Coll Cardiol 16:223, 1990.
32. Gurwitz JH, Gore JM, Goldberg RJ, et al. Recent age-related trends in the use of thrombolytic therapy in patients who have had acute myocardial infarction. National Registry of Myocardial Infarction. Ann Intern Med 124:283–291, 1996.
33. Gutmann MC, Squires RW, Pollack ML, et al. Perceived exertion–heart rate relationship during exercise testing and training in cardiac patients. J Cardiovasc Rehab 1:52, 1981.
34. Heart and Stroke Facts. 1997 Statistical supplement. Dallas: American Heart Association, 1997.
35. Hellerstein HK, Friedman EH. Sexual activity in the post-coronary patient. Arch Intern Med 125:987, 1970.
36. Kelemen MH, Stewart KJ, Gillilan RE, et al. Circuit weight training in cardiac patients. J Am Coll Cardiol 7:38, 1986.
37. Kleber FX. Slowing congestive heart failure's course with angiotensin-converting enzyme inhibition. Cardiol Rev Board 10:64, 1993.
38. Kronmal RA, Cain KC, Ye Z, et al. Total serum cholesterol levels and mortality risk as a function of age: a report based on the Framingham data. Arch Intern Med 53:1065, 1993.
39. Krum H, Schwartz B, Sackner-Bernstein J, et al. Double blind, placebo controlled study of long term efficacy of carvedilol in patients with severe heart failure treated with converting enzyme inhibitors (Abstract). J Am Coll Cardiol 21:114A, 1993.
40. Levy RI, Feinlab M. Risk factors for coronary artery disease and their management. In: Braunwald E, ed. Heart disease: a textbook for cardiovascular medicine. Philadelphia: WB Saunders, 1984.
41. Lipid Research Clinics Coronary Primary Prevention Trial Results. I: Reduction in incidence of coronary heart disease. JAMA 251:351, 1984.
42. Lorenz RL et al. Improved aortocoronary bypass patency by low-dose aspirin (100 mg daily): effects on platelet aggregation and thromboxane formation. Lancet 1:1261, 1984.
43. Manninen V, Elo O, Heikki F, et al. Lipid alterations and decline in incidence of coronary heart disease in the Helsinki Heart Study. JAMA 260:641, 1988.
44. Mark D, Froelicher V. Exercise treadmill testing and ambulatory monitoring. In: Califf R, Mark D, Wagner G, eds. Acute coronary care. St. Louis: CV Mosby, 1995;767.
45. Massie BM, Goldstein RE, Hall J, et al. Asymptomatic ventricular arrhythmias do not identify patients with severe heart failure at risk for sudden death: results of the PROMISE Trial (Abstract). J Am Coll Cardiol 21:459A, 1993.
46. Mather HG, Pearson NG, Read KLQ, et al. Acute myocardial infarction: home and hospital treatment. BMJ 1:334, 1971.
47. Meizlish JL, Berger HJ, Plankey M, et al. Functional left ventricular aneurysm after acute myocardial infarction. N Engl J Med 16:1001, 1984.
48. Milani RV, Lavie CJ, Cassidy MM. Effects of cardiac rehabilitation and exercise training programs on depression in patients after major coronary events. Am Heart J 132:726, 1996.
49. Moss AJ, Goldstein RE, Hall J, et al. Detection and significance of myocardial ischemia in stable patients after recovery from acute event. JAMA 269:2379, 1993.

49a. Moss AJ, Hall WJ, Cannom DS, et al. Improved survival with an implanted defibrillator in patients with coronary disease at high risk for ventricular arrhythmias. N Engl J Med 335:1933–1940, 1996.

50. Muller D, Topol E. Selection of patients with acute myocardial infarction for thrombolytic therapy. Ann Intern Med 113:949, 1990.

51. Multicenter Diltiazem Post-Infarction Trial Research Group. The effect of diltiazem on mortality and reinfarction after myocardial infarction. N Engl J Med 319:385, 1988.

51a. Myerburg RJ, Castellanos A. Clinical trials of implantable defibrillator. N Engl J Med 337:1621–1623, 1997.

52. Oldridge NB, Guyatt GH, Fischer ME, et al. Cardiac rehabilitation after myocardial infarction: combined experience of randomized clinical trials. JAMA 260:945, 1988.

53. Ornish DM, Scherwitz LW, Brown SC. Can lifestyle changes reverse atherosclerosis? (Abstract) Circulation 78:II-11, 1988.

54. Pfeffer M, Braunwald E, Moye L, et al. Effect of captopril on mortality and morbidity in patients with left ventricular dysfunction after myocardial infarction. N Engl J Med 327:669, 1992.

55. Plotnick GD. Approach to the management of unstable angina. Am Heart J 98:243, 1979.

56. Randomised trial of cholesterol lowering in 4444 patients with coronary heart disease: the Scandinavian Simvastatin Survival Study (4S). Lancet 344:1383–1389, 1994.

57. Randomised trial of effect of amiodarone on mortality in patients with left-ventricular dysfunction after recent myocardial infarction: European Myocardial Infarct Amiodarone Trial Investigators. Lancet 349:667–674, 1997.

58. Randomised trial of intravenous streptokinase, oral aspirin, both or neither among 17,187 cases of suspected acute myocardial infarction. ISIS-2. Lancet 2:349, 1988.

59. Randomised trial of outcome after myocardial infarction in patients with frequent or repetitive ventricular premature depolarisations. Canadian Amiodarone Myocardial Infarction Arrhythmia Trial Investigators. Lancet 349:675–682, 1997.

60. Rosati RA, Harris PJ. Acute myocardial infarction. In: Fries JF, Ehrlich GE, eds. Prognosis: contemporary outcomes of disease. Bowie, MD: Charles Press, 1981.

61. Rossouw JE, Lewis B, Rifkind BM. The value of lowering cholesterol after myocardial infarction. N Engl J Med 323:1112, 1990.

62. Russell RO Jr, Abi-Mansour P, Wenger NK, et al. Return to work after coronary artery bypass surgery and percutaneous transluminal angioplasty: issues and potential solutions. Cardiology 73:306, 1986.

63. Sacks FM, Pfeffer MA, Moye LA, et al. The effect of pravastatin on coronary events after myocardial infarction in patients with average cholesterol level. N Engl J Med 335:1001–1009, 1996.

64. Schaffer WA, Cobb LA. Recurrent ventricular fibrillation and modes of death in survivors of out-of-hospital ventricular fibrillation. N Engl J Med 293:259, 1975.

65. Schleifer SJ, Macari-Hinson MM, Coyle DA, et al. The nature and course of depression following myocardial infarction. Arch Intern Med 149:1785, 1989.

66. Schuler G, Hambrecht R, Schlierf G, et al. Regular exercise and low fat diet: effects on progression of coronary artery disease. Circulation 86:1, 1992.

67. SOLVD Investigators. Effects of enalapril on mortality and development of heart failure in asymptomatic patients with reduced left ventricular ejection fractions. N Engl J Med 32:685, 1992.

68. Stamler J. Acute myocardial infarction: progress in primary prevention. Br Heart J 33:145, 1971.

69. Stewart KJ, Effron MB, Vaeni SA, Keleman MH. Effects of diltiazem or propranolol during exercise training of hypertensive men. Med Sci Sports Exerc 22(2):171, 1990.

70. Stewart KJ, Mason M, Kelemen MH. Three year participation in circuit weight training improves muscular strength and self-efficacy in cardiac patients. J Cardiopulm Rehab 8:292, 1988.

71. Stewart KJ, McFarland LD, Weinhofer JJ, et al. No evidence for adverse clinical responses with weight training after acute MI. Med Sci Sports Exerc 27(5):S32, 1995.

72. Stewart KJ, McFarland LD, Weinhofer JJ, et al. Weight training soon after myocardial infarction. Med Sci Sports Exerc 27(5):32, 1994.

73. Sullivan MJ, Higgambotham MB, Cobb FR. Exercise training in patients with severe left ventricular dysfunction: hemodynamics and metabolic effects. Circulation 78:506, 1988.

74. Taylor JL, Copeland RB, Cousin AL, et al. The effect of isometric exercise on the graded exercise test in patients with stable angina. J Cardiopulm Rehab 1:450, 1981.

75. Theroux P, Marpole DGF, Bourassa MG. Exercise stress testing in the postmyocardial infarction patient. Am J Cardiol 52:664, 1983.

75a. The Antiarrhythmic versus Implantable Defibrillator (AVID) Investigators. A comparison of antiarrhythmic-drug therapy with implantable defibrillator in patients resuscitated form near-fatal ventricular arrhythmias N Engl J Med 337:1576–1583, 1997.

76. Thornton MA, Greventzig AR, Hollman J, et al. Coumadin and aspirin in prevention of recurrence after transluminal coronary angioplasty: a randomized study. Circulation 69:72, 1984.

77. Toffler GH, Stone PH, Muller JC, et al. Effect of gender and race in prognosis after MI: adverse prognosis for women, particularly black women. J Am Coll Cardiol 9:473, 1987.

78. Ueno M. The so-called coitus death. Jpn J Legal Med 17:330, 1963.

79. U.S. Department of Health and Human Services, Public Service Agency for Health Care Policy and Research, National Heart, Lung and Blood Institute. Clinical practice guideline. Unstable angina: diagnosis and management. AHCPR Publication No. 94-0602, No. 10, March, 1994.

80. van Ravenswaaij CMA, Kollee LAA, Hopman JCW, et al. Heart rate variability. Ann Intern Med 118:436, 1993.

81. Viscoli CM, Horowitz RI, Singer BH. Beta blockers after myocardial infarction: influence of first year clinical course on long-term effectiveness. Ann Intern Med 118:99, 1993.

82. Waters DD, Theroux P, Halphen C, Mizgala HF. Clinical predictors of angina following myocardial infarction. Am J Med 66:991, 1979.

83. Wilhelmsson C, Vedin JA, Elmfeldt D, et al. Smoking and myocardial infarction. Lancet 1:415, 1975.

84. Yusuf S, Collins R, Peto R, et al. Intravenous and intracoronary fibrinolytic therapy in acute myocardial infarction: overview of results on mortality, re-infarction and side effects from 33 randomized controlled trails. Eur Heart J 6:556, 1985.

85. Zohman LR: Beyond diet. Exercise your way to fitness and heart health. Englewood Cliffs, NJ: Mazola Products, Best Food, 1974.

C H A P T E R   59

Arrhythmias

SHELDON H. GOTTLIEB, MD
HUGH CALKINS, MD

Contraction of the heart is normally the result of a well-orchestrated electromechanical system. The orderly function of the system is maintained by the domination of the heart rate by a single pulse generator known as the pacemaker, by the relatively fast and uniform conduction of the electrical signal via specialized conduction pathways, and by the relatively long and uniform duration of the electrical signal relative to its velocity of conduction through these pathways, which ensures uniform electrical excitation and contraction of the heart. An arrhythmia is any disturbance in the normal sequence of impulse generation and conduction in the heart.

Arrhythmias may occur in the absence of heart disease, or they may be symptoms of severe disease or may themselves cause disease. Their significance and the need for treatment must be evaluated in the context of the clinical situation in which they occur. A precise etiologic diagnosis and an understanding of the pharmacology of the medications used are necessary to treat arrhythmias effectively.

PHYSIOLOGY OF IMPULSE GENERATION AND CONDUCTION

Action Potential

Muscle contraction is stimulated by an electrical impulse, the action potential. In skeletal muscle, the action potential lasts several milliseconds, and the electrical activity is essentially dissipated before the beginning of contraction. In cardiac muscle, however, the action potential lasts several hundred milliseconds, almost as long as the contraction itself (Fig. 59.1). In this way, the action potential not only stimulates contraction of the heart but also determines the duration and intensity of contraction. Furthermore, as long as the action potential is maintained, the heart cannot be stimulated to contract again.

The action potential is generated by depolarization and repolarization of the muscle cell (Fig. 59.2). In the resting state the intracellular concentration of potassium is high and that of sodium is low compared with the extracellular fluid. These gradients are maintained by metabolic activity within the cell membrane. The resting membrane potential is strongly negative (i.e., there is an electrochemical gradient across the membrane so that the inside of the membrane is negatively charged compared with the outside of the membrane). If an electrical stimulus is applied, the membrane becomes very permeable to sodium ions, which rapidly leak into the cell (phase 0). The membrane is thus depolarized (loses its negative charge) and, in fact, is transiently positively charged (overshoot). Repolarization occurs relatively slowly as chloride (phase 1), calcium ions (phase 2), and then potassium ions (phase 3) move back into the cell and thereby restore resting potential (phase 4) (Fig. 59.2) (54).

Relationship to the Electrocardiogram

In the heart the phases of rapid depolarization and overshoot correspond to the QRS complex of the electrocardiogram (ECG); phase 2 corresponds to the ST segment; and phase 3, to the T wave (Fig. 59.2). During phase 2 the membrane is absolutely and in phase 3 relatively refractory to propagation of another electrical impulse.

Fast and Slow Currents

In most cardiac tissue, excitation is propagated by the rapidly depolarizing sodium current so that the impulses are conducted rapidly. However, in

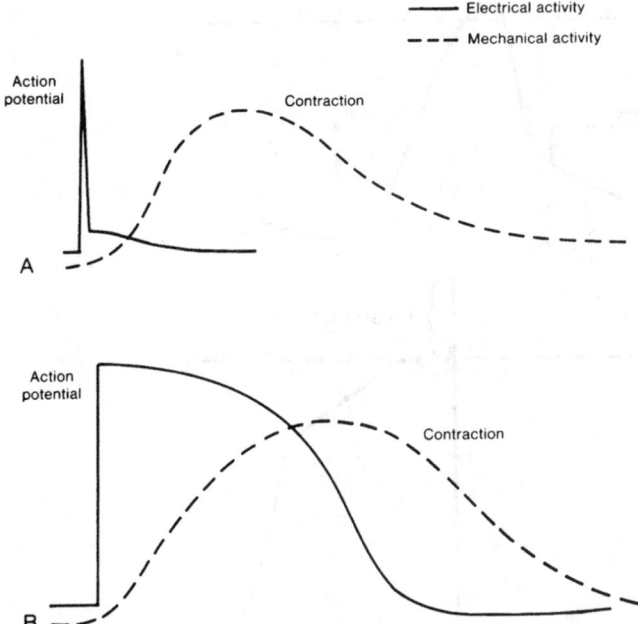

———— Electrical activity

- - - - Mechanical activity

Action potential

Contraction

A

Action potential

Contraction

B

Figure 59.1. Comparison between relative time scales of electrical *(continuous curve)* and mechanical *(interrupted curve)* activity in skeletal **(A)** and cardiac **(B)** muscle. (From Noble D. The initiation of the heart beat. Oxford, England: Clarendon Press, 1975.)

the sinoatrial node and the proximal part of the atrioventricular (AV) node, excitation is propagated by a slowly depolarizing current generated by the influx of calcium ions into the cell. Also, in diseased cardiac muscle, the sodium current may be inhibited and depolarization may occur entirely via the slow calcium current; therefore, the action potential may be conducted very slowly. This difference in conduction velocity between cells depolarized by the sodium versus the calcium current has important implications in the generation and treatment of arrhythmias (see below).

Pacemaker Generation

In most cardiac cells, an action potential is not generated until an electrical stimulus is applied. In pacemaker cells, slow spontaneous depolarization occurs until a threshold is reached, whereupon phase 0 rapidly ensues (Fig. 59.2); this process is called automaticity. In the absence of heart block, the heart rate is controlled by the pacemaker cells that depolarize most rapidly because then the action potential is conducted rapidly throughout the heart and initiates rapid depolarization of other cells, even if they already have begun spontaneous slow depolarization. Automaticity is affected by the rate of slow spontaneous depolarization and the threshold potential. Automaticity is enhanced by increased sympathetic tone, decreased vagal tone, increased catecholamine concentration in the blood, thyroid hormone, and digitalis. It is suppressed by decreased sympathetic tone, increased vagal tone, decreased thyroid hormone concentration, and various drugs (e.g., the drugs used in the treatment of arrhythmias). Antiarrhythmic drugs

may also increase automaticity under some conditions; this phenomenon is known as proarrhythmogenesis and is discussed below.

Impulse Generation and Conduction

Sinoatrial Node

The sinoatrial (SA) node is composed of pacemaker cells and is located at the junction of the right atrium and the superior vena cava (Fig. 59.3). The cells of the SA node spontaneously depolarize more rapidly than any other cells within the heart and thereby control the heart rate.

Atrioventricular Node

The AV node is the part of the specialized conduction system that carries the electrical impulse from the atrium to the ventricle. The AV node lies at the junction of the right atrium and the interventricular septum just above the tricuspid valve. Conduction through the AV node, which is mediated by calcium channels, is unique in that conduction is relatively slow, thereby resulting in a 100- to 200-msec delay between activation of the atria and ventricles. This delay is important because it ensures that ventricular contraction occurs after atrial contraction is complete, which maximizes filling of the ventricle with blood. Another unique property of the AV node is that conduction is decremental. This means that as more impulses arrive at the AV node, fewer get through, and those that do conduct through the AV node travel at a slower rate. The property of decremental conduction allows the AV node to serve as a protective gate that does not respond to extremely rapid impulses generated in the atria, thereby protecting the ventricles from rapid stimulation (e.g., during atrial fibrillation). The AV node also has intrinsic pacemaker activity, similar to that of the sinus node but slower (usually at a rate of 40 to 60 beats/minute). Because of the slower rate, the AV node may function as a subsidiary pacemaker if the SA node fails.

Bundle of His

When the action potential leaves the AV node, it enters the specialized conducting fibers known as the bundle of His. The main bundle of His divides into three branches: the right bundle branch, which runs along the right ventricular surface of the septum, the anterior superior branch, which runs along the left ventricular surface of the septum, and the posterior inferior branch, which runs along the posterior wall of the left ventricle. The action potential is conducted through the bundle branches and into the myocardium by a widespread network of smaller fibers known as Purkinje fibers.

MECHANISM OF CARDIAC ARRHYTHMIAS

There are three basic causes of disturbance in the rhythm of the heart: suppression or enhancement of initiation or propagation of the action potential,

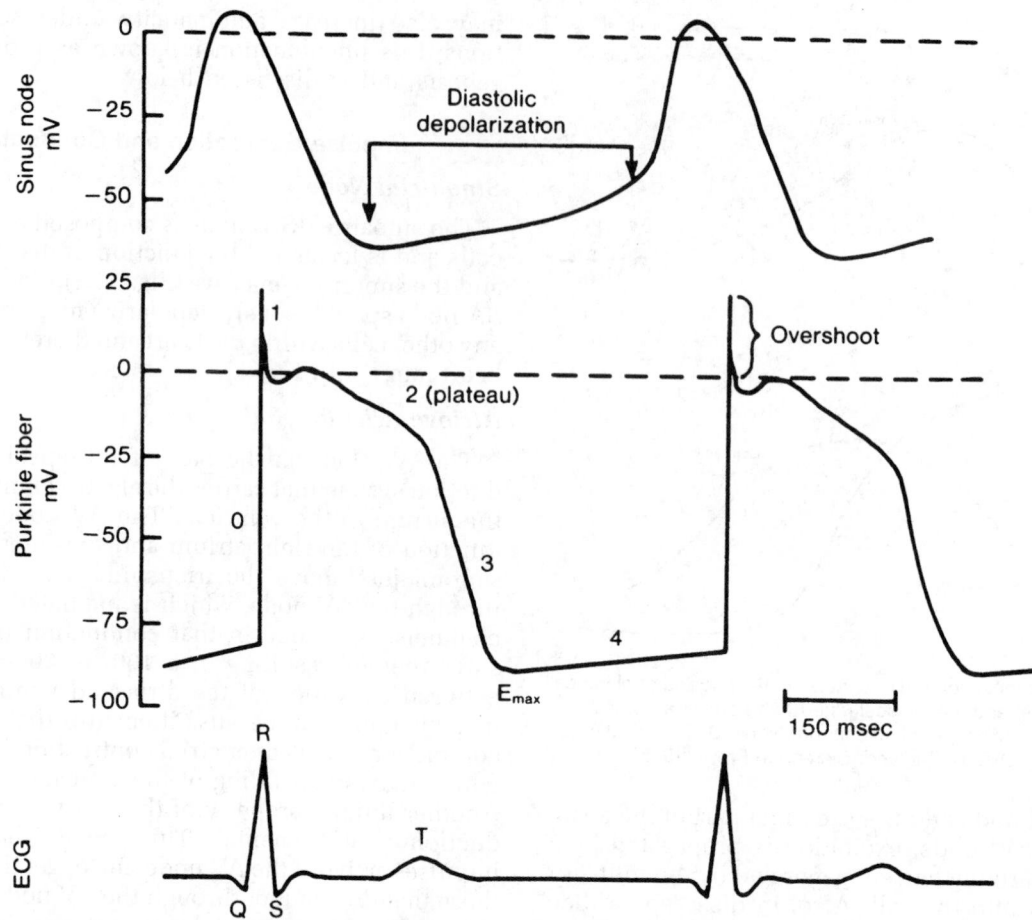

Figure 59.2.   Transmembrane potentials from the sinus node and a Purkinje fiber. Note the spontaneous diastolic depolarization in the upper panel, characteristic of pacemaker fibers. The numbers in the middle panel are explained in the text. The lower panel shows the correlation of the time sequence of changes in the action potential with the surface electrocardiogram. Alterations in depolarization are reflected in changes in the QRS duration of the surface record; those in repolarization are associated with alterations in the Q–T interval. (From Singh BN, Collett JT, Chew CYC. New perspectives in the pharmacologic therapy of cardiac arrhythmias. Prog Cardiovasc Dis 22:243, 1980.)

reentry of the action potential into a pathway through which it has already passed, and triggered activity (54). More than one of these mechanisms may be operative in producing a particular arrhythmia (e.g., ectopic supraventricular tachycardia in a patient with sinus node dysfunction).

Suppression or Enhancement of Initiation or Propagation of Action Potential

A disease process that interferes with pacemaker activity within the SA node or with the movement of the electrical impulse through the normal conduction pathways of the heart results in abnormal slowing of the heart rate (bradyarrhythmia) and/or in one of the various forms of heart block.

Enhanced automaticity of a part of the cardiac conduction system may result in the initiation of an impulse more rapidly than is normally generated by the SA node. If that happens episodically, occasional premature contractions occur, the nature of which

depends on the location of the ectopic pacemaker. On the other hand, if there is rapid sustained firing of the ectopic focus, a tachyarrhythmia ensues.

Reentry

Most clinically significant arrhythmias result from reentry (Fig. 59.4). Reentrant arrhythmias occur in the setting of two anatomically or functionally distinct conduction pathways, unidirectional conduction block in one of the pathways, and slowed conduction. When these three conditions are fulfilled, the electrical impulse may travel down one limb of the reentrant circuit and return via the second limb of the circuit, resulting in a "short circuit" or "circus" arrhythmia. The conditions needed for the development of reentrant arrhythmias often occur in the setting of structural heart disease or, less commonly, result from anatomic abnormalities such as an accessory AV connection, as in the case of the Wolff–Parkinson–White (WPW) syndrome.

Triggered Activity

Triggered arrhythmias are less common; they result from afterdepolarizations that follow an action potential and that reach threshold for triggering additional impulses (53). Examples of triggered arrhythmias include torsades de pointes, multifocal atrial tachycardia, and atrial tachycardia resulting from digitalis toxicity (see below).

DIAGNOSIS OF ARRHYTHMIAS: GENERAL CONSIDERATIONS

History

Arrhythmias may or may not cause symptoms. Symptoms are caused by an appreciation of the irregular rhythm (palpitations) or by a reduction in cardiac output (light-headedness, dizziness, presyncope, syncope, dyspnea, diaphoresis, chest pain, anxiety).

When taking a history from a patient with a suspected arrhythmia, it is important to define the onset, regularity, and duration of symptoms, and whether any factors seem to trigger symptoms (e.g., drinking coffee, smoking, exercise, emotional stress, and taking or forgetting to take medications). It may be helpful to ask the patient to tap with his or her fingers the speed and rhythm of the palpitations.

It is important to determine whether there is a history or symptoms of an underlying disease that may be associated with arrhythmia (e.g., hypertension, heart failure, ischemic or valvular heart disease, thyrotoxicosis) because the prognosis and recommended treatment depend to a large extent on the nature and severity of underlying heart disease. Patients should be asked about a family history of arrhythmias or sudden death; the taking of stimulant drugs either illicitly (see Chapter 22) or as an attempt to lose weight (see Chapter 76); and about the taking of prescription drugs that may cause arrhythmias (digitalis, theophylline, diuretics, β-blockers, β-agonists, tricyclic antidepressants, and antihypertensives).

Palpitations are heartbeats that are sensed, usually because the beats are fast or irregular. However, they do not necessarily imply a significant arrhythmia and they may represent only sinus tachycardia in an otherwise healthy person, especially if the patient is prone to somatization and hypochondriasis. In contrast, patients with paroxysmal supraventricular arrhythmias may be misdiagnosed as having a panic disorder (see

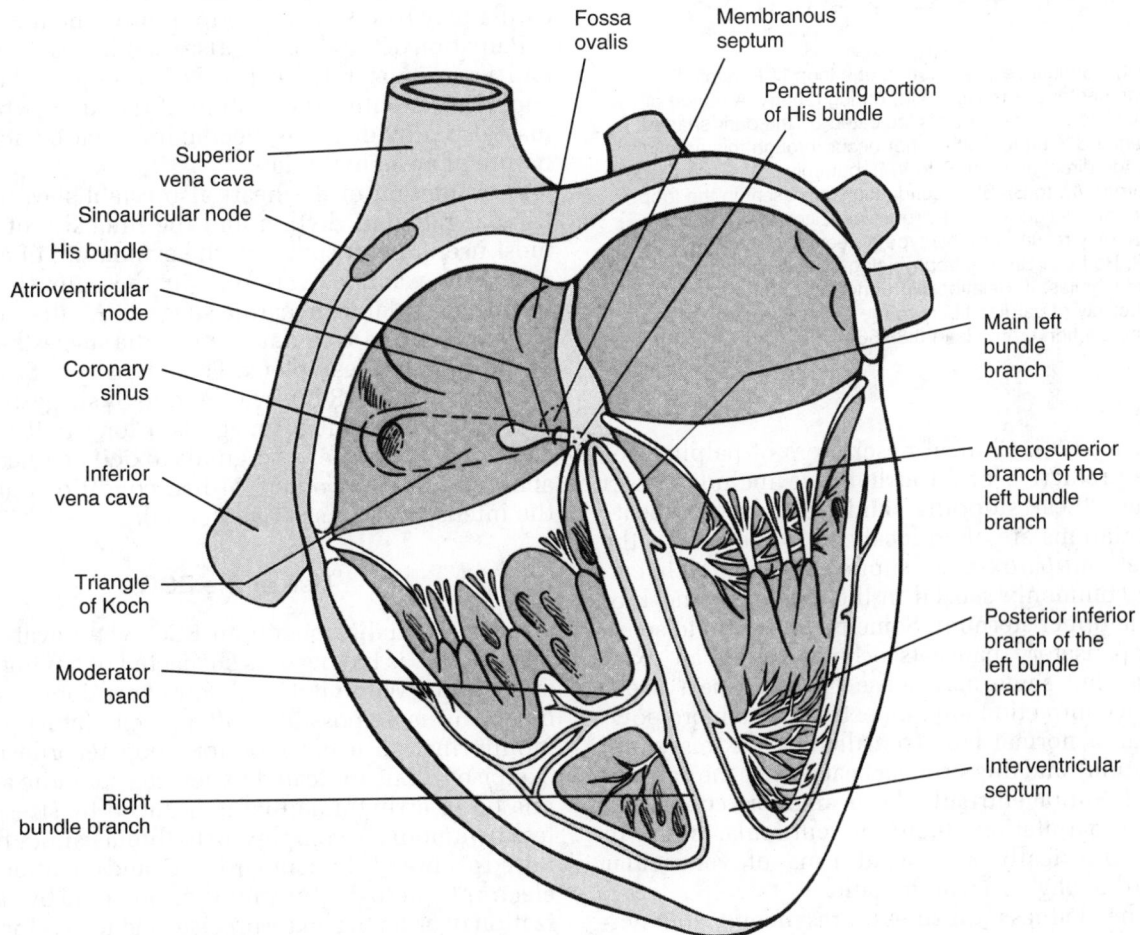

Figure 59.3. Anatomy of impulse generation.

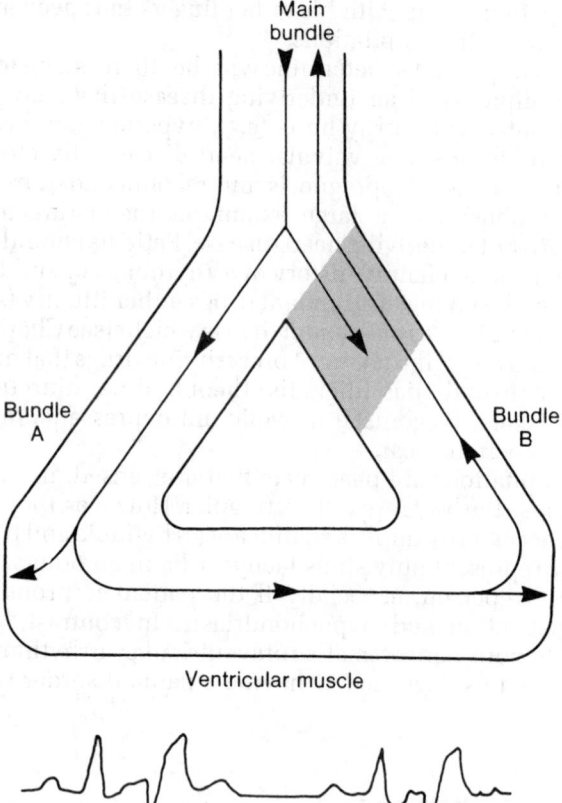

Figure 59.4. Sequence of activation of a loop of Purkinje fiber bundles and ventricular muscle *(VM)* during reentry. A region of unidirectional conduction block is indicated by the dark shaded area in branch B. Conduction cannot occur through this area in the antegrade direction (from B to VM), but only in the retrograde direction (from VM to B). Slow conduction is present in the loop. The bottom of the figure shows a possible electrocardiographic pattern that may result from this type of reentry. (From Wit AL, Rosen MR, Hoffman BF. Electrophysiology and pharmacology of cardiac arrhythmias. II. Relationship of normal and abnormal electrical activity of cardiac fibers to the genesis of arrhythmias. B. Re-entry, Section I. Am Heart J 88:664, 1974.)

Chapter 13) (26). Clinical descriptors of palpitations that are predictive of an arrhythmia include "heart fluttering," "heart stopping," and "irregular heartbeat" (1). Palpitations are often localized to the area of the apex beat, but paroxysmal supraventricular tachycardias are commonly sensed in the side of the neck or under the upper sternum. Some people seem to sense the compensatory pause (see below) after an extra heartbeat, but some may sense the extra beat itself. Often the contraction after an extra beat is more powerful than a normal beat (so-called postextrasystolic potentiation), and this stronger beat may be the one that is sensed. Supraventricular beats are more commonly sensed as palpitations than are ventricular beats; in fact, prognostically significant runs of ventricular tachycardia may be asymptomatic.

Light-headedness, dizziness, presyncope, and syncope are common symptoms of life-threatening arrhythmias, especially in the elderly. These symptoms

and the conditions associated with them are discussed in detail in Chapter 81.

Physical Examination

Paroxysmal arrhythmias are rarely present when the patient is being examined and attention should therefore be focused on obtaining orthostatic vital signs, and examining the patient for conditions associated with arrhythmia, such as hypertensive heart disease (Chapter 62), heart failure (Chapter 61), chronic obstructive lung disease (Chapter 55), ischemic heart disease (Chapter 57), or valvular heart disease (Chapter 60). These conditions can often be recognized by characteristic physical findings.

In the unusual case that a paroxysmal arrhythmia is present when the patient is being seen, or in the case of chronic or incessant arrhythmia, the characteristics of the arrhythmia are best revealed on physical examination by inspection of the jugular pulse, palpation of the arterial pulse, and auscultation of the heart.

Inspection of the jugular venous pulse may reveal atrial activity. If there is AV dissociation or complete heart block, so-called cannon waves may be seen intermittently in the jugular veins; they are caused by ejection of blood back into the veins when the right atrium contracts against a closed tricuspid valve. Atrial tachycardia may be revealed by rapid, prominent A waves.

Palpation of the arterial pulse establishes the rhythm and ventricular rate, at least of conducted beats. In conjunction with examination of the jugular pulse, it may also provide more specific information about the nature of an arrhythmia.

Auscultation of the heart also establishes the ventricular rate and rhythm and the intensity of S_1, the most useful heart sound in the evaluation of arrhythmia. For example, variation in the intensity of S_1 during a regular tachycardia suggests AV dissociation; variation during a regular bradycardia suggests second- or third-degree heart block. The intensity of S_1 is also a function of the P–R interval. A loud S_1 suggests a short P–R interval; a soft S_1 suggests a long P–R interval, caused, for example, by digitalis toxicity or electrolyte abnormalities (for other cardiac conditions affecting the intensity of S_1, see Chapter 60).

Use of the ECG

It is essential to obtain an ECG when evaluating a patient who is having or is suspected of having had an arrhythmia. Without it, with few exceptions, a specific diagnosis is impossible. Often, ambulatory (Holter) monitoring, an event monitor (loop recorder), or an exercise ECG is indicated to detect a sporadic arrhythmia or an arrhythmia that is induced by stress. Even less commonly, a complex arrhythmia cannot be diagnosed accurately by standard ECG, and an intracavitary electrophysiologic study must be obtained by catheterization in order to make a precise diagnosis. Upright tilt table testing may be necessary to differentiate presyncope or syncope caused by an arrhythmia from neurocardiogenic syncope (also called vasodepressor or vasovagal syncope). The use of this test is discussed in Chapter 81.

Surface Resting ECG

A number of features of the standard ECG must be assessed.

Atrial Activity. Atrial activity is best assessed in leads 2, 3, aVF, and V_1. The presence of P waves must be identified. If P waves are present, their configuration and their relationship to QRS complexes must be established. Normally the P–R interval is between 0.12 and 0.20 second (each 1-mm segment on the ECG = 0.04 second), and each QRS complex is preceded by a P wave whose vector is such that the P wave is upright in leads 2, 3, and aVF. If P waves are not present, other evidence of atrial activity (fibrillation or flutter waves) should be sought.

Ventricular Activity. The duration of the QRS complexes (normally less than 0.10 second) should be measured and the regularity of ventricular activity should be assessed. A basically regular rhythm may be interrupted by so-called premature beats—QRS complexes that appear before the next regular beat is expected. If premature beats are present, it should be noted whether they have a fixed relationship to the preceding normal beat and whether their configuration is the same as that of the regularly occurring complexes.

Ambulatory ECG

The ambulatory (Holter) ECG (46) records on magnetic tape the electrical activity of the heart, usually for a 24- to 48-hour period. The recording device is small and does not interfere with virtually any of the patient's activities (except bathing and swimming). The technique is useful in the following circumstances:

- Assessing whether suspicious symptoms (e.g., palpitation, light-headedness, dizziness, or syncope) in a patient with a normal resting ECG are caused by an episodic arrhythmia
- Assessing whether episodic but potentially life-threatening arrhythmias are occurring in a patient with known heart disease (e.g., ischemic heart disease or congestive heart failure)
- Assessing the efficacy of antiarrhythmic therapy or the function of a cardiac pacemaker
- Assessing whether there is episodic evidence of overt or silent ischemia

A minority of episodic arrhythmias are detected during 24 hours of Holter monitoring (22,27). If symptoms are infrequent it may be necessary to record the ambulatory ECG for 48 to 72 hours or to use an event monitor (see below). The patient should be asked to keep a record of symptoms while being monitored to determine whether those symptoms are attributable to arrhythmia. Patients should be instructed to record symptoms associated with their palpitations, including dizziness, nausea, shortness of breath, chest discomfort, or arm pain (22).

If symptoms are infrequent, an event monitor may be useful in making a diagnosis of an arrhythmia. Event monitors record 30 to 60 seconds of ECG when activated by the patient. The ECG is then transmitted via an audiotelephonic interface to a central monitor, where the rhythm strip is printed out and sent to the referring physician. Recent studies show that event monitors, when used for the diagnosis of intermittent palpitations, are more likely than Holter monitors to record diagnostic arrhythmias and do so at a lower cost (22). The cost of Holter monitoring and event monitoring is approximately 5 to 10 times that of a standard ECG.

Exercise ECG

Exercise ECG is described in detail in Chapter 57. It is a useful test in the evaluation of patients who have symptoms suggestive of an arrhythmia during or after exercise, and in those with premature ventricular contractions to determine whether they become more or less frequent during or after exercise (see below under "Ventricular Premature Beats") (41). It may also be helpful in assessing the adequacy of rate control in patients with atrial fibrillation.

GENERAL PRINCIPLES IN MANAGEMENT OF ARRHYTHMIAS

Once it has been established that a patient has a particular arrhythmia, the physician must decide whether treatment is necessary. A general principle is that treatment should be limited to symptomatic patients with prognostically significant arrhythmias and that antiarrhythmic medications should be avoided whenever possible. It must also be determined whether the arrhythmia is secondary to a noncardiac process (e.g., hypoxia, electrolyte imbalance, fever, drug toxicity) or a cardiac process (e.g., heart failure, ischemia, pericarditis, digitalis intoxication), the correction of which will restore a normal cardiac rhythm.

If specific therapy is indicated, an appropriate regimen must be selected: one or more of the antiarrhythmic drugs, electrical conversion of the arrhythmia, a cardiac pacemaker or antitachycardia device, catheter or surgical ablation of the arrhythmia focus, or a combination of these regimens. It must be determined whether the potential benefits of the proposed antiarrhythmic therapy outweigh the risk of proarrhythmia (see below) and whether the cost, side effects, and inconvenience of the therapy are justified.

An important and often difficult issue to determine is whether hospitalization is required for the initiation of therapy.

A consensus exists that antiarrhythmic therapy should be initiated in the hospital for patients with hemodynamically unstable arrhythmias, such as sustained ventricular tachycardia, or for initiation of antiarrhythmic agents, other than amiodarone, in patients with significantly compromised cardiac function as evidenced by an ejection fraction (EF) below 40%. Antiarrhythmic therapy can be initiated on an ambulatory basis in patients with functionally normal hearts in the absence of a hemodynamically compromising arrhythmia. Amiodarone may be initiated on an inpatient or ambulatory basis in patients without a hemodynamically compromising arrhythmia.

Pharmacology of Antiarrhythmic Drugs

Antiarrhythmic drugs are grouped commonly into four classes (54,57): Class I drugs, whose prototype is quinidine, interfere with the fast inward sodium current. Class II drugs, whose prototype is propranolol, affect sympathetically mediated excitability. Class III drugs, whose prototype is amiodarone, prolong the duration of the action potential by decreasing the late inward (phase 3) potassium current. Class IV drugs, whose prototype is verapamil, block calcium-mediated slow channel currents in the myocardium.

Digitalis and adenosine, both useful antiarrhythmic agents, do not fit into this classification scheme. Strictly speaking, digitalis is not an antiarrhythmic drug in that it does not have a direct effect on membrane function. It acts indirectly as an antiarrhythmic agent by increasing vagal activity, thereby increasing the refractory period of the specialized conduction tissue of the atria and slowing the velocity of the action potential through the AV node. Digitalis also increases the frequency of fibrillatory waves in atrial fibrillation, thereby presenting more impulses to the AV node, making the node refractory to conduction (this process is called concealed conduction). General considerations in the use of digitalis including dosages, choice of a preparation, and recognition and treatment of toxicity are discussed in Chapter 61. The pharmacology and use of adenosine are discussed below.

Table 59.1 shows some of the characteristics of the orally administered antiarrhythmic drugs that can be used to treat an ambulatory patient.

Most antiarrhythmic drugs have a low toxic/therapeutic ratio and some are exceedingly toxic (Table 59.2). In addition to direct toxic effects, antiarrhythmic drugs often have complex interactions with commonly used drugs such as digoxin, warfarin, and certain antihistamines and antibiotics (see below, "Torsades de Pointes") and may paradoxically induce arrhythmias and increase the incidence of sudden cardiac death, a clinical scenario called proarrhythmia. Proarrhythmic effects may include virtually any arrhythmia but often are seen as an increase in the frequency of premature ventricular contractions (PVCs) or the sudden onset of ventricular tachycardia, torsades de pointes (see below), or ventricular fibrillation. Although in the past it was believed that proarrhythmic effects of drugs are usually seen within several days after an antiarrhythmic drug is started or the dosage is changed, the results of the CAST study make it clear that these effects of drugs may be delayed (13). In general, the proarrhythmic effects of antiarrhythmic drugs are usually seen in patients with severe heart disease, as evidenced by an ejection fraction (EF) below 40% (18,38).

The risk of antiarrhythmic drug treatment has been highlighted by several clinical trials and reviews based on meta-analyses. A nearly fourfold increase in mortality has been demonstrated in patients with myocardial dysfunction and nonsustained ventricular tachycardia after a myocardial infarction when they were treated either with flecainide or encainide (13). Also, a significant increase in postmyocardial infarction mortality has been shown in patients treated with any class I antiarrhythmic agent (55). A meta-analysis of patients with atrial fibrillation treated with quinidine showed an increased mortality (8), and an analysis of antiarrhythmic drug use in the Stroke Prevention in Atrial Fibrillation Trial reported nearly a fivefold increased risk of cardiac death among patients with heart failure who were receiving an antiarrhythmic drug (15).

The safe and effective use of antiarrhythmic drugs depends on a careful assessment of the cause and physiology of an arrhythmia and a knowledge of the pharmacology of the drugs that are used. Therefore, dosages must be individualized, and drug levels should be checked periodically (at first, after a steady state has been reached [Table 59.1] and then one to three times a year, depending on the patient's response). Levels should be obtained approximately 4 hours after an oral dose of a drug that is taken every 6 to 8 hours, and approximately 8 to 12 hours after an oral dose of a drug that is taken once a day.

Class I Drugs

All class I drugs block the sodium channel (see above) but the effect on the duration of the action potential and on repolarization varies depending on the kinetics of the blockage (15,16). This has practical application in the choice of drugs for treatment of specific arrhythmias and in the use of a combination of drugs (e.g., mexiletine plus quinidine) (54), although it would be advisable to combine these drugs only after consultation with a cardiologist.

Class I drugs have been subdivided into three classes: IA, IB, and IC (Table 59.1).

Class IA Drugs. Class IA drugs prolong the duration of the action potential (Fig. 59.1) and so prolong the QRS and Q–T interval and the effective refractory period. These drugs include quinidine, procainamide, and disopyramide.

Quinidine. In addition to its direct effects on the heart, *quinidine* blocks parasympathetic stimulation by the vagus nerve and may enhance AV conduction (and the ventricular rate) in some patients. For this reason patients with supraventricular tachyarrhythmias should have their AV nodal rate controlled (e.g., with digitalis or a β-blocker) before they are given quinidine. Quinidine also is a moderately potent inhibitor of α-adrenergic activity and may cause orthostatic hypotension.

Several preparations of quinidine are available; quinidine sulfate is the recommended preparation on the basis of cost, but quinidine gluconate may have fewer gastrointestinal (GI) side effects. A sustained-release preparation containing gluconate (Quinaglute,

Table 59.1. Characteristics of Antiarrhythmic Drugs

Drug	Common Brand Name	Effects on ECG	Half-Life (hr)	Time to Steady State (days)	Available Strength (mg)	Usual Oral Dosage	Maximal Daily Dosage (mg)	Therapeutic Plasma Levels
Class IA								
Quinidine	Generic	Prolongs QRS, Q–T, and (±) P–R	6	1–2	200 (sulfate) 342 (gluconate)	200–600 mg q6–8hr	1800 (s) 2400 (g)	3–7 µg/mL
Procainamide	Pronestyl	Prolongs QRS, Q–T, and (±) P–R	3–4	1	250, 500, 750 (sustained release)	500–1000 mg q3–4hr or q6hr (sustained release)	4000	3–8 µg/mL[a]
Disopyramide	Norpace	Prolongs QRS, Q–T, and (±) P–R	6–9	1–2	100, 150	150 mg 4 times daily	1200	2–4 µg/mL
Class IB								
Mexiletine	Mexitil	Shortens Q–T	10–12	2–3	150, 200, 250	200–300 mg q8hr	1200	0.5–2 µg/mL
Class IC								
Flecainide	Tambocor	Prolongs P–R, QRS, Q–T, bradycardia	12–27	2–3	100	200 mg every day	600	0.2–1.0 µg/mL
Propafenone	Rythmol	Prolongs P–R, QRS, but not Q–T	2–10 (90% of patients) 10–32 (10% of patients)	Depends on genetically determined metabolic rate	150, 300	450–900 mg in three divided doses	900	0.2–1.5 µg/mL
Class II (Table 59.3)								
Class III								
Amiodarone	Cordarone	Prolongs P–R, QRS	53	8 days after loading dose	200	200–600 mg once daily	800	Not useful
Sotalol	Betapace	Slows HR, prolongs QTc; no effect on QRS	12	3–4	80, 160	80–160 2–3 times daily	480–640[b]	Not useful
Class IV								
Verapamil	Calan, Isoptin	Prolongs P–R	4.5–12	1–2	40, 80, 120, 180, 240 (sustained release)	80–120 mg q8hr or 120–360 mg SR once a day	480	125–400 ng/mL
Diltiazem	Cardizem	Prolongs P–R	3.5	1	30, 60, 90, 120 or 180, 240, 300 CD	30–120 mg 3–4 times daily or 120–480 mg CD once a day	480	Not useful

s, Sulfate; g, gluconate; CD, continuous delivery.

[a]It may also be important to measure, especially in patients in cardiac or renal failure, the level of the active metabolite of procainamide, N-acetylprocainamide (NAPA—therapeutic level 6–20 mg/mL).

[b]Elimination is mainly in the urine. Dosages should be lowered in patients with renal insufficiency.

Table 59.2.   Adverse Effects of Antiarrhythmic Drugs

| Drug | Cardiac | | Noncardiac | |
	Common	Uncommon	Common	Uncommon
Class IA				
Quinidine	Decreased digoxin excretion; may precipitate digitoxicity	Ventricular arrhythmias, myocardial depression, hypotension	Nausea, diarrhea, tinnitus, vertigo, rash, fever, warfarin interaction ($\uparrow$ INR)	Hepatic dysfunction, thrombocytopenia, hemolytic anemia
Procainamide	None	Myocardial depression	Nausea, vomiting	Agranulocytosis, lupuslike syndrome
Disopyramide	Myocardial depression; should be used with caution in patients with severe or poorly compensated congestive heart failure	Severe hypotension in absence of known heart disease	Anticholinergic effects, especially urinary retention, dry mouth, blurred vision, constipation, aggravation of narrow-angle glaucoma	Acute psychoses, cholestasis
Class IB				
Mexiletine	None	Increased frequency of ventricular arrhythmias	Nausea, vomiting, indigestion, dizziness, tremor	Sleep disturbances, fatigue
Class IC				
Flecainide	Increased frequency of ventricular arrhythmias, myocardial depression; use with caution in patients with ejection fraction <40%	New supraventricular arrhythmias, congestive heart failure	Dizziness, visual disturbances, dyspnea, nausea, tremor	Constipation, edema, abdominal pain
Propafenone	Conduction delay	? Congestive heart failure	Unusual taste, constipation	Nausea, blurred vision, dizziness
Class II				
Propranolol[a]	Bradycardia, myocardial depression	Anginal syndrome may worsen if drug suddenly discontinued	Fatigue, nausea, vomiting, depression, impotence, potentiates bronchospasm in patients with asthma	Peripheral vascular insufficiency, hyperglycemia, alopecia
Class III				
Amiodarone	Bradycardia, increased heart block, increased digoxin concentration	Ventricular arrhythmias	Nausea, corneal microcrystallization, thyroid function abnormalities, decreased pulmonary diffusing capacity, warfarin interaction ($\uparrow$ INR)	Blue tint of exposed skin, pulmonary fibrosis
Sotalol	Bradycardia, fatigue, increased QTc	Torsade de pointes in 3–5%	Dyspnea	—
Class IV				
Verapamil	Bradycardia, prolongation of P–R interval, peripheral edema, increased digoxin level	Precipitation of congestive heart failure or pulmonary edema, severe hypotension, heart block	Dizziness, headache, constipation, nausea	Confusion, sleep disorders
Diltiazem	Bradycardia, prolongation of P–R interval	Heart block, increased digoxin level	Dizziness, headache, constipation	Rash, itching

[a]Other β-blocking agents have the same adverse effects, although bronchospasm and peripheral vascular insufficiency may be less likely with use of cardioselective β-blockers (Table 59.3).

Duraquin) may be preferred in some patients because it can be given every 8 to 12 hours.

Table 59.1 shows the time necessary to reach a steady state after administration of usual dosages of quinidine. If a faster effect is desired, loading doses may be given (e.g., 300 mg every 3 hours for three doses); in this circumstance hospitalization is advisable, both to monitor the effect of the drug and because the arrhythmia presumably is more dangerous.

Although quinidine has been used to treat a large variety of supraventricular and ventricular arrhythmias, it is rarely used to treat arrhythmias today because of the fear of proarrhythmia (particularly in patients with structural heart disease) as well as the development of GI side effects in a large proportion of patients.

Toxicity. There are a number of possible *toxic effects* of quinidine. The most common are gastrointestinal, especially diarrhea, and occur often within hours of administering the drug. Cinchonism (tinnitus, headache, visual disturbances) should not be seen if blood levels are checked periodically and if the dosage is appropriately adjusted. Hypersensitivity reactions (e.g., rash, arthralgias, immune thrombocytopenia, or hemolytic anemia) occur occasionally. These reactions often necessitate substitution of another antiarrhythmic drug.

Cardiac toxicity is usually dose related, often signaled by a prolongation of the Q–T interval; Q–T prolongation of 50% or more beyond baseline is an indication for reduction of the dosage of quinidine. Serious toxicity is manifest by a high degree of AV block, ventricular tachycardia, torsades de pointes (see below), or ventricular fibrillation—all emergency situations that may require cardiorespiratory support and warrant immediate hospitalization. Occasionally, patients taking quinidine die suddenly, sometimes with low plasma levels of the drug. Patients with prolonged Q–T intervals before institution of therapy with quinidine may be more prone to sudden death and therefore should not be given the drug.

If patients taking quinidine are asymptomatic and have normal left ventricular (LV) function, ECGs need be recorded no more frequently than once a year; if they are symptomatic or have poor LV function (EF of 40% or less) or complain of exertional chest pain, light-headedness, or shortness of breath, more frequent tracings should be obtained (perhaps every 3 or 4 months).

Drug interactions. Because patients prescribed quinidine are commonly treated with digitalis as well, it is especially important to recognize that digoxin levels may increase significantly in patients given quinidine. Quinidine decreases the excretion of digoxin by the kidneys, so it is important to monitor serum digoxin concentrations when quinidine is first prescribed and to alter the dosage of digoxin to prevent digitalis intoxication.

Quinidine is an α-adrenergic blocker and, if it is prescribed with vasodilators (e.g., nitrates, nifedipine, hydralazine, prazosin, converting enzyme inhibitors) or with potent diuretics (e.g., furosemide), it may cause symptomatic (especially postural) hypotension.

Drugs that are metabolized by hepatic microsomal enzymes may alter the pharmacokinetics of quinidine, and conversely, quinidine may alter the kinetics of one of these drugs. For example, phenytoin may accelerate the metabolism of quinidine, shortening its effect, and quinidine may inhibit the metabolism of warfarin, prolonging its effect.

Procainamide. The suppressive effects of procainamide on the electrical activity of the heart are the same as those of quinidine; but unlike quinidine, procainamide has little effect on vagal or α-adrenergic activity.

Like quinidine, procainamide may be used to treat many supraventricular arrhythmias. Its use today is limited because of concerns about proarrhythmia as well as the very high proportion of patients who develop a lupuslike syndrome (see below) after being treated with procainamide on a long-term basis. Perhaps one of the best uses of procainamide today is in the initial treatment of patients who present with a wide complex tachycardia and are hemodynamically stable. In most of these patients, ventricular tachycardia is the cause of the wide complex tachycardia. Procainamide is much more effective than intravenous lidocaine in terminating ventricular tachycardia in this setting. Another common setting in which procainamide is used is in the treatment of atrial fibrillation after cardiac surgery. This is generally a self-limited problem, so the procainamide can often be discontinued in 1 to 2 months, thereby eliminating the concern about the development of a lupuslike syndrome.

Toxicity. The noncardiac *toxicity* of procainamide is different from that of quinidine. GI symptoms occur less often, and when they do, nausea and vomiting are more common than diarrhea. Fever, often with shaking chills, or granulocytopenia occurs occasionally.

Within 3 months, 50% of people taking procainamide develop antinuclear antibodies (ANAs), and 90% do so within 12 months (3); 20 to 30% of patients with ANAs develop a lupuslike syndrome characterized by serositis (pleuritis, pericarditis, synovitis), fever, hepatomegaly, and a positive lupus erythematosus preparation. Unlike classic systemic lupus erythematosus, vasculitis is not a manifestation of drug-induced lupus, so that renal disease, for example, does not occur; most important, the syndrome abates, usually within days, when the drug is discontinued (ANAs may persist for months). The major threat of the syndrome is hemorrhagic pericarditis, and one must watch for signs and symptoms of pericardial tamponade. For these reasons, procainamide is not recommended for long-term use.

Disopyramide. Disopyramide has direct membrane effects very much like those of quinidine and, like quinidine, blocks parasympathetic activity. It is licensed for the treatment of specific ventricular arrhythmias: unifocal or multifocal PVCs and ventricular tachycardia. Like quinidine and procainamide, disopyramide is rarely used in ambulatory practice for treatment of patients with supraventricular or ventricular arrhythmias. Perhaps the most common use of disopyramide today is in the treatment of patients with vasodepressor syncope (see Chapter 81). The effectiveness of disopyramide in the treatment of this common fainting condition is caused by its vagolytic and negative inotropic effects.

The noncardiac toxicity of disopyramide is caused mainly by its anticholinergic effects; these include dry mouth, blurred vision, urinary hesitancy, and constipation. For these reasons, it is not a useful drug for elderly patients. Nausea, vomiting, and diarrhea are less common than they are after administration of quinidine or procainamide. The cardiac toxicity of the drug is, in part, similar to that of quinidine in that it can prolong the Q–T interval and produce torsades de pointes. Disopyramide may also cause or intensify heart failure or cause profound hypotension in patients who have compromised LV function; it should not be administered to such patients.

Class IB Drugs. Class IB drugs shorten repolarization and the Q–T interval and have little effect on the duration of the QRS complex. This class includes phenytoin and mexiletine. Class IB drugs are generally not effective for supraventricular arrhythmias.

Phenytoin. Phenytoin decreases automaticity and the duration of the action potential in the Purkinje fibers of the myocardium. Its use is limited in the treatment of arrhythmias. Phenytoin toxicity is discussed in detail in Chapter 80.

Mexiletine. Mexiletine has electrophysiologic effects similar to those of lidocaine. Adverse effects include nausea, tremulousness, dizziness, and anxiety. It may be useful in combination with a class IA or class III drug (see below), but consultation with a cardiologist is advised before it is prescribed.

Class IC Drugs. Class IC drugs slow conduction and widen the QRS complex but cause only small changes in refractoriness or the Q–T interval. The class IC drugs currently available, flecainide and propafenone, are both highly effective against serious ventricular arrhythmias and may be particularly useful in treatment of supraventricular arrhythmias, especially atrial fibrillation. Because flecainide has been shown to be associated with a high incidence of sudden death (more than three times that among patients treated with placebo) when used in patients with ventricular dysfunction after myocardial infarction (MI) (13,38), it should generally not be used in patients with ischemic heart disease, particularly if the patient's ejection fraction is less than 40%. Common noncardiac side effects are nausea and epigastric pain. These are controlled largely by dosing with meals to reduce peak drug levels. These drugs should be used only in consultation with a cardiologist.

Class II Drugs (Sympathetic Blocking Agents)

These drugs block the effects of catecholamines (which may potentiate the development of arrhythmias) and slow conduction in the atria, AV node, and myocardium.

β-Blockers are used to slow the ventricular response in patients with atrial tachyarrhythmia; occasionally, in the process, they convert paroxysmal atrial tachycardia, atrial flutter, or fibrillation to normal sinus rhythm. In addition, ventricular arrhythmias initiated by exercise or ischemia (see Chapter 57) or associated with the prolonged Q–T syndrome (see below) may be prevented by these drugs. β-Blockers appear to be synergistic with digoxin, and low dosages of propranolol and digoxin, for example, may be effective in controlling heart rate in patients with atrial fibrillation, or in maintaining normal sinus rhythm in patients who have been cardioverted (see below). β-Blockers are the only antiarrhythmic medications that have been convincingly shown to reduce the incidence of sudden death after myocardial infarction (55). Their use in this regard is discussed in detail in Chapter 58.

Toxicity. β-Blockers, by blocking sympathetic tone, can precipitate heart failure in patients with poor ventricular function, and they are contraindicated in patients with bronchial asthma. Paradoxically, β-blockers may be useful in some patients with heart failure caused by systolic dysfunction if the dosage is carefully titrated (see Chapter 61). GI side effects (primarily nausea and diarrhea) occur occasionally. Most β-blockers occasionally cause hair thinning; this effect appears to be reversible when the dosage is reduced or the drug is discontinued. Peripheral vascular disease is occasionally exacerbated by nonselective β-blockers, in which case a cardioselective β-blocker such as metoprolol or atenolol should be used.

The properties of the currently available β-blocking agents are listed in Table 59.3. Propranolol crosses the blood–brain barrier and may cause such side effects as depression and sleep disturbance. Atenolol and metoprolol are long acting, do not cross the blood–brain barrier, and are cardioselective. They appear to have fewer side effects than propranolol. It is not yet clear whether any of the other available β-blockers offers significant advantages over these preparations. There is no current clear-cut cost advantage in choosing one of these drugs over another. The main advantage of the longer-acting agents is the likelihood of better compliance.

Class III (Potassium Current Blockers)

Amiodarone. Amiodarone (37) is a potent drug that effectively suppresses both supraventricular and ventricular arrhythmias. Especially at high dosages (over 300 mg/day), it is associated with a number of troublesome side effects, including photosensitivity, corneal microdeposits, hypothyroidism or hyperthyroidism, pulmonary interstitial fibrosis, hepatotoxicity, and a variety of neurologic complaints. However, the use of the drug is not associated with a high risk of proarrhythmia, and amiodarone is the only antiarrhythmic agent that has not been shown in clinical trials to be associated with an increased risk of cardiac death. Each 200-mg tablet of amiodarone contains 75 mg of iodine; the likelihood of thyroid dysfunction is very high when the drug is taken chronically (37). Amiodarone also interacts with many other drugs

Table 59.3. Currently Available β-Blockers

	Acebutolol (Sectral)	Labetalol (Normodyne Trandate)	Atenolol (Tenormin)	Metoprolol (Lopressor)	Nadolol (Corgard)	Pindolol (Visken)	Propranolol (Inderal)	Timolol (Blocadren)	Carvedilol (Coreg)ᵃ
β-Blocking plasma levels	0.2–2.0 µg/mL	0.7–3.0 µg/mL	200–500 ng/mL	50–100 ng/mL	50–100 ng/mL	50–100 ng/mL	50–100 ng/mL	5–10 ng/mL	
Eliminating half-life (hr)	3–4	5–6	6–9	3–4	14–24	3–4	3.5–6	4	7–10
Active metabolites	Yes	No	No	No	No	No	Yes	No	No
Predominant route of elimination	HM	HM	RE (mostly unchanged)	HM	RE	RE (40% unchanged) and HM	HM	RE (20% unchanged) and HM	HM (50% higher plasma levels in elderly and in CRF)
β_1-Blockade potency ratio (propranolol = 1.0)	0.3	0.3	1.0	1.0	1.0	6.0	1.0	6.0	0
Relative β_1 selectivity	+	0	+	+	0	0	0	0	0
Available strengths (mg)	200, 400	100, 200, 300	50, 100	50, 100; or 50, 100, 200 XL	40, 80, 120, 160	5, 10	10, 20, 40, 60, 80; and 60, 80, 120, 180 mg long-acting	10	3.125, 6.25, 12.5, 25.0
Usual maintenance dosage	200–600 mg twice daily	100–600 mg twice daily	50–100 mg every day	50–100 mg twice daily or 50–200 mg XL once a day	40–50 mg every day	5–20 mg 3 times daily	40–80 mg 4 times daily or 120–160 mg long-acting once a day	20 mg twice daily	25 twice daily

Modified from Frishman WH. Beta-adrenoceptor antagonists: new drugs and new indications. N Engl J Med 305:550, 1981.

RE, Renal excretion; *HM*, hepatic metabolism.

ᵃHas significant α-blocking activity; orthostasis is commonly experienced.

and, for example, may potentiate the toxic effects of digoxin and β-blocking agents. It also interferes with the metabolism of warfarin and may markedly prolong the prothrombin time (37). Because of these problems the risks and benefits of amiodarone must be considered on a patient by patient basis. Today amiodarone is one of the most commonly used drugs to treat atrial fibrillation (see below). Amiodarone is also commonly used in the treatment of patients with sustained ventricular arrhythmias. However, amiodarone has not been shown to prolong survival in patients with congestive heart failure or in high-risk patients post-MI. A cardiologist familiar with the drug should be closely involved in the patient's care. Because of a long mean half-life of nearly 2 months, the effects may persist for weeks after the drug is discontinued.

Sotalol.   Sotalol is a racemic mixture of both a class II (β-blocker, L-sotolol) and a class III agent (D-sotolol) (12). The indications for its use are the same as for amiodarone, and it has fewer side effects. However, because serious ventricular arrhythmias are seen in 3 to 5% of patients, it should be used with caution in patients with impaired ventricular function and should not be initiated on an ambulatory basis if the patient has underlying structural heart disease.

Class IV Drugs (Calcium Channel Blockers)

Calcium channel blockers (12,47) (see above) are effective and useful drugs for controlling supraventricular arrhythmias. Conduction through the AV node is dependent on calcium-mediated currents. By blocking these currents, calcium channel blockers may control the ventricular response in atrial fibrillation and may convert to sinus rhythm supraventricular arrhythmias dependent on conduction through the AV node. Verapamil may be useful in an ambulatory setting for the conversion of paroxysmal AV node reentry tachycardia (AVNRT) to sinus rhythm. Doses of 80 to 120 mg orally may be used safely in patients known to have AVNRT; conversion to sinus rhythm usually occurs in 30 minutes to 1 hour. Alternatively, a dose of 5 to 10 mg intravenously may convert AVNRT in minutes. If the drug is not effective, referral to a hospital emergency room should be considered. Oral verapamil at dosages of 240 to 360 mg/day may be used for prophylaxis against supraventricular arrhythmias. Verapamil may also be used at dosages of 240 to 360 mg/day for control of heart rate in patients with atrial fibrillation. Diltiazem at dosages of 120 to 300 mg/day may also be effective (30). These drugs are not effective for control of ventricular arrhythmias.

Verapamil is metabolized by the liver and should be used with caution in patients with impaired liver function. Both verapamil and diltiazem are available in extended-release formulations that may be taken once daily. Except perhaps for initial dosage titration, the once-daily formulations are preferred over the short-acting forms. Occasionally, elderly patients may be very sensitive to diltiazem and may require only 30 mg three times daily.

Toxicity.   The most common side effects of calcium channel blockers are headache, light-headedness, diz-

ziness, hypotension, and constipation. Both verapamil and diltiazem interfere with renal clearance of digoxin and may precipitate digitalis intoxication. All calcium channel blockers are myocardial depressants, and both verapamil and diltiazem may suppress the SA node, decrease heart rate, and prolong the P–R interval. Verapamil should be used with caution in patients with LV dilation and EF of 40% or less, although diltiazem may be used with caution in such patients. There is concern about the use of short-acting calcium channel blockers because of reports of an increased mortality rate associated with administration of these drugs (40).

Pacemaker Therapy

Implantable electrical pulse generators (pacemakers) (11,25) are the treatment of choice for patients with symptomatic bradyarrhythmias and heart block. The decision to implant a pacemaker and the type of unit to use must be determined in consultation with a cardiologist. In general, patients in atrial fibrillation who require a pacemaker (see below) require ventricular demand pacemakers. Most patients in sinus rhythm are best served by a multiprogrammable atrioventricular sequential unit. The modest increase in cost and complexity of the AV sequential units appear to be more than offset by the improved long-term physiologic response of patients. Pacemakers are less than 0.5 cm thick, weigh less than 50 g, and may function for 10 to 15 years. Pacemaker leads are easily implantable via a percutaneous transvenous technique and rarely become dislodged, even during vigorous activity. Symptoms are relieved in most patients who are symptomatic because of bradyarrhythmias and conduction block (see below).

Patient Experience. The units are implanted subcutaneously under local anesthesia in the pectoral area, and the pacemaker lead is inserted via the cephalic vein or directly with the use of a special introducer into the axillary or subclavian vein and lodged in the apex of the right ventricle or in the right-atrial appendage. The procedure takes about 1.5 hours; the patient experiences some discomfort when the anesthetic is injected and, often, an unpleasant sensation when the tissues are manipulated to create a pocket for the pacemaker unit.

After the procedure, patients, depending on their age and condition, are discharged from the hospital late on the same day, or on the next day. Patients with sedentary jobs may return to work approximately 2 weeks after pacemaker insertion, but patients with more active jobs should be kept off work for approximately 6 weeks to allow the wound to heal completely. After that, there is little or no discomfort; the unit feels like part of the chest wall and there are no restrictions on the patient's activity. Microwave ovens do not interfere with pacemaker functions but cellular phones may do so if they are held directly over the pacemaker (17). Magnetic resonance scanning is absolutely contraindicated in patients with permanent pacemakers.

Patients with implanted pacemakers require systematic, long-term follow-up. The frequency of follow-up depends on the original indication for the pacemaker. Patients who require constant pacing must be seen more often (approximately every 3 months) than do patients who require episodic pacing (approximately every 4 to 6 months). At these visits the function of the pacemaker must be assessed with a 12-lead ECG and a computerized pacemaker analyzer, which measures pacemaker parameters including battery voltage and lead resistance.

The pacemaker and its registration number should be entered into the patient's record, and the patient should keep the registration card for the pacemaker on his or her person in the event of malfunction of the instrument or an emergency intercurrent problem.

Cardioversion

The electrical conversion of atrial tachyarrhythmias is done by the application of a short burst of direct current to the chest wall. The shock is synchronized with the QRS complex of the ECG to avoid applying it during the vulnerable period of the cardiac cycle when ventricular tachycardia or fibrillation might be induced.

Cardioversion is a more reliable technique for the conversion of tachyarrhythmias than is the administration of antiarrhythmic drugs. It may be required on an emergency basis if a patient has developed severe heart failure, hypotension, or ischemia as a result of an arrhythmia. Otherwise, the procedure should be planned with the cardiologist, who will attempt the conversion.

Patients scheduled for elective cardioversion for treatment of atrial fibrillation should be anticoagulated with warfarin for at least 3 weeks before the procedure (see Chapter 52). Digitalis, if it has been prescribed, is held on the day of cardioversion. After successful cardioversion, anticoagulation should be maintained for at least 3 weeks, in case atrial fibrillation recurs and to allow atrial transport to stabilize (44). In most patients an attempt at cardioversion should be made before initiation of antiarrhythmic therapy. If atrial fibrillation recurs soon after the cardioversion, an antiarrhythmic agent can be started and the cardioversion repeated.

Patient Experience. Cardioversion is done by a cardiologist in a hospital, either with an anesthesiologist or with a nurse experienced in administering conscious sedation and with resuscitation equipment available. The patient is sedated, usually with 3 to 10 mg of intravenous midazolam given to effect. Normally the patient cannot recall afterward the details of the procedure. For atrial fibrillation, cardioversion is attempted at 100 watt-seconds; the energy level is doubled repetitively and other shocks are administered until there is conversion or until a level of 360 watt-seconds is reached. If an initial attempt using anteroposterior patch placement fails, a final attempt at cardioversion can be undertaken using an apex–base paddle position. Complications, embolism or a new arrhythmia, are unusual. After cardioversion, the patient is observed for several hours while rhythm is monitored, and then discharged if the rhythm is stable.

When to Refer a Patient for an Invasive Electrophysiologic Study

Several categories of patients should be referred for electrophysiologic (EP) study. Most of these patients are already under the care of a cardiologist. These patients include patients with a sustained wide complex tachycardia and patients who have survived an episode of sudden cardiac death, patients with nonsustained ventricular tachycardia (particularly in the setting of a prior MI) who are thought to be at increased risk of sudden cardiac death, patients with syncope of unknown origin in the setting of structural heart disease, and patients who are considered to be candidates for a curative catheter ablation procedure for treatment of a large variety of supraventricular arrhythmias (including the WPW syndrome, paroxysmal supraventricular tachycardia, atrial flutter, and atrial tachycardia) and also some types of ventricular arrhythmias (i.e., idiopathic ventricular tachycardia). Although empiric antiarrhythmic drug treatment is appropriate for many patients with paroxysmal supraventricular tachycardia and other types of supraventricular arrhythmias, many patients either fail or are intolerant to such therapy; others prefer an attempt at catheter ablation to taking drugs the rest of their lives (5,39).

Patient Experience (During EP Study). The patient's experience is similar to that during cardiac catheterization (see Chapter 57). Catheters are usually advanced through the femoral vein. The procedure takes longer than does coronary catheterization; the average diagnostic procedure takes about 1 to 2 hours, whereas a catheter ablation procedure can take up to 4 or 5 hours. The risks of a diagnostic EP procedure are slight. The risks associated with catheter ablation vary based on the target arrhythmia. There is a small risk that a permanent pacemaker will be required, because of the induction of complete heart block during an ablation procedure, in 1% or less of patients. The risk of major morbidity (e.g., stroke, MI, significant valve damage) or mortality is approximately 0.1%. Patients are usually treated with aspirin for several weeks after an ablation procedure to reduce the risk of embolization.

SPECIFIC ARRHYTHMIAS
Sinus Tachycardia

Definition and Causes

In adults the normal sinus rate is 60 to 100 beats/minute. Sinus tachycardia, a sinus rhythm at a rate greater than 100 beats/minute, is usually a physiologic rhythm in that the rate is ordinarily appropriate to the physiologic state of the patient, a state that requires an increased cardiac output to meet increased metabolic demands. The maximal sinus heart rate that can be attained varies with age but usually does not exceed 140 beats/minute unless demands are excessive (e.g., vigorous exercise; see Chapter 58, Table 58.5). The common factors that stimulate an increase in the rate of sinus rhythm, other than exercise, are fever (an increase of approximately 10 beats/minute for each Fahrenheit degree rise in body temperature), emotional stress, heart failure, hypoxia, and a variety of drugs that affect the autonomic nervous system (e.g., caffeine, aminophylline, amphetamine, alcohol, antidepressants, phenothiazines and calcium channel blockers of the dihydropyridine class, e.g., nifedipine).

Physical Findings

A regular rapid pulse and heart rate are detected, although there may be a slight variation in rate, called sinus arrhythmia. S_1 is normal and the jugular pulsations are normal.

Electrocardiogram

A P wave precedes each QRS complex; the P–R interval is normal for the rate (0.16 to 0.17 at rates over 130/minute), and the P-wave vector is normal (upright P waves in II, III, and aVF).

Treatment

In most cases persistent sinus tachycardia need not be treated; it is the underlying condition that requires therapy. Digitalis, especially, should not be used to treat a patient with sinus tachycardia unless there is associated heart failure.

In the occasional patient with an unexplained sinus tachycardia in whom a thorough evaluation fails to reveal an underlying cause, and in whom tachycardia is symptomatic, the use of small dosages of a β-blocker may be justified. Low-dose β-blockers may also be helpful in treating the anxiety and tachycardia associated with anticipated stressful situations.

Sinus Bradycardia

Definition and Causes

Sinus bradycardia is a heart rate below 60 beats/minute. Impulse generation in the sinus node is often slow in aerobically well-conditioned people (e.g., long-distance runners, heavy laborers) because of high vagal tone. Inappropriately low sinus rates are commonly caused by increased vagal tone, as is seen in association with pain, vomiting, or vasovagal syncope. A hypersensitive carotid sinus, more common in elderly people, may also result in marked bradycardia when the sinus is compressed by a tight collar or by the patient's tensing his or her neck. Parasympathomimetic drugs such as neostigmine, tranquilizers, phenothiazines, digitalis, and sympatholytic drugs such as methyldopa, clonidine, and all β-blockers also may produce sinus bradycardia. Vagally induced bradycardia may be severe and result in asystole (and loss of consciousness) when the stimulus is marked or prolonged or occurs in a hypoxic patient.

Physical Findings

A regular slow pulse and heart rate are detected. S_1 is normal and the jugular pulsations are normal.

Electrocardiogram

A P wave precedes each QRS complex; the P–R interval is normal for the rate (0.20 to 0.21) and the P-wave vector is normal (upright P waves in II, III, and aVF).

Treatment

Asymptomatic sinus bradycardia discovered as an incidental finding does not require treatment. However, patients who present with symptoms of lightheadedness or syncope and are found to have sinus bradycardia may have underlying sinus node disease or may be subject to paroxysms of tachycardia and bradycardia, the so-called sick sinus syndrome (see below). Patients with sinus bradycardia and symptoms should be evaluated with an ambulatory ECG to determine whether they have this condition. In any case, patients with symptomatic sinus bradycardia, not caused by a drug, are best treated with permanent pacemaker implantation.

Sick Sinus Syndrome

Definition and Causes

The term *sick sinus syndrome* refers to a heterogeneous group of arrhythmias involving defective impulse generation by the sinus node or abnormal impulse conduction in the atria and AV node (45). The syndrome is characterized by periods of inappropriate sinus bradycardia (often severe with rates between 25 and 40 beats/minute) that may precede or follow supraventricular tachyarrhythmias and by varying degrees of sinoatrial block, sometimes including sinus arrest. The rubrics *bradycardia–tachycardia syndrome* and *tachycardia–bradycardia* syndrome are sometimes used, depending on whether bradycardia precedes or follows a tachyarrhythmia.

The sick sinus syndrome is caused by degenerative fibrotic changes within the sinus node. It is often associated with similar abnormalities in other parts of the cardiac conduction system that result in varying degrees of atrioventricular and intraventricular block. These pathologic changes are much more common in patients over the age of 60; although their precise cause is unknown, they are often associated with hypertensive or ischemic heart disease.

Symptoms and Signs

Many patients are asymptomatic. When symptoms do occur, they are produced either by spontaneous sinus arrest or by the tachyarrhythmia itself (palpitations). If there is coexistent LV dysfunction or coronary artery disease, symptoms of heart failure or ischemia may occur.

The physical examination is often normal unless the patient is examined during an episode of bradyarrhythmia or tachyarrhythmia, in which case the findings depend on the type of arrhythmia that is present (see below). Sometimes light carotid sinus massage produces symptomatic bradyarrhythmia in a patient with sick sinus syndrome who is in normal sinus rhythm.

Electrocardiogram

The ECG may be normal or may simply reveal sinus bradycardia. Often, there are varying degrees of sinoatrial block, characterized by varying P–P intervals on the ECG. Sometimes sinus arrest occurs, manifest by absent P waves and associated, usually, with a junctional escape rhythm. Some patients have slow atrial fibrillation reflecting a concomitant AV conduction abnormality (see above). The ECG changes of the various atrial tachyarrhythmias are described below in the discussions of these entities.

If there is a history of unexplained syncope or palpitations and the resting ECG is normal, ambulatory ECG monitoring is indicated (see "Diagnosis of Arrhythmias," above).

Treatment and Course

The treatment of choice for patients with the sick sinus syndrome who are symptomatic from bradyarrhythmias is permanent pacemaker implantation (see "Pacemaker Therapy," above). Otherwise, symptoms are often progressive. Patients with minor symptoms (e.g., light-headedness or dizziness) often find that they feel significantly better after pacemaker therapy.

Tachyarrhythmias associated with the syndrome often are not prevented by electrical pacing. However, pacing does allow the use of such drugs as digitalis and β-blockers that depress the sinus node and increase the likelihood of sinus arrest or asystole. It is reasonable, after a pacemaker is implanted, to administer metoprolol 25 mg twice a day, and to increase the dosage to 50 mg or 100 mg twice a day in an attempt to prevent tachyarrhythmias. If the β-blocker is not effective, digoxin should be administered as well. If tachyarrhythmias continue, consideration should be given, in conjunction with the consulting cardiologist, to the use of an antiarrhythmic drug (see above).

Patients with sick sinus syndrome have an incidence, unaffected by pacemaker therapy, of arterial embolization of approximately 10% per year, caused by associated paroxysmal atrial arrhythmias. If tachyarrhythmias are not well controlled, these patients should be anticoagulated with warfarin (see Chapter 52). The sick sinus syndrome is not itself associated with increased mortality. Life expectancy in these patients is a function of the patient's age and comorbid conditions (45). Patients with chronic atrial fibrillation or supraventricular tachycardia as a manifestation of sick sinus syndrome should be treated with warfarin (see below) or with aspirin if the patient cannot or will not take warfarin. Warfarin may be started approximately 2 to 3 days after a permanent pacemaker is implanted.

Premature Atrial and Junctional Contractions

Definition and Causes

Premature atrial and junctional contractions (PACs and PJCs) are commonly seen in patients who are otherwise well. They often are induced by the same stimuli that produce sinus tachycardia, especially caffeine or nicotine. However, in patients with congestive heart failure or chronic pulmonary disease, PACs or PJCs may progress to atrial fibrillation or flutter.

Symptoms and Signs

Usually patients are unaware of PACs or PJCs. Occasionally they note the PAC or PJC as a palpitation; the physician, on listening to the heart or palpating the arterial pulse, is aware of a slight irregularity in the cardiac rhythm.

Electrocardiogram

PACs are reflected in the ECG by a premature morphologically abnormal P wave followed by a premature morphologically normal QRS complex. Often these impulses are not conducted (Fig. 59.5), in which case, if the P wave is buried in the preceding T wave, a false diagnosis of sinus arrest may be made. At other times the premature impulse may be aberrantly conducted, the result of relative refractoriness of one of the bundle branches (usually a right bundle branch pattern is seen after the premature atrial beat).

Premature junctional contractions are reflected in the ECG by a retrograde P wave (negatively deflected in leads II, III, and aVF) that may follow, be hidden in, or precede a morphologically normal but premature QRS complex.

Treatment

Patients with PACs who are otherwise well do not require treatment.

Rarely, it may be necessary to prescribe digoxin or a β-blocker to reduce the frequency of PACs in patients who have annoyingly frequent palpitations. In patients with underlying cardiac or pulmonary disease, digitalization may prevent the progression of PACs to atrial fibrillation. Quinidine or procainamide is also

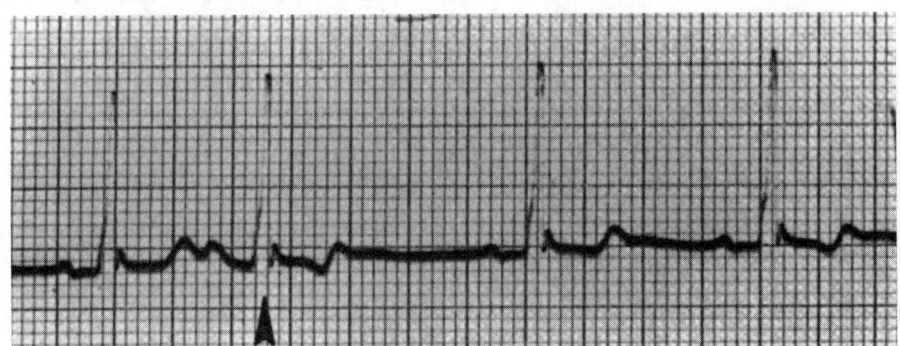

Figure 59.5. A premature atrial contraction (*arrowhead*). Note the normal configuration of the premature QRS complex.

effective in the control of PACs, but the risk associated with the use of these drugs usually is not warranted (see above) (8).

Paroxysmal Supraventricular Tachycardia

Definition and Causes

The term *paroxysmal supraventricular tachycardia* (PSVT) refers to a group of supraventricular arrhythmias that start and terminate abruptly and generally result from reentry (16). The most common cause of PSVT is *atrioventricular nodal reentrant tachycardia* (AVNRT) (accounting for two-thirds of all cases of PSVT). AVNRT occurs in the setting of two functionally distinct conduction pathways in the region of the AV node (called the fast and slow pathways). The second most common cause of PSVT is an accessory pathway–mediated tachycardia called *orthodromic AV reciprocating tachycardia*. This type of tachycardia, accounting for approximately one-third of all cases of PSVT, results from the electrical impulse traveling from the atria to the ventricles via the AV node and returning to the atria via an accessory pathway that connects the atrium and ventricle. The third, and least common cause of PSVT is a *reentrant or triggered atrial tachycardia* that is confined to the atrium (accounts for less than 5% of all cases of PSVT).

The heart rate during episodes of PSVT may vary from 130 to 240 beats/minute. In general, PSVT involving an accessory pathway tends to be more rapid and PSVT caused by an atrial tachycardia tends to be slower. However, because of a tremendous amount of overlap, the rate of the tachycardia is usually not helpful in establishing a diagnosis.

Nonparoxysmal atrial tachycardia with block (caused by gradually accelerated automaticity of an ectopic atrial focus) as a manifestation of digitalis toxicity is now rarely seen. If nonparoxysmal atrial tachycardia occurs in association with an AV conduction abnormality (commonly 2:1 block) and the patient is taking digitalis, the drug should be withheld and serum potassium concentration should be measured. If the patient is hypokalemic, potassium repletion is, of course, in order; usually this can be accomplished by administration of oral potassium salts (i.e., 20 mEq three times a day; see Chapter 46). Patients with refractory arrhythmias with block caused by digitalis toxicity should be hospitalized for more aggressive treatment.

Symptoms and Signs

PSVT can usually be suspected or diagnosed based on a careful history. The most important features of PSVT are its abrupt onset and termination and its sustained rapid and regular rate. Patients may also complain of dyspnea, diaphoresis, light-headedness, or presyncope or chest pain. Often the patient is able to terminate the arrhythmia abruptly by vagotonic maneuvers such as a Valsalva maneuver, by coughing, or by placing a cold wet towel over the face (diving reflex).

Often, polyuria is experienced for as long as the arrhythmia lasts.

Attacks often occur spontaneously but may be precipitated by physical or emotional stress, caffeine, or nicotine. They may be as short as a few seconds and as long as several weeks. The frequency of the attacks is also variable: Some people have attacks every day; some, only a few times during their entire lives.

On examination, a rapid regular arterial pulse and heart rate are noted, often faster than that measured in patients with sinus tachycardia and usually not associated with the same stimuli. When the atria and ventricles contract simultaneously, cannon waves are seen in the jugular veins.

Electrocardiogram

PSVT is characterized by a rapid regular heart rate. There is a fixed relationship of the P wave to the QRS complex. If the impulse is generated in the AV node (as in AVNRT), the P wave may be buried in the QRS complex, but the process can be identified by the normal appearance of the QRS complex and the regularity of the rate. When the P wave is visible, it may follow the QRS complex (some nodal reentry rhythms, all accessory pathway reentry rhythms). It may also precede the QRS complex and may appear morphologically normal (atrial reentry or ectopic rhythm), in which case the diagnosis can be made (by ECG) only if the rate is high enough to make sinus tachycardia unlikely. The P wave also may be hidden in the T wave, but again, the regularity of the rate and the usually normal duration of the QRS complex establish the diagnosis.

If the ECG obtained from a patient with PSVT demonstrates various degrees of AV block (Fig. 59.6), the most likely cause of the arrhythmia is an atrial tachycardia. The presence of an accessory pathway–mediated tachycardia can be completely eliminated and the possibility of AVNRT is most unlikely.

Treatment and Course

Therapy of PSVT always starts with attempts to increase vagal tone. As mentioned above (see "Symptoms and Signs"), the patient often has learned to do this. If the arrhythmia persists despite the patient's efforts, carotid sinus massage should be applied. This must be done after auscultation of the carotid arteries to ensure that there are no bruits; if there are, carotid sinus massage is contraindicated. The carotid sinus is at the point of maximal impulse of the carotid artery in the neck. The right sinus should be massaged first for up to 20 seconds; if that has no effect, the left sinus should be massaged. The two sinuses should never be massaged simultaneously. During massage, the patient's ECG should be monitored continuously, and resuscitation equipment should be available.

If carotid sinus massage fails, pharmacologic therapy is indicated. This is best done in an emergency room or a similar facility. If that is not logistically possible, the drug of choice is adenosine (which slows conduction through the AV node), 6 to 12 mg, because the effect of

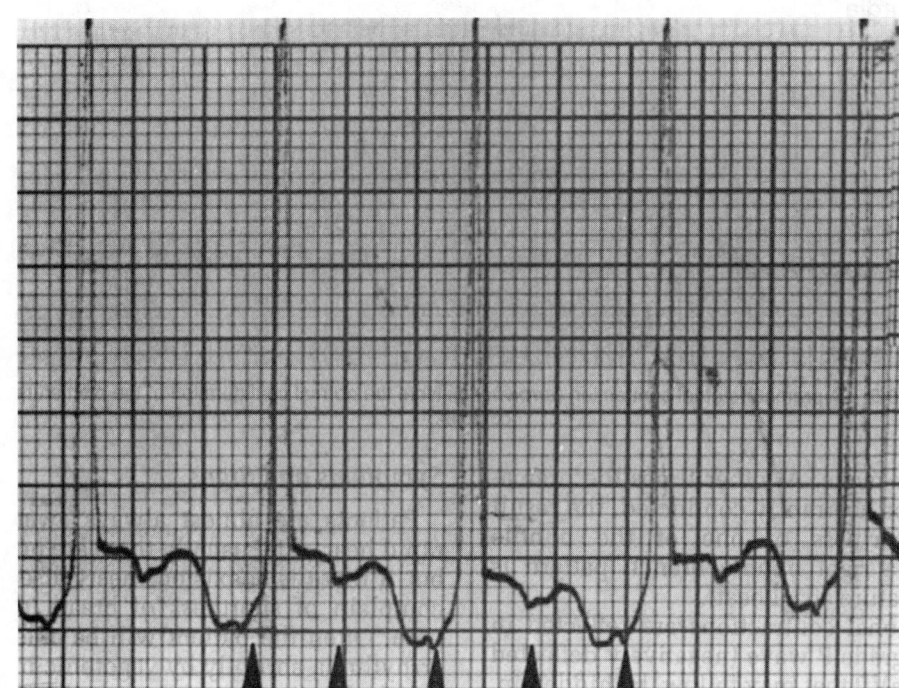

Figure 59.6. Supraventricular tachycardia with 2:1 AV block; the arrowheads point to consecutive P waves.

the drug is dissipated in only 10 to 15 seconds after intravenous administration; it usually converts the arrhythmia to normal sinus rhythm within 5 to 10 seconds. It is critical that adenosine be administered as a bolus into a rapidly flowing intravenous line. This is best accomplished by using a stopcock and immediately flushing the line with 10 mL of saline after injecting the adenosine. If PSVT persists after administration of adenosine, the patient should be transported to an emergency room for treatment. If that is not possible, verapamil (80 to 120 mg orally or 5 to 10 mg intravenously) or diltiazem (60 to 120 mg orally) can be tried (see above). Alternatively, propranolol (40 to 80 mg orally or 1 to 4 mg intravenously) may be used.

PSVT can be prevented or the number of episodes reduced with the use of a large variety of antiarrhythmic agents. If an initial episode of PSVT terminates spontaneously and is associated with mild symptoms, it would be reasonable to instruct the patient about techniques to terminate the arrhythmia and to delay initiation of antiarrhythmic therapy. On the other hand, if the patient has had multiple episodes of tachycardia, has required emergency room evaluation for termination of tachycardia, or has symptoms of hemodynamic compromise, antiarrhythmic therapy is indicated. Almost all antiarrhythmic agents may be used to treat patients with PSVT. They vary in their convenience, side effects, cost, and efficacy. Digoxin is perhaps the most convenient, best tolerated, least expensive, and least effective medication used to treat PSVT. β-Blockers and calcium channel blockers are somewhat more effective, more expensive, and when once-a-day dosing is used, equally convenient. On the other end of the spectrum are class 1C antiarrhythmic agents such as propafenone and flecainide, which are effective but more expensive and less convenient. Although amiodarone can be used to treat patients with PSVT, this drug is rarely prescribed because of the benign nature of this arrhythmia, the potential for serious side effects of the drug (see above), and the alternative of catheter ablation. Over the past 10 years catheter ablation (see above) has emerged from an experimental technique to become first- or second-line therapy for the treatment of patients with PSVT (39). Success rates exceed 90%, complications are rare (less than 1%), and the procedure is well tolerated. For this reason, patients with PSVT should be informed about the existence of a curative catheter-based procedure that can be considered as an alternative to lifelong antiarrhythmic therapy or can be used when antiarrhythmic therapy fails. Electrophysiologic testing and catheter ablation should be recommended as first-line therapy when PSVT occurs in the setting of WPW syndrome (see below). Because of the potentially life-threatening nature of WPW syndrome, these patients should be referred for electrophysiologic testing and catheter ablation (5). Similarly, if a patient with PSVT has symptoms of severe hemodynamic compromise (i.e., syncope), electrophysiologic testing and catheter ablation should be considered early in management.

Although PSVT is generally a benign arrhythmia, it rarely disappears without treatment. Once a patient has one episode of PSVT, other episodes will probably occur. In most patients the frequency of episodes of PSVT increases over time. In contrast to this generally benign course, the prognosis of patients with PSVT who have WPW syndrome, severe structural heart disease, or symptoms of hemodynamic compromise is not as favorable. For this reason, more aggressive approaches to treatment are used early in these settings.

Multifocal Atrial Tachycardia

Multifocal atrial tachycardia (MAT) is a chaotic supraventricular arrhythmia characterized electrocardiographically by varying morphology of the P waves, varying P–R intervals, and a rapid heart rate, usually 100 to 200 beats/minute; QRS morphology is normal and every QRS complex is preceded by a P wave (Fig. 59.7) (21). The arrhythmia is usually seen in patients with serious underlying disease, especially decompensated chronic obstructive pulmonary disease, and is better treated by, for example, improving ventilatory function than by attempting directly to suppress the rhythm. Digitalis does not alter this arrhythmia (which is usually well tolerated) and therefore should not be administered. Both verapamil and diltiazem may be used to control the heart rate in patients with MAT. Oral dosages of 40 to 80 mg three to four times a day of verapamil or 30 to 60 mg three to four times a day of diltiazem should be tried (21). If they are effective, a sustained-release preparation of verapamil or diltiazem at the same total daily dosage may be used.

Atrial Fibrillation

Definition and Causes

Atrial fibrillation is defined electrophysiologically as the generation of multiple reentry wave fronts by the atria. It is usually triggered by a PAC (see above) that triggers the development of these wave fronts and results in an atrial rate in excess of 300 beats/minute. These impulses enter the AV node randomly. Because of the unique conduction properties of the AV node, including slow conduction and decremental conduction, only a small proportion of the impulses are conducted to the ventricle. This results in a much slower (100 to 180 beats/minute) and irregularly irregular ventricular rate.

The prevalence of atrial fibrillation increases with age and the development of structural heart disease (19). When atrial fibrillation occurs in the absence of any evidence of structural heart disease in patients less than 50 years of age, it is called lone atrial fibrillation. In some patients, factors that trigger episodes of atrial fibrillation can be identified such as physical or emotional stress, alcohol, nicotine, or caffeine. Soaking in a hot tub while imbibing alcoholic beverages has become a recognized precipitating cause of atrial fibrillation. The major noncardiac illness associated with atrial fibrillation is hyperthyroidism; in the presence of a fast ventricular response refractory to digitalis, atrial fibrillation may be the first clue to the diagnosis.

The incidence of atrial fibrillation increases greatly with age, and often appears shortly after the onset of symptomatic coronary heart disease (19). Hypertensive and rheumatic heart disease (especially when it involves the mitral valve) also predispose to the development of atrial fibrillation, but almost every kind of myocardial disorder has been associated with it. Also, the tachyarrhythmic component of the sick sinus syndrome (see above) may be atrial fibrillation.

Symptoms and Signs

The most common symptoms of atrial fibrillation are palpitations and fatigue. If the ventricular response is fast, patients often complain of feeling disoriented, light-headed, weak, or faint as well, especially if they are elderly. Because atrial contraction normally provides approximately 20% of the total cardiac output, patients with incipient heart failure, ischemic heart disease, or valvular heart disease may develop symptoms and signs of those disorders (especially on exertion) when cardiac output is reduced as the result of atrial fibrillation.

Atrial fibrillation is characterized by an irregularly irregular heartbeat and pulse, with variation in intensity of the sounds (including murmurs) on both auscultation and palpation. It is prudent to look for signs of diseases known to be associated with atrial fibrillation (e.g., coronary heart disease, heart failure, hypertension, mitral stenosis, and hyperthyroidism), especially because those signs may be subtle or may be altered by the arrhythmia.

Electrocardiogram

The ECG shows rapid irregular fibrillatory atrial activity at rates of 300 to 500/minute; no P waves are present. The ventricular rhythm is irregularly irregular, at rates that at onset are usually 150 to 200/minute, unless there is coexistent disease in the AV node, in which case slower rates are likely (Fig. 59.8).

The QRS complex is usually morphologically normal. Occasionally there is aberrant conduction of an impulse in the ventricles, after a beat that has been preceded by a long pause. The aberrant beat usually has a right bundle branch block (RBBB) configuration. This so-called Ashman phenomenon is caused by prolonged refractoriness of the (usually) right bundle branch after the long pause. These aberrant beats must be distinguished from ventricular premature beats. Apart from their typical relationship to a preceding long R–R interval, aberrant beats are often triphasic (RSR') in lead V_1 and their initial vector is the same

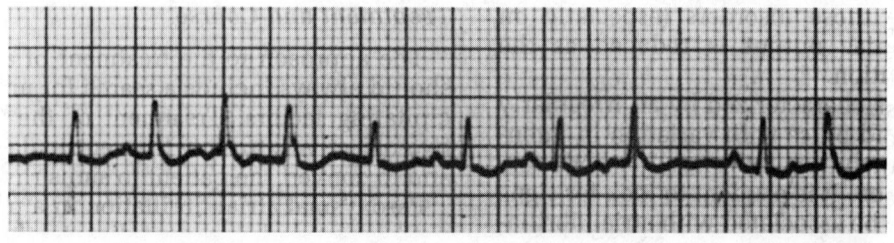

Figure 59.7. Multifocal atrial tachycardia; note the variation in the morphology of the P waves and the duration of the P–R intervals.

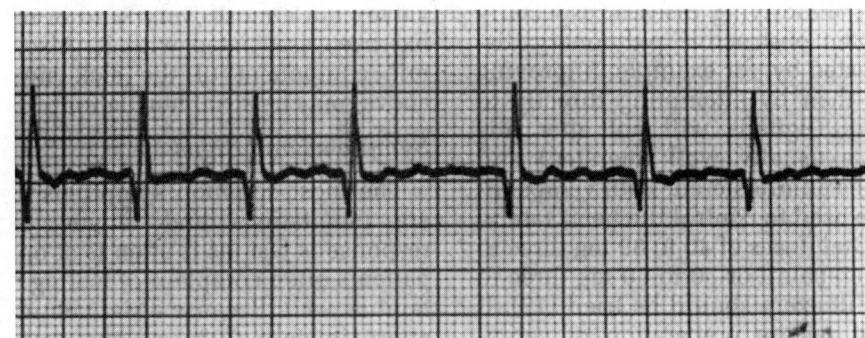

Figure 59.8. Atrial fibrillation. The ventricular rate is 90 to 100 beats/minute, indicative (because digitalis had not been administered) of an associated disorder of AV conduction.

as that of the normally conducted beats; neither of these features is characteristic of ventricular premature beats.

Other Studies

In addition to an ECG and chest x-ray, all patients presenting for the first time with atrial fibrillation should have thyroid function studies and a two-dimensional (2D) echocardiogram. Unusual causes of atrial fibrillation, such as atrial myxoma or chronic pericardial effusion, may require echocardiography for diagnosis.

Treatment and Course

The approach to the treatment of atrial fibrillation should always include a search for underlying or precipitating factors. Treatment of the arrhythmia has two objectives: to slow the ventricular rate if it is fast and to convert the patient to sinus rhythm if possible.

Paroxysmal atrial fibrillation in a patient who does not have underlying heart disease often reverts to normal sinus rhythm once precipitating factors (e.g., fever, stress, alcohol, nicotine) are controlled or removed. Specific treatment is indicated in the following circumstances: a rapid ventricular response associated with symptoms (e.g., extreme fatigue, syncope, angina, or shortness of breath), the presence of known underlying structural severe heart disease (e.g., aortic stenosis, severe mitral stenosis, ischemic heart disease, chronic congestive failure; these patients are unlikely to revert to normal sinus rhythm spontaneously), and persistent atrial fibrillation, especially if the resting ventricular rate is greater than 110 beats/minute or if the rate after moderate exercise (climbing a flight of stairs, for example) is greater than 150 beats/minute.

Symptomatic patients and patients with underlying structural heart disease generally require admission to the hospital immediately after onset of the arrhythmia for cardioversion (see above) or for pharmacotherapy. Patients with persistent atrial fibrillation of less than 6 months' duration, particularly if there is no left-atrial enlargement, should be anticoagulated for at least 3 months and then be considered for elective cardioversion. Patients with atrial fibrillation that has lasted longer than 6 months or patients with large left atria (left atrium larger than 5.0 cm on 2D echocardiogram) are likely to be refractory to cardioversion. In general, cardioversion restores normal sinus rhythm in ap-

proximately 90% of patients, but the relapse rate is high—50% in 1 year and 90% in 3 years (19)—unless the underlying disorder can be corrected or atrial fibrillation has been of short duration.

In most patients it is reasonable to restore sinus rhythm with cardioversion and to delay the initiation of antiarrhythmic therapy until a second episode of atrial fibrillation occurs. Following a second episode of sustained atrial fibrillation, antiarrhythmic therapy is often used in an attempt to maintain sinus rhythm. Because no study has demonstrated that treatment of patients with atrial fibrillation with antiarrhythmic therapy prolongs survival or reduces the incidence of strokes, the main indication of antiarrhythmic therapy should be the reduction of symptoms. An ongoing randomized study is comparing the effect on survival of anticoagulation plus rate control versus therapy to maintain sinus rhythm in patients with atrial fibrillation (36).

The selection of an appropriate antiarrhythmic agent for control of atrial fibrillation depends to a large degree on the type of underlying structural heart disease. For patients with no structural heart disease, almost any antiarrhythmic agent is safe. Class IC antiarrhythmic agents such as flecainide or propafenone or the class III antiarrhythmic agent sotalol are often used as first-line antiarrhythmic therapy in this setting. If these are ineffective, low-dose amiodarone can be considered. In contrast, the risk of proarrhythmia is high among patients with impaired ventricular function. Perhaps the most effective and safest antiarrhythmic agent in this setting is low-dose amiodarone (100 to 200 mg/day). It should be recognized that atrial fibrillation is a difficult arrhythmia to treat and that even with the most effective antiarrhythmic agents sinus rhythm can be maintained during long-term follow-up in less than 50% of patients.

If antiarrhythmic therapy fails or is poorly tolerated, the goal of treatment should be to achieve adequate rate control and to achieve effective long-term anticoagulation (48–51). When rate control is attempted, the goal should be to achieve a resting ventricular rate between 70 and 100 beats/minute and a rate after modest exercise of below 150 beats/minute. Studies show that digoxin slows the ventricular response in acute atrial fibrillation but does not enhance conversion to sinus rhythm and has limited use in controlling heart rate in chronic atrial fibrillation. This reflects the fact that most patients convert spontaneously after they are sedated and after precipitating causes such as alcohol, sympathomimetics, hypertension, and hypoxia are removed or treated, and that heart rate control is caused by increased vagal tone to the AV node, which is withdrawn during exercise (14). When used in an acute situation, 0.75 to 1.0 mg digoxin should be given by mouth, followed by 0.125 to 0.25 mg a day.

In contrast to digoxin, calcium channel blockers such as verapamil (120 to 240 mg/day, sustained release), diltiazem (120 to 240 mg/day, sustained release), or small dosages of a β-blocker (e.g. atenolol 25 to 50 mg/day, metoprolol 25 mg twice a day, or propranolol 10 to 20 mg four times a day) effectively control heart rate during exercise and are preferred to digoxin (see "General Principles in Management of Arrhythmias," above, for a discussion of the use of these drugs). Once effectiveness is demonstrated, those drugs may be taken once daily in a sustained-release form at the same total daily dosage.

If pharmacologic approaches to heart rate control are ineffective or result in intolerable side effects, the patient should be referred for electrophysiologic modification or ablation of the AV node and permanent pacemaker implantation (60).

A slow ventricular response to atrial fibrillation in untreated patients suggests an associated disorder of AV conduction. Such patients do not require specific therapy for the arrhythmia (other than anticoagulation) unless they are hemodynamically compromised (i.e., in refractory heart failure) and their heart rate is under 60 to 70 beats/minute, in which case implantation of a pacemaker may be indicated.

Anticoagulation. Patients with chronic atrial fibrillation are at increased risk of arterial embolization. For example, the Framingham study reported that, over a 24-year period, patients with chronic atrial fibrillation with and without rheumatic heart disease had a 17- and 5-fold increase, respectively, in the incidence of stroke (61). Overall the incidence of arterial embolization in patients with chronic atrial fibrillation is approximately 10% a year (48–51). In general, patients should be anticoagulated for 3 weeks before, and 3 weeks after, elective cardioversion (see above and Chapter 52). Prospective randomized trials support the use of anticoagulants in patients with chronic atrial fibrillation if there are no contraindications (31). An alternative approach is to refer the patient for transesophageal echocardiography (TEE) and, if no clots are

demonstrated, to perform cardioversion without anticoagulation (29). In patients who cannot or will not take warfarin, some studies support the use of aspirin, 325 mg/day (31,51).

Apart from the morbidity and mortality associated with atrial embolization, the prognosis of patients with atrial fibrillation depends on the nature and extent of underlying heart disease.

Atrial Flutter

Definition and Causes

Atrial flutter is a reentrant arrhythmia that is confined to the right atrium and results in an atrial rate of about 300 beats/minute. Usually there is a 2:1 AV conduction block so that the ventricular response is about 150/minute, and unlike atrial fibrillation, both atrial and ventricular responses are regular. Atrial flutter is almost always seen in patients who have underlying disease: ischemic heart disease, rheumatic heart disease, congestive cardiomyopathy, atrial septal defect, mitral valve disease, chronic obstructive pulmonary disease, and thyrotoxicosis—the same diseases often associated with atrial fibrillation. In contrast to atrial fibrillation, however, atrial flutter is rarely seen in patients who are otherwise healthy.

Symptoms and Signs

Patients are usually aware of a rapid heart rate; whether other symptoms develop depends on the severity and nature of the underlying heart disease.

A regular rapid heart rate and atrial pulse are detected. Sometimes the flutter waves are visible in the jugular pulse. An S_4 is occasionally audible (in contrast to atrial fibrillation).

Electrocardiogram

In atrial flutter, the ECG commonly shows rapid regular sawtooth flutter waves at about 300/minute (Fig. 59.9); P waves are absent. The ventricular response is regular, usually at about 150/minute, and the QRS complex is ordinarily morphologically normal. If the AV node is diseased, higher degrees of AV block may be seen, usually a multiple of 2 (4:1, 8:1, etc.). Aberrant conduction (see "Atrial Fibrillation") is unusual.

If the diagnosis is unclear, carotid sinus massage may help distinguish atrial flutter from other paroxysmal supraventricular tachyarrhythmias. It usually causes

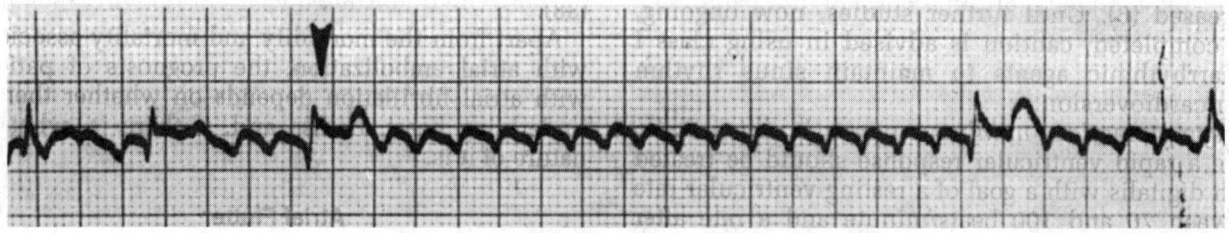

Figure 59.9. Atrial flutter. The flutter waves are clearly revealed after carotid sinus massage (arrowhead).

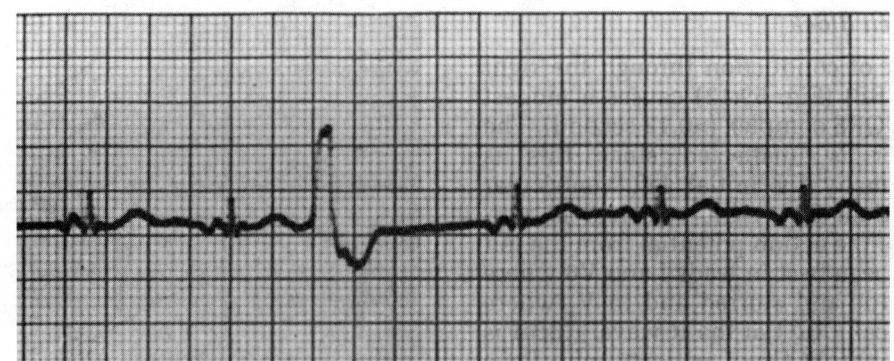

Figure 59.10. Premature ventricular beat. Note that the R–R interval between the two normal beats separated by the PVB is the same as that between two normal beats separated by another normal beat.

an abrupt temporary slowing of the rate; flutter waves, which may have been difficult to detect at a higher rate, are visible in the electrocardiogram, most commonly in leads II, III, aVF, and V_1 (Fig. 59.9). Diagnostic workup is the same as it is for atrial fibrillation.

Treatment and Course

Atrial flutter is often a chronic and very refractory arrhythmia that is difficult to treat with medical therapy. The initial goal of therapy should be to slow the ventricular response, but unlike the situation in patients with atrial fibrillation, it is often difficult to lower the ventricular rate with drugs.

If there is no contraindication, electrical cardioversion (see above) is the treatment of choice if atrial flutter persists, even if there is a high degree of AV block. Most patients can be converted to normal sinus rhythm, usually after application of a much lower energy shock than is necessary to convert atrial fibrillation. If atrial flutter recurs after cardioversion, antiarrhythmic therapy or catheter ablation should be considered.

Considerations regarding pharmacologic therapy for atrial flutter are the same as for atrial fibrillation (see above). Perhaps the only difference is that atrial flutter is even less likely to respond to antiarrhythmic therapy. Patients who have recurrent symptomatic atrial flutter despite pharmacologic treatment should be considered for an electrophysiologic study with possible catheter ablation (see below) of the reentry circuit. Catheter ablation of atrial flutter can be accomplished successfully in more than 90% of patients and with a very low incidence of complications (23,39).

Ventricular Premature Beats

Definition and Causes

Ventricular premature beats (VPBs) are impulses generated in the ventricles, usually as the result of reentry of an impulse conducted down from the atria through the AV node, but sometimes as the result of the firing of an ectopic (parasystolic) focus.

Occasional VPBs occur in many healthy people sporadically during their lives, more often in older people. However, often VPBs are associated with underlying organic heart disease (e.g., hypertensive heart disease, ischemic heart disease, cardiomyopathy, or

mitral valve prolapse). The frequency of VPBs may be increased in people both with and without heart disease by caffeine, alcohol, sympathomimetic drugs, tricyclic antidepressants, phenothiazines, hypokalemia, hypomagnesemia, hypoxia, and emotional stress. VPBs are a common manifestation of digitalis intoxication. Exercise usually abolishes VPBs in people without structural heart disease; conversely, an increase in the number of VPBs after exertion is highly suggestive of structural heart disease.

Symptoms and Signs

Patients may be unaware that they have had a VPB, but often they experience a palpitation, sensing either the premature beat itself or the more forceful normal beat that follows it after a compensatory pause.

Electrocardiogram

The ECG shows a premature ventricular response with a morphologically abnormal, often bizarre, wide QRS complex (58). No P wave precedes a VPB, but by retrograde conduction, a P wave sometimes follows it. The ST segment and the T wave have an opposite vector from the QRS complex. Typically, a VPB is followed by a compensatory pause; that is, the R–R interval between two normal beats separated by a VPB is the same as that between two normal beats separated by another normal beat (Fig. 59.10), because of retrograde conduction of the premature beat to the AV node, thereby blocking the succeeding sinus beat.

When VPBs are caused by reentry, they have a fixed temporal (coupled) relationship to the preceding normal beats. When they are caused by the firing of an ectopic (parasystolic) focus, they have no fixed relationship to the preceding normal beats but do have a regular pattern (i.e., the ectopic intervals are constant or are multiples of a constant). Ectopic beats may occasionally fuse with normal beats, producing a complex that is intermediate between the two (Fig. 59.11).

Treatment and Course

VPBs in patients with otherwise normal hearts are not harmful. However, there is an increased incidence of sudden death and myocardial infarction in patients with VPBs who have underlying ischemic heart disease (2,13). It has not been demonstrated that

Figure 59.11. Premature ventricular beats caused by the firing of an ectopic focus. The arrowhead points to a fusion beat.

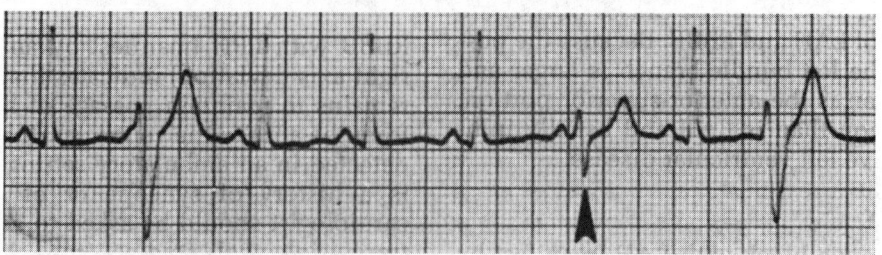

suppression of VPBs in these latter patients alters their course (52). Because all antiarrhythmic agents have potentially serious side effects (Table 59.2), the physician must consider for each patient the relative risks of treating or not treating VPBs. The following generalizations may be useful:

Apparently healthy young people with asymptomatic ventricular premature beats probably do not need treatment (2).

Apparently healthy young people with VPBs causing symptomatic palpitations also do not need pharmacologic treatment. If symptoms interfere with normal lifestyle despite reassurance, a trial of a low-dose β-blocker, such as atenolol 25 to 50 mg/day, may abolish VPBs and relieve symptoms. β-Blockers should be discontinued after several weeks. Often VPBs do not recur and no further treatment is necessary.

Patients with significant structural heart disease, evidenced by an ejection fraction below 40%, and symptomatic ventricular arrhythmias, especially symptomatic multifocal premature ventricular beats, with a frequency of greater than 10/hour or runs of ventricular tachycardia, have an increased risk of sudden death. The treatment of these patients remains highly controversial and they should be referred to a cardiologist for consideration of electrophysiologic testing or empiric treatment with a class III antiarrhythmic agent. The MADIT trial demonstrated that placement of an implantable defibrillator improves survival among patients with a prior myocardial infarction and an ejection fraction less than 35% who have inducible sustained ventricular tachycardia during electrophysiologic testing that is not suppressed with intravenous procainamide (see also Chapter 58) (6,34).

When ventricular arrhythmias occur in the setting of congestive heart failure, an attempt should be made to achieve a maximal state of cardiac compensation before instituting antiarrhythmic therapy. Hemodynamic compensation may decrease or eliminate VPBs so that specific antiarrhythmic therapy is not needed. Disopyramide and flecainide are myocardial depressants and are specifically contraindicated in patients whose hearts are enlarged and hypocontractile. Furthermore, patients in severe chronic heart failure, many of whom are taking diuretics, are more likely to experience problems such as hypokalemia, hypomagnesemia, alkalosis, hypoxemia, and digitalis toxicity, thus increasing the risk of serious side effects from antiarrhythmic agents. Such patients are best treated in consultation with a cardiologist.

Patients with structural heart disease who are symptomatic because of prognostically significant ventricular arrhythmias may be best managed with a drug regimen that is selected using intracardiac electrophysiologic techniques to assess the response to the drugs or with an implantable defibrillator (20,33). This approach requires hospitalization and consultation with a cardiologist.

General internists occasionally assume the care of new patients who are taking antiarrhythmic agents because of a history of symptomatic ventricular arrhythmias caused by structural heart disease. Consultation with a cardiologist is advisable before stopping the therapy (4).

The possibility that a patient may experience a proarrhythmic effect from an antiarrhythmic agent must always be kept in mind (see above).

Heart Block

Heart block, a delay or failure of conduction of the cardiac impulse, is categorized electrocardiographically.

Right Bundle Branch Block

A delay or block of conduction through the right bundle branch (RBBB) (Fig. 59.12) causes a modest prolongation of the QRS complex (more than 0.12 second). The initial QRS vector is unaffected because this is accounted for normally by initial LV (septal) depolarization. The right ventricle is activated by a spread of the action potential from the left ventricle, which is seen best in leads I and V_6, where the S waves are wide and slurred, and in V_1, where there is a double peak (RR') of the R wave. RBBB is sometimes seen in the ECGs of patients who have otherwise normal hearts. More often it is associated with an underlying congenital or acquired disorder (e.g., interatrial septal defect and hypertensive or ischemic heart disease). Patients with newly acquired RBBB have an increased risk of cardiovascular morbidity and death from cardiovascular disease (32,42).

Left Bundle Branch Block

A delay or block of conduction through the left bundle branch (LBBB) (Fig. 59.13) causes a marked prolongation of the QRS complex (0.14 to 0.16 second). The entire sequence of ventricular depolarization is affected so that the QRS complex is widened and the QRS axis is directed to the left and posteriorly. Abnormal repolarization is reflected in the T wave, which is always in the opposite direction of the QRS complex.

LBBB almost always signifies heart disease, usually ischemic heart disease or cardiomyopathy (32).

Hemiblocks

Left Anterior Hemiblock. When there is delay or block of the cardiac impulse in the anterosuperior

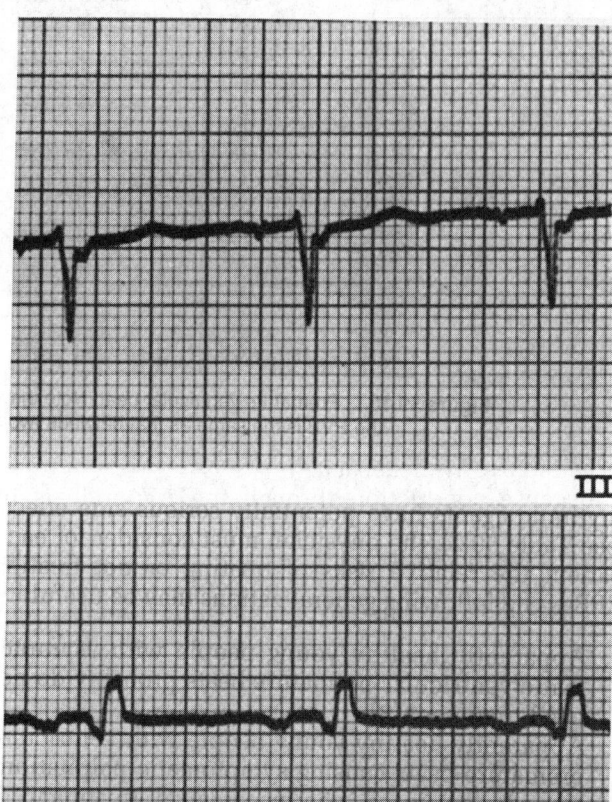

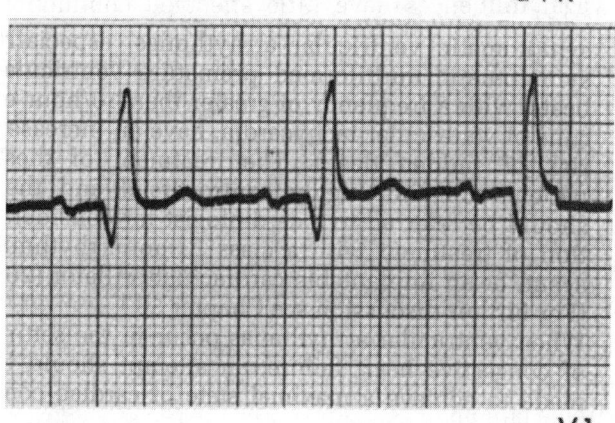

Figure 59.12. Right bundle branch block and left anterior hemiblock (bifascicular block).

portion of the left bundle branch (Fig. 59.3), the corresponding wall of the left ventricle is activated late, resulting in marked left-axis deviation on the ECG (Fig. 59.12). The duration of the QRS complex is usually normal or slightly prolonged (more than 0.10 second). The causes of left anterior hemiblock (LAH) are the same as those of LBBB. LAH is occasionally seen in patients with no discernible heart disease. Whatever the cause, LAH is not in itself a poor prognostic sign and, at least in an ambulatory setting, requires no specific therapy.

Left Posterior Hemiblock. When there is delay or block of the cardiac impulse in the posterior portion of the left bundle branch (Fig. 59.3), activation of the posterior wall of the left ventricle is delayed. The ECG pattern of left posterior hemiblock (LPH) is characterized by marked right-axis deviation (more than +110°). The causes of LPH are the same as those of LAH and LBBB. Because the posterior portion of the left bundle branch is larger and better perfused than is the anterosuperior portion, LPH is less common than is LAH and usually indicates more extensive LV disease (24,33).

Bifascicular Block

RBBB with LAH (manifest by an RBBB pattern and left-axis deviation; Fig. 59.12) or RBBB with LPH (manifest by an RBBB pattern and right-axis deviation) indicates that only one pathway remains to maintain passage of the cardiac impulse from the atria to the ventricles. If bifascicular block is detected in an ambulatory setting, especially if there is a history of syncope or light-headedness, a cardiologist should be asked to advise whether electrophysiologic studies (see above, "Diagnosis of Arrhythmias") or pacemaker implantation is indicated. The risk that unselected patients with bifascicular block will develop complete heart block is 5 to 6% a year (24,33). There is conflicting evidence, however, about the course of patients with bifascicular block: Some report no increased morbidity (24,33); others report a considerably shortened survival (9,10,20). Although there is no consensus about how to deal with the problem, the prognosis seems to be related to the extent of the underlying disease.

First-Degree Heart Block

Definition and Causes. The P–R interval normally varies with heart rate but should not exceed 0.21 second in people in normal sinus rhythm. First-degree AV block is defined as a prolonged P–R interval. The block may be caused by a prolongation of conduction in any of the structures between the SA node and the bundle of His (Fig. 59.3). Most commonly, when the QRS duration is normal, a long P–R interval is caused by a delay in conduction in the AV node. When first-degree block coincides with LBBB, it is likely that there is a delay in conduction in the His bundle. A prolonged P–R interval with RBBB may be caused by a block in the AV node or in the bundle of His.

A prolongation of the P–R interval is usually caused by degenerative, ischemic, or inflammatory changes in the AV conduction systems. It is commonly seen in

Figure 59.13. Left bundle branch block.

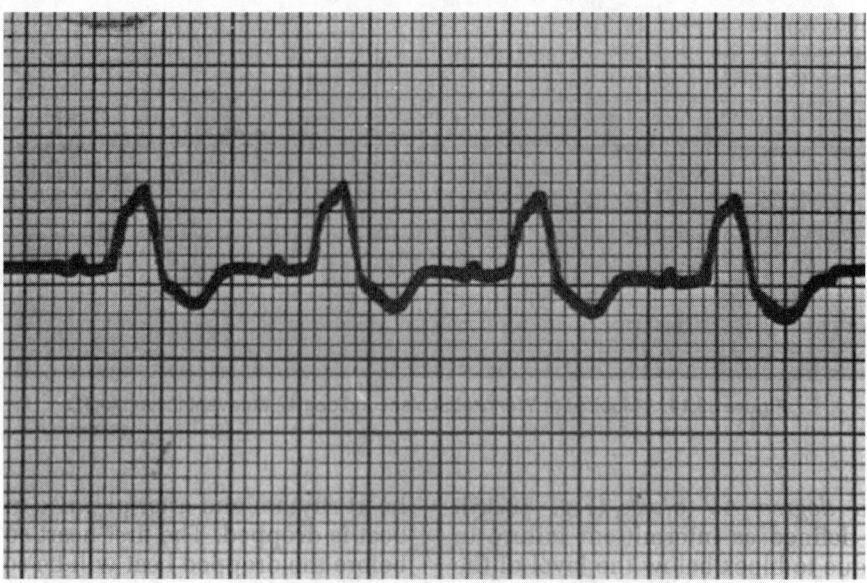

older people without other evidence of heart disease, in patients who have had an inferior wall MI, or in association with myocarditis (including acute rheumatic fever). Drugs such as digitalis, which affect vagal activity, and sympatholytic drugs also may produce a first-degree AV block.

Symptoms and Signs. First-degree AV block in itself does not produce symptoms or abnormal physical findings except a first heart sound that is reduced in intensity.

Treatment and Course. Patients with first-degree AV block who are asymptomatic and who have no other evidence of heart disease need not be treated. If patients with first-degree block complain of light-headedness or dizziness, an ambulatory ECG or event monitor should be obtained (see above, "Use of the ECG") because some of these patients may have episodic higher degrees of block.

Second-Degree AV Block

Definition and Causes. Second-degree AV block is present when some but not all P waves are followed by QRS complexes. Second-degree AV block is caused by conduction delay or block either in the AV node or in the conduction system below the AV node, most commonly caused by ischemic heart disease or idiopathic cardiomyopathy. The site of the block has important therapeutic implications (see below).

Mobitz-I or Wenckebach Second-Degree AV Block. Second-degree AV block within the AV node results in the Wenckebach phenomenon, characterized by progressive lengthening of the P–R interval with shortening of the R–R interval for several cycles until the P wave is blocked completely (Fig. 59.14); the sequence begins again, often with a normal P–R interval in the beat that follows the blocked P wave. In the absence of disease elsewhere in the conducting system, the QRS complex is normal. The degree of Wenckebach block is

characterized by the ratio of the number of P waves to the number of QRS complexes in each cycle of block. In other words, if block occurs after every third P wave, it is called 3:2 Wenckebach.

Because conduction through the AV node is influenced by vagal tone, type I—second-degree AV block—may be precipitated by anything that increases vagal tone. It therefore is sometimes seen as a transient phenomenon in people with no other evidence of heart disease. Otherwise, it is produced by the same processes that are associated with first-degree AV block.

Mobitz-II Second-Degree AV Block. Mobitz-II block is defined as intermittent failure to conduct a P wave caused by block below the level of the AV node (Fig. 59.15). The P–R interval of the conducted beat before a blocked P wave is usually normal. The block may be intermittent or may occur in a fixed 2:1 or 3:1 ratio. Coexistent bundle branch block is commonly seen. Progression to higher degrees of block or to asystole may occur rapidly.

Vagal influences have little effect on conduction below the AV node, so changes in vagal tone do not influence Mobitz-II block. However, the block may be precipitated by medications such as β-blockers, which decrease conduction through the bundle of His. The common causes of Mobitz-II block are degenerative or ischemic changes in the His–Purkinje system.

Symptoms and Signs

Mobitz-I Second-Degree AV Block. Patients are often asymptomatic but if vagal tone is increased (e.g., by digitalis or a β-blocker or central sympatholytics such as clonidine), profound bradycardia may ensue, sometimes with rates below 30/minute. Such patients may complain of light-headedness, syncope, or extreme fatigue.

Physical findings are subtle; irregularity of the heart rhythm and arterial pulse may be noted when a beat is dropped. The first heart sound of the last beat before the dropped beat is softer than that of the first beat after the pause (because of the variation in P–R interval, see Chapter 60).

Mobitz-II Second-Degree AV Block. Symptoms and physical findings are similar to those of patients with Mobitz-I block except that they are not influenced by changes in vagal activity and the intensity of the first heart sound is constant.

Treatment and Course

Mobitz-I Second-Degree AV Block. Asymptomatic patients need not be treated because the risk of rapid progression of the block and of asystole is slight. Symptomatic patients usually have pronounced bradycardia. If so, medications, which may be increasing the block, should be discontinued. If such medications are essential to the patient's management, a cardiac pacemaker should be implanted (see above, "Pacemaker Therapy").

Mobitz-II Second-Degree AV Block. Because of the high risk of rapid progression of the block and of asystole, all patients, even if asymptomatic, should be treated with a permanent cardiac pacemaker.

Patients with a history of light-headedness or dizziness who have new bundle branch block should be suspected of having had Mobitz-II block. This suspicion often can be confirmed with the use of an ambulatory ECG or event monitor (see above, "Use of the ECG"). An intracardiac ECG (see above), if necessary,

may also show prolonged conduction through the His bundle. Patients with a known history of coronary artery disease and with new or increased bundle branch blocks who have a clear-cut history of syncope must be thought to have had Mobitz-II block or complete heart block until proven otherwise.

Third-Degree (Complete) Heart Block

Definition and Causes. Complete heart block occurs when there is total failure of conduction of impulses from the atria through the AV junction to the bundle of His (or, more rarely, if all three fascicles below the His bundle are diseased). The life of the patient then depends on the escape of a ventricular pacemaker. A rhythm generated in the upper portion of the His bundle may have a QRS configuration nearly identical to that of normally conducted impulses and has a rate between 40 and 60 beats/minute (Fig. 59.16). It is more likely to be a stable rhythm than is a rhythm generated by a lower pacemaker. If the pacemaker is located more distally in the conducting system, the ventricular rate decreases, the QRS morphology becomes wider and more bizarre, and the risk of asystole increases. In children or young adults, complete heart block may occur because of congenital defects in development of the AV cushion or the conduction system itself; in such cases escape rhythms are usually generated high in the bundle of His. In older people,

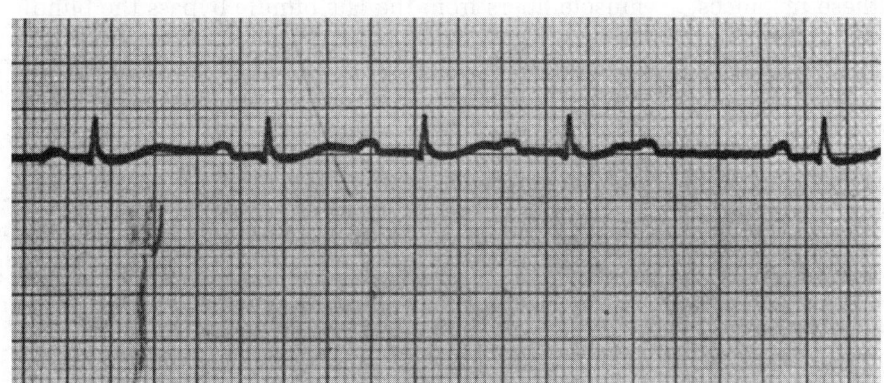

Figure 59.14. Mobitz-I or Wenckebach second-degree AV block.

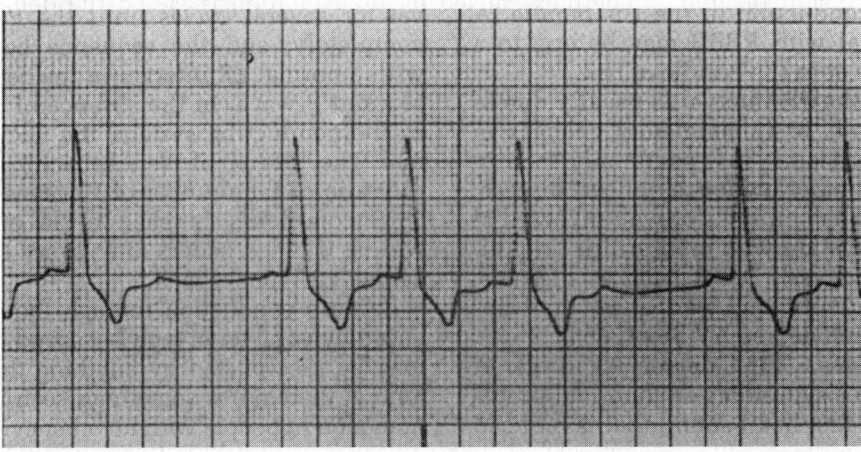

Figure 59.15. Mobitz-II second-degree AV block.

Figure 59.16.   Third-degree heart block.

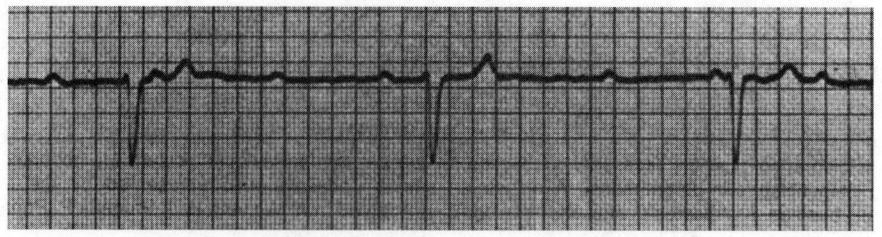

complete heart block is most commonly caused by degenerative and fibrotic changes in the conduction system. It is also seen sometimes in association with infiltrative disease of the myocardium (e.g., sarcoid or amyloid), inflammatory processes (e.g., rheumatoid arthritis), and myocardial infections (e.g., bacterial endocarditis with valve ring abscess, tuberculosis, syphilis) or ischemic heart disease. Occasionally digitalis toxicity may produce complete heart block, as may excessive dosages of β-blockers, methyldopa, and clonidine.

Complete heart block is a subcategory of *AV dissociation,* a situation in which the atria and ventricles are depolarized independently. In instances of AV dissociation, other than complete heart block, the ventricles may be paced independently because of enhancement of the rate of discharge of a latent ventricular pacemaker (e.g., ventricular tachycardia) or because of marked slowing of the rate of discharge of the ordinarily dominant atrial pacemaker. In these instances, the ventricular rate is usually greater than the atrial rate and is also usually greater than it is in patients with complete heart block.

Symptoms and Signs.   A major symptom of complete heart block is sudden loss of consciousness (a Stokes–Adams attack), the result of asystole or tachyarrhythmia (ventricular tachycardia or fibrillation). The asystole is caused by failure of the ventricular pacemaker; the tachyarrhythmia is caused by escape of another focus when the idioventricular rate falls too low (a variant of the bradycardia–tachycardia syndrome; see "Sick Sinus Syndrome," above). If the heart begins to pump effectively again within seconds, as it usually does, the patient promptly regains consciousness and is alert and oriented. If perfusion of vital organs is delayed, seizurelike activity (ordinarily not generalized) and even death may ensue. If they are unconscious for more than a few minutes, patients may not become fully alert for hours.

Complete heart block in patients with underlying myocardial disease may cause symptoms of heart failure (see Chapter 61) primarily because of further reduction in cardiac output as the result of bradycardia.

Physical findings of heart block are all attributable to the dissociation between atrial and ventricular contraction: variation in the intensity of the first heart sound, variation in systolic blood pressure, variation in the intensity of heart murmurs and of third and fourth heart sounds, and the appearance of cannon waves in the jugular pulse. The heart rate, of course, is slow.

Treatment and Course.   The treatment of complete heart block is permanent pacemaker implantation. The life expectancy of treated patients with complete heart block who have no other evidence of cardiac or systemic disease is excellent and approaches that of their age-matched cohort. Patients with complete heart block caused by coronary disease have a prognosis that is determined by the extent of their underlying coronary artery disease and their myocardial function.

Preexcitation Syndrome

Definition and Causes

The atria and ventricles are electrically isolated from each other by the AV groove, and the electrical signal from the atria is conducted to the ventricle via the AV node and conducting system. If the AV groove is short-circuited by muscle fibers, if muscle fibers from the atria enter the His bundle below the AV node, or if muscle fibers from the His bundle bypass the bundle branches, a variable portion of the right or left ventricle is depolarized early. These short-circuiting fibers are known as accessory atrioventricular, nodoventricular, and fasciculoventricular pathways—the atriofascicular bypass tract and the intranodal bypass tract, depending on their location (Fig. 59.17).

The classic example of preexcitation is *WPW syndrome,* which refers to patients with symptomatic accessory AV connections. This syndrome is characterized electrocardiographically by a short P–R interval followed by a wide QRS complex, which is a fusion beat between the ventricular myocardium that is preexcited and that which is excited via normal conduction pathways (Fig. 59.18). The portion of the complex caused by preexcitation is called the delta wave because of its resemblance to the Greek capital letter delta (Δ). If the accessory bundle connects the atria with the left ventricle, the electrocardiographic pattern resembles RBBB (type A WPW). On the other hand, if the connection is with the right ventricle, the pattern resembles LBBB (type B WPW); the negative Δwave in lead II in this situation may be taken for a Q wave, and the mistaken diagnosis of remote MI may be made.

If the atrial fibers insert into the bundle of His and short-circuit the AV node, the P–R interval is short, but no Δwave is seen because below the AV node conduction occurs along the usual pathways. This syndrome is known as the *Lown–Ganong–Levine (LGL) syndrome.* A number of other variants of preexcitation syndrome have been described but are much rarer than these two common disorders (59).

The ECG manifestations of preexcitation may vary from time to time within a given patient because, if conduction occurs through the normal anatomic pathways rather than through accessory fibers, no preexcitation is seen on the ECG. When preexcitation is facilitated because of disease in the AV node or because of drugs that suppress conduction through the AV node (e.g., digitalis, calcium channel blockers, or β-blockers), abnormalities on the ECG are seen.

Reentrant supraventricular arrhythmias are common in patients with preexcitation; estimates vary from 13 to 60%, usually paroxysmal supraventricular tachycardia, but atrial fibrillation and flutter also occur (8,39). The morphology of the QRS complex during the tachyarrhythmia depends on the direction in which the reentrant tachycardia occurs. If reentry occurs antegrade through the AV conducting system and retrograde through an accessory pathway, then the QRS duration during the tachyarrhythmia may be normal because the ventricle is depolarized in a

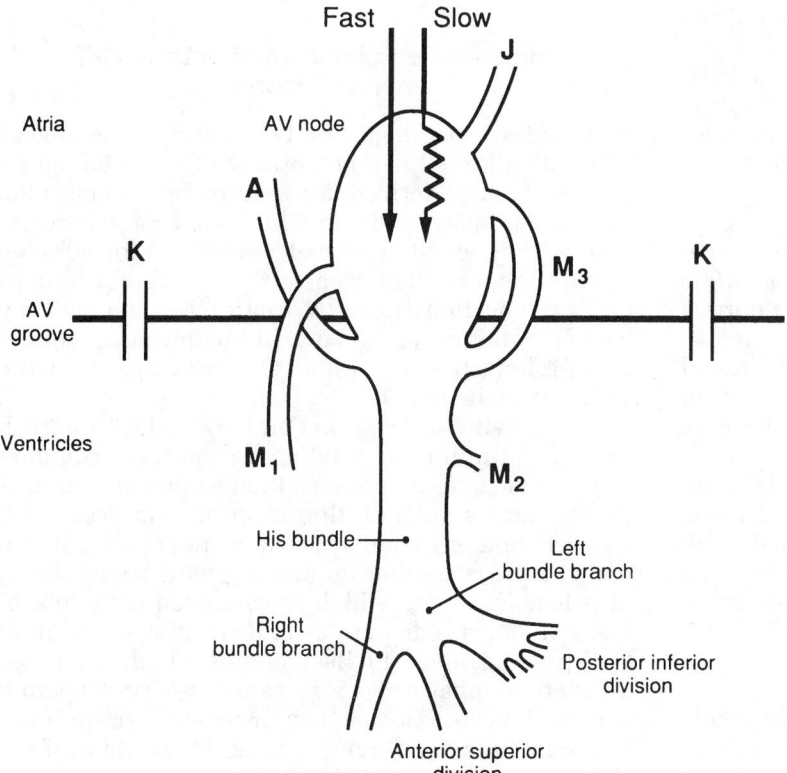

Figure 59.17. Schematic diagram of possible accessory conduction pathways. (Old eponymic nomenclature in parentheses.) *A,* Atriofascicular (atrio-Hisian) bundles; *K,* accessory atrioventricular (Kent) bundles; *J,* intranodal bypass (James) tracts; *M* (Mahaim) fibers: M_1, accessory nodoventricular; M_2, accessory fasciculoventricular; M_3, nodofascicular fibers. Dual AV node pathways are represented by the fast and slow symbols. (Adapted from Wellens HJJ, Brugada P, Penn OC. The management of preexcitation syndromes. JAMA 257:2325, 1987.)

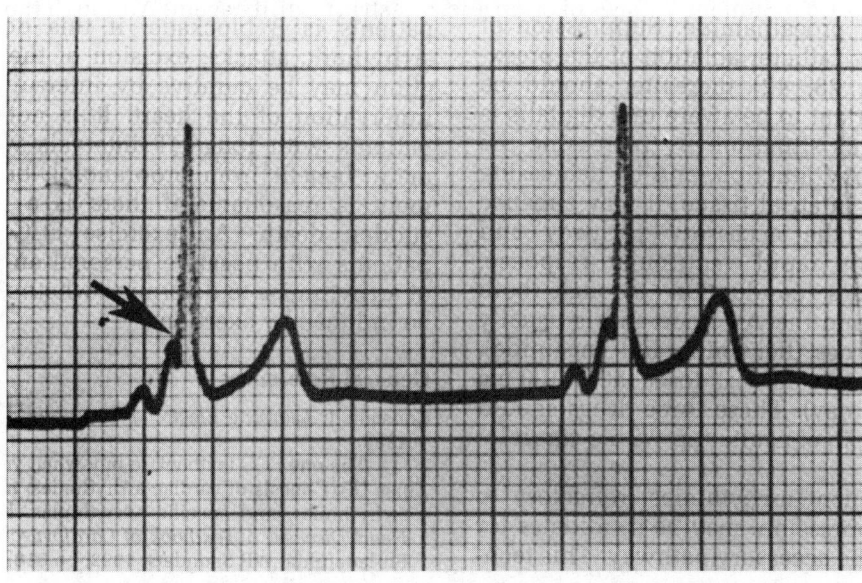

Figure 59.18. The Wolff–Parkinson–White syndrome. Note Δ wave.

normal direction through its normal specialized conducting tissue. If the circuit is established in the opposite direction, the QRS complex is wide, with a bundle branch block pattern, because most or all of the ventricle is depolarized by way of the accessory pathway, and the arrhythmia easily can be confused with ventricular tachycardia.

Symptoms and Signs

Preexcitation may be an incidental finding on an ECG or it may come to the attention of the physician because of symptoms of palpitations. Other symptoms of tachyarrhythmia depend on the nature of the arrhythmia and the presence or absence of other structural heart disease.

There are no physical findings caused by preexcitation other than occasionally a loud S_1, except during periods of tachyarrhythmia, and then the findings depend on the type of arrhythmia that is present.

Prevalence

Preexcitation syndromes are not rare. The prevalence of preexcitation is between 1 and 30/1000 people, or approximately 0.15 to 0.3% of the normal population (39,43). Accurate prevalence rates are difficult to obtain because short P–R intervals with normal QRS durations are commonly seen in people without arrhythmias so that no studies are done to determine whether a bypass tract exists.

Preexcitation syndromes occasionally may be associated with certain forms of congenital heart disease. Preexcitation of the WPW type is associated with Ebstein's anomaly of the tricuspid valve, corrected transposition of the great vessels, and hypertrophic cardiomyopathies.

Treatment and Course

The presence of preexcitation in an asymptomatic patient is associated with an annual risk of sudden cardiac death of approximately 0.1%. Because this is not markedly greater than the risk of sudden cardiac death in the general population and because treatment is associated with some risk, current guidelines recommend that asymptomatic patients who have evidence of preexcitation on their ECG not be treated. Exceptions to this rule are competitive athletes and people in high-risk occupations such as bus drivers or pilots. In these settings it is reasonable to consider performing an electrophysiologic study to determine whether the accessory pathway has the capacity to conduct rapidly (which increases the risk of sudden cardiac death fivefold) and whether a sustained arrhythmia can be induced. In these settings catheter ablation is often performed. All patients with evidence of preexcitation on their ECG should be instructed to contact their physician if symptoms subsequently develop. Because of the increased risk of sudden cardiac death among patients with WPW syndrome (preexcitation and symptoms of tachycardia), electrophysiology testing and catheter ablation is now recommended as first-line therapy. Asymptomatic patients need not be treated;

their survival is the same as that of the normal population (5).

Patients with occasional symptoms can often be taught to break the arrhythmia using vagal maneuvers. These should be tried as soon as possible after the onset of tachycardia because sympathetic tone quickly increases after the onset of tachycardia and increased sympathetic tone will interfere with the effectiveness of the maneuvers. Effective vagal maneuvers include straining against a closed glottis (Valsalva maneuver), gagging by sticking a finger down the throat, self-applied carotid sinus massage, and placing a cold wet towel over the face (the diving reflex).

Torsades de Pointes and the Long Q–T Interval Syndrome

Torsades de pointes (literally "twisting of the spikes" [QRS complexes]) is a potentially life-threatening arrhythmia characterized by a form of polymorphic ventricular tachycardia, in which the QRS axis seemingly twists about the isoelectric line. Torsades de pointes is most often seen in the setting of acquired Q–T prolongation caused by drug interactions, but may be seen with the syndrome of idiopathic or congenital Q–T prolongation, or without Q–T prolongation in the setting of ischemia (53).

Antiarrhythmic drugs that prolong the Q–T interval, such as quinidine or sotalol, are the most common cause of torsades de pointes. In most patients, predisposing factors such as diuretic use with associated hypokalemia or hypomagnesemia are present. Severe bradycardia is another important predisposing factor, as is female gender, which is associated with 70% of cases of torsades de pointes in the setting of acquired Q–T prolongation (28). Besides antiarrhythmic drugs, a variety of other drugs may cause Q–T prolongation and have been associated with torsades de pointes. These include antidepressants; antihistamines of the H_1-blocking type (astemizole and terfenadine); some antibiotics, particularly erythromycin; and high dosages of cisapride, a gastric motility agent. Although the incidence of torsades de pointes in patients taking these drugs is rare, these drugs should be used with caution in women, or in patients taking several of these drugs in combination, especially in the setting of hypokalemia or hypomagnesemia, and in patients with the long Q–T syndrome.

In contrast to the acquired long Q–T syndrome, idiopathic or congenital long Q–T syndrome is a congenital disorder in which delayed repolarization is expressed as a long Q–T interval (more than 0.45 second when corrected for heart rate) (43,56). In some families the inheritance is autosomal recessive and is associated with nerve deafness; in others, the inheritance is autosomal dominant and hearing is normal. Diagnostic criteria, using a point scale, have been published (43). The long Q–T interval predisposes to torsades de pointes, which often causes syncope and may cause sudden death, especially in the setting of acute stress (56). The Q–T interval should be measured routinely in the ECG of patients who complain of syncope for which there is no explanation.

The most effective treatment of symptomatic patients is β blockade; if this does not suppress arrhythmic attacks, excision of the left stellate ganglion may be curative, interrupting sympathetic innervation of the heart. Appropriate treatment reduces the long-term mortality from 50% to less than 5%. It is not known whether patients with long Q–T intervals who are asymptomatic benefit from antiadrenergic therapy, but certainly treatment is reasonable if there is a family history of sudden death. An exercise ECG is indicated in patients with negative personal and family histories of arrhythmias to determine whether arrhythmias can be induced by exertion (56).

ARRHYTHMIAS IN PREGNANCY

Clinically significant arrhythmias occur rarely during pregnancy, but the awareness of ventricular ectopy and ventricular tachycardia is increased (35). The most common arrhythmia, other than isolated premature atrial beats and premature ventricular beats, is PSVT caused by AV node reentry, a common arrhythmia (see above). Occasionally, nonsustained ventricular tachycardia is detected as an incidental finding in an otherwise asymptomatic patient. Antiarrhythmic treatment options are limited in pregnancy; fluoroscopy, which is necessary for catheter ablation, is contraindicated, and antiarrhythmic drug options are limited. β-Blockers, especially atenolol, have been reported to be safe during pregnancy, and quinidine and procainamide have been used as well (35). Submaximal exercise stress testing has been shown to be safe up to 25 weeks' gestation (7); ventricular arrhythmias that suppress with exercise are thought to have a benign prognosis (41). Patients with symptomatic arrhythmias should be referred to a cardiologist for evaluation.

General References*

Constant J. Learning electrocardiography. Boston: Little, Brown, 1997.
> The one ECG textbook to buy when you are buying only one.

Podrid PJ, Kowey PR, eds. Cardiac arrhythmia: mechanisms, diagnosis and management. Baltimore: Williams & Wilkins, 1995.
> A well-edited and clinically very useful and accessible textbook.

Specific References

1. Barsky AJ, Cleary PD, Barnett MC, et al. The accuracy of symptom reporting by patients complaining of palpitations. Am J Med 97:214–221, 1994.
2. Bikkina M, Larson MG, Levy D. Prognostic implications of asymptomatic ventricular arrhythmias: the Framingham Heart Study. Ann Intern Med 117:990, 1992.
3. Blomgren SE, Condemi JJ, Bignall MC, Vaughn JH. Antinuclear antibody induced by procainamide. A prospective study. N Engl J Med 281:64, 1969.

4. Cairns JA, Connolly SJ, Roberts R, Gent M. Amiodarone for patients with ventricular premature depolarizations after myocardial infarction. Is it safe to stop treatment at one year? Circulation 87:637, 1993.
5. Calkins H, Langberg J, Sousa J, et al. Radiofrequency catheter ablation of accessory atrioventricular connections in 250 patients. Abbreviated therapeutic approach to Wolff–Parkinson–White syndrome. Circulation 85:1337–1346, 1997.
6. Cardiovascular News. NHLBI stops arrhythmia study: Implantable cardiac defibrillators reduce deaths. Circulation 95:2465, 1997.
7. Carpenter MW, Sady SP, Hoegsgberg B, et al. Fetal heart rate response to maternal exertion. J Am Med Assoc 259:20, 1988.
8. Coplen SE, Antman EM, Berlin JA, et al. Efficacy and safety of quinidine therapy for maintenance of sinus rhythm after cardioversion. Circulation 82:1106, 1990.
9. Denes P, Dhingra RC, Wu D, et al. Sudden death in patients with chronic bifascicular block. Arch Intern Med 137:1005, 1977.
10. Dhingra RC, Denes P, Wu D, et al. Prospective observations in patients with chronic bundle branch block and marked HV prolongation. Circulation 53:600, 1976.
11. Dreifus LS, Fisch C, Griffin JC, et al. Guidelines for implantation of cardiac pacemakers and antiarrhythmic devices. A report of the American College of Cardiology/American Heart Association Task Force on Assessment of Diagnostic and Therapeutic Cardiovascular Procedures. J Am Coll Cardiol 18:1–13, 1991.
12. Drugs for cardiac arrhythmias. Med Lett 38:75–82, 1996.
13. Echt DS, Liebson PR, Mitchell B, et al. Mortality and morbidity in patients receiving encainide, flecainide, or placebo. The Cardiac Arrhythmia Suppression Trial. N Engl J Med 324:781, 1991.
14. Falk RH, Knowlton AA, Bernard SA, et al. Digoxin for converting recent-onset atrial fibrillation to sinus rhythm: a randomized, double-blinded trial. Ann Intern Med 106:503–506, 1987.
15. Flaker GC, Blackshear JL, McBride R, et al. Antiarrhythmic drug therapy and cardiac mortality in atrial fibrillation. The Stroke Prevention in Atrial Fibrillation Investigators. J Am Coll Cardiol 20:527–532, 1992.
16. Ganz LI, Friedman PL. Supraventricular tachycardia. N Engl J Med 332:162–173, 1995.
17. Hayes DL, Wang PJ, Reynolds DW, et al. Interference with cardiac pacemakers by cellular telephones. N Engl J Med 336:1473–1479, 1997.
18. Horowitz LN. Proarrhythmia: taking the bad with the good. N Engl J Med 319:304, 1988.
19. Jung F, DiMarco JP. Antiarrhythmic drug therapy in the treatment of atrial fibrillation. Cardiol Clin 14:507, 1996.
20. Kastor JA. Michel Mirowski and the automatic implantable defibrillator. Am J Cardiol 63:1121, 1989.
21. Kastor JA. Multifocal atrial tachycardia. N Engl J Med 322:1713, 1990.
22. Kinlay S, Leitsch JW, Neil A, et al. Cardiac event recorders yield more diagnoses and are more cost-effective than 48-hour Holter monitoring in patients with palpitations. A controlled clinical trial. Ann Intern Med 124:16, 1996.
23. Kirkorian G, Moncada E, Chevalier P, et al. Radiofrequency ablation of atrial flutter. Efficacy of an anatomically guided approach. Circulation 90:2804–2814, 1994.
24. Kulbertus HE, Demoulin JC. The left hemiblocks: significance, prognosis and treatment. Schweiz Med Wochenschr 112:1579, 1982.
25. Kusumoto FM, Goldschlager N. Cardiac pacing. N Engl J Med 334:89, 1996.
26. Lessmeier TJ, Gamperling D, Johnson-Liddon V et al. Unrecognized paroxysmal supraventricular tachycardia: potential for misdiagnosis as panic disorder. Arch Intern Med 157:537, 1997.
27. Linzer M, Pritchett EL, Pontinen M, et al. Incremental diagnostic yield of loop electrocardiographic recorders in unexplained syncope. Am J Cardiol 66:214, 1990.
28. Makkar RR, Fromm BS, Steinman RT, et al. Female gender as a risk factor for torsade de pointes associated with cardiovascular drugs. JAMA 270:2590, 1993.
29. Manning WJ, Silverman DI, Keighley CS, et al. Transesophageal echocardiographically facilitated early cardioversion from

atrial fibrillation using short-term anticoagulation: final results of a prospective 4.5-year study. J Am Coll Cardiol 25:1354–1361, 1995.

30. Maragno I, Santostasi G, Gaion RM, et al. Low and medium dose diltiazem in chronic atrial fibrillation: comparison with digoxin and correlation with drug plasma levels. Am Heart J 116:385, 1988.

31. Matchar DB, McCrory DC, Barnett HJM, et al. Medical treatment for stroke prevention. Ann Intern Med 121:41–53, 1994.

32. Mikinski M, Dunn MI. Evaluation of the patient with complete bundle branch block. ACC Curr J Rev 4:55–57, 1995.

33. Mirowski M, Reid PR, Winkle RA, et al. Mortality in patients with implanted automatic defibrillators. Ann Intern Med 98:585, 1983.

34. Moss AJ, Hall WJ, Cannom DS, et al. Improved survival with an implanted defibrillator in patients with coronary disease at high risk for ventricular arrhythmia. Multicenter Automatic Defibrillators Implantation Investigators. N Engl J Med 335:1933–1940, 1996.

35. Page RL. Treatment of arrhythmias during pregnancy. Am Heart J 130:871–876, 1995.

36. Planning and Steering Committees of the AFFIRM Study for the NHLBI AFFIRM Investigators. Atrial fibrillation follow-up investigation of rhythm management: the AFFIRM study design. Am J Cardiol 79:1198, 1997.

37. Podrid PJ. Amiodarone: reevaluation of an old drug. Ann Intern Med 122:689, 1995.

38. Pratt CM, Eaton T, Francis M, et al. The inverse relationship between baseline left ventricular ejection fraction and outcome of antiarrhythmic therapy: a dangerous imbalance in the risk–benefit ratio. Am Heart J 118:433, 1989.

39. Ruskin JN. Catheter ablation for supraventricular tachycardia. N Engl J Med 324:1660, 1991.

40. Safety of calcium channel blockers. Med Lett 39:13, 1997.

41. Sami M, Kraemer H, Harrison DL, et al. A new method evaluating antiarrhythmic drug efficacy in individual patients. Circulation 62:1171, 1980.

42. Schneider JF, Thomas HE, Kreger BE, et al. Newly acquired right bundle branch block. The Framingham study. Ann Intern Med 92:37, 1980.

43. Schwartz PJ, Moss AJ, Vincent GM, Crampton RS. Diagnostic criteria for the long QT syndrome. An update. Circulation 88:782–784, 1993.

44. Shapiro EP, Effron MB, Lima SE. Transient atrial dysfunction after conversion of chronic atrial fibrillation to sinus rhythm. Am J Cardiol 62:1202, 1988.

45. Shaw DB, Holman RR, Goiner JI. Survival in sinoatrial disorder (sick sinus syndrome). BMJ 280:139, 1980.

46. Sheffield LT, Berson A, Bragg-Remschel D, et al. Recommendation for standards of instrumentation and practice in the use of ambulatory electrocardiography. Circulation 71:626A, 1985.

47. Stone PH, Antman EM, Muller JE, Braunwald E. Calcium channel blocking agents in the treatment of cardiovascular disorders. II. Hemodynamic effects and clinical applications. Ann Intern Med 93:886, 1980.

48. Stroke Prevention in Atrial Fibrillation Investigators. Adjusted-dose warfarin versus low-intensity, fixed-dose warfarin plus aspirin for high-risk patients with atrial fibrillation. Stroke prevention in atrial fibrillation. III. Randomised clinical trial. Lancet 348:633–638, 1996.

49. Stroke Prevention in Atrial Fibrillation Investigators. Predictors of thromboembolism in atrial fibrillation. I. Clinical features of patients at risk. Ann Intern Med 116:1, 1992.

50. Stroke Prevention in Atrial Fibrillation Investigators. Predictors of thromboembolism in atrial fibrillation. II. Echocardiographic features of patients at risk. Ann Intern Med 116:6, 1992.

51. Stroke Prevention in Atrial Fibrillation Investigators. Predictors of thromboembolism in atrial fibrillation: final results. Circulation 84:527, 1991.

52. Surawicz B. Prognosis of ventricular arrhythmias in relation to sudden cardiac death: therapeutic implications. J Am Coll Cardiol 10:435, 1987.

53. Tan HL, Hou CJ, Lauer MR, Sung RJ. Electrophysiologic mechanisms of the long QT interval syndromes and torsade de pointes. Ann Intern Med 122:701–714, 1995.

54. Task Force of the Working Group on Arrhythmias of the European Society of Cardiology. The Sicilian gambit. A new approach to the classification of antiarrhythmic drugs based on their actions on arrhythmogenic mechanisms. Circulation 84:1831, 1991.

55. Teo KK, Yusuf S, Furberg CD. Effects of prophylactic antiarrhythmic drug therapy in acute myocardial infarction. An overview of results from randomized controlled trials. JAMA 270:1589, 1993.

56. Towbin JA. New revelations about the long-QT interval syndrome. N Engl J Med 333:384, 1995.

57. Vaughan Williams, EM. Significance of classifying antiarrhythmic actions since the cardiac arrhythmia suppression trial. J Clin Pharmacol 31:123,1991.

58. Wellens HJJ, Bar FW, Lie KI. The value of the electrocardiogram in the differential diagnosis of a tachycardia with a widened QRS complex. Am J Med 64:27, 1978.

59. Wellens HJJ, Brugada P, Penn OC. The management of preexcitation syndromes. JAMA 257:23, 1987.

60. Williamson BD, Man KC, Daoud E, et al. Radiofrequency catheter modification of atrioventricular conduction to control the ventricular rate during atrial fibrillation. N Engl J Med 331:910–917, 1994.

61. Wolf PA, Kannel WB, McGee DC, et al. Duration of atrial fibrillation and imminence of stroke: the Framingham Study. Stroke 14:664, 1983.

Common Cardiac Disorders Revealed by Auscultation of the Heart

EDWARD P. SHAPIRO, MD

HEART SOUNDS

First Heart Sound (S₁)

The first heart sound is a high-frequency ("clicky") sound produced by closure of the atrioventricular (AV) valves, that is, M_1 (mitral valve closure) followed by T_1 (tricuspid valve closure). Mitral valve closure is louder than tricuspid valve closure.

Abnormally wide splitting of the first heart sound is produced by delays in closure of the tricuspid valve, as in patients with right bundle branch block, ventricular ectopic beats, idioventricular rhythm, or left ventricular pacing. In mitral stenosis, mitral valve closure may be so delayed that tricuspid valve closure may actually precede mitral valve closure.

Increased intensity of the first heart sound is associated with a rapid increase in ventricular pressure, which occurs when the ventricles are presented with an increased volume (e.g., ventricular septal defect and atrial septal defect) or with a wide-open AV valve at the end of diastole, which occurs when there is shortening of the AV filling time (e.g., atrial tachycardia and conditions associated with a short P–R interval) and when AV filling time is prolonged (e.g., mitral stenosis).

Reduced intensity of the first heart sound may indi-cate an immobile valve (e.g., severe mitral regurgitation or stenosis) or a long P–R interval.

Second Heart Sound (S₂)

The second heart sound is produced by closure of the semilunar valves, that is, A_2 (aortic valve closure) followed by P_2 (pulmonic valve closure). Normal splitting of the second heart sound occurs at the height of inspiration, when the splitting may be as wide as 0.10 second and is caused by the increase in stroke volume in the right heart with the increase in venous return with inspiration. The two components of the second heart sound are synchronous and virtually single during expiration.

Abnormally wide splitting of S_2 without change in expiration is characteristic of an atrial septal defect or anomalous pulmonary venous return. S_2 is widely split but variable in patients with pulmonary stenosis. In the presence of severe aortic stenosis, A_2 is delayed beyond P_2, resulting in wide splitting during expiration with no splitting during inspiration (reversed or paradoxical splitting). Paradoxical splitting of the second heart sound also occurs in the presence of a left bundle branch block, severe hypertension, or severe left ventricular failure.

Increased intensities of A_2 and P_2 are features of aortic and pulmonary hypertension, respectively. Decreased intensities of A_2 or P_2 are features of an immobile or severely thickened aortic or pulmonic valve.

Gallops

The identification of a gallop sound affords valuable information about diagnosis, prognosis, and treatment. Gallops are diastolic sounds and appear to be related to the two periods of filling of the ventricles: the rapid filling phase (the S_3, or ventricular diastolic gallop) and the presystolic filling phase related to atrial systole (S_4, or atrial gallop).

The *atrial gallop sound,* or S_4, is a low-frequency presystolic sound and is found in patients with primary myocardial disease, coronary artery disease, systemic or pulmonary hypertension, or severe aortic or pulmonic stenosis. The atrial gallop indicates severity of the underlying disorder, and as the patient's condition improves, the sound may become fainter or disappear. With ventricular hypertrophy an S_4 is a fixed finding of no prognostic significance. An atrial gallop is commonly heard in people above the age of 65, even in the absence of heart disease or hypertension (see "Doppler Echocardiography," below).

The *ventricular gallop sound,* or S_3, is a low-frequency sound (see Chapter 61). It occurs with the same timing as the normal physiologic third sound, approximately 0.14 to 0.16 second after the second heart sound. The third sound is a normal finding in children and young adults up to the age of 30 (see "Doppler Echocardiography," below). An S_3 gallop is a feature of severe cardiac decompensation, whatever the underlying cause (e.g., hypertension, coronary artery disease, rheumatic heart disease), and indicates a poor prognosis.

Ejection Sounds (Clicks)

Ejection sounds are produced at the time of ejection of blood from the left ventricle into the aorta or from the right ventricle into the pulmonary artery. The sound may originate in a thickened valve or dilated great vessel. The aortic ejection sound is located in the area of aortic auscultation—namely, from the second right intercostal space in a straight line to the cardiac apex—and occurs 0.05 second after M_1. It is a high-frequency sound, often called a click. In the presence of systemic hypertension, the aortic ejection sound is an indication of severity. It disappears as hypertension improves. Aortic ejection clicks may also be heard in patients with aortic stenosis, aneurysm of the ascending aorta, and aortic insufficiency.

Pulmonic ejection sounds (or clicks) are often localized to the second left intercostal space and may increase in intensity with expiration. They occur immediately after M_1. Pulmonic clicks are a feature of valvular pulmonic stenosis and of pulmonary hypertension.

A *midsystolic clicking sound,* with or without a late systolic murmur, may indicate mitral valve prolapse (see below).

Opening Snaps

An opening snap occurs because of a stenotic but still mobile mitral or tricuspid valve. The mitral opening snap is best heard between the pulmonic area and the cardiac apex. It occurs 0.04 to 0.12 second after S_2 in early diastole. It is heard in patients with a thickened mitral valve. The earlier the snap, the more severe the stenosis. The tricuspid opening snap is best heard at the lower left or right sternal border and occurs immediately after S_2 in early diastole.

Murmurs

Evaluation of a heart murmur is one of the most common tasks that confronts a physician conducting a physical examination. Virtually all normal people have a systolic murmur at some time in their lives. On the other hand, a murmur may be a sign of serious underlying cardiac or noncardiac disease. It is important to be able to distinguish innocent murmurs from those that reflect an underlying disorder and to be able to appropriately select the tests that will lead to the precise diagnosis and proper management.

General Characteristics of Murmurs

A murmur is a series of audible vibrations produced by turbulence in the circulation. These vibrations can be characterized by intensity, pitch, shape, quality, and timing in the cardiac cycle, precordial location of maximal intensity, and radiation.

The *intensity or loudness* of a murmur is, by convention, graded on a scale of 1 to 6. A grade 1 murmur is audible only after concentrated auscultation. A grade 2 murmur is faint but readily audible. A grade 3 murmur is prominent but not loud. Grade 4 murmurs are loud and are often, but not always, associated with a palpable thrill. A grade 5 murmur is very loud and can be heard with only the edge of the stethoscope touching the chest wall. A grade 6 murmur is heard with the stethoscope held 1 cm above, but not actually touching, the chest wall.

The *pitch of a murmur* refers to the frequency of the sound, from high to low. High-frequency murmurs usually reflect high velocity or high pressure.

The *shape of a murmur* refers to the change in intensity throughout the duration of the sound: for example, crescendo (increasing in intensity), decrescendo (decreasing in intensity), or constant.

The *quality of a murmur* refers to the nature of the sound: harsh, blowing, musical, cooing, rumbling, etc. Although these terms are not precise, they are useful in identifying various benign and significant conditions, as described below.

The *timing of a murmur* is particularly important in establishing the cause of the sound—first, whether the murmur is systolic, diastolic, or continuous, and second, whether it is heard in early, middle, or late systole or diastole. Murmurs that last throughout systole are called holosystolic. Late diastolic murmurs are sometimes called presystolic.

The *location of a murmur* refers to the site on the chest wall where the sound is loudest. The direction of radiation refers to the other sites where the murmur, although less intense, can still be heard; those sites may be outside the chest (e.g., the back or neck). *Aortic murmurs* may be heard anywhere in a straight line from the second right interspace to the apex. *Pulmonic murmurs* are heard best at the second left intercostal space; tricuspid murmurs, at the lower left sternal border; and mitral murmurs, at the cardiac apex radiating into the axilla.

There are two kinds of systolic murmurs: ejection and regurgitant murmurs. The ejection systolic murmur may be an innocent flow murmur or it may reflect organic heart disease. The regurgitant murmur may be caused by dilation of the annulus of the valve in an otherwise normal heart or may represent organic heart disease.

The *ejection murmur* is a crescendo/decrescendo (or diamond-shaped) murmur caused by the turbulence of blood flowing through either the aortic or the pulmonic valve. The murmur is most commonly midsystolic and ends before the second or closing sound (S_2) of the valve from which the murmur was generated; that is, aortic ejection murmurs end before A_2 and pulmonic ejection murmurs end before P_2. The loudness of the murmur depends in part on the pressure gradient across the valve and in part on other factors, such as thickness of the chest and the cardiac output; the shape depends on the acceleration and deceleration of blood flow across the valve as systole proceeds. When diastole is prolonged—for example, by premature ventricular contraction or by atrial fibrillation—ejection murmurs become louder because of the passage of a large volume of blood through the valve. In general, the larger the cardiac output, the louder the murmur. Increases in cardiac output caused by hypermetabolic states, such as anemia, fever, or thyrotoxicosis, increase the loudness of the murmur. Decreases in cardiac output, as in congestive heart failure, decrease the loudness of the murmur.

Regurgitant murmurs are murmurs produced by backward flow of blood from a high-pressure chamber to a compartment of lower pressure. Intensity may be constant, as in mitral regurgitation, tricuspid regurgitation, or ventricular septal defect, or may be decrescendo, as in aortic and pulmonary regurgitation.

A number of maneuvers can be performed to alter the intensity of a systolic murmur and help determine its origin. For example, the Valsalva maneuver reduces intrathoracic venous return and softens the murmur of aortic stenosis while intensifying that of hypertrophic cardiomyopathy. Squatting, which increases venous return, has the opposite effect. Isometric handgrip, which increases blood pressure and therefore reduces forward flow, softens the murmur of aortic stenosis and intensifies that of mitral regurgitation.

Innocent Murmurs

Innocent murmurs are a series of vibrations that are produced in the absence of significant abnormalities of cardiac anatomy or function (Table 60.1).

Innocent murmurs can usually be distinguished from significant murmurs by the absence of other physical, radiologic, or electrocardiographic evidence of disease. Also, innocent murmurs are usually in early systole or midsystole, are grade 1 or 2 in intensity, and vary with respiration and position. Occasionally, echocardiography (see below) is done to clarify the cause of a murmur, but more elaborate studies, such as stress tests, radionuclide studies, and cardiac catheterization, are used only after it has been decided that a murmur is not innocent and that a more precise diagnosis is necessary.

The most common innocent *systolic murmur of childhood* and young adulthood that is clearly recognizable as benign based on the characteristics of the murmur alone is the musical or vibratory midsystolic murmur (best heard at the lower left sternal border) that is caused by the vibration of the leaflets of the pulmonary valve.

The *venous hum* is a continuous murmur, loudest in the neck, caused by altered flow through the jugular veins. It can be eliminated by turning the patient's

Table 60.1. Benign or Innocent Systolic Murmurs

Vibratory ejection systolic murmur
Continuous murmur of venous hum
Pulmonic ejection systolic murmur
Aortic ejection systolic murmur
Murmur associated with pregnancy

head, compressing the internal jugular vein on the side where the murmur is heard, or placing the patient in the supine position.

The *pulmonic ejection systolic murmur* is a systolic crescendo/decrescendo murmur generated by the flow of blood through the pulmonary valve. It is loudest in the left second intercostal space or at the midleft sternal border.

Similarly, the *aortic ejection systolic murmur* is an early systolic murmur generated by the flow of blood through the aortic valve. It is loudest in the right second intercostal space or at the apex of the heart. This innocent or flow murmur, caused by sclerosis of the aorta or the aortic valve, is the most common benign systolic murmur in middle-aged or elderly patients and may have a cooing quality. An electrocardiogram (ECG) and an echocardiogram may be necessary to rule out LV hypertrophy and aortic stenosis.

Benign flow murmurs are commonly heard in *pregnant women*. Because of the normally increased stroke volume at 28 to 30 weeks' gestation, diastolic filling sounds and systolic ejection murmurs of turbulent flow are common. In pregnant patients also, an S_3 may be prominent enough to be confused with the middiastolic murmur of mitral stenosis. The S_3 of pregnancy may be distinguished from the murmur of mitral stenosis, however, by the absence of an opening snap and by the accompanying hyperdynamic apical movement. An echocardiogram is indicated in some patients to make a precise diagnosis.

In the pregnant patient it is critical to compare the femoral and brachial pulses and the blood pressures in the presence of a heart murmur because coarctation of the aorta may present with a soft heart murmur and, if left undiagnosed, may rarely result in aortic dissection or rupture.

Clinical Applications of Echocardiography

Echocardiography is a valuable adjunct to the clinical assessment in patients suspected of having cardiovascular disease (13). This technique uses high-frequency pulsed sound waves to record echoes of cardiac structures as they move within a beam of sound directed into the chest.

To record a *transthoracic M-mode electrocardiogram*, an ultrasound transducer is placed at one point on the chest wall and rocked to inscribe an arc that encompasses several areas of the heart sequentially. The transducer serves as a source of the sound beam and a receiver of the echoes. A transthoracic *two-dimensional (2D) echocardiogram* is recorded using a pulse transducer that is automatically directed across an arc, providing a simultaneous view of the cardiac structures, which is recorded on videotape. Both modes are usually combined and reported together. These procedures do not cause discomfort, but the patient must be able to lie flat for 20 minutes for performance of the test.

Echocardiography allows visualization of all four cardiac valves, the aortic root, both atria, the right ventricle, the left ventricle including all individual wall segments (Fig. 60.1), and the pericardium. The size and function of these structures are analyzed and patterns of specific diseases may be recognized.

Two-dimensional echocardiography is particularly helpful in assessing LV function in patients with ischemic heart disease, in whom regional structure and function are most important. It should be understood that echo assessment of overall or regional LV function is usually semiquantitative. Wall motion is usually categorized as normal or as mildly, moderately, or severely depressed. If an ejection fraction is reported, this often represents a visual estimate by the echocardiographer. Small differences reported in serial studies of the same patient, therefore, may not represent an important change unless the studies have been compared side by side by the same observer. Some newer systems provide software that may allow more quantitative reporting, but their value has not yet been adequately established. The noninvasive nature of the test and its ease of performance make 2D echocardiog-

raphy extremely useful for assessing patients with cardiac decompensation.

The 2D echocardiogram is diagnostic in cases of pericardial effusion, hypertrophic cardiomyopathy, congestive cardiomyopathy, mitral valve stenosis or prolapse, aortic regurgitation, intracardiac masses, cardiomyopathy, and Ebstein's anomaly of the tricuspid valve. The technique is helpful in ischemic heart disease with regional wall motion abnormalities, aortic stenosis, infectious endocarditis, cardiac tamponade, atrial septal defect, other forms of congenital heart disease such as ventricular septal defect, tetralogy of Fallot and bicuspid aortic valve, and any other structural abnormality of the heart.

Doppler echocardiography is an extremely useful tool for the detection and quantification of the severity of valvular heart disease. High-frequency sound is directed at a column of moving red blood cells, and the reflected sound is analyzed for changes in frequency, which indicate the direction and velocity of flow. Flow velocity information is color coded and superimposed

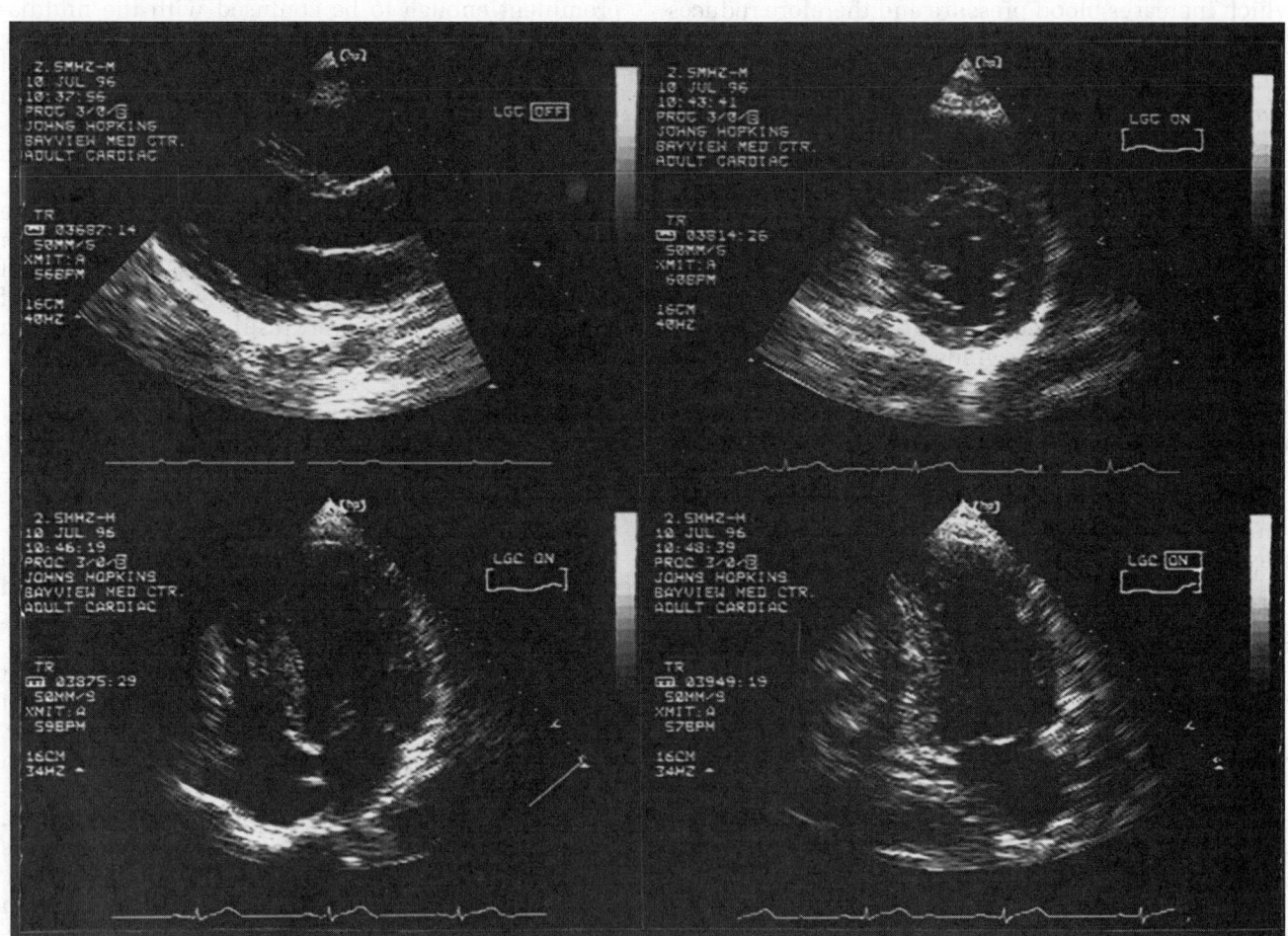

Figure 60.1. The four basic views of the 2D echocardiogram. Tomographic slices obtained from different vantage points and angles reveal valvular structure and all LV walls. *Upper left:* parasternal long axis view demonstrating septum and posterior wall. *Upper right:* parasternal short axis view displaying a "bread-loaf" slice of the left ventricle. *Lower left:* apical four-chamber view revealing septum, apex, and lateral wall. *Lower right:* apical two-chamber view, revealing inferior wall, apex, and lateral wall.

on the 2D echocardiographic image, providing visual representation of blood flow through the heart and great vessels.

In valvular stenosis a high-velocity jet of blood is detected distal to the stenosis; the higher the transvalvular gradient, the higher the velocity of the jet. The pressure gradient across a valve and the area of the aortic (20) and mitral (11,20) valves can also be calculated, providing precise quantification of the severity of aortic and mitral stenosis.

Valvular regurgitation can be detected by reverse flow and its severity estimated, usually by measuring the extent to which the regurgitant jet is detectable in the chamber proximal to the leaking valve. For example, mitral regurgitation is considered severe on a color Doppler study if the regurgitant jet occupies more than 40% of the area of the left atrium during systole (22). A small degree of regurgitation of the tricuspid valve is usually seen in normal subjects and does *not* represent disease. The presence of tricuspid regurgitation allows the estimation of right ventricular systolic pressure, which is equal to the pulmonary artery systolic pressure. This is useful in the detection and follow-up of patients with pulmonary hypertension of any cause. Very small amounts of pulmonic, mitral, and aortic regurgitation are also sometimes seen in normal people and are not a cause for concern if the echocardiographer comments that the extent is trivial or trace.

Doppler echocardiography is often used to detect "diastolic dysfunction," a frequent contributor to the development of congestive heart failure, especially in the elderly (see Chapter 61). The normal diastolic flow pattern consists of two phases: passive filling during early diastole (termed the E wave), which is aided by elastic recoil of the ventricle, and filling during late diastole (termed the A wave) due to atrial contraction. In young normal people, the left ventricle is pliable and elastic recoil during diastole is vigorous, resulting in brisk early filling, hence a large E wave. Very little filling then remains to be accomplished during late diastole, hence a small A wave. The ratio of early to late filling (the E/A ratio) therefore is high, typically about 1.5 to 2.0 in normal people in their thirties or forties. However, as the left ventricle becomes stiff, which occurs in left ventricular hypertrophy, other forms of chronic heart disease, or even the process of normal aging, the left ventricle loses its pliability. Early diastolic elastic recoil then becomes ineffective in aiding filling, and the E wave becomes small. To compensate, a substantial proportion of filling must occur during late diastole, and the A wave enlarges. The E/A ratio is thus reduced, and when it falls below 1, "diastolic" dysfunction is said to be present. Diastolic dysfunction is a normal finding in people older than 65.

However, the E/A ratio is an imperfect index of diastolic function because the velocity of early left ventricular filling depends on several factors in addition to left ventricular stiffness. For instance, a high left-atrial pressure, which occurs in congestive heart failure or restrictive cardiomyopathy, causes a high atrioventricular pressure gradient, which accelerates early filling irrespective of left ventricular stiffness, resulting in a large E wave and a high E/A ratio. This phenomenon often occurs in elderly people or in those with left ventricular hypertrophy, in whom diastolic dysfunction was previously present and is called pseudonormalization of the E/A ratio, or development of a restrictive pattern. Diastolic dysfunction will return after effective treatment of the congestive heart failure.

In patients in whom a large E wave is present, an S_3 is usually audible. These include normal people less than 30, elderly patients with congestive heart failure, and patients with constrictive cardiomyopathy, in whom the early diastolic sound is called a pericardial knock. In patients in whom a large A wave is present, an S_4 is usually audible. These include normal elderly people and patients with left ventricular hypertrophy due to hypertension or aortic stenosis.

A common limitation of standard transthoracic echocardiography is that ultrasound penetrates lung and bone poorly, and the available acoustic window is limited in many patients, resulting in poor-quality studies. The technique of *transesophageal echocardiography* (TEE) has extended the diagnostic utility of echocardiography by allowing high-quality studies, with markedly increased resolution, in all patients (9,48). Additional structures can be assessed, including the venae cavae, coronary sinus, pulmonary veins, atrial septum, atrial appendages, pulmonary artery, and ascending and descending aorta. Valve leaflets are seen with great clarity. Resolution is adequate to detect atheroma on the walls of the aorta. The method transforms a noninvasive imaging modality into a semiinvasive one; the procedure is similar to esophagoscopy and is often performed in a hospital's endoscopy unit, often on an outpatient basis. The patient is asked to fast for 6 to 8 hours and is treated with a pharyngeal topical anesthetic and intravenous sedation. The patient is then assisted in swallowing a small (i.e., 1-cm diameter) echo transducer mounted on a gastroscope-like tube. Visualization of cardiac structure from the esophagus and stomach is usually accomplished in about 20 minutes. The examination may include the intravenous injection of agitated saline, which creates ultrasonic contrast via tiny bubbles, to assess for right-to-left shunting. Complications of TEE are rare and include inability to intubate the esophagus successfully (1.9%), pulmonary difficulties such as bronchospasm (0.07%), cardiac arrhythmias (0.08%), and bleeding (0.02%) (8). Esophageal perforation is extremely rare.

The indications for TEE are evolving. The method allows visualization of almost the entire aorta and is sensitive (97.7%) and specific (76.9%) in the diagnosis of dissecting aneurysm (34). The method is much better than transthoracic echo for visualizing cardiac sources of embolus, such as thrombus in the left atrium or left-atrial appendage, sluggish blood flow in the left atrium, atrial septal aneurysm, patent foramen ovale, and complex aortic atheroma, sometimes with attached thrombus. Therefore, it is often ordered in patients with cryptogenic strokes (i.e., strokes in patients without evidence of atheroma in the carotid or vertebral systems). This is the method of choice for assessing the function of prosthetic mitral valves and for visualizing vegetations or intracardiac abscesses caused by endocarditis. TEE is sometimes indicated when transthoracic echo quality is poor and information about cardiac structure or function is deemed crucial.

SELECTED DISORDERS ASSOCIATED WITH ABNORMAL HEART SOUNDS

Aortic Stenosis

Stenosis of the aortic valve obstructs the flow of blood into the aorta and therefore raises the LV pressure above the aortic pressure. The pressure gradient across the valve is related to the severity of the stenosis. The elevated pressure results in a concentric hypertrophy of the left ventricle. Symptoms develop when the left ventricle can no longer compensate for the pressure load; the heart fails and the cardiac output declines.

Aortic stenosis may occur at any one of several levels. The most common obstruction (75% of patients) is at the aortic valve, although patients with subvalvular and supravalvular aortic stenosis may have symptoms and signs of severity similar to those of valvular disease. It is particularly important to differentiate fixed aortic outflow obstruction from idiopathic hypertrophic disease, in which the obstruction is dynamic in nature (Table 60.2; see below).

Causes and Epidemiology

In patients below the age of 30, aortic stenosis is most likely to be caused by a congenitally stenotic unicuspid valve (41). Between the ages of 30 and 65, a bicuspid aortic valve, which has become calcified and gradually more rigid over the years, is the most common cause of aortic stenosis. (In the general population, 1 or 2% have a bicuspid aortic valve, and 50% of these valves have calcified by age 50.) Rheumatic valvular disease accounts for only 6 to 27% of cases of isolated aortic stenosis in patients between the ages of 30 and 70 years. Over the age of 65, degeneration and sclerosis of the valve account for most cases of aortic stenosis. With the decline of rheumatic fever and the aging of the population, degenerative (calcific) aortic stenosis in the elderly has become the most common form of the disease that is encountered. Except in the elderly, in whom the prevalence is the same in both sexes, isolated aortic stenosis is three to four times more common in men.

Natural History and Symptoms

Patients with aortic stenosis are usually asymptomatic until late in the course of their disease. Mild to moderate obstruction does not greatly compromise LV function, and even patients with severe stenosis may compensate for years before they develop symptoms. Mortality is minimal during the asymptomatic phase of the disease. However, after the development of symptoms there is a precipitous decline in survival and if the lesion is not corrected, the average patient dies in about 4 years.

The earliest symptoms are easy fatigability and excessive dyspnea after unusual exercise. Syncope or near syncope with effort (see Chapter 81), angina (see Chapter 57), and dyspnea on usual exercise (see Chapter 61) are indicative of severe valvular obstruction. Patients with heart failure survive less long (2 years) than do patients with syncope (3 years) or angina (5 years) (43). Sudden death occurs in approximately 15% of symptomatic patients.

Physical Findings

Patients with aortic stenosis usually have a loud (grade 3 to 4) systolic ejection murmur. The maximal intensity of the murmur is at the second right intercostal space or at the cardiac apex. At the apex the murmur often has a musical cooing quality. There is usually a thrill in the suprasternal notch or the second right

Table 60.2.   Comparison of Valvular Aortic Stenosis and Hypertrophic Cardiomyopathy

	Valvular Aortic Stenosis	Hypertrophic Cardiomyopathy
Symptoms	Dyspnea, angina, syncope, or near syncope.	Dyspnea, angina, syncope, or near syncope.
Signs	Systolic ejection murmur loudest at aortic area or at apex; louder if patient squats.	Systolic ejection murmur loudest at left lower sternal border; louder if patient stands or performs a Valsalva maneuver.
	A_2 may not be audible.	A_2 is usually audible.
	S_4 is common.	S_4 is very common.
	Ejection sounds are common.	Ejection sounds are uncommon.
	Carotid upstroke is delayed.	Carotid upstroke is brisk.
ECG	LVH and strain pattern.	LVH and strain pattern; Q waves in inferior and lateral leads are common.
Chest radiograph	LVH is a late sign.	LVH may occur but unpredictably.
	Aortic valve is always calcified (may be seen only on fluoroscopy).	Aortic valve is not calcified.
	Ascending aorta may be dilated.	Ascending aorta is not dilated.
Echocardiogram	Characteristic echos of valvular calcification and valvular stenosis.	Disproportionate septal hypertrophy and systolic anterior displacement of mitral valve may be present.

LVH, Left ventricular hypertrophy.

intercostal space. However, the loudness of the murmur may not correlate with the severity of stenosis. Also, if cardiac output is reduced, as in congestive heart failure, or if the diameter of the chest is increased, the intensity of the murmur may be less than it otherwise would be. A late peak to the murmur suggests severe obstruction, but this is difficult to appreciate with a stethoscope, and absence of the peak does not mean that obstruction is not severe. Augmentation of the murmur when the patient suddenly squats and diminution of the murmur when the patient stands or performs a Valsalva maneuver are characteristic of aortic stenosis.

The systolic murmur, although it may not be loud, is an invariable sign of aortic stenosis; other cardiac sounds depend on the nature of the stenotic lesion. An early systolic ejection click is commonly heard when the valve is still mobile. The second aortic sound (A_2) is often not audible when the valve is so rigid that S_2 has only one component (P_2). Paradoxical splitting of the second heart sound, in the absence of left bundle branch block, is a sign of severity. A small pulse pressure (less than 30 mm Hg) also indicates severe obstruction (in elderly people, the pulse pressure may be normal despite severe stenosis). A slowly rising pulse—best assessed by palpation of a carotid artery—is characteristic. Under the age of 40, an S_4 is another sign of severe obstruction; over the age of 40, S_4 is common because of the high prevalence of hypertensive and ischemic heart disease and does not correlate with severity of stenosis.

The regurgitant early diastolic murmur of aortic insufficiency is heard in 30 to 40% of patients with aortic valve stenosis.

Laboratory Evaluation

An ECG, a chest x-ray, and an echocardiogram should be obtained routinely in a patient suspected of having aortic stenosis.

Electrocardiogram. The ECG is usually normal until stenosis becomes severe, at which point left ventricular hypertrophy (Table 60.3 and Fig. 60.2) and nonspecific ST depression and T-wave inversion are common, but not invariable. In older patients particularly, an abnormal ECG cannot be relied on to reflect severity because there are often other reasons why it might be abnormal.

Chest X-Ray. Calcification of the aortic valve is always present in patients with aortic stenosis who are older than 40, but often fluoroscopy is necessary to reveal it. Poststenotic dilation of the ascending aorta is also commonly seen. The heart size and configuration are usually normal until the disease is far advanced.

Echocardiogram. Echocardiography reveals immobile and usually calcified aortic valve leaflets. An increase in ventricular wall thickness on echocardiography implies severe obstruction if there is no other cause for hypertrophy. Doppler echocardiography (see above) can provide an estimate of the transaortic gradient and the aortic valve area. The valve area is generally considered a better measure of severity of

Table 60.3. Principal Electrocardiographic Features of Left Ventricular Hypertrophy

Electrocardiographic Criteria	Point System for Diagnosis[a]
Negative components of P in V₁ ≥1 mm and ≥0.4 second	3 points
QRS	
Largest limb lead R or S ≥20 mm or largest chest lead S before transition or R after transition ≥30 mm	3 points
OR	
Largest S before transition plus largest R after transition = 45 mm;	
Frontal plane axis ≥−30°	2 points
Duration in extremity lead ≥0.09 second	1 point
Intrinsicoid deflection ≥0.05 second	1 point
ST–T	
In general, opposite QRS:	
Without digitalis	3 points
With digitalis	1 point

Modified from Horan LG, Flowers NC. Electrocardiography and vectorcardiography. In: Braunwald E, ed. Heart disease: a textbook of cardiovascular medicine. Philadelphia: WB Saunders, 1980;229.

[a]Interpretation of point score: 6 points, left ventricular hypertrophy; 5 points, probable left ventricular hypertrophy; 4 points, possible left ventricular hypertrophy. If only voltage criteria are met, ECG may be designated as borderline, and left ventricular hypertrophy is suggested only by voltage and should be excluded by other clinical means.

aortic stenosis than the gradient because the gradient may be deceptively low in the presence of reduced cardiac output caused by LV dysfunction, even with severe stenosis (see below). Doppler echocardiography is helpful in distinguishing aortic stenosis from aortic valve sclerosis, in which no gradient is present.

Management

Asymptomatic patients with mild or moderate disease should be reassessed every 12 months so that signs of progressive disease can be detected promptly. Reassessment should include interval history, pertinent physical examination, ECG, chest x-ray, and echocardiogram. The asymptomatic patient with severe aortic stenosis presents a management dilemma. Although sudden death is extremely rare in asymptomatic patients, symptoms may appear suddenly and progress rapidly to sudden death (as early as 3 months after symptoms appear). The risk of that happening is 2 to 3%. Seventy percent of asymptomatic patients progress to symptoms within 3 years. Although these factors suggest that prophylactic valve replacement might be indicated in asymptomatic patients with severe disease, this must be weighed against the operative mortality (3 to 12%), the risk of prosthetic valve complications (1 to 2% per year), and the fact that many patients would be operated on needlessly (5). Patients with severe asymptomatic aortic stenosis should therefore be referred to a cardiologist. However, most cardiologists recommend that asymptomatic patients be followed extremely closely without prophylactic surgery. These issues should be discussed with the patient.

Patients should be cautioned to avoid undue exertion because acute heart failure, arrhythmia, and sudden death are more likely under such circumstances.

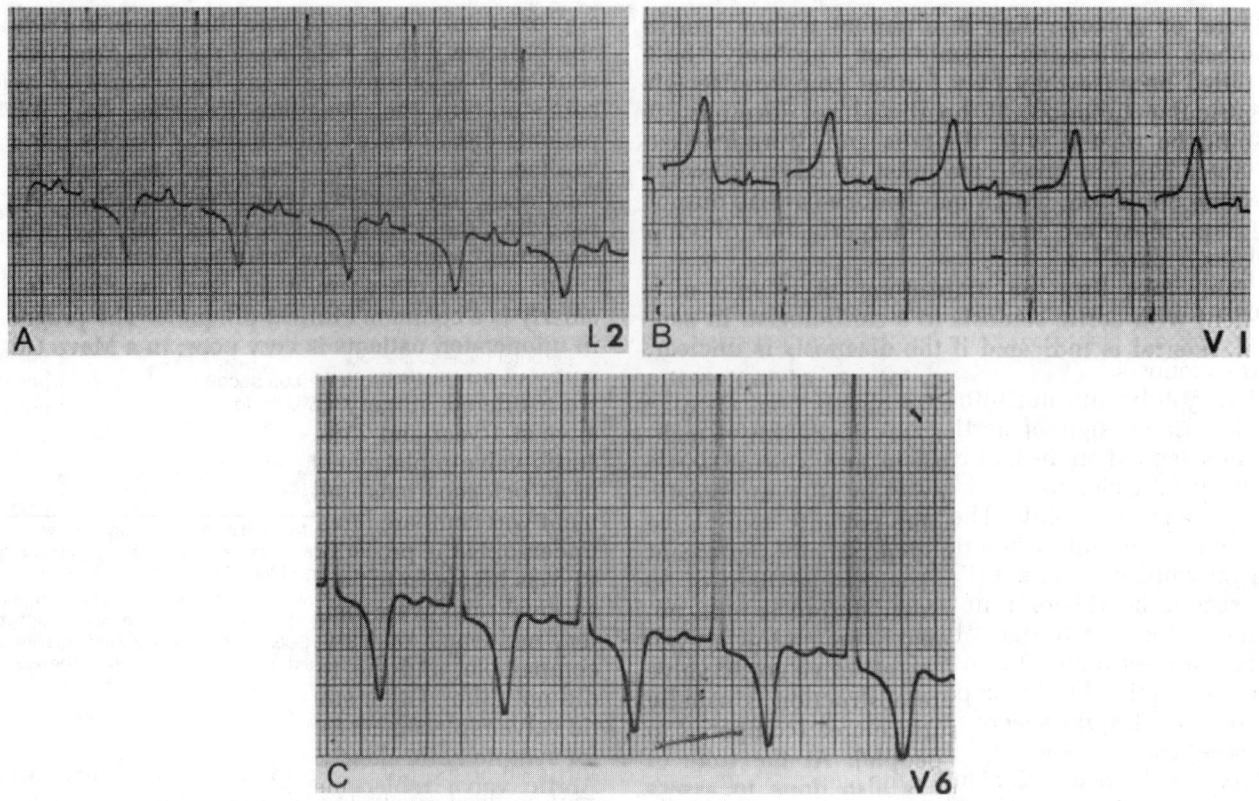

Figure 60.2. ECG of a patient with LV hypertrophy (Table 60.3).

The risk of subacute bacterial endocarditis is increased in patients with aortic stenosis and is unrelated to the severity of the stenosis (the risk is unchanged after aortic valve surgery; see below) (33). Therefore, antibiotic prophylaxis (see Chapter 86) is necessary before dental and surgical procedures.

Atrial arrhythmias are uncommon; if they occur, they must be treated aggressively (see Chapter 59) because they are more likely to cause angina, heart failure, or syncope than in a patient without aortic stenosis. β-Blocking agents are probably best avoided because they may further compromise LV function. If heart failure develops, it should be treated with digitalis and diuretics (see Chapter 61), but great care must be taken to avoid volume depletion, which may reduce cardiac output to a point where serious underperfusion of vital organs occurs.

Table 60.4 lists the indications for referral of a patient with aortic stenosis to a cardiologist. In general, referral is indicated if the diagnosis is unclear, the patient is symptomatic, or an asymptomatic patient has evidence of severe obstruction. Cardiac catheterization (see Chapter 57) is the definitive technique for assessing the severity and site of aortic stenosis. It should be performed in all symptomatic patients. Hemodynamically significant stenosis is usually associated with a gradient of 50 mm Hg or greater (unless cardiac output is reduced, in which case the gradient may be much lower even if there is severe stenosis). The effective aortic

Table 60.4. Indications for Referral of Patients with Aortic Stenosis

If there is a question about the diagnosis or severity
If the patient is symptomatic
If the asymptomatic patient has signs of severe obstruction
  Physical signs
    Small pulse pressure (<30 mm Hg)
    Late peak to systolic murmur
    Diminished A_2
    Paradoxical splitting of A_2
  ECG
    Left ventricular hypertrophy
    ST depression T-wave inversion
  Chest x-ray
    Left ventricular hypertrophy
  Echocardiogram
    Concentric left ventricular hypertrophy
    Doppler-calculated gradient greater than 50 mm Hg or valve area less than 0.75 cm^2

valve orifice in patients with severe obstruction is usually less than 0.5 cm^2 per m^2 of body surface area (compared to 1.6 to 2.6 cm^2 per m^2 in normal people). At the time of catheterization, angiography is also done to assess LV function, the patency of the coronary arteries, and the degree, if any, of aortic and mitral regurgitation.

The cardiologist is likely to recommend replacement of the stenotic aortic valve with a prosthesis in all symptomatic patients and in asymptomatic patients with signs of severe obstruction who are found to have a large gradient or evidence, on angiography, of LV dysfunction.

Operative mortality in patients without LV failure is 5 to 10%; in patients with LV failure it is 10 to 25%. The patient's postoperative health and long-term survival depend on a number of factors (including age, general health, and LV function), but overall the 5-year survival is approximately 80 to 85% and the 10-year survival is approximately 70 to 75%. Most patients experience a considerable improvement in their sense of well-being and exercise tolerance (33). When patients die, however, their death is usually caused by a cardiac complication (heart failure, myocardial infarction, or sudden death). (For further details regarding the long-term course and management of the patient with a prosthetic valve, see below.)

The proper management of *aortic stenosis in the elderly* is a common clinical challenge. The prognosis in unoperated patients is very poor; in a Mayo Clinic study of 50 patients with a mean age of 77 years who were offered surgery but refused, only 57% were alive at 1 year and 25% at 3 years (35). In a study of aortic valve replacement in the elderly (38), a group of 44 octogenarians undergoing aortic valve replacement was compared to a group of 83 younger patients undergoing the procedure. Although the early mortality was higher in the elderly (14% versus 4%), 2-year survival rates were similar (73% versus 90%, P NS), the incidence of valve-related complications was comparable, and the total duration of hospital stay did not differ. Other studies confirm that aortic valve replacement is the most appropriate therapy for symptomatic elderly patients with aortic stenosis. Aortic valve replacement should not be withheld because of age.

Percutaneous balloon valvuloplasty is a technique in which one or more balloons are placed across a stenotic aortic valve and then inflated in an attempt to reduce the severity of stenosis. This method has been applied mainly to very elderly patients or to those who are poor surgical candidates for other reasons. Although the transaortic gradient is usually reduced and initial clinical improvement is achieved, overall results have not been encouraging because high rates of death (24%) and recurrences of severe symptoms of aortic stenosis (47%) have been reported within 6 months of the procedure. Long-term survival after the procedure is dismal and resembles the natural history of untreated aortic stenosis (24). At present, aortic valvuloplasty has been abandoned at many centers and can be recommended only for severely symptomatic patients who would be at high risk were they to undergo aortic valve replacement.

Hypertrophic Cardiomyopathy

Hypertrophic cardiomyopathy (HCM) is a disease of cardiac muscle characterized by severe myocardial hypertrophy, in the absence of conditions that cause secondary hypertrophy of the heart muscle, such as hypertension and aortic stenosis. The left ventricle is hypercontractile, and during systole ejects essentially all of its blood, leaving a "clenched fist" with very high wall stress. HCM has been called a variety of names including asymmetric septal hypertrophy (because of predominant hypertrophy in the septal region) and idiopathic hypertrophic subaortic stenosis (because of the common presence of a dynamic outflow tract gradient). However, some patients with HCM do not have asymmetric septal hypertrophy, and may have either concentric hypertrophy, or only apical hypertrophy of the left ventricle. In addition, not all patients with HCM have evidence of a dynamic outflow tract gradient. In contrast to the microscopic appearance of secondary LVH, in which the fibers are enlarged but are properly oriented, the myofibrils in HCM are characterized by myofibrillary disarray.

Causes and Epidemiology

The prevalence of hypertrophic cardiomyopathy in young adults is thought to be about 2 per 1000 (31), but is higher in the elderly. The disease occurs as a familial, inherited disease in about 60% of cases and as a sporadic disease, without affected first-degree relatives, in the remainder. Men and women are equally likely to be affected. In the familial form, the mode of inheritance is autosomal dominant in about 75% of pedigrees. A variety of mutations have been identified in patients with HCM, including in the β-myosin heavy chain gene (chromosome 14), the cardiac troponin-T gene (chromosome 1), and the α-tropomyosin gene (chromosome 15).

Natural History and Symptoms

As echocardiography has become more widely used for the evaluation of patients with heart murmurs, it has become clear that most patients with hypertrophic cardiomyopathy are asymptomatic or have only mild symptoms. The prognosis in this group is excellent; one study (51) of 25 patients showed neither death nor progression of disease over a 4.4-year follow-up period.

The most common symptom of patients with hypertrophic cardiomyopathy who develop symptoms is dyspnea, but patients also often complain of angina (with or without evidence of occlusive coronary artery disease) and syncope or near syncope. These symptoms are much more likely to be induced by exertion than to occur spontaneously.

Once marked symptoms develop, some patients become rapidly worse, with progressive heart failure, angina, or arrhythmias. The most troublesome feature of the illness is its propensity to cause sudden death. The incidence of sudden death is approximately 3 to 4% per year in symptomatic patients with hypertrophic cardiomyopathy, but some families have a particularly high incidence. Unfortunately, there is no way to identify in any given patient an increased risk of sudden death; in fact, death may be the first manifestation of the disease.

Physical Findings

Clinical and laboratory features that distinguish aortic stenosis from HCM are listed in Table 60.2. The characteristic signs of the disease are a sustained left ventricular apical impulse, a loud S_4, and a harsh systolic ejection murmur, loudest at the left lower border of the sternum and often accompanied by a thrill. The location of the murmur helps to distinguish the condition from valvular aortic stenosis. Other distinguishing features are as follows: The second heart sound (A_2) is usually audible, a diastolic murmur is rare, the pulse pressure is normal, ejection sounds are uncommon, and, most important, the upstroke of the carotid pulse is brisk. In addition, the murmur of hypertrophic cardiomyopathy is augmented when the patient stands or performs a Valsalva maneuver and is diminished when the patient squats—the opposite of the findings in patients with aortic stenosis.

Laboratory Evaluation

An ECG, chest x-ray, and echocardiogram should be obtained routinely in patients suspected of having hypertrophic cardiomyopathy.

Electrocardiogram. The ECG is abnormal in most patients and is always abnormal in patients with obstruction. Typically, there is evidence of left ventricular hypertrophy (Fig. 60.2 and Table 60.3) and there is nonspecific ST depression and T-wave inversion. Q waves are often seen in the inferior and lateral leads, reflecting septal hypertrophy.

Chest X-Ray. The left ventricle is sometimes enlarged, but unpredictably so. In contrast to aortic valvular stenosis, the aortic valve is not calcified and the ascending aorta is not dilated.

Echocardiogram. Echocardiography is diagnostic; it usually demonstrates a thickened ventricular septum, hypertrophied out of proportion to the posterior wall of the left ventricle, although concentric or apical hypertrophy is sometimes present. Cavity obliteration, or near cavity obliteration, usually occurs during systole. The mitral valve apparatus moves anteriorly during systole (systolic anterior motion, or SAM), where it contributes to obstruction of the outflow tract (49). Also, the aortic leaflets may close suddenly in early systole and reopen as systole continues. (These abnormalities of the aortic valve may be present only after the patient is administered amyl nitrate.)

Management

The goal of therapy is to reduce the hypercontractile state of the left ventricle. Currently this is best done by means of the calcium channel blocker verapamil (80 to 120 mg four times a day or a sustained-release preparation once a day; Table 59.1) unless the patient has signs or symptoms of heart failure. Alternatively, a β-blocker may be prescribed (e.g., propranolol, 10 to 80 mg four times a day or a sustained-release preparation once a day). Angina, especially, is often relieved by treatment, but dyspnea also may be decreased as a result of a slower heart rate and of more time for the ventricle to fill. Although it is not clear that the risk of sudden death is reduced by therapy, most patients are symptomatically improved or at least stabilized by treatment. Disopyramide, a type 1A antiarrhythmic agent (see Chapter 59) with negative inotropic properties, has also been used successfully in patients with HCM.

Drugs that increase ventricular contractility or decrease ventricular volume (digitalis, vasodilators, β-adrenergic stimulants, and diuretics) are best avoided if possible. Patients, even if asymptomatic, should avoid undue exertion (e.g., running).

There is an increased risk of endocarditis in patients with hypertrophic cardiomyopathy, and these patients should therefore receive antibiotic prophylaxis before dental and surgical procedures (see Chapter 86).

Many patients with hypertrophic cardiomyopathy eventually become refractory to β-blockers or verapamil, or develop intolerable side effects from those medications. Until recently, the next therapeutic maneuver was surgical (see below). However, a number of reports demonstrate that dual-chamber cardiac pacing, even in the absence of bradyarrhythmias, results in a reduction in the symptoms of angina, dyspnea, and presyncope over 6 to 12 weeks. Objective measures of disease, such as exercise treadmill time and outflow tract gradient, also improve with this therapy (12). Although its use in patients on a nonexperimental basis is still controversial (30), patients with hypertrophic cardiomyopathy who show progression of symptoms or intolerance of medical treatment should be referred to a cardiologist for consideration of pacemaker therapy.

Surgical removal of a portion of the hypertrophied septum (septal myectomy) should be considered in severely symptomatic patients should other forms of therapy fail. Such a decision should be made in consultation with a cardiologist and a cardiac surgeon. Improved surgical techniques have reduced the perioperative mortality of this procedure to less than 5% (although it may be significantly higher in the elderly); symptoms are usually relieved (53) and long-term mortality is improved.

An implantable cardiac defibrillator may be placed in patients who have survived sudden death or have been observed to have life-threatening ventricular arrhythmias.

Atrial Septal Defect

Atrial septal defect of the ostium secundum type (in the midportion of the septum) is one of the most common congenital cardiac diseases that is diagnosed in adults. It causes, until late in the course (see below), a left-to-right atrial shunt with a volume overload of the right ventricle and overperfusion of the lungs.

Causes and Epidemiology

The defect is more common in females; the reported female/male ratio ranges from 1.5 to 3.5:1. Occasionally the defect is associated with other cardiac abnormalities. For example, 10 to 20% of patients with an atrial septal defect have mitral valve prolapse (23).

Natural History and Symptoms

Patients with atrial septal defect are usually asymptomatic until their third or fourth decade. Thereafter, symptoms invariably develop (usually dyspnea on exertion, fatigue, and palpitations), the result of heart failure and supraventricular arrhythmias. Less commonly, symptoms of pulmonary embolism (see Chapter 54) or paradoxical embolism (e.g., a stroke) occur. Virtually all patients are symptomatic by age 60. In fact, three-quarters of untreated patients are dead by age 50 and 90% by age 60. Increased pulmonary blood flow eventually produces pulmonary vascular disease, and consequently, pulmonary hypertension in approximately 15% of patients (7). When this happens, the left-to-right shunt first decreases and then reverses; at that point, cyanosis develops. Coexistent atherosclerotic or hypertensive cardiovascular disease may complicate the course of older patients with atrial septal defect and may make diagnosis and treatment more difficult.

Physical Findings

Atrial septal defect usually causes a wide fixed split of the second heart sound, the result of late closure of the pulmonic valve, and a soft blowing systolic pulmonic ejection murmur. A low- to medium-frequency middiastolic flow murmur across the tricuspid valve is common. The precordium may be hyperdynamic with a palpable S_3. If pulmonary hypertension has developed (see below), clubbing and cyanosis may be observed, and P_2 is accentuated. Signs of right ventricular failure (edema, distended neck veins, hepatomegaly) are common late in the disease.

Laboratory Evaluation

An ECG, a chest x-ray, and an echocardiogram should be obtained routinely in a patient suspected of having an atrial septal defect.

Electrocardiogram. The ECG displays an incomplete right bundle branch block or rSR^1 in lead V_1 90 to 95% of the time with a vertical frontal plane axis or right-axis deviation. Atrial fibrillation occurs commonly in symptomatic patients; atrial flutter and paroxysmal atrial tachycardia occur less often.

Chest X-Ray. The chest x-ray in this disease is almost invariably abnormal and shows increased pulmonary vascularity with a prominent main pulmonary artery and increased heart size (Fig. 60.3). The right pulmonary artery is usually more prominent than the left because of differential flow.

Echocardiogram. The echocardiogram demonstrates right ventricular enlargement and paradoxical motion of the ventricular septum with respect to the posterior wall of the left ventricle. These findings are also seen with other lesions that cause volume overload of the right ventricle, such as tricuspid and pulmonic regurgitation, and partial anomalous pulmonary venous return. Flow across the atrial septum can

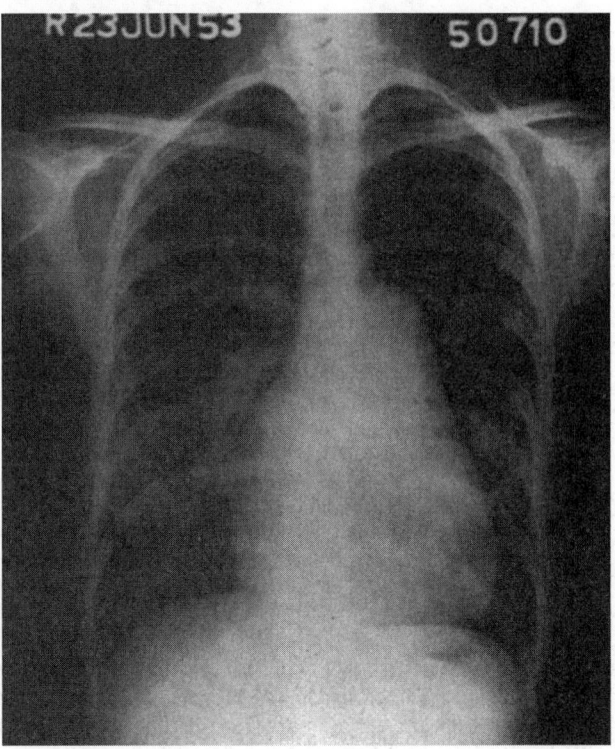

Figure 60.3. Chest x-ray of a patient with atrial septal defect.

often be visualized by using color Doppler echocardiography.

Management

Patients suspected of having an atrial septal defect should be referred to a cardiologist for definitive diagnosis. The cardiologist usually performs transesophageal echocardiography and, if the patient is over 40 years old, cardiac catheterization (see Chapter 57 for a description of the patient experience). All patients, even if they are asymptomatic, should have their defect repaired if pulmonary blood flow is more than 1.5 times systemic blood flow. The operative mortality is less than 2%, although some degree of persistent right ventricular or LV dysfunction is common in adults. If severe pulmonary hypertension has developed (pulmonary pressure equal to or greater than the systemic pressure), corrective surgery is contraindicated, but patients with lesser degrees of pulmonary hypertension may still benefit from repair of the defect. Survival after corrective surgery is influenced by the age of the patient and the degree of persistent cardiac dysfunction. Patients with otherwise normal hearts have normal survival rates after successful repair of the atrial defect and usually can resume normal activity.

Endocarditis prophylaxis is unnecessary for patients with atrial septal defect (see Chapter 86).

Mitral Regurgitation

Mitral regurgitation may develop because of an abnormality of any part of the mitral valve apparatus:

the valve leaflets, the chordae tendineae, the papillary muscles, or the annulus. Such abnormalities may result in either acute or chronic signs and symptoms, depending on the nature of the lesion.

An incompetent mitral valve allows regurgitation into the left atrium of blood from the left ventricle. The reduced load on the ventricle reduces the tension in the ventricular muscle and allows it to use more energy in contraction. Therefore, in patients with chronic mitral regurgitation, cardiac output remains normal for years until, because of age or intercurrent disease, the ventricle can no longer compensate and heart failure ensues. In patients with acute mitral regurgitation, ventricular compensation is inadequate and heart failure develops abruptly.

Chronic Mitral Regurgitation

Causes and Epidemiology. Chronic mitral incompetence in adults may occur in association with a great variety of disorders. Rheumatic fever is the cause of only 5 to 15% of cases, usually in association with some degree of mitral dysfunction. Otherwise, chronic mitral regurgitation is most often caused by papillary muscle necrosis (the result of ischemic heart disease), an inherited (e.g., Marfan's syndrome or mitral prolapse; see below) or an acquired (e.g., systemic lupus erythematosus) disorder of connective tissue, idiopathic calcification of the valve (primarily a disorder of the elderly), or congenital maldevelopment of the mitral apparatus.

Natural History and Symptoms. The left ventricle characteristically adapts to the increased preload of mitral regurgitation by adding new sarcomeres in series, which returns preload toward normal. The chamber becomes larger and more compliant, and fully compensates for the volume overload by increasing the end-diastolic volume and stroke volume. Patients may therefore remain asymptomatic for many years, even for their entire lives, if the regurgitation is not severe (14). Characteristically, when symptoms do develop, they appear gradually over years as left ventricular dysfunction slowly develops, and the ability to compensate for the loss of more than half of the stroke volume back into the left atrium is lost. Dyspnea and fatigue are the usual symptoms of LV failure. Supraventricular arrhythmias, especially atrial fibril-

lation, are likely to develop if left-atrial enlargement becomes marked, compromising somewhat the ability of the heart to compensate. Acute pulmonary edema occasionally occurs but is uncommon. Sometimes severe pulmonary hypertension develops without much enlargement of the left atrium. Early surgical correction of the lesion in patients with pulmonary hypertension and signs of right ventricular hypertrophy is important.

In a series of symptomatic patients with mitral regurgitation, 80% treated medically survived 5 years, and 60% survived 10 years (39). Moderately to severely symptomatic patients do less well; in one report 46% of patients with chronic rheumatic mitral insufficiency survived 5 years (33).

Physical Findings. A high-pitched holosystolic murmur, loudest at the apex, is characteristic of chronic mitral regurgitation (patients with mild regurgitation may have only a late systolic murmur). The holosystolic murmur is constant in intensity and radiates always to the axilla and sometimes to the back and the base of the heart. It is best heard when the patient is in the left lateral decubitus position. The murmur is diminished when the patient stands or performs a Valsalva maneuver and is intensified when the patient squats. If regurgitation is severe, the precordium is usually hyperdynamic and there is an S_3 gallop. S_1 is soft. If pulmonary hypertension has developed, an S_4 gallop, a loud P_2, and a right ventricular heave may be appreciated. Signs of right ventricular failure—edema, hepatomegaly, distended neck veins, hepatojugular reflux—may also be seen late in the course of this disease.

Laboratory Evaluation. An ECG, a chest x-ray, and an echocardiogram should be obtained routinely if a patient is suspected of having mitral regurgitation.

Electrocardiogram. The ECG shows evidence of left-atrial enlargement (Fig. 60.4 and Table 60.5) and, if present, of atrial fibrillation. The pattern of left ventricular hypertrophy (Fig. 60.2 and Table 60.3) is often seen as well, primarily in patients with severe disease. A pattern of right ventricular hypertrophy (Table 60.6) indicating pulmonary hypertension is less common and, when seen, is cause for great concern.

Chest X-Ray. Left ventricular and left-atrial enlargement are common. On a posteroanterior (PA) film, elevation of the left bronchus and prominence of the

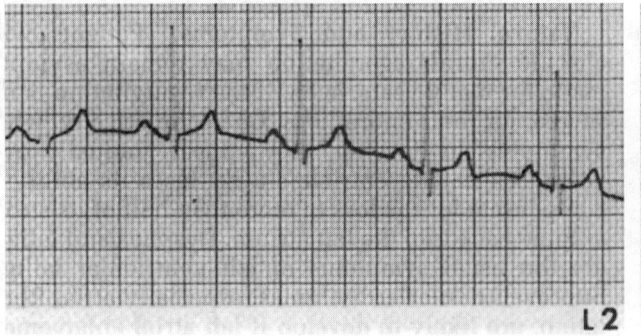
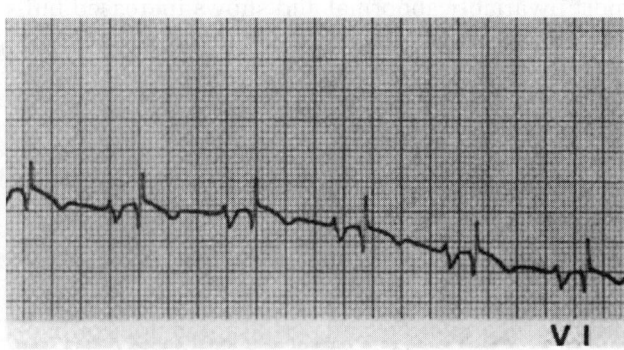

Figure 60.4.   ECG of a patient with left-atrial hypertrophy (Table 60.5).

Table 60.5. Principal Electrocardiographic Features of Left Atrial Hypertrophy

P wave	
Axis	+45° to –30°
Amplitude (II, III, aVF) duration	>0.11 second (broad)
Component (V$_1$)	
Early	Positive but inside normal
Late	Negative, ≥0.04 area units[a]

Modified from Horan LG, Flowers NC. Electrocardiography and vectorcardiography. In: Braunwald E, ed. Heart disease: a textbook of cardiovascular medicine. Philadelphia: WB Saunders, 1980;226.

[a]Area units = mm-sec. One small block on standard ECG paper = 0.04 mm-sec.

Table 60.6. Electrocardiographic Criteria of Right Ventricular Hypertrophy in Adults without Conduction Defects Known *Not* to Have Infarction

Sign	Points[a]
Ratio reversal (R/S V$_5$:R/S V$_1$ ≤0.4)	5
qR in V$_1$	5
R/S ratio in V$_1$ >1	4
S in V$_1$ <2 mm	4
R in V$_1$ + S in V$_5$ or V$_6$ >10.5 mm	4
Right-axis deviation >100°	4
S in V$_5$ or V$_6$ ≥7 mm and each ≥2 mm	3
R/S in V$_5$ or V$_6$ ≤1	3
R in V$_1$ ≥7 mm	3
S$_1$, S$_2$, and S$_3$ each ≥1 mm	2
S$_1$ and Q$_3$ each ≥1 mm	2
R' in V$_1$ earlier than 0.08 second and ≥2 mm	2
R peak in V$_1$ or V$_2$ between 0.04 and 0.07 sec	1
S in V$_5$ or V$_6$ >2 mm but <7 mm	1
Reduction in V lead R/S ratio between V$_1$ and V$_4$	1
R in V$_5$ or V$_6$ <5 mm	1

Modified from Horan LG, Flowers NC. Electrocardiography and vectorcardiography. In: Braunwald E, ed. Heart disease: a textbook of cardiovascular medicine. Philadelphia: WB Saunders, 1980;226.

[a]Interpretation of point score: 10 points, right ventricular hypertrophy; 7 to 9 points, probable right ventricular hypertrophy or hemodynamic overload; 5 to 6 points, possible right ventricular hypertrophy or hemodynamic overload. These criteria do not take into account serial ECG comparisons. Such additional data may alter the interpreter's impression of the likelihood of fixed enlargement or dynamic overload.

left-atrial appendage are the earliest signs of left-atrial enlargement; a double density is seen posteriorly when the left atrium is grossly enlarged (Fig. 60.5).

Echocardiogram. Echocardiography demonstrates left-atrial and left ventricular enlargement and hyperdynamic motion of the left ventricle, especially the septum. Two-dimensional echocardiography can usually define the etiology of the valvular disease (i.e., rheumatic, prolapsing, ischemic). Color Doppler echocardiography (see above) is sensitive in detecting mitral regurgitation and can estimate its severity.

Management. Patients who have mild disease (graded by the clinical examination and Doppler echocardiography) can be managed medically. Antibiotic prophylaxis against bacterial endocarditis should be administered before all dental and surgical procedures (see Chapter 86). If atrial fibrillation is present, restoration of sinus rhythm should be attempted unless the left atrium is greatly enlarged or mitral regurgitation has been present for many years. (A detailed discussion of the treatment of atrial fibrillation is in Chapter 59.) However, the development of atrial fibrillation may represent a marker of severe or progressive disease, the

management of which is discussed below. Likewise, the new onset of heart failure may signal either worsening of mitral regurgitation or the development of secondary LV dysfunction, and may constitute an indication for surgical intervention.

The management of moderate and severe mitral regurgitation depends on the severity of symptoms and on LV function. In patients who are symptomatic with fatigue, congestive heart failure, or arrhythmias, mitral valve replacement or repair may be indicated, and referral to a cardiologist should be made (Table 60.7). It is likely that cardiac catheterization and angiography (see Chapter 57) will be done to confirm the diagnosis, establish the severity of the lesion, and evaluate the function of the left ventricle and, often, the patency of the coronary arteries. At this point a decision is made about the value of operative repair of the lesion. Unless the patient has severe noncardiac disease, or LV function is so severely reduced that the patient would not tolerate an operation, replacement or repair of the defective valve is very likely to be recommended. The operative mortality reported from various centers is 3 to 10%.

Because mitral regurgitation is often well tolerated for years or even decades, many patients are asymptomatic. However, the long-standing chronic volume overload often results in a gradual deterioration in LV function, which greatly increases the risk and reduces the benefit of mitral valve repair or replacement when it eventually becomes necessary. Progressive LV dysfunction may be difficult to detect using the usual means of assessment of wall motion (echocardiography

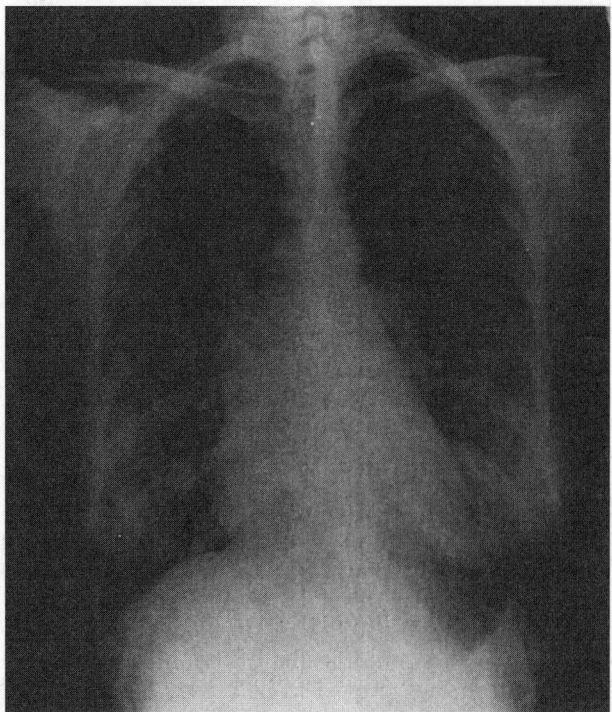

Figure 60.5. Chest x-ray of a patient with left-atrial enlargement. Note the straight left heart border and the calcification of the wall of the left atrium.

Table 60.7.   Indications for Referral of Patients with Mitral Regurgitation

Dyspnea or fatigue

Development of supraventricular arrhythmia, particularly atrial fibrillation

An asymptomatic patient with moderate or severe disease, especially if there is progressive cardiac enlargement or an ejection fraction less than 60%

Uncertainty about the diagnosis

Acute mitral regurgitation

Patients with mitral valve prolapse who have symptomatic arrhythmias; chronic, moderate, or severe mitral regurgitation; infectious endocarditis; or transient ischemic attacks

and gated blood pool scanning) because regurgitation into the low-pressure left atrium reduces the afterload of the left ventricle during ejection and results in exaggerated wall motion and falsely optimistic estimates of contractility. Many patients develop irreversible LV dysfunction before they report symptoms, even if the ejection fraction has remained within normal limits. In patients with severe mitral regurgitation caused by flail leaflet, this insidious ventricular dysfunction results in a high annual mortality rate (4.1%) even if symptoms are minimal or absent, and early surgery is associated with an improved prognosis (26). In this group, at the end of a follow-up period of 10 years, 90% of patients have either undergone surgical treatment or died. These observations, coupled with recent success in mitral valve repair procedures (see below), which avoid saddling the patient with the burdens of a prosthetic valve, suggest that surgery should be performed earlier in the course of the disease than had previously been recommended, even in patients who are asymptomatic or mildly symptomatic. The diagnosis of moderate or severe mitral regurgitation is therefore an indication for referral of the patient to a cardiologist. The recommendation may be to follow patients with ejection fractions above 60% (measured by annual echocardiograms or gated blood pool scans), looking for an increase in end-diastolic or end-systolic dimension or a reduction in wall motion. However, in patients with ejection fractions near the low end of normal (55 to 60%) or below, early surgery will probably be advised (42).

Afterload reduction by use of an arteriolar vasodilator may be particularly useful in this condition; by lowering peripheral resistance, ejection of blood into the aorta, rather than back into the left atrium, is favored. Intravenous vasodilator therapy can result in dramatic hemodynamic improvement in hospitalized patients with congestive heart failure caused by mitral regurgitation. Based on that observation, it seems reasonable to use oral vasodilators in patients with mitral regurgitation who are not yet ready for surgery. If a beneficial hemodynamic effect could be sustained, it might be possible to delay the development of LV dysfunction or symptoms, and postpone the need for surgery. Although this approach is often taken in asymptomatic patients, the efficacy of long-term va-

sodilator therapy in this regard has not been well studied, and recommendations based on randomized trials cannot be made. However, the use of vasodilators in patients with congestive heart failure caused by mitral regurgitation is well established.

The health and survival of patients who have undergone successful valve replacement depend on a number of factors (also see below). Advanced age, the presence of concomitant mitral stenosis, poor LV function (ejection fraction under 50%), and severity of symptoms preoperatively (New York Heart Association [NYHA] class III or IV; see Chapter 61) are adverse factors that reduce long-term postoperative survival. In general, patients with mitral regurgitation on the basis of ischemic heart disease do less well than patients with rheumatic heart disease. Nevertheless, even patients with one or more adverse risk factors live longer, on the average, with a prosthetic valve than they would without one (18), and most patients are able to be more active than they were before surgery. The overall 10-year survival for patients who have undergone successful mitral surgery is approximately 70% (18). Postoperatively, anticoagulation with warfarin is used routinely to prevent thromboembolic complications (see Chapter 52).

Surgical reconstruction of the incompetent mitral valve has been shown to be an excellent alternative to mitral valve replacement, particularly for valves leaking because of myxomatous degeneration (see "Mitral Valve Prolapse," below). Repair is most likely to be feasible if the etiology of the mitral regurgitation is flail posterior leaflet. Repaired valves usually maintain their competency (92%), seem not to be susceptible to infectious endocarditis, and do not require chronic anticoagulation (15). Valve repair results in better operative mortality, long-term survival, and postoperative ejection fraction than does valve replacement (10). The decision about whether to recommend valve repair or replacement depends on the availability of a surgeon who is skilled at this procedure and is usually made in consultation with the cardiologist and the cardiac surgeon.

Acute Mitral Regurgitation

Causes and Epidemiology.   Acute mitral incompetence is most often caused by rupture of the chordae tendineae, the cords that connect the valve cusps to the papillary muscles of the left ventricle. Most of the time the cause of the rupture is myxomatous degeneration of the valve (see "Mitral Valve Prolapse," below), although occasionally, acute mitral regurgitation is caused by papillary muscle rupture or dysfunction (complications of myocardial infarction) or by perforation of a mitral cusp as the result of bacterial endocarditis. The disorder is primarily encountered in middle-aged and elderly patients.

Natural History and Symptoms.   Because the left atrium is suddenly presented with a volume load to which it cannot rapidly accommodate, acute pulmonary edema is much more common in patients with acute, compared with chronic, mitral regurgitation.

Physical Findings. A harsh holosystolic murmur of constant intensity, loudest at the apex, is characteristic; if a posterior cord has ruptured, the murmur may radiate to the base of the heart and may mimic the murmur of aortic stenosis. Sometimes an early systolic or midsystolic, or even a crescendo/decrescendo, murmur is heard. An S_3 gallop is almost always heard and an S_4 gallop is common. Unlike the situation in patients with chronic mitral regurgitation, S_1 is normal or even loud. Signs of left-sided heart failure (rales) and right-sided failure (edema, distended neck veins) are also common.

Laboratory Findings

Chest X-Ray. The chest x-ray shows marked pulmonary congestion. The left atrium and the left ventricle are minimally enlarged.

Echocardiogram. Chamber enlargement is usually not seen, but increased systolic motion of the valve is common. If the chordae have ruptured, the flailing chordae or marked prolapse of the leaflets into the left atrium may be visualized by 2D echocardiography. Doppler echocardiography allows detection of the lesion, but Doppler criteria for estimating the severity of acute mitral regurgitation are not yet established.

Management. Patients suspected of having suffered acute mitral regurgitation should be hospitalized immediately for diagnosis, treatment of acute heart failure, and consideration for early operative repair.

Mitral Valve Prolapse

Causes and Epidemiology

Systolic prolapse of a leaflet of the mitral valve into the left atrium has proved to be a common phenomenon, affecting more than 5% of the population (28,56). Women are more likely to be affected than are men, although reported sex ratios vary considerably. The exact nature of this abnormality is not entirely clear, but in most cases the condition appears to be inherited (autosomal dominant), with reduced penetrance in men and children. Histologic study of prolapsing valves removed at operation shows myxomatous degeneration, a proliferation of the spongiosa layer of mucopolysaccharides into the fibrosa layer of collagen, resulting in a weakness in the supporting structure of the valve. This abnormality is also seen in a number of known disorders of connective tissue, including Marfan's syndrome and Ehlers–Danlos syndrome. However, echocardiographic prolapse is also often reported in patients with documented coronary artery disease, hypertrophic cardiomyopathy, and atrial septal defect, and these cases may represent secondary prolapse in which the valve is normal but changes in ventricular geometry cause prolapsing of the leaflets. In these secondary cases the click and associated symptoms (see below) usually are not present.

Natural History and Symptoms

Most patients are asymptomatic and the condition is identified during a routine physical examination. Less often, patients complain of palpitations, chest pain, or dyspnea. The palpitations reflect arrhythmias (see below) or, more commonly, just an awareness of sinus tachycardia. The chest pain sometimes mimics angina (or, in fact, is angina if there is concomitant ischemic heart disease) but more often is sharp lancinating pain in the left chest, unrelated to exertion, and the cause of it is unknown.

In the great majority of patients the syndrome is benign. However, in approximately 15% of patients significant mitral regurgitation occurs, and patients may complain of dyspnea caused by left ventricular failure. Approximately 3 to 4% of patients require mitral valve surgery during a follow-up period of about 8 years (57).

It is now recognized that patients with mitral valve prolapse are at risk for embolic strokes. In one study, 40% of patients under 45 who had had a stroke had mitral valve prolapse, compared with 6.8% of matched controls (1). The risk of infective endocarditis in patients with mitral valve prolapse is approximately five times that of the general population. This risk is highest in patients with mitral regurgitation.

The most feared complication of mitral valve prolapse, sudden death, is rare. The risk is higher in patients with a family history of sudden death or in patients with a prolonged Q–T interval on their ECG (see below).

The hemodynamic and infectious complications appear to be more common in men than in women, and in patients who have mitral regurgitation at the time of presentation. The echocardiographic findings of thickening and redundancy of the mitral leaflet also identify patients with mitral valve prolapse who are at higher risk (29). These findings allow targeting of prophylactic antibiotic therapy and frequent follow-up of specific groups.

Physical Findings

The characteristic finding in patients with mitral prolapse is a midsystolic click, best heard at the lower left sternal border, caused by sudden tensing of the prolapsed valve. It occurs later than the systolic ejection sound heard commonly in association with systemic hypertension (see above). Very often the click is followed immediately by a crescendo late systolic murmur that continues until A_2.

The physical findings may vary from time to time in any given patient and may also vary with the position of the patient. In those rare instances in which chronic mitral regurgitation has developed, the typical physical findings—including the holosystolic murmur—of this condition will be encountered (see above).

The mitral valve prolapse syndrome is commonly associated with skeletal abnormalities, such as scoliosis and pectus excavatum, suggesting that valve prolapse may be only one component of a generalized disease of connective tissue.

Laboratory Findings

Electrocardiogram. The ECG is usually normal, especially in asymptomatic patients. Symptomatic patients may show nonspecific ST–T wave changes, usually in the inferior leads, and sometimes prolongation of the Q–T interval.

A variety of arrhythmias may occur in patients with mitral valve prolapse. The most common are premature ventricular contractions (PVCs) and paroxysmal supraventricular tachycardia. When patients are exercised, many of them develop frequent PVCs or atrial arrhythmias.

Echocardiogram. The echocardiogram usually is diagnostic in this condition. It shows late systolic or holosystolic prolapse of one or both leaflets of the mitral valve. Sometimes, however, the echocardiogram shows no abnormalities despite the typical cardiac findings. These patients probably have minor degrees of prolapse. Mitral regurgitation, if present, can be detected by Doppler echocardiography (see above).

Management

Asymptomatic patients need no treatment but should be reassessed by interval history, physical examination, and echocardiogram every few years. Care should be taken to ensure that the diagnosis does not provide unwarranted anxiety. Patients who have a systolic murmur or echocardiographic evidence of thickening or redundancy of the mitral leaflet should receive prophylaxis against bacterial endocarditis before dental or surgical procedures (see Chapter 86). Other patients probably do not need prophylaxis.

Patients with palpitations should have ambulatory electrocardiographic monitoring or event monitoring to determine the severity of their arrhythmia, and therapy should be prescribed on the basis of the type of arrhythmia that is present (see Chapter 59). A β-blocking agent is often a drug of choice in the treatment of these patients and also in those with mitral prolapse who complain of chest pain or who have persistent palpitation caused by sinus tachycardia (e.g., long-acting propranolol, usual dosage 40 to 120 mg/day, or atenolol 25 to 50 mg/day). The mechanism of action of the drug in the relief of pain is unknown but may be explained by the fact that many untreated patients have been shown to have increased blood levels of norepinephrine and to have increased sympathetic (and vagal) tone.

Patients with symptomatic mitral regurgitation should be treated as described above.

Referral to a cardiologist is recommended at any time patients become symptomatic from arrhythmia (other than sinus tachycardia), chronic mitral regurgitation, or thromboembolism.

A pamphlet published by the American Heart Association (AHA), titled *Mitral Valve Prolapse,* provides a clear explanation of the syndrome to patients, and may help allay the anxiety that many patients with mitral valve prolapse feel regarding their risk of complications. The booklet is available through local AHA offices.

Mitral Stenosis

Stenosis of the mitral valve obstructs the flow of blood out of the left atrium and therefore raises the left-atrial pressure above the left ventricular diastolic pressure. The pressure gradient across the valve and the area of the valve orifice are measures of the severity of the stenosis. Because of the increase in left-atrial pressure, there is an increase in pressure in the pulmonary blood vessels. The pulmonary congestion accounts for most of the symptoms of the disease.

Causes and Epidemiology

By far the most common cause of mitral stenosis in adults is rheumatic fever (although a history of rheumatic fever can be elicited in only 50% of patients with pure mitral stenosis). Pure mitral stenosis occurs in 40% of all patients with rheumatic heart disease. The rest of the time there is associated mitral regurgitation, aortic valve disease, and, uncommonly, tricuspid valve disease. Two-thirds of patients with rheumatic mitral stenosis are women.

Natural History and Symptoms

On average, there is a latent period of nearly 20 years between an attack of acute rheumatic fever and the development of symptomatic mitral stenosis (47). Thus, symptoms usually do not develop before the fourth decade. The severity of symptoms is quite variable: In fact, some people are never symptomatic, some are mildly symptomatic indefinitely, and some develop progressively severe cardiopulmonary decompensation. Of the patients with progressive disease, it has been estimated that an average of 7 years elapses between the onset of symptoms and the development of total disability (class IV cardiac status; see Chapter 61). In one series the 5-year survival from that point in patients treated medically was only 15% (36).

Pulmonary congestion causes many of the symptoms of mitral stenosis: dyspnea, orthopnea, and paroxysmal nocturnal dyspnea. If left-atrial pressure rises acutely because of a sudden stress, frank pulmonary edema may occur. Hemoptysis caused by rupture of small bronchial veins or by pulmonary edema is not unusual.

As the disease progresses, pulmonary hypertension develops followed by symptoms of right heart failure: edema, distended neck veins, a tender liver, and ascites. At this point, the flow of blood into the left heart is limited and the pulmonary arterioles hypertrophy, diminishing the risk of pulmonary edema. Low cardiac output is responsible for the fatigue that is a common complaint of patients at this stage.

Atrial fibrillation (Chapter 59) complicates the course of 40 to 50% of patients with mitral stenosis. The 20% reduction in blood flow across the mitral valve by the loss of left-atrial contraction may intensify symptoms of heart failure and fatigue.

At some time in their course, 20% of patients with mitral stenosis experience symptomatic thromboembolism, most often to the brain; 80% of these patients are in atrial fibrillation.

Physical Findings

A middiastolic rumbling murmur with presystolic accentuation is characteristic of mitral stenosis. It is best heard at, and is often limited to, the cardiac apex. To hear it, it may be necessary to turn the patient to the left lateral position and to have him or her expire fully. Sometimes the patient must be exercised before the murmur is audible. The murmur is best heard with the bell of the stethoscope pressed lightly against the chest. A loud first heart sound and opening snap (see above) usually accompany the murmur when the valve is mobile.

Late in the course, signs of pulmonary hypertension (a loud P_2 and a right ventricular heave) and of right heart failure may be found.

Laboratory Findings

Electrocardiogram. The ECG shows left-atrial enlargement (Fig. 60.4 and Table 60.5) in 90% of patients who are in sinus rhythm. With the development of pulmonary hypertension, signs of right-ventricular hypertrophy appear (Table 60.6).

Chest X-Ray. Left-atrial enlargement (see above and Fig. 60.5) is seen in virtually all patients with symptomatic mitral stenosis, but the size of the left atrium does not correlate with the severity of stenosis. Late in the course right ventricular and right-atrial hypertrophy are seen as well. Symptomatic patients are also likely to show radiologic signs of pulmonary congestion, the severity of which determines the findings that are seen (see Chapter 61).

Calcification of the mitral valve is not unusual in patients with long-standing mitral stenosis, but it is better visualized by fluoroscopy or echocardiography than by a plain x-ray.

Echocardiogram. Mitral stenosis can be easily diagnosed by echocardiography. Mitral valve thickening can be seen; there is reduced excursion of the anterior leaflet of the valve and abnormal anterior motion of the posterior leaflet during diastole (it normally moves posteriorly). The severity of the stenosis can be accurately assessed by 2D and Doppler echocardiography (see above).

Management

Asymptomatic patients in normal sinus rhythm need no treatment except prophylaxis for bacterial endocarditis when they are to undergo dental or surgical procedures (see Chapter 86), and warfarin in some cases (see below). Newly diagnosed adult patients with mitral stenosis do not ordinarily require prophylaxis for β-hemolytic streptococcal infection unless they have had an attack of rheumatic fever within the last 5 to 10 years or are in a population where β-hemolytic streptococcal infection is more prevalent (e.g., military personnel or hospital workers). Patients who have received prophylaxis throughout childhood should continue to receive it indefinitely. When prophylaxis is necessary, the best regimen is 1 to 2 million units of benzathine penicillin G intramuscularly once a month.

Asymptomatic patients who develop atrial fibrillation, however, should be considered for balloon angioplasty because atrial fibrillation has its own long-term sequelae that should be avoided if possible (40). Valvuloplasty should also be considered in asymptomatic patients with moderate or severe mitral stenosis who are planning pregnancy because symptoms are likely to occur in late pregnancy and pulmonary edema may occur during labor.

Mildly symptomatic patients should be treated with diuretics and sodium restriction (see Chapter 61 for a detailed discussion of the treatment of heart failure). Because it does not affect the hemodynamic abnormality, digitalis is not useful in this situation unless rapid atrial fibrillation or flutter develops. Although the use of β-blockers has been advocated in patients with mitral stenosis in normal sinus rhythm (to reduce heart rate and prolong the diastolic filling period), randomized studies have not demonstrated a clinical benefit (52).

Warfarin anticoagulants should be administered to patients with mild mitral stenosis who have had one or more episodes of systemic or pulmonary thromboembolism (see Chapter 52), who are in atrial fibrillation, or who have echocardiographic evidence of left-atrial enlargement. All patients with moderate or severe mitral stenosis should be treated with anticoagulants.

The poor prognosis of symptomatic medically treated patients with severe or progressive disease (see "Natural History and Symptoms," above) dictates that such patients should be offered a mechanical procedure to improve transmitral flow, either *percutaneous balloon valvuloplasty* or *valve surgery*. Percutaneous valvuloplasty can be achieved using a balloon catheter passed through the venous system and then across the atrial septum to the mitral valve. This procedure is generally effective in patients who have low left ventricular end-diastolic pressures, who are not NYHA class IV, and in whom the echocardiogram shows good mitral valve mobility and minimal valvular or subvalvular thickening and calcification. In a prospective, randomized trial comparing percutaneous valvuloplasty with open surgical commissurotomy in suitable patients, after the procedure the size of the mitral valve orifice and functional class were better in the percutaneous group than in the surgical group (40). Of the patients who underwent percutaneous valvuloplasty, 72% were asymptomatic after 3 years, compared with 57% of the surgically treated patients. The better hemodynamic results, lower costs, and elimination of need for thoracotomy suggest that balloon valvuloplasty should be considered for all patients with suitable mitral valve anatomy.

In patients requiring mechanical release of mitral valve obstruction who are not suitable for percutaneous valvuloplasty, the preferred surgical procedure depends on the anatomy of the valve at the time of operation. If possible, a mitral commissurotomy is performed. The operative mortality of this procedure is low (1 to 3%) and the results are excellent for a number of years. However, after commissurotomy, 10% of patients within 5 years and 60% within 10 years require reoperation because of restenosis or because of the development of symptomatic mitral regurgitation or symptomatic aortic stenosis (21). If a prosthetic valve is implanted, the operative mortality is 3 to 10%; the course of patients who survive surgery depends on a number of factors (see below) but certainly is better than that of symptomatic patients treated medically.

Table 60.8 lists the reasons to refer patients with mitral stenosis to a cardiologist (2).

Aortic Regurgitation

An incompetent aortic valve allows regurgitation into the left ventricle of blood ejected into the aorta (16). To compensate for the increased volume load, the left ventricle dilates and hypertrophies, so the effective stroke volume may be normal for a long time. Eventually, however, the left ventricle cannot maintain the work load, and clinical signs and symptoms of heart failure ensue.

Causes and Epidemiology

Aortic regurgitation may be caused by disease of the aortic valve cusps or dilation of the aortic root.

Rheumatic fever now accounts for 29% of cases of chronic aortic valvular incompetence (37), many fewer cases than it did 20 to 30 years ago. Congenital aortic valvular incompetence caused by a bicuspid valve accounts for 12% of cases. Bacterial endocarditis is the most common cause of acute aortic valvular incompetence. Traumatic rupture of a cusp of the aortic valve is uncommon.

Chronic aortic regurgitation is caused by dilation of the aortic root in 12% of cases, most commonly idiopathic. Rare causes include rheumatoid arthritis, ankylosing spondylitis, Reiter's syndrome, congenital disorders of connective tissue (Marfan's syndrome, Ehlers–Danlos syndrome, and osteogenesis imperfecta), and syphilitic aortitis. Acute aortic regurgitation caused by dilation of the aortic root is most commonly caused by a dissecting aneurysm, usually associated with medial necrosis of the aorta. Dissection is associated with systemic hypertension in approximately 50% of cases; occasionally a primary disorder of connective tissue, such as Marfan's syndrome, can be incriminated.

Aortic regurgitation in general is more common in men than women, but there are specific exceptions (e.g., rheumatoid arthritis).

Natural History and Symptoms

In chronic aortic regurgitation, volume overload is usually tolerated for years or decades because of adaptive dilation and hypertrophy that maintains cardiac performance in or near the normal range. Patients may therefore remain asymptomatic for up to 20 years or have only mild dyspnea on exertion. However, the chronically overloaded heart eventually develops irreversible structural and functional damage, often during the asymptomatic period (50). When symptoms do develop (progressively more severe dyspnea, orthopnea, paroxysmal nocturnal dyspnea, and less often, angina), they reflect an ominous deterioration in the condition.

Patients with acute aortic regurgitation develop fulminant pulmonary edema because of the inability of the left ventricle to compensate for the sudden volume load and for the abrupt rise in left ventricular end-diastolic pressure. Marked dyspnea and weakness may be experienced virtually overnight and in most cases within 2 or 3 months. Other symptoms depend on the underlying cause: fever, for example, if it is endocarditis, severe pain in the chest or back if it is a dissecting aneurysm.

Physical Findings

Patients with chronic aortic regurgitation have a characteristic high-frequency early diastolic decrescendo murmur, best heard at the aortic area and at the left sternal border. The duration (but not the intensity) of the murmur correlates with the severity of the lesion, so the murmur is holodiastolic in patients with severe, chronic aortic regurgitation. Often there is an accompanying harsh systolic ejection murmur as well, heard at the base of the heart. Severe aortic regurgitation may also cause a loud apical diastolic murmur (the Austin Flint murmur), simulating the murmur of mitral stenosis. Unlike the situation in true mitral stenosis, however, S_1 in patients with aortic regurgitation is sometimes soft, the result of premature closure of the mitral valve, and there is no opening snap. If aortic regurgitation is moderate or severe, the pulse pressure is ordinarily wide, reflecting peripheral vasodilation. The combination of an increased systolic pressure and a reduced diastolic pressure (sometimes as low as 30 mm Hg) produces characteristic changes in the peripheral pulse (e.g., water-hammer pulse, pistol-shot sounds heard over the femoral artery) and a typical bobbing of the head with each heart beat.

Patients with acute aortic regurgitation often show signs of left- and right-sided heart failure. The regurgitant diastolic murmur is lower pitched and shorter than it is in patients with chronic aortic incompetence; S_1 is often absent and S_3, uncommon with chronic regurgitation, is usually present. The pulse pressure is normal, the result of intense peripheral vasoconstriction.

Laboratory Findings

Electrocardiogram. The ECG also reflects the severity and duration of aortic regurgitation. Patients with chronic disease show the ECG pattern of left ventricular hypertrophy (Fig. 60.2 and Table 60.3), whereas patients with acute disease do not (although

Table 60.8.   Indications for Referral of Patients with Mitral Stenosis

Asymptomatic or symptomatic patients who develop atrial fibrillation or show evidence of pulmonary hypertension
Dyspnea or recurrent attacks of pulmonary edema
Symptomatic disease of the aortic or tricuspid valve
Women, whether symptomatic or not, who wish to become or who are pregnant
Patients with chronic obstructive lung disease
Patients with angina pectoris

Modified from Brandenburg RO, Fuster V, Guiliani ER. Valvular heart disease. When should the patient be referred? Pract Cardiol 5:50, 1979.

they commonly do show nonspecific ST–T wave changes).

Chest X-Ray. The size of the heart in patients with aortic regurgitation depends on the duration and severity of the disease. Patients with chronic severe disease have very large left ventricles, but patients with acute regurgitation may have no cardiac enlargement at all.

Echocardiogram. Echocardiography with Doppler is useful in confirming the diagnosis and assessing left-ventricular function and the degree of hypertrophy. Premature mitral valve closure is helpful in confirming very severe aortic regurgitation. The severity of aortic regurgitation can also be estimated by Doppler echocardiography using a number of described criteria.

Management

Asymptomatic patients with mild aortic regurgitation need not be treated but should be assessed once or twice a year by interval history, physical examination, and chest x-ray. Yearly ECGs and echocardiograms should also be obtained. Prophylaxis for bacterial endocarditis is indicated when patients are to undergo dental or surgical procedures (see Chapter 86).

Vasodilating drugs acutely reduce the regurgitant volume and have long been known to be useful in improving hemodynamics in the short term. Recent randomized clinical trials demonstrate that long-term treatment with hydralazine (17), nifedipine (46), or enalapril (25) reduces end-diastolic and end-systolic volumes, and increases ejection fraction in asymptomatic or minimally symptomatic patients with moderate or severe aortic regurgitation. A reduction in the extent of hypertrophy can also be demonstrated. The angiotensin-converting enzymes seem to be the most potent in this regard (25), probably because suppression of the renin–angiotensin system inhibits the development of detrimental hypertrophy. These data suggest that vasodilator therapy has the potential to delay the need for valve replacement, and should be prescribed in patients with moderate or severe aortic regurgitation even if they are asymptomatic. Patients should then be assessed once or twice a year by interval history, physical examination, and chest x-ray. Yearly ECGs and echocardiograms should also be obtained. If evidence of worsening LV dilation, hypertrophy, or LV function is detected, valve repair or replacement should be considered.

Table 60.9 lists the reasons to refer patients with aortic regurgitation to a cardiologist. In general, referral is indicated in patients with chronic disease to consider whether to recommend aortic valve replacement for symptomatic patients and for asymptomatic patients with physical findings of severe disease (widened pulse pressure, holodiastolic murmur, increasing left ventricular enlargement, decreasing ejection fraction) (2). All patients with suspected acute aortic regurgitation should be seen by a cardiologist as soon as possible. The cardiologist is likely to perform cardiac catheterization (see Chapter 57) to assess the severity of the lesion, the presence of other valvular disease, and

Table 60.9. Indications for Referral of Patients with Aortic Regurgitation

Uncertainty about the diagnosis
Symptomatic chronic aortic incompetence (dyspnea, fatigue, angina)
Acute aortic incompetence
Asymptomatic patients with evidence of severe chronic aortic incompetence: widened pulse pressure, holodiastolic murmur, left ventricular hypertrophy, progressive cardiac enlargement, falling ejection fraction, or echocardiographic end-systolic valvular dimension greater than 4.5 cm

Modified from Brandenburg RO, Fuster V, Guiliani ER. Valvular heart disease. When should the patient be referred? Pract Cardiol 5:50, 1979.

the function of the left ventricle. Patients with marked left ventricular diastolic and systolic enlargement and ejection fractions of less than 50% are at high risk of requiring aortic valve replacement for symptoms of deteriorating LV function within 3 years (50).

When patients with chronic aortic regurgitation develop symptoms of congestive heart failure, 50% are dead within 2 years (32). Thus, valve replacement is warranted in all symptomatic patients, preferably before severe LV dysfunction develops. The operative mortality is 3 to 10%, but of the patients who survive surgery, 50% live 10 years or more (45) and their quality of life is usually significantly improved (see below). Symptoms of congestive heart failure are responsive to diuretics, digitalis, and vasodilators.

The Patient with a Prosthetic Valve

Although patients usually demonstrate clear improvement in symptoms and prognosis after valve replacement, they should not be considered cured. Despite refinements in design, no valve currently available is free of potential serious complications, which, because they may occur many years after surgery, dictate careful long-term follow-up of all patients who have prosthetic valves.

Many varieties of mechanical valves and tissue (bioprosthetic) valves have been developed. The most commonly used mechanical valves are the Starr–Edwards ball-in-cage series, the Björk–Shiley tilting disk valve, and the St. Jude valve, which has two semicircular tilting leaflets. The most common tissue valves are the Hancock and Carpentier–Edwards valves, which are constructed of porcine aortic valve leaflets that have been fixed in glutaraldehyde. The mechanical prosthetic valves are extremely durable but they are thrombogenic (see below) and patients who receive them require long-term anticoagulation with warfarin. Bioprosthetic valves are less thrombogenic (6) but are also less durable, often requiring late valve replacement because of structural degeneration (see below).

Potential Complications

Thromboembolic phenomena are perhaps the most common life-threatening complications of prosthetic valves and may present as sudden stroke, myocardial infarction, or peripheral arterial occlusion. Alternatively, thrombus may accumulate around the valve ring and prevent proper valve motion, resulting in gradual or sudden obstruction of flow and the development of severe congestive heart failure. Thromboembolic events have been more common with prosthetic valves in the mitral than in the aortic position. Despite treatment with full anticoagulation, the incidence of thromboembolic complications with most mechanical valves is approximately 1 to 2% per year (4). The incidence is lower with the St. Jude valve.

Perivalvular leakage resulting in regurgitation occasionally develops in the postoperative period and may require reoperation.

Prosthetic valve endocarditis develops in 2 to 3% of patients (54) and may present as a febrile illness, a new murmur of valvular regurgitation or stenosis, hemodynamic deterioration, or embolization. Because the infection is at the site of a foreign body, the prognosis for recovery with standard antibiotic therapy is worse than in native valve endocarditis. Recurrence after one trial of medical therapy is generally an indication for replacement of the valve. Prognosis is worse in infections that develop within 60 days of surgery (72% mortality), in which contamination may have occurred at operation, than in those that develop later (45% mortality), when transient bacteremia may be the source of infection.

Late valvular degeneration is a significant problem after tissue valve implantation. Histologic studies reveal fibrin deposition, tears in the leaflets, and calcification that commonly results in some degree of valvular stenosis (27) or regurgitation 5 to 15 years after operation. In some cases in which clinical deterioration occurs, reoperation is required. In a multicenter trial (19), the 11-year probability of reoperation for structural failure of bioprosthetic valves was 15% for those in the aortic position and 36% for those in the mitral position. The process of structural degeneration is greatly accelerated in children but also occurs commonly in young adults (younger than 35).

Bleeding complications are more common with the mechanical valves, which always require full anticoagulation. In the multicenter trial mentioned above (19), the 11-year probability of bleeding complications was 42% with mechanical valves and 26% with bioprosthetic valves. However, these figures may not reflect the current risk of bleeding because in the 1970s, when most patients were recruited into that study, the recommended prothrombin time ratio was 1 to 2.5 times control. Current recommendations are for less vigorous anticoagulation. Because the prothrombin time varies from laboratory to laboratory, the standard is expressed as the international normalized ratio (INR) (see Chapter 52). The current recommendation is that the INR be maintained at 2.5 to 3.5. In the event of a thromboembolic event, aspirin 160 mg/day may be added to the regimen.

Physical and Laboratory Findings

Auscultatory findings after valve replacement are variable. In general, the ball-in-cage valves produce loud opening and closing clicks. In the aortic position, therefore, there is a prominent systolic ejection click, and S_2 is loud and metallic. In the mitral position, S_1 is loud and there is a prominent systolic opening click after S_2, which is similar in timing to the opening snap of mitral stenosis. With the Björk–Shiley valve the closing sounds are loud but the opening sounds are variable. Porcine valves are the most physiological, and as in a native valve, the closing sounds are audible but opening sounds are rare. All valves in either position produce systolic ejection murmurs. Diastolic flow murmurs are common with the Björk–Shiley valve in the mitral position.

It is important to document the baseline physical examination repeatedly so that the significance of any changes that occur in association with new symptoms can be assessed. The most reliable sign of prosthetic valve dysfunction is the loss or muffling of the opening and closing clicks. New regurgitant murmurs may occur. Congestive heart failure may develop.

The 2D echocardiogram may show abnormal, delayed, or intermittent leaflet motion. Doppler echocardiography (see above) is particularly helpful (55) in accurately detecting and quantifying new valve gradients and regurgitation. Tissue valves are often well visualized and can be assessed by echocardiography. However, mechanical valves are not well seen by transthoracic echocardiography and transesophageal echocardiography is usually required to assess valve anatomy if there is clinical suspicion or Doppler evidence of impaired prosthetic valve function.

Management

Management of the patient with a prosthetic valve should begin before the valve is implanted; the selection of the proper type of valve for the individual patient is crucial. A tissue valve is most appropriate for the patient who is likely to be noncompliant with anticoagulation or who is at high risk for bleeding complications. This includes alcoholics; patients with psychiatric problems, unexplained syncope, or previous gastrointestinal bleeds; patients whose occupations put them at high risk of injury; and patients over 70 years old, who are unlikely to outlive their prosthesis. Women of childbearing age who desire future pregnancies should receive tissue valves (see below), but they should be made aware that valve replacement may have to be repeated in 8 to 10 years. Young men, or women who do not anticipate pregnancy and who will tolerate anticoagulation, are better off with the more durable mechanical valves so that reoperation is not necessary (ball-in-cage valves, the oldest type in current use, have lasted over 20 years). These decisions are usually made by the cardiac surgeon after discussing the options with the patient, but it is important that the practitioner communicate his or her opinions to the surgeon well in advance.

All patients with mechanical valves in the aortic or mitral position must be fully anticoagulated with warfarin indefinitely (see Chapter 52). The incidence of thromboembolism is 9% annually without anticoagulation, and 1 to 2% with warfarin. If an elective surgical procedure is planned, warfarin may be safely discontinued 3 days before surgery and resumed afterward (see details in Chapter 86). Antiplatelet agents (see Chapter 52) are not adequate to prevent thromboembolic complications, which occur at an annual rate of 7.5% with aspirin treatment (4). Although the routine addition of aspirin to warfarin has been advocated, this maneuver increases the incidence of bleeding complications, and a reduced rate of thromboembolism has not been conclusively demonstrated (4). Combined therapy should be reserved for patients who have already embolized to attempt to prevent recurrence.

Patients with tissue valves in the aortic position should be anticoagulated for 6 weeks after operation only, so that endothelialization of the valve may occur. Warfarin should then be discontinued. There is controversy over whether tissue valves in the mitral position require long-term anticoagulation. Many cardiologists would not prescribe indefinite anticoagulation unless atrial fibrillation were present, left-atrial enlargement were detected on echocardiogram (a common finding in mitral valve disease), or a previous thromboembolic episode had occurred. Strict antibiotic prophylaxis against endocarditis is indicated. Table 86.13 lists regimens recommended by the AHA before and after various procedures.

Prosthetic valve dysfunction is an indication for referral to a cardiologist, who will usually recommend transesophageal echocardiography and cardiac catheterization (see Table 60.10 for all of the reasons to refer a patient with a prosthetic valve to a cardiologist).

Pregnancy in a Patient with a Prosthetic Valve

Pregnancy poses a serious problem in patients with mechanical prosthetic valves. The ingestion of warfarin during pregnancy results in a definite increase in the incidence of fetal death and birth defects (see Chapter 52). The spontaneous abortion rate is approximately 30%, probably because warfarin crosses the placenta barrier and predisposes the fetus to intrauterine hemorrhage. Between 8 and 16% of the liveborn infants have various birth defects, most commonly nasal hypoplasia with stippled epiphysis (a specific warfarin embryopathy), as well as optic atrophy, microcephaly, and mental retardation.

On the other hand, the risk of thromboembolism is greater during pregnancy, and discontinuation of anticoagulation greatly increases the danger of systemic embolism. In one study (44), systemic embolism was seen in 31% of such patients despite antiplatelet therapy. Most of the patients had Starr–Edwards valves.

Table 60.10.   Indications for Referral of Patients with Prosthetic Valves

Progressive symptoms of congestive heart failure
Progressive cardiac enlargement
Changes in prosthetic heart sounds
Pregnancy or the desire to become pregnant
Embolization
Endocarditis

There is no consensus regarding the management of early pregnancy when a mechanical prosthetic valve is in place. Some authors recommend substituting full-dose heparin, which does not cross the placenta, for warfarin during the first trimester of pregnancy. However, such therapy requires prolonged hospitalization, and the incidence of fetal death appears to be high with this regimen as well (see Chapter 52). Many pregnant patients with mechanical valves are treated with subcutaneous heparin, which the patient learns to self-administer. The safety and efficacy of this regimen are not clearly established (see Chapter 52). The proper management of anticoagulation at the end of pregnancy is more clearly defined. If warfarin has been given, it should be replaced by heparin 2 weeks before delivery is expected. Heparin can then be stopped at the onset of labor to prevent peripartum hemorrhage. Aspirin is not effective in preventing thromboembolism in these patients.

Most clinicians strongly counsel patients with mechanical prosthetic valves to avoid pregnancy. Patients with valves should be well aware of the risks if pregnancy is contemplated. Pregnancy or the desire to become pregnant is an indication for referral to both a cardiologist and an obstetrician specializing in high-risk patients.

Pregnancy for the patient with a tissue (bioprosthetic) valve is much safer because anticoagulation can be avoided. It is uncertain whether antiplatelet agents have a role here. Unfortunately, pregnancy may accelerate the structural degeneration of these valves, and some patients require reoperation within a year of successful pregnancy (3).

The best approach to these problems is to avoid valve replacement in women in whom future pregnancy is likely; if possible, mitral stenosis should be managed medically, with percutaneous valvuloplasty, or with surgical commissurotomy, and mitral regurgitation with medical therapy or valve repair. If valve replacement is necessary in such a patient, the surgeon should be strongly urged to use a bioprosthesis rather than a mechanical valve, and the patient should be aware that eventual reoperation will probably be necessary.

General References*

Braunwald E, ed. Heart disease: a textbook of cardiovascular medicine. 5th ed. Philadelphia: WB Saunders, 1997.
    Encyclopedic review of cardiac physical examination, heart sounds, and cardiac graphic techniques.
Carabello BA, Crawford FA Jr. Valvular heart disease. N Engl J Med 337:32, 1997.
    An up-to-date overview.
Constant J. Bedside cardiology. Boston: Little, Brown, 1976.
    The best teaching text for understanding the physiological basis of heart sounds and how to hear and describe them.
Tavel ME. The systolic murmur: innocent or guilty? Am J Cardiol 39:757, 1977.
    Concise characterization of the most commonly heard murmurs in ambulatory practice.

*Bold print (general references) and bold numerals (specific references) denote published controlled clinical trials, meta-analyses, or consensus-based recommendations.

Specific References

1. Barnett JHM, Boughner DR, Taylor DW, et al. Further evidence relating mitral valve prolapse to cerebral ischemic events. N Engl J Med 302:139, 1980.
2. Brandenburg RO, Fuster V, Giuliani ER. Valvular heart disease. When should the patient be referred? Pract Cardiol 5:50, 1979.
3. Budduke BR, Jamieson WRE, Miyagishima RT, et al. Pregnancy and childbearing in a population with biologic valvular prostheses. J Thorac Cardiovasc Surg 102:179, 1991.
4. Cannegieter SC, Rosendaal FR, Briet E. Thromboembolic and bleeding complications in patients with mechanical heart valve prostheses. Circulation 89:635,1994.
5. Carabello BA. Indications for valve surgery in asymptomatic patients with aortic and mitral stenosis. Chest 108:1678, 1995.
6. Cohn LH, Koster GK, Mee RBB, Collins JJ Jr. Long term follow-up of the Hancock bioprosthetic heart valve. A six-year review. Circulation 60(Suppl 2):93, 1979.
7. Craig RJ, Selzer A. Natural history and prognosis of atrial septal defect. Circulation 37:805, 1968.
8. Daniel WG, Erbel R, Kasper W, et al. Safety of transesophageal echocardiography. Circulation 83:817, 1991.
9. Daniel WG, Mugge A. Transesophageal echocardiography. N Engl J Med 332:1268,1995.
10. Enriquez-Sarano M, Schaff HV, Orszulak TA, et al. Valve repair improves the outcome of surgery for mitral regurgitation. A multivariate analysis. Circulation 91:1022,1995.
11. Faletra F, Pezzano A Jr, Fusco R, et al. Measurement of mitral valve area in mitral stenosis: four echocardiographic methods compared with direct measurement of anatomic orifices. J Am Coll Cardiol 28:1190,1996.
12. Fananapazir L, Cannon RO, Tripodi D, Panza JA. Impact of dual-chamber permanent pacing in patients with obstructive hypertrophic cardiomyopathy with symptoms refractory to verapamil and β-adrenergic blocker therapy. Circulation 85: 2149, 1992.
13. Feigenbaum H. Echocardiography. 5th ed. Philadelphia: Lea & Febiger, 1994.
14. Gaasch WH, John RM, Aurigemma GP. Managing asymptomatic patients with chronic mitral regurgitation. Chest 108:842, 1995.
15. Galloway AC, Colvin SB, Baumann FG, et al. Long-term results of mitral valve reconstruction with Carpentier techniques in 148 patients with mitral insufficiency. Circulation 78(Suppl I):97, 1988.
16. Goldschlager N, Pfeifer J, Cohn K, et al. The natural history of aortic regurgitation. A clinical and hemodynamic study. Am J Med 54:577, 1973.
17. Greenberg B, Massie B, Bristow JD, et al. Long-term vasodilator therapy of chronic aortic insufficiency. A randomized double-blinded, placebo-controlled clinical trial. Circulation 78(1):92, 1988.
18. Hammermeister KE, Fisher L, Kennedy JW, et al. Prediction of late survival in patients with mitral valve disease from clinical, hemodynamic, and quantitative angiographic variables. Circulation 57:341, 1978.
19. Hammermeister KE, Sethi GK, Henderson WG, et al. A comparison of outcomes in men 11 years after heart-valve replacement with a mechanical valve or bioprosthesis. N Engl J Med 328:18, 1993.
20. Hatle L, Angelsen B. Doppler ultrasound in cardiology, physical principles and clinical applications. Philadelphia: Lea & Febiger, 1985.
21. Heger JJ, Wann LS, Weyman AE, et al. Long-term changes in mitral valve area after successful mitral commissurotomy. Circulation 59:443, 1979.
22. Helmcke F, Nanda NC, Hsiung MC, et al. Color Doppler assessment of mitral regurgitation with orthogonal planes. Circulation 75:175, 1987.
23. Leachman RD, Cokkinos DV, Cooley DA. Association of ostium secundum atrial septal defects with mitral valve prolapse. Am J Cardiol 38:167, 1976.
24. Lieberman EB, Bashore TM, Hermiller JB, et al. Balloon aortic valvuloplasty in adults: failure of procedure to improve long-term survival. J Am Coll Cardiol 26:1522,1995.
25. Lin M, Chiang HT, Lin SL, et al. Vasodilator therapy in chronic asymptomatic aortic regurgitation: enalapril versus hydralazine therapy. J Am Coll Cardiol 24:1046, 1994.
26. Ling LH, Enriquez-Sarano M, Seward JB, et al. Clinical outcome of mitral regurgitation due to flail leaflet. N Engl J Med 335:1417, 1996.
27. Lipson LC, Kent KM, Rosing DR, et al. Long term hemodynamic assessment of the porcine heterograft in the mitral position. Late development of valvular stenosis. Circulation 64:397, 1981.
28. Markiewicz W, Stoner J, London E, et al. Mitral valve prolapse in one hundred presumably healthy young females. Circulation 53:464, 1976.
29. Marks AR, Choong CY, Sanfilippo AJ, et al. Identification of high-risk and low-risk subgroups of patients with mitral-valve prolapse. N Engl J Med 320:1031, 1989.
30. Maron BJ. Appraisal of dual-chamber pacing therapy in hypertrophic cardiomyopathy: too soon for a rush to judgment? J Am Coll Cardiol 27:431,1996.
31. Maron BJ, Gardin JM, Flack JM, et al. Prevalence of hypertrophic cardiomyopathy in a general population of young adults. Echocardiographic analysis of 4111 subjects in the CARDIA Study. Coronary Artery Risk Development in (Young) Adults. Circulation 92(4):785,1995.
32. Massell BF, Ameccua FJ, Czohiczer G. Prognosis of patients with pure or predominant aortic regurgitation in the absence of surgery. Circulation 34(Suppl 2):164, 1966.
33. Munoz S, Gallardo J, Diaz-Gorrin JR, Medina O. Influence of surgery on the natural history of rheumatic mitral and aortic valve disease. Am J Cardiol 35:234, 1975.
34. Nienaber CA, von Kodolitsch Y, Nicolas V, et al. The diagnosis of thoracic aortic dissection by noninvasive imaging procedures. N Engl J Med 328:1, 1993.
35. O'Keefe JH Jr, Vlietstra RA, Bailey KR, Holmes DR. Natural history of candidates for balloon aortic valvuloplasty. Mayo Clin Proc 62:986, 1987.
36. Oleson KH. The natural history of 271 patients with mitral stenosis under medical treatment. Br Heart J 24:349, 1962.
37. Olson LJ, Subramanian R, Edwards WD. Surgical pathology of pure aortic insufficiency: a study of 225 cases. Mayo Clin Proc 59:835, 1984.
38. Olsson MA, Granstrom L, Lindblom D, et al. Aortic valve replacement in octogenarians with aortic stenosis: a case-control study. J Am Coll Cardiol 7:1512, 1993.
39. Rapaport E. Natural history of aortic and mitral valve disease. Am J Cardiol 35:221, 1981.
40. Reyes VP, Raju BS, Wynne J, et al. Percutaneous balloon valvuloplasty compared with open surgical commissurotomy for mitral stenosis. N Engl J Med 331:961,1994.
41. Roberts WC. Anatomically isolated aortic valve disease: a case against its being of rheumatic etiology. Am J Med 49:151, 1970.
42. Ross J Jr. The timing of surgery for severe mitral regurgitation. N Engl J Med 335:1456–1458, 1996.
43. Ross J Jr, Braunwald E. Aortic stenosis. Circulation 38(Suppl 5):61, 1968.
44. Salazar E, Zajarias A, Gutierrez N, Iturbe I. The problems of cardiac valve prostheses, anticoagulants and pregnancy. Circulation 70(Suppl 1):169, 1984.
45. Samuels DA, Curfman GD, Friedlich AL, et al. Valve replacement for aortic regurgitation: long-term follow-up with factors influencing the results. Circulation 60:647, 1979.
46. Scognamiglio R, Fasoli G, Ponchia A, et al. Long-term nifedipine unloading therapy in asymptomatic patients with chronic severe aortic regurgitation. J Am Coll Cardiol 16:424, 1990.
47. Selzer A, Cohn K. Natural history of mitral stenosis: a review. Circulation 45:878, 1972.
48. Seward JB, Khandheria BK, Edwards WD, et al. Biplanar transesophageal echocardiography: anatomic correlations, image orientation, and clinical applications. Mayo Clin Proc 65:1193, 1990.
49. Sherrid MV, Chu CK, Delia E. An echocardiographic study of the fluid mechanics of obstruction in hypertrophic cardiomyopathy. J Am Coll Cardiol 22:816,1993.
50. Siemienczuk D, Greenberg B, Morris C, et al. Chronic aortic

insufficiency: factors associated with progression to aortic valve replacement. Ann Intern Med 110:587, 1989.

51. Spirito P, Chiarella F, Carratino L, et al. Clinical course and prognosis of hypertrophic cardiomyopathy in an outpatient population. N Engl J Med 320:749, 1989.

52. Stoll BC, Ashcom TL, Johns JP, et al. Effects of atenolol on rest and exercise hemodynamics in patients with mitral stenosis. Am J Cardiol 75:482, 1995.

53. ten Berg JM, Suttorp MJ, Knapen PJ, et al. Hypertrophic obstructive cardiomyopathy. Initial results and long-term follow-up after Morrow septal myectomy. Circulation 90:1781, 1994.

54. Watanakunakorn C. Prosthetic valve endocarditis. Prog Cardiovasc Dis 22:181, 1979.

55. Weinstein IR, Marbarger JP, Pérez JE. Ultrasonic assessment of the St. Jude prosthetic valve: M-mode, two dimensional, and Doppler echocardiography. Circulation 68:897, 1983.

56. Wooley CF, Baker PB, Kolibash AJ, et al. The floppy, myxomatous mitral valve, mitral valve prolapse, and mitral regurgitation. Prog Cardiovasc Dis 33:397, 1991.

57. Zuppiroli A, Rinaldi M, Kramer-Fox R, et al. Natural history of mitral valve prolapse. Am J Cardiol 75:1028, 1995.

CHAPTER 61

Heart Failure

SHELDON H. GOTTLIEB, MD

DEFINITION

The amount of blood that the heart pumps per minute (the cardiac output) is normally precisely adjusted to meet the metabolic needs of the body. The cardiac output may increase twofold or threefold as a person goes from rest to exercise. An increase in cardiac output may occur within the space of one heartbeat by a decrease in vagal tone, which causes an increase in heart rate. After several seconds of exercise, sympathetic tone increases, which causes a further increase in cardiac output by increasing the heart rate and the amount of blood pumped per heartbeat (the stroke volume). The increased cardiac output soon brings about an increase in the amount of blood returning to the right side of the heart (the venous return); also, the heart further increases its output in response to the stretch in the heart muscle that results from the increased volume of venous return (the Frank–Starling principle). If the heart is unable to pump enough blood to maintain tissue perfusion pressure and thereby to meet the metabolic needs of the body, compensatory neural and hormonal mechanisms are brought into play. These adjustments cause symptoms and signs recognized as the syndrome of heart failure. *Acute heart failure,* manifest usually by pulmonary edema (recognized by the abrupt onset of extreme breathlessness and evidence of alveolar edema by physical and radiologic examination), warrants immediate hospitalization for diagnosis of the underlying or precipitating cause and for treatment. However, *chronic heart failure* can usually be managed in an ambulatory setting.

EPIDEMIOLOGY

The incidence of heart failure is approximately 0.3/1000 per year under age 45, remains constant at approximately 3/1000 per year in the middle-age groups, and increases to 10/1000 in patients over the age of 65 (23). The incidence among men is slightly higher than among women in the 45- to 84-year-old range but is higher among women in the 85- to 94-year-old range (23).

The prevalence of heart failure increases greatly in patients over 60 years old (Fig. 61.1) and is at least 25% greater among the African-American population than among the white population (20). Over the age of 70, women with congestive heart failure (CHF) outnumber men. This is true despite the higher incidence in men and probably reflects the earlier mortality among men from coronary artery disease (24).

In 1990, there were 720,000 hospital discharges for heart failure (20). Between 1973 and 1995, the annual hospitalization rates for CHF among patients over age 65 more than tripled, from approximately 60 per 10,000 people to more than 200 per 10,000, probably reflecting in part improved treatment because the

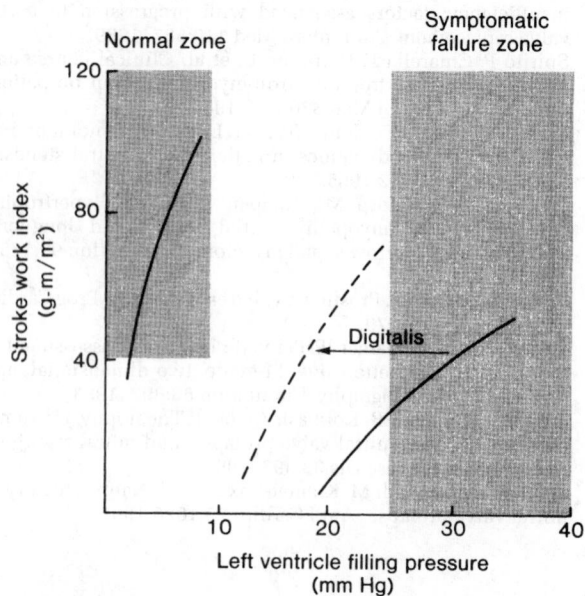

Figure 61.2.   Ventricular function curves showing the relationship between LV filling pressures and stroke work. The position of the curve defines the inotropic state of the heart. Note that for a given curve (i.e., a given inotropic state), the function of the heart, or the amount of work the heart is capable of performing, varies with the LV filling pressure. (Adapted from Weisfeldt ML. Congestive heart failure: pathophysiology and the evaluation of ventricular function. In: Harvey AM, Johns RJ, McKusick VA, et al, eds. The principles and practice of medicine. New York: Appleton-Century-Crofts, 1984.)

percentage of hospitalized CHF patients who died fell from 11.3% in 1981 to 6.1% in 1993 (38).

PHYSIOLOGY
The Heart as a Pump

Length–Tension Relationship: Frank–Starling Principle and Preload

As heart muscle is stretched, it develops increased tension. The relationship of length to tension defines the *compliance* of heart muscle; the inverse of compliance is *stiffness*. If the ventricle is distended with blood, pressure develops within the cavity. A higher pressure is needed to distend the ventricle to a given volume in a less compliant (i.e., stiffer) ventricle. The pressure needed to stretch the ventricle to a given end-diastolic volume is called the *preload*, clinically measured as the *left ventricular end-diastolic pressure* (LVEDP). The relationship between the volume of the ventricle just before contraction and the force developed during contraction defines the Frank–Starling principle (33). If the LVEDP is plotted against stroke work (the stroke volume times the mean blood pressure), a ventricular function curve is defined (Fig. 61.2). It can be seen from this relationship that the normal ventricle is compliant: It develops an adequate amount of force during contraction with a low preload. However, the failing ventricle requires a higher preload to increase its stroke work (Fig. 61.2). The implications of this relationship are discussed below.

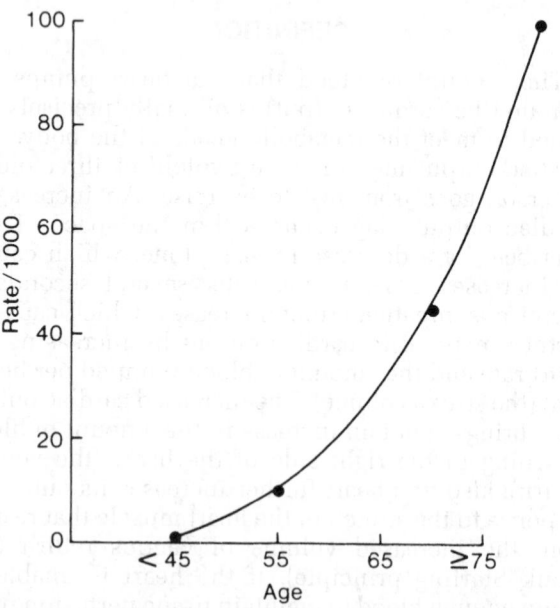

Figure 61.1.   The prevalence of heart failure reported from physicians' offices as a function of patient age. Note the marked increase in the sixth and seventh decades. Between 10 and 20% of patients older than age 60 followed regularly by a physician have a history of heart failure. (From McKee P, Castelli W, McNamara P, Kannel W. The natural history of congestive heart failure: the Framingham study. N Engl J Med 285:1441, 1971.)

Afterload

Afterload is the dynamic resistance against which the heart contracts. It determines the degree of stress within the myocardium. Systolic blood pressure closely approximates and is clinically the most useful indicator of afterload. Afterload determines the ease or speed of ventricular contraction; hence, the ejection fraction (the portion of the ventricular volume that is ejected with each beat) is a function of afterload (Fig. 61.3).

Contractility and Inotropic State

The relationship of preload to stroke work defines the functional state of cardiac muscle (see above). The relative position of the curve defines the inotropic state of the muscle (Fig. 61.2). For example, infusing the heart with an inotropic substance such as digitalis causes the ventricular function curve to shift to the left, to perform a higher stroke work at a given preload, assuming that afterload is kept constant. In other words, the contractility of the heart is increased.

Relationship Between Preload, Afterload, and Inotropic State

The relationship between the preload, afterload, and inotropic state is summarized in Figure 61.3. If preload is kept constant, an increase in afterload or decrease in inotropic state causes a depression in ventricular func-

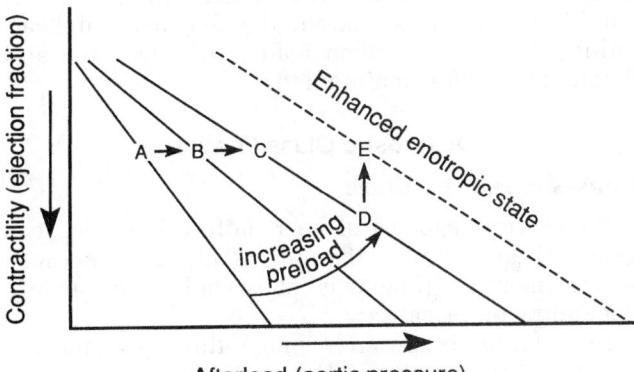

Figure 61.3. The relationship between preload, afterload, and inotropic state. The three solid lines are a family of curves at different levels of preload but with inotropic state kept constant. Taken together, they represent ventricular function as a function of both preload and afterload. Note that if preload is kept constant, an increase in afterload causes a decrease in contractility as measured by the ejection fraction (when afterload is decreased to 0, the preload curves converge because the inotropic state of the muscle is unchanged). As afterload increases, the ejection fraction may be maintained by increasing preload (shifting from point **A** to **B** to **C**). When preload reaches the point (**C**) at which an increase will cause pulmonary congestion (the preload reserve), any further increase in afterload will decrease the ejection fraction (point **C** to **D**). The ejection fraction may then be increased only by measures such as digitalization that enhance the inotropic state (point **D** to **E**). Patients are most sensitive to changes in afterload when their filling pressures are at the preload reserve because any further increase in preload leads to pulmonary congestion. (Adapted from Ross J Jr. Afterload mismatch and preload reserve: a conceptual framework for the analysis of ventricular function. Prog Cardiovasc Dis 18:255, 1976.)

tion, as measured clinically by the ejection fraction. Thus, if afterload or blood pressure increases, ventricular function or ejection fraction (normally 50 to 75%) decreases. In response, the LVEDP, or preload, increases, and restores the ventricular function to baseline. A further increase in afterload leads to a further depression in ventricular function, which again may be restored by an increased preload (i.e., by increasing LVEDP). The *preload reserve* is the LVEDP above which the pulmonary capillary oncotic pressure is exceeded; fluid passes into the alveoli, and pulmonary congestion, with symptoms of cough and dyspnea, occurs. Any increase in afterload that occurs when the preload reserve is reached causes a decrease in ventricular function and a worsening in symptoms of congestion. The preload reserve varies with the compliance of the ventricle. If heart muscle is made stiffer or less compliant by a chronic disease process such as hypertension or aortic stenosis, or by an acute process such as ischemia, a higher filling pressure is necessary to set the level of ventricular function by means of the Frank–Starling principle, and the preload reserve is reached at a lower level of stroke work. The only ways to improve ventricular function when the preload reserve is reached are to decrease the afterload or change the inotropic state of the muscle. The clinical significance of these relationships is discussed at greater length under "Management."

Biochemical Basis for Altered Contractility in the Failing Heart

The contractile unit of heart muscle is the sarcomere, which consists of fibers of protein called actin and myosin. *Actin* and *myosin* interact with each other by an interlocking protein, called *troponin.* The interlocking mechanism is facilitated by adenosine triphosphate (ATP) and magnesium. An inhibitory protein, *tropomyosin,* is present on the myosin fibers. Tropomyosin inhibits the interaction between actin and myosin and allows the muscle to relax. Calcium inhibits the tropomyosin complex, frees the interlocking troponin, and allows actin and myosin to interact and to develop tension. Calcium is therefore necessary for myocardial contraction to take place. Large amounts of calcium are stored within the heart in the *sarcoplasmic reticulum.* Excitation–contraction coupling takes place in heart muscle when an action potential causes a release of calcium from the sarcoplasmic reticulum, thereby initiating contraction. In classic heart failure, there appears to be decreased energy available for cardiac contraction (27). This leads to *decreased systolic function* and to slow transport of calcium back into the sarcoplasmic reticulum after contraction, which causes a delay in relaxation (lusitropy) of cardiac muscle (27). There is a reduction in early diastolic filling and an increased dependence on atrial pumping for ventricular filling. Abnormalities in calcium transport may also predispose the failing heart to develop arrhythmias (27,32).

In approximately 30% of patients with heart failure, systolic function as judged by the ejection fraction is normal but diastolic function is markedly impaired (35). This leads to inadequate LV filling; any compensatory increase in heart rate shortens diastole disproportionately more than systole, which leads to a further reduction in both LV filling and the time available for calcium uptake; therefore, both systolic function and diastolic compliance worsen (35).

Compensatory Mechanisms

Heart Rate

The neural and hormonal responses to heart failure lead to an increase in heart rate in an attempt to maintain cardiac output. This may lead to rapid deterioration in systolic and diastolic function because of the disproportionate shortening of diastole relative to systole as heart rate increases (see above).

Hypertrophy and Dilation

Left ventricular hypertrophy (LVH) and dilation may allow compensation of the failing heart to be maintained for many years. The stress in the wall of the heart varies with the radius of the ventricular cavity. If the heart is subjected to a *volume load,* it dilates to accommodate the load and to increase its ability to eject the load (the Frank–Starling principle; see above). However, ventricular dilation causes an increase in ventricular wall stress, which stimulates ventricular hypertrophy. Eventually the heart becomes both dilated and hypertrophied, and the ratio of wall thickness to cavity size returns to normal, which normalizes wall stress; therefore, a state of compensated ventricular dilation is achieved (27). The response to a *pressure overload* is different. An increase in wall stress in the absence of volume overload leads to cellular hypertrophy; wall stress per unit area returns to normal, but the cavity size is unchanged (27).

Activation of the Neurohormonal System

The neurohormonal activation triggered by the inability of the failing heart to maintain blood pressure and tissue perfusion is a major cause of the syndrome of heart failure. Neurohormonal activation leads to an increase in peripheral vascular resistance, a redistribution of cardiac output (maintaining flow to the heart and brain and reducing it to the kidneys, skin, splanchnic organs, and skeletal muscle), and the retention of salt and water. In less severe heart failure, when the resting cardiac output is normal, redistribution occurs only during exercise. In severe heart failure, when the resting cardiac output is significantly decreased, redistribution occurs at rest. The decrease in blood flow is functionally most important in the kidneys. Decreased renal blood flow causes a release of renin from the juxtaglomerular apparatus, which leads to increased plasma angiotensin activity. *Angiotensin* is a potent vasoconstrictor and acts both directly on smooth muscle and indirectly by increasing norepinephrine release from vascular nerve endings. Norepinephrine and angiotensin may directly damage myocardial cells. Prolonged increased plasma norepinephrine levels

lead to a decreased density of β_1-adrenergic receptors on cardiac myocytes and thereby may decrease the normal myocardial response to sympathetic stimulation (17). The increase in angiotensin activity leads to an increase in aldosterone production, which causes an increase in sodium resorption from the distal nephron, thereby increasing plasma volume. The renal resorption of sodium is also facilitated by an increased filtration fraction at a given glomerular filtration rate, which causes increased sodium reabsorption in the proximal nephron. Paradoxically, hyponatremia may result from increased thirst and consumption of free water, triggered by increased levels of circulating renin, angiotensin, aldosterone, and antidiuretic hormone, and by a decreased renal responsiveness to atrial natriuretic peptide. The importance of these compensatory responses to neurohormonal activation in the management of patients with heart failure is discussed below.

DIAGNOSTIC PROCESS

No symptoms, signs, or laboratory tests are pathognomonic of heart failure. The significance of symptoms and signs must be inferred based on the patient's overall condition and the stage at which the patient appears to be in the natural history of his or her disease. Clinical criteria for the diagnosis of heart failure are listed in Table 61.1 (24). In ambulatory practice, a patient often presents to a new physician with the diagnosis of heart failure and is taking medicine for this condition. In this situation, the diagnosis of heart failure should be verified before it is accepted and before treatment is maintained.

Diagnostic Classification

Causes of Heart Failure

When the diagnosis of heart failure is made, it is essential to determine the most likely cause because the treatment and prognosis of heart failure vary greatly depending on its cause.

Heart failure is caused by one of three basic mechanisms: an increased work load to which the heart cannot accommodate, a disorder of the myocardium so that it is unable to accommodate normal work loads, or a restriction of ventricular filling so that an adequate stroke volume cannot be achieved. Table 61.2 lists selected examples of these conditions. In this country, the most common condition associated with heart failure is hypertension, followed closely by ischemic heart disease (34).

The most common precipitating causes of heart failure (Table 61.3) are noncompliance with medication or diet in a patient with previously compensated heart failure, acute myocardial ischemia or infarction, poorly controlled hypertension, and pneumonia. In patients for whom the precipitating cause is not obvious, it is important to consider arrhythmia (Chapter 59), covert ischemia (Chapter 57), and pulmonary embolism (Chapter 54). In addition, it is important to inquire about psychosocial stress, which may lead

Table 61.1. Diagnostic Criteria for Heart Failure

Major Criteria
Paroxysmal nocturnal dyspnea
Jugular venous distension
Crackles at the lung bases
Cardiothoracic ratio >0.5
History of acute pulmonary edema
S_3 gallop
Hepatojugular reflux

Minor Criteria
Bilateral ankle edema
Nocturnal cough
Dyspnea on ordinary exertion
Hepatomegaly
Pleural effusion
Decrease in vital capacity by one-third from maximum value
    recorded
Tachycardia (rate >120)

Major or Minor Criteria
Weight loss >4.5 kg in 5 days in response to treatment of heart
    failure

The diagnosis of heart failure required that two major or one major and two minor criteria be present concurrently. Minor criteria were acceptable only if they could not be attributed to another medical condition (24).

Table 61.2. Causes of Heart Failure

Increased Work Load to Which the Heart Cannot Accommodate
High-output states
    Hyperthyroidism[a]
    Anemia[a]
    Systemic arteriovenous fistulas[a]
    Certain dermatologic disorders (e.g., psoriasis, erythroderma)[a]
Valvular regurgitation or left-to-right shunts[a]
Increased impedance to injection
    Systemic hypertension[a]
    Pulmonary hypertension
    Pulmonic or aortic stenosis[a]

Disorders of Myocardium so that the Heart is Unable to Accommodate Normal Work Loads
Cardiomyopathies (viral, familial, drug induced [cytotoxic chemo-
    therapy, chronic use of amphetamines, cocaine])
Myocardial infarction

Restriction of Ventricular Filling
Pericardial constriction or effusion[a]
Atrial myxoma
Mitral and tricuspid valvular stenosis[a]
Increased ventricular stiffness
    Infiltrative myocardial disease (e.g., amyloid, hemochromatosis)
    Ventricular hypertrophy
    Hypertrophic cardiomyopathy

Adapted from Weisfeldt ML. Congestive heart failure: pathophysiology and the evaluation of ventricular function. In: Harvey AM, Johns RJ, McKusick VA, et al, eds. The principles and practice of medicine. New York: Appleton-Century-Crofts, 1984.
[a]Indicates causes of heart failure that are potentially treatable by specific therapy.

to increased energy demands and is often associated with increased salt and water intake.

Right- and Left-Sided Heart Failure

Heart failure may be classified as *right sided* (e.g., as evidenced by jugular venous congestion, hepatic enlargement, ascites, or peripheral edema; see below) or *left sided* (as evidenced by signs and symptoms of pulmonary congestion; see below) depending on which chamber or chambers are compromised.

Functional Classification

The amount of physical activity that a patient can perform without symptoms of heart failure determines functional class. Several classification schemes that are useful in categorizing patients in this regard are presented in Tables 61.4 and 61.5. Correctable disease may be present despite severe symptoms, so the functional classification provides useful prognostic information only within selected subsets of patients. Functional class is best determined by questioning the patient regarding performance during daily activities. For example, a patient may be asked how many stairs can be climbed or how many blocks can be walked before having to stop and rest, or how heavy a load can be carried and what household or work activities have had to be modified (see Chapter 58 for metabolic requirements of daily activities).

History

The most common symptoms of heart failure are dyspnea and fatigue. *Dyspnea* in heart failure is a symptom of increased LVEDP with pulmonary venous and capillary congestion. Increased pulmonary congestion causes decreased lung compliance and vital capacity. The work of breathing increases and breathing becomes rapid, shallow, and forced. *Fatigue*, caused by low cardiac output, is often described as a general sense of weakness or "lack of ambition." Some patients may complain of fatigue rather than dyspnea.

Table 61.3. Precipitating Causes of Heart Failure

Factors Decreasing Myocardial Efficiency
Myocardial infarction
Ischemia
Arrhythmia
Hypoxia
Alcohol and other toxic substances
Recent initiation of a β-blocking drug
Discontinuation of a cardiac glycoside
Myocardial depressant drugs (e.g., verapamil, disopyramide [Norpace], adriamycin)
Pericardial tamponade
Myocardial infections (e.g., bacterial endocarditis, myocarditis, parasitic infection)
Vasculitis

Factors Increasing Cardiac Load
Noncompliance with low-salt diet
Uncontrolled systemic hypertension
Systemic infection
Psychological stress
Exercise, especially in extremes of heat or humidity
Discontinuing diuretics, antihypertensive drugs, or afterload-reducing agents
Drugs that retain or contain sodium
Infection
Anemia
Pulmonary embolism
Thyrotoxicosis
Acute valvular dysfunction

Table 61.4.   Assessment of Functional Capacity

New York Heart Association Classification[a]	Severity of Symptoms[b]	Max. Oxygen Uptake (mL/mm/kg)[b]	Goldman's Specific Activity Scale (METs)[c,d]
I Patients with cardiac disease but without resulting limitations of physical activity. Ordinary physical activity does not cause undue fatigue, palpitations, dyspnea, or anginal pain.	None to mild	>20	10
II Patients with cardiac disease resulting in slight limitation of physical activity. They are comfortable at rest. Ordinary physical activity results in fatigue, palpitations, dyspnea, or angina pain.	Mild to moderate	16–20	5–6
III Patients with cardiac disease that results in marked limitation of physical activity and causes fatigue, palpitations, dyspnea, or anginal pain.	Moderate to severe	10–16	3.6–4.2
IV Patients with cardiac disease that results in inability to carry on any physical activity without discomfort. Symptoms of cardiac insufficiency or of the anginal syndrome may be present even at rest. If any physical activity is undertaken, discomfort is increased.	Severe	<10	2–2.3

[a]The Criteria Committee of the New York Association, Inc. Diseases of the heart and blood vessels, nomenclature and criteria for diagnosis. 6th ed. Boston: Little, Brown, 1964.
[b]Adapted from Weber KT, Janiski JS. Cardiopulmonary exercise testing. Philadelphia: WB Saunders, 1986.
[c]Adapted from Goldman L, Hashimoto B, Cook EF, Loscalzo A. Comparative reproducibility and validity of systems for assessing cardiovascular functional class: advantages of new specific activity scale. Circulation 64:1227, 1981.
[d]METs, Metabolic equivalents of activity, where 1 MET = 3.5 mL of O_2/kg/min at rest.

Table 61.5.   Goldman's Specific Activity Scale[a]

	Any Yes	No
1. Can you walk down a flight of steps without stopping? (4.5–5.2 METs[b])	Go to #2	Go to #4
2. Can you carry anything up a flight of eight steps without stopping (5–5.5 METs) or can you	Go to #3	Class III
a. Have sexual intercourse without stopping (5–5.5 METs)		
b. Garden, rake, weed (5.6 METs)		
c. Roller skate, dance foxtrot (5–6 METs)		
d. Walk at a 4 miles/hr rate on level ground (5–6 METs)		
3. Can you carry at least 24 pounds up eight steps (10 METs) or can you	Class I	Class II
a. Carry objects that are at least 80 pounds (8 METs)		
b. Do outdoor work—shovel snow, spade soil (7 METs)		
c. Do recreational activities such as skiing, basketball, touch football, squash, handball (7–10 METs)		
d. Jog/walk 5 miles/hr (9 METs)		
4. Can you shower without stopping (3.6–4.2 METs) or can you	Class III	Go to #5
a. Strip and make bed (3.9–5 METs)		
b. Mop floors (4.2 METs)		
c. Hang washed clothes (4.4 METs)		
d. Clean windows (3.7 METs)		
e. Walk 2.5 miles/hr (3–3.5 METs)		
f. Bowl (3–4.4 METs)		
g. Play golf (walk and carry clubs) (4.5 METs)		
h. Push power lawn mower (4 METs)		
5. Can you dress without stopping because of symptoms? (2–2.3 METs)	Class III	Class IV

[a]See legend to Table 61.3.
[b]METs, Metabolic equivalents of activity, where 1 MET = oxygen consumption at rest (3.5 mL O_2/kg/min).

Fatigue may be a symptom of low cardiac output with hypotension caused by overaggressive diuresis, especially when there is concomitant use of converting enzyme inhibitors. A complaint of dyspnea or fatigue may be difficult to interpret because effort intolerance may bear little or no relationship to objective measures of circulatory, ventilatory, or metabolic dysfunction during exercise; factors other than the degree of hemodynamic dysfunction may be important. These include musculoskeletal status, muscle deconditioning, body composition, obesity, motivation, and tolerance of discomfort (55).

Orthopnea is dyspnea in the recumbent position. It is often experienced by patients with heart failure, although it may also be a symptom of patients with obstructive lung disease or obesity. Blood normally pools in the lower extremities when a person is upright. When the patient who is in heart failure lies down, there is an increase in venous return to the heart, which increases LVEDP and pulmonary venous congestion. The severity of orthopnea is often assessed by the number of pillows the patient must use to be able to breathe comfortably in the recumbent position.

Patients in heart failure often have a nonproductive cough, especially when they are in the recumbent position; at times this is the patient's premonitory symptom of decompensated heart failure and may precede the development of dyspnea. The cough is caused by pulmonary venous congestion and usually improves with diuresis. A nonproductive, hacking cough also develops in 2 to 10% of patients treated with converting enzyme (CE) inhibitors (30,31); it may occur within days to months after the patient begins to take these drugs. Some patients may tolerate the cough when they understand its cause and the importance of the CE inhibitor for the treatment of their heart failure. In many cases, however, the cough is sufficiently disruptive to justify switching the patients to angiotensin receptor–blocking drugs, which appear to have many of the benefits of CE inhibitors but do not cause cough (see below).

Paroxysmal nocturnal dyspnea (PND) is characteristic of poorly compensated heart failure; it occurs approximately 2 hours after falling asleep and is relieved by sitting up in bed or by getting out of bed and sitting in a chair. Because PND often is associated with wheezing, it must be distinguished from the nocturnal shortness of breath sometimes experienced by people with obstructive lung disease (see Chapter 55). Periodic, or Cheyne–Stokes breathing, is a symptom of severe heart failure with low cardiac output; during the hyperpneic phase this respiratory pattern may be confused with PND and it also may need to be distinguished from obstructive sleep apnea (see Chapter 85).

A history of *edema* or weight gain (from retention of salt and water) is often elicited from patients in heart failure. Many also give a history of having taken digitalis, diuretics, or a CE inhibitor in the past for a "heart problem."

Chest pain caused by myocardial ischemia is common in patients in heart failure (see Chapter 57). Decompensated heart failure caused by salt and water overload may cause ischemic chest pain due to LV dilation with increased LV oxygen demands. Heart failure caused by systolic or diastolic dysfunction (see below) may rapidly decompensate because of ischemia, especially if there is associated paroxysmal mitral regurgitation caused by acute papillary muscle dysfunction. This may happen in association with exercise in patients with stable ischemic heart disease or may occur paroxysmally and at rest in patients with unstable ischemic heart disease (see Chapter 57). The symptomatic response to nitroglycerin does not by itself differentiate between dyspnea caused by ischemia with acute LV dysfunction and dyspnea caused by chronic heart failure; sublingual nitroglycerin may relieve symptoms of congestion caused by either condition (see below).

Nocturia, a common symptom of heart failure, often occurs early in the illness. It is caused by the redistribution in cardiac output that occurs in the recumbent position, restoring in part blood flow to the kidney that, in the upright position, has been diverted to other organs; the circadian pattern of atrial natriuretic peptide release may also be disturbed (see above) (37).

Decreased cardiac output by itself, or in association with disturbed sleep patterns caused by orthopnea, PND, and Cheyne–Stokes respirations, or with concomitant cerebrovascular disease, may lead to *impairment in mental function,* ranging from mild confusion to overt psychosis. However, the most common neuropsychiatric complaints are mild chronic anxiety and depression; these may be the presenting complaints, especially in elderly patients with previously undiagnosed heart failure.

Symptoms of *gastrointestinal congestion* may be seen in patients with chronic, poorly compensated heart failure. Chronically increased right heart pressure may cause passive congestion of the liver, with swelling and discomfort in the right upper quadrant of the abdomen.

Physical Findings

The physical findings in heart failure depend on its cause, the degree to which neurohumoral compensatory mechanisms are invoked (see above), and whether the heart failure is uncompensated or compensated.

Uncompensated Heart Failure

In chronic uncompensated or poorly compensated heart failure, there are signs of an attempt at cardiac compensation (increased heart size and heart rate) and signs of increased renin, angiotensin, and aldosterone activity (vascular redistribution and evidence of cardiac, pulmonary, and peripheral congestion) (27). Congestion is manifest by a ventricular gallop sound (S_3), pulmonary crackles, jugular venous distension, hepatojugular reflux, and peripheral pitting edema (22,36).

Increased heart size may be recognized by inspection, palpation, and percussion of the precordium. The precordium should be palpated with the patient in the supine and the left lateral position. The location, quality, and size of the point of maximal impulse (PMI) should be noted. The PMI of a dilated and enlarged heart is displaced laterally and caudally and is heaving and diffuse. The PMI of a concentrically enlarged heart is not displaced but may be thrusting or sustained.

Sinus tachycardia, defined as a resting heart rate in an adult greater than 100 beats/minute, is a sensitive but nonspecific sign of heart failure; it is a compensatory mechanism to increase cardiac output (see below). In patients with poorly compensated heart failure, a relative tachycardia of 85 to 95 beats/minute may be seen. The tachycardia shortens diastolic filling time and may lead to further deterioration in function (see above). Low-dose β-blockers, often as little as 12.5 mg/day of sustained-release metoprolol, may lower heart rate and thereby improve function in such patients (see below) (17).

The second pulmonic sound (P_2) is often accentuated in patients in left ventricular (LV) failure because of increased pulmonary artery pressure. *Paradoxical splitting of the second heart sound,* an indication of prolonged LV ejection time, may be heard in patients with chronic heart failure and is often associated with a left bundle branch block (LBBB).

The *ventricular or S_3 gallop sound* is the most specific sign of heart failure (22). The sound is heard shortly after the second heart sound (S_2) and is caused by sudden restriction of filling in a noncompliant left ventricle. It is usually heard directly over the PMI and may be audible only when the patient is in the left lateral position. The sound is low pitched and often may be sensed by the cadence of the heart sounds rather than specifically heard. The cadence closely approximates the word *Kentucky* (pronounced kyn-TUC-ky). The middle syllable is accentuated to represent the loud second heart sound caused by increased pulmonary artery pressure in patients in heart failure. The timing of the last syllable closely approximates the timing of the third heart sound, when the word is repeated at a rate of 85 to 100 times/minute.

Crackles (formally called rales) are high-pitched sounds (similar to the sound of a clump of hair rubbed between the fingers) produced by the sudden filling with air of fluid-filled alveoli. They are a sign of moderately to severely decompensated left heart failure.

Neck vein distension and hepatojugular reflux are insensitive but specific findings of heart failure (7). In chronic heart failure, right ventricular filling pressure usually increases as the LVEDP increases. With time, the right ventricle becomes less compliant; as heart size increases, the pericardium may also restrain the heart and thereby limit filling (14).

Neck vein distension is assessed while the patient is semirecumbent, with a small pillow supporting the neck and the head turned slightly away from the examiner. Ideally, the internal rather than the external jugular vein is inspected because the latter contains valves and may not reflect accurately the right heart pressure. Internal jugular venous distension is seen as a broad-based filling in the anterior cervical triangle. However, because the external jugular venous system is often more easily identified, it may be used as an index of the pressure in the superior vena cava if the physician examines the neck properly. If the external jugular is compressed in the supraclavicular fossa and the examining finger then strips the vein cephalad, blood rises in the more proximal (caudal) portion of the vein and the height of this volume of blood reflects the central venous pressure. An arbitrary reference point may be chosen (e.g., 10 cm anterior to the posterior axillary line; this approximates in many the level of the right atrium), and the column of blood above this point may be measured without regard for the angle of elevation of the thorax. The value of this observation is that accurate serial assessments are possible, permitting the physician to confirm worsening failure (increasing jugular venous pressure) or to recognize a too vigorous diuretic response (abnormally low jugular venous pressure).

Hepatojugular reflux is assessed by having the patient lie supine and semirecumbent at 45°. The patient is asked to breathe normally and is warned that the examiner will apply pressure over the right upper quadrant of the abdomen. Patients so warned comply and do not hold their breath or perform the Valsalva maneuver, which distends the jugular vein and makes the sign impossible to elicit. The pressure on the vena cava causes right ventricular end-diastolic pressure and right-atrial pressure to rise and to remain elevated; this is seen as jugular venous distension (7).

Peripheral pitting edema is a common but not specific sign of heart failure. It occurs in the dependent portions of the body, which in ambulatory patients means the feet and lower legs. Edema in heart failure is caused by increased resorption of salt and water by the kidney. An increase in weight may precede pitting edema as an early objective manifestation of decompensated heart failure. Patients should be encouraged to weigh themselves daily, or at least three times a week, and they should record the values and bring the weight record with them at each visit.

It is worth noting that calcium channel blockers (see below) are a common cause of pitting edema, so if a patient is taking one of these drugs, peripheral edema is not necessarily caused by heart failure.

Because of low cardiac output and vascular redistribution, patients' extremities may be cool and their nail beds may be cyanotic. Delayed capillary filling in the skin of the abdomen may be apparent when the examiner's hand is removed after assessing hepatojugular reflux.

Compensated Heart Failure

In contrast to the findings in patients with acute or chronic uncompensated heart failure, there may be few or no specific physical findings in patients with compensated heart failure at rest other than signs of increased heart size (27). A presystolic gallop or fourth heart sound (S_4) can be heard in most patients with long-standing high blood pressure or ischemic heart disease who are in normal sinus rhythm. The fourth heart sound is thought to be caused by atrial contraction into a stiff ventricle (see also below). A soft systolic murmur, approximately grade 1–2/6, is commonly heard at the PMI or along the left sternal border in patients with chronic compensated heart failure. This murmur usually represents a minor degree of mitral or tricuspid insufficiency.

Laboratory Diagnosis

Chest X-Ray

The chest x-ray is a useful diagnostic procedure for the evaluation of suspected heart failure (22,36). The radiologic signs of heart failure are cardiac enlargement and pulmonary congestion.

A number of factors influence heart size on the chest x-ray. These include body build, the depth of inspiration when the film is taken, and the chambers that are enlarged. Nevertheless, determination of the ratio of the transverse diameter of the heart to the greatest diameter of the chest, the cardiothoracic ratio (CTR), is a reliable and valid measurement of heart size and should be part of the database of every patient who is thought to have or to have had heart failure. The normal cardiothoracic ratio is less than 0.5.

The pulmonary vasculature should be examined, and signs of vascular redistribution, caused by pulmonary venous hypertension, and of enlarged hilar vessels, caused by acute or chronic pulmonary hypertension, should be noted.

Normally, the lower lobes of the lungs are better perfused than the upper lobes. The earliest radiologic sign of pulmonary congestion is reduction of blood flow to the lower lobes caused by compression of vessels by extravascular fluid that has gravitated to the lung bases. In early heart failure, there is simply an equalization of the size of the vessels to the upper and lower lobes; as congestion increases, the vessels to the upper lobes become more prominent, the so-called cephalization of flow. More severe failure is manifest by signs of interstitial edema and ultimately by alveolar edema and a transudative pleural effusion (see Chapter 54).

Electrocardiogram

No changes in the electrocardiogram (ECG) are diagnostic of heart failure. However, the ECG may reflect an underlying disease (e.g., left ventricular hypertrophy caused by hypertension; Q waves or ST–T wave changes caused by infarction) or the presence of an unstable rhythm (e.g., atrial fibrillation with rapid ventricular response) that has caused heart failure. A normal ECG is almost never seen in patients with chronic LV dysfunction.

Patients with hypertrophy of the heart may show only minor nonspecific ST–T wave changes. Grossly abnormal changes are commonly seen in the ECG of patients who have both dilation and hypertrophy of the left ventricle. The most common manifestations of left ventricular hypertrophy are *left axis deviation, increased QRS voltage and QRS duration, and ST–T wave changes.* Although there are numerous ECG criteria for LVH, a clinically useful criterion is the index of Lewis: net positivity in lead 1 plus net negativity in lead 3 equals 2.0 mV or more (see also Table 60.3, Chapter 60). Also, an R wave greater than 11 mm in aVL is highly specific for LVH.

Conduction abnormalities are common in patients in heart failure, especially LBBB. LBBB may be an early sign of congestive cardiomyopathy, especially when it occurs in young patients. It is nearly always a sign of organic heart disease.

Left-atrial enlargement is diagnosed by the presence of a negative P wave with an area of greater than 1 mm^2 in lead V_1. It commonly is seen in the ECG of a patient with acute heart failure and may disappear as the patient is treated and the volume of the heart decreases.

Right ventricular hypertrophy is most reliably diagnosed in adults by a shift of the QRS axis toward the right greater than 90° in combination with altered precordial R-wave progression (see also Table 60.6, Chapter 60).

Certain ECG changes suggest a decreased ejection fraction, especially in patients with heart failure caused by ischemic heart disease. These include Q waves in leads 1, aVL, and V_1 through V_4 with persistently upward coving of the ST segments in the precordial leads (seen in patients with extensive anterior wall infarctions with aneurysms) and deep Q waves in both inferior and precordial leads with QRS duration greater than 0.1 second (suggesting ischemic cardiomyopathy) [15].

Low QRS voltage (less than 10 mm in precordial leads and less than 5 mm in limb leads) is commonly caused by pericardial effusion, hypothyroidism, or infiltrative disease of the heart (e.g., amyloid) but also may be seen in patients with severe emphysema or marked obesity.

Echocardiography

The two-dimensional (2D) echocardiogram with Doppler is a reliable technique for determining ventricular size and thickness, the presence of valvular and structural abnormalities, the evaluation of systolic and diastolic function, and the presence or absence of pericardial effusion. Echocardiography should be considered for patients with suspected valvular or pericardial disease or for patients in whom the cause of heart failure is unclear. In the primary care setting, echocardiography is unlikely to be useful in the evaluation of patients with suspected heart failure in patients with a normal ECG and a chest x-ray showing a CTR below 0.5 [15]. (The use of echocardiography in the diagnosis of valvular heart disease is discussed more fully in Chapter 60.)

Two-dimensional echocardiography with color flow Doppler is useful in estimating the ejection fraction and detecting valvular stenosis or regurgitation. Pulmonary artery pressures may be estimated accurately but only in patients who have tricuspid regurgitation; this includes most patients with heart failure. Two-dimensional echocardiography with pulsed Doppler evaluation of mitral valve flow velocity is also useful in differentiating between systolic and diastolic dysfunction [1].

Radionuclide Angiography

Radionuclide angiography (gated blood pool scan or multigated acquisition study [MUGA]) is a technique for visualizing the cardiac chambers throughout the cardiac cycle. The major advantages of this technique over echocardiography are that good images may be obtained even in patients who are obese or who have severe chronic lung disease, and the ejection fraction may be determined precisely.

Radionuclide angiography is an effective tool to evaluate LV wall motion abnormalities, including ventricular aneurysm, and to evaluate LV function and diastolic compliance. The general physician does not ordinarily consider radionuclide angiography without the advice of a cardiologist. In most institutions echocardiography has largely replaced radionuclide angiography as a diagnostic tool because it provides much more information without radiation.

Cardiac Catheterization and Myocardial Biopsy

Cardiac catheterization (see Chapter 57) should be considered in any patient in chronic heart failure in whom an etiologic and anatomic diagnosis has not been made by noninvasive techniques. The sudden onset of heart failure with cardiomegaly in a previously healthy patient is an indication for immediate referral to a cardiologist. Cardiac catheterization may be the only way to diagnose pericardial disease. Myocardial biopsy may be useful in young patients suspected of having a cardiomyopathy, who have the sudden onset of heart failure of uncertain cause. Approximately one-third of patients with chronic dilated cardiomyopathy are found, by cardiac catheterization, to have severe diffuse coronary disease. The procedure should be considered in all cases with dilated cardiomyopathy of uncertain origin, especially in diabetic patients, who may have severe coronary heart disease with no symptoms of chest pain.

Exercise Testing

It is often difficult to determine the functional status of patients with heart failure, and functional limitation is often overestimated or underestimated. Studies show that the most precise determination of functional classification is given by exercise testing with assessment of oxygen consumption (25). The protocol used should be one in which the level of exercise is increased in small increments (see Chapter 57). The test should be obtained in consultation with a cardiologist or a pulmonologist and only if functional classification cannot be satisfactorily determined by clinical means. The 6-minute walk test, in which the distance that the patient is able to walk in 6 minutes is measured, correlates well with function assessed by measurement of oxygen consumption, and also with prognosis; it is a useful, inexpensive tool for the assessment of functional status (5).

Systolic Versus Diastolic Dysfunction

The clinical signs and symptoms of heart failure may result from systolic or diastolic dysfunction of the myocardium (see above); it is important to determine whether one or both of these mechanisms are operative to prescribe appropriate treatment.

In patients with heart failure caused by *systolic dysfunction,* the heart is dilated, often hypertrophied, and the inotropic state of the heart is impaired relative to the afterload so that the ejection fraction, and often the blood pressure, is decreased. A reduced ejection fraction, detected by echocardiography or gated blood pool scan, and an S_4 on auscultation may be the only signs of compensated systolic dysfunction. In uncompensated systolic dysfunction, an S_3 may also be heard. The heart is usually enlarged on chest x-ray and Q waves or left bundle branch block may be present on the ECG (3).

In patients with signs and symptoms of heart failure caused by *diastolic dysfunction,* the ventricle is less compliant (i.e., stiffer) and early diastolic passive filling of the left ventricle is decreased. Therefore, immediately before atrial systole, the atrium has a greater than normal volume and pressure and by the Frank–Starling principle, the force of atrial contraction is increased. Clinically, this may be detected by a palpable presystolic apical filling wave, or heard as a loud S_4. On pulsed Doppler echocardiography diastolic dysfunction may be diagnosed by the increased velocity of the atrial component of diastolic filling relative to the peak velocity of the early diastolic rapid filling phase (1).

The diagnosis of diastolic dysfunction is more difficult to make clinically than is that of systolic dysfunction. The diagnosis should be suspected in patients with evidence of increased filling pressure (jugular venous distension and pulmonary redistribution of blood flow) and concomitant elevation of blood pressure (3).

MANAGEMENT

The goal of therapy is not merely to control symptoms but to treat specifically the underlying causes of heart failure if possible (Table 61.2). If the underlying disease cannot be effectively treated, an attempt should be made to increase the capacity of the heart to do work

or to decrease the amount of work that the heart has to do. Table 61.6 shows the various measures that can be used to accomplish these goals in ambulatory patients. These measures are discussed in detail below.

General Principles

Lifestyle

It is not always possible to improve the function of the failing heart, but it usually is possible to decrease the metabolic needs of the body by encouraging a patient to stop smoking (see Chapter 20), to avoid emotional stress, and to get an adequate amount of rest (Table 61.7). A thorough understanding of the patient's home and work environment and the relationship of the patient to his or her supporting family members and caregivers is important. When possible, the recommended treatment regimen should be discussed with the patient and the patient's family.

The ambulatory patient should be encouraged to exercise (see Chapter 58), but to take care to avoid exertion to the point of causing further symptomatic cardiac decompensation. Sometimes this simply means performing the same activities more slowly.

There is a decreased stimulus to renin, angiotensin, and aldosterone production during supine rest, and even severely disabled patients may be able to lead socially useful and satisfying lives if they rest in the afternoon and in the early evening or before social or business engagements. Strict bed rest, which causes muscle weakness and deconditioning, should be strongly discouraged.

It is important that the temperature and humidity of the patient's home and work environment be controlled. Patients should be encouraged to have air conditioners for the summer months to reduce the extra demand placed on the heart by hot, humid weather.

Diet

There is surprisingly little experimental evidence that a severely salt-restricted diet is of long-term benefit in controlling heart failure in patients who respond well to moderate dosages of diuretics. It is commonly observed, however, that sudden increases in salt intake

Table 61.6.   Measures Used in Ambulatory Treatment of Heart Failure

Increasing Capacity of Heart to Do Work
Digitalis
Antiarrhythmic drugs (Chapter 59)
Pacemaker (Chapter 59)

Decreasing Amount of Work that Heart has to Do
Rest
Low-sodium diet
Diuretics
Vasodilator drugs
Home oxygen
Exercise training in selected patients

Table 61.7. Suggested Topics for Patient, Family, and Caregiver Education and Counseling

General Counseling
Explanation of heart failure and the reason for symptoms
Cause or probable cause of heart failure
Expected symptoms
Symptoms of worsening heart failure
What to do if symptoms worsen
Self-monitoring with daily weights
Explanation of treatment/care plan
Clarification of patient's responsibilities
Importance of cessation of tobacco use
Role of family members or other caregivers in the treatment/
   care plan
Availability and value of qualified local support group
Importance of obtaining vaccinations against influenza and
   pneumococcal disease

Prognosis
Life expectancy
Advance directives
Advice for family members in the event of sudden death

Activity Recommendations
Recreation, leisure, and work activity
Exercise
Sex, sexual difficulties, and coping strategies

Dietary Recommendations
Sodium restriction
Avoidance of excessive fluid intake
Fluid restriction (if required)
Alcohol restriction

Medications
Effects of medications on quality of life and survival
Dosing
Likely side effects and what to do if they occur
Coping mechanisms for complicated medical regimens
Availability of lower-cost medications or financial assistance
Importance of compliance with the treatment/care plan

may precipitate acute pulmonary edema in patients who have moderately well compensated chronic heart failure. Holiday seasons are particularly dangerous in this regard, probably also because of the increased activity and emotional stress. The various types of salty food that the patient is likely to eat should be anticipated, based on the patient's cultural background. Examples of frequently eaten salty food include breakfast meats such as sausage, bacon, scrapple, deli meats including "low-salt" ham, salt pork or fatback in cooking vegetables, and many foods prepared by traditional ethnic cooks. Many patients attempt to substitute condiments in place of salt and are not aware that ketchup, hot sauce, soy sauce, and other sauces have high salt concentrations. Homebound patients may eat prepared foods such as frozen pancakes and waffles, or frozen convenience dinners, or they may have fast food brought to their home by family and neighbors; most patients are unaware of the high sodium content of these foods. A no-added-salt diet, which contains approximately 2 to 3 g of sodium, suffices for most patients in compensated heart failure. Patients with poorly compensated heart failure may require a diet

that contains 500 mg to 1 g of sodium, along with a restriction of volume intake to 1.5 L or less. The caregiver must take the time to give specific, concrete advice about diet and nutrition.

A high-soluble-fiber diet may help avoid constipation and straining (see Chapter 39). Referral to a dietitian may be essential for patients with frequent episodes of cardiac decompensation caused by noncompliance with advice about salt and fluid restriction. Guidelines for planning these diets and a list of foods to be avoided by patients being treated for heart failure are given in Tables 62.12 and 62.13 in Chapter 62.

Patients with heart failure may wish to know whether they can continue to drink alcoholic beverages. Alcohol increases blood pressure and impairs cardiac function. In any patient with a cardiomyopathy apparently related to prolonged heavy alcohol use, total abstinence from alcohol is essential. In other patients, alcohol use should be discouraged, or at least restricted to no more than the equivalent of 1 to 2 oz of alcohol per day.

Drugs that Promote Positive Sodium Balance

A number of drugs can promote a positive sodium balance: Renal sodium retention may be caused by corticosteroids, estrogens, and nonsteroidal antiinflammatory agents other than aspirin; and some antacid preparations contain a significant amount of sodium. Patients with heart failure should not receive these drugs, or if the drugs are necessary, the patients should be monitored closely for symptoms of increased heart failure or electrolyte disturbance.

Drugs that May Directly or Indirectly Impair LV Function

Calcium channel blockers depress LV function and should be avoided in patients with systolic dysfunction. Second-generation drugs (felodipine and amlodipine) (see below) may be an exception. The antiarrhythmic agents disopyramide and flecainide should not be used in patients with systolic dysfunction.

Drug Therapy

The goal of drug therapy for heart failure is to relieve symptoms, improve function, and prolong life (Table 61.6). Clinical trials demonstrate that it is possible to achieve these goals in most patients with chronic heart failure (18).

There are important differences in the therapeutic approach to patients whose heart failure is caused by systolic dysfunction (dilated left ventricle with decreased ejection fraction) as opposed to patients whose heart failure is caused primarily by diastolic dysfunction (hypertrophied, stiff heart with a normal or increased ejection fraction) (see above). For example, a young patient with heart failure caused by viral myocarditis (primarily systolic failure) will be treated with diuretics, an angiotensin-converting enzyme (ACE) inhibitor, and digitalis. A middle-age patient with ischemic cardiomyopathy is likely to have both systolic dysfunction and variable degrees of diastolic dysfunction; treatment may include diuretics and an ACE inhibitor, a long-acting nitrate, digitalis, or a β-blocker. Elderly patients with long-standing hypertension often experience heart failure caused by diastolic dysfunction with cardiac hypertrophy and an increased ejection fraction. Vasodilators (other than ACE inhibitors) and digitalis are contraindicated in these patients, who respond best to diuretics, verapamil or diltiazem, and β-blockers (Fig. 61.4). ACE inhibitors, which are associated with a reduction of LVH, may also be useful for control of blood pressure and edema in these patients.

Diuretic Drugs

Diuretic drugs are used when it is impossible to treat the underlying cause of heart failure or when signs and symptoms of heart failure persist despite treatment of the underlying condition. Although diuretic drugs have not been shown to prolong life, they relieve symptoms and improve function in most patients with

heart failure, so most patients with heart failure are treated with a diuretic agent. Diuretics reduce symptoms of circulatory congestion by increasing sodium and water excretion.

The goal of diuretic therapy is to reach and maintain the patient's ideal weight. Physiologically, this is the weight at which signs of peripheral congestion are substantially relieved and the left ventricular filling pressure remains near the preload reserve (i.e., function is optimized via the Frank–Starling principle). Clinically, this is the weight at which peripheral edema is no more than a trace, jugular venous distension is absent, hepatojugular reflux, if present, is no more than a few centimeters above the clavicle, and the blood urea nitrogen and creatinine determinations are at, or slightly above, baseline. After diuresis to the ideal weight, the decrease in ventricular wall stress (i.e., afterload) and the improvement in ventricular contraction brought about by a decrease in heart size and peripheral vascular resistance often lead to a prompt improvement in ventricular function and, in hypertensive patients, a reduction in blood pressure.

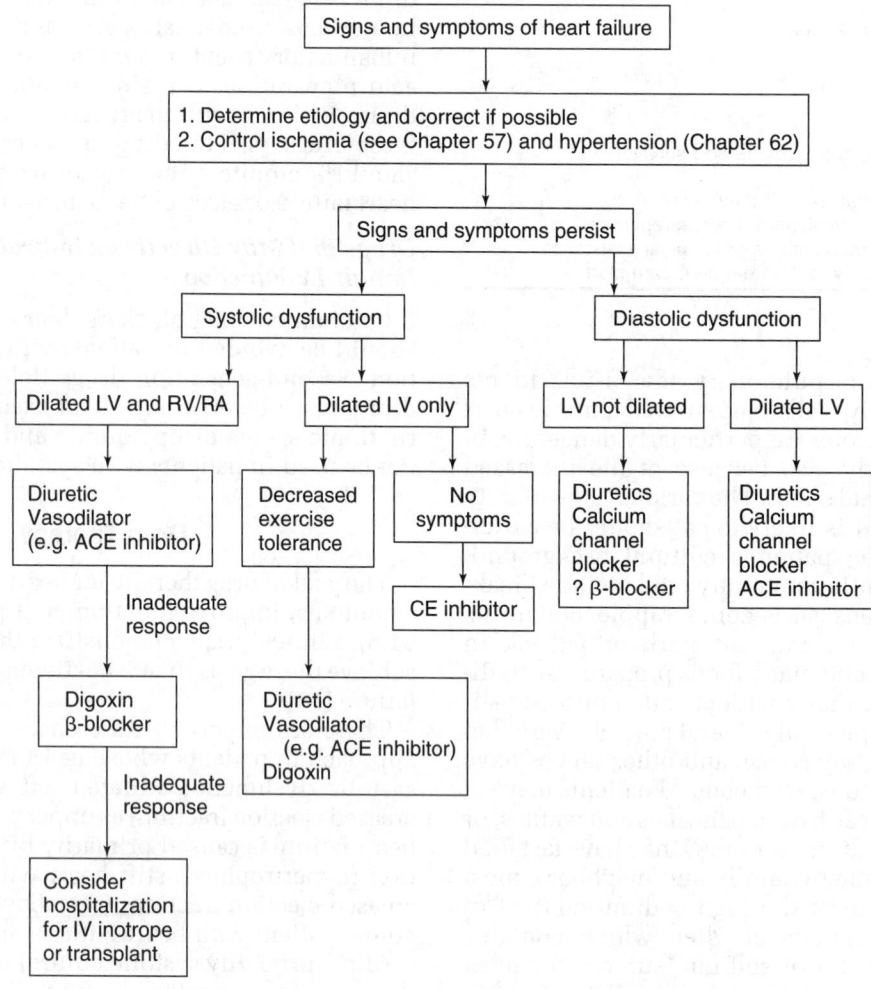

Figure 61.4. Algorithm for treatment of heart failure.

Table 61.8.   Characteristics of Selected Diuretic Drugs

Generic Name	Brand Name	Available Preparations	Usual Daily Dosage (mg/day)	Frequency of Dosing (per day)	Onset of Effect	Peak Effect	Duration
Hydrochlorothiazide	Generic, Hydro-Diuril, Esidrix	25-, 50-, 200-mg tablet	25–100	1–2	2 hr	4 hr	12 hr or more
Chlorthalidone	Generic, Hygroton	50-, 100-mg tablet	50–100	1	2 hr	6 hr	24 hr
Metolazone	Zaroxolyn	2.5-, 5-, 10-mg tablet	2.5–10	1	1 hr	2 hr	12–14 hr
Indapamide	Lozol	2.5-mg tablet	2.5–5.0	1	1 hr	2 hr	28 hr
Furosemide	Lasix	20-, 40-, 80-mg tablet	20–160	1–2	1 hr	1–2 hr	6 hr
Ethacrynic acid	Edecrin	50-mg tablet	50–100	1–2	30 min	2 hr	6–8 hr
Bumetanide	Bumex	0.5-, 1-mg tablet	0.5–2	1–2	30 min to 1 hr	1–2 hr	4 hr
Torsemide	Demadex	20-, 40-mg tablet	20–40	1	30 min to 1 hr	3 hr	12 hr
Triamterene	Dyrenium	100-mg capsule	100–300	1–2	2 hr	6–8 hr	12–16 hr
Spironolactone	Aldactone	25-mg tablet	50–400	1–2	Gradual onset	2–3 days after initiation of therapy	2–3 days after cessation of therapy
Amiloride	Midamor	5-mg tablet	5–10	1	2 hr	6–10 hr	24 hr

There are three classes of diuretics in common use: thiazides (hydrochlorothiazide) and thiazidelike agents (e.g., metolazone, chlorthalidone), the so-called loop diuretics (e.g., furosemide, bumetanide, and torsemide), and the potassium-sparing diuretics (spironolactone, triamterene, and amiloride) (Table 61.8) (see also Chapter 46).

The *thiazides* and the *thiazidelike diuretics* act on the early portion of the distal convoluted tubule of the nephron; they cause a moderate increase in the excretion of sodium and chloride. Potassium and hydrogen losses are accentuated because of the increased delivery of solute to the terminal portion of the distal tubule, where potassium secretion occurs and is modulated by aldosterone. Thiazidelike agents such as metolazone act on both the proximal and distal convoluted tubules of the nephron and may be particularly effective in patients with very low renal blood flow.

The *loop diuretics* inhibit tubular resorption of chloride and sodium in the ascending limb of the loop of Henle. These diuretics are potent and result in a substantial increase in the excretion of sodium, chloride, and water. Like thiazides, the loop diuretics increase the delivery of solute to the more distal portion of the nephron, where potassium and hydrogen secretion is accentuated.

Potassium-sparing diuretics act on the terminal portion of the distal convoluted tubule, where only a small proportion of sodium is reabsorbed; by themselves they are only weak diuretics. However, they may be especially useful in combination with a thiazide or loop diuretic in preventing hypokalemia or when a patient becomes refractory to the more potent diuretics. The effect of thiazides and loop diuretics may be dampened by the resorption of sodium in the terminal portion of the distal convoluted tubule because they act proximal to the portion of the distal nephron where aldosterone influences sodium resorption. *Spironolactone* is structurally similar to aldosterone and competitively inhibits aldosterone binding to cellular receptors. *Triamterene* and *amiloride* block sodium resorption and potassium excretion but do not compete with aldosterone or even depend on its presence to be effective. These diuretics may cause life-threatening increases in the serum potassium level. Patients should usually not receive potassium supplementation while taking them. Also, patients with renal failure or patients taking an ACE inhibitor are at increased risk for developing hyperkalemia if given these diuretics. Serum potassium must be monitored carefully when these agents are used.

Use of Diuretic Drugs.   When used in the treatment of heart failure, diuretics should always be prescribed with another agent (e.g., an ACE inhibitor). Therapy should start with the lowest effective dosage of a thiazide compound (Table 61.8). Generic hydrochlorothiazide is the drug of choice. Many patients with mild heart failure may effectively control symptoms by use of the drug every other day or three times a week. Patients with progressive disease may become resistant gradually to the effect of thiazides and may require dosages of 50 to 100 mg of hydrochlorothiazide a day for control of edema and dyspnea. Patients become resistant to thiazides when there is significant renal failure (e.g., when the serum creatinine is above 2.5 to 3 mg/dL) or when renal blood flow is decreased markedly, as it may be in severe heart failure. There is no evidence that if one thiazide has failed, another will be effective. However, thiazidelike agents (Table 61.8) may be effective in such circumstances, even in patients with very low renal blood flow (28).

When a patient becomes resistant to thiazides or has complications of thiazide therapy (see below), a loop diuretic—furosemide, bumetanide, torsemide—should be prescribed (Table 61.8) (ethacrynic acid is no longer widely used). These drugs are often effective in low oral dosages. Furosemide and bumetanide are available in generic forms. Bumetanide and torsemide are less ototoxic than furosemide and their bioavailability orally is higher than that of furosemide. However, furosemide is still the most popular of these drugs, in part because of cost. Furosemide should be started at a dosage of 20 mg/day and increased as necessary for control of symptoms. Although a single dose of furosemide or bumetanide is commonly administered each day, these drugs are short acting (half-life of 1 to 1.5 hours), and patients with moderate to severe heart failure may require a second dose given in the late afternoon to effect a negative sodium balance. Torsemide has a longer half-life and may be effective given once daily, even in patients with moderately severe heart failure.

Dosages of furosemide higher than 160 to 240 mg/day are rarely required and may cause ototoxicity. If so, at this point (if not previously prescribed for potassium control) a potassium-sparing diuretic, triamterene or spironolactone, should be added to the drug regimen or bumetanide or torsemide should be substituted for furosemide. The addition of a thiazide diuretic in modest dosages (12.5 to 25 mg of hydrochlorothiazide or 2.5 to 5 mg of metolazone) may markedly potentiate the effect of loop diuretics, leading to a rapid mobilization of fluid, and thereby allow these patients to be treated in an ambulatory setting and without the use of intravenous diuretics. Careful monitoring of electrolyte levels is essential, and the diuretic dosage should be reduced when the dry weight is achieved.

Side Effects of Diuretics

Hypokalemia. The thiazide and loop diuretics have marked kaliuretic effects, and especially in edematous patients, hypokalemia is a common complication of the use of diuretic therapy. Hypokalemia may lead to fatigue, muscle cramps, and depression and often precipitates arrhythmias or digitalis toxicity. A high-sodium diet predisposes to hypokalemia in patients taking loop diuretics because of aldosterone-mediated sodium–potassium exchange in the distal tubule. Patients with persistent hypokalemia should be encouraged to adhere to a very-low-sodium diet. The justification for sodium restriction must be explained to the patient in concrete terms. If hypokalemia persists despite a low-sodium diet and treatment with an ACE inhibitor, a potassium-sparing diuretic such as triamterene or spironolactone should be used in preference to potassium salts. Potassium supplementation should be discontinued before the administration of a potassium-sparing diuretic and the patient's electrolyte concentration must be monitored carefully when these medications are started, when the dosage is adjusted, or when there is a change in the severity of the heart failure. The serum potassium should be measured again 3 days to 1 week later; the goal is to maintain serum potassium concentration within the normal range. The usual dosage of triamterene is 50 to 100 mg one to three times a day, and of spironolactone, 12.5 to 100 mg once or twice daily. The indications for and use of potassium salts in patients taking diuretics are fully discussed in Chapter 46.

Hyponatremia. The loop diuretics and the thiazides may occasionally be associated with hyponatremia by impairing free water clearance, so caution is especially appropriate in patients who tend to consume large quantities of fluid. These diuretics also may be associated with hyponatremia when the extracellular volume has become contracted (a potent stimulus to the release of antidiuretic hormone) and fluid intake has not been restricted. Usually the hyponatremia may be corrected by restricting water intake to less than 1 L/day (50). Finally, the thiazides may be associated rarely with hyponatremia in euvolemic patients who also are severely potassium depleted. This situation clinically resembles the syndrome of inappropriate secretion of antidiuretic hormone, although the exact mechanism of the complication is not fully known. The drug must be withdrawn until hyponatremia is corrected.

Contraction of the Extracellular Volume. Diuretics exert their therapeutic effect by causing a net loss of sodium, chloride, and water. If the response is excessive, depletion of the extracellular fluid compartment (the maintenance of which depends on sodium and chloride) occurs. This may have catastrophic consequences such as postural hypotension, sometimes with loss of consciousness, or precipitation of ischemia caused by changes in cerebral, coronary, or renal blood flow. This complication is especially common when loop diuretics are used but may occur after the use of thiazides or combination diuretics, especially in patients also taking an ACE inhibitor. The patient should be monitored carefully, therefore, for evidence of excessive contraction of extracellular volume by daily self-assessment of weight and the presence or absence of edema and frequent assessment by the caregiver of the degree of fullness of the neck veins and of orthostatic changes in the blood pressure and pulse.

Acid–Base Disturbance. By their different actions on the nephron, diuretics have an effect on acid–base balance. The thiazides and the loop diuretics are often associated with the generation and maintenance of a metabolic alkalosis. This usually requires no therapy. To correct the alkalosis, the associated volume and potassium deficiency would have to be corrected. If the volume were replenished, the effect of the diuretic would be negated. Therefore usually only potassium-sparing diuretics or potassium chloride supplements are given (see Chapter 46). If the alkalosis is thought to be detrimental, for example in patients with respiratory failure, the diuretic should be discontinued or the dosage reduced.

Potassium-sparing diuretics may be associated with diminished hydrogen ion excretion and therefore with a mild metabolic acidosis. This is usually of no consequence and requires no treatment.

Hyperuricemia. Thiazides and loop diuretics commonly elevate the concentration of serum urate by blocking urate secretion by the proximal renal tubules or enhancing resorption through contraction of extracellular volume. However, symptomatic gout is not usual, nor is the elevation of uric acid likely to cause renal injury or stone formation. Therefore, unless gout does occur, routine measurement of uric acid and treatment are unnecessary.

Hyperglycemia. Thiazides and, less commonly, loop diuretics may cause glucose intolerance. Hypoglycemic therapy may be required (or changed, in diabetic patients already receiving a hypoglycemic agent) if the diuretic is to be continued (see Chapter 72).

Lipid Abnormalities. Thiazides may increase triglyceride concentrations in the blood. In patients with lipid abnormalities, a loop diuretic at low dosages (10 to 20 mg) may be preferable to a thiazide.

Other Effects. Thiazides are occasionally associated with a hypersensitivity-induced small vessel vasculitis (Chapter 51), thrombocytopenia (Chapter 51), and hypercalcemia (Chapter 74) and may be associated with impotence. Furosemide at high dosages has been associated with the development of interstitial nephritis and renal failure, especially in patients with marked proteinuria. Spironolactone, which structurally is related to estrogen, may cause gynecomastia and may reduce libido in men or cause impotence; these side effects usually resolve within a few weeks of discontinuing the drug.

Even when diuretics have substantially relieved the signs and symptoms of CHF, other medications are usually necessary to optimize function and prolong life.

Digitalis

Digitalis may help restore cardiac compensation by increasing the inotropic state, or contractility, of cardiac muscle, thereby increasing the ejection fraction at a given preload and afterload, as described above. It appears to act by increasing the delivery of calcium to the contractile apparatus of the heart. Digoxin is the only positive inotropic agent that has been convincingly shown both to improve function and quality of life and not to increase mortality in patients with symptomatic heart failure (16). Because digoxin is indicated only for patients with heart failure caused by systolic dysfunction, it is ordinarily used in patients treated also with a diuretic and an ACE inhibitor (see below).

Indications for Use of Digitalis Drugs. Digitalis has been shown in several large studies to reduce symptoms of heart failure and to decrease the hospitalization rate for heart failure (8,16,41,52). Digitalis improves ventricular performance by moderating the heart rate of patients in atrial fibrillation or atrial flutter and by improving contractility in patients with systolic dysfunction heart failure. However, the degree to which digitalis preparations increase ventricular contractility is modest and the toxic to therapeutic ratio is small. Furthermore, the indiscriminate use of digitalis as a first-line medication for control of heart failure has led to its use in many patients in whom heart failure is not caused primarily by a decrease in the inotropic state of myocardial muscle. Such patients include those whose heart failure is caused by systemic hypertension, those with diastolic dysfunction or restriction to LV filling, and those in whom symptoms of fatigue are caused by a decreased cardiac output induced by excessive diuresis. In a recent definitive study, overall mortality was not higher with digitalis than with placebo (16), and digitalis was most beneficial in patients who were most symptomatic and had marked LV dysfunction.

Recommendations for Use of Digitalis Compounds. Digitalis glycosides should be prescribed only for patients with symptomatic CHF caused by systolic dysfunction (EF 35% or lower, cardiothoracic ratio 0.5 or higher). It is also a useful drug for certain types of arrhythmias (see Chapter 59).

The practitioner should use the purified glycoside, digoxin, exclusively. The Glaxo–Burroughs–Wellcome preparation of digoxin, Lanoxin, has a bioavailability of approximately 75% and an intermediate duration of action (half-life of 36 to 48 hours). Digitalis elixir in capsules, Lanoxicaps (0.05-, 0.10-, and 0.20-mg capsules), has a bioavailability of nearly 100% and is useful when careful titration of the dosage is important, as in small elderly patients. Digitalization is best accomplished in an ambulatory patient by daily administration of the drug at the maintenance dosage (see below). Within four or five half-lives of the drug (approximately 7 days), full digitalization is ordinarily achieved.

The effect of digitalis on the patient's condition should be monitored and reassessed periodically. If there is no objective decrease in heart size or improvement in exercise capacity after a 1- or 2-month trial of digitalis therapy, the drug should probably be discontinued. However, serum digoxin concentration (see below) should be measured first to be certain that adequate blood levels are being attained. Digitalis should be used cautiously in older patients and in any patient known to have impaired renal function. There is no evidence that elderly patients are intrinsically more sensitive to digitalis compounds, but they have a smaller body mass, often have impaired renal excretion of the drug, and have higher serum levels for a given oral dosage of the drug.

The average dosage of digoxin in patients below age 60 with normal renal function is 0.25 mg/day (of Lanoxicap, 0.20 mg/day). In patients older than 65 years or in patients with known impairments of renal function, dosages of 0.125 mg/day of digoxin (0.1 mg of Lanoxicap) should be prescribed, and the drug should be taken only 6 days a week.

Digitalis may interact with other medications, and because of its low therapeutic ratio, the possibility of an interaction should be considered when any medication is added to the regimen of a patient already taking digoxin. The administration of quinidine causes a decreased renal excretion of digoxin, which may lead to digitalis toxicity; similar effects have been seen when digitalis is prescribed along with either of the calcium channel blockers, verapamil or diltiazem (but not with nifedipine). The antiarrhythmic agent amiodarone may increase bioavailability of digoxin; the dosage of digoxin must be reduced and levels monitored when these drugs are used concomitantly. The use of thiazides and loop diuretics may lead to digitalis toxicity either because of increased retention of digoxin secondary to decreased renal blood flow or because of increased sensitivity to digitalis as the result of hypokalemia or hypomagnesemia. Cholestyramine and neomycin and some antacids impair digoxin absorption and may result in a subtherapeutic effect. The use of nonsteroidal anti-inflammatory agents may decrease renal function and thereby cause digitalis toxicity, especially in elderly patients.

Recognition and Treatment of Digitalis Toxicity. Digitalis toxicity commonly is caused by administration of too much digitalis, overdiuresis (often with associated hypokalemia and/or hypomagnesemia), intercurrent development of renal insufficiency, or administration of drugs that interact with digitalis to increase its plasma concentration. Digitalis toxicity is especially common in older patients in an ambulatory practice. In a recent large trial, 2% of the digitalized patients required hospitalization for suspected digitalis toxicity (16). Approximately 10% of patients in the seventh and eighth decades being seen regularly by a physician are taking digitalis (47).

The manifestations of digitalis toxicity may be difficult to recognize in older patients and in patients whose normal baseline level of function is not familiar to the practitioner. They include changes in the cardiovascular system, gastrointestinal tract, and central nervous system. The most common cardiac manifestations of digitalis toxicity are progressive slowing and regularization of the heart rate (i.e., development of a nodal rhythm) of patients in atrial fibrillation, and frequent premature ventricular contractions (PVCs). Digitalis toxicity should be suspected in any patient who is taking digitalis and has PVCs or in any patient in atrial fibrillation whose heart rate falls below 60 and becomes regular. Because digitalis both increases automaticity and decreases conduction through the AV node, paroxysmal atrial tachycardia (PAT) with block may be seen. The peripheral pulse in PAT with block is usually 100 to 120 beats/minute (see Chapter 59). Cardiac toxicity may occur in the absence of other signs or symptoms of digitalis overdose.

Gastrointestinal side effects are common manifestations of digitalis intoxication. They include anorexia, mild nausea, and occasionally vomiting and diarrhea.

Digitalis may cause changes in the sensorium ranging from mild confusional states to frank delirium and psychosis. In an older patient it may be difficult to determine, without stopping the drug, whether these symptoms are caused by primary cerebral disease or digitalis excess.

Digitalis is structurally related to estrogen and may cause gynecomastia, decreased libido, or impotence in men.

The diagnosis of digitalis toxicity is based on clinical and laboratory findings. If symptoms compatible with digitalis toxicity are present, especially in elderly patients, the drug should be stopped immediately. The patient should be reassessed in approximately 3 to 5 days. If symptoms have abated, a presumptive diagnosis of digitalis intoxication is warranted.

At the time of presentation, it is reasonable to measure the serum digoxin concentration. That is done by use of a radioimmunoassay. An adequately digitalized patient has a serum digoxin concentration of approximately 0.8 to 1.2 ng/mL; most toxic patients have concentrations above 1.8 ng/mL. However, if a patient has symptoms compatible with digitalis toxic-

ity and his or her serum digoxin level is within the normal range, toxicity has not been ruled out because at therapeutic digoxin levels, hypokalemic, hypomagnesemic (or hypercalcemic) patients may develop digitalis toxicity. Most patients with digitoxicity can be treated by temporary withdrawal of the medication and reinstitution of it at a lower dosage. Often, diuretic therapy must also be modified or potassium or magnesium supplements administered. However, patients with symptomatic arrhythmias are best hospitalized for a few days so that they can be monitored closely.

It is appropriate for all patients taking digitalis, and certainly for those who develop toxicity, to have the indications for digitalis therapy carefully reviewed, to be sure that the patient clearly has systolic dysfunction or requires the drug for control of atrial arrhythmias (see Chapter 59).

Vasodilator Therapy

Physiologic Rationale for Vasodilator Therapy. The signs and symptoms of heart failure are caused by the compensatory responses triggered by the inadequate response of the left ventricle to demands for a cardiac output adequate to maintain tissue perfusion (see above). Neurohumoral compensatory mechanisms result in an increase in left ventricular preload and afterload. In the setting of left ventricular dysfunction, these compensatory mechanisms lead to a further deterioration of cardiac function (Figs. 61.3 and 61.5). The judicious use of vasodilator agents may optimize cardiac function, prevent further deterioration of LV function, improve the patient's functional state, and prolong the life of patients in chronic heart failure (12,13,18,48,49,53).

The hemodynamic effects of drugs that are predominantly *venodilators*, such as nitroglycerin preparations, and diuretics are essentially the same. Both classes of drugs cause a decrease in preload, thereby relieving symptoms of vascular congestion (Fig. 61.3). Venodilators are most useful in patients with severe heart failure in whom preload reserve is exceeded during exercise, which leads to an increase in LVEDP

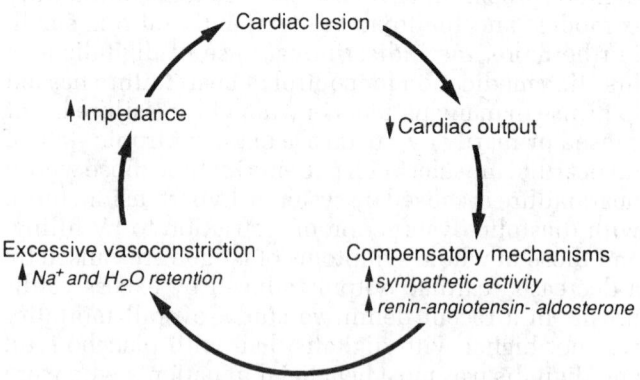

Figure 61.5. Vicious circle in congestive heart failure. (From Wester PO, Dyckner T. Intracellular electrolytes in cardiac failure. Acta Med Scand 219(Suppl 707):33, 1986.)

Table 61.9.   Vasodilators Useful in Treating Heart Failure

Site of Action	Drugs	Venodilation/ Arteriolar Dilation	Available Tablet Strength	Usual Dosage	Effectiveness After 1 Year
Smooth muscle	Isosorbide dinitrate (Isordil)	+++/+	10, 20, 40 mg	20–60 mg q6hr	?
	Nitroglycerin dermal patches[a]	+++/+	0.1, 0.2, 0.4, and 0.6 mg/hr	0.2–0.6 mg/hr	
	Hydralazine (Apresoline)	0/+++	10, 25, 50, 100 mg	25–50 mg q6hr	1+
	Hydralazine plus long-acting nitrate	+++/+++		As above, in combination	+++
Calcium channel blockers	Nifedipine (Procardia)	+/+++	10, 20 mg	10–30 mg q6hr	?
	Felodipine (Plendil)	+/+++	5, 10 mg	5–10 mg q24hr	?
	Amlodipine (Norvasc)	+/+++	2.5, 5, 10 mg	5–10 mg q24hr	?
	Diltiazem (Cardizem)[b]	+/++	120, 180, 240, 300, 360 mg—all sustained release	120–360 mg q24hr	?
	Verapamil (Calan, Isoptin)[b]	+/++	120, 180, 240, 300, 360 mg—all sustained release	120–360 mg q24hr	?
Converting enzyme inhibitors	Captopril (Capoten)	++/+++	12.5, 25, 50 mg	6.25–50 mg TID	+++
	Enalapril (Vasotec)	++/+++	2.5, 5, 10, 20 mg	5–20 mg q24hr	+++
	Lisinopril (Zestril, Prinivil)	++/+++	5, 10, 20 mg	5–20 mg q24hr	+++
	Benazepril (Lotensin)	++/+++	5, 10, 20 mg	5–20 mg q24hr	+++
Angiotensin-receptor blockers	Losartan (Cozaar)		50 mg	25–100 mg q24hr	+++
	Valsartan (Diovan)		80 mg	80–160 mg q24hr	+++
	Irbesartan (Avapro)		75, 100, 300 mg	100 mg q24hr	+++

[a]To avoid development of tolerance, an 8- to 12-hr period without topical nitrates should be scheduled daily. Usually, this means applying nitroglycerin patches upon awakening and removing them at bedtime.

[b]Should be used only in patients with heart failure caused by diastolic dysfunction or when ischemia is a major reason for LV decompensation. Short-acting preparations are not recommended, and available tablet strengths refer only to sustained-release preparations.

and to pulmonary vascular congestion. This also may occur at rest in association with ischemia in patients with ischemic heart disease or in association with progression of disease in patients with cardiomyopathy or valvular heart disease. Venodilators should not be used in patients with heart failure caused by restriction to ventricular filling (e.g., hypertrophic cardiomyopathy) or in patients with aortic stenosis in whom a reduction in preload may lead to a marked decrease in cardiac output.

Arteriolar vasodilators increase cardiac output by decreasing afterload (i.e., decreasing ventricular wall stress during contraction), thereby allowing the myocardium to contract more efficiently (Fig. 61.3). These medications are most effective in patients with severe peripheral and central congestion who have signs of peripheral hypoperfusion, such as cool hands and acrocyanosis. It is important to note that arteriolar vasodilators increase cardiac output only if preload remains near the preload reserve (Fig. 61.3). With afterload reduction the left ventricle unloads more efficiently, and volume shifts from the thorax to the abdomen and the peripheral venous circulation, thereby lowering preload. However, if preload drops significantly, cardiac output cannot be maintained, and the blood pressure falls. Thus, in an ambulatory setting vasodilators must be used with caution and often with a concomitant adjustment of diuretic dosage.

Three classes of arteriolar vasodilators are available: drugs that block angiotensin-converting enzyme, drugs that act directly on smooth muscle, and drugs that act by blocking calcium channels (Table 61.9). The choice of an appropriate agent and the effective use of that agent depend on an understanding of the physiologic properties of these drugs.

Converting Enzyme Inhibitors.   As discussed, the syndrome of heart failure is caused in large part by the stimulation of the renin–angiotensin–aldosterone system by the kidney. ACE inhibitors block the conversion of angiotensin I to angiotensin II, a potent vasoconstrictor and a regulator of renin and aldosterone production. They cause a marked decrease in angiotensin II levels approximately 30 minutes to 2 hours after administration. ACE inhibitors also inhibit the degradation of bradykinin, a potent vasodilator. ACE inhibitors are thus effective vasodilators; they also block aldosterone-mediated salt and water retention.

ACE inhibitors appear to be the most effective vasodilators currently available for the treatment of heart failure: They retain their effectiveness after long-term use (30), have been shown to decrease the rate of progression of LV dysfunction and to decrease the rate of hospital admission in patients with heart failure (20,53), and are the only class of drugs that has been shown convincingly to prolong life in patients with LV systolic dysfunction (13,20,43). ACE inhibitors are first-line agents for treatment of heart failure caused by systolic dysfunction. All such patients should be prescribed an ACE inhibitor, unless a significant contraindication to its use, such as a history of allergic reactions to the drug or significant renal failure, is present.

Patients with systolic dysfunction and an EF 35% but without symptomatic heart failure should probably be taking an ACE inhibitor because this class of drugs has been shown to reduce the likelihood of progression to symptomatic heart failure in these patients (53).

The currently available ACE inhibitors approved for use in CHF and their dosage ranges are shown in Table 61.9. Captopril is most useful for initiating ACE inhibitor therapy because of its short half-life, rapid onset of action (approximately 30 minutes), and wide dosage range. In patients with obvious signs of circulatory congestion, a dose of 12.5 mg of captopril should be given and the blood pressure checked in 1 hour. The usual effective dosage of captopril for heart failure is 12.5 to 50 mg three to four times a day. Patients who are hyponatremic or at their dry weight, or who are known to have significant renal vascular disease, should be started at 6.25 mg (one-half of a 12.5-mg cross-scored tablet) and their diuretic dosage should be decreased (because the danger of symptomatic hypotension is greater in such situations). Patients who are stable and have mild heart failure (EF 30 to 40%; creatinine 3 or less) may respond well to enalapril 2.5 to 20 mg/day or lisinopril 2.5 to 20 mg/day in one dose. Both of these are prodrugs and their onset of action is approximately 2 to 4 hours. Symptomatic improvement is usually seen in several days, with maximal benefit after 3 months, although further improvement is often seen with longer treatment (18).

Because ACE inhibitors block the effect of aldosterone, potassium-sparing diuretics or supplementation may need to be decreased and potassium levels and renal function should be monitored 3 to 7 days after initiation of therapy and again at 2 to 4 weeks and periodically thereafter. ACE inhibitors also block angiotensin-mediated vasoconstriction, which may maintain renal perfusion pressure in patients with renal insufficiency. If creatinine rises after the initiation of ACE inhibitor therapy, diuretic dosages should be halved; the dosage of inhibitor may need to be reduced and titrated upward more gradually. Consultation with a cardiologist or nephrologist may be helpful in this situation. Some studies suggest that aspirin, especially at high dosages, may interfere with the vasodilating effects of ACE inhibitors (10); this effect does not seem to be clinically important at the usual dosages of aspirin (81 to 325 mg) used in patients with concomitant coronary heart disease and heart failure. It seems prudent, however, to use the lowest effective dosage of aspirin in these patients.

Side Effects.   The most common side effect of ACE inhibitors is cough. A persistent nonproductive, hacking cough is seen in 2 to 10% of patients treated with these drugs. Decreasing the dosage or switching to a different converting enzyme inhibitor is only occasionally helpful. The cough is thought to be caused by the stimulation of vagal afferents that trigger the cough reflex by bradykinin, the levels of which are increased by these drugs. Patients who have had significant symptomatic relief of heart failure after ACE inhibitor therapy may wish to try continuing the drug at a lower dosage or to learn to live with the cough. Often, the drug must be discontinued, in which case therapy with a related class of medication, angiotensin receptor blockers (ARBs), should be considered (see below). If medication cost is paramount, hydralazine and long-acting nitrates may be tried. Because cough may itself be a symptom of heart failure (see above) or of a number of other conditions (see Chapter 54), the practitioner should be as certain as possible that the drug has caused the cough before discontinuing it.

Other side effects are uncommon. The ones most often seen are skin rash in patients taking captopril and angioedema in patients taking long-acting inhibitors (enalapril, lisinopril). These side effects warrant stopping the drug. Taste alteration and neutropenia are rarely seen. Rarely, ACE inhibitors may cause an interstitial nephritis with sudden and profound decrease in renal function. This complication requires immediate consultation with a nephrologist.

Angiotensin Receptor Blockers.   This new class of drugs binds directly to the angiotensin II receptor. ARBs share many important effects with ACE inhibitors, with some important differences (2). They do not increase bradykinin levels and do not cause cough. They may affect renal perfusion less than ACE inhibitors. Preliminary clinical trials suggest that they are equipotent to the inhibitors in relieving symptoms of heart failure. Three ARBs are currently available: losartan, Valsartan, and irbesartan, any of which may be given once a day (Table 61.9). A recent double-blind randomized study reports that, in an elderly population with heart failure, losartan was better tolerated, and was associated with lower mortality, than was captopril (44). The same cautions apply as for ACE inhibitors with regard to dosing; side effects, except for cough, appear to be similar.

Smooth Muscle Dilators.   Nitroglycerin in various formulations is an effective venodilator at the low end of the dosage range and a mixed venodilator and arteriolar dilator at higher dosages. The practitioner should be familiar with the use of nitrates in several forms (see Chapter 57): short-acting sublingual nitrates, long-acting nitrates taken orally, and nitroglycerin dermal patches. *Sublingual nitroglycerin* is generally used in a dosage of 0.4 mg. The medication is sensitive to body heat, light, and moisture and must be kept in a sealed dark glass or metal container. Patients should be encouraged to purchase new sublingual nitroglycerin every 6 months to ensure that the medication is active. Sublingual nitroglycerin may be used liberally to control symptoms of pulmonary congestion during normal physical activity such as walking up stairs, shopping, and so forth. Small bottles of 25 tablets may be prescribed and should be kept in strategic locations in the patient's home, car, and workplace. An effective *long-acting medication* is isosorbide dinitrate (generic, Isordil, Sorbitrate) in dosages of 5 to 20 mg orally, two to three times a day. If symptoms have not improved within a few days, the dosage should be increased. Dosages as high as 40 to 60 mg orally, four times a day, may be used safely depending on the patient's blood pressure response. Before and after each increase in the dosage, the patient should be checked for orthostatic hypotension. If there is a drop of more than 15 to 20 mm Hg systolic blood pressure 3 minutes after rising from the supine to the standing position, the dosage should be decreased slightly. *Nitroglycerin dermal patches* give sustained high blood levels of nitrate. Tolerance to the effect of sustained levels of nitroglycerin develops after 7 to 10 days of continuous use of nitroglycerin patches, and patients should be advised to remove the patch at bedtime and reapply a fresh patch upon awakening. The usual dosage is a 0.2 to 0.6 mg/hour patch, applied in the morning and removed at bedtime. The patient need not be concerned about having the patch in contact with water during bathing or swimming; if it does fall off, however, a new one should be applied.

All nitrate preparations must be prescribed to allow a dose-free interval of 12 to 14 hours a day to avoid the development of tolerance to the drug.

The most common side effects of nitrate therapy are headache and nausea. Skin irritation is occasionally seen with the use of dermal patches. Headache can usually be controlled by aspirin or acetaminophen, and it usually abates after several days of nitrate therapy. Gastrointestinal side effects of long-acting oral nitrates can occasionally be eliminated by switching to a different preparation of long-acting nitroglycerin or switching to nitroglycerin patches. Rubbing alcohol should be used to remove nitroglycerin dermal patches. If skin irritation develops, a different brand of patch should be tried.

Hydralazine is an effective direct arteriolar vasodilator. In properly selected patients and when used in effective dosages, hydralazine may increase the cardiac output as much as twofold. This improved cardiac output may persist chronically in patients who respond initially. The combination of hydralazine and long-acting nitroglycerin has been shown to prolong survival in patients with severe heart failure treated concomitantly with diuretics and digitalis (12). Their use has been largely superseded by the ACE inhibitors (see above), which have fewer side effects and have been shown to be more effective (18).

The major complication of hydralazine is a reversible lupuslike syndrome. However, this syndrome usually does not become apparent until 18 to 24 months of treatment with hydralazine in dosages above 200 mg/day. Because of the severity of their heart disease, most patients who require such large dosages of hydralazine for treatment of CHF do not live long enough to develop a lupuslike syndrome. Additional information about the properties of hydralazine and other vasodilators is provided in Chapter 62.

Hydralazine with nitrate is now used chiefly in patients who are unable to tolerate any of the ACE inhibitors (see above) or in whom the modest cost advantage of generic hydralazine and nitrates is an important consideration.

Calcium Channel Blockers. These drugs interfere with contractility of smooth muscle by blocking the entry of calcium into muscle cells, resulting in vasodilation, especially of the arterioles. All of the currently available calcium channel blockers also depress myocardial contractility, although with calcium channel blockers of the *nifedipine* class afterload reduction caused by vasodilation may offset the direct cardiac depressant effects and cardiac output may be maintained or may increase. The second-generation drugs *felodipine* and *amlodipine* 2.5 to 20 mg/day may be effective in some patients with cardiomyopathy (42) because of their vasodilatory properties. In such patients afterload reduction is predominant, but these drugs should still be used with caution in patients with severe LV dysfunction (EF 30% or less). *Verapamil* is an arteriolar vasodilator that has a significant negative effect on cardiac contraction and relaxation. It may be particularly useful, at dosages of 120 to 360 mg/day (in sustained-release preparations), in patients with heart failure caused by diastolic dysfunction, but because of its negative inotropic effect, it should not be used in patients who have a congestive cardiomyopathy or an ejection fraction less than 45%. *Diltiazem,* in sustained-release dosages of 120 to 360 mg/day, may also be used for treatment of angina or hypertension in patients with heart failure caused by diastolic dysfunction. Common side effects of calcium channel blockers include headache, hypotension, nausea, constipation, and pedal edema (not caused by volume overload). Short-acting calcium channel blockers have been associated with increased mortality in patients in heart failure and their use should be avoided.

General Recommendations for Use of Afterload Reduction Therapy in an Ambulatory Setting. Select patients whose heart failure is caused by decreased LV function, with evidence of both central and peripheral congestion.

ACE inhibitors are the most effective agents for long-term use in an ambulatory setting. When medication cost is paramount, hydralazine plus a long-acting nitrate (isosorbide dinitrate, nitroglycerin patch) may be used at approximately one-half the cost of a full dose of an ACE inhibitor. In patients who cannot tolerate inhibitors, the hydralazine–nitrate combination or an angiotensin receptor blocker may be substituted.

The patient's weight should be measured daily; signs of circulatory congestion (dependent edema, jugular venous distension and hepatojugular reflux, liver enlargement) should be assessed each time the physician sees the patient.

Symptomatic postural hypotension is a common complication of vasodilator therapy in patients in whom diuresis has been excessive; if this happens, the dosage of diuretic, not that of the vasodilator, should be reduced.

β-Blocker Therapy

Activation of the neurohormonal system in heart failure leads to a chronic increase in sympathetic stimulation of the heart. This is facilitated by the resetting of aortic and cardiac baroreceptors that lose their inhibitory effectiveness. Chronic sympathetic stimulation of the heart leads to the down-regulation of β_1 adrenergic receptors and may directly damage cardiac myocytes, thereby leading to further deterioration of myocardial function in CHF. A series of clinical trials shows convincingly that the cautious use of β-blockers may lead to improvement in LV function and clinical status in patients with idiopathic dilated cardiomyopathy. The ability of β blockade to improve LV function and to decrease the frequency of arrhythmias suggests that β-blockers may also improve survival; clinical trials to test this hypothesis are currently under way. The effects of β blockade may be additive to those of standard therapy (diuretics, digitalis, vasodilators) in CHF (17).

Potential candidates for β blockade therapy are patients with CHF who remain tachycardic and symptomatic despite treatment with diuretics, digitalis, and vasodilators, and who are not overdiuresed. The usual protocol is to begin with dosages of metoprolol (the β-blocker of choice) 12.5 mg twice daily and to titrate the dosage gradually upward to 50 to 100 mg twice daily. In patients with cardiomyopathy, the use of long-acting microencapsulated metoprolol (Toprol-XL) in very low dosages, 12.5 mg/day (¼ tablet) may be safe and effective, and the drug is inexpensive. Carvedilol, a β-blocker with vasodilator properties, has been shown to improve symptoms of heart failure, and may also decrease mortality (40). It has been approved by the FDA for use in both hypertension and CHF. Its use requires careful dosage titration, and it is expensive. Consultation with a cardiologist is recommended before beginning β-blocker therapy in patients with CHF.

β Blockade may also be useful in the treatment of heart failure caused by the following conditions: thyrotoxicosis, severe hypertension responsive to β-blockade therapy, hypertrophic cardiomyopathy, and in patients with failure caused by recurrent ischemia. The combination of β-blockade therapy with nitrate therapy may be effective in patients with ischemic cardiomyopathy and chest pain. In these cases, β-blockade therapy is given until the resting heart rate falls below 70 beats/minute and does not show a significant increase with mild to moderate exercise. This may require careful titration to high dosages of metoprolol (e.g., 100 to 200 mg/day in divided doses). Lower dosages may be effective in patients with depressed hepatic blood flow or function caused by CHF. The possible adverse effects of β-blockers are described in Chapter 59.

Importance of Hypertension Control in Patients in Heart Failure

Hypertension increases ventricular wall stress, and therefore the afterload on the heart, and reduces the cardiac output, especially as the heart begins to fail (34). It is essential, therefore, that hypertension be controlled in patients in heart failure. This subject is discussed in detail in Chapter 62.

Home Oxygen Therapy

Patients with severe end-stage heart failure and arterial oxygen desaturation at rest caused by low cardiac output or concomitant pulmonary disease may feel more comfortable, especially while sleeping, with the use of low-flow nasal oxygen. Patients who require home oxygen therapy because of CHF rarely survive for more than 6 months to a year, and oxygen therapy has been associated with a deterioration in LV function in some studies (21). The most efficient way to supply oxygen for therapy at home is by means of an oxygen generator, which is usually rented. The presence of oxygen desaturation should be documented (most easily done by use of a pulse oximeter) before oxygen is prescribed.

Anticoagulation Therapy

Patients with chronic severe CHF are at increased risk for pulmonary and peripheral emboli. Studies show an incidence of peripheral arterial embolization in these patients that ranges from 2 to 18% per year (4). A patient with a markedly dilated LV cavity or a patient with a left ventricular aneurysm, especially if in atrial fibrillation, should be considered for treatment with warfarin anticoagulants (see Chapters 52 and 59). Some expert panels advise against the routine use of warfarin anticoagulation in patients in heart failure with normal sinus rhythm (4,29) and no controlled trials of anticoagulation in such patients have been done. Warfarin therapy may be hazardous in patients with severe heart failure who may have wide swings in prothrombin time caused by hepatic dysfunction and multiple drug interactions. In such circumstances, the prothrombin time should be checked more frequently, perhaps every few weeks, or within 3 days to 1 week after a medication known to interact with warfarin has been introduced or the dosage of warfarin or an interacting medication is changed.

Control of Arrhythmias in Heart Failure

One of the cardinal features of CHF is a tendency to develop arrhythmias (27,32). Between 30 and 50% of patients with chronic heart failure die suddenly, presumably of ventricular tachyarrhythmias, although some studies show bradyarrhythmias to be as likely a cause of death. Holter monitoring is seldom useful in evaluating patients without symptomatic arrhythmias. Patients with symptomatic arrhythmias should be referred to a cardiologist for evaluation.

Clinical trials suggest that amiodarone (see Chapter 59) improves symptoms in patients with arrhythmias who are in CHF, but it is not clear that survival is improved (6,46). Amiodarone interacts with digitalis and may precipitate digitalis toxicity; it may also markedly potentiate the effect of warfarin anticoagulants. Consultation with a cardiologist is recommended before using amiodarone in patients with CHF.

Operative Correction of Problems Causing Heart Failure

The most commonly encountered surgically correctable problems in patients with chronic congestive failure include ischemic heart disease with revascularizable lesions or with resectable ventricular aneurysm, valvular heart disease, and atrial septal defect (see Chapter 60). Any patient who is in heart failure caused by a surgically correctable cause of myocardial dysfunction should be considered for operative correction, and consultation with a cardiologist should be obtained.

Heart transplants should be considered for patients in severe refractory heart failure. The procedure is being performed in specialized centers throughout the United States. There are a number of contraindications to transplantation, including age of 70 or greater; irreversible severe renal, hepatic, or pulmonary disease; severe peripheral or cerebral vascular disease; insulin-requiring diabetes mellitus; and psychiatric impairment, so the proportion of eligible patients with heart failure is small. Even so, because of the scarcity of donated cadaver organs, the wait for an available compatible heart can be many months, during which time the patient may succumb to his or her disease.

Coronary Artery Bypass Graft Surgery and Congestive Heart Failure

Patients with chronic CHF and angina pectoris or silent ischemia (see Chapter 57) may benefit from coronary artery revascularization using coronary artery bypass graft surgery or percutaneous transluminal coronary angioplasty. Patients with symptoms and signs of heart failure and ischemia should be referred for cardiology consultation.

Community Health Services

Many community health services are available to help the caregiver deal with the patient and the patient deal with the illness.

Home Visits

In two situations, home visits by the patient's physician or a visiting nurse should be considered in the management of a patient in heart failure: when the patient has repeatedly returned to the office or has been readmitted to the hospital with heart failure caused by dietary neglect or to failure to use medications correctly (see below) and when the homebound patient's symptoms are so severe (NYHA class IV, Table 61.4) that he or she is unable to come for an office visit without becoming exhausted.

Information Booklets

The American Heart Association has useful free booklets that describe low-salt diets and the management of CHF for the patient and family. These booklets may be obtained from local chapters of the American Heart Association. Extensive, authoritative guidelines for physicians treating CHF have been published by the Agency for Health Care Policy and Research (29). Copies of these booklets are available free by calling 202-512-1800. Extensive information, which is occasionally pertinent and useful, is also available on numerous world wide web sites.

Exercise Programs

Graduated regular exercise may improve exercise tolerance and increase daily activities and general well-being in some patients with heart failure, even in patients with severe LV dysfunction caused by ischemic heart disease (see Chapter 58) (11). The improvement in function is thought to be caused by improved efficiency of the skeletal muscles; there is no evidence that myocardial function can be improved by exercise. Patients may also develop a sense of increased confidence in their ability to function (39).

Patients with class I to III CHF may be trained to exercise to 60% of their maximal heart rate for 20 minutes a day, 3 days a week. Exercise may be contraindicated entirely in patients who are in uncompensated left heart failure or whose heart failure is caused by valvular heart disease. Isometric exercise should be prescribed with caution in patients in heart failure because of the extra afterload this form of exercise imposes on the heart. However, muscle toning exercises using 1-kg hand weights are usually safe and they may be safely used to help maintain function in all but the most frail patients with heart failure.

PROGNOSIS

The prognosis in heart failure is related clinically to the LV ejection fraction, the functional status of the patient, the initial response to treatment, the patient compliance with the treatment regimen, the patient age, and the cause of the heart failure. Physiologically, prognosis is related most importantly to LVEDP (51) and to the degree of neurohumoral activation (43). Most patients in chronic CHF die suddenly, presumably from ventricular arrhythmia (24). Other common causes of death are progressive heart failure and cerebral and peripheral embolization. In the Framingham study, which included heart failure from all causes, the probability of dying within 5 years of onset of heart failure was 62% for men and 42% for women (24,26). The median survival after the onset of heart failure was 1.7 years in men and 3.2 years in women (24). The cause of heart failure in most of these patients was hypertension or ischemic heart disease. Heart failure complicating uncorrected aortic stenosis is a particularly ominous sign, and most of these patients die within 3 years (see Chapter 60) unless aortic valve surgery is performed.

In general, prognosis is related to the patient's functional class (Table 61.4). Patients in functional class I have an annual mortality of approximately 10%. Patients in functional class IV have an annual mortality of approximately 50% (24). It is important that the practitioner not give a prognosis to the patient and family until the optimal level of response to therapy has been achieved (the advent of vasodilators has improved the mortality rate of these patients) (48,49). However, it is appropriate to discuss advance directives and living wills with the patient early in the course of treatment (29).

It has been shown in asymptomatic patients that the development of symptomatic heart failure may be predicted by the finding of cardiac enlargement on echocardiography (53). The prognosis of these patients may be improved by treatment with ACE inhibitors, which may delay the development of overt heart failure in patients with a low EF (18,53).

Over the 40-year period from 1948 to 1988 (before the widespread use of vasodilator drugs) there was no improvement in survival for patients with heart failure (24). However, over the past 9 years, the treatment of CHF in the ambulatory setting has evolved rapidly and the outlook for these patients, although guarded, is no longer as grim (51).

Hospital Readmission

Patients discharged from the hospital with the diagnosis of heart failure have a 44% readmission rate within 1 year (9). Factors associated with readmission to the hospital include poor compliance with medications, inadequate treatment of associated hypertension and ischemic heart disease, and underuse of ACE inhibitors (9). The risk for readmission for heart failure may be much higher for African-American than for white patients, probably due to their greater prevalence of hypertension and diabetes (19). Comprehensive outpatient programs, which include intensive education of the patient and family, social service support, titration of medications, and close follow-up, have demonstrated reductions in hospitalization rates of up to 87%, associated with clinically significant decreases in sodium intake from 3400 to 2100 mg/day, and increases in the daily dosages of ACE inhibitors (45,54).

General References*

Baker DW, Konstam MA, Bottorff M, Pitt B. Management of heart failure. I. Pharmacologic treatment. JAMA 272:1361, 1994.
> A summary of the recommendations of the Expert Panel for the Agency for Health Care Policy and Research Heart Failure Guideline.

Cohn JN. The management of chronic heart failure. N Engl J Med 335:490, 1996.
> Authoritative, concise review.

Katz AM. Cardiomyopathy of overload. A major determinant of prognosis in congestive heart failure. N Engl J Med 322:200, 1990.

Specific References

1. Aguirre FV, Pearson AC, Leeven MK, et al. Usefulness of Doppler echocardiography in the diagnosis of congestive heart failure. Am J Cardiol 63:1098, 1989.
2. Awan NA, Mason DT. Direct selective blockade of the vascular angiotensin II receptors in therapy for hypertension and severe congestive heart failure. Am Heart J 131:177, 1996.
3. Badgett RG, Lucey CR, Muhow CD. Can the clinical examination diagnose left-sided heart failure in adults. JAMA 277:1712, 1997.
4. Baker DW, Wright RF. Management of heart failure IV. Anticoagulation for patients with heart failure due to left ventricular systolic dysfunction. JAMA 272:1614, 1994.
5. Bittner V, Weiner DH, Yusef S, et al. Prediction of mortality and morbidity with a 6-minute walk test in patients with left ventricular dysfunction. SOLVD Investigators. JAMA 270:1702, 1993.

---

*Bold print (general references) and bold numerals (specific references) denote published controlled clinical trials, meta-analyses, or consensus-based recommendations.

6. Breithardt G. Amiodarone in patients with heart failure. N Engl J Med 333:121, 1995.
7. Butman SM, Ewy GA, Standen JR, et al. Bedside cardiovascular examination in patients with severe chronic heart failure: importance of rest or inducible jugular venous distension. J Am Coll Cardiol 22:968, 1993.
8. Captopril Multicenter Research Group. A placebo-controlled trial of captopril in refractory chronic congestive heart failure. J Am Coll Cardiol 2:755, 1983.
9. Chin MH, Goldman L. Factors contributing to the hospitalization of patients with congestive heart failure. Am J Public Health 87:643, 1997.
10. Cleland JG, Bulpitt, CJ, Falk RH, et al. Is aspirin safe for patients with heart failure? Br Heart J 74:215, 1995.
11. Coats AJS. Exercise rehabilitation in chronic heart failure. J Am Coll Cardiol 22(4 Suppl A):172A, 1993.
12. Cohn JN, Archibald DG, Ziesche S, et al. Effect of vasodilator therapy on mortality in chronic congestive heart failure. Results of a Veterans Administration cooperative study. N Engl J Med 314:1547, 1986.
13. Consensus Trial Study Group. Effects of enalapril on mortality in severe congestive heart failure. N Engl J Med 316:1429, 1987.
14. Dauterman K, Pak PH, Maughan WL, et al. Contribution of external forces to left ventricular diastolic pressure. Implications for the clinical use of the Starling law. Ann Intern Med 122:737, 1995.
15. Davie AP, Francis CM, Love MP, et al. Value of the electrocardiogram in identifying heart failure due to left ventricular systolic dysfunction. BMJ 312:222, 1996.
16. Digitalis Investigation Group. The effect of digoxin on mortality and morbidity in patients with heart failure. N Engl J Med 336:525, 1997.
17. Eichorn EJ. The paradox of beta-adrenergic blockade for the management of congestive heart failure. Am J Med 92:527, 1992.
18. Garg R, Yusuf S. Overview of randomized trials of angiotensin-converting enzyme inhibitors on mortality and morbidity in patients with heart failure. Collaborative Group on ACE Inhibitor Trials. JAMA 273:1450, 1995.
19. Ghali JK, Kadakia S, Cooper R, Ferlinz J. Precipitating factors leading to decompensation of heart failure. Traits among urban blacks. Arch Intern Med 148:2013, 1988.
20. Gillum RF. Epidemiology of heart failure in the United States. Am Heart J 126:1042, 1993.
21. Haque WA, Boehmer J, Clemson BS, et al. Hemodynamic effects of supplemental oxygen administration in congestive heart failure. J Am Coll Cardiol 27:353, 1996.
22. Harlan W, Oberman A, Grimm R, Rosati R. Chronic congestive heart failure in coronary artery disease: clinical criteria. Ann Intern Med 86:133, 1977.
23. Ho KK, Pinsky JL, Kannel WB, Levy D. The epidemiology of heart failure: the Framingham study. J Am Coll Cardiol 22(4 Suppl A):6A, 1993.
24. Ho KKL, Anderson KM, Kannel WB, et al. Survival after the onset of congestive heart failure in Framingham study patients. Circulation 88:107, 1993.
25. Jennings GL, Esler MD. Circulatory regulation at rest and exercise and the functional assessment of patients with congestive heart failure. Circulation 81(1 Suppl):II-5, 1990.
26. Kannel WB, Plehn JF, Cupples LA. Cardiac failure and sudden death in the Framingham study. Am Heart J 115:869, 1988.
27. Katz AM. Cardiomyopathy of overload. A major determinant of prognosis in congestive heart failure. N Engl J Med 322:100, 1990.
28. Kiyingi A, Field M, Pawsey C, et al. Metolazone in treatment of severe refractory congestive cardiac failure. Lancet 335:29, 1990.
29. Konstam MA, Dracup K, Bottorff MB, et al. Heart failure: management of patients with left-ventricular systolic dysfunction. Quick Reference Guideline for Clinicians No. 11. AHCPR Publication No. 94-0613. Rockville, MD: Agency for Health Care Policy and Research, Public Health Service, US Department of Health and Human Services, June 1994.
30. Kostis JB. Angiotensin-converting enzyme inhibitors. I. Pharmacology. Am Heart J 116:1580, 1988.

31. Kostis JB. Angiotensin-converting enzyme inhibitors. II. Clinical use. Am Heart J 116:1591, 1988.

32. Lakatta EG. Chaotic behavior of myocardial cells: possible implications regarding the pathophysiology of heart failure. Perspect Biol Med 32:421, 1989.

33. Lakatta EG. Starling's law of the heart is explained by an intimate interaction of muscle length and myofilament calcium activation. J Am Coll Cardiol 10(5):1157, 1987.

34. Levy D, Larson MG, Vasan RS, et al. The progression from hypertension to congestive heart failure. JAMA 275:1557, 1996.

35. Litwin SE, Grossman W. Diastolic dysfunction as a cause of heart failure. J Am Coll Cardiol 22(4 Suppl A) 49A, 1993.

36. Marantz PR, Alderman MH, Tobin JN. Diagnostic heterogeneity in clinical trials for congestive heart failure. Ann Intern Med 109:55, 1988.

37. Michell AR. Effective blood volume: an effective concept or a modern myth. Perspect Biol Med 39:471, 1996.

38. National Heart, Lung, and Blood Institute. Data fact sheet: congestive heart failure. Washington, DC: US Department of Health and Human Services, September 1996.

39. Oka RK, Gortner SR, Stotts NA, Haskell WL. Predictors of physical activity in patients with chronic heart failure secondary to either ischemic or idiopathic dilated cardiomyopathy. Am J Cardiol 77:159, 1996.

40. Packer M, Bristow MR, Cohn JN, et al. The effect of carvedilol on morbidity and mortality in patients with chronic heart failure. N Engl J Med 334:1349, 1996.

41. Packer M, Gheorghiade M, Young JB, et al. Withdrawal of digoxin from patients with chronic heart failure treated with angiotensin-converting-enzyme inhibitors. N Engl J Med 329:1, 1993.

42. Packer M, O'Connor CM, Ghali JK. Effect of amlodipine on morbidity and mortality in severe chronic heart failure. N Engl J Med 375:1107, 1996.

43. Pfeffer MA, Braunwald E, Moye LA, et al. Effect of captopril on mortality and morbidity in patients with left ventricular dysfunction after myocardial infarction. N Engl J Med 327:669, 1992.

44. Pitt B, Segal R, Martinez FA, et al. Randomized trial of losartan versus captopril in patients over 65 with heart failure (Evaluation of Losartan in the Elderly Study, ELITE). Lancet 349:747, 1997.

45. Rich MW, Beckham V, Wittenberg C, et al. A multidisciplinary intervention to prevent the readmission of elderly patients with congestive heart failure. N Engl J Med 333:1190, 1995.

46. Singh SN, Fletcher RD, Fisher SG, et al. Amiodarone in patients with congestive heart failure and asymptomatic ventricular arrhythmia. Survival Trial of Antiarrhythmic Therapy in Congestive Heart Failure. N Engl J Med 333:77, 1995.

47. Smith TW. Digitalis. Mechanisms of action and clinical use. N Engl J Med 318:358, 1988.

48. SOLVD Investigators. Effect of enalapril on mortality and the development of heart failure in asymptomatic patients with reduced left ventricular ejection fractions. N Engl J Med 327:685, 1992.

49. SOLVD Investigators. Effect of enalapril on survival in patients with reduced left ventricular ejection fractions and congestive heart failure. N Engl J Med 325:293, 1991.

50. Sonnenblick M, Friedlander Y, Rosin AJ. Diuretic-induced severe hyponatremia. Review and analysis of 129 reported patients. Chest 103:601, 1993.

51. Stevenson LW. Modern management of heart failure. Hosp Pract (Office Edition) 31:103, 109, 1996.

52. Uretsky BF, Young JB, Shahidi FE, et al. Randomized study assessing the effect of digoxin withdrawal in patients with mild to moderate chronic congestive heart failure: results of the PROVED trial. J Am Coll Cardiol 22:955, 1993.

53. Vasan RS, Larson MG, Benjamin EJ, et al. Left ventricular dilatation and the risk of congestive heart failure in people without myocardial infarction. N Engl J Med 336:1350, 1997.

54. West JA, Miller NH, Parker KM, et al. A comprehensive management system for heart failure improves clinical outcomes and reduces medical resource utilization. Am J Cardiol 79:58, 1997.

55. Wilson JR, Rayos G, Yeoh TK, et al. Dissociation between exertional symptoms and circulatory function in patients with heart failure. Circulation. 92:47, 1995.

C H A P T E R   62

Hypertension

L. RANDOL BARKER, MD

High blood pressure (HBP), or hypertension, is the most common problem addressed at office visits to internists and general practitioners (see Table 1.3). The ambulatory management of this condition is a longitudinal process requiring skill in enlisting the patient's cooperation and in selecting, monitoring, and adjusting treatment. Hypertension has been studied extensively by epidemiologists and clinicians. The recommended care of patients with hypertension is based on the findings from numerous clinical and epidemiologic studies.

EPIDEMIOLOGY

Incidence and Prevalence

Incidence. It has been estimated that 1.8 million adults in the United States develop hypertension each year (69).

Prevalence. As shown in data from the 1988–1991 Health and Nutritional Examination Survey (NHANES) (Table 62.1), the *prevalence* of hypertension increases with age in all gender and race/ethnic subgroups. In this survey, hypertension was defined as a mean systolic blood pressure (BP) on a single occasion of 140 mm Hg or greater, a mean diastolic BP of 90 mm Hg or greater, or current treatment for hypertension with prescribed medication. Because it has been shown that some survey subjects are normotensive at repeat visits (17), the figures from NHANES overstate the prevalence of *sustained hypertension*.

Isolated systolic hypertension (ISH) is seen mainly in the elderly. The prevalence of ISH is approximately 6% in those aged 60 to 69 and approximately 18% in those aged 80 and older (13).

Of those individuals with hypertension, approximately 75% have *stage 1 hypertension*, which is defined as systolic 140 to 159 mm Hg or diastolic 90 to 99 mm Hg (see "Clinical Classification," below) Thus, in a typical practice, decisions must be made most often for patients with stage 1 hypertension.

Secular Trends

Two secular trends in the United States probably reflect the beneficial impact of widespread attention to

Table 62.1. Prevalence of High Blood Pressure (SBP ≥140 mm Hg or DBP ≥90 mm Hg or Taking Antihypertensive Medication) by Age and Race/Ethnicity for Men and Women, U.S. Population 18 Years of Age and Older

	African American[a]	White[b]	Mexican American
Men			
18–29	6.8	4.4	2.8
30–39	20.9	12.8	9.3
40–49	36.8	23.4	22.4
50–59	55.9	41.8	36.0
60–69	63.6	51.3	53.8
70–79	68.0	60.3	52.1
80 and older	62.4[c]	60.3	70.5[c]
Women			
18–29	2.0[c]	0.6[c]	1.0[c]
30–39	11.3	4.6[c]	6.2
40–49	30.5	12.7	10.6
50–59	47.9	36.8	33.5
60–69	77.8	50.9	59.3
70–79	72.6	66.9	67.0
80 and older	80.5[c]	74.3	71.0[c]

From Burt VL, et al. Prevalence of hypertension in the US adult population: results from the Third National Health and Nutrition Examination Survey, 1988–1991. Hypertension 23(3):305–313, 1995.

[a]Excludes Hispanic blacks.

[b]Excludes Hispanic whites.

[c]Estimate is based on sample size not meeting minimum requirement of NHANES III design or relative standard error is greater than 30%.

hypertension and other cardiovascular risk factors in the past three decades (81):

- *The prevalence of hypertension in adults has decreased.* This may reflect lifestyle changes that are known to prevent BP increase (see "Primary Prevention").
- *The age-adjusted mortality rates from the two major consequences of hypertension have decreased.* Between 1972 and 1990, stroke mortality decreased by nearly 60%, and coronary heart disease mortality decreased by approximately 50%.

Other recent trends are a cause for concern (81):

- *There has been an increase in the age-adjusted incidence of stroke and end-stage renal disease and the prevalence of congestive heart failure (CHF)—* three problems for which hypertension is commonly an antecedent risk factor.
- *Levels of awareness, proportion being treated, and proportion controlled decreased* modestly in the most recent national survey (Table 62.2).

PRIMARY PREVENTION

Many subgroups in the population have an increased risk of developing sustained hypertension (e.g., people who are overweight or sedentary, have high-normal BPs, consume excessive amounts of salt or alcohol, are African American, or have a family history of hypertension). Clinical trials have shown that weight reduction, regular exercise (aerobic and low intensity), reduced salt or alcohol intake, and a diet rich in vegetables and fruits but low in animal fat can prevent

the development of hypertension and reduce BP (4,64,91). Other lifestyle changes that have been evaluated in clinical trials have been found to have inconsistent or unproved efficacy in the prevention of hypertension; these include stress reduction and increased intake of potassium, fish oil, magnesium, and dietary fiber (64).

The widespread adoption of measures known to help prevent hypertension and of other measures known to protect cardiovascular health (e.g., not smoking) would reduce significantly the cardiovascular morbidity in the population. In addition to public health approaches, physicians can help by recommending these measures to all patients and especially to those who have a family history of hypertension or have high-normal BPs (see below). A subsequent section of this chapter describes practical details regarding nonpharmacologic measures for controlling or preventing hypertension.

RISKS AND RISK REDUCTION
Risks Attending Untreated Hypertension
Risk from HBP

For a patient and a physician, the single most important concept in approaching hypertension is that high BP increases the risk of symptomatic cardiovascular disease (stroke, coronary artery disease, CHF, renal insufficiency) during the patient's entire life. This concept has been elucidated best by the longitudinal observations on subjects in the Framingham study (43). A number of other longitudinal studies have corroborated the major findings of this study (50).

In the *Framingham study*, adult subjects ranging in age from 45 to 74 years who entered the study in 1951 through 1953 were followed for 18 years or more. For practical purposes, Framingham subjects at entry can be likened to patients making their first office visit to a physician, at ages ranging from 45 to 74. Based on the average of BPs taken on three separate visits, these subjects were subgrouped into three BP subgroups: 140/90 or less, 141/91 to 159/94, and 165/95 or more. During follow-up, an intense effort was made to detect each new cardiovascular event. This study established three points:

Table 62.2. Trends in the Awareness, Treatment, and Control of High Blood Pressure in Adults: United States, 1976–1994[a]

	NHANES II (1976–1980)	NHANES III (Phase I) 1988–1991	NHANES III (Phase 2) 1991–1994
Awareness	51.0%	73.0%	68.4%
Treated	31.0%	55.0%	53.6%
Controlled[b]	10.0%	29.0%	27.4%

From Burt VL, et al. Prevalence of hypertension in the US adult population: results from the Third National Health and Nutrition Examination Study, 1988–1991. Hypertension 23(3):305–313, 1995.

[a]Adults age 18 to 74 years with SBP ≥140 mm Hg or DBP ≥90 mm Hg or taking antihypertensive medication.

[b]SBP <140 mm Hg and DBP <90 mm Hg.

- Risks rise progressively with both systolic and diastolic BP.
- The annual risk of major cardiovascular events is higher for older patients, as a function of both age and BP at entry.
- At all ages and BPs, the annual incidence of events is somewhat higher for men than for women.

Baseline Target Organ Damage

In addition to age and BP level, *coexisting cardiovascular abnormalities* (target organ damage) increases the size of the risk. This is illustrated in Table 62.3, which summarizes findings in subgroups of placebo-treated subjects from the Veterans Administration Therapeutic Trial.

Coexisting Cardiovascular Risk Factors

One or more other treatable risk factors are present in many subjects with hypertension. These risk factors may affect a patient's prognosis far more than hypertension (1). This is illustrated by the fact that two hypothetical patients with the following risk-factor profiles have similar long-term cardiovascular risks:

Age	Cigarettes per Day	Total Cholesterol	Diastolic Blood Pressure
50	0	180 mg/day	125 mm Hg
50	30	220 mg/dL	95 mm Hg

Risk Reduction by Treatment of Hypertension

Relative Risk Reduction

A number of placebo-controlled clinical trials completed between 1970 and 1985 demonstrated that pharmacologic treatment reduces risks in *middle-age adults with diastolic hypertension* (20). Table 62.4 summarizes for each of the major trials (6,39,57,97,98) the principal characteristics and crude percent reduction in expected morbidity and mortality. Six placebo-controlled clinical trials reported between 1985 and 1997 (3,22,49,77,83,86) showed convincingly that pharmacologic treatment also reduces morbidity and mortality in *older persons with HBP, including those with isolated systolic hypertension* (ISH). The principal characteristics and results of these trials are summarized in Table 62.5.

Aggregate analysis of trial results has shown that *in the first few years of treatment,* there is a 42% reduction in expected stroke incidence and fatality (95% confidence interval 33 to 50%) and a 14% reduction in coronary heart disease incidence and fatality (95% confidence interval 4 to 22%) (20). Recent analyses of clinical trial results have shown that treatment of HBP reduces the incidence of CHF by more than 50% (61) and that the largest impact is in older patients with ISH and evidence of a previous myocardial infarction (MI) (47). Treatment also prevents the onset or worsening of renal insufficiency, although population-based data suggest that in African Americans satisfactory BP control may not protect renal function as effectively as in Caucasians (69).

The impact of HBP treatment according to gender was the focus of a recent meta-analysis of clinical trials that included both men and women (35a). Relative risk reduction was similar for both groups.

Table 62.3. Placebo-Treated Subjects, Veterans Administration Trial: Impact of Blood Pressure, Age, and Cardiovascular Abnormalities on Attack Rate

Risk Factor at Entry	Number Randomized	Attack Rate[a]
Cardiovascular and Renal Abnormalities[b] and Diastolic Blood Pressure (mm Hg):		
Without abnormality		
90–104	36	0.145
109–114	51	0.173
With abnormality		
90–104	48	0.352
105–114	50	0.426
Age and Diastolic Blood Pressure (mm Hg):		
<50 yr		
90–104	43	0.121
105–114	56	0.413
50+ yr		
90–104	41	0.413
104–114	54	0.459

Adapted from Veterans Administration Cooperative Study Group on Antihypertensive Agents. Effects of treatment on morbidity in hypertension. III. Influence of age, diastolic pressure, and prior cardiovascular disease; further analysis of side effects. Circulation 45:991, 1972.

[a]Rate observed during 3 years.

[b]Presence of any of the following: grade 2 or greater hypertensive retinopathy, cardiomegaly on chest x-ray, left ventricular hypertrophy on ECG, evidence of renal damage, myocardial infarction, congestive heart failure, cerebrovascular accident.

Table 62.4. Clinical Trials in Adults with Diastolic Hypertension

	VA (Mild)	VA (Severe)	Australian[a]	Oslo	MRC
No. of patients randomized	380	143	3,427	785	17,354
Average age	51	51	50	45	51 (male) 53 (female)
% female	0	0	37	0	48
Range of diastolic BP at entry (mm Hg)	90–104	115–129	95–109	90–109	90–109
Principal medications	•TZ, R, H	•TZ, R, H	•TZ or BB •M •C	•TZ or BB •M	•TZ or BB •M or BB •TZ or C
Approximate % reduction in cardiovascular morbidity and mortality	35	75	30	25	19

VA, Veterans Administration; *MRC,* Medical Research Council (British); *TZ,* thiazide diuretic; *R,* reserpine; *H,* hydralazine; *BB,* β-blocker; *M,* methyldopa; *C,* clonidine.
[a]Control group got no treatment (all other control groups got placebo).

Table 62.5. Clinical Trials in Older People with Hypertension

	EWPHE	Coope and Warrender	STOP-Hypertension	MRC	SHEP	SYST-EUR
No. of patients randomized	840	884	1627	4396	4736	4695
Average age (range)	72 (60–97)	69 (60–79)	75 (70–84)	70 (65–74)	72 (60–80 or more)	70
% female	70	70	63	58	57	66
Mean BP at entry (mm Hg)	182/101	197/100	195/102	185/91	170/77	174/87
Principal medications	•TZ •TZ/TRIAM •M	•AT •TZ •M	•TZ/AMIL •AT, METOP •PIND	•TZ/AMIL •AT	•CTHAL •AT	•NITREND •ENAL •TZ
Approximate % reduction in cardiovascular morbidity and mortality	29	24	40	17	32	31

EWPHE, European Working Party on High Blood Pressure in the Elderly; STOP-Hypertension, Swedish Trial in Old Patients with Hypertension; MRC, Medical Research Council (British); SHEP, Systolic Hypertension in the Elderly Program; SYST-EUR, Systolic Hypertension in Europe; BP, blood pressure; CAD, coronary artery disease; CHF, congestive heart failure; CVD, cardiovascular disease; TZ, thiazide; TRIAM, triamterene; M, methyldopa; AT, atenolol; CTHAL, chlorthiadone; AMIL, amiloride; METOP, metoprolol; NITREND, nitrendipine; PIND, pindolol; ENAL, enalapril.

Absolute Risk and Benefit

As noted, the absolute risk of cardiovascular disease is much higher in the elderly and in people with target organ damage and multiple risk factors. Figure 62.1 shows the combined impact of these patient characteristics on absolute risk. The absolute benefit of treatment is also much higher when patients with these characteristics are treated. Bearing in mind the approximate one-third reduction in morbidity and mortality that has been found in the trials summarized in Tables 62.4 and 62.5 and using the information summarized in Figure 62.1, one can discern that the absolute benefits attending treatment for groups of patients with similar BPs differ greatly. For example:

- *A 70-year-old man with three major risk factors and a BP of 160/90* has approximately a 45% ten-year risk of a major cardiovascular event. A one-third reduction in risk would mean that about 15 of an expected 45 events would be prevented in a group of 100 such patients treated for 10 years. Stated otherwise, the *number needed to treat* (NNT) for 10 years to prevent one event would be 6 or 7.
- *A 40-year-old man with a BP of 160/90 and no major risk factors* has approximately a 10% ten-year risk of a major cardiovascular event. A one-third reduction in risk would mean that about 3 of an expected 10 events would be prevented in a group of 100 such patients treated for 10 years. In this instance the NNT for 10 years to prevent one event would be about 33.

Absolute risk reduction differs by type of cardiovascular event in men and women (35a). In women, the major benefit is reduction in stroke. In men, treatment prevented as many coronary disease events as cerebrovascular events. This difference is thought to reflect the greater absolute risk of coronary events in untreated men.

Nonpharmacologic Measures

In clinical trials, nonpharmacologic measures (weight reduction; salt restriction; physical exercise; high-vegetable, low-fat diet) have been shown to reduce BP in hypertensive subjects (81). Although these

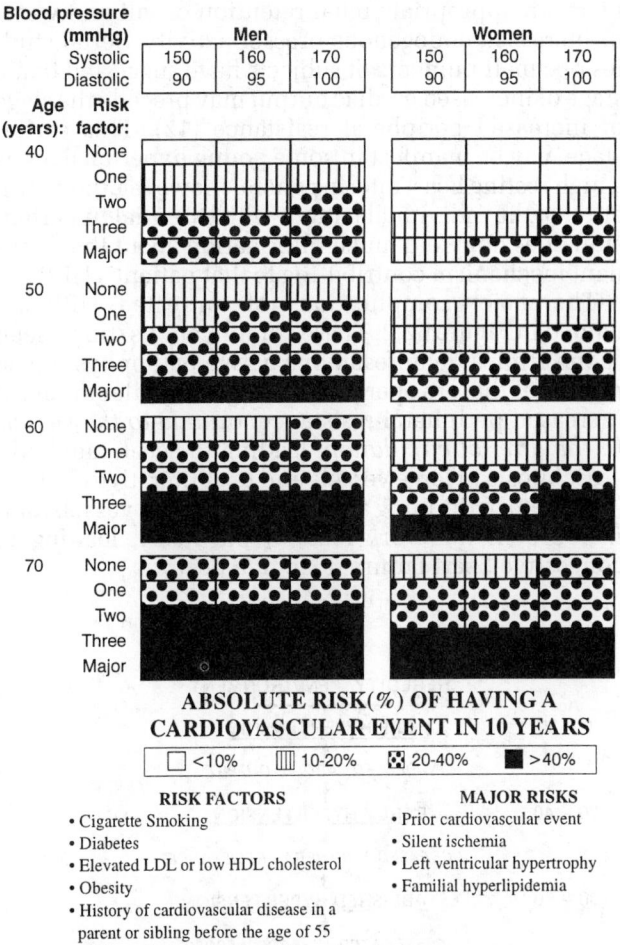

ABSOLUTE RISK(%) OF HAVING A CARDIOVASCULAR EVENT IN 10 YEARS

□ <10%   ▥ 10-20%   ▨ 20-40%   ■ >40%

RISK FACTORS
- Cigarette Smoking
- Diabetes
- Elevated LDL or low HDL cholesterol
- Obesity
- History of cardiovascular disease in a parent or sibling before the age of 55
- Male gender or postmenopausal
- Age over 60

MAJOR RISKS
- Prior cardiovascular event
- Silent ischemia
- Left ventricular hypertrophy
- Familial hyperlipidemia

Figure 62.1. Matrix developed to help in decisions regarding the active treatment of hypertension. (Shading patterns shown in box represent absolute risks during 10 years.) (From Jackson R, Barham P, Bills J, et al. Management of raised blood pressure in New Zealand: a discussion document. BMJ 307:107, 1993.)

trials were not designed to detect the impact of nonpharmacologic measures on symptomatic cardiovascular morbidity, it is likely that they are efficacious (91,92).

PATHOPHYSIOLOGY AND NATURAL HISTORY OF ESSENTIAL HYPERTENSION

It is estimated that 95 to 99% of hypertensives do not have an identifiable cause for their hypertension. Their problem has been designated *essential hypertension*, a condition whose antecedents are probably a mix of genetic and environmental factors (81). Several abnormal physiologic characteristics have been demonstrated in essential hypertension; these provide a conceptual basis for understanding the clinical consequences of hypertension and the mechanisms of action of antihypertensive drugs.

As indicated in Figure 62.2, the patient with established essential hypertension has an increase in peripheral arterial resistance; this is hypothesized to be the final consequence of either or both of two mechanisms: inappropriate renal retention of salt and water or increased endogenous pressor activity. Serial studies on small numbers of subjects have suggested that a stage of increased cardiac output may precede the stage of increased peripheral resistance (12). This earlier stage may be manifest in some young hypertensives as a high resting heart rate. In general, however, the evaluation of the individual patient with essential hypertension does not yield much information about the dominant mechanism contributing to that patient's HBP.

The major complications of untreated HBP are named in Figure 62.2. These complications can be seen as the clinical manifestations of two pathophysiologic processes that are operating during many silent years of increased peripheral resistance: *trauma to the vessels in the arterial circulation*, leading to accelerated atherosclerosis in large vessels and to obliterative changes (Fig. 62.3) or thinning and rupture in small vessels, and *increase in the work load of the heart*, leading to congestive heart failure or angina pectoris.

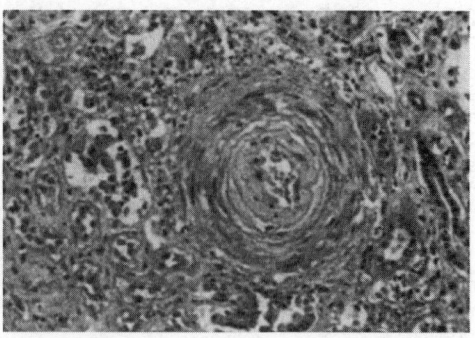

Figure 62.3. Hyperplastic arteriosclerosis in renal tissue from a patient with essential hypertension.

MEASURING THE BLOOD PRESSURE

Standard Practices

A number of factors can affect the level of the BP that is measured using a sphygmomanometer (8). To ensure the validity of the measured BP and to ensure that comparable information is obtained in repeated observations, the following standard practices should be followed at each visit (68,71,81):

- *Ensure that the patient has not smoked, chewed or snuffed tobacco, eaten a meal, or ingested caffeine within 30 minutes* before measurement. Nicotine and caffeine cause a transient rise in BP, and eating can cause a transient decrease in BP, especially in elderly persons.
- *Select an appropriate-size cuff*: The width of the rubber bladder in the cuff should be 40 to 50% of upper arm circumference. The ratio of bladder length to width is 2:1 in most adult cuffs, meaning that a bladder that encircles approximately 80% of the arm will have the right width. When bladder dimensions are too small for the patient's arm, the measured BP obtained may be higher than the actual BP (Fig. 62.4). Overestimation of the BP because of small cuff size can be minimized by using large adult cuffs (bladder dimensions about 30 ³/₁₅ cm) for all adult patients.
- *Apply the cuff to the subject's arm* so that the lower margin is 2.5 cm above the antecubital space and the middle of the inflatable bladder is aligned with the brachial artery pulse.
- *Have the patient sit with back supported in a chair for a few minutes. Measure the BP with the arm passively supported across the chest or resting on a table* so that the stethoscope head is placed over the brachial artery pulse at the level of the heart (about the level of the junction of the fourth intercostal space with the lower left sternal border). Sitting unsupported or actively holding one's arm across the chest may cause the systolic and diastolic pressures to increase 5 to 10 mm Hg. Standing (in the untreated patient) may cause an increase and recumbency a decrease in the BP.
- *In a new patient, measure the pressure in each arm.* If a difference between arms is noted and confirmed

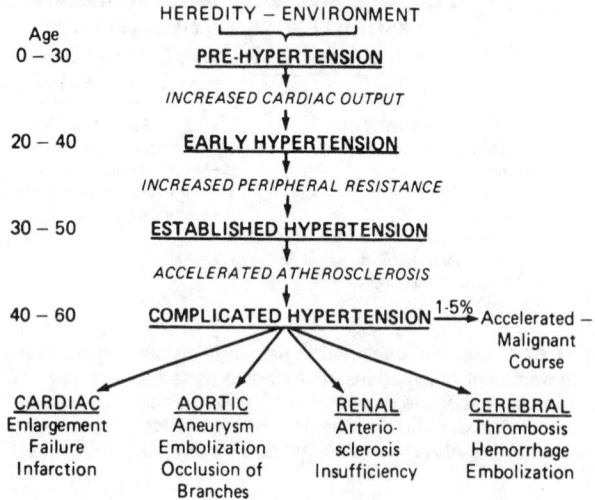

HEREDITY – ENVIRONMENT

Age	
0 – 30	**PRE-HYPERTENSION**
	INCREASED CARDIAC OUTPUT
20 – 40	**EARLY HYPERTENSION**
	INCREASED PERIPHERAL RESISTANCE
30 – 50	**ESTABLISHED HYPERTENSION**
	ACCELERATED ATHEROSCLEROSIS
40 – 60	**COMPLICATED HYPERTENSION** ——1-5%→ Accelerated – Malignant Course

CARDIAC	AORTIC	RENAL	CEREBRAL
Enlargement	Aneurysm	Arterio-	Thrombosis
Failure	Embolization	sclerosis	Hemorrhage
Infarction	Occlusion of	Insufficiency	Embolization
	Branches		

Figure 62.2. A representation of the natural history of untreated essential hypertension. (From Kaplan N. Clinical hypertension. 6th ed. Baltimore: Williams & Wilkins, 1994;110.)

on repeated measurement, take all subsequent BPs in the arm with the higher pressure. The most common cause of arm-to-arm difference, which occurs in occasional patients with atherosclerotic disease, is partial occlusion of blood flow proximal to the brachial artery.

- *Record the first Korotkoff sound (KS) for systolic pressure.* The cuff pressure should be high enough to obliterate the radial pulse; by ensuring that this occurs, one will avoid reading a falsely low systolic pressure due to the *silent auscultatory gap* that occasionally occurs between the first and second Korotkoff sounds.
- *Deflate the cuff slowly (about 2 mm Hg/second).* This prevents underestimation of the systolic pressure and overestimation of the diastolic pressure. Both may occur with too rapid deflation, especially in a patient with a relatively slow resting heart rates. Underestimation of systolic pressure may occur if the patient has an auscultatory gap (silence between KS_1 and KS_3).
- *Record the fifth Korotkoff sound (disappearance) for diastolic pressure.*
- *Wait 1 to 2 minutes* before repeating measurement in the same arm to permit the return of the blood that has transiently filled the veins distal to the inflated cuff.
- *Orthostatic pressure. To detect orthostatic hypotension before initiating antihypertensive treatment and after starting or increasing antihypertensive drugs,* record the BP with the patient standing for at least 1 minute. In treated patients, consider also measuring the BP after a standard exercise (e.g., 10 steps on a footstool or walking a fixed distance) because the orthostatic effect of drugs is often more pronounced after exercise.
- *Record BP, pulse rate, position, arm, and cuff size* (if large cuff used), thereby ensuring that these conditions will be duplicated when BPs are measured at subsequent visits.

Special Situations

In patients with atrial fibrillation, whose beat-to-beat stroke volume and BP differ because of varying intervals between ventricular beats, record the average of several systolic and diastolic pressures.

Pseudohypertension. When the wall of the brachial artery is rigid from calcification, the cuff pressure needed to compress the artery may greatly exceed the intra-arterial pressure, and a very high cuff pressure may be assumed, incorrectly, to be the actual BP. This condition, which has been called pseudohypertension, can be tentatively diagnosed by the finding that the (presumably calcified) radial artery does not collapse when the pulse is obliterated during cuff inflation; there is substantial intraobserver and interobserver variability in the interpretation of this maneuver (94). Definitive diagnosis of pseudohypertension requires arterial catheterization to measure directly the BP, which is then compared with the cuff pressure. It is important to consider pseudohypertension in the evaluation of patients—usually older patients who have widespread atherosclerosis—who describe hypotensive symptoms despite apparently normal or high cuff pressures. A practical approach to management when pseudohypertension is suspected is described below ("Orthostatic Symptoms").

White-coat hypertension and white-coat effect. Of patients with stage 1 hypertension (see Table 62.7), 20% or more have elevated average office BPs and normal average daytime BPs (69a). This pattern is referred to as white-coat hypertension. Many patients with apparent white-coat hypertension have normal BPs when measurement is repeated after having the patient rest quietly in the office. The white-coat effect refers to an average office-measured BP that is higher than the average daytime BP. This effect is largest in patients with stage 2 and stage 3 HBP (96). Clinical decisions for patients who demonstrate these patterns are discussed in a subsequent section ("Treatment: General Considerations").

Ambulatory Monitoring and Home Measurement

Ambulatory monitoring and home measurement by the patient or someone else are two ways in which the snapshot type of information obtained at office visits can be expanded. Critical assessment of experience with these two methods yields the following conclusions (5,7,81):

- Neither method has been used to classify the subjects in the observational studies and the clinical trials,

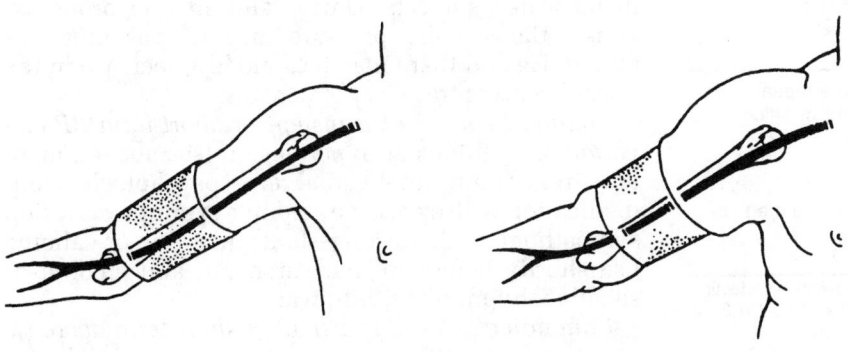

Figure 62.4. On right, bladder width is small for arm, and full cuff pressure is never applied to artery. An erroneously high pressure results. On left, bladder width is adequate for arm, and full cuff pressure is applied to brachial artery. (Reproduced with permission from the American Heart Association.)

described above, that are the basis for current treatment guidelines. Therefore neither method is recommended for routine assessment and management of patients.

- The findings from cross-sectional and prospective studies have shown that target organ disease (e.g., left ventricular hypertrophy [LVH]) and long-term risks correlate better with automated ambulatory BPs than with office BPs.

- Both self-measurement and automated ambulatory monitoring can be helpful when office BPs do not seem to be sufficient for making clinical decisions (Table 62.6) or when patients wish to be more involved in monitoring the status of their BPs.

Home *measurement devices.* Many devices are available, ranging from inexpensive ($20 to $30) simple units that require auscultation with a stethoscope to more expensive ($50 to $150) electronic units that display the BP digitally. These devices are reviewed periodically to help consumers select among them (21). *Finger monitors* are not accurate (65). When a patient decides to measure BPs at home, it is essential to confirm at periodic office visits that the patient's technique is satisfactory and that similar pressures are obtained with the home monitoring device and the office unit. Home readings of 135/85 mm Hg or more ("high normal"; see Table 62.7) should be considered elevated (81).

Automated ambulatory monitoring devices. These are portable devices that measure cuff pressures frequently for 24-hour periods. Patients are instructed to hold the arm still during automatic cuff inflation and to keep a diary (e.g., to report dizziness, headache, or other symptoms of interest). Reports display average daytime, nighttime, and 24-hour pressures; frequencies and temporal distribution of selected pressures; and in some cases, the *BP load* (e.g., percentage of waking pressures more than 140/90 mm Hg and sleeping pressures more than 120/80 mm Hg). Because there are no standard recommendations for the use of these types of aggregate data in decision making, automated ambulatory monitoring is mainly useful in selected patients (Table 62.6). The charge for 24-hour monitoring may range from $150 to $450.

One clinical trial comparing treatment decisions

Table 62.6.   Situations in Which Self-Measurement Devices or Automated Noninvasive Ambulatory Blood Pressure Monitoring Devices May Be Useful for Clinical Decisions

"Office" or "white-coat" hypertension; blood pressure repeatedly elevated in office setting but repeatedly normal out of office
Evaluation of apparent drug resistance
Evaluation of nocturnal blood pressure changes
Episodic hypertension
Hypotensive symptoms associated with antihypertensive medications or autonomic dysfunction
Carotid sinus syncope and pacemaker syndromes[a]

From The Sixth Report of the Joint National Committee on Prevention, Detection, Evaluation, and Treatment of High Blood Pressure. Arch Intern Med 157:2413, 1997.

[a]Along with ECG monitoring.

Table 62.7.   Classification of Blood Pressure for Adults Age 18 Years and Older[a]

Category	Systolic (mm Hg)		Diastolic (mm Hg)
Optimal[b]	<120	and	<80
Normal	<130	and	<85
High-normal	130–139	or	85–89
Hypertension			
Stage 1[c]	140–159	or	90–99
Stage 2[c]	160–179	or	100–109
Stage 3[c]	≥180	or	≥110

From The Sixth Report of the Joint National Committee on Prevention, Detection, Evaluation, and Treatment of High Blood Pressure. Arch Intern Med 157:2413, 1997.

[a]Not taking antihypertensive drugs and not acutely ill. When systolic and diastolic blood pressures fall into different categories, the higher category should be selected to classify the individual's blood pressure status. For example, 160/92 mm Hg should be classified as stage 2 hypertension, and 174/120 mm Hg should be classified as stage 3 hypertension. Isolated systolic hypertension is defined as SBP ≥140 mm Hg and DBP <90 mm Hg and staged appropriately (e.g., 170/82 mm Hg is defined as stage 2 isolated systolic hypertension). In addition to classifying stages of hypertension on the basis of average blood pressure levels, clinicians should specify presence or absence of target organ disease and additional risk factors. This specificity is important for risk classification and treatment (see Table 62.10).

[b]Optimal blood pressure with respect to cardiovascular risk is <120/80 mm Hg. However, unusually low readings should be evaluated for clinical significance.

[c]Based on the average of two or more readings taken at each of two or more visits after an initial screening.

based on average office BPs to decisions based on average daytime ambulatory BPs concluded that the latter decisions led to less intensive BP treatment and a better sense of well-being but did not reduce the overall cost of treatment (82).

Blood Pressure Variability

There are a number of psychologic, biologic, and pharmacologic causes of BP variability. When deciding what the measured BP means in an individual patient, these factors should be considered, in addition to following the standard approach to measuring the BP described above.

Normal patterns. In a 24-hour period, the average person's resting BP fluctuates (systolic, 20 to 40 mm Hg; diastolic, 10 to 20 mm Hg). The lowest BPs occur during sleep. These ranges occur in patients with normal BP and in hypertensive patients who are or are not taking antihypertensive drugs. During low-level dynamic exercise (e.g., walking), there may be a slight increase in both the systolic and diastolic pressures in untreated subjects. During and after vigorous exercise, the systolic pressure may rise as much as 60 mm Hg and there may be a modest decrease in the diastolic pressure.

Common causes of transient or short-term BP elevation are white-coat hypertension (see above); mental stress, both intellectual and psychologic; self-medication with excessive amounts of nonprescription sympathomimetic decongestants; nicotine or caffeine use shortly before BP measurement; and alcohol or sedative–hypnotic withdrawal.

Common causes of transient or short-term decrease in a patient's BP are eating a meal (especially in sedentary older persons); volume contraction from intercurrent illness that causes fluid losses or reduced intake; bed rest for several days; and hospitalization with or without strict bed rest (40).

EVALUATION OF THE HYPERTENSIVE PATIENT
Clinical Classification

In its 1997 report, the Joint National Committee (JNC) on Detection and Evaluation of High Blood Pressure revised the national standards for clinical classification of adult patients with high BP (81). The new classification (Table 62.7) differs in two ways from that published in 1993 (31):

1. *A new clinical category has been added: optimal BP (i.e., 120/80 mm Hg or less).*
2. *There are now three instead of four stages, according to BP level.* Old stage 4 (210 or greater systolic BP or 120 or greater diastolic BP) has been eliminated because of the relative infrequency of stage 4.

The JNC classification gives equal weight to the risks that attend systolic and diastolic hypertension and promotes decision making that takes into consideration coexisting factors that increase the patient's cardiovascular risks (target organ disease and other risk factors).

The treatment section contains the JNC's guidelines for treatment of patients with stage 1, 2, or 3 HBP based on the burden of coexisting risk factors (Fig. 62.1) and target organ disease (see Table 62.10 below).

The classification of patients should be addressed using standard methods for BP measurement (see above) on two or more occasions after initial detection of HBP. This approach is important because being labeled hypertensive may lead to increased sick days, to increased life insurance premiums, or to employment restrictions (37); and a variable characteristic such as BP will regress to the person's usual level, which will be normal in some subjects whose initial BP is high. Two research findings underline the latter point: First, a sizable proportion of people who are found to be hypertensive at an initial screening visit do not have HBP at follow-up visits (17); second, systolic and diastolic BPs predictably decrease when daily measurements are made over several weeks (28).

Clinical Presentation

There are several ways in which patients with high BPs present to physicians.

History of Hypertension

On their initial visits, many patients state that they have hypertension. For some of these patients, recorded BPs from other sources will be available. Some will be taking antihypertensive drugs, presumably for sustained hypertension. Based on this information, BP recordings made at the initial and follow-up visits, and clinical and laboratory data regarding target organs, the patient's hypertension can usually be classified with confidence.

High Initial Blood Pressure

In practice, patients found to have one elevated systolic or diastolic BP should have their BP remeasured within 2 months for stage 1 (SBP 140 to 159 or DBP 90 to 99), 1 month for stage 2 (SBP 160 to 179 or DBP 100 to 109), and 1 week for stage 3 (SBP 180 or greater or DBP 110 or greater (81). Even very high initial BPs, especially when they are measured in emergency departments, may represent transient elevations.

Because patients with transient high BPs or with high-normal BPs are at increased risk for developing sustained hypertension, they should have their BP checked once each year (81). Such patients must understand that they do not have sustained hypertension. In addition, however, they should be advised to avoid excess salt and to follow other practices that reduce the likelihood of developing hypertension (see "Primary Prevention," above).

Options for evaluating patients with *suspected white-coat hypertension* are described above ("Ambulatory Monitoring and Home Measurement").

Chronic Hypertension

Hypertension is chronic if the average systolic or diastolic pressure at multiple visits is more than 140 or 90 mm Hg, respectively. At a patient's first visit, there may be evidence of chronic hypertension (e.g., a preexisting electrocardiogram that shows left ventricular hypertrophy, or fundal hemorrhages or exudates found on physical examination). Eye ground findings indicative of arteriolosclerosis (grade 1: narrowing of arteriolar lumen; grade 2: arteriovenous crossing changes) are less specific indicators of chronic hypertension and should not be substituted for BP measurements on multiple occasions. Most patients with chronic hypertension are in JNC stages 1 and 2 (Table 62.7) when they first present.

The prognosis of untreated chronic hypertension and the benefits of treatment are summarized above ("Risks and Risk Reduction").

Accelerated Hypertension

Hypertension is accelerated when there is clinical evidence of severe arteriolosclerosis, meaning either *grade 3 or 4 hypertensive retinopathy* (grade 3: hemorrhages or fresh exudates; grade 4: papilledema), or *renal insufficiency* for which there is no apparent cause except the hypertension. Before developing evidence of accelerated hypertension, most of these patients have had very high BPs (i.e., JNC stage 3; Table 62.7) for several years.

The prognosis in *untreated accelerated hypertension* is poor: approximately 95% of subjects die of cardiac, renal, or central nervous system (CNS) complications within 5 years of initial presentation. Control of BP and (for those with end-stage renal disease) dialysis, have dramatically improved the prognosis in these individuals.

Hypertensive Emergency

A hypertensive emergency exists when marked elevation of the BP will predictably cause a catastrophic outcome within hours or days. Patients with two types of hypertensive emergency—hypertensive encephalopathy and dissecting aneurysm of the thoracic aorta—may present initially in an office setting. When either of these diagnoses is suspected, the patient should be transported immediately to a hospital emergency department for evaluation and treatment.

Hypertensive encephalopathy is the result of cerebral edema that develops gradually over 1 day or more in a patient with severe hypertension. In such a patient, global cerebral symptoms, such as headache, confusion, and irritability, have usually been present and progressive for hours or days. Papilledema may be present. Hypertensive encephalopathy should not be diagnosed until intracerebral mass or hemorrhage, which may also present with hypertension, has been excluded by computed tomographic scanning. Diffuse or focal white matter edema in the supratentorial compartment will usually be seen on the scan (99).

Thoracic aortic dissection results from an expanding hematoma in the wall of the aorta. The patient with acute dissection usually has a history of known hypertension and presents with a story of sudden anterior chest pain or tearing pain in the back. Two noninvasive imaging modalities—computerized tomography and magnetic resonance imaging—are very sensitive and specific diagnostic tests for dissection. By definition, a *proximal dissection* involves the aorta between the aortic root and the left subclavian artery (palpated pulse intensity and BP levels may be decreased in either arm; there may be a murmur of aortic regurgitation) and a *distal dissection* involves only that part of the aorta distal to the left subclavian artery.

The prognosis in encephalopathy and aortic dissection—when either condition is diagnosed before there has been irreversible damage—depends on prompt hospitalization for antihypertensive treatment and, for some patients with dissection, surgery. Despite the overwhelming threat to life without treatment, good outcomes can be achieved with appropriate intervention.

Hypertensive Urgency

The term *hypertensive urgency* is often used to categorize patients with severe hypertension (e.g., systolic 210 mm Hg or more or diastolic 120 mm Hg or more) who may have evidence of target organ disease but are asymptomatic. Some authors advocate lowering of the BP within a few hours, using doses of oral medications with prompt onset of action. There is no evidence for benefit—and there is anecdotal evidence for harm (35)—to asymptomatic patients whose BP is treated hourly until their urgent hypertension responds. As discussed below under "Treatment," using currently available drugs it is usually possible, and more appropriate, to control severe hypertension within a few days.

Baseline Evaluation: Overview

The baseline evaluation of patients with sustained hypertension has five objectives:

1. To assess the status of *target organs* affected by hypertension
2. To identify clues to the presence of a *treatable etiology* for the hypertension
3. To guide the selection of *initial treatment*
4. To establish the *pretreatment status* of the patient's electrolytes, renal function, and other characteristics that may be affected by antihypertensive drugs
5. To detect the presence of additional *cardiovascular risk factors*

Table 62.8 lists by source the information that is recommended to accomplish these five objectives at baseline. These recommendations match the recommendations of the 1997 JNC report (81).

Target Organ Status

At baseline evaluation, most patients with sustained hypertension, including those with accelerated hypertension, have no symptoms attributable to their hypertension. In the past, it was thought that headache, tinnitus, epistaxis, and dizziness were common symptoms of hypertension, but community-based studies have demonstrated that these symptoms are not more prevalent in hypertensive than in normotensive subjects (100).

The major morbidity of HBP is due to cardiac, cerebral, and renal disease. Baseline information about the target organs affected by HBP often helps one to make decisions in follow-up care of a patient (see "Recommendations Regarding Initial Treatment," below).

Heart

A history of symptoms caused by congestive heart failure or by coronary artery disease will occasionally be obtained at baseline evaluation. Auscultation of the heart commonly reveals accentuation of the aortic second sound and a systolic ejection murmur. Infrequent auscultatory findings include a systolic ejection sound at the base of the heart, paradoxical splitting of the second heart sound, or a short, high-pitched diastolic murmur at the base. Evidence of LVH may be found at baseline evaluation, either on physical examination (left ventricular [LV] heave or fourth heart sound) or on the ECG. Evidence of left-atrial abnormality is the earliest change on the ECG, reflecting atrial contraction against a left ventricle with decreased compliance during diastole. The electrocardiographic criteria for LVH are summarized elsewhere (see Chapter 60, Table 60.3). The concentric hypertrophy typical of hypertension causes only a modest increase in the LV silhouette on the chest x-ray, and the plain film of the chest is much less sensitive than the ECG in identifying changes from LVH.

The *functional abnormalities associated with LVH* have been studied extensively in recent years. In some

Table 62.8. Recommended Baseline Evaluation of the Patient with Sustained Hypertension

Information	End-Organ Status	Etiology Screening	Selecting Treatment	Factors Modified by Treatment	Additional Cardiovascular Risk Factors
Interview, Old Records					
Age and race		X	X		
Blood pressure levels		X	X	X	
Hypertension treatment, results, side effects		X	X		
Family history		X	X		X
Congestive heart failure	X		X		
Angina	X		X		
Transient ischemic attack or cerebrovascular accident	X				
Renal disease	X	X	X		
Comprehension of hypertension			X	X	
Diet (Na, K, fats)		X	X	X	X
Exercise habits			X		X
Current medications[a]		X	X	X	X
Alcohol use		X	X		
Tobacco use					X
Current life stresses		X	X		X
Coexisting conditions[b]		X	X		
Periodic sympathetic symptoms		X			
Physical Examination					
Weight		X	X	X	
Blood pressure (right, left, resting, standing)		X	X	X	
Heart rate and rhythm		X	X	X	
Eye grounds	X		X		
Peripheral pulses	X	X	X		
Heart	X				
Lungs			X		
Abdomen (mass, bruit)		X			
Neurological	X				
Laboratory					
Complete blood count				X	
Calcium level		X		X	
Creatinine level	X	X	X	X	
Potassium level		X	X	X	
Sodium level				X	
Fasting glucose level			X	X	
Cholesterol (total, high-density lipoprotein) level[c]				X	X
Uric acid level			X	X	
Urinalysis		X		X	
ECG	X		X		

[a]Identify medications that may cause hypertension or may counteract antihypertensive drugs (e.g., oral contraceptives, tricyclic antidepressants, sympathomimetic decongestants, appetite suppressants, corticosteroids, nonsteroidal anti-inflammatory drugs, cyclosporine, erythropoietin, monoamine oxidase inhibitors, venlaxapine).

[b]See Table 62.16.

[c]Recommendations of the National Cholesterol Education Program: nonfasting total and high-density lipoprotein (HDL) cholesterol. If total cholesterol is ≥240 mg/dL or if HDL is ≤35 mg/dL, obtain fasting lipoprotein analysis (see Chapter 75).

asymptomatic patients, the resting ejection fraction (measured by echocardiogram) is normal but the ejection fraction shows a subnormal increase during exercise. In hypertensive patients with symptoms of LV failure, echocardiographic studies have revealed that some have global LV dysfunction; some have functional subaortic stenosis; some have a hyperkinetic left ventricle with a normal or high ejection fraction and diminished relaxation during diastole; and some in the latter group (usually older patients) have cavity obliteration during diastole (78). Because appropriate drug therapy for patients in these groups differs in important ways (see below), it is recommended that hypertensive patients with signs and symptoms of heart failure should have echocardiograms to ensure that the drugs selected for them are likely to improve rather than worsen the heart failure.

Most symptoms of *coronary artery disease* in hypertensive patients are related to occlusive disease of the coronary arteries. Some hypertensive patients who describe exertional angina and who have normal coronary arteriograms may have ischemia caused by increased resistance of the microvasculature of the myocardium (15).

Kidney

Simple tests of kidney status (urinalysis and serum creatinine concentration) are normal in the majority of hypertensives at baseline. In patients with a high baseline BP, the finding of an elevated creatinine concentration, proteinuria (sometimes more than 1 g/24 hours), or microscopic hematuria may signify accelerated hypertension. In such patients, other forms of renal or urologic disease should be excluded before these findings are attributed to hypertension.

Central Nervous System

A history of stroke or transient ischemic attacks, an asymptomatic carotid bruit, or neurologic findings of a remote stroke may be present at baseline evaluation, but most patients will not have evidence of cerebrovascular disease when they are first evaluated.

Eye

Ophthalmic symptoms attributable to HBP (decreased acuity from retinal hemorrhages or retinal detachment) are uncommon. However, examination of the retina has been emphasized in the evaluation of hypertensive patients because it offers direct inspection of blood vessels affected by hypertension. Most patients with chronic hypertension have evidence of arteriolosclerosis (grade 1 or 2 hypertensive retinopathy), but these findings have little practical value because they are not specific for hypertension, and there is significant interobserver and intraobserver variability in detecting them. Grade 3 retinopathy should be sought in patients with stage 3 baseline BPs (Table 62.7); these changes are specific for accelerated hypertension.

Evaluation for Secondary Hypertension

Information obtained at baseline evaluation or during follow-up will identify those patients who may have hypertension secondary to a reversible cause. Because surgically curable causes of HBP are uncommon, only highly selected patients should undergo the costly evaluations needed to diagnose these problems (81).

Chronic Alcoholism

In some individuals, heavy, *chronic alcohol use* causes sustained hypertension. For patients found to have both HBP and alcoholism at the baseline evaluation, BP control should be attempted initially through detoxification and treatment of the alcoholism (see Chapter 21). The BP becomes normal in those with alcohol-induced hypertension within about 1 week after discontinuation of alcohol.

Current Use of a Medication that May Cause HBP

This cause of HBP should be considered in any patient concurrently using one of the medications that occasionally cause BP elevation (see list in footnote to Table 62.8). Although there is a detectable increase in the BP in most women who take *oral contraceptives*, the BP usually remains within the normal range with preparations that contain less than 50 µg of estrogen, the amount contained in currently prescribed products (see Chapter 93 for practical considerations related to oral contraceptives). *Estrogen* in the doses used for postmenopausal replacement therapy (about one-sixth of the amount in oral contraceptives) usually does not cause the BP to rise (25), but because estrogen may occasionally cause hypertension, women who take it should have their BP monitored at several visits during their first year on estrogen replacement.

To confirm that a medication is the cause of a patient's hypertension, there should be evidence that the patient had a normal BP before use of the medication, and the patient's BP should become normal within a few weeks after discontinuation of the medication (if this can be done safely).

Renovascular Hypertension (RVH)

It is estimated that 0.5% or less of all hypertensive patients have renovascular hypertension (hypertension caused by unilateral stenosis of the main or of a segmental renal artery) (24). In patients under 40, the cause is usually fibromuscular hyperplasia of the renal artery; in older patients, atherosclerosis of the renal artery is the usual cause. There is probably no racial or sexual predominance in the population of patients with RVH (87). Smoking is more common in all groups of patients with RVH (67).

A number of clinical findings increase the probability that the patient has RVH.

- The presence of a unilateral high-pitched abdominal bruit radiating to the flank
- Well-documented recent (span of 1 or 2 years) change from normal BP to stage 2 or 3 hypertension (Table 62.7)
- A very high baseline diastolic pressure (e.g., 115 mm Hg or more) in a person under 30 years of age
- Evidence of accelerated hypertension (i.e., grade 3 or 4 hypertensive retinopathy or renal insufficiency caused by hypertension) in any patient
- Hypertension that is refractory to maximal tolerated doses of multiple antihypertensive drugs
- Unexplained renal failure, especially with a normal urinary sediment
- Unexplained refractoriness to previously effective drugs
- Doubling of the patient's serum creatinine concentration after initiation of an angiotensin-converting enzyme (ACE) inhibitor (suggests bilateral renal artery stenosis)

If a patient has one or more of these findings and is a candidate for surgery, the following choices can be presented:

1. *Use medication to control the hypertension*, including drugs not previously tried in those patients who seem to be refractory to maximal doses of multiple drugs. This choice is supported by the findings that RVH generally responds to medical therapy and that many patients with RVH caused by atherosclerosis (the most common cause of RVH) need to resume drug treatment within 1 year or more of surgery (24). Because control of systemic HBP will not prevent progressive renal failure caused by bilateral reno-

vascular disease, patients whose renal function worsens on treatment should be considered for vascular evaluation (63).

2. *Undergo evaluation for renal artery stenosis (RAS).* Before undergoing tests for RAS, the patient should declare an interest in accepting angioplasty or surgery if testing shows RAS. Also the patient should understand that if RAS is found, the only way to establish whether renovascular HBP is present is to undergo angioplasty or vascular surgery and then to await the BP response to the procedure. There are two generally accepted *criteria for confirmed RVH* (24):

   - Stable postangioplasty/surgery cure (BP of 140/90 or less, off medicine) or significant improvement (systolic or diastolic pressure reduced by at least 15% without a change in medication)

   or

   - Much less medication needed to maintain a normal BP

Functional evaluation followed by anatomic diagnosis. Noninvasive evaluation for functional evidence of RVH, which eliminates the risk of arteriography, is reasonable for patients in whom the clinical suspicion of RVH is moderately high (i.e., 5 to 15% pretest probability of RVH; Table 62.9). Patients with positive findings are then referred for renal arteriography. Of the several noninvasive techniques available, *captopril scintirenography* has excellent performance characteristics (sensitivity approximately 93% and specificity approximately 95%). Based on published experience (54), in a patient with an estimated 15% pretest probability of having RVH, a positive captopril scan would increase to approximately 77% the probability (positive predictive value) that the patient has RVH; a negative test would increase from 85 to approximately 99% the probability (negative predictive value) that the patient does not have RVH. *Duplex scanning* of renal arteries and *magnetic resonance angiography* have characteristics comparable to those of captopril scintirenography (63).

Patient Experience and Description of Test: Captopril Scintirenography. The patient receives an injection of tracer material and undergoes scintigraphic scanning twice: before and after receiving a standard dose of captopril. The two-stage procedure takes about 3 hours. If the patient is currently taking an ACE inhibitor or an angiotensin receptor–blocking drug, it should be held on the day of the test. Other current antihypertensive medications may be continued. The test measures quantitative and/or qualitative changes in renal flow or filtration to detect asymmetry between the two kidneys. The test depends on the influence of captopril upon renal handling of radioactive tracers: in a kidney with significant RAS, there is angiotensin II–mediated constriction of the postglomerular arterioles; captopril reduces or eliminates this, thus lowering glomerular pressure/filtration and leading to a change in the renal handling of tracer materials.

Anatomic diagnosis. For an interested patient in whom the clinical suspicion of RVH is high (i.e., 25% or higher pretest probability; Table 62.9), it is reasonable to refer the patient directly for renal arteriography. Noninvasive study with intravenous digital subtraction angiography usually does not provide adequate detail to make a decision for intervention; most patients with positive findings need to have a second study, conventional renal arteriography or intra-arterial digital subtraction angiography (63).

If unilateral RAS is found and the patient has fibromuscular hyperplasia or focal nonostial atherosclerotic RAS, percutaneous transluminal renal angioplasty (PTRA) may yield results equal to those of surgery. Neither PTRA nor surgery has produced very satisfactory long-term results if RAS from more extensive atherosclerosis is present. In some patients with the triad of HBP resistant to medical therapy, renal insufficiency, and atherosclerosis causing either bilateral renal artery stenosis or renal artery stenosis in a single functioning kidney, surgery or PTRA may control the HBP and stabilize or improve the renal function (63). The use of a stent following PTRA may afford the best long-term results (36).

Patient Experience: Renal Arteriography. The patient experience is similar to that described for cerebral arteriography in Chapter 78. For both studies femoral artery catheterization is used, and when a small catheter is used, the patient does not need hospital admission.

Kidney Disease

Kidney disease should be suspected as a possible cause of HBP in patients with a history of hematuria, stones, or recurrent pyelonephritis; or in patients in whom large kidneys (e.g., from obstruction or to polycystic disease) or a large bladder (after voiding) are palpated; or when the urinalysis suggests acute or chronic glomerulonephritis (i.e., proteinuria and/or many casts, especially red cell casts). If obstructive uropathy is suspected, a sonogram should be obtained. In patients with established chronic renal failure and small kidneys, it is usually impossible to determine whether the hypertension or the renal disease was the initial problem.

Table 62.9. Clinical Index of Suspicion (Pretest Probability) for Renovascular Hypertension

Moderate Suspicion (5–15%)
Very severe diastolic hypertension (≥120 mm Hg) at baseline
Change over 1 to 2 years from normal blood pressure to severe diastolic hypertension (≥110 mm Hg) in patients <20 or >50 years old
Hypertension refractory to pharmacologic treatment

High Suspicion (≥25%)
Severe diastolic hypertension (≥110 mm Hg) with either progressive renal insufficiency or grade 3 or 4 hypertensive retinopathy plus resistance to aggressive pharmacologic treatment
Severe diastolic hypertension (≥110 mm Hg) with incidentally detected asymmetry of kidney size

Adapted from Mann SG, Pickering TG. Detection of renovascular hypertension: state of the art—1992. Ann Intern Med 117:845, 1992.

Primary Hyperaldosteronism

The most common clue to this cause is a baseline potassium level significantly below normal for which there is no explanation, such as diuretic use or gastrointestinal fluid loss. Hypertensive patients with this finding should be asked about excess consumption of licorice, which contains glycyrrhetinic acid, a moiety with mineralocorticoidlike activity; there are case reports of hypertension that abated when the patient discontinued consuming large amounts of licorice. The ambulatory evaluation of the patient with suspected primary hyperaldosteronism is discussed in detail in Chapter 45 ("Hypokalemia").

Pheochromocytoma (53)

Clues to the presence of pheochromocytoma are a history of a hypermetabolic state (which may resemble hyperthyroidism) or of paroxysms of symptoms caused by increased sympathetic nervous system activity (tachycardia, palpitations, diaphoresis), with associated severe headaches. The absence of such symptom clusters virtually excludes the presence of pheochromocytoma. Paroxysms last from minutes to several hours, but usually less than 1 hour. In approximately 75% of patients with pheochromocytoma, paroxysms occur at least once per week; the remaining patients either experience multiple attacks on most days or only experience an attack every few months. These symptoms are especially important when there is no evidence for more common causes for them; that is, hyperthyroidism (see Chapter 73), reactive hypoglycemia (see Chapter 74), migraine or cluster headaches (see Chapter 79), or panic attacks and other anxiety disorders (see Chapter 13).

Paroxysmal and persistent hypertension are equally common in patients with pheochromocytoma. Orthostatic hypotension, with or without symptoms, is present in some patients, presumably because of vasodilation caused by predominant β_2-sympathetic activity.

Additional findings that increase the prior probability of pheochromocytoma are a marked change in BP or heart rate in response to minor injury, parturition, or general anesthesia; a neurocutaneous syndrome (von Recklinghausen's disease or von Hippel–Lindau syndrome); a blood relative with a pheochromocytoma; and type II multiple endocrine neoplasia (medullary carcinoma of the thyroid or parathyroid adenoma, or both, with symptoms suggesting pheochromocytoma).

Screening tests. Because pheochromocytoma is uncommon, the best practice is to screen only those patients in whom clinical suspicion is high and to refer for costly diagnostic evaluation only those patients with positive screening tests. Measurement of 24-hour urinary excretion of one or more of the three markers for increased pressor synthesis (catecholamines, metanephrines, and vanillylmandelic acid) is a screening test that has satisfactory performance characteristics. When used in a patient with an estimated 5% pretest probability of having a pheochromocytoma (a hypertensive patient who reports paroxysms of headache, tachycardia, and/or diaphoresis), excess excretion of any of the three markers would increase to 35 to 45% the probability (positive predictive value) that the patient has pheochromocytoma, and normal results would increase from 95 to approximately 99% the probability (negative predictive value) that the patient does not have pheochromocytoma (103).

Screening procedures. For the 24-hour urine tests, the patient is given a plastic container that contains a fixed amount of a strong acid and is instructed to collect a 24-hour specimen. The same specimen can be used to screen for catecholamines, metanephrines, and vanillylmandelic acid. With modern assay techniques, no foodstuffs and only a small number of drugs interfere with test results (measured *catecholamines* may be increased by methyldopa, labetalol, rapid withdrawal of clonidine, ethanol, tetracycline, erythromycin, L-dopa, theophylline, hypoglycemia, isoproterenol, and prochlorperazine; measured *metanephrines* may be increased by monoamine oxidase inhibitors, labetalol, ethanol, clonidine withdrawal, and occasionally methyldopa; measured *vanillylmandelic* acid may be decreased by monoamine oxidase inhibitors and clofibrate, and it may be increased by nalidixic acid, levodopa, labetalol, and clonidine withdrawal). In patients who have normal BPs between paroxysms of hypertension, the urine specimen should be taken when the patient is hypertensive. In a patient with especially concerning symptoms whose marker excretion is normal, it is reasonable to repeat the test one or more times.

Diagnostic tests. Patients with positive screening tests should undergo definitive diagnostic testing to localize the presumed tumor. This process has been improved by the availability of radioisotope scanning using labeled iodobenzylguanidine, followed by computerized tomographic scanning or magnetic resonance imaging of the site that takes up this substance. Almost all pheochromocytomas are located in the adrenal glands; 1 to 3% may be located in the posterior mediastinum. Of these tumors, 90% can be totally removed at surgery. Up to 10% are found to be malignant at surgery.

Coarctation of the Aorta

Clues to the presence of this condition are hypertension in a relatively young patient (most will be recognized in the pediatric age group); decreased BP in the lower extremities, suggested by diminished or absent femoral pulses and corroborated by auscultation over the popliteal artery, using a large cuff; and evidence of collateral arterial circulation either on inspection of the trunk or on the plain chest x-ray, which may also show poststenotic dilation of the aorta. In a minority of patients, the coarctation occurs proximal to the left subclavian artery, and the BP is high only in the right arm. To confirm the presence of a coarctation, the patient must be hospitalized for aortography.

Status of Factors Modified by Treatment

Table 62.8 lists factors that should be addressed or documented at baseline because they may be modified as part of the treatment plan or as a consequence of treatment. These include information obtained in the history (patient's understanding of hypertension, usual diet, alcohol consumption, current medications), in the physical examination (weight, BP, heart rate and rhythm, edema), and in the laboratory examination (creatinine, electrolytes, fasting glucose, complete blood count, uric acid, cholesterol, and urinalysis).

Status of Other Cardiovascular Risk Factors

Coexisting cardiovascular risk factors are common in patients with hypertension (1); they affect greatly long-term probability of morbidity and mortality (Fig. 62.1). Therefore, the baseline evaluation of a hypertensive patient should include checking for other risk factors and these factors should be considered in planning the overall management of the patient. These include gender, family history of premature cardiovascular disease, tobacco use, high-cholesterol diet, hypercholesterolemia, sedentary living, stressful lifestyle, overweight, and diabetes mellitus.

TREATMENT OF HYPERTENSION: GENERAL CONSIDERATIONS

Goals of Treatment

When sustained hypertension has been confirmed, the goal of treatment is to reduce the patient's risk of future cardiovascular disease by restoring the BP to normal. Normal BP is defined as a systolic pressure below 140 mm Hg and a diastolic pressure below 90 mm Hg (81). For patients in whom it is impossible to achieve these levels, partial reduction of the BP has been shown to reduce risks (88).

For all diabetic patients and for patients with congestive heart failure or chronic renal failure, a BP below 130/85 mm Hg is now recommended (see details below) (63,81).

These BP goals are shown in the strategy summarized in Figure 62.5 (see p. 863).

White-coat hypertension and white-coat effect (see "Measuring the Blood Pressure," above). There are preliminary and conflicting data regarding the risks associated with these patterns of BP elevation and the advisability of treatment (32,82,96). At least one large study showed similar 4-year rates of cardiovascular morbidity in patients with high office BPs (stages 1 to 3) who did or did not manifest a "white-coat" effect (lower, often still high daytime BPs) and were treated on the basis of office BPs (96). The current consensus is that home BPs of 135/85 mm Hg or greater should be considered elevated, meaning that the goal BP for these and other patients' home BPs should be below these levels (81).

Timetable. In patients who choose a nonpharmacologic regimen (see below), a trial of this approach for 6 months to 1 year is usually needed to evaluate its impact on the BP. When drug treatment is selected, a goal of satisfactory BP control without significant drug side effects can usually be achieved within 1 to 3 months.

Other risk factors. A second goal in the care of any hypertensive patient is the control of other treatable cardiovascular risk factors.

J-curve hypothesis. Analysis of data from the major clinical trials in middle-age adults has suggested that increased risks of MI attend drug-induced lowering of the resting diastolic pressure to less than 85 mm Hg, particularly in patients with preexisting coronary artery disease (30). Because of this finding, some authorities have recommended that the diastolic pressure not be reduced below 85 mm Hg; others point out that no J-curve pattern was reported in the Systolic Hypertension in the Elderly Program (SHEP) in which the average diastolic pressure was 68 mm Hg in treated subjects (77). A clinical trial that is in progress (the Hypertension Optimal Treatment, or "HOT," trial) will establish the relative benefit of on-treatment diastolic pressures of 90 or less, 85 or less, and 80 mm Hg or less (42).

Treatment According to Risk Stratification

The 1997 JNC report recommends treatment according to the stratification shown in Table 62.10 (risk groups A, B, C). *Initial treatment with antihypertensive drugs is recommended for all patients with sustained diastolic BP of 100 mm Hg or more or sustained systolic BP of 160 mm Hg or more (stage 2 or 3 hypertension).* As pointed out earlier, the absolute risk and absolute benefit of treatment is related to the burden of and modification of associated risk factors as well as to the patient's BP (see "Risks and Risk Reduction").

For stage 1 hypertension (systolic BP 140 to 159 mm Hg or diastolic BP 90 to 99 mm Hg), an individualized approach to initial treatment is recommended. The presence at baseline of *multiple major cardiovascular risk factors* (smoking, hypercholesterolemia, diabetes, age over 60, male gender, postmenopause, a strong family history of cardiovascular morbidity), or *target organ disease* (TOD, see Table 62.11) are characteristics that favor initial drug treatment for such patients. Figure 62.1 shows the graded impact of risk factors, TOD, and BPs on the 10-year prognosis of patients with stage 1 hypertension. For patients with stage 1 hypertension who do not have these associated characteristics, it is reasonable to try nonpharmacologic treatment for up to 1 year (risk group A: no risk factors or TOD) or 6 months (risk group B: one risk factor, not including diabetes), especially in those patients who voice a strong preference to try this approach.

Special considerations for the treatment of hypertension in *adolescents, elderly persons, and pregnant women* are discussed in subsequent sections of this chapter.

Table 62.10.   Risk Stratification and Treatment[a]

	Risk Group A	Risk Group B	Risk Group C
	No risk factors[b] No TOD/CCD[c]	At least one risk factor, not including diabetes No TOD/CCD[c]	TOD/CCD[c] or diabetes, with or without other risk factors
Blood pressure stages (mm Hg):			
High-normal (130–139/85–89)	Lifestyle modification	Lifestyle modification	Drug therapy[e]
Stage 1 (140–159/90–99)	Lifestyle modification (up to 12 months)	Lifestyle modification[d] (up to 6 months)	Drug therapy
Stages 2 and 3 (≥160/≥100)	Drug therapy	Drug therapy	Drug therapy

For example, a patient with diabetes and a blood pressure of 142/94 mm Hg plus left ventricular hypertrophy should be classified as having stage 1 hypertension with target organ disease (left ventricular hypertrophy) and with another major risk factor (diabetes). This patient would be categorized as *stage 1, risk group C,* and recommended for immediate initiation of pharmacologic treatment.
From The Sixth Report of the Joint National Committee on Prevention, Detection, Evaluation, and Treatment of High Blood Pressure. Arch Intern Med 157:2413, 1997.
[a]Lifestyle modification should be adjunctive therapy for all patients recommended for pharmacologic therapy.
[b]Major risk factors (see Figure 62.1).
[c]*TOD/CCD,* Target organ disease/clinical cardiovascular disease (see Table 62.11).
[d]For patients with multiple risk factors, clinicans should consider drugs as initial therapy plus lifestyle modifications.
[e]For those with heart failure or renal insufficiency or those with diabetes.

Table 62.11.   Manifestations of Target Organ Disease

Organ System	Manifestations
Cardiac	Clinical, ECG, or radiologic evidence of coronary artery disease; LVH or "strain" by ECG or LVH by echocardiography; left ventricular dysfunction or cardiac failure
Cerebrovascular	Transient ischemic attack or stroke
Peripheral vascular	Absence of one or more major pulses in extremities (except for dorsalis pedis) with or without intermittent claudication; aneurysm
Renal	Serum creatinine ≥130 μmol/L (1.5 mg/dL); proteinuria (1+ or greater); microalbuminuria
Retinopathy	Hemorrhages or exudates, with or without papilledema

From The Fifth Report of the Joint National Committee on Detection, Evaluation, and Treatment of High Blood Pressure (JNC V). Arch Intern Med 153:154, 1993.

Nonpharmacologic Treatment

A number of nonpharmacologic modalities prevent the development of HBP (see "Primary Prevention," above) or lower BP. Although there have not been clinical trials of the impact of these measures upon symptomatic cardiovascular disease, there is evidence that nonpharmacologic control of HBP may be as effective as pharmacologic control in preventing LVH (84). Those individual measures for which there is evidence for effectiveness include reducing weight, reducing daily intake of sodium chloride, increasing physical exercise, and limiting alcohol intake (81). Each of these has been shown to produce long-term reduction of BP in some patients and to add to the BP-lowering effect in patients who take antihypertensive drugs.

Recently, *a diet that is rich in fruits and vegetables and low in saturated and total fat* also has been shown to reduce BP independently of exercise, salt reduction, and weight reduction (4). The effect on BP occurred during 8 weeks. Long-term impact probably persists. Because this multifactor diet reduces other risk factors, it should be recommended to motivated patients in conjunction with other nonpharmacologic measures.

Nonpharmacologic measures require significant changes in lifestyle, and it is generally more difficult to achieve long-term adherence to them than to drug treatment. Nevertheless, for motivated patients with stage 1 hypertension, one or more of these can be tried as primary treatment (Table 62.10), and they should be recommended, when pertinent, to all patients who are beginning treatment with antihypertensive drugs.

Weight Reduction

Practical approaches to weight reduction are described in Chapter 76 ("Obesity"). A decrease in BP may occur after only modest weight loss (e.g., about 10 pounds) (81).

Sodium Restriction (60)

Limitation of daily sodium intake to 100 mmol (about 2 g) of elemental sodium, which is equivalent to 4 to 6 g of salt, should be recommended to all patients with hypertension. The impact of salt reduction occurs over weeks. If BP decreases to and remains at normal levels, salt limitation should be maintained as definitive therapy.

Tables 62.12 and 62.13, which can be copied for distribution to patients, summarize what patients need to know to follow a low-salt diet. When giving this information to a patient, it is important to point out that approximately 75% of one's daily intake of salt usually comes in processed foods ("What Not to Eat" column, Table 62.13) and that there are many ways to make food tasty without adding salt (Table 62.12).

Salt use and diuretics. As discussed below, when a patient continues to ingest a large amount of salt while taking diuretics, potassium wasting is increased. Therefore salt restriction may both prevent excessive potassium loss and facilitate BP reduction in patients taking diuretics.

Physical Exercise

Both *low-intensity exercise* (e.g., gardening, walking, or cycling at approximately 40 to 60% of

Table 62.12.   Information for Patients Who Are Advised to Follow a 2-g Sodium Diet

Americans eat about **20 times more sodium** than they need, most of which comes from salt, which is one source of sodium.

Sodium is:

found naturally in foods, even those that do not taste salty.

added to food by manufacturers in food processing.

added in cooking in the form of salt, baking powder, baking soda, or seasonings such as monosodium glutamate (MSG).

added as salt to food at the table.

Add New Flavors to Your Food!
☐ Herbs and spices can give new zest to your unsalted cooking.
☐ A little herb goes a long way. If you are making your own substitution without the benefit of a recipe, try ¼ teaspoon of dried herb or spice to:

a recipe for 4 servings,

a pound of meat, poultry, fish, or vegetable or 2 cups of sauce.

If you are using red pepper or garlic powder start with only ⅛ teaspoon. Taste and add a little more depending on your preference.

☐ If you use fresh herbs use four times the amount of dried herb. Instead of ¼ teaspoon of dried herb use 1 full teaspoon of fresh herb.
☐ Add dried herbs to soups and stews during the last hour of cooking.
☐ Use whole spices in slow-cooking dishes and add them at the beginning of the cooking period.

Beware of Hidden Sodium!
Processed Foods

Salt is added to many packaged, convenience, "fast," and canned foods. Examples are packaged dinners (e.g., macaroni and cheese), packaged coatings and "helpers," combination dinners (e.g., frozen meals and casserole dishes), canned soups, dried soups, canned vegetables, and frozen vegetables with sauces.

"Fast Foods"

Generally, meals served at "fast food" places are high in sodium. A typical meal of a hamburger, french fries, and a vanilla shake can total more than 1000 mg of sodium—more than half of your total daily allowance. Remember pizza, hot dogs, burgers, fried chicken, fried fish, omelettes, and tacos served at fast food places are usually high in sodium. Just one whole dill pickle contains 1900 mg of sodium, almost the total allowed in this diet.

Read labels carefully. Foods that list salt or sodium as ingredients should be avoided. Compare different brands of the same product. It is unnecessary to purchase special dietetic foods. Many dietetic foods contain sodium or salt, **so read the labels carefully.**

Some Tips on Eating Out!
☐ Select restaurants that offer à la carte service.
☐ For breakfast, order from the allowed cereals. Poached or boiled eggs with toast may be ordered at most restaurants.
☐ For lunch, try fruit or tossed salads; roast beef, sliced chicken, or turkey breast sandwich; and fruit for dessert.
☐ At dinner, try fruit (fresh, canned, or frozen), fruit juice, or fruit cup as an appetizer.
☐ If you select broiled meats, fresh fish, or chicken, you may request that no salt or other condiments like garlic salt or onion salt be added before or after broiling.
☐ Inside cuts of roast beef, lamb, pork, veal, chicken, and turkey have less sodium than outside cuts. Trim off the edges that would have been salted. Ask that it be served without gravy or sauce.

To Sum It Up
☐ Using less salt is advisable for almost everyone, even children, so let the whole family join in.
☐ Avoid shaking salt on your food. Substitute a blend of herbs for your salt shaker.
☐ Cook without salt. Try leaving it out of recipes.
☐ Experiment with new flavors by using herbs and spices. Fine restaurants rely on herbs, spices, and the natural flavor of food, *not salt,* for good taste.
☐ Avoid fast foods and other processed foods high in sodium.
☐ Read the labels of foods and medicines to find "hidden" sodium. Look for the symbol: Na^+; look for the words: salt, sodium, soda, brine.
☐ Become familiar with foods that are high in sodium.

In the body, sodium acts like a sponge to hold water in the body tissues. Sometimes the body cannot get rid of enough of the sodium. High blood pressure may result. If not controlled, high blood pressure leads to stroke, kidney failure, and heart disease.

Using no salt in cooking or at the table and eliminating highly salted food cuts down the sodium level of the food you eat to about **2000 mg day**.

☐ When using ground spices, add them 15 minutes before the end of the cooking period. If adding them to uncooked dishes, add them several hours before serving. As a start, try one or a combination of the following popular herbs:

Basil	Rosemary
Celery seed	Sage
Marjoram	Savory
Mint	Thyme

Additives

Sodium may be added to food as a preservative; for quick cooking; to soften or loosen skins of fruits and vegetables; to cure meats, fish, sausage; to stop growth of molds. Additives that contain sodium include:

Monosodium glutamate (MSG)
Baking soda
Disodium phosphate
Sodium alginate
Sodium benzoate
Sodium hydroxide
Sodium nitrate
Sodium propionate
Sodium sulfite

☐ In ordering rice, ask if it has been cooked in salted water. Some restaurants cook rice without salt. Rice pilaf is usually prepared with salt.
☐ You can count on baked potato. For toppings use butter, margarine, or sour cream.
☐ If in doubt about cooked vegetables, order sliced tomatoes or a salad such as tossed salad, lettuce wedge, or fruit salad. Try lemon or oil and vinegar for the dressing. Ask the waiter to leave off the croutons!
☐ Help yourself to the bread basket, but avoid salted breadsticks and crackers with salted tops.
☐ For dessert select fruit, sherbet, ice cream, or plain yogurt.
☐ Most airlines provide "special meals." A low-sodium meal may be ordered at no extra cost when you make your flight reservation.
☐ Fast food menu items (except for the salad bar where you can select low-sodium items) have usually been salted. If food can be prepared to order, request that no salted seasonings be added.

☐ Low-sodium salt, such as "Lite Salt," is a combination of sodium and potassium. Do not be misled that it is free of sodium. It has about half the sodium content of regular salt.
Use of low-sodium salt and salt substitutes can be dangerous because of the very high potassium content. It is **essential** that you ask your doctor if you may use them. Also ask **how much** you may use each day.

Modified from "Health Is In—Salt is Out," courtesy of The Maryland High Blood Pressure Coordinating Council.

Table 62.13.   Food List for Patients Who Are Advised to Follow a 2-g Sodium Diet (Shows What to Eat and What Not to Eat)[a]

Category	What to Eat	What Not to Eat
Vegetables	**Fresh and Most Frozen Vegetables** Artichoke, Asparagus, Avocado, Bamboo shoots, Bean sprouts, Beets, Broccoli, Brussels sprouts, Cabbage, Carrots, Cauliflower, Celery, Chicory, Collards, Corn, Cucumber, Dried beans, Dried peas, Eggplant, Endive, Escarole, Green beans, Kale, Kohlrabi, Leeks, Lettuce, Lima beans, Mixed vegetables, Mushrooms, Mustard greens, Okra, Onion, Parsley, Parsnips, Peas, Peppers, Potato, sweet, Potato, white, Pumpkin, Radishes, Rutabaga, Scallions, Soybeans, Spinach, Squash, summer, Squash, acorn winter, Tomato, Tomato juice, low sodium, Turnip, V-8 Juice, low sodium, Water chestnuts, Watercress, Wax beans, Yams *Note:* Low-sodium canned vegetables may be used.	Canned vegetables, Canned tomato juice, Canned vegetable juice, Frozen peas, Frozen lima beans, Frozen vegetables with seasoned sauce, Olives, Pickled vegetables, Pickles, Sauerkraut, Seaweed
Breads	**Breads** Cracked wheat, French, Hamburger roll, Hot dog roll, Italian, Raisin, Rye, Vienna, White, enriched, Whole wheat	Danish pastries, Muffins, Pancakes, Pizza, Spoonbread, Stuffing mix, Sweet rolls, Waffles
Crackers	**Crackers** Matzoh, Melba toast, Rusk, Rye Krisp, Zwieback	**Crackers/Snack Foods[a]** Crackers with salted tops, Pretzels, Soda crackers, Consider crackers, chips, pretzels to be high in sodium unless labeled as "unsalted"
Cereals	**Cereals** Barley, Cream of Wheat, regular, Cornmeal, Granola, Grits, regular, Oatmeal, regular, Petijohns, Popcorn, unsalted, Puffed Rice, Puffed Wheat, Ralston, Rice, Shredded Wheat, Special K, Tapioca, Wheatena	**Cereals** Dry cereals, except those listed under "What to Eat", Instant grits, Instant hot cereals, Salted popcorn
Pastas	**Pastas, Cooked Without Salt** Macaroni, Noodles, Spaghetti	**Pastas** Chow mein noodles, Prepackaged meals, such as macaroni, noodle, or spaghetti dinners
Protein Foods	**Lean Fresh Meat** Beef, Lamb, Liver, Pork, Veal	Bacon, Canned meats, Corned beef, Dried chipped beef, Ham, cured or "low salt", Hotdogs, Luncheon meats, Salt pork, Sausage, Scrapple, Smoked meats, Salted or pickled meats, Meat extenders and "helpers", TV and frozen meat dinners, "Fast food" meats
Fruits	**Fresh, Frozen, Canned, or Dried Fruit** Apple, Apple juice, Applesauce, Apricots, Banana, Berries, Cantaloupe, Cherries, Cranberries, Dates, Figs, Grapefruit, Grapefruit juice, Lemon, Nectarine, Orange, Orange juice, Peach, Pear, Pineapple, Pineapple juice, Plums, Prunes, Prune juice, Raisins, Raspberries, Rhubarb	Dried fruits that contain sodium preservative

Foods to Use	Foods to Avoid
Fresh Fish Bass Bluefish Carp Cod Flounder Haddock Hake Halibut Ocean perch Pike Pollack Pompano Porgy Red snapper Rockfish Salmon Shad Sole Swordfish Trout Tuna Whitefish	Anchovy Canned fish Commercially frozen fish "Fast food" fish Herring Salted fish Sardines Smoked or pickled fish TV and frozen fish dinners
Fresh Shellfish Crab Lobster Oysters* Shrimp *If from saltwater bed, rinse saltwater out with fresh water.	Crabs, prepared with salty seasoning Mussels Scallops
Peanut Butter	
Dried Beans, Cooked Without Salt, Salt pork, or Ham	Canned beans
Lean Fresh Poultry Capon Chicken Cornish hen Duck Goose Turkey	Canned chicken Canned turkey Commercial fried chicken TV dinners Turkey roll Frozen turkey or chicken casseroles/pies Frozen omelet Frozen souffle Frozen quiche
Beverages Alcoholic beverages, in moderation Club soda Cocoa Coffee—ground, instant, decaffeinated Soft drinks Sugar-free beverages, in moderation Tea—loose, teabags, instant Tonic water Wine	
Breads, Crackers **Breads** Cinnamon Corn and molasses **Crackers** Any crackers with unsalted tops	**Breads** Biscuits Cornbread Croutons, packaged
Desserts Grapes Grape juice Honeydew Strawberries Tangerine Watermelon Custard, homemade Fruit Fruit cake Fruit cobbler Gelatin desserts, all flavors Ice cream Ice milk Lady fingers Sherbert Sponge cake, homemade Yogurt, plain	**Commercially Prepared** Cake Cookies Donuts Pie Pudding mixes Sweet rolls
Seasonings Garlic, fresh or powdered Herbs and spices Horseradish, fresh or prepared Lemon, juice and peel Onion, fresh, powdered, or flaked Pepper Tabasco sauce Vanilla extract Vinegar Wine Worcestershire sauce (used sparingly)	Barbeque sauce Catsup Celery salt Chili sauce Cooking wine (has salt added) Garlic salt Lemon pepper seasoning Meat tenderizers Monosodium glutamate (MSG) Onion salt Pickle relish Prepared mustard Salt, seasoned or plain Sea salt Soy sauce Steak sauce
Dairy Products Skim milk Dry milk Evaporated milk Yogurt, plain Brie Cheddar Colby Cottage Gruyere Monterey Jack Mozzarella Muenster Natural Swiss Neufchatel Port du Salut Ricotta Cheese labeled "low sodium" or "unsalted"	Buttermilk (commercial) Condensed milk "Fast food" shakes Bleu Camembert Cheezola Edam Feta Gouda Limburger Parmesan Processed cheese, American and Swiss Processed cheese foods Processed cheese spreads Provolone Roquefort Romano Slim Line cheese Tilsit

Adapted from "Health Is In—Salt Is Out," courtesy of The Maryland High Blood Pressure Coordinating Council.

aUseful conversions: 100 mg of sodium = 4.35 mEq of sodium.
100 mg of sodium = 250 mg of salt.
1 teaspoon of salt = 6 g of sodium.

maximum oxygen consumption) and the high-intensity exercise needed to attain cardiac conditioning have BP-lowering effects. A typical low-intensity exercise program would be walking briskly for a distance of 3 miles four or more times per week. Chapter 58 provides details regarding low-intensity exercise and exercise programs needed to achieve cardiovascular conditioning.

Physical activities while taking antihypertensive drugs. Most patients want to be informed about the implications of hypertension and antihypertensive drug therapy for ordinary physical activity. Subjects with untreated hypertension have the same patterns of BP fluctuation during exercise as normotensive subjects, only at higher pressures: with vigorous exercise, the systolic pressure rises (as much as 60 mm Hg) while the diastolic pressure may rise or fall slightly. Similar patterns are usually found in patients treated with antihypertensive drugs. The effects of a number of antihypertensives and other cardiovascular drugs on BP during exercise are summarized in Chapter 58, Table 58.10. Overall, it is reasonable to inform patients that their hypertension does not make them different and to reassure them that they can engage in all of their usual activities after beginning treatment for hypertension.

Moderation or Discontinuation of Alcohol Intake

Limiting alcohol intake by social drinkers to 2 ounces/day (e.g., 2 cans of beer, 2 glasses of wine, 2 one-jigger drinks) and treating alcoholism have both been shown to be efficacious as the only treatment or as adjunctive treatment for some hypertensive patients. Approaches useful in the detection and treatment of alcoholism are described in Chapter 21.

Dietary Potassium (101)

Consuming a diet with substantial potassium content may facilitate the BP-lowering effects of weight reduction, sodium restriction, or antihypertensive drugs. Increased potassium intake usually occurs as a consequence of changing to a low-sodium diet, which tends to contain more potassium-rich natural foods (e.g., fresh fruits and vegetables) in place of processed food. Because potassium deficiency may cause the BP to increase, maintenance of a normal potassium concentration (3.5 mEq/L or more) probably facilitates the BP-lowering effect of diuretics.

Cognitive and Behavioral Techniques

Cognitive and behavioral techniques include biofeedback, stress management, meditation, and muscle relaxation techniques (38). Critical assessment of clinical trials of these techniques does not support the efficacy of any of them as a primary method for decreasing BP (26,81). Motivated patients may wish to use one of these techniques as an adjunct to another primary treatment strategy. Muscle relaxation tech-

niques useful for stress reduction are described in Chapter 13.

Other Substances and Nutrients

Adequate intake of *calcium and magnesium* may promote BP reduction, but there is no evidence that increased amounts of either of these nutrients should be recommended. Although *fish oils* may lower BP, they are associated with adverse effects that counterbalance the small benefit. *Caffeine and nicotine* may transiently raise BP, but elimination of these does not lower BP. The amount of nicotine patches and other smoking cessation aids described in Chapter 20 does not usually raise BP (45).

Pharmacologic Treatment: General Recommendations

To date, objective methods for selecting the most appropriate antihypertensive drug for an individual patient have not been developed. Therefore drug treatment for most patients should be initiated and adjusted using the strategies recommended in the algorithm from the 1997 JNC Report (Fig. 62.5). The JNC continues to recommend initial treatment with a diuretic or a β-blocker because these remain the two classes of drugs that have been shown to reduce morbidity and mortality in randomized controlled trials (73). In older patients with isolated systolic hypertension, a long-acting nondihydropyridine (nitrendipine) has also been shown to be efficacious (83). As indicated in the algorithm and discussed below ("Individualizing Drug Selection"), a number of considerations may be helpful when selecting drugs for individual patients.

The impact of most antihypertensive drugs on the BP occurs within 1 day to 1 week. For patients with stage 1 or stage 2 HBP, it is reasonable to evaluate the response to medications within 1 month. Patients with stage 3 hypertension (e.g., systolic BP 180 mm Hg or more or diastolic BP 110 mm Hg or more) should be evaluated frequently until there is evidence that the BP is responding to the drug(s) or dosage(s) prescribed.

Because drugs from each class of antihypertensives are available in preparations that are effective for 24 hours or longer, it is prudent to attempt to control patients' BPs with a *once-a-day medication schedule*.

Monotherapy

Classes

Antihypertensive drugs belong to one of the following classes listed in Table 62.14: diuretics, adrenergic inhibitors, direct vasodilators, calcium antagonists, ACE inhibitors, or angiotensin II receptor blockers.

Initial monotherapy with a low dosage of a diuretic (e.g., 12.5 to 25 mg of hydrochlorothiazide daily) or a β-blocker (e.g., 25 to 50 mg of atenolol daily) is appropriate for many or most patients (81). The rationale for this recommendation is that drugs from one of these two classes—but not from the newer classes of drugs—were the principal drugs in each of the

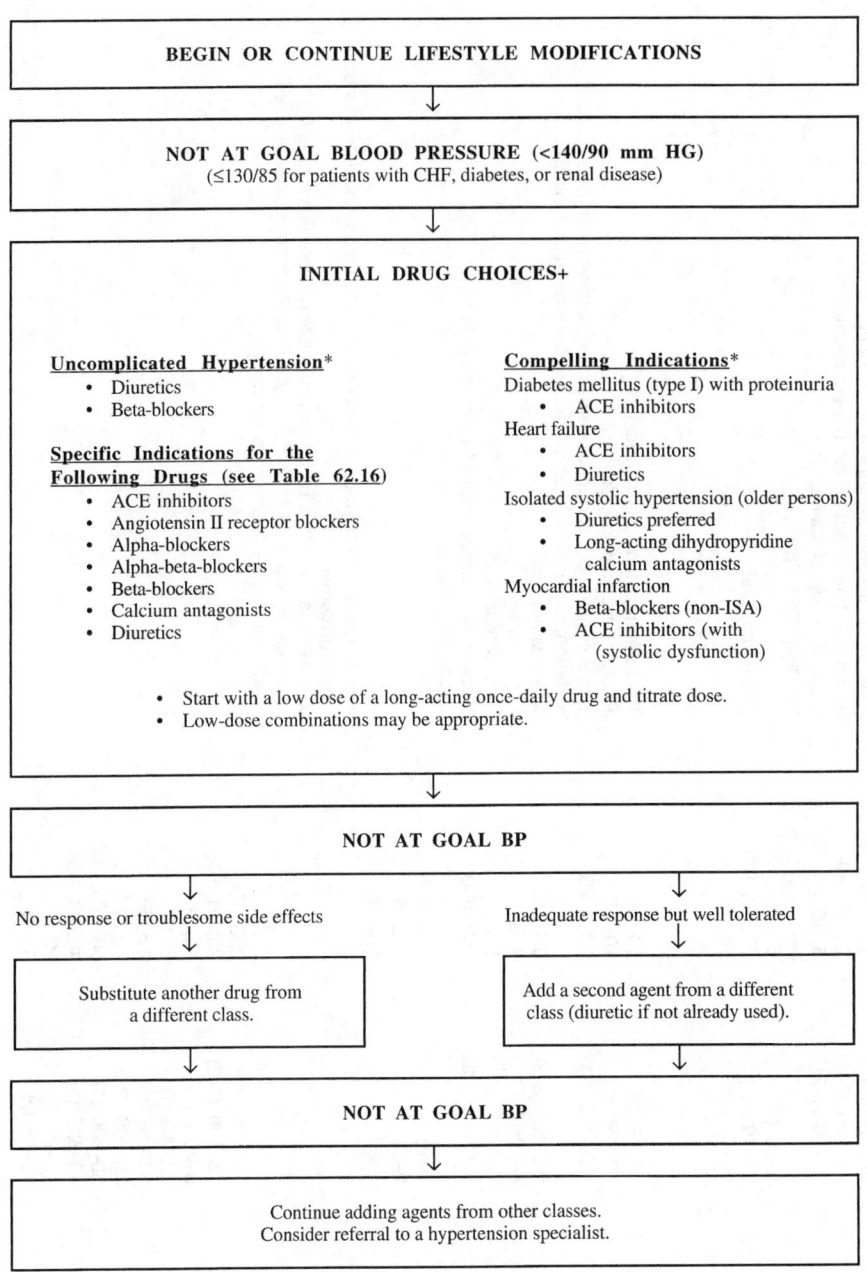

Figure 62.5. Treatment algorithm. (Adapted from The Sixth Report of the Joint National Committee on Detection, Evaluation, and Treatment of High Blood Pressure [JNC VI]. Arch Intern Med 157:2413, 1997.)

placebo-controlled trials that showed that treatment decreases mortality and major morbidity (73). Tables 62.4 and 62.5 summarize features of the major placebo-controlled trials.

Because drugs from each of the classes of antihypertensive drugs effectively reduce BP (55,90), monotherapy with most of them can be chosen initially; exceptions are two vasodilators—hydralazine and minoxidil—that usually require cotreatment with an adrenergic inhibitor to prevent reflex tachycardia. For most patients, it is reasonable to assess the response to monotherapy after 2 to 4 weeks. In systematic studies,

it has been shown that 50% or more of patients will respond to low-dose monotherapy alone (55,90). Increasing the dosage of the initial drug, substituting another drug, or adding a drug or drugs from another class are strategies that lead to control in most patients who do not respond to or tolerate the initial regimen (Fig. 62.5).

To establish whether drugs from other classes of antihypertensives are superior to diuretics and β-blockers, at least eight large clinical trials are in progress. End points in all are cardiovascular events. Most compare monotherapy with one or more

Table 62.14.   Oral Antihypertensive Drugs[a]

Drug Classes and Drugs	Trade Name	Usual Dose Range in Total mg/day[a] (Frequency per Day)	Available Strengths (mg)	Selected Side Effects and Comments[a] (Parentheses = Individual Drug Effect; All Others Are Class Effects)
DIURETICS (PARTIAL LIST)				
Thiazide and thiazidelike diuretics				Short-term: ↑ cholesterol, ↑ glucose / Biochemical abnormalities: ↓ potassium, ↓ sodium, ↑ uric acid, ↑ calcium, ↓ magnesium / Rare: blood dyscrasias, photosensitivity, pancreatitis, hyponatremia
Chlorthalidone (G)[b]	Hygroton	12.5–50 (1)	25, 50	
Hydrochlorothiazide (G)	Hydrodiuril, Microzide, Esidrix	12.5–50 (1)	25, 50	
Indapamide	Lozol	1.25–5 (1)	2.5	(Less or no hypercholesterolemia)
Metolazone	Mykrox	0.5–1.0 (1)	0.5	
	Zaroxolyn	2.5–10 (1)	2.5, 5	
Loop diuretics				
Bumetanide (G)	Bumex	0.5–4 (2–3)	0.5, 1	(Short duration of action, no hypercalcemia)
Ethacrynic acid	Edecrin	25–100 (2–3)	50	(Only nonsulfonamide diuretic, ototoxicity)
Furosemide (G)	Lasix	40–240 (2–3)	20, 40, 80	(Short duration of action, no hypercalcemia)
Torsemide	Demadex	5–100 (1–2)	5, 10, 20, 100	(Long duration of action)
Potassium-sparing agents				
Amiloride (G)	Midamor	5–10 (1)	5	Hyperkalemia
Spironolactone (G)	Aldactone	25–100 (1)	25, 50, 100	(Gynecomastia)
Triamterene (G)	Dyrenium	25–100 (1)	50, 100	
ADRENERGIC INHIBITORS				
Peripheral-acting agents				
Guanadrel	Hylorel	10–75 (2)	10, 25	(Postural hypotension, diarrhea)
Guanethidine	Ismelin	10–150 (1)	10, 25	(Postural hypotension, diarrhea)
Reserpine (G)[c]	Serpasil	0.05–0.25 (1)	0.1, 0.25	(Nasal congestion, sedation, depression, activation of peptic ulcer)
Centrally acting				
Clonidine (G)	Catapres	0.2–1.2 (2–3)	0.1, 0.2	Sedation, dry mouth, bradycardia, withdrawal hypertension
Guanabenz (G)	Wytensin	8–32 (2)	4, 8	(More withdrawal)
Guanfacine (G)	Tenex	1–3 (1)	1, 2	(Less withdrawal)
Methyldopa (G)	Aldomet	500–3000 (2)	250, 500	(Hepatic and "autoimmune" disorders)
α-blockers				
Doxazosin	Cardura	1–16 (1)	1, 2, 4, 8	Postural hypotension
Prazosin (G)	Minipress	2–30 (2–3)	1, 2, 5	
Terazosin (G)	Hytrin	1–20 (1)	1, 2, 5, 10	
β-Blockers				Bronchospasm, bradycardia, heart failure, may mask insulin-induced hypoglycemia / Less serious: impaired peripheral circulation, insomnia, fatigue, decreased exercise tolerance, hypertriglyceridemia (except agents with intrinsic sympathomimetic activity)
Acebutolol[d,e]	Sectral	200–800 (1)	200, 400	
Atenolol (G)[d]	Tenormin	25–100 (1–2)	25, 50, 100	
Betaxolol[d]	Kerlone	5–20 (1)	10, 20	
Bisoprolol[d]	Zebeta	2.5–10 (1)	5, 10	
Carteolol[e]	Cartrol	2.5–5 (1)	2.5, 5	
Metoprolol (G)[d]	Lopressor	50–300 (2)	50, 100	
	Toprol-XL	50–300 (1)	50, 100, 200	
Nadolol (G)	Corgard	40–320 (1)	40, 80, 120	
Penbutolol[e]	Levatol	10–20 (1)	20	
Pindolol (G)[e]	Visken	10–60 (2)	5, 10	

Drug	Trade Name	Usual Dose Range in mg/day (Doses per Day)	Dose Strengths (mg)	Selected Side Effects and Comments
Propranolol (G)	Inderal	40–480 (2)	10, 20, 40, 60, 80	
Timolol (G)	Inderal LA	40–480 (1)	80, 120, 160	
	Blocadren	20–60 (2)	5, 10, 20	
Combined α- and β-blockers				Postural hypotension, bronchospasm
Carvedilol	Coreg	12.5–50 (2)	3.125, 6.25, 12.5, 25	
Labetalol (G)	Normodyne, Trandate	200–1200 (2)	100, 200, 300	
DIRECT VASODILATORS				Headaches, fluid retention, tachycardia
Hydralazine (G)	Apresoline	50–300 (2)	10, 25, 50, 100	(Lupus syndrome)
Minoxidil (G)	Loniten	5–100 (1)	2.5, 10	(Hirsutism)
CALCIUM ANTAGONISTS				
Nondihydropyridines				Conduction defects, worsening of systolic dysfunction, gingival hyperplasia
Diltiazem	Cardizem SR	120–360 (2)	60, 80, 120	(Nausea, headache)
	Cardizem CD, Dilacor XR, Tiazac	120–360 (1)	120, 180, 240, 300	
Mibefradil (T channel calcium antagonist)	Posicor	50–100 (1)	50, 100	(No worsening of systolic dysfunction; contraindicated with terfenadine, astemizole, and cisapride, lovastatin, simvistatin)
Verapamil	Isoptin, Calan	40, 80, 120 (3)	120, 180, 240	(Constipation)
	Isoptin SR, Calan SR	90–480 (2)	120, 180, 240, 360	
	Verelan, Covera HS	120–480 (1)		
Dihydropyridines				Ankle edema, flushing, headache, gingival hypertrophy
Amlodipine	Norvasc	2.5–10 (1)	2.5, 5, 10	
Felodipine	Plendil	2.5–20 (1)	5, 10	
Isradipine	DynaCirc	5–20 (2)	2.5, 5	
	DynaCirc CR	5–20 (1)	5, 10	
Nicardipine	Cardene SR	60–90 (1)	20, 30	
Nifedipine	Procardia XL, Adalat CC	30–120 (1)	30, 60, 90	
Nisoldipine	Sular	20–60 (1)	10, 20, 30, 40	
ACE INHIBITORS				Common: cough
Benazepril	Lotensin	5–40 (1–2)	5, 10, 20, 40	Rare: angioedema, hyperkalemia, rash, loss of taste, leucopenia
Captopril (G)	Capoten	25–150 (2–3)	12.5, 25, 50, 100	
Enalapril	Vasotec	5–40 (1–2)	2.5, 5, 10, 20	
Fosinopril	Monopril	10–40 (1–2)	10, 20	
Lisinopril	Prinivil, Zestril	5–40 (1)	5, 10, 20, 40	
Moexipril	Univasc	7.5–15 (2)	7.5, 15	
Quinapril	Accupril	5–80 (1–2)	5, 10, 20, 40	
Ramipril	Altace	1.25–20 (1–2)	1.25, 2.5, 5, 10	
Trandolapril	Mavik	1–4 (1)	1, 2, 4	
ANGIOTENSIN II RECEPTOR BLOCKERS				Angioedema (very rare), hyperkalemia
Losartan	Cozaar	25–100 (1–2)	25, 50	
Valsartan	Diovan	80–320 (1)	80, 160	
Irbesartan	Avapro	150–300 (1)	150, 300	

From The Sixth Report of the Joint National Committee on Prevention, Detection, Evaluation, and Treatment of High Blood Pressure. Arch Intern Med 157:2413, 1997.

a These dosages may vary from those listed in the *Physicians' Desk Reference*, which may be consulted for additional information. The listing of side effects is not all-inclusive, and clinicians are urged to refer to the package insert for a more detailed listing.

b G = generic available.

c = also acts centrally.

d = cardioselective.

e = has intrinsic sympathomimetic activity.

nondiuretics to diuretic or β-blocker monotherapy. Results for most of these trials will not be known until 1999 or later. The largest trial ALLHAT (The Antihypertensive and Lipid-Lowering Treatment for the Prevention of Heart Attack Trial) will enroll 40,000 patients 60 years and older and will measure the impact of a diuretic (chlorthalidone), a calcium blocker (amlodipine), an α-blocker (doxazosin), and an ACE inhibitor (lisinopril) on coronary artery disease (102).

Many proprietary antihypertensive drugs are substantially more expensive than *generic preparations*. Generic preparations are available for each class of drug except the newest class, the angiotensin II receptor blockers (Table 62.14).

Additional properties of drugs in each class are described in detail below (see "Selected Properties of Individual Drugs").

Drug Combinations

Combinations of antihypertensive drugs from most classes have been studied (29,56,81). The principal advantage of combining agents is successful BP control—often with relatively low dosages of drugs from different classes—in patients whose BP is not controlled with monotherapy. This advantage has been demonstrated in a number of studies, including one that randomly allocated nonresponding patients to two-drug combinations of drugs from each of the following classes: diuretic (hydrochlorothiazide), β-blocker (atenolol), ACE inhibitor (captopril), α-blocker (prazosin), calcium antagonist (diltiazem-SR), and central-acting α-agonist (clonidine) (56).

Adding a Diuretic

The addition of a diuretic has been shown to enhance the antihypertensive effect of all nondiuretic drugs. This synergy may be due to reversal of the sodium retention that frequently accompanies BP lowering by nondiuretic antihypertensives, a response that may attenuate their antihypertensive effects. Therefore, in a patient who does not achieve control with one of the nondiuretic drugs, the *addition of a low dosage of a thiazide diuretic* should be considered, especially if the patient gains weight or develops edema despite instructions to limit salt intake. More potent diuretic regimens or the addition of potassium-sparing diuretics may be needed in some patients.

Fixed-Dose Combination Tablets

Drugs from two or more classes of antihypertensive drugs (usually a low-dose thiazide diuretic plus one or two nondiuretics) are available in the fixed-dose combinations listed in Table 62.15. The appropriate combination tablets may provide additional convenience at no additional cost. Examples are thiazide/potassium-sparing diuretic, β-blocker–diuretic, ACE inhibitor–diuretic, calcium antagonist–ACE inhibitor, angiotensin II receptor antagonist–diuretic combinations, and the combination of low-dose reserpine, hydralazine, and hydrochlorothiazide. An especially potent

regimen—the combination of a loop diuretic (e.g., furosemide) with a low dosage of a diuretic active at the distal convoluted tubule (e.g., a thiazide or metolazone)—may occasionally be needed to control volume overload in a patient whose hypertension is related to this (27).

Special Advantages of Drug Combinations

Several antihypertensive drug combinations have been shown to have advantages in addition to control of BP:

- ACE inhibitor plus nondihydropyridine calcium blocker: may enhance impact of ACE inhibitor on preservation of renal function in patients with diabetes nephropathy
- ACE inhibitor added to thiazide or loop diuretic: may prevent diuretic-induced hypokalemia
- Adrenergic inhibitor (β-blocker or central-acting α-agonist) plus vasodilator (hydralazine or minoxidil): the former prevents reflex tachycardia induced by a vasodilator, enabling patient to take the latter potent antihypertensive drug

Individualizing Drug Selection

A number of factors may be helpful in choosing initial drugs for individual patients.

Demographic Characteristics

In general, *African-American subjects* respond less often than whites to ACE inhibitor and β-blocker monotherapy and more often to monotherapy with diuretics; calcium antagonists and α–β-blockers are also effective as monotherapy. A large proportion of *older patients* with diastolic or isolated systolic hypertension respond to low-dose diuretic monotherapy; long-acting nondihydropyridine calcium antagonists have also been shown to be effective in controlling the BP in older patients. *Gender* has not been correlated with selected advantages or disadvantages of any classes of antihypertensive drugs. Because the potent vasodilator minoxidil causes marked hirsutism, it is not an acceptable medication for women. Additional considerations in managing hypertension in *adolescents*, *older patients*, and *pregnant patients* are discussed in later sections of this chapter.

Coexisting Medical Conditions

Coexisting medical conditions may influence the selection of antihypertensive drugs. Figure 62.5 and Table 62.16 list as *compelling indications* several conditions for which there is evidence for drug-specific benefits from randomized controlled trials:

- Type 1 diabetes with proteinuria: ACE inhibitors
- Heart failure (systolic dysfunction): ACE inhibitors, diuretics
- Isolated systolic HBP in older persons: diuretics, long-acting dihydropyridines
- MI: β-blockers (non-ISA), ACE inhibitors (if systolic dysfunction)

Table 62.15.   Combination Drugs for Hypertension

Drug	Trade Name
β-Adrenergic Blockers and Diuretics	
Atenolol 50 or 100 mg/chlorthalidone 25 mg	Tenoretic
Bisoprolol 2.5, 5, or 10 mg/hydrochlorothiazide 6.25 mg	Ziac[a]
Metoprolol 50 or 100 mg/hydrochlorothiazide 25 or 50 mg	Lopressor HCT
Nadolol 40 or 80 mg/bendroflumethiazide 5 mg	Corzide
Propranolol 40 or 80 mg/hydrochlorothiazide 25 mg	Inderide
Propranolol (extended release) 80, 120, or 160 mg/hydrochlorothiazide 50 mg	Inderide LA
Timolol 10 mg/hydrochlorothiazide 25 mg	Timolide
ACE Inhibitors and Diuretics	
Benazepril 5, 10, or 20 mg/hydrochlorothiazide 6.25, 12.5, or 25 mg	Lotensin HCT
Captopril 25 or 50 mg/hydrochlorothiazide 15 or 25 mg	Capozide[a]
Enalapril 5 or 10 mg/hydrochlorothiazide 12.5 or 25 mg	Vaseretic
Lisinopril 10 or 20 mg/hydrochlorothiazide 12.5 or 25 mg	Prinzide, Zestoretic
Angiotensin II Receptor Antagonists and Diuretics	
Losartan 50 mg/hydrochlorothiazide 12.5 mg	Hyzaar
Calcium Antagonists and ACE Inhibitors	
Amlodipine 2.5 or 5 mg/benazepril 10 or 20 mg	Lotrel
Diltiazem 180 mg/enalapril 5 mg	Teczem
Verapamil (extended release) 180 or 240 mg/trandolapril 1, 2, or 4 mg	Tarka
Felodipine 5 mg/enalapril 5 mg	Lexxel
Other Combinations	
Triamterene 37.5, 50, or 75 mg/hydrochlorothiazide 25 or 50 mg (G)	Dyazide, Maxide
Spironolactone 25 or 50 mg/hydrochlorothiazide 25 or 50 mg (G)	Aldactazide
Amiloride 5 mg/hydrochlorothiazide 50 mg	Moduretic
Guanethidine 10 mg/hydrochlorothiazide 25 mg	Esimil
Hydralazine 25, 50, or 100 mg/hydrochlorothiazide 25 or 50 mg	Apresazide
Methyldopa 250 or 500 mg/hydrochlorothiazide 15, 25, 30, or 50 mg	Aldoril
Reserpine 0.125 mg/hydrochlorothiazide 25 or 50 mg	Hydropres
Reserpine 0.10 mg/hydralazine 25 mg/hydrochlorothiazide 15 mg (G)	Ser-ap-es
Clonidine 0.1, 0.2, or 0.3 mg/chlorthalidone 15 mg	Combipres
Methyldopa 250 mg/chlorthiazide 150 or 250 mg	Aldochlor
Reserpine 0.125 or 0.25 mg/chlorthalidone 25 or 50 mg	Demi-Regroton
Reserpine 0.125 or 0.25 mg/chlorothiazide 250 or 500 mg	Diupres
Prazosin 1, 2, or 5 mg/polythiazide 0.5 mg	Minizide

From The Sixth Report of the Joint National Committee on Prevention, Detection, Evaluation, and Treatment of High Blood Pressure. Arch Intern Med 157:2413, 1997.
[a]Approved for initial therapy.

Table 62.16 also lists antihypertensives from certain classes that may either have *favorable or unfavorable effects on coexisting conditions.*

Nondiabetic Renal Disease. Based on findings from a number of animal models of renal insufficiency and on preliminary results from human studies, it appears that ACE inhibitors may have renoprotective effects independent of BP-lowering effects (63). On the other hand, BP reduction with drugs from all classes has delayed the progression of chronic renal failure. The level of 130/85, or lower, has been associated with optimal renoprotection; this finding was especially true in patients with 1 g/day or more of proteinuria, including African Americans, a group at high risk of developing end-stage renal disease (63). Therefore any antihypertensive drug or drug combination that controls the BP to 130/85 or less is appropriate for patients with renal disease.

Diabetes Mellitus. Because elevated BP accelerates the development of diabetic nephropathy, a goal BP of 130/85 or less is now recommended for all diabetic patients (81). All classes of antihypertensives, with the exception of β-blockers and high-dose diuretics, are reasonable (β-blockers may prolong hypoglycemia and mask its symptoms; high-dose diuretics may cause worsening glucose tolerance). In clinical trials in which control of HBP in diabetic patients protected renal function (48a) and reduced the incidence of cardiovascular events (22a), low-dose diuretics were included in the treatment regimen for most patients.

Pretreatment and posttreatment *standing BPs* should always be measured in diabetic patients; when orthostasis is found, presumably caused by neuropathy, the standing pressure should be followed and used in treatment decisions.

In *diabetic patients with nephropathy* (30 mg/day or more urine albumin), ACE inhibitors should be used because they have been shown to reduce proteinuria and delay loss of renal function even in nonhypertensive diabetic patients (9). The addition of a nondihydropyridine calcium antagonist, in patients with BP above 130/85 who are already taking an ACE inhibitor, may further decrease the proteinuria and loss of function (63). It is not yet known whether angiotensin II receptor blockers will confer specific renoprotection in diabetics who cannot tolerate ACE inhibitors.

Table 62.16. Considerations for Individualizing Antihypertensive Drug Therapy

Compelling Indications Unless Contraindicated[a]		May Have Favorable Effects on Comorbid Conditions[a]		May Have Unfavorable Effects on Comorbid Conditions[a,b]	
Diabetes mellitus (type 1) with proteinuria	ACE I	Angina	β-Blockers CA	Bronchospastic disease	β-Blockers[c]
Heart failure	ACE I Diuretics	Atrial tachycardia and fibrillation	β-Blockers CA (non-DHP)	Second or third-degree heart block	β-Blockers[c] CA (non-DHP)[c]
Isolated systolic hypertension (older patients)	Diuretics (preferred) CA (long-acting DHP)	Cyclosporine-induced hypertension (caution with the dose of cyclosporine)	CA	Depression	β-Blockers Centrally-acting α-agonists Reserpine[c]
Myocardial infarction	β-Blockers (non-ISA) ACE I (with systolic dysfunction)	Diabetes mellitus (type 1 and 2) with proteinuria	ACE I (preferred) CA	Diabetes mellitus type 1 and 2	β-Blockers High-dose diuretics
		Diabetes mellitus (type 2)	Low-dose diuretics	Dyslipidemia	β-Blockers (non-ISA) Diuretics (high-dose)
		Dyslipidemia	α-Blockers	Gout	Diuretics
		Essential tremor	β-Blockers (non-CS)	Heart Failure	β-Blockers (except carvedilol) CA (except amlodipine; felodipine)
		Heart failure	Carvedilol Losartan	Liver disease	Labetalol Methyldopa[c]
		Hyperthyroidism	β-Blockers	Peripheral vascular disease	β-Blockers
		Migraine	β-Blockers CA (non-DHP)	Pregnancy	ACE I[c] Angiotensin II receptor blockers[c]
		Myocardial infarction	Diltiazem Verapamil	Renal insufficiency	Potassium-sparing agents
		Osteoporosis	Thiazides	Renovascular disease	ACE I Angiotensin II receptor blockers
		Preoperative hypertension	β-Blockers		
		Prostatism (BPH)	α-Blockers		
		Renal insufficiency (caution in renovascular hypertension and creatinine ≥3 mg/dL)	ACE I		

From The Sixth Report of the Joint National Committee on Prevention, Detection, Evaluation, and Treatment of High Blood Pressure. Arch Intern Med 157:2413, 1997.

ACE I, ACE inhibitors; *BPH*, benign prostatic hyperplasia; *DHP*, dihydropyridine; *ISA*, intrinsic sympathomimetic activity; *MI*, myocardial infarction; *non-CS*, noncardioselective; *CA*, calcium antagonists.

[a]Conditions and drugs are listed in alphabetical order.

[b]These drugs may be used with special monitoring unless contraindicated.

[c]Contraindicated.

Left Ventricular Hypertrophy. When the baseline electrocardiogram shows LVH, this finding is an independent predictor of cardiovascular morbidity. LVH may be reduced by weight reduction or salt restriction, and by antihypertensive drugs from all classes except direct vasodilators (76). The following two unanswered questions are being tested in multicenter clinical trials: (a) Are agents that interrupt the renin–angiotensin system especially effective in causing LVH reversal? and (b) Does reversal of LVH offer health benefits beyond those associated with BP reduction? (23). In the subset of patients with the combination of electrocardiographic LVH, symptoms of heart failure and echocardiographic evidence for *diastolic dysfunction*, a calcium channel blocker or a β-blocker may provide symptom relief because of a modest decrease in contractility (78); these drugs do not appear to decrease the late-diastolic stiffness that is present in these patients (44).

Cost of Antihypertensive Drugs

The charge for a 1-month supply of starting doses of most brand-name nondiuretic antihypertensive drugs is between $25 and $60. This may explain why studies have shown that up to 35% of Americans with hypertension report that they have difficulty affording their prescribed medications (52).

When *generic preparations* are available, the cost is substantially lower. The least expensive regimens (less than $10 per month) are monotherapy with a generic thiazide diuretic, β-blocker (atenolol or propranolol), short-acting α-blocker (prazosin), ACE inhibitor (captopril), short-acting nondihydropyridine (verapamil), or reserpine.

When combination therapy is needed, a *combination product* may be less expensive than the component drugs purchased separately (Table 62.15).

Drug–Drug Interactions

Table 62.17 provides drug interaction information that may be important in selecting and monitoring both antihypertensive drugs and other drugs. This information is not exhaustive. Today, pharmacists usually can provide prompt responses to queries about drug interactions.

Drug Side Effects: Overview

The most common side effects for each class or subclass of antihypertensive drugs are listed in Table 62.14. Additional details are found below ("Selected Properties for Individual Drugs").

Modification of the regimen may be needed when drugs control the hypertension but cause troublesome side effects. After any drug has been initiated, the patient should be encouraged to discuss any drug-associated disturbances, such as reduced mental alertness, mood change, or impairment in physical exercise or sexual activity. From 5 to 20% of subjects discontinue therapy in the trials of most antihypertensive drugs because of such side effects, and many subjects notice minor side effects as long as they are taking antihypertensive drugs. Even taking a placebo for hypertension is associated with side effects, and for many side effects, the frequency is similar in active-drug and placebo patients. Table 62.18 summarizes the frequency of some of the side effects that were systematically enumerated in patients taking a prototypic drug from each of the principal classes or a placebo.

Recently, *quality of life indices* have been used to measure the impact of antihypertensive drugs on patients' energy levels, mental health, physical abilities, and social functioning. In one study, patients on each of the major classes of drugs and on placebo reported modest improvement in most of these measures four years after starting treatment (34).

Because *orthostatic exaggeration of the BP-lowering effect* can occur with any antihypertensive drug, patients should be asked about orthostatic symptoms and should have a standing BP measured to check for asymptomatic orthostasis after every change in the regimen. For those with an orthostatic fall in systolic pressure of more than 15 mm Hg, a standing BP should also be measured after exercise (e.g., 10 steps on a footstool or walking a fixed distance) because exercise may exacerbate drug-induced orthostatic hypotension. For patients who report that they have orthostatic symptoms shortly after taking their daily medication, the standing BP should be measured when symptoms are present—either at home by the patient or in the office—because profound but transient orthostatic hypotension may occur in some patients.

Impact on serum lipid concentrations. Although thiazide diuretics at high dosages may cause short-term increase in total and LDL cholesterol and β-blockers may decrease HDL cholesterol, these unfavorable effects were not seen in a 4-year study of monotherapy that compared a low-dose thiazide diuretic, a β-blocker, an ACE inhibitor, a nondihydropyridine calcium antagonist, and a long-acting α-blocker (33). The JNC consensus recommendations are to address any lipid abnormality according to current recommendations (see Chapter 75) and to use antihypertensive drugs, including low-dose diuretics, according to the scheme in Figure 62.6. Because α-blockers may actually lower cholesterol concentrations, this property should be considered in a patient whose lipid levels are hard to control.

Step-Down Therapy

Patients who are taking multiple drugs or a high dosage of a single drug may want to know whether they can expect to reduce the total amount of antihypertensive medicine that has been prescribed. Based on the results of preliminary clinical trials (85), it is reasonable to try to reduce the regimen in patients whose BP has been controlled for 1 year, at several consecutive visits, especially patients who have made lifestyle changes (e.g., salt restriction, weight reduction) that favor BP lowering.

Table 62.17. Selected Drug Interactions with Antihypertensive Therapy (For Initial Drug Therapy Recommendations, See Fig. 62.8)

Class of Agent	Increase Efficacy	Decrease Efficacy	Effect on Other Drugs
Diuretics	Diuretics that act at different sites in the nephron (e.g., furosemide + thiazides)	Resin-binding agents NSAIDs Steroids	Diuretics raise serum lithium levels. Potassium-sparing agents may exacerbate hyperkalemia due to ACE inhibitors.
β-Blockers	Cimetidine (hepatically metabolized β-blockers) Quinidine (hepatically metabolized β-blockers) Food (hepatically metabolized β-blockers)	NSAIDs Withdrawal of clonidine Agents that induce hepatic enzymes, including rifampin and phenobarbital	Propranolol induces hepatic enzymes to increase clearance of drugs with similar metabolic pathways. β-Blockers may mask and prolong insulin-induced hypoglycemia. Heart block may occur with nondihydropyridine calcium antagonist. Sympathomimetics cause unopposed α-adrenoceptor–mediated vasoconstriction. β-Blockers increase angina-inducing potential of cocaine.
ACE inhibitors	Chlorpromazine or clozapine	NSAIDs Antacids Food decreases absorption (moexipril)	ACE inhibitors may raise serum lithium levels. ACE inhibitors may exacerbate hyperkalemic effect of potassium-sparing diuretics.
Calcium antagonists	Grapefruit juice (some dihydropyridines) Cimetidine or ranitidine (hepatically metabolized calcium antagonists)	Agents that induce hepatic enzymes, including rifampin, phenytoin, and phenobarbital	Cyclosporine levels increase[a] with diltiazem, verapamil, mibefradil, or nicardipine (but not felodipine, isradipine, or nifedipine). Nondihydropyridines increase levels of other drugs metabolized by the same hepatic enzyme system, including carbamazepine, digoxin, quinidine, sulfonylureas, and theophylline. Verapamil may lower serum lithium levels.
α-Blockers			Prazosin may decrease clearance of verapamil.
Centrally acting α₂-agonists and peripheral neuronal blockers		Tricyclic antidepressants (and probably phenothiazines) Monoamine oxidase inhibitors Sympathomimetics or phenothiazines antagonize guanethidine or guanadrel Iron salts may reduce methyldopa absorption	Methyldopa may increase serum lithium levels. Severity of clonidine withdrawal may be increased by β-blockers. Many agents used in anesthesiology are potentiated by clonidine.

From The Sixth Report of the Joint National Committee on Prevention, Detection, Evaluation, and Treatment of High Blood Pressure. Arch Intern Med 157:2413, 1997.
See *Physicians' Desk Reference* and Frishman WH, Sonnenblick EH. Cardiovascular pharmacotherapeutics. New York: McGraw-Hill, 1997.
NSAIDs, nonsteroidal anti-inflammatory drugs.

[a]This is a clinically and economically beneficial drug–drug interaction because it both retards progression of accelerated atherosclerosis in heart transplant recipients and reduces the required daily dosage of cyclosporine.

Promoting Compliance with Pharmacologic Treatment

Compliance with treatment as a generic feature of ambulatory care is discussed in detail in Chapter 4. Because poor compliance is so common in hypertensive patients, the problem has been studied extensively (46). Nonjudgmental statements such as the following have been shown to be effective in eliciting accurate information from patients for whom antihypertensive drugs are prescribed: "People often have difficulty taking their medicines for one reason or another and we are interested in finding out any problems that occur so that we can understand them better." After this statement, patients are asked whether they ever miss tablets

and are encouraged to discuss any problems they are having with taking medicine.

Certain strategies have been shown to improve compliance with antihypertensive treatment. Several of these should be used routinely. More intensive strategies should be used for those patients who appear to be especially noncompliant.

Strategies recommended for all patients include the following:

- Ensure that the patient knows several critical facts about hypertension: that it increases the risk of disabling illness (stroke, heart disease, kidney failure) or premature death; that it is usually asymptomatic when initially detected; that treatment reduces the risk of illness or premature death by one third or more; and that treatment is continuous for life. This information is covered well in patient information pamphlets available from the American Heart Association. One of these pamphlets should be offered to each hypertensive patient as an adjunct to a verbal summary of this information, and the patient's comprehension of the fundamentals of hypertension should be ascertained periodically. (For further information on techniques for effective patient education, see Chapter 4.)

- Prescribe drugs that can be taken once per day (see schedules for all drugs in Table 62.14).
- Have patients state how they are taking their medication at each visit (including what they have taken "today" and, for drugs with a duration of action under 12 hours, when the last dose was taken). Patients taking multiple drugs should be encouraged to bring their bottles of medicine to every visit.
- Ensure that supervision is provided frequently enough. During the first year of treatment, this should probably be at least every 3 months, at scheduled visits.
- Ensure that the practice is planned to maximize convenience for the patient, meaning that waiting time is brief, telephone access to the practice is easy, requests for appointment changes are accommodated, and prescription renewals are easy to obtain.

For patients who admit poor compliance, the reason should be explored and addressed (see practical approaches for detecting and addressing noncompliance in Chapter 4).

For patients with uncontrolled hypertension in whom poor compliance is suspected but not admitted, the following strategies have been shown to help:

- Have the adult with whom the patient has the most contact (usually the spouse) become an active participant in promoting compliance. This other adult should know the treatment regimen and should be asked to provide specific reinforcement for medication taking. Sometimes it is helpful to have a visiting nurse provide initial education and check BPs in the patient's home.
- Have the patient or another person take BPs at home and bring the record to office visits. When this is done, the home measuring technique should be observed periodically, using the equipment that is used at home.
- Observe the patient's BP response for several hours after the prescribed medication is taken under supervision in the office (10).
- Have the patient participate in group meetings with other hypertensive patients, coordinated by someone skilled in promoting group support mechanisms.

SELECTED PROPERTIES OF INDIVIDUAL DRUGS

The foregoing sections summarize for each class of antihypertensive drugs information about available products, dosages, and common side effects (Tables 62.14, 62.15, and 62.18); and selective advantages and disadvantages according to patient characteristics, coexisting conditions (Table 62.16), and common drug–drug interactions (Table 62.17). This section provides individual drug information about mechanism of

Table 62.18. TOMHS[a] Participants Attending the 12-Month Visit Who Reported a Worsening or New Condition Through the 12-Month Visit

Condition	No. (%)					
	Acebutolol	Amlodipine Maleate	Chlorthalidone	Doxazosin Mesylate	Enalapril Maleate	Placebo
Tiredness or fatigue	45 (36.3)	36 (30.8)	43 (34.7)	38 (31.1)	33 (26.8)	72 (33.8)
Weakness	21 (16.9)	18 (15.3)	20 (16.3)	15 (12.3)	17 (13.8)	38 (17.8)
Trouble falling asleep	21 (16.8)	14 (11.9)	22 (17.7)	19 (15.8)	22 (17.9)	43 (20.2)
Nightmares	12 (9.6)	10 (8.5)	8 (6.5)	10 (8.2)	2 (1.6)	18 (8.5)
Nervousness	12 (9.7)	17 (14.4)	14 (11.3)	18 (14.8)	18 (14.6)	43 (20.2)
Feeling depressed	23 (18.4)	21 (17.8)	19 (15.4)	20 (16.4)	24 (19.5)	41 (19.2)
Decreased frequency of sex	22 (17.7)	23 (19.5)	24 (19.5)	16 (13.2)	27 (22.0)	27 (12.7)
Decreased interest in sex	14 (11.3)	16 (13.6)	19 (15.4)	14 (11.6)	20 (16.3)	24 (11.3)
Drowsiness or sleepiness	30 (24.2)	31 (26.3)	37 (29.8)	29 (24.0)	33 (26.8)	47 (22.1)
Faintness, dizziness	23 (18.4)	22 (18.6)	24 (19.4)	28 (23.0)	28 (22.8)	44 (20.7)
Light-headedness when standing up	21 (16.8)	19 (16.1)	23 (18.5)	35 (28.7)[b]	36 (29.3)[b]	8 (3.8)
Headaches	27 (22.1)	27 (22.9)	26 (21.7)	38 (31.4)	31 (25.2)	72 (34.3)
Numbness or tingling	23 (18.4)	28 (23.9)	24 (19.4)	29 (24.0)	19 (15.4)	34 (16.0)
Stuffy nose	42 (33.9)	38 (32.5)	34 (27.4)	48 (40.0)	57 (46.3)	77 (36.3)
Dry mouth	23 (18.4)	22 (18.6)	26 (21.0)	24 (19.7)	27 (22.0)	41 (19.2)
Rash	13 (10.4)	14 (11.9)	22 (17.7)	22 (18.2)	29 (23.8)	39 (18.3)
Cough	29 (23.2)	34 (28.8)	28 (22.6)	32 (26.2)	35 (28.7)	48 (22.6)
Swelling of feet, ankles	14 (11.2)	16 (13.6)	11 (8.9)	13 (10.7)	14 (11.4)	31 (14.6)
Nausea or vomiting	9 (7.2)	10 (8.5)	16 (13.1)	12 (9.8)	10 (8.1)	33 (15.5)
Muscle pain or cramps	31 (24.8)	35 (29.9)	31 (25.6)	34 (27.9)	31 (25.2)	69 (32.7)
Increased urination	41 (32.8)	35 (29.7)	37 (30.1)	43 (35.2)	45 (36.6)	63 (29.6)

From Treatment of Mild Hypertension Research Group. A randomized, placebo-controlled trial of a nutritional-hygienic regimen along with various drug monotherapies. Arch Intern Med 151:1413,1991.

[a]TOMHS, Treatment of Mild Hypertension Study.

[b]$p < .01$ for comparison with placebo group.

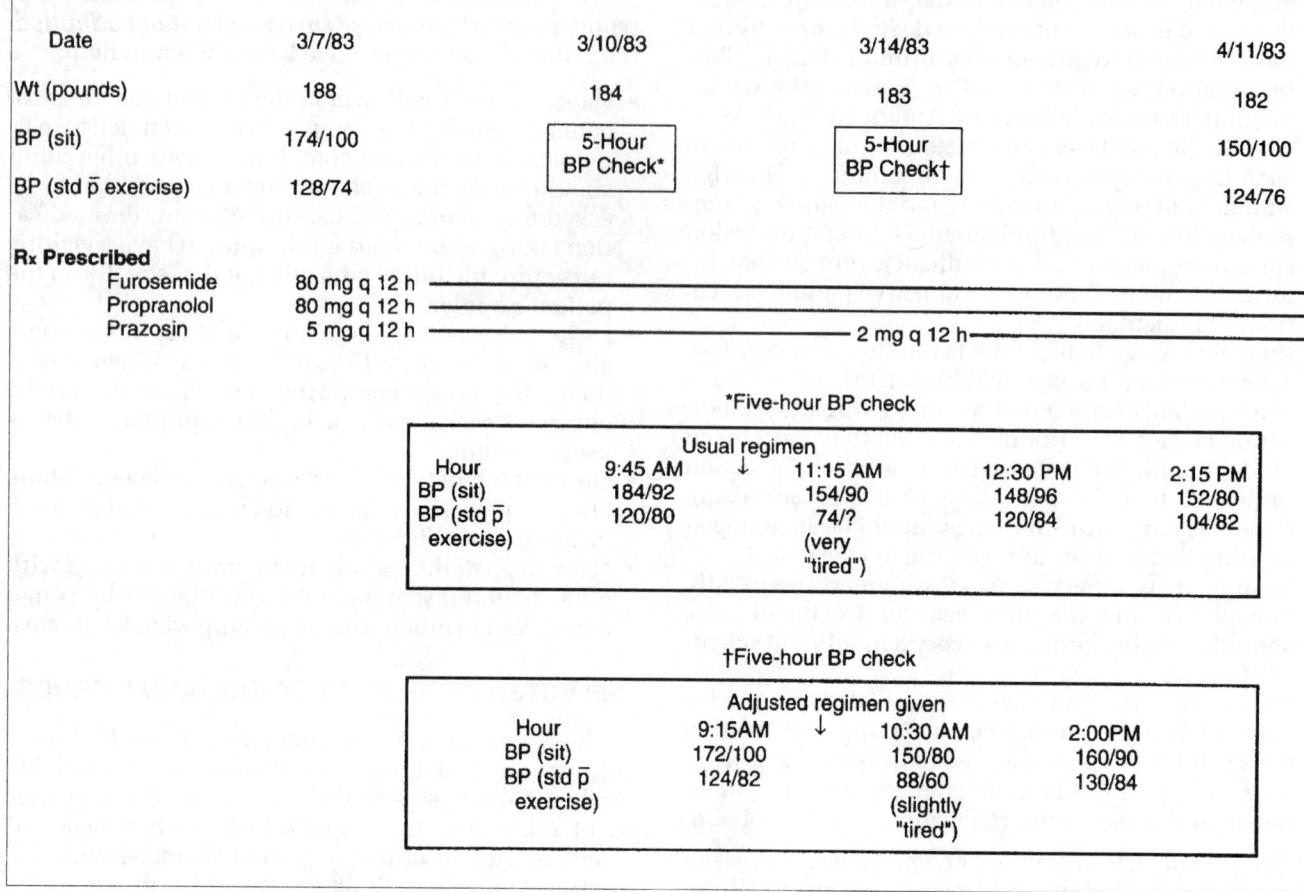

Date	3/7/83	3/10/83	3/14/83	4/11/83
Wt (pounds)	188	184	183	182
BP (sit)	174/100	5-Hour BP Check*	5-Hour BP Check†	150/100
BP (std p̄ exercise)	128/74			124/76

Rx Prescribed

Furosemide	80 mg q 12 h			
Propranolol	80 mg q 12 h			
Prazosin	5 mg q 12 h		2 mg q 12 h	

*Five-hour BP check

Usual regimen

Hour	9:45 AM	↓	11:15 AM	12:30 PM	2:15 PM
BP (sit)	184/92		154/90	148/96	152/80
BP (std p̄ exercise)	120/80		74/? (very "tired")	120/84	104/82

†Five-hour BP check

Adjusted regimen given

Hour	9:15AM	↓	10:30 AM	2:00PM
BP (sit)	172/100		150/80	160/90
BP (std p̄ exercise)	124/82		88/60 (slightly "tired")	130/84

Figure 62.6. Office evaluation of a 54-year-old woman who had severe hypertension at baseline (230/140) and who complained of transient "tiredness" after taking her medicine each day. The tiredness was not present when she came for routine afternoon visits. Office evaluation confirmed that the tiredness was due to orthostatic hypotension that occurred for 1 to 2 hours after her morning dose of prazosin. (From Barker LR. Five-hour blood pressure check to assess hypertension not responding to conventional therapy. Md Med J 35[2]:94, 1986.)

action and additional detail regarding some of the properties listed in the tables in the foregoing sections.

Diuretics

Thiazide and Loop Diuretics

Mechanism. Thiazide and loop diuretics probably lower BP by decreasing modestly the circulating blood volume and by decreasing peripheral resistance. An increase in plasma renin activity has been demonstrated in diuretic-treated patients; this provides indirect evidence that the decrease in circulating volume persists as long as the patient is taking the diuretic.

Selected Properties. Table 62.14 lists practical information about these drugs.

Doses and response times. For monotherapy or combined diuretic–nondiuretic therapy, a once-daily schedule is satisfactory, and the patient can select the time of day that is most convenient (e.g., after rather than before work because of dieresis). Recommended starting and maximal doses for diuretics are the equivalent of 12.5 to 25 mg and 50 mg of hydrochlorothiazide; in most patients, the principal antihypertensive effect of diuretics occurs at these dosages, and higher dosages increase the likelihood of unwanted metabolic consequences. The major antihypertensive response is seen within 1 to 2 weeks of initiating or increasing a diuretic. Full reversal of antihypertensive effect occurs within 1 to 2 weeks of discontinuing the drug.

Special situations. High doses of loop diuretics (furosemide, bumetanide) may be necessary in an occasional patient who requires large doses of one or more nondiuretic drugs. These more potent diuretics may also be needed to control hypertension in patients who have edema that does not respond to thiazides or restricted salt use; the serum potassium concentration should be monitored closely in such patients (e.g., within 1 or 2 weeks of adding or increasing a loop diuretic) because precipitous potassium depletion may occur.

Patients with moderate renal insufficiency (e.g., creatinine concentration of 2.5 mg/dL or more) who have *volume-dependent hypertension* that does not respond to thiazide diuretics may require a high-potency diuretic (metolazone or indapamide), loop diuretic (furosemide, bumetanide, or ethacrynic acid), or combined metolazone and a loop diuretic (27).

Precautions. Mild side effects, such as increased urination and transient orthostatic symptoms, are common when diuretics are initiated. Sexual impotence is an important, although uncommon, side effect of diuretics.

Of the *other side effects*, those seen most commonly because of metabolic effects of diuretics are the following: hypokalemia, hyponatremia, gout related to hyperuricemia, impaired glucose tolerance, and a small increase in low-density lipoprotein cholesterol and triglyceride levels (thiazides and chlorthalidone). Most of these do not occur when low dosages of diuretics are used. A modest reduction in total body potassium may occur and frank hypokalemia (3.5 mEq/L or less) occurs in some patients. In nonedematous patients taking thiazide diuretics, restriction of sodium intake (Table 62.12 and 62.13) and the use of the equivalent of 25 mg of hydrochlorothiazide, and adequate potassium intake or less will prevent most hypokalemia. Because ventricular ectopy may be precipitated by hypokalemia, patients should be monitored for hypokalemia after starting or increasing a diuretic (at 2 to 4 weeks; if greater than 3.5 mEq/L, twice yearly) and the hypokalemia should be treated whenever it is detected. In nonedematous patients with hypokalemia, potassium supplements do not restore a normal potassium level as reliably as potassium-sparing diuretics (see the next section). Chapter 46 ("Hypokalemia") provides additional details regarding diuretics and potassium balance.

If *diabetes mellitus is found at the baseline evaluation* or if new diabetes develops in the course of long-term diuretic therapy, strict calorie and sodium restriction should be prescribed instead of diuretic therapy, and nondiuretic antihypertensives should be used if dietary modification fails to control the BP. With these measures, glucose tolerance does not deteriorate (or returns to normal) in many patients.

Contraindications. Apart from allergy and a number of uncommon coexisting conditions (e.g., psychogenic polydipsia, hypercalcemia, history of hyponatremia from inappropriate antidiuretic hormone excretion), there are no absolute contraindications to diuretics in hypertension. Because thiazides cause an increase in renal *reabsorption of lithium*, it is advisable to select an alternative drug for hypertension in patients who are taking lithium.

Potassium-Sparing Diuretics

Mechanism. The potassium-sparing diuretics (amiloride, spironolactone, and triamterene) have modest antihypertensive effects when used alone in some patients with essential hypertension. They are useful chiefly in combination with other diuretics, to avoid or reverse hypokalemia (see Chapter 46). They may also enhance diuretic action in patients who remain edematous while taking thiazide or loop diuretics in combination with nondiuretic antihypertensives.

Selected Properties. *Precautions.* To avoid iatrogenic hyperkalemia, potassium-sparing diuretics should not be prescribed for patients with renal insufficiency; should not be given concurrently with potassium supplements or with ACE inhibitors and probably angiotensin-receptor blockers (see below); and should be used with caution in diabetic patients because some diabetics have an increased risk of developing hyperkalemia when they take these diuretics. Spironolactone has a number of undesirable endocrine side effects (especially gynecomastia, which may be irreversible, and impotence). Therefore either amiloride or triamterene is preferable to spironolactone in male subjects.

Adrenergic Inhibitors

β-Blocking Drugs

Mechanism. One or more of the following mechanisms probably accounts for the antihypertensive effect in patients who respond to β-blocking agents: blockade of cardiac β_1-receptors causing decreased cardiac output, blockade of renal β-receptors causing inhibition of renin release, blockade of CNS β-receptors causing decreased sympathetic outflow, or blockade of presynaptic β-receptors causing decreased release of catecholamines. Evidence of some cardiac β-receptor blockade (heart rate of 64 beats/minute or less at rest and less than 80 beats/minute after brief exercise in the office) is present in many but not all patients whose hypertension responds to these drugs. However, there is no clinically useful way to determine which blocking mechanism is dominant in responders.

Selected Properties. Table 62.14 lists practical information about each of these drugs. The major theoretical advantage of a *cardioselective β-blocker* is the relative lack of β_2-receptor blockade. β_2-Receptors mediate bronchodilation, dilation of resistance vessels, and the sympathetic response to hypoglycemia (tachycardia, sweating). Those β-blockers—that have *intrinsic sympathomimetic activity* (ISA)—are less likely to cause bradycardia, bronchospasm, or heart failure in patients whose baseline respiratory or cardiac function is partly dependent on β-sympathetic stimulation.

Doses and response times. Most β-blockers may be useful over a broad dose range (Table 62.14). Atenolol, however, produces little or no additional BP reduction when the daily dosage exceeds 100 mg. For all of the β-blocking drugs (except for those drugs with ISA), slowing of heart rate and some BP response occur within 2 to 4 hours of taking an initial dose, but the full antihypertensive effect may not be seen until the patient has taken the drug for 1 week. The principal antihypertensive effect of these drugs resolves within 1 to 2 days of discontinuing the drug.

Precautions. Whenever a short-acting β-blocking agent is being discontinued after prolonged use, it should be tapered over 1 to 2 weeks rather than abruptly stopped because of the possibility of precipitating angina, acute rebound to pretreatment BP levels, or a number of other withdrawal symptoms (e.g., anxiety, tachycardia, palpitations, tremor, perspiration, or increase in headaches in patients with migraine).

The most common side effects are nausea, abdominal cramps, diarrhea, mild sedation, fatigue, nightmares, cool extremities, and asymptomatic bradycardia. Sexual impotence has been reported occasionally. Hypertensive athletes usually tolerate β-blocking agents well.

With certain coexisting conditions, the β-blocking properties of these drugs may cause serious side effects. *Absolute contraindications* to the use of β-blockers are baseline marked bradycardia (heart rate less than 50), impaired LV function from dilated cardiomyopathy, high-degree heart block, symptomatic asthma or chronic obstructive pulmonary disease, and severe peripheral vascular disease (e.g., gangrene, skin necrosis, severe or worsening claudication). For patients with mild asthma or chronic obstructive pulmonary disease, stable peripheral vascular disease, or stable insulin-requiring diabetes, it is reasonable to try a low dosage of a cardioselective β-blocker or a β-blocker with ISA if other antihypertensive regimens have been unsuccessful.

Modest decreases in glucose tolerance may accompany long-term use of propranolol; and those β-blockers that do not have ISA cause small increases in serum triglyceride and decreases in high-density lipoprotein concentrations in some patients. The significance of these changes has not been established.

Combinations. The addition of a diuretic usually enhances the antihypertensive effect of a β-blocker. The addition of a vasodilator, calcium antagonist, or an α-blocker may be effective in patients not controlled with β-blocker monotherapy.

α–β-*Blockers*

Mechanism. *Labetalol* and *carvedilol* combine nonselective β blockade with α_1-adrenergic blockade. During *labetalol treatment*, control of hypertension is usually accompanied by a modest reduction in resting and postexercise heart rate. The cardiac index and peripheral resistance are reduced during the first year of treatment, but after several years, cardiac index returns to normal, whereas total peripheral resistance remains lower. *Carvedilol* has been used chiefly as an adjunct to other drugs to improve control of CHF. In these patients, the drug causes a decrease in LV size and increase in ejection fraction (18).

Selected Properties. Table 62.14 lists practical information about these drugs. Labetalol is effective as monotherapy in somewhat more than 50% of patients with stage 1 or 2 hypertension and in about one third of patients with severe hypertension. It seems to be equally effective in African-American and white subjects.

Doses and response times. The dose range for *labetalol* is large (200 to 1200 mg/day or higher). The drug must be taken twice a day because the full impact of a dose occurs within 1 to 3 hours, the dosage can be

adjusted rapidly. Most responders are controlled with 200 to 400 mg twice a day. Abrupt discontinuation does not appear to cause a withdrawal state similar to that observed occasionally with short-acting β-blockers.

In the United States, *Carvedilol* has not been used or marketed for uncomplicated hypertension. When added to a CHF regimen, it is initiated at a dosage of 3.125 mg twice a day and can be increased to 25 mg twice a day. To prevent hypotensive responses, it should be taken with food to slow the rate of absorption (18).

Precautions. The most common side effects seen with *labetalol* are fatigue, nausea, dyspepsia, dizziness, nasal stuffiness, and pruritic rash. Impotence has been the most common reason for early termination of labetalol. Like other nonselective β-blockers, it should not be given to patients with asthma. It is contraindicated in patients with greater than first-degree heart block.

Carvedilol, in studies of patients with CHF, commonly causes symptomatic hypotension during the first week of use (18). It can also cause each of the side effects described above for nonselective β-blockers.

Combinations. As is true of all antihypertensives, diuretics may enhance the effect of α–β-blockers on BP.

α_1-*Adrenergic Inhibitors*

Mechanism. These drugs block postsynaptic α_1-receptors in arterioles and venules, presumably decreasing BP by impairing sympathetic tone at both sites. They do not block presynaptic α-receptors. This may explain why they do not predictably cause tachycardia and renin release because both of these adaptive responses to BP lowering are inhibited by activation of presynaptic α-receptors.

Selected Properties. Table 62.14 lists practical information about each of these drugs.

Doses and response times. Because of the broad range of doses that may be needed to control blood pressure in different patients, each of these drugs may require more dosage changes than other antihypertensive drugs in patients who do not respond to an initial low dosage.

The usual schedule for *prazosin* is twice daily. Studies have shown that some patients may have to follow a three-times-daily schedule, whereas others may be able to take prazosin once a day. It is helpful to check the BP just before the next scheduled dose to determine the most appropriate schedule for prazosin. The major antihypertensive response to a dose of prazosin occurs within 1 to 2 hours and remits entirely after 24 hours.

The properties of *doxazosin* and *terazosin* are identical to those of prazosin except that both have a longer duration of action, meaning that they can be taken once per day.

All α-blockers lower slightly the serum concentration of low-density lipoprotein cholesterol. In male patients with benign hypertrophy of the prostate gland, a controlled trial has shown that these drugs may yield long-term decrease of obstructive symptoms, which are partly due to reversible bladder outlet obstruction (see details in Chapter 49).

Precautions. The most common side effects from these drugs are postural hypotension, headache, drowsiness, dry mouth, and palpitations. Sexual dysfunction is uncommon. *Postural hypotension,* usually without tachycardia and at times asymptomatic, occurs as a transient problem in up to half of patients during the first few days they take prazosin. Syncope occurring within 30 minutes to several hours after the initial dose is an uncommon but severe side effect. It may occur after taking a 1-mg dose or after an increase in dosage. Warning and reassurance about postural symptoms (for the first few days) are important whenever this drug or a long-acting α-blocker is prescribed. In addition, patients should be instructed to take the first dose at bedtime, so that they will be recumbent during the initial adjustment to the drug.

There are no absolute contraindications to the use of the α-blockers.

Centrally Acting Adrenergic Inhibitors

Mechanism. *Centrally acting α-agonists* (clonidine, guanabenz, and guanfacine). These drugs are α₂-adrenergic receptor agonists. Their locus of action is thought to be the medulla oblongata where, through a feedback effect, sympathetic outflow to the peripheral vasculature is reduced. In addition, these drugs suppress renin release, but a relationship between this property and the antihypertensive effect of the central α-agonists has not been established.

Methyldopa. There is evidence that the derivative of methyldopa, methylnorepinephrine, displaces norepinephrine in the CNS and that the hypotensive effect of methyldopa is related to this effect. Methyldopa also suppresses renin release from the kidney, but a relationship of this property to its antihypertensive action has not been clearly established.

Selected Properties. *Doses and response times.* Table 62.14 lists practical information about each of these drugs. The major antihypertensive response to *clonidine* occurs within 1 hour and remits after 8 to 16 hours. Therefore the usual schedule is twice per day. Because of its rapid onset of action, oral clonidine can be given hourly in doses of 0.1 or 0.2 mg to determine quickly the dose needed to treat an individual patient. This property has been exploited to lower the BP over several hours in symptom-free patients with very high pressures (so-called hypertensive urgencies). However, apart from hypertensive emergencies requiring hospitalization and parenteral treatment (see "Hypertensive Emergencies," above), there are no indications for such rapid lowering of the BP.

Clonidine is also available in a *sustained-release patch* (the Catapres Transdermal Therapeutic System [TTS]), which lasts 7 days. In addition to the advantage of once-a-week application, the TTS delivers a smaller dose of the drug and may therefore cause fewer side effects; also blood levels subside slowly at the end of a week, eliminating the risk of rebound hypertension from abrupt termination of clonidine. The patch is available in three sizes, delivering 0.1, 0.2, and 0.3 mg/day, respectively. The major antihypertensive effect is not seen until the third day after applying the initial TTS or after applying a new patch containing a higher dosage. About two-thirds of patients with stage 1 hypertension have been well controlled; however, up to 20% of patients have had to discontinue the clonidine TTS because of skin irritation at the site of the patch.

Guanfacine has a longer duration of action than oral clonidine and guanabenz, so it can be taken once per day. Patients should be instructed to take guanfacine at bedtime to minimize problems caused by the sedating effect of the drug.

Methyldopa. The BP response to methyldopa occurs within hours and remits after 1 to 2 days. It usually must be taken twice a day, although once-daily dosing at bedtime may suffice. This previously widely-used drug is still regarded as an important drug for the treatment of chronic hypertension during pregnancy (see below).

Precautions. Rebound to pretreatment or higher than pretreatment BP, with accompanying symptoms of increased sympathetic nervous system activity (tachycardia, perspiration, headache, palpitations), may follow within 1 to 2 days the abrupt discontinuation of oral clonidine, guanabenz, or guanfacine. Treatment for this problem is reinstitution of the drug. If a patient is taking a β-blocker in addition to an α-agonist, selective abrupt cessation of the α-agonist can lead to an exaggerated withdrawal state because of unopposed stimulation of α-receptors. Because there is no way to recognize prospectively patients who are at risk of developing α-agonist withdrawal symptoms, all patients must be regarded as at risk. When selecting antihypertensive drugs, patients known to be erratic in taking medication should thus not receive these drugs, and all patients for whom they are prescribed should be warned explicitly not to discontinue the drug abruptly.

The most common side effects of the *central α-agonists* are sedation, dry mouth, constipation, and orthostatic symptoms. Impotence has been reported. There are no absolute contraindications to the use of these agents.

The most common side effects of *methyldopa* are orthostatic symptoms, sedation, mood alteration, impotence, and diarrhea (soft stools, two to four times daily). After 6 to 12 months, approximately 10% of patients taking methyldopa develop a positive direct Coombs' test, and rarely there is associated hemolysis. Because methyldopa may cause hepatitis, it is contraindicated in patients with active liver disease.

Combinations. Clonidine has been used with hydralazine to prevent the reflex sympathetic response to hydralazine (see below). This combination is useful in patients needing a vasodilator who cannot take the more widely studied combination of β-blocking drugs and hydralazine, such as patients with a history of bronchospasm. Synergy between clonidine and prazosin has also been demonstrated.

Peripheral-Acting Adrenergic Inhibitors

Mechanism. *Reserpine* depletes the stores of catecholamines in many tissues, probably by impairing the uptake of essential precursors. The antihypertensive effect is attributed to impaired uptake both *centrally and peripherally* of dopamine, a precursor for the intracellular synthesis of norepinephrine.

Guanadrel and guanethidine prevent release of and deplete stores of norepinephrine in *peripheral tissues* but not in the CNS. Their hypotensive action is ascribed to the loss of sympathetic regulation of vessel tone in the venous and arterial circulation. Because their hypotensive effect depends predominantly on impaired venous tone, the effects of guanethidine and guanadrel are always more pronounced (often very pronounced) when patients are standing, particularly after exercise.

Selected Properties. Table 62.14 lists practical information about these drugs.

Doses and response times. The major antihypertensive response to *reserpine* occurs 1 to 2 weeks after initiating treatment and remits within 1 to 2 weeks after stopping the drug. Most responders require 0.25 mg of reserpine per day or less; at this dosage, reserpine alone or in combination with a diuretic has been found to be as effective as other nondiuretic antihypertensive drugs (52). The principal advantages of reserpine are the once-a-day schedule and low cost.

The major antihypertensive effect of *guanadrel* occurs within 4 to 6 hours of the first dose and lasts 12 to 24 hours. The major effect of *guanethidine* is seen after 3 to 5 days of initiating treatment and remits within 1 to 2 weeks after discontinuing the drug.

Precaution with reserpine. Frank *depression* occurs in some patients taking reserpine, and slight decrease in mental alertness is common. Both are dose related and occur chiefly at dosages higher than the recommended range (0.1 to 0.25 mg) (52). Nasal and gastric hypersecretion occurs at therapeutic dosages and may produce nasal stuffiness or dyspepsia. Two definite *contraindications* for reserpine are active peptic ulcer and a history of depression.

Reserpine may interact unfavorably with a number of drugs. Because it releases stored norepinephrine, a hypertensive crisis may occur if it is given with a monoamine oxidase inhibitor. Reserpine plus digitalis may cause cardiac arrhythmias (ventricular ectopy and atrial arrhythmias, similar to those caused by digitalis toxicity). Tricyclic antidepressants can reduce the BP-lowering effect of reserpine. The CNS depressant effects of many drugs may be increased by reserpine. Finally, reserpine antagonizes the antiparkinsonian effect of L-dopa.

Precautions with guanadrel and guanethidine. Orthostatic exaggeration of the hypotensive response severely limits the usefulness of these drugs. Most patients show one of two unsatisfactory patterns: a normal resting pressure and an unacceptably low pressure after exercise, or a high resting pressure and a normal pressure after exercise (11). In addition, sexual dysfunction in male patients (impairment of erection or ejaculation) and diarrhea are common. Because of the frequency of orthostatic hypotension and because of the availability of well-tolerated, potent drugs (e.g., minoxidil), the use of guanethidine or guanadrel can almost always be avoided in the management of hypertension. Patients who currently take either of these drugs should be monitored carefully, and an alternative regimen should be considered whenever there is any suggestion that the exaggerated orthostasis is producing symptoms.

Combinations. In the landmark Veterans Administration clinical trial, which confirmed for the first time the benefits of BP control, the combination of *reserpine, hydralazine, and hydrochlorothiazide* was used (98). These three drugs are available in a fixed-dose combination tablet (Ser-Ap-Es or a less expensive generic preparation) that contains small amounts of each drug (i.e., 0.10 mg of reserpine, 25 mg of hydralazine, and 15 mg of hydrochlorothiazide). This preparation, which must be taken twice per day, may be effective in patients who do not respond to or comply with other regimens.

Calcium Antagonists

Mechanism

Calcium antagonists block or alter cell membrane calcium flux, thereby reducing BP through one or more of the following mechanisms: decreased vascular smooth muscle contractility in both the arterial and venous circulation, negative inotropic and chronotropic effects (slows atrioventricular nodal conduction) on the heart, and inhibition of secretion of catecholamines. The *dihydropyridines* lower BP chiefly via arteriolar and venous vasodilation. The *nondihydropyridines* are less potent vasodilators; they probably lower BP via combined peripheral vasodilation and a negative inotropic effect. These differences in mechanism may be important in drug selection (Table 62.16).

Selected Properties

Table 62.14 lists practical information about these drugs.

Each of the calcium channel blockers has been shown to be effective for monotherapy. All decrease myocardial contractibility, but this property is most pronounced in the nondihydropyridines. Two dihydropyridines, nifedipine and nicardipine, predictably cause initial and in some patients chronic, reflex increase in heart rate when used for monotherapy (59).

Doses and response times. Short-acting preparations of the dihydropyridines are no longer recommended for the treatment of hypertension because of a statistically significant association to use of these drugs with occurrence of MI (72). Multiple strengths of long-acting preparations of all calcium antagonists are available for once or twice daily use. The major antihypertensive effects are seen within several hours of an initial dose.

When the liquid contents of a 10-mg nifedipine capsule are given sublingually, the patient's BP may drop within minutes. In the past, this property was exploited to lower the BP promptly in symptom-free patients with very high pressures (so-called hypertensive urgencies). Accumulated reports of harm due to acute hypotension have been cited to support the discontinuation of this use of nifedipine (35). Apart from hypertensive emergencies requiring hospitalization and parenteral treatment, there are no indications for such rapid lowering of the BP.

Precautions. Side effects commonly reported with the dihydropyridines are nausea, flushing, headache, and tachycardia. Vasodilator effects (flushing and headache) are less common with verapamil and diltiazem. All of these drugs may cause orthostatic symptoms, ankle edema (not caused by salt retention), and palpitations. Verapamil may cause marked constipation, especially when large doses are used, and nifedipine occasionally causes diarrhea.

Because of their cardiodepressive effects, *diltiazem and verapamil* are contraindicated in patients with bradycardia, atrioventricular conduction disturbances, or uncontrolled heart failure. Because the cardiodepressive effects of these two drugs may be additive to the cardiodepressor effects of β-blocking drugs, such combinations should be avoided. Although their cardiodepressor actions are much less pronounced, the dihydropyridines should also be used with caution in patients with underlying dilated cardiomyopathy. On the other hand, calcium antagonists may be useful in treating LV failure in that subgroup of patients with severe hypertension and well-preserved cardiac function, whose heart failure is due to poor diastolic phase relaxation associated with LVH (78).

Mibefradil is a recently approved nondihydropyridine selective T-channel blocker. T-type (transient) calcium channels are found in vascular smooth muscles and myocardial conducting tissue but usually not in myocardium. Mibefradil's purported advantage over the other nondihydropyridines is that it does not have a negative inotropic effect on the heart and does not cause reflex tachycardia (93). Because of its effect on conducting tissue, mibefradil may slow or suppress sinuatrial node activity; it is contraindicated in elderly patients with a pretreatment sinus rate below 55 beats/minute and generally should not be used with other drugs that slow the sinus node (β-blockers, digitalis, and the nondihydropyrine calcium antagonists). In addition, mibefradil is contraindicated in patients taking terfenadine, astemizole, cisapride, lovastatin, or simvastatin because of an increased risk of rhabdomyolysis.

Combinations. The combination of a dihydropyridine and a β-blocker has been shown to be effective in some patients with severe hypertension. In addition to its synergy, the β-blocker blunts the reflex tachycardia that may occur with some dihydropyridines. Nondihydropyridines may add to the renoprotective effects of ACE inhibitors when they are used together.

Drugs that Affect the Renin–Angiotensin Axis

Mechanisms

Angiotensin I is the product of the interaction between the proteolytic enzyme renin and an α_2-globulin, renin substrate. The ACE inhibitors block the enzymatic conversion of angiotensin I to the potent vasoconstrictor angiotensin II; their antihypertensive effect has been attributed to this action. Because *ACE inhibitors* also inhibit the enzymatic degradation of the potent vasodilator bradykinin, there is controversy regarding their mechanism of action. The *angiotensin II receptor blockers* block binding of angiotensin II to vascular receptors. None of these drugs crosses the blood–brain barrier; their antihypertensive action is therefore strictly peripheral.

ACE Inhibitors

Selected Properties. Table 62.14 lists practical information about these drugs.

Doses and response times. The major antihypertensive effect of ACE inhibitors occurs within a few hours of a dose. The full impact of a dose is seen after 1 to 2 weeks at that dosage. Because a profound fall in BP (and occasional syncope) may follow the first dose of an ACE inhibitor, patients should begin treatment with the lowest available dosage and they should be warned about orthostatic symptoms.

The many available ACE inhibitors are similar to *captopril*—the prototype, now available in an inexpensive generic product—except that the duration of action of these drugs is longer than that of captopril. All are effective for 24 hours in most patients, so a once-a-day schedule can be tried in most patients. Captopril must be taken two or three times per day.

Precautions. The most common side effects that may be seen with all of the ACE inhibitors are nonproductive cough, maculopapular rash, and dysgeusia (decreased, totally lost, or altered taste). These effects occur within the first 1 to 2 months of use and remit with either a decrease in dosage or discontinuation of the drug. The option to substitute an angiotensin II receptor blocker in patients with these side effects is discussed below. Serious, although rare, adverse reactions are neutropenia and angioedema. The first occurs within the first 1 to 2 months of treatment and are reversible. *Angioedema*, which may be life threatening if it affects the upper airway, often occurs more than 1 month after initiation of ACE inhibitor use and recurs when an ACE inhibitor is inadvertently readministered at a later time (14).

Because *renal function* may depend on the action of angiotensin on postglomerular arterioles in patients with bilateral renal artery stenosis, renal artery stenosis in a solitary kidney, or in renal transplant patients with stenosis of the transplanted renal artery, the ACE inhibitors may cause acute renal failure in patients with these conditions. The type of patients most likely to have the former two problems are those with widespread atherosclerosis, manifested by multiple bruits and diminished peripheral pulses. An increase in the serum creatinine concentration in such patients occurs within 1 or 2 days of initiating treatment and remits within days after discontinuation of the ACE inhibitor. In patients who do not have stenotic renal arteries, ACE inhibitors do not cause renal insufficiency. However, reversible increase in the creatinine concentration may occur in patients who do not have renal artery stenosis but do have preexisting renal insufficiency from hypertension (89). In the latter patients, the creatinine change is usually associated with relative hypotension and can usually be managed by dosage reduction.

Because of their *teratogenic effects* during the last two trimesters, ACE inhibitors are contraindicated in pregnant patients and must be regarded as potentially harmful in women of childbearing age who are not using birth control.

Combinations. The action of ACE inhibitors is enhanced predictably by *adding a diuretic.* A low-dose diuretic/low-dose ACE inhibitor regimen may be effective and well tolerated in patients who do not respond to monotherapy with either drug.

ACE inhibitors *may reduce or reverse the aldosterone secretion* by the adrenal glands that is stimulated by angiotensin II. This property has two important implications regarding diuretics: *(a)* diuretic-induced hypokalemia, a problem that is caused partly by increased aldosterone secretion, is less likely to occur during concurrent treatment with an ACE inhibitor; potassium supplements should be given to patients taking this combination only for well-documented hypokalemia, with careful monitoring to avoid hyperkalemia; and *(b)* potassium-sparing diuretics should be used with caution, if at all, in conjunction with ACE inhibitors because this combination increases the risk of hyperkalemia.

Combination of an ACE inhibitor with a *calcium antagonist* is a second strategy in patients who fail to respond to monotherapy. In diabetic patients with proteinuria, this combination may be additive in reducing proteinuria and delaying loss of renal function (63).

ACE inhibitors should be used cautiously with agents that affect sympathetic activity because the sympathetic nervous system may be especially important in supporting the BP in the event of acute hypotension. Despite this concern, β-blockers have been used in conjunction with captopril in patients whose BP did not respond to captopril alone.

Angiotensin II Receptor Blockers

Selected Properties. Table 62.14 lists practical information about these drugs.

Doses and response times. Their major antihypertensive effect occurs within a few hours after the first dose.

Because experience with these drugs is still limited, it is unknown whether they have a renoprotective effect in patients with diabetic nephropathy (63). There is evidence from one clinical trial for an equal or greater favorable impact on patients with heart failure caused by systolic dysfunction (70).

Precautions. These drugs are well tolerated. They do not seem to cause cough, the major reason for discontinuing ACE inhibitors. Angioedema may occur, rarely.

The manufacturers of losartan and Valsartan warn that acute renal failure may be expected to occur in patients with bilateral renal artery stenosis, based on the physiologic mechanism described for ACE inhibitors above. The implications of these drugs' effects on potassium excretion are similar to those described above for ACE inhibitors.

Direct Vasodilators

Hydralazine

Mechanism. Hydralazine directly relaxes smooth muscle in resistance vessels (arterioles and small arteries); it has a similar but lesser effect on capacitance vessels (venules and small veins). Secondary effects are stimulation of renin release and reflex increase in activity of the sympathetic nervous system that may cause tachycardia, palpitations, headache, or increased angina. Because of this latter effect, hydralazine is not recommended for monotherapy but should be used in combination with an adrenergic inhibitor.

Selected Properties. Table 62.14 lists practical information about hydralazine.

Doses and response times. The daily dosage range is 20 to 300 mg. An upper limit of 200 mg is sometimes recommended because of the increased risk of hydralazine-induced lupus at higher dosages. However, 400 mg or more may be effective and appropriate in patients with severe hypertension who are difficult to control and who do not tolerate other drugs.

Hydralazine must be taken twice daily. The major antihypertensive response occurs within 2 to 4 hours and remits within 12 to 24 hours. If there is evidence that an individual patient's response does not persist for 12 hours, a three-times-daily schedule may be required. Hydralazine should be taken with meals because absorption is maximal with food and BP response may be erratic if the drug is taken irregularly.

Precautions. The most common side effects (headache, palpitations, tachycardia) occur when hydralazine is given without an adrenergic inhibitor. The uncommon but widely publicized *lupuslike hydralazine syndrome* has the following features in most affected subjects: it occurs after 6 months or more of exposure to 200 mg/day or more, begins as new arthritis or arthralgia, rarely affects the kidneys, stimulates the production of antinuclear antibodies, and remits entirely within a few months of discontinuing hydralazine (rarely, a patient may have persistent rheumatologic symptoms or antinuclear antibodies long after discontinuation of hydralazine). Another uncommon, reversible side effect is *peripheral sensory neuropathy* presenting as paresthesias and numbness and responding to pyridoxine, 50 mg/day, or to discontinuation of the drug.

Except for a history of systemic lupus erythematosus, there are no absolute contraindications to hydralazine when used in combination with an adrenergic inhibitor.

Combinations. When hydralazine is added to any adrenergic inhibitor, the hypertension responds well in most patients who are not controlled with the adrenergic inhibitor alone. In the past, the addition of hydralazine to a β-blocking agent (and usually a diuretic) was widely practiced, both because of the effectiveness of this combination and the protection against reflex sympathetic activity that the β-blockers provide.

Minoxidil

Mechanism. Minoxidil is a potent peripheral arteriolar vasodilator. Like hydralazine, it stimulates renin release and induces reflex hyperactivity of the sympathetic nervous system. Therefore the patient should always be taking an adequate dose of an adrenergic inhibitor (usually a β-blocker) before minoxidil is initiated.

Selected Properties. Table 62.14 lists practical information about minoxidil.

Doses and response times. The daily dose range is 2.5 to 100 mg. Because of its extraordinary potency, minoxidil should be initiated at a trial dose of 2.5 mg; dosage increases can be made daily until a response occurs. The major antihypertensive effect occurs within 1 to 3 hours and remits within 1 to 2 days.

Minoxidil can be given once or twice daily. When minoxidil is being substituted for another drug (e.g., hydralazine), this drug should be continued until response to minoxidil occurs; then the other drug should be gradually discontinued while the minoxidil dosage is increased if necessary.

Precautions. Fluid retention, sometimes marked, occurs in most patients as a consequence of the hypotensive action of the drug; and furosemide or another potent loop diuretic should be given in a dose adequate to eliminate the problem. Most patients also develop *hirsutism* within 1 month of starting minoxidil. In addition, darkening of facial pigment and thickening of facial features may occur (so-called leonine facies). These effects, which may require up to 1 year to remit after discontinuation of minoxidil, make minoxidil unacceptable to most women. No other common side effects occur. A minority of patients (estimated at 3% of those not receiving dialysis) develop a *pericardial effusion* (transudate) after prolonged use of minoxidil; rarely cardiac tamponade occurs. The effusion usually resolves or decreases with added diuretic treatment; it resolves entirely if minoxidil is discontinued. The development of *anasarca*, which remits when the drug is stopped, has been seen in an occasional patient taking minoxidil.

Combinations. Minoxidil should always be used in conjunction with a diuretic and an adrenergic inhibitor that will prevent reflex tachycardia. The addition of an ACE inhibitor to a minoxidil β-blocker diuretic regimen has been shown to control refractory hypertension.

For patients with severe hypertension, a once-daily regimen of minoxidil, a long-acting β-blocker, and a diuretic is highly effective and increases the likelihood that the patient will not forget a dose.

PROBLEMS IN THE COURSE OF TREATMENT

Four problems that occur during the long-term treatment of many patients with hypertension are the need for adjustment of the antihypertensive regimen, instability in BP control, orthostatic symptoms, and intercurrent illness.

Medication Adjustment

Within 3 months of initiating pharmacologic treatment, most patients should have satisfactory BP control without significant medication side effects. In the ensuing months and years, minor or major changes in the medical regimen will be needed for some patients. Each medication change brings the possibility for medication error. Therefore, whenever a medication adjustment is contemplated, the reason should be well established. Whenever medication adjustments affect one or more of the medications that the patient is already taking, it is important to write down the new instructions for the patient.

Instability in Blood Pressure Control

General Approach

Most patients in whom satisfactory control has been achieved will have either uncontrolled HBP at some follow-up visits or, less often, overcontrolled BP. At those visits, one can usually identify the probable cause and design a plan to restore satisfactory control. In assessing loss of BP control for which the cause is unclear, it is always useful *to check the BP in both arms* (to rule out pseudocontrol in an arm that may have a stenotic artery proximal to the brachial artery) and to *review the information recorded at the most recent visit when the BP was controlled and ask, "What is different today?"* The differential diagnosis of instability in BP control is summarized in Table 62.19, divided into common and uncommon causes. Before revising a patient's regimen, a prompt follow-up visit should usually be scheduled to determine whether the loss of control is persistent.

Home monitoring of the BP, either by the patient or by someone else, can be useful in assessing apparent loss of response to antihypertensive drugs. If this strategy is used, the patient should obtain and document the following information: BP, arm, position, heart rate, time since last dose of each medication. The

Table 62.19. Differential Diagnosis of Instability in Blood Pressure Control

Common Causes	Uncommon Causes
Noncompliance	Concurrent medications[a]
Increased salt consumption	Tolerance
Weight gain	Sleep apnea
Psychological stress	Refractory hypertension
Increased use of or withdrawal from ethanol	
Intercurrent illness[b]	

[a]See footnote to Table 62.8 and Table 62.17.
[b]See text (p. 881).

currently marketed home monitoring devices range from inexpensive devices that require skill in auscultation to more expensive electronic devices that give digital readouts (21). If one plans to rely on data from home monitoring, it is advisable to have the patient (or family member) bring the device to the office periodically to check technique and accuracy.

Noncompliance

Noncompliance, or overcompliance, can often be identified by nonjudgmental inquiry, as described above ("Promoting Compliance") and in Chapter 4. When patients have deliberately discontinued medications, they will often explain their reasons.

At certain times, patients simply omit their medications on the day of the visit. On the other hand, they may be taking medications consistently but incorrectly. Because this may be due to an error in dispensing of medication, patients who report that they are complying should be asked to telephone the office and read the information on their medication bottles or to bring their medication bottles to the next visit.

If patients with uncontrolled BPs report taking their medication correctly, this can be further evaluated by having them take their medicine under supervision in the office and then measuring the BP response for several hours (10).

Changes in Salt Consumption or Weight Gain

Increase in salt consumption may lead to a positive sodium balance, which can blunt the effects of antihypertensive drugs. Because of increased thirst, this problem is not uncommon in the summer months. The converse situation—negative sodium balance from inadequate replacement of sweat—may cause overresponse to antihypertensive drugs. Increased salt consumption should be suspected whenever loss of BP control is associated with a weight gain of 2 to 3 lb (1 kg) or more, with or without edema. Brief review of the patient's current diet often helps support this hypothesis. Management consists of having the patient resume moderate sodium restriction or substituting more potent diuretic treatment. Temporary use of furosemide (e.g., 20 to 40 mg daily for a few days) to eliminate excess sodium is often useful in this situation. For patients in whom sodium overload is a recurrent problem, furosemide in dosages adjusted by the patient to maintain a stable weight is effective.

If the patient's weight gain is associated with increased caloric intake, reduced caloric intake, leading to weight reduction, may restore response to antihypertensive medications.

Psychologic Stress

In a patient who is adhering faithfully to treatment, intercurrent psychologic stress may explain failure to respond as usual to antihypertensive drugs. This is probably because of the increase in sympathetic nervous system activity that may accompany psychologic stress.

Stress may be associated only with visits to a physician's office (white-coat hypertension), especially if the patient is being seen by a new physician, and the rise in BP may be strictly transient. This problem can be minimized by ensuring that the patient is at ease before taking the BP and by repeating the measurement later in the visit if the initial pressure is high. When stress is suspected as the reason for elevated office BPs, home BP measurements may provide better information for judging the effectiveness of treatment and may spare patients from inappropriate increases in antihypertensive drugs and the associated side effects.

Psychologic stress may also be caused by a serious job- or family-related crisis. Brief inquiry may reveal additional stress-related symptoms, such as headache, dyspepsia, sleeplessness, and irritability. In such patients, management consists of supportive counseling (see Chapter 11) and, if deemed appropriate, short-term prescription of an anxiolytic medication (see Chapter 13).

Excess Alcohol or Withdrawal from Alcohol

Because hypertension may occur as a manifestation of excessive alcohol intake or of alcohol withdrawal, it is important to check for alcohol abuse in a patient who has previously had controlled hypertension (see Chapter 21). Unstable BP control caused by alcohol withdrawal is probably most common in patients whose medical appointments occur after a weekend.

Concurrent Medications

A number of prescribed and over-the-counter (OTC) medications may attenuate the response to some or most antihypertensive drugs (see Table 62.17 and footnote to Table 62.8). Some drugs can potentiate the response to antihypertensive medications (Table 62.17). Antagonism of antihypertensives has been assessed for two common classes of drugs, both available in OTC and prescription formulations: (a) *decongestants* containing phenylpropanolamine, which may raise the BP in patients but do not impair the response to not receiving treatment antihypertensives when the recommended OTC dosage is taken (48); and (b) *nonsteroidal anti-inflammatory drugs*, some of which have been shown to interfere with the response to antihypertensives (74).

Sleep Apnea

Sleep apnea may cause HBP or explain instability in response to antihypertensive treatment in some patients. This has two implications for patient care: to inquire about the symptoms of sleep apnea in nonresponding patients (see Chapter 85) and to consider effective treatment of sleep apnea as an explanation for easier to control HBP in those patients whose sleep problem is identified and treated (56a).

Hypertension that Becomes Refractory to Treatment

Rarely, a patient's BP may become refractory to previously effective drugs, and none of the above causes will be found. In such patients, two questions must be answered:

1. *Is the hypertension really refractory to a previously effective regimen?* This question can be answered best by direct observation of medication taking and measurement of the BP response for 2 to 5 hours in the office (10). Although there is little published information on the subject, it is likely that confirmed loss of response can be caused either by tolerance to an antihypertensive drug or by progression of the physiologic factors that underlie the patient's HBP. Increased doses of the current regimen or change to another is indicated when this explanation is hypothesized.
2. *If refractoriness is confirmed, what is the reason?* This question is especially important for the occasional patient whose refractory hypertension is confirmed and who does not respond to other antihypertensive drugs. This situation is unusual (2) and suggests that one of the causes of secondary hypertension may be present, especially new renovascular hypertension (see "Secondary Hypertension," above).

Resistant Hypertension

Occasionally, a newly-diagnosed patient fails to respond to a variety of antihypertensive drugs at high dosages. Apparently resistant hypertension can also be assessed by direct observation of response to drugs during several hours in the office (10). Regimens that may be particularly effective in controlling resistant hypertension, each of which can be given in forms that allow only once-a-day dosing, are as follows:

- Minoxidil or nifedipine with a β-blocker and a diuretic
- An ACE inhibitor in conjunction with a calcium channel blocker or in combination with a minoxidil–β-blocker–diuretic regimen
- High-dose furosemide in conjunction with two potent nondiuretic drugs
- High-dose prazosin or terazosin plus a diuretic

If no regimen controls the BP in a patient with resistant hypertension, evaluation for a surgically treatable cause of hypertension, especially RVH, is indicated.

Orthostatic Symptoms

Many patients taking antihypertensive drugs describe brief orthostatic dizziness or faintness, particularly when they first stand up in the morning. Either sitting for a few minutes before standing or a modest reduction in drug dose usually alleviates the problem.

At times a patient who has satisfactory BPs at office visits will describe orthostatic symptoms lasting an hour or more after taking medicine. In this situation, it is important to reduce or discontinue the medication promptly. If such a patient has severe hypertension when not taking medicine, it is helpful to evaluate objectively the orthostatic symptoms before reducing medications (see case example, Fig. 62.6).

Occasionally a patient—usually an older person—will describe orthostatic symptoms related to medications at a time when the standing BP is measured as normal or high. In patients with known atherosclerosis (e.g., carotid bruits), this may be due to *positional cerebral ischemia* (58). In such patients, the problem may also be due to pseudohypertension, a measurement artifact caused by a difficult-to-compress calcified brachial artery (see "Measuring the Blood Pressure," above). For practical purposes, when either positional cerebral ischemia or pseudohypertension is suspected, a trial of less (or no) antihypertensive drugs is appropriate; if the patient's symptoms improve, it is reasonable to withhold antihypertensive drugs or to prescribe doses that do not cause the symptoms.

Intercurrent Illness

During long-term treatment, most hypertensive patients develop acute or chronic conditions that require adjustment of their antihypertensive drugs. One of the most common situations in which less medication may be needed to control hypertension is *elective or nonelective hospitalization* for any reason (40). For patients with selected chronic conditions, one or more antihypertensive drugs may be advantageous or inappropriate, as summarized in Table 62.16. Several common intercurrent problems require extra caution with any antihypertensive drug regimen.

Acute Illness

All patients with hypertension have intercurrent acute illnesses. The following factors, which *increase a person's sensitivity to antihypertensive drugs*, may accompany some of those intercurrent illnesses:

- Reduced intake of food, including salt
- Bed rest (In previously healthy individuals, bed rest for more than a few days produces a modest reduction in recumbent BPs and may cause a marked reduction in standing BP.)
- Volume loss caused by vomiting, diarrhea, or hyperglycemia
- Vasodilation caused by febrile illness

If lower BPs are documented or if the patient describes orthostatic symptoms, short-term decrease or withholding of antihypertensive drugs will protect such patients from the additional morbidity brought by hypotension or electrolyte depletion. The patient's usual antihypertensive regimen should be resumed gradually as the BP returns to hypertensive levels. In some situations (e.g., after major surgery), the previous regimen may not be needed for 1 month or more.

New Stroke or Myocardial Infarction

In patients who remain hypertensive after completed strokes, controlled studies of antihypertensive treatment have shown both a reduction or no reduction in the occurrence of second strokes (see details Chapter 83). These studies have not reported the impact of treatment on other morbidity from hypertension in poststroke patients, particularly CHF, a problem that should be prevented by antihypertensive treatment.

Patients who remain hypertensive after their neurologic status has stabilized should therefore be treated.

The hypertensive patient who has had a recent MI may have a normal BP or less severe hypertension during convalescence. Because this fall in BP may be transient, the BP should be evaluated at least monthly in the first 3 to 4 months after discharge.

Preplanned Surgery (see Chapter 86)

HYPERTENSION IN SELECTED SUBGROUPS
Hypertension in Adolescence

Epidemiology

There are no longitudinal or clinical-trial data relating BP level or treatment of HBP to health outcomes in adolescents and children.

In young adults (18 to 29), the crude prevalence of hypertension, defined as 140/90 mm Hg or more, varies from 0.6% (white women) to 6.8% (African-American men) (Table 62.1). Both prevalence and incidence of HBP are higher in adolescents who are overweight or become overweight. The prevalence of hypertension in children 17 years and younger has been arbitrarily established by defining as HBP the 95th percentile BP for each age and gender group, according to height (Table 62.20). The cut off levels for systolic and diastolic BP are higher for taller adolescents (80,95).

Recommendations

In 1996, the U.S. Task Force Report on High Blood Pressure in Children and Adolescents recommended the following approach for adolescents with systolic or diastolic BP levels approaching or above the 95th percentile (Table 62.20) (95):

- Measure BPs on at least three separate occasions before classifying the BP.
- Advise weight reduction, if needed.
- Advise avoidance of markedly elevated salt intake.
- Encourage physical activity.
- Encourage discontinuing smoking cigarettes (nonsmokers should be discouraged from starting the habit).
- Examine for other risk factors (e.g., serum lipids, glucose).

For patients whose BPs remain above the 95th percentile despite nonpharmacologic measures, pharmacologic treatment is recommended. The goal is a BP below the 95th percentile for the patient's age and height. The baseline evaluation and the principles for selecting individual antihypertensive drugs for adolescents are essentially the same as those described above for adults. However, because of their teratogenic effects, ACE inhibitors and angiotensin II receptor blockers should not be used in pregnant or sexually active teenage girls.

Because of the psychologic and social stresses associated with adolescence, the care of a chronic condition such as hypertension requires special considerations in this age group (see Chapter 5).

Hypertension in the Elderly

Hypertension is common in older patients (Table 62.1), and the risks associated with systolic and diastolic hypertension increase substantially with each decade of life and with the coexistence of other major risk factors (Fig. 62.1). There is evidence that an elevated pulse pressure (systolic BP minus diastolic BP) may be a stronger predictor of morbidity than BP level in older persons (51).

Recommendations

The recommendations for older patients in the 1997 report of the JNC (81) are based on the findings from clinical trials (3,22,49,77,83,86); five of these are summarized in Table 62.5. The most recent, the Syst-Eur trial for patients with isolated systolic HBP, showed that nitrendipine, a long-acting dihydropyridine calcium antagonist, had an effect similar in magnitude to regimens used in earlier trials (83). The principal JNC recommendations for older patients are the following:

- For older persons with sustained diastolic pressures of 90 mm Hg or greater, reduction of the pressure to less than 90 mm Hg is recommended.
- For older persons with a systolic pressure greater than 140 mm Hg, reduction of the pressure to less than 140 mm Hg is now recommended; an interim goal of 160 mmHg or less is regarded as appropriate in patients with very high pretreatment systolic pressures.
- A trial for up to 1 year of nonpharmacologic measures before drugs is regarded as appropriate initial treatment for older patients with stage 1 hypertension (Table 62.7), particularly those without target organ disease.

Several general points about the clinical trials in older patients are helpful in making decisions for individual patients:

- *Stage 1 hypertension* (140 to 159/90 to 100). Although the JNC now recommends BP reduction in older persons with stage 1 HBP, this recommendation is made recognizing that (a) the clinical trials were enrolled in older patients and showed benefits for patients with stage 2, not stage 1, HBP and (b) on-treatment BPs were not as low as those currently recommended.
- *Demographic features*: The clinical trial populations were comprised of healthy people who were genuinely older (mean ages 70 to 75 years old). Women, whose hypertension-related morbidity and mortality is similar to that in men after age 60, were heavily represented. Notably, African-American subjects were not included in three U.S. trials and were underrepresented in the fourth (Systolic Hypertension in the Elderly [SHEP]).
- *Antihypertensive medications*: Low-dose diuretic treatment was used as first-line treatment in five of the six trials summarized in Table 62.5, and in at least one trial (British Medical Research Council) benefit accrued to the diuretic-treated subjects but not to subjects treated with a β-blocker (atenolol) (49).

Table 62.20.   95th Percentile of Blood Pressure in Boys and Girls 3 to 17 Years of Age, According to Height[a]

Blood Pressure	Age (yr)	Height Percentile for Boys (mm Hg)				Height Percentile for Girls (mm Hg)			
		5th	25th	75th	95th	5th	25th	75th	95th
Systolic	3	104	107	111	113	104	105	108	110
	6	109	112	115	117	108	110	112	114
	10	114	117	121	123	116	117	120	122
	13	121	124	128	130	121	123	126	128
	17	132	135	138	140	126	127	130	132
Diastolic	3	63	64	66	67	65	65	67	68
	6	72	73	75	76	71	72	73	75
	10	77	79	80	82	77	77	79	80
	13	79	81	83	84	80	81	82	84
	17	85	86	88	89	83	83	85	86

Adapted from Sinaiko AR. Hypertension in children. N Engl J Med 335:1968–1973, 1996.

[a]The height percentiles were determined with standard growth curves (see Fig. 5.1). Data are adapted from those of the Task Force on High Blood Pressure in Children and Adolescents.

- *Morbidity and mortality*: Treatment reduced morbidity and mortality in subjects with either isolated systolic hypertension or the combination of systolic and diastolic hypertension.
- *Size of the benefit*: The absolute benefit—not just the percent reduction in events—was substantial. During 5 years, stroke, MI, or cardiovascular death was prevented in 50 to 150 of 1000 subjects. A meta-analysis has shown that the benefits of treatment may be smaller in the oldest age groups (41).

Caveats Regarding Drug Treatment

Several special characteristics of older persons should be considered in deciding how to treat their hypertension.

Orthostatic hypotension unrelated to drugs is fairly common in elderly patients (16). An increase in sedentary activity or blunting of autonomic reflexes may explain this. Thus, it is particularly important to obtain baseline and follow-up standing BPs (including standing after walking) in older patients taking antihypertensive drugs.

Both *pseudohypertension* and *white-coat hypertension* (see "Measuring the Blood Pressure," above) may be more prevalent in older persons, especially those who describe orthostatic symptoms despite apparent high pressures at office visits and those who have not target organ disease.

Other characteristics of older subjects that increase the risk of antihypertensive drugs include the following:

- Salt and fluid intake may vary significantly from week to week.
- Concomitant large vessel atherosclerosis (kidneys, brain, heart) may increase the risk of ischemic damage resulting from drug-induced hypotension.
- Errors in taking medication may be increased.
- Drug excretion rates are generally reduced as a function of aging.

Three precautions minimize the risks of antihypertensive drugs in older patients: using the lowest recommended dosage and increasing the dosage very slowly, keeping the drug schedule simple, and promptly decreasing or discontinuing drugs if there are signs or symptoms of significant orthostatic hypotension or other annoying side effects.

Hypertension in Pregnancy

This section addresses BP and HBP assessment and management in women when they are pregnant and when they are lactating. For *nonpregnant women*, longitudinal studies have delineated the risks of HBP, and clinical trials have demonstrated the benefits of treatment (Tables 62.4 and 62.5). The negligible impact on BP of oral contraceptives and estrogen replacement in most women is addressed above ("Evaluation for Secondary Hypertension").

Normally, the systolic BP does not change during pregnancy but the diastolic BP *falls about 10 mm Hg during the first and second* trimesters and reverts to the prepregnancy level in the third trimester. The maximal fall occurs between the 13th and 20th weeks. It is probably caused by the general vasodilation that accompanies pregnancy. An increase in renin and aldosterone levels also occurs in normal pregnancy.

Hypertension is present or develops in 10 to 12% of pregnancies in the United States. Most women with hypertension during pregnancy are primigravidas who develop preeclampsia (104).

Based on previous records or history from the patient, it should be possible at the first prepartum visit to decide for most women whether they are usually normotensive or have chronic hypertension. This decision is helpful in managing the following *three categories of hypertension* in pregnancy: chronic hypertension, gestational hypertension, and preeclampsia–eclampsia.

This recently-recommended classification differs from that issued previously (62) by naming gestational hypertension as a distinct category.

Chronic Hypertension in Pregnancy

Chronic hypertension is defined as a systolic pressure of 140 mm Hg or greater or a diastolic pressure of 90 mm Hg or greater diagnosed before pregnancy or appearing before the 20th week of pregnancy. It is more common in pregnant women who are in their 30s because the prevalence of hypertension increases with age (Table 62.1).

There are two important questions to consider in patients with chronic hypertension:

1. *Should a woman with chronic hypertension avoid pregnancy?* In the woman with uncomplicated stage 1 or stage 2 HBP (Table 62.7), there is a small increase in the risk to the mother or to the infant. However, in women with stage 3 HBP or evidence of target organ disease (cardiomegaly, renal impairment, or eye ground changes of accelerated hypertension), infant mortality is greatly increased; these women should be advised to avoid pregnancy.

2. *How should chronic hypertension be treated during pregnancy?* Current recommendations (79) are that a patient who becomes pregnant while taking a nondiuretic antihypertensive medication should substitute methyldopa (labetalol or hydralazine if methyldopa is not tolerated) for her usual medication and should continue treatment unless she becomes hypotensive during the pregnancy. A patient who becomes pregnant while taking a diuretic for hypertension can continue this treatment. In these patients, it is important to confirm that chronic hypertension was documented before drug treatment was initiated.

For patients with chronic hypertension who are not already taking antihypertensives, treatment should be considered for the hypertension. Controlled-trial data are limited and inconsistent, but the evidence favors treatment for women with long-standing stage 2 HBP or already-present target organ disease. Untreated women with uncomplicated stage 1 HBP have pregnancy outcomes similar to normotensive women. The recommendation to select methyldopa is based on the finding of improved fetal survival in a single controlled trial of methyldopa treatment (without diuretics) for women with chronic hypertension (75) and on the fact that methyldopa, hydralazine, labetalol have been found to be safe during pregnancy. ACE inhibitors and β-blockers (specifically atenolol) should be avoided because fetal abnormalities have been reported with these classes of drug. The long-term effects of calcium antagonists on the fetus are unknown.

Gestational Hypertension

Gestational hypertension is defined as the development of HBP after the 20th week of pregnancy without other manifestations of preeclampsia. In some it may be an early manifestation of preeclampsia, in others previously-unrecognized chronic HBP. Without treatment, the outcome of pregnancy in women with this form of HBP is usually good (79).

Preeclampsia

Pathophysiology. Preeclampsia is a pregnancy-induced syndrome in which the clinical data must be carefully considered before making the diagnosis, in particular to distinguish it from preexisting chronic hypertension and gestational hypertension. Preeclampsia occurs in 5 to 10% of all pregnancies, and a number of factors increase the risk of developing it (Table 62.21). Untreated preeclampsia is associated with a high incidence of fetal mortality and with maternal morbidity, especially the convulsive syndrome known as eclampsia. The major pathophysiologic derangements in preeclampsia are placental hypoperfusion caused by abnormal implantation of the trophoblast; this state leads to endothelial damage, which initiates the release of compounds that cause generalized vasospasm, reduced plasma volume and cardiac output, decreased glomerular filtration rate, and compromised perfusion of the placenta, kidneys, liver, and brain (104).

Diagnosis. The criteria for the diagnosis of preeclampsia are as follows:

- *Development of new hypertension after the 20th week of pregnancy.* The recommended criteria for hypertension in this instance are *(a)* systolic BP increases of 30 mm Hg or greater or *(b)* diastolic BP increases of 15 mm Hg or greater from early values (average of values before 20 weeks' gestation). If previous BP is unknown, readings of 140 mm Hg or greater systolic or 90 mm Hg or greater diastolic after 20 weeks' gestation are considered sufficiently elevated to satisfy the BP criteria of preeclampsia. Many young pregnant women meet the BP criterion for preeclampsia at levels below 140/90 mm Hg.

and

- *The development of new proteinuria*, in the absence of urinary tract infection, during the last trimester (two clean-catch specimens at least 4 hours apart that reveal 1+ proteinuria by dipstick or more than 300 mg of protein in a 24-hour specimen).

or

- The development of hyperuricemia (serum urate 3.5 mg/100 mL or more). The development of new, generalized edema during the last trimester is another manifestation of preeclampsia. Dependent edema alone is not a predictor of preeclampsia; it is seen in approximately one third of pregnant women whose BP remains normal.

Treatment. Fortunately, most preeclampsia develops late in the third trimester, when the fetus is mature and delivery, the definitive treatment, can be planned promptly. The usual management for preeclampsia,

Table 62.21. Risk Factors for Preeclampsia

Primigravida
Familial history of preeclampsia/eclampsia
Diabetes mellitus
Multiple gestation
Extremes of age
Preexisting hypertensive vascular or renal disease
Hydatidiform mole
Fetal hydrops, but not isoimmunization per se
Previous history of preeclampsia/eclampsia

under the supervision of the patient's obstetrician, is hospital admission, modified bed rest, frequent monitoring of maternal BP and fetal status, and antihypertensive drugs. Clinical trials completed in recent years have not shown clear benefits from any of these measures (79).

Preeclampsia resolves within 6 weeks of delivery. Approximately 25% of primigravidas with preeclampsia develop it during a future pregnancy. However, epidemiologic studies have shown that women with a history of preeclampsia do not have an increased risk of developing chronic hypertension (19).

Prevention. No measures have been shown convincingly to prevent preeclampsia. Salt restriction and aspirin, previously thought to be efficacious, have been shown in large clinical trials to be no better than placebo. This is also true for calcium supplementation, although it may decrease the risk of one component of preeclampsia, hypertension (79).

Management of Hypertension During Lactation

Because breast-feeding is practiced widely, some women who need antihypertensive drugs will seek advice regarding breast-feeding (66). Most drugs appear in breast milk, but the calculated dose consumed by the suckling infant ranges from 0.001 to 5% of the standard therapeutic dose tolerated by infants without toxicity. Based on what is known of antihypertensive drugs, the following drugs, if needed, are regarded as compatible with lactation: atenolol, propranolol, methyldopa, captopril, and hydrochlorothiazide.

General References*

The Sixth Report of the Joint National Committee on Detection, Evaluation, and Treatment of High Blood Pressure. Arch Intern Med 157:2413, 1997.
> 1997 update of specific recommendations, based on the consensus of a national panel of experts. Well-referenced coverage of all aspects of hypertension.

Loggie JMN. Pediatric and adolescent hypertension. Boston: Blackwell Scientific, 1992.
> Definitive text on hypertension in adolescents.

Kaplan NM. Clinical hypertension. 7th ed. Baltimore: Williams & Wilkins, 1998.
> Monograph covering in detail what the clinician needs to know about essential and secondary hypertension.

Specific References

1. Alderman MH. Blood pressure management: individualized treatment based on absolute risk and the potential for benefit. Ann Intern Med 119:329, 1993.
2. Alderman MH, Budner N, Cohen H, et al. Prevalence of drug resistant hypertension. Hypertension 11(Suppl II):II-71, 1988.
3. Amery A, Birkenheager W, Brixko P, et al. Mortality and morbidity results from the European Working Party on High Blood Pressure in the Elderly trial. Lancet 1:1349, 1985.
4. Appel LJ, Moore TJ, Obarzanek E, et al. for the DASH Collaborative Research Group. A clinical trial of the effects of dietary patterns on blood pressure. N Engl J Med 336:1117–1124, 1997.
5. Appel LJ, Stason WB. Ambulatory blood pressure monitoring and blood pressure self-measurement in the diagnosis and management of hypertension. Ann Intern Med 118(11):867, 1993.
6. The Australian therapeutic trial in mild hypertension. Lancet 1:1261, 1980.
7. American College of Physicians. Automated ambulatory blood pressure devices and self-measured blood pressure monitoring devices: their role in the diagnosis and management of hypertension. Ann Intern Med 118(11):889, 1993.
8. Baker RH, Ende J. Confounders of auscultatory blood pressure measurement. J Gen Intern Med 10:223–231, 1995.
9. Bakris GL. Angiotensin-converting enzyme inhibitors and progression of diabetic nephropathy. Ann Intern Med 118(8):643, 1993.
10. Barker LR. Five-hour blood pressure check to assess hypertension not responding to conventional therapy. Md Med J 35(2):94, 1986.
11. Barker LR. Guanethidine, exercise, and hypotension. Lancet 2:1297, 1976.
12. Birkenhager WH, Krauss XH, Schalekamp MADH, Kolsters G. Consecutive haemodynamic patterns in essential hypertension. Lancet 1:560, 1972.
13. Borhani NO, Applegate WB, Cutler JA, et al. Systolic Hypertension in the Elderly Program (SHEP): baseline characteristics of the randomized sample. I: Rationale and design. Hypertension 17(Suppl II):2, 1991.
14. Brown NJ, Ray WA, Snowden M, Griffin MR. Black Americans have an increased rate of angiotensin converting enzyme inhibitor associated angioedema. Clin Pharmacol Ther 60:8–13, 1996.
15. Brush JE Jr, Cannon RO III, Schenke WH, et al. Angina due to coronary microvascular disease in hypertensive patients without left ventricular hypertrophy. N Engl J Med 319:1302, 1988.
16. Caird FI, Andrews GR, Kennedy RD. Effect of posture on blood pressure in the elderly. Br Heart J 35:527, 1973.
17. Carey RM, Reid RA, Ayers CR, et al. The Charlottesville blood-pressure survey. Value of repeated blood-pressure measurements. JAMA 236:847, 1976.
18. Carvedilol for heart failure. Med Lett 39:89–91, 1997.
19. Chesley LC, Annitto JE, Cosgrove RA. The remote prognosis of eclamptic women: sixth periodic report. Obstetrics 124:446, 1976.
20. Collins R, Peto R, MacMahon S, et al. Blood pressure, stroke, and coronary heart disease. Part 2, short-term reductions in blood pressure: overview of randomized drug trials in their epidemiological context. Lancet 335:827, 1990.
21. Consumer Reports. Blood-pressure monitors: convenience doesn't equal accuracy. Consumer Reports 61:50, 53–55, 1996.
22. Coope J, Warrender TS. Randomised trial of treatment of hypertension in elderly patients in primary care. BMJ 293:1145, 1986.
22a. Curb JD, Pressel SL, Cutler JA, et al. Effect of diuretic-based antihypertensive treatment on cardiovascular disease risk in older diabetic patients with isolated systolic hypertension. JAMA 276(23):1886–1892, 1996.
23. Devereaux RB. Regression of left ventricular hypertrophy: how and why? JAMA 275(19):1517–1518, 1996.
24. Detection, evaluation, and treatment of renovascular hypertension. Working Group on Renovascular Hypertension. Arch Intern Med 147:820, 1987.
25. Effects of estrogen or estrogen/progestin regimens on heart disease risk factors in postmenopausal women: the postmenopausal estrogen/progestin interventions (PEPI) trial. The Writing Group for the PEPI Trial. JAMA 273(3):199–208, 1995.
26. Eisenberg DM, Delbanco TL, Berkey CS, et al. Cognitive behavioral techniques for hypertension: are they effective? Ann Intern Med 118(12):964, 1993.
27. Ellison DH. The physiologic basis of diuretic synergism: its role in treating diuretic resistance. Ann Intern Med 114:886–894, 1991.
28. Engel BT, Gaarder KR, Glasgow MS. Behavioral treatment of high blood pressure. I. Analyses of intra- and interdaily variations of blood pressure during a one-month, baseline period. Psychosom Med 43:255, 1981.

---

*Bold print (general references) and bold numerals (specific references) denote published controlled clinical trials, meta-analyses, or consensus-based recommendations.

29. Epstein M, Bakris G. Newer approaches to antihypertensive therapy: use of fixed-dose combination therapy. Arch Intern Med 156:1969–1978, 1996.

30. Farnett L, Mulrow CD, Linn WD, et al. The J-curve phenomenon and the treatment of hypertension: is there a point beyond which pressure reduction is dangerous? JAMA 265:266, 1991.

31. The Fifth Report of the Joint National Committee on Detection, Evaluation, and Treatment of High Blood Pressure (JNC V). Arch Intern Med 153:154, 1993.

32. Glen SK, Elliott HL, Curzio JL, et al. White-coat hypertension as a cause of cardiovascular dysfunction. Lancet 348:654–657, 1996.

33. Grimm RH Jr, Flack JM, Grandits GA, et al. Long-term effects on plasma lipids of diet and drugs to treat hypertension. JAMA 275:1549–1556, 1996.

34. Grimm RH Jr, Grandits GA, Cutler JA, et al, for the TOMHS Research Group. Relationships of quality-of-life measures to long-term lifestyle and drug treatment in the treatment of mild hypertension study. Arch Intern Med 157:638–648, 1997.

35. Grossman E, Messerli FH, Grodfzicki T, Kowey P. Should a moratorium be placed on sublingual nifedipine capsules given for hypertensive emergencies and pseudoemergencies? JAMA 276:1328–1331, 1996.

35a. Gueyffier F, Boutitie F, Boissel JP, et al. Effect of antihypertensive drug treatment on cardiovascular outcomes in women and men: a meta-analysis of individual patient data from randomized, controlled trials. Ann Intern Med 126:761–767, 1997.

36. Harden PN, MacLeod MJ, Rodger RSC, et al. Effect of renal-artery stenting on progression of renovascular renal failure. Lancet 349:1133–1136, 1997.

37. Haynes RB, Sackett DL, Taylor DW, et al. Increased absenteeism from work after detection and labeling of hypertensive patients. N Engl J Med 299:741, 1978.

38. Health and Public Policy Committee, American College of Physicians. Philadelphia: Biofeedback for hypertension. Ann Intern Med 102:709, 1985.

39. Helgeland A. Treatment of mild hypertension: a five-year controlled drug trial. The Oslo study. Am J Med 69:725, 1980.

40. Hossmann V, Fitzgerald GA, Dollery CT. Influence of hospitalization and placebo therapy on blood pressure and sympathetic function in essential hypertension. Hypertension 3:113, 1981.

41. Insua JT, Sacks HS, Lau TS, et al. Drug treatment of hypertension in the elderly: a meta-analysis. Ann Intern Med 121:355–362, 1994.

42. Julius S. The Hypertension Optimal Treatment (HOT) study in the United States. J Hypertens 9:41S–44S, 1996.

43. Kannel WB, Sorlie P. Hypertension in Framingham. In: Paul O, ed. Epidemiology and control of hypertension. Miami: Symposia Specialists, 1975.

44. Kass DA, Wolff MR, Ting CT, et al. Diastolic compliance of hypertrophied ventricle is not acutely altered by pharmacologic agents influencing active processes. Ann Intern Med 119(6):466, 1993.

45. Khoury Z, Comans P, Keren A, et al. Effects of transdermal nicotine patches on ambulatory ECG monitoring findings: a double-blind study in healthy smokers. Cardiovasc Drugs Ther 10:179–184, 1996.

46. Klein LE. Compliance and blood pressure control. Hypertension II(Suppl II):II-61, 1988.

47. Kostis JB, Davis BR, Cutler J, et al. Prevention of heart failure by antihypertensive drug treatment in older persons with isolated systolic hypertension. 278:212–216, 1997.

48. Kroenke K, Omori DM, Simmons JO, et al. The safety of phenylpropanolamine in patients with stable hypertension. Ann Intern Med 111:1043, 1989.

48a. Lewis EJ, Hunsicker LG, Bain RP, Rohde RD. The effect of angiotensin-converting-enzyme inhibition on diabetic neuropathy. N Engl J Med 329:1456–1462, 1993.

49. MRC Working Party. Medical Research Council trial of treatment of hypertension in older adults: principal results. BMJ 304:405, 1992.

50. MacMahon S, Peto R, Cutler J, et al. Blood pressure, stroke, and coronary heart disease. Part 1, prolonged differences in blood pressure: prospective observational studies corrected for the regression dilution bias. Lancet 335:765, 1990.

51. Madhavan S, Ooi WL, Cohen H, Alderman MH. Relation of pulse pressure and blood pressure reduction to the incidence of myocardial infarction. Hypertension 23:395–401, 1994.

52. Magarian GJ. Reserpine: a relic from the past or a neglected drug of the present for achieving cost containment in treating hypertension? J Gen Intern Med 6:561, 1991.

53. Manger WM, Gifford RW Jr. Pheochromocytoma: current diagnosis and management. Cleve Clin J Med 60(5):365, 1993.

54. Mann SJ, Pickering TG. Detection of renovascular hypertension: state of the art—1992. Ann Intern Med 117:845, 1992.

55. Materson BJ, Reda DJ, Cushman WC, et al. Single-drug therapy for hypertension in men. N Engl J Med 326:914, 1993.

56. Materson BJ, Reda DJ, Cushman WC, Henderson WG. Results of combination anti-hypertensive therapy after failure of each of the components. J Human Hypertens 9:791–796, 1995.

56a. Becker JM, Brandenburg U, Penzel T, et al. Blood pressure and sleep apnea: results of long-term nasal continuous positive airway pressure therapy. Cardiology 79:84–92, 1991.

57. Medical Research Council Working Party. MRC trial of treatment of mild hypertension: principal results. BMJ 291:97, 1985.

58. Meyer JS, Leiderman H, Denny-Brown D. Electroencephalographic study of insufficiency of the basilar and carotid arteries in man. Neurology 6:455, 1956.

59. Michalewicz L, Messerli FH. Cardiac effects of calcium antagonists in systemic hypertension. Am J Cardiol 79(10A):39–46, 1997.

60. Midgley JP, Matthew AG, Greenwood CMT, Logan AG. Effect of reduced dietary sodium on blood pressure: a meta-analysis of randomized controlled trials. JAMA 275:1590–1597, 1996.

61. Moser M, Hebert PR. Prevention of disease progression, left ventricular hypertrophy and congestive heart failure in hypertension treatment trials. J Am Coll Cardiol 27:1214, 1996.

62. National High Blood Pressure Education Program Working Group on High Blood Pressure in Pregnancy. Working Group report on high blood pressure in pregnancy. Am J Obstet Gynecol 163:1689, 1990.

63. National High Blood Pressure Education Program Working Group. 1995 update of the working group reports on chronic renal failure and renovascular hypertension. Hypertension 29:744–750, 1997.

64. National High Blood Pressure Education Program Working Group. Report on primary prevention of hypertension. Arch Intern Med 153:186, 1993.

65. Nesselroad JM, Flacco VA, Phillips DM, Kruse J. Accuracy of automated finger blood pressure devices. Fam Med 28:189–192, 1996.

66. Newton ER. Lactation and its disorders. In: Mitchell GW Jr, Bassett LW, eds. The female breast and its disorders. Baltimore: Williams & Wilkins, 1990.

67. Nicholson JP, Alderman MH, Pickering TG, et al. Cigarette smoking and renovascular hypertension. Lancet 1:765, 1983.

68. Perloff D, Grim C, Flack J, et al, for the Writing Group. Human blood pressure determination by sphygmomanometry. Circulation 8:2460–2467, 1993.

69. Perneger TV, Klag MJ, Whelton PK. Projections of hypertension-related renal disease in middle-aged residents of the United States. JAMA 269(10):1272, 1993.

69a. Pickering TG, James GD, Boddie C, et al. How common is white coat hypertension? JAMA 259:225–228, 1988.

70. Pitt B, Segal R, Martinez FA, et al. Randomised trial of losartan versus captopril in patients over 65 with heart failure (Evaluation of Losartan in the Elderly Study, ELITE). Lancet 349:747–752, 1997.

71. Prisant LM, Alpert BS, Robbins CS, et al. American National Standard for nonautomated sphygmomanometers: summary report. Am J Hypertens 8:210–213, 1995.

72. Psaty BM, Heckbert SR, Koepsell TD, Siscovick DS. The risk of myocardial infarction associated with antihypertensive drug therapies. JAMA 274:620–625, 1995.

73. Psaty BM, Smith NL, Siscovick DFS, et al. Health outcomes associated with antihypertensive therapies used as first-line agents: a systematic review and meta-analysis. JAMA 277: 739–745, 1997.

74. Radack K, Deck C. Do nonsteroidal anti-inflammatory drugs interfere with blood pressure control in hypertensive patients? J Gen Intern Med 2:108, 1987.

75. Redman CWG, Beilin LJ, Bonnar J, Ounsted MK. Fetal outcome in trial of antihypertensive treatment in pregnancy. Lancet 2:753, 1976.

76. Schmieder RE, Martus P, Klingbeil A. Reversal of left ventricular hypertrophy in essential hypertension: a meta-analysis of randomized double-blind studies. JAMA 275:1507–1513, 1996.

77. SHEP Cooperative Research Group. Prevention of stroke by antihypertensive drug treatment in older persons with isolated systolic hypertension. JAMA 265:3255, 1991.

78. Shepherd RFJ, Zachariah PK, Shub C. Hypertension and left ventricular diastolic function. Mayo Clin Proc 64:1521, 1989.

79. Sibai BM. Treatment in hypertension in pregnant women. N Engl J Med 335(4):257–265, 1996.

80. Sinaiko AR. Hypertension in children. N Engl J Med 335: 1968–1973, 1996.

81. The Sixth Report of the Joint National Committee on Prevention, Detection, Evaluation, and Treatment of High Blood Pressure. Arch Intern Med 157:2413, 1997.

82. Staessen JA, Byttebier G, Buntinx F, et al. Antihypertensive treatment based on conventional or ambulatory blood pressure measurement: a randomized controlled trial. JAMA 278:1065–1072, 1997.

83. Staessen JA, Fagard R, Thijs L, et al, for the Systolic Hypertension—Europe (Syst-Eur) Trial Investigators. Morbidity and mortality in the placebo-controlled European Trial on Isolated Systolic Hypertension in the Elderly. Lancet 350:757, 1997.

84. Stamler R, Grimm RH Jr, Dyer AR, et al. Cardiac status after four years in a trial of nutritional therapy for high blood pressure. Arch Intern Med 149:661, 1989.

85. Stamler R, Stamler J, Grimm R, et al. Nutritional therapy for high blood pressure: final report of a four-year randomized controlled trial—the Hypertension Control Program. JAMA 257:1484, 1987.

86. Swedish Trial in Old Patients with Hypertension (STOP-Hypertension). Morbidity and mortality in the Swedish Trial in Old Patients with Hypertension. Lancet 338:1281, 1991.

87. Svetkey LP, Kadir S, Dunnick NR, et al. Similar prevalence of renovascular hypertension in selected blacks and whites. Hypertension 17:678, 1991.

88. Taguchi J, Freis ED. Partial reduction of blood pressure and prevention of complications in hypertension. N Engl J Med 291:329, 1974.

89. Toto RD, Mitchell HC, Lee HC, et al. Reversible renal insufficiency due to angiotensin converting enzyme inhibitors in hypertensive nephrosclerosis. Ann Intern Med 115:513, 1991.

90. Treatment of Mild Hypertension (TOMH) Research Group. A randomized, placebo-controlled trial of a nutritional-hygienic regimen along with various drug monotherapies. Arch Intern Med 151:1413, 1991.

91. Trials of Hypertension Prevention Collaborative Research Group. The effects of nonpharmacologic interventions on blood pressure of persons with high normal levels. Results of Trials of Hypertension Prevention, phase 1. JAMA 267:1213, 1992.

92. Trials of Hypertension Prevention Collaborative Research Group. Effects of weight loss and sodium reduction intervention on blood pressure and hypertension incidence in overweight people with high-normal blood pressure: Trials of Hypertension Prevention, Phase II. Arch Intern Med 157:657–667, 1997.

93. Triggle DJ. Pharmacologic and therapeutic differences among calcium channel antagonists: profile of Mibefradil, a new calcium antagonist. Am J Cardiol 78(Suppl 9A):7–12, 1996.

94. Tsapatsaris NP, Napolitana GT, Rothchild J. Osler's maneuver in an outpatient setting. Arch Intern Med 151:2209, 1991.

95. Update on the 1987 Task Force Report on high blood pressure in children and adolescents: a working group report from the National High Blood Pressure Education Program. Pediatrics 98(4):649, 1996.

96. Verdecchia P, Schillaci G, Borgioni C, et al. Prognostic significance of the white coat effect. Hypertension 29:1218–1224, 1997.

97. Veterans Administration Cooperative Study Group on Antihypertensive Agents. Effects of treatment on morbidity in hypertension: results in patients with diastolic blood pressures averaging 115 through 129 mm Hg. JAMA 202:116, 1967.

98. Veterans Administration Cooperative Study Group on Antihypertensive Agents: II. Effects of treatment on morbidity in hypertension: results in patients with diastolic blood pressures averaging 90 through 114 mm Hg. JAMA 212:1143, 1970.

99. Weingarten KL, Zimmerman RD, Pinto RS, Whelan MA. Computed tomographic changes of hypertensive encephalopathy. AJNR 6:395, 1985.

100. Weiss NS. Relation of high blood pressure to headache, epistaxis, and selected other symptoms: the United States Health Examination Survey of Adults. N Engl J Med 287:631, 1972.

101. Whelton PK, He J, Cutler JA, et al. Effects of oral potassium on blood pressure: meta-analysis of randomized controlled clinical trials. JAMA 277:1624–1632, 1997.

102. Wright JT Jr. The Antihypertensive and Lipid Lowering Heart Attack Prevention Trial (ALLHAT). Am J Hypertens 8:27A, 1995.

103. Young MJ, Dmuchowski C, Wallis JW, et al. Biochemical tests for pheochromocytoma: strategies in hypertensive patients. J Gen Intern Med 4:273, 1989.

104. Zuspan FP, Samuels P. Preventing preeclampsia. N Engl J Med 329(17):1265, 1993.

Musculoskeletal Problems

CHAPTER 63

Shoulder Pain

DAVID E. KERN, MD, MPH

Shoulder pain is common. Its prevalence ranges from 8 to more than 20% in the population age 30 and above; it is most prevalent in middle and older age (2,3,9). It represents the seventeenth and twenty-ninth most common reasons why patients consult their internist and family physician, respectively (24). Usually the general physician can establish the correct diagnosis and direct appropriate therapy without orthopedic or rheumatologic consultation. This chapter reviews the major causes of shoulder pain and provides a basis for diagnosis and treatment of these conditions.

ANATOMY AND FUNCTION

To enable accurate diagnosis and treatment of disorders of the shoulder, it is necessary to understand the anatomy and function of the shoulder structures (Figs. 63.1 and 63.2; Table 63.1). Normal shoulder motion depends on the smooth, integrated movement of the glenohumeral, acromioclavicular, and sternoclavicular joints and the scapulothoracic articulation.

The shoulder structures themselves are organized in four layers (Fig. 63.1).

1. The most superficial layer of the shoulder consists of the deltoid (abducts the shoulder), pectoralis major and minor (adducts the shoulder), and trapezius muscles (elevates and rotates the scapula). The acromion, coracoacromial ligament, and deltoid muscle form a roof overlying the deeper structures.

2. Beneath the superficial layer is the *subacromial or subdeltoid bursa,* which assists free movement of underlying structures in relation to the roof.

3. Beneath the bursa lies the *rotator cuff,* a group of muscles and their tendons, which consists of the supraspinatus superiorly, the infraspinatus and teres minor posteriorly, and the subscapularis anteriorly. The rotator cuff muscles stabilize the humeral head in the glenoid fossa. *Abduction* of the shoulder is accomplished by the coordinated action of the deltoid (which initially elevates, or shrugs, the glenohumeral joint, then abducts the arm at the glenohumeral joint) and the rotator cuff muscles, especially the supraspinatus (which hold the humeral head in the glenoid fossa while abducting). In addition, the rotator cuff muscles assist in internal and external rotation of the shoulder. Repetitive impingement of these structures between the acromion or coracoacromial ligament and the greater tuberosity of the humerus during abduction is thought to lead to inflammatory and degenerative changes within the cuff that are the most common cause of nontraumatic shoulder pain.

4. Beneath the rotator cuff are the ligamentous capsule and the glenohumeral *joint space.* The tendon of the long head of the biceps runs through the joint capsule and along the bicipital or intertubercular groove of the humerus on its way from its origin on the superior aspect of the glenoid fossa to its muscular attachment on the proximal radius; its major function is to supinate the flexed forearm and to flex the supinated forearm. Also, it has a modest involvement in flexion of the arm at the shoulder.

The joint is formed by the articulation of the humeral head with the shallow glenoid fossa of the scapula, the diameter and depth of which are increased by the fibrocartilaginous glenoid labrum. The shallowness of the fossa enables nearly hemispheric motion of the arm, but this wide range of motion is achieved at the price of joint stability. Stability of the shoulder joint depends primarily not on bony structures, but on the integrity of supporting soft tissue structures including the labrum, capsule, and rotator cuff.

DIAGNOSTIC APPROACH

Pain about the shoulder usually originates from one of three sites: periarticular structures (e.g., the rotator cuff), the glenohumeral joint, or sites distant from the shoulder. The causes of shoulder pain arranged by their relative frequencies are listed in Table 63.2.

History and Physical Examination

History and physical examination are usually sufficient to establish a working diagnosis and direct effective treatment. For these reasons, among joints, examination of the shoulder has been called the most rewarding (Cyriax, 1982, "General References"). History is less useful than physical examination in estab-

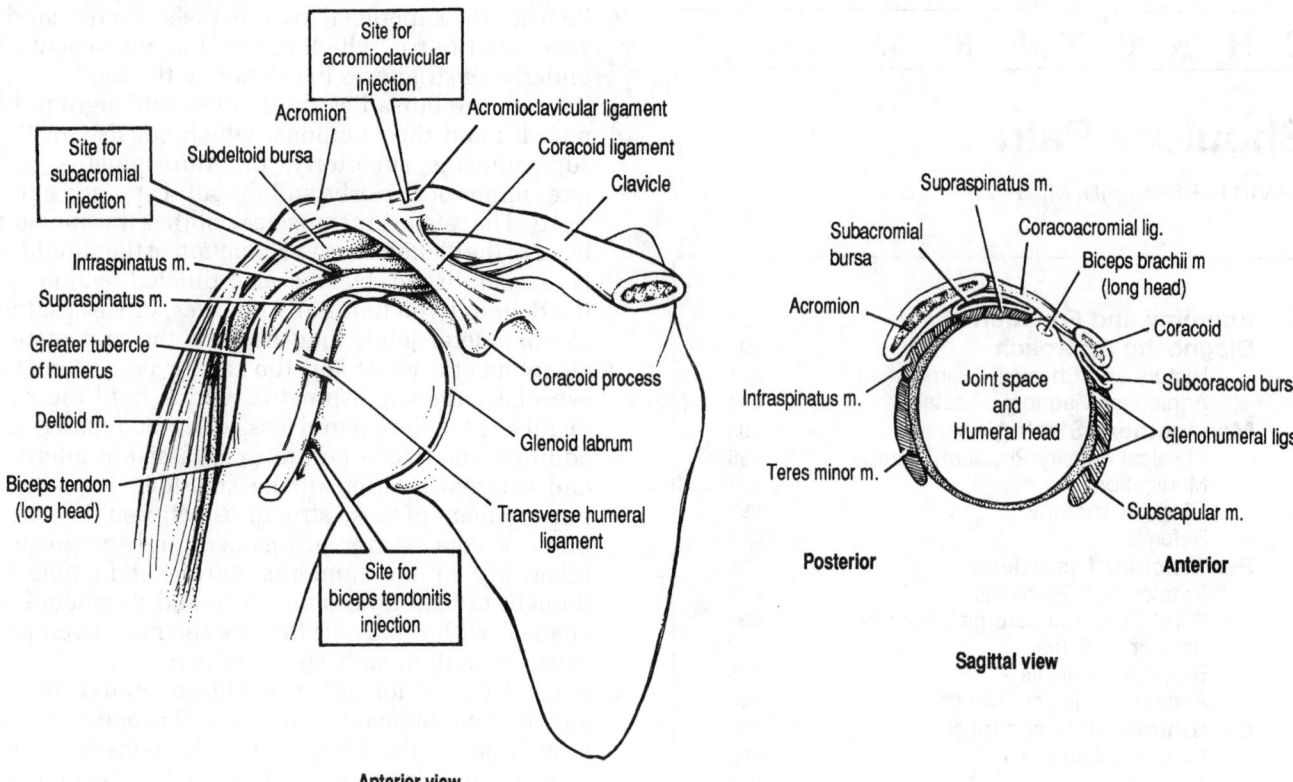

Figure 63.1. Structures of the shoulder and their relationships. Note that the subdeltoid bursa lies next to the supraspinatus tendon, but separate from the shoulder joint. Note the acromion and the coracoacromial ligaments, which may impinge on the supra-

spinatus tendon upon abduction of the arm. Note the location for subacromial injection into the bursa and about the rotator cuff tendons. (Sagittal section adapted from Pansky B. Review of gross anatomy. New York: Macmillan, 1979.)

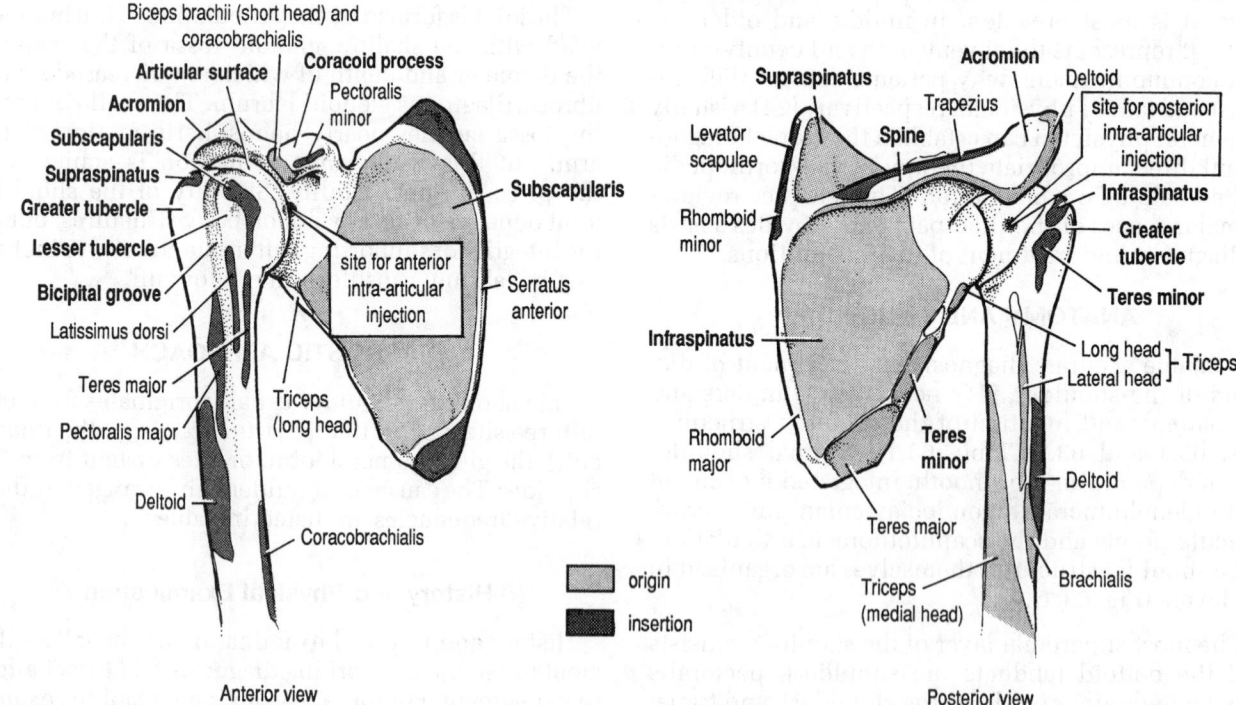

Figure 63.2. Humerus and scapula showing attachments of muscles. The insertions of the triceps and biceps onto the ulna and radius, respectively, are not shown. (Adapted from Agur AMR,

Lee MJ, eds. Grant's atlas of anatomy. Baltimore: Williams & Wilkins, 1991.)

Table 63.1.   Muscles Acting on the Shoulder Joint

Flexion	Extension	Abduction	Adduction	Medial Rotation	Lateral Rotation
Pectoralis major (clavicle head)	Latissimus dorsi	Deltoid (as whole)	Pectoralis major (as whole)	Pectoralis major (as whole)	Infraspinatus[a]
	Teres major	Supraspinatus[a]			Teres minor
Deltoid (anterior fibers)	Deltoid (posterior fibers)		Latissimus dorsi	Latissimus dorsi	Deltoid (posterior fibers)
Coracobrachialis	Triceps (long head)		Teres major	Teres major	
Biceps[a] (long head)			Subscapularis	Subscapularis[a]	
			Triceps (long head)	Deltoid (anterior fibers)	

Modified from Pansky B. Review of gross anatomy. 4th ed. New York: Macmillan, 1979.

[a]Muscles (rotator cuffs and biceps) most commonly associated with shoulder pain.

Table 63.2   Differential Diagnosis of Shoulder Pain in Primary Care Adult Patients

Most Common
Rotator cuff tendinitis (supraspinatus, infraspinatus–teres minor, subscapularis)

Common
Rotator cuff tears (partial more common than complete)
Subdeltoid/subacromial bursitis

Intermediate
Adhesive capsulitis/frozen shoulder

Occasional
Acromioclavicular arthritis/strain
Biceps (long head) tendinitis
Cardiac (referred pain)
Carpal tunnel syndrome (referred pain)
Cerebrovascular accident with hemiparesis (see Chapter 83)
Cervical/neck disorders (referred pain)
Degenerative/osteoarthritis (often posttraumatic)
Dislocation
Fracture (neck of humerus, greater tuberosity)
Glenohumeral instability/subluxation
Glenoid labral tears
Neoplasm (local or referred pain)
Rheumatoid arthritis

Rare
Arthritis, other causes (e.g., gout, pseudogout, psoriasis, neuropathic, ankylosing spondylitis)
Infection (intra-articular or extra-articular)
Nerve entrapment: axillary and suprascapular nerves (referred pain)
Osteonecrosis (avascular or aseptic necrosis)
Polymyalgia rheumatica
Reflex sympathetic dystrophy/shoulder–hand syndrome
Sickle cell crisis
Thoracic outlet syndrome (referred pain)
Visceral (referred from sources other than neck or heart, e.g., pleural irritation by lung cancer or other cause; irritation to phrenic nerve or diaphragm by pathologic process such as subdiaphragmatic abscess, ruptured viscus, or disease of the mediastinum, pericardium, liver, spleen, or gallbladder; dissecting aortic aneurysm)
Other traumatic or periarticular soft tissue problems

lishing the anatomic problem, but is nevertheless helpful. *Perceived location* of the pain is usually not helpful because most sources of pain (e.g., rotator cuff tendon, subdeltoid bursa, glenohumeral joint space) share a fifth (or sixth) cervical derivation and cause pain in the upper arm only. More severe lesions tend to cause pain radiating down the arm and forearm, usually along the anterolateral aspect. Pain confined to the point of the shoulder, however, suggests a lesion of the acromioclavicular joint, which has a fourth cervical derivation. Involvement of other joints suggests a generalized arthritic process. *Asking about recent trauma and briefly reviewing the patient's problem list, medication list, and past medical history* may be helpful in raising the suspicion for certain less common causes of shoulder pain, such as dislocation (e.g., from trauma), neoplasm (e.g., a history of breast or lung cancer), or osteonecrosis (e.g., from corticosteroid use). Dislocation of the glenohumeral joint should be suspected with major injuries to the arm, especially if the shoulder is abducted and externally rotated at impact, whereas injury to or separation of the acromioclavicular joint usually results from a direct blow to the acromion. Asking *what precipitates or makes the pain worse* is also helpful. Pain referred to the shoulder from a distant site should not be exacerbated by movement of the shoulder. In contrast, pain with active or passive movement of the shoulder suggests a shoulder or periarticular problem. A history of *occupational* (17) *and sports activities,* such as working with hands elevated, lifting heavy objects, carrying loads supported by the shoulders, hand–arm vibration, pitching baseballs, swimming, or serving tennis balls, can identify exacerbating factors that may both suggest a cause and direct the attention of the clinician to an activity of the patient that should be modified as part of the treatment plan, especially in a patient with chronic or recurrent shoulder pain.

Physical examination is usually successful in identifying the source of the pain. The uninvolved shoulder should be used as a control to confirm any questionable abnormality found on examination of the symptomatic shoulder. *Inspection* is the least helpful part of the examination, but it may reveal evidence of atrophy or displacement of bony landmarks. The approach of Cyriax (1982, "General References") is most useful, and widely accepted, for the rest of the examination. First, the *location of pain origin* is surveyed through a brief examination of the neck, scapula, shoulder, elbow, and wrist, usually involving a combination of active and resisted movements (see below). The suspected abnormal site is then examined in depth. If the shoulder appears normal but another site is abnormal on the survey, the shoulder pain is probably referred from the abnormal site. If the survey reveals no abnormalities, the pain may be referred or an abnormality in the shoulder may still be present. The shoulder is examined in the following way.

Active motion is studied by having the patient perform a few simple maneuvers. The patient is asked to elevate the arm as far as possible (normal is 180°). External and internal rotation is assessed with the elbow at the patient's side and the forearm held at a right angle in the anteroposterior plane (normal values are 40° to 45° and 55° to 60°, respectively). Internal rotation is usually limited by the patient's body and can be further evaluated by having the patient touch his or her back from below. Alternatively, external and internal rotation can be assessed with the patient's arm in 90° abduction. Adduction is assessed by placement of the patient's hands on the opposite shoulders.

Passive range of motion is then examined and compared with the active range. About 90° of arm elevation is accomplished through abduction at the glenohumeral joint, 60° by rotation of the scapula by the serratus anterior and upper half of the trapezoid, and 30° by adduction and external rotation, which increases the articulating surface of the humeral head and turns the surgical neck away from the tip of the acromion. Glenohumeral abduction can be isolated by immobilizing the scapula or observing for scapular movement with one's fingers on the inferior angle of the scapula.

Next, *resisted movements* are examined, as this helps elicit pain from the deep muscles of the rotator cuff. These are accomplished without movement of the shoulder joint, with the elbow at the patient's side, and with the forearm at a right angle in the anteroposterior plane. Abduction is tested by having the patient press outward at the elbow against the examiner's braced hand so that movement does not occur. Adduction is tested by having the patient press in, flexion forward, and extension backward at the elbow against the examiner's hand. External rotation is tested by having the patient press laterally and internal rotation medially at the wrist against the examiner's braced hand, again without movement and with the elbow kept at the side. Resisted flexion and supination of the elbow are assessed with the arm in the same position in order to test for a lesion of the biceps tendon. Strength and the elicitation of pain are noted.

Finally, *palpation* is performed. Palpation is less useful than the combination of active movements, passive range of motion, and resisted movements because pain from palpation is common and nonspecific and because some structures are difficult or impossible to palpate. However, differential tenderness, compared with the control side, can help confirm disorders at the acromioclavicular joint, the bursa, or the biceps tendon in the bicipital groove.

Interpretation of the physical examination (Table 63.3). Both articular and periarticular disorders can cause pain and limitation on active movements. If both active and passive ranges of motion of the shoulder are limited, a disorder of the glenohumeral joint, adhesive capsulitis, or bursitis should be suspected. Limited range of motion with a *capsular pattern* (lateral rota- tion more impaired than abduction, internal least impaired) suggests adhesive capsulitis or gleno- humeral arthritis. A *noncapsular pattern* (abduction limited with little limitation to either rotation) suggests subdeltoid bursitis. When passive range of motion is normal or exceeds the active range and when passive movements are not painful or less painful than active ones, a *periarticular cause* is likely. Pain on resisted movements identifies the anatomic location of the disorder (i.e., some element of the muscle or adjacent tissue, e.g., a bursa, that is being tensed). Weakness on resisted movements suggests a muscle or tendon tear or neurologic compromise. Sometimes strength cannot be accurately assessed because of pain, unless the shoul- der is examined after the appropriately placed injec- tion of a local anesthetic.

Additional Diagnostic Tests

Additional diagnostic tests should be used selec- tively to confirm or further define, for therapeutic purposes, a diagnosis suspected on the basis of history and physical examination. Depending on the circum- stances, additional diagnostic tests may include a complete blood cell count, erythrocyte sedimentation rate, serologic tests for rheumatologic disorders, diag- nostic arthrocentesis, plain x-ray of the shoulder or neck, and further imaging modalities. All have impor- tant roles in selected patients (see below). Acute epi- sodes of shoulder pain caused by rotator cuff tendini- tis, bursitis, or biceps tendinitis should usually be managed without any additional testing.

Plain shoulder x-rays should usually be ordered in the presence of significant trauma, suspected arthritis (limited range of motion in the capsular pattern on physical examination), suspicion of neoplasm, or sus- picion of osteonecrosis, or with chronic, recurrent, or unexplained symptoms. Standard views consist of anteroposterior (AP) films in external and internal rotation. Additional views can be helpful in specific circumstances. An axillary lateral view (which permits accurate evaluation of the glenohumeral articulation but requires that the arm be held in abduction) or a scapular Y view (a lateral view that displays the scapula on end) will detect a posterior dislocation, which may not be noticed on routine AP views. A caudal tilt view can help identify subacromial spurs, which may contribute to a chronic impingement or rotator cuff syndrome. A true AP view, in which the patient is turned 40° to 45° toward the symptomatic shoulder, provides a tangential view for evaluation of the glenohumeral joint space in a patient with arthritis. Plain x-rays, although useful in detecting fracture, dislocation, bone destruction, advanced osteonecrosis, calcific tendinitis, and arthritis, are insensitive in the diagnosis of early osteonecrosis and, at best, are only suggestive in the diagnosis of rotator cuff tear and other soft tissue disorders. For all of these reasons, a detailed explanation of the reason for the x-ray will guide the radiologist to obtain the appropriate views.

Further imaging studies are best ordered in consul-

Table 63.3.   Interpretation of the Physical Examination

| | Rotator Cuff Lesions | | | | | | | |
L = Limited P = Pain W = Weak ( ) = Variably present	Supraspinatus tendinitis	Supraspinatus tear	Infraspinatus tendinitis	Subscapularis tendinitis	Subacromial/subdeltoid tendinitis	Adhesive capsulitis/arthritis	Biceps tendinitis/arthritis	Acromioclavicular joint
Active range of motion	(L)[a]	(L)[a,c]	(L)[a]	(L)[a]	L[d] P	L[e] P		P[f]
Passive range of motion					L[d] P	L[e] P		P[f]
Painful arc	P[b]	P[b]	P[b]	P[b]	P			
Resisted *abduction*	P	(P)[b,c] W						
Resisted external rotation			P					
Resisted internal rotation				P				
Resisted flexion/ supination of elbow							P	
Full passive *adduction*								P[f]

[a]Range of motion may be limited by pain.

[b]Pain may be absent in deep or musculotendinous lesions.

[c]When the tear is complete, initiation of abduction may be impossible and pain may be absent.

[d]Limitation is in a noncapsular pattern, with marked limitation of abduction and little restriction of external rotation.

[e]Limitation is in a capsular pattern, with limitation of exernal rotation greatest, abduction intermediate, and internal rotation least.

[f]Pain is usually felt at A–C joint or point of shoulder (C4). For all other lesions, pain is usually felt in anterolateral aspect of upper arm (C5), with or without radiation to the forearm.

tation with a specialist when referral or the possibility of surgery is being considered. *Ultrasonography* (about 1.2 to 4 times more expensive than plain x-rays) can demonstrate even partial rotator cuff tears, but it requires skilled interpretation. Reported sensitivities and specificities (compared with arthrography, magnetic resonance imaging [MRI], or direct visualization at surgery) are variable, ranging from 58 to more than 90% and from 50 to 96%, respectively. The diagnostic accuracy of ultrasonography for tendon tears ranges from 77 to 95% in recent reports (Smith and Campbell, "General References"). *Arthrography* (3 to 8 times more expensive than plain x-rays) is both sensitive (approximately 92%) and specific (approximately 98%) for detecting rotator cuff tears (8), but causes patient discomfort and may miss partial tears, particularly those on the bursal side. Communication of dye between the glenohumeral joint and the subacromial space unequivocally confirms a full-thickness tear. Arthrography can also confirm a diagnosis of adhesive capsulitis when clinical findings are equivocal. *Arthrography combined with computerized tomography (arthro-CT)* is of value in detecting soft tissue lesions (e.g., partial tendon tears) and intra-articular pathology (e.g., labral tears, capsular tears, loose bodies, chondral defects), especially in cases of recurrent subluxation/ dislocation (18). *Computerized tomography (CT)* (4 to 8 times the expense of plain x-rays) and *MRI* (7 to 17 times the expense of plain x-rays) are noninvasive but expensive techniques for the evaluation of soft tissue lesions. MRI better defines capsule anatomy, supraspinatus tendon integrity, the site of impingement, and bursal anatomy than does CT. It is equal to arthrography and superior to ultrasound in detecting rotator cuff tears (sensitivity 75 to 100%, specificity 84 to 100%) (6,8). It is the imaging technique of choice in the diagnosis of early osteonecrosis (18).

MANAGEMENT STRATEGIES

Specific management varies depending on the disorder responsible for the pain. However, some management strategies are broadly applicable.

Physical Activity/Physical Therapy

In the treatment of acute pain, the patient may benefit from a brief period (2 to 3 days) of rest with the arm in a sling. Many patients can begin range-of-motion movements immediately to maintain mobility, while avoiding aggressive exercise or overuse. Prolonged immobilization of the shoulder should be avoided whenever possible because contracture of the shoulder capsule and periarticular structures, known as adhesive capsulitis or frozen shoulder, may result. When glenohumeral range of motion remains restricted after the acute pain has diminished, specific exercises, such as pendular and wall-climbing exercises (Fig. 63.3), should be prescribed for 5 to 10 minutes two to four times per day to maintain joint mobility. Patients with impingement disorders (e.g., rotator cuff lesions and subdeltoid bursitis) should avoid repetitive tasks with their arms overhead or their elbows above midtorso height, especially if the condition is recurrent or chronic. A program of balanced isometric or isotonic exercise to strengthen the

rotator cuff musculature may also help prevent recurrences.

The effectiveness of adjunctive physical therapy measures, such as heat or ultrasound, has not been adequately demonstrated (14,26). Nevertheless, on empiric and theoretical grounds, local cooling is generally recommended after acute injury to relieve pain and to limit hemorrhage and edema. Similarly, local superficial heat or ultrasound can be recommended to decrease pain and promote tissue extensibility in the subacute and chronic stages, respectively (31).

Referral to a physical therapist is recommended when patients require a supervised exercise program after surgery or when satisfactory understanding of prescribed exercises or improvements in range

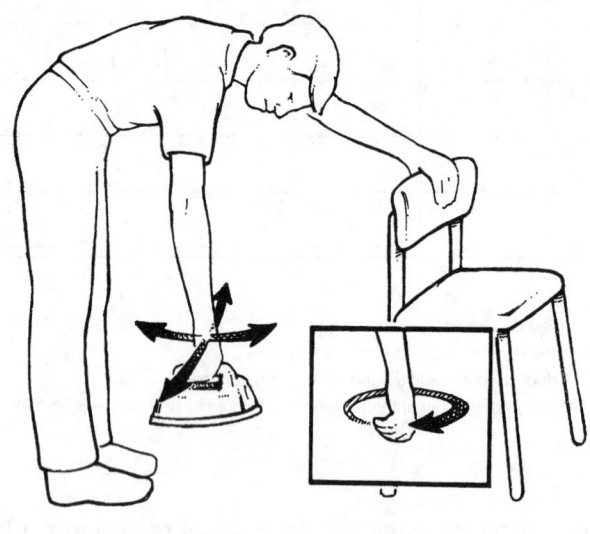

A. Pendular Exercise

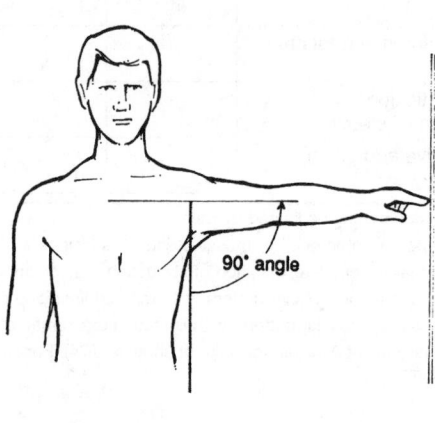

B. Normal Abduction

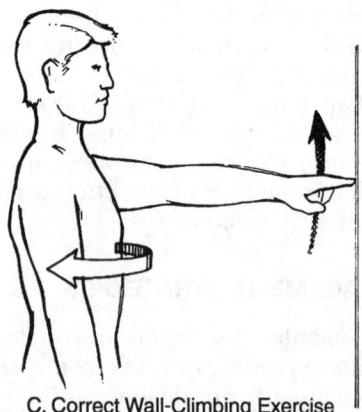

C. Correct Wall-Climbing Exercise

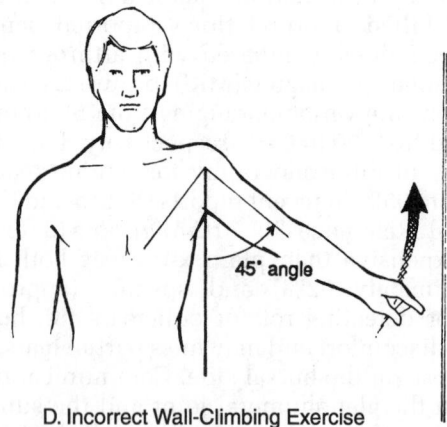

D. Incorrect Wall-Climbing Exercise

Figure 63.3. Range-of-motion exercises of the shoulder. **A.** Pendular exercise can be done with a weight, which facilitates the pendular movement. The arm is moved back and forth in the sagittal and frontal planes, then circumducted in the clockwise and counterclockwise directions in increasingly large circles. **B** and **C.** Wall-climbing exercise done correctly. The wall climb can be started facing the wall. The body is then turned until the patient is at a right angle to the wall. The shoulder movement is at the glenohumeral joint. **D.** Wall-climbing exercise done incorrectly, with shrugging of the scapula. (Redrawn from Cailliet R. Shoulder pain. Philadelphia: FA Davis, 1981.)

of motion have not been achieved after physician counseling.

Medication

Nonsteroidal anti-inflammatory drugs (NSAIDs) appear to be more effective than placebo but somewhat less effective than steroid injections in decreasing pain and restoring function in periarticular disorders (1,27,35,38). Generally, a 2-week course of one of these agents is prescribed for acute disorders (see Chapter 70 for a full discussion of NSAIDs). The effectiveness of NSAIDs for this purpose, compared with analgesics such as acetaminophen, has not been adequately studied (35), although NSAIDs have a theoretical advantage because of their anti-inflammatory properties. Some concern has been expressed regarding their gastrointestinal (peptic disease with bleeding or perforation) or renal (proteinuria and failure) toxicity, particularly in the elderly (32).

Injection Therapy

Based on studies using injections of lidocaine only, placebo oral drugs, NSAIDs/analgesics, heat, ultrasound, exercise, and acupuncture, injections of depocorticosteroid appear to reduce pain and speed functional recovery in patients with rotator cuff tendinitis/bursitis and are probably more effective than NSAIDs/analgesics (1,4,22,27,29,36). A second or even third injection is sometimes required. Based on controlled and uncontrolled studies (7,12,21,23,30,33,34,37), steroid injections (often several), combined with an exercise program that is designed to increase range of motion, appear to be more effective than analgesic or no therapy (16,28) in reducing pain and speeding the recovery of patients with adhesive capsulitis.

A 60 to 90% success rate can be expected after steroid injections for the treatment of bursitis and tendinitis of the shoulder. In one study, injection, after diagnosis by the physical examination strategies described above, was shown to be much more effective than tender or trigger point injections (20% success rate) (19). Serious complications of treatment (infection, degenerative changes after multiple injections, weakening or rupture of tendons) are rare (less than 1%). They can be minimized by using sterile technique, observing contraindications to intra-articular injection (Table 63.4), following the procedures for injection described in Chapter 66, limiting the number of injections into an area over a given period, and avoiding the injection of a volume greater than 1 to 2 mL or of solutions that are not diluted at least 1:1 with lidocaine directly into tendons. Instead, the diluted steroid can be injected around the length of the affected tendon. Subcutaneous tissue atrophy occasionally occurs and may be caused by inappropriately superficial injections. Postinjection flares of pain are uncommon (approximately 2% of injections), begin 6 to 12 hours after injection, last up to 72 hours, and can be treated with local cooling and

Table 63.4. Contraindications to Arthrocentesis or Injection into the Shoulder or Periarticular Structures

Diagnostic and Therapeutic
Overlying soft tissue infection
Bacteremia
Clotting disorder (relative)

Therapeutic (Corticosteroid Injection)
Septic arthritis
Unstable joint
Osteonecrosis
Neurotrophic joint
Marked juxta-articular osteoporosis
Intra-articular fracture

analgesics or NSAIDs. Systemic absorption of locally injected steroid does occur and may cause transient suppression of the hypothalamic–pituitary–adrenal axis, and this must be considered in certain situations, as in a diabetic patient in whom the blood sugar could become unusually elevated.

Injection techniques. Because of the frequency of shoulder pain and the apparent efficacy of steroid injections in treating a number of the most common causes, primary care physicians should become proficient in these techniques. Depending on the number and type of sites to be injected, 1 to 10 mL of a short-acting local anesthetic (e.g., 1% lidocaine) is mixed in a syringe with a variable amount of long-acting (depo) corticosteroid preparation (20 to 80 mg of triamcinolone [Kenalog 10 or 40], betamethasone [Celestone], or methylprednisolone [Depo-Medrol]). Injection is then accomplished, observing sterile technique and universal precautions, with a 1.5- to 2-inch 22- or 25-gauge needle; an 18- or 20-gauge needle is used if joint aspiration is required. For patient comfort, the steroid injection may be preceded by superficial and deep infiltration of a local anesthetic using a 25- to 30-gauge needle. Patients should be told that pain may return 1 to 4 hours after injection, when the effect of the short-acting local anesthetic wears off, but that the pain should improve again as the anti-inflammatory actions of the corticosteroid take effect (several hours or more after injection).

Rotator cuff lesions and subdeltoid bursitis are generally treated with a *subacromial injection* (Fig. 63.1) of 20 to 40 mg of triamcinolone or its equivalent in 4 to 6 mL of local anesthetic. The local anesthetic provides an adequate volume for the medication to diffuse through the bursa or along the rotator cuff tendons. The needle is inserted medially along the groove between the midpoint of the lateral acromion and the head of the humerus until grittiness and resistance to depression of the plunger are appreciated, as the needle enters the rotator cuff tendon. The needle is then slowly withdrawn while the plunger is depressed lightly, until resistance lessens and some of the solution can be injected. The needle is then partially withdrawn and redirected anteriorly and then posteriorly to deposit the remaining solution. This technique probably results in deposition of solution both in the subacromial portion of the bursa and along the rotator cuff tendon. When bursitis is the predominant finding and there is marked tenderness over the lower portion of the bursa, the injection should be directed toward this area as well. Cyriax (1984, "General References") describes techniques for injecting around the insertion of the specifically involved tendons, but the therapeutic trials described above generally use the subacromial fan distribution for injection.

Adhesive capsulitis is treated with *intra-articular injection* of 20 to 40 mg of triamcinolone or its equivalent in local anesthetic. A posterior or anterior approach may be used (Fig. 63.2). If the *posterior approach* is used, the patient should rotate the shoulder medially, which turns the articular surface posteriorly and presents a larger target. This position can be fixed, if necessary, by having the patient lie prone, with the forearm under the upper abdomen. The physician places an index finger on the point of the coracoid process and thumb on the point where the acromion and spine of the scapula meet at right angles, punctures the skin just inferior to the thumb, and directs the needle along the line joining the fingers, which crosses the glenoid cavity. Once impingement against cartilage is felt and there is resistance to depression of the plunger, the syringe is minutely withdrawn and the injection accomplished. A 2-inch needle is usually required. If the *anterior approach* is used, the patient is asked to sit with the shoulder externally rotated. The needle is inserted at a point just medial to the head of the humerus and slightly inferiorly and laterally to the coracoid process. It is directed posteriorly and slightly superiorly and laterally. Passage into joint space should be unobstructed. If bone is hit, the needle should be withdrawn and directed at a slightly different angle.

When bicipital tendinitis is the diagnosis, the *bicipital tendon* is identified by palpating it in its groove as the arm is rotated internally and externally with the elbow held in 90° of flexion. Twenty milligrams of triamcinolone or its equivalent in local anesthetic is injected along the length of the affected tendon.

The *acromioclavicular joint* (Fig. 63.1) may be palpated as a groove at the lateral end of the clavicle just medial to the shoulder. A ⅝- to 1-inch needle is directed inferiorly from the superior aspect of the joint. If the needle hits bone at less than 1-cm or ⅜-inch depth, the tip probably does not lie intra-articularly and slightly different spots should be tried until the needle slips in to about 2 cm length. Triamcinolone (Kenalog) 4 to 10 mg in a small volume of local anesthetic is then injected about the joint space. Alternatively, the needle can be inserted from an anterior approach, with the tip of the needle slightly inferior to the joint.

Because the glenohumeral joint capsule juxtaposes the rotator cuff tendons and rotator cuff tendon disorders may accompany adhesive capsulitis, subacromial and intra-articular injections are often combined at one session. This is particularly true for the treatment of adhesive capsulitis. Because intra-articular injections are not consistently successful in entering the joint space, the posterior and anterior approaches are sometimes used sequentially at the same or separate sessions.

Use of a short-acting local anesthetic with or without steroid allows the physician to assess immediately after injection the accuracy of an injection by asking the patient whether the pain is gone and by repeating the examination. Also, strength and range of motion, now uninhibited by pain, may be assessed more accurately if the injection was effective.

Because pain may be completely relieved, patients may be tempted to resume full activity of their shoulder immediately after injection. Common sense suggests that the patient should rest the arm briefly after injection in the case of periarticular disorders, avoid heavy use (or use of the type that may have precipitated the disorder) for several weeks while healing occurs, and take appropriate precautions to prevent recurrence.

Referral

Occasionally, the patient needs to be referred to an orthopedist, rheumatologist, or physical medicine and rehabilitation specialist. Indications for referral include dislocation, fracture, functionally significant rotator cuff tear or rupture, suspected neoplasm, inability to perform indicated steroid injection therapy, nonresponsiveness to therapy, chronic or recurrent symptoms despite appropriate management, or uncertainty regarding the diagnosis or treatment.

PERIARTICULAR DISORDERS
Rotator Cuff Tendinitis

Rotator cuff tendinitis is the most common cause of shoulder pain (9,19,29). The tendinous fibers of the rotator cuff muscles undergo degenerative changes with advancing age. The tendons, particularly the supraspinatus, which is the most superior, are thought to be worn down by repetitive excursion between the greater tuberosity of the humerus and the acromion and acromioclavicular ligament. Edema, hemorrhage, and inflammation associated with repeated trauma cause pain that may lead the patient to seek medical attention. Inflammation of the subacromial bursa may also occur in this manner. The *impingement syndrome* and *pericapsulitis* are less specific terms that are applied to these degenerative and inflammatory disorders of the tendons and bursa. Risk factors for rotator cuff tendinitis include repetitive overhead work or activities and increasing age. The physical examination is characterized by pain on resisted abduction (supraspinatus, most common), lateral rotation (infraspinatus), and/or medial rotation (subscapularis, least common). In the most common lesions, which involve the superficial distal end of the tendons, there is a *painful arc;* that is, pain occurring between 60° and 120° of shoulder abduction (or 60° to 90° of glenohumeral abduction) where the impingement occurs, but resolving with further elevation as the shoulder is flexed, externally rotated, and adducted and the impingement is relieved. An *impingement sign* (pain) can also be elicited by forcibly flexing/elevating the arm to 130° while immobilizing the scapula. In isolated rotator cuff tendinitis, muscle strength is normal; passive range of motion is normal or exceeds active range of motion, which may or may not be limited by pain. The indications for obtaining an x-ray are stated above. When rotator cuff tendinitis is the only problem, the x-ray is normal. However, periarticular calcification in the supraspinatus tendon or subacromial bursa is occasionally seen. Its clinical significance is uncertain because the majority of patients with this radiographic finding do not have symptoms; calcium deposits may disappear spontaneously and generally require no specific treatment (15). However, when these calcium deposits are associated with chronic or recurrent symptoms, removal of the deposit by lavage and aspiration or surgery may occasionally be successful. An orthopedist should be consulted in this situation for consideration of the performance of these procedures.

Treatment of patients with rotator cuff tendinitis is described above under "Management Strategies." Most patients improve over the course of a few weeks. Relief usually occurs immediately after injection therapy. However, recurrences and eventually the development of chronic symptoms are common (3,10), underscoring the importance of preventive counseling, based on a careful history of occupational and other activities. Persistent symptoms, despite appropriate treatment, suggest the possibility of a continued impingement, a tear, or instability (see below).

Subdeltoid (Subacromial) Bursitis

Bursitis may involve the subacromial or subdeltoid portion of the bursa and may accompany rotator cuff tendinitis. Its onset is often abrupt. The disorder is characterized by pain, often severe, with a noncapsular limitation (see above) of both active and passive ranges of motion. Active range of motion is usually more limited than passive range of motion. Abduction is significantly more limited than lateral or medial rotation. The bursa is tender to palpation; the area of tenderness may be used to direct the injection of corticosteroids. A painful arc may not be demonstrable until the patient recovers sufficient range of motion. Treatment is described above under "Management Strategies."

Rotator Cuff Tear

By the sixth decade, degenerative changes in the rotator cuff are seen almost universally and are thought to be secondary to diminished blood flow. Tears and ruptures of the cuff may then occur even in the absence of significant trauma. In younger patients, trauma (e.g., falling on an outstretched hand), injuries with subluxation or dislocation, and overuse are usually involved.

Most tears occur just proximal to the insertion of the supraspinatus tendon. A small tear may be indistinguishable from rotator cuff tendinitis on physical examination. Larger tears are characterized by weakness on resisted abduction. In complete tears (ruptures), the patient is unable to initiate abduction or lower the arm to the side smoothly *(drop arm test)* because the supraspinatus is necessary in stabilizing the humeral head and assisting the deltoid in the initial phase of abduction. X-rays are indicated when symptoms are recurrent or persistent, despite treatment (see "Diagnostic Approach," above). An uncommonly seen radiologic sign, narrowing of the space between the acromion and humerus (abnormal is 5 mm or less), suggests a tear, as does proximal subluxation of the humeral head and erosive changes in the anterior aspect of the acromion. The techniques of arthrography, CT, ultrasonography, and MRI are more useful than x-rays in confirming partial or complete tears (see "Diagnostic Approach," above); an orthopedic surgeon should be consulted at least by telephone to discuss the approach to establishing the diagnosis. In general, minor tears can be treated conservatively in the manner described for rotator cuff tendinitis. The decision to treat a patient with a large tear medically or surgically depends on the severity of symptoms, the functional disability, and the functional demands of each patient. The patient, the family, the general physician, and an orthopedist are optimally involved in making decisions. Indications for surgery remain somewhat unclear because of uncertainty about short- and long-term benefits versus risks in the absence of well-designed controlled trials. However, when a complete tear is diagnosed, early surgical intervention seems to be preferable to delayed intervention (25). The traditional surgical approach involves the resection of the anterior acromion (acromioplasty) and repair of the rotator cuff tendon. The recovery period is more protracted after surgery (6 to 9 months of painful or restricted movement) than after conservative therapy (typically 8 weeks of painful or restricted movement). Arthroscopic repair may shorten the recovery period compared with open surgical techniques. Because immobilization of the shoulder joint after surgery may lead to adhesive capsulitis, early and regular postoperative passive range-of-motion exercises under orthopedic or physical therapy supervision must be done. Complete pain relief and return to full function are uncommon after surgery.

Bicipital Tendinitis

With aging, the biceps tendon, like the rotator cuff tendons, is subject to inflammation, erosion, and rupture. Because the biceps tendon runs through the joint space and next to the rotator cuff and subacromial bursa, bicipital tendinitis may coexist with inflammation of these structures. However, attrition or chronic subluxation of the tendon in the bicipital groove of the humerus is more often responsible for symptoms. Pain on resisted supination *(Yergason's test/sign)* and flexion of the elbow are the characteristic findings on physical examination. When the glenoid origin is involved, the pain may be felt purely under the acromion. More often, pain is elicited in the upper arm, and the biceps tendon of the involved arm is tender to palpation in the bicipital groove. If bicipital tendinitis is isolated, active and passive ranges of motion of the shoulder are painless and full. X-rays are not necessary or diagnostic, but if done for other reasons, they may show degenerative changes in the wall of the bicipital groove on tangential views. Treatment is described above ("Management Strategies"). Subacromial or intra-articular injection should suffice when this portion of the tendon is involved; otherwise, injection is directed along (but not into) the tendon in the bicipital groove.

Rupture of the biceps tendon, which occurs rarely, is evident on physical examination as a mass of contracted muscle midway between the shoulder and elbow *(Popeye sign).* Rupture is accompanied by a sudden painful popping sensation, usually during a lifting effort. The upper arm remains painful and tender for several days following the rupture. Surgical repair, if desired (e.g., in an athlete or if an occupation demands maximal biceps function), is best accomplished within 7 days; otherwise the tendon is likely to be contracted or fibrosed, precluding effective repair. Conservative management is an acceptable alternative. With regular exercise the strength of forearm flexion and supination gradually returns; however, a 5 to 10% deficit in these movements usually persists.

Acromioclavicular Disorders

The acromioclavicular joint is formed by the articulation of the distal part of the clavicle and the acromion. Osteoarthritis is common in this joint during middle age and later life. Subluxation or dislocation may result from trauma, such as a fall on or a direct blow to the shoulder or acromion, which forces the scapula down and applies stress to the acromioclavicular and coracoclavicular ligaments. Laborers who lift heavy objects overhead or carry weights on their shoulders and athletes who compete in contact sports or weight lifting often sustain repetitive trauma to this joint. Injuries are classified as grade I, injury without subluxation; grade II, subluxation; and grade III, complete dislocation.

Pain is usually localized to the exact site of the acromioclavicular joint or to the point of the shoulder (acromial area). There is little or no radiation of pain into the upper deltoid area. On physical examination, active and passive ranges of motion are generally normal. Pain may be felt at the extreme limits of passive motion. *Full passive adduction* of the arm across the front of the upper thorax is often the most painful movement. Local tenderness is present when the superior ligament is involved. In grade III separation, the acromion is displaced inferiorly and anteriorly, in front of the clavicle. Plain x-rays are indicated in situations of severe trauma. When obtained, osteoarthritic changes are common but also are often present in asymptomatic patients. Alleviation of pain after injec-

tion of a short-acting anesthetic directly into the joint confirms this site as the source of pain. When a severe injury is suspected, the radiologic technician should be asked to obtain anteroposterior x-rays with the patient holding weights in both hands to help reveal grade II and grade III separations.

Treatment of pain caused by degenerative arthritis is discussed above ("Management Strategies") and includes the use of NSAIDs or nonnarcotic analgesics. Local injection of corticosteroid/anesthetic solution may relieve symptoms in arthritic or low-grade traumatic conditions. In patients in whom pain from trauma in which subluxation or complete dislocation is suspected cannot be controlled with conservative measures over a few days, referral to an orthopedist should be obtained for consideration of surgery. However, one caveat should be considered before considering surgery: Several prospective studies of grade III injuries that compared conservative management with strapping or a sling versus open reduction and internal fixation have failed to demonstrate improved results from surgical treatment. Therefore, conservative treatment of shoulder separations of all grades is currently recommended by most orthopedists (13). Conservative management consists of treatment with an analgesic and a sling until the acute pain subsides. The patient should be aware that there will be a permanent prominence of the distal clavicle in grade III separations and a 5 to 10% loss of shoulder strength, which for most people is functionally insignificant. Surgery may be considered in the rare person whose occupation depends on continuous overhead activity (e.g., painters and some athletes) and in whom conservative treatment has failed to control pain.

GLENOHUMERAL DISORDERS
Adhesive Capsulitis

Adhesive capsulitis, or *frozen shoulder,* is a condition of unknown (but likely multiple) causes in which progressive restriction of shoulder motion occurs. It is commonly seen in diabetic patients. Often, an underlying painful condition of the shoulder, such as rotator cuff tendinitis or subdeltoid bursitis, precedes the development of adhesive capsulitis. However, this disorder may also occur in association with a cerebrovascular accident (especially hemiparesis, in which case it affects the paretic side), myocardial infarction, cervical radiculopathy, and other conditions. The common underlying factor in these diverse conditions appears to be prolonged immobility of the arm. Eventually, the adhesive capsulitis may represent a greater disability than the initial cause of immobilization. Thickening of the joint capsule and capsular adhesions to the underlying humeral head develop. However, inflammatory findings in the capsule or synovial lining of the joint are not constant findings. It remains unclear, therefore, whether contracture of the shoulder capsule is a passive process related to lack of motion or an active process caused by inflammation.

Adhesive capsulitis is somewhat more common in

women than in men and generally occurs in the fifth decade or later. The patient characteristically complains of the insidious onset of diffuse pain and limitation of motion in the shoulder. In particular, the patient notes difficulty in performing tasks that require overhead arm motion, such as combing the hair and grasping objects from high shelves. Physical examination reveals pain at the extremes of motion and markedly reduced active and passive ranges of motion of the glenohumeral joint in a *capsular pattern* (see "Diagnostic Approach," above). Injection of an anesthetic agent into the glenohumeral joint may reduce the pain but does not result in an improved range of motion. A plain x-ray (see above for indications), if adhesive capsulitis is the only problem present, is generally normal. Arthrography, although usually unnecessary, is diagnostic; it shows a markedly reduced joint capacity, intact tendons, and an absence of inflammatory arthritic changes. If an arthrogram is done, corticosteroid injection by the orthopedist or radiologist can be accomplished at the same time, with accurate placement of solution.

The primary aims of treatment of adhesive capsulitis are pain relief, restoration of motion, and correction of any contributing cause. Treated only with analgesics, most patients recover within 2 to 3 years (16,28), but residual slight restriction of movement is common and severe restriction occasional at 3 to 4 years (5,16,28). In controlled and uncontrolled trials, intra-articular and periarticular corticosteroid injection, usually combined with a progressive exercise program designed to increase range of motion, has been associated with shortened recovery periods of 4 to 8 weeks (6,12,21,23,30,33,34,37). Typically, injections are repeated weekly for several weeks until the patient's pain is controlled and progress in mobility is being made. Capsular distension or rupture may actually speed recovery (21,30). In this regard, an exercise program should be started as soon as the acute pain subsides. This may be limited initially to passive range-of-motion exercises, performed at home with a trained family member. Active range of motion can often begin after injection, with pendular and then wall-climbing exercises (Fig. 63.3). Too aggressive mobilization may actually be associated with less satisfactory outcomes (5). Referral to a physical therapist is indicated when there is poor patient understanding, noncompliance, or lack of progress within a few weeks. In the past, referral to an orthopedist for manipulation of the shoulder under anesthesia to free capsular adhesions had been recommended for patients who do not improve with conservative management. The efficacy of this treatment has not been studied in a controlled fashion. Now it is generally not recommended and should be considered only in recalcitrant cases.

Trauma

Because of its instability, the shoulder is the joint most commonly dislocated. Dislocation occurs most often in active young to middle-aged adults. *Anterior dislocation* (95% of shoulder dislocations) usually follows a fall on an outstretched hand, with forceful abduction, extension, and external rotation of the shoulder. On physical examination, the contour of the shoulder, which is normally convex below the acromion because of the humeral head, is flattened. The tip of the acromion is now the most lateral point of the shoulder region, and a noticeable prominence, caused by the displaced humeral head, is seen and felt inferior to the clavicle. Standard anteroposterior x-rays confirm the diagnosis.

Posterior dislocation (5% of shoulder dislocations) is less obvious and more likely to be overlooked on examination and x-ray. It results from direct or indirect trauma that forces the humeral head posteriorly out of the glenoid fossa, and may follow an electrical shock or convulsion. On physical examination, the arm is held adducted and fixed in internal rotation. Anteriorly, there is flattening of the shoulder contour and prominence of the coracoid process. Posteriorly, there is prominence and rounding of the shoulder. The findings on standard anteroposterior x-ray are subtle (slight increase in space between the anterior glenoid rim and the medial humeral head, failure on the external rotation [see above] view to see the normal club-shaped humeral head with its greater tuberosity prominent at the superolateral margin, because the shoulder is locked in internal rotation). An axillary lateral or scapular Y view (see "Diagnostic Approach," above), however, reveals the posterior displacement of the humeral head relative to the glenoid fossa.

Treatment of dislocations requires prompt reduction and usually involves immediate referral to an orthopedist or emergency department. Postreduction management includes a period of immobilization of variable duration, followed by an intensive physical therapy program to restore range of motion and strengthen the appropriate anterior or posterior muscle groups in the hope of preventing recurrence. Dislocations may be accompanied by rotator cuff injury, neurovascular compromise (commonly the axillary nerve in anterior dislocation), or fracture, so pretreatment and posttreatment physical examination and x-ray should be done to evaluate these complications and to ensure the adequacy of the reduction.

Recurrent dislocation may follow the acute dislocation. It is especially common in younger patients (more than 50% in patients 25 years of age or younger) (20,39). Each subsequent dislocation may require less force; eventually dislocation may occur even during routine tasks such as combing the hair. A variety of surgical procedures are available to treat this condition.

A syndrome of *glenohumeral instability, with subluxation* without dislocation, is often seen in athletes, particularly in the dominant arm of baseball pitchers, racket sport players, and swimmers. Anterior subluxation, with secondary impingement, can be an additional cause of rotator cuff tendinitis. In addition to pain, patients may describe a sense of instability, weakness, or even radicular symptoms. This syndrome can be difficult to diagnose. Occasionally, pain may be reproduced by placing the arm in an evocative position, or the arm may be excessively subluxed by the application of force in one direction on physical examination. A *sulcus sign,* or subacromial indentation, may occur because of subluxation of the arm inferiorly with longitudinal traction or weights. Plain x-rays are usually normal, but may show subluxation with the patient holding a weight while relaxing the shoulder musculature. Special x-rays may demonstrate a *Bankart's lesion* (avulsion of the anterior inferior glenoid rim) or a *Hill–Sachs lesion* (osteochondral defect of the posterior humeral head) apparently caused by recurrent subluxation of the humeral head in front of the anterior glenoid rim. An arthrogram–CT scan may demonstrate a glenoid labral tear, laxity of the glenohumeral ligaments, or a Hill–Sachs lesion. Treatment first involves a program of shoulder strengthening exercises. If conservative treatment fails or if help is needed in making the diagnosis, referral to an orthopedist is appropriate. Surgery is directed toward tightening the capsular structures and stabilizing the joint.

Glenoid labral tears most commonly follow a fall on an outstretched arm with the shoulder in abduction and forward flexion. They also occur in people involved in throwing sports, racket sports, and swimming. The diagnosis may be confused with rotator cuff tendinitis or bicipital tendinitis. It can be confirmed by arthro-CT, double-contrast arthrotomography, or arthroscopy. If the diagnosis is suspected, referral to an orthopedist is indicated. If the tear is associated with instability, the conservative or surgical treatments described above may be required. Treatment may involve arthroscopic debridement or stapling.

Fractures of the proximal humerus occur most commonly in the elderly, usually after a fall, although they may accompany traumatic dislocation in patients of any age. The neck and the greater tuberosity are most often involved. Extensive bruising of the upper and middle arm may appear 1 to 2 days after fracture of the neck. Plain x-ray establishes the diagnosis. Referral to an orthopedist is generally advised for definitive treatment, which varies depending on the type of fracture and the presence or absence of displacement of the segments.

Arthritic and Other Conditions

Arthritic conditions are distinguished by pain and limitation in a capsular pattern on active and passive range of motion (see "Diagnostic Approach," above). Plain x-rays may show chronic arthritic changes but be normal in early or acute arthritis. Radiologic changes must always be interpreted with the clinical information on hand. Monoarticular arthritis uncommonly is the cause of shoulder pain. *Primary osteoarthritis* of the shoulder is rare, although secondary osteoarthritis may occur as a result of recurrent dislocation, complete rotator cuff tear (cuff tear arthropathy), fracture, neuropathy (Charcot joint), osteonecrosis, hemoglobinopathy, or inflammation (see

Chapter 68). In chronic *inflammatory arthritides,* such as rheumatoid arthritis, the shoulder is usually involved as part of a constellation of articular complaints (see Chapter 70). A septic (usually gonococcal or staphylococcal, less commonly streptococcal or Gram-negative) or microcrystalline (see Chapter 69) process should be suspected if the shoulder is the site of monoarticular arthritis of acute onset. Joint aspiration should be performed promptly to obtain fluid for culture and fluid analysis, including cell count and examination for crystals by polarization microscopy (see Chapter 69). The patient with a septic arthritis should be hospitalized and treated with intravenous antibiotics and drainage, usually by percutaneous but occasionally by surgical means.

Osteonecrosis (also called avascular or aseptic necrosis) of the humeral head should be suspected in the patient with a history of fracture of the humeral head or of prolonged corticosteroid therapy. Diagnosis is confirmed by plain x-ray or occasionally an MRI (see "Diagnostic Approach"), if necessary. Treatment includes range-of-motion exercises, analgesics or NSAIDs, and limitation of stress, as discussed above under "Management Strategies." Patients with significant loss of function or severe pain who do not respond to conservative management over several months may be considered for replacement of the humeral head or total joint replacement, and an orthopedist should be consulted.

REFERRED PAIN

Occasionally, pain in the shoulder area is referred from other regions of the body. Referred pain should be suspected when *(a)* the initial physical examination reveals another source for the pain; *(b)* active, passive, and resisted movements and palpation of the shoulder fail to elicit or exacerbate pain; or *(c)* the pain is in an atypical distribution (see "Diagnostic Approach"). The common causes of referred pain are discussed below.

Visceral sources of referred pain may be suggested by a review of the patient's problem list or medical history and the absence of another cause for the referred pain. Irritation of the phrenic nerve or diaphragm may arise from pathologic processes abutting these structures such as subdiaphragmatic abscesses, ruptured viscus, or diseases involving the mediastinum, pericardium, liver, spleen, and gallbladder. In addition, ischemic heart disease, apical or superior sulcus tumors of the lung (Pancoast tumor; see Chapter 56), and dissecting aortic aneurysms all may be causes of referred pain (usually acute) to the shoulder.

Reflex sympathetic dystrophy, or *shoulder–hand syndrome,* is a poorly understood condition that may be a cause of referred shoulder pain. It is characterized by stiffness and swelling, without pitting edema, of the hand, which is warm and pink. The syndrome may occur in association with trauma or surgery of the involved extremity, acute myocardial infarction, or cerebrovascular accident. It is discussed further in Chapter 83.

Nerve compression or irritation that is manifested clinically by shoulder pain may originate at the level of the cervical spine, wrist, or shoulder. In addition to pain, the patient may occasionally complain of paresthesias, numbness, muscular weakness, or atrophy. Neurologic examination often delineates the nerves or nerve roots affected. *Cervical nerve root* irritation is a common cause of shoulder pain. The pain is often felt above the shoulder, rather than in the upper arm, and may or may not be accompanied by neck pain. Characteristically the pain is exacerbated by movement of the neck but not of the shoulder. The diagnosis and management are discussed in Chapter 64. Compression of the median nerve in the carpal tunnel of the wrist *(carpal tunnel syndrome)* is occasionally associated with pain about the shoulder. Usually, the pain originates in the wrist and radiates to the upper arm or shoulder. This condition is discussed in Chapter 84. Irritation or compression of the *axillary* or *suprascapular nerve* may also result in pain referred to the shoulder.

Thoracic outlet syndrome is an uncommon but serious condition in which pain in the shoulder is a common complaint. Neck pain may also be present. The thoracic outlet consists of a series of narrow, fixed passages within which the neurovascular supply of the upper extremity (brachial plexus and subclavian vessels) can become compressed as it exits the neck and thorax to enter the axilla (Fig. 63.4). Compression of the neural or vascular structures results most often from mechanical traction caused by muscle weakness, obesity, heavy breasts or arms, poor posture, or the carrying of heavy loads on one's shoulders. Symptoms may also develop from periods of prolonged overhead work or sleeping with the arms hyperabducted. Only a minority of cases are caused by anatomic abnormalities such as a cervical rib (enlargement of the transverse process of C7), anomalies of the clavicle or first rib, cervical bands, hypertrophy of the omohyoid or scalene muscles, or subclavian artery aneurysms. The presenting complaint depends on the predominant structure that is compressed. If it is neural in origin, the patient complains of pain, often extending from the neck or shoulder area to the forearm or hand and accompanied by paresthesias or numbness, usually along an ulnar distribution. Muscle weakness and atrophy may be noted on physical examination. If it is vascular in origin, the patient may complain of an alteration in color or temperature, swelling of the affected hand, or a Raynaud-like phenomenon.

On physical examination, the force of the patient's radial pulse is palpated during the following maneuvers: *(a)* The patient holds his or her breath in full inspiration while rotating the extended (posterior) neck toward the side that is being examined (*Adson test;* a modified Adson test also includes arm elevation and a Valsalva maneuver), *(b)* the patient abducts the arm 180° in external rotation *(hyperabduction maneuver),* and *(c)* the patient assumes an exaggerated military posture with the shoulder braced posteriorly and inferiorly *(costoclavicular maneuver).* Because a substantial percentage of normal patients manifest a decrease or obliteration of their radial pulse with these maneuvers (38, 54, and 68%, respectively) (11), reproduction of symptoms in parallel with the change in arterial pulse at the wrist is necessary to properly interpret these physical findings. Only a minority of patients have discoloration, temperature changes, or edema as a result of arterial or venous compression. Plain films of the neck, chest, and shoulder should be obtained when referred pain is suspected. Noninvasive Doppler studies of the vascular structures of the upper extremity can be performed at rest and during the maneuvers listed above when a vascular impingement is considered likely. Subclavian arteriography is occasionally needed to confirm stenosis, to identify an anatomic abnormality such as an aneurysm, or as a prelude to surgical intervention.

Management of a patient with the thoracic outlet syndrome depends on the underlying cause. For most

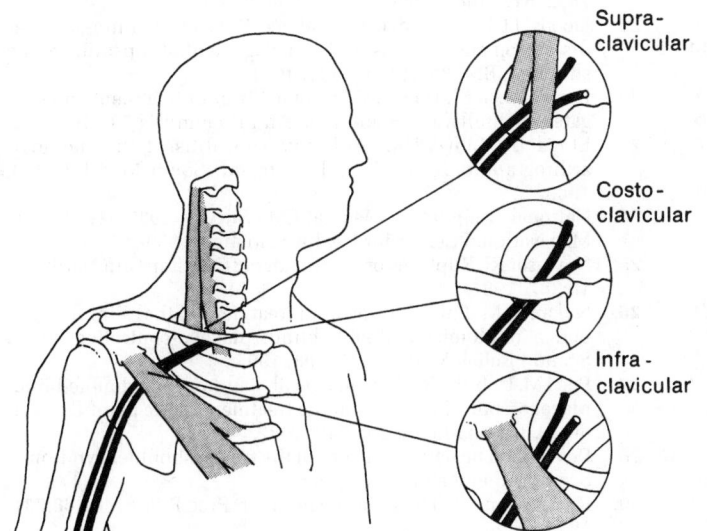

Figure 63.4. Points of neurovascular compression in the thoracic outlet syndrome. (From Steinberg GC, Akins CM, Baran DT, eds. Ramamurti's orthopaedics in primary care. Baltimore: Williams & Wilkins, 1992.)

Supra-clavicular

Costo-clavicular

Infra-clavicular

conditions, conservative management is beneficial and this involves the identification and elimination (or reduction) of aggravating factors and the implementation of an appropriate exercise and postural program. Such conservative measures provide relief in 50 to 90% of patients (see Sheon, "General References"). An occupational (if functional guidance is necessary) or physical therapist (if exercise guidance is necessary) should be consulted in initiating the exercise program. Occasionally, patients with severe or refractory pain may be helped by surgical intervention, which can involve resection of the first rib, a portion of the scalene muscles, or an abnormal constricting structure such as a cervical rib. Consultation with a surgeon should be considered in such situations.

General References*

Cyriax JH. Textbook of orthopaedic medicine. Vol. 1: diagnosis of soft tissue lesions. 8th ed. London: Bailliere-Tindall, 1982.
> Source of most commonly accepted and useful approach to physical examination. Otherwise somewhat dated.

Cyriax JH. Textbook of orthopaedic medicine. Vol. 2: treatment by manipulation, massage and injection. 11th ed. London: Bailliere-Tindall, 1984.
> Good quick reference to diagnosis and injection techniques.

Cyriax JH, Cyriax PJ. Cyriax's illustrated manual of orthopaedic medicine. 2nd ed. Oxford: Butterworth-Heinemann, 1993.
> Abbreviated, well-illustrated but unreferenced version of the above two texts.

Goss TP. Shoulder and upper arm. In: Steinberg GG, Akins CM, Baran DT, eds. Ramamurti's orthopaedics in primary care. 2nd ed. Baltimore: Williams & Wilkins, 1992.
> Basic, general chapter on shoulder and upper arm disorders that includes sprains, dislocations, and fractures.

Kozin F. Painful shoulder and the reflex sympathetic dystrophy syndrome. In: Koopman WJ, ed. Arthritis and allied conditions: a textbook of rheumatology. 13th ed. Baltimore: Williams & Wilkins, 1997;1887–1922.
> Comprehensive, up-to-date, well-referenced chapter with a large section on reflex sympathetic dystrophy.

Owen DS Jr. Aspiration and injection of joints and soft tissue. In: Kelley WN, Harris ED Jr, Ruddy S, Sledge CB, eds. Textbook of rheumatology. 5th ed. Philadelphia: WB Saunders, 1997;591–608.
> Good general source of injection technique.

Sheon RP, Moscowitz RW, Goldberg VM. Soft tissue rheumatic pain: recognition, management, prevention. 3rd ed. Philadelphia: Lea & Febiger, 1996;79–146.
> Good source for advice on joint protection and for additional shoulder exercises.

Smith DL, Campbell SM. Painful shoulder syndromes: diagnosis and management. J Gen Intern Med 7:328, 1992.
> Well-referenced, practical recent review.

Thornhill TS. Shoulder pain. In: Kelley WN, Harris ED Jr, Ruddy S, Sledge CB, eds. Textbook of rheumatology. 5th ed. Philadelphia: WB Saunders, 1997;413–438.
> Comprehensive, up-to-date, well-referenced chapter that includes discussions of surgical approaches to treatment.

Specific References

1. Adebajo AO, Nash P, Hazleman BL. A prospective double blind dummy placebo controlled study comparing triamcinolone hexacetonide injection with oral diclofenac 50 mg TDS in patients with rotator cuff tendinitis. J Rheumatol 17:1207, 1990.

2. Allender E. Prevalence, incidence, and remission rates of some common rheumatic diseases or syndromes. Scand J Rheumatol 3:145, 1974.
3. Bergenudd H, Lindegarde F, Nilsson B, Petersson CJ. Shoulder pain in middle age: a study of prevalence and relation to occupational work load and psychosocial factors. Clin Orthop 231:234, 1988.
4. Berry H, Fernandes L, Bloom B, et al. Clinical study comparing acupuncture, physiotherapy, injection, and oral anti-inflammatory therapy in shoulder-cuff lesions. Curr Med Res Opin 7:121, 1980.
5. Binder AI, Bulgen DY, Hazleman BL, Roberts S. Frozen shoulder: a long-term prospective study. Ann Rheum Dis 43:361, 1984.
6. Boorstein JM, Kneeland JB, Dalinka MK, et al. Magnetic resonance imaging of the shoulder. Curr Probl Diagn Radiol 3, Jan/Feb 1992.
7. Bulgen DY, Binder AI, Hazleman BL, et al. Frozen shoulder: prospective clinical study with an evaluation of three treatment regimens. Ann Rheum Dis 43:353, 1984.
8. Burk DL, Karasick D, Kurz AB, et al. Rotator cuff tears: prospective comparison of MR imaging with arthrography, sonography, and surgery. AJR 153:87, 1989.
9. Chard MD, Hazleman BL, King RH, Reiss BB. Shoulder disorders in the elderly: a community survey. Arthritis Rheum 34:766, 1991.
10. Chard MD, Sattelle LM, Hazleman BL. The long-term outcome of rotator cuff tendinitis: a review study. Br J Rheumatol 27:395, 1988.
11. Conn J Jr. Thoracic outlet syndromes. Surg Clin North Am 54:155, 1974.
12. Dacre JE, Beeney N, Scott DL. Injection and physiotherapy for the painful stiff shoulder. Ann Rheum Dis 48:322–325, 1989.
13. Dias JJ, Steingold RF, Richardson RA, et al. The conservative treatment of acromioclavicular dislocation. J Bone Joint Surg 68B:719, 1987.
14. Downing DS, Weinstein A. Ultrasound therapy of subacromial bursitis: a double-blind trial. Phys Ther 66:194–199, 1986.
15. Faure G, Daculsi G. Calcified tendinitis: a review. Ann Rheum Dis 42(Suppl):49, 1983.
16. Grey RG. The natural history of idiopathic frozen shoulder. J Bone Joint Surg 60A:564, 1978.
17. Hales TR, Bernard BP. Epidemiology of work-related musculoskeletal disorders. Orthop Clin North Am 27:679–709, 1996.
18. Heron CW. Imaging the painful shoulder. Clin Radiol 41:379, 1990.
19. Hollingworth GR, Ellis RM, Hattersley TS. Comparison of injection techniques for shoulder pain: results of a double blind, randomized study. BMJ 287:1339, 1983.
20. Hovelius L, Augustini BG, Fredin H, et al. Primary anterior dislocation of the shoulder in young patients. J Bone Joint Surg 78A:1677–1684, 1996.
21. Jacobs LGH, Barton MA, Wallace WA, et al. Intra-articular distension and steroids in the management of capsulitis of the shoulder. BMJ 302:1498–1501, 1991.
22. Lee PN, Lee M, Haz AMMM, et al. Trial of treatments investigated by multivariate analysis. Ann Rheum Dis 33:116, 1974.
23. Lloyd JA, Lloyd HM. Adhesive capsulitis of the shoulder: arthrographic diagnosis and treatment. South Med J 76:879, 1983.
24. National Ambulatory Medical Care Survey, 1985. Hyattsville, MD: National Center for Health Statistics, 1989.
25. Neviaser RJ. Ruptures of the rotator cuff. Orthop Clin North Am 18:387, 1987.
26. Nykanen M. Pulsed ultrasound treatment of the painful shoulder: a randomized, double-blind, placebo-controlled study. Scand J Rehab Med 27:105–108, 1995.
27. Petri M, Dobrow R, Neiman R, et al. Randomized, double-blind, placebo-controlled study of the treatment of the painful shoulder. Arthritis Rheum 30:1040, 1987.
28. Reeves B. The natural history of the frozen shoulder syndrome. Scand J Rheumatol 4:193, 1975.
29. Richardson AT. The painful shoulder. Proc R Soc Med 68:731, 1975.

---

*Bold print (general references) and bold numerals (specific references) denote published controlled clinical trials, meta-analyses, or consensus-based recommendations.

30. Rizk TE, Gavant ML, Pinals RS. Treatment of adhesive capsulitis (frozen shoulder) with arthrographic capsular distension and rupture. Arch Phys Med Rehabil 75:803–807, 1994.

31. Rocks JA. Intrinsic shoulder pain syndrome: rationale for heating and cooling in treatment. Phys Ther 59:153, 1979.

32. Roth SH. Nonsteroidal anti-inflammatory drugs: gastropathy, deaths, and medical practice. Ann Intern Med 109:353, 1988.

33. Roy S, Oldham R. Management of painful shoulder. Lancet 1322, June 19, 1976.

34. Steinbrocker O, Argyros TG. Frozen shoulder: treatment by local injections of depo corticosteroids. Arch Phys Med Rehabil 55:209, 1974.

35. van der Windt DAWM, van der Heijden GJMG, Scholten RJPM, et al. The efficacy of non-steroidal anti-inflammatory drugs (NSAIDs) for shoulder complaints: a systematic review. J Clin Epidemiol 48:691–704, 1995.

36. Vecchio PC, Hazleman BL, King RH. A double-blind trial comparing subacromial methylprednisolone and lignocaine in acute rotator cuff tendinitis. Br J Rheum 32:743–745, 1993.

37. Weiss JJ, Ting YM. Arthrography-assisted intra-articular steroids in treatment of adhesive capsulitis. Arch Phys Med Rehab 59:285, 1978.

38. White RH, Paull DM, Fleming KW. Rotator cuff tendinitis: comparison of subacromial injection of a long acting corticosteroid versus oral indomethacin therapy. J Rheumatol 13:608, 1986.

39. Yu J. Anterior shoulder dislocations. J Fam Pract 35:567–576, 1992.

C H A P T E R 64

Neck Pain

FREDERICK A. LENZ, MD, PhD

Neck pain is a common problem. Nearly 50% of people over 50 years of age experience neck pain at some time. Because there are many structures in the neck that, when diseased, may cause pain, as well as multiple sources of referred pain, patients who complain of new or persistent neck pain should be systematically evaluated. This chapter provides a review of the skeletal structures of the neck, the method of evaluation for complaints of neck pain, a description of common problems and their treatment, and guidance for referral of selected patients with neck pain.

ANATOMY OF THE NECK AND SOURCES OF PAIN

The cervical spine consists of seven vertebral bodies connected by facet joints, interspinous ligaments, and an anterior and a posterior longitudinal ligament (Fig. 64.1). These ligaments provide stability when the neck is flexed and extended. The vertebral bodies are joined by intervertebral discs composed of a gel-like material (the nucleus pulposus) that absorbs increased pressure applied to the spine. The nucleus pulposus is contained within an annulus fibrosus, a fibrous structure ringing the outer margin of the disc. During the fourth decade of life, both the nucleus pulposus and the annulus fibrosus undergo progressive degeneration, seen microscopically as a loss of the fibrous pattern and the collagen alignment. As a result, the ability of the disc to absorb shocks is reduced. Facet joints are found between vertebral elements posteriorly, one on each side of the spine; they are apophyseal (projecting) joints with a synovium-lined capsule. It is within these small joints in the posterior spine that osteoarthritis, a breakdown of the articular cartilage within the joints, can occur. The intervertebral neural foramina, located on either side of the vertebral bodies, are the canals through which the nerve roots emerge from the spinal

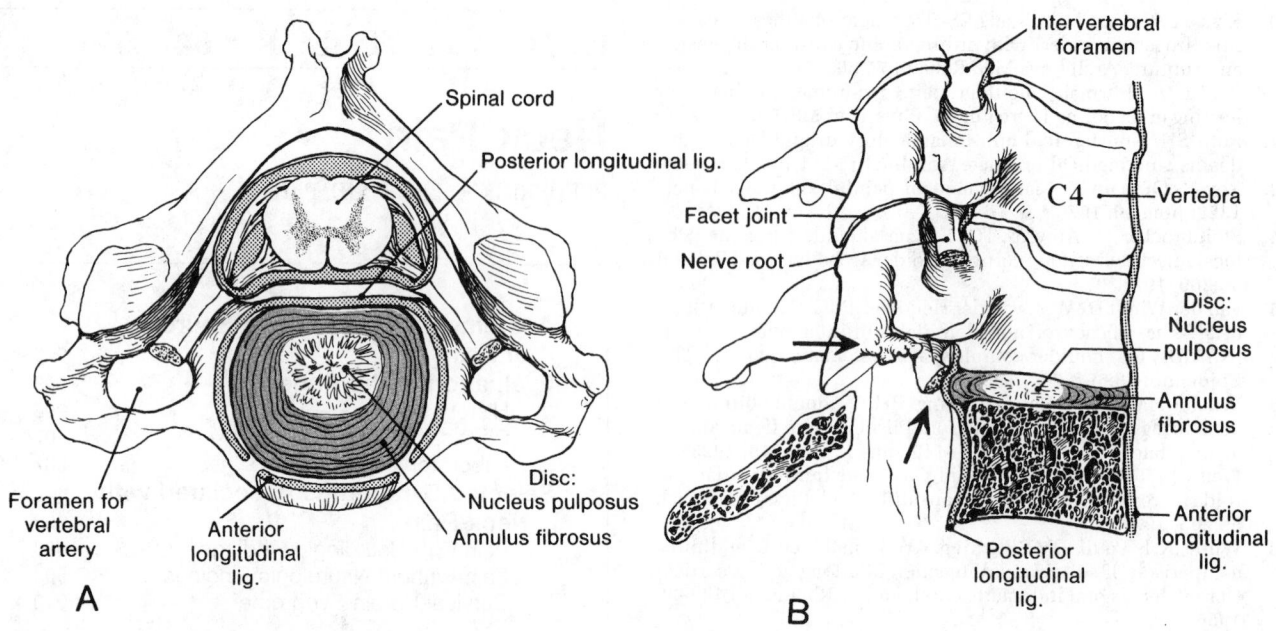

Figure 64.1. Anatomy of disc and ligaments of the cervical spine. **A.** Superior view. Note relationship of anterior and posterior longitudinal ligament to the intervertebral disc. **B.** Lateral view. Note relationship of intervertebral foramen to the intervertebral disc and facet joint. Bulging of the intervertebral disc or bone spurs forming from the facet joint may cause compression of the nerve root within the intervertebral foramen *(arrows)*.

canal. The spinal canal and the foramina can be encroached on by a bulging intervertebral disc or an osseous proliferation (bony spur) originating in a vertebral body, by a facet joint, or from the bony margin of a neural foramen (Fig. 64.1). When the encroachment involves a nerve root, pain in the distribution of that root (radicular pain) may occur. The facet joint capsules and the intervertebral disc are innervated by fine nerves that have simple nerve endings. When these nerve endings are stimulated by degenerative disease within the disc or joint capsules, the patient may experience pain, which is referred to the posterior aspect of the neck at any level. The pain felt in the neck may not be at the cervical level from which the nerve is arising. In addition, stimulation of the nerves can cause pain to be referred to the interscapular area, superiorly and laterally over the shoulders. Spasm of any of the many muscles of the neck region is also a common source of pain.

EVALUATION OF THE PATIENT

History

The date of onset of the patient's symptoms and any associated trauma should be ascertained. Often, knowledge of the specific activity the patient was performing at the onset of pain is helpful in establishing the cause of the pain. Prolonged extension of the neck, as occurs in people doing overhead work, is a common occupational situation that can give rise to pain in the cervical region. Another common occupational cause of neck pain is prolonged sitting with the neck flexed in one position. This occurs commonly in computer operators or typists. The sustained position causes spasm of the neck muscles, which results in pain. Also, patients commonly sustain minor twisting injuries or trauma to the neck but do not experience neck pain within the first 24 hours, after which pain may begin to appear and progress. Reproduction or increase of pain by neck motion is helpful in localizing the problem to the cervical spine rather than to a referred source (Table 64.1). It is also important to know whether the pain is felt outside the neck as well, such as in the head, posteriorly between the scapulae, about the shoulder, down the arm, or in the hand. The patient should be asked about decreased sensation in the hands and, if possible, to say specifically which fingers are involved. If the pain and numbness are felt in a dermatome distribution (see dermatome map, Chapter 78, Fig. 78.2), this indicates nerve compression (Table 64.2). Muscle weakness in the shoulder, arm, and hand should be elicited to help identify potential nerve compression. Pain associated with motion of the shoulder is not characteristic of cervical spine disease and suggests that the problem is within the shoulder joint (see Chapter 63). Symptoms such as dizziness, visual changes, and ataxia brought on by neck motion (usually rotation) are not usually caused by nerve root compression or degenerative disc disease, but they may be found when bony spurs encroach on the vertebral foramina and compress the vertebral arteries. These rare symptoms usually occur when the neck is in a certain position, and they are usually of short duration.

Physical Examination

Anterior and posterior inspection of the head, neck, shoulders, and upper extremities should be done initially. Any abnormal posture such as torticollis (wry neck) or muscle atrophy will be noticed. Next, the patient should be asked to demonstrate active range of motion of the neck, including flexion to touch the chin to the chest, extension, rotation to touch the chin to the shoulder on both sides, and lateral bending to touch the ear to the shoulder on both sides. Normally, the chin can be placed easily upon the anterior chest and the neck can be extended so that the patient is looking directly above. Normally, there is almost 90° of rotation of the neck to both sides. Simple hyperextension of the neck commonly exacerbates the pain caused by cervical disc degeneration. The patient should be asked to extend the neck and to maintain this position for 30 seconds to determine whether the pain is made worse. Putting direct compression on top of the head also may produce or exacerbate pain in the patient with degenerative disc disease, especially if the head is compressed while the neck is extended. The posterior neck muscles are palpated for muscle spasm, which may be asymmetric and may give the patient the appearance of torticollis (wry neck). Next, the shoulder should be subjected to a range of motion to see whether this elicits pain within the shoulder itself.

Selected neurologic tests (see Chapters 78 and 84) are important in the evaluation of the patient with neck pain whenever there is any suggestion of nerve root involvement or cord compression. These tests include reflex testing of the upper and lower extremities, muscle strength testing of the upper extremities, and sensory testing of the upper extremities. The reflex testing should include the biceps, triceps, brachioradial, quadriceps, and gastrocnemius tendons, and the plantar. Muscle strength in the upper extremities should include the biceps (flexion of elbow), triceps (extension of elbow), wrist extensors and flexors, hand and finger flexors, and intrinsic muscles of the hand. A sensory examination is then performed. An objective sensory deficit is one that conforms to a dermatomal distribution (see Chapters 78 and 84).

Cervical spine problems can cause cervical myelopathy when a bone spur forms posteriorly at the margin of an intervertebral disc and then impinges on the spinal cord, producing signs of cord compression: increased reflexes in the upper and lower extremities with a positive Babinski sign. Intradural or other extradural lesions at this level could give similar findings.

Laboratory Assessment

If the history reveals severe, progressive pain or an episode of recent trauma or if the neurologic examination reveals abnormalities, a complete set of cervical

Table 64.1. Sources of Referred Pain in the Neck[a]

Source	Referred Location
Disorders of the Head	
Migraine or tension headache	Anterior or posterior
Sinus infection	Most often anterior but occasionally posterior
Temporomandibular joint problem	Usually anterolateral
Oral problems (see Chapter 101) such as a pharyngeal or tonsillar abscess	Middle of the neck
Distant Lesions	
Irritation of the surface of the diaphragm innervated by the phrenic nerve (C3, 4, and 5)	Often shoulder as well as low neck pain, but medial diaphragmatic lesion may be associated with neck pain
Shoulder problems (see Chapter 63) such as arthritis or periarticular inflammation	May be referred to the lateral part of the neck
Thoracic outlet syndrome from the compression of vascular and neural structures between the rib and the clavicle or between the scalene muscles	May be noticed in the lateral aspect of the neck
Lung problems such as superior sulcus tumor (Pancoast's tumor)	Initially may be located in the lateral aspect of the neck and shoulder
Cardiovascular problems such as a heart attack or an aneurysm of the thoracic aorta	May be localized to the base of the neck

[a]The clue to referred pain is the absence of any tenderness in the neck or of exacerbation of symptoms with manipulation of the neck.

Table 64.2. Characteristic Findings at Individual Cervical Nerve Root Levels

Nerve Root	Disc Level	History	Examination[a]
C3	(C2–3)	Pain into the back of the neck to the pinnae and the angle of the jaw	No reflex changes
C4	(C3–4)	Pain into the back of the neck to the levator scapulae to anterior chest	No reflex changes
C5	(C4–5)	Pain into side of the neck to the superior lateral shoulder, numbness over the deltoid muscle	Deltoid muscle atrophy and weakness of shoulder abduction
C6	(C5–6)	Pain to the lateral aspects of the arm and forearm and into the thumb and index finger, with numbness of thumb and dorsum of hand	Weak biceps and brachioradial muscles and decreased biceps and brachioradial tendon reflexes
C7	(C6–7)	Pain into the midforearm to middle and ring fingers	Triceps muscle weakness with decreased triceps muscle reflex
C8	(C7–T1)	Pain to the medial aspect of the forearm into the ring and small fingers, with numbness of the ulnar border and small finger	Triceps weakness with weakness of intrinsic muscles of the hand

[a]Sensory testing usually shows abnormalities in dermatome of the affected nerve root (see Chapter 78, Fig. 78.2).

spine x-rays should be obtained. These films should include an assessment of levels C1 through C7–T1 with oblique and open-mouth odontoid views. These x-rays will help in assessing the patient for fracture or metastatic disease. However, there is not a good correlation between clinical symptoms or signs and degenerative abnormalities on x-ray. In fact, in asymptomatic people after age 40, cervical degenerative changes (spondylosis) are common and are evident in more than 90% of people over 50 (1). On the other hand, there may be serious cervical disease with minimal or no changes on x-ray.

Computerized tomographic (CT) myelography is also useful in the evaluation of problems of the upper cervical spine. Magnetic resonance imaging (MRI) is especially useful when evaluating patients suspected of having abnormalities of the soft tissue such as metastatic cancer or a primary disc problem. CT myelography is more effective for assessment of abnormalities of bone such as osteophytes.

SELECTED SYNDROMES ASSOCIATED WITH NECK PAIN

Many problems of the neck may result in neck pain (Table 64.3). Because the most common problems—herniated cervical disc and cervical spondylosis (degenerative changes)—may have similar manifestations, they are discussed together based on the presence or absence of neurologic findings (see below).

Pain with Neurologic Findings

Diagnosis

Patients with neurologic findings can have either nerve root or spinal cord compression (upper motor neuron syndrome, see Chapter 78). The objective signs of nerve root compression are muscle weakness, a decreased deep tendon reflex, and decreased sensation in a dermatome distribution.

Patients with nerve root compression present with the acute or gradual onset of posterior neck pain that radiates to the shoulder and down one arm into the lower arm and often into the hand itself. The pain often radiates into a finger that corresponds to the dermatome of the nerve root involved. The pain may be made worse by movement of the neck and extreme neck positions. In addition, the patient may complain of decreased sensation and paresthesias in the arm and hand. A patient may have nerve root compression from the cervical spine but have little or no neck and arm pain, and instead have arm weakness and loss of sensation. Nerve root compression can be caused by impingement of the nerve by a cervical disc—most common in younger patients—or by osseous proliferation that can impinge on the nerve as it exits through its foramen—most common in patients over 50 (Fig. 64.1B). Also, the thoracic outlet syndrome may be confused with cervical disease associated with nerve root compression, and this syndrome should be ruled out (see Chapter 63).

Table 64.3.   Selected Problems of the Neck that May Result in Neck Pain

Problem	Comment
Arthritis	Especially rheumatoid (see Chapter 70) and degenerative joint disease (see text and Chapter 68).
Disc disease	See text.
Fibromyalgia	See Chapter 66.
Infection	Osteomyelitis or soft tissue infection; look for point tenderness (see Chapter 31).
Neoplasia	Myeloma or metastatic disease is associated with point tenderness and x-ray (or bone scan in the case of metastases) abnormalities.
Neuritis	Any nerve may be involved. A common one is the spinal accessory nerve. Look for tenderness over the nerve, lateral aspects of upper one-third of sternomastoid muscle.
Platybasia	A congenital disorder that may not manifest symptoms before age 40 or a complication of Paget's disease; x-rays show characteristic changes (i.e., invagination of the base of the skull).
Sprain	Cervical sprain syndrome caused by whiplash and other forms of trauma (see text).
Structures in neck	Any organ or structure located in the neck may become a source of neck pain. Careful examination will detect abnormalities such as thyroiditis, lymphadenitis, pharyngitis, sialadenitis, or tender carotid artery (carotodynia).
Tendinitis	Any tendon may be involved but occipital and sternomastoid are particularly common. Local tenderness is a clue.
Torticollis (wry neck)	Diagnosis is usually obvious by observation. An underlying structural problem could produce reflex muscle spasm; therefore, with an initial episode an underlying problem (e.g., tumor or infection) should be considered.
Trauma	Because of the danger of cord injury, trauma associated with neck pain should be carefully evaluated.
Vascular	Arteritis or dissection may cause neck pain.

Patients with spinal cord compression may have numb, clumsy hands or spastic paraparesis. The complaint of neck pain need not be prominent and radicular symptoms may be present. The presence of radicular findings of weakness and fasciculations raises the possibility of motor neuron disease. In a younger patient, medical causes of myelopathy, such as multiple sclerosis, must be excluded.

Management

Patients with evidence of *myelopathy* (i.e., involvement of the spinal cord) must be referred to a neurologist or neurosurgeon to establish the cause. Investigation usually includes MRI or CT myelogram. If the myelopathy is secondary to a cervical disc or cervical spondylosis, surgery is often indicated—either laminectomy or anterior cervical fusions. Symptoms of myelopathy, particularly chronic myelopathy, may not remit after decompression, so the goal of surgery is to prevent progression.

Patients with *nerve root compression* should be referred to an orthopedist or to a neurosurgeon for more complete examination and follow-up, particularly if muscle weakness and sensory impairment are present. If the neurologic deficit would be unacceptable if permanent, the consultant will evaluate these patients further with CT, MRI, or myelography. If the neurologic deficit would be acceptable if permanent, conservative therapy is an option and has a good chance of success (6).

If the pain is severe, bed rest may be necessary. A *cervical collar* may be beneficial. It is helpful to place a small pillow under the nape of the neck to provide proper positioning. If muscle spasm is present, moist or dry heat applied to the neck may give symptomatic relief. Analgesia using a nonsteroidal anti-inflammatory drug (NSAID) (see Chapter 70) or acetaminophen may help. If a stronger analgesic becomes necessary, codeine, 30 to 60 mg orally three or four times daily, may be added. Although not a first-line agent, a muscle relaxant may be helpful (see Chapter 65, "Low Back Pain") if symptoms persist after 3 or 4 days.

The acute phase usually lasts only 1 or 2 weeks. When symptoms become recurrent or chronic (lasting more than 2 to 3 weeks) *cervical traction* may provide relief. This is performed initially by a physical therapist, after x-rays of the cervical spine have been shown to rule out instability. For 30 minutes, 15 to 20 lb of chin halter traction are applied to the neck. The neck must be positioned in slight flexion; extension, which could worsen symptoms, must be avoided. After several sessions, the patient can be instructed in the use of a home cervical traction unit that can be applied for 30 minutes at a time, up to three times a day, for several months. If symptoms persist for more than 2 or 3 weeks, a brief course of steroids may also be beneficial. Prednisone 60 mg/day is administered for 3 days followed by a 4-day taper. Even when symptoms and signs subside there is a high rate of recurrence of symptoms. It is therefore important to educate the patient in activities or positions that should be avoided and in exercises that may help relieve muscle spasm (Figs. 64.2 and 64.3).

If the acute symptoms do not subside or if new signs develop, referral to an orthopedist or a neurosurgeon is necessary for confirmation of the diagnosis and consideration of surgery (usually discectomy and anterior interbody fusion). The current standard of care is that surgery should be performed to relieve compression of neural structures as demonstrated by symptoms, signs, and radiologic findings (5). A trial of conservative therapy is indicated in all cases except those with evidence of myelopathy, functionally significant weakness, or instability. In some patients, neurologic deficits can take months to resolve postoperatively and may never resolve, particularly in the case of myelopathy.

Pain Without Neurologic Findings

Diagnosis

Most patients with neck pain have no objective neurologic findings. The patient may present either with an acute onset of pain (most of the time a disc herniation) or with a slowly progressive discomfort (most often from osteoarthritis) that has been building over several months. In the acute disc herniation syndrome, the patient experiences rather sudden onset of neck pain that is associated with decreased range of motion of the cervical spine, bilateral muscle spasm, or occasionally asymmetric muscle spasm that produces torticollis (wry neck). The patient may have pain in the shoulder or arm but have no objective weakness or sensory findings on examination.

Treatment

Initial treatment is basically the same as that outlined above for patients with neurologic findings. The neck may be "immobilized" with a cervical collar (2); several cervical collars are available, but a soft collar is often prescribed first, although it may serve only as a reminder to the patient not to move the neck too quickly or too far. Local heat and analgesics or NSAIDs (see Chapter 70) also may give symptomatic relief. Muscle relaxants (see Chapter 65) may be tried if symptoms persist after 3 or 4 days of initial treatment. In patients who have a chronic, more insidious onset of pain, it is helpful to examine the patient's occupational situation more closely to see whether there are exacerbating circumstances. Any activity that creates a prolonged extension of the neck, such as overhead work (e.g., painting), or prolonged flexion of the neck, such as sitting at a computer or typewriter, may aggravate a preexisting problem. If after initial treatment pain lasts more than 2 or 3 weeks, x-rays of the cervical spine should be obtained. The treatment is based on the severity of the symptoms. An oral, rapidly acting anti-inflammatory agent, such as piroxicam (Feldene), 20 mg once a day, may be tried over a course of 2 or 3 weeks. (Alternative NSAIDs, including aspirin, may be tried also; see Chapter 70.) When cost is a factor, aspirin is preferred; however, a daily dosage of 3 to 6 g is needed for 7 to 10 days to achieve an anti-inflammatory effect. Shorter courses and lower dosages of aspirin provide analgesic benefit. The patient should be informed that symptoms often may be chronic or recurrent and should be advised about how to avoid recurrences (Fig. 64.2).

If an acute severe episode of neck pain does not respond to treatment within a few weeks, the patient should be referred. When the symptoms are more mild and chronic, a trial of treatment for several months would be reasonable before referral. In the absence of neurologic signs or symptoms, the symptomatic level is difficult to define. Provocative discography is sometimes used in this situation in an attempt to define the levels producing the patient's neck pain. Provocation of the patient's pain by injection of saline into the disc

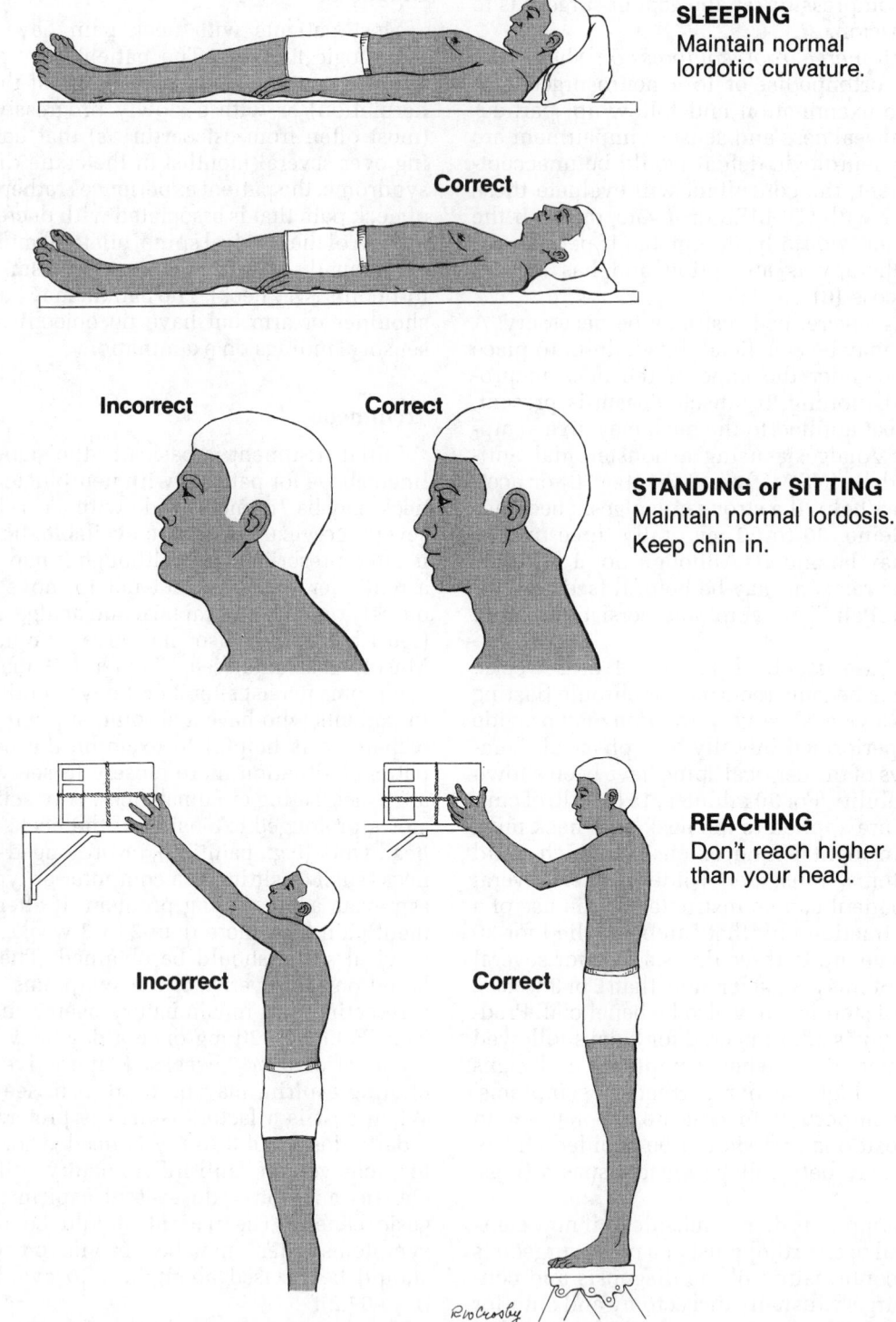

Incorrect

Correct

SLEEPING
Maintain normal
lordotic curvature.

Incorrect   **Correct**

STANDING or SITTING
Maintain normal lordosis.
Keep chin in.

Incorrect   **Correct**

REACHING
Don't reach higher
than your head.

Figure 64.2.   Positions to prevent recurrence of neck pain.

space and relief of the pain by injection of local anesthetic is assumed to implicate a particular level in producing the patient's pain. Anterior cervical fusions carried out on the basis of positive discograms are sometimes effective in treating patients with neck pain without neurologic symptoms.

Cervical Sprain Syndrome

Mechanism

Cervical sprain syndrome is a term given to acute injuries of the neck caused by sudden extension of the cervical spine *(whiplash)*. Patients involved in rear-end automobile accidents may have such acute hyperextension injuries to the neck. In experiments, monkeys subjected to acute hyperextension forces can show tearing of sternocleidomastoid and longus colli muscles in the absence of injuries to the anterior longitudinal ligament or disc. This injury is thought to form the basis of the cervical sprain syndrome. Neck pain from more mild forms of injury that result from repeated hyperextension, such as movements associated with painting a ceiling, usually resolves in a day or two and is not known to be associated with pathologic

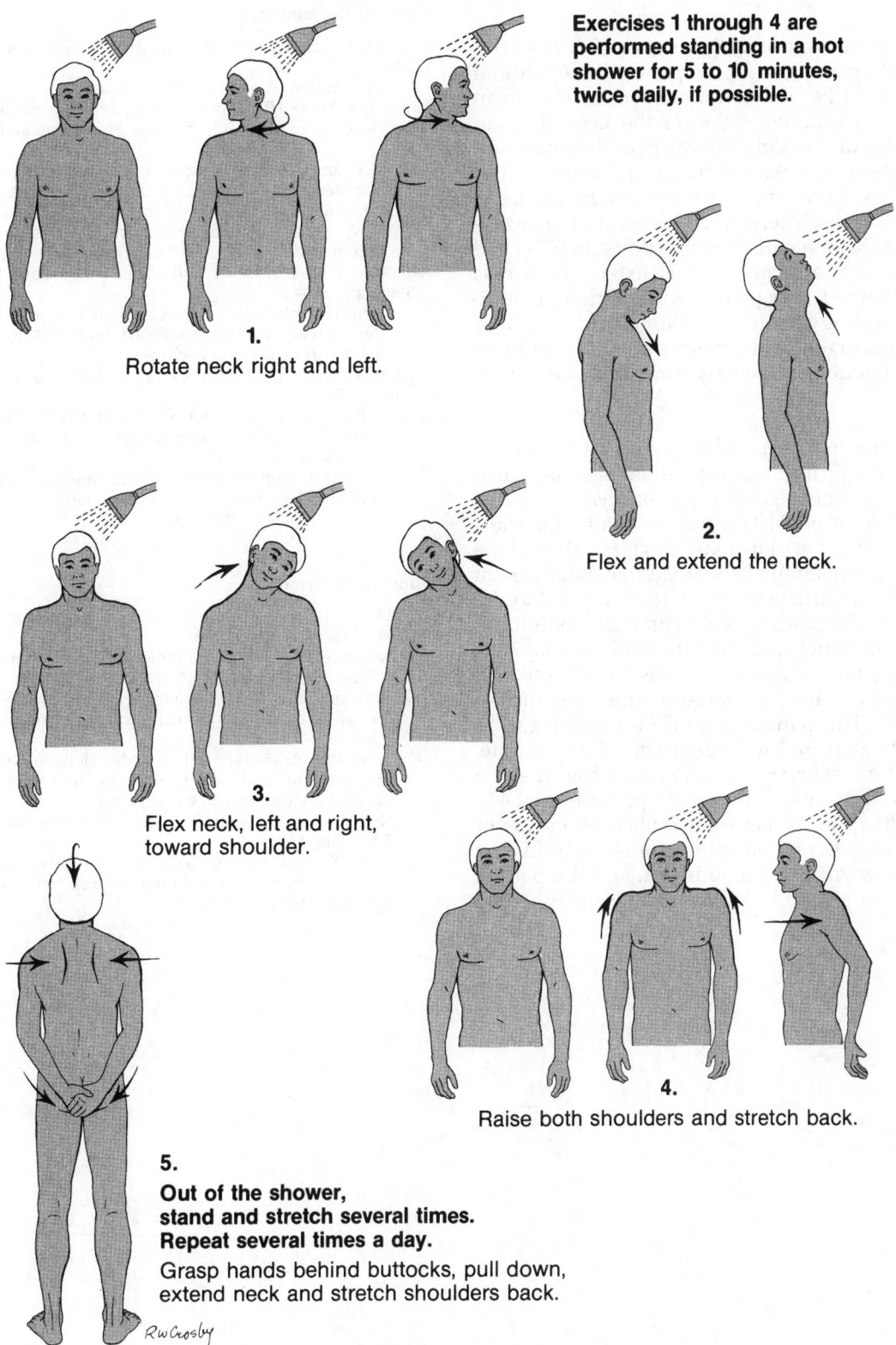

Exercises 1 through 4 are performed standing in a hot shower for 5 to 10 minutes, twice daily, if possible.

1.
Rotate neck right and left.

2.
Flex and extend the neck.

3.
Flex neck, left and right, toward shoulder.

4.
Raise both shoulders and stretch back.

5.
Out of the shower, stand and stretch several times. Repeat several times a day.

Grasp hands behind buttocks, pull down, extend neck and stretch shoulders back.

Figure 64.3.   Exercises to rehabilitate the neck.

changes. The reason that this syndrome can become persistent is unclear. A recent prospective study found that the presence of stress unrelated to the accident was a better predictor of persistent symptoms than clinical findings (3), suggesting that psychologic variables are important.

Diagnosis

Although patients usually have pain after the accident, it is not uncommon for the patient to be without discomfort initially. The patient experiences pain in the posterior or anterior region of the neck. It commonly radiates to the occipital aspect of the head, and it may radiate to the shoulders. Occipital headaches often occur. Disc herniation fracture or subluxation can occur in this setting. Therefore, it is essential to visualize the cervical spine radiologically down to C7–T1. If plain x-rays are normal, flexion extension x-rays should be obtained. Any patient with neurologic findings in this setting should be immobilized in a hard collar and seen urgently by a neurosurgeon or orthopedic surgeon before flexion extension x-rays are taken.

Treatment

If muscle spasm or limitation of motion is present without neurologic findings, the patient may be placed in a cervical collar (see above). Analgesics such as acetaminophen or NSAIDs (or occasionally, for short periods, codeine), at adequate dosages, should be given. The patient should be warned that extension of the neck will exacerbate the pain. Heat applied to the cervical spine, either moist or dry, may give symptomatic relief but does not speed healing. Patients may seek manipulation for treatment of this condition and should be aware that the value of this modality is uncertain (4). The patient should be encouraged to perform daily work and activities as much as possible. If the patient has severe pain and muscle spasm at the initial injury, the clinical course will probably last 4 to 6 weeks. When the patient's pain subsides and he or she has full range of motion without muscle spasm, the collar can be gradually discontinued, and the patient should also be advised of the methods of relieving muscle spasm and preventing recurrent symptoms (Figs. 64.2 and 64.3). If there are no symptoms of nerve root compression, the patient with persistent symptoms should be treated for a long time, perhaps a year, before consideration of further workup.

General References

Adams R, Victor M. Principles of neurology. New York: McGraw-Hill, 1993.
>A standard comprehensive textbook.
Bailey RW, Sherk HH, Dunn EJ, et al, eds. The cervical spine. The Cervical Spine Research Society. Philadelphia: JB Lippincott, 1983.
>A comprehensive textbook with in-depth and well-illustrated chapters on all problems of the cervical spine.
Cailliet R. Neck and arm pain. Philadelphia: FA Davis, 1981.
>A very practical, concise, and well-illustrated manual covering the common causes of neck pain.
Carette S. Whiplash injury and chronic neck pain. N Engl J Med 330:1083, 1994.
>This editorial outlines succinctly the magnitude of the problem of whiplash injury and reviews the treatment of chronic neck pain, which may follow.
Frymoyer JW, ed. The adult spine. Principles and practice. New York: Raven, 1991.
Nakano KK. Neck pain. In: Kelley WN, Harris ED, Ruddy S, Sledge CB, eds. Textbook of rheumatology. 5th ed. Philadelphia: WB Saunders, 1997.
>An excellent discussion of the anatomy and biomechanisms and the diagnosis, treatment, and differential diagnosis of common cervical spine problems.

Specific References

1. Elias F. Roentgen findings in the asymptomatic cervical spine. NY J Med 58:3300, 1958.
2. Johnson RM, Hart DL, Simmons EF, et al. Cervical orthoses. J Bone Joint Surg 59:332, 1977.
3. Karlsborg M, Smed A, Jespersen H, et al. A prospective study of 39 patients with whiplash injury. Acta Neurol Scand 95:65, 1997.
4. Koes BW, Assendelft WJ, van der Heijden GJ, et al. Spinal manipulation and mobilization for back and neck pain: a blinded review. BMJ 303:1298, 1991.
5. Rothman RH, Simeone FA, eds. The spine. Philadelphia: WB Saunders, 1992.
6. Saal JS, Saal JA, Yurth EF. Nonoperative management of herniated cervical intervertebral disc with radiculopathy. Spine 21:1877, 1996.

C H A P T E R   65

Low Back Pain

DAVID G. BORENSTEIN, MD

Low back pain is one of the most common human afflictions. Between 70 and 80% of the population experience back pain sometime during their lives. The prevalence of back pain ranges, in reports, from a low of 10% of adults during a 2-year period to a high of 20% of the population of a Western industrial society during a 2-week period (21,38). Although as many as 30% of people with back pain do not seek medical evaluation, the remainder eventually request medical advice. The office is the appropriate setting for the evaluation of these patients. A review of three time periods (1980–1981, 1985, and 1989–1990) studied by the National Ambulatory Medical Care Survey revealed mechanical low back pain (defined below) as the fifth most common reason for all physician office visits. Nonspecific low back pain was the most common diagnosis, accounting for 56.8% of these cases (23). Most patients with low back pain have underlying conditions that can be diagnosed and treated in the ambulatory setting. Most patients do not require hospitalization or surgery. The task is to separate the few who require more aggressive assessment from those who will recover with only office evaluation and conservative management.

ANATOMY AND BIOMECHANICS OF THE LUMBOSACRAL SPINE AND ASSOCIATED STRUCTURES

The structure of the lumbosacral spine is complex (Fig. 65.1A–C). The lumbar spine is composed of five vertebrae with interposed intervertebral discs that consist of a gelatinous nucleus pulposus and a surrounding annulus fibrosus. The vertebrae and discs are supported by strong ligamentous structures and paraspinous muscles. The posterior aspects of the vertebrae surround the spinal canal, form the neural foramina, and interlock to form apophyseal joints (facet joints) whose main purpose is motion (Fig. 65.1A and B). The sacrum is the part of the spine that interdigitates with the iliac bones to form part of the pelvis.

An understanding of the nerve supply to the lumbosacral spine is essential in recognizing the patterns of pain associated with disease processes that affect components of the back (15). The *sinuvertebral nerve* (Fig. 65.1C) is the major sensory nerve supplying structures in the lumbar spine. The nerve arises from the corresponding spinal nerve before it divides into anterior and posterior branches. The nerve enters the intervertebral foramen and divides into ascending, descending, and transverse branches that anastomose with the contralateral side and with sensory nerves at adjacent levels above and below. The sinuvertebral nerve supplies the posterior longitudinal ligament, superficial annulus fibrosus, epidural blood vessels, anterior dura mater, dural sleeve, and posterior vertebral periosteum. The posterior rami of the spinal nerves supply the apophyseal joints above and below the nerve and the paraspinous muscles at multiple levels. The complex innervation of lumbar spine structures helps explain the diffuse nature of pain associated with a wide variety of disorders.

A number of organs are situated in the retroperitoneum, anterior to the lumbar spine. The kidneys, ureters, aorta, inferior vena cava, pancreas, and periaortic lymph nodes are retroperitoneal organs. Diseases that affect these organs may result in referred pain that is localized to the lumbar spine.

In the upright position with a normal spinal curvature (lordosis), the ligamentous structures maintain the position of the spine with little need for contraction of the paraspinous muscles or for weight bearing by the apophyseal (facet) joints (Fig. 65.1A). However, if the normal curve is flattened or accentuated, the paraspinous muscles contract and the apophyseal (facet) joints become weight bearing. This change in body mechanics results in pain.

The lumbar vertebrae are exposed to tremendous forces. This is caused principally by the magnification of stresses that result from the lever effect of the arm in lifting and by vertical forces associated with the human upright position. Figure 65.2 demonstrates how lifting an object away from the body introduces the lever magnification phenomenon, resulting in a marked increase in forces on the vertebral bodies and discs. Because each intervertebral disc is a fluid system, hydraulic pressure is created whenever a load is placed

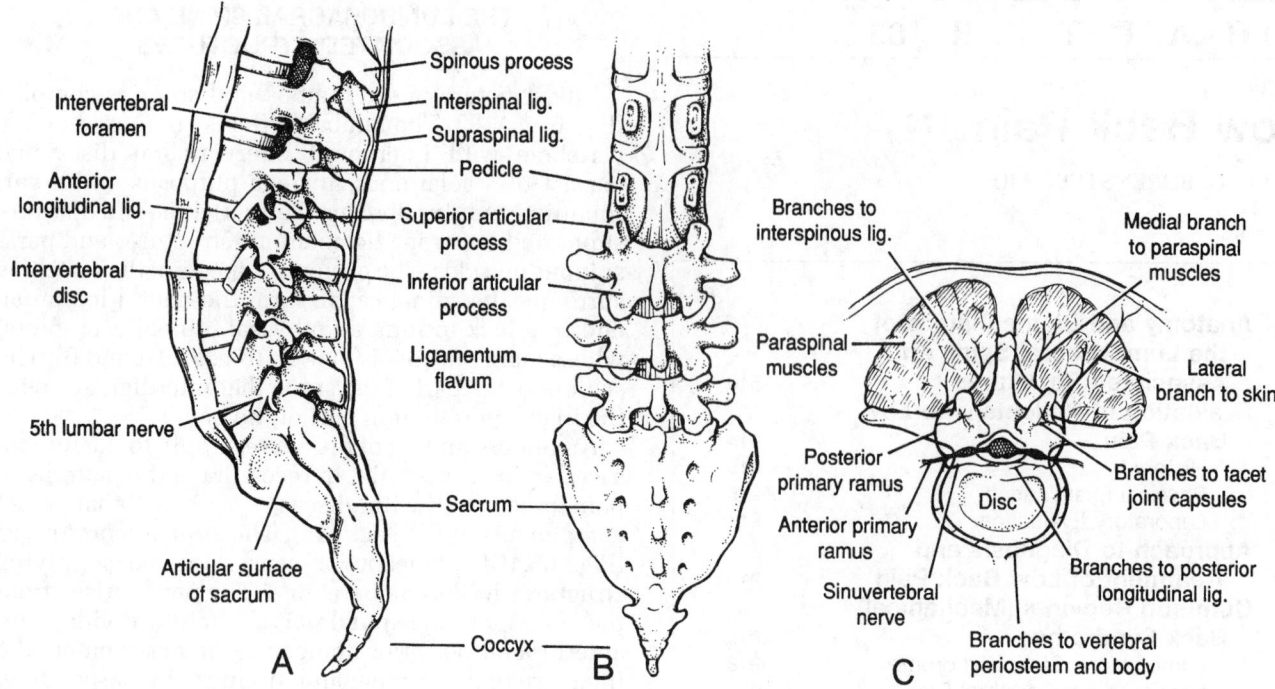

Figure 65.1. Anatomic relationships of the lumbosacral spine. **A.** Lateral view. **B.** Posterior view. **C.** Cross-sectional view.

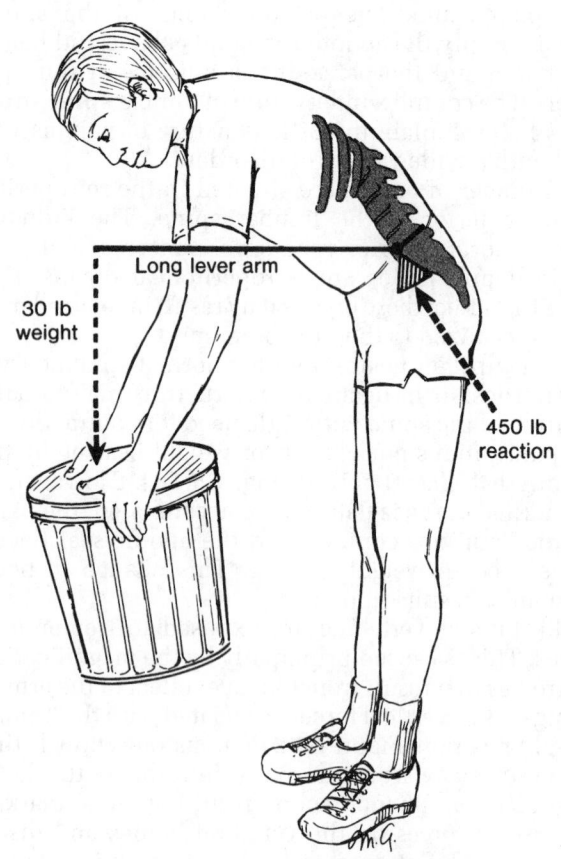

Figure 65.2. Forces in the lumbar area.

on the axial skeleton. This hydraulic pressure magnifies three to five times the force that occurs on the annulus fibrosus. This force is akin to the hoop stress that occurs in a barrel when pressure is applied to its liquid content. The ability of the annulus fibrosus to withstand stress decreases significantly with age, and by 60 years many people have only 50% of the strength in these fibers that they had at age 30.

However, the lumbar spine is not just an isolated structure. Much support is obtained by the muscles and ligaments of the spine and by the muscles of the thoracic and abdominal cavities. These latter structures act as a sort of muscular cylinder that helps decrease the load on the axial skeleton by as much as 30% in the lumbar area and 50% in the thoracic spine.

EVALUATION OF PATIENTS WITH LOW BACK PAIN

Certain facts pertaining to the causes and natural history of back pain influence the evaluation and treatment of patients with this symptom. Back pain is most often associated with a mechanical cause, although it sometimes has a nonmechanical (called medical or systemic in this text) cause. Mechanical low back pain may be defined as pain secondary to overuse of a normal anatomic structure (e.g., muscle strain) or deformity of an anatomic structure (e.g., herniated nucleus pulposus). Medical back pain syndromes are simply the manifestation, in the area of the lower back, of a systemic disorder. These are defined more fully below, under "Approach to Diagnosis and Treatment of Low Back Pain." A majority of patients with mechanical back pain do not have an associated history of acute trauma, lifting, or strain (26). Most low back pain problems are self-limited. Of patients evaluated by physicians, 40 to 50% are better in 1 week, 51 to 86% in 1 month, and 92% within 2 months (14). Most patients with low back pain do not require surgery.

History

Questions about back pain should concentrate on a history of episodes, and for the current episode, the onset, duration, frequency, location, radiation, time of day, quality, intensity, and the aggravating and alleviating factors. A history of motor or sensory nerve root irritation or sphincter (bladder or rectal incontinence) or sexual dysfunction is important in identifying patients with *cauda equina compression* (see below). Occupational history may reveal predisposing factors associated with recurrent episodes of back injury.

Patients should also be questioned about systemic symptoms that are indicative of a medical (systemic) cause of their back pain. Patients with fever, weight loss, pain with recumbency, extended morning stiffness, acute bone pain, or viscerogenic pain should be evaluated for a systemic illness. Patients who are over 60 years of age are also at greater risk of a medical (systemic) cause for their pain.

Physical Examination

Physical Examination of the Lumbosacral Spine and Associated Musculoskeletal Areas

Abnormalities of the spine may be discovered while the spine is stationary or in motion. The patient should be examined in an orderly fashion that evaluates the function of musculoskeletal and neurologic structures of the lumbosacral spine (22).

Initially, the patient is examined in a gown while *standing* barefoot or wearing only socks. The spinal column is examined from all directions to check for excessive kyphosis, lordosis, or scoliosis. The presence of scoliosis is best determined by having the patient flex at the waist with arms extended in front. Any asymmetry of the height of the shoulders can be appreciated. Any deviation of a spinous process from the midline is noted. Firm palpation of the paravertebral muscles and of each vertebral spine is performed. Isolated tenderness over a bone suggests a localized problem such as tumor, infection, or compression fracture. Firm paraspinous muscles result from spasm secondary to local injury or referred pain.

Mobility of the spine is assessed by having the patient bend forward and attempt to touch the toes (normal is about 50° to 80°). However, the hip joints also participate in the movement. Range of flexion can be determined by quantifying the expansion of a 10-cm line measured from the lumbosacral junction superiorly during maximal flexion (*Schober test,* see Chapter 71) or noting the distance of the fingertips from the floor. During this movement the normally smooth rhythm of the reversal of the lumbar lordosis is noted. If the rhythm is interrupted or hesitant, an abnormality of the apophyseal joints or of paraspinous structures may be present.

Lateral flexion (normal is to about 30°) and extension (normal is to about 30°) are then assessed. Lateral flexion is usually preserved in disc disease but may be limited in patients with a spondyloarthropathy (i.e., a joint problem of the spine). Increased discomfort with extension suggests disease of the apophyseal joints or spinal stenosis.

The patient is then examined *bent forward* over the examining table. In this position, the inferior portion of the sacroiliac joints, ischial tuberosities, and sciatic notch are more easily palpated.

The *gait of the patient* should be observed. Patients with back pain may walk in a stiff, guarded fashion or may favor one leg if a radiculopathy is present.

The patient is next examined *sitting with the legs dangling.* The deep tendon reflexes of the knees (L4) and ankles (S1) are elicited to test the integrity of the reflex arcs. An absent reflex may signify nerve root impingement secondary to a herniated nucleus pulposus. While seated, the patient extends each knee The flexion of the hip and extension of the knee stretch the lumbar nerve roots. Radicular pain that radiates from the back to below the knee is associated with nerve root impingement. The origin of the pain from the nerve root can be confirmed by lowering the leg just to the point where the pain disappears and then reproducing the pain by dorsiflexing the foot. This sign, if positive, suggests a herniated intervertebral disc or, less commonly, bony impingement of a nerve root caused by arthritis affecting the apophyseal joints, lumbar stenosis, or, rarely, a tumor of the spinal cord or surrounding structures. This *distracted straight leg raising* (SLR) test helps confirm the organic source of pain and identify patients who may exaggerate their symptoms. Patients with functional complaints have no discomfort with a distracted SLR test but may describe excruciating pain when the SLR test is done in the supine position. Not all patients with a herniated disc have a positive SLR test. A patient, especially over age 30 years, may have a herniated disc that is too small or in the wrong location to irritate the nerve roots.

Next, the patient assumes the *supine* position, so that a *standard* SLR test can be performed. The examiner fully extends the knee and slowly flexes the lower extremity at the hip. Normally the hip can be flexed to 80° without pain, except for discomfort in the thigh or behind the knee secondary to hamstring muscle tightness. A positive test is manifested by radicular pain that radiates below the knee on the affected side or bilaterally. The nerve root and surrounding dura do not move in the neural foramen until an elevation of 30° or greater of the lower extremity has been reached. Therefore, radicular pain that is elicited at an elevation less than 30° is suspect. After the SLR test, the unaffected lower extremity should be raised, thus performing the *crossed SLR test* (25). This procedure causes tension and stretch of the nerve roots of the opposite (affected) lower extremity and reproduces the radicular pain caused by SLR in that lower extremity. When this test is positive, there is a strong but not absolute correlation with disc herniation (44,48).

Next, *sensory assessment* of the buttock, perineum, and lower extremities should be performed. Figure 78.2 (Chapter 78) shows the relevant sensory dermatomes that can be evaluated by pinprick and touch. Abnormalities help localize a lesion and help the physician to determine the need and urgency of an orthopedic or neurosurgical consultation. An important component of the sensory assessment is the search for signs compatible with a *cauda equina syndrome* (a syndrome of neurologic dysfunction from compression of the nerves at the L4–5 level and inferior to the spinal cord proper, often secondary to a central disc herniation). The signs of compression of the cauda equina include saddle anesthesia, loss of anal sphincter tone (assessed by rectal examination), bilateral *sciatica* (pain in the distribution of the sciatic nerve), lower extremity motor weakness, and a history of bowel, bladder, or sexual dysfunction. This syndrome, if present, is an indication for immediate referral to a neurosurgeon or orthopedic surgeon for hospitalization and surgical decompression of the spinal cord.

A detailed assessment of *motor function* of the lower extremities also helps localize a lesion in the patient in whom neurologic involvement is suspected (see Table 84.7 in Chapter 84). This assessment can be done while the patient is supine, sitting, or standing. Muscles tested include hip flexors (L2–3) and extensors (L4–5), the knee extensors (L3–4), the dorsiflexors of the foot (L4–5), the knee flexors (L5–S1), and the plantar flexors of the foot (S1–2). Subtle weakness may be elicited by having the patient walk on his or her toes (gastrocnemius muscle group, S1–2) and heels (tibialis anterior muscles, L4–5).

While the patient is in the supine position, an assessment of the hip, sacroiliac, and knee joints is done. The hip and knee joints are assessed by moving these joints through a normal range of motion when they are unweighted. Pain with motion suggests an articular cause of leg pain. The *sacroiliac joint* is tested by the Patrick or FABER (flexion, abduction, external rotation) test. The test is done by positioning the lateral malleolus of the tested leg on the patella of the opposite leg. Downward pressure is then placed on the medial aspect of the knee while stabilizing the pelvis by placing a hand on the contralateral anterior superior iliac spine. Pain associated with a quick pulse or downward pressure is usually localized to the lateral aspect of the lumbar spine and originates in the sacroiliac joint. Slow pressure may elicit groin pain indicative of hip joint dysfunction.

In the *lateral* position, the sacroiliac joint and muscles of hip abduction (L2–3) are tested. Pressure is applied to the iliac wing, compressing the sacroiliac joints. Pain felt in the sacroiliac joint suggests an intra-articular process or a strain of the posterior sacroiliac ligaments. The muscles of hip abduction are tested as the patient elevates the upper leg against downward pressure applied below the knee by the examiner.

In the *prone* position, the symmetry of the buttocks is assessed (gluteus maximus, L5, S1–2). A femoral stretch test (i.e., extending the hip joint) elicits pain in the anterior thigh (L2–3) or the medial aspect of the leg (L4) in patients with corresponding herniated intervertebral discs.

To evaluate the rare patients suspected of *malingering* or of a psychiatric origin for their back pain, Waddell et al. identified five physical signs associated with functional disorders (45). First, overreaction during examination was found to be the single most important sign indicating a nonorganic cause. Overreaction may take the form of collapsing, sweating, tremor, muscle tension, bizarre facial expression, or disproportionate verbalization. Second, simulation testing may be used to elicit nonorganic pain. Two useful examples are axial loading and rotation. In the first example, with the patient standing, low back pain is reported in overreactors (but not in others) on vertical loading by pressing down on the patient's head. Neck pain is common during this examination in all and does not constitute a positive sign. In the hip rotation test, the patient stands with feet together and arms fixed firmly to the lateral sides of the body at the hip level by the examiner's hands. In this manner, the torso (and the spine) is passively rotated on the hips. Because the units of the spine itself are not moved, reports of low back pain are a positive sign of a nonorganic cause. However, in the presence of true radiculopathy, leg pain may be produced because there is movement at the hip joint and nerve roots may be stretched. Third is the use of distraction testing. This consists of observing the patient during the course of the examination for variable findings when the patient is unaware of being observed or tested, such as during the *distracted SLR* (see above). Fourth, superficial, nonanatomic or variable tenderness is also a nonorganic sign. A useful technique is Magnuson's test, in which tender areas are subtly marked and later examined again for reproducibility. Fifth, motor or sensory findings that are not explained by an anatomic lesion provide clues that the problem is psychiatric in origin. Also, sudden giving away or flaccidity of a muscle during strength testing of the symptomatic area supports a nonorganic problem. A finding of three or more of the five types of signs is clinically significant.

Examination of Other Regions

Patients with constitutional symptoms or with symptoms not attributed to a local process in the back (e.g., abdominal pain) should undergo a focused physical examination. The physical examination including pelvic and rectal, and breast examinations in women, is particularly important in patients who describe new back pain and are 50 years of age or older.

Common origins of metastatic cancer to the spine are the breast, lung, prostate, thyroid, kidney, and rectum. Referred pain from cancer or other lesions may also be felt in the back. For example, pancreatic tumors or duodenal ulcers cause pain to be referred to the high lumbar or low thoracic vertebral region. Bowel or urinary tract cancer may cause pain to be referred to the mid- or low lumbar region, and a disease process located in the pelvis may cause lower lumbar or sacral pain. Also, neoplasia primarily affecting the bones, especially multiple myeloma, is an important consideration in the elderly.

Important also is the assessment of the adequacy of the arteries of the lower extremities. Vascular abnormalities may cause pain due to ischemia in the back, buttock, or lower extremities during exertion. In addition to diminished pulses and bruits over arteries, cutaneous signs of ischemia (ulcers, loss of hair or nails) should be sought in the legs or feet (see Chapter 87). Sudden change in a pain pattern associated with an abdominal aneurysm or an episode of hypotension should alert one to the possibility of impending extension or rupture of the aneurysm.

Although the physical examination adds essential information for the evaluation of low back pain, the reproducibility of findings can vary widely among examiners and at different times. In one study of the physical examination of patients with low back pain, McCombe et al. evaluated the reproducibility of a number of signs (35). They conclude that precise examination, careful measurement of locations of pain and tenderness and degrees of movement of the back and legs, and careful documentation of this was most important to accurately reproduce a patient's findings. Certain caveats relevant to this examination were developed. The most important among these were as follows: Bony tenderness is more reproducible and of greater diagnostic significance than soft tissue tenderness, pain on hip flexion and external rotation is reproducible and valuable, heel and toe standing are not an accurate method of assessing muscle strength, straight leg raising is reliable and reproducible if there is precise measurement and documentation of the extent of pain radiation, and measurements of the range of flexion and lateral bend are reliable. A study by Jensen of the accuracy of certain signs in predicting a precise cause and location of a problem showed a reasonable but imperfect correlation of disturbed sensory and motor function with anatomic abnormalities confirmed at surgery in 52 patients with lumbar disc herniations (28). The time of day of the examination also may have an effect on physical findings. Ensink reports the measured lumbar spine motion in 29 patients with chronic back pain in the morning and afternoon. Flexion was increased to the greatest degree at the end of the day and extension was independent of time of measurement (17). The sum of all these studies is that careful examination and precise measurements of dysfunction and pain location are important in evaluating back pain. However, no sign is absolutely diagnostic or perfectly reproducible and some signs are frankly unreliable. The entire constellation of findings must therefore be considered in developing a proper approach to a patient.

With information obtained from the history and physical examination, a working diagnosis may be generated based on first defining the pain as mechanical or nonmechanical (medical or systemic) in nature. Patients with mechanical disorders may be treated without additional laboratory or radiographic tests during the initial visit. On the other hand, those believed to have a nonmechanical (medical or systemic) problem should undergo further diagnostic testing.

Laboratory Evaluation

Radiographic Tests

A *plain x-ray of the lumbar spine* is not a necessary part of the initial evaluation of patients with back pain unless they have a history of recent major trauma or acute constitutional symptoms. Patients with back pain of a mechanical origin often have normal x-rays. In addition, many patients with abnormal x-rays may be entirely asymptomatic (47). By age 50, 67% of normal people have evidence of disc disease characterized by narrowing of one or more disc spaces or disc calcifications; an additional 20% of people have lumbar osteophytes. In fact, only 13% of 50-year-olds have normal x-rays. Two-thirds of patients with roentgenographic evidence of lumbar disc degeneration are asymptomatic. Osteoarthritis of the apophyseal (facet) joints is not correlated with symptoms (33). In addition, plain films may not be sensitive enough to identify bony lesions unless 50% of the medullary portion of the bone has been destroyed (3). Therefore, plain x-rays of the lumbar spine should be obtained only in patients who have failed a course of conservative therapy, persist with pain, have reflex asymmetry, have point vertebral tenderness, or are elderly and have new onset pain (because of the higher incidence of a fracture or a systemic cause of their symptoms) (20).

Other radiographic techniques that are useful in the evaluation of patients with back pain include *bone scan* (infection, tumor [but multiple myeloma is notoriously missed], arthritis, fracture), *computerized tomography* (disc herniation, spinal stenosis, myeloma, retroperitoneal structures), and magnetic resonance imaging (disc herniation, intraspinal tumors). Each should be highly selected on the basis of the history and physical examination and often a consultation from a radiologist, neurosurgeon, or orthopedist is helpful in deciding the approach. *Magnetic resonance imaging* (MRI) is able to detect specific anatomic lesions in the lumbar spine with greater sensitivity than any other radiographic technique (1,37). MRI detects degenerative intervertebral disc disease and spinal stenosis and is an excellent method for detecting medical disorders affecting the lumbar spine, including primary and metastatic malignancies and osteomyelitis (2). Computerized tomography (CT) is especially valuable for the definition of trabecular architecture of bone. Benign and malignant tumors, and infectious lesions, may be differentiated by CT. Radiographic findings become significant only when the history, physical examination, and radiographic findings agree. These more expensive imaging techniques are confirmatory, not diagnostic, tests. Nearly one-third of asymptomatic patients have identifiable abnormalities that are of no significance (8,27,46).

Other Laboratory Evaluations

Most patients with low back pain do not require laboratory studies with their initial evaluation. Patients who are elderly, have constitutional symptoms, or have failed conservative therapy may benefit from a laboratory evaluation (see above). The laboratory evaluations that may be useful include complete blood count and erythrocyte sedimentation rate (inflammatory and neoplastic disorders), serum calcium concentration and alkaline phosphatase activity (diffuse bone disease), serum and urine electrophoresis (multiple myeloma), prostate-specific antigen (metastatic prostate cancer), urinalysis (renal disease), and occult blood in the stool (ulcers, gastrointestinal tumors). All such evaluations should be based on distinct diagnostic possibilities based on the history and physical examination.

APPROACH TO DIAGNOSIS AND TREATMENT OF LOW BACK PAIN

In describing various conditions that result in back pain, it is useful to place them into two categories: regional (mechanical) and medical (systemic or nonmechanical). Both are defined above, under "Evaluation of Patients with Low Back Pain." Differentiating medical back pain syndromes from a mechanical cause can be difficult when the back is the only anatomic area in which symptoms are manifest. This difficulty is most commonly experienced when evaluating elderly patients. Systemic conditions that typically affect the low back region, including infections and tumors, are discussed below.

Most patients with an acute onset of low back pain have a regional (mechanical) cause for their symptoms. Up to 90% of these patients respond to a course of conservative medical therapy. Serial observation is very important in management of patients with back pain. If on reassessment there are symptoms or signs of progression or of an incomplete response to treatment,

evaluation for an alternative diagnosis is indicated. The follow-up contact should occur 3 to 4 weeks after the initial visit for all patients because by this time most patients with nonserious disorders causing their symptoms are markedly improved. The follow-up visit is also important for patients whose back pain has resolved so that they have an opportunity to be educated in regard to recurrent symptoms and advised regarding prophylactic measures.

COMMON REGIONAL (MECHANICAL) BACK SYNDROMES

Lumbosacral Strain Syndrome

Lumbosacral strain is the most common cause of low back pain. The cause of back strain is not always clear but may be related to muscular, ligamentous, or fascial strain secondary to either a specific traumatic episode or continuous mechanical stress. People between the ages of 20 and 40 years are at greatest risk of developing muscle strain. Predisposing factors include failure to use good techniques in lifting, obesity, abnormal forward pelvic tilt (accentuated lordosis, most usually an acquired posture resulting from abdominal obesity), and leg length discrepancy (43).

Diagnosis

The patient complains of pain that may be severe in the back, buttock, or one or both thighs. Usually symptoms follow a recent increase in physical activity for that patient, such as gardening, lifting, or an infrequently played sport. Usually the patient experiences no (or minimal) discomfort during or immediately after the activity. Within the next 12 to 36 hours, as the soft tissues swell, pain develops and is associated with a feeling of muscular stiffness. The patient complains of pain that is accentuated by standing and bending and alleviated by lying. Table 65.1 provides information useful in the differential diagnosis of mechanical low back pain.

Examination of the back may show nonspecific signs of muscle spasm and loss of lumbar lordosis, but characteristically there is no evidence of nerve root impingement. Pain radiating to the low back from an inflamed ischial or trochanteric bursa is occasionally

Table 65.1. Information Useful in the Differential Diagnosis of Mechanical Low Back Pain

Characteristics	Lumbosacral Strain	Herniated Nucleus Pulposus	Osteoarthritis	Spinal Stenosis
Age (yr)	20–40	30–50	>50	>60
Pain characteristics				
Location	Back (unilateral)	Back and leg (unilateral)	Back (bilateral)	Leg (bilateral)
Onset	Acute	Acute (prior episodes)	Insidious	Insidious
Standing[a]	+	−	+	+
Sitting[a]	−	+	−	−
Bending[a]	+	−	−	−
Straight leg raising test	−	+	−	+
				(stress, i.e., after walking)
Plain x-ray	−	−	+	+

Adapted from Borenstein DG, Wiesel SW. Low back pain: medical diagnosis and comprehensive management. Philadelphia: WB Saunders, 1989.
[a]+, Exacerbating; −, alleviating.

seen, but marked tenderness over the inflamed bursa should reveal the correct diagnosis (see Chapter 66).

Management

In December 1994, the Agency for Health Care Policy and Research (AHCPR) published a Clinical Practice Guideline booklet concerning the diagnosis and management of acute low back pain (6). The booklet included the recommendations of a 23-member panel that critically reviewed 3918 published scientific articles. The recommendations are listed in Table 65.2. The reviewed articles related to management were rated from A to D, ranging from studies with strong research-based evidence to studies in which the design did not meet inclusion criteria. The final recommendations were based on the strength of evidence, risk–benefit ratios, and cost of each intervention. In the absence of controlled trials, the potential benefit of an intervention had to outweigh its possible risks to be considered cost-effective.

In general the guidelines encourage early return of function. The recommended medications have mild toxicities and little abuse potential. Invasive therapies are limited to patients who fail to improve over 4 to 12 weeks. The guidelines do have limitations: The recommendations are options and not the sole method for treating low back pain; they are based on a small number of studies (although many were reviewed), and they are made for acute low back pain and do not apply to patients with chronic low back pain.

The conservative therapy of low back pain from lumbosacral strain includes controlled physical activity (low stress, gradually increasing aerobic and back-strengthening exercises), physical therapy, nonsteroidal anti-inflammatory drugs, and muscle relaxants. To minimize back motion and provide support, the bed should be firm but comfortable. A bed board cut from ⅝-inch particle-board or plywood (more expensive but will last for years) placed between the mattress and box spring is usually effective. Avoiding strenuous activity for most patients is appropriate, and even for those with severe pain, a minimal period of strict bed rest as short as 2 days has been shown to be adequate in relieving back pain (13). Controlled physical activity allows injured tissues to rest, permitting a greater opportunity for healing without reinjury. Pushing this concept further, Malmivaara reported on the efficacy of ordinary activity as tolerated in comparison with efficacy of bed rest for 2 days and back-mobilizing exercises (34). Better recovery, improved function, and fewer missed work days were associated with ordinary activity. Also, Faas points out the absence of significant benefit from exercise taught and monitored by a physiotherapist in the resolution of low back pain (19). In this study of 473 patients, flexion and stretching exercises were only minimally better at decreasing the duration of low back pain recurrences and had no other benefit compared with placebo interventions, which consisted of ultrasonography by a physiotherapist and usual care. The important lesson for the physician from these studies is to encourage the patient to do gentle

Table 65.2. AHCPR Guidelines for Management of Acute Low Back Pain

I. Patient education
Patients with acute low back problems should be given accurate information about the following (strength of evidence = B):
  A. Expectations for both rapid recovery and recurrences of symptoms based on natural history of low back symptoms.
  B. Safe and effective methods of symptom control.
  C. Safe and reasonable activity modifications.
  D. Best means of limiting recurrent low back problems.
  E. The lack of need for special investigations unless danger signs are present (see text).
  F. Effectiveness and risks of commonly available diagnostic and further treatment measures to be considered should symptoms persist.
II. Medications
Acetaminophen and nonsteroidal anti-inflammatory drugs (NSAIDs)
  A. Acetaminophen is reasonably safe and is acceptable for treating patients with acute low back problems (strength of evidence = C).
  B. NSAIDs, including aspirin, are acceptable for treating patients with acute low back pain (strength of evidence = B).
  C. NSAIDs have a number of potential side effects. The most common complication is gastrointestinal irritation. The decision to use these medications can be guided by comorbidity, side effects, cost, and patient and provider preference (strength of evidence = C).
III. Physical treatments
Spinal manipulation
  A. Manipulation can be helpful for patients with acute low back problems without radiculopathy when used within the first month of symptoms (strength of evidence = B).
  B. A trial of manipulation in patients without radiculopathy with symptoms longer than a month is probably safe, but efficacy is unproven (strength of evidence = C).
IV. Activity modification
Activity recommendations for bed rest and exercise
  A. A gradual return to normal activities is more effective than prolonged bed rest for treating acute low back problems (strength of evidence = B).
  B. Prolonged bed rest for more than 4 days may lead to debilitation and is not recommended for treating acute low back problems (strength of evidence = B).
  C. Low-stress aerobic exercise can prevent debilitation due to inactivity during the first month of symptoms and thereafter may help to return patients to the highest level of functioning appropriate to their circumstances (strength of evidence = C).

Ratings for strength of evidence: A = Strong research-based evidence (multiple relevant and high-quality studies); B = Moderate research-based evidence (one relevant, high-quality or multiple adequate studies); C = Limited research-based evidence (one adequate scientific study); D = Studies did not meet inclusion criteria.

activity as tolerated early in the course of acute low back pain when the cause is felt secondary to lumbosacral strain.

Physical therapy modalities, in the form of cold (ice massage) initially or heat subsequently, may decrease pain and diminish spasm. The application of dry heat by a heating pad for 20 to 30 minutes several times a day (on low or medium setting with a protective towel between skin and pad to prevent burns) is preferred by some patients. Others prefer moist heat, which is accomplished by using hot towels, or a heat pack, which produces sustained heat for up to 30 minutes (available at pharmacies).

Nonnarcotic analgesics in the form of nonsteroidal anti-inflammatory drugs (NSAIDs) are helpful in making patients comfortable while their injury heals.

NSAIDs with a rapid onset of action such as diclofenac (Cataflam) or naproxen (Anaprox) are most appropriate. Other nonsteroidals that are useful include aspirin, 600 mg four times a day, ibuprofen (Motrin) 600 to 800 mg three times a day, diflunisal (Dolobid) 500 mg twice a day, or ketoprofen 200 mg once a day (Oruvail). In general, all nonsteroidal analgesics should be used for a limited time (e.g., 2 to 6 weeks) in treating patients with mechanical back pain. The choice of any of these nonsteroidal drugs must be made in consideration of both patient and drug characteristics. For example, some patients prefer twice-a-day drug administration whereas a few prefer more frequent dosing. Some groups of patients are especially vulnerable to the side effects of these drugs. Particularly important are the gastrointestinal and renal toxicity that occur often in elderly patients, especially women, who take NSAIDs. These drugs must be used with great caution or avoided in this population. For the older patient, pain control with acetaminophen alone (or occasionally with small doses of a narcotic for a short time) is preferred. NSAID use is described in detail in Chapter 70. *Muscle relaxants* are not first-line therapeutic agents but should be considered for the patient with significant muscle spasm on physical examination. Cyclobenzaprine (Flexeril) is more efficacious than placebo in the treatment of intractable pain syndromes associated with muscle spasm (9). Most patients have a beneficial response to the drug at a dosage of 10 mg once a day. The dosage may be increased up to 10 mg three times a day, but this is associated with a greater frequency of drowsiness and dry mouth. Taking the drug 2 hours or more before bedtime may limit early morning drowsiness. This efficacy of cyclobenzaprine may be judged after a 7- to 10-day trial. Other muscle relaxants that may be useful, if cyclobenzaprine is ineffective, include methocarbamol (Robaxin) 750 mg four times a day, chlorzoxazone (Parafon DSC) 500 mg four times a day, or orphenadrine citrate (Norflex) 100 mg twice a day (16). Diazepam (Valium) is no more effective than placebo in improving back spasm (4). This drug should not be used for patients with low back pain.

Neither biofeedback nor acupuncture is recommended by the AHCPR (6) for the treatment of patients with acute low back pain.

During the recovery period, the patient should be advised to avoid activities that greatly increase the forces applied to the lower spine (e.g., lifting, pushing, force on outstretched upper extremity, as in making beds or vacuuming, lurching, or bending). If the patient fails to respond or pain recurs, the patient should be reexamined 3 to 4 weeks later to investigate the possibility of a medical (systemic) cause of back pain. If a mechanical cause remains the most likely diagnosis, a modification in drug therapy (prescribing an alternative nonsteroidal and, if needed, muscle relaxant drug) is indicated.

For the patient who is recovering satisfactorily, various exercise programs have been advocated. One simple back strengthening exercise program combines isometric gluteal and abdominal muscle contractions and pelvic tilt (Fig. 65.3). These exercises, which are performed standing with the back against a wall, should be recommended as soon as tolerated (see above). These exercises strengthen the muscles that support the spine and may relieve current symptoms and help prevent future episodes of back pain. The exercises should be performed for a few minutes four to six times a day. Exercises designed to strengthen the abdominal musculature, such as sit-ups with the knees flexed or straight leg raising, increase intradiscal pressure, may exacerbate symptoms and are not recommended (however, see below for management of intercritical period).

Braces are reserved for the occasional patient with persisting back pain who must remain active while healing continues. However, only limited data support their use. Lumbosacral supports theoretically help relieve back pain by increasing intra-abdominal pressure, which results in greater support of the vertebral column, allowing paraspinous muscles to relax. The lumbosacral support may be a cloth corset fitted with metal stays posteriorly or a smaller cloth brace with a molded plastic insert. The patient obtains a prescription for the corset or brace from the physician and is fitted by an orthotist or physical therapist. The patient should use the support while working and then remove the appliance. The use of a lumbosacral support weakens supporting back muscles, so patients should be weaned gradually but steadily from their supports. It is important for this group of patients to return gradually to full activity because an abrupt return may cause a recurrence of low back pain.

Herniated Intervertebral Disc

The intervertebral disc is composed of the annulus fibrosus and the nucleus pulposus. The annulus fibrosus maintains pressure on the contents of the nucleus pulposus, allowing the intervertebral disc to cushion the forces placed on the spine. Tears in the annulus fibrosus allow the contents of the nucleus pulposus to herniate beyond their normal confines. Tears in the annulus may be associated with transient episodes of low back pain. Herniation of the nucleus may result in sudden severe pain if neural elements are compressed and inflamed by the nuclear contents (Fig. 65.4). A sudden pressure placed on the lumbar spine that may occur with flexion (e.g., bending over to lift a heavy object, lifting with the arms extended away from the body, a sudden lurch, or even a sneeze or cough) can precipitate the rupture. However, many patients who have a herniated disc do not give a history of injury or of a sudden increase in pressure. Lumbar disc disease is most common at the L4–5 and L5–S1 levels and is less common between the other vertebral bodies.

Diagnosis

Patients with herniated intervertebral discs complain of sharp, lancinating pain. The pain radiates from

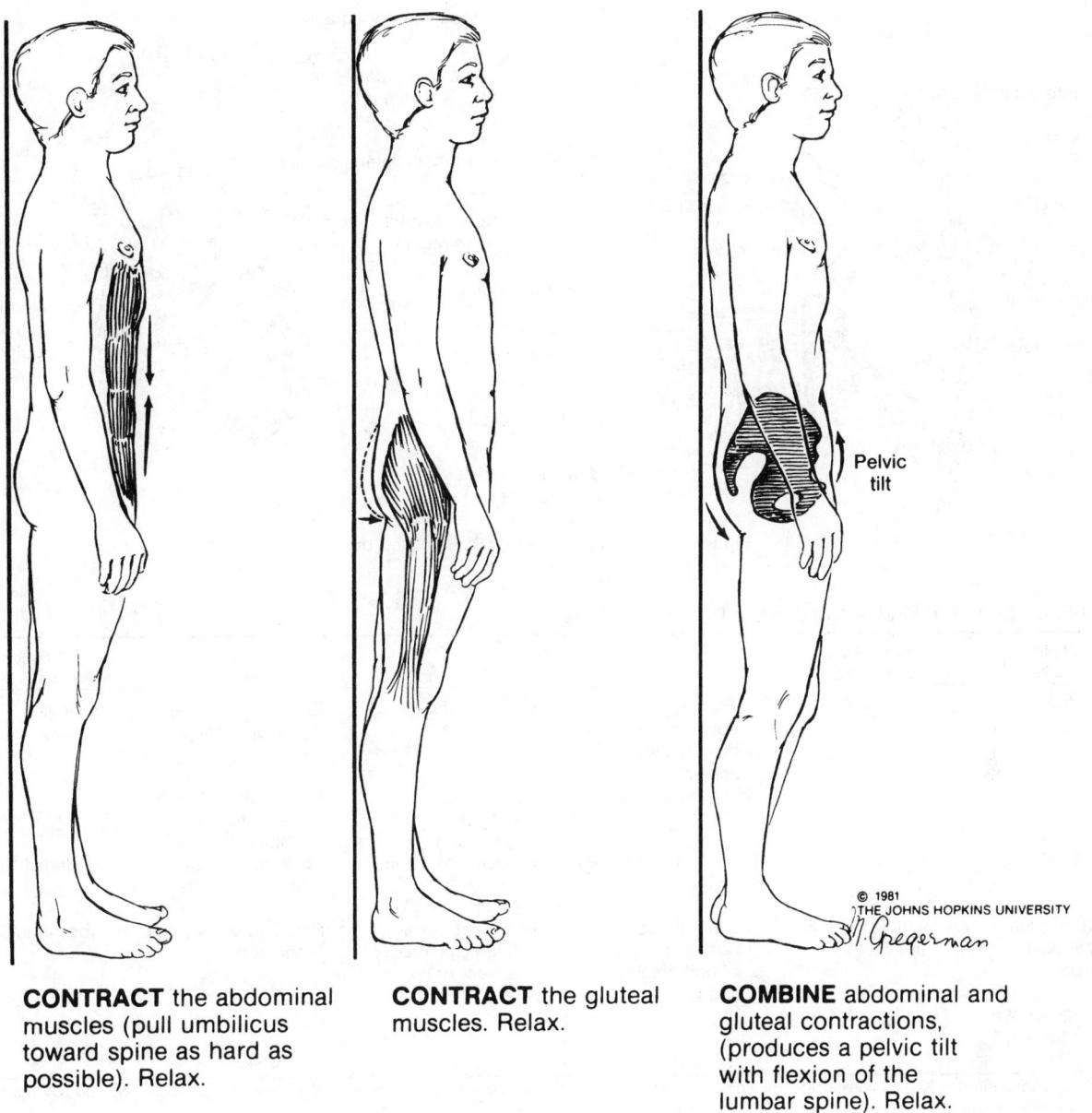

CONTRACT the abdominal muscles (pull umbilicus toward spine as hard as possible). Relax.

CONTRACT the gluteal muscles. Relax.

COMBINE abdominal and gluteal contractions, (produces a pelvic tilt with flexion of the lumbar spine). Relax.

Figure 65.3. Exercises: abdominal muscles and pelvic tilt.

the back down the leg in the anatomic distribution of the affected nerve root. The pain may be so severe that the patient resists examination and splints the back in an awkward position of lateral lumbar flexion and hip flexion. Patients with bilateral sciatica (pain in the distribution of the sciatic nerve L5–S1 roots [buttocks, posterior thighs, and extending below the knees]), progressive muscle weakness, or bladder or bowel incontinence should be evaluated for cauda equina compression (see above). The diagnosis of acute intervertebral disc herniation is most likely when physical examination reveals signs of nerve root compression with either a loss of motor function, loss of deep tendon reflexes, or a localized sensory deficit. Specific disc herniations may result in well-defined motor, sensory,

and reflex deficits that aid in their diagnosis (Table 65.3). Patients with progressive neurologic deficits, particularly muscle weakness, should be referred to an orthopedist or neurosurgeon for close observation. These patients may benefit from early surgical intervention before a course of conservative therapy.

Documentation of the anatomic abnormality associated with radicular pain is necessary for patients who have continued pain despite a 3- to 4-week course of conservative therapy. A number of radiographic techniques may be useful for demonstrating disc herniation. In the past CT and myelography were the preferred techniques to identify herniated discs. MRI readily identifies the location of herniated discs without the need for myelographic dye or radiation

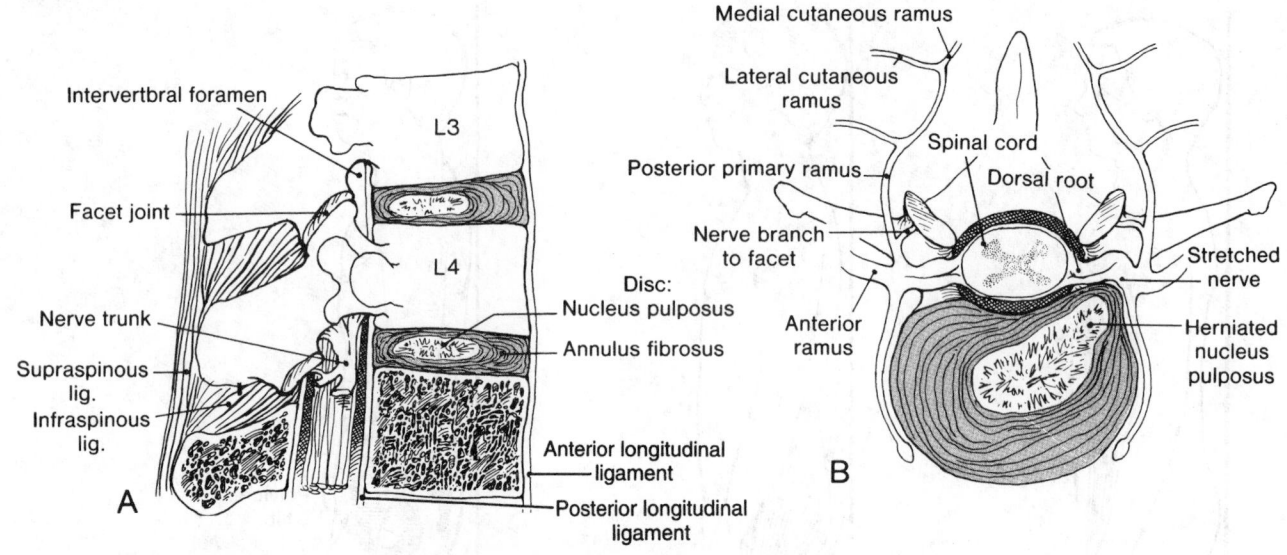

Figure 65.4. **A.** Normal disc. **B.** Herniated disc.

Table 65.3. Common Findings in Lumbar Disc Herniations

Level of Disc Herniation	Nerve Root Compressed	Pain	Numbness[a]	Weakness	Reflexes (Decreased or Absent)
L3–4	L4	Sacroiliac joint, hip, posterolateral thigh, anterior aspect of leg	L4 dermatome	Extension of knee (quadriceps)	Knee jerk
L4–5	L5	Sacroiliac joint, hip	L5 dermatome (includes great toe)	Dorsiflexion of great toe (extensor hallucis longus)	
L5–S1	S1	Lateral aspect of leg and foot	S1 dermatome (includes lateral toes)	Unusual (plantar flexion of foot)	Ankle jerk
Massive midline lumbar disc herniation	Multiple roots in dural sac	Midline of back, posterior aspect of both thighs and legs	Perineum, posterior thighs, plantar aspect of feet	Paralysis of feet and sphincters	Absent ankle jerk
Cauda equina syndrome (usually L4 or L5)					

Adapted from Vanden Briuk KD, Edmonson AS. The spine. In: Edmonson AS, Crenshaw AH, eds. Campbell's operative orthopaedics. St. Louis: CV Mosby, 1980.
[a]See Figure 78.2, Chapter 78.

exposure (7). Therefore, in most circumstances MRI examination has replaced the myelogram as the current preferred test by most surgeons for documenting disc herniation. *Electromyography* (EMG) is occasionally necessary for demonstrating the nerve root level associated with denervation of leg muscles. EMG may also be able to differentiate by the pattern of muscle involvement patients with herniated disc and those with peripheral sciatic nerve abnormalities secondary to another problem such as trauma or tumor. Its use is recommended only after consultation with an orthopedist, neurosurgeon, or neurologist.

Management

The treatment for most patients with a herniated disc is nonoperative because 80% of them respond to conservative therapy (see below) and are completely free of pain within 2 months. In patients whose pain and other neurologic abnormalities remit without surgical reduction of the disc, an adjustment of the annulus and posterior longitudinal ligament to the presence of the herniated disc fragment is the most likely reason for the diminution of edema, inflammation, back pain, and leg pain. Also, desiccation of the fragment may play a role in resolution of symptoms.

Conservative therapy consists of limiting physical activity with the patient at bed rest in the semi-Fowler's position (hips and knees flexed, supported by pillows) for several days. Nonsteroidal anti-inflammatory analgesics and muscle relaxants, as described above, and narcotic analgesics (if the pain is severe) should be prescribed. However, patients whose symptoms are so pronounced that narcotics are required beyond 2 to 3 days should be hospitalized until pain control is satisfactory, and an orthopedist or neurosurgeon should be consulted. Physical therapy is usually unnecessary in treating patients with acute disc herniations. Active exercise programs may intensify acute symptoms and should be avoided. Therapy such as ultrasound, shortwave, diathermy, heat, or cold packs may provide short-term pain relief only (as they do in lumbosacral pain) but do not alter disc lesions or have any long-term effect on symptoms. Lumbar traction has not been shown to be more effective than bed rest in the treatment of lumbar disc disease and is not indicated (12). Patients should be prescribed such a conservative regimen for 3 to 4 weeks, and if this fails, they should consider epidural corticosteroid injection performed by a neurosurgeon, orthopedist, or rheumatologist. A series of 3 injections over 3 to 6 weeks may improve back and leg pain (41). Surgical decompression of the appropriate disc space is indicated for persistent pain resistant to conservative therapy. The size of the disc herniation does not correlate with a lack of response to conservative management. Large herniated discs are more likely to decrease in size as documented by CT scan (42). For management of the intercritical period, see "Management of the Intercritical Period," below.

Osteoarthritis and Spinal Stenosis

The lumbar spine is one of the common locations for osteoarthritis, the most common form of arthritis. This noninflammatory joint disease is associated with joint pain, stiffness, deformity, and limitation of motion. Alterations over time secondary to osteoarthritis result in loss of disc volume, increased pressure on apophyseal joints, and hypertrophy of soft tissue and bony structures resulting in a decrease in the size of the spinal canal. Osteoarthritis is discussed fully in Chapter 68.

Diagnosis

Initially, patients may complain of pain after repeated episodes of hyperextension that traumatizes the apophyseal (facet) joints, resulting in a stretching or tearing of the ligamentous capsule of the apophyseal joint. Typically, back flexion (bending forward) relieves the pain whereas hyperextension (e.g., a painter working overhead) exacerbates it. Patients may also experience back pain related to gradual degeneration of the intervertebral disc or the development of osteophytes, either of which may impinge on a nerve root. Patients with lumbar osteoarthritis or degenerative disc disease describe back, buttock, or unilateral lower extremity pain. Examination usually reveals evidence of irritation of a specific nerve root resulting in loss of a localized motor or sensory neurologic function or of an absent deep tendon reflex (L5–S1 disc, ankle; or L3–4 disc, knee). The SLR may be positive. Many of these patients respond to conservative therapy because

the anti-inflammatory action of the nonsteroidal drugs is effective in diminishing the swelling of the soft tissues, which causes nerve impingement.

As patients grow older, particularly during the fifth to seventh decade, back symptoms become suggestive of impingement of multiple nerve roots at different levels on both sides of the spinal cord. Spinal stenosis occurs most commonly in men, who complain of chronic low back pain with unilateral or bilateral lower extremity discomfort, exacerbated by extension of the spine while standing. They also may develop frank hypesthesia or dysesthesias (Table 65.1). There also may be a history of disc surgery. Many patients with spinal stenosis have symptoms mimicking those of peripheral vascular insufficiency (claudication) (31). These patients develop lower extremity pain while standing or walking, or hyperextension of the spine in the absence of any evidence of peripheral vascular disease. Painful paresthesias are present in the feet or legs and may radiate to the hip girdle or lower trunk. Patients may experience lower extremity numbness and weakness. These symptoms are relieved by rest or flexion of the spine (the patient may report relief by bending forward as if to tie shoelaces). Physical examination may show no abnormalities until the patient is asked to walk. In this regard, the patient suspected of having spinal stenosis should be walked until pain develops—sometimes this requires many minutes—and then examined in the sitting position; abnormal motor or sensory deficits may be present only after such increased activity.

Plain x-rays show degenerative changes in the apophyseal joints (facet joints) and decreased anteroposterior canal diameter. CT is the best diagnostic radiographic technique for spinal stenosis (36). CT shows the narrowed canal or the impingement of osteophytes on the intervertebral foramina.

Management

Most patients with spinal stenosis can be treated nonsurgically. Activities that bring on pain should be discouraged. Patients may respond to NSAIDs or a course of epidural corticosteroid injections (administered by a consulting rheumatologist or orthopedist). Operative therapy for spinal stenosis is reserved for patients who are severely incapacitated by their condition. Surgery for spinal stenosis requires decompression of the bony impingement of the spinal cord and nervi erigentes. If vertebral instability is documented before surgery, fusion of the vertebral bodies is accomplished also. Postoperative relief of pain is seen within a week or so and full recovery, when surgery is successful, within a month. Patients treated successfully with surgery have a more rapid and greater improvement in neurogenic claudication than medically treated patients. However, only two-thirds of patients describe improvement with initial decompressive surgery (24). Also, medically treated patients have no severe deterioration of neurologic function. Therefore, medical treatment for 2 to 3 years before considering surgery seems to be a good approach for the majority of patients with spinal stenosis (29).

MEDICAL (SYSTEMIC) BACK PAIN SYNDROMES
Spondyloarthropathies

Patients with spondyloarthropathies (ankylosing spondylitis, Reiter's syndrome, psoriatic spondylitis, enteropathic spondylitis) often complain of low back, buttock, or leg pain. These patients have morning stiffness as a major component of their symptom complex. Although back pain is the first symptom in a number of young patients, it is often associated with other symptoms and signs of the specific disorder (iritis, conjunctivitis, or skin rash). A clue to the presence of a spondyloarthropathy on physical examination is tenderness with percussion over the axial skeleton or sacroiliac joints. The sacroiliac joints may be painful when stressed while the patient is in the prone or supine position. Conditions affecting the axial skeleton and sacroiliac joints are discussed in Chapter 71.

Infections

Although rare, infections of the axial skeleton (osteomyelitis, discitis, or septic arthritis) must be considered in any patient with back pain (32). Osteomyelitis is an infection of the vertebral bodies. Discitis is an infection of the intervertebral disc (49). Septic arthritis of the back is an infection of the sacroiliac joints. These conditions are discussed in detail in Chapter 31.

Vertebral Fractures

Vertebral compression fractures are common, especially among the elderly, and usually the result of a flexion injury when the spine is abruptly flexed as it is, for example, during jumping. Fractures conceivably could be classified as a regional (mechanical) cause of back pain. It is arbitrarily classified as a medical (systemic) cause of low back pain because it most typically occurs in the elderly and often it is a manifestation of a systemic disorder such as osteoporosis. The thoracic spine is most commonly involved. The force needed to compress a vertebral body in healthy bone is considerable. However, when the bone is diseased, as it is with osteoporosis, multiple myeloma, metastatic cancer, or hyperparathyroidism, the injury may be insignificant. Pain is usually localized and immediate, although it may be delayed for several days after the fracture. Often tenderness over a single vertebra indicates the presence of a fracture, but an x-ray is necessary to confirm the diagnosis.

Other radiographic techniques are useful for identifying the locations of fractures that may not be detected by plain x-rays. A bone scan is often useful in demonstrating whether there are single or multiple fractures. CT, MRI, or myelography (the selection determined in consultation with an orthopedist and radiologist) is indicated for patients with compression fractures who also have neurologic deficits. These techniques can lo-

calize abnormalities associated with nerve impingement. Not all processes that weaken bone are detected by bone scan (e.g., multiple myeloma). Blood chemistries, including the concentration of serum proteins, and the serum and urine electrophoretic pattern of proteins are helpful in identifying patients with myeloma.

With lumbar or thoracic vertebral compression fractures, management includes rest, adequate analgesia, and gradual ambulation when the patient is free from severe pain. A lumbosacral support or, for the patient with a thoracic vertebral fracture, a chair-back or hyperextension brace may be helpful in alleviating pain. These may be obtained by prescription from an orthopedic appliance shop. The pain from a vertebral fracture may persist for several months, although the severe and incapacitating component is usually of only 2 to 3 weeks' duration.

Tumors

Tumors of the lumbar spine are unusual causes of back pain; however, these diseases are associated with the highest morbidity, mortality, and dysfunction. Patients with tumors of the lumbar spine usually have back pain as their initial complaint. Commonly, patients with tumor-associated pain have increased discomfort with recumbency. Physical examination demonstrates localized tenderness as well as neurologic dysfunction if the spinal cord or a nerve root is compressed. Although laboratory evaluation often yields nonspecific results, radiographic evaluation is useful in identifying the location and type of neoplastic lesion. In general, benign tumors are located in the posterior elements of vertebrae (spinous, transverse process), and malignant (both primary and metastatic) tumors are located in the anterior components of vertebrae (body). The definitive diagnosis of a tumor must be

Table 65.4. Medical Causes of Low Back Pain

Systemic: Constitutional symptoms, severe localized pain, morning stiffness are clues suggestive of generalized disorder.
   Rheumatologic: spondyloarthropathies, polymyalgia rheumatica, fibromyalgia
   Infectious; vertebral osteomyelitis, Pott's disease (tuberculosis of spine), discitis, septic arthritis, epidural abscess, herpes zoster
Neoplastic:
   Benign: osteoid osteoma, osteochondroma, giant cell tumor
   Malignant: metastatic, multiple myeloma, chondrosarcoma, chordoma, lymphoma, retroperitoneal sarcoma, neural tumor
   Neurologic–psychiatric: neuropathic (Charcot) joints, femoral neuropathy, depression, hysteria
   Miscellaneous: vertebral sarcoidosis, Paget's disease, retroperitoneal fibrosis
Referred pain: The absence of any tenderness, limitation of motion, or aggravation of pain or spasm during the physical examination is suggestive of referred pain (see Table 65.5 for dermatome to which pain from various visceral structures may be referred).
Lower thoracic and upper lumbar pain from an upper abdominal disease process (e.g., pancreas)
Low lumbar pain from a lower abdominal disease process (e.g., aortic aneurysm)
Sacral pain from a pelvic problem (e.g., endometriosis, prostate cancer)

Table 65.5.   Dermatome to Which Pain from Various Visceral Structures May Be Referred

Dermatome[a]	Viscera
L1	Kidney, ureter, body of uterus, abdominal aorta, small intestine
L2	Bladder, abdominal aorta, ascending colon
L3	Abdominal aorta
L4	Abdominal aorta
L5, S1, S2	—
S3	Rectum, anus, lower portion of bladder, cervix, upper vagina, prostate
S4	Rectum, anus, base of bladder, cervix, upper vagina, prostate
S5	—

Modified from Borenstein DG, Wiesel SW. Low back pain. Philadelphia: WB Saunders, 1989;33.

[a]See Figure 78.2, Chapter 78, for cutaneous pattern of dermatomes.

derived from histologic examination of biopsy material obtained from the lesion. The most effective therapy for both benign and malignant tumors is removal of the lesions that are accessible to surgical excision. When excision is impossible, partial resection, radiation therapy, corticosteroids, or chemotherapy may be indicated to control symptoms and compression of the spinal cord and nerve roots.

Referred Pain

Disease processes that affect organs in the retroperitoneum not only may cause pain locally but may refer pain in the distribution of the sensory nerve supplying the diseased tissue. Diseases of the vascular, genitourinary, and gastrointestinal systems may refer pain to the lumbar spine. Characteristically, referred pain is unaffected by the physical position of the patient. Patients usually have symptoms in the affected organ, raising the possibility of a medical cause of the patient's back pain (Tables 65.4 and 65.5).

MANAGEMENT OF THE INTERCRITICAL PERIOD

Although most patients with low back pain have a complete remission of symptoms within 3 to 4 weeks, many patients experience a recurrence (10). Patients should return to the physician's office even if they have had a resolution of their pain. The purpose of these visits is to discuss ways to prevent recurrent attacks of back pain. Areas of discussion include posture, weight control, exercise, and work activities.

Figure 65.5 shows some correct and incorrect postures and practical advice that may be useful to give to patients who have experienced low back pain. Weight reduction is desirable in the obese patient because excessive weight directly increases the load on the lower vertebral column and its supporting structures. Exercise initiated as soon as the acute pain subsides (usually 2 to 4 days after its onset) improves function and decreases pain (18). At a minimum, such exercises alert patients to their back problem, which increases the likelihood of performing daily activities in a way

that may allow them to avoid reinjury. Certainly, prolonged bed rest weakens back muscles and should be avoided. Furthermore, certain advice to the patient regarding lifting is prudent. Sudden loading of the spine when the back is flexed and the knees are straight markedly increases forces placed on the lumbar spine (Fig. 65.2) compared with when the knees are bent and the back is straight. Exercises that strengthen the quadriceps (extend knees) are theoretically sound for anyone who may have to lift at all. These exercises include swimming, cycling, or jogging on a flat, even surface. The patient should be advised to exercise only if it does not initiate or increase back pain. In addition, because the abdominal muscles are important in supporting the spine when a weight is brought to bear on it, exercises that strengthen the abdominal muscles (Fig. 65.3) are helpful. Patient education is an effective component in the treatment of all patients who have experienced back pain. Education about such matters may improve a patient's lifestyle and the likelihood of returning to work (39). So-called back schools have been organized in many worksites. These are generally conducted by physical therapists. However, a large controlled trial of an educational program to prevent low back injuries organized as a back school for postal workers failed to prevent work-associated back injury in employees with or without a history of back injury, although the knowledge of safe behavior was increased by the training (10a).

Spinal manipulation has been recommended by the practice guidelines published by the AHCPR (6) but these guidelines do not specifically recommend that manipulation be done by a chiropractor. Initial evaluation of low back pain by a *chiropractor* often does not include screening evaluation with history and physical examination for systemic disorders. Also, chiropractors generally do not offer additional therapies beyond those offered by an experienced physical therapist. Patient satisfaction with chiropractors is related to the chiropractor's willingness to listen to a patient's concerns (10,30). Too often physicians and physical therapists do not show such a level of concern and even minimize the patient's problems. Furthermore, studies of manipulation of the back do not define precisely what is done during a manipulation, making comparisons impossible.

The patient may need to modify *work or athletic activities* once an episode of back pain occurs. It should be noted, however, that there is no convincing evidence to support the concept that heavy labor or lifting predisposes to the development of the initial episode of back pain (40). Certain factors do predispose patients to injury. These include improper technique in lifting, sitting for prolonged periods or not at all during the workday, and sudden maximal physical activity (e.g., participation in an occasional vigorous game without conditioning). Furthermore, back pain occurs more often in people who consider their occupation to be physically hard and in those who believe their work to be stressful to the spine or who are dissatisfied with their work (5,11).

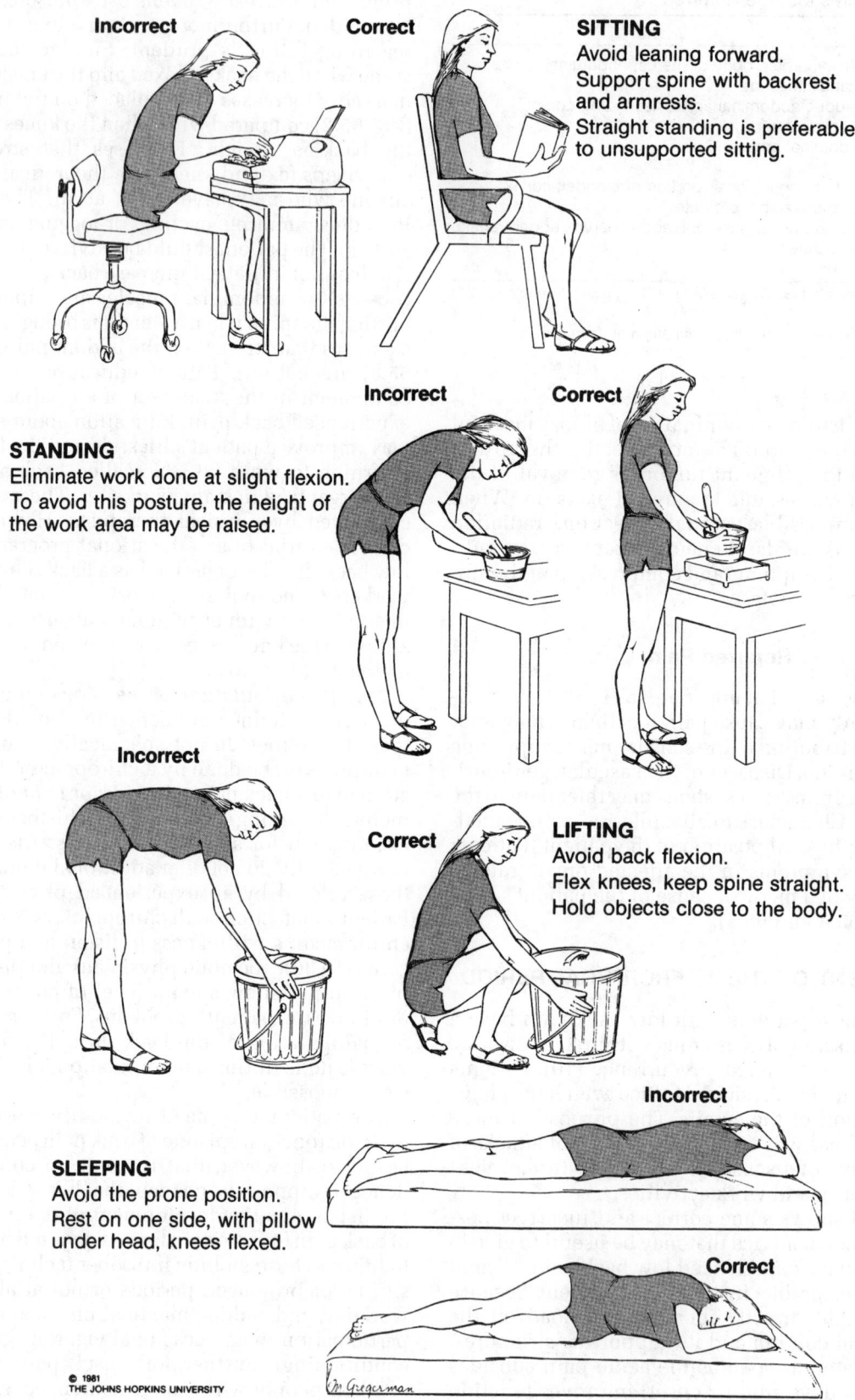

Incorrect   **Correct**

SITTING
Avoid leaning forward.
Support spine with backrest
and armrests.
Straight standing is preferable
to unsupported sitting.

Incorrect   **Correct**

STANDING
Eliminate work done at slight flexion.
To avoid this posture, the height of
the work area may be raised.

Incorrect

Correct

LIFTING
Avoid back flexion.
Flex knees, keep spine straight.
Hold objects close to the body.

Incorrect

SLEEPING
Avoid the prone position.
Rest on one side, with pillow
under head, knees flexed.

Correct

© 1981
THE JOHNS HOPKINS UNIVERSITY

M Gregerman

Figure 65.5.   Incorrect and correct postural attitudes.

General References*

Borenstein DG, Burton JR. Lumbar spine disease in the elderly. J Am Geriatr Soc 41:167, 1993.
> A clinical review of back pain as commonly encountered in the elderly.

Borenstein DG, Wiesel SW, Boden SD. Low back pain: medical diagnosis and comprehensive management. 2nd ed. Philadelphia: WB Saunders, 1995.
> A reference for all causes of low back pain.

Hall S, Bartleson JD, Onofrio BM, et al. Lumbar spinal stenosis. Ann Intern Med 103:271, 1985.
> A review of 68 patients with this condition.

Hoffman RM, Wheeler KJ, Deyo RA. Surgery for herniated lumbar discs: a literature synthesis. J Gen Intern Med 8:487, 1993.
> A review reiterating that the long-term benefit of surgery is no greater than conservative therapy.

Macnab I, McCulloch JA. Backache. 2nd ed. Baltimore: Williams & Wilkins, 1989.
> A well-illustrated monograph of mechanical disorders of lumbar spine.

Nordin M, Anderson GBJ, Pope MH, eds. Musculoskeletal disorders in the workplace: principles and practice. St. Louis: CV Mosby, 1997.
> A well-referenced encyclopedic text with a very good section on low back pain.

Rothman RH, Simeone FA. The spine. 3rd ed. Philadelphia: WB Saunders, 1992.
> A detailed and well-referenced encyclopedic text of techniques used for spinal surgery.

Steinberg GG, Akins CM, Baran DT, eds. Ramamurti's orthopaedics in primary care. 2nd ed. Baltimore: Williams & Wilkins, 1992.
> An orthopedic-focused text that is practical and helpful.

Specific References

1. Albeck MJ, Hilden J, Kjaer L, et al. A controlled comparison of myelography, computed tomography, and magnetic resonance imaging in clinically suspected lumbar disc herniation. Spine 20:443, 1995.
2. Alexander AR. Magnetic resonance imaging of the spine and spinal cord tumors. Spine State Art Rev 2:499, 1988.
3. Ardan GM. Bone destruction not demonstrable by radiography. Br J Radiol 24:107, 1951.
4. Basmajian JV. Cyclobenzaprine hydrochloride effect on skeletal muscle in the lumbar region and neck: two double blind controlled clinical and laboratory studies. Arch Phys Med Rehabil 59:58, 1978.
5. Bigos SJ, Battie MC, Spengler DM, et al. A prospective study of work perceptions and psychosocial factors affecting the report of back injury. Spine 16:1, 1991.
6. Bigos SJ, Bowyer O, Braen G, et al. Acute low back problems in adults. Clinical Practice Guideline No. 14. AHCPR Publication No. 95-0642. Rockville, MD: Agency for Health Care Policy and Research, Public Health Service, US Department of Health and Human Services, December 1994.
7. Boden SD. The use of radiographic imaging studies in the evaluation of patients who have degenerative disorders of the lumbar spine. J Bone Joint Surg 78A:114–124, 1996.
8. Boden SD, David DO, Dina T, et al. Abnormal magnetic resonance scans of the lumbar spine in asymptomatic subjects: a prospective investigation. J Bone Joint Surg 72A:403, 1990.
9. Brown BR Jr, Womble J. Cyclobenzaprine in intractable pain syndromes with muscle spasm. JAMA 240:1151, 1978.
10. Cherkin DC, MacCornack FA. Patient evaluations of low back pain care from family physicians and chiropractors. West J Med 150:351, 1989.
10a. Daltroy LH, Iversen MD, Larson MG, et al. A controlled trial of an educational program to prevent low back injuries. N Engl J Med 337:332, 1997.

11. Dehlin O, Hedenrud B, Horal J. Back symptoms in nursing aides in a geriatric hospital. Scand J Rehabil Med 8:47, 1976.
12. Deyo RA. Conservative therapy for low back pain. Distinguishing useful from useless therapy. JAMA 250:1057, 1983.
13. Deyo RA, Diehl AK, Rosenthal M. How many days of bed rest for acute low back pain? N Engl J Med 315:1064, 1986.
14. Dillane JB, Fry J, Kalton G. Acute back syndrome: study from general practice. BMJ 3:82, 1966.
15. Edgar MA, Ghadially JA. Innervation of the lumbar spine. Clin Orthop 115:35, 1976.
16. Elenbaas JK. Centrally acting oral skeletal muscle relaxants. Am J Hosp Pharmacol 37:1313, 1980.
17. Ensink F, Saur PMM, Frese K, et al. Lumbar range of motion: influence of time of day and individual factors on measurements. Spine 21:1339, 1996.
18. Estlander AM, Mellin G, Vanharanta H, Hupli M. Effects and follow-up of multimodal treatment program including intensive physical training for low back pain patients. Scand J Rehabil Med 23:97, 1991.
19. Faas A, Chavannes AW, van Eijk JTM, Gubbels JW. A randomized, placebo-controlled trial of exercise therapy in patients with acute low back pain. Spine 18:1388, 1993.
20. Frazier LM, Carey TS, Lyles MF, et al. Selective criteria may increase lumbarsacral spine roentgenogram use in acute low-back pain. Arch Intern Med 149:147, 1989.
21. Frymoyer JW, Pope MH, Costanza MC, et al. Epidemiologic studies of low back pain. Spine 5:419, 1980.
22. Hall H. Examination of the patient with low back pain. Bull Rheum Dis 33:1, 1983.
23. Hart LG, Deyo RA, Cherkin DC. Physician office visits for low back pain: frequency, clinical evaluation, and treatment patterns from a US national survey. Spine 20:11, 1995.
24. Herno A, Airaksinen O, Saari T, Sihoven T. Surgical results of lumbar spinal stenosis: a comparison of patients with or without previous back surgery. Spine 20:964, 1995.
25. Hudgins WR. The crossed-straight leg-raising test. N Engl J Med 297:1127, 1977.
26. Hult L. Cervical, dorsal and lumbar spinal syndromes. Acta Orthop Scand Suppl 17:1, 1954.
27. Jensen MC, Brant-Zawadski MN, Obuchowski N, et al. Magnetic resonance imaging of the lumber spine in people without back pain. N Engl J Med 331:69, 1994.
28. Jensen OH. The level-diagnosis of a lower lumbar disc herniation: the value of sensitivity and motor testing. Clin Rheumatol 6:564, 1987.
29. Johnsson K, Uden A, Rosen I. The effect of decompression on the natural course of spinal stenosis: a comparison of surgically treated and untreated patients. Spine 16:615, 1991.
30. Kane RL, Leymaster C, Olsen D, et al. Manipulating the patient. A comparison of the effectiveness of physician and chiropractor care. Lancet 1:1333, 1974.
31. Karayannacos PE, Yashon D, Vasko JS. Narrow lumbar spinal canal with vascular syndromes. Arch Surg 111:803, 1976.
32. Kornberg M, Eismont FJ. Discitis: an elusive infection. Infect Surg 2:818, 1983.
33. Lawrence JS, Bremmer JM, Bier F. Osteo-arthrosis. Prevalence in the population and relationship between symptoms and X-ray changes. Ann Rheum Dis 25:1, 1966.
34. Malmivaara A, Hakkinen U, Aro T, et al. The treatment of acute low back pain: bed rest, exercises, or ordinary activity? N Engl J Med 332:351, 1995.
35. McCombe PF, Fairbank JCT, Cockersole BC, Pynsent PB. Reproducibility of physical signs in low back pain. Spine 14:908, 1989.
36. Modic MT, Masaryk T, Boumphrey F, et al. Lumbar herniated disk disease and canal stenosis: prospective evaluation by surface coil MR, CT, and myelography. Am J Neuroradiol 7:709, 1986.
37. Modic MT, Ross JS. Magnetic resonance imaging in the evaluation of low back pain. Orthop Clin North Am 22:283, 1991.
38. Nervill RLM, Turner JG. Orthopaedic disorders in general practice. Boston: Butterworth, 1985;35.
39. Rainville J, Ahem DK, Phalen L, et al. The association of pain

---

*Bold print (general references) and bold numerals (specific references) denote published controlled clinical trials, meta-analyses, or consensus-based recommendations.

with physical activities in chronic low back pain. Spine 16(Suppl):S198, 1991.

40. Rowe ML. Low back pain in industry. J Occup Med 11:161, 1969.
41. Spaccarelli KC. Lumbar and caudal epidural corticosteroid injections. Mayo Clin Proc 71:169, 1996.
42. Thelander U, Fagerland M, Friberg S, Larsson S. Straight leg raising test versus radiologic size, shape, and position of lumbar disc hernias. Spine 17:395, 1992.
43. Turek SL. Orthopaedics: principles and their application. Philadelphia: JB Lippincott, 1984;1483.
44. Vaz M, Wadia RS, Gokhale SD. Another cause of positive crossed-straight-leg-raising test. N Engl J Med 295:779, 1978.
45. Waddell G, McCulloch JA, Kummel E, et al. Nonorganic physical signs in low-back pain. Spine 5:117, 1980.
46. Wiesel SE, Tsourmas N, Feffer H, et al. A study of computer assisted tomography. 1. The incidence of positive CAT scan in an asymptomatic group of patients. Spine 9:49, 1984.
47. Witt I, Vestergaard A, Rosenklint A. A comparative analysis of x-ray findings of the lumbar spine in patients with and without lumbar pain. Spine 9:298, 1984.
48. Woodhall B, Hayes GJ. The well-leg raising test of Fajersztajn in the diagnosis of ruptured lumbar intervertebral disc. J Bone Joint Surg 32A:786, 1950.
49. Zimmernman B, Lally EV. Infectious diseases of the spine. Semin Spine Surg 7:177–186, 1995.

C H A P T E R 66

Nonarticular Rheumatic Disorders

DAVID B. HELLMANN, MD

BURSITIS
General Considerations

Definition

Bursitis, the inflammation of a bursal sac, is a common problem. Bursal sacs are structures lined with synovial membrane that secretes and absorbs liquid. The bursae thereby provide a lubricating mechanism between structures such as bones, ligaments, tendons, muscles, and skin. Although usually isolated, occasionally they are in communication with a joint space. There are more than 150 such structures in the body, but the number is not fixed and a new bursa may appear whenever there is friction between structures.

Bursitis is usually easy to diagnose and treat in the office. Occasionally, physicians face the challenge of distinguishing bursitis from arthritis or other conditions. Also, it is important to quickly recognize and treat the few patients who have septic bursitis. When the diagnosis remains uncertain or the usual treatments are unsuccessful, referral to an orthopedist or rheumatologist may be necessary.

Causes

The most common cause of bursitis is minor trauma, as may occur to the subdeltoid bursa from repetitively throwing a baseball or to the prepatellar bursa from prolonged kneeling on a concrete floor. Because the development of bursitis is a function of both physical stresses and the condition of the bursa and surrounding tissues, bursitis is rare before the age of 20 and is particularly common in middle-aged and older people. Less often, bursitis is caused by systemic disorders such as rheumatoid arthritis or gout. Septic bursitis after trauma is a special concern in patients with superficial bursitis (e.g., olecranon or prepatellar bursitis) (8). Basic calcium phosphate crystals are known to be associated with calcific periarthritis, tendinitis, and bursitis, but little is understood about the exact mechanism of calcium crystal deposition.

Manifestations

Patients with acute bursitis experience abrupt onset of localized pain that is aggravated by any movement of the structures adjacent to the bursa. The pain is usually described as a deep, aching discomfort. How well the patient can localize the discomfort depends on whether the bursa is superficial or deep to the skin, and on whether the affected region has extensive or exiguous sensory nerve fibers. Thus, when asked, "Where does it hurt?" the patient with anserine bursitis often uses a fingertip to pinpoint the location, whereas a patient with trochanteric bursitis usually waves the entire hand over the general region of pain.

Bursitis near the knee, hip, elbow, or shoulder can mimic arthritis of those structures. Features that suggest bursitis include sudden onset after some repetitive physical activity; swelling, redness, or tenderness localized to the bursa and not the joint (see below); absence of pain on passive motion of the joint; and, if necessary, a normal joint x-ray.

Infection is suggested by fluctuant swelling of the bursa in association with redness and heat of the overlying skin (8,9,25). Fever should always suggest infection but can also complicate gouty bursitis. The absence of fever does not exclude infection; for example, only one-third of patients with olecranon septic bursitis demonstrate fever (8,9). A large bursal swelling can compress other structures or even rupture, thus explaining why bursitis around the knee or the hip can present as diffuse leg swelling (mimicking thrombophlebitis), an inguinal hernia, or a pelvic mass (19).

Aspiration of Bursae

Aspiration is usually easily accomplished by the general physician, especially when the bursa is superficial (Table 66.1). The chief indication for aspirating a bursa is to rule out infection. Analysis of bursa (or joint) fluid can also reveal whether the fluid is inflamed or contains crystals (usually from gout).

The laboratory tests performed on bursal (or joint) fluid depend on the clinical questions (Table 66.2). A bursal or joint fluid white blood cell count of greater than 1,000 indicates inflammation; fewer than 1,000 white blood cells is characteristic of traumatic fluid (Table 66.2). Bursal infection tends to give very high white blood cell counts, averaging approximately 75,000 for olecranon bursitis (9), but rheumatoid arthritis and gout can also occasionally produce markedly elevated bursal fluid white blood cell counts. Gram's stains and cultures are the specific tests for

Table 66.1. Technique for Aspiration of Superficial Bursae (or Joints) and Analysis of Bursal (or Synovial) Fluid

1. Determine by palpation the area of maximal tenderness or fluctuance and outline with indelible pen.
2. Clean the skin with iodine solution such as povidone (Betadine).
3. Anesthetize the skin with lidocaine in the area of planned aspiration.
4. Use an 18-gauge needle to aspirate.
5. Grossly inspect the fluid and analyze for the following:
   a. Cell count and differential; fluid must be in a tube containing heparin or ethylenediamine tetra-acetate (EDTA).
   b. Type of crystals (see Chapter 69).
   c. Gram's stain and culture using transport media (even in the absence of a high white cell count).

infection. Similarly, examining the fluid with a microscope equipped with polarizing lenses is the only way to identify the crystals that are specific for gout (see Chapter 69). Therefore, most bursal fluid can be characterized by the white blood cell count, the Gram's stain plus culture, and the analysis for crystals. Glucose, protein, mucin clot, and other (e.g., enzymes, complement) determinations are not specific and are not needed.

Treatment

Treatment of septic bursitis requires administering antibiotics and draining the bursal sac. The Gram's stain of the bursal fluid (see below) should guide initial antibiotic choice. Most cases of septic bursitis are caused by *Staphylococcus aureus,* but the Gram's stain is positive in only 65% (9). If the Gram's stain shows no bacteria or if Gram-positive cocci are found, a penicillinase-resistant antistaphylococcal drug should be used. If Gram-negative organisms are found, blood cultures should be obtained and an extrabursal site of infection should be sought. The antibiotic choice should be based on the most likely organism causing the extrabursal infection. The need for hospitalization depends on both the severity of the infection and the degree of compromise of the host. Patients with high fever and chills, intense surrounding cellulitis, deep bursal involvement, extrabursal infection, or suspicion of an uncommon organism should be hospitalized for parenteral antibiotics (9). Hospitalization should also be considered for patients who are compromised by alcoholism, diabetes mellitus, or immunosuppression, almost regardless of the intensity of bursal inflammation (25). Patients who are less ill and less frail can be treated as outpatients with oral antibiotics. Repeated bursal aspiration is also required until the fluid stops accumulating. On average, successful treatment of septic olecranon bursitis, for example, requires two to three aspirations over a week or two. The timing of these repeat aspirations is made solely on the clinical response (or absence thereof) of the patient (8). The duration of antibiotic therapy averages 3 to 4 weeks but should be individualized according to the clinical response and the character of aspirated fluid. Antibiotics should be

Table 66.2. Patterns of Bursal (or Joint) Fluid Findings in Common Problems

	Normal	Trauma	Sepsis	Rheumatoid Inflammation	Microcrystalline Inflammation
Color of fluid	Clear yellow	Bloody, xanthochromic	Yellow to cloudy	Clear yellow to cloudy	Clear yellow to cloudy
WBC, RBC	0–200/0	<1,000/many	1,000–200,000/few	1,000–20,000[a]/few	1,000–20,000[a]/few
Crystals	–	–	–	–	+[b]
Culture	–	–	+	–	–

[a]Cell count in noninfected inflammatory fluid may sometimes be as high as it is with sepsis, thus the need for culture.
[b]Gout, negatively birefringent sodium urate (see Chapter 69). Pseudogout, positively birefringent sodium pyrophosphate (see Chapter 69).

continued for 5 additional days after the bursal fluid has cleared or has become sterile (8).

Gout, pseudogout, or rheumatoid arthritis should be treated with anti-inflammatory agents (see Chapter 69).

Usually *traumatic bursitis* resolves spontaneously if the area of inflammation is rested. However, the spontaneous resolution requires several weeks and therapy shortens this period considerably. Therefore, if sepsis and gout are ruled out, the treatment outlined in Table 66.3 is indicated.

If there is no initial response to treatment with a nonsteroidal anti-inflammatory agent (see Chapter 70 for a description), the patient should be treated by an injection into the inflamed bursa of a mixture of lidocaine and depoglucocorticoid (Table 66.4). Immediate and dramatic but transient relief of pain secondary to lidocaine indicates that the proper site has been injected. The anti-inflammatory effect of the steroid injection is seen in approximately 72 hours. If a satisfactory response has not occurred, the bursa may be reinjected in approximately 2 weeks. Waiting 2 weeks before reinjection provides ample time to rule out iatrogenic sepsis, which rarely occurs after a steroid injection. Depending on the location, other modalities such as ultrasound, heat or cold application, and physical therapy may be used as adjuncts. If a bursitis does not respond to two steroid injections, rheumatologic consultation to rule out associated systemic disease may be necessary. Rarely, definitive treatment by surgical excision of the bursa may be necessary.

Specific Forms

Several forms of bursitis are particularly common; their unique aspects are described here.

Olecranon Bursitis

This common form of bursitis—also called student's or miner's elbow—is characterized by a goose-egg–like swelling located just behind the olecranon process of the ulna (see Chapter 67, Fig. 67.14). An effusion of the elbow joint itself, in contrast, causes diffuse swelling. Another feature that distinguishes olecranon bursitis from elbow joint inflammation is that passive extension and flexion of the elbow are nearly painless when the only problem is olecranon bursitis. Important features of olecranon bursitis are that it is often associated with systemic disease, such as rheumatoid arthritis or gout; symptoms often are chronic, in that they have been present for 2 or 3 weeks before a patient

sees a physician; and it is a common site for septic bursitis after trauma and may be associated with surrounding cellulitis (8,9). If rheumatoid arthritis or gout is present, it is important to realize that sepsis sometimes coexists. Traumatic olecranon bursitis is usually hemorrhagic, although xanthochromic fluid may be present.

Swelling in the area of the olecranon bursa should be aspirated if symptomatic (Tables 66.1 and 66.2) and a Gram's stain, culture, white blood cell count, and crystal identification with polarizing microscopy should be obtained.

Therapy. Therapy depends on the characteristics of the fluid (15). If monosodium urate crystals are present, specific therapy for gout is indicated (see Chapter 69). Traumatic bursitis responds to simple removal of fluid; however, if the fluid reaccumulates, a steroid injection (Table 66.4) should be given. If sepsis is identified, the patient should be treated with an antibiotic and bursal aspiration as outlined above. An x-ray of the elbow should be obtained to rule out osteomyelitis or a foreign body if the process has been present for more than 2 weeks.

Prepatellar Bursitis

Prepatellar bursitis (housemaid's or carpenter's knee) is a common form of bursitis, easily recognized by its location overlying the inferior portion of the patella (see Chapter 67, Fig. 67.1B). It is particularly common in carpet layers, plumbers, and carpenters. It is most often caused by trauma from kneeling, but it may also be a site of sepsis, and the bursa, for this reason, should always be aspirated, even if it feels dry (8).

Anserine Bursitis

The anserine bursa is fan shaped and lies between the confluence of tendons of the sartorius, gracilis, and semitendinosus muscles and the tibia at the anterior medial aspect of the knee just below the joint space (see Chapter 67, Fig. 67.1B) (10). Anserine bursitis is most often seen in patients with arthritis, especially overweight middle-aged women with osteoarthritis of the knee, and is recognized by its location; the pain is typically produced when the knee is flexed and is particularly troublesome at night. The patient often seeks comfort by sleeping with a pillow between the thighs.

If there is surrounding erythema or if the patient is febrile, aspiration should be attempted because sepsis, although uncommon, may be present. Therapy depends on the findings (Tables 66.2 and 66.3). When injection therapy is used, the solution should be injected in a fan-shaped pattern so that the entire bursa is treated.

Ischial Bursitis

The ischial bursa is located over the ischial tuberosity, close to the sciatic nerve and the posterior femoral cutaneous nerve (17). When a person is sitting, the ischial bursae are covered only with subcutaneous tissue and skin; when a person is standing, the gluteus maximus also covers the bursa.

The most common reason for inflammation of this bursa is trauma, as may occur in bicycling. It is rarely a site of sepsis.

Usually the inflammation results in an abrupt onset of pain, but occasionally the onset is more insidious. The patient often has exquisite pain when sitting or lying. Because of the close proximity of the sciatic nerve to the bursa, there may be an associated neuritis resulting from pressure on the nerve, which causes sciatic pain to radiate into the leg (see Chapter 65). Direct pressure over the ischial tuberosity causes sharp pain and the patient may hold the painful buttock elevated when sitting. In addition, the pain is intensified when the patient is supine and the hip is passively flexed. The patient has difficulty standing on tiptoe on the affected side.

The differential diagnosis of symptoms suggestive of ischial bursitis includes lumbar spine disease, thrombophlebitis, and inflammatory back disease or sacroiliitis (see Chapter 71). Localization of the pain over the ischial tuberosity and the finding of induration near the ischial tuberosity on rectal examination establish the diagnosis of ischial bursitis.

Aspiration of the bursa, even when it is inflamed, is discouraged because it is often difficult to localize, and the surrounding structures, especially the sciatic nerve, may be injured. If aspiration is indicated because there is associated fever and, therefore, the possibility of septic bursitis, the patient should be referred to an orthopedist for immediate evaluation.

The patient may obtain some comfort when sitting by using a pillow that allows pressure to be eliminated from the ischial tuberosity underlying the inflamed bursa.

Table 66.3.   Treatment of Bursitis

1. Splint where feasible (especially effective in the hand and fingers).
2. Application of heat or cold may be of benefit in some patients.
3. Anti-inflammatory agents: A nonsteroidal anti-inflammatory agent with rapid onset of action is preferred (see Chapter 70 for a full discussion of NSAIDs).
4. Improvement is usual in several days, but the anti-inflammatory agent should be continued an additional 4–5 days to prevent recurrence.
5. If no significant response is noted in 5–7 days and sepsis has been ruled out, the bursa may be injected with lidocaine or a steroid preparation (see Table 66.4).

Table 66.4.   Methods of Injection of Bursae or Joints with Lidocaine or Depoglucocorticoid Preparations

1. Be certain sepsis has been ruled out (Tables 66.1 and 66.2).
2. Prepare the skin carefully with an iodine-containing solution such as povidone (Betadine).
3. Anesthetize the skin with intradermal 1–2% lidocaine.
4. Mix 2–3 mL of 1–2% lidocaine with 20–40 mg of a depoglucocorticoid (such as Celestone, Aristocort, or Kenalog) and inject the bursa with 1–3 mL of this mixture using a 22-gauge needle.

Notes of caution: Injection into the skin will cause atrophy and thus should be avoided; the patient should understand that there is a possibility of this complication. Injection into tendons themselves may cause degeneration and, in time, rupture; these structures should be avoided by careful palpation.

Standard therapy (Table 66.3) with a nonsteroidal anti-inflammatory agent usually provides dramatic improvement within 2 to 3 days; however, if there has been associated leg pain or weakness from sciatic nerve inflammation, those symptoms may persist for several months.

Ultrasound therapy, administered by a physical therapist, may be effective and it should be considered if initial therapy has not relieved the symptoms within several days.

If the diagnosis is unclear, there is a question of sepsis, and the patient does not respond within a week to therapy, consultation with a rheumatologist or orthopedist is recommended. If the diagnosis is confirmed, the consultant may aspirate the bursa and, if sepsis is ruled out, inject it with lidocaine and depoglucocorticoid, which often results in dramatic improvement.

Semimembranosus-Gastrocnemius Bursitis (Baker's Cyst)

The semimembranosus-gastrocnemius bursa, commonly called a cyst, lies in the posterior medial aspect of the knee behind the femoral condyle (see Chapter 70, Fig. 70.2, photo of arthrogram) and in 50% of patients is continuous with the knee joint (3). The cyst is best seen and palpated when the patient is standing. Swelling of this bursa is commonly associated with other knee problems such as internal derangements, rheumatoid arthritis, or degenerative arthritis. The bursa is rarely infected. Often, a Baker's cyst is asymptomatic. With a large cyst the patient may note a vague discomfort or fullness behind the knee. Many Baker's cysts produce symptoms only when they rupture, causing acute swelling, pain, and redness of the calf and lower leg (the syndrome of pseudothrombophlebitis). The possibility that a patient with acute calf swelling has pseudothrombophlebitis from a ruptured Baker's cyst is strongly suggested by finding swelling of the knee joint. When in doubt, a study to exclude thrombophlebitis should be done (see Chapter 52). Sonography, magnetic resonance imaging, and arthrography can visualize a ruptured cyst but are usually not needed if the clinical picture is consistent and thrombophlebitis has been excluded (13). Rarely, an unruptured Baker's cyst can compress deep veins and cause thrombophlebitis.

The differential diagnosis of a posterior knee fullness includes an aneurysm of the popliteal artery.

Therefore, it is important to palpate any fullness for pulsations.

Management of an uncomplicated Baker's cyst includes aspiration and instillation of a corticosteroid–anesthetic mixture. Usually this can be accomplished by aspirating and injecting the joint space (see Chapter 67 for discussion). Rarely the cyst may need to be aspirated/injected from the posterior approach. Because of the important structures in the popliteal fossa (artery, nerve, and vein), aspiration of the bursa posteriorly should be done by an orthopedist. Weight bearing should be minimized for several days. The response to this therapy is usually excellent. Management of a ruptured cyst consists of bed rest, heat, and elevation. Although there are no data to confirm this recommendation, an elastic bandage around the knee when treating a Baker's cyst is not recommended because it may cause the cyst to compress more severely the venous system, increasing the chance of a thrombophlebitis. Instillation of corticosteroids into the joint that has an effusion may be helpful. Nonsteroidal anti-inflammatory agents may also help; after symptoms have begun to abate, ambulation can slowly be increased.

Iliopectineal Bursitis

The iliopectineal bursa lies anterior to the hip joint, with which it communicates in approximately 15% of people. It lies between the inguinal ligament and the iliopsoas muscle just lateral to the femoral artery. It may be inflamed from running or other similar trauma. Pain in the anterior pelvis, groin, and thigh is the most common manifestation of iliopectineal bursitis; swelling may result in a bulge resembling a femoral hernia (see Chapter 91) below the inguinal ligament. Bursitis may be present in conjunction with intrinsic inflammatory joint disease such as rheumatoid arthritis. Extension of the hip (e.g., during walking) intensifies the pain, so the patient often limits the stride of the affected side. The anterior crural nerve (the largest branch of the lumbar plexus) lies just below the bursa and it may be irritated from bursal inflammation; resulting neuritis causes pain in the thigh, which often is also intensified by walking, and there may also be weakness of anterior muscles of the thigh. When a bursa is enlarged it may compress the femoral vein, resulting in edema in the affected leg.

If a hernia can be ruled out (see Chapter 91), the bursa should be aspirated by an orthopedist. Aspiration and injection with lidocaine and usually a corticosteroid result in lasting improvement.

Trochanteric Bursitis

The trochanteric bursa lies in the lateral aspect of the thigh over the greater trochanter of the femur and is closely associated with tendons of the glutei muscles (16). The problem affects primarily older people. Most cases are of unknown cause, although many are thought to result from osteoarthritis. Infection of the bursa is rare. The onset of pain may be abrupt, subacute, or chronic. Patients with trochanteric bursitis often misinterpret their lateral buttock pain to be caused by hip arthritis (which more characteristically produces groin pain). At times, the discomfort mimics that of lumbar spine disease (see Chapter 65). Occasionally, trochanteric bursitis can cause pain that radiates to the knee or even to the groin. Discomfort is intensified by movement from the sitting to the standing position, going up and down stairs, or sleeping on the affected side.

On examination there is point tenderness over the bursa with reproduction of the pain. Patrick's test (external rotation of the hip combined with abduction) is often painful, whereas internal rotation, flexion, and extension of the hip are usually pain free. Any remaining concern about the knee or the lumbar spine causing the pain is eliminated by the normal physical examination of these structures. X-rays of the bursa, which sometimes reveal calcifications, are usually not necessary.

Therapy, as outlined in Table 66.3, is usually effective. In addition, it is important for the patient to sleep with a small pillow under the involved buttock to keep weight shifted off the bursa.

Subdeltoid Bursitis

Subdeltoid bursitis is discussed in Chapter 63.

TENOSYNOVITIS

As with bursae, there are many sites of potential tenosynovial inflammation. Tendinitis and tenosynovitis generally occur simultaneously. The synovial-lined tendon sheath is usually the site of maximal inflammation.

Inflammation of a sheath of a tendon is a common problem. For the most part, only long tendons have sheaths. Tenosynovitis most often occurs from exercise, especially when a tendon has been used repetitively in an improperly conditioned person (see Chapter 67). Tenosynovitis also may be part of a generalized inflammatory process. Sometimes tenosynovitis is the first manifestation of this process.

Tenosynovitis often affects the dorsal extensor tendons of the wrist. It is manifest most commonly by pain that is intensified with hand extension. In the acute stage, swelling and pain over the dorsal aspect of the wrist or over the dorsal radioulnar joint may occur. Occasionally, a friction rub is felt or heard when the appropriate muscle is contracted.

When tenosynovitis is identified in the absence of trauma, a systemic disease should be suspected. If present, specific therapy for that disease is obviously important. Gonorrhea should be suspected in sexually active people if inflammation involves the tendons of the ankle or wrist in the setting of a monarthritis, fever, and skin rash. Using Transgrow media, culture of the endocervical canal and rectum in women and of the urethra in men is indicated (see Chapters 27 and 94).

If the tenosynovitis has developed because of trauma, such as exercise or overuse, or for unknown reasons, nonspecific therapy with a nonsteroidal anti-inflammatory agent, as for bursitis (Table 66.3), is appropriate. The fingers should be splinted in the position of function (see Chapter 67, Fig. 67.17). If symptoms persist after 3 or 4 days of conservative therapy, the peritenon (loose tissue surrounding the tendon) should be injected with lidocaine and a corticosteroid (e.g., Celestone, Aristocort, or Kenalog) (Table 66.4). To avoid injuring the tendon or causing skin atrophy, only small doses of depoglucocorticoid (i.e., about 0.5 mL of steroid mixed with an equal amount of lidocaine depending on the site) should be injected. To avoid injecting directly into the tendon, one should never inject if the syringe plunger cannot be depressed easily. Occasionally, symptoms are recurrent, in which case referral to a rheumatologist or orthopedist is indicated.

Tenosynovitis and tendinitis involving specific tendons are also discussed in Chapters 63 ("Shoulder Pain"), 67 ("Exercise-Related Musculoskeletal Problems"), and 102 ("Common Problems of the Feet").

STENOSING TENOSYNOVITIS

Stenosing tenosynovitis is not a complication of tenosynovitis; rather, it occurs primarily when trauma is severe and localized. In stenosing tenosynovitis, either a nodule forms on a tendon or an actual stenosis of a tendon sheath of a long tendon develops. This results in the affected part sticking in a fixed position that is sometimes painful. When this affects the flexor tendons of the fingers, it is called *trigger finger.* The patient is unable to flex a digit fully or, once it is flexed, the digit locks and literally must be straightened by external force until it suddenly snaps free. When stenosing tenosynovitis is present in the abductor or extensor tendon of the thumb, it is called *De Quervain's disease,* the most common form of stenosing tenosynovitis. In this problem, the thumb usually still has motion and does not always lock like a trigger finger. To evaluate for De Quervain's tenosynovitis, the patient should make a fist by curling the fingers over the flexed thumb, then passively deviate the fist in an ulnar direction. Exquisite pain over the base of the thumb with this maneuver *(Finkelstein's test)* confirms the diagnosis. Stenosing tenosynovitis is usually caused by repeated trauma (e.g., prolonged use of a screwdriver), but it is occasionally seen in association with rheumatoid arthritis, amyloidosis, pregnancy, and myxedema.

The treatment is identical to that of bursitis as outlined in Tables 66.3 and 66.4. Splinting is especially helpful in the treatment of tenosynovitis of the hands and fingers. If the patient does not respond to several weeks of conservative therapy, surgical release may be necessary. When a nodule is palpable, it should be injected with a small amount of corticosteroid (e.g., 10 mg of Celestone, Aristocort, or Kenalog) and lidocaine. Often, the condition resolves in several days to weeks.

DUPUYTREN'S CONTRACTURE

The palmar fascia may undergo nodular, hypertrophic fibroplasia of unknown cause. This results over many years in the development of a flexion contracture (Dupuytren's contracture). The process causes the skin to be fixed to the underlying fascia by adhesive bands, resulting in a fixed, puckered appearance. A Dupuytren's contracture is almost always painless but may result in significant functional disability. Although all digits may be involved, the fourth and fifth are affected most commonly. The condition affects primarily middle-aged or older men and, in nearly 40%, it is bilateral. It is more common in epileptics and alcoholics, but the majority of affected patients have neither condition. Once the condition is present, passive extension of the fingers does not retard the process; in fact, it may accelerate it. If functional disability is present, the patient should be referred to an orthopedic surgeon for consideration for surgery. Oral anti-inflammatory agents and local cortisone injections are not effective in retarding the process.

GANGLIONS

Ganglions, cystic swellings arising from the synovium of a joint or tendon sheath, are the most common benign tumor of the hand (18). They tend to occur more often in women from the teens through age 50. Onset may be sudden or gradual and the cyst may change over time, sometimes disappearing and then recurring. The swellings are usually smooth, tense, and fixed to the deep tissues. The most common site is the dorsum of the wrist between the extensor tendon of the thumb and the extensor tendon of the index finger. They may also occur on the volar aspect of the foot (the tarsal area) and ankle. There may be associated aching or weakness of the involved area. Nonoperative treatment in symptomatic patients (generally asymptomatic ganglions are left untreated), consisting of aspiration or cortisone injection, may be successful. Recurrences may need to be treated by operative excision.

FIBROMYALGIA

Fibromyalgia (commonly called *fibrositis*) is a syndrome of widespread, chronic musculoskeletal pain, chiefly affecting young women, that is unaccompanied by any objective findings except for increased tenderness at specific anatomic sites known as tender points (5,6,23,24). The diagnosis is purely clinical; no laboratory tests establish the diagnosis of fibromyalgia. The cause of fibromyalgia is unknown, but speculations center on disturbances in rapid eye movement sleep, chronic viral infections, psychologic disorders, and metabolic muscle defects (5,6,23). Usually fibromyalgia is primary, occurring in the absence of other medical conditions. A minority of patients have secondary fibromyalgia, which is diagnosed when the syndrome accompanies another disorder, most commonly hypothyroidism or rheumatoid arthritis.

Fibromyalgia is important to recognize for three reasons: Fibromyalgia is common, affecting 3 to 10% of the general population and accounting for 20 to 30% of all patients referred to rheumatologists; fibromyalgia responds, albeit imperfectly, to treatment; and failure to diagnose and treat fibromyalgia often subjects the patient to multiple consultations and needlessly expensive laboratory testing.

Manifestations

Ninety percent of patients with fibromyalgia are women. Most experience the gradual onset of symptoms between the ages of 20 and 45. The cardinal features of fibromyalgia are widespread soft tissue aching and stiffness, essentially daily, although varying in severity, often involving the axial skeleton and the shoulder and pelvic girdles, of more than 3 months' duration. Typically the pain is chronic, persisting for years. The condition may be aggravated by fatigue, tension, excessive work, immobilization, and changes in the weather. Although pain is the predominant symptom, most patients with fibromyalgia have many other symptoms, including fatigue, recurrent headaches, sore throat, depression, fitful sleep, difficulty concentrating, alternating constipation and diarrhea, numbness, swollen glands, and subjective sense of fever or joint swelling (5,6,23,24). In fact, a careful history to rule out depression (see Chapter 15) and somatization (see Chapter 12) is important.

Characteristically in fibromyalgia, the rich history of complaints contrasts starkly with the poverty of physical findings. Objective adenopathy, weakness, and joint inflammation or weakness are notably absent. Indeed, the only physical finding in fibromyalgia is tender points. Although the exact number and location of these tender points are somewhat controversial, nine paired tender points most commonly found, along with four control points, are illustrated in Figure 66.1. Nearly 90% of patients with fibromyalgia have tenderness at least 11 of the 18 (9 paired) tender point sites (24).

Laboratory tests in primary fibromyalgia are normal. The purpose of the laboratory tests and physical examination is to exclude other causes of diffuse musculoskeletal pain, which include polymyalgia rheumatica (a condition of elderly people), Parkinson's syndrome, polymyositis, endocrine disorders (especially hypothyroidism, but also hyperthyroidism, Addison's disease, hyperparathyroidism, and panhypopituitarism), cancer, renal tubular acidosis, and chronic fatigue syndrome (see Chapter 53) (considered by many experts to be a variant of fibromyalgia). Laboratory testing need not be extensive. Basic laboratory tests should include complete blood cell count, erythrocyte sedimentation rate, thyroid function tests, and muscle enzyme levels. By definition, all of these studies are normal in patients with primary fibromyalgia, so any abnormalities should warrant a further search for an underlying disorder.

The approach to the diagnosis of fibromyalgia is summarized in Table 66.5. The two criteria for the diagnosis—widespread pain and mild or greater tenderness in 11 or more of 18 tender point sites—are 88% sensitive and 81% specific (24). The diagnosis of fibromyalgia should not be made too quickly or too slowly. Because the diagnosis depends on excluding objective abnormalities, it is rarely wise to diagnose primary fibromyalgia on the patient's first visit. Documenting the absence of fever, weight loss, or any other abnormality takes time and increases the certainty of the diagnosis. Because fibromyalgia rarely begins after age 50, great caution should be exercised in considering the diagnosis in older patients. On the other hand, there is no benefit to delaying the diagnosis in a typical host with a compatible clinical picture. Indeed, such delays often prompt unnecessary consultations and redundant laboratory investigations.

Treatment

The cornerstone of treatment is education. Explaining to the patient that a distinct, recognizable syndrome is present reduces significantly the frustrations that may have built up over months, and sometimes years, of previously unproductive medical evaluations. Patients also take solace in learning that fibro-

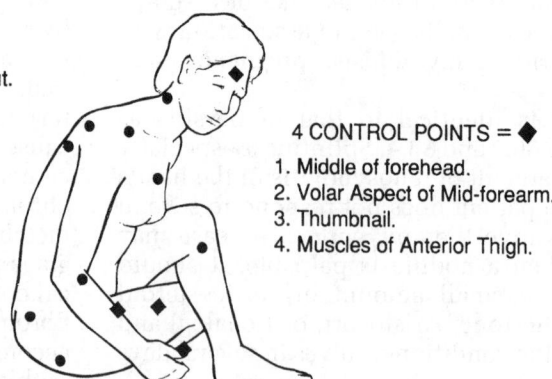

9 PAIRED TENDER POINTS = ●

1. Insertion of Nuchal Muscles into Occiput.
2. Upper Trapezius (mid-point).
3. Pectoralis Muscle - just lateral to second costo-chondral junction.
4. 2 cm below Lateral Epicondyle.
5. Upper Gluteal Region.
6. 2 cm posterior to Greater Trochanter.
7. Medial Knee in area of Anserine Bursa.
8. Paraspinous, 3 cm lateral to midline at the level of mid-scapula.
9. Above the Scapula spine near medial border.

4 CONTROL POINTS = ◆

1. Middle of forehead.
2. Volar Aspect of Mid-forearm.
3. Thumbnail.
4. Muscles of Anterior Thigh.

Figure 66.1.   The tender point locations in fibromyalgia are remarkably constant from patient to patient. Multiple location have been described; the 9 paired tender points shown represent frequently occurring points in a wide distribution. Most patients with fibrositis usually have 11 or more tender points. Control points are not unduly tender; their examination should be interspersed with that of the tender points. (Modified from Bennett RM. The fibromyalgia syndrome. In: Kelly WN, Harris ED, Ruddy S, Sledge CB, eds. Textbook of rheumatology. 5th ed. Philadelphia: WB Saunders, 1997.)

Table 66.5. Initial Examination of a Patient with Possible Fibromyalgia Syndrome

Diagnostic Step	Finding
Consider diagnosis	In any patient with chronic, poorly defined, generalized musculoskeletal pain; most patients have been studied previously, with normal test results; most often women, aged 20–50 yr; rule out depression and somatization by careful history.
Obtain positive response to most of the following	Chronic fatigue; chronic neck, shoulder, hip, and back pain; disturbed sleep; feeling unrefreshed and stiff in morning; hypersensitivity to cold, heat; history consistent with tension headaches, irritable bowel syndrome; subjective paresthesias and swelling of hands and feet without objective abnormalities.
Confirm presumptive diagnosis with physical examination	General physical examination findings normal and no evidence of arthritis or myositis (unless coexistent illness such as rheumatoid arthritis or hypothyroidism is present); tender point examination demonstrates multiple tender points at characteristic locations; associated diffuse muscle spasm and skin hypersensitivity may be present.
Laboratory tests	Complete blood cell count, erythrocyte sedimentation rate, thyroid function tests, and muscle enzyme levels should be normal.

From Goldenberg DL. Fibromyalgia syndrome. An emerging but controversial condition. JAMA 257:2782, 1987.

myalgia does not shorten life or cause crippling deformities, and that the cause and treatment of fibromyalgia are under active investigation (5,6).

Patients should know that symptoms of fibromyalgia, although chronic, can be improved. The medications shown to be somewhat effective (approximately one-third of patients showing moderate to marked improvement) are the tricyclic antidepressants, amitriptyline (e.g., Elavil, Endep, or generic, 10 to 50 mg at bedtime), and cyclobenzaprine compounds, structurally related to the tricyclic antidepressants (e.g., Flexeril or generic, 5 to 30 mg at bedtime) (2). Fluoxetine (Prozac) 20 mg a day has also been demonstrated to be effective (7); it is the only selective serotonin reuptake inhibitor studied in this situation. Nonsteroidal anti-inflammatory medications are generally not effective (24). Corticosteroids and narcotics have no role in the treatment of fibromyalgia. Because of the modest efficacy of pharmacologic therapy, treatment may often include other modalities as well. These include physical therapy (relaxation, heat, massage) and a graded exercise program to maintain a good general level of aerobic fitness (11). Attempts should also be made to modify other aggravating factors such as mechanical, physical, and psychologic stresses.

MYOFASCIAL PAIN SYNDROMES

Related problems, possibly distinct from fibromyalgia, are the myofascial pain syndromes (MPS) (1). They are characterized by the presence of deep tender points also. However, in MPS, the tender point is termed a *trigger point* because firm palpation of the point produces pain in a referred distribution. A second feature distinguishing MPS from fibromyalgia is the presence of just one or a regional clustering of points in MPS in contrast to the widespread distribution of symptoms and tender points in any given patient with fibromyalgia. A wide array of clinical syndromes in many different anatomic areas have been ascribed to MPS.

The pathogenesis of MPS is unknown. Patients with MPS may be helped by passive stretching of involved muscles after injection of the trigger point with a local anesthetic or use of a vapocoolant spray (e.g., ethyl chloride). Attention should also be directed to elimination of any possible aggravating factors such as overuse or repetitive injury to involved muscle areas.

RAYNAUD'S PHENOMENON

Definition

Raynaud's phenomenon is a syndrome characterized by episodic vasospasm of the digital vessels in response to cold or emotional stress. Classically, a triphasic response occurs: First cutaneous pallor extends from the fingertips to the mid-fingers; then mottling of the skin and cyanosis rapidly follow as venous blood refluxes back into an empty cutaneous capillary bed (this pallor or cyanosis persists until rewarming of the digits); finally, the recovery phase occurs over 15 to 20 minutes, resulting in intense hyperemia (21). Vasospasm is usually triggered by an abrupt change in ambient temperature, so it may occur even in the summer when a patient moves into air-conditioned or refrigerated areas. One or two digits may have more intense vasospasm, but generally the episodes are bilateral and symmetric. Also, the feet and other acral parts (e.g., the ears or nose) may be involved. Patients often do not describe spontaneously the classic phases of Raynaud's phenomenon but commonly note deep cyanosis associated with numbness, a pins-and-needles sensation, or frank pain on cold exposure.

Causes and Prevalence

Raynaud's phenomenon most commonly occurs in an idiopathic or primary form, Raynaud's disease, in which no underlying abnormality can be defined. Raynaud's phenomenon may also occur secondary to a defined vascular abnormality or in association with a specific disease process (Table 66.6). Primary Raynaud's phenomenon is thought to be common, occurring principally in women aged 20 to 30 years. The true prevalence of Raynaud's phenomenon is unknown, but it has been estimated to be 2 to 6% of the general population and up to 20% of the selective population of young women (12). Patients with primary Raynaud's phenomenon are otherwise healthy, generally have infrequent attacks (one to four episodes weekly), and rarely develop local cutaneous complications, such as digital pitting, ulcerations, or loss of hand function. Patients with primary Raynaud's

Table 66.6.   Classification of Raynaud's Phenomenon

A. Primary: Idiopathic Raynaud's, Raynaud's disease
B. Secondary: Disorders associated with Raynaud's phenomenon

	Percentage of Patients with Stated Disorder Who Also Have Raynaud's Phenomenon
1. *Connective tissue diseases*	
a. Systemic sclerosis	90
b. Systemic lupus erythematosus	20
c. "Mixed" connective tissue disease	75
d. Dermatomyositis/polymyositis	20
e. Rheumatoid arthritis	10
2. *Neurovascular compression*	
a. Thoracic outlet syndrome (e.g., cervical ribs, scalenus anticus syndrome)	
b. Carpal tunnel syndrome	
3. *Arterial disease*	
a. Arteriosclerosis	
b. Arteritis (thromboangitis obliterans)	
4. *Hematologic disorders*	
a. Paraproteinemia	
b. Cryoglobulinemia	
c. Polycythemia	
d. Hyperviscosity syndrome	Unknown
5. *Occupational*	
a. Vibratory tools (white finger syndrome)	
b. Polyvinyl chloride exposure	
6. *Drugs*	
a. Ergot-containing drugs (such as ergotamine)	
b. β-Adrenergic blockers	
c. Sympathomimetic agents (such as Actifed)	
d. Methysergide (Sansert)	
e. Chemotherapy (bleomycin, vinblastine)	
7. *Miscellaneous*	
a. Primary pulmonary hypertension	30
b. Migraine headache	10

phenomenon usually have an uncomplicated course with gradual decrease over a number of years in the frequency of episodes. Estimates suggest that 8 to 19% of patients believed initially to have the primary form will develop a defined secondary form (usually a connective tissue disease) (20).

In approximately 40% of patients who present to a general physician with Raynaud's phenomenon, it is secondary to an underlying condition, the most common being a connective tissue disease (Table 66.6). Raynaud's phenomenon occurs in more than 90% of patients with systemic sclerosis and may be the initial symptom, preceding the other features of the disease by years. Approximately 40% of patients with systemic lupus erythematosus, and 10% of patients with rheumatoid arthritis may also have associated Raynaud's phenomenon. Raynaud's phenomenon may be a presenting feature in patients who have a systemic vasculitis. Disturbances of the axillary or cervical neurovascular bundle also can lead to Raynaud's phenomenon. Patients with neurovascular compression syndromes (cervical rib, scalenus anticus syndrome) and proximal

vascular lesions (atherosclerosis) may present with unilateral Raynaud's phenomenon. Hematologic abnormalities, such as cryoglobulinemia, paraproteinemia, or cold hemagglutinins, may present as typical Raynaud's phenomenon. Ergot-containing drugs, such as ergotamine, and β-blocking agents may be causative or potentiating agents. Occupational injury (vibration white finger syndrome) causing the syndrome occurs in a high proportion of workers operating vibratory tools (e.g., lumberjacks, shipyard workers, or meat cutters).

Initially it may be difficult to determine whether a patient has a primary or secondary form of Raynaud's phenomenon. Clues that suggest a secondary form include onset during childhood, male sex, onset in a woman after age 30, unilateral Raynaud's, Raynaud's affecting a single digit, fingertip ulcers, digital gangrene, or symptoms or signs of a systemic disorder.

Evaluation

Every patient with Raynaud's phenomenon should have a focused history (including a drug review) and physical examination looking for diseases associated with Raynaud's phenomenon. An extension of the examination, evaluation of the nail bed with an ophthalmoscope (using approximately a 20+ diopter), may reveal small telangiectasias or abnormal cutaneous capillary loops; these small vessel changes may be the earliest findings in an associated underlying connective tissue disease, primarily systemic sclerosis (4). The presence of ulcers on the digits indicates that the Raynaud's is very severe and that the patient is likely to have a secondary form of Raynaud's phenomenon. Patients with unilateral Raynaud's phenomenon should be carefully evaluated for a local vascular lesion, including bilateral blood pressure determination, auscultation over major vessels to determine the presence or absence of vascular bruits, and assessment of the peripheral pulses. Special testing for possible neurovascular compression syndrome (see Chapter 63) and consideration for chest x-ray and a noninvasive evaluation of the peripheral circulation (Doppler studies or digital plethysmography) are appropriate when only unilateral Raynaud's phenomenon is present. Angiography may be necessary in cases in which a correctable occlusive vascular lesion is strongly suspected. Carpal tunnel syndrome has been implicated in both unilateral and bilateral Raynaud's phenomenon, and nerve conduction studies may be appropriate when the history and physical examination suggest this nerve compression syndrome (see Chapter 84).

If the patient is a woman with onset between the ages of 20 and 30 who has mild bilateral Raynaud's, does not have nail fold capillary changes, and exhibits no other manifestations of a connective tissue disease, primary Raynaud's is the likely diagnosis (21). For such a patient, the laboratory evaluation can be limited to verifying a normal complete blood count and testing renal and liver function to screen for collagen disease affecting these organs. If the patient is suspected of having secondary Raynaud's, antinuclear antibody (ANA) screen, cryoglobulins, Westergren erythrocyte sedimentation rate, and serum protein electrophoresis are indicated. Referring the patient to a rheumatologist for any additional evaluation is appropriate. Even when a systemic illness is not identified, the patient should be followed expectantly because an underlying illness may emerge several years later.

Treatment

The principal mode of treatment in patients in which a correctable cause cannot be found is to avoid the cold and stay warm. This includes wearing mittens or gloves and avoiding a general chill of the body by wearing a hat and loose-fitting warm clothing in winter months. Smoking aggravates Raynaud's phenomenon and should be stopped (see Chapter 20). Emotional stress should be assessed and controlled by appropriate measures (see Chapter 11). Patients with mild Raynaud's phenomenon often improve with education about the cause and nature of these episodes. Biofeedback therapy, usually offered by behavioral psychologists, is available in some communities and may provide partial benefit in patients with mild primary Raynaud's phenomenon. The nonpharmacologic treatment of patients with Raynaud's phenomenon is summarized in Table 66.7. Most patients, particularly those with primary Raynaud's phenomenon, do not need and should not be treated with drugs. Rather, pharmacologic treatment should be limited to patients with repeated attacks who limit their daily activities or who have significant loss of nutritional blood flow such that skin breakdown or ulceration may occur. There is no evidence that decreasing the number of episodes of Raynaud's phenomenon will alter the progressive changes that may occur in patients with scleroderma or another connective tissue disease.

A wide variety of vasoactive agents have been used in patients with Raynaud's phenomenon, but few agents have been proven of definite benefit. Many of these patients are young women who have childbearing potential; therefore, unproven treatment that may have a teratogenic effect should be avoided.

The calcium channel blockers nifedipine and diltiazem, but not verapamil or nicardipine, have been demonstrated to be effective in several prospective, controlled, and double-blind studies (14). These agents relax smooth muscle, reduce peripheral vascular resistance, and increase peripheral blood flow. Patients with primary Raynaud's tend to respond better than patients with Raynaud's phenomenon secondary to a connective tissue disease, especially systemic sclerosis. The major side effects of these agents are secondary to their vasodilatory activity and include hypotension, dizziness, headache, and peripheral edema. Approximately 40 to 50% of patients experience some lightheadedness caused by hypotension and flushing on initiation of the calcium channel blockers; however, these side effects are usually transient, lasting 1 to 2 days, and do not require the discontinuation of the medication. For this reason, the orthostatic blood pressure should be periodically measured. Calcium channel blockers should never be used during pregnancy or in a patient planning to become pregnant because they have been shown in animal models to be teratogenic.

The calcium channel blocker that has been most extensively studied, and the drug of first choice, is nifedipine. The initial dosage is usually 30 mg of a sustained released preparation once daily. The patient should be encouraged to assume usual activities and to keep a diary of the number and intensity of Raynaud's attacks. The patient should be monitored for important orthostatic hypotension (a symptomatic decrease in systolic pressure of 20 mm Hg or greater below baseline, or a fall below 90 mm Hg). If needed to improve control of Raynaud's, the dosage of nifedipine can be increased by 30 mg sustained release every 2 weeks to a maximum of 90 mg sustained release daily. Thereafter, monitoring every 2 to 4 months is important because the initial response may be transient and side effects, such as esophageal reflux, may limit the usefulness of the drug. If nifedipine fails or is not tolerated, diltiazem at a dosage of 30 mg four times a day may be tried as an alternative calcium channel blocker. The dosage may be advanced by 30 mg/day every 3 to 4 days until the symptoms improve or a maximum of 120 mg four times a day is reached. Patients generally have resolution or a dramatic reduction in the intensity and number of episodes of Raynaud's phenomenon in the summer. For this reason, medication should be discontinued unless repeated cold exposure or active Raynaud's phenomenon is documented.

Other drugs that have been used for the treatment of Raynaud's are reserpine, phenoxybenzamine (Dibenzyline), and in the past, guanethidine (Ismelin). These agents have been generally disappointing, with both unproven long-term control and intolerable side effects (orthostatic hypotension, reflex tachycardia, impotency, lassitude), so they are not recommended.

Table 66.7. Nonpharmacologic Management of Patients with Raynaud's Phenomenon

Education and reassurance
  Establish precipitating factors (e.g., refrigerator/freezer, air conditioning, emotional stress).
  Provide emotional support (e.g., assurance of the mild nature of the disease in most patients may reduce some of the stress that can precipitate attacks).
Avoidance of precipitating factors
  Wear gloves before reaching into refrigerator or freezer.
  Wear warm body clothing to avoid cold exposure when dressing.
  Keep head covered to avoid heat loss.
  Keep extremities warm and body well covered in cool weather or in air-conditioned environments.
  Be aware that stress can cause Raynaud's attacks.
Avoidance of certain drugs that precipitate attacks
  β-Blockers (e.g., propranolol)
  Ergot-containing drugs (i.e., ergotamine)
  Sympathomimetic agents (e.g., isoproterenol, Actifed, or other cold remedies)
  Nicotine (smoking)
  Oral contraceptives

Prazosin (Minipress) has been studied in controlled trials and may occasionally be of benefit if tolerated (2 to 8 mg/day in two or three divided doses). Topical nitroglycerin paste applied to the digits or nitroglycerin patches have been used with some success, but their indications are not established and consultation with a rheumatologist is suggested before prescribing them. Intravenous iloprost has been shown to be moderately effective for severe Raynaud's in patients with scleroderma (22).

Surgical sympathectomy was once popular for the treatment of Raynaud's phenomenon but is now rarely performed, primarily because of the high relapse rate (40 to 50%) and frequency of significant postural hypotension. Selective digital sympathectomy may be done in centers where microsurgery is available; however, long-term controlled studies of this procedure are lacking. Sympathectomy should be considered only for short-term relief from an intractable course complicated by digital ulceration that has failed medical treatment. All patients who have had such a severe course or who have ulcers on their digits should be seen in consultation by a vascular surgeon or a rheumatologist. Local digital block performed by a vascular surgeon or rheumatologist has been used for temporary treatment of patients with significant digital tissue compromise; also, a good response may predict which patient may have a good effect from digital or cervical sympathectomy. A patient who has severe disease with digital ulcers is susceptible to developing secondary soft tissue infection. Local debridement and antimicrobial treatment may be necessary if ischemic ulcerations become infected. Whirlpool treatment is the most effective method of ulcer debridement. In instances of secondary complications, consultation with a vascular surgeon or a rheumatologist is advised.

General References*

Bennett RM. The fibromyalgia syndrome. In: Kelley WN, Harris ED, Ruddy S, Sledge CB, eds. Textbook of rheumatology. 5th ed. Philadelphia: WB Saunders, 1997.

Hellmann DB. Arthritis and musculoskeletal disorders. In: Tierney LM, McPhee SJ, Papadakis MA, Schroeder SA, eds. Current medical diagnosis and treatment. Norwalk, CT: Appleton & Lange, 1998.

Owen DS Jr. Aspiration and injection of joint and soft tissues. In: Kelley WN, Harris ED, Ruddy S, Sledge CB, eds. Textbook of rheumatology. 5th ed. Philadelphia: WB Saunders, 1997.

Schumacher HR. Synovial fluid analysis and synovial biopsy. In: Kelley WN, Harris ED, Ruddy S, Sledge CB, eds. Textbook of rheumatology. 5th ed. Philadelphia: WB Saunders, 1997.

*Bold print (general references) and bold numerals (specific references) denote published controlled clinical trials, meta-analyses, or consensus-based recommendations.

Specific References

1. Campbell SM. Regional myofascial pain syndromes. Rheum Dis Clin North Am 15:31, 1989.
2. Carette S, McCain GA, Bell DA, Fam AG. Evaluation of amitriptyline in primary fibrositis: a double-blind, placebo controlled study. Arthritis Rheum 29:655, 1986.
3. Doppman JL. Baker's cyst and normal gastrocnemius-semimembranosus bursa. AJR 94:646, 1965.
4. Fitzgerald O, Hess EV, O'Connor GT, et al. Prospective study of the evaluation of Raynaud's phenomenon. Am J Med 84:718, 1988.
5. Goldenberg DL. Fibromyalgia syndrome: an emerging but controversial condition. JAMA 257:2782, 1987.
6. Goldenberg DL. Treatment of fibromyalgia syndrome. Rheum Dis Clin North Am 15:61, 1989.
7. Goldenberg D, Mayskiy M, Mossey C, et al. A randomized double-blind crossover trial of fluoxetine and amitriptyline in the treatment of fibromyalgia. Arthritis Rheum 39:1852, 1966.
8. Ho G, Mikolich DJ. Bacterial infection of the superficial subcutaneous bursae. Clin Rheum Dis 12:437, 1986.
9. Ho G, Tice AD, Kaplan SR. Septic bursitis in the prepatellar and olecranon bursae: an analysis of 25 cases. Ann Intern Med 89:21, 1987.
10. Larsson L-G, Baum J. The syndromes of bursitis. Bull Rheum Dis 36:1, 1986.
11. McCain GA, Bell DA, Mai FM, Halliday PD. A controlled study of the effects of a supervised cardiovascular fitness training program on the manifestations of primary fibromyalgia. Arthritis Rheum 31:1135, 1988.
12. Olsen N, Nielsen SL. Prevalence of primary Raynaud's phenomenon in young females. Scand J Clin Lab Invest 37:761, 1978.
13. Pathria MN, Zlatkin M, Sartoris DJ, et al. Ultrasonography of the popliteal fossa and lower extremities. Radiol Clin North Am 26:77, 1988.
14. Rodeheffer RJ, Rammer JA, Wigley F, Smith CR. Controlled double-blind trial of nifedipine in the treatment of Raynaud's phenomenon. N Engl J Med 303:880, 1983.
15. Smith DL, McAfee JH, Lucas LM, et al. Treatment of nonseptic olecranon bursitis: a controlled, blinded prospective trial. Arch Intern Med 149:2527, 1989.
16. Spear IM, Lipscomb PR. Noninfectious trochanteric bursitis and peritendinitis. Surg Clin North Am 32:1217, 1952.
17. Swartout R, Compere E. Ischiogluteal bursitis: the pain in the arse. JAMA 227:551, 1974.
18. Turek S. The wrist in orthopedics. 4th ed. Philadelphia: JB Lippincott, 1984.
19. Underwood PL, McLeod GA, Ginsburg WW. The varied clinical manifestations of iliopsoas bursitis. J Rheumatol 15:1683, 1988.
20. Velogos E, Robinson H, Porcluncula F, Masi A. Clinical correlation analysis of 137 patients with Raynaud's phenomenon. Am J Med Sci 262:347, 1971.
21. Wigley FM, Flavahan NA. Raynaud's phenomenon. Rheum Dis Clin North Am 22:765, 1996.
22. Wigley FM, Wise RA, Seibold JR, et al. Intravenous iloprost infusion in patients with Raynaud phenomenon secondary to systemic sclerosis: a multicenter placebo-controlled, double-blind study. Ann Intern Med 120:199, 1994.
23. Wolfe F. Fibromyalgia. The clinical syndrome. Rheum Dis Clin North Am 15:1, 1989.
24. Wolfe F, Smythe HA, Yunus MB, et al. The American College of Rheumatology 1990 criteria for the classification of fibromyalgia. Arthritis Rheum 33:160, 1990.
25. Zimmerman B III, Mikolich DJ, Ho G Jr. Septic bursitis. Semin Arthritis Rheum 24:391, 1995.

CHAPTER 67

Exercise-Related Musculoskeletal Problems

RONALD P. BYANK, MD
WILLIAM E. BEATIE, MD

Activities such as jogging, marathon running, golf, tennis, softball, and bowling are an integral part of the lives of millions of Americans. (See Chapter 58 for a discussion of physical conditioning from the standpoint of the cardiovascular system.) Fitness has become a common goal, and health and exercise clubs are extremely popular. These can often overstress recreational athletes. Consequently, physicians are contacted frequently by patients with exercise-related problems. This chapter describes for a number of common exercise-related syndromes the mechanism of injury, usual signs and symptoms, treatment, indications for referral, and methods of preventing recurrences. *Most of the injuries associated with exercise also may occur in nonexercising people who suffer injury caused by falls, missteps, overactivity, or minor motor vehicle accidents.* Evaluation and management are similar for exercising and nonexercising patients with these injuries.

PROBLEMS OF THE KNEE

Knee Structure and Function

The knee is the largest joint in the body. It has both hingelike motion and rotatory motion (of the tibia on the femur) during flexion and extension. The principal components of the knee and their functions are the following (Fig. 67.1):

- *Three articulations* that have a common articular cavity: the lateral and medial tibiofemoral articulations, each of which has an important cartilaginous buffer; the lateral and medial menisci; and the patellofemoral articulation. Weight-bearing stresses are seen in all three areas.
- Several *muscles* control the motion of the knee: *Flexors* are the hamstring muscles, which arise from the ischium and diverge to form tendons that insert into the tibia and the fibula, and the gastrocnemius muscle, which arises from the distal posterior femur and inserts on the calcaneus through the Achilles tendon. *Extensors* are the quadriceps muscles, which originate at the ilium and the femur and converge distally as the common quadriceps tendon, which attaches to the superior aspect of the patella, continuing on as the patellar tendon to insert into the tibia.
- Several *external tendons and ligaments* support the knee: the patellar tendon, a continuation of the common tendon of the quadriceps that joins the patella to the tibial tuberosity and makes possible extension of the knee joint; and the collateral ligaments, which give stability to the joint. The lateral connects the lateral femoral condyle to the fibula, and the medial connects the medial femoral condyle to the medial condyle and surface of the tibia.
- *The cruciate ligaments,* which are located inside the joint and stabilize the joint in the anteroposterior plane: the anterior cruciate ligament, which is attached anteriorly to the intercondylar eminence of the tibia and posterosuperiorly to the lateral femoral condyle; and the posterior cruciate ligament, which is attached posteriorly to the posterior intercondylar fossa of the tibia and to the lateral meniscus and anterosuperiorly to the medial femoral condyle.
- The *bursae of the knee,* which provide lubrication between the many dynamic components of the knee. These consist of the suprapatellar, prepatellar, superficial patellar tendon, retropatellar tendon, and pes anserinus.

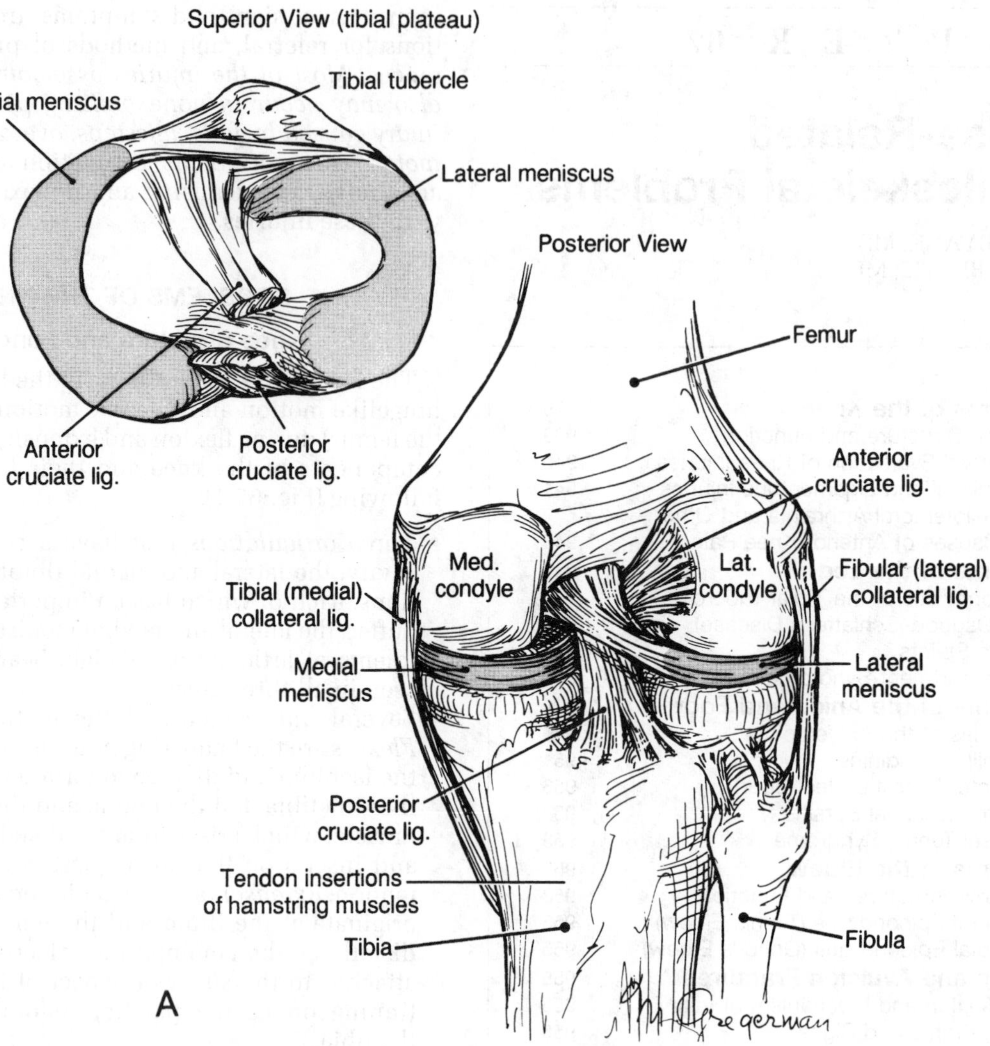

Superior View (tibial plateau)

Figure 67.1. **A.** Important structures of the knee.

General Evaluation of Knee Injuries

Traumatic knee injury may be caused by a single event in which the knee is suddenly stressed or by chronic, repetitive stress. When there is no history of sudden trauma, two features are especially helpful in evaluating knee pain: identification of any recently initiated physical activities or a sudden change in type or intensity of physical activities and identification of problems elsewhere in the lower extremity that may cause inappropriate stresses on the structure of the knee (e.g., excessive pronation of the feet, see Chapter 102). When there is no clear-cut history of trauma and physical examination does not indicate injury to one or more anatomic structures, conditions that may cause spontaneous knee pain or referred pain should be considered (see Chapter 66, "Nonarticular Rheumatic Disorders"; Chapter 68, "Osteoarthritis"; Chapter 69, "Crystal-Induced Arthritis"; and Chapter 70, "Rheumatoid Arthritis").

Knee pain may be caused by injury to any one of the structures described above. Except when there is a large effusion, the structures responsible for the pain can usually be identified by systematic examination. Focal tenderness to palpation is present when pain is caused by structural inflammation (e.g., bursitis) or ligament, meniscus, or muscle injury. Specific tests for meniscal injury, ligamentous injury, and patellofemoral arthralgia are described below.

Examination for a small or moderate *knee joint effusion* is done in one of two ways:

- *By inspection,* with the patient seated and both knees flexed 90°; if there is an effusion in the symptomatic knee, there will be a bulge on either side of the patellar ligament that is not seen in the normal knee.
- *By ballottement* (Fig. 67.2), with the patient supine and the knee fully extended; the knee is compressed above and on either side of the patella to localize any fluid under the patella; then the patella is pressed against the joint with an examining finger to determine whether it is ballotable.

Meniscal and Ligamentous Injuries

Definition and Mechanism of Injury

Tears of the medial or lateral meniscus (a disc-shaped fibrous cartilage) of the knee are common. When a rotary force is applied to the flexed knee joint, the meniscus can be trapped between the femur and the tibia; when the knee is extended, the cartilage may be torn (17). Tears of the medial meniscus are about 10 times as common as those of the lateral meniscus, probably because the medial meniscus is less mobile than the lateral meniscus. This problem is encountered especially in people who play football, soccer, basketball, and lacrosse as well as in bowlers, golfers, and baseball players. A simple twisting motion of the femur on the tibia with the foot planted can cause a meniscal injury and often a traumatic event is not identified.

Sprains or tears of the collateral ligaments and the cruciate ligaments are caused by a combination of angulating forces at the knee with rotational forces that cause rotation of the leg at the knee. The forces that most often cause ligament injuries are those that produce abduction of the leg at the knee (e.g., a direct blow to the lateral aspect of the leg with foot planted and

fixed). In these injuries all four of the major stabilizers of the knee are at risk: medial collateral ligament, anterior cruciate ligament, posterior cruciate ligament, and lateral collateral ligament.

Symptoms and Signs

Meniscus Injury. The patient with a torn meniscus usually describes a twisting flexion injury of the knee followed by pain and inability to flex the knee fully or to bear weight. Examination usually reveals knee joint effusion and tenderness over the joint line (located just above the tibial plateau), either medially (medial meniscus injury) or laterally (lateral meniscus injury). Sometimes the onset is insidious and the patient notes episodes of knee effusion or clicking or locking of the knee in a partially flexed position (which may last for several minutes or several hours). Examination of patients who have this more chronic condition often reveals only minimal joint line tenderness. Quadriceps muscle wasting from disuse can be the only positive physical finding in this situation. Certain maneuvers are helpful in the diagnosis of meniscal injury; they are more likely to be diagnostic in patients with acute

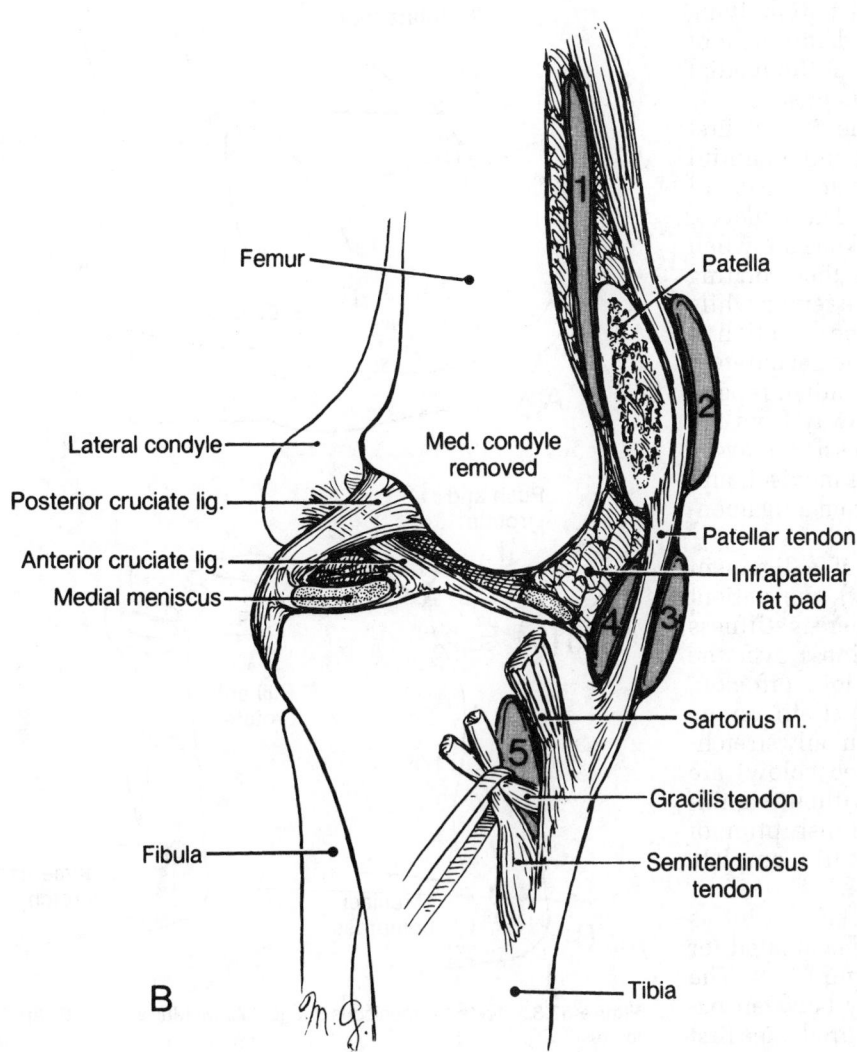

Figure 67.1 B. Five bursae of the knee: *1,* suprapatellar; *2,* prepatellar; *3,* superficial patellar tendon; *4,* retropatellar tendon; *5,* pes anserinus.

Femur

Lateral condyle

Posterior cruciate lig.

Anterior cruciate lig.

Medial meniscus

Fibula

Med. condyle removed

Patella

Patellar tendon

Infrapatellar fat pad

Sartorius m.

Gracilis tendon

Semitendinosus tendon

Tibia

B

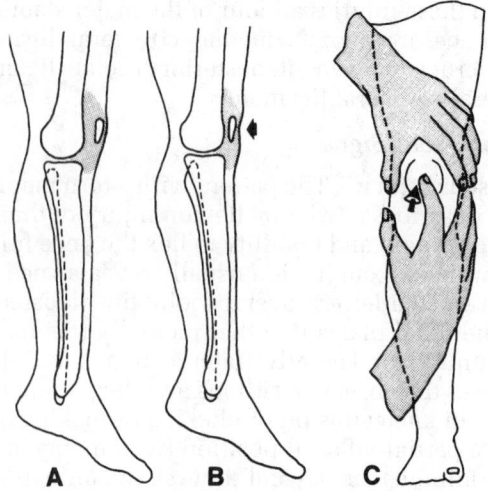

Figure 67.2. Examination for knee joint effusion. Patient is in supine position. **A.** Patella forced away from the femur by the effusion. **B.** Patella forced downward into the femur by the ballottement maneuver (lateral view). **C.** Illustration of the ballottement maneuver (anterior view).

symptoms than in patients with chronic symptoms. The *McMurray test* is performed with the patient lying supine with the hip and knee fully flexed and the foot rotated outward to its full capacity to test the medial meniscus and inward to test the lateral meniscus (Fig. 67.3A). The knee is extended, with the foot at first rotated out and again with it rotated in, and a painful click in the knee indicates a positive test. Not all meniscal tears result in a positive test. The *Apley or grinding test* is performed by flexing the knee 90° when the patient is in the prone position, and then rotating the tibia internally and externally on the femur while compressing the leg against the femur (the direction of the rotation that produces pain does not accurately predict the meniscus that is injured), and then repeating the rotation while pulling the leg away from the femur (Fig. 67.3B). Pain during compression may be caused by a tear of the lateral or medial menisci, and pain while pulling the leg is probably from a ligamentous injury.

Ligament Injuries. With a sprain of a ligament (usually the medial collateral ligament), the patient describes pain at the time of injury and there is stiffness of the knee, tenderness, and often fullness over the ligament. Occasionally there is a serous joint effusion, as opposed to a sanguineous effusion. (A strain, on the other hand, is a milder injury resulting in only stretching of a muscle.) Ligament sprains (see below) are classified as grade I (stretching fibers without significant structural damage), grade II (partial disruption of fibers with increased laxity), and grade III (complete tearing of ligamentous tissues).

When injury to a ligament of the knee joint is suspected, the joint should be carefully evaluated for ligament instability, as illustrated in Figure 67.4. The laxity of ligaments varies tremendously between patients; therefore, assessment of the uninjured knee first

is important in evaluating an injured knee. The stability of the collateral ligaments should be tested with the patient supine and the knee in about 20° of flexion. Varus stress is applied to test the lateral collateral ligament (Fig. 67.4A), and valgus stress is applied to test the medial collateral ligament (Fig. 67.4B). If there is a grade I sprain, the affected ligament is painful and tender, but there is no instability, as there would if the ligament were ruptured. With grade II or III injuries, the lateral or medial joint space of the knee widens when stress is applied to the leg with the thigh fixed. The integrity of the anterior and posterior cruciate ligaments is tested with the knee at 15° and 90° of flexion (see Lachman and Drawer tests, Fig. 67.4C–E). Grasping the leg, the examiner exerts pressure posteriorly to test the posterior cruciate and then anteriorly to test the anterior cruciate. Instability in the direction of pressure indicates a tear of the cruciate ligament being

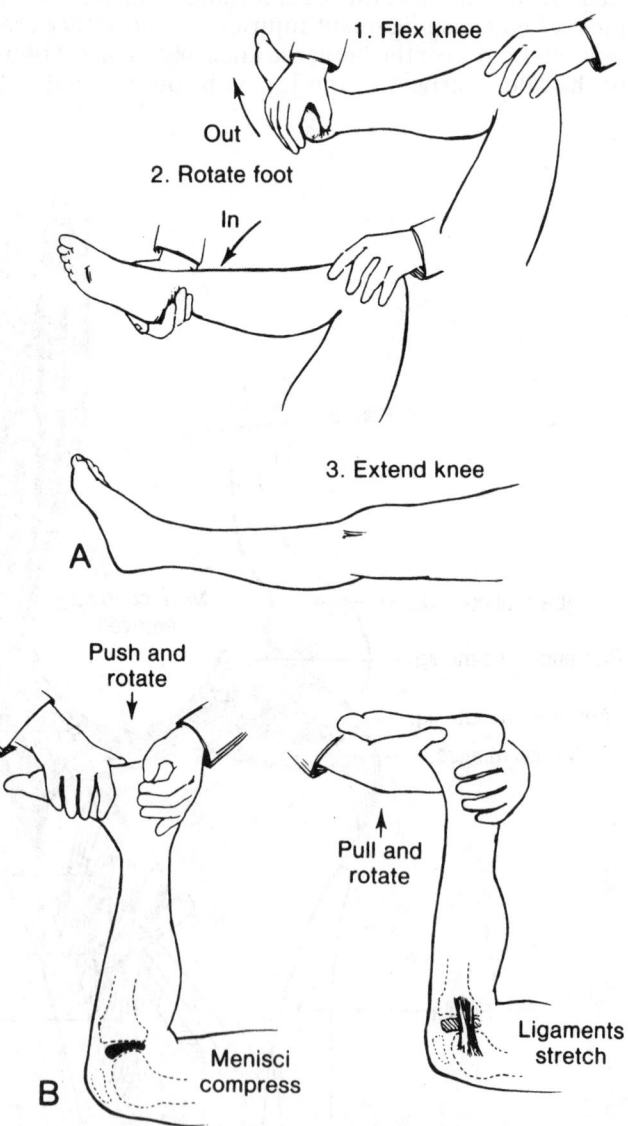

Figure 67.3. Tests for meniscus injuries. **A.** McMurray test. **B.** Apley test.

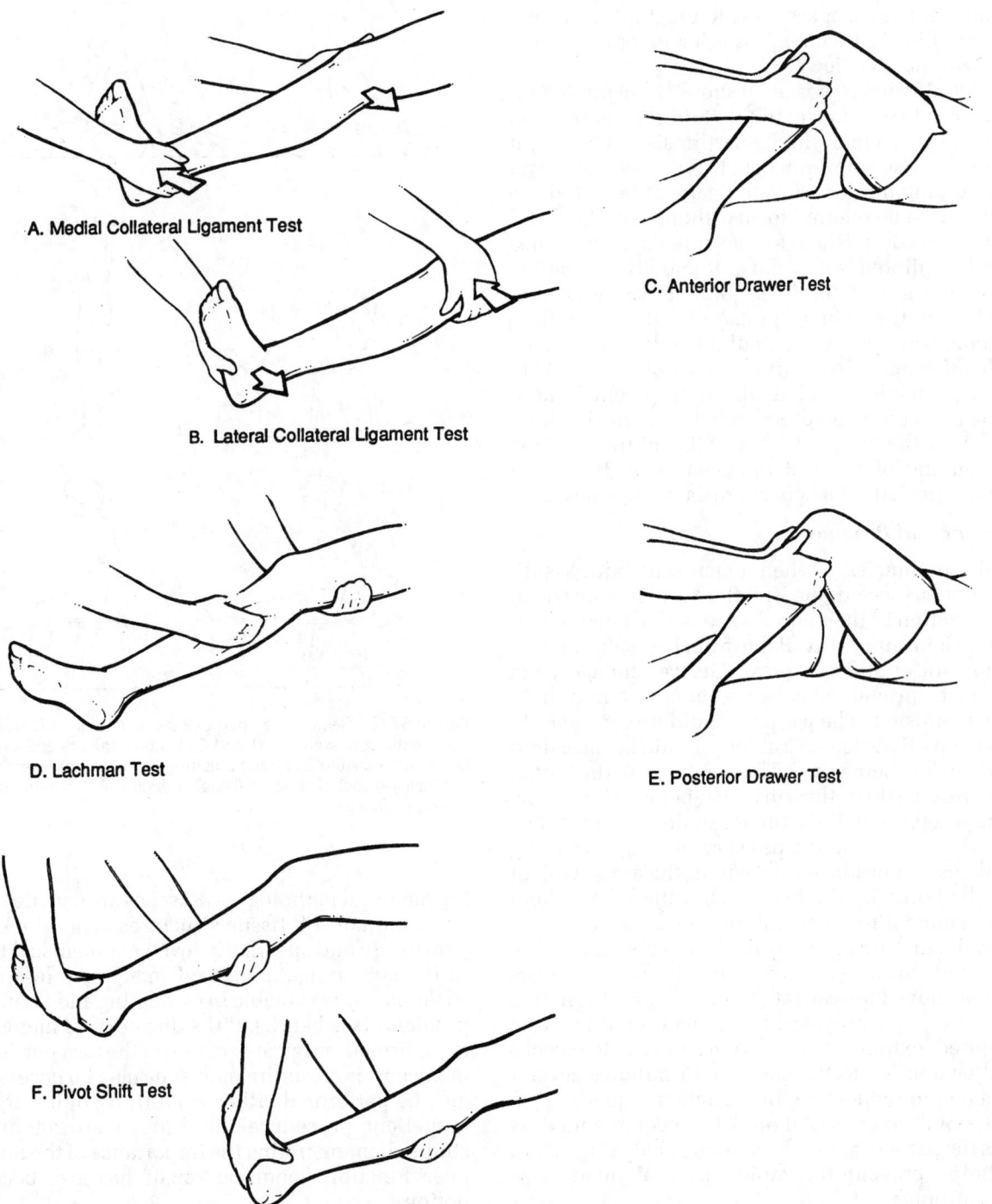

A. Medial Collateral Ligament Test

B. Lateral Collateral Ligament Test

C. Anterior Drawer Test

D. Lachman Test

E. Posterior Drawer Test

F. Pivot Shift Test

Figure 67.4. Examination for collateral and cruciate ligament injuries. **A.** Medial collateral ligament test. **B.** Lateral collateral ligament test. **C.** Anterior drawer test. **D.** Lachman test. **E.** Posterior drawer test. **F.** Pivot shift test. (Modified and redrawn from Scott WN, Nisonson B, Nicholas JA, eds. Principles of sports medicine. Baltimore: Williams & Wilkins, 1984.)

tested. The most sensitive test of the anterior cruciate ligament is the *Lachman test,* in which the knee is flexed to 15° and the tibia is pulled anteriorly on the femur. The test is defined as positive if there is anterior laxity. A partial tear usually has laxity with a firm endpoint, whereas a complete tear does not have a firm endpoint. Another important test to determine anterior cruciate ligament instability is *the pivot shift test* (Fig. 67.4F). With the foot internally rotated, the proximal tibia subluxes anteriorly with knee extension when the anterior cruciate ligament is not fully intact.

Additional Evaluation.   X-rays of the knee should always be obtained to exclude other problems, such as loose bodies within the knee, osteochondritis dissecans, fractures, or arthritis. Radiographic evaluation should include anteroposterior, lateral, tunnel, and sunrise patella views.

If a large effusion is present, it should be aspirated for two reasons: first, removal of the fluid results in relief of discomfort; second, if a hemarthrosis is present, it may indicate a serious injury such as an osteochondral fracture or an anterior cruciate ligament tear, and the patient should be referred to an orthopedist. If referral cannot be accomplished for several days, the knee should be splinted with a knee immobilizer (see below). Aspiration of the knee joint is easily accomplished after the skin is prepared with an iodine-containing solution (e.g., Betadine) and anesthetizing it with lidocaine. Generally the easiest approach to aspiration is medially or laterally at the patellofemoral joint. The needle should be angled posteriorly about 20° to follow the posterior slope of the midpoint of the patellofemoral joint. An 18- or 20-gauge needle should be used, especially if a hemarthrosis is suspected.

Treatment and Prognosis

Meniscus Injuries.   When a meniscus injury is diagnosed or suspected, the initial treatment consists of immobilization of the injured knee with a knee immobilizer (a rigid support available from large pharmacies or orthopedic appliance stores). An Ace bandage is not sufficient to provide stability, although it may help diminish effusion. The patient should use *crutches* to keep weight off the knee. Crutches should be measured properly before being used. The upper end of the crutch should rest against the ribs just below the axilla. Bearing weight with the crutches in the axilla must be avoided because it could cause nerve damage, resulting in weakness, hypesthesia, or pain in the arms. Weight should be borne by the hands, with the elbows kept fully extended. Proper technique should be taught by the physician, nurse, or physical therapist before the patient starts to ambulate with crutches. Both crutches should be moved forward at the same time, alternating with the weight-bearing leg. The patient should elevate the injured extremity when lying down. Ice packs should be applied to the knee for 15 minutes several times a day to reduce swelling. Isometric quadriceps-strengthening exercises should be recommended as soon as the patient can do these comfortably (Fig. 67.5). This helps prevent the rapid onset of quadriceps muscle atrophy.

Most often symptoms subside within 14 days; if symptoms resolve, the prognosis is variable. In the instance of a small tear, complete healing may occur without subsequent symptoms. On the other hand, a larger tear may result in recurrent symptoms after initial improvement. Therefore, if symptoms persist beyond 2 weeks with conservative treatment or if they recur after return to normal activity, an orthopedic referral is indicated for consideration of magnetic resonance imaging (11) or arthroscopy to establish the diagnosis. *Magnetic resonance imaging* (MRI) is a noninvasive procedure and a good method of evaluat-

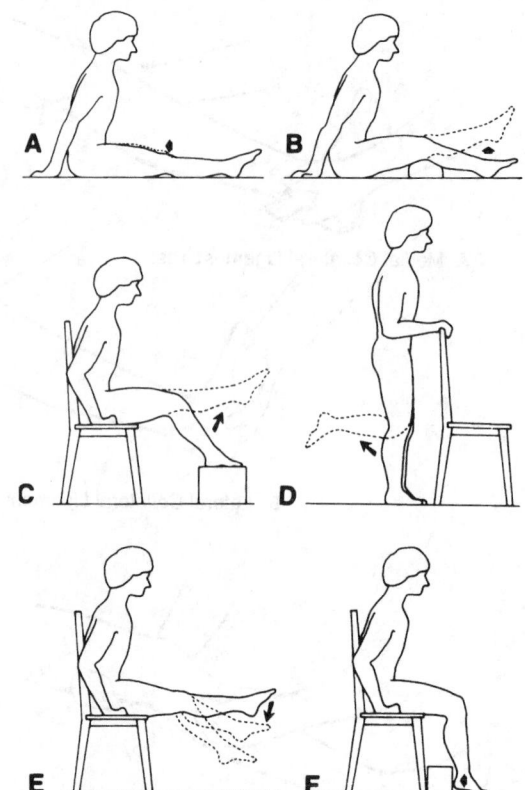

Figure 67.5.   Restorative knee exercises. **A.** Isometric quadriceps (knee extensor) exercise. **B and C.** Isotonic quadriceps exercises. **D.** Gravity-resisted isotonic hamstring (knee flexion) exercise. **E.** Gravity-assisted isotonic flexion exercise. **F.** Isometric knee flexion exercise.

ing meniscal pathology. MRI scans are excellent for the evaluation of soft tissue structures about the knee (4). Sensitivity and specificity levels for meniscal tears are in the 90% range. Ligament imaging is less reliable. *Arthroscopy* is valuable in evaluating and treating knee problems (see below). If the diagnosis of meniscal tear is confirmed, surgical excision of the torn portion of the meniscus or the entire meniscus may be necessary and may be performed either via arthroscopic surgery (an outpatient procedure) or through arthrotomy. With studies demonstrating the importance of the menisci to knee function, meniscal repair has also become an option.

After surgery for a torn meniscus, the patient is often able to return to light sports activity within 6 to 8 weeks, but it may be 3 months or longer before such activities as running or tennis can be resumed. A proper postoperative conditioning period of supervised physical therapy is important and consists of strengthening the quadriceps and hamstring muscles (Fig. 67.5) and range-of-motion exercises to ensure normal mobility of the knee. Proprioceptive training helps regain position sense of the joint and decreases the chance of reinjury. Joint space narrowing and arthritic change almost always follow meniscectomy but may not limit a patient's activity significantly. The menisci are extremely valuable for knee stability, distribution of weight-bearing loads, and smooth range of motion; therefore, it is imperative to treat meniscal tears aggressively to avoid further damage (1,6).

Ligament Injuries. If a ruptured ligament is suspected, the patient's knee should be immobilized in a posterior splint or rigid knee immobilizer, and the patient should be referred immediately to an orthopedist.

If a grade I collateral ligament sprain (see above) is diagnosed, a patient with minor symptoms can be permitted to increase activity gradually over the succeeding 1 to 2 weeks. For more pronounced symptoms, the knee should be immobilized with a knee immobilizer (see above), and the patient should use crutches for 5 to 10 days. Ice packs and isometric quadriceps-tensing exercises should be recommended, as for meniscus injuries. When the knee brace is removed, the patient can progressively increase activity and should begin isotonic quadriceps exercises (Fig. 67.5) and range-of-motion exercises.

Prevention

Acute meniscus injury occurs by chance when a rotational force is applied to the knee when it is in the flexed position; it cannot be prevented by conditioning. Ligamentous injuries can be prevented to some degree by proper conditioning. Prophylactic braces (those placed on the normal knee to prevent ligamentous injury) are being used less often because their effectiveness is controversial (18). Because they may preload the ligaments and make them more prone to injury, braces are not recommended.

Patellofemoral Arthralgia and Other Causes of Anterior Knee Pain

Definition and Mechanism of Injury

Patellofemoral arthralgia is pain originating from the patellofemoral joint. The patellofemoral joint is the most common source of painful symptoms encountered by athletes, with 30% of exertion-related conditions involving this joint. It is often associated with changes in the articular cartilage of the patella. *Anterior knee pain* can occur without cartilage changes as well. When the cartilage does become soft, it can break down, causing crepitus and pain. This condition is called *chondromalacia* (10). Anterior knee pain can also occur secondary to instability of the patellofemoral joint, most often *lateral subluxation* or hypermobility of the patella. This can be caused by an increased angle between the quadriceps and patellar tendon (Q angle), *patella alta,* or muscle and bony imbalances in the lower extremity (7). The normal Q angle is up to 20°; if it is greater than this, increased lateral displacement of the patella results (Fig. 67.6). An abnormal Q angle is sometimes associated with excessive pronation of the feet (flat feet, see Chapter 102). Patella alta is an anatomic variant in which the patella rides more proximally than usual, so that it becomes hypermobile.

Patella alta can be identified on a lateral x-ray when the patellar tendon length exceeds the maximum length of the patella by more than 1 cm (Fig. 67.7). Normally, the lengths of these two structures are equal. Patients with a variation in hip joint anatomy that results in compensatory external tibial torsion (external rotation of lower leg in axial plane, slew foot) also have lateral displacement of the patella and excess wear of the patellofemoral joint.

Anterior knee pain is a common disorder, especially in adolescent athletes. This can be caused by alignment problems, as discussed above, or overuse syndromes related to improper conditioning or stretching. The source of the pain may be the extensor mechanism (quadriceps muscle, quadriceps tendon, or patellar tendon), in the patella itself, or outside the knee (see below). If stress on the articular cartilage is allowed to continue (whether secondary to subluxation or malalignment), cartilage breakdown, chondromalacia, may result as described above. With

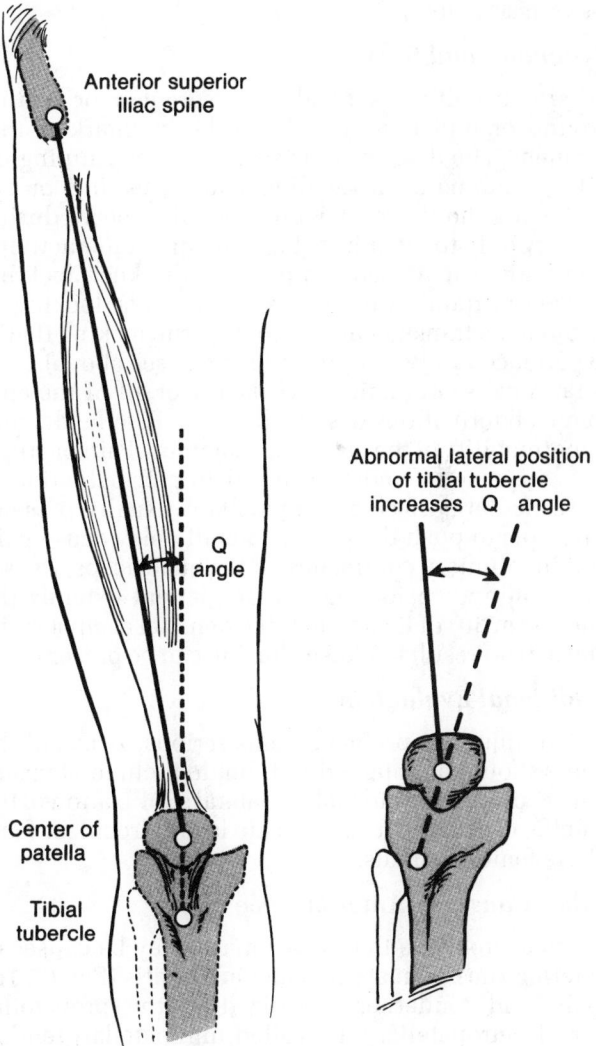

Figure 67.6.   Q angle.

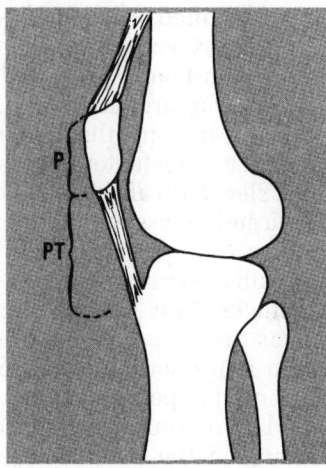

Figure 67.7. Patella alta. The ratio of PT to P is normally less than 1.2. In this case PT:P is 1.5, so this is patella alta. *P*, patella; *PT*, patellar tendon.

appropriate treatment, this can be avoided in many cases (see below).

Symptoms and Signs

Pain, usually described as a soreness or aching around or under the patella, is the hallmark of this problem. The discomfort is aggravated by running up hills, climbing or descending stairs, kneeling, or hyperflexing the knee (9). Pain often disappears during activity only to recur just at the end of or after activity. The patient may also complain of the knee locking; however, upon careful questioning, this locking is found to be transient and is not the true locking that is experienced in tears of the meniscus (see above).

Physical examination reveals any or all of the anatomic abnormalities described above. Patella alta and hypermobility of the patella are common. Pain or crepitus with patellofemoral manipulation or palpation of the articular surface of the patella is usually present. Attempts to push the patella laterally may cause pain and involuntary contracture of the quadriceps, the so-called apprehension sign. If the patient extends the knee from 30° of flexion to full extension against resistance, pain results. A knee effusion can be present.

Additional Evaluation

If an injury or problem seems serious, x-rays of the knees should be obtained and should include a tangential or sunrise view to look for lateral subluxation of the patella, often with a hypoplastic lateral trochlear facet of the femoral sulcus.

Other Causes of Anterior Knee Pain

Other problems that occasionally may be causes of anterior knee pain are prepatellar bursitis (Fig. 67.1B) (pain and tenderness localized to the prepatellar bursa), retropatellar (also called infrapatellar) tendon bursitis (Fig. 67.1B) (pain and tenderness localized to the area below the patella and behind the tendon), pes anserinus bursitis (Fig. 67.1B) (pain and tenderness in

the bursa that lies deep to the combined insertion of the sartorius, gracilis, and semitendinosus tendons into the proximal medial tibial metaphysis), fat pad syndrome (trauma-related inflammation of the infrapatellar fat pad) (Fig. 67.1B), meniscal injury (see above), ligamentous instability of the knee (see above), arthritis, and osteochondritis dissecans (necrosis within the condylar epiphysis characterized by insidious onset of knee ache at rest, worsened by weight bearing and confirmed by x-ray). Hip or pelvic disease is associated with referred pain from sciatic nerve root irritation. These problems can be differentiated by careful radiologic and physical examination (including test of ligament stability and palpation of bursae, ligaments, and joint margin); if there is any doubt, referral to an orthopedic surgeon is appropriate.

Treatment and Prognosis

Therapy is initiated as soon as possible after the appearance of symptoms. The use of crutches for up to 7 days to rest the knee is important; and the application of ice to the knee for approximately 15 minutes several times a day helps to decrease swelling. In addition, analgesic medications should be prescribed, such as enteric coated aspirin 600 mg four times a day or acetaminophen 650 mg four times a day. Nonsteroidal anti-inflammatory drugs (NSAIDs) also are effective, but they should be used cautiously and only for a short period. The patients should be warned of the potential symptomatic as well as asymptomatic side effects (see Chapter 70 for a full discussion of NSAIDs) (2).

After the initial inflammation has subsided, the application of ice may be discontinued and heat may be applied for 15 to 20 minutes several times a day. The patient should avoid vigorous sports activities until symptoms subside, which often takes several weeks. Progressive resistance exercises of the quadriceps should be supervised by a physical therapist (especially one experienced in sports medicine, if available) to maximize quadriceps strength and stability (Fig. 67.5). Stretching to increase flexibility is extremely important, especially in the hip flexors, quadriceps, and hamstring muscle groups (see "Stretching Exercises," below). The course of this problem is unpredictable. Orthopedic referral is usually necessary if the patient has been forced to abandon a major sport for more than a few weeks, or if the problem recurs. Intra-articular corticosteroid injections may alleviate symptoms, but this treatment must be restricted because it increases cartilage deterioration if done repeatedly (5). The treatment, including the injection of corticosteroid for bursitis around the knee, is discussed in Chapter 66. Correction of the tracking problem in the patellofemoral joint may require the use of an orthotic to correct excess pronation of the foot (see Chapter 102) or the use of a cartilage knee brace (a heavy elastic brace containing a horseshoe-shaped pad to stabilize the patella, available from large pharmacies or orthopedic appliance stores without prescription). Occasionally, when anterior knee pain progresses to cartilage damage, surgical treatment is necessary if conservative treatment fails. Surgery is designed to prevent subluxation of the patella or decrease stress in the patellofemoral articular cartilage. Results vary, depending on the extent of the problem and the type of surgery, but occasionally the patient may not be able to return to sports that place stress on the knee.

Prevention

Prevention of anterior knee pain and chondromalacia requires the use of proper foot gear (see Chapter 102), often including the use of orthotics, and proper conditioning of the athlete by gradually increasing his or her level of activity and performing stretching exercises (see below).

PROBLEMS OF THE LEG

Apophysitis of the Tibial Tubercle (Osgood–Schlatter's Disease)

Osgood–Schlatter's disease is a common cause of knee pain in adolescents. This condition is usually self-limited, and symptoms generally cease when skeletal growth stops. It is thought to be caused by repetitive avulsions or stress fractures caused by traction of the patellar tendon where it inserts into the growth plate of the tibial tubercle. This repetitive trauma causes inflammation and pain at the insertion point of the tendon.

The patient describes the insidious onset of pain of the tibial tubercle with activity. This condition is often bilateral. On examination the tubercle and adjacent tendon are enlarged and tender. There may be quadriceps atrophy from decreased activity, which often occurs because of the pain experienced with physical activity involving the leg. There may also be tightness of the quadriceps and hamstring muscle groups.

The adolescent with Osgood–Schlatter's disease should be instructed to avoid activities that entail resisted knee extension, such as climbing, running, and kicking, until pain has resolved (usually 6 to 8 weeks). Range of motion and stretching (see "Stretching Exercises," below) should be stressed early in the course of treatment. If pain persists after ossification is complete, surgical excision of heterotopic bone at the tibial tubercle and reattachment of the patellar tendon are sometimes necessary.

Shin Splints

Definition and Mechanism of Injury

Shin splints (16) are the occurrence of pain over the anteromedial aspect of the mid- to distal portion of the lower leg (Fig. 67.8, site A). They are caused by overuse of the muscles of this region as may occur with running, jogging, or sustained walking. The pain is thought to result from tendinitis of the posterior tibial tendon and periostitis from the pulling of this muscle from its bony attachment along the medial aspect of the tibia, interosseous membrane, and fibula.

Shin splints develop most often in patients who are not properly conditioned, do not warm up or stretch properly, run on hard or uneven surfaces, wear improper foot gear, or have anatomic abnormalities such as variation in the anatomy of their hip joint with resultant excessive tibial torsion (external rotation of the tibia in the axial plane, or slew feet) and hyperpronation of the feet (flat feet).

Symptoms and Signs

Shin splints are characterized by pain, usually gradual but occasionally abrupt in onset, that occurs during or just after exercise. Athletes often continue to exercise despite the discomfort, but occasionally the pain is so severe that the exercise must be stopped. Examination reveals only the presence of tenderness along the medial aspect of the tibia.

Differential Diagnosis

If the area of tenderness is localized, a stress fracture may have occurred, although pain from a stress fracture is present immediately on starting activity. A compartment syndrome is similar to shin splints, but the location of pain and tenderness is different (see below). Occasionally fascial hernias, tenosynovitis, or tears of the interosseous membrane may produce symptoms suggesting shin splints; for this reason, an orthopedic consultation should be requested if symptoms persist after 3 weeks of therapy (see below) or if symptoms recur. The orthopedist confirms the diagnosis and looks for anatomic abnormalities that predispose to this condition (see below). Also, an x-ray (indicated when symptoms are prolonged or recurrent) of the leg in the case of shin splints occasionally shows irregular bone formation of the tibia or fibula as a result of periostitis. A radionuclide bone scan is more sensitive than an x-ray in the diagnosis of shin splints and may be necessary if the diagnosis is uncertain. A positive bone scan shows increased uptake of radionuclide by the tibia, fibula, or interosseous membrane.

Treatment and Prognosis

Ice packs should be applied several times a day for 15 minutes at a time to reduce swelling and inflammation. In severe cases, the patient should avoid, for several weeks, the exercise that has precipitated the problem. The use of an elastic wrap on the lower leg provides some comfort. The prescription of analgesic agents is the same as described in the section on anterior knee pain (see above).

Acute shin splints should resolve with rest in 3 weeks; after this, conditioning is necessary before the patient can return to the sport. Stretching (see "Stretching Exercises," below) may help in the therapy of this condition, and if symptoms persist, formal evaluation of foot and lower extremity biomechanics is indicated. The syndrome rarely recurs if conditioning has been correct.

Prevention

To help prevent shin splints, the patient should try stretching exercises before physical activity (see below); running or walking on soft, level surfaces and

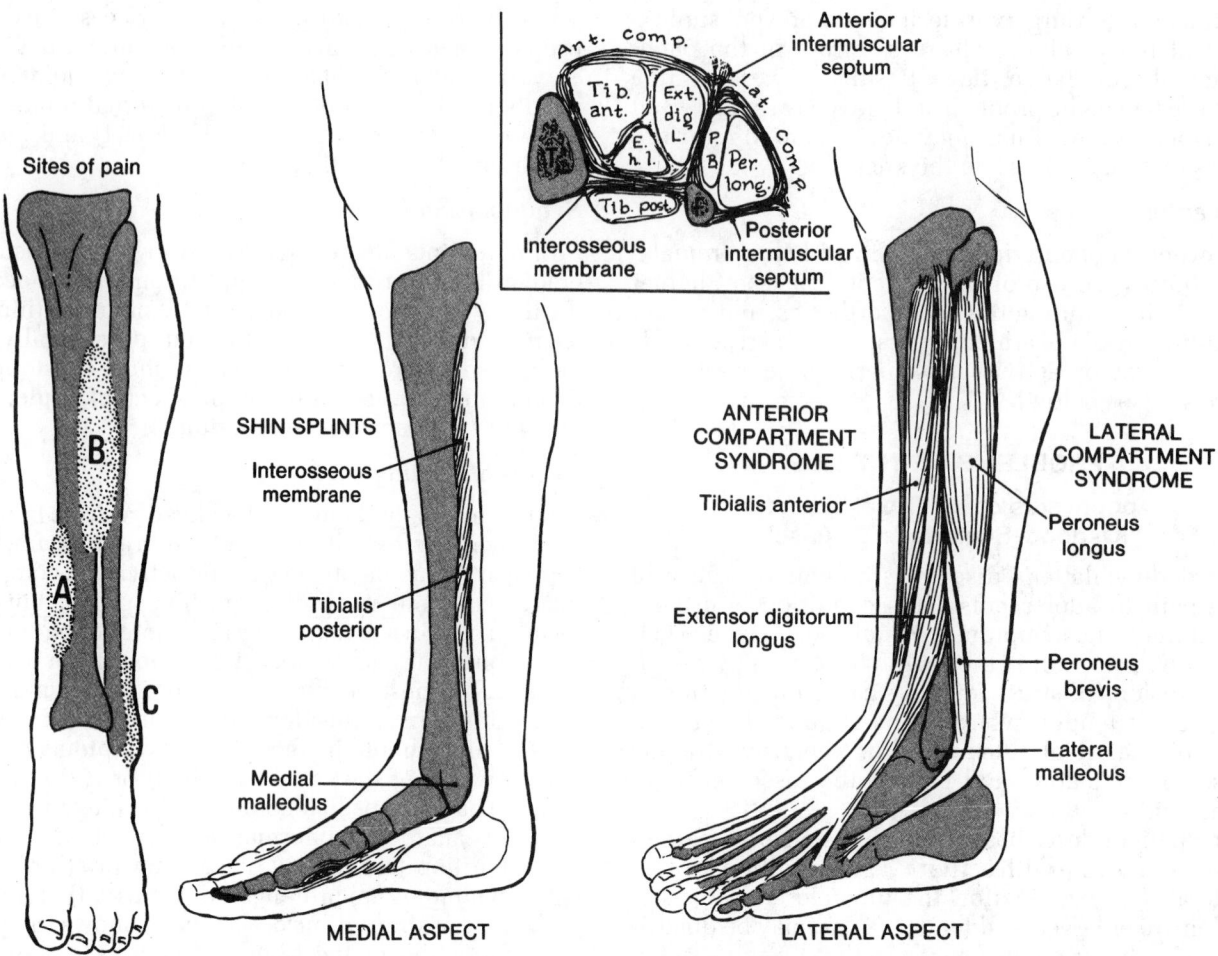

Figure 67.8. Sites of pain and relevant anatomy of (**A**) shin splints, (**B**) anterior compartment syndrome, and (**C**) lateral compartment syndrome.

use of proper shoes (see Chapter 102) also are important. An orthotic device may also be prescribed by an orthopedist or podiatrist if hyperpronation of the feet or excessive tibial rotation is present. These also are helpful in preventing recurrences.

Compartment Syndromes

Definition and Mechanism of Injury

Two compartments in the leg are prone to injury and subsequent swelling: the anterior (tibial) compartment and the lateral (peroneal) compartment. The anterior compartment syndrome is also called lateral shin splints and occurs when an athlete runs to excess on his or her toes or on a hill, or runs with shoes with overly flexible soles. Activity can cause muscles to hypertrophy and repeated contraction can cause tissue edema. These factors lead to overswelling in the compartment, and blood supply to muscles and nerves can be compromised. This causes the symptoms during exercise and can lead to permanent damage.

Compartment syndromes are usually seen in competitive runners, and they are much less common than shin splints.

Symptoms and Signs

Anterior Compartment Syndrome. The patient notices pain in the foot dorsiflexor muscles of the leg and in the lower leg, ankle, and foot. Discomfort usually occurs during or just after exercise. Examination reveals tenderness and often swelling of the anterior compartment, which is located over the midlateral aspect of the lower leg (Fig. 67.8, site B). Weakness of toe extensors and ankle dorsiflexors can also be seen.

Lateral Compartment Syndrome. In this situation the pain is located in the posterolateral aspect of the ankle above and behind the lateral malleolus (Fig. 67.8, site C); this is the area where the peroneal tendons are located. Often the patient feels as if the ankle has given out. This syndrome is caused by excessive pronation of the foot (flat foot) and ankle (eversion) in runners with hypermobile ankles (weak ankles).

Treatment and Prognosis

Initially, ice should be applied for 15 minutes several times a day, and the patient must rest from exercise for 3 to 4 weeks. Anti-inflammatory agents are helpful in controlling the inflammatory response. An anti-inflammatory agent with a rapid onset of action is suggested; naproxen (Naprosyn) 375 to 500 mg twice daily and piroxicam (Feldene) 20 mg once a day are effective. If cost is a factor, enteric coated aspirin is recommended, although it takes 7 to 10 days at a dosage of 3 to 4 g/day to achieve an anti-inflammatory effect. Once symptoms subside, the patient should begin a conditioning program before returning to full exercise. In this effort, preexercise stretching (see below), especially of the muscles that are involved, may be beneficial, and the patient should return to running gradually. The patient should have well-designed running shoes (see Chapter 102), avoid toe running, and always run on a level surface.

In the management of the lateral compartment syndrome an orthopedist or podiatrist should be consulted to evaluate the use of an orthotic device or heel wedge to prevent hyperpronation, which predisposes to recurrence of the problem.

The prognosis for patients with these compartment syndromes is excellent if the patient is properly conditioned. If symptoms persist, pressure elevation within the compartment can become a chronic and persistent problem and fasciotomy may be required.

Differential Diagnosis

If symptoms do not respond within 7 to 10 days, an x-ray of the area should be obtained to rule out other causes, such as a stress fracture or osteoid osteoma. A compartment syndrome also can be confused initially with thrombophlebitis, cellulitis, or vascular insufficiency, and these should all be investigated by means of serial observations and appropriate specific diagnostic procedures.

Prevention

Stretching exercises (see below) before running, especially of the musculature involved in each of the compartments, and the use of good quality running gear, often including orthotics, may help prevent compartment syndromes.

PROBLEMS OF THE ANKLE AND FOOT
Injuries of the Ankle Joints

Ankle Structure and Function

The ankle joint consists of articulations between the distal tibia and fibula, which form an arch, or mortise, and the talus, which fits into the mortise (Fig. 67.9). The talus fits tightly into the mortise during dorsiflexion of the foot and is mobile during plantar flexion. The stability of the ankle is provided by the various ligaments shown in Figure 67.9.

Mechanism of Injury

Ankle injuries occur when there is sudden stress on one or more of the supporting ligaments. Such injuries may occur during vigorous activity or as a consequence of inadvertently stepping onto an uneven surface or off an unnoticed curb's edge. Figures 67.10 and 67.11 illustrate the spectrum of ankle ligament injuries and

the stresses that cause them. The most commonly sprained ankle ligament is the anterior talofibular ligament. The grades of ligament injury (sprain) are defined above (see "Problems of the Knee").

Signs and Symptoms

The patient usually can recall the position of the foot and whether there was a sensation or sound of tearing at the ankle. Immediate pain is noted, and if there has been a sprain, the patient is aware of instability with weight bearing. Swelling over the injured ligament occurs within 1 hour of the injury, and it may be followed later by diffuse swelling of the foot and by an ecchymosis if there has been a significant ligament tear.

Examination of the strained or sprained ankle reveals marked tenderness over the injured ligament, made worse by replicating the stress that led to the injury (most commonly inversion of the foot). If there is not tense swelling, joint instability (e.g., obvious looseness or tilting of the talus with inversion of the foot) can be demonstrated when there has been a significant ligament tear. When the ankle cannot be easily manipulated to test for instability, a stress x-ray, under block anesthesia if needed, provides definitive diagnosis of severe sprain (see example, Fig. 67.12).

Treatment, Prognosis, and Prevention

Promptly after injury, the ankle should be immobilized (elastic bandage, no walking), ice packs (or ice

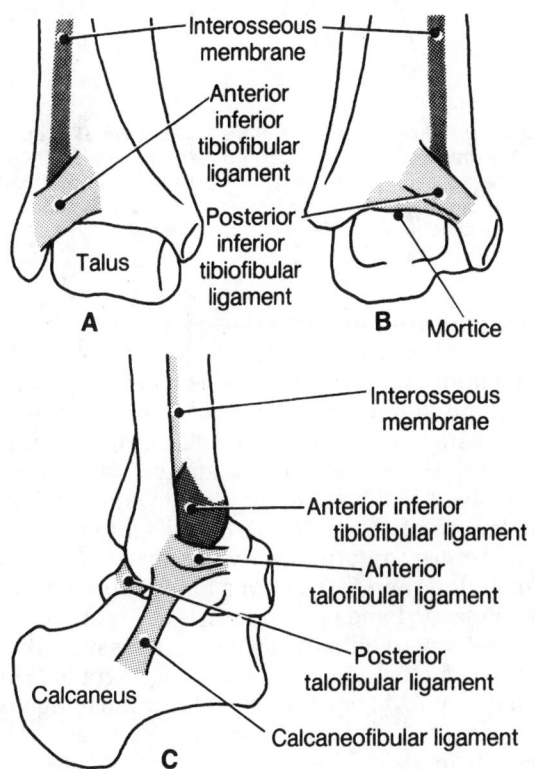

Figure 67.9. Distal tibiofibular joint and tibiotalar joint. **A.** Anterior view. **B.** Posterior view. **C.** Lateral view. (From Ramamurti CP, Tinker RV. Orthopaedics in primary care. Baltimore: Williams & Wilkins, 1979.)

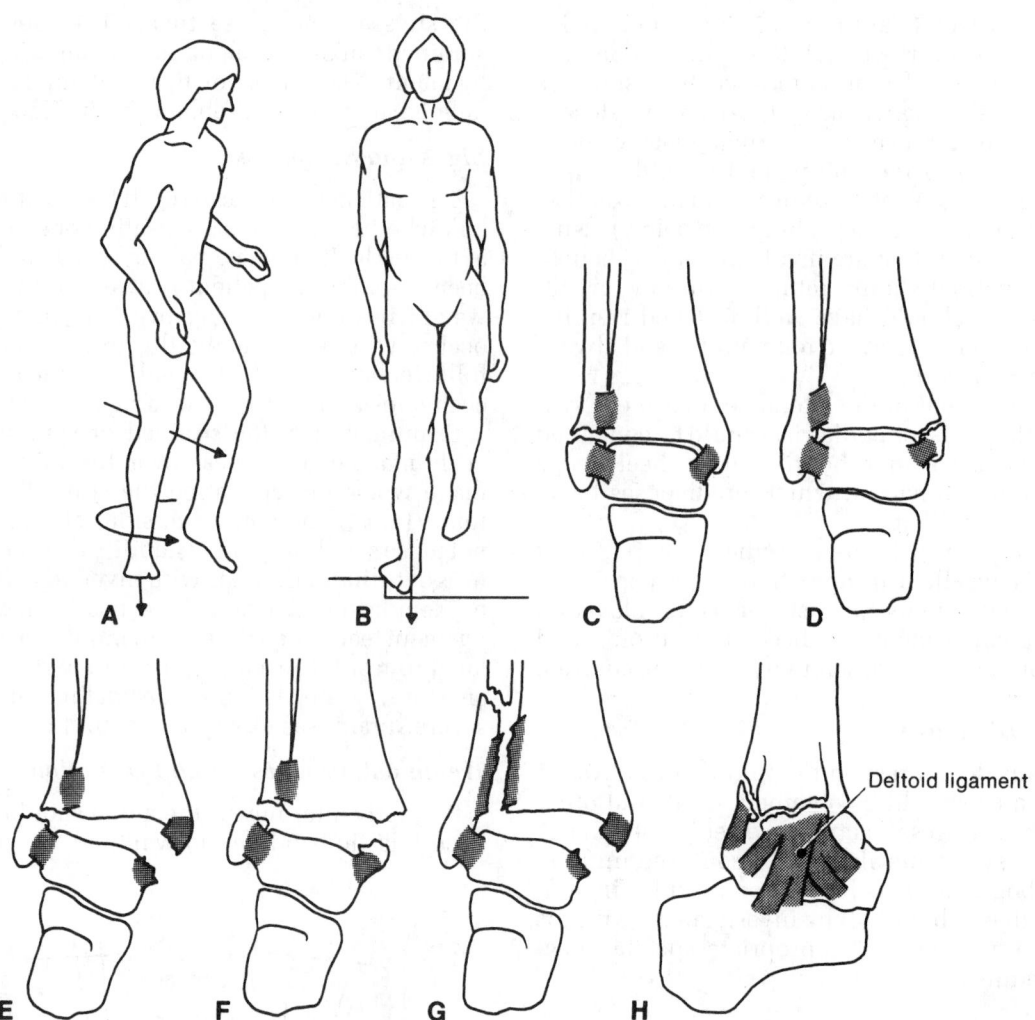

Figure 67.10.   Pronation injuries of the ankle. **A** and **B**. Modes of injury. **A**. Extremity rotates internally on the fixed foot. **B**. The foot is forced into pronation by weight taken on the lateral aspect of the forefoot. **C** and **D**. Brief forces of lesser severity may fracture a malleolus without tearing a ligament. **E–G**. Forces of greater severity destroy the mortice in one of three ways. **H**. When forward displacement of the tibia accompanies severe pronation forces, the posterior margin of the tibial articular surface may be fractured as well.

water immersion) should be used for 10 to 15 minutes, and the leg should be elevated. If examination suggests that the injury represents a grade I sprain (i.e., stretching without significant structural damage, with only modest pain, tenderness, and swelling, and no obvious instability), the ankle can be managed with an elastic bandage for 1 to 3 weeks, rest and elevation whenever possible, use of a cane for partial weight bearing, and gradual return to normal activities over 2 to 4 weeks. The technique and instructions for wrapping the ankle with an elastic bandage are shown in Figure 67.13.

If there is marked pain, swelling, or instability, it is likely that the patient has a significant (grade II or III) sprain (i.e., partial or complete disruption of ligament) of one or more ligaments, or, in the case of an eversion injury, an avulsion fracture (Figs. 67.10 and 67.11). Referral to an emergency room or an orthopedic surgeon's office for definitive diagnosis and management is indicated. For these patients, treatment consists of immobilization with a rigid ankle splint for usually no

more than 3 weeks and no weight bearing (i.e., use of a crutch) for 2 weeks, followed by progressive return to weight bearing. To ensure optimal long-term outcome, convalescence from a significant ankle sprain should be planned and supervised by an orthopedic surgeon if the general physician is inexperienced in their treatment. For severe injuries and for instability that does not improve with conservative management, surgical realignment or repair may be necessary.

Prevention

Recurrent ankle sprain is common. Muscle rehabilitation and proprioceptive training are important for full return to function. Proprioceptive training can aid in regaining agility and normal strength, and it plays a major role in the prevention of recurrent injuries. Exercises consist of several positioning tasks for the foot: inversion and eversion resistance with surgical tubing and sliding on a teeter-totter are two examples. There are also commercially made teeter boards to improve ankle agility. Referral to a sports medicine physical therapist is appropriate for patients progressing slowly after ankle injuries. The optimal method for preventing recurrent injury, especially for an athlete with lax ankle joints, is to tape the ankle before engaging in exercise involving running. Alternatively, the patient can use a commercially available elastic ankle support when exercising; these supports permit full range of motion but prevent the foot from falling into excessive inversion when it is not touching the ground (15).

Achilles Tendinitis

Definition and Mechanism of Injury

Achilles tendinitis is inflammation of the heel tendon and surrounding tissue and is caused by overuse. The problem is most often caused by repetitive

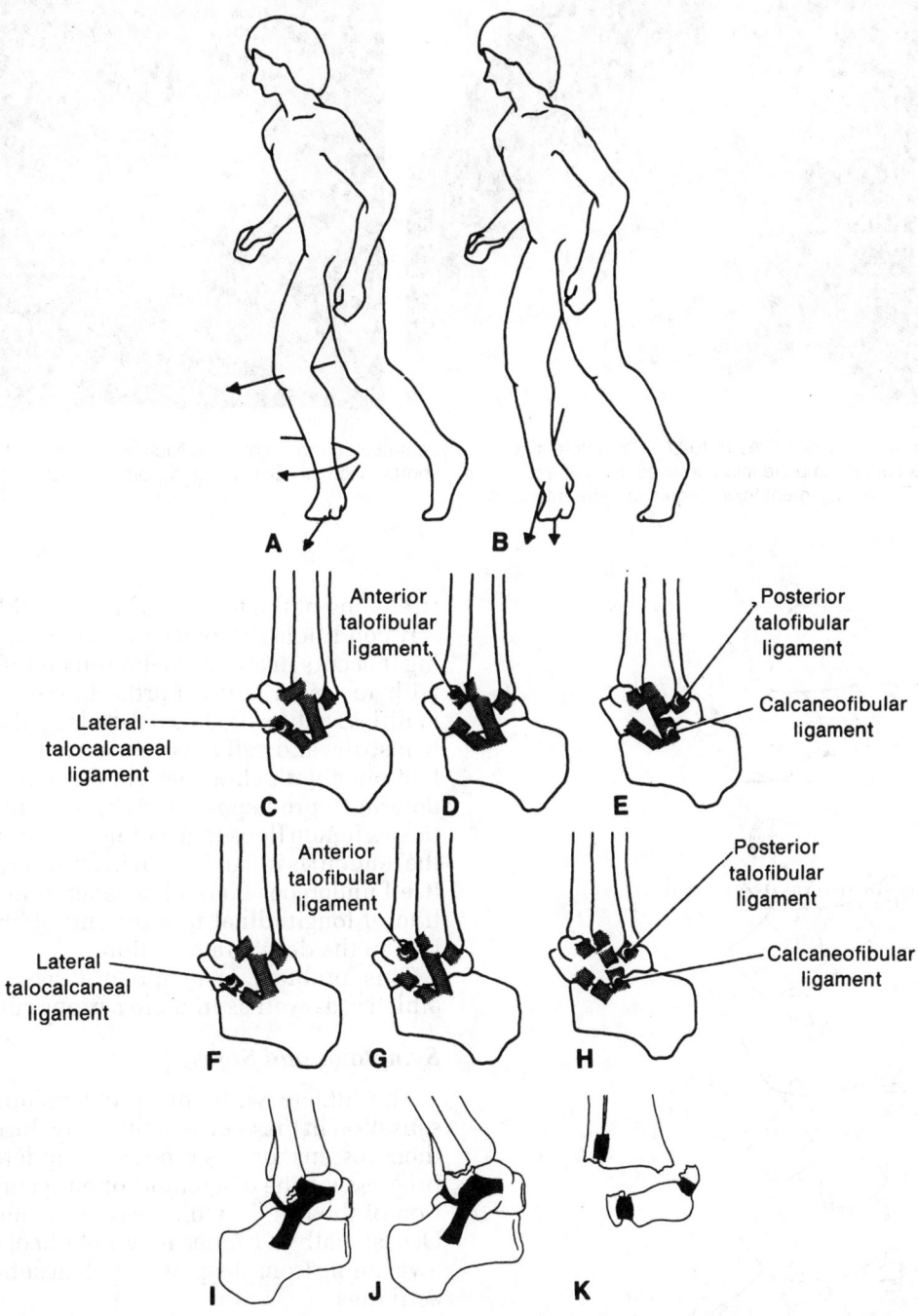

Figure 67.11. Supination injuries to the ankle. **A** and **B**. Modes of injury. **A**. Extremity rotates externally on the fixed foot. **B**. Plantar-flexed foot is forced into supination. **C–E**. Sequence of injuries. Lateral talocalcaneal ligament (**C**) is injured before the anterior talofibular (**D**), which is injured before the calcaneofibular (**E**). **F–H**. When the injuring force is sufficient, the ligaments tear completely and in the same sequence. **I–K**. Rather than tear the lateral ligaments, the injuring force may avulse a flake of fibula (**I**), fracture off the end of the fibula (**J**), or fracture off both the end of the fibula and the medial malleolus (**K**).

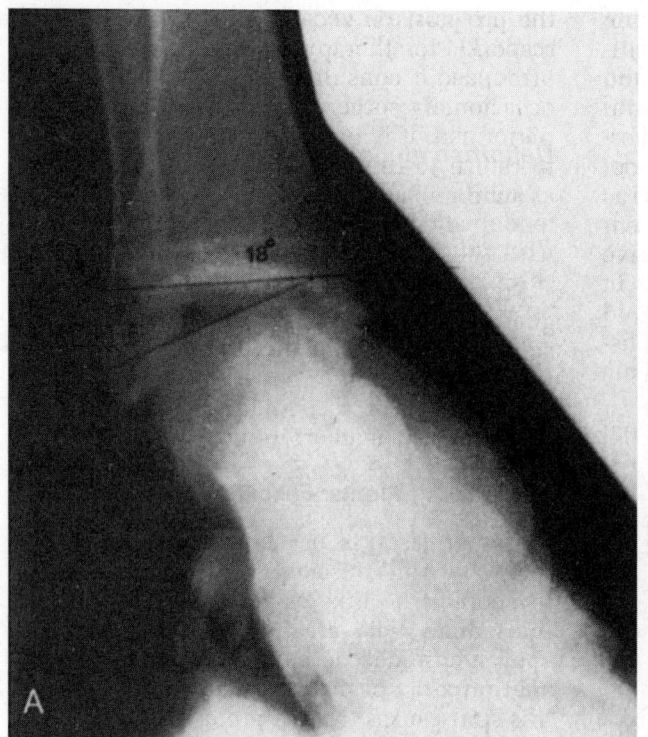
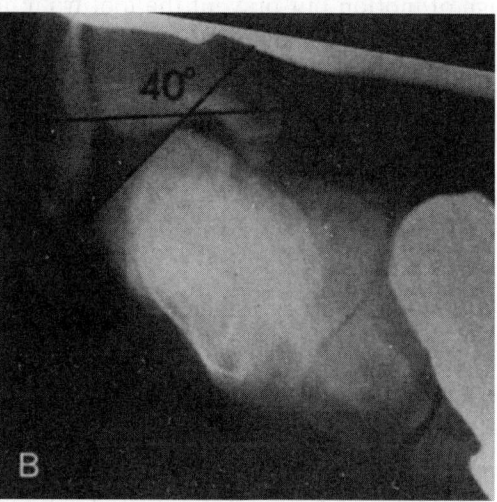

Figure 67.12. Examples of talar tilt. **A**. 15 to 20°. Complete single-ligament tear with partial or complete injury to second ligament. **B**. Greater than 25°. Double-ligament injury requiring more intensive treatment. (From Scott NW, Nicholas JA, eds. Principles of sports medicine. Baltimore: Williams & Wilkins, 1984.)

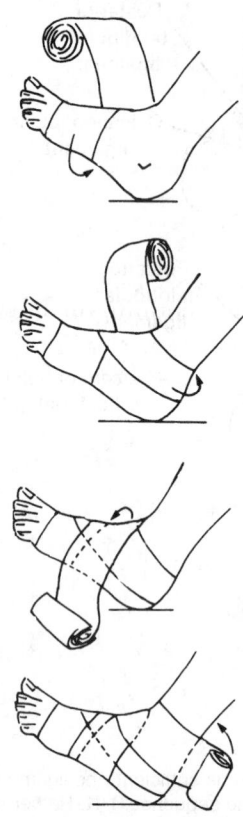

Figure 67.13. Technique for wrapping the ankle.

stretching of the tendon when the athlete is not properly conditioned. However, even with good conditioning it occurs in athletes who run on hills or wear shoes with too rigid soles. Furthermore, structural abnormalities such as tibia vara (bowlegged deformity), tight hamstring and calf muscles, a cavus foot (high arched foot often with claw toes), and a varus (inverted) heel deformity predispose to Achilles tendinitis. Initially, the peritenon (loose soft connective tissue surrounding the tendon) is inflamed, but in chronic cases the tendon itself undergoes mucoid degeneration with the formation of longitudinal fissures and often nodule formation in the degenerate tendon.

This problem is commonly seen in recreational athletes, as well as in more serious runners.

Symptoms and Signs

The athlete with this problem notices a burning sensation in the heel, usually early during a run, which then lessens or disappears completely as running progresses. The discomfort often recurs upon completion of the run, in which case it is often more severe. Occasionally a runner may note heel pain soon after awakening from sleep, which then subsides with daily activities.

On examination there is local or diffuse tenderness in the Achilles tendon; when the condition is chronic, there may be a tender nodule in the tendon, crepitus, and swelling. This condition should be distinguished from retrotendinous and retrocalcaneal bursitis (see below).

Treatment and Prognosis

The application of an ice pack to the area for 15 minutes several times a day provides comfort and reduces swelling. Analgesic agents such as aspirin, acetaminophen, or NSAIDs should be used as described above in the section on anterior knee pain (see Chapter 70 for a full discussion of NSAIDs). The runner should rest for several days, then reduce his or her running mileage and avoid hills until symptoms have been absent for 10 to 14 days. Exercises that gently stretch the tendon may help condition the runner (see below) and prevent recurrences. If symptoms persist, a rest from exercise for 3 to 4 weeks or longer may be necessary to permit healing. Corticosteroid injections are not recommended for refractory cases because the incidence of tendon rupture is high. In general, steroid injections should not be used to treat tendinitis of major extensor tendons (i.e. triceps, patellar, and Achilles tendons; Achilles tendinitis, if chronic, may lead to increased risk of rupture).

In resistant cases, physical therapy, especially ultrasound, is helpful. A removable heel lift inserted into the shoe also may provide relief. In addition, when the syndrome is severe, splinting or casting of the ankle joint and the use of crutches are necessary to immobilize the Achilles tendon. In mild cases, with initial treatment and then proper conditioning, the prognosis is excellent. If the condition does not respond to therapy within 1 to 2 weeks, an orthopedic consultation should be obtained because occasionally surgery is necessary. If surgery must be performed, it is unlikely that the athlete will be able to return to running, although other exercises, such as swimming or cycling, may be readily performed.

Prevention

Prevention of this problem requires the use of good running shoes (see Chapter 102) with flexible soles, a well-molded Achilles pad, and a rigid heel wedge. If the runner has a cavus foot (see above) an orthopedist or a podiatrist should be consulted about the use of an orthotic device.

Plantar Fasciitis (Heel Spur)

Plantar fasciitis, or heel spur syndrome, is the most common cause of heel pain; it occurs most often in people who hike or run, but it may also occur in people who are not athletic. The name *heel spur syndrome* derives from the finding of a bone spur on x-ray of the calcaneus, but it is unlikely that this spur causes the symptoms in most patients. This problem is fully discussed in Chapter 102.

Retrocalcaneal Bursitis

Inflammation of the bursae that overlie the calcaneus (heel bone) may produce symptoms similar to those of Achilles tendinitis. Bursitis of the heel affects runners, but it may also occur at the upper border of the area just anterior to the Achilles tendon and just superior to the calcaneus, when tight-fitting shoes rub the heel with ordinary walking. On examination, there is focal tenderness confined to the calcaneus. Heel bursitis is managed with rest, properly fitted shoes, and, in runners, a heel pad (see Chapter 102).

Tarsal Tunnel Syndrome

Tarsal tunnel syndrome can occur in runners. It is caused by entrapment of the posterior tibial nerve in the fibro-osseous canal posterior to the medial malleolus. This problem is discussed fully in Chapter 84 ("Peripheral Neuropathy," under "Compression and Entrapment Neuropathies").

PROBLEMS OF THE ELBOW

Elbow Structure and Function

The elbow joint consists of articulations between the distal humerus, the proximal radius, and ulna. Flexion and extension occur at the humeroulnar joint, whereas supination and pronation occur at the humeroradial joint. The stability of the elbow is provided by various ligaments shown in Figure 67.14. This figure identifies important structures of the elbow and provides an orientation to the common conditions seen there.

Lateral Epicondylitis (Tennis Elbow)

Definition and Mechanism of Injury

The term *tennis elbow* refers to inflammation in the region of the lateral epicondyle of the humerus at the origin of the common extensor muscles; it is a common exercise-related syndrome. It is caused by activities that combine excessive pronation and supination of the forearm with an extended wrist. The predominant muscle involved is the extensor carpi radialis brevis. Although the mechanism causing tennis elbow is unknown, the actual cause of pain may be radiohumeral synovitis or bursitis, tendinitis of the common extensor origin, traumatic epicondylitis or periostitis of the lateral epicondyle, or entrapment by scarring of a branch of the radial nerve in this region.

This problem is common in people performing activities such as tennis, badminton, and bowling, as well as with many non–sports-related activities such as using a screwdriver or a wrench repetitively.

Symptoms and Signs

The onset of symptoms is usually gradual. Physical examination reveals tenderness over the lateral epicondyle or radiohumeral joint (Fig. 67.14). The proximal common extensor muscle is often tender to palpation, and on occasion, there is swelling in this area. The elbow usually has a normal flexion and extension, although the latter may sometimes be temporarily painful. Supination (palms up) and especially pronation (palms down) of the arm may be painful if

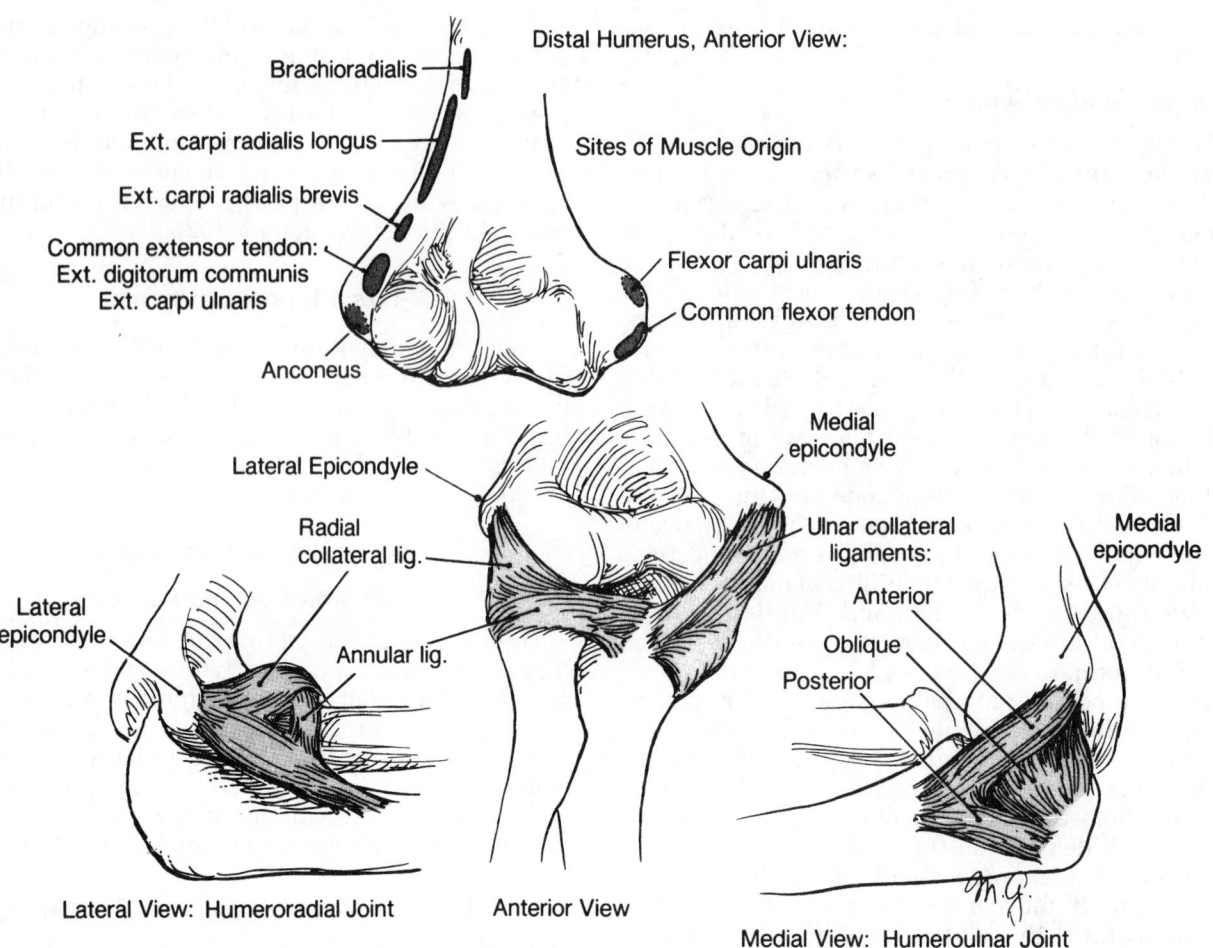

Figure 67.14. Important structures of the elbow.

performed against resistance. Pain can be elicited by stretching the wrist extensors by holding the elbow fully extended with the forearm pronated and the wrist maximally palmar flexed (Fig. 67.15).

Additional Evaluation

The history and physical examination are diagnostic, and further studies are not indicated unless symptoms fail to improve with treatment. In that case, an x-ray of the elbow should be obtained; on occasion, there may be calcium deposits noted at the lateral epicondyle of the humerus. Entrapment of the radial nerve in the proximal forearm should always be included in the differential diagnosis.

Treatment and Prognosis

The painful arm should initially be immobilized in a sling or, if symptoms are severe, immobilized in a long arm splint with the wrist held in dorsiflexion to rest the extensor tendons. Analgesics may be helpful (see discussion of anterior knee pain, above). Injection of the area at the point of tenderness with a mixture of 3 mL 1 to 2% lidocaine and 1 mL glucocorticoid suspension (e.g., Aristocort, Celestone, or Kenalog) using a 22- or 25-gauge needle followed by the use of a sling for 1 or 2 weeks often provides dramatic relief of pain. A second injection may be repeated in approximately 3 weeks if symptoms fail to improve or if they recur during this period.

The prognosis is variable and depends to a large extent on the patient's activities. Tennis elbow may recur even in patients who are conscientious about their activity. If symptoms recur or fail to respond promptly to treatment, an orthopedic consultation is indicated. Surgery may occasionally be required (13). The type of surgery depends on the problem, and occasionally a return to the vigorous activity that precipitated the problems may not be possible.

Prevention

Prevention of tennis elbow requires conditioning of the muscle groups in the forearm and wrist through an exercise program. This program often must be specialized, and a physical therapist should be consulted. Often the use of a tennis elbow strap (available at sports stores) in the area of the muscle mass of the proximal portion of the forearm is helpful because it decreases strain of the common extensor origin at the lateral epicondyle. Racket size, weight, and tension can also be a factor, along with proper technique (avoid using wrist motion at ball impact).

Medial Epicondylitis (Golfer's Elbow)

Definition and Mechanism of Injury

Medial epicondylitis of the elbow is caused by inflammation of the tissues in the area of the medial epicondyle (Fig. 67.14) where the muscles that flex and pronate the wrist originate. It is caused by overuse of these muscles.

This problem is less common than tennis elbow and is seen in people performing repetitive pronation exercises, as occur in golf, or in people who carry things with their elbows flexed.

Symptoms and Signs

The manifestations of this problem are similar to those of tennis elbow except that the location is in the area of the medial, rather than the lateral, epicondyle. The inflammation in this area can involve the ulnar nerve, so a careful neurologic examination is required. With ulnar neuritis, splinting and rest are the treatment of choice and an orthopedist should be consulted.

Treatment, Prognosis, and Prevention

These aspects are similar to those of tennis elbow.

SPRAINS AND AVULSION FRACTURES

Definition and Mechanism of Injury

A *strain* is defined as overstretching a muscle, although it sometimes is applied also to a tendon or ligament, without actual disruption of tissue. Strains occur during mild stress, as when one overuses muscle groups that have not been exercised regularly. The pain of muscle strain resolves after 1 or 2 days.

A *sprain* is defined as a partial or complete rupture of the fibers of a ligament, as well as a stress injury to the joint capsule.

Avulsion fractures occur when the ligament is strong and it does not rupture, but a chip of bone is avulsed from the insertion of the ligament. These injuries are most common around the ankle, knee, elbow, and fingers. Violent muscle action in athletes, especially adolescents, may avulse a traction epiphysis (apophysis), usually at one of three sites on the pelvis: anterior superior iliac spine from sartorius avulsion, anterior inferior iliac spine from rectus femoris avulsion, and ischial tuberosity from avulsion of the hamstring (Fig. 67.16). Also, injuries to the joint capsules and ligaments of the fingers are particularly common.

As described for ligament injuries above, strains and sprains are classified as grade I, grade II, or grade III depending on the amount of fiber involvement and the amount of instability created. Grade I injuries generally involve minor stretching or tearing of small numbers of fibers. Symptoms are usually minimal. Grade II injuries involve more tissue tearing and increased laxity is present. Grade III injuries involve complete tissue tearing and significant instability.

Sprains and related injuries of the ligaments of the knees and ankles are discussed above.

Sprains and avulsion fractures result from sudden forceful muscle contraction and are common in athletes.

Symptoms and Signs

The hallmark of a sprain or avulsion fracture is pain in the area of the injury. Physical examination reveals swelling and stiffness of the involved joint, with increased pain as the patient attempts to use it.

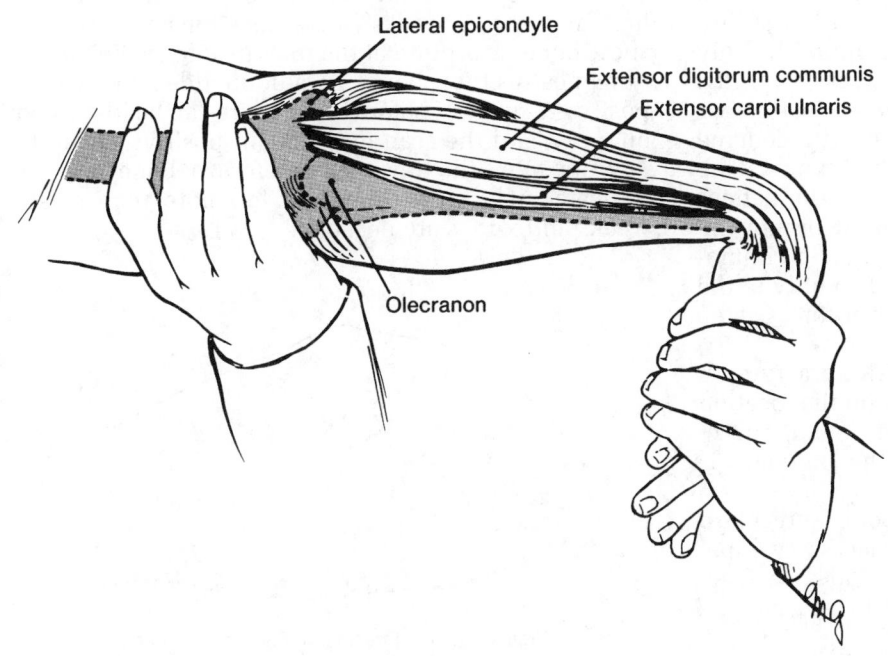

Lateral epicondyle
Extensor digitorum communis
Extensor carpi ulnaris
Olecranon

Figure 67.15. Test for tennis elbow. The wrist is extended against resistance from a fully flexed position and the patient notices pain at the lateral epicondyle. This usually mimics the patient's symptoms if the diagnosis is correct.

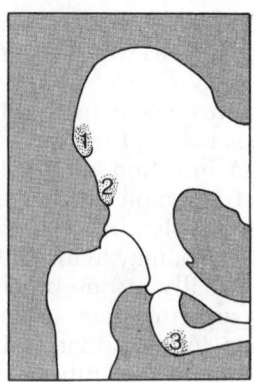

Figure 67.16. Common sites of avulsion fracture: *1,* anterior superior iliac spine; *2,* anterior inferior iliac spine; and *3,* ischial tuberosity.

The joint may be unstable if the ligament rupture is complete. Maximal swelling and tenderness are usually localized at the area of the sprain or fracture, especially if it is superficial, as in the ankle, knee, or finger.

Additional Evaluation

X-rays of an injured area must be done to establish the diagnosis of an avulsion fracture.

If joint instability is found on examination, a consultation from an orthopedic surgeon should be requested. Also, stress x-rays, especially of the ankle, knee, and finger, are often done by the orthopedic surgeon under local or general anesthesia to evaluate the degree of instability of the joints.

Treatment and Prognosis

The initial treatment of sprains or avulsion fractures consists of immobilization of the area with a splint, elevation, and application of ice for approximately 15 minutes several times a day to decrease swelling, and the prescription of analgesics such as aspirin or acetaminophen alone or in combination with codeine 30 to 60 mg or oxycodone 5 mg, every 4 to 6 hours. If the injury is in the area of the ankle or knee, the patient must keep his or her weight off the injured joint by the use of crutches (see above). A finger should be immobilized for no more than 3 weeks and then only in the position of function to avoid permanent stiffness of the joints (Fig. 67.17).

The prognosis for sprains and avulsion fractures is variable and depends to a large extent on the location of the injury; with proper treatment and subsequent conditioning of the patient, the outcome is generally good.

Surgical intervention by the orthopedic surgeon to repair joint instability is occasionally necessary, especially in injuries in the area of the ankle and knee. Even after surgery, an athlete is often unable to return to the activity that resulted in the injury.

Prevention

The prevention of sprains and avulsion fractures requires proper conditioning, especially by the performance of stretching exercises (see below) before exertion and the use of proper foot gear and protective equipment.

STRESS FRACTURES

Definition and Mechanism of Injury

A stress fracture is a hairline crack, sometimes minute, that can occur in almost any bone that has been repetitively subjected to impact. The most common sites of stress fractures are the metatarsal shafts, especially the second and third metatarsals, the distal fibula, the proximal tibia, and the symphysis pubis. However, stress fractures may occur in other bones, such as the lumbar vertebrae, the sacroiliac joint, the distal femur, the femoral neck (8), the tarsal navicula (19), the distal aspect of the tibia, the lateral malleolus, and the pubis ramus (14). The most serious stress fracture involves the femoral neck.

Stress fractures occur most commonly from walking or running, usually when an athlete has tried to do too much too fast, used improper shoes, or exercised on hard surfaces. Stress fractures occur in both poorly conditioned and highly conditioned people.

Symptoms and Signs

A patient who has sustained a stress fracture notices the gradual onset of aching of the affected bone during or just after exercising. Examination reveals localized tenderness and occasional swelling.

Additional Evaluation

The diagnosis depends on the symptoms and signs because x-rays of the affected area are usually normal at first; after 2 to 4 weeks (sometimes longer) they may show bone resorption at the fracture site or the formation of callus (new bone). A radionuclide bone scan is positive, however, before the fracture can be identified on x-ray, and the scan may remain positive for up to 2 years after the injury. Therefore a bone scan is indicated if symptoms persist for more than a few weeks and x-rays are negative.

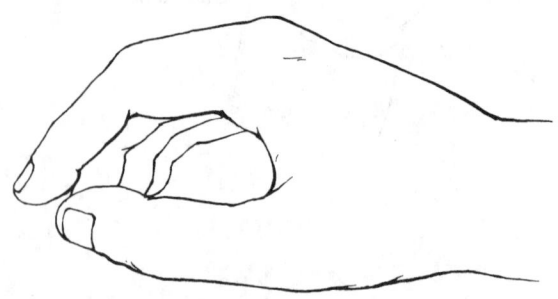

Figure 67.17.   Position of function of fingers.

Differential Diagnosis

Tibial stress fractures may be confused with pes anserinus bursitis, shin splints, and bone tumors, especially osteoid osteoma. If there is uncertainty about the correct diagnosis, a consultation should be requested from an orthopedist.

Treatment and Prognosis

The treatment of stress fractures involves complete immobilization of the injured part in a splint. If the injury is in a lower extremity, the patient should not bear weight on it. The injured part should also be elevated, and ice should be applied initially for approximately 15 minutes several times a day until the swelling subsides, which usually occurs in 24 to 36 hours. After the swelling has subsided, heat may be applied for 15 minutes several times a day; this should be discontinued if the discomfort is made more severe, which occasionally occurs. Pain should be controlled with aspirin or acetaminophen alone or combined with codeine 30 to 60 mg or oxycodone 5 mg, every 4 to 6 hours as needed.

Metatarsal stress fractures should be treated initially with a cast, which should be left on 4 to 8 weeks. (If the physician is unfamiliar with the application of a short leg cast, referral to an orthopedist is indicated.) What appears to be a stress fracture of the proximal fifth metatarsal may actually be a Jones fracture. It is important for the general physician to recognize a Jones fracture because of an 80% nonunion rate. The fracture often occurs in athletes and usually there is a history of trauma. The fracture is transverse and occurs at the metaphyseal/diaphyseal junction. A non–weight-bearing short leg cast is applied for approximately 8 weeks. If healing has not occurred by that time, the patient should be referred to an orthopedic surgeon. In most of those cases, surgical screw fixation is usually recommended (12). Stress fractures of the tibia and fibula require more prolonged periods of immobilization and may require a cast for 12 weeks or longer. All patients with suspected stress fractures of the tibia or fibula should be seen by an orthopedist. Patients who can bear weight without symptoms may be treated with rest of the injured extremity and avoidance of impact loading. The risk in stress fracture treatment is that the fracture will become a complete fracture and in areas such as the tibial shaft, femoral neck, and femoral shaft, these stress fractures can require surgical stabilization if they become complete.

With proper treatment and appropriate conditioning, the prognosis is excellent and most patients are able to return to normal sports activities. Occasionally bone grafting is required to obtain healing.

Prevention

Prevention of stress fractures requires proper conditioning with preexercise stretching, proper footwear, and avoidance of hard surfaces and too rapid acceleration of physical activity.

STRETCHING EXERCISES

It has been pointed out that the occurrence (and recurrence) of some of the problems described in this chapter may be prevented by several measures: selecting good shoes (see Chapter 102 for a description), not increasing the amount of stress on the musculoskeletal system too rapidly, and stretching the major muscle groups of the lower extremity before participating in sports. Four stretching exercises that may be helpful if practiced routinely are illustrated in Figure 67.18. Each exercise should be done for both sides for 15 to 30 seconds each for a few minutes before engaging in sports activities.

ARTHROSCOPY

Arthroscopic technique has progressed rapidly over the last 20 years and has greatly improved methods of diagnosis and treatment of joint problems.

Arthroscopic evaluation can now be carried out effectively in the hip, knee, ankle, shoulder, elbow, and wrist. Surgical techniques through the arthroscope often enable the orthopedist to avoid opening of the joint (arthrotomy). When arthrotomy is required, recovery time, rehabilitation, and complications are increased tremendously. To evaluate the interior of a joint, the arthroscope is fitted with fiberoptic light cables to illuminate and multiple lenses to identify and magnify all intra-articular structures.

Arthroscopy has had its greatest advances, both diagnostic and therapeutic, in the knee. Arthroscopy of the knee is indicated for diagnostic purposes in acute injury or chronic knee pain where diagnosis has been difficult. The ligaments, articular cartilage, synovium, bony surfaces, and menisci can be accurately evaluated. Often meniscal injuries can be treated with partial meniscectomy or cartilage repair arthroscopically. Ligament reconstruction is performed with arthroscopic assistance to decrease morbidity and shorten rehabilitation.

Also, the hip can be viewed arthroscopically; loose body removal and synovial biopsy have been performed in the hip. The joint capsules in the hip and wrist are small and somewhat tight, but as instrumentation advances arthroscopy is expected to have a larger role in evaluating and treating problems in these joints.

The ankle has long been a difficult joint in which to diagnose intra-articular pathology because the joint capsule is smaller and tighter. Nevertheless, an experienced arthroscopic surgeon can adequately evaluate and treat various ankle problems. Chronic ankle pain has been treated effectively with arthroscopic synovectomy. Osteochondritis dissecans (transchondral talar dome fractures), loose bodies, chondromalacia, rheumatologic disorders, and infections have all been evaluated or treated in the ankle joint using arthroscopic methods. More recently, arthroscopic techniques have been applied to lateral instability and ankle fusions.

Arthroscopy has also been applied to the upper

extremity in the shoulder, elbow, and wrist. In the shoulder joint, arthroscopy allows complete evaluation of the humeral head, glenoid, rotator cuff, anterior stabilizing structures, and subacromial space. Many athletes with vague shoulder complaints and nonspecific physical findings can be placed on proper rehabilitation or treatment programs after arthroscopic evaluation. Other areas where arthroscopy can be useful include the arthritides, dislocations, subluxations, loose bodies, rotator cuff lesions, labral tears, and frozen shoulders. Newer operative techniques allow subacromial decompression and anterior shoulder stabilization procedures to be performed arthroscopically. These procedures reduce recovery time and postoperative rehabilitation dramatically because the musculature surrounding the shoulder (deltoid, pecto-

ralis major, supraspinatus, infraspinatus) is not disrupted, as it is with open techniques.

The elbow offers fewer diagnostic and therapeutic problems amenable to arthroscopic techniques. The ulnar, median, and radial nerves are in close proximity to the joint capsule, and anatomic knowledge is critical. The anterior and posterior compartments of the elbow can be evaluated with the arthroscope. The greatest value of arthroscopy of the elbow is in the diagnosis and treatment of loose bodies, osteochondrotic lesions, or an articular cartilage problem.

Arthroscopy of the wrist is also advancing, and patients with subtle carpal instabilities, chronic pain, and small chondral fractures have been diagnosed and treated by arthroscopy.

Arthroscopy is a surgical procedure and com-

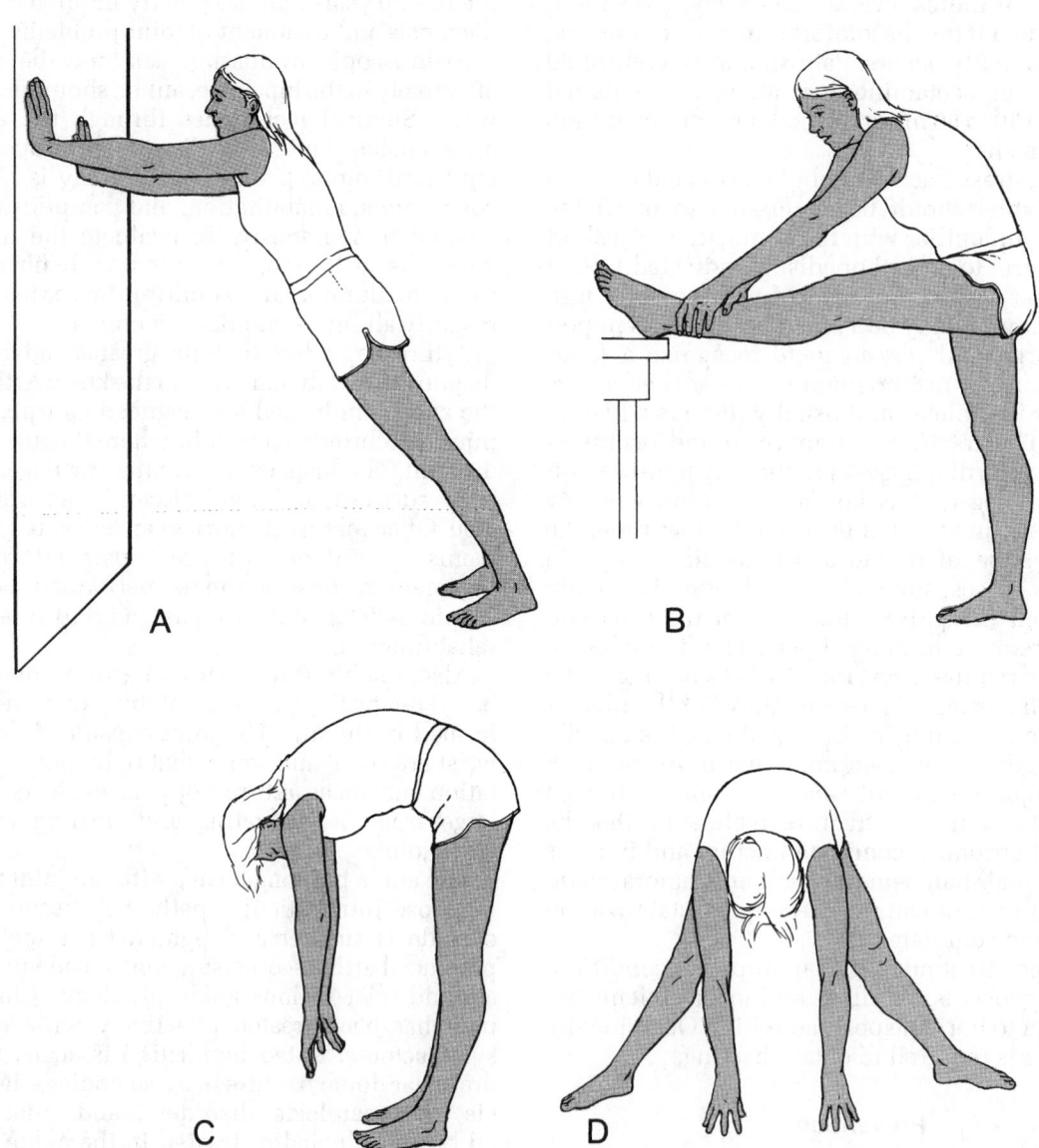

Figure 67.18. **A**. Stretch the Achilles tendon by leaning forward with the feet flat and placed at least 4 feet from the wall. **B**. Stretch the hamstring and gastrocnemius muscle groups by elevating the leg and bending forward as far as possible. **C**. Stretch the ham-string and back muscles by touching the toes slowly; bouncing should be avoided. **D**. Stretch the adductor muscle by gradually spreading the legs as far apart as possible; place the fingers on the floor for support.

plications may occur. These complications include iatrogenic damage to intra-articular or extra-articular structures, hemarthrosis, thrombophlebitis, infection, synovial fistula, reflex sympathetic dystrophy, and instrument breakage (leaving intra-articular fragments).

Although arthroscopy is not a panacea for all sports injuries, there are many advantages to arthroscopic techniques, especially in the athlete. As noted above, there is greatly reduced postoperative morbidity, and patients can often return to work or the playing field quickly. This is because of a decreased inflammatory response, smaller incisions, less disruption of muscles and other tissues, and decreased immobilization. Arthroscopy improves diagnostic capabilities, especially in the athlete with troublesome symptoms and a nonspecific physical examination. The complication rate, length of hospital stay, and even pain are often less than with open procedures. In addition, in many areas the arthroscope provides a better view of intra-articular structures and pathology than open surgery provides.

Anterior cruciate ligament reconstructions are often done using arthroscopic techniques. This allows inspection of the menisci for tears because there is a 35 to 76% incidence with anterior cruciate ligament tears. Inspection of the articular cartilage helps determine whether arthritis is involved, and the ligaments can also be visualized to help determine the extent of the tear (partial versus complete) (3).

Patient Experience. Arthroscopy may be accomplished using local, regional, or general anesthesia. The arthroscope is usually 3 to 5 mm in width and is inserted through a stab wound in the joint. A sterile solution is infused to irrigate and distend the joint. (Therefore, in serious injury in which the joint capsule is disrupted, arthroscopy is difficult or even contraindicated because the fluid may dissect out of the joint into the tissue of the leg.) The procedure may be accomplished in 30 to 45 minutes. After the procedure the patient should rest the joint (and not bear weight) for 2 to 3 days. Mild analgesics for a few days are usually necessary to relieve discomfort.

General References

American Academy of Orthopaedic Surgeons. Knee braces: seminar report. Chicago: American Academy of Orthopaedic Surgeons, 1985.
> A report that extensively reviews all types of knee braces: their indications, functions, and costs. Prepared by the Sports Medicine Committee of the AAOS.

Crenshaw AH, ed. Campbell's operative orthopaedics. 8th ed. St. Louis: CV Mosby, 1992.
> A standard surgically oriented text.

Leadbetter WB, Buckwater JA, Gordon SL. Sports-induced inflammation: clinical and basic science concepts. Naperville, IL: American Academy of Orthopaedic Surgeons, 1992.
> This book discusses fundamental principles of athletic injuries as viewed from many different perspectives.

McGinty JB, Caspari RB, Jackson RW, Poehling GG. Operative arthroscopy. New York: Raven Press, 1991.
> An excellent description of arthroscopic indications and techniques.

Minhoff J, Sherman OH, eds. Arthroscopy. Clin Sports Med 6(3), July 1987.
> A collection of review articles covering arthroscopic procedures in the knee, ankle, wrist, elbow, and shoulder.

Nordin M, Andersson GBJ, Pope MC, eds. Musculoskeletal disorders in the workplace: principles and practice. St. Louis: CV Mosby, 1997.
> Very detailed and valuable text.

Paty JG. Diagnosis and treatment of musculoskeletal running injuries. Semin Arthritis Rheum 18(1), August 1988.
> Good review of the biomechanics, physical examination, injury types, and treatment of running injuries.

Rockwood CA Jr, Green DP, Bucholz RW, Heckman JD. Fractures in adults. 4th ed. Philadelphia: JB Lippincott, 1996.
> An excellent description of knee ligament and cartilage injuries including history, diagnosis, and treatment.

Specific References

1. Allen PR, Denhan RA, Swan AV. Late degenerative changes after meniscectomy. Factors affecting the knee after operation. J Bone Joint Surg 66B:666, 1984.
2. Berger RG. Nonsteroidal anti-inflammatory drugs: making the right choices. J Am Acad Ortho Surg 2(5):255–260, 1994.
3. Buss DD, Warren RF, Wickiewicz TL, et al. Arthroscopically assisted reconstruction of the anterior cruciate ligament with use of autogenous patellar-ligament grafts. Results after 24 to 42 months. J Bone Joint Surg 75-A(9):1346–1355, 1993.
4. Cues JV III. Magnetic resonance imaging of sports injury. Techn Orthop 7:71, 1992.
5. Fadale PD, Wiggins ME. Corticosteroid injections: their use and abuse. J Am Acad Orthop Surg 2(3):133–140, 1994.
6. Fairbank TJ. Knee joint changes after meniscectomy. J Bone Joint Surg 30B:644, 1948.
7. Ficat RP, Hungerford DS. Disorders of the patello-femoral joint. Baltimore: Williams & Wilkins, 1977.
8. Fullerton LR, Snowdy HA. Femoral neck stress fractures. Am J Sports Med 16:365, 1988.
9. Grana WA. Runner's injury. Techn Orthop 5:64, 1990.
10. Insall J. Chondromalacia patellae. J Bone Joint Surg 58A:1, 1976.
11. Jackson DW, Jennings LD, Maywood RM, Berger PE. Magnetic resonance imaging of the knee. Am J Sports Med 16:29, 1988.
12. Mindrebo N, Shelbourne KD, vanMeter CD, Rettig AC. Outpatient percutaneous screw fixation of the acute Jones fracture. Am J Sports Med 21(5):720–723, 1993.
13. Nirschl RP, Pettrone FA. Tennis elbow. The surgical treatment of lateral epicondylitis. J Bone Joint Surg 61A:832, 1979.
14. Pavlov H, Nelson TL, Warren RF, et al. Stress fractures of the pubic ramus. J Bone Joint Surg 64A:1020, 1982.
15. Rovene GD, Clarke TS, Yates CS, Burley K. Retrospective comparison of taping and ankle stabilizers in preventing ankle injuries. Am J Sports Med 16:228, 1988.
16. Slocum DB. The shin splint syndrome: medical aspects and differential diagnosis. Am J Surg 114:875, 1967.
17. Slocum DB, Larson RL. Rotatory instability of the knee. J Bone Joint Surg 50A:211, 1968.
18. Teitz CC, Henmarson BK, Krommal RA, Diehr PH. Evaluation of the use of braces to prevent injury to the knee in college football players. J Bone Joint Surg 69A:2, 1987.
19. Torg JS, Pavlov H, Cooley LH, et al. Stress fractures of the tarsal navicular. J Bone Joint Surg 64A:700, 1982.

C H A P T E R 68

Osteoarthritis

ALEXANDER S. TOWNES, MD

The common occurrence, the chronic and often benign course, and the lack of definitive treatment of osteoarthritis or degenerative joint disease have generated a general apathy and disinterest on the part of many physicians about this disease. A common attitude among patients is that this form of arthritis is an inevitable consequence of aging and must be accepted as such. Advances in understanding of the pathophysiology of osteoarthritis, especially in the past decade, have accomplished a great deal in dispelling these undeserved attitudes. As a result, a better perspective of the multiple etiologic factors potentially involved in this disease and a better understanding of the clinical problems presented by patients with this disorder have developed.

Osteoarthritis is particularly important to the general physician who sees ambulatory adult patients. Estimates indicate that approximately half of all visits to physicians for joint disease are for this diagnosis. Osteoarthritis is the most common arthritis diagnosed in a general practice (49). It accounts for as much physical disability in the lower extremity as any other disease diagnosis (33). The economic impact of disease-specific indirect and nonmedical costs of the disease are substantial, as demonstrated in a controlled community-based sample (29).

PREVALENCE

Prevalence of osteoarthritis increases with advancing age, beginning perhaps as early as the third decade of life and being almost ubiquitous as detected by radiography or biochemical changes in articular cartilage in the seventh and eighth decades and beyond. It is fortunate and important, however, that clinical symptoms are not necessarily associated with structural changes, so estimates of prevalence based on these findings exceed the magnitude of the clinical problem. Thus, symptoms and clinical findings of degenerative joint disease are not an inevitable accompaniment of aging. However, symptoms and findings are uncommon below age 35 and are more common above age 65, with perhaps as much as 30 to 40% of the population aged 65 and above having some symptoms related to this diagnosis. A survey of osteoarthritis of the knee in subjects aged 63 to 94 indicated an increasing prevalence of radiographic evidence of osteoarthritis with age to the level of 44% of subjects aged 80 or older and a higher proportion of symptomatic disease in women (11%) than in men (7%) (23). New onset of radiographic and symptomatic osteoarthritis of the knee continued to develop in elderly patients at the rate of 1 to 2% per year, again more in women than in men (26).

PATHOPHYSIOLOGY

The pathogenesis of osteoarthritis is multifactorial (20); however, the final common pathway is believed to be injury to articular cartilage, which then undergoes a sequence of changes resulting eventually in progressive depletion of the collagen and proteoglycan matrix and proliferation of underlying bone with osteophyte formation. Under normal conditions, chondrocytes regulate the extracellular matrix with a balance between the synthesis of its structural components and their degradation. In osteoarthritis there is a disequilibrium between the degradation and repair processes, with abnormal production of metalloproteases, collagenase, cytokines, and growth factors so that the structure is weakened and damage occurs. Susceptibility to cartilage damage increases with age and may be the result of abnormal biomechanics leading to excessive stress or defective matrix components and alteration of the normal structure. Impact loading and repetitive stress are more important than frictional wear. Changes are most severe in or may be confined entirely to areas of maximal stress on the articular cartilage, most striking in weight-bearing areas of the large joints. Synovitis is usually minimal in the early stages but may contribute to joint damage in advanced disease. Change in the hardness of bone as a result of microfractures and loss of ability of cartilage to absorb stress as a primary mechanism in osteoarthritis has also been proposed (59). The role of bone in the progression of the disease has also been suggested by observations that dietary intake and serum levels of vitamin D may predispose to progression of osteoarthritis in the elderly (50). The increased prevalence of disease in women and the progression sometimes seen after menopause also suggests the possibility of hormonal influences that are as yet poorly understood. Crystalline deposits of calcium pyrophosphate, hydroxyapatite, or basic calcium salts may play a role in the synovial inflammatory response (38) or destructive arthropathy (19) in certain patients, especially those with more advanced osteoarthritis (38) (see Chapter 69).

Because there are no nerve fibers in articular cartilage, no symptoms are caused by early changes in the joints. There are multiple sources of pain, however, as the disease progresses. Periosteal irritation as a result of proliferating bone, denuded bone, compression of soft tissues by osteophytes in confined spaces, microfractures of subchondral bone, stress on ligaments as a result of loss of cartilage and joint incongruity, low-grade synovitis, effusion, and spasm of surrounding muscles are all potential sources of pain in osteoarthritis.

CAUSES AND PREDISPOSING FACTORS

The precise cause of osteoarthritis is unknown. It is likely that there are multiple causes and many factors that may influence disease expression, some of which are listed in Table 68.1.

Because of multiple etiologic mechanisms in the

Table 68.1. Factors Contributing to Development of Osteoarthritis

Aging
Diminished proteoglycan aggregation
Diminished resistance of cartilage to fatigue fracture (?defective collagen network)
Decreased resiliency of soft tissues
Loss of normal anatomic relationship (hip)

Heredity
Heberden's nodes
Primary generalized osteoarthritis (female gender)
Postural or developmental defects (e.g., scoliosis, slipped capital femoral epiphyses, Legg–Calvé–Perthes disease)
Procollagen gene (COL2A1) defects
Metabolic defects (ochronosis, Wilson's disease)

Abnormal Distribution of Mechanical Stress
Postural or developmental defects
Joint instability or hypermobility
Local incongruity of joint surfaces posttraumatic, after meniscectomy, prolonged immobilization
Obesity

Excessive Repetitive Stress
Occupational
Sports related
Associated with neuropathy

Crystalline Deposit Disease
Calcium pyrophosphate
Hydroxyapatite

Previous Inflammatory Joint Disease

Metabolic Abnormalities
Ochronosis
Wilson's disease
Acromegaly

pathogenesis of osteoarthritis, the history should seek to determine specific factors that may be implicated in each patient. Heredity is clearly important, with influence on some patterns of disease development more evident than others, for example in the hands and knees of women (66) but not in the hips (72). A family history of onset in the fourth or fifth decades of osteoarthritis in the proximal and distal interphalangeal joints is often associated with the development of generalized osteoarthritis. However, development of distal joint involvement (Heberden's nodes) in older patients is likely to be benign and result in little functional impairment in the aging hand (55). Drawing attention of patients with the new appearance of bony enlargements of the distal joints to the occurrence of this abnormality in elderly family members and its benign course may reassure them.

Hereditary abnormalities in structural components of cartilage have also been implicated in the development of osteoarthritis. A syndrome, inherited as a mendelian dominant, is related to a single base mutation in the type II procollagen gene (COL2A1) resulting in mild chondrodysplasia and premature osteoarthritis, often in the fourth decade (1). Type II collagen is a major structural protein in articular cartilage and important in maintaining its integrity during mechanical stress. Further studies indicate that this is probably a rare cause of osteoarthritis (61). Although osteoarthritis may dominate the clinical picture, evidence of mild, often late-onset spondyloepiphysial dysplasia is evident. Whether heterogeneity or mutations of alleles of this or other genes coding for cartilage matrix constituents may play a role in predisposition to cartilage injury in other forms of osteoarthritis remains to be determined. Additional studies searching for genetic defects in collagen or proteoglycan have so far been nonproductive (47), but further research is needed.

Obesity is an obvious risk factor for osteoarthritis, but its extent and duration are important in assessing potential damage to weight-bearing joints, especially the knees. The association of obesity with osteoarthritis of the hands suggests the possibility of influences other than mechanical factors (13). Preceding trauma may be important in subsequent development of degenerative arthritis in a joint damaged by ligamentous instability or meniscal tear in the knee joint. Traumatic episodes with sufficient damage to induce these abnormalities are likely to be severe enough to be recalled, for example, as severe sprains with swelling lasting several days or longer after a sports-related or other injury. Jogging without preceding injury or joint pain does not significantly predispose to osteoarthritis (54). Moreover, people regularly engaging in vigorous running or other aerobic activities have lower mortality rates and slower development of disability than the general population (28). Studies in elite female athletes indicate a mild increase in prevalence of radiographic osteoarthritis in hips and knees (67). Males engaging in mixed sports and power sports were more at risk than those in endurance sports and at an earlier age (45). In a prospective study of elderly patients in their seventies, the risk of development of knee osteoarthritis was higher in patients with a high level of physical activity than in those who were remarkably sedentary (25). However, in a careful study of 462 randomly selected community volunteers over age 65, lesser strength in the quadriceps muscle significantly correlated with radiographic and symptomatic osteoarthritis of the knee, suggesting that quadriceps weakness may be a risk factor for developing osteoarthritis of the knee (9,65). Postural defects with abnormal distribution of stress (e.g., valgus or varus knee deformities) induce osteoarthritic changes at the site of weight bearing. Prior joint surgery with removal of a meniscus in the knee is also a predisposing factor to osteoarthritis of the knee, with age over 35 at the time of surgery a major risk factor (53). Thus, repetitive stress and minor trauma may predispose to development of osteoarthritis, and may account for osteoarthritis at sites not commonly affected (e.g., elbows of baseball pitchers and upper limbs of air hammer operators). Because abnormalities such as varus or valgus deformities of the knees may also occur as a result of osteoarthritic damage to the joint, the history is important in determining which came first.

Osteoarthritis may also be associated with other disease states: preceding inflammatory arthritis; metabolic diseases, such as ochronosis, with deposition of metabolites in cartilage; diseases predisposing to chondrocalcinosis, such as hemochromatosis and hyperparathyroidism; and acromegaly.

GENERAL CLINICAL FEATURES

History

Characteristically, one or a few joints are involved in osteoarthritis. Joints commonly affected and those usually spared are shown in Table 68.2. Because the presentations of patients may differ, depending on the pattern of joints involved and predisposing factors, some of these presenting symptoms are highlighted separately after a general discussion of the symptoms and findings in this disease.

Osteoarthritis usually begins insidiously and progresses slowly. Aching discomfort early in the course characteristically increases in severity with use of the joint; therefore, it tends to reach a peak after the activity of the day and is relieved by rest. Pain is often aching in character and may be difficult for the patient to localize precisely. It is usually felt in the areas surrounding the involved joint. However, hip pain may be referred to the medial aspect of the thigh, the lateral portion of the buttock, or the knee. Morning stiffness and stiffness after rest may be absent, or if present may last only 15 to 20 minutes or less, in contrast to a longer duration in inflammatory joint disease such as rheumatoid arthritis. However, in advanced disease stiffness may be more profound, and pain may occur at rest. When joint destruction is marked, the patient may be kept awake at night by the pain.

As the disease progresses, large pieces of degenerated cartilage may shed into the joint, producing loose

Table 68.2.   Distribution of Joint Involvement in Osteoarthritis

Commonly Affected
Hands
  Distal interphalangeal (Heberden's nodes)
  Proximal interphalangeal (Bouchard's nodes)
  Carpometacarpal of the thumb (joints between first metacarpal and greater multangular and between greater multangular and navicular)
Knees
Hips
Spine
  Cervical
  Lumbar
  Thoracic
Feet
  Metatarsophalangeal (especially first)

Usually Spared
Ankles
Hands
  Metacarpophalangeal
  Carpometacarpal (except first)
Wrists
Elbows
Shoulders

bodies that may cause the joint to lock or give way.

There are no systemic symptoms in osteoarthritis. This is an important negative feature of the history that helps differentiate this disease from other forms of arthritis.

The influence of psychologic factors on the level of pain and disability is an important consideration in evaluation and treatment of the patient with osteoarthritis. A study of patients with symptoms and objective clinical findings of osteoarthritis of the hip and knee demonstrate that psychologic variables account for a far greater percentage of the variation observed in both functional impairment and severity of pain than do objective estimates of disease severity (69). Thus in osteoarthritis, as in other chronic diseases in which chronic pain may occur, it is essential in taking the history to learn as much as possible about the patient and his or her environment to appropriately interpret findings and plan the most effective approach to treatment.

Physical Findings

Early in the disease there may be no physical findings. Most patients who have symptoms have some pain on passive motion of the involved joints or on motion against resistance. There is often a sense of crackling or crepitus as the joint is moved, probably caused by joint surface incongruities and irregularities of opposing cartilaginous or bony surfaces. Crepitus may be exaggerated by movement with weight bearing or by manual compression of the joint during movement (e.g., compression of the patella against the condyle of the femur when patellofemoral arthritis is present). In patients with painful knees, crepitus transmitted to the tibia during a stress maneuver, although not a sensitive test, was able to localize the affected compartment of the joint with surprising specificity in disease of the medial and lateral compartments of the knee as assessed by direct observation with needle arthroscopy (39). In more advanced disease, joint motion may be limited and gross deformities may develop. Tenderness along the joint line is common but may be mild or absent. In contrast to most inflammatory joint diseases, soft tissue swelling is usually absent or minimal in osteoarthritis except in its most advanced stages. Bony enlargement and irregularity are common, especially in the hands at the distal interphalangeal joints (Heberden's nodes) and less commonly in the proximal interphalangeal joints (Bouchard's nodes). Joint effusions are uncommon compared with more inflammatory forms of joint disease. However, they may occur, especially in the knees. There is usually no detectable heat or redness over involved joints, although some warmth may be present as the disease progresses and chronic synovitis develops. With involvement of the hip or knee, gait may be altered and patients may be noted to have a noticeable limp.

Physical examination of the patient with osteoarthritis should always include a careful evaluation of the anatomically relevant components of the neurologic system, peripheral vascular system, and soft tissues because disease in these systems may produce pain or limited motion in an extremity that may be erroneously attributed to osteoarthritis (see "Diagnosis and Differential Diagnosis"). Because most of these patients are older, they often have other diseases concomitantly that may influence the interpretation of findings and influence decisions of management.

Laboratory Findings

Osteoarthritis is characterized by normal laboratory tests unless it is associated with some other disease process. In particular, acute phase reactants, including the erythrocyte sedimentation rate (ESR) and the C-reactive protein as usually measured, are characteristically normal, in contrast to the inflammatory arthritides. Mild and transient elevation of ESR may occasionally be associated with the acute inflammatory events described below or may be caused by intercurrent disease elsewhere. With the use of a highly sensitive radioimmunoassay to measure C-reactive protein, slight elevations were observed in patients with osteoarthritis and increased levels predicted progression of disease in a 4-year follow-up study (68). Recent efforts to measure products of cartilage breakdown show some promise but are not practical currently (46). Further research for a marker of disease activity or progression since assessment of preventive measures or treatment efficacy now requires long-term studies, which are difficult to accomplish (34).

Examination of synovial fluid is helpful when effusion is present in a large joint. Synovial fluid in osteoarthritis is usually of the noninflammatory type (i.e., white blood cells below 2000/mm^3 and, if performed, a protein content below 4 g/dL and glucose concentration approximately equal to a simultaneous serum glucose concentration; see Chapter 66, Table 66.1). A more inflammatory fluid with elevated white cell count may occur especially when crystals of calcium pyrophosphate or hydroxyapatite are present (see Chapter 69, Fig. 69.1 and Table 69.1).

Imaging

Radiographic findings, especially in the lower extremity, are important in the diagnosis and differential diagnosis of osteoarthritis because certain abnormalities are characteristic of this disorder. Therefore, plain x-rays of the affected joints are indicated in the evaluation of patients who have persistent symptoms to confirm the diagnosis and determine the extent of abnormalities present. An x-ray is always indicated if an effusion is present (e.g., in the knee) to be certain that an injury is not present. However, in early disease, x-rays may be normal, and even with characteristic findings of joint narrowing and proliferation of subchondral bone with spur formation, symptoms may be absent. Hence, the importance of relating radiographic findings to the history and physical examination cannot be overemphasized. Standard x-rays are commonly used as a measure of prevalence of disease or progression over time. A set of standard criteria of the degree of radiologic disease graded on a scale of 1 to 4 was developed by Kellgren and Lawrence (41) and is widely used in clinical and epidemiologic studies. In general, the more severe the radiographic changes, the more likely the patient is to have symptoms and findings of osteoarthritis. Radiographic findings from the earliest to the most advanced changes are listed in Table 68.3, and examples of x-rays are shown in Figure 68.1.

For evaluation of hands, a single anteroposterior (AP) view of both hands is sufficient in most cases. Both hips can be visualized on a single AP film of the pelvis; more specific films including laterals and obliques may be required if an abnormality is detected or if findings do not correlate with the clinical picture. AP and lateral films are required for adequate evaluation of the knee joint. Films made with the patient standing may better demonstrate advanced changes. Special views of the

Table 68.3. X-Ray Findings in Osteoarthritis

Earliest
No abnormality

Early
Slight loss of articular cartilage thickness (narrowing of radiologic joint space)

Moderate
Marginal osteophyte formation

Late
Loss of cartilage space (often focal in weight-bearing joints)
Sclerosis of subchondral bone
Subchondral cyst formation
Loose bodies
Subluxation or deformity

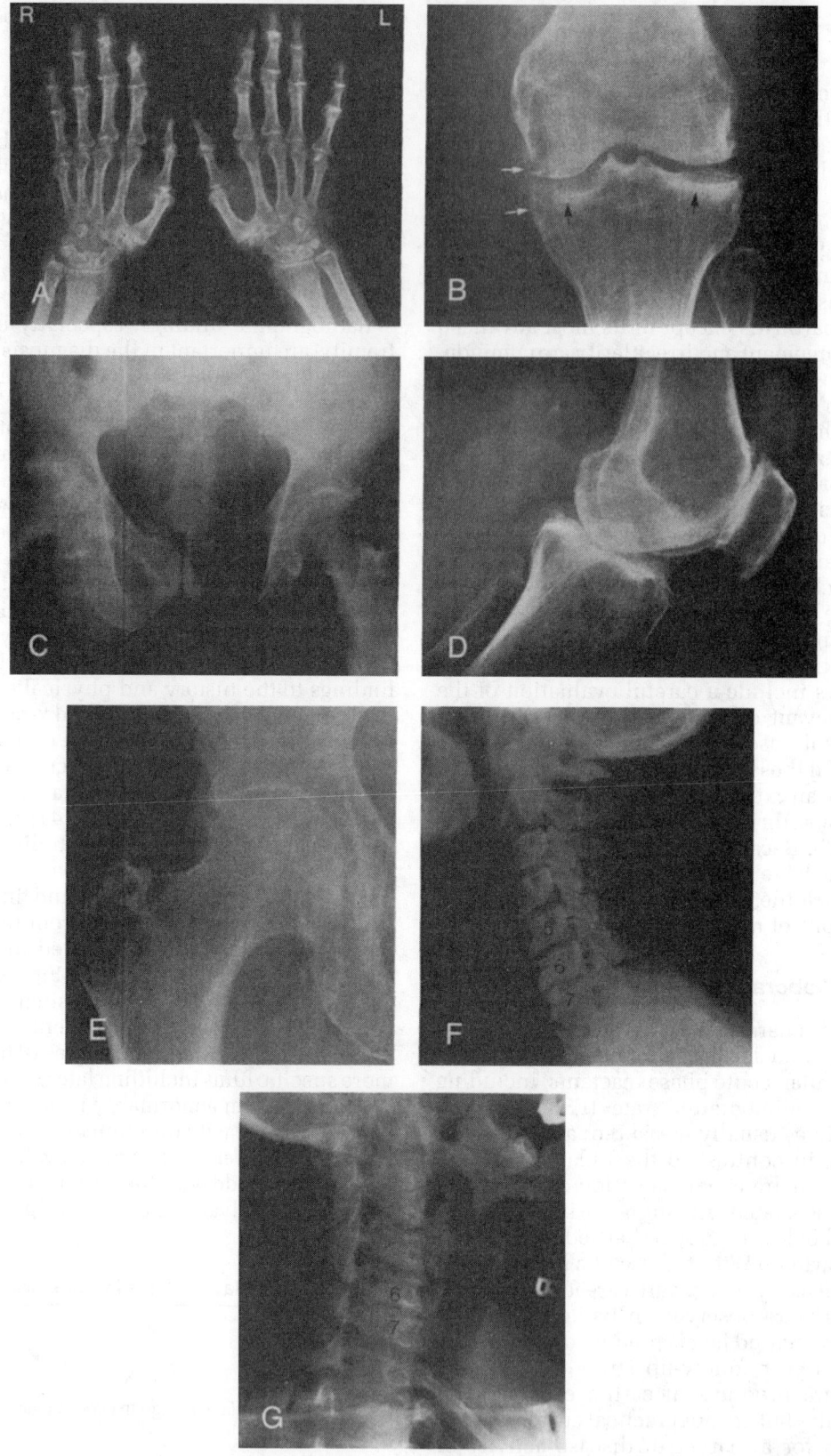

Figure 68.1. A. Hands of patient with degenerative joint disease. Note soft tissue enlargement on right over the second interphalangeal (DIP) joint (Heberden's node); the loss of joint space and bony proliferation of all DIP joints, especially 2 and 3 in the right hand and 3 in the left hand; involvement of carpometacarpal joint of both thumbs with narrowing and increased density of subchondral bone; and normal metacarpophalangeal joints and wrist joints. **B.** X-ray of knee showing degenerative joint disease with loss of joint space (cartilage) especially in medial compartment, sclerotic subchondral bone, subchondral cysts, and early marginal spurs especially on lateral side. **C.** Pelvic film of a patient with advanced degenerative joint disease in the right hip. Notice the joint space narrowing and proliferation of subchondral bone. The left hip shows the minimal change of marginal sclerosis. **D.** Lateral x-ray of same knee in **B** illustrating involvement of patellofemoral joint with narrowing and spur formation superiorly. **E.** X-ray of a hip showing early degenerative joint disease. Notice the narrowed joint space and spur formation of femoral head at upper margin of acetabulum. **F.** X-ray of the lateral cervical spine showing degenerative joint disease. Note narrowing of C5–6 and, especially, C6–7 interspace with anterior lipping and spur formation. **G.** Oblique x-ray view of cervical spine of same patient (**F**) showing osteophytes encroaching on neural foramina C5–6, C6–7.

patella (skyline view) may also be required to demonstrate the extent of patellofemoral arthritis. In evaluating the spine, AP, lateral, and oblique views are needed, the latter to visualize the neural foramina and the localization of nerve root compression by bony spurs.

In patients with degenerative disease of the spine, computerized tomography (CT) scans or magnetic resonance imaging (MRI) may demonstrate encroachment of osteophytes or disc material on nerve roots. MRI is particularly useful in delineating soft tissue detail (e.g., in differentiating the annulus fibrosus from the nucleus pulposus of the intervertebral disc). However, abnormal findings on CT scan and MRI in the absence of symptoms or equivocal findings despite significant symptoms and signs occur commonly. Thus, as with plain x-rays, careful correlation of findings with clinical symptoms is imperative. In general, CT and MRI scans and myelography are reserved for patients in whom conservative management has failed and in whom surgery or alternative causes of pain or radiculopathy are being strongly considered. It is usually advisable to consult with a rheumatologist or radiologist before deciding which of these procedures should be done.

CT and MRI scans can also demonstrate lesions in peripheral joints but should be used only as an adjunct to conventional radiography. MRI has all but replaced CT in specialized imaging of peripheral joints. It avoids CT radiation exposure and is particularly helpful in demonstrating soft tissue structures including cartilages, which are not shown on conventional x-rays. On the other hand, MRI may not show small calcific densities. Performance and interpretation of these procedures require experience and expertise. Because MRI may identify early changes, caution must be used in overinterpreting their usefulness in diagnosis and therapy (6). In moderate to severe disease, physical examination and routine x-rays provide sufficiently sensitive and specific information. For this reason and because of the expense of MRI procedures, they are best performed by the rheumatologist or orthopedic consultant on patients referred because of uncertain diagnosis or for consideration of arthroscopy or surgery after careful evaluation, including standard x-rays (32).

CLINICAL PATTERNS OF OSTEOARTHRITIS

Heberden's Nodes

These bony enlargements of the distal interphalangeal joints occur more often in women and commonly begin to appear in the fifth or sixth decade of life. They are often asymptomatic but a source of concern on the part of many patients, who may view them as an outward sign of aging or the beginning of a more serious and disabling arthritic disorder. This has been documented in two studies of elders in whom there was no correlation of osteoarthritis of the hands with objective measures of hand function, yet there was a definite correlation with subjective perception of functional limitation (5,55). Thus, one must be aware of and prepared to deal with the emotional investment of the patient who may focus concerns about declining functions on an obvious change in physical appearance such as Heberden's nodes. With a curt dismissal, no explanation of the true significance of this abnormality, and no opportunity for the patient to ventilate personal concerns, the physician misses an important therapeutic opportunity.

Primary Generalized Osteoarthritis

The term *primary generalized osteoarthritis* was applied by Kellgren and Moore (42) to a group of patients whom they characterized as having osteoarthritis involving the distal interphalangeal (DIP) and proximal interphalangeal joints (PIP) and the carpometacarpal joint of the thumb in addition to multiple other joints (hips, knees, metatarsophalangeal, and spine). The radiologic appearance of the involved joints is similar to the usual changes of osteoarthritis, but the pattern suggests this syndrome. This pattern of osteoarthritis affects mostly middle-age women who have a positive family history of a similar disorder of joint involvement. It is an uncommon pattern of osteoarthritis. Occasionally in early phases they have had some inflammatory symptoms with an elevated ESR and an episodic course. It is suggested that these patients constitute a subgroup of patients with a heritable form of osteoarthritis that involves multiple joints and perhaps has some distinctive radiologic features. It is important to recognize the syndrome clinically, primarily to differentiate it from rheumatoid arthritis and other polyarticular diseases (10).

Erosive Osteoarthritis of Hands

The term *erosive osteoarthritis* has been applied to patients with severe osteoarthritis of the hands (DIP and PIP joints) in which extensive erosion of subchondral bone occurs, with eventual deformity and some limitation of motion of the finger joints. These patients also may have episodes of acute inflammation in these joints and their surrounding tissues. X-rays reveal the extensive bony erosion and subchondral cyst formation that may be interpreted incorrectly as rheumatoid or gouty erosions. The distribution of involvement in DIP and first carpometacarpal joints, sparing the metacarpophalangeal joints and wrists, should easily establish the true nature of the process. From the clinical view, this syndrome is important because of the severity of symptoms and physical findings, which are uncommon in milder forms of osteoarthritis of the hands. Functional status is not as favorable as in patients with nodal disease without erosions, but is still surprisingly little affected (55).

Hip

Hip involvement is potentially the most painful and disabling joint abnormality in osteoarthritis. It is more often unilateral. Developmental defects in the structure of the hip, including congenital hip dysplasia, slipped capital femoral epiphysis, or unrecognized avascular necrosis, may have gone undetected but have predisposed the patient to develop osteoarthritis; with age, disturbance of the normal anatomic relationship between femoral head and acetabulum may also predispose to osteoarthritis. In contrast to osteoarthritis of the knee, obesity is not a major causal factor in osteoarthritis of the hip.

Pain, which early in the disease is associated with weight bearing and movement, may become severe even at rest, and night pain is common in advanced disease. Patients may walk with a limp or abnormal gait. Pain and limitation of motion during internal rotation and extension are early physical signs, and subsequently all motions may be painful and restricted. Clear identification of pain on motion of the hip is important in differentiating hip disease from bursitis (trochanteric and ischial; see Chapter 66), peripheral neuropathy (see Chapter 84), and other causes of pelvic pain (51). Flexion and adduction contracture and shortening may occur as disability progresses. Most patients who are symptomatic have characteristic changes of osteoarthritis on radiographic films of the hip. MRI may be useful to detect and differentiate early aseptic necrosis from osteoarthritis. Progression of osteoarthritis is variable but perhaps more likely to occur rapidly in the hip than in other joints.

Knee

The knee (see "Anatomic Relationships," Chapter 67, Fig. 67.1) is the most common symptomatic joint in osteoarthritis. Chronic and slowly progressive pain with ambulation is the hallmark. There is a definite relationship to obesity, and the weight-bearing areas of the medial compartment are most often involved. Patellofemoral joint involvement is also common. The causative role of obesity in the development of osteoarthritis of the knee has been clearly shown in epidemiologic studies. The association of obesity with osteoarthritis of the knee is stronger in women than in men, and the relative risk of osteoarthritis of the knee in obese African-American women is twice that of white women (2). In addition, evidence indicates that osteoarthritis of the knee is a consequence of and not a risk factor for obesity (17). Quadriceps muscle weakness was found to be a risk factor for knee osteoarthritis in both men and women over age 65 in both overweight and average-weight subjects (65).

Knee pain (especially with activities performed in flexion such as running or stair climbing) is a common symptom of *patellofemoral dysfunction*. This may arise from one or more factors resulting in abnormal knee mechanics (57) and may eventually lead to chondromalacia patellae (see Chapter 67, "Exercise-Related Musculoskeletal Problems"). One technique is useful in treating this problem. Forcing the patella medially with strong taping to hold it in place for a few days resulted in better tracking of and thereby relief of pressure on the lateral aspect of the patella with movement. This produced pain relief in a short-term

study of patients with patellofemoral arthritis with predominant changes in the lateral facet (16). Chondromalacia patellae usually occurs in younger people (second, third, and fourth decades), probably resulting from trauma and shearing forces against the patella as it contacts the femur in midflexion. Knee effusion is often associated with this syndrome. In younger patients with knee effusion who do not respond to rest or palliative aspiration (see Chapter 66), arthroscopy (see details in Chapter 67) may be indicated and shows characteristic changes. The relationship of this rather common syndrome to osteoarthritis is not entirely clear. Osteoarthritis of the patellofemoral joint may eventually develop in some cases.

Spinal Syndromes

Osteoarthritis can result in neck or back pain that may be acute or chronic (see Chapters 64 and 65). Particularly in cervical spine involvement, symptoms may be more related to referred pain than to neck pain. These syndromes can also result in pain without obvious nerve root compression or neurologic abnormalities (75). Low cervical spine involvement can cause pain that is usually aching or burning in quality and referred to the upper anterior chest, to the lower border of the scapula, and radiating down the arm to the elbow. Confusion with anginal pain may occur, but the history usually makes it clear that pain is localized to one side and occurs at rest, particularly during the night or in the early morning after sleep (probably caused by positioning of the head during sleep). Although it may also be exacerbated by activity during the day, pain related to cervical arthritis does not subside rapidly with rest and is not related to specific exertion. Physical examination usually can reproduce the pain on extremes of movement of the neck or with manual compression of the cervical segments in hyperextension, rotation, or lateral flexion. Impingement by osteoarthritis of the cervical spine on the spinal cord itself rather than nerve roots is uncommon. Central disc protrusion or extensive anterior osteophyte formation (especially when associated with cervical kyphosis, which may cause additional narrowing of the spinal canal) is an occasional cause of cord compression with neurologic sequelae of weakness or spasticity from impingement on centrally located cerebrospinal tracts. Degenerative arthritis of the thoracic spine also can cause radicular pain in the thoracic area, but this is surprisingly uncommon in contrast to frequent radiologic findings of spur formation in the thoracic spine, probably because of the anterior position of most of these bony abnormalities. Lumbar stenosis caused by osteoarthritis is strongly suggested by a history of lower extremity pain with standing or walking that is considerably relieved or absent when seated. It is often associated with a slightly wide-based gait, no pain on flexion, and thigh pain within 30 seconds of lumbar extension (40).

Another spinal syndrome, the relationship of which to osteoarthritis is unclear, is *diffuse idiopathic skel-*

etal hyperostosis (DISH). Differing from the usual findings in osteoarthritis, the intervertebral disc height is relatively preserved despite extensive hyperostosis and osteophytic bony bridging between the vertebral bodies. In contrast to ankylosing spondylitis, motion and function may be less impaired because the apophyseal joints are usually spared. This syndrome is chiefly important because of its impressive radiographic appearance (Fig. 68.2), the diffuse bony changes with hyperostosis, and the importance of distinguishing it from ankylosing spondylitis (see Chapter 71).

Acute Exacerbations of Osteoarthritis

Patients with osteoarthritis may occasionally have acute or subacute painful episodes with swelling of the affected joint. These episodes are usually superimposed on more typical preceding symptoms and signs of osteoarthritis, but they may precipitate an initial visit to the physician. In these patients there may be evidence of inflammation with pain, swelling, warmth, and some erythema on occasion. When the knee is involved, there may be a joint effusion. The episodes, which may be precipitated by minor trauma, probably are caused by sudden release into the joint of large amounts of cartilaginous debris or microcrystalline deposits contained therein, and rarely by complicating sepsis. In a study by Huskisson et al. (38), calcium pyrophosphate or hydroxyapatite crystals were found in a high proportion of knee effusions of patients with

such episodes, but these were also found in a significant proportion of unselected patients with osteoarthritis of the knee with effusion. Thus, the concurrence of crystalline deposit disease and osteoarthritis seems to be well established, although the relationship of cause and effect is unclear. From the clinical standpoint, however, this relationship provides a better understanding of these acute inflammatory episodes that punctuate the course of otherwise typical osteoarthritis (see Chapter 69, "Crystal-Induced Arthritis"). Sepsis may occasionally complicate an osteoarthritic joint, but it is a much less common event than occurs in a rheumatoid arthritic joint.

For these reasons a patient with established osteoarthritis who develops an acutely swollen, painful, hot joint should have the joint aspirated (see Chapter 67 for technique) and the fluid analyzed because of the possibility of a complicating microcrystalline-induced or septic arthritis.

DIAGNOSIS AND DIFFERENTIAL DIAGNOSIS

The diagnosis of osteoarthritis is based on the history and physical findings related to the joints, the absence of systemic signs, and typical radiologic findings. Differentiation from other forms of arthritis is usually easy, with the possible exception of some of the more unusual diffuse or inflammatory patterns of involvement described above. Consideration of the age of the patient, the distribution of the joints involved, and the radiologic findings usually lead to the correct

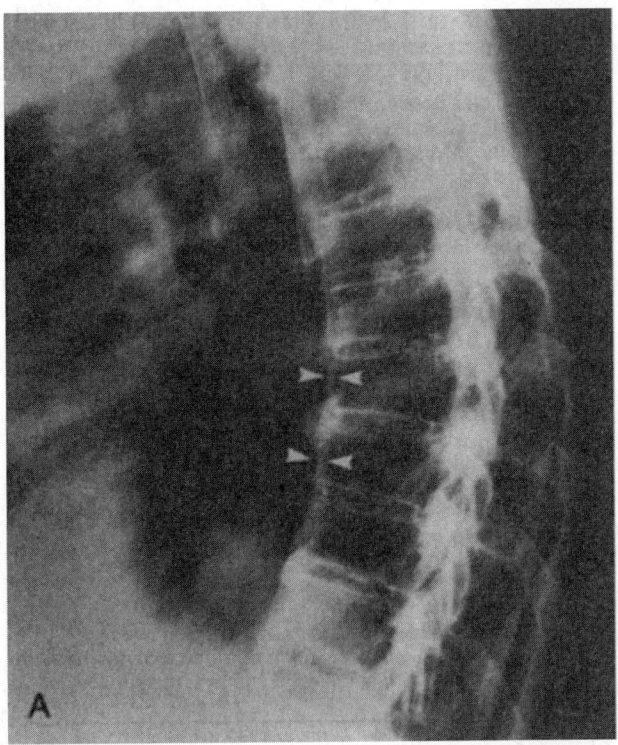 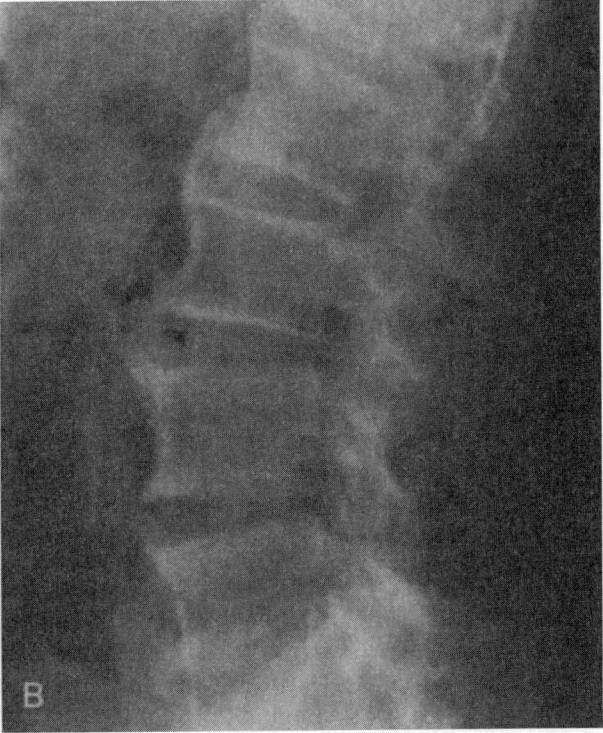

Figure 68.2. **A.** Lateral x-ray of thoracic spine of patient with diffuse idiopathic skeletal hyperostosis. **B.** Lateral x-ray of lumbar spine of patient with diffuse idiopathic skeletal hyperostosis. Prominent bony fusion and lipping anteriorly are seen.

Table 68.4. Differential Diagnosis of Osteoarthritis: Extra-Articular Causes of Pain or Restricted Movement

Bone Disease
Osteopenia or osteoporosis (see Chapter 74)
Malignancy: myeloma, metastatic
Paget's disease
Osteomyelitis (see Chapter 31)

Periarticular Soft Tissue Abnormalities
Soff tissue contractures (Dupuytren's, postcerebrovascular accident, or debilitating disease with disuse)
Tendinitis or bursitis (see Chapters 63 and 66)
Ligament strain (see Chapter 67)
Reflex sympathetic dystrophy

Neuromuscular Diseases
Neuropathy (diabetes, alcoholism, B_{12} deficiency) (see Chapter 84)
Parkinsonism (see Chapter 82)
Tardive dyskinesias (see Chapters 16 and 82)
Senile dementia with rigidity (see Chapters 17 and 82)

Vascular Diseases (See Chapter 87)
Atherosclerosis
Diabetes
Vasculitis

diagnosis. Criteria for classification and reporting of osteoarthritis of the hip (4) and knee (3) have been reported by an expert panel of rheumatologists.

The most common errors in differential diagnosis occur in attributing symptoms of pain or restricted movement to osteoarthritis when the problem is not the joints. This is a particularly common mistake in the evaluation of knee pain (ligament injury; see Chapter 67), hip pain (bursitis; see Chapter 66), and shoulder pain (periarticular problem; see Chapter 63). Because x-rays may demonstrate changes of osteoarthritis in asymptomatic or mildly symptomatic patients, one must rely on a careful history and physical examination to localize the disease to the joints. Table 68.4 lists other disorders, also common in older patients, that often give rise to pain and to painful or restricted movement and that may be erroneously attributed to osteoarthritis unless a careful examination is done.

MANAGEMENT

There is no cure for osteoarthritis and no therapy yet available that can be directed toward the specific pathophysiology of cartilage degeneration. However, experience indicates that much can be done to relieve symptoms, minimize disability, and perhaps delay progression of the disease. Certainly a nihilistic approach to therapy is not justified. Objective studies to establish therapeutic efficacy of interventions require large numbers of patients and long-term follow-up, so that one must often rely on subjective and incomplete data in deciding the best management of patients with this disorder (34). Recent concerns regarding the risks, especially in elderly patients, and lack of long-term benefit of nonsteroidal drugs have generated renewed interest in traditional and nonme-

dicinal modes of therapy. Objective evidence of the benefits of these measures as demonstrated in controlled trials has recently been reviewed (58). The importance of measures other than drug therapy cannot be overemphasized.

General Measures

Patient Education

Explaining to the patient the nature of the disease, that other joints are not likely to be involved, that progression of disease is slow, and that preservation of function is likely reassures most patients. For the patient with Heberden's nodes or mild disease in other joints, this reassurance and understanding are the most important therapeutic step in management. The physician should suggest some reading material for the patient such as *Learning to Live with Osteoarthritis,* published by Medicine in the Public Interest, Inc. (Suite 720, 600 New Hampshire Ave. NW, Washington, DC 20037). The importance of education and rapport with patients has been emphasized in recent studies using lay personnel to conduct monthly telephone interviews with patients. Improvement in pain and functional status occurred in patients who had this added contact with providers as compared with those with routine clinic visits only (60). This intervention was also cost-effective (74).

Rest

Pain and discomfort of osteoarthritis are often exacerbated by use, especially continuous use or weight bearing. Furthermore, excessive use of joints already damaged by osteoarthritis may accelerate cartilage degeneration. Therefore rest is an important treatment modality for osteoarthritis. Short periods of rest through the day are usually more effective than are less frequent longer periods. With weight-bearing joints, rest is particularly important. Many patients, especially elderly ones, believe that use of a joint becomes limited if it is rested too much, so needless overuse is common. When an understanding of the value of rest balanced with appropriately directed exercise and reassurance about function are given, patients often quickly learn to live within their own limitations without undue restrictions of activity and with improvement in symptoms.

Use of Canes, Crutches, and Walkers

In more severe disease, rest from weight bearing and stability when walking may be partially achieved by the use of a crutch, cane, or walker. The patient's attitude about the use of such assistive devices is an important consideration here because some interpret their cane as a sign of infirmity and fail to use it, whereas others carry it proudly as a badge of dependency even when it is not needed. Instruction in proper use of a cane, crutch, or walker should be given by the physician or a physical therapist. The object is to take some of the weight off the affected limb; thus, a cane or a crutch should be used on the opposite side and used simultaneously with the affected limb for weight bearing. Also, a cane of the proper length (e.g., from the floor to the bend of the wrist) should be held tightly and close to the body. Proper use is ensured by pressing the handle against the good hip. To completely prevent bearing weight on an affected limb, a crutch is required; it is used on the affected side, or two crutches are used (see Chapter 67 for a discussion of the proper use of crutches). A walker does not provide this type of unilateral support, but it may be needed in patients with bilateral knee pain or in patients whose instability requires more support than that provided by a cane or a crutch.

Correction of Postural or Mechanical Strain

This is an important consideration in patients with poor body mechanics. Thus, patients with pronated feet (see Chapter 102, "Common Problems of the Feet") have excessive stress on the knees and low back. Genu varus or valgum stresses the lateral or medial compartment excessively. The use of a wedged insole to compensate for valgus stress in mild knee disease in an uncontrolled trial was effective in relieving pain and improving function (62). Instruction in proper lifting and avoidance of unnecessary strain on certain joints or muscles by occupational or other activities may also need attention, such as use of a cervical pillow in the patient with neck involvement (see also Chapter 64, "Neck Pain," and Chapter 65, "Low Back Pain").

Physical Therapy

Simple measures can be prescribed for home use without the need for referral to a physical therapist in patients with mild disease. However, one must be sure that the patient understands directions. Reinforcement on subsequent visits is also important to ensure compliance. Patients with more advanced disease should be referred to a physical or occupational therapist for more extensive instruction in an exercise program, joint protection maneuvers, use of assistive devices, gait training, and similar measures.

Heat. No controlled trials establish beneficial effects of the external application of thermal therapy. However, experience and precedent suggest that application of heat often provides symptomatic relief of pain, reduces muscle spasm, and facilitates performance of an exercise program. Most patients prefer moist heat, which can be applied for 15 to 20 minutes via bathtub, hot towels, or commercially manufactured packs. Electric heating pads may also be used. Paraffin wax baths (available from large pharmacies) may be useful in patients with extensive hand involvement. With all modalities of heat therapy, temperatures that are very hot (above 110°F [43°C]) and prolonged or uninterrupted use should be avoided, to prevent skin damage. This is especially important with electric heating pads and patients should always be instructed to use the low temperature setting and place a towel between the skin and pad. Use of diathermy, ultrasound, heat cabinets, and other modalities offers little additional benefit but increase cost, and generally are

not recommended. Cold packs may be more effective in relieving pain and reducing swelling, especially after minor trauma or after exercise to relieve muscle soreness. Limiting application to no more than 20 to 30 minutes is again important.

Exercise. Goals of an exercise program are to maintain or improve function by preserving range of motion and improving muscle strength. The latter is important to help stabilize the joint and, by maintaining soft tissue cushioning of stress, to reduce the stress applied to the joint. Gradual conditioning is important so that muscle pain and soreness are not aggravated. Pain is often relieved as strength is gained and mechanical advantage is restored. Exercise should be graded according to the ability of the patient and carried out at least three times a day for optimal effect. In general, if muscle soreness or joint pain is worse after exercise, the intensity of the exercise should be reduced or progression halted until symptoms subside. Although walking may induce knee pain in patients with symptomatic osteoarthritis, supervised fitness walking accompanied by light stretching and strengthening exercises and educational sessions improves pain and physical fitness while reducing medication requirement (44). Aerobic exercise is highly desirable to maintain strength and general fitness. Exercise in a pool is a valuable means of aerobic exercise that does not involve weight-bearing stress (52). Bicycling with stationary arm or leg equipment also provides exercise with less weight-bearing stress than walking.

Maintenance of quadriceps strength is particularly important in osteoarthritis of the knee (48). This can be accomplished by beginning with slow full extension of the knee against gravity and then, as symptoms and progress allow, by extension with progressively increasing weight attached to the lower leg. (A bag with a strap to which are added canned goods of specific weight from the pantry shelf will suffice, although graded weights may be purchased from a sports store or provided by a physical therapist.) In patients whose pain prevents active quadriceps strengthening, isometric exercises are useful. With the knee extended the patient is instructed to tighten the quadriceps maximally so that the patella becomes fixed, hold for 10 to 15 seconds by count, release, and repeat. For patients who have difficulty rising from a seated position because of hip or knee disease, standing exercise from a high to a progressively lower stool may be useful in restoring function. The importance of maintaining muscle strength and conditioning is emphasized by studies measuring the energy expenditure of walking in patients with symptomatic arthritis of the hip or knee (73). The markedly increased energy requirement results in excessive fatigue that discourages mobility and may begin a cycle of progressive functional impairment in the frail elderly patient. Because of the importance of proper exercise in patients with arthritis, a consultation with a physical therapist is usually beneficial (11).

Other Measures. Other nonmedicinal treatments have been shown to be useful in treatment of osteoarthritis, particularly in relieving pain. These include transcutaneous nerve stimulation, acupuncture, low-energy laser, and pulsed electrical stimulation (58). In most studies of these therapies, pain relief rather than functional status or progression of disease have been assessed, with modest benefit as compared with controls. The use of topical capsaicin cream (0.025%) applied four times a day was effective in pain relief in a double-blind trial in knee osteoarthritis (18). Continued application for 2 to 4 weeks is necessary to achieve benefit. Initial discomfort from the application tends to disappear with continued use. Use of a stronger preparation (0.25%) applied twice daily was somewhat more effective but with more discomfort, especially at the initiation of treatment (63). Many patients report relief of stiffness and discomfort with a sense of joint protection through the use of elastic supports around the joint. Such devices used at the knee, however, should be fitted appropriately to avoid obstruction of venous circulation in the leg. Splints may be useful when the first carpometacarpal joint is involved or with finger deformities caused by erosive disease. Wearing nylon stretch gloves (e.g., Isotoner gloves, available in department stores) may provide relief for some patients with extensive hand involvement (22).

Diet

Control of obesity (see Chapter 76) is important in osteoarthritis of the knees, hips, and metatarsophalangeal joints. Logic would dictate that weight loss for the obese patient would be beneficial and is recommended, but no controlled trials support its efficacy in relieving symptoms. Patients should be cautioned against food fads and unwarranted claims of relationship of diet and osteoarthritis. Recent attention has been given to the use of dietary supplements of glucosamine and chondroitin sulfate (available in health food stores at a cost of about $50 a month) as a result of a few studies in animals and trials in humans, mostly in Europe. The efficacy of this therapy has not been established, however, despite recent articles in the reputable lay press prompted by a book written by a physician touting it as a cure (71). (For an informative review of this topic and sound nutritional advice, see Reference 31). The possible association of low serum levels and intake of vitamin D in progression of disease (50) indicates the prudence of ensuring an adequate dietary intake of this vitamin especially in elderly subjects.

Drug Therapy

There has been a minor revolution in the therapeutic use of drugs in the treatment of osteoarthritis. Drug therapy should be viewed as an adjunct to the general measures described above. For a long time the mainstay of treatment, nonsteroidal anti-inflammatory drugs (NSAIDs) including aspirin have come into disfavor for several reasons. Because of their effects on the gastrointestinal mucosa and kidneys, they add increased risks of unwanted and potentially serious

side effects with long-term use, especially in elderly patients. In addition, because of variable effects on cartilage metabolism through the prostaglandin system, some NSAIDs have apparently contributed to progression of disease, and none has demonstrated prevention of progression. Because osteoarthritis is a largely noninflammatory condition, analgesic drugs are usually sufficient. In controlled trials, analgesic dosages of acetaminophen have been as effective as analgesic dosages of NSAIDs with fewer risks and side effects (7,76). Therefore, the current recommended guideline for analgesic drug therapy is to begin with acetaminophen up to 1 g four times a day (35,36).

However, some patients, especially those with advanced disease and an inflammatory component, clearly respond better to NSAIDs. The patient should take the lowest dosage that provides symptomatic relief, and intermittent use or drug-free periods rather than long-term continuous use should be considered. Ibuprofen 1800 to 2400 mg/day in divided doses is a reasonable first choice because of lower rates of side effects and low cost. Naproxen 375 to 500 mg twice daily is a longer-acting and cost-effective drug. Efficacy and side effects of the many available NSAIDs vary among patients and the choice must be individualized. In patients at high risk of serious gastrointestinal side effects, the concomitant use of misoprostol has been shown to be effective in preventing gastric and duodenal ulcers (43), and in one study was judged to be cost-effective (30). Side effects of abdominal discomfort and diarrhea are common and dyspepsia is not relieved. Histamine 2-receptor antagonists have been shown to be effective in preventing duodenal but not gastric ulcers. However, in a recent study high-dose famotidine (40 mg twice daily) was effective in both without side effects (70). This adds considerable expense and complexity to the treatment. Narcotic analgesics are best avoided but may be used occasionally on a short-term basis for pain relief. In general they are not more effective than acetaminophen or NSAIDs and are not suitable for long-term use in this chronic condition.

Results of studies in experimental models of osteoarthritis suggest that some agents might modify the pathophysiology of cartilage degradation to prevent or slow disease progression (8,27). The potential availability of chondroprotective or disease-modifying drugs is a fruitful area for research and a promise for the future. A few human trials of drugs or biologicals have yielded early positive results, but none is yet proven effective or available for clinical use.

Because many patients with osteoarthritis have other medical conditions for which they are receiving therapeutic drugs, one must be alert to problems of interactions with NSAIDs. For example, NSAIDs may mitigate the therapeutic effect of agents that depend on prostaglandins to mediate a response, such as the natruretic and antihypertensive effects of furosemide, thiazides, or captopril, or may exacerbate asthma. These and other characteristics of NSAIDs are more fully discussed in Chapter 70.

Corticosteroids

Intra-articular injection of suspensions of corticosteroids (see Chapter 66, Table 66.4) has been shown to be useful in the management of osteoarthritis, especially when associated with effusions in large joints such as the knee (21). The removal of joint fluid (without corticosteroid injection) when an effusion is present in osteoarthritis usually does not improve symptoms unless a microcrystalline arthritis is superimposed (see Chapter 69). In an experimental model of osteoarthritis in dogs, intra-articular corticosteroid had both a prophylactic and therapeutic effect (56). However, in patients the effect is variable and often short lived. If prolonged relief lasting several months is not achieved with one or two injections, this therapy should not be continued. The risk of serious side effects including enhanced destruction of the joint and infection may follow repeated injections, which should therefore be avoided.

There is absolutely no indication for systemic administration of corticosteroids in the management of osteoarthritis.

Orthopedic Surgery

An orthopedist should be consulted in the treatment of patients with osteoarthritis who have a problem of malalignment or major instability in weight-bearing joints, for symptoms or findings of loose bodies in the joint, and for intractable pain with advanced disease of the hips or knees. Osteotomy may correct malalignment. Arthroplasty to improve instability and remove loose bodies, meniscal fragments, and perhaps large spurs may be useful in some patients. This procedure has been largely replaced by arthroscopic surgery, which can accomplish much of the same result and is a much more tolerable procedure. It is useful particularly in knees that are not subject to undue stress in elderly patients (64). However, a randomized trial of closed needle lavage of the joint has been equally effective in most patients in the absence of meniscus tears, and is less costly (14). An indication of the infrequency with which this procedure is indicated is the large number of patients referred who responded to exercise and medications and were therefore excluded from the trial. In another randomized trial involving patients with more advanced disease, debridement was superior to washout with follow-up of 1 to 5 years (37). When pain or disability is refractory to treatment and joint destruction of a hip or a knee is advanced, consideration should be given to total joint replacement. Disabling pain is the principal indication for this procedure. Contraindications include neuromuscular or sensory deficits, severe peripheral vascular disease, marked obesity, dementia, and lack of motivation or inability to cooperate with a postoperative rehabilitation program. Results of joint replacement in osteoarthritis of the hip are generally excellent. In patients with functionally significant osteoarthritis undergoing hip replacement, evaluation of function, short-term and long-term costs indicate that the procedure improved quality adjusted life years and was cost-effective (15). Knee replacement in the past has been somewhat less successful, but results demonstrated in a meta-analysis of 130 reports indicate that with new prostheses and in the hands of experienced surgeons, good to excellent results were obtained in 90% of patients (12) with relief of pain and functional improvement. Arthrodesis (i.e., surgical fusion of the joint) is usually reserved for patients with failed joint replacement. Major complications of joint replacement are postoperative thrombophlebitis and infection. Elimination of potential foci of infection is important preoperatively, and prophylactic antibiotics are advocated by some (see Chapter 32) after joint replacement surgery and during dental or urinary tract procedures that might produce bacteremia. Although the continued improvement in synthetic materials and surgical techniques has prolonged the durability of an artificial joint, most rheumatologists do not refer patients with hip or knee arthritis for surgery until symptoms are pronounced or functional impairment is considerable. Because prostheses wear out and must be replaced after 10 to 15 years, surgery is usually reserved for patients in their sixth decade or beyond.

PREVENTION

Because the cause of osteoarthritis is uncertain, so is its prevention. However, recognition of predisposing factors and elucidation of normal physiology of articular cartilage suggest certain prudent steps that can be recommended.

Immobilization with avoidance of joint stress gives rise to biochemical changes in cartilage similar to early lesions in osteoarthritis. Thus, normal stress and functioning of joints are important in maintenance of normal cartilage physiology. Perhaps one can abstract from this that a sedentary and inactive life is not good for the integrity of articular cartilage. Furthermore, because strong periarticular muscles lend stability and help absorb stress applied to joints, it seems logical that physical conditioning to maintain muscle strength and a lean habitus may be important in prevention of osteoarthritis. Because quadriceps weakness has been suggested as a risk factor for osteoarthritis of the knee, there is a need for a controlled trial to determine whether strengthening this muscle group will prevent or halt progression of osteoarthritis of the knee (9,65). That weight loss reduces the risk for symptomatic knee osteoarthritis in women has been demonstrated (24). Soft tissues tend to lose mobility with advancing age and such changes have been shown to increase impact stress of joints. Physical activity may retard this loss of mobility and therefore should be encouraged.

At the same time it is evident that repetitive stress, especially when abnormally applied, or when resulting in injury or structural damage, is a strong predisposing factor to osteoarthritis. Thus, correction of abnormal mechanical forces from developmental or postural defects, avoidance of unusual occupational stress, and avoidance of traumatic injury to joints are important in prevention of osteoarthritis and preservation of good muscle strength and tone. Maintenance of good nutrition with adequate intake of vitamin D in elderly patients may be of benefit (50).

General References*

Buckwalter JA. Current concepts review: operative treatment of osteoarthritis. J Bone Joint Surg 76A: 1405, 1994.
> A good review of current practice and future developments.

Dalinka MK, ed. Radiographic imaging in orthopedics. Orthop Clin North Am 21(3):405, 1990.
> The entire volume is dedicated to modern imaging techniques in orthopedics and is well illustrated.

Dieppe P, Altman R, Lequesne M, et al. Osteoarthritis of the knee: report of a task force of the International League of Associations for Rheumatology and the Osteoarthritis Research Society. J Am Geriatr Soc 45:850, 1997
> Current status referable to diagnosis, therapy, and outcomes.

Hamerman D. Aging and osteoarthritis: basic mechanisms. J Am Geriatr Soc 41:760–770, 1993.
> An excellent review of basic biology and pathophysiology.

Jones A, Doherty M. ABC of rheumatology. Osteoarthritis. BMJ 310:457–460, 1995.
> A concise review of essentials with no references.

Kelley WN, Harris ED, Ruddy S, Sledge CB, eds. Textbook of rheumatology. 5th ed. Philadelphia: WB Saunders, 1997.

Koopman WJ, ed. Arthritis and allied conditions. 13th ed. Baltimore: Williams & Wilkins, 1997.
> Kelley et al. and Koopman are two excellent multiauthored textbooks of rheumatology, with sections on osteoarthritis providing more detailed presentation of the topic and extensive bibliographies.

Liang MH, Fortin P. Management of osteoarthritis of the hip and knee. N Engl J Med 325:125, 1991.
> An excellent editorial that accompanies Bradley et al. (7) and summarizes the issues regarding management of osteoarthritis of the knee and hip.

Ling SM, Bathon JM. Osteoarthritis in older adults. J Am Geriatr Soc 46:216, 1998.
> A good review of osteoarthritis in the elderly.

Moskowitz RW, Howell DS, Goldberg VM, Mankin HJ, eds. Osteoarthritis, diagnosis and management. 2nd ed. Philadelphia: WB Saunders, 1992.

Peter JB, Pearson CM, Marmnor L. Erosive osteoarthritis of the hands. Arthritis Rheum 9:365, 1966.
> The original description of this concept.

Resnick D, Niwazama G. Diagnosis of bone and joint disorders. 3rd ed. Philadelphia: WB Saunders, 1995.
> A 6-volume set with extensive coverage of radiography of all forms of arthritis.

Specific References

1. Ala-Kokko L, Baldwin CT, Moskowitz RW, et al. Single base mutation in the type II procollagen gene (COL2A1) as a cause of primary osteoarthritis associated with mild chondrodysplasia. Proc Natl Acad Sci U S A 87:6565, 1990.

2. Anderson JJ, Felson DT. Factors associated with osteoarthritis of the knee in the first national health and nutrition survey (HANES I). Evidence for an association with overweight, race and physical demands of work. Am J Epidemiol 128:179, 1988.

3. Altman R, Alarcon G, Appelrouth D, et al. The American College of Rheumatology criteria for classification and reporting of osteoarthritis of the hip. Arthritis Rheum 35:505, 1991.

4. Altman R, Asch E, Black D, et al. Development of criteria for the classification and reporting of osteoarthritis of the knee. Arthritis Rheum 29:1039, 1986.

5. Baron M, Dutil E, Berkson L, et al. Hand function in the elderly: relation to osteoarthritis. J Rheumatol 14:815, 1987.

6. Black WC, Welch HG. Advances in diagnostic imaging and overestimations of disease prevalence and benefits of therapy. N Engl J Med 328:1237, 1993.

7. Bradley JD, Brandt KD, Katz BP, et al. Comparison of an antiinflammatory dose of ibuprofen, an analgesic dose of ibuprofen, and acetaminophen in the treatment of patients with osteoarthritis. N Engl J Med 325:87, 1991.

8. Brandt KD. Toward pharmacologic modification of joint damage in osteoarthritis. Ann Intern Med 122:874, 1995.

9. Brandt KD. Putting some muscle into osteoarthritis. Ann Intern Med 12:154, 1997.

10. Buchanan WW, Park WM. Primary generalized osteoarthritis: definition and uniformity. J Rheumatol 10:S4, 1983.

11. Bunning RD, Materson RS. A rational program of exercise for patients with osteoarthritis. Semin Arthritis Rheum 21(Suppl 2):33, 1991.

12. Callahan CM, Drake BC, Heck DA, Ditters RS. Patient outcomes following tricompartmental knee replacement. JAMA 217:1349, 1994.

13. Carman WJ, Sowers MF, Hawthorne VM, Weissfeld LA. Obesity as a risk factor for osteoarthritis: a prospective study. Am J Epidemiol 139:119, 1994.

14. Chang RW, Falconer J, Stulberg JG, et al. A randomized controlled trial of arthroscopic surgery versus closed needle lavage for patients with osteoarthritis. Arthritis Rheum 36:289, 1993.

15. Chang RW, Pellisier JM, Hazen GB. A cost effective analysis of total hip arthroplasty for osteoarthritis of the hip. JAMA 275:858, 1996.

16. Cushnagan J, McCarthy C, Dieppe P. Taping the patella medially: a new treatment for osteoarthritis of the knee joint? BMJ 308:753, 1994.

17. Davis MA, Ettinger WH, Neuhaus JM, Hauck WC. Sex differences in osteoarthritis of the knee. The role of obesity. Am J Epidemiol 127:1019, 1988.

18. Deal CL, Schnitzer TJ, Lipstein E, et al. Treatment of arthritis with topical capsaicin: a double blind trial. Clin Ther 13:383, 1991.

19. Dieppe PA, Doherty M, McFarlane DG, et al. Apatite associated destructive arthritis. Br J Rheumatol 23:84, 1984.

20. Dieppe P, Kirwan J. The localization of osteoarthritis. Br J Rheumatol 33:201, 1994.

21. Dieppe PA, Sathapatayavongs B, Jones H, et al. Intraarticular steroids in osteoarthritis. Rheum Rehabil 19:212, 1980.

22. Ehrlich GE, DiPiero AM. Stretch gloves: nocturnal use to ameliorate morning stiffness in arthritic hands. Arch Phys Med Rehabil 52:479, 1971.

23. Felson DT, Naimark A, Anderson J, et al. The prevalence of knee osteoarthritis in the elderly. The Framingham osteoarthritis study. Arthritis Rheum 30:914, 1987.

24. Felson DT, Zhang Y, Anthony JM, et al. Weight loss reduces the risk for symptomatic osteoarthritis in women. Ann Intern Med 116:535, 1992.

25. Felson DT, Zhang Y, Hannan MT. Risk factors for incident radiographic knee osteoarthritis in the elderly. The Framingham study. Arthritis Rheum 40:728, 1997.

26. Felson DT, Zhang Y, Hannan MT, et al. The incidence and natural history of knee osteoarthritis in the elderly. The Framingham osteoarthritis study. Arthritis Rheum 38:1500, 1995.

27. Fernandes JC, Caron JP, Martel-Pelletier J, et al. Effects of tenidap on the progression of osteoarthritic lesions in a canine experimental model. Suppression of metalloprotease and interleukin-1 activity. Arthritis Rheum 40:284, 1997.

28. Fries JF, Singh G, Morfeld D, et al. Running and the development of disability with age. Ann Intern Med 121:502, 1994.

29. Gabriel SE, Crowson C, O'Fallon M. Costs of osteoarthritis: estimates from a geographically defined population. J Rheumatol 43(Suppl):23, 1995.

30. Gabriel SE, Jaakkimainen RL, Bombardier C. The cost-effectiveness of misoprostol for nonsteroidal antiinflammatory drug-associated adverse gastrointestinal events. Arthritis Rheum 36:447, 1993.

31. Gershoff S, ed. Special report: is there an arthritis cure? Tufts U Diet Nutr Lett 15(2), April 1997.

---

*Bold print (general references) and bold numerals (specific references) denote published controlled clinical trials, meta-analyses, or consensus-based recommendations.

32. Gramas DA, Antounian FS, Peterfy CG, et al. Assessment of needle arthroscopy, standard arthroscopy, physical examination, and magnetic resonance imaging in knee pain. A pilot study. J Clin Rheumatol 1:26, 1995.

33. Guccione AA, Felson DT, Anderson JJ, et al. The effect of specific medical conditions on the functional limitation of elders in the Framingham study. Am J Public Health 84:351, 1994.

34. Herman JH, Hess EV. Therapeutic impasse in osteoarthritis. Br J Rheumatol 33:1098, 1994.

35. Hochberg MC, Altman RD, Brandt KD, et al. Guidelines for the medical management of osteoarthritis. Part I. Osteoarthritis of the hip. Arthritis Rheum 38:1535, 1995.

36. Hochberg MC, Altman RD, Brandt KD, et al. Guidelines for the medical management of osteoarthritis. Part II. Osteoarthritis of the knee. Arthritis Rheum 38:1541, 1995.

37. Hubbard MJS. Articular debridement versus washout for degeneration of the medial femoral condyle. J Bone Joint Surg 78B:217, 1996.

38. Huskisson EC, Dieppe PA, Tucker AK, Channel LB. Another look at osteoarthritis. Ann Rheum Dis 38:423, 1979.

39. Ike RW, O'Rourke KS. Compartment directed physical examination of the knee can predict articular cartilage abnormalities disclosed by needle arthroscopy. Arthritis Rheum 38:917, 1995.

40. Katz JN, Dalgus M, Stucki G, et al. Degenerative lumbar spinal stenosis: diagnostic value of the history and physical examination. Arthritis Rheum 38: 1236, 1995.

41. Kellgren JH, Lawrence JS. Atlas of standard radiographs: the epidemiology of chronic rheumatism. Oxford, UK: Blackwell Scientific, 1963;2.

42. Kellgren JH, Moore R. Generalized osteoarthritis and Heberden's nodes. BMJ 1:181, 1952.

43. Koch M, Dezi A, Capurso L. Prevention of nonsteroidal antiinflammatory drug-induced gastrointestinal injury. A meta-analysis of randomized controlled trials. Arch Intern Med 156:2321, 1996.

44. Kovar PA, Allegrante JP, McKenzie CR, et al. Supervised fitness walking in patients with osteoarthritis of the knee. Ann Intern Med 116:529, 1992.

45. Kujala UM, Kaprio J, Sarna S. Osteoarthritis of weight bearing joints of the lower limbs in former elite male athletes. BMJ 308:231, 1994.

46. Lohmander LS. Molecular markers to monitor outcome and intervention in osteoarthritis (promises, promises). Br J Rheumatol 34:599–601, 1995.

47. Loughlin J, Irven C, Fergusson C, Sykes B. Sibling pair analysis shows no linkage of generalized osteoarthritis to the loci encoding type II collagen, cartilage link protein or cartilage matrix protein. Br J Rheumatol 33:1103, 1994.

48. Marks R. Quadriceps strength training for osteoarthritis of the knee. A literature review and analysis. Physiotherapy 79:13, 1993.

49. Marsland DW, Wood M, Mayo F. Content of family practice. I. Routine order of diagnosis by frequency. II. Diagnosis by disease category and age/sex distribution. J Fam Pract 8:37, 1976.

50. McAlindon TE, Felson DT, Zhang Y, et al. Relation of dietary intake and serum levels of vitamin D to progression of osteoarthritis of the knee among participants in the Framingham study. Ann Intern Med 125:353, 1996.

51. Merlo IM, Poloni TE, Alfonsi E, et al. Case report: sciatic pain in a young sportsman. Lancet 349:846, 1997.

52. Minor MA, Hewett JE, Webel RR, et al. Efficacy of physical conditioning exercise in patients with rheumatoid arthritis and osteoarthritis. Arthritis Rheum 32:1396, 1989.

53. Neyret P, Donnell ST, Dejour H. Osteoarthritis of the knee following meniscectomy. Br J Rheumatol 33:267, 1994.

54. Panush RS, Hanson CS, Caldwell JR, et al. Is running associated with osteoarthritis? An eight-year follow-up study. J Clin Rheumatol 1:35, 1995.

55. Pattrick M, Aldridge S, Hamilton E, et al. A controlled study of hand function in nodal and erosive osteoarthritis. Ann Rheum Dis 48:978, 1989.

56. Pelletier JP, Di Battista JA, Raynauld JP, et al. The in vivo effects of intraarticular steroid injections on cartilage lesions, stromelysin, interleukin-1, and oncogene protein synthesis in experimental osteoarthritis. Lab Invest 72:578, 1995.

57. Post WR, Fulkerson JP. Anterior knee pain. A symptom, not a diagnosis. Bull Rheum Dis 42:5, 1993.

58. Puett DW, Grifiths MR. Published trials of nonmedicinal and noninvasive therapies for hip and knee osteoarthritis. Ann Intern Med 121:133, 1994.

59. Radin EL, Burr DB, Caterson B, et al. Mechanical determinants of osteoarthritis. Semin Arthritis Rheum 21(Suppl 2):12, 1991.

60. Rene J, Weinberger M, Mazzuca SA, et al. Reduction of joint pain in patients with knee osteoarthritis who have received monthly telephone calls from lay personnel and whose medical treatment regimens have remained stable. Arthritis Rheum 35:511, 1992.

61. Ritvaniemi P, Korkko J, Bonaventure J, et al. Identification of COL2A gene mutations in patients with chondrodysplasias and familial osteoarthritis. Arthritis Rheum 38:999, 1995.

62. Sasaki T, Yasuda K. Clinical evaluation of the treatment of osteoarthritic knees using a newly designed wedge insole. Clin Orthop 221:181, 1987.

63. Schnitzer TJ, Posner M, Lawrence ID. High strength capsaicin cream for osteoarthritis pain: rapid onset of action and improved efficacy with twice daily dosing. J Clin Rheumatol 1:268, 1995.

64. Schonholtz GJ. Arthroscopic debridement of the knee joint. Orthop Clin 20(2):257, 1989.

65. Slemenda F, Brandt KD, Heilman DK, et al. Quadriceps weakness and osteoarthritis of the knee. Ann Intern Med 127:97, 1997.

66. Spector TD, Cicuttini F, Baker J, et al. Genetic influences on osteoarthritis in women: a twin study. BMJ 312:940, 1996.

67. Spector TD, Harris PA, Hart DJ, et al. Risk of osteoarthritis associated with long term weight-bearing sports. A radiologic survey of the hips and knees in female ex-athletes and population controls. Arthritis Rheum 39:988, 1996.

68. Spector CD, Hart DJ, Nandra D, et al. Low level increases of C-reactive protein are present early in osteoarthritis and predict progressive disease. Arthritis Rheum 40:723,1997.

69. Summers MN, Haley WE, Reveille JD, Alarcon G. Radiologic assessment and psychological variables as predictors of pain and functional impairment in osteoarthritis of the knee or hip. Arthritis Rheum 31:204, 1988.

70. Taha AS, Hudson N, Hawkey CJ, et al. Famotidine for the prevention of gastric and duodenal ulcers caused by nonsteroidal antiinflammatory drugs. N Engl J Med 334:1435, 1996.

71. Theodosakis J, Adlery B, Fox B. The arthritis cure. New York: St. Martin's Press, 1997.

72. Villiaumey J. Is the hip involved in generalized osteoarthritis? Br J Rheumatol 32:85, 1993.

73. Waters RL, Perry J, Conaty P, et al. The energy cost of walking with arthritis of the hip and knee. Clin Orthop 214:278, 1987.

74. Weinberger M, Tierney WM, Cowper PA, et al. Cost effectiveness of increased telephone contact for patients with osteoarthritis. Arthritis Rheum 36:243,1993.

75. Weinstein JN. The role of neurogenic and non-neurogenic mediators as they relate to pain and the development of osteoarthritis. Spine 17:S356, 1992.

76. Williams HJ, Ward JR, Egger MJ, et al. Comparison of naproxen and acetaminophen in a two year study of treatment of osteoarthritis of the knee. Arthritis Rheum 36:1196, 1993.

C H A P T E R 69

Crystal-Induced Arthritis

ALEXANDER S. TOWNES, MD

Gout was the first form of arthritis that was recognized to be caused by the deposition of (urate) crystals in the joints and periarticular tissues. It is now known that other crystalline substances—most commonly calcium pyrophosphate dihydrate (CPPD), hydroxyapatite, and basic calcium phosphates—also are implicated in the pathogenesis of certain kinds of arthritic disease. Although disorders associated with these various crystals differ in cause and specific characteristics, they have in common the deposition of crystals in and around joints, the propensity to episodes of acute inflammatory arthritis, and sometimes the development of a destructive arthropathy. It is therefore appropriate to consider these varied clinical disorders together under the unifying concept of crystal-induced arthritis.

MECHANISMS OF CRYSTAL-INDUCED ARTHRITIS

Crystals such as monosodium urate and CPPD, when experimentally injected into joints, produce an acute inflammatory response. The mechanisms involved in this response are complex but perhaps are as well studied as any of the stimuli that produce arthritis. By the nature of their electrostatic surface characteristics, crystals attract and bind many plasma proteins including fibronectin, IgG, C-reactive protein, and complement. Crystals are phagocytized by synovial lining cells, probably as a result of binding of crystal-bound IgG (32), complement, or other proteins to membrane receptors. This initiates formation or release of leukotrienes, prostaglandins, lysosomal enzymes, and other mediators that increase vascular permeability and promote the influx of polymorphonuclear neutrophils (PMNs), which are essential for the inflammatory reaction to continue. Phagocytosis of crystals by PMNs is accompanied by the release of a potent chemotactic glycopeptide that further amplifies the PMN response. PMNs release lysosomal enzymes in the process of crystal phagocytosis and as a result of the membranolytic effect of urate crystals themselves on phagolysosomes after digestion of proteins from the crystal surface. In this process crystals are again released into the synovial fluid for further phagocytosis. Urate crystals also stimulate macrophages and synovial lining cells to produce interleukin-1 (IL-1), tumor necrosis factor–α (TNF-α) (11), interleukin-6 (IL-6) (23), and interleukin-8 (IL-8) (67), a potent neutrophil chemotactic factor. The precise sequence of release and the essentialness of these inflammatory mediators is unknown. The dissemination of cytokines including IL-1, TNF-α, and IL-6 is probably responsible for the systemic effects of fever, leukocytosis, and acute phase reactants sometimes observed in acute crystal-induced arthritis (21,40).

Crystals may be identified in synovial fluid and synovial membrane with low levels of phagocytosis in asymptomatic people (2,58), and may contribute to joint damage in the absence of acute attacks (46). The events that trigger acute inflammation are not entirely clear. It is likely that the precipitation from fluid phase or release of a sufficient volume of crystals from soft tissue deposits begins the cycle of crystal phagocytosis and inflammation. In patients with gout, there is an association of acute attacks with rapid changes in serum urate concentration, as may occur with dietary indiscretion, alcohol ingestion, rapid weight loss, or initiation of therapy with drugs that lower serum urate. In CPPD deposit disease, release of crystals from tissue deposits in cartilage or soft tissues may result from trauma or enzymatic digestion of matrix.

The invariable association between phagocytosis of crystals and the acute inflammatory response is important clinically because demonstration of crystals within leukocytes from synovial fluid is a convenient method of making a definitive diagnosis in patients with acute inflammatory crystal-induced arthritis.

The acute inflammatory response in crystal-induced arthritis is self-limited. The complex mechanisms that terminate the attack are not well understood but may involve TGF-β and lipoproteins. TGF-β, present in gouty effusions (18), markedly inhibits the leukocyte response in an in vivo model (39). Lipoproteins that coat crystal surfaces during the subsiding phase of inflammation displace IgG (45), reduce their adherence to cell membranes, and inhibit phagocytosis and thereby may blunt or terminate the inflammatory response (66).

Although gouty arthritis and other crystal-induced diseases are usually characterized by symptoms and signs of acute inflammation, the persistence of crystals in the joint with mild chronic inflammation may contribute to chronic joint damage eventually. Sometimes a progressive destructive arthropathy occurs with little evidence of inflammation. In these patients (a few with CPPD and others with mixed CPPD, hydroxyapatite, and other basic calcium phosphate crystals), the PMN response is for some reason markedly reduced, but extensive destruction of bone and soft tissues occurs. Release of protease and collagenase enzymes was demonstrated and postulated to produce disruption of additional crystal deposits into the joint with continuation of the cycle of destruction (42). Others have not found collagenase (10) and have proposed other bone resorbing agents, including prostaglandin E_2 (3).

Crystal Identification

The identification of crystals in synovial fluid or periarticular tissue is fundamental to the diagnosis and treatment of patients with crystal-induced arthritis. Crystals of monosodium urate are best identified by placing a drop of aspirated tissue fluid directly on a glass slide and examining the wet preparation through a microscope under polarized light (49). Although specialized equipment is ideal, crystals can be demonstrated adequately in the physician's office by placing a plastic polarizing lens (e.g., made from an old pair of sunglasses) between the light source and the microscopic stage, and by placing another lens in the body or the eyepiece of the microscope. When one lens is rotated so that the field becomes dark, the negatively birefringent urate crystals (i.e., crystals capable of bending light rays in two planes; the notation of negativity is an arbitrary term used by physicists to describe the direction of bend), dimly seen in ordinary light, stand out brightly and can be identified within the cytoplasm of polymorphonuclear leukocytes. If a red plate compensator is placed between the light source and the stage of the microscope (one can be fabricated by wrapping a glass slide longitudinally with two or more layers of transparent tape) (14), the crystals are even more easily identified because the field turns red and crystals parallel to the axis of the compensator appear yellow, whereas those perpendicular to the axis appear blue. Monosodium urate crystals are usually needle or rod shaped. The size varies, but some large crystals equal to or larger than the diameter of the leukocyte are usually seen. A wet slide of joint fluid prepared in this manner may be kept for a few hours at room temperature; however, once the cells die and lyse, evaluation is less valid. If the aspirated fluid cannot be examined immediately, urate crystals may be preserved overnight by refrigeration in a plain test tube. However, CPPD crystals may dissolve within a few hours even at refrigerator temperatures (34).

Monosodium urate crystals (which are usually present in abundance) are pathognomonic of gout (Table 69.1 and Fig. 69.1). Absence of crystals in an inflamed joint is strong evidence against the diagnosis and, especially if leukocytosis is significant, infection or another diagnosis should be considered.

Monosodium urate is usually easily distinguished from CPPD on the basis of morphology and characteristics of the crystals under polarized light (Table 69.1 and Fig. 69.1). CPPD crystals vary much more in size and shape from rodlike to rhomboid and irregular forms, are usually much shorter, and are never needle-like. They are usually refractile without polarized light and do not increase appreciably in brilliance when the light is polarized. They are weakly positively birefringent and change color in the opposite direction to urate when the red plate compensator is placed between the polarizing lens (i.e., blue when parallel to the axis and yellow when perpendicular).

Because CPPD crystals are small and do not stand out in polarized light, they are overlooked more often by the occasional observer. Routine reports from nonspecialized clinical laboratories are often falsely negative. A method for long-term preservation of crystals for quality-control slides has been described (61).

Other crystalline materials that may be seen include

Table 69.1.   Identification of Crystals in Synovial Fluid

Monosodium Urate
Morphology
    Rod or needle shaped
    Length often approaches diameter of PMN leucocyte
Polarized light
    Stand out brightly when field is dark
    Strongly negative birefringent
Red plate compensator
    Yellow crystals parallel and blue crystals perpendicular to axis

Calcium Pyrophosphate Dihydrate
Morphology
    Rhomboid, rod, or irregular rhomboid shape
    Length variable, often smaller than one lobe of a PMN nucleus
Polarized light
    No increase in refractile appearance when field is dark
    Weakly positively birefringent
Red plate compensator
    Blue crystals parallel and yellow crystals perpendicular to axis

Hydroxyapatite and Basic Calcium Phosphates
Not usually seen with ordinary or polarized light microscopy except as large aggregates that are not birefringent.
    Aggregates of BCP may occasionally be seen as "shiny coin" refractile bodies.
Stain nonspecifically with alizarin red S (available in histology laboratories) as clusters of crystalline material. Useful as a screening test.
Requires electron microscopy, x-ray diffraction, or microprobe analysis for more definite identification.

Calcium Oxalate
Morphology
    Polymorphic, irregular squares, short rods, bipyramidal; may appear in clumps
Polarized light
    Variable, most not birefringent, some strongly positively birefringent

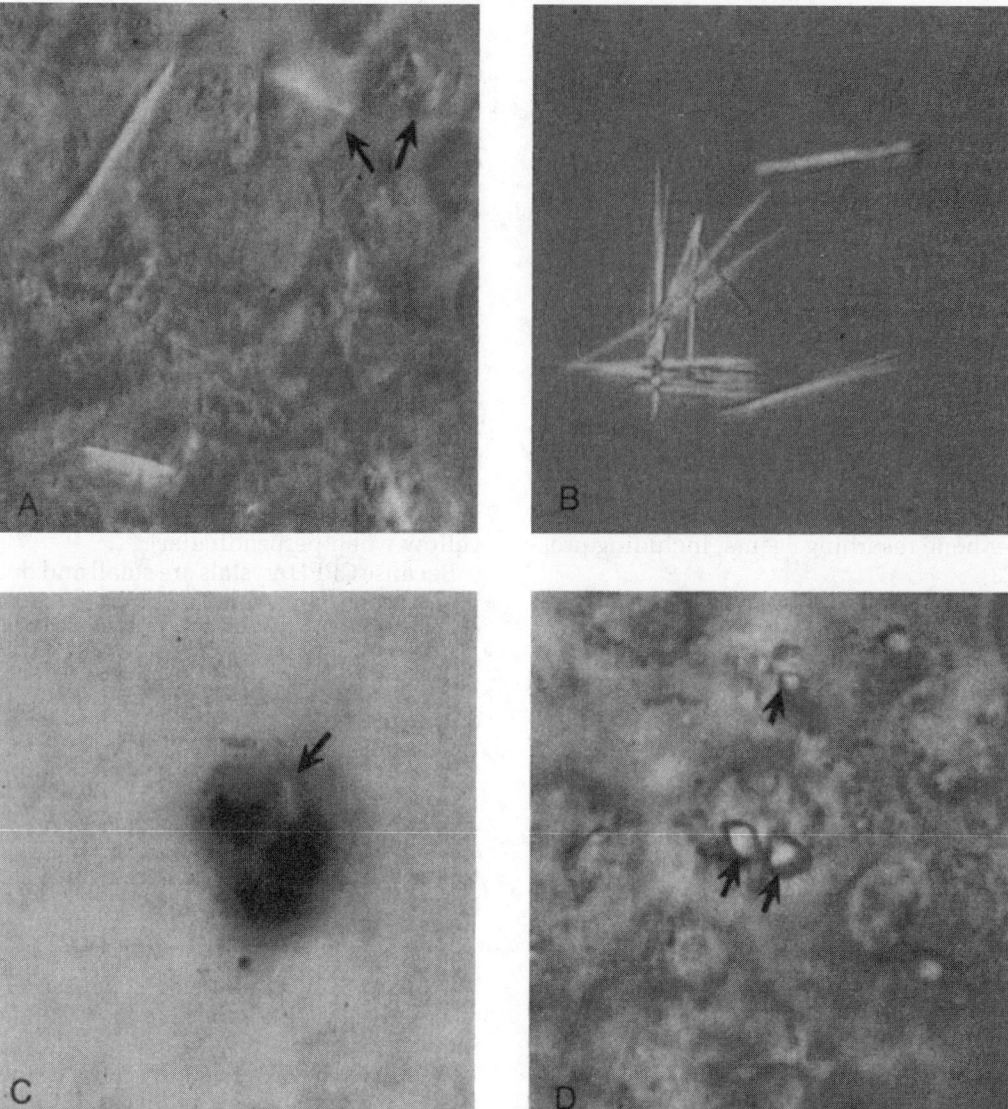

Figure 69.1.   A. Urate crystals in synovial fluid examined by polarized light microscopy. Note the needle shape and variable size *(arrow),* but many have larger diameter than white blood cells *(arrow;* oil immersion). **B.** Urate crystals from tophus examined by polarized light with red plate compensator (oil immersion). **C.** CPPD crystal in white blood cell found on Gram's stain (oil immersion). Note the shape and size relative to nucleus and cytoplasm. Gram's stain is not the usual method of demonstration, but it is occasionally useful. **D.** Wet preparation of synovial fluid demonstrating varied size and shape of CPPD crystal phagocytized by white blood cell (oil immersion lens, polarized light). Size and shape vary from squat rhomboid to rod shaped. Note several crystals in some cells.

those from previously injected corticosteroids (which appear as crystals of varying and unusual configuration) and occasionally cholesterol crystals, which are easily distinguished from all of the above (resembling a folded envelope). Contaminating crystalline or refractile substances, such as ethylenediaminetetraacetic acid (EDTA) anticoagulant, and talc, can be avoided by use of careful technique.

GOUT

Pathophysiology

Gout is a word derived from Latin meaning "a drop." It is applied to this form of arthritis because of the false belief, in ancient times, that the disease was caused by drops of bad humor. Gout is caused by an alteration in purine metabolism, the end product of which is uric acid. This alteration results in hyperuricemia and the deposition of urate crystals in various tissues. Periodic attacks of acute inflammatory arthritis, characteristic of gout, are caused by the deposition of urate crystals in and about joints. Primary gout is caused by an inborn error in the production or excretion of uric acid. Secondary gout is caused by an increased breakdown of nucleic acids in association with one of a variety of acquired diseases or by impaired excretion of urate as a consequence of acquired renal disease (Table 69.2).

Most patients with primary gout (approximately

90%) have, usually for unknown reasons, an elevated renal threshold for the excretion of uric acid. The rest (approximately 10%) overproduce urate, some as a result of recognized genetic abnormalities in purine metabolism with increased purine biosynthesis, as occurs in hypoxanthine phosphoribosyl transferase deficiency (74). Onset of gout before the age of 35 with a positive family history should suggest the possibility of a condition causing overproduction of urate. To assess production and excretion of urate, measurement in a 24-hour sample of urine may be indicated. Normally less than 600 mg/day is excreted if the diet for 5 days has been free of foods rich in purines. Because this diet is impractical for most patients, a reasonable estimate can be made on a regular diet. Urinary excretion exceeding 1000 mg/day is clearly abnormal and 800 to 1000 mg/day is borderline (33). An alternative method to screen for increased urate excretion on a regular diet is to measure urate and creatinine in serum and in spot midmorning urine samples, calculating the urate excretion normalized to a glomerular filtration rate of 100 mL/minute (62). Because overproduction related to a genetic defect is an uncommon cause of primary gout, the measurement of urinary urate is unnecessary for the management of most patients with gout unless a secondary cause of overproduction is suspected or uric acid stones have developed.

Normal levels of serum urate vary widely in the population, with a range of 3 to 8 mg/dL; also, there may be spontaneous variation within individual patients. The upper limit of normal for serum urate measured by the uricase method usually is considered to be 7.0 mg/dL for adult males and 6.0 mg/dL for females. Ranges may be higher by 1 mg/dL or more if automated colorimetric methods are used.

Table 69.2.   Causes of Hyperuricemia

With Increased Urinary Urate	With Normal or Low Urinary Urate
10% or primary gout (defects usually unknown)	90% of primary gout (defects unknown)
Specific enzyme defects	
HGPRTase deficiency, partial	
PP-Ribose-P synthetase	
variants	
Secondary causes	Secondary causes
Myeloproliferative disease	Renal insufficiency
Lymphoproliferative disease	Lead nephropathy
Obesity	Drugs
Glycogen storage disease	Diuretics
Psoriasis	Salicylates (low dose)
Vigorous exercise	Cyclosporine
	Pyrazinamide
	Ethambutol
	Nicotinic acid
	Others
	Obesity
	Fasting
	Hypothyroidism
	Sarcoidosis

Modified from Wyngaarden JB, Kelly WN. Gout and hyperuricemia. New York: Grune & Stratton, 1976.

Epidemiology

Gout is estimated to occur at a lifetime frequency of 3/1000 population in the United States. A recent study in England suggested an increase in prevalence to perhaps 10/1000 (27). Obesity and excessive weight gain were important risk factors for the development of gout in a prospective study of white men (59). However, in a later follow-up study including both white and black men, body mass index at enrollment was not a significant risk factor. However, the incidence of gout in black men was significantly higher than in white men and associated with systolic blood pressure at baseline and subsequent development of hypertension (28). Gout in all of its forms is 10 times more common in males and is rare in premenopausal females. Gout is rare below age 30 and increases in frequency to a plateau at about age 60. Age at onset is probably related to the duration and severity of preceding hyperuricemia. Gout is more common in obese or hypertensive people, although the relationships are complex. The frequency of gout in hypertensive subjects, for example, is magnified by treatment with thiazide diuretics, and this was not excluded as a cofactor in the incidence in black men noted above. Gout is also more common in patients with a chronically high alcohol intake, especially if they also are obese or have mildly impaired renal function. Gout may result from nephropathy caused by lead exposure, as exemplified by saturnine gout following ingestion of contaminated moonshine (6). More recently, the possibility that chronic environmental exposure to lead may occur more widely than suspected has been raised as the result of studies demonstrating increased levels of mobilization and excretion of lead following administration of the chelating agent EDTA (calcium disodium edetate) in industrial workers. An increased incidence of asymptomatic interstitial nephritis in addition to hyperuricemia, gout, and hypertension was observed to correlate with abnormally high levels of mobilized lead excretion (7). Hypertriglyceridemia is often present in patients with gout (75 to 80%), but whether this is related to alcohol, diet, obesity, or genetic factors is unclear (65). Data from the Framingham population study have confirmed the long-held clinical impression of an increased incidence of coronary heart disease (especially angina pectoris) in males with gout. A 60% greater prevalence of coronary heart disease was observed in men with gout than in men without gout in this population. Interestingly, this was independent of other measured risk factors, and as reported in other studies, there was no significant difference in the prevalence of diabetes mellitus or elevated serum cholesterol in the gouty men and in men without gout in the population studied over a 14-year period (1). The association of hyperuricemia and gout with hypothyroidism has been demonstrated in a study of 54 patients with gout tested with a sensitive TSH assay. Overall, 20% (15% of men and 40% of women) were shown to have hypothyroidism that was often subclinical or unrecognized (13).

Clinical Features

Acute Arthritic Attack

The acute arthritic attack is the hallmark of gout (Table 69.3). It is characterized by the onset of pain, swelling, and discomfort that progress rapidly to a peak level of intensity within 24 to 36 hours after onset. The pain is often severe enough to prevent use of the affected joint or even for the patient to bear the weight of bed clothing. The metatarsophalangeal joint of the great toe is the most commonly affected joint, followed by the forefoot, heel, ankle, knee, wrist, fingers, and elbow. The great toe is affected at some time during the course of perhaps 90% of gouty subjects. Usually a single joint is involved early in the course of the disease but pauciarticular arthritis (two or three joints) may occur; polyarticular (more than three joints) onset is rare. Polyarticular gout is more common in late disease associated with soft tissue tophi. Recurrent acute arthritis is more common in previously affected joints.

Several events may trigger an acute attack of gout: trauma, an acute illness such as an acute myocardial infarction, dietary indiscretion, overuse of alcohol, fasting, and recent administration of drugs that lower serum urate concentration. Most of these events are associated with rapid changes in serum urate concentration, and it has been postulated that such changes cause dissolution of tissue deposits with discharge of crystalline material locally to induce the acute attack.

A family history of gout may be present in patients with primary gout, and especially in patients who excrete excess amounts of uric acid in whom a specific enzyme defect may be suspected. However, a positive family history is obtained in less than half of gouty subjects, so a negative history is of no differential diagnostic value.

On physical examination of the patient with acute gouty arthritis there is often erythema overlying or adjacent to the affected joints, especially when small joints are involved. The erythema often involves only a localized area rather than the entire joint. The intensity of the inflammatory reaction often results in a mistaken diagnosis of cellulitis, a diagnosis that may appear to be supported by a fever that may reach 101°F (38°C), although temperature in this range or higher is uncommon in acute gout. Joint swelling usually is marked and joint effusion is also common. Tenderness on palpation or motion of the affected part usually is marked.

The intensity and severity of these classic acute signs and symptoms may vary from one attack to another. Early in the disease, milder episodes lasting only a few days may be passed off by the patient as being caused by minor trauma. The outward evidence of inflammation also may be less evident when a large joint such as the knee is involved, especially in elderly patients and in patients with polyarticular gout. However, the history almost always indicates rapid progression to a peak intensity within 24 to 36 hours, an important feature in differential diagnosis. A history of episodes of similar events is also helpful.

Laboratory findings may include a mild leukocytosis and an elevated erythrocyte sedimentation rate. Serum uric acid almost always is elevated but is of limited diagnostic value because of the frequency of hyperuricemia in the absence of gout, and because the acute attack, which is related principally to the concentration of tissue urate, may occur at a time when the serum urate may be normal as a result of previous drug administration or spontaneous variation. Examination of the synovial fluid provides diagnostic findings in almost all instances in which it can be obtained. There is a leukocytosis in the joint fluid with polymorphonuclear leukocytes that, when examined under polarized light, can be seen to contain phagocytized urate crystals (see "Crystal Identification"). The technique of aspiration of joint fluid is described in Chapter 66. The physician should be experienced in this technique before attempting it or the patient should be referred to a rheumatologist. The first metatarsophalangeal joint is a particularly painful joint to tap, especially during an acute attack, and this is not recommended without considerable experience.

The acute attack is self-limited and even without treatment it subsides in several days to weeks. Early in the disease, once the acute attack subsides or is treated, there are no residual joint symptoms—another important point in the differential diagnosis.

Recurrent acute attacks are usual: Approximately 75% of patients have a second gouty attack within 2 years of their first and most of these occur within the first year; occasionally 10 years or more may elapse between attacks (76).

Intercritical Gout

Between acute attacks of gout, patients are totally asymptomatic with no abnormal physical findings

Table 69.3. Clinical Features of Gout

Epidemiology
Sex: Males 10 to 1; rare in premenopausal women
Age: Usually middle age or older (peak age 60)

Acute Gout
History
 Acute attacks, recurrent, with disease-free intervals
 Rapid progression to peak severity within 24 hours
Physical findings
 Usually monoarticular with swelling, tenderness, erythema, and intense inflammation
 Big toe metatarsophalangeal joint commonly involved (podagra)
 Forefeet, heels, ankles, knees, wrists, fingers, elbows, and other joints may be affected
 Occasionally polyarticular
 Fever may occur
Laboratory
 Joint aspiration with leukocytosis and identification of urate crystals is diagnostic

Intercritical Gout
No symptoms or findings except hyperuricemia

Chronic Gout
Often polyarticular
Symptoms may persist between attacks
Tophi are common (approximately 90–95%)
Deformities may develop

unless tophi are present or unless the disease has progressed to the chronic phase. If the patient's first visit to the physician is at this stage, a presumptive diagnosis can be made on the basis of a history of a typical attack, especially if there have been multiple attacks, and on the basis of hyperuricemia. Aspiration of the great toe during intercritical gout demonstrates urate crystals in many (70%) patients with gout, but crystals rarely may be found in patients with asymptomatic hyperuricemia or renal failure (58,69,72). Knee joint aspiration also yielded urate crystals in patients with intercritical nontophaceous gout. The yield was much higher (97%) in fluid from previously inflamed but asymptomatic knees in patients who had not received urate-lowering drugs (46). Although urate crystals are highly specific for gout, the difficulty of obtaining synovial fluid in asymptomatic patients in the absence of overt inflammation or effusion suggests that these procedures have limited usefulness in clinical practice.

Chronic Gout

Chronic gout is rare, especially since the advent of effective therapy to control hyperuricemia. Patients with chronic gout often have some persistent symptoms (e.g., morning stiffness) and manifest signs of synovial tissue thickening and some joint deformity. Acute exacerbations are still common and are often polyarticular. Tophi (soft tissue deposits of sodium urate) are present in 90 to 95% of patients with chronic gout. The rate of formation of tophi seems to be a direct function of the level and duration of hyperuricemia. Tophi are chalky or pinkish, gritty, usually superficial deposits that are palpable in joints or over tendons, in pressure points, or in the pinnae of the ears. Tophi in fingerpads were found in 30% of 36 patients with tophaceous gout attending hospital outpatient clinics (29).They are usually painless but after palpation they may be tender. Large tophi may look like bulbous swellings of the joints or, when they are located over the extensor surface of the forearm or in the ulnar bursa, may be mistaken for rheumatoid nodules. The distribution of tophi may be different in females, with elbows and feet less common sites than in males (52). The coincident occurrence of proven gout in distal interphalangeal joints associated with nodal osteoarthritis, especially in elderly patients on diuretic therapy for hypertension, has been reported (17). In such circumstances, aspiration or biopsy of tophi with demonstration of urate crystals confirms the diagnosis of chronic gout. The actual concurrence of gout and rheumatoid arthritis is extremely rare (70).

Extra-Articular Manifestations

It has long been known that gout may be associated with renal disease in three forms: *chronic urate nephropathy, nephrolithiasis,* and *acute uric acid nephropathy.*

Chronic urate nephropathy develops after many years of hyperuricemia and results from the deposition in the interstitial medullary tissue of sodium urate crystals that cause, ultimately, an interstitial nephritis.

In patients with asymptomatic hyperuricemia regardless of the level, the risk of developing nephropathy does not warrant treatment to lower the serum urate as a prophylactic measure. At one time, the frequency of the complication of chronic urate nephropathy in gouty subjects was assumed to be high. However, controlled studies indicate that the incidence of renal insufficiency solely from gout and hyperuricemia is low and that renal dysfunction is usually mild; most often renal failure in patients with gout can be attributed to other causes such as vascular disease or primary renal disease (8,76). Renal failure from primary gout and hyperuricemia is usually silent and suspected only because of the identification of a mild abnormality of the blood urea nitrogen or serum creatinine concentration. Some patients have slight proteinuria; only a few are found to have peripheral tophi. The evaluation and management of patients who have renal failure are discussed in Chapter 48.

Uric acid nephrolithiasis accounts for only a small number of patients who have urinary calculi (see Chapter 47). However, approximately 20% of patients with gout develop calculi, although the stones may antedate acute gouty arthritis by years. From a different perspective, approximately 25% of patients with uric acid calculi have an abnormal serum urate concentration. The prevalence of uric acid calculi increases proportionately to the concentration of serum urate or the excretion of uric acid whether or not gout is present. In one study, in which a cohort of men was followed for 12 years, serum levels of urate of 7 to 8, 8 to 9, and more than 9 mg/dL were associated with renal stones in 12.7, 22, and 40%, respectively (24). Also in gouty patients, urinary excretion rates of less than 300, 300 to 700, 701 to 1100, and more than 1100 mg uric acid per 24 hours were associated with an incidence of renal stones of 11, 21, 35, and 50%, respectively (77). The development of uric acid calculi is related not only to uric acid excretion but also to urinary pH and concentration. This subject is more fully discussed in Chapter 47. An effective scheme for ambulatory evaluation of nephrolithiasis has been presented in detail (37).

Acute uric acid nephropathy is associated with a sudden increase in urate production and a marked rise in uric acid excretion, resulting in the formation of microcrystals in the renal tubules. This most often occurs in patients with lymphoproliferative or myeloproliferative disorders, especially during treatment. Preventive measures to lower urate production are effective and acute uric acid nephropathy is rarely encountered in ambulatory practice.

Differential Diagnosis

During the acute attack gout must be differentiated principally from acute infectious arthritis, bursitis related to a bunion (see Chapter 102), or other forms of crystal-induced arthritis. Therefore, it is important to aspirate joint fluid for smear and culture (see Chapter 66 for technique and finding in the synovial fluid) as well as for crystal identification. Infectious arthritis is associated with a very low synovial fluid glucose, not found in gouty fluids. Rarely, acute gout and infectious arthritis coexist (4). Fever above 101°F (38°C) or lack of prompt defeverescence in response to anti-inflammatory drugs should raise suspicion of infection or an alternative diagnosis.

X-Rays

In the early course of gout, x-rays are normal except for acute soft tissue swelling (Fig. 69.2). As the disease progresses, lucent areas of urate deposits may be seen in bone adjacent to the joints. These lesions may be mistaken for the erosions that are seen in rheumatoid or other arthritides but may be distinguished from them in that osteoporosis and bony sclerosis, which are common in other erosive diseases, are not present. Overhanging margins of bone are said to be characteristic of gouty erosions but are not often found. Therefore, only occasionally are x-rays indicated as an aid to diagnosis or differential diagnosis of patients suspected of having gout. Tophi appearing as capsular or intra-articular opaque masses were identified on CT scan of the knee in 5 of 16 patients with advanced crystal proven gout, sometimes in the absence of subcutaneous tophi (20).

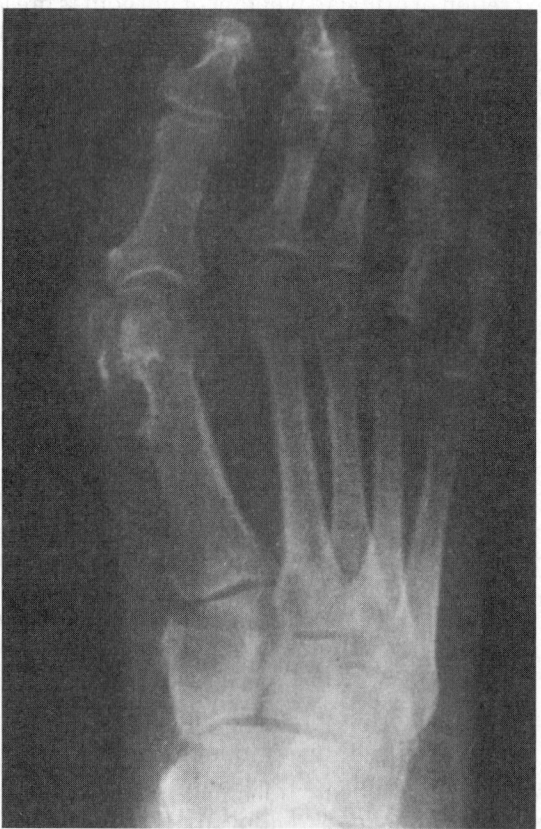

Figure 69.2. X-ray of the foot in patient with gout showing soft tissue swelling over the first metatarsophalangeal joint and typical gouty erosion; away from joint margin, punched out with overhanging edge and no osteoporosis.

Management

If the diagnosis of gout can be established with certainty by the demonstration of urate crystals, the treatment is simple and straightforward. Unless there is a complicating illness, hospitalization is not required. Even the most severe case can be effectively managed on an ambulatory basis. The key elements in management are control of the pain of the acute attack and patient education to ensure compliance with therapy administered to reduce serum urate concentration and prevent recurrent attacks and progression to chronic tophaceous gout.

Management of the Acute Attack

If the diagnosis of acute gout is established or if gout has been diagnosed previously by the identification of urate crystals in the affected joints, rapid relief can be obtained in almost all cases by the administration of nonsteroidal anti-inflammatory drugs (NSAIDs) in appropriate dosages. Indomethacin (Indocin) 50 mg (two 25-mg capsules) every 6 hours for six to eight doses is dramatically effective in reducing pain, often within a few hours. In the absence of moderate to severe compromise of renal function, there are few side effects if the dosage is quickly reduced to 25 mg every 6 to 8 hours after the pain and inflammation begin to wane and maintained until the attack is completely resolved, usually no more than 5 to 7 days. Alternatively, other NSAIDs may be used (see Chapter 70 for a full discussion of NSAIDs) and are apparently equally effective, although few comparative studies are available. The plasma concentration and therapeutic effect of indomethacin (and of naproxen but apparently not of other NSAIDs) are potentiated by an unknown mechanism by the simultaneous administration of probenecid (see below). Although the clinical significance of this interaction is unclear, especially with short-course therapy, the manufacturer recommends that the dosage of the nonsteroidal drug be reduced in patients who also are taking probenecid. Caution should also be used in patients with impaired renal function or reduced renal blood flow caused by cardiovascular disease because NSAIDs may acutely reduce renal function and precipitate acute renal failure or hyperkalemia (see Chapter 48). This is especially important in frail elderly patients with low muscle mass in whom the degree of renal impairment may not be immediately evident from the level of serum creatinine.

Colchicine is the time-honored drug for treatment of acute gout, but its efficacy is limited by side effects that are almost invariable if an adequate dosage is administered orally. The usual regimen is 0.6 mg every 1 to 2 hours up to 16 doses until relief is obtained or until side effects, usually diarrhea, nausea, or vomiting, develop. The dosage should be reduced in patients with impaired renal or hepatic function. It is no longer necessary to subject a patient to severe diarrhea when he or she already has a very painful joint, so oral colchicine has largely been replaced by other agents that are as effective and have fewer side effects. The exception is in the well-instructed patient who immediately after recognizing the onset of an acute attack of gout can institute oral colchicine and in doing so can abort the attack with a few doses and with minimal side effects.

Intravenous administration of colchicine rapidly provides a therapeutic plasma level of the drug and does not cause gastrointestinal side effects. It is useful in treatment of acute gout when the patient cannot take medication by mouth and in the patient with peptic ulcer disease, or with another contraindication to the use of nonsteroidal agents or corticosteroids. Two milligrams colchicine (available in ampules containing 1 mg in 2 mL) diluted with isotonic saline to 20 mL and given over 10 minutes intravenously usually provides relief within 6 to 8 hours and, if necessary, may be followed by one or two doses of 1 mg in 20 mL isotonic saline intravenously in 12 to 24 hours, not to exceed 4 mg in 24 hours. Reduced dosage is necessary in patients with impaired renal or hepatic function and in the frail elderly patient with apparently normal renal function or in patients with neutropenia. Care must be used to prevent extravasation of colchicine into the soft tissues because it may cause necrosis. Intravenous colchicine should not be used if the patient has recently received a course of oral colchicine or if there is combined renal and hepatic disease, creatinine clearance below 10 mL/minute, or extrahepatic biliary obstruction. No additional colchicine should be given by any route for 7 days after a full intravenous dose (41). Because of the potentially serious toxicity of intravenous colchicine (53,71), its rare indication, and lack of knowledge by practitioners about its use and limitations, some medical centers have proscribed its use.

A therapeutic response of a typical attack of gout in the great toe to oral colchicine has often been advocated to make a presumptive diagnosis of gout in the absence of crystal identification. Such a trial has limited value, however, because acute gout of several days' duration may not respond rapidly to colchicine and because pseudogout caused by CPPD-induced arthritis and occasionally other forms of arthritis may occasionally affect this joint and respond.

Because the patient or the inexperienced physician may be wary of attempting aspiration of this joint when it is exquisitely painful with acute inflammation, a presumptive diagnosis of gout can be made on clinical grounds and the patient treated with nonsteroidal or other agents. A raised serum uric acid would further support the diagnosis of gout but is neither specific nor always present. A strong suspicion of infection would mandate a diagnostic aspiration.

Corticosteroids provide another therapeutic alternative for acute gout in the patient who has a contraindication to therapy with NSAIDs. Aspiration and intra-articular injection of corticosteroid suspension is useful when a single large joint is involved. For patients requiring parenteral therapy, intramuscular or intravenous injections of adrenocorticotrophic hormone (ACTH) or soluble corticosteroid preparation is effective. Intramuscular ACTH 40 to 80 units every 6 to 12 hours for up to 3 days, intravenous methylprednisolone 100 to 150 mg repeated as needed, and triamcinolone acetonide 60 mg intramuscularly per day for 2 to 3 days are equally effective (15). A single dose is effective in some patients, especially early in the attack (73). Moderately high initial dosages of oral corticosteroids are usually required (30 to 60 mg/day of prednisone tapered slowly over 7 to 10 days) for complete resolution without recrudescence (22).

Drugs administered to lower serum urate have no place in the treatment of the acute gouty attack. In fact, these agents may exacerbate acute attacks by the associated changes in plasma urate levels (see above).

Intercritical Gout

The efficacy of colchicine in dosages of 0.6 mg one, two, or three times daily (dosage frequency depends on control; most patients tolerate two doses a day without side effects) in reducing the frequency of acute attacks of gout has been well established (48,76). Thus, prophylactic colchicine is indicated for patients who have had more than one episode of acute gout in a year or when therapy to lower urate is initiated. Caution again is required in patients with impaired renal function. Reversible myopathy and neuropathy have been observed in some patients whose serum creatinine was above 1.6 mg/dL even with two tablets per day (35). Infertility or azoospermia was also reported with the use of long-term prophylactic colchicine in 4 of 19 young men with familial Mediterranean fever (12). In elderly patients without tophi (nontophaceous gout), with infrequent acute attacks and only mild hyperuricemia (i.e., below 8 to 9 mg/dL), prophylactic colchicine may be all that is required. Some patients who have nontophaceous gout with infrequent attacks of arthritis (e.g., fewer than one or two a year) and who have mild hyperuricemia (i.e., below 8 to 9 mg/dL) may elect not to take regular colchicine prophylaxis; in this instance, the episodic use of an NSAID such as indomethacin (Indocin; see above) is appropriate to control acute attacks. However, in most patients with gout and with persistent hyperuricemia of 9 mg/dL or higher, the serum urate concentration should be reduced to prevent recurrent gout and to reverse the accumulation of urate in the tissues. In this instance, colchicine prophylaxis should be continued until the patient has been free of attacks for at least 1 year after the concentration of serum urate has returned to normal. As an alternative in patients intolerant of colchicine, NSAIDs can also be used in prophylaxis but may have more serious toxic effects than colchicine. Omitting prophylactic therapy and treating acute attacks early if they occur may be an alternative for some patients with rare attacks.

Two classes of drugs that lower serum urate concentration are available: *uricosuric agents* promote urinary excretion of urate by blocking tubular urate resorption, and *allopurinol* (Zyloprim) decreases production of urate through inhibition of purine metabolism. Indications for the use of allopurinol are a history of urinary calculi or the presence of renal dysfunction, of chronic tophaceous gout, or excessive basal urinary uric acid excretion (i.e., more than 750 mg/24 hours), or of high levels of serum urate associated with secondary gout. Uricosuric agents are most effective in patients with nontophaceous gout with normal renal function (creatinine clearance of at least 60 to 80 mL/minute) and normal uric acid excretion (i.e., less than 750 mg/24 hours). In most patients clinical evidence identifying one of the causes of impaired urinary excretion rather than overproduction of urate (as noted in Table 69.2) is obvious. When there is uncertainty, evaluation of urinary uric acid excretion is important not only as a clue to the mechanism of hyperuricemia (Table 69.2) but in the choice of therapy.

Probenecid (Benemid) is the uricosuric agent of choice because of its well-established safety and its long duration of effect. An initial dosage of 0.5 g twice daily should be increased to 1.5 g daily or to a maximum of 2 g/day (in two or three divided doses) to achieve a serum urate concentration consistently below 6.5 mg/dL, the level required to produce a urate gradient from tissue to plasma and to prevent further deposition of urate. To minimize the chance of precipitating a recurrent arthritic attack, the uricosuric agent should not be initiated until at least a week after an acute attack of gout has subsided and only after colchicine prophylaxis (see above) has been initiated for 3 or 4 days. The principal side effect of probenecid is gastrointestinal distress (which is uncommon), but there is a risk of the formation of uric acid calculi in the renal tubules in the first week of therapy, especially when there is a large basal uric acid excretion (i.e., 600 to 800 mg/day); this risk can be minimized if the patient drinks 2 to 3 L of fluid/day and takes an alkalinizing agent such as sodium bicarbonate or citrate salt (polycitrate), 0.5 to 1 mEq/kg of body weight in five or six doses a day, to keep the urine pH (measured from time to time with pH paper) above 6.0 or 6.5 for the first week of uricosuric therapy. Small dosages of aspirin (2.4 g/day) block the effect of probenecid on renal excretion of urate and should be avoided. Probenecid may reduce the excretion of other drugs, including NSAIDs and penicillin, and prolong their half-life. Probenecid may also give a false-positive test for glucose in the urine.

Sulfinpyrazone (Anturane) is a more potent uricosuric agent but has more potential for adverse effects. It can be given beginning with 50 to 100 mg twice daily and increasing gradually to 600 to 800 mg/day if required to achieve the desired serum urate level (below 6 mg/dL). This agent, which is an analog of phenylbutazone, may cause gastric ulceration and platelet dysfunction. It may also interact with sulfonamides or sulfonylureas to increase their hypoglycemic effect. For these reasons, it should be used principally when probenecid or allopurinol (see below) is not tolerated.

Allopurinol (Zyloprim) is a potent agent that reduces the concentration of serum urate. Because it blocks urate production by inhibition of xanthine oxidase, it is particularly useful in patients with renal dysfunction or with uric acid calculi and in patients with long-standing gout with tophi. Serious side effects of rash, fever, leukopenia, hepatitis, and occasionally a generalized vasculitis occur in less than 2% of patients. These symptoms are most likely to occur within the first 2 months after initiation of therapy, so patients should be kept under close surveillance during this period. Toxicity is enhanced in patients with severe renal compromise or when the drug is administered concomitantly with ampicillin or thiazide diuretics (26). Allopurinol (Zyloprim, available in 100- and 300-mg tablets) should be started at a dosage of 200 mg/day and increased over 2 or 3 weeks until the serum urate is consistently below 6.0 mg/dL; no more than 300 mg should be administered as a single dose. Prolonged use of dosages in excess of 300 mg twice a day increases the risk of toxicity; however, dosages of 400 to 600 mg/day are commonly required initially for effective control of serum urate and reduction of tissue urate load.

In patients with chronic tophaceous gout, concomitant use of allopurinol and probenecid has been advocated (60). These agents seem to have an additive effect in lowering serum uric acid. However, use of a single agent is preferable if possible.

Compliance is the major factor in the effective therapy of intercritical gout. Patients feel well between attacks, and continued compliance with medications requires reinforcement in patient education and follow-up visits to ensure maintenance of normal serum levels of urate.

In general, therapy should be lifelong to prevent recurrent attacks or further accumulation of urate in the tissues. Continued treatment with drugs to lower serum urate was estimated to be cost-saving if the patient has 2 attacks per year and cost-effective if one per year occurs (19).

Dietary advice to patients with gout should be kept simple. High-purine foods (organ meats, seafood, all meats, meat gravies and extracts, lentils, peas, asparagus, yeast, and beer) are common in Western diets and strict avoidance is neither practical nor necessary in the treatment of most patients with gout. Patients should be aware of these high-purine foods and avoid excesses of intake. More important dietary advice is to avoid alcohol (beer especially because it also adds to the purine load) and to avoid fasting beyond 24 hours because both these situations may be associated with an acute increase of serum urate concentration, which may precipitate an attack of gout.

Chronic Gout

Compliance with appropriate therapy should eliminate this phase of gout except in a few patients with severe disease who are intolerant of one or more drugs used in treatment. Continuous or intermittent use of NSAIDs may be required in some of these patients for adequate control of inflammation and chronic symptoms. Effective reduction in serum urate for months or years results in dissolution of tophi and general improvement. However, very large tophi may require surgical removal. After prolonged therapy and resolution of tophi, consideration has been given to discontinuation of therapy with urate-lowering drugs. However, acute attacks and tophi are likely to recur (68) so that stopping therapy is not recommended.

Patients with severe chronic tophaceous gout and renal insufficiency often have recurrent polyarticular gout and present a difficult management problem if they develop cutaneous reactions to allopurinol (Zyloprim). Success in desensitizing some patients was reported by administering gradually increasing dosages of the drug, beginning with as little as 5 mg/day (16), but patients with severe reactions such as toxic epidermal necrolysis, hepatitis, or acute interstitial nephritis were excluded from this study. Anturane as a potent uricosuric agent is most likely to be a successful alternative if renal function permits.

Asymptomatic Hyperuricemia

Hyperuricemia (more than 7 mg/dL in males and more than 6 mg/dL in females) is a common laboratory finding in asymptomatic patients evaluated in a variety of clinical settings. In most patients, clinical findings point to an obvious cause and no other therapy is required unless gout or nephrolithiasis develops (9,38). If the cause is unclear or the level of serum urate is near 11 mg/dL, further evaluation to estimate urinary excretion and identify secondary causes of excessive urate production (Table 69.2) should be initiated (33).

Hyperuricemia Secondary to Diuretics

The renal tubular handling of uric acid is complex: There is complete glomerular filtration followed by tubular resorption, tubular secretion, and further tubular resorption. The resorption of uric acid is in part modulated by the volume of extracellular fluid (expansion increases excretion and contraction decreases excretion). Diuretics modify the renal handling of uric acid by their effect on volume, and some diuretics may directly affect urate transport. Thiazides regularly cause a dosage-related rise of the serum urate level. This elevation is reversed upon withdrawal of the agent. The increase in concentration averages 1 to 2 mg/dL but occasionally may be 4 to 5 mg/dL. Furosemide also is often associated with a rise in concentration of serum urate; less commonly ethacrynic acid, acetazolamide, and rarely triamterene are associated with hyperuricemia. Spironolactone per se is not associated with hyperuricemia.

The incidence of gout after the initiation of a diuretic is a complex issue. Other factors that affect the incidence of gout, such as hypertension and obesity, are often present in patients treated with diuretics. Approximately 10% of hypertensive patients with hyperuricemia secondary to diuretic therapy develop gout. This risk increases in patients with known gout and patients with diseases associated with elevation of serum urate, such as myeloproliferative disorders or psoriasis. Also in association with diuretic therapy,

uric acid excretion is diminished and there is no increase in the incidence of urinary calculi. The risk of developing urate nephropathy is minimal (see above). For these reasons, expectant management of patients with asymptomatic hyperuricemia secondary to diuretics is appropriate.

Should acute gout develop, treatment as described above may be initiated. Intercritical gout is managed similarly to primary gout; prophylactic colchicine and uricosuric therapy with probenecid (if there is no renal failure) or allopurinol to decrease production of urate may be used. Reducing the dosage or stopping the diuretic is usually associated with a slight fall in the plasma urate concentration, but many patients continue to have attacks of gout. Therefore, if a patient develops gout while taking diuretics and the need for the diuretic continues, it is best to treat the gout as discussed above and to continue the use of the diuretic at the minimally effective dosage. In the management of hypertension, the use of angiotensin-converting enzyme inhibitors and long-acting calcium channel blocking agents, which have no effect on urate excretion, may allow discontinuation of diuretics in some patients (36).

CALCIUM PYROPHOSPHATE DIHYDRATE–INDUCED ARTHRITIS
Pathophysiology

Pseudogout is a syndrome caused by the deposition of CPPD in fibrocartilage (chondrocalcinosis) and joint tissue and in ligaments and tendons, with an occasional resulting inflammatory response. It most often is idiopathic but may be associated with certain other diseases (see below).

Inorganic pyrophosphate is an important metabolite in many biosynthetic reactions, where it is removed from macromolecules through the action of pyrophosphatases. It is adsorbed to hydroxyapatite and is probably involved in the regulation of mineralization, both in the accretion from amorphous calcium phosphate and in the dissolution of crystalline hydroxyapatite.

Epidemiology

Chondrocalcinosis increases in frequency with age; it is present in approximately 5% of the adult population at the time of autopsy and in 20 to 30% of people above age 80, most of whom are asymptomatic. The exact prevalence of CPPD deposit disease is unknown. In one series of consecutive patients with newly diagnosed crystal-induced arthritis, CPPD deposit disease accounted for about one-third of the cases. Men are probably affected more than women, with a male/female ratio of 1.5:1 (41).

Causes

Familial cases with an autosomal-dominant inheritance have been described (56) in which chondrocalcinosis appears at an earlier age. These families are uncommon, and many of these patients remain asymptomatic for many years; the metabolic defect has not been identified, however. Early onset of osteoarthritis and chondrocalcinosis has been linked to chromosome 8q (5). Most cases of CPPD deposit disease are sporadic and idiopathic; a few are associated with one of a variety of metabolic diseases (43). Many of the diseases associated with deposits of CPPD involve metabolic abnormalities in connective tissues, but the precise mechanisms of CPPD crystallization are unknown. A list of these associated diseases is presented in Table 69.4.

Clinical Features

Patients are usually middle-age to elderly at the time of onset of arthritic symptoms (Table 69.5). There are several possible patterns of presentation: About one-quarter have *self-limited acute goutlike attacks (pseudogout)* predominantly affecting the knees and wrists, but occasionally involving other joints, including rarely the first metatarsophalangeal joint. Monarticular attacks are the rule, but involvement of symmetric joints and polyarthritis may occur rarely. Symptoms are often less intense than they are in gout, but the presentation is variable and some attacks may be severe. Systemic symptoms, including fever to 101°F (38°C) or more, may occur as in gout, and patients are often misdiagnosed as having infection. In some elderly patients, the fever may be the dominant symptom and the joint abnormalities subtle and overlooked (54). Attacks are often exacerbated by trauma and by acute illness. Long intervals (sometimes years) between attacks are common.

In about half the patients, and especially in women, the presentation resembles osteoarthritis with bilateral involvement, especially of the knees. The wrists, the metacarpophalangeal (MCP) joints, hips, shoulders, elbows, or ankles also may be affected. Acute exacerbations occur in about half of these patients with features that resemble osteoarthritis, except that the disease is more progressive and destructive. Varus or valgus knee deformities are common, and extensive calcification around the patella may be seen on x-ray. Flexion contractures may occur also. The relationship to ordinary osteoarthritis is still unclear, except that the involvement of joints not usually affected in osteoarthritis (MCP joints, wrists, shoulders, elbows) suggests a different pathogenesis. However, this is controversial. Use of a new, sensitive technique to measure calcium crystals along with light and elec-

Table 69.4. Diseases Associated with CPPD Deposition Disease

Hemochromatosis–hemosiderosis	Hereditary hypophosphatasia
Gout	Hypothyroidism
Osteoarthritis	Neurogenic arthropathy
Hyperparathyroidism	Osteochondrodysplasia
Hypomagnesemia	Synovial chondromatosis

Table 69.5. Clinical Features of CPPD Deposit Disease

Epidemiology
Age: middle aged or elderly

Site
Knee and wrist most common joints involved
Metacarpophalangeal joints, hips, shoulders, elbows, ankles may be affected
Arthritis usually monoarticular

Pattern
Acute goutlike attacks with symptom-free intervals in 25%
Osteoarthritislike disease in 50%, with superimposed acute attacks in half of these patients
Rheumatoidlike polyarthritis in 5%
Neuropathiclike arthritis without neurologic damage (rare)
Asymptomatic chondrocalcinosis in 20% (found on x-ray)

Laboratory
Synovial fluid shows leukocytosis and characteristic CPPD crystals

tron microscopy allowed CPPD or basic calcium phosphate crystals to be demonstrated in 11 of 12 patients with typical osteoarthritis of the knee when they were not always detected by usual methods (see Chapter 68) (64).

In a few patients, persistent subacute inflammation with fatigue, morning stiffness, and synovial swelling in multiple joints lasting weeks or months resembles rheumatoid arthritis.

A few patients also have been reported with severely *destructive arthritis* resembling the Charcot joints of neuropathic arthropathy but associated with a normal neurologic examination. CPPD deposit disease may also be associated with a true neuropathic arthritis caused by tabes dorsalis.

Laboratory Findings

Patients may have peripheral leukocytosis and an elevated erythrocyte sedimentation rate in association with acute or subacute attacks of arthritis. The synovial fluid shows polymorphonuclear leukocytosis that may exceed $50,000/mm^3$ in acute pseudogout but is more commonly in the range of 15,000 to 25,000. Crystal identification is the key to diagnosis (see above). In the absence of acute or subacute inflammation, leukocyte counts may be low (below $2,000/mm^3$) and crystals may be largely extracellular.

Because of the occasional association with other potentially treatable disorders (Table 69.4) and the ease of these determinations, the patient's serum calcium, phosphorus, magnesium, alkaline phosphatase, and uric acid concentrations should be measured, although they usually are normal (41). Seven patients with familial Bartter's syndrome and associated chondrocalcinosis were reported to have hypokalemia and hypomagnesemia, with excessive urinary excretion of these ions and hypocalciuria. Of interest in pathogenesis is that magnesium supplementation resulted in a striking reduction of chondrocalcinosis over a

10-year period (63). Because pseudogout may be the presenting manifestation of hemochromatosis and because of the importance of early diagnosis in this disorder, measurement of serum ferritin is also indicated if there is any suspicion of this diagnosis (31).

Radiographic Findings

The typical radiographic findings of CPPD deposit disease are punctate and linear calcifications (chondrocalcinosis), seen most often in the fibrocartilage of the menisci of the knee, usually bilaterally (Fig. 69.3). Other fibrocartilages may show similar changes, including the disc in the distal radioulnar joint, the symphysis pubis, the lip of the acetabulum, or the glenoid fossa or intervertebral discs. Hyaline cartilage may also be involved with similar punctate linear calcifications that may be identified as a dense line parallel to the subchondral bone. Calcification in the soft tissues of the joint capsule and occasionally in ligaments and tendons may also be seen but is less characteristic. In patients with the type of CPPD deposit disease that resembles osteoarthritis, subchondral cyst formation with bony collapse may be prominent. Osteophyte formation is variable and inconsistent.

These radiographic findings may be helpful in suggesting or confirming the diagnosis of CPPD deposit disease. However, it may not be possible to visualize the extent of deposits radiographically, and their absence does not exclude the diagnosis if typical crystals can be demonstrated in synovial fluid or in biopsy material.

Management

No therapy influences the deposition or resolution of tissue deposits of CPPD. In the acute episode, diagnostic aspiration (see Chapter 67 for technique) of synovial fluid with removal of crystals and leukocytes may provide significant clinical improvement. Local injection of depocorticosteroid is often effective and avoids potential side effects of systemic drug therapy (see Chapter 66 for technique). Efficacy of colchicine has been debated, and although it is sometimes effective, the use of indomethacin (Indocin) or other NSAIDs is generally preferred as described above for acute gout. Because many of these patients are elderly (and may therefore have an impaired glomerular filtration rate), caution regarding renal toxicity of these agents should be exercised (see Chapter 48). A brief course of systemic corticosteroids as in the treatment of acute gout is an alternative, but because a single joint is usually affected, intra-articular steroid is preferred. In patients with only recurrent acute attacks, no therapy is indicated between attacks, but early administration of anti-inflammatory agents on exacerbation may minimize or abort attacks. Therapy for patients with more subacute inflammation or for those with osteoarthritis-like disease is similar to that described for osteoarthritis (see Chapter 68), except that anti-inflammatory levels of drugs may be required for optimal symptomatic control.

HYDROXYAPATITE-INDUCED ARTHRITIS

The capacity of hydroxyapatite crystals to induce an inflammatory response was first appreciated in some

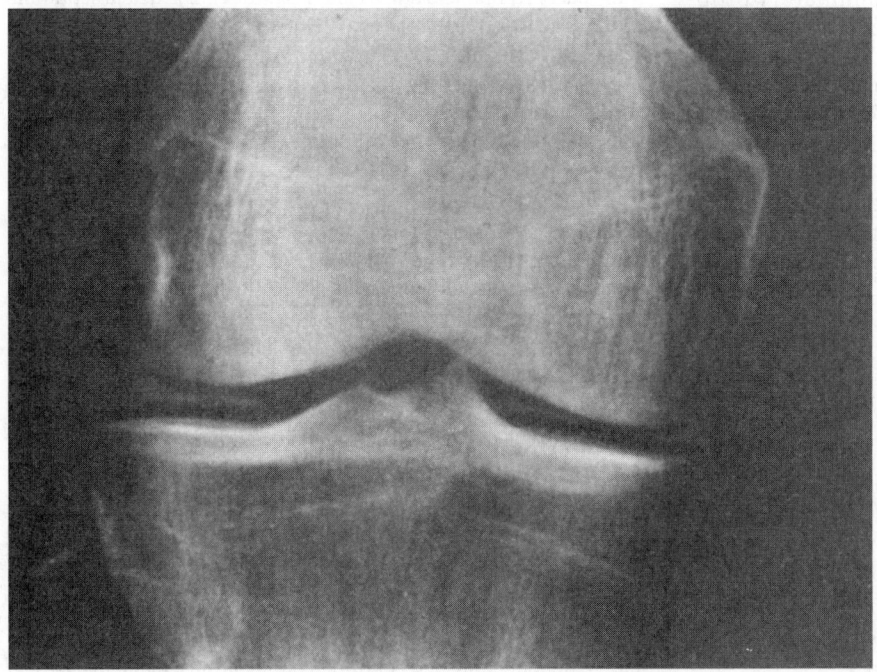

Figure 69.3. X-ray of knee of patient with chondrocalcinosis. Stippled calcification of the medial and lateral menisci is easily identified.

patients with acute tendinitis (50). More recently, hydroxyapatite crystals have been identified in patients with osteoarthritis, especially in association with acute inflammatory episodes (30) and in patients with destructive arthropathy of the shoulder joint (25,42). The latter, called *Milwaukee shoulder,* is associated with painful limited shoulder motion, complete disruption of the rotator cuff, and extensive degenerative changes in the bone. In these conditions (see Chapter 63 for discussion), crystals of other basic calcium salts including octacalcium phosphate and tricalcium phosphate in addition to hydroxyapatite have sometimes been identified. This has prompted the use of the term *BCP (basic calcium phosphate)* deposit disease to describe these syndromes (25). The capacity of the various crystals to induce inflammation varies according to crystal type, surface area, and calcium/phosphate ratio (51). CPPD crystals may also be found in addition to BCP crystals in these syndromes. Alizarin red S dye (available from scientific supply houses) may be used to stain wet preparations of synovial fluid to screen for the presence of hydroxyapatite crystals, which appear with ordinary light microscopy as red-stained clumps of crystalline material (47). Because all other calcium-containing crystals and even noncrystalline calcium salts stain with this dye, specific identification of BCP crystals requires techniques not usually available, such as electron microscopy, microprobe analysis, or x-ray diffraction. It is now clear that BCP crystals alone or in combination with CPPD are broadly associated with calcinosis in soft tissue, tendons, and bursae as well as in joints. These deposits may be secondary in some instances to trauma, neurologic injury, collagen disease, or chronic renal failure. In any of these locations an acute goutlike inflammation or a more chronic and sometimes destructive tissue response may ensue. One need only be aware of the potential inflammatory properties of this crystalline material and consider its implication in the above clinical situations. The patient may be treated with the aspiration, from a joint or soft tissue, of the crystalline material and with the subsequent local injection of lidocaine/corticosteroids solution (see Chapter 66) or treatment using an NSAID (see Chapter 70). These modalities should provide symptomatic relief in acute inflammatory arthritis or tendinitis associated with BCP crystal deposits. When symptoms become chronic or when extensive destructive arthropathy is present, rheumatologic or orthopedic referral is indicated.

ARTHRITIS ASSOCIATED WITH CALCIUM OXALATE

Another crystal-associated arthritis has been demonstrated in patients on long-term dialysis (usually hemodialysis but also seen with peritoneal dialysis) for end-stage renal disease. Extensive deposits of calcium oxalate in soft tissues occur in this setting, and these deposits may cause acute arthritis, destructive arthropathy, tenosynovitis, or bursitis (55,57). These patients are difficult to treat because of the presence of extensive and continuing deposits and incomplete response to colchicine, nonsteroidal agents, and corticosteroids.

General References*

Emmerson BT. Drug therapy: the management of gout. N Engl J Med 334:445, 1996.

A thorough and current exposition of the topic with extensive bibliography.

Kelley WN, Wortman RL. Gout and hyperuricemia. In: Kelley WN, Harris ED Jr, Ruddy S, Sledge CB, eds. Textbook of rheumatology. 5th ed. Philadelphia: WB Saunders, 1997.

Probably one of the most thorough reviews available on purine metabolism, hyperuricemia, and gout, with 297 references.

Reginato AJ, Reginato AM. Diseases associated with deposition of calcium pyrophosphate or hydroxyapatite. In: Kelley WN, Harris ED Jr, Ruddy S, Sledge CB, eds. Textbook of rheumatology. 5th ed. Philadelphia: WB Saunders, 1997.

An excellent review.

Schumacher HR. Crystal-induced arthritis. An overview. Am J Med 100(Suppl 2A):46S, 1996.

A brief review with good color photographs of urate and pyrophosphate crystals.

Schumacher HR Jr, Reginato AJ. Atlas of synovial fluid analysis and crystal identification. Philadelphia: Lea & Febiger, 1991.

Steinbroker O, Neustadt PH. Arthritis and musculoskeletal disorders. Hagerstown, MD: Harper & Row, 1972.

This is a very practical manual to aid the physician in the techniques of joint aspiration.

Uri DS, Dalinka MK. Imaging of arthropathies. Crystal disease. Radiol Clin North Am 34:359,1996.

Excellent reproductions of x-rays of these disorders.

Specific References

1. Abbott RD, Brand FN, Kannel WB, Castelli W. Gout and coronary heart disease. The Framingham Study. J Clin Epidemiol 41:237, 1988.
2. Agudelo CA, Schumacher HR. The synovitis of acute gouty arthritis. A light and electron microscopic study. Hum Pathol 265, 1973.
3. Alwan WH, Dieppe PA, Elson CJ, Bradfield JWB. Hydroxyapatite and urate crystal induced cytokine release by macrophages. Ann Rheum Dis 48:476, 1989.
4. Baer PA, Tennenbaum J, Fam AG, Little H. Coexistent septic and crystal arthritis. Report of four cases and literature review. J Rheumatol 13:604, 1986.
5. Baldwin CT, Farrer LA, Adair R, et al. Linkage of early-onset osteoarthritis and chondrocalcinosis to chromosome 8q. Am J Hum Genet 56:692, 1995.
6. Ball GV, Morgan JM. Chronic lead ingestion and gout. South Med J 61:21, 1968.
7. Batuman V. Lead nephropathy, gout and hypertension. Am J Med Sci 305:241, 1993.
8. Berger L, Yu TF. Renal function in gout. Am J Med 59:605, 1975.
9. Campion EM, Glynn RJ, DeLabry LO. Asymptomatic hyperuricemia, risks and consequences in the normative aging study. Am J Med 82:421, 1987.
10. Dieppe PA, Cawston T, Mercer E, et al. Synovial fluid collagenase in patients with destructive arthritis of the shoulder joint. Arthritis Rheum 31:882, 1988.
11. di Giovine FS, Malawista SF, Thornton E, et al. Urate crystals stimulate production of tumor necrosis factor alpha from human blood monocytes and synovial cells. Cytokine messenger RNA and protein kinetics and cellular distribution. J Clin Invest 87:1375, 1991.
12. Ehrenfeld M, Levy M, Margolioth EJ, Eliakim M. The effects of long-term colchicine therapy on male fertility in patients with familial Mediterranean fever. Andrologia 4:420, 1986.

*Bold print (general references) and bold numerals (specific references) denote published controlled clinical trials, meta-analyses, or consensus-based recommendations.

13. Erickson AR, Enzenauer RJ, Nordstrom DM, Merenich JA. The prevalence of hypothyroidism in gout. Am J Med 97:231, 1994.

14. Fagan TJ, Lidsky MD. Compensated polarized light microscopy using cellophane adhesive tape. Arthritis Rheum 17:256, 1974.

15. Fam AG. Current therapy of acute microcrystalline arthritis and the role of corticosteroids. J Clin Rheumatol 3:35, 1997.

16. Fam AG, Lewtas J, Stein J, Paton TW. Desensitization to allopurinol in patients with gout and cutaneous reactions. Am J Med 93:299, 1992.

17. Fam AG, Stein J, Rubenstein J. Gouty arthritis in nodal osteoarthritis. J Rheumatol 23:684, 1996.

18. Fava R, Olsen N, Keski-Oja J, et al. Active and latent forms of transforming growth factor beta activity in the synovial effusions. J Exp Med 169:291, 1989.

19. Ferraz MB, O'Brien B. A cost effective analysis of urate lowering drugs in non-tophaceous recurrent gouty arthritis. J Rheumatol 22:908, 1995.

20. Gerster JL, Landry M, Duvoisin B, Rappaport G. Computed tomography of the knee joint as an indication of intraarticular tophi in gout. Arthritis Rheum 39:1406, 1996.

21. Gordon TP, Terkeltaub R. Gout: crystal induced inflammation. In: Gallin JI, Goldstein IM, Synderman R, eds. Inflammation. Basic principles and clinical correlates. New York: Raven Press, 1988.

22. Groff GD, Frank WA, Raddatz DA. Systemic steroid therapy for acute gout: a clinical trial and review of the literature. Semin Arthritis Rheum 19:329, 1990.

23. Guerne PA, Terkeltaub R, Zuraw B, Lotz M. Inflammatory microcrystals stimulate interleukin-6 production and secretion by human monocytes and synoviocytes. Arthritis Rheum 32:1443, 1989.

24. Hall AP, Barry PE, Dawber TR, et al. Epidemiology of gout and hyperuricemia. Am J Med 42:27, 1967.

25. Halverson PB, McCarty DJ, Cheung HS, Ryan LM. Milwaukee shoulder syndrome: eleven additional cases with involvement of the knee in seven (basic calcium phosphate crystal deposition disease). Semin Arthritis Rheum 14:36, 1984.

26. Hande KR, Noone RM, Stone WJ. Severe allopurinol toxicity: description and guidelines for prevention in patients with renal insufficiency. Am J Med 76:47, 1984.

27. Harris CM, Lloyd DC, Lewis J. Prevalence and prophylaxis of gout in England. J Clin Epidemiol 48:1153, 1995.

28. Hochberg MC, Thomas J, Thomas DJ, et al. Racial differences in the incidence of gout. The role of hypertension. Arthritis Rheum 38:628, 1995.

29. Holland NW, Jost D, Beutler A, et al. Finger pad tophi in gout. J Rheumatol 23:690, 1996.

30. Huskisson EC, Dieppe PA, Tucker AK, Cannell LB. Another look at osteoarthritis. Ann Rheum Dis 38:423, 1979.

31. Jones AC, Chuck AJ, Arie EA, et al. Diseases associated with calcium pyrophosphate dihydrate deposition disease. Semin Arthritis Rheum 22:188, 1992.

32. Kam M, Perl-Travis D, Addadi L. Antibodies against crystals. FASEB J 6:2608, 1992.

33. Kelley WN, Wortman RL. Gout and hyperuricemia. In: Kelley WN, Harris ED Jr, Ruddy S, Sledge CB, eds. Textbook of rheumatology. 5th ed. Philadelphia: WB Saunders, 1997;1332.

34. Kerolus G, Clayburne G, Schumacher HR Jr. Is it mandatory to examine synovial fluids promptly after arthrocentesis? Arthritis Rheum 32:271, 1989.

35. Kuncl RW, Duncan G, Watson D, et al. Colchicine myopathy and neuropathy. N Engl J Med 316:1562, 1987.

36. Leary WP, Reyes AJ. Angiotensin converting enzyme inhibitors and the renal excretion of urate. Cardiovasc Drug Ther 1:29, 1987.

37. Levy FL, Adams-Huet BA, Pak CYC. Ambulatory evaluation of nephrolithiasis. An update of a 1980 protocol. Am J Med 98:50, 1995.

38. Liang MH, Fries JF. Asymptomatic hyperuricemia: the case for conservative management. Ann Intern Med 88:666, 1978.

39. Liote F, Prudhommeaux F, Schiltz C, et al. Inhibition and prevention of monosodium urate monohydrate crystal-induced inflammation in vivo by transforming growth factor B1. Arthritis Rheum 39:1192, 1996.

40. Malawista SE, Duff GW, Atkins E, et al. Crystal induced endogenous pyrogen production. A further look at gouty inflammation. Arthritis Rheum 28:1039, 1985.

41. McCarty DJ. Pseudogout and pyrophosphate metabolism. Adv Intern Med 25:363, 1980.

42. McCarty DJ, Halverson PB, Carrera GF, et al. "Milwaukee shoulder": association of microspheroids containing hydroxyapatite crystals, active collagenase and neutral protease with rotator cuff defects. I. Clinical aspects. Arthritis Rheum 24:464, 1981.

43. McCarty DJ, Silcox DC, Coe F, et al. Diseases associated with calcium pyrophosphate dihydrate crystal deposit disease. A controlled study. Am J Med 56:704, 1974.

44. Moreland LW, Ball GV. Colchicine and gout. Arthritis Rheum 34:782, 1991.

45. Ortiz-Bravo E, Sieck MS, Schumacher HR Jr. Changes in the proteins coating monosodium urate crystals during active inflammation. Immunogold studies of synovial fluids from patients with gout and fluid obtained using the rat subcutaneous air pouch model. Arthritis Rheum 36:1274–1285, 1993.

46. Pascual E. Persistence of monosodium urate crystals and low grade inflammation in the synovial fluid of patients with untreated gout. Arthritis Rheum 34:141, 1991.

47. Paul H, Reginato AJ, Schumacher HR Jr. Alizarin red staining as a screening test for calcium compounds in synovial fluid. Arthritis Rheum 26:191, 1983.

48. Paulus HE, Schlosstein LH, Godfrey RG, et al. Prophylactic colchicine therapy of intercritical gout. A placebo controlled study of probenecid-treated patients. Arthritis Rheum 17:609, 1974.

49. Phelps P, Steele AD, McCarty DJ Jr. Compensated polarized light microscopy. JAMA 203:508, 1968.

50. Pinals RS, Short CL. Calcific periarthritis involving multiple sites. Arthritis Rheum 9:566, 1966.

51. Prudhommeaux F, Schiltz C, Liote F, et al. Variation in the inflammatory properties of basic calcium phosphate crystals according to crystal type. Arthritis Rheum 39:1319, 1996.

52. Puig JG, Michán AD, Jiménez ML, et al. Female gout. Clinical spectrum and uric acid metabolism. Arch Intern Med 151:726, 1991.

53. Putterman C, Ben-Cherit E, Caraco Y, Levy M. Colchicine intoxication, risk factors, features and management. Semin Arthritis Rheum 3:143, 1991.

54. Rahman M, Shenberger KN, Schumacher HR Jr. Initially unrecognized calcium pyrophosphate dihydrate deposition disease as cause of fever. Am J Med 89:115, 1990.

55. Reginato AJ, Kurnick BRC. Calcium oxalate and other crystals associated with kidney diseases and arthritis. Semin Arthritis Rheum 18:198, 1989.

56. Reginato A, Valenzuela F, Martinez V, et al. Polyarticular and familial chondrocalcinosis. Arthritis Rheum 13:197, 1970.

57. Rosenthal A, Ryan LM, McCarty DJ. Arthritis associated with calcium oxalate crystals in an anephric patient treated with peritoneal dialysis. JAMA 260:1272, 1988.

58. Rouault T, Caldwell DS, Holmes EW. Aspiration of the asymptomatic metatarsophalangeal joint in gout patients and hyperuricemic controls. Arthritis Rheum 25:209, 1982.

59. Roubenouff R, Klag, MJ, Mead LA, et al. Incidence and risk factors for gout in white men. JAMA 266:3004, 1991.

60. Rundles RW, Metz EN, Silberman JR. Allopurinol in the treatment of gout. Ann Intern Med 64:229, 1966.

61. Schumacher HR Jr, Sieck M, Clayburne G. Development and evaluation of a method for preservation of synovial fluid wet preparations for quality control testing of crystal identification. J Rheumatol 17:1369, 1990.

62. Simkin PA, Hoover PL, Paxon CS, Wilson WF. Uric acid excretion quantitative assessment from spot midmorning serum and urine samples. Ann Intern Med 91:44, 1979.

63. Smilde TJ, Haverman JF, Schipper P, et al. Familial hypokalemia/hypomagnesemia and chondrocalcinosis. J Rheumatol 21:1515, 1994.

64. Swan A, Chapman B, Heap P, et al. Submicroscopic crystals in osteoarthritis synovial fluid. Ann Rheum Dis 53:467, 1994.

65. Takahashi S, Yamamoto T, Moriwaki Y, et al. Impaired

lipoprotein metabolism in patients with primary gout. Influence of alcohol intake and body weight. Br J Rheumatol 33:731, 1996.

66. Terkeltaub R, Smeltzer D, Curtiss LK, Ginsberg MH. Low density lipoprotein inhibits the physical interaction of phagocytic crystals and inflammatory cells. Arthritis Rheum 29:363, 1986.

67. Terkeltaub R, Zachariae C, Santoro D, et al. Monocyte-derived neutrophil chemotactic factor/interleukin-8 is a potential mediator of crystal-induced inflammation. Arthritis Rheum 34:894, 1991.

68. Van Lieshout-Zuidema MF, Breedveld FC. Withdrawal of long term anti-hyperuricemic therapy in tophaceous gout. J Rheumatol 22:1383–1385, 1993.

69. Wall B, Agudelo CA, Tesser JRP, et al. An autopsy study of the prevalence of monosodium urate and calcium pyrophosphate dihydrate crystal deposition in the first metatarsophalangeal joints. Arthritis Rheum 26:1522, 1983.

70. Wallace DJ, Klinenberg JR, Morhaim D, et al. Coexistent gout and rheumatoid arthritis. Case report and literature review. Arthritis Rheum 22:81, 1979.

71. Wallace SL, Singer JZ. Systemic toxicity associated with IV administration of colchicine. Guidelines for use. J Rheumatol 15:495,1988.

72. Weinberger A, Shumaker HR, Agudelo CA. Urate crystals in asymptomatic metatarsophalangeal joints. Ann Intern Med 91:56–57, 1979.

73. Werlen D, Gabaz C, Vischer TL. Corticosteroids for the treatment of acute attacks of crystal-induced arthritis: an effective alternative to nonsteroidal antiinflammatory drugs. Rev Rheum, Engl ed 63:248–254, 1996.

74. Wilson JM, Young AB, Kelley WN. Hypoxanthine–guanine phosphoribosyl transferase deficiency. The molecular basis of the clinical syndrome. N Engl J Med 309:900–910, 1983.

75. Yu T-F, Berger L. Renal function in gout: its association with hypertensive vascular disease. Am J Med 72:95–100, 1982.

76. Yu T-F, Gutman AB. Efficacy of colchicine prophylaxis in gout. Prevention of recurrent gouty arthritis over a mean period of five years in 208 gouty subjects. Ann Intern Med 55:179–192, 1961.

77. Yu T-F, Gutman AB. Uric acid nephrolithiasis in gout. Predisposing factors. Ann Intern Med 67:1133–1148, 1967.

C H A P T E R 70

Rheumatoid Arthritis

ALAN K. MATSUMOTO, MD
FREDRICK M. WIGLEY, MD

Rheumatoid arthritis is a chronic inflammatory systemic disease of unknown cause that has a predilection for involvement of the peripheral joints. The articular inflammation has a variable course, but the primary clinical problem is an additive, progressive, symmetric polyarthritis leading to joint destruction, deformity, and loss of function. Extra-articular features and systemic symptoms are recognized as an integral part of the disease and may antedate the onset of inflammatory arthropathy.

In the past few decades, it has been recognized that the spectrum of inflammatory arthritis can be separated into a number of distinct disease processes. Prognosis, course, and treatment can differ among these different disease processes and a clinician must develop a comprehensive diagnostic and therapeutic approach that encompasses the history, physical examination, and appropriate laboratory studies.

EPIDEMIOLOGY

Population surveys have used somewhat different criteria for the diagnosis of rheumatoid arthritis, making accurate assessments of prevalence difficult. Most agree that it has a worldwide distribution with important geographic and ethnic/racial variations. In Caucasian populations it has an estimated prevalence of 1 to 2%. Native Americans have a high prevalence of 3.5 to 5.3%, and in rural South African blacks and Japanese, the prevalence is 0.1% (7).

Prevalence increases with age, approaching 5% in women over age 55. The average annual incidence in the United States is about 70/100,000 annually (7). Both incidence and prevalence of rheumatoid arthritis are two to three times greater in women than in men. Although rheumatoid arthritis may present at any age, it most commonly affects patients in the third to sixth decades. Women tend to have a more severe articular disease, whereas extra-articular features are more common in men.

Genetic influences on disease frequency and severity are suggested by increased incidence of human class II histocompatibility antigens HLA-DR4 and HLA-DR1 in patients with rheumatoid arthritis compared with a matched control population (16). The HLA-DR molecule consists of an α and β chain with the various HLA-DR specificities determined by heterogeneity at the three hypervariability regions of the HLA-DRβ chain. The molecular basis for the HLA association is defined by the presence of a shared amino acid sequence from amino acids 70 to 74 in the third hypervariable region of the DRβ chain in patients with rheumatoid arthritis. The presence of this shared structural element or "susceptibility cassette" increases the risk of developing rheumatoid arthritis and correlates with greater disease severity (27).

PATHOGENESIS

Normal joint architecture consists of a fibrous capsule that surrounds a 1– to 3–cell layer lining of synovial cells. Synovial cells bear markers of fibroblast and macrophage lineage and, among many functions, secrete joint lubricants such as hyaluronic acid. The area beneath the synovial lining cells is acellular. The pathologic hallmark of rheumatoid arthritis is the infiltration of the subsynovia of affected joints by lymphocytes, plasma cells, and macrophages, and the proliferation of synovial lining cells and blood vessels into a tumorlike structure called the pannus (6). The

event or factor triggering the recruitment of inflammatory cells to the joint remains unknown. Local production of rheumatoid factor–containing immune complexes activates complement and attracts inflammatory cells. The predominance of CD4-positive T cells in the rheumatoid synovium suggests an antigen-driven, cell-mediated inflammatory process. The inflammatory process is amplified by a number of macrophage- and fibroblast-derived cytokines found in large quantities in the rheumatoid joint including tumor necrosis factor (TNF-α), interleukin-1 (IL-1), interleukin-6 (IL-6), and platelet-derived growth factor (PDGF) (3). These cytokines drive the recruitment of additional inflammatory cells and subsequent release of destructive enzymes. Enzymes such as collagenase and stromelysin destroy cartilage and bone, leading to loss of normal joint architecture.

HISTORY

The presentation of the disease (Table 70.1) varies from situations in which the diagnosis is obvious to ones in which the presentation is so atypical that it suggests other conditions. The typical case of rheumatoid arthritis begins insidiously, with the slow progressive development of signs and symptoms over weeks to months. Occasionally, patients experience an explosive polyarticular onset occurring over 24 to 48 hours. Sometimes an acute presentation appears to be associated with either emotional or physical stress, such as loss of a loved one or a recent injury.

Arthritic signs and symptoms provide the definitive clues to a specific diagnosis. Often the patient first notices stiffness (see below) in one or more joints, usually accompanied by pain on movement and by tenderness in the joint. Unlike a patient with gout (see Chapter 69), a patient with rheumatoid arthritis can bear weight and move the inflamed joint but has a persistent, deep, gnawing discomfort. Severe pain in a patient with established rheumatoid arthritis should suggest a superimposed infection or an acute structural problem. The number of joints involved is highly variable, but almost always the process is eventually polyarticular, involving five or more joints. Rheumatoid arthritis is an additive polyarthritis, with the sequential addition of involved joints, in contrast to the migratory or evanescent arthritis that can be seen in systemic lupus erythematosus or the episodic arthritis seen in gout. The American College of Rheumatology, in its revised criteria for the diagnosis of rheumatoid

Table 70.1. Symptoms and Signs of Rheumatoid Arthritis

Symptoms		Signs	
Extra-Articular	Articular[a]	Extra-Articular	Articular
Fatigue	Morning stiffness	Rheumatoid nodules	Pain on passive motion
Depression	Pain and tenderness	Lymphadenopathy	Tenderness
Malaise	Swelling	Splenomegaly	Swelling
Anorexia		Ocular disease	Heat
		Entrapment neuropathies	Typical deformity

[a]Persistence (6 weeks or more) and symmetric nature of signs and symptoms are important, but not invariable, diagnostic features.

arthritis (2), emphasizes the importance of persistent symmetric swelling or fluid in the joints for longer than 6 weeks. Any joint may be involved but there is a predilection for peripheral joints with a sparing of the axial skeleton. The joints involved most often are the proximal interphalangeal (PIP) and metacarpophalangeal (MCP) joints of the hands, the wrists (particularly at the ulnar–styloid articulation), shoulders, elbows, knees, ankles, and metatarsophalangeal (MTP) joints. Involvement of non–weight-bearing joints— shoulders, elbows, and wrists especially—should raise suspicion for rheumatoid arthritis. The distal interphalangeal (DIP) joints are generally spared.

Morning stiffness may be a feature of any inflammatory arthritis but is especially characteristic of rheumatoid arthritis. Virtually all patients complain of morning stiffness, and its duration is a useful gauge of the inflammatory activity of the disease. Significant morning stiffness is defined as stiffness, predominantly over joints, that persists for more than 1 hour but often lasts several hours. Similar stiffness can occur after long periods of sitting or inactivity (gel phenomenon). In contrast, patients with degenerative arthritis complain of stiffness lasting but a few minutes (see Chapter 68).

Nonspecific systemic symptoms, primarily fatigue, malaise, and depression, are common but not invariable and may precede other symptoms of the disease by weeks to months. Usually the patient does not feel tired upon awakening but complains of severe fatigue 4 to 6 hours later. Fever occurs occasionally and is almost always low grade (37° to 38°C; 99° to 100°F). A higher fever suggests another illness, and infectious causes must be considered.

It is typical of patients with rheumatoid arthritis that their symptoms wax and wane, especially at the beginning of the illness. Because of this and because objective signs may not be present at first, it is not unusual that the diagnosis is delayed for months. Diagnosis may be complicated by the fact that rheumatoid arthritis patients may present with nonspecific complaints or signs and symptoms that mimic other musculoskeletal disorders. Atypical presentations include intermittent joint inflammation that can be confused with gout or pseudogout (see Chapter 69), proximal muscle pain and tenderness mimicking polymyalgia rheumatica (see Chapter 79), or diffuse musculoskeletal pain as seen in fibromyalgia (see Chapter 66).

During the time of diagnostic uncertainty, the physician can best serve the patient by providing reassurance, taking careful interval histories, performing periodic physical examinations (see below), and if appropriate, performing selected tests (see below). Symptomatic treatment with anti-inflammatory drugs may be instituted during this period (see below).

PHYSICAL EXAMINATION

The performance of an initial complete physical examination and then a limited examination every 3 to 6 months is important in patients with suspected rheumatoid arthritis, not only to make the diagnosis but to establish a baseline against which to assess the possible later development of both articular and extra-articular disease.

However, the primary focus of examinations in the physician's office is the joints. Serial joint examinations should be performed with careful records of the status of affected joints, determined by history and previous examinations.

Joints

Swelling is the most measurable change that occurs in a joint affected by rheumatoid arthritis. Symmetric joint swelling, although not invariable, is characteristic of rheumatoid arthritis. The first change is usually periarticular soft tissue swelling. Eventually, increased amounts of fluid within the joint space produce more readily recognizable and often persistent changes. In the hands, where the disease is often first manifested, typical fusiform swelling of the PIP joints commonly occurs (Fig. 70.1). The MCP joints and the wrists swell even more often and are more specific for an inflammatory arthropathy. Careful palpation of the joints can help to distinguish the swelling of joint inflammation from the bony enlargement seen in osteoarthritis. The elbows, knees, ankles, and MTP joints are other common sites of disease where swelling may be readily apparent.

In contrast to gout (see Chapter 69) or septic arthritis, redness of affected joints is not a prominent feature of rheumatoid arthritis.

Pain on passive motion, although not specific for rheumatoid arthritis, is the most sensitive indicator of joint inflammation. When examining a joint, it is important to apply gentle but firm pressure at the joint line so that tenderness caused by inflammation is elicited, but not so much pressure that a normal joint is inappropriately symptomatic. Inflamed joints are also usually warmer than normal joints and are best assessed by feeling them with the back of the fingers.

The *range of motion* of the joint may be limited by inflammation, structural deformity, or both. To institute proper therapy (see below), it is important to determine which of these processes is the major factor limiting joint function.

Weakness is a common feature of patients with rheumatoid arthritis, but like range of motion, it is difficult to assess. Patient perception of weakness and objective testing is influenced by pain limiting movement of joints. The fatigue produced by the illness may contribute to an overall sense of weakness. Chronic, uncontrolled joint inflammation can have systemic effects, mediated by inflammatory cytokines, resulting in marked decrease in lean body mass (19). Weakness of one or more extremities may be caused by muscle atrophy, a result of joint deformity and disuse.

Permanent deformity is an unwanted result of the inflammatory process. Joint damage occurs at the level of the bone, cartilage, and periarticular soft tissues. Persistent tenosynovitis and synovitis leads to the formation of synovial cysts and to displaced or rup-

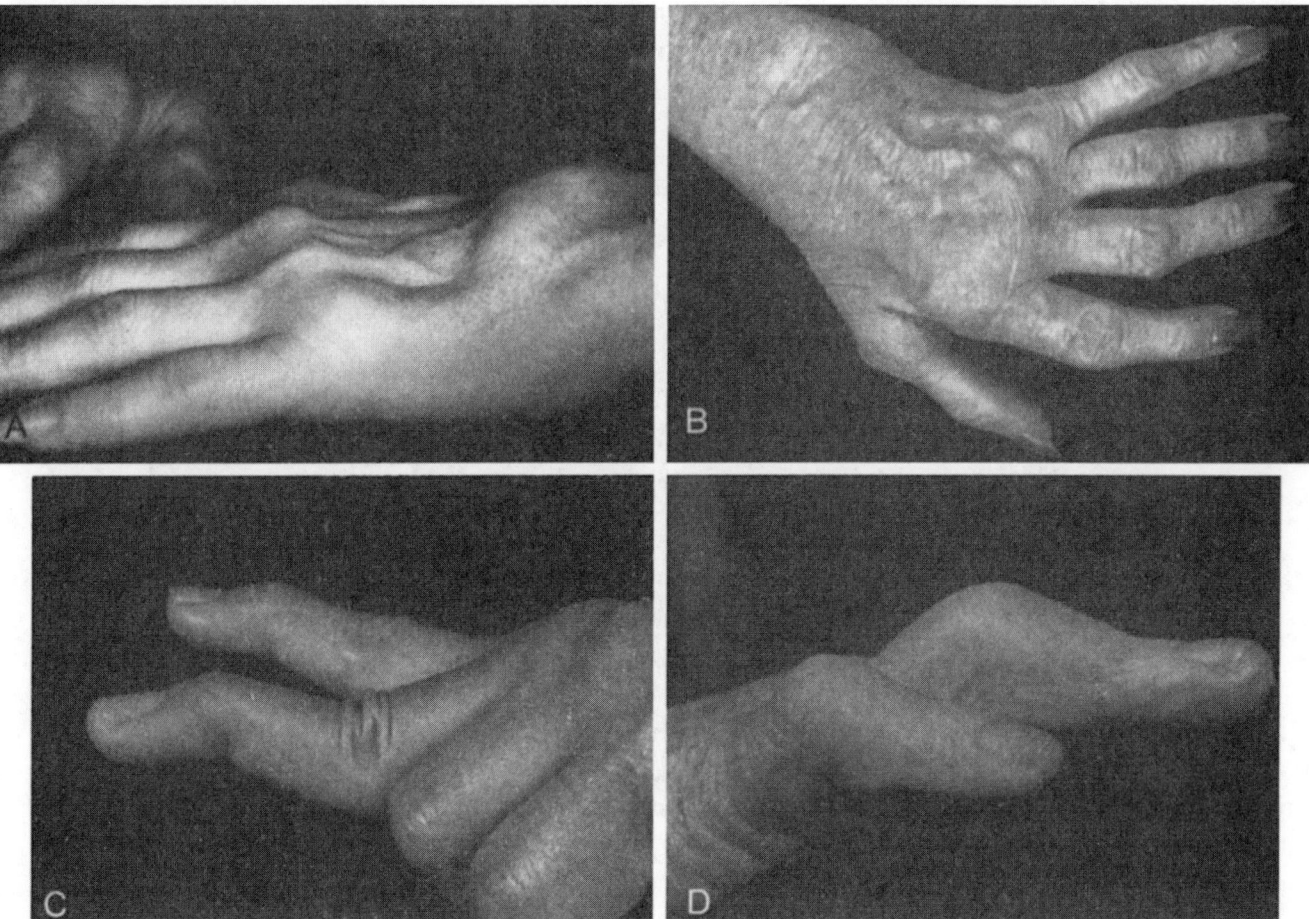

Figure 70.1. Hand deformities in rheumatoid arthritis. **A.** Typical fusiform swelling of the PIP joints; note also the synovial swelling of the wrist and MCP joints. **B.** Ulnar deviation of the fingers. **C.** Swan-neck deformity (hyperextension of the PIP joint). **D.** Boutonnière deformity (flexion contracture of the PIP joint).

tured tendons. Extensor tendon rupture at the dorsum of the hand is a common and disabling problem. Cartilage damage and joint space narrowing occur early in the disease. Bony erosions seen at the margins of the joint, at the attachment of the synovium, are the hallmark of rheumatoid arthritis. Erosions occur rapidly within the first 2 years of the disease (25). These anatomic changes result in limitations in range of motion, flexion contractures, and subluxation (incomplete dislocation) of articulating bones. Typical visible changes (Fig. 70.1) include ulnar deviation of the fingers at the MCP joints, hyperextension or hyperflexion of the MCP and PIP joints, flexion contractures of the elbows, and subluxation of the carpal bones. Ankylosis (fusion) of the carpal and tarsal joints can occur but ankylosis of other joints is rare. Commonly, displaced toes (cocked-up) with hallux valgus formation (angulation of the great toe laterally) lead to prominence of the metatarsal heads at the plantar aspect of the foot, resulting in pain with ambulation and ulcer formation.

Synovial cysts are common in patients with rheumatoid arthritis and can be readily seen and palpated overlying the joints with which they communicate.

Synovial cysts of the popliteal space (Baker's cysts) may develop in patients with a variety of disorders of the knee but are especially prevalent in patients with rheumatoid disease (Fig. 70.2). If popliteal cysts rupture, the signs and symptoms mimic those of acute thrombophlebitis with calf swelling, tenderness, and a positive Homans's sign. A magnetic resonance imaging (MRI) scan or ultrasound of the popliteal space is a noninvasive technique to confirm the diagnosis. Noninvasive vascular studies of the lower extremities (see Chapter 52) are recommended to rule out deep vein thrombosis if the diagnosis is unclear. Symptoms can usually be relieved effectively by decompressing the cyst by aspiration of synovial fluid from either the joint or the cyst and injecting a corticosteroid into the joint (see below).

LABORATORY TESTS

Baseline diagnostic laboratory information in patients with suspected rheumatoid arthritis should include a complete blood count and differential, erythrocyte sedimentation rate, urinalysis, and rheumatoid factor titer. In the absence of adverse drug reactions,

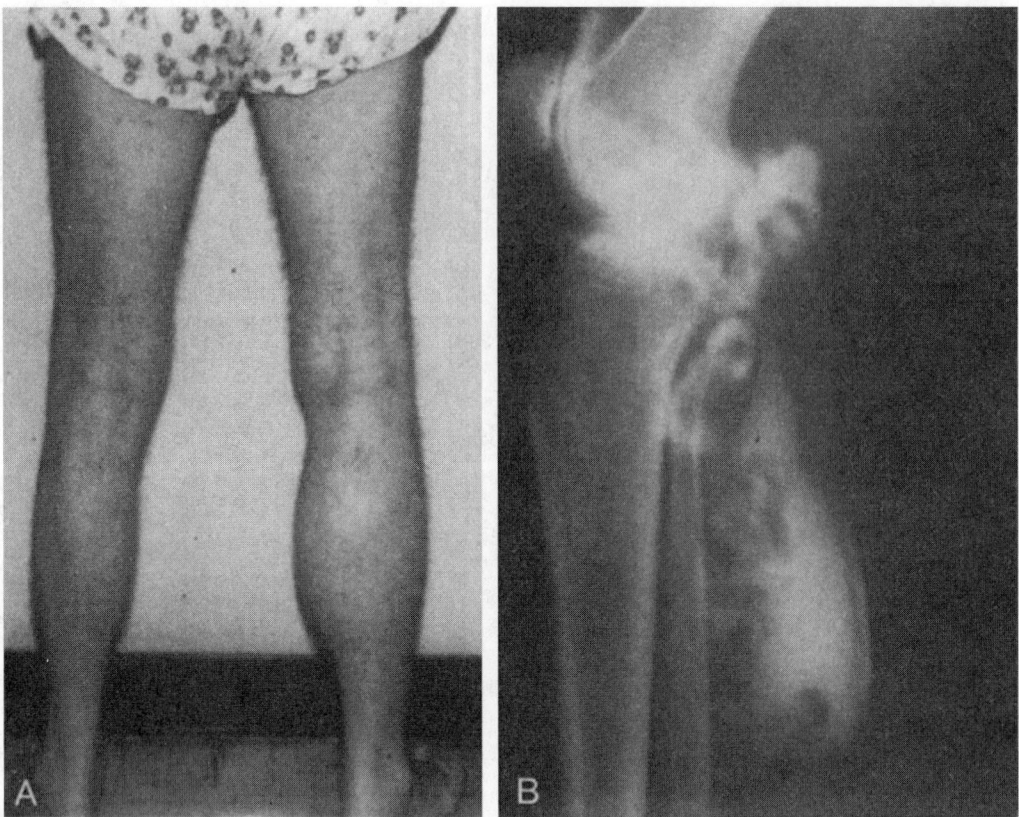

Figure 70.2.   Baker's cyst. **A.** Swelling of the calf secondary to dissection of the cyst. **B.** Arthrogram of the knee demonstrating the cyst.

renal disease is rare in rheumatoid arthritis and an abnormal urinalysis should alert the clinician to alternative diagnoses. Baseline values of electrolytes, creatinine, and liver function tests should also be established before initiating the use of drugs in the treatment of rheumatoid arthritis. In selected patients, synovial fluid analysis, additional serologic studies, and appropriate x-rays are also important (see below).

Hematology

A mild anemia with hematocrit values in the range of 30 to 34% occurs in approximately 25 to 35% of patients with rheumatoid arthritis. In most cases, the reduced red cell mass is caused by the anemia of chronic disease (see Chapter 50), a normocytic–normochromic process characterized by a low concentration of serum iron, a low serum iron-binding capacity, and a normal or increased serum ferritin concentration. However, occasionally true iron deficiency anemia can develop secondary to intercurrent blood loss. The inflammation of rheumatoid arthritis inhibits erythropoiesis, making it difficult to differentiate anemia secondary to chronic blood loss from the anemia of chronic disease without an iron stain of the bone marrow. Nonsteroidal anti-inflammatory drugs (NSAIDs) used to treat the disease increase the risk of gastrointestinal (GI) bleeding from peptic ulcer disease and gastritis, particularly in the elderly. In patients over the age of 40, it is especially important to monitor for GI blood loss and consider other causes of blood loss such as colonic lesions (see Chapter 38).

The white cell count is usually normal in patients with rheumatoid arthritis, but can be mildly elevated secondary to inflammation. Similarly, the platelet count is usually normal but thrombocytosis occurs in response to inflammation. Drug reactions and Felty's syndrome are rare causes of leukopenia or thrombocytopenia (see below).

The erythrocyte sedimentation rate (ESR), most reliably measured by the Westergren method, is usually elevated in patients with rheumatoid arthritis and in some patients is a helpful adjunct in following the activity of the disease.

Serology

Rheumatoid Factor

Rheumatoid factors are antibodies directed against the Fc portion of immunoglobulin G (IgG). Although these antibodies may belong to any of the three major classes of immunoglobulin (IgG, IgM, and IgA), rheumatoid factors, as measured for clinical purposes, are IgM. A positive test for rheumatoid factor is by no means pathognomonic of rheumatoid arthritis, but is present in 70 to 90% of patients with the disease (29). A significant titer of rheumatoid factor is 1:80 or greater by latex fixation method and over 20 IU/mL by the

ELISA method. In early disease, the rheumatoid factor may be negative but becomes positive within the first 6 months of active disease. The titer does not correlate with the activity of disease, but patients with a high titer rheumatoid factor are more likely to have erosive joint disease, extra-articular manifestations, and greater functional disability.

Rheumatoid factors are also detectable in the serum of many patients without rheumatoid arthritis. Most of these patients have had demonstrated or presumed chronic antigenic stimulation, such as prolonged infection (bacterial endocarditis, tuberculosis, cytomegalovirus, human immunodeficiency virus [HIV], viral hepatitis), collagen vascular disease, chronic lung disease (pulmonary fibrosis, sarcoidosis, asthma), or dysproteinemia (myeloma, macroglobulinemia, mixed cryoglobulinemia). Also, transient appearance of rheumatoid factors may occur in patients who have been recently vaccinated or who have had a self-limited viral infection. Finally, low titers of rheumatoid factors may be detected in the serum of apparently normal people, especially over the age of 70, where its prevalence is anywhere from 10 to 25% (21).

Antinuclear Antibodies

Antinuclear antibodies (ANAs), measured by immunofluorescent techniques, are present in approximately 20 to 30% of patients with rheumatoid arthritis. ANAs are more common in patients with extra-articular manifestations of disease and in patients with a high titer of rheumatoid factor. In comparison with systemic lupus erythematosus (SLE), the titer of antinuclear antibodies is low in patients with rheumatoid arthritis, and antibodies to native deoxyribonucleic acid (DNA) or other specific nuclear antigens are unusual. The ANA test is generally unnecessary in a patient with typical rheumatoid arthritis unless the diagnosis is in doubt or other systemic symptoms are noted.

Serum Complement

Serum hemolytic complement ($C'H_{50}$) and complement components C_3 or C_4 are generally normal or increased in patients with rheumatoid arthritis. It may be low in an occasional patient with severe disease or systemic vasculitis. The test is most useful in helping distinguish the patient with early rheumatoid arthritis from patients with immune complex–mediated disease such as SLE, in whom serum complement components are often markedly decreased.

Synovial Fluid

Synovial fluid should be analyzed (Table 70.2) in a patient with monarthritis or with polyarthritis and fever, or in any patient with a joint effusion in whom the diagnosis is in doubt. Also, patients with known rheumatoid arthritis who develop disproportionate pain and swelling of one joint should have fluid aspirated from that joint to rule out infection. If the physician is unfamiliar with the technique of arthrocentesis (see Chapter 66, Table 66.1) or is uncomfortable about tapping a joint, the patient should be referred to a rheumatologist or to an orthopedic surgeon.

There is increased susceptibility of the rheumatoid joint to infection, usually by streptococcal or staphylococcal organisms. Whenever a single joint flares up or such a flare-up is accompanied by fever or follows a recent invasive procedure, synovial fluid examination is essential to rule out infection.

Recommended studies on fluid aspirated from the joint include cell count and differential, Gram's stain, culture, and crystal examination. Joint fluid should be added immediately to a tube containing EDTA (purple top) or heparin to prevent clotting and cell lysis. If quantity of fluid is limited, priority is given first to culture, then to Gram's stain, and finally to crystal examination. There is considerable variation in the total white cell count and neutrophil count in synovial fluid of rheumatoid joints, but in general, the total white cell count in an inflamed joint exceeds 2,000 cc/mm, predominantly neutrophils. Occasionally, white cell counts exceed 75,000, but values in this range should raise concern about infection. Other analyses such as protein, glucose, enzymes, complement, immune complexes, rheumatoid factor, ANA, viscosity, turbidity, or mucin clot are not recommended, as they are neither specific nor sensitive.

Radiology

Roentgenograms are occasionally necessary in the diagnosis of rheumatoid arthritis to exclude diseases that mimic rheumatoid arthritis (gout, pseudogout, sarcoidosis). However, radiographic changes require sufficient time (months) to evolve into a characteristic pattern, limiting their usefulness early in the course of the disease. Significant cartilage damage caused by inflammation occurs before radiographic changes can be observed. X-rays should be obtained if there is suspicion of structural or traumatic damage to the bone or joint. Also, x-rays are of value in determining the course of the erosive process (Fig. 70.3). However, it is not recommended that the primary care physician

Table 70.2. Synovial Fluid Findings in Various Arthritides

Synovial Fluid Finding	Normal	Rheumatoid Arthritis	Noninflammatory Arthritis	Septic Arthritis
Color	Clear	Yellow	Clear-yellow	Variable
Clarity	Transparent	Turbid	Transparent	Opaque
White cells (per mm^3)	<150	2,000–75,000	<2,000	>75,000
Polymorphonuclear leukocytes (%)	<25	>70	<25	>75

See Chapter 66, Table 66.2 also.

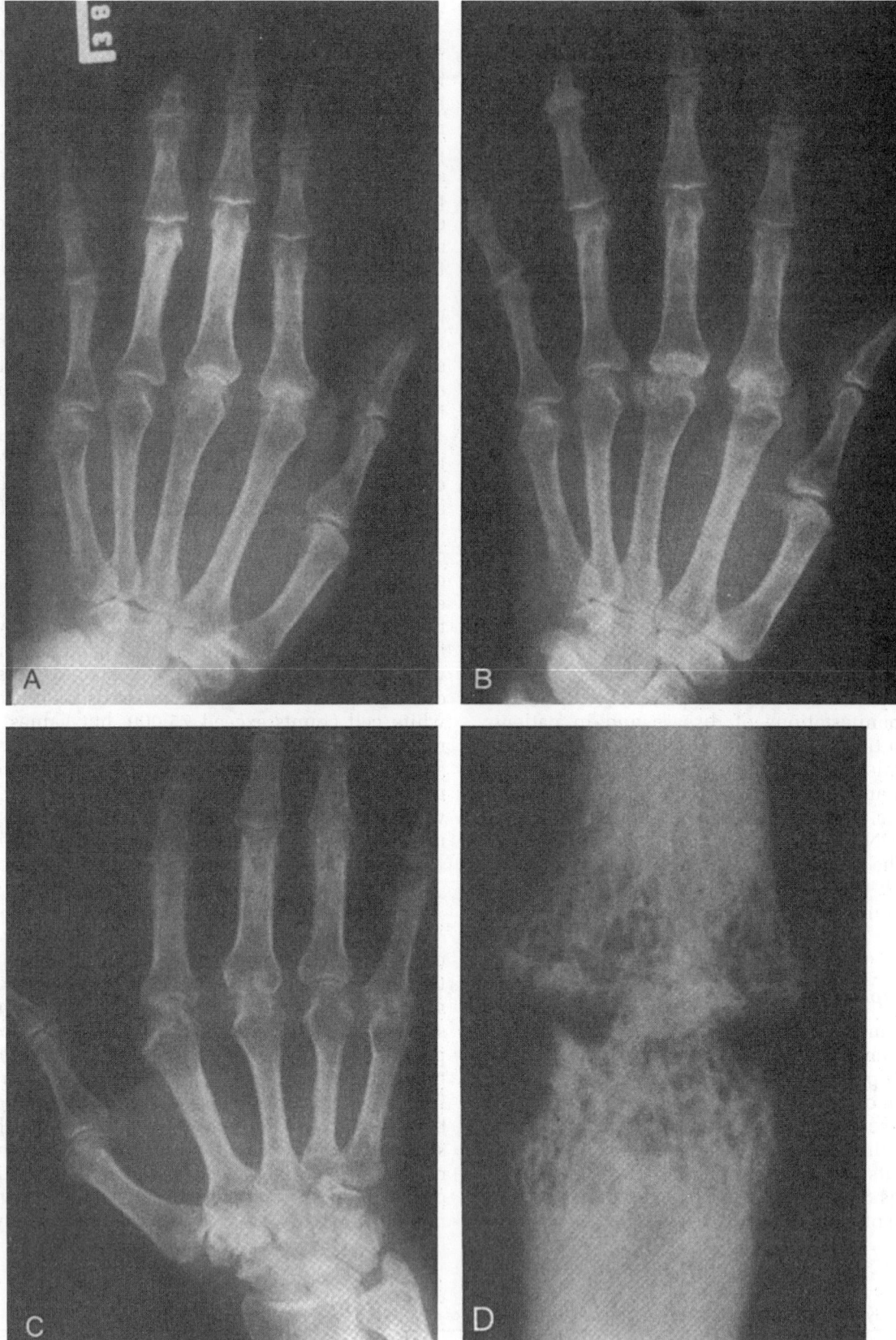

Figure 70.3.   Radiographic changes in rheumatoid arthritis.
A. Early joint space narrowing in the second and third MCP joints.
B. Cystic changes, erosions, and further bony proliferation in the second and third MCP joints. **C.** Periarticular osteoporosis, most noticeable in the interphalangeal joints, and numerous marginal erosions and cysts in the carpal bones and metacarpal heads.
D. Juxta-articular erosions in a PIP joint.

obtain routine serial x-rays of joints because it is controversial whether they are useful in guiding therapeutic decisions.

Radiologic findings vary in rheumatoid arthritis depending on the duration and severity of the illness. Early in the disease x-rays may show nothing other than soft tissue swelling. Thereafter, periarticular osteopenia may develop, most noticeable in the small joints of the hands, wrists, and feet. With progression of the disease, narrowing of the joint space is caused by loss of cartilage, and juxta-articular erosions appear, generally at the point of attachment of the synovium. In end-stage disease, large cystic erosions of bone may be seen. Bony proliferation may occur because of degenerative changes that follow inflammation, and the marked deformities that are visible to the naked eye (see above) are also visible radiologically. These changes are in contrast to the bony hypertrophy (osteophytes), sclerosis, and fusion seen in patients with osteoarthritis (see Chapter 68).

Special radiologic studies are helpful in certain situations. *MRI* is useful to define possible internal joint derangement or injury to a supporting structure, such as a torn rotator cuff of the shoulder, or meniscal tears of the knee. MRI has largely replaced arthrography for the diagnosis of these problems. MRI is also a sensitive method to detect aseptic necrosis of bone. Computerized tomography (CT) or MRI is important in evaluation of cord compression secondary to atlantoaxial (C1/C2) subluxation.

Biopsies

Although the histology of rheumatoid arthritis is characteristic, synovial biopsy is rarely necessary in the diagnosis of the disease. Similarly, biopsy of a nodule (see below) is indicated only to distinguish it from another process (e.g., a tumor).

EXTRA-ARTICULAR DISEASE

Although the joints are almost always the principal focus of the rheumatoid arthritis, other organ systems may also be involved (8). Extra-articular manifestations of rheumatoid arthritis occur most often in seropositive patients with more severe joint disease. Interestingly, extra-articular manifestations can occur in later stages of the disease when there is little active synovitis ("burnt-out" disease). In contrast to the predilection of rheumatoid arthritis for women, extra-articular manifestations of the disease (Table 70.3) are more common in men.

Rheumatoid Nodules

Although not specific for rheumatoid arthritis (nodules with identical pathology may be seen in patients with SLE or rheumatic fever), the subcutaneous nodule is the most characteristic extra-articular lesion of the disease (Fig. 70.4). Nodules occur in 20 to 30% of cases, almost exclusively in seropositive patients. They vary

Table 70.3.   Systemic Manifestations of Rheumatoid Arthritis (Rheumatoid Disease)

I. General
  A. Fever
  B. Fatigue, malaise, diffuse stiffness
  C. Adenopathy
  D. Splenomegaly
II. Pulmonary
  A. Pleuritis (± effusion)
  B. Intrapulmonary nodules
  C. Interstitial pneumonitis
  D. Rheumatoid pneumoconiosis (Caplan's syndrome)
  E. Pulmonary fibrosis
  F. Arteritis (rare)
III. Cardiovascular
  A. Heart
    1. Pericarditis, effusion, tamponade, constriction
    2. Myocarditis
    3. Endocarditis, including valvulitis
    4. Rheumatoid nodule (conduction defects)
  B. Peripheral
    1. Vasculitis or arteritis
IV. Nervous system
  A. Peripheral neuropathy (mononeuritis multiplex) (sensory, motor, or both)
  B. Central nervous system
    1. Spinal cord lesion
      a. Vascular thrombosis
      b. Rheumatoid nodule
    2. Intracranial
      a. Arteritis (rare)
      b. Rheumatoid nodule (rare)
V. Ocular
  A. Keratoconjunctivitis (Sjögren's syndrome)
  B. Episcleritis (simple or nodular)
  C. Scleritis
    1. Diffuse
    2. Nodular (scleromalacia perforans)
    3. Necrotizing
VI. Hematologic
  A. Anemia (chronic disease)
  B. Neutropenia (Felty's syndrome)
  C. Thrombocytosis
  D. Eosinophilia
VII. Skin
  A. Palmar erythema
  B. Nodules
  C. Vasculitic lesions
  D. Leg ulcers (Felty's syndrome)
VIII. Others
  A. Sjögren's syndrome
  B. Osteoporosis
  C. Hyperviscosity
  D. Lymphoma (Sjögren's syndrome)
  E. Secondary amyloidosis (controversial)

in size from a few millimeters to several centimeters and are either fixed to surrounding tissue or freely movable beneath the skin. They are located most commonly on the extensor surfaces of the arms and elbows but are also prone to develop at pressure points on the feet and knees. Rheumatoid nodules may arise within tendons or ligaments and can cause joint dysfunction or tendon rupture. Rarely, nodules may arise in visceral organs, such as the lungs, the heart, or the sclera of the eye. Wherever their location, nodules usually persist, but occasionally regress, even with a remission of activity of the overall disease. Generally

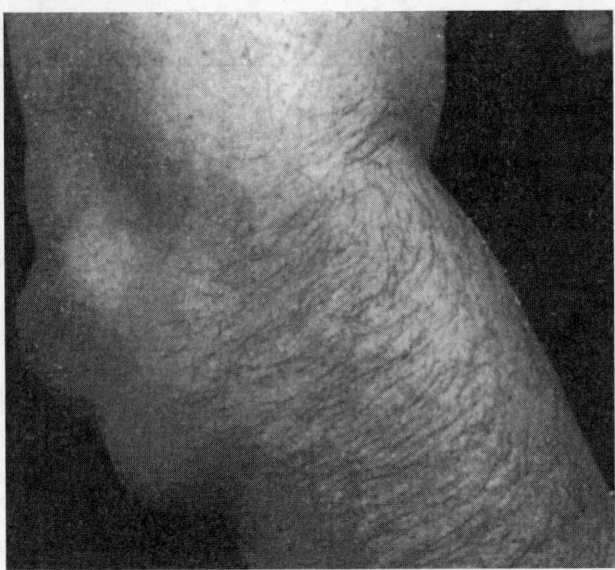

Figure 70.4. Rheumatoid nodules along the extensor surface of the forearm.

asymptomatic, occasionally subcutaneous nodules can become painful, erode underlying bone, or ulcerate, and require surgical excision.

Pleuropulmonary Disease

There are several pulmonary manifestations of rheumatoid arthritis, including pleurisy with or without effusion, intrapulmonary nodules, rheumatoid pneumoconiosis (Caplan's syndrome), diffuse interstitial fibrosis, and rarely, bronchiolitis obliterans, pneumothorax, or pulmonary arteritis (9). On pulmonary function testing, there commonly is a restrictive ventilatory defect with reduced lung volumes and a decreased diffusing capacity for carbon monoxide. Although the issue is controversial, most rheumatologists believe that rheumatoid arthritis does not cause intrathoracic obstructive airway disease. Extrathoracic upper airway obstruction may occur secondary to involvement of the cricoarytenoid joints of the larynx.

Pulmonary involvement may precede by months the onset of arthritis. Pleurisy, the most common problem, is clinically apparent in 5% of patients, but pleural thickening and inflammation is found at 50% of autopsy cases. Pleural effusions, either unilateral or bilateral, are usually exudates. Even in transudates the glucose concentration of the fluid is usually low (less than 30 mg/100 mL), a finding otherwise seen only in pleural space infections. The first approach to the management of a pleural effusion includes a diagnostic aspiration and pleural biopsy to exclude infection and malignancy.

Rheumatoid nodules in the lung are usually asymptomatic, but cavitation simulating cancer or infection may occur. Therefore appropriate diagnostic steps should be taken to ensure that an isolated pleural or pulmonary nodule is in fact rheumatoid in origin.

Interstitial pneumonitis or a fibrosing mononuclear alveolitis precedes progressive pulmonary fibrosis, the most severe form of rheumatoid lung disease. Fine dry rales are heard on auscultation of the lung and reticulonodular infiltrates are seen on chest x-rays. This process is more common among patients who smoke.

To date, no regression of rheumatoid lung disease has been shown with conventional modes of treatment. Patients with symptomatic pleural or pulmonary manifestations of rheumatoid arthritis should be followed in consultation with a rheumatologist and pulmonologist.

Cardiac Disease

Pericarditis is the most common cardiac manifestation of rheumatoid arthritis (11). Echocardiographic studies demonstrate pericardial effusion in 55% of patients with subcutaneous nodules and 15% of patients who do not have nodules. Symptomatic pericarditis usually presents with fever, chest pain, and a pericardial rub that resolve spontaneously. Recurrent or persistent pericardial disease, complicated by tamponade or constriction, is rare. Other unusual cardiac manifestations include nonspecific valvulitis, nodule formation in a valve cusp, myocarditis, and conduction abnormalities secondary to nodule formation in the heart. The treatment of patients with symptomatic cardiac disease is best done in consultation with a rheumatologist and cardiologist.

Ocular Disease

Keratoconjunctivitis of Sjögren's syndrome is the most common ocular manifestation of rheumatoid arthritis (see below and Chapter 99). Episcleritis occurs occasionally and is manifested by mild pain and intense redness of the affected eye. Ordinarily, episcleritis is a self-limited process of a few weeks' duration. Scleritis and corneal ulcerations are rarer but more serious problems. Unlike episcleritis, scleritis is a slowly progressive, often bilateral process that may lead to perforation and loss of vision. It is characterized by nodularity, intense redness, and often severe pain. The distinction between episcleritis and scleritis is difficult (see Chapter 99), and all patients with a red, painful eye should be referred to an ophthalmologist.

Neurologic Disease

The most common neurologic manifestation of rheumatoid arthritis is a mild, primarily sensory *peripheral neuropathy,* usually more marked in the lower extremities. Entrapment neuropathies (e.g., carpal tunnel syndrome and tarsal tunnel syndrome) sometimes occur in patients with rheumatoid arthritis because of compression of a peripheral nerve by inflamed edematous tissue (see Chapter 84). Cervical myelopathy secondary to atlantoaxial subluxation is an uncommon but particularly worrisome complication potentially causing permanent, even fatal neurologic damage. Approximately 30% of patients with rheumatoid arthritis followed in a referral practice have atlantoaxial subluxation without symptoms, and very few of them develop neurologic dysfunction (see Kelly et al., "General References"). Specific studies of the cervical spine such as CT scan and MRI are not indicated unless symptoms (pain, paresthesias, weakness) or neurologic signs are present. However, cervical spine studies and neurosurgical consultation should be sought at the first sign of cord compression. A patient with rheumatoid arthritis who may have sustained cervical injury or is at risk for a neck manipulation (e.g., during general anesthesia) should have flexion/extension cervical spine x-rays so that special caution can be exercised if subluxation, even without symptoms, is present.

Lymphoid Hyperplasia

Lymphadenopathy, either local or generalized, occurs in 25% or more of patients with rheumatoid arthritis. The nodes are nontender, firm, and freely movable. Although the diagnosis of lymphoma is sometimes considered, the process almost always proves to be benign. When examined by biopsy, the nodes show a proliferation of normal plasma cells. Splenomegaly occurs more rarely (5 to 10% of patients), usually in association with lymphadenopathy.

Felty's Syndrome

Felty's syndrome is characterized by rheumatoid arthritis, splenomegaly, and leukopenia—predominantly granulocytopenia (18). Patients with this syndrome usually are older and have a high titer of rheumatoid factor, often a positive ANA, severe arthritis, and other extra-articular manifestations of the disease. Recurrent bacterial infections and chronic refractory leg ulcers are the major complications. Patients suspected of having Felty's syndrome should see a rheumatologist urgently because therapy is difficult and must be aggressive (see below).

Rheumatoid Vasculitis

Evidence of vasculitis is found in 10 to 25% of autopsy patients with rheumatoid arthritis. The most common clinical manifestations of vasculitis are small digital infarcts along the nailbeds. In less than 1% of patients, a syndrome of accelerated vasculitis is seen characterized by distal cutaneous ulcerations, gangrene, peripheral polyneuropathy, and visceral (intestinal, renal, cardiac, cerebral) ischemia. The abrupt onset of an ischemic mononeuropathy (mononeuritis multiplex) or progressive scleritis is typical of rheumatoid vasculitis. The syndrome ordinarily emerges after years of seropositive, persistently active rheumatoid arthritis; however, vasculitis may occur when joints are inactive. Immediate consultation with a rheumatologist and immunosuppressive therapy (see below) is usually indicated.

Sjögren's Syndrome

Approximately 10 to 15% of patients with rheumatoid arthritis, mostly women develop Sjögren's syndrome, a chronic inflammatory disorder characterized by lymphocytic infiltration of lacrimal and salivary glands. This leads to impaired secretion of saliva and tears and results in the *sicca complex:* dry mouth (xerostomia) and dry eyes (keratoconjunctivitis sicca). Patients should use lubricating eye drops and be followed by an ophthalmologist to prevent corneal ulcerations and be followed closely by a dentist to prevent dental caries.

Patients with Sjögren's syndrome have a variable expression of disease in other exocrine glands. This is manifested clinically as dry skin, decreased perspiration, dry vaginal membranes, or a nonproductive cough. Commonly, there is also a polyclonal lymphoproliferative reaction, characterized by lymphadenopathy and occasionally splenomegaly. This can mimic and rarely transform into a malignant lymphoma. Sjögren's syndrome may also be associated with a number of other systemic manifestations, including vasculitis, peripheral neuropathy, and thyroiditis. Other consequences of the polyclonal gammopathy include diffuse hypergammaglobulinemia (sometimes causing renal tubular acidosis), cryoglobulinemia, an elevated titer of antinuclear antibodies, and a number of tissue-directed autoantibodies.

COURSE

The course of rheumatoid arthritis, like most chronic diseases, cannot be predicted in a given patient. Several patterns of activity have been described: a spontaneous remission particularly in the seronegative patient, recurrent explosive attacks followed by periods of quiescence most commonly in the early phases, and the usual pattern of persistent and progressive disease activity that waxes and wanes in intensity.

A self-limited course with spontaneous remission is thought to occur in fewer than 10% of patients and is unlikely to occur after 6 months of active disease. Rarely, the inflammatory process is rapidly destructive, leading to early loss of function and disability. A few patients have a course that is characterized by remissions and exacerbations, often with months or even years during which they are asymptomatic. Most patients develop a more typical sustained progressive course with persistent symptoms that vary in intensity. Paradoxically, patients who have an abrupt onset of their disease have a better prognosis than the patient with an indolent presentation. Patients almost always go into remission during pregnancy, but usually disease activity returns several weeks after the childbirth. Although current medications are helpful to control the inflammatory process, fewer than 2% of patients demonstrate a sustained remission attributable to drugs. Patients with persistent signs of inflammation develop radiologic signs of joint space narrowing within a 2-year period.

Significant morbidity from rheumatoid arthritis has long been recognized. Approximately 60% of the patients with rheumatoid arthritis were unable to work 10 years after the onset of their disease (32). However, only recently have studies demonstrated an increased mortality in rheumatoid patients. Median life expectancy was shortened an average of 7 years for men and 3 years for women compared to control populations, and in more than 5000 patients with rheumatoid arthritis from four centers, the mortality rate was two times greater than in the control population (31). Patients at *higher risk* for shortened survival are those with systemic extra-articular involvement, low functional capacity, low socioeconomic status, low education, and prednisone use.

DIFFERENTIAL DIAGNOSIS

The difficulty of diagnosing early rheumatoid arthritis emphasizes the importance of a systematic approach to patients with arthritis (Table 70.4). Epidemiologic studies have clarified that the age, sex, ethnic background, and family history of the patient influence the likelihood of disease expression. Therefore a clear definition of host features forms a framework to begin the evaluation of a patient with arthritis. Table 70.5 outlines examples of the differential diagnosis of polyarthritis based on prevalence of disease expression defined by age and sex. Other important factors include the patient's occupation, habits, drug usage, and medical history (Table 70.6). Finally, the characteristics of the arthritis itself provide important clues to the differential diagnosis (Tables 70.7 and 70.8).

MANAGEMENT

General Principles

Rheumatoid arthritis is a chronic disorder for which there is no known cure. It therefore requires a comprehensive program that combines medical, social, and emotional support for the patient. An understanding of each patient's specific problems is essential. Serial observations (Table 70.9) and in-depth investigation of the impact of the disease on both the patient and the patient's family provide the basis for effective management.

The major goals of treatment of the arthritis are to reduce pain and discomfort, prevent deformities and loss of joint function, and maintain a productive and active life. To achieve these goals, an understanding of the cause of pain and joint destruction is important. In rheumatoid arthritis pain and dysfunction are caused by acute inflammation and subsequent mechanical and structural abnormalities. Each of these processes warrants a different therapeutic approach. Often both are present, although depending on the stage of disease, one process may predominate. Acute inflammation is always the major problem in early disease. Mechanical and structural abnormalities do not ordinarily develop until later in the course of the disease.

Management begins with effective communication

Table 70.4. Outline of Diagnostic Approach to Polyarthritis

A. Define the host features
  1. Age, sex, and ethnic background
  2. Family history
  3. Environmental factors
B. Describe the joint involvement
  1. Number
  2. Patterns
  3. Specific joints
  4. Intensity of pain
  5. Course
C. Characteristics of extra-articular features
D. Supporting laboratory studies
E. Response to therapeutic trial

Table 70.5. Differential Diagnosis of Polyarthritis Based on Age and Sex

	Male	Both Sexes	Female
Childhood (1–15)	Juvenile ankylosing spondylitis (Chapter 71) Kawasaki's syndrome[a] Hemophilia (Chapter 51)	Juvenile rheumatoid arthritis, systemic onset (Still's disease)[a] Rheumatic fever[a] Leukemia[a]	Juvenile rheumatoid arthritis[a] Pauciarticular arthritis[a] Juvenile rheumatoid arthritis, polyarthritis onset[a]
Young adult (15–30)	Ankylosing spondylitis (Chapter 71) Reiter's syndrome (Chapter 71) "Reactive" arthritis[a] Behçet's syndrome[a]	Psoriatic arthritis (Chapter 100) Lyme disease (Chapter 30) Inflammatory bowel disease (Chapter 39)	Systemic lupus erythematosus[a] Gonococcal arthritis (Chapter 27) Scleroderma[a]
Middle years (30–60)	Gout (Chapter 69) Palindromic rheumatism[a] Whipple's disease[a]	Seronegative polyarthritis (Chapter 70) Hypersensitivity reactions (Chapter 23) Vasculitic syndromes[a] Relapsing polychondritis[a]	Rheumatoid arthritis Sjögren's syndrome Sarcoidosis[a] Polymyositis[a] Erosive osteoarthritis (Chapter 68)
Elderly (60+)	Diffuse idiopathic skeletal hyperostosis (DISH) (Chapter 68) Hypertrophic pulmonary osteoarthropathy (HPO) (Chapter 56)	Pseudogout (Chapter 69) Polymyalgia rheumatica (Chapter 79) Tumor-related syndromes Secondary osteoarthritis (Chapter 68) Metabolic disorders	Primary generalized osteoarthritis (Chapter 68)

[a]These conditions are not discussed in this book. Information about them is contained in the General References at the end of this chapter.

Table 70.6. Examples of Environmental Factors in Diagnosis of Arthritis

	Disease
Occupation	
Bartender (lead exposure)	Gout (Chapter 69)
Health worker	Hepatitis (Chapter 43)
Athlete	Secondary osteoarthritis (Chapter 68)
Outdoor worker	Lyme disease (Chapter 30)
Gardener	Sporotrichosis[a]
Deep sea diver	Aseptic necrosis of bone[a]
Habits	
Alcohol abuse	Gout (Chapter 69), aseptic necrosis[a]
"Moonshine" ingestion	Saturnine gout (Chapter 69)
Smoking	Hypertrophic osteoarthropathy (Chapter 56)
Intravenous drug abuse	Septic arthritis, hepatitis, vasculitis
Sexual promiscuity	Gonococcal arthritis (Chapter 27), hepatitis (Chapter 43), Reiter's syndrome (Chapter 71)
Drugs	
Diuretics	Gout (Chapter 69)
Corticosteroids	Aseptic necrosis[a]
Hydralazine, procainamide	Systemic lupus erythematosus[a]
Any drug	Hypersensitivity reactions (Chapter 23)

[a]These conditions are not discussed in this book. Information about them is contained in the General References at the end of this chapter.

between physician and patient. It is essential that the patient and the patient's family be educated about the nature and course of the disease; the specific causes of the pain; and the goals, problems, and expectations of treatment. Chronic arthritis is a major emotional and physical stress that often requires a major change in lifestyle. A misunderstanding about the disease and the setting of inappropriate goals leads to frustration and depression.

In addition to laboratory testing and physical examination, a simple self-report questionnaire has been shown to be an effective, inexpensive method to assess the patient's status and response to treatment (17) (Fig. 70.5). The questionnaire can assess functional status, which reflects both mechanical and inflammatory problems.

Treatment options include reduction of joint stress, physical and occupational therapy, drug therapy, and surgical intervention.

Reduction of joint stress is accomplished by a number of practical measures that do not depend on the use of drugs. Because obesity stresses the musculoskeletal system, ideal body weight should be achieved and maintained. Rest, in general, is an important feature of management. Eight to nine hours' sleep at night and a 2-hour rest period in the middle of the day are reasonable recommendations for everyone with active disease. When the joints are actively inflamed, vigorous activity (heavy work, brisk exercise) should be avoided because of the danger of intensifying joint inflammation or causing traumatic injury to structures weakened by inflammation. On the other hand, patients should be urged to maintain a modest level of activity to prevent joint laxity and muscular atrophy. Splinting of acutely inflamed joints, particularly at

night, and the use of walking aids (canes, walkers) are all effective means of reducing stress on specific joints. Specially designed furniture and household utensils can help not only to relieve stress on joints but also to maintain independent function. Such aids are provided on recommendation of the consultant rheumatologist, orthopedist, physiatrist, physical therapist, or occupational therapist and are obtained from an orthotics appliance store.

A consultation with a *physical* and an *occupational therapist* is recommended early in the course of treating a patient with rheumatoid arthritis. Therapists can effectively design a program of balanced rest and activity that is appropriate for the stage of the disease. Passive exercise (moving the joints through a full range of motion) is used when inflammation is active and poorly controlled. An active exercise program, when tolerated, can be designed to prevent contractures and muscular atrophy. The application of local heat, the use of various supporting aids, education in joint protection, and maintenance of good joint function are all part of the therapist's role.

Wet or dry local heat gives transient symptomatic relief of pain and stiffness, particularly to patients with chronic synovitis. A hot shower in the morning, coupled with passive warm-up exercises, may relieve stiffness and help the patient to get the day started.

Drug Treatment

Three general classes of drugs are commonly used in the treatment of rheumatoid arthritis: NSAIDs, corticosteroids, and remittive agents or disease-modifying antirheumatic drugs (DMARDs). NSAIDs and corticosteroids have a short onset of action, whereas DMARDs can take several weeks or months to demonstrate a clinical effect. DMARDs include antimalarials, methotrexate, gold salts, sulfasalazine, d-penicillamine, cyclosporine, cyclophosphamide, and azathioprine.

In the past these drugs were prescribed in a stepwise fashion, starting with less toxic, generally less potent agents and moving to more toxic and potent agents. In general, even today, patients with mild disease are usually first prescribed NSAIDs; DMARDs are added only if the clinical response is not optimal (Fig. 70.6). However, because NSAIDs appear to have little effect on the progression of the disease and cartilage damage and bony erosions often occur within the first 2 years, rheumatologists now move more aggressively to a DMARD agent, often in combination with low-dose (less than 10 mg/day of prednisone) corticosteroids. However, the physician should always try to lower the dosage of prednisone to the minimum consistent with control of synovitis.

The inflammatory process of rheumatoid arthritis involves complicated interactions of immunologic and inflammatory mediators. No single therapeutic agent currently exists to interrupt these interactions permanently. Even DMARDs have been disappointing: Only approximately 2% of patients have an initial remission of rheumatoid arthritis in response to a DMARD, and

Table 70.7. Assessment of Joint Involvement

Number

Monarthritis	Oligoarthritis (2–4)	Polyarthritis (≥5)
Septic arthritis[a]	Reiter's syndrome	Rheumatoid arthritis
Gout	Inflammatory bowel disease	Systemic lupus erythematosus[a]
Pseudogout	Psoriatic arthritis	Serum sickness
Other crystals	Rheumatic fever[a]	Psoriatic arthritis
Local tumor[a]	Juvenile rheumatoid arthritis[a]	Tophaceous gout

Patterns

Symmetric	Asymmetric
Rheumatoid arthritis	Psoriatic arthritis
Serum sickness	Reiter's syndrome
Systemic lupus erythematosus[a]	Gout, pseudogout

Intensity of Pain

Severe	Moderate
Septic arthritis[a]	All others, including rheumatoid arthritis
Microcrystalline arthritis	

Course

Acute	Infection, gout, pseudogout
Chronic	Psoriatic arthritis, rheumatoid arthritis, ankylosing spondylitis
Additive	Rheumatoid arthritis
Migratory	Rheumatic fever,[a] systemic lupus erythematosus[a]
Evanescent	Systemic lupus erythematosus,[a] viral[a]
Episodic	Gout, pseudogout, palindromic rheumatism[a]

[a]These conditions are not discussed in this book. Information about them is contained in the General References at the end of this chapter.

Table 70.8. Diagnostic Clues Provided by Arthritis of Specific Joints

First metatarsal (podagra)	Gout
Knee (acute, episodic)	Pseudogout
Distal interphalangeal	Psoriatic arthritis
	Osteoarthritis
Metacarpals, wrist, metatarsals	Rheumatoid arthritis
Sausaged digits	Reiter's syndrome
	Psoriatic arthritis
	Sarcoidosis
Sacroiliac	Ankylosing spondylitis
	Reiter's syndrome
	Psoriatic arthritis
	Inflammatory bowel disease
Sternoclavicular	Septic arthritis
	Polymyalgia rheumatica
Heel/ankle	Reiter's syndrome

Table 70.9. Observations to be Made Serially in Patients with Rheumatoid Arthritis

Duration of morning stiffness
Degree of fatigue
Limitations of function
Patient assessment of pain
Number of joints that are painful on passive motion or tender
Degree of swelling of affected joints

only approximately 10% of those patients stay in remission for more than 3 years.

Rheumatoid arthritis has a major impact on earning, functional capacity, and life span (see above). Each therapeutic decision must be weighed in light of the potential risks and benefits, both in the long and the short term. Consultation with a rheumatologist is important so that an appropriately aggressive drug treatment program is established in the early phases of the disease (Fig. 70.6). Decisions must be made jointly with

the patient. It must also incorporate patient expectations, comorbid medical problems, and the preservation of function. Detailed reviews of all drugs used in treating patients with rheumatoid arthritis are available (see Kelly et al., "General References").

Nonsteroidal Anti-Inflammatory Drugs

In the presence of acute or chronic inflammation, it is appropriate first to prescribe NSAIDs. These drugs should always be used in conjunction with the general modalities of rest, heat, and joint protection discussed above. The major effect of these agents is to reduce acute inflammation, thereby decreasing pain, improving function, and ideally, preventing joint destruction. All of these drugs have mild to moderate analgesic properties independent of their anti-inflammatory effect.

Aspirin is the oldest drug of the nonsteroidal class, and it remains an economical, effective choice. However, because of its higher rate of GI toxicity, the narrow window between toxic and anti-inflammatory serum levels, and the inconvenience of multiple daily doses, aspirin as the initial choice of drug therapy has largely been replaced by the newer NSAIDs. The increasing generic and over-the-counter preparations of NSAIDs has further eroded the economic advantage of aspirin. Nonacetylated salicylates (Disalcid, Trilisate) are less potent anti-inflammatory agents but have the advantage of less GI toxicity, lack of inhibition of platelet aggregation, and decreased incidence of NSAID-induced angioedema reactions. Nonacetylated salicylates can be considered in patients with a significant risk of GI bleeding, particularly the elderly, and in patients on anticoagulation therapy. However, nonacetylated salicylates may displace warfarin from protein binding and patients must be monitored closely.

There are now a large number of NSAIDs from which to choose (Table 70.10), and at full dosage all may be equally effective. Likewise, the toxicities of the currently available NSAIDs are similar. However, there is a great deal of variation in tolerance and response to a particular NSAID. Long-acting NSAIDs that allow daily or twice-daily dosing improve compliance and help with morning stiffness.

Mechanism. NSAIDs inhibit prostaglandin synthesis by blocking cyclooxygenase enzymes, COX-1 and COX-2. Prostaglandins are important mediators of pain and inflammation.

Dosage. If there is active inflammation, a full dosage of an NSAID should be prescribed (Table 70.10). A lower dosage should initially be used if inflammation is mild, mechanical pain is the major problem, the patient is elderly, or the patient suffers from conditions that increase the risk for toxicity (see below). If a particular preparation is ineffective after a 4-week trial or is not tolerated, another NSAID can be initiated. No one NSAID has been demonstrated to be better than another for the treatment of rheumatoid arthritis (see Table 70.10 for NSAIDs approved for use in rheumatoid arthritis). An individual patient's response to NSAIDs in both tolerance and effectiveness is unpredictable and varied. One should become familiar with a few of these agents rather than trying to master all available NSAIDs. Combinations of NSAIDs should be avoided because studies show that combinations do not increase effectiveness and toxicities are additive.

Usual Time to Maximal Effect. Although these agents have a maximal anti-inflammatory effect within hours, a reasonable trial period is 1 month.

Side Effects. The most common toxicity of NSAIDs is GI disturbance (1,23,24) (Table 70.11). The term *NSAID gastropathy* describes a variety of gastric lesions, including mucosal erythema, gastric erosions, and frank ulcerations. NSAIDs also increase the risk of lower GI bleeding. Life-threatening bleeding may occur and does so more commonly in elderly patients (5). The gastropathy is caused by dose-related direct damage to the gastric mucosa and the blocking of locally pro-

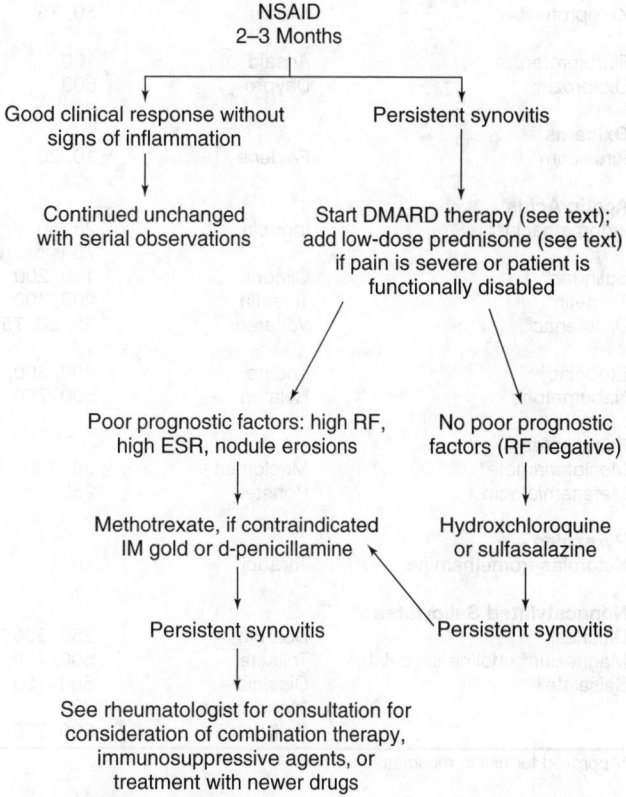

Figure 70.6. Suggested approach to anti-inflammatory drug treatment in rheumatoid arthritis.

	Without Any Difficulty	With Some Difficulty	With Much Difficulty	Unable to Do
A. Dress yourself, including tying shoelaces and doing buttons?	_____	_____	_____	_____
B. Get in and out of bed?	_____	_____	_____	_____
C. Lift a full cup or glass to your mouth?	_____	_____	_____	_____
D. Walk outdoors on flat ground?	_____	_____	_____	_____
E. Wash and dry your entire body?	_____	_____	_____	_____
F. Bend down to pick up clothing from the floor?	_____	_____	_____	_____
G. Turn regular faucets on and off?	_____	_____	_____	_____
H. Get in and out of a car?	_____	_____	_____	_____

Figure 70.5. Self-report questionnaire used to quantitatively assess the functional capacity of the patient to accomplish activities of daily living.

Table 70.10.   Nonsteroidal Anti-Inflammatory Drugs

Generic Names	Trade Names	Available Strengths (mg)	Recommended Dosage and Schedule	Maximal Daily Dosage (mg/day)
Propionic Acid Derivatives				
Ibuprofen[a]	Motrin, Rufen, IBU Nuprin, Advil	300, 400, 600, 800 200	600–800 mg 3–4 times a day	3200
Naproxen[a]	Naprosyn Anaprox, Aleve	250, 375, 500 275	500 mg twice a day	1000
Fenoprofen[a]	Nalfon, Fenopron	200, 300, 600	600 mg 3 times a day	2400
Ketoprofen[a]	Orudis	50, 75	50 mg 3–4 times a day or 75 mg 3 times a day	300
Flurbiprofen[a]	Ansaid	100	100 mg 2–3 times a day	300
Oxaprozin[a]	Daypro	600	600–1200 mg once daily	1200
Oxicams				
Piroxicam[a]	Feldene	10, 20	10–20 mg/day	20
Acetic Acids				
Indomethacin[a]	Indocin	25, 50 75 (slow release)	50 mg 3–4 times a day 1–2 times a day	150–200
Sulindac[a]	Clinoril	150, 200	150–200 mg twice a day	400
Tolmetin[a]	Tolectin	200, 400	400 mg 3–4 times a day	2000
Diclofenac[a]	Voltaren	25, 50, 75	50 mg 2–3 times a day or 75 mg twice a day	150
Etodolac[a]	Lodine	200, 300, 400, 500	200–400 mg 3 times daily	1200
Nabumetone[a]	Relafen	500, 750	1000–2000 mg once daily	2000
Fenamates				
Meclofenamate[a]	Meclomen	50, 100	50–100 mg 3–4 times a day	400
Mefenamic acid	Ponstel	250	250 mg q6hr	Use only short periods
Pyrazoles				
Ketorolac tromethamine	Toradol	10	10 mg q4–6hr	Use only short periods
Nonacetylated Salicylates				
Diflurisal	Dolobid	250, 500	250–500 mg twice daily	1000
Magnesium choline salicylate[a]	Trilisate	500, 750, 1000	1500 mg twice daily	3000
Salsalate[a]	Disalcid Mono-gesic Salflex	500, 750 750 500, 750	1500 mg twice daily	3000

[a]Approved for use in rheumatoid arthritis.

duced protective prostaglandins. The patient should be carefully monitored for GI symptoms and evidence of GI blood loss. The lowest effective dosage of the NSAID is recommended. In general, at equivalent dosages, no one NSAID has been shown to be conclusively less toxic to the GI tract. Newer NSAID agents now in clinical trials that selectively block the COX-2 enzyme, which is upregulated in inflammatory states but preserves COX-1 activity, promise to provide safer alternatives.

A cytoprotective agent (see Chapter 37) should be prescribed to patients who are at increased risk of an NSAID-induced gastropathy. Included in this group are patients with a history of peptic ulcer disease, patients with a history of GI bleeding, and the elderly (more than 70 years old). Misoprostol (Cytotec), a prostaglandin analog, has been shown to decrease endoscopic NSAID gastropathy (22). However, the drug is often associated with abdominal cramping and diarrhea. Although they improve GI tolerance and decrease dyspepsia, sulcrafate and H₂ blockers do not appear to significantly decrease the risk of GI bleeding.

Renal Side Effects.   Because prostaglandins play a role in the regulation of renal blood flow and maintenance of glomerular filtration, NSAIDs can impair renal function in certain patients. The patients at highest risk are those with fluid imbalances or compromised renal function (e.g., heart failure, diuretic use, cirrhosis, dehydration, and renal insufficiency) (28). If NSAIDs are prescribed in such patients, renal function should be monitored soon after starting NSAID therapy with serial measurements of serum creatinine. Urinalysis is usually normal. The drugs should be stopped if there is a rise in serum creatinine or increased edema. Usually, the creatinine level returns to normal within 1 or 2 weeks. Rarely, an interstitial nephritis can develop in association with a sustained rise in serum creatinine and eosinophiluria.

Less than 5% of patients develop a hypersensitivity reaction, usually a rash, to an NSAID. This reaction is generally specific to a particular drug, so another NSAID of a different class can be substituted. Rarely, an anaphylactoid reaction occurs (see Chapter 23) that can be intrinsic to the mechanism of prostaglandin inhibition. If anaphylaxis to an NSAID occurs, subsequent exposure to all classes of nonsteroidal anti-inflammatory agents (including aspirin) is contraindicated. If NSAID therapy is deemed essential, an allergy consultation is recommended for evaluation and possible desensitization.

Some side effects are more common with a particular NSAID. Indomethacin is more commonly associated than other NSAIDs with GI side effects and neurologic symptoms, including frontal headache, dizziness, vertigo, light-headedness, and mental confusion. Its long-term usefulness is therefore limited, particularly in elderly patients. Fenoprofen causes acute interstitial nephritis more often than have other NSAIDs, meclofenamate may cause diarrhea, and diclofenac sodium requires periodic monitoring of liver function tests because of reversible elevation of liver transaminases.

Significant drug interactions can occur with any of the NSAIDs (Table 70.12) and must be anticipated.

Corticosteroids

Corticosteroids have both anti-inflammatory and immunoregulatory activity. Whether they can induce actual remission of rheumatoid arthritis or have disease modifying effects is controversial. They can be given systemically or can be injected intra-articularly, depending on the clinical situation. If patients continue to have active inflammation and functional disability despite the use of an NSAID, a low dosage of a corticosteroid (e.g., prednisone less than 10 mg/day orally) can be started at the same time a DMARD is

Table 70.11. Side Effects of Nonsteroidal Anti-Inflammatory Drugs

	Approximate Incidence
Gastrointestinal	10–20%
Epigastric pain, nausea	
Anorexia, dyspepsia, peptic ulceration	
Overt or occult bleeding	<1%
Hypersensitivity reactions	1–5%
Rashes, rarely Stevens–Johnson syndrome	
Very rarely, anaphylactoid reactions	
Aggravation of allergic rhinitis or asthma	10% of sufferers
Renal effects	>5%
Transient renal failure	
Water and salt retention	
Hypokalemia, inhibit diuretic action	
Interstitial nephritis, nephrotic syndrome	>1%
Hepatic effects	5–15%
Cholestatic hepatitis	
Central nervous system	>5%
Tinnitus/deafness	Primarily aspirin
Headache, vertigo, confusion	Higher with indomethacin
Others	
Diarrhea	10–15% (mefenamic acid, other fenamates)
Aggravation of congestive heart failure, angina	>1%
Toxic amblyopia	<1% (ibuprofen)

Table 70.12. Nonsteroidal Anti-Inflammatory Drugs: Drug Interactions

Antacids	Reduce rate and extent of absorption of NSAIDs; variable effect.
Anticoagulants	Aspirin, and potentially all NSAIDs, increases the risk of bleeding of an anticoagulant patient.
Oral hypoglycemic drugs	NSAIDs may potentiate the activity of sulfonylurea drugs.
Digoxin	NSAIDs may increase serum concentration.
Antihypertensive/ diuretics	NSAIDs may attenuate the effect of diuretics, β-blockers, hydralazine, prazosin, angiotensin-converting enzyme inhibitors.
Lithium	Elevation of plasma lithium level may occur, particularly with indomethacin and diclofenac.
Methotrexate	Salicylate inhibits the renal clearance of methotrexate, and toxic levels may occur.
Phenytoin	NSAIDs may displace phenytoin from albumin and increase the concentration of free drug.
Probenecid	Inhibits renal clearance of several NSAIDs.
Combination of NSAIDs	Should be avoided.

begun (see above and Fig. 70.6). Although prednisone can be started at higher dosages (15 to 20 mg/day), attempts should be made to taper the dosage over a few weeks to less than 10 mg/day. Once started, corticosteroid therapy is difficult to discontinue and even at low dosages. Tapering of prednisone should be done slowly over a few weeks and symptoms may reoccur with small changes in the prednisone dosage. At low dosages of prednisone, patients often notice a worsening of symptoms with reductions of 1 to 2 mg in the daily dosage of prednisone.

Weight gain and cushingoid appearance is a common problem and source of patient complaints. Recent studies have raised concern over the increased cardiovascular risk and accelerated osteoporosis associated with low-dose prednisone, particularly at dosages above 10 mg/day (20). Because osteoporosis is more common in both men and women with rheumatoid arthritis, patients with and without osteoporosis risk factors on low-dose prednisone should undergo bone densitometry to assess fracture risk. Hormone replacement therapy (in women) and bisphosphonates (in men and women) are recommended to prevent cardiovascular events and osteoporosis, respectively. A DMARD agent should be added if prednisone is unable to be tapered below 10 mg/day, if concern exists about the morbidity of low-dose prednisone, or if significant poor prognostic factors (nodules, high titer rheumatoid factor, radiographic erosions) are present.

Higher dosages of prednisone are rarely necessary unless there is a life-threatening systemic disease and, if used for prolonged periods, lead to unacceptable steroid toxicity. Although a few patients can tolerate every-other-day dosing of corticosteroids, which may reduce side effects, most require corticosteroids daily to avoid symptoms. Once-a-day dosing of prednisone is associated with fewer side effects than the equivalent dosage given two or three times a day. Repetitive short courses of high-dose corticosteroids, intermittent intramuscular injections, adrenocorticotropic hormone injections, and the use of corticosteroids as the sole therapeutic agent are all to be avoided. The use of pulse therapy (methylprednisolone 100 mg intravenously daily on three consecutive days) for management of very difficult cases is controversial and should be reserved for patients failing other therapy who are experiencing a great deal of functional disability. Pulse therapy always should be initiated in conjunction with a rheumatologist because other treatment modalities should be initiated concurrently. Clinical trials show no advantage of 1 g of intravenous methylprednisolone over 100-mg pulse treatments.

Intra-articular corticosteroids (e.g., 40 mg triamcinolone in a knee, 20 mg in a shoulder, or 2 mg in a finger) are effective for controlling a local flare in one or two joints without changing the overall drug regimen (see Chapter 66 for details about the technique of injection). Intra-articular injections of steroids into symptomatic joints can help limit systemic side effects. Joint fluid should always be obtained and cultured at the time of injection to exclude a complicating infection. The injection should be administered by a rheumatologist or orthopedist if the primary physician is inexperienced with the techniques. Generally, the same joint should not be injected with steroid more than twice a year because of the danger of inducing deterioration of intra-articular cartilage, although it must be recognized that uncontrolled joint inflammation can also cause rapid deterioration of cartilage.

Disease-Modifying Antirheumatic Drugs (Agents with Delayed Onset of Action)

Although both NSAIDs and DMARD agents improve symptoms of active rheumatoid arthritis, DMARD agents may alter the disease course and improve long-term outcomes, although this effect has been difficult to prove conclusively because of disagreements on study design and the necessity of long-term patient follow-up. In any case, DMARDs have an effect on rheumatoid arthritis that is different and more delayed in onset than that of NSAIDs or corticosteroids. Once persistent disease activity (chronic synovitis) is established, a DMARD agent should be given (Fig. 70.6). Persistent disease is defined as continued joint swelling, warmth, and tenderness for 2 to 3 months despite an optimal trial of an NSAID with or without low-dose prednisone. The development of erosions or joint space narrowing on x-rays of the involved joints is a clear indication for DMARD therapy, but one should not wait for radiographic changes to occur. The decision to use a DMARD is difficult because of the need for frequent monitoring, expense, and potential toxicity related to drugs of this class (Table 70.13). The currently available drugs include hydroxychloroquine, sulfasalazine, gold, d-penicillamine, cyclosporine, azathioprine, cyclophosphamide, and most popularly methotrexate.

Hydroxychloroquine and sulfasalazine have the advantage of low toxicity and therefore are generally the first DMARD agents used. Although these agents are well tolerated, most patients have a modest beneficial response, with very few patients having a complete remission. Thus, hydroxychloroquine and sulfasalazine are most useful in patients with mild disease who are rheumatoid factor negative and lack other poor prognostic risk factors. Either drug is usually used in combination with an NSAID, corticosteroids, or other DMARD.

Methotrexate has become the most popular DMARD agent because of its early onset of action (4 to 6 weeks), ease of administration, and high patient tolerability. Methotrexate is the only DMARD agent in which most patients continue on therapy after 5 years (30). Methotrexate is best used in patients with persistent, active disease who may have poor prognostic factors such as the presence of rheumatoid factor, rheumatoid nodules, poor functional status, young age, or erosions on x-ray.

Intramuscular gold salts were until recently the most often used DMARD agents, but because of toxicity (see

Table 70.13.   Toxicities and Monitoring of Commonly Used Disease Modifying Anti-Rheumatic Drugs

Drug	Common Toxicities	Monitoring
Hydroxychloroquine	Macular damage	Ophthalmology examination every 6 months
Sulfasalazine	Myelosuppression, hepatotoxicity	CBC, LFTs every month for first 3 months then every 3 months
Methotrexate	Myelosuppression, hepatotoxicity, interstitial pneumonitis, alopecia, oral ulcers	CBC, LFTs, creatinine every 2–3 weeks until dosage stable then every 4–8 weeks
Gold, intramuscular	Myelosuppression, nephropathy, rash, oral ulcers	CBC, urine dipstick for protein before each injection
d-Penicillamine	Myelosuppression, nephropathy, autoimmune syndromes	CBC, urine dipstick for protein every 2 weeks until dosage stable then every 1–2 months
Azathioprine	Myelosuppression, secondary hepatotoxicity possible	CBC, LFTs every 1–2 weeks until dosage stable then every 1–2 months
Cyclophosphamide	Myelosuppression, hemorrhagic cystitis, alopecia, secondary malignancy (bladder cancer, myeloproliferative disorders), premature ovarian failure	CBC every 1–2 weeks until dosage stable then every 1–2 months. Urinalysis every 1–2 months. Urinalysis and urine cytology every 6–12 months after cessation.
Cyclosporine	Hypertension, renal insufficiency	Electrolytes, creatinine every 1–2 weeks until dosage stable then monthly; CBC, LFTs every 3 months

below), they are now used only after failure of methotrexate. In addition, patients dislike the requirement of weekly visits for injections during the first 4 months of therapy. Oral gold is ineffective and is no longer recommended. d-Penicillamine also has multiple toxicities (see below) and, like injectable gold, is prescribed primarily for patients with persistent aggressive disease who have failed to achieve remission with less toxic agents. Gold injections or d-penicillamine may be the only alternative in patients with significant liver disease (see below). Persistent signs of synovitis dictate a change in the regimen of anti-inflammatory and DMARD agents. Consultation with a rheumatologist early in the course of disease in a patient with resistant or progressive disease is indicated to help in choosing the appropriate regimen.

Cytotoxic drugs, other than methotrexate (e.g., azathioprine, cyclophosphamide) or cyclosporine, are used only in patients who have aggressive disease or extra-articular manifestations such as systemic vasculitis. Consultation with a rheumatologist is recommended before starting cytotoxic agents.

Combinations of DMARD agents are often used, but only now are careful studies being done to determine safety and efficacy compared to single-drug therapy. The combination of methotrexate/sulfasalazine/hydroxychloroquine was superior to methotrexate alone in a recent controlled trial and the addition of low-dose cyclosporine (2.5 to 5 mg/kg per day) to methotrexate benefited patients who were failing methotrexate therapy. Some advocate that combination therapy should be started early in patients with aggressive or persistent disease. However, it is recommended that combination therapy be reserved for patients with disease resistant to usual treatment, then used only after rheumatology consultation.

Analgesic Drugs

Pain caused by inflammation is best treated with an anti-inflammatory drug (see above), although occasionally the addition of acetaminophen can be helpful. Chronic narcotic therapy should be avoided because of side effects such as diminished mental status, hypersomnolence, and constipation, particularly in the elderly. Dependency and addiction occur infrequently, but the clinician must be alert to these behavior patterns. Mechanical pain secondary to structural changes, including joint space narrowing, subluxation, muscle atrophy, and weakness, is best approached through nonpharmacologic modalities such as splints, joint protection, and surgery.

Characteristics of Individual Drugs

Antimalarials. Antimalarials are rapidly absorbed, safe, well tolerated, and often effective remittive agents in the treatment of rheumatoid arthritis, particularly mild to moderate disease.

Mechanism. The mechanism of action of antimalarials in the treatment of patients with rheumatoid arthritis is unknown.

Dosage. Hydroxychloroquine (Plaquenil, 200-mg tablets) is the drug of choice among antimalarials. Chloroquine is no longer recommended because of its greater ocular toxicity. The initial dosage is 400 mg/day (6 mg/kg) and should not be exceeded. Normally it is prescribed as a single nighttime dose to avoid GI symptoms. If a good clinical response is noted, the dosage can be lowered to a maintenance dosage of 200 mg/day.

Usual Time to Maximal Effect. A period of 3 to 6 months is usual. A 6-month period without clinical effect should be considered a drug failure.

Side Effects. The most important toxicities are ocular: corneal deposits, extraocular muscular weakness, loss of accommodation, and a retinopathy that may progress to irreversible visual loss. At the dosage recommended, these toxicities are rare, but a baseline ophthalmologic examination and a follow-up examination every 6 months are mandatory during the period of treatment. GI upset, pigmentation changes, leukopenia, and a variety of neurologic side effects can also rarely be seen.

Sulfasalazine (Azulfidine EN-Tabs 500 mg). Sulfasalazine offers an option for mild disease. Sulfapyridine is linked to salicylic acid to create salicylazosulfapyridine, the currently used agent.

Mechanism. The mode of action is unknown. Studies comparing sulfapyridine (sulfonamide) with 5-aminosalicylic acid (anti-inflammatory) suggests that the active moiety in rheumatoid arthritis is the sulfonamide.

Dosage. Toxicities are dose related, with most occurring at the higher dosages of sulfasalazine. The best results are found at a dosage of 40 mg/kg body weight. It is suggested to begin at 500 mg/day and to increase the dosage every week in evenly divided intervals to 2 g/day. The maximal dosage of the enteric coated preparation is 2 to 3 g/day.

Usual Time to Maximal Effect. Clinical trials show improvement within 2 months of reaching full maintenance dosages. A 4- to 6-month trial is suggested.

Side Effects. Approximately 30% of patients receiving this drug experience side effects. These may be lessened by slow upward dosing. The most common side effects are GI, including nausea, vomiting, anorexia, heartburn, and epigastric distress. These symptoms can be reduced by stopping the medication and adjusting the dosage downward. The enteric coated preparation is better tolerated. GI symptoms are often accompanied by central nervous system symptoms, including headache and dizziness. Rare but more serious side effects may occur in the first 3 months of treatment, including bone marrow suppression, mucocutaneous eruptions, and hepatotoxicity. Reversible infertility can occur secondary to oligospermia. Hypersensitivity reactions can be violent, and the drug should not be used in patients with known sulfa allergy.

Monitoring should include complete blood counts and liver function tests at 2- to 4-week intervals for

3 months, then every 6 to 12 weeks for 6 months and thereafter every 3 months.

Methotrexate. Methotrexate is a folic acid antagonist and is the best tolerated and most efficacious DMARD available. Methotrexate therapy should be considered in patients with active disease with risk factors for poor prognosis (see above). Rheumatology consultation is suggested to help with the decision to start methotrexate, guide dosage titration, and establish a monitoring schedule.

Mechanism. Although the immunosuppressive and cytotoxic effects of methotrexate are caused by the inhibition of dihydrofolate reductase, the anti-inflammatory effects in rheumatoid arthritis appear to be unrelated to this mechanism of action. This is evidenced by the continued efficacy despite supplementation with folic acid (15). The anti-inflammatory mechanism remains unclear but may be caused by increases in extracellular adenosine, a potent inhibitor of inflammation.

Dosage. Methotrexate (available as a 2.5-mg tablet) is prescribed in an initial dosage of 7.5 mg once weekly. Rarely, some patients prefer to use 2.5 mg every 12 hours for three doses to reduce GI side effects. If no effect is noted in 6 to 8 weeks, then the dosage can be increased to 15 mg once weekly. The dosage can be increased to 10 to 12.5 mg weekly in the elderly or in partial responders. The maximal dosage is 25 mg weekly. Some patients who experience intolerable GI side effects can be changed to self-administered IM injections (methotrexate is available as 25-mg/mL solution). Patients should be excluded if they have renal insufficiency, acute or chronic liver disease, alcohol abuse, leukopenia, thrombocytopenia, or untreated folate deficiency. Obesity, diabetes, and history of hepatitis B or C are factors that have been suggested but not confirmed to increase methotrexate hepatotoxicity. Salicylates (and probably other NSAIDs) and trimethoprim (Bactrim, Septra) block the renal excretion of methotrexate and lead to higher serum levels and potential toxicity. If alternatives exist, concomitant use of methotrexate and trimethoprim is to be avoided. NSAIDs and methotrexate are often used together, but methotrexate toxicity monitoring should be done more often when NSAIDs are added or changed while the patient is on methotrexate therapy.

Usual Time to Maximal Effect. The onset of action is 3 to 6 weeks, with 70% of patients having some response (4). A trial of 3 to 6 months is suggested.

Side Effects. Fortunately the most serious complications of methotrexate therapy (hepatic cirrhosis, interstitial pneumonitis, and severe myelosuppression) are rare (26). Stomatitis, mild alopecia, and GI upset may occur and are related to folic acid antagonism and can be improved with folic acid supplementation (15). Folic acid 1 mg/day has been shown not to diminish the efficacy of methotrexate. Before starting methotrexate, baseline studies should include complete blood count (CBC), liver chemistries, serum creatinine, hepatitis B and C serologies, and chest radiography. Routine toxicity monitoring should include a CBC, liver transaminases, serum albumin, and serum creatinine every 4 to 8 weeks.

Hepatotoxicity is not significant if patients with preexisting liver disease, alcohol abuse, or hepatic dysfunction are excluded from treatment. Patients are instructed to stop all use of alcohol. Baseline or surveillance liver biopsies are not indicated unless preexisting liver disease is suspected. Elevated liver enzymes do not directly correlate with toxicity but therapy should be stopped if transaminases are elevated to three times the upper limit of normal. Liver biopsy should be done if elevated liver enzymes persist or if methotrexate therapy is to be continued.

Interstitial pneumonitis is rare (2%), but the clinician should be alert to symptoms of cough or shortness of breath that may herald the onset of this severe complication. Methotrexate pneumonitis may occur at any time during therapy and is not dose related. A baseline chest x-ray is useful for comparison. Patients with poor pulmonary reserve from other causes may be excluded from therapy over concerns of increased morbidity if methotrexate pneumonitis occurs.

Myelosuppression is also rare at the low dosages of methotrexate used for rheumatoid arthritis. Increased renal insufficiency from other causes, or use of trimethoprim (Bactrim, Septra), often raises methotrexate levels and causes myelosuppression.

In the absence of leukopenia, no conclusive information links methotrexate use in rheumatoid arthritis with increased risk of infection. The exception is a slight increased risk of localized herpes zoster infection.

Although there are case reports of lymphoma associated with methotrexate therapy, including a case in which the lymphoma resolved after cessation of therapy (10), increased occurrence of malignancy has not been found in large population-based studies (12), nor have there been noted effects on sperm production or ovarian function. Women of childbearing potential or men with partners of childbearing potential must understand that methotrexate has potential for teratogenesis and should practice effective birth control. Women must discontinue methotrexate for one ovulatory cycle before attempting conception, and men should wait 3 months.

Gold (Myochrysine, Solganal). Gold is effective in the treatment of rheumatoid arthritis when it is given intramuscularly. Side effects and the need for initial weekly injection visits are factors limiting its use. An oral gold compound (Auranofin) is also available but is not recommended.

Mechanism. A number of mechanisms have been postulated, but how gold works in patients with rheumatoid arthritis remains unknown.

Dosage. Myochrysine or Solganal therapy is started at 10 mg intramuscularly, 25 mg is then given the second week, then 50 mg is given weekly until a response has occurred or until a total of 1 g has been given. If there is a favorable response, therapy is tapered to 50 mg every 2 weeks for 3 months, then every 3 weeks for 3 months, and then finally to a maintenance monthly dosage. No response after a total of 1 g should be considered a treatment failure. Monthly gold should be continued indefinitely.

Usual Time to Maximal Effect. Maximal effect is achieved within 4 to 6 months or after administration of 1 g of gold.

Side Effects. Approximately 35% of patients receiving gold therapy experience side effects, and this often leads to discontinuation of the drug. Before each gold injection, patients should have a CBC and urine test for protein.

The most common reaction is a rash, which can vary from a simple pruritic erythematous patch to a severe exfoliative dermatitis. Ulcerations and mucositis of the mouth, tongue, and pharynx can occur. If a mild mucocutaneous eruption occurs, therapy should be interrupted. If the eruption abates, therapy can be restarted at 10 to 15 mg weekly, titrating upward to 50 mg weekly, monitoring carefully for further rash.

Up to 10% of patients have mild proteinuria that can progress to the nephrotic range because of a gold-induced membranous glomerulonephropathy. Patients with a positive urine qualitative measurement for protein should be evaluated with a 24-hour urine collection and gold therapy stopped if proteinuria exceeds 500 mg/24 hours. Mild proteinuria generally resolves with the cessation of therapy. Occasionally patients have isolated microscopic hematuria on gold therapy. If monitored closely, gold therapy can be continued but other causes of hematuria must be excluded (see Chapter 45).

Immune thrombocytopenia, granulocytopenia, and aplastic anemia occur uncommonly but are absolute indications for cessation of gold therapy. Myochrysine, and less often Solganal, can produce a nitritoid reaction (flushing, dizziness, or fainting) occurring immediately after the gold injection. Rarely, there is a paradoxic increase in musculoskeletal pain that requires discontinuation of treatment.

d-Penicillamine. Dimethylcysteine, a product of hydrolysis of penicillin, is named penicillamine. It has remitting effects in the treatment of rheumatoid arthritis similar to those of gold.

Mechanism. Penicillamine chelates metals, interferes with cross-linking of collagen fibrils, and disrupts sulfhydryl–disulfide bonds, but the mechanism of the beneficial effect in patients with rheumatoid arthritis is unknown.

Dosage. Penicillamine (Cuprimine, Depen) is available in 125- and 250-mg capsules. Toxicity is reduced by starting at a low dosage, 250 mg taken on an empty stomach, and increasing the dosage every 3 months by 125 to 250 mg/day until clinical benefit is observed or maximal dosage of 750 to 1000 mg once a day is reached.

Usual Time to Maximal Effect. Maximal effect from initiation of therapy or change in dosage is noted within 4 to 6 months, with the earliest response to changes in therapy taking 8 to 12 weeks. If there is no clear benefit after 9 to 12 months, treatment should be stopped.

Side Effects. d-Penicillamine monitoring consists of a CBC and urine dipstick for protein every 2 weeks during adjustment of dosage and then every 1 to 2 months when the dosage is stable. Common early toxicities include skin rash, loss of taste, metallic taste, and GI upset. These early side effects may be dose dependent and transient. After 3 to 4 months of treatment, mouth ulcers, thrombocytopenia, and renal toxicity (proteinuria, nephrotic syndrome) become potential problems. Patients who have a history of gold-induced nephrotoxicity are more likely to have a nephrotoxic reaction to d-penicillamine. Several cases have been reported of unusual autoimmune syndromes secondary to penicillamine, including Goodpasture's syndrome, SLE, myasthenia gravis, polymyositis, and pemphigus. One or more of these side effects may occur in up to 30% of patients taking the drug, in which case treatment must be stopped.

More Toxic Agents Used for Refractory Disease. The most commonly used drugs in this category are azathioprine (Imuran), cyclophosphamide (Cytoxan), and cyclosporine. Because the potential of high toxicity, these agents are used for life-threatening extra-articular manifestations or severe articular disease refractory to other therapy. It is recommended that these agents be used under the direction of a rheumatologist.

Azathioprine is a purine analog that can cause severe bone marrow suppression, particularly in patients with renal insufficiency or when used concomitantly with allopurinol or angiotensin-converting enzyme inhibitors. A CBC should be initially monitored every 2 weeks then monthly if the dosage remains stable. Increased risk of secondary malignancy caused by azathioprine is controversial.

Cyclophosphamide is an alkylating agent with serious toxicities, including bone marrow suppression, hemorrhagic cystitis, premature ovarian failure, infection, and secondary malignancy, particularly an increased risk of bladder cancer. For these reasons it is not often used in the treatment of uncomplicated rheumatoid arthritis. Cyclophosphamide is used in rheumatoid vasculitis or lung disease.

Cyclosporine is an immunosuppressive agent approved for use in preventing renal and liver allograft rejection. It inhibits T-cell function by inhibiting transcription of interleukin-2. Main toxicities include infection and renal insufficiency.

Treatment During Pregnancy

Rheumatoid arthritis therapy during pregnancy is complicated by the fact that *none of the drugs discussed above has been shown to be safe in pregnant women* with adequate, controlled studies. Although joint symptoms often remit during pregnancy, this effect is not universal. Treatment decisions require careful consideration of the risks and benefits to the mother and fetus.

All DMARD therapy should be stopped in women planning to conceive and in pregnant and lactating women. Evidence of the risks of these agents to the fetus either exists or cannot be ruled out. Methotrexate, because of evidence of potential teratogenicity, should be stopped in men and women planning conception (see above).

Although safety has not been proven in controlled trials, no evidence exists for risks to the fetus of low-dose *prednisone* (less than 20 mg/day) or NSAIDs used in the first two trimesters. If necessary, joint symptoms are best managed with the lowest possible dosage of prednisone. Potential prednisone complications include worsening of maternal gestational diabetes, hypertension, and intrauterine growth retardation. NSAIDs should be avoided in the third trimester because of the potential for premature closure of the ductus, prolonged labor, and peripartum hemorrhage. Although both NSAIDs and prednisone are excreted in the breast milk, both are considered compatible with breast-feeding by the American Academy of Pediatrics.

Treatment of Felty's Syndrome

The treatment of patients with Felty's syndrome is especially complicated and their management should be coordinated with a consulting rheumatologist. These patients should be treated with a remittive agent; methotrexate and injectable gold are the most commonly used agents. If patients develop Felty's syndrome while on a remittive agent, another remittive agent should be tried. Asymptomatic patients who remain neutropenic despite remittive therapy should be monitored closely for infection, but no further therapy prescribed. The treatment benefits of splenectomy and granulocyte colony-stimulating factor are mixed and consist largely of uncontrolled case reports. Therefore these therapies should be reserved for patients with persistent neutropenia and recurrent or severe infections.

Experimental Treatments

Limitations in the tolerability and efficacy of current therapy highlight the need for new approaches to the treatment of rheumatoid arthritis. Years of basic research in inflammation and immunology have yielded many promising agents currently in clinical trials. The goal is to develop therapy that is well tolerated, relieves symptoms, and most important, preserves joint function and prevents disability.

Biologics

Although the T cell is a likely cellular target for intervention, the intense efforts over the past several years to use monoclonal antibodies directed against T cells have been disappointing (13). More promising are soluble cytokine receptors to inhibit TNF-α and IL-1, inflammatory cytokines found in high levels in the rheumatoid joint (see "Pathogenesis"). These promising agents are entering the late stages of clinical trials (14). Approaches that stimulate normal pathways of immune regulation such as oral tolerance with type II collagen and T-cell receptor peptide vaccination therapy also hold promise.

Metalloproteinase Inhibitors

Matrix metalloproteinases (MMP) are a family of proteinases, which include the gelatinases, stromelysins, and collagenases, that are capable of degrading cartilage. They are produced by macrophages, neutrophils, lymphocytes, and chondrocytes and mediate the joint destruction in rheumatoid arthritis. These MMP inhibitors, many of which are analogs of normally occurring inhibitors of MMPs, show great promise in preventing inflammatory damage to the joints but are still in late stages of development. Tetracycline antibiotic analogs such as minocycline, which is available now, have MMP-inhibiting activity and have been shown to have efficacy in early clinical trials but are not recommended for treatment without consultation from a rheumatologist.

Nonsteroidals

Current NSAIDs inhibit both the COX-1 and COX-2 forms of cyclooxygenase (see above). COX-2 is the cyclooxygenase form upregulated in inflammatory conditions and COX-1 is constitutively produced. Newer NSAIDs capable of selectively inhibiting COX-2 are in the final stages of testing and promise to provide anti-inflammatory activity without the gastrointestinal and renal toxicity that limit current NSAID use.

Surgery

Although rheumatoid arthritis is generally an inflammatory process of the synovium, structural or mechanical derangement is a common cause of pain or loss of joint function. Pain and joint mobility may be improved by a surgical approach. The primary physician, the rheumatologist, and the orthopedist all help the patient understand the risks and benefits of the surgical procedure. The decision to have surgery is a complex one that must take into consideration the motivation and goals of the patient, the patient's ability to undergo rehabilitation, and the patient's general medical status.

Synovectomy is ordinarily not recommended for patients with rheumatoid arthritis, primarily because relief is only transient. However, an exception is synovectomy of the wrist, which is recommended if intense synovitis persists despite medical treatment over 6 to 12 months. Persistent synovitis involving the dorsal compartments of the wrist can lead to extensor tendon sheath rupture, resulting in severe disability of hand function.

Total joint arthroplasties, particularly of the knee, hip, wrist, and elbow, are highly successful. Arthroplasty of the MCP joints also can reduce pain and improve function. Other operations include release of nerve entrapments (e.g., carpal tunnel syndrome), arthroscopic procedures, and occasionally, removal of a symptomatic rheumatoid nodule.

Table 70.14. Indications for Referral of Patients with Rheumatoid Arthritis for Consultation

To a Rheumatologist

If there is any question about the validity of the diagnosis.

During the early phase of the disease to develop a management program.

If the therapeutic regimen requires the use of remitting agents (see the text).

If there are severe manifestations of extra-articular disease.

If arthrocentesis is indicated and the primary physician is not comfortable in performing the procedure (an orthopedist can also do this procedure).

For advice about splinting (an orthopedist can also provide this advice).

If there is any consideration of corrective surgery (an orthopedist can also provide this advice).

To an Orthopedist

For advice about splinting.

If there is any consideration of corrective surgery.

To a Physical and Occupational Therapist

Soon after diagnosis to advise and institute appropriate physical therapy.

Summary of Indications for Referral

The indications for consultation are listed in Table 70.14.

General References*

American College of Rheumatology Ad Hoc Committee on Clinical Guidelines. Guidelines for the management of rheumatoid arthritis. Arthritis Rheum 39:713, 1996.

American College of Rheumatology Ad Hoc Committee on Clinical Guidelines. Guidelines for monitoring drug therapy in rheumatoid arthritis. Arthritis Rheum 39:723, 1996.

Canoso JJ. Rheumatology in primary care. Philadelphia: WB Saunders, 1997.

    A well-illustrated and practical text covering rheumatoid arthritis and many other important and common forms of arthritis and nonarticular rheumatic conditions.

Cash JM, Klippel JH. Second-line drug therapy for rheumatoid arthritis. N Engl J Med 330:1368, 1994.

Harris ED Jr. Rheumatoid arthritis. Philadelphia: WB Saunders, 1997.

Kelly WN, Harris ED Jr, Ruddy S, Sledge CB, eds. Textbook of rheumatology. 5th ed. Philadelphia: WB Saunders, 1997.

McCarty DJ, Koopman WJ, eds. Arthritis and allied conditions. 12th ed. Philadelphia: Lea & Febiger, 1993.

Schumacher HR, Kippel JH, Koopman WJ. Primer on the rheumatic diseases. 10th ed. Atlanta: Arthritis Foundation, 1988.

Sjögren's syndrome. Rheum Dis Clin North Am 16:3, 1992.

Weisman MH, Weinblatt ME, eds. Treatment of the rheumatic diseases, companion to the textbook of rheumatology. Philadelphia: WB Saunders, 1995.

Specific References

1. Allison FC, Howatson MD, Torrance MB, et al. Gastrointestinal damage associated with the use of nonsteroidal anti-inflammatory drugs. N Engl J Med 327:749, 1992.
2. Arnett FC, Edworthy SM, Bloch DA, et al. The American Rheumatism Association 1987 revised criteria for the classification of rheumatoid arthritis. Arthritis Rheum 31:315, 1988.

*Bold print (general references) and bold numerals (specific references) denote published controlled clinical trials, meta-analyses, or consensus-based recommendations.

3. Firestein GS, Alvaro-Garcia JM, Maki R. Quantitative Analysis of cytokine gene expression in rheumatoid arthritis. J Immunol 144:3347, 1990.
4. **Furst DE, Kremer JM. Methotrexate in rheumatoid arthritis. Arthritis Rheum 31:305, 1988.**
5. Griffin MR, Ray WA, Schaffner W. Nonsteroidal anti-inflammatory drug use and death from peptic ulcer disease in elderly persons. Ann Intern Med 109:359, 1988.
6. Harris ED Jr. Rheumatoid arthritis. Pathophysiology and implications for therapy. N Engl J Med 322:1277, 1990.
7. Hochberg MC, Spector TD. Epidemiology of rheumatoid arthritis: update. Epidemiol Rev 12:151, 1990.
8. Hund ER. Extraarticular manifestations of rheumatoid arthritis. Semin Arthritis Rheum 8:151, 1979.
9. Hyland RH, Gordon DA, Broden I, et al. A systematic controlled study of pulmonary abnormalities in rheumatoid arthritis. J Rheumatol 10:395, 1984.
10. Kamel OW, van de Rijin J, Weiss LW, et al. Reversible lymphomas associated with Epstein Barr virus occurring during methotrexate therapy for rheumatoid arthritis and dermatomyositis. N Engl J Med 328:1317, 1993.
11. Lebowitz WB. The heart in rheumatoid arthritis (rheumatoid disease). A clinical and pathological study of sixty-two cases. Ann Intern Med 58:102, 1963.
12. Moder KG, Tefferi A. Hematologic malignancies and the use of methotrexate in rheumatoid arthritis: a retrospective study. Am J Med 99:276, 1995.
13. Moreland LW, Heck LW, Koopman WJ. Biologic agents for treating rheumatoid arthritis. Arthritis Rheum 40:397, 1997.
14. **Moreland LW, Baumgurtner SW, Schiff MH, et al. Treatment of rheumatoid arthritis with a recombinant human tumor necrosis factor receptor (p75)–Fl fusion protein. N Engl J Med 337:141, 1997.**
15. **Morgan SL, Baggott JE, Vaughn WH. Supplementation with folic acid during methotrexate therapy for rheumatoid arthritis. Ann Intern Med 121:833, 1994.**
16. Ollier W, Thomson W. Population genetics of rheumatoid arthritis. Rheum Dis Clin North Am 18:741, 1992.
17. Pincus T, Callahan LF, Brooks RH, et al. Self-report questionnaire scores in rheumatoid arthritis compared with traditional physical, radiographic, and laboratory measures. Ann Intern Med 110:259, 1989.
18. Rosenstein ED, Kramer N. Felty's and pseudo-Felty's syndrome. Semin Arthritis Rheum 21:129, 1991.
19. Roubenoff R, Roubenoff RA, Cannon JG, et al. Rheumatoid cachexia: cytokine driven hypermetabolism accompanying reduced body cell mass in chronic inflammation. J Clin Invest 93:2379, 1994.
20. Saag KG, Koehnke R, Caldwell JR, et al. Low dose long term corticosteroid therapy in rheumatoid arthritis: an analysis of serious adverse events. Am J Med 96:115, 1994.
21. Schmerling RH, Delbanco TL. The rheumatoid factor: an analysis of clinical utility. Am J Med 91:528, 1991.
22. **Silverstein FE, Graham DY, Senior JR, et al. Misoprostol reduces serious gastrointestinal complications in patients with rheumatoid arthritis receiving nonsteroidal anti-inflammatory drugs. Ann Intern Med 123:241, 1995.**
23. Simm LS. Nonsteroidal anti-inflammatory drug toxicity. Curr Opin Rheumatol 5:265, 1993.
24. Soll AH, Weinstein WM, Kurata J, McCarthy D. Nonsteroidal anti-inflammatory drugs and peptic ulcer disease. Ann Intern Med 114:307, 1991.
25. van der Heijde DMFM, van Leeuwen MA, van Riel PLCM, et al. Biannual radiographic assessments of hands and feet in a three year prospective followup of patients with early rheumatoid arthritis. Arthritis Rheum 35:26, 1992.
26. **Weinblatt ME, Kaplan H, Germain BF, et al. Methotrexate in rheumatoid arthritis: a five year prospective multicenter study. Arthritis Rheum 37:1492, 1994.**
27. Weyand CM, Hicok KC, Conn DL, et al. The influence of HLA-DRB1 genes on disease severity in rheumatoid arthritis. Ann Intern Med 117:801, 1992.
28. Whelton A, Hamilton CW. Nonsteroidal anti-inflammatory drugs: effects on kidney function. J Clin Pharmacol 31:588, 1991.

29. Wolfe F, Cathey MA, Roberts FK. The latex test revisited: rheumatoid factor testing in 8287 rheumatic disease patients. Arthritis Rheum 34:951, 1991.

30. Wolfe F, Hawley DJ, Cathey MA. Termination of slow acting antirheumatic therapy in rheumatoid arthritis: a 14-year prospective evaluation of 1017 consecutive starts. J Rheum 17:994, 1990.

31. Wolfe F, Mitchell DM, Sibley JT, et al. The mortality of rheumatoid arthritis. Arthritis Rheum 37:481, 1994.

32. Yelin E, Meenan R, Nevitt M, Epstein W. Work disability in rheumatoid arthritis: effects of disease, social, and work factors. Ann Intern Med 93:551, 1980.

C H A P T E R 71

Sacroiliitis, Ankylosing Spondylitis, and Reiter's Syndrome

FRANK C. ARNETT, JR, MD

SACROILIITIS

Chronic inflammation of the sacroiliac joints, *sacroiliitis,* may occur as an isolated clinical syndrome or a component feature of several other chronic rheumatic disorders, which are classified within a family called *spondyloarthropathies* (4). Osteoarthritis may affect the sacroiliac joints in older people, but these are radiologic changes that are usually readily differentiated from inflammatory sacroiliitis and are typically unassociated with symptoms. Sacroiliitis is considered the sine qua non for early *primary ankylosing spondylitis;* however, this latter diagnosis should be applied only when symptoms or signs indicate progression of inflammation into additional segments of the axial skeleton. *Secondary forms of sacroiliitis* or

spondylitis may complicate the clinical course in 10% of patients with inflammatory bowel disease (ulcerative colitis and Crohn's disease), 20% of those with psoriatic arthritis, and 20% of those with Reiter's syndrome (also called reactive arthritis). The dominant clinical problems that bring the patient with primary spondylitis to a physician and require careful management over many years are pain, limitation of motion, and deformity of the spine. In secondary spondylitis the same principles of diagnosis and management of the axial problem apply but must be accompanied by attention to the cutaneous, gastrointestinal (GI), genitourinary (GU), ocular, and peripheral articular manifestations of the primary disorders.

The pathogenesis of spinal inflammation is unknown; however, there is a strong hereditary component marked by the histocompatibility antigen HLA-B27 (18). This genetic marker is strongly associated with sacroiliitis and spondylitis regardless of clinical setting (Table 71.1). More than 90% of patients with primary ankylosing spondylitis have HLA-B27. Conversely, if normal subjects with HLA-B27 are carefully assessed, clinical or radiographic evidence of disease can be found in only 2% (21). Transgenic rats possessing the human HLA-B27 gene develop nearly all the clinical features of spondyloarthropathies and have confirmed the direct participation of this gene in disease pathogenesis (12). In addition to genetic predisposition, certain environmental agents appear to be associated with these diseases in the B27-positive host. There is evidence that normal bacterial flora in the GI tract participate in the pathogenesis of primary ankylosing spondylitis (4,18), as well as in the disease seen in HLA-B27 transgenic animals (18). Reiter's syndrome (reactive arthritis) is known to be triggered by certain specific GI, GU, or other infections (see "Reiter's Syndrome," below).

ANKYLOSING SPONDYLITIS

Prevalence

The prevalence of ankylosing spondylitis parallels the frequency of HLA-B27 in different populations in the United States and in other regions of the world. This gene occurs in 8 to 10% of Caucasian Americans, and the disease occurs in 0.1 to 0.2% of the white population (21). African Americans have a much lower frequency of both disease and the HLA-B27 gene. On the other hand, there is a high frequency of spondylitic disease and of HLA-B27 in certain Native American and Eskimo groups. Ankylosing spondylitis is common in Europeans and most Asian groups but is found rarely in African blacks and in Japanese, again reflecting the relative frequency of the B27 marker.

Histopathology

The spondylitic diseases are characterized by chronic inflammation of *synovial* joints, especially those in the axial skeleton; *fibrous* joints such as

Table 71.1.   Classification of Spondylitis and Frequency of HLA-B27[a]

Classification	HLA-B27 Positive
Primary	
Isolated sacroiliitis	70–90%
Ankylosing spondylitis	>90%
Secondary	
Spondylitis of inflammatory bowel disease	50%
Psoriatic spondylitis	50%
Reiter's disease with spondylitis	90%
Infectious	
Sacroiliitis	Not increased
Discitis	Not increased
Osteomyelitis	Not increased
Degenerative spondylosis	Not increased

[a]Found in 8 to 10% of normal white subjects and 2 to 4% of African Americans.

sacroiliacs and symphysis pubis; and nonarticular bony areas where tendons and fascia have their insertions (enthesopathy) (4). The chronic inflammatory infiltrates are nonspecific and histologically indistinguishable from those of rheumatoid arthritis. On the other hand, unlike the rheumatoid process in which there is cartilaginous and bony destruction, this inflammatory process tends to promote new bone formation across previous articulations. This ossification of the articular and ligamentous structures of the spine results in eventual fusion and gives rise to the characteristic radiographic findings.

History

The typical patient with sacroiliitis or ankylosing spondylitis is a young white man under the age of 40 years (Table 71.2). Occasionally the diagnosis of ankylosing spondylitis is made in older patients but careful questioning often reveals that symptoms began years earlier. However, the impression that women are affected less often than men (ratio 1:3) may be caused by underrecognition of the disease in women. The initial symptoms of the disorder in women may be peripheral or cervical joint arthritis, and low back involvement may be absent or overshadowed by these complaints. Many are misdiagnosed and labeled seronegative rheumatoid arthritis (1) (see Chapter 70). Therefore the physician should be mindful of these differences between men and women and must consider an emerging spondylitic process in young women who present with a seronegative arthritis. Similarly, children with ankylosing spondylitis are also more likely to develop a peripheral oligoarticular lower extremity arthropathy including severe hip disease, and symptoms in the axial skeleton may not develop for many years, if ever. Their illness is often inappropriately labeled juvenile rheumatoid arthritis (1,5).

The usual presenting symptoms of sacroiliitis or ankylosing spondylitis are pain and stiffness in the low back or buttocks. These symptoms begin insidiously, and the patient has usually noticed them for at least 3 months before seeking medical advice. Unlike mechanical low back syndromes, the pain and stiffness of inflammatory disease are usually worsened by rest and improved by exercise. The patient is unable to rest at night or sit for prolonged periods and must arise and stretch to obtain relief. As in discogenic disease, however, symptoms of shooting pains into the buttocks and down the posterior or lateral thighs may mimic sciatica. These pains are usually transient and not associated with any demonstrable neurologic deficits. Often, patients already have been treated conservatively or surgically for presumed disc disease.

With time, the disease progresses into the lumbar and thoracic regions. Chest wall radicular pain occurs often and may mimic pleuritic, pericardial, or anginal pain syndromes. Progressive limitation of spinal movements ensues, and patients may note more difficulty in bending forward, the development of a stooped posture, and actual loss of height. Finally, the disease process reaches the cervical spine, and if appropriate preventive measures are not taken, the neck may become fused in a flexed position. Although peripheral joints are uncommonly affected, the root joints (hips and shoulders) eventually become involved in 50% of patients. Occasionally, fusion of the back may be entirely asymptomatic, and the patient develops complaints only when the disease reaches the cervical spine, hips, or shoulders.

Additional important historical facts should be sought in the assessment of the patient. In 16% of patients, the family history is positive for a first-degree relative with spondylitis (21). The history should seek prior episodes of peripheral arthritis, perhaps beginning in childhood, or even an episode of Reiter's syndrome. Acute anterior uveitis (iritis) may have been a harbinger of the articular syndrome, and at least 25% of patients have had iritis at some time before or during their course of illness. The review of systems as well as the family history should seek symptoms or diagnoses of psoriasis or inflammatory bowel disease in the patient or in family members. Patients with spondylitis may have relatives with psoriasis or inflammatory bowel disease but may never manifest these disorders themselves (9).

Physical Examination

A complete physical examination initially and every 4 to 6 months is important in patients with suspected inflammatory axial skeletal disease. Although the primary focus of examinations is the musculoskeletal system, especially the axial skeleton, shoulders, hips, and peripheral joints, additional attention must be

Table 71.2.   Clues to Early Ankylosing Spondylitis

A young man (less often a woman)
Pain/stiffness in buttocks, low back, chest wall
   Worse with rest
     Better with exercise
Sciaticlike pains
Family history of spondylitis
History of iritis

directed toward the eyes, heart, skin, and GI tract. This practice ensures the diagnosis and provides the baseline with which the physician can assess future articular or extra-articular complications or the superimposition of unrelated systemic or musculoskeletal disorders. It must be emphasized that ankylosing spondylitis is a disease that requires management over decades, and each new complaint cannot necessarily be ascribed to the basic disease process.

Articular Features

There are few measurable abnormalities in patients with early spondylitis (Table 71.3). In fact, the patient with sacroiliitis may have an entirely normal physical examination, despite significant symptoms of pain and stiffness in the low back region. At most, there may be tenderness on direct palpation of these joints in the buttocks or upon compression of the pelvis. Stressing the sacroiliac joint to elicit pain (see Chapter 65, "Low Back Pain") may also be useful.

Abnormalities that eventually appear in the patient with progressive disease relate to loss of range of motion and deformity in mobile structures. After evaluation of the sacroiliac regions the physician should direct attention to the lumbar spine. The patient with lumbar involvement has often lost the normal lordosis, and there is flattening of that segment of the back. In addition, there is loss in range of motion when the patient attempts to bend forward and touch toes. It should be recalled that hip motion accounts for 90° of the flexion of the trunk on the lower extremities and that the lumbar spine provides the remaining stretch by reversing its lordosis and becoming kyphotic. Serial measurements of the distance between the patient's fingertips and the floor with maximal forward bending should be obtained (because of variation between individuals, isolated measurements are not interpretable). Another objective measurement of lumbar motion is the Schober test. With the patient standing erect, a horizontal line is drawn at the L5–S1 region and another line 10 cm above that. With forward flexion, the distance between these two points should increase to 15 cm in the normal lumbar spine. This test is best applied and interpreted in the young patient because lumbar motion normally decreases with age. Lateral bending and extension of the lumbar spine should also be assessed at the same time.

Involvement of the *thoracic spine* is determined subjectively by the patient's complaints of pain or stiffness in that region and by demonstrable tenderness along the vertebral column and paravertebral muscles. Compression of the rib cage laterally and over the sternum may also elicit pain. Objective determination of fusion of the costovertebral joints is obtained by measuring the chest expansion. A tape measure is placed around the patient's chest wall at the nipple line or fourth intercostal space, and the change in circumference from full expiration to full inspiration is measured. Less than 3 cm is considered abnormal. Chest expansion in normal people also decreases with increasing age.

The range of motion of the cervical spine should be determined for extension, right and left rotation, lateral flexion, and forward flexion. Loss of extension is usually the earliest abnormality, and as the disease progresses, the patient tends to develop fixed deformity in the forward flexed position. Therefore another rough estimate of developing cervical kyphosis is the occiput-to-wall measurement. This is obtained with the patient placing both heels against the base of the wall and attempting to extend the neck fully to touch the wall with the back of the head. This is normally readily accomplished.

Examination of the range of motion and elicitation of any pain on motion of both shoulders and hips is important because one-third to one-half of patients develop involvement of these joints some time during the course of the disease. Less often, peripheral joints become inflamed, but usually only transiently. The joints most commonly involved are the knees, ankles, and wrists. Approximately 10% of patients with ankylosing spondylitis complain of pain in the heels either at the Achilles tendon insertion or over the attachment of the plantar aponeurosis in the sole of the foot (enthesopathies). Swelling is usually not apparent in these areas, but tenderness to direct palpation is found.

Extra-Articular Features

Cardiac abnormalities occur in less than 5% of patients with ankylosing spondylitis (Table 71.4) (3). The most common, first-degree atrioventricular (AV) block, can be determined only electrocardiographically. A history of palpitations or syncope and the finding of a slow or irregular pulse on examination should alert the physician to higher degrees of AV block. At times a cardiac pacemaker is required for serious arrhythmias or complete AV dissociation. Aortic regurgitation caused by inflammatory thickening of the aortic valve and root is another serious cardiac complication. Once the diastolic murmur becomes apparent, there is usually cardiac decompensation requiring valve replacement in 1 to 2 years.

Table 71.3. Physical Examination in Ankylosing Spondylitis

Sacroiliac Joints	Thoracic Spine
Tenderness	Increased kyphosis
Pain with compression/stress	Tenderness
	Pain with rib cage compression
Lumbar Spine	Decreased chest expansion
Tenderness	(<3 cm)
Paravertebral muscle spasm	
Loss of lordosis	**Cervical Spine**
Decreased flexion: Schober	Tenderness
test (<5 cm) (see text)	Pain on motion
Abnormal finger-floor	Muscle spasm
Decreased lateral motion and	Decreased motion
extension	Kyphosis, decreased lordosis
	Occiput to wall movement
Hips, Shoulders	(see text)
Pain on motion	
Decreased range	

Table 71.4.   Extra-Articular Manifestations and Complications of Ankylosing Spondylitis

Cardiac	5%
First-degree AV block	
Second- and third-degree AV block	
Aortic regurgitation	
Ocular	25%
Acute iritis	
Chronic iritis	
Neurologic	Rare
Cauda equina syndrome	
Cord injury caused by fractures	
Renal	Rare
IgA nephropathy	
Amyloidosis	4%
Pulmonary fibrosis	Rare

Iritis occurs in approximately 25% of patients with ankylosing spondylitis and does not necessarily parallel the course of the articular disease. It may occasionally be the sentinel symptom. Its onset is usually abrupt and unilateral, with intense pain, redness, and photophobia as the cardinal symptoms. Immediate ophthalmologic attention is required to prevent serious damage to the anterior chamber of the eye. Local corticosteroids are usually successful in abating an acute episode; however, frequent slitlamp examinations determine the response and help determine whether systemic steroids are required.

The *cauda equina syndrome* is a rare but serious neurologic complication of spondylitis (see Chapter 65). It is believed to be related to entrapment of exiting lumbar and sacral nerves through the inflamed spinal column; however, compressive inflammatory lesions within the spinal column may be found in some cases and are surgically remediable. Patients with ankylosing spondylitis should be questioned regularly about paresthesias and pain or weakness in the legs, as well as about symptoms of bladder or bowel sphincter dysfunction. Other neurologic sequelae of the disorder include injuries to the spinal cord from fracture dislocation of a rigid and brittle spine. The neck is especially prone to fracture, and paraplegia or quadriplegia may result (13).

Secondary amyloidosis can be found in approximately 4% of patients with ankylosing spondylitis, usually after many decades of persistent inflammatory disease. Proteinuria and nephrotic syndrome indicate renal involvement, which is usually the most serious manifestation of amyloidosis. *IgA nephropathy* has been reported as another cause of proteinuria and renal dysfunction in this disease.

Apical pulmonary fibrosis, sometimes with cavity formation, is rare and usually of no clinical consequence. This radiographic abnormality may mimic tuberculosis, and vice versa.

Laboratory Tests

Radiographic evaluation of the sacroiliac joints is the single most specific test for this disorder. Although a diagnosis of sacroiliitis/spondylitis can be suspected based on the history and physical examination, definitive diagnosis cannot be established without radiographic findings. A single anteroposterior view of the pelvis may be adequate to define sacroiliitis; however, at times Ferguson's or oblique views are necessary to evaluate fully the integrity of the sacroiliac joints (20). The earliest radiographic change is usually bony sclerosis on the iliac sides of the joint margins. Thereafter, bony erosions occur (Fig. 71.1). There is eventual fusion across the joint space with subsequent loss of the early sclerotic changes (Fig. 71.2). Sacroiliitis is often confused with the radiographic anomaly *osteitis condensens ilii,* in which there is symmetric sclerosis on the iliac side of each sacroiliac joint without any erosions. This finding is most common in young women who have borne children.

An early radiographic finding on lateral lumbar spine films is squaring of the vertebral bodies. This phenomenon may also be seen in the thoracic and cervical regions. The apophyseal joints of the spine become fused and, presumably because of immobility, diffuse osteoporosis ensues. Calcification and ossification of the ligamentous structures between vertebral bodies result in the characteristic syndesmophytes seen on x-ray (i.e., the bamboo spine) (Fig. 71.2). Large "flowing" syndesmophytes, typically most prominent in the right thoracic spine but also common in the lumbar and cervical areas, are seen in another disease, diffuse idiopathic skeletal hyperostosis (DISH), which may clinically and radiographically mimic ankylosing spondylitis. Such patients can usually be discriminated by disease onset in late middle age and the absence of sacroiliitis.

Radionuclide scanning (scintigraphy) of the sacroiliac joints is not useful if there is bilateral disease and is probably of most value in localizing pyogenic infections in the sacroiliac joints and other spinal structures. Computerized tomography and magnetic resonance imaging of the sacroiliac joints are more sensitive than conventional x-rays in early disease but are also more expensive (5,20). Typing for HLA-B27 may be a more practical diagnostic approach when x-rays are not definitively abnormal (14) (see below). The cost of simple HLA-B27 typing was approximately $25 to $50 in 1997.

Hematologic studies are usually normal. In patients with severe disease, however, there may be a mild normocytic–normochromic anemia reflective of chronic disease. The white blood cell count is usually normal, as is the platelet count, although again patients with highly inflammatory disease may demonstrate mild thrombocytosis. The erythrocyte sedimentation rate is usually elevated. *Serologic studies* for rheumatoid factor and antinuclear antibodies are negative, and serum complement levels are normal.

On tissue typing, HLA-B27 occurs in more than 90% of patients with sacroiliitis or spondylitis. This genetic marker also occurs in 8 to 10% of the normal white American population. Recently, HLA typing by many commercial laboratories has become available to practicing physicians and, when properly used, may be a

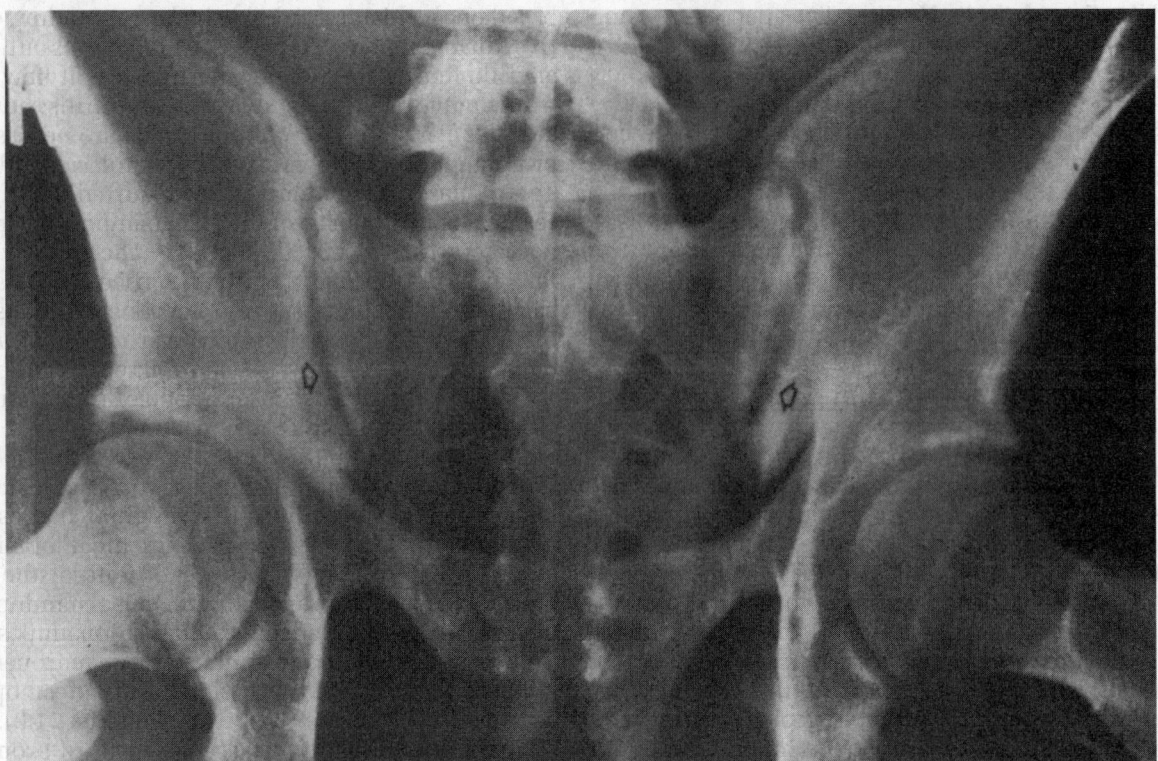

Figure 71.1. Early radiographic changes of sacroiliitis indicated by bony sclerosis on both sides of the joint margins, especially on the left *(arrows)*. Joint space erosions, a later manifestation of the disease, are present on both sides also.

helpful diagnostic aid in the assessment of a patient with low back symptoms or seronegative peripheral arthritis (14). It must be emphasized, however, that indiscriminate HLA typing cannot be substituted for a thorough clinical and radiographic evaluation of the patient. In fact, determination of B27 is rarely needed in making the diagnosis of spondylitis (see above). There are unusual circumstances, however, in which the patient gives a strong history suggestive of inflammatory axial skeletal disease but the x-rays are not yet diagnostic of sacroiliitis. In such situations, HLA typing may be helpful, as well as in children and women with early or atypical disease (1). Even then, a positive B27 does not establish a diagnosis of sacroiliitis but only provides supporting data for the diagnosis when the most specific finding (radiographic sacroiliitis) is not present.

Many patients already know their B27 status or wish to have the test performed because of the hereditary impact of disease on their family. In these circumstances, the physician must offer proper genetic counseling. The facts should be simply presented to the patient as they are currently known. It should be emphasized that spondylitis is not usually a lifethreatening or crippling disorder and that symptoms can be controlled medically in most patients. The likelihood that a family member will develop inflammatory back disease is low. Because HLA antigens, including B27, are inherited in a Mendelian dominant fashion, the risk of inheriting this tissue type is 50% for each of a patient's children (this assumes that the patient is heterozygous and the other parent is negative for B27). Even if a child inherits this tissue type, the likelihood of developing arthritis is only around 20% (21). Therefore, without any knowledge of HLA status, every child of a patient with B27-positive spondylitis has roughly a 10% (50% times 20%) chance of developing spondylitis. The 90% probability of never developing this form of arthritis must be emphasized to patients concerned about this hereditary factor.

Diagnostic Criteria

The diagnostic criteria for ankylosing spondylitis are summarized in Table 71.5.

Course

It is impossible to predict the ultimate course of any patient with sacroiliitis. The inflammatory process may remain confined to these isolated joints or it may progressively ascend into the lumbar, thoracic, and cervical spinal segments. Likewise, the duration of time from onset of symptoms to fusion of higher spinal segments is highly variable (6). Thus, each patient should understand the nature of this illness and the need for *continued medical surveillance,* as well as the principles of physical and pharmacologic management of the disorder (Table 71.6).

Management

Pharmacologic

Nonsteroidal anti-inflammatory drugs (NSAIDs) are used to relieve the pain and stiffness of the disease and to promote the patient's ability to perform the physical exercises so important to maintaining a good posture (7). It is unclear whether these drugs actually affect the natural history of the disease because no long-term controlled studies are available. It seems likely, however, that they do alter and improve overall functional capacity. Most often their use is required throughout the patientís life, but occasionally when symptoms completely remit, the NSAID may be tapered over several weeks and reinstituted if symptoms recur. Silent progress of the disease may occur; therefore the physician should closely monitor these patients even when they are not taking medication.

Indomethacin (Indocin) is especially effective therapy in many patients in dosages up to 75 to 150 mg/day. A number of side effects are important to consider, and these are discussed in detail in Chapter 70. Additional NSAIDs such as tolmetin (Tolectin), sulindac (Clinoril), and naproxen (Naproxyn) are also useful in those

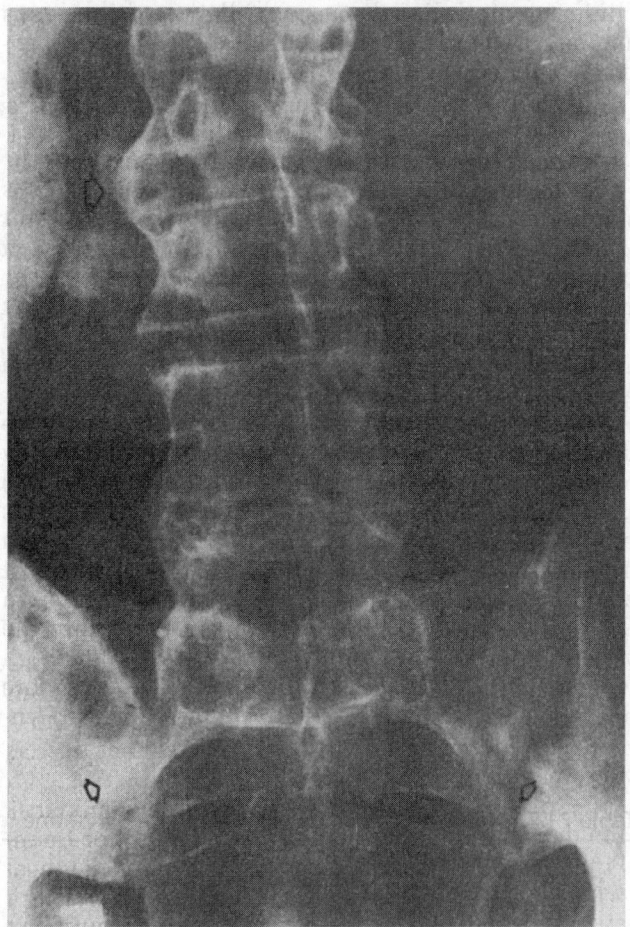

Figure 71.2. Late radiographic changes of sacroiliitis showing complete bony fusion of the joint spaces *(small arrows)*. Bridging syndesmophytes also are present in the lumbar spine *(large arrows)*.

Table 71.5. New York Diagnostic Criteria for Ankylosing Spondylitis[a]

Clinical

Limitation of motion of the lumbar spine in all three planes: anterior flexion, lateral flexion, and extension
History or presence of pain at the dorsolumbar junction *or* in the lumbar spine
Limitation of chest expansion to 2.5 cm (1 inch) or less, measured at the level of the fourth intercostal space

Radiographic

Sacroiliitis: grade 3 (sclerosis and erosions of the joint margins) or grade 4 (fusion across the joint)

From Bennet PH, Burch TA. New York symposium on population studies in the rheumatic diseases: new diagnostic criteria. Bull Rheum Dis 17:453, 1967.
[a]Definite ankylosing spondylitis = grade 3 or 4 bilateral sacroiliitis with at least one clinical criterion *or* unilateral grade 3 or 4 or bilateral grade 2 (sclerosis or joint margins) sacroiliitis with clinical criterion 1 *or* with both clinical criteria 2 and 3.

Table 71.6. Principles of Management in Ankylosing Spondylitis

Ensure patient understanding of disease process and objectives in management.
Alleviate pain and stiffness with anti-inflammatory drugs.
Use physical measures to maintain posture and range of motion in affected areas.

intolerant of indomethacin. Other NSAIDs may be tried when these drugs are ineffective (see Chapter 70). Aspirin is usually ineffective. Low-dose prednisone (10 mg/day or less) may occasionally be necessary, especially in patients with peripheral arthritis or enthesopathy, but should not be used in the long term.

Sulfasalazine (Azulfidine), a drug used for inflammatory bowel disease, has recently been found to be effective therapy for ankylosing spondylitis, especially early in the disease, and it may have disease-modifying potential (7,8). Its mechanism of action is unknown but is presumed to be anti-inflammatory or antimicrobial. An enteric coated preparation should be given starting at 500 mg/day for 1 week and gradually increased thereafter to total dosages of 2 to 3 g/day (1 g two to three times a day). Adverse reactions are common and include anorexia, headache, nausea, vomiting, gastric distress, and reversible oligospermia in men. Serious blood dyscrasias (aplastic anemia, agranulocytosis, thrombocytopenia), hypersensitivity reactions, hepatic or renal damage, and central nervous system reactions occur occasionally, and complete blood counts and urinalyses should be monitored. Absorption of folic acid and digoxin are both reduced by sulfasalazine. Consultation with a rheumatologist should be obtained before using this agent.

Radiation therapy to the spine was once an effective means of relieving pain. This form of treatment is no longer recommended because of the risk of subsequent leukemia.

Physical Measures

Although anti-inflammatory agents relieve the pain and stiffness of spondylitis, an equally important function is their promotion of the patient's ability to perform the physical therapy necessary to prevent spinal deformity and loss of motion in the joints. In fact, such a program usually cannot be instituted until symptoms have been brought under control. The natural history of the disease should be explained so that the patient understands the rationale for the exercise program that must be followed (and that the physician must reinforce) over many years. An erect posture when sitting or standing should be encouraged. The patient's bed should be firm or should be supported by a bed board. Use of a pillow should be avoided, or the smallest possible pillow should be used to prevent flexion of the neck. Sleeping in the prone position is most efficacious in promoting spinal extension, but the supine position is adequate if there is good support. The patient should refrain from sleeping on a side in a curled up position.

An active exercise program to promote extension of the back and increase range of motion of the axial and peripheral joints, as well as breathing exercises to maintain chest expansion, should be performed two to three times a day. Referral to a physical therapist to provide specific instructions and determine that the patient is performing well is a good investment. Swimming is an excellent recreational exercise for the patient with ankylosing spondylitis.

If spinal structures undergo complete ankylosis, the danger of spinal fracture after even minor trauma is increased. This is especially true in the neck, where whiplash types of injury occur. Thus, the spondylitic patient should take special precautions to prevent injury, including the use of a soft cervical collar when riding in an automobile or walking on slippery surfaces.

Prognosis

The prognosis for patients with ankylosing spondylitis is excellent. Most patients can be treated successfully by pharmacologic and physical means. Most continue to lead productive lives and change in vocational plans is usually not indicated (6). The morbidity from articular and extra-articular complications is low, and life span is not reduced significantly, if at all. In many instances pain in an affected area of the spine disappears after that segment has fused, and often disease halts at a particular segment and does not proceed to others. Although these facts should be optimistically presented to the patient, they are not cause for laxity in following the postural and exercise program and in maintaining close medical surveillance.

REITER'S SYNDROME

Definition

Reiter's syndrome is a reactive arthritis that occurs following certain genitourinary or GI infections. Recently, studies have demonstrated bacterial antigens from the triggering microbe in the synovial fluid and tissue of patients with Reiter's syndrome. Moreover, there is increasing evidence for persistence of dormant microorganisms known to be associated with reactive arthritis (see below) in the gut, genitourinary tract, and even the joints in patients with this disease (11,19).

Unlike ankylosing spondylitis, Reiter's syndrome is primarily a peripheral arthritis. However, it shares with ankylosing spondylitis a predisposition to affect young people and a tendency for sacroiliitis or spondylitis, inflammation of tendon and fascial attachments, uveitis, the same cardiac complications, and a strong association with HLA-B27 (60 to 75% positive). Although it is classically defined as the triad of nongonococcal urethritis, conjunctivitis, and arthritis, it has been found that most patients do not express the classic triad and that approximately 40% of patients have arthritis as the only feature of the triad. This latter group has been called incomplete Reiter's syndrome and more recently reactive arthritis, and diagnosis depends on recognition of the typical pattern of arthritis, the presence of mucocutaneous lesions, and other features that are discriminating (2). The diagnosis and management of the disease focus primarily on symptoms and signs referable to the joints and nonarticular musculoskeletal structures. The diagnosis is made on clinical grounds based on a constellation of symptoms and signs. Typing for HLA-B27 may be a useful diagnostic aid in the incomplete or atypical case (2,14).

History and Examination

The principal clues to the diagnosis of Reiter's syndrome are summarized in Table 71.7. The patient with Reiter's syndrome is usually a young white person between puberty and age 40. Rarely it occurs in older patients. African Americans and Japanese (but not other Asians) are affected far less commonly, presumably because of the low frequency of HLA-B27 in these groups.

The disorder occurs in two main settings. First, the disease may follow an episode of diarrhea caused by *Shigella, Salmonella, Yersinia,* or *Campylobacter* (17) (see Chapter 26). Second, the endemic form results primarily from venereal exposure, and *Chlamydia trachomatis* (see Chapters 27 and 94) is the most common causative agent (16). The sex ratio is equal in the postenteric form, but men appear to acquire the venereal form more often than women, although women with the disease are being recognized more often. The prevalence of postvenereal Reiter's syn-

Table 71.7. Clues to the Diagnosis of Reiter's Syndrome

A young person with arthritis
Symptoms
    Preceding diarrhea, urethritis, or conjunctivitis
    Lower extremity oligoarthritis (knee, ankle, foot)
    Heel pain or sausaging of digits
    Rash on soles, penis; painless oral ulcers; dystrophic nails
    Fever, weight loss, leukocytosis
HLA-B27 antigen

drome has probably fallen over the last decade because of safer sexual practices.

In the classic form, urethritis, usually painless or with mild dysuria and a mucopurulent discharge, is usually the first symptom. It generally lasts only 1 to 2 weeks. *Conjunctivitis* usually follows shortly. This is most often mild with redness, weeping, and morning crusting. Generally the conjunctivitis lasts only a few days. Photophobia is unusual, and its presence suggests uveitis (see below). Arthritis is usually the last feature of the triad to appear, usually from several days up to 1 month after the onset of urethritis. The *arthritis* is typically in the lower extremities, involving only one to four joints, most commonly the knees, ankles, and small joints of the feet. The patient notes pain, swelling, heat, and erythema over the joints. In addition to arthritis, more than 50% of patients have *nonarticular musculoskeletal pain* caused by inflammation of the insertion of tendons or fascia (enthesopathy). Heel pain caused by inflammation of the plantar aponeurosis or of the Achilles tendon insertion is one of the most prominent symptoms of the disease and may be one of the most disabling (10). Diffuse swelling of digits (sausaging), especially the toes, also occurs in more than 50% of patients and indicates involvement not only of the joints but of tendons and periosteal structures.

The *mucocutaneous features* of Reiter's syndrome are often asymptomatic and must be sought on physical examination. These include painless shallow oral ulcers, usually on the tongue and palate; circinate balanitis (Fig. 71.3) manifested by shallow moist painless ulcers on the glans penis in uncircumcised men or a dry scaling eruption on the glans in the circumcised; keratoderma blennorrhagica, a papulosquamous skin eruption usually beginning on the palms or soles (Fig. 71.4) and closely resembling pustular psoriasis; and onychodystrophy (Fig. 71.5). These lesions last for a highly variable period (several days to several months).

Additional features include fever in approximately one-third of patients, weight loss, and uveitis. The disease may begin abruptly and run a toxic course or begin insidiously and pursue an indolent one. Often, heel pain (see Chapter 102) is the first symptom, and this complaint should raise the question of emerging Reiter's syndrome.

Laboratory Tests

Hematologic studies usually demonstrate a mild normocytic–normochromic anemia characteristic of chronic disease. The hematocrit value rarely falls below 30%. A modest leukocytosis in the range of 10,000 to 15,000/mm³ with a mild shift to the left is common in those with an acute toxic presentation. Thrombocytosis with platelet counts in the range of 400,000 to 600,000/mm³ is found in approximately one-third of patients. The erythrocyte sedimentation rate is usually elevated.

Serologic studies for rheumatoid factor and antinuclear antibodies are negative. Serum complement is

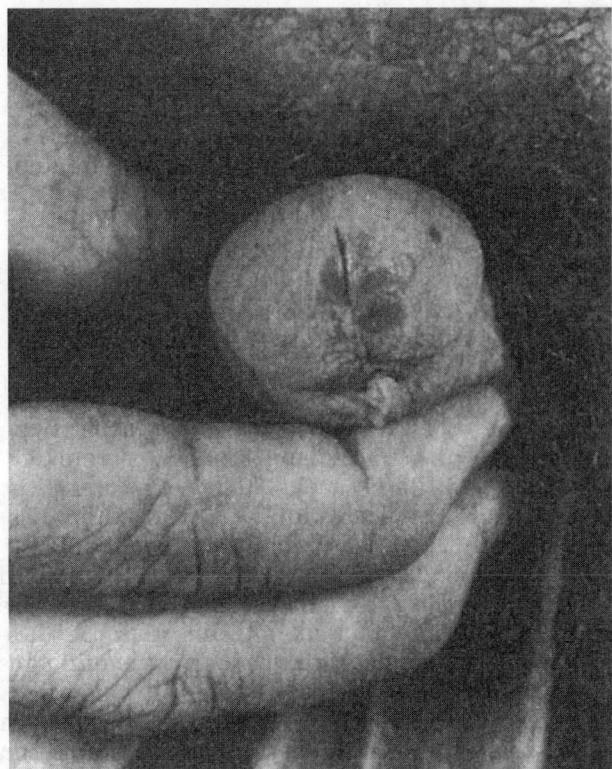

Figure 71.3. Moist, shallow circular lesions on the glans penis characteristic of circinate balanitis.

typically normal or elevated as an acute phase reactant. HLA typing reveals the B27 antigen in 60 to 75% of cases but is rarely required in diagnosing the disease. *X-rays* are typically normal early in the course of the disease; however, over time, periostitis may be seen involving the calcaneus or along the shafts of swollen digits. If sacroiliitis appears (it does in approximately 20% of cases), it is more likely to be unilateral in this disease than in ankylosing spondylitis. This may be detected by examination (see above) and confirmed by x-ray if there is doubt. In severe disease cartilage may be lost in joint spaces, and bony ankylosis may ensue.

Synovial fluid has the characteristics of a moderate inflammatory process with a poor mucin clot, white blood cell counts ranging from 5,000 to 50,000/mm³, elevated protein, normal glucose, and a high complement (as opposed to the reduced complement in the synovial fluid of patients with rheumatoid arthritis). Routine bacterial cultures are negative but newer methods, such as polymerase chain reaction (PCR), have detected bacterial deoxyribonucleic acid (DNA) or ribonucleic acid (RNA) in synovial fluid (11,16,19). Synovial biopsy demonstrates an acute and chronic inflammatory process that is nonspecific and indistinguishable from that of many other inflammatory synovitides, and therefore it is not usually necessary. A urinalysis performed on the first voided specimen in the morning is a useful way to identify asymptomatic urethritis. *Urethral stains* and cultures are negative for gonococci in the majority, although the concurrence of

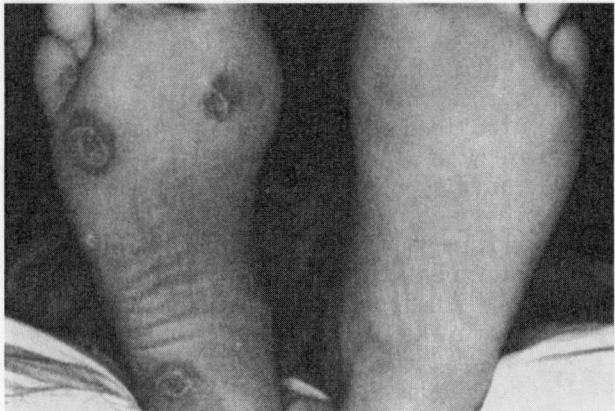

Figure 71.4. Typical keratoderma blennorrhagica involving the sole.

gonococcal urethritis with Reiter's syndrome has been documented. Therefore this culture should not be overlooked. *Chlamydia trachomatis* infection by urethral cultures or molecular probes or serum antibodies can be found in 30 to 50% of cases.

It is mandatory that HIV infection be considered in patients with sexually transmitted disease and, when appropriate, excluded by serologic testing (22) (see Chapter 34).

Course and Prognosis

Reiter's syndrome follows a self-limited course and completely resolves in 3 months to 1 year in most cases, although annoying arthralgias may persist for many years. Approximately 15% of patients have relapses and it is unclear whether these are caused by reinfection. Less commonly, a chronic progressive course ensues, resulting in articular destruction and fusion of peripheral and usually axial skeletal joints. Disability results primarily from severe heel pain, deformities of the feet, visual loss caused by uveitis, and less commonly, cardiac complications. Approximately 10% of patients become permanently disabled and unable to work (10).

Management

Treatment is directed toward suppressing the inflammatory process in joints and tendon insertions, preventing deformity, and managing the extra-articular manifestations. In addition, recent studies support the rationale for eradicating a persisting microorganism with the use of antibiotics (15). When it appears that the disease was caused by *C. trachomatis* (positive urethral cultures/probes or serum antibodies), a 3-month course of tetracycline (or doxycycline 100 mg twice a day) has been shown to shorten the course of Reiter's syndrome (15). In those with a postdysenteric onset, identification of the initiating organism is often impossible because stool cultures are usually negative and serologic detection of the specific enteric pathogen

often is unreliable. In such cases, a course of sulfasalazine is a rational approach (8). Patients who have had Reiter's syndrome who plan travel to areas endemic for the GI pathogens probably should receive prophylactic antibiotics. Even early antibiotic therapy for gastroenteritis does not appear to prevent the subsequent reactive arthritis (17).

Indole NSAIDs (indomethacin, tolmetin, or sulindac) are effective in suppressing inflammation and relieving pain in most cases of Reiter's syndrome. Aspirin is helpful in a minority of patients. Systemic corticosteroids may be necessary to treat severe uveitis or inflamed joints that have been unresponsive to NSAIDs, and in these instances consultation with a rheumatologist also is suggested. At times, intra-articular corticosteroid injection (usually performed by a rheumatologist) may be useful when systemic therapy has not completely suppressed the inflammatory process. Only occasional patients with extensive cutaneous or articular disease require more radical therapy with cytotoxic drugs, and consultation with a rheumatologist should be sought in these circumstances. Anti-inflammatory agents are generally continued for as long as inflammatory signs, pain, and stiffness persist.

Physical measures are important adjuncts in the management of this disorder as they are in ankylosing

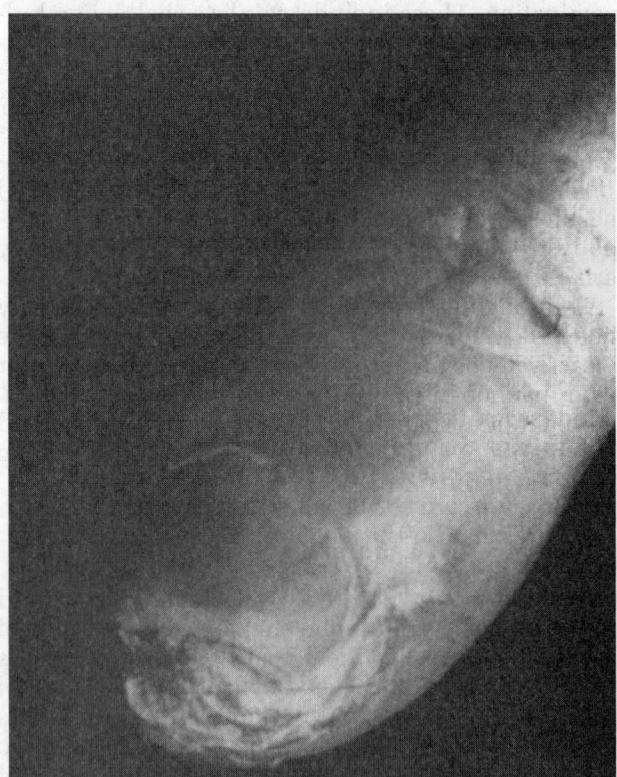

Figure 71.5. Opacification and onychodystrophy of a fingernail in Reiter's syndrome. (Taken with permission from Arnett FC. Reiter's syndrome. In: Fitzpatrick TB, Eisen AZ, Wolf K, et al, eds. Dermatology in general medicine. 3rd ed. New York: McGraw-Hill, 1985.)

spondylitis. There is a tendency for fusion of affected peripheral and axial joints. During acute inflammatory episodes, rest is important, and severely inflamed joints should be splinted to ensure comfort for the patient. As soon as inflammation can be brought under control with drugs, the affected joints should be exercised to maintain their ranges of motion. At first, passive range of motion should be encouraged in all affected joints. Later, more active range of motion and strengthening exercises should be prescribed as the patient improves.

Painful feet, especially heels, may be helped by shoe inserts that shift weight bearing to nonaffected areas (see Chapter 102).

Urethritis does not require specific therapy unless *C. trachomatis* (or gonococci) are identified. Patients should be counseled about ways to prevent reinfection with venereal and enteric pathogens (e.g., use of condoms and treatment of conjugal partner). Conjunctivitis responds to compresses or astringent drops (see Chapter 99). Uveal tract involvement, if present, requires close follow-up by an ophthalmologist to prevent permanent visual loss. The skin lesions are usually self-limited and require no therapy, or only the use of local corticosteroid creams. Rarely, extensive psoriasislike lesions or even erythroderma develop and require more intensive management by a dermatologist.

General References*

Arnett FC. Spondyloarthropathies. In: Rich RR, ed. Clinical immunology: principles and practice. St. Louis: CV Mosby, 1996;1166–1184.

Khan MA, ed. Spondyloarthropathies. Rheum Dis Clin North Am 81:1–282, 1992.

Specific References

1. Arnett FC, Bias WB, Stevens MB. Juvenile-onset chronic arthritis: clinical and roentgenographic features of a unique HLA-B27 subset. Am J Med 69:369–376, 1980.
2. Arnett FC, McClusky OE, Schacter BZ, Lordon RE. Incomplete Reiter's syndrome: discriminating features and HL-A W27 in diagnosis. Ann Intern Med 84:8–12, 1976.
3. Bergfeldt L, Insulander D, Linbolm D, et al. HLA-B27: an important genetic risk factor for lone aortic regurgitation and severe conduction system abnormalities. Am J Med 85:12–18, 1988.

4. Braun J, Sieper J. The sacroiliac joint in the spondyloarthropathies. Curr Opin Rheumatol 8:275–287, 1996.
5. Burgos-Vargos R, Pineda C. New clinical and radiographic features of the seronegative spondyloarthropathies. Curr Opin Rheumatol 3:562–574, 1991.
6. Carette S, Graham D, Little H, et al. The natural disease course of ankylosing spondylitis. Arthritis Rheum 26:186–190, 1983.
7. Cuellar ML, Espinoza LR. Management of spondyloarthropathies. Curr Opin Rheumatol 8:275–287, 1996.
8. Dougados M, van der Linden S, Leirsalo-Repo M, et al. Sulfasalazine in the treatment of spondyloarthropathy. A randomized, multicenter, double-blind, placebo-controlled study. Arthritis Rheum 38:618–627, 1995.
9. Enlow RW, Bias WB, Arnett FC. The spondylitis of inflammatory bowel disease. Arthritis Rheum 23:1359–1365, 1980.
10. Fox R, Calin A, Gerber RC, Gibson D. The chronicity of symptoms and disability in Reiter's syndrome. Ann Intern Med 91:190–193, 1979.
11. Granfors K, Jalkanen S, von Essen R, et al. Yersinia antigens in synovial-fluid cells from patients with reactive arthritis. N Engl J Med 320:216–221, 1989.
12. Hammer RE, Maika SD, Richardson JA, et al. Spontaneous inflammatory disease in transgenic rats expressing HLA-B27 and human β_2-m: an animal model of HLA-B27–associated human disorders. Cell 63:1099–1112, 1990.
13. Hunter T, Dudo HI. Spinal fractures complicating ankylosing spondylitis. A long-term followup study. Arthritis Rheum 26:751–758, 1983.
14. Khan MA, Khan MK. Diagnostic value of HLA-B27 testing in ankylosing spondylitis and Reiter's syndrome. Ann Intern Med 96:70–76, 1982.
15. Lauhio A, Leirisalo-Repo M, Lühdevirta J, et al. Double blind, placebo-controlled study of three-month treatment with lymecycline in reactive arthritis, with special reference to chlamydia arthritis. Arthritis Rheum 34:6–14, 1991.
16. Li F, Bulbul R, Schumacher HR Jr, et al. Molecular detection of bacterial DNA in venereal-associated arthritis. Arthritis Rheum 39:950–958, 1996.
17. Locht H, Kihlström E, Lindström FD. Reactive arthritis after salmonella among medical doctors: study of an outbreak. J Rheumatol 20:845–848, 1993.
18. López-Larrea C, Gonzalez-Roces S, Alvarez V. HLA-B27 structure, function, and disease association. Curr Opin Rheumatol 8:296–308, 1996.
19. Nanagara R, Li F, Beutler A, et al. Alteration of *Chlamydia trachomatis* biologic behavior in synovial membranes. Arthritis Rheum 38:1410–1417, 1995.
20. Ryan LM, Carrera GF, Lightfoot RW Jr, et al. The radiographic diagnosis of sacroiliitis. A comparison of different views with computed tomograms of the sacroiliac joint. Arthritis Rheum 26:760–763, 1983.
21. van der Linden S, Valkenburg HA, DeJongh BM, Cats A. The risk of developing ankylosing spondylitis in HLA-B27 positive individuals. A comparison of relatives of spondylitic patients with the general population. Arthritis Rheum 27:241–249, 1984.
22. Winchester R, Bernstein DH, Fisher HD, et al. The co-occurrence of Reiter's syndrome and acquired immunodeficiency. Ann Intern Med 106:19–26, 1987.

*Bold print (general references) and bold numerals (specific references) denote published controlled clinical trials, meta-analyses, or consensus-based recommendations.

Metabolic and Endocrinologic Problems

CHAPTER 72

Diabetes Mellitus

ROBERT I. GREGERMAN, MD

DEFINITION AND CLASSIFICATION

Diabetes mellitus is characterized by an abnormal increase in the concentration of blood glucose. It is not a single distinct disease entity. The most common varieties of diabetes mellitus are known to be associated with abnormalities of insulin secretion and concentration, cellular resistance to insulin action, and the development after many years of vascular damage to various organs, especially the kidneys, eyes, cardiovascular system, and nervous system.

Until recently the classification and terminology proposed by the National Diabetes Data Group of the National Institutes of Health in 1979 (based on insulin dependence) (58) were widely followed. In 1997, the Expert Committee on the Diagnosis and Classification of Diabetes Mellitus developed the new classification (33) (Table 72.1), followed in this chapter, that is based on etiology.

Type 1 Diabetes Mellitus (Formerly Insulin-Dependent Diabetes Mellitus—IDDM)

Type 1 diabetes, which accounts for approximately 10 to 12% of cases in the United States, generally has its onset in childhood, often near puberty, and was in fact once called juvenile onset diabetes mellitus. However, that designation was misleading because this type of diabetes also can develop in adulthood (43). Its essential characteristic is that insulin dependence is absolute; without insulin therapy, ketosis–acidosis usually ensues rapidly. Recent studies focus on type 1 diabetes mellitus as a chronic autoimmune disease (29), characterized by destruction of β cells in pancreatic islets and, therefore, by failure of those cells to synthesize insulin. A variety of autoantibodies (e.g., to islet cells and to insulin) have been identified in animal models and in humans early in the course of the illness. There is clearly a genetic susceptibility to this process (see below), but environmental influences also play a role. Those influences are not yet well defined. There have been claims, for example, that viral infection (85) or antibodies to bovine albumin (42) may be important triggers, but the precise pathogenesis of type 1 disease has not been established (4).

Inheritance

The precise genetics of type 1 diabetes is unclear, and prediction of the occurrence of diabetes in offspring of diabetic parents is presently impossible; even statistical estimates are crude. The prevalence of overt diabetes in offspring of conjugal diabetic parents is remarkably low, ranging from 3 to 12% in most reports. Only 2% of siblings of type 1 diabetic patients develop diabetes; when tested initially, these people may show only impaired glucose tolerance but eventually develop overt type 1 diabetes. Increased or decreased frequency of certain histocompatibility antigens, abnormal immune responses and autoimmunity, and antibodies to islet cells have been demonstrated in

Table 72.1.   Classification and Clinical Characteristics of Diabetes Mellitus

Type of Diabetes	Former Terminology	Clinical Characteristics
Type 1	Insulin-dependent diabetes mellitus (IDDM) Juvenile diabetes Juvenile onset type diabetes Ketosis-prone diabetes Brittle diabetes	Onset usually in youth but occurs at any age. Insulin deficiency requires exogenous insulin to prevent ketosis–acidosis. Non–insulin-dependent phases may occur during natural history. 10–12% of all cases.
Type 2	Non–insulin-dependent diabetes mellitus (NIDDM) Adult-onset diabetes, maturity onset diabetes (MOD), stable diabetes, nonketosis-prone diabetes; in young people, called maturity onset diabetes of youth (MODY)	Onset generally after age 40, but may occur in young; not insulin dependent or ketosis prone, but may need insulin for control of persistent hyperglycemia; periods of ketosis–acidosis may occur during stress or illness; weight control of obese subtypes may ameliorate disease. 80–90% of all cases.
Other Types		
Diabetes mellitus associated with	Secondary diabetes	Diagnosis demands usual abnormalities of glucose handling and documentation of associated condition.
Pancreatic exocrine disease Hormone excess caused by endocrine disease or hormone treatment (steroids of glucocorticoid type) Drug use (e.g., thiazide diuretics, nicotinic acid) Insulin receptor abnormalities		Usually associated with acanthosis nigricans; rare, familial.
Genetic syndromes		
Gestational diabetes mellitus (GDM)	Gestational diabetes	Glucose intolerance has onset during pregnancy; does not include diabetic who becomes pregnant; increased risk of perinatal complications and future diabetes.

Modified from (33).

type 1 diabetes. None of these findings is currently useful in a diagnostic sense.

If expression of disease in type 1 diabetes were based entirely on genetics, one would expect 100% concordance for diabetes in monozygotic twins. However, this is not the case: Both members of pairs become diabetic only about one-third of the time (59). Thus, environmental factors must be important as well (48).

Parents who have an insulin-dependent diabetic child often wish to know the risk to future offspring. Prenatal HLA typing of fetal cells obtained at amniocentesis could be compared with that of the diabetic sibling; a fetus with the same HLA identity would increase the risk, but the accuracy of the prediction would still be only approximately 50%. The imprecise nature of this assessment is in contrast to the nearly 100% certainty of predicting Tay–Sachs disease or Down's syndrome. Thus, even with an accurate family history and pedigree, together with chemical assessment of diabetes (glucose tolerance testing), only crude predictions can be made for a couple who wish to know their own chances of developing diabetes and the risk for their offspring.

At this point, only a few generalities seem safe. Prospective parents should not be told to avoid procreation merely because one parent is diabetic. Even when both parents are diabetic, the risk seems low. If avoidance of pregnancy is decided on, a diabetic woman may be at increased risk from several commonly used contraceptive measures, although the evidence for this increased risk is not firm. Use of high-

dose estrogen-based contraceptives may be unwise because of possibly increased risk in the diabetic of vascular thrombosis and hyperlipidemia. Low-dose estrogen or progestogen alone would theoretically be safer. Intrauterine devices may produce infection more often in a diabetic. Thus, mechanical means of contraception such as the diaphragm or condom seem to be the safest methods (see Chapter 93).

Type 2 Diabetes Mellitus (Formerly Non–Insulin-Dependent Diabetes Mellitus—NIDDM)

Type 2 diabetes is the most common form of diabetes mellitus and accounts for approximately 80 to 90% of patients presenting with an abnormality of glucose metabolism. More than 10 million people in the United States are affected. Patients with type 2 disease are ordinarily neither absolutely dependent on treatment with insulin nor ketosis prone. Nonetheless, patients being treated with oral hypoglycemic drugs (see below) may require insulin to control hyperglycemia or ketoacidosis during stress; other patients may become refractory to oral agents. Most patients are over age 40 at the time of diagnosis, but this type of disease is also seen in young people, and it is for this reason that older terms such as *maturity onset type diabetes* have been abandoned.

A current concept (64) of the evolution of the disease is as follows: Insulin resistance of unknown cause develops first and triggers the subsequent course of the disease. At this stage, fasting and postabsorptive blood glucose may be normal; hyperinsulinemia is present and can be considered compensatory. A defect of first-phase insulin secretion ensues (56), at least in obese patients, along with impaired glucose tolerance. Hyperglycemia (i.e., overt diabetes) is now present, as is hyperinsulinemia. After hyperglycemia becomes more severe and long-standing, hyperinsulinemia eventually diminishes, the result of progressive impairment in the patient's ability to secrete insulin. The degree of β-cell "exhaustion" is related in part to the duration of the illness. Some patients ultimately become insulin-openic to the point that they become totally dependent on exogenous insulin and are at risk of developing ketoacidosis if stressed.

Included in the group of type 2 diabetic patients are those who develop the disease before they reach adulthood (formerly known as maturity onset diabetes of the young, or MODY). These young adults (or older children) have what was once considered a variant of type 2 diabetes but has been shown to be a heterogeneous disorder. Many such patients have a familial genetic disorder in which the gene for glucokinase in liver and pancreatic islets is defective because of a variety of mutations.

Behavioral and possibly environmental factors appear to be involved in the onset of type 2 diabetes. Especially prominent is the role of excessive caloric intake and subsequent obesity in 60 to 90% of cases. Although it is clear that obesity somehow aggravates the metabolic abnormalities in diabetes and that weight loss often ameliorates them, it is not clear whether the obesity is primary or even secondary (e.g., to hyperinsulinemia). In this type of diabetes, association with certain histocompatibility antigen (HLA) subtypes and with antibodies to islet cells has not been found. Blood insulin levels are variable (see above) and, depending on the evolutionary stage of the disease, may be supranormal, normal, or subnormal. Insulin resistance is the rule, but measurement of insulin concentration has no clinically diagnostic usefulness.

Inheritance

Type 2 diabetes mellitus is clearly a genetically and clinically heterogeneous disorder (41). It has a much more obvious familial pattern of expression than does type 1 disease (see below). Glucose metabolism is commonly abnormal in the first-degree relatives of patients with type 2 disease even when their oral glucose tolerance is normal.

Studies of ethnic groups show distinctive patterns of inheritance of type 2 diabetes and superimposed geographic (environmental) effects on these patterns. The most easily apparent correlate is obesity. Certain Native American tribes (e.g., Pima, Navajo) show a remarkably high prevalence of diabetes, with about one-half of the adults having the disease; obesity appears to be the major factor in expression of diabetes in these groups. The Hispanic population (Mexican American) of the southwestern United States also shows similar but less frequent expressions of obesity and diabetes. In terms

of the patterns of disease, in South Africa, black and Indian (south Asian) populations have similar environments and diets, but only the black diabetic patients are prone to ketosis. In contrast, the Indians have more frequent vascular disease. In nonnative populations in the United States, no such distinctive ethnic or racial patterns in the pathology of type 2 diabetes have been recognized to date. In contrast to type 1 diabetes mellitus, there is essentially complete concordance for diabetes in monozygotic twins (6).

Other Types of Diabetes

Sometimes diabetes is associated with another disease (Table 72.2); usually the association is infrequent but more common than in the general population. This heterogeneous group includes some disorders in which there is a clear relationship between the associated disease and the diabetes (e.g., chronic pancreatitis) and many others in which an association has been noted but is not well understood (e.g., primary hyperaldosteronism).

Problems in Classification of Individual Patients

On occasion, classification may be difficult. For example, an adult with ketoacidosis may be erroneously classified as a type 1 diabetic when in fact the diabetes is type 2, with insulin dependence having been precipitated by the stress of infection. Similarly, the process of distinguishing between a patient with type 1 diabetes and a thin patient with type 2 disease for whom insulin has been prescribed may require discontinuation of the insulin therapy, a maneuver that may be impractical. Diagnostic procedures necessary to exclude the possibility that the diabetes is one of the other types (e.g., Cushing's syndrome, hemochromatosis) may not have been performed. In addition, for patients in whom diagnosis was based on an abnormality of glucose tolerance, diagnostic criteria may not have been met or may have been equivocal (see below). In these situations, classification should be considered tentative.

CLINICAL PRESENTATION

Most diagnoses of diabetes mellitus are now made at an asymptomatic stage of the disease as a result of

Table 72.2. Diseases Associated with Diabetes Mellitus

Obesity	Autoimmune Disorders
	Adrenal insufficiency (Addison's
Endocrine Disorders	disease)
Acromegaly	Thyroid disease
Aldosteronism	Hypoparathyroidism
Glucocorticoid excess	Myasthenia gravis
(Cushing's syndrome;	Pernicious anemia
iatrogenic)	Polyglandular failure (adrenals,
Pheochromocytoma	gonads, thyroid)
Thyrotoxicosis from any cause	Primary hypothyroidism
Somatostatinoma	Graves's hyperthyroidism

routine blood tests that reveal elevation of plasma glucose concentration. When the diagnosis is actively sought, glucose tolerance tests (GTT) reveal additional cases because up to one-quarter of patients with a diagnostic GTT have a normal fasting plasma glucose concentration. Of patients who are symptomatic at time of diagnosis, most complain of increased frequency of urination (polyuria), excessive thirst with increased fluid intake (polydipsia), and if the disease is very severe, increased appetite and increased food consumption (polyphagia) associated with weight loss. All of these symptoms are manifestations of excessive blood sugar and secondary glucosuria. Other symptomatic manifestations include blurred vision, vaginitis (usually caused by monilial infection), and skin infections. Furuncles and carbuncles, once common, are now rarely seen, but intertriginous candidiasis is common in the obese. Oral candidiasis is uncommon.

Usually, these symptoms are present for weeks or months before medical attention is sought. The onset of symptoms is often insidious and may be attributed by the patient, or even by the physician, to emotional factors or a common problem such as a urinary tract infection. Indeed, the diagnosis may be missed for a time because the physician believes that the patient is not diabetic on the basis of previous evaluation.

Many patients with type 2 diabetes present with minimal or no symptoms of hyperglycemia and glucosuria but have already developed complications such as neuropathy or, more commonly, vascular disease. Also, it is common to encounter patients who believe that their long-standing diabetes is "mild" only to find themselves with severe complications of the disease. However, only occasionally will a patient be completely unaware of having diabetes and yet present with retinopathy or nephropathy.

DIAGNOSIS

Elevation of blood sugar concentration is the hallmark of diabetes mellitus. Glucosuria alone is not a pathognomonic finding because rare patients may have a renal tubular glucose leak (renal glucosuria) at normal concentrations of blood sugar. Often, patients show diagnostically elevated blood sugar levels before glucosuria develops.

Criteria for Diagnosis of Diabetes Mellitus

The following revised criteria have been recently established by the Expert Committee of the American Diabetes Association (ADA) (see above) (33): (a) unequivocal elevation of plasma glucose (PG) concentrations associated with classic symptoms of diabetes mellitus, or (b) elevation of fasting plasma glucose (FPG) on more than one occasion (see below), or (c) elevation of PG following an oral glucose challenge (standardized oral glucose tolerance test) on more than one occasion (see below). A single elevated FPG or a single oral glucose tolerance test never establishes the diagnosis.

In most modern laboratories, glucose is determined in plasma or serum. Plasma and serum values are identical, but both are 5 to 15% higher than those obtained in whole blood from which they are derived. Portable devices for measuring blood glucose are not sufficiently accurate to be used in diagnosis.

The diagnostic standards are not arbitrary but have been derived from many studies and numerous considerations, including prospective studies conducted in the United States and Europe over the past 25 years. Although some disagreement inevitably exists on all standards, perhaps the most important point is that no single value of fasting glucose or combination of values in glucose tolerance tests sharply divides diabetic from nondiabetic patients. Most populations exhibit a continuous unimodal distribution of values, usually skewed to the higher end. An exception is the Pima Indian population, in which bimodal distribution of both fasting and 2-hour postglucose values is seen (45). The current criteria (33) are derived from prospective observations of the development of complications in people whose glucose concentrations fall within certain ranges.

Fasting Plasma Glucose

The latest cutpoint for making a diagnosis of diabetes is 126 mg/dL, (Table 72.3), which is a lower value than that previously accepted (140 mg/dL). Two values of 126 mg/dL (7.0 mol/L) or greater are needed for a definitive diagnosis. Values above 110 and less than 126 mg/dL are considered to represent impaired fasting glucose (IFG), see below.

FPG may be elevated transiently by stress or illness. When that occurs, it is usually unclear whether a diabetic state has been unmasked or a reversible disturbance of carbohydrate metabolism has occurred. Long-term follow-up may be necessary to provide the answer. In the interim the patient may be deemed to have impaired fasting glucose (IFG) (see below). Such terms as *subclinical, preclinical, chemical, latent,* and *borderline diabetes* should be avoided, both because of

Table 72.3. Interpretation of Values for Plasma Glucose

Test	Value (mg/dL)	Interpretation
Fasting PG (no caloric intake for at least 8 hr)	<110	Normal
	110–125	Impaired fasting glucose (IFG) (see text)
	≥126	Provisional diagnosis of diabetes mellitus[a]
Oral glucose tolerance test[b] (OGTT), 2-hr PG	<140	Normal
	140–199	Impaired glucose tolerance (IGT) (see text)
	≥200	Provisional[a] diagnosis of diabetes mellitus

[a]The diagnosis must be confirmed on another day according to the criteria described in the text.

[b]OGTT is performed in fasting patients by administration of 75 g of glucose dissolved in water following the standards of the World Health Organization (83; also see text).

their uncertain meaning and because of the psychologic trauma and economic penalties (e.g., insurance ratings, job qualifications) that are often needlessly created.

The Oral Glucose Tolerance Test

The oral glucose tolerance test (OGTT), for many years an accepted diagnostic standard for the diagnosis of type 2 diabetes, is no longer recommended for routine clinical use. It is less convenient, more costly, and more variable than the FPG. It may have some utility when there is a need to prognosticate for a sibling of a diabetic the chances of developing diabetes. The test still has a place in diagnosis during pregnancy (see below).

Diagnostic criteria for the OGTT are listed in Table 72.3. The test may be falsely abnormal in people who have had a recent stressful illness, have had a reduced food intake (less than 150 g of carbohydrate a day), or who have been taking one of a variety of drugs (e.g., glucocorticoids, most diuretics). Even smoking or caffeine can cause an abnormal test result. Also, the values in the OGTT tend to increase with age; that is not true of the FPG.

Measurement of the 2-hour postprandial blood sugar should never be done for screening purposes; it has low sensitivity, specificity, and reliability.

Impaired Fasting Glucose (IFG) or Glucose Tolerance

Patients whose fasting plasma glucose levels or whose levels obtained during an OGTT fall between normal and diabetic (Table 72.3) are now classified into a group (impaired fasting glucose [IFG] or impaired glucose tolerance [IGT]) separate from those with overt glucose intolerance who meet the diagnostic criteria for diabetes mellitus.

Both IFG and IGT are risk factors for the development of diabetes. In this combined group, one can expect 1 to 5% per year to develop diagnosable diabetes mellitus. On the other hand, many patients eventually show normalization of glucose tolerance, and still others remain in the IFG or IGT range. The higher the blood sugar within the range of IGT, the greater the tendency for tolerance to deteriorate.

Perhaps the most convincing evidence on IGT progression has come from long-term studies of Pima Indians (45). The risk of progression to overt diabetes in this group is clearly related to the level of glucose within the range of 160 to 200 mg at 2 hours (three times the risk of that of people with lower values). In this group, however, the rate of decompensation to overt diabetes is still only 3% per year.

Treatment of patients with IFG or IGT with oral antidiabetic (hypoglycemic) agents probably has no effect on the eventual development of diabetes, and there is no risk of microvascular complications (retinopathy or nephropathy) in people with IGT or, presumably, IFG unless they develop overt diabetes.

Significance of IFG or IGT for Development of Cardiovascular Disease

Although morbidity and mortality from cardiovascular disease are unequivocally increased in patients with clinical diabetes mellitus, the impact of IFG or IGT on that disease is uncertain. The National Diabetes Data Group Study in 1979 concluded that morbidity and mortality from atherosclerotic disease appeared to be significantly increased in patients with IGT, although to a lesser degree than the twofold to threefold increase seen in overt diabetes (58). On the other hand, no such conclusion could be drawn from other studies in 15 populations of the impact of IGT on development of coronary artery disease (74). In some of these studies, a strong relationship was found between IGT and coronary heart disease death rates, but in others no such relationship was evident. No satisfactory explanation is available for these discrepancies. Nevertheless, at this time IFG and IGT are generally conceded to be risk factors for cardiovascular disease, perhaps through a linkage to the insulin resistance syndrome (67) (see below).

Previous and Potential Abnormalities of Glucose Tolerance

According to the currently accepted scheme, people with a normal OGTT who previously showed either IGT or overt diabetic hyperglycemia should be classified as having previous abnormality of glucose tolerance (PrevAGT). These people are not to be considered diabetic and should no longer be labeled with the terms *prediabetic* or *latent diabetic*. The economic and psychosocial stigmata of such labels are not justified.

The term *potential abnormality of glucose tolerance* (PotAGT) should never be used as a diagnostic label for any person. The term is useful only in research.

Gestational Diabetes

The term *gestational diabetes mellitus* (GDM) refers only to women who meet the diagnostic criteria (Table 72.10) during pregnancy (see "Diabetes During Pregnancy," below). Women who are known to have diabetes and who become pregnant are not included. Most gestational diabetic patients return to a state of normal glucose tolerance postpartum. GDM occurs in 1 to 14% of all pregnancies, depending on the prevalence of diabetes in the population. Such patients are at increased risk (approximately 30%) for developing diabetes within 5 to 10 years after parturition.

TREATMENT OF DIABETES MELLITUS

Patient Education

Of the chronic conditions that are common in ambulatory practice, diabetes stands apart because of the broad scope and the critical importance of patient education and long-term management. For all diabetic patients, the following factors are important: the impact of diet and patterns of eating on diabetes, the implications of having diabetes on ordinary activities and the reverse, recognition of the signs of worsening diabetes, the importance of proper foot care, and the clarification of misconceptions about diabetes. For patients receiving insulin, the following additional factors are important: correct administration of insulin, the unique constraints that insulin therapy places on dietary management and changes of activity, recognition of the symptoms of hypoglycemia, and adjustment of insulin dosage during intercurrent illness.

The patient's response to being informed of a diagnosis of diabetes varies widely. Many patients have already suspected the diagnosis as the result of previous observations of similar symptoms in family members. These patients are often aware of the complications of the disease (loss of vision, amputations) and the use of the needle (insulin self-administration). Transient or even prolonged anxiety or depression is common and should be anticipated by the physician. Similar problems at this time are commonly seen in close relatives or friends of the patient. Management of these minor mood disturbances is described in Chapter 11.

Many patients are reluctant to accept the need for self-injection of insulin, and many physicians are unwilling to press the issue. The result is poor control, inappropriate use of oral hypoglycemic drugs, or both. Reluctance of both patient and physician may stem from unfamiliarity with the techniques of insulin injection. In fact, insulin injection is simple and almost without discomfort. A firm attitude on the part of the physician and input from nurses and, if necessary, other diabetic patients overcomes patient reluctance in almost all cases. The use of disposable syringes has eliminated the inconvenience of sterilization, and the modern thin, very sharp, plastic-hubbed or syringe-attached needles render the injections practically painless. Aspects of technique are described below.

A substantial proportion of new diabetic patients quickly reveal a noncompliant pattern of handling their particular chronic illness. These patterns are usually difficult to alter. Perhaps the best way to prevent the development of poor compliance is to educate the patient and other members of the patient's household from the outset (see Chapters 3 and 4 for a detailed discussion of patient education and compliance-promoting strategies).

Educational Process

The educational process should be as frank and authoritative as possible because much misinformation is apt to deluge the patient. Misconceptions should be explained and countered. The physician cannot undertake and continue this process in the detail it deserves; therefore, a nurse or other trained person should be available whenever possible to instruct the newly diagnosed diabetic and to continue the educational process as necessary. Excellent booklets are available from the American Diabetes Association (ADA) and pharmaceutical manufacturers as adjuncts to personal instruction, as are a variety of teaching films and newsletters dealing with all aspects of diabetic care (see "General References"). In all aspects of management, the need for reinforcement and continuing patient education must be stressed. Even the most intelligent patient often needs reiteration of treatment principles and procedures.

The goal of such instruction is correct patient self-care. When possible, even such procedures as altering the dosage of insulin to conform to changing needs should be taught. Successful management is never possible without such education. On the other hand, all patients need assistance from time to time. Telephone contact with a physician or a nurse should be available and encouraged. Many problems (e.g., adjustment of insulin dosage) should be handled by telephone to avoid excessive use of office time and unnecessary expense and loss of work time for the patient. Finally, the need for education of key members of the patient's family should not be forgotten. Alterations of diet and eating patterns are not often made easily and may not be made at all if a spouse is unaware, for example, that punctual meals are essential for the patient receiving conventional insulin therapy. The distinctions between *minimal, standard, and intensive* therapy (including therapy using insulin pumps) are described below. The various programs impose different demands on patients. Standard therapy is the most demanding in terms of the need for punctual meals; intensive therapy actually allows more flexibility in the timing of meals.

Diet Therapy

Different diet strategies guide therapy for diabetes, depending on whether one is dealing with an obese type 2 diabetic patient or a patient of appropriate weight who has type 1 disease. For the obese type 2 diabetic, the immediate and long-term goal is weight reduction (see Chapter 76). Ideally, diet composition should approximate that shown in Table 72.4. Most obese diabetic patients are not symptomatic and do not require immediate therapy with insulin or oral hypoglycemic agents for control of symptoms; rather, diet therapy is instituted for correction of hyperglycemia and weight. The blood sugar may fall rapidly on initiation of a diet (i.e., within a few days). This effect is caused by caloric restriction and occurs before significant weight loss is seen. Oral agents, if used along with diet, have the advantage that they do not usually produce hypoglycemia, but simultaneous institution of a weight reduction program and treatment with insulin can lead to hypoglycemia and must be done cautiously. No attempt at tight control should be made until active efforts to lose weight have ended.

Population studies indicate that most type 2 diabetes is either made manifest by obesity in genetically predisposed persons or is actually caused by obesity; studies in various animal models confirm this concept. Overt diabetes in obese patients is potentially preventable or can be ameliorated by weight reduction, provided that the diabetes has not been present for more than a few years. The potential importance and efficacy of weight reduction for ameliorating the diabetic state

Table 72.4.   Distribution of Major Nutrients in Diabetic Diets (United States)

	Nutrients (Percentage of Total Calories)						
				Fat			
	Starch and Other Complex Polysaccharides	Sugars and Dextrins	Total Carbohydrates	Total	% Monounsaturated or Polyunsaturated	Protein	Alcohol
Typical American diet	25–35	20–30	45–50	35–45	30	12–20	1–10
Current diabetic diets[a]	40[b]	10	50	30	50	20	—
Diet suggested by recent research	30	5	35	50	40 (monounsaturated or polyunsaturated) ≥10 (saturated)	15–20	1–10

Modified from West KM. Diet therapy of diabetes: an analysis of failure. Ann Intern Med 79:425, 1973.

[a]The recommended diet of the American Diabetic Association also provides <300 mg cholesterol and 28 g dietary fiber.

[b]Even higher levels of starch and lower levels of fat might be desirable, but are seldom possible in Western societies because they differ too much from the traditional diets of these cultures.

in the obese diabetic thus cannot be disputed; sometimes loss of even 5 or 10 pounds has a salutary effect. However, the problem is that most patients are unable to achieve or maintain a weight that will reverse overt diabetes, even though they are made aware of the necessity for doing so. Moreover, diabetologists grossly overstate the case that weight loss is likely to be successful or permanent.

A guiding principle for formulating diabetic diets should be the recognition that individual food preferences must be respected whenever possible. The dietitian should obtain the patient's preferred dietary history and then should attempt to construct the diet around these preferences. Such an approach is demanding for the dietitian, but the issuance of a standardized American diet to a diabetic from an ethnic minority simply guarantees noncompliance. Chapter 76 on obesity, Chapter 3 on patient education, and Chapter 4 on compliance deal with this problem in greater detail.

Prevention of Atherosclerosis

A goal of diet therapy, beyond weight reduction, is the prevention of atherosclerotic disease. This problem is both more prevalent and accelerated in all types of diabetes and accounts for approximately 25% of deaths among type 1 diabetic patients with onset before age 20. Adults with type 2 diabetes are at least twice as likely as those in the general population to die from coronary artery disease. A large portion of this excess mortality is undoubtedly caused by the abnormalities of lipids that are so common in diabetes mellitus.

Role of Diet. The evidence that atherosclerosis in the diabetic may be preventable is based to a large degree on comparisons of the prevalence of atherosclerotic disease in different populations with widely varying diets (79,80). The diabetic subjects in the United States who followed conventional high-fat, low-carbohydrate diabetic diets—at least until about 1970—had the highest rate of coronary disease seen anywhere in the world (three times the rate of the general population). For this reason and because of the evidence from population studies, the ADA recommended that its old standard diabetic diets be abandoned. Currently it advocates a diet high in carbohy-

drates (50% of calories) and low in fat (30%), a diet similar to that recommended by the American Heart Association (AHA) for nondiabetic people (Table 72.4). Although such diets have been successfully used in diabetic patients studied on metabolic wards, their reported beneficial effects on blood lipids may result from other factors: control of caloric intake with concomitant weight reduction, very low cholesterol content, high fiber content, and absence of sucrose. Several studies in which patients with type 2 diabetes received such diets resulted in unchanged low-density lipoprotein (LDL) cholesterol, lowered high-density lipoprotein (HDL) cholesterol, and increased triglyceride levels (15,18), as well as in accentuated postprandial lipemia with accompanying potential for increased atherogenicity. Thus, the AHA diet widely recommended by the ADA does not appear to be ideal and may actually be harmful. In contrast, another study used a high monounsaturated fat diet (50% of calories) low in carbohydrates (35%). The result was improved PG, triglycerides, and HDL cholesterol compared with the ADA diet (35). A later report comparing a high-carbohydrate (60% of calories) with a high-fat diet (40% of calories) rich in monounsaturates saw no differences in lipid profiles between these regimens (9). It is unclear whether seemingly small differences of carbohydrate and monounsaturated fat are critical or whether other factors are involved. The optimal diet for the control of blood lipids and glucose in the diabetic must still be considered unsettled, but it is reasonable currently to recommend 50% of calories from fat that is high in monounsaturates and 35% of calories from carbohydrates.

Role of Hyperglycemic Control. At a minimum and before hypolipidemic drug therapy is considered, efforts to control hyperlipidemia in diabetic patients must include at least near-normalization of the fasting blood glucose (along with initiation of the standard AHA diet [see above] for at least 3 months). At present, no evidence is available that favors insulin or oral hypoglycemic drugs to achieve this goal, although a theoretical advantage for glipizide (see below) has been suggested (75). Treatment of coexisting diseases that can cause hyperlipidemia (e.g., hypothyroidism) is also necessary.

Hypolipidemic Drug Therapy. It is inappropriate and usually ineffective to introduce hypolipidemic drug therapy (see Chapter 75) if hyperglycemia is not controlled. However, gross elevations of triglycerides (above 1000 to 1500 mg/dL) can predispose to the dreaded complication of acute pancreatitis. Early institution of drug therapy (usually gemfibrozil) is indicated under these circumstances (i.e., even before sugar control is achieved).

Fiber

In the past few years, diets containing large quantities of nonabsorbable plant fibers have been explored for use in diabetic patients. Fiber-rich foods decrease blood glucose after glucose loads or meals in both normal persons and patients with type 2 diabetes, and chronic ingestion of high-fiber, high-carbohydrate diets decreases fasting blood glucose and may permit decreased dosages of oral hypoglycemic drugs or lower insulin requirements. The mechanisms of these effects are not fully understood. Although delayed carbohydrate absorption probably accounts for most of the acute effect, increased sensitivity to insulin seems also to be involved. Abnormalities of blood lipids often improve. However, a role for high-fiber diets in routine therapy has not been established. In many patients these diets produce a variety of unpleasant side effects, including increased frequency of stools, diarrhea, abdominal pain, and flatulence. The formulation of fiber-rich diets (see Chapter 39, Table 39.2) is difficult, and most patients do not accept the major alterations of diet that are necessary to produce the desired effects on blood glucose levels.

Estimation of Caloric Needs

Caloric requirements for maintenance of weight vary considerably from person to person and are influenced by activity level. Required calories are approximately 40 kcal/kg or 20 kcal/lb per day for an adult with normal activity. Thus, a person of 70 kg may require 2800 kcal, although some lean men performing ordinary activities may require as much as 3000 to 3500 kcal/day. Individuals who perform manual labor may need 4000 or more kcal, whereas sedentary people may need only 2000 kcal or less.

In prescribing diets, caloric requirements are often underestimated. Physicians commonly prescribe an 1800-kcal diet for maintenance even if it is grossly inadequate for a particular patient's caloric needs. Prescription of such a diet leads to frustration and noncompliance. Overzealous decreases of calories for weight reduction may be equally defeating. When maintenance of weight is the goal, a careful dietary history by a skilled dietitian may be a good starting point for establishment of a patient's needs; the prescribed diet should then become simply a modification of that patient's ordinary pattern.

Diet During Standard Insulin Therapy

Any patient who receives insulin faces a special problem. Unlike patients who are not receiving insu-

lin, who require no special timing of meals and whose total intake can vary from day to day, patients receiving standard therapy with insulin require rigid patterns of food intake; greater flexibility is possible with intensive conventional therapy (see below). Total caloric intake must be distributed among the meals of the day, which usually include mid-afternoon and bedtime snacks as well, so that insulin dosage can be adjusted according to the patient's needs. The reverse procedure, selection of an insulin dosage and adjustment of total caloric intake to this dosage, is unphysiologic and should never be used. Occasional patients strive to reduce insulin dosage by senseless restriction of intake, incorrectly assuming that insulin dosage has some relationship to severity of their disease. Needless to say, patients must be dissuaded from such practices.

The exact composition of the diet for the patient with type 1 diabetes is less important in blood sugar control than is the constancy of distribution of the amount of food at each meal from day to day. Insulin effect (duration, intensity), even for a particular type of insulin, varies from patient to patient. Accordingly, avoidance of extremes of blood sugar concentration (hypoglycemia and hyperglycemia) requires some adjustment of food apportionment for each patient. However, one should attempt to simulate as closely as possible the patient's usual and preferred pattern of food intake. The main modification is usually to add between-meal snacks. Once an acceptable food pattern has been established and insulin dosage adjusted to that pattern, the patient must adhere to the program if extremes of blood sugar are to be avoided. Patients learn by trial and error how much latitude they can tolerate. Problems, not easily solved, are encountered in individuals who engage in strenuous sports or work that varies from day to day. Such people may have to eat more on some days than others or make frequent adjustments of their insulin dosage. Rigid control of blood sugar by use of conventional insulin therapy is not possible in such cases. Intensive conventional therapy (see below) allows for better control of blood sugar and greater variation in the level of physical activity.

The major adaptive problem with diet in patients treated with conventional insulin therapy (see below) is the need for most of them to eat in a programmed fashion (i.e., by the clock). No longer can the person wait for hunger to prompt a meal, nor can dining out at a restaurant be approached with indifference to the time the meal will be served. To do so is to court a major hypoglycemic episode. However, delay of a meal may be unavoidable. To prevent hypoglycemia in this circumstance, about 10 g of carbohydrate per half hour should be ingested. This can be provided by 4 to 6 oz (180 mL) of a sugar-containing soda (soft drink) or 4 oz orange juice, palatable premeal alternatives to glucose tablets, Life Savers, or a candy bar (see "Hypoglycemia During Insulin Therapy," below).

Exchange Lists and Special Foods. After a dietitian estimates the constituents that will be acceptable to a patient, joint discussion should be held with the spouse or other involved family members. Cooperation and participation of a spouse in the process may be essential for successful adaptation, which, for practical reasons, may require that both partners participate in the diet modifications.

The intelligent use of diet exchange lists (food equivalents) is helpful for many patients. Such lists are available from the ADA, the American Dietetic Association, and most hospital dietetic units.

Special diabetic or dietetic foods are expensive and usually are unnecessary. Some such foods do contain less free sugar than is ordinarily the case, but the patient must read the labels carefully to avoid deception.

Exercise as Therapy

Historically, exercise was recommended for control of hyperglycemia as part of a basic program of diet and insulin for type 1 patients, but conclusive data indicating such a benefit are not available. Although diabetics, like others, derive health benefits from regular exercise, the complexities of avoiding hypoglycemia during exercise in type 1 patients makes blanket recommendations tenuous (see, "Exercise During Insulin Therapy," below). The case for exercise is better in type 2 diabetes. Regular exercise may actually help prevent the emergence of type 2 diabetes (38). The conditioning effect of regular exercise also decreases insulin resistance and can improve hyperglycemia. In patients with type 2 diabetes who receive sulfonylurea drugs, the likelihood of provoking hypoglycemia by an exercise program is not great, but obese patients on low-calorie weight-reduction diets who exercise at high intensity may be severely limited by lack of muscle glycogen unless they consume additional carbohydrates immediately before exercising. Walking or cycling may be the least threatening form of exercise for these patients; attention to a period of adaptation is vital. All patients must avoid exercise that aggravates latent or existing problems (e.g., foot trauma that can lead to ulceration). It should be assumed that patients with long-standing diabetes who may have occult cardiac disease must be especially cautious when initiating an exercise program. A stress electrocardiogram is a prudent measure in such patients. The clearest rationale for exercise as therapy is as an adjunct to weight reduction programs. With weight loss, sensitivity to endogenous insulin may be restored in obese, insulin-resistant patients, and normoglycemia may ensue, sometimes obviating the need for oral agents or insulin. The blood-sugar–lowering effect of exercise often antedates significant weight loss.

Exercise During Insulin Therapy

Exercise has an insulinlike but insulin-independent effect on blood glucose that can be as strong as the maximal effect produced by insulin. The pattern of glycemic response to exercise varies. Some patients may require an anticipatory reduction of insulin (e.g., 30%) to prevent hypoglycemia. Others may need additional food before moderate activity. In some pa-

tients, especially those who exercise sporadically, prolonged exercise may result in severe hypoglycemia some 6 to 15 hours after cessation of exercise (52); again, an anticipatory reduction of insulin dosage or extra food may be needed. Modest exercise (walking 3.5 miles in 1 hour) may utilize 350 extra calories, but only 10 to 20 g of carbohydrates, a fraction of these extra calories, may be sufficient to prevent hypoglycemia. Similar considerations guide management of more vigorous exercise. The hypoglycemic effect of exercise may be greater if the insulin has been injected into an extremity that is being exercised. Many patients ordinarily prefer to inject insulin into the thigh, but some who engage in vigorous exercise (jogging, other sports, manual labor) may have to use abdominal or arm injection sites to avoid excessive insulin effect caused by exercise-induced rapid absorption.

Selection of Patients for Insulin Therapy or Oral Hypoglycemic Drugs

Type 1 Diabetes

Many patients with type 1 diabetes are started on insulin during an episode of ketoacidosis. By the time the patient is seen in an ambulatory mode, he or she will have been switched from short-acting insulin, used in the treatment of the acute phase, to an intermediate- or long-acting preparation. The insulin dependence has been established by the occurrence of the acute episode. Unless this acute event was precipitated by stress in a type 2 diabetic patient, insulin dependence is usually absolute and permanent. Occasionally in adults (more often in children), the insulin requirement may decrease or even disappear over several months, but relapse is the rule in such cases. Many nonobese adults were in the past considered to have type 2 disease when first diagnosed because they had not developed ketoacidosis on presentation. The presence of type 1 diabetes can be suspected from the lack of obesity, lack of response to sulfonylurea, and a low level of insulin C–peptide (a marker for endogenous insulin secretion).

Type 2 Diabetes

A therapeutic approach to patients with type 2 diabetes is shown in Table 72.5. As noted, the initial approach to the obese non–insulin-dependent patient should be weight reduction. Such therapy, if successfully followed, can be expected to reduce blood sugar within a few weeks. However, caloric restriction sometimes can induce a marked fall in the blood sugar within a few days, well before significant weight loss has occurred. If FPG is less than 200 to 250 mg/dL, hyperglycemia and glucosuria will not ordinarily produce enough symptoms to be troublesome during this period and no additional drug therapy (oral hypoglycemics or insulin) is needed. Even an FPG of 300 may be tolerated. These patients are not prone to ketosis; no urgency exists for instituting drug therapy. On the other hand, symptomatic hyperglycemia or glucosuria, persisting for weeks despite efforts at (or actual) weight

Table 72.5. Initial Therapeutic Approach to Patients with Type 2 Diabetes Mellitus

Fasting Plasma Glucose (mg/dL)	Age of Patient (yr)			
	20	40	60	80
Obese patient (initial dietary treatment)				
110–125	DIET	DIET	DIET	Diet or do nothing
126–199	ORAL AGENT[a] or insulin	ORAL AGENT or insulin	ORAL AGENT	Oral agent or diet
200	INSULIN or oral agent	INSULIN or ORAL AGENT	ORAL AGENT or insulin	Oral agent, insulin, or diet
Nonobese patient (initial dietary treatment)				
110–125	INSULIN or oral agent	ORAL AGENT or insulin	ORAL AGENT	Oral agent or diet
126–199	INSULIN	INSULIN or ORAL AGENT	ORAL AGENT or INSULIN	ORAL AGENT or INSULIN
200	INSULIN	INSULIN or ORAL AGENT	INSULIN or oral agent	INSULIN or oral agent

Modified from ADA Physician's Guide to Non–insulin-Dependent Type II Diabetes. Diagnosis and treatment. 2nd ed. Alexandria, VA: ADA, 1988.

This table presents results of a poll involving specialists in diabetes. However, it does not represent the opinion of all experts. Treatment must be *individualized* for all patients. When two therapeutic approaches are listed, if both are capitalized, slight preference is given to the first one listed. If the second approach is in lowercase letters, the first approach is strongly preferred. If both approaches are in lowercase letters, no clear-cut preference can be stated. Evening insulin plus a daytime sulfonylurea is another option, recently promulgated (see text).

[a]Oral agent is a sulfonylurea, metformin or a combination.

loss, should not be ignored. In this case, drug therapy is indicated for symptomatic relief and can be discontinued if weight reduction is successful.

Most patients with symptomatic type 2 diabetes are treated initially with oral hypoglycemic drugs, although some require insulin (see below). However, even asymptomatic patients have in the past also been treated for only modest elevations of FPG or even for abnormal glucose tolerance, and such treatment may indeed improve or normalize glucose tolerance. Extrapolation of results from patient surveys relating abnormalities of glucose tolerance to development of complications of diabetes suggests that such treatment might be beneficial. However, no evidence exists to support this hypothesis in patients with type 2 disease.

The official recommendation of the ADA, the American Medical Association Council on Drugs, and the FDA is that oral agents be limited to patients with symptomatic type 2 diabetes that cannot be controlled by diet (within 3 to 4 months) and in whom addition of insulin is impractical or unacceptable. This stand may be inappropriately conservative; in fact, Table 72.5, from a publication of the ADA, suggests a more liberal approach.

The indications for use of insulin in patients with *asymptomatic* type 2 diabetes are unclear. Although evidence is clear that modest elevations of blood sugar do indeed relate to at least the microvascular complications of diabetes (24,28,33), no prospective studies are as yet available to demonstrate that insulin therapy for type 2 diabetes with asymptomatic hyperglycemia is beneficial (see "Implications of the DCCT for Type 2 Diabetes," below). Such studies are currently under way. Insulin therapy is certainly indicated for control of symptomatic diabetes (see above) in type 2 diabetes that cannot be controlled with diet or diet plus oral agents.

Determination of hemoglobin A_{1c} in cases of modest elevation of blood sugar is an important guide to therapy (33,57) (see below). Using the best available methodology (high-performance liquid chromatography, HPLC) for measurement, the normal mean HbA$_{1c}$

is approximately 5% and the upper limit of normal is 6.5% (3 standard deviations). A near-normal value (e.g., below 7.0%) might deter a recommendation for drug or insulin therapy, whereas an elevated value would suggest that long-term benefit might outweigh the possible risks or inconvenience of treatment. Recommendations for or against therapy under these circumstances are currently determined not only by the clinical circumstances including lipid abnormalities, but by the physician's concerns over the long-term deleterious effect of hyperglycemia (see "Normoglycemia as a Goal of Therapy," below).

Other Circumstances Requiring Insulin Therapy

Some patients who are not, strictly speaking, insulin dependent also need insulin therapy. Patients with type 2 diabetes may be prescribed oral hypoglycemic drugs to control blood glucose but may be unresponsive with an initial attempt (primary failures). Others, adequately controlled by oral hypoglycemic drugs for a time, become unresponsive to these agents (secondary failures). Insulin therapy may become essential in such cases. Other patients with type 2 disease develop grossly uncontrolled hyperglycemia during stress (trauma, infection, surgery). Whether or not ketosis ensues, the gross hyperglycemia may produce severe osmotic diuresis and its sequelae. Obviously, such patients require control of hyperglycemia with insulin therapy, which may be discontinued as soon as the situation warrants. Most young people of normal weight who develop diabetes require insulin, even though they are not especially prone to ketosis. Children or young adults formerly termed MODY (see above) are also candidates for insulin, although some may be treated with diet alone.

Occasional adults, usually thin and not necessarily exhibiting much glucosuria, may exhibit unexplained weight loss and lack of well-being. Such patients may show dramatic improvement with insulin.

Some patients receive insulin therapy needlessly. Typically these are obese, often elderly patients with type 2 diabetes who have already developed an array of medical problems, usually cardiovascular. The management of such patients is difficult and the goals of therapy are often uncertain. The blood sugar control, even with large amounts of insulin (e.g., 100 units a day), may be poor. Although aggressive use of insulin will certainly normalize blood glucose, hypoglycemia becomes a risk in such people. On the other hand, abrupt discontinuation of insulin often results in no worsening of control and reveals that no significant insulin effect was manifest at the prescribed dosage. Such patients may do better with combination therapy (sulfonylurea plus metformin; sulfonylurea plus insulin [65]).

Normoglycemia as a Goal of Therapy

The results of a National Institutes of Health (NIH)-sponsored multicenter study, the Diabetes Control and Complications Trial (DCCT), were released in 1993. The study's definitive results have profoundly altered the goals of clinical practice in patients with type 1 diabetes and have provoked new efforts to control blood glucose in type 2 diabetes

The DCCT enrolled only patients with minimal evidence of complications at entry, and the beneficial results were striking. The following is excerpted and minimally modified from the initial policy statement (24) of the American Diabetes Association on the implications of the DCCT results.

The DCCT was designed to test the proposition that the complications of diabetes mellitus are related to elevation of the plasma glucose concentration. Previous studies, for example, of patients who had received pancreas or islet cell transplants had suggested that the incidence of renal disease could be reduced in euglycemic patients (70). In this trial, 1441 patients with type 1 diabetes were studied; no patients with type 2 diabetes were included. Two groups of patients were followed long term: one treated conventionally (two injections of insulin daily, with a goal of clinical well-being; called standard treatment group) and another treated intensively (with a goal of normalization of blood glucose; called intensive treatment group). The intensive treatment group was clearly distinguished from the standard treatment group in terms of glycated hemoglobin levels and capillary blood glucose values throughout the study. Normalization of glucose values could not be achieved in every individual in the intensively treated group: Mean glucose values for the group were approximately 40% above normal limits. Nevertheless, over the study period, which averaged 7 years, there was approximately a 60% reduction between the intensive treatment group and the standard treatment group in the incidence of diabetic retinopathy, nephropathy, and neuropathy. Intensive therapy resulted in a delay in the onset and major slowing of the progression of these three complications. The benefits of intensive therapy were seen in all categories of subjects regardless of age, gender, or duration of diabetes, although all patients were under age 30.

A computer model that used the DCCT data projected considerable gains for patients with type 1 diabetes who maintain over their lifetimes a near-normal blood sugar: an extra 5 years of longevity, 8 years of sight, and 6 years' delay of renal failure, amputations, and neuropathy. The cost of the required intensive therapy is about $4500 per patient per year (versus $1700 for conventional therapy). The DCCT is the longest and largest prospective study showing that lowering blood glucose concentration slows or prevents the development of diabetic complications. As such, it has major therapeutic implications for health care providers and their patients. However, its results apply only to type 1 diabetes; relevance to type 2 diabetes is discussed below. Many questions remain unanswered, but the following conclusions appear warranted.

A primary treatment goal in type 1 diabetes should be blood glucose control at least equal to that achieved in the intensively treated cohort of the DCCT. This goal may not apply to all patients with type 1 disease and must be based on clinical judgment. Of importance, intensively treated patients had a threefold greater risk of hypoglycemia than did patients in the control group. Because serious hypoglycemia is dangerous and may not be avoidable, tight control goals may have to be abandoned for some patients.

There is no favored form of treatment to achieve tight control of blood glucose levels in type 1 diabetes. However, the goal is not achievable in most type 1 diabetic patients by use of single-dose or even two-dose insulin regimens. The decision to use multiple injections of insulin versus an insulin pump (see below) depends on patient preference and the ability of the health care team to provide the necessary resources and support, but even with these regimens normoglycemia can be achieved in only about half of the patients.

Young patients with type 1 diabetes in the early years of their disease stand to gain the most from normalization of blood sugar (tight control) because prevention of complications is the goal. Patients with type 1 disease who already have advanced complications of diabetes will not benefit at all because such complications are irreversible and probably cannot even be stabilized.

At what point in the course of type 1 diabetes should physicians consider initiation of intensive therapy? After an initial period of conventional therapy for several months (see below), the issue of tight control should be considered and discussed with patients who are suitable candidates. In those to whom tight control is suggested, the physician must explain the current view that maintained normoglycemia prevents the long-term complications of diabetes mellitus. The magnitude of the effort that is necessary to maintain normoglycemia must also be explained, including the need for self-monitoring of blood glucose. One of the frequent-dose, intensified conventional insulin therapy schemes or its alternative, infusion pump delivery of insulin, must also be presented (see below). If the patient understands and accepts the problems and effort required, the physician may consider a program of tight control. However, serious consideration should be given to referral of the patient to an endocrinologist familiar with such a program because the process is difficult, very demanding of the physician's time, and usually requires a team approach using a specially trained physician's assistant or nurse. The demands on the patient and the physician are greatest at onset of intensive therapy. The effort should be made only when the schedules of all parties permit the undertaking.

When is standard glycemic control rather than intensive therapy appropriate in type 1 diabetes? Often intensive therapy proves to be less than intensive, regardless of the initial intent. Standard therapy attempts to achieve near-normalization of *fasting* plasma glucose, as opposed to near-normalization of blood sugar throughout the day (see p. 1039). Even this degree of control is simply not possible using standard therapy. Many physicians, failing to realize the limitation of one- or two-dose schedules, nonetheless still go through an agonizing trial of standard therapy with such patients, only to have the effort end in failure and produce frustration for all involved. In such futile efforts, several types and mixtures of insulin are often tried along with both one- and two-dose schedules. At this point, the options include acceptance of a simplified treatment scheme that merely avoids excessive symptomatic glucosuria with resultant symptoms and prevents development of ketoacidosis (minimal therapy), or reconsideration of institution of intensive conventional therapy.

Implications of the DCCT for Type 2 Diabetes Mellitus

The results of the DCCT and its implications for type 1 diabetes (62) can be extrapolated to the treatment of type 2 diabetes only with serious reservations. The major conclusion that control of hyperglycemia in type 2 diabetic patients prevents *microvascular complications* is almost certainly correct, and is a worthwhile goal. Although at this time only a few small studies involving small numbers of patients bear on the issue of prevention of microvascular disease in type 2 disease, these studies show that control of blood sugar can indeed prevent microvascular complications (49).

Young or even middle-age patients with type 2 diabetes may stand to gain as much from tight control as do young patients with type 1 disease. On the other hand, in the elderly, whose life expectancy is limited by age, complications of diabetes, or concurrent disease, the problems associated with tight control should strongly influence the physician to avoid this approach because prevention of complications is not an issue and progression of complications cannot be prevented.

A major problem in type 2 diabetes is *macrovascular (atherosclerotic) disease.* Whereas hyperglycemia per se may directly contribute to the development of atherosclerosis, the evidence is weak and other factors are clearly operative. Although the DCCT trial produced a favorable trend for type 1 diabetes, the data

were not statistically significant in this regard. In fact, DCCT was so small and was conducted in such young patients (less than age 30) that it could not have been expected to yield useful information on slowing atherosclerotic disease involving the coronary arteries, cerebral vessels, and peripheral vasculature. Studies are currently under way to examine the best ways to treat patients with type 2 diabetes (e.g., the United Kingdom Prospective Diabetes Study, or UKPDS) and others are being planned. Unfortunately, the ongoing UKPDS was not designed to compare the effects of intensive insulin therapy of type 2 diabetes with standard therapy using insulin and therefore will not yield definitive data in this regard. The only information currently available is from a feasibility study of 153 patients over 27 months by a Department of Veterans Affairs (VA) group (17). Results were contrary to expectation. Among men without a previous cardiovascular event, 25% of patients given intensive therapy had a new cardiovascular event, compared to only 4% of those treated with standard therapy. The differences were not statistically significant, but the data, limited as they are, must deter or give physicians serious pause in their aggressive use of insulin for type 2 diabetes. Funding for a larger study of this type is still pending, and useful information on this issue is years away.

Insulin Therapy

Three major characteristics distinguish the various preparations of insulin: *(a)* onset and duration of action; *(b)* purity, important as it relates to cost and, rarely, to insulin allergy and resistance; and *(c)* species of origin, because this also affects cost. A significant recent realization is that some of the newer human (recombinant origin) insulin preparations have a shorter duration of action than that of animal insulins.

Most preparations now in use are suspensions of insulin that have been modified to prolong their action after subcutaneous injection. The characteristics of these insulins are summarized below.

Rapidly Acting Insulin

Regular Insulin (Crystalline Zinc Insulin). Regular insulin is the completely dissolved (clear) preparation that has long been used intravenously in hospitalized patients for acute therapy of ketoacidosis. In the treatment of ambulatory patients, regular insulin is used subcutaneously, often in mixtures with other insulins. The onset of action of subcutaneously injected regular insulin is 20 minutes; peak action is at 2 to 4 hours, and the duration of action is 4 to 6 hours. In occasional patients receiving one dose of intermediate-acting insulin daily, regular insulin may be given as the second dose. Regular insulin also is used for continuous subcutaneous injection with portable infusion pumps and is increasingly used in combination with Ultralente insulin in intensive control schemes; the long-acting preparation provides the equivalent of background activity provided by the basal infusion rate of a pump, whereas superimposed injections before meals are equivalent to the bolus injections of the pump (see below) (Fig. 72.1).

Insulin Lispro. Insulin lispro, an amino-acid-modified recombinant human insulin, was marketed recently. It has a slightly more rapid onset of action than ordinary regular insulin and a somewhat shorter duration of action. In theory, its faster onset permits injection, or administration in a bolus by a pump, closer to a meal, but that feature is of marginal usefulness at best (40).

Neutral Protamine Hagedorn Insulin

Neutral protamine Hagedorn (NPH) insulin is a standardized crystalline suspension prepared from regular insulin and protamine zinc insulin (PZI). NPH is the most commonly used intermediate-acting insulin in the United States. Although considered to be intermediate-acting, NPH in fact exhibits rather rapid onset of action and a duration of action that begins to wane after about 12 hours but may last up to 20 hours. Ideally, with a single injection of NPH, the short-acting component provides insulin effect during the day when meals are elevating the blood glucose, whereas the long-acting component of PZI provides insulin effect through the night. For most patients the achieved ratio of insulin effects is inadequate. Nonetheless, in the United States, many physicians continue to prescribe a single daily injection of NPH, a practice that has long been discontinued in Europe, where NPH is almost always given in two doses. Recently, NPH has been increasingly used in combination with sulfonylureas (see below). Mixtures of

NPH and regular insulin (70:30) are now marketed (see "Insulin Injection Technique," below) and are useful in some patients in controlling the postprandial increase in blood sugar.

The Lente Insulin Series

The Lente insulin series was devised to avoid the use of protamine. Controlled addition of zinc was used to prepare an amorphous, rapidly absorbed, and rapidly acting material (Semilente insulin) and another crystalline product with much slower absorption and longer action, Ultralente insulin. These insulins avoided the use of a foreign protein, protamine, and could be mixed in varying proportions. In some geographic areas, in both the United States and abroad, the Lente insulins are used almost exclusively.

Semilente insulin is similar to regular insulin in onset and duration of action, although its effects are somewhat slower in onset and more prolonged. Semilente is always given subcutaneously. The chief use of Semilente is in mixtures with Ultralente or as a supplementary dose in conventional therapy schemes. Semilente is little used in the United States.

Ultralente insulin has a duration of action exceeding 24 hours. It may occasionally be used alone. However, the main use of Ultralente is as the long-acting component in the mixture that is known as Lente insulin. Ultralente insulin has recently become the backbone of intensified conventional therapy. The prolonged effect of this preparation provides the background activity equivalent to the basal infusion rate of an insulin pump (see below).

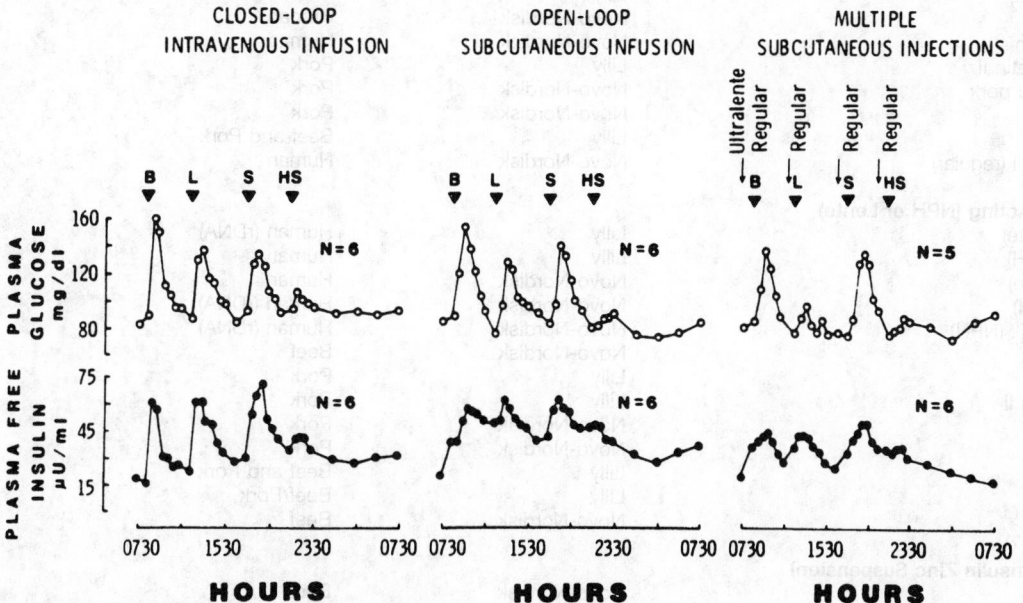

Figure 72.1. Plasma glucose and free insulin levels in patients with type 1 diabetes treated by three methods: closed-loop intravenous infusion (PG sensor-controlled apparatus), open-loop subcutaneous injections (insulin pump), and multiple subcutaneous injections (intensive conventional therapy). *B,* Breakfast; *L,* lunch; *S,* supper; *HS,* bedtime snacks. Note that the results are essentially the same with all methods used. (Modified from Rizza R,

Gerich JE, Haymond MD, et al. Control of blood sugar in insulin-dependent diabetes: comparison of an artificial endocrine pancreas, continuous subcutaneous insulin infusion, and intensified conventional insulin therapy. N Engl J Med 303:1313, 1980; Schade DS, Santiago JV, Skyler JS, Rizza RA. Intensive insulin therapy. Garden City, NY: Medica Examination Publishing, 1983;138.)

Lente insulin is an intermediate-acting preparation. It is a mixture of amorphous (Semilente) and crystalline (Ultralente) insulins. Although it is commonly thought to be equivalent to NPH, the duration of action of Lente insulin is significantly longer, usually exceeding 24 hours. If a single daily dose of insulin is the treatment goal, Lente is the insulin of choice.

Mixtures of Insulins

The usual goal of conventional insulin therapy is a single injection once daily. If this goal is to be reached, insulin effect must be prolonged sufficiently to produce normoglycemia in the morning and at the same time provide adequate daytime control of the increases of blood glucose that occur postprandially. However, the duration of action of NPH is usually too short for this goal and Lente, although a better choice, is often unsatisfactory as well. One of two scenarios is observed. In the first, the excessive daytime hyperglycemia and glucosuria dictate the need for additional rapidly acting insulin. Thus, regular insulin is added to NPH or Lente, or Semilente is added to Lente (see "Insulin Injection Technique," below). In the second, the single injection of NPH or Lente controls daytime hyperglycemia and glucosuria, but the total duration of action is inadequate, resulting in hyperglycemia at the beginning of the next day. Under these circumstances,

an additional long-acting component is needed. If Lente is used, Ultralente can be added, or a mixture of Semilente and Ultralente can be used with a ratio of 20:80 or 10:90. However, most diabetologists in the United States use NPH; their only option is to give an additional dose before dinner or at bedtime. This scheme has been called a split-dose program (see below). A bedtime dose of NPH can be added to a sulfonylurea regimen (see below).

Commercial Insulin Preparations

Nearly 40 commercial insulins are available; many of the various types, species of origin, and suppliers are listed in Table 72.6. Clearly, no physician needs to memorize this ever-changing list. However, even though most physicians write prescriptions for insulin without specifying the brand, it is important to be able to recognize the product that the pharmacist has dispensed. Not all preparations are available in a given region; pharmacies often supply the products of particular manufacturers according to local profit considerations.

At present, two companies market insulin in the United States: Lilly and Novo-Nordisk. Both produce reliable, clinically comparable products within a particular category. Although no uniform terminology is established, these insulins can be grouped into grades,

Table 72.6. Insulins Currently Sold as of June 1997 in the United States

Trade Name	Manufacturer	Form	Cost Index
Rapid-Acting (Regular)			
Humulin R	Lilly	Human (rDNA)	1.5
Humalog (Lispro)	Lilly	Human (rDNA; modified)	1.9
Novolin R	Novo-Nordisk	Human	1.5
Velosulin human	Novo-Nordisk	Human	1.5
Pork Regular Iletin II	Lilly	Pork	1.9, 1.0[a]
Regular Purified pork	Novo-Nordisk	Pork	1.7
Regular insulin	Novo-Nordisk	Pork	1.1
Regular Iletin I	Lilly	Beef and Pork	1.2
Novolin R Penfill (regular)	Novo-Nordisk	Human	3
Intermediate-Acting (NPH or Lente)			
Humulin L (Lente)	Lilly	Human (rDNA)	1.5
Humulin N (NPH)	Lilly	Human	1.5
Novolin L (Lente)	Novo-Nordisk	Human	1.5
Novolin N (NPH)	Novo-Nordisk	Human (rDNA)	1.5
Novolin N Penfill (NPH)	Novo-Nordisk	Human (rDNA)	3
Lente Insulin	Novo-Nordisk	Beef	1.1
Lente Iletin II	Lilly	Pork	1.9
Pork NPH Iletin II	Lilly	Pork	1.9
NPH-N	Novo-Nordisk	Pork	1.7
Lente	Novo-Nordisk	Pork	1.7
Lente Iletin I	Lilly	Beef and Pork	1.2
NPH Iletin I	Lilly	Beef/Pork	1.2
NPH Insulin	Novo-Nordisk	Beef	1.1
Long-Acting (Insulin Zinc Suspension)			
Ultralente U	Novo-Nordisk	Beef	1.1
Humulin U (Ultralente)	Lilly	Human	1.8
Mixtures (NPH/Regular)			
Novolin 70:30	Novo-Nordisk	Human	1.5
Novolin 70:30, Penfil	Novo-Nordisk	Human	3
Humulin 70:30	Lilly	Human (rDNA)	1.8
Humulin 50:50	Lilly	Human (rDNA)	NA

Modified from American Diabetes Association Physician's guide to insulin-dependent (type I) diabetes. Diagnosis and treatment. 2 ed. Alexandria, VA: ADA, 1988.
[a]All insulins are now marketed in a single strength (100 units per mL, U100) with the exception of this form, which can also be obtained as U500.

not to be confused with the various types of insulin already described (e.g., NPH, Lente). The principal determinant of which grade to prescribe is whether a clinical need exists for insulin more highly purified than standard-grade material. The other major considerations are cost, which varies considerably between grades, and use of animal-derived versus human insulin (obtained via recombinant technology or chemical modification of pork insulin).

Most of the problems caused by impurities in insulin in the past disappeared with the introduction of the more pure standard insulins two decades ago. Allergic reactions and lipoatrophy were the two most troublesome events; both appear to have been related to impurities and now are rarely seen.

Standard grades of insulin (Lilly, Novo Nordisk) are derived from the pancreases of pigs or beef cattle; Lilly's material (Iletin I) is a variable mixture of the two species, mostly beef, whereas Novo Nordisk insulin is solely of beef origin. These standard animal insulins are the least expensive preparations and are satisfactory for use in almost all patients.

Purified animal insulin of pig origin is about as expensive as human insulin and is of a comparable degree of purity. *Human insulins* are available in almost all types: regular, NPH, Lente, and Ultralente. Lilly's human insulin (Humulin) is actually of recombinant origin and is prepared from bacteria *(E. coli)* that have been modified to contain and express the human insulin gene. Bacterial protein contaminants are not present and have not been a clinical problem. Comparable *human semisynthetic insulins,* prepared by chemical modification of pork insulin, are available from Novo-Nordisk. The least expensive standard insulin costs approximately 50% as much as human or purified pork insulin; the most expensive preparations are those packaged for use with special injectors (about three times the cost of standard insulin).

Although some physicians are inclined to use the most highly purified animal insulins or human insulin, standard insulin is nearly always satisfactory and is much less costly. The rare patients who prove to be allergic to standard insulin (see below) should be switched to purified pork or human insulin. In the past, insulin resistance was often ascribed to antibody formation, but little evidence exists to document significant immunogenic differences or clinical improvement as the result of switching insulins. Human insulin is certainly immunogenic in humans, as is purified pork insulin. The various types of human insulin do differ from the products of animal origin by somewhat more rapid onset and peak of action and shorter duration of effect. Given the variability of onset and duration shown under clinical conditions (86), these differences may not be particularly important, especially in a multidose program. However, long-acting Ultralente human insulin has a maximal duration of action in many patients of less than 24 hours, making control impossible with a single dose. Attempts to produce a satisfactory fasting (overnight) blood sugar with a large single daily dose could lead to excessive daytime or evening effect and to hypoglycemia.

Trade Names, Unit Designations, and Syringes

All insulin (Table 72.6), regardless of type or source, is standardized at a specific concentration per milliliter. The symbol *U* refers to the insulin concentration in units per milliliter. All insulins are marketed at a concentration of 100 units/mL (U100) except pork regular Iletin II (500 units/mL). Although long-term storage is best done by refrigeration, insulin is stable for weeks at room temperature, and vials need not be refrigerated after opening. When insulin is used during travel, extremes of temperature should be avoided, as in a sun-exposed automobile or next to a stove or heating element.

Several sizes of syringes are available for use with U100. A 1-mL syringe can be used for all doses up to 100 units, but most accurate dispensing of less than 30 units is made when syringes of 0.5-mL (50 units) capacity are used. The bores of these syringes are smaller and the scales are consequently expanded. Some patients require more than 100 units for a single injection. For such use, 2-mL syringes (200-unit capacity) are manufactured, but these are in short supply and are difficult to obtain. No syringe is calibrated for use with U500.

The use of disposable plastic syringes with attached needles has greatly simplified use of insulin and is preferred by almost all patients. Many patients reuse disposable syringes without obvious harm, but the practice should be discouraged. Reusable glass syringes requiring detachable needles are also available. Special syringes are available for use by patients with severe impairment of vision that prevents them from accurately measuring a dose. However, a simple solution to this problem is often possible. Disposable syringes can be prefilled with ordinary sterile precautions by an able person (relative, friend) and safely stored in a refrigerator for at least a week.

Insulin Injection Technique

After initial instruction the patient should be observed during self-administration of insulin to be certain that the correct volume is being drawn into the syringe and that the proper injection technique is used. Sterilization of the skin with an alcohol wipe is not necessary, although the injection site should be clean. If the injection is made through skin that is wet with alcohol, unnecessary burning discomfort is produced. Injections with disposable needles are essentially painless. Repeated punctures of the rubber diaphragm of vials of insulin with the same needle dulls the point and leads to painful injections.

In ambulatory patients, insulin preparations should always be given subcutaneously. Most needles in present use are one-half inch in length. Unless the patient is very thin, the best technique involves insertion of the needle at 90° to the skin surface. If the patient is very thin, the needle is ⅝ inch in length, or the site is covered by thin skin, the needle may be inserted at approximately 45° to avoid intramuscular injection. After injection, the area should not be massaged because that may accelerate absorption.

The choice of injection region is important because

the rate of insulin absorption, and hence the duration and magnitude of insulin effect, varies considerably between anatomic locations (86). Absorption is slowest from the thigh, fastest from the anterior abdominal wall, and intermediate from the arm. In addition, absorption from an exercising extremity is accelerated (see above). The long-used technique of rotation of sites is unwise and may contribute to erratic control. On the other hand, the repeated use of precisely the same spot within a region should be avoided.

Regular and NPH insulins can be mixed in the same syringe in all proportions without affecting the onset and duration of action of the separate components, although the net effects overlap. In the United States, 70:30 and 50:50 mixtures of NPH and regular are now sold; in Europe a series of such mixtures (e.g., 90:10, 80:20) have long been available.

Regular and Lente insulins cannot be mixed and allowed to stand for more than a few minutes before injection; delay of injection results in blunting of the action of the rapidly acting regular insulin.

Insulin Injection Devices

A variety of devices are of variable utility in facilitating injections of insulin. Buttonlike injection ports are devices that can be left in place, usually over the abdomen, all day and decrease the number of skin punctures when multiple injections are being given. Needleless injectors that use a high-pressure jet are used by some patients, but they are not always painless, and absorption may be more rapid than with ordinary injections. Fountain pen–shaped injectors use a cartridge containing insulin; the needle need not be changed for several days. Delivery is with a push button or a preset dial. These devices are especially useful for diabetic patients taking more than one injection daily, who are eating meals in a restaurant or are traveling. The cost of the insulin in the cartridges used with these devices is high.

Initiation of Insulin Therapy: Setting the Goal

At the time of initiation of therapy with insulin (or other agents), the physician should establish a clear goal for the degree of control of glycemia. The blood glucose ranges that can be considered are the following: (a) hyperglycemia that is sufficient to avoid gross symptoms (minimal therapy), (b) approximation of a normal fasting plasma glucose with the expectation that postprandial blood sugar will be elevated (standard therapy), and (c) near-normalization of glucose over the entire day (intensive therapy). Obviously, many intermediate gradations of blood glucose may be achieved, but the goals are important for avoiding many management difficulties. Methods of monitoring are described below.

Minimal Therapy. In this approach the goals are (a) avoidance of the extremes of symptomatic hyperglycemia and hypoglycemia; (b) use of the least amount of insulin that is effective, usually in a single AM or PM dose; (c) minimal testing of blood or urine, usually urine, with the first morning urine specimen negative

to two plus, and a blood hemoglobin A_{1c} (HbA_{1c}) that corresponds to an average blood sugar of 230 to 310 mg/dL, or 9.5 to 12% (nondiabetic mean, 5%; range, 3.8 to 6.3%). Diet is prudent (less than 30% as calories from fat, less than 10% from saturated fat, less than 300 mg of cholesterol). Exercise is according to patient preference.

Standard Therapy. An attempt is made to approach a nearly normal fasting (prebreakfast) blood sugar, using one or two doses of insulin, usually mixed with added regular insulin. The prebreakfast blood sugar should range from 70 to 140 mg/100 mL and the mean glucose 160 to 230 mg/100 mL, corresponding to an $HgbA_{1c}$ of 7.5 to 9.5%. Self-monitoring of blood glucose is necessary, usually daily but sometimes up to three times a day.

Institution of insulin therapy coincides with or follows the establishment of a diet (see above). As pointed out earlier, relative constancy of food intake is essential. If such modest dietary compliance cannot be ensured, the goals of insulin therapy should be minimal (i.e., the avoidance of symptomatic hyperglycemia and ketoacidosis). Attempts to manipulate insulin dosage while diet is varying widely will unquestionably result in hypoglycemic episodes. In any case, insulin therapy cannot possibly achieve normoglycemia when diet is varying greatly.

First attempts at blood sugar control in almost all ambulatory patients treated by the conventional approach should be done with an intermediate-acting insulin (NPH or Lente). However, use of NPH usually requires two doses. Although initial dosages are often calculated as units per kilogram, the range of requirements is so large that one might just as well begin with the following dosages, ignoring the weight: a safe initial dosage for a diabetic who has not received previous insulin therapy is 15 units for a nonobese patient and 25 units for an obese patient. Many experts recommend addition of 5 to 10 units of regular insulin to the NPH or Lente to help normalize the postbreakfast blood sugar during the morning. Because of this common practice, several manufacturers market mixtures of insulin (ratio of NPH to regular, 70:30).

Previously treated patients often require higher initial dosages. Insulin-dependent patients ordinarily have been started on insulin therapy while in the hospital, but the scheme below can be used for further dosage adjustment for both types of patient.

Continuing to Adjust Insulin Dosage. The patient can be instructed to increase the initial dosage of insulin (see above) by 5 units every 3 days until satisfactory control is approached. Usually, such a program brings the patient under control within a few weeks. Increments of 10 units every 3 days are also safe as long as the patient is not markedly symptomatic or if no effect is apparent within a week. During this time the patient should at least monitor urine glucose, although blood glucose monitoring is preferred (see "Monitoring Insulin Therapy," below). A telephone call to the physician, nurse, or physician's assistant can be made every week or more, but at least when a single-dose program is being established, the patient should be encouraged to proceed with the dosage adjustments as planned and should not require or expect a physician's instructions at every dosage increment. Unnecessary dependence is thus discouraged, and the patient's involvement in management is enhanced.

When glucosuria begins to subside, or when aglucosuria begins to be seen in the first morning specimen, the dosage of insulin should be held constant until FPG can be obtained. Sometimes glucosuria first subsides during the day rather than in the morning. If this pattern develops, the dosage of insulin should be held constant until both FPG and the PG at the aglucosuric time are measured. When the PG is measured, a double-voided urine sample should be obtained and glucosuria should be measured simultaneously. A few such determinations allow an estimate of the patient's renal threshold; thereafter, the physician can approximate elevations of the PG for that particular patient from the glucosuria. Progressing from the point of development of aglucosuria during some portion of the day to the eventual targeted level of control requires continued adjustment of insulin dosage, almost always upward, and adjustment of the patient to the diet and the routine of monitoring. During this time the patient should be reassured that the period of close dependency on the physician will soon come to an end. Every effort must also be made to avoid rigidly scheduled visits to the physician's office or the clinical laboratory that interfere with the patient's livelihood or important personal affairs. Such intrusions only discourage the patient and promote future noncompliance. On the other hand, achievement of the targeted level of control should not be prolonged and should be possible within a few weeks. If months pass and the patient's control remains irregular, seems to follow no pattern, or is marked by many hypoglycemic episodes, the problem is either noncompliance (see Chapter 4), usually dietary, or improper prescription or administration of insulin. Noncompliance in the use of insulin can sometimes be ascertained by the equivalent of a pill count, by comparison of the volume of insulin used with the predicted volume of insulin use. For example, a 10-mL vial of U100 insulin contains 1000 units; if the patient was supposed to receive 50 units daily, a vial should last 20 days (1000/50).

Evolution to a Two-Dose Program. Many patients cannot be controlled with a single dose of intermediate-acting insulin (NPH or Lente; see "Types of Insulin," above). In these patients, a single dose will improve hyperglycemia and glucosuria; the late morning or afternoon glucose measurements are the first to show a tendency to normalize. However, the long-acting component of the insulin preparation is insufficient to ensure normoglycemia in the fasting state (i.e., in the early morning). Two maneuvers can be tried. Usually, a predinner or bedtime dose of the same intermediate-acting insulin can be added, sometimes requiring a concomitant reduction of the morning dose. For example, if such a patient is receiving 60 units daily, up to 15 units may be given in the

evening—usually before dinner—and the morning dose can be reduced to 50 units. Additional increments of 5 units may then be made to either dose, depending on whether the fasting or postprandial glucose is too high. Patients using such a split-dose schedule often receive 40 units or more daily, with 50 to 70% of total daily dose in the morning and the remainder in the evening. A two-thirds morning, one-third evening split is common.

To avoid a two-dose schedule, the alternative approach of increasing the long-acting component can be instituted. In this case, the Lente insulins are preferred (see "Types of Insulin," above). If the patient is already receiving NPH, a switch to the same dosage of Lente is made. Ultralente insulin may then be mixed with Lente in increments of 5 to 10 units. Because Lente insulin is already a mixture of Semilente and Ultralente in a proportion of 30:70, addition of Ultralente merely alters this ratio in favor of the longer-acting component, thus providing a greater likelihood that early morning PG will be controlled without producing midday hypoglycemia. To some extent, addition of a more long-acting component effects a lowering of glucose even during the day and may prompt a decrease of the morning dosage. In any case, some patients can be controlled on a single injection of mixed insulins in this way. For the patient who does not want a second daily injection, this approach is worthwhile.

Much effort can be expended in attempts at fine tuning. Once the FPG is normalized (see above), efforts to attain normalization during the day with these approaches are rarely successful and usually end in unacceptable hypoglycemic episodes. Because normalization of blood sugar is usually impossible by the schemes described, one should avoid machinations of this type. Normalization of blood daytime sugar or tight control is simply unachievable in most diabetic patients treated with conventional therapy using one or two daily doses of insulin.

Evening Insulin Therapy for Type 2 Diabetes, Alone or in Combination with Sulfonylurea. A number of investigators report improved control of hyperglycemia using intermediate, active insulin (NPH) given in the evening (before dinner or at bedtime) rather than as conventionally used, in the morning. The insulin can be given alone or added to a sulfonylurea (65) if insulin alone is inadequate (36,84). Part of the rationale includes a need for increased insulin action during the night to suppress the normal tendency for hepatic glucose output to increase during the early morning. Even patients with severe obesity are candidates for this type of therapy. Improved metabolic control has been claimed for this approach (36), but advantages of this kind of combined therapy are not widely accepted (66).

Intensive Therapy. This approach is an attempt to normalize not only FPG but also preprandial levels (39). It requires a maximal effort by the patient, the physician, and a team of support personnel (trained nurse or practitioner or dietitian). An insulin pump or three or four daily doses of insulin are used. In the multiple-dose regimen, a long-acting form of insulin is required (Ultralente, possibly of animal origin because of its longer duration of action compared with human insulin) to provide background insulin activity; boluses of regular or Lispro insulin are given before meals to anticipate postmeal rises. The diet should contain as close to a constant total of calories from carbohydrate at each meal as possible.

The goal for preprandial sugars should be 70 to 120 mg/dL. Occasional postprandial blood sugars are measured and should not exceed 180 mg. Weekly 3 AM levels should be determined to detect nocturnal hypoglycemia. Diet must be optimized and home blood glucose monitoring practiced before any program of intensive therapy with insulin is initiated.

On such a program one can expect a mean glucose of 155 mg/dL and a HbA_{1c} of 7.2% (24,28). These values compare to a normal mean blood glucose of 110 mg/dL and HbA_{1c} of less than 5.0%. Thus, even with the best possible motivation and supervision, the mean blood glucose will still be on average 40% greater than normal, yet severe hypoglycemic attacks can be expected to occur some three times more often than during conventional therapy.

It must be stressed that these are mean (average) glucose values for the treatment groups of the DCCT. Some patients fare better in terms of the degree of control, and others do not do as well; the same is true of the frequency of hypoglycemia. For patients who can achieve the mean or lower values for control, the benefits in terms of prevention of complications are obvious. However, these patients must decide whether the effort is personally worthwhile; the treating physician's role can only be that of a supportive advisor. A significant number of patients who try intensive therapy are not able to achieve a satisfactory degree of control because of lack of motivation or skill, but for others, despite maximal cooperation the goal is not attainable, presumably because of their particular metabolic makeup. For such patients, continuing intensive therapy is to no advantage and may be harmful.

Continuous subcutaneous insulin infusion using a pump was first reported in 1978. In the past few years, many efforts attest to the efficacy and advantages of this approach and have defined the complications and risks of this method of therapy. Not as generally appreciated is the demonstration that identical success at normalization can be achieved by multiple-dose programs that do not use a pump but do use a similar principle: delivery of insulin continuously from a subcutaneous depot site with additional doses of short-acting insulin given in bolus form (see above) (Table 72.7 and Fig. 72.1). Approximately 50 to 60% of the total daily dosage of insulin is given as the long-acting depot injection in the morning or before bed; the remainder is divided and given before meals as bolus injections of regular insulin. Regular insulin can be mixed with the long-acting form before breakfast, but two or three later injections of short-acting insulin are necessary (69).

If a physician decides to institute therapy with a

Table 72.7. Algorithm for Multidose Intensive Insulin Therapy

Target: Blood glucose 70–125 mg/dL AM fasting, before meals, at bedtime, and not below 50 mg/dL at 3 AM.

Insulin Regimen

Insulin	Before		
	B	L	D
Regular	10	6	8
Ultralente	10	0	10

Algorithm

Blood Glucose Before Meals (mg/dL)	Inject Regular Insulin as Below
60 mg/dL or less	2 units less
70–140 mg/dL	Usual dosage
141–200 mg/dL	2 units extra
201–250 mg/dL	4 units extra
251–300 mg/dL	6 units extra
Over 300 mg/dL	8 units extra

All dosages are illustrative and must be adjusted as appropriate for each patient. *B*, Breakfast; *L*, lunch; *D*, dinner.

pump, referral to a specialist familiar with one of these devices is usually necessary. Selection of a suitable current model of pump (cost of $1500 to $3000) and initiation of therapy are best made by a team active in this specialized field, although if necessary the continuation of therapy can be supervised by the general physician.

Current pumps have fail-safe devices and alarms to guard against runaway pump action, power (battery) failure, empty insulin reservoir, and inadvertent turnoff. The insulin is administered through a 25-gauge scalp-vein needle attached to the pump via a piece of plastic tubing and inserted into the subcutaneous tissue of the abdomen. The needle is replaced every day or two. Insulin reservoirs vary greatly in size and can accommodate one to several days' supply. Pumps must be worn almost continuously, being removed for only short periods (15 to 30 minutes) to allow showering, bathing, or swimming. Some patients need a respite from the pump (e.g., in anticipation of sexual activity); in that case a dose of intermediate-acting insulin can be used at bedtime and the pump used during the day. Other physical activities, including sports, are performed with the pump in operation.

Initiation of therapy can be expected to take about 2 weeks, generally during at least a brief hospitalization in which the patient becomes familiar with pump operation as the dosage schedule is adjusted. Despite the apparent inconvenience of wearing the device, acceptance of the pump is remarkable. Many patients have continued pump therapy for 5 years or more. Patients, observing the improved blood glucose levels, are gratified by a sense of control of their destinies. In addition, they experience a normalization of activities by being freed from the tyranny of a clock-oriented existence because meals no longer need be taken at fixed times but can be taken at will without great concern over the possible development of hypoglycemia. However, hypoglycemia does occur even in the best-managed cases. The concentrations of lipids and lipoproteins, often abnormal in diabetic patients with even modest elevations of blood sugar, may fall, in theory decreasing the increased risk of atherosclerosis of conventionally treated patients.

A number of problems with pump therapy have become obvious. Pump failure, caused by failure of the pump itself or clogging of its infusion line, sometimes occurs. Diabetic ketoacidosis (DKA) rapidly ensues, often overnight, when the insulin infusion is interrupted. Local infection at the needle site also predisposes to ketoacidosis caused by poor absorption of insulin, and it may be severe enough to require antibiotic therapy and hospitalization. The approximate frequency of DKA has been estimated at one episode per 100 patient months; infection at one per 40 patient months; and severe hypoglycemia at one per 30 patient months.

Multidose intensive conventional insulin therapy has the advantage over the pump approach of lower initial cost and freedom from the hazards of DKA and local infection, but the disadvantage of multiple injections. In crossover studies, an equal number of patients prefer one or the other form of therapy. Both forms of intensive therapy require extraordinary commitment by the patient, the family, and the physician's team.

Hypoglycemia During Intensive Therapy. Intensively treated patients lose their early-warning system of adrenergic symptoms of hypoglycemia and develop neuroglycopenic symptoms instead, and at a lower level of blood sugar (1,2,6,20–22). Indeed, the 1980s saw an epidemic of frequent and severe hypoglycemia, a byproduct of the then-new popularity of intensive therapy. So far, intensively treated adults subject to hypoglycemia have not shown decreased psychomotor function, although this was a problem in children and in young adults in earlier studies of frequent, severe hypoglycemic episodes.

Obstacles to Successful Intensive Therapy. Even with renewed efforts at tight control triggered by the DCCT, one must recall that considerable experience with intensive therapy programs has been available for some time. Initial enthusiasm that diabetic complications could be prevented or stabilized has often given way to discouragement as patients and families realize the intense demands of such therapy. The logistics and mechanics of multiple blood sampling, wearing a pump, cost, and the constant reminder of the presence of chronic illness all cause many patients eventually to abandon pump therapy. Moreover, in some patients blood sugars vary widely despite meticulous adherence to the rules of the intensive therapy program. Sometimes patients assume that they are at fault and stop reporting the truth about their glycemic control. Periodic monitoring with HgbA$_{1c}$ measurement is useful in defining the true state of control (see below and Fig. 72.2).

Monitoring Insulin Therapy

The rational approach to day-to-day monitoring depends on whether the treated patient has type 1 or type 2 diabetes, and whether conventional or intensive therapy is being used. Frequent determinations of PG are not essential—or even desirable—in type 2 patients receiving conventional therapy. The simplest approach is to use urine glucose monitoring supplemented by self-monitoring of blood glucose (SMBG). Patients with type 1 diabetes receiving conventional therapy should be monitored by frequent SMBG, but unless insulin dosage is being adjusted as a function of the results of SMBG, multiple daily measurements are unnecessary.

Efficacy of treatment in the conventionally treated ambulatory patient should be monitored, if possible, by measuring FPG. Normalization of FPG represents the basic or coarse adjustment of insulin dosage. Preprandial and postprandial normalization can be viewed as fine adjustments, both of which are difficult to attain. No useful purpose is served by attempts to adjust preprandial PG before normalization of the FPG is achieved; only thereafter should PG be monitored at mid-afternoon or before the evening meal. The availability of techniques for self-monitoring of blood glucose (SMBG; see below) have made blood glucose much easier to track.

Urine glucose monitoring is no longer advocated by most diabetologists. Yet urine glucose monitoring remains simple and inexpensive and provides considerable information. As a sole technique for monitoring it is inadequate but clearly preferable to no monitoring at all, or to inaccurately performed blood monitoring.

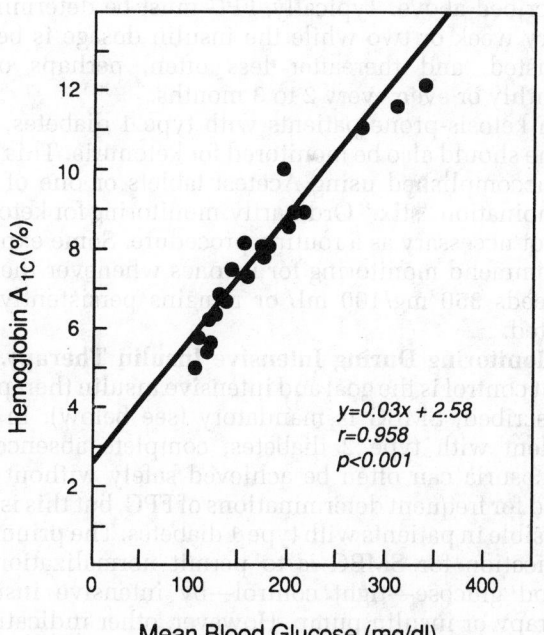

Figure 72.2. Relationship between HbA$_{1c}$ and mean blood glucose. Twenty-one subjects performed SMBG four to six times per day for 8 weeks. The arithmetic mean of those values as compared to the HbA$_{1c}$ value determined at the end of the 8-week period. (From Nathan DM, Singer DE, Hurxthal K, et al. The clinical information value of the glycosylated hemoglobin assay. N Engl J Med 310:341, 1984.)

Two drawbacks are the variability among patients of the renal threshold (normal range, 160 to 250 mg/dL) and the inability to detect hypoglycemia. Nevertheless, even two daily determinations of urine glucose can be a useful guide and may be complementary to blood monitoring.

Double-voiding technique should be used when possible, especially for the first morning specimen, if the patient has not voided during the night. When heavy daytime glucosuria is still present, no useful purpose is served by additional frequent monitoring of PG. On the other hand, when afternoon (before dinner) glucosuria has cleared, PG determination—like that of FPG—becomes essential to determine whether the PG has reached or is approaching hypoglycemic levels. Of course, the development of such episodes indicates the need for adjustment of the treatment program.

Upward titration of insulin to the point of abolishing morning glucosuria can be accomplished without risk of hypoglycemia if the dosage escalation is stopped when glucosuria first disappears. The patient almost always is still hyperglycemic at this point. Further reductions of glycemia require blood glucose determinations. Monitoring blood sugar in the poor or homeless diabetic patient is often impossible, but urinary glucose measurement may still be practical and helpful.

The optimal frequency of monitoring of FPG or urinary glucose must be determined for each patient. During initiation of therapy, determination of the degree of glucosuria four times daily (first voided morning specimen, prelunch, predinner, and at bedtime) is essential if insulin is to be varied (increased) as described above. Typically, FPG must be determined every week or two while the insulin dosage is being adjusted, and thereafter less often, perhaps only monthly or even every 2 to 3 months.

In ketosis-prone patients with type 1 diabetes, the urine should also be monitored for ketonuria. This can be accomplished using Acetest tablets or one of the combination "stix." Ordinarily, monitoring for ketones is not necessary as a routine procedure. Some experts recommend monitoring for ketones whenever the PG exceeds 350 mg/100 mL or remains persistently elevated.

Monitoring During Intensive Insulin Therapy.   If tight control is the goal and intensive insulin therapy is prescribed, SMBG is mandatory (see below). In the patient with type 2 diabetes, complete absence of glucosuria can often be achieved safely without the need for frequent determinations of FPG, but this is not possible in patients with type 1 diabetes. The principal indication for SMBG is to permit normalization of blood glucose—tight control—by intensive insulin therapy or insulin pump. However, other indications include patients with unusually low or high renal threshold for glucose, many patients with type 1 diabetes treated conventionally, all patients prone to hypoglycemic episodes, pregnant patients, and some patients with type 1 diabetes who, despite an inability to master effective therapy, seem to find SMBG more satisfying than the simpler and less expensive procedures of testing urine.

The process of SMBG should be initiated as a prelude to tight control because, unless the patient is able to master the technique and accept it as an ongoing necessity, the effort at tight control will fail. SMBG does not eliminate the need for dietary compliance. Recent studies indicate that within the wide range of what is grossly considered normal, neither intelligence, socioeconomic status, nor personality type has any predictive value for success with SMBG. Patients of limited financial means may drop out of such a program because of its high cost (approximately $100 per month; see below).

With programs of intensive therapy blood glucose may need to be monitored up to seven times daily: 1 hour before and after breakfast, lunch, and dinner, and before bedtime. Testing may be reduced to two to four times daily once a pattern of normalization is achieved. Patients who monitor less than four times daily are unlikely to maintain near-normalization of blood glucose.

The basis for all SMBG methods is a paper strip impregnated with an enzyme reagent (glucose oxidase) and suitable dyes. When placed in contact with a drop of capillary blood, the change of color intensity indicates the glucose concentration. Some strips are read only visually (without a reflectance meter) (e.g., Chemstrip bG), others either visually or with a reflectance photometer (e.g., Glucostix), still others only with a photometer (e.g., Glucofilm). Accuracy of strips properly examined visually is adequate for monitoring control, except when the goal is intensive therapy with normalization of the blood sugar. For many patients a meter is not necessary, but most feel more secure with machine readings.

In the United States several meters are in widest use. Accu-Check, which uses Chemstrips bG, and Lifescan are particularly popular. All machines are reliable, portable, battery operated, and cost between $10 and $50 with rebates (3), depending on whether they have memory for previous determinations. The manufacturers have reduced the prices to promote sale of the matching strips, the retail cost of which is approximately $0.70 each. If four are used daily, the monthly cost is more than $80.

Capillary blood is most commonly obtained from the tip of the finger, although some patients prefer the earlobe. The required drop of blood is obtained almost painlessly using a spring-triggered device such as the Autolet (about $30). Disposable Monolet lances are used to produce the puncture. At a current cost of $0.10 per Monolet, the monthly cost is approximately $12.

Blood flow from the finger can be enhanced before puncture by holding the hand in warm (not hot) water for 30 seconds. The skin should be quickly dried. Puncturing the thumb is least painful, but the ring finger has the best blood supply. Puncturing the lateral aspect of the fingertip (distal phalanx) is less painful than puncturing the ball. Pain is also less when sufficient pressure to produce erythema is applied to the palmar surface (ball) of the distal phalanx; an opposing digit of the same hand is used to apply the pressure. The first drop of blood produced suffices; the presence of extravascular fluid does not affect the result. An ideal puncture produces a 5-mm drop. The finger is inverted and the drop is allowed to fall to the strip; timing is begun. The strip usually is blotted or wiped, following directions of the supplier, and the glucose level is read. If the earlobe is used, a second or third sample can subsequently be obtained on the same day without repuncture if the site is rubbed with an alcohol wipe and allowed to dry, and the earlobe is flipped with the finger. This procedure is preferred by some patients.

Glycosylated Hemoglobins. Chronic elevation of blood glucose results in an increase in the concentration of glycosylated hemoglobins, a major component of which is $HgbA_{1c}$ (13). Determination of the level of either the total glycosylated $HgbA_1$ or $HgbA_{1c}$ gives essentially the same information, an integrated estimate of the degree of hyperglycemia over 5 weeks to 2 months (Fig. 72.2). The normal range of $HgbA_{1c}$ is 3.8 to 6.3% of total hemoglobin (normal range of total glycosylated hemoglobin is slightly higher, e.g., 5.3 to 7.9%) and may rise to 15% with chronic hyperglycemia postprandially. Values of less than 7.5% suggest excellent control with fasting and 1-hour postprandial sugars in the range of 70 to 120 and 100 to 140 mg/100 mL, respectively. With 120 to 140 mg/100 mL fasting and 141 to 160 mg/100 mL postprandial, one might see HbA_{1c} at 7.5 to 9%. At 140 to 160 mg/100 mL fasting and 160 to 200 mg/100 mL postprandially, values of 9.1 to 11% are common, whereas minimal control gives values of greater than 11%. Glycosylated hemoglobin levels fall slowly with reduction of mean glucose because circulating red blood cells containing high levels of glycosylated hemoglobin disappear normally in approximately 120 days. If euglycemia is established, glycosylated hemoglobins subsequently normalize in 4 to 6 weeks. Conversely, persistent hyperglycemia must be present for 1 to 4 weeks before elevated levels of glycosylated hemoglobins are seen. Short periods of hyperglycemia (6 to 24 hours' duration) may result in disproportionate elevations because some methods include measurement of unstable glycosylated derivatives. Other conditions render interpretations of glycosylated hemoglobin values uncertain, including any in which red cell life span is low (bleeding; hemolysis) or in which hemoglobin F is increased (some hemoglobinopathies).

The measurement of glycosylated hemoglobins is a useful clinical adjunct in the assessment of the efficacy of control of hyperglycemia. However, proteins other than hemoglobin that also undergo glycosylation exist in nerve, retina, ocular lens, kidney, and cell membranes. Of great importance is the realization that glucose is not an inert substance but one that can produce postsynthetic modification of many proteins. Some of these alterations may be harmful and provide a possible biochemical mechanism by which hyperglycemia per se may result in deleterious alterations of tissue structure and function and produce long-term complications of the diabetic state (13).

Factors Affecting Insulin Requirement

Mechanisms of Insulin Resistance in Type 2 Diabetes Mellitus. Insulin resistance is a hallmark of type 2 diabetes, but the mechanisms are still being elucidated (8). Free fatty acids (FFA) have long been shown to interfere with glucose utilization. Because obesity and diabetes are often associated with elevations of plasma FFA, a major role in insulin resistance for FFA was postulated. Indeed, a specific role for increased FFA flux from the central body (intra-abdominal) fat depots has been postulated to result in increased hepatic glucose output and elevation of blood sugar (7).

In addition to the FFA hypothesis, recent work linking obesity and insulin resistance has focused on the secretion by adipose tissue of the cytokine tumor necrosis factor-α (TNF-α) as a metabolic messenger that induces insulin resistance. The inhibitory effects of TNF-α on insulin action and experiments in animals support this concept, but very recently when obese diabetic patients were given antibodies to TNF-α for a month, no effect was seen. Nonetheless, this is an active area of research (8).

Classically, the term *insulin resistance* refers to a state in which the requirement for insulin exceeds 200 units daily. This extreme type of insulin resistance is only occasionally caused by the development of antibodies to insulin (see below). Ordinarily, resistance to insulin occurs independently of antibodies to insulin. This resistance—or decreased sensitivity to insulin—is most apparent in type 2 diabetes that is associated with obesity. Even nondiabetic obese patients who maintain normal levels of blood sugar do so by secreting supranormal amounts of insulin (i.e., they are in a state of compensated insulin resistance).

Although obese diabetic patients are insulin resistant in terms of their glucose homeostasis and certain aspects of lipoprotein metabolism, their metabolic state is not so deranged that it allows ketoacidosis to develop. In most insulin-resistant diabetic patients, weight reduction at least partially reverses the insulin resistance. Glucose tolerance often improves to (or toward) normal, and the need for insulin to control hyperglycemia may decrease or disappear. In contrast, some nonobese patients with type 2 diabetes have lower than normal levels of plasma insulin. Such patients comprise a spectrum of combinations of insulin resistance and insulin deficiency.

Current evidence suggests that sulfonylurea compounds, in addition to their action in facilitating insulin release, may act by returning insulin sensitivity toward normal, perhaps by increasing insulin receptors. However, the use of these drugs is dictated by other considerations (see below).

Insulin Requirement Increases Caused by Stress. The stress of infection or trauma may increase insulin requirements quickly. Usually the site of any infection that is severe enough to produce this effect is obvious, or at least there is good evidence of an infectious process (fever, leukocytosis). The mechanisms by which infections increase insulin requirement are not understood completely but appear to relate to the interference of insulin action by cytokines (e.g., TNF-α) produced in excess during the infection. In addition, stress hormones such as cortisol may also increase insulin requirement by increasing insulin resistance.

Only rarely does a search for a hidden focus of infection provide an explanation for changing insulin requirements or even for the development of ketoacidosis. Although most type 2 diabetic patients are not prone to the development of overt ketoacidosis during metabolic stress, occasional patients are. African-American type 2 diabetic patients seem especially prone to this type of response. After the acute episode is over, they may return to their baseline state. These patients may have been controlled by diet, oral agents, or insulin. Most episodes of ketoacidosis that are not related to stress are not caused by an increased insulin requirement. Rather, such episodes are usually related to noncompliance in type 1 diabetic patients, although this may be unintentional, as when the patient mistakenly omits insulin. Illness that produces anorexia leads the patient to fear hypoglycemia if insulin use is continued when food intake has been decreased. Rather than omitting insulin completely, patients need to reduce their dosage, perhaps by one-third, but only as appropriate and as guided by SMBG. Insulin requirement tends to increase after the end of the first trimester of pregnancy (see below).

Insulin Resistance Caused by Insulin Antibodies. A slow increase of insulin requirement (for the commonly used insulin of beef–pork origin) occurring over months may be related to development of insulin antibodies of the immunoglobulin G (IgG) type. Usually the patient may be stabilized at a new, higher dosage. Under these circumstances, the duration of action of short-acting insulin is often prolonged, whereas that of intermediate- or long-acting insulins may be shortened. Insulin requirement may exceed 200 units/day and administration may become a problem. In patients who develop resistance while taking beef or beef–pork insulin, a switch to purified pork or human insulin may result in up to a 30% decrease in requirement. Occasionally, a short course of glucocorticoid therapy is necessary to effect reduction in insulin dosage. Prednisone (40 to 60 mg/day), rather than producing an increase in insulin requirement, usually produces a dramatic fall in insulin requirement after 7 to 10 days, although the response may occur after only a few days. Hospitalization should be considered after several days of such therapy in anticipation of development of hypoglycemia and rapid decrease of insulin dosage. When the decrease occurs, glucocorticoid therapy can be abruptly discontinued. Recurrence of the resistant state is infrequent but may occur after months or years.

Decreases of Insulin Requirement. Vigorous exercise reduces blood glucose and, in anticipation of such activity, the dosage of insulin may need to be reduced (see above). During *pregnancy,* insulin requirement drops during the first trimester, rises and may double during the second and third trimesters, and falls suddenly at delivery (see below). Diabetic patients who develop *nephropathy* often show a decreased insulin

requirement. (Patients receiving long-term dialysis may develop severe hypoglycemia, even after insulin is discontinued, an ominous prognostic sign, presumably caused by failure of gluconeogenesis.) A tendency to normoglycemia or even hypoglycemia develops occasionally in patients previously requiring insulin who develop *chronic congestive heart failure.* Development of *adrenal* or *pituitary insufficiency* in a diabetic patient results in a decreased insulin requirement, but such cases are rare.

Effect of Anorexia

When a patient with type 1 diabetes develops anorexia because of mild short-term illness (cold, flu, gastroenteritis), insulin should not be discontinued, but a reduction of the normal dosage by one-third to one-half may be needed. More severe illness (e.g., a marked febrile state) may require continuation of the usual dosage or even an increase in the dosage. Every effort should be made to ensure intake of 50 g of carbohydrate in every 8-hour period to prevent starvation ketosis and hypoglycemia. Careful monitoring of urine ketones (and blood glucose) during such periods with prompt adjustment of insulin dosage may prevent a hospitalization for ketoacidosis.

Hypoglycemia During Insulin Therapy: Recognition, Prevention, and Treatment

Hypoglycemia is an inevitable effect of an excessive insulin dosage. Especially when severe, hypoglycemia causes central nervous system symptoms ranging from headache, subtle disturbances of mental function, confusion, and visual disturbances to personality change, seizures, unconsciousness, and transient hemiparesis. When hypoglycemia occurs during waking hours and is accompanied by the usual symptoms of epinephrine release (tremor, sweating, tachycardia, and palpitations), there is no problem in recognizing the condition. However, in some poorly controlled diabetics, as in some normal people, even mild reductions of blood glucose to levels (50 to 70 mg/100 mL) not clearly identifiable as hypoglycemia can sometimes produce epinephrine release with its resulting symptoms (see Chapter 74). Under these circumstances, documentable hypoglycemia is not present and the clinical situation may be confusing.

Perhaps the most common cause of hypoglycemia in the diabetic patient receiving insulin therapy is failure of the patient to eat at normal times. Despite repeated warnings many patients not only miss meals, but obfuscate the treatment program further by denying that they have done so. The physician must be ever on guard but tactful in considering this possibility.

Diabetic patients may develop defects in mechanisms that normally counterregulate hypoglycemia (1,2,20–22). This pathophysiologic state may occur within a few years of onset of the disease. Absolute deficiency of glucagon secretion is common in type 1 diabetes and sometimes occurs in type 2 diabetes. Defective counter-regulation caused by impaired secretion of epinephrine is also common early in type 1 disease and may become marked in patients with autonomic (adrenergic) neuropathy late in the course of the illness. Other patients may have defective counter-regulation caused by impairment of epinephrine action as a result of treatment with β-adrenergic–blocking drugs. In addition, such agents may mask many of the symptoms of epinephrine excess. Regardless of their precise mechanisms, these defective counterregulatory responses undoubtedly contribute in many diabetic patients to their high risk of developing severe hypoglycemia during therapy with insulin, especially during intensive therapy (1,20). In addition, many intensively treated patients appear to develop tolerance to hypoglycemia and remain asymptomatic with markedly subnormal concentrations of glucose (10). Defective glucagon responsiveness to hypoglycemia in type 1 diabetes is not normalized (reversed) by establishment of tight control (1). In contrast, poorly controlled diabetic patients may develop symptoms of hypoglycemia at higher levels of glucose than do people without diabetes (11).

Nocturnal or Early Morning Hypoglycemia. Excessive insulin action often occurs during the night or early morning hours. The hypoglycemia-induced release of epinephrine and other counter-regulatory hormones (cortisol, growth hormone, glucagon) then causes rebound hyperglycemia, glucosuria, and ketonuria *(Somogyi phenomenon)*. If the physician notes an elevated blood sugar and prescribes still more insulin, the result is further hypoglycemia, perpetuation of the cycle, and possible serious consequences.

To detect this phenomenon all insulin-receiving patients should be questioned carefully for clues to the presence of nocturnal hypoglycemia (e.g., nightmares, night sweats, and headache during the night or on arising), although these symptoms may not be present. The point at which epinephrine release is secreted and produces sweating and other symptoms is quite variable; some diabetic patients trigger secretion at glucose concentrations as high as 50 mg/dL; others do not have counterregulatory release until the blood sugar falls to as low as 30 to 40 mg/dL, and still others have defective counter-regulation (see above) and only neuroglycopenic symptoms.

Increasing the intake of carbohydrate in the late evening or reducing insulin dosage by 10% in type 1 diabetes and up to 20 to 30% in type 2 diabetes often corrects the situation. In the latter patients, such a brief and substantial reduction in insulin dosage can be made with impunity. If the situation cannot be resolved by such maneuvers, frequent blood glucose monitoring, including measurements during the night and early morning hours, is necessary (see "Monitoring," above).

The classic Somogyi phenomenon must be distinguished from two other possibilities: waning of insulin action and the dawn phenomenon. *Waning of insulin action* occurs when the patient is receiving an insufficient amount of intermediate- or long-acting insulin; either a single morning dose is not carrying into the next day, or the second dose, given before dinner or at bedtime, is inadequate. The *dawn phenomenon* is an increase of blood sugar between 3 and 7 AM that occurs despite continuous subcutaneous infusion or background insulin action from Ultralente. An increased amount of insulin is necessary to overcome the action of growth hormone, which is secreted in pulsatile fashion during the night with considerable interindividual variation and, unfortunately, variation from day to day as well. Because of this variation, an amount of insulin that is sufficient one day may be inadequate the next.

Obviously, patients with waning insulin action or the dawn effect need more insulin, whereas the Somogyi effect requires that less be given. The simplest way to distinguish these is by SMBG with samples at 9 PM, midnight, 3 AM, and 7 AM. Several nights and more frequent sampling may be needed. The differing patterns are shown in Figure 72.3. Constantly rising glucose indicates waning insulin. A plateau followed by a rise indicates the dawn phenomenon. A drop during the night to a clearly hypoglycemic level points to the Somogyi effect. If SMBG cannot be done, cautious reduction of the dosage of (evening) insulin should be attempted. Although the existence of the Somogyi phenomenon has been repeatedly challenged (77), other evidence convincingly points to its contribution to the problem of glucose regulation (61).

Daytime Hypoglycemia. The immediate therapy of daytime hypoglycemia in a conscious patient is ingestion of food, preferably sugar. Patients should carry a ready carbohydrate source, such as candy, and must realize that a tiny piece of such material will not suffice. Five or six Life Savers provide the minimum necessary 10 g of carbohydrate, as does a piece of fruit. Glucose

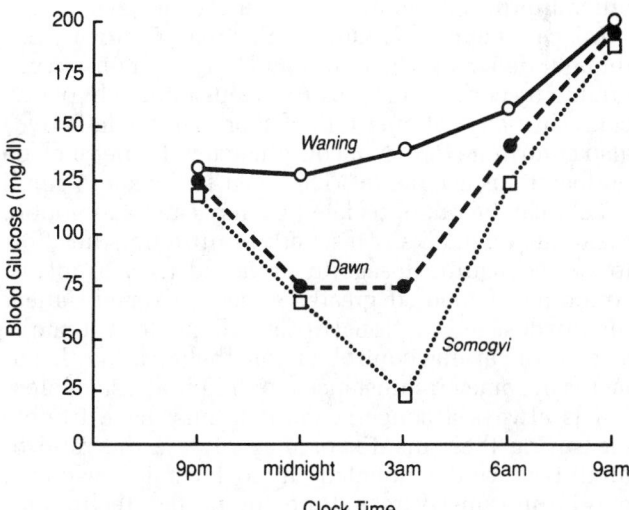

Figure 72.3. Idealized patterns of blood glucose concentrations during the night. The three patterns represent waning insulin action, the dawn phenomenon, and the classic Somogyi effect. All result in fasting hyperglycemia but are distinguished by the patterns of blood glucose concentration in the preceding hours.

tablets (5 to 10 g glucose/tablet) are now available; at least two are recommended. If available, 4 to 6 oz sweetened juice or a nondiet soft drink are most satisfactory. A tablespoon of sugar may be added to fruit juice or dissolved in one-half cup of water. Relief should be obtained in 10 to 20 minutes. Family members or friends should be instructed in the treatment of such an emergency and should not waste time attempting to reach medical assistance before administering sugar. Although emergency medical care may be sought after sugar is given, the problem is usually resolved by the time medical assistance can be obtained. If no obvious cause is apparent for the episode of hypoglycemia—such as a missed meal that is subsequently eaten—the patient should be on guard for recurrence over the next few hours, during which time repeated ingestion of sugar, at hourly intervals, may be advisable.

Most patients treated with less than intensive therapy never require emergency medical assistance for treatment of hypoglycemia. However, occasional patients are prone to this problem and sometimes cannot be treated by the simple means described. Either because of a hypoglycemia-related alteration of mental status resulting in an uncooperative state or even combativeness or because of unconsciousness, such patients cannot take oral sugar. A safe and effective emergency therapy is administration of 1 mg of glucagon subcutaneously by a person instructed in this technique (glucagon augments the breakdown of hepatic glycogen to glucose). Glucagon is readily available in single-dose form (1-mg vial) and should be kept available during initiation of insulin therapy and in hypoglycemia-prone patients. About 10 to 15 minutes are required for an obvious effect on the sensorium. As soon as possible, oral sugar should then be given. An effort should always be made to identify the cause of the hypoglycemic episode and to reduce dosage or take other appropriate action to prevent recurrence.

Miscellaneous Factors Affecting Control. Although defects of counterregulatory responses undoubtedly contribute to recurrent episodes of hypoglycemia in many patients, other factors in their daily lives also contribute (63). Noncompliance with diet may be deliberate or accidental. The need to consume small snacks can be unappreciated or they can be forgotten. Meals are often taken off schedule, upsetting the effort to adjust insulin dosage to preferred time of meals. Amounts of food, if greatly varied, adversely affect insulin dosage. Emotional upset, difficult to evaluate as a cause of varying control, is nonetheless a significant factor in some circumstances. Injudicious use of alcohol is always a concern. Patients may have trouble measuring their insulin or may reverse the ratio of mixtures. Undocumented hypoglycemic reactions may be improperly treated and unreported. Techniques of blood monitoring are often at fault; patients misread directions or introduce variations that lead to errors of measurements. Not to be ignored is the effect of exercise (see above).

Allergic Reactions to Insulins

Allergy to insulin is rare. When it occurs, it is most commonly a local reaction at the site of injection. Local redness, swelling, heat, and itching occur within minutes to an hour after injection and persist for a few hours to a day, often with formation of an area of induration. Such reactions, no longer common, occur during the first few weeks of therapy and usually disappear as therapy is continued. Similar reactions can develop many hours or up to a day after injection (delayed hypersensitivity). Local reactions, misinterpreted as allergic, may also be caused by improper injection technique, the presence of preservatives in a particular brand, or even the injection of cold insulin.

Systemic allergic reactions, with or without a local reaction, are vanishingly rare; they are manifest by urticaria, angioedema, and even anaphylactic shock (IgE mediated; see Chapter 23). Such reactions seem to occur most often in patients who have previously received insulin and appear during reinstitution of therapy after a lapse of months or years. Local reactions may progress to systemic ones; if this seems to be occurring, one should treat the patient before anaphylaxis occurs. The first maneuver involves a trial of highly purified insulin. If this approach fails, drugs such as antihistamines and glucocorticoids are helpful, but persistent insulin allergy is best treated by *desensitization.* With the patient receiving no antihistamines or steroids and no insulin in the preceding 12 to 24 hours, the procedure involves injection of 0.1-mL volumes of insulin that have been diluted 1:100 in 0.1% human serum albumin to prevent adsorption losses onto glass. An initial dose (0.001 unit) is given intradermally. Subsequent doses of 0.1 mL contain doubling amounts (units). After several intradermal injections at 30-minute intervals, the subcutaneous route is used. If a reaction occurs, epinephrine may be administered; the dosage of insulin is reduced, but the process is continued. This procedure requires a series of solutions of insulin. These may be prepared by the physician or pharmacist but are also available by telephone request to Eli Lilly Co., Indianapolis. Special kits and instructions for desensitizing patients who have delayed hypersensitivity reactions are also available from the same source.

Lipoatrophy and Lipohypertrophy

Insulin lipoatrophy is now an uncommon event. Harmless but disfiguring localized atrophy of subcutaneous fatty tissue occurs around the site of insulin injections and is sometimes seen simultaneously with insulin allergy. The process may be related to impurities in insulin preparations rather than to insulin itself because preparations of high purity are much less likely to produce this problem.

Insulin lipohypertrophy is even less common than insulin atrophy. This phenomenon is probably caused by an intrinsic action of insulin and has not been improved by use of purer insulins. Repeated injections into the same area do appear to predispose to lipohypertrophy.

Oral Hypoglycemic Drugs

Sulfonylureas

Within a few years after their introduction some 40 years ago, sulfonylureas came into wide use for the treatment of type 2 diabetes. The acute hypoglycemic effects of the sulfonylureas appear to be mediated through insulin release. However, in chronic administration, during which blood glucose has been lowered or even normalized, no increase of plasma insulin is apparent. Studies of the mechanisms of action of these drugs show both an increase in the number of insulin receptors and a potentiation of insulin action. Numerous effects other than the desired hypoglycemic action of the sulfonylureas have been studied in connection with drug interactions of these compounds (see below).

Current Place in Therapy. Although sometimes used to good purpose for treatment of symptomatic hyperglycemia, sulfonylureas were often administered to patients with type 2 diabetes who could have been treated with diet (i.e., by weight reduction). Many patients with minimal fasting or postprandial hyperglycemia or other abnormalities of glucose tolerance were also treated.

A multicenter long-term cooperative study (UGDP) attempted to assess the usefulness of these agents in asymptomatic diabetic patients by comparing tolbutamide with diet and insulin treatment. The study began a vitriolic controversy in 1970, when it was reported that tolbutamide-treated patients fared no better than those given placebo and indeed had a higher cardiovascular (but not overall) death rate. After that report, diabetologists became divided concerning the usefulness (or dangers) of these agents. On reanalysis of the data, the harmfulness of these agents seems to be open to serious question. A number of other studies of this issue concluded that sulfonylureas do not result in harmful effects, and the use of these drugs therefore increased. By 1979, the ADA recommended that restrictions on the use of sulfonylureas were unwarranted.

The results of the UGDP indicated that insulin treatment sufficient to reduce hyperglycemia did not reduce morbidity or mortality over 10 years but it is certain that the original UGDP study was too brief and involved too few patients to have permitted answers to questions concerning mortality or prevention of complications. Over the next 10 years a new generation of diabetologists and professional groups therefore issued statements that attempts to lower blood sugar aggressively would probably be beneficial (see above).

Candidates for Therapy with a Sulfonylurea. Obese type 2 diabetic patients who have not responded to a weight reduction diet within 3 to 4 months or who, having started on a diet, need interim symptomatic relief from hyperglycemia that is producing osmotic diuresis (polyuria, polydipsia) may benefit from an oral hypoglycemic drug (Table 72.8). Typically these patients are over age 40 and are more likely to respond if their diabetes has been present for only a few years. Other candidates are those who are unwilling to accept insulin therapy or in whom the risks of hypoglycemia

Table 72.8. Characteristics of Oral Hypoglycemic Drugs

Compound	Generic Available	Trade Name	Tablet Size	Daily Dosage Range	Duration of Action (hr)	Doses/ Day	Route of Inactivation
Sulfonylureas							
Tolbutamide	Yes	Orinase	0.5 g	1–3 g	12	2–3	100% in liver
Chlorpropamide	Yes	Diabinese	0.1 g 0.25 g	0.1–0.5 g	24–72	1	100% excretion by kidney: as intact drug, 30%, plus less active metabolites, 70%
Tolazamide	Yes	Tolinase	0.1 g 0.25 g 0.5 g	0.25–1.0 g	12–24	1–2	Partial liver metabolism; partial excretion via kidney
Glyburide	Yes	Micronase, Diabeta	1.25 mg 2.5 mg 5 mg	1.25–20 mg	16–24	1–2	100% metabolized to inactive compounds
		Glynase PresTab	1.5 mg 3 mg 6 mg	0.75–12 mg			
Glipizide	Yes	Glucotrol, Glucotrol XL extended-release tablets	5 mg 10 mg	2.5–40 mg	12–24	1–2	100% metabolized to inactive compounds
Glimeparide	No	Amaryl	1, 2, 4 mg	1–8 mg	24	1	100% metabolized to less active compounds
Metformin	No	Glucophage	500 mg 850 mg	1000–3000 mg	24	2	100% excretion of active compound by kidney
Acarbose	No	Precose	50 mg 100 mg	75–300 mg	NA	3	<2% of active drug is absorbed
Troglitazone	No	Rezulin	200 mg 400 mg	200–600 mg	24	1	100% metabolized by the liver and excreted in the feces

seem unacceptable. The latter might include patients with occupations involving hazardous conditions (vehicle or dangerous equipment operators). Still others include nonobese patients in whom insulin therapy is unacceptable, but for whom persistent hyperglycemia is a risk factor for microvascular disease.

Oral agents should not be prescribed for certain patients: those with a history of ketoacidosis, unless the latter has developed in relation to stress (see below); those with a history of severe toxic reaction to a sulfonylurea; and those with severe hepatic or renal disease, although correct choice of an agent may make such therapy possible (Table 72.8).

Effectiveness. In optimally selected patients, about one-half can be expected to experience normalization of fasting blood sugar and about one-third do not respond. In others, some drug effect is evident, perhaps to a degree that permits symptomatic relief. Maximal drug effect can be expected within a few days to a week. Those who do not respond during initial therapy are considered to be primary sulfonylurea failures. In other cases, following a month or more of good response, the drug seems to become ineffective (secondary sulfonylurea failure). The frequency of this response has been estimated at 3 to 10% per year, so by 15 years of treatment almost all patients are refractory. Some apparent secondary failures are in fact caused by noncompliance. Only rarely in secondary failure is a switch from a maximal dosage of one agent to another successful.

Dosing. In initiating therapy, an average dosage is usually appropriate. A single adjustment upward or downward by a factor of two may then be made as indicated by the blood sugar response after a suitable interval (see below). When switching from insulin to an oral agent, initial dosage can usually safely be at the maximum recommended level for the particular oral agent, or at least in its middosage range. Before switching from one sulfonylurea to another or one oral agent to another, the first should have been tried at a maximal recommended dosage for at least 1 week; trials of more than 2 weeks are not indicated. In changing from a first- to a second-generation sulfonylurea, similar time intervals pertain.

Therapeutic Effects Versus Side Effects. No doubt exists that short-term symptomatic relief of hyperglycemia and its sequelae can be obtained in most type 2 diabetic patients treated with sulfonylureas. This result can be gratifying in properly selected patients. For example, patients who may have difficulty in self-administering insulin because of visual or other physical disabilities may benefit symptomatically from use of sulfonylureas. On the other hand, the use of sulfonylureas is not totally without risk because of their intrinsic pharmacologic action in lowering blood glucose and because of a number of toxic effects. Hypoglycemia can occur and may be both severe and protracted, especially in the elderly or in patients with decreased hepatic or renal function. Other complications of these drugs in elderly patients are described below (p. 1049).

Choice of Sulfonylureas

The First-Generation Sulfonylureas. *Tolbutamide* was the only sulfonylurea studied in the UGDP. Although the admonitions of the FDA concerning other oral agents were extrapolated from this study of tolbutamide, it may be useful to remember that the related available drugs might have fared better or worse. This caveat aside, for patients with normal hepatic and renal function, there is little to lead one to choose among the first- or second-generation agents (Table 72.8) except for cost and convenience of dosing in that the longer-acting drugs need not be taken as often. The frequency of toxicity with any of these drugs is very low. *Chlorpropamide* should never be used at a dosage greater than 500 mg/day, above which hepatic toxicity becomes common and additional therapeutic effect is not seen. Because of the ability of chlorpropamide to produce a syndrome of drug-induced water intoxication (SIADH), this drug should be avoided in the elderly, in whom this effect has been seen almost exclusively. *Tolazamide* was introduced 25 years ago but has never been marketed vigorously.

The Second-Generation Sulfonylureas. Second-generation sulfonylureas have been in wide use in the United States and abroad for many years. *Glyburide* (Micronase, Diabeta) and *glipizide* (Glucatrol) are both safe agents, but no long-term studies of the UGDP type are available for them. Although all sulfonylureas improve the second phase of insulin secretion, claims have been made that only glipizide in response to glucose stimulation improves both first- and second-phase responses. The second-generation sulfonylureas are more potent on a per milligram basis, but only rarely, if ever, are effective when a first-generation agent fails. Slow-release forms of glipizide (Glucotrol-XL) and glyburide (Glynase Prestab) have been heavily marketed in the recent past, but have not been a significant advance. The latest entry to the U.S. market is *glimepiride* (Amaryl); the drug has no advantage over older agents. Glibenclamide and other sulfonylureas are widely used outside the United States.

Transfer from Insulin to a Sulfonylurea. Type 2 diabetics receiving insulin can be abruptly switched, provided that they do not need more than 40 units of insulin a day. Patients who require such dosages are unlikely to respond well to a sulfonylurea. Patients with a history of ketoacidosis are ordinarily not candidates for a transfer from insulin. If the patient has manifested ketosis in the past (e.g., during stress) but is otherwise thought to be a candidate for a switch to an oral agent, the dosage of insulin may be cut in half as the drug is started. Subsequent monitoring over the next few days will show whether the oral agent can control hyperglycemia or must be abandoned. A history of hyperosmolar nonketotic coma does not preclude a successful change from insulin. Patients with no tendency to ketosis, but whose diabetes is so severe that it has produced weight loss, may not respond to sulfonylureas given as initial therapy but may respond after hyperglycemia has been controlled for a short time with insulin.

Comparative Cost. At present, the approximate monthly retail cost of therapy with these drugs has a very wide range, from $4 to $80 depending on the dosage and the agent used. Three of the drugs, tolbutamide, chlorpropamide, and tolazamide, are currently available in their generic forms at one-half to one-third the price of the trade name products. The cost of insulin therapy may be significantly less than that with the oral agents, depending on the dosage and the grade of insulin used, as well as the choice of oral agents.

Instruction to the Patient. The obese patient must be made to realize that weight reduction is the mainstay of therapy and is not simply a general health measure; weight loss has a specific beneficial effect in diabetes. Drug therapy is an adjunct, not a substitute, for weight reduction. The possible risks and goals of therapy should be clearly outlined. Although hypoglycemia is uncommon with the sulfonylureas, when it does occur, it is likely to be both severe and prolonged. Chlorpropamide and glyburide are the two drugs most likely to produce this problem. The symptoms of hypoglycemia should be clearly described to the patient, and whoever is in close contact with the patient, usually family or friends, and corrective measures outlined and understood (see "Insulin Therapy"). The possibility of drug interactions (see below) should be mentioned lest another physician prescribe a drug that potentiates or decreases the effectiveness of the sulfonylureas, or vice versa.

The sulfonylureas are most effective when administered about 30 minutes before breakfast or dinner.

Monitoring Therapy with Sulfonylureas. The frequency and type of monitoring (see above) should be determined by the severity of the diabetes and the goal of treatment. For patients whose FPG becomes normal or reaches an acceptable level, monitoring can be simple because patients receiving sulfonylurea drugs are not ketosis prone and have fairly stable diabetes. Similar considerations apply to patients being treated with diet alone. No compelling indication exists for SMBG (see above) in most such patients. Patients who have FPG in or near the normal range exhibit little or no fasting glucosuria but may show glucosuria in the postprandial state. If clinically stable, such patients can check their overnight (early morning) urine samples for glucose as infrequently as once a week or even every 2 weeks. More important, they should understand that development or worsening of glucosuria where none was evident is an indication for prompt contact with a physician. Similarly, these patients must be taught that if they develop symptoms and signs of uncontrolled hyperglycemia (heavy glucosuria, polyuria, polydipsia, blurred vision), prompt advice from a physician is absolutely necessary. Routine testing for urinary acetone is unnecessary unless the patient has new onset of persistent glucosuria or at some earlier time had an episode of ketoacidosis, perhaps during stress.

FPG should be determined every few months in most patients, but the best means of monitoring

sulfonylurea-treated patients who respond to treatment with normalization of blood sugar is by determination of glycosylated hemoglobin. Development of frank hypoglycemia or excessive lowering of FPG below 70 mg/dL (which may be detected before symptoms develop) is an indication for downward adjustment of drug dosage.

When dosages are changed or when drugs are added or removed, monitoring should be done more often, perhaps daily, with SMBG.

Special Considerations in Treatment of the Geriatric Patient. Many elderly patients are best treated with oral agents. Simple, symptomatic therapy may be the foremost consideration for these patients. Insulin therapy may present special problems for elderly diabetics (because of poor vision or poor manipulative skill) that make self-administration of insulin difficult. On the other hand, many elderly patients can manage insulin therapy, especially of the type that is not excessively aggressive, and age alone should not deter the physician from instituting insulin therapy. As noted earlier, insulin syringes can be prefilled and stored in the refrigerator for 1 to 2 weeks; this plan is useful for the older person who cannot accurately draw up the correct amount of insulin. The elderly are especially likely to have multiple diseases and to use multiple drugs. The risk of drug interactions in this group is therefore greater than in younger people (see below); insulin therapy avoids this problem. A recent study of various insulin regimens in the elderly, as well as of insulin–sulfonylurea combinations concluded that twice-daily insulin administration was the simplest, most effective, and most cost-effective regimen (82).

The elderly are also especially prone to development of severe and prolonged hypoglycemia with use of the sulfonylureas (73), which may be related, in part, to the decrease of renal function that normally accompanies aging and may be worse in the diabetic. Decreased renal function (glomerular filtration rate, creatinine clearance) is often present in the elderly even when the serum creatinine is normal because creatinine production decreases with age as muscle mass decreases. Thus, sulfonylureas that are disposed of exclusively by excretion (acetohexamide) or in part by this route (chlorpropamide, tolazamide) might be expected to be more likely to produce hypoglycemia when renal function decreases. In fact, no data are available to support this notion. Clinically, chlorpropamide and glyburide appear to be responsible for most instances of hypoglycemia in the elderly.

Chlorpropamide is also capable of inducing enhanced endogenous antidiuretic hormone action and inducing a water intoxication syndrome, a phenomenon seen almost exclusively in elderly diabetic patients (78). Tolazamide has not been associated with this problem, but the second-generation sulfonylureas can be. Tolbutamide and tolazamide are probably the safest first-generation sulfonylureas for use in the elderly. Initial dosages should be low and increases should be made cautiously. Second-generation drugs seem to be prescribed much more often than first-generation drugs, probably because of intense marketing, despite their much higher cost and despite glyburide's propensity to produce hypoglycemia.

Drug Interactions. Various drugs enhance the hypoglycemic action of sulfonylureas, and others decrease their effect. The magnitude of this effect varies with the different sulfonylureas. Several mechanisms are involved, some of which are known. Among the more commonly used drugs, salicylates, some sulfonamides, chloramphenicol, phenylbutazone and its derivatives, and warfarin all enhance the hypoglycemic action of the sulfonylureas. Nonspecific β-blockers may mask the hypoglycemia-induced release of epinephrine and thus prolong and intensify hypoglycemic reactions. β-Blockers may also block insulin release. Clonidine (Catapres), like β-blockers, may mask the signs and symptoms of hypoglycemia. Acute ingestion of alcohol can enhance hypoglycemia; chronic alcohol use accelerates metabolic disposal of sulfonylureas and antagonizes their hypoglycemic action. Sulfonylureas, especially chlorpropamide, interfere with the metabolism of alcohol and may produce a disulfiram-like (Antabuse) effect (see Chapter 21). Diuretics (the thiazides, chlorthalidone, and loop diuretics) may produce hyperglycemia even in normal people and antagonize the sulfonylureas. Another commonly used drug, the anticonvulsant phenytoin (Dilantin), also has an antagonist action. Numerous other drugs may enhance or negate the effect of the sulfonylureas; equally important, the sulfonylureas themselves produce numerous alterations of drug action. These problems should not be overstated, but the physician should be aware of these possibilities and interactions, especially in the elderly, who may be receiving many drugs. Therapy with insulin prevents these problems. A pharmacist with access to a computerized system for monitoring drug interactions can be of great assistance.

Other Oral Agents: Metformin, Acarbose, and Troglitazone

Metformin (Glucophage), a biguanide, was approved for use in the United States several years ago, after decades of use in Europe and elsewhere (5,19,23). The drug's lowering of blood sugar is probably the result of multiple actions; it does not enhance insulin secretion. Another biguanide, *phenformin,* was at one time in wide use but was withdrawn because of occasional cases of fatal lactic acidosis. Metformin causes this problem much less often (see below). The drug is effective as monotherapy, producing a 50 to 60 mg/100 mL fall of PG (decrease of HbA$_{1c}$ of 1 to 1.5%). Data on overall efficacy are scarce; primary failures occur in 10 to 15% of patients and secondary failures in about 5%. Metformin is often used in combination with a sulfonylurea, as an add-on after failure of the latter. If the combination is effective, an attempt to reduce or withdraw the sulfonylurea can be made after a month. After another month, the need for readministration of the sulfonylurea can be determined. Small decreases of LDL cholesterol and triglycerides are common, as is minimal weight loss (1 to 3 kg). Metformin is not

well tolerated by all patients: Nausea, anorexia, and diarrhea are fairly common side effects. These symptoms can be minimized by starting at a once-daily dose (500 mg) and increasing the dosage at weekly intervals until a maximum dosage of 2500 mg in divided doses is reached. Lactic acidosis is very rare in younger patients, but if the patient has renal or cardiopulmonary disease with hypoxia, a significant risk is present. Metformin is not metabolized and is disposed of by renal excretion. It should not be used if renal function is decreased (serum creatinine above 1.5 mg). The drug should be used with great caution in the elderly because their renal function is often compromised even when the serum creatinine is normal.

Acarbose (Precose) is a recently introduced agent for treatment of type 2 diabetes. Monotherapy can be expected to produce only minimal effect on the FPG (15 to 20 mg/100 mL) and then only in patients with no more than modest hyperglycemia. A greater effect is seen on postprandial than on fasting glucose (a reduction of 30 to 60 mg/100 mL), not a surprising finding because the drug is a nonabsorbable α-glucosidase inhibitor that acts by inhibition of the enzymes in the mucosal cells of the small intestine that digest complex carbohydrates. Abdominal fullness, flatulence, and less commonly, diarrhea are the side effects, all of which tend to abate with time. Acarbose should be considered as an expensive adjunctive drug ($50 to $70 per month), which is only occasionally useful as monotherapy. The drug (50 to 100 mg) is taken at the beginning of each meal.

Troglitazone (Rezulin) is the latest addition to a growing list of antidiabetic drugs (72). It is representative of a class of agents known as thiazolidinediones ("glitazones") that decrease insulin resistance by enhancing insulin activity at cellular receptor sites. Troglitazone is unimpressive as monotherapy in type 2 diabetes, producing at most only a modest decrease of blood glucose and failing to have any effect at all in up to 25% of patients. However, the drug has recently been approved as an adjunct to the insulin therapy of patients with type 2 diabetes mellitus who require high dosages of insulin. Under these conditions, the dosage of insulin can often be reduced even as glycemic control is improving. The cost is considerable. At $160 per month (wholesale; 400 to 600 mg/day) the drug is usually considerably more expensive than the amount of insulin replaced. Troglitazone is not approved for use in combination with other oral agents, but the manufacturer strongly suggests that it can be added safely to the regimen of a patient taking a sulfonylurea. The manufacturer recently has warned of possible hepatotoxicity with this drug and suggests measuring the patient's liver enzymes before prescribing the drug and then measuring them every 2 to 3 months thereafter.

Treatment of Other Types of Diabetes Mellitus (Secondary Diabetes)

Drug-induced diabetes (e.g., diabetes induced by thiazides) and diabetes associated with the use of glucocorticoids are usually not characterized by ketosis and ordinarily resemble type 2 diabetes. Treatment with a sulfonylurea may be tried, but insulin is often necessary. Withdrawal of the offending agent does not always ameliorate the diabetic state. The possibility of precipitating diabetes in patients with a strong family history should not deter the physician from the judicious use of diuretics or glucocorticoids when these agents are clinically indicated. Similarly, a diabetic who is already receiving insulin should not be denied diuretic therapy (e.g., when hypertension develops) or glucocorticoids for fear of aggravating the diabetes. If such aggravation occurs, usually only an increase of insulin dosage is necessary to reestablish the previous state of glycemic control.

Diabetes secondary to chronic pancreatitis or pancreatectomy should be treated with insulin. The insulin requirement is usually 20 to 40 units/day. The patients should be instructed to follow the dietary strategy outlined for insulin-dependent diabetes in Table 72.4. Alcoholic patients with this form of diabetes are particularly difficult to manage if they continue to drink heavily and to eat erratically.

COMPLICATIONS OF DIABETES MELLITUS

Diabetes mellitus is a leading cause of death in the United States today. Most of these deaths are caused by the complications of the disease, primarily those associated with accelerated atherosclerosis and chronic renal failure (16) (Fig. 72.4). The risk of both atherosclerotic heart disease and atherosclerotic peripheral vascular disease is approximately three times higher in diabetics and is a function of the duration of disease in patients with both type 1 and type 2 diabetes (see below). Atherosclerotic disorders are also discussed in Section 8 and in Chapters 83 and 87; chronic renal failure is discussed in Chapter 48.

Hyperlipidemia

Nature of the Lipid Abnormalities

The kinds of lipid abnormalities in type 1 and type 2 diabetic patients differ (26,47). In patients with type 1 diabetes whose blood sugar is very well controlled and who have normal renal function, the serum lipoproteins are not very different from those in normal subjects: LDL is usually normal, and HDL may even be higher than normal. Oxidized LDL is not ordinarily measured but is thought to be more atherogenic than normal LDL and is often increased. In contrast, patients with type 2 disease have increased levels of intermediate-density lipoproteins (β-VLDL, IDL), and HDL is often low. LDL has increased glycation, which, like oxidation, increases its atherogenicity. A direct contribution of hyperinsulinemia to the atherogenic process is also strongly suspected.

Hyperlipidemia of Type 2 Diabetes Mellitus and Syndrome X (Metabolic Syndrome)

The type 2 diabetic state is so commonly associated with other problems that the constellation has been

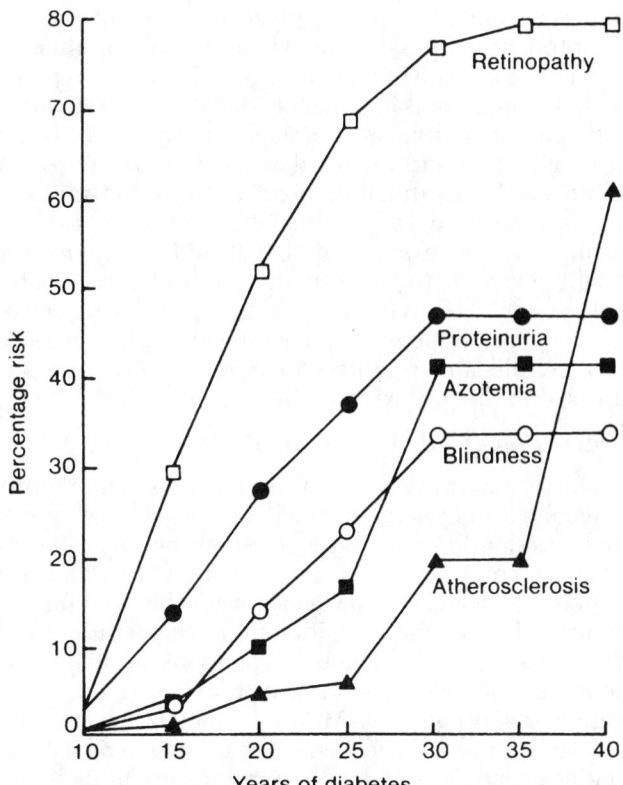

Figure 72.4. Complications of diabetes mellitus as a function of duration of the disease. (From Davidson MB. The continually changing "natural history" of diabetes mellitus. J Chronic Dis 34:5, 1981.)

given the name *syndrome X* or *metabolic syndrome* (67). The components of the syndrome are insulin resistance, hypertension, obesity of the central (visceral) type, combined hyperlipidemia, and atherosclerosis. Since the original report, thousands of papers have appeared on the subject. The pathogenesis of the syndrome is unclear. Genes closely linked to the ones that cause hyperglycemia have been considered most likely to account for hyperlipidemia and its atherosclerotic consequences, whereas the hypertension, it has been argued, may be a result of the hyperinsulinemia invariably seen in the earlier phases of diabetes. Neither of these hypotheses is well supported (see below).

Type 1 diabetes exhibits certain of these features (dyslipidemia, atherosclerosis), but syndrome X is not a feature of type 1 diabetes. Insulin resistance, for example, is not a major part of type 1 diabetes, although some degree of insulin resistance may result from hyperglycemia per se; with effective therapy this type of insulin resistance subsides. The gross hyperlipidemia of type 1 diabetes usually responds to conventional control of hyperglycemia. LDL cholesterol (LDL-C) is usually normalized, although detailed lipid studies show the presence in plasma of small high-density LDL-C, and HDL-C is often low. Triglycerides are usually not elevated if hyperglycemia is controlled.

In patients with syndrome X, hyperlipidemia may improve somewhat with effective lowering of hyperglycemia, but even euglycemia may not abolish the problem. A possible explanation, and an alternative to the multiple associated genetic defect hypothesis, is that the same factor that leads to insulin resistance and hyperglycemia is responsible. Thus, although lipids are lowered when hyperglycemia is controlled by insulin, the resistance factor continues to act, interfering with insulin's effect on lipid metabolism. It has been speculated that additional insulin might overcome the abnormality of lipid metabolism, but testing this hypothesis is not possible because unacceptable hypoglycemia would ensue. The therapy of the lipid abnormalities in type 2 diabetes is addressed in the following section and in Chapter 75.

Prevention of Atherosclerotic Disease

The serum lipid abnormalities that persist after optimal control of hyperglycemia in both type 1 and type 2 diabetes should be treated aggressively because atherosclerotic complications are very common in diabetic patients, indeed several times greater than in nondiabetics. The general considerations that guide such therapy are given in Chapter 75 and most apply to diabetic patients. However, a few points need emphasis here. Statin drugs (the HMG Co-A reductase inhibitors lovastatin and its successors) may actually be first-choice agents, even when hypertriglyceridemia is the most obvious abnormality, a situation where fibrates (gemfibrozil, clofibrate) would normally be considered first. Individual patient responses vary greatly, so the two classes of drugs should be tried successively for 3 to 4 months each and compared. Determinations of total, LDL, and HDL cholesterol should be made monthly, and the mean values compared. Unfortunately, the combination of gemfibrozil and lovastatin (or other statins) is potentially dangerous; severe rhabdomyolysis has been reported when the drugs are given in combination, especially to patients in chronic renal failure. The combination of long-acting nicotinic acid and lovastatin is extremely effective for lowering LDL-C and elevating HDL-C; low HDL-C is a common problem in type 1 diabetes. This combination is safe in nondiabetics and is very well tolerated, although no series of diabetic patients treated in this fashion has been reported. A bile acid sequestrant (cholestyramine, colestipol) in combination with nicotinic acid or a statin is also very effective. Sequestrants can occasionally induce hypertriglyceridemia even in nondiabetic patients, and this may occur more often in diabetic patients. These agents are unpleasant to take; only about one-half of patients tolerate them. It is reasonable to consider even triple therapy (a statin, nicotinic acid, and a bile-acid sequestrant) in selected high-risk patients.

The presence of renal failure may preclude successful attempts to normalize blood lipids. Indeed, lipid-lowering agents, especially combinations, may be dangerous in such patients. Diabetic renal transplant patients receiving immunosuppression (cyclosporine) also are at high risk from complications of lipid-lowering agents. If nephrotic syndrome is present, gross hyperlipidemia is not readily manageable, even with drugs.

Hypertension and Its Therapy

Hypertension in diabetic patients requires aggressive therapy (see Chapter 62). Hypertension accelerates diabetic retinopathy and diabetic renal disease and is a major risk factor for coronary atherosclerosis and probably other large vessel atherosclerotic disease. Indeed, control of hypertension has been shown to slow the progression of both eye and renal disease. The choice of a specific antihypertensive drug or combination of drugs is influenced by the type of diabetes present and the stage of complications (see below).

In uncomplicated type 1 or type 2 diabetes, *thiazides* are still useful, although until recently concern over their tendency (at dosages of 50 to 100 mg of hydrochlorothiazide per day) to worsen glucose intolerance often deterred their use. In type 2 diabetic patients, the dosage of insulin could be increased slightly to compensate for this adverse effect. In contrast, patients with type 2 disease sometimes showed enough of a change of glucose tolerance to compromise what was acceptable therapy with an oral agent. These concerns are probably no longer valid since the realization that minidosages of thiazides (e.g., 10 to 15 mg/day of hydrochlorothiazide) are to be preferred. Not only are low dosages of thiazides just as effective as larger dosages, but the problem of potassium depletion, which probably contributes to glucose intolerance and adverse cardiac events, is avoided. The risk of increased mortality in hypertensive diabetic patients treated with higher dosages of thiazides is probably no longer a concern when these lower dosages are used. Worsening hyperlipidemia can also occur with these agents. Loop diuretics resemble the thiazides in their adverse action on glucose tolerance.

Agents that promote orthostatic changes (e.g., α-blockers; methyldopa) may be unacceptable in a diabetic patient who has autonomic dysfunction and already tends to have orthostatic changes. On the other hand, the use of α-blockers in diabetic patients is becoming popular, perhaps in part because they have also been shown to reduce proteinuria (see below). The *β-adrenergic–blocking agents* are useful in many cases, despite some concerns. The nonselective β-blocking agents (propranolol, pindolol, nadolol, timolol) are best avoided because of possible worsening of glucose tolerance (inhibition of insulin release in type 2 diabetes) and interference with recovery from hypoglycemia, masking of hypoglycemic symptoms, and occasional promotion of hyperkalemia. However, the selective β_1-blockers (atenolol, metoprolol) can be used because they are unlikely to produce these problems at conventional dosages. Concern over aggravation of hyperlipidemia by this class of drugs is unwarranted because, unlike the nonspecific propranolol, which gave rise to these concerns, the more selective agents actually have only trivial effects on blood lipids.

The angiotensin-converting enzyme (ACE) inhibitors are also useful, especially in patients with nephropathy (see Chapters 44 and 48). Despite the occasional production of proteinuria in some nondiabetic patients, ACE inhibitors actually decrease proteinuria and slow progress of disease in diabetic patients with nephropathy. Other problems with antihypertensive drugs that may be especially troublesome in diabetic patients are impotence (diuretics, α- or β-adrenergic blockers) and hyperkalemia (triamterene, ACE inhibitors), presumably in relation to the subclinical hyporeninemic hypoaldosteronism often present in these patients. Recent work raises doubt about the relative safety of calcium channel blockers in diabetic patients.

Neuropathy

The prevalence of neurologic deficits in diabetic patients is unknown, although it is clear that in most patients the occurrence and severity of involvement are related to duration of the disease. Usually, many years pass before the process becomes obvious, but occasionally even severe neuropathy can have an early onset (71). (See Chapter 84 for a general discussion of peripheral neuropathy.)

The most commonly appreciated abnormality is that which affects peripheral sensory nerves. Several types of sensation are involved (pain, proprioception, vibration, light touch) and can lead to unsteadiness, ataxic gait, and such uncommon but striking disorders as neuropathic arthropathy. Less well appreciated are the autonomic disorders that give rise to disturbances of cardiovascular function (postural hypotension, resting tachycardia), genitourinary function (impotence, bladder dysfunction), and gastrointestinal function (nocturnal diarrhea, fecal incontinence). Motor deficits are much less common but may occur with striking suddenness. Weakness is distal (neuropathic) rather than proximal (myopathic), although a specific type of myopathy also occurs in diabetic patients (see "Diabetic Myopathy," below). Some authors use the term *distal symmetric sensorimotor polyneuropathy* to describe the most common form of diabetic polyneuropathy.

Peripheral Sensory Neuropathy

Classically, the deficit is distal, with the lower extremities affected first, followed by the upper extremities. The term *stocking–glove distribution* is appropriate. The disorder is a symmetric polyneuropathy with a proximal–distal gradient of dysfunction. In severe cases, even the sensory innervation of the trunk is involved; in this instance the most distal fibers are those of the anterior abdomen and lower thorax. Rarely, even the distal portions of the cranial nerves are affected (e.g., the distal sensory portion of the trigeminal nerve). The patterns of loss are not specific for diabetes mellitus and can be seen in such diverse states as amyloid neuropathy and toxic (e.g., lead) neuropathies.

The nerve damage may at first be asymptomatic, although subtle symptoms may be revealed with careful questioning of the patient. Alternatively, the patient may first complain of hyperesthesia and dysesthesia, including tingling and burning sensations. Later, various symptoms are experienced, including sensations of numbness or heaviness. Patients often complain that their feet feel dead or that they have a sensation of walking on a soft or nonexistent surface. Loss of ability to perceive temperature and firmness gives rise to these complaints. Severe, spontaneous, short-lived stabbing leg pains and cramps are common. Often, these pains are most troublesome at night.

On neurologic testing, skin hypesthesia is the most common finding (pinprick, two-point discrimination, light touch). *The nylon monofilament test* may be better for screening (68). The hypesthesia and loss of temperature perception lead to unappreciated skin trauma and predispose to infection. The sensory loss in the fingertips can prevent the blind diabetic from learning braille. Deep tendon reflexes, especially that of the Achilles tendon, are lost, often in the early stages of the neuropathy.

Peripheral Motor Neuropathy

Much less common and less well recognized are the motor function abnormalities that occur as part of diabetic neuropathy. The intrinsic muscles of the feet are those most commonly involved. Interosseous atrophy produces inability to separate toes but, more important, allows the foot to assume abnormal positions. When claw or hammer toe develops, new pressure points appear at the tips of the toes and along the dorsal aspects; hyperkeratosis, callus formation, and ulceration follow. The interosseous atrophy that may affect the hands does not lead to total loss of function but does result in weakness of grip. Diffuse weakness of the legs and upper extremities may also occur.

Therapy of Painful Peripheral Neuropathies

Until recently, medical therapy was limited to the acute and chronic treatment of pain with analgesics such as codeine. Although this approach will no doubt continue to be needed, relief of pain and discomfort can now be offered by use of amitriptyline and desipramine, shown to be effective in several well-designed trials (53). Amitriptyline may have more side effects than desipramine and may be less desirable for use in elderly diabetic patients. The mean effective dosage of drug is 100 mg/day. The mechanism of action of these drugs in the relief of pain does not appear to be an effect on mood.

Capsaicin (Zostrix) applied to the skin as a cream three to four times a day has been shown to be effective in some patients in the treatment of painful diabetic neuropathy, including radiculopathy, and results in improvement in daily activities. The agent is well tolerated.

A number of other drugs (phenytoin, carbamazepine, and diphenhydramine) have been recommended for treatment of pain in peripheral neuropathy, but there have been no controlled trials to test their efficacy (see Chapter 84 for additional details). Transcutaneous electrical nerve stimulation has been said to be useful. Vitamin therapy is often given but is almost certainly useless for this purpose. Aldose reductase inhibitors, once promising, are still experimental drugs, as is aminoguanidine, under investigation as a prophylactic agent.

Mononeuropathies

Mononeuropathy (mononeuritis simplex and multiplex) may occur in any superficial nerve (simplex) or asymmetric simultaneous combination (multiplex). The lower extremities are more commonly involved (femoral, lateral femoral cutaneous, sciatic, peroneal) than are the upper (e.g., ulnar, radial). Onset is usually sudden with intense, often cramping and lancinating pain (see Chapter 84, Tables 84.6 and 84.7). Typically, the pain is worse at night and, when the lower extremities are involved, may be relieved by pacing about. When the pain is radicular (trunk or abdomen) intrathoracic or intra-abdominal disease may be misdiagnosed.

At onset, diagnosis can only be surmised, although tenderness along a nerve trunk is suggestive. Herpes zoster may be suspected, especially when hyperesthesia occurs, but when no vesicles appear and muscle weakness and atrophy are eventually evident, the diagnosis becomes obvious. The prognosis is good, with complete recovery within a few months the rule.

Cranial and Oculomotor Neuropathies

Cranial and oculomotor neuropathies are distinguished from other mononeuropathies mainly by their location. Pain and headache may be present. The most common nerves involved are III (palpebral ptosis, pupillary function undisturbed), VI (inward deviation of eye, diplopia), and IV (inward and upward deviations, diplopia). Recovery within 3 months is almost universal. When the facial nerve is involved, distinction from Bell's palsy is impossible (see Chapter 84), although the diabetic variety tends to be less severe and recovery is usually complete.

Neuropathic Foot Ulcers

Long thought to be the result of vascular disease, especially the probably nonexistent "small vessel disease," foot ulcers are now considered to be primarily the manifestations of diabetic neuropathy. Although the diabetic is certainly prone to vascular (arterial) insufficiency as well as neuropathy and although the presence of vessel disease often contributes, the origin of the problem is primarily the sensory deficit. Neuropathy often is asymptomatic until an ulcer develops. Because the patient does not perceive pain normally, unappreciated trauma occurs, for example from new or poorly fitting shoes that produce pressure points that go unrelieved and end in penetrating abrasions. Wounds can also result from skin penetration by foreign materials or from inept self-trimming of toenails. In addition to the sensory deficit, simultaneous motor weakness of extensor or flexor muscles together with proprioceptive defects can also contribute to anatomic deformity that in turn produces pressure points and ulceration.

Typically, foot ulcers are plantar and occur at the point where weight bearing is greatest. Altered motor nerve function leads to muscle atrophy and tendon shortenings, which result in chronic toe flexion and finally hammertoe deformity. This anatomic change shifts weight from the padded ball of the foot to the metatarsal heads, where calluses form and contribute to the formation of new pressure points. The calluses themselves may develop fissures, which further promote ulceration. A recently recognized contributor to the problem is loss of adipose tissue from the padded areas of the foot. This padding normally distributes weight of the foot; loss of this tissue is a major anatomic destabilizer.

Therapy of Ulceration. Decreased weight bearing usually is essential as part of treatment. Infection is invariably present and is almost always a mixture of aerobic, facultatively anaerobic, and anaerobic organisms (81). Antibiotics of choice and their method of administration are discussed under "Infections," below (50,81). Intravenous antibiotics and hospitalization have been standard therapy for many years, but recently oral antibiotics in a home-based setting have been shown to be effective for most patients. Because callus formation aggravates the tendency to increase local pressure and worsens ulceration, regular debridement is essential. Some patients can be taught debridement techniques, which may at least delay the intervals between visits to the physician for this purpose, but usually periodic professional assistance is essential. Such care is often best provided by podiatrists (see Chapter 102). Fitting of custom-made molded shoes is helpful and is essential in some cases for prevention of ulceration. Remarkably, with proper treatment the ulcer may heal completely and not recur. However, recurrence is likely as long as the anatomic distortion or continued point pressure is unchanged.

Increasing emphasis is being placed on the prevention of neuropathic ulcers. A simple nylon filament touch perception test (see above) allows detection of the presence of sensory impairment, which is a major predictor of the risk of foot ulceration. Patients who cannot feel the filament are at about 10 times greater risk of ulceration and 17 times greater risk for amputation (68). Identification of such patients and institution of preventive measures may be useful in avoiding amputations, although no data are available.

Neuropathic Arthropathy (Charcot's Joint, Diabetic Charcot's Foot)

Neuropathic arthropathy, a complication of diabetes, is often unrecognized or misdiagnosed. The disorder, preceded by a sensory neuropathy, is a progressive, degenerative change of the bony structure of the foot, most often involving the tarsal and tarsometatarsal joints (60%), but also the metatarsophalangeal joints (30%) and the ankle (10%). The prevalence has been estimated at 1 in 680 cases, but the disorder is probably more common. The patient presents with a swollen foot, often attributed to or associated with recent trauma. The foot may be painful or may be remarkably free of pain, considering the appearance. Examination shows moderate to gross deformity of the foot with rocker-bottom subluxation of the midtarsal region or subluxation of the metatarsophalangeal joints. Usually the foot is erythematous and warm to the touch. An infected neuropathic ulcer may be present. More often than not, the pulses are intact. Physicians unfamiliar with this presentation are likely to diagnose some other type of inflammatory arthritis or osteomyelitis, and their impression may be apparently verified by radiographic findings. In these early stages, the x-rays often show severe osteoarthritis, but as the disease progresses, there is complete destruction of the involved joints with resorption of the metatarsal heads and phalangeal diaphyses. Various other bony changes occur, including fractures, joint effusions, and subluxations. When these changes are at the maximal stage (i.e., when soft tissue involvement is most prominent), the diagnosis of osteomyelitis is often entertained, especially when there is an associated, often infected ulcer. Synovial biopsy showing a thickened synovium containing osseous debris may provide the correct diagnosis and avoid the necessity of embarking on a prolonged and difficult course of antibiotic therapy for suspected osteomyelitis.

Diabetic Charcot's foot may also be confused with the changes associated with osteoarthritis and gouty, rheumatoid, and psoriatic arthritis. Consultation by an orthopedic surgeon, rheumatologist, or podiatrist to confirm the diagnosis and assist with therapy is almost always indicated.

Treatment is based on the cessation of further trauma to the affected area, which is best accomplished by elimination of weight bearing. Hospitalization may be necessary for this purpose. Reduction of edema and signs of inflammation may take several weeks. Immobilization with a cast may be helpful but should not be undertaken in the acute stage and, if used, should be done with great care to ensure the integrity of the areas covered by the cast. Simpler bootlike devices may also be used. Crutches can be used at this point, followed eventually by a walking cast. Up to 4 months of treatment may be required. Thereafter, molded or contoured shoes are essential to proper long-term management. Surgical intervention is inadvisable, although occasionally a stabilization procedure may be required if conservative therapy fails. Amputation is not indicated unless osteomyelitis unequivocally coexists or the entire process fails to respond to prolonged conservative efforts. Despite the discouraging appearance of the foot at its worst stages, sufficient healing and stabilization to produce a useful foot can be anticipated.

Neuropathic Cachexia

Another rare complication is known as neuropathic cachexia. Seen in both men and women, the typical case is a man in his 60s with anorexia and profound weight loss. The extremities are painful and bilateral neuropathy is common. Spontaneous recovery in about 1 year can be expected in most cases.

Autonomic Neuropathy

Abnormal Sweat Production. Almost always associated with other evidence of diabetic autonomic neuropathy, this complication in its typical form produces heat intolerance and increased sweating (hyperhidrosis) of the upper half of the body with decreased or absent sweating (anhidrosis) below the midtrunk. In other cases, anhidrosis is generalized and recognition of the complication may be difficult. In women the condition may be confused with menopausal sweats.

Affected patients have decreased thermoregulatory reserve and are predisposed to hyperthermia and heat stroke. Another consequence of impaired sweating includes failure to recognize hypoglycemia (see "Hypoglycemia During Insulin Therapy," above). This is a serious problem because one of the warning signals of insulin reaction is lost. Many elderly patients, including those without diabetes mellitus, already have impaired sympathetic responses as a result of aging rather than diabetes.

Cardiovascular Autonomic Neuropathies. In addition to abnormalities of innervation that result in abnormal cardiovascular reflexes (see below), diabetic cardiac denervation apparently accounts for the phenomenon of painless myocardial infarction, which is said to occur in more than 30% of diabetic patients who experience an acute event. Diagnosis is difficult unless acute electrocardiographic changes are present. Precipitation of unexplained ketoacidosis or myocardial failure may divert attention to these secondary events.

Resting Tachycardia. Heart rates of 90 to 100 beats/minute are common in patients with autonomic neuropathy; occasionally even higher rates are observed. Normal sleep-related bradycardia is absent. Parasympathetic damage is the apparent explanation; the sympathetics appear to be less affected. A β-blocker is useful if therapy is needed. In severe cases, the tachycardia "improves" over the years as denervation becomes more complete and the sympathetics are also lost.

Several noninvasive tests are available to assess the presence of autonomic cardiovascular dysfunction. These include the Valsalva maneuver, beat-to-beat heart rate variation, and the lying-to-standing heart rate response. Such assessments are more subtle indicators of the presence of autonomic dysfunction than is postural hypotension. These tests are rarely of use clinically but do allow objective assessment. The consequences—or at least the associations—of these abnormal cardiovascular reflexes in diabetic patients are important. Once they have developed, there is a marked decrease of 5-year survival. Sudden death, not attributable to myocardial infarction, has been described in many such patients (32).

Postural Hypotension. The most readily recognized, troublesome cardiovascular abnormality is postural hypotension (see Chapter 81). The patient may complain merely of dizziness or faintness on standing, or the problem may be more severe, with visual disturbances and syncope. These symptoms may be confused with episodes of hypoglycemia. Remarkably, some patients with fairly marked postural hypotension are asymptomatic.

On initial examination, every diabetic patient should be checked for a postural decrease in blood pressure. In addition, a check for postural hypotension should be made whenever a potentially aggravating condition occurs. The onset or aggravation of postural hypotension is often associated with the beginning of therapy with a variety of drugs often used in diabetic patients such as antihypertensive drugs, including diuretics, vasodilators/antispasmodics such as nitroglycerin (glyceryl trinitrate), antidepressants (tricyclic), and phenothiazines. Occasional diabetic patients may be unable to tolerate effective dosages of these drugs because of this problem.

The mechanism of this disorder is thought to reside in the efferent limb of the baroreceptor arc secondary to damaged sympathetic vasoconstrictor fibers in the splanchnic bed, muscles, and skin. Diminished plasma renin responses to postural change have been noted in such patients, as have abnormalities of plasma norepinephrine, but the role of these defects is unclear.

Various mechanical maneuvers, including the use of antigravity or space suits, have been recommended but are not useful. Drug therapy with clonidine, vasopressors such as phenylephrine, or combinations of tyramine or amine-containing cheeses and monoamine oxidase inhibitors have had their advocates, but none of these has been consistently effective. For patients with severe postural hypotension, the most useful drug has been the mineralocorticoid fludrocortisone (Florinef). In dosages of 0.1 to 1.0 mg/day, the drug is often helpful, but because one of its actions is to expand fluid volume, it can precipitate cardiac failure or produce severe hypertension in the recumbent state. Refractoriness may eventually occur. Recently, the α-adrenergic agonist midodrine (ProAmatine) has been marketed for the treatment of orthostatic hypotension caused by a variety of causes, including diabetes. The drug requires careful dosing (starting at 2.5 mg twice a day) but seems useful (51). In mild cases, the simple advice that the patient assume upright positions slowly by sitting on the edge of the bed after recumbency may help avoid syncopal episodes, whereas continuing postural hypotension, although readily documented, may not be especially symptomatic and may not warrant therapy (also see Chapter 81).

Miscellaneous Foot Problems

In addition to neuropathic disorders, a number of common foot problems (e.g., bunions, calluses, corns, fungal infections, and ingrown toenails) can lead to devastating complications in diabetic patients. Prevention through proper foot care and early recognition and treatment are important considerations in the long-term care of every diabetic patient. These problems are discussed in detail in Chapter 102.

Digestive System Dysfunction

Most of the disorders of the gastrointestinal tract in diabetes are related to disturbances of motility. Esophageal motor dysfunction can be demonstrated on testing but is usually not a clinical problem.

Atony of the stomach (gastroparesis diabeticorum) is often asymptomatic but may be troublesome. Symptoms include anorexia, early satiety, postprandial fullness and bloating, and occasionally, vomiting. Delayed and unpredictable emptying of the stomach may pro-

duce irregular diabetic control in already difficult to manage patients with type 1 diabetes. Diagnosis is apparent—sometimes as an incidental finding—on barium x-ray of the upper gastrointestinal tract. Metoclopramide (Reglan) 10 mg three times daily is helpful (see Chapter 37). Cisapride (Propulsid), 10 to 20 mg three or four times daily, is also effective in some cases.

Small bowel dysfunction is common and symptomatic, leading to diabetic diarrhea. Typically the diarrhea is nocturnal. Fecal incontinence, a result of impaired sensation of rectal distension, may occur and is very distressing. The disorder tends to be episodic, with attacks lasting from a few days to weeks or rarely months. Watery brown diarrhea, usually without steatorrhea, is typical. On barium x-ray of the small bowel, the findings are those of disturbed motility. Despite the distressing symptoms, the patient appears well; weight loss is uncommon. When steatorrhea occurs, pancreatic exocrine insufficiency and sprue syndrome, more common in diabetic patients than in the general population, should be considered. Fully developed sprue is associated with gross evidence of malabsorption. A trial of antibiotic therapy (e.g., tetracycline, 250 mg four times a day for 2 weeks) may improve the diarrhea and the malabsorption if the latter is caused by small bowel stasis and bacterial colonization. Symptomatic treatment with antispasmodics (e.g., Lomotil) may be useful, especially when attacks of diarrhea are short lived.

Large bowel complaints, especially of constipation, are common in the elderly. It does not appear that diabetic patients are especially prone to any additional problems in this regard.

Patients with poorly controlled diabetes may develop *fatty changes of the liver.* Hepatomegaly or elevations of liver enzymes may occur and prompt a fruitless search for other diseases. Effective control of blood sugar results in disappearance of these abnormalities.

Bladder Dysfunction (Neurogenic Bladder)

The symptoms of bladder dysfunction in diabetic patients are often overlooked (12). Onset is insidious and occurs over many years. Most patients (80%) have clinical evidence of neuropathy affecting other systems. The first clinical manifestation of bladder dysfunction is an increase in the interval between voidings until urine is passed only twice or even once daily. A need to strain, slow stream, dribbling, and sensation of incomplete voiding may be present. These symptoms should be routinely solicited from diabetic patients, especially when there are symptoms or signs of peripheral neuropathy.

Demonstration of residual urine is the hallmark of clinically symptomatic cystopathy, but many diabetic patients, when studied by cystometric techniques, have objective evidence of neurogenic involvement and a grossly enlarged bladder well before symptoms are evident (12). At this stage, residual urine is not present and other urinary tract abnormalities (recurrent infections) are not evident. If large volumes of residual urine do develop, patients become prone to infection (see Chapter 27) and incontinence (see Chapter 6).

Patients suspected to have cystopathy should be referred to a urologist for evaluation and recommendations about treatment.

Sexual (Erectile) Dysfunction

The frequency of erectile dysfunction, formerly termed impotence, is high in diabetic men, perhaps 50 to 60% overall. This complication, like many others in diabetic patients, is related to duration of disease. The problem is usually caused by a type of autonomic neuropathy involving the pelvic parasympathetic nerves, but impaired blood flow is the cause in some cases.

The problems leading to *erectile dysfunction* must be included in the differential diagnosis in the diabetic (46). Psychogenic factors probably account for a large fraction of nondiabetic cases. Although no evidence suggests that psychogenic problems are more common in diabetic patients, they are not immune to psychogenic disturbances. The onset of erectile dysfunction usually is slow (6 months to several years), often associated with retrograde ejaculation; impotence eventually becomes complete. Despite this, libido is characteristically retained. Although patients with psychogenic impotence often report nocturnal erections and emissions and may retain masturbatory activity, all of these are absent in diabetic impotence.

An important point on clinical examination is that testicular sensitivity to pressure sufficient to cause pain is retained in men with psychogenic impotence but is often greatly diminished or lost in the diabetic in whom accompanying sensory neuropathy is common.

Endocrinologic causes of impotence (see Chapters 18 and 77) should be considered because they are potentially treatable, but it is rare to find an endocrine basis for impotence in the diabetic. Testosterone secretion, easily verified by plasma testosterone measurement, is invariably normal in diabetic patients; therefore, as one would expect, testosterone therapy is useless.

A variety of drugs, especially ones that are often used in diabetics, may cause erectile dysfunction. The most common offenders are the nondiuretic antihypertensives (see Chapter 62).

Several studies report that sexual function in diabetic women appears to be unaffected by the disease. Others assert that many diabetic women lose the ability to achieve orgasm (30).

The differential diagnosis and therapy of impotence (46) are discussed in detail in Chapter 18. Considerable success has been achieved in diabetic patients by the implantation of prosthetic devices that cause erection, but these operations are less popular than they once were. Intrapenile injections of papaverine, papaverine plus phentolamine, or prostaglandin E plus phentolamine are also effective in many cases. Recently, self-administration of intraurethral prostaglandin E (al-prostadil) has been reported to be an effective, albeit expensive therapy (about $20 per dose) for erectile dysfunction in diabetic and nondiabetic men (60). The overall success rate is approximately 70%. Because of its simplicity, this form of therapy should probably be tried first, before initiating an extensive workup.

Myopathy (Amyotrophy or Proximal Asymmetric Motor Neuropathy)

Myopathy is a rare but devastating complication of diabetes mellitus that is thought by some to be a proximal motor neuropathy. Severe asymmetric proximal muscle weakness and pain usually affect the pelvic girdle and thigh muscles, although upper truncal musculature can also be involved. The typical patient is an elderly, type 2 diabetic with mild disease. Men are affected more often than are women. Onset may be fairly rapid, and low-grade fever and elevated erythrocyte sedimentation rate may be present. Cerebrospinal fluid protein may be very high. Muscle biopsy shows fiber degeneration. Electromyography shows a pattern typical of motor denervation. Prognosis for spontaneous improvement over 2 to 6 months is good, but significant residual effects are common.

Nephropathy

Progressive renal failure is a major, life-threatening complication of diabetes. The relationship between hyperglycemia and the development of microangiopathy with eventual nodular glomerulosclerosis (Kimmelstiel–Wilson disease) now seems to be unequivocally established, as strong clinical and experimental evidence has accumulated in favor of such a relationship. Certainly the cause is either hyperglycemia per se or some other factor in the internal milieu of the diabetic that is responsible for the development of *diabetic renal disease* because kidney transplants from nondiabetic donors in diabetic patients often develop typical lesions of diabetes. One of the earliest indications of incipient diabetic nephropathy is proteinuria, first manifest as microalbuminuria. The detection and significance of proteinuria and of microalbuminuria in diabetic patients are discussed in Chapter 44 and under "Hypertension and Its Therapy," above.

Diabetic patients with even minimal elevations of serum creatinine above 1.1 mg/dL, but not those with normal renal function, are at increased risk of acute renal failure from contrast media used in various radiographic procedures. Although the risk is only moderately increased (approximately 10 to 15% in the highest-risk patients versus 5% in low-risk patients and less than 2% in those with no renal disease and in nondiabetic subjects), these procedures can often be replaced by others with less risk (magnetic resonance imaging, sonography). If contrast media are to be used, the dosage should be minimal and the patient well hydrated.

The clinical course of diabetic nephropathy and the impact of failing renal function on insulin requirement and on the dosage of oral hypoglycemic drugs are discussed in Chapter 48.

Infections

It is a long-time clinical observation that diabetic patients are more prone to infections than are nondiabetics. Clinicians often encounter patients who have experienced repeated bacterial or fungal skin infections (carbuncles, furuncles, external otitis, moniliasis) or gastrointestinal moniliasis at some time before the diagnosis of diabetes was made or in association with uncontrolled hyperglycemia. Once established, infections in the diabetic are difficult to treat and patients are prone to develop complications. Experimentally, hyperglycemia (blood glucose levels above 250 mg/100 mL) inhibits the phagocytic activity of granulocytes and the immune function of lymphocytes, factors that may contribute to lowered host resistance. Control of blood sugar, therefore, should be part of any treatment program for an infection.

Urinary tract infections are an especially troublesome problem in diabetic patients. Although infections are not clearly increased in incidence, a greater prevalence of complications is obvious. Half of all cases of papillary necrosis occur in diabetics. Diabetic patients also seem prone to develop infections with unusual pathogens. However, no statistical case has been made for the desirability of suppression of asymptomatic bacteriuria in diabetics. Development of pyelonephritis is an indication for immediate hospitalization and vigorous antibiotic treatment; the risk of a renal abscess is a special hazard for the diabetic.

Skin infections caused by *Candida* are common in diabetics, especially those with type 2 disease who are obese, and require therapy with a local antifungal agent (see Chapter 100) as well as control of hyperglycemia.

Major soft tissue infections in diabetic patients require prompt hospitalization and treatment with systemic antibiotics. However, most of the infections encountered involve the lower extremities, usually the feet, and are not complicated by serious conditions such as osteomyelitis or gangrene (see "Neuropathic Foot Ulcers," above). Until recently such uncomplicated infections were treated by hospitalization and a combination of systemic antibiotics, often for several weeks. Such an approach can be expected to cost $5,000 to $10,000 per hospitalization. It is now clear that most of these less severe infections can be treated just as well with an oral antibiotic and without hospitalization (50).

Most *infections of the feet* (over half) are acute, with concomitant skin ulceration; others are acute infection of a previously uninfected chronic foot ulcer whereas a lesser number are abscesses (often paronychias) or cellulitis. Although cultures of such lesions are of limited usefulness, they can be obtained by swab, aspiration, or curettage, the latter being more likely to reveal anaerobes. Aerobic Gram-positive organisms are present in more than 50% of lesions, aerobic Gram-negative organisms in 15 to 25%. On average, slightly more than two organisms are isolated, and anaerobes are present in 15% of cases. *Staphylococcus* is the most common organism, followed by *Streptococcus;* in addition to the common Gram-negative organisms *(Klebsiella, Pseudomonas, Proteus). Corynebacteria* should not be considered contaminants; they are the only organism present in many cases.

Choice of Antibiotic

Clindamycin or cephalexin given orally cures 75% of these infections clinically and bacteriologically, even when treatment is without reference to culture results. Another 15 to 20% of infections are greatly improved, and some 5 to 15% are treatment failures (50). Other antibiotic regimens yield similar results (81). The use of topical antibiotic preparations (povidone–iodine; silver sulfadiazine) is controversial (14).

It must be emphasized that such results can be expected only in these less severe infections. Gangrene, severe ischemia, crepitus, and persistent fever are indications for hospitalization. Also to be emphasized is the need for proper adjunctive local care of the foot: elevation of the affected extremity, limitation of ambulation, proper foot hygiene, and, of course, surgical drainage, if appropriate.

Retinopathy

Diabetic retinopathy has become one of the leading causes of blindness in the United States. In type 1 diabetic patients, some degree of retinopathy can be detected by the most sensitive technique, angiography, after as little as 1 to 2 years in 10% of patients. By 10 years, retinopathy is evident in 50% of cases by ophthalmoscopy, with a 70% prevalence by angiography. At 25 years, nearly all patients can be shown to have some degree of retinopathy. By the time diabetes has been present for 15 to 20 years, about one-third of patients have severe disease and another one-half have obvious but lesser degrees of progressive retinal involvement. Remarkably, not all cases of early retinopathy are progressive.

Type 2 diabetic patients also develop retinopathy, apparently with less frequency, but when retinopathy does develop in this older group, the process seems to progress even more rapidly than it does in type 1 diabetic patients. Hyperglycemia, as indirectly measured by glycosylated hemoglobin, clearly predicts the incidence and progression of diabetic retinopathy in type 2 diabetes (31,44). Early reports failed to demonstrate slowing of the progression of retinopathy with intensive therapy, but the DCCT trial and a number of others have clearly shown the value of intensive insulin treatment (see above) in the prevention of retinopathy in patients with type 1 disease. The effect of such therapy takes at least 3 years to be demonstrable.

Blindness in Diabetic Retinopathy

The visual loss in diabetic retinopathy is potentially even more severe than in blindness due to other causes.

Many people who are legally blind (defined as visual acuity less than 20/200 in both eyes) from causes other than diabetes have slow onset of visual loss, thus allowing time for adaptation. In addition, they often retain reasonably full visual fields and visual acuity at or close to the legal limit. Such patients can see well enough to ambulate independently and perform a variety of common activities (self-care, housework). With the aid of special devices they may even be able to read newsprint and to engage in some occupations. In contrast, the visual loss from diabetic retinopathy is often caused by sudden hemorrhage or retinal detachment and often leaves the patient with only light perception. In addition, the diabetic often already has other complications of the disease when blindness develops.

Although total blindness afflicts only a minority of diabetic patients, a larger number have some degree of loss of visual acuity caused by macular edema, the most common cause of visual loss in diabetics (see below).

Ocular Symptoms

Diabetic patients who experience symptoms of visual disturbance are not necessarily experiencing a catastrophic complication and deserve reassurance along these lines. Like others, diabetic patients develop changes of visual acuity such as a change in refractive error and astigmatism. In addition, they can experience decreased visual acuity as a result of marked changes in blood sugar (e.g., as the lens swells during acute normalization of blood sugar after prolonged hyperglycemia). However, sudden or persistent change of visual acuity requires examination by an ophthalmologist, especially when advanced retinal disease, proliferative diabetic retinopathy (PDR), is present. A common cause of visual loss in PDR, macular edema (see below), is not readily detectable by the direct ophthalmoscopy available to internists and requires stereoscopic examination by an ophthalmologist.

Sudden, painless loss of vision in PDR demands urgent ophthalmologic consultation. This symptom is often caused by hemorrhage from proliferating new vessels or from retinal detachment. Lesser degrees of hemorrhage may cause floaters or cobwebs. Another complication in PDR is outflow obstruction of the aqueous humor produced by fibrous scar tissue extending into the angle of the anterior chamber, causing a marked rise in intraocular pressure and acute (neovascular) glaucoma with severe pain. Loss of vision occurs unless emergency therapy is given.

Types of Retinal Disease in Diabetic Patients

The current classification of diabetic retinal disease is nonproliferative (or background, BDR), preproliferative (PPDR), and proliferative diabetic retinopathy (PDR). The latter, more advanced stage is the point at which sudden and massive visual loss becomes a problem.

Nonproliferative and Preproliferative Retinopathy. The earliest lesions—readily visible with an ordinary ophthalmoscope—are in the region of the macula: microaneurysms, punctate retinal hemorrhages, hard exudates, soft exudates (cotton wool), and so-called intraretinal microvascular anomalies (IRMAs). Both *microaneurysms* and *small dot intraretinal hemorrhages* appear as red dots, and both tend to fade within months. *Blot hemorrhages* are larger. Distinction can best be made by fluorescein angiograms, in which only microaneurysms light up. This procedure, performed by an ophthalmologist, often identifies extensive intraretinal disease when only a few abnormalities are evident by ophthalmoscopy.

Hard exudates are glistening yellow or white lipid deposits located in the outer retinal layers. If they are greater than one disc diameter from the macula, they are not ominous. *Soft exudates* are areas of ischemia or infarction of the nerve fiber layer; they disappear within a few months. *IRMAs* are dilated, hypercellular vessels that are thought to represent either dilated capillaries or intraretinal vascular proliferation. These abnormal vessels are identifiable using the green filters of an ordinary ophthalmoscope but are best seen in the secondary phase of fluorescein angiograms, during which they leak dye into the retina. IRMAs occur adjacent to areas of capillary closure. Their identification is not essential in the routine examination.

Whereas changes of background retinopathy indicate capillary damage and leakage, preproliferative changes (many soft exudates, extensive hemorrhages, IRMAs, and venous bleeding from enlarged dilated [beaded, sausage-link] retinal veins) indicate areas of intraretinal vascular occlusion with resulting nonperfusion. Decreased visual acuity at this stage requires an ophthalmologist's examination to determine with stereoscopic techniques whether macular edema is present. It is not usually appreciated by general physicians that even without proliferative disease, macular edema may result in visual loss as severe as the 20/200 level. Spontaneous improvement is not common but may occur. Visual acuity can also become poor because of lack of proper perfusion of the perifoveal capillaries. In this instance, visual acuity may be as low as 20/200 in the absence of macular edema. Fluorescein angiography reveals the cause of poor visual acuity to be due to the lack of perfusion of the perifoveal capillaries. In the absence of accompanying proliferative disease, patients at this stage can usually ambulate freely and can engage in some occupations. Ability to read a newspaper, except with a vision aid, is unlikely, and the patient will have to stop driving.

Eyes with retinal ischemia and moderate to severe preproliferative changes have a 50% chance of developing new vessel proliferation (neovascularization) within 1 year.

Proliferative Retinopathy. At this stage of retinal disease, new vessels and accompanying fibrous tissue extend from the retinal substance and grow along the inner retinal surface and the posterior surface of the vitreous gel, often causing contraction of the gel and traction on the vessels and the retina. This process creates the conditions for retinal detachment and hemorrhage into the vitreous.

In addition, in advanced PDR, growth of new vessels and scar tissue into the angle of the eye may cause acute glaucoma (see "Ocular Symptoms," above). When the new blood vessels grow out of the surface of the optic nerve heads, they are called new vessels on the disc (NVD); elsewhere in the retina, usually extending from large vessels, they are called new vessels elsewhere (NVE).

The National Diabetic Retinopathy Study (DRS) not only established the efficacy of photocoagulation therapy (see below) but also defined high-risk characteristics as follows: NVD greater than 25% of the optic disc area; any NVD with preretinal or vitreous hemorrhage; or NVE equal to or exceeding 50% of the disc area with preretinal or vitreous hemorrhage. The presence of high-risk characteristics increases the chance of blindness to 30 to 50% within 3 to 5 years unless appropriate photocoagulation therapy is given.

Treatment of Diabetic Retinopathy

Two forms of surgical therapy are now available for the treatment of proliferative retinopathy and its complications. Photocoagulation is of proven value in the prevention of visual loss caused by proliferative disease, and vitrectomy restores and appears to stabilize vision after hemorrhage and/or retinal detachment.

Photocoagulation Therapy. Argon laser therapy reduces severe visual loss by nearly 60% over 5 years in patients with proliferative disease. Multiple (1200 to 1600) 500-μm burns are placed in the retinal periphery. The Early Treatment Diabetic Retinopathy Study (ETDRS) evaluated panretinal photocoagulation (and laser photocoagulation using 450- to 650-μm widely spaced burns) to determine whether such therapy affects the course of disease in eyes with high-risk characteristics or PPDR. Considerable benefit has been shown.

Diabetic *macular edema* is also treated with photocoagulation therapy. Leaking microaneurysms and other lesions in the macula are treated with 50- to 100-μm burns. ETDRS showed a reduction of visual loss due to macular edema of 50% over 3 years.

Patient Experience. Photocoagulation therapy is an office procedure, usually performed in several sessions. Ordinarily only topical (corneal) anesthesia is necessary. Occasionally, some discomfort may be experienced, in which case a local anesthetic is injected into the retro-orbital tissues to allow a completed, pain-free procedure.

Vitrectomy for Proliferative Retinopathy. Hemorrhage into the vitreous is the usual indication for vitrectomy, a procedure that removes old blood and opaque vitreous and can be combined with cataract extraction. Retinal detachment resulting from traction bands that are formed in the vitreous is another indication for vitrectomy. Other repair procedures can be attempted. The results of vitrectomy can be dramatic in restoring sight after vitreous hemorrhage. Currently, however, vitrectomy is used only in severely diseased eyes. Recovery of near-normal vision is the exception

rather than the rule, but the results are definitely worthwhile in many patients.

Every effort should be made to control hypertension in an attempt to prevent retinal hemorrhages. Lifting of heavy objects, jarring exercise, and exposures to high altitudes may also increase the risk of hemorrhages and should be avoided, but commercial airline travel presents no increased risk.

Role of the Internist Versus that of the Ophthalmologist: Indications for Referral

The primary care physician should perform regular examinations of the eyegrounds of diabetic patients in order to ensure prompt and appropriate referral to an ophthalmologist (Table 72.9). Because most diabetic retinopathy occurs within several disc diameters of the macula, most lesions are visible by examination with the direct ophthalmoscope after dilation of the pupils. Nonophthalmologists often defer this examination out of concern over precipitating acute angle-closure glaucoma. Such reluctance is not warranted because this complication is rare at any age and is hardly ever seen before age 40. A drop of dilating solution (2.5% phenylephrine; 1% tropicamide) in each eye is sufficient and causes only sensitivity to bright light (requiring dark glasses) that lasts but a few hours. In addition to examining the retina, the physician should note the condition of the lens because senile cataracts occur prematurely in diabetic patients and metabolic cataracts result from chronic elevation of blood glucose levels.

If only minimal nonproliferative diabetic retinopathy is present, the patient need not be referred immediately if visual acuity is normal. Early preproliferative changes (see above) warrant prompt referral, whereas more extensive changes and proliferative changes should be followed by an ophthalmologist who is expert in photocoagulation. Periodic checks of intraocular pressure to detect glaucoma, especially important in diabetic patients, are part of routine health

---

Table 72.9. Reasons for Referral of Patients with Diabetes Mellitus to an Ophthalmologist

High-Risk Patients
Neovascularization covering more than one-third of optic disc
Vitreous or preretinal hemorrhage with any neovascularization, particularly on optic disc
Macular edema (suspect from hard exudates in macula)

Symptomatic Patients
Blurry vision persisting for more than 1 to 2 days or not associated with a change in blood glucose; suspect macular edema
Sudden loss of vision in one or both eyes
Black spots, cobwebs, or flashing lights in field of vision

Asymptomatic Patients
Yearly examinations (an optometrist can check pressures if no retinal changes or if only BDR is present)
Hard exudates near macula
Any preproliferative or proliferative characteristics
Pregnancy

Modified from ADA physician's guide to non–insulin-dependent (type II) diabetes. Diagnosis and treatment. 2nd ed. Alexandria, VA: ADA, 1988.

maintenance but can be made by an optometrist (see Chapter 98). Recommendations for follow-up are given above (Table 72.9) and in detail elsewhere (25).

DIABETES DURING PREGNANCY AND GESTATIONAL DIABETES

Overt diabetes (grossly elevated fasting and postprandial blood sugars) already under therapy with insulin in type 1 diabetics or untreated in type 2 diabetics has long been associated with adverse outcomes for both mother and fetus. No question remains that such patients should be treated with insulin in a fairly intensive manner; the result is a great reduction in perinatal mortality and morbidity. However, the implications of what is called gestational diabetes (i.e., much lower levels of blood sugar than meet standard diagnostic criteria during pregnancy) are uncertain. Clearly, with a spectrum of severity of these abnormalities of blood sugar, it is no surprise that treatment would be controversial. Moreover, in populations that have a high prevalence of impaired glucose tolerance and type 2 diabetes (e.g., Mexican Americans), gestational diabetes is clearly associated with increased perinatal morbidity and mortality, which can be reduced with treatment. In other populations an adverse influence of gestational diabetes is much less obvious. The contrasting outcomes in different populations without doubt account for some of the differences of physicians' attitudes toward treatment. The issues involved in initiating therapy are important and still unresolved: Great emotional impact, expense, inconvenience, and potential adverse events (including low–birth weight babies) are often associated with intensive insulin therapy. A well-tempered assessment of gestational diabetes has recently been presented (27).

Diagnosis During Pregnancy

The American Diabetes Association recommended in 1985 that all pregnant women be screened for diabetes between the 24th and 28th weeks of pregnancy using a 50-g oral glucose load and a single blood sample 1 hour later. If the value exceeds 140 mg/dL, a glucose tolerance test is performed using 100 g of glucose. (The World Health Organization recommends a 75-g dose of glucose for the OGTT; no validation of this test through outcomes studies is available.) Criteria for a diagnosis of gestational diabetes are given in Table 72.10; they were not changed by the Expert Committee that promulgated new standards for diagnosis of diabetes (see above). The screening procedure identifies 80 to 90% of diabetic patients but has 15 to 20% false positives.

Implications for Pregnancy of OGTT-Diagnosed Glucose Intolerance

A study of the effect of glucose intolerance, not overt diabetes, diagnosed by glucose tolerance test reported

Table 72.10. Diagnosis of Gestational Diabetes by the OGTT[a,b]

	Venous Plasma[b] (mg/dL)
Fasting	105
1 hr	190
2 hr	165
3 hr	145

[a]See text for indications.
[b]Test positive for diabetes mellitus: two or more of the values must be met or exceeded.

significant stepwise increases of macrosomia, congenital abnormalities, perinatal mortality, prematurity, toxemia, and cesarean section as the 2-hour plasma glucose increased from 100 to 164 mg/dL (76). These observations have been challenged (54). However, on the basis of this report and others, many obstetricians initiate therapy with insulin that is designed to maintain fasting and postprandial blood sugars that are normal for pregnancy (i.e., lower than the nonpregnant state). Such an approach demands self-monitoring of blood glucose (SMBG). Many physicians, especially internists, remain skeptical of this approach as overly aggressive. Large studies of such intervention are not yet available. However, one can be certain that such therapy will be attended by many episodes of hypoglycemia. In numerous earlier studies, the prognosis for the pregnant state and the perinatal morbidity of infants born of mothers with an abnormal OGTT but with essentially normal FPG did not differ from normal. This has led some to advocate diet therapy alone, so long as maternal fasting and postprandial glucose levels remain within the range of normal for the nonpregnant state. Ten years ago an authoritative view was that pregnant women with abnormalities of blood glucose should probably be vigorously treated (34). Today a more conservative view is emerging that takes into account severity of the glucose intolerance, population characteristics, and the long-term medical impacts on mothers and their children.

Counseling the Diabetic Woman: Risks of Pregnancy

The complexity of diabetic management is not likely to deter pregnancy. On the other hand, the possibility of diabetes in the newborn or young child is often of great concern; this issue has already been discussed (see "Inheritance"). Other questions concern maternal and fetal mortality. Although the diabetic mother without overt complications has little or no increased risk, the fetal issues must be presented with candor. Of special importance beyond that of infant survival is the problem of an increased risk of congenital abnormalities (see below) and long-term neurologic abnormalities in children of diabetic mothers (37). Therefore preconception patient education and intensive therapy are extremely important for young diabetic women who plan to become pregnant.

Whether complications of diabetes are accelerated by pregnancy is unclear, although nephropathy and retinopathy may worsen, as discussed above. The long-term survival of the diabetic with microvascular disease is already significantly compromised and an honest prognosis in this regard may deter pregnancy, not necessarily because of concern over acceleration of the diabetic complications, but out of concern for the future welfare of a child born to a mother whose health may be poor and whose survival is threatened.

Pregnancy in the diabetic woman presents a major challenge to the physicians involved in the care of the mother and the fetus. Ideally, the medical team should include both an experienced internist/diabetologist and an obstetrician who cooperate actively in the management of the pregnancy. Others in the team may include an experienced teaching nurse and, ultimately, a pediatrician/neonatologist.

The course of the pregnancy in a diabetic woman and its impact on the fetus depend on the type of diabetes and the stage of the disease at which the pregnancy occurs. Unless these are defined, it is impossible to address the issues of management and outcome; generalizations tend to be meaningless. Thus, when pregnancy occurs in the type 1 diabetic without diabetic complications, who is already under close medical supervision and is practicing intensive insulin therapy, management of the diabetes consists of continuation of therapy with institution of even lower limits for blood glucose and special attention to avoidance of nocturnal hypoglycemia (see below). When pregnancy occurs in a diabetic woman with vascular disease, the mother is in danger of an adverse outcome. Nephropathy may worsen, at least temporarily, especially if hypertension is present. Premature delivery and smaller than normal infants occur with even modest increases of serum creatinine (above 1.5 mg/dL) and with proteinuria. Diabetic retinopathy, especially if already proliferative, or if hypertension is present, may progress rapidly and result in loss of visual acuity. Under these circumstances, various questions must be asked. Should an abortion be considered? Does the woman fully understand the risks of continuing the pregnancy?

Most experts are now convinced that modern optimal management of diabetes during pregnancy has reduced perinatal infant mortality to that of nondiabetic women. However, the treatment of most pregnant diabetic women is in fact less than optimal. It is the exceptional baby that is conceived in a mother whose diabetes is under rigorous control by intensive therapy, whose physical and emotional health is uncompromised by the diabetes, and whose physicians always provide unerring exemplary advice and care.

Fetal Mortality and Congenital Malformations

The view that the more severe the diabetic state, the worse the perinatal survival was definitively substantiated by a multicenter study (55) that showed that overtly diabetic women with nearly normal blood glucose levels are at no greater risk of having a spontaneous abortion than are nondiabetic women (83% successful outcome). In contrast, those with elevated blood glucose and elevated glycosylated hemoglobin in the first trimester have additional risk, estimated to be increased by 3% for each standard deviation (elevation of HbA_{1c} of approximately 0.5%) above the upper limit of the normal range (approximately 6.5%). In contrast to earlier reports, patients classified according to White Class scale rating (severity of diabetes based on age at onset, duration of disease, and presence of complications) showed no difference between groups (54). Ketoacidosis occurs in 2 to 10% of diabetic pregnancies and is associated in these cases with fetal losses of 80 to 100%.

The incidence of significant congenital abnormalities in nondiabetic women is approximately 2 to 3% but rises to 8 to 12% in infants born to type 1 diabetic patients and reaches 25% when control is poor, as evidenced by grossly elevated glycosylated hemoglobin. Almost all authorities now agree that hyperglycemia during the early weeks of pregnancy (gestational weeks 3 to 7 when embryogenesis occurs) appears to account for the increased incidence of congenital malformations. Near-normalization of blood sugar before conception and continued normalization through the critical first weeks have been reported to reduce this increased incidence to normal.

Maternal Mortality and Morbidity

Maternal mortality during pregnancy is definitely increased and at 0.5% is about 20 times that in nondiabetics. Most deaths are caused by ketoacidosis or hypoglycemia, the latter usually occurring in the first trimester or immediately postpartum, times at which insulin requirements often decrease. Obviously, optimal management could eliminate most or all of these deaths. Some deaths that may not be preventable include infections after cesarean section or hemorrhage after traumatic delivery of a large infant. Diabetics with overt heart disease (ischemic heart disease, congestive heart failure) have a high mortality (75%) when allowed to go to term. Such patients should never become pregnant or should have an abortion if pregnancy occurs.

Maternal morbidity also increases during the diabetic pregnancy. Polyhydramnios occurs in 25% of pregnancies (10 times greater incidence than expected). Asymptomatic bacteriuria (20%) and frank pyelonephritis (7%) occur three times more often than in the general population. Pyelonephritis is said to occur in 25% of bacteriuric diabetic patients and is associated with a high rate of fetal loss.

Management of Overt Diabetes During Pregnancy

Insulin Therapy: Monitoring Control

Patients with overt diabetes, including gestational diabetes, who are receiving insulin therapy should be monitored to establish optimal control of blood sugar.

Although some obstetricians still favor hospitalization with frequent daytime blood sugar determinations (glucose panel) as an aid to establishment of optimal control, the procedure is useless unless patient compliance can be foreseen after the hospitalization.

Several studies report that near-normalization of blood sugar (tight control) is associated with reduction of fetal loss from 25% to 3 or 4%. On the basis of this information, the goal of insulin and diet therapy should be the closest approximation of normalization of blood sugar that is possible using SMBG while avoiding therapeutic heroics (i.e., multiple and prolonged hospitalizations solely for the purpose of blood sugar control). Normal fasting blood sugar (not exceeding 90 mg/dL), preprandial blood sugar less than 105 mg/dL, and 2-hour postprandial blood sugars that do not exceed 120 mg/dL are considered tight control. However, some obstetricians using standard therapy with insulin strive for blood sugar levels averaging 100 mg/dL, a goal probably impossible to achieve without prolonged hospitalizations and excessively frequent hypoglycemia. If near-normalization of blood sugar is attempted, either *intensified conventional therapy* or an insulin pump should be used in conjunction with SMBG (see "Monitoring During Intensive Insulin Therapy," above). Intensified therapy is probably to be preferred because ketoacidosis and infection are significant risks with pump therapy; either complication could be lethal to the fetus.

Most patients managed with standard therapy require at least two doses of intermediate-acting insulin or mixtures of intermediate- and short-acting insulin. A few patients with type 2 diabetes may have satisfactory control on a single dose of insulin. The safety of oral agents in the therapy of pregnant type 2 diabetics is uncertain because of lack of data; most physicians advise against their use. It should be kept in mind that insulin requirements often decrease in the first trimester, only to increase during the third trimester by up to 50% and to fall again after delivery. Patients on intensive therapy should monitor their glucose in the fasting (overnight) state, before each meal, and, possibly, 2 hours after meals. In addition, monitoring during the night (2 to 3 AM) may be necessary because nocturnal hypoglycemia is common during pregnancy, especially in the first and third trimesters. Frequent monitoring of glucosuria and ketonuria remains an invaluable adjunct to ambulatory management, but only SMBG with frequent determinations can provide optimal management. Because of the disastrous effect of ketoacidosis during pregnancy, daily monitoring of urine for ketones is strongly advised. Minor ketonuria caused by carbohydrate lack is common but can usually be distinguished from ketoacidosis by rough quantitation of the ketonuria, minimal or absent glucosuria, and measurement of the blood sugar at less than 200 mg/dL. Determination of plasma bicarbonate and plasma ketones (negative when ketonuria is caused by carbohydrate lack) should be made if any doubt still exists. The development of ketoacidosis is an indication for immediate hospitalization.

Diet Therapy

Diet therapy is often modified slightly to include increased protein intake. Weight gain of about 25 lb (11.5 kg) is expected and acceptable in both normal and diabetic pregnancies. Severe weight control, previously advocated by some, has been abandoned.

Timing of Delivery

This issue is decided by the obstetrician (and neonatologist) and has been argued for decades, since it was recognized that the incidence of stillbirths in diabetic women increases beyond the 36th week. However, attempts to deliver infants early (before 40 weeks) resulted in a high rate of cesarean section and a high rate of neonatal loss caused by neonatal respiratory distress syndrome (RDS). Currently, if fetal surveillance is normal, delivery is delayed to term when it is induced if the cervix is favorable or if spontaneous labor occurs. However, if the pregnancy has been complicated by vascular disease or poor control of glucose, or if there are other adverse factors such as a prior stillbirth, delivery may be performed at 38 weeks in an effort to prevent late fetal death. Such early delivery is predicated upon finding suitable values for amniotic fluid phospholipids (lecithin/sphingomyelin [LS] ratio and the presence of phosphatidylglycerol), biochemical markers of fetal pulmonary maturation. RDS is highly unlikely if LS is greater than 2.0. Delivery despite fetal pulmonary immaturity may be necessary if the pregnant patient worsens (preeclampsia, renal failure) or there is other evidence of fetal distress.

General References*

Textbooks

Kahn CR, Weir GC, eds. Joslin's diabetes mellitus. 13th ed. Philadelphia: Lea & Febiger, 1994.

> A major textbook, already dated and heavy with accumulated information and references. If one wishes to find the old material of the field, as well as the new, this is the book.

Porte D Jr, Sherwin RF, Ellenberg M, Rifkin H, eds. Ellenberg & Rifkin's diabetes mellitus. 5th ed. East Norwalk, CT: Appleton & Lange, 1997.

> The most current major textbook available in the United States, by the most prominent people in the field. Well-printed, well-edited, and up-to-the moment clinical material.

Books for Physicians

American Diabetes Association (ADA). A series of 6 authoritative, multiauthored mini-textbooks in paperback, approximately $30–$40 each. Sold singly or as a set. Can be ordered at 800-232-6733. *Medical Management of Non-Insulin Dependent (type II) Diabetes,* 112 pp.; *Medical Management of Insulin-Dependent Diabetes Mellitus (type I),* 176 pp.; *Medical Management of Pregnancy*

---

*Bold print (general references) and bold numerals (specific references) denote published controlled clinical trials, meta-analyses, or consensus-based recommendations.

Complicated by Diabetes; Therapy for Diabetes Mellitus and Related Disorders, 384 pp.; *Intensive Diabetes Management,* 128 pp.; *The Health Professional's Guide to Diabetes and Exercise,* 352 pp. The ADA also sells slides for teaching lectures and books on the vital statistics and costs of diabetes.

Journals for Professionals

Diabetes (monthly); *Diabetes Reviews* (quarterly), *Diabetes Care* (monthly), and *Diabetes Spectrum* (nurses, dietitians, educators; quarterly).

Primarily for Educators and Patients

The American Diabetes Association publishes many first-rate materials in English and Spanish at nominal prices: *Practical Psychology for Diabetes Clinicians; Life with Diabetes; Facilitating Lifestyle Change: A Resource Manual; Diabetes Education Goals; Single-Topic Diabetes Resources,* reproducible handouts on a variety of topics; *Right from the Start; Gestational Diabetes;* and many small books on nutrition, exercise, and costs of care. A *Diabetes Resource Catalog for Health Professionals* is available. Call 800-232-6733 or fax 770-442-9742, or write to American Diabetes Association, Order Fulfillment Department, P.O. Box 930850, Atlanta, GA 31193-0850.

Miller-Fenwick, Inc. specializes in video materials for patient education (approximately $20 per tape). Spanish versions are available. Production is with the American Association of Diabetes Educators; call 800-432-8433 or fax 410-352-6316, or write to Miller-Fenwick, Inc., 2125 Greenspring Drive, Timonium, MD 21093.

Specific References

1. Amiel S. Glucose counter-regulation in health and disease: current concepts in hypoglycemia recognition and response. Q J Med 80(293):707, 1991.
2. Amiel SA, Tamborlane WV, Simonson DC, Sherwin RS. Defective glucose counter-regulation after strict glycemic control of insulin-dependent diabetes mellitus. N Engl J Med 316:1376, 1987.
3. Anonymous. Meters for glucose monitoring. Med Lett 34(886): 115, 1992.
4. Atkinson MA, Bowman MA, Kao KJ, et al. Lack of immune responsiveness to bovine serum albumin in insulin-dependent diabetes. N Engl J Med 329:1853, 1993.
5. Bailey CJ, Turner RC. Metformin. N Engl J Med 334:574, 1996.
6. Barnett AH, Eff C, Leslie RDG, Pyke DA. Diabetes in identical twins: a study of 200 pairs. Diabetologia 20:87, 1981.
7. Bjorntorp P. Visceral obesity: a "civilization syndrome." Obesity Res 1:206, 1993.
8. Boden G. Role of fatty acids in the pathogenesis of insulin resistance and NIDDM. Diabetes 46:3, 1997.
9. Bonanome A, Visona A, Lusiani L, et al. Carbohydrate and lipid metabolism in patients with non–insulin-dependent diabetes mellitus: effects of a low-fat, high-carbohydrate diet vs. a diet high in monosaturated fatty acids. Am J Clin Nutr 54:586, 1991.
10. Boyle PJ, Kempers SF, O'Connor AM, Nagy RJ. Brain glucose uptake and unawareness of hypoglycemia in patients with insulin-dependent diabetes mellitus. N Engl J Med 333:1726, 1995; Bolli GB, Fanelli CG. Unawareness of hypoglycemia (Editorial). N Engl J Med 333:1771, 1995.
11. Boyle PJ, Schwartz NS, Shah SD, et al. Plasma glucose concentrations at the onset of hypoglycemic symptoms in patients with poorly controlled diabetes and in nondiabetics. N Engl J Med 318:1487, 1988.
12. Bradley WE. Diagnosis of urinary bladder dysfunction in diabetes mellitus. Ann Intern Med 92(2):323, 1980.
13. Brownlee M, Cerami A, Vlassara H. Advanced glycosylation end products in tissue and the biochemical basis of diabetic complications. N Engl J Med 318:1315, 1988.
14. Caputo GM, Cavanagh PR, Ulbrecht JS, et al. Assessment and management of foot disease in patients with diabetes. N Engl J Med 331:854, 1994.
15. Chen Y-DI, Swami S, Skowronski R, et al. Effect of variations in dietary fat and carbohydrate intake on postprandial lipemia in patients with noninsulin dependent diabetes mellitus. J Clin Endocrinol Metab 76:347, 1993.
16. Clark CM Jr, Lee DA. Prevention and treatment of the complications of diabetes mellitus. N Engl J Med 332:1210, 1995.
17. Colwell JA. The feasibility of intensive insulin management in non–insulin-dependent diabetes mellitus. Implications of the Veterans Affairs cooperative study on Glycemic Control and Complications in NIDDM. Ann Intern Med 124:131, 1996.
18. Coulston AM, Hollenbeck CB, Swislocki ALM, et al. Deleterious metabolic effects of high-carbohydrate, sucrose-containing diets in patients with non–insulin-dependent diabetes mellitus. Am J Med 82:213, 1987.
19. Crofford OB. Metformin (Editorial). N Engl J Med 333:588, 1995.
20. Cryer PE. The metabolic impact of autonomic neuropathy in insulin-dependent diabetes mellitus (Editorial). Arch Intern Med 146:2127, 1986.
21. Cryer PE, Gerich JE. Glucose counterregulation, hypoglycemia, and intensive insulin therapy in diabetes mellitus. N Engl J Med 313:232, 1985.
22. Cryer PE, White NH, Santiago JV. The relevance of glucose counterregulatory systems to patients with insulin dependent diabetes mellitus. Endocrinol Rev 7:131, 1986.
23. DeFronzo RA, Goodman AM, and the Multicenter Metformin Study Group. Efficacy of metformin in patients with non–insulin-dependent diabetes mellitus. N Engl J Med 333:541, 1995.
24. Diabetes Control and Complications Trial Research Group. The effect of intensive diabetes treatment on the development and progression of long-term complications in insulin-dependent diabetes. N Engl J Med 329:977, 1993.
25. Diabetic retinopathy. A booklet prepared by the Retina Panel, Quality of Care Committee, the American Academy of Ophthalmology, 1989. P.O. Box 7424, San Francisco, CA 94120-7424.
26. Dinneen S, Gerich J, Rizza R. Carbohydrate metabolism in non–insulin-dependent diabetes mellitus. N Engl J Med 327: 707, 1992.
27. Dornhorst A, Girling JC. Management of gestational diabetes mellitus (Editorial). N Engl J Med 333:1281, 1995.
28. Eastman RC, Siebert CW, Harris M, Gorden P. Clinical review 51. Implications of the Diabetes Control and Complications Trial. J Clin Endocrinol Metab 77:1105, 1993.
29. Eisenbarth GS. Type I diabetes mellitus. A chronic autoimmune disease. N Engl J Med 314:1360, 1986.
30. Ellenberg M. Sexual dysfunction in diabetic patients. Ann Intern Med 92(2):331, 1980.
31. Emanuele N, Klein R, Abraira C, et al. Evaluations of retinopathy in the VA Cooperative Study on Glycemic Control and Complications in Type II Diabetes (VA CSDM). A feasibility study. Diabetes Care 19:1375, 1996.
32. Ewing DJ, Campbell IW, Clarke BF. Assessment of cardiovascular effects in diabetic autonomic neuropathy and prognostic implications. Ann Intern Med 92(2):308, 1980.
33. Expert Committee on the Diagnosis and Classification of Diabetes Mellitus. Report. Diabetes Care 20:1183, 1997.
34. Gabbe S. Gestational diabetes mellitus (Editorial). N Engl J Med 315:1025, 1988.
35. Garg A, Bonanome A, Grundy SM, et al. Comparison of a high-carbohydrate diet with a high monounsaturated-fat diet in patients with non–insulin-dependent diabetes mellitus. N Engl J Med 319:829, 1988.
36. Garrison CR, Riddle MC. Evening insulin therapy for type II diabetes. Pract Diabetol 9:1, 1990.
37. Haworth JC, McRae KN, Dilling LA. Prognosis of infants of diabetic mothers in relation to neonatal hypoglycemia. Dev Med Child Neurol 18:471, 1976.
38. Helmrich SP, Ragland DR, Leung RW, et al. Physical activity and reduced occurrence of non–insulin-dependent diabetes mellitus N Engl J Med 325:147, 1991.
39. Hirsch IB. Implementation of intensive diabetes therapy for IDDM. Diabetes Rev 3:288, 1995.
40. Holleman F, Hoekstra JBL. Insulin lispro. N Engl J Med 337:176, 1997.

41. Kahn CR, Vicent D, Doria A. Genetics of non–insulin-dependent (type II) diabetes mellitus. Ann Rev Med 47:509, 1996.

42. Karjalainen J, Martin JM, Knip M, et al. A bovine albumin peptide as a possible trigger of insulin-dependent diabetes mellitus. N Engl J Med 327:302, 1992.

43. Karjalainen J, Salmela P, Ilonen J, et al. A comparison of childhood and adult type I diabetes mellitus. N Engl J Med 320:881, 1989.

44. Klein R, Klein BE, Moss SE, et al. Glycosylated hemoglobin predicts the incidence and progression of diabetic retinopathy. JAMA 260:2864, 1988.

45. Knowler WC, Saad MF, Pettitt DJ, et al. Determinants of diabetes mellitus in the Pima Indians. Diabetes Care 16:216, 1993.

46. Korenman SG. Advances in the understanding and management of erectile dysfunction. J Clin Endocrinol Metab 80:1985, 1995.

47. Kostner GM, Karadi I. Lipoprotein alterations in diabetes mellitus. Diabetologia 31:717, 1988.

48. Kumar D, Gemayel NS, Deapen D, et al. North American twins with IDDM. Genetic, etiological, and clinical significance of disease concordance according to age, zygosity, and the interval after diagnosis in first twin. Diabetes 42:1351, 1993.

49. Laasko M. Glycemic control and the risk for coronary heart disease in patients with non–insulin-dependent diabetes mellitus. The Finnish studies. Ann Intern Med 124:127, 1996.

50. Lipsky BA, Pecoraro RF, Larson, SA, et al. Outpatient management of uncomplicated lower-extremity infections in diabetic patients. Arch Intern Med 150:790, 1990.

51. Low PA, Gilden JL, Freeman R, et al. Efficacy of midodrine vs placebo in neurogenic orthostatic hypotension. A randomized, double-blind multicenter study. JAMA 277:1046, 1997.

52. MacDonald MJ. Postexercise late-onset hypoglycemia in insulin-dependent diabetic patients. Diabetes Care 10:584, 1987.

53. Max MB, Lynch SA, Muir J, et al. Effects of desipramine, amitriptyline, and fluoxetine on pain in diabetic neuropathy. N Engl J Med 326:1250, 1992.

54. Mills JL, Knopp RH, Simpson JL, et al. Lack of relation of increased malformation rates in infants of diabetic mothers to glycemic control during organogenesis. N Engl J Med 318:671, 1988.

55. Mills JL, Simpson JL, Driscoll SG, et al. Incidence of spontaneous abortion among normal women and insulin-dependent diabetic women whose pregnancies were identified within 21 days of conception. N Engl J Med 319:1617, 1988.

56. Mitrakou A, Kelley D, Mokan M, et al. Role of reduced suppression of glucose production and diminished early insulin release in impaired glucose tolerance. N Engl J Med 326:22, 1992.

57. Nathan DM, Singer DE, Hurxthal K, et al. The clinical information value of the glycosylated hemoglobin assay. N Engl J Med 310:341, 1984.

58. National Diabetes Group. Classification and diagnosis of diabetes mellitus and other categories of glucose tolerance. Diabetes 28:1039, 1979.

59. Olmos P, A'Hern R, Heaton DA, et al. The significance of the concordance rate for type 1 (insulin-dependent) diabetes in identical twins. Diabetologia 31:747, 1988.

60. Padma-Nathan H, Hellstrom WJ, Kaiser FE, et al. Treatment of men with erectile dysfunction with transurethral alprostadil. Medicated Urethral System for Erection (MUSE) Study Group. N Engl J Med 336:1, 1997.

61. Perriello G, DeFeo P, Torlone E, et al. The effect of asymptomatic nocturnal hypoglycemia on glycemic control in diabetes mellitus. N Engl J Med 319:1233, 1988.

62. Pollet RJ, El-Kebbi IM. The applicability and implications of the DCCT to NIDDM. Diabetes Rev 2:413, 1994.

63. Polonsky K, Bergenstal R, Pons G, et al. Relation of counter-regulatory responses to hypoglycemia in type I diabetics. N Engl J Med 307:1106, 1982.

64. Polonsky KS, Sturis J, Bell GI. Non–insulin-dependent diabetes mellitus: a genetically programmed failure of the beta cell to compensate for insulin resistance. N Engl J Med 334:777, 1996.

65. Pugh JA, Wagner ML, Sawyer J, et al. Is combination sulfonylurea and insulin therapy useful in NIDDM patients? A metaanalysis. Diabetes Care 15:953, 1993.

66. Raskin P. Combination therapy in NIDDM. N Engl J Med 327:1453, 1992.

67. Reaven GM. Role of insulin resistance in human disease. Diabetes 37:1595, 1988.

68. Rith-Najarian SJ, Stolusky T, Gohdes DM. Identifying patients at high risk for lower-extremity amputation in a primary health care setting. A prospective evaluation of simple screening criteria. Diabetes Care 15:1386, 1992.

69. Rizza RA, Gerich JE, Haymond MW, et al. Control of blood sugar in insulin-dependent diabetes: comparison of an artificial endocrine pancreas, continuous subcutaneous insulin infusion and intensified conventional insulin therapy. N Engl J Med 303:1313, 1980.

70. Robertson RP. Pancreatic and islet transplantation for diabetes: cures or curiosities? N Engl J Med 327:1861, 1992.

71. Said G, Goulon-Goeau L, Slama G, Tchobroutsky G. Severe early-onset polyneuropathy in insulin-dependent diabetes mellitus. A clinical and pathological study. N Engl J Med 326:1257, 1992.

72. Saltiel AR, Olefsky JM. Thiazolidinediones in the treatment of insulin resistance and type II diabetes. Diabetes 45:1661, 1996.

73. Shorr RI, Ray WA, Daugherty JR, Griffen MR. Incidence and risk factors for serious hypoglycemia in older persons using insulin or sulfonylureas. Arch Intern Med 157:1681, 1997.

74. Stamler R, Stamler J, eds. Asymptomatic hyperglycemia and coronary heart disease. A series of papers by the International Collaborative Group, based on studies in fifteen populations. J Chronic Dis 32:683, 1979.

75. Stolar MW. Atherosclerosis in diabetes: the role of hyperinsulinemia. Metab Clin Exp 37(Suppl 1):1, 1988.

76. Tallarigo L, Giampietro O, Penno G, et al. Relation of glucose tolerance to complications of pregnancy in nondiabetic woman. N Engl J Med 315:989, 1986.

77. Tordjman KM, Havlin CE, Levandowski LA, et al. Failure of nocturnal hypoglycemia to cause fasting hyperglycemia in patients with insulin-dependent diabetes mellitus. N Engl J Med 317:1552, 1987.

78. Weissman PN, Shenkman L, Gregerman RI. Chlorpropamide hyponatremia: drug-induced inappropriate antidiuretic-hormone activity. N Engl J Med 284:65, 1971.

79. West KM. Diet therapy of diabetes: an analysis of failure. Ann Intern Med 79:425, 1973.

80. West KM. Diet and diabetes. Postgrad Med 60:209, 1976.

81. Wheat LJ, Allen SD, Henry M, et al. Diabetic foot infections. Bacteriologic analysis. Arch Intern Med 146:1935, 1986.

82. Wolffenbuttel BH, Sels J-PJE, Rondas-Colbers GJ. Comparison of different insulin regimens in elderly patients with NIDDM. Diabetes Care 19:1326, 1996.

83. World Health Organization. Diabetes mellitus: report of a WHO Study Group. Geneva: World Health Organization, 1985 (Tech. Rep. Series no. 727).

84. Yki-Jarvinen H, Kauppila M, Kujansuu E, et al. Comparison of insulin regimens in patients with non–insulin-dependent diabetes mellitus. N Engl J Med 327:1426, 1992.

85. Yoon JW. Role of viruses in the pathogenesis of IDDM. Ann Med 23:437, 1991.

86. Zinman B. The physiologic replacement of insulin. An elusive goal. N Engl J Med 321:363, 1989.

CHAPTER 73

Thyroid Disorders

ROBERT I. GREGERMAN, MD

Disturbances of thyroid growth and function are among the most common endocrinologic disorders encountered in ambulatory practice. Excessive production of the iodine-containing thyroid hormones thyroxine (T_4) and triiodothyronine (T_3) (Fig. 73.1) results in *hyperthyroidism* or *thyrotoxicosis;* decreased hormone production results in *hypothyroidism.* Generalized enlargement of the thyroid, regardless of cause, is termed *goiter.* Focal enlargement of the thyroid is termed a *nodule* and is usually benign. Either goiter or focal enlargement may be associated with abnormal thyroid function. Goiter can produce anatomic changes ranging from simply cosmetic to obstruction of contiguous structures such as the trachea and esophagus.

THYROID PHYSIOLOGY

Thyroid Regulatory Mechanisms

The principal regulatory mechanism of the thyroid is the hypothalamic–pituitary–thyroid negative feedback control system. The hypothalamus secretes thyrotropin-releasing hormone (TRH), which travels via the hypophyseal portal system to the pituitary, where it stimulates release of thyroid-stimulating hormone (TSH). TSH stimulates many aspects of thyroid activity, including hormone synthesis, thyroid growth, and the release of thyroid hormones. Secretion of TSH by the pituitary is inhibited by the thyroid hormones—thus the term *negative feedback loop.*

The thyroid hormones are unique because they are the only substances in the body that contain the trace element iodine. Iodide from plasma is concentrated by an active process (iodide "pump") that can maintain a thyroid/plasma iodide ratio as high as 500 to 1. Iodide is thereafter converted through a series of enzymatic steps resulting in the formation of T_4 and T_3 within the thyroglobulin sequence. The iodide pump transports a

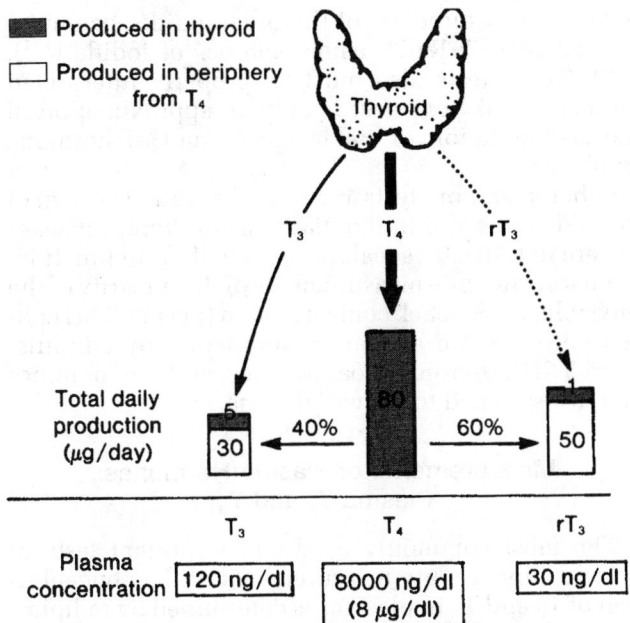

- ■ Produced in thyroid
- □ Produced in periphery from T_4

Thyroid

T_3 T_4 rT_3

Total daily production (µg/day)

5 / 30   ←40%— 80 —60%→   1 / 50

T₃   T₄   rT₃

Plasma concentration: | 120 ng/dl | | 8000 ng/dl (8 µg/dl) | | 30 ng/dl |

Figure 73.1. Production rates by the thyroid and in the periphery of thyroid hormones and their mean concentrations in the plasma.

number of anions other than iodide, a phenomenon that has been exploited diagnostically and therapeutically. For example, the pertechnetate anion, TcO_4^-, as the radioactive isotope ^{99m}Tc, has been widely used for thyroid imaging, although ^{123}I is now preferred.

The minimal daily requirement of iodide is only about 100 to 200 µg, an amount that is determined by obligatory loss, mainly through the kidney. In the United States and in most of the developed countries, the minimal daily requirement is enormously exceeded by dietary intake because of the addition of iodide to the dietary salt ("iodized salt"); for example, iodized salt provides about 1000 µg in a normal 10-g daily intake. Thus, iodide deficiency and its concomitant iodide-deficiency goiter is no longer seen in the United States but is still a major problem in many parts of the world (34) (see also "Goiter").

Any chemical substance that interferes with thyroid hormone function or release may lower blood hormone concentration and induce compensatory hypertrophy of the gland (goiter) via stimulation of TSH secretion. Certain substances are known to prevent iodide accumulation by impairment of the iodide pump. Other substances interfere with hormone synthesis or inhibit hormone release. Clinically useful agents that have been used for therapeutic effects in states of excess hormone production (hyperthyroidism) are known to act at one or another of these points. Perchlorate, now used therapeutically only occasionally, inhibits the iodide pump. The thiocarbamide "antithyroid" drugs (e.g., propylthiouracil, methimazole) interfere with hormone synthesis by blockade of incorporation of iodide into the tyrosines (organification) and with coupling reactions in iodothyronine formation, but they have more effect on coupling than on organifica-

tion. Lithium ion (currently in wide use for the treatment of affective disorders, see Chapter 15), interferes with thyroglobulin proteolysis and hormone release and may result in goiter and, occasionally, hypothyroidism. Lithium also interferes with the action of TSH on the thyroid, and therefore some cases of hypothyroidism caused by lithium are not associated with goiter. Iodide itself in pharmacologic amounts interferes with hormone formation and release and in some individuals is a goitrogen.

Metabolic Effects of Thyroid Hormone

The thyroid hormones exert their actions through a variety of mechanisms. A classic thyroid hormone effect is on metabolic rate. Measurement of *basal metabolic rate* (BMR) was the basis for the first laboratory method for clinical assessment of thyroid status. The numerous known actions of thyroid hormones range from specific stimulation of mitochondrial oxidative metabolism to the nuclear regulation of protein synthesis. Thyroid hormones also exert specific regulatory effects on membrane function (e.g., potentiation of catecholamine effects). This action of thyroid hormones explains the signs of exaggerated sympathetic activity in hyperthyroidism and the effectiveness of the therapy of this condition by β-adrenergic blockade.

Hormone Transport

The thyroid hormones in the blood are T_4 and a much smaller quantity of T_3. Both hormones are tightly but reversibly bound to several plasma proteins, mainly thyroid hormone–binding globulin (TBG). In the normal person, 65 to 70% of the thyroid hormones are bound to TBG, approximately 15% to the secondary carrier, transthyretin (TTR), formerly called thyroxine-binding prealbumin (TBPA), and approximately 15% to albumin. Variations of TBG occur in many clinical states and account for most of the changes in T_4 concentration in plasma that are seen in a variety of diseases, including hypothyroidism and hyperthyroidism. Small quantities of T_4 (0.03%) and T_3 (0.3%) are not protein bound but are free and in rapid equilibrium with the protein-bound fraction.

The concentrations of free T_4 and T_3 in plasma are thought to reflect the amount of hormone exerting an effect on tissues. Clinical status in a number of conditions correlates with free T_4 rather than with total hormone in plasma. A good example of this correlation is the normal pregnant state in which total T_4 is high but in which there is no clinical or laboratory evidence of free thyroid hormone excess. Much of the elevation is due to increased glycosylation (sialation) and binding capacity of TBG, as well as to an increase in the protein concentration.

In some pathologic states that affect the quantity of TBG in plasma (Table 73.1), and hence the total T_4, the absolute concentration of free T_4 may not adjust to a normal value. During a variety of nonthyroidal illnesses, undefined factors in plasma other than the

Table 73.1. Factors Affecting Thyroxine-Binding Globulin (TBG)

TBG Increased	TBG Decreased
Estrogens	Androgens
Exogenous	Anabolic steroids
Pregnancy	Cirrhosis
Hypothyroidism	Glucocorticoids
Acute hepatitis	Nephrotic syndrome
Cirrhosis	Severe chronic nonthyroidal
Genetic TBG excess	illness
Acute intermittent porphyria	Cushing's syndrome
Perphenazine (Trilafon)	Genetic TBG deficiency

concentration of TBG and TTR (TBPA) appear to determine the free hormone concentration, presumably by decreasing the affinity of the interaction of binding proteins with T_4 (see "Free T_4" and "Estimates of TBG," below).

Metabolism and Interconversion of Thyroid Hormones

Practically all tissues metabolize and degrade the thyroid hormones, but the liver is quantitatively most important as a site at which regulation of hormone degradation occurs. T_4 metabolism is the major source (80%) of circulating T_3 in the normal individual. The normal thyroid secretes mainly T_4 and only a small amount of T_3 (Fig. 73.1). Only in hyperthyroidism, iodine deficiency, and certain other pathologic circumstances is T_3 sometimes the predominantly secreted hormone.

Approximately 85% of the T_4 secreted is ultimately deiodinated and further degraded. The physiologically most important pathway involves conversion of approximately 35% of the T_4 to metabolically active T_3, which is itself further deiodinated. About an equal amount of T_4 is converted to reverse T_3 (rT_3) (Fig. 73.1). Although not active in calorigenesis, rT_3 does antagonize a number of the effects of T_3 and thus may have some physiologic importance. In a variety of pathologic states, the formation of T_3 is inhibited, whereas that of rT_3 is reciprocally enhanced. Measurement of rT_3 has some usefulness in the differential diagnosis of the "euthyroid sick syndrome" (see "Differential Diagnosis" under "Hypothyroidism").

LABORATORY TESTS OF THYROID FUNCTION AND OF THYROID DISEASE

Most thyroid function tests assess secretory activity of the thyroid gland indirectly. Measurements of blood hormone concentrations, the most commonly used tests, cannot be equated directly with the rate of hormone production, although they reflect that rate when plasma binding of hormones is normal. However, various illnesses, drugs, and alterations of physiologic state affect plasma binding. Accordingly, proper interpretation of plasma hormone concentrations demands concomitant assessment of plasma binding. Thyroid gland function can be assessed somewhat more di-

rectly by measurement of thyroidal iodide accumulation ("uptake"; RaIU) using isotopes of iodide (^{131}I, ^{123}I). These tests also must be properly interpreted because uptake of tracer is only an approximation of the accumulation of stable iodide and of hormone synthesis.

Other laboratory tests are useful in the assessment of thyroid status and in the diagnosis of thyroid disease but are not, strictly speaking, tests of thyroid function. Such tests include measurements of the integrity of the physiologic feedback control system (plasma TSH concentration before and after stimulation by administered TRH), thyroid autoantibodies, and the immunoglobulins related to Graves' disease.

Measurements of Plasma Hormones: Plasma T_4 and T_3

The most commonly used and important tests of thyroid function are measurements of the concentration of T_4 and T_3 in plasma, as determined by radioimmunoassay or other specific methods. rT_3 is occasionally also used in differential diagnosis, especially of ill patients. The concentration of T_4 in plasma is certainly the single most important measurement in clinical evaluation of thyroid disease. However, interpretation of a given value (concentration) must consider whether T_4 binding to plasma proteins is normal. Accordingly, T_4 must be measured in conjunction with assessment of hormone binding to plasma proteins or with determination of TBG. In practice this is done by determining the free T_4 or the free T_4 index (see below). Normal values of the common tests are given in Table 73.2.

Free T_4: Measurement of Non–Protein-Bound Thyroid Hormone in Plasma

The free T_4 of plasma is estimated by separate measurements of the percentage of non–protein-bound T_4 (usually by equilibrium dialysis—using isotopic T_4, added to the serum) and the total T_4; their arithmetic product equals the free T_4 in ng%. The dialyzable (non–protein-bound) T_4 normally approximates only 0.03% of the total. New methods are beginning to be used in which free T_4 is measured directly, by a sensitive assay.

The free T_4 hypothesis (see above) has been helpful as a physiologic concept. Determination of the free T_4 for clinical purposes is often useful. In some clinical states, such as pregnancy or during estrogen therapy, both T_4 and TBG are elevated and thyroid status is accurately reflected by the free T_4: the dialyzable fraction is decreased, but because the T_4 is elevated, the free T_4 is normal. In hyperthyroidism, free T_4 reflects thyroid status better than total T_4 because the altered metabolic state of hyperthyroidism itself lowers TBG; in some cases a normal or borderline elevation of T_4 is associated with a clearly elevated free T_4. In hypothyroidism, TBG is often elevated and the free T_4 is decreased more than is the total T_4.

Problems of interpretation of the free T_4 arise in

many seriously ill patients. A variety of nonthyroidal diseases ranging from acute infections to liver disease can result in elevation of the free T_4. In these situations, the patient is usually euthyroid with a normal T_4; the free T_4 is elevated only because the dialyzable fraction is increased. An explanation for this phenomenon is not readily available. Altered concentrations of neither TBG nor TTR account for the increased free T_4. The appearance of a factor in plasma that interferes with protein binding of T_4 has been demonstrated. Thus, an elevated free T_4 is not a specific finding related solely to thyroid status. Moreover, the test is several times more expensive than the free T_4 index, which is preferred as the single most effective screening test of thyroid function (see below).

Estimates of TBG: T_3 Resin Uptake and Free T_4 Index (FTI)

The T_3 uptake test (T_3U) is not to be confused with the concentration of T_3 in plasma. The T_3U is not a thyroid function test but merely provides an indirect estimate of the concentration of plasma TBG. To some extent, T_3U is also influenced by the quantity of T_4 in plasma (i.e., by the degree of saturation of the T_4 [and T_3] binding sites on TBG). The T_3U may eventually be replaced by direct quantitation of TBG. Technically, the T_3U is measured by adding a tracer quantity of T_3 and a nonspecific T_3 binding absorbent (resin) to the sample of plasma to be tested. The tracer distributes itself between nonspecific binding sites on the resin and specific binding sites on TBG. Resin-bound tracer is therefore reciprocally related to the quantity of TBG in the plasma. The test result is expressed either as a percentage or as a ratio of the test sample to that of the laboratory's control plasma (T_3U ratio).

The usefulness of the T_3U is in interpreting a given level of T_4. A high (or low) T_4 can be interpreted as reflecting increased or decreased T_4 secretion only if the plasma binding of T_4 is normal (i.e., only if the TBG [T_3U] is normal). Otherwise, to reach a proper conclusion about thyroid function, disturbance of binding must be considered along with the high (or low) T_4. For convenience the T_4 and T_3U have been combined to give a so-called free T_4 index (FTI) by simply multiplying one number times the other (the index is sometimes designated the "T_7" or "T_{12}"). This widely used index compensates for the high or low T_4 value that results from the abnormality of TBG concentration. In most, but not all, cases, FTI closely parallels free T_4.

In severely ill patients of the type more likely to be hospitalized than to be ambulatory, the FTI may be misleading. In such cases the resin uptake is elevated, not because TBG is low but as the result of the appearance in plasma of a nonspecific inhibitor of hormone binding that affects the distribution of tracer T_3 between sites in plasma and sites on the resin. Both the free T_4 and FTI tests must be interpreted with caution in any patient with severe nonthyroidal illness.

Tests of the Negative Feedback System

Thyroid-Stimulating Hormone

Plasma TSH is invariably elevated in primary hypothyroidism because of reduced feedback inhibition by the decreased concentrations of the thyroid hormones. The measurement of plasma TSH is important both in the diagnosis of primary hypothyroidism and in monitoring the adequacy of thyroid hormone replacement therapy (see below). Elevation of plasma TSH is the most sensitive indicator of hypothyroid status, but not every elevated TSH indicates hypothyroidism (see below). Elevations of TSH were for many years reliably measured by radioimmunoassay, but the available assays were not sufficiently sensitive to detect *suppression* of TSH. Newer immunoradiometric (second generation) and chemiluminescent (third generation) assays have been introduced that can quantitate TSH within the normal and subnormal range. As a result, the determination of TSH has become an important diagnostic measurement and alternative to measurement of TRH testing (see below) when blood levels of T_4 and T_3 are only borderline. Another use for the sensitive TSH assay is in assessing replacement therapy with T_4 (see below). Recent evidence indicates that suppression or even modest elevation of TSH may be seen in, or during the recovery phase of, a variety of nonthyroidal illnesses, at least in hospitalized patients. Thus one should be cautious in interpreting these assays (including third-generation assays) even in ambulatory patients when they are seriously ill (23).

Most important, the newer assays for TSH have been widely but often inappropriately used as single tests for the diagnosis of hyperthyroidism. Although they have a high degree of sensitivity, they are not specific. Thus, the TSH assays must be interpreted in the context of the clinical circumstances and along with simultaneous measurements of the circulating thyroid hormones. Modest elevations of TSH (20 µU/mL or less) similarly should not be overinterpreted (26). Such elevations are

Table 73.2. Thyroid Function Tests[a]

	Plasma T_4 (µg/dL)	Plasma T_3 (ng/dL)	T_3 Resin Uptake (T_3U) (%)	T_3 Resin Uptake Ratio (T_3UR)	TSH (µU/mL)	Free T_4 (FT$_4$) (ng/dL)	Free T_4 Index (FTI)[b]
Normal mean	8	120	30	1		1.5	8.0
Normal range	5–12	80–160	25–35	0.85–1.15	0.3–5	1.0–2.0	5.8–10.6
Confidence limits	±1	±20	±2	±0.05		±0.3	

[a]See the text for limitations of interpretation of normal ranges. Confidence limits (95%) of a single value are approximate and depend on both the laboratory and the level within the range.

[b]The FTI on any sample is calculated as $T_4 \times T_3UR$, but the normal range for the FTI is determined empirically. The units of the FTI depend on whether the percentage T_3 resin update or the T_3 resin uptake ratio is multiplied times T_4.

common in healthy elderly people, especially women, and in the recovery phase of acute illness; they do not necessarily indicate hypothyroidism (see "Subclinical Hyperthyroidism; Subclinical Hypothyroidism" and "Screening for Thyroid Disease").

TRH Test

Parenterally administered TRH produces release of TSH from the pituitary. Response to TRH is abnormal in several clinical circumstances and can be diagnostically useful.

The TRH test remains occasionally useful in the diagnosis of primary hypothyroidism. In minimal clinical hypothyroidism, the serum T_4 may be within the lower part of the normal range and the TSH may be borderline or only minimally elevated, even after repeated testing. In such cases an exaggerated plasma TSH response to TRH is seen. In normal people the increment of TSH after TRH administration does not usually exceed 30 µU/mL, but elevations several times this amount may be seen in cases of borderline hypothyroidism.

Until a few years ago, the most common use of the TRH test was in the diagnosis of suspected hyperthyroidism. The advent of sensitive assays for TSH (see above) makes the TRH test obsolete, for this purpose. In the absence of severe illness, lack of significant increase of TSH suggests hyperthyroidism. However, if a second- or preferably third-generation TSH assay is not available or is equivocal, a TRH test can be done. The TRH test is also occasionally useful in the differential diagnosis of severely ill patients with low plasma T_4 (see "Hypothyroidism Versus Euthyroid Sick Syndrome," below). The test is of limited use in the elderly in whom lack of response to TRH can be normal.

The test is performed by injecting 500 µg of TRH intravenously. Plasma TSH is measured before injection and at 20 and 30 minutes after. A significant response is an increase of more than 1 microunit/mL. The general physician can easily perform the TRH test in the office. (The TRH [Thypinone] can be bought through any commercial pharmacy.)

Thyroidal Radioiodide Uptake (RaIU) Tests

The rate of tracer iodide accumulation (^{131}I, ^{123}I) in the thyroid can be measured by using times ranging from a few minutes to the plateau of accumulation (24 hours). These procedures, although still in wide use, have been rendered almost obsolete by the simpler and less expensive measurements of hormone concentrations in plasma. The diagnostic usefulness of the RaIU in the United States is also seriously limited by the saturation of the diet with iodide from table salt. This has resulted in RaIU values that are too low to discriminate normal function from hypofunction, so the test is now useless for the diagnosis of hypothyroidism. It is still of diagnostic usefulness in hyperthyroidism, although because results are normal in up to 50% of cases of proven hyperthyroidism, a normal RaIU does not exclude the diagnosis. One important

use of the test is in patients with hyperthyroidism associated with thyroiditis. If this condition is suspected, an RaIU is important; a low value deters inappropriate therapy. Determination of the RaIU is sometimes used in the selection of dosage in RaI therapy. The RaIU is subject to interference by various chemical agents, especially iodide-containing drugs and the radiographic media used in pyelograms, cholecystograms and in computerized tomography (CT) contrast imaging. Certain clinical states also produce false-positive or false-negative results.

Immunologic Tests

Assay of antibodies to thyroidal constituents (thyroglobulin, microsomes), so-called thyroid autoantibodies, is useful in determining the presence of autoimmune thyroiditis, in the differential diagnosis of goiter and in predicting the significance of elevations of TSH (see "Hypothyroidism" and "Goiter," below). The term *microsomal antibodies* is synonymous with TPO (thyroid peroxidase) antibodies. Assays for thyroid-stimulating immunoglobulin (TSI) (see "Graves' Disease," below) are not yet readily available. TSI measurements are useful in the pregnant hyperthyroid patient because high levels are associated with an increased likelihood of neonatal hyperthyroidism. A fall in TSI is a good indicator of remission in Graves' disease. The original test for TSI, a bioassay called the long-acting thyroid stimulator (LATS) test, still performed in some laboratories, is useless.

Other Tests: Fine-Needle Aspiration, Needle Biopsies, and Imaging

Fine-needle aspiration (FNA) for cytologic examination or biopsy of the thyroid for the diagnosis of nodules (see "Thyroid Nodules," below) and other enlargements is now routine in many centers. Although the procedure may fail to distinguish benign adenomas from well-differentiated follicular carcinomas (38), it may help avoid many operations and may provide much needed reassurance for the patient. Unfortunately, pathology reports that lack definitiveness or that routinely end with a statement such as "... carcinoma cannot be excluded" merely ensure that surgery will be done. *FNA* (25-gauge needle) with cytologic examination is the usual procedure of choice because it is simple, virtually painless, and without complications (see "Thyroid Nodules"). The procedure is performed by an endocrinologist or another trained specialist. A few centers use *needle biopsy* (aspiration or cutting), usually performed only if the simpler FNA is not sufficiently informative. In the hands of an appropriate operator, needle biopsy is probably more definitive and, because it is performed with local (cutaneous) anesthesia, is ordinarily painless. The only significant complication is local hemorrhage, but this is an uncommon problem and usually is of minor degree. Ultrasound or CT guidance is sometimes used.

Various *imaging techniques* are available to delineate the anatomy of the thyroid and to distinguish functional from nonfunctional tissue, a consideration in the differential diagnosis of thyroid neoplasms. These include radioisotopic scanning (scintiscan), CT scanning, and magnetic resonance imaging (MRI). The isotope most widely used is ^{99m}Tc pertechnetate (TcO_4^-), but ^{123}I is the isotope of choice. (Some tumors accumulate pertechnetate, thereby obscuring the diagnosis.) *Ultrasonography* is now a routine procedure for distinguishing cystic from solid nodules, an important point in differential diagnosis of these lesions. Moreover, ultrasonography can accurately assess the size of nodules, providing an objective basis for evaluation of changes in the size of the nodule and of medical therapy. Both imaging and ultrasonography can determine whether a nodule is truly single or is in fact one of many in a multinodular gland. CT and MRI add nothing to sonography except that these techniques may be useful in evaluating substernal extension of goiters and in follow-up of patients with thyroid cancer.

Nonspecificity of Thyroid Function Tests in Nonthyroidal Illness

Thyroid function tests may be nonspecifically altered in many nonthyroidal diseases (9,56,58); that is, these tests are not specific when severe illness is present (Table 73.3). Moreover, a variety of drugs affect both thyroid function and the function tests (Tables 73.1 and 73.4). Some examples are presented below.

Effects of Gonadal and Adrenal Hormones on Thyroid Function

Estrogens (pregnancy, contraceptives) raise and androgens lower T_4 by altering plasma TBG. Glucocorticoids inhibit thyroid activity acutely by interfering with TSH secretion and affecting the pituitary's responsiveness to TRH. The plasma T_4 is lowered during chronic glucocorticoid therapy, mainly because of a decrease of TBG.

Table 73.3. Nonthyroidal Illness: Effects on T_4, Free T_4, TBG, and TSH in Plasma[a,b]

	T_4	Free T_4	TBG	TSH
Liver Disease				
Active hepatitis	↑	↔↑	↑	
Cirrhosis, other chronic diseases	↑↓	↔↑	↑↓	↔↑
Cholangitis	↑	↔↑	↑	
Renal Disease				
Nephrotic syndrome	↔↓	↔	↔↓	
Uremia, chronic	↔↓	↔↓	↔↓	
Infections	↓	↑	↔	
Malnutrition	↔↓	↔↑	↔↓	
Severe Acute Illness[c]	↑↓	↔↑	↔	↑↓

[a]Most illnesses and even such minor alterations of physiological state as decreased food intake will produce a decrease of plasma T_3.

[b]Changes of TSH not likely in ambulatory patients.

[c]Not likely to be seen in ambulatory patients.

Table 73.4. Drug and Hormone Effects on T_4, Free T_4, TBG, and TSH

Gonadal Hormones	T_4	Free T_4	TBG	TSH
Estrogens	↑	↔↓	↑	
Exogenous				
Pregnancy				↓
Androgens	↓	↔		
Testosterone		↑		
Anabolic steroids				
Glucocorticoids	↓	↔	↓	
Cushing's syndrome				
Pharmacologic uses				
Psychotropic Drugs				
Perphenazine (Trilafon)	↑	↔	↑	
Amphetamines	↑	↑	↔	
Anticonvulsants				
Phenytoin (Dilantin)	↓	↔↓	↔	↔↑
Heparin	↔	↑	↔	
Adrenergic Blockers				
Propranolol (Inderal)	↔ (↓T_3)	↔	↔	
Antiarrhythmic Drugs				
Amiodarone	↑	↑	↔	
Gallbladder Dyes				
Iopanoic acid	↑↔ (↓T_3)	↔↑	↔↑	↔↑
Ipodate	↑↔ (↓T_3)	↔↑	↔	↔↑
Opiates	↑		↑	
Miscellaneous				
Clofibrate	↑		↑	
5-Fluorouracil	↑		↑	

Liver Diseases

Various alterations of thyroid function tests are produced by liver disease. Early in infectious hepatitis, the T_4 level is elevated secondary to an increase of TBG. Chronic liver disease produces many abnormalities in an unpredictable fashion. T_4 may be increased or decreased in parallel with TBG and the T_3U. Free T_4 is often elevated with no obvious relationship to the TBG. T_3 is usually low. A frequent and unexplained abnormality is elevation of TSH, although the response to TRH is not exaggerated as it is in hypothyroidism. RaIU is often elevated in acute alcoholic hepatitis with or without cirrhosis and in some cases of cholangitis. These changes have been attributed to both iodide depletion and acceleration of T_4 metabolism.

Renal Diseases

The nephrotic syndrome is often associated with depressed T_4, but the decrease is not always explained by a lowering of the TBG. In chronic renal disease, the group means of T_4, TBG, and the FTI are not significantly different from normal, but the range is greater and values may exceed the usual normal limits. Some patients with severe chronic renal failure receiving long-term dialysis show a progressive decrease of T_4. As expected in any chronic illness, the plasma T_3 is often depressed.

Infections, Malnutrition, and Drugs

The T_4 may drop early in the course of acute infection and free T_4 may rise. Neither change is accounted for by an alteration of TBG. During starvation, plasma T_3 falls. Free T_4 is often increased without relation to the TBG. Plasma T_3 is often decreased in the elderly, a change that has been attributed to aging but may in large part be caused by diminished food intake and nonspecific illness. Closely correlated alterations of T_3U and plasma TBG have been reported in protein-calorie malnutrition. Some pharmacologic agents affect the thyroid hormones of plasma (2) (Table 73.4). Phenytoin (Dilantin) lowers the T_4 and free T_4, often into the hypothyroid range. Although plasma TSH may be somewhat elevated, clinical hypothyroidism is not seen. Heparin acutely elevates the free T_4. The mechanisms of these changes are unknown. β-Adrenergic blockers decrease plasma T_3 by inhibition of the normal T_4 deiodination route; rT_3 is increased. A similar decrease of T_3 through reduced hepatic metabolism of T_4 is produced by propylthiouracil, dexamethasone, amiodarone, and the radiopaque contrast media used for visualization of the gallbladder. In the case of the latter agents, additional mechanisms are operative because these compounds also elevate T_4 and TSH, an effect attributed to their inhibition of conversion of T_4 and T_3 in the pituitary and the periphery. Amphetamine abuse may increase plasma T_4, presumably by central stimulation of TSH release (9).

Altered Plasma T_4 Caused by Inherited and Other Abnormalities of Protein Binding

In addition to those disease states in which T_4 levels are related to altered hormone binding to TBG, other situations that are explicable in terms of altered protein binding include inherited disorders of TBG excess, TBG deficiency, increases of concentration of TBPA, and increases in the number of T_4 binding sites on an albumin variant (familial dysalbuminemic hyperthyroxinemia). The first two conditions are X-linked. The latter two conditions, inherited as autosomal dominants, are rare. All of these conditions can produce diagnostic difficulties, however, because they are not detected by the T_3 resin uptake; and the free T_4 index is accordingly elevated, although the free T_4 is normal (9), if measured by equilibrium dialysis. If a newer method of measurement of T_4 is used, the T_4 may be spuriously elevated.

Alterations of Plasma T_4 in Nonthyroidal Illness Not Caused by Abnormalities of Protein Binding

Elevations of T_4 that are unexplained by changes in thyroxine binding are common. These situations are most difficult to distinguish from hyperthyroidism. Included are the elevation of T_4 seen in acute nonthyroidal illness, in psychiatric disease, and as the effect of some drugs. The stress of serious illness may also lower T_4 and simulate hypothyroidism, but such severe illness is rarely encountered in ambulatory patients. An exception may be seen in patients receiving dialysis for chronic renal failure. Abnormal thyroid hormone levels in these situations and diseases that are regularly associated with such changes (9,56,58) are described briefly below.

Increase of Plasma T_4 During Nonspecific Illness. Although the phenomenon of decreased T_4 during

severe illness is now widely recognized (see above), the frequent occurrence of increased T_4 (and FTI) caused by illness is not generally appreciated. The increase of T_4 is modest, and the T_4 generally does not exceed about 15 μg. This problem is commonly seen in severely ill elderly patients in whom it raises the issue of hyperthyroidism (26). Similar findings have been reported in hyperemesis gravidarum.

Acute Psychiatric Illness. Restlessness, hyperactivity, tachycardia, and tremor are often seen as part of severe, acute psychiatric illness. Clinical suspicion of hyperthyroidism leads to thyroid function tests and laboratory results consistent with this diagnosis. Such patients may have elevated T_4, FTI, and T_3. In some series, up to one-third of acutely hospitalized psychiatric patients have an elevated T_4. Although the phenomenon is documented only in hospitalized patients, it may be encountered in any severely disturbed person. The T_4 returns to normal within 1 to 2 weeks of clinical improvement of the psychiatric disturbance.

Increased Plasma T_4 Caused by Resistance to Thyroid Hormones. Rare but well-recognized cases of increased T_4 unaccompanied by binding protein abnormalities are seen with peripheral resistance to thyroid hormones. Originally described as a familial syndrome of increased T_4, goiter, deaf mutism, and some degree of hypothyroidism with delayed bone maturation and epiphyseal stippling, the most common situation is actually that of elevated T_4 in a phenotypically normal person without evidence of hyperthyroidism. The abnormality occurs both sporadically and in familial form and is probably part of a heterogeneous group of disorders with variable inheritance (59). Most cases are due to abnormal (mutant) thyroid hormone receptors.

Interpretation of Thyroid Function Tests: Statistical Considerations

No single numerical value divides normal from abnormal in any thyroid function test. The upper and lower limits of normal for plasma T_4, free T_4 index, and T_3 are set at ±2 standard deviations from the mean. By definition, therefore, 2.5% of normal people will have abnormal values at each end of the distribution. To complicate the issue, a small number of hyperthyroid or hypothyroid patients have values that fall within the normal range. In addition to the statistical overlap, both biological day-to-day variation and unavoidable analytical error further obscure the dividing line between normal and abnormal. For example, 95% confidence limits of a single T_4 test are ±1 μg/dL at the upper and lower limits of the normal range. For all of these reasons and because of the occasional instance of laboratory or reporting error, a single determination can neither establish nor exclude a diagnosis with anything more than reasonable statistical certainty. Therefore all abnormal values should be confirmed before therapy is undertaken, and borderline values should be repeated several times before drawing conclusions. Occasionally it will be impossible to determine with certainty whether one is dealing with a normal value or an evolving clinical state.

HYPERTHYROIDISM (THYROTOXICOSIS)

Hyperthyroidism is the clinical state resulting from an excess of thyroid hormone. Although essentially the same clinical picture results from any of several distinct pathologic processes (Table 73.5), selection of proper therapy demands that the correct diagnosis be established. The most common variety of hyperthyroidism is *Graves' disease*, an autoimmune process also known as *diffuse toxic goiter*. Only slightly less common is hyperthyroidism caused by a hyperfunctioning multinodular goiter (toxic nodular goiter). Occasionally hyperthyroidism is caused by a *solitary hyperfunctioning adenoma*. Hyperthyroidism also has been seen with increasing frequency as a transient phenomenon in the evolution of *thyroiditis* (28,40). In addition, the induction of hyperthyroidism by iodide and iodide-containing drugs (e.g., amiodarone) and contrast media should be considered for those patients who have had such exposures (22). The other causes of hyperthyroidism listed in Table 73.5 are so rare that they are not usually encountered in ordinary practice.

Graves' Disease

Graves' disease is a complex disorder comprising toxic goiter, ophthalmopathy, and occasionally dermopathy. At any given time during the course of the disease, one of these manifestations may be an isolated finding. Graves' ophthalmopathy and Graves' dermopathy can occur independently of thyroid hormone excess. It is generally accepted that ophthalmopathy and dermopathy are closely related but separate and overlapping immunologic disorders.

Table 73.5. Causes of Hyperthyroidism[a]

Common
Graves' disease
Toxic nodular goiter
   Multinodular
   Uninodular
Hyperthyroidism in association with thyroiditis
Postpartum hyperthyroidism
Iodide induced (iodide, iodine-containing drugs and contrast media)

Rare to Vanishingly Rare
Thyrotoxicosis caused by TSH or TSH-like stimulator
   Choriocarcinoma or hydatidiform mole
   Embryonal cell carcinoma of testis
   Pituitary tumor with TSH excess
   Idiopathic TSH excess
Toxic thyroid carcinoma
Hyperthyroidism caused by exogenous thyroid hormone
   Factitia
   Medicamentosa (iatrogenic)
Toxic struma ovarii

[a]Listed in approximate decreasing order of frequency.

Various abnormal immunoglobulins are found in the plasma of patients with Graves' disease. Some of these immunoglobulins have TSH-like activity and are designated thyroid-stimulating immunoglobulins (TSIs); they are antibodies to the normal receptor sites for TSH. The reasons for development of abnormal immunoglobulins in Graves' disease are not clearly understood. Recent thinking views Graves' disease as a failure of T-cell surveillance rather than as a response to thyroid antigens released from a thyroid damaged by unknown causes.

The plasma of some patients with Graves' *ophthalmopathy* contains a factor (exophthalmos-producing substance [EPS]) that produces exophthalmos and other abnormalities of orbital tissues in suitable test animals. In Graves' ophthalmopathy, the extraocular muscles show interstitial edema, increased connective tissue, fatty infiltration, and infiltration with lymphocytes. Eventually, gross degenerative changes such as fibrosis may occur (see "Ophthalmopathy of Graves' Disease," below).

Dermopathy, a unique, albeit unusual, finding in Graves' disease, consists of more or less circumscribed areas of mucopolysaccharide deposition, typically over the shins—hence the term *pretibial myxedema*. This unfortunate designation unjustifiably suggests a relationship between the very different type of generalized mucopolysaccharide deposition in hypothyroidism and the localized deposition in Graves' disease. No relationship exists between these processes.

Clinical Presentation and Diagnosis of Hyperthyroidism

Historical Features

The presentation of the patient with hyperthyroidism is highly variable (Table 73.6). The severity of the thyrotoxic aspect is determined by not only the degree of hormone excess but also its rapidity of onset, its duration, and the age of the patient. The "typical" patient has one or more of the following spontaneous complaints: nervousness, weight loss, palpitations (which at first may be intermittent), enlarging neck mass (goiter), change in appearance of eyes (Graves' disease), or symptoms of heart failure. These symptoms usually have been present anywhere from a few weeks to up to a year or longer.

As the disease progresses in severity, *skeletal muscle wasting* occurs, which tends to involve especially the limb girdle musculature, producing a proximal myopathy. This problem may result in weakness, expressed, for example, as great difficulty in climbing stairs or, on examination, in arising from a squatting position. Exertional dyspnea without evidence of cardiac failure is common and may be related to the myopathy.

The so-called *nervousness* is typically irritability, inability to concentrate, restlessness, or overt emotional lability, but it is the tremor that most often leads the patient to express this complaint. Impairment of normal sleep pattern with frequent wakening is common.

Table 73.6.   Signs and Symptoms of Hyperthyroidism

Organ or System	Signs and Symptoms
Adrenergic manifestations	Excess sweating, heat intolerance, palpitations, tachycardia, tremor, lid lag, stare, nervousness, and excitability
Hypermetabolism and catabolism	Increased appetite, weight loss
One system predominance	
Eyes[a]	Periorbital edema, exophthalmos (proptosis), chemosis, ophthalmoplegia, papilledema
Cardiac	Arrhythmia, congestive heart failure
Muscle	Fatigue and weakness, muscle wasting, proximal myopathy, periodic paralysis
Gastrointestinal	Increased frequency of bowel movements, pernicious vomiting
Bone	Acropachy, osteoporosis, hypercalcemia
Reproductive	Infertility, abortion, scanty menses, testicular atrophy, gynecomastia
Mental	Anxiety, irritability, psychosis, insomnia
Skin	Onycholysis, "pretibial" myxedema, hyperpigmentation

[a]Graves' disease only.

The *weight loss* classically occurs in the face of increased appetite, although often no obvious change in appetite is noticed or there may actually be anorexia, especially in elderly patients. The only prominent gastrointestinal symptom is increased frequency of bowel movements, but true diarrhea is not seen.

The *heat intolerance* of hyperthyroidism is often apparent only on questioning. Commonly the patient admits to having reduced the number of covers used on the bed at night or to the development of new and unusual habits, such as sleeping in the nude or with feet extended from under the blankets. Sweating is increased but is not usually a spontaneous complaint.

Skin changes are hardly ever noticed by the patient, and silky skin or hair is only occasionally seen on examination. Hair loss is common, usually noticed as thinning of the scalp hair by women. Other skin changes include occasional cases in white people of diffuse hyperpigmentation with darkening noted mostly over extensor surfaces of elbows, knees, and small joints. In African-American patients, darkening of skin is common.

Physical Findings

The thyroid is visibly or palpably enlarged in almost all young patients with hyperthyroidism, but in the elderly the thyroid may not be enlarged. Asymmetric enlargement is common, especially in patients with toxic nodular goiter. Extreme vascularity of the gland may result in palpable or audible blood flow, a bruit, usually heard over the enlarged lobes but occasionally best heard more rostrally over the superior thyroidal arteries. A bruit over the thyroid of a hyperthyroid patient is usually diagnostic of Graves' disease; this finding is not present in patients with toxic nodular goiter.

The *cardiovascular findings* include sinus tachycardia, systolic flow murmurs, and wide pulse pressure commonly, and atrial fibrillation occasionally. It is a common belief that most patients with hyperthyroidism have at least a tachycardia, but in fact only 50% of patients, regardless of age, have an increased heart rate. The apex impulse is often prominent and forceful. Cardiac failure may develop in severe cases of long duration, especially in the elderly.

The *eye findings* can be separated into those that occur as a result of thyroid hormone excess and those that are part of the ophthalmopathy of Graves' disease (4). Excessive thyroid hormone enhances sympathetic tone. The innervation of the eyelids is partially under sympathetic control. Lid retraction with increased scleral visibility above and below the iris, along with infrequent blinking, leads to the stare so commonly seen. Failure of the lid to follow movements of the globe (lid lag) is another manifestation of the same process. When Graves' ophthalmopathy is present, there is forward protrusion of the globe. This process may be unilateral at first and is often asymmetric. The protrusion represents true proptosis and contributes an additional component to the stare produced by increased sympathetic tone. Extraocular muscle weakness results in limitation of ability to converge and to perform extreme movements of gaze. Strabismus and diplopia are more severe manifestations. The most serious complications of Graves' ophthalmopathy are infiltrative disease and optic neuritis (see below).

The *dermopathy* of Graves' disease occurs most commonly on the legs (pretibial myxedema) but also can be seen on the dorsum of the foot or on the back, the hands, or even the face. The plaque usually has a sharp, raised margin and may have an orange-peel–like appearance. The affected areas are often intensely pruritic.

Clubbing of the fingers and toes is rare (thyroid acropachy) and is distinguishable radiographically from that seen in pulmonary disease. A common sign is separation of the distal portion of one or more fingernails from their nail bed (onycholysis; "dirty fingernail" sign).

A postural tremor, usually of the hands, is a common physical finding (see Chapter 82).

Diagnosis

Recognition of Graves' disease in a typical case is not difficult, but because of its frequently insidious onset, an absence of eye findings or of an overtly enlarged thyroid, or because of involvement of one or relatively few organ systems, the diagnosis may be missed for months or years.

The usual thyroid function tests substantiate the

diagnosis in most cases. If the results of the T_4 and free T_4 index (or free T_4) are borderline or normal, the plasma T_3 must be measured because hyperthyroidism may be due to elevation of T_3 alone. However, T_3 *toxicosis* (see below) occurs in less than 5% of cases. Occasionally, all of the tests of thyroid hormone levels are borderline. If the clinical suspicion of thyrotoxicosis is strong, every effort should be made to obtain laboratory confirmation by multiple, serial determinations of T_4 and T_3 and by assay of TSH. Hyperthyroidism is an evolving disease—thus the need for serial measurements. It is sometimes reasonable to treat the symptoms with a β-adrenergic antagonist (see below) while following the laboratory measurements, which may become diagnostic only after months. Clinical trials of antithyroid drugs should be avoided.

Differential Diagnosis

In some patients, particularly elderly ones, the clinical picture may not suggest hyperthyroidism. Such patients may have only unexplained weight loss or weakness. Occult neoplasm may first be suspected, and the diagnosis of hyperthyroidism may be missed entirely or considered only after extensive evaluation fails to yield a diagnosis. These are the patients often labeled *apathetic hyperthyroidism*. The term implies lethargy—which is not often present—but should rather be used to denote that group of patients who for unclear reasons lack the signs of sympathetic hyperactivity and hence do not exhibit tachycardia, lid retraction, tremor, etc.

Congestive heart failure, atrial fibrillation, or new-onset or worsening *angina pectoris* may be the presenting manifestation. So-called thyrocardiac patients have been incorrectly thought to be resistant to ordinary doses of digitalis. This is occasionally true, but a normal response to conventional therapy for cardiac failure or an arrhythmia should not be considered incompatible with a diagnosis of hyperthyroidism.

Some patients with *anxiety* may experience tachycardia, tremor, irritability, and weakness simulating hyperthyroidism. The anxiety of thyrotoxicosis is more likely to appear as irritability and hyperkinesis than as an expressed feeling of anxiety. Primary anxiety disorders are either related to identifiable stresses, coexist with symptoms of depression, or have distinctive characteristics that make them recognizable (see Chapter 13). In depression, weight loss is invariably accompanied by anorexia, a relatively unusual symptom of hyperthyroidism (see above).

The characteristic *ophthalmopathy* of Graves' disease may offer the first clue to the diagnosis (4). However, ophthalmopathy may not be accompanied by hyperthyroidism and may be unilateral. TSH measurement, the T_3 suppression test, or the TRH test will substantiate the diagnosis in most but not all cases of euthyroid Graves' ophthalmopathy. Without evidence of either thyroid hyperfunction, disturbance of the negative feedback system (suppression of TSH), or dermopathy, the diagnosis of Graves' ophthalmopathy cannot be made with absolute assurance. Indeed, other diseases of the orbit or retro-orbital space must be considered. Computerized axial tomography of the skull and the orbital contents and high-resolution sonography are useful diagnostic tools. These procedures can visualize the enlarged extraocular muscles of Graves' ophthalmopathy, although such enlargement is also seen in pseudotumor. In many cases of Graves' ophthalmopathy without hyperthyroidism, other aspects of Graves' disease eventually become apparent.

When hyperthyroidism is found in a patient without goiter or exophthalmos, suspicions of *factitious hyperthyroidism* may be warranted. An RaIU test and scan establish whether the thyroid is functional, and a sonogram may give evidence for enlargement that is not palpable. A very low uptake and a normal-size gland on sonogram suggests ingestion of thyroid hormone or the presence of thyroiditis with hyperthyroidism (see below).

Therapy

Hyperthyroidism caused by Graves' disease is often a self-limited process that terminates within a year or two in about half of patients. This natural history strongly influences selection of therapy. Other therapeutic considerations relate to the age of the patient and the presence or absence of complications.

Because there is currently no means of controlling the underlying cause of the disease, presumably TSI production, therapy is designed to interfere with thyroid hormone synthesis by drugs or by ablation of thyroid tissue by radioiodide or surgery. Opinions differ on approaches, but the views expressed here closely approximate those of conservative medical opinion in the United States. Each form of therapy has advantages and disadvantages; none provides a simple, definitive solution and none is truly curative. The objective of therapy is to ensure minimal morbidity from both the therapy and the disease. The therapy of hyperthyroidism attributable to causes other than Graves' disease is discussed separately. It is clear that any of the three forms of therapy when properly exercised results in a satisfactory outcome as shown in a recent prospective randomized trial (52).

Antithyroid Drugs

Antithyroid drugs predictably control excessive production of thyroid hormone in essentially all cases, although in only about half or less of cases will a permanent remission of the hyperthyroidism be seen. It is not generally appreciated that of these latter cases, about half will become hypothyroid in between 15 to 20 years after successful treatment. Relapses may occur within 6 months to a year or even longer after apparent remission, but such relapses are uncommon except in postpartum patients.

Restoration of the clinically euthyroid state requires at least 4 to 8 weeks, although clinical improvement is usually seen much sooner. Antithyroid drugs are ordinarily the preferred initial treatment for children, some young adults without complications or other medical problems, and pregnant patients. The antithyroid drugs are also routinely used as preliminary therapy in patients who are to be treated by surgery (see below). The objective in these cases is to ensure euthyroid status at the time of operation. Patients who are to be treated with radioiodide (see below) are also commonly treated with an antithyroid drug before and/or after ablation. Radioiodide in less than thyroid-ablating doses is slow in producing its effect and may have to be given repeatedly; use of an antithyroid drug before or after such therapy is therefore a temporary but useful adjunct.

In the United States, only two thiocarbamide drugs are available: propylthiouracil and methimazole (Tapazole). Other equally effective thiocarbamides are used in other countries. Propylthiouracil may have an advantage when speed in restoration of euthyroid status is an urgent consideration. *Propylthiouracil,* unlike methimazole, in addition to its effects in inhibiting thyroid hormone synthesis, also inhibits conversion of T_4 to T_3 in peripheral tissues. On the other hand, *methimazole* is longer acting than propylthiouracil and may be given on a less frequent dosage schedule, thus facilitating compliance. In most adults with hyperthyroidism, 100 to 150 mg of propylthiouracil (available in 50-mg tablets) every 8 hours or 20 to 30 mg of methimazole (available in 5- and 10-mg tablets) every 12 hours usually suffices as initial therapy, whereas maintenance is often possible with 50 to 100 mg of propylthiouracil twice daily or 5 to 10 mg of methimazole once or twice daily. The T_4 level should be measured after a month of treatment and every 2 to 3 months thereafter. If at these relatively low maintenance dosages of antithyroid drug the plasma T_4 falls below normal, efforts to titrate the dosage further are often tedious and unsuccessful and should be avoided. A euthyroid state can be achieved under these circumstances by the addition of oral thyroxine, usually at somewhat less than full replacement dose. A simple program is to initiate treatment with methimazole alone and, when the T_4 has become normal, to institute maintenance with a single daily dose of 60 mg of methimazole (an amount that normally completely halts thyroid hormone formation) plus 0.10 to 0.125 mg of thyroxine.

This combined therapy has long been advocated by some for both convenience and simplicity, and a report from Japan suggests (31) that such therapy is associated with a much better remission rate. Needless to say, this report rekindled interest in long-term drug therapy of hyperthyroidism, but several attempts in the United States to replicate these results have failed. Moreover, this therapy will never induce permanent remission in toxic nodular goiter (see below), which is the diagnosis in about half the thyrotoxic patients over age 55 years.

Although the recommended dosages of antithyroid drugs control the disease in most cases, some individuals clearly need higher dosages. Severely ill patients should be given larger doses from the beginning. The risk of an adverse drug effect may be increased, but this is not established and should not be a consideration

under such circumstances. To achieve total blockade of hormone synthesis, as much as 200 mg of propylthiouracil every 4 hours may be necessary. Because methimazole has a longer duration of action, it need not be given so often, but 30 to 40 mg three times daily may be needed in rare cases.

Duration of Therapy

Therapy should continue for 12 to 24 months before discontinuation of the drug is considered, although conflicting evidence suggests that lasting remission may not be related to duration of therapy beyond the point at which the patient becomes euthyroid. A few indicators are helpful in predicting success or failure of the outcome of a course of antithyroid drug therapy. Patients who have continued to require large doses of drugs are almost certain not to have achieved remission. On the other hand, reduction of thyroid size during therapy is often predictive of lasting clinical remission. For determination of short-term status, neither the TSH nor the TRH test is of any use, but a *suppression test* using T_3 or T_4, although not accurately predictive of the long term, may nonetheless be helpful in establishing the clinical status at the time of discontinuation of drug therapy. Such testing is not in vogue at present, and most endocrinologists simply discontinue therapy and observe the patient (see below). To perform the suppression test, the antithyroid drug is withheld through the period of the test. The patient is given 75 µg of T_3 (Cytomel) as a single dose daily for 7 days or one 3-mg dose of T_4. RaIU is then determined 1 week after initiation of T_3 administration (or after the single dose of T_4). Low postsuppression 24-hour uptake (less than 10%) indicates accurately that the patient is in remission at the time of the test. More significantly, an uptake above the normal range almost invariably indicates continuation of active disease. Intermediate values are not useful. If on clinical grounds, or as a result of testing, continued disease activity seems to be present, discontinuation of therapy is inadvisable and almost certainly will result in clinical relapse and needless morbidity. Measurement of titers of TSI may be useful in predicting relapse, but such measurements are not widely available and also are not accurate predictors.

If the clinical status indicates that remission may have been reached, antithyroid drug therapy is terminated and the patient is observed. Routine determination of plasma T_4 every 3 to 4 weeks for 3 to 6 months allows early recognition of return of thyroid overactivity. If the status is ambiguous and especially if there is evidence of continued disease activity, the antithyroid drug dosage may be reduced to one half the maintenance level for 3 to 6 months in the expectation that if recurrence occurs, it will be blunted. Prophylactic use of a β-adrenergic–blocking drug (see below) during withdrawal of antithyroid drugs is a useful maneuver that prevents emergence of symptoms of overt hyperthyroidism should relapse occur.

If the hyperthyroid state recurs, treatment with an antithyroid drug may be reinitiated for another year or alternative therapy may be undertaken (^{131}I or surgery). A second course of antithyroid drug has a significant chance of inducing remission. In selected patients, prolonged or even indefinite drug therapy is reasonable, but with most patients such an approach is undesirable.

Minor side effects of drug therapy occur in 1 to 5% of patients. Skin rashes, the most common side effect, are usually seen in the first months of therapy and often disappear even if therapy is continued. Antihistamine drugs are useful in controlling these rashes and the sometimes associated urticaria and pruritus. Neutropenia is not uncommon but is usually not severe and is dose related. If the absolute number of polymorphonuclear neutrophils falls below 2000, the dosage should be reduced; but the drug need not be immediately discontinued. The white blood cell count should be monitored after several weeks of therapy and after increases of drug dosage. If the side effects are not tolerated, a switch to another agent allows continuation of therapy in about half of the cases. Major complications of drug therapy occur in less than 0.1% of cases. Agranulocytosis is the most dreaded complication. Unlike neutropenia, thiocarbamide-induced agranulocytosis from antileukocyte antibodies is not dose related and is of such sudden onset that routine blood counts are of no help in prevention. However, the patient should be instructed to contact the physician promptly if severe sore mouth or sore throat and fever occur. Immediate hospitalization is probably indicated. Fortunately, most patients with agranulocytosis recover, albeit after a stormy course. Other toxic reactions include drug fever, arthralgias, and hepatitis. Elevations of alkaline phosphatase activity are commonly seen in patients receiving propylthiouracil. If other liver enzymes are normal, the drug may be continued, but persistent laboratory evidence of hepatocellular damage indicates a need to discontinue therapy. Liver enzymes should be measured every 3 to 6 months.

Adjunctive Drug Therapy

Iodide.   Nonradioactive iodide in the treatment of hyperthyroidism should be reserved for patients with severe illness. Occasionally, iodide therapy produces severe dermatitis. Use of iodide may preclude for many weeks the use of radioactive iodide, the uptake of which by the thyroid will be greatly diminished.

Iodide is the best agent available for inhibiting hormone release and is useful in patients who need rapid correction of the hyperthyroid state. Iodide also has a time-honored place in preoperative preparation (see below) for thyroidectomy to reduce vascularity of the gland. When given for several weeks after radioiodide therapy, iodide seems especially effective in accelerating restoration of euthyroid status.

The standard dosage of iodide is one drop of a saturated solution of potassium iodide (40 mg) diluted in several ounces of water or juice once daily; higher dosages are often given but are unnecessary because a dose of only 5 mg produces a maximal effect. Lugol's solution is an obsolete pharmacologic concoction, containing iodine and iodide, and has no virtue over iodide alone.

Adrenergic Antagonists.   The symptoms and signs of thyrotoxicosis that are related to sensitization of the sympathetic nervous system are in large measure abolished by β-adrenergic–blocking drugs. The current agent of choice is propranolol. Other newer, more selective β-adrenergic antagonists are probably equally effective, although no clear advantage has been demonstrated over propranolol. Some of these agents have intrinsic sympathomimetic activity (acebutolol, penbutolol, pindolol) and are inappropriate for use in hyperthyroidism. The indications for use of propranolol are severe tachycardia, tremor, sweating, and agitation. Propranolol is effective for relief of these manifestations of hyperthyroidism but does not appreciably affect excessive metabolic rate or reverse the catabolic state of severe cases. Propranolol has occasional undesirable side effects and is relatively contraindicated in some individuals (e.g., those with asthma). Concern is often expressed that patients with heart disease may be thrown into congestive heart failure or that heart failure, if present, may worsen. On the other hand, some patients with congestive heart failure respond well to the drug when excessive heart rate is a major contributing factor. Other uses for propranolol are in the prevention of symptoms during trial withdrawal of an antithyroid drug and while awaiting the effects of ^{131}I therapy. Most patients require propranolol at dosages of at least 160 mg/day (40 mg every 6 hours or 80 mg every 12 hours in a sustained-release form), but doses up to 720 mg may be necessary. The drug should be discontinued as soon as the patient is rendered euthyroid (T_4 normal) by other therapy.

Radioactive Iodine (Iodide) Therapy

Radioactive iodide (^{131}I) is uniformly effective therapy; it is simple to administer and inexpensive. In the United States, and unlike in Japan and Europe, it is the preferred form of therapy for most adults with Graves' disease and is much preferred over surgery. The rapidity of response is dose dependent and dependent also on the size of the gland, but improvement is often apparent in a few weeks and euthyroidism (or hypothyroidism, see below) is achieved on the average within a few months.

The single disadvantage of radioactive iodide is that hypothyroidism is a common consequence. For many years, concern was expressed over the possibility of producing carcinoma of the thyroid, leukemia, or genetic damage in the future offspring of women in their childbearing years. All of these concerns have been shown to be groundless. Although low dosages of external radiation or radioiodide produce carcinoma of the thyroid, the higher dosages used for treatment of hyperthyroidism do not. Long-term follow-up of treated patients over the past 30 years has failed to substantiate any such risk or any increased risk of leukemia. The amounts of radiation to the ovaries from therapeutic doses of radioiodide used for therapy of hyperthyroidism are lower than those delivered by diagnostic radiographic procedures and can be expected to produce no genetic effects. Thus, radioiodide therapy for hyperthyroidism can be considered for any adult patient, including women of childbearing age who plan to have children.

Hypothyroidism follows radioiodide therapy in the immediate few months after therapy in a more or less dose-related fashion. Large doses predictably eliminate hyperthyroidism with certainty but totally ablate the thyroid with great regularity. Small, single doses render the patient euthyroid with 50 to 70% likelihood but unavoidably still produce hypothyroidism within a year in approximately 10% of cases. Furthermore, of the patients rendered euthyroid, 3 to 4% per year develop hypothyroidism over the ensuing 20 years.

One may question whether the high frequency of posttreatment hypothyroidism constitutes a significant disadvantage of radioiodide therapy. The answer is that for the majority of those who become hypothyroid, replacement therapy with thyroxine is a trivial inconvenience. For these patients, the advantages of radioiodide therapy far outweigh the one disadvantage. Unfortunately, a few patients, despite warnings to the contrary, discontinue their required lifelong replacement therapy, become lost to follow-up, and suffer all of the consequences of long-standing hypothyroidism and myxedema.

Some physicians, including the author, advocate the use of deliberately ablative doses of ^{131}I. This approach to therapy certainly greatly simplifies patient management, accelerates restoration of the euthyroid state, and is reasonable in view of the high probability of eventual posttherapy hypothyroidism regardless of dose. Nonetheless, most physicians do not advocate deliberate ablation unless the patient is elderly, has experienced a major complication of hyperthyroidism (e.g., severe heart disease), has complicating medical problems that demand prompt control, or has severe ophthalmopathy (13). In young patients who are tolerating their disease reasonably well, some physicians prefer to use small doses of ^{131}I, repeated if necessary, until the patient is euthyroid. Such an approach does not, of course, guarantee that hypothyroidism will be avoided.

As discussed below, larger doses of ^{131}I are appropriate initially in the treatment of toxic nodular goiter.

In the past, elaborate schemes have been used to estimate the required dose of ^{131}I. Unfortunately, none has proven helpful because the variability of the thyroid's sensitivity to radiation—the most important determinant of effect—is not measurable. Currently, in a typical low-dose treatment scheme patients with small glands are given 3 to 5 mCi, whereas those with moderately enlarged to large glands are given 7 to 10 mCi (1 mCi equals 37 MBq). Ablative doses approximate 15 mCi. Because of the unpredictable response with nonablative doses, antithyroid drugs are often used initially to render the patient euthyroid. Antithyroid therapy is then interrupted for 48 hours before the

^{131}I is given and reinstituted 24 hours afterward. Alternatively, an antithyroid drug can be initiated 24 to 48 hours after therapy with ^{131}I, although that does not in fact appear to hasten recovery from the hyperthyroid state. Similar approaches combining antithyroid drug and ^{131}I are almost routinely used in patients with severe or complicated hyperthyroidism (e.g., thyrocardiac disease).

Radioactive iodide can be administered only by an appropriately licensed physician—usually a nuclear medicine physician or an endocrinologist. A few precautions are necessary. In women of childbearing age, a negative test for pregnancy must be obtained by the therapist immediately before the therapy dose is given because exposure of a fetus to radiation is unacceptable. In the United States, women who have a young child at home are given no more than 8 mCi and are instructed to avoid prolonged close contact (e.g., sharing a bed) for a week.

The undocumented notion has long persisted that radiation thyroiditis may produce excessive release of thyroid hormones 7 to 14 days after therapy, with the possibility of consequent worsening of the clinical state. This complication, if it occurs at all, must be rare. Nonetheless, prudence dictates a conservative approach in precarious patients (e.g., those in congestive heart failure), who are best brought to euthyroid status or who are at least significantly improved by antithyroid drug therapy before ablation with ^{131}I. At 3 months after ^{131}I therapy, when the short-term radiation effect becomes maximal, the antithyroid drug can be discontinued or tapered, provided that the laboratory and clinical evidence indicates return to euthyroid status. Adjunctive therapy with propranolol is useful at this point to ameliorate possibly emerging symptoms when the preceding dose of ^{131}I has been inadequate. If the laboratory evidence indicates continuing hyperthyroidism, another dose of ^{131}I is required.

Therapy with ^{131}I is always successful if enough ^{131}I is given. "Failure" after one or more doses is never an indication for surgery or indeterminate therapy with antithyroid drug. Rather, additional ^{131}I should be given to complete the process.

Surgical Therapy

For many years surgical ablation of the thyroid (e.g., subtotal thyroidectomy) was the main therapy for hyperthyroidism. This procedure still has its advocates, especially for young adults and for children who cannot be successfully treated with antithyroid drugs. In the hands of experienced surgeons, subtotal thyroidectomy is effective therapy, attended by minimal morbidity. However, complications include the small but real risk of anesthesia/operative mortality, recurrent laryngeal nerve damage with vocal cord paralysis, permanent hypoparathyroidism, and most commonly, hypothyroidism. The latter two complications are unavoidable to a certain extent and are not merely the consequence of poor surgical technique. In addition to about a 10% occurrence of immediate postsurgical hypothyroidism, 2 to 3% of patients become hypothyroid each year after surgery, a figure only slightly lower than that after therapy with ^{131}I. A higher complication rate must be expected when the operation is performed by surgeons with limited experience in thyroid surgery. Surgery also is followed by a significant (5%) rate of recurrent hyperthyroidism, sometimes occurring many years later. In this case, even the most enthusiastic supporters of surgical treatment agree that recurrent hyperthyroidism should never be treated by a second operation because the frequency of major complications rises to an unacceptable level.

Treatment of Hyperthyroidism During Pregnancy

Hyperthyroidism during pregnancy, almost invariably caused by Graves' disease, should be treated with an antithyroid drug (45). Surgery has been used successfully during pregnancy but has no advantage and may be associated with increased fetal losses. Radioactive iodide is contraindicated. Therapy with antithyroid drugs during pregnancy is guided by two considerations. First, the antithyroid drugs freely cross the placenta and, in large doses, can produce goiter and hypothyroidism in the infant. Second, thyroid hormones do not cross the placenta from mother to fetus. The dosage of antithyroid drugs should be the minimal amount adequate to control the hyperthyroidism. A dose of drug that totally blocks hormone synthesis along with a replacement amount of thyroxine is inappropriate during pregnancy. When ordinary doses of antithyroid drug are used, the fetus is usually born without goiter, but as a precaution, the dosage is often reduced, if possible, during the last month of pregnancy. Iodide should not be used during pregnancy because the fetal thyroid is especially susceptible to the goitrogenic effect of iodide. Monitoring the plasma hormone level requires determination of free T_4 or the free T_4 index because T_4 is normally elevated during pregnancy in association with the increased TBG.

TSIs (see above) of Graves' disease cross the placenta and enter the fetal circulation. Occasionally, the newborn infant is hyperthyroid as a result of this passive transfer of antibodies. The physician who will care for the newborn should always be alerted to this possibility.

Ophthalmopathy of Graves' Disease (4)

The exact frequency of ophthalmopathy in Graves' disease is unknown, but most patients have either no obvious infiltrative eye involvement or show only minimal to moderate proptosis, which generally stabilizes at a tolerable level. Severe exophthalmos occurs in no more than a few percentage of cases of Graves' disease. Proptosis becomes more than a cosmetic concern when the eyelids fail to close, especially when the patient is sleeping, setting the stage for exposure keratitis or corneal ulceration. Paresis of the extraocular muscles producing diplopia can also be troublesome and may require use of an eye patch or corrective surgery. The most disturbing but fortunately uncommon eye involvement is severe chemosis (marked

inflammation and edema) of the conjunctivae and periorbital soft tissues. Ophthalmopathy of this severity is termed malignant or infiltrative exophthalmos. Rarely, optic neuritis leading to blindness occurs.

Graves' ophthalmopathy follows a temporal course such that the eye disease and thyroid hyperactivity often coincide; in 85% of cases, the two occur within 2 years. However, the ophthalmopathy may occur years before or after the onset of hyperthyroidism. Occasionally, the thyroid may become autonomous (nonsuppressible) with function still within the normal range but TSH suppressed.

Despite claims to the contrary, no form of treatment of hyperthyroidism has been shown to have any consistent advantage for control of the ophthalmopathy. However, recent evidence supports the long-held belief that induction of hypothyroidism may aggravate exophthalmos. Development of clinical hypothyroidism should therefore be avoided, especially when exophthalmos is present. The cornea becomes exposed and may dry out when proptosis prevents the lids from closing completely. This problem may be relieved by the application of liquid tears (available over-the-counter) and the wearing of eye patches at night and sunglasses in bright sunlight or on windy days. Treatment of severe ophthalmopathy is best given by an endocrinologist, in consultation with an ophthalmologist who has experience with the problem. Corticosteroids (e.g., prednisone, 60 mg a day for 1 to 2 weeks, tapered over 6 to 8 weeks) are useful for patients with severe periorbital and conjunctival edema and inflammation. Other therapy, if warranted, includes orbital radiation and radioactive-iodide ablation of the thyroid (with or without orbital radiation). Surgical decompression is only rarely needed and is reserved for patients with severe proptosis. There is considerable controversy (13) about which therapy is optimal.

Hyperthyroidism Associated with Thyroiditis (Lymphocytic Thyroiditis with Spontaneously Resolving Hyperthyroidism, Postpartum Thyroiditis with Hyperthyroidism, Silent Thyroiditis)

Classical subacute thyroiditis (see below) has long been known to be associated occasionally with short-lived, self-limited hyperthyroidism. The explanation for this phenomenon has been that the destructive inflammatory process causes release of preformed thyroid hormone. The hyperthyroidism invariably disappears within a few months (see "Postpartum Thyroid Dysfunction," below).

Another apparently distinct variant of the thyroiditis–hyperthyroidism syndrome has been recognized—*lymphocytic thyroiditis*. These patients have a modestly enlarged, nontender thyroid gland. No history of viral illness can be obtained. The radioiodide uptake is very low, as it is in subacute thyroiditis, whereas the T_4 and T_3 levels are high. About half of cases have significant elevations of thyroid antibodies, and about half of these high titers subside within a few months. A propensity of the condition to occur in the postpartum period has been noted, sometimes in successive pregnancies and sometimes followed by the development of hypothyroidism. On biopsy the changes seen differ from those of the peak phase of classical subacute thyroiditis, but the latter, in its late stages of evolution, may be indistinguishable from that of lymphocytic thyroiditis. Whether lymphocytic thyroiditis with spontaneously resolving hyperthyroidism (silent thyroiditis) is a new disease, as has been suggested by some, or is a newly recognized variant of subacute thyroiditis is a matter of debate (28,40,41).

A radioiodide uptake measurement should be obtained in all patients with hyperthyroidism who do not clearly have Graves' disease (i.e., who do not have associated eye findings) or toxic nodular goiter. A very low radioiodide uptake establishes the diagnosis of hyperthyroidism associated with thyroiditis and allows the physician to avoid inappropriate therapy (radioiodide or surgery). Treatment with an antithyroid drug may be useful; propranolol (see above) affords symptomatic relief and may be all the treatment that is necessary.

Long-term follow-up studies on these patients show that about half persist in having some degree of thyroid abnormality: antithyroid antibodies or goiter, recurring bouts of hyperthyroidism, elevation of TSH (decreased thyroid reserve), and occasionally, hypothyroidism (41).

Hyperthyroidism Associated with Multinodular Goiter (Toxic Nodular Goiter) or with a Solitary ("Hot") Nodule

Toxic nodular goiter is usually seen in adults in midlife or in the elderly. Although the typical patient with Graves' disease usually relates symptoms extending over a few months to a year, the history in toxic nodular goiter is often much longer. Many years may pass before diagnosis. Because of the patient's age and the duration of illness, severe cardiac or musculoskeletal involvement is common.

Toxic nodular goiter appears to arise in the pathologic evolution of some cases of nodular goiter. Most nodular goiters (see below) are initially TSH dependent (i.e., suppressible with exogenous thyroid hormone). Eventually, some of these goiters develop autonomous areas, with other regions of relatively decreased activity. Nodular goiters at this stage of evolution do not secrete enough hormone to produce clinical hyperthyroidism but in 20% of cases show nonsuppressible function. A few of these autonomously functioning goiters evolve to a stage in which excessive production of hormone and clinical hyperthyroidism ensue.

If the usual laboratory tests (T_4, FTI) are borderline, special tests such as measurement of TSH suppression (see above) by use of a second- or third-generation assay for TSH and measurement of T_3 should be performed. Many multinodular goiters occur in the elderly, who may already have low TSH. A normal response to TRH excludes a diagnosis of hyperthyroidism at any age, but failure to respond is common in normal elderly people.

Therapy of toxic nodular goiter is best accomplished with [131]I. Rather large doses, in the range of 15 to 30 mCi, are usually necessary and may have to be repeated. Hypothyroidism occurs much less commonly after ^{131}I therapy for nodular goiter than for Graves' disease. If the clinical situation demands prompt relief of the hyperthyroidism, an antithyroid drug can be used after the therapeutic dose of ^{131}I because the response to radioiodide is often slow and multiple doses may be needed. Otherwise, ^{131}I given alone is simple therapy, without side effects, and easily monitored by measurements of plasma T_4. With ablative therapy (large doses), thyrotoxicosis may be controlled in several weeks; with smaller doses, in several months. Other therapeutic considerations including the use of adjunctive therapy follow those outlined for the therapy of Graves' disease with one exception. In hyperthyroidism due to toxic nodular goiter, antithyroid drugs alone, although effective while administered, will not produce a lasting remission. The same is true for hyperthyroidism due to a "hot" nodule (see "Management of the Hot Nodule," below).

Hyperthyroidism Caused by Excessive Secretion of T₃; T₃ Toxicosis

In most cases of hyperthyroidism, the thyroid secretes excessive quantities of both T_4 and T_3. However, in perhaps 5% of cases, T_3 is the predominant hormone secreted. T_3 toxicosis may occur in hyperthyroidism due to Graves' disease, toxic multinodular goiter, or autonomous adenoma. The patient who appears clinically hyperthyroid but whose T_4 is normal should have plasma T_3 measured. T_3 toxicosis sometimes occurs early in the course of hyperthyroidism due to Graves' disease and can develop during therapy with an antithyroid drug, in which case the dosage should be increased. Continuing clinical findings of hyperthyroidism during such therapy—despite a normal or low T_4—should raise the possibility that T_3 toxicosis is now present and that more, rather than less, antithyroid drug is needed. The treatment of T_3 toxicosis is the same as is that of other forms of hyperthyroidism.

Hyperthyroidism (and Hypothyroidism) Caused by Iodide

Iodide from a variety of sources can induce hyperthyroidism (22). The agent currently most likely to produce hyperthyroidism is the antiarrhythmic drug amiodarone (see Chapter 59). This drug contains nearly 40% iodine and can exert a number of effects on thyroid function. The drug inhibits conversion of T_4 to T_3; coincidentally increases of serum T_4 and free T_4 occur. Although this circumstance per se does not cause clinical hyperthyroidism, amiodarone can cause either overt hyperthyroidism or hypothyroidism, the dominant dysfunction apparently depending on regional iodine intake. In Europe some 10% of patients receiving the drug develop hyperthyroidism, whereas in the United States, hypothyroidism is much more common at nearly 20%. Most of the latter cases are presumably iodide induced in susceptible people with preexisting Hashimoto's thyroiditis. The diagnosis of hyperthyroidism caused by amiodarone depends on demonstration of an elevated T_3 and suppression of TSH. This type of hyperthyroidism cannot be treated with radioiodide (low thyroidal radioiodide uptake) and is often resistant to standard antithyroid drug therapy. The combination of propylthiouracil or methimazole plus perchlorate is effective. An endocrinologist should be consulted in such cases. Treatment of hypothyroidism requires only ordinary replacement with T_4.

Subclinical Hyperthyroidism

The term *subclinical hyperthyroidism* has been applied to the combination of a TSH suppressed state in the presence of normal free T_4 and free T_3 concentrations (48,49,53). In one large series, this situation was associated with a threefold increased risk of developing atrial fibrillation over 10 years in people 60 years or older (49). Otherwise, there is no clear-cut risk of the condition, and in fact, when identified, it may spontaneously abate (i.e., the TSH normalizes) (53) (see "Screening for Thyroid Disease," below). Very few patients with low TSH go on to develop clinical hyperthyroidism with elevation of T_4 or T_3 concentrations. Thus, the term *subclinical hyperthyroidism* may be a misnomer. This is in contrast to subclinical hypothyroidism (see below), which is, at least for some cases, a phase in the longitudinal development of hypothyroidism.

Thyroid Storm (Thyrotoxic Crisis)

Thyroid storm, a complication of hyperthyroidism, is now only rarely encountered. When thyroid storm does occur, it is usually in the setting of a severe medical or surgical stress imposed on a patient with uncontrolled or unrecognized hyperthyroidism. Clinical features of full-blown thyroid storm include fever, sometimes to the level of extreme hyperpyrexia, marked tachycardia, great irritability, diarrhea, and hypotension. Thyroid storm often progresses rapidly to delirium and coma. Any such severe exacerbation of hyperthyroidism demands hospitalization and urgent consultation with an endocrinologist.

Surgery in the Patient with Hyperthyroidism

This problem is discussed in Chapter 86.

HYPOTHYROIDISM

Hypothyroidism, the metabolic state resulting from deficient thyroid hormones, is common. Most cases can be diagnosed even when symptoms and signs are minimal, provided that the physician considers the diagnosis and seeks appropriate laboratory confirmation. The manifestations of hypothyroidism are varied and to a large measure age dependent. *Myxedema* is a severe form of hypothyroidism that results in deposition of mucopolysaccharides in the skin and other tissues, producing a characteristic appearance and a constellation of physical findings. The term *myxedema* is commonly but incorrectly used interchangeably with *hypothyroidism. Primary hypothyroidism* is a term used to indicate that the hormone deficiency results from a disease or other process within the thyroid gland. *Secondary hypothyroidism*, much less common, results from lack of thyrotropin (TSH) secretion, a result of pituitary or, rarely, hypothalamic disease. The thyroid is usually smaller than normal and not palpable. Plasma TSH, using a second- or third-generation assay, is usually low, but experience with TSH assays in this situation is limited, and biologically inactive TSH may be produced so that the TSH can be low, normal, or even slightly elevated (42). Almost invariably the hypothyroidism is part of a decrease in pituitary function involving tropic hormones in addition to TSH with consequent hypogonadism or adrenal insufficiency. Causes include postpartum necrosis, pituitary tumor, pituitary apoplexy, and granulomatous disease, or possibly part of an autoimmune process involving failure of other endocrine glands. Some cases occur without identifiable cause and are termed idiopathic (see also Chapter 74).

Etiology

Throughout the world, the most common cause of hypothyroidism remains dietary *iodide deficiency*. However, in those parts of the developed world, including the United States, where iodide deficiency no longer exists because iodide is added to dietary salt, most cases of hypothyroidism are due to *autoimmune destruction* of the thyroid, either with or without goiter (see below). Goitrous autoimmune hypothyroidism is also called *Hashimoto's thyroiditis*. The remaining cases are iatrogenic, the result of therapy of hyperthyroidism (see above).

Autoimmune destruction of the thyroid may occur in association with other autoimmune glandular disorders, especially adrenal insufficiency (Schmidt's syndrome) and autoimmune ovarian failure (polyglandular failure) as well as with diseases such as pernicious anemia. High titers of antibodies to thyroid antigens (thyroglobulin, microsomes) are seen in 90% of cases. An easily overlooked form of hypothyroidism is that which occurs *postpartum* (see "Postpartum Thyroid Dysfunction," below). *External radiation of the neck* (e.g., for nonthyroidal neoplastic disease) can also cause thyroid atrophy and subsequent hypothyroidism.

A classification of the causes of hypothyroidism is given in Table 73.7.

Drug-Induced Hypothyroidism

A variety of drugs can produce hypothyroidism—invariably associated with goiter formation. Only a few in current use have such an effect. Lithium, currently in wide use for the treatment of manic–depressive illness (see Chapter 15), is one such agent. If goiter occurs,

Table 73.7. Clinical Classification of Hypothyroidism[a]

Hypothyroidism Without Goiter (Decrease of Thyroid Tissue Mass)
Postablative for hyperthyroidism (radioiodide therapy or surgery)
Autoimmune atrophy
Postpartum
External radiation
Developmental defect (congenital)
Pituitary or hypothalamic disease

Hypothyroidism with Goiter
Autoimmune (Hashimoto's disease)
Postpartum
Drug induced (e.g., antithyroid drugs, iodide, lithium[b])
Iodide deficiency (many geographic areas)
Genetic biosynthetic defects

[a]Hypothyroidism in the United States is now most commonly the consequence of therapy for hyperthyroidism. Hypothyroidism from idiopathic atrophy of the thyroid is second in frequency. Developmental defects (e.g., lingual thyroid) are rare. Hypothyroidism with goiter is nearly always caused by Hashimoto's thyroiditis, rarely by a drug. Genetic biosynthetic defects are rare and usually become manifest in childhood.

[b]Hypothyroidism from chronic lithium therapy may occur without goiter.

lithium need not be stopped; addition of thyroxine relieves the hypothyroidism and causes regression of the goiter. Overtreatment of hyperthyroidism with an antithyroid drug will, of course, produce hypothyroidism. Iodide in pharmacologic amounts is an antithyroid drug and also occasionally produces goiter and hypothyroidism as in patients given long-term iodide therapy for asthma or other chronic lung disease. However, most adults who are susceptible to the antithyroid action of iodide have an underlying thyroid abnormality, such as Hashimoto's thyroiditis (see below) or radioiodide-treated Graves' disease. Amiodarone, an antiarrhythmic agent, contains iodine and can produce hypothyroidism in up to 20% of patients treated with this drug (see "Hyperthyroidism (and Hypothyroidism) Caused by Iodide," above). One should also keep in mind the possibility of inapparent iodide administration during hospitalizations (contrast media, including those used in conjunction with CT scanning) with development of thyroid dysfunction some months later.

Clinical Features

Hypothyroidism in the adult is highly variable in presentation. Usually, onset is insidious, often occurring over many years, with the result that the symptoms go unappreciated by patient and physician alike. The nonspecificity of the symptoms also contributes to the delayed diagnosis. No predictable progression of symptoms is apparent, but easy fatigability, lethargy, increased sleep requirement (and sometimes, sleep apnea—see Chapter 85), cold intolerance, muscle aching, and stiffness are perhaps the most common early symptoms. The skin is dry and scaling. Hair loss is common. The eyebrows become sparse, the face is "puffy" (i.e., full) because of cutaneous deposition of mucopolysaccharides, with edema of the periorbital areas. The voice often becomes low pitched and rough.

Constipation is common and may be severe enough to produce megacolon; sometimes the diagnosis is suggested by the radiologist from the results of a barium enema. Diminished hearing, especially in older persons, is easily overlooked or is attributed to aging. Ordinarily, the affected individual becomes abnormally placid, but agitation or frank psychosis may occur. In the elderly, depression is the most common psychiatric accompaniment of hypothyroidism. Dementia from hypothyroidism is rare, if it occurs at all, but the association of the two processes in the elderly is not uncommon. Paresthesias and pain in the hands from carpal tunnel syndrome, may occur. Diminished sexual function is the rule. Women often experience menorrhagia. Rarely, galactorrhea may be seen in women of childbearing age. Fertility is diminished, but pregnancy may occur and normal delivery is possible. The newborn is euthyroid, unless the mother's hypothyroidism is drug related or the hypothyroidism is of the rare familial athyrotic variety.

Subclinical Hypothyroidism

The most common stage of hypothyroidism likely to be encountered in ambulatory patients is mild hypothyroidism, commonly termed subclinical hypothyroidism. This condition, which is strongly age and gender dependent (26), occurs with an overall prevalence of 2 to 7%. The condition is defined by a paucity of nonspecific but suggestive symptoms and few clinical findings, serum thyroid hormone levels that are within the normal range, but an elevation of thyrotropin (TSH). One study suggests that some of these patients are clinically improved after therapy with L-thyroxine (11). Older women often show modest elevations of TSH (6 to 15 μU) despite normal levels of T_4 (see "Screening for Thyroid Disease," below). Only those with elevated thyroid autoantibodies are likely to develop hypothyroidism (50% over 5 years).

Severe Hypothyroidism with Myxedema

In spontaneous cases of hypothyroidism, only with severe, long-standing disease does extensive deposition of mucopolysaccharide occur, producing the clinical state of myxedema. Rarely, myxedema may develop rapidly after radioiodide therapy or after surgical ablation of the thyroid for hyperthyroidism.

In myxedema, a variety of manifestations can be appreciated on physical examination and, of course, they vary with the severity and duration of the disease. The skin, in addition to being dry and scaling, is typically cool. The scaling may be extensive, and large flakes may be shed from the elbows and knees. The subcutaneous tissues may be infiltrated by mucopolysaccharides so the skin appears to be "thickened" or "doughy." In the elderly, atrophy of the epidermis may occur simultaneously, producing a stiff, translucent, parchmentlike appearance. Yellow-orange discoloration of the skin from carotene may be evident, especially in the palms. The presence of edema is not obvious because pitting is not noted except in extreme cases complicated by hypoproteinemia. An exception is the collection around the eyes of "bags of water" (lymphedema). This finding is not, however, specific for hypothyroidism. The tongue is sometimes enlarged. The heart rate is usually slow (sinus bradycardia). The heart may appear enlarged, because of either dilation of the myocardium or pericardial effusion. Pleural effusions and ascites may also be present, sometimes even in cases that are otherwise not clinically severe. Dilutional hyponatremia, clinically indistinguishable from the syndrome of inappropriate antidiuretic hormone excess, may be present. The deep tendon reflexes characteristically show a delay in their relaxation phase, the so-called hung-up reflex. This is a highly suggestive finding but may be seen occasionally in other diseases. Mental functioning is slowed, as reflected in the characteristically slow speech. The reading speed may be greatly reduced. Hearing loss may be severe or of a degree apparent only on audiometric testing. Cerebellar dysfunction, if present, is usually evident only on extensive neurologic testing, but in rare cases is grossly apparent as ataxia.

Myxedema Coma

Myxedema coma is a severe, often fatal, event that is an uncommon complication of long-standing disease and is typically seen in the elderly patient. Myxedema coma is often associated with or precipitated by pneumonia, peritonitis, or some other serious infection, the presence of which may not be immediately apparent. Severe respiratory failure is a major feature and can be due to a variety of factors ranging from upper airway obstruction to impaired chest wall mechanics.

Because elderly patients often become hypothermic on exposure to cold or during sepsis, the diagnosis of myxedema coma is more commonly considered than actually confirmed. Any of these events demands hospitalization.

Laboratory Findings

In primary hypothyroidism, the combination of low plasma T_4, FTI index (or free T_4), and high TSH is diagnostic. Difficulties in diagnosis are encountered only in occasional cases. The plasma T_3 is usually low, but because T_3 decreases in a variety of nonthyroidal illnesses ranging from malnutrition to liver disease, its measurement is not useful for diagnosis of hypothyroidism. Furthermore, it is normal in many patients with mild hypothyroidism. In hypothyroidism caused by pituitary or hypothalamic disease, the TSH should be low in the new sensitive assays. However, TSH may be low in severely ill patients with nonthyroidal illness also (see above). The TRH test is ordinarily unnecessary for diagnosis of primary hypothyroidism but can be helpful when the T_4 and TSH are borderline. In this situation, an exaggerated response to TRH may be seen (TSH increment greater than 30).

In addition to the definitive diagnostic tests, various other laboratory abnormalities are encountered, although they serve no useful diagnostic purpose. A common laboratory finding is elevation of plasma enzymes that originate in skeletal muscle: creatine kinase (CK), serum aspartate aminotransferase (AST), serum alanine aminotransferase (ALT), and lactic dehydrogenase (LDH). Fractionation studies show that when these enzymes are elevated in hypothyroidism, they do not originate in cardiac muscle. Virtually all of the phenotypic abnormalities of hyperlipoproteinemia have been observed in hypothyroid patients and are reversible when thyroid hormone is replaced (see Chapter 75). Other abnormalities include electrocardiographic changes (e.g., flattened or inverted T waves, minor ST-segment depressions, and low amplitude QRS complexes) and abnormalities of blood gas measurements caused by hypoventilation. Anemia (see Chapter 50), usually normocytic and normochromic, may be present, as may macrocytic anemia of coexistent vitamin B_{12} deficiency (pernicious anemia). An abnormality of red cell shape (spiculation) also has been described in hypothyroidism.

Differential Diagnosis

The most difficult problem in diagnosis is the simple clinical appreciation of the possibility that the patient may be hypothyroid. Once suspected, the subsequent history, physical examination, and particularly, laboratory findings will easily establish the diagnosis in all but a few cases. However, some special problems may be encountered. Any elderly patient who is sick, pale, and puffy faced becomes a suspect for the diagnosis, especially if an adequate history cannot be obtained. A patient with atypical chest pain, nonspecific electrocardiographic abnormalities, and elevated CK, AST, or ALT is occasionally labeled as having ischemic heart disease and myocardial infarction; the proper diagnosis may be hypothyroidism. A patient with the nephrotic syndrome might be mistaken for one having hypothyroidism. However, although the plasma T_4 may be low (TBG is low in many nephrotic patients), the FTI (or free T_4) is normal, as is the TSH. More important, the patient with the nephrotic syndrome has features characteristic of that disorder (i.e., massive proteinuria and hypoalbuminemia and gross hyperlipidemia) (see Chapter 44).

Diagnosis of Hypothyroidism in Patients Already Receiving Thyroid Hormone Therapy

Patients are often encountered who, having been diagnosed as hypothyroid at some time in the past, are receiving replacement therapy when first seen. Lack of documentation may lead one to question the original diagnosis. Alternatives include continuation of therapy despite an uncertain diagnosis, or discontinuation of therapy, a maneuver that will confirm or refute the need for continued treatment. In many instances, continuation of therapy may be simpler, less expensive, and more appropriate than an attempt to resolve the issue, but this can often be easily accomplished, even after many years of treatment, by abrupt discontinuation of hormone therapy. After 5 weeks, determination of plasma T_4 (and FTI) is made. If the value is normal, the patient is considered euthyroid and the original diagnosis is discarded. In contrast, a low T_4 (and a subsequently determined high TSH) verifies a diagnosis of hypothyroidism.

Occasional euthyroid patients who were inappropriately treated with thyroid hormone for long periods and most hypothyroid patients become grossly symptomatic toward the end of the 5-week period of withdrawal. An occasional inappropriately treated patient can show a delay of several additional weeks in return of normal thyroid function. If the physician wishes to avoid the possibility of the development of symptoms as a result of withdrawal, a rapid but expensive way to determine thyroid status while the patient continues to receive full hormone replacement is to administer human recombinant TSH (hrTSH) intramuscularly followed 18 hours later by an RaIU test (see above). A normal or elevated RaIU post-TSH injection indicates normal thyroid function and a previously inappropriate diagnosis of primary hypothyroidism.

Hypothyroidism Versus "Euthyroid Sick Syndrome"

The diagnosis of hypothyroidism in severely ill patients presents special problems (56,58). Patients with the simulating euthyroid sick syndrome are usually elderly and often have sepsis. The T_4 and T_4 indexes are low; TSH may be low, normal, or moderately elevated (up to 20 µU/mL), depending on the stage of the illness (23); and response to TRH is normal or blunted. Plasma rT_3 is often elevated.

Although to date this euthyroid sick syndrome has been clearly recognized only in hospitalized, severely ill patients, it probably also occurs in less dramatic form in chronically ill, nonhospitalized people. Many patients with chronic renal failure undergoing hemodialysis appear to fall into this group. The mechanisms underlying this phenomenon appear to involve a combination of factors including accelerated T_4 metabolism, impairment of TSH secretion (23,58), and impairment of T_4 binding to plasma proteins. Most of these pathophysiologic abnormalities are probably due to the cytokines that are produced in excess during severe illness.

Treatment

It has been clear for many years that thyroxine is the best preparation for ordinary use, but the subject is still being discussed (42). Thyroxine—levothyroxine, sodium L-thyroxine, Synthroid, Levothroid, Levoxine—is available in color-coded tablets of 25, 50, 75, 88, 100, 112, 125, 137, 150, 175, 200, and 300 µg. T_3 (liothyronine, Cytomel—available in 5-, 25-, and 50-µg tablets) is also effective and may possibly be more effective for treatment of goiter. However, it has no special advantage for routine therapy of hypothyroidism and has the distinct disadvantage that one cannot monitor the plasma T_4 or T_3 to determine adequacy of replacement. Combinations of T_4 and T_3, thyroglobulin

preparations, and desiccated thyroid should no longer be used.

Traditionally, initiation of thyroid hormone replacement therapy has been cautious and conservative and has used dosage schedules that ensure slow restoration of a normal metabolic state. Although the principle is rational, the practice is often faulty. Therapy should be adjusted to the individual case, with several points in mind. If the patient is not elderly and has never had overt cardiac disease, overcautious initiation of therapy will result only in needless prolongation of the hypothyroid state with its attendant morbidity. If the patient has evidence of preexisting cardiac disease or is frail and elderly, therapy should be started at low dosage (see below), but unnecessary delay should be avoided. Only rarely will serious heart disease, such as angina pectoris, prevent at least partial therapy sufficient to eliminate myxedema, if not full correction of hypothyroidism.

The usual hypothyroid patient, without complicating medical problems, may be started on full daily replacement dosage. Even with this therapeutic schedule, the clinical response will be slow. One can expect several months to pass before restoration of the normal metabolic state. If the patient is elderly or has known cardiovascular disease, a daily dosage of 12.5 to 25 µg of T_4 should be started, with 25-µg increases at 4-week intervals.

The objective of therapy is to restore the clinically euthyroid state. Enough thyroxine is given daily to maintain the plasma T_4 at the mid to upper range of normal, or, ideally, to the lowest level of T_4 at which the TSH is restored to normal (see below). Most people need about 125 µg (0.125 mg) per day; only rarely is as much as 200 µg (0.2 mg) necessary, and more is hardly ever needed. A single weekly dose of T_4 can be used; the dosage is slightly more than 7 times the daily dosage (25). Elderly patients often require only 100 µg/day for maintenance; often as little as 50 or 75 µg may suffice. The T_4 requirement during pregnancy is increased by about one-third (57).

Some concern has been expressed over whether treatment with thyroid hormone leads to osteoporosis. The concern is clearly unwarranted. T_4-treated patients show no evidence of an increase in bone-mineral loss, except for patients with a history of hyperthyroidism, suggesting that previous thyrotoxicosis may have produced this effect, not merely the slightly increased levels of T_4 that often result from replacement (6,36) (see "Thyroid Hormone Suppression Therapy for Benign Nodule Disease," below).

The T_4 alone is the least expensive way to follow the titration phase of replacement; use of the TSH is unnecessary at this stage. It is usually not helpful to measure the T_4 any sooner than every 8 weeks after a change of dosage. When the T_4 reaches the middle of the normal range to the upper end of normal, the TSH can be measured as a fine adjustment. Third-generation assays are not necessary for this purpose; their cost may exceed that of a T_4 by eightfold to tenfold ($80 for a third generation TSH is not unusual).

The "ideal" laboratory endpoint of therapy is a T$_4$ and TSH that are within the normal range. However, attaining such precision is expensive and probably unnecessary, especially the precise normalization of the TSH (42). Take as an example a patient receiving a replacement dose of 0.1 mg of T$_4$ who has reached a serum T$_4$ of 9 µg% and who has at this point a TSH slightly elevated at 8 µU/mL (normal up to 5). It is unlikely that such a patient will derive any benefit if the dosage of T$_4$ is increased slightly (e.g., by 12 or 25 µg so that the T$_4$ reaches 11 µg% and the TSH falls to normal at 3 µU/mL). Similarly, if the TSH is found to be low (e.g., 0.1 µU/mL [lower limit of normal 0.5]), with a T$_4$ within the normal range, it is unlikely that any clinically useful result will follow from a minor downward adjustment of the replacement dosage of T$_4$. Much effort and expense is expended in such fine tuning, the benefits of which are presently unprovable. Once a plateau of the serum T$_4$ is reached, repeat measurements at yearly intervals should suffice. Determination of serum T$_3$ during therapy with T$_4$ is unnecessary.

It should be noted that patients who receive replacement T$_4$ to an endpoint defined by a normal (not elevated) TSH reach a serum T$_4$ plateau that is on average approximately 25% higher than the mean for normals. At this point, their T$_3$ is normal. If a normal TSH is the goal, the physician should expect a serum T$_4$ that is above the upper limit of normal in approximately 20% of patients.

Concern has been expressed over the bioavailability of hormone in certain generic preparations and even lack of standardization of certain brands of thyroxine, but clinically significant problems are not likely to be encountered with any of the preparations from the suppliers of the named brands. Use of generic thyroxine should be avoided.

Surgery in the Hypothyroid Patient

Patients with grossly evident hypothyroidism who require surgery are poor risks until their thyroid status is at least partially corrected (see Chapter 86), a process that requires 3 to 4 weeks with ordinary oral therapy. Elective surgery is best delayed in such patients. In an urgent situation, an intravenous dose of T$_4$ is probably warranted to prepare the patient for surgery in a few days. The increased susceptibility of severely hypothyroid patients to respiratory depression by conventional doses of many central nervous system (CNS) active drugs should be borne in mind. This increased drug sensitivity has been responsible for precipitation of myxedema coma. On the other hand, recent studies indicate that patients with minimal hypothyroidism appear to tolerate ordinary surgical stress (e.g. elective cholecystectomy) well.

POSTPARTUM THYROID DYSFUNCTION (POSTPARTUM THYROIDITIS)

Postpartum thyroid dysfunction is common, occurring in some 17% of women in one study (24). Both hyperthyroidism and hypothyroidism can occur; in some cases one state follows the other (1,57). The hypothyroid variation may be transient, lasting only 1 to 4 months, and is most likely to occur in the first 8 months postpartum. However, in 30% of cases the hypothyroidism is permanent. Many of the cases that are not permanent are caused by the transient occurrence of thyroid-blocking antibodies (vanishing hypothyroidism). Most cases show antimicrosomal (thyroid peroxidase [TPO]) antibodies; antithyroglobulin antibodies are uncommon. In the United States, the hyperthyroid variety has been associated with postpartum lymphocytic thyroiditis (see "Hyperthyroidism Associated with Thyroiditis," above). Postpartum hypothyroidism is often misdiagnosed as postpartum depression. Some women have repeated bouts of thyroidal illness with successive pregnancies. The disease also has other long-term implications as a risk factor for later development of both Graves' disease and especially hypothyroidism (17% of patients over 5 to 16 years in one series; 23% in 2 to 4 years in another [57]). Of special interest is the increased incidence (25%) in women with type 1 diabetes, a threefold increase over nondiabetic patients. Because of this high incidence, 3 month follow-up (TSH and TPO antibodies) is recommended postpartum for all type 1 diabetic patients (1). The disorder is often familial.

SCREENING FOR THYROID DISEASE (HYPERTHYROIDISM AND HYPOTHYROIDISM)

Because thyroid diseases are common and clinical diagnosis can be difficult (see also "Subclinical Hyperthyroidism" and "Subclinical Hypothyroidism," above), a rational argument can be made in favor of attempting to detect clinically inapparent thyroid disease by laboratory tests in individuals without overt symptoms (3,32). Experienced clinicians have long held that modest degrees of hypothyroidism or hyperthyroidism are essentially impossible to detect by routine clinical means, and several careful studies have recently confirmed this impression (16). However, the screening of asymptomatic populations by laboratory testing has been shown not to be cost-effective. Most investigators favor a case-finding approach—that is, testing only patients who are seeing a physician for symptoms—although there is not uniform agreement (12,27). In patients who exhibit any clinical findings that could conceivably be attributable to thyroid disease, laboratory testing should be done, but this approach should probably not be termed screening.

Most studies that have attempted to detect thyroid disease during screening (or case finding) have focused on evaluation of "sensitive" (second-generation) assays for TSH (see above) and their use as a single screening test. These are 10 times more sensitive than earlier assays (first-generation) and, unlike the earlier assays, can recognize low (suppressed) values—those which are below the lower limit of the normal range (0.3 to 5 µU/mL). In these assays, the TSH is undetectable in patients with hyperthyroidism.

Unfortunately this finding is sensitive but not specific; many sick people and even normal elderly patients are found to have low levels of TSH (17,43). Thus, used alone, second-generation assays *cannot establish* a diagnosis of hyperthyroidism, whether in community populations or in sick patients at any age. A normal TSH *can* be useful in *excluding* a diagnosis of hyperthyroidism, but so can a normal T_4 (or FT_4 index), at lower cost. Third-generation assays are no more specific in this regard (23).

The results of screening for thyroid disease, using second-generation TSH tests and appropriate follow-up of abnormal values are remarkably consistent in various populations (16,20,32,43). Approximately 1% of apparently healthy individuals, all ages included, are found to be hypothyroid. Many fewer individuals are shown to be hyperthyroid (0.1 to 0.2%). Women over 40 have the most thyroid disease; young men have essentially none. Asymptomatic patients with elevated or depressed levels of TSH may have subclinical hypothyroidism (p. 1082) or subclinical hyperthyroidism (p. 1081).

GOITER

A goiter is an enlarged thyroid gland. The term implies nothing about the functional state of the gland. Goiter is the most common thyroid abnormality. *Diffuse goiter*, also called simple goiter, is a gland that is uniformly and symmetrically enlarged without apparent irregularities. (Some use the term *simple goiter* to denote any nontoxic or nonhyperfunctioning gland, regardless of its anatomy.)

In some areas of the world, thyroid enlargement is so prevalent that it is termed *endemic goiter*. Before the widespread introduction of iodized salt, endemic goiter was common in the United States, but this is no longer the case. Endemic goiter, for practical purposes synonymous with iodine deficiency goiter, is now found principally in geographically isolated areas of the underdeveloped world, but some of these areas are vast, such as much of China and central Asia. Moreover, some parts of Europe such as Germany—which never iodized its salt supply—and parts of Italy, Switzerland, Denmark, etc. are still areas of low iodide intake and, therefore, of goiter. The term *sporadic goiter* refers to thyroid enlargement as now encountered in the United States and other developed areas. Sporadic goiter is now seen in a small percentage of the population and increases in frequency with age.

Any process that prevents the synthesis of normal quantities of thyroid hormones may produce goiter. If impairment of hormone synthesis is severe enough, goiter formation is associated with reduction of blood hormone levels, eventually to be followed by clinical hypothyroidism. The mechanism of the thyroid enlargement in this situation is increased pituitary TSH secretion via activation of the feedback system. The resulting increased thyroid mass is a compensatory mechanism that may allow sufficient hormone synthesis to occur so that the patient remains euthyroid.

Drugs that interfere with thyroid hormone synthesis (e.g., thiocarbamides, lithium, iodides) can lead to goiter. Withdrawal of a goitrogenic drug results in regression of the goiter, as will administration of enough T_4 or T_3 to suppress endogenous TSH secretion.

Only one well-defined naturally occurring "goitrogen" is known: L-5-vinyl-2-thiooxazolidone. This substance, with a mechanism of action much like that of the thiocarbamides, is in cabbage, turnips, soybeans, and several other vegetables. Other poorly characterized goiter-producing substances have been detected in the food and water supplies of some areas. No environmental factor has been widely incriminated, however, as a cause of sporadic goiter, the etiology of which remains obscure.

Recognition

A mass in the base of the neck is the usual mode of presentation of goiter. Occasionally, especially in the elderly, an enlarged thyroid is neither visible nor readily palpable but is incidentally found by x-ray of the chest or esophagus when either a retrosternal mass is noted or the trachea or esophagus is found to be deviated. Confirmation of the nature of a neck mass as an enlarged thyroid gland and precise determination of its size are now most economically and accurately performed by ultrasonic examination (sonography). Although radionuclide scintigraphy ("scanning") was previously used for this purpose, it is not as accurate and fails to show nodularity with comparable clarity. CT is also accurate in delineating the relationship of a goiter to contiguous structures but is much less useful in defining the thyroid itself.

Except in subacute thyroiditis, pain is not a usual symptom but can develop during cyst formation or hemorrhage, a fairly common event, usually accompanied by rapid and sometimes painful enlargement of a portion of the gland. Obstruction of the trachea or esophagus can be produced by goiter, but dysphagia should not be readily attributed to minor degrees of thyroid enlargement. Hoarseness may occur because of involvement of the recurrent laryngeal nerve, but this is rare in benign enlargement and its occurrence suggests thyroid malignancy.

Differential Diagnosis

Clinical and laboratory assessment of thyroid function should be made in all cases of goiter. The functional state may change with time, sometimes rather rapidly, and hence the precise diagnosis may not be possible on a single examination. Goiter in association with hyperthyroidism suggests Graves' disease, toxic nodular goiter, or a hyperfunctioning (hot) nodule. Hypofunction in association with goiter is likely to represent Hashimoto's thyroiditis (see "Hypothyroidism," above), but other possibilities, such as drug ingestion, may have to be excluded. Rarities such as an infiltrative process (amyloid disease, metastatic neoplasm) and the inherited defects of hormone synthesis (organification or coupling defects) have to be kept in mind (Table 73.7).

If the clinical and laboratory assessments indicate normal thyroid function, the diagnosis of euthyroid goiter is made. Multinodular enlargement almost always indicates a process of many years' standing. Differentiation of diffuse enlargement from nodular enlargement may require ultrasonic examination because small nodules may be missed on physical examination, whereas ultrasound may detect nodules as small as 0.5 cm. If the ultrasound image is not helpful, an optimally performed scintiscan may show irregular ("patchy") uptake of tracer, but even the best technique can delineate nodules of only about 0.5 cm in size. A goiter composed of many such small nodules may appear to represent a nonnodular thyroid. Antithyroglobulin or antimicrosomal antibodies in serum are readily determined commercially and should be routinely sought in all cases of goiter. Titers of such antibodies are elevated in the blood of 90% of patients with goiters caused by Hashimoto's thyroiditis. A proper history will point to possible drug-related goiter. Rapidity of enlargement may help differentiate benign from malignant lesions, and the presence or absence of pain will help identify inflammatory thyroiditis (see below).

Treatment: Suppression Therapy

Although thyroid enlargement is idiopathic in sporadic goiter, the process nevertheless depends on the presence of TSH. Administration of a physiologic quantity of thyroid hormone results in suppression of TSH release. When TSH secretion is chronically suppressed in this manner, the enlarged thyroid often regresses, at least partially, or at least ceases to enlarge. The larger and more long-standing the goiter, the less likely is regression to occur. Suppression therapy may be accomplished with T_4 (sodium L-thyroxine) or T_3 (liothyronine, Cytomel). The dosage (see available dosages above) should not be excessive. T_4 at a dose of 125 µg/day is usually ample. T_3 is given at a dose of 25 ± 5 µg/day. Some evidence suggests that T_3 may be effective in a greater proportion of cases.

Suppression therapy is often properly performed for cosmetic reasons. Suppression therapy is also clearly indicated for individuals with many years of life expectancy during which time mechanical problems may develop. However, little is to be gained by treatment of patients whose glands are known not to have changed in size over many years and who are, therefore, unlikely to develop difficulties. Until recently, a clear and unequivocal indication for therapy was the patient who had already had surgery for goiter. Recurrence of goiter was believed to be common in such people and thought to be predictably prevented with suppression therapy; this information has been challenged (10).

To avoid iatrogenic hyperthyroidism, suppression therapy must be monitored by determination of both the serum TSH *and* the T_4, which should not exceed the upper limit of normal during therapy. The importance of monitoring the T_4 is that one must be certain that the production of T_4 by the gland is suppressible; however, 20% of nontoxic nodular goiters are autonomous. In these cases the TSH may fall with T_4 therapy but the T_4 could rise into the hyperthyroid range as the exogenous T_4 adds to that being produced by the thyroid. Some nonsuppressible goiters may represent inapparent euthyroid Graves' disease. These patients may, if not monitored, also develop iatrogenic hyperthyroidism from the exogenous thyroid hormone. Monitoring of therapy also ensures that an adequate amount of hormone is being given. Although regression of goiter is evidence of adequacy of therapy, the physician should be certain that the dose is adequate in those cases that do not show obvious regression. In suppression therapy with T_3, the plasma T_4 falls to a level below normal if suppression is adequate. With either T_4 or T_3, adequacy of suppression can be determined by a low TSH in a second- or third-generation assay. Minimally, subnormal TSH in the morning indicates incomplete suppression of TSH secretion; in this circumstance, the normal nocturnal surge of TSH usually persists and the suppression is inadequate.

If the treated gland is diffusely enlarged, obvious regression by 6 months can be expected in about one-half of cases. Nodular glands are less likely to respond, and any response that occurs is slower. Even if complete regression is not accomplished, prevention of further glandular enlargement is a reasonable goal and makes the process worthwhile. A baseline ultrasound examination (not necessary in every case) and follow-up visits at 6-month or yearly intervals provide objective assessment of the therapeutic responses but are not always necessary.

Several years may be necessary to discern regression of a long-standing multinodular goiter, and during that time, one or more nodules may become more easily palpable as the relatively normal portions of the gland regress. Some confusion may occur if that is interpreted as a progression of the disease or as the development of a malignant nodule. Serial ultrasonic examinations will help avoid this error.

Once started, suppression therapy is usually continued indefinitely but can be terminated or withdrawn if regression occurs. Some goiters do not recur; in those that do, therapy can be reinstituted. Suppression therapy does not lead to permanent loss of TSH secretion, even after decades of thyroid hormone administration, although rare individuals may manifest a brief period of hypothyroidism when prolonged therapy is withdrawn.

Goiters large enough to produce not only tracheal deviation but also significant tracheal compression, as assessed by plain x-ray views or CT scan of the trachea, or by flow-loop respirometry (see Chapter 55), or large enough to interfere with swallowing, are now uncommon. In these cases, surgery, although attended by significant morbidity, should be considered. Radioiodide therapy also can be considered an option in these cases, especially in the elderly or in patients with other serious medical problems. Doses of 20 to 100 mCi are necessary. Although the response is slow, useful reduction in the size of the goiter can be achieved.

The frequency of carcinoma in multinodular goiter has been debated for years. Unwarranted concern has resulted in countless unnecessary operations (see below).

THYROID NEOPLASMS

Thyroid Nodules

One of the most common abnormalities of the thyroid is a localized area of enlargement commonly known as a nodule. The evaluation and treatment of a nodule are controversial among thyroidologists. In evaluating a thyroid nodule, the possibility of malignancy is the main concern. However, approximately 90% are benign adenomas or cysts; the remaining ones are lesions of varying degrees of malignancy, almost all of low grade. Even those that are termed malignant on histologic grounds behave clinically as benign lesions; clinically aggressive thyroid carcinoma is rare. Nodules are usually discovered by the patient as a visible or palpable lump, or incidentally by a physician or dentist during a physical examination. As with most newly discovered masses, the immediate concern is whether the lump is a cancer. Immediate reassurance of the patient is the correct response: first, the lump is unlikely to be a cancer (less than 10% chance); second, if it is a cancer, it is very unlikely to require either intensive therapy or involve a fatal outcome because most thyroid "cancers" are not at all like the frequently lethal varieties familiar to most patients.

Most solitary nodules are true adenomas and are encapsulated. Although most such benign adenomas are relatively hypofunctioning, follicular adenomas may exhibit normal or greater than normal function (i.e., they take up iodine and elaborate thyroid hormone, sometimes enough to produce hyperthyroidism). Adenomas that are functional but independent of TSH are termed autonomous. The growth of most benign adenomas, hypofunctional although they may be, depends on endogenous TSH.

Benign thyroid nodules are present in up to 50% of the population, depending on age and on how they are detected (i.e., by palpation or by sonography) (37). In a group of more than 200 patients with thyroid nodules identified in the Framingham study (4% of 5000 patients examined only by palpation, ages 30 to 60) and followed for 15 years, none developed clinically evident malignancy. In that population, new thyroid nodules continued to appear at a rate of about 1 in 1000 people per year, about twice as frequently in women as in men (54). Actually, nodules are much more common than one would suspect from studies that detect them only by palpation. When ultrasound is the detection method, between ages 30 and 60 some 20 to 40% of individuals have nodules (37). Whether a relatively small nodule (less than 1.5 cm diameter) is detected by palpation is largely a matter of chance, in turn reflecting the skill and effort of the examiner, the self-awareness of the patient, and the anatomy of the individual's neck.

Management

General Considerations. The major concern with most nodules is malignancy. The diagnostic workup and therapeutic approach to these lesions should be determined by a number of considerations, including the biological potential of the nodule and the age of the patient (29). In the elderly, even more than in the young, a conservative approach is necessary because thyroid nodules are common in older persons (37) (see above).

Because most cold nodules—variously estimated at 75 to 95% of all nodules encountered—are benign lesions, the overall risk of malignancy is small. The risk is smaller still when it is realized that the remaining lesions are almost always clinically nonaggressive papillary or follicular carcinomas. These lesions are usually nonlethal (see below) and slow growing, so a conservative course is always reasonable. Nonetheless, some patients become extremely anxious when faced at this point with the possibility of cancer and may wish to proceed directly to excision. Such patients should be strongly dissuaded from this course because immediate and indiscriminate excision of all thyroid nodules is irrational and cannot be justified (see above).

Once the "solitary" nodule has been discovered, what does one do next? There are four options: FNA, scintiscan, ultrasound, or suppression therapy with thyroxine; all are acceptable. The choices are described below, along with their advantages and limitations.

The issue of whether to perform a biopsy on nodules or to treat them conservatively with initial suppression has received a detailed decision analysis and statistical treatment. The conclusion is that no best approach exists and that continued arguments over this issue will be futile. The decisions to operate, suppress, or aspirate have equal validity, dependent in the individual case on such subjective factors as psychologic disability, relative cost, and attitudes toward operative risk and long-term medical therapy (39).

The issue logically arises: Why not simply follow most solitary nodules that are not unsightly and have not rapidly enlarged using periodic examination (palpation), or serial sonograms? Given the statistics, a calm patient, and a calm, experienced physician, this approach would certainly seem reasonable and is low risk. On the other hand, these conditions are only rarely encountered. The words *cancer* or *possible cancer,* no matter how indolent that cancer might be, are usually extremely anxiety-provoking for most patients or their physicians; thus, some action is usually thought to be required. Moreover, follow-up alone would not be considered the standard of practice in most communities. Finally, one cannot equate suppression therapy with no therapy at all (39).

The Next Step: Fine-Needle Aspiration (FNA), Scintiscan, or Ultrasonogram?   In most cases, no nodes are present, thyroid function is normal, and the nodule is not part of Hashimoto's thyroiditis (antibodies are negative; see above). For many years the next step would have been immediate surgical excision or, in a more conservative mode, radionuclide scanning to determine whether the nodule was functioning. Although a hyperfunctioning, or hot, nodule would be found in only a small percentage of cases, hot nodules are almost invariably (99.8%) benign. In contrast, a hypofunctioning, or "cold," nodule would be considered suspect and warrants immediate surgery to rule out carcinoma. Immediate surgery is certainly obsolete, but so is a thyroid scan in the opinion of most, but not all, experts because of the advent of FNA biopsy of the thyroid. However, other initial approaches are appropriate, perhaps even preferable. The author prefers to start with ultrasonography.

Ultrasonography as the First Step.   The main advantage of obtaining an ultrasonogram as the first diagnostic maneuver after discovery of a nodule is that—even in expert hands—many "solitary" nodules turn out to be only one of many in a multinodular goiter. Obviously, the expertise of the examiner in palpating the thyroid will strongly influence the results, but most physicians are not expert in the examination of nodular thyroids. The ultrasonogram is objective and excludes the need for further workup of the many instances in which the "solitary" nodule turns out to be a multinodular gland. Although some still believe that "dominant" nodules in a multinodular gland should be suspect, the chance that one is dealing with clinically significant thyroid carcinoma in a multinodular gland is low. If one subscribes to this view, the workup may be terminated upon identification of a multinodular goiter. Cysts will also be discovered by ultrasonogram, another advantage, because again further workup is unnecessary. Of course, cysts are also identified when FNA is the first procedure.

If with ultrasound the nodule is truly solitary, and is not cystic, one can proceed to FNA, suppression therapy with thyroxine, or, if the patient insists, surgical excision.

Fine-Needle Aspiration (FNA) as the First Step

Patient Experience. FNA with a 25-gauge needle is essentially painless, but cutaneous anesthesia is preferred by some. Multiple aspirations are made, often through a single skin puncture. No significant bleeding is likely to occur, although ecchymoses often result, and complications are not seen. Other types of needle biopsy (aspiration, cutting) use much larger needles. These are more formidable procedures, require cutaneous anesthesia, and occasionally result in local hemorrhage, usually easily controlled with local pressure.

The argument that FNA helps avoid unnecessary operations is correct if one considers that some physicians have long erroneously held and acted on the premise that excision of all newly discovered nodules is indicated. However, when physicians have an initial approach that is conservative, universal institution of needle aspiration probably *increases* the number of unnecessary operative excisions. Reasons include frequently indeterminate histologic diagnoses and discovery of papillary carcinomas that might have been adequately treated by suppression (see "Therapeutic Consideration in Thyroid Carcinoma," below).

FNA with cytologic examination, because of its simplicity and safety, has largely replaced biopsy by use of a conventional cutting needle in the differential diagnosis of a solitary thyroid nodule (37,55). It is probably possible under optimal conditions to make an accurate diagnosis (concerning possible malignancy) in more than 90% of cases with FNA, although it is difficult or impossible to distinguish benign adenomas from many well-differentiated follicular carcinomas (30,38), an important limitation of the technique. Multiple aspirations (six have been recommended as ideal) should be obtained to assure adequate sampling for cytology (30). If inadequate material is obtained, the FNA should be repeated. However, it must be strongly stressed and is not generally appreciated that the most important consideration in the use of needle aspiration is the expertise of the pathologist who examines the biopsy material. If a specifically trained cytopathologist *who regularly examines such specimens from the thyroid* is not available, FNA should be avoided. Slides, however, can be sent to a trained person with ongoing experience regardless of geographic distance, to conform to this essential requirement of expert examination of material obtained at FNA. Similarly, if the patient is reluctant to have FNA, or refuses to undergo the procedure, one of the other approaches can be taken, including suppression therapy with thyroxine (see below).

If FNA reveals a cancer (papillary or follicular), no further diagnostic studies are indicated and treatment should be instituted (see below). If the aspiration yields cystic fluid (clear or "chocolate" brown indicating old hemorrhage), follow-up physical examination every 6 months is adequate. If FNA reveals a benign adenoma and if thyroid function tests are normal (see "The Autonomous (Hot) Nodule," below), no treatment is necessary unless the nodule increases in size. Of course, suppression therapy can be used for cosmetic considerations.

Scintiscan as the First Step: Hot, Warm, and Cold Nodules.   Most patients will be evaluated initially by FNA or ultrasound but a scintiscan may be done as the next step. It will identify a hot, warm, or cold nodule and, sometimes a multinodular goiter (although ultrasonography is a better technique to demonstrate multinodularity). The scan should not be combined with a thyroidal radioiodide uptake, a procedure that adds no useful information but increases the cost of the workup.

The Autonomous (Hot) Nodule.   If uptake of isotope is exclusively concentrated in the nodule, the nodule is considered to be autonomous. When an adenoma produces an amount of hormone equal to or greater than that of the output of the normal gland, TSH becomes suppressed; the remaining normal tissue then becomes relatively inactive and may not be visible, or may be only poorly visible, by scintiscan.

Management of a hot nodule depends on whether an excessive amount of thyroid hormone is being produced. If the amount of hormone produced by the adenoma considerably exceeds normal, thyrotoxicosis may be clinically apparent, at least in retrospect. Usually T_4 and T_3 are produced in excess. However, hyperthyroidism caused by T_3 alone (T_3 toxicosis) is fairly common with such hyperactive nodules (28), and so the usual screening thyroid function tests (suppressed TSH) should have indicated this situation.

The natural history of the hot nodule is variable. Over a 10-year interval, about one-third show little change, one-third become frankly hyperactive, and the remainder become cold, sometimes with obvious hemorrhagic infarction and cystic degeneration. Treatment of the hot nodule that is producing hyperthyroidism can be satisfactorily accomplished with surgery or radioactive iodine, although hypothyroidism may result. In recent years, several studies have shown that hot nodules can be safely and effectively ablated nonsurgically by injection with ethanol. The advantage over radioiodide is that hypothyroidism does not occur (35). Prophylactic ablative therapy is not indicated if thyroid function (T_4 and T_3) is not elevated. Suppression therapy with thyroid hormone is, of course, ineffective and leads to iatrogenic hyperthyroidism. An antithyroid drug will control the excessive thyroid hormone production but must be continued indefinitely and is a poor choice.

The Warm Nodule. On the initial scan, some nodules are not unequivocally cold or hot; instead, they appear to take up some tracer, but not to the exclusion of the remainder of the gland. Their status can be further defined by repeating the scan after several weeks of suppression. Some prove to be autonomous and can be managed as a hot nodule; others prove to be cold and should be managed as described below.

The Cold Nodule. If the scan shows no accumulation ("uptake") of isotope in the nodule (a marker should be used), it is considered to be nonfunctional (i.e., cold). Most nodules fall into this category; although most cold nodules are in fact benign, these are the lesions that are considered suspect, and thus need to be subjected to FNA or ultrasound or treated with suppression.

Thyroid Hormone Suppression Therapy for Benign Nodular Disease

Efficacy. The effectiveness of suppression therapy for benign nodular disease has until recently been widely accepted. However, in the past few years, several studies have questioned this approach (10). The published data support the following: *(a)* Both single nodules, simple (nonnodular) goiters, and multinodular glands do respond to suppression therapy, but the reported response rates are variable; approximately 25% show complete regression; another 25%, moderate regression; and the remainder, no apparent response. *(b)* Studies that purport to show no responses at all are probably the result of inadequate duration of therapy or inadequate dosage. Experienced clinicians have long been impressed that the regression of nodular disease can be slow and may take years; studies using 6 month trials are simply too brief. *(c)* The current notion that the TSH should be suppressed only to the lower limits of normal (10) in "sensitive" assays (second- or third-generation) is unsupported. There are no data that indicate that this degree of suppression is sufficient to induce regression. The basis for the concern about overtreatment is a desire to avoid the long-term consequences of osteoporosis or cardiac toxicity. These issues are discussed below.

Safety. The fears of inducing demineralization of bones are unfounded. Patients treated with suppressive doses of T_4 are not at risk, provided their TSH is suppressed by an amount of T_4 that is the minimal amount necessary to accomplish this goal (6,36). Only patients with a history of overt hyperthyroidism show demineralization.

Recent evidence suggests that TSH-suppressive doses of T_4 given for treatment of thyroid cancer (TSH less than 0.05 µU/L) can produce objective evidence of cardiac abnormalities by echocardiogram (left ventricular hypertrophy, diastolic dysfunction), in 40% of patients, but the clinical significance of the finding is unclear (33). Only patients who had T_4-related symptoms clearly showed echocardiographic abnormalities. The patients were not apparently individually titrated with T_4 to suppress TSH. Certainly, the extensive experience of many thyroid experts does not suggest that adverse clinical consequences are likely to occur (29). For the occasional patients who do develop some symptoms of adrenergic hyperactivity, simultaneous administration of a β-adrenergic blocker abolishes symptoms and reverses cardiac dysfunction and hypertrophy detectable by echocardiogram (7,8,19). This form of combination therapy seems to be reasonable when the goal of therapy is prevention of recurrence of thyroid cancer, but whether it is worth the theoretical risk in treating benign thyroid disease is unclear (10). More to the point is that whether these abnormalities would ever develop in patients whose TSH is suppressed by individually titrated minimal doses of T_4 is unknown.

Course. Regression of a nodule over a 6-month period of suppression of TSH with thyroxine indicates clinically benign disease; such nodules can be followed indefinitely with continued suppression therapy. Some endocrinologists are satisfied that benign disease is present when a nodule at least does not grow larger during suppression therapy over the initial 6 months, after which suppression can continue. Regression of some TSH-dependent malignant nodules will no doubt occur. Physicians should not be dismayed by this statement because suppression therapy is the mainstay of postoperative therapy of such lesions and there is no reason to believe that the delay in diagnosis—if the diagnosis is ever made—will be harmful (39).

Treatment of Thyroid Cysts. If a predominantly cystic nodule is identified on sonogram, aspiration or suppression therapy can be considered. Some cystic nodules require several aspirations, but most eventually disappear with this approach. Suppression therapy after aspiration is rational because most cysts arise in benign adenomas, but its usefulness is not established. The sonogram provides an objective and accurate measurement of size of cold nodules (both cystic and noncystic) so that regression or progression of the lesion can be followed during suppression therapy.

Thyroid Carcinomas

General Considerations

Approximately 95% of thyroid carcinomas are of the papillary or follicular variety; of these, 80 to 90% are papillary carcinomas. Anaplastic and medullary carcinomas probably account for no more than 5% of the total. The relative frequency of the various types of thyroid carcinomas is markedly age dependent (see below).

Occult thyroid carcinoma (defined as lesions with the histologic appearance of carcinoma, but less than 1.5 cm in diameter) is found in 5 to 10% of U.S. and European populations and in 30% of Japanese samples at autopsy. Death from thyroid carcinoma is as rare in Japan as in the United States. Clearly, occult carcinoma behaves as a benign disease and does not warrant aggressive management.

In the United States, about 10,000 new cases of thyroid carcinoma are seen each year, but only about 1,000 persons die. Most of these deaths result from the aggressive forms of the disease, that is, anaplastic lesions (50%), the unusually aggressive follicular carcinomas, and a few from the very uncommon aggressive papillary lesions. A few deaths are also attributable to medullary carcinoma.

Therapeutic Considerations in Thyroid Carcinoma

Papillary Carcinoma. Enough information is now available to provide support for a middle-of-the-road initial approach, one that falls between that which advocated thyroid hormone suppression therapy without surgery and that which has employed radical surgery alone. Long-term observations have now also reasonably defined the role of radioiodide ablation therapy (37,46).

Surgery for papillary carcinoma. Follow-up at 10 years indicates a recurrence rate of approximately 20% for subtotal resection versus 10% for total removal of the gland. Deaths caused by carcinoma are 1.5 and 0.5%, respectively. This small difference is reported for one retrospective study to be statistically significant and currently strongly influences the surgical approach. However, the complication rate for total thyroidectomy (hypoparathyroidism, vocal cord paralysis) remains high. As a result, many surgeons have now adopted a modified or near-total thyroidectomy. In this procedure the affected side is completely removed; most of the contralateral lobe is also removed but the posterior capsule is left, together with the tip of the upper pole. Whether this approach will succeed remains to be established. Meanwhile, conservative surgeons call anew for more limited surgery (5). Visibly involved lymph nodes are always removed, but radical neck dissection is not justified even in the presence of obviously involved nodes (37,46).

The presence of cervical node metastases at operation or the extent of lymphadenectomy does not seem to influence either recurrence or death rate. The death rate in lesions under 2.5 cm without local invasion and without evident distant metastases at the time of surgery is less than 1% in 10 years and is 4 to 8% in the less favorable categories (37,46).

Postoperative Therapy: TSH Suppression and Ablation with Radioiodide. Postoperative therapy with full replacement doses of thyroxine (see above) suppresses endogenous TSH, reduces recurrence, and is routine in all cases. In addition, postsurgical ablative therapy with radioactive iodide has a role, although not all cases of localized disease need such therapy. The patient with a minimal papillary lesion needs no such therapy, but the patient with a large, locally invasive lesion should receive ablative therapy with ^{131}I. In cases with an intermediate-size lesion, without invasion of the thyroid capsule, and without lymph node metastases, the recurrence rate is greatly reduced by treatment with radioiodide, and deaths from recurrent disease may be completely abolished. The hesitation to use radioiodide routinely stems from the unwarranted fear of radiation-induced leukemia. Doses of ^{131}I smaller than those customarily recommended may be equally effective. In contrast to the constraints on radioiodide therapy of localized disease, known metastatic disease should always be treated vigorously (18).

Follicular Carcinoma. Follicular carcinoma can be more aggressive than papillary carcinoma, tends to be angioinvasive, and may metastasize to bones and lungs. The tumor may bypass regional lymph nodes, a marked difference from papillary disease. The most important prognostic feature is invasion, either through the tumor capsule or into blood vessels. At least one report suggests that unlike papillary carcinoma, primary tumor size at presentation does not appear to influence prognosis (60). In contrast, in another series not a single patient under 45 with an intrathyroidal tumor less than 2.5 cm in diameter died (14).

The clinical presentation may be very different from that of papillary disease; the patient may have metastatic disease involving lungs, bone, brain, or spinal cord. In these cases the primary tumor may be relatively small and initially overlooked. Only rarely do the metastases produce sufficient thyroid hormones to cause thyrotoxicosis.

The surgical approach to follicular carcinoma should be that taken for papillary carcinoma. Suppression therapy with thyroid hormone replacement is routine. Postoperative ablative therapy with radioiodide appears warranted (14), especially for those patients with overtly invasive disease. However, the case for routine postoperative use of ^{131}I ablation therapy in the treatment of follicular carcinoma is not statistically established (60).

Anaplastic Carcinoma. Anaplastic carcinoma is fortunately distinctly uncommon; its frequency depends on the age of the population. Anaplastic carcinoma is rare in children and in adults under the age of 35. By age 50, as many as 10% of cases of thyroid carcinoma are due to anaplastic disease, and by age 80, by which time the overall incidence of thyroid carcinoma has fallen markedly, nearly half of the cases that do occur are of this variety. The disease is locally invasive in a highly aggressive fashion and quickly produces pain, dysphagia, hemoptysis, and hoarseness. Death usually occurs within 6 to 12 months. However, surgically resectable disease without evidence of metastases, even if it has extended outside the thyroid capsule, can be associated with long-term survival (20 to 30%). It is important to distinguish the small cell type from lymphoma of the thyroid. This rare disease, unlike anaplastic carcinoma, is radiosensitive and amenable to chemotherapy.

Medullary Carcinoma. Medullary carcinoma accounts for 1 to 2% of all thyroid cancers. The tumors arise from the parafollicular or C cells and produce thyrocalcitonin. Both sporadic and familial varieties are known. The sporadic case typically presents as a solitary nodule, whereas the familial variety is often multifocal and part of a multiple endocrine adenomatosis syndrome. Diarrhea occurs in some patients. Thyrocalcitonin in plasma is elevated in the basal state or after stimulation with calcium or pentagastrin infusion. Some authorities advocate obtaining at least a plasma thyrocalcitonin level as part of the evaluation of all nonfunctional thyroid nodules (15). When surgical excision is performed before regional nodes have become involved, 90% of patients survive for 10 years. Once the nodes are involved, only 40% survival can be expected. Medullary carcinoma does not appear to respond to suppression therapy with thyroid hormone.

The Question of Carcinoma in the Multinodular Thyroid

The risk of clinically significant carcinoma in a nontoxic nodular goiter is low. Occult carcinoma is found in a significant proportion of such cases. However, the approach to such occult lesions is no different from that to occult carcinoma in the nonnodular gland. Demonstration of multinodularity by palpation or sonogram or its suggestion by scan leads some physicians, including the author, to a firm recommendation against surgical intervention. Suppression therapy is recommended, but only for prevention of further gland enlargement or to induce regression of symptomatic goiters and not out of concern for malignancy. Others believe that large nonfunctioning nodules within multinodular goiters should be treated with suppression therapy for 6 months. Failure to regress is considered an indication for surgical excision. However, because most large nodules in multinodular goiters do not regress within such a period, while a significant number may actually become more prominent as less abnormal tissue regresses, this approach is certain to result in unnecessary surgery. Serial sonographic estimates of nodule size may prove useful in such cases.

Radiation-Associated Thyroid Carcinoma

Low-dose irradiation of the thyroid is a stimulus to thyroid carcinogenesis, with a latency period of one to several decades (50). The radiation may be from an external source or from radioiodide as has occurred following nuclear bomb fallout or the nuclear reactor accident at Chernobyl. Public Health authorities recommend stockpiling stable iodide for distribution to exposed persons in case of a nuclear plant accident. A single dose of 50 mg of sodium iodide would suffice to protect the thyroid in such an event.

In recent years thyroid carcinomas have been reported to occur in increased incidence in patients who received radiation therapy some years earlier for conditions such as enlarged tonsils or adenoids, or an enlarged thymus, or for acne. A distinction must be made between treatment with penetrating external radiation and local irradiation with point sources (radium rod and plaque treatment). It has not been possible to relate thyroid carcinoma to such limited exposure.

No relationship has been seen between the radiation and the development of medullary or anaplastic carcinoma (47), but radiation-induced cancers appear to present more often with dissemination than those occurring spontaneously, an argument for early detection (47). Accordingly, high-resolution thyroid scintiscans or sonograms should be part of the follow-up, because nonpalpable lesions can be detected. The only blood test of value is determination of serum thyroglobulin, elevation of which predicts the development of nodules (51).

The approach to the patient with a history of irradiation to the head and neck is not currently standardized. Examination of the patient at 2- to 3-year intervals should suffice. Routine isotopic scintigraphy or sonographic examination of the thyroid to detect patients with nonpalpable lesions is probably indicated. Many nonpalpable lesions (0.5 to 1.0 cm) can be detected by these methods. Although lesions too small to be palpable are clinically, if not pathologically, benign and should be managed conservatively, reports that carcinomas that are radiation induced may disseminate more readily than those occurring spontaneously should not be ignored. Thyroid suppression with thyroxine is recommended even for patients with nodules detected only by scintigraphy or sonography. If careful follow-up reveals an increase of nodule size despite suppression, surgery should be performed. A widespread, aggressive approach to nodules in these patients is not warranted.

Surgical therapy should involve the same approach as that for nonirradiated patients (i.e., near-total thyroidectomy, although a plea for a return to the earlier practice of lobectomy has been made (5). All patients who have had surgery for benign or malignant nodules should receive suppression therapy with thyroid hormone. Recurrence of benign nodules, but not malignant ones, is greatly reduced (21).

Radiation of the head and neck predisposes patients not only to thyroid cancer but to salivary gland tumors with a ratio of benign to malignant lesions similar to that of thyroid. The incidence of benign neural tumors (neurilemomas, acoustic neuromas) and parathyroid adenomas is also increased. External radiation can also ablate thyroid tissue and produce hypothyroidism. This has been seen for example in mantle irradiation for Hodgkin's disease and can occur after combined surgery and irradiation for head and neck cancers such as those of the larynx.

THYROIDITIS

Pyogenic (Suppurative) Thyroiditis

Pyogenic or suppurative thyroiditis, also known as acute thyroiditis, is rare, and most physicians will never encounter a case. The thyroid infection usually follows bacteremia but can occur as an isolated, primary event. The gland shows typical signs of an acute inflammatory process.

Riedel's Thyroiditis

Riedel's thyroiditis is another rare but indolent and painless form of thyroiditis. The intense induration associated with this process makes the clinical differentiation from infiltrating neoplasm difficult.

Hashimoto's Thyroiditis

Hashimoto's thyroiditis is common (see "Hypothyroidism," "Goiter," and Table 73.7). The process is painless and usually produces only modest enlargement of the thyroid. Nodularity is the rule. Distinction from nontoxic nodular goiter is made by the presence of high titers of thyroid autoantibodies in the serum of 80 to 90% of patients with Hashimoto's thyroiditis.

Subacute Thyroiditis

Subacute thyroiditis, also known as granulomatous or de Quervain's thyroiditis, is common. Many mild cases are probably never diagnosed. The term *subacute* is often deceiving and sometimes inappropriate. Although the onset may be insidious, it is perhaps just as often acute over several days. Many patients give a history of recent antecedent upper respiratory tract infection.

The earliest symptoms may be referred pain, usually to the ear, but pain can appear to originate in the jaw or occiput. This phase may last a few hours or days before tenderness and discomfort in the thyroid area become apparent. Rarely, the patient is concerned only with the referred pain and is unaware of thyroidal tenderness

until examination makes it apparent. When the onset is acute, the symptoms and signs are more likely to be severe. Initially, pain and swelling of the thyroid are often unilateral, but the process usually does not remain localized for more than a few days. Systemic symptoms include fever, especially in acute cases, and a sensation of intense fatigue and malaise. The course may be protracted with symptoms persisting for months, although usually they subside within a week or two.

Erythrocyte sedimentation rate is elevated. Early in the disease, the thyroidal radioiodide uptake is depressed, and plasma T_4 may be elevated. Mild cases have no or only borderline abnormalities of the tests. Significant titers of thyroid autoantibodies are not common but can be seen. The radioiodide uptake test is not likely to be useful diagnostically because in many normal people the uptake is low (see above).

Clinical hyperthyroidism is occasionally seen with subacute thyroiditis (see above). Rarely, hypothyroidism occurs and lasts for several months. Permanent hypothyroidism is unusual. A variant of this syndrome has been described in which neither hypothyroidism nor hyperthyroidism is present but symptoms of severe systemic illness with fever and weight loss dominate (44). Blood tests of thyroid function are normal except for minimal elevation of free T_4 in a few. Thyroidal radioiodide uptake is low. Thyroid autoantibodies are not present. The thyroid is modestly enlarged and nontender in most cases, but even this clue is absent in some. Biopsies are typical of lymphocytic thyroiditis. Patients respond to anti-inflammatory therapy (see below).

Therapy

Therapy for subacute thyroiditis is symptomatic. The patient should be strongly reassured concerning the benign, self-limited character of the disorder. Thyroid tenderness often responds within several days to aspirin in doses sufficient to maintain therapeutic (anti-inflammatory) blood levels. Codeine should be added if neck discomfort is severe. In less than 10% of cases, the process may be severe enough to require glucocorticoid therapy (30 to 60 mg of prednisone daily or equivalent). A glucocorticoid produces prompt relief of pain and tenderness but, if the disease is severe enough to require its use, will usually be necessary for weeks to several months. Relapse is common when therapy is discontinued, and retreatment may be necessary.

Lymphocytic Thyroiditis (Silent Thyroiditis)

Lymphocytic thyroiditis is an important process that occurs in association with both hyperthyroidism and hypothyroidism and is discussed earlier, under "Hyperthyroidism Associated with Thyroiditis and with Postpartum Thyroid Dysfunction."

General References*

Braverman LE, Utiger RD, eds. Werner and Ingbar's the thyroid. 7th ed. Philadelphia: JB Lippincott, 1996.
  Comprehensive textbook on all aspects of the subject.
Felig P, Baxter JD, Frohman LA, eds. Endocrinology and metabolism. 3rd ed. New York: McGraw-Hill, 1995.
Wilson J, Foster D, Larson R, Kronenberg H, eds. Williams' textbook of endocrinology. 9th ed. Philadelphia: WB Saunders, 1998.
  Standard textbooks containing excellent chapters on the thyroid.
Hamburger JI. The thyroid gland: a book for thyroid patients. Boston: The Thyroid Foundation of America, Inc. (Telephone: 617-726-8500).
Wood LC, Cooper DS, Ridgeway EC. Your thyroid: a home reference. Boston: The Thyroid Foundation of America, Inc. (Telephone: 617-726-8500).
  These 2 books are written for patients with thyroid disease.

Specific References

1. Alvarez-Marfany M, Roman SH, Drexler AJ, et al. Long-term prospective study of postpartum thyroid dysfunction in women with insulin dependent diabetes mellitus. J Clin Endocrinol Metab 79:10, 1994.
2. Anonymous. Effects of drugs on thyroid function tests. Med Lett 23:30, 1981.
3. Bagchi N, Brown TR, Parish RF, et al. Thyroid dysfunction in adults over age 55 years: a study in an urban US Community. Arch Intern Med 150:785, 1990.
4. Bahn RS, Heufelder AE. Mechanisms of disease: pathogenesis of Graves' ophthalmopathy. N Engl J Med 329:1468, 1993.
5. Baker RR, Hyland J. Papillary carcinoma of the thyroid gland. Surg Gynecol Obstet 161:546, 1985.
6. Baran DT. Detrimental skeletal effects of thyrotropin suppressive doses of thyroxine: fact or fantasy? J Clin Endocrinol Metab 78:816, 1994.
7. Biondi B, Fazio S, Carella C, et al. Cardiac effects of long term thyrotropin-suppressive therapy with levothyroxine J Clin Endocrinol Metab 77:334, 1993.
8. Biondi B, Fazio S, Carella C, et al. Control of adrenergic overactivity by β-blockade improves the quality of life in patients receiving long term suppressive therapy with levothyroxine. J Clin Endocrinol Metab 78:1028, 1994.
9. Borst GC, Eil C, Burman KD. Euthyroid hyperthyroxinemia. Ann Intern Med 98:366, 1983.
10. Cooper DS. Thyroxine suppression therapy for benign nodular disease. J Clin Endocrinol Metab 80:331, 1995.
11. Cooper DS, Halpern R, Wood LC, et al. L-Thyroxine therapy in subclinical hypothyroidism. A double-blind, placebo-controlled trial. Ann Intern Med 101:18, 1984.
12. Danese MD, Powe NR, Sawin CT, Ladenson PW. Screening for mild thyroid failure at the periodic health examination. A decision and cost-effectiveness analysis JAMA 276:285, 1996.
13. DeGroot LJ, Gorman CA, Pinchera A, et al. Radiation and Graves' ophthalmopathy. J Clin Endocrinol Metab 80:339, 1995.
14. DeGroot LJ, Kaplan EL, Shukla MS, et al. Morbidity and mortality in follicular thyroid cancer. J Clin Endocrinol Metab 80:2946, 1995.
15. Dunn JT. When is a thyroid nodule a sporadic medullary carcinoma? J Clin Endocrinol Metab 78:824, 1994.
16. Eggertsen R, Petersen K, Lundberg PA, et al. Screening for thyroid disease in a primary care unit with a thyroid stimulating hormone assay with a low detection limit. BMJ 297:1586, 1988.
17. Ehrmann DA, Sarne DH. Serum thyrotropin and the assessment of thyroid status. Ann Intern Med 110:179, 1989.
18. Emerson CH, Colzani R, Braverman LE. Epithelial cell thyroid cancer and thyroid stimulating hormone—when less is more. J Clin Endocrinol Metab 82:9, 1997.

19. Fazio S, Biondi B, Carella C, et al. Diastolic dysfunction in patients on thyroid-stimulating hormone suppressive therapy with levothyroxine: beneficial effect of β-blockade. J Clin Endocrinol Metab 80:2222, 1995.
20. Finucane P, Rudra T, Church H, et al. Thyroid function tests in elderly patients with and without an acute illness. Age Aging 18:398, 1989.
21. Fogelfeld L, Wiviott MBT, Shore-Freedman E, et al. Recurrence of thyroid nodules after surgical removal in patients irradiated in childhood for benign conditions. N Engl J Med 320:835, 1989.
22. Fradkin JE, Wolff J. Iodide-induced thyrotoxicosis. Medicine 62:1, 1983.
23. Franklyn JA, Black EG, Betteridge J, et al. Comparison of second and third generation methods for measurement of serum thyrotropin in patients with overt hyperthyroidism, patients receiving thyroxine therapy, and those with nonthyroidal illness. J Clin Endocrinol Metab 78:1368, 1994.
24. Fung HYM, Kologlu M, Collison K, et al. Postpartum thyroid dysfunction in Mid Glamorgan. BMJ 296:241, 1988.
25. Grebe SKG, Cooke RR, Ford HC, et al. Treatment of hypothyroidism with once weekly thyroxine. J Clin Endocrinol Metab 82:870, 1997.
26. Gregerman RI, Katz MS. Thyroid diseases. In: Hazzard R, Bierman EL, Blass JP, et al, eds. Principles of geriatric medicine. 3rd ed. New York: McGraw-Hill, 1994;807.
27. Goldmann DR. Subclinical hypothyroidism revisited. When is not enough really not enough? J Gen Intern Med 11:771, 1996.
28. Hamburger JI. Pitfalls in the laboratory diagnosis of atypical hyperthyroidism. Arch Intern Med 139:96, 1979.
29. Hamburger JI. The autonomously functioning thyroid nodule: Goetsch's disease. Endocrinol Rev 8:439, 1987.
30. Hamburger JI. Diagnosis of thyroid nodules by fine needle biopsy: use and abuse. J Clin Endocrinol Metab 79:335, 1994.
31. Hashizume K, Ichikawa K, Sakurai A, et al. Administration of thyroxine in treated Graves' disease. Effects on the level of antibodies to thyroid-stimulating hormone receptors and on the risk of recurrence of hyperthyroidism. N Engl J Med 324:947, 1991.
32. Helfand M, Crapo IM. Screening for thyroid disease Ann Intern Med 112:840, 1990.
33. Ladenson PW. Thyrotoxicosis and the heart: something old and something new. J Clin Endocrinol Metab 77:332, 1993.
34. Laurberg P. Iodine intake—what are we aiming at? J Clin Endocrinol Metab 79:17, 1994.
35. Lippi F, Ferrari C, Manetti L, et al. Treatment of solitary autonomic thyroid nodules by percutaneous ethanol injection: results of an Italian multicenter study. J Clin Endocrinol Metab 81:3261, 1996.
36. Marcocci C, Golia F, Bruno-Bossio G, et al. Carefully monitored levothyroxine suppressive therapy is not associated with bone loss in premenopausal women. J Clin Endocrinol Metab 78:818, 1994.
37. Mazzaferri EL. Management of a solitary thyroid nodule. N Engl J Med 328:553, 1993.
38. Miller JM, Hamburger MD, Kini S. Diagnosis of thyroid nodules. Use of fine needle aspiration and needle biopsy. JAMA 241:481, 1979.
39. Molitch ME, Beck JR, Dreisman M, et al. The cold thyroid nodule: an analysis of diagnostic and therapeutic options. Endocrinol Rev 5:185, 1984.
40. Nikolai TF, Brosseau J, Kettrick MA, et al. Lymphocytic thyroiditis with spontaneously resulting hyperthyroidism (silent thyroiditis). Arch Intern Med 140:478, 1980.
41. Nikolai TF, Coombs GJ, McKenzie AK. Lymphocytic thyroiditis with spontaneously resolving hyperthyroidism and subacute thyroiditis. Long-term follow-up. Arch Intern Med 141:1455, 1981.
42. Oppenheimer JH, Braverman LE, Toft A, et al. Thyroid hormone treatment: when and what? J Clin Endocrinol Metab 80:2873, 1995.
43. Parle JV, Franklin JA, Cross KW, et al. Prevalence and follow-up of abnormal thyrotrophin (TSH) concentrations in the elderly in the United Kingdom. Clin Endocrinol 34:77, 1991.
44. Rotenberg Z, Weinberger I, Fuchs J, et al. Euthyroid atypical

---

*Bold print (general references) and bold numerals (specific references) denote published controlled clinical trials, meta-analyses, or consensus-based recommendations.

subacute thyroiditis simulating systemic or malignant disease. Arch Intern Med 146:105, 1986.

45. Roti E, Minelli R, Salvi M. Management of hyperthyroidism and hypothyroidism in the pregnant woman. J Clin Endocrinol Metab 81:1679, 1996.

46. Samaan NA, Schultz PN, Hickey RC, et al. The results of various modalities of treatment of well differentiated thyroid carcinoma: a retrospective review of 1599 patients. J Clin Endocrinol Metab 75:714, 1992.

47. Samaan NA, Schultz PN, Ordonez NG, et al. A comparison of thyroid carcinoma in those who have and have not had head and neck irradiation in childhood. J Clin Endocrinol Metab 64:219, 1987.

48. Sawin CT, Geller A, Kaplan MM. Low serum thyrotropin (thyroid-stimulating hormone) in older persons without hyperthyroidism. Arch Intern Med 151:165, 1991.

49. Sawin CT, Geller A, Wolf PA, et al. Low serum thyrotropin concentrations as a risk factor for atrial fibrillation in older persons. N Engl J Med 331:1249, 1994.

50. Schneider AB, Recant W, Pinsky SM, et al. Radiation-induced thyroid carcinoma. Clinical course and results of therapy in 296 patients. Ann Intern Med 105:405, 1986.

51. Schneider AB, Shore-Freedman E, Ryo UY, et al. Prospective serum thyroglobulin measurements in assessing the risk of developing thyroid nodules in patients exposed to childhood neck irradiation. J Clin Endocrinol Metab 61:547, 1985.

52. Torring O, Tallstedt L, Wallin G, et al. Graves' hyperthyroidism: treatment with antithyroid drugs, surgery, or radioiodine—a prospective randomized study. J Clin Endocrinol Metab 81: 2986, 1996.

53. Utiger RD. Subclinical hyperthyroidism—just a low serum thyrotropin concentration, or something more? N Engl J Med 331:1302, 1994.

54. Vander JB, Gaston EA, Dawber TR. The significance of nontoxic thyroid nodules. Final report of a 15-year study of the incidence of thyroid malignancy. Ann Intern Med 69:537, 1968.

55. Van Herle AJ, Rich P, Britt-Marie EL, et al. The thyroid nodule. Ann Intern Med 96:221, 1982.

56. Wartofsky L, Burman KD. Alterations in thyroid function in patients with systemic illness: the "euthyroid sick syndrome." Endocrinol Rev 3:164, 1982.

57. Weetman AP. Insulin-dependent diabetes mellitus and postpartum thyroiditis: an important association. J Clin Endocrinol Metab 79:7, 1994.

58. Wehmann RE, Gregerman RI, Burns WH, et al. Suppression of thyrotropin in the low-thyroxine state of severe nonthyroidal illness. N Engl J Med 312:546, 1985.

59. Wortsman J, Premachandra BN, Williams K, et al. Familial resistance to thyroid hormone associated with decreased transport across the plasma membrane. Ann Intern Med 98:904, 1983.

60. Young RL, Mazzaferri EL, Rahe AJ, Dorfman SG. Pure follicular carcinoma: impact of therapy in 214 patients. J Nucl Med 21:733, 1980.

C H A P T E R   74

Selected Endocrine Problems: Disorders of Pituitary, Adrenal, and Parathyroid Glands; Pharmacologic Use of Steroids; Hypocalcemia and Hypercalcemia; Water Metabolism; Hypoglycemia; and Hormone Use of Unproven Value

ROBERT I. GREGERMAN, MD

PITUITARY DISEASES

Disorders of the pituitary gland are manifest by disturbance of function (hypersecretion or hyposecretion of trophic hormones), by anatomic encroachment on adjacent structures (enlargement of tumors), or by a combination of these processes. Many of the cases of hormone hypersecretion are due to benign tumors—often clinically inapparent microadenomas.

Clinical Presentations

When a patient presents with evidence of decreased endocrine function, routine evaluation must include consideration of whether the process is primary (i.e., in the end organ) or is due to pituitary disease (i.e., secondary gland failure). For example, in most patients with hypothyroidism, thyroid-stimulating hormone (TSH) is elevated because of failure of normal inhibition of the negative feedback loop. However, if TSH is not elevated in the face of hypothyroidism, the possibility of hypopituitarism must then be further evaluated. Similarly, in patients with hypogonadism an easy differential diagnosis can be made because levels of follicle-stimulating hormone (FSH) and luteinizing hormone (LH) are invariably elevated when there is primary end-organ failure. In patients with adrenal insufficiency, however, the plasma adrenocorticotropic hormone (ACTH) does not always clearly differentiate primary from secondary disease. In cases of endocrine hyperfunction, pituitary function may also be evaluated but not necessarily routinely (see "Hyperthyroidism," Chapter 73; and "Adrenocortical Hyperfunction," below).

Not infrequently, the issue of pituitary disease is raised inadvertently. The patient's complaints lead to radiologic examination of the skull because of headaches, suspected sinusitis, injury, or other reasons. An enlarged or an abnormal sella turcica is noted. The issue then arises concerning further evaluation of what may be an incidental finding, a so-called pituitary "incidentaloma" (32). Referral to an endocrinologist is appropriate at this point, but further evaluation by the nonspecialist is also possible (as described below).

Evaluation of the Sella Turcica

The sella turcica as seen in ordinary x-rays of the skull may appear deceptively normal or may appear abnormal when it is not. Computerized tomography (CT) with contrast and magnetic resonance imaging (MRI) have almost totally replaced older techniques for evaluating the sella. In major medical centers, MRI is used almost exclusively because of its better resolution, even for initial examinations, but for this purpose CT is less expensive, more readily available, and completely satisfactory for the demonstration of 50 to 60% of lesions, most of which are intrasellar microadenomas. If a microadenoma cannot be demonstrated by CT or if suprasellar extension proves to be present on CT, MRI (gadolinium enhanced) should then be obtained; an additional 20% of microadenomas will be demonstrated. In a few centers, venous sampling techniques for ACTH can lateralize many of the nonvisualizable adenomas that are the cause of Cushing's disease, thus facilitating hemisectioning at surgery. In addition, if suprasellar extension is present, the patient should be referred for ophthalmologic examination of the visual fields, preferably with a red dot, the most sensitive technique for detection of field defects produced by suprasellar masses.

Empty Sella Syndrome

An enlarged sella does not always mean that a pituitary tumor is present. Extensive evaluation commonly leads to demonstration of an empty sella turcica. Such patients are often discovered during evaluation of skull x-rays obtained for reasons other than suspected hypopituitarism—usually headache—and, indeed, usually have no clinical endocrine disease. The cause of the empty sella syndrome is unknown, but open communication of cerebrospinal fluid through a defect in the diaphragma sellae and a ruptured cyst have been postulated. In most cases, a rim of nonvisualizable normal pituitary tissue remains, and pituitary function, which should be routinely evaluated, is normal; in some there is minimal hypopituitarism or a visual field defect for reasons that are not clear but that could represent a previous cyst. The diagnosis can be suspected from CT that fails to show enhancement, but definitive diagnosis and differentiation from intrasellar tumor requires MRI or, if MRI cannot be done, use of radiopaque dye; pneumoencephalography for this purpose is now obsolete.

Pituitary Tumors

When a pituitary tumor is large enough to produce increased pressure within the sella turcica, enlargement and erosion of the bony walls of that structure either produce no symptoms or may cause headache. Tumor enlargement superiorly leads to encroachment on the adjacent optic chiasm and may produce visual field defects. Pituitary tumors large enough to be anatomically apparent are often associated with failure of hormone secretion (hypopituitarism), a process that results in end-organ failure (hypoadrenalism, hypogonadism, or hypothyroidism). The pituitary may also be affected by a wide variety of systemic illnesses, including granulomatous, infectious, vascular, and neoplastic processes, but all are extremely uncommon causes of hypopituitarism.

A related problem is that of *craniopharyngioma*. This developmental abnormality may simulate pituitary tumor. The lesion is usually outside the pituitary and presents as a suprasellar mass lesion readily evident on CT or MRI. Most cases are manifest during childhood.

Chromophobe Adenomas

Chromophobe adenomas, the most common of the pituitary tumors, account for approximately 85% of cases; most occur between ages 30 and 60, often in association with parathyroid or pancreatic islet cell adenomas and, sometimes, with the Zollinger–Ellison syndrome (see Chapter 37). These associations constitute the syndrome of multiple endocrine adenomatosis (MEA type I). When the pituitary is not involved, but pheochromocytoma, medullary thyroid carcinoma, and occasionally parathyroid adenomata occur together, the syndrome is termed MEA type II.

Chromophobe adenomas are usually noninvasive but may infiltrate local structures and on rare occasions even behave as locally malignant lesions. Long thought to be functionless, many are now known to be prolactinomas (see below). A few produce growth hormone (GH) and, even fewer, gonadotropins. The term *chromophobe adenoma* belongs to the era in which pituitary tumors were classified by their histologic staining characteristics (chromophobe, eosinophile, and basophile). A more precise classification that is based on the secretory product of the tumor (e.g., somatotrope tumor, GH producing) can now be constructed, but the old terms persist.

Pituitary function remains clinically normal until more than 75% of the normal pituitary has been destroyed by the adenoma. Hypogonadism is usually the earliest evidence of a hormone deficiency state (60 to 80% of cases), but hypothyroidism as an initial manifestation is almost as common. Adrenal insufficiency is usually the last problem to develop and is often inapparent except on laboratory testing. In approximately 10% of cases, diabetes insipidus develops.

Prolactinomas: Prolactin and Galactorrhea

In the female, unilateral or bilateral galactorrhea may be the first clue to the presence of a prolactin-secreting adenoma (prolactinoma). In many cases, discharge from the breast is minimal and may be apparent only on physical examination when a few drops of milk may be expressible. Breast enlargement may occur in the male, but prolactin excess is an uncommon cause of gynecomastia (see Chapter 77). Galactorrhea in the male, a rare event, is diagnostic of a prolactinoma. Prolactin secretion appears to inhibit the secretion of gonadotropins and hence may also be associated with evidence of hypogonadism, including impotence and amenorrhea (see Chapter 77).

However, most cases of galactorrhea in women are not caused by a tumor but by functional disturbance of prolactin secretion, which in turn is either spontaneous or related to the use of certain drugs. In either case, the hallmark of galactorrhea is an increase of the concentration of prolactin in plasma. Radioimmunoassays for prolactin are widely available and present no special problems of interpretation except for the demonstration of a high-molecular-weight form of prolactin in some amenorrheic women. The significance of this material is unknown. The drugs most commonly incriminated in the production of galactorrhea are estrogens (oral contraceptives), phenothiazines, tricyclic antidepressants, α-methyldopa (Aldomet), and reserpine. If no drugs are involved, a functional disorder is still likely, but some cases are caused by chromophobe adenoma. Rarely, galactorrhea occurs secondary to hypothyroidism.

The degree of prolactin elevation is strongly suggestive of the cause of the disorder. Levels of prolactin greater than 200 ng/mL are essentially diagnostic of tumor, even in the absence of changes in the sella. Low levels of prolactin (less than 50 ng/mL) are much more likely to be due to a functional disorder or a drug, but in many cases, differentiation is impossible by quantification of the prolactin level.

Treatment (33). Many cases of galactorrhea, with or without microadenoma, can be treated successfully with the drug bromocriptine (Parlodel), which often lowers the prolactin level, abolishes the galactorrhea, and restores normal menses. Bromocriptine not only reduces prolactin secretion but in many cases causes the tumor to shrink so that even visual field defects can be reversed. A favorable response occurs in 80% of cases. The drug is now commonly given preoperatively, even when a large tumor is present, because surgical removal is thereby facilitated. Long-term drug therapy is an alternative to surgery in most cases (24,25,33). Treatment with bromocriptine can be undertaken by the nonspecialist provided that tumor is unlikely: 2.5 mg Snaptabs and 5 mg capsules; the initial

dosage is 1.25 to 2.50 mg/day; the dosage may be increased by 2.5 mg every 3 to 7 days until an optimum response is achieved—usually 5 to 7 mg/day; patients requiring higher dosages should be referred to an endocrinologist. Adverse effects—especially nausea, headache, dizziness, fatigue—are common. If prolactin levels are very high, if radiographic evidence of tumor is present, or if the condition is unresponsive to bromocriptine, an endocrinologist should be consulted. Alternative drugs that can be useful in bromocriptine refractory cases are available.

Until recently the indications for surgical intervention (transsphenoidal; see "Acromegaly," below) were mainly related to the size of the tumor. Visual field impairment has in the past been the major indication for urgent surgery, but extensive experience indicates that even patients with significant visual loss can be successfully treated with bromocriptine. With transsphenoidal surgery, microadenomas can often be removed successfully and normal pituitary function restored. With marked suprasellar extension, a transfrontal surgical approach may be needed. This is a much more formidable procedure. In many cases a large tumor cannot be completely removed; postoperative radiation therapy prevents clinical recurrence in these instances.

Acromegaly

Pituitary tumors that produce an excess of growth hormone (GH) result in the clinical state termed acromegaly. If the GH excess occurs before cessation of growth, gigantism occurs. When GH excess begins in the adult, the most common clinical feature suggesting the presence of acromegaly is insidious alteration of facial appearance over many years. Old photographs may be useful in helping identify such changes. The various physical findings include enlargement (lengthening) of the mandible, sometimes with separation of the teeth; coarsening of facial features because of both overgrowth of frontal, malar, and nasal bones and soft tissue overgrowth producing widening of the nose and protrusion of the lips; enlargement of the hands and feet, often noted by increasing glove and shoe size; and dermatologic changes that include skin thickening and sebaceous gland enlargement (hydradenitis). Commonly, patients present with a nerve entrapment (carpal tunnel) syndrome. Osteoarthritis and diabetes mellitus, although often seen in this disorder, are too common to provide a clue to the presence of acromegaly. Tumors large enough to produce sellar enlargement may lead to headache; suprasellar extension may result in visual field defects.

The laboratory diagnosis is simple in overt cases but may be difficult in mild cases. GH varies rapidly during the day in the serum of acromegalic patients, so single samples of blood may not be helpful. The best test for screening is probably the determination of serum insulinlike growth factor-I (IGF-I). This product of GH action varies little and correlates well with the 24-hour integrated serum GH level, the most definitive test.

Unfortunately, the accurate laboratory determination of IGF-I cannot be assumed. If GH is measured directly in screening, elevation of serum GH in the fasting, basal state to values consistently greater than 10 ng/mL strongly suggests the diagnosis. However, stress and physical activity may also elevate the GH levels. Elevated values must therefore be confirmed with a test of the ability of glucose to suppress the GH. During a standard glucose tolerance test (see Chapter 72), the GH—determined simultaneously with the glucose—should normally fall to a value less than 2 ng/mL. Most acromegalics show no fall of GH, and a few exhibit a paradoxical rise during the test. Laboratory evidence of elevated and nonsuppressible GH warrants referral to an endocrinologist, as does the presence of equivocal clinical or laboratory findings.

Treatment of Acromegaly. Treatment should be directed by an endocrinologist (30). Irradiation of the pituitary, usually by external high-voltage techniques, has been standard treatment for years. Such therapy is effective but is usually extremely slow in its effect and may take several years to produce maximal suppression of hormone production. Surgery is indicated when rapid reduction of the elevated GH is needed (e.g., for cosmetic reasons in a young woman with early disease; visual field loss; or intractable headache). Transsphenoidal operation is now standard for most cases and should, if at all possible, include an attempt at selective removal of a microadenoma. The transsphenoidal operation involves minimal morbidity, a very low rate of complications, and essentially no mortality, but recurrences are common, leading some authorities to continue to advocate radiation therapy as the first approach for uncomplicated cases. The somatostatin analog, octreotide (a potent GH antagonist), is effective long-term medical therapy but should only be prescribed by an endocrinologist. The drug requires multiple subcutaneous injections. Long-acting depot preparations, already available in Europe, may soon be marketed in the United States (37).

Cushing's Disease

When evidence is obtained for overproduction of glucocorticoids and testing suggests the presence of adrenal hyperplasia (see "Adrenal Diseases," below), evaluation of the sella turcica is in order. Most cases of Cushing's disease with adrenal hyperplasia are caused by a basophilic microadenoma of the pituitary that can be visualized preoperatively, in 80% of cases, with an optimal MRI examination (see below).

Other Secretory Pituitary Tumors

Although quite rare, pituitary tumors that secrete thyrotropin (TSH) and produce hyperthyroidism do occur. Even rarer are cases of hypersecretion of TSH without demonstrable tumor. Patients with tumors have been successfully treated with a somatostatin analog (25). Tumors that produce excessive amounts of gonadotropins are very rare.

Pituitary Failure (Hypopituitarism)

Idiopathic Causes

Patients are occasionally encountered in whom pituitary failure occurs without evidence of pituitary tumor or of another anatomical defect demonstrable by current techniques. Some are eventually found to have infiltrative processes (sarcoidosis, histiocytosis, lymphoma, benign lymphocytic infiltration [hypophysitis]). Hypopituitarism is diagnosed by the demonstration of end-organ failure that occurs in the absence of the expected elevation of trophic hormone. Isolated deficiencies of trophic hormones also occur but are rare. Among these, the most likely to be encountered is hypogonadotropic hypogonadism in the male, sometimes associated with anosmia *(Kallmann's syndrome)*. In these patients, no anatomic basis is apparent.

Sheehan's Syndrome (Postpartum Pituitary Failure)

Massive uterine hemorrhage occurring at delivery occasionally results in pituitary infarction and panhypopituitarism. In this syndrome, failure of postpartum lactation and absence of menses are attended by development of debility and other evidences of end-organ failure. Because of improvements in obstetric care (prompt treatment of hemorrhage), such cases are now rare.

Pituitary Apoplexy

Rarely hemorrhagic infarction of a pituitary tumor leads to severe headache and/or signs of a rapidly expanding intracranial abnormality. Radiographic examination of the sella turcica is abnormal. Another rare phenomenon is that of pituitary infarction (apoplexy) occurring during the course of a febrile illness, presumably viral. Intense headache lasts for days and is usually but not always severe enough to require hospitalization. The acute febrile illness subsides with symptomatic therapy and without specific clinical or radiographic findings, only to be followed later by the development of hypopituitarism. Both men and women can be affected.

Hormone Replacement Therapy of Hypopituitarism

Pituitary insufficiency, regardless of the cause, is treated with thyroid hormone (thyroxine, see Chapter 73), adrenal glucocorticoid (cortisol, see below), and gonadal hormone (testosterone [Chapter 77] or an estrogen [Chapter 77]). GH has recently been used to restore muscle mass. Other pituitary trophic hormones are not used routinely. Occasionally, young women may be candidates for therapy with gonadotropins to produce ovulation and restore fertility. Such therapy may be effective but is available at only a few centers. In men, normal libido and sexual performance consistent with age can be ensured with testosterone therapy. Restoration of fertility in the male is also possible with the use of a combination of gonadotropins, but such therapy is not generally available.

Disturbances of Pituitary Function Caused by Nonendocrine Disease

Much more common than decreased pituitary function resulting from intrinsic pituitary disease is altered gonadotropin secretion on a functional basis. Many illnesses can affect the functional integrity of the hypothalamic–pituitary–end-organ axis. This phenomenon is most obvious as disturbance of menstruation in women and, less often, impotence in men (see Chapter 77). Any disease that results in *malnutrition* can produce decreased gonadotropins and (secondary) amenorrhea or impotence. *Alcoholism* is an outstanding example. Liver disease need not be present in alcoholism to produce amenorrhea or impotence, but various liver diseases are themselves associated with loss of menses. The common factor seems to be malnutrition.

The classic example of nonendocrine illness that simulates an endocrine disturbance is *anorexia nervosa* (see Chapter 5). In this psychiatric disturbance, which results in severe malnutrition with resultant weight loss, the most marked disturbance of endocrine function is cessation of menses resulting from a decrease of gonadotropins. Other trophic hormones are not affected. Thyroid function is usually normal. Axillary and pubic hair are retained, giving important clinical evidence for the preservation of adrenal function. Although cortisol secretion is low (urinary steroid excretion is decreased), this results from slow metabolic disposal of cortisol rather than decreased ability to increase ACTH secretion appropriately; plasma cortisol is normal. GH concentration may be elevated, a consequence of starvation due to any cause. The diagnosis of anorexia nervosa should be based on the association of psychiatric abnormalities and obvious decrease in food intake. The tests described will serve merely to support the diagnosis.

Other diseases may also result in secondary amenorrhea because of failure of gonadotropin secretion. These include such diverse conditions as severe emotional disturbances, marked obesity, poorly controlled diabetes mellitus, and severe chronic infections.

ADRENAL DISEASES

Adrenocortical Insufficiency (Addison's Disease)

In ambulatory patients the clinical presentation of adrenocortical insufficiency is related to a number of chronic complaints that are nonspecific in character. Although being suspicious will certainly result in far more tests than positive diagnoses, detection of this rare problem demands such an approach. The alternative is needless morbidity culminating in acute hospitalization for full-blown disease (i.e., vascular collapse with Addisonian crisis).

Etiology and Association with Other Autoimmune Diseases

Adrenocortical insufficiency is now most commonly the result of *autoimmune disease* and is associated with the presence of antibodies to adrenal tissue. Most other cases are secondary to *pituitary disease.* Tuberculosis, once a common cause, now only rarely produces adrenocortical insufficiency, probably because of decreased frequency of *tuberculosis* and effective therapy. Many cases of autoimmune adrenocortical insufficiency are associated with autoimmune thyroiditis, although the two problems may develop years apart. The simultaneous occurrence of autoimmune thyroid and adrenal disease is termed *Schmidt's syndrome.* Rarely, autoimmune adrenocortical insufficiency, autoimmune hypothyroidism, and autoimmune gonadal failure occur in the syndrome of *polyglandular failure.* There is also an association of autoimmune adrenocortical insufficiency with pernicious anemia and Sjögren's syndrome, and probably with systemic lupus erythematosus. Other rare causes of adrenocortical insufficiency include histoplasmosis and sarcoidosis.

Clinical Presentation

Chronic symptoms include anorexia, weight loss, weakness, and decreased physical endurance. Vomiting may occur, and abdominal pain, sometimes resembling that of peptic ulcer disease, can be a presenting feature. Other symptoms include mental sluggishness, irritability, and symptoms of either postural hypotension or of hypoglycemia. In primary adrenal insufficiency, increasing pigmentation (white patients) or further darkening of skin (African-American patients) may be noted. Loss of axillary and pubic hair—an important finding when present—may occur in women. Such hair loss is commonly overlooked on physical examination and is rarely volunteered as part of the history.

Physical examination often shows postural hypotension. Pigmentation is diffuse but in addition is especially evident in creases of the hands, the areolae, over pressure areas (knuckles, elbows), and in new scars. Pigmentation of buccal mucous membranes is a pathognomonic finding in white patients but is a normal finding in blacks. Lymphadenopathy is occasionally seen. When the adrenal insufficiency is secondary to pituitary disease, additional findings may relate to the manifestations of a pituitary tumor (headache, visual loss; see above), to hypothyroidism (see Chapter 73), or to hypogonadism (see Chapter 77).

Laboratory Evaluation

Classically, hyponatremia associated with hyperkalemia and some degree of azotemia provided the clues to the diagnosis. These latter abnormalities are manifestations of severe disease and are usually absent in the less severe cases that are likely to be encountered in an ambulatory practice. Various other nonspecific abnormalities occur, occasionally including anemia, lymphocytosis, and eosinophilia.

Laboratory diagnosis of adrenal insufficiency must be made or excluded by determination of plasma cortisol. Determinations of plasma cortisol made without prior adrenal stimulation by injected ACTH have many limitations. In this regard both the normal diurnal rhythm of cortisol and the high degree of variability of plasma cortisol in normal people must be kept in mind. Plasma cortisol can be initially measured at any time of the day, and a robust normal value (15 to 25 µg/dL) will exclude the diagnosis. However, afternoon determinations may be low simply because of the normal evening drop, and even the fasting morning cortisol is highly variable. Values lower than 5 µg/dL at any time are highly likely to be due to adrenal insufficiency. Intermediate values (5 to 10 µg/dL) may be seen in less severe cases and may overlap those of normals. Thus, measurement of unstimulated plasma cortisol is useful, especially in excluding the diagnosis, but may fail to detect mild cases or may yield indeterminate values.

Evaluation of the significance of low or borderline values of plasma cortisol should always be made by administering exogenous ACTH and then measuring plasma cortisol again—after the adrenal stimulation. The ease with which such testing is performed—and the common failure of unstimulated plasma cortisol values to give definitive information—provides a cogent argument for use of ACTH stimulation as the preferred screening procedure for adrenal insufficiency. Many variations of *ACTH stimulation tests* have been advocated. A simple and reliable procedure is the bolus intravenous injection of 0.25 mg of synthetic ACTH (Cortrosyn) (see below). Plasma cortisol obtained 2 to 3 hours after injection will normally increase two to four times over baseline and should rise to be above the normal baseline range (to at least 18 to 20 µg/dL). Patients with adrenocortical insufficiency do not show a response. If the test is positive (no response), confirmation should be made with an *8-hour intravenous infusion of ACTH* (Cortrosyn, 0.25 mg in 500 to 1000 mL of saline or glucose) and at least two plasma cortisol measurements obtained between 6 and 8 hours. Expected increments of cortisol are somewhat greater after ACTH infusion than after bolus injection.

Rapid 1-hour screening tests with ACTH are widely recommended but should be avoided because the increment of cortisol is less than when a longer period is used. The 1-hour test is therefore more difficult to interpret and less reliable. ACTH can be given by intramuscular injection, but if there is no response, the test must be repeated by intravenous administration.

Tests of adrenal function based on *urinary excretion of steroid metabolites* (17-ketogenic [17-KGS] or 17-hydroxysteroids [17-OHS]) should be avoided as initial tests for adrenal insufficiency. These tests offer no advantage over plasma cortisol measurements and often yield artificially low values because of incomplete collection of urine. After stimulation with ACTH, determinations of urinary steroids can, however, provide useful confirmation of the plasma cortisol response. The adrenal response to ACTH is slow in secondary adrenal insufficiency and requires stimulation for up to 3 days. However, other tests of pituitary function are available (e.g., FSH, LH, TSH assay) and

serve better to identify the presence of adrenal insufficiency resulting from pituitary disease (18).

Plasma ACTH can be determined by immunoradiometric assay. An elevated level (above 100 pg/mL) is seen in primary adrenal insufficiency because of the lack of inhibition of the negative feedback system. Plasma ACTH is an adjunct to diagnosis; its major usefulness is in establishing a diagnosis of secondary (pituitary) adrenocortical insufficiency.

Although the adrenal mineralocorticoid *aldosterone* may be low in adrenal insufficiency, the hormone is secreted by the zona glomerulosa rather than the more central portion of the adrenal cortex and may be relatively unaffected by processes that destroy much of the adrenal. Therefore measurements of plasma and urinary aldosterone have no place in routine diagnosis of adrenocortical insufficiency.

Treatment of Addison's Disease

The Addisonian patient should be made to realize the importance of taking hormone therapy regularly and of understanding self-care during situations of stress. Unless both patient and physician cooperate in this effort, the life of the Addisonian patient becomes a series of hospitalizations requiring emergency therapy for crises, most of which should be avoidable.

Steroid Replacement Therapy. Recommended dosage schemes vary. Under normal circumstances patients are given 15 to 20 mg of cortisol (or equivalent) daily. The simplest and least expensive therapy is 12.5 mg (one-half of a 25-mg cortisone tablet) taken twice daily. In another scheme, 10 to 15 mg of cortisol (hydrocortisone) is used on the same schedule. Some authorities prefer to simulate the normal diurnal rhythm of cortisol secretion, although no evidence indicates that this scheme is of any special benefit. In this approach, 10 to 15 mg of cortisol is given on arising and 5 to 10 mg in the evening. Many physicians still prescribe 30 mg of cortisol (hydrocortisone) per day, an amount that exceeds physiologic replacement and should be avoided. Hydrocortisone is not readily available in pharmacies; as a result, noncompliance is more likely to result than with the use of other glucocorticoids (cortisone acetate, prednisone, dexamethasone) that are routinely kept in stock.

Equivalent doses of prednisone or another glucocorticoid (Table 74.1) may be used but have no advantage. Their use may, indeed, dictate a requirement for additional mineralocorticoid therapy because glucocorticoids such as prednisone and dexamethasone have much less mineralocorticoid activity than does cortisol (or cortisone). Overtreatment with glucocorticoids should be avoided. Frequently increasing the dosage for treatment of nonspecific complaints is a common practice but is to be deplored because iatrogenic Cushing's syndrome is a real hazard to the long-term well-being of patients with Addison's disease. The response to replacement therapy varies: Weakness and lassitude ordinarily abate within hours to days, but other symptoms may diminish somewhat more slowly.

The requirement for glucocorticoids (cortisol) is

Table 74.1.   Commonly Used Glucocorticoids[a]

Generic Name	Common Trade Name(s)	Equivalent Potency (mg)[b]	Sodium Retention Relative to Cortisol
Cortisol (hydro-cortisone)	Cortef	20	—
Cortisone[c]	—	25	1
Prednisone	Deltasone Meticorten Delta Cortef	5	0.1
Prednisolone	Meticortelone Sterane	4	0.1
Methylprednisolone	Medrol	4	0
	Aristocort, Kenacort	4	0
Dexamethasone[d]	Decadron	0.75	0
Betamethasone[d]	Celestone	0.6	0
For Parenteral Use			
Cortisol	Solu-Cortef		
Methylprednisolone	Solu-Metrol		
Triamcinolone	Aristocort		
Dexamethasone	Decadron		
Betamethasone	Celestone		
For Topical Use			
Triamcinolone	Aristocort, Kenalog		
Fluocinolone	Synalar		
Methamethasone	Valisone		
For Inhalation and Intranasal Use			
Beclomethasone and others (see Chapters 23 and 55)	Vanceril		

[a]Most of the compounds listed are available in generic forms. All are marketed as ester derivatives or salts of esters (e.g., cortisol sodium hemisuccinate [Solu-Corte]). For practical purposes, only cortisol and cortisone have significant salt-retaining (mineralocorticoid) action.

[b]Also equivalent to daily physiologic replacement when given in divided doses.

[c]Cortisone acetate has long been given parenterally (intramuscular route) as well as orally; however, this compound is unpredictably absorbed from injection sites and cannot be relied on to produce adequate blood levels.

[d]This compound has a relatively long duration of action and should not be used for alternate day glucocorticoid therapy.

increased during stress. In the ambulatory patient, minor stress can be handled by a properly instructed and motivated patient. Telephone contact with the physician is also useful—or even essential—on many such occasions, especially in the early months of therapy before the patient's ability to deal with these episodes has been demonstrated. The most common stress for the ambulatory patient is an infection, often a viral, febrile illness. Ordinarily, a febrile response to approximately 101°F (38°C) that is unaccompanied by vomiting or diarrhea can be handled by simply increasing the cortisol dose to 50 to 75 mg/day in divided doses. A more severe episode (e.g., bronchitis) may require 100 mg. The occurrence of vomiting or significant diarrhea requires contact with a physician and may demand the use of parenteral glucocorticoids.

The need for hospitalization during stress must be determined by the physician and depends on the circumstances. It is obviously prudent to be cautious, but in this long-term chronic illness, frequent and precipitous hospitalizations should be avoided. Many minor events can be handled by judicious increase of steroid dosage. Perioperative management is described in Chapter 86.

Although not all patients with fully developed adrenal insufficiency require mineralocorticoid therapy in addition to cortisol replacement, such therapy is usually started when the diagnosis is made. The initial dose is 0.1 mg of fludrocortisone daily (Florinef, 0.1-mg tablets). Aldosterone is not available for therapy of Addison's disease. Only rarely will patients require more than 0.1 mg of fludrocortisone. In the past, dosages as high as 0.2 mg/day were used, but hypertension and edema were common. A maintenance dosage of 0.05 mg is average, and some individuals require as little as 0.05 mg every other day. Adequacy of therapy can be judged by determinations of serum sodium and potassium and clinical observations, including normalization of blood pressure without postural hypotension. When, during stress, the dosage of cortisol is increased beyond 50 to 75 mg/day, fludrocortisone therapy becomes unnecessary because the mineralocorticoid activity of cortisol is sufficient to maintain salt balance when taken in greater than baseline physiologic amounts.

Patient education. The patient and members of the patient's household should be educated about the symptoms of Addisonian crisis and how to respond in emergencies. In addition, the patient should carry an identification document or wear an inscribed bracelet that identifies the Addisonian state and contains instructions for therapy. Appropriate information in addition to name, address, and telephone number should read approximately as follows:

I am a patient with adrenal insufficiency (Addison's disease). If I am seriously injured, found unconscious, or am vomiting, I should be given an injection of dexamethasone, as emergency treatment for Addisonian crisis. A filled syringe is with my belongings. Notify my physician (name, telephone number) or other medical authority immediately.

Syringes containing dexamethasone phosphate (4 mg in 1 mL of water) are available for patients and can be conveniently carried.

All patients with Addison's disease should eat a diet that contains a liberal quantity of sodium (100 to 150 mEq/day), regardless of whether mineralocorticoids are used. In the event of intercurrent diarrhea or profuse sweating, additional salt should be consumed. Electrolytes should be checked periodically (every 3 to 4 months during the critical first year of therapy). Mineralocorticoid therapy should be cautiously reduced if edema, hypertension, or hypokalemia is noted, and salt or mineralocorticoid should be increased if postural hypotension, hyponatremia, or hyperkalemia appears. Overtreatment with glucocorticoids should be carefully avoided. Over the long-term, it should be borne in mind that, if the Addison's disease is idiopathic (i.e., autoimmune), related diseases and their own manifestations may appear at any time (hypothyroidism, hypoparathyroidism, hypogonadism).

Adrenocortical Hyperfunction: Cushing's Syndrome and Adrenal Androgen Excess

The adrenals produce several steroid products: glucocorticoids (chiefly cortisol), mineralocorticoids (chiefly aldosterone), and so-called adrenal androgens (a group of steroids collectively termed 17-ketosteroids [17-KS]). Clinical disorders are known that affect predominantly the secretion of one or other of these hormones. Table 74.2 lists these disorders of adrenal hyperfunction. Most are rather uncommon or rare, but some essentially functional disorders are commonly encountered. The approach presented here is predominantly oriented to the recognition—or exclusion—and initial evaluation of these diseases in ambulatory patients. Once the practitioner is reasonably certain that a problem exists, detailed evaluation often requires consultation with an endocrinologist and sometimes hospitalization for special procedures. However, many relatively simple tests to define the situation can and should be performed on an ambulatory basis. It must be appreciated that details of diagnostic workups vary widely even among specialists and are in constant evolution as new hormone assays and tests emerge.

Cushing's Syndrome (Glucocorticoid Excess)

Etiology. In this syndrome a supraphysiologic amount of glucocorticoid (cortisol) is secreted along with varying amounts of adrenal androgens. Most cases are due to *hypersecretion of ACTH from the pituitary* with resultant adrenal hyperplasia (Cushing's disease). In recent years it has become apparent that almost all of these cases are caused by *pituitary microadenomas* that produce excessive amounts of ACTH (see "Pitu-

Table 74.2. Adrenocortical Hyperfunction

Glucocorticoid Excess Predominates
Adrenal hyperplasia (60–70% of all cases)
1. Pituitary microadenoma secreting ACTH (most cases of adrenal hyperplasia)
2. Endocrine tumor (pheochromocytoma, medullary carcinoma of thyroid, others secreting ACTH in addition to other hormones [rare])
3. Nonendocrine tumor secreting ACTH (rare)
Adrenal neoplasm (30–40% of all cases)
1. Adrenal adenoma
2. Adrenal carcinoma (about equal in frequency)

Adrenal Androgen Excess Predominates (Hirsutism/Virilism)
Some adrenal adenomas
Some adrenal carcinomas
Partial adrenogenital syndrome[a]

Aldosterone Excess
Primary aldosteronism
1. Adrenal adenoma
2. Adrenal nodular hyperplasia
Secondary aldosteronism
1. Salt and volume depletion, including diuretic use and various disease states causing increased production of renin
2. Juxtaglomerular cell hyperplasia or tumor (rare)

[a]Complete enzymatic defects in steroid synthesis are rare and are invariably manifest early in life as adrenal insufficiency and abnormalities or genital development. In ambulatory adults, partial defects of synthesis of cortisol lead to compensatory adrenal hyperplasia with production of excessive quantities of adrenal steroids with weak androgenic activity. Hirsutism, with or without virilism, ensues (see Chapter 77).

itary Diseases," above). A smaller number are caused by *adrenal adenomas* or *carcinomas.* Cushing's syndrome may also occasionally be caused by *ectopic production of ACTH* by malignant tumors. Of these tumors, small cell carcinoma of the lung is most commonly involved. When a tumor causes Cushing's syndrome, the malignancy is usually obvious, although rarely a small neoplasm may be inapparent when the evidence of glucocorticoid excess first appears.

Clinical presentation. The severity of the signs and symptoms depends on the magnitude of the steroid excess, the rapidity with which it develops, and the degree to which androgen production is increased. The signs and symptoms of glucocorticoid excess are familiar to all physicians who have seen the entire picture of this disease emerge as the result of long-term treatment of patients with prednisone and similar drugs. Glucocorticoid excess produces increased deposition of subcutaneous fat in the face *(moon facies),* and deposition of fat in the upper body produces *buffalo hump* and *truncal obesity.* Skin changes include *telangiectasia* over the face, atrophy and thinning of the skin with easy or spontaneous bruising, ecchymoses, and development of purplish *abdominal striae.* Hyperpigmentation is sometimes seen. *Muscle weakness* results from so-called steroid myopathy (often associated with elevated creatine phosphokinase activity in the blood) and is especially prominent in the shoulder and pelvic girdle areas. The extremities become thin as muscle wasting occurs. Eventually bone mineral loss occurs, producing *osteoporosis* with its resultant back pain. Crush fractures of the vertebrae are common and often spontaneous, and hip or wrist fractures may occur after minimal trauma. *Hypertension* and diabetes mellitus are common. Hypokalemia may occur. Probably less well recognized are the *psychiatric disturbances* that result from chronic glucocorticoid excess. Lability of mood, depression, mania, and frank psychoses may all be precipitated by glucocorticoid excess.

Androgenic effects occur from both the intrinsic properties of the glucocorticoids and the associated production of adrenal androgens. With glucocorticoid excess alone, only mild signs are usually evident: hirsutism (facial, extremities, truncal) and acne. More profound androgen effects that include virilization suggest adrenal tumor. These signs include frontal baldness in women, oligomenorrhea, increase in muscle mass, and enlargement of the clitoris. Androgenic effects cannot, of course, be appreciated in men.

Differential Diagnosis

Obesity and Hirsutism. In women, obesity is often associated with hirsutism, hypertension, and diabetes mellitus. When weight gain is rapid, striae may appear. These findings often raise the possibility of Cushing's syndrome and provoke laboratory screening for this disorder. Few such patients are found to have Cushing's syndrome.

Half of obese people have increased cortisol production, which is a phenomenon resulting from the obese state. In these people the urinary excretion of steroid metabolites is increased and falls into the range of that seen in Cushing's syndrome. However, in distinction from Cushing's syndrome, such obese people have plasma cortisol concentrations that are normal rather than elevated. Furthermore, the suppressibility of the pituitary–adrenal axis in obesity is also normal (see "Laboratory Diagnosis," below). The obesity-related increase of urinary steroid metabolite excretion is one of several reasons why such measurements are to be avoided for screening purposes.

Psychiatric Illness. Psychiatric symptoms are common in Cushing's syndrome. However, it has also been appreciated that severe depressive illness may be associated with markedly excessive production of glucocorticoids and lack of suppressibility with dexamethasone (see below). These patients do not appear clinically to have full-blown Cushing's syndrome, but at least some clinical features suggest the diagnosis and lead to laboratory investigation. Differentiation from true Cushing's syndrome may be difficult at first, but the differential diagnosis eventually becomes clear because remission of the psychiatric disturbance results in disappearance of the abnormal laboratory findings.

Laboratory Diagnosis

General. The tests of adrenal and pituitary function fall into two groups: static measurements of blood or urine steroids or dynamic testing of the pituitary–adrenal axis. Both procedures are useful and may be combined. With regard to the measurements themselves, in blood both plasma cortisol and ACTH can be assayed. In urine, assays are available for cortisol (free cortisol), two different groups of cortisol metabolites (17-OHCS and 17-KGS), and the adrenal androgens (17-KS), which also include some cortisol metabolites.

Screening for Suspected Cushing's Syndrome. *Suppression tests.* Many patients with Cushing's syndrome have mild disease. Steroid production in such individuals is not greatly increased and there is considerable overlap with normal values. Accordingly, determination of plasma cortisol or urinary steroid excretion is not likely to be helpful. Screening can best be performed with an abbreviated suppression test with use of dexamethasone. A single oral dose of 1 mg is given between 11 PM and midnight, and the plasma cortisol is measured at 8 to 9 AM. Normal people show suppression of cortisol to less than 5 µg/dL. If the test is abnormal, a more involved but more reliable suppression test is performed in which dexamethasone is given orally at a dosage of 0.5 mg every 6 hours for 2 days. Plasma cortisol, urinary 17-OHCS, or both can be monitored by this test. The plasma cortisol at the end of the suppression period should be suppressed to less than 3 µg/dL. Urinary 17-OHCS during the second 24 hours should not exceed 2.5 mg. Suppression is normal in obesity but may be abnormal in patients with psychiatric illness.

Other Screening Procedures. An alternative screening procedure is measurement of the 24-hour urinary excretion of cortisol (free cortisol). This test is relatively sensitive. Minimal elevations of plasma cortisol result in marked increases of urinary cortisol. The test is not affected by obesity but may be altered in patients with psychiatric illness.

The normal diurnal rhythm of plasma cortisol tends to be obliterated in Cushing's syndrome. In normal individuals, the 4-PM cortisol is on an average 50% of that obtained in the early morning. Although widely advocated for diagnosis, determination of this rhythm by measurement of morning and evening cortisol is an unreliable screening procedure.

Interpreting tests and additional diagnostic maneuvers. Unfortunately, both false-positive and false-negative screening tests occasionally are seen. If the tests are equivocal and the clinical features strongly suggestive, referral to an endocrinologist is appropriate. In expert hands, a variety of maneuvers can usually establish or exclude the diagnosis and differentiate among the causes of Cushing's syndrome, but familiarity with the specialized test procedures is essential. Often a degree of laboratory precision is required that is not always achieved by ordinary commercial laboratories. Useful tests likely to be used in such consultations, in addition to those described, include multiple samplings of plasma cortisol throughout the day and night (integrated blood levels), determinations of urinary excretion of steroids on multiple occasions, variations of the dexamethasone suppression test with the use of different doses of the steroid, and plasma ACTH measurements.

Until strong laboratory evidence is at hand to indicate that steroid production is abnormal, procedures such as CT or MRI of the sella turcica and of the adrenal areas are not justified. These procedures are not useful in screening, although they are important in determining the locus and cause of steroid excess once this phenomenon has been established.

Treatment of Cushing's Syndrome

Surgery remains the treatment of Cushing's syndrome caused by an adrenal adenoma. Although surgical removal of the adrenals (bilateral adrenalectomy) was accepted for years as the most effective therapy for Cushing's disease (adrenocortical hyperfunction caused by ACTH excess), this treatment has been abandoned. Induction of permanent adrenal insufficiency, the risk of development of an enlarging pituitary adenoma accompanied by hyperpigmentation *(Nelson's syndrome),* and significant operative mortality and morbidity are drawbacks of adrenalectomy for this condition. Over the past decade, it has been appreciated that most cases of Cushing's disease can be treated by transsphenoidal surgical removal of a pituitary microadenoma, and this approach has become the preferred therapy (4,26). However, a significant number (estimates range from 5 to 25%) of patients treated in this manner experience recurrence within a short time despite apparently successful removal of a microadenoma. Medical therapy with an inhibitor of adrenal steroid synthesis is effective for these cases, either alone or in combination with pituitary irradiation. The current drug of choice may be ketoconazole

(600 to 800 mg/day) (43), but older inhibitors (mitotane o,p'-DDD, metyrapone, and aminoglutethimide) are also effective. The selection of the therapeutic approach for the individual patient should be made by an endocrinologist.

Adrenal Androgen Excess

If evidence of Cushing's syndrome coexists with signs of androgen excess, the 24-hour excretion of 17-KS should be measured along with 17-OHCS or 17-KGS. However, the 17-KS measurement is of no use in routine screening for Cushing's syndrome. Elevated values do occur but do so less often than the other indices of cortisol production. However, an argument can be made for including a single 24-hour determination of urinary 17-KS in the initial screening workup for Cushing's syndrome, if there is clinical evidence of androgen excess. When adrenal tumor is present, measurement of urinary 17-KS may be the most abnormal test. Some adrenal tumors (benign adenomas or carcinomas) produce enormous amounts of 17-KS. In suspected cases of adrenal tumor, measurement of 17-KS is specifically indicated. Serum testosterone also is elevated in women but not in men (see "Adrenal Mass Lesions," below).

Hirsutism. Hirsutism without virilism (androgen-dependent hirsutism) is common (see Chapter 77). The combination of hirsutism plus virilism, which is rare, is invariably associated with elevated 17-KS. When such a patient is encountered, referral to an endocrinologist is the most appropriate course. In adults, most cases prove to be caused by adrenal tumors. Other causes, such as entities like congenital adrenal hyperplasia (female pseudohermaphroditism, isosexual precocity in men, hypertension, and salt loss), all become apparent in childhood. Only a few cases (due to 21-hydroxylase deficiency) have ever been seen in adults.

Other Adrenal Diseases

Mineralocorticoid Excess

The classical condition resulting from mineralocorticoid excess is primary aldosteronism due to a benign adrenocortical adenoma (Conn's syndrome). Clinical features include hypertension and the manifestations of hypokalemia. A significant number of cases are due to bilateral adrenocortical nodular hyperplasia. The evaluation of this condition is described in Chapter 46.

Mineralocorticoid Deficiency

Aldosterone deficiency is part of classical adrenal insufficiency (Addison's disease) but may also occur as a selective, functional deficiency state in the syndrome of hyporeninemic hypoaldosteronism. The identifying feature is hyperkalemia. The syndrome is described in Chapter 48.

Pheochromocytoma

Pheochromocytoma is a rare catecholamine (epinephrine, norepinephrine)-producing tumor that is usually considered in relationship to the evaluation of hypertension. This tumor is described in Chapter 62.

Adrenal Mass Lesions, Incidentally Identified

Adrenal masses were in the past occasionally discovered during intravenous pyelography, but such lesions are now commonly recognized during CT of the upper abdomen (17,19). When such a lesion is discovered, consideration should be given to the possible presence of Cushing's syndrome, of mineralocorticoid or catecholamine excess producing intermittent or sustained hypertension (pheochromocytoma, aldosteronism), of hirsutism and virilization, and of feminization. Biochemical testing should be initiated as appropriate (36).

Most lesions incidentally encountered during CT are benign, clinically silent adenomas, but a major concern is whether the mass represents a carcinoma. Three considerations are relevant in attempting to make this distinction: biochemical activity, size of the lesion, and the relative incidence rates. Most carcinomas produce biochemically measurable products (e.g., an excess of 17-KS); a few produce 17-KGS but produce normal 17-KS; and rarely only testosterone or aldosterone levels are increased. Benign adenomas may also produce excess quantities of steroids. Nevertheless, tumors producing biochemical products generally should be removed.

If no biochemical abnormality is demonstrable, the size of the lesion gives some indication of whether it is benign or malignant. When discovered, most adenomas are small (less than 6 cm diameter), and most carcinomas are large (more than 6 cm diameter). However, a conservative approach to all such biochemically silent lesions is warranted because even with tumors over 6 cm, more than 60 operations would be necessary to remove one carcinoma, whereas more than 4000 operations would be needed to remove a single carcinoma if one considers all lesions of diameter greater than 1.5 cm.

Occasionally, the adrenal mass is cystic. Large cystic masses can be aspirated by needle puncture; clear fluid indicates a benign lesion, but bloody fluid is indeterminate and cytology is not helpful. Similarly, needle aspiration biopsy is usually not useful in distinguishing benign from malignant cystic lesions.

In follow-up of biochemically silent adrenal masses, CT scans at 2, 6, and 18 months are indicated. Clear evidence of progressive enlargement is an indication for excision. Lesions that are stable at 18 months can be considered to be benign and should not be removed (12).

PHARMACOLOGIC USES OF STEROIDS AS ANTI-INFLAMMATORY AND IMMUNOSUPPRESSIVE DRUGS

Most steroid (glucocorticoid) use is related to treatment of diseases other than adrenal insufficiency. The dosages used exceed those of physiologic output and are best termed supraphysiologic or, simply, pharmacologic. The anti-inflammatory and immunosuppressive properties of these drugs constitute an invaluable part of the modern therapeutic armamentarium, but such uses, at least when prolonged, are invariably associated with side effects. Short-term uses are much safer, if not entirely innocuous. Although the glucocorticoid and mineralocorticoid actions of steroids have been chemically dissociated, no such separation has been possible for desired versus undesired effects. All available glucocorticoids share these properties to an equal degree, although potency (effectiveness per milligram) varies widely (Table 74.1). Despite this fact, certain glucocorticoid compounds have tended to become associated with the treatment of particular conditions (e.g., dexamethasone for treatment of cerebral edema). Often no secure pharmacologic base supports such practices. On the other hand, legitimate pharmacologic differences between available preparations do exist that include different rates of absorption, metabolic disposal, and solubility. Exploitation of such properties is seen in dermatologic use. Triamcinolone and fluocinolone acetonides appear to be much more effective than hydrocortisone for topical use, a phenomenon apparently related to properties of absorption. Another example is the use of beclomethasone (Vanceril) as an aerosol in the treatment of asthma (see Chapter 55) and allergic rhinitis (see Chapter 23).

Adverse Effects

Untoward effects of glucocorticoids are listed in Table 74.3. These problems are related to dose and, equally important, duration of therapy (13,29). No contraindication ever exists to a single dose of glucocorticoid, regardless of the size of that dose. Thus, treatment of an allergic reaction with one or a few doses carries no risk. Long-term therapy, however, should be instituted only after consideration of the risk/benefit ratio. Therapy that is not intended as long term may become so. For example, asthmatic patients may be so impressed by relief afforded by systemic steroids that other modalities are abandoned and the patient becomes totally dependent on glucocorticoids.

Side effects of steroids are closely related to desired effects. Anti-inflammatory effects are obviously desirable when treating a disease such as rheumatoid arthritis. However, many inflammatory responses are beneficial, as for example the inflammatory responses associated with bacterial infection. In this situation, glucocorticoids may inhibit a useful inflammatory response that otherwise would serve to localize the process. Thus, one ordinarily avoids pharmacologic doses of glucocorticoids when infection requiring an antibiotic is necessary. However, patients receiving glucocorticoids commonly develop an infection. Ordinarily, steroid therapy is not discontinued; rather, vigorous antibiotic therapy is instituted and the dosage of steroid is kept at as low a level as the clinical situation allows, thus preventing clinical evidence of adrenal insufficiency and the development of nonspecific but serious symptoms (see "Steroid Withdrawal Syndrome," below).

Adverse effects of steroids are related to not only duration of therapy but the dosage used. Obviously,

Table 74.3.   Untoward Effects of Chronic Glucocorticoid Therapy

Acute
Fluid/electrolyte disturbances
   Sodium retention
   Fluid retention
   Potassium depletion
   Hypokalemic alkalosis
Gastrointestinal
   Peptic ulcer (hemorrhage, perforation)
   Ulcerative esophagitis
Endocrine
   Precipitation of diabetes mellitus
Ophthalmic
   Glaucoma
Neurologic
   Mood swings
   Acute psychosis
   Convulsions

Chronic
Fluid/electrolyte disturbances
   See above, plus hypertension
Musculoskeletal
   Muscle weakness
   Muscle atrophy
   Steroid myopathy
   Osteoporosis/pathologic fractures
   Aseptic necrosis of femoral or humeral heads
   Tendon rupture
Gastrointestinal
   Pancreatitis
Dermatologic
   Impaired wound healing
   Atrophy of skin (fragility)
   Ecchymoses
   Increased sweating
Neurologic
   Convulsions
   Increased intracranial pressure
   Insomnia
   Euphoria
   Depression
Endocrine
   Menstrual irregularities
   Carbohydrate intolerance/diabetes mellitus
   Adrenal atrophy/disruption of normal response to stress
      (iatrogenic Addison's disease)
Ophthalmic
   Cataracts
   Glaucoma
Hematologic
   Thromboembolism
Other
   Weight gain
   Increased susceptibility to infections

one should attempt to use a minimally effective dosage. Nonetheless, some people seem especially vulnerable to unwanted side effects. Poorly nourished, debilitated, and elderly patients are all more prone to the muscle-wasting effects of steroids (steroid myopathy). Postmenopausal women (already prone to develop osteoporosis) are especially vulnerable to the demineralization that accompanies steroid use. Genetically predisposed individuals may develop overt diabetes mellitus when given glucocorticoids. Peptic ulcer disease may be reactivated, and complications such as bleeding or perforation may be precipitated.

Tuberculosis, clinically inapparent except for a positive tuberculin test, may become active. The role of isoniazid prophylaxis in this situation is described in Chapter 29. A gamut of psychiatric problems may be seen in patients who receive corticosteroids—emotional lability, depression, euphoria—which may necessitate adjustment of the dosage.

Topical Therapy

When steroids can be used locally, such use is preferred, especially when long-term treatment is involved. Although absorption may be complete from a local site, the amount of steroid required is often far less when use is local. One thus avoids, to some extent, systemic effects, side effects, and pituitary–adrenal suppression. In addition to dermatologic use of topical steroids, treatments of some ophthalmologic conditions, allergic rhinitis, asthma, and localized joint disease are examples of this principle.

Intermittent Therapy

Usually, severe disease requires initiation of steroid therapy given as multiple daily doses. When the disease intensity has waned (e.g., 1 to 2 weeks), conversion to alternate-day therapy can be made. Intermittent therapy of this type should always be considered when long-term use is contemplated. Such therapy is to be preferred because pituitary–adrenal suppression is not likely, and the adverse effects of glucocorticoids are minimized (13,29). When initiating intermittent therapy, the daily divided dose is given as a single morning dose. After this dose has been shown to be tolerated for several days, the single daily dose may be doubled and given as a single dose every other day. Thereafter, the dose given every other day can be reduced slowly, as clinically indicated. The off day, particularly when alternate-day therapy is first started, may result in the patient becoming symptomatic. To handle this situation small doses of glucocorticoid may be given on this day. Nonsteroidal anti-inflammatory agents may also be helpful in ameliorating symptoms at this time and in easing the transition.

Use of Adrenocorticotropic Hormone

The clinical indications for use of ACTH rather than a glucocorticoid are practically nonexistent. ACTH was available for clinical use even before cortisone was. It is clear that in sufficient amounts (100 units), long-acting preparations (gel or zinc suspensions) given once daily are capable of stimulating adrenal secretion of up to 300 mg of cortisol daily. However, disadvantages are multiple: the route is parenteral, magnitude of response is unpredictable, mineralocorticoid effects (salt and fluid retention, potassium wasting) are considerable, and response in patients previously treated with glucocorticoids is slow and unpredictable. The only advantage is that adrenal responsiveness is maintained during therapy. Com-

bined ACTH–glucocorticoid therapy has been advocated for this reason, as has the occasional injection of ACTH to prevent adrenal atrophy. The advantage of such an approach over that of intermittent glucocorticoid therapy is unclear. Moreover, when ACTH is used alone at high dosages for a prolonged period, pituitary suppression occurs even though adrenal suppression does not. Another disadvantage of ACTH therapy is failure to produce more than the equivalent of 300 mg of cortisol (60 mg of prednisone) despite maximal stimulation of the adrenals. Such a dosage, although considerable, may be insufficient to produce the desired anti-inflammatory effect. The only current, fairly widespread (but diminishing) use of ACTH is in the treatment of acute exacerbations of multiple sclerosis.

Withdrawal from Acute or Chronic Glucocorticoid Therapy

Treatment with glucocorticoids (e.g., cortisone, hydrocortisone, prednisone) produces suppression of the hypothalamus–pituitary–adrenal (HPA) axis; the output of ACTH falls, and there is subsequent adrenal atrophy and an inability to respond to stress with increased cortisol output. The time required for initial suppression is highly variable (see "Recovery from HPA Suppression," below). Patients receiving daily pharmacologic doses of glucocorticoids for more than 1 week should be presumed to have a suppressed response to stress (7,9,44). If stressed by surgery, trauma, or severe infection, these patients should be treated with replacement glucocorticoids as if they had Addison's disease. On the other hand, glucocorticoids may be discontinued abruptly after 2 to 4 weeks of pharmacologic steroid therapy provided that the patient is not under stress, because baseline—as opposed to stress-related—adrenal function is almost always adequate. Patients who have been treated with alternate-day steroid therapy are not at risk because pituitary–adrenal function seems well preserved in these individuals (13,29).

When it becomes desirable to terminate glucocorticoid therapy, the question arises of how to accomplish this goal while avoiding adrenal insufficiency. In the presence of active underlying disease, for which the glucocorticoids may have been given in the first place, a dilemma quickly becomes apparent. The nonspecific symptoms of adrenal insufficiency may be similar or identical to those of the disease that was under treatment. In addition, the occurrence of the "steroid withdrawal syndrome" (see below) may further compound the issue.

Withdrawal Schedule

No single scheme can solve this difficult clinical problem, although many have been proposed (5). However, a few general points can be made. First, even after prolonged therapy, in the absence of active underlying systemic disease, symptoms of true adrenal insufficiency will not occur until the daily dose of glucocorticoid drops below physiologic replacement

(20 mg of cortisol, 5 mg of prednisone, or equivalent; see Table 74.1) although symptoms similar to those of adrenal insufficiency may occur as the daily dose is being reduced (see "Steroid Withdrawal Syndrome," below). Most patients will not be symptomatic if they take a single 20- to 30-mg daily dose of cortisol (or 5 to 7.5 mg of prednisone). Continuation of 20 mg of cortisol a day for 2 months should ensure some degree of recovery of pituitary–adrenal function. Further withdrawal begins to reestablish the normal pituitary–adrenal relationship. Additional reductions of 5 mg of cortisol can be made every 2 to 3 weeks over the next 2 months, or alternatively, an every-other-day program can be tried over the same period; the glucocorticoid can then usually be stopped without producing symptoms. A laboratory assessment of the functional status of the patient's adrenals at this point is described elsewhere (see "Recovery from Pituitary–Adrenal Suppression," below).

Steroid Withdrawal Syndrome

Abrupt withdrawal of pharmacologic doses of glucocorticoids, even after months of therapy, does not always produce chemical evidence of adrenal insufficiency. Nonetheless, the patient may experience many of the symptoms of adrenal insufficiency (e.g., lethargy, malaise, anorexia, nausea, vomiting, myalgias, fever, and in severe cases, desquamation of skin in a manner resembling exfoliative dermatitis). Less than abrupt withdrawal may result in similar but not as severe symptomology (9). Such patients may be found to have normal or elevated levels of cortisol. This phenomenon is not simply adrenal insufficiency but rather is a pharmacologic withdrawal syndrome. Symptoms subside promptly with reinstitution of glucocorticoid therapy (1).

Recovery from Hypothalamic–Pituitary–Adrenal Suppression

Recovery of the HPA axis after 1 week of "steroid burst therapy" (e.g., 40 mg of prednisone for 3 days, followed by a 4-day taper) appears complete within 1 week (7), but the rate of recovery is unpredictable after withdrawal from longer courses of therapy. After long-term glucocorticoid therapy (pharmacologic doses for a year or more), recovery of normal pituitary–adrenal responsiveness does not occur for at least several months, even if the patient receives no exogenous steroid therapy during that time. In the first month after withdrawal, both pituitary and adrenal function remain depressed (low plasma ACTH and low plasma cortisol). Over the following 4 months, pituitary function recovers (plasma ACTH is elevated), but adrenal function remains subnormal (plasma cortisol is lower than normal). Eventually, adrenal function recovers (plasma cortisol levels normalize) and elevated plasma ACTH returns to normal. The entire process may require up to 9 months. During this interval the patient may fare well, provided there is no stress, but replacement therapy with glucocorticoids may become necessary at any time. Accordingly,

no patient should be considered to have normal pituitary–adrenal function unless at least 1 year has elapsed after complete withdrawal of chronic glucocorticoid therapy. Occasional patients seem never to recover normal responsiveness. Ideally, therefore, all patients with a history of long-term steroid therapy should be tested for normal responsiveness 1 year after withdrawal.

Assessment of a glucocorticoid-treated patient's adrenal function under baseline conditions is easy. Both plasma cortisol measurements and urinary excretion of steroid metabolites give a reasonable estimate of such baseline function. However, predicting the response to stress is more difficult. Because hypothalamic–pituitary function usually recovers first, followed by adrenal function, a normal response to exogenous ACTH usually indicates recovery of the entire axis (see "Laboratory Evaluation" in the section on Addison's disease, above, for details of testing with ACTH). A more complete assessment of the integrity of the axis can be made by induction of hypoglycemia with insulin (insulin tolerance testing). Hypoglycemia triggers ACTH release and the cortisol secretory response of the adrenal. A normal insulin tolerance test essentially ensures that if the patient is subjected to stressful circumstances, replacement therapy with steroids will not be necessary. Administration of corticotropin-releasing hormone (CRH) has been advocated as an alternative to the insulin-induced hypoglycemia test. The endpoint is plasma cortisol response. This procedure is certainly easier and safer than an insulin tolerance test. However, the correlation between the two is only fair and the magnitude of the response is only a 1.5-fold mean increase in plasma cortisol, requiring a laboratory with optimal accuracy. Ideally, neither an insulin tolerance test nor a CRH stimulation test should be done by other than an endocrinologist. As a practical matter, empirical short-term corticosteroid administration (coverage) during stress in these patients is probably the simplest, safest, and cheapest way of handling the uncertainty (9).

HYPOCALCEMIC STATES

Hypocalcemia is an uncommon problem in ambulatory patients. The classic cause of hypocalcemia is idiopathic hypoparathyroidism, but most cases encountered are a consequence of inadvertent surgical ablation of the parathyroids during thyroidectomy or of a metabolic disturbance such as renal failure. The causes of hypocalcemia (20) are listed in Table 74.4.

Clinical Manifestations of Hypocalcemia

The symptoms of hypocalcemia are primarily neuromuscular and are not usually evident until the serum calcium falls below about 8 mg/dL and often considerably lower. Mild but very real symptoms are totally nonspecific and include psychologic manifestations (irritability, mood changes, depression), paresthesias, and muscle cramps. More severe symptoms are de-

Table 74.4.   Causes of Hypocalcemia[a]

Hypocalcemia with High Serum Phosphate
Renal failure
Postablative hypoparathyroidism (postthyroidectomy)
Idiopathic hypoparathyroidism

Hypocalcemia with Low or Normal Serum Phosphate
Malabsorption (vitamin D deficiency)
Magnesium deficiency (alcoholism)
Renal rickets (renal tubular acidosis; phosphate diabetes;
    cystinosis; Fanconi's syndrome; vitamin D–resistant rickets)
Medullary carcinoma of thyroid

[a]The serum alkaline phosphatase activity is elevated when severe metabolic bone disease is present. Parathyroid hormone levels are depressed in magnesium deficiency. Parathyroid hormone levels are regularly elevated in renal failure and in pseudohypoparathyroidism. Urine calcium is depressed in most hypocalcemic states, except when the rare renal tubular calcium-wasting syndromes are responsible for the hypocalcemia.

lirium, psychosis, tetany (including laryngeal stridor), and seizures. Neuromuscular irritability can often be demonstrated by the twitching, which is induced by tapping over the facial nerve just anterior to the ear. A positive response is contraction of the facial muscles around the lip *(Chvostek's sign).* Another clinical maneuver is compression of the upper arm by a blood pressure cuff with the pressure elevated above the systolic pressure. A positive response is spasm of the hand induced within 3 minutes *(Trousseau's sign).* Signs of chronic hypocalcemia include patchy hair loss, scaling of skin, atrophy and brittleness of fingernails, and cataract formation. Candidiasis is common. Calcification of the basal ganglia may be seen on radiographic examination of the skull. Either osteosclerosis or osteopenia may occur depending on the cause of the hypocalcemia.

Laboratory Findings

Hypocalcemia can be said to be present when the serum calcium falls below 8.5 mg/dL. However, because almost half of serum calcium is protein bound, reduction of serum protein by 1 g/dL lowers the serum calcium by about 0.8 mg/dL. The level of serum calcium must, therefore, always be evaluated in the context of the serum protein concentration; the serum magnesium concentration should also be evaluated at the same time (see "Other Causes of Hypocalcemia," below). Plasma parathyroid hormone (PTH) levels are low or nondetectable in idiopathic or postablative hypoparathyroidism and in some cases of hypocalcemia due to magnesium deficiency, but they are elevated in pseudohypoparathyroidism, renal failure, malabsorption, and vitamin D deficiency. The interpretation and indications for determination of PTH levels are discussed below.

Idiopathic Hypoparathyroidism

Idiopathic hypoparathyroidism is rare. Although most patients are diagnosed in childhood, some do not exhibit the disease until adult life. Occasionally familial, the idiopathic disease is autoimmune, often associated with high titers of antibodies to parathyroid tissue, and may be seen in association with other autoimmune endocrine diseases (adrenal insufficiency, Hashimoto's thyroiditis) and pernicious anemia.

Postthyroidectomy Hypoparathyroidism

Probably the most common cause of hypoparathyroidism, postthyroidectomy hypoparathyroidism is a complication of surgical thyroidectomy. The hypocalcemic state may become evident immediately after surgery but often takes many years to develop, presumably because of slowly progressive interference with the blood supply to the parathyroids. Routine screening of serum calcium in patients who have had thyroidectomy reveals many asymptomatic patients. Most of these patients seem to need no therapy, but in view of the subtle neuromuscular changes that can result from hypocalcemia, careful consideration should always be given to this issue. Hypoparathyroidism is vanishingly rare after radioiodide therapy of thyroid disease. Only a very few cases have been reported.

Pseudohypoparathyroidism

Pseudohypoparathyroidism is a rare disorder of genetic origin (X-linked dominant trait). In addition to hypocalcemia and its manifestations, there are associated skeletal developmental defects that result in short stature, shortening of metacarpals and metatarsals, and round face. Clinical manifestations attributable to hypocalcemia may not appear until adult life. The biochemical basis of the hypocalcemia is end-organ resistance to the action of PTH. The combination of hypocalcemia, elevated level of parathyroid hormone, and typical skeletal abnormalities is virtually diagnostic.

Treatment of Hypoparathyroidism and Pseudohypoparathyroidism

The treatment of all forms of hypoparathyroidism is similar. A few patients with idiopathic or postablative PTH deficiency can be managed with calcium supplements alone. The dosage is 1 to 2 g of calcium daily. Because calcium gluconate and lactate contain only approximately 10% calcium, one must administer 10 to 20 g of these salts; the carbonate contains 40% calcium. Numerous tablets must be taken; patient compliance is a common problem. Every effort should be made to work out an acceptable, palatable, and economic program with a consistently available preparation for what is invariably lifelong therapy.

The second mainstay of therapy is *vitamin D.* The most commonly used preparation in the past has been *ergocalciferol* (vitamin D$_2$, Calciferol). The dosage is usually 50,000 or 100,000 units daily, although higher doses may be necessary. The compound is available in 50,000-unit (1.25-mg) capsules. The sole advantage of ergocalciferol is cost; it is by far the least expensive form of vitamin D therapy. The disadvantage of ergocalciferol is somewhat unpredictable toxicity with resultant hypercalcemia and all of its manifestations (see below). Because vitamin D is fat soluble, toxicity may last for many weeks or even months after discontinuation of therapy. Glucocorticoids are effective therapy for hypercalcemia caused by vitamin D toxicity.

A preferable vitamin D preparation is its synthetic analog *dihydrotachysterol* (DHT, Hytakerol). The dosage varies from 0.2 to 2 mg/day. The compound is available as tablets and as a solution. The advantage of therapy with DHT is more rapid onset of action than D_2 and more rapid reversal of toxicity on withdrawal of the drug. The only disadvantage of DHT is its relatively high cost. Yet another effective compound is *1,25-dihydroxyvitamin D_3* (calcitriol, Rocaltrol), the natural, active form of vitamin D. This compound is more rapid than DHT in onset and has a shorter duration of effect but has the disadvantage of even greater cost. The dosage is 0.25 to 1.0 μg/day.

The approach to long-term therapy of hypoparathyroidism is institution of a relatively fixed calcium intake at a total level of about 2 g, which is about 1 g over regular dietary intake. Thus, a patient whose normal daily calcium intake approximates 1 g needs an additional 1 g of calcium in the form of supplementary calcium salts (see above). Instruction of the patient by a dietitian is essential. Vitamin D, in whatever form is selected, is given simultaneously, with adjustments of dosage at weekly or biweekly intervals depending on the serum calcium level. The goal of therapy is a serum calcium concentration of 8.5 to 9.5 mg/dL. Hypercalcemia is to be avoided. Once a stable level of serum calcium is reached (1 to 2 months), the patient can be monitored at monthly intervals and eventually every 3 to 4 months. The possibility of toxicity from hypercalcemia is always to be kept in mind. Even mild hypercalcemia predisposes to nephrocalcinosis and nephrolithiasis in these patients.

Hypocalcemia from Other Causes

When hypocalcemia is related to malabsorption, efforts to correct that situation should be undertaken, but simultaneous treatment with vitamin D and calcium may be indicated.

One common cause of hypocalcemia is alcoholism with resultant *magnesium deficiency*. Overt malnutrition need not be present. The mechanisms by which alcohol abuse produces magnesium depletion include decreased dietary intake and alcohol-facilitated renal excretion of magnesium. Magnesium depletion results in both impaired secretion of PTH and impaired PTH action. Intramuscular magnesium therapy normalizes the serum calcium within hours.

Other diseases associated with hypocalcemia include osteomalacia (vitamin D or calcium deficiency) and variants of Fanconi's syndrome (a spectrum of renal tubular abnormalities). The hypocalcemia associated with renal failure is described in Chapter 48.

HYPERCALCEMIC STATES

Routine, automated blood analyses include determinations of serum calcium so that many cases of hypercalcemia (in most laboratories, serum calcium greater than 10.5 mg/dL) are thereby detected, most of them mild and asymptomatic. The demonstration of hypercalcemia always requires investigation.

Etiologies

In an ambulatory setting the most common cause until recently of minimal, asymptomatic hypercalcemia may have been that associated with use of *thiazide diuretics*, although the precise prevalence was unknown. The problem is encountered less often now that dosages of thiazides are generally lower than in the past, and in any case, it is fully reversible upon withdrawal of the drug. Once established as the cause of the hypercalcemia, thiazide therapy may be continued or its dosage decreased if otherwise clinically indicated, if the hypercalcemia is minimal, and if the patient is truly asymptomatic (see "The So-Called Asymptomatic Patient," below). If the serum calcium exceeds 11 mg/dL, one should switch to an alternative, nonthiazide diuretic.

The most common cause of benign hypercalcemia (1 of 1000 people screened) in ambulatory patients probably is *hyperparathyroidism*, due to a small, indolent parathyroid adenoma (21). The approach to such patients is described below.

Some ambulatory patients who are found to have hypercalcemia have weight loss, anorexia, etc. A calcium elevation in this setting is ominous. Because minimal elevations of calcium (10.2 to 11.5 mg/dL) are ordinarily asymptomatic, the patient's symptoms are more likely attributable to the underlying disease rather than to the incidental and associated, but minimal, hypercalcemia. However, hypercalcemia suggests a malignancy (e.g., carcinoma of the lung or breast). These patients should be promptly evaluated and treated (34).

When malignancy is not apparent, the differential diagnosis includes primary hyperparathyroidism (see below). At this point, determination of PTH concentration is useful in elucidating the cause of the hypercalcemic state. However, one should not rely on only a PTH assay to determine the cause of the hypercalcemia. A normal PTH level on repeated determinations usually excludes a diagnosis of hyperparathyroidism (see below), but an elevated PTH level does not necessarily indicate its presence. PTH assays do not always reliably differentiate between hypercalcemia from hyperparathyroidism and that from a PTH-producing tumor. Although tumor-produced hormone is not identical to normal PTH, the antibodies used to quantitate PTH may fail to distinguish between these substances. However, improvements in PTH assays with more specific antibodies and radioimmunometric techniques have improved diagnostic accuracy to a high degree of specificity. Information concerning specificity should be available from the laboratory (see below).

Various other circumstances produce hypercalcemia. These are listed in Table 74.5.

Therapy of Hypercalcemia

The treatment of hypercalcemia from hyperparathyroidism is discussed below (see "Primary Hyperparathyroidism," below).

Therapy to control hypercalcemia that results from a cause other than hyperparathyroidism is not commonly initiated in ambulatory patients. Most often the hypercalcemia or its underlying cause has required initial therapy in a hospital (3,34). However, when the acute symptoms of hypercalcemia have been controlled during hospitalization, long-term palliative therapy may be needed for the ambulatory patient.

Treatment of hypercalcemia of malignancy is usually begun in the hospital; the current drug of choice is the *bisphosphonate* pamidronate (Aredia) (34). Once the problem is controlled, therapy may be continued on an ambulatory basis by administration of intravenous pamidronate, 60 to 90 mg, over a 2- to 4-hour period every 2 weeks. (If this dosage is inadequate or if severe hypercalcemia—calcium above 12.5 mg/100 mL—occurs, the patient may need to be hospitalized again.) Alternatively, the oral bisphosphonate alendronate may be prescribed, but it is not yet approved for this purpose by the FDA and is associated with considerably more toxicity (e.g., oral and esophageal ulcers) than is pamidronate. Other drugs (e.g., glucocorticoids, mithramycin, calcitonin) that have been used in the treatment of malignancy are less effective or potentially more toxic than pamidronate and are prescribed less often today. If possible, the hypercalcemia of malignancy is best dealt with by an oncologist.

Glucocorticoids are often effective in lowering hypercalcemia caused by sarcoidosis and vitamin D intoxication. Mild hypercalcemia in elderly postmenopausal women may sometimes respond to physiologic amounts of estrogen (11,39). Treatment of hypercalcemia with phosphates administered orally is sometimes possible, especially in mild hyperparathyroidism (see below). Often partial control of hypercalcemia is sufficient to relieve symptoms; complete normalization of calcium level is often neither desirable nor necessary.

Primary Hyperparathyroidism

The term *primary hyperparathyroidism* refers to autonomous hyperfunction of one or more parathyroid glands. Hypercalcemia is the hallmark of this disorder. Secondary hyperparathyroidism, on the other hand, is a physiologic or pathophysiologic homeostatic response to situations that lower blood calcium.

The most common cause of primary hyperparathyroidism is a solitary benign adenoma (85% of patients). In a small proportion of patients, more than one adenoma is present, and in the remainder, the cause is idiopathic hyperplasia. Carcinoma of the parathyroid is rare (less than 1% of patients). Hyperparathyroidism may be familial and may occur as part of the syndrome of MEA (see "Chromophobe Adenomas," above).

Diagnosis

Most cases are now detected by routine automated analysis of blood electrolytes. The symptoms (Table 74.6) or sequelae of hypercalcemia may also alert the physician to the diagnosis, but unlike the situation in the past, symptomatic hyperparathyroidism is now a rarity, except for a history of kidney stones in perhaps 20% of cases (41). Once the diagnosis is suspected, however, the presence of hypercalcemia must be established beyond a doubt. Multiple determinations of serum calcium should be made in a laboratory where a high degree of precision is ensured. Because of spontaneous fluctuations of the serum calcium and because of analytic error, values that are only minimally elevated (10.2 to 11.5 mg/dL) must be repeated several times. The resulting mean level should be used for diagnostic purposes, not the last—sometimes normal—value obtained.

Once hypercalcemia is established as being present (greater than 10.2 mg/dL on multiple determinations), the next (or simultaneous) step is to determine the likelihood of the presence of other causes of hypercalcemia (Table 74.5). Finally, assay of PTH in blood should be performed (see below).

Other laboratory findings may include low serum phosphorus concentration and, very rarely in severe cases with bone involvement, elevation of serum alkaline phosphatase activity. Other abnormalities in

---

Table 74.5. Causes of Hypercalcemia

Condition	Comment
Common Causes	
Thiazide drugs	Mild elevation (not >12.5 mg/dL); requires 2 weeks or more to subside
Hyperparathyroidism	Often asymptomatic; commonly discovered on routine blood test
Malignancy (including myeloma)	Most common cause in hospitalized patients; may lead to initial encounter in ambulatory patients
Spurious	Inappropriate technique while drawing blood (venous stasis produces hemoconcentration)
Rare Causes	
Milk alkali syndrome	Requires use (abuse) of both alkali ($NaHCO_3$) and large quantities of milk or calcium salts
Hypervitaminosis D	Usually 50,000 units or more daily
Thyrotoxicosis	Severe disease is evident
Paget's disease of bone	Immobilization is necessary
Immobilization	Body cast in adolescent males; patients with Paget's disease of bone; quadriplegia
Sarcoidosis	Hyperglobulinemia usually present
Chronic renal failure	Uncommon; may exacerbate after transplantation or during hemodialysis
Adrenal insufficiency	Hemoconcentration present
Idiopathic elevation	Mild elevation in postmenopausal women; may revert to normal with physiologic estrogen therapy

Table 74.6.   Symptoms and Signs of Hypercalcemia

Short-Term (Readily Reversible)
General: weakness, anorexia, weight loss, fatigue
Gastrointestinal: nausea, vomiting, constipation
Genitourinary: polyuria, azotemia
Musculoskeletal: bone aches
Neurologic: lethargy, sleepiness, difficulty concentrating, confusion, psychosis
Cardiovascular: bradycardia, electrocardiographic abnormalities (short QT, arrhythmias, digitalis toxicity)
Ophthalmologic: difficulty focusing
Dermatologic: pruritis

Long-Term (Irreversible or Slowly Reversible)
Gastrointestinal: peptic ulcer, pancreatitis
Genitourinary: renal calculi (colic, hematuria); nephrocalcinosis; polyuria
Skeletal: bone loss (osteopenia); subperiosteal resorption, bone cysts, pseudogout
Neuromuscular: muscle atrophy
Ophthalmologic: band keratopathy; conjunctival calcifications (usually require slitlamp examination)

laboratory tests occur but are not useful for screening or in differential diagnosis because they occur nonspecifically. Patients with hypercalcemia, regardless of cause, usually show hypercalciuria, but hypercalciuria may also occur without hypercalcemia. Increased excretion of hydroxyproline-containing peptides occurs, as it does in other bone diseases.

In severe cases of long duration, radiographic studies of various bones reveal a variety of changes suggestive but not diagnostic of hyperparathyroidism. Demineralization (osteopenia) and subperiosteal resorption are most obvious in the clavicles and the hands, and the lamina dura of the teeth may be resorbed. Cystic changes occur in skull and long bones. None of these changes is likely to be seen in cases with minimal hypercalcemia (10.2 to 11.5 mg/100 mL). Radiographic studies are not useful for screening purposes.

Parathyroid hormone assays. Radioimmunoassays are useful but have several limitations. Specificity of the assay varies among laboratories because of the use of different antibodies. Some laboratories offer several different PTH assays, each of which has its own advantages and limitations. The most commonly used procedure until recently, the so-called C-terminal assay, measures a peptide fragment derived from PTH. This assay, as performed on peripheral venous blood (plasma or serum), may be the most sensitive test for detecting hyperparathyroidism, but it is also elevated by impaired renal function, partly because of decreased peptide fragment excretion, and is often elevated in normal elderly patients, especially women over age 65. The elevations seen in primary hyperparathyroidism are often only modest (e.g., 50% greater than the upper limits of normal). Accordingly, at least two or three assays should ordinarily be obtained. The assay also measures PTH-like materials produced by tumors.

Several other widely available assays measure intact hormone or N-terminal fragments. Although these assays are more specific and less likely to be elevated in

cases of ectopic (tumor) production of PTH, they are also less sensitive in detecting primary hyperparathyroidism, being normal in nearly half of cases, albeit inappropriately so for the degree of hypercalcemia. In patients with chronic renal failure, in whom secondary hyperparathyroidism is invariably present, the intact hormone assays are not artificially raised by retention of PTH fragments, as are the C-terminal assays, and more or less reflect the degree of secondary hyperparathyroidism.

Recently introduced immunoradiometric assays for PTH (IRMAs) are replacing the older radioimmunoassays. IRMAs have improved sensitivity and appear to be superior for detecting hyperparathyroidism. Moreover, they show a high degree of specificity and do not detect the PTH-like peptides produced by tumors. Recently, assays have become available that measure the tumor-produced PTH-like peptides but not PTH. The evaluating physician is obliged to know the specificity of the assay used in the laboratory.

Steroid suppression test. Although most cases of hyperparathyroidism and other hypercalcemic states can be diagnosed by the means described, the cause of occasional cases of hypercalcemia remains in doubt. In these, a short course of prednisone therapy (30 to 40 mg/day for 10 to 14 days) may help diagnostically. The hypercalcemia of hyperparathyroidism does not respond to such therapy. Although only about half of cases of hypercalcemia due to malignancy respond, hypercalcemia from diseases that are not always apparent, such as sarcoidosis, and vitamin D intoxication, responds consistently. Daily determinations of blood calcium should always be obtained during such a test.

Further evaluation. Having established the presence of hypercalcemia and elevation of PTH and having excluded by appropriate means malignancy, impaired renal function, and other conditions listed in Table 74.5, the diagnosis of hyperparathyroidism is reasonably well established. However, the urinary excretion of calcium should be determined at this point because patients with *benign familial hypercalcemia* from parathyroid hyperplasia do not have hypercalciuria or other complications of minimal hypercalcemia and do not need surgical intervention. In most cases of hyperparathyroidism, referral to an endocrinologist should be made if the diagnosis is in doubt or if surgery is contemplated.

The So-Called Asymptomatic Patient

A common dilemma in demonstrated hyperparathyroidism is the so-called asymptomatic patient with mild hypercalcemia (10,35). If the patient is truly asymptomatic, a conservative, expectant approach is appropriate given the nonspecific nature of the symptoms. However, most cases of hyperparathyroidism are in fact associated with psychiatric and neuromuscular disturbances that are often not spontaneously articulated. Correlation with the degree of hypercalcemia is poor. The prominent symptoms include anxiety, nervousness, indecision, daytime sleepiness, loss of energy, and typical manifestations of depression such as crying easily, excessive worrying, irritability, and lack of interest. Somatic symptoms are not increased. These psychiatric symptoms are reversible with relief of the hypercalcemia; indeed they may justify a decision in favor of surgery (22).

Therapy

In diagnosed patients the main question is whether surgical intervention is warranted (27). The rate of development of complications (neuromuscular disease, bone disease, decreased renal function) in patients with asymptomatic hypercalcemia is low, with the exception of nephrolithiasis, which develops in approximately 20% of patients (41). Conditions classically associated with hyperparathyroidism such as hypertension, peptic ulcer disease, and pancreatitis, may not be associated with it at all (41). However, the decision for or against surgery will obviously be based not only on the presence of complicating problems, but on such factors as patient age, associated medical illness, and the presence or absence of neuropsychiatric dysfunction (21). In many patients, medical management of the hyperparathyroidism may be indicated (see below).

Surgical Versus Conservative Therapy. In 1990, the National Institutes of Health convened a Consensus Development Conference on the Management of Asymptomatic Primary Hyperparathyroidism (35). The Conference established guidelines for consideration of surgical treatment: *(a)* serum calcium concentration greater than 12 mg/100 mL; *(b)* hypercalciuria, greater than 400 mg/24 hr; *(c)* nephrolithiasis, cystic bone disease, or overt neuromuscular disease; *(d)* markedly reduced cortical bone density; *(e)* reduced renal function as determined by creatinine clearance in the absence of other causes; and *(f)* age less than 50 years. Whether all of these guidelines (e.g., age) are equally important is unclear (41).

A major concern is whether conservative medical management permits progression of bone disease as measured by longitudinal changes in bone mineral density or biochemical indices. When a group of 66 patients were followed for 7 years (24 met guidelines for surgical intervention), no progressive changes were seen. Thus, conservative medical management appears safe (42).

If a decision is made to treat the patient surgically, referral to a surgeon experienced in parathyroid/thyroid exploration is warranted. In such experienced hands, an adenoma, if present, will be located and easily removed in 90 to 95% of cases. Parathyroid hyperplasia, which accounts for 10% of cases of hyperparathyroidism, is usually easily identified. In such cases, the surgeon should be prepared to perform a nearly-total parathyroidectomy. Second neck explorations are technically difficult and may result in unnecessary morbidity (damage to the recurrent laryngeal nerve). Accordingly, any hyperplastic parathyroid tissue that is left behind should be identified with clips. As an alternative, many surgeons are now removing all parathyroid tissue from the neck and transplanting a portion of one hyperplastic gland to an accessible location, usually a sternocleidomastoid muscle or into the forearm.

Failure to identify an adenoma and absence of hyperplasia may require partial thyroidectomy—the adenoma may be embedded in the thyroid—or exploration of the anterosuperior mediastinum. This procedure may be performed at the time of initial surgery or at some time later. Such details obviously involve the surgeon's preference and experience but should be considered and discussed before surgery. If the neck has already been explored unsuccessfully, a selective venous catheterization study with sampling of PTH levels is a useful procedure for preoperative localization of the tumor. Only a few major medical centers can perform this procedure but it is probably worthwhile to avoid unnecessary morbidity when a second operation is performed. Such localization studies are not indicated before initial surgery.

Medical Therapy. The medical therapy of hyperparathyroidism with phosphate is ordinarily limited to those patients in whom surgery is not desirable but who require therapy (35). Although intravenous phosphate therapy carries the risk of soft tissue calcium deposition that problem is much less likely when phosphate is given orally. Sodium–potassium phosphate salts given orally (K-Phos, Neutra-Phos) may produce diarrhea. Dosage should be titrated upward as tolerated. A sodium-free preparation is also available (Neutra-Phos-K) for use in patients whose sodium intake should be restricted. Asymptomatic patients with mild hypercalcemia probably should not be treated with phosphate.

Estrogen has been recommended as an alternative to surgery for uncomplicated hyperparathyroidism. Because many patients with asymptomatic hyperparathyroidism are postmenopausal women, this approach has considerable appeal. Unfortunately, not all patients respond and even in those who do, some abnormalities of bone persist. Norethindrone, a progestogen, has a similar effect to that of estrogen in occasional patients (39).

DISORDERS OF WATER METABOLISM

The combination of excess thirst, increased intake of water, and increased output of urine is a common clinical presentation of a number of conditions (Table 74.7). In most of these, the symptoms are related to some event that results in excessive loss of fluid via the kidney. For example, *hyperglycemia* results in a large solute load (glucose) being presented to the renal tubules; an obligatory loss of water (osmotic diuresis) ensues. *Hypercalcemia* produces abnormalities of renal tubular function that result in impaired ability to concentrate urine. *Lithium*, widely used for treatment of bipolar affective disorders (manic–depressive illness), impairs the action of antidiuretic hormone (ADH) and thereby produces water loss.

A noteworthy disorder of water metabolism in ambulatory patients is that of *psychogenic water drinking*.

Table 74.7.   Causes of Polyuria[a]

Disorder	Mechanism
Glucosuria (diabetes mellitus)	Osmotic diuresis
Excessive intake of water	Psychogenic
Various drugs	Often due to anticholinergic effects producing dryness of mouth; possible central effects
Decreased ADH effect	Deficiency of ADH secretion (idiopathic diabetes insipidus or due to pituitary–hypothalamic disease); nephrogenic diabetes insipidus
Renal disease, plus renal effects of potassium depletion, hypercalcemia, and lithium therapy	In all of these disorders, impairment of renal concentrating ability is present
Hyperthyroidism	Impairment of urinary concentrating ability; decreased salivary flow

[a]Disorders associated with increased urine volume.

In this disorder, the patient's psychiatric state alters normal behavior in such a way as to produce compulsive water drinking. Many of these patients have poorly defined psychiatric disorders, but some are overtly psychotic (15). Studies in these patients have identified unequivocal defects in urinary dilution, the osmoregulation of water intake, and the secretion of vasopressin, but the precise causes of these abnormalities remain unexplained (14). Occasional people begin excessive water intake on the mistaken impression that drinking large quantities of water is healthful. Regardless of the cause, once such behavior is started, a compulsive pattern tends to persist and is reinforced by a pathophysiologic mechanism. Whatever the cause, large urine output, if it persists for a long time, produces a reversible impairment of urine-concentrating ability due to washout of renal medullary solutes. Thus, the behavior pattern, although basically of psychogenic origin, may become self-perpetuating. Attempts to have the patient restrict water intake when urinary concentrating ability is impaired under these conditions lead to continued water loss, and the resulting hyperosmolality leads to intense thirst. Weaning from excessive water intake may be difficult.

A rare disorder of water metabolism in ambulatory patients is *diabetes insipidus*, a deficiency of ADH (arginine vasopressin [AVP]). This condition is either idiopathic—in which case it is unassociated with other evidence of pituitary–hypothalamic disease—or, more commonly, is secondary to pituitary disease (tumor) or other disease in the hypothalamic–pituitary stalk-pituitary area (craniopharyngioma, aneurysm). Other rare causes include a variety of infiltrative diseases (sarcoidosis, tuberculosis), head trauma—especially with basal skull fracture or neurosurgical procedures—and central nervous system infections. The most common illness mimicking diabetes insipidus is the drug-related disorder that results from use of *lithium* for bipolar affective illness. Another rare condition resembling lack of ADH results from an inherited renal tubular resistance to antidiuretic hormone, *nephrogenic diabetes insipidus*.

Approach to the Patient with Polydipsia and Polyuria

The history should be corroborated by family or friends if possible. Important historical points are rapidity of onset of symptoms, a preference for use of iced water, and nocturnal drinking habits. Sudden onset and preference for iced water are classical for diabetes insipidus. Numerous spontaneous awakenings at night to drink and urinate also strongly suggest this diagnosis, whereas absence of such events is in favor of functional disease. A careful psychiatric and pharmacologic history is important.

Initial laboratory workup should be simple. A morning serum glucose, sodium or osmolality determination along with serum potassium, calcium, urea nitrogen, and creatinine determinations should be made. The patient should collect all urine over one or two 24-hour periods. The sample should be examined to determine the volume, osmolality, total urine glucose excretion, and total creatinine excretion, the latter serving as a marker for completeness of the collection. Measurement of urine specific gravity is obsolete and should not be done.

These preliminaries define the problem and provide an insight into the diagnosis. Unless considerable glucosuria is present, the patient's problem is not caused by uncontrolled diabetes mellitus, even if blood glucose concentration is incidentally elevated. The presence of a normal serum sodium or osmolality indicates only that the process is not severe enough to have overwhelmed the ability to excrete water or the homeostatic (thirst) mechanism. Elevated serum osmolality strongly suggests diabetes insipidus; reduced osmolality indicates psychogenic water drinking. Normal serum calcium and potassium concentrations exclude several metabolic problems, whereas abnormalities of calcium, potassium, or renal function make it clear that the problem is not primarily one of water metabolism (Table 74.7).

At this point, most patients have normal findings in serum but a large volume of urine with low osmolality. Normal urine volume ranges up to 2500 mL; urine osmolality is decidedly low when the value is well below that of serum (less than 300 mOsm/kg; the urine is maximally dilute at 50 to 70 mOsm/kg). In both diabetes insipidus and psychogenic water drinking, urine volume usually exceeds 4 L/day. Values less than 5 to 6 L/day do not distinguish between these possibilities but do indicate less than complete diabetes insipidus, in which urine volumes approach 10 to 12 L/day, as they may also in cases of severe psychogenic water drinking. If the serum sodium/osmolality is low and the urine volume is large with low osmolality, a diagnosis of psychogenic water drinking is essentially established.

Diabetes Insipidus Versus Psychogenic Water Drinking

If there is a large urine volume of low osmolality and normal serum electrolyte concentrations, additional testing is necessary to establish a diagnosis. Referral to an endocrinologist or nephrologist is appropriate, although under optimal conditions further efforts to establish the diagnosis in the ambulatory patient may be undertaken before referral (see below). Hospitalization for testing under metabolic conditions is nearly always to be preferred in these cases.

The first additional test is that of water deprivation. Best performed during the day when monitoring is possible, the patient remains recumbent and refrains from fluid intake; all urine is collected in hourly batches for 6 hours. Volumes and osmolalities are determined on each sample. Body weight is determined hourly. When the urine volume and osmolality seem to have stabilized after several hours, ADH (Pitressin) is given (5 units, aqueous, subcutaneously). Urine osmolality and volume are then determined every 30 minutes for an additional 90 to 120 minutes. If at any point, a drop in body weight exceeds 3%, the ADH should be injected and the test terminated over the next 90 minutes.

In the normal individual, urine volume falls and osmolality rises over several hours. Urine osmolality exceeds 500 mOsm/kg. Administration of ADH produces an additional increase in urine osmolality, but the increase is small if the level is already high. In the patient with partial diabetes insipidus, the plateau is at 300 mOsm/kg, with an increase to at least 500 mOsm/kg after ADH; some patients do not respond maximally (osmolality 1000 mOsm/kg). Patients with nephrogenic diabetes insipidus do not respond to ADH. A prompt fall of urine volume and an increase of urine osmolality may not occur in some patients with psychogenic water drinking. These patients are often overhydrated and may not reach plateau levels for as long as 12 hours. If the diagnosis is still doubtful at this point, referral for consultation should be made. Further tests can be performed to provoke ADH release by infusion of hypertonic saline. Administration of intravenous ADH and other special maneuvers may be necessary. CT scans of the area of the sella turcica, although usually negative, are important in cases of diabetes insipidus to rule out space-occupying lesions. Anterior pituitary function must be assessed when diabetes insipidus is diagnosed.

Treatment

The treatment of *psychogenic water drinking* involves psychiatric counseling. These patients are difficult to manage, especially if they become severely hyponatremic. Weaning such patients from water may also be a slow process not only because of the profound nature of their psychiatric disturbance, but because of their acquired inability to concentrate urine, a process that is only slowly reversible.

The treatment of *diabetes insipidus* involves use of ADH in some form. Until several years ago, Pitressin Tannate in oil given intramuscularly was the preferred agent, but this material is no longer marketed. For ambulatory patients, ADH is available in a nasal solution as the synthetic analog desmopressin (DDAVP). This material acts for 12 hours or longer. Nasal absorption may be impaired by rhinitis or respiratory tract infections, during which treatment with injectable ADH (Pitressin) may be necessary. Patients with partial diabetes insipidus can sometimes be managed with chlorpropamide (Diabinese, 250 to 500 mg/day), a drug that potentiates endogenous ADH. However, hypoglycemia is a significant hazard. Nephrogenic diabetes insipidus, both idiopathic and secondary to lithium, is partially responsive to thiazide diuretics (31).

Syndrome of Inappropriate Secretion of Antidiuretic Hormone (SIADH)

The clinical manifestations of the syndrome of inappropriate secretion of antidiuretic hormone (SIADH) are due to hyponatremia and the diagnosis is based on that finding. The causes are multiple. Classically, the disturbance was related to ectopic production of ADH by a neoplasm. The tumor most likely to produce this syndrome is a small cell (oat cell) carcinoma of the lung, but many other tumors have also been shown to produce the same syndrome. The presence of a tumor is usually obvious but occasionally may be clinically occult. In addition, a variety of acute and chronic diseases of the central nervous system can produce SIADH. Drugs, acting centrally, may also produce ADH hypersecretion (morphine, barbiturates [31]). The best described drug-related SIADH that is likely to be encountered in an ambulatory patient is that due to chlorpropamide (Diabinese) during the therapy of diabetes mellitus (see Chapter 72). In this case, the disturbance is due to potentiation of ADH action, although increased ADH release may also be involved. Drug-related SIADH should always be considered; many drugs have now been implicated.

Treatment

The treatment of SIADH is usually that which is related to the underlying disease or involves withdrawal of drug therapy (e.g., chlorpropamide; see Chapter 72). Water restriction is effective but is difficult to maintain in an ambulatory setting. Lithium has been occasionally useful. Demeclocycline, a tetracycline analog, is an ADH antagonist and is effective in some cases. An ADH peptide analog that blocks ADH action has been developed, is effective, and offers promise for therapy (38), but the agent is not yet available for clinical use.

HYPOGLYCEMIA

Because the symptoms of hypoglycemia are rather nonspecific, hypoglycemia is probably more often suspected than present. Chemical hypoglycemia, defined as a plasma sugar concentration of less than 50 mg/dL, may not be symptomatic, although levels less than 30 mg/dL are nearly always associated with symptoms.

Hypoglycemia produces symptoms by two mechanisms: by triggering the release of epinephrine, one of several homeostatic responses that tend to normalize a low blood sugar; and by deprivation of the nervous system of its essential energy source.

The causes of hypoglycemia are numerous, but by far the most common is a benign functional disturbance of insulin secretion that is temporally associated with absorption of food from the gastrointestinal tract. Most other hypoglycemic events are seen in diabetic patients being treated with insulin or, occasionally, an oral sulfonylurea. Rarely, some other drug produces hypoglycemia (Table 74.8). A few other conditions that produce hypoglycemia are associated with insulin overproduction, the rarest of which is an insulinoma. In most situations hypoglycemia is due not to insulin excess but to disturbances of glucose production, as in ethanol ingestion, or rarely to glucose overutilization, as in the presence of certain extrapancreatic tumors. The causes of hypoglycemia are listed in Table 74.8.

Clinical Diagnosis

Presentation of the Problem

In some patients the history suggests to the physician that the patient is experiencing periodic hypoglycemia. Other patients will themselves suggest to their physician that hypoglycemia accounts for the symptoms. Much has been written in the lay literature about hypoglycemia, and many books attribute the entire range of human miseries to this disorder. Needless to say, the case has been overstated. The physician encountering such a patient may find mere reassurance ineffective, so convincing is some of the lay literature on this subject and so obsessed are some patients. However, the physician inevitably embarks on a search, to either confirm or refute the suspected diagnosis. Verification of the presence of hypoglycemia, or more precisely its exclusion, can be attempted by instructing the patient in the use of a glucose oxidase strip (e.g., Chemstrips bG). The strip can be brought or sent to the physician or laboratory within 1 week for confirmation of the reading. Unfortunately, failure to document the presence of hypoglycemia may not serve to dispose of the issue, and generation of dubious or equivocal results with a meter may merely serve to prolong the preoccupation, initiate useless diets, or even delay diagnosis of serious but unrelated disease.

"Nonhypoglycemia"

The frequency with which self-diagnosis of hypoglycemia occurs depends on the population, but in some populations the problem is common (46). The condition has been termed *nonhypoglycemia* and extends the concept of "nondisease," as it originates from misattributes of the physician, such as misinterpretation of laboratory values, or misattributes of the patient. Identification of such individuals is important, as is their reeducation (6). The ready acceptance by patients of hypoglycemia as a diagnosis is perhaps related to its social acceptability, the comfort received from attributing vague symptoms (e.g., fatigue, mental fogginess) to a real disease, the satisfaction of an escape into dietary rituals, and possibly relief from the anxiety that life-threatening or at least serious disease may be lurking.

The recognition of nonhypoglycemia requires a careful history that fails to demonstrate the legitimate symptoms of hypoglycemia as well as a clear demonstration that glucose metabolism is normal (see below). Exclusion of other organic disease is routine (Table 74.8). Distinction from the idiopathic postprandial syndrome must be made (see below). Finally, psychiatric disease must be considered, based on positive findings rather than merely on an exclusion of organic illness.

If the evaluation fails to establish the presence of bona fide hypoglycemia, the issue of the therapy of nonhypoglycemia remains. This difficult problem includes at least three steps that have been termed disattribution, explanation and ventilation, and reattribution (46). Disattribution involves confrontation of the patient with the results of the test procedure. For some patients the mechanics or ritual of the procedure itself is impressive and therefore helpful. If the patient clings to the diagnosis of hypoglycemia despite strong evidence to the contrary, an attempt should be made to explore the reason for the patient's need to do so. During this process, an effort should be made to have the patient fully explain his notions about hypoglycemia and verbalize what might happen if those notions are challenged. Finally, an alternate explanation must be provided for the symptoms—reattribution—along with a treatment plan or a willingness to assist the patient in accepting an uncertain and ambiguous situation. Unless grossly apparent emotional problems

Table 74.8.   Causes of Hypoglycemia in Ambulatory Adults

Postprandial State
Reactive (idiopathic)
Early diabetes mellitus
Ethanol ingestion
Postgastrectomy state

Fasting State
Insulin excess
  1. Insulin injection
  2. Sulfonylurea ingestion[a]
  3. Miscellaneous drugs and poisons[b]
  4. Insulinoma
  5. Autoimmune hypoglycemia (very rare)
Alcohol ingestion
Hormonal deficiencies
  1. Glucocorticoid
  2. Growth hormone
Fasting in normal young women (24–48 hr)
Malnutrition
Liver disease
Extrapancreatic tumors
Renal failure (chronic end stage)
Congestive heart failure

[a]Many drugs, including such diverse compounds as anti-inflammatory agents, antibiotics, and lipid-lowering agents, potentiate the effects of sulfonylureas and may cause hypoglycemia.

[b]Haloperidol, propoxyphene, salicylates, etc.

become evident during this process, psychiatric referral should be made after considerable deliberation and only after an effort has been made to resolve the problem. (Chapters 10 and 11 describe in detail interviewing and psychotherapeutic techniques for working with patients such as these.)

Defining Hypoglycemic Symptoms

Because laboratory confirmation may be difficult in some cases, an extraordinarily careful history is essential. The degree to which the history is convincing determines the vigor with which a rather nebulous diagnosis is to be pursued. Two issues guide the process. First, what exactly are the symptoms? Second, do the symptoms occur postprandially or in the fasting state?

Adrenergic versus neuroglycopenic symptoms. Two groups of symptoms and signs are associated with hypoglycemia. Many of the symptoms of hypoglycemia relate to stimulation by low blood glucose of the release of epinephrine. These comprise the first group and are termed adrenergic or sympathetic. Usually these symptoms are of rapid onset, and more than one is ordinarily present. Typically they last only 15 to 30 minutes and include sweating, tremor (shakiness), a sensation of hunger, and anxiety. Irritability and palpitations are often mentioned but are rarely spontaneous or prominent complaints.

The second group of symptoms is related to glucose deprivation of the central and, to a lesser extent, peripheral nervous systems. These symptoms may be termed neuroglycopenic and, when severe, mimic those of central nervous system hypoxia. Minimal symptoms are headache, mental dullness, and sudden fatigue. Confusion and visual disturbances (blurring, dimming of vision) are associated with moderate to severe hypoglycemia, whereas unconsciousness and seizures are indications of very severe hypoglycemia.

Adrenergic symptoms are mainly postprandial and neuroglycopenic symptoms, especially those of severe variety, and are seen in association with fasting hypoglycemia. Minor neuroglycopenic symptoms may also be seen in the postabsorptive state, but symptoms severe enough to cause loss of consciousness are rare and should not be readily attributed to this condition. When severe symptoms do occur in the postprandial state, great difficulty in establishing a diagnosis may be encountered. The duration of this type of hypoglycemia is so short that by the time the patient is seen by a physician and a blood sugar determination is obtained, the glucose concentration has often returned to normal.

Postprandial reactive ("food stimulated") versus fasting (food deprived) hypoglycemia. An accurate history is essential to identify the hypoglycemia as either postprandial or fasting. The subsequent evaluation and the diagnostic possibilities segregate clearly once this distinction is made. If a distinction can be made based on the history, the alternate type of hypoglycemia should no longer be considered because the two types do not coexist.

Postprandial hypoglycemia. In this situation the patient has no problem on arising and before breakfast.

Similarly, no difficulty is experienced if the patient sleeps late. The symptoms usually develop 2 to 5 hours after a meal.

Inquiry concerning the patient's dietary habits may be revealing. Some patients restrict carbohydrate intake intermittently. When this is done and a large carbohydrate meal follows, hypoglycemia may be precipitated. A history of previous gastrointestinal surgery (gastrectomy) is also important. The amount of alcohol consumed should be noted because ethanol ingestion may precipitate hypoglycemia, even in the nonfasting patient (see below). Often the patient may recall milder symptomatic episodes experienced over a long period because the intensity of postprandial hypoglycemia tends to wax and wane over the years. A family history of diabetes mellitus should be sought. Postprandial hypoglycemia can be an early manifestation of type 2 diabetes mellitus (see Chapter 72). Although symptoms and signs of anxiety or depression may be present, they have no diagnostic usefulness.

General physical examination can be expected to be negative. Even when early diabetes mellitus is found by glucose tolerance testing to be the cause of the hypoglycemia, complications of diabetes that can be found on physical examination (retinopathy, neuropathy) will not be present.

Postprandial Hypoglycemia

Laboratory Evaluation

As discussed above, an attempt can be made to determine the presence or absence of hypoglycemia by instructing the patient in the use of a glucose measuring strip. However, unless such a simple maneuver eliminates the problem, an unlikely outcome, laboratory evaluation will be necessary. The only practical and standardized test for detection of postabsorptive hypoglycemia is the glucose tolerance test, although some have abandoned this procedure because of its unreliability in establishing the diagnosis. For this purpose, the test as described for diagnosis of diabetes mellitus (see Chapter 72) is modified to include more frequent sampling (30-minute intervals) and a longer period (5 hours). The patient is observed during the entire test. Correlation of blood sugar values with clinical symptoms is essential. If the patient develops hypoglycemia associated with typical adrenergic symptoms and signs that reproduce those ordinarily experienced, a diagnosis of postabsorptive hypoglycemia can be considered established. A more precise diagnosis depends on the type of curve observed (see below). If symptoms without signs occur in the absence of hypoglycemia, the diagnosis is psychiatric. If hypoglycemia is seen but no symptoms occur, the hypoglycemic response may simply not have been severe enough to have triggered symptoms. The diagnosis then remains presumptive. A repeated test may succeed in reproducing the clinical situation.

Criteria for Diagnosis of Hypoglycemia. Plasma glucose values are greater than 50 mg/dL during glucose tolerance testing in 75% of normal, asymptomatic people. However, some normal individuals show values that fall to 50 mg/dL or somewhat lower and may exhibit hypoglycemic symptoms during the test, even though they never have such symptoms spontaneously. Thus, even a finding of hypoglycemia during testing should not be used to explain atypical symptoms. In addition, occasional normal individuals may reach levels below 35 mg/dL without any symptoms at all. In individuals who develop typical adrenergic symptoms and signs during the glucose tolerance test, without evidence of hypoglycemia, an increase of plasma epinephrine can sometimes be documented even though the glucose concentration never reaches a diagnostic level for hypoglycemia (8). This phenomenon appears to provide an objective criterion for what has been termed *idiopathic postprandial syndrome* (see below).

Determinations of plasma insulin, GH, glucagon, and norepinephrine concentrations in connection with the glucose tolerance test are of no particular use in interpreting the results. Variability is great, and results are in no sense diagnostic.

Types of Hypoglycemic Response During Glucose Tolerance Testing

Early Diabetes Mellitus. When the cause of hypoglycemia is early diabetes mellitus, the fasting glucose concentration is normal. In the first 2 hours, values diagnostic of diabetes mellitus are reached. Although the highest values are usually between 200 and 250 mg/dL (see Chapter 72), thereafter, between 3 and 4 hours, the glucose concentration falls to its lowest value and below 50 mg/dL.

Postgastrectomy State. Plasma glucose concentration rises rapidly and may reach a peak over 300 mg/dL by 1 hour, after which a rapid decline occurs. The lowest value is seen at 2 to 3 hours.

Idiopathic. In this response the blood glucose values in the first 2 hours are normal, but at about 3 hours a fall to hypoglycemic levels occurs. Values usually return to baseline by 5 hours.

Management of Hypoglycemia

Early Diabetes Mellitus. If the patient is obese, weight reduction may normalize the glucose tolerance and abolish the hypoglycemic episodes. If the patient is not obese, dietary manipulation can be attempted, but no standardized approach is available. The diet most likely to succeed is one that simulates the diet now recommended for diabetes generally (i.e., a diet that contains a high proportion of complex carbohydrates rather than simple sugars) (see Chapter 72). Also important is the distribution of food intake into small meals—often as many as six. Alcohol may be an aggravating factor in producing hypoglycemia and should be restricted, at least on a trial basis. Caffeine (coffee, tea) need not be restricted. Sulfonylurea drugs are not useful.

Postgastrectomy State. As many as 75% of asymptomatic patients who have had a partial gastrectomy show reactive hypoglycemia during a glucose toler-

ance test. The therapy of symptomatic patients is similar to that described above: frequent small meals and restriction of simple sugars. The anticholinergic drug propantheline (Pro-Banthine), 7.5 mg taken 30 minutes before meals, may be helpful. This drug inhibits gut motility and delays gastric emptying. At this dosage, side effects (blurred vision, dry mouth) are minimal. Propranolol (Inderal) often blocks symptoms but does little to affect hypoglycemia and therefore may be hazardous.

Idiopathic Hypoglycemia. The course of this disorder is obscure. Some patients may have anxiety or depression in association with onset of hypoglycemic symptoms. Although diet manipulation or propantheline therapy as described above may ameliorate the hypoglycemia, additional treatment may be needed for the psychologic aspects. Recent introduction of high-protein, low-carbohydrate diets for weight reduction has also led to difficulties in some patients. Carbohydrate restriction followed by carbohydrate ingestion leads to the hypoglycemia in these individuals. Ethanol (doses of 3 ounces of gin or equivalent) may potentiate reactive hypoglycemia in normal subjects (see below).

Idiopathic Postprandial Syndrome

In this situation patients complain of typical adrenergic symptoms and show objective signs, but during glucose tolerance testing (see above) never achieve diagnostic levels of hypoglycemia. This condition has been termed idiopathic postprandial syndrome. Plasma epinephrine has been shown to increase abnormally in such persons. In these individuals, or in some diabetics (see Chapter 72, under "Hypoglycemia During Insulin Therapy"), the release of epinephrine appears to be triggered at levels of blood glucose (50 to 70 mg/dL) not ordinarily considered to be in the hypoglycemic range. Determination of plasma epinephrine levels during the performance of the glucose tolerance test has been proposed as an objective criterion for this disorder (8). Whether release of epinephrine is caused by change of blood glucose concentration or some other mechanism is unclear. It should be stressed that affected individuals have typical adrenergic symptoms and signs; their complaints are not to be confused with the vague symptoms of nonhypoglycemia (see above).

Fasting Hypoglycemia

The classical entity associated with fasting hypoglycemia is the insulinoma, but such insulin-secreting tumors are rare, and other causes of fasting hypoglycemia should be eliminated before embarking on the difficult task of establishing the presence of an insulinoma.

Fasting hypoglycemia in a well-nourished or obese person suggests insulinoma, drug (sulfonylurea) ingestion, or insulin self-administration. Debilitation suggests hepatic disease (most often related to chronic alcohol abuse) or, rarely, extrapancreatic tumor. The history, physical examination, and routine laboratory studies readily identify patients with chronic congestive heart failure or chronic renal disease, two other conditions occasionally associated with fasting hypoglycemia. Other aspects of these problems as well as endocrine deficiencies and alcohol abuse as causes of hypoglycemia are discussed below.

Laboratory Evaluation

As already noted, an attempt can be made to verify the presence or absence of hypoglycemia with the use of a reagent strip. However, if hypoglycemia remains a concern, determination of serum glucose concentration needs to be confirmed in a controlled setting.

When symptoms of hypoglycemia occur in the fasting state (usually overnight but in any case longer than 4 hours after a meal), a number of diagnostic possibilities more serious than those associated with postprandial hypoglycemia must be considered. However, the first step in evaluation of the problem is to establish the existence of hypoglycemia. Assuming that the symptoms are not so profound as to have caused coma, in which case hospitalization is mandatory, an overnight fast followed by determination of plasma glucose is the simplest screening procedure. This procedure may have to be repeated several times. If hypoglycemia cannot be documented in this way, the period of fasting may have to be extended to 24, 48, or even 72 hours. Hospitalization and close monitoring are necessary under these circumstances.

A sex difference in response to fasting is well established. Normal men may fast for up to 72 hours and will not show fasting plasma glucose (FPG) below 50 mg/dL. In contrast, women often exhibit a progressive fall in the concentration of plasma glucose during prolonged fasting. At 72 hours, most premenopausal women have a concentration of glucose less than 50 mg/dL and some as low as 25 mg/dL. Thus, prolonged fasting to establish the diagnosis of fasting hypoglycemia is not always useful because so many normal women become hypoglycemic.

Insulinoma

This pancreatic tumor occurs with equal frequency in men and women and at any age. Symptoms of headache on arising, confusion before breakfast, or nocturnal or early morning seizures may be present for years before the diagnosis is suspected. Hyperinsulinism may produce abnormal hunger, weight gain, and obesity. Neuropsychiatric symptoms may lead to neurologic or psychiatric evaluations or to hospitalizations. In some of these cases, permanent neurologic deficits have been seen and are presumably related to long duration of symptomatic hypoglycemia before diagnosis.

Diagnosis. In addition to the demonstration of hypoglycemia, the simultaneous determination of plasma insulin activity remains the most definitive diagnostic test (16). During fasting in normal people, both glucose and insulin levels decline and the ratio of immunoreactive insulin (IRI) to glucose (G) is maintained at less than 0.3 (milliunits of IRI/mg of G/dL). In many patients with insulinoma an abnormally high IRI/G ratio is apparent after overnight fasting. These determinations should be made repeatedly because fasting hypoglycemia and an abnormal IRI/G ratio often occur only intermittently even in patients with subsequently proven insulinomas. In addition, a single abnormal ratio never establishes the diagnosis. Insulin/glucose ratios may be misinterpreted if the glucose concentration is not at hypoglycemic levels (41). The physician should be cautious in accepting the accuracy of IRI values obtained from commercial laboratories. Proinsulin levels are elevated in 85% of patients with insulinoma and can be a useful adjunct, especially in those whose insulin levels are low (16). A variety of other useful procedures should, if necessary, be conducted by an endocrinologist. If fasting fails to provoke hypoglycemia (see above), the patient should exercise as vigorously as tolerable. Up to 2 hours of exercise should be completed with sampling of plasma glucose every 15 to 20 minutes before concluding that hypoglycemia has not developed. An exercise bicycle, jogging, or vigorous calisthenics may be used. Exercise raises glucose levels in normal people but lowers plasma concentration further in patients with insulinoma. Provocative tests of insulin secretion (tolbutamide, leucine, glucagon) can be used with appropriate caution. Suppression of endogenous insulin C-peptide is another useful procedure in difficult cases, but it requires induction of hypoglycemia by infusion of insulin under controlled conditions, a procedure that must be performed by an endocrinologist in a hospital. The localization procedure of choice is ultrasonography of the pancreas. CT and MRI are apparently not useful. Celiac axis arteriography may be useful for localizing lesions smaller than 2 to 3 cm (i.e., those that can be expected to be seen with sonography) (40). These procedures must not be used as alternatives to the tests described above but should be performed after demonstration of abnormal secretion of insulin. The definitive treatment of an insulinoma is surgical.

Insulin and Sulfonylurea Self-Administration

Occasional nondiabetic patients, usually family members of diabetics or people with medically related occupations, engage in surreptitious insulin administration. Examination may reveal needle marks. Other clues can be provided by the presence of antibodies to insulin, which are present only in persons given insulin or by the measurement of insulin C-peptide. In people who are secreting insulin, C-peptide is also produced concomitantly, but C-peptide is not present in commercial insulin and will be very low or absent when hypoglycemia is induced by exogenous insulin.

Oral hypoglycemic drugs (sulfonylureas; see Chapter 72), like insulin, may occasionally be abused and cause fasting hypoglycemia. The drug can be detected by analysis of the blood, although only specialized laboratories perform these measurements.

Alcohol Abuse

Alcohol abuse probably produces hypoglycemia more commonly than any other single cause. As stated above, ingestion of ethanol can produce postprandial hypoglycemia in normal, well-nourished people who engage in social drinking. However, fasting hypoglycemia related to ethanol ingestion occurs in chronic alcohol abusers and especially in those who are malnourished. The situation most likely to provoke hypoglycemia is cessation of food intake and continued ingestion of ethanol over the ensuing 10 to 20 hours. Under these circumstances, ethanol intoxication (i.e., drunkenness) may mistakenly be thought to be responsible for the symptoms.

Liver Disease, Chronic Congestive Heart Failure, and End-Stage Renal Disease

Although hypoglycemia can be seen in the course of severe, acute hepatitis or as a result of chronic passive congestion in long-standing congestive heart failure, liver disease does not usually produce hypoglycemia. Patients with severe cirrhosis may occasionally have fasting hypoglycemia, but the development of hypoglycemia in such a patient should suggest the presence of a hepatoma. In patients with well-differentiated hepatoma, hypoglycemia may be an early symptom. The phenomenon of hypoglycemia that develops in the course of chronic dialysis therapy for end-stage renal disease is described in Chapter 72.

Endocrine Disease

Glucocorticoids and growth hormone are important regulators of glucose metabolism. Thus, either pituitary insufficiency or adrenal insufficiency (primary or secondary to hypopituitarism) can result in hypoglycemia as a presenting manifestation. The diagnosis of these disorders is described elsewhere in this chapter.

Autoimmune Hypoglycemia

There are rare conditions in which autoantibodies develop to insulin receptors. Patients have no history of insulin use. The hypoglycemia is often severe and refractory. These conditions are unlikely to be encountered in an ambulatory setting.

HORMONE USE OF UNPROVEN VALUE

The lay press and the media regularly carry news of the use of various hormones for common problems. Health food stores are allowed to sell these substances as food additives, the term used by this industry, which is unregulated by the FDA under current law. Although most of these substances are probably relatively innocuous, they do pose some risk because they are not subjected to the rigorous drug testing that attends the approval of ordinary pharmaceuticals.

DHEA (Dehydroepiandrosterone)

DHEA and its metabolite, DHEA sulfate, are produced in amounts (25 to 50 mg/day) that far exceed daily secretion of any other adrenal steroid. It is not, however, classified as a hormone by the FDA and so can be sold as an uncontrolled substance. Its physiologic function is uncertain. Because its secretion rate falls off dramatically with increasing age in many people and because of evidence, primarily in aged rodents, but also in older humans, of improvement in cellular immunologic function, a belief has taken hold in the lay population that DHEA can retard and perhaps even reverse the aging process (2). There is no evidence to support this belief (45); but also, the safety of DHEA is not established. Because it is metabolized to androgens and estrogen, it could conceivably exacerbate benign prostatic hypertrophy, prostate cancer, sleep apnea, and hyperlipidemia in men, and heart disease and breast or gynecologic cancer in women.

Melatonin

Melatonin, a secretory product of the pineal gland, has been touted to be a regulator of circadian rhythms, and so has been used to induce sleep and prevent or facilitate recovery from time-zone changes (jet-lag). The agent is also promoted to slow aging and to enhance libido and as an antioxidant. No controlled studies are available to support any of these claims, nor have dosages or toxicity been studied.

Testosterone

Although long promoted as a libido and sex-performance enhancer, little if any evidence supports its usefulness in men with normal endogenous circulating levels. Some evidence supports a role for this agent in the minority of men who at advanced age show decreased circulating levels. The drug and other androgenic anabolic agents (synthetic steroids) have been widely used also to enhance muscle mass in male and female athletes and are probably effective for this purpose, but may also have adverse effects (e.g., hepatic toxicity, exacerbation of prostatic cancer or of coronary artery disease).

Growth Hormone

Human recombinant growth hormone (rhGH) is readily available but not approved for purposes other than enhancing the height of GH-deficient children. Like testosterone, or in combination with it, rhGH has been used to enhance muscle mass in athletes. Its effectiveness for this purpose is not established and its long-term toxicity has not been studied. Because GH levels are low in at least half of elderly patients, rhGH has been used in clinical trials with the hope that it will restore muscle mass and reduce adiposity in the elderly. So far, the results, largely unpublished, are not encouraging (23). Complications have included pseudotumor cerebri, carpal tunnel syndrome, and peripheral edema. This hormone is clearly no panacea for the problems of aging (28).

General References*

DeGroot LJ, Besser GM, Cahill GF, et al, eds. Endocrinology. 3rd ed. Philadelphia: WB Saunders, 1995.
> A comprehensive, multivolume text.

Felig P, Baxter JD, Frohman LA, eds. Endocrinology and metabolism. 3rd ed. New York: McGraw-Hill, 1995.
> An authoritative textbook of manageable size.

Wilson JD, Foster D, Larson R, Kronenberg, eds. Williams' textbook of endocrinology. 9th ed. Philadelphia: WB Saunders, 1998.
> The longtime standard textbook for the field.

Specific References

1. Amatruda TT Jr, Hurst MM, D'Esopo ND. Certain endocrine and metabolic facets of the steroid withdrawal syndrome. J Clin Endocrinol Metab 25:1207, 1965.
2. Baulieu EE. Dehydroepiandrosterone (DHEA): a fountain of youth? J Clin Endocrinol Metab 81:3147, 1996.
3. Bilezekian JP. Management of hypercalcemia. J Clin Endocrinol Metab 77:1445, 1993.
4. Bochicchio D, Losa M, Buchfelder M. Factors influencing the immediate and late outcome of Cushing's disease treated by transsphenoidal surgery: a retrospective study by the European Cushing's Disease Survey Group. J Clin Endocrinol Metab 80:3114, 1995.
5. Byyny RL. Withdrawal from glucocorticoid therapy. N Engl J Med 295:30, 1976.
6. Cahill GF Jr, Soeldner JS. A noneditorial on nonhypoglycemia. N Engl J Med 291:905, 1974.
7. Carella MJ, Srivastava LS, Gossain VV, Rovner DR. Hypothalamic-pituitary-adrenal function one week after a short burst of steroid therapy. J Clin Endocrinol Metab 76:1188, 1993.
8. Chalew SA, McLaughlin JV, Mersey JH, et al. The use of the plasma epinephrine response in the diagnosis of idiopathic postprandial syndrome. JAMA 251:612, 1984.
9. Christy NP. Pituitary-adrenal function during corticosteroid therapy. Learning to live with uncertainty. N Engl J Med 326:266, 1992.
10. Coe FL, Favus MJ. Does mild, asymptomatic hyperparathyroidism require surgery? N Engl J Med 302:224, 1980.
11. Coe FL, Favus MJ, Parks JH. Is estrogen preferable to surgery for postmenopausal women with primary hyperparathyroidism? N Engl J Med 314:1508, 1986.
12. Copeland PM. The incidentally discovered adrenal mass. Ann Intern Med 98:940, 1983.
13. Fauci AS, Dale DC, Balow JE. Glucocorticosteroid therapy: mechanisms of action and clinical considerations. Ann Intern Med 84:304, 1976.
14. Goldman MB, Luchins DJ, Robertson GL. Mechanisms of altered water metabolism in psychotic patients with polydipsia and hyponatremia. N Engl J Med 318:397, 1988.
15. Goldman MB, Robertson GL, Luchins DJ, Hedeker D. The influence of polydipsia on water excretion in hyponatremic, polydipsic, schizophrenic patients. J Clin Endocrinol Metab 81:1465, 1996.
16. Gordon P, Skarulis MC, Roach P, et al. Plasma proinsulin-like component in insulinoma: a 25-year experience. J Clin Endocrinol Metab 80:2884, 1995.
17. Griffing GT. A-I-D-S: the new endocrine epidemic. J Clin Endocrinol Metab 79:1530, 1994.
18. Grinspoon SK, Biller BM. Laboratory assessment of adrenal insufficiency. J Clin Endocrinol Metab 79:923, 1994.
19. Gross MD, Shapiro B. Clinically silent adrenal masses. J Clin Endocrinol Metab 77:885, 1993.
20. Guise TA, Mundy GR. Evaluation of hypocalcemia in children and adults. J Clin Endocrinol Metab 80:1473, 1995.
21. Heath H III, Hodgson SF, Kennedy MA. Primary hyperparathyroidism. Incidence, morbidity, and potential economic impact in a community. N Engl J Med 302:189, 1980.
22. Joborn C, Hetta J, Lind L, et al. Self-rated psychiatric symptoms in patients operated on because of primary hyperparathyroidism and in patients with longstanding mild hypercalcemia. Surgery 105:72, 1989.
23. Johannsson G, Mårin P, Lönn L, et al. Growth hormone treatment of abdominally obese men reduces abdominal fat mass, improves glucose and lipoprotein metabolism, and reduces diastolic blood pressure. J Clin Endocrinol Metab 82:727, 1997.
24. Johnston DG, Prescott RWG, Kendall-Taylor P, et al. Hyperprolactinemia. Long-term effects of bromocriptine. Am J Med 75:868, 1983.
25. Kohler PO. Treatment of pituitary adenomas (Editorial). N Engl J Med 371:45, 1987.
26. Lamberts SW, van der Lely AJ, deHerder WW. Transsphenoidal selective adenomectomy is the treatment of choice in patients with Cushing's disease. Considerations concerning medical treatment and the long-term follow-up. J Clin Endocrinol Metab 80:3111, 1995.
27. Marcus R. Bones of contention: the problem of mild hyperparathyroidism. J Clin Endocrinol Metab 80:720, 1995.
28. Marcus R, Reaven GM. Growth hormone—ready for prime time? J Clin Endocrinol Metab 82:725, 1997.
29. Melby JC. Systemic corticosteroid therapy: pharmacology and endocrinologic considerations. Ann Intern Med 81:505, 1974.
30. Melmed S, Ho K, Klibanski A, et al. Recent advances in pathogenesis, diagnosis, and management of acromegaly. J Clin Endocrinol Metab 80:3395, 1995.
31. Miller M, Moses AM. Drug-induced states of impaired water excretion. Kidney Int 10:96, 1976.
32. Molitch ME. Evaluation and treatment of the patient with a pituitary incidentaloma. J Clin Endocrinol Metab 80:3, 1995.
33. Molitch ME, Thorner MO, Wilson C. Management of prolactinomas. J Clin Endocrinol Metab 82:996, 1997.
34. Mundy GR, Guise TA. Hypercalcemia of malignancy. Am J Med 103:134, 1997.
35. NIH Conference. Diagnosis and management of asymptomatic primary hyperparathyroidism: Consensus Development Conference Statement. Ann Intern Med 114:593, 1991.
36. Osella G, Terzolo M, Borretta G, et al. Endocrine evaluation of incidentally discovered adrenal masses (incidentalomas). J Clin Endocrinol Metab 79:1532, 1994.
37. Robbins RJ. Depot somatostatin analogs—a new first line therapy for acromegaly. J Clin Endocrinol Metab 82:15, 1997.
38. Saito T, Ishikawa S, Abe K, et al. Acute aquaresis by the nonpeptide arginine vasopressin (AVP) antagonist OPC-31260 improves hyponatremia in patients with syndrome of inappropriate secretion of antidiuretic hormone (SIADH). J Clin Endocrinol Metab 82:1054, 1997.
39. Selby PL, Peacock M. Ethinyl estradiol and norethindrone in the treatment of primary hyperparathyroidism in postmenopausal women. N Engl J Med 314:1481, 1986.
40. Service FJ. Clinical review 42. Hypoglycemias. J Clin Endocrinol Metab 76:269, 1993.
41. Silverberg SJ, Bilezekian JP. Evaluation and management of primary hyperparathyroidism. J Clin Endocrinol Metab 81:2036, 1996.
42. Silverberg SJ, Gartenberg F, Jacobs TP, et al. Longitudinal measurements of bone density and biochemical indices in untreated primary hyperparathyroidism. J Clin Endocrinol Metab 80:723, 1995.
43. Sonino N. The use of ketoconazole as an inhibitor of steroid production. N Engl J Med 317:812, 1987.
44. Spielgel RJ, Vigersky RA, Oliff AI, et al. Adrenal suppression after short-term corticosteroid therapy. Lancet 1:630, 1979.
45. Wolf OT, Neumann O, Hellhammer DH, et al. Effects of a two-week physiological dehydroepiandrosterone substitution on cognitive performance and well-being in healthy elderly women and men. J Clin Endocrinol Metab 82:2363, 1997.
46. Yager J, Young RT. Non-hypoglycemia is an epidemic condition. N Engl J Med 291:907, 1974.

---

*Bold print (general references) and bold numerals (specific references) denote published controlled clinical trials, meta-analyses, or consensus-based recommendations.

C H A P T E R   75

Clinical Implications of Abnormal Lipoprotein Metabolism

M. JANETTE BUSBY-WHITEHEAD, MD
MARC R. BLACKMAN, MD

Interest in plasma lipids, lipoproteins, and apoproteins stems from their strong relationship to the development of atherosclerosis (7,8,44). At a time when it is possible to reduce the frequency of premature death and disability from atherosclerotic disease, the physician should be knowledgeable about and capable of diagnosing and treating the major abnormalities of lipoprotein metabolism.

LIPOPROTEIN NOMENCLATURE AND COMPOSITION

Lipids are insoluble in the aqueous plasma medium. They circulate in plasma as component parts of macromolecules that consist of a nonpolar hydrophobic lipid core of cholesterol esters and triglycerides and a polar hydrophilic monolayer surface coat of protein, phospholipid, and unesterified cholesterol (Fig. 75.1). These macromolecules, which are made miscible in plasma by their surface coat, are called lipoproteins.

Lipoproteins have traditionally been classified as a family of molecules containing the same basic constituents, but in different proportions (Table 75.1). The major classes of lipoproteins can be separated from each other by differences in density (ultracentrifugation), net surface charge (electrophoresis), size, and composition. Ultracentrifugation, which provides the most useful means of classification, separates lipoproteins into five principal classes. From the least dense and largest to the most dense and smallest, these are the *chylomicrons, very low-density lipoproteins* (VLDLs), *intermediate-density lipoproteins* (IDLs), *low-density lipoproteins* (LDLs), and *high-density lipoproteins* (HDLs) (47).

Each lipoprotein contains characteristic proportions of lipids and type-specific apoproteins (apos) such that, with increasing lipoprotein density, the relative amount of lipid decreases and that of (apo)protein increases (Table 75.1). Thus, triglyceride is the major lipid component in chylomicrons and VLDL, whereas cholesterol is the major component of LDL. Intermediate-density, or remnant lipoproteins, are catabolic products of chylomicrons and VLDLs and contain similar amounts of both lipids and apos (see "Normal Physiology of Lipoprotein Transport," below). The HDLs are the densest lipoproteins; they contain the most apos and ordinarily consist of 15 to 25% cholesterol and a small amount of triglyceride in the core. HDLs are further subdivided into HDL_2 and HDL_3. The former is more buoyant, as reflected by its higher lipid to protein ratio and richer apo A–I and apo C and E content, relative to the more dense HDL_3, which has a lower lipid to protein ratio and a higher apo A–II than A–I composition. There is a strong inverse relationship of coronary risk to plasma concentrations of HDL_2 and apo A–I related to the heightened capacity of the latter molecules to transport cholesterol from cells (51) (see below).

A LIPOPROTEIN PARTICLE

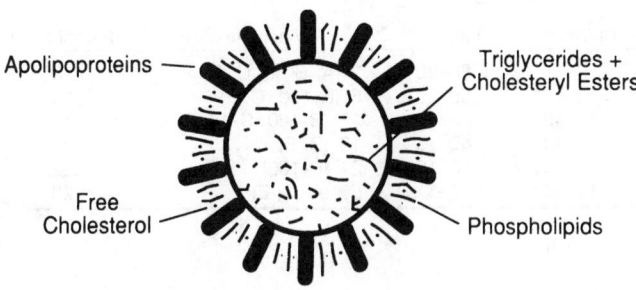

Figure 75.1. Structure of the lipoprotein macromolecule with the nonpolar lipids, cholesterol ester and triglyceride, in the lipoprotein core surrounded by a monolayer composed of specific apolipoproteins, proteins and the polar lipids, unesterified cholesterol and phospholipid. (From The Johns Hopkins Physicians Lipid Education Program. 2nd ed. Baltimore: The Johns Hopkins University, 1988;11.)

PLASMA LIPOPROTEINS AS RISK FACTORS FOR ATHEROSCLEROSIS

The risk factor concept, which developed as an outgrowth of the Framingham study and other large epidemiologic studies, is based on the strong association between certain characteristics in people and the increased likelihood of developing cardiovascular disease (40). Among the risk factors for atherosclerotic vascular disease, the most clearly established ones are plasma total cholesterol levels (and plasma LDL and HDL content), hypertension, and cigarette smoking. Each has been clearly implicated and makes a sizable independent contribution to the overall risk of developing coronary artery disease (CAD). Other identified risk factors that have more modest associations with cardiovascular disease include diabetes mellitus, central obesity, and physical inactivity.

Evidence from several large prospective and retrospective epidemiologic studies among diverse populations has demonstrated that variations in plasma levels of certain lipids and lipoproteins are associated with an increased likelihood of developing or having CAD. *Hypercholesterolemia*, for example, is strongly associated with the subsequent development of CAD. The relationship is uniformly consistent, dose related, and independent of sex. The predictive value of the plasma level of total cholesterol is somewhat limited, however, by the fact that it reflects the opposing influences of LDL and HDL cholesterol. Levels of LDL correlate positively, whereas those of HDLs are inversely related to CAD risk. The negative correlation between HDL levels and CAD depends mainly on its subfraction HDL$_2$, which may provide, along with its major protein component, apo A–I, a better index of risk than the total plasma level of HDL (51). Over the range of plasma levels of total cholesterol or of HDL cholesterol levels found in an average American population, the risk of CAD varies roughly fivefold. Although the impact of cardiovascular risk factors declines after age 75, they

are still predictive of CAD in older people. The relative risks of CAD associated with any particular risk factor (i.e., cholesterol levels) decrease with aging because of the increased prevalence of multiple risk factors; however, the absolute risk of morbidity and mortality increases markedly (43). Most, but not all, studies (42) indicate that plasma levels of total cholesterol retain predictive value in the "old old," that is, in men aged 75 to 95 years (12,70,82). Moreover, HDL cholesterol levels and the ratio of LDL to HDL cholesterol remain useful predictors in this age group.

The relationships of plasma levels of total cholesterol, LDL cholesterol, and HDL cholesterol with CAD are independent ones, in that the associations remain significant even after statistical adjustment for the contributions of other risk factors. Current information suggests that a low concentration of HDL cholesterol is a stronger independent risk factor for CAD than is either total cholesterol or LDL cholesterol (44).

Elevated fasting levels of plasma *triglyceride* and its major lipoprotein transporter, VLDL, also correlate with an increased risk of atherosclerotic disease. The consensus from most large epidemiologic studies is that the association is not an independent one (13), even though in the earlier Framingham Heart Study, the plasma triglyceride level was found to be an independent risk factor for CAD (11). The conclusion that the fasting triglyceride level is not an independent predictor of CAD in healthy people is supported by a recent National Institutes of Health (NIH) Consensus Development Conference. However, in certain subgroups of patients (e.g., those with familial combined hyperlipoproteinemia or familial dysbetalipoproteinemia), the hypertriglyceridemia may reflect altered lipoprotein and apoprotein composition and metabolism (69) and seems causally related to the development of premature atherosclerosis (8). In addition, hypertriglyceridemia may be prognostically important in patients with diabetes mellitus (78) or end-stage renal disease (23).

Not only do these lipoprotein and apoprotein abnormalities seem to increase one's predisposition to CAD, but there also is a parallel increased risk for cerebrovascular disease (32,40) and peripheral vascular disease as well (32).

A number of lipid fractions are even more strongly related to CAD than are total, LDL, and HDL cholesterol or apo A–I, and measurements of these fractions may become more useful in cardiovascular and cerebrovascular risk factor assessments (44). Elevated plasma concentrations of LDL apo B appear to discriminate between patients with and without atherosclerosis of the coronary and peripheral vasculature, even in the presence of normal plasma levels of total cholesterol and LDL cholesterol (8,10,69). The determination of plasma LDL apo B concentrations may also prove useful in assessing risk in hypertriglyceridemic patients (8,69). It is now known that LDL consists of several lipoprotein subclasses that differ in size and core lipid content, and that LDL subclass pattern B, characterized by small, dense LDL particles, is

Table 75.1.   Classification of Plasma Lipoproteins by Physical and Chemical Characteristics

Lipoprotein Fraction (Ultracentrifugation)	Density (g/mL)	Migration (Electrophoresis)	Composition as Percentage of Total Mass			
			Cholesterol	Triglyceride	Apoprotein	Phospholipid
Chylomicron	0.95	Origin	2–7	80–90	2 (A, B-48, C, E)	3
Very low density (VLDL)	<1.006	Pre-β	10–22	50–70	6 (B-100, C, E)	14
β-Very low density (β-VLDL or VLDL₂)	<1.006	β	30–40	45	12 (B-100, B-48, C, E)	15
Intermediate density or remnant (IDL)	1.006–1.019	Slow pre-β	30–40	40	18 (B, E)	22
Low density (LDL)	1.019–1.063	β	45–50	5–10	21 (B-100)	22
High density (HDL)	1.063–1.21	α	15–25	3–5	50 (A, C, E)	28

associated with a threefold increased risk of myocardial infarction (MI), independent of age, gender, and body weight (2).

In addition, MI, the progression of angiographically documented CAD, postangioplasty restenosis, and cerebrovascular disease are strongly associated with the lipoprotein (a) [Lp(a)] blood pattern, particularly in patients with elevated levels of LDL cholesterol (58). Current evidence (77) suggests that Lp(a) consists of a circulating complex of LDL and apo(a) that is more atherogenic than LDL, and that apo(a) exists in more than 30 isoforms, accounting for the great interperson variability in the plasma concentrations of Lp(a). Moreover, Lp(a) is structurally similar to plasminogen and inhibits the conversion of plasminogen to plasmin, thus attenuating fibrinolysis. Finally, Lp(a) appears to be directly involved in the formation of atherosclerotic plaques, perhaps because of its susceptibility to oxidative alteration in the arterial wall. However, at present there is no evidence from clinical trials to support routine measurement of Lp(a).

A number of investigations have demonstrated that tissue oxidative damage to LDL, and the subsequent interactions between damaged LDL and vascular endothelium, smooth muscle, macrophages, and monocytes, elicit more atherogenic activity than occurs with native LDL (73). Research in animals indicates that use of exogenous antioxidants retards the progression of experimentally induced atherogenesis by 30 to 80%. Several epidemiologic studies suggest that use of various antioxidants (e.g., probucol, ascorbic acid, vitamin E, β-carotene) may reverse this process and reduce risk of CAD. In this context, two large-scale epidemiologic reports, one in women and the other in men, revealed substantial cardiovascular protection in people who consumed large doses of vitamin E (62,72). A subgroup analysis of individuals in the Cholesterol Lowering Atherosclerosis Study in whom antioxidant vitamin E and C intake was nonrandomized revealed an association between supplementary vitamin E intake and angiographically demonstrated reduction in the progression of CAD lesions (33). Also, a study comparing the effect on endothelium-dependent coronary vasomotion of antioxidant therapy (lovastatin plus probucol) versus cholesterol lowering therapy (lovastatin plus cholestyramine) versus AHA Step 1 diet revealed that the greatest improvement in the vasoconstrictor response occurred in the lovastatin–probucol group

(1). Measurements of oxidized LDL and other oxidized lipoproteins are not currently part of the routine profile for CAD risk assessment.

In *familial dysbetalipoproteinemia*, a genetic disorder characterized by elevated plasma levels of IDL and an abnormally migrating β-VLDL (52), there is an increased risk of both peripheral and coronary atherosclerotic disease. In contrast, *fasting chylomicronemia* is associated with recurrent episodes of abdominal pain and pancreatitis, but not with the early development of atherosclerosis.

In several epidemiologic studies, plasma levels of total cholesterol below 180 to 195 mg/dL have been associated with an increased risk of cancer, especially cancer of the colon. The evidence does not, however, suggest a significant causal link because *(a)* in most studies the association was strongest in the first year of follow-up, then attenuated and disappeared in subsequent years, suggesting that preclinical cancer might have lowered levels of plasma cholesterol rather than vice versa; *(b)* studies comparing populations have shown a positive association between dietary fat intake and risk for major cancers, such as breast, prostate, and colon cancer; and *(c)* the relationship was generally weak, present in a minority of studies, and demonstrated no consistent relation between cholesterol level and cancer risk (46).

RATIONALE FOR DIAGNOSIS AND TREATMENT

Despite the fact that many risk factors linked with coronary and other atherosclerotic vascular disease have been identified and targeted for intervention, atherosclerotic disease constitutes the leading cause of death and disability in western industrialized societies. In the United States, approximately 725,000 individuals die annually from atherosclerotic disease, 550,000 of them from CAD. The economic costs are formidable, with more than $80 to $100 billion being spent annually in direct health care costs, lost wages, and decreased productivity.

To control this problem, major risk factor identification and prevention programs, primarily targeting hyperlipidemia, hypertension, and smoking, have been promulgated during the past 15 years and mortality from CAD did decline steadily in the 1980s. A recent study used a computerized algorithmic model to assess the degree to which preventive and therapeutic interventions now used in the United States have contributed to the decline in mortality (35). This model revealed that risk factor identification and associated treatment accounted for virtually all of the decline in mortality, with medical and surgical treatment of existing CAD or acute MI accounting for 43% of this trend. Primary prevention, or risk factor modification in people without CAD, contributed to 25% of the decrease in mortality, whereas secondary prevention, or risk factor modification reduction in people with CAD, accounted for 29%. Lipid management had the greatest impact of all risk factor interventions.

A large and increasing body of data derived from pathologic, genetic, metabolic, epidemiologic, animal, and clinical studies has demonstrated that certain abnormalities in plasma lipoproteins (in particular elevated levels of total cholesterol and LDL cholesterol and reduced HDL cholesterol) actually promote or cause atherosclerosis. It is equally well established that both exogenous factors (e.g., imprudent diet, drugs, lack of exercise, and cigarette smoking) and endogenous metabolic factors (which are genetically determined and may be affected by various diseases) determine plasma levels of lipids and lipoproteins.

The "lipid (or cholesterol) hypothesis," based on the data described above, also postulates that favorable alterations of plasma lipoprotein levels by diet, drugs, or other therapy reduce the risk of atherosclerosis in humans. The first conclusive evidence supporting the lipid hypothesis was supplied by the Lipid Research Clinics Coronary Primary Prevention Trial (48). This prospective, randomized, double-masked, multi-institutional trial compared cholestyramine and diet treatment with placebo and diet administration in 3806 healthy hypercholesterolemic men aged 35 to 59 followed for an average of 7.4 years. The cholestyramine group experienced a 19% reduction in the frequency of definite CAD death and/or definite nonfatal MI (the primary end points). There was a 2% reduction in overall CAD risk for each 1% reduction in plasma level of total cholesterol; thus in men compliant with the prescribed dose of cholestyramine (24 g/day), a 25% decrease in total cholesterol level resulted in a 50% decrease in overall CAD risk.

In the Helsinki Heart Study (20), approximately 4000 asymptomatic, middle-age men with elevated levels of total and LDL cholesterol were randomized to a diet plus gemfibrozil therapy or diet and placebo. After 5 years, the gemfibrozil group exhibited average decreases in total and LDL cholesterol of 9%, an increase in HDL cholesterol levels of 8%, and a decrease in triglyceride levels of 35%. The changes in lipoprotein levels were accompanied by decreases in the frequencies of nonfatal MIs of 37%, and of definite coronary deaths of 26%, for an overall reduction in the incidence of CAD end points of 34%.

In these two studies, cholesterol-lowering drug treatment was not associated with a significant decrease in all-cause mortality. An unexplained, nonsignificant excess of violent and accidental deaths in both studies was noted. Treatment of hypercholesterolemia as primary prevention for CAD has therefore remained controversial. In a more recent study, however, 6596 men with a mean plasma total cholesterol level of 272 mg/dL and no history of MI were randomized to receive either pravastatin (4 mg/day) and diet or placebo plus diet for a mean follow-up period of 4.9 years (67). The relative risk reduction for definite coronary events (nonfatal MI or death from CAD) with pravastatin was 31%. The overall reduction in the relative risk for death in the treated group was 22%. The number needed to treat to prevent one death was 111. No excess deaths from noncardiac causes were reported.

In contrast to primary prevention trials, secondary prevention trials have conclusively shown that cholesterol-lowering drugs can decrease CAD progression as well as the incidence of new and recurrent CAD-related events without an associated increase in total mortality. A double-masked, 5-year prospective, randomized study examined the effect of cholestyramine plus diet versus placebo plus diet on the angiographic progression of CAD in 116 hypercholesterolemic patients with prior angiographic evidence of CAD (4). The cholestyramine group exhibited a suggestive decrease in definite CAD progression and a significant decrease in definite and probable CAD progression in patients with coronary artery occlusion of 50% or more. Favorable alterations in the ratios of plasma levels of total (or LDL) cholesterol to HDL cholesterol correlated significantly with a decrease in CAD progression, however defined.

A combination of niacin and clofibrate was used to lower cholesterol and triglycerides in the Stockholm Secondary Prevention Study. Both overall mortality and recurrent coronary heart disease were significantly decreased. In the "4S" (Scandinavian Simvastatin Survival Study) Study, 4444 men and women were randomized to receive 20 mg simvastatin or placebo. Over a 5-year period, a 42% decline in coronary mortality and a decline of 35% in total mortality were observed (63). Thus, the evidence supporting secondary prevention of CAD by lipid-lowering medications is strong.

NORMAL PHYSIOLOGY OF LIPOPROTEIN TRANSPORT

Plasma lipoproteins arise from both exogenous dietary sources and endogenous hepatic sources (Fig. 75.2). They carry lipids in three distinct but interacting pathways: The exogenous pathway consists primarily of chylomicrons; the endogenous pathway consists mostly of VLDL, IDL, and LDL; and the reverse cholesterol transport pathway consists mostly of HDL activity.

After the ingestion of fat, dietary triglycerides are hydrolyzed in the gut and absorbed by intestinal enterocytes. Triglyceride-containing chylomicrons, formed in these cells, are secreted into lymphatic vessels and subsequently enter the venous system via the thoracic duct. Chylomicrons function as a system of

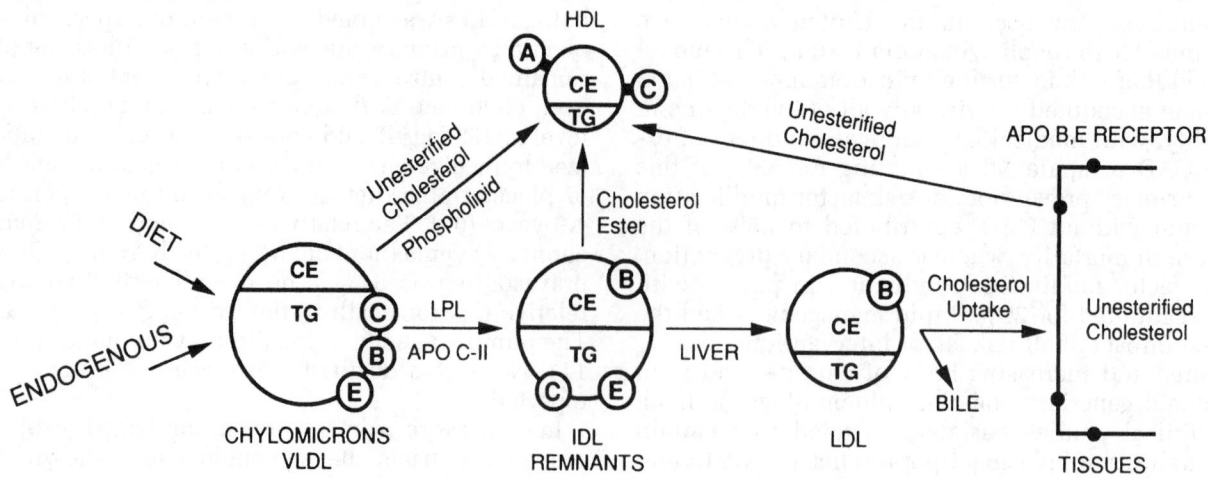

Figure 75.2. The normal physiology of lipoprotein transport is illustrated schematically.

high-energy caloric transport, allowing the calories ingested in excess of the immediate needs of the body to be transferred to sites of storage between meals. Absorbed dietary cholesterol is also esterified and transported in chylomicrons.

Other triglyceride-rich lipoproteins are synthesized from endogenous sources by the liver and intestine. Cholesterol synthesis from acetate also occurs in the liver and is regulated by the enzyme hydroxymethylglutaryl (HMG) CoA reductase. Triglycerides synthesized in the liver combine with cholesterol ester and are enveloped in a lipoprotein monolayer before being secreted into the hepatic venous outflow system as endogenous triglyceride-rich VLDLs.

Chylomicrons and VLDLs are transported to adipose tissue and muscle for storage and utilization. The uptake and storage of triglyceride are regulated by *lipoprotein lipase* (LPL). LPL is secreted by cells in virtually all parenchymal tissues and migrates to the endothelial cells of local capillary beds where it is activated by the apo C–II peptide normally found on chylomicrons, VLDL, and HDL. It hydrolyzes triglyceride and surface components from chylomicrons and VLDL to transform them into *remnant lipoproteins* (Fig. 75.2). The fatty acids released during this reaction migrate to muscle cells for combustion or to adipose cells for resynthesis and storage as triglyceride (55). The remnant lipoproteins are smaller, denser, and relatively enriched in cholesterol, apo B, and apo E compared with the chylomicrons and VLDL from which they derive. They are taken up by apo B–E (LDL) receptors in the liver. The chylomicron remnants are further degraded, and the VLDL remnants are processed into IDL and cholesterol-rich LDL (Fig. 75.2). Apo C–II and apo C–III, and the phospholipids and free cholesterol released during the LPL reaction, are transferred to HDL for utilization. The surface material generated by LPL-mediated removal of core triglyceride from VLDL and chylomicrons is the substrate (apo A–I is the cofactor) for the enzyme *lecithin-cholesterol acyl transferase* (LCAT), which converts nascent HDL

to mature spherical HDL and plays a major role in reverse cholesterol transport (see below).

Hepatic triglyceride lipase, like LPL, is released into plasma by heparin administration, hence the term *postheparin lipolytic activity* (PHLA). Hepatic lipase and LPL differ in composition; yet both are involved in the regulation of the plasma concentration of HDL_2 and in the catabolism of triglyceride-rich lipoproteins. Hepatic lipase promotes the hepatic removal of phospholipids and cholesterol from HDL_2 to form either HD_3 (which reenters the circulation) or irreversible catabolic products of HDL.

The LDLs are the principal carriers of cholesterol in plasma. Cholesterol is a major structural component of all cell membranes and is a precursor for steroid hormone synthesis by the adrenal glands and gonads. The LDL cholesterol-rich particles are derived mainly from VLDL and their catabolic remnants via the action of LPL and hepatic lipase. The principal removal of LDL occurs in the periphery by cells having a specific cell surface receptor (7) that recognizes all forms of apo B and is currently referred to as the apo B–E (LDL) receptor (Fig. 75.2). After specific cell receptor binding, LDLs are internalized by receptor-mediated endocytosis and carried to lysosomes, where apo B is irreversibly degraded to amino acids and LDL cholesterol ester is hydrolyzed to free cholesterol. The free cholesterol is transported to an intracellular cholesterol pool where it regulates, by a cellular feedback pathway, the resynthesis of cholesterol, cholesterol ester, and apo B–E (LDL) receptors (31).

The cholesterol content of the cell is also regulated by a removal system involving HDL as a vehicle for cholesterol transport from peripheral to hepatic cells for catabolism and excretion into bile directly or after conversion to bile acid (31,56). This reverse cholesterol transport system provides an efficient mechanism for the transfer of esterified cholesterol to LDL and VLDL, the absorption of free cholesterol from vascular endothelial cells, and the removal of cholesterol arising from cell membrane turnover and cell death.

Continued LDL catabolism in excess of that performed by hepatic and other parenchymal cells occurs in macrophages via a *scavenger pathway*. The observation that oxidatively modified LDLs are efficiently taken up by the scavenger pathway receptors, and subsequently influence macrophage and monocyte motility, served as the basis for proposing the current oxidative theory of atherogenesis (73). Abnormalities in oxidative metabolism of LDL are considered to account for the dyslipidemia in persons with homozygous familial hypercholesterolemia (7).

An apparent antiatherogenic alteration in both the lipoprotein and apoprotein composition of HDL, the formation of HDL_2, occurs during high-cholesterol feeding and represents one pathway by which the body can enhance its capacity to clear excess cholesterol from cells (31).

Apoproteins occupy specific domains on the three-dimensional structures of the individual lipoproteins. Alterations in lipid-protein interactions occur during the normal metabolism of lipoproteins, resulting in changes in the association of apoproteins with lipoproteins. Abnormalities in lipoprotein transport occur when the domains of apoproteins are altered by substitutions or deletions in amino acids. For example, the abnormal recognition of β-VLDL by the apo B–E receptor on cells occurs due to an abnormality in apo E in dysbetalipoproteinemia (see "Pathophysiology of Lipoprotein Disorders," below), and abnormalities in the apo B–E receptors are responsible for the defect in familial hypercholesterolemia (7,52).

HYPERLIPOPROTEINEMIA

Definition

Hyperlipoproteinemia is the excessive accumulation in the blood of one or more of the lipoprotein classes of lipid-transporting macromolecules. The diagnosis of hyperlipoproteinemia is sometimes based on plasma levels of lipids or lipoproteins above the 95th percentile of those found in a reference population. The distributions of plasma levels of total cholesterol, LDL cholesterol, total triglyceride, VLDL triglycerides, and HDL cholesterol among North American participants in the Lipid Research Clinics Prevalence Study have been published (50,61,76). Although the participants in that study did not represent a random sample of the entire North American population, they did encompass a broad range of sociodemographic groups and thus provide the best available reference values for lipoproteins. Because lipoprotein values vary with age, sex, and race, these factors must be considered when assigning a range of normal or a percentile to an individual's lipid levels (Table 75.2).

Based on the results of some treatment trials (48), the arbitrary use of a 95th percentile cutoff point in the diagnosis of hyperlipoproteinemia has some utility in suggesting the need for drug therapy in hypercholesterolemic patients. However, it should not be considered the dividing point between diseased and healthy individuals because CAD risk increases continuously over a broad range of lipid values. Furthermore, lipid distributions vary among and within populations. For example, levels of total and LDL cholesterol (and the prevalence of CAD) are much higher in North American and Northern European populations than they are in the Japanese population. Many people diagnosed as normolipidemic in the United States would probably be classified as hyperlipidemic in Japan.

Decreased and increased plasma levels of certain lipoproteins can also pose a threat of atherosclerosis. Specifically, plasma levels of HDL cholesterol and apo A–I are inversely correlated with the risk for CAD, so the 5th rather than 95th percentile can be used as the arbitrary cutoff point to distinguish those at greatest risk (Table 75.2).

The Adult Treatment Panel II (ATPII) of the National Cholesterol Education Program (NCEP) categorizes patients by measurements of serum levels of total cholesterol and HDL cholesterol (see "Indications for Evaluation," below). Once a patient is found to have an abnormal blood cholesterol concentration, decisions regarding possible diet, drug, or other therapy are made after a more detailed lipoprotein analysis, including calculation of the LDL cholesterol level (see below), and determination of other CAD risk factors.

Classification

Primary Versus Secondary

For clinical purposes, hyperlipoproteinemic states should be classified as primary (hereditary or sporadic genetic disorders of metabolism), secondary, or both. Secondary hyperlipoproteinemia is associated with an identifiable disease or condition and is reversible with control or eradication of that disease or condition. The major causes of secondary hyperlipoproteinemia are listed in Table 75.3.

Phenotypic Versus Genotypic and Pathophysiologic

In the 1960s, it was popular to classify the various hyperlipidemic states *phenotypically*, based on specific concentrations of lipids and lipoproteins and electrophoretic patterns (Table 75.4). Although the phenotypic classification describes in abbreviated fashion the plasma lipoproteins that are present in elevated or low concentrations, it does not reflect the genetic mechanisms or pathophysiology of the lipoprotein disorders. It is desirable to classify patients *pathophysiologically* and *genotypically* (Table 75.4) to diagnose and treat lipoprotein disorders accurately. Because apoproteins, enzymes, and cellular receptors are the major regulators of lipoprotein metabolism, it is appropriate to categorize lipoprotein disorders whenever possible in terms of pathophysiologic defects in the structure, function, and metabolism of these molecules, rather than by using a rigidly fixed phenotypic classification. Often, the pathophysiologic and genotypic classification can be surmised from a patient's phenotypic pattern, medical history, family history, and physical examination. Sometimes family members must be studied or more sophisticated

Table 75.2.   Fasting Plasma Concentrations (mg/dL) of Lipoprotein Lipids in North Americans[a]

Caucasians[b]

	Men											Women											
	TC[a]			LCL-C			TG			HDL-C			TC[a]			LCL-C			TG			HDL-C		
Age	5th%	Mean	95th%	5th%	Mean	95th%	5th%	Mean	95th%	5th%	Mean	95th%	5th%	Mean	95th%	5th%	Mean	95th%	5th%	Mean	95th%	5th%	Mean	95th%
15–19	118	153	191	62	94	130	38	78	143	30	46	63	118	159	207	59	96	137	36	73	126	35	52	74
20–24	118	162	212	66	103	147	44	89	165	30	45	63	121	170	237	57	104	159	37	87	168	33	53	79
25–29	130	179	234	70	117	165	45	104	204	31	45	63	130	179	231	71	110	164	42	87	159	37	56	83
30–34	142	193	258	78	126	185	46	122	253	28	46	63	133	179	228	70	111	156	40	86	163	36	56	77
35–39	147	201	267	81	133	189	52	141	316	29	43	62	139	190	249	75	120	172	45	98	205	34	55	82
40–44	150	205	260	87	136	186	56	152	318	27	44	67	146	198	259	74	125	174	44	98	191	34	58	88
45–49	163	213	275	98	144	202	56	143	279	30	45	64	148	206	268	79	129	186	53	113	223	34	59	87
50–54	156	213	274	89	142	197	63	153	313	28	44	63	163	217	281	88	138	201	59	116	223	37	62	92
55–59	161	215	280	88	146	203	60	134	261	28	48	71	167	229	294	89	146	210	57	133	279	37	62	91
60–64	163	217	287	83	146	210	56	131	240	30	52	74	172	232	300	100	152	224	56	132	256	38	64	92
65–69	166	221	288	98	150	210	54	139	256	30	51	78	167	234	291	92	154	221	60	137	260	35	63	98
70+	144	210	265	88	143	186	63	133	239	31	51	75	173	225	280	96	149	206		128	289	33	61	92

African Americans

Men

	TC[c,d]			TG[d]			HDL-C[e]	
Age	5th%	Mean	95th%	5th%	Mean	95th%	Age	Mean ± SD
10–19	120	160	205	31	59	102	15–19	53 ± 11
20–29	—	179	—	—	81	—	20–24	—
30–39	138	192	253	42	107	224	25–29	58 ± 15
40–49	148	207	—	52	126	294	30–34	54 ± 13
50–59	—	207	—	—	142	—	35–39	53 ± 16
60+	—	221	—	—	109	—	40–44	58 ± 20

Women

	TC[c,d]			TG[d]			HDL-C	
Age	5th%	Mean	95th%	5th%	Mean	95th%	Age	Mean ± SD
10–19	124	165	211	36	65	110	15–19	54 ± 11
20–29	124	177	235	38	77	137	20–24	—
30–39	132	185	243	38	80	150	25–29	57 ± 10
40–49	146	202	268	43	99	188	30–34	60 ± 13
50–59	—	217	—	—	104	—	35–39	59 ± 15
60+	—	234	—	—	120	—	40–44	62 ± 19

[a] 5th%, 5th percentile; 95th%, 95th percentile; TC, total cholesterol; LDL-C, low-density lipoprotein cholesterol; HDL-C, high-density lipoprotein cholesterol; TG, total triglycerides.
[b] Adapted from Reference 49, visit 2.
[c] Levels determined routinely by clinical laboratories are often higher (up to 30 mg/dL or more) than those determined by a standard laboratory (e.g., Centers for Disease Control). Check how your laboratory is standardized.
[d] Adapted from Reference 47, visit 1.
[e] Adapted from References 47 and 76.

Table 75.3. Causes of Secondary Lipoprotein Disorders

Exogenous	Alcohol, oral contraceptives, estrogens, androgens, corticosteroids, diuretics (thiazides, chlorthalidone), β-adrenergic–blocking agents, obesity, nutrition (diet high in cholesterol/saturated fat)
Endocrine-metabolic	Diabetes mellitus, hypothyroidism, Cushing's disease, Addison's disease, acromegaly, hypopituitarism, growth hormone deficiency
Hepatic	Obstructive or parenchymal disease, hepatoma
Renal	Nephrotic syndrome, chronic renal failure, hemodialysis
Acute stress situations	Acute myocardial infarction, sepsis, burns
Pregnancy	
Pancreatitis	
Dysgammaglobulinemias	Multiple myeloma, macroglobulinemia
Systemic lupus erythematosus	
Gout	
Viral infections, including AIDS	
Other	Glycogen storage disease, lipodystrophies, progeria, acute intermittent porphyria, anorexia nervosa, Klinefelter's syndrome

laboratory analyses performed, necessitating referral to a specialist in endocrinology and metabolism.

PATHOPHYSIOLOGY OF LIPOPROTEIN DISORDERS

The abnormal accumulation of lipoproteins in plasma results from their excessive production, defective removal, or both. Lipoprotein disorders may be primary (usually genetic), may be secondary to certain diseases (especially diabetes mellitus, chronic renal disease, hypothyroidism, dysglobulinemia) or drugs (corticosteroids, estrogens, thiazide diuretics), or may represent an interaction between primary and secondary factors. Abnormalities can occur in triglyceride-rich lipoprotein synthesis, lipoprotein lipase-mediated triglyceride catabolism, remnant lipoprotein catabolism, cholesterol-rich lipoprotein catabolism, and cholesterol-rich lipoprotein (LDL cholesterol) synthesis and absorption.

Increased Triglyceride Synthesis

Most triglyceride input is from the diet in normal individuals. However, abnormalities in the regulation of the endogenous production of triglyceride-rich VLDLs are fairly common and are the most common causes of hypertriglyceridemia. They are associated with an increase in plasma levels of VLDL (type IV) or VLDL plus chylomicrons (type V). The underlying metabolic cause for endogenous hypertriglyceridemia is usually related to hyperinsulinemia and insulin resistance, due most often to obesity, diabetes mellitus, the ingestion of excessive calories or alcohol, or the use of estrogens or corticosteroids.

The primary forms of endogenous hypertriglyceridemia, familial hypertriglyceridemia, and primary familial combined hyperlipidemia also appear to be related to an increase in the synthesis of triglyceride-rich lipoproteins. *Familial hypertriglyceridemia* results in an increase in the endogenous synthesis of large triglyceride-rich VLDL. Many such patients are obese and exhibit mild glucose intolerance, hyperinsulinemia, and clinical evidence of diabetes mellitus, conditions that contribute to the excessive hepatic production of VLDL triglyceride.

In contrast, patients with *familial combined hyperlipidemia* (multiple lipoprotein-type hyperlipidemia) exhibit an increase in the production of apo B, which can appear in VLDL, LDL, or both. Various lipoprotein types (IIA, IIB, or IV) are found in patients with familial combined hyperlipidemia, and the presenting sign can be an increase in either VLDL triglyceride, LDL cholesterol, or both. The clinical expressions of this disorder vary among individual patients depending on diet, the degree of obesity, the level of physical activity, and the concomitant use of other drugs.

Familial hypertriglyceridemia and familial combined hyperlipidemia are inherited as separate autosomal-dominant disorders, each occurring in approximately 1% of the general population. Familial hypertriglyceridemia is not associated with xanthomas unless hyperchylomicronemia supervenes. Basal concentrations (after a 12-hour fast) of total triglycerides and VLDL triglycerides are characteristically elevated, but plasma levels of total and LDL cholesterol are normal or low unless levels of VLDL cholesterol are also increased. Familial hypertriglyceridemia is not associated with an increased incidence of premature CAD; however, patients with familial combined hyperlipidemia are at high risk, primarily because of their increased plasma levels of apo B and abnormalities in the composition of HDL, reduced levels of apo A–I and HDL$_2$ (8). Familial combined hyperlipidemia may be present in as many as 10% of the survivors of MI under the age of 60 and thus represents a common and important risk for atherosclerosis.

The diagnosis of these disorders of lipoprotein metabolism and their exact definition can be established only by family studies. A strongly positive family history of atherosclerosis favors the diagnosis of familial combined hyperlipidemia in hypertriglyceridemic patients in whom secondary causes for hyperlipidemia have been excluded. Differentiating between these two disorders of lipoprotein metabolism is important in the evaluation of a patient with hyperlipidemia, particularly with regard to deciding whether therapeutic intervention is warranted for the prevention of CAD and its complications.

Occasionally, patients have marked *hypertriglyceridemia* and *hyperchylomicronemia* (triglyceride levels greater than 1000 mg/dL), pancreatitis, eruptive xanthomas, and lipemia retinalis. Coexistence of familial hypertriglyceridemia or familial combined hyperlipidemia with either obesity, uremia, untreated

Table 75.4.   Classification of Lipoprotein Disorders by Phenotypes and Genotypes and Corresponding Clinical Manifestations

Phenotype	Lipoprotein in Excess	Plasma Lipid Levels		Plasma Appearance[a]	Genotype	Age of Onset (Primary Form)	Xanthomas[b]	Other Clinical Manifestations
		Cholesterol	Triglyceride					
I	Chylomicrons	Normal or ↑	↑↑↑ lipemia	Clear plasma, creamy supernatant	Familial lipoprotein lipases deficiency, apo C–II deficiency	Infancy or childhood	Eruptive, tubero-eruptive	Recurrent abdominal pain, other gastrointestinal symptoms, lipemia retinalis, hepatosplenomegaly
IIA	LDL	↑↑↑	Normal	Clear	Familial hypercholesterolemia; Familial combined hyperlipidemia; Polygenic and sporadic hypercholesterolemia	Childhood for homozygous FHC,[c] late childhood to middle age for heterozygous FHC, adulthood for others	Tendinous, xanthelasma, tuberous; planar (homozygous)	Premature CAD,[c] arcus cornae, aortic stenosis (homozygous FHC), arthritic symptoms
IIB	LDL + VLDL	↑↑	↑	Clear	Familial combined hyperlipidemia; Familial hypercholesterolemia			
III	β-VLDL, IDL	↑↑	↑↑	Slightly turbid	Familial dysbetalipoproteinemia	Adulthood (occasionally late adolescence)	Planar (especially palmar), tuberous	Premature CAD and peripheral vascular disease, male > female, obesity, abnormal glucose tolerance, hyperuricemia, aggravated by hypothyroidism, good response to therapy
IV	VLDL	Normal or ↑[d]	↑↑	Turbid	Familial hypertriglyceridemia; Familial combined hyperlipidemia; Sporadic hypertriglyceridemia	Early to late adulthood	Usually none; rarely eruptive, or tubero-eruptive	CAD and peripheral vascular disease, obesity, abnormal glucose tolerance, hyperuricemia, arthritic symptoms, gallbladder disease
V	Chylomicrons + VLDL	Normal or ↑	↑↑↑	Turbid plasma, creamy supernatant	Homozygous familial hypertriglyceridemia	Childhood to middle age, usually adulthood	Eruptive, tubero-eruptive	Recurrent abdominal pain, other gastrointestinal symptoms, lipemia retinalis, hepatosplenomegaly, peripheral paresthesias, abnormal glucose tolerance, hyperuricemia

[a] Plasma obtained after 12 hours of fasting, left undisturbed in refrigerator overnight.
[b] Seen only in a minority of patients, but the frequency increases as plasma lipid levels rise.
[c] FHC, Familial hypercholesterolemia; CAD, coronary artery disease.
[d] Cholesterol normal if triglycerides are less than 400 mg/dL.

diabetes mellitus, chronic alcoholism, or the use of corticosteroids, thiazide diuretics, or estrogens can result in this syndrome. The chylomicronemia syndrome requires immediate treatment with elimination of dietary fat, nasogastric suction, and treatment of the secondary causes. Prevention is the primary means to avoid recurrences, and patients with primary hypertriglyceridemia often receive lipid-lowering agents prophylactically (31).

Decreased Lipoprotein Lipase-Mediated Triglyceride Catabolism

LPL is the rate-limiting enzyme for the uptake and storage of triglyceride by adipose tissue or muscle tissue and for the processing of triglyceride-rich lipoproteins to chylomicrons and VLDL remnants. In patients with the autosomal-recessive trait of apo *C–II deficiency*, LPL activity is normal, but marked hypertriglyceridemia is present (31). In contrast, in the more commonly encountered (yet also rare) autosomal-recessive syndrome of *familial LPL deficiency*, marked hypertriglyceridemia and chylomicronemia are both evident and LPL activity is absent. The type I phenotypic pattern is more likely to occur in patients with the familial form of LPL deficiency, rather than in those with apo C–II deficiency; yet both conditions manifest themselves in childhood with episodes of eruptive xanthomas and with the acute abdominal pain of pancreatitis.

Most adult patients who have an acquired impairment in LPL function usually have moderately severe type 1 diabetes mellitus, hypothyroidism, end-stage renal disease, or dysgammaglobulinemia, or are receiving corticosteroids or thiazide diuretics. The severity of the lipoprotein abnormality seems to be directly related to the decrease in LPL activity in postheparin plasma and adipose tissue.

The hypertriglyceridemia can be controlled by restriction of dietary fat and substitution of carbohydrates or medium-chain triglycerides as energy sources. Effective treatment of diabetes mellitus with diet, insulin, or an oral sulfonylurea usually normalizes LPL activity and plasma triglyceride levels within several months. Similar beneficial changes are seen after appropriate therapy of hypothyroidism with thyroxine or of uremia with renal transplantation.

LPL also plays a role in the formation of HDL_2 (see "Normal Physiology of Lipoprotein Transport," above). LPL appears to mediate the increase in HDL_2 seen in endurance-trained athletes (16) and in patients with primary hypercholesterolemia treated with colestipol. Hence, diseases associated with abnormalities in LPL often have concomitant reductions in HDL cholesterol.

Defective Remnant Lipoprotein Catabolism and Dysbetalipoproteinemia

Excessive accumulation of lipoprotein remnants in plasma is usually caused by a defect in their removal due to an autosomal-recessive derangement in the structure of apo E (52). Apo E3, the predominant form of apo E in the normal population, is absent in patients with the classic form of dysbetalipoproteinemia (type III hyperlipoproteinemia). The mutation causing this syndrome results in the occurrence of an abnormal form of apo E. Of the 1% of people homozygous for this condition, only 1 to 2% exhibit hyperlipoproteinemia clinically.

Dysbetalipoproteinemia (remnant removal disease or broad β disease) has served as a prototype for the study of remnant lipoprotein metabolism. It appears that several defects in lipoprotein metabolism are required before excessive accumulation of IDL and of cholesterol-enriched β-VLDL can occur. The diagnosis is suggested by the initial findings of β-VLDL (rather than pre-β–VLDL) and similarly elevated plasma concentrations of cholesterol and triglyceride. It is made more likely by the finding of an abnormally cholesterol-rich VLDL fraction (ratio of VLDL cholesterol to VLDL triglyceride above 0.42). The presence of tuberous and planar xanthomas (Fig. 75.3) is highly characteristic of the disorder. Definitive diagnosis, however, requires analysis of VLDL to demonstrate the absence of apo E3. A strong association between this lipoprotein disorder and atherosclerosis of the coronary arteries and peripheral vessels has been reported, and vasculopathy appears to diminish during treatment.

The accumulation of remnants in plasma is also found in certain patients with hypothyroidism, end-stage renal disease, and liver disease. The latter disorders are associated with an increase in the activity of the enzyme hepatic lipase, suggesting that a relationship may exist between this enzyme and the catabolism of remnant lipoproteins by the liver.

Increased Cholesterol Synthesis

The accumulation of cholesterol-rich LDL can occur as a result of an increased input of cholesterol into the plasma from dietary or endogenous sources. The latter occurs because of an increase in HMG CoA reductase activity and enhanced synthesis of cholesterol, or as a consequence of a primary genetic increase in the hepatic synthesis of apo B and cholesterol. The presence of apo B–enriched VLDL suggests a genetic disorder of overproduction of apo B, compared with the overproduction of VLDL triglyceride in familial hypertriglyceridemia.

The overproduction of apo B–containing LDL and VLDL leads to an increased propensity for the development of atherosclerosis (8). Moreover, the coexistence of obesity promotes the overproduction of apo B–enriched VLDL and cholesterol in these individuals. Finally, the augmented intake of dietary cholesterol usually contributes to the hypercholesterolemia characteristic of these patients.

Primary (sporadic) forms of hypercholesterolemia, with a genetic defect in the steps controlling the rate of hepatic synthesis of cholesterol from acetate, lead to an

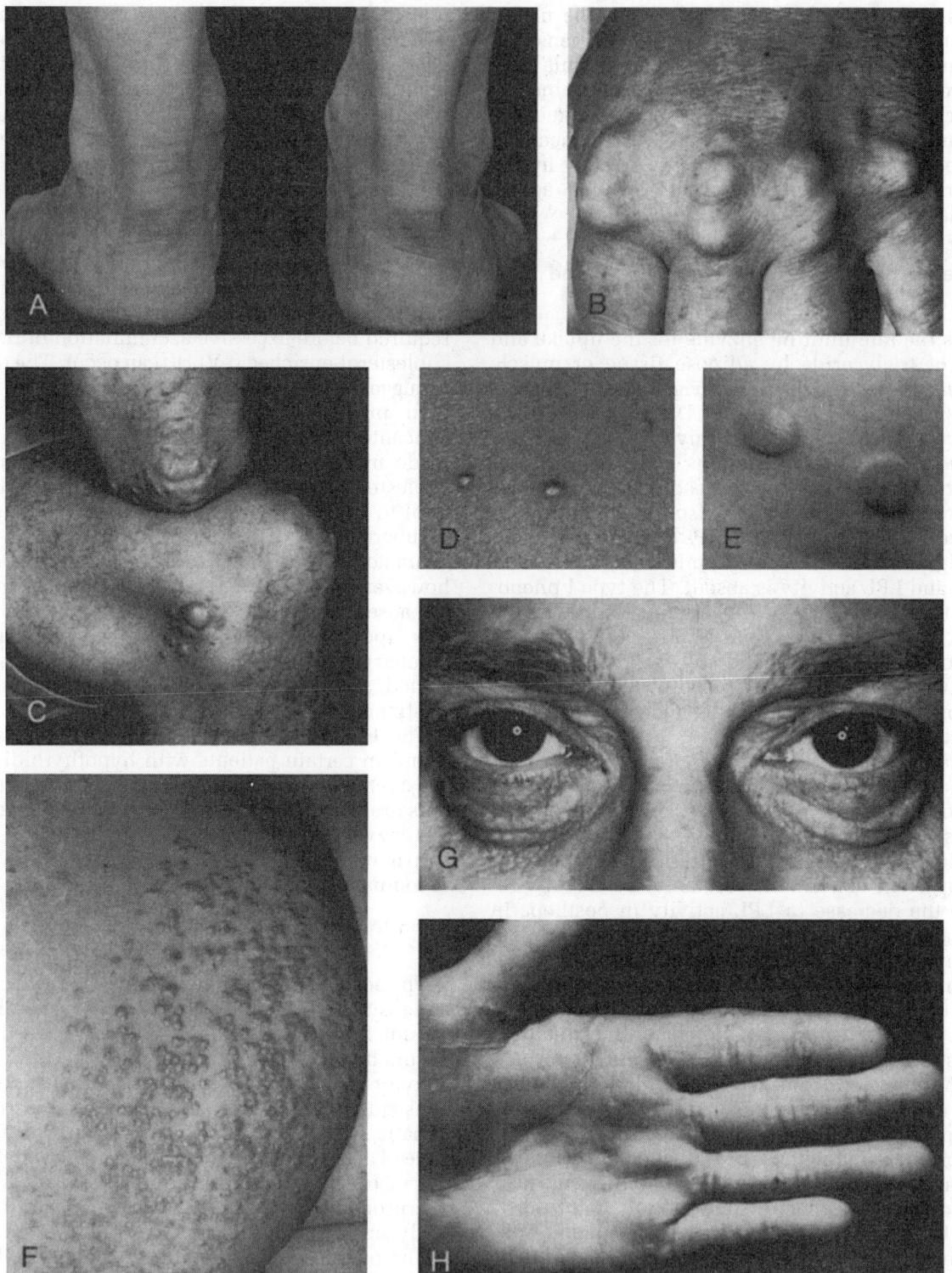

Figure 75.3. Dermatological manifestations of lipid disorders. **A.** Tendinous xanthomas. **B.** Tuberous xanthomas. **C.** Tuberous xanthomas. **D.** Eruptive xanthomas. **E.** Planar xanthomas. **F.** Erup-tive xanthomas. **G.** Planar xanthomas on eyelids (xanthelasma). **H.** Planar xanthomas confined to palm creases (xanthoma striata palmaris).

overproduction of cholesterol and resultant hypercho-lesterolemia. Usually dietary therapy involving an increase in polyunsaturated fat and a reduction in sucrose and simple carbohydrates is helpful in the treatment of these disorders; less often, drugs are required. Hypercholesterolemia in obese hyperin-sulinemic patients with type 2 diabetes mellitus is decreased by hypocaloric diets and the return of body weight toward normal. In patients noncompliant with dietary measures, therapy with cholestyramine or nicotinic acid is usually effective in lowering plasma levels of cholesterol.

Defective Removal of Low-Density Lipoproteins

Isolated primary elevations of plasma LDL or combined elevations of LDL and VLDL can be seen in affected members of families with familial hypercholesterolemia (7). Although the cells of some homozygous patients may be totally lacking in identifiable LDL (apo B–E) receptors, in other patients these receptors are present but functionally defective. Individuals heterozygous for familial hypercholesterolemia exhibit more than a 50% reduction in LDL receptor number or a 50% defect in receptor-mediated catabolism; commonly their plasma levels of LDL cholesterol are elevated above 400 mg/dL regardless of their level of cholesterol synthesis. In homozygous patients, plasma levels of LDL cholesterol may reach 1000 mg/dL (31). Documentation of abnormal receptor binding in cultures of skin fibroblasts is necessary for the precise diagnosis of individuals with familial hypercholesterolemia.

Although primary causes (including familial combined hyperlipoproteinemia) predominate, secondary causes for increased concentrations of LDL cholesterol occur in patients with hypothyroidism, nephrotic syndrome, multiple myeloma, obstructive liver disease, and porphyria and in patients who have ingested excessive amounts of dietary cholesterol. Whatever the cause of the LDL accumulation in the plasma, the primary forms are associated with marked susceptibility to CAD and a high frequency of complications associated with early mortality, such as MI, stroke, and severe peripheral vascular disease. The hallmark of these disorders is the tendon xanthomas that often affect the Achilles tendon or the extensor tendons of the forearm and hand (Fig. 75.3). Patients with secondary hypercholesterolemia appear not to develop atherosclerosis at as high a rate as people with the primary disorders.

COMMON SECONDARY DISORDERS OF LIPOPROTEIN METABOLISM

Several disease states are commonly associated with increased plasma levels of VLDL, elevated levels of both VLDL and LDL, or decreased levels of HDL cholesterol.

Diabetes Mellitus

Abnormalities in fat transport are often noted in patients with diabetes mellitus and are related to abnormalities in insulin action or insulin availability that lead to increased production or decreased removal of plasma lipoproteins. For example, patients with type 2 diabetes mellitus who are often obese, hyperinsulinemic, and insulin resistant exhibit both an en-

hanced production and reduced plasma clearance of triglycerides. These patients also have abnormalities in HDL cholesterol. In contrast, the hypertriglyceridemia that occurs in patients with insulin-dependent (type 1) diabetes mellitus is due to markedly reduced levels of LPL activity, as insulin is required for normal synthesis of the enzyme (31). The diabetic lipemia syndrome is characterized by low or absent levels of LPL in the plasma and tissues of these patients. Although the underlying enzyme deficiency can be reversed after insulin repletion, normalization of the lipoprotein abnormalities can take several months.

In the treated diabetic patient, variability in plasma levels of lipoprotein lipids is primarily related to dietary factors, the amount and distribution of body fat, physical activity, and the degree of glycemic control. If glucose tolerance deteriorates because of inadequate insulin administration or increased insulin resistance, severe hypertriglyceridemia may ensue and alter the concentrations of other classes of lipoproteins. In well-treated type 1 diabetic patients, plasma levels of HDL cholesterol are increased; in contrast, even patients with well-treated type 2 diabetes usually have low plasma levels of HDL cholesterol. Regardless of the specific treatment or type of diabetes mellitus, women ordinarily exhibit higher plasma levels of VLDL triglyceride and LDL cholesterol, and lower levels of HDL cholesterol, than do diabetic men (78). This may explain the increased prevalence of atherosclerosis in diabetic women and the disappearance of the usual preponderance of atherosclerotic disease in men compared with premenopausal women (40).

Hypercholesterolemia, with increased plasma concentrations of LDL cholesterol and apo B, also can occur in patients with either type 1 or type 2 diabetes mellitus and is usually induced by diet. Intensive therapy with diet, exercise, and insulin usually normalizes lipoprotein levels unless a genetic lipoprotein disorder coexists.

Hyperlipidemia in the patient with diabetes mellitus increases the risk for the major complications of atherosclerosis, CAD, cerebrovascular disease, and peripheral vascular disease. The severity of peripheral vascular disease has been associated with the lipoprotein abnormalities in diabetic women. Whether treatment of the lipid abnormalities in diabetic patients will decrease their risk for CAD and other arteriosclerotic complications remains to be ascertained.

Chronic Uremia and Treatment with Dialysis

Many patients with chronic uremia have increased plasma levels of VLDL triglycerides and decreased levels of HDL cholesterol (23). These abnormalities persist during maintenance hemodialysis or peritoneal dialysis. The accelerated atherosclerosis observed in white versus African-American men undergoing long-term hemodialysis appears to be related to the abnormal composition of HDL_2 cholesterol in the plasma of white men. A sedentary lifestyle, obesity, high-fat diets, or treatment with corticosteroids, β-blockers, or androgens worsens the lipoprotein profiles in these patients, whereas effective reversal of these secondary causes improves the lipid profile (23).

Hypothyroidism

Adequate levels of thyroid hormone appear to be necessary for the homeostatic maintenance of lipoprotein physiology. Decreases in LDL receptor function, abnormalities in LPL and hepatic lipase-mediated metabolism of triglycerides and HDL, and reduced LCAT activity have been demonstrated in some patients with hypothyroidism. Consequently, increased plasma levels of VLDL, IDL, and LDL and reduced levels of HDL cholesterol have all been reported in patients with this disease. Treatment with thyroid hormone improves LDL receptor function, increases the activity and function of LPL and LCAT, and normalizes lipoprotein profiles.

Other Common Secondary Causes of Hyperlipidemia

Patients with the *nephrotic syndrome* commonly lose apo C–II in the urine, thus decreasing LPL-mediated triglyceride clearance. The hypoalbuminemia that accompanies the nephrotic syndrome increases hepatic VLDL synthesis, thereby elevating plasma levels of VLDL triglyceride and LDL cholesterol. Treatment of the primary disease causing the nephrotic syndrome usually corrects the lipoprotein abnormalities, but drug and diet (low fat) therapy may be required.

Hypercortisolemia of endogenous or exogenous origin increases hepatic synthesis of VLDL, LDL, or both. Kidney transplant recipients treated with high dosages of corticosteroids often exhibit elevated plasma levels of both VLDL and LDL as well as reduced levels of HDL cholesterol. The atherosclerosis that develops in such patients is probably related to these lipid abnormalities, which should be treated accordingly.

Obesity, *alcohol ingestion*, and *androgen administration* tend to increase hepatic lipoprotein synthesis but have different effects on levels of HDL cholesterol and LDL cholesterol. In obese people, plasma levels of VLDL triglyceride and LDL cholesterol are increased, whereas those of HDL are decreased. Mild alcohol ingestion (up to 2 ounces/day) increases levels of VLDL triglyceride and HDL cholesterol but lowers levels of LDL cholesterol. Exogenous androgens raise levels of LDL cholesterol and lower HDL cholesterol levels.

Diseases affecting the liver, such as hepatitis or cholelithiasis, alter lipoprotein metabolism. Diseases causing an obstruction in the hepatobiliary system tend to elevate plasma LDL, IDL, and remnant lipoproteins and cause abnormal lipoproteins (Lp X) to accumulate in plasma.

Inflammatory processes usually lower levels of HDL and LDL cholesterol and raise VLDL, depending on the nutritional state of the patient.

Drugs used to treat hypertension, particularly thiazide diuretics and β-adrenergic blockers, raise levels of VLDL and LDL and lower levels of HDL cholesterol. Weight loss or the discontinuation of these drugs usually normalizes lipoprotein profiles.

Hyperlipidemia occurs in patients with *systemic lupus erythematosus* or *dysgammaglobulinemia*. This may be related to interactions among amyloid protein, certain immunoglobulin fractions, and various steps in the lipoprotein cascade.

Table 75.3 lists common causes for secondary lipoprotein disorders. Table 75.5 lists several exogenous and endogenous factors that affect plasma levels of HDL cholesterol.

CLINICAL MANIFESTATIONS OF LIPOPROTEIN DISORDERS

Adverse clinical sequelae of the lipoprotein disorders most commonly manifest themselves as disorders of the vascular, dermatologic, and gastrointestinal systems. The clinical manifestations associated with each of the major disorders of lipoprotein metabolism are outlined in Table 75.4.

Vascular

As discussed previously, elevated levels of total cholesterol, LDL cholesterol, apo B–enriched lipoproteins, oxidized LDL, and Lp(a) and decreased levels of HDL cholesterol, HDL_2, and apo A–I contribute to the development of atherosclerotic disease. The earlier the onset of symptomatic disease of the coronary, cerebral, or peripheral vasculature, the more likely it is that a lipoprotein abnormality or another major risk factor (cigarette smoking, hypertension, diabetes) is present (40). In the most severe form of hypercholesterolemia, *homozygous familial hypercholesterolemia*, plasma levels of total cholesterol vary from 600 to 1200 mg/dL, CAD generally develops in childhood, and very few patients survive past age 30. In *heterozygotes*, plasma levels of total cholesterol vary from about 270 to 550 mg/dL, and the time of onset of CAD varies between

Table 75.5. Factors that Affect HDL Cholesterol Levels

Increase	Decrease
Exercise	Androgens (male sex, drugs)
Oral estrogens (female sex)	In males, puberty
Alcohol (moderate)	In females, menopause
Familial (hyperalphalipoproteinemia)	Obesity
Leanness	Hypertriglyceridemia
Antihyperlipidemic drugs:	Type 2 diabetes mellitus
Nicotinic acid, colestipol, clofibrate, lovastatin, gemfibrozil	Familial hypoalphalipoproteinemia (Tangier's disease)
Insulin	Cigarettes
IV heparin	Sedentary lifestyle
	Probucol
	Uremia
	Vegetarian diet
	Progestogens

early adulthood and late middle age, with approximately 50% of men and women becoming symptomatic by age 50 and 60, respectively. Patients with *monogenic familial combined hyperlipoproteinemia* exhibit elevated levels of VLDL, LDL, or both, as well as abnormalities in HDL, apo A, and apo B; most patients manifest symptoms of CAD by age 60. Individuals with *familial dysbetalipoproteinemia* develop premature peripheral vascular disease and CAD at about equal rates, with a mean age of onset in both men and women of about 40. Such patients seem to be especially responsive to therapy. Individuals with *monogenic familial hypertriglyceridemia* or with *fasting chylomicronemia* do not appear to be at increased risk for CAD unless other risk factors for atherosclerosis are also present.

Dermatologic

Xanthomas may occur in all of the hyperlipidemias; however, they are present in a minority of hyperlipidemic patients. They occur with increasing frequency as the plasma lipid levels rise. They are present predominantly in the primary forms of hyperlipoproteinemia: familial hypercholesterolemia, familial dysbetalipoproteinemia, and familial LPL deficiency. Xanthomas are cutaneous or subcutaneous papules, plaques, or nodules characterized histopathologically by localized collections of lipid-laden histiocytes (foam cells). The presence or absence of xanthomas should always be noted. If present, their appearance (see below) can provide useful information about the nature of the underlying lipid disorder (Table 75.4). Unless tendons (especially the Achilles tendon) are palpated, tendon thickening characteristic of tendon xanthomas may be missed. Xanthomas are divided morphologically into several types:

1. *Tendinous* (Fig. 75.3A)—firm subcutaneous masses that arise in tendons and occasionally in ligaments, fascia, or periosteum. They characteristically move in concert with the associated tendon and can appear as diffuse thickenings of the tendon. They most often occur on the Achilles tendons and the extensor tendons of the hands, knees, and elbows. The overlying skin is normal in color.
2. *Tuberous* (Fig. 75.3B and C)—soft cutaneous and subcutaneous nodules that may harden with age and increasing fibrosis. Occasionally, they occur as superficial extensions of tendon xanthomas. They can also form from the confluence of eruptive xanthomas, and an intermediate stage is called tuberoeruptive xanthomas. They occur most often on extensor surfaces and areas subjected to trauma, such as the elbows, the knees, the dorsa of the hands, the heels, and the buttocks. The overlying epidermis can be normal in color or have a yellow or orange hue.
3. *Eruptive* (Fig. 75.3D and F)—small (1 to 4 mm) cutaneous papules, that tend to appear in crops, often coincident with an abrupt rise in plasma

triglyceride levels. Compared with the other types of xanthomas, they contain more inflammatory cells, free fatty acids, and triglycerides and fewer foam cells and cholesterol esters. They most often occur over pressure areas, such as the buttocks, parts of the trunk, elbows, and knees. They often have a yellow center and red halo.
4. *Planar* (Fig. 75.3E, G, and H)—flat, slightly elevated cutaneous lesions that occur most often in skin folds and scars but can be more widely distributed. When present on the eyelids, they are called *xanthelasma*. When located on the palms, they are called palmar xanthomas, and when confined to the palmar creases, *xanthoma striata palmaris*. They tend to be yellow or yellow-brown.

Hypercholesterolemia is associated with tendinous, planar, and tuberous xanthomas. Severe hypertriglyceridemia and chylomicronemia are associated with eruptive and occasionally tuberoeruptive or tuberous xanthomas. Palmar xanthomas are characteristic of familial dysbetalipoproteinemia and florid obstructive liver disease. Planar xanthomas on the body or palms in the presence of a type II lipid profile suggest homozygous monogenic familial hypercholesterolemia. The presence of tendinous or tuberous xanthomas or premature xanthelasma with a type II lipid profile suggests either heterozygous or homozygous monogenic familial hypercholesterolemia, as opposed to the polygenic or nongenetic forms. Tendon xanthomas are found in one-third to one-half of heterozygotes, whereas tuberous xanthomas are seen most often in patients with familial dysbetalipoproteinemia.

Occasionally, xanthomas appear in the absence of a hyperlipidemic state. For example, xanthelasma occur commonly in normolipidemic older individuals and in nonwhites, and planar xanthomas can occur in patients with lymphoma, leukemia, or myeloma. Studies in normolipidemic individuals with xanthelasma have revealed abnormalities in apo B and E suggestive of familial dysbetalipoproteinemia and/or elevated levels of LDL apo B, suggesting that these individuals may be at an increased risk of developing atherosclerosis.

Differences exist in the responses to treatment of the various hyperlipidemia-associated xanthomas. Thus, tendon xanthomas are the most resistant to treatment and, in practice, seldom disappear. In contrast, eruptive and planar xanthomas can disappear within a few weeks after plasma lipid levels return to normal.

Gastrointestinal

As many as 35 to 55% of patients with fasting chylomicronemia experience episodes of recurrent abdominal pain. Symptoms are ordinarily associated with marked elevations of plasma triglyceride levels (greater than 1000 to 2000 mg/dL). Abdominal pain may be so severe that it prompts unnecessary surgery, particularly if the lipid disorder is not suspected. The pain is often associated with pancreatitis, although the responsible pathogenetic mechanism is not well understood. Routine serum amylase determinations are often subject to technical artifacts when hyperlipidemia is present because of the presence of an amylase-inhibiting factor that may or may not be triglyceride. In such cases, a more reliable estimate of the serum amylase value can be obtained by determining amylase levels on serial dilutions, until the value obtained no longer changes with further dilution. Another cause of abdominal pain may be rapid hepatic or splenic enlargement with capsular distension from triglyceride deposition in reticuloendothelial cells. Often the cause is unclear. Gastrointestinal symptoms other than abdominal pain, such as nausea, vomiting, borborygmi, and diarrhea, also occur.

Other Clinical Associations

Other clinical concomitants of hyperlipidemia include the following: premature arcus corneae (grayish-white corneal ring caused by lipid droplets) in hypercholesterolemia (elevated LDL); aortic stenosis in homozygous monogenic familial hypercholesterolemia; Achilles tendinitis in heterozygous monogenic familial hypercholesterolemia; obesity, glucose intolerance, hyperinsulinemia, hyperuricemia, and perhaps cholelithiasis in association with hypertriglyceridemia and elevated VLDL; recurrent polyarthralgias, arthritis, tenosynovitis, and siccalike syndromes in hypertriglyceridemia (elevated VLDL) or hypercholesterolemia (elevated LDL); lipemia retinalis (cream-colored retinal vessels) in chylomicronemia (evident when plasma triglycerides rise above 3,000 mg/dL; obvious when they exceed 10,000 mg/dL).

DIAGNOSIS

Indications for Evaluation

Controversy persists regarding the optimal, cost-effective approach to the identification of hyperlipidemic patients at high risk for CAD (5,34,45,71). Many authorities believe that routine screening of healthy young adult men and women who have no CAD risk factors, family history, or clinical evidence of CAD is unwarranted because the benefits of case finding may be outweighed by the long-term risks of treatment (34). At present, the most widely used guidelines for case findings are those issued by the Adult Treatment Panel of the National Cholesterol Education Program (NCEP), which updated its recommendations for the detection, evaluation, and treatment of high blood cholesterol in adults in 1993. As in the 1988 report (see "General References"), the NCEP emphasizes LDL as the primary target of cholesterol-lowering therapy; the role of the clinical approach to primary prevention of CAD; and dietary therapy as the initial treatment, with hypolipidemic drug therapy reserved for patients at high risk for CAD. The current guidelines, however, emphasize CAD risk status as a major determinant for the type and intensity of treatment, pay more attention to HDL as a risk factor, and underscore the importance of including physical activity and weight loss as com-

ponents of dietary therapy. With regard to assigning risk factor status, the revised NCEP report places patients with existing CAD or other atherosclerotic disease at highest risk, establishing lower target levels of LDL cholesterol in these patients; adds age to the list of major risk factors (45 years or older in men, 55 years or older in women); recommends delaying drug therapy in most young adult men and premenopausal women with high LDL cholesterol levels who are otherwise at low short-term CAD risk; and encourages consideration of drug therapy for high-risk postmenopausal women and old patients who are in good general health. *The panel also recommends that HDL cholesterol above 60 mg/dL be considered a negative risk factor; and that HDL levels be used in deciding on drug therapy.*

Interpretation of the Results of Initial Screening

The panel recommends that levels of total cholesterol should be measured in all adults 20 years of age or older at least once every 5 years, assuming blood cholesterol levels are below 200 mg/dL, and that HDL should be measured at the same time if accurate results are available (see below). An HDL level below 35 mg/dL is considered to be a low value. Measurements of total cholesterol and HDL for screening purposes can be obtained from nonfasting people. However, final classification of abnormal lipid profiles requires lipid determinations in subjects who have been fasted overnight (see below). The NCEP classifies individuals by measurements of serum levels of total, LDL, and HDL cholesterol. In this schema, serum levels of total cholesterol less than 200 mg/dL are considered to represent a *desirable blood cholesterol*; levels from 200 to 239 mg/dL, to indicate a *borderline-high blood cholesterol*; and levels 240 mg/dL or above, to signify a *high blood cholesterol*. Data from numerous epidemiologic studies reveal that the relationships between serum levels of total (or LDL) cholesterol and CAD risk are continuous and that CAD risk at a cholesterol value of 240 mg/dL is nearly double that at 200 mg/dL and rises rapidly at levels above 240 mg/dL. Total cholesterol levels of 240 mg/dL or more correspond to the uppermost 20% of cholesterol values in the entire population 20 years of age and older. Patients with levels of total serum cholesterol between 200 and 239 mg/dL and either an HDL cholesterol less than 35 mg/dL, known CAD, or two or more known risk factors for CAD (Table 75.6) are considered to have high blood cholesterol values.

Evaluation of the Patient with Hypercholesterolemia

Once a patient is found to have a high blood cholesterol level or physical stigmata of hypercholesterolemia (e.g., dermatologic signs), decisions regarding possible diet, drug, or other therapy are made after a more detailed lipoprotein analysis, including measurements of triglyceride levels on a blood specimen obtained after an overnight fast, calculation of the LDL cholesterol level (see below), and determination of

Table 75.6. CAD Risk Factors as Defined by the 1993 NCEP Adult Treatment Guidelines

Positive Risk Factors

Age
  Male ≥45 yr
  Female ≥55 yr or premature menopause without estrogen re-
  placement therapy
Family history of premature CHD (definite myocardial infarction or
  sudden death before 55 yr of age in father or other male first-
  degree relative, or before 65 yr of age in mother or other female
  first-degree relative)
Current cigarette smoking
Hypertension (blood pressure ≥140/90 mm Hg or taking antihyper-
  tensive medication)
Low HDL cholesterol (<35 mg/dL [0.9 mmol/L])
Diabetes mellitus

Negative Risk Factor

High HDL cholesterol (≥60 mg/dL [1.6 mmol/L])

From Summary of the Second Report of the National Cholesterol Education Program (NCEP) Expert Panel on Detection, Evaluation, and Treatment of High Blood Cholesterol in Adults (Adult Treatment Panel II). JAMA 269:3015, 1993.

other CAD risk factors. An LDL cholesterol level of 160 mg/dL or more is considered to represent a *high-risk LDL cholesterol*, whereas levels of LDL cholesterol from 130 to 159 mg/dL signify *borderline-high risk* and LDL levels less than 130 mg/dL are considered *desirable*. In patients with known CAD or two or more major CAD risk factors (Table 75.6), LDL cholesterol levels from 130 to 159 mg/dL are considered *high-risk*. The NCEP considers an HDL level less than 35 mg/dL to be an independent risk factor for CAD. Thus, decisions regarding both the implementation and goals of therapy are based not on ratios of LDL (or total) cholesterol to HDL cholesterol but on absolute levels of LDL and HDL cholesterol. Such decisions are also influenced by the presence or absence of other CAD risk factors.

It is important to emphasize that assignment of risk levels using total, LDL, and HDL cholesterol cutoff values, and the therapeutic actions that are based upon these values (see below), derive from studies in middle-age men and have not yet been proved to be applicable to young and elderly men or to women (5,45). Nonetheless, given the strong evidence favoring the lipid (or cholesterol) hypothesis, most authorities believe it is appropriate to apply the diagnostic guidelines described above to all adult population groups.

Triglycerides. Both the current NCEP guidelines and an NIH Consensus Development Conference (see "General References") classify fasting triglyceride levels less than 200 mg/dL as normal; levels from 200 to 400 mg/dL as *borderline-high*; values from 400 to 1000 mg/dL, as *high*; and values greater than 1000 mg/dL as *very high*. As already noted, although fasting hypertriglyceridemia is not an independent risk factor for CAD, there is a complex link between hypertriglyceridemia and CAD, which is explained in part by the association between high triglycerides and low HDL and/or unusually atherogenic forms of LDL. Moreover, elevated triglycerides often reflect increased triglyceride-rich remnant lipoproteins that have atherogenic potential.

Currently, it is recommended that fasting triglycerides be measured only in patients at high risk for CAD, and not as a routine screening measure in healthy people.

Measurement of plasma levels of total cholesterol, HDL cholesterol, and fasting triglyceride and calculation of the level of LDL cholesterol (see below) are desirable when abnormalities are detected on screening or conditions coexist that could cause secondary abnormalities in lipoprotein metabolism (Table 75.3). Although the frequencies with which certain drugs (e.g., thiazide diuretics, antihypertensives, oral contraceptives) adversely affect lipoprotein metabolism are unknown and direct causal interrelationships between such drug-associated lipid abnormalities and premature atherosclerosis are unproved, it seems prudent also to consider the more complete evaluation before therapy is initiated with these drugs.

Laboratory Evaluation

Serum levels of total cholesterol are not appreciably influenced by acute dietary intake and thus can be obtained from patients in the nonfasting state and at any time of the day. Cholesterol levels can also be measured in plasma, but the results should be multiplied by 1.03 to obtain the equivalent serum value. There is considerable biological variability in total cholesterol levels, with repeated measurements on the same person showing a standard deviation of as much as 18 mg/dL (81). Thus, the 95% confidence interval of a patient with a total cholesterol value of 220 mg/dL would be 184 to 256 mg/dL. In addition, both intralaboratory and interlaboratory errors in measurement are common. Current estimates are that as many as one-half of all laboratory determinations of total cholesterol vary by 5% or more from the correct value, although several groups have proposed methods to reduce these errors in accuracy and precision to approximately 3% within the next several years. Thus, it remains important to obtain blood for cholesterol measurements from a nonstressed patient, to send the blood for measurement to a reliable laboratory, and to average the results of at least two to three measurements before final classification of the patient by total cholesterol level. Results from one recent study suggest that there is also seasonal variation in cholesterol measurements in men, but not in women (59). Using the NCEP cutoff value of 240 mg/dL, the age-adjusted prevalence of hypercholesterolemia detected in men in the winter was double that found in the summer. The implications of this observation for the detection and treatment of patients with hypercholesterolemia remain to be determined.

Levels of total (and LDL) cholesterol fall during the first few days after MI (26), so cholesterol determinations either should be made within 24 hours of a severe acute MI (when they are still valid) or should be postponed until 3 to 4 weeks after recovery. Fasting triglyceride (and VLDL) levels tend to rise slowly after an MI, peaking at 3 to 4 weeks and returning to baseline by 8 to 12 weeks. Triglyceride levels should therefore be obtained either within 24 hours of the acute event or after 8 to 12 weeks.

Because measurements of HDL cholesterol depend on the prevailing level of triglycerides, HDL cholesterol levels should be determined in patients after a standard 12- to 15-hour overnight fast. The *determination of HDL cholesterol* is the measurement most subject to laboratory error. The precision of its measurement was inadequate in most clinical laboratories surveyed by the Centers for Disease Control and Prevention. It is therefore important for each physician periodically to assess the performance of an individual laboratory against one that is rigidly standardized (a list of CDC-approved lipid laboratories is available from regional and national offices of the American Heart Association). Repetition of the baseline measurement provides a further safeguard. Such measures to enhance validity are important because there is a relatively narrow range of HDL cholesterol values within which even small differences are prognostically important. For example, a reduction in the level of HDL cholesterol of 5 mg/dL from 40 to 35 mg/dL increases the risk for CAD by approximately 25%. When triglyceride levels exceed 400 mg/dL, the standardized techniques for the precipitation of VLDL and LDL are ineffective and HDL cholesterol levels are unreliable. The plasma can be ultrafiltered to remove the interfering VLDL. If this is required, the physician should consult the laboratory.

Calculation of LDL level. Despite these problems, the level of HDL cholesterol represents a strong index of CAD risk, an aid to diagnosis, and an important measure to follow during therapy. It also allows one to calculate LDL cholesterol (LDL-C) levels (provided triglyceride level is below 400 mg/dL) by the formula: LDL-C = TC − (TG/5 + HDL-C), where *TC* is the plasma level of total cholesterol, *TG* is the fasting plasma triglyceride level, and *HDL-C* is the level of HDL cholesterol (21).

Observation of a fasting plasma sample, which has been left undisturbed overnight in a refrigerator at 4°C, is indicated in the presence of a significantly elevated fasting plasma triglyceride level. Elevated levels of total (or LDL) cholesterol do not affect the appearance of plasma, whereas hypertriglyceridemia associated with increased levels of VLDL imparts uniform turbidity to plasma, and hypertriglyceridemia associated with chylomicronemia is characterized by a creamy supernatant fraction that floats on the top of plasma.

A marked abnormality in plasma lipid levels, especially marked hypertriglyceridemia (triglyceride greater than 2000 mg/dL), can affect the validity of other laboratory tests. Marked hypertriglyceridemia has an inhibitory effect on the plasma amylase assay, interferes with the measurement of liver enzymes (aspartate aminotransferase, alanine aminotransferase) and calcium by autoanalyzer, and causes artifactual reductions in the serum concentration of molecules restricted to the aqueous phase, such as sodium. Ultracentrifugation of plasma, with the removal of chylomicrons, permits these measurements to be performed accurately; but sometimes serial dilutions of the plasma are necessary, particularly for the measurement of amylase.

Clinical Evaluation

Clinical data contribute substantially to the diagnosis of specific lipoprotein disorders and to decisions about treatment when abnormalities are found. History, physical examination, and indicated laboratory evaluation are required to rule out secondary causes of hyperlipidemia (Table 75.3). A positive family history, the presence of premature atherosclerotic disease, and the presence of specific dermatologic manifestations may permit the diagnosis of a primary form of hyperlipoproteinemia (Table 75.4).

Referral

When laboratory and clinical evaluations do not result in a clear-cut diagnosis of a lipoprotein disorder, referral to a specialist in endocrinology and metabolism is indicated. Such specialists can perform (or readily obtain) and interpret more sophisticated tests, such as ultracentrifugal quantification of lipoprotein levels, apoprotein measurement, receptor analysis, and determination of LPL activity. They may also assist in the evaluation of family members, so that the presence of a genetic disorder can be accurately diagnosed.

TREATMENT

General Considerations

The first step in the management of a lipoprotein disorder is accurate diagnosis. Causes of secondary lipoprotein disorders should be identified (Table 75.3) and treated. If the cause of a secondary disorder is not reversible or a primary disorder exists, treatment may be required that is specifically directed at the abnormal lipoprotein pattern.

Such treatment should be part of the comprehensive management of other coexisting CAD risk factors (e.g., cigarette smoking, hypertension, diabetes mellitus, obesity, and inactivity). It will likely require behavioral change on the part of the patient and lifelong management, emphasizing the need for a positive patient–physician relationship, appropriate patient education, and skill on the part of the physician in promoting patient compliance (see Chapters 3 and 4). The long-term follow-up and monitoring of various parameters in such patients are necessary to enhance compliance, assess the effectiveness of therapy, and detect drug toxicity or the effect of concomitant therapy on plasma lipids (e.g., diuretics and other antihypertensive agents).

Patients without CAD who are classified as having a *desirable* total cholesterol level (less than 200 mg/dL) and an HDL cholesterol level above 35 mg/dL are usually instructed on the principles of a prudent diet and healthy lifestyle, educated about CAD risk factors

(Table 75.6), and advised to have their total cholesterol levels rechecked at least once every 5 years. If the HDL cholesterol level is less than 35 mg/dL, patients should have a full lipoprotein analysis, which consists of measurement of total cholesterol, HDL cholesterol, and fasting triglycerides and calculation of LDL cholesterol level (see "Laboratory Evaluation"). Patients with high total cholesterol levels (240 mg/dL or more) should undergo lipoprotein analysis and are advised about specific therapy depending upon their LDL cholesterol levels. Patients with *borderline-high cholesterol values* (200 to 239 mg/dL) who have an HDL cholesterol level of 35 mg/dL or greater and fewer than two other CAD risk factors should also receive education about diet, exercise, and lifestyle modification and should have total and HDL cholesterol levels rechecked in 1 to 2 years. If the HDL cholesterol level is below 35 mg/dL or at least two risk factors are present (Table 75.6), or if the total cholesterol level is 240 mg/dL or greater, a lipoprotein profile should be done. LDL cholesterol levels are labeled as *desirable* (less than 130 mg/dL), *borderline-high* (130 to 159 mg/dL) or *high* (greater than 160 mg/dL). Patients who have desirable or borderline-risk LDL cholesterol levels and fewer than two CAD risk factors should receive diet and exercise information and be evaluated in 5 years or 1 year, respectively. Those with *borderline-high* LDL levels and two or more risk factors or *high* LDL levels should receive clinical evaluation and should be placed on a Step 1 diet (see below).

Treatment of hypercholesterolemia is based on the results of lipoprotein analyses and determinations of LDL cholesterol levels. It is suggested that two or three measurements be performed 1 to 8 weeks apart and that decisions about definitive therapy be based on the average of these LDL cholesterol values. Patients with a desirable LDL cholesterol (less than 130 mg/dL) are treated as if the total blood cholesterol is also in the desirable range. Patients with LDL cholesterol values between 130 and 159 mg/dL and with CAD or two or more CAD risk factors and individuals with LDL cholesterol values greater than 160 mg/dL should be evaluated first for possible causes of secondary hypercholesterolemia (see above) before being advised about specific dietary or drug therapy. In addition, first-degree family relatives should be screened for hypercholesterolemia.

Management of patients with isolated reductions in HDL levels (less than 35 mg/dL) should emphasize nonpharmacologic approaches, such as weight loss, aerobic exercise, and discontinuation of cigarette smoking (see below). Although certain drugs used for treatment of elevated levels of LDL cholesterol or of triglycerides may also raise HDL levels, at present no data support their use in the patient whose only lipid abnormality is a reduction in the level of HDL.

Management of hypertriglyceridemia must be individualized. When familial combined hyperlipidemia or familial dysbetalipoproteinemia is diagnosed, specific treatment is required. Patients with fasting triglyceride levels above 500 mg/dL sometimes accumulate chylomicrons and develop pancreatitis. The risk becomes substantial when triglyceride levels exceed 1000 mg/dL. The plasma triglyceride level should therefore be lowered in these patients. Patients with familial hypertriglyceridemia or fasting triglyceride levels in the 250 to 500 mg/dL range in the absence of other CAD risk factors do not seem to be at increased risk of CAD or pancreatitis. Treatment is recommended only when risk factors coexist, such as a family history of premature CAD; abnormal levels of total (or LDL) cholesterol, HDL cholesterol, or apoproteins; concomitant CAD, diabetes, end-stage renal disease, smoking, or obesity; and young age. Isolated fasting triglyceride levels below 250 mg/dL do not require treatment.

Nonpharmacologic Therapy

Diet (Tables 75.7 and 75.8)

It is now well established that plasma lipid levels can be altered by dietary manipulations. Under strictly controlled conditions (e.g., in a metabolic unit), elevated plasma levels of total (or LDL) cholesterol may be reduced by as much as 30% or more and levels of triglyceride or VLDL (in the presence of marked elevations) by as much as 80% or more. Fasting chylomicronemia can also be eliminated. Under ambulatory conditions, in which diets tend to be less restrictive and noncompliance more common, reductions in lipid levels are less dramatic. For example, among prospective studies of cholesterol-lowering diets, the decrease in plasma cholesterol averaged 15% (range, 8.5 to 22%).

Single-Diet Approach (Table 75.7). The second report of the Adult Treatment Panel II (NCEP) (see "General References") continues to highlight dietary therapy as the first line of treatment of elevated blood cholesterol levels. In primary prevention trials to date, dietary therapy has not been associated with decreased all-cause mortality. There is little evidence to support treatment of healthy normolipidemic individuals with restrictive diets. Recent studies have shown little change in the lipid profiles of healthy subjects with intake of either a high- or low-cholesterol diet. Dietary

Table 75.7.   Dietary Therapy of High Blood Cholesterol

Nutrient	Recommended Intake	
	Step 1 Diet	Step 2 Diet
Total fat	Less than 30% of total calories	
Saturated fatty acids	Less than 10% of total calories	Less than 7% of total calories
Polyunsaturated fatty acids	Up to 10% of total calories	
Monounsaturated fatty acids	10 to 15% of total calories	
Carbohydrates	50 to 60% of total calories	
Protein	10 to 20% of total calories	
Cholesterol	Less than 300 mg/day	Less than 200 mg/day
Total calories	To achieve and maintain desirable weight	

From The Expert Panel Report of the National Cholesterol Education Program Expert Panel on Detection, Evaluation and Treatment of High Blood Cholesterol in Adults. Arch Intern Med 148:36, 1988.

Table 75.8. Dietary Guidelines to Lower Blood Cholesterol

Food	Recommended	Avoid or Use Sparingly
Fish, Shellfish, Poultry, Shrimp, Lean Red Meats		
Up to 6 to 7 oz are recommended per day (limit shrimp to 3 oz)	Fish; skinless chicken, turkey, Cornish hen; very lean cuts of beef, lamb, pork and veal; low-fat lunchmeats with 3 g fat or less per oz. Dry beans or tofu may be used as a substitute for fish, poultry, and meat.	Any fatty cuts of meat; lunchmeats; sausages; scrapple, bacon; hot dogs; caviar, fish roe; deep-fried meats, fish, and poultry; organ meat; duck; goose
Fats and Oils		
Up to 6 to 7 tsp may be used per day, including fat used in cooking	Unsaturated oils: safflower, sunflower, corn, soybean, sesame, olive, rapeseed (canola); margarine with first ingredient a liquid unsaturated oil listed above; 4 to 6 nuts or 3 olives count as 1 teaspoon of oil. Mayonnaise; salad dressing made with unsaturated oils listed above (2 teaspoons count as 1 teaspoon oil).	Butter; lard; palm kernel oil; meat fat; salt pork; bacon fat; coconut oil; palm oil; hydrogenated or solid shortenings; gravy; cream sauce; salad dressing made with cream, cheese, or sour cream
Milk and Yogurt		
2 or more cups recommended per day	Skim or 1% milk, including evaporated and powdered milk; buttermilk; nonfat and low-fat yogurt.	Whole milk, including evaporated and condensed milk; eggnog; yogurt; cream; sour cream; half and half; coconut milk
Cheese		
1 oz of recommended cheese or ¼ cup cottage cheese may be substituted for 1 oz of fish, poultry, or lean red meat	Low-fat cottage cheese; low-fat cheese with 4 g of fat or less per oz.	High-fat cheeses containing more than 4 g of fat per oz
Eggs		
Egg yolks should be limited to 2 per week, including those used in cooking	Egg whites (2 egg whites will substitute for 1 whole egg in recipes); cholesterol-free egg substitutes.	Egg yolks in excess of 2 per week
Vegetables and Fruits		
4 or more servings are recommended per day. Include at least 1 serving of citrus fruit or other source of vitamin C per day	Fresh, frozen, canned, or dried.	Vegetables in cream, cheese, or butter sauces, deep-fried vegetables, french fries
Breads and Cereals		
4 or more servings recommended per day	Loaf bread and bagels (except egg); English muffins, pita bread; most sandwich and dinner rolls; Melba toast; water crackers; soda crackers; rice cakes; rye crisp; matzo, pretzels, breadsticks (made without cheese). All cereals except as noted. Pasta (except egg); all grains, including rice, barley, buckwheat, bulgur, corn, millet, rye, and oats.	Croissants, biscuits, and other rich rolls; pastries; doughnuts; egg breads; commercial baked products; high-fat crackers; cereals with added oils and coconut, such as granola-type; egg pasta
Desserts and Sweets		
Foods high in sugar are best used in small amounts. They should be used infrequently by persons with high triglycerides or excess weight.	Fruit Sugar, jelly; cocoa powder, gelatin, Italian ice; frozen fruit bars; frozen low-fat yogurt; pudding made with skim milk; angel food cake; sherbet; sorbet; low-fat cookies; homemade baked products made with skim or low-fat milk, egg whites, and small amounts of unsaturated fat.	Chocolate; ice cream; coconut; cream desserts; egg custard; commercial baked products
Miscellaneous		
	Bouillon; fat-free broths. Air-popped popcorn or popcorn made with small amounts of unsaturated oil; pretzels, chestnuts. Vinegar, spices, herbs, mustard, fat-free salad dressing.	Cream or other fatty soups; high-fat snack foods such as potato chips, corn chips, granola bars, microwave popcorn, non-dairy creamers, and whipped toppings made with coconut or palm oil

From The Johns Hopkins Physicians Lipid Education Program. 2nd ed. Baltimore: The Johns Hopkins University, 1988;26.

therapy has more impact in those who are dyslipidemic and have risk factors for CAD. It is now appreciated that one diet can be used to treat all of the common forms of hyperlipoproteinemia. Using the principle of graduated regimen implementation (see Chapter 4), the diet can be introduced in two steps, with the second step introducing further restrictions in dietary total fat, saturated fat, and cholesterol (Table

75.7). Step 1 represents the American Heart Association (AHA) *prudent diet*, which is recommended for the entire American population. When severe chylomicronemia is present, dietary fat must be more severely restricted (see below).

The AHA and other organizations publish useful booklets on this diet for the patient, physician, and nutritionist (see "General References"). Most patients with hyperlipoproteinemia benefit from referral to a suitably trained dietitian.

The single diet actually incorporates several nutritional strategies, each of which tends to have a selective effect on plasma lipoprotein levels. It is helpful to consider each strategy separately.

Cholesterol Reduction (Tables 75.7 and 75.8). The Step 1 diet to lower serum cholesterol levels is characterized by a restriction of dietary cholesterol to less than 300 mg/day and reductions in daily total and saturated fat intake to less than 30 and 10% of caloric intake, respectively. The Step 2 diet further decreases cholesterol intake to less than 200 mg/day and the intake of saturated fat to less than 7% of daily caloric intake. Caloric allowance is adjusted to ensure loss of excess weight or maintenance of ideal body weight (see Chapter 76). Restrictions in dietary cholesterol and saturated fats independently contribute to the reduction in plasma cholesterol levels. A modest increase in dietary polyunsaturated fat results in further, although less marked, reduction in plasma cholesterol level.

The two major categories of *polyunsaturated fatty acids* are the omega-6 and omega-3 types. Linoleic acid is the principal omega-6 fatty acid and, when consumed in large amounts, can decrease levels of total cholesterol. Lecithin, a phospholipid derived from soybeans, is a widely publicized popular remedy for hypercholesterolemia and is commonly sold in health food stores. Because it is not absorbed as such from the gastrointestinal tract, any hypocholesterolemic effect probably derives from its high content of linoleic acid. Vegetable oils rich in linoleic acid, such as safflower oil, soybean oil, sunflower oil, and corn oil, are the preferred dietary sources of the omega-6 fatty acids.

The major sources of the omega-3 fatty acids are the fish oils. Taken as dietary supplements, high dosages of fish oil lower elevated triglyceride levels but do not reduce levels of total or LDL cholesterol. In patients with nephrotic syndrome, dietary supplementation with omega-3 fatty acids is associated with an increase in LDL cholesterol levels (29). Recent evidence suggests that use of fish oil capsules may worsen hyperinsulinemia, insulin resistance, and glucose tolerance in patients with non–insulin-dependent diabetes mellitus (22,64).

Data from prospective epidemiologic studies (41) support the recent findings from the Chicago Western Electric Study, which show an inverse relationship between fish consumption and death from CHD, especially nonsudden death from MI (15). Although the cause is unclear, there is no evidence to date that this results from intake of omega-3 fatty acids. In fact, high dietary levels of polyunsaturated omega-3 fatty acids may increase LDL oxidation. Thus, at present, the use of fish oil capsules containing omega-3 fatty acids is discouraged, particularly in patients with non–insulin-dependent diabetes mellitus.

The typical North American diet has an unfavorable polyunsaturated to saturated fat (P/S) ratio of 0.4. On the other hand, there is no historical precedent that attests to the safety of diets very rich in polyunsaturated fats (e.g., P/S ratio of 1.5 or more). It does appear that the latter diets can promote the formation of lithogenic bile and actually increase the incidence of symptomatic biliary tract disease. Although there was a concern that such diets are associated with an increased risk of malignant disease, this finding was not supported when data from several trials were pooled (18). Another disadvantage to substantially increasing dietary intake of polyunsaturated fat is that the resultant high caloric intake might promote obesity. Finally, it should be noted that diets with very high P/S ratios (e.g., 3 or more) may decrease HDL levels and lead to an unfavorable increase in the LDL/HDL ratio. For all of these reasons, a P/S ratio of about 1.0 is recommended in most hypocholesterolemic diets.

Recent evidence suggests that *monounsaturated fatty acids*, principally oleic acid, found in canola oil, olive oil, and certain forms of safflower and sunflower seed oil, lower levels of LDL cholesterol as effectively as do polyunsaturated fatty acids such as linoleic acid. Thus, it is now recommended that both the Step 1 and Step 2 diets contain approximately 10 to 15% monounsaturated fatty acids, derived mainly from these vegetable oils.

The influence of *dietary fiber* on plasma cholesterol levels is complex, dependent on the type of fiber, and somewhat controversial. Guar, pectin, and unprocessed high-fiber food, such as legumes and oats, lower plasma total cholesterol levels, whereas other fibers, such as wheat bran, do not. Effects on levels of HDL cholesterol and triglyceride are minimal. In the amounts consumed in a palatable diet, fiber plays a minor role compared to control of dietary fats and cholesterol.

Goals of dietary therapy. The goals of dietary therapy are to reduce levels of LDL cholesterol to less than 160 mg/dL in patients who have neither CAD nor evidence of two or more CAD risk factors, to less than 130 mg/dL in patients without CAD but with two or more CAD risk factors, and to less than 100 mg/dL in patients with CAD. The Adult Treatment Panel II (NCEP) suggests that levels of LDL cholesterol be used for classification of patients and decisions regarding dietary (and drug) therapy, but that levels of total cholesterol be used for assessment of the efficacy of diet therapy. In patients with normal levels of HDL cholesterol and triglycerides, a total cholesterol of 240 mg/dL corresponds to an LDL cholesterol value of 160 mg/dL, whereas a total cholesterol of 200 mg/dL corresponds to an LDL cholesterol of 130 mg/dL. The level of LDL cholesterol should be monitored in patients with abnormal levels of HDL cholesterol or triglycerides to decide whether the goals of dietary therapy have been achieved and whether to pursue drug therapy.

Monitoring and adjusting diet. Results of the Step 1 diet should be monitored after 4 to 6 weeks and again at 3 months, when the effects should be maximal. In general, formal consultation with a dietitian is not required during implementation of the Step 1 diet, and the physician and other health care providers should serve as the primary sources of education and compliance monitoring of and encouragement for the patient. It is important to emphasize to all patients that diet therapy of hypercholesterolemia implies permanent, rather than temporary, changes in eating behavior. If the goals of diet therapy are not met after 3 months, it is recommended that the patient continue on the Step 1 diet for another 3 months or progress to a Step 2 diet, which leads to a reduction of saturated fatty acid intake from 10% to less than 7%, and of dietary cholesterol from less than 300 mg/day to less than 200 mg/day. Ordinarily, implementation of the Step 2 diet requires consultation with a registered dietitian. Decisions regarding the use of hypocholesterolemic drug therapy should not usually be made until the patient has undergone an adequate 6-month trial of diet therapy and has failed to meet the target LDL cholesterol goals.

Dietary and drug therapy. Dietary therapy alone is often sufficient in the approximately 85% of hypercholesterolemic patients with polygenic or nonhereditary forms of hypercholesterolemia. Numerous studies indicate that dietary therapy alone is less effective in lowering total or LDL cholesterol levels than the combination of dietary therapy and drug treatment. For example, in a multicenter trial comparing the separate and combined effects of intensive dietary therapy and low-dose lovastatin in outpatients with moderate hypercholesterolemia, a low-fat diet alone reduced LDL cholesterol by 5%, whereas lovastatin alone lowered LDL by 27%, and lovastatin plus dietary therapy reduced LDL by 32% (36). Whereas selected patients may achieve a decrease in total cholesterol by 30 to 40 mg/dL with the Step 1 diet and by an additional 15 mg/dL with the Step 2 diet, many high-risk patients require concomitant drug therapy. In elderly patients with hypercholesterolemia, the benefits of diet therapy should be weighed against the possibility of inadequate nutrition. For this reason, aged patients at high risk should generally be treated only with the Step 1 diet and not with the more restrictive Step 2 diet.

Triglyceride Reduction. Diets designed to reduce plasma triglyceride and VLDL levels emphasize the loss of excess weight by total caloric restriction. Plasma triglyceride levels usually fall, often to normal, after a few days of caloric restriction. The reduction is maintained as long as weight loss continues at a rate of 1 to 2 lb (0.5 to 1 kg) per week. If normal weight is attained and maintained, further therapy may not be necessary. If hypertriglyceridemia persists or occurs in individuals of normal weight, a cholesterol-lowering diet, as outlined above, may be effective. Alcohol intake should be restricted because it can cause a striking rise in triglyceride levels in some patients with hypertriglyceridemia. Although extreme increases in the carbohydrate content of a diet can cause transient and, rarely, sustained hypertriglyceridemia, there is no firm evidence to suggest that total carbohydrate restriction is helpful in the treatment of hypertriglyceridemia. There are conflicting data regarding the effect on plasma triglyceride level of excessive intake of sucrose (common sugar) and simple sugars. In most studies, especially in patients who are already hypertriglyceridemic, they do raise plasma levels of triglycerides and lower those of HDL cholesterol, but the effect is small. The rationale for dietary restriction of sugar is based more on the need to avoid excessive caloric intake (and to prevent caries) than on its having a direct effect on plasma lipids. Like alcohol, sucrose provides empty calories in that it contains none of the valuable nutrients, such as protein, fiber, minerals, or vitamins. Therefore the substitution of complex (e.g., starches) for simple carbohydrates in the diet is recommended. A triglyceride-lowering diet should favorably affect plasma HDL cholesterol levels in most individuals because obesity and triglyceride levels are inversely correlated with the levels of HDL cholesterol, and since plasma HDL levels usually rise during weight reduction. Plasma levels of total (and LDL) cholesterol often fall with loss of excess weight; when they rise, familial combined hyperlipoproteinemia may be present.

Chylomicron Reduction.   Treatment of fasting chylomicronemia (type I) involves the restriction of dietary fat intake to 5 to 20% of total calories (0.5 g of fat per kilogram of body weight is a reasonable starting point). The fat deficit should be corrected predominantly by substitution of complex carbohydrates. Because medium-chain triglycerides (available as MCT oil) are transported directly from the intestine to the liver in the portal circulation without incorporation into chylomicrons, they may be added to the diet to provide calories. The recommended dose of MCT oil (available at most pharmacies) is 1 tablespoonful three to four times daily, mixed with foods. Five grams of vegetable fat rich in polyunsaturates should be included to prevent essential fatty acid deficiency.

Dietary fat is severely restricted until fasting chylomicronemia is eliminated and clinical symptoms are prevented or reduced in frequency; dietary fat is then chronically restricted to whatever degree is necessary to prevent fasting chylomicronemia. The efficacy of fat restriction in preventing recurrent abdominal pain is supported by clinical observations in individual patients.

When fasting chylomicronemia is accompanied by elevation of VLDL triglyceride levels, therapy is initiated with restriction of dietary fat intake and correction of coexistent secondary causes for the disorder. Once chylomicronemia has been eliminated, a triglyceride-lowering diet with a modest reduction in total fat intake (to approximately 30% of total calories) is all that is usually required to prevent recurrence. Total abstinence from alcohol is usually necessary.

Diets to raise levels of HDL. Some studies have reported that low-fat, low-cholesterol diets have resulted in decreased HDL cholesterol levels (14), whereas others have found increased HDL values (79). The dietary approach to the patient with an HDL cholesterol level below 35 mg/dL should incorporate loss of excess weight with an aerobic exercise program. Although moderate alcohol consumption (2 to 3 ounces/day) is positively correlated with HDL cholesterol level and negatively correlated with CAD, it is discouraged for three reasons: excessive use (more than two or three drinks/day) increases the overall risk of morbidity and mortality, its use may interfere with attempts to control obesity and hypertriglyceridemia, and evidence is not conclusive that modest intake results in an overall health advantage.

Exercise

During the past decade, evidence has accumulated that regular isotonic exercise enhances fatty acid oxidation and glycogen storage, thus increasing HDL formation, triglyceride clearance, and insulin sensitivity. These metabolic changes favorably affect plasma lipid levels. Most of the exercise programs that have been evaluated, including jogging, rapid walking, swimming, bicycling, cross-country skiing, and mountain climbing, have involved 30 minutes or more of continued effort at 70 to 85% of maximal heart rate at least three times weekly. In most studies, levels of HDL cholesterol have been shown to rise (approximately 20%) and triglyceride levels to fall (approximately 25%) with exercise (16). Although levels of LDL cholesterol usually do not fall in normal subjects, reductions of as much as 10% may occur in individuals with elevated levels of total and LDL cholesterol.

Resistive training programs conducted in normolipidemic individuals have resulted in increases in HDL cholesterol levels of 10 to 15% and decreases in LDL cholesterol levels of 5 to 39% (38). In contrast, in one well-controlled prospective study of resistive training in subjects at risk for CAD (37), no changes in lipid profiles were observed after 20 weeks. Both aerobic and resistive exercise training improve glucose tolerance and insulin sensitivity, reduce blood pressure, and improve body composition (24,25).

To date, most prospective exercise studies have been performed in men. A meta-analysis of the existent longitudinal exercise investigations in women revealed an overall decrease in levels of total cholesterol and triglycerides, with little or no change in values of HDL or LDL cholesterol (75). Gender-related differences in the lipoprotein response to exercise may reflect the generally higher endogenous levels of HDL cholesterol in women or differences in metabolic factors such as levels of sex steroids or regulatory enzymes.

It has been demonstrated in both cross-sectional and longitudinal epidemiologic studies that people who exercise regularly are at a reduced risk for CAD. Exercise also improves glucose metabolism, assists in weight reduction, and may reduce blood pressure (28,57).

Thus, exercise counseling (see Chapter 58) is an important part of the management of patients with abnormalities in lipoprotein metabolism.

Smoking Cessation

Plasma levels of HDL cholesterol have been found to be lower and levels of VLDL triglyceride higher in people who smoke cigarettes than in nonsmokers or ex-smokers. Moreover, an inverse relationship exists between the number of cigarettes smoked daily and the level of HDL cholesterol. Smoking cessation has been associated with a modest rise in plasma HDL level. It is not known what proportion of the increased risk of CAD associated with smoking is mediated through alteration in the plasma lipids or via other mechanisms. There is, however, substantial evidence that smoking cessation reduces CAD risk. There is also evidence that counseling of patients increases cessation rates. Therefore, all patients who smoke cigarettes should be counseled, regardless of their lipoprotein profile (see Chapter 20).

Drugs

For primary prevention, drug therapy is now recommended by the Adult Treatment Panel II (see "General References") only after a minimum of 6 months of intensive dietary intervention with inadequate results, unless the patient has an LDL cholesterol level of 220 mg/dL or greater. Candidates for drug therapy should always continue dietary intervention (see above), as the effects of each mode of treatment are often additive. For all patients, hygienic interventions such as weight control, habitual exercise, and cessation of cigarette smoking should be maximized. Information on lipid-lowering drugs is provided in Table 75.9.

Hypercholesterolemia

In general, the NCEP guidelines suggest a need for drug therapy (Table 75.10) when, despite dietary intervention, LDL cholesterol level is above 190 mg/dL in patients without, or is above 130 mg/dL in patients with, CAD or two or more known risk factors. Patients with marked elevations of LDL cholesterol (greater than 220 mg/dL), in whom dietary therapy alone is unlikely to normalize LDL cholesterol levels, should be considered for drug therapy after only 3 months of an adequate dietary trial. In patients without CAD the minimal goals of drug treatment should be the same as those for dietary therapy (i.e., an LDL cholesterol level less than 160 mg/dL for patients without, and a level less than 130 mg/dL for patients with, two or more CAD risk factors). Evidence exists that reducing LDL cholesterol levels to as low as 100 mg/dL leads to a further reduction in CAD risk, and this level is now the treatment goal for patients with known CAD. A recent AHA Consensus Panel Statement supports the initiation of lipid-lowering therapy in CAD patients with LDL-C levels between 100 and 130 mg/dL (68). To monitor drug therapy, LDL cholesterol levels should be

Table 75.9.   Commonly Used Lipid-Lowering Drugs

Bile Acid Sequestering Resins (Cholestyramine, Colestipol)

Mechanism: Anion exchange resins that bind bile acids, resulting in increased hepatic synthesis of cholesterol and bile acids, increased apo B catabolism, increased fecal excretion of cholesterol, increased LDL receptor activity, and usually a net reduction of plasma cholesterol levels.

Efficacy: Decreases total and LDL cholesterol up to 25–40% (onset 4–7 days, maximal effect within 1–3 weeks). In the LRC trial, mean reductions in experimental group of total and LDL cholesterol were 13.4 and 20.3%. Apo B level falls, while HDL level rises slightly. VLDL is unchanged or increased.

Pharmacokinetics: Not absorbed, but may bind other drugs (e.g., thiazides, digitalis preparations, anticoagulants, phenobarbital, thyroxine, phenylbutazone, propranolol, iron).

Side Effects: (a) Common: unpleasant sandy/gritty preparations, gastrointestinal (e.g., constipation in 10–20%, nausea, heartburn, abdominal discomfort, flatulence) often resolve with continued therapy or treatment of constipation), lowered serum folate levels; (b) uncommon: gastrointestinal (steatorrhea), hyperchloremic acidosis (small patients on high dosages), fat-soluble vitamin deficiency; increased alkaline phosphatase and amino transferase (usually transient).

Administration: (a) Cholestyramine: 12–32 g/day given two to four times daily before or during meals; supplied as Questran 9-g packets each containing 4 g of active drug; (b) Colestipol: 15–30 g/day, given two to four times daily before or during meals; supplied as Colestid in 5-g packets or 500-g bottles.

Preparations should be taken in water or juice to prevent esophageal irritation or blockage. Other medicines should be taken 1 hour before or 4 hours after dosage. Monitor serum folate levels and consider supplemental multivitamins with folic acid.

Clinical Use: Drugs of first choice in the treatment of hypercholesterolemia, because of their relative safety and efficacy. Well tolerated in combination with niacin or lovastatin. Contraindications include marked hypertriglyceridemia and severe constipation. Poor compliance limits use.

Nicotinic Acid (Niacin, and preparations such as Nicobid (time-released), 125, 250, or 500 mg)

Mechanism: Diverse effects on lipid metabolism: decreases LDL and apo B synthesis by decreasing hepatic synthesis of VLDL, increases synthesis of HDL, inhibits lipolysis in adipose tissue, increases lipase activity.

Efficacy: Decreases VLDL triglycerides within 1–4 days (mean 26% in Coronary Drug Project, range up to 80% depending on pretreatment levels); decreases LDL cholesterol, onset 5–7 days, maximal effect 3–5 weeks (mean decrease of 10% in total cholesterol in Coronary Drug Project, range up to 30%). Favorable impact on total and LDL cholesterol, triglyceride, VLDL, HDL (increases up to 35%), apos A–I and B.

Pharmacokinetics: Absorbed by mouth; peak concentrations in 20–70 minutes; at the high dosages used it is partially metabolized in liver and partially excreted unchanged in urine; plasma half-life is about 45 minutes.

Side Effects: (a) Common: cutaneous flushing and pruritis, which diminish after several weeks of therapy; gastrointestinal (nausea, diarrhea, abdominal pain, abnormal liver function); (b) less common: dermatologic disorders (e.g., increased pigmentation); activation of peptic ulcer; arrhythmia; gout; urinary frequency and dysuria; glucose intolerance; etc. Sustained release forms are associated with irreversible chronic liver disease and fulminant hepatic failure.

Administration: (100-, 250-, 300-, 400-, and 500-mg tablets). Gradual increase over 1–3 weeks from 100–200 mg/day to 2–9 g/day; given in three times daily dosage; give with meals to diminish side effects. Flushing may be ameliorated by pretreatment with aspirin, one half to one 324-mg tablet 30 minutes before each dose. Generic form is inexpensive compared with time-release form (Nico-Bid); the latter may reduce the frequency of flushing, but increase the frequency of gastrointestinal side effects. Nicotinic acid should be administered with caution in presence of coronary artery disease.

Clinical Use: First-line (despite side effects) effective drug in the treatment of elevated LDL cholesterol or VLDL triglyceride or low HDL. Well tolerated in combination with bile acid binding resins and statins. Contraindications include peptic ulcer disease, arrhythmia, liver disease, diabetes mellitus, hyperuricemia, and gout.

HMG-COA Reductase Inhibitors (lovastatin, pravastatin, simvastatin, fluvastatin, atorvastin)

Mechanism: Competitively inhibits HMG-CoA reductase, the rate-limiting enzyme in the synthesis of cholesterol, decreases production of LDL, increases LDL receptor activity in the liver and the rate of removal of LDL from the plasma.

Efficacy: Decreases total cholesterol (20–37%), LDL cholesterol (20–48%), LDL apo B (20–37%), VLDL cholesterol (27–40%), and triglycerides (7–27%). Provides variable and modest increases in HDL cholesterol (4–12%) and apo A–I and A–II.

Pharmacokinetics: Incompletely absorbed (average 30%); extensive first pass extraction by the liver with less than 5% reaching systemic circulation; inactive lovastatin converted to several active metabolites; peak plasma concentrations of active metabolites within 2–6 hours; steady state concentrations of total inhibitors achieved within 2–3 days; 83% of radiolabeled dose eliminated in feces (represents unabsorbed drug and active and inactive metabolites excreted in bile) and 10% in urine (as inactive metabolites).

Side Effects: (a) Generally well tolerated, discontinuation required in 1–2% of patients because of adverse effects; reasonable safety well established; (b) occasional: headache (9% of patients), gastrointestinal (flatulence, abdominal pains or cramps, diarrhea, constipation, nausea, dyspepsia—usually mild and transient [4–6%]); elevation in liver aminotransferases, and uncommonly, alkaline phosphatases usually within 3–16 months (≥3 times increase in 2%), reverses over several weeks after discontinuation of drug; mild increase in creatinine kinase (11%); myalgias (3%); rash and pruritis (5%); (c) uncommon: gastrointestinal (heartburn, dysgeusia), dizziness, insomnia, malaise, fatigue, myopathy (0.5%, but up to 30% in patients taking immunosuppressant drugs or gemfibrozil—also reported in patients taking nicotinic acid or erythromycin), renal failure from rhabdomyolysis.

Administration: Lovastatin (Mevacor, 20, 40 mg)—20–80 mg/day once daily with evening meal or twice daily with meals (administration with food results in 50% higher plasma concentrations of total inhibitors, effectiveness greater when given as evening dose, perhaps because cholesterol synthesis occurs mainly at night); pravastatin (Pravachol, 10 and 20 mg)—10–40 mg once a day at bedtime; simvastatin (Zocor, 5, 10, 20, and 40 mg) 5–40 mg once a day in the evening; Fluvastatin (Lescol, 20, 40 mg), 20–40 mg once a day at bedtime; 40 mg twice daily if no response; absorption not affected by food. Atorvastatin (Lipitor, 10, 20, 40 mg), 10 mg once a day; up to 80 mg once a day if no response. Obtain baseline liver function tests, then at 6, 12 weeks, and semiannually. Discontinue if aminotransferase rise more than 3 times normal. Because of the development of cataracts in animals receiving very high dosages, baseline and yearly slitlamp examinations are currently recommended.

Clinical Use: First-line drugs, effective and well tolerated drugs for the treatment of hypercholesterolemia. When response to a single drug is inadequate, statins are effective in combination with a bile acid sequestering agent or nicotinic acid. Each drug contributes separately to reductions in lipoprotein concentrations.

Fibric Acid Derivatives (Gemfibrozil, Fenofibrate)

Mechanism: Increases clearance of VLDL by enhancing lipolysis, may increase lipoprotein lipase activity, reduces hepatic cholesterol synthesis, and increases cholesterol excretion in the bile.

Efficacy: Gemfibrozil lowers triglycerides to a greater extent, raises HDL more consistently and is less likely to raise LDL than clofibrate. In familial combined hyperlipoproteinemia, however, use of any fibric acid analog is likely to raise LDL cholesterol.

Pharmacokinetics: Gemfibrozil and fenofibrate: completely absorbed; peak concentration within 2 hours; half-life 1.5 hours; undergoes enterohepatic circulation; metabolized in liver and excreted in urine. May enhance action of oral anticoagulants, phenytoin, and hypoglycemic agents, and of furosemide by displacing them from albumin-binding sites.

Side Effects: (a) Usually: well tolerated; (b) occasional: (sixfold) increase in the incidence of cholelithiasis (may be less with gemfibrozil and newer analogs); other gastrointestinal (nausea, abdominal pain, diarrhea, weight gain); reduced libido, impotence; unusual flulike syndrome; (c) uncommon: rash, alopecia, breast tenderness, reversible abnormality in liver function, hepatomegaly, myositis, increased plasma glucose, etc; (d) unknown: (?)thromboembolism, (?)intermittent claudication, (?)arrhythmia, (?)neoplasia.

Administration: Gemfibrozil (Lopid, 300, 600 mg): 600 mg twice daily (30 minutes before meals). Fenofibrate 300 mg/day in three divided doses taken with meals. Dosage reduction required in renal failure patients. Some recommend periodic monitoring of asparate aminotransferase (formerly SGO-T), alanine aminotransferase (formerly SGP-T), and creatinine kinase (formerly CPK).

Clinical Use: Gemfibrozil is the drug of choice in the treatment of elevated VLDL triglyceride; it can also be used to lower total and LDL cholesterol and to raise HDL cholesterol, of particular utility in type III. Fenobrate is more effective in lowering LDL. Use with caution in the presence of hepatic or renal insufficiency.

Table 75.10. NCEP Guidelines for Treating Adults with Elevated LDL with Drugs[a,b]

	Start Treatment LDL (mg/dL)	Goals of Treatment LDL (mg/dL)
Without CAD or without 2 or more risk factors (Table 75.6)	≥190	<160
Without CAD but with 2 or more risk factors	≥160	<130
With CAD	≥130	≤100

[a]A trial of dietary modification should be attempted first.

[b]In certain groups of patients treatment should be delayed.

checked at 4 to 6 weeks and at 3 months. Once target levels have been achieved, patients should be evaluated with measurement of total serum cholesterol at least every 4 months, and a full lipoprotein analysis should be performed yearly.

Drug therapy should be delayed in the following groups of patients: men less than 35 years old, premenopausal women without other risk factors whose LDL cholesterol levels are between 190 and 220 mg/dL, those without two other risk factors and LDL cholesterol levels between 160 and 190 mg/dL, and patients with two other risk factors and LDL cholesterol levels in the range of 130 to 160 mg/dL on adequate dietary therapy.

Cholesterol-lowering drugs are categorized into two groups: (a) first-choice agents, such as bile acid sequestrants and nicotinic acid, which are effective in lowering total and LDL cholesterol levels, reduce CAD risk and are generally safe for long-term use (HMG CoA reductase inhibitors are now considered appropriate for initial therapy, as they are extremely effective in lowering LDL cholesterol and are relatively safe and well tolerated by patients, particularly in combination with other drugs); and (b) other drugs, such as gemfibrozil and probucol, which lower LDL cholesterol levels.

Before drug therapy is initiated, two or three serum lipid measurements performed at 1- to 2-week intervals and a baseline liver enzyme "safety profile" and serum creatinine phosphokinase level should be obtained. Follow-up biochemistry safety profile and serum lipoprotein levels should be checked twice, at 1- to 2-month intervals, then every 3 to 4 months. In secondary prevention, these laboratory values should be checked every 4 to 6 weeks during the first 6 months to maximize drug safety and efficacy and minimize morbidity (17).

Bile Acid Sequestering Resins

The bile acid binding resins *cholestyramine* and *colestipol* remain the drugs of first choice for patients with primary hypercholesterolemia. They are particularly useful for primary prevention therapy of young men and of premenopausal women without other risk factors, with moderately elevated LDL cholesterol levels. They enhance LDL catabolism and excretion and prevent intestinal absorption by diverting cholesterol and bile acids into the feces. They also increase levels of triglycerides and HDL, particularly HDL_2. At dosages of 20 to 24 g/day, a 20 to 30% reduction in LDL cholesterol may be achieved, but the expense is high ($50.00/month). Although these resins may be the safest of all of the hypolipidemic drugs, compliance is a problem because taste and gastrointestinal side effects prevent many patients from taking a full dose. As many as 30% of clinical trial participants admit to taking less than half of the prescribed dosage of bile acid binding resins (48). Gradual increase of dose, continuation of therapy, and concomitant symptomatic management of constipation may diminish side effects. The resins are better tolerated when used at lower dosages in combination with other lipid lowering agents.

Nicotinic Acid (Niacin)

Nicotinic acid (3 to 6 g/day) significantly lowers plasma levels of LDL and VLDL while raising the level of HDL cholesterol. It is thus the drug of first choice for patients with concomitant elevations in LDL cholesterol and triglycerides. It is the first lipid-lowering drug that has been shown to lower levels of Lp(a) (10). There is evidence in secondary prevention trials that nicotinic acid may reduce total mortality. Its use is often limited, however, by unpleasant side effects and the frequent presence of coexisting contraindications. Therapy should be discontinued if gout, hyperglycemia, or hepatotoxicity develops (17). By starting at a very low dosage of 100 to 200 mg/day and gradually increasing the dosage of the drug and adding aspirin, increased tolerance often develops to the common side effects of cutaneous flushing, rashes, hives, and pruritus. Nicotinic acid is inexpensive, with monthly costs averaging $5.00 at a dosage of 2 to 4 g/day. Sustained-release forms of nicotinic acid were initially thought to produce fewer side effects than immediate release forms. However, because of reports of irreversible chronic liver disease and fulminant hepatic failure with sustained-release nicotinic acid, immediate release forms are strongly preferred (19,53) (Table 75.9).

HMG CoA Reductase Inhibitors

The *statins* (lovastatin, simvastatin, pravastatin, fluvastatin, and atorvastatin) are specific, potent, competitive inhibitors of HMG CoA reductase, the rate-limiting enzyme in cholesterol biosynthesis. These drugs increase hepatic LDL receptor activity and LDL clearance from the circulation and, in addition, decrease production of LDL (27). More than 10 years of clinical experience with this class of drugs has confirmed their effectiveness in reducing levels of total and LDL cholesterol by 20 to 50%, in decreasing triglyceride levels slightly, and in modestly increasing the levels of HDL cholesterol in some patients (27,74). They appear to be equally effective in individuals with familial and nonfamilial hypercholesterolemia. When compared with bile acid and nicotinic acid in the treatment of patients with type 2a hyperlipidemia, lovastatin elicits a greater reduction in LDL cholesterol levels and better compliance.

A 5-year study demonstrated lovastatin to be comparable in safety to the other major cholesterol-lowering drugs (49). The safety profiles are similar for lovastatin, pravastatin, simvastatin, fluvastatin, and atorvastatin, with drug-related adverse events occurring in approximately 2 to 3% of patients. Side effects include increase in transaminases, myopathy, insomnia, myalgia, arthralgia, and gastrointestinal disturbances. No study has shown a significant increase in the development of lens opacities; therefore, routine ophthalmologic monitoring is no longer required. Periodic tests of liver function are now suggested before initiation of therapy, at weeks 6 and 12, and then semiannually. At average dosages, lovastatin and pravastatin cost about the same; simvastatin is currently more expensive than these two drugs and atorvastatin is cheaper.

Fibrates

Gemfibrozil is the most commonly used drug in this class in the United States. *Clofibrate*, rarely used since the World Health Organization Cooperative trial reported significantly increased all-cause mortality in patients taking the drug (80), and the newer *fenofibrate* are also available in the United States, whereas bezafibrate and ciprofibrate are available in Europe. Although gemfibrozil is approved for the treatment of hypertriglyceridemia, data from the Helsinki Heart Study (20) have revealed it to be effective as well in lowering LDL cholesterol, raising HDL cholesterol, and reducing the morbidity and mortality from CAD. In general, gemfibrozil is not considered as useful for secondary prevention as other drugs such as the statins because it does not achieve maximal reductions in LDL cholesterol. Diabetic patients with elevated triglyceride levels and patients with type 3 hyperlipoproteinemia are excellent candidates for treatment with this drug. However, in patients with primary hypertriglyceridemia, gemfibrozil may increase LDL cholesterol levels, whereas in patients with elevations of both cholesterol and triglycerides, this drug can cause either an increase or a decrease in LDL cholesterol levels. The newer fibrates may lower LDL-C more effectively than does gemfibrozil (66). A significant side effect of gemfibrozil is its tendency to increase bile lithogenicity. At a dosage of 1.2 g/day, gemfibrozil costs about $30.00/month.

Probucol

Probucol remains a second-line drug for the treatment of hypercholesterolemia. It appears to lower LDL cholesterol levels by a receptor-independent mechanism and by an increase in LDL catabolism. In addition, it inhibits the oxidative metabolism and tissue deposition of LDL. Probucol use leads to a reduction in total and LDL cholesterol levels of 8 to 15% and a concomitant reduction of HDL cholesterol levels by as much as 25%. The significance of the consequent reduction in the LDL/HDL ratio remains uncertain. To date, there are no reported studies of its efficacy in reducing CAD risk or of its long-term safety. The electrocardiogram (ECG) should be monitored in patients taking probucol, as the drug can cause prolon-gation of the QT interval (at which point the drug should be discontinued). At a dosage of 1 mg/day, probucol costs about $30.00/month.

Combination Drug Therapy

When the response to one of the first-line drugs proves to be inadequate, combined therapy with two drugs should be considered. In general, one should choose drugs with complementary or synergistic mechanisms of action (65) and should consult with a specialist in lipid disorders. The use of a bile acid sequestrant in combination with either nicotinic acid or lovastatin (39) can lower levels of LDL cholesterol by 45 to 60% in patients with hypercholesterolemia and normal triglyceride levels. These regimens have been well tolerated, with synergistic effects on LDL cholesterol without an additive effect on drug-related toxicity. Probucol or gemfibrozil may also be used in combination with a bile acid sequestering resin, although these regimens are less effective. The reported occurrence of rhabdomyolysis with the combination of lovastatin and nicotinic acid contraindicates their use together (60). The combination of a statin and gemfibrozil also causes an increased risk of myopathy and is contraindicated.

Two placebo-controlled studies of intensive lipid lowering therapy utilizing combined colestipol and niacin therapy or combined lovastatin and niacin treatment for men with documented CAD have shown reduced frequency of progression of coronary lesions, increased frequency of regression, and reduced incidence of cardiovascular events in the active drug groups (3,6). Patients with homozygous familial hypercholesterolemia may respond less well to treatment with drugs and diet than do patients with heterozygous monogenic, polygenic, or nonhereditary hypercholesterolemia.

Other Hypocholesterolemic Drugs

The use of *estrogen replacement therapy* (ERT) in postmenopausal women has a number of effects on cholesterol metabolism (see Chapter 77). Treatment with oral estrogens usually lowers levels of LDL cholesterol and raises those of HDL cholesterol, but the dosages required for these effects probably exceed those for physiologic replacement therapy. In contrast, administration of nonoral (e.g., transdermal) estrogens usually results in lower LDL cholesterol levels but unaltered levels of HDL cholesterol. Both oral and transdermal ERT have been shown to significantly lower Lp(a) levels (31% versus 16%, respectively) in postmenopausal women. Concomitant use of the progestin medroxyprogesterone acetate (Provera) with either form of ERT appears not to influence either form of ERT adversely. Epidemiologic evidence suggests that ERT in women may reduce the risk for CAD (54). Although clinical trial data with heart disease endpoints are limited, estrogens may be particularly beneficial in postmenopausal women with preexistent CAD. The primary side effect of unopposed estrogen is the increased risk of endometrial cancer, a risk that is greatly attenuated by cotreatment with progestogens (see Chapter 77).

Hypertriglyceridemia

Drugs that decrease hepatic production of VLDL and apo B, enhance VLDL clearance by stimulating LPL activity, or both are generally effective in treating hypertriglyceridemia. Gemfibrozil and nicotinic acid do both.

Although *nicotinic acid* may be most efficacious, its use is limited by its side effects and the presence of coexisting contraindications. The fibric acid derivative *gemfibrozil* is therefore the drug most commonly used. Although gemfibrozil is generally well tolerated, an acute myositis, which is occasionally associated with renal failure, may occur, particularly in patients with impaired renal clearance or hypoalbuminemia. Either the drug should not be used or the dosage should be reduced by 70 to 90% in azotemic patients. Periodic monitoring of muscle enzymes (creatine kinase, aldolase) is required to avoid toxicity. When the level of LDL cholesterol rises in a patient taking gemfibrozil, the diagnosis of familial combined hyperlipoproteinemia should be considered.

In compliant patients who remain hypertriglyceridemic with diet and a single drug, combined therapy with a fibric acid drug and nicotinic acid may be useful. Rarely, after consultation with a specialist in lipid disorders, the progestational agent norethindrone acetate or the androgenic anabolic steroid oxandrolone may be required to treat persistent hypertriglyceridemia plus chylomicronemia in women or men, respectively.

Dysbetalipoproteinemia

The decreased remnant catabolism characteristic of this clinically uncommon disorder can be corrected or improved by drug therapy. *Gemfibrozil* appears to normalize lipid levels and to enhance remnant clearance in patients with dysbetalipoproteinemia. It is the drug of choice in this disorder. *Ethinyl estradiol* has a similar and even more dramatic effect, but at dosages that greatly exceed those used for postmenopausal replacement therapy. Hence, its use requires careful monitoring for possible adverse estrogenic effects that would necessitate discontinuation of the drug. *Nicotinic acid* is the drug of second choice.

Surgery and Other Therapies

More experimental forms of therapy (e.g., ileal bypass, portacaval shunt, plasma exchange, extracorporeal hemoperfusion, and liver transplantation) exist for the severely hypercholesterolemic patient who is resistant or only partially responsive to diet, exercise, and lipid-lowering drugs. Patients with drug-resistant nephrotic syndrome from focal segmental glomerulosclerosis have shown improvement in renal function and proteinuria when treated with LDL apheresis combined with pravastatin (30). These therapies

should be implemented only in consultation with a specialist in lipid disorders.

Obtaining Consultation

The Lipid Metabolism Branch of the National Heart, Lung and Blood Institute (National Institutes of Health, Bethesda, MD 20205) can provide the names of research centers in each geographic area where sophisticated evaluation of lipoprotein abnormalities, consultation services, and experimental forms of therapy are offered.

Additional information for the management of patients with hyperlipoproteinemia and other risk factors for CAD is available from both regional and national offices of the AHA. This agency can provide information about diet, drugs, and exercise in the treatment of hyperlipidemia, hypertension, cigarette smoking, and obesity.

General References*

Eating for a Healthy Heart, Dietary Treatment for Hyperlipidemia. American Heart Association Booklets for patients on the American Heart Association (AHA) single-diet approach to improving plasma lipoprotein levels.
Counseling the Patient with Hyperlipidemia. Short booklet for the physician or nutritionist on implementing the AHA diet.
Heart to Heart, Nutrition Counseling for the Reduction of Cardiovascular Disease Risk Factors. Detailed book for the physician or nutritionist on counseling patients regarding the AHA diet.
NIH Consensus Development Panel on Triglyceride, High-Density Lipoprotein, and Coronary Heart Disease. JAMA 269:505, 1993. Up-to-date compendium of information assessing the controversies between abnormalities of triglyceride and HDL cholesterol metabolism, and CAD risk.
Summary of the Second Report of the National Cholesterol Education Program (NCEP) Expert Panel on Detection, Evaluation, and Treatment of High Blood Cholesterol in Adults (Adult Treatment Panel II). JAMA 269:3015, 1993. Updated recommendations for the detection and management of elevated levels of total and LDL cholesterol, and reduced levels of HDL cholesterol, in adults beyond 20 years of age.
The Expert Panel. Report of the National Cholesterol Education Program Expert Panel on Detection, Evaluation and Treatment of High Blood Cholesterol in Adults. Arch Intern Med 148:36, 1988. Original, highly influential report outlining an approach to the detection and management of elevated levels of total and LDL cholesterol in the adult population beyond 20 years of age.

Specific References

1. Anderson TJ, Meredith IT, Yeung AC, et al. The effect of cholesterol-lowering and antioxidant therapy on endothelium-dependent coronary vasomotion. N Engl J Med 333:324, 1995.
2. Austin MA, Breslow JL, Hennekens CH, et al. Low-density lipoprotein subclass patterns and risk of myocardial infarction. JAMA 260:1917, 1988.
3. Blankenhorn DH, Nessim SA, Johnson RL, et al. Beneficial effects of combined colestipol-niacin therapy on coronary atherosclerosis and coronary venous bypass grafts. JAMA 257:3233, 1987.

*Bold print (general references) and bold numerals (specific references) denote published controlled clinical trials, meta-analyses, or consensus-based recommendations.

4. Brensike JF, Levy RI, Kelsey SF, et al. Effects of therapy with cholestyramine on progression of coronary arteriosclerosis: results of the NHLBI type II coronary intervention study. Circulation 69:313, 1984.

5. Brett AS. Treating hypercholesterolemia: How should practicing physicians interpret the published data for patients. N Engl J Med 321:676, 1989.

6. Brown G, Albers JJ, Fisher LD, et al. Regression of coronary artery disease as a result of intensive lipid-lowering therapy in men with high level of apo lipoprotein B. N Engl J Med 323:1289, 1990.

7. Brown MS, Goldstein JL. How LDL receptors influence cholesterol and atherosclerosis. Sci Am 251:58, 1984.

8. Brunzell JD, Sniderman AD, Albers JJ, Kwiterovich PO Jr. Apoproteins B and A-1 and coronary artery disease in humans. Arteriosclerosis 4:79, 1984.

9. Campeau L, Enjalbert J, Lesperance J, et al. The relationship of risk factors to the development of atherosclerosis in saphenous-vein bypass grafts and the progression of disease in the native circulation: a study 10 years after aortocoronary bypass surgery. N Engl J Med 311:1329, 1984.

10. Carlson LA, Hamsten A, Asplund A. Pronounced lowering of serum levels of Lp(a) in hyperlipidemic subjects treated with nicotinic acid. J Intern Med 226:271, 1989.

11. Castelli WP. The triglyceride issue: A view from Framingham. Am Heart J 112:432, 1986.

12. Corti M-C, Guralnik JM, Salive ME, et al. Clarifying the direct relation between total cholesterol levels and death from coronary heart disease in older persons. Ann Intern Med 126:753, 1997.

13. Criqui MH, Heiss G, Cohn R, et al. Plasma triglyceride level and mortality from coronary heart disease. N Engl J Med 328:1220, 1993.

14. Dattilo AM, Kris-Etherton PM. Effects of weight reduction on blood lipids and lipoproteins: A meta-analysis. Am J Clin Nutr 56:320, 1991.

15. Daviglus ML, Stamler J, Orencia AJ, et al. Fish consumption and the 30 year risk of fatal myocardial infarction. N Engl J Med 336:1046, 1997.

16. Dufaux B, Assmann G, Hollman W. Plasma lipoproteins and physical activity: a review. Int J Sports Med 3:123, 1982.

17. Dujovne CA, Moriarty PM. Clinical pharmacological concepts for the rational selection and use of drugs for the management of dyslipidemia. Clin Ther 18:392, 1996.

18. Ederer F, Leren P, Turpeinin O, Frantz ID Jr. Cancer among men on cholesterol-lowering diets. Lancet 2:203, 1971.

19. Etchason JA, Miller TD, Squires RW, et al. Niacin-induced hepatitis: A potential side effect with low-dose time-release niacin. Mayo Clin Proc 66:23, 1991.

20. Frick MH, Elo O, Haapa K, et al. Helsinki Heart Study: primary prevention trial with gemfibrozil in middle-aged men with dyslipidemia. N Engl J Med 317:1237, 1987.

21. Friedewald WT, Levy RI, Fredrickson DS. Estimation of the concentration of low-density lipoprotein cholesterol in plasma, without use of the preparative ultracentrifuge. Clin Chem 18:499, 1972.

22. Glauber H, Wallace P, Griver K, et al. Adverse metabolic effect of omega-3 fatty acids in non-insulin-dependent diabetes mellitus. Ann Intern Med 108: 663, 1988.

23. Goldberg AP. Lipid abnormalities in hemodialysis: prevalence, implications and treatment. Perspect Lipid Disord 2:17, 1984.

24. Goldberg AP. Aerobic and resistive exercise modify risk factors for coronary heart disease. Med Sci Sports Exerc 21:669, 1989.

25. Goldberg LE, Elliot DL, Shutz RW, Kloster FE. Changes in lipid and lipoprotein levels after weight training. JAMA 252:504, 1984.

26. Gore JM, Goldberg RJ, Matsumoto AS, et al. Validity of serum total cholesterol level obtained within 24 hours of acute myocardial infarction. Am J Cardiol 54:722, 1984.

27. Grundy S. HMG-CoA Reductase inhibitors for treatment of hypercholesterolemia. N Engl J Med 319:24, 1988.

28. Hagberg JM. Exercise, fitness, and hypertension. In: Bouchard C, Shepard RJ, Stephens T, et al, eds. Exercise, fitness and health. Champaign, IL: Human Kinetics, 1990;455.

29. Hall AV, Parbtani A, Clark WF, et al. Omega 3 fatty acid supplementation in primary nephrotic syndrome: effects on plasma lipids and coagulopathy. J Am Soc Nephrol 3:1321, 1992.

30. Hattori M, Ito K, Kawaguchi H, et al. Treatment with a combination of low-density lipoprotein aphaeresis and pravastatin of a patient with drug resistant nephrotic syndrome due to focal segmental glomerulosclerosis. Pediatr Nephrol 7:196, 1993.

31. Havel RJ, ed. Symposium on lipid disorders. Med Clin North Am 66:319, 1982.

32. Heiss G, Johnson NJ, Reiland S, et al. The epidemiology of plasma HDL cholesterol levels. The Lipid Research Clinics Prevalence Study. Summary. Circulation 62(Suppl 4):116, 1980.

33. Hodis HN, Mack WJ, La Bree L, et al. Serial coronary angiographic evidence that anti-oxidant vitamin intake reduces progression of coronary artery atherosclerosis. JAMA 273:1849, 1995.

34. Hulley SB, Newman TB, Grady D, et al. Should we be measuring blood cholesterol levels in young adults? JAMA 269:1416, 1993.

35. Hunink MG, Goldman L, Tosteson AN, et al. The recent decline in mortality from coronary heart disease, 1980–1990. JAMA 277:535, 1997.

36. Hunninghake DB, Stein EA, Dujovne CA, et al. The efficacy of intensive dietary therapy alone or combined with lovastatin in outpatients with hypercholesteremia. N Engl J Med 328:1213, 1993.

37. Hurley BF, Hagberg JM, Goldberg AP, et al. Resistive training can reduce coronary risk factors without altering VO_2 max or percent body fat. Med Sci Sports Exerc 20:150, 1988.

38. Hurley BF. Effects of resistive training on lipoprotein-lipid profiles: a comparison to aerobic exercise training. Med Sci Sports Exerc 21:689, 1989.

39. Illingsworth DR. Mevinolin plus colestipol in therapy for severe heterozygous familial hypercholesterolemia. Ann Intern Med 101:598, 1984.

40. Kannel WB, Schatzkin A. Risk factor analysis. Prog Cardiovasc Dis 26:309, 1983.

41. Kromhout D, Katan MB, Havekes L, et al. The effect of 26 years of habitual fish consumption on serum lipid and lipoprotein levels (the Zutphen Study). Nutr Metab Cardiovasc Dis 6:65, 1996.

42. Krumholz HM, Seeman TE, Merrill SS, et al. Lack of association between cholesterol and coronary heart disease mortality and morbidity and all-cause mortality in persons older than 70 years. JAMA 272:1335, 1994.

43. LaRosa J. Dyslipidemia and coronary artery disease in the elderly. Clin Geriatric Med 12:33, 1996.

44. Lavie CJ. Lipid and lipoprotein fractions and coronary artery disease. Mayo Clin Proc 68:618, 1993.

45. Leaf A. Management of hypercholesterolemia: are preventive interventions advisable? N Engl J Med 321:680, 1989.

46. Levy RI. Consideration of cholesterol and nonvascular mortality. Am Heart J 104:324, 1982.

47. Lindgren FT, Jensen LC, Hatch FT. The isolation and quantitative analysis of serum lipoproteins. In: Nelson GJ, ed. Blood lipids and lipoproteins: quantitation, composition, and metabolism. New York: John Wiley & Sons, 1972;181.

48. Lipid Research Clinics Program. The Lipid Research Clinics Coronary Primary Prevention Trial results: II. The relationship of reduction in incidence of coronary heart disease to cholesterol lowering. JAMA 251:365, 1984.

49. Lovastatin Study Group I-IV. Lovastatin 5-year safety and efficacy study. Arch Intern Med 153:1079, 1993.

50. U.S. Department of Health and Human Services, Public Health Service, National Institutes of Health: Lipid Research Clinics Populations Studies Data Book, vol I. The Prevalence Study. NIH publication no. 80-1527, 1980.

51. Maciejko JJ, Holmes DR, Kottke BA, et al. Apolipoprotein A-I as a marker of angiographically assessed coronary artery disease. N Engl J Med 309:385, 1983.

52. Mahley RW, Angelin B. Type III hyperlipoproteinemia: recent

insights into the genetic defect of familial dysbetalipoproteinemia. Adv Intern Med 29:385, 1984.

53. McKenney JM, Proctor JD, Harris S, Chenchili VM. A comparison of the efficacy and toxic effects of sustained vs immediate release niacin in hypercholesterolemic patients. JAMA 271: 672, 1994.

54. Nabulsi A, Folsom AR, White A, et al. Association of hormone-replacement therapy with various cardiovascular risk factors in postmenopausal women. N Engl J Med 328:1069, 1993.

55. Nilsson-Ehle P. Regulation of lipoprotein lipase: triacylglycerol transport in plasma. In: Carlson LA, Pernow B, eds. Metabolic risk factors in ischemic cardiovascular disease. New York: Raven Press, 1982;49.

56. Oram JF, Brenton EA, Bierman EL. Regulation of high density lipoprotein activity in cultured human skin fibroblasts and human arterial smooth muscle cells. J Clin Invest 72:1611, 1983.

57. Paffenberger RS, Hyde RT, Wing AL, Steinmetz CH. A natural history of athleticism and cardiovascular health. JAMA 252: 491, 1984.

58. Rader DJ, Brewer HB Jr. Lipoprotein (a): clinical approach to a unique atherogenic lipoprotein. JAMA 267:1109, 1992.

59. Rastam L, Hannan PJ, Luepker RV, et al. Seasonal variation in plasma cholesterol distributions: implications for screening and referral. Am J Prev Med 8:360, 1992.

60. Reaven P, Witztum JL. Lovastatin, nicotinic acid and rhabdomyalysis. Ann Intern Med 109:597, 1988.

61. Rifkind BM, Segal P. Lipid Research Clinics Program reference values for hyperlipidemia and hypolipidemia. JAMA 250:1869, 1983.

62. Rimm EB, Stampfer MJ, Ascherio A, et al. Vitamin E consumption and the risk of coronary disease in men. N Engl J Med 328:1450, 1993.

63. Scandinavian Simvastatin Survival Study Group. Randomised trial of cholesterol lowering in 4444 patients with coronary heart disease: The Scandinavian Simvastatin Survival Study (4S). Lancet 344:1383, 1994.

64. Schectman G, Kaul S, Cherayil GD, et al. Can the hypotriglyceridemic effect of fish oil concentrate be sustained? Ann Intern Med 110:346, 1989.

65. Schectman G, Hiatt J, Hartz A. Evaluation of the effectiveness of lipid-lowering therapy (bile acid sequestrants, niacin, psyllium, and lovastatin) for treating hypercholesterolemia in veterans. Am J Cardiol 71:759, 1993.

66. Schonfeld G. The effects of fibrates on lipoprotein and hemostatic coronary risk factors. Atheroclerosis 11:161, 1994.

67. Shepherd J, Cobbe SM, Ford I, et al. Prevention of coronary heart disease with pravastatin in men with hypercholesterolemia. West of Scotland Coronary Prevention Study Group. N Engl J Med 333:1301, 1995.

68. Smith SC Jr, Blair SN, Criqui MH, et al. Preventing heart attack and death in patients with coronary disease. Circulation 92:2, 1995.

69. Sniderman AD, Wolfson C, Teng B, et al. Association of hyperbetalipoproteinemia with endogenous hypertriglyceridemia and atherosclerosis. Ann Intern Med 97:833, 1982.

70. Sorkin JD, Andres R, Muller DC, et al. Cholesterol as a risk factor for coronary heart disease in elderly man. Ann Epidemiol 2:59, 1992.

71. Sox HC Jr: Screening for lipid disorders under health system reform. N Engl J Med 328:1269, 1993.

72. Stampfer MJ, Hennekens CH, Manson JE, et al. Vitamin E consumption and the risk of coronary disease in women. N Engl J Med 328:1444, 1993.

73. Steinberg D. Antioxidant vitamins and coronary heart disease. N Engl J Med 328:1487, 1993.

74. The Lovastatin Study Group II. Therapeutic response to lovastatin in nonfamilial hypercholesterolemia. A multicenter trial. JAMA 256:2829, 1986.

75. Tran EVT, Weltman A. Differential effects of exercise on serum lipid and lipoprotein levels seen with changes in body weight: a meta-analysis. JAMA 254:919, 1985.

76. Tyroler HA, Hess G, Schonfeld G, et al. Apoprotein A-I, A-II and C-II in black and white residents of Evans County. Circulation 62:249, 1980.

77. Wade DP. Lipoprotein (a). Curr Opin Lipidol 4:244, 1993.

78. Walden CE, Knopp RH, Wahl PW, et al. Sex differences in the effect of diabetes mellitus and lipoprotein triglyceride and cholesterol concentrations. N Engl J Med 331:953, 1984.

79. Watts GF, Lewis B, Brunt JHN, et al. Effects on coronary artery disease of lipid-lowering diet or diet plus cholestyramine in the St. Thomas Atherosclerosis Regression Study. Lancet 339:563, 1992.

80. W.H.O. Clofibrate Trial. W.H.O cooperative trial on primary prevention of ischaemic heart disease using clofibrate to lower serum cholesterol: mortality follow-up. Lancet 2:379, 1980.

81. Wyngaarden JB. Variability in individual cholesterol level clouds risk assessment. JAMA 260:759, 1988.

82. Zimetbaum P, Frishman WH, Ooi Wl, et al. Plasma lipids and lipoproteins and the incidence of cardiovascular disease in the very elderly: The Bronx Aging Study. Arterioscler Throm 12:416, 1992.

CHAPTER 76

Obesity

MARC R. BLACKMAN, MD

Obesity, defined as an excess of total body fat, is one of the most prevalent chronic medical disorders in the world. Moreover, its incidence and prevalence appear to be increasing, particularly in the highly industrialized nations (see below). Recent research has increased our understanding of the numerous complex interactions among predisposing genetic and environmental factors that influence the initiation, development, and persistence of excess adiposity. Although controversy exists about the exact health risks associated with mild obesity (3,27,55), in more obese patients, morbidity and mortality vary directly with the amount and topographic distribution of excess body fat, as well as with certain associated medical and behavioral abnormalities. Newer classification schemes need to be devised so that rational therapeutic interventions can be targeted more specifically toward those obesity syndromes associated with increased risk for morbidity and mortality. In so doing, perhaps both short- and long-term treatment results will improve substantially. In addition, there remains an urgent need to promote a variety of effective societal and individual approaches for prevention of excess adiposity.

DEFINITION

Obesity Versus Overweight

Obesity must be distinguished from overweight, which refers to an increase in body weight from increased bone, muscle, or fat. Although the two terms are often used synonymously, errors do occur in equating obesity with overweight, as for example in the muscular athlete with normal or decreased body fat. Because body composition and, in particular, body fat normally vary with age, sex, diet, physical activity, and population group, it is important to compare measurements of body fat in individual patients with those derived from appropriate control groups.

Methods for Quantifying Adiposity

Numerous methods exist for assessing and quantifying the amount and distribution of body fat. Although hydrostatic densitometry has been considered the gold standard technique for measurement of total fat mass, recent studies suggest that dual energy x-ray absorptiometry (DEXA) scanning, a less cumbersome method, may provide even more accurate estimates of total and regional fat (28). DEXA scans are especially useful in older people, in whom hydrodensitometry often leads to overestimates of total fat. Nonetheless, the simplest, most common, and most reliable clinical approaches to date involve either determination of relative weight or measurement of skinfold thickness. In the former approach, a patient's weight is expressed as a percentage or ratio of an ideal, desirable, or acceptable weight, such as that issued in the Metropolitan Life Insurance Company's Build and Blood Pressure Study (56) and updated in the Metropolitan's Height and Weight Tables of 1983 (40). Of the various indices of weight and height tested, the body mass index (BMI; weight [kg]/height^2 [m^2]) has the highest correlation with other measures of body fat (Fig. 76.1). Although measurements of skinfold thickness (using standardized calipers) are useful in assessing body fat in population studies, the technique is often less reliable in individual patients than are direct measurements of weight and height.

The topographic distribution of body fat is most conveniently and reliably estimated by determining the waist/hip ratio (WHR), which is measured as the ratio of the minimal circumference at the waist to the maximal circumference at the hips with the patient in the standing position (Fig. 76.2). The criteria for and significance of normal and abnormal WHRs are discussed below. Although measurements of the WHR do not discriminate between subcutaneous and intra-abdominal fat, they nonetheless correspond closely to more quantitative measures of central adiposity, such as quantitative computed tomography or magnetic resonance imaging of the abdomen.

CLASSIFICATION

The heterogeneous nature and the many approaches to evaluation and management of the obesity syndromes have made classification schemes necessary but nonuniform. Thus, various classification systems might serve different purposes, as for example (a) to identify subpopulations of obese individuals at risk for increased morbidity and mortality, in whom therapeu-

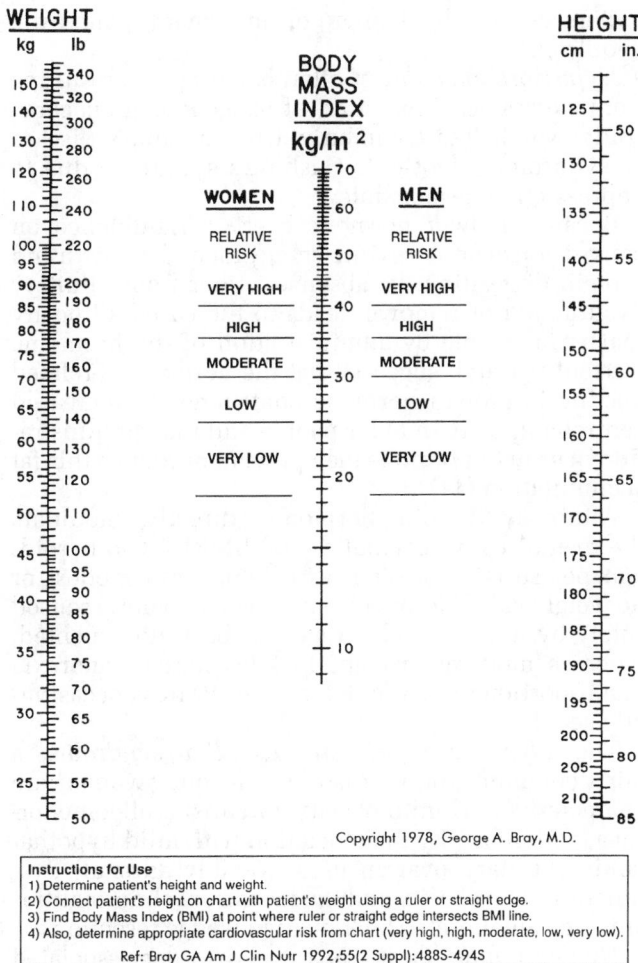

Copyright 1978, George A. Bray, M.D.

Instructions for Use
1) Determine patient's height and weight.
2) Connect patient's height on chart with patient's weight using a ruler or straight edge.
3) Find Body Mass Index (BMI) at point where ruler or straight edge intersects BMI line.
4) Also, determine appropriate cardiovascular risk from chart (very high, high, moderate, low, very low).

Ref: Bray GA Am J Clin Nutr 1992;55(2 Suppl):488S-494S

Figure 76.1. Nomogram for body mass index.

tic interventions might be beneficial; and *(b)* to distinguish among primarily genetic, environmental, and combined genetic plus environmental causes. With regard to the former, recent research suggests that patients with predominantly upper-body obesity (i.e., increased fat in the back of the neck, shoulder areas, and intra-abdominal depots) exhibit an increased frequency of metabolic concomitants of obesity and an enhanced risk for developing diabetes mellitus, hyperlipidemia, and cardiovascular disease (19,32,36,45). In contrast, patients with predominantly lower-body obesity (i.e., increased fat in the hips, thighs, and buttocks) are metabolically stable and are not at significantly enhanced risk for such diseases. Further research is needed to discern whether therapeutic interventions should be targeted mostly toward patients with upper-body obesity and whether doing so will improve short- and long-term treatment results. In this regard, a study conducted in healthy, sedentary, obese old men demonstrated significant decreases in intra-abdominal fat by computerized tomography (CT) following a 6-month trial of moderate endurance exercise training (52). The physiologic and clinical significance of this observation remains to be clarified.

Numerous studies comparing monozygotic twins

reared separately or together have suggested an important genetic influence on some types of human obesity (57) and on indices of human energy metabolism such as the resting metabolic rate, the thermic effect of food, and the energy cost of submaximal exercise (7). The recent identification of several different genetically mediated obesity syndromes in rodents has prompted a search for similar genetic markers of human obesity. In this regard, considerable investigative attention is now focused on elucidating the possible pathophysiologic significance of alterations in the genes for leptin (a newly discovered adipocyte derived protein that contributes importantly to appetite regulation and energy expenditure [66]; see below), the leptin receptor, and the β_3-adrenergic receptor (4,14,62). With regard to the latter classification scheme, categorization can be conveniently based on anatomic/developmental and etiologic criteria.

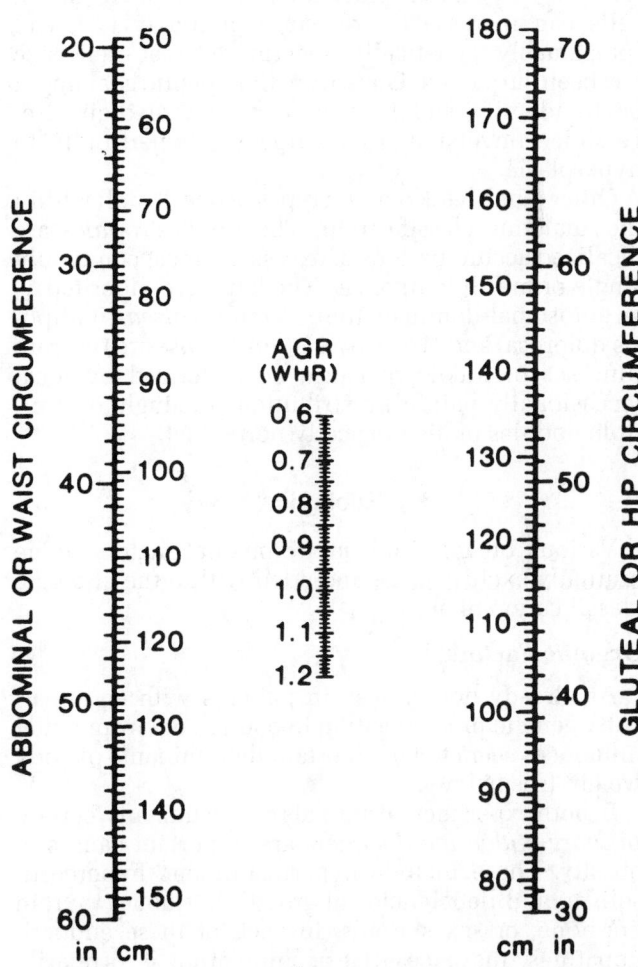

Figure 76.2. Nomogram for determining abdominal (waist) to gluteal (hips) ratio. Place a straight edge between the column for waist circumference and the column for hip circumference and read the ratio from the point where this straight edge crosses the AGR or WHR line. The waist or abdominal circumference is the smallest circumference below the rib cage and above the umbilicus, and the hips or gluteal circumference is taken as the largest circumference at the posterior extension of the buttocks. (George A. Bray, copyright 1988.)

Anatomic/Developmental

It was once thought that the number of fat cells in healthy people increased steadily through the first few years of life, again increased slightly during the peripubertal years, and remained fixed thereafter. Subsequent gains or losses of body fat in adulthood were considered to result solely from corresponding increases or decreases in fat cell size. As confirmation of this hypothesis, it was recognized that patients with youth-onset (less than 15 to 20 years old) obesity more often had generalized obesity with both hyperplasia and hypertrophy of their adipocytes, whereas patients with adult-onset (greater than 15 to 20 years old) obesity more often had a centripetal distribution of excess fat and adipocyte hypertrophy without an increase in the number of fat cells (26).

With the increasing awareness of the considerable overlap between these two groups, the concept of hyperplastic versus hypertrophic obesity has undergone further revision. Thus, it is currently appreciated that, in any given individual, the number of fat cells can increase at any stage of life if a critical (presumably genetically determined) fat cell size has been surpassed. One future therapeutic goal might be to identify and treat patients before their irreversible conversion from adipocyte hypertrophy to hyperplasia.

Other much less common types of obesity fall within the anatomic classification. The *lipodystrophies* are localized accumulations of excess fat, most commonly single or multiple lipomas. The latter are inherited as an autosomal-dominant trait. *Dercum's disease* (adiposis dolorosa) and *Weber–Christian disease* are two rare illnesses of unknown cause characterized by focal (occasionally painful) distributions of single or multiple nodules of histologically normal fat.

Etiologic

Various organic and environmental factors, none mutually exclusive, are included within the etiologic classification of obesity.

Organic Factors

As already noted, even in patients with an apparently genetic predisposition to obesity, environmental influences seem to be important determinants of body weight (see below).

In both experimental animals and in humans, certain *primary endocrine disorders* are important causes of obesity. These include hyperinsulinism, hypercortisolism, and deficiencies of growth hormone, thyroid hormone, or sex steroids. In each of these endocrinopathies, the excess fat accumulation is primarily upper body in distribution and may contribute to enhanced cardiovascular risk. Moreover, the possible contribution to these syndromes of pathophysiologic alterations in leptin or its receptor remain to be clarified.

Hyperinsulinemia can result from appropriate or surreptitious use of exogenous insulin, or from insulin hypersecretion by benign or malignant pancreatic neoplasms.

Hypercortisolism most often is iatrogenic, resulting from excess administration of exogenous glucocorticoids. Much less commonly, true Cushing's disease or syndrome, or pseudo-Cushing's syndrome due to depression, is responsible.

Because *growth hormone* exerts an influence on conversion of fat stores into energy for body growth and protein deposition, its absence, either from pituitary dysfunction or removal, leads to increased adiposity that is reversible by administration of the hormone. Current research suggests that the normal age-related decline in growth hormone contributes to increased central adiposity in older people and that administration of growth hormone may prevent or reduce this fat accumulation (44).

Although thyroid hormones directly modulate the overall basal metabolic rate (BMR), hypothyroidism per se is most often associated with modest or no weight gain. Morbid obesity (defined below) caused solely by hypothyroidism has not been documented, whereas moderate weight loss because of anorexia disproportionate to the decrease in BMR is occasionally seen.

The *polycystic ovary (Stein–Leventhal) syndromes*, a fairly common group of disorders in young women, are characterized by mild obesity, hirsutism, oligomenorrhea, and infertility in association with mild hypothalamic–pituitary–ovarian (and possibly adrenal) dysfunction. The obesity and the menstrual abnormalities are often ameliorated after ovarian wedge resection.

Hypothalamic obesity is a rare disorder associated most often with the presence of a craniopharyngioma or, less often, with other neoplastic or inflammatory diseases near the hypothalamic ventromedial nuclei, sites in the brain that appear to be involved in the control of normal feeding and satiety.

Of uncertain cause, but increasingly recognized, are the *primary eating disorders* of *bulimia* (binge eating) and *anorexia nervosa* (self-induced starvation). Although the true incidence and prevalence of these conditions are unknown, bulimia is thought to occur in as many as 20 to 70% of obese people applying to a weight loss program, and is more common in those who are actively gaining weight. It is even more common in patients with anorexia nervosa. It is generally refractory to most forms of medical, surgical, and psychiatric management.

In addition to insulin and glucocorticoids, other pharmacologic agents induce increases in food intake and in body fat. The most commonly used are phenothiazines, oral contraceptives, anticonvulsives (e.g., valproic acid), and the antihistamine cyproheptadine (Periactin). Weight gain associated with the latter drug probably results from its antiserotoninergic properties.

Most chronic cigarette smokers weigh less than age- and sex-matched nonsmokers but gain weight after they stop smoking. The weight gain often leads to resumption of smoking with its attendant risks for developing cardiovascular disease, emphysema, or cancer. Although the mechanisms responsible for weight loss during active cigarette smoking remain unknown, there is a strong positive correlation between the activity of the enzyme adipose tissue lipoprotein lipase in the fasting state and the amount of weight regained during the first 2 to 3 weeks after smoking cessation (12). Cigarette smoking also is associated with an increase in the WHR, despite its tendency to decrease body weight and BMI (54).

Environmental Factors

In view of the obvious imbalance between energy input and expenditure in obese people, it is not surprising to find numerous clinical studies that document the importance of nutritional habits and patterns of physical activity in the development of excess adiposity. The adverse effects of an absolute or relative excess in total caloric intake, of a maldistribution of foodstuffs (especially too much fat or carbohydrate), and of the general increase in sedentary lifestyles are particularly important.

In contemporary affluent societies, obesity is most often associated with behavioral and psychologic determinants that affect both the circumstances and substance of food intake. Although numerous studies have sought to identify the obese persona, it appears that no such diagnostic personality profile exists. Nonetheless, a major distinction between youth- and adult-onset obesity may reside in the distorted perception of body image that is commonly associated with obesity in childhood and adolescence. Thus, in the latter group, those affected often believe that their body habitus and weight are normal, a phenomenon rarely encountered in adult-onset obesity. Moreover, in contrast to certain commonly held notions, it appears that obese people are often depressed, are unhappy about being fat, and are relieved by successful and sustained weight loss.

Socioeconomic factors exert strong influences on the development and persistence of obesity in people as well as in population groups. In the United States, obesity is more common in children and adults from the lower socioeconomic groups, African-American versus white women, white versus African-American men, and first-generation Americans versus their descendants. Women born later in this century are less heavy than women born in the early 1900s; the opposite trend appears true for men. The reason for this is unclear but may be related to the steadily increasing fashion consciousness and emphasis on exercise among American women, and to the generally more sedentary work habits and lifestyles of men.

Morbid Obesity

The term *morbid obesity* has been used to define a subset of patients who are 50 to 100%, or 100 lb (45.5 kg), above their ideal, desirable, or acceptable body weights. This criterion, taken from the 1983 Metropolitan Life Insurance tables, has been shown to have a high sensitivity and low specificity, suggesting that overweight people may occasionally be misclassified as obese. Using a BMI value greater than 39 has been suggested as an alternative criterion for morbid obesity. Based on the NHANES II data of 1976 to 1980, about 2 million adults in the United States aged 20 to 79 were defined as morbidly obese, with women affected nearly five times more often than men (33). A predominantly genetic origin, with onset of disease in youth; a generally relentless progression through life; and a long-term cure rate of less than 5% are characteristic. In contrast, the onset and progression of the usual forms of mild to moderate adult-onset obesity are influenced more by psychosocial factors, although current research suggests a contributory role for genetic factors as well. Whereas patients with youth-onset morbid obesity often have distorted perceptions of body image, this has not been true of patients with adult-onset morbid obesity. However, the latter group has been characterized as generally lacking in internal cues that control food intake, thus being more susceptible to external, environmental eating cues. This observation, confirmed in numerous psychologic studies, has exerted a major influence on the philosophy and design of behavior modification programs.

EPIDEMIOLOGY

Before the epidemiology of obesity in any population group can be ascertained, several general methodologic concerns must be addressed. *(a)* A practical, standardized definition of obesity or overweight must be available and used. *(b)* The study population should be representative of the larger population group of which it is a part. *(c)* The presence and significance of coexistent morbid diseases or other conditions that may affect body weight must be known. *(d)* The effects of sex, age, socioeconomic status, religion, ethnicity, and other related factors must be considered. *(e)* The effects of confounding variables, such as cigarette smoking, should be analyzed. *(f)* Both cross-sectional and long-term longitudinal data should be collected. *(g)* Methods used for quantifying body fat in epidemiologic studies, such as relative weight (e.g., BMI), should be further refined to more closely approximate the most accurate known measures of adipose tissue mass. *(h)* The prevalence and significance of topographic variations in the distribution of body fat (i.e., upper versus lower-body obesity) need to be assessed. Although many excellent, large scale demographic surveys have been reported, to date no single study has satisfied all of the above criteria.

Comparative data on weight and height derived from the first three major cross-sectional surveys of the U.S. population published by the National Center for Health Statistics reveal that for both men and women, weights and heights were greater in the periods from 1971 to 1974 and from 1976 to 1980 than they were from 1960 to 1962. These findings have been replicated in numerous studies, particularly in the Build Study of 1979 (11), a survey of 4.2 million generally healthy, middle class people insured by 25 U.S. and Canadian insurance companies. Data from this latter study have been widely publicized by the Metropolitan Life Insurance Company as the 1983 Metropolitan Height and Weight Tables (40) and have led to upward revisions of the widely used desirable weights previously derived from the Build Study of 1959 (56). Because weights in these latter tables were not derived from a representative sample of the North American population, they should not be considered desirable and are therefore not labeled as such.

The usually high incidence and prevalence of obesity and its adverse sequelae in certain minority populations, such as Mexican Americans (25) and Native Americans (10), are of great medical, sociocultural, and political concern. Therefore, in the fourth and most recent cross-sectional survey of the U.S. population published by the National Center for Health Statistics, NHANES III, Phase I (1988 to 1991), estimates of prevalence of overweight, or obesity, were based on measures of BMI in 8620 adults 20 years of age and older (34). NHANES III differed from earlier surveys in that there was no upper limit of age eligibility, and it was designed to oversample Mexican Americans, African Americans, young children, and the elderly. During the 10-year period between NHANES II (1976 to 1980) and NHANES III, Phase I (1988 to 1991) U.S. adults aged 20 to 74 years exhibited an overall increase in prevalence of overweight of 31%, from 25.4% to 33.3%. There was a 49% increase in obesity in men aged 50 to 59 years, and a 53% increase in men aged 60 to 74 years. The increase in prevalence of obesity occurred among women and men at every decade, even after adjustment for the declining incidence of cigarette smoking. Increased research is clearly needed to elu-

cidate the underlying genetic and environmental determinants of these population differences so that more effective preventive and management strategies can be used.

There is now widespread recognition that with advancing age, physiologic alterations occur both in body weight (which increases gradually until the fifth to sixth decade, then tends to plateau) and body composition (with progressive loss of lean body mass and absolute or relative increase in total and intraabdominal body fat). Table 76.1 (3) illustrates comparative weight-for-height data derived from the 1983 Metropolitan Height and Weight Tables (uncorrected for age) and from the Baltimore Longitudinal Study of Aging, conducted at the Gerontology Research Center of the National Institute on Aging. Perusal of these data reveals that, for most of the heights reported, the Metropolitan optimal weights for men and women are similar to those for the age-adjusted weights of individuals in their thirties and forties. Therefore the Metropolitan tables overestimate the norms for younger adults but underestimate the corresponding norms for elderly people. In the age-adjusted data from the Gerontology Research Center, there is an increased weight allowance of about 10 lb/decade. More recent studies using various anthropometric ratios (including the WHR) have demonstrated an age-related increase in upper and central body adiposity. The ratios are independently influenced by BMI and are higher in men than in women despite a postmenopausal acceleration in the trend in women (53).

Data accrued from the three NHANES studies reveal a clear-cut and progressive increase in the prevalence of obesity and overweight among U.S. children and

Table 76.1. Comparison of the Weight for Height Tables from Actuarial Data (*Build Study,* 1979): Non–Age-Corrected Metropolitan Life Insurance Company and Age-Specific Gerontology Research Center Recommendations

Height		Metropolitan 1983 Weights (lb)[a]		Gerontology Research Center[a]				
		Men	Women	Age-Specific Weight Range for Men and Women (lb)				
Feet	Inches	25–59 yr		25 yr	35 yr	45 yr	55 yr	65 yr
4	10		100–131	84–111	92–119	99–127	107–135	115–142
4	11		101–134	87–115	95–123	103–131	111–139	119–147
5	0		103–137	90–119	98–127	106–135	114–143	123–152
5	1	123–145	105–140	93–123	101–131	110–140	118–148	127–157
5	2	125–148	108–144	96–127	105–136	113–144	122–153	131–163
5	3	127–151	111–148	99–131	108–140	117–149	126–158	135–168
5	4	129–155	114–152	102–135	112–145	121–154	130–163	140–173
5	5	131–159	117–156	106–140	115–149	125–159	134–168	144–179
5	6	133–163	120–160	109–144	119–154	129–164	138–174	148–184
5	7	135–167	123–164	112–148	122–159	133–169	143–179	153–190
5	8	137–171	126–167	116–153	126–163	137–174	147–184	158–196
5	9	139–175	129–170	119–157	130–168	141–179	151–190	162–201
5	10	141–179	132–173	122–162	134–173	145–184	156–195	167–207
5	11	144–183	135–176	126–167	137–178	149–190	160–201	172–213
6	0	147–187		129–171	141–183	153–195	165–207	177–219
6	1	150–192		133–176	145–188	157–200	169–213	182–225
6	2	153–197		137–181	149–194	162–206	174–219	187–232
6	3	157–202		141–186	153–199	166–212	179–225	192–238
6	4			144–191	157–205	171–218	184–231	197–244

From Andres R. Mortality and obesity. The rationale for age-specific height-weight tables. In: Andres R, Hazzard WR, Bierman E, eds. Principles of geriatric medicine. New York: McGraw-Hill, 1985.

[a]Values in this table are for height without shoes and weight without clothes.

adolescents. Using age- and gender-specific 85th and 95th percentile cutoff values for BMI developed during the NHANES II study, increases in the prevalence of overweight were detected in all age ranges and in both sexes (60). Using the 85th percentile criterion, the prevalence of overweight among boys aged 6 to 11 years increased from 15.2% during the NHANES I survey to 22.3% during the NHANES III evaluation. The corresponding increases for girls were from 15.2 to 22.7%. Using the 95th percentile BMI cutoff values, the prevalence of overweight increased from 5.2 to 10.8% in boys, and from 5.2 to 10.7% in girls. Among adolescents aged 12 to 17 years, using the 85th percentile criterion, the prevalence of overweight increased from 15.1 to 21.7% in boys, and from 15.2 to 21.2% in girls. The corresponding increases using the 95th percentile cutoff were from 5.2 to 12.8% in boys, and from 5.2 to 8.8% in girls. As with adults, most of the increase in prevalence of overweight among children and adolescents occurred between the NHANES II and NHANES III studies. In general, the progressive increases in prevalence of overweight among African-American and Hispanic children and adolescents, and their relationships with patterns of weight increases among comparably aged Caucasians, mirror those of their adult counterparts.

The Seven Country Study of Keys (30) (Table 76.2) provided comparative data on obesity and overweight using criteria of skinfold thickness and relative weight; by either criterion, men from the United States were among the most corpulent examined. More recent studies have revealed that the prevalence of overweight in U.S. women and men is higher than that in people from England, France, the Netherlands, and Italy, despite the increasing trend toward overweight in those countries.

PATHOGENESIS

Energy Intake

In the United States, the typical diet is composed of approximately 40 to 45% carbohydrate, 35 to 40% fat, and 15 to 20% protein. Energy intake that exceeds energy expenditure is the cardinal pathogenetic mechanism promoting an increase in body fat. Although much evidence supports the idea that, in healthy people, body weight is closely regulated over long periods, body composition changes considerably with age, as noted previously. The numerous genetic and environmental factors controlling normal food intake and distribution, storage, and expenditure of energy represent a complex, highly integrated series of events, as yet only partially understood.

It has long been thought that normal control of hunger and satiety in humans resided in certain nuclei of the lateral and medial hypothalamus, respectively, and that other neural, nutritional, endocrine–metabolic, gastrointestinal, and psychologic factors exerted their influences by impinging upon these sites. The recent discovery in rodents that secretion of leptin, the adipocyte-derived protein product of the ob gene,

Table 76.2. Prevalence of Overweight and Obesity in Groups of Men from Seven Countries

| | Percentage of Sample | |
Country	Overweight[a]	Obese[b]
Japan	2	2
Greece	11	11
Finland	15	14
Yugoslavia	19	29
Italy	33	28
Netherlands	13	32
United States	32	63

Data adapted from Keys and Bray GA. The obese patient. In: Smith LH. Major problems in internal medicine. Vol 9. Philadelphia: WB Saunders, 1976.
[a]Overweight = men 10% or more over standard weight.
[b]Obesity = men with sum of triceps and subscapular skinfold greater than 28 mm.

inhibits appetite and increases energy expenditure via receptor-mediated effects in the hypothalamus provides an important opportunity to advance our pathophysiologic understanding of, and design better pharmacologic treatments for, obesity (66). Numerous clinical studies suggest that circulating leptin levels are increased in obese people, are positively correlated with various measures of body fat, and decrease after successful weight loss (16). Studies in monozygotic twins discordant for obesity reveal leptin levels to be elevated in obese versus nonobese siblings (49). The possibility that leptin resistance may contribute to some syndromes of human obesity is supported by the observation of a decreased cerebrospinal fluid/serum ratio of leptin in obesity (13). Thus, the leptin/leptin receptor system may serve a lipostatic role in the development of human obesity (see below).

The continued application of contemporary techniques of cell, tissue, and organ culture has allowed for novel approaches to examine directly the basic cellular, biochemical, and molecular processes occurring in various tissues and cells (e.g., adipocytes, hepatocytes, neuroendocrine cells) known to be affected by metabolic derangements in obesity, in both humans and experimental animals. Data derived from such studies will continue to provide important new information pertinent to understanding the pathophysiologic derangements in cellular uptake, storage, and expenditure of energy in human obesity.

Energy Expenditure

Even after adjustments for differences in age, sex, and body weight, energy expenditure varies considerably among normal adults. Under resting conditions, there are adaptations to the amount and type of food ingested that allow for increased or decreased utilization of nutrients and that maintain a stable weight in most people. For example, after increased food intake above that required for maintenance of normal weight, healthy people exhibit an initial increase in weight followed by a new plateau of weight despite continued overeating, a phenomenon referred to as luxuskonsumption, or dietary-induced thermogenesis (DIT).

Current evidence favors the hypothesis that DIT is an important factor in regulating body weight, but whether the missing energy is burnt off in brown fat, metabolically more active than the usual white fat, is somewhat uncertain.

For many people in our sedentary society, physical exercise plays a minor role in energy expenditure. Nonetheless, evidence exists that energy expenditure differs in obese people during exercise and during ingestion of food, which contributes to the genesis of obesity. For example, studies in southwestern Native Americans suggest that a low rate of 24-hour energy expenditure contributes to the familial aggregation of obesity in that group (48). In addition, as noted above, there appears to be considerable genetic variation in such components of energy expenditure as resting metabolic rate, the thermic effect of food, and the energy cost of submaximal exercise (8). Recent studies suggest that genetically-acquired alterations in the β_3-adrenergic receptor of the sympathetic nervous system may account for the lower resting metabolic rate, reduced energy expenditure, and proclivity towards early development of obesity and non–insulin-dependent diabetes mellitus in diverse populations (4,14,62).

Short-term vigorous exercise, such as weight lifting or competitive contact sports, often leads to increases in dietary intake, utilization of muscle glycogen stores, and muscle mass. In contrast, frequent, sustained, moderate aerobic exercise, such as jogging or swimming, mobilizes fat stores, and in elderly people may decrease intra-abdominal fat (52).

Despite the apparent long-term control of general energy balance and body weight in normal people, and the discovery of the leptin-leptin receptor system, there is no conclusive evidence of an endogenous set-point (e.g., glucostatic, lipostatic, or thermostatic) that modulates adipose tissue mass. However, Schwartz and Brunzell have reported that the activity of adipose tissue lipoprotein lipase (LPL), the rate-limiting enzyme in the uptake and storage of lipoprotein triglyceride in adipose tissue, is increased in obese Caucasians and that enzyme activity increases, rather than decreases, after weight loss (51). Moreover, there appear to be demographic and genetic differences in the occurrence of this phenomenon. These authors have proposed that adipose tissue LPL may exert a counterregulatory role in preventing deviation from a set-point for fat cell size or mass, thus predisposing to a return to the original obese state (51). As noted above, the correlation between baseline adipose tissue LPL activity and the amount of weight gained after cessation of cigarette smoking further supports this hypothesis.

Certain indices of cellular sodium potassium adenosine triphosphatase (ATPase) activity have been reported to be increased (8), decreased (17), or unchanged (6) in red blood cells or liver from obese subjects, as compared with controls. Further investigation is needed to clarify whether genetic or environmental alterations in the activity of this critical cellular enzyme contribute to the pathophysiologic mechanisms by which cellular thermogenesis, and therefore the efficiency of energy expenditure, might be perturbed in human obesity.

The observation that most obesity in adult men is upper body in distribution, whereas that in most adult women is lower body in distribution, suggested that sex hormones might influence body fat topography and function. Increased androgenic activity has been reported in the blood of premenopausal women with upper- versus lower-body obesity and has been shown to correlate with abnormalities in fat cell size and biochemical function (19). Moreover, abdominal adipocytes from patients with upper-body obesity are metabolically active, whereas abdominal adipocytes from patients with lower-body obesity, and thigh adipocytes from patients with upper- or lower-body obesity, are metabolically relatively stable. The clinical implications of alterations in regional adiposity have recently been reviewed (46) and are discussed below.

NATURAL HISTORY

Much information has been adduced to show that obese infants and children become obese adults more often than do their lean counterparts. In addition, youth onset obesity tends to be more severe and persistent, and more resistant to treatment, than the usually milder forms of later onset. This may be because of the fact that weight loss and decrease in adiposity per se result predominantly from a decrease in adipocyte size and not number, so adipose hyperplasia (regardless of age of onset) (see above) is ordinarily irreversible. A recent analysis of the long-term effects of obesity in 508 adolescents 13 to 18 years old, enrolled in the Harvard Growth Study of 1922 to 1935, revealed that, after an average of 55 years of follow-up there were increased risks of both cardiac (2.3-fold) and all-cause (1.8-fold) mortality in men, but not in women. The risks of colorectal carcinoma and gout were also increased in men, whereas the risk of arthritis was augmented in women (42). These findings are consistent with previous reports conducted in larger numbers of people for much shorter periods. In contrast, there is greater therapeutic promise for the more common adult onset obese population, who have a normal number of adipocytes.

Metabolic Concomitants

Although the exact roles of all organic and environmental factors in the pathogenesis of obesity remain to be elucidated, certain metabolic concomitants of excess adiposity, particularly upper-body obesity, have been characterized. Numerous studies document the close association between obesity and diabetes mellitus and suggest that obesity per se is diabetogenic. Obesity leads to increased pancreatic insulin production and *hyperinsulinemia*, both basally and after stimulation by ingestion of glucose, amino acids, and so on. Evidence exists that the hyperinsulinemia and concurrent glucose intolerance are caused by *insulin resistance* at the tissue level (e.g., liver, adipose tissue, and skeletal muscle), which results from a decrease in the number of cell surface receptors for insulin and/or from aberrant, insulin-dependent intracellular glucose metabolism. Finally, it has been proposed that chronic hyperinsulinemia leads to a further decrease in the number of cell surface insulin receptors (i.e., down-regulation), the latter serving as an adipocyte response to prevent episodes of hypoglycemia.

There is also a significant association between obesity and the presence of *hyperlipidemia*, especially hypertriglyceridemia. This latter relationship probably results, at least in some patients, from the hyperinsulinemia-induced increase in hepatic triglyceride synthesis and formation of triglyceride-rich very-low-density lipoproteins (VLDL). Increased endogenous cholesterol synthesis is also more common in obese patients, leads to increased circulating concentrations of total cholesterol and low-density lipoprotein (LDL) cholesterol and decreased concentrations of high-density lipoprotein (HDL and HDL_2) cholesterol, and results in increased risk of coronary artery disease and, probably, cholesterol gallstones.

Many patients with adult-onset upper-body obesity appear cushingoid. Simple obesity is associated with an increased cortisol production rate leading to increased hepatic steroid metabolism and increased urinary excretion of certain steroid conjugates. Such patients typically have increased urinary 17-hydroxycorticoids; however, plasma cortisol, urinary free cortisol, and overnight dexamethasone suppression tests are usually normal.

Salt and water retention is a common problem in obese patients, and it is in part mediated by increases in aldosterone secretion induced by dietary carbohydrate and, to a lesser extent, protein intake.

Onset of normal menarche does not occur until a critical body weight is reached (usually 40 to 45 kg), a finding that explains the earlier menarche in women with youth onset obesity. Menstrual abnormalities such as dysfunctional uterine bleeding, amenorrhea, and infertility are also more common in obese women and are often associated with aberrant cyclical reproductive hormone function (subnormal levels of follicle-stimulating hormone [FSH] in the follicular phase, and of progesterone on the luteal phase).

Other important endocrine or metabolic sequelae of obesity include increased androgenicity, especially in women; augmented sympathoadrenal activity; decreased spontaneous and stimulated (e.g., by growth hormone-releasing hormone) growth hormone release; and hyperuricemia. In women with the polycystic ovarian syndrome, hyperandrogenism and sympathoadrenal excess contribute to obesity-related hyperinsulinemia, insulin resistance, glucose intolerance, and dyslipidemia. In patients with growth hormone deficiency, decreased availability of this lipolytic hormone permits excess accumulation of total body and intra-abdominal fat. The increased prevalence of hyperuricemia in obese individuals is responsible for their increased prevalence of gout.

Risks

A large body of research and anecdotal data has suggested that obesity and overweight are graded phenomena and that there is strong positive correlation between the degree of excess adiposity and increased morbidity and mortality, the latter particularly from cardiovascular and cerebrovascular diseases. It now appears that this hypothesis must be somewhat modified.

Critical analysis of data derived from retrospective life insurance studies suggested that there was no significant increase in mortality until body weight rose to values greater than 30% above ideal body weight. Data from a large number of prospective studies also suggest that severe to extreme, but not mild to moderate, obesity is associated with decreased longevity. More recent reanalyses of data from various large-scale epidemiologic studies have led several investigators to conclude that the "mortality-for-weight curves" are often J or U shaped, in that the highest mortality rates occur at both extremes of relative weight, whereas the lowest mortality rates occur at intermediate weights (55). Andres has demonstrated that the BMI associated with lowest mortality itself increases with advancing age, both in men and in women, and has thus emphasized the need for age-specific weight-height tables (3). It is also evident, as noted above, that the risks of obesity vary not only with the amount but with the topographic distribution of excess body fat. Finally, data published as part of a 26-year follow-up of subjects in the Framingham study (27) reveal that obesity per se is an independent risk factor for premature dying. Current evidence favors the view that hyperinsulinemia is the common pathogenetic mechanism by which upper-body obesity influences known cardiac risk factors, such as hyperlipidemia, diabetes mellitus (29,45), and hypertension, although the significance of the hyperinsulinemia–hypertension link has been questioned (41). It seems likely that public health and other officials, as well as individual physicians, will become more cautious in their advice regarding evaluation and management of patients with mild to moderate obesity, particularly if it is lower body in distribution.

Medical Consequences

The major physiologic and medical concomitants of moderate to extreme obesity are depicted in Table 76.3. Although a direct pathophysiologic link between obesity and these conditions has not been unequivocally established, in each instance the morbidity associated with the condition is proportional to the degree of excess adiposity and is partially or totally reversed after successful weight loss. In addition, obesity, particularly when severe, often exacerbates or complicates

Table 76.3.   Possible Medical Consequences of Obesity

Endocrine–Metabolic
Hyperglycemia, hyperinsulinemia, insulin resistance
Hypertriglyceridemia, hypercholesterolemia ($\uparrow$ VLDL, $\uparrow$ LDL, $\downarrow$ HDL)
$\uparrow$ Cortisol production but normal plasma cortisol, diurnal rhythm, urine free cortisol, and overnight dexamethasone suppression
Early menarche, menstrual abnormalities, hirsutism
$\downarrow$ Sympathoadrenal activity
$\downarrow$ SHBG and $\uparrow$ total or free androgens
$\downarrow$ Growth hormone, basally and after provocative stimuli
Hyperuricemia, gout

Cardiovascular
Hypertension
Coronary artery disease
Congestive heart failure
Varicose veins
Cerebrovascular disease

Pulmonary
Hypoventilation (e.g., pickwickian) syndromes
Sleep apnea syndrome
Chronic respiratory infections

Gallbladder
Cholelithiasis (cholesterol gallstones)

Musculoskeletal
Osteoarthritis
Chronic orthopedic problems
$\downarrow$ Ambulation

Renal
Nephrotic syndrome (normal or nonspecific biopsy)

Oncologic
Endometrial, breast carcinoma (postmenopausal women), prostate, colon

Dermatologic
Acanthosis nigricans
Chronic skin infections

Psychosocial
Depression, loss of self-esteem
$\downarrow$ Employability

Pregnancy
Worsen underlying hypertension, diabetes mellitus
$\uparrow$ Maternal mortality

Surgery (Especially Under General Anesthesia)
Increased perioperative morbidity and mortality

the course of a variety of other conditions; for example, by delaying surgical procedures, enhancing perioperative risks, prolonging convalescence from many illnesses, worsening pregnancy-associated problems, and exacerbating unstable behavioral patterns.

EVALUATION AND MANAGEMENT

Evaluation

The history usually indicates whether the patient has youth- or adult-onset obesity, and it often provides important information regarding usual or unusual dietary practices, as well as patterns of physical activity. It is particularly important to identify any medical or psychologic factors that may motivate the patient to lose weight or that militate for or against certain treatment plans. The physical examination should include an assessment of whether the patient has primarily upper- or lower-body obesity by measuring the ratio of the minimal circumference at the waist to the maximal circumference at the hips with the patient in the standing position. A WHR greater than 0.85 indicates definite upper-body obesity, whereas a WHR less than 0.75 indicates lower-body obesity.

Although secondary obesity is rare, its importance lies in its reversibility after identification and specific therapy of the underlying medical or pharmacologic disorder. Special emphasis should therefore be placed on screening an obese patient for any contributing endocrine–metabolic process and on obtaining a history of medication use (see above).

Evidence of glucose intolerance should be sought by obtaining fasting blood glucose levels with the patient on a regular (or, preferably, high-carbohydrate) diet, and comparing the results with those from age- and sex-matched controls. The oral glucose tolerance test is not ordinarily necessary to make the diagnosis of type 2 diabetes mellitus. Hypercortisolemia should be suspected in any plethoric, hypertensive patient with upper-body obesity, hypokalemia, and glucose intolerance. A normal overnight dexamethasone suppression test (1 mg of oral dexamethasone given at 11 PM, followed by an 8-AM plasma cortisol of less than 5 µg/dL) or a normal value for 24-hour urinary free cortisol excretion (less than 100 µg/24 hours) ordinarily eliminates the diagnosis of endogenous hypercortisolemia with a reasonable degree of certainty. Clinically significant hypothyroidism can usually be ruled out when the free thyroxine (T_4) index (i.e., serum $T_4 \times$ resin triiodothyronine [T_3] uptake) is normal. On occasion, hyperthyroid patients outeat their increased BMR and complain to the physician of weight gain. The finding of menstrual irregularities, mild hirsutism (but not virilization), and central obesity in a young woman prompts suspicion of the polycystic ovarian syndrome, a diagnosis made more likely by the additional findings of a mildly elevated serum testosterone level (60 to 100 ng/dL), flat basal body temperature curve (i.e., no ovulation), and palpable abnormalities on pelvic examination. Diseases of the hypothalamic–pituitary region should be considered in obese patients with otherwise unexplained neuroendocrine abnormalities. Certain rare syndromes, such as the Prader–Willi syndrome (obesity, short stature, hypogonadism, and mental retardation), are usually recognized in childhood by their characteristic clinical presentations.

In addition to the above, fasting blood samples should be sent for determinations of triglyceride, total cholesterol, HDL cholesterol, and uric acid levels. Most patients with hyperlipidemia have acquired (secondary), not genetic (primary), hyperlipidemias and will respond to appropriate diet regimens (see Chapter 75). Finally, in patients with clinically apparent or suspected hypoventilation syndromes or sleep-disordered breathing, pulmonary function and polysomnographic profiles should be tested.

One evaluation of 234 obese women and 27 obese men led to detection of the following significant abnormalities: hypertension (16%), hypertriglyceridemia (25%), glucose intolerance (25%), hypercholesterolemia (11%), and hyperuricemia (7%). In 2 of 57 patients studied, T_4 values were abnormal: One was high and one low (9).

Management of Mild to Moderate Obesity

Based on the initial assessment of the patient, the type (adult-onset versus childhood-onset), topographic distribution, and degree of obesity should be ascertained, including the medical or psychologic urgency for weight loss, the patient's motivation and readiness for weight loss, and the most suitable treatment plan. Because the usual form of simple adult onset, mild to moderate *lower*-body obesity appears not to carry an increased risk of morbidity or mortality (see above), it should probably not be treated at all. On the other hand, until the possible risks of mild to moderate *upper*-body obesity are more clearly defined, it would seem prudent to treat it with a combination of moderate diet, regular exercise, and patient-motivated nutritional education and behavioral relearning. There is no justification for the use of anorexigenic drugs in the treatment of this problem. If the patient asks for them, the physician should explain that they are modestly effective; they are of little, no, or uncertain help in maintaining long-term weight loss; and many of them are potentially dangerous (see below). Moreover, the patient should be cautioned against the purchase of patent medicines. It is now clear that several lay organizations for weight reduction (e.g., Weight Watchers, Take Off Pounds Sensibly [TOPS], Diet Center, and NutriSystem) are as capable as health professionals in effecting weight loss in this category of obese patient.

General nutritional guidelines for reducing the risk of diet-related chronic disorders, including obesity, have been published by the National Research Council (Table 76.4). For most adults, a balanced diet containing 1500 to 1800 calories/day is necessary for maintenance of optimal body weight under conditions of basal activity. Thus, modest caloric restriction to 900 to 1200 calories/day for women and 1200 to 1500 calories/day for men is appropriate, with small increases proportionate to increases in levels of physical activity. It is often useful to advise patients who are motivated to diet to purchase one of the readily available, inexpensive calorie counters and to use the information to limit their daily diet to a specific number of calories. In general, daily modest exercise programs should be tailored to the individual patient's ability and enjoyment. Regular physical conditioning facilitates weight loss and decreases or abolishes obesity-associated hyperinsulinemia, insulin resistance, glucose intolerance, hypertriglyceridemia, hyperuricemia, and systolic and diastolic hypertension; it also improves cardiovascular, respiratory, and musculoskeletal prob-

lems. A goal of a loss of 1 or 2 pounds (0.5 to 1 kg) a week is appropriate whenever a patient embarks on a weight reduction program.

Improved nutritional understanding often results from effective and practical dietary and behavioral counseling. As part of behavior modification, it is usually helpful to ask participants about their previous efforts to lose weight and why they failed. Diet sheets and booklets that set forth recommendations that are easy to understand and follow, particularly when attuned to the sociocultural and economic characteristics of the patient, are especially valuable. Improved patterns of eating behavior should be encouraged. Specific suggestions should include smaller, more frequent, or regular meals, eaten more slowly, in defined surroundings. Use of food diaries is especially helpful (Fig. 76.3), particularly in assisting both patients and their physicians to identify abnormal behavioral patterns that lead to excess food intake. For the patient who makes a significant effort, reinforcement of the improved eating behavior by his or her physician is important in maintenance of weight reduction. Usually, formal consultation with a professional

Table 76.4. Recommended Dietary Guidelines

1. Reduce total fat intake to 30% or less of calories, saturated fatty acid intake to less than 10% of calories, and cholesterol intake to less than 300 mg/day. The intake of fat and cholesterol can be reduced by substituting fish, poultry without skin, lean meats, and low- or nonfat dairy products for fatty meats and whole-milk dairy products; by choosing more vegetables, fruits, cereals, and legumes; and by limiting oils, fats, egg yolks, and fried and other fatty foods.
2. Every day eat five or more servings of a combination of vegetables and fruits, especially green and yellow vegetables and citrus fruits. Also, increase intake of starches and other complex carbohydrates by eating six or more daily servings of a combination of breads, cereals, and legumes. An average serving is equal to a half cup for most fresh or cooked vegetables, fruits, dry or cooked cereals or legumes, one medium piece of fresh fruit, one slice of bread, or one roll or muffin.
3. Maintain protein intake at moderate levels (less than 1.6 g/kg body weight for adults).
4. Balance food intake and physical activity to maintain appropriate body weight.
5. The committee does not recommend alcohol consumption. For those who drink alcoholic beverages, the committee recommends limiting consumption to the equivalent of less than 1 ounce of pure alcohol in a single day. This is the equivalent of two cans of beer, two small glasses of wine, or two average cocktails. Pregnant women should avoid alcoholic beverages.
6. Limit total daily intake of salt to 6 g or less. Limit the use of salt in cooking and avoid adding it to food at the table. Salty, highly processed salty, salt-preserved, and salt-pickled foods should be consumed sparingly.
7. Maintain adequate calcium balance. The potential benefits of calcium intakes above the RDAs (recommended daily allowances) to prevent osteoporosis or hypertension are not well documented and do not justify the use of calcium supplements.
8. Avoid taking dietary supplements in excess of the RDA in any one day.
9. Maintain an optimal intake of fluoride, particularly during the years of primary and secondary tooth formation and growth.

Adapted from Diet and Health. Implications for reducing chronic disease risk. Committee on Diet and Health. Food and Nutrition Board. Commission on Life Sciences. National Research Council. Washington, DC: National Academy Press, 1989.

JOHNS HOPKINS BAYVIEW MEDICAL CENTER
WEIGHT CONTROL PROGRAM

Name: _____ Date: _____

Day: Mon.   Tues.   Wed.   Thurs.   Fri.   Sat.   Sun.   (circle one)

Exercise or activity: A. Type_____   Minutes_____   B. Type_____   Minutes_____

Time	Minutes	Food Type	Amount	Meal/ Snacks	Hunger Yes No	Body Position	Activity while Eating	Location of Eating	Eating (with Whom)	Feeling

Time: starting time for a meal or snack; Meal/snack: indicate type of eating by the appropriate letter—M (meal) or S (snack). Hunger: check yes or no.

Figure 76.3. Food diary for identification of abnormal behavioral patterns leading to excess food intake.

behavioral therapist is not required. Chapters 3 (section on patient education), 4 (compliance-improving strategies), and 11 (psychotherapy in ambulatory practice) describe generic approaches to behavior modification that can be used in office visits.

Management of Morbid Obesity

Morbid obesity (see above), particularly of the upper body, is associated with a measurably increased morbidity and mortality, as well as with a generally poor response to conventional methods of moderate caloric restriction. Although hazards are associated with each of the more intensive forms of treatment, in many severely obese patients, the risks and disadvantages of being overweight greatly exceed those of treatment. In many individuals, behavioral modification (see below), alone or in combination with other therapies, may offer an effective and safe management option. It is now recognized that obesity should be treated as a chronic condition, and that various therapeutic strategies are more effective when continued for longer periods and when coupled with one another.

Diet

Total Fasting. Significant weight loss (up to 5 to 6 kg/week) can be achieved by prolonged (4 to 8 weeks) starvation of motivated, hospitalized morbidly obese patients. Within 1 to 2 years after such treatment, however, fewer than 30% of these patients have maintained their initial weight loss, and in the long-term, fewer than 5% attain and maintain their ideal body weight. A major hazard of such treatment is the extensive loss of lean body mass, and thus negative nitrogen balance, that occurs predictably within the first 1 or 2 weeks of starvation and continues at a somewhat lower rate thereafter. Other complications of this technique include orthostatic hypotension, ketoacidosis, electrolyte and vitamin deficiencies, weakness, decreased libido and impotence, menstrual irregularities, hyperuricemia and acute gout, renal uric acid calculi, emotional disturbances, and rarely, sudden death. Despite these potential disadvantages, the need for hospitalization, and the high incidence of recidivism, in selected patients total fasting appears to be a generally safe and efficacious technique for inducing significant short-term (e.g., presurgical) weight loss when supervised by physicians experienced in the technique.

Supplemented Fasting. Supplemented fasting techniques or very *low-calorie diets* (VLCDs) exploit in an ambulatory setting several of the advantages of total fasting, particularly those of significant short-term weight loss and high patient adherence. In general, patients consume 1 to 1.5 g of protein/kg of desirable body weight—enough to prevent loss of lean body mass in a hypocaloric (e.g., 300 to 500 calories/day) diet supplemented by adequate hydration, potassium salts, and other vitamins and minerals. In one study of nearly 1200 patients who were followed clinically and biochemically at frequent intervals, approximately 75 to 80% of the patients lost more than 40 lb (18 kg) (21). Moreover, hypertension and glucose intolerance, as well as the need for appropriate medications, disappeared or diminished in most affected patients; other benefits, such as improved exercise tolerance, ambulation, pulmonary function, and psychosocial and employment status, also became evident. The disadvantages of the technique are similar to but of lesser magnitude than those described above for total fasting; there also have been several sudden cardiac deaths in patients without known preexisting heart disease. A major problem with supplemented fasting is that the initial success rate drops to approximately 25% on subsequent attempts at fasting after major weight regain. Improved responsivity to VLCDs results not only from enrollment of highly motivated, younger people with upper-body obesity and significant obesity-related comorbidity, but also from the combination of this dietary approach with long-term behavioral modification techniques (47).

Liquid Protein Diets. A variant of the supplemented fast—the liquid protein diet—has been widely used in this country and consists of a poor quality protein, collagen hydrolysate, supplemented with tryptophan. Because of the ready commercial availability of this diet, many obese patients have consumed it without appropriate vitamin or mineral supplementation or medical supervision. In one report (61), more than 60 sudden cardiac deaths were documented during or shortly after discontinuation of this diet. Although electrocardiograms often showed prolonged QT intervals, decreased QRS voltages, and refractory ventricular arrhythmias, electrolyte abnormalities such as hypokalemia and hypocalcemia were not invariably present. Some autopsy studies have revealed a nonspecific cardiac muscle atrophy similar to that seen in protein-calorie malnutrition states in humans and experimental animals. Also, transient, potentially life-threatening cardiac arrhythmias were detected by 24-hour Holter monitoring, but not by standard 12-lead electrocardiograms, in three of six morbidly obese hospitalized patients followed for 40 days on a commercially available liquid protein diet (35). In none of the six patients was there an antecedent history of cardiac disease, and in all of the patients Holter monitoring was normal before and after the study diet. Except for mild hypokalemia in one of the affected patients, none of many routine chemical or metabolic measurements distinguished between patients with and without cardiac abnormalities. In a subsequent related study, six additional morbidly obese but otherwise healthy patients were hospitalized and fed for 40 days with a markedly hypocaloric (470 kcal/day) experimental diet containing 60% high-quality protein, 25% carbohydrate, and 15% fat and supplemented with the Recommended Daily Allowances or more of all essential minerals, trace elements, vitamins, and essential fatty acids (2). No arrhythmias were detected on 24-hour Holter monitoring, nitrogen balance remained positive, and the previously noted electrolyte abnormalities were reversed or decreased. The results of the latter study suggested that appropriate supplementation of even a markedly hypocaloric diet was safer than the nutritionally inadequate

liquid protein diet, and a model was thus provided for several popular diet programs, such as Optifast and Medifast. The FDA requires that warning labels be placed on all protein-supplemented diets and has suggested restricting such diets to certain people, all of whom should be aware of the potential hazards and should be followed by physicians experienced in using such diets. However, in view of the above observations, it appears prudent to discontinue use of liquid protein diets until the mechanisms of their cardiac toxicity are elucidated.

Numerous palatable balanced and unbalanced low-calorie diets are commonly used. Many patients find it easier to follow regimens that limit caloric intake by eliminating entire food groups, such as carbohydrates, or by providing nutritionally adequate food homogenates. Perhaps the benefits of these approaches derive both from a perception that they are more medicinal and from diminution in external feeding cues.

Diets that are very low in calories (fewer than 800 calories/day) and carbohydrates are usually ketogenic. They are particularly popular because of the commonly held ideas that nutritional ketosis exerts an anorexic effect, greater weight loss ensues than after a balanced diet containing an equal number of calories, and such diets spare body protein better than balanced diets. There are no unequivocal data to support the first two notions. Although low-carbohydrate, low-calorie diets do generally cause a more profound early (1- to 2-week) diuresis of salt and water than do balanced diets, the rate of fat loss is no greater. Moreover, hypocaloric, low-carbohydrate diets, like fasting and supplemented fasting, are associated with weakness, dehydration, postural hypotension, and occasional hyperuricemia and acute gout.

The safest diets are balanced and contain more than 800 calories/day.

Table 76.5 illustrates several popular *fad diets* that are nutritionally unbalanced or hypocaloric. Use of these and the numerous other related fad diets that are hypocaloric and unbalanced, particularly when medically unsupervised, should be avoided.

Olestra, a nondigestable fat substitute, has received a great deal of popular attention and has been approved by the FDA as a food additive. It is alleged by its manufacturer to be effective in allowing calorie consumption without weight gain. However, to date there have been no controlled clinical trials that validate the utility of this preparation.

Effectiveness of Diet. How effective are dietary attempts at long-term weight loss? Although quantitation of successful weight loss has been defined differently by various investigators, numerous studies confirm that at most, only 10 to 20% of obese patients who initially lose significant amounts of weight on diets maintain or increase that weight loss several years later. This is unfortunate, as even modest weight reduction (approximately 10% or less) can ameliorate obesity-related medical complications and improve longevity (22). Although all factors that promote such success or failure remain unknown, it has been shown

Table 76.5.   Characteristics of Several Widely Used Fad Diets

Diet	Composition	Deficiencies	Side Effects and Potential Hazards	Other Comments
High-Protein/Keto-genic Diets Dr. Atkin's Revolution-ary Diet The Drinking Man's Diet The Scarsdale Diet Dr. Stillman's Quick-Weight-Loss Diet	High protein Moderate to high fat Low carbohydrate Caloric intake varies from 1000–2000 calories	Likely deficiencies: Dietary fiber Calcium Riboflavin Folic acid Vitamins A, C Thiamine Iron	Potential exists for: Ketosis, anorexia, fa-tigue, dehydration, postural hypotension, hypokalemia/sodium loss, hyperlipidernia, hyperuricemia, consti-pation, halitosis	Long-term maintenance unre-alistic. NOT RECOM-MENDED especially during pregnancy, in kidney dis-ease, diabetes mellitus, lipid disorders. Can precipi-tate an acute attack of gout. Effectiveness due to high satiety values of foods consumed in diet. Large initial weight loss felt to be due to loss of body water. No greater actual fat loss than with balanced diet of equal calories.
Protein-Sparing Modi-fied Fast (PSMF) Liquid Protein Diet The Last Chance Diet Cambridge Diet	Variation of total fast; maxi-mize fat loss but minimize lean body mass lost by adding 1.0 to 1.5 g of vari-able quality protein/kg of ideal body weight ~400 calories (300–700 calories) For example, 330 calories/day 31 g of protein 44 g of carbohydrate 2 g of fat and vitamin and mineral supplements	If poor biological quality protein, tryptophan deficiency Likely deficiencies in poorly supplemented regimens: Potassium Phosphorus Calcium Magnesium Vitamin A Riboflavin	Ketosis Dehydration Hypokalemia Postural hypotension Cold intolerance Constipation Rarely—sudden death, felt to be secondary to cardiac arrhythmias	Unrealistic for long-term maintenance. Not recom-mended for ambulatory management since needs careful medical monitoring. Tolerated more by morbidly obese than by mildly to moderately overweight indi-viduals. Some programs do include instructions on nu-trition, exercise, mental conditioning, lifestyle modi-fications.
Pritikin Diet	80% complex carbohydrate 10% fat 10% protein 650–1000 calories/day	Likely to be deficient in calcium, B_{12}, iron (slightly); does not meet FDA's require-ment for protein (es-pecially high-quality protein)	Dry skin, flatulence, gas-tric distress secondary to high fiber content	Long-term compliance un-likely because of extreme change from average American diet. Exercise is encouraged.
Fasting	Fluid/electrolytes/vitamin and mineral supplementation	Extensive	Extensive	Inappropriate for ambulatory management. Needs to be done on metabolic ward only.

that ability to continue in a diet program (nearly 25% of patients drop out within the first few weeks) and emotional stability are important. The appearance of pathologic depression during or after dietary weight loss is well recognized and is more common in juvenile-onset obese patients, in whom the baseline distortion of body image is often accompanied, para-doxically, by a perception of larger body size with progressive weight loss. Data from the Framingham study suggest that obese patients who undergo repeti-tive cycles of dietary-induced weight loss followed by weight regain are at increased risk for cardiac disease and total mortality and that the magnitude of the risk is similar to that for obese patients generally (38). Thus, weight cycling, a common behavior in obese people, may be dangerous. It is hoped that improved classifi-cation schemes will better identify subpopulations of obese patients more amenable to specifically defined therapeutic programs.

Exercise

Numerous studies have assessed the efficacy of exercise interventions, alone and in concert with other treatments, in reducing body weight and body fat in obese people. Several meta-analyses have suggested that, by itself, modest to moderate aerobic exercise training, such as walking, running, or cycling, leads to modest reductions in weight (about 0.1 kg/week) and body fat (about 1.0 kg/week) in moderately obese, physically sedentary individuals (5,20). Exercise-induced weight loss appears to depend on initial body (fat) mass and the frequency and energy expenditure of the exercise. Not surprisingly, high energy exercise training, as in military inductees, promotes more sig-nificant losses of weight and fat (37). As noted above, regular aerobic exercise improves many obesity-associated metabolic abnormalities, thus reducing car-diac risk. Moderate endurance training for 6 months decreases HDL and HDL_2 catabolism, thus increasing

HDL levels (52); moreover, the beneficial effects on HDL levels and cardiac risk can be achieved by as little as 10 miles of jogging per week (58). The observation that, in elderly obese men, moderate aerobic exercise reduces excess intra-abdominal fat accumulation suggests one mechanism for the ameliorative metabolic effects of endurance training (52). Recent studies suggest that resistive (i.e., strength) training may also exert beneficial effects on the metabolic sequelae of obesity and thereby may also reduce cardiac risk. Of note is that diet generally exerts a faster and nearly threefold greater loss of weight than does exercise training alone (20).

Behavior Modification

The basis for behavior modification therapy in the management of obesity rests on the finding that many patients, particularly those with adult-onset obesity, respond predominantly to external rather than to internal feeding cues. Thus, the focus of treatment is to alter daily habits, such as eating behaviors and attitudes, social supports, exercise, nutrition, and other factors related to eating (65). A governmental panel has underscored the importance of initiating treatment for obesity with lifestyle behavioral changes (43). Weight loss resulting from behavior modification, unlike that produced by dietary, pharmacologic, or surgical therapy, has not been associated with serious adverse side effects. Although these techniques offer great therapeutic promise, particularly when used for extended durations in conjunction with highly structured diet and exercise programs, or pharmacotherapy, not all obese individuals will respond, even in the short-term, to this form of therapy, a fact that underscores the need for improved categorization and prognostication of obesity subtypes.

The short- and long-term efficacy of group therapy for obesity has also been examined and appears to be similar to that of individual therapy, a finding that should prompt more effective use of trained therapists. Data published by two of the most popular lay self-help groups that advertise success at weight reduction, Weight Watchers and TOPS, confirm prior anecdotal impressions by experienced therapists that these groups achieve short-term results as good as, and long-term results as poor as, those in medically supervised programs. Currently, nearly all of the major commercial weight management programs include some component of behavioral therapy. Overeaters Anonymous, a 12-step program modeled after Alcoholics Anonymous (see Chapter 21), uses the donated services of previously obese people to modify behavior of currently obese people. The short- and long-term success of this program remains to be demonstrated.

Pharmacologic Therapy

Increasing interest in the use of medications for the treatment of obesity stems from the rapidly advancing state of knowledge regarding the biological basis of obesity, from the recognition that the aggregate impact of dietary, exercise, and behavioral therapies has not altered the increasing rate of weight gain in the United States and in many other populations, and from the consideration that obesity is a chronic disorder that requires long-term treatment. The initial, widely publicized report of safe and effective maintenance of weight loss for up to 3.5 years in some patients enrolled in a program of drug therapy combined with dietary and behavioral modification (64) further stimulated scientific, public, and commercial interests in the possible benefits of anti-obesity drugs. Nonetheless, to date there remains no known pharmacologic agent for the treatment of obesity that is reliably effective, devoid of short- and long-term adverse effects, inexpensive, and readily available. Moreover, the clinician is faced with the absence of clear guidelines related to the selection of patients for, management of patients on, and information regarding the long-term safety and efficacy of anti-obesity pharmacotherapy. In the absence of such guidelines, pharmacotherapy should be considered only in patients with moderate to severe obesity and obesity-related complications in whom nonpharmacologic approaches have failed.

The anorexigenic derivatives of phenylethylamine (Table 76.6) include the amphetamines, phenylpropanolamine and other noradrenergic agents, such as fenfluramine and dexfenfluramine. All possess certain

Table 76.6.   Appetite-Suppressing Drugs

Generic and Proprietary Names	Common Trade Names	Dosage (mg)	Administration[a] (mg)
Over-the-Counter			
Phenylpropanol- amine	Acutrim, Dexatrim	75	75 once a day
Schedule IV			
Diethylpropion	Tenuate, Propion	25, 75	25 before meals (TID) 75 in morning
Mazindol	Sanorex, Mazanor	1, 2	1 before meals 2 in morning
Phentermine	Ionamin	15, 30	15 (TID) 30 in morning
Schedule III[b]			
Phendimetrazine	Plegine, Obalan	35	35 before meals
Benzphetamine	Didrex	25, 50	25–50 before meals
Schedule II[b]			
Dextroamphet- amine	Dexedrine	5, 10, 15	5–10 before meals (TID)
Methamphet- amine	Desoxyn	5, 10, 15	2.5 or 5 before meals (TID) 10 or 15 in morning
Phenmetrazine	Preludin	25, 50, 75	25 (BID or TID)

[a]BID, Twice a day; TID, three times daily.

[b]The Federal Controlled Substance Act of 1970 places the prescription anorexiants into three of five schedule categories. Appetite suppressants in schedule II are most likely to be abused; those in schedule IV have little or no risk of abuse. The schedules of the Controlled Substance Act are numbered in order of decreasing potential for abuse; drugs in Schedule II (amphetamine, methamphetamine, and phenmetrazine) are the most restricted. The currently scheduled drugs are all derivatives of amphetamine.

pharmacologic properties like those of epinephrine and norepinephrine; however, their various chemical modifications have led, to differing extents, to decreased cardiovascular and central nervous system toxicity and to preservation of anorexigenic properties. Despite their similarities in chemical structure, these agents exert their effects via different mechanisms of action and, consequently, exhibit different side effect profiles (see below).

Phenylpropanolamine (Acutrim, Dexatrim) is an over-the-counter noradrenergic drug used as both an appetite suppressant and a decongestant. A review of placebo-controlled trials using this agent concluded that weight loss was less than that achieved with prescription noradrenergic agents, but greater than that with placebo (63). It appears to be safe, albeit modestly effective, when used at dosages of 75 mg/day or less.

In a prior detailed analysis of the safety and efficacy of the noradrenergic group of drugs and fenfluramine, the FDA examined clinical data from nearly 10,000 patients reported in a large number of double-blind and two-drug comparison studies. At the end of 20 weeks, patients taking either drug or placebo had equal dropout rates, whereas patients taking drugs averaged about 0.5 lb (0.25 kg)/week greater weight loss. There were no significant differences in weight loss when any drugs in this class were used. Intermittent therapy (2 to 4 weeks on, 1 to 2 weeks off) was often as effective as uninterrupted treatment, except with fenfluramine, which sometimes led to depression after the drug was stopped.

Until recently, both fenfluramine (Pondimin) and dexfenfluramine (Redux) had been available as non-scheduled prescription drugs. Their prior widespread use was based on early trials showing substantial efficacy with minimal side effects (23), and the major obstacle to their more widespread use was thought to be their potential for inducing neurotoxicity and psychobehavioral abnormalities, which, although reported in animal studies, had yet to be documented in humans. However, these drugs have recently been associated with a number of severe adverse effects. The report that use of fenfluramine or its derivatives (especially dexfenfluramine) for more than 3 months was associated with a 23-fold increase in the occurrence of primary pulmonary hypertension raised appropriate concern regarding one major possible side effect of this class of drugs (1), although it was suggested that the health risks of developing this uncommon but serious condition were far outweighed by the health gains to be achieved by proper use of these agents in selected obese patients (39). More recently, significant cardiac valvular dysfunction was reported in 24 women evaluated an average of 12 months after initiation of fenfluramine plus phentermine cotherapy (15). Both right- and left-sided functional valvular abnormalities were noted. Histopathologic findings were consistent with those reported in patients with carcinoid and ergotamine-induced valvular disease. Eight of the women also exhibited pulmonary hypertension. A number of similar case reports, including several apparent drug-

related deaths, were rapidly filed with the FDA. Because of the uncertainty regarding the frequency of these serious adverse pulmonary and cardiac events and because of the consequent public health implications of these reports, both fenfluramine and dexfenfluramine were removed from the U.S. market in September, 1997. This action did not limit use of phentermine, although it effectively ended further use of the popular, but non-FDA approved, "fen-phen" combination, for which there were more than 18 million prescriptions in 1996. The experience with fenfluramine and dexfenfluramine further underscores the need for caution in the pharmacotherapeutic management of obesity.

For the noradrenergic agents, the most common side effects are mild and consist primarily of insomnia, dry mouth, and restlessness, to which tolerance tends to develop after several weeks. Noradrenergic agents are contraindicated in patients taking monoamine oxidase inhibitors, in whom hypertensive crises may occur. They may be used in hypertensive patients whose blood pressure is controlled on medication.

It is evident that individual patients exhibit considerable variations in short- and long-term responsivity to anorexigenic drugs and that patients often derive improved benefit, and avoid tolerance to the drug, after even small increases in dosage. Thus, there seems to be a role for the judicious use of these anorexigenic agents in carefully selected patients followed in medically supervised, comprehensive, therapeutic programs that include diet, exercise, and so on. However, as noted, exact guidelines for the optimal use of these drugs remain to be determined.

Although the 1997 Physicians Desk Reference still lists several amphetamines with indications for their use in promoting weight loss, these drugs should not be used for treatment of obesity because of their high risk for abuse.

There is considerable interest in pursuing the therapeutic potential of the anorexigenic properties of the antidepressant drugs *fluoxetine* (Prozac) and *sertraline* (Zoloft). These drugs exert their effects by blocking neuronal reuptake of serotonin in the central nervous system. Neither fluoxetine nor sertraline exerts any significant adverse effects on the heart. In addition, sertraline, unlike fluoxetine, does not significantly inhibit the hepatic microsomal enzyme system, thus minimizing the frequency of drug interactions. Clinical trials are currently under way to assess the efficacy and safety of these agents in the treatment of obesity.

Sibutramine is an FDA-approved drug that blocks presynaptic reuptake of both noradrenaline and serotonin, and thus may exert an effect on appetite regulation like that of combination drug therapy. Early trials have revealed a dose-responsive reduction in weight in otherwise healthy obese patients, with dosages of 30 mg/day (5-, 10-, and 15-mg capsules) leading to average weight losses of 6 to 7 kg after 24 weeks (50). Side effects reported include dry mouth, constipation, and insomnia, as well as modest increases in heart rate and blood pressure.

Orlistat, another investigational drug, is a gastric and pancreatic lipase inhibitor that decreases intestinal triglyceride hydrolysis and subsequent fat absorption. At dosages of 180 to 360 mg/day for 12 weeks, modest weight loss has occurred (18). Side effects include mild decrease in absorption of fat soluble vitamins and fecal soiling, which latter may limit its use.

Further advances in the development of anorexigenic and other drugs for inducing weight loss may derive from increased understanding of the molecular basis of altered energy intake and expenditure in the obesity syndromes, including the leptin/leptin receptor and β_3-adrenergic receptor systems (see above).

Surgical Therapy

Because of the increased morbidity and mortality associated with extreme degrees of obesity, and the generally unsatisfactory results produced by more conservative therapies, several surgical techniques have been devised to effect substantial weight loss in massively obese patients. Although some controversy exists regarding optimal selection criteria, surgery generally should be reserved for psychologically stable, highly motivated patients with massive obesity (usually 100 pounds [45 kg] or more above ideal body weight [40]) and repeated failures on strict diet and other therapies; severe medical consequences of obesity (e.g., hypertension, diabetes mellitus, hyperlipidemia, orthopedic problems) refractory to conventional therapy alone; and severe obesity-related despair, loss of self-esteem, and poor quality of life.

In the past, the most commonly used procedure was *jejunoileostomy*, performed by anastomosing the distal jejunum to the terminal ileum either as an end-to-side or end-to-end procedure; in the latter approach, the defunctionalized bowel was drained with an ileocolonic anastomosis. The major benefits from successful surgery were permanent (if no reanastomosis) weight loss varying from 10 to 15 to 100 kg within 1 to 3 years postoperatively, resulting primarily from a marked decrease in food intake (despite normal appetite), and only secondarily from an iatrogenic chronic malabsorption syndrome; substantial improvement in blood pressure, hyperinsulinemia, glucose intolerance, hyperlipidemia, and so on; and dramatic improvement in sense of well-being and self-esteem.

Unfortunately, the list of adverse effects associated with the intraoperative or postoperative course of jejunoileostomy patients grew progressively more formidable. Even in large medical centers with experienced personnel, the overall mortality rate after surgery varied from 3 to 5%. Serious perioperative complications included pulmonary embolus, renal failure, wound infection, gastrointestinal bleeding, and pancreatitis. Among the adverse long-term effects were chronic diarrhea and flatulence, malabsorption with electrolyte and vitamin imbalance, cholelithiasis, urinary tract stones (calcium oxalate), hyperuricemia, polyarthralgias, intestinal bacterial overgrowth (pseudoobstructive megacolon and bypass enteropathy), and progressive hepatic dysfunction leading to hepatic

failure. In one large series (24), 58% of patients experienced potentially life-threatening complications or major reoperations; 17% of patients required surgical reversal of reanastomosis, usually because of severe hepatic cirrhosis and failure.

Gastric bypass surgery and its variants (e.g., gastroplasty), currently more popular than jejunoileostomy (31), induce significant weight loss by promoting decreased oral food intake while preserving normal gastrointestinal absorptive and digestive function. In the gastric bypass procedure, the proximal 10% of the stomach is fashioned into a 15- to 30-mL pouch by anastomosis to the jejunum through a 0.9- to 1.2-cm channel, thus producing rapid gastric filling, slow emptying, and prolonged satiety. One year postoperatively, weight loss in one review (31) of approximately 1500 reported patients averaged 30 to 35% of baseline weight, with one-third of patients losing 50 kg or more. Although carbohydrate and bile acids are absorbed normally after gastric bypass, glucose intolerance and hyperlipidemia (especially hypertriglyceridemia) are, nonetheless, substantially improved; in addition, liver function does not worsen, and malabsorption and kidney stones do not occur. Deficiencies of calcium or of iron, or B_{12} hypovitaminosis, occur occasionally. By taking frequent small feedings of high-calorie foods, it is possible for patients to "outeat" the bypass (the soft calorie syndrome). Within the first postoperative month, vomiting occurs two to three times weekly in nearly 65 to 70% of patients. However, this complication becomes progressively less frequent, so that by 2 years postoperatively it occurs in less than 10% of patients. Other complications of the procedure include channel ulcers or obstruction, bile reflux, and the dumping syndrome. In centers with experienced personnel, the overall mortality rate has been reduced from 3 to 1% but remains as high as 8 to 10% in patients over 50 years old. Reoperation necessitated either by surgical complications or unsatisfactory weight loss appears to be uncommon, and takedown of the gastric bypass has been described in less than 1% of patients.

The common *gastric restrictive operations*, such as vertical banded gastroplasty, create a 10- to 15-mL stapled proximal gastric pouch that limits receptive capacity. The opening between this pouch and the remainder of the stomach is externally banded to create an inner diameter of about 1 cm to delay emptying of solid food. Thus, the distal 80 to 90% of the stomach is no longer excluded from the flow of nutrients, and gastrointestinal continuity is maintained. Difficulties with gastric restrictive operations include distension of the wall of the proximal pouch, rupture of the staple line, or erosion of the band into the stomach. As with the gastric bypass procedures, postoperatively some patients exhibit the soft calorie syndrome or vomiting.

Although more research is needed to determine the long-term efficacy and safety of gastric bypass surgery and its variants, it appears that these procedures may be of considerable benefit in the treatment of selected morbidly obese patients. In contrast, the striking complication rates associated with jejunoileal bypass procedures militate strongly against use of this technique in all but the most extreme instances.

A recent National Institutes of Health Consensus Development Panel recommended that gastric bypass or restrictive procedures could be considered for well-informed and motivated severely obese patients in whom the operative risks were acceptable; that patients who are candidates for surgical procedures should be selected carefully after evaluation by a multidisciplinary team with medical, surgical, psychiatric, and nutritional expertise; that surgery be performed by a surgeon who has substantial experience in the particular procedure and who works in a clinical setting with adequate support for all aspects of management and assessment; and that patients undergo lifelong medical, psychologic, and nutritional surveillance after surgery.

PREVENTION OF OBESITY

Current rapid advances in understanding the biological bases for the obesity syndromes suggest that future therapies will be more specifically and effectively targeted toward preventing, as well as reversing, the underlying pathophysiologic abnormalities leading to excess body fatness. Nonetheless, as is evident from the preceding discussion, psychologic and sociocultural factors play prominent roles in the development and maintenance of nearly all types of obesity, and lifestyle modifications should be incorporated into all preventative and treatment strategies. The finding that behavior modification techniques can benefit not only individual obese patients but also groups of such people, even in commercially run weight-reducing programs, is provocative and suggests that this approach to weight reduction may have much wider application.

General References*

Bray GA, ed. Obesity. Endocrinol Metabol Clin North Am 25(4), 1996.
  Excellent contemporary compendium of information on obesity-related research and clinical practice.
Diet and health. Implications for reducing chronic disease risk. Committee on Diet and Health. Commission on Life Sciences. National Research Council. Washington, DC: National Academy Press, 1989.
  Comprehensive, critical assessment of the roles of the major macronutrients and micronutrients as risk factors for diet-related chronic illnesses.
Foster WR, Burton BT, Hubbard VBS, eds. Gastrointestinal surgery for severe obesity. Proceedings of an NIH Consensus Development Conference. Am J Clin Nutr 55(Suppl 2), 1992.
  Excellent account of a multidisciplinary approach to evaluation and management of the obese patient.
Rosenbaum M, Leibel RL, Hirsch J. Obesity. N Engl J Med 337:396, 1997.
  A recent authoritative review.

---

*Bold print (general references) and bold numerals (specific references) denote published controlled clinical trials, meta-analyses, or consensus-based recommendations.

Specific References

1. Abenheim L, Moride Y, Brenot F, et al. Appetite-suppressant drugs and the risk of primary pulmonary hypertension. N Engl J Med 335:609, 1996.
2. Amatruda JM, Biddle TL, Patton ML, Lockwood DH. Vigorous supplementation of a hypocaloric diet prevents cardiac arrhythmias and mineral depletion. Am J Med 74:1016, 1983.
3. Andres R. Mortality and obesity: the rationale for age-specific height-weight tables. In: Hazzard WR, Bierman EL, Blass JP, et al, eds. Principles of geriatric medicine and gerontology. New York: McGraw-Hill, 1994;844.
4. Arner P. The beta 3-adrenergic-receptor—a cause and cure of obesity? N Engl J Med 333:382, 1995.
5. Ballor DL, Keesey RE. A meta-analysis of the factors affecting exercise-induced changes in body mass, fat mass, and fat-free mass in males and females. Int J Obesity Related Metab Disorders 15:717, 1991.
6. Beutler E, Kuhl W, Sacks P. Sodium-potassium-ATPase activity is influenced by ethnic origin and not by obesity. N Engl J Med 309:756, 1983.
7. Bouchard C, Despres JP, Tremblay A. Genetics of obesity and human energy metabolism. Proc Nutr Soc 50:139, 1991.
8. Bray GA, Kral JG, Bjorntorp P. Hepatic sodium-potassium-dependent ATPase in obesity. N Engl J Med 304:1580, 1981.
9. Bray GA, Teague RJ. An algorithm for the medical evaluation of obese patients. In: Stunkard AJ, ed. Obesity. Philadelphia: WB Saunders, 1980.
10. Broussard BA, Johnson A, Himes JH, et al. Prevalence of obesity in American Indians and Alaska Natives. Am J Clin Nutr 53:1535S, 1991.
11. Build Study 1979. Chicago, Society of Actuaries and Association of Life Insurance Medical Directors of America, 1980.
12. Carney RM, Goldberg AP. Weight gain after cessation of cigarette smoking: a possible role for adipose-tissue lipoprotein lipase. N Engl J Med 310:614, 1984.
13. Caro JF, Kolacynski JW, Nyce MR, et al. Decreased cerebrospinal-fluid/serum leptin ratio in obesity: a possible mechanism for leptin resistance. Lancet 348:159, 1996.
14. Clement K, Vaisse C, Manning BS, et al. Genetic variation in the beta 3-adrenergic receptor and an increased capacity to gain weight in patients with morbid obesity. N Engl J Med 333:352, 1995.
15. Connolly HM, Crary JL, McGoon MD, et al. Valvular heart disease associated with fenfluramine-phentermine. N Engl J Med 337:581, 1997.
16. Considine RV, Sinha, Heiman ML, et al. Serum immunoreactive-leptin concentrations in normal-weight and obese humans. N Engl J Med 334:292, 1996.
17. DeLuise M, Blackburn GL, Flier JS. Reduced activity of the red-cell sodium-potassium pump in human obesity. N Engl J Med 303:1017, 1980.
18. Drent ML, Larsson I, William-Olssen T, et al. Orlistat (RO 18-0647), a lipase inhibitor, in the treatment of human obesity: a multiple dose study. Int J Obesity 19:221, 1995.
19. Evans DJ, Hoffman RG, Kalkhoff RK, Kissebah AH. Relationship of androgenic activity to body fat topography, fat cell morphology and metabolic aberrations in premenopausal women. J Clin Endocrinol Metab 57:304, 1983.
20. Garrow J, Summerbell C. Meta-analysis on the effect of exercise on the composition of weight loss. Int J Obesity Related Metab Disorders 18:516, 1994.
21. Genuth SM, Castro JH, Vertes V. Weight reduction in obesity by outpatient semistarvation. JAMA 230:987, 1974.
22. Goldstein DJ. Beneficial health effects of modest weight loss. Int J Obesity 16:397, 1992.
23. Guy-Grand B, Apfelbaum M, Crepaldi G, et al. International trial of long-term dexfenfluramine in obesity. Lancet 26:1142, 1989.
24. Haverson JD, Wise L, Wazna MF, Ballinger WF. Jejunoileal bypass for morbid obesity. A critical appraisal. Am J Med 64:461, 1978.
25. Hazuda HP, Mitchell BD, Haffner SM, Stern MP. Obesity in Mexican-American subgroups: findings from the San Antonio Heart Study. Am J Clin Nutr 53:1529S, 1991.

26. Hirsch J, Batchelor B. Adipose tissue cellularity in human obesity. Clin Endocrinol Metab 5:299, 1976.

27. Hubert HB, Feinleib M, McNamara PM, Castelli WP. Obesity as an independent risk factor for cardiovascular disease: a 26 year follow-up of participants in the Framingham heart study. Circulation 67:968, 1983.

28. Hymsfield SB, Wang J, Heshka JJ, Pierson RN. Dual-photon absorptiometry: comparison of bone mineral and soft tissue mass measurements in vivo with established methods. Am J Clin Nutr 49:1283, 1989.

29. Kaplan NM. The deadly quartet. Upper body obesity, glucose intolerance, hypertriglyceridemia, and hypertension. Arch Intern Med 149:1514, 1989.

30. Keys A, ed. Coronary heart disease in seven countries. American Heart Association Monograph No. 29, 1970.

31. Kral JG. Surgical treatment of obesity. Med Clin North Am 73:251, 1989.

32. Krotkiewski M, Bjorntorp P, Sjostrom L, Smith U. Impact of obesity on metabolism in men and women—importance of regional adipose tissue distribution. J Clin Invest 72:1150, 1983.

33. Kuczmarski RJ. Prevalence of overweight and weight gain in the United States. Am J Clin Nutr 55:495S, 1992.

34. Kuczmarski RJ, Flegal KM, Campbell SM, Johnson CL. Increasing prevalence of overweight among US adults: the National Health and Nutrition Examination Surveys, 1960 to 1991. JAMA 272:205, 1994.

35. Lantigua RA, Amatruda JM, Biddle TL, et al. Cardiac arrhythmias associated with a liquid protein diet for the treatment of obesity. N Engl J Med 303:735, 1980.

36. Larson B, Svardsudd K, Welin L, et al. Abdominal adipose tissue distribution, obesity, and risk of cardiovascular disease and death: 13 year follow-up of participants in the study of men born in 1913. BMJ 288:1401, 1984.

37. Lee L, Kumar S, Leong L. The impact of five-month basic military training on the body weight and body fat of 197 moderately to severely obese Singaporean males aged 17-19 years. Int J Obesity Related Metab Disorders 18:105, 1994.

38. Lissner L, Odell PM, D'Agostino RB, et al. Variability of body weight and health outcomes in the Framingham population. N Engl J Med 324:1839, 1991.

39. Manson JE, Faich GA. Pharmacotherapy for obesity—do the benefits outweigh the risks? N Engl J Med 335:659, 1996.

40. Metropolitan Height and Weight Tables, 1983. Stat Bull Metrop Life Found 64(Jan–June):2, 1983.

41. Muller DC, Elahi D, Pratley RE, et al. An epidemiological test of the hyperinsulinemia-hypertension hypothesis. J Clin Endocrinol Metab 76:544, 1993.

42. Must A, Jacques PF, Dallal GE, et al. Long-term morbidity and mortality of overweight adolescents—a follow-up of the Harvard Growth Study of 1922 to 1935. N Engl J Med 327:1350, 1992.

43. NIH Technology Assessment Conference Panel. Methods for voluntary weight loss and control. Ann Intern Med 119:764, 1993.

44. O'Connor KO, Stevens TE, Blackman MR. GH and Aging. In: Juul A, Jorgensen JOL, eds. Growth hormone in adults. Cambridge, UK: Cambridge University Press, 1996;323.

45. Peiris AN, Sothmann MS, Hoffman RG, et al. Adiposity, fat distribution, and cardiovascular risk. Ann Intern Med 110:867, 1989.

46. Peiris AN, Gustafson AB, Kissebah AH. Health and regional adiposity: implications for the clinician. Yearbook of endocrinology. Chicago: Yearbook Medical Publishers, 1989.

47. Pi-Sunyer FX. The role of very-low-calorie diets in obesity. Am J Clin Nutr 56:240S, 1992.

48. Ravussin E, Lillioja S, Knowles WC, et al. Reduced rate of energy expenditure as a risk factor for body weight gain. N Engl J Med 318:467, 1988.

49. Ronnemaa T, Karonen S-L, Rissanen A, et al. Relation between plasma leptin levels and measures of body fat in identical twins discordant for obesity. Ann Intern Med 126:26, 1997.

50. Ryan DH, Kaiser P, Bray GA. Sibutramine: a novel new agent for obesity treatment. Obesity Res 3(Suppl 4):553s, 1995.

51. Schwartz RS, Brunzell JD. Increase of adipose tissue lipoprotein lipase activity with weight loss. J Clin Invest 67:1425, 1981.

52. Schwartz RS, Shuman WP, Larson V, et al. The effect of intensive endurance exercise training on body fat distribution in young and older men. Metabolism 40:545, 1991.

53. Shimokata H, Tobin JD, Muller DC, et al. Studies in the distribution of body fat: I. Effects of age, sex, and obesity. J Gerontol 44:M66, 1989.

54. Shimokata H, Muller DC, Andres R. Studies in the distribution of body fat. III. Effects of cigarette smoking. JAMA 261:1169, 1989.

55. Simopoulos AP, Van Itallie TBV. Body weight, health, and longevity. Ann Intern Med 100:285, 1984.

56. Society of Actuaries. Build and blood pressure study. Vol 1. Chicago: The Society, 1959.

57. Stunkard AJ, Sorensen TIA, Hanis C, et al. An adoption study of human obesity. N Engl J Med 314:193, 1986.

58. Superko HR. Exercise training, serum lipids, and lipoprotein particles: is there a change threshold? Med Sci Sports Exerc 23:677, 1991.

59. Thompson PD, Cullinane EM, Sady SP, et al. High density lipoprotein metabolism in endurance athletes and sedentary men. Circulation 84:140, 1991.

60. Troiano RP, Flegal KM, Kuczmarski RJ, et al. Overweight prevalence and trends for children and adolescents. The National Health and Nutrition Examination Survey. Arch Pediatr Adolesc Med 149:1085, 1995.

61. Van Itallie TB. Liquid protein mayhem. JAMA 240:144, 1978.

62. Walston J, Silver K, Bogardus C, et al. Time of onset of non-insulin–dependent diabetes mellitus and genetic variation in the beta 3-adrenergic-receptor gene. N Engl J Med 333:343, 1995.

63. Weintraub M. Phenylpropanolamine as an anorexiant agent in weight control: a review of published and unpublished studies. Clin Pharmacol Ther 5:53, 1985.

64. Weintraub M, Sundaresan PR, Cox C. Long-term weight control study VI. Clin Pharmacol Ther 51:619, 1992.

65. Williamson DA, Perrin LA. Behavioral therapy for obesity. Endocrinol Metabol Clin North Am 25(4):943, 1996.

66. Zhang Y, Proenca R, Maffei M, et al. Positional cloning of the mouse obese gene and its human homologue. Nature 372:425, 1994.

CHAPTER 77

Common Problems in Reproductive Endocrinology

S. MITCHELL HARMAN, MD, PhD
MARC R. BLACKMAN, MD

INTRODUCTION

Relatively few physicians are entirely comfortable investigating and managing sexual and reproductive problems. This is partly because medical school curricula and postgraduate training have generally not dealt adequately with reproductive medicine and partly because sexuality and gender identity are psychologically "loaded" issues, with the potential to produce acute feelings of embarrassment in both patient and physician. Thus, many physicians regard complaints involving the reproductive system as esoteric, to be referred immediately to an appropriate specialist. On the contrary, however, sexual and reproductive dysfunction is far from rare. For example, nearly 50% of men will experience some degree of impotence between the ages of 20 and 50 (27); up to 10% of married couples have trouble conceiving; and approximately 1 in 400 males is born with Klinefelter's

syndrome (XXY sex chromosomes). Also the constant outpouring of articles and programs dealing with human sexuality in the popular media has led to a general expectation of "normal" sexual function as part of a healthy lifestyle. Thus, sexual dysfunction, even in the elderly, is likely to be perceived as a health problem. It is therefore important that generalists have adequate knowledge of reproductive and sexual disorders and of related history taking, physical diagnosis, and laboratory testing to allow them to distinguish patients who require only reassurance or simple treatment from those who should be referred to a specialist for more complex testing or therapy.

SEXUAL AND REPRODUCTIVE PHYSIOLOGY

Levels of Sexual Differentiation

Sexual differentiation can be viewed as two parallel continua, the first proceeding in time from conception to adulthood and the second in biological "depth" from genetic to psychologic to social as follows: (a) genetic sex is determined at conception when the egg, bearing an X chromosome, is fertilized by a sperm bearing either a Y (XY = male) or an X (XX = female) chromosome. The Y chromosome contains a gene that specifies a product essential for differentiation of the primal gonad into a testis, but, because the X chromosome carries genes that regulate Y chromosome function, the testis differentiation genes are only expressed normally in the presence of a single X chromosome. Active function of two X chromosomes, in the absence of a Y chromosome, must occur during fetal life in order to produce differentiation of the fetal gonad into an ovary. Thus, genetic sex determines (b) gonadal (or somatic) sex. The presence or absence of testicular function determines (c) primary (or phenotypic) sex, which is defined by the development of the genitalia. This is because the embryonic testis produces two critical molecules. The first is testosterone, the major male sex steroid, which causes the development of the undifferentiated external genitalia into a penis and scrotum and of the wolffian (primitive mesonephric) duct system into epididymis, vas deferens, prostate, and seminal vesicles. The second is a peptide, müllerian-inhibiting substance (MIS), which mediates the regression of the primitive müllerian duct structures. In the absence of MIS the müllerian ducts develop into a vagina, uterus, and fallopian tubes; without the action of testosterone, female external genitalia (labia and clitoris) form. Thus, normal infantile female genitalia will develop in the absence of both ovaries and testes. It is the primary sex characteristics (appearance of the external genitalia) that identify an individual's apparent gender at birth. Further sexual development, defined as (d) secondary sex, occurs at puberty as a result of greatly increased secretion by the gonads of sex steroid hormones. In males, growth of male pattern body and pubic hair and beard, as well as increase in muscle mass, deepening of voice, and onset of male libido with ejaculations and increased frequency of erections are characteristic effects of testosterone. In females, rounding of body contours with breast growth and subcutaneous deposition of fat in the hips and buttocks, and also the onset of menses, are effects of cyclic estrogen secretion, whereas growth of pubic and axillary hair (and probably libido) are manifestations of adrenal and, to a lesser extent ovarian, androgen secretion. Both sexes experience a period of accelerated increase in height at puberty, which is followed by closure of the epiphyses and cessation of growth of long bones. It is the hormone-dependent secondary sex characteristics that help define adult sexual identity and that stabilize the individual's *(e) tertiary (or psychologic) sex* which is the way in which an person identifies himself or herself. Only a handful of mammalian species have a level of sexual dimorphism as overt as that of humans (e.g., lions, baboons, gorillas). The extent to which the physical differences between the sexes were reinforced by survival versus sexual "signaling" functions in our own and other species during evolution remains controversial. What is clear is that, in humans, identification as a man or a woman is crucial to balanced psychologic and social function and is a critical component of self-image and quality of life. It should be borne in mind that any condition that alters a patient's perceived masculinity or femininity is felt as profoundly threatening, well beyond its biological manifestations.

Male Reproductive Physiology

Activity of the male reproductive system is regulated by the neurosecretory cells contained in the hypothalamus. The axons of these cells end on capillaries of the median eminence into which, at irregular intervals of 60 to 120 minutes, they secrete surges of a decapeptide, *gonadotropin-releasing hormone (GnRH)*. Rather than returning blood directly to the heart, these vessels collect into the pituitary portal veins that ramify as sinusoidal capillaries within the pituitary gland. Thus GnRH reaches the pituitary in high concentrations where it stimulates gonadotropic cells to secrete luteinizing hormone (LH) and follicle-stimulating hormone (FSH). LH and FSH are large heterodimeric glycoprotein molecules, each of which consists of a common (identical for both hormones as well as for thyroid-stimulating hormone [TSH]) α subunit and a hormone-specific β subunit.

FSH acts directly on the Sertoli (support) cells of the seminiferous tubules to initiate and maintain early stages of maturation of the male germ cells (i.e., spermatogenesis). Induction of male fertility depends on the presence of FSH. FSH-stimulated Sertoli cells in turn secrete a peptide hormone called *inhibin* that downregulates pituitary production of FSH, forming a closed loop negative feedback system (Fig 77.1).

LH acts on the Leydig (interstitial) cells of the testis to stimulate testosterone secretion. Testosterone has effects within the testis to promote spermatogenesis and is also the major circulating steroid that produces

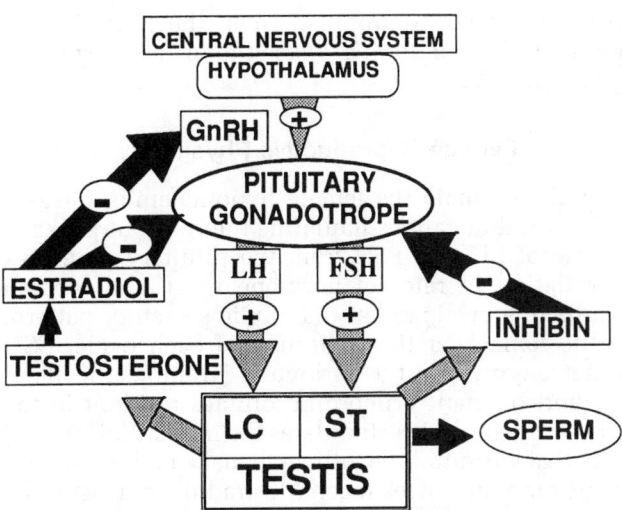

Figure 77.1. Reproductive endocrinology in the male. A variety of central nervous system inputs, from both exogenous (e.g., environmental stress) and endogenous (e.g., biorhythms) sources, act via neurotransmitters and neuropeptides to influence the amplitude and frequency of pulsatile hypothalamic neuronal output (secretion = light gray arrows) of gonadotropin releasing hormone (GnRH) into the pituitary portal system. GnRH stimulates pituitary gonadotropic cells to release LH and FSH. LH induces the Leydig cell (LC) compartment of the testis to secrete testosterone (T). FSH and T act together to stimulate spermatogenesis in the seminiferous tubule compartment (ST). T acts via negative feedback (dark gray arrows) to inhibit gonadotropin and GnRH secretion, probably after aromatization locally to estradiol. Inhibin, produced by the ST in response to FSH, also acts by negative feedback to decrease FSH release.

and maintains male secondary sex characteristics (see above). In plasma, testosterone is partially bound to a protein, *sex hormone–binding globulin (SHBG)* that decreases the testosterone clearance rate. SHBG bound testosterone is not directly available to target cells but provides a circulating hormone reservoir in equilibrium with the free or bioactive fraction. This free fraction correlates better than does total plasma testosterone with peripheral androgenic effects. Whether a cell responds to androgens depends on whether it contains androgen receptor protein. In the cells of hair follicles, pubic skin, prostate gland and other male sex organs testosterone is reduced by a cytoplasmic enzyme, 5 α-reductase, to 5 α-dihydrotestosterone (DHT). It is DHT that binds specifically to the androgen receptors of these organs. In certain other tissues (e.g., skeletal muscle), androgen action is mediated directly by testosterone without reduction to DHT. Physiologic functions of testosterone include stimulation of growth and secretory activity of the prostate and seminal vesicles. Androgens also exert important systemic effects such as promoting positive nitrogen and calcium balance (with increased muscle and bone formation) and augmenting function of apocrine and sebaceous glands of the skin, which may result in comedones and acne. Testosterone also exerts negative "feedback" at the hypothalamus and pituitary to inhibit secretion of gonadotropins. Thus, the reproductive hormones in men form a "closed-loop" autoregulated system (Fig 77.1).

Female Reproductive Physiology

As in the male the female hypothalamus releases GnRH rhythmically, stimulating intermittent peaks of release of LH and FSH from the pituitary. Complex modulation of rates of hormone release in women results in a cyclic rather than tonic secretory pattern. In the female, at the beginning of each cycle, FSH initiates growth of the periovular (granulosa) cells of a cohort of small primordial follicles resident in the ovary from birth. LH stimulates the interstitial (thecal) cells that surround the follicle to make androgens and small amounts of estrogens (estradiol and estrone). The granulosa cells convert thecal androgens to estradiol. Estradiol in concert with FSH, produces further growth of follicles by proliferation of the granulosa cells. A dominant (Graafian) follicle emerges in each cycle as the major source of estradiol secretion, while adjacent follicles undergo atresia (degeneration). Rising estrogen secretion in this early or follicular phase of the cycle induces proliferation of the uterine endometrium, and by a "positive feedback" effect, causes a sudden surge of LH secretion around day 14 of the cycle. This LH surge causes the follicle to release the ovum (ovulation). LH then induces the follicle to become a functioning corpus luteum, producing both estradiol and progesterone during the latter half (luteal phase) of the cycle. Progesterone acts on the uterus to produce a secretory endometrium, rich in glycogen and, in concert with estrogen, causes a negative feedback effect that gradually reduces the secretion of LH and FSH. With loss of gonadotropic stimulation, the corpus luteum involutes, steroid secretion diminishes, and the endometrium, left without estrogen and progesterone support, sloughs off as the menstrual flow. At this point, with estradiol and progesterone negative feedback at low levels, FSH and LH begin to rise, a new cohort of small follicles is recruited, and the stage is set for the next cycle. Ovarian estradiol is the major estrogen in cycling women. Estrone, a weaker estrogen, is mainly formed peripherally in fat, liver, kidney, and other tissues by conversion of adrenal and ovarian androgenic precursors. The secretion of androgens also increases at puberty in the female. Female reproductive hormone relationships are illustrated in Figure 77.2.

Male and Female Hormones and Libido

The reader is referred to Chapter 18 ("Sexual Disorders") for a description of the stages of the sexual response that characterize sexual physiology in men and women. Experimental evidence demonstrates that endogenous testosterone (20) stimulates sexual behavior in the male. Recently, endogenous dihydrotestosterone has been shown to play a role as well (47). Observations on men who are acutely deprived of

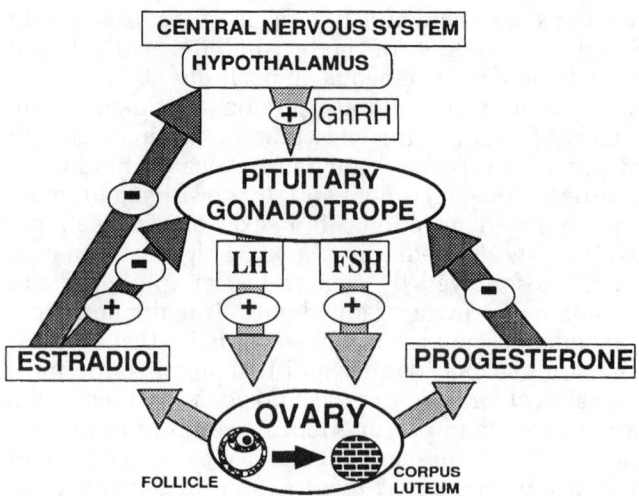

Figure 77.2. Reproductive endocrinology in the female. The central nervous system releases neurotransmitters and neuropeptides which influence the amplitude and frequency of pulsatile hypothalamic neuronal secretion (secretion = light gray arrows) of gonadotropin-releasing hormone (GnRH) into the pituitary portal system. GnRH stimulates pituitary gonadotropic cells to release LH and FSH. LH stimulates the thecal cells of the ovary to make androgens (e.g., androstenedione) which are converted into estrogens, mainly estradiol (E_2), by the follicular granulosa cells. Estradiol and FSH act together to promote follicular growth and maturation. At midcycle a sudden increase in secretion of LH induces ovulation and conversion of the follicle to a corpus luteum which secretes both E_2 and progesterone (P). E_2 initially exerts positive feedback control on LH secretion leading to the ovulatory peak. Later in the cycle, E_2 and P act together to inhibit gonadotropin secretion.

testosterone by inhibition of the hypothalamic–pituitary axis with a GnRH analog reveal variable degrees of loss of interest in sexual activity in as little as 2 to 4 weeks (45). Men who are chronically androgen deficient experience reduced arousal in response to sexual cues (e.g., female nudity) as well as less frequent erections and ejaculation. In a study of men with varying degrees of chronic hypogonadism (13), findings suggested the existence of two thresholds for serum testosterone: a level below which the sexual response to erotic stimuli is reduced but nocturnal erections remain intact, and a lower level below which erections are also impaired. Many hypogonadal men also report heightened emotional sensitivity, weepiness, and loss of aggressive interest, focus, and drive. In women, the relationship between libido and sex hormones is less obvious, but it has been reported that women are more likely to initiate sexual contact during phases of the menstrual cycle when androgen activity is highest (1), that adolescent girls' initiation of coital activity is correlated with plasma testosterone levels (35), and that the addition of androgen to estrogen replacement in postmenopausal women results in higher levels of sexual interest and activity (64). Clinicians also find that women with androgen hypersecretion often report heightened sex drive and increased sexual content of dreams and fantasies. By contrast, the pituitary hormone prolactin, which in women is responsible for lactation, is an "antisexual" hormone that appears to reduce libido in both women and men. In women, estrogens are necessary to maintain the vagina and the external genitalia in their mature reproductive states. In the absence of adequate estrogen, genital atrophy may result in pain during intercourse, with resultant loss of interest in sexual activity.

SEXUAL AND REPRODUCTIVE DYSFUNCTION IN MEN
Hypogonadism

Etiologies

Failure of the testes to secrete adequate amounts of testosterone for development or maintenance of male secondary sex characteristics, body composition, and libido results in the syndrome of male hypogonadism. Although, for purposes of diagnosis and classification a level of 300 ng/dL of total serum testosterone or 120 ng/dL of free or "bioactive" testosterone are usually (depending on the assays employed) used as the cutoff points for diagnosis of hypogonadism, the clinician should bear in mind that these thresholds are derived from the 95% confidence limits around the mean for a population of young healthy men. Thus, the definition of hypogonadism they provide is statistical rather than functional. There are no good experimental data that define the actual levels of total or free testosterone below which testosterone effect is suboptimal for various organ systems. Therefore hypogonadism in a patient should be approached with the entire complex of signs and symptoms in mind and not rigidly defined by a threshold level of a single hormone.

It is helpful to classify male hypogonadism along each of the three axes shown in Figure 77.3. These axes describe, respectively, the locus of the underlying lesion *(central, gonadal, or peripheral);* the type of

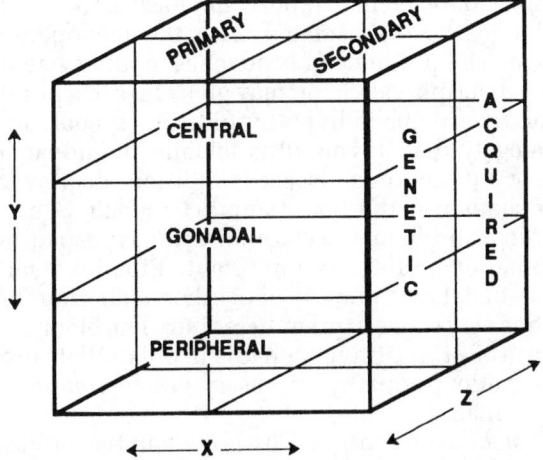

Figure 77.3. Each axis of the cube represents a different way of classifying hypogonadism. There are 12 possible categories and, hence, 12 "compartments" in the cube. The *y* axis represents anatomical location (central, gonadal, peripheral); the *z* axis etiology (genetic, acquired); and the *x* axis time of onset (primary, secondary).

Table 77.1.   Classification of Male Hypogonadism

Classification	Criteria
According to Location of Lesion	
Central (hypothalamic or pituitary)	Gonadotropins ↓ or →
	Testosterone ↓
Gonadal (testis)	Gonadotropins ↑
	Testosterone ↓
Peripheral (failure of end-organ response)	Gonadotropins ↑
	Testosterone ↑ or →
According to Etiology	
Genetic	History (especially family history)
	Buccal smear, karyotype
Acquired	History, physical examination, radiology
	Evidence of infection, trauma, neoplasia, etc.
According to Time of Onset	
Primary (failure of pubertal development)	History, physical examination
Secondary (loss of previously developed libido and secondary sex characteristics)	

underlying pathophysiology *(genetic or acquired),* and whether the onset of clinical manifestations occurs before *(primary)* or after *(secondary)* puberty. Criteria for classification are shown in Table 77.1. Use of this system of classification narrows the range of possibilities and helps one to arrive more quickly at the correct diagnosis. Examples of the classification of various hypogonadal conditions follow.

Central hypogonadism is dysfunction primarily at the level of the pituitary or the hypothalamus. It is characterized by deficient gonadotropin secretion. One example is *Kallmann's syndrome,* which is associated with hyposmia or anosmia, and is due to defective forebrain development leading to absent hypothalamic GnRH secretion. Kallmann's is also *genetic* (i.e., an inherited condition), and *primary,* in that it is expressed as a failure to mature sexually. *Acquired* hypothalamic failure may also occur, usually from diencephalic tumors or granulomatous disease. Occasionally, pituitary hypogonadism is congenital (i.e., *genetic*), but more commonly it is acquired. The etiology may be infectious (e.g., tuberculosis or systemic mycosis), traumatic, vascular (as in infarction with pituitary apoplexy), or most commonly, neoplastic (usually either a nonsecreting adenoma, or a craniopharyngioma). *Central* hypogonadism may also be associated with functioning pituitary tumors, including those that secrete prolactin (prolactinoma), growth hormone (acromegaly), or adrenocorticotropin (Cushing's disease). Rarely, apparently nonsecreting pituitary adenomas may produce a gonadotropin (usually FSH) or a β subunit thereof leading to confusion of central with gonadal hypogonadism, which is characterized by elevated FSH levels.

Gonadal. The most common cause of *genetic, gonadal* hypogonadism in phenotypic males is Klinefelter's syndrome, which, in its classic form, is caused by chromosomal nondisjunction producing XXY genetic sex. These patients have small, firm testes and gynecomastia. They usually enter puberty but fail to progress fully and present with a "eunuchoid habitus" (see below). They typically have relative impotence, small phallus, and often, some degree of gender confusion. Testosterone levels are generally in the low to low normal range (200 to 350 ng/dL). *Genetic, gonadal* hypogonadism may also occur if one or more critical enzymes in the sex steroid synthetic pathway is missing or reduced in activity. Usually such defects involve enzymes common to the adrenal gland and testis and produce ambiguous genitalia or female phenotypic sex in XY individuals. *Acquired* causes of *gonadal* hypogonadism include trauma, infection (usually viral such as mumps orchitis or granulomatous, as in urogenital tuberculosis), and autoimmunity. Autoimmune damage to the testis may occur either alone or as part of a complex of multiple endocrine failure (Hashimoto's thyroiditis, idiopathic Addison's disease, adult-onset diabetes mellitus, hypoparathyroidism, or pernicious anemia). Occasionally, a varicocele will produce partial hypogonadism. Whether these entities result in *secondary* or *primary* hypogonadism depends on the time of life at which the damage occurs.

Peripheral. Peripheral hypogonadism is always *genetic* and is due to absence or dysfunction of androgen receptor protein. It is expressed as a continuum from complete androgen insensitivity or "testicular feminization" in which the phenotype is female (affected patients have female external genitalia at birth and normal estrogenization at puberty, but lack a uterus, and hence menses), through varying degrees of partial androgen sensitivity, in which midline fusion of labioscrotal structures is highly variable (Reifenstein's syndrome), producing gender confusion, and ending with minor defects such as hypospadias and cryptorchidism, in which phenotypic gender is still clearly male. In all cases, the genetic sex is male (i.e., XY).

Approach to the Patient

The approach to the patient with symptoms suggestive of hypogonadism should be directed first at determining whether hypogonadism truly exists, then at its classification as discussed above, next at discovering its specific cause, and finally at providing appropriate therapy and/or referral for the condition diagnosed.

Patient presentations. Primary hypogonadism may present before puberty as genital intersexuality. A finding of hypospadias, cryptorchidism, or ambiguous genitalia in a patient with symptoms or signs of hypogonadism should lead to further diagnostic procedures. These patients are usually identified at birth and referred to an appropriate specialist so that they rarely present as a diagnostic problem for the primary care practitioner. However, boys are often brought to the attention of physicians by parents concerned with failure of pubertal onset or progression (see Chapter 5).

Primary hypogonadism is more commonly expressed as failure of secondary sex characteristics to appear at an appropriate age. It may stem from almost any of the causes cited above and must be differentiated from constitutional delayed puberty, which is a common, idiopathic, self-limited, familial condition. A strong family history of late blooming and a finding of beginning enlargement of the testicles are reassuring in this regard. A set of standards for pubertal development of adolescent boys is available (see Chapter 5, Table 5.5). In general, any boy reaching 16 years of age without signs of pubertal onset or who begins but does not complete puberty by age 18 deserves further investigation. The index of suspicion should be heightened if the patient has a history of childhood genital abnormalities (e.g., hypospadias or undescended testes) or signs or symptoms of a disease that can produce hypogonadism (e.g., severe headaches, indicating intracranial tumor).

The gradual loss of male secondary sex characteristics and libido (i.e., *secondary* hypogonadism) is a third presentation of male hypogonadism. This may be so insidious that it is taken for normal by the patient, especially in a man progressing from middle age toward old age. Sometimes hypogonadism is recognized only during investigation of some related condition, such as hypothyroidism, adrenal failure, severe headaches, or renal tuberculosis. Finally, and probably most common, is the complaint of impotence, which may be the earliest manifestation of hypogonadism, but is also seen in various other physical and psychologic conditions. Impotence is discussed more completely below and also in Chapter 18.

History. A proper history should include a chronicle of pubertal progression, with time of appearance of pubic hair, beard growth, voice change, growth spurts, erections, and ejaculations. Of critical interest are loss or diminution of libido and erections or ejaculations, slowing of beard growth, thinning of body and pubic hair, changes in the breast (i.e., swelling or tenderness), and loss of aggressive impulse or drive. Severely hypogonadal men may report "hot flashes" and sweats similar to those associated with the menopause in women. The presence of headaches, double vision, or reduced peripheral vision may give clues to a pituitary tumor. Symptoms of hypothyroidism, adrenal failure, acromegaly, diabetes mellitus, anemia, pulmonary disease, or autoimmune disease (conditions dealt with in other chapters of this book) should be sought. A history of urologic problems, cryptorchidism, hypospadias, or episodes of orchitis is important. Finally, a family history of delayed puberty or of other endocrine abnormalities may suggest either hereditary late blooming in the case of *primary* hypogonadism, or familial autoimmune endocrinopathy in cases with *secondary* hypogonadism.

Physical examination. The body habitus and facies should be evaluated first. Does the patient look mature or babyish? masculine or feminine? A lower body segment (femoral greater trochanter to floor) longer than the upper segment (femoral greater trochanter to crown) and arm span greater than height comprises "eunuchoid" proportions and suggests pubertal or prepubertal hypogonadism. Good muscle mass and axillary hair militate against long-standing hypogonadism. Male pattern baldness is an androgen-dependent process. The presence of comedones, especially in the tragus of the ear, is a good sign of androgen activity. Complexion should be noted because increased pigmentation suggests primary adrenal failure; and dry flaky skin, hypothyroidism. Vital signs should always be evaluated. The presence of hypertension may indicate an adrenal enzyme defect or Cushing's disease whereas postural hypotension may alert the physician to Addison's disease. Special attention should be paid to the eyes to look for limitation of extraocular movements, papilledema, or restriction of visual fields, all suggestive of an intracranial tumor. Examination of the male breast should include careful palpation for the subareolar thickening and nodularity that may be the only evidence of gynecomastia (see below). Squeezing of the nipple may elicit galactorrhea, which, although rare in males, is pathognomonic of a prolactinoma. Examination of the genitals is critical. Pubic hair pattern should extend up the linea alba to the umbilicus in a diamond shaped pattern (the so-called male escutcheon); a triangular pattern, cut off at the pubis, suggests androgen deficiency as does sparse or excessively fine pubic hair. Penis size and location of urethral meatus, scrotal rugosity and pigmentation, and size and turgor of the testicles should all be noted. The normal adult testis should be no less than 15 mL in volume (approximately 4.0×3.0 cm) and should have the resistance to palpation of a firm ripe plum. An "overripe" softer feeling is a sign of testicular atrophy. Careful palpation of the left side of the scrotum while the patient performs a Valsalva maneuver may reveal the presence of a varicocele, which is nearly always on the left side. Approximately 5% of varicoceles are associated with reduced testosterone production from both testes (venous drainage from the left testis crosses over to the right). Rectal examination should assess prostate size because the prostate shrinks with testosterone deficiency. Careful neurologic examination should include testing of the sense of smell to look for Kallmann's syndrome.

Differential Diagnosis

The tests that give the most information about suspected male hypogonadism are serum testosterone and gonadotropin (LH and FSH) measurements. Table 77.1 shows the hormonal patterns typical of *central*, *gonadal*, and *peripheral* hypogonadism in males. These determinations are readily available from most commercial laboratories and are generally accurate within 20%. Ninety-five percent of adult males will have morning serum testosterone levels between 300 and 1200 ng/dL (with most between 450 to 700 ng/dL). Borderline values between 250 and 350 ng/dL should be considered suspicious. It is important that testosterone levels be determined in the morning because the diurnal variation in testosterone can produce an afternoon and evening decrement in testosterone concentration of as much as 200 ng/dL.

Abnormal or ambiguous determinations should be repeated at least once for confirmation because there is considerable variability both in radioimmunoassay determinations and, from time to time, within patients. Because total plasma testosterone is affected by variation in plasma SHBG levels in states such as aging, obesity, and liver disease, if testosterone levels are repeatedly in the borderline range, it may be helpful to obtain a "bioactive" (non-SHBG bound) testosterone determination. This level should be greater than 120 ng/dL.

In normal men, serum LH varies from 2 to 30 mlU/mL and FSH from 2 to 16 mlU/mL, but different assays will have different ranges of normal. Low or normal LH and FSH in the presence of subnormal testosterone defines *central* hypogonadism. Elevated gonadotropin levels with low testosterone indicate gonadal failure, except in rare cases of an FSH secreting pituitary adenoma. Central hypogonadism caused by prolactin (PRL) secreting pituitary tumors (prolactinomas) will usually be accompanied by plasma PRL levels of 100 ng/mL or more. Impotence is an especially prominent symptom in hyperprolactinemic hypogonadism.

Peripheral hypogonadism (resistance to testosterone action) is a form of hypogonadism characterized by normal or elevated testosterone levels. Gonadotropin levels are high or normal. Because, as noted above, these patients suffer from some degree of intersexuality at birth, they are rarely a diagnostic problem. High gonadotropin and normal testosterone levels may also be seen in evolving *secondary gonadal* hypogonadism when an increase in pituitary gonadotropin secretion is still able to compensate for the testicular failure.

Further investigation and initiation of treatment of patients with proven hypogonadism should probably be undertaken by a specialist in endocrinology. Table 77.2 lists various investigative procedures and types of patients for whom they are pertinent.

Referral to a urologist for testicular biopsy may be

Table 77.2. Additional Investigations Useful in the Evaluation of Hypogonadism

Type of Failure	Radiologic Procedure	Hormone Measurements	Other Tests
Central	Skull film	Prolactin	Visual fields (formal)
	Computerized tomography scan with contrast	T_4	Clomiphene test
	Magnetic resonance scan	TSH	Luteinizing hormone-releasing hormone test
	Cerebral angiogram	Cortisol (morning)	
		Growth hormone (with glucose tolerance test)	
Gonadal	Bone age (if primary)	T_4	Buccal smear
		Cortisol (morning)	Karyotyping Gonad biopsy

helpful in diagnosing traumatic or infectious damage. Biopsy also shows a diagnostic form of shrinkage and hyalinization of tubules in Klinefelter's syndrome. The procedure can often be done on an ambulatory basis under local anesthesia; however, it may cause hemorrhage and considerable pain. About a week is required for full recovery. Therefore it usually should be undertaken only after consultation with an endocrinologist to confirm that the procedure is necessary to provide useful diagnostic information.

Therapy

There are three aims of therapy in patients with *central* hypogonadism. The first is to suppress or remove any intracranial mass whose size or extent threatens vision or brain function. This may sometimes be accomplished by medical therapy (e.g., use of a synthetic dopamine agonist in prolactinoma), but it usually requires neurosurgery or radiation therapy, depending on the type and size of the lesion. The second aim is to suppress abnormal hormone secretion. In patients with prolactinomas, treatment with synthetic dopamine agonists has proven effective in not only lowering serum prolactin, increasing gonadotropins and testosterone, and restoring libido but also shrinking tumor mass and improving vision. Bromocriptine, the drug that has been used the longest is associated with a high incidence of gastrointestinal side effects (dyspepsia, nausea, vomiting, cramping, or diarrhea in 10 to 15% of patients), some of which may be ameliorated by administration of the drug in divided doses with food or an antacid. High dosages of bromocriptine have also been associated with depression and bizarre dreams or nightmares. Bromocriptine usually is started at a dosage of one 2.5 mg tablet/day and increased by one tablet/day each week up to a maximum of three/day to obtain the desired effect. Dosages as high as 16 to 24 mg/day are sometimes necessary, but they are associated with frequent side effects. Recently, a new long-acting dopamine agonist more specific for the D_2 receptor cabergoline (Dostinex) has been approved in the United States. Although dosages from 0.25 up to 1 mg twice weekly are recommended, the agent may also be effective given only once weekly in dosages from 0.5 to 3 mg (9). Cabergoline has a lower incidence of adverse effects than does bromocriptine (73) and may work well in patients in whom bromocriptine does not (16).

The third aim of therapy is to replace deficient androgen, which may be necessary in patients with either central or gonadal hypogonadism. Many issues having to do with androgen replacement therapy have been recently reviewed (7). The reasons for replacing testosterone in male hypogonadism are multiple. The most pressing reason is to ameliorate or reverse the symptoms of testosterone deficiency such as hot flashes, reduced libido, erectile dysfunction, and emotional lability and to restore male secondary sex characteristics such as beard growth and pubic hair. Beyond this however, it has become increasingly apparent from a variety of clinical studies that testosterone deficiency in

adults is associated with negative nitrogen balance, loss of lean body mass and muscle strength (32), loss of bone calcium with reduced bone mineral density (i.e., osteoporosis), and an increase in percent body fat with greater central fat distribution. The latter is, in turn, accompanied by deterioration of serum lipid pattern (increased LDL cholesterol and triglyceride) and insulin resistance, hence presumably with increased risk of cardiovascular disease. Testosterone replacement can improve or reverse the hypogonadal changes in body composition and function (8,12).

Options for testosterone replacement include transdermal patches (either scrotal or nonscrotal), topical creams, and implantable pellets (oral preparations are hepatotoxic and should not be used). The "tried and true" method is injection of testosterone enanthate (e.g., Delatestryl), cypionate, or other esters in oil. Effective therapy requires deep intramuscular injection at regular intervals. Therapy may be started at 200 mg every 4 weeks or 200 mg every 2 weeks. The dosage and interval should be adjusted depending on duration of the therapeutic (enhanced libido, sexual potency) effect and the testosterone level measured at the midpoint between injections. This type of injection therapy inevitably produces unphysiologically high-plasma testosterone levels immediately after injection that may fall to deficient levels before the subsequent injection, depending on the dosage and interval. It also suffers from the limitation that the injections are moderately painful and require regular visits to the physician's office or clinic. Two forms of transdermal testosterone patches are now approved in the United States. Both appear equally effective at relieving the symptoms and improving body composition, etc. in male hypogonadism. One preparation (Testoderm) requires daily application of a single patch to the scrotal skin, which usually must be shaved. A potential limitation on use of this product is insufficient size of the scrotum in pubertal failure or long-standing hypogonadism. The second product (Androderm) currently requires application of two patches daily for most patients (although a single patch system is under development). These may be applied to any skin surface that does not have underlying bony projections (back, thigh, chest, buttocks). These transdermal delivery systems produce more physiologic levels of plasma testosterone, with patterns of diurnal variation similar to the natural variation, if applied at bedtime. Both are associated with a relatively high incidence of skin irritation and occasionally with severe skin reactions. The scrotal patches may be somewhat better in this regard. Scrotal patches, however, produce unphysiologically elevated levels of circulating dihydrotestosterone (DHT) because of the high concentration of the 25-α-hydroxylase enzyme in scrotal skin. Whether this may lead to increased growth of prostate tissue is currently unknown.

It must be remembered that the replacement of testosterone may fail to restore sexual competence in hyperprolactinemic patients because of the antisexual effects of prolactin itself. In these cases either surgery to remove the prolactinoma or a prolactin-lowering drug (see above) may be required for potency to be restored.

A fourth treatment goal in hypogonadal patients may be to restore or improve fertility. Patients with gonadal hypogonadism may or may not be infertile, depending on the underlying lesion. Infertility that is primarily gonadal is generally resistant to medical intervention. Moreover, replacement of testosterone, by whatever means, suppresses LH and FSH causing reduced sperm counts and testicular atrophy.

In patients with *central* hypogonadism (i.e., LH or FSH deficiency) infertility as well as deficient testosterone levels may be treated with gonadotropins. Human chorionic gonadotropin (hCG) may be used for its LH-like activity (human LH is unavailable). Injections of 2000 to 4000 IU of hCG (e.g., Pregnyl or Follutein) three times weekly will normalize testosterone levels, generally within a month of initiation of therapy, and may also stimulate spermatogenesis. In patients with *primary* central failure, agents with both LH (hCG) and FSH-like activity may be required to initiate spermatogenesis. Because of the requirement for more frequent injections as compared with testosterone, use of gonadotropin injections probably should be restricted to those patients with central hypogonadism who are concerned about fertility.

Follow-up of treated patients should include questions about sexual function, assessment of habitus, beard growth, and in patients with failure of pubertal development, assessment of growth in stature, growth of phallus, and depth of voice. Libido and potency usually return within a few weeks of initiating treatment, whereas secondary sex characteristics improve gradually after 6 months to 1 year. Determination should be made of whether gynecomastia or prostate enlargement with symptoms of urethral obstruction are occurring as side effects of therapy. In older patients, it is a good idea to initiate therapy with a short-acting form of testosterone, either a transdermal system or, if injections are to be used, 20 mg of aqueous testosterone propionate (duration, approximately 3 days). Then, if prostate complications (e.g., acute urethral outlet obstruction) ensue, the effect will be short lived.

Gynecomastia

Importance

Significant enlargement of the male breast requires a physician's attention so that those cases with a serious hormonal or neoplastic cause can be distinguished from the common benign idiopathic forms.

Etiologies

Gynecomastia is common as plasma sex steroid hormone levels rise during early adolescence (occurring in up to 65% of boys age 14), but breast enlargement regresses spontaneously and is present in less than 15% of boys age 17. Prevalence of gynecomastia increases again in the twenties, remains stable at around 25%, and increases gradually to approximately 60% of men age 50 and older. This mild idiopathic

gynecomastia is nearly always less than 5 cm in diameter and causes no symptoms. Noticeable gynecomastia of greater than 5 cm in diameter may be the first clue to the presence of a benign or malignant adrenal or testicular neoplasm or to a pituitary prolactinoma. In the case of adrenal tumors, there are usually associated symptoms and signs of Cushing's syndrome. Malignancies of the testis, lung, stomach, and occasionally, other cancers, may secrete chorionic gonadotropin, which can overstimulate testicular steroid production and thus lead, indirectly, to gynecomastia. Hypothyroidism and hyperthyroidism have also been associated with breast enlargement. The taking of exogenous estrogen either purposely (by individuals with gender confusion or with prostate carcinoma) or accidentally because of estrogenic activity of various medications (e.g., diazepam, cimetidine, spironolactone, digitalis glycosides) should always be considered. Another iatrogenic cause is peripheral conversion to estrogens of excess androgens during testosterone or hCG therapy. Gynecomastia is also common in liver failure, in which hepatic metabolism of endogenous androgens is impaired. Finally, true gynecomastia must be differentiated from the "gynecoid" breast, seen in obesity and old age, which contains increased fatty tissue, but not glandular breast tissue, and also from carcinoma of the male breast. Approximately 1% of all breast carcinomas occur in men.

Approach to the Patient

History. The duration and age of onset of breast swelling is important; for example, recent onset of breast swelling in a 30 year old male would be of more concern than in an adolescent or than gradual breast enlargement in a man of 70. The presence of tenderness or discharge and the quality of the discharge (clear, turbid, bloody) should be noted. Any symptoms of hypogonadism (see above) should be elicited, as should symptoms of hypothyroidism (see Chapter 73) or Cushing's disease (see Chapter 74). Careful medication history and sexual history may reveal an exogenous cause.

Physical examination. In general the examination should be the same as for hypogonadism (see above) with the addition that signs of Cushing's disease and thyroid disease should be emphasized. Deep palpation of the upper abdomen may reveal an adrenal tumor or downward displacement of the kidney by such a tumor. Careful bimanual palpation of the testicles may detect a secretory tumor (androblastoma). A useful formal system for staging breast development has been described by Marshall and Tanner in adolescent girls (see Chapter 5), but it is equally useful for staging gynecomastia. Briefly, at stage I there is minimal proliferation of glandular tissue just beneath the areola. At stage II a flat pad of glandular tissue spreads beyond the bounds of the areola (i.e., greater than 5 cm). At stage III, this pad rounds up, lifting the breast area forward from the chest wall in a cone shape with the nipple at the tip. At stage IV the areola spreads laterally as subareolar gland proliferation gives the breast a double-contoured appearance. Finally further maturation with increase in fatty tissue results in the mature single contour of stage V. The examiner needs to differentiate between proliferation of glandular breast tissue (firm, slightly lobulated, and symmetrically distributed from the nipple outward with a limited boundary); fat (softer, diffusely distributed, and with no clear separation from surrounding subcutaneous adipose); and tumor (hard, nodular, frequently tender, often fixed to skin or underlying muscle, and eccentrically located with regard to the nipple). Milky nipple discharge on firm squeezing suggests prolactinoma; clear or bloody discharge suggests breast cancer. Unilateral breast enlargement should increase the suspicion of neoplasia, but asymmetry occurs in 10 to 15% of patients with idiopathic gynecomastia. The decision whether further investigation is required depends on the age of the patient, the rapidity of enlargement of the breast, and the degree of such enlargement. Men between 18 and 45 years of age with recent onset of rapidly enlarging mammary glands, or glandular breast tissue diameter greater than 5 cm, or with symptoms or signs suggesting hypogonadism, hypothyroidism, or Cushing's disease should receive further attention.

Diagnostic Procedures

Determinations of serum levels of estradiol, testosterone, gonadotropins (LH and FSH), serum prolactin, and hCG-β subunit are indicated. If the serum estradiol is greater than 50 pg/mL and if the testosterone/estradiol ratio is reduced to less than 100:1, the diagnosis of estrogen-secreting testicular tumor is strongly suggested. Elevation of 24-hour urinary 17-ketosteroids indicates an adrenal cause in which case adrenal hyperfunction should be investigated with the diagnosis of adrenal neoplasm in mind (see Chapter 74). Gynecomastia in late adolescence or young adulthood accompanied by testicular atrophy (small, very firm testes) and low or low normal testosterone levels with elevated FSH and LH suggests the diagnosis of Klinefelter's syndrome (XXY trisomy). Elevated serum hCG should prompt a search for occult malignancy with particular attention to gonads, lungs, and gastrointestinal tract. Elevated prolactin levels could be associated with use of certain medications (especially major tranquilizers) or with a pituitary prolactinoma (see Chapter 74 and Table 77.2). The possibility of hypothyroidism should be evaluated by thyroxine (T_4), triiodothyronine (T_3), and TSH determinations. Finally, patients with firm, nodular, unilateral or notably eccentric enlargement should be referred for mammography or surgical biopsy of the breast.

Therapy

Drug-induced gynecomastia remits gradually (in several months) if the drug is discontinued. Treatment of primary endocrine disease (e.g., prolactinoma, adrenal tumor, hCG-secreting carcinoma) should be undertaken by an appropriate specialist once the diagnosis is clear. Remission of the accompanying gynecomastia depends on the success of the treatment and the stage of advancement of breast development. When idiopathic gynecomastia is a cosmetic problem, plastic surgical excision of breast tissue is usually the therapeutic method of choice. It is important to bear in mind that breast development that has progressed beyond Tanner stage II (see Chapter 5) will never fully regress even if the proximate cause is corrected and therefore will require surgical intervention if complete cosmetic correction is desired.

Impotence

In this section, impotence and loss of libido are considered only as they relate to endocrine disorders. For a more general treatment of sexual dysfunction see Chapter 18. Briefly, impotence is the inability to achieve or maintain erection satisfactorily to effect penetration and ejaculation. Transient or occasional impotence is common and not necessarily evidence of a medical problem, but a pattern of repeated (greater than 25% of opportunities) episodes over more than a month should be investigated. Impotence may or may not be accompanied by loss of libido, depending on the cause.

Etiologies

A disorder of any of the systems that maintain the sexual response and apparatus may lead to impotence. Etiologies may therefore be *(a) psychologic* (see Chapter 18); *(b) vascular:* this may be of the arterial type, with diminished blood supply to the corpora cavernosa (e.g., congenital vascular anomaly, traumatic injury to vessels, large vessel atherosclerosis, or disease of smaller peripheral vessels), or it may be due to venous incompetence, in which partial erections occur but blood drains off because of "venous leak"; *(c) neuropathic:* damage to the peripheral pelvic autonomic nerves (e.g., diabetic neuropathy, heavy metal poisoning, or nerve trauma) or disease of the spinal cord or brain (e.g., tumor, multiple sclerosis) may inhibit or obliterate the erectile response; *(d) toxic:* substances of abuse (e.g., alcohol, opiates, major tranquilizers) can acutely and chronically diminish sexual ability, and many medications that affect the autonomic and central nervous system (e.g., tranquilizers and sympatholytic antihypertensives) are associated with impotence; *(e) debilitative:* various severe and chronic medical illnesses (e.g., malignancy, renal failure) are accompanied by loss of sex drive and/or impotence; and *(f) endocrine: hypogonadism* and prolactinoma (see above) have been discussed as causes of impotence.

Other endocrine diseases that commonly produce sexual dysfunction are hyperthyroidism and hypothyroidism, Cushing's syndrome, and acromegaly. In one series of patients referred to a major diagnostic center for persistent symptoms without apparent psychiatric cause, 35% were found to have an endocrine disorder (66).

Approach to the Patient

History. The duration of symptoms, the frequency with which intercourse is attempted, and the percentage of attempts ending in erectile failure should be recorded to determine whether the impotence is absolute or relative and if it is progressing. Impotence unaccompanied by loss of libido suggests a neurologic or vascular problem, whereas loss of interest in sexual activity is consistent with either hypogonadism or a psychologic cause. The history should include the patient's marital situation, whether there are sex partners other than the spouse, the perceived level of partners' desire, and a social and work history to determine whether there is excessive stress. Situational impotence (i.e., experienced with one partner but not another) is good evidence of a psychologic problem. Normal men often awaken in the morning with an erection. This is a local response to a full bladder; detumescence follows urination. Preservation of morning erections is good evidence against vascular or neuropathic disease; however, in the cited series (66), 14% of patients with an endocrine cause maintained morning erections. A history of medication use and substance abuse should be diligently sought. Heavy smoking is often associated with a peripheral vascular cause of impotence. The patient should be asked about symptoms of hypothyroidism or hyperthyroidism, Cushing's disease, and diabetes, peripheral neuropathy (paraesthesia, hyperesthesia, burning or shooting pains) or central nervous system disease, and vascular disease (claudication, angina, cold extremities, skin ulcers).

Physical examination. The physical examination should be conducted with particular attention to the manifestations of hypogonadism described above, to signs of thyroid or adrenal disease (see Chapters 73 and 74), and also to signs of peripheral vascular disease (peripheral pulses, skin temperature, skin atrophy, or hair loss) (see Chapter 87) and central or peripheral neuropathy (see Chapter 84).

Diagnostic Procedures

Hormone determinations should be used to investigate for hypogonadism or prolactinoma (see above). If historical or physical findings lead to a suspicion of thyroid or adrenal disease, appropriate tests should be done (see Chapters 73 and 74). A fasting blood sugar should always be obtained to screen for diabetes mellitus (see Chapter 72). Spontaneous erection during sleep (nocturnal penile tumescence) tends to be intact in psychogenic impotence but reduced when there is an organic cause. Nocturnal penile tumescence may be tested by the patient at home using a "snap gauge," but for definitive measurement, studies should be conducted using quantitative instrumentation in a sleep laboratory. Intracavernous injection of prostaglandin-E_1 (PGE_1) (see below) is often used as a diagnostic test to differentiate between vascular (in which response is reduced or absent) versus psychogenic or neurologic dysfunction. However, lack of full erection may occur in patients without vascular disease due to stress related to the procedure, and a positive response does not completely rule out vascular disease. Definitive diagnosis of vascular disorders may require Doppler studies of penile blood flow or selective angiography; venous incompetence may be revealed by dynamic cavernosography, all procedures used by urologists specializing in the diagnosis and treatment of impotence. If peripheral neuropathy seems a likely cause, this can often be confirmed by referral to a urologist for bladder manometrics and to a neurologist for nerve conduction velocity measurements (see Chapter 84).

Therapy

Therapeutic efforts should be directed at the specific cause of the impotence, whenever one can be found. Psychologic impotence may respond to various therapeutic modalities depending on its severity and associated problems (see Chapter 18). Vascular disease may respond to medication or to surgical revascularization. Caution should be exercised in this regard in that whereas good results are often obtained with surgery in young patients with traumatic or congenital abnormalities, results are nearly always disappointing in older patients with atherosclerotic disease, perhaps because of the involvement of smaller peripheral vessels in the process. Neuropathic impotence is occasionally reversible with removal of the inciting lesion (e.g., spinal cord tumor) but, if irreversible, may also be treated with local measures (see below). Drug-induced impotence is usually reversed if the offending agent can be discontinued. Therapy of hypogonadism has been discussed above. If sexual function does not improve within 6 weeks after specific therapy for an organic cause has been instituted, consideration should be given to the possibility that the experience and expectation of sexual failure are inhibiting the response (so-called performance anxiety) even though the primary cause is no longer present. Such secondary psychologic impotence may respond to psychologic or behavioral therapy (see Chapter 18).

There are also nonspecific approaches to therapy that may succeed in restoring sexual function despite an irremediable (e.g., vascular or neuropathic) cause. These therapies generally require urologic consultation. Implantable penile prostheses have been used extensively but, because of local complications, are no longer as popular as they once were. Implants come in two basic types: those that are permanently stiff or semiflexible, and more complex devices that inflate by means of a pump and valve mechanism. Another option is the use of a device that draws blood into the penis by negative pressure, then retains it there with an occlusive ring applied to the base of the penis. A number of different types of suction devices are available. Although earlier reports stressed the satisfactory results obtained in selected patients, continuing experience with these devices has been less positive. For example, one retrospective study found that 81% of men using vacuum devices abandoned this therapy reporting that "it did not work," and that patients' attitudes to the device were unfavorable overall (24).

Currently, a more popular approach is injection of vasoactive agents directly into the corpus cavernosum. Various combinations have been used. Most effective is PGE_1 (alprostadil) or papaverine combined with phentolamine. A recent study concluded that papaverine plus phentolamine is about as effective as PGE_1 with similar rates of overly prolonged erections but significantly less pain (4). Cavernosal injection therapy generally produces erections lasting 30 minutes to several hours. Although highly effective, especially in neuropathic impotence of diabetes mellitus, injection therapy should be supervised by a urologist familiar with its use because priapism is a potentially serious and fairly common (2 to 4%) acute complication. A long-term, but rare, complication is gradual fibrosis of the corpora cavernosa with loss of responsiveness. A promising new modality, recently approved by the FDA, is alprostadil administered as a urethral suppository (MUSE). Studies show efficacy and adverse effect rates comparable to injection therapy (37,57), but experience with this method is still relatively limited.

Aging

A series of early investigations found that men's testosterone levels declined with age and that protein binding of testosterone to sex hormone-binding globulin (SHBG) increased with age, resulting in a profound decrease in mean free (bioavailable) testosterone. In these same reports, the changes in androgens were generally accompanied by an increase in circulating estrone and estradiol and in gonadotropins. Further studies, in which older men were carefully selected to match the younger men in terms of health, obesity, alcohol intake, social class, and so on, revealed total testosterone to decrease less steeply than originally reported. Decreases in free or bioactive testosterone remained disproportionate because of significant increases in SHBG. No convincing longitudinal studies of the effects of age on sex steroids have been published to date, but large cross-sectional studies (more than 1500 carefully studied men of various ages) demonstrated a significant decrease with age in both total testosterone and in the free testosterone index (31). The number or proportion of men who develop truly hypogonadal levels of total or free testosterone during normal aging remains unknown. Therefore the issue of "male menopause" in healthy men remains controversial. Regardless of changes in levels of sex steroids, numerous studies in healthy men have revealed a steady decrease both in sexual interest and ability with decreases in frequency of intercourse from an average

of two to three events a week to less than two a month by age 70 to 75 (49). This decrease does not appear to be directly related to hypogonadism, but probably reflects changes in other (i.e., nervous and vascular) systems occurring with age. There are no data to support a beneficial effect of administration of androgens to aging men whose testosterone levels are normal; however, it is the anecdotal observation of many andrologists that some men with symptoms of hypogonadism and free or total testosterone levels in the low normal range appear to benefit from androgen replacement therapy. Therefore several studies that are designed to determine the possible benefits and risks of androgen treatment of older men with low to low normal testosterone levels are under way. Until definitive data become available showing a positive benefit/risk ratio, androgen replacement in older men should be limited to research investigations. However, older men with truly abnormally low testosterone levels should be investigated in the same way as are other men with suspected hypogonadism (see above) and treated appropriately.

SEXUAL AND REPRODUCTIVE DYSFUNCTION IN WOMEN

Hirsutism and Virilization

Growth of coarse dark hair (terminal hairs) in various body areas (besides the scalp and eyebrows) depends on the action of androgens. The pattern of hair growth reflects the relative sensitivity of different zones of the skin to androgen effect. Whereas pubic and axillary hair appear in both sexes, further hair growth diverges because of different androgen levels. Although male patterns vary, maximum expression of androgen effect includes terminal hair development over the face, limbs, chest, superior pubic triangle, linea alba, and back. In those carrying genes for male-pattern baldness, high levels of androgens are also associated with loss of scalp hair, with hair receding first at the temporal hairline ("widow's peak") and later at the crown.

Most women (80%) develop some degree of dark hair growth over the legs and forearms but not much facial hair. About one-third have small amounts of hair on the chest and abdomen (extending along the linea alba). Abnormally high levels of plasma androgens can result in male distribution of hair growth, the state of hirsutism. Over time, very high levels of androgen production also lead to virilization, defined as increased muscle mass, redistribution of fat from subcutaneous depots in hips and breasts to abdominal and intra-abdominal areas ("male habitus"), clitoral enlargement (greater than 2.0 cm), deepening of the voice, male-pattern baldness, development of acne, and increased perspiration odor from activation of sebaceous glands.

Excess body hair without signs of virilization is termed simple hirsutism. Hirsutism with virilization is rare and is usually from diagnosable causes, the most common of which are adrenal or ovarian tumor, congenital adrenal hyperplasia, male pseudohermaphroditism, or use of exogenous androgen (e.g., female athletes and body builders). Therefore truly virilized women should generally be referred directly to an endocrinologist for detailed diagnostic investigation.

Hirsutism without virilization. Although simple hirsutism may be an early manifestation of Cushing's syndrome or of an adrenal or ovarian neoplasm, most cases fall into a group termed idiopathic or constitutional hirsutism. The prevalence of simple hirsutism has been estimated to be as high as 10% in adult North American women. It typically develops during the late teens, although progression may be so slow that troublesome amounts of hair do not appear for 10 or more years after onset of menses.

In one-half to two-thirds of hirsute patients, excessive ovarian production of androgens (testosterone or androstenedione) is demonstrable and is often associated with oligomenorrhea and decreased fertility. Ovarian structure may show hyperthecosis (overgrowth of interstitial tissue) or multiple cyst formation (polycystic ovary syndrome, or PCOS). *PCOS is the most common endocrine disorder in women of reproductive age.* Recent estimates suggest that 5 to 10% of premenopausal women have the full-blown syndrome of hyperandrogenism, chronic anovulation, and polycystic ovaries (22). The associated decrease in ovulation rate in patients with PCOS causes varying degrees of infertility. Women with this syndrome secrete excessive quantities of androgenic steroids from the ovaries and often from the adrenal glands as well. Ovarian production of estrogens is usually sufficient to produce plasma estradiol and estrone levels in the normal range. These women often have increased ratios of LH to FSH in plasma. In approximately 50% of patients, hyperandrogenism is accompanied by carbohydrate intolerance and elevated levels of insulin and insulin-like growth factor-I (26). Studies of patients with PCOS suggest that they are two etiologically distinct subpopulations (51). Insulin-resistant patients tend to be more obese, with a greater waist/hip ratio, to be more hirsute, and to have higher levels of plasma testosterone and lower levels of sex hormone–binding globulin. The finding that the drug troglitazone improves insulin sensitivity and also lowers free testosterone and SHBG levels in patients with insulin resistant PCOS suggests that the insulin resistance may be the underlying cause of the gonadal dysregulation (23). Finally, a unique insulin receptor defect has been identified in approximately 50% of women with PCOS (22). In contrast, the non–insulin-resistant patients have higher LH/FSH ratios than do the insulin-resistant patients, suggesting that the former group has a primary problem with neuroendocrine regulation.

In about half of all patients with simple hirsutism, elevated serum testosterone levels are not demonstrable. However, approximately half of patients with normal total testosterone have been shown to have increased plasma "free" (i.e., nonprotein bound) testosterone due to reduced SHBG. Increased hair follicle conversion of testosterone to the more potent dihydrotestosterone has been demonstrated in some of the remaining cases and other causes of increased sensitivity of hair follicles to androgens have been postulated.

Racial and ethnic factors are also important determinants of hair growth. Women of Asian ancestry and Caucasian women of northern European origins usually have relatively little terminal hair on face, torso, or extremities. In contrast, Caucasian women of Mediterranean origin often develop mustache, beard, or sideburn hair and have dark hair on legs and arms. Constitutional hirsutism also tends to run in families. Thus, a patient with moderate hirsutism who is of Mediterranean origin, who has a mother with excessive facial hair, and has normal menses is unlikely to have identifiable endocrine disease. The timing of onset of hirsutism is also important. For example, sudden development of hirsutism many years after menarche is likely to be due to a tumor of the ovary or adrenal rather than a functional cause.

Transitory hirsutism may occur during pregnancy and occasionally during menopause. A number of pharmacologic agents, including glucocorticoids, phenytoin (Dilantin), minoxidil, diazoxide, and phenothiazines, can produce hirsutism. Drug-induced hirsutism is characterized by increased hair growth that is not limited to the androgen-sensitive areas of the skin. Rare causes include chronic local skin trauma and porphyria cutanea tarda.

Besides polycystic ovarian disease, the other major cause of adult-onset simple hirsutism, sometimes with disturbance of menstrual pattern, is *congenital adrenal hyperplasia (CAH)*. CAH is produced by a deficiency of one of the several enzymes in the steroid synthetic pathway. Although such defects are usually manifest in childhood as ambiguous genitalia with salt loss (21-hydroxylase deficiency) or salt retaining hypertensive syndromes (11-hydroxylase deficiency), patients with partial 21- or 11-hydroxylase defects can manifest hirsutism with onset in puberty or adult life without symptomatic disturbances of salt and water balance.

Approach to the Patient

A careful ethnic and family history is essential. The temporal evolution of the problem should be noted, including the menstrual history. On physical examination, one should carefully note the distribution and density of terminal hairs in the sideburn and mustache areas, the periareolar and midsternal regions, and over the back and buttocks. Particular attention should be paid to the pattern of pubic hair. In the female, the pubic hair forms an inverted triangle in the inferior pubic region only. The male escutcheon is a rhomboid space with terminal hairs filling the superior pubic triangle and extending up the linea alba to the umbilicus. A male type escutcheon in a female is a good presumptive sign of hyperandrogenism. Physical signs of virilization (see above) should be sought. Cases with virilism require urgent referral to an endocrinologist, whereas those with severe ovarian dysfunction may require the attention of a gynecologist for treatment of abnormal menstruation or impaired fertility. Finally, symptoms and signs of Cushing's syndrome (in which hirsutism and even virilization may occasionally be more prominent than the classic "Cushingoid" changes) should also be sought. Obesity with acanthosis nigricans is highly suggestive of the insulin-resistant variant of PCOS.

The decision to proceed with laboratory testing depends on the history and severity of the hirsutism. Laboratory studies can be performed sequentially if financial considerations are dominant or simultaneously if speed is of the essence. Serum testosterone, which is of ovarian and rarely of adrenal origin, is measured first. A normal serum testosterone level suggests idiopathic hirsutism and excludes major ovarian disorders. Not excluded are mild cases of ovarian hyperthecosis/polycystic ovaries with abnormal androstenedione production or decreased sex hormone–binding globulin (increased free or bioavailable androgen). The uncovering of such borderline cases usually is not worthwhile because management would be unaffected. If the testosterone level is elevated to between 85 and 200 ng/dL, a diagnosis of ovarian hyperthecosis or polycystic ovaries is most likely. Increased LH and low normal or reduced FSH is highly suggestive of polycystic ovary disease but does not occur in all patients. Pelvic sonography usually reveals multiple cysts or thickening of the cortex and enlargement of the ovaries. Levels of testosterone greater than 200 ng/dL suggest a diagnosis of ovarian neoplasm and further diagnostic workup should be directed by specialists. This may include sonography, computerized axial tomography, laparoscopy with ovarian biopsy, or ovarian vein catheterization.

If testosterone levels are normal, excess production of weak androgens (e.g., androstenedione, dehydroepiandrosterone) by the adrenal remains a consideration and can be confirmed by appropriate assays. In 21-hydroxylase deficiency, which is the most common type of CAH producing adult hirsutism, serum 17α-OH progesterone and urinary pregnanetriol may be elevated. Unfortunately, in about half the patients with this syndrome these steroid levels will be significantly increased only after stimulation with exogenous adrenocorticotropic hormone (ACTH). Therefore, if CAH is suspected, endocrine specialty referral is appropriate. Large increases in serum dehydroepiandrosterone-sulfate or 24-hour urinary excretion of 17-ketosteroids suggests adrenal neoplasia (adenoma or carcinoma) and should be evaluated by an endocrinologist.

Therapy

Treatment of hyperandrogenism and hirsutism has been recently reviewed (42). The therapy of simple hirsutism usually is local and essentially cosmetic, even when there is a hormonal abnormality, because medical reduction of androgen excess does not rapidly affect the presence of existing hair and is often incomplete.

Local measures include bleaching, wax stripping, shaving, plucking (tweezing), using hair removal creams (depilatories), and performing electrolysis. Contrary to popular belief, such measures do not accelerate the growth rate of remaining hair. Plucking

may cause local infection. Wax applications or hair removal creams are effective but may be irritating and must be used with care. All of these procedures must be repeated at intervals. Electrolysis and thermolysis are effective procedures for permanent removal of hair, but are expensive and uncomfortable. Effectiveness and safety (avoidance of burns, scarring, and infection) depend on the technique of the operator. Referral of the patient requires that the physician be familiar with the electrologist's skill. Under the best of circumstances, electrolysis is generally successful in destroying approximately 50% of the follicles treated at one time. Thus, many repetitions are invariably required.

Patients with hyperandrogenic hirsutism (PCOS or CAH) often respond to medical therapy. Such patients should be cautioned not to expect rapid results because dedifferentiation of androgenized follicles may require 6 to 18 months, even when androgen excess is totally eliminated. The immediate benefit to be expected is prevention of progression of the hirsutism, with variable degrees of reversal occurring only as therapy is continued. Medical therapy is directed toward the suppression of androgen production, the blocking of peripheral androgen action, or both. Although such therapy appears more rational when androgen excess is demonstrable, patients with idiopathic hirsutism may occasionally respond. Adrenal suppression with low dosages of dexamethasone, although introduced on the erroneous assumption that adrenal androgens were responsible for most cases of hirsutism, is nonetheless effective in about one-third of cases. This seems to be due to an accompanying reduction of ovarian androgen secretion, which is either directly dependent on ACTH or indirectly dependent via ovarian conversion of circulating adrenal steroids. Adrenal suppression is, of course, effective in cases of congenital adrenal hyperplasia. This form of therapy is simple and usually free from side effects. Dexamethasone can be given as a single dose of from 0.1 to 0.3 mg (as a pediatric solution) orally at bedtime. At these low dosages, neither glucocorticoid excess (i.e., iatrogenic Cushing's syndrome) nor chronic adrenal suppression with adrenal insufficiency is likely to occur, but levels of both plasma or urinary cortisol and adrenal androgen should be monitored and the dosage of dexamethasone adjusted to keep both in the normal range. Side effects of dexamethasone therapy include occasional insomnia and appetite stimulation.

The most appropriate treatment for ovarian hyperandrogenism is suppression of ovarian androgen production. The first line of treatment is use of a cyclically administered estrogen–progestin combination (oral contraceptive). This is effective in about half of cases. Estrogens, especially when given orally, also increase concentration of plasma sex hormone–binding globulin, reducing the concentration of circulating free androgens. Because progestins have some intrinsic androgen like activity on hair follicles, a combination that minimizes the content of progestational agent may be the most appropriate. Agents containing 2 mg or less of norethindrone or 0.5 mg or less of norgestrel are acceptable. When used, oral contraceptives (OCs) should be given on the usual schedule recommended for fertility control for the particular preparation (see Chapter 93).

Disadvantages of OCs include their potential for cardiovascular, thrombogenic, and other undesirable effects. These disadvantages have probably been overstated and are less often seen with the low-dose contraceptives of today than with their high-dose predecessors; nonetheless, possible adverse effects must be weighed carefully when they are to be prescribed for an essentially benign problem. Combined adrenal–ovarian suppression may be used if neither alone is effective.

Suppression of ovarian androgen production by OCs precludes pregnancy. Thus, therapy must be interrupted when fertility is desired and the drug withheld until pregnancy is terminated. Hirsutism may recur during this time. Where fertility is at issue, an antiestrogen, clomiphene citrate (Clomid) 50 to 100 mg/day, may be administered to induce ovulation. Success rates in patients with the PCOS are favorable (greater than 60% of patients pregnant in three cycles). Clomiphene administration should always be managed by a specialist experienced in the use and monitoring of fertility drugs.

Several other agents have been used successfully for the medical therapy of hirsutism. Medroxyprogesterone acetate (Provera), 100 mg intramuscularly every 2 weeks, or 30 to 40 mg orally reduces testosterone production and interferes with testosterone action at the tissue level. A variety of side effects may be encountered, and this mode of therapy is not recommended. There is evidence that implanted progestin-only contraceptives (i.e., Norplant) may also reduce acne and hirsutism. Spironolactone (Aldactone), at a generally well-tolerated dosage of 25 to 50 mg twice daily, suppresses ovarian androgen production and antagonizes androgen action at the hair follicle. Spironolactone is a well-accepted and relatively safe drug, and the combination of spironolactone with an oral contraceptive is often effective in more severe cases of hirsutism or those that are unresponsive to ovarian and/or adrenal suppression alone. Contraindications to spironolactone include concomitant use of potassium supplements or renal insufficiency, either of which may predispose to hyperkalemia.

Cyproterone acetate and flutamide are competitive inhibitors of androgen that block peripheral androgen receptors and have been used successfully in the treatment of hirsutism. Finasteride (Proscar), which inhibits the enzyme (5α-reductase) mediated conversion of testosterone to the active form, DHT, in prostate also appears to be effective in skin and hair follicles. Studies of finasteride in the treatment of idiopathic hirsutism (14) and polycystic ovary disease (72) have shown it to be reasonably effective and well tolerated. Although none of the latter agents is currently FDA approved for the treatment of hirsutism in women, it is not unreasonable to try one of them alone or in combination with ovarian or adrenal suppression in resistant patients.

Finally, suppression of the reproductive system using a GnRH antagonist such as Buserelin has also been found to be effective in reducing severe ovarian hyperandrogenism with hirsutism (6).

Dysmenorrhea

Dysmenorrhea (painful menstruation) is a common problem. It is considered *primary* when it appears within a year or two of the menarche. When painful menstruation appears for the first time or suddenly intensifies in a mature women, it is referred to as *secondary* dysmenorrhea and is nearly always a result of a specific pathologic process, such as uterine myomas, endometriosis, pelvic inflammatory disease, or an intrauterine contraceptive device. Therefore, in secondary dysmenorrhea, one should seek an initiating cause. Patients with secondary dysmenorrhea generally should be referred to a gynecologist. Typical primary dysmenorrhea consists of the development within 1 or 2 days of the onset of menstruation of either crampy or sustained lower abdominal and pelvic pain that may radiate into the legs and that can be associated with nausea, vomiting, irritability, diarrhea, or abdominal distension. In a few patients, symptoms may be so severe that performance of usual daily activities is impaired or prevented. Usually the discomfort is most severe during the initial several hours of menstrual flow, fades gradually, and disappears within 2 or 3 days. The episodes tend to become less severe with increasing age and often disappear spontaneously within 5 or 10 years after the menarche or after the first pregnancy. Occasionally, idiopathic dysmenorrhea reappears (or makes its first appearance) in the perimenopausal period. The hormonal pattern leading to primary dysmenorrhea is not completely understood, but it requires ovulation and disappears if ovarian hormones are suppressed. The proximal cause of symptoms appears to be increased or sustained myometrial contractions, possibly from excess formation of uterine prostaglandins.

Mild forms of dysmenorrhea require only analgesic therapy, such as aspirin or acetaminophen, and reassurance from the physician. A number of preparations are available without prescription and are marketed for menstrual cramps. Most are combination tablets, and none is proven to be more effective than aspirin or acetaminophen alone. Examples of these combination tablets are Femcaps (aspirin, phenacetin, citrate, ephedrine, and atropine) and Midol (aspirin, caffeine, and cinnamedrine). Analgesics work best when taken promptly at or slightly before the onset of menses and continued regularly (every 4 to 6 hours), rather than taken only when pain is perceived.

When symptoms are more severe or incapacitating, therapy should be tried with nonsteroidal anti-inflammatory drugs (NSAIDs) that have antiprostaglandin activity greater than that of aspirin; these will be effective in approximately half of patients.

Ibuprofen (e.g., Motrin 400 mg four times daily for 5 to 6 days), mefenamic acid (Ponstel 250 mg four times daily for 5 to 6 days), and naproxen (Naprosyn 500 mg two times daily for five doses) have been approved by the FDA for use in dysmenorrhea. Other NSAIDs such as indomethacin (Indocin 25 mg four times daily for six doses) are effective in the treatment of dysmenorrhea but have not been approved for this purpose. NSAIDs are most effective if given just before menstrual flow begins and continued for 2 to 3 days thereafter. However, because of the uncertainty of the effects of these agents in early pregnancy, it is suggested that their use be delayed until the beginning of menstrual flow in those patients who are sexually active and who are not using effective means of birth control. The patient should use one agent as a trial for three cycles, and then this agent should be discontinued if there has been an inadequate response in controlling the symptoms. It is currently unknown whether one NSAID might be effective when another has failed.

Steroidal contraceptive agents, either oral or implantable (Norplant), suppress ovarian hormone production and therefore usually control dysmenorrhea; these agents occasionally may be necessary for management of this problem when it is severe. The use of oral contraceptive agents is discussed fully in Chapter 93.

The unusual patient who does not respond to any of these therapies should be seen by a gynecologist for evaluation for an undetected problem causing secondary dysmenorrhea or to provide more experienced guidance in the drug therapy of primary dysmenorrhea.

Premenstrual Tension Syndrome

The premenstrual tension syndrome is an ill-defined complex of signs and symptoms that occurs to some degree in approximately 30% of women of reproductive age. Symptoms include irritability and increased aggressiveness, cravings for sweet or salty foods, nervousness, depression, tearfulness, mood swings, difficulty in concentrating, headaches, fullness and tenderness of the breasts, fatigue, and abdominal bloating. A significant minority of affected women find such symptoms severely disruptive to their lives. Any or all of the symptoms may be present, and the characteristic complaints vary among patients, but the hallmark of the syndrome is that these problems appear during the latter half (luteal phase) of the menstrual cycle, disappear with the onset of menstruation, and are absent during the first part (follicular phase) of the cycle.

Investigations of the cause of this entity have not been rewarding. Most investigations have found no typical pattern of hormone or electrolyte changes that distinguishes symptomatic women from asymptomatic women. Nonetheless, although progesterone supplementation does not eliminate symptoms, the suppression of ovarian cyclicity medically (e.g., GnRH analogs) or surgically effectively eliminates premenstrual syndrome, and sex steroid hormone replacement in suppressed patients does not restore symptoms. It

therefore seems most likely that the symptoms stem from an "abnormal" physical response to a more or less normal pattern of steroid hormone fluctuations during the menstrual cycle.

There is at this time no truly specific treatment for the premenstrual tension syndrome. Although pyridoxine, minor tranquilizers, and thiazide diuretics have all been tried, their effectiveness has not been substantiated in clinical trials, nor is there a definite rationale for the use of any of these agents. It is advisable to treat symptoms of mild premenstrual syndrome empirically, while reassuring the patient that she is not mentally ill, but rather the victim of a common, hormonally related malady with no serious physical consequences. In severe cases, a trial of ovarian suppression with steroid hormone replacement may be warranted, but such treatment should be implemented only by a medical or gynecologic endocrinologist.

Abnormal Vaginal Bleeding Before Menopause

During the 35 to 40 years of menstruation, most women experience occasional variations in bleeding pattern. In women approaching menopause, irregularity of the menstrual cycle is typical, as described below. In younger women, most changes in bleeding pattern are of the type called dysfunctional uterine bleeding (DUB), which is defined as abnormal bleeding for which no anatomic source can be found. Most DUB is related to anovulation, generally as a manifestation of alterations in pituitary–gonadal physiology that may be related to hypothalamic oligomenorrhea (see below). DUB may also be seen in the hirsutism anovulation syndrome (i.e., PCOS). A variety of physical and emotional stressors can precipitate DUB. In a few patients, abnormal vaginal bleeding is related to unsuspected pregnancy or to anatomic problems.

Women often describe abnormal menstrual bleeding first to their general physician and are often concerned about cancer. Therefore it is important to have a systematic approach to this problem. With careful history taking and a limited evaluation, a working diagnosis and plan can usually be developed in the office. Table 77.3 lists the various causes of abnormal vaginal bleeding in the premenopausal woman.

Table 77.3. Causes of Abnormal Vaginal Bleeding in the Premenopausal Woman

Dysfunctional uterine bleeding (hypothalamic idiopathic anovulation)
Perineal causes: bladder pathology, hemorrhoids
Vulvar causes: infection, laceration, tumor
Vaginal causes: infection, laceration, tumor, foreign body
Cervical causes: infection, erosion, polyp, carcinoma
Uterine causes: infection, polyp, leiomyomata, carcinoma, intrauterine device
Ovarian causes: infection, polycystic ovary (Stein-Levinthal syndrome)
Pregnancy: threatened abortion, complete abortion, ectopic pregnancy
Oral contraceptives
Systemic medical conditions: for example, bleeding diathesis (especially thrombocytopenia), thyroid disease

History

The patient should be asked how the abnormal bleeding differs from that which occurs during her normal cycle in terms of amount, timing, and quality, and when the normal pattern changed. *Menorrhagia* refers to menstruation occurring at the expected time or extended by only a few days but with blood loss greater than usual (e.g., the patient has to change pads more frequently, or pads contain more blood than usual). Menorrhagia is consistent with DUB, leiomyomata uteri (i.e., fibroid uterus), endometrial polyps, or an underlying medical problem (e.g., hypothyroidism). *Metrorrhagia* is the term for vaginal bleeding (usually spotting) in the interval between otherwise normally spaced periods. Metrorrhagia may be found with leiomyomata, polyps, or local vulvar vaginal problems, but carcinoma of the endometrium or cervix and breakthrough bleeding related to OCs may also present this way. *Menometrorrhagia* is a term used to indicate the occurrence of both menorrhagia and metrorrhagia. *Polymenorrhea* is the occurrence of menstruation at intervals of less than 21 days. *Oligomenorrhea* refers to infrequent menses (intervals greater than 35 days) or missed periods. The latter two patterns are more commonly associated with alterations in hormone balance (i.e., DUB) and may be precipitated by physical or emotional stress.

The history can also provide evidence about whether ovulation is occurring. This may be helpful because DUB is often associated with failure to ovulate. Features indicating ovulation include *mittelschmerz* (mild or moderate lower abdominal or pelvic pain at midcycle), which indicates rupture of an ovarian follicle; *increased midcycle mucus* (due to the secretory effect of progesterone); *premenstrual molimina* (abnormal fullness, headaches, and irritability immediately preceding the onset of bleeding); *dysmenorrhea*; and a *biphasic basal body temperature pattern*; at time of ovulation, the temperature usually rises 1°F (½°C) and remains elevated until the onset of bleeding.

Sexually active women should be asked what type of contraception they are using and questioned about symptoms suggesting pregnancy. Breakthrough bleeding (metrorrhagia) is not uncommon in women using OCs, especially during the first year of use. Pregnancy related bleeding is a problem in the first trimester, when it may be difficult to determine clinically whether the patient is pregnant. Almost always, the patient will have missed the most recent period, and she may have morning sickness, frequent urination, breast tenderness, and other early symptoms of pregnancy. Bleeding in the pregnant patient may be due to one of several conditions. Leakage of small amounts of blood from the cervical os is referred to as *threatened abortion*. This occurs in approximately 10% of pregnancies, but only half of these women will ultimately abort. *Spontaneous abortion* is characterized by intense cramping and bleeding with passage of clots. The abortion may be complete (the uterus is empty and no further management may be needed) or incomplete (partial loss of uterine contents and need for prompt

attention by a gynecologist). *Ectopic pregnancy* is another cause of first trimester bleeding and is a life-threatening medical emergency. It is characterized by a missed period followed by bleeding that may range from spotting to frank hemorrhage. There is often associated unilateral pelvic pain. When there is any question of ectopic pregnancy, women should be urgently referred for pelvic sonography, which is nearly always diagnostic.

In patients with menorrhagia, polymenorrhea, or oligomenorrhea, the history should include information about abnormal vaginal discharge or other symptoms of pelvic infection or irritation (see Chapter 94) because chronic pelvic infection may cause any of the abnormal bleeding patterns described above. Questions should also be asked about symptoms of other medical conditions. Severe thrombocytopenia may cause menorrhagia. The patient with abnormal vaginal bleeding from thrombocytopenia will usually have other manifestations of this problem (see Chapter 51). Other coagulation abnormalities, including anticoagulant therapy, rarely cause abnormal vaginal bleeding. Hypothyroidism may cause menorrhagia, whereas hyperthyroidism tends to be associated with oligomenorrhea (see Chapter 73).

When dysfunctional uterine bleeding is suspected (absence of features of ovulation and lack of evidence for other causes), the patient should be asked about recent changes in her general health and in her daily activities. Among the factors that may precipitate DUB are dieting, weight gain or loss, and emotional stress. Oligomenorrhea or amenorrhea is especially common in association with eating disorders (bulimia, anorexia). It may also be related to jogging or other strenuous exercise, sleep loss, mental strain, chronic medical conditions, and alcohol or illicit drug use.

Physical Examination

All patients complaining of abnormal vaginal bleeding should have a pelvic examination to look for obvious anatomic causes of the bleeding. It is important not to defer the examination because of the bleeding. Hemorrhoids, vulvar conditions, vaginitis and cervicitis, cervical polyp or cervical erosion, and leiomyomata uteri are the principal anatomical problems that may be identified. Vulvovaginal and cervical sources of bleeding should be suspected, especially in patients who describe metrorrhagia or postcoital bleeding. In an actively bleeding patient, orthostatic blood pressure and heart rate should be checked to detect severe anemia. The patient should also be examined for ecchymoses and petechiae, especially on the lower extremities, and for physical signs of thyroid disease.

Laboratory Tests

A hemoglobin concentration or a hematocrit value should always be obtained. In addition, every woman with a change in her bleeding pattern should have a Pap smear evaluated (see Chapter 95). Sexually active women should always have a pregnancy test. The presence of ectopic pregnancy will nearly always be detected by pelvic sonography, which should be undertaken immediately whenever this diagnosis is suspected.

If the history or physical examination suggests the possibility of a bleeding diathesis, a platelet count, bleeding time, prothrombin time, and partial thromboplastin time should be obtained (see Chapter 51). Thyroid function tests should be obtained if thyroid disease is suspected on clinical grounds.

Working Diagnosis and Management

Anatomic causes. The general evaluation described above is nearly always sufficient to identify the anatomic causes for abnormal bleeding in the premenopausal woman. A history consistent with regular ovulation increases the likelihood that the bleeding is due to an anatomic problem or a local medical condition rather than hormonal dysregulation. Because uterine problems (e.g., fibroid tumors, and much less commonly, endometrial cancer) are more common in women over 35, these patients should be evaluated by a gynecologist if they develop any unexplained change that persists for more than two cycles. With the exceptions of vaginitis and cervicitis, which may be treated by the general physician (see Chapter 94), pelvic disease or pregnancy should be referred promptly to a gynecologist. The evaluation that a gynecologist will perform for possible gynecologic cancer is described in Chapter 95. When a primary medical condition seems to explain the patient's problem, this condition should be managed appropriately (thrombocytopenia, see Chapter 51; thyroid disorders, see Chapter 73).

Dysfunctional uterine bleeding. For the large number of women in whom the working diagnosis is DUB, the general physician may elect to manage the problem or to refer the patient to a gynecologist. The most common cause of DUB is anovulation. In this case no corpus luteum is formed, so a progesterone primed endometrium is not produced. If levels of estrogen are fairly high, the endometrium will continue to proliferate, will become hyperplastic, and then break down irregularly and bleed. Two objective findings that help confirm the absence of ovulation are the lack of a biphasic basal body temperature pattern described above and a failure of serum progesterone to rise during the latter half of the patient's menstrual cycle. These data should be obtained if possible before referral. In some women in whom the data indicate ovulation, DUB may still be the correct diagnosis.

When dysfunctional bleeding has been a problem for a brief period (e.g. two to four cycles), appropriate management consists of explaining the problem to the patient and having her modify obvious precipitating factors when possible. If menorrhagia is particularly heavy and is interfering with usual activities, the problem can usually be controlled promptly by prescribing a 21-day package of a combination oral contraceptive. The patient should be given written instructions to take the first three tablets immediately, then one tablet twice daily for the next 9 days. Within 24 hours, the current bleeding will be suppressed, and the patient will then have withdrawal bleeding at the end of the 9-day course. Patients with persistent DUB, especially those in whom there is a problem of infertility, should be referred to a gynecologist or a reproductive endocrinologist. An endometrial biopsy will often be performed by the consulting gynecologist. A biopsy can confirm either the absence of ovulation (the endometrium will be proliferative, indicating only an estrogen effect) or the presence of ovulation (the endometrium will be secretory, reflecting a progesterone effect, or it may show a mixture of proliferative and secretory changes). Depending on these findings and additional investigations, the gynecologist/endocrinologist will develop a management plan for the patient.

Oligomenorrhea and Hypogonadism

Gonadal hypofunction in women nearly always presents as alteration of the menstrual pattern, either irregular and infrequent menses (oligomenorrhea) or cessation of menses (amenorrhea). Female hypogonadism may be classified by the locus of the lesion *(central, gonadal, peripheral, or exogenous)*; the type of underlying pathophysiology *(congenital or acquired)*, whether the onset of clinical manifestations occurs before *(primary)* or after *(secondary)* puberty, and finally as *juvenile, feminized, or masculinized* (see Table 77.4 for definitions of terms).

Primary

Primary central amenorrhea with maturational failure suggests idiopathic or genetic gonadotropin deficiency of pituitary or hypothalamic origin. A patient with primary *gonadal* failure is most likely to have

Table 77.4. Classification of Female Hypogonadism (i.e., Oligomenorrhea)

Classification	Criteria
According to Time of Onset	
Primary (no onset of menses)	History
Secondary (cessation of established menses)	
According to Somatotype	
Maturation failure (juvenile)	Physical examination
Feminized (normal secondary sex)	
Masculinized (hirsute, deep voice, increased muscle mass, clitoromegally)	
According to Location of Lesion	
Central (hypothalamic or pituitary):	Gonadotropins ↓ or →
a. Without galactorrhea	
b. With galactorrhea	
Gonadal (ovarian failure)	Gonadotropins ↑
Exogenous (disruption of menses by drugs, stress, or illness of other than reproductive organs)	History, physical examination, various laboratory and radiologic tests
According to Etiology	
Genetic (chromosomal or familial)	History, buccal smear, karyotype
Acquired (infectious, neoplastic, traumatic, surgical, hemorrhage or infarction, autoimmune)	History, physical examination, radiology, other special procedures

Turner's syndrome (XO sex chromosomes and no ovaries). *Primary amenorrhea* with *normal maturation* may be due to peripheral causes as simple as imperforate hymen with obstruction of menses, or as serious as congenital uterine agenesis. A special case of this latter kind is testicular feminization in which androgen receptors are absent or nonfunctional (see above).

Secondary

Feminized patients with *central secondary amenorrhea* may have brain tumors or anorexia nervosa, but most commonly they have hypothalamic amenorrhea. Although this may have an *exogenous* cause (see below), it is often idiopathic with no explanation even after thorough examination. Pituitary amenorrhea is usually *acquired* and is often accompanied by deficiencies in other hormone axes (adrenal, thyroid). Etiologies are the same as in the male (see above).

Gonadal secondary amenorrhea refers to loss of function of the ovary itself after puberty. This can be due to infection (e.g., tuberculosis), neoplasm (e.g., Krukenberg tumor—metastasis of a gastrointestinal neoplasm to an ovary), trauma, surgery, or an autoimmune disorder. This latter category is often associated with a syndrome of polyglandular failure that may include thyroid (Hashimoto's thyroiditis), adrenal (primary Addison's disease), Type 1 diabetes mellitus, and rarely, autoimmune hypophysitis. Autoimmune ovarian failure is the most common cause of idiopathic premature menopause.

Exogenous

Exogenous amenorrhea may be caused by other systemic disease such as hyperthyroidism or hypothyroidism, liver failure, renal failure, or other nonendocrine illness. *Hypothalamic (secondary, central, acquired) amenorrhea* is also often *exogenous* in that there is a proximate cause such as weight loss (especially in anorexia nervosa), pathologic obesity, vigorous exercise (e.g., runners or ballet dancers), or severe stress, as in grief reactions or mental illness. Another form of *exogenous* interruption of menses may come from consumption of substances of abuse (opiates, alcohol) or prescribed medications (major tranquilizers, estrogens).

Galactorrhea

Galactorrhea (see above) refers to the production of milk (confirmed by demonstrating fat after staining the fluid with Sudan stain) in a woman who is not recently postpartum or nursing a baby. *Secondary central amenorrhea* is often (15%) accompanied by galactorrhea. In approximately 40% of cases, galactorrhea/amenorrhea is due to a prolactin-secreting pituitary adenoma that may or may not be readily detectable by imaging procedures (macro- versus microadenoma). Other causes of galactorrheic amenorrhea include medication (isoniazid, phenothiazines), recent pregnancy, hypothyroidism, and idiopathic hypothalamic dysfunction. Occasionally, a woman who has nursed may have mild persistent galactorrhea (without amenorrhea) for up to 5 years after weaning. In these cases prolactin levels are usually normal (less than 30 ng/mL).

Diagnosis of Female Reproductive Dysfunction

The diagnostic approach to female reproductive disturbances is aimed at classifying the kind of disorder (see above), identifying or eliminating specific disease entities that require medical or surgical treatment, and having done this, determining to what extent the remaining symptoms represent a problem to the patient and treating these problems appropriately.

History

The physician should determine whether the problem is primary or secondary. A chronicle of pubertal events should be recorded including earliest budding of breast tissue (thelarche), pubic hair darkening and lengthening (pubarche), onset of menstrual flow (menarche), and time of growth spurt and its cessation. A menstrual history includes the average interval between menses, their regularity and when any irregularity developed, date of last period and previous period before that, the duration of flow and its magnitude, the presence of ovulatory pain (mittelschmerz), premenstrual tension, and dysmenorrhea (the latter three findings suggest ovulatory cycles). A pregnancy and nursing history (mature and premature deliveries, abortions, success with and duration of lactation, and living children's ages) and history of gynecologic surgery (including dilation and curettage) are pertinent. A history of breast changes (swelling, tenderness, discharge) should be determined. The physician should ask whether the patient is troubled by growth of excessive hair and, if so, the duration of symptoms, the location and severity of the problem, and any treatment used. Also of interest are symptoms of virilization (see above), which may include increased libido with greater sexual appetite, or increased sexual dreaming and fantasies. Symptoms of estrogen deficiency (hot flashes, vaginitis, dyspareunia, breast atrophy) are important. A careful history of medication and drug use, including oral contraceptive agents, may be helpful. A further general history should include weight gain or loss, dietary habits (especially rigorous dieting), strenuous exercise (e.g., running, ballet, gymnastics), symptoms of diabetes mellitus, adrenal or thyroid disease, and history of tuberculosis or hepatic, renal, or neurologic problems. A family history should include ethnic origin and familial occurrence of reproductive and other endocrine dysfunctions (e.g., hirsutism, oligomenorrhea, hypothyroidism, Type 1 diabetes mellitus).

Physical Examination

On inspection the physician should note body habitus (obese or wasted, mature or childlike, masculine or feminine). The presence or absence of pubic and axillary hair; distribution of coarse dark hair on chest (periareolar, midsternal), abdomen, buttocks, and extremities; and the density of such hair must be noted. The quality of the patient's voice should be evaluated. Examination of breasts and pubic hair should include an estimate of their stage of maturity based on available standards (see Chapter 5, Fig. 5.2 and Table 5.4). Nipples should be squeezed to assess for expressible galactorrhea. On pelvic examination it is important to look for clitoromegaly (greater than 2.0 cm in length), state of the vaginal mucosa (dry versus moist, thick and rugose versus thin and atrophic), discharge, presence or absence and size and consistency of cervix and uterus. Bimanual examination should be done to estimate whether ovaries are enlarged (cystic) or not. In primary amenorrhea without maturation, signs of Turner's syndrome (wide set eyes, shield chest, wide set nipples, "webbing" of neck, short fourth metacarpal, and signs of aortic coarctation) should be sought. The remainder of the general physical examination (e.g., eyes, abdomen) should be as described in the evaluation of male hypogonadism (see above), looking especially for signs of an intracranial mass lesion and thyroid or adrenal disease.

Diagnostic Procedures

All women with secondary amenorrhea should be considered pregnant until proven otherwise (even if sexual activity is not admitted, as may be the case in adolescents). Specific hCG assay is the most sensitive test for pregnancy (see Chapter 93). Further testing should be delayed until pregnancy is ruled out.

Serum estrogen radioimmunoassays have now improved to the point that one can generally distinguish low normal from definitely low (values less than 40 pg/mL are suspect and less than 25 pg/mL are severely deficient), but estrogen status may also be assessed by vaginal cytology and by the provocation of withdrawal bleeding. Cells for vaginal cytology should be obtained at the time of pelvic examination so that a maturational index can be estimated (see Chapter 94). A progesterone withdrawal test (7 days of 10 mg of medroxyprogesterone acetate [Provera] orally or a single 100-mg dose of progesterone in oil intramuscularly) will result in withdrawal bleeding within a few days (2 to 5 days if oral and 7 to 10 days if intramuscular) if estrogen levels are adequate. If there is no bleeding, a 21-day course of estrogen (1.25 mg of conjugated estrogen, e.g., Premarin, a day) with 5 to 10 mg of medroxyprogesterone acetate (Provera) for the last 7 days should be administered. Absence of vaginal bleeding at this point indicates an absent or severely damaged endometrium, sometimes secondary to previous overvigorous dilation and curettage (Asherman's syndrome).

Serum or urinary gonadotropins are used to classify hypogonadism as gonadal (LH and FSH elevated) or central (LH and FSH low or normal). The investigation of central hypogonadism should include a serum prolactin level, especially if galactorrhea is present. Prolactin values between 30 and 100 ng/mL are elevated and are consistent with a prolactinoma, but they may be due to other causes such as hypothalamic (idio-pathic) galactorrhea or drug effects. Values greater than 100 ng/mL nearly always mean that a prolactinoma is present. Further testing should be undertaken by appropriate specialists and is similar to that outlined for patients with male hypogonadism (Table 77.2). If hirsutism is present, the serum testosterone and urinary 17-ketosteroids should be measured (see above).

Treatment of Women with Oligomenorrhea Syndrome

Absence of Menses

Amenorrhea is disturbing to some women, but not to others. Women with idiopathic oligomenorrhea who desire regular periods can be treated with low-dose estradiol plus progestin regimens in cyclic fashion as outlined below. When fertility is an issue, appropriate referral to a specialist should be made.

Galactorrhea

Women with hyperprolactinemia due to a prolactinoma can be treated by transsphenoid removal of the tumor or by suppression with a dopamine agonist. Such treatment suppresses prolactin levels and may also restore libido (see "Frigidity and Female Endocrine Dysfunction," below), decrease lactation, restore menses and fertility, and shrink the mass of a prolactinoma. Bromocriptine is the drug with the longest clinical experience. When tolerated, this agent is 85 to 90% effective; however, it often causes gastroenteric side effects, with dyspepsia, nausea, vomiting, cramping, and diarrhea in 10 to 15% of patients. These adverse effects may be ameliorated by administration of the drug in divided doses with food or an antacid. High dosages of bromocriptine have also been associated with symptoms of depression and bizarre dreams or nightmares. Bromocriptine is usually started at a dosage of one 2.5-mg tablet per day and increased by one tablet per day each week up to a maximum of three/day to obtain the desired effect. Recently, a new long-acting dopamine agonist more specific for the D_2 receptor, cabergoline (Dostinex), has been approved in the United States. Although dosages from 0.25 up to 1 mg twice weekly are recommended, the agent may also be effective given only once weekly in dosages from 0.5 to 3 mg (9). Cabergoline causes fewer adverse effects than bromocriptine (73) and may work well in patients who do not respond adequately to bromocriptine (16). Surgery (transsphenoidal adenomectomy) is successful, in experienced hands, in restoring menses and reducing or eliminating galactorrhea in approximately 80% of cases. Risks of surgery include meningitis and cerebrospinal fluid (CSF) leakage into the sphenoid sinus, or permanent damage to the pituitary gland (hypogonadism in approximately 5%, abnormalities of other hormone axes, less than 2%), as well as the usual anesthetic and hemorrhagic risks of any surgical procedure. Other causes of hyperprolactinemia can be treated either by eliminating the proximal cause (e.g., drugs, excessive manual breast stimulation) or with a dopamine agonist.

Intracranial Tumor

If vision or brain function is threatened, surgery or radiotherapy is indicated. The exception to this maxim is the prolactin-secreting adenoma, which may decrease in size in response to dopamine agonists. In these cases, the volume (but not the number) of cells is reduced. Dopamine agonist therapy may be helpful, even in patients with suprasellar extension of tumor and visual symptoms, and may be used as emergency therapy before surgery. In patients with macroprolactinomas and no neurophthalmologic complications, bromocriptine or cabergoline may be used as the initial, and sometimes as the sole, therapeutic modality. Clinically evident tumor shrinkage occurs in more than 50% of cases, most often during the first 6 to 8 weeks of treatment. If the tumor is small (microadenoma), it may be sufficient simply to follow visual fields and serial head computerized tomography (CT) or magnetic resonance imaging (MRI) scans at intervals of 6 months to 1 year and to treat any hormone deficiency appropriately.

Estrogen Deficiency State

Estrogen deficiency is an uncommon occurrence in young women with *central secondary amenorrhea,* but may occur in some women, especially those with hyperprolactinemia. It may be defined by a failure to develop withdrawal bleeding after progestin administration, by serum estrogen levels less than 25 pg/mL, or by failure to ovulate and menstruate after being given clomiphene citrate (Clomid) 50 to 100 mg/day for 5 days. Estrogen deficiency is invariable in gonadal hypogonadism. Symptoms, complications, and therapy are discussed in the section on menopause (see below).

Female Sexual Dysfunction (Frigidity and Dyspareunia)

Definition

As in the male, female hyposexuality can be divided into reduced sexual interest or appetite (inhibition of desire), failure of arousal (inhibition of excitement), and anorgasmia (for a more complete discussion, see Chapter 18). The discussion below is limited to physical and especially to endocrine etiologies.

Etiologies

Organic etiologies of female hyposexuality include diabetes mellitus with peripheral neuropathy, hyperprolactinemia, hypogonadism with estrogen deficiency, and organic disease of the vagina, uterus, fallopian tubes, or ovaries with resultant dyspareunia. Various endocrine (e.g., hyperthyroidism or hypothyroidism) and other systemic debilitating diseases can also cause loss of interest in sexual activity.

History

Questions should be the same as those asked of the woman with hypogonadism (see above). Additional questions should be asked about dyspareunia.

If there is pain or discomfort on intercourse, it is important to know if it occurs with attempts at penetration (suggesting local vaginal or vulvar problems) or only after deep penetration (suggesting pelvic disease—e.g., leiomyoma, endometriosis, salpingitis). The physician should determine whether there was a previous history of satisfactory sexual activity and, if so, the time and circumstances of onset of its deterioration. Careful questioning should reveal to what extent the problem is one of loss of interest, excitation (lubrication and heightened pelvic blood flow), or orgasm. A history of symptoms of diabetes mellitus or peripheral neuropathy and of thyroid, adrenal, or other serious systemic disorders should be obtained. Knowledge of medication use (tranquilizers, OCs) and substance abuse (opiates, alcohol) is also important.

Physical Examination

The physical examination should be conducted in the same way as for patients with female hypogonadism (see above). Careful attention should be given to the genitalia, uterus, and adnexa for evidence of infection, atrophy, or neoplasia. Endometriosis, a common cause of dyspareunia, is sometimes detected on rectovaginal examination by palpation of nodules in the space between the rectum and vagina (pouch of Douglas). Neurologic examination should include testing of peripheral sensation and position sense and deep tendon reflexes.

Diagnostic Procedures

If evidence of hypogonadism exists, appropriate tests should be made (see above) to classify the syndrome and diagnose the underlying condition. Measurement of serum prolactin level may be helpful even in patients without apparent galactorrhea or amenorrhea (see above). Patients with pelvic disease should be referred to a gynecologist for further evaluation and therapy.

Therapy

Therapeutic efforts should be directed at the specific organic cause whenever possible. Estrogen deficiency should be corrected (see below), and hyperprolactinemia should be treated surgically or medically (see above). When no organic cause is evident after careful examination, consideration of various modes of psychologic diagnosis and treatment is appropriate (see Chapter 18).

Problems of Menopause

Definition

Menopause is the irreversible cessation of the female reproductive cycle and menses that follows from a permanent loss of ovarian response to gonadotropins. This change generally occurs spontaneously between the ages of 45 and 55 in American women, with an average age of 51. Destruction or cessation of function of the ovary before age 40 is referred to as premature menopause. Hysterectomy terminates menstrual bleeding, but not ovarian function, and hence, does not constitute a true menopause. In any year up to 2000, there will be approximately 30 million women of postmenopausal age (roughly one-third of the female population in the United States). With continued improvements in health care and longevity in our population, the absolute and relative numbers of women in the postmenopausal age range will increase steadily well into the next century. Thus, an understanding of the medical problems of the menopausal period is important for the primary caregiver.

Physiology

Although it has long been known that the menopausal ovary is nearly depleted of primary follicles, the hormonal events of the perimenopausal transition have still not been completely elucidated. After age 35 to 40, serum estradiol levels tend to decrease, probably reflecting a reduction in the responsive cohort of follicles at the onset of a cycle. This results in less feedback inhibition, which raises FSH levels and leads to a shortened follicular phase of the cycle (earlier ovulation), so women in their late thirties to early forties may go from a regular 28 or 29 day menstrual interval to one lasting 25 to 27 days. In the late forties, the luteal phase may also become inadequate with lower progesterone levels and early dissolution of the corpus luteum, resulting in further shortening of the cycle. Estradiol levels continue to decline. Next, anovulatory cycles and "missed" cycles, with long quiescent periods in which gonadotropins are high and estradiol very low, begin to occur. For a year or two, menses are irregular and occur less frequently, although occasional ovulatory cycles are seen. Finally, cyclic bleeding ceases. FSH and LH levels become greatly elevated in serum and urine. Usually the FSH increase is greater. The ovary may still contain a few follicles, but these do not respond to gonadotropin. Estradiol levels become extremely low (10 to 25 pg/mL) and adrenal estrone becomes the major circulating estrogen.

Psychologic Symptoms

The psychologic response to the menopause may range from little or none to profound alteration of affect and personality, depending on the woman. Symptoms vary from minor irritability and emotional lability to severe depression and withdrawal from usual activities. Sexuality is also commonly affected, with some women reporting an increase in libido attendant on release from worries about conception, whereas other women have a reduction in sexual interest, usually associated with a perceived loss of attractiveness and femininity. Epidemiologic and clinical studies have shown that there is no increase in definable mental illness attributable to menopause per se and that, in particular, women who develop depression during the menopausal years do not have a distinct syndrome but rather are characterized by a previous history of depressive illness or symptoms and/or the presence of situational factors (e.g., late life divorce, the empty nest) commonly associated with depressive episodes.

Although not conclusive, a number of studies have suggested that significant relief of psychologic symptoms and an overall increase in sense of well-being and ability to concentrate may occur when estrogen replacement is undertaken (64,75). Beneficial effects of estrogen replacement on measures of cognitive function or memory have been difficult to document in normal women (3,60), but a preventive effect against senile dementia appears highly likely (10).

It has also been suggested that the addition of low dosages of androgen to estrogen replacement therapy (ERT) may further increase sexual desire (but not performance) and sense of well-being (64). Routine replacement of androgen along with estrogen therapy is discouraged because of the high probability of undesirable androgenic side effects. However, a cautious trial of low dosages of androgen (30 mg of testosterone enanthate by injection every 3 weeks) may be attempted in cases of extreme decrease of libido at the menopause. Such therapy should probably be supervised by a specialist.

In addition, there are many cultural misapprehensions about the menopausal period (e.g., expectations of loss of sexual interest and ability and of an increased incidence of mental illness), and these beliefs may propagate feelings of inadequacy, somatic symptoms such as fatigue, and other complaints. Thus, some women who have previously been emotionally stable will still have psychologic symptoms associated with the "change of life." For the most part, these will be minor and self-limited and will resolve with sympathetic support from the physician and the family. The organic changes of the menopause may reinforce these symptoms, and many women have had their symptoms worsened even further by the comment from a physician that the phenomenon is "an expected part of aging."

The physician should try to educate each patient about the menopause and should evaluate her for any underlying psychologic disturbances. In some cases a short course of a minor tranquilizer or an antidepressant may be justified. Women who develop significant psychologic problems during the menopause should be managed appropriately, as described in the chapters in Section 2 of this book. In more severe cases, psychiatric consultation is warranted.

Estrogen Deficiency State

Ovarian estrogen production is minimal after the menopause. Ovarian interstitial and hilus cells still retain some secretory capacity but produce mainly small amounts of testosterone and androstenedione. Most estrogen is therefore formed from peripheral conversion of androgen, 75% of which comes from the adrenal. There is considerable evidence that this rate of conversion is greater in obese women, who therefore tend to have higher estrogen levels postmenopausally. Estrogen deficiency results in various symptomatic manifestations in approximately 70% of postmenopausal women.

Hot flashes. Nearly 50% of menopausal women complain of sudden sensations of flushing and extreme warmth, followed by profuse sweating and sometimes shaking or tremor. These episodes occur at irregular intervals from a few to many times a day and may awaken the patient at night. In approximately 15% of women, they are severe enough to limit normal daily activities. It is important to remember that this and other menopausal symptoms may have their onset before actual cessation of the menses because estrogen levels fall progressively in the perimenopausal period. Investigations have shown that these episodes, objectively identifiable by altered skin and core temperature and skin resistance, are closely related temporally to episodic gonadotropin secretion by the pituitary gland. Hot flashes precede LH and FSH secretory rises by just a few minutes. LH and FSH secretory episodes are generally increased in amplitude, but not frequency, during the menopause, probably reflecting derepression of neurosecretory activity of the hypothalamus by loss of estrogen feedback. It is theorized that this exaggerated excitation of neurosecretory nuclei may spread to the adjacent thermoregulatory centers in the hypothalamus, setting off the hot flash (which is thus a form of "hypothalamic seizure").

Genital and breast atrophy. The female reproductive organs undergo striking changes at the time of the menopause. Pubic hair becomes sparse and lank, and may turn gray. The labia majora lose their fullness as subcutaneous adipose is withdrawn from them and the mons veneris, thus exposing the labia minora. The skin and mucous membranes of the genitalia become thin and dry. The vaginal pH becomes more alkaline as glandular secretion of glycogen is lost. This change and the mucosal atrophy may result in a chronic vaginitis with itching, discharge, and local tenderness (see Chapter 94). Many women report decreased lubrication at intercourse and complain of dyspareunia. The cervix, uterus, and fallopian tubes also shrink. Estrogen deprivation is implicated in the relaxation of pelvic ligaments and muscles that may result in uterine or bladder prolapse and contributes to the disturbing symptom of stress incontinence. At the same time glandular breast tissue atrophies, and the breasts lose adipose and become shrunken and pendulous. There is a decrease in the erectile response of the nipple.

Osteoporosis

It has been estimated that if a Caucasian woman lives to be 90 years of age, she has a 32% chance of sustaining a hip fracture. About 1 million bone fractures occur annually in women over 45 years of age, of which 150,000 are hip fractures. The death rate within 3 months of hip fracture is 12 to 20%, usually from complications of surgery or prolonged hospitalization. Repeated fractures are all too likely in survivors as is loss of independent ambulatory ability. With approximately 30 million women at risk annually in the United States until the year 2000, and the number rising there-

after, osteoporotic fractures will continue to be a major contributor to morbidity and mortality in postmenopausal women. Thus, it is exceptionally important that caregivers appreciate the link between hypogonadism (especially in the menopause) and osteoporosis.

Bone is a metabolically active tissue that is constantly being remodeled. Old bone is reabsorbed by large multinuclear cells called osteoclasts, and new bone is deposited by osteoblasts. Whether net bone loss or accretion occurs depends on the balance between the activities of these two kinds of cells. Osteoporosis, better described by the term *diffuse osteopenia*, is a condition of generally reduced bone mass resulting from a relatively long period of negative imbalance in the remodeling process. Loss of calcium from bone may begin as early as age 30. The rate of mineral loss is highly variable but is greater in women (approximately 1% per year) than in men. An accelerated rate of demineralization (2 to 5% per year) occurs at the menopause (or with any other cause of severe estrogen deficiency) and has been well documented in a number of studies (39). Current evidence suggests that estrogen acts on estrogen receptors in osteoblasts to prevent local production of cytokines (e.g., interleukins-1 and -6, and tumor necrosis factor). These factors stimulate osteoclastic cells to resorb bone (56). Thus, estrogens act mainly to inhibit bone resorption rather than to enhance deposition.

During the first 5 years after the menopause, calcium loss is primarily from trabecular bone (e.g., vertebrae), whereas later, calcium loss occurs nearly equally from trabecular and cortical bone (e.g., hip and long bones). Eventually, fractures may occur. Crush fractures of the vertebral bodies initially predominate, causing back pain, loss of height, and stooped posture (dowager's hump). Later in the course, fractures of the hip and forearm (e.g., distal radius or Colles') are common. The incidence of fractures is greater in Caucasian than in African-American women, probably reflecting greater peak bone mass at maturity in African Americans. Clinically significant fractures are five to eight times more common in women than in men. Besides female sex and menopause, risk factors for osteoporosis include a positive family history of osteoporosis, slender body structure (i.e., low peak bone mass at maturity), sedentary lifestyle, prolonged bed rest, cigarette smoking, alcohol abuse, nulliparity, diabetes mellitus, and chronic glucocorticoid therapy.

A number of investigations have revealed that dual x-ray photon absorptiometry (DEXA) and quantitative computerized tomographic (QCAT) scanning have the capacity to measure local bone density accurately in the regions most susceptible to fracture. However, DEXA measurements may be inaccurate for vertebral assessment when significant spinal osteoarthritis has led to proliferative changes (e.g., vertebral "lipping"). Current evidence suggests that these techniques can help predict whether a patient is at high risk for fracture (55); however, it is likely that single determinations will be less accurate in this regard than measurements repeated at intervals to identify those patients losing bone at more rapid than average rates. QCAT is more precise than DEXA and has the advantage of elucidating structure more clearly (11). Unfortunately, QCAT requires relatively high levels of radiation exposure that, combined with its greater expense, limits it for the present to use for research purposes. On the other hand, DEXA scanning is increasingly accepted as a reliable method for helping identify postmenopausal women at presumed high risk for osteoporotic fractures. In addition, new and more accurate biochemical methods for assessing rates of bone resorption (e.g., urinary or serum levels of pyridinoline cross-links) and bone deposition (e.g., serum osteocalcin and procollagen type I) are being investigated to learn whether they add to the ability to prognosticate fracture risk. Most recently, determination of urinary N-telopeptides has been shown to correlate well with rates of bone loss (48). Nonetheless, there is no universally accepted method for predicting osteoporotic fracture risk to determine which women are the best candidates for ERT. Recommendations for general use of these techniques await the results of further investigations.

Atherosclerosis and Plasma Lipids

Before the menopause, rates of myocardial infarction, angina, and sudden cardiac death are significantly lower in women than in men, even after accounting for known risk factors, such as blood pressure and cigarette smoking. These rates increase during the sixth through eighth decades to become equal to or slightly greater than those of age-matched men, suggesting that premenopausal estrogen levels may be the protective factor. Further evidence for this hypothesis comes from the Framingham study, which found that the level of coronary artery disease (CAD) risk is higher in postmenopausal women than in cycling women of the same age (30).

It is well established that plasma lipoprotein patterns predict risk of CAD (see Chapter 75). In particular, the lower the total cholesterol and the greater the percentage of total cholesterol present in the high-density lipid (HDL) fraction, and accordingly the less cholesterol in the low-density (LDL) fraction, the lower the risk of CAD. Cross-sectional measurements in normal men and women of various ages (Fig. 77.4) have shown that mean levels of HDL cholesterol are considerably higher in women than in men at every age and decrease little if at all (50) in women at the time of the menopause. In contrast, LDL levels (Fig. 77.4) are lower in young women than in age-matched men and increase gradually with age in both sexes, but between ages 45 and 55 (i.e., at the menopause), LDL cholesterol in women increases substantially and actually exceeds the LDL level in men after age 50. Another circulating lipid factor that is associated with a higher risk of coronary disease is Lp(a), a variable fraction of LDL lipid tightly bound to apoprotein(a) (see Chapter 75). The amount of Lp(a) appears to be genetically determined, is generally lower in women, and rises after the menopause.

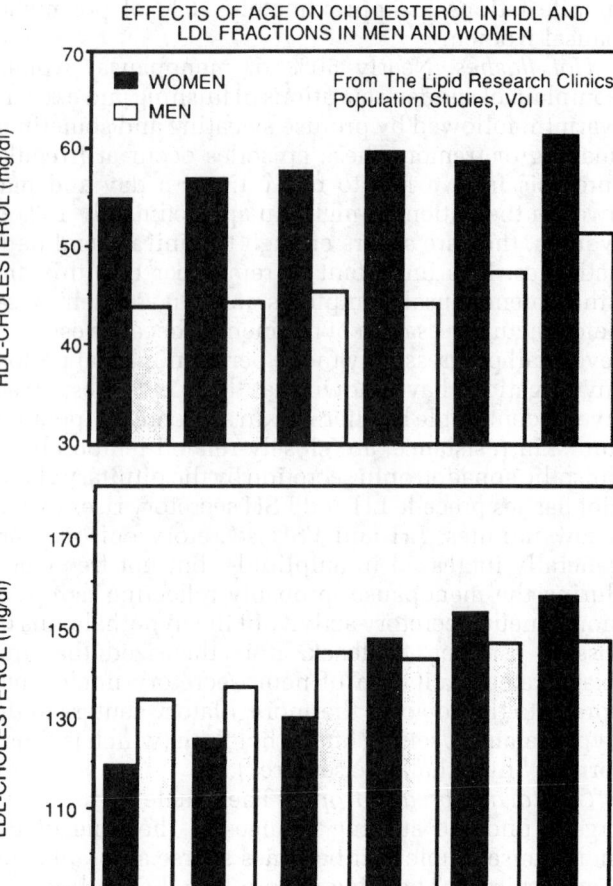

Figure 77.4. This figure, taken from data of the Lipid Research Clinics Population Study, shows plasma levels of HDL cholesterol (upper panel) and LDL cholesterol (lower panel) in women (not using oral estrogens) and men by 5 year age intervals from 35 to 64. Menopause may be assumed to occur between ages 45 and 55. Note that during the perimenopausal period there is little change in HDL cholesterol, but a relatively large increment in LDL cholesterol. (From The Lipid Research Clinics. Population studies data book. Vol 1. The prevalence study. US Department of Health and Human Services, National Institutes of Health Publication No. 80-1527, 1980.)

Most studies strongly support a protective role of estrogen replacement against coronary vascular disease and cardiac death (33). However, the magnitude of this protection exceeds that expected from the documented effects on HDL and LDL cholesterol by 40 to 60% (2). There is considerable evidence to demonstrate potentially cardioprotective effects of estrogens beyond their effects on lipoprotein profile. These include vasodilation (18) due to local endothelial release of vasoactive substances such as nitric oxide by the endothelium (70) and prevention of thrombus formation and accelerated fibrinolysis (43).

Endometrial Hyperplasia and Carcinoma

With loss of regular progesterone-induced maturation and subsequent shedding of the endometrium, the incidence of endometrial hyperplasia, due to the unopposed tonic effects of residual (adrenal) estrogen, begins to rise. This lesion is rarely seen in cycling premenopausal women but commonly occurs in those young women with a pattern of irregular anovulatory bleeding because these women also lack progesterone. Hyperplasia also appears to be more common in obese postmenopausal women, probably because of increased aromatization of androgens to estrogens in fatty tissue. Endometrial hyperplasia, especially the atypical adenomatous pattern characteristic of unopposed estrogens, appears to be a precursor of endometrial carcinoma. It is therefore not surprising that carcinoma of the uterus is also more common in young anovulatory and postmenopausal obese women.

The incidence of endometrial carcinoma begins to rise at age 45, reaches a peak at about 0.08% (80/100,000) at age 70, and decreases thereafter. It is usually first suspected by the finding of postmenopausal vaginal bleeding, is invasive (into myometrium and vessels) in approximately 10% of cases, and has a relatively good prognosis if treated promptly by hysterectomy. It results in very few deaths because it is relatively rare and often is curable.

Estrogen Replacement Therapy

Benefits. Use of estrogen is highly effective, compared with placebo, in suppressing the symptoms of the hot flash. Even low dosages (0.01 mg/day of ethinyl estradiol [Estinyl] or 0.625 mg/day of Premarin), which have little effect on circulating serum gonadotropins, are effective. Such therapy is often given for 6 months to a year and then tapered; hot flashes recur in approximately 50% of cases, however. In this instance, a more prolonged course of low-dose estrogens or of cyclic or progestin-opposed estrogen therapy (see below) may be useful. Genital atrophy, vaginitis, and dyspareunia are all relieved by estrogen therapy, which may be systemic or local (by means of estrogen-containing cream). This latter form of therapy is not necessarily advantageous for preventing systemic effects of estrogen because estrogens are taken up through the vaginal mucosa in unpredictable but significant amounts.

In estrogen-deficient/postmenopausal women, hormone replacement has been shown to be effective in reducing calcium loss and in preserving bone density (39), even at low dosages. Moreover, estrogen replacement reduces the number of fractures in estrogen-deficient women by 60 to 70% (15,74). Osteoporotic fractures are a major contributor to morbidity and mortality in postmenopausal women and their incidence is increasing (61,62). Therefore prevention of osteoporosis and its complications is one of the persuasive indications for long-term postmenopausal ERT.

Sex steroid hormones have specific and highly significant effects on circulating lipoproteins (see below). In general, exogenous estrogens have beneficial effects, raising HDL (when taken orally) and lowering LDL cholesterol. Numerous epidemiologic studies have shown that postmenopausal women taking ERT have a 40 to 60% reduction in their risk of coronary events

(33,52), in CAD-related death (33,67), and on all-cause mortality (25) compared to women not taking estrogen. Moreover, the longer the duration of estrogen treatment, the higher the level of cardiovascular protection (36). In one prospective study, estrogen replacement showed synergistic effects on LDL reduction and raised HDL levels, even in patients simultaneously taking a "statin" lipid lowering agent (21). Finally, of the available lipid-lowering drugs, only estrogen and, to a lesser extent, nicotinic acid are effective in reducing Lp(a) levels (68).

Controversy regarding the cardioprotective effects of estrogen centers around the facts that a few studies have shown no apparent protection, that women taking estrogen in population studies may already be those at lower risk (e.g., less obese, more likely to exercise, less likely to smoke), and that there has never been a large randomized, controlled, prospective study of this question. Nonetheless, if estrogen can reduce the risk of coronary artery disease by as much as 60% (as seems the case), then prevention of CAD represents an even more compelling indication for ERT than does osteoporosis because coronary artery disease is a much more common cause of disability and death in postmenopausal women.

Most recently, evidence has been accumulating from both epidemiologic and experimental studies that estrogen may help protect women from neurodegenerative disease leading to dementia, in particular, Alzheimer's disease (10,58,71). Neither the exact mechanisms nor the precise degree of protection is known.

Risks. One risk of estrogen therapy of potential concern is endometrial carcinoma (see above). A number of studies have demonstrated that postmenopausal estrogen therapy, as formerly practiced in the United States (i.e., 1.25 to 2.5 mg of oral conjugated estrogens [Premarin] given daily without interruption) is associated, after 2 or more years of therapy, with a sixfold to eightfold increase in the incidence of endometrial carcinoma. However, it has been demonstrated (40) that monthly interruption (see below) of therapy reduces the relative risk of invasive carcinoma to about 1.3 (not statistically significant). Furthermore, the addition of an oral progestin for 7 to 10 days of the cycle to mature the endometrium eliminates excess risk of endometrial hyperplasia or carcinoma (19,29). Women treated for up to 10 years with cycles of combined estrogen–progestin for birth control have not shown an increased rate of development of endometrial carcinoma, despite the high dosages of estrogen used. Thus, cyclic, progestin-opposed estrogen therapy is free of endometrial carcinoma risk and has now become the accepted practice in the United States. There is no reason why regular monthly bleeding in a 60-year-old woman should be alarming, if one is aware that the patient is taking cyclic estrogen–progestogen therapy. As in a younger woman, it is intermenstrual spotting or unexpectedly heavy flow that should alert the caregiver to the necessity for investigation. Current practice does not require routine endometrial biopsy when starting ERT in healthy women without a history of abnormal intermenstrual bleeding, but this procedure should be performed if bleeding occurs at other than the expected withdrawal periods.

Resumption of regular monthly bleeding is considered undesirable by a significant proportion of postmenopausal women and frequently leads to discontinuation of hormone therapy. Recently, regimens combining daily low-dose estrogen (e.g., 0.625 mg of conjugated estrogens) with low-dose progestin (e.g., 2.5 mg of medroxyprogesterone acetate) given continuously rather than cyclically have also been shown to be safe and effective. This practice eliminates regular withdrawal bleeding but is associated with a 30% incidence of sporadic vaginal bleeding or spotting, especially in the first 6 months. In most cases, the endometrium becomes atrophic and remains so as long as treatment is continued. Although there are no long-term data on the rates of endometrial cancer in patients treated with this constant combined regimen, the histology of the endometrium suggests that protection should be excellent. Another alternative is cycling with progestogen at less frequent intervals (e.g., 90 days). Experience with this modality is not sufficient to determine whether risk of endometrial cancer would be greater than with monthly cycles.

Although numerous investigations have been conducted (41,59), it remains uncertain whether estrogens used for postmenopausal replacement therapy are associated with a significantly increased incidence of breast cancer. Post hoc epidemiologic studies are difficult to interpret because women who take estrogen may differ from nonestrogen users with regard to various risk factors for breast cancer. Because women taking estrogen are more likely to be examined by physicians, there is also a potential for detection bias. In a randomized prospective study (17), the risk of breast cancer was significantly elevated among current but not past users of ERT, but there was no effect of increasing duration of use. The authors interpreted their data to mean that past long-term use of estrogen is not related to risk of breast cancer but that current use may modestly increase risk. Recently, several large meta-analyses have been published, some of which include post hoc analysis of the preexisting risk factors mentioned above (65,69). The overall conclusion of such studies is that, at worst, the use of postmenopausal estrogen replacement carries a relative risk of 1.2 to 1.5, compared with that in untreated women, and that the death rates from breast cancer do not differ significantly in the treated versus the control group.

With regard to the effects of added progestogen, an unconfirmed study (28) suggested that the use of cyclic progestin in combination with estrogen might reduce the incidence of breast cancer. In contrast, an epidemiologic study of 23,000 women (5) reported an increase of about twofold in breast cancer risk after 8 years in women using estradiol but not conjugated estrogens, and a fourfold increased risk after 6 years in women taking cyclic therapy with estrogen plus Provera. The conclusions of both these studies are doubtful because of the small numbers of cancer cases

and the fact that statistical significance was borderline or absent. Finally, one prospective investigation of estrogen–progestin therapy has shown no increase in breast cancer risk in the treated group (53), but this study also had a small number of subjects and relatively few cases of breast cancer.

The high dosages of estrogen in OCs cause a number of side effects, including increase in the incidence of hypertension and thromboembolic disease (fully discussed in Chapter 93). These effects are due in part to portal absorption of orally administered steroid, which results in supraphysiologic levels in the liver on first pass, and increased hepatic protein (e.g., renin substrate, clotting factors) synthesis. No dose of oral estrogen will provide physiologic replacement without increasing hepatic protein synthesis. Even though only one hepatic-related complication (gallbladder disease) has been shown to increase in women taking ERT (as opposed to those on OCs), these effects are a legitimate consideration. Dermal patches (Estraderm) which supply 50 or 100 µg of estradiol (E_2) per day are also available. These patches provide slow constant release directly into the systemic circulation and, unlike oral estrogens, produce physiologic blood levels and ratios of E_2 and estrone (E_1). They do not cause elevations of hepatic proteins (thyroid hormone–binding globulin [TBG], SHBG, renin substrate) and presumably will not increase risks of hypertension, thromboembolic disease, or cholelithiasis. Results obtained to date suggest that transdermal estrogens exert beneficial effects on calcium excretion and bone density comparable to those of oral estrogens (38). In a prospective study, transdermal estrogen reduced the occurrence of vertebral fractures (46), but large epidemiologic studies evaluating effects on fracture rates or hip fractures are not yet available.

It has also become apparent that the route of sex steroid administration influences the pattern of lipoprotein effects observed. When estrogens are given orally, there is a 10 to 30% increase in plasma HDL cholesterol levels and a significant reduction in LDL cholesterol values. Mechanisms for these effects include hepatic first pass increase in synthesis of apo A_1C, the major apolipoprotein of the HDL subfraction. In addition, there may be estrogen effects on hepatic lipoprotein receptors and on the enzyme, hepatic lipoprotein lipase, all of which tend to increase HDL. If estrogens are given by a nonoral route (e.g., by injection or transdermally), the HDL effect is not observed; however, prolonged (but not short-term) transdermal estrogen administration will lower LDL cholesterol. There also appears to be less effect of transdermal compared to oral estrogen on Lp(a) levels. Thus, use of nonoral exogenous estrogens produces a lipoprotein pattern resembling that seen before the menopause, whereas oral estrogen use exerts an additional pharmacologic effect to increase HDL beyond the characteristic high female levels. Because normally cycling premenopausal women are significantly protected from CAD risk, it is reasonable to suppose that transdermal estrogen confers a similar degree of protection; however, currently available data showing protection against cardiovascular disease are derived from studies of oral therapy. Whether the greater HDL or lower Lp(a) levels produced by oral estrogens lead to greater benefit is not known, nor will it be known until long-term studies comparing CAD rates in patients treated with oral versus parenteral estrogens are carried out.

The final consideration involves the use of progestogen. As noted above, cyclic progestogen appears to provide good protection against estrogen-induced endometrial hyperplasia and carcinoma. Progestogens, however, are weak androgens, antagonizing the beneficial effects of estrogens on LDL and HDL cholesterol during first pass through the liver, thus possibly interfering with their cardioprotective action. It has been said that 21-carbon progestogens (Provera or progesterone) have less androgenic effect than do the 19-carbon compounds (e.g., norethindrone, levonorgestrel). However, at the low dosages of progestogen needed, this difference may be inconsequential. It is reassuring that epidemiologic studies have found no attenuation of the cardioprotective effects of estrogen replacement in women taking progestogen (33,52). To further complicate matters, Provera has been implicated in possibly increasing the risk of breast cancer (see above), and some data suggest that progestogen may attenuate the positive effects of estrogen on mood and affect (63). Thus, determination of risk/benefit ratios for ERT must factor in the route of estrogen administration, whether to use progestogen and the type of progestogen to use.

A number of overall estimates of the risk/benefit ratio of hormone replacement therapy have been published. In a follow-up study of more than 121,000 women (34), data analysis demonstrated a gradually diminishing rate of protection against mortality over 10 years of continuous hormone replacement therapy, probably because of the increasing rate of breast cancer deaths in treated women. Even at 10 years, however, the mortality rate remained lower in treated women. There was

no apparent interaction of estrogen replacement with family history of breast cancer. Benefits appeared greatest in women at high risk for coronary vascular disease. This and most other such studies have focused on mortality and have not included the morbidity associated with nonfatal fractures, coronary events, or the potential prevention of dementia in their calculations of benefit. Thus, current evidence still favors the use of ERT after the menopause, especially in women with premature loss of ovaries (under age 40), in Caucasian women, particularly those at high risk for osteoporosis (see above), and in women with unfavorable lipid patterns or strong family histories of CAD. Estrogen therapy is contraindicated in patients with known breast cancer and in women with a high risk of breast cancer (see Chapter 89). Oral estrogen probably should not be administered to women who have suffered from stroke, phlebitis, or pulmonary emboli. The use of progestogen is not indicated in those women who have had a hysterectomy. A regimen of 24 days of 1 or 2 mg of micronized estradiol (Estrace), 0.625 mg of conjugated estrogens (Premarin and others), or 50 or 100 µg Estraderm by transdermal patch can be used. The routine addition of a progestogen (e.g., 10 mg of Provera) for the last 10 days provides protection against endometrial cancer and is now considered standard of practice. Each cycle should be followed by 5 to 6 days without therapy before initiation of the next cycle. Alternatively, one may use daily administration of estrogen, at the dosages described above, as well as a low dosage (2.5 mg/day) of Provera. The various methods of therapy, with their advantages, and disadvantages are summarized in Table 77.5. Current cost for the oral regimen is approximately $20 to $25 per month and for transdermal patches $35 to $50 per month.

The addition of androgens to ERT is controversial. Increase in libido and other subjective beneficial effects of androgens have been described in some studies. However, all androgens carry the risk of

Table 77.5. Regimens of Estrogen Replacement Therapy

Type	Method	Advantages	Disadvantages
Continuous estrogen[a]	Estrogen given daily without interruption	Easily remembered No regular menses No progestogen lipid effect	Risk of endometrial cancer increased Irregular bleeding frequent
Cyclic estrogen	Estrogen for 21–24 days; off for 7 days	Less risk of endometrial cancer No progestogen lipid effect	Risk of endometrial cancer increased Withdrawal bleeding may occur
Cyclic progestogen[b] Opposed estrogen	Estrogen for 21–24 days; add progestogen for last 10–12 days; then off both for 4–7 days	No excess risk of endometrial cancer Irregular bleeding infrequent	Regular withdrawal bleeding Progestogen effect on lipids
Interrupted progestogen Opposed estrogen	Estrogen for 90–180 days; add progestogen for last 12–14 days; off both for 7 days	Probably less risk of endometrial cancer Withdrawal bleeding less common Progestogen lipid effect insignificant	Level of cancer protection unknown Irregular bleeding may occur
Continuous progestogen Opposed estrogen	Estrogen and progestogen[c] both given daily without interruption	Probably no excess cancer risk No withdrawal bleeding Easily remembered	Level of cancer protection unknown Irregular bleeding frequent, especially in first 3 months Progestogen effect on lipids

[a]Conjugated estrogens (e.g., Premarin) 0.625 to 1.25 mg/day; micronized estradiol (e.g., Estrace) 1 to 2 mg/day; transdermal estradiol (e.g., Estraderm) 50 to 100 µg/day.

[b]Medroxyprogesterone acetate (e.g., Provera) 5 to 10 mg/day; norethindrone 350 µg/day.

[c]Medroxyprogesterone acetate (e.g., Provera) 2.5 mg/day, increase to 5 mg/day for bleeding.

virilization; and because oral androgens lead to a deterioration of lipoprotein pattern as well as a high risk of hepatotoxicity, the routine addition of androgens to ERT is not recommended.

Although phytoestrogens, available from health food stores, recently have become popular, there are no data to support their use as replacement therapy in postmenopausal women.

Alternatives to Estrogen Therapy

There is no good alternative to use of estrogens for genital atrophy or hot flashes. As noted above, local estrogen cream produces unpredictable systemic estrogen absorption and thus has no advantages over systemic therapy.

Calcium and vitamin D have been proposed as alternative prophylactic agents against osteoporosis. Because older women often consume calcium deficient diets (400 to 600 mg/day), many are in a state of markedly negative calcium balance. In addition, there may be an age-related decrease in the efficiency of calcium absorption by the gastrointestinal tract. Consequently, a National Institutes of Health (NIH) Consensus Conference has recommended that postmenopausal women increase their daily dietary calcium intake to a minimum of 1500 mg/day. Although there is evidence both for and against a beneficial effect of calcium supplementation, there are, to date, no conclusive studies showing that oral calcium decreases the risk of osteoporotic fractures in postmenopausal women. The National Research Council has concluded that the benefits of calcium intake above the recommended dietary allowance (RDA) are not documented and do not justify the use of calcium supplements (54). Another recommended mode of therapy has been supplementation of the diet with vitamin D (1000 units/day). However, in older patients vitamin D can increase resorption of calcium from bone, despite its stimulatory effect on calcium uptake from the gut. The net effect of vitamin D supplementation in the elderly remains unknown. Therefore supplemental vitamin D above minimum daily requirements is not recommended in postmenopausal women at present. On the other hand, weight-bearing exercise (e.g., walking, but not swimming) has shown significant benefit in reducing bone loss and should be encouraged.

There are other effective nonestrogenic therapies for the treatment and prevention of osteoporosis. These include the bisphosphonates and calcitonin. Like estrogen, these agents exert their beneficial effects on bone primarily by inhibiting bone resorption.

The bisphosphonates comprise a class of synthetic, long-lived analogs of pyrophosphate, a naturally occurring inhibitor of bone resorption. The newest congeners are nearly 10,000 times more potent than the originally described compound etidronate (Didronel). The bisphosphonates are most useful in patients with diseases of high bone turnover, such as osteoporosis and Paget's disease. They are also useful in preventing bone loss in glucocorticoid-treated and immobilized patients. Clinical trials with alendronate (Fosamax),

one of the newest bisphosphonates, indicate that at an oral dosage of 10 mg/day, there is a 48% reduction (3.2% versus 6.2% in the placebo group) in the risk of developing new radiographic evidence of vertebral fractures over 3 years in postmenopausal women with low bone mass and preexisting vertebral fractures (44). The orally active bisphosphonates should be taken in the morning, 1 hour before eating, with at least 8 ounces of water. When taken properly, adverse effects of bisphosphonates are relatively few, mild and transient, and tend to be limited to abdominal discomfort, nausea, dyspepsia, constipation, and diarrhea. Esophageal ulcerations have been reported to be an uncommon complication, occurring almost exclusively in patients who did not adhere to the specific treatment of recommendations.

Use of calcitonin should also be considered in patients with established osteoporosis, especially those intolerant of estrogen or bisphosphonates. Its mechanism of action is to reduce calcium resorption from bone by inhibiting the metabolism of osteoclasts and inducing osteoclast cell death by apoptosis. Because salmon calcitonin is about 40 to 50 times more potent than human calcitonin and is relatively nonimmunogenic, it is the preferred form for use in humans. Originally, calcitonin was given by daily or thrice weekly subcutaneous injections, but recently calcitonin nasal spray has become available. The dosage of the latter for established osteoporosis is 200 IU/day. Calcitonin effectively inhibits loss of bone mineral at the hip and spine in patients with established osteoporosis, but data on efficacy in fracture prevention are not yet available. The dosage for prevention of postmenopausal osteoporosis has not been established. Calcitonin exerts analgesic effects and may be of special benefit to the patient symptomatic with acute vertebral fracture or chronic bone pain. Calcitonin may also be protective against corticosteroid-induced osteoporosis, but results from studies in patients on therapeutic steroids are mixed. To date, there are few studies comparing the bisphosphonates with calcitonin or other antiosteoporotic therapies. Clearly, more comparative trials of these agents need to be conducted, and the benefits and risks, as well as costs, of long-term treatments need to be further defined. Of importance is that neither bisphosphonates nor calcitonin provides the protection against coronary vascular or neurogenerative disease, which are putative benefits of estrogen replacement therapy.

Postmenopausal Bleeding

Postmenopausal bleeding is defined as any vaginal bleeding that occurs in a woman who has had no menstrual periods for at least 1 year (and is not on cyclic ERT).

Postmenopausal bleeding must always be investigated because approximately 10% of women with such bleeding will be found to have a malignant process of some kind. The remainder have various problems such as endometrial hyperplasia, polyps, infections, and traumatic lacerations. It is important that patients be educated that any bleeding after 1 year of menopause is abnormal and needs to be reported to the physician.

History

The management of postmenopausal bleeding begins with a careful review of the history with respect to duration, frequency, and the characteristics of the bleeding in terms of color, amount, and flow. The presence or absence of hormone therapy is important. Even if cyclic hormones are being used, heavy bleeding or bleeding at unexpected times in the cycle may still need to be investigated.

Physical Examination

A careful physical examination should be undertaken. The abdomen must be evaluated for suprapubic masses and lower abdominal tenderness. The external genitalia should be inspected for neoplasia and atrophic changes. Examination of the vaginal mucosa may reveal atrophy or lacerations. The cervix must be visualized and a Pap smear obtained if needed. The examiner should note the size, shape, and position of the uterus and evaluate the adnexa for enlargement or tenderness. A rectal examination may reveal the presence of hemorrhoids or fissures. Samples of stool and of urine should be obtained for analysis for occult blood. These latter procedures may suggest the rectum or bladder rather than the uterus or genitals as the source of bleeding.

Diagnostic Procedures

Patients with obvious lesions of the vulva, vagina, or cervix should have a direct biopsy taken for histologic evaluation. When there is no obvious lesion of the cervix, colposcopy (rather than biopsy) is indicated. Patients with significant adnexal disease should be further investigated by flat plate of the abdomen, intravenous pyelogram, barium enema, sonography, CT, or MRI as appropriate. Bleeding from nonmalignant causes such a atrophic vaginitis, or traumatic lacerations secondary to intercourse, should not postpone the next and most important step, namely referral of the patient to a gynecologist for endometrial biopsy (if the uterus is present).

Cervical biopsies are indicated only if the Pap smear is borderline or abnormal. Using modern techniques, endometrial brush biopsy or suction curettage can be carried out successfully in most postmenopausal patients with a minimum of pain. Anesthesia is rarely required.

General References*

Blackman MR, Elahi D, Harman SM. Endocrinology and aging. 3rd ed. In: DeGroot et al, eds. Endocrinology. Philadelphia: WB Saunders, 1995;3:2702.

> Comprehensive review of effects of aging on hormone balance, including the male and female reproductive systems.

---

*Bold print (general references) and bold numerals (specific references) denote published controlled clinical trials, meta-analyses, or consensus-based recommendations.

McLachan RI, McClure N, Healy DL, Burger HG. The ovary: basic principles and concepts; B. Clinical. 3rd ed. In: Felig P, Baxter JD, Broadus AE, Frohman LA, eds. Endocrinology and metabolism. New York: McGraw-Hill, 1995;1016.

> Thorough exposition of diagnosis and management of disturbances of female reproductive system from puberty through menopause.

Santen RJ. The testis. 3rd ed. In: Felig P, Baxter JD, Broadus AE, Frohman LA, eds. Endocrinology and metabolism. New York: McGraw-Hill, 1995;885.

> Excellent discussion of the physiology and pathology of the male reproductive system.

Specific References

1. Adams DB, Gold AR, Burt AD. Rise in female-initiated sexual activity at ovulation and its suppression by oral contraceptives. N Engl J Med 299:1145, 1978.
2. Barrett-Connor E, Bush TL. Estrogen and coronary heart disease in women. JAMA 265:1861–1867, 1991.
3. **Barrett-Connor E, Kritz-Silverstein D. Estrogen replacement therapy and cognitive function in older women. JAMA 269: 2637–2641, 1993.**
4. Bechara A, Casabé A, Chéliz G, et al. Comparative study of papaverine plus phentolamine versus prostaglandin E1 in erectile dysfunction. J Urol 157:2132, 1997.
5. Bergkvist L, Adami H-O, Persson I, et al. The risk of breast cancer after estrogen and estrogen-progestin replacement. N Engl J Med 321:293, 1989.
6. **Bertoli A, Fusco A, Magnani A, et al. Efficacy of low-dose GnRH analogue (Buserelin) in the treatment of hirsutism. Exp Clin Endocrinol Diabetes 103:15, 1995.**
7. Bhasin S, Bremner WJ. Clinical review 85: emerging issues in androgen replacement therapy. J Clin Endocrinol Metab 82:3, 1997.
8. **Bhasin S, Storer TW, Berman N, et al. Testosterone replacement increases fat-free mass and muscle size in hypogonadal men. J Clin Endocrinol Metab 82(2):407, 1997.**
9. **Biller BM, Molitch ME, Vance ML, et al. Treatment of prolactin-secreting macroadenomas with the once-weekly dopamine agonist cabergoline. J Clin Endocrinol Metab 81:2338, 1996.**
10. Birge SJ. Is there a role for estrogen replacement therapy in the prevention and treatment of dementia? J Am Geriatr Soc 44:865, 1996.
11. Block JE, Smith R, Glueer CC, et al. Models of spinal trabecular bone loss as determined by quantitative computed tomography. J Bone Mineral Res 4:249, 1989.
12. **Brodsky IG, Balagopal P, Nair KS. Effects of testosterone replacement on muscle mass and muscle protein synthesis in hypogonadal men—a clinical research center study. J Clin Endocrinol Metab 81:3469, 1996.**
13. Carani C, Granata AR, Fustini MF, Marrama P. Prolactin and testosterone: their role in male sexual function. Int J Androl 19:48, 1996.
14. Castello R, Tosi F, Perrone F, et al. Outcome of long-term treatment with the 5 alpha-reductase inhibitor finasteride in idiopathic hirsutism: clinical and hormonal effects during a 1-year course of therapy and 1-year follow-up. Fertil Steril 66:734, 1996.
15. Cauley JA, Seeley DG, Ensrud K, et al. Estrogen replacement therapy and fractures in older women. Ann Intern Med 122:9, 1995.
16. **Colao A, Di Sarno A, Sarnacchiaro F, et al. Prolactinomas resistant to standard dopamine agonists respond to chronic cabergoline treatment. J Clin Endocrinol Metab 82:876, 1997.**
17. **Colditz GA, Stampfer MJ, Willett WC, et al. Prospective study of estrogen replacement therapy and risk of breast cancer in postmenopausal women. JAMA 264:2648, 1990.**
18. Collins P. Vascular aspects of oestrogen. Maturitas 23:217, 1996.
19. Creasy GW, Kafrissen ME, Upmalis D. Review of the endometrial effects of estrogens and progestins. Obstet Gynecol 47:654–678, 1992.
20. Davidson JM. Hormones and sexual behaviour in the male. Hosp Pract 10:126, 1975.

21. Davidson MH, Testolin LM, Maki KC, et al. A comparison of estrogen replacment, pravastatin, and combined treatment for the management of hypercholesterolemia in postmenopausal women. Arch Intern Med 157:1186, 1997.

22. Dunaif A. Hyperandrogenic anovulation (PCOS): a unique disorder of insulin action associated with an increased risk of non-insulin-dependent diabetes mellitus. Am J Med 98:33S, 1995.

23. Dunaif A, Scott D, Finegood D, et al. The insulin-sensitizing agent troglitazone improves metabolic and reproductive abnormalities in the polycystic ovary syndrome. J Clin Endocrinol Metab 81:3299, 1996.

24. Earle CM, Seah M, Coulden SE, et al. The use of the vacuum erection device in the management of erectile impotence. Int J Impot Res 8:237, 1996.

25. Ettinger B, Friedman GD, Bush T, Quesenberry CP Jr. Reduced mortality associated with long-term postmenopausal estrogen therapy. Obstet Gynecol 87:6, 1996.

26. Falsetti L, Eleftheriou G. Hyperinsulinemia in the polycystic ovary syndrome: a clinical, endocrine and echographic study in 240 patients. Gynecol Endocrinol 10:319, 1996.

27. Frank E, Anderson C, Rubinstein D. Frequency of sexual dysfunction in normal couples. N Engl J Med 299:111, 1978.

28. Gambrell RD, Maier RC, Sanders BI. Decreased incidence of breast cancer in postmenopausal estrogen-progesterone users. Obstet Gynecol 62:435, 1983.

29. Gambrell RD, Massey FM, Castaneda TA. Reduced incidence of endometrial cancer among postmenopausal women treated with progestogens. J Am Geriatr Soc 27:389, 1979.

30. Gordon T, Kannel WB, Hjortland MC, McNamara PM. Menopause and coronary heart disease, The Framingham Study. Ann Intern Med 89:157–161, 1978.

31. Gray A, Feldman HA, McKinlay JB, Longcope C. Age, disease, and changing sex hormone levels in middle-aged men: results of the Massachusetts Male Aging Study. J Clin Endocrinol Metab 73:1016, 1991.

32. Griggs RC, Kingston W, Jozefowicz RF, et al. Effect of testosterone on muscle mass and muscle protein synthesis. J Appl Physiol 66:498, 1989.

33. Grodstein F, Stampfer MJ, Manson JE, et al. Postmenopausal estrogen and progestin use and the risk of cardiovascular disease. N Engl J Med 335:453, 1996

34. Grodstein F, Stampfer MJ, Colditz GA, et al. Postmenopausal hormone therapy and mortality. N Engl J Med 336:1769, 1997.

35. Halpern CT, Udry JR, Suchindran C. Testosterone predicts initiation of coitus in adolescent females. Psychosom Med 59:161, 1997.

36. Heckbert SR, Weiss NS, Koepsell TD, et al. Duration of estrogen replacement therapy in relation to the irsk of incident myocardial infarction in postmenopausal women. Arch Intern Med 157:1330, 1997.

37. Hellstrom WJ, Bennett AH, Gesundheit N, et al. A double-blind, placebo-controlled evaluation of the erectile response to transurethral alprostadil. Urology 48:851, 1996.

38. Hillard TC, Whitcroft SJ, Marsh MS, et al. Long-term effects of transdermal and oral hormone replacement therapy on postmenopausal bone loss. Osteoporosis Int 4:341, 1994.

39. Horsman A, Gallagher JC, Simpson M, et al. Prospective trial of estrogen and calcium in postmenopausal women. BMJ 2:789, 1977.

40. Hulka B, Kaufman DG, Fowler WC, et al. Predominance of early endometrial cancers after long-term estrogen use. JAMA 244:2419, 1980.

41. Kaufman DW, Palmer JR, DeMouzon J, et al. Estrogen replacement therapy and the risk of breast cancer: results from the case-control surveillance study. Am J Epidemiol 134:1375, 1991.

42. Knochenhauer ES, Azziz R. Advances in the diagnosis and treatment of the hirsute patient. Curr Opin Obstet Gynecol 7:344, 1995.

43. Koh KK, Mincemoyer R, Bui MN, et al. Effects of hormone-replacement therapy on fibrinolysis in postmenopausal women. N Engl J Med 336:683, 1997.

44. Liberman UA, Weiss SR, Broll J, et al. Effect of oral alendronate on bone mineral density and the incidence of fractures in postmenopausal osteoporosis. The Alendronate Phase III Osteoporosis Treatment Study Group. N Engl J Med 333:1437, 1995.

45. Loosen PT, Purdon SE, Pavlou SN. Effects on behavior of modulation of gonadal function in men with gonadotropin-releasing hormone antagonists. Am J Psychiatry 151:271, 1994.

46. Lufkin EG, Wahner HW, O'Fallon WM, et al. Treatment of postmenopausal osteoporosis with transdermal estrogen. Ann Intern Med 117:1, 1992.

47. Mantzoros CS, Georgiadis EI, Trichopoulos D. Contribution of dihydrotestosterone to male sexual behaviour. BMJ 310:1289, 1995.

48. Marshall LA, Cain DF, Dmowski WP, Chestnut CH III. Urinary N-telopeptides to monitor bone resorption while on GnRH agonist therapy. Obstet Gynecol 87:350, 1996.

49. Martin CE. Sexual activity in the aging male. In: Money J, Musaph N, eds. Handbook of sexology. New York: Elsevier North Holland, 813, 1977.

50. Matthews KA, Meilahn E, Kuller LH, et al. Menopause and risk factors for coronary heart disease. N Engl J Med 321:641, 1989.

51. Meirow D, Yossepowitch O, Rosler A, et al. Insulin resistant and non-resistant polycystic ovary syndrome represent two clinical and endocrinological subgroups. Human Reproduction 10:1951, 1995.

52. Nabulsi AA, Folsom AR, White A, et al. Association of hormone replacement therapy with various cardiovascular risk factors in postmenopausal women. N Engl J Med 328:1069, 1993.

53. Nachtigall MJ, Smilen SW, Nachtigall RAD, et al. Incidence of breast cancer in a 22 year study of women receiving estrogen-progestin replacement therapy. Obstet Gynecol 80:827, 1992.

54. National Research Council Committee on Diet and Health: Implications for reducing chronic disease risks: executive summary. Washington, DC: National Academy Press, 1989; 111.

55. Overgaard K, Hansen MA, Riis BJ, Christiansen G. Discriminatory ability of bone mass measurements (SPA and DEXA) for fractures in elderly postmenopausal women. Calcif Tissue Int 50:30, 1992.

56. Pacifici R. Estrogen, cytokines, and pathogenesis of postmenopausal osteoporosis. J Bone Mineral Res 11:1043, 1996.

57. Padma-Nathan H, Hellstrom WJ, Kaiser FE, et al. Treatment of men with erectile dysfunction with transurethral alprostadil. Medicated Urethral System for Erection (MUSE) Study Group. N Engl J Med 336:1, 1997.

58. Paganini-Hill A, Henderson VW. Estrogen replacement therapy and risk of Alzheimer disease. Arch Intern Med 156(19):2213, 1996.

59. Palmer JR, Rosenberg L, Clark EA, et al. Breast cancer risk after estrogen replacement therapy: results from the Toronto Breast Cancer Study. Am J Epidemiol 134:1386, 1991.

60. Phillips SM, Sherwin BB. Effects of estrogen on memory function in surgically menopausal women. Psychoneuroendocrinology 17:485, 1992.

61. Randell A, Sambrook PN, Nguyen TV, et al. Direct clinical and welfare costs of osteoporotic fractures in elderly men and women. Osteoporos Int 5(6):427, 1995.

62. Riggs BL, Melton L III. The worldwide problem of osteoporosis: insights afforded by epidemiology. Bone 17(Suppl 5):505S, 1995.

63. Sherwin BB. The impact of different doses of estrogen and progestin on mood and sexual behavior in postmenopausal women. J Clin Endocrinol Metab 72:336, 1991.

64. Sherwin BB. Sex hormones and psychological functioning in postmenopausal women. Exp Gerontol 29(3–4):423, 1994.

65. Sillero-Arenas M, Delgado-Rodrigues M, Rodriguez-Canteras R, et al. Menopausal hormone replacement therapy and breast cancer: a meta-analysis. Obstet Gynecol 79:286, 1992.

66. Spark RF, White RA, Connolly PB. Impotence is not always psychogenic. Newer insights into hypothalamic-pituitary-gonadal dysfunction. JAMA 243:750, 1980.

67. Stampfer MJ, Colditz GA. Estrogen replacement therapy and coronary heart disease: a quantitative assessment of the epidemiologic evidence. Prev Med 20:47, 1991.

68. Stein JH, Rosenson RS. Lipoprotein Lp(a) Excess and Coronary Heart Disease. Arch Intern Med 157:1170, 1997.
69. Steinberg KK, Thacker SB, Smith SJ, et al. A meta-analysis of the effect of estrogen replacement therapy on the risk of breast cancer. JAMA 265:1985, 1991.
70. Sudhir K, Jennings GL, Funder JW, Komesaroff PA. Estrogen enhances basal nitric oxide release in the forearm vasculature in perimenopausal women. Hypertension 28(3):330, 1996.
71. Tang MX, Jacobs D, Stern Y, et al. Effect of oestrogen during menopause on risk and age at onset of Alzheimer's. Lancet 348:429, 1996.
72. Tolino A, Petrone A, Sarnacchiaro F, et al. Finasteride in the treatment of hirsutism: new therapeutic perspectives. Fertil Steril 66:61, 1996.
73. Webster J. A comparative review of the tolerability profiles of dopamine agonists in the treatment of hyperprolactinaemia and inhibition of lactation. Drug Saf 14:228, 1996.
74. Weiss NS, Ure CL, Ballard JH, Williams AR Jr. Decreased risk of fractures of the hip and lower forearm with postmenopausal use of estrogen. N Engl J Med 303:1195, 1980.
75. Wiklund I, Berg G, Hammar M, et al. Long-term effect of transdermal hormonal therapy on aspects of quality of life in postmenopausal women. Maturitas 14:225, 1992.

Neurologic Problems

Neurologic Problems

CHAPTER 78

Evaluation of the Patient with Neurologic Symptoms

CONSTANCE J. JOHNSON, MD

This chapter describes approaches to history taking, physical examination, and laboratory evaluation that are most useful in ambulatory patients with neurologic symptoms. One or more of these approaches is appropriate in patients with each of the neurologic problems discussed in subsequent chapters (headache, seizures, dizziness, vertigo, syncope, tremor, Parkinson's disease, cerebrovascular disease, and peripheral neuropathy).

NEUROLOGIC HISTORY AND PHYSICAL EXAMINATION

General Principles

To proceed with appropriate diagnostic and therapeutic actions, one must localize the lesion in the nervous system and determine the probable cause of the signs and symptoms. This requires knowledge of the presentation, epidemiology, and temporal profile of neurologic diseases. For example, new-onset central paralysis of an arm in a 20-year-old could be multiple sclerosis, whereas in a 60-year-old stroke is far more

likely; if the pattern is peripheral, then traumatic nerve injury is likely in the young whereas tumor is an important consideration in the old. Figures 78.1 and 78.2 summarize facts that are often needed for anatomic localization. Additional details regarding the anatomic relationships of peripheral nerves are shown in Table 64.2 (cervical nerve roots) and Table 65.2 (lumbar nerve roots) and in Figures 84.1 (upper extremity) and 84.2 (lower extremity).

Most individual neurologic symptoms or signs are not specific for one functional or anatomic disturbance or for one cause (e.g., loss of a reflex is not necessarily due to motor nerve damage, a hemiparesis is not necessarily due to cerebrovascular disease, and a resting tremor is not necessarily due to Parkinson's disease). The constellation of findings from the history and physical examination, however, is often quite specific. Therefore, a thorough history and physical examination are adequate for making a working diagnosis for most neurologic problems encountered in office practice.

Depending on the hypotheses one is entertaining, a brief, general neurologic evaluation may be required; more often, only selected areas of the nervous system needs evaluation.

Components of a General History

Higher Functions and Consciousness

Handedness. Is the patient right-handed or left-handed? Regardless of handedness, most people are left-hemisphere dominant for language; however, some left-handers are right- or mixed-hemisphere dominant. A knowledge of handedness is useful when localizing cortical versus subcortical lesions. A patient with right hemiparesis and intact language who is right handed has a subcortical lesion. A patient with left hemiparesis and intact language who is left handed may have a cortical or subcortical lesion.

Language. Has the patient had any problems with thinking or speech? Minor difficulty in finding words is common in normal people, as are brief lapses of memory.

Memory. How is the patient's memory? What kind of things are forgotten? (To the family: Have any problems with concentration, memory, or general abilities been noted?)

Acute cerebral dysfunction. Has the patient ever fainted, lost consciousness, felt dizzy, or had a seizure (fit, convulsion)? Does the patient have frequent or severe headaches? How often?

Mood. How are the patient's spirits? Feel depressed? Worrying a great deal? How does the patient feel about the future? About self (confident, hopeless, helpless, guilty)?

Hallucinations/delusions. Has the patient seen or heard things that are unusual or things that are not there? Does the imagination seem to play tricks? What feels wrong? Does he or she perceive being controlled by anything or anybody?

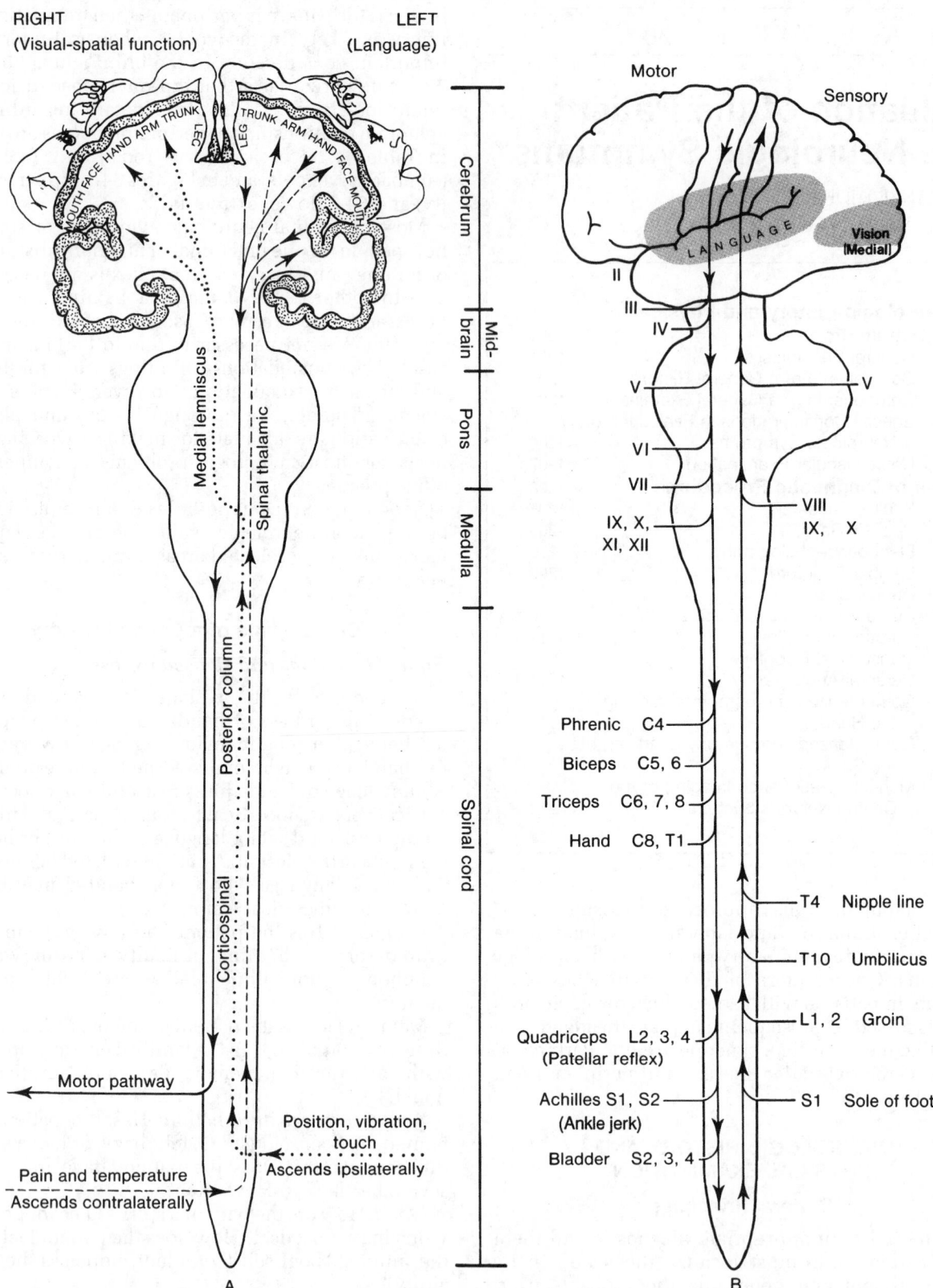

Figure 78.1. Schematic of neurologic localization. Anterior **(A)** and lateral **(B)** schematics of central nervous system localization. Upper motor neuron signs and nonradicular sensory signs can define only the side of the lesion **(A)**; in general, they do not reveal the level of the lesion. The presence or absence of other neurologic signs or symptoms can help to specify the level of a localized neurologic problem **(B)**. (Courtesy of Barry Gordon, MD, PhD.)

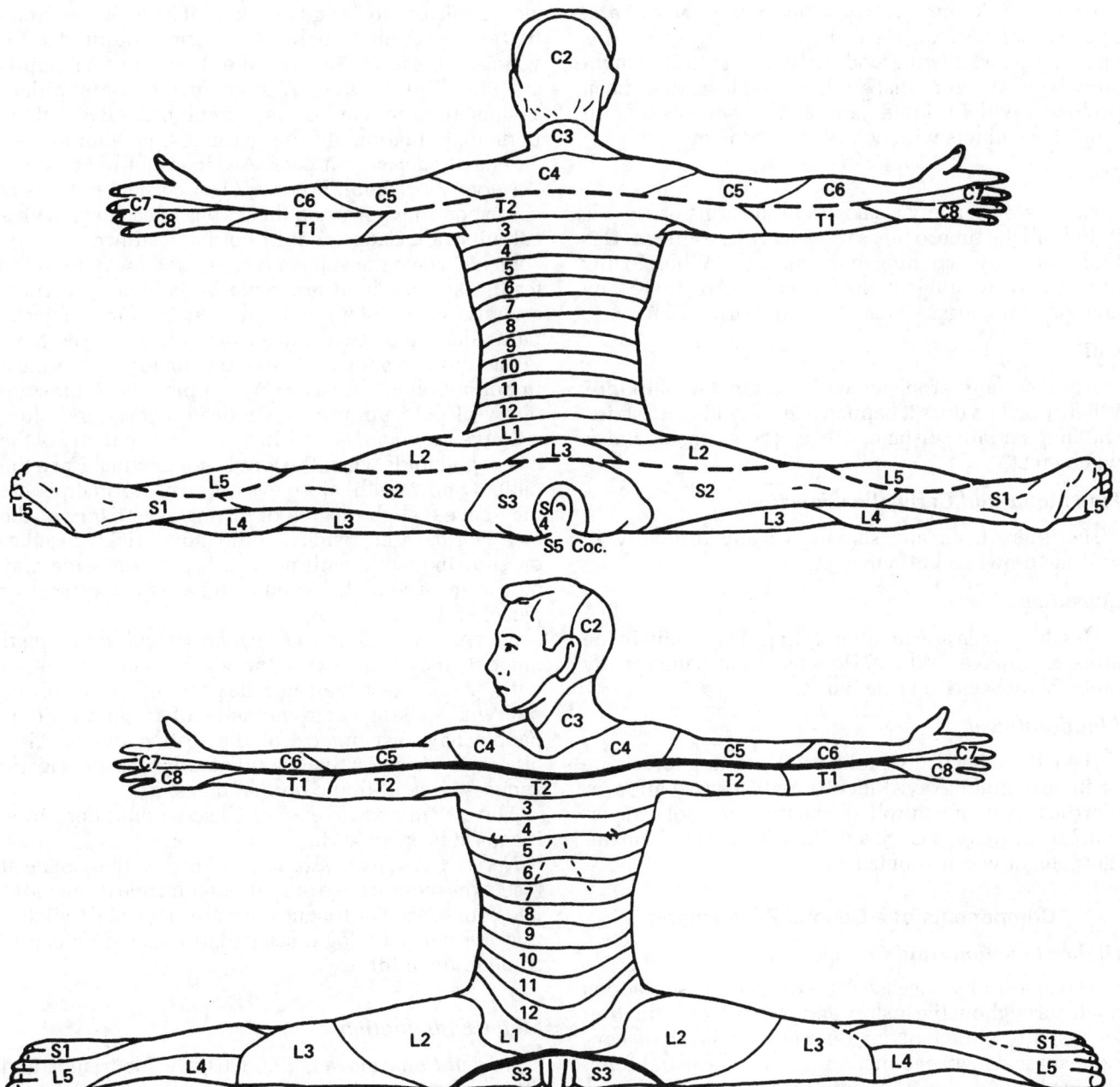

Figure 78.2. Cutaneous innervation areas of dermatomes. The numbers correspond to the spinal cord level of the dermatome. *C,* Cervical; *T,* thoracic; *L,* lumbar; *S,* sacral. (From Haymaker W, Woodhall B. Peripheral nerve injuries. 2nd ed. Philadelphia: WB Saunders, 1962.)

Cranial Nerves

Nerve I (olfactory). Not tested in brief history and physical unless patient specifically mentions a loss of smell or has a history of head trauma with loss of consciousness.

Nerve II (optic nerve and vision). Is there impaired vision? Do things seem blurred or are there patches where it is hard to see? Has vision ever been lost in one eye or has there been trouble seeing out of one side or in one direction?

Nerves III, IV, and VI (extraocular motions). Has there ever been double vision?

Nerve V (trigeminal nerve). Has there been numbness over the face or difficulty chewing?

Nerve VII (facial nerve). Has there been any weakness in the face or paralysis of the face?

Nerve VIII (auditory–vestibular nerve). How is the patient's hearing? Has there been any ringing in the ears or difficulty hearing out of one side? Any loss of balance, spinning sensations, or dizziness?

Nerves IX, X, and XII (glossopharyngeal, vagal, and hypoglossal nerves). Have there been any problems chewing or swallowing food? Does it seem to get caught anywhere? Where? What kinds of food have there been problems with? (Liquids are often the most difficult foods for patients with neurologic problems.)

Motor

Has there been any weakness in the arms or legs? Is it there all the time, or does it seem to come and go? Has there been any twitching in the muscles? Where? How often? Any wasting of the muscles? Are there any cramps in the legs? Under what circumstances?

Gait

Are there any problems with walking? What kind? Where or when does it happen (e.g., climbing up stairs, walking certain distances,)? Is there unsteadiness when erect?

Fine Motor and Cerebellar Function

Has there been any shaking or any difficulty in writing, drawing, buttoning, etc.?

Sensation

Has there been any numbness, tingling, or pain in the arms, legs, or feet? Where? Does position change or any other factor seem to bring it on?

Bladder/Bowel

Have there been any problems in starting to urinate or in urinating? Any difficulty with constipation or diarrhea? Any uncontrolled urination or stool evacuation? If so, was it associated with the urge to urinate/defecate, or was it spontaneous?

Components of a General Examination

Higher Functions and Consciousness

The questions suggested above plus observations made throughout the history and physical examination are usually sufficient for determining level of consciousness, language functioning, visual–spatial functioning, mood, level of intelligence, and memory. Systematic mental status examinations appropriate for patients with psychiatric problems and for patients with suspected cognitive impairment are described in Chapters 10 and 17, respectively.

Cranial Nerves

Nerve II (optic nerve and vision). Check vision (make sure that patients wear their glasses, if needed) with the use of the Snellen chart or by having the patient read from a newspaper; test each eye separately. Check fields by confrontation (each eye separately) using finger wiggle. Examine fundi.

Nerves III, IV, and VI (extraocular movement and pupils). Have the patient move the eyes into all principal positions of gaze (horizontal, vertical, diagonal), observe for dysconjugate movements, and ask, while testing, about diplopia. Look for nystagmus and lid lag also. Look for ptosis and check pupils for size, symmetry, and reaction to light. The normal pupil size for young adults is 3 to 5 mm. In the elderly, normal pupils are often 2 to 3 mm. A slight degree of pupillary asymmetry, 1 mm or less, is present in about 5% of the normal population; it usually varies from hour to hour and day to day, and it decreases in bright light.

Nerve V (trigeminal nerve). Test corneal reflexes at corresponding points on the cornea of each eye with a cotton swab. Gauze should not be used because it is abrasive. Have the subject look up and away from the testing swab. There are wide variations in corneal sensitivity among normal individuals; some subjects, particularly those who have worn contact lenses, have virtually no response at all. Asymmetry is the most important clue to disease. With a pin, check for symmetry of perception over forehead, cheek, and chin.

Nerve VII (facial nerve). Inspect for asymmetry of the nasolabial folds when the face is not moving. Have the patient show teeth, close eyes, frown. Normal people may have a slight degree of resting asymmetry of the face. Normally both sides should move briskly together on showing teeth, smiling, etc. Lag on one side may be a sign of a slight seventh nerve palsy, central or peripheral.

Nerves IX and X (glossopharyngeal and vagus nerves). Inspect the uvula for position and for motion with "Ahh." Test the gag reflex on both sides of the pharynx, looking for asymmetry of response. Some people have asymmetry of the resting uvula. Also, bilaterally hyperactive to bilaterally absent gag responses are within the normal range.

Nerve XI (accessory nerve). Observe shoulder shrug; it should be symmetric.

Nerve XII (hypoglossal nerve). Inspect the tongue at rest in the mouth; have the patient protrude it and move it to both sides. The tongue normally has small twitches that are not pathologic fasciculations; it should protrude in the midline.

Motor Examination

Adventitious movements. Observe for tremor and other spontaneous movements. (See additional details in Chapter 82, "Common Disorders of Movement.")

Bulk. Examine for asymmetries of muscle mass. Denervation will cause loss of muscle bulk, reaching a maximum by 4 months; disuse over months to years will also cause a decrease in muscle bulk (e.g., in the legs of patients who are permanently bedridden).

Muscle tone (resistance to passive motion). Test tone by passively flexing and extending the upper and lower extremities. (Normal tone is a slight firmness of muscles and slight resistance to passive motion. In hypotonia, the muscles are flaccid, without resistance to passive motion. This may mean lower motor neuron or cerebellar disease.)

There are several subtypes of *hypertonia:*

- *Rigidity* is increased resistance to passive motion throughout the whole range of motion around a joint.

- In *spasticity,* the initial passive motion is easy, but then there is a tightening of the muscle (spastic catch) possibly followed by a sudden release (clasp-knife effect). Spasticity usually affects only one set of muscles around a joint (in the upper extremities, the biceps, forearm pronators, and finger flexors; in the lower extremities, the quadriceps, hamstrings, and plantar flexors).
- In *gegenhalten or paratonia,* resistance is present in all directions but varies with the examiner's force and speed. It often seems to be voluntary (fighting back). (Gegenhalten is seen normally in infants, but it appears pathologically in adults with dementias or with frontal lobe disease.)

Voluntary strength. Test voluntary strength in several major muscle groups. Survey proximal and distal muscles in each extremity. An adequate screen includes testing shoulder abduction, elbow extension and flexion, wrist and finger extension, grip strength (with two fingers), hip flexion (with patient sitting), knee flexion, knee extension, and foot dorsiflexion. Also observe the patient's gait (see below).

For precise documentation, the following rating scale can be used: 0 = no movement, 1 = flicker, 2 = able to move with gravity eliminated (e.g., lateral motion of arm when recumbent), 3 = able to move against gravity, 4 = able to move against resistance, 5 = normal strength.

In conversion reactions and malingering, strength on formal testing is usually jerky or giving. With sudden passive motions in the opposite direction, the examiner may find that the muscles produce normal resistive force. The examiner may find that the subject can do some voluntary activities (e.g., combing hair, reaching for objects, getting up or sitting down) with muscles that the patients states are too weak to use for such motions on formal testing.

Reflexes

The most important reflexes to test are the biceps (C5–6), triceps (C6–8), patellar (L2–4), Achilles tendon (S1–2), and plantar flexion. Activity of the reflexes varies widely among patients and can vary depending on a patient's emotional state and ability to relax muscles. As in the rest of the examination, asymmetries between two sides generally carry more weight than symmetric reflex changes; comparison must be made with the muscles relaxed to a similar degree and with the two extremities in identical positions. A decrease in the reflex or reflexes is generally caused by disruption of the sensory or motor nerves of the reflex loop itself. Sometimes decreased reflexes are seen immediately after a cerebrovascular accident, in which case interpretation does not depend on the reflexes alone. Increased reflexes mean upper motor neuron (UMN) disease located anywhere from just above the anterior horn cell to the cerebral cortex. A Babinski sign is dorsiflexion of the big toe after plantar stimulation, which may be associated with dorsiflexion and spreading of the other toes and dorsiflexion of the foot. The classic Babinski response is slow and deliberate. Nonspecific withdrawal may resemble the Babinski reflex, but it is usually rapid and the patient usually complains of subjective distress; a reliable Babinski sign can and should occur in the absence of any patient discomfort from the stimulus. A Babinski sign may be found as the sole indicator of UMN disease.

Sensation

The patient should be tested for symmetry and for differences in proximal and distal perception, in all four extremities. Light touch (posterior columns) is not a well-delineated modality and can be normal when abnormalities of pinprick (lateral spinothalamic tract) or proprioception/vibration (posterior columns) are present; therefore, it should not be used as the sole screen of sensory function. Sensitivity to pinprick, proprioception, and vibratory sense should be tested. There are normal differences in pinprick perception over different areas of the body (e.g., it is decreased over the beard area), but patients generally ignore these differences. Particularly introspective or anxious patients can give very confusing responses and must be told to ignore small subjective differences. Repeated testing is often important to determine the reliability of a patient's response. Vibration sense should be tested with a 128-Hz tuning fork. Proprioception is tested in the most distal joint of the fingers and toes by moving the digit approximately 30° to 45° and then asking the patient to report the direction in which the digits have moved.

The Romberg test (patient stands with feet together and closed eyes and the ability to maintain balance is assessed) is a test of integrity of vibration, proprioception, and the posterior columns through which they are conveyed. Nonetheless, the ability to stand with eyes closed must be integrated with caution in patients with cerebellar ataxia. If the patient cannot stand steady with eyes open then there is cerebellar ataxia and the Romberg test can be altered to allow testing of posterior columns by having the patient stand with a wide base (compensates for cerebellar ataxia) and then close the eyes. If the posterior columns are intact, the patient will not waver more than a slight amount.

Fine Motor and Cerebellar

The patient should be told to touch the thumb sequentially to each of the fingers of each hand separately and the speed, effort, and rhythm should be observed. Finger-to-nose-to-finger should be tested (subject has to touch examiner's moving finger, then touch his or her own nose, then touch the examiner's finger again, etc.) for speed, rhythm, intention tremor, and inaccuracy (dysmetria). The subject should be asked to tap each foot separately, and differences in speed, ease, and rhythm should be observed. In these tests, normal subjects show equal ability with either side or are slightly better on the side of their preferred hand. Slowness and subjective effort on repetitive movements, without a loss of rhythm, are characteristic of UMN lesions. Preserved speed with erratic movements and loss of rhythm may be seen in cerebellar disease. Finger–nose–finger testing may be affected by tremor of various types, as described in Chapter 82.

Station and Gait

Any tendency to list or any need for support while sitting, standing, or walking should be observed. The patient should be asked to walk normally and to walk on the heels and toes (tests strength and balance). Tandem gait testing (walking heel to toe) requires the patient to narrow the base of support and reveals abnormalities of balance in patients with ataxia not detected with normal walking.

In *cerebellar disease,* there is a wide base (legs widely separated), unsteadiness, and lateral reeling. Lateral reeling can be evaluated by having the patient walk around a chair in both directions; he or she will tend to walk into the chair when it is on the affected side and to veer away from the chair when it is on the unaffected side. Because of fundamental abnormality of motor coordination, the patient with cerebellar disease that affects the lower extremities cannot participate in a standard Romberg test, which requires standing with the two feet together; a modified Romberg test for such patients is described above.

In *sensory ataxia* (loss of proprioception), there is uncertainty, slapping or stamping of the feet, and a positive Romberg test (the patient loses balance with eyes closed but can avoid falling when the eyes are open because of visually mediated vestibular or cerebellar compensation).

In a *spastic gait* (in UMN disease), the leg does not flex but circumducts, and there is foot dragging (the toe of the sole of the patient's shoe becomes disproportionately worn); there is also loss of arm swinging on the spastic side.

In a *parkinsonian gait,* there is unilateral or bilateral loss of arm swinging, the patient is bent forward, and there is rigidity, shuffling, and festination (the upper part of the body advances ahead of the lower extremities; gait becomes faster as if to catch up).

In *lower motor neuron (LMN)* paralysis of the pretibial and peroneal muscles, there is foot-drop; hip flexion is preserved, and the patient lifts the foot very high, advances it by swinging it forward, then slaps it down.

In *frontal lobe disease,* gait may be wide based, shuffling, and slow, and turning is slow, but there is no weakness or loss of sensation.

Special Considerations in Evaluation of Neurologic Symptoms

The neurologic symptoms seen in ambulatory patients are often less florid than are those of patients hospitalized for neurologic disease, and many of these symptoms are related to prior acute neurologic events. Two important considerations in the evaluation of ambulatory patients with neurologic symptoms are the variability in performance over time and the difference between the manifestations of UMN and LMN lesions.

Variability over Time

In patients who have abnormalities of the peripheral nerves, spinal cord, and brainstem, symptoms and signs remain about the same after the basic problem has stabilized; subsequently, alterations of the findings usually reflect a change in the patient's disease. On the other hand, the performance of patients with ostensibly stabilized cerebral disease may vary greatly from minute to minute, hour to hour, or day to day. The variability affects the psychomotor domain (e.g., performance of everyday tasks, memory, speech and language, and mood). For example,

- The patient may be able to dress, fix breakfast, and bring in the mail one morning, be incapable of these tasks the next morning, and perform them correctly on the third morning.
- The patient may remember his or her spouse's name in the morning but not in the evening of the same day.
- The aphasic patient may be able to say something one minute and be unable to say it several minutes later.
- The stroke survivor's affect may vary from depressed to euphoric from hour to hour and day to day.

As a result of this type of variability, members of the patient's family may become confused and angry; they may inquire whether a change in behavior means that the disease is getting worse, or they may conclude that the patient is capable of doing certain tasks but just not trying sometimes. When the pattern is clearly one of waxing and waning, the family should be reassured that, just as they have their good days and bad days, the patients will also, but in exaggerated and different ways. The evaluation and management of behavioral changes of patients with cerebral damage are discussed in more detail in Chapters 17 (dementia) and 83 (stroke).

Difference Between Upper Motor Neuron and Lower Motor Neuron Symptoms

The manifestations and the course of UMN and LMN damage differ fundamentally. UMN lesions affect the pathways that bring a command from the cortex to the anterior horn cell. UMN function depends on integrity of the cortex and the corticospinal and corticobulbar tracts. LMN lesions affect the final common pathway for muscle movements. LMN function depends on the integrity of the anterior horn cell in the spinal cord and its nerve fiber for carrying impulses to the muscle cell. A number of points are helpful in recognizing or distinguishing these two patterns of motor abnormality when they are not overt, which is often the case in patients seen in office practice.

UMN Lesion Syndrome. If a UMN lesion is total, movements are absent. However, there may be preservation of involuntary movements, such as those associated with yawning, laughing, crying, or anger.

When there is weakness (paresis) rather than paralysis caused by UMN damage, the following patterns of weakness are seen.

In the face, the lower muscles are usually involved. There is variable but often some involvement of the orbicularis oculi, producing a widened palpebral fissure and weakness of eye closure, but the forehead is completely spared. This is in contrast to LMN (peripheral) seventh nerve damage, in which usually both the upper and lower facial muscles are involved, although sometimes mild peripheral seventh nerve weakness (e.g., early Bell's palsy, an LMN lesion) can mimic a UMN pattern. One additional differential point is that the LMN lesion will produce the same amount of weakness with both a voluntary and an involuntary movement (e.g., laughing). A UMN seventh nerve paresis (from a stroke, for example) may not be apparent when the patient is laughing or crying involuntarily and may be present only when the patient is asked to smile voluntarily.

In the arm and leg, distal muscles are affected by UMN lesions much more than proximal muscles. In addition, some specific motor functions are affected more than others: in the arm, shoulder abduction and external rotation; in the forearm, extension and supination; in the wrist and finger, extension; in the hip, flexion; in the knee, flexion; and in the foot and toe, dorsiflexion.

Whether or not the muscles are weak in a UMN lesion, voluntary movements are typically slowed and require greater effort than usual, and the ability to make fine movements with the affected limb is lost. A patient with a very mild hemiparesis may be able to squeeze the examiner's hand with normal strength, but movements are slower and clumsier than usual; the patient may be unable easily to use fingers individually. Also, when the patient is asked to extend both arms with the eyes closed, there may be downward and inward drift of the weak arm (pronator sign). In the lower extremity, a patient with such a mild defect may be able to dorsiflex the foot voluntarily. However, the same patient may not be able to do this very rapidly (as revealed on attempted foot tapping), and the movement may not be automatically coordinated with walking, resulting in a foot drop.

Typically (but not invariably), UMN lesions are accompanied by spasticity and hyperreflexia.

LMN Lesion Syndrome. Weakness resulting from a permanent LMN lesion is fixed and unchanging. Only the muscles served by the involved spinal cord segment or peripheral nerve are weak. There are none of the widespread effects characteristic of a UMN lesion. Atrophy is usually apparent within several weeks after an LMN lesion, in contrast to UMN lesions, where atrophy is slight and late (many months). Pathologic fasciculations may be present in affected muscle groups, distinguishable from benign occasional muscle twitching by the fact that they are frequent and occur only in the denervated muscles. Muscles are usually flaccid and hyporeflexic or areflexic. If a peripheral nerve has been involved, there may be associated hypesthesia or anesthesia.

In some situations, UMN and LMN lesions may occur together. For instance, spinal cord injury typically gives signs of a LMN lesion at the level of the injury, caused by localized destruction of the anterior horn cells and their nerve roots; below the level of the injury, there may be a partial or complete UMN syndrome with spasticity, hyperreflexia, and preserved involuntary reflexes. Likewise, amyotrophic lateral sclerosis, an idiopathic degenerative disease, affects both pyramidal tract cells and anterior horn cells. Along with LMN type weakness, fasciculations, and wasting, these patients have hyperreflexia and may have Babinski signs.

Neurovascular Examination

This examination is especially important in patients in whom cerebrovascular disease or an increased risk of cerebrovascular disease is the problem (see Chapter 83). The examination includes an assessment of the heart and peripheral vasculature, with emphasis on the vessels of the head and neck.

Heart and Peripheral Vessels

The radial arteries should be simultaneously palpated at the wrists to determine any asymmetry in pulse amplitude or timing (pulse delay). The brachial arterial blood pressure should be measured in the supine, sitting, and standing positions. Blood pressure should be measured in both arms to check for asymmetry. Unequal blood pressure in the two arms (20 mm Hg or more difference in systolic and greater than 10 mm Hg in diastolic pressure) suggests a stenotic lesion of the subclavian or innominate artery on the side with the lower pressure. Orthostatic hypotension, defined as a fall in systolic pressure of greater than 15 mm Hg on moving from a supine to an upright position, may be important in explaining symptoms in patients with severe stenotic lesions of carotid or vertebral–basilar arteries.

A detailed cardiac examination can provide evidence of cardiomegaly, valvular disease, or arrhythmia, each of which may predispose a patient to a stroke. Finally, a complete assessment of the peripheral vasculature, for evidence of widespread atherosclerosis, should include palpation and auscultation of the femoral arteries and palpation of the arterial pulses in the feet.

Vessels of Head and Neck

Evaluation of the vessels of the head and neck may include inspection, palpation, and auscultation.

Inspection. Prominence of the superficial temporal artery with erythema and, occasionally, ulceration of the overlying skin in a patient with persistent malaise is suggestive of giant cell arteritis, an inflammatory process that can lead to retinal or cerebral infarction (see Chapter 79).

Dilation of the *episcleral arteries* of an eye can result from occlusion of the ipsilateral internal carotid artery; in this instance, the hemisphere on the side of the occlusion is being supplied in a retrograde fashion by the external carotid artery through dilated ophthalmic arteries. The funduscopic examination allows direct visualization of the retinal vessels, and changes resulting from atherosclerosis, hypertension, or diabetes mellitus can be detected. Moreover, the absence of an expected change can be informative, as in the case of the hypertensive patient with normal retinal vessels on the side of a severely stenosed carotid artery; in this instance, occlusive disease of the ipsilateral carotid artery protects the retina from the effects of chronic hypertension. A detailed funduscopic examination may also demonstrate emboli, seen as white or refractile elements in the retinal arterioles (see Fig. 83.1). These emboli may be composed of cholesterol, platelets and fibrin, or calcium and are suggestive of atherosclerotic carotid occlusive disease or cardiac valve disease.

Palpation. Reports of embolic stroke after firm palpation of a diseased carotid artery have left some clinicians with a sense of trepidation regarding manipulation of this vessel. The current consensus, however, is that gentle palpation of the carotid artery can be performed with limited risk and occasionally provides useful information about the status of the vessel. Perhaps more valuable, and without risk, is palpation of the superficial temporal and facial arteries, which are branches of the external carotid artery. A weak or absent pulse in these arteries on one side of the head is suggestive of ipsilateral occlusive disease of the external or common carotid artery. In contrast, an increase in pulsation in these vessels may result from stenosis or occlusion of the ipsilateral internal carotid artery causing collateral flow through the external system. Finally, the finding of a tender superficial temporal artery with decreased pulsation may support other data consistent with the diagnosis of giant cell arteritis (see Chapter 79).

Auscultation. After auscultation of the heart to check for transmitted cardiac murmur, the examiner should proceed to the supraclavicular regions over the subclavian arteries and to the carotid arteries up to their bifurcation at the angle of the jaw; a cervical bruit is suggestive, but not diagnostic, of atherosclerotic occlusive disease. Auscultation may at times be useful over the occipital, temporal, and parietal regions of the cranium, and over the orbits. The finding of a cephalic bruit in an adult raises the possibility of an arteriovenous malformation; an orbital bruit suggests intracranial internal carotid artery disease.

USE OF DIAGNOSTIC PROCEDURES

Patients may be referred for any of a number of diagnostic procedures in evaluating a neurologic problem. The principles described in Chapter 1 are especially important in deciding which of these procedures to select. Costs of neurodiagnostic tests vary widely from region to region and within a region because fee profiles are individually determined. Charges for many of these tests are in the $200 to $2000 range; however, practitioners should become aware of costs in their own regions. For most of the procedures currently available for ambulatory application, the definition, principal indications, limitations, and a description of

the patient experience are provided here. Chapter 84 provides this information for nerve conduction tests and electromyography.

Skull X-Rays

Definition of Procedure

The term *routine skull x-rays* refers to a set of films that include three standard views: lateral, anteroposterior (AP), and inclined AP. Many other views are possible and may be indicated in specific conditions (e.g., basal skull views for a patient with atypical trigeminal neuralgia).

Principal Indications

The principal indications are suspected skull fracture and suspected problems involving the bones, such as metastatic tumor (osteoblastic or osteolytic), myeloma, or Paget's disease.

Limitations

The skull x-ray has little value as a screening or diagnostic test for intracranial disease because few intracranial neurologic conditions are associated with bony changes.

Patient Experience. The patient will be asked to keep his or her head in several uncomfortable positions for short periods of time; accurate positioning might be impossible for elderly patients or those who have neck problems.

Spine X-Rays

Definition of Procedure

Standard spine films are usually AP and lateral views; oblique and flexion/extension views usually must be ordered specifically.

Principal Indications

- Suspected cervical spondylitic radiculopathy; in this case, oblique films are necessary to examine the intervertebral foramina through which the roots pass.
- Suspected cervical or lumbar stenosis, spondylolisthesis, luxation, subluxation.
- Suspected vertebral fracture.
- Suspected metastatic tumor.
- To check for evidence of other problems, such as tumor, fracture, and infection, in patients with suspected spondylosis or disc disease.

Limitations

Asymptomatic cervical spondylosis and interspace narrowing caused by disc degeneration are so common after age 40 (see Chapter 64) that their presence has limited usefulness in the absence of more specific findings from the history and physical examination. Negative films provide good evidence against spondylosis as the cause of radicular symptoms.

X-rays do not show soft tissue or the actual status of the cord and nerve roots; these must be inferred. In patients with herniated intervertebral discs, films are usually normal or show only nonspecific intervertebral narrowing. However, patients with congenitally small bony canals (cervical or lumbar stenosis) are at high risk for neurologic problems occurring secondary to degenerative changes in the disc and ligaments; the radiologist should be specifically asked about these possibilities if they are important diagnostic considerations.

Patient Experience. The patient must cooperate for several views. Patients with neck problems and those who are elderly may be unable to position themselves for adequate cervical spine films.

Electroencephalography

Definition of Procedure

This is a record of the (1- to 50-mV) electrical rhythms of the brain.

Principal Indications

- Known or suspected seizure disorders (see Chapter 80). Recording during sleep or after sleep deprivation significantly increases the chances of a useful diagnostic examination; for complex partial seizures, nasopharyngeal leads record from the medial temporal regions where some of these seizures originate and, therefore, can increase the yield of the study.
- Confirmation of focal brain lesions in the absence of other evidence (e.g., in the diagnosis and localization of brain tumor, stroke, abscess, and other mass lesions).
- Confirmation of diffuse brain disease, such as dementia, delirium, cerebral vasculitis, and drug effect or withdrawal. Because the general criteria for normal are broad, serial EEGs on the same subject are most helpful in these situations to confirm/disprove an abnormal condition. The EEG may at times be helpful in the differentiation of the dementia syndrome of depression from organic dementia (see Chapter 17).
- Sleep disorders (see Chapter 85); routine and special EEG recording techniques are often indicated.

Limitations

The EEG records cortical activity and, although sensitive for processes affecting the cortex, is not useful for delineation of subcortical processes. However, this property can be useful in investigating vascular lesions when a cortical lesion cannot be distinguished from a subcortical lesion by other criteria.

Negative EEG. A single negative EEG is not convincing evidence for the absence of a seizure disorder. For example, up to 50% of patients with known epilepsy have normal interictal records. Serial or repeated negative EEGs may be far more significant (see Chapter 80). A normal EEG in a patient with suspected delirium suggests psychiatric illness.

"Mildly abnormal" EEG. Depending on the reader and the classification scheme, some (5 to 30% or more)

adult EEGs can be classified as minimally or mildly but nonspecifically abnormal. The relevance of these interpretations must be judged in the context of the patients' problems but should not be given undue weight because of the broad range of normal. This is particularly true in infancy, childhood, adolescence, and old age. For instance, temporal slow activity (usually on the left, occasionally on the right or bilaterally) is present after age 40 in as many as 30 to 40% of subjects; it may be confused with the slowing produced by a focal brain lesion.

Patient Experience. Subjects are asked to lie down or recline while surface electrodes are attached with electrode paste. The total procedure takes an average of 40 to 60 minutes, with 20 to 30 minutes of actual recording time. For most of the actual recording, the patient is simply asked to lie calmly with eyes closed. Additional studies that most laboratories routinely perform include recording during hyperventilation (for 3 to 5 minutes) and photic simulation with a repetitive flash. For many tracings, subjects are encouraged to fall asleep. Some laboratories induce sleep with oral chloral hydrate if permitted by the referring physician; if this is planned in advance the patient should be told to bring someone who will drive home.

The EEG is extremely sensitive to patient movement, sweating, or muscle tension; any of these may make a tracing uninterpretable.

For sleep-deprived EEGs, the patient is asked to stay up the night before, and the EEG is done in the laboratory first thing in the morning.

Nasopharyngeal leads are applied through the nostrils after local anesthesia of the nasopharynx by spray; they may be annoying and they may interfere with nasal breathing, but they should not hurt.

Lumbar Puncture

Definition of Procedure

Lumbar puncture (LP) is performed to obtain cerebrospinal fluid for analysis and to measure intracranial pressure. A normal opening pressure does not exceed 200 mm Hg. Normal cerebrospinal fluid is crystal clear and contains no more than five mononuclear cells; the normal glucose is two-thirds that of a simultaneously determined serum glucose, and the protein is less than 45 mg/dL. Xanthochromia is a yellowish discoloration of the spinal fluid present with red cell breakdown (indicating previous subarachnoid hemorrhage), hyperbilirubinemia, and extreme elevations of protein.

Principal Indications

- Measurement of intracranial pressure: Elevated pressure must be documented to diagnose pseudotumor cerebri (see Chapter 79). The low-pressure headache syndrome (see Chapter 79) can be documented by LP but may be exacerbated by the procedure.
- Evaluation of patients with suspected meningitis.
- Evaluation of patients with suspected or known chronic infections of the central nervous system such as syphilis, acquired immunodeficiency syndrome

(AIDS), Lyme disease, cryptococcus, and tuberculosis.

- Evaluation for subarachnoid hemorrhage.
- Evaluation of patients with suspected demyelinating or inflammatory disease such as multiple sclerosis, and inflammatory neuropathy (e.g., Guillain–Barré syndrome).
- Evaluation of patients with undiagnosed central nervous system disease.

Limitations

The opening pressure depends on the intracranial pressure, which can be elevated by measures that increase venous pressure such as straining and tightening of the abdominal musculature. A tense patient with an elevated opening pressure should be encouraged to relax and pressure should be remeasured before fluid is removed. The closing pressure depends on the pressure/volume dynamics, which are influenced by the amount of fluid removed and the intracranial compliance. Abnormalities of cerebrospinal fluid are nonspecific; however, when they are interpreted in the context of the clinical presentation and further evaluation in the laboratory, diagnostic accuracy can be increased.

The procedure is completely safe if infection of the skin overlying the puncture site, an intracranial mass lesion, and bilateral brain edema are ruled out. Neurologic consultation and computerized tomography (CT) or magnetic resonance imaging (MRI) of the brain (see below) before the lumbar puncture will eliminate the potential for complications caused by the latter two coexisting problems. If papilledema is present, an imaging study to rule out a mass lesion before LP is always mandatory in an outpatient.

Patient Experience. Patients are often reluctant to undergo LP, based on widespread belief that it is dangerous and very painful. The patient should be reassured that, after neurologic evaluation or an imaging study, the procedure is safe. Under adequate local anesthesia, the discomfort is mild. When LP is done properly under aseptic conditions, the most common complication is a post-LP headache (see Chapter 79). The probability of post-LP headache can be decreased by using the smallest gauge needle practical, a 20 gauge in most adults. Newer blunt-tipped "atraumatic" LP needles are postulated to result in a smaller dural hole, and have been demonstrated to reduce post-LP headache. However, flow rate through the needle may be compromised with the 22 gauge or higher, but is adequate with the 20 gauge. For most patients a 20-gauge atraumatic needle would be ideal. Performing the tap with the patient in a sitting position also increases the likelihood of a first-pass nontraumatic tap; however, the lateral decubitus position is necessary to obtain a precise opening pressure measurement. After the LP the patient is instructed to lie flat for about an hour and to drink copious amounts of fluid over the ensuing 6 hours. A minority of patients complain of pain at the puncture site that may be treated with nonnarcotic analgesics.

Duplex Scan

Definition of Procedure

Duplex scanning combines B-mode ultrasonic scanning of the carotid bifurcation with spectral analysis of a Doppler signal to assess plaque disease. The extent of plaque is classified into categories that vary with the laboratory, but generally approximate the following categories: 0 to 15%, 16 to 40%, 41% to 60%, 61 to 80%, 81 to 99%, and occluded. The percentage of stenosis approximates angiographic measurements; however, some discrepancy occurs as duplex scanning approximates area, whereas angiography is usually a linear measurement. Plaque characteristics such as calcification, hemorrhage, and ulceration can be determined. Plaque distribution in common, internal, and external carotid arteries is delineated.

Principal Indications

This noninvasive screening technique may be used in the evaluation of patients with asymptomatic carotid bruits, transient ischemic attacks (TIAs), and stroke. With use of this procedure, stroke-prone patients may be selected for arteriography (see Chapter 83).

Limitations

No more than 3 cm of the internal carotid artery can be imaged above the bifurcation. The proximal common carotid is imaged for a variable distance, depending on its tortuousity. This technique cannot distinguish complete occlusion from a very high-grade stenosis. No information about intracranial disease is obtained.

Patient Experience. A comprehensive duplex examination of the carotid arteries takes approximately 45 minutes. The transducer head is held over the carotid bifurcation at the angle of the mandible. There is no appreciable discomfort or risk.

Supraorbital Carotid Doppler

Definition of Procedure

The carotid Doppler examination is an ultrasonic study of blood flow in the supraorbital artery, with and without superficial temporal artery compression. The supraorbital artery is a branch of the internal carotid, with anastomotic connections with the external carotid system via the superficial temporal artery. With a patent internal carotid, flow through the supraorbital artery should be unaffected by compression of the temporal artery. The direction of flow may transiently reverse as the internal carotid supply compensates. However, with significant compromise of the internal carotid circulation, supraorbital artery flow becomes totally dependent on the superficial temporal artery supply and is abolished or markedly reduced by compressing it. Therefore, this study depends on both a hemodynamically significant alteration of flow in the internal carotid and the normal pattern of vascular supply to the supraorbital artery.

Principal Indications

To confirm suspected significant internal carotid artery stenosis (carotid bifurcation), a supraorbital Doppler (SOD) study has approximately 90% sensitivity and specificity as an indicator of significant (greater than 80%) carotid bifurcation stenosis. Its principal use has been to complement findings in the duplex scan; however, the SOD may be positive when the duplex is negative in distal (intracranial) internal carotid artery disease.

Limitations

This procedure is useful for determining high-grade internal carotid stenosis. It is normal if there is less than 80% occlusion. It does not reveal plaque ulceration or intracranial vascular disease in the middle cerebral artery. A negative study does not completely rule out significant stenotic disease; 10% of even highly stenotic lesions are missed by SOD because of variations in collateral flow. It is never a substitute for thorough investigation of suspected cerebrovascular disease. It is not useful for the investigation of vertebral–basilar disease.

Patient Experience. The patient sits or reclines with eyes closed while an ultrasound-conducting gel is applied to the supraorbital region. An ultrasonic probe is then held over the artery for a few minutes while the temporal artery is compressed and released. There is no discomfort or risk.

Carotid Blood Flow

Definition of Procedure

While carotid duplex scanning and angiography delineate anatomy, the quantitated carotid blood flow study measures actual blood flow in the common carotid artery in milliliters/second. An angle-independent A-mode ultrasonic probe is used to determine intima to intima vessel diameter and velocity, from which flow is calculated. This unique technique detects abnormalities of flow in the common carotid artery as well as upstream intracranial blood flow changes. When used in conjunction with an imaging technique (duplex, angiography), the significance of stenotic lesions can be assessed.

Principal Indications

In patients with cerebrovascular disease (TIA, stroke, bruit) this technique is useful to evaluate the hemodynamic significance of stenotic lesions and in the detection of collateral flow patterns. Compensatory flow patterns in the carotid free of a high-grade stenotic lesion may also be monitored. Bilateral abnormalities of flow are seen in dementia and in low cardiac output states.

Limitations

Carotid flow patterns remain normal in most patients until a 70 to 80% stenosis occurs; therefore, lower-grade lesions cannot be followed serially.

Patient Experience. The carotid blood flow study is similar to duplex scanning except that the probe is held just cephalad to the clavicle. The study involves no discomfort or risk and takes about 20 minutes.

Transcranial Doppler

Definition of Procedure

An ultrasound system is used to measure blood velocity in the ophthalmic, middle, anterior, posterior, vertebral, and basilar arteries.

Principal Indications

TCD can be used in patients with TIA and stroke to screen for intracranial disease and to identify abnormal blood flow patterns suggestive of intracranial carotid disease. It is most useful in patients where middle cerebral artery or basilar stenosis is suspected.

Limitations

This is a new technique with low sensitivity and specificity. Blood flow cannot be directly measured and velocity–flow correlations are not exact; therefore, TCD (at present) can confirm a clinical impression but cannot rule out structural disease.

Patient Experience. The patient lies on a stretcher while the ultrasound-conducting gel is applied to the bony windows and the arteries to be evaluated. There is no discomfort.

Cerebral Angiography

Definition of Procedure

Cerebral angiography provides imaging by intra-arterial injection of a contrast agent or by the magnetic resonance technique (magnetic resonance angiography [MRA]).

For intra-arterial angiography a flexible catheter is placed in an artery, usually the femoral artery, and passed to the aortic arch, where it is selectively advanced into the arteries of interest, including the common carotid or vertebral arteries, which are then injected with a contrast agent. Serial x-rays are taken.

MRA is a noninvasive procedure that uses radiofrequency signals to construct images of the cerebral vessels.

Principal Indications

Cerebral angiography can be used in the delineation of a number of intracranial processes. Since the advent of CT and MRI (see below), the principal indication for angiography has been the definitive diagnosis of cerebrovascular diseases including extracranial and intracranial arterial stenosis, vascular malformations, aneurysms, and vasculitis.

Limitations

Intra-Arterial Angiography.   Adequate renal function is a prerequisite. Serious complications (approximately 1 to 2% of patients) occur related to femoral puncture, manipulation of the catheter, and reactions to the contrast agent. Serious complications include femoral artery clot with embolization, strokes, and anaphylactoid reaction to the contrast agent. The ionic load of the contrast agent may precipitate heart failure in susceptible patients.

Magnetic Resonance Angiography.   Resolution with MRA is not yet as acute as with intra-arterial angiography; this limitation is related to disturbances of laminar flow and to the multiplanar course of cerebral vessels. The hazards associated with MRA are the same as those listed below for MRI.

Patient Experience. For intra-arterial angiography, the patient lies on an x-ray table and a femoral artery puncture is made after local anesthesia with Lidocaine. The major discomfort is a burning sensation, which can be intense, felt with the injection of contrast. Less stressful reactions are a metallic taste in the mouth, itching, and occasionally hives. Mild or severe bronchospasm, although uncommon, can occur. The patient must be able to lie still for the x-rays. After the procedure, patients are instructed to drink a large amount of fluid, limit activity, and monitor for signs of bleeding or obstruction at or distal to the site of arterial puncture. Instructions usually include limiting ambulation, no lifting or other strenuous activity for 24 hours, and no bathing for at least 12 hours. For MRA the patient experience is the same as MRI (see below).

Computerized Tomography Scanning of the Head

Definition of Procedure

CT uses narrow x-ray beams to exploit the differences in x-ray absorption between different kinds of intracranial tissues. Without contrast, the CT scanner can differentiate between the density of bone, calcified tissue, blood, gray matter, white matter, cerebrospinal fluid (CSF), and air. Its resolving power is proportional to the differences in the densities of these tissues; modern CT scanners can reveal hematomas only several millimeters wide and infarcts 1 to 1.5 cm wide. Although CT scan results are typically presented as horizontal slices through the brain, present technology allows slices to be reconstructed in the vertical or in any other plane to give a better perspective on abnormal findings.

Intravenous injection of contrast is used to enhance the x-ray contrast of vascular lesions; contrast material diffuses into an area where the blood–brain barrier has broken down to increase the x-ray absorption density.

CT scanning is highly sensitive and often diagnostic; thus, it has a place in both screening and specific investigation.

Principal Indications

Evaluation of patients with intracranial problems where structural alteration is known or suspected,

such as tumor, ischemic cerebrovascular disease, hemorrhagic cerebrovascular disease, atrophic degenerative disease (Alzheimer's, Huntington's), hydrocephalus, subdural hematoma, or unexplained headache. Many conditions can be screened for without the use of radiographic contrast; this should be strongly considered when patients have conditions for which the most common causes do not require contrast for visualization (i.e., dementia, remote stroke) and in the elderly, in whom the risks of contrast studies are somewhat greater.

Limitations

A negative CT scan does not exclude structural damage. The damage may not have caused enough change in local absorption density to contrast with its surroundings. This is not uncommon in cerebral infarction a week or so after the initial insult, when the original edema has cleared and new vessel formation and phagocytosis have not yet begun to affect brain density. A CT scan can also be negative because the damage is in an area of the brain that is poorly seen, such as the brainstem or spinal cord. In addition, a CT scan is typically negative after transient ischemia; this finding does not detract from the significance of the event and the need for further study.

When done without contrast injection, CT scanning is essentially free of risk. When done with contrast, the risk is that of the contrast material itself, often a warm flush in the face, nausea, and sometimes vomiting. In approximately 1 case in 100,000 there is the possibility of death from anaphylaxis. The serum creatinine concentration should be measured before the infusion of contrast. If it is abnormal, the risks and precautions related to renal insult from contrast media must be considered (see details, Chapter 48).

Patient Experience. The patient is asked to lie down with his or her head inside what looks somewhat like a large doughnut. Straps are usually applied over the forehead to prevent motion. The procedure takes 5 to 20 minutes, depending on the scanner. Contrast material may be given intravenously, by single bolus, or by intravenous drip.

Computerized Tomography Scanning of the Spine

Definition of Procedure

See "Computerized Tomography Scanning of the Head," above.

Principal Indications

CT is an important diagnostic modality for studying the spine; it shows both the osseous and soft tissues of the spine better than conventional radiographic techniques, including myelography, without morbidity and without excess cost or exposure to radiation. Indications for primary CT of the spine include suspected disc herniation, spinal dysraphism, and facet joint pathology. Because 90% of herniated lumbar intervertebral discs occur at L4–5 or L5–S1, a CT scan of these two levels can be performed quickly. In cases of spinal fractures it may demonstrate lesions missed by conventional tomography besides showing traumatic injuries of the spinal soft tissues. Spinal stenosis, narrowing of the spinal canal, or narrowing of the neural foramen and lateral recess may be most accurately diagnosed with CT.

Limitations

If the spinal region to be studied spans three or more vertebrae, myelography or MRI is more practical than CT because the former studies can visualize the entire spine (myelography) or its segments (MRI) with one test. Diagnostic accuracy of CT presupposes use of a localizer image for accurately selecting the plane and angle of the slice, as well as a thin slice and optimal resolution. CT diagnosis of a herniated disc may be inaccurate in patients with a previous laminectomy. If clinical criteria do not permit the selection of appropriate levels for scanning, CT may be a less satisfactory technique than myelography for examining the cervical spine. Arteriovenous malformation, syringomyelia, spinal neoplasms, and inflammatory processes are more accurately evaluated with MRI.

Patient Experience. See "Computerized Tomography Scanning of the Head," above.

Magnetic Resonance Imaging of the Central Nervous System

Definition of Procedure

MRI is a noninvasive imaging technique that gives better contrast and sensitivity for most central nervous system lesions than does x-ray CT. It uses radio waves of a specific (resonance) frequency. No ionizing radiation is required. MRI studies usually are substantially more expensive than CT studies.

Principal Indications

Many central nervous system abnormalities can be demonstrated with MRI, including intracranial and extracranial tumors (especially posterior fossa), early cerebral infarctions, vascular malformations, hydrocephalus, sinusitis, white matter disease (multiple sclerosis), and spinal cord abnormalities.

In several aspects of brain imaging, MRI has shown itself to be superior to CT. First, MRI provides better imaging of the posterior fossa than does CT because the surrounding bone causes no streak artifacts. Second, the soft tissue contrast with MRI is better than that with CT. As a result, gray matter and white matter are better delineated in magnetic resonance images, and the extent of certain diseases is better appreciated. For example, MRI can reveal many more of the lesions of multiple sclerosis than can CT. Third, coronal and sagittal plane views can be made directly with MRI,

rather than requiring the reformatting of serial transverse plane views, as required in CT. Fourth, major blood vessels can be identified with MRI without the need for contrast media because the flowing blood, as a result of its velocity, appears dark. The common carotid, internal carotid, external carotid, vertebral, and basilar arteries are easily seen. Aneurysms of the internal carotid artery have been detected and a thrombus in the lumen of the artery can be identified.

Limitations

MRI has high sensitivity for disease detection in the central nervous system but is limited and may be less useful than CT in evaluating acute hemorrhages, calcified lesions, and bony structures, each of which is easily detected by CT.

The known hazards of MRI result from the force and torque exerted by the field on ferromagnetic objects brought into the vicinity of the magnet and on patients' prostheses, such as surgical clips, pacemakers, cochlear implants, metal in the eye, and joint replacements. Cardiac pacemaker function can be disrupted and false signals produced, and ferromagnetic metal clips, such as those on cerebral aneurysms, may be dislodged.

Patient Experience. The patient lies down on a table identical to the CT scanner, but the head holder consists of a plastic coil that passes very close to the patient's nose. The entire table is then moved into a larger tunnel. The patient may experience claustrophobia. A knocking sound is heard during data collection, at which time the patient must remain absolutely still. The test lasts about 45 minutes. Because the scanning time is longer than that for CT studies, MRI studies are more subject to artifact caused by patient motion.

General References

Baker AB, Baker LH, eds. Clinical neurology. 3 vols. New York: Harper & Row, published since 1976, with yearly updates.
  Contains excellent detailed reviews of the neurologic examination and neurodiagnostic tests.
Carson D, Serpell M. Choosing the best needle for diagnostic lumbar puncture. Neurology 47:33, 1996.
  Excellent discussion of pros and cons of various LP needles.
Edelman RR, Warach S. Magnetic resonance imaging. N Engl J Med 328:708, 1993.
  Well-referenced review (this part covers the use of MRI for the nervous system).
Health and Public Policy Committee, American College of Physicians. Diagnostic evaluation of the carotid arteries. Ann Intern Med 835, November 1988.
  Specific recommendations for the use of tests in screening and diagnosis.
Heinz ER. Neuroradiology. In: Rosenberg RN, Grossman RG, Heinz ER, Willis WD, eds. The clinical neurosciences. Vol. 4. New York: Churchill Livingstone, 1984.
  Comprehensive description of neuroradiologic procedures, including all of the newer techniques covered in this chapter. Good background reading for a more thorough understanding of the technologic advances made in this field.

C H A P T E R   79

Headaches and Facial Pain

CONSTANCE J. JOHNSON, MD

EPIDEMIOLOGY

Although epidemiologic surveys of headache are not always comparable or consistent with one another, all agree on the magnitude of the problem: 80 to 90% of the U.S. population reports a history during adulthood of recurrent headache, and in 30 to 50% headaches are described as severe at times. Women suffer disproportionately from headaches, both in terms of numbers affected and in severity of headaches; the reported prevalence in women varies from slightly higher to as much as three times higher than in men (3,13,14,23,32). Most patients presenting to the office have patterns that meet the criteria for tension headache or migraine. A small percentage will have organic syndromes such as temporal arteritis, glaucoma, acute

sinusitis, or intracranial infection, tumors, or hemorrhage (5). Recent findings suggest that withdrawal from caffeine may be a particularly common cause of transient headache (24). Most headache sufferers depend on self-care with over-the-counter remedies rather than on visits to their doctors to deal with their headache problems.

In *surveys of visits to physicians,* headache has been named by patients as the principal reason for the visit at approximately 2 to 4% of all visits to internists, general practitioners, and family practitioners (18). Table 79.1, adapted from the National Ambulatory Care Survey (NAMCS), indicates the differences in visit rate for headache with respect to age group and sex of patients. Table 79.2 shows the distribution of duration of new headache reported by these patients; almost 50% of visits were for headache of less than 1 week's duration. An important additional finding from this study was the low frequency of recurrent headache in people 65 and older. In this age group, 57% of men and 43% of women report themselves as headache free, and only 18 to 30% report disabling or severe headaches. On the other hand, as indicated in Table 79.1, the frequency of visits to physicians by those who do have headache increases with age.

CLASSIFICATION

This chapter uses the diagnostic criteria for headache syndromes defined in 1988 by the *International Headache Society* (10). These criteria are widely used for clinical decisions as well as research. The term *muscle contraction headache* has been replaced by the term *tension headache.* Debate within the neurologic community continues about the practical difference between tension and migraine headache; individual patients often have both types of headache. Some patients with frequent tension headache respond to drugs used for migraine, and some with typical migraine respond to regimens recommended for tension headache. Most patients presenting to the office have patterns that meet the criteria for one of these two types of headache. A small percentage have headache caused by drugs or toxins, infection (e.g., meningitis), traction on pain-sensitive intracranial structures (e.g., tumor, hemorrhage, edema), inflammatory disease (e.g., vasculitis), and diseases of the eye, ear, sinuses, teeth, and facial nerves and structures.

GENERAL APPROACH TO THE PATIENT WITH HEADACHE

History

The history provides by far the most useful information for evaluating headache, particularly a careful account by the patient of the current or most recent episode. The most useful aspects of the history in determining cause are the temporal profile, associated symptoms, and family history; the least specific aspects are the character and location of the pain. Undue emphasis should not be placed on differentiating, for

Table 79.1. Average Annual Rate of Office Visits for Headache, by Sex and Age of Patients: United States 1977–1978

Sex and Age (yr)	Average Annual Visit Rate/1000 Persons
Both Sexes	
All ages	43.2
Under 15	17.6
15–24	31.4
25–44	53.8
45–64	60.2
65 and over	63.9
Female	
All ages	55.4
Under 15	15.8
15–24	40.8
25–44	67.0
45–64	82.0
65 and over	81.8
Male	
All ages	30.3
Under 65	19.4
15–24	21.7
25–44	39.7
45–64	36.3
65 and over	38.4

Adapted from Cypress BK. Headache as the reason for office visits, National Ambulatory Medical Care Survey: United States, 1977–1978. Advance data, vital and health statistics of the National Center for Health Statistics. Number 67, Jan 7, 1981.

example, throbbing pain from pressure pain because the subjective interpretation of headache pain is so variable. The following questions are helpful in the differential diagnosis of headache (the interpretation of the patient's answers to these questions is discussed in detail in the sections on specific headache syndromes).

Associated factors. Is there any warning of the attack (prodromal feeling, focal numbness or weakness, or visual symptoms including the fortification hallucinations of migraine)? Is the patient aware of any factors that can bring on these headaches (withdrawal from caffeine, alcohol ingestion, vasodilator use, psychosocial stress, perimenstrual period, foods, drug use, position, sexual orgasm, exertion, tobacco)? What drugs is the patient taking for other conditions? To what does the patient attribute the headache? Does the patient fear a dreaded cause such as a tumor?

Temporal features. When did the patient first experience this type of headache? How does the headache begin (suddenly, or by building up slowly over a period of several hours or days)? When does the headache occur? Does it waken the patient from sleep or is it present on awakening? Does it recede after the patient is up for several hours? What is the frequency of headaches? (Have the patient recount the past month's and the past year's pattern.) How long do the headaches last (maximum, minimum, average)? Have there been intervals of weeks or months without the headache?

Character and location of pain. What kind of pain is the patient experiencing with the current headaches (band-like, squeezing, pressure, pounding, or throb-

bing)? Where is the pain located (one side of the head, all over the head, in the eyes, radiating up the back of the neck)? Does the pain radiate anywhere or seem to spread during the course of attack? How severe can the headaches be (on a scale of 1 to 10)? How does the patient rate this headache pain to the pain of other headaches or other situations (e.g., is it the worst headache ever or the worst pain in my life)?

Aggravating and alleviating factors. Does anything make the headache pain worse (bending, standing, sneezing, straining, coughing)? What factors reduce the headache (lying down, pressing on the temples, avoidance of work, simple analgesics, narcotics, or other medications)? How is the patient currently treating the headache?

Environmental exposures. Does the headache occur predictably after exposure to an environment that may have elevated carbon monoxide levels (e.g., a closed room heated by a space heater)? Did the headache start after the patient began work (or activities at home) that entails exposure to fumes or dust containing lead? These and other environmental exposures that may cause headache are listed in Chapter 7, Table 7.2.

Associated neurologic symptoms. Does the patient have associated symptoms during the headaches such as spots before the eyes (common in both tension and migraine headaches); inability to tolerate light, sound, touch, or movement; nausea or vomiting; focal numbness or weakness; or vertigo? Did the patient have motion sickness as a child? Does the patient note scalp tenderness? (All of these symptoms are common in migraine.)

Prior evaluation. Has the patient been evaluated for the headaches and what were the results of this evaluation? It is important to request previous records for all patients who give a history of severe, disabling headache, irrespective of the reported duration of the present headache problem or the nature of the previous evaluation; sometimes just requesting the records reminds the patient of a 10- or 20-year history of severe headache and multiple visits, and sometimes the previous records confirm this despite a patient's poor recall. In either case, this information can be particularly valuable in evaluating a patient who describes recent onset of severe headaches.

Functional impact. How are the headaches currently affecting the patient (work and social relationships)?

Family and household history. Is there a history of

Table 79.2. Percentage of Office Visits with Headache as a New Problem, by Sex of Patient and Time Since Onset: United States, 1977–1978

Time Since Onset	Female (%)	Male (%)
Less than 1 week	43.9	49.3
1–3 weeks	16.3	22.7
1–3 months	16.1	13.6
More than 3 months	20.5	13.7

Adapted from Cypress BK. Headache as the reason for office visits, National Ambulatory Medical Care Survey: United States, 1977–1978. Advance data, vital and health statistics of the National Center for Health Statistics. Number 67, Jan 7, 1981.

headaches in the parents, siblings, children, or other people living in the patient's household? What type?

Physical and Laboratory Examination

In most cases the history suggests the probable basis for a patient's headache. Appropriate physical examination and laboratory examination are described under each type of headache below. The appropriate extent of these objective aspects of the examination may vary from a limited physical examination (e.g., in a patient with headache after vasodilator therapy), to an examination focused on structures that may be the source of the headache (e.g., teeth), to a complete neurologic examination plus imaging studies or laboratory tests (e.g., the patient with new onset or marked change in prior headache pattern, the patient with headache and a new focal neurologic abnormality such as weakness, the patient whose presentation suggest giant cell arteritis).

The role of imaging studies in the patient with headache and a normal neurologic examination was addressed by a 1994 practice guideline issued by the American Academy of Neurology (9). Based on a review of all relevant publications, there was sufficient information to be explicit in recommending *against* the routine use of imaging in such patients with migraine, including migraine with aura. Because of the absence of published evidence, the guideline makes no explicit recommendations for patients other than those with migraine. To inform clinical decisions, however, the discussion that accompanies the guidelines cites one available study of a large HMO population in which it was estimated that a tumor will be found less than 1 in 10,000 patients with headaches as the only symptom and with a normal neurologic examination. Table 79.3 summarizes other information from the guideline that may be useful in decision making about costly imaging studies in such patients.

Table 79.3. Abnormal CT or MRI in Migraine and Unspecified Headache

Migraine

Total Scans	Tumor	AVM
897	3	1
100%	0.3%	0.1%

Total potentially treatable lesions:
4/897 = 0.4%

Unspecified Headache

Total Scans	Tumor	AVM	Hydrocephalus	Aneurysm	Subdural Hematoma
1825	21	6	8	3	5
100%	1%	0.3%	0.4%	0.2%	0.3%

Total potentially treatable lesions:
All studies   43/1825 = 2.4%
Without studies 9 and 10   3/725 = 0.4%

From Frishberg BM. The utility of neuroimaging in the evaluation of headache in patients with normal neurologic examinations. Neurology 44:1191–1197, 1994.
Note: Studies 9 and 10 were done in the early CT era and addressed any kind of headache at referral centers.

Principles of Initial Treatment

Most patients with a headache history consistent with tension or migraine and a normal examination can be treated presumptively for tension or migraine headache, as described below. A more extensive investigation should be carried out in patients who show either of the following situations after initial treatment: *patients who fail to respond to treatment of the presumed condition* (even in this situation, the extent of the evaluation should be tempered by the circumstances) and *patients who show significant changes in complaints or physical findings* that point to one of the less common causes of headache discussed below.

Treatment Expectations

When the issue of expectations of physicians and patients has been studied, the majority of the physicians have expected that their patients would demand pain relief and not care much about getting an explanation of their problem; in contrast, only 31% of the patients have stated that pain relief was most important, and 46% rated an explanation of their problem as their most important concern (19).

When the usual tension or migraine headache syndrome is treated, total relief of headache pain often is not possible. The patient must be helped to understand the limitations of drug therapy and the potential for drug side effects that, in some cases, can be more distressing than the headaches. Selection of a treatment regimen is complicated by the high placebo response rate (20 to 40%) and the variable natural history of headaches. Because of this variability, a detailed baseline history of the patient's headache problems is important for subsequent assessment of the patient's response to treatment.

SPECIFIC HEADACHE SYNDROMES
Tension Headache

Classification and Diagnostic Criteria

In the absence of any rigorous criterion or physiologic markers, the term *tension headache* has been applied to what is probably a heterogeneous group of headache syndromes. The 1988 international classification delineates two subtypes of tension headache: *episodic headache* (fewer than 180 episodes per year) and *chronic headache* (more than 180 episodes per year, including continuous chronic headache) (10). Additional consensus criteria for *episodic tension headache* include the following:

1. Duration 30 minutes to 7 days.
2. At least two of the following pain characteristics:
   a. Pressing/tightening (nonpulsating) quality.
   b. Mild or moderate intensity.
   c. Bilateral location.
   d. No aggravation by walking stairs or similar routine physical activity.

3. Both of the following:
   a. No nausea or vomiting (anorexia may occur).
   b. Photophobia and phonophobia are absent, or one but not the other is present.

Recurrent tension headaches are usually similar in quality and location. Patients with *chronic tension headache* often have associated depression or anxiety. Occasionally a patient with chronic tension headache complains of headaches that have been unremitting for years.

Physical examination of the patient with tension headache is normal except for neck or scalp muscle tenderness in some patients.

Pathogenesis

The symptoms of tension headache are presumed to be a somatic consequence of psychosocial stress in the patient's life, although the stress cannot always be identified. Neither increased muscle tension nor precipitating stress is specific for tension headaches; both are also common in migraine, which is the prototype of vascular headache (see below). Table 79.4 summarizes the data on the frequency of several characteristics in a large number of patients and shows considerable overlap between tension and migraine headaches (8). The pathogenesis may be the same (see below). Depression or anxiety, which may be masked, is usually associated with chronic tension headache. The causal relationship between headache and depression and anxiety is controversial; some believe these to be causal whereas others consider them to be secondary to headaches.

Treatment

Patients with intermittent headache that is not severe usually respond to simple over-the-counter analgesics. Most of these patients do not seek medical attention for their headaches but admit to headaches on review of systems. Patients with continuous daily headache of months' or years' duration usually have depression or anxiety states. These patients describe constant headache that lacks any localizing characteristics and is refractory to analgesics and migraine prophylaxis with the exception of the antidepressants.

Nonpharmacologic. It is usually helpful to explain to the patient that the mechanism of pain is unknown but that it may be related to stress. Emphasis on the benign nature of the headache is important to relieving patient concerns over more serious pathology such as a brain tumor. As explained elsewhere (see Chapter 11), concerned listening often helps to reduce somatic symptoms caused by stress as does encouragement for any effort made by the patient to reduce stressful situations. For patients seeking nonpharmacologic relief of symptoms, massage of the scalp and neck muscles by another person or use of relaxation techniques (see Chapter 13) can be recommended; in addition, any other procedure that the patient may have found helpful should be encouraged.

Table 79.4. Characteristics of Migrainous and Tension Headaches

	Migraine (%)	Tension (%)
Age at onset		
<20 years	55	30
>20 years	45	70
Premonitoring symptoms	60	10
Frequency		
Daily	3	50
<Weekly	60	15
Duration		
Constant, daily	0	20
1–3 days	35	10
Throbbing pain	80	30
Location		
Unilateral	80	10
Bilateral	20	90
Vomiting with attacks	50	10
Family history of headache	65	40

Adapted from Raskin NH, Appenzeller O. Headache. Philadelphia: WB Saunders, 1980; as modified from Friedman AP et al. Neurology 4:773, 1954.

Pharmacologic. Symptomatic treatment with drugs is an important adjunct to the general measures just described; for selected patients, prophylactic drug treatment can also be tried. Most patients have used headache remedies containing aspirin or acetaminophen before consulting their physician about treatment. For mild to moderate headaches, however, an additional trial of these mild analgesics should be recommended if they have not been taken at the usual effective dosage (650 mg every 4 to 6 hours). If these remedies fail to help, a trial of nonsteroidal anti-inflammatory drugs (NSAIDs) other than aspirin is indicated.

A number of drugs are widely prescribed for patients with moderately severe episodic headaches unresponsive to acetaminophen, aspirin, or other nonsteroidal agents. These drugs include codeine sulfate, propoxyphene (Darvon), and two products that contain combinations of analgesics, sedatives, and caffeine (butalbital/caffeine plus aspirin or acetaminophen, and oxycodone plus aspirin or acetaminophen). Each of these drugs can lead to dependency. Therefore, it is unwise to initiate treatment with them unless there is a strict contractual agreement regarding limited use (see Chapter 22).

Prophylaxis is warranted for the patient whose tension headaches are severe or frequent. The best results have been obtained with the tricyclic antidepressants such as nortriptyline, given in daily doses of 50 to 100 mg at bedtime. (A detailed discussion of the use of the tricyclics is found in Chapter 15.)

Migraine

Classification and Diagnostic Criteria

The classification of migraine headache was revised in 1988 from "common" and "classic" migraine to *migraine without* aura and *migraine with aura* (10).

Consensus criteria for the syndrome of *migraine without aura* include the following:

A. The patient has had at least five attacks of fulfilling B–D.
B. Headache attacks last 4 to 72 hours (untreated or unsuccessfully treated).
C. Headache has at least two of the following characteristics:
   1. Unilateral location
   2. Pulsating quality
   3. Moderate or severe intensity
   4. Aggravation by walking stairs or similar routine physical activity
D. During headache at least one of the following:
   1. Nausea or vomiting
   2. Photophobia and phonophobia

Unilateral head pain during a migraine attack usually increases gradually, reaching a peak in several hours and lasting for several hours to a day in typical cases. Attacks lasting 2 to 3 days are not uncommon, and some migraine attacks last 1 to 2 weeks. The pain may be described as pounding or throbbing, but the quality of the pain is variable and may be aching or stabbing. Although headaches are typically unilateral at the beginning of a single attack, they often generalize and most patients have attacks on both sides of the head; however, in a minority of patients, headaches are always on the same side.

The additional criteria for the syndrome of *migraine with aura* are the following:

A. The patient has had at least two attacks fulfilling B.
B. At least three of the following four characteristics:
   1. One or more fully reversible aura symptoms indicating focal cerebral cortical or brainstem dysfunction.
   2. At least one aura symptom develops gradually over more than 4 minutes, or two or more symptoms occur in succession.
   3. No aura symptom lasts more than 60 minutes. If more than one aura symptom is present, accepted duration is proportionally increased.
   4. Headache follows aura with a free interval of less than 60 minutes. (It may also begin before or simultaneously with the aura.)

Headaches with aura are subdivided into typical, prolonged, familial hemiplegic, basilar, aura without headache, and acute onset aura.

Migraine with typical aura (the most common form with aura) has one of the following types of aura symptoms:

• Homonymous visual disturbance
• Unilateral paresthesias or numbness
• Unilateral weakness
• Aphasia or unclassifiable speech difficulty

Fortification hallucinations are almost specific for migraine; these are slowly enlarging scotomata that are surrounded by luminous angles and that slowly change shape and appear to move across the visual fields (Fig. 79.1). Rarely, occipital lobe tumors or arteriovenous malformations may produce the same effects.

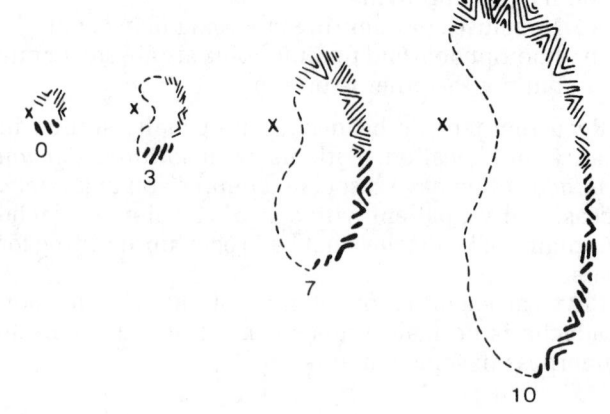

Figure 79.1. Lashley's maps of the progression of his own fortification spectra at varying time intervals after the onset of a migrainous attack. The X in each instance indicates the visual fixation point. The numbers represent minutes. (From Raskin NH, Appenzeller O. Headache. Philadelphia: WB Saunders, 1980; as appeared in Lashley KS. Arch Neurol Psychiatry 46:331, 1941.)

Further types of migraine include ophthalmoplegic, retinal, childhood periodic syndromes, complications of migraine (infarction, status migrainosis), and unclassified.

Migraine is more common than is generally appreciated, and many patients with recurrent moderate to severe migraine headaches are misdiagnosed as having tension headache. Failure of analgesics in an emotionally healthy patient with recurring headaches justifies a revised diagnosis of migraine.

In the *differential diagnosis of migraine,* the most important considerations are transient ischemic attacks (TIAs) or other cerebrovascular events, particularly in middle-age and older patients (see Chapter 83 for details). *Migrainous ischemia* usually occurs in patients with a history of similar attacks, often in young adulthood; the family history in these cases tends to be particularly strong. Symptoms of migrainous ischemia typically last for a half hour to several hours; TIAs usually last minutes to several hours. Headaches should be a prominent component of the migrainous ischemic event; although headache may occur in up to 25% of patients with transient ischemic events, it is usually mild and transitory. Older patients with suspected migrainous ischemic events, particularly those with migraine equivalents (ischemic symptoms without headache), should be evaluated for TIA (see Chapter 83) before their symptoms are attributed to migraine.

Pathogenesis

For many years, the symptoms of a migraine headache have been attributed to sequential changes affecting intracranial and extracranial arteries. An initial stage of vasoconstriction, producing brain ischemia, is thought to be responsible for the fortification hallucinations (see below), transient hemiparesis or hemiparesthesias, confusion, vertigo, and other focal neurologic manifestations that can be seen in migraine with aura. Although vasoconstriction presumably also occurs in migraine without aura, it is thought to be below the threshold necessary to produce obvious symptoms. Vasoconstriction is thought to last from a half hour to several hours in a typical migraine attack. In the sequential theory, the initial vasoconstriction is thought to be followed by vasodilation of the affected vessels, resulting in typical vascular headache pain that throbs in unison with the pulse. Some patients report dilated, throbbing, aching vessels over one side of the scalp during an episode, tenderness of the scalp, and some relief during the attack by pressure on the temples, presumably decreasing blood flow to the dilated temporal arteries.

The vascular theory of migraine does not adequately account for many aspects of the migraine syndrome such as malaise, autonomic components (nausea, vomiting, diarrhea, bloating, fluid retention), and the postheadache elation or sense of well-being many patients describe. Other theories include electrical depression, an imbalance in sympathetic nervous system regulation, dysautonomia of the trigeminal nerve, and dysregulation of the ascending brainstem serotonergic system. Increasing evidence now makes it clear that migraine is an organic illness, not psychologically based.

Epidemiology and Natural History

The lack of a simple, specific test for migraine headache and variations in the definition of migraine headache make it difficult to determine the prevalence and natural course of this condition. However, it is estimated that about 23 million people in the United States (approximately 18% of adult women and 6% of adult men) have migraine and that more than 4 million of these have one or more attacks per month. More than half of working people with migraine report that they miss more than 2 days of work per month (25).

From 20 to 50% of migraine headache sufferers have a positive family history for migraine, usually in one parent. This seems to be particularly true with patients who have migraine with aura. Many patients report motion sickness and vertigo as a child, with vertigo persisting into adulthood.

The onset of migraine is most common between the ages of 15 and 25; however, onset can occur throughout the adult life span. Recurrence is a hallmark of migraine headache. The majority of migraine sufferers have several attacks each year; some have one or more episodes per week and some have only rare episodes or even only a single typical episode in their lives. Migraine episodes usually become less frequent and less severe with age.

Possible precipitating factors. The perimenstrual period (particularly before the onset of bleeding, when levels of estradiol are falling), oral contraceptives (particularly off-days, presumably because of falling estrogen levels), and menopause (frank estrogen deficiency) are associated with migraine headaches. The following substances may initiate headaches in susceptible subjects: vasodilators (nitrates and antihypertensives);

alcohol; chocolate; cheeses, wines, and other foods containing tyramine; and monosodium glutamate. Withdrawal of caffeine or ergotamine can also cause headaches. An unusually long period of sleep, such as sleeping in on weekends, may provoke migraine. Attacks tend to occur also during periods of relaxation, such as weekends, holidays, and vacations. The patient should be asked about these associations and any others that may have been noted.

Nonpharmacologic Treatment

Most migraine sufferers can be helped by treatment, principally pharmacologic treatment. A number of nonpharmacologic measures may help also.

The most useful nonpharmacologic treatment is *avoidance of known trigger factors,* when this is possible. Common drugs that may trigger an attack are nitrates, vasodilators, and oral contraceptives. Other trigger factors that can be eliminated are alcohol, irregular sleep habits, excess caffeine use, and caffeine withdrawal. There are no consistently implicated dietary trigger factors; however, each patient should be encouraged to try eliminating any dietary component or other trigger factor that can be identified.

During an established attack, a patient usually feels better reclining in a dark room with a cool compress or an ice pack applied to the head. This is the only practice other than drug treatment that appears to be helpful.

Abortive Pharmacologic Treatment

Because migraine attacks can be debilitating, migraine sufferers are usually motivated to learn the optimal use of medications to control attacks; most learn readily the regimen that works best for them. Recent advances have added important new options for the pharmacologic approach to migraine. This section describes abortive treatment of migraine attacks. The following section describes preventive treatment of migraine. It is important to emphasize that migraines are usually not cured, but can be controlled.

Patients with a history of *mild migraine attacks* often obtain relief from analgesics including acetaminophen, aspirin, or another NSAID, used as described above under "Tension Headache." Commonly used agents and dosages of these plus a number of products that combine analgesics, barbiturate, or caffeine are listed in Table 79.5.

At the start of an attack in a patient with *moderate to severe migraine,* ergotamine tartrate, sumatriptan, or an NSAID may be used. Because both ergotamine and sumatriptan are vasoconstrictors, they should not be used together during the treatment of a migraine episode.

Ergotamine.   The action of ergotamine has traditionally been attributed to its vasoconstrictor properties; however, its effect may be related to its serotonin receptor agonist properties. Ergotamine is available in preparations that permit administration by multiple routes (Table 79.5). It provides effective symptom control in approximately 50% of migraine sufferers

Table 79.5. Drugs for Acute Migraine Attacks

Drug	Route	Trade Name	Dosage[a]
Nonprescription Analgesic			
Aspirin	Oral		650 mg q4hr PRN
Acetaminophen	Oral	Tylenol	650 mg q4hr PRN
Ibuprofen	Oral	Advil, Nuprin, etc.	200 mg 1 to 4 q4–8hr PRN
Naproxen	Oral	Aleve	275 mg, one q6hr PRN
Prescription Analgesics			
Naproxen (or other NSAID)[b]	Oral	Anaprox DS	550 mg q12hr PRN
		Naprosyn	500 mg q12hr PRN
Ketorolac	Oral, IM	Toradol	10-mg tablets: 2 initially then 1 q6hr
			Prefilled syringes: 15, 30 mg
			30–60 mg, then 30 mg q6hr
Isometheptene, acetominophen and dichloralphenazone	Oral	Midrin	2 capsules, then 1 qhr (up to 5 capsules/12 hr)
Butalbital, acetaminophen	Oral	Phrenilin	1–2 q4hr PRN (up to 6/day)
Butalbital, acetaminophen, and caffeine	Oral	Fioracet, Esgic	1–2q4h PRN
	Oral	Fiorinol	1–2 q4h PRN (up to 6/day)
Butorphanol	Nasal spray	Stadol NS	1 mg (1 spray), may repeat this sequence in 3–4 hr as needed
Prescription Nonanalgesics			
Ergotamine	Oral[c]	Cafergot Wigraine	2 mg at onset, 1 mg q0.5hr (up to 6 tablets/day; 10 tablets/wk)
	Suppository[c]	Cafergot	2 mg at onset, may repeat in 1 hour (up to 5/wk)
	Sublingual	Ergostat	2 mg at onset and q0.5hr (up to 3 tablets/day, 5/wk)
Dihydroergotamine	Intramuscular or intravenous	D.H.E. 45	1 mg IM or IV and qhr (3/day. IM, 2/day IV, 6/wk)
Sumatriptan[d]	SC	Imitrex	6 mg may repeat in 1 hr (up to 2/24 hr)
	Oral	Imitrex	25 mg or 50 mg. Repeat if no improvement after 2 hr (max. cumulative dosage 300 mg)
	Nasal spray	Imitrex	5- or 20-mg spray; may repeat in 2 hr (up to 40 mg/24 hr)

[a]Information given in quantities of available strengths unless otherwise described in parentheses.
[b]See list of NSAIDs and available strengths in Chapter 70.
[c]These ergotamine products also contain caffeine (100 mg per dose), which enhances gastrointestinal absorption.
[d]Note: Additional selective serotonin antagonist, with properties similar to sumatriptan, are available.

and is generally recommended as the most cost-effective first choice among the nonanalgesic agents. Dihydroergotamine, given intravenously or intramuscularly, is useful chiefly for treating refractory migraine in an emergency department or in hospitals.

The ideal route for administering ergotamine is one that is convenient, leads to prompt absorption of the drug, and is not affected by vomiting. Suppository and sublingual preparations meet these criteria. Ingested tablets may be vomited and are therefore less reliable. The traditional recommended schedules for ergotamine administration are summarized in Table 79.5. The objective of these schedules is to attain a total dosage that is effective but is below the dosage that produces nausea and vomiting. Traditionally this has been accomplished by taking additional doses at 30 and 60 minutes if the first dose is ineffective. An alternative strategy may increase the likelihood of prompt attenuation of headaches: Patients can determine the dosage that produces nausea for them (the nauseating dosage) by following the traditional schedule on a headache-free day. The cumulative dosage attained just before the nauseating dosage is the appropriate total therapeutic dosage (the subnauseating dosage) for that patient to take all at once at the onset of future attacks.

A number of points are important in instructing a patient about the use of ergotamine. Above all, the patient should understand that ergotamine is not a pain killer but that it is used to interrupt the events causing migraine pain, and that for maximal benefit one must take ergotamine at the onset of prodromal symptoms or headache (waiting for the headache to become well established is a common problem in patients who report no benefit from ergotamine). In order to ensure immediate access to their medicine, patients should be advised to carry some with them at all times. They should be informed that taking more than the recommended maximum daily dosage (Table 79.5) carries the risk of peripheral vasoconstriction in addition to nausea and vomiting. Because ergotamine preparations have a short shelf life, patients should obtain a new supply if they fail to obtain benefit from their medicine or if they have not used it for many months.

Occasionally the patient has *side effects* from ergotamine even when taken at the subnauseating dosage. These include abdominal cramps, vertigo, diarrhea, and distal paresthesia; less commonly, syncope, tremor, angina pectoris, and claudication may occur. However, most patients tolerate the drug well.

Serious adverse effects, including mental changes, edema, peripheral vascular occlusion, and distal gangrene, can occur if the daily dosage of ergotamine exceeds 6 mg or the weekly dosage exceeds 10 mg on a chronic basis. Patients should therefore be warned not to use ergotamine more than twice in the same week and no more than 10 mg in 1 week, to avoid both the aforementioned side effects and tolerance to the drug's effects.

The principal *contraindications* to ergotamine use are established angina, history of myocardial infarction, and symptomatic peripheral arterial disease. Ergotamine should not be used in combination with sumatriptan. Traditionally, hypertension has been named as a contraindication, but the risk has probably been overemphasized. When there is concern about the effect of ergotamine on the blood pressure of an individual patient, the blood pressure response to ergotamine can be measured in the physician's office, following the protocol for determining the subnauseating dosage of ergotamine outlined above.

Sumatriptan. Sumatriptan succinate, which was introduced in 1993, is a serotonin receptor agonist that aborts or significantly reduces moderate or severe migraine symptoms even if the headache has been present for many hours (26). Controlled trials have shown that 25, 50, or 100 mg of sumatriptan taken *orally* at the onset of aura or headache produces relief of headache symptoms within 2 hours in approximately 55% of patients and within 4 hours in about 70% of patients. Similar responses to placebo occur in 20% or less of patients (6). Administration of a single 6-mg dose *subcutaneously* yields symptom relief in about 75% of patients within 1 hour and in over 80% within 2 hours (30). Sumatriptan also relieves nausea, vomiting, and other disabling symptoms of migraine with few side effects. The unique advantage of sumatriptan compared with ergotamine is that the drug is effective when taken at any time during a migraine headache, whereas ergotamine must be given at the beginning of an attack. The incidence of recurrence of migraine within the ensuing 24 hours is higher with sumatriptan than with ergotamine, although this has not been a significant limitation. The drug is more expensive than ergotamine ($10 to $15 per pill and about $35 per injected dose), but it may save patients office visits or emergency room fees.

Available Preparations. Sumatriptan (Imitrex) is available for administration orally and subcutaneously.

Tablets are manufactured in two strengths: 25 and 50 mg. In controlled trials, the response rates were similar with initial doses of 25, 50, or 100 mg (6). If a patient has had no improvement after 2 hours, the initial oral dose should be repeated at that time (maximum cumulative dosage of 100 mg in 2 hours). The cumulative dosage needed for relief in an individual patient can be taken as the initial dose for future attacks. For return of headache on the same day, treatment can be repeated up to 300 mg in the same day.

A *self-injection* kit that does not require skill in subcutaneous injection makes this an acceptable option for aborting migraine headaches. The dose in this kit is 6 mg. A second 6-mg dose may be repeated at 1 hour if the patient has had a partial response. Efficacy has not been demonstrated for a second dose in patients who did not respond initially.

Because both are vasoconstrictors, ergotamine and sumatriptan should not be used on the same day.

Side Effects. The most common side effects are transient paresthesias, tingling, dizziness, and, after subcutaneous administration, injection-site reactions (pain, erythema lasting about 1 hour). One or more transient side effects occur in approximately 50% of patients after oral administration (25% with placebo) and approximately 70% after injection (40% with placebo). Up to 5% of patients describe transient chest tightness. Many patients respond to a lower injected dosage (3 or 4 mg), which may be prescribed if side effects limit usefulness. This requires use of the multidose vial, which means that the patient must be instructed in sterile technique. Because in large dosages sumatriptan is embryolethal in rabbits and because there has been no trial to establish the safety of sumatriptan in pregnant women, its use in pregnancy is proscribed. This warning may be revised as experience with the drug increases. No adverse age-related effects have accrued in patients over 60 who participated in clinical trials. Sumatriptan is not recommended in patients with hemiplegic or basilar artery migraine and is contraindicated in patients with known coronary artery disease.

Nonsteroidal Anti-Inflammatory Drugs. NSAIDs often help at the onset of an acute attack and should be used in full doses (Table 79.5). These drugs are generally more efficacious than simple analgesics (aspirin, acetaminophen) and narcotics (propoxyphene, low-dose codeine) and may be used for acute attacks alone or in conjunction with ergotamine or sumatriptan.

Narcotic Analgesics. For an established, severe migraine headache not responsive to NSAIDs, ergotamine, or sumatriptan, simple analgesics do not help. For this reason, reliable patients may be given small supplies of either codeine (60 mg) or an equipotent narcotic analgesic (see Chapter 19, Table 19.1) to be taken as needed. This measure may save a patient many unnecessary trips to the physician's office or an emergency department.

Nausea and Vomiting. These migraine symptoms can be treated with prochlorperazine suppositories (25 mg), which patients can easily self-administer. Because of the likelihood of vomiting, oral antiemetics are of limited usefulness but can be tried in patients who prefer not to take suppositories. Intravenous metoclopramide is also effective but not practical for self-administration by patients.

Prophylactic Pharmacologic Treatment

Prophylactic drug therapy for migraine should be considered when the patient has two or more attacks per week or less frequent attacks that cannot be controlled with abortive therapy and that disrupt employment or social life. Importantly, known precipitating factors described above should be eliminated when possible as the initial step in prevention.

The decision regarding prophylaxis must be the patient's, after the distinction between abortive and prophylactic therapy has been explained clearly. Even a patient who has not had adequate relief from routine measures may forego prophylactic treatment because of the need to take medicine daily. For each of the drugs used prophylactically for migraine, a long trial period (1 month or more) may be necessary to assess effectiveness, and trials with a number of drugs may be necessary. Patients should understand that during the trial of prophylaxis they can continue the usual measures for treating their migraine attacks.

Drugs that have been effective in migraine prophylaxis, together with daily dosage ranges, are listed in Table 79.6. Recently, divalproex sodium (Depakote) was approved for migraine prophylaxis. Of patients taking divalproex sodium in dosages to achieve levels of 70 to 120 mg/L (500 to 1500), 48% reported headache frequency reduced by 50%, compared to 14% of patients taking placebo (17). Despite this comparable efficacy profile, serious side effects are more likely than with β-blockers, tricyclic antidepressants, and calcium channel blockers. Patients who are not helped by these drugs can be referred to a neurologist or other specialist in migraine to learn of other options.

The following general conclusions can be drawn about migraine prophylaxis (30):

- At least 50% of patients report some improvement in their migraine syndrome during the first year, compared with a reported improvement in 25% or less of control patients. During the second year of prophylaxis, the response rate may be lower.
- Most of the improvement consists of a decrease in frequency or severity of headaches; complete freedom from headaches occurs in only a minority of patients.
- Each of the drugs that has been tried (Table 79.6) gives similar results; failure of a drug from one class does not predict response to another from that class or to a drug from another class. Therefore, a sequential trial of different drugs is reasonable.
- The drugs that one knows best should be tried first for at least 2 to 3 months (e.g., β-blockers, tricyclics, and

Table 79.6. Prophylactic Therapy for Migraine

Drugs	Dose/Day (mg)
β-Blockers	
Propranolol	80–320
Metoprolol	100–250
Atenolol	50–100
Timolol	10–60
Nadolol	40–240
Calcium channel blockers	
Verapamil	240–480
Tricyclic antidepressants	
Amitriptyline	10–150
Nortriptyline	10–150
Doxepin	10–100
Anticonvulsants	
Divalproex	500–1500

Most of these drugs are now available in generic forms. Most are available in forms that can be taken once per day. Text of Chapter 62 ("Hypertension") and Table 62.11 contain information regarding side effects, trade names, available strengths, and dosing schedule for β-blockers and calcium channel blockers; information is found for tricyclic antidepressants in Chapter 15 ("Affective Disorders") and Table 15.5.

calcium channel blockers). To facilitate compliance, it is helpful to select agents that can be taken once per day.

- Failure to give an adequate dosage (i.e., up to the maximal dosages listed in Table 79.6) is a common reason for failure of migraine prophylaxis.

Each patient who chooses prophylactic therapy should be asked to keep a log in which to record the frequency and severity of headaches and the nature of any associated factors.

Patients with Intractable Migraine Headaches

A small number of migraine sufferers have intractable and disabling headaches for which no effective regimen can be found despite trials of all available pharmacologic regimens. For a further assessment and consideration of other therapeutic options, these patients should be referred to a neurologist.

Cluster Headache

Classification and Diagnostic Criteria

Cluster headache is classified separately from migraine because of its distinct clinical characteristics and different therapy (10). It has previously been designated by a number of names, such as *Horton's headache, histamine headache* (a misnomer), and *migrainous cranial neuralgia*. The 1988 international consensus criteria for the diagnosis of cluster headache are the following:

A. The patient has had at least five attacks fulfilling B–D.
B. Severe unilateral orbital, supraorbital, or temporal pain lasting 15 to 180 minutes untreated.
C. Headache is associated with at least one of the following signs, which must be present on the pain side:
   1. Conjunctival injection
   2. Lacrimation
   3. Nasal congestion
   4. Rhinorrhea
   5. Forehead and facial sweating
   6. Miosis
   7. Ptosis
   8. Eyelid edema
D. Frequency of attacks: from one every other day to eight per day.

Attacks occur in clusters extending over days to weeks, thus giving the syndrome its name. Most cluster episodes last from 4 to 6 weeks and are followed by long pain-free intervals. The intervals between episodes range from 3 months to 5 years, and occasionally longer. However, most patients have one or two episodes/year. Eventually the problem ceases altogether.

A typical attack begins with sudden stabbing or burning pain in the eye, orbit, and cheek on one side. The pain is usually excruciating. Unlike patients with migraine, patients with cluster headaches are usually agitated and they often pace the floor during the attack.

Characteristically, the patient also describes at least one of the other symptoms listed above. Usually the same side is involved during a cluster of attacks. Attacks may last from a few minutes to 2 hours (most often 30 to 40 minutes), and they tend to occur at the same time each day, most commonly in the evening just after the patient has gone to bed. In some patients, alcohol may be a potent trigger factor. Nitrates and vasodilator drugs may also induce attacks. Therefore, patients should be asked about concurrent use of alcohol and drugs.

The above characteristics describe the diagnostic features for the typical syndrome of cluster headache. Some patients have less well-defined episodes, whereas other patients may have almost daily attacks of pain for a number of years, a syndrome known as *chronic paroxysmal hemicrania* (20).

Except during an attack, when the unilateral findings described above are present, the physical examination in patients with cluster headache is unremarkable.

Differential Diagnosis.   Cluster headache must be distinguished from tic douloureux (see below), acute glaucoma (by the presence of miosis, normal tonometry, no lasting visual impairment), sinusitis (by lack of history of upper respiratory infection, lack of purulent rhinorrhea or sinus tenderness, and negative x-rays), peripheral dental abscess (by the absence of tenderness on tooth percussion), and atypical facial neuralgia (see below).

Epidemiology

Cluster headache is much less common than migraine in the population. It occurs predominantly in middle-age men and is associated with being thin and smoking cigarettes. Onset usually occurs between the age of 20 and 50. There is no evidence for a familial basis for cluster headache.

Treatment

Abortive.   Because attacks may be short, lasting only 30 to 40 minutes, oral drug treatment may be ineffective in ameliorating an acute episode. When available, *100% oxygen,* administered for approximately 15 minutes at a flow rate of 7 L/minute, may abort attacks. In a double-blind trial, about half of the subjects were helped within 10 minutes by 100% oxygen but not placebo (room air) given by nonrebreathing face mask (7). The therapeutic effect of oxygen may result from its vasoconstrictor action. *Ergotamine,* administered sublingually, may also be effective abortive therapy for cluster headaches. A sublingual preparation of ergotamine containing 2 mg (Table 79.5) may be given at the beginning of the attack and repeated twice at 30-minute intervals. No more than 6 mg should be taken in a 24-hour period, nor more than 10 mg/week. *Subcutaneous sumatriptan,* used as described above for migraine, has been shown to decrease the severity of headache in approximately 75% of attacks as compared with placebo (27).

Prophylactic.   Other drugs, taken at the onset of a cluster episode and continued for several weeks, may be helpful for terminating an episode after the first headache occurs. Those drugs include verapamil, β-blockers, and tricyclic depressants, in dosages similar to those described above for migraine prophylaxis. *Prednisone,* beginning at 60 to 80 mg/day and tapering over 2 to 4 weeks, shortens the duration of a cluster episode and decreases the severity and frequency of the attacks (4). A maximal effect occurs within 2 or 3 days after initiation of therapy. (See additional information on prescribing and tapering of corticosteroids in Chapter 74.)

For patients who suffer from almost *daily cluster headaches (chronic paroxysmal hemicrania),* lithium carbonate has been used successfully. The use of this drug is described in detail in Chapter 15. Patients who respond to lithium seem to be controlled at serum levels below 0.8 mEq/L. If lithium fails to control daily cluster headache, the addition of ergotamine tartrate or methysergide (either alone or with ergotamine) may help.

The patient for whom neither treatment nor prophylaxis with the above regimens helps should be referred for further empiric treatments to a neurologist or an internist with wide experience in headache management.

Sinus Headache

The pain of *acute sinusitis* may be described by the patient as headache. The diagnosis is based on the other manifestations of acute sinusitis and the reproduction or exacerbation of the patient's headache by applying pressure to affected sinuses (see Chapter 28 for a full account).

Chronic sinusitis is often cited by patients as the reason for their headaches; it is actually an uncommon cause for recurrent headache. Chronic sinusitis can present diagnostic difficulties, particularly when it involves the sphenoid sinus (causing a dull boring pain behind the eyes). The diagnosis of sinus headache is most likely when there is a history of preceding acute sinusitis, especially if there is not a long history of headache. The diagnosis and management of chronic sinusitis are discussed in Chapter 28.

Acute Exertional Headache (Orgasm, Cough, Sneeze)

The features of acute exertional headache are that it is of sudden (or almost instantaneous) onset and it is directly related to exertion of some kind (e.g., orgasm, coughing, sneezing, straining, bending, running, lifting). It may last from minutes to one-half hour, rarely longer. In 90% of patients the headache is presumed to be caused by transient intracranial–spinal pressure dissociations, and the course is benign. In about 10% of patients significant organic disease has been found (Arnold–Chiari malformation, hydrocephalus, tumor, or subarachnoid hemorrhage) (21).

Exertional headache must be differentiated chiefly from the headache of *subarachnoid hemorrhage.* The headache of subarachnoid hemorrhage is usually far more persistent and is often associated with fever, stiff neck, progressive clouding of consciousness, and focal neurologic signs. Exertional headaches may be quite severe, but they are brief and recur with the trigger activity. Because it may be impossible to distinguish the first episode of exertional headache from a minor subarachnoid hemorrhage, and because of the 10% risk of another organic basis for the headache, computerized tomography (CT), with and without contrast because of the possibility of tumor or arteriovenous malformation, or a magnetic resonance imaging (MRI) scan (see "Patient Experience," Chapter 78) should be considered when patients initially report the problem. If imaging findings are normal, the benign nature of the condition should be explained to the patient. The patient usually finds ways to avoid some of the activities that produce headache. In addition, an NSAID (Table 79.5) or α-blocker (Table 79.6) can be tried for prophylaxis when the patient plans to engage in a headache-provoking activity.

Sudden-Onset Unprovoked Severe Headache

Sudden-onset, unprovoked severe headache is uncommon but alarming. In a single large prospective study based in general practice, 37% of patients with this presentation had serious CNS disease (25% had subarachnoid hemorrhage, SAH). Less than 10% of those with SAH had a history of "sentinel" severe headaches. In 1 year of follow-up, none of those with undiagnosed sudden headache experienced SAH (15). Patients with sudden-onset headache (peak pain within 1 minute, duration at least 1 hour) should be evaluated promptly for intracranial disease.

Headache Caused by Medications

Headache is an occasional side effect of many drugs. Among the commonly used drugs for which headache is more than an occasional side effect are indomethacin (Indocin), nalidixic acid (NegGram), trimethoprim–sulfamethoxazole (Bactrim, Septra), oral contraceptives, and vasodilators. Therefore, as noted earlier, it is important to ask the patient routinely about new drugs when evaluating a headache of recent onset.

A throbbing vascular-type headache often occurs shortly after initiation of treatment (or a dosage increase) with a *vasodilator* drug. The most common offenders are the short- and long-acting nitrates, dihydropyridine, calcium channel blockers, and the vasodilators used to treat hypertension (hydralazine and minoxidil). The management of this problem depends on the indications for the drug and the severity of the headache. Some patients, if informed in advance of the possibility of headache, choose to take the drug anyway; this is particularly true of sublingual nitrates administered for angina. For the long-acting nitrates, dosage reduction may effectively reduce headache for some patients, whereas alternative antianginal treatment is needed for others (see Chapter 57). The head-

ache associated with antihypertensive vasodilators can usually be prevented by treating the patient with a β-blocker before the vasodilator is added (see Chapter 62).

Headache in Acute Febrile Illnesses

Acute febrile illnesses may cause vascular-type throbbing headaches that remit when the illness resolves. A febrile patient in whom the headache is the major symptom and in whom nuchal rigidity or other manifestation of meningeal irritation is present requires a cerebrospinal fluid examination to exclude meningitis (see "Patient Experience," Chapter 78).

Giant Cell Arteritis and Polymyalgia Rheumatica

Giant cell arteritis (GCA) is a vasculitis that affects large arteries throughout the body. However, clinical manifestations are usually caused by involvement of extracranial branches of the carotid artery, and the most common syndrome is headache. GCA has also been called *temporal arteritis* because temporal headaches and a positive temporal artery biopsy are the findings that are most typical of the disease. The cause of GCA is unknown.

Polymyalgia rheumatica (PMR) is a debilitating condition of older people that presents with stiffness and aching of the neck and shoulder muscles and pelvic girdle. It precedes, accompanies, or follows the onset of GCA in approximately 50% of patients with GCA. In approximately 75 to 80% of patients with PMR in the United States and Europe, GCA does not occur (8). In patients who develop both GCA and PMR, the two syndromes may occur at the same time or GCA may begin months to years after the onset of PMR symptoms. In some patients GCA may precede PMR.

Epidemiology

GCA and PMR are almost exclusively diseases of people over the age of 50; the average age of onset is 65 to 70. Both are uncommon in African Americans, Hispanics, and Asians. They are most common in people of northern European descent, and they are more common in women than in men. In Minnesota, where there is a large northern European population, a community-level study of GCA found a yearly incidence in people over 50 of 17/100,000 and a prevalence of 223/100,000 (11,16). There are no other population-based studies of frequency of GCA or PMR in the United States; however, it is estimated that the incidence and prevalence rates of PMR are about two or three times higher than the rates for GCA.

Manifestations (31)

The headache of GCA does not have specific features that distinguish it clearly from other headaches. It is temporal in more than 50% of patients; however, it may be frontal, occipital, parietal, or holocephalic. The patient usually reports that it involves the surface and is not intracranial. It may be made worse by hair brushing, resting the head on a pillow, and, at times, by exposure to cold. It is usually not described as throbbing. It is often described as being worse at night and building up gradually over a number of hours. Because these symptoms are not specific, the most important factors in suggesting the diagnosis of GCA are a number of associated findings, listed in Table 79.7. It is important to inquire specifically about pain (claudication) associated with chewing, swallowing, and arm or tongue motion, as these symptoms are highly suggestive of GCA. The combination of one or more of the findings listed in Table 79.7 with a new headache in an older patient is sufficient to suspect GCA.

PMR is insidious in onset. The chief complaints are aching and stiffness of the shoulder girdle and, less commonly, of the thigh muscles. These symptoms may make it particularly hard for the patient to get up in the morning. Associated low-grade fever, weight loss, and anorexia are common. On physical examination, there may be some tenderness of the shoulder and neck muscles, but there is no significant loss of muscle strength.

Diagnosis

When GCA or PMR is suspected, the erythrocyte sedimentation rate (ESR) measured by the Westergren method is the most useful screening test. The vast majority of patients have a markedly elevated ESR (often 100 or greater). Because the upper limit of normal for people over 60 may be as high as 40, an ESR of 40 to 60 is less informative than is a very high ESR. Unlike other chronic inflammatory diseases, GCA and PMR are not associated with autoantibody production or abnormalities in complement factors or immunoglobulin levels.

Definitive diagnosis of GCA is made with a temporal artery biopsy. Because the typical histologic changes (inflammatory cells, edema, and giant cells) are patchy in distribution, examination of serial sections of the resected segment of artery is essential; in occasional patients with GCA, even extensive sampling of one temporal artery does not yield a positive biopsy and the other artery must also be examined by biopsy.

Patient Experience. A temporal artery biopsy can be done in an ambulatory surgery facility (by a general surgeon, ophthalmologist, vascular surgeon, plastic surgeon, or neurosurgeon). The scalp hair is shaved, the skin is anesthetized with Xylocaine, and a large segment of artery (4 to 6 cm) is excised. The entire procedure requires about one-half hour. There are no serious sequelae.

The *diagnosis of PMR* is based on the combination of the typical symptoms, a high ESR, and exclusion of other explanations for the patient's symptoms. Normocytic anemia is common. Muscle enzyme levels, electromyography, and muscle histology are all normal. If a patient with typical PMR has manifestations suggesting GCA (Table 79.7), a temporal artery biopsy is indicated because the recommended dosages of corticosteroids for the two conditions are different.

Course and Treatment

Both GCA and PMR are thought to be self-limited conditions in most patients, lasting up to 2 years. There have been no randomized controlled trials of treatment. Recommendations are based on the comparison of untreated patients with patients treated with corticosteroids. Treatment with corticosteroids appears to prevent almost entirely the most serious complication of GCA (unilateral or bilateral blindness caused by ischemic optic neuropathy, which occurs in 20 to 30% of untreated patients). Although the symptoms of both GCA and PMR may respond to aspirin and other NSAIDs, these agents have not been shown to prevent the progressive vasculitis in GCA that may lead to blindness.

If the diagnosis of GCA is strongly suspected, treatment should be initiated immediately and the temporal artery biopsy should be obtained within 3 to 4 days. The initial treatment is prednisone (40 to 60 mg once per day) for 4 to 6 weeks. Within 1 to 3 days, symp-

Table 79.7. Clinical Features of Giant Cell Arteritis

Common Features (Approximate % of Patients with Features at Initial Evaluation)		Less Common but Characteristic Features
Headache	(85)	Raynaud's phenomenon of limbs or tongue
Temporal artery tenderness	(70)	Tender scalp nodules
Jaw claudication	(65)	Thick, tender occipital arteries
Lingual, limb, or swallowing claudication	(20)	Necrotic lesions of scalp, tongue
Brachiocephalic bruits	(50)	Carotid artery tenderness
Thickened or nodular temporal artery	(45)	Swelling of the hands
Pulseless temporal artery	(40)	Taste, smell disturbances
Visual symptoms	(40)	Distended, beaded retinal veins
Fixed blindness, partial or complete	(15)	
Polymyalgia rheumatica	(50)	Diminished or absent radial artery pulses
Weight loss >6 kg	(40)	Mononeuropathy (median, peroneal, cervical root)
Erythrocyte sedimentation rate		
>50 mm/hr	(95)	
>100 mm/hr	(60)	
Fever (>37.7°C)	(20)	
Abnormal liver function	(50)	
Anemia (hematocrit level <35%)	(50)	

Adapted from Raskin NH, Appenzeller O. Headache. Philadelphia: WB Saunders, 1980.

toms usually remit entirely and there is a significant decrease in the ESR. After 4 to 6 weeks, the prednisone should be tapered every 1 to 2 weeks by approximately 10% until a dosage of 10 to 15 mg daily has been reached. Further tapering and duration of treatment depend on the clinical response and ESR (see Chapter 74 for details regarding long-term corticosteroid therapy and practical strategies for tapering corticosteroids). A 2-year course of prednisone is generally recommended. Some authors, who documented GCA relapse after discontinuing treatment, recommend lifelong maintenance treatment with low-dose prednisone, especially in patients who have no intolerable side effects from treatment (1,2).

If the patient has *isolated PMR*, the treatment is 10 to 20 mg of prednisone daily, tapered to a daily maintenance dosage of 5 to 7.5 mg daily after several weeks. Treatment is continued for approximately 2 years, with gradual discontinuation at the end of that time. The symptoms of PMR, and the ESR, respond to this regimen dramatically, often within the first 24 hours. In general, the ESR does not provide a useful guide to the activity of PMR, and it is reasonable to taper the prednisone without regard to the ESR. PMR recurs in some patients, within months to years of discontinuing prednisone; these patients usually respond to a second course of treatment.

Benign Intracranial Hypertension (Pseudotumor Cerebri)

Benign intracranial hypertension is a condition of unknown cause characterized by headache, papilledema, and elevated intracranial pressure in the absence of a mass lesion or venous sinus thrombosis (12). Headache in this condition is presumably caused by stretching of the dura and perhaps the large vessels. Papilledema is a direct result of the increased pressure. The paucity of focal neurologic symptoms and signs is caused by the global increase in intracranial pressure. Those focal signs that do appear (e.g., sixth nerve palsies producing horizontal diplopia) are probably related to stretching of the involved structure.

This condition may occur de novo or it may appear in association with a number of purported contributing factors (obesity, menstrual irregularity, steroid therapy or steroid withdrawal, oral contraceptives, nalidixic acid, and vitamin A intoxication).

Manifestations

The prototypical patient is an obese young woman who develops progressively more severe headaches, nausea, vomiting, dizziness, and transiently blurred vision. In approximately 50% of patients, onset is abrupt; the rest develop symptoms progressively over several weeks or months. The headache always precedes visual symptoms. It is usually generalized, constant, and often more severe in the morning, and is aggravated by coughing, straining, or changing position. The diagnosis is suggested strongly by these historical characteristics coupled with a physical ex-

amination that shows papilledema without focal neurologic signs. Visual fields may be constricted and the blind spot enlarged. Rarely the papilledema involves the macular area, resulting in blindness (22).

The diagnosis of pseudotumor is always one of exclusion, as its name implies. The most important considerations in the *differential diagnosis* are intracranial mass lesion, hydrocephalus, hypertensive encephalopathy, and venous sinus thrombosis. To exclude an intracranial mass or hydrocephalus, a CT or MRI scan (see "Patient Experience," Chapter 78) should be obtained. In pseudotumor, the scan may show small ventricles, but there is no evidence of a mass lesion. After a negative scan, a lumbar puncture should be performed (see "Patient Experience," Chapter 78). In pseudotumor, the cerebrospinal fluid (CSF) pressure is high (200 to 400 mm H_2O or more), the content of CSF protein is normal or low, and the cell count is normal. The diagnosis of hypertensive encephalopathy should be made if the patient has the typical clinical features of pseudotumor, severe diastolic hypertension (above 120 mm Hg), and a negative CT scan. In a very obese woman with a history of amenorrhea for many months, it is also important to consider pregnancy-induced hypertension (toxemia), which is ruled out by a negative pregnancy test (see Chapter 93).

For less clear-cut cases, such as a typical clinical presentation in an older male patient, or when the spinal fluid is abnormal, referral to a neurologist is indicated.

Treatment and Course

Most patients recover completely from pseudotumor within several weeks or months; however, some patients require ongoing therapy to control headaches and prevent visual loss. In a very obese patient, weight reduction is recommended, although this may not directly affect the course.

The goal of therapy is to reduce intracranial pressure in order to reduce the risk of loss of vision. At the time of the initial lumbar puncture, enough fluid should be removed to reduce the closing pressure to 100 mm H_2O or less (usually about 25 to 35 mL CSF). Acetazolamide (Diamox), as 500 mg sustained-release capsules, is then begun on a twice-daily schedule with periodic check of serum electrolytes. If the patient remains asymptomatic and the papilledema clears, acetazolamide can be discontinued. For patients with continued headache, visual impairment, and papilledema, repeated lumbar punctures should be performed with removal of adequate volumes of CSF with each tap, and acetazolamide should be continued.

The use of corticosteroids to treat pseudotumor cerebri is controversial. Should the patient remain symptomatic after repeated lumbar punctures and acetazolamide, CSF shunting via a lumboperitoneal shunt or surgical incision of the optic nerve sheath should be considered. Treatment of these patients is difficult and requires the consultation of neurologists and neurosurgeons experienced in handling this disorder.

Posttraumatic (Postconcussive) Headache

Manifestations

Head trauma, with or without loss of consciousness, may be followed by a number of symptoms that are collectively called the postconcussive syndrome: headache, vertigo (often positional, see Chapter 81), light-headedness or giddiness, poor concentration and memory, lack of energy, irritability, and anxiety. There is convincing evidence that these varied symptoms may be organic consequences of the injury, although their exact causal mechanism is not understood.

Headache is the most common and often the most troubling manifestation of this syndrome. It typically begins within 24 hours of the trauma as a dull, constant, generalized aching discomfort that may wax and wane through the day or become concentrated at different points on the head (bifrontal or unilateral). During exacerbations, the pain typically has a throbbing quality. Headache may be worsened by sneezing, coughing, stooping, straining, or rapid head motions and changes in body position; it may be accompanied by nausea and vomiting.

Typically, these headaches worsen over days to weeks, then resolve over weeks or months; in some patients (roughly 15%) headache and other postconcussive symptoms continue for more than a year. It is now appreciated that minor head trauma in patients with no headache history may lead to chronic recurrent headaches typical of migraine, with or without aura.

Differential Diagnosis

Subdural hematoma and other expanding mass lesions. Although postconcussive syndrome is a far more likely explanation of posttraumatic headache and ill-defined intellectual impairments than subdural hematoma, the seriousness of this possibility and the ease of ruling it out with CT scan make it an important consideration.

Posttraumatic dysautonomic cephalgia. Predominantly throbbing headache pain associated with sweating of one side of the face, pupillary dilation, and, sometimes, carotid bifurcation tenderness may represent a lesion of the carotid sympathetic plexus produced by whiplashlike injury (28). This condition may respond well to propranolol (Table 79.6).

Preexisting migraine or chronic tension headaches must be excluded by history; furthermore, posttraumatic headaches may make a preexisting headache condition temporarily worse. (For details regarding cervical spine injury, see Chapter 64.)

Objective Tests

In addition to the neurologic history and examination, a number of objective tests may be helpful for confirming the diagnosis of postconcussive syndrome: electroencephalography, vestibular function tests, electronystagmography, and auditory and visual evoked potentials. Abnormal results, although indicative of organic disease, are nonspecific. Negative test results do not exclude an organic basis for the patient's symptoms.

Treatment

In most patients, the course of the illness is self-limited even though fairly lengthy. Treatment similar to that used for tension headache may be successful. Propranolol or amitriptyline used alone or in combination (Table 79.6) dramatically reduces the frequency and severity of the headaches in some patients who develop typical migraine headaches following head trauma (29).

Low-Pressure (Post–Lumbar Puncture or Positional) Headache

Low-pressure headache from persistent leakage of CSF occurs most commonly after lumbar puncture. Less commonly, it is caused by a CSF fistula caused by blunt trauma to any part of the neural axis (i.e., closed head or spine trauma); occasionally no causal event can be identified. The headache is markedly positional, brought on by sitting or standing and relieved almost entirely by lying down. Nausea and dizziness are common nonspecific accompaniments. There are no focal neurologic symptoms or signs, and the patient is afebrile.

The majority of post–lumbar puncture and posttraumatic leaks close spontaneously, signified by resolution of the headache, within a few days; occasionally the problem does not resolve for several weeks. Appropriate management is essential for rapid healing of the leak: The patient is instructed to remain recumbent for several days, after which usual activities can be resumed. The rare patient with persistent, typical post–lumbar puncture headache should be referred to an anesthesiologist for epidural instillation of autologous blood; the blood will clot, forming a patch, at the site of the leak. Because of the risk of meningitis, any patient with a suspected persistent CSF fistula (i.e., a patient with a typical low-pressure headache that persists after blunt trauma) should be referred to a neurologist or neurosurgeon for complete evaluation.

Characteristics of Headache Caused by a Mass Lesion

For both the headache sufferer and the physician, concern about the possibility of a brain tumor often dominates the situation. The most important clue to the presence of an intracranial lesion is the simultaneous onset of headache and focal neurologic signs/symptoms or a change in mental status. In a person over the age of 50, the onset of persistent headache for the first time is also very worrisome.

A number of other features, none of them specific, may be clues to the presence of an intracranial mass lesion:

- Although the headache associated with a mass lesion can initially be intermittent, mild, and responsive to mild analgesics, typically it becomes more continuous and intense and, at the same time, less responsive to analgesics.

- The headache awakens the patient from sleep or is present on awakening every day, decreasing after the patient has been up for several hours. True sinus headache may also be worse in the morning because of lack of postural drainage during the night.
- Coughing, sneezing, and straining aggravate a persistent headache caused by a mass lesion, presumably by transiently increasing intracranial pressure and accentuating the stretching of pain-sensitive structures.
- Anorexia, nausea, and vomiting may accompany the headache.

Except when there are focal neurologic signs or symptoms, the decision to evaluate a patient for a mass lesion is usually made after an initial period of observation and a trial of analgesics. A CT scan with contrast, or brain MRI, which is more expensive (see special advantages of both CT and MRI, and "Patient Experience," Chapter 78), is the diagnostic procedure of choice when the decision is made to evaluate for a mass lesion. When the CT scan or MRI is positive for intracranial disease, the patient should be referred to a neurologist or neurosurgeon for definitive care.

FACIAL PAIN SYNDROMES
Idiopathic Trigeminal Neuralgia (Tic Douloureux)

Manifestations

Trigeminal neuralgia is seen almost exclusively in patients over the age of 40, most of them elderly. It has several distinguishing features: The pain is severe, paroxysmal, and lancinating, and it lasts only a few seconds to a minute. The patient's face usually contorts with the pain, and the patient may find it impossible to control his or her emotional response. Between attacks the patient is usually pain free, although some patients may have a dull ache in the area. The interval between paroxysms is usually at least 2 or 3 minutes. The frequency of paroxysms is highly variable; some patients have hundreds each day.

The pain is usually felt in the structures innervated by the second and third divisions of the trigeminal nerve (lips, gums, cheek, chin). The pain is typically unilateral in a single attack, and in 95% of patients it remains unilateral. It is uncommon for attacks to involve both sides of the face simultaneously.

The patient often can identify trigger points on the face or in the mouth that, when touched (even by contact with a gust of cold air) or moved, precipitate pain.

A few patients with idiopathic trigeminal neuralgia have some areas of slightly decreased sensation that may be difficult to distinguish from normal; however, there is generally no objective decrease in sensation.

Other less common syndromes with paroxysms of lancinating pain include glossopharyngeal neuralgia (pharynx pain) and occipital neuralgia (posterior head pain).

Differential Diagnosis

A syndrome identical or similar to idiopathic trigeminal neuralgia can be produced by a number of known conditions (secondary trigeminal neuralgia), such as multiple sclerosis, acoustic neurinoma, aneurysms, trigeminal neuromas, meningiomas, and others. These conditions should be considered, particularly if the patient is less than 40 years old and has any of the following: pain predominantly in the upper division of the trigeminal nerve (forehead and eye), bilateral pain, or evidence of bilateral sensory loss or associated motor signs (e.g., weak jaw, facial weakness, swallowing difficulty).

Treatment

In a patient with a typical clinical presentation, medical therapy (see below) can be initiated without further workup. If medical therapy is ineffective, or if there are any atypical features, referral to a neurologist is appropriate. The consultant usually requests imaging studies helpful in evaluating the divisions of the trigeminal nerve that are clinically most involved (for the first division, the superior orbital fissure; for third division, the foramen ovale).

Advances in drug therapy have made the treatment of idiopathic trigeminal neuralgia effective. The initial treatment is *carbamazepine* (Tegretol, 200-mg tablets) one-half tablet (100 mg) twice daily, with meals, increasing every 2 to 3 days to a three-times-daily schedule and a total daily dosage of 300 to 600 mg. An occasional patient may need dosages as high as 1200 mg/day; in these cases, blood levels should be monitored to confirm the adequacy of the drug trial. Most patients can expect excellent to satisfactory relief with carbamazepine. Benign side effects of the drug include nausea, vomiting, ataxia, vertigo, and transient leukopenia. The most serious side effects are persistent leukopenia and aplastic anemia. Patients must be informed of these possible risks, the frequency of which is unknown but appears to be quite low. Because of these risks, patients should have serial hemograms performed after 1 week, 6 weeks, 3 months, and on a periodic basis. Because trigeminal neuralgia may remit spontaneously after 6 months to a year, discontinuation of drug therapy should be tried after treatment for 6 months to a year.

If the patient fails to improve with carbamazepine or fails to tolerate the drug, two alternative medications can be tried: a *tricyclic antidepressant* (e.g., amitriptyline progressing over several weeks from 25 to 150 mg at bedtime) or the muscle relaxant *baclofen* (a trial of several weeks, progressing from 10 to 40 mg twice daily). A patient whose symptoms cannot be controlled medically should be offered consultation with a neurosurgeon for possible percutaneous radiofrequency treatment of the trigeminal ganglion on the affected side.

Atypical Facial Pain

Atypical facial pain is a collective term for a variety of painful facial symptoms that do not meet the diagnostic criteria for a recognized entity. If untreated, most patients with this problem continue to complain of it for many years. The management of these patients involves excluding all reasonable possibilities; a one-time referral to a dentist and to an otolaryngologist should be part of this evaluation.

Most of these patients whose workup is negative improve with treatment with a tricyclic antidepressant (17).

Temporomandibular Joint Syndrome

On history and examination, some patients complaining of headache have the stigmata of this common syndrome: pain brought on by motion of the jaw and tenderness of the temporomandibular joint. The epidemiology, course, and management of this syndrome are described in Chapter 101.

General References*

Davidoff RA. Migraine: manifestations, pathogenesis, and management. Philadelphia: FA Davis, 1995.
> Excellent up-to-date information on the science and practical issues of headache.

Delassio DJ, ed. Wolff's headache and other head pain. 5th ed. New York: Oxford University Press, 1987.
> The most recent edition of the classic reference work on headache.

Specific References

1. Andersson R, Malmvall BE, Bengtsson BA. Long-term corticosteroid treatment in giant cell arteritis. Acta Med Scand 220:465, 1986.
2. Beevers DG, Harpur JE, Turk KAD. Giant cell arteritis: the need for prolonged treatment. J Chronic Dis 26:571, 1973.
3. Cook NR, Evans DA, Funkenstein HH. Correlates of headache in a population-based cohort of elderly. Arch Neurol 46:1338, 1989.
4. Clinical Conferences at the Johns Hopkins Hospital. Cluster headache. Johns Hopkins Med J 150:246, 1982.
5. Dhopesh V, Anwar R, Herring C. A retrospective assessment of emergency department patients with complaint of headache. Headache 19:37, 1979.
6. Edmeads J. Advances in migraine therapy: focus on oral sumatriptan. Neurology 45(Suppl 7):S1, 1995.
7. Fogan L. Treatment of cluster headache. Arch Neurol 42:362, 1985.
8. Friedman AP, von Storch TJC, Merritt HH. Migraine and tension headaches: a clinical study of 2,000 cases. Neurology 4:773, 1954.
9. Frishberg BM. The utility of neuroimaging in the evaluation of headache in patients with normal neurologic examinations. Neurology 44:1191, 1994.
10. Headache Classification Committee of the International Headache Society. Classification and diagnostic criteria for headache disorders, cranial neuralgias and facial pain. Cephalalgia 8(Suppl 7):1, 1988.
11. Huston KA, Hunder GG, Lie JT, et al. Temporal arteritis: a 25-year epidemiologic, clinical and pathologic study. Ann Intern Med 88:162, 1978.
12. Johnston I, Patterson A. Benign intracranial hypertension. Brain 97:289, 1975.
13. Lance JW, Curran DA, Anthony J. Investigations into the mechanism and treatment of chronic headache. Med J Aust 2:909, 1965.
14. Linet MS, Stewart WF, Celentani DD. An epidemiologic study of headache among adolescents and young adults. JAMA 261:2211, 1989.
15. Linn FHH, Mijdicks EFM, Graaf Y, et al. Prospective study of sentinel headache in aneurysmal subarachnoid haemorrhage. Lancet 344:590, 1994.
16. Machado EBV, Michet CJ, Ballard DJ, et al. Trends in incidence and clinical presentation of temporal arteritis in Olmsted County, Minnesota, 1950–1985. Arthritis Rheum 31:745, 1988.
17. Mathew NT, Saper JR, Silberstein SD, et al. Migraine prophylaxis with Divalproex. Arch Neurol 52:281, 1995.
18. Office visits to internists: National Ambulatory Medical Care Survey, United States, 1975. Advance Data, No. 16, February 7, 1978.
19. Packard RC. What does the headache patient want? Headache 19:370, 1979.
20. Price RW, Posner JB. Chronic paroxysmal hemicrania: a disabling headache syndrome responding to indomethacin. Ann Neurol 3:183, 1978.
21. Rooke ED. Benign exertional headache. Med Clin North Am 52:801, 1968.
22. Rush JA. Pseudotumor cerebri, clinical profile visual outcome in 63 patients. Mayo Clin Proc 55:541, 1980.
23. Schnarch DM, Hunter JE. Migraine incidence in clinical versus nonclinical populations. Psychosomatics 21:314, 1980.
24. Silverman K, Evans S, Strain EC, Griffiths RR. Withdrawal syndrome after the double-blind cessation of caffeine consumption. N Engl J Med 327(16):1109, 1992.
25. Stewart WF, Lipton RB, Celentano DD, Reed ML. Prevalence of migraine headache in the United States: relation to age, income, race, and other sociodemographic factors. JAMA 267:64, 1992.
26. Subcutaneous Sumatriptan International Study Group. Treatment of migraine attacks with sumatriptan. N Engl J Med 325:316, 1991.
27. Sumatriptan Cluster Headache Study Group. Treatment of acute cluster headache with sumatriptan. N Engl J Med 325:322, 1991.
28. Vijayan N, Dreyfus PM. Post-traumatic dysautonomic cephalgia. Arch Neurol 32:649, 1975.
29. Weiss H, Stern BJ, Goldberg J. Chronic migraine after minor head trauma. Ann Neurol 16:113, 1984.
30. Welch KMA. Drug therapy of migraine. N Engl J Med 329(20):1476, 1993.
31. Weygaud CM, Gorozny JJ. Polymyalgia rheumatica and giant cell arteritis. In: Koopman WJ, ed. Arthritis and allied conditions: a textbook of rheumatology. 13th ed. Philadelphia: Lea & Febiger, 1997.
32. Ziegler DK, Hassasein RW, Cough JR. Characteristics of life headache histories in a nonclinic population. Neurology 27:265, 1977.

*Bold print (general references) and bold numerals (specific references) denote published controlled clinical trials, meta-analyses, or consensus-based recommendations.

CHAPTER 80

Seizure Disorders*

PETER W. KAPLAN, MBBS, FRCP

About 2 million people in the United States may have epilepsy. An even larger number seek medical advice for treatment of seizures, generating approximately 5% of visits to physicians and 20% of visits to

*Robert S. Fisher, MD, PhD contributed to this chapter in previous editions of this book.

neurologists (24). This chapter addresses the basic principles that should guide the diagnosis and management of seizures in office practice.

DEFINITION AND CLASSIFICATION OF EPILEPTIC SEIZURES

Any paroxysmal disturbance in consciousness, behavior, or motor activity may be called a spell, fit, or seizure, but this chapter addresses primarily *epileptic seizures.* These may be defined as the clinical manifestations of an abnormal, usually brief, excessive or hypersynchronous neuronal discharge in the cerebral cortex or deep limbic structures. A seizure has a definite start and finish. Seizures are associated with characteristic electrical abnormalities of the brain. Most patients are normal and their electroencephalograms (EEGs) are often normal between seizures (the interictal period).

The term *epilepsy* refers to a chronic neurologic condition causing spontaneous, recurrent seizures. Therefore, single or even multiple seizures arising during transient systemic insult such as fever, infection, toxic (e.g. alcohol), or metabolic disturbances should not be labeled as epilepsy and are called *reactive seizures.*

The basic mechanisms underlying epileptic seizures are still uncertain, although much is known about predisposing conditions. The most widely accepted classification is based on behavioral and electroencephalographic aspects (Table 80.1) (11).

CLINICAL MANIFESTATIONS OF DIFFERENT SEIZURE TYPES

The clinical manifestations of seizures vary according to the degree of maturity of the nervous system, the initial seizure focus, and the pattern of ictal spread (9). A seizure focus in the motor cortex produces jerking of the corresponding contralateral parts of the body, seizures in sensory regions result in abnormal sensations, and seizures in areas of higher cortical function may produce complex cognitive and behavioral manifestations (Fig. 80.1). Certain types of seizures present with sudden changes in vigilance or consciousness rather than with focal motor or sensory signs or symptoms.

Generalized Tonic–Clonic Seizures (Grand Mal)

Generalized tonic–clonic seizures (GTCSs) occur when ictal discharges involve most of the cortex. They may arise in the context of primary, *idiopathic generalized (genetic) epilepsies* (IGEs), in which seizure activity appears synchronously over both hemispheres, or may also result from *secondarily generalized seizure* discharges arising from a unilateral focus. Generalized tonic–clonic seizures may be called *major motor seizures,* although the now-disused term *grand mal* referred to bilateral generalization of seizure activity.

Idiopathic generalized epilepsies may appear at any age, although onset is rare after age 35. Frequency may

Table 80.1. Classification of the Epilepsies

Primary Generalized Epilepsy (Idiopathic Generalized Epilepsy, IGE)
Tonic–clonic (grand mal) (GTC)
Absence (petit mal)
Myoclonic
Atonic, others

Secondarily Generalized Seizures

Partial (Focal) Epilepsy
With elementary symptomatology
Focal motor
Focal sensory
Vegetative
Psychic
Mixed
With complex symptomatology
Complex partial (psychomotor) (CPS)

Unclassifiable Seizures

Adapted from Dreifuss FE. Proposal for revised clinical and electroencephalographic classification of epileptic seizures. Epilepsia 22:489, 1981.

range from two seizures in an entire lifetime to several seizures a day. Symptomatic epilepsies giving rise to focal and secondarily generalized tonic–clonic seizures may occur throughout life, caused by developmental abnormalities, perinatal insults, infection and head trauma, and strokes, particularly in the elderly.

GTCs typically begin with an arrest of activity and sudden loss of consciousness, followed by trembling, tonic extension of the arms and legs, and then clonic rhythmic but progressively slower limb jerking, followed by flaccidity, stupor, and labored, deep breathing. Seizures usually last less than 2 minutes and are followed by lethargy lasting for minutes to hours. During the seizures, consciousness is always lost, so a history of the utterance of meaningful speech, the presence of purposeful eye movements, or a memory of the seizure itself excludes the diagnosis. Although malaise may precede GTCs, a definite sensory, autonomic, psychic, or motor prelude suggests a *focal onset with subsequent generalization* (secondarily generalized tonic–clonic seizures). Tonic–clonic seizures may be accompanied by incontinence, sweating, tachycardia, elevated blood pressure, minor cardiac arrhythmias, and biting of the lip, cheek, and lateral aspect of the tongue.

The EEG that is typical in IGEs shows a pattern of bilateral synchronous spike-and-wave discharges, whereas patients with generalized seizures that arise from a lateralized focus may show focal epileptiform discharges over the affected cortical zone.

Generalized Absence Seizures (Petit Mal)

Typical absence seizures are also generalized seizures; they occur in *childhood absence epilepsy* (CAE), a type of *idiopathic generalized epilepsy* (IGE). Absence seizures may also occur in Lennox–Gastaut syndrome and juvenile myoclonic epilepsy (JME). CAE constitutes approximately 5% of childhood epilepsy.

The onset is usually between 4 and 12 years of age. Most affected children (75%) have absence seizures that remit by the age of 20 years, although about half (especially with atypical absence) may later develop tonic–clonic seizures.

Because of the previous classification of generalized seizures into "petit mal" and "grand mal," some patients incorrectly continue to believe that these two entities are different severities of the same seizure type (although both can occur with IGEs). There is often confusion also between the staring component of absence seizures and the initial staring phase of partial complex seizures (see below). Finally, "petit mal" was often incorrectly used by patients to refer to partial seizures with a motor component, or minor motor seizures. Such confusions in classification may lead to incorrect diagnosis, prognosis, and antiepileptic drug (AED) therapy.

Typical absence seizures in CAE, consisting of lapses of vigilance or awareness, usually last about 3 to 20 seconds. There is no tonic–clonic phase or loss of posture. Slight rhythmic twitching of the mouth and periorbital musculature or upgaze may be observed. With atypical absence seizures, duration may be prolonged, leading to confusion with complex partial seizures arising from the temporal or other lobes. In CAE, there is a rapid recovery of awareness following absence seizures, but amnesia for events during the seizure persists. Absence seizures typically can occur up to 100 times per day. Children who have such frequent seizures may be labeled as being inattentive, daydreamers, or slow learners until the correct diagnosis is made.

Both clinical and EEG findings should be used to secure a diagnosis of CAE; neither alone is diagnostic. The EEG during an absence seizure shows a characteristic bilateral synchronous three-per-second spike-and-wave pattern; between seizures, the EEG may be normal, but brief 3/second bursts usually persist in the absence of AED therapy. Often, hyperventilation or stimulation with regularly flashing lights (intermittent photic stimulation) induces an absence seizure. Three-per-second spike-and-wave patterns on EEG may be

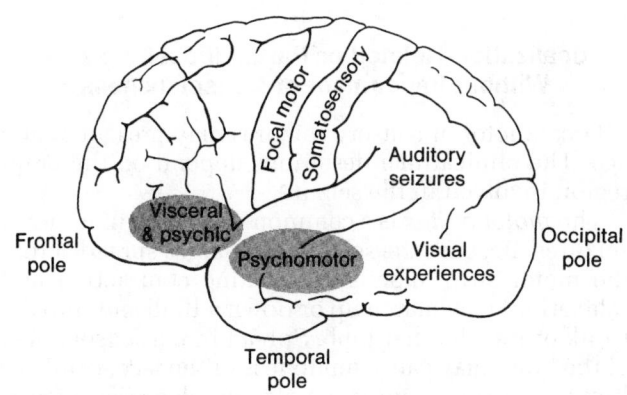

Figure 80.1. Relationship of local seizure phenomena to brain topography.

seen in asymptomatic close relatives of patients with CAE as well as in other seizure types (e.g. tonic–clonic seizures).

Myoclonus and Myoclonic Seizures

Myoclonus is the predominantly synchronous, involuntary, nonrhythmic jerking of limbs, trunk, or head. Epileptic myoclonus arises from paroxysmal discharges of the central nervous system (CNS) above the brainstem. Conditions in which nonepileptic myoclonus (segmental myoclonus) may occur are conditions affecting the brainstem and the spinal cord.

Myoclonic seizures are most often seen after severe, diffuse cortical injury from cerebral ischemia and anoxia; these seizures are difficult to suppress and carry a poor prognosis. When myoclonic seizures arise from hypoglycemia, severe renal or hepatic failure, or drug toxicity, they are often self-limited and resolve with correction of the underlying disturbance. Primary neurologic diseases, such as viral encephalitis, Jakob–Creutzfeldt disease, Huntington's chorea, Wilson's disease, and ceroid lipofuscinoses may also include myoclonic seizures. Myoclonic seizures are also seen in IGEs, benign myoclonic epilepsy of childhood, JME, the Lennox–Gastaut syndrome (triad of multiple seizure types, psychomotor retardation, and a characteristic EEG pattern, seen mainly in children), progressive myoclonic epilepsies, and a wide variety of seizures from toxic and metabolic causes.

Myoclonic seizures consist of brief and violent muscular contractions, usually bilateral, that do not affect consciousness. Myoclonic contractions may be single or multiple, lasting for seconds to hours. Contractions may be rhythmic or irregular. When the upper limbs are involved, patients may drop or toss objects. When the legs or trunk are involved, the patient may suddenly fall. Myoclonic seizures may be spontaneous or may be induced by flashes of light, more rarely by other triggering stimuli.

The usual EEG correlate of myoclonic seizures is generalized or multifocal spikes, polyspikes, and slow waves. Scalp-recorded EEG discharges may be seen in the case of cortical myoclonus but may not be seen in the case of subcortical myoclonus.

Localization-Related or Partial (Focal) Seizures Without Impairment of Consciousness

Focal motor or sensory seizures may present at any age. The clinical manifestations depend on the brain region involved in the seizure.

The *motor cortex* is a common site of origin for focal seizures. Because the seizure discharges spread across the motor strip, clonus (alternating contraction and relaxation) may march up or down a limb and into the trunk or into another limb. Spread into a sensory area of the brain may cause numbness in the face, trunk, or limbs. *Sensory seizures* can also involve areas of special sensation such as sight or hearing. A focus in or near the visual cortex or its association areas may cause

the patient to see spots, lights, or geometric shapes, similar to the experience of patients with classic migraine. Perception of buzzing, clicking, or ringing sounds may be generated from a focus in the superior and mesial temporal lobe. Gustatory and olfactory sensations, usually unpleasant, are components of partial seizures involving mesial temporal lobe structures. Seizures dominated by vestibular symptoms (e.g., dizziness, vertigo) are rare.

Retention of some degree of consciousness is characteristic of focal seizures, so patients may, for example, walk and talk during a seizure—activities that would be impossible during a generalized seizure. However, a large focus in the dominant hemisphere may generate seizures that blunt awareness.

After a focal motor seizure, there may be *focal weakness of a limb, or Todd's paralysis,* which usually resolves within a few hours or, rarely, after a few days. Distinction between cerebrovascular ischemic events with associated seizures and seizures with Todd's paralysis may be difficult without clues from the patient's history. A Todd's paralysis has localizing value and is good evidence of the focality of a seizure.

EEG does not necessarily reveal a seizure focus, especially if the seizure is small (e.g., motor seizure involving the leg, in which case the focus lies deep within the interhemispheric fissure), and particularly if it is obtained between seizures.

Complex Partial Seizures

The category of complex partial seizures (CPSs) is important for several reasons: The condition is common in the adult population, the seizures are often misdiagnosed, and correct diagnosis leads to a search for potentially correctable lesions and effective AED therapy. CPSs are classified with focal or localization-related seizures because of clinical evidence linking these seizures with focal as opposed to generalized epileptiform discharges. CPSs are largely synonymous with the older term *psychomotor seizures,* but are not synonymous with temporal lobe seizures because they may arise from any brain region. Although CPSs may begin at any age, the majority begin before age 20. An adult onset of CPS carries the same significance as does a new onset of any focal seizure; a treatable structural lesion should be sought after. Patients with CPS who come to surgery or to postmortem may either show no histologic abnormality of the brain or have tumors, infarcts, granulomas, or infections; often with temporal lobe origin there is gliosis of the mesial temporal lobe. It is not known whether gliosis causes temporal lobe CPSs or results from them.

CPSs impair attention or consciousness through focal seizure activity. This is why they are called complex. The presentation of these seizures is more varied than that of the other seizure types and may include autonomic, psychic, visceral, sensory, or motor symptoms. Seizures often begin with an aura, which is, in fact, a simple partial seizure. The classic aura, usually consisting of an unpleasant olfactory or gustatory hallucination, is less common than is an aura of poorly described unpleasant visceral sensations or malaise. In general, there is no clear boundary between the aura and the seizure itself, particularly when seizures feature distorted visual or auditory sensations, or vertigo or unsteadiness. Arrest of motor activity, rigid posturing of the head and eyes, and slow repetitive limb movements may occur and are easily distinguished in most cases from the tonic–clonic sequence of convulsive attacks. Autonomic instability, including fluctuating heart rate or blood pressure, flushing, sweating, salivation, or changes in pupillary reactions, may occur in patients with complex partial seizures. Patients often say that they feel strange or as if in a dream, or experience inappropriate emotions such as intense dread or strange serenity. If they can talk during a CPS, patients may portray what appears to be a psychiatric disturbance. The distinction between CPSs and psychosis may be further obscured in patients with psychologic or psychiatric problems between seizures. Such patients can be misdiagnosed as schizophrenic.

In a condition whose presentation may range from apparent appendicitis to apparent schizophrenia, special efforts should be made to elicit a detailed history of a spell and, when possible, to observe one. CPSs should have a definite start and finish, they should be associated with some impairment in ability to register and process information during the seizure, and they should be stereotyped from episode to episode. Observations of automatic behavior, such as repetitive lip licking or smacking, raising and lowering the arm, fidgeting or buttoning and unbuttoning clothing, stroking or rubbing movements, or pacing in circles, may secure the diagnosis of a CPSs because such automatisms are common in CPS but are uncommon in other seizure types.

The routine EEG is abnormal in less than half the patients with partial seizures, but positive tracings may be found in 80 to 90% of patients by recording EEGs during sleep and, in the case of temporal lobe origin, by using special electrodes positioned closer to temporal lobe structures.

Complex electrophysiologic mechanisms determine whether seizure discharges remain localized, spread along particular anatomic pathways, or involve much of the brain. AEDs can limit the spread of a focal seizure and prevent generalization. It is unknown how often tonic–clonic seizures are caused by spread from occult primary foci.

Unclassifiable Seizures

With an adequate history, most seizures should be classifiable by the scheme given above. Unfortunately, the history is often lacking, as the event may not have been witnessed, or observers might report the patient falling down and shaking but cannot describe the full sequence of events. In these instances it is best to list the seizure as unclassifiable or to use descriptive terms that are not otherwise used to classify seizure types, such as *jerks, convulsions,* or *staring spells,* until a specific seizure type can be identified.

CLASSIFICATIONS OF EPILEPSY SYNDROMES

Seizures are observable phenomenon with symptoms or signs that last a finite time. An *epilepsy syndrome* is a cluster of signs and symptoms occurring together and constituting a chronic condition of recurrent seizures. There is no single known cause or pathology for epilepsy. Features of a particular epilepsy syndrome include cause, family history, age of onset, seizure frequency, typical course, precipitating factors, imaging studies, and the EEG. Thus, damage to the temporal lobe may result in a condition of recurrent seizures characterized by an aura, unresponsiveness with automatisms, and tonic–clonic movements. This would represent a syndrome in which there is a progression of seizure types from simple partial to complex partial to secondarily generalized tonic-clonic seizures. If clinical data point to damage in the temporal lobe (EEG focus, imaging findings), the epilepsy syndrome is that of symptomatic temporal lobe epilepsy. This is also true with idiopathic generalized epilepsies (called primary generalized epilepsies). For example, absence seizures can be seen in a number of epilepsy syndromes (e.g., childhood absence epilepsy), each of which may have a different constellation of signs and symptoms and carry a different prognosis.

The importance of establishing a syndromic classification of epilepsy is that the particular prognosis in this chronic condition is tied to the epilepsy syndrome rather than the seizure type. Furthermore, the success in the use of antiepileptic drugs or even seizure surgery is also predicated more by the epilepsy syndrome classification than by the seizure type (6).

EPIDEMIOLOGY

The annual incidence rate of epilepsy is approximately 40 to 70 per 100,000 population, and the reported prevalence rates are between 1.5 and 57 in 1,000 (38). Partial epilepsies constitute about two-thirds, one-fifth are generalized, and the remainder are unclassified (47). In adults, CPSs may constitute approximately 40%, GTCSs about 40%, and simple partial (focal motor or sensory) seizures approximately 15% (47). For younger age groups, partial seizures are less prevalent and generalized absence seizures are correspondingly more common.

NATURAL HISTORY AND PROGNOSIS

The natural course of epilepsy is difficult to determine because modern studies include a mixture of treated and untreated patients. Comparison of prevalence and incidence ratios suggests a crude mean for the duration of epilepsy of approximately 12 to 13 years (3), not taking into consideration the age of onset of epilepsy, the clinical type, or the response to treatment.

After a first unprovoked seizure the cumulative risk of recurrence at 3 to 5 years has been estimated to be 40% (5,21). Until further data are available, a 40% crude risk for recurrence within a few years of a spontaneous tonic–clonic seizure is a reasonable estimate. Of adults who have a recurrence of tonic–clonic seizures, approximately 60% have recurrence in the first year and 70% by 3 years (22). Risk factors that increase the risk of recurrence and decisions about treatment are discussed in a later section ("The Patient with a First Seizure"). If a person has a second, unprovoked seizure, the risk for further seizures is higher, and after several unprovoked seizures it exceeds 75%.

Once two spontaneous seizures have occurred, epilepsy is considered to exist, and the epidemiologic focus switches to the possibility for remission. Before the development of AEDs, the spontaneous remission rate for all types of epilepsy was approximately 10 to 32%. Reported remission rates for epilepsy with or without treatment vary between 10 and 82% (4,42), according to when the study was done, retrospective versus prospective methodology, and the length of follow-up. Studies on prognosis have not yet clarified the role of treatment in the long-term outcome. The probability of going 5 years without seizures is approximately 40% at 1 year and 50% at 2 years after diagnosis of epilepsy (4). From 50 to 82% of patients are in remission after 2 to 5 years (10,17). The probability of remission at 20 years is 80 to 85% for idiopathic generalized epilepsies, but only 65% for localization-related epilepsies. After being free from seizures for 5 years, almost 50% of patients relapse after tapering AEDs, usually in the first year and particularly in the first 6 months (31).

Prognostic factors include age of onset, severity of epilepsy, number of seizures before treatment, number of types of seizures, history of status epilepticus, number of medications required to control the disease, and length of time before attainment of seizure control. CPSs without secondary generalization are the most difficult seizure type to control (26,35).

Epilepsy that has not been controlled after 2 years of treatment represents a significant risk for chronic epilepsy. Some authorities believe that the long-term risk may be decreased by early treatment of seizures; however, this concept remains controversial. An abnormal EEG during AED withdrawal increases the chance of relapse in patients with CPSs (40), but a normal EEG CPS does not exclude a relapse (83 versus 54%) (45). The presence of neurologic or psychiatric problems worsens the prognosis.

It is generally possible to reassure a person with epilepsy that the long-term prognosis for remission is good; however, except for CAE, which usually remits before young adulthood, the attainment of remission can be expected to require many years.

CAUSES OF SEIZURES

Classification of seizures requires clinical observation, and classification of an epilepsy syndrome often requires clinical, EEG, and imaging data. Because a seizure represents a symptom of cerebral dysfunction, a primary cause should be sought.

Epilepsy that arises from *definable causes* has also been called symptomatic as opposed to essential or idiopathic. Symptomatic epilepsies often arise from identifiable brain lesions, as from infections, trauma, tumors, or strokes. With IGEs, however, patients have a normal examination, normal screening laboratory tests (see below), an EEG often showing a generalized spike-and-wave pattern, and a family history for similar seizures. Such patients would not be exhaustively studied for underlying causes.

Table 80.2 lists *specific causes* that should be considered for different types of seizures at various ages; the causes are listed from top to bottom in approximate order of frequency. It is worth emphasizing that many of the partial epilepsies may display secondarily generalized seizures, and that the focal onset may be obscured. Therefore, causes of focal seizures should be sought even in apparently generalized seizures.

Special issues are raised by *seizures that are manifested for the first time in the elderly*. First, most seizure disorders have onset in the first three decades of life, and onset of the IGEs almost never occur after this age. Second, cerebrovascular disease accounts for 30 to 60% of all new seizures in the elderly population. Tumors, the major cause of focal seizures in middle-age, have been found to be the cause of 2 to 30% of seizures in elderly patients (41); brain tumors in this age group are likely to be malignant. No cause is found in about half of elderly patients with seizures. When an elderly patient presents with seizures, a special effort should be made to find treatable conditions such as carotid artery stenosis, cardiac arrhythmias, infection, and toxic–metabolic derangements.

Posttraumatic Seizures

New-onset seizures after head trauma are usually partial (focal) in onset, and often secondarily generalized seizures may occur after serious head injuries. There is little risk of seizures after mild head trauma with brief unconsciousness or amnesia, whereas severe injuries with intracranial hematomas, focal neurologic signs, and unconsciousness for more than 24 hours result in epilepsy in about 10% of patients. Moderately severe injuries (skull fractures or unconsciousness for 30 minutes to 24 hours) impose an intermediate risk. Injuries over the vertex are more epileptogenic.

The value of *prophylactic therapy* to prevent the onset of posttraumatic seizures has not been firmly established. Until more data are available, the following approaches are recommended: Patients with minor scalp lacerations or brief loss of consciousness should not be considered to have a significantly increased risk of epilepsy. A single seizure occurring early (during the first 2 weeks after head injury), or while the patient is still suffering from the acute effects of injury, should not be an indication for long-term therapy; a second seizure in this setting might be grounds for treatment.

Table 80.2. Causes of Seizures with Onset at Various Ages

Adolescent (12–21 yr)	Adult (21–65 yr)	Elderly (65+ yr)
Common Causes		
Genetic (g)	Alcohol withdrawal (g)	Cerebrovascular (m)
Mesial temporal sclerosis (f)	Toxins or drugs (g)[b]	Thrombotic
Infection (m)	Drug withdrawal (g)	Embolic
Meningitis	Tumor (f)	Hemorrhagic
Viral encephalitis	Trauma (f)	Cardiac arrhythmia
Abscess	Scar	Trauma (f)
TORCHS[a]	Subdural hematoma	Scar
Parasites	Mesial temporal sclerosis (f)	Subdural hematoma
Psychogenic (m)	Genetic (g)	Tumor (f)
Toxins or drugs (g)[b]	Psychogenic (m)	Infection (m)
Drug withdrawal (g)	Infection (m)	Meningitis
	Meningitis	Viral encephalitis
	Viral encephalitis	Abscess
	Abscess	Syphilis
	Syphilis	Parasites
	Parasites	
Occasional Causes		
Metabolic (g)	Metabolic (g)	Alcohol withdrawal (g)
Hypoglycemia	Hypoglycemia	Toxins or drugs (g)[b]
Hyponatremia	Hyponatremia	Drug withdrawal (g)
Hypocalcemia	Hypocalcemia	Hypoxia (g)
Porphyria	Hypomagnesemia	Metabolic (g)
Trauma (f)	Hypoxia (g)	Hypoglycemia
Scar	Cerebrovascular (m)	Hyponatremia
Subdural hematoma	Thrombotic	Hypocalcemia
Tumor (f)	Embolic	
Arteriovenous malformation (f)	Hemorrhagic	
Subarachnoid hemorrhage (m)	Cardiac arrhythmia	
Eclampsia (m)	Renal failure (g)	
Renal failure (g)	Eclampsia (m)	
Rare Causes		
Collagen disease (m)	Collagen disease (m)	Hypertensive encephalopathy (m)
Hepatic failure (g)	Hypertensive encephalopathy (m)	Hyperosmolar (m)
Multiple sclerosis (f)	Hyperosmolar (m)	Renal failure (g)
	Multiple sclerosis (f)	Hepatic failure (g)
	Degenerative (m)	Degenerative (g)
		Factitious (m)
Idiopathic	Idiopathic	Idiopathic

f, Usually focal; *g,* usually generalized; *m,* often mixed.

[a]TORCHS, toxoplasmosis, rubella, cytomegalovirus, herpes, syphilis.

[b]See list of occupational exposures that may cause seizures, Table 7.3.

Some patients with brain injuries should be considered for a 2- to 4-year course of prophylactic phenytoin, especially with severe, penetrating, or vertex injuries. A patient with a seizure occurring more than 2 weeks after a head injury should be evaluated and managed as one would evaluate any other patient with new-onset seizures, and the seizure should not be attributed to a recent or remote episode of head trauma until other treatable causes of seizures have been excluded.

Alcohol-Related Seizures

Alcohol withdrawal is a common cause of seizures; almost all of them occur within the first 48 hours of abstinence or after marked reduction in alcohol intake, and most of them are generalized. In some series, up to 25% of withdrawal seizures have been focal, presumably because of an old cortical scar from trauma, infection, or vascular disease. The risk of epilepsy in the alcohol abuser is related to the amount of alcohol

that was consumed (no longer being consumed at time of seizure) (20), but may be increased by the higher likelihood of head trauma and intracranial infection in this population. If a known alcohol abuser has had a prior withdrawal seizure, presents a typical picture of a generalized seizure without focal features, and has a normal examination and no complications, then investigations may be limited. More often, the history is imprecise and findings are equivocal, or the patient has a fever or an elevated leukocyte count. In these instances, lumbar puncture, EEG, and continued observation are indicated. A computerized tomographic (CT) scan may be indicated with new-onset focal seizures, focal neurologic deficits, fever, neck stiffness, or signs of acute head trauma.

The use of AEDs to prevent alcohol withdrawal seizures is controversial. Some investigators recommend the use of AEDs for recent seizures or clusters of seizures during alcohol withdrawal (37), but others argue that alcohol withdrawal seizures are self-limited

(50), and some studies show that treatment is usually ineffective (2). During alcohol withdrawal, hospitalized patients with a history of epilepsy may be given a 5-day course of phenytoin (300 mg/day) to try to prevent seizures and the attendant risks of aspiration pneumonia and falls. Long-term therapy with AEDs is not recommended.

Alcohol abusers may abuse other drugs. Concurrent benzodiazepine or barbiturate withdrawal may cause fulminant seizures. Occasionally, seizures may occur during periods of alcohol consumption, as distinct from the period of alcohol withdrawal (33).

Seizures and Brain Tumors

Brain tumor is an uncommon cause of epilepsy, but epilepsy is a common symptom of brain tumors. About one-third of intracranial and one-half of intrahemispheric tumors are associated with seizures. Our present understanding of epilepsy secondary to tumors has been completely changed with the advent of CT and magnetic resonance imaging (MRI) head scanning (32). More and more often, tumors present with a single seizure leading to early investigation and diagnosis with CT head scan or MRI. From 1 to 16% of patients with epilepsy are found to have tumors. The probability varies according to age group: In adolescents it is approximately 1%; in young adults, 12 to 16%; and in older people, approximately 10% (1,23). *Young and middle-aged adults with new onset of focal seizures* have the greatest chance of having a tumor (35%) (47). Nonetheless, CT or MRI scanning is not indicated in the investigation of patients with IGEs who have diagnostic EEG patterns and in previously investigated patients who present with repeated seizures of unchanged character.

Seizures may be generalized tonic–clonic or partial. Diverse and changing clinical features are highly indicative of neoplasia. The following features suggest that seizures may be associated with a brain tumor: onset after 20 years of age, presence of persistent focal neurologic signs, signs of increased intracranial pressure, and focal unilateral slow waves on the EEG. Seizure frequency varies according to tumor location and histology: Frequent seizures are seen with supratentorial tumors, especially in the rolandic, temporal, or parietal cortical regions. Slow-growing tumors appear to be more epileptogenic.

Seizures and Cerebrovascular Disease

Cerebrovascular disease and epilepsy are the two most common causes of serious neurologic illnesses, and often occur in the same patient. Ischemia damages brain and can lead to an epileptic focus. The incidence of early seizures (within the first 2 weeks of stroke onset) is approximately 5% in patients with nonembolic stroke (44). The seizures are more likely to be focal (80%) than generalized, and the distribution depends on stroke location. Only a small proportion of stroke patients develop recurrent seizures (i.e., epilepsy): 2.5% of those with intracranial hemorrhage and 3% of

those with ischemic stroke (44). In ischemic stroke, although the highest incidence of seizures is shortly after stroke onset (19), epilepsy is most common in patients with late-onset (greater than 2 weeks) seizures (90%) rather than those with early-onset seizures (35%). Consequently, early seizures after stroke do not mandate antiepileptic drugs; late recurrent seizures should be treated as epilepsy.

As previously mentioned, seizures in the elderly should raise the suspicion of cerebrovascular disease and may herald transient ischemia or impending stroke. In young patients, cerebral vascular disease is uncommon, but a seizure may lead to a diagnosis of an arteriovenous malformation, an aneurysm, collagen vascular disease, or a rare case of cortical thrombophlebitis.

Seizures and Infections

A seizure may be an early sign of bacterial meningitis, particularly in the very young and in the very old patient in whom the classic signs of meningitis may be lacking. Less fulminant forms of meningitis, such as cryptococcal or tuberculous meningitis, produce seizures that recur over weeks or months. Viral encephalitides, including herpes simplex encephalitis, the childhood exanthems, and the equine viruses may also produce seizures. Human immunodeficiency virus (HIV) infection (see Chapter 34) is increasingly of concern as a cause of neurologic and systemic disease; most seizures in association with acquired immunodeficiency syndrome (AIDS) result from secondary complications such as cerebral toxoplasmosis, other atypical infections, or CNS lymphoma (29). Any meningoencephalitis may scar the cerebral cortex, resulting in an epileptic focus that can persist after resolution of the infection.

For reasons that are poorly understood, *systemic infections* may trigger seizures in susceptible patients, even if the infection does not directly involve the CNS. However, when a patient presents with a seizure and signs of infection, especially if the seizure is focal or if focal signs are detected on neurologic examination, the possibility of brain abscess must be explored using a head CT scan or MRI, often with contrast.

EVALUATION OF A PATIENT WITH SEIZURES

In the evaluation of a patient with a history of one or more episodes of self-limited disturbance of consciousness or behavior, three questions must be addressed: First, was (were) the event(s) epileptic seizure(s)? Second, if so, what type of seizure(s) (Table 80.1)? Third, are there clues in the history, physical examination, or laboratory tests that point to a cause for the epileptic seizure(s) (Table 80.2) or toward another cause?

Differential Diagnosis of Seizurelike Behavior

Determination of the nature of a seizurelike episode is often difficult (Table 80.3). Unless the physician has

Table 80.3. Differential Diagnosis of Seizurelike Behavior

Condition	See Chapters
Syncope	81
Cerebrovascular disease	83
Migraine	79
Narcolepsy	85
Fluctuating delirium	17
Paroxysmal vertigo	81
Breath-holding spells	
Episodic movement disorders	82
Malingering, factitious illness	12
Conversion disorder	12
Panic attack	13

observed an attack, the patient or witnesses must be asked for information about the sequence of behavioral events with attention to specific signs of neurologic dysfunction. Inquiry should be directed at establishing whether there were tonic–clonic features, with or without tongue, lip, or cheek biting, head and eye deviation, urinary or fecal incontinence, rhythmic face or limb jerking, or speech and motor arrest followed by automatisms. *Syncope* not caused by a seizure is characteristically associated with prodromal malaise, dizziness and light-headedness, often with pallor, sweating, palpitations, and upright posture (see Chapter 81); if an observer notes sudden loss of consciousness and tone without convulsions and with brief postictal confusion, syncope is a much more likely diagnosis than is seizure. However, syncopal events can include some arrhythmic limb jerking, occasionally accompanied by incontinence and brief confusion. Transient numbness, weakness, speech or vision problems, or dizziness may occur with *cerebrovascular events* (see Chapter 83), including transient ischemic attacks, stroke, bleeding from an arteriovenous malformation or from an aneurysm, or a classic migraine (see Chapter 79). Precipitating factors such as postural changes, changes in antihypertensive medication, and the sequence of seizure characteristics may help distinguish epileptic seizures from cerebrovascular insufficiency. Particularly in the elderly, where the two conditions may be linked, a firm diagnosis may have to be deferred.

Hypoglycemia (see Chapter 74) is most commonly seen in alcoholics, diabetics, and patients who have had gastrointestinal (GI) surgery and often presents with presyncopal symptoms.

Narcolepsy (see Chapter 85) is a rare disorder characterized by the sudden lapse into REM (rapid eye movement) sleep or with episodes, when alert, of brief inhibition of muscle tone (cataplexy). These patients can be aroused from their sleep, often report that they dreamed during the attack, and deny postictal confusion.

In the elderly, a waxing and waning delirium with fluctuating agitation, lethargy, and occasional motor manifestations (see Chapter 17) occurring with intercurrent illness (e.g., renal failure, drug intoxication, or infection) may superficially resemble a seizure but usually lacks both the stereotypical aspects of a seizure and a clear start and finish.

Vertigo, caused by disease of the inner ear, can present paroxysmally and may be confused with epilepsy (see Chapter 81).

Certain adults may have *face or limb tics,* which, unlike most epileptic seizures, can be partially controlled by volition and often occur at predictable times.

Psychogenic Seizures

In some patients, the greatest challenge is to distinguish between epileptic and psychogenic events. Misdiagnosis of an epileptic seizure may result in incorrect treatment of the actual underlying condition and the possible social stigma and consequences of being labeled an epileptic. *Panic attacks* can produce recurrent, fulminant, and moderately stereotyped symptoms, all of which may be seen in patients with partial complex seizures (see Chapter 13). Because epileptic seizures may have emotional concomitants (e.g., an aura of extreme fear) and may be triggered by stressful situations, distinction may be difficult. If a diagnosis of psychogenic illness can be supported on other grounds, if the attacks are strongly linked to preceding anxiety, and if automatisms are lacking, a panic attack becomes a more likely diagnosis.

Patients with seizures caused by a *conversion disorder* may manifest inattention, staring, deep unresponsiveness, and tonic and clonic movements that closely resemble epileptic events. These psychogenic seizures are involuntary events and must be differentiated from *malingering* and *factitious seizures,* which are produced deliberately by the patient. However, patients with nonepileptic events often also have epilepsy, and the management of epileptic events may be complicated by nonepileptic ones. Thrashing, asynchronous limb movements, crying, screaming, pelvic thrusting, and rapid side-to-side head turning have traditionally been ascribed to nonepileptic events but may also be seen with epileptic seizures. Observation of a generalized attack may reveal features atypical of an epileptic event, such as retention of protective reflexes such as the blink reflex, a breathing effort when the airway is briefly occluded, coherent speech, or directed eye movements. Other features include the variability and nonstereotypy of each event, emotional precipitants, the usual presence of witnesses, recall after the event, biting of the tip of the tongue, forced eye closure, and the absence of postictal confusion (14). The motor activity may lack the organized tonic–clonic stages seen with generalized seizures, unless the patient is sophisticated and has observed seizures before. Psychogenic partial complex seizures may be the most difficult to diagnose.

As a general rule, purposeful, goal-directed behavior such as driving, shopping, talking in full sentences, or coordinated acts of violence should not be considered to be part of an epileptic seizure unless there is strong supporting evidence. Some of these features may be seen in the postictal state. Other features typical of a conversion disorder—presence of secondary gain, la belle indifference, inappropriate reactions to stress—may contribute to a correct diagnosis. Consultation among primary physician, neurologist, and psychiatrist may be required for proper diagnosis and management (see also Chapter 12).

Initial Determination of Seizure Type and Cause

The identification of seizure type (Table 80.1) should be made at the time of diagnosis of epilepsy. Features of the clinical onset should be especially addressed because a brief focal onset or an aura may be the only indication that a seizure was secondarily rather than primary generalized.

The history usually provides the main clues to the cause of the seizure. Contributory factors may include birth trauma or perinatal illness, head trauma, previous cerebral infarction or intracranial hemorrhage, encephalitis or meningitis, malignancies, and prior seizures. A family history of seizures may be pertinent because there is increased risk, particularly with IGEs, for seizures in relatives of people with epilepsy. There should be inquiry into the use of alcohol, benzodiazepines, barbiturates, and other proconvulsants such as cocaine, amphetamine, neuroleptic medications, tricyclic antidepressants, bupropion, and theophylline. Patients may volunteer accounts of precipitating events such as flashing lights or hyperventilation. In some epilepsies, patients may identify particular stimuli such as games, music, eating, laughing, or the touching of certain regions of skin. These *reflex seizures* may be avoided by avoiding the offending stimulus.

A general physical examination and neurologic examination (see Chapter 78) may reveal asymmetries or provide evidence for a structural, metabolic, or other cause of the seizure disorder. Some findings—for example, focal paralysis—may be postictal, indicating focal onset (Todd's paralysis), or conversely may be suppressed, warranting reexamination in a few hours or days.

Investigations in a Patient with Seizures

Laboratory tests are usually not very helpful in determining whether a seizure has taken place, but they may be useful in establishing an underlying cause, in epilepsy classification, and in patient management.

Laboratory Tests

Depending on one's diagnostic hypotheses, investigations may include a full blood count, blood urea nitrogen or serum creatinine, serum glucose, and serum electrolytes. In evaluating test results, it should be remembered that *striking abnormalities may appear transiently immediately after a seizure* (e.g., metabolic acidosis, marked leukocytosis). If clinically indicated, blood gases, liver function tests, and a screen for proconvulsive drugs should be obtained. A baseline electrocardiogram may show arrhythmias or ischemia, although immediately after a seizure these changes also may be the results, rather than causes, of the seizure.

At times, measurement of a *serum prolactin level* helps in the evaluation of a patient with a suspected psychogenic seizure. Commonly, the prolactin levels may rise two to three times after an epileptic but not a psychogenic tonic–clonic event. In a lesser percentage of patients (45%), CPSs may cause serum prolactin increases as may syncope (34), but most simple partial (epileptic) seizures (85%) cause no rise (51). PCSs of temporal lobe origin are more likely to cause prolactin increases than those from the frontal lobe (30). Because this transient rise is present for 10 to 60 minutes after the event, positive findings are helpful, but negative findings, especially measured after an hour, are inconclusive.

Electroencephalography

The EEG is the most useful laboratory study in the diagnosis of seizure disorders. An EEG may show generalized or focal epileptiform activity or, even in the absence of such activity, may demonstrate asymmetries of basic rhythms, focal slow waves, or diffuse slowing, all of which may give direction to further investigation. The appearance of epileptiform discharges on an EEG performed within a week of a *first seizure* predicts an 83% recurrence rate within 2 years, versus a 41% recurrence in patients without them (49). In general, the EEG should be relied on not to make a diagnosis of a seizure but to confirm a clinical impression derived from the history. When history and EEG are at variance, primacy should go to the history. Patients should not be treated for epilepsy because of an abnormal EEG alone because interictal pattern epileptiform discharges may be seen in 0.4% of the healthy population, in 2.2% of patients with nonepileptic neurologic disease, and in 3.5% of asymptomatic relatives of people with epilepsy (16). Conversely, one should not be dissuaded from a clinical impression of a seizure disorder just because of a normal EEG.

When EEG confirmation of seizure activity is needed (e.g., when the history is equivocal, or when seizures occur during sleep or drowsiness), repeated studies with sleep deprivation or sleep induction, hyperventilation or intermittent photic stimulation, use of other scalp or semi-invasive electrodes (nasopharyngeal or sphenoidal leads), or eventually the use of prolonged video monitoring with EEG recording may be indicated. Many hospitals have epilepsy monitoring units specializing in the diagnosis and treatment of epilepsy. Referral to such units is sometimes the most effective way to elucidate the nature of spells not delineated by more routine maneuvers.

Epileptiform EEG discharges can usually be observed in the presence of AEDs, although some generalized discharges may be suppressed. Therefore, medications should not be altered for the first EEG. If tracings are repeatedly negative and the diagnosis of epilepsy is suspect, then the patient can be admitted to a hospital for rapid tapering of AEDs and concurrent EEG and video monitoring to look for epileptic activity. However, abrupt withdrawal of barbiturates or benzodiazepines may precipitate seizures even in normal subjects. Among patients with epilepsy, the pattern of generalized EEG slowing without seizure discharges is fairly common, usually resulting from underlying diffuse cortical dysfunction, medication effects, or a postictal state.

Because EEGs may stay abnormal for several weeks after a tonic–clonic seizure, any findings should be reevaluated with repeated studies. An EEG is without risk, barring an injudicious interpretation (see "Patient Experience" in Chapter 78).

Cerebrospinal Fluid Examination

Certain illnesses that lead to seizures may require examination of cerebrospinal fluid (CSF) to secure a diagnosis; suspected acute or chronic meningitis or subarachnoid hemorrhage are examples. The yield of CSF studies in patients with various seizure types is unknown, and the indication for these studies should be considered on a case-by-case basis. The CSF examination is not indicated in a normal child with classic absence epilepsy or with EEG evidence of focal rolandic spikes, and is contraindicated in a patient in whom a mass lesion is strongly suspected. Most other patients with focal or generalized seizures of uncertain cause should undergo spinal fluid analysis (see "Patient Experience" in Chapter 78).

After prolonged generalized seizures, the CSF may show a pleocytosis of up to 100 cells, presumably from a transient breakdown of the blood–brain barrier (39). Clearly, however, infection must be excluded or temporarily considered in this setting.

Cerebral Imaging

CT head scans (see "Patient Experience" in Chapter 78) of patients with primary generalized seizures are abnormal (excluding nonspecific atrophy) in approximately 10% of instances. Scans of patients with focal motor or secondarily generalized seizures show a focal abnormality in 65%. Patients with CPSs show abnormalities about one-third of the time. An abnormal and asymmetric neurologic examination has a high correlation with focal abnormalities on the head CT scan. Studies of patients with seizures show that MRI of the head (see "Patient Experience" in Chapter 78) has a higher diagnostic yield than CT scanning (8), but is not a procedure needed for all patients.

Adults with new-onset focal or secondarily generalized seizures should have an MRI or CT scan with contrast if possible unless the EEG shows a pattern of a genetic disorder. Patients with an abnormal neurologic examination should also be imaged. In patients with a normal examination and in children, this decision should be individualized. Subsequent imaging may also be indicated when there is a change in seizure pattern or neurologic examination.

Other Diagnostic Tests

Skull x-rays, radionuclide brain scans, pneumoencephalography, and arteriography have largely been replaced by newer imaging studies. Several techniques show promise for definition of seizure foci, but are still considered experimental: imaging of brain metabolism and chemistry by positron emission tomograph (PET) scanning, single-photon emission computerized tomography (SPECT, which examines cerebral blood flow at particular time points), and magnetoencephalographic (MEG) recording of brain activity.

TREATMENT OF EPILEPSY

Except in unusual instances, epilepsy cannot be cured. In about three of four patients, it can be controlled so that patients experience few or no seizures. Much attention has been focused on the pharmacologic management for seizures, but the importance of a comprehensive approach cannot be overemphasized: A patient who is seizure free, but so toxic from medicines that employment is impossible, is at best a dubious success. Employment problems and other social aspects of managing epilepsy are considered below. General measures of therapy should not be neglected. Removal of precipitating factors for seizures, reduction of stress, and provision for adequate amounts of rest can all be important in the control of epilepsy and are also discussed below. Patients should be advised to wear *medical alert bracelets or medallions.*

The Patient with a First Seizure

In deciding whether to treat a first seizure, one should recall that a single seizure does not constitute epilepsy or necessarily require treatment. In patients with *"provoked"* or acute symptomatic seizures such as those following alcohol withdrawal, cocaine intake, or tricyclic overdose, identification and removal of the precipitating cause usually prevents further seizures. AEDs are rarely indicated. In addition, single or early seizures (i.e., within 2 weeks) after head trauma or stroke do not require chronic AED therapy.

In about a third of patients with first seizures, the seizures *are unprovoked.* Such patients may be so frightened by the possibility of having another seizure, with potential repercussions on employment, social relations, and license to drive, that they are willing to accept the inconvenience and morbidity of chronic medication. Most patients first present to a physician after having had several unprovoked seizures. In this group, more than three-fourths are expected to have further seizures. This contrasts with the finding from prospective studies that approximately 16 to 36% of patients who present after their first unprovoked seizure have a recurrence within 1 year, and in the aggregate 27 to 50% have recurrent seizures within 3 years (5,21). Retrospective studies suggest higher recurrence rates.

Because for a given patient the probability of further seizures over a 5-year period might vary from 30 to 80%, it is important to consider the following *risk factors that increase the probability of additional seizures:* an identifiable cause for the first seizure, such as CNS infection or recent stroke or head injury; the presence of EEG epileptiform abnormalities; occurrence of the initial seizure at night; previous febrile seizures; status epilepticus or multiple seizures in the same day; Todd's paralysis; and partial seizures (21,26). With genetic epilepsies typically with childhood onset in which the EEG shows epileptiform activity, there is an increased risk of seizure reoccurrence in the short term. Many of these epilepsy syndromes are age-dependent, and remit after several years.

In one prospective study, addressed to the issue of treatment following a first unprovoked tonic–clonic seizure, the rate of recurrent at 1 year in patients randomized to AED treatment was 18 versus 38% for those who were not started immediately on treatment (15). Depending on the antiepileptic drug used, the incidence of side effects severe enough to warrant discontinuation of treatment ranges from less than 1% to approximately 6%. These figures are usually not used in deciding whether a patient should be offered a specific AED. Rather, the efficacy profile, overall side effect profile, and frequency with which the medication must be taken govern the institution of the drug (see below).

General Principles of Drug Therapy

Many patients who have monthly or more frequent generalized seizures are probably undertreated. In contrast, other patients may be taking an unnecessary polypharmacy or incorrect regimens of AEDs. General principles for the planning of drug therapy are summarized in Table 80.4. Prospective observations show that with adequate AED treatment, the prognosis for seizure control during the first 12 months varies according to seizure type: Generalized tonic–clonic 60 to 70%, mixed (predominately GTC) 50 to 53%, complex partial 21 to 28% (26).

To select the appropriate AED, it is important to know the type of epilepsy under consideration. Table 80.5 represents a general but not unanimous consensus on drugs of choice and alternatives for the principal types of seizures and epilepsy. One large controlled trial compared the effectiveness of four AEDs (carbamazepine, phenobarbital, phenytoin, and valproic acid) for the treatment of *partial seizures* or *secondarily generalized tonic–clonic seizures* (25). Both carbamazepine and phenytoin were highly effective and are recommended as drugs of choice for these two common types of seizures. Valproic acid is generally recommended as the drug of first choice for IGEs. *Childhood absence epilepsy* (CAE) may be treated with either

Table 80.4. Principles of AED Therapy

Decide whether to treat.
Select the proper drug for the particular form of epilepsy.
Start drugs slowly and build up levels gradually to avoid toxicity.
Start with one drug, and use it to effect or toxicity before adding another.
Choose the simplest regimen possible.
Suspect compliance problems in treatment failures.
Monitor blood levels in problem cases.
Withdraw medications gradually.
Decide how long to treat.

Table 80.5. Drugs of Choice for Monotherapy According to Seizure Type

Seizure Category	Drugs of Choice	Alternatives
Primary generalized, tonic–clonic	Valproate	Carbamazepine Phenytoin Primidone Phenobarbital
Primary generalized, absence	Ethosuximide Valproate	Clonazepam
Primary myoclonic	Valproate Clonazepam	Phenytoin Phenobarbital
Partial simple and complex and secondarily generalized epilepsy	Carbamazepine Phenytoin	Valproic acid Phenobarbital Primidone
Mixed forms	Valproate Clonazepam	Carbamazepine Phenytoin Phenobarbital

ethosuximide or valproic acid, although the former does not prevent concurrent tonic–clonic seizures. *Myoclonic seizures* are best treated with valproate acid or clonazepam. A certain percentage of IGEs with GTCS respond to monotherapy with carbamazepine (although absence seizures may worsen), and a certain percentage of partial seizures respond to valproic acid monotherapy. In several instances, more than one drug may be considered the drug of choice in terms of efficacy, in which case the selection can be made on the basis of personal familiarity with the drug, convenience of dose scheduling, or the relative risk and spectrum of side effects. For example, some practitioners prefer carbamazepine to phenytoin to avoid possible gum hyperplasia and hirsutism, even though these side effects are seen in only approximately 10% of patients. With phenytoin, the convenience of a simpler dosage regimen, lower cost, and availability of a parenteral preparation may offset these considerations. Several reviews compare controlled trials of AEDs (18,46). Dosages, half-lives, serum levels, and principal side effects of the drugs are given in Table 80.6.

Drugs should be initiated at one-quarter or one-half of the anticipated maintenance dosage (except for phenytoin and phenobarbital; see below), and the dosage should be increased over several weeks to avoid early side effects that might discourage the patient from continuing with treatment. Because some AEDs remain in the blood for some time, it may take several days to weeks before the effects of a dosage adjustment are manifested.

Although initial treatment *with more than one AED,* typically phenytoin and phenobarbital, was once common, there was little evidence that two drugs at subtherapeutic dosages are better tolerated or more effective than one drug at higher dosages. In fact, 90% of new-onset seizures that are controlled can be controlled with one drug. When one drug is unsuccessful, addition of a second helps in only approximately 36% of patients (43).

Compliance is a major factor in the success of drug therapy for epilepsy (see Chapter 4). Every effort should be made to simplify the dosage regimen and choose the best-tolerated drug. Phenobarbital and certain formulations of phenytoin can be given in a once-daily dose. The complexity of providing carbamazepine, primidone, or valproic acid, which must be given in divided doses, should be offset by a better-suited profile of side effects for the individual patient. At each visit the patient (or the responsible person) should be asked to report on the exact medication regimen and encouraged to bring the most recent medicine bottles with them. All too often, inquiry indicates a need for clearer oral and written communication with the patient. If necessary, the drug regimen should be written out for the patient's use.

Familiarity with cost of medicines is important because patients may be hesitant to buy an expensive medicine unless the need is clearly explained. *Generic brands* are less expensive, but for several AEDs, such as carbamazepine, primidone, phenytoin, and valproic acid, bioavailability is variable. Generally, generic brands should be avoided in patients with seizures that are difficult to control. If generic brands are prescribed, the same brand should be encouraged; drug levels may have to be checked more often if seizures or toxicity appear.

The optimal dosage of an AED may vary severalfold among different patients. Determination of serum levels (Table 80.6) is a reliable way to measure how much medication is circulating, but such measurements should not be ordered routinely. If a patient's seizures are controlled on the regimen that is initiated and there is no toxicity from that drug regimen, measurement of a drug serum level might lead one to alter a successful regimen inappropriately. If control is not optimal, drug levels can help detect inadequate compliance or absorption. The levels may also provide guidance for patients with symptoms that might be caused by drug intoxication. Ideally, blood specimens obtained to monitor side effects should be taken at times of peak serum levels; specimens obtained to monitor drug efficacy should be taken at times of trough serum levels. It is important to know that for some AEDs, particularly phenytoin, drug dosage and drug level are not linearly related: A saturation point is reached above which small increments in daily dosage (e.g., increasing from 400 to 500 mg of phenytoin a day) may lead to marked increases in serum level and side effects. A level is most informative if measured in the steady state (Table 80.6), which

Table 80.6. Major Antiepileptic Drugs (AEDs)

Medication[a] (Brand Name)	Available Preparations and Strength (mg)	Typical Adult Dose, Schedule, Range	Half-Life (hr)	Target Levels (mg/L)[b]	Major Side Effects
Phenytoin (Dilantin)[c]	30, 100 capsules 30/5 mL and 125/5 mL suspension 50 chewable tablets	300 mg QD[d,e] (200–500 mg)	22[e]	10–20	Ataxia Cosmetic changes (gum hyperplasia, hirsutism) osteoporosis
Fosphenytoin IV sodium (Cerebyx)	IV preparation 2 mL (100 mg PE) and 10 mL (500 mg PE)	150 mg PE/min diluted in 0.9 saline or 5% dextrose before infusion	15 min	10–20	Pruritis Paresthesia Dizziness Headache Somnolence Ataxia Nystagmus
Carbamazepine[c] (Tegretol)	200 tablets (100 chewable) 100/5 mL suspension	200 mg TID or QID (400–2000 mg)	10–25	4–12	Gastrointestinal (GI) distress Ataxia Blurred vision Blood changes Hepatotoxicity
Carbamazepine extended release (Tegretol XR)	100, 200, 400 tablets	200–1000 mg BID			Same as carbamazepine
Valproic acid[c] (Depakene)	250 capsules 250/5 mL syrup	50–4000 mg 250 mg BID to QID (500–4000 mg)	8–12	50–100	GI distress Drowsiness Ataxia
(Depakote)	125, 250, 500 tablets 125 sprinkles	Same as above			Alopecia Tremor Blood changes Rare liver toxicity Rare pancreatitis
Valproate IV (Depacon)	IV preparation 5 mL single-dose vials equal to 100 mg per mL	60-min infusion but not >20 mg/min	16 ± 3	50–100	Same as valproic acid
Phenobarbital[c] (Luminal)	15, 30, 60, 100 tablets	100 mg QD	72	15–40	Sedation Hyperactivity Confusion Mood change
Primidone (Mysoline)	50, 250 scored tablets and suspension	250 mg TID or QID (500–1500 mg)	3–12[f] 72[g]	6–12[f] 15–40[g]	Sedation Hyperactivity Mood change

PE, Phenytoin equivalents.

Table 80.6—*continued.*   Major Antiepileptic Drugs (AEDs)

Medication[a] (Brand Name)	Available Preparations and Strength (mg)	Typical Adult Dose Schedule, Range	Half-life (hr)	Target Levels (mg/L)[b]	Major Side Effects
Felbamate (Felbatol)	400, 600 tablets 600/5 mL suspension	1200–3600 mg/day in three or four divided doses	20–23	Unknown	Aplastic anemia Acute liver failure ↑ ALT Insomnia Headache
Gabapentin (Neurontin)	100, 300, 400 capsules	1800–3600/day in three divided doses	5–7	Unknown	Somnolence Ataxia Dizziness Fatigue Nystagmus
Lamotrigine (Lamictal)	25, 100, 150, and 200 tablets	300–500 mg BID	12–14	1.4–4.8	Rash Dizziness Ataxia Somnolence Headache Blurred vision Nausea Vomiting
Topiramate (Topamax)	25, 100, 200 tablets	100–400 mg/day in two divided doses	12–15 with other AED 21–24 as mono-therapy	Unknown	Somnolence Dizziness Ataxia Psychomotor slowing Kidney stones
Tiagabine (Gabitril)	4 mg, 12, 16, 20 mg	32 to 56 mg in 2–4 divided doses		Unknown	Dizziness Confusion Tiredness GI upset
Ethosuximide (Zarontin)	250 capsules 250/5 mL syrup	250 mg BID to QID (500–1500 mg)	30	50–100	GI distress Sedation Headache Dizziness
Clonazepam (Klonopin)	0.5, 1, 2 tablets	2 mg TID (2–20 mg)	20–40	0.05–0.7	Drowsiness Ataxia Behavior changes Dizziness

[a]Generic products are available but there have been reports of bio-inequivalence between brand name and generic products.

[b]Laboratory may report same figures as micrograms per milliliter.

[c]Generic product available.

[d]These doses are usually attained gradually over days to weeks. The ranges are relatively rough guidelines; because absorption varies, serum levels are better guides to dosage.

[e]Only for Dilantin capsules (Kapseals).

[f]For primidone.

[g]For phenobarbital.

requires a stable dosage for at least about five half-lives before measurement.

Many patients with severe and long-standing epilepsy have endured a gradual increase in AED dosage. Excessive polypharmacy may be ineffective, produce marked side effects, and even limit the ability to increase a single potentially effective AED to the maximum dosage. In this circumstance, one should consider reduction in AED dosage or number of medications over several months. Other side effects may prompt discontinuation of AEDs.

Although several AEDs may cause modest rises in *liver enzyme levels,* only moderate to marked abnormalities (more than 2 times baseline) necessitate stopping the drug. Conversely, serious hepatotoxicity may not be heralded by changes in liver function tests. Symptoms may include anorexia, malaise, tiredness, and jaundice, usually appearing 2 to 16 weeks after starting treatment. Carbamazepine may cause mild *leukopenia and thrombocytopenia,* but a rapid, pro-

gressive leukocyte decline, typically below 3000/mm^3 with a total neutrophil count of less than 1000/mm^3 would warrant concern (14). *Nystagmus* should not be used as an indication of toxicity, but rather as a marker of AED therapy. Conversely, ataxia, unacceptable somnolence, cognitive impairment, and malaise may indicate the need for modification of therapy.

Duration of Treatment

The determination of how long to maintain treatment with AEDs may be difficult because seizures remit over time, and thus freedom from seizures may not be caused by the medicine. About one-half to two-thirds of patients are entirely seizure free for 2 years with therapy. If an adult patient is seizure free for about 5 years on medication and stops treatment by gradual tapering, there is a 30 to 50% chance of relapse in the next 5 years (7,13,31). Approximately 90% of the relapses occur within the first 2 years after discontinuing medication.

As with the decision to initiate therapy, the decision to terminate AED therapy must be individualized. A patient with seizures that were initially very difficult to control who has an underlying structural lesion or a persistently abnormal EEG may benefit from lifelong therapy. In contrast, a patient with idiopathic epilepsy who has been seizure free for 2 to 5 years and is willing to accept an increased risk of having a seizure may be a candidate for drug withdrawal. Certain patients who have attained seizure control over a long period of time do not wish to stop treatment. In these instances, potential benefits and risks of medication reduction should be discussed, but patients should not be forced off medications for the sake of principle. If more than one drug has been prescribed, the medications should be tapered one at a time, each over a period of several months, and reinstated rapidly if seizures recur. The least effective medication or the most toxic may be chosen as the candidate for initial reduction.

An example of a cautious tapering schedule for a patient who has been taking carbamazepine 400 mg (two 200 mg tablets) three times daily would be a reduction by one tablet per day every 2 weeks. During tapering and in the first few months after the tapering of all AEDs, it is prudent for the patient to refrain from driving.

Ambulatory Follow-Up

Seizure frequency, medication side effects, and social factors determine the pattern for outpatient follow-up. Patients who are free from seizures for more than a year and who have no intercurrent problems may be seen yearly. Conversely, patients with frequent seizures, significant side effects, or social problems may need to be seen every few weeks during problem periods. Visits may be necessary every 2 to 4 weeks during adjustment of the drug regimen. For appropriate management and monitoring of therapeutic changes, a patient should be seen no sooner than five AED half-lives.

Specific Antiepileptic Drugs

Carbamazepine (Tegretol)

Carbamazepine has been used for over two decades for the treatment of seizures and chronic neuropathic pains. Carbamazepine is one of the drugs of choice in partial complex epilepsy. Studies comparing carbamazepine with other AEDs for the treatment of partial epilepsy have shown the highest rates of complete remission for patients taking carbamazepine (although mean seizure frequency was similar for patients taking carbamazepine, phenytoin, or phenobarbital) (25). The adult dosage is 400 to 2000 mg/day. Tablets come in 200-mg or 100-mg chewable preparations. A 100-mg/5 mL suspension is also available. It is advisable to initiate therapy with no more than 200 to 400 mg/day, increasing to the full dosage over a week or two. The half-life is about 10 to 25 hours, and dosage should be divided into three- or four-times-a-day regimens. A newer long-acting preparation, Tegretol XR, is available in 100-, 200-, and 400-mg tablets, with ports that allow slow release. This form can be taken twice daily. It is now the preparation indicated in all patients treated with Tegretol. Total daily dosage remains the same, meaning that conversion to the more convenient form is simple, but more even blood levels are obtained. Patients should be warned that the tablet shell may appear in the stool, but does represent inadequate release of contents. Patients must be instructed not to chew XR tablets but to swallow them whole. Recommended target serum levels with all preparations of carbamazepine are 4 to 12 mg/L. In 1997, a typical 1-month supply of generic carbamazepine cost about $17 versus $45 for Tegretol. Because of erratic absorption of the generic preparation, it should not be continued in any patient who takes it and continues to have seizures.

Because carbamazepine in tablet form may lose one-third or more of its effectiveness if stored in humid conditions, patients should be advised to keep their tablet containers in a dry location, away from the bathroom. Recently, manufacturers have been asked by the FDA to package carbamazepine in moisture-proof containers.

The *side effects* of carbamazepine include fatigue, nystagmus, diplopia, dizziness, ataxia, dysarthria, rash (including, rarely, Stevens–Johnson syndrome), inappropriate secretion of antidiuretic hormone, occasionally abnormal liver function tests, and an infrequent lupuslike syndrome. GI distress is the most common side effect, particularly if the medication is initiated too rapidly. Reversible leukopenia or thrombocytopenia is seen in 5 to 10% of patients, so blood counts should be monitored weekly for the first few weeks after the start of therapy. This drug has had a reputation for causing aplastic anemia, based largely on six cases of this complication that were reported in the 1960s (even though a causal relationship to carbamazepine was not established). The actual incidence of aplastic anemia is unknown, but it is thought to be very small (the warning provided by the manufacturer reports a general population incidence of potentially fatal blood dyscrasia of 8 per million and an incidence associated with carbamazepine of about 40 per million).

Phenytoin (Diphenylhydantoin, DPH, PHT, Dilantin)

Since its introduction in 1938, phenytoin has been one of the major drugs used to treat seizures. It is most useful in IGEs and in epilepsies with simple and complex partial seizures, with or without secondary generalization. Phenytoin may make absence seizures worse.

Phenytoin is absorbed from the GI tract in 4 to 8 hours. Without a loading dose, a full week is required to reach therapeutic levels, but a load of three times the daily maintenance dose, given in the first day, achieves immediate therapeutic levels. This rapid dosing scheme is likely to induce transient side effects and is useful chiefly for initiating treatment in a patient who has seized repeatedly (e.g., in an emergency department).

The mean half-life of phenytoin is 22 hours, with a range from 7 to 42 hours. It is 90% protein bound, so *low serum albumin* can lead to an increased concentration of the free agent and to increased toxicity. The drug is metabolized in the liver and is not excreted by the kidney. In renal failure, drug-binding proteins may be deficient, resulting in a low measured total serum level with an adequate free drug serum level. Dosage should be lowered only in renal failure to compensate for a decrease in serum protein, and then approximately a 25% reduction usually suffices. Phenytoin is partially removed by hemodialysis.

The usual starting dosage of phenytoin is 100 mg/day for 3 to 5 days, increasing by 100 mg at similar intervals to 300 mg/day. If seizures are not controlled at this dosage, it is prudent to increase by increments of 50 mg/day because small increases in dosage may cause large increases in serum levels. Phenytoin (as Dilantin) comes in 30- and 100-mg capsules, suspension (30 mg/5 mL and 125 mg/5 mL), and chewable 50-mg tablets. This medication can be given once a day if it is given as Dilantin capsules because this preparation is manufactured as a slow-release form. Other preparations are fast-release capsules; they are less expensive but must be given in divided doses (100 mg three times a day). A new parenteral formulation of phenytoin is fosphenytoin sodium injection (Cerebyx), which can be given intramuscularly or intravenously. It is dosed in phenytoin equivalents and can be given more rapidly intravenously at up to 150 mg/minute. A target range for phenytoin is generally between 10 and 20 mg/L (toxicity usually occurs over 20 mg/L, but patients show fairly wide individual susceptibility to side effects). The lethal dose may range from 2 to 20 g.

Several drugs elevate phenytoin plasma levels: disulfiram and isoniazid commonly, and warfarin, chloramphenicol, methylphenidate, phenothiazines, benzodiazepines, and propoxyphene less often. Other drugs may lead to *increased phenytoin metabolism,* resulting in decreased phenytoin levels: alcohol, folic acid, pyridoxine, theophylline, and occasionally carbamazepine, cimetidine, oral contraceptives, and sulfonamides. *Other drug interactions* may occur with concurrent use of amiodarone, cimetidine, diazoxide, fluconazole, folic acid, isoniazid, phenacemide, phenylbutazone, rifampicin, trimethoprim, ibuprofen, metronidazole, miconazole, and several others. These potential drug interactions may be managed best by patient and physician awareness and by observation of serum drug levels during times of medication changes.

There are many potential *undesirable effects of phenytoin.* Dose-related *acute effects* include ataxia (usually above 30 mg/L), lethargy, depression, paradoxic tendency to increased seizures at higher toxic levels (usually above 40 mg/L), and allergic reactions. *Chronic side effects* of phenytoin are generally manifested after a few months to several years of daily ingestion. Chronically progressive cosmetic changes can be vexing in young women. Gum hyperplasia occurs in approximately 30%; it may be forestalled by good oral hygiene, but once established may regress only partially; hirsutism is seen in 5% overall, but in 30% of young women. Even more disconcerting are facial changes caused by thickening of subcutaneous tissue about the nose and eyes, the so-called leonine facies. Cosmetic side effects can be avoided or even reversed by switching to a less well-known hydantoin, ethotoin (Peganone), given in dosages of 500 to 1000 mg three times a day (up to 3 g total per day). Skin rash occurs in 2 to 10% of users of phenytoin, with a peak incidence about 2 weeks into the course. Stevens–Johnson syndrome occurs rarely. Lymphadenopathy develops in 2 to 5%, sometimes in association with fever, arthralgia, eosinophilia, and hepatosplenomegaly, presenting a picture of pseudolymphoma and, rarely, true lymphoma. Hepatitis and a variety of blood dyscrasias have been reported. Megaloblastic anemia may occur, which responds to folate. Many patients develop measurable antinuclear antibodies in the serum; a tiny minority of this group progress to symptomatic systemic lupus erythematosus, which remits entirely within days to weeks after discontinuing phenytoin. Peripheral neuropathy with loss of muscle stretch reflexes has been alleged to occur in approximately 20% of long-term users. The rare pulmonary infiltrates and fibrosis have given rise to the term *Dilantin lung.* Phenytoin can induce liver enzymes, thereby secondarily affecting metabolism of numerous hormones and drugs. Induced inactivation of vitamin D leads to radiologic or biochemical evidence of bone disease in one of every three chronically treated patients. Teratogenic effects of phenytoin are strongly suspected (see below).

Valproic Acid (Depakene), Sodium Valproate (Depakote)

The antiseizure effect of valproic acid was discovered in 1963, but it is a recent addition to the list of major drugs used to treat seizures. Its effectiveness is broad, but it is thought to be particularly valuable for absence seizures and CAE, for idiopathic and symptomatic generalized epilepsies, and as a second-line agent for partial epilepsies (27).

Valproic acid is a fatty acid, structurally dissimilar from all other common AEDs. It is usually prescribed as sodium valproate/valproic acid (Depakote), purported by the manufacturer to cause less GI upset than pure valproic acid (Depakene). It is available in 125-, 250-, and 500-mg tablets and in 125-mg sprinkle capsules. Valproic acid is also available in generic form (approximately $15 versus $80 for a monthly supply of Depakote in 1997). Peak serum levels are reached in 1 to 4 hours after ingestion, and the half-life is about 8 to 12 hours. The drug is metabolized in the liver and excreted in the urine in modified form. Serum levels may be measured but at present have limited utility. The approximate therapeutic range is 50 to 100 mg/L. The manufacturer suggests initiation of therapy with a dosage of about 10 to 15 mg/kg per day, to be increased at weekly intervals by about 5 to 10 mg/kg per day to a maximal dosage of 60 mg/kg per day. A common final regimen is 250 to 500 mg orally, two to four times/day.

In studies on several thousand patients abroad, before the release of the drug in the United States in 1978, valproic acid proved to be quite safe. About one in five patients had significant side effects, commonly GI upset, drowsiness, rash, reversible hair loss, weight loss or gain, ataxia, tremor, or hyperactivity. A limited number of studies suggest that valproic acid inhibits platelet aggregation and may prolong the bleeding time, but this effect is poorly documented. Less commonly, valproate may produce frank thrombocytopenia. The health risk from the use of valproate that has received the greatest attention is *hepatic* toxicity. Thirty-seven fatalities from hepatic failure associated with use of valproic acid were reported in the United States between 1978 and 1984 (12). Among patients receiving valproate as monotherapy, the calculated rate of fatality from hepatic injury was 1 per 37,000. This rate was much higher for children less than 2 years old and for children receiving polytherapy. These two risk factors together resulted in a fatality rate from hepatic injury of 1 per 500 children. In contrast, no fatalities from hepatic injury were reported in patients over 10 years of age receiving monotherapy. Several patients have developed serious episodes of pancreatitis while taking valproic acid. Because of these recently discovered toxicities, and because of high cost, valproic acid has not yet replaced ethosuximide as the drug of choice for absence epilepsy unless there are concurrent atypical absence attacks or tonic–clonic seizures. There may be drug interactions with aspirin, warfarin, cimetidine, phenothiazines, antacids, and the benzodiazepines.

Phenobarbital

In past decades phenobarbital was a drug of choice for generalized tonic–clonic seizures. It is now a second-line agent for a variety of seizure types. Phenobarbital is particularly useful in the pediatric age group, where it may be better tolerated than phenytoin because it does not cause cosmetic side effects; however, it may cause significant behavioral side effects (hyperactivity in up to 40% of children).

Phenobarbital is a long-lasting drug. The GI absorption is slow, so it takes 10 to 12 hours for levels to reach their peak after an oral dose, compared with 20 minutes after an intravenous dose. The drug is detoxified by the liver and excreted by the kidney, but the dosage need be only slightly reduced in renal failure. The serum half-life is about 72 hours, ranging from 37 to 96 hours. Therapeutic levels are 15 to 40 mg/L. Phenobarbital is a potent inducer of liver enzymes and leads to rapid tolerance, as well as to alteration of kinetics of numerous other medications. The dosage of phenobarbital is 1 to 3 mg/kg per day, or about 100 mg/day for the average adult. Little justification can be made for giving it in divided doses. Available tablet strengths are 15, 30, 60, and 100 mg.

The main *acute side effect* of phenobarbital in adults is sedation. After a few weeks, partial tolerance to the sedation usually develops. In elderly patients, phenobarbital can cause confusion and respiratory depression. Subtle or overt personality changes caused by phenobarbital probably occur more often than is generally recognized, especially in the elderly. Ataxia and nystagmus are common in all patients at high dosages. Occasionally, there is idiosyncratic allergy, with accompanying dermatitis or GI symptoms. Phenobarbital must not be administered to potential drug or alcohol abusers or to unreliable patients who might precipitously discontinue their medicine. There are drug interactions with warfarin, β-blockers, and corticosteroids, and possible interactions with acetaminophen, chloramphenicol, chlorpromazine, cimetidine, cyclosporin, desipramine, furosemide, haloperidol, meperidine, methadone, methyldopa, phenacemide, prochlorperazine, propoxyphene, rifampicin, thioridazine, tricyclic antidepressants, and verapamil.

Primidone (Mysoline)

Primidone is a barbiturate used for treatment of CPSs and other partial epilepsies (usually as a second choice after carbamazepine). It has also been used in place of phenobarbital for treatment of generalized tonic–clonic or focal seizures and epilepsies, when the latter drug has failed, but it should not be a drug of first choice for these conditions. Primidone is excreted in part unchanged and is in part metabolized to phenobarbital and to phenylethylmalonic acid (PEMA). Primidone and PEMA are cleared in hours, whereas phenobarbital persists for days. Serum levels of primidone and PEMA can be ascertained, but it often suffices just to confirm that a therapeutic steady-state level of phenobarbital is present. To benefit from the short-lived primidone and PEMA, each of which has some antiepileptic action, primidone must be given in three or four divided doses. A therapeutic dosage is usually around 250 mg orally three or four times a day, but the initial dosages should be much lower to avoid inducing extreme sedation. A test dose of 50 mg should be given to rule out a hypersomnolence reaction. If none occurs, then it is reasonable to start with 125 to 250 mg daily, with increments each week, until therapeutic effect, therapeutic levels, unacceptable sedation, or the maximal dosage of 2 g/day is reached. If patients are taking other antiepileptic drugs, it is better to start with a dosage of 100 to 125 mg/day. The dosage should be reduced by about half in patients with significant renal failure. Strengths available are 50- and 250-mg tablets and suspension.

Side effects of primidone parallel those of phenobarbital, except that primidone tends to be more sedating.

Ethosuximide (Zarontin)

Ethosuximide is the drug of choice for treatment of absence epilepsy in children (CAE) when there are concerns for potential hepatotoxicity from valproic acid. It is as effective as valproic acid in controlling absence seizures. It has little efficacy in other types of seizures, and patients with mixed seizure types may respond better to valproic acid. Peak plasma levels are reached 3 to 7 hours after oral ingestion in children and 2 to 4 hours after ingestion in adults. It is only minimally protein bound, with a volume of distribution of

70% of body weight; it has minimal interaction with other AEDs. The half-life is about 30 hours in children, rising to 60 hours in adults, taking 6 to 12 days, respectively, to reach steady state. Elimination is primarily by metabolism, with urinary excretion of the metabolites. Absence seizures appear to be controlled by blood levels of about 25 to 165 mg/L, and an average of about 60 mg/L. Levels of 150 mg/L may be needed and tolerated. Dose-related side effects include anxiety, depression, behavioral and psychiatric disturbances, nausea, vomiting, anorexia, fatigue, headache, lethargy, and dizziness. Liver function tests and complete blood counts are recommended monthly for 6 months and occasionally thereafter. Ethosuximide is supplied as syrup (250 mg/5 mL) and as capsules (250 mg).

Clonazepam (Klonopin)

Clonazepam is a benzodiazepine, closely related to diazepam, that is used principally for treatment of myoclonus. It is not approved for treatment of partial seizures but has been used effectively for these conditions in Europe. Clonazepam is an oral medicine, with a serum half-life of 20 to 40 hours. Serum levels vary from 0.05 to 0.7 mg/L and correlate only very roughly with clinical effect. Because of the sedative effect of the medicine, therapy is usually initiated very gradually, beginning with 0.01 to 0.15 mg/kg, increased each third day to clinical effect or to maintenance at 0.1 to 0.2 mg/kg per day. In adults the daily maximal dosage is 20 mg. Clonazepam commonly produces drowsiness, ataxia, and behavioral changes and can also cause dizziness and decreased muscle tone. Strengths available are 0.5-, 1-, and 2-mg tablets.

New Antiepileptic Drugs

After more than a decade without new antiepileptic drugs on the market, several new agents have become available in the United States. Experience with these medications has been gained predominantly in European and American trials. These drugs are likely to be recommended when a patient requires consultation for difficult-to-control epilepsy, but they are gaining popularity for use earlier in the treatment of epilepsy because of their *lower side effect profiles*. They are usually more expensive.

Felbamate (Felbatol)

Felbamate (FDA approved in 1993) is a new drug that has been tested as add-on therapy for drug-resistant CPSs with or without secondary generalization and in patients with Lennox–Gastaut syndrome in several European and American trials.

An oral dose has a half-life of about 20 hours as monotherapy, or 14 hours in patients receiving polypharmacy, and a volume of distribution of 0.8 L/kg.

Typical dosing regimens vary from 2400 to 3600 mg/day. Felbamate may increase phenytoin levels but decrease carbamazepine levels. Little effect has been noted on valproate levels.

Side effects include mild problems such as weight loss, nausea, blurred vision, diplopia, headache, and ataxia, as well as severe problems including aplastic anemia (31 reported cases, 10 deaths), and primary hepatotoxicity (liver failure reported in 19 patients with 8 deaths). At present the drug is largely restricted to use in patients with epilepsy that cannot be controlled by other AEDs, and in whom the morbidity from epilepsy is believed to outweigh the morbidity risk from felbamate.

γ-Vinyl-GABA (Vigabatrin, Sabril)

γ-Vinyl-GABA (not FDA approved as of March 1998) was specifically synthesized to act as an irreversible GABA-transaminase inhibitor, thus potentiating the accumulation of GABA. GABA is the major inhibitory neurotransmitter in the brain. Clinical trials show that one-third to two-thirds of patients have a 50% decrease in predominantly CPSs with or without secondary generalization when this agent is *added to* regimens of other AEDs. There is little evidence for an effect on absence seizures.

Taken orally, it is absorbed in 0.5 to 2 hours, has a half-life of 6 to 9 hours, has negligible protein binding and hepatic enzyme induction, is excreted by the kidneys, and has a volume of distribution of 0.8 L/kg. Concurrent use with phenytoin may decrease the levels of the latter.

Preliminary concern about microvascular changes in myelin in animal toxicology studies has not been borne out, and it is generally considered to be a safe drug. The most important side effects are behavioral changes and psychoses, which may occur in approximately 7% of patients. It may also cause sedation, fatigue, depression, confusion, GI upset, and, rarely, a rash. Hematologic depression occurs at very high dosages.

Gabapentin (Neurontin)

This GABA analog (FDA approved in 1994) was developed and used as an AED based on the GABAergic theory of epileptogenesis; however, it probably does not work via a GABAergic mechanism. Gabapentin is not protein bound, does not alter other antiepileptic drug levels, and is not metabolized. The half-life is 5 to 7 hours.

Clinical trials so far have been as *an add-on AED* in refractory partial epilepsies with or without secondary generalization. There are usually few if any side effects.

Lamotrigine (Lamictal)

Lamotrigine is structurally unrelated to any other AED in current use. Its antiepileptic action is probably related to its inhibitory effect on glutamate release and stabilization of neuronal membrane voltage-sensitive sodium channels.

It appears to be effective in patients with intractable CPSs with or without secondary generalization who are already taking other AEDs; patients with primary generalized tonic–clonic seizures, atypical absences, or nonconvulsive status epilepticus; and some patients with Lennox–Gastaut syndrome (see above).

The pharmacokinetics in normal human subjects

show complete bioavailability, a very long plasma half-life (24 ± 5 to 7 hours), linear kinetics, and approximately 60% protein binding.

Enzyme-inducing AEDs reduce its half-life; valproic acid increases it, sometimes twofold, but lamotrigine does not appear to alter other AED levels. The drug is well tolerated and side effects are few: Skin rashes, sometimes severe, but reversible, occur in 2 to 5% of patients. The incidence of skin rashes falls the more gradually the drug is started. Diplopia, dizziness, nausea and vomiting, drowsiness, and headache also occur in a small percentage. It may be used in women taking an oral contraceptive.

The drug may be started at 50 mg at night for 2 weeks, 50 mg twice daily for 2 weeks, then 100 mg twice daily, increasing in steps of 50 mg every 2 weeks until seizure control, clinical toxicity, or a maximum of 600 to 700 mg/day is encountered. In patients also taking valproic acid or valproate, lamotrigine should be started at 25 mg every other day, increasing by 25 mg every 2 weeks to so as minimize the incidence of rash. Lamotrigine serum levels do not clearly correlate with clinical response ("therapeutic level") but may be used as markers of patient compliance.

Oxcarbazepine

Oxcarbazepine is a 10-keto analog of carbamazepine and is active as a prodrug, having similar efficacy to carbamazepine. It is effective against partial seizures. It is not yet available in the United States.

Tiagabine (Gabitril)

Tiagabine was approved in late 1997 for adjunctive therapy in partial-onset seizures in adults and children 12 years and older. Tiagabine was specifically designed to inhibit the uptake of γ-aminobutyric acid and prolong its action after synaptic release. Clinical trials have shown it to be effective as an *add-on drug* for patients with intractable focal seizures; 26% of patients have a 50% or greater reduction in focal seizures (36). A reduction of 50% or more of complex partial seizures was seen in 20 to 30% of patients. Tiagabine should be started at 4 mg once daily and increased 4 mg the first week and 8 mg weekly thereafter to 32 to 56 mg/day. It should be taken with food, in divided doses (two to four times) with the largest dose at bedtime. Tablets are available in 4-, 12-, 16-, and 20-mg strengths. Side effects include dizziness, confusion, tiredness, and GI upset.

Topiramate (Topamax)

Topiramate was approved in early 1997 for use as *adjunctive therapy* in partial-onset seizures in adults. It probably has multiple mechanisms of action, including modulation of sodium channels, enhancing the effect of GABA and decreasing the excitability of brain cells. As of February 1997, more than 6000 patients had taken it, with a greater than 50% reduction in seizures in 35 to 44% patients on 400 mg/day. Topiramate has a T_{max} of about 2 hours, a bioavailability of approximately 80% unaffected by food, and little plasma

protein binding (13 to 17%). It has linear pharmacokinetics, is not extensively metabolized, and is predominantly excreted by the kidneys. It has limited pharmacokinetics interactions and its half-life makes it suitable for twice-daily dosing. Clinical studies show that it has no effect on carbamazepine but may increase phenytoin levels in some patients. The side effect profile is similar to those of most other AEDs and most are not serious. They occur in the first weeks of therapy and usually resolve by the fourth month in most patients. Side effects are predominantly CNS related, including dizziness, drowsiness, and problems with coordination. There is a 1.5% incidence of kidney stones. Oral contraceptive effectiveness may be affected. The medication is available in 25-, 100-, and 200-mg tablets. Therapy should be initiated at a dosage of 50 mg/day and gradually increased over several weeks to a recommended dosage of 200 mg to 400 mg/day in two divided doses.

Other Antiepileptic Drugs

No attempt has been made here to catalog all of the agents used as AEDs; only the major drugs of choice for the common types of seizures have been discussed. Ineffectiveness of the standard agents, when they have been applied in accordance with the general therapeutic principles given previously, is certainly an indication for specialty referral and for possible trials of the more unusual therapies. Practitioners often use diazepam, clorazepate, or chlordiazepoxide to treat seizures under certain circumstances. Benzodiazepines (other than clonazepam and clorazepate) have drawbacks for long-term therapy; AED effects tend to diminish as sedative effects accumulate.

REFERRAL TO A NEUROLOGIST

The role of a consulting neurologist to help with the evaluation and management of epilepsy depends on the experience of the primary physician. Common problems for which referral may be helpful are listed in Table 80.7.

HOSPITALIZATION

Few general statements can be made about the need for hospital admission for seizure patients because the availability of monitoring systems, emergency room holding rooms, and inpatient beds varies from locale to locale. A set of reasonable guidelines is shown in Table 80.7. Patients brought to offices or emergency rooms after a first seizure are usually admitted to facilitate the diagnostic workup and observe the patient in case a serious underlying cause (e.g., meningitis or subdural hematoma) is present. This principle has exceptions. A young patient with a normal examination and a reliable family may be evaluated in an ambulatory setting. Any patient with new focal signs on examination should be admitted, as should obtunded patients, febrile patients, or those whose postictal lethargy persists for over 30 minutes. A patient with a crescendo pattern of

Table 80.7.   When to Refer or Hospitalize the Patient with Seizures

Diagnostic Issues for Referral
Question about whether a seizure took place
Abnormal physical examination
Questionable focal neurologic findings
Focal seizures
Focality on the EEG
Need for special diagnostic investigations (e.g., lumbar puncture, CT or MRI scan)
Uncertainty about cause

Therapeutic Issues for Referral
Complex medication adjustments
Patient does not respond to a drug of choice
Patient has significant medication side effects
Patient wishes to become pregnant
Patient wishes to taper off medication
Significant change in the pattern of seizures

When to Hospitalize
Most new-onset seizures
New focal signs on examination
Obtunded or prolonged postictal patients
Febrile patients
Crescendo pattern of seizures
All cases of status epilepticus
Barbiturate and benzodiazepine withdrawal seizures
Possibility of rapidly expanding mass lesion
Seizures after recent head trauma
Need for special inpatient studies
Consideration for neurosurgery
Monitoring of compliance

seizures, with several in one day, especially if tonic–clonic, should be admitted to a hospital immediately. *Status epilepticus,* when continuous or back-to-back seizures occur without intervening return of consciousness, is a medical emergency and requires immediate hospitalization. Barbiturate withdrawal seizures may become fulminant; therefore, patients having seizures in this setting should be admitted. If the possibility exists of a rapidly expanding mass lesion, such as tumor, abscess, or possible hematoma after head trauma, then admission should not be delayed. Reasons for elective admissions include a need for special inpatient studies (arteriography, continuous monitoring), evaluation for possible neurosurgical procedures for intractable epilepsy, and, lastly, trials of supervised drug management to check for noncompliance as a factor in treatment failure.

Admission is usually not needed for patients who are known to have chronically recurrent seizures, whose pattern of seizures is stable, whose cause is established or is thought to be idiopathic on the basis of a prior thorough workup, who have fully recovered from recent seizures, who have normal examinations (or static documented old deficits), and who are reliable enough to return for follow-up.

SOCIAL ISSUES AND PATIENT EDUCATION

Once a serious underlying cause has been ruled out, there is a tendency for physicians to view epilepsy as a benign disease. From the viewpoint of the patient, this is often far from the case. Seizures are distressing for every patient and for the patient's family. Fear of having a seizure can cause people with epilepsy to withdraw from society, and those who are willing to compete may be faced with nearly insurmountable discrimination.

The Commission for the Control of Epilepsy and Its Consequences (1977) found that the unemployment rate among those with epilepsy is twice the national average, and the underemployment rate is even higher. Suspension of a driver's license (see below) may make it nearly impossible to get to work. Children may be denied participation in sports or moved unnecessarily to special sections in school. People with epilepsy marry less often than matched subjects. A significant fraction of the public believe that people with epilepsy are likely to be physically unattractive. Because of these and other social stigmata associated with epilepsy, it is important to focus on the patient's overall functioning rather than simply on seizure control. The patient and family should be counseled regularly to help them address the concerns that limit full participation in society.

Patients should be told that epilepsy is a medical illness because too many believe that it is a punishment for some past abuse. Whereas a single seizure should not be labeled as epilepsy, definite epilepsy should not be mislabeled as something else in an attempt to avoid facing the diagnosis. The patient should know that individual seizures do not cause measurable brain damage and that the condition does not lead to mental deterioration. Numerous historical figures, including Julius Caesar, Holy Roman Emperor Charles V, Fyodor Dostoyevsky, Gustave Flaubert, Napoleon Bonaparte, Jonathan Swift, George Frederick Handel, and President William McKinley, achieved high stations while suffering from frequent seizures. The prognosis for most patients with epilepsy is good.

Restrictions of Activity

Patients often ask for guidelines about what they can and cannot do. Clearly, if identifiable precipitants such as sleep deprivation, flashing lights, alcohol, or particular medicines can be avoided, the patient should be so advised. Maximal activity consistent with avoidance of risk of personal injury should be the goal. The specifics must be formulated by a physician familiar with the individual patient and the patient's pattern of seizures. Patients with nocturnal seizures need not be restricted during the day. Contact sports are safe for people with infrequent seizures. Common sense dictates limits on activities during which a seizure could be fatal—for example, piloting an airplane, rock climbing, or scuba diving. Some potentially hazardous activities, such as swimming, may be acceptable if provisions can be made for proper supervision. Seizures are not contraindications to strenuous activities, including sex. Alcohol consumption (in moderation) can be enjoyed by most with impunity (28).

Driving a Motor Vehicle

Overall, motor vehicle accident rates for people with epilepsy are about twice the rates in control subjects. The actual proportion of all traffic accidents caused by people with epilepsy has been estimated at 1/10,000 accidents (48). It is estimated that 6/10,000 of all deaths at the wheel are from natural causes, including epilepsy, and that 5,000/10,000 are caused by alcohol use. Approximately 12 to 20% of accidents involving people with epilepsy occur with the patient's first seizure. As indicated by these statistics, seizures at the wheel do occur and can represent both personal and public dangers. The key element of increased risk is blunting or loss of consciousness. Seizures without this element (e.g., partial simple motor seizures) do not affect the risk of driving, and affected patients are usually exempted from restrictions.

Some states require that physicians directly report occurrence of seizures to the Department of Motor Vehicles; others require only documentation in the medical record that the patient has been informed of the risks for traffic accidents and has been instructed to contact the Motor Vehicle Department for a hearing. Patients and physicians should be honest in their communications; both are potentially liable for consequences of inaccurate or incomplete information. In general, the physician should address the medical facts of a case and leave the final determination of licensing to the state authorities. Often, if an applicant has regular lapses of consciousness, the license will be suspended until a period of 3 months to 2 years without seizures has elapsed (depending on the state); the recent national trend has been to consider shorter periods of suspension.

Employment

It is illegal to discriminate against handicapped people, including people with epilepsy, in the job market. If a person with seizures is unemployed or dissatisfied with work, one should consider prompt referral to a vocational rehabilitation agency for possible retraining, patient and employer education, or advice on legal action. *The Epilepsy Foundation of America* (4351 Garden City Drive #406, Landover, MD 20785, telephone 301-459-3700) is a central nonprofit organization that can serve as a source for information and action on social and occupational aspects of epilepsy; at least one chapter exists in each state. Their training and placement service (TAPS) has been effective in training people with epilepsy for work and in finding them employment, either in the general work pool or in sheltered workshops. The same local organizations may further aid patients with regular group counseling for those who cannot live independently, or in providing for regular home visits by visiting nurses and other medical personnel.

Some patients with difficult-to-control seizures should be advised to apply for *medical disability under Social Security* (see criteria in Table 9.4).

Pregnancy

Special problems are raised by a woman with epilepsy who is, or wishes to become, pregnant (52). Approximately 0.4% of all pregnancies occur in mothers with seizures. In women with epilepsy, childbearing carries an above-average risk for eclampsia, vaginal hemorrhage, and complicated labor. The rate of premature births and perinatal deaths is elevated. Seizures become more difficult to control during pregnancy in approximately 30 to 50% of cases, easier to control in approximately 10 to 30%, and unchanged in the rest. Rarely, pregnancy can induce a new onset of recurring idiopathic seizures. AEDs—phenytoin, carbamazepine, valproic acid, and to a lesser extent all of the other agents—are believed to be *teratogenic.* The teratogenic effects of the newer AEDs are unknown. Studies suggest that the incidence of congenital abnormalities, particularly cleft lip, cleft palate, and cardiac defects, is two to six times higher in offspring of drug-treated mothers with epilepsy. Valproate has specifically been associated with a 1 to 2% risk of neural tube closure defects.

Unfortunately, no study has delineated the relative contributions of medication and of epilepsy itself to this increased incidence of congenital abnormalities. Authorities agree that tonic–clonic seizures can produce anoxic, ischemic, or traumatic damage to a fetus and that this risk must be balanced against the teratogenic potential of medication. The best solution to this dilemma is *careful planning.* Physicians should ask their patients not only to plan pregnancies but also to alert the physician to the plan months in advance. Before pregnancy, special efforts can be made to taper medications or to switch to phenobarbital or carbamazepine, which may be less teratogenic than phenytoin or valproate. However, most authorities agree that the AED to be used in pregnancy should be the one best suited for the patient and her epilepsy. Switching drugs after conception when the patient discovers that she is pregnant usually is not recommended, partly because the greatest vulnerability of the developing fetus is early in the pregnancy. Brief CPSs or absence seizures pose no known risk to a fetus, and a decision may be made by the patient to tolerate them during pregnancy rather than take medication. If pregnancy is unexpected, an ongoing successful regimen of AEDs should probably be continued, to avoid the possibility of fulminant withdrawal seizures during a critical obstetric stage. Ultimately, all of these relative risks must be discussed among primary and specialist physicians, patient, and husband, so that a mutually satisfactory plan can be derived. The problems of childbearing are increased for mothers with epilepsy, but not greatly, and only the severely disabled epileptic woman should be flatly discouraged from having children.

Mothers taking AEDs who wish to breast-feed may do so because the amount of AEDs excreted in breast milk is low.

Potential parents wonder about the *likelihood that their child will have epilepsy* if they or one of their children have epilepsy. Although there are methodologic problems in performing studies to answer this question, it can generally be said that there is a risk of about 1 in 40 of transmitting idiopathic generalized epilepsy from the mother. When seizures result from head trauma, tumor, drug withdrawal, or other identified causes, then the risk of heritability is not increased.

Family Education

Families must be told how to *behave during a seizure;* too often, frantic efforts to treat the seizure result in extreme anxiety and broken teeth. Seizures should be allowed to run their course; unless convulsions become nearly continuous (status epilepticus) they are not dangerous, and no first aid can shorten them. The mouth should not be forced open so that matchbooks, pencils, or other objects can be pushed in. The family should be informed that it is impossible to swallow the tongue. The person undergoing a seizure should be moved away from sharp corners and heights and turned on his or her side to decrease the risk of aspiration. Forcible restraint during a tonic–clonic phase is of no value, and during the automatisms of CPSs restraints may increase agitation. There is little need to fear behavior during automatisms, because directed violence is extremely rare.

Concerned family members may be very helpful in *promoting improved seizure control.* They should be encouraged to discuss compliance, the cost of a medicine regimen, and how the seizures or drug toxicities affect school, work, and social relations. Patients should be encouraged to keep a log of their seizures, medication times, side effects, and possible precipitating stresses. Perfect control of epilepsy with no toxicity is an ideal attained in only a minority of cases; in the remainder, patient, family, and physician can decide in concert how to balance the inconvenience of seizures against the unpleasant side effects of medication and thereby achieve the best possible results.

Medicolegal Issues

In addition to conducting discussions of the diagnosis, management, and prognosis of epilepsy, it is important to document in the patient's record the principal points that have been addressed with the patient and the family. One should ensure that patients have written information advising them of driving laws and warning them to avoid dangerous activities and occupations. They should also have full written records of medications and their side effects, in lay terms, and instructions to contact the physician for any worrisome side effects. In addition, all women of childbearing age should be counseled regarding fetal teratogenicity, possible change in maternal seizure frequency, and the need or lack of a need for AED therapy (see above). Many of these essential facts are covered well in patient education literature available from the Epilepsy Foundation of America (see address above).

Attention to these aspects of patient and family education in addition to a close, compassionate, and open doctor–patient relationship are sound ways to limit malpractice exposure.

General References*

Dam M, Gram M, ed. Comprehensive epileptology. New York: Raven Press, 1990.

French J. The long-term therapeutic management of epilepsy. Ann Intern Med 120:411, 1994.
   Review article based on literature 1964–1993.

Greenberg MK, Barsan WG, Starkman S. Neuroimaging in the emergency patient presenting with seizure. Neurology 47:26–32, 1996.

Hauser WA, ed. Current trends in epilepsy: a self-study course for physicians. Landover, MD: Epilepsy Foundation of America, 1988.

Kaplan PW, Loiseau P, Fisher RS, Jallon P. Epilepsy A to Z: a glossary of epilepsy terminology. New York: Demos Vermande, 1995.
   One- to two-page condensed information, with references, on most practical aspects of epilepsy.

Kaplan PW, Schachter SC. The role of neurologist in the management of epilepsy: guidelines and tools for patient care. Neurologist 2:302–314, 1996.
   Comprehensive approach to longitudinal care of epileptic patients with special attention to patient education.

Levy RH, Dreifuss FE, Mattson RH, et al, eds. Antiepileptic drugs. 4th ed. New York: Raven Press, 1995.
   A compendium of antiseizure medications.

Temkin O. The falling sickness: a history of epilepsy from the ancient Greeks to the beginnings of modern neurology. Baltimore: Johns Hopkins University Press, 1971.
   The definitive history of epilepsy from ancient to modern times.

Wyllie E, ed. The treatment of epilepsy. principles and practice. Baltimore: Williams & Wilkins, 1997.

Specific References

1. Aicardi J. Epilepsies as a presenting manifestation of brain tumors. In: Epilepsy in children. New York: Raven Press, 1986.
2. Alldredge BK, Lowenstein DH, Simon RP. Placebo-controlled trial of intravenous diphenylhydantoin for short-term treatment of alcohol withdrawal seizures. Am J Med 87:51, 1980.
3. Anderson DW, McLawsin RL. The national head and spinal cord injury survey. J Neurosurg 53:51, 1980.
4. Annegers JF, Hauser WA, Elveback LR. Remission of seizures and relapse in patients with epilepsy. Epilepsia 20:729, 1979.
5. Annegers JF, Shirts SB, Hauser WA, Kurland LT. Risk of recurrence after an initial unprovoked seizure. Epilepsia 27: 43–50, 1986.
6. Benbadis SR, L‚ders H. Epileptic syndromes: an underutilized concept. Epilepsia 37:1029–1034, 1996.
7. Callaghan N, Garrett A, Goggin T. Withdrawal of anticonvulsant drugs in patients free of seizures for two years: a prospective study. N Engl J Med 318(15):942, 1988.
8. Conlon P, Trimble MR, Rogers D, Callicott C. Magnetic resonance imaging in epilepsy: a controlled study. Epilepsy Res 2:37, 1988.
9. Delgado-Escueta AV. Epileptogenic paroxysms: modern approaches and clinical correlations. Neurology 29:1014, 1979.
10. Delgado-Escueta AV, Treiman DM, Wahs GO. The treatable epilepsies (second of two parts). N Engl J Med 308:15, 1983.
11. Dreifuss FE. Proposal for revised clinical and electroencephalographic classification of epileptic seizures. Epilepsia 22:489, 1981.
12. Dreifuss FE, Santilli N, Langer DJ, et al. Valproic acid hepatic fatalities: a retrospective review. Neurology 37(3):379, 1987.
13. Emerson R, D'Souza BJ, Vining EP, et al. Stopping medication in

---

*Bold print (general references) and bold numerals (specific references) denote published controlled clinical trials, meta-analyses, or consensus-based recommendations.

children with epilepsy: predictors of outcome. N Engl J Med 304:1125, 1981.

14. Engel JE Jr. Seizures and epilepsy. Philadelphia: FA Davis, 1989.

15. Bleck TP. Recurrence of tonic–clonic seizures after antiepileptic drugs. Neurology 43:478–483, 1993.

16. Gastaut H, Tassinari CA. Epilepsies. In: Remand A, ed. Handbook of EEG and clinical neurophysiology. Vol. 13, part A. Amsterdam: Elsevier, 1975.

17. Goodridge DMG, Shorvon SD. Epileptic seizures in a population of 6,000. BMJ 287:641, 1983.

18. Gram L, Bentsen KD, Parnas J, Flachs H. Controlled trials in epilepsy: a review. Epilepsia 23:491, 1982.

19. Gupta SR, Naheedy MH, Elias D, Rubino FA. Postinfarction seizures. A clinical study. Stroke 19:1477, 1988.

20. Hauser WA, Ng SKC, Brust JCM. Alcohol, seizures and epilepsy. Epilepsia 29(2):S66, 1988.

21. Hauser WA, Rich SS, Annegers YF, Anderson VE. Seizure recurrence after a first unprovoked seizure: an extended follow-up. Neurology 40:1163, 1990.

22. Hopkins A, Garman A, Clarke C. The first seizure in adult life. Value of clinical features, electroencephalography, and computerized tomographic scanning in prediction of seizure recurrence. Lancet 1:721–726, 1988.

23. Luhdorf K, Jensen LK, Plesner AM. Epilepsy in the elderly: etiology of seizures in elderly. Epilepsia 27:458, 1986.

24. Masland RL. Commission for the control of epilepsy. Neurology 28:861, 1978.

25. Mattson RH, Cramer JA, Collins JF, et al. Comparison of carbamazepine, phenobarbital, phenytoin, and primidone in partial and secondarily generalized tonic–clonic seizures. N Engl J Med 313:145, 1985.

26. Mattson RH, Cramer JA, Collins, JF et al. Prognosis for total control of complex partial and secondarily generalized tonic clonic seizures. Neurology 47:68–76, 1996.

27. Mattson RH, Cramer JA, Williamson PD, Novelly RA. Valproic acid in epilepsy: clinical and pharmacological effects. Ann Neurol 3:20, 1978.

28. Mattson RH, Sturman JK, Gronowski ML, Goici H. Effects of alcohol intake in non-alcoholic epileptics. Neurology 25:361, 1975.

29. McArthur JC. Neurologic manifestations of AIDS. Medicine (Baltimore) 66:407, 1987.

30. Meierkord H, Shorvon S, Lightman S, Trimble M. Comparison of the effects of frontal and temporal lobe partial seizures on prolactin levels. Arch Neurol 49:225, 1992.

31. MRC Antiepileptic Drug Withdrawal Study Group. Randomised study of antiepileptic drug withdrawal in patients in remission. Lancet 337:1175–1180, 1991.

32. Morris HH, Estes ML, Gilmore R, Van Ness PC, et al. Chronic intractable epilepsy as the only symptom of primary brain tumor. Epilepsia 34:1038–1043, 1993.

33. Ng SK, Hauser WA, Brust JC, Susser M. Alcohol consumption and withdrawal in new-onset seizures. N Engl J Med 319:666, 1988.

34. Oribe E, Rohullah A, Nissenbaum E, Boal B. Serum prolactin concentrations are elevated after syncope. Neurology 47:60–62, 1996.

35. Reynolds EH, Elwes RCD, Shorvon SD. Why does epilepsy become intractable: prevention of chronic epilepsy. Lancet 2:952, 1983.

36. Richens A, Chadwick DW, Duncan JS, et al. Adjunctive treatment of partial seizures with Tiagabine; a placebo-controlled trial. Epilepsia Res 21:37–42, 1995.

37. Sampliner R, Iber FL. Diphenylhydantoin control of alcohol withdrawal seizures: results of a controlled study. JAMA 230:1430, 1974.

38. Sander JWAS, Shorvon SD. Epidemiology of the epilepsies. J Neurol Neurosurg Psychiatry 61:433–443, 1996.

39. Schmidley JW, Simon RP. Postictal pleocytosis. Ann Neurol 9:81, 1981.

40. Schmidt D. Prognosis of chronic epilepsy with complex partial seizures. J Neurol Neurosurg Psychiatry 47:12, 1984.

41. Schold C, Yarnell PR, Earnest MP. Origin of seizures in elderly patients. JAMA 238:1177, 1977.

42. Shorvon SD. The temporal aspects and prognosis in epilepsy. J Neurol Neurosurg Psychiatry 4:1157, 1984.

43. Shorvon SD, Chadwick D, Galbraith AW, Reynolds EH. One drug for epilepsy. BMJ 1:474, 1978.

44. Sung CY, Chu NS. Epileptic seizures in thrombotic stroke. J Neurol 237:166, 1990.

45. Tinuper P, Avoni P, Riva R, et al. The prognostic value of the electroencephalogram in antiepileptic drug withdrawal in partial epilepsies. Neurology 47:76–78, 1996.

46. Treiman DM. Efficacy and safety of antiepileptic drugs: a review of controlled trials. Epilepsia 28(3):S1, 1987.

47. Treiman DM. Seizure types and causes of epilepsy. Semin Neurol 1:65, 1981.

48. van der Lugt PJ. Traffic accidents caused by epilepsy. Epilepsia 16:747, 1975.

49. van Donselaar CA, Schimsheimer R-J, Geerts AT, Declerck AC. Value of the electroencephalogram in adult patients with untreated idiopathic first seizures. Arch Neurol 49:231, 1991.

50. Victor M, Brausch V. The role of abstinence in the genesis of alcoholic epilepsy. Epilepsia 8:1, 1967.

51. Wyllie E, Luders H, MacMillan JP, Gupta M. Serum prolactin levels after epileptic seizures. Neurology 34:1601, 1984.

52. Yerby MS. Problems and management of the pregnant woman with epilepsy. Epilepsia 3(28):S29, 1987.

C H A P T E R   81

Dizziness, Vertigo, Motion Sickness, Syncope and Near Syncope, and Disequilibrium

STEPHEN D. SISSON, MD
PHILLIP D. KRAMER, MD

DIZZINESS

Dizziness is the ninth most common chief complaint in ambulatory settings (29). However, the word *dizzy* is a very inexact term. It can mean uncertainty of one's position or motion in relation to the environment or spatial disorientation. Sometimes patients are referring to fatigue, dysphoric mood, lightheadedness, ataxia, disequilibrium, or other subjective states. Hispanic patients often use the word *dizzy* to mean sick. A correct diagnosis is often possible on the basis of the history and physical examination. A limited number of diagnostic studies can aid the evaluation of selected patients, but these can be in-terpreted properly only in the light of information gained from the patient.

Categorizing a Patient's Dizziness

Evaluation of the dizzy patient starts with categorizing the patient's symptoms. Categorization of symptoms usually can determine the involved system and give focus to the differential diagnosis. The major categories of dizziness are *vertigo,* the illusion that the patient or the environment is moving or rotating; *near syncope or syncope,* a sensation of impending faint or actual loss of consciousness; and *disequilibrium,* a sensation of impaired balance or ataxia (46). When patients have ill-defined dizziness that cannot be readily classified, the patient should be asked to *use words more specific than dizziness,* and should be asked to *describe a discrete recent episode.* Typical words they may use and potential categories are listed in Table 81.1. If the patient's brief account is too vague, the following questions may help:

- Is there actually the sensation of movement or rotation of you or the environment? (Positive response favors vertigo.)
- Is it a sensation that you might black out? (Positive response favors near syncope.)
- Is it a sensation of unsteadiness on your feet? A sensation that you are not sure where your hand or body is and that you cannot quite keep your balance? (Positive response favors disequilibrium.)

Questions about associated auditory, neurologic, or cardiac symptoms may help classify the patient's problem more specifically.

The patient who claims to be dizzy "right now" while sitting before the physician should be checked for hypotension, first while seated, then standing; observed for hyperventilation (slow, hyperpneic breathing, not overt tachypnea); and examined for nystagmus (see below).

A patient who produces dizziness by turning his or her head should be asked to elaborate on the symptoms; vertigo (positional) and near syncope (caused by compromise of cerebral blood flow) are the two problems most likely to be described.

In some cases, *asking whether the patient can reproduce the symptoms* may be more efficient than exhaustive questioning. If the patient reports typical dizziness on rising from a chair, orthostatic hypotension (or possibly benign paroxysmal positional vertigo) is likely; hypotension can be confirmed by measuring supine and standing blood pressure. If the patient demonstrates gait ataxia (see Chapter 78) or reports dizziness on turning while walking (as opposed to turning their head while sitting), the problem may be disequilibrium rather than vertigo.

As part of the preliminary inquiry, it is important to ask the patient whether dizziness has interfered with usual activities, especially driving a motor vehicle. This information will be important in management regardless of the cause of dizziness.

Table 81.1. Potential Categorization of Terms Used by Patients to Describe Dizziness

Vertigo	Syncope or Presyncope	Disequilibrium
Spinning of self	Fainting	Imbalance
Spinning of environment	Light-headedness	Tilting
Swaying	Woozy	Poor equilibrium
Twisting	Blackout	Impeding fall
Moving	Pass out	Unsteady
Weaving		Staggering
Rocking		Drunk
Rolling		Listing
Tilting		

VERTIGO

Vertigo is an illusion of movement and may be described either as a sensation as if the external world were turning around the patient or as if the patient were turning in place. This sensation is similar to that experienced after being on a merry-go-round or after spinning in place for several seconds.

It has been estimated that half of the patients who visit physicians for dizziness have vertigo (28). For most of these patients, vertigo is caused by conditions affecting labyrinthine structures or the vestibular nerve *(peripheral vertigo)* (see Chapter 96, Fig. 96.1). Although these conditions may be distressing and disabling, they usually are self-limited (43). In about one-fifth of these patients (28), vertigo is a manifestation of progressive disease of the central nervous system *(central vertigo)* or is a secondary manifestation of a *systemic condition.* The major causes of vertigo in these three categories are listed in Table 81.2.

Evaluation of the Undiagnosed Patient

A systematic approach to the history and physical examination should be used for all patients with vertigo. Even when a working diagnosis of a self-limited peripheral vertigo is made, follow-up is needed for confirmation because there is overlap in the symptoms and signs produced by peripheral and central vertigo.

History

Several questions about the quality of the vertigo are useful for differentiating between diseases. *Ten of the most useful questions* are outlined in Table 81.3. *Additional questions are*

- How often do symptoms occur?
- Are symptoms brought on by noise (Tulio's phenomenon)?
- Are symptoms brought on by stress?
- Is there anything that makes symptoms better or worse?
- Does the patient tend to fall, and to which side? (Patients tend to fall in the direction of the canal with the lower function.)
- Are symptoms severe, moderate, or mild? Is there

associated nausea or vomiting? (Peripheral lesions often have more severe vertigo.)
- Is there an associated sensation of tilt or linear movement? (This suggests a lesion of the otolith.)

Because the peripheral vestibular structures are so closely associated with *peripheral auditory structures,* there are often corresponding hearing changes. This is especially true of Ménière's disease.

Associated Auditory Symptoms

- Is hearing impaired in one or both ears?
- Is tinnitus present (pulsatile or constant)?
- Is there a history of ear infections or draining ears?
- Is there a sensation of aural pressure?
- Is there a history of head or neck trauma, recent barotrauma, or recent viral illness?
- Has the patient been exposed to any ototoxic drugs (e.g., aspirin, aminoglycoside, high dosage of a loop diuretic)?

Associated *neurologic symptoms* suggesting central (C) or peripheral (P) causes

- Is there diplopia? (C)
- Is there numbness of face or extremities? (C)
- Is there weakness in arms or legs? (C)

Table 81.2. Major Causes of Vertigo

Peripheral Causes of Vertigo
Benign positional vertigo
Posttraumatic vertigo
Peripheral vestibulopathy (labyrinthitis, vestibular neuronitis)
Vestibulotoxic drug-induced vertigo (aminoglycosides)
Ménière's syndrome (endolymphatic hydrops)
Inflammatory labyrinthitis (syphilis, vasculitis)
Other focal peripheral disease (acute and chronic otitis media, cholesteatoma, tumor, fistula, genetic anomalies, rarely focal ischemia and others)

Central Causes of Vertigo
Migraine
Brainstem ischemia and infarction
Cerebellopontine angle tumor (e.g., acoustic neurinoma, meningioma, metastatic tumor)
Demyelinating disease (multiple sclerosis, postinfectious demyelination, remote effect of carcinoma)
Cranial neuropathy with focal involvement of eighth nerve
Intrinsic brainstem lesions (tumor, arteriovenous malformation, trauma)
Other posterior fossa lesions (primarily intrinsic or extra-axial masses of the posterior fossa, such as meatoma, metastatic tumor, and cerebellar infarction)
Seizure disorder (temporal lobe epilepsy)
Heredofamilial disorders (spinocerebellar degenerations: Friedreich's ataxia, olivopontocerebellar atrophy, etc.)

Systemic Causes of Vertigo and Dizziness
Drugs (anticonvulsants, hypnotics, antihypertensives, alcohol, analgesics, tranquilizers)
Infectious disease (meningitis and systemic infection)
Endocrine disease (diabetes mellitus and hypothyroidism particularly)
Vasculitis (systemic lupus erythematosus, giant cell arteritis, and drug-induced vasculitis)
Other systemic conditions (erythrocytosis, anemia, dysproteinemia, Paget's disease of the bone, sarcoidosis, granulomatous disease, and systemic toxins)

Adapted from Troost BT. Dizziness and vertigo in vertebrobasilar disease. Curr Concepts Cerebrovasc Dis 14:21, 1979.

Table 81.3.   Questions Useful in the Differential Diagnosis of Vertigo

Question Content	BPPV	H/A	EH	Labyr	CVA	TIA	Fistula	AN	MVC
Sudden onset	+++		a	++	+++	+++	+++	+	+++
Gradual onset		+++	++	+				+	
Constant		b		c	c			+	
Episodic	+++	+++	+++			+++	+++	+	+++
Duration	<1 min	30 minutes–days	30 minutes–hours	Days	Days	2–5 minutes	Seconds	Seconds	Seconds–minutes
Caused by head movement with respect to gravity	+++							+	++
Caused by valsalva, cough, laugh, straining, air travel	d	+					+++		+
Tinnitus or ear pressure associated with the vertigo			+++				+	+	+
A single or very few major episodes				+++	+++				
Multiple episodes	+++	++	++			e	+++	+	+++

BPPV, Benign paroxysmal positional vertigo; *H/A*, migraine; *EH*, endolymphatic hydrops (Ménière's); *Labyr*, labyrinthitis/vestibular neuritis; *CVA*, stroke; *TIA*, transient ischemic attack; *AN*, acoustic neuroma; *MVC*, microvascular compression; *+*, may occur; *++*, common; *+++*, less common.

[a]A form of Ménière's disease, otolithic crisis of Tumarkin, has extremely sudden onset.

[b]Vestibular migraine can present as a constant vague dizziness as well as an episodic vertigo.

[c]A stroke and labyrinthitis usually produce a constant vertigo that improves over days to weeks.

[d]Only if caused by a corresponding head movement.

[e]A very large number of TIAs without a complete stroke is unlikely.

- Is there clumsiness in the arms or legs? (C)
- Is there confusion or loss of consciousness? (C)
- Is there slurring of speech? (C)
- Is there difficulty with swallowing? (C)
- Is there blurring of vision? (C or P)
- Are there flashing lights? (P)
- Is there an associated headache? (C or P)

Examination

Examination includes inspection of external auditory canal and tympanic membrane (see Chapter 96), simple office assessment for hearing impairment (see Chapter 96), observation for spontaneous nystagmus (see below), tests for positional vertigo and nystagmus (see below), evaluation of the vestibulo-ocular reflex (VOR) (see below), and selective neurologic and neurovascular examination (cranial nerves, particularly V and VII; cerebellar, gait, Romberg; and motor testing—see Chapter 78 for recommended brief neurologic and neurovascular examination).

Evaluation of Nystagmus

Nystagmus is an involuntary rhythmic movement of the eyes and is almost always present with vertigo. (Vertigo caused by a cortical lesion can theoretically occur without nystagmus.) *Jerk nystagmus* (having a slow and a quick component) is typically a sign of vestibular disease. Every patient complaining of vertigo should be checked for this type of nystagmus. It is important to know how to recognize and test for jerk nystagmus because it may be the only objective indicator of vestibular dysfunction. Jerk nystagmus is most easily understood and remembered when one understands the *vestibulo-ocular reflex*.

The Vestibulo-Ocular Reflex. The purpose of the vestibulo-ocular reflex (VOR) is to keep the image of an object stationary on the retina despite head movement so as to maintain clear vision. This can be demonstrated by comparing the ability to read a page held at arm's length and moved quickly back and forth from left to right to holding it at arms length and rotating one's head left and right. In the later case the VOR uses information from the semicircular canals to detect rotational movements of the head and generate appropriate compensatory eye movements. All reflex arcs between the vestibular sensory structures and the central nervous system (CNS) use the vestibular branch of the eighth cranial nerve and the four vestibular nuclei of the brainstem.

When the head is stationary the hair cells of the semicircular canals fire at a tonic rate. When the head is rotated toward a canal the hair cells of that canal increase their firing rate. Conversely, when the head is rotated away from a canal, the hair cells of that canal decrease their firing rate. When the head is rotated in any direction, to keep the eyes pointed at an object, the eyes must move in the opposite direction. Whenever there is an imbalance in the firing rates received by the vestibular nuclei, the CNS commands eye movements away from the side with the higher firing rate.

These principles are most easily understood with a physiologic example: horizontal head movements. Head motion to the right increases the firing rate of the hair cells of the right horizontal canal and decreases the firing rate of the hair cells of the left horizontal canal, resulting in a slow-phase eye movement to the left.

Impairment of the normal VOR can be caused by a lesion that causes canal hyperactivity or canal hypoactivity or interferes with transmission along the eighth nerve. Thus peripheral lesions can cause inappropriate eye movements that are the slow phases of jerk nystagmus. The slow phase of jerk nystagmus is the pathologic phase. The fast phase is a correction. Because it is easier to see, the direction of the fast phase is used to describe the nystagmus (e.g., left horizontal for a leftward fast phase and a rightward slow phase).

Localization of the Lesion (Central Versus Peripheral). In patients with peripheral or central vestibular dysfunction, nystagmus may be present with the eyes in midposition and the head upright *(spontaneous nystagmus)*. The nystagmus may be detected even when the patient is not experiencing vertigo. During an episode of vertigo, there should usually be accompanying nystagmus if the vertigo is caused by organic disease. Spontaneous nystagmus that is caused by a peripheral lesion typically increases in amplitude with gaze in the direction of the quick phase, and decreases or reverses with gaze in the opposite direction (Alexander's law) (38). *Visual fixation tends to suppress the spontaneous nystagmus of peripheral vestibular disease.* Therefore, if spontaneous nystagmus is not observed, the patient should close his or her eyes (to eliminate visual fixation) and be observed for nystagmus through the eyelids. Preferably, the patient can be examined with eyes open through Frenzel lenses (special 10-diopter lenses that distort the patient's view, making fixation impossible). Fixation also can be eliminated by viewing the optic fundus of one eye with an ophthalmoscope while covering the other eye. Nystagmoid movements of the optic disc may be visualized with this method. Because the back of the eye is being viewed, the direction of horizontal and vertical nystagmus will appear to be opposite its true direction. If spontaneous nystagmus is present with the eyes open, the patient should be asked to fixate on a nearby object; suppression of nystagmus with fixation favors peripheral vestibular disease, whereas persistence or enhancement of the nystagmus is typical of central disease. It should be noted, however, that nystagmus caused by peripheral disease may not be suppressed with fixation until 24 hours after onset of the disease. Features that distinguish peripheral from central spontaneous nystagmus are summarized in Table 81.4.

Gaze-evoked nystagmus (GEN) is elicited when the eyes are held eccentrically in the orbit, and consists of slow phases directed toward the center, followed by quick phases in the direction of gaze. GEN is most often caused by drugs, such as phenytoin and diazepam, but may also occur with brainstem and cerebellar lesions.

When nystagmus is *pendular* (to and fro movements about equal in amplitude and speed), it is inevitably caused by disturbance of the CNS.

Positioning nystagmus (and vertigo) is produced by a sudden change in head position. The patient with positional vertigo usually gives a history of symptoms brought on by lying back in bed, turning the head while lying, arising from bed, bending over, or looking upward, but not when the head is stationary. The purposes of provocative testing are to replicate the patient's symptoms, elicit positioning nystagmus, and determine whether the nystagmus is fatigable.

The Dix–Hallpike maneuver (also called the *Bárány maneuver*), used to detect positional vertigo, is illustrated in Figure 81.1. The patient sits close enough to one end of the examining table so that the head would be over the edge if the patient were lying down. The patient is asked to keep the eyes open during the maneuver and to report any sensations (e.g., vertigo, nausea) that are experienced. Frenzel lenses are used, if available, to prevent suppression of the nystagmus. The patient's head is turned 45° to one side. Then, while the examiner supports the head and shoulders, the patient is quickly brought to a reclining position with the head still rotated to one side and hanging over the end of the table. This position should be maintained for 30 seconds and the examiner should observe the patient's eyes for nystagmus. If nystagmus appears, the examiner should note its time of onset (relative to the start of the maneuver), the direction of eye motion (left, right, up, down, rotatory [CW or CCW], or mixed), the nature of associated symptoms, the adaptability of nystagmus (does it disappear despite maintaining the same head position?), and its fatigability on repeated testing. The maneuver should then be repeated with the head turned in the opposite direction. In particular, if nystagmus is present in one position, one should note any change in its direction or amplitude when tested in the opposite direction.

Features that distinguish benign positional vertigo, the most common cause of peripheral nystagmus, from central positional nystagmus are summarized in Table 81.5.

With *bilateral labyrinthine damage,* which is often a result of ototoxic drugs (see below), patients usually do not complain of vertigo, and they often do not have nystagmus. They usually have disequilibrium that worsens with the eyes closed (positive Romberg sign).

Evaluation of the VOR. When normal VOR function is lost, images move across the retina when the head moves and this leads to symptoms of visual blurring and image movement (2). When it is indicated to make a clinical decision, assessment of the VOR at the bedside can be done with the following three maneuvers:

- *Dynamic visual acuity.* Measure the patient's visual acuity with the head still and during passive horizontal and vertical head oscillation. In normal subjects, acuity decreases by at most one line on the Snellen chart when the head is oscillated (30).

Table 81.4.   Features of Spontaneous Nystagmus, According to Anatomic Location of the Cause

Feature	Peripheral	Central
Direction	Usually horizontal–rotatory Never purely vertical	Any direction May be purely vertical
Direction of fast component	Away from side with disease	Toward side with disease (or direction changing)
Effect of visual fixation	Suppressed	Not suppressed
Usual anatomic location of problem	Labyrinth or vestibular nerve	Brainstem or cerebellum

- *Head thrust.* Rapidly rotating the patient's head 20° to 30° while the eyes fixate on the examiner's nose (the eyes should remain still in space). A rapid corrective eye movement (saccade) after the head thrust indicates an abnormal VOR (17). The maneuver should be performed in all six directions (left, right, up, down, CW, or CCW).
- *Head shaking nystagmus.* With the patient wearing Frenzel lenses the head is oscillated horizontally (in a head shaking "no" fashion) at approximately 2 Hz. The head is then stopped and the eyes observed for nystagmus with the fast phase beating away from the side of a hypoactive lesion.

Laboratory Tests

If no clear cause of vertigo is identified from the initial history and physical examination, certain laboratory tests should be considered. Because syphilitic labyrinthitis and hypothyroidism can cause peripheral vertigo, a serologic test for syphilis (FTA-ABS, because nontrepoemal tests may be negative in tertiary syphilis; see Chapter 30) and a thyroid-stimulating hormone (TSH) level should be obtained on patients with peripheral vertigo. In addition, hematocrit and fasting

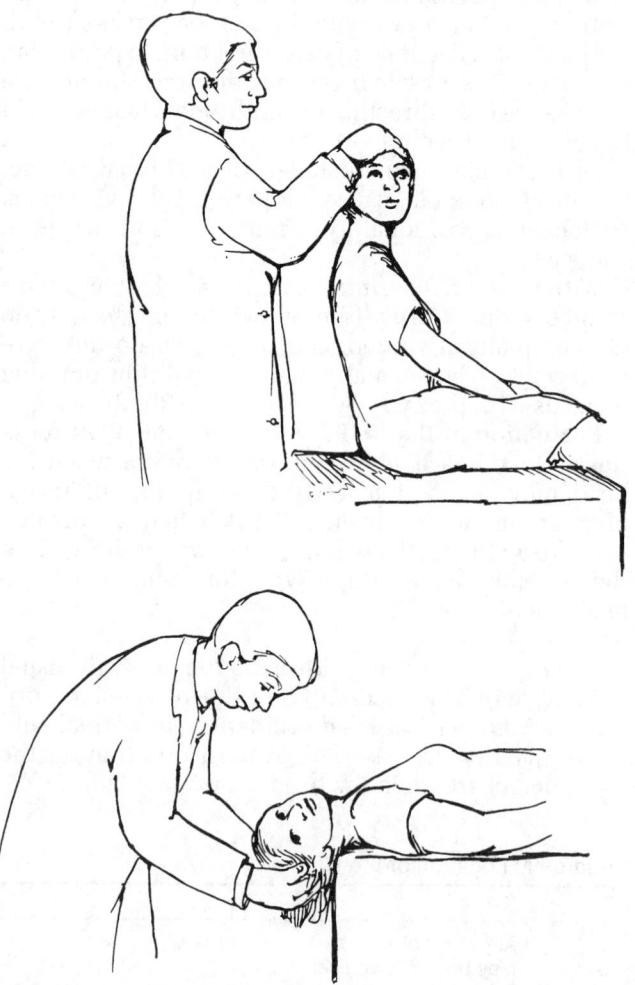

Figure 81.1. Bárány maneuver for testing a patient for positional vertigo and nystagmus.

blood glucose levels should be ordered to check for anemia and diabetes mellitus. Autoimmune disease can be screened for with an antinuclear antibody and erythrocyte sedimentation rate can screen for vasculitis. There are no other routinely indicated screening tests in the initial office evaluation of vertigo. Several tests of vestibular and audiologic function may be used by a consulting otolaryngologist (see below).

Most of the systemic causes of vertigo listed in Table 81.2 present with other symptoms. Rarely, vertigo and decreased hearing may be the only symptoms described by a hypothyroid patient. If there is a neuropathy on examination, vitamin B_{12} and E levels should be checked.

Peripheral Causes of Vertigo

Benign Paroxysmal Positional Vertigo

Benign paroxysmal positional vertigo (BPPV) is the most common cause of vertigo in adult patients (1,28). It occurs at all ages but is most common after the fourth decade and in persons with recent head trauma. BPPV results from pathology in the posterior semicircular canal approximately 95% of the time but can occur in any canal. It is usually caused by inappropriate activation of the canal by calcium carbonate particles, which are normally found in the macula of the utricle and saccule.

Vertigo is noted when the patient lies down, gets up from a recumbent position, rolls over in bed, looks up while standing, or bends forward. The episodes of vertigo always last less than 1 minute and are brought on only with a *change in head position relative to gravity.* If the vertigo is related to trauma (see below), it may begin immediately after the trauma or days to weeks later. Typically, patients with BPPV do not complain of tinnitus or hearing impairment. However, they may have nausea or vomiting during episodes of vertigo. Between episodes patients may be slightly unsteady.

On examination, spontaneous nystagmus (see above) is not present. A positive Dix–Hallpike (Bárány) test (Table 81.5 and Fig. 81.1) with the absence of other otologic or neurologic findings supports the diagnosis of BPPV. The key finding on examination that allows one to distinguish BPPV from other types of positional vertigo is the direction of the nystagmus. As shown in Figure 81.2, patients with BPPV demonstrate nystagmus with quick phases directed upward and torsionally toward the abnormal ear (i.e., counterclockwise as viewed by the examiner when the right ear is abnormal and clockwise when the left ear is abnormal) (1). In the Dix–Hallpike maneuver, this is elicited by turning the abnormal ear down.

BPPV is usually self-limited to about 2 weeks; however, symptoms may persist for months or years, and episodes recur in 20% of patients. Because positional vertigo is observed in conditions other than BPPV (Table 81.3), it is important to reevaluate the patient serially, following the systematic approach used initially and looking for ancillary evidence for one of the other causes of vertigo listed in Table 81.2. Any patient

Table 81.5. Features of Positional Nystagmus Elicited by the Bárány Maneuver

Feature	Peripheral (BPV)	Central
Time to onset after quick position change (latency)	3–20 seconds	Immediate
Duration	Less than 1 minute (often only a few seconds)	Persists longer than 1 min
Fatigability	Marked (may not be present on immediate repetition)	None
Subjective vertigo	Often marked	Often minimal or absent
Nystagmus direction	Upward and torsional toward abnormal ear	Changing with change in head position

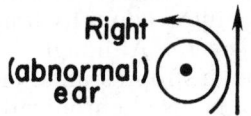 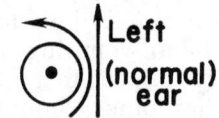

Figure 81.2. Pathognomonic nystagmus of BPPV. The pathognomonic nystagmus consists of quick phases directed upward (with respect to the head), and torsionally toward the abnormal ear. In this example, the torsional element is counterclockwise toward the abnormal right ear.

whose course is atypical should be seen in consultation by an otolaryngologist or a neurologist.

Treatment. If BPPV persists or recurs, two specific maneuvers can be used to treat it (symptomatic treatment with drugs is described below): *Positional exercises* (Brant–Daroff) often lead to a remission of BPPV within 2 weeks. The patient is instructed to sit at the edge of a bed, and then to lie down quickly on one side with the symptomatic ear down (6). After the vertigo resolves, the patient sits up. This exercise is repeated multiple times until symptoms are no longer elicited. The exercises should be performed three times a day until the patient has two consecutive days without vertigo. The *canal repositioning (Epley) maneuver* is a physical maneuver that can be performed in the office and is very effective (15). It usually eliminates the patient's symptoms after being performed once. This therapy requires the expertise of an otolaryngologist.

It is common for BPPV to coexist with Ménière's disease. Rarely, an acoustic neuroma (see below) can mimic BPPV. Therefore if BPPV is refractory to treatment, a contrast-enhanced MRI of the head should be obtained.

People with BPPV who work at heights (e.g., builders, roofers) may have to curtail these activities until the symptoms have abated.

Posttraumatic Vertigo

Vertigo is common after both blunt head trauma and whiplash (flexion–extension) injury to the neck (19). The basis for the vertigo may be dislocation of particles in the macula (leading to BPPV), damage to the membranous labyrinth, hemorrhage into the endolymph or eighth nerve, fracture of the bony labyrinth (leading to a perilymph fistula), or fracture of the temporal bone with resulting damage to the eighth nerve. Clinically, it may be impossible to determine which of these mechanisms is responsible for a patient's symptoms. However, typical patterns may suggest the dominant problem.

The first pattern is *immediate posttraumatic vertigo,* with associated spontaneous nystagmus (beating away from the side of injury), nausea and vomiting, and conductive or sensorineural hearing loss. This pattern suggests temporal bone fracture and is typical of moderately severe trauma to the temporal bone or occiput. A history of brief unconsciousness, the presence of Battle's sign (postauricular ecchymosis), and bleeding in the external auditory canal are other findings that suggest this diagnosis. Computerized tomographic scanning of the temporal bone is needed to detect the fracture. Because there is the possibility of finding surgically correctable damage, these patients should always be evaluated immediately by an otolaryngologist. Based on this evaluation, an exploratory tympanotomy may be recommended. These patients must be carefully examined for facial nerve paralysis also. In general, immediate palsy requires immediate decompression, whereas delayed palsy may be followed conservatively, as in Bell's palsy (see Chapter 84). A perilymph fistula (see below) can be caused by head trauma.

In most patients with immediate nonspecific posttraumatic vertigo, the vestibular symptoms improve rapidly over the first few days and are gone entirely within 6 to 12 weeks. Symptomatic treatment (see below) may be helpful.

Another common pattern is that of *delayed onset* (latent period of days to weeks) of posttraumatic positional vertigo, which presents with the characteristics of BPPV. This pattern is more typical of minor head injury, whiplash, or even high-impact aerobics. The course and management of posttraumatic positional vertigo are identical to those of BPPV. Ménière's syndrome (see below) may also result from head trauma, and typically presents with spontaneous episodes of vertigo and audiologic symptoms that may begin weeks or months after the trauma.

Some patients with posttraumatic vertigo may have a *combination of the features of immediate and delayed-onset vertigo.* After systematic examination, these patients should be treated symptomatically (see below) because it is likely that their vertigo will be self-limited.

Trauma, especially when there is a loss of consciousness, can result in a postconcussive syndrome that includes *migrainelike phenomenon* or a vaguely described dizziness. It is usually treated in manner similar to migraine (see Chapter 79).

Perilymph Fistula

Perilymph fistula can be the sequela of head trauma or barotrauma (air travel with a head cold or sneezing while holding one's nose). It typically presents with episodes of vertigo and hearing loss precipitated or exacerbated by Valsalva maneuvers (e.g., coughing) or by changes in barometric pressure (e.g., air travel). If vertigo and nystagmus can be provoked by a Valsalva maneuver (straining against a closed glottis) or by altering the pressure in the middle ear (by compressing the tragus against the external auditory canal), a fistula is the probable diagnosis. The majority of fistulas heal spontaneously, but surgical intervention may be necessary for intractable cases (42).

Peripheral Vestibulopathy (Acute Viral Labyrinthitis and Vestibular Neuronitis)

The collective term *peripheral vestibulopathy* has been used for a number of benign conditions for which the pathologic basis is chiefly conjectural. Because these conditions often follow viral upper respiratory or gastrointestinal infections, they are thought to be caused by inflammation of the vestibular end organ (labyrinthitis) or the vestibular nerve (neuronitis). They are most common in the third to the fifth decade but may occur at any age. Occasionally, a cluster of cases occurs *(epidemic vertigo)*. The working diagnosis of peripheral vestibulopathy is based on typical clinical features that are not pathognomonic; therefore, consideration of one of the progressive causes of central vertigo listed in Table 81.2 must be kept in mind in follow-up.

Typically, there is a sudden onset of moderate to severe *spontaneous vertigo*. Often there is accompanying nausea and vomiting, and symptoms are made worse by any change in position. The initial symptoms usually persist for several days, when they may be incapacitating. There is generally no complaint of hearing loss or tinnitus with vestibular neuronitis, but these symptoms are commonly present with labyrinthitis. There may be a tendency for the patient to fall when trying to walk.

On examination, *spontaneous nystagmus with peripheral features* (Table 81.4) is present. This is an important feature differentiating peripheral vestibulopathy from BPPV in which spontaneous nystagmus is not present. Because involvement is usually unilateral, there may be a typical nystagmus pattern in which the fast component is away from the side of the lesion when the patient is asked to look away from the lesion and the nystagmus may lessen or cease when the patient looks toward the side of the lesion. Caloric testing after recovery from the acute episode (see below) shows an absent or decreased response on the affected side, but this test is not needed routinely.

The vertigo of peripheral vestibulopathy *usually resolves within 6 weeks,* although nystagmus may be demonstrated for several months, especially if electronystagmography (ENG) is performed (see below). In occasional patients, the vertigo may also persist for more than 6 weeks. Such patients should be systematically reexamined for evidence of a central cause of vertigo, particularly acoustic neuroma and brainstem or inferior cerebellar infarction (see below).

There is no specific treatment. Patients should be told that the worst symptoms will last only a few days, that all symptoms usually resolve within 4 to 6 weeks, and that they should adjust their usual activities according to how they feel (during the first few days, many patients require strict bed rest for symptomatic relief). Antivertigo drugs may be helpful (see below). Clonazepam (Klonopin) 0.25 to 0.5 mg two or three times a day may also be useful in patients with peripheral vestibulopathy. An occasional patient may require hospital admission for intravenous hydration if nausea and vomiting are severe. Although it was formally believed that vestibular suppressants, such as benzodiazepines, should not be used chronically because they inhibited vestibular compensation and delayed symptomatic recovery, recent research has shown that these drugs do not interfere.

A neurologic examination is needed to rule out vertigo caused by a CVA but even this cannot rule out end organ/peripheral ischemia.

Vertigo Caused by Vestibulotoxic Drugs

Ototoxicity is an occasional complication of aminoglycosides, salicylates, ethacrynic acid, and furosemide (21). Often these drugs are cochleotoxic and produce sensorineural hearing loss and tinnitus (see Chapter 96). Two aminoglycosides, streptomycin and gentamycin, are vestibulotoxic. The basis for aminoglycoside ototoxicity seems to be that these drugs are concentrated in the inner ear. Pathologically, there is destruction of the sensory hair cells of either the cochlea or the labyrinth. The labyrinth is often more sensitive to gentamycin than is the cochlea. Therefore it is possible to develop imbalance without hearing loss. Ototoxicity caused by an aminoglycoside has occurred with serum concentrations within the therapeutic range and after a short duration of therapy (18).

In office practice, vestibular toxicity may be seen shortly after discharge in a patient who has been treated with an aminoglycoside while in the hospital. Because these drugs produce bilateral, symmetric damage, the patient usually does not describe frank vertigo but has a reduction in VOR function (see above), unsteadiness, and intolerance to motion, and may describe difficulty walking in the dark. The pathologic changes produced by aminoglycosides are *permanent,* and the symptoms usually persist indefinitely. Vestibular exercises may reduce the patient's symptoms by maximizing compensatory mechanisms of gaze and posture stabilization. Most patients with vestibular toxicity adjust to their problem, and hearing aids may help those with cochlear toxicity.

Nowadays, *gentamycin* leads to ototoxicity far more than any other agent. Ototoxicity (and litigation) risks can be reduced by using gentamycin only as a last resort, performing a dynamic visual acuity test daily in the awake patient, and immediately stopping the gentamycin if the dynamic visual acuity test is positive. Because of the risk of ototoxicity, the case can be made that cost-effectiveness is not a sufficient reason for choosing gentamycin over another drug of equal or better efficacy.

Mild vertigo or disequilibrium may occur as a side effect of a number of drugs (Table 81.2) that do not produce permanent pathologic damage; these side effects remit promptly after stopping the drug.

Ménière's Syndrome (Endolymphatic Hydrops)

Ménière's syndrome is described in Chapter 96. This condition should always be considered in the differential diagnosis of a patient with the acute onset of severe vertigo with peripheral characteristics. The features that distinguish it from other causes of vertigo are the spontaneous onset of recurrent attacks, the limited duration of symptoms during each discrete attack (minutes to hours, not 1 day or more as seen with peripheral vestibulopathy), associated tinnitus, ear discomfort and sensorineural hearing loss, recruitment on audiometric studies, and normal brainstem and cerebellar function. A relative loss of low-frequency hearing is common with Ménière's syndrome but is unusual with other otologic disorders. Episodic vertigo with aural symptoms and degradation of hearing is the hallmark of Ménière's. After repeated attacks the diagnosis of Ménière's disease should be made reluctantly if there is no hearing loss. The treatment is Diamox 250 mg four times a day (starting at 250 mg daily and increasing by 250 mg a day every 4 days to 1 week). The patient should be given a 1.5-g sodium diet (see Table 62.12). Patients may require potassium supplement. Diamox therapy increases the risk of kidney stones. Cases refractory to this treatment may require labyrinthectomy, neurectomy, or transtympanic gentamycin to oblate vestibular function on that side.

Inflammatory Labyrinthitis

Labyrinthitis may occur, although rarely, as a manifestation of secondary or tertiary *syphilis*. It is always important to consider this cause because it may mimic other forms of peripheral vertigo and requires antibiotic treatment. Typically, the patient has a combination of sensorineural hearing loss, which may be unilateral or bilateral and fluctuating or sudden; impaired ability to understand speech (loud enough but not clear); and peripheral-type vertigo. Every patient with new peripheral-type vertigo should be checked routinely for syphilis with a serologic test (always including an FTA-ABS). If the test is positive, the patient should have a cerebrospinal fluid FTA-ABS determination and be treated according to the stage of the disease (see Chapter 30). Lyme disease may present in a similar manner.

Systemic lupus erythematosus, polyarteritis nodosa, and other causes of vasculitis may present with vertigo or loss of hearing. Nearly always other manifestations of the disease are also apparent.

Bilateral vestibular damage may occur following bilateral vestibular neuronitis, as a consequence of autoimmune disease of the inner ear (i.e., Cogan's syndrome), or idiopathically (2).

Central Causes of Vertigo

Table 81.2 lists the principal central causes of vertigo. Most (excluding migraine) are uncommon. The important clues to the presence of one of these conditions are the finding of associated neurologic signs and symptoms, the presence of nystagmus with central characteristics (Tables 81.4 and 81.5), or deviation of the patient's presentation and course from that expected for the common peripheral causes of vertigo. When a central cause for vertigo is suspected, the patient should be referred for evaluation to a neurologist or otolaryngologist. When the onset of symptoms is acute or there is evidence of rapidly progressive neurologic symptoms, the patient should be hospitalized. It is often impossible at the bedside to distinguish acute labyrinthitis from an ischemic event.

The principal manifestations of the three causes of central vertigo that a generalist is most likely to see are described here.

Migraine

Vestibular migraine is common. It is diagnosed in approximately 20% of patients presenting to a "dizziness" referral practice and is by far the most commonly diagnosed central cause of vertigo and general dizziness. Just as migraine can cause visual changes if the occipital lobe is affected or a paralysis if the parietal lobe is affected, it can cause frank vertigo if vestibular structures are affected. The onset and duration of episodes of vertigo are similar to those of the headache or aura of migraine. Vertigo can occur with or separate from the headache and can occur in patients without headache. The patient should have a current, past, or strong family history of migraine. Another presentation is a near constant vague, difficult to describe dizziness in a patient with a history of migraine. The neurologic examination should be normal but the may be unilateral vestibular hypofunction on testing. Treatment is identical to that of migraine (see Chapter 79).

Cerebellopontine Angle Tumor

Acoustic neuroma, the most common cerebellopontine (CP) angle tumor, is described in Chapter 96. The usual manifestations of these tumors are compression of the auditory component of the eighth nerve (sensorineural hearing loss) and, much later, compression of adjacent structures (the fifth and seventh cranial nerves in particular). Frank vertigo and nystagmus are present in a minority of patients. However, a vague complaint of unsteadiness is present in almost half of the patients when they are first seen. Most patients complain of unilateral hearing loss and tinnitus but vestibular symptoms may appear first. They generally have a great deal of difficulty in understanding speech in the affected ear. The ENG (see description below) usually shows a markedly decreased or absent response in the affected ear. The symptoms of CP angle tumor typically are insidious in onset (usually confined to sensorineural hearing loss for a prolonged interval), constant, and progressive. This time course distinguishes them from the periodic or severe symptoms typical of most peripheral vertigo and of the central vertigo of transient ischemia. Occasionally, onset of vertigo may be acute, but even then hearing loss is apparent earlier. Thirty seconds of hyperventilation may produce nystagmus. Occasionally symptoms mimic BPPV and this diagnosis should be considered in patients with BPPV refractory to treatment.

Consultation with an otolaryngologist (see Chapter 96) is the most appropriate plan for a patient who may have a CP angle tumor. The consultant should determine which of a large variety of otoneurologic tests is appropriate in pursuing this diagnosis.

Vertebrobasilar Arterial Disease

Cerebrovascular disease may cause vertigo in two ways. When vertigo is caused by ischemia of the brainstem or cerebellum, there are almost always other symptoms or signs of brainstem involvement, such as clumsiness, weakness, vision loss, diplopia, perioral numbness, ataxia, dysarthria, or drop attacks. When vertigo is caused by ischemia of only the labyrinth (through occlusion of its blood supply from a branch of the basilar artery), there usually is unilateral hearing loss but no symptoms or signs of brainstem involvement (36). It may be indistinguishable from an acute labyrinthitis or vestibular neuritis.

When vertigo with central symptoms is transient, it may be caused by a transient ischemic attack (TIA) (see Chapter 83), compromise of the vertebrobasilar circulation (Fig. 81.3) brought on by rotation of the neck (detected either in the history or by having the patient replicate symptoms in the office), or diversion of blood from the brainstem to an arm during use of that arm, or subclavian steal syndrome (suspected on the basis of

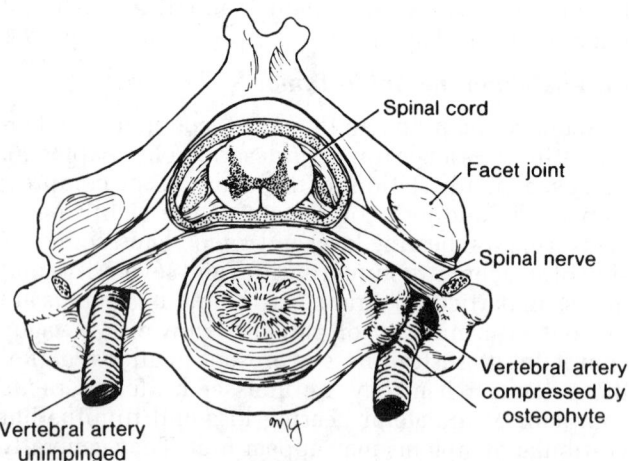

Figure 81.3. Anatomic relationship of the vertebral artery in a transverse foramen. The artery lies alongside the uncinate portion of the vertebra, the most common site of degenerative changes caused by cervical spondylosis with osteophyte formation. (From Sheehan S, Bauer RB, Meyer JS. Vertebral artery compression in cervical spondylosis. Neurology 10:968, 1960.)

history and the finding of a subclavian artery bruit or decreased blood pressure in the symptom-provoking arm). When the symptoms are abrupt in onset and persistent, they may be caused by infarction of the brainstem or cerebellum. Insidious onset of persistent symptoms is more suggestive of tumor. Acute cerebellar infarction in the distal territory of the posterior inferior cerebellar artery (PICA), an uncommon problem, may initially mimic acute vestibulopathy, presenting as sudden marked vertigo, nausea, and vomiting. Usually infarction caused by PICA occlusion involves the brainstem, so that other neurologic signs are present (ipsilateral loss of pain and temperature sense of the face and contralateral loss of these sensations in the rest of the body, ataxia, or ipsilateral Horner's syndrome).

Symptomatic Treatment of Vertigo

When the working diagnosis is peripheral vertigo of any type, treatment with one of the *antivertigo antihistamines* may provide symptomatic relief. It is hypothesized that these agents work by suppressing the vestibular end organ receptors and inhibiting activation of vagal responses. The major side effects of the antihistamine antivertigo drugs are dry mouth and sedation. Commonly recommended drugs in this group are listed in Table 81.6. A benzodiazepine can also be used to control vertigo. One with a long half-life is preferred so that fluctuation in blood levels can be avoided. Klonopin 0.25 to 0.5 mg once to three times daily is often useful. The typical precautions of other benzodiazepines apply (see Chapter 13). Because peripheral vertigo from common causes is usually self-limited, the patient should be instructed to take an antivertigo agent only for a few weeks and then to try discontinuing the drug.

When nausea and vomiting are pronounced, in either peripheral or central vertigo, an *antiemetic* can be tried. It is hypothesized that these agents work by suppressing central vestibular pathways that activate vagal responses. The commonly recommended antiemetic prochlorperazine is listed in Table 81.6. The major side effect occurring with short-term use is sedation; acute dystonias may occur in occasional patients taking prochlorperazine (see Chapter 16 for a full discussion of phenothiazine side effects).

Patients with persistent and disabling vertigo should be referred to an otolaryngologist for definitive evaluation and management. For permanent relief of symptoms, some patients require surgery, which may consist of sectioning of the vestibular nerve, repair of an inner ear fistula, or labyrinthectomy. These procedures may produce unilateral deafness.

Tests Used in Evaluation of Vertigo

When a patient with vertigo that is difficult to diagnose is referred to a neurologist or an otolaryngologist, one or more of the studies listed in Table 81.7 is

Table 81.6.   Drugs for Symptomatic Treatment of Vertigo

Type of Action	Generic (Trade Name)	Available Preparations	Dosage and Schedule
Labyrinthine suppressants			
Antihistamines	Meclizine (Antivert, Bonine)	12.5 and 25 mg	12.5–25 mg BID–QID
Benzodiazepines	Clonazepam (Klonopin)	0.5 mg	0.25–0.5 mg QD–TID
Antiemetic	Prochlorperazine (Compazine)	5-, 10-mg tablets	5–10 mg q4hr PRN
		10-, 25-mg suppositories	10 mg QID, 25 mg BID

Table 81.7.   Tests Used in the Evaluation of Vertigo

Audiometry (e.g., pure-tone, speech, tone decay, brainstem evoked potentials)
Caloric tests
Electronystagmography
Rotatory tests
Skull x-rays
Mastoid x-rays
Polytomogram of temporal bone and internal auditory canal
Computed tomography scan or magnetic resonance imaging

usually conducted. A combination of results from several tests may support a specific diagnosis.

Audiometry

A number of audiologic tests are usually performed in evaluating vertigo (e.g., pure-tone audiometry, speech audiometry, tone decay testing, acoustic reflex testing). Typically, there is no audiometric abnormality in the most common forms of peripheral vertigo (BPPV and peripheral vestibulopathy), whereas there are typical patterns of hearing loss in Ménière's syndrome (low-frequency hearing loss), acoustic neurinoma (high-frequency hearing loss, with poor discrimination), and a variety of middle ear disorders (conductive hearing loss).

Patient Experience. These tests are performed in a small soundproof testing room. There is no significant discomfort for the patient. Complete testing may take up to 1 hour.

Caloric Stimulation

The test is based on the fact that the intact labyrinth responds to caloric stimulation with a typical pattern (i.e., warm water induces horizontal nystagmus with the rapid phase toward the stimulated ear, and cool water produces nystagmus in the opposite direction). Vertigo may be induced with both hot and cold stimulation. ENG is used (see below) in addition to direct observation during caloric stimulation. Ideally, the water temperatures are set at 30° and 44°C, which are equidistant from normal body temperature, constitute equal stimuli, and produce less distress than more extreme temperatures. Absence of the normal caloric response or deviation from the normal response may be helpful in diagnosis. Vestibular neuronitis and acoustic neurinoma are examples of conditions in which the normal response to caloric stimulation is absent or decreased on the involved side.

Patient Experience. The patient lies on one side with the head positioned comfortably at an angle of about 30°. Flowing water is introduced into the external auditory canal for 30 seconds. During caloric stimulation, the patient will experience vertigo. An absent caloric response signifies vestibular disease.

Electronystagmography

Electronystagmography (ENG) records changes in the electrical potential between the cornea and the retina; when the eye moves, characteristic changes in electrical potential can be sensed (and recorded) in the skin adjacent to the eye (39). ENG's advantages are that it is more sensitive than simple inspection and provides a quantitative assessment. The principal value of ENG is in picking up subtle spontaneous nystagmus and in differentiating peripheral from central nystagmus, usually by caloric stimulation.

Patient Experience. The patient is recumbent. Small electrodes are taped to the skin on either side of the eye. Nystagmus is measured under a number of conditions, including caloric stimulation (see above), optokinetic testing (the patient is asked to follow the stripes on a rotating drum), and others. The entire procedure may take up to 1 hour. The major discomfort is that associated with caloric stimulation (vertigo and occasionally mild otalgia).

Rotatory Testing

In this test, the patient sits in a chair that rotates, while eye movements are measured with ENG. Head rotation induces nystagmus, which is quantitatively analyzed and may suggest the presence of unilateral or bilateral labyrinthine dysfunction, or a lesion in the brainstem or cerebellum (31).

Patient Experience. The patient is seated in a chair and has electrodes attached to the skin around the eyes. The chair rotates briefly in the dark and may evoke a sensation of vertigo or nausea.

PSYCHOGENIC DIZZINESS RESEMBLING VERTIGO

Psychogenic dizziness is the working diagnosis for about one-fifth of patients in a vestibular clinic (7). These patients have significant comorbidity and disability (10,45) and require an interdisciplinary evaluation (9,10,45).

MOTION SICKNESS

Motion sickness is experienced by most normal people when they are exposed to conditions analogous to those of severe storm conditions at sea. About one-third of people experience some symptoms when exposed to the equivalent of moderate sea conditions such as may occur with automobile travel and air travel, as well as with boating. A minority of people experience the symptoms of motion sickness after returning to land from a sea voyage (mal de debarquement) (8,16). Normal vestibular function is necessary for a person to experience motion sickness. Visual stimuli are contributory but not necessary for the experience of motion sickness (e.g., looking out of the window of a vehicle on a curving or undulating road).

The symptoms of motion sickness vary from person to person, but an individual usually experiences the same symptoms each time. Malaise and nausea are always present, and vomiting is common. Other symptoms may include drowsiness, yawning, salivation, swallowing, hyperventilation, headache, flushing, and diaphoresis. There is a major psychologic component in motion sickness; for example, some people develop their typical symptoms in anticipation of an air flight or a boat ride. *Vertigo is usually not present.*

Most people adapt fairly rapidly to motion. After the first few days of a sea voyage, for example, they can tolerate the motion that made them ill at the beginning of the voyage.

In tests simulating sea conditions, a number of drugs have been shown to be effective in preventing motion sickness (40). These drugs are much less effective if taken after the onset of symptoms. Because *all drugs that prevent motion sickness are sedating,* people should not operate cars, boats, planes, or potentially dangerous machines while taking these drugs.

Meclizine (Antivert requires a prescription; Bonine does not) 25 to 50 mg or dimenhydrinate (Dramamine, prescription) 50 to 100 mg can be used. For people who routinely get moderate or marked motion symptoms, taking one of these drugs about 1 hour before embarking in a car, plane, or boat may be helpful. Although prophylactic use is preferable, dimenhydrinate, with its rapid onset of action, can decrease symptoms that have already started. The protective effect from meclizine lasts from 12 to 24 hours, whereas that from dimenhydrinate lasts only 4 hours. The principal side effect is drowsiness; because this is more prominent with dimenhydrinate, meclizine is the better choice for people who wish to remain alert during travel; others may prefer the greater sedating property of dimenhydrinate. Scopolamine patches are no longer commercially available in the United States. A low-dose scopolamine tablet recently has been issued (scopace 0.4 mg); if taken on an empty stomach 1 hour before departure, it provides several hours of protection from motion sickness with only modest drowsiness and/or dry mouth.

SYNCOPE AND NEAR SYNCOPE

Definitions and Pathophysiology

Syncope is "a sudden transient loss of consciousness associated with a loss of postural tone, with spontaneous recovery" (23). Syncope typically lasts from seconds to minutes; longer episodes are classified as stupor or coma. *Unconsciousness* implies that both cerebral hemispheres have become impaired or that certain critical structures in the brainstem have failed. In general, unilateral diseases of the cerebral hemispheres do not lead to unconsciousness unless the brain becomes more generally affected.

There are three major pathophysiologic mechanisms of syncope (41):

- *Acute decrease in cerebral blood flow.* This may be caused by cardiac disorders, pulmonary vascular disorders, failure of venous return, cerebrovascular disease, loss of peripheral vascular tone, and vasodepressor syncope. This last mechanism is thought to result from a triggering of a neural reflex resulting in an episode of hypotension in the setting of bradycardia and peripheral vasodilation. It is thought to be a common cause of syncope, and carries a good prognosis.
- *Chemical aberration of blood flowing to the brain.* Examples include hypoglycemia, hypocapnia, and hypoxia.
- *Neural or psychologic causes.* These include nonconvulsive seizures, carotid sinus syncope, and hysteria.

Syncope must be differentiated from presyncope and other disorders that may, on initial history-taking, sound similar to syncope. *Many types of "spells" are not syncope;* a spell is "a sudden onset of a symptom or symptoms that are recurrent, self-limited, and stereotypic in nature" (47). Such spells are not necessarily syncope, and may be caused by endocrine, cardiovascular, psychologic, pharmacologic, neurologic, or other miscellaneous disorders. Carcinoid syndrome and pheochromocytoma are classic examples of disorders in which patients describe spells that are distinct from syncope.

Presyncope, or near syncope, is the sense of imminent loss of consciousness without frank syncope. It may be a prelude to true syncope or it may be related to a spell or to unexplained dizziness.

Incidence and Mortality

In the longitudinal community-based Framingham study, one or more episodes of syncope per year was reported in 3% of men and 3.5% of women. Framingham subjects ranged in age from 30 to 62; the mean age of an initial episode of syncope was 52 in men and 50 in women (14). The incidence of syncope increased with increasing age, and in patients aged 65 or older, syncope occurred at an annual rate of 6%. More than 75% of the patients with syncope had no evidence of neurologic or cardiovascular disease and isolated syncope was not associated with increases in morbidity or mortality. Thirty percent of men and 27% of women who experienced syncope had more than one episode of syncope.

Morbidity and mortality in patients with syncope differ according to the underlying cause of the syncopal event. Studies of patients with syncope report a 1-year mortality of 18 to 33% for patients with a cardiovascular cause of syncope, 0 to 12% for patients with a known noncardiovascular cause, and 6% for patients with an unknown cause of syncope (21). A study of patients with inducible ventricular tachycardia showed that they are the subgroup with the highest mortality; those taking a drug that effectively suppressed ventricular tachycardia did slightly better (4). Patients with underlying heart disease who have a history of syncope do not have a higher mortality than patients with the same extent of heart disease who do not have a history of syncope (25).

Differential Diagnosis

The vasovagal faint is thought to be the most common cause of syncope, especially if there is no evidence of a cardiovascular cause (5). However, the differential diagnosis of disorders presenting as syncope is broad. Table 81.8 lists causes, classified as hypotension, cardiac disease, metabolic conditions, intracranial conditions, or psychiatric disorders. Depending on the diagnostic criteria used, *an underlying cause will not be found for approximately 38 to 42% of patients evaluated for syncope* (23). In a recent study of psychiatric illnesses in patients with syncope, of patients who did not have an underlying medical explanation found for their syncopal episode, 20% met diagnostic criteria for at least one psychiatric disorder (24). In this same study, approximately half of the psychiatric disorders were not recognized by the patient's physicians. Somatization, panic disorder, generalized anxiety, major depression, and alcohol dependence were prevalent in this group of patients with unexplained syncope; these patients had higher rates of syncope recurrence during follow-up than patients with unexplained syncope who did not have underlying psychiatric disorders.

Of patients for whom the cause of syncope is determined, hypotension is the cause in 20 to 50%, cardiac disease in 10 to 25%, metabolic disorders in less than 5%, intracranial disease in less than 5%, and psychiatric disorders in up to 30% (33). In many patients, no cause can be clearly discerned on initial evaluation. For patients with syncope of unknown origin, additional testing or prolonged follow-up may be necessary, but often a diagnosis is never established.

In a classic prospective evaluation of 204 patients presenting with syncope, 25% had the cause diagnosed on the basis of the history and physical examination (26). In this study population, in which approximately 50% of patients eventually received a diagnosis, the importance of the history and physical examination was well illustrated. Table 81.9 lists the diagnostic

Table 81.8. Differential Diagnosis of Syncope/Near Syncope

Hypotension	Cardiac Disease
Vasovagal or neurocardiogenic syncope	*Arrhythmia (heart block, bradyarrhythmias, and tachyarrhythmias)*
Vasodilating drugs	Drugs associated with torsades de pointes
Angiotensin-converting enzyme inhibitors	Quinidine
Calcium channel blockers	Procainamide
Nitroglycerine preparations	Disopyramide
Vasodilator antihypertensives	Flecainide
	Encainide
Drugs affecting autonomic function	Amiodarone
Sympatholytic antihypertensives	Sotalol
Neuroleptics	Terfenadine
Tricyclics and monoamine oxidase inhibitors	Astemizole
Levodopa	*Outflow obstruction*
Cholinergic agents	Aortic stenosis
Autonomic neuropathy	Idiopathic hypertrophic subaortic stenosis
Peripheral neuropathy	Aortic dissection
Postsympathectomy	Myxoma
Tabes dorsalis and diabetic pseudotabes	*Acute myocardial infarction*
Parkinsonism (Shy–Drager syndrome)	*Mitral valve prolapse*
Idiopathic	*Cyanotic congenital heart disease*
Decreased blood volume	*Cardiac tamponade*
Hemorrhage	
Salt and water deficit	**Metabolic Conditions**
Fasting	*Hypoglycemia or hyperglycemia*
Adrenal insufficiency	*Hyponatremia, hypokalemia, or hypocalcemia*
Hypoalbuminemia	*Hypocapnia (hyperventilation)*
Diuretics	*Hypoxia*
Venous pooling	Anemia
Prolonged immobility while standing	Airway obstruction
Severe varicose veins	Carbon monoxide
Late pregnancy	Change to moderate/high altitude
After exercise	*Hyperviscosity*
Mobilization after bed rest	Drug overdose (sedatives and ethanol)
Orthostasis of aging	
Valsalva maneuver	**Intracranial Conditions**
Tussive	*Seizure disorder*
Micturition	*Subarachnoid hemorrhage*
Defecation (with straining)	*Cerebral embolism or thrombosis*
Intermittent positive-pressure breathing	*Migraine*
Compromise of cerebral blood flow caused by cervical osteoarthritis or subclavian steal	*Acutely increased intracranial pressure*
	Tumor
	Trauma
	Ventricular obstruction
	Hypertensive encephalopathy
Carotid sinus hypersensitivity	*Brainstem compression*
	Cervical or odontoid fractures
Pulmonary embolism	Metastasis
	Cysts or anomalies of the posterior fossa
	Platybasia
	Psychiatric Disorders
	Panic disorder
	Generalized anxiety disorder
	Major depression
	Somatization disorder
	Conversion disorder

Modified from Lee JE, Killip T, Plum F. Episodic unconsciousness. In: Baron JA, ed. Diagnostic approaches to presenting syndromes. Baltimore: Williams & Wilkins, 1971.

studies (including history and physical) that demonstrated the cause in patients for whom a cause was identified. This study was done before the widespread use of tilt table testing (see below).

Table 81.9. Diagnostic Studies that Demonstrated the Cause of Syncope in 107 of 204 Patients in Whom Exhaustive Study Established a Cause

Study	No. of Patients
History and physical	52
Electrocardiography	12
Electrocardiographic monitoring	29
Electrophysiologic studies	3
Cardiac catheterization	7
Cerebral angiography	2
Electroencephalography	1
Total	106[a]

From Kapoor WN, Karpf M, Wieand S, et al. A prospective evaluation and follow-up of patients with syncope. N Engl J Med 309:197, 1983.

[a]In one additional patient a diagnosis of aortic dissection was made at autopsy, 7 days after the patient presented with syncope.

General Approach to the Patient

Most patients who come to a physician after an episode of syncope or near syncope do so after their symptoms have resolved. The history should be obtained both from the patient and from anyone who observed the episode. The inquiry should focus on the events immediately preceding and following the attack, associated problems that may have been present for days to weeks before the episode, and evidence of trauma, neurologic deficit, or aspiration complicating the current episode of syncope. The objectives of these initial steps are to reach a working diagnosis or decide what further evaluation is needed and to decide on initial management for the patient. Appropriate management may range from reassurance (e.g., the patient with vasovagal syncope), to volume expansion (e.g., the patient with a diarrheal illness), to hospital admission for observation, prompt diagnostic testing, and necessary treatment (e.g., the patient with a history suggesting life-threatening arrhythmias or the patient with a major fracture complicating syncope).

Details regarding the critical features of many of the causes of syncope listed in Table 81.8 are described below.

History

Current Episode. The patient should always be questioned about his or her situation and body position immediately before the attack. If there was psychologic stress (e.g., an argument or fear about a medical procedure) or prodromal autonomic symptoms (nausea, pallor, diaphoresis), vasovagal syncope should be considered. If exercise preceded the attack, a number of cardiopulmonary abnormalities are possible, including aortic stenosis, hypertrophic cardiomyopathy, arrhythmia, and pulmonary hypertension. If syncope was associated with micturition, coughing, or defecation, the episode may have been caused by an associated Valsalva-induced decrease in venous return. Syncope from most causes does not occur unless the patient is in the upright position. If the attack occurred when the patient first stood up, orthostatic hypotension caused by venous pooling, loss of intravascular volume, or autonomic failure should be considered.

Syncope that occurs when the patient is seated or recumbent suggests hypoglycemia, carotid sinus hypersensitivity, cardiac arrhythmia, hyperventilation, seizure, or a psychiatric disorder. Syncope or dizziness occurring with position change while recumbent should always be distinguished from BPPV (see above).

The patient also should be asked *whether consciousness was lost completely* and whether a fall or any injury occurred. Although patients with many different causes of syncope may recall feelings of dizziness, heaviness of the limbs, or dimming of vision before loss of consciousness, other associated symptoms may suggest a diagnosis. Nausea is characteristic of vasovagal syncope but may also occur with bradyarrhythmias, myocardial ischemia, and loss of intravascular volume. Palpitations may suggest an arrhythmia, whereas chest pain and diaphoresis suggest myocardial ischemia. Headache and characteristic visual changes suggest a migraine. Incontinence and tonic–clonic movements of the extremities suggest a seizure. Hemiparesis, paraparesis, diplopia, and dysarthria may occur with transient occlusion of the basilar artery or vasospasm associated with migraine. The presence of multiple nonspecific associated complaints should raise suspicion of a psychiatric disorder.

Observations made by others who witnessed the period of unconsciousness. Particular attention should be paid to the duration of the spell, whether a convulsion occurred, the sequence of events, and how the patient seemed during the period of recovery. In general, recovery of consciousness is swift. If recovery of clear consciousness takes more than 5 minutes, one should suspect a seizure, hypoglycemia, or occluded intracranial vessel.

History Preceding the Current Episode. Information about the patient during the hours, days, or weeks preceding syncope/near syncope is often helpful in the differential diagnosis. In particular, one should determine the frequency of any previous episodes of syncope or near syncope, as the frequency of episodes influences decisions regarding the urgency of obtaining diagnostic studies. Frequent episodes without injury, especially if the syncope typically is preceded by nonspecific prodromal symptoms, should raise suspicion of a psychiatric disorder. Other circumstances surrounding previous episodes of dizziness or syncope may help develop a working diagnosis for the current episode of syncope. For example, a patient may report that previous episodes of dizziness or near syncope occurred after taking a new antihypertensive medication. A patient convalescing from recent illness may relate the symptoms to being up and around after bed rest.

Some patients describe prior episodes of frank syncope, without prodromal near syncope. Most often, these patients have a history, often long-standing, of syncope caused by vasovagal attack brought on by psychologic or physical stress. A history of recurrent syncope without the features of vasovagal attacks warrants consideration of arrhythmia, transient cerebrovascular occlusion, or a seizure disorder.

A patient with known organic heart disease, especially a patient with depressed left ventricular function or a history of ischemic heart disease, is at high risk of syncope caused by an arrhythmia.

Physical Examination

General Examination. The physical examination should include a search for abnormalities that may confirm a diagnosis suggested in the history or may reveal an unexpected cause. In particular, the heart rate and blood pressure should be measured after the patient has been recumbent for a few minutes and again after standing for 1 to 2 minutes. Very different blood pressures in the two arms would raise the possibility of aortic dissection or subclavian steal. The strength and upstroke of the carotid pulses should be appraised, and any bruits should be noted. The pulse should be palpated for 1 to 2 minutes to look for irregularities. The heart should be examined for murmurs, clicks, or gallops. Abdominal examination may reveal a large bladder or signs of a visceral catastrophe. If orthostatic hypotension has been found, a rectal examination should be performed to check the stool for occult or gross blood.

Carotid Massage. For patients with episodes suggestive of carotid sinus hypersensitivity (see below), or older patients with recurrent syncope and a nondiagnostic evaluation, carotid massage can be performed. However, it should be performed only when there is intravenous access, electrocardiographic and blood pressure monitoring, and atropine at hand, and only after checking the adequacy of the carotid pulses. When performed, carotid massage involves application of digital pressure over each carotid sinus separately, for up to 5 seconds. A resulting carotid asystole of more than 3 seconds or a systolic blood pressure drop of more than 50 mm Hg is considered abnormal.

Neurologic Examination. A brief examination of the major components of the nervous system (see Chapter 78) may reveal evidence of preexisting neurologic disease or of an acute insult. One should note the patient's orientation, speech, memory (for general information and the episode itself), and judgment. The fundi may reveal microemboli (see Chapter 83, Fig. 83.1) or subhyaloid hemorrhages (a sign of subarachnoid hemorrhage). Involvement of the midbrain, pons, or medulla is suggested by nystagmus, ophthalmoplegia, and other abnormalities of the cranial nerves. Weakness, sensory abnormalities, and pathologic reflexes may indicate a lesion elsewhere in the CNS. Any neurologic abnormalities should raise the suspicion of cerebrovascular disease, intracranial mass, subarachnoid hemorrhage, seizure, or CNS infection. If trauma has occurred in the recent past or if a fall was sustained during the syncopal episode, subdural or epidural hemorrhage should be considered.

Significance of Seizures and Neurologic Deficits. Seizure activity may occur after syncope with a variety of causes, including the simple faint, hyperventilation, orthostatic hypotension, or venous pooling. This is not surprising because unconsciousness signifies a major disruption in normal brain function. A single tonic convulsion is the most common type of postsyncopal seizure; less often a focal seizure or a generalized convulsion may occur. In all three of these instances, the patient's evaluation should include routine tests for a seizure focus (see Chapter 80).

Minor neurologic signs, such as slight focal weakness, reflex asymmetries, or pathologic reflexes, may be found after syncope from any cause, particularly if the patient is examined immediately after recovering consciousness. Such findings rarely persist for more than a few minutes. If such signs persist, are more profound, or occur in a constellation that suggests a particular anatomic lesion, they warrant further pursuit. However, one should not be surprised if a source is not found because minor neurologic signs are not uncommon after general ischemic or metabolic insults to the brain.

Diagnostic Tests

The history and physical examination lead to a diagnosis in at least 25% of patients with syncope (26). For these patients, no additional diagnostic tests are necessary. For the remaining patients, however, several diagnostic tests should be considered.

Electrocardiogram. An ECG, with a rhythm strip, is indicated in all patients with syncope if the cause is not obvious from the history and physical examination. Although the ECG shows some abnormality in a large proportion of patients with syncope, it confirms a diagnosis in a much smaller number (Table 81.9). Specific diagnostic workups may be prompted by certain ECG abnormalities. For instance, sinus bradycardia in the absence of a β-blocker should prompt concern for sick sinus syndrome or sinus arrest. Sinus tachycardia may be present in patients with dehydration, congestive heart failure (CHF), or pulmonary embolus. Left ventricular hypertrophy may be caused by aortic stenosis or hypertrophic cardiomyopathy, and a prolonged QT interval increases susceptibility to ventricular tachycardia. Left bundle branch block could be caused by cardiomyopathies or myocardial infarction, and bifascicular block is associated with increased risk for complete heart block (see details in Chapter 59, "Arrhythmias").

ECG Monitoring. The *Holter monitor* is the most commonly used diagnostic test in patients with syncope, but it is nondiagnostic in more than 90% of patients with a history of syncope (32). The clinical significance of asymptomatic arrhythmias found on Holter monitoring is unknown. Holter monitoring is indicated particularly in patients whose history suggests a cardiac basis for syncope; and in any older patient in whom the evaluation for syncope leads to an uncertain diagnosis.

The value of Holter monitoring in patients with symptoms of dizziness or syncope was assessed in a meta-analysis of seven studies; Holter monitoring was nondiagnostic in 78% of cases (13). Interestingly, only one quarter of patients with symptoms during monitoring had simultaneous arrhythmias, meaning that most patients (i.e., those experiencing symptoms without evidence of an underlying arrhythmia) undergoing Holter monitoring have the diagnosis of arrhythmia excluded by the findings.

The duration of Holter monitoring affects the diagnostic yield. In a study comparing the diagnostic yields of 24- 48-, and 72-hour Holter, a "major abnormality" was noted in 15% of patients within the first 24 hours, and 11% of patients who had a negative 24-hour Holter had a positive finding in the second 24 hours. Only 4.2% of patients with a negative 24- and 48-hour Holter had abnormalities documented in the third 24-hour period. None of the arrhythmias found after the first 24 hours were associated with symptoms (3).

There are other methods to monitor patients for arrhythmias for longer periods, including an implantable device (27) and a simpler *loop recorder,* which saves several minutes of rhythm retroactively when activated by a patient while symptoms are experienced. A study of 57 patients with unexplained syncope who underwent at least 24 hours of Holter monitoring without a diagnosis, who then underwent 1 month of monitoring with a loop electrocardiographic recorder, demonstrated a 25% diagnostic yield in this group (32). This type of testing may be useful in patients in whom arrhythmia is felt to be likely, who have a negative Holter monitor, and who have mild enough symptoms so that they can activate the recorder. It is less expensive than Holter monitoring. Typically, a 24-hour Holter with interpretation costs $200 to $300, whereas a 1-month loop recorder with interpretation costs approximately $100.

Arrhythmias detected during Holter monitoring but not accompanied by symptoms are difficult to interpret. Although some believe that these arrhythmias, even if unaccompanied by symptoms, may provide a working diagnosis, others disagree. Some arrhythmias, such as sinus arrest and nonsustained ventricular tachycardia, can be seen in normal people. Therefore the results of the Holter must be interpreted with caution, with consideration paid to the severity of the detected arrhythmia and the presence of any underlying heart disease.

Electrophysiologic Testing. Although the diagnostic yield of electrophysiologic (EP) studies varies among the populations studied, EP studies are considered the final step in the evaluation when arrhythmia is strongly suspected and noninvasive testing is nondiagnostic. *Indications* (23) for EP testing include

- Structural or ischemic heart disease, CHF, valvular disease, or hypertrophic cardiomyopathy
- Abnormalities on ECG such as bundle branch block or Wolff–Parkinson–White syndrome
- Abnormalities on ambulatory monitoring, such as nonsustained ventricular tachycardia

EP testing is most likely to produce abnormal findings in patients with underlying heart disease. In a study of 111 patients with *unexplained syncope* referred for EP testing, 50% of those with underlying heart disease had positive findings on EP testing, whereas 16% of those without underlying heart dis-

ease had positive findings (12). Because other studies have failed to identify clinical predictors that correlate with positive findings on EP studies (11) and because EP findings may lead to treatment that decreases episodes of syncope (4), there are no clear-cut guidelines for excluding EP testing for patients with unexplained syncope.

The most common abnormal finding in patients undergoing EP testing is ventricular tachycardia, followed by conduction disturbances and supraventricular tachycardia, with the percentage of patients with abnormal findings depending on the population studied. As with Holter monitoring, certain abnormalities detected, especially conduction abnormalities and even certain tachyarrhythmias, have questionable clinical significance.

Tilt Table Testing. Tilt table testing is the most recent addition to diagnostic testing in patients who have had syncope. It is used *to document susceptibility to vasovagal syncope.* In the tilt table test, the patient is secured to the tilt table in a supine position, tilted to a 60° to 80° angle within 10 to 15 seconds, and kept in this position for 15 to 60 minutes, while blood pressure and heart rate are monitored. A tilt table test is deemed positive if either hypotension or bradycardia develops and the patient experiences syncope or presyncope considered severe enough that syncope is felt to be inevitable. Positive objective findings are not always correlated with symptoms, and equivocal findings may be difficult to interpret. That is why the tilt table test is said to test for the *susceptibility* to vasovagal syncope.

In 1996, the American College of Cardiology published a consensus document on indications for tilt table testing in the assessment of patients with syncope (Table 81.10) (5).

Guidelines for Admission to a Hospital

Patients should be considered for admission to a hospital for initial evaluation and treatment if there is a high risk of injury from a recurrent event or a high risk of a life-threatening arrhythmia. Assessment of the risk of injury should be based on the degree of injury sustained in the current episode, the frequency of episodes, and the fragility of the patient. Assessment of the risk of an arrhythmia should be based on the status of any underlying heart disease and the presence of any current or previous ECG abnormalities.

Syncope from Hypotension or Circulatory Failure

Because of autoregulation, cerebral blood flow is protected over a wide range of systemic blood pressure. In normal people, a critical decrease in CNS blood flow (producing near syncope or syncope) does not occur until the mean blood pressure is below 50 mm Hg. Under a number of circumstances (e.g., sympatholytic drug treatment, cerebrovascular disease), however, the minimal tolerated blood pressure may not be this low. Thus, symptomatic failure of the systemic circulation may occur over a wide range of blood pressures.

Table 81.10. Summary of Principal Indications for Tilt Table Testing for Evaluation of Syncope (5)

Tilt Table Testing is Warranted
Recurrent syncope or single syncopal episode in a high-risk patient, whether or not the medical history is suggestive of neurally mediated (vasovagal) origin, and
No evidence of structural cardiovascular disease, or
Structural cardiovascular disease is present, but other causes of syncope have been excluded by appropriate testing
Further evaluation of patients in whom an apparent cause has been established (e.g., asystole, atrioventricular block), but in whom demonstration of susceptibility to neurally mediated syncope would affect treatment plans
Part of the evaluation of exercise-induced or exercise-associated syncope

Conditions for Which Reasonable Differences of Opinion Exist Regarding Utility of Tilt Table Testing
Differentiating convulsive syncope from seizures
Evaluating patients (especially the elderly) with recurrent unexplained falls
Assessing recurrent dizziness or presyncope
Evaluating unexplained syncope in the setting of peripheral neuropathies or dysautonomias
Follow-up evaluation to assess therapy of neurally mediated syncope

Tilt Table Testing Not Warranted
Single syncopal episode, without injury and not in a high-risk setting with clear-cut vasovagal clinical features
Syncope in which an alternative specific cause has been established and in which additional demonstration of a neurally mediated susceptibility would not alter treatment plans

Potential Emerging Indications
Recurrent idiopathic vertigo
Recurrent transient ischemic attacks
Chronic fatigue syndrome
Sudden infant death syndrome

Vasovagal (Neurocardiogenic, Vasodepressor) Syncope (Simple Faint)

The simple faint (vasovagal episode) has long been known to afflict young people; it is apt to occur in the setting of anxiety, fatigue, or pain and especially during venipuncture or other painful procedures. The simple faint is not just a disease of the young but can occur in older patients in identical settings. Improved understanding of the pathophysiology of vasovagal syncope has led to the term *neurocardiogenic or vasodepressor syncope.* Episodes are believed to be triggered when venous pooling or catecholamine release leads to increased ventricular contractions and activation of cardiac mechanoreceptors; this causes reflex increase in parasympathetic and decrease in sympathetic nervous system activity, resulting in symptomatic bradycardia or hypotension (21). Vasovagal attacks nearly always occur while the patient is upright, but they may occur while seated; consciousness is nearly always regained promptly when the patient lies down. Typically there is a prodromal warning period, lasting up to 5 minutes, when the patient feels dizzy or flushed, with mild nausea and occasionally palpitations or throat tightness. If the subject lies down during this stage, loss of consciousness may be avoided. An observer will note

cold hands, pale skin, and tachycardia just before the patient loses consciousness. After the faint, a flush replaces the pallor. If the patient is unable to lie flat, recovery may be prolonged; an occasional death has been noted if the person is held upright during the spell. Bradycardia may persist for up to 30 minutes after a simple faint. During this time the patient should remain lying down. The examination is otherwise normal unless there has been trauma or aspiration.

Vasovagal syncope is often selected as a diagnosis of exclusion because the history and physical examination are often nondiagnostic. As noted above ("Diagnostic Tests"), standardized *tilt table testing* can be used to confirm susceptibility to vasovagal syncope in patients for whom this information is needed to make a clinical decision.

Vasovagal syncope may be prevented by treatment with β-blockers, disopyramide, theophylline, or measures to increase intravascular volume (e.g., high-salt diet, supportive stockings, or fludrocortisone), but such treatment is necessary only for patients with frequent or disabling symptoms (21).

Autonomic Impairment

Syncope/near syncope caused by autonomic impairment is always associated with orthostatic hypotension. To document this problem, blood pressure must be taken while the patient is supine, and again while standing. In some patients, exercise while standing (e.g., walking for a few minutes) may be required for a significant orthostatic drop (20 mm Hg systolic) to occur.

The most common cause of this problem is *antihypertensive drug use;* most syncope caused by these drugs is preventable if the drugs are prescribed cautiously and the standing blood pressure, after exercise, is monitored routinely. Other drugs may also produce orthostatic hypotension (Table 81.8). The management of drug-induced orthostasis requires discontinuation or reduced dosage of the drug.

Orthostatic hypotension can also be caused by *autonomic neuropathy.* In patients suspected of having this problem, the integrity of the autonomic nervous system can be tested by noting the size and reaction of the pupils, the distribution of sweating, and the response to a Valsalva maneuver. The *Valsalva maneuver* is performed by having the patient expire against a closed glottis for 20 to 30 seconds, then release air from the chest (Table 81.11). This maneuver creates a sudden reduction in cardiac output, stimulating vagal (afferent) and sympathetic (efferent) responses. Absence of the reflex tachycardia (phase II) or absence of the blood pressure overshoot and reflex bradycardia (phase IV) indicate autonomic impairment.

Sympathetic failure commonly occurs late in diabetic peripheral neuropathy (see Chapter 72) and may be the presenting feature of amyloidosis or the neuropathy associated with various neoplasms. The Shy–Drager syndrome, which occurs in late life, is caused by failure of central autonomic neurons and causes orthostatic hypotension, parkinsonism, and

Table 81.11. Four Phases of a Normal Valsalva Maneuver

Onset	*Phase I:* A *sharp rise* in systolic pressure caused by an abrupt increase in intrathoracic pressure and emptying of the pulmonary bed during forced expiration against a closed glottis.
(20–30 seconds)	*Phase II:* A *gradual fall* in systolic pressure and a concomitant narrowing of peripheral pulse pressures caused by decrease in pulmonic and systemic venous return. *Heart rate increases* during this phase.
Release	*Phase III:* A sudden *further drop* in blood pressure occurs. Pulse pressure may be very narrow for the few beats during refilling of pulmonary venous reservoir.
	Phase IV (overshoot): Cardiac output increases with the increase in ventricular filling. Within 30 seconds of release of intrathoracic pressure, blood pressure *rises above its original level* because of reflex vasoconstriction initiated by small pulse pressure during phase III. The pressoreceptor stimulation in phase IV results in *transient bradycardia.*

other autonomic symptoms in varying combinations. Sympathectomy, particularly when done bilaterally or in the lumbar segments, may be followed immediately by orthostatic hypotension and syncope, although usually venous tone recovers several weeks after the operation. Tabes dorsalis and more commonly diabetic pseudotabes may present with lightning pains and autonomic failure. The management of orthostasis caused by autonomic neuropathy is symptomatic; it is summarized in Chapter 84.

Decreased Intravascular Volume

Decreased intravascular volume caused by hemorrhage or to salt and water loss (e.g., from gastroenteritis, heat exposure, or diuretics) is recognized by the combination of orthostatic hypotension and an associated basis for the volume deficit. Hot weather and exercise predispose to volume depletion and thereby to syncope, particularly after vigorous exercise. Prolonged fasting, as in anorexia nervosa or with fad diets, also may produce syncope through volume depletion. Adrenal insufficiency caused by pituitary or adrenal disease may produce syncope through the combination of chronic volume deficit and a loss of vascular tone; the syncope is often precipitated by an intercurrent illness. Hypoalbuminemia caused by liver disease, enteropathies, or chronic disease can also lead to syncope/presyncope caused by volume deficit. Volume expansion, either by increased salt and water ingestion or by intravenous fluids, is the initial treatment; the choice of ambulatory or hospital management and the planning of definitive treatment depends on the severity and cause of the volume deficit.

Venous Pooling

Venous pooling prevents return of blood to the heart, lowering cardiac output, at times sufficiently to produce near syncope or syncope. Symptoms may occur after prolonged standing in one position, particularly after exercise, as in recruits standing at attention. Severe dependent varicose veins or the compression of pelvic veins by a fetus or a large abdominal mass may produce symptoms through a similar mechanism. Syncope 15 to 30 minutes after exercise has been attributed to dilation of the splanchnic circulation before blood flow to the skeletal muscles has completely returned to normal. Management of these conditions involves chiefly avoidance of the precipitating factors. Supportive elastic stockings may be helpful for patients with marked pooling in varicose veins (see Chapter 88).

Orthostatic Syncope/Near Syncope After Bed Rest

This problem is caused by the combined effects of venous pooling, relative hypovolemia, and probably to some degree lowered sensitivity of the baroreceptor system. It is very common at all ages, but especially among the elderly, and should be anticipated in any person who has been at bed rest for more than a few days; moreover, it may persist for 1 or 2 weeks or longer after mobilization begins. Orthostatic symptoms may be minimized or prevented by having the patient gradually stand only after several minutes of sitting on the bed with the legs dependent. Practical exercises that may help convalescing patients in overcoming postural weakness and hypotension are illustrated in Figure 81.4. These patients should be encouraged to be out of bed for at least 2 hours a day, including morning, afternoon, and evening.

Orthostasis of Aging

Transient orthostatic dizziness and hypotension occur in many healthy older people. A significant fall in systolic blood pressure also is common in elderly patients immediately after eating, even in a seated position (34), which may make them especially susceptible to syncope when standing up after a meal. The physiologic basis for orthostatic symptoms in the elderly is often multifactorial, and may be related not only to postural hypotension but also cerebral ischemia, vestibular dysfunction, visual impairment, and abnormal proprioception. The orthostasis of aging is important because it increases the risk associated with drugs that may cause orthostatic hypotension. Clearly, older patients should have their standing blood pressure checked whenever they complain of even mild orthostatic symptoms, and they should be monitored similarly whenever a drug in one of the groups listed in Table 81.6 is prescribed. Those who are troubled by orthostatic symptoms should be advised to follow the steps recommended above for patients rising after bed rest.

Micturition Syncope

Micturition syncope, defined as syncope occurring at the beginning of, during, at the end of, or immediately after urination, occurs typically in several types of subjects: young men who are otherwise healthy, in whom the Valsalva mechanism (see above) and direct vagal stimulation have been hypothesized as the basis for this form of syncope; older men and women, many of whom have baseline orthostasis related to drugs or to aging; and older men with prostate gland hypertrophy, which can predispose to a Valsalva response when the patient strains to urinate. Alcohol, because it causes venous pooling, may also be a predisposing factor, especially in young men. Patients with micturition syncope should be evaluated for orthostasis, and when this is found any factors contributing to it should be modified. In addition, all patients with recurrent micturition syncope should be advised to sit while urinating and to remain seated for a minute after urination.

Leg Exercises

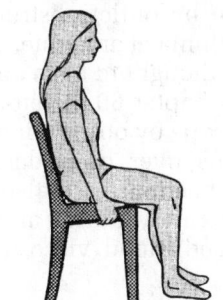 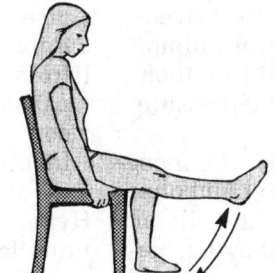 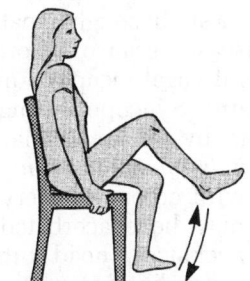

Starting position: Sitting in chair, exercise one leg at a time.

Raise leg up and down. Repeat 10 times.

Keeping knee bent, raise leg up and down.

Arm Exercises: To increase effectiveness, hold a soup can in each hand for weight.

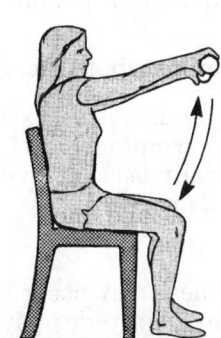 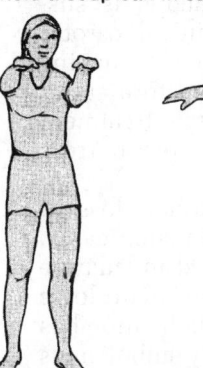 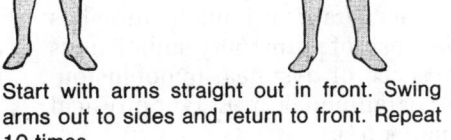

Start with arms straight out in front. Raise arms up and down, only to chin level. Repeat 10 times.

Start with arms straight out in front. Swing arms out to sides and return to front. Repeat 10 times.

Rising Exercise

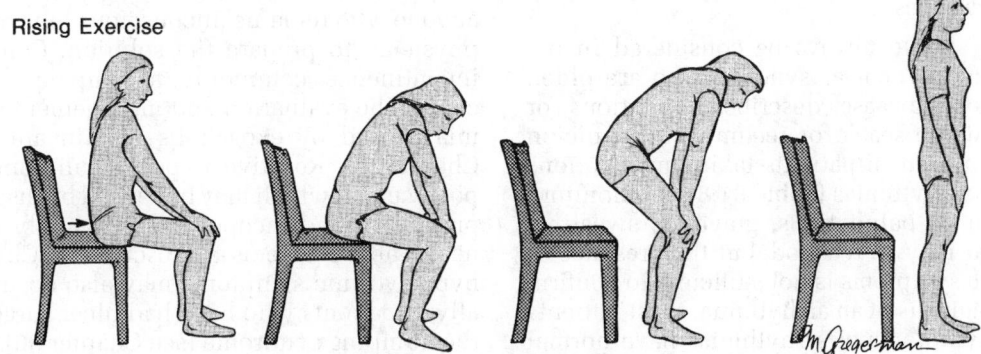

Slide to front of chair, keeping legs apart.

Place hands on knees and push yourself to straight stand. Sit down, using hands on knees to help.

Repeat 3–5 times using hands less and legs more each time. Repeat exercise without using hands to help.

Figure 81.4. Exercise for weakness and orthostatic hypotension after prolonged bed rest. Patient must be out of bed 2 hours a day, morning, afternoon, and evening. Exercises are done three times a day. (Courtesy of Karen Ryder, Registered Occupational Therapist.)

Other Forms of Syncope Related to Systemic Circulation

Tussive syncope may follow a prolonged bout of coughing in otherwise normal people or in patients with chronic cough (see Chapter 54), including cough due to gastroesophageal reflux (37). In these patients, the syncope is thought to be caused by the Valsalva mechanism (see above). Tussive syncope may also occur after only a slight cough in patients with obstructive airway disease because abnormalities of pulmonary and pleural vagal receptors may aggravate their tendency to faint. Syncope during positive-pressure breathing occurs by similar mechanisms.

Hypersensitivity of the carotid sinus is common in older men with coronary artery disease or hypertension, and may be exacerbated by tight collars, cumbersome necklaces, head turning, shaving, or large neck masses, but is an uncommon cause of syncope. Syncope may result when stimulation of the baroreceptors in the carotid sinus leads to an increase in vagal activity with resulting bradycardia or leads to sympathetic relaxation with resulting hypotension (44). If carotid sinus syncope is suspected, one should consider performing a carotid massage (see above). Patients diagnosed as having carotid sinus syncope should be referred to a cardiologist for consideration of anticholinergic treatment or pacemaker insertion, if the symptoms are recurrent or severe.

Pulmonary embolism may cause sudden loss of consciousness in up to 10% of cases. In such cases, unconsciousness may be brief or prolonged and may be accompanied by a small seizure or minor neurologic abnormalities, even when paradoxic embolization has not occurred. The diagnosis of pulmonary embolism is suggested by the presence of dyspnea, hypotension, tachycardia, or acute cor pulmonale by ECG or physical examination (see Chapter 52).

Syncope from Cardiac Abnormalities

Rhythm Disturbances

Arrhythmias should always be considered in patients with syncope or near syncope who are older, have known heart disease, describe palpitations, or have syncope while seated or recumbent. Suspicion should also be raised in patients taking medications that may cause arrhythmias (Table 81.8). Premonitory symptoms such as palpitations, grayouts, sweating, nausea, and fear may be recalled, but the presence or absence of these symptoms is not sufficient to confirm or refute the diagnosis of an arrhythmia. Most patients with cerebral symptoms of arrhythmias have normal resting ECGs. In general, at least 24 hours of ECG monitoring should be performed to identify potentially important arrhythmias in patients with syncope that is not explained by the initial history, physical examination, and 12-lead ECG (see "ECG Monitoring" above) and some should have electrophysiologic testing (see above).

Outflow Obstruction

An obstruction to ventricular outflow caused by rheumatic or calcific aortic stenosis may lead to syncope. It nearly always follows exertion and is often associated with chest pain. Unconsciousness may be prolonged and may be followed by neurologic abnormalities. Similarly, hypertrophic cardiomyopathy may lead to syncope by outlet obstruction after exercise or by an arrhythmia at any time. The diagnostic approach to patients thought to have outflow obstruction is described in Chapter 60. A left-atrial myxoma (rare) may cause syncope by obstruction of blood flow when a patient leans over or undergoes exertion. Cyanotic congenital heart disease also leads to syncope after exercise or, rarely, during an airplane flight. Hypoxia and increased blood viscosity are contributing factors.

Myocardial Infarction

Acute myocardial infarction may present with syncope, which may result from an arrhythmia, low cardiac output, or severe pain. Embolization from a mural thrombus should be considered when syncope occurs during recovery from myocardial infarction.

Syncope from Metabolic Abnormalities

The initial history and physical examination should seek to identify any symptoms or signs of metabolic derangement, especially because some derangements may lead to lasting damage.

Hypoglycemia

Loss of consciousness may occur in hypoglycemic adults, although rarely in older patients, when the blood glucose level is below 40 mg/100 mL. Hunger, palpitations, sweating, and anxiety nearly always occur 5 to 15 minutes before the patient loses consciousness. Because the brain can survive for only about 10 minutes with a blood glucose of 20 mg/100 mL, the prophylactic administration of glucose is warranted in anyone who remains unconscious long enough for the physician to prepare the solution. Convulsions and incontinence commonly accompany hypoglycemic coma. The evaluation and management of hypoglycemia caused by exogenous insulin are described in Chapter 72. Reactive hypoglycemia and fasting hypoglycemia (which may be caused by insulinoma) may produce near syncope but only rarely unconsciousness. These problems are described in Chapter 74. Mild hypoglycemic symptoms may also occur postprandially in patients who have had ulcer surgery, as part of the dumping syndrome (see Chapter 36).

Hypocapnia (Hyperventilation)

Hypocapnia caused by hyperventilation leads to syncope, near syncope, or ill-defined dizziness by decreasing cerebral blood flow through vasoconstriction of small arterioles throughout the brain. A P_{CO_2} of 25 mm Hg is sufficient to lower cerebral blood flow to levels at which symptoms may occur; such a value may be produced in some people by a few very deep breaths. Athletes preparing to race, musicians playing wind instruments, or anyone who is fearful or anxious may develop transient symptoms in this way. Tetany or carpopedal spasm may or may not precede the cerebral symptoms. Recovery is prompt if ventilation is slowed. Hyperventilation may be a contributing factor in many patients with *chronic dizziness* (28). The diagnosis and management of hyperventilation related to anxiety, the most common cause of this problem, are described in Chapter 13.

Hypoxemia

Hypoxemia caused by any primary cause may predispose to syncope/near syncope. Severe anemia (see Chapter 50) may sufficiently deprive the brain of oxygen to lead to syncope after exercise; it may also predispose to syncope from any other cause. Asphyxiation caused by obstruction of the upper airway should be considered in small children, patients with bad teeth, or patients with masses in the neck. The "café coronary" caused by laryngeal aspiration of food is usually betrayed by sudden collapse at the table. However, patients with esophageal diverticula may choke hours after a meal. Poisoning with *carbon monoxide* is suggested by a history of exposure to products of combustion (e.g., poorly ventilated space heaters, gas-burning engines in closed spaces). Manifestations may include prodromal headache and confusion plus bright pink color and prolonged unconsciousness. Short-term exposure to moderate or *high altitude,* even in healthy young adults, may lead to syncope, possibly mediated by a decrease in arterial oxygen saturation (35).

Seizures are common in patients with acute hypoxemia, and neurologic sequelae are the rule after unconsciousness lasting more than 1 or 2 minutes. The management of hypoxemic syncope depends entirely on prompt and accurate diagnosis to prevent recurrence or worsening of the hypoxemia.

Drug Overdose

Overdose of some drugs may cause syncope/near syncope due to orthostatic hypotension. These drugs include sedatives, which may produce venous pooling (particularly chloral hydrate, paraldehyde, and ethanol, and less often benzodiazepines and barbiturates) and all of the drugs listed as potential causes of autonomic impairment in Table 81.8. However, overdose of most drugs is more likely to cause stupor or coma from their sedating effects than to cause syncope or near syncope from orthostatic hypotension.

Syncope from Intracranial Abnormalities

Seizure

Seizure as a cause of syncope is a diagnosis that is thought to be made easily from historical details. However, as noted above, clonic movements are seen in some patients who have syncope unrelated to sei-zure, with the duration of clonic movements being brief. In the prospective evaluation of patients presenting with syncope mentioned above, 50% of patients underwent EEG testing, and this confirmed an underlying seizure disorder in only 1.5% (26). It has been demonstrated that the best discriminating finding distinguishing seizure from syncope was orientation immediately after the event, as reported by an eyewitness. A seizure was found to be five times more likely if the patient was reported to be disoriented after the seizure. In the absence of an eyewitness, the age of the patient was the most useful discriminator; a seizure was three times more likely if the patient was younger than 45. Incontinence and trauma were not discriminative findings (20).

The diagnosis and management of seizure disorders are described in detail in Chapter 80.

Subarachnoid Hemorrhage

A brief period of unconsciousness at the beginning of subarachnoid hemorrhage is the rule. This diagnosis is strongly suggested when the constellation of headache, confusion, and neck stiffness follows shortly after a syncopal episode. Any patient who is confused and develops headache during initial evaluation should be admitted for observation and evaluation, even if meningismus has not yet developed.

Embolism or Thrombosis

Cerebral embolism or thrombosis may cause brief (TIA) or prolonged (cardiovascular accident) unconsciousness if the basilar artery is affected. Rarely, a carotid occlusion may cause unconsciousness initially, even if the remaining vessels are patent. A carotid occlusion likewise may cause loss of consciousness if the contralateral carotid is already occluded; in this instance, the period of unconsciousness is usually prolonged and seizures may occur; neurologic symptoms and signs nearly always are present. The diagnosis and management of cerebrovascular disease are described in Chapter 83.

Migraine

Migraine (see Chapter 79) may produce syncope/near syncope by spasm of the basilar artery or of the posterior cerebral arteries. Syncope that occurs with migraine is more often caused by hyperventilation or a vasovagal mechanism than by a central abnormality.

Increased Intracranial Pressure

Increased intracranial pressure, whether caused by a brain tumor, trauma, or an obstruction to the ventricular system, may result in syncope when a Valsalva maneuver is performed such as during straining at defecation or bending over. The hallmarks are preexisting symptoms, papilledema, and neurologic signs.

Brainstem Compression

Rarely, brainstem compression caused by metastatic tumors, cystic anomalies, or a displaced fracture of C1 or of the odontoid process may lead to syncope with movement of the neck because of transient compression of critical structures of the brainstem. Patients with severe rheumatoid arthritis also may develop cervical instability leading to compression of the brainstem with neck motion (see Chapter 70). Associated neurologic abnormalities are often present. Patients thought to have this problem require prompt hospital admission for diagnosis and treatment.

Syncope from Psychiatric Disorders

As many as 25% of patients with syncope or near syncope may have a psychiatric diagnosis (33). The most common psychiatric diagnoses in patients with unexplained syncope are panic disorders and major depression. However, anxiety disorders, somatization, and conversion disorders also may be frequent causes of syncope or near syncope. The diagnosis and management of these disorders are described in Chapters 12, 13, and 15.

Selected Conditions that May Mimic Syncope

Hysterical Faint

Sudden, dramatic fainting was said to be common in the 19th century, especially in women. Today fainting caused by conversion disorder or other forms of somatization is more common. Usually the fainting occurs in a manner to avoid injury, an important distinguishing feature from true syncope. The patient crumples to the ground with a limp body and shallow respirations. Recovery is usually immediate. Often, the faint may be embellished with movements that resemble seizures but more often voluntary movements are the rule. Hyperventilation or coaxing may reproduce the spell. Chapter 12 provides additional detail regarding the evaluation and management of such patients, whose physical symptoms are often caused by emotional factors.

Drop Attack

Older patients, especially men, may report sudden and unprovoked falls to the ground. Consciousness is not lost, and the patients can usually remember the entire episode. The history of maintenance of consciousness distinguishes drop attacks from syncope. Ischemia of the lower brainstem is thought to cause drop attacks, and occasionally patients report other concurrent symptoms that suggest vertebrobasilar ischemia. Management is identical to that of TIAs occurring in the posterior circulation (see Chapter 83).

Cataplexy

Cataplexy is a special kind of drop attack, not caused by ischemia, that occurs as part of the syndrome of narcolepsy (see Chapter 85). The patient falls suddenly to the ground because of a loss of extensor muscle tone but without loss of consciousness. These spells are usually provoked by a sudden startle, a joke, laughing, or sneezing. They may be effectively managed by tricyclic agents. *Sleep paralysis* (paralysis of the limbs for a minute or two upon awakening) and peculiar visual hallucinations on awakening or before falling asleep may also accompany narcolepsy. (See Chapter 85 for additional details.)

DISEQUILIBRIUM OF MISCELLANEOUS ORIGINS

Some patients with persistent dizziness do not have manifestations that make it possible to classify their problem as vertigo or near syncope. Many of these patients have disequilibrium, or a sense of imbalance, that may be caused by cerebellar ataxia (see Chapter 78); multiple sensory deficits (e.g., partial hearing, visual, and proprioceptive impairment); lower extremity weakness (e.g., from an old stroke or from disuse after a period of bed rest); pain in a weight-bearing joint; recently initiated drugs, especially anxiolytics, hypnotics, or neuroleptics; or the onset of a progressive CNS disease such as parkinsonism (see Chapter 82), normal pressure hydrocephalus (see Chapter 17), or CP angle tumor (see Chapter 96). These problems often occur in older patients, debilitated patients (particularly chronic alcoholics), or patients with long-standing diabetes mellitus. In these patients, cerebrovascular disease or autonomic neuropathy may cause periodic vertigo and near syncope to be superimposed on their day-to-day problem with imbalance.

The evaluation of patients describing imbalance consists chiefly of obtaining a history of the duration, progression, and day-to-day characteristics of the problem, focusing on the limitations imposed on their usual activities and on any falls or near accidents that may have occurred. In the physical examination, it is important to determine which of the many problems listed above may be contributing to the patient's symptoms.

Depending on the individual patient, management by the generalist may include referring the patient for correction of any impairment in hearing or vision (see Chapters 96 and 97), consulting a neurologist if unexplained progressive symptoms are found (e.g., cerebellar ataxia in an otherwise healthy person), consulting a physical therapist if weakness or the need for selecting a cane or walker is apparent, and discontinuing drugs that may be contributing to the patient's symptoms and avoiding drugs that may worsen symptoms (Tables 81.2 and 81.8).

CHRONIC DIZZINESS: GENERAL MEASURES IN MANAGEMENT

Patients with chronic dizziness, vertigo, syncope, or disequilibrium have a far better prognosis if their home environments are safe and others in their households are aware of risks that should be avoided and devices that may be helpful. A number of general measures to recommend include using night-lights, tacking down loose carpeting and floorboards, installing special railings in the bathroom, selecting proper footwear, and learning to assume an upright posture gradually. These measures can be accomplished most effectively if the physician or a visiting nurse evaluates the patient's home. In some patients with unsteady gait, a cane or a walker may be helpful; a physical therapist can be very helpful in selecting the best assistive device.

General References*

Baloh RW, Honrubia V. Clinical neurophysiology of the vestibular system. Philadelphia: FA Davis, 1991.
> Excellent review of vertigo.

Brandt T. Vertigo: its multisensory syndromes. London: Springer-Verlag, 1991.
> Excellent review of vertigo.

Linzer M, Yang EH, Estes M III, et al. **Clinical guideline—diagnosing syncope. Part 1: Value of history, physical examination, and echocardiography.** Ann Intern Med 126:989–996, 1997.

Linzer M, Yang EH, Estes M III, et al. **Clinical guideline—diagnosing syncope. Part 2: Unexplained syncope.** Ann Intern Med 127:76–86, 1997.

Specific References

1. Baloh RW, Honrubia V, Jacobson K. Benign positional vertigo: clinical and oculographic features in 240 cases. Neurology 37:371, 1987.
2. Baloh RW, Jacobson K, Honrubia V. Idiopathic bilateral vestibulopathy. Neurology 39:272, 1989.
3. Bass EB, Curtiss EI, Arena VC, et al. The duration of Holter monitoring in patients with syncope. Arch Intern Med 150: 1073, 1990.
4. Bass EB, Elson JJ, Fogoros RN, et al. Long-term prognosis of patients undergoing electrophysiologic studies for syncope of unknown origin. Am J Cardiol 62:1186, 1988.
5. Benditt DG, Ferguson DW, Grubb BP, et al. Tilt table testing for assessing syncope. J Am Coll Cardiol 28:263, 1996.
6. Brandt T, Daroff RB. Physical therapy for benign paroxysmal positional vertigo. Arch Otolaryngol 106:484, 1980.
7. Brandt T, Huppert D, Dieterich M. Phobic postural vertigo: a first follow-up. J Neurol (abstract) 241:191, 1994.
8. Brown JJ, Baloh RW. Persistent mal de debarquement syndrome: a motion-induced subjective disorder of balance (Abstract). Am J Otolaryngol 8:219, 1987.
9. Clark MR. Chronic dizziness: an integrated approach. Hosp Pract 29:57, 1994.
10. Clark MR, Sullivan MD, Katon WJ, et al. Psychiatric and medical factors associated with disability in patients with dizziness. Psychosomatics 34:409, 1993.
11. Denes P, Uretz E, Ezri MD, Borbola J. Clinical predictors of electrophysiologic findings in patients with syncope of unknown origin. Arch Int Med 148:1922, 1988.
12. Denniss AR, Ross DL, Richards DA, Uther JB. Electrophysiologic studies in patients with unexplained syncope. Int J Cardiol 35:211, 1995.
13. DiMarco JP, Philbrick JT. Use of ambulatory electrocardiographic (Holter) monitoring. Ann Intern Med 113:53, 1990.
14. Farrehi PM, Santinga JT, Eagle KA. Syncope: diagnosis of cardiac and non-cardiac causes. Geriatrics 50:24, 1995.
15. Fife TD. Bedside cure for benign positional vertigo (Abstract). BNI Q 10:2, 1994.
16. Gordon CR, Spitzer O, Shupak A, Doweck I. Survey of mal de debarquement (Abstract). BMJ 304:545, 1992.
17. Halmagyi GM, Curthoys IS. A clinical sign of canal paresis. Arch Neurol 45:737, 1988.
18. Halmagyi GM, Fattore CM, Curthoys IS, Wade S. Gentamicin vestibulotoxicity. Otolaryngol Head Neck Surg 111:571, 1994.
19. Hart CW. Evaluation of post-traumatic vertigo. Otolaryngol Clin North Am 6:157, 1973.
20. Hoefnagels WAJ, Padberg GW, Overweg J, et al. Transient loss of consciousness: the value of the history for distinguishing seizure from syncope. J Neurol 238:39, 1991.
21. Hybels RL. Drug toxicity of the inner ear. Med Clin North Am 63:309, 1979.
22. Kapoor WN. Evaluation and management of the patient with syncope. JAMA 268:2553, 1992.
23. Kapoor WN. Workup and management of patients with syncope. Med Clin North Am 79:1153, 1995.
24. Kapoor WN, Fortunato M, Hanusa BH, Schulberg HC. Psychiatric illnesses in patients with syncope. Am J Med 99:505, 1995.
25. Kapoor WN, Hanusa BH. Is syncope a risk factor for poor outcomes? Comparison of patients with and without syncope. Am J Med 100:646, 1996.
26. Kapoor WN, Karpf M, Wieand S, et al. A prospective evaluation and follow-up of patients with syncope. N Engl J Med 309:197, 1983.
27. Krahn AD, Klein GJ, Norris C, Yee R. The etiology of syncope in patients with negative tilt table and electrophysiological testing. Circulation 92:1819, 1995.
28. Kroenke K, Lucas CA, Rosenberg ML, et al. Causes of persistent dizziness: a prospective study of 100 patients in ambulatory care. Ann Intern Med 117:898, 1992.
29. Kroenke K, Mangelsdorff AD. Common symptoms in ambulatory care; incidence, evaluation, therapy and outcome. Am J Med 86:262, 1989.
30. Langridge HS, Mallinson AI. The dynamic illegible E-test. Acta Otolaryngol (Stockholm) 103:273, 1987.
31. Leigh RJ, Zee DS. The neurology of eye movements. Philadelphia: FA Davis, 1991.
32. Linzer M, Pritchett ELC, Pontinen M, et al. Incremental diagnostic yield of loop electrocardiographic recorders in unexplained syncope. Am J Cardiol 66:214, 1990.
33. Linzer M, Varia I, Pontinen M, et al. Medically unexplained syncope: relationship to psychiatric illness. Am J Med 92(Suppl 1A):18S, 1992.
34. Lipsitz LA, Nyquist RP, Wei JY, Rowe JW. Postprandial reduction in blood pressure in the elderly. N Engl J Med 309:81, 1983.
35. Nicholas R, O'Meara PD, Calonge N. Is syncope related to moderate altitude exposure? JAMA 268:904, 1992.
36. Oas JG, Baloh RW. Vertigo and the anterior inferior cerebellar artery syndrome. Neurology 42:2274, 1992.
37. Puetz TR, Vakil N. Gastroesophageal reflux–induced cough syncope. Am J Gastroenterol 90:2204, 1995.
38. Robinson DA, Zee DS, Hain TC, et al. Alexander's law: its behavior and origin in the human vestibulo-ocular reflex. Ann Neurol 16:714, 1984.
39. Rubin W. Electronystagmography and its value in the diagnosis of vertigo. Otolaryngol Clin North Am 6:95, 1973.
40. Ruckenstein MJ, Harrison RV. Motion sickness: helping patients tolerate the ups and downs. Postgrad Med 89:139, 1991.
41. Savage DD, Corwin L, McGee DL, et al. Epidemiologic features of isolated syncope: the Framingham Study. Stroke 16:626, 1985.
42. Singleton GT, Karlan MS, Post KN, Bock DG. Perilymph fistulas. Diagnostic criteria and therapy. Ann Otolaryngol Rhinolaryngol 87:1, 1978.
43. Slater R. Vertigo: how serious are recurrent and single attacks? Postgrad Med 84:58, 1988.
44. Sugrue DD, Wood DL, McGoon MD. Carotid sinus hypersensitivity and syncope. Mayo Clin Proc 59:637, 1984.
45. Sullivan M, Clark MR, Katon WJ, et al. Psychiatric and otologic diagnoses in patients complaining of dizziness. Arch Intern Med 153:1479, 1993.
46. Warner EA, Wallach PM, Adelman HM, Sahlin-Hughes K. Dizziness in primary care patients. J Gen Intern Med 7:454, 1992.
47. Young WF, Maddox DE. Spells: in search of a cause. Mayo Clin Proc 70:757, 1995.

---

*Bold print (general references) and bold numerals (specific references) denote published controlled clinical trials, meta-analyses, or consensus-based recommendations.

C H A P T E R   82

Common Disorders of Movement: Tremor and Parkinson's Disease

STEPHEN G. REICH, MD

TREMOR

Definition and Classification

Tremor is defined as the involuntary rhythmic or semirhythmic oscillation of a body part, resulting from alternating or simultaneous contractions of antagonistic muscle groups. Despite extensive clinical study, the pathophysiology of different tremor types is poorly understood, so the differential diagnosis centers on clinical observation. Tremor is conveniently classified by its relationship to the conditions of rest, postural maintenance, and movement. The three major clinical types of tremor are thus resting, postural, and kinetic (intention) (21). Accurate classification of tremor type is important because each type points to a group of specific underlying conditions (Table 82.1), each with specific therapy.

Tremor can usually be distinguished from other hyperkinetic movement disorders by its rhythmicity and the presence or absence of other neurologic signs. A brief review of the characteristics of other involuntary movement disorders will help prevent diagnostic errors. *Chorea* consists of rapid, often distal, nonrhythmic, nonstereotyped movements that often coexist with the slower, writhing movements called *athetosis*. In its extreme, when it is violent or flinging and more proximal, choreoathetosis merges with *ballismus*. *Myoclonus* refers to rapid, brief muscle jerks that affect random body parts, are usually nonrhythmic, may persist during sleep (unlike tremors and other hyperkinetic movement disorders), and commonly occur in the setting of a metabolic or toxic encephalopathy. *Asterixis,* sometimes called negative myoclonus, consists of brief lapses of posture (flapping) of the dorsiflexed hands caused by inhibition of agonist muscle groups; like myoclonus, asterixis most often occurs in the setting of an encephalopathy. *Motor tics* can be distinguished from tremor by their lack of rhythmicity, erratic appearance in different body parts, complexity of movement, and onset in childhood or adolescence, and often by associated vocalizations and behavioral disturbances. Tics are often preceded by a buildup of inner tension that subsides after the tic. Patients may be able temporarily to suppress a tic, whereas most other abnormal movements lack such a degree of voluntary control. *Dystonia* refers to sustained, often proximal twisting movements that lack regular oscillations, although tremorlike movements of the head may occur in spasmodic torticollis, a form of dystonia.

Evaluation of the Patient with Tremor

The history and physical examination are fundamental in the diagnosis of tremors (Table 82.2), and in almost all cases no further workup is necessary. The differential diagnosis, in general practice, is almost always between Parkinson's disease and essential tremor.

History

Important historical information includes the temporal onset of the tremor, associated neurologic symptoms, family history, a survey of medications and other medical illnesses, and whether the tremor is suppressed by alcohol. Almost all varieties of tremor increase in amplitude under stress, diminish with relaxation, and disappear during sleep. The impact of the tremor on the patient determines whether treatment is indicated. Some patients do not find their tremor disabling and seek medical attention only for diagnostic purposes; young patients with essential tremor often just need reassurance that their tremor is benign and that they do not have Parkinson's disease or another degenerative disorder. However, most patients find the tremor physically or emotionally problematic.

Emphasis should be placed on the *activities of daily living* (ADLs). Patients with tremor typically have trouble with tasks requiring fine motor control such as buttoning, feeding, shaving, brushing their teeth, writing, and cooking. Embarrassment is often an unvoiced source of disability, and patients should be questioned about social isolation caused by the tremor. The ADLs also provide objective parameters for judging the effectiveness of therapy.

Table 82.1.   Conditions Associated with the Three Major Types of Tremor

Resting Tremor
Parkinson's disease
Secondary parkinsonism: postencephalitic, toxic (neuroleptics, reserpine, carbon monoxide, manganese, carbon disulfide, MPTP), tumor, trauma, vascular, metabolic (hypoparathyroidism, chronic hepatocerebral degeneration)
Heterogeneous disorders with parkinsonian features: striatonigral degeneration, olivopontocerebellar atrophy, progressive supranuclear palsy, Wilson's disease

Postural Tremor
Exaggerated physiological tremor
　Anxiety, fright, fatigue, exercise
Endocrine: thyrotoxicosis, hypoglycemia, pheochromocytoma
Drugs: any sympathomimetics, amiodarone, caffeine, theophylline, L-dopa, lithium, tricyclic antidepressants, neuroleptics, thyroid hormone, hypoglycemic agents, withdrawal from alcohol and sedative-hypnotic drugs
Essential tremor
　Familial (autosomal dominant)
　Sporadic
　With other neurologic disorders: parkinsonism, torsion dystonia, spasmodic torticollis, neuropathy

Kinetic or Intention Tremor (Cerebellar Dysfunction)
Cerebellar degeneration, infarction
Multiple sclerosis
Wilson's disease
Drugs and toxins: phenytoin, barbiturates, lithium, alcohol, mercury, 5-fluorouracil
Miscellaneous cerebellar and cerebellofugal lesions

Adapted from Jankovic J, Fahn S. Physiologic and pathologic tremors: diagnosis, mechanism, and management. Ann Intern Med 93:460, 1980.
MPTP, 1-methyl-4-phenyl-1,2,3,6-tetrahydropyridine.

Physical Examination

The objectives of the physical examination are to determine the anatomic localization, frequency, and conditions of maximal activation of the tremor and to search for associated neurologic signs. Patients should be examined with their hands resting on their laps, with their arms held outstretched, and while performing finger-to-nose and heel-to-shin maneuvers. Samples of handwriting and a drawing of a spiral should also be obtained. Observations while the patient is drinking from a cup or using a fork or spoon are also helpful in assessing functional impairment.

The *resting tremor of parkinsonism* is characterized by 3- to 6-Hz flexion–extension at the metacarpophalangeal joints, abduction–adduction of the thumb, and pronation–supination of the forearm; these produce the so-called pill-rolling tremor. Resting tremor is often brought out by having the patient walk or by distracting the patient with conversation or mental arithmetic. Early in its course, the parkinsonian tremor is almost always unilateral, which is one of the most helpful signs distinguishing it from essential tremor. Essential tremor almost always begins bilaterally, although it may be asymmetric.

Postural tremor is characteristic of essential tremor and consists of 6- to 12-Hz symmetric flexion–extension at the wrists and shoulders. It is brought on by having the patient assume an antigravity posture of the upper extremities (i.e., outstretched arms), and it is not present when the arms are resting against the body or on a surface. Essential tremor may persist during finger-to-nose testing, leading to the misdiagnosis of a cerebellar tremor.

Kinetic tremor (*also called intention tremor*) is encountered most commonly in cerebellar disease and is characterized by 3- to 5-Hz irregular oscillations as the limb approaches a target. This type of tremor is often accompanied by inaccuracies in movement direction

Table 82.2.   Principal Features of Different Tremor Types and Their Treatment

	Resting (Parkinsonian)	Postural (Essential)	Kinetic or Intention (Cerebellar)
History			
Age at onset	60 yr and older	All ages, more common after age 60	All ages
Family history	Negative	Often positive (autosomal dominant)	Rarely positive
Response to alcohol	No effect	Often suppresses tremor	No effect
Physical Examination			
Frquency	3–6 Hz[a]	6–12 Hz	3–5 Hz
Symmetry	Almost always begins unilaterally	Symmetric	Either symmetric or asymmetric
Body part(s) affected	Arms > legs	Hand > head > voice	Arms > legs > trunk/head
Associated signs	Bradykinesia, rigidity, postural instability	None	Dysarthria, nystagmus, broad-based gait
Treatment			
	Anticholinergics	Primidone	Stereotactic surgery
	Amantadine	Propranolol	
	L-dopa	Alprazolam	
	Bromocriptine	Stereotactic surgery	
	Pergolide		
	Selegiline		
	Stereotactic surgery		

[a]H$_z$ (Hertz), cycles per second.

(dysmetria). In acquired cerebellar diseases, such as strokes and multiple sclerosis, kinetic tremors are often asymmetric, whereas heredofamilial and sporadic degenerative diseases involving the cerebellum produce bilateral, symmetric tremor. Conditions that may mimic this aspect of cerebellar disease include marked essential tremor (which may impair purposeful movements) and proprioceptive loss; careful assessment of all of the patient's signs and symptoms usually makes it possible to distinguish these conditions from true cerebellar dysfunction (see Table 82.3, which compares cerebellar and proprioceptive incoordination). Unlike patients with Parkinson's disease or essential tremor, patients with cerebellar impairment rarely present complaining only of tremor. Additional signs pointing toward the cerebellum include gait ataxia, dysarthria, and nystagmus.

COMMON CONDITIONS PRESENTING WITH TREMOR
Parkinson's Disease

The typical resting tremor of Parkinson's disease is discussed below.

Physiologic and Exaggerated Physiologic Tremor

Most people have a barely perceptible postural tremor, so-called physiologic tremor, that may be best appreciated by placing a piece of paper over the outstretched hands. Although asymptomatic, this tremor may be transiently exacerbated during systemic illness, metabolic derangements, stress, and by the use or withdrawal of certain drugs or alcohol (Table 82.1).

The most important step in management is identification and removal of the offending cause; resolution of the tremor confirms the diagnosis of exaggerated physiologic tremor. Although discontinuation of tremorogenic drugs usually leads to prompt resolution of the tremor, it may take 1 to 2 weeks for the tremor to resolve after resolution of a systemic illness or a severe metabolic abnormality.

If the underlying condition cannot be eliminated (e.g., in patients requiring lithium for manic–depressive illness), the tremor can often be suppressed using medications for essential tremor. For patients subject to situational anxiety, manifested by exaggerated physiologic tremor, prophylactic treatment with propranolol (20 to 40 mg) taken 1 hour before an anxiety-producing situation (e.g., public speaking) may be helpful.

Essential Tremor

Essential tremor (ET), the most common form of postural tremor, affects more than 1 million Americans (13,20). Essential tremor is synonymous with heredofamilial tremor, benign essential tremor, and senile tremor. No neuropathologic abnormalities have been identified in ET, but physiologic evidence suggests that both the central and peripheral nervous systems are involved. The onset is insidious and may begin as early as childhood, but ET characteristically presents in adulthood, usually after age 50. Unlike the tremor of Parkinson's disease, which typically makes the patient seek medical attention within months of onset of the tremor, patients with ET often give a history of tremor going back many years. At least 50% of patients with ET give a positive family history; the inheritance is autosomal dominant.

In its prototypical form, ET is characterized by a bilateral and symmetric tremor of the hands, but it may also affect other body parts either in isolation, commonly the head or voice, or combined with a hand tremor. At least half of patients with ET notice a beneficial effect from small amounts of alcohol (19). Although its regular use to suppress tremor should be discouraged, when used sparingly alcohol is an effective treatment for ET, particularly when exacerbated by situational stress. There does not seem to be an increased prevalence of alcoholism among patients with ET (30).

Treatment

When ET begins to interfere with the ADLs or causes significant embarrassment, treatment is indicated. Before starting medication, patients should be told that the goal of treatment is not to abolish the tremor, which

Table 82.3. Characteristics of Cerebellar and Sensory (Proprioceptive) Incoordination

Observation or Examination	Cerebellar	Sensory
Influence of vision	Elimination of visual aid (night, eyes closed) does not affect symptoms or signs	Symptoms and signs markedly increased by eliminating visual aid
Sensation	No necessary sensory problems (although may be superimposed, as in alcoholic cerebellar degeneration and sensory neuropathy)	Impaired position and vibration sense is sine qua non for diagnosis
Finger–nose–finger or toe–finger testing of coordination	Could be marked intention tremor and dysmetria (inaccuracy); affected limbs depend on site of lesion	Marked intention tremor and dysmetria (inaccuracy), usually most marked in legs
Gait	Wide-based, asynchronous limb movements (depending on nature of the lesion)	Wide-based, high-stepping foot-slapping (steppage) gait (often caused by foot drop from motor neuropathy)
Romberg testing	Patient equally unsteady with eyes open or closed	Patient can find a stable position with eyes open, but becomes markedly unsteady with eyes closed (positive Romberg)

is rarely possible, but instead to reduce its severity and allow them to function better. The patient's ADLs should be used as a gauge to determine the effectiveness of treatment.

The two medications most effective for ET are propranolol (Inderal or generic) and primidone (Mysoline). The drugs are equally effective and may be synergistic (32).

Propranolol is started at 10 mg twice per day in elderly patients and gradually increased, depending on the beneficial response and appearance of side effects, to a maximum of 320 mg/day. Once a stable dosage has been reached, patients can be converted to Inderal LA, as the once-daily administration is preferred by most patients (31). In younger patients, treatment can be started with Inderal LA, with a gradual escalation of the dosage. Although other β-blockers have also been shown to be effective for ET, none is superior to propranolol (26,35). Metoprolol has the theoretical advantage of being a β_1-selective blocker and therefore safer to use in patients with ET and asthma, but at higher dosages the β_1 selectivity is diminished. In general, β-blockers should be avoided in the presence of bronchospastic disease, second- or third-degree heart block, congestive heart failure, or insulin-dependent diabetes. Additional practical details about β-blockers are found in Chapter 62 ("Hypertension").

Primidone, an anticonvulsant, was found by serendipity to improve ET. The mechanism of action of primidone is unknown, but its effect does not appear to result from either of its metabolites, phenylethylmalonamide and phenobarbital (33). Primidone is available as scored tablets in two strengths, 50 and 250 mg. The starting dosage must be very low (e.g., 25 mg/day) because occasional patients, especially the elderly, develop severe side effects after even a single small dose, known as the first-dose phenomenon. Symptoms include dizziness, lethargy, confusion, nausea, sedation, and ataxia, which usually diminish with continued use. The dose is initially given at bedtime and then gradually escalated to a maximum of 250 mg three times per day as tolerated. In general, if patients show no response to low dosages (250 mg/day), it is rare for higher dosages to be effective.

If there is a beneficial but suboptimal response to either propranolol or primidone used alone, the two should be combined beginning at low dosages and increasing in small increments, watching carefully for side effects, particularly in elderly patients. Blood levels of primidone or phenobarbital are not helpful (unless toxicity or noncompliance is suspected) because they do not correlate with its tremor-suppressing effect.

The *benzodiazepine alprazolam* (Xanax) has also been shown to be effective in the treatment of ET (23). The maintenance dosage is 0.75 to 3.0 mg/day, in divided doses. Its rapid onset of action and intermediate half-life, in comparison with other benzodiazepines, allow for its intermittent use when situational stress temporarily exacerbates ET (13). Practical de-

tails regarding alprazolam are found in Chapter 13 ("Anxiety").

The most recent drug shown to be effective for some patients with ET is *methazolamide* (Neptazane), a carbonic anhydrase inhibitor; its effectiveness has not been uniform and further testing is under way (5,40).

When ET is disabling and poorly controlled with optimal medical therapy, consideration should be given to referral to a neurosurgeon for *stereotactic thalamotomy.* When carried out at a center experienced in the procedure, stereotactic thalamotomy has a high success rate with minimal morbidity (18,41). Patients with severe essential tremor should be encouraged to join the International Tremor Foundation, which serves as a resource for education and support (833 West Washington Blvd., Chicago, IL 60607).

Tremor Caused by Cerebellar Dysfunction (Kinetic or Intention Tremor)

Tremor is rarely the sole presenting sign of cerebellar dysfunction, and most often, the underlying disease is already known or readily apparent (multiple sclerosis, stroke, drug intoxication, long-standing alcoholism, or head trauma). Occasionally, severe essential tremor may be exacerbated with action, giving the impression of cerebellar disease, but the faster frequency, prominent postural component, and lack of associated cerebellar signs usually suffice to distinguish the ET from cerebellar dysfunction.

With the exception of drug-induced cerebellar tremor (Table 82.1), which should be managed by discontinuation or reduction of the dosage of the offending drug, a patient with newly diagnosed cerebellar tremor should be referred to a neurologist. Unless the underlying disease is amenable to treatment, there is little that can be done medically for cerebellar tremor. Adding weights to the affected limbs may offer a small amount of improvement but seldom enough to translate into a functional change. As is the case with severe essential tremor, stereotactic thalamotomy is a viable solution for disabling cerebellar tremor (41).

Primary Writing Tremor and Orthostatic Tremor

Two uncommon but distinct types of tremor are primary writing tremor (28) and primary orthostatic tremor (22).

Primary writing tremor is one variant of a group of task-specific tremors. These are characterized by maximal activation during a specific task. Primary writing tremor occurs exclusively when patients attempt to write. It probably is related to ET but may share some features in common with dystonic writer's cramp (50). Writing tremor may respond to drugs used to treat essential tremor (see above) or anticholinergics used to treat dystonia (see below).

Primary orthostatic tremor is characterized by rapid shaking of the legs, only with standing, and it may respond to clonazepam (0.5 to 3.0 mg/day).

PARKINSON'S DISEASE AND "PARKINSONISM"

History

In 1817 James Parkinson, a London general practitioner, published his *Essay on the Shaking Palsy,* based on observations of six patients (44). Although much has subsequently been learned about the pathology, pathophysiology, and treatment of what later became known as Parkinson's disease (PD), little has been added to Parkinson's original clinical description of the movement disorder: involuntary tremulous motion, with lessened muscular power, in parts not in action and even when supported; with a propensity to bend the trunk forward and to pass from a walking to a running pace. However, Parkinson did not appreciate the muscular rigidity or the high frequency of depression and cognitive impairment associated with the disease.

Epidemiology

PD is one of the most common neurologic diseases in the ambulatory setting. Epidemiologic studies demonstrate varying incidence and prevalence rates among different geographic, socioeconomic, and racial groups, but no one group has been found to be unaffected by PD. In the United States, the *prevalence rate* is approximately 100 per 100,000 for people under 50 years of age and more than 600 per 100,000 for people over 70. The overall *annual incidence* in the general population is approximately 18 per 100,000; in the 70 to 79 age group the annual incidence is 1 to 2 cases per 1,000. The average age of onset is 60 years, with equal distribution between sexes. Young-onset of PD has been described in a review article (17).

Causes

The cause of PD has remained elusive despite tremendous advances in understanding other aspects of the disease. Interest has focused on three main areas: infectious disease, genetics, and environmental toxins. A *viral cause* for PD was suggested by the occurrence of a permanent parkinsonian syndrome after the epidemic of encephalitis lethargica (1918 to 1922) plus the appearance of transient parkinsonian features after other encephalitides. Attempts to identify viral inclusions or serologic markers of prior viral infection have been unsuccessful, as have attempts to transmit PD to nonhuman primates. A *genetic basis* for PD seems unlikely because there is not a higher prevalence of PD among first-degree relatives of patients when compared with those of the spouse, and twin studies have not demonstrated a higher-than-expected concordance rate. Recently, however, there has been a resurgence of interest in a genetic predisposition to PD, possibly caused by an intrinsic mitochondrial defect, although results are conflicting (43,52).

More recently, enthusiasm has focused on the possibility of an *environmental toxin* after the discovery that 1-methyl-4-phenyl-1,2,3,6-tetrahydropyridine (MPTP), an impurity of synthetic heroin, produced an outbreak of a severe, permanent parkinsonian syndrome in intravenous drug abusers (4,34). Although neither MPTP nor its active metabolite, MPP+, is known to occur naturally in the environment, the discovery that a toxin can selectively destroy the pigmented dopaminergic cells of the substantia nigra has opened new avenues of research and has also produced an animal model of PD. A current working hypothesis is that PD results from a subclinical toxic exposure leading to an acceleration of the normal aging process of the brain, which includes loss of nigral neurons and depletion of brain dopamine (6) in a genetically susceptible host (27).

Diagnosis and Differential Diagnosis

The cardinal signs of PD include tremor at rest, bradykinesia, muscular cogwheel rigidity, and postural instability. Common symptoms include impaired handwriting (micrographia); trouble walking; falling; poor coordination; trouble arising from a deep chair, couch, or the toilet; drooling; and trouble turning in bed. When the syndrome is fully developed, the diagnosis is straightforward. Errors in diagnosis are uncommon but are most often encountered when the clinical picture is dominated by a severe tremor, in which case essential tremor may be mistakenly diagnosed; when tremor is absent in a patient with unilateral rigidity and bradykinesia (pseudohemiplegic PD), in which case diagnoses of upper or lower motor syndromes are entertained; and when patients are younger than 50, an age at which PD may not be considered in the differential diagnosis.

Although idiopathic Parkinson's disease is the most common diagnosis among patients presenting with parkinsonian signs, a number of other conditions should be considered in the differential diagnosis (Table 82.4) (25). It has been estimated that as many as 20% of patients who carry the diagnosis of PD actually have another parkinsonian syndrome. The initial clue that a patient may have another parkinsonian syndrome is usually failure to respond to L-dopa. Other indicators are summarized in Table 82.5.

Although a discussion of each of the parkinsonian syndromes in Table 82.4 is beyond the scope of this chapter, three deserve special mention. *Neuroleptic-induced parkinsonism,* described in Chapter 16, may be clinically indistinguishable from idiopathic PD and can be diagnosed only retrospectively when parkinsonian signs resolve after discontinuation of the offending drug. In some patients signs may take as long as 1 year to resolve completely, emphasizing the periodic need to reassess antiparkinsonian therapy. In patients whose signs never resolve, it is likely that the neuroleptic simply uncovered a case of latent PD (56).

Progressive supranuclear palsy is the most common nonpharmacologic mimic of PD. It is distinguished by impaired vertical eye movements, although early in its

Table 82.4. Differential Diagnosis of Parkinsonism

Toxins
Manganese
Carbon monoxide
Carbon disulfide
Cyanide
Methanol
MPTP

Drug-Induced
Neuroleptics
Metoclopramide (Reglan)

Multisystem Degenerations
Progressive supranuclear palsy
Shy–Drager syndrome
Olivopontocerebellar atrophy
Striatonigral degeneration
Amylotrophic lateral sclerosis–PD–dementia complex of Guam

Primary Dementing Illnesses
Alzheimer's disease
Creutzfeldt–Jakob syndrome

Heredofamilial Diseases
Wilson's disease
Juvenile Huntington's disease
Hallervorden–Spatz

Multi-Infarct State

Calcification of the Basal Ganglia
Idiopathic
Hypoparathyroidism

Postencephalitic

Trauma
Dementia pugilistica

course ocular motility may be full with the only clinical clue being slow vertical saccades. Other distinguishing features include neck extension as opposed to the flexion seen in PD, early dysarthria and dysphagia, early and prominent balance and gait impairment with associated falls, greater axial than appendicular rigidity (axial dystonia), progression to severe disability in 5 to 10 years, and limited response to antiparkinsonian medications (24,47).

Wilson's disease (hepatolenticular degeneration) is an autosomal-recessive condition characterized by copper accumulation throughout the body. Parkinsonian features in a young patient should prompt an investigation for this condition. Liver disease may be present at the onset of neurologic disease, but normal liver studies should not deter one from pursuing the diagnosis. The diagnosis is confirmed by demonstrating Kayser–Fleischer rings (green or golden deposits of copper in the Descemet's membrane of the cornea), low blood ceruloplasmin, and elevated urinary copper excretion (2,53).

Natural History of Parkinson's Disease

Although treatment diminishes the manifestations of PD, the condition is slowly progressive. Neverthe-

less, patients can be reassured that the life span is rarely shortened in PD and that most patients remain functional and fairly independent throughout the course of the illness. Although some patients become incapacitated after many years of PD, this is the exception rather than the rule.

Manifestations

Resting Tremor

Tremor is the presenting complaint in at least 70% of patients with PD. The tremor is maximal when the limb is at rest and has a frequency of 3 to 6 Hz. It consists of flexion–extension at the metacarpophalangeal joints, abduction–adduction of the thumb, and pronation–supination of the forearm, producing the typical pill-rolling morphology. The tremor may affect the legs, lips, tongue, or chin but virtually never affects the head; a tremor of the head suggests essential tremor. The parkinsonian tremor is accentuated by stress and distraction, diminishes with relaxation, and disappears during sleep. Although there may be an associated postural tremor in PD, typically the resting tremor suppresses with posture and movement, which helps to distinguish it from essential tremor (see above).

Rigidity

Rigidity is defined as abnormal plastic resistance to passive movement. There is a ratchety quality throughout the entire range of motion, producing the cogwheel phenomenon.

Patients rarely complain of rigidity per se and instead notice stiffness or often describe the abnormal tone as weakness. Cogwheel rigidity is best felt at the elbow, wrist, or neck and may be demonstrated or enhanced by having the patient perform a maneuver with the contralateral limb such as opening and closing the fist or drawing a circle in the air.

Bradykinesia and Akinesia

Patients with PD have difficulty initiating movements, and their movements are slow and performed with much greater conscious effort. Speech gradually becomes soft, slow, and monotonal. The blink rate is diminished, as is facial expression (hypomimia), producing the so-called masked face. Because rigidity and

Table 82.5. Clinical Features Suggesting a Parkinsonian Syndrome Rather than Idiopathic Parkinson's Disease

Little or no response to L-dopa
Young onset
Early-onset dementia
Rapid progression
Early-onset dysarthria or dysphagia
Prominent and early dysautonomia
Early falling
Impaired ocular motility
Positive family history
Lower motor neuron, cerebellar, or pyramidal signs

akinesia can occur independently of each other, akinesia is not caused solely by rigidity. This becomes apparent when treatment markedly decreases a patient's rigidity but has little or no effect on akinesia.

Gait and Postural Abnormalities

Patients with PD are flexed at multiple joints (neck, hips, knees, elbows, and fingers), producing the typical stooped posture. Arising from a chair is often accomplished only with difficulty; patients may need to rock back and forth several times and eventually push off from arm rests. The gait is slow and shuffling, with diminished associated movements. Turning is done en bloc, with the entire body moving as the feet slowly rotate. There is a tendency to progress involuntarily from walking to running (festination), seemingly in an attempt to catch up with the body's center of gravity thrown forward by the flexed posture. A patient may describe festination as like chasing your shadow. Patients have difficulty maintaining balance and are often unable to correct for a rapid postural displacement, particularly backward. The combination of the flexed posture, bradykinesia, freezing, festination, and impaired postural righting reflexes leads to one of the major problems in the latter stages of PD: falling.

Other Associated Symptoms or Signs

Seborrhea and excessive perspiration and facial oiliness are both common, and although often attributed to inadequate hygiene caused by physical impairment, they are more likely an intrinsic part of the disease process.

Dysphagia often surfaces in the latter stages of the disease when it contributes significantly to morbidity and mortality caused by inanition and aspiration pneumonia. Although not completely understood, swallowing abnormalities have been demonstrated at various levels: the voluntary muscles of the oral cavity plus the involuntary muscles of the pharynx and esophagus. Solids are usually more of a problem than liquids. If patients with advanced PD are unable to maintain sufficient caloric intake, a discussion of the pros and cons of tube feeding should be held with the patient and family.

Sialorrhea is probably the result of decreased initiation of swallowing rather than overproduction of saliva; this can be treated with a low dosage of an anticholinergic (see below).

Autonomic dysfunction may occur in PD itself and as a side effect of antiparkinsonian medication. When the clinical picture is dominated by severe dysautonomia, particularly when accompanied by cerebellar and lower motor neuron signs, with rapid progression and poor response to drugs for PD, this is known as the Shy–Drager syndrome (54). Orthostatic hypotension and constipation are the most common autonomic signs in PD, but bladder dysfunction and impotence are also encountered. In each case, medications may be at fault and a search for other causes should be carried out before the defects are ascribed to PD.

Unvoiced Symptoms in Parkinson's Disease

Some of the most bothersome problems in Parkinson's disease are never discussed by the patient, spouse, or physician. A helpful mnemonic to remember these problems is the ABCs and the DEFs of Parkinson's disease.

A stands for *amorous activity.* Impotence is common in Parkinson's disease and women may also experience sexual dysfunction (3). Levodopa may cause increased and often inappropriate sexual interest or activity.

B stands for *burden.* Many patients are paralyzed more by the fear of losing their independence than by the paralysis of the disease itself.

C stands for *caregiver.* Parkinson's disease places a burden not only on the patient but also on the caregiver. Caregivers may experience anger, resentment, frustration, fatigue, guilt, and loneliness. During each office visit, caregivers should be asked how they are holding up.

D stands for *depression,* which is discussed below.

E stands for *embarrassment.* This is particularly common in patients who have large-amplitude tremors and often leads to social isolation. Many patients are reticent to admit how embarrassed they are.

Finally, *F* stands for *fear of the future.* Many patients spend considerable time worrying about their future and often ask themselves, "Will I die of Parkinson's? Will I go into a nursing home? Will I need a wheelchair? Will I lose my mind?" Yet these fears are often unvoiced. Patients can be reassured that today, with treatment, most patients can expect to lead a normal life-span and, generally, maintain their independence. Only a small minority of patients with Parkinson's end up severely disabled, in nursing homes, or dying of complications of immobility.

Treatment

The treatment of PD can be divided into patient and family education and pharmacologic treatment.

Patient and Family Education

Education consists of explaining to the patient and to family members the nature of PD, particularly its very slow progression and the fact that with treatment most patients can expect to remain functional and maintain a normal lifestyle. Patient-oriented books such as *Parkinson's Disease: A Guide for Patient and Family* (see "General References") and support groups are often helpful, sometimes as much to the caregiver as to the patient, but these should be recommended with caution in the early stages of the disease because patients often concentrate only on the worst prognosis. Patients should know that their goals for social, professional, and physical activity will be used to guide decisions about when to initiate treatment and to make changes in the dosing regimen. Before starting treatment it should be emphasized to patients that the goal is not to eliminate all of the symptoms and signs of PD but rather to maintain an acceptable degree of functioning.

Physical activities should be encouraged, particularly walking. However, activities that can be dangerous if balance is impaired or motor response is delayed should be avoided (e.g., skiing, bicycling, driving in heavy traffic, using power tools).

Soft or slow speech and poverty of facial expression can produce the impression of lack of interest during a conversation. Therefore, patients should be advised tactfully to make a conscious effort to let others know that they are interested, despite their lack of facial expression. Having patients practice speech by reading aloud and by recording and listening to their voice may help to overcome their reticence to speak.

Fear of falling is experienced by virtually all parkinsonian patients. Walking with hands clasped behind the back or, when symptoms are advanced, using a standard walker or one on wheels (but not a cane) may improve stability. A rolling walker is often more helpful than a standard walker. Two tests often predict success with a rolling walker: first, if the patient feels more secure walking behind a grocery cart, and second, if the patient is more secure when observed walking behind a wheelchair, holding onto the handles. Patients' living environments should be free of obstacles that may cause them to stumble, and they should avoid walking in places where they are apt to encounter obstacles (e.g., rocky terrain).

When the patient becomes progressively disabled, the assistance of others is necessary to avoid as much as possible the complications of bradykinesia and sedentary living. Such assistance includes periodic change in the patient's position to avoid skin breakdown, passive range of motion of the limbs and digits to avoid flexion contractures, and as much mobility and social and intellectual stimulation as possible.

Pharmacologic Treatment

General Principles. Pharmacologic treatment is based on what is known of the neurotransmitter defect in PD. Two major neurotransmitters found in the basal ganglia are dopamine and acetylcholine. In PD, loss of the dopaminergic cells in the substantia nigra leads to *depletion of dopamine* in the striatum and a relative *excess of acetylcholine.* The two main classes of antiparkinsonian drugs currently available work either by increasing dopamine activity directly or indirectly (dopaminergic drugs) or by decreasing acetylcholine activity (anticholinergic drugs) (see details regarding available strengths, recommended dosages, and schedules in Table 82.6).

Stepwise Initiation and Adjustment of Medication. The pharmacologic regimen for each patient must be individualized, but the general rule is to use the least amount of medication needed to achieve reasonable control of the symptoms and signs of PD. Early, when there is no significant impairment of ADLs or of occupational or social functioning, symptomatic treatment is generally withheld unless the tremor or other signs cause embarrassment.

During the course of PD, it is necessary to use a stepwise approach to prescribing, assessing, and adjusting antiparkinsonian medications as follows:

- As symptoms progress, it has been recommended traditionally that *monotherapy* should be initiated with either an anticholinergic or amantadine alone. Because neither of these drugs alleviates symptoms as predictably as L-dopa, L-dopa monotherapy should be offered to any patient for whom reliable symptom control may be crucial (e.g., a draftsperson whose occupation is at stake).

Table 82.6.   Drugs Used for Parkinson's Disease

Drug	Available Preparation (mg)	Schedule	Starting Dose (mg)	Maintenance Dose (mg)
Anticholinergic Agents (Representative Examples)				
Trihexyphenidyl (Artane, generic)	Scored tablets: 2, 5 Elixir: 2 mg/5 mL	3–4 times daily	2	2–10
	Time-release capsules: 5	Once daily	(May be substituted for regular Artane after maintenance dose is determined)	(May be substituted for regular Artane after maintenance dose is determined)
Benztropine mesylate (Cogentin, generic)	Tablets: 0.5, 1, 2	Once or twice daily	1	0.5–6
Dopaminergic Agents				
Carbidopa L-dopa (Sinemet, generic)	Scored tablets: 10/100, 25/100, 25/250	2–4 times daily	50/200 in 2 divided doses	400–500 L-dopa
Sinemet CR	Scored tablets: 50/200	2–4 times daily	50/200 twice daily	500–1000 L-dopa
Bromocriptine (Pariodel)	Scored tablets: 2.5 Capsules: 5.0	2–3 times daily	1.25 daily	7.5–30
Pergolide (Permax)	Scored tablets: 0.05, 0.25, 1.0	3 times daily	0.05 daily	1–3
Selegiline[a] (Eldepryl)	Tablets: 5.0	2 times daily	5 daily	10
Anticholinergic or Dopaminergic Activity				
Amantadine (Symmetrel, generic)	Capsules: 100	2 times daily	200 daily	200

[a]Alternative generic name: deprenyl.

- Almost all patients eventually require *levodopa* (L-dopa), but there is controversy about the optimal time to begin this drug. Proponents for early treatment cite studies indicating that this leads to decreased morbidity and mortality (11). On the other hand, the length of time a patient is on L-dopa may be a risk factor for later motor complications (10,12). The current consensus is that clinical status is determined mainly by disease duration and that early initiation of L-dopa does not have a major adverse effect on the patient's course (8). A reasonable approach is to explain to the patient the options above for initial monotherapy. For patients not treated initially with L-dopa, this drug should be added when PD begins to limit function.
- Once the patient has responded to L-dopa, an attempt should be made gradually to *reduce the dosage of other antiparkinsonian medications* and, if possible, discontinue them. Some patients deteriorate as this is attempted, necessitating continued polypharmacy.
- As the disease progresses and L-dopa alone is insufficient to control the symptoms and signs, a *direct-acting dopamine receptor agonist* such as bromocriptine or pergolide or the monoamine oxidase (MAO) inhibitor deprenyl, which prevents catabolism of dopamine, should be added. Some evidence suggests that beginning with a combination of L-dopa and an agonist or beginning with an agonist alone is associated with a reduced incidence of later motor fluctuations including on–off and dyskinesias (see below). The following agents may also preserve L-dopa's effectiveness in late PD: two dopamine agonists (ropinirole and pramipexole, both were approved by the FDA in 1997), which may have fewer side effects than bromocriptine and pergolide; and two catechol-o-methyltransferase inhibitors (tolcapone and entacapone), which prolong carbidopa/L-dopa activity but have not yet been approved.

Anticholinergics. In some patients, anticholinergics are helpful in the early stages of PD, particularly when tremor is a predominant sign. Although a number of different preparations are available, none has clear superiority. They generally take 2 to 4 weeks before the maximal effect is observed. Side effects are common and may be unacceptable. They include dry mouth (which may help sialorrhea), blurred vision, urinary retention, constipation, memory loss, and confusion. Narrow angle glaucoma is a contraindication to these agents. Anticholinergics should be avoided or used cautiously in very elderly or demented patients, who are often more sensitive to the side effects of these medications.

Amantadine (Symmetrel). Originally marketed as an anti-influenzal drug, amantadine was found to help some patients with PD. Its exact mechanism of action is not known but it has been shown to have both anticholinergic and dopaminergic activity. The full impact of amantadine may not be seen for 2 weeks. Although amantadine is helpful in the early stages of PD, the beneficial effect of this drug is generally short-lived, approximately 6 months. Once L-dopa has been added, it is often possible to taper off amantadine without any clinical deterioration. Side effects include pedal edema, confusion, hallucinations, and livedo reticularis. In the latter stages of PD, when the effect of L-dopa wanes or motor fluctuations appear, the addition of amantadine occasionally produces temporary improvement.

L-Dopa (as Sinemet) The hallmark of PD is depletion of dopamine in the striatum, and replacement of dopamine is the mainstay of treatment. Dopamine does not cross the blood–brain barrier and is given instead in the form of its precursor, L-dopa, which does cross the blood–brain barrier. To avoid the extracerebral conversion of L-dopa to dopamine by peripheral dopa decarboxylase, L-dopa is combined with carbidopa, a decarboxylase inhibitor, as Sinemet or now-available generic preparations. Scored tablets combine 10 mg carbidopa with 100 mg of L-dopa, or 25 mg of carbidopa with either 100 or 250 mg of L-dopa. The controlled-release preparation, Sinemet CR (7), combines 50 mg of carbidopa with 200 mg of L-dopa; because of its diminished bioavailability, less than the full 200 mg is absorbed. *At least 75 mg of carbidopa per day* is required to inhibit dopa decarboxylase. At lower dosages of carbidopa, nausea and vomiting caused by dopamine are more likely. Because it does not provide enough carbidopa, the 10/100 preparation of Sinemet is useful only for adding L-dopa to a regimen that already contains 75 mg of carbidopa.

The usual starting dosage is one tablet (25/100) twice per day, but in the elderly it is best to begin with half tablets. De novo treatment with Sinemet CR is generally equally efficacious, beginning with one tablet per day and shortly thereafter increasing to twice per day. Although Sinemet is absorbed best on an empty stomach, this also usually leads to an increased incidence of nausea; therefore Sinemet is initially prescribed with meals and, once tolerated, can be taken 0.5 hour earlier. Although some patients have an immediate beneficial effect, it may take several weeks before a change is noticed. After that time, if there is no improvement, the dosage is gradually increased every few days to three to four times daily, using full or half-tablet increments, until the patient has shown significant improvement or a total daily dosage of 400 to 600 mg of L-dopa per day has been reached.

After about 5 years of treatment, the previously consistent response to Sinemet wanes and fluctuations in motor function begin to appear in at least 50% of patients (38,49). Initially, these fluctuations follow a predictable pattern: The beneficial effect of a dose of Sinemet is noted within about 0.5 hour and lasts from 1 to 3 hours; then there is another 0.5 to 1 hour of loss of effect. This is referred to as *end-of-dose wearing off.* The initial treatment for wearing off of Sinemet is to decrease the dosing interval, often using half-tablets without increasing the total daily dosage, or to change to Sinemet CR (42). Previously, the total dosage of L-dopa was advanced to at least 1 g/day, but a more recent approach has been gradually to increase the dosage to no more than 400 to 600 mg and to start a dopamine receptor agonist early. This approach is based on the observation that as the disease progresses, patients become more sensitive to the dyskinesias caused by L-dopa (see below).

Less predictable response fluctuations, called *the "on–off" phenomenon,* are manifested by frequent and often rapid changes in parkinsonian signs with freezing, hesitation when initiating movements, and akinesia. This class of fluctuations proves much more difficult to treat, but the addition of an agonist or conversion to Sinemet CR may help.

Drug-induced dyskinesias (choreiform movements of the limbs, face, or trunk) initially appear during peak level, approximately 1.5 to 2 hours after Sinemet is taken. They can be reduced by decreasing the Sinemet dosage and making up the difference with an agonist or converting to Sinemet CR. Like "off" periods, dyskinesias may also occur unpredictably, and it is not uncommon in the late stages of the disease for patients to have a complex mix of "off" time, "on" time, and dyskinesias. When this mix of motor fluctuations begins to occur, consultation with a neurologist experienced in treating PD is suggested.

The reasons for fluctuations in response to Sinemet may include erratic gastric emptying and duodenal absorption, competition with dietary amino acids for transport across the intestine and blood–brain barrier, inability of the remaining nigral dopaminergic neurons to metabolize and store dopamine, and alterations in the number and sensitivity of postsynaptic dopamine receptors. "Off" time may diminish if dietary protein is limited during the day to less than 7 g, and the balance is made up during the evening meal. This change eliminates the competition between large dietary amino acids and Sinemet for transport across the intestine and blood–brain barrier. Although the amount of time "off" has been found to diminish with this technique, dyskinesias may increase, necessitating a decrease in the dosage of Sinemet (48). Improvement in erratic motor fluctuations has also been attained with delivery of a constant amount of levodopa directly into the duodenum with an infusion pump (51).

Drug holidays were once advocated when the effectiveness of Sinemet diminished. This method has fallen out of favor because of the common complications encountered as patients deteriorated while off treatment and because of the transient nature of the improvement when Sinemet was restarted.

Although most patients tolerate Sinemet well, *side effects* are common, particularly in the elderly or in patients with dementia (see below). These include confusion, hallucinations, hypersexuality, and fluid retention. *Orthostatic hypotension* is common; because this is often a finding in untreated PD, supine and standing blood pressure should be checked before starting Sinemet and after each dosage increase. All side effects decrease with reduction of the dosage.

Direct Dopamine Receptor Agonists. These drugs have the theoretical advantage of acting directly on postsynaptic dopamine receptors and therefore bypassing the ineffective nigral dopaminergic neurons. As mentioned above, they are useful adjuncts to Sinemet, particularly when its effectiveness wanes and when there are motor fluctuations. When one of these drugs is added, the Sinemet dosage is maintained. In the United States, the currently available agonists include the ergot derivatives bromocriptine (Parlodel), pergolide (Permax), and two recently approved dopamine agonists pramipexole (Mirapex) and ropinirole (Requip) (46a).

Bromocriptine is available as scored 2.5-mg tablets and 5-mg capsules. The starting dosage is 1.25 mg at night, and the dosage is gradually increased, every 3 to 5 days, in 1.25-mg increments, aiming for a maintenance dosage of 7.5 to 30 mg/day in two or three divided doses.

Pergolide is available as scored 0.05-, 0.25-, and 1.0-mg tablets. It is started at 0.05 mg/day for 2 days and increased gradually (about every 3 days) to a maintenance dosage of 1 to 3 mg/day in two or three divided doses. Although pergolide is at least 10 times more potent than bromocriptine, at present there does not appear to be any compelling advantage of one over the other (36), although some patients may find one more tolerable or beneficial than the other.

The *side effects* of bromocriptine and pergolide are similar to those of Sinemet, but there is a much lower incidence of drug-induced dyskinesias. Both drugs are tolerated poorly in the elderly and should be avoided in demented patients because of their propensity to cause confusion, hallucinations, and psychosis.

Selegiline (Eldepryl). Selegiline (also called deprenyl) is a MAO B inhibitor that prevents the catabolism and reuptake of dopamine. It has been shown to be an effective adjunct to Sinemet for patients with response fluctuations (16,37). Because only the B form of MAO, which exists exclusively in the central nervous system, is inhibited, it is not necessary to restrict dietary tyramine to prevent systemic hypertension. Although dyskinesias may be exacerbated, necessitating a reduction in the Sinemet dosage, deprenyl otherwise has few side effects. Reported side effects include nausea, dry mouth, dizziness, psychosis, and confusion. After a brief trial of 5 mg/day the patient should advance to a maintenance dosage of 5 mg twice a day. Because it may cause insomnia, both doses should be given early in the day.

Treatment to Delay the Progression of PD

In addition to providing symptomatic treatment for PD, it was once thought that *selegiline* slowed disease progression. This tentative conclusion was based on results indicating that in patients with early PD who were treated with selegiline, the progression of PD was slower than in placebo-treated patients (45,57). Follow-up of the DATATOP cohort indicated that some of the "prophylactic" effect of selegiline is caused by symptomatic improvement rather than a delay in the progression of the disease (46). The possible prophylactic effect of selegiline therefore remains controversial.

Vitamin E (tocopherol), another agent that has been tested to delay the progression of PD, is not effective (46).

Surgical Treatment

Stereotactic *thalamotomy* or *pallidotomy,* when performed at a center specializing in the procedure, is a safe, effective treatment for parkinsonian patients with disabling tremor unresponsive to medical therapy, severe fluctuations with dyskinesias, or waning response to L-dopa (29).

In addition to stereotactic surgery for PD, *tissue implantation* also holds promise (1). The original report of improvement following adrenal-to-caudate implantation led to a flurry of clinical trials. Because the results were disappointing, adrenal transplantation has been abandoned in favor of fetal nigral implantation. Recent studies indicate that this procedure, which can be performed with very low morbidity and mortality, improves objective parameters used to assess PD (14,55,58). A large clinical trial now in progress should establish whether fetal nigral cell implantation is efficacious.

Dementia and Depression in Patients with Parkinson's Disease

Dementia

The estimated frequency of dementia in patients with PD varies widely, depending on the population studied, the definition of dementia, and the instruments used to assess cognitive performance. A conservative estimate is that at least 15 to 20% of patients with PD develop dementia (15). Although the incidence of dementia in PD is higher than in nonparkinsonian age-matched controls, it is crucial to appreciate that dementia is not an inevitable feature of PD and thus must be approached with the same search for remediable causes used in nonparkinsonian patients (see Chapter 17). All medications used to treat PD have cognitive and behavioral side effects, particularly the anticholinergics; when cognitive abnormalities occur, an attempt should be made to reduce the dosages of these drugs or, if possible, to discontinue them.

Dementia in patients with PD is occasionally complicated by bothersome hallucinations, agitation, psychosis, insomnia, or a reversal in the sleep–wake cycle. If these problems do not respond to reduction of the dosage of antiparkinsonian medications or use of a mild sedative, a very low dosage of a neuroleptic (see Chapter 16) may be required; it must be recognized that worsening of parkinsonian signs may result but the suppression of intolerable behavior usually leads to an overall improvement in the patient's condition and eases the burden of the caregiver.

Depression

Depression is common in PD, occurring in as many as 50% of patients (9,39). It is not clear to what extent it is the result of an intrinsic neurochemical defect or a depressive reaction to the disability of the disease. Both PD patients and their physicians commonly fail to recognize depression and often mistakenly attribute a decline in motor function to PD when in reality it is the result of depression-induced psychomotor slowing; a rapid decline in a patient's functional status is often a clue to depression.

Depression in PD can be treated very effectively with tricyclic antidepressants or selective serotonin reuptake inhibitors (SSRIs). SSRIs are contraindicated in patients taking selegiline. As depression resolves there is often concurrent improvement in parkinsonian symptoms and signs. In severe cases, particularly when compounded by delusions, agitation, severe anxiety, or psychosis, tricyclics and SSRIs may be either ineffective or not tolerated; in these patients electroconvulsive therapy is the treatment of choice. Chapter 15, "Affective Disorders," contains details about these forms of treatment for depression.

General References*

Tremor

Capildeo R, Findley LJ, eds. Movement disorders: tremor. London: Macmillan, 1984.

Elble RJ, Koller WC, eds. Tremor. Baltimore: Johns Hopkins University Press, 1990.

Jankovic J, Fahn S. Physiologic and pathologic tremors: diagnosis, mechanism, and management. Ann Intern Med 93:460, 1980.

Koller WC. Diagnosis and treatment of tremors. In: Jankovic J, ed. Neurologic clinics. Philadelphia: WB Saunders, 1984;2:449.

Watts RL, Kaller WC. Movement disorders: neurologic principles and practice. New York: McGraw-Hill, 1997.
    Comprehensive text covering all movement disorders.

Parkinson's Disease

Duvoisin RC. Parkinson's disease. A guide for patient and family. 3rd ed. New York: Raven Press, 1991.

Jankovic J, Tolosa E, eds. Parkinson's disease and movement disorders. 2nd ed. Baltimore: Williams & Wilkins, 1993.

Koller WC, ed. Handbook of Parkinson's disease. New York: Marcel Dekker, 1987.

Nadeau SE. Clinical decisions: Parkinson's disease. J Am Geriatr Soc 45:233–240, 1997.

Nutt JG, Hammerstad JP, Gancher ST, eds. Parkinson's disease. St. Louis: CV Mosby, 1992.

Specific References

1. Ahlskog JE. Cerebral transplantation for Parkinson's disease: current progress and future prospects. Mayo Clin Proc 68:578, 1993.
2. Brewer GJ, Yuzbasiyan-Gurkan V. Wilson's disease. Medicine 71:139, 1992.
3. Brown RG, Jahanshahi M, Quinn N, et al. Sexual function in patients with Parkinson's disease and their partners. J Neurol Neurosurg Psychiatry 53:480, 1990.

*Bold print (general references) and bold numerals (specific references) denote published controlled clinical trials, meta-analyses, or consensus-based recommendations.

4. Burns RS, LeWitt PA, Ebert MH, et al. The clinical syndrome of striatal dopamine deficiency. N Engl J Med 312:1418, 1985.
5. Busenbark K, Pahwa R, Hubble J, et al. Double-blind controlled study of methazolamide in the treatment of essential tremor. Neurology 43:1045, 1993.
6. Calne DM, Langston JW. Aetiology of Parkinson's disease. Lancet 2:1457, 1983.
7. Cedarbaum JM. The promise and limitation of controlled-release levodopa administration. Clin Neuropharmacol 12:147, 1989.
8. Cedarbaum JM, Gandy SE, McDowell FH. "Early" initiation of levodopa treatment does not promote the development of motor response fluctuations, dyskinesias, or dementia in Parkinson's disease. Neurology 41:622–629, 1991.
9. Cummings JL. Depression and Parkinson's disease: a review. Am J Psychiatry 149:443, 1992.
10. de Jong GJ, Meerwaldt JD, Schmitz PIM. Factors that influence the occurrence of response variations in Parkinson's disease. Ann Neurol 22:4, 1987.
11. Diamond SG, Markham CH, Hoehn MM, et al. Multi-center study of Parkinson mortality with early versus late dopa treatment. Ann Neurol 22:8, 1987.
12. Duvoisin RC. To treat early or to treat late? Ann Neurol 22:2, 1987.
13. Findley LJ, Koller WC. Essential tremor: a review. Neurology 37:1194, 1987.
14. Freed CR, Breeze RF, Roserberg NL, et al. Survival of implanted fetal dopamine cells and neurological improvement 12 to 46 months after transplantation for Parkinson's disease. N Engl J Med 327:1549, 1992.
15. Gibb WRG. Dementia and Parkinson's disease. Br J Psychiatry 154:596, 1989.
16. Golbe LI. Deprenyl as symptomatic therapy in Parkinson's disease. Clin Neuropharmacol 11:387, 1988.
17. Golbe LI. Young-onset Parkinson's disease: a clinical review. Neurology 41:168, 1991.
18. Goldman MS, Ahlskog JE, Kelly PJ. The symptomatic and functional outcome of stereotactic thalamotomy for medically intractable essential tremor. J Neurosurg 76:924, 1992.
19. Growdon JH, Shahani BT, Young RR. The effect of alcohol on essential tremor. Neurology 25:259, 1975.
20. Haerer AF, Anderson DW, Schoenberg BS. Prevalence of essential tremor. Arch Neurol 39:750, 1982.
21. Hallett M. Classification and treatment of tremor. JAMA 266:1115, 1991.
22. Heilman KM. Orthostatic tremor. Arch Neurol 41:880, 1984.
23. Huber SJ, Paulson GW. Efficacy of alprazolam for essential tremor. Neurology 38:241, 1988.
24. Jankovic J. Progressive supranuclear palsy: clinical and pharmacological update. In: Jankovic J, ed. Neurologic clinics. Vol. 2 of 3. Philadelphia: WB Saunders, 1984.
25. Jankovic J. Parkinsonism-plus syndromes. Mov Disord 4(Suppl 1):S95, 1989.
26. Jefferson D, Jenner P, Marsden C. Beta-adrenoreceptor antagonists in essential tremor. J Neurol Neurosurg Psychiatry 42:904, 1979.
27. Jenner P, Schapira AH, Marsden CD. New insights into the cause of Parkinson's disease. Neurology 42:2241, 1992.
28. Kachi T, Rothwell JC, Cowan JMA, et al. Writing tremor: its relationship to benign essential tremor. J Neurol Neurosurg Psychiatry 48:545, 1985.
29. Kelly PJ, Ahlskog JE, Goerss SJ, et al. Computer assisted stereotactic ventralis lateralis thalamotomy with microelectrode recording control in patients with Parkinson's disease. Mayo Clin Proc 62:655, 1987.
30. Koller WC. Alcoholism in essential tremor. Neurology 33:1074, 1983.
31. Koller WC. Long-acting propranolol in essential tremor. Neurology 35:108, 1985.
32. Koller WC, Biary N, Cone S. Disability in essential tremor: effect of treatment. Neurology 36:1001, 1986.
33. Koller WC, Royce JL. Efficacy of primidone in essential tremor. Neurology 36:121, 1986.
34. Langston JW, Ballard P, Tetrud JW, et al. Chronic parkinsonism in humans due to a product of meperidine-analog synthesis. Science 219:9789, 1983.
35. Larson TA, Teravainen H. Beta-blockers in essential tremor. Lancet 2:533, 1981.
36. Lewitt PA, Ward CD, Larsen TA, et al. Comparison of pergolide and bromocriptine therapy in parkinsonism. Neurology 33:1009, 1983.
37. Lieberman AN, Gopinathan G, Neophytides A. Deprenyl versus placebo in Parkinson's disease. NY State J Med 87:646, 1987.
38. Marsden CD, Parks JD. Success and problems of long-term levodopa therapy in Parkinson's disease. Lancet 1:345, 1977.
39. Mayeux R. A current analysis of behavioral problems in patients with idiopathic Parkinson's disease. Mov Disord 4(Suppl 1):S48, 1989.
40. Muenter MD, Daube JR, Caviness JN. Treatment of essential tremor with methazolamide. Mayo Clin Proc 66:991, 1991.
41. Narabayashi H. Surgical approach to tremor. In: Marsden CD, Fahn S, eds. Movement disorders. London: Butterworths, 1982; 292.
42. Pahwa R, Busenbark K, Huber SJ, et al. Clinical experience with controlled-release carbidopa/levodopa in Parkinson's disease. Neurology 43:677, 1993.
43. Parker WD Jr, Boyson SB, Parks JK. Abnormalities of electron transport chain in idiopathic Parkinson's disease. Ann Neurol 26:719, 1989.
44. Parkinson J. An essay on the shaking palsy. London: Wittingham and Rowland, 1817; Chicago: American Medical Association Press, 1959.
45. Parkinson Study Group. Effect of deprenyl on the progression of disability in early Parkinson's disease. N Engl J Med 321:1364, 1989.
46. Parkinson Study Group. Effects of tocopherol and deprenyl on the progression of disability in early Parkinson's disease. N Engl J Med 328:176, 1993.
46a. Pramipexole and ropinirole for Parkinson's disease. Med Lett 39(1014):109–110, 1997.
47. Reich S. Progressive supranuclear palsy. In: Johnson RT, Grifin JW, eds. Current therapy in neurologic disease. 4th ed. St. Louis: BC Decker, 1993.
48. Riley D, Lang AE. Practical application of a low-protein diet for Parkinson's disease. Neurology 38:1026, 1988.
49. Riley DE, Lang AE. The spectrum of levodopa-related fluctuations in Parkinson's disease. Neurology 43:1459, 1993.
50. Rosenbaum F, Jankovic J. Focal task-specific tremor and dystonia: categorization of occupational movement disorders. Neurology 38:522, 1988.
51. Sage JI, Trooskin S, Sonsalla PK, et al. Long-term duodenal infusion of levodopa for motor fluctuations in parkinsonism. Ann Neurol 24:87, 1988.
52. Schapira AHV, Holt IJ, Sweeny M, et al. Mitochondrial DNA analysis in Parkinson's disease. Mov Disord 5:294, 1990.
53. Scheinberg IH, Sternlieb I. Wilson's disease. Philadelphia: WB Saunders, 1984.
54. Shy GM, Drager GA. A neurological syndrome associated with orthostatic hypotension: a clinical–pathological study. Arch Neurol 2:511, 1968.
55. Spencer DD, Robbins RJ, Naftolin F, et al. Unilateral transplantation of human fetal mesencephalic tissue into the caudate nucleus of patients with Parkinson's disease. N Engl J Med 327:1541, 1992.
56. Stephen PJ, Williamson J. Drug-induced parkinsonism in the elderly. Lancet 2:1082, 1984.
57. Tetrud JW, Langston JW. The effect of deprenyl on the natural history of Parkinson's disease. Science 245:519, 1989.
58. Widner H, Tetrud J, Rehncrona S, et al. Bilateral fetal mesencephalic grafting in two patients with Parkinsonism induced by 1-methyl-4-phenyl-1,2,3-tetrahydropyridine (MPTP). N Engl J Med 327:1556, 1992.

C H A P T E R 83

Cerebrovascular Disease

CONSTANCE J. JOHNSON, MD

OVERVIEW

Epidemiology

Cerebrovascular disease is a major cause of disability and the third leading cause of death in the United States. According to 1997 American Heart Association (AHA) estimates, the annual cost is greater than $18 billion, and there are almost 4 million stroke survivors in this country (2). Approximately 80% of strokes are caused by thrombotic or embolic cerebral infarction, 12% by cerebral hemorrhage, and 8% by subarachnoid hemorrhage. Approximately 28% of strokes occur in people under age 65. The annual death rate from stroke is higher in African Americans (men, 52/100,000; women 40/100,000) than in whites (men, 27/100,000; women 23/100,000) (2).

The death rate from stroke declined by 19.8% from 1984 to 1994 (2). Studies in the 1980s showed that stroke incidence had decreased nationwide and world-wide (20,45). Factors that may have contributed to the decline include more aggressive treatment of hypertension, more effective and early delivery of health care, and better management and recognition of the cardiogenic sources of cerebral embolization. Some community-based studies in the 1980s indicated a later stabilization of the decline; some also showed a possible increase in stroke incidence, a finding that may have resulted from the earlier detection of stroke

because of the introduction of new imaging techniques such as computerized tomography (CT) in the 1980s (6).

Cerebrovascular disease presents two major challenges in ambulatory practice : the prevention of stroke in the large number of people with risk factors that make them stroke prone, and the optimal care of the many stroke survivors in each community.

Risk Factors

A major goal of patient evaluation in ambulatory practice is the identification of the patient with an increased risk of stroke. Patients who have previously had a stroke are an important subgroup of this high-risk population. Community-based data on the natural history of stroke show that the first-year recurrence rate among survivors of a first stroke is approximately 10% and that the 5-year recurrence rate is approximately 20% (32). In addition to a history of stroke and aging, other factors that predispose a patient to stroke are transient episodes of focal cerebral dysfunction of vascular origin called transient ischemic attacks (TIAs), hypertension, certain cardiac disorders, cigarette smoking, diabetes mellitus, and hyperlipidemia.

Transient Ischemic Attacks

Approximately one-third of patients with a TIA subsequently develop a stroke, and the TIA provides a significant warning of impending infarction. The cause, natural history, and treatment of TIAs are discussed in detail later in this chapter.

Hypertension

Data accumulated during the Framingham study indicate that the risks of both nonhemorrhagic and hemorrhagic stroke are strongly related to hypertension. Atherothrombotic brain infarction occurred in hypertensive subjects (blood pressure greater than 160/95) four times more often than in normotensive subjects (27). Evidence from controlled trials shows that stroke risk and other cardiovascular disease risk is significantly reduced by the treatment of hypertension in all patients, including those with a history of cerebrovascular disease (4,7,41–44). The evaluation and long-term management of hypertension are discussed in detail in Chapter 62.

Cardiac Impairment

Patients with cardiac impairment are clearly predisposed to stroke, either directly because of emboli from the heart that lodge in cerebral arteries and lead to cerebral infarction, or indirectly because chronic atherosclerotic cardiac disease is associated with atherothrombotic cerebral disease. Cardioembolic stroke accounts for 15 to 30% of all ischemic strokes and is highly associated with cardiac arrhythmias, particularly atrial fibrillation with or without valvular disease, and with valvular disease, recent myocardial infarction (MI), and dilated cardiomyopathy (8). Data from the Framingham study identified cardiac impairment as a significant risk factor in the occurrence of the more common nonembolic atherothrombotic brain infarction (ABI) (47). Subjects with electrocardiographic evidence of left ventricular hypertrophy (LVH) were nine times more likely to develop ABI than those without this abnormality. Patients with coronary artery disease (CAD) had five times the risk of ABI, and those with radiographic evidence of cardiomegaly had three times the risk. When the contribution of concomitant hypertension was eliminated, LVH and CAD were each associated with a threefold increase in the risk of ABI; the contribution of cardiomegaly on x-ray was not found to be significant when other variables were controlled. On the basis of these findings it was concluded that cardiac impairment, especially if associated with hypertension, significantly heightens the risk of stroke occurrence.

Other Factors

A number of other factors have been associated with an increased incidence of stroke: family history of vascular disease, elevated serum glucose concentration, elevated serum lipid levels, cigarette smoking, elevated blood hematocrit levels, and the presence of a cervical bruit. To date, definitive studies have not been done to establish whether modification of any of these risk factors reduces the likelihood of stroke. With regard to diabetes mellitus, prospective data from the Framingham study indicate an increased risk of cerebral infarction in subjects with even a modest abnormality of glucose tolerance (25). This study also demonstrated that elevated serum lipid levels were associated with increased stroke risk but only in subjects under age 50. A recent meta-analysis of clinical trials has suggested that HMGcoA reductase inhibitors prevent strokes in hyperlipidemic patients (6a). Cigarette smoking clearly increases the risk of ischemic stroke and is a predictor of the presence of significant intracranial and extracranial vascular stenosis (8). The duration of cigarette smoking is predictive of extracranial carotid artery stenosis as detected by duplex scanning (46). Elevated blood hemoglobin and hematocrit levels have also been implicated as possible risk factors, but a cause-and-effect relationship has not been established (26). Oral contraceptive use is associated with a fivefold to tenfold increase in the risk of vascular diseases, including stroke (see details in Chapter 93). For postmenopausal women, hormone replacement therapy (HRT) is protective of the vasculature. Epidemiologic studies demonstrate a decreased risk of ischemic stroke for HRT users (34). Finally, it is generally accepted that the presence of an asymptomatic cervical bruit correlates with an increased incidence of subsequent stroke, but there is controversy regarding the approach to patients with this finding (see below).

ASYMPTOMATIC CAROTID STENOSIS

Asymptomatic carotid stenosis is detected by the presence of a cervical bruit or because a vascular screening test was performed. Bruits occur in 4.5% of the population over 45 years of age (23). A bruit is not pathognomonic of underlying stenosis (see Table 83.1 for other causes). A duplex scan (see description in Chapter 78) can define which patients with bruits have carotid stenosis and require further evaluation. Stenosis exceeding 75 to 80% of the lumen is associated with an annual risk of ipsilateral stroke of 2 to 3% (22). A large controlled trial (ACAS) demonstrated that for asymptomatic patients with more than 60% stenosis of the carotid artery, the combination of medical management (risk factor reduction and 325 mg of aspirin per day) and carotid endarterectomy (CEA) was superior to medical management alone (14). Over 5 years, the projected incidence of morbid events (perioperative death or stroke) was 5.1% for CEA patients, and the incidence of ipsilateral stroke was 11.0% for patients treated medically (an aggregate risk reduction of 53%). Patients to whom CEA is offered should be told that in ACAS there was approximately a 3% risk of perioperative stroke or death with CEA and that the benefit found in the ACAS trial accrued over 5 years.

Patients with excess cardiac risk were excluded from the ACAS trial. Medical management alone would probably benefit the latter group. Information about the symptoms of TIA should be given to any patient with a cervical bruit so that the patient does not ignore this warning should it occur. The American Heart Association has excellent patient education materials on TIA.

CLASSIFICATION OF CEREBROVASCULAR EVENTS

Type of Event

Symptoms and signs of vascular origin are characterized by the rapid onset of deficits referable to a vascular distribution. The following classification has been developed based on duration.

A *TIA* is defined as a transient episode of focal cerebral dysfunction, rapid in onset (from none to maximal symptoms in less than 5 minutes), that usually lasts from 2 to 15 minutes but always resolves completely within 24 hours.

A *reversible ischemic neurologic deficit* (RIND) is defined as an episode of focal cerebral dysfunction that lasts longer than 24 hours but resolves completely within 3 weeks. This type of event is sometimes called a minor stroke.

Table 83.1. Possible Causes of Cervical Bruit

Physiologic murmur
Venous hum
Transmitted cardiac murmur
Atherosclerosis and stenosis of carotid, vertebral, subclavian, or
    innominate artery
Loops, kinks, inflammation, fibromuscular dysplasia of carotid artery
Arteriovenous fistula
Angiomatous malformation
Intracranial neoplasm
Paget's disease of the skull

A *completed stroke* is defined as an episode of focal cerebral dysfunction that has stabilized and may have improved but has not resolved completely after 3 weeks. The most characteristic pattern is the abrupt occurrence of a neurologic deficit that improves or worsens, sometimes repeatedly, over minutes to hours to days and then becomes a fixed deficit.

The term *stroke in evolution* is used to describe a vascular syndrome that is acute in onset and progressively worsens during the period of observation.

Vascular Territory

Cerebrovascular events are also classified on the basis of the vascular territory involved. Symptoms and signs referable to the two major vascular territories are listed in Table 83.2. There is overlap in the symptom complexes, making the distinction between carotid and vertebrobasilar disease difficult at times. However, the history alone often provides the evidence necessary to identify the arterial territory involved.

A subgroup of ischemic events, called *lacunar syndromes*, is caused by occlusion of penetrating non-anastomosing branches of the major cerebral arteries. The pathology of the involved vessels has been characterized; occlusion is caused either by miniature atherosclerotic plaques at the origin of vessels 400 to 1000 μm in diameter or, more commonly, by a degenerative process called lipohyalinosis affecting vessels 200 μm or less in diameter. These changes correlate strongly with the presence of hypertension. At least 20 clinical lacunar syndromes have been described (16); lacunar infarctions may also be silent, identified only by CT scan. The common syndromes are the following:

- *Pure motor hemiparesis* (internal capsule or pons): hemiplegia or hemiparesis involving the face, arm, and leg without sensory deficit, dysphasia, or hemianopsia
- *Pure sensory stroke* (thalamus): numbness of the face, arm, and leg on one side without weakness or hemianopsia
- *Ataxic hemiparesis* (internal capsule or pons): cerebellar ataxia, weakness, and pyramidal signs involving the limbs on the same side, the lower extremity more than the arm
- *The dysarthria or clumsy hand syndrome* (internal capsule or pons): dysarthria, facial weakness, clumsiness of the hand with little or no weakness, a slight imbalance, and a Babinski sign on the affected side
- *Multi-infarct dementia*: a dementia syndrome characterized by stepwise progression (see description of dementia in Chapter 17)

SYMPTOMATIC PATIENTS

TIA and Stroke

Most TIAs and strokes are caused by artery-to-artery embolization or cardiogenic embolus. The distinction

Table 83.2. Clinical Features of Ischemia Involving the Major Vascular Territories

Carotid Artery Disease
Paresis (mono- or hemi-)
Sensory loss or paresthesias (mono- or hemi-)
Speech or language disturbances
Loss of vision in one eye or part of one eye (amaurosis fugax)
Homonymous hemianopsia
Cognitive impairment

Vertebrobasilar Arterial Disease
Vertigo, diplopia, dysphagia, or dysarthria when two occur together or when one occurs with any of the following:
Paresis (any combination of the extremities)
Sensory loss or paresthesias (any combination of the extremities)
Ataxia
Homonymous hemianopsia (unilateral or bilateral)

between TIA and stroke is becoming less important because a rigorous search for cause is indicated in both and many patients with TIA have evidence of brain infarction on imaging. Treatment is based on cause of the event regardless of whether the patient has had a TIA or stroke. Both events signal brain ischemia; stroke occurs when blood supply from collateral vessels is insufficient or the occluding thrombus is too large to be rapidly cleared.

For patients with TIA, other transient neurologic events described elsewhere, such as seizure (Chapter 80), hypoglycemia (Chapter 74), syncope (Chapter 81), and migraine (Chapter 79) must be considered. A Todd's paralysis (transient focal weakness following a focal motor seizure or secondarily generalized tonic–clonic seizure) is diagnosed when it is established that the primary event was a seizure. Transient episodes with altered consciousness are almost never vascular in nature. Migraine occurs primarily in younger patients, is associated with headache, and must conform to defined criteria (see Chapter 79). A mass lesion such as a tumor or subdural hematoma may present with transient neurologic symptoms; however, these patients usually have persistent signs and symptoms; CT or magnetic resonance imaging (MRI) scanning (see Chapter 78) is diagnostic. Occasionally, an acute exacerbation of multiple sclerosis may mimic TIA; however, these patients are usually younger and have had multiple episodes with nonvascular localization (for example, optic neuritis).

Evaluation

Initial evaluation of the patient with TIA or stroke may be in the hospital (the patient who presents within hours or days of the event) or in the ambulatory setting (the patient who presents within weeks of the event). A detailed history is essential, to identify risk factors for cerebrovascular disease and to delineate and classify the focal symptoms (Table 83.2). The physical examination should include assessment for hypotension, hypertension, cardiac disease, cerebrovascular and peripheral vascular disease, and any persisting neurologic abnormality. The patient should also have a careful funduscopic evaluation to assess the status of the retinal vessels and to detect emboli (Fig. 83.1) that suggest atherothrombotic carotid occlusive disease or cardiac disease. For all patients, a noncontrast brain CT or MRI scan (see Chapter 78) should be considered to localize the event, evaluate for previous silent events, and rule out other causes of neurologic symptoms that mimic cerebrovascular disease.

If there is clinical evidence of heart disease, in particular a murmur, atrial fibrillation, or left ventricular dysfunction, a transthoracic echocardiogram should be obtained to look for an intracardiac source of arterial emboli. Transesophageal echocardiography should be considered in patients for whom no source can be found. Patients with heart disease should also have Holter monitoring to check for cardiac arrhythmias.

Screening tests to check for treatable causes of occlusive cerebrovascular disease include a serologic test for syphilis, hematocrit measurement (polycythemia), and erythrocyte sedimentation rate (vasculitis).

Patients with initial carotid territory events should have a noninvasive carotid evaluation, using the available technique with the best performance characteristics. Decision analysis of the various available procedures shows that the preferred noninvasive technique is duplex ultrasonography (1). The characteristics of duplex ultrasonography and the patient experiences associated with it and other noninvasive diagnostic tests are described in Chapter 78.

Cerebral angiography (see description in Chapter 78)

should be considered in most patients who do not have a definite cardiac source of brain embolus. Although a duplex scan can rule out carotid stenosis, intracranial vascular disease cannot be identified conclusively by noninvasive means. A transcranial Doppler (TCD) scan can be useful to follow a patient known to have intracranial disease or to detect disease, but a normal TCD does not rule out disease. A noninvasive evaluation only (duplex, TCD) in patients with no cardiac source can be justified if the patient's event was so devastating that further evaluation and treatment are precluded.

Early Management

Atherothrombotic Events

Patients with atherothrombotic events, either cortical or lacunar, may be treated medically or surgically.

Medical Therapy. This aspect of management includes risk factor modification and anticoagulant and antiplatelet drugs.

Antihypertensive therapy. In a small controlled study of hypertensive patients who had sustained a nonembolic ischemic stroke, 44% of the untreated patients, compared with 20% of the treated patients, suffered another major stroke; and at the end of a 2- to 5-year follow-up period, 46% of the untreated patients and 26% of the treated patients had died (7). Although the number of recurrent strokes was too small to allow a valid comparison, the difference in mortality was statistically significant in favor of the treated group. No

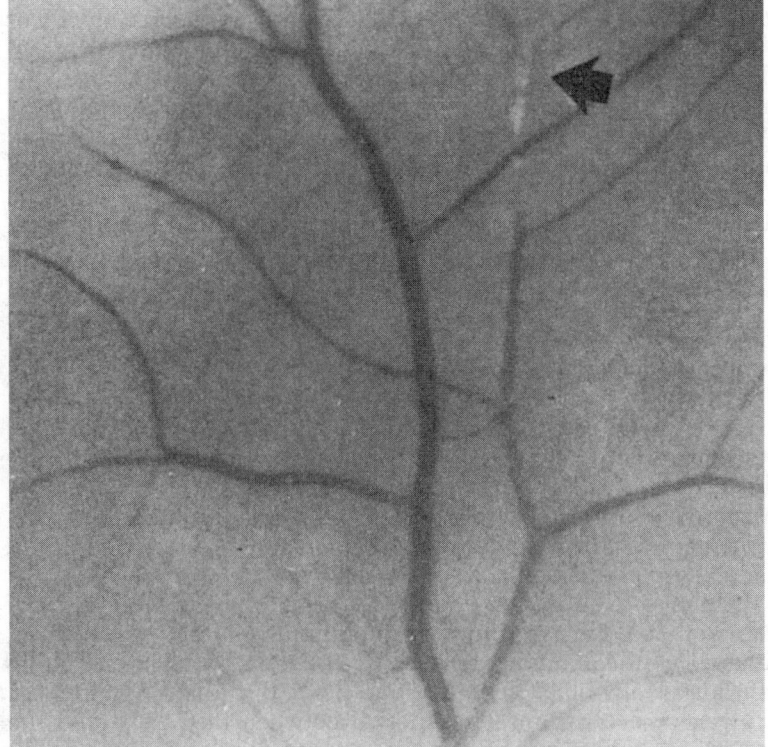

Figure 83.1. Atheromatous debris embolus lodged in retinal arteriole *(arrow)* in patient with recurrent hemisphere TIA and amaurosis fugax. These emboli persist for hours to weeks, and even permanently, whereas the platelet–fibrin emboli are fleeting and are gone within a few minutes. (From Meyer JS, Shaw T. Diagnosis and management of stroke and TIAs. Baltimore: Williams & Wilkins, 1982.)

treated patient sustained a neurologic complication as a result of a documented hypotensive episode. Subsequent studies of the effect of antihypertensive treatment on stroke recurrence included patients with hemorrhagic as well as ischemic strokes. In a noncontrolled study, patients with good, fair, and poor control of hypertension respectively, had recurrence rates of 16%, 32%, and 55% (4). A placebo-controlled study did not demonstrate a significant reduction in stroke recurrence in treated patients, although the incidence of congestive heart failure was reduced (24). Despite the differences in these study findings, it is reasonable to conclude that antihypertensive medication can be safely administered to hypertensive stroke survivors and that it is indicated for these patients to reduce recurrent cerebrovascular events and other cardiovascular morbidity. (See Chapter 62 for details on the treatment of hypertension.)

The *antiplatelet drugs* aspirin and ticlopidine are effective in reducing the recurrence of TIA or stroke. Although the dosage of aspirin effective in secondary prevention is not yet unequivocally established for cerebrovascular disease, 650 mg twice daily (1300 mg) is known to be efficacious (10). Enteric coated tablets are recommended to decrease gastrointestinal symptoms. Ticlopidine (Ticlid) is an antiplatelet agent with a slight statistical advantage over aspirin for efficacy (17 versus 19% occurrence of stroke or death from any cause at 3 years, a 12% risk reduction) (21). The dosage is 250 mg twice daily. The neutrophil count must be monitored every 2 weeks for 3 months, as fatal neutropenia has been reported. Other, more common side effects are rash and diarrhea. Expense is a factor for ticlopidine (it is much more expensive than aspirin). Additional details regarding the use of and efficacy of antiplatelet drugs are in Chapter 52.

Anticoagulant therapy with warfarin has not been proven to be effective for atherothrombotic disease, but it has been recommended for symptomatic patients (post-TIA or stroke) with known high-grade intracranial stenosis or preocclusive extracranial carotid bifurcation disease that cannot be addressed surgically (e.g., in patients who have had a recent myocardial infarction) (13) (see details regarding anticoagulation in Chapter 52).

The *impact of aspirin is being compared with the impact of warfarin* on the recurrence of stroke in an ongoing clinical trial (44).

A role for *cholesterol lowering* in preventing stroke has not been established in stroke survivors; however, a meta-analysis has shown that the HMGcoA reductase inhibitors may reduce stroke incidence when these agents are prescribed to patients with established coronary artery disease (9).

Surgical Therapy. *Carotid endarterectomy* (CEA) can be recommended to patients with hemispheric or retinal TIAs or nondisabling stroke with ipsilateral 70% or greater stenosis at the carotid bifurcation. This recommendation is supported by a large clinical trial (NASCET) in which 9% of CEA patients versus 26% of patients receiving antiplatelet treatment experienced an ipsilateral stroke during the 2 years after initiation of treatment (33). For symptomatic patients with less than 70% stenosis, the efficacy of surgery is still under investigation in a second stage of the same clinical trial. Patients who have undergone CEA are usually continued on long-term antiplatelet therapy to prevent restenosis.

In patients with *intracranial carotid and middle cerebral artery stenosis,* extracranial–intracranial bypass surgery has been shown in randomized controlled trials to confer no benefit beyond aspirin's effect (11).

In patients with *severe basilar vertebral insufficiency* with a history of recurrent TIAs or strokes in the basilar vertebral territory and arteriographic evidence of bilateral vertebral artery compromise or high-grade basilar artery stenosis, bypass procedures and angioplasty have been undertaken. The efficacy of these procedures has not yet been established.

Because the guidelines for the treatment of patients with TIAs and survivors of stroke are still evolving, the advice of a neurologist who specializes in cerebrovascular disease should be sought.

Cardioembolic Events

Patients with cardioembolic events who benefit from anticoagulation with warfarin include those with atrial fibrillation (both valvular and nonvalvular disease), recent MI, dilated cardiomyopathy, and rheumatic and prosthetic valves (8). Clinical trials consistently show that there is approximately a two-thirds reduction in expected events in anticoagulated patients with atrial fibrillation; for those who have had a TIA or minor stroke the annual incidence of a new event is reduced from 12% to 4%; for those with no history of TIA or stroke the annual incidence is reduced from approximately 5% to 2% (3). Whether aspirin is as effective as warfarin for younger patients with nonvalvular atrial fibrillation is unknown. Specific aspects of anticoagulant therapy to prevent CVA are described in Chapter 52 and in chapters that cover postinfarct mural thrombi (Chapter 58), atrial fibrillation (Chapter 59), and valvular heart disease (Chapter 60).

For patients with both a cardiac source and high-grade carotid stenosis (70% or higher) proximal to the territory of a TIA or stroke, carotid endarterectomy should be considered.

STROKE PROGNOSIS

Morbidity in Stroke Survivors

A number of studies have evaluated stroke survivors on the basis of the degree of neurologic, functional, and psychosocial impairment.

Table 83.4 shows the spectrum and frequency of neurologic impairments found in stroke survivors in the Framingham study (19). Study subjects were living at home or in institutions at the time of functional evaluation. The interval between the stroke and the functional assessment ranged from 6 months to 33 years (mean, 7 years). It is notable that half of these

Table 83.3. Percentage Distribution of Stroke Survivors by Age Group

Age Group	Onset	Percentage Surviving								
		Days				Years				
		30	60	90	180	1	2	3	4	5
Under 65	100.0	73.7	71.1	69.4	65.9	63.2	57.6	57.6	52.0	49.2
65–74	100.0	75.6	69.5	65.2	63.1	59.4	52.9	46.1	42.7	34.5
75–84	100.0	68.1	62.1	57.6	52.4	45.7	37.2	30.0	23.1	21.9
85+	100.0	52.4	45.8	37.2	33.0	27.8	20.7	15.1	9.2	7.4

From National Survey of Stroke, U.S. Department of Health, Education and Welfare, Public Health Service, National Institutes of Health, NIH pub. no. 80-2069, January 1980.

Table 83.4. Prevalence of Neurologic Deficits in the 123 Survivors of Completed Stroke, Framingham Study (1972–1974)

Type of Peripheral Motor Deficit	Survivors	No. Surviving with			
		Sensory Deficit	Hemianopsia	Dysarthria	Dysphasia
No motor deficit	63	3	5	2	10
Left hemiparesis	28	13	6	3	2
Right hemi-paresis	27	10	5	13	9
Bilateral motor deficit	4	4	3	2	1
No data	1	1	1	1	1
Total survivors	123	31	20	21	23

From Gresham E, Fitzpatrick TE, Wolf PA, et al. Residual disability in survivors of stroke: the Framingham study. N Engl J Med 293:954, 1975.

°patients (63 of 123) had no motor deficit. These findings are probably representative of the situation in other communities.

In a classic study of overall function, Katz et al. (28) found that of patients who survive a stroke, approximately 50% are independent 2 years later and can ambulate and perform activities of daily living with minimal or no assistance. Spontaneous improvement is most rapid in the first few months after the stroke and is rarely noted after 2 years. Only a small percentage of stroke survivors remain bedridden and completely dependent. These findings were corroborated by results from the Mayo Clinic, where only 4% of the community-dwelling survivors of a stroke required total care at 6 months; 36% had some degree of neurologic deficit, yet were able to work; and 29% were functioning normally (32). On the basis of the authors' assessment, 54% of their patients may have benefited from rehabilitative care, including the 10% who were aphasic.

The Framingham study provided information on the equally important *social and psychologic sequelae* of stroke (19). A significant decrease in the levels of vocational function and socialization outside the home was noted among stroke survivors compared with age- and sex-matched controls (Table 83.5), and the decrease exceeded that anticipated based on the levels of neurologic deficit. In a prospective study in Monroe County, New York, the social and psychologic difficulties facing the stroke survivor were evaluated in more detail (15). Within the first 6 months after hospital discharge, 37% of the patients demonstrated moderate or severe depression, 32% anger or anxiety, 56% social isolation, 43% reduction in community involvement, 46% economic strain causing lifestyle alteration, and 52% disruption of normal family functions. Additional studies have confirmed the high incidence of moderate or severe depression in the first year after stroke and have shown that the risk of depression is particularly high in patients with damage in the left frontal hemisphere (37,38). Longitudinal studies show that post-stroke depression lasts up to 2 years. Recent studies suggest two types of depression: a major depressive syndrome and a minor or dysthymic depression. Patients with the major depressive syndrome respond well to tricyclic antidepressants (see below).

Recognition and treatment of the psychosocial problems of the stroke patient and family are discussed in more detail below.

Mortality in Stroke Survivors

The *death rate among stroke survivors* is significantly greater than that expected for the general population matched for age and sex. The 5-year cumulative mortality is approximately 50 to 60%, with the greatest number of deaths occurring in the first year. With time, however, the mortality rate approaches that of the general population, and in at least one study the increased rate of death after a stroke subsided completely after 24 to 30 months (28).

National data from the 1970s (Table 83.3) illustrate the dramatic impact of *age* on survival following stroke.

Studies that classified strokes on the basis of *type of vascular pathology* indicate that the early prognosis is much better for thrombotic or embolic disease than for hemorrhage (32). There is evidence that the type of pathology is a less reliable predictor of late prognosis. Eisenberg et al. (12) report that patients with cerebral hemorrhage who lived 1 month had a 5-year survival equal to or better than patients with cerebral thrombosis.

The leading cause of death in stroke survivors is cardiovascular disease, with cardiac-related deaths exceeding deaths attributed to cerebrovascular disease by a factor of 2 to 1. Because cardiac disease is a major contributor to the cause of the stroke, stroke recurrence, and the survival from stroke, thorough

Table 83.5. Prevalence of Four Types of Functional Disability in 119 Survivors of Completed Stroke and in 119 Controls, Framingham Study (1972–1974)

Type of Disability	Survivors		Matched Controls[a]		p Value
	No.	%	No.	%	
All persons examined for functional disability	119	100	119	100	—
Dependent in activities of daily living	37	31	9	8	<0.0001
Dependent in mobility	24	20	6	5	<0.0001
Decrease in level of vocational function[b]	85	71	49	41	<0.0001
Decrease in socialization	74	62	37	31	<0.0001

From Gresham E, Fitzpatrick TE, Wolf PA, et al. Residual disability in survivors of stroke: the Framingham study. N Engl J Med 293:954, 1975.

[a]Matched for age and sex.

[b]Either stopped working or incomplete resumption of homemaking activities.

evaluation and management of cardiac disease are of great importance in the care of stroke survivors.

LONG-TERM MANAGEMENT

Management of the patient who has survived a stroke involves the evaluation and treatment of any physical and psychosocial sequelae and the selection of appropriate therapy to lessen the risk of recurrence. Once the patient has been discharged from the hospital, the patient's personal physician plays a critical role in coordinating care. Reduction in a patient's disability and dependency often requires the concerted efforts of the patient's family; physical, occupational, and speech therapists; and occasionally a psychiatrist. Patients with significant deficits persisting for 3 months or longer may qualify for *disability insurance under Social Security* (see Table 9.3).

Role of the Family

At the time of discharge from the hospital, appropriate education is especially important for the stroke survivor and the patient's family. At this juncture, patients are confronted with the full extent of their functional loss. By dispelling myths regarding stroke and supplanting them with accurate information, physicians and therapists can ensure that the actions of well-meaning family members do not foster the patients' feelings of inadequacy. The AHA has produced a series of invaluable booklets that discuss stroke and its sequelae in lay terms and provide guidelines for the home management of the stroke patient. The titles of these publications are listed in Table 83.6.

The following general suggestions can be helpful for the family of a stroke patient with residual disability:

- Divide duties so that the full burden of care does not fall on one person.
- Help the patient take responsibility for exercising regularly.
- Allow the patient to take on responsibilities for self-care and other activities gradually and by easy

steps. It calls for fine judgment to encourage independence and not to frustrate a patient with over-difficult tasks, and to stimulate progress without encouraging unrealistic expectations.

- Praise any successful efforts that are made; do not be discouraged by failures. Recovery from a severe stroke is a slow process.
- Have the patient participate in as many family activities and as much family planning as possible. Feeling useful is a tremendous morale builder.
- Help him or her keep in contact with the world.
- Do not relegate the patient to the sidelines and leave him or her with only television and radio. Encourage the patient to develop a hobby. Spend time with him or her and encourage visitors if warranted. Make him or her feel wanted and a part of the social picture.
- Get in touch with the doctor if things are not going as you think they should.

Role of Rehabilitation

Success in stroke rehabilitation often depends on the extent of permanent central nervous system damage and the patient's ability to use *alternative methods of function* to compensate for fixed deficits. As noted above, spontaneous improvement in the stroke survivor may continue to occur for the first 6 to 12 months after the stroke, yet the mechanisms underlying such gains remain obscure. In studies to determine whether intensive rehabilitation results in functional gains after the period of spontaneous improvement, it has been found that even significantly impaired patients admitted to a rehabilitation program 12 months after a stroke may show marked improvement in dressing skills, bladder and bowel function, and walking (29). These findings form the basis for the conclusion that a program of rehabilitation does improve the outcome of the stroke survivor. It is estimated that the savings derived in returning a patient to the family or to independent living more than equals the costs of rehabilitation (29).

It is clear that not all patients in a rehabilitation program show significant functional improvement. A number of patient characteristics correlate with poor rehabilitation results, including bowel and bladder incontinence, low self-care status on admission, right hemispheric involvement, intellectual and perceptual

Table 83.6. Booklets Published by the American Heart Association

Recovering from a Stroke is a booklet written for the patient and the patient's family on ways in which the patient can regain activities of daily living.

How Stroke Affects Behavior is a detailed booklet providing recommendations for the care of the patient who has completed most of his or her spontaneous recovery of higher functions and has major residual deficits (see Table 83.7).

Caring for a Person with Aphasia explains many of the problems in aphasia and suggests practical ways in which the family can help the aphasic patient.

Available without charge from local AHA chapters.

deficits, heart failure, signs of generalized arteriosclerosis, and lower educational levels (5,30). However, because none of these factors correlates strongly with poor outcome, the best approach is to offer rehabilitation services when possible to each stroke survivor with significant functional impairments.

It is generally agreed that, except for patients with evidence of subarachnoid bleeding, for whom bed rest and mild sedation are indicated, a *program of functional rehabilitation* should begin as soon as possible after a stroke occurs. There are several reasons for the early initiation of a program of rehabilitation. First, it is generally accepted that patients who are provided with rehabilitation services early are likely to experience greater long-term functional improvement. Second, early transfer from bed to chair coupled with physical therapy reduces the complications that can develop in the immobile bedridden patient and that can subsequently limit the extent of functional recovery. Stretching of tight muscles, passive range of motion, and active or resistive exercises minimize the degree of muscle atrophy and prevent the development of contractures. In addition, even limited mobility of the patient reduces the risk of circulatory complications such as thrombophlebitis, postural hypotension, and pressure sores. Third, early rehabilitation is of particular benefit to the patient who demonstrates an impaired ability to communicate because of either dysphasia or dysarthria. Approximately one-third of stroke patients exhibit some form of communication disorder, and many of these remain severely impaired beyond the period of spontaneous recovery (40). Such patients may feel desperately isolated because of their loss of ability to communicate. Therapists who specialize in speech and hearing are skilled in the evaluation and management of these problems and play an integral role in daily interactions with the patient and in recommending appropriate strategies to the patient's family and physician.

Everyone involved in the rehabilitation process must appreciate the significance of the functional losses sustained by the patient, so the losses must be viewed from the patient's perspective. This requires an awareness of the patient's usual activities before the stroke; this essential information should be obtained in conjunction with a social worker who can evaluate the patient's role at home before the stroke and can project how the stroke will alter that role when the patient returns home.

The rehabilitation initiated in the hospital (usually in a unit dedicated to intensive short-term rehabilitation) is always designed to be continued after the patient gets home. Most communities have physical, occupational, and speech therapists available for both home and ambulatory follow-up. For patients meeting eligibility criteria, these services are covered by third-party payers. The patient and family should be acquainted with the goals and plans for continued rehabilitation before discharge. Chapter 9 provides information about home health services. The comprehensive text of Brandstater and Basmajian (see

"General References") provides details about the many individualized approaches available for rehabilitation.

Management of Psychologic and Behavioral Sequelae

The high incidence of psychologic and behavioral problems among stroke survivors has been noted above. These problems often hinder rehabilitation efforts. Fear of a second stroke and depression caused by loss of functional ability are readily understandable in the context of the patient's predicament. Appropriate counseling of the patient and family (as outlined above), coupled with participation in an active rehabilitation program, are the best ways to minimize the adverse psychologic reactions to a stroke.

A number of stroke survivors experience *mood disturbances* that do not correlate with the level of functional disability, and there is evidence that for many patients the mood disorder is a specific complication of cerebral damage rather than simply a reaction to functional loss (17,37,38). This mood disorder may augment the cognitive impairment of the patient or on occasion may be expressed as an apparent cognitive impairment (pseudodementia of depression, described in Chapter 17). Response in such patients to antidepressant treatment may be dramatic. Earlier observations suggested that the type of mood disorder depends on the side of the brain affected by the stroke (36). Gainotti (18) reported that behavior denoting a catastrophic reaction (see Chapter 17) and anxious depressive orientation of mood (anxiety reactions, bursts of tears, provocative utterances, depressed renouncements, or sharp refusals to go on with the examinations) are more common among patients with *left* (dominant) hemisphere damage. Symptoms denoting an opposite emotional reaction (denial of illness, minimization, indifference reactions, and tendency to joke) and expressions of hate toward the paralyzed limbs are more common among patients suffering from a lesion of the *right* (minor) hemisphere. Most authorities agree, however, that both psychologic and physiologic factors contribute to the development of mood disorders after strokes. Tricyclic antidepressants have been shown to benefit patients with poststroke depression (36–38). Practical information about these drugs is found in Chapter 15.

The AHA booklet *How Stroke Affects Behavior* is particularly helpful for the family and for health care professionals caring for the patient who has survived a major stroke involving the cerebral cortex. Table 83.7 contains summaries of the recommendations for dealing with permanent behavioral problems in these patients.

Management of Late Complications

A number of complications may occur during the months to years after a stroke.

Table 83.7. Recommendations for Dealing with Behavioral Problems Associated with Permanent Loss of Higher Functions in Stroke Patients

Left Hemisphere Damage	**One-Sided Neglect**
Right hemiplegics often have difficulties with speech and language. They also tend to be somewhat cautious, anxious, and disorganized when attempting a new task. Keep in mind the following suggestions:	One-sided neglect is a problem that involves more than a simple visual field cut or hearing loss. It can occur in both right and left hemiplegics but seems to be more common and more persistent among left hemiplegics. When dealing with a neglect problem, you should:
• Do not underestimate the patient's ability to learn and communicate even if he or she cannot use speech.	• Keep the unimpaired side toward the action unless specifically working with neglected side.
• If he or she cannot use speech, try other forms of communication. Pantomime and demonstration are often useful.	• Avoid trapping the patient in an unnecessarily confined environment.
• Do not overestimate his or her understanding of speech and overload him or her with "static."	• Avoid nagging but give frequent cues to aid orientation.
• Do not shout. Keep messages simple and brief.	• Provide reminders of the neglected side.
• Do not use special voices.	• Arrange the environment to maximize performance.
• Divide tasks into simple steps.	
• Give much feedback and many indications of progress.	**Memory Problems**
	Some memory problems can be expected in most stroke patients. When working with memory deficits, you can often increase the patient's ability to perform if you:
Right Hemisphere Damage	• Establish a fixed routine whenever possible.
If the patient is having difficulty with self-care activities, you can expect spatial–perceptual deficits. He or she will tend to talk better than he or she can actually perform. The patient may be impulsive or careless. Remember, when working with the patient who has significant spatial–perceptual deficits:	• Keep messages short enough to fit retention span.
	• Present new information one step at a time.
	• Allow the patient to finish one step before proceeding to the next.
• Do not overestimate abilities. Spatial–perceptual difficulties are easy to miss.	• Give frequent indications of effective progress; the patient may forget past successes.
• Use verbal cues if he or she has difficulty with demonstration.	• Train in settings that resemble, as much as possible, the setting in which the behavior is to be practiced.
• Break tasks into small steps and give much feedback.	• Use memory aids such as appointment books, written notes, and schedule cards whenever possible.
• Watch to see what he or she can do safely rather than taking the patient's word for it.	• Use familiar objects and old associations when teaching new tasks.
• Minimize clutter.	
• Avoid rapid movement around the patient.	
• Highlight visual reference points.	

Adapted from *How Stroke Affects Behavior,* American Heart Association.

Shoulder Problems

The painful shoulder is one of the most disturbing complications encountered in the patient with a residual hemiparesis. Shoulder pain is often caused by increased traction on the shoulder capsule secondary to abnormal positioning of the paralyzed arm. The normal alignment of the joint can be restored through the use of a sling and proper positioning of the arm at night. Physical therapy, after initial symptomatic treatment with analgesics and the application of heat, can limit the extent of permanent structural damage (see Chapter 63 for additional details).

The *shoulder–hand syndrome* (reflex sympathetic dystrophy) occurs in approximately 5% of stroke patients. It is characterized by the occurrence of a painful shoulder associated with stiffness and swelling of the hand and fingers. Onset is acute or subacute (developing over 3 to 6 months) and may involve the hand and shoulder simultaneously or one followed by the other. Although a number of conditions can result in shoulder discomfort, the dystrophic changes in the hand are characteristic of the shoulder–hand syndrome. There is swelling below the wrist but no pitting edema, and the skin of the hand is warm and pink. With time, the intrinsic muscles of the hand atrophy and extension deformities in the metacarpophalangeal joints develop. At this stage radiographic examination of the hand often shows spotty demineralization of the carpal bones. The severe pain associated with this condition greatly hinders rehabilitation efforts. Therefore,

early recognition and treatment are important. The following plan is recommended for the management of this condition: Begin treatment with a nonsteroidal anti-inflammatory drug and with heat to the shoulder, then carefully initiate and gradually increase abduction and external rotation exercises of the arm (described in Chapter 63). If there is no significant improvement after 1 month, the patient should be referred to a neurosurgeon for consideration of stellate ganglion block (39).

Complications of Inactivity

The partially paralyzed stroke survivor often leads a sedentary existence. This lifestyle is conducive to the development of vascular complications such as thrombophlebitis and pressure sores. Use of elastic stockings and frequent repositioning of the immobile patient by an informed family member minimizes these problems.

Neurologic Complications

Prolonged pressure on a paralyzed limb may lead to a peripheral nerve lesion, which may be difficult to recognize when superimposed on brain damage resulting from the stroke. An awareness of this potential complication can expedite its recognition, and electrodiagnostic studies can confirm the lower motor neuron damage (see Chapter 84). Once a diagnosis is made, prompt initiation of physical therapy limits the degree of functional loss resulting from this usually reversible lesion.

Approximately 2.5 to 5% of stroke survivors develop focal or generalized recurrent *seizures* (epilepsy) as a late complication. Patients with damage to their sensorimotor cortex are the most likely to develop epilepsy, with the first seizure usually occurring 6 to 12 months after the stroke (31,35). Transient neurologic dysfunction after a seizure in a stroke survivor is often attributed to a second stroke. The rapid resolution of symptoms and electroencephalographic (EEG) evidence of an epileptogenic focus point to seizure activity rather than ischemia as the cause. Recurrent seizures in the stroke survivor confirm the diagnosis of epilepsy. Seizure control can usually be achieved through the use of anticonvulsant medication (see Chapter 80).

Finally, *stroke-related deficits may transiently worsen* when the patient develops a major intercurrent illness such as pneumonia or MI. In this instance, neurologic status returns to baseline after resolution of the intercurrent illness. (See discussion of upper motor neuron symptoms in Chapter 78.)

General Surgery

The approach to general surgery in patients who have a history of stroke is addressed in Chapter 86.

General References*

Benton AL, ed. Behavioral changes in cerebrovascular disease. New York: Harper & Row, 1970.
> A detailed account of psychological problems complicating stroke.

Brandstater M, Basmajian J, eds. Stroke rehabilitation. Baltimore: Williams & Wilkins, 1987.
> A detailed, well-illustrated, and extensively referenced resource on all aspects of the rehabilitation of stroke patients.

Caplan LR. Stroke: a clinical approach. 2nd ed. Boston: Butterworth-Heinemann, 1993.
> An excellent source for clinicians with practical, up-to-date information on diagnosis and treatment.

Feussner JR, Matchar DB. When and how to study the carotid arteries. Ann Intern Med 109:805, 1988.
> Detailed review of the literature and use of decision analysis to determine the relative value of diagnostic strategies.

Specific References

1. American College of Physicians Health and Public Policy Committee. Diagnostic evaluation of the carotid arteries. Ann Intern Med 109:835, 1988.
2. American Heart Association. 1997 heart and stroke facts statistical update. Dallas: American Heart Association, 1997.
3. Anticoagulants for atrial fibrillation (Commentary). Lancet 342:1251, 1993.
4. Beevers DG, Fairman MJ, Hamilton M, Harpur JE. Antihypertensive treatment and the course of established cerebrovascular disease. Lancet 1:1407, 1973.
5. Bourestom NC. Predictors of long term recovery in cerebrovascular disease. Arch Phys Med Rehabil 48:415, 1967.
6. Broderick JP, Phillips SJ, Whisnant JP, et al. Incidence rates of strokes in the eighties: the end of the decline in stroke? Stroke 20:577, 1989.
6a. Bucher HC, Griffith LE, Guyatt GH. Effect on HMGcoA reductase inhibitors on stroke: a meta-analysis of randomized, controlled trials. Ann Intern Med 128:89–95, 1998.
7. Carter AB. Hypertensive therapy in stroke survivors. Lancet 1:485, 1970.
8. Caplan LR. Stroke: a clinical approach. Boston: Butterworth-Heinemann, 1993.
9. Crouse III JR, Byington RP, Hoen HM, Furberg CD. Reductase inhibitor monotherapy and stroke prevention. Arch Intern Med 157:1305–1310, 1997.
10. Dyken ML, Barnett HJM, Easton JD. Low-dose aspirin and stroke: it ain't necessarily so. Stroke 23:1395, 1992.
11. EC/IC Bypass Study Group. Failure of extracranial–intracranial arterial bypass to reduce the risk of ischemic stroke: results of an international randomized trial. N Engl J Med 313:1191–1200, 1985.
12. Eisenberg H, Morrison JT, Sullivan P, Foote FM. Cerebrovascular accidents: incidence and survival rates in a defined population. Middlesex County, Connecticut. JAMA 189:883, 1964.
13. Estol CJ, Pessin MS. Anticoagulation: is there still a role in atherothrombotic stroke? Curr Concepts Cerebrovasc Dis Stroke 25:1–6, 1990.
14. Executive Committee for the Asymptomatic Carotid Atherosclerosis Study. Endarterectomy for asymptomatic carotid artery stenosis. JAMA 273(18):1421–1428, 1995.
15. Feibel JH, Berk S, Joynt RJ. The unmet needs of stroke survivors. Neurology 29:592, 1979.
16. Fisher CM. Lacunar strokes and infarcts: a review. Neurology 32:871, 1982.
17. Folstein MF, Maiberger R, McHugh PR. Mood disorders as a specific complication of stroke. J Neurol Neurosurg Psychiatry 40:1018, 1977.
18. Gainotti G. Emotional behavior and hemispheric side of the lesion. Cortex 8:41, 1972.
19. Gresham GE, Fitzpatrick TE, Wolf PA, et al. Residual disability in survivors of stroke: the Framingham study. N Engl J Med 293:954, 1975.
20. Hachinski V. Decreased incidence and mortality of stroke. Stroke 15:376, 1984.
21. Hass WK, Easton JD, Adams HP. A randomized trial comparing ticlopidine hydrochloride with aspirin for the prevention of stroke in high-risk patients. N Engl J Med 321:501, 1989.
22. Hennerici M, Hulsbomer HB, Hefter H, et al. Natural history of asymptomatic extracranial arterial disease. Brain 110:777, 1987.
23. Heyman A, Wilkinson WE, Heyden S, et al. Risk of stroke in asymptomatic persons with cervical arterial bruits: a population study in Evans County, Georgia. N Engl J Med 302:838, 1980.
24. Hypertensive-Stroke Cooperative Study Group. Effects of antihypertensive treatment on stroke recurrence. JAMA 229:409, 1974.
25. Kannel WB. Current status of the epidemiology of brain infarction associated with occlusive arterial disease. Stroke 2:295, 1971.
26. Kannel WB, Gordon T, Wolf PA, McNamara PM. Hemoglobin and the risk of cerebral infarction: the Framingham study. Stroke (Baltimore) 3:409, 1972.
27. Kannel WB, Wolf PA, Verter J, McNamara PM. Epidemiologic assessment of the role of blood pressure in stroke. JAMA 214:301, 1970.
28. Katz S, Ford AB, Chinn AB, Newill VA. Prognosis after strokes. II. Long-term course of 159 patients. Medicine 45:236, 1966.
29. Lehmann JF, DeLateur BJ, Fowler RS, et al. Stroke: does rehabilitation affect outcome? Arch Phys Med Rehabil 56:375, 1975.
30. Lehmann JF, DeLateur BJ, Fowler RS, et al. Stroke rehabilitation: outcome and prediction. Arch Phys Med Rehabil 56:383, 1975.
31. Louis S, McDowell F. Epileptic seizures in nonembolic cerebral infarction. Arch Neurol 27:414, 1967.
32. Matsumoto N, Whisnant JP, Kurland LT, Okazaki H. Natural

---

*Bold print (general references) and bold numerals (specific references) denote published controlled clinical trials, meta-analyses, or consensus-based recommendations.

history of stroke in Rochester, Minnesota, 1955 through 1969: an extension of a previous study, 1945 through 1954. Stroke 4:20, 1973.

33. North American Symptomatic Carotid Endarterectomy Trial Collaborators. Beneficial effect of carotid endarterectomy in symptomatic patients with high-grade carotid stenosis. N Engl J Med 325:445, 1991.

34. Paganini-Hill, A. Estrogen replacement therapy and stroke. Prog Cardiovasc Dis 38(3):223–242, 1995.

35. Richardson EP Jr, Dodge PR. Epilepsy in cerebral vascular disease: a study of the incidence and nature of seizures in 104 consecutive autopsy-proven cases of cerebral infarction and hemorrhage. Epilepsy 3:49, 1954.

36. Robinson RG, Balduc PL, Price TR. Two-year longitudinal study of post stroke mood disorders: diagnosis and outcome at one and two years. Stroke 18:837, 1987.

37. Robinson RG, Starr LB, Kubos KL, Price TR. A two-year longitudinal study of post-stroke mood disorders: findings during the initial evaluation. Stroke 14:736, 1983.

38. Robinson RG, Starr LB, Lipsey JR, et al. A two-year longitudinal study of post-stroke mood disorders: dynamic changes in associated variables over the first six months of follow-up. Stroke 15:510, 1984.

39. Ross GS, Chipman M. The neuralgias. In: Baker AB, Baker LH, eds. Clinical neurology. Vol. 3. Hagerstown, MD: Harper & Row, 1974.

40. Sarno MT. Disorders of communication in stroke. In: Licht S, ed. Stroke and its rehabilitation. Baltimore: Williams & Wilkins, 1975.

41. SHEP Cooperative Research Group. Prevention of stroke by antihypertensive drug treatment in older persons with isolated systolic hypertension. JAMA 265:3255, 1991.

42. VA Cooperative Study Group on Antihypertensive Agents. Effects of treatment on morbidity in hypertension. Results in patients with diastolic blood pressures averaging 115 through 129 mm Hg. JAMA 202:1028, 1967.

43. VA Cooperative Study Group on Antihypertensive Agents. Effects of treatment on morbidity in hypertension. II. Results in patients with diastolic blood pressure averaging 90 through 114 mm Hg. JAMA 213:1143, 1970.

44. WARSS, APASS, PICSS, HAS and GENESIS Study Groups. The feasibility of a collaborative double-blind study using an anticoagulant. Cerebrovasc Dis 7:100–112, 1997.

45. Whisnant JP. The decline of stroke. Stroke 15:160, 1984.

46. Whisnant JP, Homer D, Ingall TJ. Duration of cigarette smoking is the strongest predictor of severe extracranial carotid artery atherosclerosis. Stroke 21:707, 1990.

47. Wolf PA, Kannel WB, McNamara PM, Gordon T. The role of impaired cardiac function in atherothrombotic brain infarction: the Framingham study. Am J Public Health 63:52, 1973.

CHAPTER 84

Peripheral Neuropathy

ANDREA M. CORSE, MD
RALPH W. KUNCL, MD, PhD

DEFINITIONS AND PATHOPHYSIOLOGY

Peripheral neuropathies result from disease processes that involve the peripheral nervous system (PNS). The PNS includes cranial nerves III through XII, dorsal and ventral spinal roots, dorsal root ganglia, spinal nerves, and most autonomic ganglia and nerves.

Peripheral nerves consist of a bundle of fibers called *axons;* the large- and medium-size axons are normally covered with a layer of myelin. Most peripheral nerves are mixed nerves that carry both incoming sensory information (afferent fibers) and outgoing motor and autonomic impulses (efferent fibers). Large-diameter afferent fibers convey information about position and vibration; large-diameter efferent fibers innervate the muscles themselves. Small-diameter, often unmyelinated fibers convey pain and temperature sensation as well as autonomic information.

Based on the primary site of involvement of the peripheral nerves, peripheral neuropathies can be classified into three categories: neuronopathies, axonopathies, and myelinopathies. *Neuronopathies* result from processes affecting primarily the sensory cell bodies in the dorsal root ganglia or motor neuron cell bodies in the spinal cord. By convention, because motor neuron cell bodies are in the central nervous system (CNS), motor neuronopathies are not usually classified among the peripheral neuropathies. *Axonal neuropathies* result from processes affecting primarily the axon, whereas *myelinopathies* (also called demyelinating neuropathies) result from processes affecting primarily the myelin sheath. In some chronic disorders such as diabetes mellitus, irrespective of the primary pathologic process, the interdependence between axon and myelin produces secondary changes that, on biopsy, reveal a mixed pathologic picture. The etiologic diagnosis of peripheral neuropathies, therefore, depends on both the clinical features and the supportive laboratory and pathologic findings.

Three major anatomic patterns of peripheral nerve disease may be distinguished by clinical presentation: mononeuropathy, mononeuropathy multiplex (multifocal neuropathies), and polyneuropathy. *Mononeuropathies* are lesions of individual nerve roots or peripheral nerves; they usually are due to local causes such as trauma or entrapment (compression of a nerve by adjacent structures). *Mononeuropathy multiplex* refers to involvement of two or more named nerves, usually asymmetrically and not contiguously, either at the same time or sequentially. This less common pattern is usually caused by systemic diseases such as the necrotizing vasculitides (e.g., polyarteritis nodosa) or diabetes mellitus, which may affect several nerves focally. *Polyneuropathy* is the result of a generalized disease process affecting many peripheral nerves, often in a symmetric distribution.

In both axonal and demyelinating diseases the longer, larger nerves are generally involved earlier and more severely than the shorter nerves. In demyelinating neuropathies, this vulnerability of the longer axons may reflect the increased number of potential sites for demyelination; in axonal neuropathies, the longer axons require more metabolic support and, therefore, may be more susceptible to disruption of this support. As a result, symptoms of axonal and demyelinating types of neuropathies tend to appear first in the feet and then in the hands. Most polyneuropathies indiscriminately affect both the sensory and the motor nerve fibers (mixed polyneuropathies or sensorimotor neuropathies); some affect peripheral autonomic nerves. However, clinically (and occasionally pathologically) in some patients there is a predilection for the sensory nerves (sensory neuropathies), motor nerves (motor neuropathies), or autonomic nerves.

APPROACH TO THE PATIENT
History and Physical Examination

Symptoms of peripheral neuropathy include reduced sensitivity to stimuli (hypesthesia), spontaneous unusual sensations such as tingling, burning, or pain (paresthesias or dysesthesias), weakness, and muscle cramps. If autonomic nerves are involved, impotence, urinary retention or overflow incontinence, constipation or diarrhea, diminished sweating, and orthostatic hypotension are common symptoms. In patients with polyneuropathy, paresthesias in the feet are the most common presenting complaint. Often, patients are bothered by nonnoxious sensory stimuli such as light touch perceived as pain (allodynia) and may report that symptoms are relieved by pacing the floor or by firm massage. Complaints of heaviness or coldness of the extremities are also common. Diminished joint position sense (proprioception) may be reported as unsteady gait, particularly on uneven surfaces or in the dark.

The *major signs of peripheral neuropathy* are sensory loss, weakness, muscle atrophy, diminished or absent tendon reflexes, and if autonomic nerves are involved, trophic changes in the skin. The most common sensory modalities affected in polyneuropathy are pain and vibration, in a symmetric stocking–glove distribution. Thermal sensation is usually affected, but this is harder to document in the clinical setting. In polyneuropathies the weakness is most often distal, affecting the intrinsic muscles of the feet (e.g., inability to spread or extend the toes). In long-standing neuropathies the muscle imbalance causes high arched feet and hammer toes. Eventually the shin may appear prominent because of atrophy of the tibialis anterior muscle (sharp shin sign), and there may be striking wasting of the small muscles of the hand. The skin of the lower extremities may appear shiny, scaling, and atrophic, although similar changes can be seen with vascular insufficiency. Marked loss of proprioception in the feet may be manifest as unsteadiness, ataxia, or a positive Romberg test (see Chapter 78 for additional details about neurologic signs).

Causes and Distinctive Features

Whereas a limited number of conditions produce mononeuropathy and mononeuropathy multiplex (Table 84.1), there are many causes of polyneuropathy (Table 84.2). Diagnosis often depends on obtaining a thorough history (e.g., of alcoholism or of occupational exposure to toxins) or finding a relevant systemic condition (e.g., diabetes mellitus). Table 84.3 lists the three features most useful in the differential diagnosis of a polyneuropathy—time course, selective functional involvement, and distribution—and the causes associated with these features.

Time Course

Mononeuropathies are often acute in onset; that is, the patient remembers the time of onset. The most common of the acute polyneuropathies, the

Table 84.1.   Common Causes of Mononeuropathy and Mononeuropathy Multiplex

Mononeuropathy
Trauma: direct (occupational, recreational, e.g., ulnar or peroneal nerve), compression, and entrapment (e.g., carpal tunnel, root compression)
Infection: herpes zoster
Vascular: vasculitis, diabetes mellitus
Neoplasm: neurofibroma, lymphoma

Mononeuropathy Multiplex
Diabetes mellitus
Vasculitis

Guillain–Barré syndrome, and other processes—metabolic, vasculitic, or toxic—may cause rapid onset of severe neurologic dysfunction, sometimes within hours. Most toxic neuropathies (lead poisoning, for example) develop more slowly (within weeks), as do neuropathies associated with malnutrition (e.g., thiamine deficiency). The most common of the chronic neuropathies (gradual progression over months to years) are associated with diabetes mellitus (see Chapter 72) and alcoholism (see below); in an unselected population, these are the most common polyneuropathies.

Patients with *hereditary neuropathies* sometimes may be unaware that they have a long-standing progressive disorder. A history of a lack of athletic ability in school or problems fitting shoes may be useful clues. Irreducibly high-arched feet and hammer toes reflect long-standing disease occurring during foot development and may therefore suggest a hereditary process.

Patterns of Involvement

Mononeuropathy usually produces both motor and sensory involvement in the distribution of the affected nerve root or peripheral nerve (see below, Tables 84.6 and 84.7).

Most *polyneuropathies* produce both sensory and motor disturbances. Polyneuropathy with *predominantly sensory involvement* suggests diabetes mellitus, carcinoma, amyloidosis, and dysproteinemia. Occasionally, sensory losses are dissociated, that is, the patient has diminished pain and temperature sensation but preserved vibration and joint position sense; this pattern is typical of small fiber neuropathies. When position and vibratory sense are lost but pain sense is preserved, vitamin B_{12} deficiency (usually pernicious anemia) or, much more rarely, Friedreich's ataxia should be considered. In polyneuropathy, *predominantly motor involvement* suggests inflammatory demyelinating neuropathy, hereditary neuropathies, lead intoxication, or acute intermittent porphyria. *Predominantly autonomic involvement* suggests diabetes mellitus, amyloidosis, familial dysautonomia, or dysproteinemia.

INVESTIGATIONS

Clinical Laboratory

The cause of a peripheral neuropathy must be identified because often neurologic dysfunction persists unless the underlying disease can be treated. The common causes of polyneuropathy (shown in italics in Table 84.3) may be obvious to a patient's physician, but sometimes even these require direct questioning (concerning alcoholism, for example) or specific laboratory tests (e.g., measurement of glycosylated hemoglobin) before they are appreciated. If the cause of the neuropathy is not obvious, one should consider the following *screening tests* that may point to a cause: erythrocyte sedimentation rate, fasting blood glucose level, glycosylated hemoglobin, serum creatinine concentration, a complete blood count (CBC), serum B_{12} level, a chest x-ray, and a serum and urine immunofixation electrophoresis. Many unusual conditions may be associated with neuropathy, but an extensive screening program to rule out all of these processes would be expensive and almost always unrewarding unless there is some

Table 84.2.   Polyneuropathy: Causes and Modes of Predominant Involvement

	Predominant Involvement
Metabolic	
Diabetes mellitus	
Polyneuropathy	S, SM, A
Mononeuropathy	SM
Lumbar plexopathy (diabetic amyotrophy)	M > S
Alcohol with vitamin deficiency	SM
Uremia	SM
Porphyria	M > S
B_{12} deficiency	S > M
Toxic (see Table 84.5)	
Lead	M > S
Pyridoxine	S
Cis-platinum	S
Most other drugs and toxic agents	SM
Infectious	
Diphtheria	M
Leprosy	S
Lyme disease	SM
Human immunodeficiency virus	S, SM, M
Inflammatory and Collagen–Vascular	
Guillain–Barré syndrome	M
Chronic inflammatory demyelinating polyneuropathy	M
Noncarcinomatous sensory neuropathy (e.g., Sjögren's)	S
Systemic lupus erythematosus	SM
Polyarteritis nodosa	SM
Sjögren's syndrome	SM, S
Rheumatoid arthritis	SM
Neoplastic	
Carcinomatous	S, SM
Paraproteinemia, plasma cell dyscrasias	S, SM, A
Benign monoclonal gammopathy	S, SM
Waldenström's macroglobinemia	SM, M
Cryoglobinemia	SM
Hereditary	
Hereditary motor and sensory neuropathies	M > S
Amyloidosis	S > M, A
Dysautonomia (Riley–Day)	S, A
Tomaculous neuropathy	SM
Tangier (Bassen–Kornzweig)	S
Fabry	S

A, Autonomic; *M*, motor; *S*, sensory.

Table 84.3.   Polyneuropathy: Differential Diagnosis

Time Course	**Predominately sensory**
Acute (days)	Global sensory loss
Guillain–Barré syndrome	*Diabetes mellitus*
Porphyric neuropathy	Carcinomatous sensory neuropathy (ganglioradiculitis)
Vasculitic neuropathy	Paraproteinemic and cryoglobulinemic neuropathy
Some toxins (e.g., triorthocresyl phosphate)	Tabes dorsalis
Subacute (weeks)	Dissociated loss of pain and thermal sensibility
Many toxins and drugs (see Table 84.5)	Diabetes (small fiber type)
Nutritional neuropathies	Amyloidosis
Carcinomatous neuropathies	Hereditary sensory neuropathies
Diabetic amyotrophy	Lepromatous leprosy
Uremic neuropathy	Dissociated loss of joint position and vibration sensibility
Relapsing	Subacute combined degeneration
Chronic inflammatory demyelinating polyneuropathy	Friedreich's ataxia
Refsum's disease	**Autonomic neuropathy**
Porphyria	*Diabetes*
Chronic (many months or years)	*Amyloid*
Diabetic motor and sensory neuropathy	Acute, chronic, and relapsing pandysautonomia
Alcoholic neuropathy	Dysautonomia (Riley–Day)
Chronic inflammatory demyelinating polyneuropathy	
Very chronic (childhood onset)	**Distribution**[b]
Hereditary, motor and sensory neuropathies (e.g.,	Proximal weakness
Charcot–Marie–Tooth disease)	Guillain–Barré syndrome
	Porphyria
Selective Functional Involvement[a]	Diabetic amyotrophy
Predominantly motor	Carcinomatous neuropathy with proximal weakness ("carcinomatous
Guillain–Barré syndrome	neuromyopathy")
Chronic inflammatory demyelinating polyneuropathy	Proximal sensory loss
Acute intermittent porphyria	Porphyria
Lead neuropathy	Tangier disease (analphalipoproteinemia)
Hereditary motor and sensory neuropathies (e.g.,	Temperature-related distribution
Charcot–Marie–Tooth)	Lepromatous leprosy
Diphtheritic neuropathy	

Modified from Griffin JW, Cornblath DR. Peripheral neuropathies. In: Harvey AM, et al, eds. Principles and practice of medicine. 22nd ed. New York: Appleton & Lange, 1988.

The most common causes are set in *italic*.

[a]Most polyneuropathies produce sensory and motor disturbances.

[b]Most polyneuropathies produce distal involvement.

clue in the history or physical examination to warrant a particular test (e.g., measurement of blood lead levels in a patient with a possible history of occupational exposure). If no cause of the process is identified on evaluation, consultation with a neurologist should be considered.

Nerve Conduction Studies

The measurement of nerve conduction is useful as an *initial diagnostic screen* because it can distinguish major categories of disease (axonal versus demyelinating) and can localize entrapments and other mononeuropathies. A baseline measurement makes it possible to differentiate progression of the peripheral neuropathy from other clinical conditions in the future.

Nerve conduction measurements involve stimulating a nerve at one point and recording the response, either at the muscle (motor nerve) or at some distance along the nerve (sensory nerve). The results of nerve conduction studies usually include latency of response, conduction velocity, and amplitude of response. The *latency of response* refers to the time elapsed between the start of the stimulus and the muscle response (muscle fiber depolarization) or nerve response (sensory nerve action potential). The *conduc-*

tion velocity between two points along the nerve is expressed in meters per second.

Conduction disturbances of the peripheral nerve may be localized, as in an entrapment syndrome, or may involve nerves more diffusely, as in polyneuropathies. In general, early axonal degenerations are associated with normal conduction and the presence of denervation on electromyography (EMG; see below), whereas early demyelination is characterized by slowing of nerve conduction and normal EMG studies. Nerve conduction velocities are normal and sensory nerve action potentials are spared in cervical or lumbar disc disease with radiculopathy, because the potential site of nerve root compression at the neural foramina is proximal to the sensory cell body in the ganglion and therefore does not cause degeneration of the distal sensory nerve fiber. This is an important point because spondylotic radiculopathy is common and may mimic polyneuropathy (see Chapters 64 and 65).

The procedure has several *limitations*. First, nerve conduction studies test directly only the portion of the nerve between the two sites; they generally do not detect damage more distal than (e.g., intramuscular nerve) or more proximal to (e.g., nerve root) the segment tested. F waves may detect proximal segment disease. Second, electrophysiologic studies measure the speed of conduction in the largest and fastest conducting fibers of peripheral nerves. Therefore, nerve conduction studies are most sensitive in diseases that involve such fibers.

When ordering electrophysiologic studies, the clinical problem and question to be addressed should be specified as precisely as possible; stating only "numbness in the upper extremities" or "test nerves in lower extremities" without any specific guidance is unlikely to be productive.

Patient Experience. With the patient comfortably positioned, conducting gel is applied and electrodes are taped over the appropriate muscles and nerves to be tested. The shocks are mildly unpleasant. Usually the nerves on both sides of the body are compared. Testing takes approximately 20 to 60 minutes.

Electromyography

One important use of EMG is to help define entrapment neuropathies (e.g., radial nerve entrapment) and differentiate these from more proximal radicular compression (e.g., apparent carpal tunnel syndrome that is actually caused by C6 radiculopathy). The EMG can recognize denervation in muscles that are difficult to assess on physical examination. EMG is not often helpful in patients with diffuse peripheral neuropathy. However, it may detect the early denervation changes of axonal neuropathy before striking changes are recognized on nerve conduction studies. EMG can also help differentiate the muscle wasting of neuropathic or myopathic disorders from disuse atrophy. Table 84.4 summarizes the changes found in denervation and myopathic conditions.

EMG involves the insertion of needles into a muscle to record electrical activity directly. With the muscle at rest, no electrical activity should be observed. Spontaneous *fibrillation potentials* are the action potentials of single myofibers that are twitching spontaneously. Fibrillation potentials and positive waves are usually, but not invariably, a good indication of denervation (they also occur in polymyositis and more rarely in other myopathic processes). *Fasciculations* are the spontaneous firings of whole motor units (all of the muscle fibers innervated by a single motor neuron and its branches). Fasciculations may be seen in normal subjects, although they are more frequent and likely to be more polyphasic in states of denervation. Therefore

the presence of fasciculations is only moderately useful in diagnosing denervation.

Voluntary motor unit potentials (MUPs) are examined individually by asking the patient to contract a given muscle slightly. Long-duration, large-amplitude polyphasic potentials suggest a denervating process. Brief, small-amplitude polyphasic potentials are associated with myopathic processes.

Graded increasing effort is used to analyze the orderly recruitment of MUPs, including their number and firing rates. Recruitment of a reduced repertoire of large-amplitude MUPs firing at rapid rates is indicative of denervation and reinnervation. Early recruitment of numerous brief, small-amplitude MUPs indicates a myopathic process.

The EMG electrodes mildly inflame the muscles into which they have been inserted (note that serum creatine phosphokinase activity is rarely altered substantially by this procedure). Thus, if there is a possibility that a muscle biopsy will be required, the muscle to be biopsied should not be tested by EMG. The need for EMG in patients with bleeding tendencies or at risk from recurrent infection should be carefully reviewed with a neurologist.

Patient Experience. There is usually discomfort with the initial insertion of the recording needles and during movement of the muscles when the needles are in place. Because the needles are very thin and penetrate only skin and muscle, the risks of infection or hemorrhage are almost nil. The procedure takes 30 to 60 minutes.

Nerve Biopsy

Nerve biopsy is a useful last step that should be reserved for patients in whom a specific histologic diagnosis, and a management decision that may help the patient, are possible (e.g., amyloidosis, demyelination, inflammation, or necrotizing vasculitis). Its use should be guided by the history and electrophysiology. The nerve studied by biopsy is almost always a sensory nerve (the sural) and sometimes may not reflect a disease process that appears to affect only the motor nerves. The biopsy always leads to a fixed numbness in the distribution of the excised nerve (usually the sural distribution on the lateral heel and ankle) but rarely may lead to painful sequelae such as neuroma formation. If a nerve biopsy is done, it should be done at a center where it is performed frequently, where plastic embedded nerve histopathology and electron micros-

Table 84.4. Electromyography: Patterns Typical of Nerve and Muscle Disorders

Disorder	Insertional Activity	Complete Rest (Spontaneous Activity)	Motor Unit Potentials	Recruitment
Neuropathic[a]	Increased	Fibrillations, positive sharp waves, fasciculations	Long duration, high amplitude, polyphasic	Reduced
Myopathic				
Myopathy	Normal	Normal or rare fibrillations	Brief duration, small amplitude, polyphasic	Early
Myositis	Increased	Fibrillations, positive sharp waves	Brief duration, small amplitude, polyphasic	Early

[a]Neuropathy or radiculopathy.

copy are routinely available, and where a pathologist with special expertise in nerve morphology can interpret it, so that maximum information can result from this invasive procedure. Consultation with a neurologist is helpful in determining whether a nerve biopsy is indicated.

COMMON PROBLEMS
Diabetic Neuropathy

Diabetic neuropathy is one of the most common neuropathies seen in primary care settings (7,24). The diabetic neuropathies have protean manifestations, capable of presenting as chronic sensorimotor polyneuropathy, autonomic neuropathy, acute amyotrophy, mononeuropathy multiplex, or nerve entrapment. The problem is discussed in detail in Chapter 72 ("Diabetes Mellitus") and in the section on femoral neuropathy below.

Alcoholic Neuropathy

The neuropathy associated with alcoholism and related vitamin deficiencies is a sensorimotor polyneuropathy (3). The presenting symptoms are often pain and paresthesias in the feet and legs reflecting a distal, symmetric sensorimotor axonopathy. Many patients are asymptomatic. Examination often shows diminished ankle jerks and a stocking–glove pattern of decreased sensation to all modalities. Autonomic features, including impotence, bladder dysfunction, and orthostatic hypotension, may rarely be seen. Electrodiagnostic studies commonly reveal reduced amplitudes of the sural sensory nerve action potentials and abnormal H reflexes. Sural nerve sections show primary axonal degeneration. Malnutrition and vitamin deficiencies (particularly thiamine deficiency) probably make a major contribution to the neuropathy, although there is evidence that alcohol has a direct toxic effect on peripheral nerves.

Treatment is aimed toward improved nutrition and vitamin replacement as well as effective treatment for the alcoholism (see Chapter 21). The paresthesias of a mild neuropathy can be expected to improve with good nutrition and abstinence from alcohol. However, with moderate to severe sensorimotor and autonomic neuropathy, significant residual symptoms and findings will persist.

Carcinomatous Neuropathy

The most common form of neuropathy associated with malignancies is a distal sensorimotor polyneuropathy. Compression or infiltration of nerves by tumor or a pure sensory neuronopathy occurs less commonly. Both the distal sensorimotor neuropathy and pure sensory neuronopathy are most often associated with carcinoma of the lung, and the onset of the neuropathic symptoms can either precede, follow, or coincide with the diagnosis of the malignancy (15,26).

Distal Sensorimotor Neuropathy

Distal sensorimotor neuropathy is primarily an axonal process with sensory loss and weakness appearing initially in the feet. It is more common in men, develops over weeks or months, and is generally progressive in its course. If the underlying cancer responds to treatment, the neuropathy may improve.

Carcinomatous Sensory Neuropathy

Carcinomatous sensory neuropathy has a distinctive pattern beginning subacutely, often with pain and paresthesias involving legs, arms, or, rarely, face. Over many weeks a profound proprioceptive sensory loss develops, accompanied by pseudoathetosis (seemingly purposeless movements caused by loss of position sense). Areflexia is common. The patient may be unable to stand or walk unassisted despite normal strength. Nerve conduction studies may show reduced or unobtainable sensory potentials. It occurs more typically in women (15). The underlying tumor is most often small cell carcinoma of the lung, but this neuropathy also may accompany breast, ovarian, uterine, and gastrointestinal tract tumors. The neuropathy is usually progressive. A common chemotherapeutic agent for the treatment of ovarian cancer, cis-platinum, produces a similar picture.

Paraproteinemic Neuropathies

An association between peripheral neuropathies and monoclonal gammopathies has been increasingly recognized. In patients with idiopathic peripheral neuropathy a monoclonal gammopathy can be identified in nearly 10%; in half of these a plasma cell dyscrasia is diagnosed, whereas in the other half the monoclonal gammopathy is of undetermined significance (MGUS) and an association with the neuropathy is unclear (16).

Peripheral neuropathy may be the presenting symptom in plasma cell dyscrasias, such as in primary amyloidosis or the rare osteosclerotic form of myeloma. Neuropathic symptoms typical in primary amyloidosis are prominent burning dysesthesias and autonomic dysfunction. It is generally an axonal neuropathy that, like the amyloidosis, does not respond to treatment. Nearly 50% of patients with osteosclerotic myeloma have a neuropathy characterized as a symmetric, demyelinating, primarily motor neuropathy. Although the course is usually one of steady progression, improvement in the neuropathy occurred in nearly 50% of patients in one series in response to successful treatment of osteosclerotic myeloma (19).

Neuropathy Caused by Toxins and Drugs

Toxic neuropathies, including those caused by drugs, are becoming increasingly recognized. Toxic neuropathies are potentially reversible if the toxin can be identified and the exposure to the toxin eliminated. The diagnosis may be made easily if there is a history of drug exposure (e.g., colchicine, isoniazid, hydralazine, vincristine) or industrial exposure (Table 84.5). Because these neuropathies have no distinguishing features on routine history or physical examination, a detailed history of exposure to drugs and the patient's occupation and recreational habits is important. Axonal involvement in the spinal cord may also occur and be masked by the toxic neuropathy. In these cases, a residual spastic paraparesis becomes apparent when the peripheral neuropathy has resolved. Toxic neuropathies are classically associated with chronic low-dose exposure (months to years), although they may appear within days to weeks with high-level exposure. The syndrome of proximal muscle weakness and axonal polyneuropathy caused by colchicine may appear after the patient has taken this drug for years, usually because of elevated drug levels caused by altered renal function. A delayed neuropathy associated with organophosphates develops 10 to 14 days after exposure, whereas Vacor, a rodenticide, produces an acute toxic neuropathy within 2 to 3 days.

Toxicity caused by megadose pyridoxine (vitamin B_6) consumption produces a gradually progressive sensory ataxia with profound distal limb impairment of position and vibratory sense (23). General public acceptance of vitamin B_6 therapy makes direct questioning about vitamin habits necessary. Neuropathy has been reported in patients consuming dosages as low as 200 mg/day.

HIV Infection

There are many peripheral nervous system manifestations of human immunodeficiency virus (HIV) infection (4). A *painful sensory neuropathy*, usually confined to the feet, affects 30% of patients with the acquired immunodeficiency syndrome (AIDS), often late in the course. Nerve conduction studies show reduced or absent sensory potentials. Histologic studies demonstrate a reduction in the number of small, unmyelinated fibers. Treatment is currently limited to symptomatic relief using tricyclic antidepressants such as amitriptyline (Elavil) or carbamazepine (Tegretol), described below.

Multiple *mononeuropathies* have been described, most often in HIV-infected patients who have not yet developed AIDS.

Both acute and chronic inflammatory demyelinating polyneuropathies have been seen, usually in the early stages of HIV infection, in otherwise asymptomatic seropositive patients. Treatment has been tried with plasmapheresis, as in seronegative cases of demyelinating neuropathy.

Chapter 34 provides a detailed account of the ambulatory care of patients with HIV infection.

Compression and Entrapment Neuropathies

When a peripheral neurologic abnormality occurs in one upper or lower extremity, the abnormality is usually caused by nerve entrapment or compression caused by anatomic abnormalities or trauma, although polyneuropathy and mononeuropathy multiplex may present initially as a focal deficit in one extremity. With clinical evaluation, it is usually possible to determine

Table 84.5.   Toxins and Drugs Associated with Peripheral Neuropathies

Industrial[a]
Pesticides: organophosphates, dichlorophenyoxyacetate (2,4-D), Vacor rodenticide
Metal work: lead, arsenic, mercury, thallium, methyl bromide
Plastics, synthetic fabrics: *n*-hexane, methyl, *n*-butyl ketone, acrylamide, carbon disulfide, perchlorethylene, trichlorethylene, dimethylaminoproprionitrile
Gases: carbon monoxide, ethylene oxide

Euphorants
Glue sniffing: *n*-hexane, solvents
Nitrous oxide inhalation: whipped cream dispensers, dental offices

Pharmacotherapeutic Agents
Antimicrobial: isoniazid, nitrofurantoin, metronidazole
Cardiovascular: hydralazine, procainamide, amiodarone
Other: phenytoin, colchicine, disulfiram, pyridoxine, vincristine, cis-platinum, taxol, thalidomide

[a]See also Chapter 7, Table 7.2.

Table 84.6.   Comparative Data on Root and Nerve Lesions in the Upper Extremity

Roots →	C5	C6	C7	C8	T1
Sensory loss[a,b]	Lateral upper arm	Dorsolateral forearm and thumb	Mid-dorsal forearm and middle finger	Medial forearm, ring and small fingers	Medial arm, axilla
Motor loss[b]	Deltoid, some biceps, infraspinatus and supraspinatus	Biceps, brachioradialis, some deltoid	Triceps, wrist and finger extensors	Thenar eminence and interossei of hand	Thenar eminence and interossei of hand
Tendon reflex	Biceps, brachioradialis	Biceps, brachioradialis	Triceps	Triceps, finger jerk	Finger jerk

Peripheral Nerves →	Axillary	Musculocutaneous	Radial	Median (Carpal Tunnel)	Ulnar (Cubital Tunnel)
Sensory loss	Over deltoid	Radial forearm	Dorsal lateral hand	First 3½ digits	4th and 5th digits
Motor loss	Deltoid	Biceps, brachialis	Triceps, wrist and finger extensors	Thenar: abductor pollicis brevis, opponens	Hypothenar: abductor digiti minimi, first dorsal interosseus
Tendon reflex	None	Biceps	Triceps, brachioradialis	Finger jerk	Finger jerk
Pain	Over deltoid	Lateral forearm	Dorsal lateral forearm and hand	Nocturnal in forearm, lateral hand, and first 3½ digits	4th and 5th digits and tenderness at elbow

[a]See dermatomal pattern, Table 78.1.

[b]Pain usually radiates from the neck to the distal area of sensory loss.

Table 84.7.   Comparative Data on Root and Nerve Lesions in the Lower Extremity

Roots →	L2	L3	L4	L5	S1
Sensory loss[a]	Upper and medial thigh	Anterior thigh	Lateral thigh to medial leg	Lateral leg to dorsum of foot	Posterior leg to plantar foot
Motor loss	Iliopsoas (hip flexion)	Quadriceps (knee extension), adductor	Quadriceps, tibialis anterior (dorsiflexion of foot)	Great toe extensor, tibialis anterior, tibialis posterior	Gastrocnemius, gluteus maximus (hip extension)
Tendon reflex	Adductor	Adductor, knee jerk	Knee jerk	Medial hamstring	Achilles

Peripheral Nerves →	Obturator	Femoral	Lateral Femoral Cutaneous (Meralgia Paresthetica)	Sciatic Peroneal Division	Sciatic Tibial Division
Sensory loss, pain area	Medial thigh	Anterior medial thigh	Upper lateral thigh usually to 10–12 inches below the iliac crest	Dorsum of foot and lateral leg	Plantar foot (with burning pain), tips of toes
Motor loss	Adductors	Quadriceps (knee extension)	N/A	Tibialis anterior (dorsiflexion of ankle), extensor digitorum brevis (toe extension)	Gastrocnemius
Tendon reflex	Adductor	Knee jerk	N/A	None	Achilles

[a]See dermatomal pattern, Table 78.1.

whether the patient's problem is caused by nerve root damage or damage to a peripheral nerve or one of its branches. Tables 84.6, 84.7, 84.8, and Figures 84.1 and 84.2 summarize the information needed to make this distinction: distribution of sensory, motor, and reflex deficits; common causative factors; and critical anatomic relationships.

Several common compression and entrapment neuropathies and specific approaches to treatment are discussed here. Working diagnoses and decisions regarding conservative management can usually be accomplished without costly electrodiagnostic studies. The latter are useful for unclear diagnosis and for supporting the decision to recommend surgery. Additional general aspects of prognosis and treatment are described in a later section ("Therapeutic Principles"). Root compression symptoms caused by cervical and lumbar spine disease are discussed in Chapters 64 ("Neck Pain") and 65 ("Low Back Pain").

Median Nerve (Carpal Tunnel Syndrome)

Causes.   Carpal tunnel syndrome (CTS) is the most common of all the entrapment neuropathies. In CTS, symptoms and signs result from compression by neighboring anatomic structures on the median nerve as it passes from the forearm to the palm (Fig. 84.1). The median nerve and nine digital flexor tendons pass through the carpal tunnel, a rigid compartment formed by the concave arch of the carpal bones and roofed by the transverse carpal ligament. Conditions that cause a decrease in the size of the carpal tunnel (e.g., Colles's fracture, rheumatoid arthritis, congenital carpal tunnel stenosis), enlargement of the median nerve (e.g., amyloid, neuroma, endoneural edema in diabetes mellitus), or increase in the volume of other structures within the tunnel (e.g., tenosynovitis, ganglion, lipoma, urate deposits in gout, hematoma, fluid retention in pregnancy) may all result in compression of the median nerve. Many cases previously classified as idiopathic are explained by occupational factors. CTS

Table 84.8.   Entrapment Neuropathies: Common Causative Factors

Nerve, Location	Causative Factors
Median	
At wrist	Meat processing, upholstering, knitting, painting, weight lifting, using vibrating tools, pregnancy, musical instruments
At forearm	Repeated pronation (e.g., screwdriver), weight lifting
Ulnar	
At wrist	Bicycling, leaning on a walker, using pliers, using palm as a hammer
At elbow	Injury to elbow, chronic flexion of elbow (e.g., sitting in wheelchair or lying in bed), leaning on elbow on tables and desks
Radial	
At forearm	Lipoma, tennis, trauma
At arm	Saturday night palsy, bridegroom's palsy, crutches, pneumatic tourniquets
Axillary	Fracture/dislocation of shoulder, deep injections into deltoid muscle
Musculocutaneous	Weight lifting, shoulder dislocations
Tibial	
At knee	Chronic standing
At ankle	Trauma, weight gain, or edema
Peroneal	
At knee	Ankle sprains, crossed legs, after weight loss, squatting, kneeling
At ankle	Tight shoes, trauma
Femoral	Inguinal surgery, childbirth, psoas hemorrhage, dorsal lithotomy position
Lateral femoral cutaneous	Ascites, overweight, pregnancy, utility belts, blunt sports injury to anterior iliac spine
Obturator	Pelvic fracture, hip surgery, childbirth, retroperitoneal hematoma, malignancy
Sciatic	Hip surgery, pelvic fracture, injections, endometriosis, retroperitoneal hematoma, lipoma

in the workplace is associated with occupations in which the wrist position deviates from the normal straight alignment and with occupations involving the use of greater hand force in all wrist positions (e.g., meat processing, fruit packing, upholstering, and

The most frequently encountered
causes of damage at the
various sites are indicated

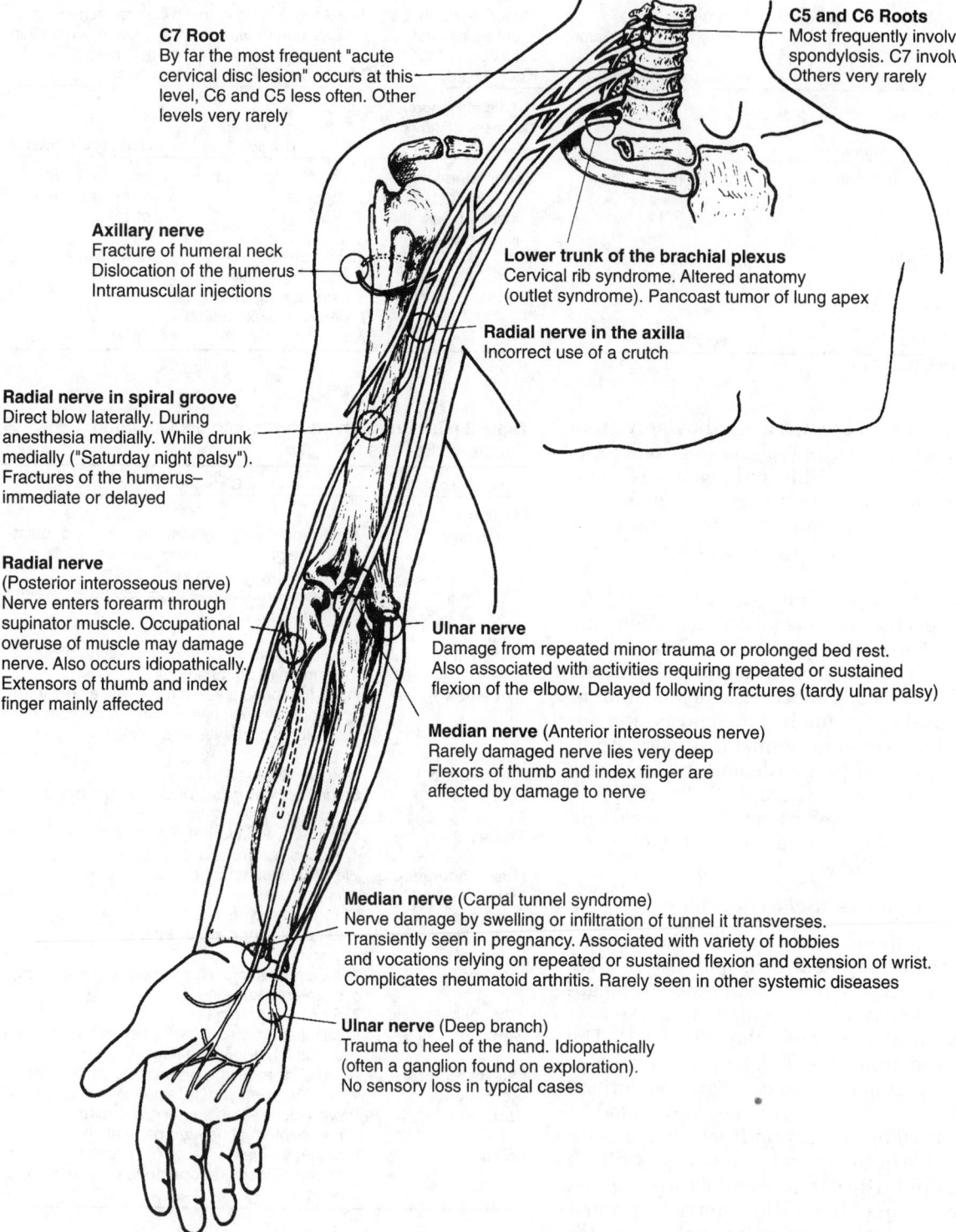

C7 Root
By far the most frequent "acute
cervical disc lesion" occurs at this
level, C6 and C5 less often. Other
levels very rarely

C5 and C6 Roots
Most frequently involved roots in cervical
spondylosis. C7 involved occasionally.
Others very rarely

Axillary nerve
Fracture of humeral neck
Dislocation of the humerus
Intramuscular injections

Lower trunk of the brachial plexus
Cervical rib syndrome. Altered anatomy
(outlet syndrome). Pancoast tumor of lung apex

Radial nerve in the axilla
Incorrect use of a crutch

Radial nerve in spiral groove
Direct blow laterally. During
anesthesia medially. While drunk
medially ("Saturday night palsy").
Fractures of the humerus–
immediate or delayed

Radial nerve
(Posterior interosseous nerve)
Nerve enters forearm through
supinator muscle. Occupational
overuse of muscle may damage
nerve. Also occurs idiopathically.
Extensors of thumb and index
finger mainly affected

Ulnar nerve
Damage from repeated minor trauma or prolonged bed rest.
Also associated with activities requiring repeated or sustained
flexion of the elbow. Delayed following fractures (tardy ulnar palsy)

Median nerve (Anterior interosseous nerve)
Rarely damaged nerve lies very deep
Flexors of thumb and index finger are
affected by damage to nerve

Median nerve (Carpal tunnel syndrome)
Nerve damage by swelling or infiltration of tunnel it transverses.
Transiently seen in pregnancy. Associated with variety of hobbies
and vocations relying on repeated or sustained flexion and extension of wrist.
Complicates rheumatoid arthritis. Rarely seen in other systemic diseases

Ulnar nerve (Deep branch)
Trauma to heel of the hand. Idiopathically
(often a ganglion found on exploration).
No sensory loss in typical cases

Figure 84.1.   Anatomic relationships of nerves to the upper extremity. (Modified from Patten J. Neurological
differential diagnosis. 2nd ed. New York: Springer-Verlag, 1995.)

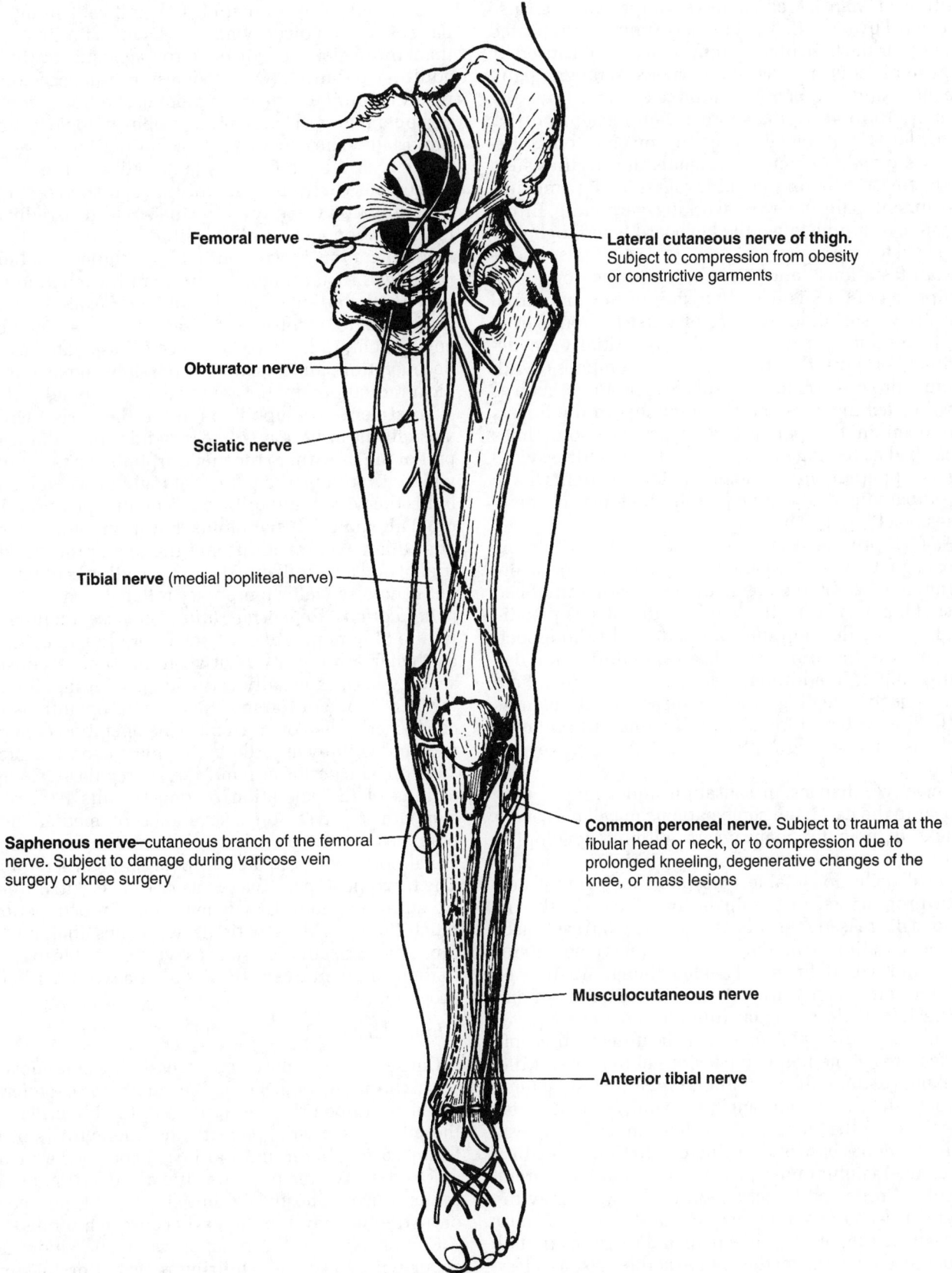

Femoral nerve

Lateral cutaneous nerve of thigh. Subject to compression from obesity or constrictive garments

Obturator nerve

Sciatic nerve

Tibial nerve (medial popliteal nerve)

Saphenous nerve—cutaneous branch of the femoral nerve. Subject to damage during varicose vein surgery or knee surgery

Common peroneal nerve. Subject to trauma at the fibular head or neck, or to compression due to prolonged kneeling, degenerative changes of the knee, or mass lesions

Musculocutaneous nerve

Anterior tibial nerve

Figure 84.2. Anatomic relationships to nerves to the lower extremity. (Modified from Patten J. Neurological differential diagnosis. 2nd ed. New York: Springer-Verlag, 1995.)

waiting on tables). Median nerve compression can also be caused by tasks that require a sustained or repeated stress over the base of the palm, such as that caused by the use of tools such as screwdrivers, scrapers, paint brushes, and buffers. Vibration exposure (low frequency, 10 to 40 Hz) is another well-recognized risk factor for CTS (typically from air-powered tools). Repetitive wrist and hand movements in activities such as knitting, crocheting, hooking rugs, playing a musical instrument, painting, woodworking, gardening, lifting weights, or typing when the keyboard is too high may also lead to CTS.

Manifestations and Evaluation. The onset of symptoms of CTS is usually insidious and nocturnal because of sustained posture of wrist flexion during sleep. Symptoms in the hand may initially be described as episodic tingling and numbness with gradual progression to more severe symptoms, such as burning, aching, or a painful numbness in the fingers and deep in the palm. The fingers are sometimes described as feeling swollen, even though little swelling is apparent on inspection. Many patients have accompanying dull aching pain in the forearm, sometimes reaching the shoulder.

As CTS progresses, the nocturnal pain and tingling may begin to wake the patient after a few hours' sleep. Relief may be obtained by hanging the arm out of bed or shaking or rubbing the hand. At this stage episodic tingling may develop during the day, but the associated pain in the arm occurs less often during the day than at night. In addition to sensory symptoms, there is a subjective feeling of uselessness and clumsiness in the fingers with difficulty performing certain tasks, such as unscrewing bottle tops, turning a key, or crocheting.

Objective changes in sensation and strength may appear in the hand, but some patients may have severe attacks of pain for many years without developing neurologic signs. Sensory signs within the median nerve distribution (Table 84.6) are first evident and most pronounced in the fingertips. Occasionally, instead of decreased sensation, there is an overreaction to cutaneous stimuli in the median innervated lateral three and a half fingers. Isolated thenar wasting or isolated sensory impairment in the distribution of one of the lateral three digital (thumb and digit #2, #3, lateral half of digit #4) nerves may be unusual presenting features of median nerve lesions at the wrist. Mild weakness of the abductor pollicis brevis (to test, patient abducts thumb at right angle to palm, against resistance) or of the opponens pollicis muscle (to test, patient touches base of little finger with thumb, against resistance) is often present with no visually apparent atrophy. Prolonged hyperflexion of the wrist may reproduce sensory symptoms *(Phalen's sign)*. *Tinel's sign,* consisting of shocklike pain and tingling elicited by percussion of the median nerve at the wrist, is a less specific finding.

Electrodiagnostic studies (see details above). Although abnormalities of the *nerve conduction studies* in CTS are more likely to be found when physical signs

are evident on examination, a significant number of patients with typical symptoms have no findings other than those detected on electrodiagnostic testing. In addition, because CNS or root lesions can occasionally result in similar sensory symptoms, confirmation of a peripheral nerve lesion by electrophysiologic testing is important. The most common finding on nerve conduction studies in CTS is abnormality in the median sensory nerve studies, including a segmental reduction in conduction velocity across the wrist and a reduction in the action potential amplitude. Abnormalities of median motor nerve conduction studies, including prolonged distal motor latency, are less common but important findings. Needle electrode examination is important to confirm localization of median nerve entrapment, to look for evidence of associated axonal degeneration, and to rule out possible coexistent cervical radiculopathy (double crush syndrome).

Treatment. Immobilization of the wrist with a close-fitting *anterior splint* (extends from the upper part of the forearm to the metacarpophalangeal joints), which is worn by the patient at night or when resting, holds the wrist immobilized in a neutral position. This often alleviates all symptoms, but if symptoms persist after a few weeks, additional therapy is indicated. A trial of oral anti-inflammatory medication is often used but generally yields temporary relief at best.

Indications for carpal tunnel release include the failure of nonoperative treatment or clinical evidence of thenar atrophy. A relative indication is constant sensory loss, especially if it is long-standing. Surgery for CTS is one of the most successful operations that can be performed on the hand. The operation demands care and skill by an orthopedic, plastic, or neurologic surgeon who performs hand surgery regularly. Complications of the operation or poor results (i.e., reflex sympathetic dystrophy, severance of median nerve branches, hypertrophic scar, adherent flexor tendons) are almost always related to poor surgical technique. The usual postoperative recovery time is 6 to 8 weeks. An additional month may be needed for occupational rehabilitation. Most patients with jobs that involve repetitive wrist motion such as typing are able to return to their preoperative activities after a work-hardening program.

Ulnar Nerve

Causes. Ulnar nerve compression occurs most often at the elbow (Fig. 84.1). The *cubital tunnel* refers to the area of potential entrapment of the ulnar nerve at the elbow as it runs beneath the aponeurosis of the flexor carpi ulnaris muscle just distal to the medial epicondyle. Minor pressure directly over the cubital tunnel during anesthesia, intoxication, stupor, coma, or by trauma may subsequently cause symptoms.

Compression of the ulnar nerve at the elbow may occur with activities requiring repeated or sustained flexion of the elbow because the cubital tunnel is at its smallest when the elbow is at 90% flexion. Hypermobility of the ulnar nerve can result in subluxation over the medial epicondyle and repeated trauma.

Manifestations and Evaluation. Patients may awaken at night with elbow pain, shooting pain in the hand or fifth digit, and paresthesias and hypesthesia in the ulnar nerve distribution. These symptoms usually improve with elbow extension. The amount of pain and paresthesia varies, and for some the sensory loss is not bothersome. Patients usually see a physician when they experience motor dysfunction, such as weakness of grasp and pinch or loss of dexterity.

Ulnar sensory loss (Table 84.6) is easiest to establish with two-point discrimination over the distal two phalanges of the little finger. Transition between the ulnar territory over the hypothenar eminence and the medial antebrachial cutaneous nerve (branch from the brachial plexus) of the forearm is often detected at the skin crease at the wrist. Motor disability is usually manifested as decreased grip and pinch strength, which is related to the degree of atrophy of the involved intrinsic muscles, especially the palmar and dorsal interossei and flexor digitorum profundus to the fourth and fifth digits. One of the earliest signs of ulnar nerve entrapment is weakness of fifth finger adduction with a tendency to catch the finger (e.g., on a pants pocket).

Ulnar neuropathy distal to the elbow occurs at the wrist or in the hand and must be considered if there is no weakness in the flexor digitorum profundus. This is most often caused by a ganglion, rheumatoid arthritis, or trauma (e.g., long-distance bicycling). Often lesions in the wrist or hand produce no paresthesias or sensory loss. Depending on the level of entrapment at the wrist, either all of the ulnar innervated muscles may be weak or there may be selective preservation of hypothenar function (i.e., abductor digiti minimi).

Electrodiagnostic study (see details above). Focal slowing of the ulnar motor or sensory nerve conduction across the elbow is useful in localizing the nerve damage, depending on the severity. False-positive findings may be obtained, so close correlation with the clinical findings is mandatory. Increased distal latencies are found with entrapment at the wrist but must be correlated with EMG (see above) to determine the actual site of the lesion.

Treatment. Nonsurgical treatment is indicated for the patient with intermittent symptoms, acute or chronic mild neuropathy, or mild neuropathy associated with an occupational cause. For a mild ulnar neuropathy, wearing elbow pads during the day and *splinting the elbow* at night in an extended position may be helpful. An easy way to splint the elbow during sleep is to strap a pillow around it. Elbow protection should be continued for 2 to 3 months, especially if the symptoms are intermittent or show improvement. For ulnar compression at the wrist, whether caused by a single traumatic event or by chronic trauma, conservative treatment with a wrist splint (see under "Carpal Tunnel Syndrome") is generally adequate.

Surgical intervention is not necessary as long as symptoms do not progress and especially as long as there is no motor involvement or objective sensory loss. Surgical approaches to lesions of the ulnar nerve at the elbow depend on the cause and the surgeon. These include simple release of the cubital tunnel, medial epicondylectomy, and anterior transposition of the nerve. Complications from any of the surgical approaches include persistent or recurrent symptoms caused by inadequate surgery or recurrent scarring around the nerve.

Radial Nerve

Causes. Radial nerve lesions are the least common of the major upper extremity nontraumatic compression neuropathies and usually involve the nerve at or proximal to the elbow (Fig. 84.1).

Besides traumatic conditions such as humeral fractures, more proximal radial nerve injuries can occur when the arm has been held in a hyperabducted position that causes traction to the nerve, as in surgery or sleep. Proximal nerve injury may also follow axillary pressure caused by incorrect use of a crutch. The middle third of the nerve is compressed against the humerus in the so-called Saturday night palsy, as when an intoxicated person sleeps with the arm draped over a chair. Compression of the posterior interosseous nerve (branch of radial nerve in the forearm) can result from a variety of masses, such as lipomas, fibromas, or calluses from old fractures.

Manifestations and Evaluation. The radial nerve is predominantly a motor nerve. Depending on the location of a high radial compression, the triceps function (elbow extension) may or may not be affected. Elbow flexion and supination may be slightly affected by brachioradialis weakness. The most obvious finding in a radial palsy is wrist drop and digital extensor paralysis (finger drop). A lesion of the posterior interosseous nerve results in finger drop alone.

High radial nerve lesions may produce sensory loss over the dorsum of the hand. Pain and tenderness in the area of nerve damage may be present. Nerve conduction studies and EMG (see above) can be helpful in localizing and quantifying radial nerve compression. For example, acutely, a Saturday night palsy can cause focal slowing of conduction at the site of pressure injury but normal motor and sensory conduction below this lesion.

Treatment. The treatment of traumatic radial nerve compression is generally conservative and recovery of function occurs within a few weeks to months. To prevent flexor contractures, a *cock-up splint for the wrist joint* should be accompanied by a *spring-loaded extensor brace for the fingers* if the weakness is severe and long lasting. Individually constructed splints made by an occupational therapist are superior to those obtained from a surgical supply house. For compression of the posterior interosseus nerve with no obvious cause, imaging of the nerve should be performed to investigate for possible masses. If no mass is identified, surgical exploration is indicated if there has not been spontaneous recovery within 2 to 3 months.

Peroneal Nerve

Causes. The most common site of compression of the peroneal nerve is at the fibular head (Fig. 84.2). Such compression may result from improperly applied plaster casts or tight stockings and garters, or from falling asleep with the side of the leg resting against a protruding object, as in a drug- or alcohol-induced stupor or in the weakened bedridden patient. Prolonged leg crossing, squatting, or kneeling may also result in peroneal compression. Entrapment of the peroneal nerve can also occur in the *fibular tunnel* formed by the peroneus longus muscle.

Manifestations and Evaluation. Symptoms of peroneal palsy consist of painless weakness of ankle dorsiflexion (foot drop) and foot eversion and sensory loss over the lateral calf and dorsum of the foot.

Electrodiagnostic studies (see details above). Nerve conduction studies can detect focal slowing or conduction block in the peroneal nerve segment across the fibular head. The superficial peroneal sensory potential may be absent. EMG may demonstrate denervation in peroneal innervated muscles with sparing of the short head of the biceps femoris muscle, the most distal of the peroneal innervated muscles above the fibular head.

Peroneal palsy with loss of motor function and no clear history of trauma or external compression should be investigated with appropriate physical examination and imaging of the popliteal fossa to rule out a mass lesion.

Treatment. Mild compressive peroneal lesions can be treated conservatively. Patients should be advised to avoid potentially injurious positions for the nerve (e.g., leg crossing, squatting). A custom-fitted *ankle–foot orthotic* (AFO) is recommended for increased ankle stability and prevention of plantar flexion contractures. Most patients with a transient compressive insult recover peroneal function within weeks to months. Surgical exploration should be considered in severe cases with no clear cause.

Tibial Nerve (Tarsal Tunnel Syndrome)

Causes. The *tarsal tunnel* is located at the inferoposterior margin of the medial malleolus (Fig. 84.2) and is formed by bones of the ankle and the flexor retinaculum (fibrous sheath from medial malleolus posteroinferior to the medial side of the calcaneus). In addition to the posterior tibial nerve the tunnel contains the posterior tibial artery and three long flexor tendons (10).

Enlarged tortuous veins within the tarsal tunnel, fracture or dislocation at the ankle, and tenosynovitis may lead to compression of the tibial nerve trunk. Prolonged standing and walking often aggravate the pain, indicating that stasis or engorgement within the tunnel is likely to play some role. Also, sensory symptoms are made worse by the venous stasis and engorgement that occur at night during sleep. Except for a high prevalence in jockeys, no common occupational factors have been identified.

Manifestations and Evaluation. The primary symptom of tarsal tunnel syndrome is pain and dysesthesia in the sole of the foot. The burning pain (description by patient may vary, e.g., walking on knives or pins, sole feels very thick) worsens with rest after a day of activity. Nocturnal pain is characteristic. Any or all of the three terminal divisions of the tibial nerve (medial plantar, lateral plantar, and calcaneal) may be affected, resulting in sensory disturbance over the entire plantar surface or only one portion of it.

Tinel's sign, consisting of shooting pain to the plantar surface produced by gentle percussion over the tarsal tunnel, may be present. Sensory loss, if present, is localized to the plantar surface of the foot and over the tips of the toes (the sural and peroneal territories on the dorsum of the foot do not include the tips of the toes). Weakness in the intrinsic muscles of the foot may lead to a change in configuration of the foot and to instability of the phalanges, which impairs the pushing-off phase of walking. Tarsal tunnel syndrome is usually unilateral.

Electrodiagnostic studies (see details above). In the tarsal tunnel syndrome, sensory nerve conduction studies of medial and lateral plantar nerves are the most sensitive electrodiagnostic measures, showing reduced sensory nerve action potential amplitudes or absent responses. Reduced motor or sensory conduction velocities across the flexor retinaculum are found less commonly. EMG demonstrates chronic partial denervation in the tibial innervated intrinsic muscles of the feet (e.g., abductor hallucis and abductor digiti quinti).

Treatment. It is important to identify and remove any source of external pressure at the flexor retinaculum. Definitive treatment of tarsal tunnel syndrome is surgical release of the flexor retinaculum, which can result in dramatic relief of symptoms.

Femoral Nerve

Causes. The femoral nerve may be injured by stab wounds to the groin or hip, pelvic fractures, inguinal surgery (inguinal hernia, vascular repair, node resection), angiography, or retraction during pelvic surgery (Fig. 84.2). Stretch injuries can occur with prolonged lithotomy position or with hyperextension during gymnastics or dance. Pressure on the femoral nerve can also be produced at the psoas muscle by hematoma or abscess.

Manifestations and Evaluation. The patient often complains about buckling of the knee (quadriceps weakness), and falls are common. Pain in the groin radiating into the thigh may be severe. Sensory loss is present in the anterior medial thigh and medial leg. Weakness of the quadriceps (knee extension) and loss of the knee jerk are noted on examination. Weakness of hip flexors indicates a more proximal lumbar plexus or root lesion. EMG helps differentiate these problems.

Femoral neuropathy is to be distinguished from *diabetic lumbar plexopathy* (diabetic amyotrophy). The latter disorder, seen most commonly in diabetics over 50 years of age, begins abruptly with severe pain in the thigh and progresses over days to produce weakness, often most severe, in the femoral nerve distribution. With EMG a wider distribution of involvement can be appreciated. Sensory signs are mild. The prognosis for recovery over 2 to 6 months is good (see Chapter 72, "Diabetes Mellitus").

Treatment. Treatment depends on accurate diagnosis (e.g., discontinuation of anticoagulants when a psoas hematoma has been identified as the cause of the neuropathy). Physiotherapy may be required to maintain the mobility of the hip joint. The outcome and extent of rehabilitation measures are determined by the cause and extent of injury.

Saphenous Nerve

The saphenous nerve is one of three sensory branches of the femoral nerve (Fig. 84.2). It is most often injured at Hunter's canal (10 cm proximal to the medial condyle of the femur). Vein stripping and knee surgery are common causes. A small medial nerve branch can be injured by knee surgery. The patient has pain and numbness at the medial aspect of the knee and leg. The pain may worsen with walking and climbing. Manual pressure over Hunter's canal produces pain that radiates. If the pain becomes chronic, local anesthetic can be injected to the area of injury.

Sciatic Nerve

Causes. The sciatic nerve is often injured as a complication of trauma involving structures that the nerve traverses (Fig. 84.2), including hip fractures, dislocations, and arthroplastic surgery. Compression of the nerve can occur in comatose or chronically bedridden patients, or after sitting on a hard edge. Hematoma, endometriosis, lipoma, and aneurysms of the gluteal artery are other causes of compression. Injections into the buttock are now less common causes of sciatic nerve injury. Benzylpenicillin and diazepam are particularly potent damaging agents. Injections usually cause immediate dysfunction with poor recovery.

Manifestations and Evaluation. Symptoms of sciatic nerve compression may mimic L5–S1 radiculopathy caused by disc disease (see Chapter 65). The lateral trunk or peroneal division of the sciatic nerve is often affected more severely than the tibial division. Therefore, the distinction between a proximal sciatic injury and a more distal peroneal injury (e.g., after awakening from hip surgery) may be difficult. EMG studies may be particularly helpful in this clinical situation.

Lateral Femoral Cutaneous Nerve (Meralgia Paresthetica)

The lateral femoral cutaneous nerve may be compressed or stretched at the anterior superior iliac spine at the lateral end of the inguinal canal (see lateral cutaneous nerve of the thigh, Fig. 84.2), causing burning pain, paresthesia, and decreased sensation over the lateral thigh. The sensory involvement is more lateral than that in femoral neuropathy, which causes sensory loss in the anterior medial aspect of thigh, and there is no motor involvement or loss of patellar reflex. Point tenderness can usually be elicited at the passage of the nerve at the ipsilateral anterior iliac crest. Common causes include obesity, acute abdominal enlargement (ascites, pregnancy), external mechanical trauma (girdle, utility belt, climbing with body against utility pole), and diabetes mellitus. The nerve compression may be relieved by weight loss or correction of the aggravating condition. Pain may respond to medical management (see below), but generally resolves spontaneously over months. If the pain is severe, local injection of an anesthetic may provide relief for long periods; sectioning of the ligament over the canal or sectioning of the nerve is rarely needed. Paresthesias and pain usually disappear gradually, but a painless sensory loss in the lateral thigh may persist.

Bell's Palsy

Paralysis of the facial muscles caused by inflammation and swelling of the seventh (the facial) cranial nerve (Bell's palsy) is seen occasionally in a general medical practice. One large series reported an incidence of 23 cases per 100,000 population per year (14). There is no predilection for a particular sex, age group, or race. In most patients, the cause of the condition is unknown. Two specific causes for seventh nerve neuropathy that have been recognized in recent years are Lyme disease (8,13) (see Chapter 30) and HIV infection (see Chapter 34).

Manifestations

Usually patients note the sudden onset, within hours, of a unilateral paralysis of a facial nerve: the eyebrow sags, the eye cannot be closed, the nasolabial fold disappears, and the mouth is drawn to the unaffected side. Less commonly, there is loss of taste on the anterior two-thirds of the tongue and there is hyperacusis (an accentuation of sounds) in the affected ear. There may be pain behind the ear. Most patients recover spontaneously within weeks to a few months; approximately 15% recover incompletely, but severe residual weakness is rare (14). Patching of the unclosed eye may be needed to avoid corneal injury. In those who do not recover completely, there is a considerable risk of synkinesis (a contraction of all of the facial muscles on the affected side when the patient attempts to move just one or a few of them) caused by aberrant reinnervation.

Management

Corticosteroids appear to reduce the incidence of incomplete recovery (1,27) in patients with Bell's palsy. When the palsy has been present less than 4 days, it is moderately severe, and there is no strong contraindication to steroids (e.g., uncontrolled diabetes mellitus, hypertension, or active peptic ulcer disease), it is reasonable to begin a 10-day tapering course of prednisone beginning with 60 mg for 3 days and tapering by 10 mg each day thereafter. If pain behind the ear recurs during the tapering, the prednisone should be increased and a neurologist should be consulted. The use of surgical decompression for treatment of this condition has largely been abandoned.

LESS COMMON PROBLEMS

Hereditary Motor and Sensory Neuropathies

Of the heritable disorders affecting the PNS, the hereditary motor and sensory neuropathies (HMSN) are the most common. HMSN are a heterogeneous group of neuropathy syndromes affecting an estimated 1 per 2500 people (see "General References"). HMSN are classified into three types: HMSN type I, or Charcot–Marie–Tooth disease; HMSN type II, or the neuronal form of Charcot–Marie–Tooth disease; and HMSN type III, or Dejerine–Sottas disease. The most common type, HMSN type I, is characterized by slowly progressive distal weakness, muscle wasting, foot abnormalities, including pes cavus and hammer toe, and mildly diminished distal sensation. Symptoms are usually manifest by the fourth decade; however, many patients have few or no symptoms. Sensory symptoms are rarely the presenting complaint and when present suggest an acquired rather than inherited neuropathy.

Physical examination demonstrates a wide range of clinical severity and may include distal weakness, thin peroneal muscles, diminished deep tendon reflexes in the legs, characteristic abnormalities of the feet (see above), and mildly reduced distal sensation. Occasionally, enlarged nerves can be palpated. Electrophysiologic studies of sensory and motor nerves show diffuse involvement, with severely reduced conduction velocities uniformly along the nerve segment. Nerve pathology shows onion bulb formation composed of redundant Schwann cell processes resulting from recurrent demyelination and remyelination. Diagnosis is established by identifying a history of childhood onset and by physical examination, characteristic electrophysiologic findings, electrodiagnostic evaluation of family members, and genetic testing. In most families, HMSN type I is transmitted as an autosomal-dominant pattern, and the abnormal gene has been localized to chromosome 17. The most common treatment required is the use of custom-fitted ankle–foot orthotics.

Guillain–Barré Syndrome

Guillain–Barré syndrome or acute inflammatory polyradiculoneuropathy is a rapidly progressive paralytic syndrome affecting all ages. Evidence is strong for an immune-mediated pathogenesis. Most cases of Guillain–Barré syndrome follow a mild viral illness (by 10 to 12 days) (22). The syndrome also may be associated with pregnancy, the postoperative period, recent influenza immunization, and HIV infection. A link between *Campylobacter jejuni* and Guillain–Barré syndrome is particularly strong; it is estimated that 20% of cases of Guillain–Barré syndrome follow *Campylobacter* infection (see Dyck and Griffin et al., "General References"). More severe cases of Guillain–Barré syndrome are associated with *Campylobacter* infection. Diagnosis of *C. jejuni* infection is based on isolation of *C. jejuni* from stool. The *differential diagnosis* in patients with the rapid onset of a polyradiculopathy includes acute intermittent porphyria, botulism, diphtheria, poliomyelitis, Lyme disease, and toxic neuropathies (arsenic, thallium).

Manifestations

There is rapid progression of ascending, symmetric weakness (usually moving from the lower extremities to the upper extremities) accompanied by loss of deep tendon reflexes. Although acute pain or paresthesias in the back and proximal limbs may be prominent early symptoms, objective evidence of sensory loss is generally limited to mild impairment of distal joint position sense and vibratory sensation. Cranial muscle weakness may be present, with bilateral facial nerve palsy in 40% of patients. Nerve conduction studies (see above) show changes of demyelination (prolonged distal motor and F-wave latencies and reduced motor conduction velocities). The cerebrospinal fluid may show an increased protein concentration with normal cell counts (cytoalbumin dissociation).

Management and Course

Because of rapid progression of the disease, patients suspected of having this disorder should be admitted to the hospital for close monitoring for potential respiratory failure and autonomic instability (hypotension, hypertension, cardiac arrhythmias, or hyperpyrexia occur in two-thirds of patients with Guillain–Barré syndrome). Treatment with either plasmapheresis or intravenous human immunoglobulin early in the course shortens the period of disability, and the combination is no better than either treatment alone (21). Recovery is complete in approximately 50% of patients (although it may take 6 to 18 months); most of the remainder have only mild residual deficits, but 10% have severe permanent disability. Splints (to prevent contractures) and physiotherapy should be used until the recovery period is complete.

Chronic Inflammatory Demyelinating Polyneuropathy

Chronic inflammatory demyelinating polyneuropathy (CIDP) is an acquired motor and sensory neuropathy of unknown cause but with strong evidence for an immune-mediated pathogenesis. CIDP can occur in the absence of systemic disease or, less commonly, in association with such disorders as systemic lupus erythematosus, HIV infection, or dysproteinemias. Clinically, CIDP is a predominantly *motor polyneuropathy*. It may affect all ages, and may have either a chronic progressive or relapsing course. Weakness typically develops over at least 2 months (distinguishing CIDP from acute inflammatory demyelinating neuropathy, so-called Guillain–Barré syndrome) and generally begins in the legs. Sensory involvement is variable. The majority of patients experience some degree of numbness or paresthesia; occasionally, there may be painful dysesthesias. On examination, weakness may be both proximal and distal, and the tendon reflexes are reduced or absent in all four limbs.

Electrodiagnostic studies demonstrate features of demyelination, including prolonged distal and F-wave latencies, reduced conduction velocities variably along nerve segments, abnormal temporal dispersion, and conduction block. Cerebrospinal fluid protein is often elevated. Sural nerve pathology may show evidence of demyelination and remyelination with onion bulb formation, subperineurial and endoneurial edema, and mononuclear cell infiltration.

Management

Common practice is to begin treatment with prednisone 1 mg/kg per day (6) and to use either plasmapheresis or intravenous human immunoglobulin as adjuvants (5). Each of these immunomodulating therapies has been demonstrated to be effective in randomized, placebo-controlled trials, and the great majority of patients respond. Long-term corticosteroid therapy usually is effective, but it is limited by side effects. The effect of either plasmapheresis or human immunoglobulin is large and of equal likelihood, but for most patients is short-lived and requires continued intermittent treatment (5). For plasmapheresis, improved motor conduction velocities and reversal of conduction block predict improvement in motor function (11). Plasma exchange treatments should be given two to three times per week until improvement is established, then tapered in frequency; concurrent immunosuppressive drug treatment is usually required (11). Human immunoglobulin treatment is effective in about two-thirds of patients, most often in patients with acute relapse or disease duration less than one year (12). Improvement after a dose of 2 g/kg lasts a median 6 weeks and is reproducible, so that follow-up pulses of 1 g/kg as single infusions can maintain a stable benefit (12). Of the two adjuvants, both are extraordinarily expensive, but intravenous immunoglobulin infusion may be preferable because it does not require expensive medical devices and can be given at home (5).

Multifocal Motor Neuropathy

Patients with multifocal motor neuropathy have progressive, predominantly distal, asymmetric weakness that usually begins in the arms. Early in the disease course, multifocal motor neuropathy can mimic CIDP or the lower motor neuron presentation of amyotrophic lateral sclerosis. Nerve conduction studies show multiple areas of persistent partial motor conduction block, and many patients have high IgM anti-GM1 ganglioside antibody titers. Most patients with multifocal motor neuropathy respond to immunosuppressive therapy with human immune globulin or Cytoxan (2). Corticosteroids are ineffective.

THERAPEUTIC PRINCIPLES

General Measures that Improve Nerve Function

Treatment of peripheral neuropathies first requires identifying and treating any underlying cause, if possible. For type 1 diabetes mellitus, for example, it is now known that intense efforts at tight glucose control dramatically reduce the incidence of neuropathy (see Chapter 72). Efforts should be made also to prevent further damage; for example, patients with an underlying generalized polyneuropathy are more prone to pressure palsies, and it is important to educate them about habits that could be injurious (e.g., leaning on elbows or crossing legs). The daily administration of multivitamins is necessary only in patients whose nutrition may be poor. For entrapment and compression neuropathies, eliminating pressure on the affected nerve is the primary mode of treatment. Pain and paresthesias may be relieved rapidly within hours or days. The prognosis for recovery depends on the pathophysiology of the nerve injury. When little or no denervation is demonstrated by EMG, which suggests that the predominant pathophysiology is edema or demyelination, recovery of function over weeks is expected. In more severe cases with marked denervation indicating axonal injury, recovery is more prolonged (months).

The most important *prognostic indicators for traumatic nerve injuries* are the site, mechanism, and completeness of the injury. Traumatic injuries can occur at the level of the root, plexus, or peripheral nerve. Root avulsion has the worst prognosis. Electrodiagnostic studies are helpful in localizing the site of injury; however, because denervation may not be evident for at least 14 days, EMG studies should be done approximately 3 to 4 weeks after injury. Complete nerve transections caused by sharp penetrating injury, although rare, more often benefit from early primary anastomosis than do complicated nerve injuries such as gunshot wounds. Physical therapy, particularly range of motion exercises, should be initiated early after injury to prevent contractures. The onset of spontaneous recovery can vary from weeks to 6 months or more after injury. In cases of persistent loss of function or severe pain, surgical exploration should be considered.

Symptomatic Treatment for Irreversible Damage

Polyneuropathy is often irreversible and progressive. Symptomatic therapy and rehabilitative measures are therefore fundamental in helping these patients.

Motor Neuropathies

In most polyneuropathies, weakness usually affects ankle dorsiflexors early (causing foot drop); ambulation can be greatly improved by a custom-fitted ankle–foot orthotic (AFO), such as a rigid plastic splint worn in the shoe or a spring-loaded brace attached to the shoe. Fine motor weakness in the hands can be aided by special tools, such as large-handled utensils and other devices, provided by occupational therapists.

Sensory Neuropathies

Small, hard objects (keys, faucet handles) can be built up with soft materials. Occupational therapists can make useful suggestions in this regard. Anesthetic limbs are vulnerable to repeated, unrecognized trauma. The patient should always check the temperature of bath water, pot handles, and so on with parts of the body that have normal sensation. Meticulous care should be given to feet and toenails to prevent ulceration or infection (see Chapter 102). Moisturizing cream for dry, insensitive skin will reduce serious abrasions (see details, Chapter 100).

Pain associated with sensory neuropathies is usually chronic and difficult to treat. Simple analgesics (aspirin), whirlpool, and massage may help relieve mild pain. Outside pain treatment centers, narcotics should probably be avoided because of the potential for addiction. Tricyclic antidepressants (e.g., amitriptyline or nortriptyline, 25 to 75 mg at bedtime) are most often effective (see details, Chapter 15). Carbamazepine (Tegretol) 200 to 1000 mg/day in divided doses may provide relief of refractory pain and is worth a therapeutic trial. This drug is started at 100 mg two or three times a day and is increased slowly (200 mg every 4 days in divided doses), to yield a serum level of 8 to 12 µg/mL. Once a therapeutic daily dosage has been established, conversion to the sustained-release form of Tegretol allows a more convenient twice-daily schedule. Intolerance to carbamazepine (ataxia, drowsiness, and nausea) is especially likely in the older patient. Hematologic values and liver function tests must be checked periodically. If Tegretol has been maintained in the therapeutic range for 2 to 4 weeks and still proves unsuccessful, it should be discontinued and phenytoin (Dilantin) 300 to 500 mg/day to yield a serum level of 15 to 20 µg/mL should be tried. Details regarding carbamazepine and phenytoin are found in Chapter 80.

Autonomic Neuropathies

Autonomic dysfunctions should also be approached symptomatically (18). The *hypotonic bladder* may be treated by drugs that increase bladder tone (Urecholine, 10 to 25 mg every 8 hours), by self-catheterization, or occasionally with surgery to decrease resistance to bladder emptying. Details regarding the evaluation and management of the hypotonic bladder are in Chapter 6. For *male sexual impotence,* penile prostheses and pharmacologic erections produced by intracavernous injection or intraurethral suppositories have represented significant advances (see Chapter 18). The knowledge that sexual dysfunction has a neurologic basis may relieve the anxiety that often accompanies the problem. A check for medications that may be contributing to impotence is important (see Chapter 18).

Orthostatic hypotension may be treated with salt supplementation and a volume-expanding mineralo-corticoid (fludrocortisone 0.1 to 0.2 mg/day) in patients without congestive heart failure or hypertension. A recently released, expensive α_1-adrenergic agonist, midodrine (proamaine), has been shown to help patients with orthostatic hypotension. The dosage is 10 mg three times per day. Contraindications are the same as those for fludrocortisone (17). Support stockings with pressure gradients may be helpful to prevent venous pooling, but many patients do not tolerate these stockings well. Arising slowly from recumbent or sitting positions, maintaining active ambulation, and sleeping with the head of the bed elevated on blocks (to stimulate renin release) are other measures that may help. Table 84.9 summarizes the practical ways to manage orthostatic hypotension caused by autonomic dysfunction.

OTHER PROBLEMS

Restless Legs Syndrome

Restless legs syndrome is common, affecting perhaps 5% of the general population. It is an important cause of insomnia (see Chapter 85). Patients complain of an aching or painful crawling sensation deep inside the legs at rest, especially in the evening or in bed. Walking provides some relief but the dysesthesias often return quickly upon resting (9,25).

The exact pathophysiology has not been elucidated; both peripheral and central mechanisms have been proposed. The syndrome has been related in some patients to the peripheral neuropathies of diabetes mellitus and uremia. An association has also been found with iron and folate deficiency anemias, calcium and potassium deficiency, pregnancy, post–gastric surgery state, excessive caffeine, sedative drug withdrawal, and exposure to neuroleptic medication. An idiopathic form is associated with periodic movements during sleep and a positive family history.

These patients should be evaluated for associated

Table 84.9.   Measures that May Help Patients with Orthostatic Hypotension Caused by Autonomic Neuropathy

Avoid sudden changes in position
Avoid excessive intake of alcohol
Avoid diuresis
Correct hypovolemia
Discontinue or reduce the dosage of drugs known to cause orthostatic hypotension:
   Antihypertensive drugs
   Nitroglycerin
   Diuretics
   Neuroleptics
   Tricyclic antidepressants
   CNS depressants (opiates, alcohol)
   Levodopa
Prescribe mineralocorticoid (if no congestive heart failure or hypertension)
Supplement diet with salt
Tilt up the head of the bed (may stimulate renin release)
Use elastic support stockings

conditions for specific treatment. Restricting caffeine use and performing regular exercise before bedtime may be helpful recommendations. Simple analgesics (aspirin, acetaminophen) at bedtime may help early symptoms. In other patients, nonsedating dosages of clonazepam (Klonopin, 0.5 to 2 mg) or triazolam (Halcion, 0.125 mg) may relieve nocturnal symptoms. The drug of choice for people with severe restless leg syndrome is Sinemet (a combination of L-dopa and carbidopa) at dosages of one-half to two 25/100 mg tablets at bedtime. If the patient is typically awakened later during the night, the controlled-release form of Sinemet is preferable. Sinemet is generally well tolerated (see details in Chapter 82).

Muscle Cramps

Cramps are localized involuntary painful contractions of skeletal muscles that produce a visible, palpable, hard, and bulging muscle. They must be distinguished from the sensation of cramp such as that described with intermittent claudication; the latter is not associated with a palpable hard and bulging muscle.

Ordinary muscle cramps are common and may be stopped by stretching the affected muscles. Frequent cramps are most often associated with denervating diseases, fatiguing exercises, salt depletion, dehydration, pregnancy, hypothyroidism, alcoholism, uremia, or hypomagnesemia (20). Patients with frequent daytime cramps related to exercise or fasting should be referred to a neurologist for evaluation for one of the rare muscle enzymatic defects (e.g., myophosphorylase, phosphofructokinase, or carnitine palmityltransferase deficiency). If no correctable associated condition exists, these patients may be given a therapeutic trial of phenytoin, carbamazepine, or amitriptyline (see above for dosages) (20).

Nocturnal cramps occur in 15% of healthy young adults and are even more common in the elderly. One drug reported to be effective is single-dose clonazepam, 0.25 to 0.5 mg at bedtime.

General References*

Dawson DM. Current concepts: entrapment neuropathies of the upper extremities. N Engl J Med 329:2013, 1993.
Dawson DM, Hallett M, Millender LH. Entrapment neuropathies. 2nd ed. Boston: Little, Brown, 1990.
Dyck PJ, Thomas PK, Asbury AK, et al. Diabetic neuropathy. Philadelphia: WB Saunders, 1987.
   A thorough review of pathophysiologic and clinical aspects of diabetic neuropathy.
Dyck P, Thomas PK, Griffin JW, et al, eds. Peripheral neuropathy. 3rd ed. Philadelphia: WB Saunders, 1993.
   An excellent comprehensive review.

*Bold print (general references) and bold numerals (specific references) denote published controlled clinical trials, meta-analyses, or consensus-based recommendations.

Medical Research Council. Aids to the examination of the peripheral nervous system. London: Bailliere-Tindall, 1986.
   Well-illustrated guide to the physical examination for testing all peripheral nerves.
Midroni G, Bilbao JM. Biopsy diagnosis of peripheral neuropathy. Stoneham, MA: Butterworth, 1995.
Schaumburg HH, Berger AR, Thomas PK. Disorders of peripheral nerves. 2nd ed. Philadelphia: FA Davis, 1992.
   A short work organized by disease processes that involve peripheral nerves.
Stewart JD. Focal peripheral neuropathies. 2nd ed. New York: Raven Press, 1993.

Specific References

1. Adour KK, Wingerd J, Bell DN, et al. Prednisone treatment for idiopathic facial paralysis (Bell's palsy). N Engl J Med 287:1268, 1972.
2. Azulay J-P, Rihet P, Pouget J, Cador F, et al. Long term follow up of multifocal motor neuropathy with conduction block under treatment. J Neurol Neurosurg Psychiatry 62:391, 1997.
3. Behse F, Buchthal F. Alcoholic neuropathy: clinical, electrophysiological and biopsy findings. Ann Neurol 2:95, 1977.
4. Cornblath DR. Treatment of the neuromuscular complications of human immunodeficiency virus infection. Ann Neurol 2:S88, 1988.
5. Dyck PJ, Litchy WJ, Kratz KM, et al. A plasma exchange versus immune globulin infusion trial in chronic inflammatory demyelinating polyradiculoneuropathy. Ann Neurol 36:838, 1994.
6. Dyck PJ, O'Brien PC, Oviatt KF, et al. Prednisone improves chronic inflammatory demyelinating polyradiculoneuropathy more than no treatment. Ann Neurol 11:136, 1982.
7. Ewing DJ, Clarke BF. Diabetic autonomic neuropathy: present insights and future prospects. Diabetic Care 9:648, 1986.
8. Finkel M. Lyme disease and its neurologic complications. Arch Neurol 45:99, 1988.
9. Gibb WRG, Lees AJ. The restless leg syndrome. Postgrad Med J 62:329, 1986.
10. Goodgold J, Kopell HP, Spielholz NI. The tarsal tunnel syndrome. N Engl J Med 273:742, 1965.
11. Hahn AF, Bolton CF, Pillay N, et al. Plasma-exchange therapy in chronic inflammatory demyelinating polyneuropathy: a double-blind, sham-controlled, cross-over study. Brain 119: 1055–1066, 1996.
12. Hahn AF, Bolton CF, Zochodne D, Feasby TE. Intravenous immunoglobulin treatment in chronic inflammatory demyelinating polyneuropathy: a double-blind, placebo-controlled, cross-over study. Brain 119:1067–1077, 1996.
13. Halperin JJ, Little BW, et al. Lyme disease: cause of treatable peripheral neuropathy. Neurology 37:1,700, 1987.
14. Hauser WA, Karnes WE, Annis J, Kurland LT. Incidence and prognosis of Bell's palsy in the population of Rochester, Minnesota. Mayo Clin Proc 46:258, 1971.
15. Horwich MS, Cho L, Porro RS, Posner JB. Subacute sensory neuropathy: a remote effect of cancer. Ann Neurol 2:7, 1977.
16. Kissel J, Mendell JR. Neuropathies associated with monoclonal gammopathies. Neuromusc Disord 6:3, 1996.
17. Low PA, Gilden JL, Freeman R, et al. Efficacy of Midodrine vs placebo in neurogenic orthostatic hypotension: a randomized, double-blind multicenter study. JAMA 277(13):1046–1051, 1997.
18. McCleod JG, Tuck RR. Disorders of the autonomic nervous system. II. Investigation and treatment. Ann Neurol 21:519, 1987.
19. Miralles GD, O'Fallon JR, Talley NJ. Plasma-cell dyscrasia with polyneuropathy. The spectrum of POEMS syndrome. N Engl J Med 327:1919, 1992.
20. Moxley R. Cramps. In: Johnson RT, ed. Current therapy in neurologic disease. Philadelphia: BC Decker, 1990;3:410.
21. Plasma Exchange/Sandoglobulin Guillain–Barré Syndrome Trial Group. Randomized trial of plasma exchange, intravenous immunoglobulin, and combined treatments in Guillain–Barré syndrome. Lancet 349:225–230, 1997.

22. Ropper AH, Wijdicks EFM, Truax BT. Guillain–Barré syndrome. Philadelphia: FA Davis, 1991.
23. Schaumberg H, Kaplan J, Windebank A, et al. Sensory neuropathy from pyridoxine abuse, a new megavitamin syndrome. N Engl J Med 309:445, 1983.
24. Vinik A, Mitchell B. Clinical aspects of diabetic neuropathies. Diabetes Metab Rev 4:223, 1988.
25. Walters A, Hening W. Clinical presentation and neuropharmacology of restless legs syndrome. Clin Pharmacol 10:225, 1987.
26. Wilkinson M, Croft PB, Urich H. The remote effects of cancer on the nervous system. Proc R Soc Med 60:683, 1967.
27. Wolf SM, Wagner JH, Davidson S, Forsythe A. Treatment of Bell's palsy with prednisone: a prospective, randomized study. Neurology 28:158, 1978.

C H A P T E R 85

Sleep Disorders

DAVID N. NEUBAUER, MD
PHILIP L. SMITH, MD
CHRISTOPHER J. EARLEY, MD, PhD

EPIDEMIOLOGY

In recent years, disorders of sleep and wakefulness have been recognized increasingly as pervasive throughout our society. The magnitude of the public health implications was emphasized in the 1992 report of the National Commission on Sleep Disorders Research (16). It noted that about 40 million Americans have chronic sleep–wake disorders, and that many of those people are undiagnosed and untreated. Furthermore, the report emphasizes the vital role of primary care physicians in recognizing, treating, and helping educate the vast majority of those patients experiencing symptoms related to their sleep–wake cycles. Even though sleep-related complaints are common in general medical practice, a 1991 Gallup survey (8) showed that only a small minority of sleep-disturbed people bring their concerns to the attention of their physicians.

The sleep disorders represent a wide spectrum of symptoms. The inability to sleep at the desired time and the inability to remain awake during appropriate hours make up the majority of patient concerns. Abnormal behaviors and movements also may be associated with sleep. The American Sleep Disorders Association (4) recognizes more than 70 individual sleep disorders, involving intrinsic and extrinsic processes, as well as sleep disturbances associated with other medical and psychiatric illnesses.

Appropriate diagnosis and effective treatment of sleep disorders can result in significant improvement in the quality of life for patients. In addition, this may allow a reduction in the tremendous morbidity and mortality associated with excessive sleepiness. An exploration of sleep–wake patterns and possible sleep disorders is an important component of any general review of systems. Sleep disturbances can exacerbate other medical conditions, and conversely, many medical illnesses and medications can affect sleep patterns.

BASIC SLEEP PHYSIOLOGY

Daytime alertness and nighttime sleepiness are natural drives for most people leading normal lives. The fundamental sleep–wake cycle is maintained by at least two physiologically distinct control mechanisms:

- The *homeostatic mechanism* establishes a balance between wake and sleep time over several days. This time balance varies greatly with species but for adult humans is set at one-third sleep and two-thirds waking. Sleep deprivation leads to increased sleepiness; however, the relationship is not exactly linear. Many people have had the experience of getting a second wind of alertness the morning after a night without sleep. This phenomenon is caused by the prominent circadian rhythm driving sleepiness and alertness.

- The *circadian oscillator* establishes a sleep tendency variation over the normal 24-hour day. This oscillator also modulates core temperature and the activity levels of a large number of physiological functions (e.g., certain neurotransmitters and hormone levels). Without time cues, especially the day/night light/dark cycle, this circadian mechanism has a periodicity slightly greater than 24 hours, and therefore must be reset daily. Light exposure during the daytime and darkness at night synchronize the rhythm. Neural pathways including the retina, suprachiasmatic nucleus, and pineal gland are well established.

These mechanisms promote the cycle of sleepiness and alertness, and usually are in stable harmony. Although homeostatic sleepiness increases throughout the day, circadian alertness peaks in the evening. Under normal circumstances these rhythms allow us to remain alert for 16 hours and then fall asleep rapidly at our habitual bedtime.

Normal sleep includes two major physiologically distinct states: *rapid eye movement* (REM) sleep and *non–rapid eye movement* (NREM) sleep. Initially, sleep may consist of the four successively deeper stages of NREM sleep. During each of these four stages, there is decreased fluctuation in heart rate, blood pressure, and respiration. This contrasts with REM sleep, where greater lability is noted. The presleep wake stage and the NREM sleep stages have additional distinctive clinical and electroencephalographic (EEG) characteristics.

Presleep wake (sleep latency period). As a person begins to fall asleep, eye blinks, limb movements, and moderate tone in skeletal muscles are accompanied by either low-voltage, mixed frequency EEG or the characteristic α pattern (basic posterior rhythm).

Stage 1. This represents light sleep with slow rolling eye movements. The α pattern disappears with lower frequency and usually higher voltage than the wake EEG. Sudden limb jerks normally may occur episodically, particularly during early stage 1 sleep.
Stage 2. Eye movements become infrequent or absent and muscle tone usually is reduced. The EEG shows the stage-defining sleep spindle bursts, vertex sharp waves, K complexes, and some slow waveforms.
Stages 3 and 4. EEG high-voltage, slow-wave activity predominates. These stages are defined according to the percentage of slow-wave activity present. Muscle tone is variable. Arousal is difficult from these deeper sleep stages.

REM sleep. At 1 to 2 hours after sleep onset, the first period of REM sleep occurs, with a characteristic marked decrease in muscle tone and bursts of rapid eye movements. During REM sleep there is a paralysis of major skeletal muscles punctuated by occasional episodes of muscle twitches, hypercapnic and hypoxic respiratory drive are decreased, thermoregulation is decreased, heart rate and blood pressure are extremely variable, and penile erections occur. Dreaming is also most closely related to REM sleep but may occur, usually less vividly, at other times.

On a typical night, a subject passes through three to five cycles of NREM and REM sleep. Typical sleep patterns for healthy young adults and elderly people are shown in Figure 85.1. With aging, generally there is a decrease in slow-wave sleep (stages 3 and 4), an earlier sleep onset and waking time, and more frequent awakenings during the night. The apparently decreased arousal threshold in older people is the most prominent difference between sleep at age 50 and that at age 80. During the day, young adults require 10 to 15 minutes to fall asleep for a nap; older adults fall asleep more easily. As discussed later in this chapter, the recognition and deviations from the normal sleep

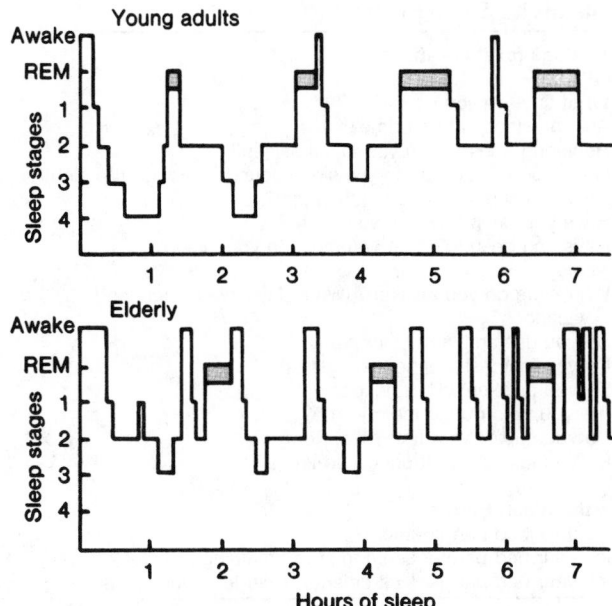

Figure 85.1.   Normal sleep cycles in healthy young and elderly subjects. Darkened area indicates REM sleep. (Adapted from Kales A, Kales JD. Sleep disorders: recent findings in the diagnosis and treatment of disturbed sleep. N Engl J Med 290:487, 1974.)

cycles are helpful at times in establishing the correct diagnosis for a sleep disorder.

HISTORY

The full evaluation of sleep complaints requires a general consideration of the patient's sleep–wake cycle, as well as specific questions that focus on the presenting symptoms. Table 85.1 lists questions that may yield information that supports a diagnostic hypothesis.

COMMON CLINICAL PRESENTATIONS

Insomnia

Insomnia is the perception of not sleeping well, and it is the most common sleep complaint. It is estimated that one in three people in the United States has frequent or chronic difficulty with insomnia. Almost everyone experiences some degree of insomnia during their lifetime. People of all ages may experience disrupted sleep; however, there is a general increase in frequency with age. Men and women are affected equally until middle age. From the mid-40s on, women are much more likely to complain of difficulty sleeping (8).

Insomnia may involve difficulty falling asleep, awakening too early, or experiencing disrupted sleep throughout the night. The presentation also may include the report of unrefreshing sleep. Often, the patient complains of fatigue, poor concentration, and low productivity.

In properly diagnosing complaints of poor sleep, it is important to realize that insomnia is a symptom that

Table 85.1.   Sleep History

Questions for the Patient

Nighttime
What time do you go to bed?
Are you sleepy at that time?
How long does it take you to fall asleep?
Once you fall asleep, do you sleep soundly through the night?
Do you feel restless during the night?
Have you been told that you snore?
Have you been told that you move in your sleep?

Daytime
What time do you awaken? (Work days, weekends, and vacations?)
Do you use an alarm clock?
Do you feel rested when you get up?
Do you awaken with a headache?
Are you tired during the daytime?
Do you nap? (What time? How long?)
Do you fall asleep at undesired times?

For the Sleep Partner

Does your bed partner snore?
Does your bed partner seem to stop breathing at times?
Does your bed partner kick or jerk his/her legs during sleep?

may result from a wide variety of processes. An important initial consideration is the duration of the disturbance.

Transient insomnia, by definition, lasts a few days and often is associated with a recognizable stimulus, such as anxiety, grief, or anticipation. Changes in the sleep schedule caused by travel or work also can promote brief sleep disturbances.

A sleep disturbance up to 3 weeks in duration is considered *short-term insomnia.* Again, environmental stressors may be evident, but typically the stimulating factors are more severe, such as the loss of a loved one or a job, or a physical or emotional problem.

Chronic insomnia, by definition, lasts longer than 3 weeks. An initial precipitant often is recognizable in the history; however, other perpetuating factors promote the persistent symptoms (24). Complaints of marked sleep difficulty that have continued for several years are not uncommon. Although the cause of chronic insomnia is often multifactorial, it is useful to consider the individual factors that may be associated with long-standing symptoms (Table 85.2).

Most *psychiatric disorders* can cause disturbed sleep. Symptoms of depression and anxiety often are associated with insomnia and may be precipitating and perpetuating causes. Early morning awakening is a characteristic of major depressive disorder; however, difficulty falling and staying asleep commonly is present as well. Difficulty sleeping is typical of patients with generalized anxiety disorder, posttraumatic stress disorder, panic disorder, schizophrenia, personality disorders, and dementia. Acute sleep changes often are seen with adjustment disorders. Each of these psychiatric disorders is described in detail in Section 2 of this book ("Psychiatric and Behavioral Problems").

A broad range of *physical conditions* can cause difficulty sleeping. Pain and discomfort are common factors; however, other pathophysiologic processes may play important contributory roles. The more common medical problems associated with chronic insomnia are arthritic disorders, peptic ulcer disease and gastroesophageal reflux, asthma and chronic obstructive pulmonary disease, cardiovascular disease, hyperthyroidism, and renal failure. Orthopnea and nocturia cause fragmented sleep. Patients with fibromyalgia (see Chapter 66) often complain of unrefreshing sleep. Insomnia is common during normal physiologic stress such as pregnancy, especially during the last trimester.

Among the *neurologic disorders* more commonly associated with insomnia are Parkinson's disease and other movement disorders, stroke, epilepsy, and cerebral degenerative processes. Head trauma may cause long-standing sleep disturbance.

Several hundred *medications* may cause insomnia. Stimulants, ranging from caffeine to amphetamines, predictably decrease the ability to sleep. Correspondingly, withdrawal from sedating medications, including hypnotics, can be associated with a temporary sleep disruption. Long-term use of sedatives may cause tolerance and a worsening of insomnia. Bronchodilators, corticosteroids, and some antihypertensives, antiarrhythmics, calcium channel blockers, antiparkinson agents, anticonvulsants, antidepressants, and nonsteroidal anti-inflammatory drugs may cause insomnia. It is important to consider over-the-counter preparations as causes of disrupted sleep, particularly diet and cold/allergy products because these may contain stimulating compounds such as caffeine, ephedrine, pseudoephedrine, and phenylpropanolamine.

Substance abuse can promote acute and chronic disturbances of sleep. Cocaine and other stimulants inhibit or fragment sleep. Paradoxically, narcotics such as heroin and morphine can have arousing effects that disturb sleep. The acute sedating effect of alcohol is well known; however, although sleep onset may be enhanced, the withdrawal-related catecholamine release often causes sleep disruption. This may occur after a single episode of moderate drinking. Heavier drinking can impair sleep markedly. Symptoms may persist during months to years of abstinence.

The influence of *circadian rhythms* on the sleep–wake cycle most readily is apparent transiently with acute changes in the sleep schedule. Rapid transmeridian travel causes symptoms of jet lag, and changes in shift-work schedules may promote acutely disturbed sleep. Constantly changing work shifts or permanent night work schedules often inhibit effective entrainment and thereby can cause chronic insomnia.

Table 85.2.   Causes of Chronic Insomnia

Psychiatric disorders
Medical and neurologic illnesses
Medications
Substance abuse
Circadian rhythm disturbances
Other sleep disorders
Environmental factors
Poor sleep hygiene and behavioral patterns

Delayed sleep phase syndrome is a disorder of circadian rhythms characterized by great difficulty attaining sleep until 3 to 6 AM. The natural tendency of affected people is to sleep until late morning or early afternoon. Occupational or educational requirements may demand a more socially acceptable wake-up time that effectively truncates the sleep period and causes chronic sleep insufficiency. These people feel out of synchronization with the rest of society and usually come to the physician because of their inability to fall asleep at a more conventional hour. Less common are people with *advanced sleep phase syndrome*. They may sleep from 6 PM until 2 AM, and complain of an inability to remain asleep throughout the night. Generally, the delayed pattern is more common among young people, whereas the advanced pattern occurs more in the elderly. A rare circadian rhythm disturbance occurs in some completely sightless people who are not entrained to a 24-hour cycle. They move in and out of phase with the day/night cycle and thus have periodic symptoms of insomnia every few weeks.

Symptoms of insomnia may be associated with other sleep disorders in which the primary problems are breathing irregularity or excessive body muscle movements during sleep (see below).

Consideration of the *sleeping environment* is an important component of the evaluation of patients with insomnia. Excessive light or noise may be arousing. Living near an airport or another source of loud noise may be detrimental to sleep in vulnerable patients. Temperature extremes may disrupt sleep continuity. Discomfort in bed may result from a poor mattress or a snoring bed partner. Household (e.g., loud televisions) and neighborhood (e.g., city noises) characteristics also may be significant. A sense of insecurity or fear may promote sleeplessness.

Issues related to sleep hygiene (see Table 85.7) are important for all patients with insomnia complaints. Even when there is another reason that sleep is disturbed, behavioral patterns that affect sleep commonly play a role in perpetuating the disorder. Irregularity of bedtime and wake time may undermine the underlying circadian drive for sleepiness and alertness at the appropriate hours. Patients may have unrealistic expectations of their ability to change their sleep schedule markedly and then sleep effectively. Some patients nap in the daytime to make up for lost nighttime sleep, and thereby further diminish their propensity to fall asleep at the desired hour.

Chronic insomniacs may spend excessive amounts of time in bed with hopes of maximizing their total sleep time, thereby further fragmenting their sleep. Remaining in bed during extended sleepless periods may reinforce the association between being in bed and being awake. Often, frustration and anxiety are integral to this repeated experience, and thereby prolong wakefulness. Subsequently, sleep becomes less attainable.

In *psychophysiologic insomnia*, perpetuating factors predominate after the initial stimulating precipitants have subsided. A conditioned pattern of anxiety and tension has become established. The patient may report increasing tiredness during the evening, but tortured wakefulness upon getting in bed. Alternatively, what might have been a minor nighttime awakening becomes an exaggerated emotional response that further inhibits a rapid return to sleep.

In summary, the history may identify one or more precipitating or perpetuating conditions that promote chronic insomnia. *Practical approaches to the management of these conditions are described below.*

Excessive Daytime Sleepiness

Clinical Features

Up to 5% of the population has problems with excessive daytime sleepiness (EDS) or related symptoms (Table 85.3). The younger and older age groups tend to experience more EDS than the middle-age group. Also, shift workers complain more of being tired and of various other problems associated with EDS than nonshift workers. Unfortunately, some patients do not perceive that their problems are sleep-related and therefore may not mention being sleepy during the day. The degree or severity of reported sleepiness can be judged by identifying which situations are most likely to produce sleep, by determining how often and how pervasively sleepiness occurs throughout the day, and by learning how disruptive this is to family, job, and personal well-being.

In determining the severity of sleepiness, one needs to ask patients under what conditions they are most likely to fall asleep. Table 85.4 lists how severe the problem is according to the situations in which sleep may occur. If the situations listed are not associated with falling asleep, it is unlikely that EDS is the problem. If patients awaken from sleep feeling tired, further questioning about their nighttime sleep habits is needed. Patients' perceptions of sleepiness vary. They depend on the environment, level of activity, and degree of motivation. Sitting in a dark room or listening to an uninteresting lecture may unmask sleepiness. Some people may be so busy and active all day, they may have no sense of tiredness despite the fact they have not slept in over 36 hours. As noted in Table 85.3, such people may not complain of being tired but may have problems with concentration or stamina. They may be fatigable or forgetful, or have decreased motivation. They may have accidents either on the job or on the highway. Their job performance may suffer. In-

Table 85.3. Symptoms Associated with the Complaint of Excessive Daytime Sleepiness

Sleepiness
Fatigue
Decreased motivation
Forgetfulness
Poor concentration
Increased aggressive behavior
Depression and irritability
Motor vehicle accidents or near-accidents
Workplace mistakes

Table 85.4. Sleepiness Scale

Severity	Falls Asleep While
Mild	Watching television
	Reading
	Attending lectures
	Riding in car
	Sitting in church
Moderate	Visiting family and friends
	During working day
	During extended driving
Severe	During local driving or at stop light
	Eating a meal

creased irritability or depression may be noted by family or friends.

Animal and human studies show that with insufficient sleep, the EEG identifies brief but frequent disturbances in the ongoing wakeful state. If frequent, these brief intrusions may lead to inattention and poor concentration before sleepiness is perceived. The problems of EDS often are insidious. However, EDS can be identified if specifically explored with appropriate direct questions.

Differential Diagnosis

Once it is established that the patient has EDS, the cause must be identified. One first needs to determine whether drugs (e.g., alcohol, benzodiazepines, antidepressants, neuroleptics, antihistamines, some antihypertensive drugs) or medical conditions (e.g., chronic renal failure, cirrhosis, hypothyroidism) might be the cause of EDS. A common cause of transient daytime fatigue is cessation of low to moderate caffeine consumption (19). After considering these causes, one should attempt to identify patients with disturbed nocturnal sleep. Disorders likely to cause sleep disruption and therefore EDS are discussed in the section on insomnia (see above). Chronic insufficient sleep, chronic fatigue, narcolepsy, and idiopathic hypersomnia are discussed in this section. The sleep apneas are discussed in the next section.

Chronic Insufficient Sleep. The most common cause of EDS is chronic insufficient sleep. The primary problem is that the patients do not have enough sleep to satisfy their body's requirements. The most common causes are personal lifestyles (e.g., shift workers, medical/surgical residents) and poor sleep habits (e.g., watching television until midnight, then getting up for work at 6 AM). Such people rarely have problems falling asleep or staying asleep. They may wake up feeling tired and may have symptoms of EDS. A detailed history of the amount of sleep per night over the past several months is important. If someone is getting 7 hours a night and is tired, 8 or 9 hours may be needed on a regular basis. Questioning these patients about weekend or holiday patterns of sleep, or about how they slept when they were younger or had different lifestyles, may help determine what the normal amount of sleep is for them. To establish the diagnosis and treat the problem, an 8-hour sleeping pattern must be established. Patients need to *keep a written record* of when they go to sleep (not when they go to bed but when they think they fall asleep) and when they awaken. This should be done for at least 1 month and then, with the diary in hand, the patient should return for reassessment. If the patient is feeling better after the forced 8-hour sleep schedule, the diagnosis of chronic insufficient sleep is established. If the patient still complains of EDS and the diary indicates 8 or more hours of sleep per night, a referral to a sleep specialist should be offered.

Chronic Fatigue. Psychiatric disorders, especially depression and certain life events (e.g., death of family member, divorce, job loss, or marital discord) often are associated with insomnia. On occasions, there is no clear-cut insomnia but only what appears to be symptoms of EDS. The person may complain of increased fatigue, lack of motivation, poor concentration, or feeling tired all the time. These patients may sleep in the afternoon, but if they consistently sleep for long periods during the day, they invariably will have disturbed sleep at night and thus experience insomnia. The severity of sleepiness (Table 85.4) is important in differentiating fatigue from sleepiness. Although there may be complaints of tiredness, often there are no clear and consistent episodes of falling asleep. More often, the complaints are more severe than the actual degree of reported sleepiness. Finally, when lack of motivation overshadows all other complaints, one should consider chronic fatigue syndrome (see Chapter 53) or depression (see Chapter 15). There is no defined treatment for chronic fatigue other than treating the underlying problem. If a clear distinction between sleepiness and fatigue cannot be made, referral to a sleep specialist is appropriate.

Narcolepsy. The prevalence of narcolepsy in this country is approximately 0.05 to 0.09%. The disorder may start in childhood but the peak incidence is in the second decade. The diagnosis is made on clinical grounds; however, a daytime sleep laboratory study (see multiple sleep latency test [MSLT], below) may be valuable when the clinical picture is not clear. Objective support for the diagnosis of narcolepsy is established with a median sleep latency on the MSLT of less than 5 minutes and the presence of two or more REM onsets occurring during the naps that occur during the test (1). Normal results from this testing include a median sleep latency greater than 15 minutes and no REM sleep during these daytime naps.

Several clinical features constitute the syndrome of narcolepsy (Table 85.5). The most common of these is a state of chronic daytime sleepiness and the occurrence of episodes of falling asleep. The sleepiness is similar to that experienced by normal people after sleep deprivation. In a patient with narcolepsy, no amount of normal sleep leads to a state of full alertness. It should be appreciated that sleepiness may be the only symptom the patient exhibits. Alternatively, patients may complain of memory difficulties, problems in maintaining attention during certain tasks, blurred vision, or difficulty focusing. They may report saying and doing things for which they have absolutely no memory (automatic behavior). One therefore should not view narcolepsy as strictly a disorder of excessive sleepiness, but also as a disorder of decreased alertness and attentiveness.

Cataplexy and sleep paralysis are present in some patients with narcolepsy. Both of these conditions are associated with loss or absence of muscle tone and strength. Cataplexy occurs when the patient is awake. There is a sudden loss of muscle strength precipitated by an emotional response (i.e., laughter, fear, anger). It can affect any muscle group in the face, trunk, or limbs. There is full alertness during these episodes. Sleep paralysis occurs just before falling asleep or just after awakening. The person usually cannot move or speak; however, breathing is not disturbed. There may be a high degree of anxiety or terrifying hallucinations. The paralysis lasts seconds or minutes and resolves spontaneously. Cataplexy occurs only with narcolepsy. Accordingly, a history of cataplexy and excessive daytime sleepiness leads to the diagnosis of narcolepsy. Sleep paralysis may occur alone as an idiopathic condition and therefore does not confirm the presence of narcolepsy.

Another cardinal feature of narcolepsy is *hypnagogic hallucinations.* These are vivid and sometimes very realistic sensory experiences before falling asleep. The experiences may be in any sensory modality (e.g., visual, auditory, tactile) and may range from simple to complex in presentation. For example, there may be a sense of something crawling on the legs, a well-formed visual hallucination, or an out-of-body experience. The phenomenon is comparable with dreaming with one's eyes open and being fully alert. Some patients have hypnagogic hallucination and no other components of the narcolepsy syndrome. This symptom also may exist independently of EDS.

Disturbed nocturnal sleep often is seen with narcolepsy. The most common complaint is that after sleeping for 3 to 4 hours, the patient awakens fully alert. After about 45 to 60 minutes, the patient becomes tired and falls back to sleep. Sometimes there are multiple awakenings throughout the night. Patients may experience vivid dreams or hallucinations with these awakenings. The vivid dreams may be terrifying and nightmarish in content. The patient starts the day tired and unrested and this only worsens the underlying daytime problems.

Idiopathic Hypersomnia. This syndrome presents as excessive daytime sleepiness; however, the other clinical features seen with narcolepsy (Table 85.5) are absent in this disorder. Most patients have no difficulty sleeping throughout the night. However, often they wake up tired and remain tired throughout the day. They may be very difficult to arouse and, when awake, may stumble around in a semistuporous state, sometimes called sleep drunkenness. Naps are long and unrefreshing, which is the opposite to that seen in narcolepsy. The patient may demonstrate automatic behaviors or have amnesia for various events throughout the day. Daytime sleep studies (see "MSLT," below) demonstrate very short sleep latencies, as seen with narcolepsy, but there are no REM episodes during these naps.

Breathing Problems During Sleep (Sleep Apneas)

Definitions

These are by far the most serious disorders associated with sleep. They are characterized by breathing abnormalities that vary from reduction to complete cessation of air flow (hypopnea and apnea, respectively). The sleep apneas include central apnea, which is associated with cessation of respiratory effort, and obstructive apnea, which is associated with occlusion of upper airway and continued respiratory effort. Importantly, the various types of sleep-related apnea can be associated with hypoxemia and sleep fragmentation that lead to right ventricular heart failure alterations and cognitive dysfunction.

Epidemiology

A 1993 study of healthy men and women reported a prevalence of clinically significant sleep apnea in 4% of women and 9% of men (27). This prevalence may even be higher in obese people. Because of increased public awareness and the availability of diagnostic facilities, breathing problems during sleep are now being recognized in the very young and very old. The typical patient who presents with obstructive sleep apnea is a middle-age, mild to moderately obese man. Obstructive apneas occasionally are associated with specific abnormalities of the upper airway or with metabolic dysfunction (Table 85.6). One reversible cause that should be considered is *hypothyroidism,* especially in hypothyroid patients who describe their tiredness as daytime somnolence. By contrast, central sleep apnea occurs most commonly in infants or patients over 65 (10). Often, central apnea may occur as a result of major cerebral disease, brainstem and spinal disorders, or cardiovascular disease (Table 85.6).

Presentation

Characteristically, patients with obstructive apnea present with significant snoring or daytime hypersom-

Table 85.5.   Clinical Features of Narcolepsy

Altered Levels of Alertness and Attentiveness
Sleepiness
Poor concentration
Memory difficulty
Automatic behavior
Blurred or poorly focused vision

REM-Related Disturbances
Cataplexy
Sleep paralysis
Hypnagogic hallucinations

Sleep Disturbances
Frequent awakenings
Vivid dreams
Sleep terrors

Table 85.6.   Disorders Associated with Sleep Apnea

Obstructive Sleep Apnea
Narrowing of upper airway
  Nasal abnormalities (deviation, polyps)
  Oral abnormalities (tonsillar hypertrophy, acromegaly)
  Bony abnormalities (micrognathia)
  Shy–Drager syndrome
  Myotonic dystrophy
Hypothyroidism

Central Sleep Apnea
Cerebral disorders (stroke)
Brainstem–spinal disorder (polio, infarction, neoplasia, surgery)
Congestive heart failure (increased circulation time)

nolence (20). The snoring is loud, intermittent, and often punctuated by respiratory efforts unaccompanied by obvious air flow. A *bed partner* can document that the apneas are associated with a struggling effort (obstructive apnea) or a lack of effort (central apnea). Because apnea, or any form of periodic breathing, usually is associated with both oxyhemoglobin desaturation and a brief arousal, sleep becomes fragmented, leading to daytime sleepiness. Initially, the patient may experience a subtle decrease in alertness toward the end of the day or when engaged in sedentary activities. As the apnea progresses in severity because of weight gain or age, more obvious signs of hypersomnolence such as napping in the daytime, difficulties driving a car, and even severe sleepiness during normal waking activities may occur (Table 85.4). Because most patients are unaware of their breathing pattern and often underestimate the severity of daytime hypersomnolence, it is essential that a bed partner or other observer be questioned regarding the patient in whom sleep apnea is suspected. Additional clinical features such as choking, gasping episodes at night, evidence of systemic or pulmonary hypertension, and in severe cases, cor pulmonale may also suggest the underlying diagnosis. In general, the presenting symptoms of patients with both obstructive and central apnea are indistinguishable. Patients seldom have pure central or pure obstructive apneas.

The *physical examination* usually is not diagnostic in patients with obstructive apnea, although patients with narrowing of the upper airway are at significantly higher risk. In particular, children and adults who demonstrate a compatible history and marked tonsillar hypertrophy or retrognathia should be suspected of having this disorder. In elderly patients with central apnea, the physical examination is normal, whereas patients with neurologic or cardiovascular pathology usually demonstrate obvious localizing neurologic signs (e.g., stroke) or cardiomegaly.

Course

The course of obstructive sleep apnea is chronic and progressive because of the typical weight gain seen in a sedentary aging population. Some patients develop progressive cardiopulmonary decompensation manifested by worsening hypercarbia and hypoxemia,

which can be associated with cor pulmonale and life-threatening arrhythmias. Nevertheless, these complications are the exception and tend to occur in the more severely obese patients after many years of disease. By contrast, the course of central apnea is determined by the underlying pathologic process. Thus, if reversible central nervous system or cardiovascular disease exists, central apnea may resolve entirely. In normal elderly patients with central apnea, the course and prognosis are unknown.

Diagnosis

A working diagnosis of sleep apnea can be made by direct observation of the patient during sleep, either at home or in a general hospital. The occurrence of 10 or more apneic episodes per hour lasting at least 10 seconds is the usual criterion for the diagnosis. However, even with ideal observation, clinically significant apnea may not be appreciated (11). Definitive diagnosis requires a sleep study (see below). Other laboratory studies such as arterial blood gases and routine pulmonary function provide information about mechanical abnormalities or problems with gas exchange that may be useful in therapy but not in diagnosis. Flow-volume curves (see Fig. 55.2) may demonstrate fluttering during expiration associated with evidence of variable extrathoracic obstruction in patients with obstructive apnea. However, this test is neither specific nor sensitive; therefore, it is not recommended to screen patients. Although computerized tomography or MI scanning may demonstrate narrowing of the upper airway in patients with obstructive sleep apnea, it is unclear at present how this information can best be used in the management of these patients.

Sleep-Associated Leg Discomfort and Movements

Sleep-associated leg discomfort and movements generally represent *restless leg syndrome* (RLS) and isolated periodic leg movement (PLM) of sleep (6). The cause of RLS and PLM is unknown in the majority of patients. There does appear to be a familial component to the disorders. It is estimated that 25 to 30% of people over 65 years of age have RLS or PLM. RLS is seen in association with iron-deficiency anemia, dialysis, and the use of dopamine antagonists. PLM is seen with the use of most antidepressants. Disorders of the spinal cord or peripheral nerves may precipitate or augment RLS or PLM.

There are two major clinical components to RLS: a primary sensory disturbance while awake and a motor disturbance while asleep. The *sensory component has three primary features.* First, there is a sensation that usually is characterized as a deep, uneasy feeling. This offending sensation occurs in one or both legs, either independently or concomitantly. The feeling may be reported as aching, as something moving, as little insects, as crazy legs, etc. The description of the feeling is highly variable but is not that of pain. Along with this deep, uneasy feeling is a compulsion or urge to move (*akathisia*, literally "inability to sit still"). This is focal (single area on the leg) or segmental (the whole leg). Therefore the person is constantly moving or rubbing the legs or walking to relieve the sensation. The second feature of the sensory component is that the sensation worsens with rest and relaxation, and improves with movement and walking. The third feature is that the akathisia is at its worst in late evening. Commonly, the akathisia is not present at all during the day. It appears as soon as the person tries to relax in the late evening or upon getting into bed at night. Because of this sensory disturbance, the affected person cannot rest comfortably. He or she often cannot travel by any means that would limit movement. The patient commonly cannot relax long enough to sit through a movie or to read without having to shuffle or pace compulsively. At night, the akathisia prevents sleep. Some sufferers spend several hours at night pacing, until finally they are exhausted enough to fall asleep.

The second major component of RLS is the *motor movement that occurs during sleep.* On observation of the sufferer during sleep, brief, periodic leg and foot movements are evident. They may occur in one or both legs, either independently or simultaneously. These leg movements have been called *sleep-related myoclonus* or PLM of sleep. The major problem created by PLM is that, if frequent enough, it is associated with brief but repeated arousals from sleep. The person usually has no awareness of the arousals but complains of having awakened feeling tired and of being excessively sleepy during the day. Sometimes the leg kicks cause complete awakening several times throughout the night. These patients rarely know that it is the leg movements that are waking them. The usual response is that they awaken to go to the bathroom. Some people have little if any symptoms suggestive of the sensory disturbance or akathisia but suffer significantly with PLM. However, those with RLS (akathisia plus PLM) and those with just PLM probably have the same underlying problem and are treated similarly.

RLS is diagnosed on the clinical history of akathisia, whereas PLM is identified either by history given by the bed partner or by polysomnographic (PSG) recording made in the sleep laboratory (see below). Thus the PSG can be used to support the clinical suspicion of RLS, or to make the diagnosis of PLM in the absence of any clear history of akathisia. The deep, uneasy feelings of RLS must be differentiated from arthralgia, myalgia, or sensory neuropathy. The absence of frank pain, the history of relief with movement, the compulsion to move, and a normal neurologic, muscle, and joint examination should help in the differentiation. The presence of an initial sensory component and the voluntary nature of the movements should differentiate the restless, secondary movements of RLS from myoclonus or dyskinesia. Nocturnal seizures, sleep-related dystonia, myoclonus, sleep apnea, primary insomnia, and isolated PLM are part of the differential diagnosis when a patient presents with a history of disturbed sleep associated with movements during sleep. If the clinical history is insufficient to establish the diagnosis, the person should be referred to a sleep disorder clinic.

Abnormal Behaviors Emanating from Sleep (Parasomnias)

Restful sleep may be punctuated by behaviors that may or may not awaken the patient. The behaviors may range from the benign to the dramatic and may be violent. Several distinct syndromes have been recognized. Factors that can help distinguish the causes include the timing of the behavior, likelihood of awakening from the episode, degree of confusion present, and memory of the events. Sleep laboratory recordings may associate the types of episodes with different sleep stages.

Arousal Disorders

Three types of sleep-related behaviors are classified as arousal disorders (4): sleepwalking, sleep terrors, and confusional arousals. They share an association with *slow-wave sleep,* and thereby tend to occur during the first third of the night. The prevalence is greatest in childhood, but these disorders may persist in adulthood. A familial association has been noted in some cases. The frequency of episodes may range from several times per night to less than once a year. Commonly *there is amnesia for the event. Typically the person does not awaken spontaneously and is difficult to arouse.* The person may become aware of the events because of residual evidence such as relocated furniture or food left out on a table. Resistance to full awakening is characteristic, and marked confusion may be evident. Behaviors may be inappropriate, such as urinating in a closet or searching for nonexistent intruders.

Sleepwalking most commonly is simple, in that the person typically walks around the room or house but rarely goes outside. Generally sleepwalkers do not put themselves or others in a dangerous situation; however, dramatic exceptions have been reported. In some cases there may be an overlap with sleep terror symptoms, in which the person aggressively attempts to escape from or protect against an imagined threat.

By definition, *sleep terrors* are dramatic events. Evidence of autonomic discharge may be pronounced. Often, the person will sit up and scream loudly and commonly is unarousable. He or she may return to sleep after several minutes and have no recollection of the incident the following morning. If the person does awaken, he or she will report an intense sense of fear. The person may describe a distinct threat, but generally does not offer a lengthy dreamlike narrative. The sleep terror may lead to forceful escape behavior, which may cause injury to the person or someone else perceived to be an obstacle. Injury may result from leaping out of bed or colliding with furniture. Rarely, people have jumped through windows attempting to escape.

Confusional arousals involve persistent disorientation and incomplete awakening after an arousing stimulus while the person was in slow-wave sleep. Behaviors and speech content may be meaningless or inappropriate. A typical example would be a person responding to a ringing telephone 1 hour after sleep onset. The person may reach for other objects or may make little sense when talking. Amnesia for these episodes is common. Factors promoting deeper sleep increase the likelihood of such incomplete awakening. These may include sleep deprivation and sedating substances, such as alcohol and central nervous system (CNS) depressants.

Nightmares

Nightmares usually result in full awakenings and generally are not associated with prolonged confusion or sleep-related behaviors. Typically the person can recount an extended dream narrative and can describe the frightening aspects of the story. In contrast to arousal disorders, nightmares are most common during REM sleep and tend to occur during the latter part of the night. Nightmares also are more likely to be remembered in the morning.

Dreams may be related to physical activity during sleep in the rare *REM behavior disorder* (4). Normally there is skeletal muscle atonia during REM sleep; however, in this disorder the active inhibition of motor impulses is incomplete. The dreamer may physically act out dream content. Physical activity may include kicking or punching, and the person may leap from the bed. Violent behaviors causing injury to the person or bed partner have been reported. This disorder is more common in the elderly. Most cases are idiopathic; however, neurologic diseases, toxic and metabolic processes, and medications have been implicated in promoting the symptoms.

Summary

The differential diagnosis of sleep-related behaviors usually can be broken down into the slow-wave sleep and REM-associated symptom complexes. In rare instances, sleep-related behaviors have been attributed to complex partial seizures. *Nocturnal enuresis* is not associated with a particular sleep stage.

MANAGEMENT

Insomnia

A comprehensive sleep history from a patient with insomnia establishes the duration of the symptoms and explores possible predisposing, precipitating, and perpetuating factors. *Multifactorial causes are common* with insomnia. Treating the primary cause of the insomnia may be important, but reinforcing factors should also be addressed. Identified medical and psychiatric illnesses must be treated. Attention to sleep hygiene, behavioral programs, relaxation techniques, psychotherapy, environmental manipulations, and the use of hypnotic medications may play important roles in management. The objective of treatment is development by the patient of new behaviors and routines that allow a renewed sense of confidence in the ability to sleep effectively. This is achieved by a therapeutic

alliance where the patient plays an active role in exploring potential sleep-inhibiting factors. Considerable experimentation may be necessary.

Although the quality of clinical studies has been highly variable, critical reviews of the published literature support the conclusion that both behavioral and pharmacologic approaches reduce the time it takes to fall asleep by 15 to 30 minutes and the number of awakenings by one to three per night (see review by Kupler and Reynolds, "General References").

Sleep Hygiene Measures

Recommendations about sleep hygiene are beneficial to most patients with insomnia, regardless of the duration of their symptoms (Table 85.7). These basic guidelines address factors that directly cause disturbed sleep and inhibit recovery. They take into account fundamental physiological and psychological understanding of the sleep process.

It is important to *take full advantage of the underlying circadian rhythm,* described above, that promotes nighttime sleepiness and daytime alertness. Attempts to sleep at various times throughout the 24-hour cycle may perturb the rhythm. Daytime or evening napping can inhibit the onset of sleep at night. A consistent wake-up time is important because this is when the system is most sensitive to daily reinforcement.

Some people with insomnia spend excessive time in bed (e.g., 9 PM to 9 AM) in hopes of getting a little more sleep. Generally this is counterproductive. Physiologically there may be less effective support of the circadian pattern. Because continuous sleep is unlikely, the person is creating a situation in which failure is inevitable. Extended wakeful periods may be self-reinforcing. Sleep restriction therapy (see below) is a treatment modality that specifically addresses this problem.

It is useful to consider the *extent to which a patient develops negative associations with the bed and bed-*

Table 85.7.   Sleep Hygiene Measures

Try to maintain a regular sleep–wake schedule. It is particularly important to get up at about the same time every day.

Avoid afternoon or evening napping if you have difficulty getting to sleep at night.

Allow yourself enough time in bed for adequate sleep duration (e.g., 11 PM to 7 AM). Do not spend excessive time in bed hoping to get more sleep.

Spend some idle time reflecting on the day's events before going to bed. Make a list of concerns and how you might solve them.

Avoid alcohol and caffeine in the evening.

Reserve the bed for sleep and sex. Do not do homework or pay bills in bed.

Avoid stressful activities at bedtime. Develop a relaxing and enjoyable routine before retiring to bed (e.g., reading, television).

Minimize annoying noise, light, or temperature extremes.

Consider a light snack before bedtime.

Exercise regularly, but not late in the evening.

Do not try harder and harder to fall asleep. If you are unable to sleep, do something else, out of bed and in a room other than the bedroom if possible.

Avoid smoking.

time routines. Good general advice includes reserving the bed for sleeping and sexual relations. Anxiety-provoking activities performed in bed may promote residual tension when sleep is attempted. Stressful behaviors may include studying for tests, paying bills, having domestic discussions, or watching violent television drama or news programs. These negatively stimulating activities should be replaced with relaxing behaviors.

Some people find significantly improved sleep with the *elimination of stimulants,* such as nicotine and caffeine. This especially is true during the hours leading up to bedtime. Late evening alcohol should be avoided because of the potential for stimulation related to withdrawal later in the night.

A *comfortable bedroom environment* is important. Temperature extremes, particularly a warm room, can promote sleep disruption. Outside noises may be blocked out by white noise machines or wax ear plugs. Generally people should not try to fall asleep with the television or radio playing. This tends to inhibit deep sleep and can cause awakenings.

Dietary habits may need to be addressed. Late heavy meals may produce abdominal discomfort or reflux symptoms. On the other hand, hunger may interfere with sleep onset. A light snack may be an appropriate solution.

Regular exercise (see Chapter 58) is recommended to promote improved sleep at night (13). However, aerobic exercises should be avoided in the hours leading up to bedtime to prevent excessive stimulation. For this reason, patients should be warned against trying to wear themselves out at night with hopes of falling asleep quickly.

Behavioral Management

Behavioral approaches are the primary treatment for chronic insomnia. *Relaxation techniques* may have a permissive effect by reducing arousal and thereby allowing sleep onset (24). Relaxation may be achieved through the use of progressive relaxation, meditation, and biofeedback (see techniques described in Chapter 13). Two other techniques, stimulus control therapy and sleep restriction therapy, involve specific instructions regarding nighttime routines and sleep–wake schedule hours.

Stimulus Control Therapy. Conditioned arousal is an important perpetuating factor in many people with chronic insomnia (2). The goal of stimulus control therapy is to reestablish the connection between the bedroom and sleeping. The fundamental strategy is to eliminate the nightly reinforcement of the anxiety and arousal that have become associated with the act of going to bed or awakening during the night. Basic sleep hygiene measures (Table 85.7) are pointed out as the necessary elements in a stimulus control plan. The purpose of these measures is to minimize the time that the patient is sleepless in bed. Chronic insomniacs often overvalue their time in bed and find the prospect of being out of bed abhorrent. They do not want to miss the opportunity for any potential sleep. The prescription of this technique should be framed positively so that the patient can view the time out of bed as an investment in better future sleep. Considerable discipline in following the guidelines is required for a positive result; however, many patients respond very well to this approach.

Sleep Restriction Therapy. The excessive time some chronic insomniacs spend in bed can undermine their recovery. Sleep may occur intermittently over a long period. Maximal reinforcement of the circadian influence is reduced. Sleep restriction therapy (25) attempts to consolidate sleep by limiting time in bed to specific hours. The schedule depends on the patient's perception of total sleep time. For example, patients reporting only 5 hours of sleep at night may be told that they may be in bed only from 3 AM until 8 AM. As sleep efficiency increases during this restricted time, the bedtime hour gradually is advanced. The wake-up time remains constant to promote regularity in the circadian pattern. The efficacy of this method has been confirmed in at least one clinical trial (7).

Circadian Manipulations

Successful treatment of insomnia may require paying attention to fundamental circadian principles. Transient insomnia secondary to jet lag can be minimized with the appropriate timing of activity and bedtime before and after the travel. Generally it is advisable to begin following the day/night pattern of the new time zone as quickly as possible. This allows more rapid entrainment as advantage is taken of external reinforcing stimuli, particularly sunlight. In some cases, problems associated with shift work also can be decreased to a limited extent with strategic manipulation of sleeping hours and light exposure (3).

Basic recommendations include regularity in timing of the sleep–wake cycle to maximize circadian reinforcement. Specific guidelines about bedtime, wake-up time, and bright light exposure are advisable in selected cases. Delayed sleep phase syndrome (see above) may be treated with varying degrees of success with a program of gradually advancing the wake-up time. Exposure to bright light (sunlight or therapeutic light boxes) soon after the wake-up time should help in resetting the underlying circadian clock. Bright light late in the day should be avoided. Advanced sleep phase syndrome may be treated with evening bright light exposure.

Hypnotic Medications

Hypnotic medications may play a valuable role in the treatment of selected patients. The use of hypnotics should always be part of an integrated approach that includes measures to promote sleep hygiene and psychotherapeutic support. The hypnotics may be used to help the patient during a stressful period and thereby hasten a return to a normal sleep–wake pattern. Hypnotics also may be beneficial in reestablishing a regular sleep cycle following time zone and work schedule shifts. A recent meta-analysis of clinical trials confirmed the efficacy of benzodiazepines and zolpidem for the short-term treatment of insomnia in adults younger than 65 (17a).

Prescription hypnotics are indicated *for short-term use* (e.g., for no more than 3 or 4 weeks). Accordingly, they are helpful mostly for patients with transient and short-term insomnia. The lowest effective dosage should be prescribed for the shortest possible duration. These medications may be used nightly from several days to 3 weeks; however, intermittent use (e.g., 2 to 4 nights per week) should be encouraged for most patients. Rarely is it necessary to recommend a dosage higher than the standard available strengths.

Medications from several classes have been used for their hypnotic effects. The predominant ones have been the barbiturates (secobarbital, amobarbital, and pentobarbital) and related compounds (chloral hydrate, ethchlorvynol, and methyprylon); the benzodiazepines and related compounds (Table 85.8); sedating antidepressant medications (see Chapter 15); and over-the-counter antihistaminic preparations (5).

The *barbiturates* were the mainstay of prescription hypnotic use until the introduction of the benzodiazepines in the 1960s and 1970s. The *benzodiazepines* are much safer (decreased toxicity and potential for lethal overdose, less residual sedation, fewer and less severe withdrawal effects, and reduced potential for abuse and dependence). There is no reason to use the barbiturates in the routine management of insomnia. Of the prescription *nonbenzodiazepine nonbarbiturate* hypnotic agents, chloral hydrate (500-mg tablet) has the best safety profile.

Sedating antidepressants with minimal anticholinergic action, such as trazodone and nefazodone, have been used successfully as hypnotics. They are especially helpful for depressed patients who have markedly disturbed sleep. Some nondepressed patients with insomnia respond well to low dosages of these medications.

The *over-the-counter antihistaminic agents* (diphenhydramine, hydroxyzine, doxylamine, and pyrilamine) are used widely because of easy access and effective marketing. Their hypnotic efficacy is limited compared with that of the benzodiazepines, but they are safer. Consideration must be given to possible anticholinergic effects and next-day "hangover" sedation. The constituents of several popular products are listed in Table 85.9.

Table 85.8. Benzodiazepine and Related Hypnotic Medications

Generic Name	Brand Name	Available Strengths and Dosage Ranges (mg)
Shorter-Acting		
Triazolam	Halcion	0.125–0.25
Zolpidem[a]	Ambien	5–10
Intermediate-Acting		
Estazolam	ProSom	1–2
Temazepam	Restoril	7.5–15–30
Longer-Acting		
Flurazepam	Dalmane	15–30
Quazepam	Doral	7.5–15

[a]A nonbenzodiazepine agent.

Table 85.9. Constituents of Commonly Used Over-the-Counter Sleep Remedies

Product Name	Constituent	
Miles Nervine[a]		
Sleep-Eze	Pyrilamine maleate[b]	25 mg
Sominex[c]		
Nytol		
Unisom Night-time Sleep Aid	Doxylamine succinate[d]	25 mg
Benadryl	Diphenhydramine	25 mg

[a]This product no longer contains bromine.
[b]Antihistamine of the ethylenediamine class.
[c]This product no longer contains scopolamine.
[d]Antihistamine of the ethanolamine class.

Benzodiazepine hypnotics and zolpidem (allosteric modulators of the GABA-A receptor complex) are among the most widely prescribed of all medications. All are classified as Schedule IV drugs under the federal Controlled Substance Act. Their proper use requires a knowledge of their onset and duration of action. All benzodiazepines marketed as hypnotics are rapidly absorbed and thereby have an acceptable onset of action. The duration of action depends on several factors, including volume of distribution, solubility in fat, half-life, and presence of active metabolites. The age of the patient also may be a factor; elderly patients have extended elimination periods. This also may be true in patients with liver impairment.

The benzodiazepines and related hypnotics can be categorized according to their duration of action (Table 85.8). The advantages and disadvantages to the shorter- and longer-acting medications should be considered in hypnotic selection.

A gradually tapered dosage often is useful in discontinuing a benzodiazepine hypnotic in order to minimize *withdrawal symptoms.* This helps reduce patient discomfort following extended hypnotic usage. Patients may confuse physiologically predictable withdrawal insomnia symptoms with the belief that they inherently are unable to sleep without the sleeping pill. Patient education is vital to successful treatment. *The longer-acting hypnotics* tend to be associated with less pronounced withdrawal symptoms than are the shorter-duration compounds. An exception may be the reported minimal withdrawal symptoms associated with the short-acting nonbenzodiazepine agent zolpidem (Ambien). When withdrawal insomnia is present, it tends to occur earlier with the shorter-acting agents. Withdrawal from longer-acting hypnotics may be delayed for several days following discontinuation. A pronounced *rebound insomnia syndrome* has been reported with sudden discontinuation of triazolam, which has an especially short half-life.

Shorter-acting hypnotics (short and intermediate duration) have the advantage of producing minimal *residual daytime sedation.* Excessive daytime sleepiness can be a major problem with longer-acting agents, particularly flurazepam. In addition, impairment of daytime performance and an increased propensity for falls among the elderly may be associated with the longer-duration hypnotics. On the other hand, the longer-acting medications may be useful when a daytime anxiolytic or sedative effect is desired.

Less common side effects of benzodiazepines include dizziness, headache, and disinhibited or bizarre behaviors. Ataxia, slurred speech, or confusion may be seen at higher dosages. Interdose anxiety and anterograde amnesia have been reported with triazolam in rare cases. Caution is advised in using benzodiazepines in patients with hepatic, renal, or respiratory impairment. Additionally, they should be avoided during pregnancy and lactation. Cumulative effects with other CNS depressants always must be considered.

The question of abuse often influences the decision to initiate hypnotic treatment. This issue was examined in a task force report by the American Psychiatric Association (26). It was concluded that most patients who take benzodiazepines do so for limited periods of time, according to the prescription guidelines. It was noted that benzodiazepine abuse occurs most commonly in patients who are concurrently abusing other substances (see Chapters 21 and 22). Accordingly, particular caution is recommended with such patients.

In summary, benzodiazepines and related hypnotics can be used effectively in selected patients when prescribed as part of an overall treatment plan. The pattern of the patient's sleep disturbance helps guide hypnotic selection. *Sleep onset insomnia* may respond well to a short-acting agent. A *sleep continuity problem* may be helped more by a medication of short or intermediate duration.

Narcolepsy and Idiopathic Hypersomnolence

In the management of narcolepsy there are pharmacologic and nonpharmacologic approaches to excessive daytime sleepiness (1). Nonpharmacologic treatments (Table 85.10) should be used by all narcoleptic patients whenever possible. The first of these approaches is *activity*. As long as narcoleptic patients continue some level of physical activity, a reasonable level of alertness usually can be maintained. Adding exercise to the daily schedule further enhances the alertness. Brief *naps* (10 to 30 minutes), preferably taken on a scheduled basis (e.g., work breaks and lunchtime), are a valuable strategy to maintaining alertness throughout the day. *Caffeinated beverages* may be used for a short and quick pick-me-up, whereas food may attenuate alertness. These various approaches can be used alone or in combination for the best effect. For example, at lunchtime a light meal may be taken or avoided altogether. This can be followed by a brief nap and 30 minutes of mild to moderate activity. Use of a brief nap followed by caffeinated beverage may be used just before a conference or just before driving to or from work. In fact, narcoleptic patients should be *instructed about the dangers of driving.* If they feel tired while driving, they should not push themselves but should pull off as soon as possible. They can take a brief nap, get out of the car and walk around, or get a cup of coffee. The final concern is *nocturnal sleep.* Extra nighttime sleep has no effect on daytime alertness and sleepiness. However, disturbed sleep at night produces greater problems during the day. Narcoleptic patients need to maintain normal sleep habits when possible. Staying out late at night, working two jobs, doing shift work, or living on 4 or 5 hours of sleep does not work for most people and it definitely does not work for narcoleptic patients.

The pharmacologic treatment of daytime sleepiness and diminished alertness involves the use of *stimulant medication* (Table 85.11). Attempts to completely normalize a patient with narcolepsy are fraught with many problems, often marked frustration and frequent failure. It is important to identify specific difficulties for targeted use of stimulants (i.e., falling asleep while driving or during meetings, inability to concentrate while at work or during the afternoon). Both pharmacologic and nonpharmacologic treatment must be structured to suit the problems that have been identified. The same amount of medication does not need to be given every day or at the same time each day. Drug holidays on weekends with amphetamine and methylphenidate should be established as often as possible. A persistent increase in heart rate and blood pressure is not uncommon with these medications. Pemoline may cause increases in liver enzymes in children and rarely in adults. Liver function studies should be performed once or twice a year while pemoline is being taken. If elevations occur, changing to another drug may be the most prudent approach. Addiction to amphetamine or methylphenidate may occur in rare cases. Weight loss, agitated behavior, tachycardia, hypertension, diaphoresis, end-of-dose depression, and high expectation or strong social pressure to be normal are characteristics of psychophysiologic dependence. In patients who exhibit these characteristics, efforts should be made to withdraw the medication under optimal conditions. This might include support from a chemical dependence service and a specialist in narcolepsy.

The *cataplexy* in narcolepsy may improve when either pharmacologic or nonpharmacologic therapies are used in the management of excessive daytime somnolence. Many people with cataplexy make adaptive changes in their personal and social lifestyles. These changes may reduce or eliminate emotional precipitants in the environment. However, even with the above therapies and lifestyle adaptations, cataplexy may remain a significant problem. Previously, tricyclic antidepressants were the primary medication used for this problem. For many patients *fluoxetine* 20 to 60 mg/day or another SSRI may be as effective as the tricyclics and without many of the side effects.

Table 85.10. Nonpharmacologic Treatment of Narcolepsy

Brief daytime naps as needed
Light meals during the day
Remain active, if at all possible
If sleepy, get up, walk around, take a break
Avoid sedative medication
Use caffeinated beverages as needed
Add exercise to the daily routine

Table 85.11. Stimulant Medication

Generic Name	Brand	Initial Dosage (mg)	Maximum Dosage (mg)	Available Strengths (mg)
Pemoline	Cylert	18.75 QD	75 mg BID	18.75, 37.5, 75
Methylphenidate	Ritalin	5 TID	30 QID	5, 10, 20
Dextroamphetamine	Dexedrine	5 BID	40 BID/TID	5, 10, 15

Protriptyline may be started at 5 mg in the morning and, if necessary, increased to 10 mg twice a day. If anticholinergic side effects or sedation are troublesome, one can try nortriptyline 25 to 100 mg in a single or divided dose. If these medications do not fully benefit the patient, then referral to a sleep disorder clinic is the best option.

The tricyclic antidepressants can be used to treat *sleep paralysis* and *hypnagogic hallucinations.* Protriptyline, 5 mg, can be given about an hour before bed if the paralysis or hallucinations occur near sleep onset. Otherwise, the medication can be given at bedtime.

The *management of idiopathic hypersomnia* is less clear-cut than that for narcolepsy. The stimulant medications outlined in Table 85.11 are used, but with less predictable benefits. The use of nonpharmacologic methods, as outlined for narcolepsy, is even less beneficial in this condition. These patients have moderate to severe disabilities from the excessive daytime tiredness.

Sleep Apnea and Other Breathing Disorders

The treatment of *obstructive sleep apnea* continues to evolve. Management options for an individual patient are recommended by the consultant who has evaluated the patient with a formal sleep study (see below). Table 85.12 summarizes a number of the approaches that have been used. Initial management should emphasize correcting associated medical conditions such as hypothyroidism (18), severe tonsillar hypertrophy, and obesity. CNS depressants, if prescribed, should be discontinued. Although the mechanism is still unknown, it is clear that as little as 10 to 15% weight loss may markedly improve the severity of the sleep apnea (21). Because most patients are 30 to 40% above ideal body weight, the minimal amount of weight reduction expected does not represent an unrealistic goal (see "Practical Approaches" in Chapter 76).

Continuous positive airway pressure (CPAP) remains the mainstay of therapy for patients with moderate to severe disease. The patient is fitted with a cuplike mask that forces air, usually from a stationary unit in the bedroom, into the nasal airway. The pressure from the continuous air flow prevents upper airway collapse during sleep. Careful adjustment of pressure is important because patient compliance depends on elimination of apnea and symptom improvement. Patients experience a pressure sensation in the upper airway and the ears when first using the mask. Drying of the mucosal membranes and rhinorrhea can be reduced by adding a humidifier to the inspired air, and nasal congestion is improved by the addition of deconges-

Table 85.12. Approaches to Management of Obstructive Sleep Apnea

Most Effective
General
  Avoid CNS depressants
  Weight loss
Upper airway measures
  Continuous positive airway pressure (CPAP)
  Tracheostomy
  Palatopharyngoplasty

Least Effective
Medications
  Medroxyprogesterone
  Protriptyline
  Oxygen

tants. Most patients experience immediate and dramatic improvement in their daytime sleepiness. If this does not occur, compliance may be inadequate; otherwise, inadequate sleep or another concomitant sleep disorder should be suspected (14).

Selection of *surgical measures* to alter upper airway anatomy requires consultation with an otolaryngologist. Although tracheotomy was used regularly in the past for the treatment of this syndrome, it is rarely performed now because of the newer forms of medical therapy and the associated psychosocial adjustments and physical discomfort of tracheotomy. Palatopharyngoplasty generally is considered after medical therapy has been tried because the rate of treatment success approaches 40 to 50%.

Medications such as medroxyprogesterone and protriptyline have been used to treat obstructive sleep apnea, but it is still unclear which patients will respond to pharmacologic therapy (22). In general, protriptyline has been shown more consistently to reduce the snoring and the frequency of deoxygenation, and to improve daytime hypersomnolence in people with mildly severe obstructed apnea. The initial dosage is 5 to 10 mg given at bedtime or early in the morning if sleep onset is delayed as a result of the medication. Approximately 30% of patients experience side effects that include dry mouth and constipation. Because protriptyline is a mild appetite suppressant, it may facilitate weight reduction.

Only patients with significant cor pulmonale appear to benefit from *oxygen therapy.* These patients usually have evidence of hypoxemia both when awake and when asleep; therefore, continuous 24-hour oxygen therapy usually is indicated. As a general rule, drugs or oxygen reduces but does not eliminate episodes of obstructive sleep apnea (23).

Currently, no therapies for central apnea consistently reduce the frequency of events. However, administration of oxygen almost always reverses any associated hypoxemia and bradyarrhythmias (23). CPAP and various respiratory stimulants have produced conflicting results. However, the central sleep apnea associated with Cheyne–Stokes respiration appears to respond to CPAP or theophylline as well as treatment of the underlying heart failure that commonly is associated (9,12).

Restless Legs and Periodic Leg Movements

Nonpharmacologic methods to improve the symptoms of RLS or PLM have not been effective consistently (15). Exercise and prolonged soaking in a hot bath usually eliminate the symptoms, and there may be attenuation of the symptoms for a brief period of time after the person stops exercising or gets out of the hot bath. This reprieve may be sufficient to allow the person to fall asleep. However, it has little effect on subsequent development of nighttime leg movements.

For patients who ask for treatment, a *pharmacologic approach* to managing the symptoms is the most consistently successful strategy. The first line of treatment is dopaminergic medication. One can start with one-half tablet of Sinemet 25/100 at bedtime. Adjustments can be made every 3 or 4 days by increments of one-half tablet. The increments are based on benefits versus side effects. The single most common side effect is an augmentation of the symptoms. The augmentation is considered to be a temporal redistribution of the underlying akathisia. The late night symptoms become early evening symptoms. If the dosage is increased further, RLS symptoms may begin in the early afternoon. Attempts to modify the treatment schedule rarely succeed. The outcome of such treatment plans is a worsening of the symptoms between doses and a shortening of the effectiveness of the Sinemet. If augmentation occurs then the Sinemet should be discontinued and the patent started on *pergolide.* It is recommended that one start with 0.05-mg tablets taken 2 hours before bedtime. Increments are made every 3 to 4 days, if necessary, by one tablet. Most patients reach satisfactory treatment at dosages of 0.25 mg or less. The management of RLS can be sufficiently complicated that referral to a sleep disorder center may be warranted. Practical details regarding all classes of dopaminergic medications are found in Chapter 82.

Many drugs have been tried over the years for RLS, many of them without proven efficacy. The opiates, usually propoxyphene, are the second choice after a dopamine agonist. These may be given alone or in combination with a dopamine agonist to achieve symptomatic relief. Benzodiazepines and anticonvulsants may provide another line of treatment if opiates and dopamine agonists fail. However, at this stage, the patient should be assessed by a sleep disorder specialist.

Sleepwalking, Sleep Terrors, and Confusional States

These arousal disorders are viewed as emanating from slow-wave sleep. Sleep deprivation for any reason enhances slow-wave sleep on recovery nights, and increases the likelihood of these events in vulnerable people. Accordingly, appropriate recommendations always include minimizing situations that increase sleep loss. Vulnerable people also are more likely to experience episodes during stressful periods. Stress reduction techniques may be helpful for some patients, and psychotherapy may be indicated in selected cases. In some cases, presleep suggestions are beneficial. In a relaxed state at bedtime, the patient can focus on anticipated sleep-related behavior and can reaffirm that he or she will be safe and will do no harm. The sleepwalker can gradually limit the boundaries of wandering in this manner.

Severity in these disorders may be reflected in the frequency of the events and the dangerousness of the behaviors. Particularly severe cases (e.g., multiple episodes per week or less frequent incidents resulting in injury) may be appropriate for *pharmacologic treatment.* In theory, substances that decrease the intensity and duration of slow-wave sleep should decrease the symptoms. This seems to be the case with the benzodiazepines. Successful extended treatment has been accomplished with clonazepam 0.5 mg at bedtime. REM behavior disorder, although not associated with slow-wave sleep, often responds well to this medication.

Enuresis

Primary enuresis in the adult warrants urologic evaluation. The absence of demonstrable organic pathology should not discourage treatment attempts. Several strategies used in children also may be beneficial for adults. Behavioral management is the initial treatment of choice. Conditioning of the urge to urinate and going to the bathroom can be developed with pad and alarm systems (Wet-Stop, Palco Laboratories, Santa Cruz, CA). Standard medication trials have included tricyclic antidepressants. Intranasal desmopressin has been used successfully in many cases (17).

SLEEP CENTER REFERRAL

For a number of the problems discussed in this chapter, referral for expert evaluation and management is recommended. The evaluation of patients with sleep disorders often includes consideration of referral for sleep laboratory evaluation. Because sleep laboratories are now more accessible, it is possible to refer the patient either directly to a laboratory for specific sleep studies or to an expert at a sleep center who may be useful in determining the specific type of sleep test to be conducted. Often, a consultant may recommend adjustments in medications or in the sleep–wake cycle before suggesting a sleep study. More importantly, interpretation of the sleep laboratory results and an explanation to the patient must be made by someone familiar with these studies. Currently there are over 250 sleep disorders centers accredited by the American Sleep Disorders Association (ASDA). The ASDA can supply the locations of these centers (ASDA, 1610 14th St. NW, Suite 300, Rochester, MN 55901-2200; telephone: 507-287-6008).

Patient Experience. When patients are evaluated at a sleep center, they undergo a careful historical review of their sleep problem and a general physical examination. An all-night sleep study (polysomnogram) may be scheduled in order to evaluate sleep objectively. The polysomnogram is performed using noninvasive simultaneous measurements of a number of physiological activities during sleep: eye movements, brain activity by EEG, submental and anterior tibialis muscle activity, respiratory air flow and effort, cardiac rhythm, and continuous blood oxyhemoglobin saturation. Sometimes additional parameters are recorded such as rectal temperature, esophageal pH, and penile circumference.

Multiple sleep latency test (MSLT), a day test with four to five repeated 20-minute naps spaced 2 hours apart, may also be scheduled. For this nap test, patients stay in their usual sleeping clothes and are asked to stay awake between the naps. A full-sleep EEG is recorded as is done for the polysomnogram, except the respiration and oxygen saturation measurements either are not made or are used in a limited form because the primary question addressed by this test is the degree of the patient's excessive sleepiness. The time it takes the patient to fall asleep (sleep latency) during these naps provides the measure of the patient's sleepiness. The nap test usually is scheduled for the day after the nighttime polysomnogram. A typical schedule for the patient in the sleep lab is 9:30 PM to 8 AM for the polysomnogram and 8 AM to 4:30 PM for the nap tests.

General References*

Diagnostic Classification Steering Committee, Thorpy MJ, Chairman. International classification of sleep disorders: diagnostic and coding manual. Rochester, MN: Sleep Disorders Association, 1990.
> This classification manual lists all recognized sleep disorders. Clinical features and diagnostic criteria are outlined.

Kryger M, Roth T, Dement WC, eds. Principles and practice of sleep medicine. 2nd ed. Philadelphia: WB Saunders, 1994.
> This comprehensive textbook covers basic science and clinical issues in sleep disorders medicine.

Kupfer DJ, Reynolds CF III. Management of insomnia. N Engl J Med 336(5):341, 1997.
> Up-to-date review. Authors' summary assessments of clinical trials of published behavioral and pharmacologic interventions are included.

Strollo PJ Jr, Rogers RM. Current concepts: obstructive sleep apnea. N Engl J Med 334(2):99, 1996.
> Recent well-referenced review article.

Specific References

1. Aldrich MS. Narcolepsy. Neurology 42(Suppl 6):34, 1992.
2. Bootzin RR, Nicassio PM. Behavioral treatments for insomnia. Progress in behavioral modification. Vol 7. San Diego: Academic Press, 1978.
3. Czeisler CA, Kronauer RE, Allan JS, et al. Bright light induction of strong (type 0) resetting of the human circadian pacemaker. Science 244(4910):1328, 1989.
4. Diagnostic Classification Steering Committee. International classification of sleep disorders: diagnostic and coding manual. Rochester, MN: Sleep Disorders Association, 1990.
5. Drugs used for anxiety and sleep disorders. In: Drug evaluation subscription. Chicago: American Medical Association, I/PSY-1, Spring 1993.
6. Dyken ME, Rodnitzky RL. Periodic, aperiodic, and rhythmic motor disorders of sleep. Neurology 42(Suppl 6):68, 1992.
7. Friedman L, Bliwise DL, Yesavage JA, Salom SR. A preliminary study comparing sleep restriction and relaxation treatments for insomnia in older adults. J Gerontol Psychol Sci 46:1–8, 1991.
8. The Gallup Organization, Inc. The Gallup survey. Sleep in America. 1991.
9. Granton JT, Naughton MT, Benard DC, et al. CPAP improves inspiratory muscle strength in patients with heart failure and central sleep apnea. Am J Respir Crit Care Med 153:277, 1996.
10. Guilleminault C, Eldridge FL, Dement WC. Insomnia with sleep apnea: a new syndrome. Science 181:856, 1973.
11. Haponik EF, Smith PL, Myers DA, Bleecker ER. Evaluation of sleep disordered breathing: is polysomnography necessary? Am J Med 77:671, 1984.
12. Javaheri S, Parker TJ, Wexler L, et al. Effects of theophylline on sleep-disordered breathing in heart failure. N Engl J Med 335(8):562, 1996.
13. King AC, Oman RF, Brassington GS, et al. Moderate-intensity exercise and self-rated quality of sleep in older adults. JAMA 277(1):32, 1997.
14. Kribbs NB, Pack AI, Kline LR, et al. Objective measurement of patterns of nasal CPAP use by patients with obstructive sleep apnea. Am Rev Respir Dis 147:887, 1993.
15. Montplaisir J, Lapierre O, Warnes H, Pelletier G. The treatment of the restless leg syndrome with or without periodic leg movements in sleep. Sleep 15(5):391, 1992.
16. National Commission on Sleep Disorders Research. Report of the National Commission on Sleep Disorders Research, DHHS Publication, Washington, DC: US Government Printing Office, 1992.
17. Nino-Murcia G, Keenan SA. Enuresis and sleep. In: Guilleminault C, ed. Sleep and its disorders in children. New York: Raven Press, 1987.
17a. Nowell PD, Mazumdar S, Buysse DJ, et al. Benzodiazepines and zolpidem for chronic insomnia: a meta-analysis of treatment efficacy. JAMA 278(24):2170–2177, 1997.
18. Rajagopal KR, Abbrecht PH, Derderian SS, et al. Obstructive sleep apnea in hypothyroidism. Ann Intern Med 101:491, 1984.
19. Silverman K, Evans SM, Strain EC, Griffiths RR. Withdrawal syndrome after the double-blind cessation of caffeine consumption. N Engl J Med 327:1109, 1992.
20. Smith PL. Evaluation of patients with sleep disorders. In: White DP, ed. Seminars in respiratory medicine. New York: Thieme Stratton, 1988;534.
21. Smith PL, Gold AR, Myers DA, et al. Weight loss in mildly to moderately obese patients with obstructive sleep apnea. Ann Intern Med 103:850, 1985.
22. Smith PL, Haponik EF, Allen RP, Bleecker ER. The effects of protriptyline in sleep-disordered breathing. Am Rev Respir Dis 127:8, 1983.
23. Smith PL, Haponik EF, Allen RP, Bleecker ER. The effects of oxygen in patients with sleep apnea. Am Rev Respir Dis 130:958, 1984.
24. Spielman AJ, Caruso LS, Glovinsky PG. A behavioral perspective on insomnia treatment. Psychiatr Clin North Am 10(4):541, 1987.
25. Spielman AJ, Saskin P, Thorpy MJ. Treatment of chronic insomnia by restriction of time spent in bed. Sleep 10:45, 1987.
26. Task Force on Benzodiazepine Dependency. Benzodiazepine dependence, toxicity, and abuse: a task force report of the American Psychiatric Association. Washington, DC: American Psychiatric Association, 1990.
27. Young T, Palta M, Dempsey J, et al. The occurrence of sleep-disordered breathing among middle-aged adults. N Engl J Med 328:1230, 1993.

*Bold print (general references) and bold numerals (specific references) denote published controlled clinical trials, meta-analyses, or consensus-based recommendations.

Selected General
Surgical Problems

C H A P T E R 86

Preoperative Planning for Ambulatory Patients

RICHARD J. GROSS, MD

PREOPERATIVE PLANNING: OVERVIEW

Preoperative planning for elective surgery is now done almost entirely in the ambulatory setting, as most surgery is now performed in outpatient surgical units or patients are admitted on the day of surgery for inpatient surgery. The general physician invests substantial time initially in establishing a diagnosis for the initial complaint, arriving at the decision to recommend surgery, and discussing the findings with the patient and family; the physician then evaluates the medical risks from factors unrelated to the primary surgical problem and consults on the care of the patient's medical problems in the perioperative period.

The *principal reasons for office-based preoperative assessment* are that health care insurers now reimburse only for same-day surgery for many procedures, insurers do not reimburse for admission the day before surgery for preoperative assessment, office assessment eliminates the costs and inconvenience associated with unanticipated cancellation of surgery after the patient has been admitted, and better planning of care and higher patient satisfaction are often achieved.

In general, the surgeon expects the referring physician to have made an independent assessment of the need for surgery and of the patient's general fitness for surgery. Although the surgeon obtains the actual consent for the surgical procedure, the patient's decision is based in part on the counseling provided by the personal physician. The referral itself is usually understood by a patient and the family as an endorsement of a surgical opinion and of the consulting surgeon. For these reasons, it is important for referring physicians to know the place of surgery in the management of a broad array of conditions.

General guidelines on eligibility for same-day ambulatory surgery, based on the patient's medical status, are summarized in Table 86.1 (2,11).

Laparoscopic techniques, though more comfortable to the patient, do not necessarily carry a lower medical, anesthetic, or surgical risk.

In counseling the patient and family, the patient's physician, as well as the consulting surgeon, should explain clearly the objective, potential complications, and expected outcome of the operation. This is especially important for surgical procedures that are undertaken for asymptomatic conditions (e.g., elective cholecystectomy) and for procedures that may be disfiguring (e.g., mastectomy or amputation). Preoperative counseling should be documented in the patient's record, including any special issues raised by the patient and how they were resolved (e.g., obtaining additional consultations or providing supportive counseling).

Approximately 50% of adults who undergo surgery are ostensibly in good general health; the other 50% have various medical problems (the percentages vary depending on the age of the population). In perhaps 5 to 10% of patients, new medical problems are identified during preoperative evaluation; a small proportion of these problems have implications for the planning of surgery. Whenever surgery is planned, the patient's referring physician should complete an appropriate preoperative evaluation (see below), ensure that existing medical conditions that may affect the outcome of surgery are optimally controlled, and communicate specific recommendations to the surgeon regarding the care of the patient's medical problems during the perioperative period. This chapter provides guidelines for these steps in the management of patients with a number of common medical problems.

GENERAL PREOPERATIVE EVALUATION

There is no consensus on the makeup of a general preoperative evaluation. For adult patients undergoing general or spinal anesthesia, most physicians perform a history and physical examination and order a number of routine laboratory tests (e.g., chest x-ray and electrocardiogram in patients over 40 and complete blood count, tests of hemostasis, electrolytes, glucose, measurement of serum urea nitrogen or creatinine, and urinalysis in all adults). This complete workup has been criticized for having a low yield and being unnecessarily costly (2). The large number of factors that

influence the preoperative evaluation make a consensus unlikely. The patient's age, the nature of the planned surgery (major or minor), the type of anesthesia to be used (general, spinal, regional, or local), and the interval since the patient's last comprehensive evaluation are relevant in the preoperative evaluation of every patient. In addition, one or more of the following considerations are often pertinent: estimating operative risk, establishing a baseline for expected postoperative changes or possible complications, avoiding harm to other patients or medical personnel (e.g., hepatitis, tuberculosis, or human immunodeficiency virus [HIV] infection), documenting selected information for medicolegal reasons, determining drug dosage, and detecting rare but potentially catastrophic circumstances (e.g., thrombocytopenia in a patient scheduled for a craniotomy).

A practical approach for the individual patient is to select one of the two general types of preoperative evaluation as summarized in Table 86.2 (i.e., a limited or a comprehensive workup). Guidelines for choosing between these alternatives are summarized in Table 86.3. Selected screening tests should be added to either workup to avoid potential catastrophes associated with certain high-risk situations (Table 86.4). Routine HIV screening of preoperative patients is currently not recommended; instead, the universal precautions described in Chapter 34 are recommended.

Another approach is to recommend fewer tests as part of the basic limited or comprehensive workup, and to use a grid to select tests based on individual patient characteristics and type of surgery (27). A number of such grids have been published but recommendations are not uniform (2).

Commonly overlooked aspects of evaluation and planning in the assessment of the outpatient presurgical patient are listed in Table 86.5.

Table 86.1. General Guidelines on Patient Eligibility for Ambulatory Surgery Based on Medical Condition (Not Considering Type of Surgery)

American Society of Anesthesiologists class 1–2 (some class 3 for minor procedures).

Class 1: There is no physiological, biochemical, or psychiatric disturbance. The pathologic process for which operation is to be performed is localized and not conductive to systemic disturbance. *Examples:* A fit patient with inguinal hernia; fibroid uterus in an otherwise healthy woman.

Class 2: Mild to moderate systemic disturbance caused either by the condition to be treated surgically or by other pathophysiologic processes. *Examples:* Presence of mild diabetes mellitus, essential hypertension, or anemia.

Class 3: Rather severe systemic disturbance from whatever cause, even though it may not be possible to define the degree of disability with finality. *Examples:* Severe diabetes mellitus with vascular complications, moderate to severe degrees of pulmonary insufficiency, angina pectoris or healed myocardial infarction.

Stable chronic medical problems well controlled by medicines; absence of acute medical problems.

No recent myocardial infarction or unstable cardiac disease.

No decompensated lung disease.

If diabetic, not taking insulin; if taking insulin; stable and capable of self-monitoring (insulin-dependent diabetics should be operated upon in the morning).

Adapted from Gross RJ, Gaputo GM, eds. Medical consultation: the internist on surgical, obstetric, and psychiatric services. 2nd ed. Baltimore: Williams & Wilkins, 1998;37.

CURRENT MEDICATIONS AND KNOWN ALLERGIES

All drugs that a patient is taking and any known drug allergies should be specified at the time of referral for surgery. Planning should be initiated at that time to avoid possible interactions with anesthetic agents and possible complications during surgery, manage the patient when an essential drug cannot be administered orally during the perioperative period, and avoid exposure to drugs to which the patient is allergic. The patient should be asked specifically about nonprescription drug use that, although common, is often not mentioned spontaneously (particularly aspirin-containing compounds and nonsteroidal anti-inflammatory drugs [NSAIDs], which may potentiate postoperative bleeding, and sedatives, which may interact with anesthetic drugs); other anticoagulants (coumadin, ticlopidine); prior allergic reactions to drugs for medical conditions (especially penicillin and other antibiotics that may be indicated postoperatively at a time when a patient is unable to provide information) and to local and general anesthetic agents (e.g.,

Table 86.2. Two Types of General Preoperative Evaluation

Component of Workup	Limited Workup[a]	Comprehensive Workup[a]
History	HPI, medical history, allergies, medications, brief ROS (heart, lungs, hemostasis, endocrine, family history of surgical/anesthesia problems and new symptoms, especially upper respiratory infection)	HPI, medical history, social history, family history, allergies, medications, complete ROS
Physical examination	Vital signs, oral cavity, chest, heart, and abdomen	Complete physical examination
Laboratory[a]	Hematocrit, urinalysis (dipstick only), ECG (some cases >age 35), serum potassium concentration some cases, pregnancy test[b]	Chest radiograph, ECG (>age 35), complete blood count, serum urea nitrogen or serum creatinine, serum glucose, serum electrolytes, urinalysis, pregnancy test[b]

HPI, History of present illness; ROS, review of symptoms.

[a]Basic evaluation for screening and baseline data. Other tests may be added to evaluate known disease in a patient or to follow up findings in the preoperative history and physical examination; see also Table 86.4.

[b]Women in childbearing age group.

Table 86.3. Guidelines for Selecting the General Preoperative Evaluation

Limited Workup	Comprehensive Workup
Age <40 yr	Age >40 yr (especially >60 yr)
Recent comprehensive physical examination	No, old, or inadequate data base
Well patient	Patient with moderate or severe major organ disease
Local, regional, or spinal anesthesia	General anesthesia
Established patient; previously examined by physician	New patient, unknown to physician
Minor procedure	Major procedure (especially thoracic, abdominal, neurosurgical)

halothane); use of corticosteroids within the past year (particularly patients with obstructive airway disease or seasonal allergy); prior reactions to blood products; and current use of recreational substances that may affect the patient's course during or after surgery (alcohol, tobacco, illicit drugs).

For patients taking one or more medications regularly, specific perioperative recommendations regarding those medications should be communicated to the surgeon (Table 86.6). Modification of chronic medications for surgery is best done well before surgery to allow time to detect unanticipated effects. Most medications have a duration of action between 6 and 12 hours, and omission of one or more doses may precipitate symptoms. For patients who are expected to be awake and to be able to take oral medications within this time span, it is appropriate to recommend giving a dose, with a small amount of water (1 ounce or less), in the morning before the induction of anesthesia and resuming the medication orally 6 to 12 hours later. When oral medications cannot be continued throughout the perioperative period, alternate medications or routes of administration should be recommended.

PREOPERATIVE DONATION FOR AUTOLOGOUS TRANSFUSION

Self-donation of one or more units of blood for autologous transfusion for elective surgery is now widely practiced. The risks of autologous transfusion are lower than the risks with bank blood but bacterial contamination and error remain small possibilities.

Current blood preservation methods limit autologous donation to about 3 units. Single units are donated beginning about 4 weeks before surgery, at weekly intervals. In preoperative planning, it is important to leave sufficient time for donation of the required units but not so much time that the units expire if there is a minor delay in the scheduled surgery. Usually this is arranged by the surgeon, but the patient's primary physician may want to discuss this option with the patient, including the time necessary (depending on the number of units needed) and any medical contraindications or limitations in autologous donations.

Medical problems that are potential contraindications or that limit the number of units donated (depending on the severity of the situation) include anemia, cardiovascular disease, hypertension and antihypertensive medication, lung disease with significant hypoxia, orthostatic hypotension, certain infectious diseases (including hepatitis and HIV infection), and very frail or debilitated patients. Despite this list of limitations, most patients are able to donate for autologous transfusion, including most elderly patients with chronic diseases. The patient's physician may want to plan for partial volume repletion with saline at the time of donation for some patients who may be very sensitive to the volume loss. Most patients are placed on iron (see Chapter 50) beginning about 1 week before the first donation and continuing for 2 to 3 months after donation (depending on the number of units donated).

SURGERY IN THE ELDERLY PATIENT

Size of the Risk

The mortality risk associated with anesthesia and surgery is increased in the elderly. However, the risk in elderly patients has fallen substantially over the past 10 to 20 years. The overall mortality risk for major surgery in patients under 65 is approximately 1%; the risk is approximately 5% between ages 65 and 80. Patients over age 80 have a 10% risk, although mortality as low as 6 to 8% has been reported (2,7,19).

Several factors are more important than age itself in increasing surgical risk in older patients (16). The most important of these factors are general overall health,

Table 86.4. Additional Preoperative Screening Tests for Common High-Risk Situations

High-Risk Situation	Screening Tests
Patient undergoing neurosurgical, cardiac, vascular, or major abdominal procedure	Tests of hemostasis: platelet count, prothrombin time, partial thromboplastin time
Patient on diuretics, with vomiting/diarrhea, other abnormal fluid loss, cardiac disease, renal disease	Electrolytes
Patient with increased risk of active liver disease (e.g., alcoholism, drug addiction, homosexuality, dialysis, high-risk medications) who is undergoing general or spinal anesthesia	Liver function tests: serum aminotransferases, alkaline phosphatase, bilirubin, hepatitis-associated antigen
Patient with increased risk of chronic pulmonary disease (e.g., smoker with ≥10 pack years) who is undergoing general anesthesia	Pulmonary function tests (spirometry)
Patient with increased risk of tuberculosis (e.g., known exposure, HIV positive, underprivileged population)	Chest x-ray, purified protein derivative skin test for TB
Patient with increased risk of coronary artery disease (i.e., smoker, hypertensive, strong family history, diabetic, hyperlipidemia)	ECG
Malnourished patient or prolonged inability to eat	Nutritional assessment

Table 86.5. Commonly Forgotten or Underestimated Items in the Office Evaluation and Management of the Surgery Patient

Evaluation
One disease (review the problem list)
The generally sick patient
Inquiry about current medications (include aspirin and other over-the-counter)
Blood tests indicated by specific medical disease or medications (e.g., drug levels, potassium for diuretics)
Inquiry about abnormal bleeding or knowledge that the patient is a bleeder
Inquiry about history of transfusion or transfusion reactions
Inquiry about current use of alcohol or illicit drugs
Pregnancy test (serum qualitative human chorionic gonadotropin)
Spirometry (smoker who may have unrecognized COPD)
Echocardiogram (evaluation of murmur regarding subacute bacterial endocarditis prophylaxis)

Management
Tell patient to report even minor intercurrent illnesses between physical and day of surgery
Stop smoking, alcohol, illicit drugs, OTC medications (no new OTC medications)
Medications (see Table 86.6): whether to take medications the morning of surgery and when to restart postoperatively. Discontinue certain medications (such as aspirin, coumadin). Coverage for corticosteroids if indicated
Subacute bacterial endocarditis prophylaxis
Teach patient what to expect preoperatively and postoperatively; call if unexpected problems arise
Tell the patient about, and plan several weeks in advance, banking of one or more units of blood for autologous transfusion

Adapted from Gross RJ, Caputo GM, eds. Medical consultation: the internist on surgical, obstetric, and psychiatric services. 2nd ed. Baltimore: Williams & Wilkins, 1998;38–39.

nutrition, type of surgery (body cavity versus non–body cavity; emergency versus elective), type of anesthesia, coexisting conditions (cardiac, infectious, renal, pulmonary, central nervous system [CNS]), and psychosocial status (attitude toward surgery, will to live, cognitive level, social situation).

The conditions associated with *very high surgical mortality in elderly patients* are uncorrectable surgical lesions such as infarcted bowel or ruptured aneurysm. The next most important cause of death is coexisting cardiac disease, followed by infections (especially pneumonia), renal disease, and pulmonary disease. In

the preoperative evaluation, attention should be focused on these problems because they account for most perioperative deaths.

Certain common procedures can be performed at low risk in the elderly, often without general anesthesia. These low-risk operations include cataract surgery, simple hernia repair, and transurethral prostate resection. The risks of some major surgical procedures in the elderly have fallen greatly over the past few years; examples include elective abdominal aortic aneurysm repair and repair of hip fractures. Laparoscopic surgery, such as for cholecystectomy, produces less medical morbidity but has not yet been shown to have a lower mortality than traditional surgery in the elderly.

Preoperative Planning

Office Evaluation

The elderly patient undergoing major surgery should have a comprehensive preoperative evaluation (Table 86.2) because of the wide variety of coexisting, often unrecognized medical conditions found in older patients. The workup should be reviewed specifically for the risk factors listed above. Any major preoperative risks must be weighed against the benefits of the operation, with attention to the fact that quality of life may be as important as longevity in this age group. An accurate estimation of average future longevity for the patient's age group is important; this is often underestimated.

Preoperative cardiac evaluation is discussed below. Manifestations of infection (including simple upper respiratory infections) should be carefully sought because classic signs may not be present in the elderly. Spirometry should be performed in patients over age 65 if there is pulmonary disease, because of the increased incidence of pulmonary complications in older patients. It should be remembered that serum creatinine may be falsely low in elderly patients because of their reduced muscle mass; therefore, a creatinine clearance should be obtained if the state of the patient's renal function is not certain, because of the importance in determining drug dosages. Finally, a baseline mental status examination (see Chapter 17) should be completed because postoperative changes in mental status are common in the elderly. If there is hearing impairment caused by cerumen impaction preoperatively, this problem should be corrected.

Recommendations to the Surgeon

Elderly patients often have limitations of understanding because of memory deficits and hearing prob-lems. Because these are often known to the primary physician, communication to the surgeon of these limitations improves the effectiveness of the surgeon's explanation of the procedure. Explanation of what to expect during hospitalization and surgery is even more important in the elderly to avoid fear and confusion and because of outdated conceptions of the nature of surgery among the elderly.

Table 86.6.   Recommendations to the Surgeon Regarding the Patient's Regular Medications[a]

Drug Class	Anticipated Problems	Recommendations to Surgeon for Perioperative Period
Cardiovascular		
Antihypertensives[b]	Interaction with anesthetics, hypotension	Inform anesthesiologist of use.
	Inability to give orally	Plan postoperative regimen with alternative agents if needed.
Antiarrhythmics[b]	Inability to give orally	ECG monitor in operating room and postoperatively, use alterantive parenteral agents.
β-Blockers[b]	Myocardial depression, bradycardia	Continue intravenously, taper to lower dosage, or discontinue depending on circumstances.
Digitalis[b]	Toxicity	Obtain serum levels preoperatively.
	Inability to give orally	Give 75% of daily oral dosage of digoxin intravenously each day.
Long-acting oral nitrates[b]	Inability to give orally	Substitute transdermal nitroglycerine.
Gastrointestinal		
Antacids[b]	Inability to give orally	Intravenous H_2 blockers, nasogastric suction (if patient has active peptic ulcer disease).
Antibiotics		
Tetracycline	Risk of renal failure if given with methoxyflurane	Use alternative antibiotic or anesthetic.
Corticosteroids[b]	Adrenal insufficiency	Plan coverage (with intravenous corticosteroids) adequate for the stress of surgery.
	Poor wound healing	Discuss with surgeon.
Neurologic		
Levodopa/carbidopa[b]	Interaction with anesthetics (hypertension or hypotension), inability to give orally	Inform anesthesiologist of use; resume orally as soon as possible after surgery.
Barbiturates	Increased CNS depression by anesthesia, inability to give orally	Inform anesthesiologist of use; give daily dosage intramuscularly.
Dilantin	Inability to give orally	Give daily dosage slowly intravenously (or substitute phenobarbital before admitting patient for surgery).
Bronchodilators		
Theophylline[b]	Inabiltiy to give orally	Switch to intravenous aminophylline.
β₂-Sympathomimetics[b]	Inability to give orally	Switch to aerosolized or subcutaneous β₂-agent.
Psychiatric		
Antidepressants[b]	Hypotension or hypertension, arrhythmias	Inform anesthesiologist of use; withhold monoamine oxidase inhibitors 2 weeks preoperatively; selectively withhold other agents 24 hours preoperatively.
Neuroleptics (i.e., phenothiazines and haloperidol)[b]	Arrhythmias, enhancement of neuromuscular blocking agents, hypotension	Inform anesthesiologist of use; withhold 24 hours preoperatively in some cases.
Benzodiazepines	Increased CNS depression by anesthesia	Inform anesthesiologist of use.
Lithium[b]	Myocardial depression, hypernatremia	Inform anesthesiologist of use; determine blood levels; withhold 24 hours preoperatively; avoid diuretics and NSAIDs; follow electrolytes closely.
Analgesics		
Narcotics	Decreased cough reflex, increased CNS depression by anesthesia, hypotension	Inform anesthesiologist of use.
Aspirin compounds[b]	Increased bleeding	Discontinue 1–2 weeks before surgery.
NSAIDs	Gastrointestinal tract bleeding	Discontinue 1 day or more preoperatively.
Anticoagulants, Antiplatelet		
Warfarin[b]	Increased bleeding	Discontinue 4–7 days before surgery, vitamin K_1 if needed, check prothrombin time before operation.
Aspirin, other NSAIDs, ticlopidine[b]		Discontinue aspirin and other NSAIDs 1 week before surgery; ticlopidine 2 weeks before surgery.

Table 86.6—continued.   Recommendations to the Surgeon Regarding the Patient's Regular Medications[a]

Drug Class	Anticipated Problems	Recommendations to Surgeon for Perioperative Period
Diuretics	Electrolyte abnormalities, hypotension, inability to give orally	Obtain electrolytes and check blood pressure (lying, standing) within 24 hours preoperatively, use intravenous furosemide if needed.
Gout		
Benemid, allopurinol	Inability to give orally	Observe, treat acute gout with intravenous colchicine.
Diabetes		
Oral hypoglycemics[b]	Inability to give orally	Switch to insulin preoperatively in selected patients.
Insulin[b]	Risk of hyperglycemia or hypoglycemia	Give one-third to one-half of usual dosage preoperatively.
Thyroid Therapy		
Thyroid hormone[b]	Inability to give orally	Usually can be discontinued for up to 7–10 days.
Antithyroid drugs[b]	Inability to give orally	Use parenteral iodides or propranolol if necessary.
Lipid Lowering		
Lovastatin, other hydroxymethylglutaryl-CoA reductase inhibitors	Rhabdomyolysis	? Discontinue preoperatively.
Gemfibrozil	Rhabdomyolysis	? Discontinue preoperatively.
Topical Drugs for Glaucoma		
Timolol	Systemic β blockage	Notify anesthesiologist preoperatively.
Phospholine iodide	Prolonged muscle relaxant activity	Discontinued 7–10 days preoperatively.
Recreational Drugs		
Alcohol	Affect drug metabolism, drug interactions, withdrawal syndrome, impaired respiratory function	If possible, have patient discontinue use 1 or more weeks before admission for surgery; inform anesthesiologist and surgeon of recent use.
Illicit drugs		
Tobacco[b]		

[a]If the patient will be able to take medication orally within 12 hr postoperatively, most maintenance drugs can be given at that time. If a shorter interval is crucial, a maintenance drug can be given with less than 1 oz of water, several hours before anesthesia (e.g., 6 AM), and the drug can be resumed orally after surgery.
[b]See additional details in subsequent section of this chapter.

Simple measures that can be planned before admission may help reduce the high incidence of *postoperative confusion* in older patients. These measures include planning to allow family members to stay beyond visiting hours, avoid placing the patient unnecessarily in an intensive care unit, return the patient to the same room postoperatively, allow the presence of familiar objects, leave a night light on, and avoid unnecessary instrumentation. Tranquilizers, sedatives, hypnotics, and pain medications should be used in reduced dosages and for appropriate indications, not routinely.

Postoperative mobilization of the elderly patient should be planned, and anticipated by the patient, preoperatively. In general, the patient should expect to resume ambulation as early as possible.

SURGERY IN THE PREGNANT PATIENT

Size of the Risk

Up to 2% of women require nonobstetric surgery during pregnancy. Risks posed to the mother and fetus include complications from the surgical problem, effects of anesthesia and medication (including teratogenicity), and precipitation of premature labor. Because of these problems, women of childbearing age who are not known to be pregnant should be screened for pregnancy before surgery. History, pelvic examination, and sensitive serum human chorionic gonadotropin

pregnancy tests usually suffice, but very early pregnancy may still be missed. If it is uncertain whether a woman is pregnant, nonurgent surgery should be postponed for 2 to 3 weeks until the situation is clarified; more urgent surgery requires judgment on an individual basis.

Physiologic alterations in pregnancy that may complicate anesthetic and surgical management are listed in Table 86.7. Two common changes of pregnancy should be taken into account when evaluating the patient preoperatively: The normal serum creatinine concentration is lower in pregnancy and an S_3 gallop, systolic murmur, or edema is commonly present in the pregnant patient without cardiac disease.

Fetal risks include teratogenicity of drugs and anesthetics, risk of diagnostic x-rays, premature labor, and fetal death. No definitive evidence exists that any one inhalational anesthetic is safer than another for the fetus.

Preoperative Planning

Preoperative planning for the pregnant surgical patient involves a number of complex issues. Considerations should include the following:

- *Urgency of the surgery.* Can it be postponed until after delivery or is it urgent (e.g., acute appendicitis), when delay will increase fetal–maternal mortality? In general, emergency surgery should not be delayed because of pregnancy, and totally elective surgery should be postponed until the postpartum period. In intermediate situations, the duration and risk to the mother of waiting must be balanced against the risk of immediate surgery.

- *Testing.* Tests should be carefully planned to allow a precise diagnosis with minimal risk, especially risk from x-ray exposure. Whenever possible, other tests should be substituted for radiologic procedures (e.g., gallbladder sonogram instead of oral cholecystogram in suspected cholelithiasis). Routine x-rays, such as chest films or flat abdominal films, should be avoided. When these x-rays are unavoidable, use of lead screening, collimated equipment with minimal exposure, and few films can minimize fetal exposure. Avoidance of x-ray exposure should be continued in the postoperative as well as the preoperative period.
- *Medications.* Drugs required during the perioperative period should be anticipated. The potential effects on the fetus should be ascertained from obstetric colleagues or available reference sources, and the least toxic alternative should be used. Routine drugs prescribed postoperatively should be avoided unless they are believed to be absolutely necessary.
- *Anesthesia.* A decision on the type of anesthesia must be left to the anesthesiologist and obstetrician. Local or regional anesthesia would presumably be safer than general or spinal anesthesia, but no data exist to support this impression.
- *Monitoring of fetal status* by the obstetrician should be planned throughout the perioperative period.

PROBLEMS AFTER DISCHARGE

Miscellaneous Problems

During the weeks and months after surgery, patients often have questions about incisional pain, various symptoms in the system that was operated on, and restrictions of activity. These questions are best answered by the surgeon. In addition, patients who have major surgery often complain of postoperative fatigue, a problem that can usually be handled by the patient's regular physician.

Postoperative Fatigue

Patients with postoperative fatigue may describe any of a number of symptoms: the need for increased sleep, weakness of the arms and legs when resuming usual activity, symptoms of orthostatic hypotension, and loss of interest in resuming usual activities (29). The physiologic changes responsible for these symptoms have not been well defined.

Although the symptoms of postoperative fatigue often last for 1 month or more, it is important that each symptom be evaluated carefully to identify drugs or underlying medical problems that may be contributing to the problem. Sleepiness may be related to sedatives, tranquilizers, or analgesics prescribed at the time of discharge and may improve with discontinuation of these drugs. The patient with orthostatic symptoms may have had a drug prescribed that can produce this problem (diuretics, antihypertensives, long-acting nitrates, antidepressants); because bed rest alone may cause orthostasis, these drugs should be resumed cautiously in a patient who has had recent major surgery and blood pressure should be checked in the lying,

Table 86.7.   Physiologic Alterations in Pregnancy and Their Relevance to the Surgical Patient

System	Change	Clinical Implications
Cardiovascular	Uterine compression of vena cava and aorta in supine position	Decreased cardiac output and uterine perfusion; avoid supine recumbency; tilt hip 15° in perioperative period.
	Decrease in blood pressure in early- to midgestation	Altered criteria for diagnosis of hypotension.
	Presence of dyspnea, third heart sound, and edema	No known increased risk, and such findings are not an indication for diuretic therapy or delay of surgery.
Respiratory	Decreased arterial P_{O_2} when patient is in the supine position	Avoid supine recumbency.
	Decreased pulmonary functional residual capacity and increased O_2 consumption	Increased risk of hypoxia perioperatively; avoid hypoventilation and increase inspired O_2 content before procedures inducing apnea (intubation or tracheal suctioning).
	Arterial P_{CO_2} and serum HCO_3 decrease to 30 mm Hg and 20 mmol/L, respectively	Maternal and fetal acidosis may occur in patient ventilated to "normal," nonpregnant values of arterial P_{CO_2}; normal values for pregnancy should be used to guide diagnosis and therapy of acid–base disturbances.
Hematologic	Decreased venous flow in legs and increased levels of clotting factors	Increased risk of thromboembolism; avoid supine position and consider use of support stockings or pneumatic compression device.
	Proximity of fetal and maternal circulations	Risk of isoimmunization; $Rh_0(D)$ immune globulin should be considered when uterine trauma is likely.
Gastrointestinal	Decreased gastric motility and reduced competency of gastroesophageal sphincter	Increased risk of aspiration; preoperative antacids should be considered.
Renal	Dilation of urinary collecting system	Increased risk of urinary infection, so catheterization should be avoided when possible.
	30 to 50% increase in glomerular filtration rate and renal plasma flow with a concomitant decrease in serum creatinine and urea nitrogen to 0.5 and 9 mg/dL, respectively	Serum creatinine above 0.8 mg/dL may reflect impaired renal function; the clearance of many drugs is increased, and dosage schedules may require alteration.

From Barron WM. The pregnant surgical patient: medical evaluation and management. Ann Intern Med 101:683, 1984.

Table 86.8. Summary of Perioperative Cardiovascular Risk in Patients with Ischemic Heart Disease

Patient Status (Preoperative)	% Mortality (Range) Total	% Mortality (Range) Cardiac	Postoperative Myocardial Infarction (%)
No "cardiac disease"[a]	3 (0.2–10)	?[b]	0.8 (0.1–2)
"Cardiac disease" present[a]	11 (5–20)	?	5 (2–8)
Angina (stable)	4 (4–12)	?	4 (?)
Past myocardial infarction			
All	5–15	5	7
Within 3 months	25–40 ⎫	?	35 ⎫
Between 3 and 6 months	5–20 ⎬ 15–25[c]	?	17 ⎬ 25[d]
More than 6 months	2.5 ⎭	?	5 ⎭
Unknown	?	?	10

From Kammerer WS, Gross RJ. Medical consultation: the internist on surgical, obstetric, and psychiatric services. 2nd ed. Baltimore: Williams & Wilkins, 1990.

[a]Cardiac disease data based mostly on patients with ischemic heart disease.

[b]?, data not available or uncertain.

[c]Recent figures show that postoperative mortality may be less.

[d]Recent studies indicate that current risk of reinfarction may be approximately 2–6%, using modern hemodynamic monitoring and anesthesia.

sitting, and standing positions. Dosage reduction or discontinuation of the drug should be considered where orthostatic hypotension is documented or orthostatic symptoms persist. Loss of interest may also be secondary to drugs prescribed after surgery (see list of drugs that may cause a depressed mood, Table 15.4). Alternatively, this symptom may represent a minor mood disturbance in a patient who has had similar problems at previous times of stress (see Chapter 12), or it may represent a reactive depression, similar to a grief reaction (see Chapter 15), that is related to disfiguring surgery. Because other medical problems related to surgery may occasionally cause postoperative fatigue, a hematocrit, serum urea nitrogen or creatinine, electrolytes, and liver enzymes should be checked if history suggests a problem that testing would identify or if fatigue is prolonged.

When evaluation of postoperative fatigue does not disclose contributing factors that can be treated, patients should be reassured that the problem will gradually resolve; they should also be given a rough timetable for a return to regular activities that is realistic in terms of both the surgical procedure and the fact that postoperative fatigue may take a number of months to resolve entirely. Simple exercises for patients convalescing from bed rest are illustrated in Figure 81.4. For selected patients, these or similar exercises can be recommended during the period of recovery from postoperative fatigue.

PATIENTS WITH CARDIOVASCULAR DISEASE

Overview

Most forms of general anesthesia can cause cardiovascular stresses (decreased myocardial contractility, peripheral vasodilatation, arrhythmias, hypotension), and spinal or epidural anesthesia can cause hypotension. These factors and the stresses associated with surgery itself probably account for the greatly increased risk of surgery for patients with underlying cardiovascular disease (10).

Ischemic Heart Disease

Size of the Risk

Ischemic heart disease poses two major risks perioperatively in the patient undergoing general anesthesia: myocardial infarction (MI) and death. These risks depend on the patient's preoperative status. Overall, the risks for patients with arteriosclerotic heart disease are two or three times those of patients of the same age without cardiac disease.

The increased risk posed by ischemic heart disease is dependent on *preoperative cardiac status* (Table 86.8). Stable mild to moderate angina pectoris alone represents only a small increase in risk. The risk attending severe or unstable angina cannot be estimated accu-

Table 86.9A. Cardiac Risk Index in Surgical Patients

Risk Factors	Points for Cardiac Risk Index (Table 86.9B)
History	
Myocardial infarction in past 6 months	10
Age >70	5
Physical	
S_3 gallop or jugular venous distension	11
Significant aortic stenosis	3
ECG	
Rhythm other than sinus or premature atrial contractions on last preoperative ECG	7
>5 premature ventricular contractions/minute any time preoperatively	7
Other Organ Systems	
Po_2 <60 mm Hg, Pco_2 >50 mm Hg	
K <3.0 mEq/dL, HCO_3 <20 mEq/dL	
BUN >50	
Creatinine conc. >3.0 mg/dL	3 (each factor)
Signs of chronic liver disease or elevated aminotransferase	
Bedridden from noncardiac causes	
Operation	
Intraperitoneal or intrathoracic	3
Emergency	4
Total Possible	53

Adapted from Goldman L, Caldera DL, Nussbaum SR, et al. Multifactorial index of cardiac risk in noncardiac surgical procedures. N Engl J Med 297:845, 1977.

Table 86.9B. Cardiac Risk Index (Based on a Prospective Study of Patients at the Massachusetts General Hospital)

Class	Point Total[a]	No or Moderate Complication (N = 943)[b] (%)	Life-Threatening Complication (N = 39)[c] (%)	Cardiac Deaths (N = 19)[d] (%)
I	0–5	99	0.7	0.2
II	6–12	93	5	2
III	13–25	86	11	2
IV	≥26	22	22	56

Adapted from Goldman L, Caldera DL, Nussbaum SR, et al. Multifactorial index of cardiac risk in noncardiac surgical procedures. N Engl J Med 297:845, 1977.

[a]See Table 86.9A.

[b]New or worsened heart failure without pulmonary edema, supraventricular tachyarrhythmia, or intraoperative or postoperative ischemia (as indicated by chest pain or ECG changes) without documented myocardial infarction.

[c]Documented intraoperative or postoperative myocardial infarction, pulmonary edema, or ventricular tachycardia without progression to cardiac death.

[d]Deaths from arrhythmia or to low-output heart failure.

rately because of varying definitions and the small number of patients reported in the medical literature, but there is a significantly increased risk. An MI during the 6 months preceding surgery represents a high risk, particularly an MI 3 months or less before surgery. There is some evidence (23,26) that aggressive perioperative management may significantly lower cardiovascular risk (e.g., reduce recurrent MI risk from 30 to 4%). Even 6 months after an infarction, the risk of a perioperative MI is considerably larger than the risk in a control population.

In addition to a recent MI, a number of factors contribute to the risk of perioperative cardiac complications or mortality. The most important of these factors are decompensated congestive heart failure (CHF), arrhythmias, and significant chronic obstructive lung disease. These and other factors were incorporated in 1977 into a *Cardiac Risk Index (Goldman Index)* (Table 86.9A and B), which has been validated (6,14,15). More recently, the *American College of Physicians (ACP) published its "Guidelines for Assessing and Managing Perioperative Risk from Coronary Artery Disease"* (see "General References"). This report was based on critical review of the literature from 1977 to 1996. The ACP recommendations, summarized in Figures 86.1 and 86.2, use point scores for cardiac and noncardiac risk factors, similar to those used in the Goldman index, for stratification of patients into *three groups with different risks of perioperative cardiac events: low risk* (below 3%), *intermediate risk* (3 to 15%), and *high risk* (above 15%). Practical guidelines for management are recommended for each risk category, as shown in Figures 86.1 and 86.2.

A joint *American College of Cardiology/American Heart Association (ACC/AHA) Task Force also recently issued guidelines for perioperative evaluation* (1). They contain less quantitative information for risk stratification than the ACP guidelines. They add the information in Table 86.10, which stratifies the *risk of cardiac death or MI according to type of noncardiac surgical procedure;* procedures are listed as high risk (above 5%), intermediate risk (below 5%), and low risk (below 1%).

Clinical assessment of the cardiac patient is approximately 75% sensitive for detecting high-risk patients. In intermediate- or high-risk *vascular surgery patients,* dipyridamole–thallium or other types of stress tests can accurately identify those with ischemia who have an increased operative risk (9); the usefulness of preoperative stress testing has not been demonstrated for risk assessment before other types of surgery (1). Detailed discussion of the use of noninvasive testing for preoperative decision making is contained in the ACP guidelines and other recent publications (1,10).

Preoperative Planning

Office Evaluation. Patients with established ischemic heart disease should have a comprehensive preoperative evaluation (Table 86.2). Noninvasive tests of cardiac function including echocardiography, nuclear scanning, and stress tests should generally be reserved for situations where the evidence for the presence or severity of cardiovascular disease is questioned or in certain high-risk situations such as vascular surgery (see above).

Based on the preoperative evaluation, the risk of general anesthesia and surgery should be estimated for each patient. For patients with recent MI (within less than 6 months), unstable angina, or less severe coronary artery disease and multiple other risk factors (Fig. 86.1), only urgent lifesaving surgery should be undertaken until the risk is lowered. Surgery may be done 3 months after infarction when the risk of waiting the additional 3 months is thought to be significant (e.g., recurrent cholecystitis). Patients with stable angina or uncomplicated recovery from MI more than 6 months previously have a small increase in risk that does not decline further with time; thus, there is no need to postpone necessary operations.

Coronary artery bypass surgery or angioplasty should be considered before elective noncardiac surgery, in consultation with a cardiologist, in patients who have other indications for coronary revascularization (see Chapter 57).

Recommendations to the Surgeon. A *baseline electrocardiogram* (ECG) should be obtained before surgery for all patients with known coronary artery disease and for all patients over approximately age 35 to 40. Routine postoperative ECGs should be obtained only in high-risk patients (e.g., all patients with known coronary artery disease and any adults who develop hypotension during surgery) because the yield of useful information from them is low.

For patients taking a long-acting oral nitrate for angina, the drug should be administered on the morning of surgery with a sip of water. If the patient is unable to take medications orally, nitroglycerin paste or a transdermal patch should be substituted; if there is no simple way to determine the paste dosage equivalent to the oral nitrate, an intermediate dose equivalent to 1 to 2 inches of Nitrol paste every 4 to 6 hours should be recommended.

For patients taking a β-blocking agent for angina, intravenous small dosages of propranolol (1 to 2 mg every 6 hours or a continuous infusion of 0.5 to 3 mg/hour [this is not an FDA-approved method of administration]) should be substituted, given by a physician, while the patient is unable to take medications by mouth. This should protect the patient from the risk of acute cardiac ischemia, which occasionally follows abrupt cessation of β-blocking agents. Patients able to resume oral intake within 12 to 24 hours usually can be observed without intravenous propranolol.

Perioperative β-blocker treatment. For patients who are not already taking a β-blocking agent and who have coronary artery disease, a β-blocker should be considered during the perioperative period. In a controlled trial, this regimen reduced significantly the 6-month morbidity and mortality of treated patients but not the immediate perioperative mortality (8). See details in the footnote to Figure 86.1.

Calcium blocking agents should usually be given on the morning of surgery. Another type of antianginal medication must be used postoperatively until the

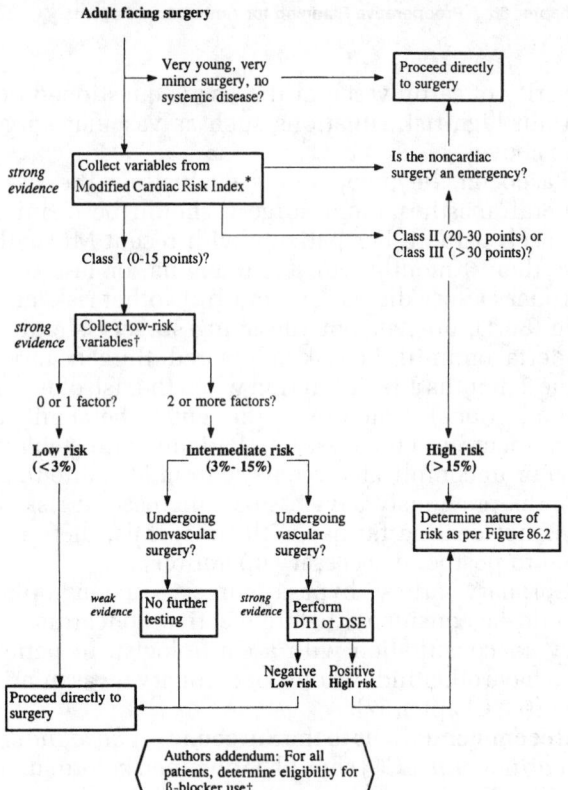

Figure 86.1. Suggested algorithm for the risk assessment and management of patients at *low or intermediate risk* **for perioperative cardiac events,** usually myocardial infarction and death. Boxed phrases indicate recommended actions. The italicized words beside the boxes indicate the level of evidence supporting the recommendation. If no italicized word is present, no evidence exists for or against use. *DTI,* Dipyridamole thallium imaging; *DSE,* dobutamine stress echocardiography. (From American College of Physicians. Guidelines for assessing and managing the perioperative risk from coronary artery disease associated with major noncardiac surgery. Ann Intern Med 127:309–312, 1997.)

*Modified Cardiac Risk Index§

Variable	Points, *n*
Coronary artery disease	
Myocardial infarction <6 months earlier	10
Myocardial infarction >6 months earlier	5
Canadian Cardiovascular Society angina classification	
Class III	10
Class IV	20
Alveolar pulmonary edema	
Within 1 week	10
Ever	5
Suspected critical aortic stenosis	20
Arrhythmias	
Rhythm other than sinus or sinus plus arterial premature beats on electrocardiogram	5
>5 premature ventricular contractions on electrocardiogram	5
Poor general medical status, defined as any of the following: Po_2 <60 mm Hg, Pco_2 >50 mm Hg, K^+ level <3 mmol/L, blood urea nitrogen level >50 mmol/L, creatinine level >260 μmol/L, bedridden	5
Age >70 years	5
Emergency surgery	10

§ Class I = 0 to 15 points; class II = 20 to 30 points; class III = more than 30 points.

‖ Canadian Cardiovascular Society classification of angina: 0 = asymptomatic; I = angina with strenuous exercise; II = angina with moderate exertion; III = angina with walking 1 to 2 level blocks or climbing 1 flight of stairs or less at a normal pace; IV = inability to perform any physical activity without development of angina.

† Low-Risk Variables

Criteria of Eagle et al. (9)	Criteria of Vanzetto et al. (33)
Age >70 years	Age >70 years
History of angina	History of angina
Diabetes mellitus	Diabetes mellitus
Q waves on electrocardiogram	Q waves on electrocardiogram
History of ventricular ectopy	History of myocardial infarction
	ST-segment ischemic abnormalities during resting electrocardiography
	Hypertension with severe left ventricular hypertrophy
	History of congestive heart failure

‡ Criteria used by to define eligibility for β-blocker use were coronary artery disease (defined as a previous myocardial infarction, typical angina, or atypical angina with positive results on a stress test) or risk for coronary artery disease (defined as the presence of at least two of the following: age ≥65 years, hypertension, current smoking, serum cholesterol level ≥240 mg/dL [6.2 mmol/L], and diabetes mellitus). Administration of the drug at each time point required that the heart rate be at least 55 beats/min and the systolic blood pressure be at least 100 mm Hg with no evidence of congestive heart failure, third-degree heart block, or bronchospasm. Patients received two 5-mg doses administered of intravenous atenolol, each over 5 minutes 30 minutes before surgery and again immediately after surgery. After surgery, patients were given oral atenolol, 100 mg (if heart rate was ≥65 beats/min) or 50 mg (if heart rate was 55 to 64 beats/min). If the patient was unable to take oral medication, two 5-mg doses were given intravenously every 12 hours. Atenolol was given until hospital discharge (maximum, 7 days).

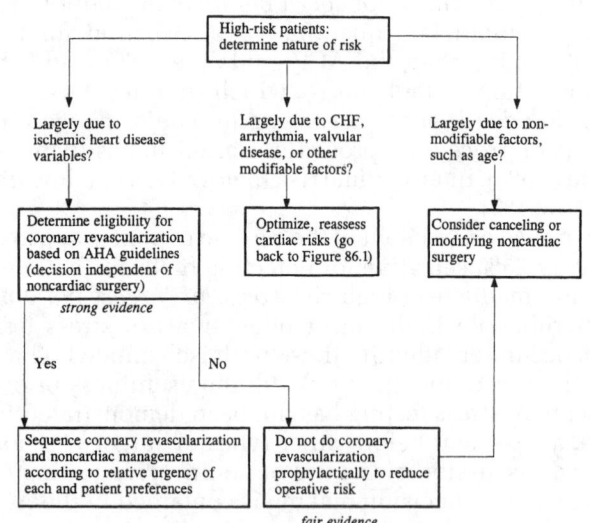

Figure 86.2. Suggested algorithm for the management of patients at *high risk* **for perioperative cardiac events.** Boxed phrases indicate recommended actions. The italicized words below the boxes indicate the level of evidence supporting the recommendation. If no italicized word is present, no evidence exists for or against use. *AHA,* American Heart Association; *CHF,* congestive heart failure. (From American College of Physicians. Guidelines for assessing and managing the perioperative risk from coronary artery disease associated with major noncardiac surgery. Ann Intern Med 127:309–312, 1997.)

Table 86.10. Cardiac Risk[a] Stratification for Noncardiac Surgical Procedures

High (Reported Cardiac Risk Often >5%)
Emergent major operations, particularly in the elderly
Aortic and other major vascular
Peripheral vascular
Anticipated prolonged surgical procedures associated with large fluid shifts or blood loss

Intermediate (Reported Cardiac Risk Generally <5%)
Carotid endarterectomy
Head and neck
Intraperitoneal and intrathoracic
Orthopedic
Prostate

Low[b] (Reported Cardiac Risk Generally <1%)
Endoscopic procedures
Superficial procedure
Cataract
Breast

From ACC/AHA Task Force. Guidelines for perioperative cardiovascular evaluation for noncardiac surgery. J Am Coll Cardiol 27:910–948, 1996; with permission.
[a]Combined incidence of cardiac death and nonfatal myocardial infarction.
[b]Do not generally require further preoperative cardiac testing.

patient can resume oral intake. Diltiazem and verapamil are available in intravenous form, but maintenance regimens are not established.

Intensive intraoperative monitoring using Swan–Ganz and radial artery catheters should be planned in consultation with the anesthesiologist for patients who are very sensitive to volume changes, such as those in CHF (see below), for operations when loss and replacement of large volumes of fluid are expected (e.g., aneurysm repair), and for patients with a recent MI (less than 6 months) or severe, unstable coronary disease.

Hypertension

Size of the Risk

Controversy still exists about whether mild to moderate hypertension (diastolic 110 mg Hg or lower) increases anesthetic and surgical risks. The only prospective study showed no correlation between uncontrolled diastolic pressures in this range and the risk of perioperative cardiac, renal, or cerebrovascular events (13). Patients in this study often had other cardiac risk factors that did correlate with the inci-

dence of perioperative cardiac morbidity (Tables 86.9 and 86.11).

Too few patients have been studied to define adequately the risk for patients operated on when their diastolic pressure exceeds 110 mm Hg, but there is probably an increased risk (17). Likewise, control of hypertension may be more important in selected patients with significant cardiac, renal, or cerebrovascular disease.

Preoperative Planning

Office Evaluation. The basic preoperative evaluation in the hypertensive patient should establish whether there is end-organ damage (renal: serum creatinine concentration and urinalysis; cerebrovascular: history, neurologic and neurovascular examination; and cardiovascular: history, cardiac examination, chest x-ray, and ECG). Blood pressure and pulse measurements should be made with the patient lying or sitting and standing (after brief exercise, to identify the maximal orthostatic fall in patients taking antihypertensive drugs); the preoperative status of blood pressure control may then be classified as untreated, hypertensive despite therapy, or controlled.

Patients who are controlled, or patients who are partially controlled and have diastolic pressures 110 mm Hg or lower, should be continued on their prescribed antihypertensive medication. Three exceptions to this rule are reserpine, guanethidine, and monoamine oxidase inhibitors. A patient taking either of these infrequently used drugs should be switched to a different drug during the 2 weeks preceding surgery because each of these drugs may cause markedly labile blood pressure during anesthesia.

Untreated patients with diastolic pressures 110 mm Hg or lower may undergo surgery, with institution of antihypertensive therapy after convalescence from surgery, if there are no other complicating cardiovascular risks.

Individual judgments must be made about patients with *diastolic pressures that are repeatedly above 110 mm Hg,* depending on the severity and duration of hypertension, the presence of end-organ damage, and the extent of planned surgery. Most patients with diastolic blood pressure above 110 mm Hg should have their blood pressure at least partly controlled before admission for nonurgent surgery, although there are no

Table 86.11. Risk of Perioperative Cardiac Complications in Patients with Mild to Moderate Hypertension

Preoperative Characteristics	Mean Point Total[a] (± SEM)	Patients with No Cardiac Complication (%)	Patients with Minor Complications Only[b] (%)	Patients with Major Nonfatal Complications[c] (%)	Patients with Cardiac Death[c] (%)
Normal blood pressure, no history of hypertension	4.3 ± 0.3	89	9	2	0.2
Hypertension controlled, taking antihypertensive drug(s)	6.9 ± 0.6	76	15	8	1
Hypertensive					
Taking antihypertensive drug(s)	4.4 ± 0.5	93	8	—	1
Not taking antihypertensive drug(s)	5.5 ± 0.6	88	9	1	1

Adapted from Goldman L, Caldera DL. Risks of general anesthesia and elective operation in the hypertensive patient. Anesthesiology 50:285, 1979.
[a]See Table 86.9A.
[b]New or worse heart failure, supraventricular tachycardia, or intraoperative or postoperative ischemia (typical chest plain or ECG changes).
[c]Fatal events or life-threatening events (pulmonary edema, myocardial infarction, ventricular tachycardia).

studies proving that such control modifies risks. Attempts to control blood pressure too rapidly (e.g., rapid increases in diuretic treatment over several days) may result in volume depletion, hypokalemia, or hypotension at the time of surgery. Therefore these patients should have their blood pressure stabilized during the 1 to 2 weeks before admission for surgery.

Recommendations to the Surgeon. For all hypertensive patients, the surgeon should be advised to avoid significant intravascular volume expansion or contraction because these conditions may either cause a significant rise in blood pressure (volume expansion) or fall in blood pressure (volume contraction, especially in the patient who is taking antihypertensive drugs).

Current antihypertensive medications should be continued through the morning of surgery (diuretics are usually withheld the morning of surgery) and resumed postoperatively when the patient is stable and can take oral medications. Because bed rest and inactivity during convalescence can lower blood pressure, some patients require less antihypertensive medication postoperatively and during the first few weeks after major surgery. Relatedly, because antihypertensive effects may be amplified when the postoperative patient's position changes from recumbent to sitting or standing, blood pressure should be measured in the latter positions after antihypertensive treatment has been instituted or resumed.

In some patients, the diastolic pressure exceeds 110 mm Hg postoperatively before oral medication can be resumed. For such patients, the surgeon should know that there are several regimens that reliably control the blood pressure when carefully administered and adjusted. The available intravenous antihypertensive medications include propranolol (1 to 2 mg intravenously every 4 to 6 hours or a continuous infusion of 0.5 to 3 mg/hour; this is not an FDA-approved method of administration) plus hydralazine (10 to 50 mg intravenously every 4 to 6 hours); transcutaneous clonidine (one or more patches, lasting up to 7 days), especially for patients who were taking clonidine before surgery and are at risk of rebound hypertension and tachycardia caused by clonidine withdrawal; enalapril (0.625 to 1.25 mg intravenously every 6 hours); labetalol (dosage recommendations for intravenous maintenance are not available); diuretics (furosemide 20 to 40 mg, or bumetanide 0.5 to 1 mg/day); methyldopa (250 to 500 mg every 6 hours); and nitroprusside (0.25 to 5 µg/kg per minute; start with nitroprusside 50 mg in 500 to 1000 mL of compatible intravenous fluids, not higher concentrations) or nitroglycerin (5 to 100 µg/minute).

Valvular Heart Disease

Size of the Risk

The risk of surgery in the patient with valvular heart disease varies with the valve affected (aortic versus mitral), the nature (stenosis versus insufficiency), and the severity of the lesion (10,15). The severity of valvular lesions as judged clinically by New York Heart Association (NYHA) classification (see Table 61.4A) provides a reasonable indication of surgical risk except in patients with aortic stenosis.

Valvular heart disease poses two major surgical risks: cardiac death and CHF. The presence of aortic stenosis of any degree of hemodynamic significance poses a high risk of surgical mortality. Mild to moderate mitral lesions or aortic insufficiency pose only slightly increased risk of cardiac death; however, hemodynamically severe valvular disease (NYHA class 3 or 4) caused by these lesions creates major risks. In addition to increasing the risk of perioperative mortality, significant valvular disease poses an increased risk of decompensated heart failure.

Little specific information exists regarding the risks associated with *prolapsed mitral valve* or *hypertrophic cardiomyopathy.* It is reasonable to assume that the risk in patients with prolapsed mitral valve depends on the

Table 86.12. Subacute Bacterial Endocarditis Prophylaxis: Recommendations for Procedures in the Respiratory, Gastrointestinal, and Genitourinary Tracts (See Recommended Antibiotic Regimens, Table 86.13)

Endocarditis Prophylaxis Recommended
Respiratory tract
  Tonsillectomy or adenoidectomy
  Surgical operations that involve respiratory mucosa
  Bronchoscopy with a rigid bronchoscope
Gastrointestinal tract[a]
  Sclerotherapy for esophageal varices
  Esophageal stricture dilation
  Endoscopic retrograde cholangiography with biliary obstruction
  Biliary tract surgery
  Surgical operations that involve intestinal mucosa
Genitourinary tract
  Prostate surgery
  Cytoscopy
  Urethral dilation

Endocarditis Prophylaxis Not Recommended
Respiratory tract
  Endotracheal intubation
  Bronchoscopy with a flexible bronchoscope, with or without biopsy[b]
  Tympanostomy tube insertion
Gastrointestinal tract
  Transesophageal echocardiography[b]
  Endoscopy with or without gastrointestinal biopsy[b]
Genitourinary tract
  Vaginal hysterectomy[b]
  Vaginal delivery[b]
  Cesarean section
  In uninfected tissue
    Urethral catheterization
    Uterine dilation and curettage
    Therapeutic abortion
    Sterilization procedures
    Insertion or removal of intrauterine devices
Other
  Cardiac catheterization, including balloon angioplasty
  Implanted cardiac pacemakers, implanted defibrillators, and coronary stents
  Incision or biopsy of surgically scrubbed skin
  Circumcision

Reprinted with permission from Dajani AS, Taubert KA, Wilson W, et al. Prevention of bacterial endocarditis: recommendations by the American Heart Association. JAMA 277:1794–1801, 1977.

[a]Prophylaxis is recommended for high-risk patients; optional for medium-risk patients.

[b]Prophylaxis is optional for high-risk patients.

Table 86.13. Prevention of Bacterial Endocarditis in Patients with Valvular Heart Disease, Prosthetic Heart Valves, and Other Abnormalities of the Cardiovascular System

Situation	Agent	Regimen[a]
Dental, Oral, Respiratory Tract, or Esophgeal Procedures		
Standard general prophylaxis	Amoxicillin	Adults: 2.0 g; children: 50 mg/kg orally 1 hr before procedure
Unable to take oral medications	Ampicillin	Adults: 2.0 g IM or IV; children: 50 mg/kg IM or IV within 30 min before procedure
Allergic to penicillin	Clindamycin *or*	Adults: 600 mg; children: 20 mg/kg orally 1 hr before procedure
	Cephalexin or cefadroxil[b] *or*	Adults: 2.0 g; children: 50 mg/kg orally 1 hr before procedure
	Azithromycin or clarithromycin	Adults: 500 mg; children: 15 mg/kg orally 1 hr before procedure
Allergic to penicillin and unable to take oral medications	Clindamycin *or*	Adults: 600 mg; children: 20 mg/kg IV within 30 min before procedure
	Cefazolin[b]	Adults: 1.0 g; children: 25 mg/kg IM or IV within 30 min before procedure
Genitourinary, Gastrointestinal (Excluding Esophageal) Procedures		
High-risk patients[c]	Ampicillin plus Gentamicin[d]	Adults: ampicillin 2.0 g IM or IV plus gentamicin 1.5 mg/kg (not to exceed 120 mg) within 30 min of starting the procedure; 6 hr later, ampicillin 1 g IM/IV or amoxicillin 1 g orally
		Children: ampicillin 50 mg/kg IM or IV (not to exceed 2.0 g) plus gentamicin 1.5 mg/kg within 30 min of starting the procedure; 6 hr later, ampicillin 25 mg/kg IM/IV or amoxicillin 25 mg/kg orally
High-risk patients allergic to ampicillin/amoxicillin[c]	Vancomycin plus Gentamicin[d]	Adults: vancomycin 1.0 g IV over 1–2 hr plus gentamicin 1.5 mg/kg IV/IM (not to exceed 120 mg); complete injection/infusion within 30 min of starting the procedure
		Children: vancomycin 20 mg/kg IV over 1–2 hr plus gentamicin 1.5 mg/kg IV/IM; complete injection/infusion within 30 min of starting the procedure
Moderate-risk patients[c]	Amoxicillin or ampicillin	Adults: amoxicillin 2.0 g orally 1 hr before procedure, or ampicillin 2.0 g IM/IV within 30 min of starting the procedure
		Children: amoxicillin 50 mg/kg orally 1 hr before procedure, or ampicillin 50 mg/kg IM/IV within 30 min of starting the procedure
Moderate-risk patients allergic to ampicillin/amoxicillin[c]	Vancomycin[c]	Adults: vancomycin 1.0 g IV over 1–2 hr; complete infusion within 30 min of starting the procedure
		Children: vancomycin 20 mg/kg IV over 1–2 hr; complete infusion within 30 min of starting the procedure

Reprinted with permission from Dajani AS, Taubert KA, Wilson W, et al. Prevention of bacterial endocarditis: recommendations by the American Heart Association. JAMA 277:1794–1801, 1997.

[a]Total children's dosage should not exceed adult dosage.

[b]Cephalosporins should not be used in individuals with immediate-type hypersensitivity reaction (urticaria, angioedema, or anaphylaxis) to penicillins.

[c]*High risk:* prothestic heart valve, history of endocarditis, complex cyanotic congenital heart disease. *Moderat risk:* Uncorrected congenital conditions (patent ductus, ventricular septal defect, coarctation, bicuspid aortic valve; rheumatic valve disease; hypertrophic cardiomyopathy; prolapsing or leaking mitral valve (i.e., audible click and murmurs or Doppler-confirmed mitral insufficiency).

[d]No second dose of vancomycin or gentamicin is recommended.

degree of mitral regurgitation. Patients with hypertrophic cardiomyopathy may be very sensitive to volume contraction and are probably best managed with a Swan–Ganz catheter in place during major procedures associated with rapid volume changes.

Endocarditis risk. Patients with artificial heart valves, patients with any evidence of valvular heart disease (including mitral prolapse and hypertrophic cardiomyopathy), and patients with congenital structural defects (e.g., patent ductus arteriosus, ventricular septal defect) have a small but definite risk of acquiring bacterial endocarditis when they undergo procedures in the oral cavity and upper respiratory, gastrointestinal, or genitourinary tracts (5).

Preoperative Planning

Office Evaluation. The basic cardiac evaluation should delineate the nature and severity of the valvular disease and should identify any associated cardiac conditions. The uses of echocardiography and cardiac catheterization to evaluate valvular heart disease are described in Chapter 60. Patients with severe valvular disease should have corrective cardiac surgery followed by a period of convalescence before they undergo major elective noncardiac operations.

Recommendations to the Surgeon. The preoperative management of CHF, arrhythmia, or anticoagulant therapy (in patients with artificial valves) is described in subsequent sections of this chapter.

Endocarditis prophylaxis. Patients undergoing procedures attended by a risk of endocarditis should receive antimicrobial prophylaxis as summarized in Tables 86.12 (recommendations regarding procedures in the respiratory, gastrointestinal, and genitourinary tracts) and 86.13. The information in these tables was updated in the 1997 recommendations of the American Heart Association on the basis of an exhaustive review of the literature between 1936 and 1996. The information in Table 86.13 is available from the AHA in a wallet-size card for patients. The authors emphasize that these recommendations are not based on randomized controlled trials and that they should not be substituted for clinical judgment in some situations (5). For the most common indication, dental procedures, there are several changes: antibiotics are recommended only preprocedure, erythromycin is no longer recommended as a substitute for amoxicillin, and antibiotic prophylaxis is not recommended for procedures not associated with bleeding.

Congestive Heart Failure

Size of the Risk

Information on the risk of developing CHF perioperatively is limited because of the few studies available. However, the best prospective studies (15) closely correspond to general clinical experience. The most significant risk factors for postoperative CHF are decompensated failure preoperatively and, to a lesser extent, prior CHF that is clinically stable preoperatively (Table 86.14). However, only 40% of patients who develop perioperative CHF have had prior failure. The best predictors for the other 60% of patients are age greater than 60, major surgery (especially abdominal aortic aneurysm repair or major abdominal surgery), and nonspecific ECG abnormalities.

Patients with postoperative pulmonary edema have a high total mortality (20 to 57%), most of which is cardiac. Patients who develop less severe postoperative CHF do not have an increased risk of postoperative cardiac death, although the overall mortality from all causes is increased. Most postoperative CHF occurs during or within several hours of surgery.

Preoperative Planning

Office Evaluation. Patients with compensated CHF should have a comprehensive preoperative evaluation (Table 86.2). This evaluation should include an assessment of volume status (lying and standing blood pressures, inspection of neck veins, determination of whether edema is present) and examination for cardiac gallops and rales. Laboratory data should include BUN, creatinine, electrolytes, and a digoxin level if that drug is being administered. Noninvasive methods for assessing left ventricular function (see Chapter 61) may be useful when the degree of cardiac dysfunction is uncertain.

Although there are no definitive perioperative studies in this regard, it is prudent to administer digitalis to patients with a confirmed history of moderate or severe dilated congestive cardiomyopathy, ideally during the week before admission. Most controversy about preoperative digitalization has concerned the patient who has a history of no or minimal CHF yet has a risk of developing CHF because of an enlarged heart or because the surgery will involve major volume shifts; most experts do not recommend digitalis in this situation (1).

Patients with decompensated CHF should have all but lifesaving surgery postponed until the failure is controlled, either in the office or in the hospital.

Recommendations to the Surgeon. Patients with controlled CHF should be maintained on their usual oral regimen until midnight before surgery and maintained with intravenous diuretics and digoxin (75% of the oral dosage) during the immediate postoperative period. Perioperative monitoring with a Swan–Ganz catheter should be considered in advance in situations

Table 86.14. Risks of Developing CHF in the Perioperative Period

Patient Characteristics	All CHF (%)	Pulmonary Edema (%)
No prior CHF	4	2
Past CHF:		
All—now compensated	16	6
Past pulmonary edema (regardless of current status)	32	23
Decompensated CHF preoperatively	21	16
Preoperative physical findings:		
S$_3$ gallop	47	35
Jugular venous distension	35	30
NYHA class preoperatively (see Table 61.3)		
Class 1	5	3
Class 2	7	7
Class 3	18	6
Class 4	31	25

Adapted from Goldman L, Caldera DL, Southwick FS, et al. Cardiac risk factors and complications in non-cardiac surgery. Medicine (Baltimore) 57:357, 1978.

Table based on 1001 consecutive patients undergoing general surgery, orthopedic surgery, or urologic surgery (transurethral resection of the prostate omitted because of existing evidence of its safety even in elderly patients).

where large volume shifts are anticipated during surgery, or the heart failure is severe or decompensated.

Arrhythmias

The arrhythmias that are most common in ambulatory patients are described in detail in Chapter 59.

Size of the Risk

Patients with arrhythmias before surgery have significantly increased risks of cardiac morbidity and death. These risks have not been quantified for subgroups of patients with specific arrhythmias, except as indicated in the cardiac risk indices shown in Table 86.9 and Figure 86.1. Patients with complete heart block, Mobitz type II second degree block, and a few patients with sick sinus syndrome (see Chapter 59) have a significant risk of complications during anesthesia if a pacemaker is not inserted. On the other hand, there is little or no increased risk associated with bifascicular or trifascicular block on ECG in patients who are asymptomatic.

Arrhythmias do occur in approximately 20% or more of adult patients during general anesthesia; however, most of these patients do not have preoperative arrhythmias. Most intraoperative arrhythmias are supraventricular, transient, and related to specific anesthetic or surgical manipulation, and do not require specific therapies. The number of arrhythmias that are detected clinically, without the use of continuous monitoring, is lower: supraventricular arrhythmias are detected clinically in 4% of patients and other arrhythmias in 11% (12,15).

Preoperative Planning

Office Evaluation. Patients with arrhythmias should have the comprehensive preoperative evaluation (Table 86.2) expanded in several ways. The probable cause of the arrhythmia should be delineated (see

Chapter 59). If the arrhythmia is intermittent or control is uncertain, 24-hour Holter monitoring should be done. Levels of antiarrhythmic drugs that are being administered should be obtained. This evaluation should be accomplished before admission for surgery.

Patients with *supraventricular arrhythmias* should have their ventricular rates controlled or should be converted to more stable rhythms. Except for atrial fibrillation, this usually means conversion either to normal sinus rhythm or atrial fibrillation because other supraventricular arrhythmias are hemodynamically unstable or give an unpredictable ventricular response even with appropriate drug therapy. Patients with atrial fibrillation should have their rates slowed but should be able to accelerate their heart rate under stress as indicated by their ability to raise their pulse rate more than 10 points by mild exercise.

Established indications for *preoperative digitalis administration* in patients with arrhythmias are control of rate in atrial fibrillation and prophylaxis of supraventricular arrhythmias in selected patients (e.g., patients with past histories of supraventricular arrhythmias, especially atrial fibrillation or flutter, who remain at high risk for recurrence; and patients with significant mitral stenosis).

Patients with *ventricular premature beats* (VPB) or other ventricular arrhythmias should be treated according to the criteria outlined in Chapter 59.

Recommendations to the Surgeon. Antiarrhythmic drugs should be continued orally through the morning before surgery, after which the following intravenous treatment should be substituted until the patient can take oral medications again: intravenous digoxin (75% of the oral dosage) for patients taking digoxin, and intravenous lidocaine or procainamide for patients taking quinidine, procainamide, or disopyramide for ventricular arrhythmias.

There is general agreement that patients undergoing general anesthesia should have a *prophylactic or therapeutic pacemaker* inserted for the following conditions:

- Symptomatic or significant dysfunction of the sinoatrial node
- Idioventricular rhythm
- Current or past history of third-degree or Mobitz type II second-degree atrioventricular (AV) block
- Occasional instances of Mobitz type I (Wenckebach) second-degree AV block
- Occasional patients with trifascicular block (right bundle branch block plus left anterior hemiblock plus first-degree AV block; alternating left and right bundle branch block; or left bundle branch block and first-degree AV block) especially in the presence of severe valvular disease, ischemic disease, or CHF
- A history of Stokes–Adams attacks

Patients with a history suggesting symptomatic bradyarrhythmias (especially a history of syncope or near syncope and an underlying ECG abnormality) probably should have a temporary pacemaker recommended if a full workup to evaluate the cause of the symptoms cannot be performed preoperatively. Isolated conditions for which a pacemaker is more controversial, but generally not indicated, include bifascicular block, bundle branch block, first-degree AV block, and asymptomatic sinus bradycardia.

PATIENTS WITH PULMONARY DISEASE

Overview

Patients with significant pulmonary disease have an increased mortality and morbidity during surgery. The increased risks are caused chiefly by the following physiologic changes produced by the effects of anesthesia, sedatives, and analgesics: abnormalities of pulmonary gas exchange, causing hypoxemia; depression of the cough reflex and decrease in clearance of respiratory tract secretions; respiratory depression; and loss of sighing and normal lung inflation. Each of these changes increases the risk of atelectasis and pneumonia. In addition, normal breathing and voluntary coughing are decreased after surgery because of pain and discomfort, especially after upper abdominal and thoracic surgery. Optimal preoperative treatment of pulmonary disease can reduce perioperative morbidity and mortality.

Chronic Obstructive Pulmonary Disease

Size of the Risk

The precise risk of perioperative death from pulmonary causes for patients with chronic obstructive pulmonary disease (COPD) is not known because of the lack of information regarding patients with mild lung disease. In patients with moderate to severe COPD, pulmonary deaths occur in approximately 4% (versus 0 to 2% of unselected patients) and pulmonary complications in 36% (versus 9% of unselected patients) (21,23).

The *presence of a smoking history, dyspnea, cough, or abnormal spirometry* increases the risk of minor postoperative pulmonary complications (i.e., atelectasis or infection without significant respiratory compromise). The risk of respiratory failure requiring vigorous postoperative respiratory therapy is increased in patients with a forced expiratory volume in 1 second (FEV_1) less than 1.5 L. An FEV_1 less than 1.0 L or a Pco_2 greater than 45 mm Hg predicts a substantial increase in perioperative pulmonary mortality and in the incidence of postoperative respiratory failure requiring prolonged mechanical ventilation. However, no study has definitively shown that any pulmonary function test, including FEV_1 or arterial blood gases, predicts major pulmonary complications (respiratory failure, need for mechanical ventilation, or death) with enough precision to establish a prohibitive criteria for surgery. The decision for surgery in the presence of pulmonary disease requires consideration of all clinical and laboratory data.

A number of *nonpulmonary factors* are helpful in predicting postoperative pulmonary complications in patients with COPD (Table 86.15). The greatest risks are in patients who are older than 60, who undergo upper

Table 86.15. Nonpulmonary Factors that Increase Pulmonary Risks During General Surgery

Most Important	Other
Age over 60	General anesthesia lasting more than 3 hours
Upper abdominal or thoracic operation	Obesity
Repeat operations within 1 year	Abnormal ECG
	Poor patient effort/cooperation
	Narcotic analgesics
	Upper respiratory infection

abdominal and thoracic operations or operations under general anesthesia lasting more than 3 hours, or who have repeated operations within 1 year. A much lower risk is posed by operations on the extremities, back, breast, and central nervous system. Lower abdominal surgery represents an intermediate risk. Combining these factors with the pulmonary factors listed above increases the physician's ability to predict operative morbidity.

The *type of anesthesia* may affect the risk of pulmonary complications. Local anesthesia creates very little risk; if the patient is also sedated ("conscious sedation"), however, there may be temporary deterioration in respiratory control and there may be a suppression of the cough reflex. Spinal anesthesia has been reported to be associated with a low mortality rate in patients with COPD (31) in some studies. However, because of the simultaneous use of sedatives and because the patient must ventilate in the supine position, spinal anesthesia creates a significant risk of intraoperative and postoperative respiratory complications; this is especially true of obese patients with chronic pulmonary disease. Because of these problems, general anesthesia, which permits control of ventilation and clearance of secretions, is often preferable to spinal anesthesia in patients with moderate or severe COPD.

Preoperative Planning

Office Evaluation. Patients with known COPD should have a comprehensive preoperative evaluation (Table 86.2) and additional evaluation focused on the status of their pulmonary disease (32). If they are taking aminophylline, they should have measurement of the serum aminophylline concentration and adjustment of the dosage if it is above or below the therapeutic range. Any history of smoking, chronic or intermittent sputum production, recent upper respiratory infection, dyspnea on effort, or concomitant cardiovascular disease is particularly pertinent. Ideally, smokers should stop smoking 8 weeks before admission for surgery to be performed under general or spinal anesthesia, and patients with upper respiratory infections should have surgery postponed at least 2 weeks, regardless of how minor the episode.

Table 86.16 summarizes for patients undergoing general or spinal anesthesia the principal *indications for preadmission spirometry alone* (forced vital capacity [FVC] and FEV_1) or for spirometry plus lung volumes and arterial blood gases. Unfortunately, major operations are often performed without pulmonary function testing, despite the fact that even experienced

clinicians sometimes misjudge the severity of obstructive lung disease. Spirometry clarifies the presence and severity of lung disease in questionable cases.

Pulmonary consultation should be obtained for patients whose FEV_1 is less than 1.0 L, those whose P_{CO_2} is above 45 mm Hg, and those with less severe pulmonary disease who are being evaluated for thoracic or upper abdominal surgery.

Recommendations to the Surgeon. Preoperatively, the patient should be instructed on coughing and deep breathing exercises, as well as on the use of devices such as an incentive spirometer that will be used postoperatively. Patients already taking bronchodilators should continue their regimen through the morning of surgery; patients who have a history of intermittent airway obstruction should be started on an inhaled bronchodilator or theophylline compound before surgery. To prevent bronchospasm, especially in the immediate postoperative period, inhaled β_2-sympathomimetics and intravenous aminophylline should be administered, and the serum aminophylline level should be kept in the therapeutic range (10 to 20 mg/L) while the patient cannot take oral medications. Patients who have received corticosteroids for more than 2 weeks during the year before surgery should be appropriately covered for stress with parenteral steroids (see below). Patients with chronic purulent sputum production should receive a 5- to 7-day course of broad-spectrum antibiotics (tetracycline, amoxicillin, trimethoprim–sulfamethoxazole, azithromycin, or clarithromycin) to decrease the quantity and purulence of secretions. Finally, arterial blood gases should be checked in all patients with moderate to severe COPD before and, as needed, after surgery. There is some dispute about the efficacy of most of these individual measures. However, controlled trials show that the combination, preoperatively, of bronchodilators, antibiotics, lung expansion, and mobilization of secretions decreases the number of perioperative complications (31).

Lung Resection and COPD

Overall mortality rates for lung resection are about 5% for lobectomy and approximately 15% for total pneumonectomy. The mortality and morbidity rates

Table 86.16. Indications for Pulmonary Function Test in Preoperative Patients with Pulmonary Disease

Spirometry Only (FEV_1 and FVC)
Smokers (>10 pack years)
Any pulmonary symptoms (e.g., dyspnea, wheezing, cough, or sputum production)
Upper abdominal surgery
Age >60
Repeat surgery within 1 year
Multiple other risk factors (obesity, recent upper respiratory infections, narcotics abuse, abnormal ECG)

Spirometry, Lung Volumes, and Arterial Blood Gases
Thoracic surgery
Upper abdominal surgery and pulmonary disease
Patients with restrictive lung disease
Patients with chronic obstructive pulmonary disease with FEV_1 <1.0 L

for lung surgery vary widely depending on patient factors (particularly age and pulmonary function), type of operation (pneumonectomy, lobectomy, segmental resection), and experience and skill of the surgical team.

Assessment of pulmonary function in the patient with COPD who has an indication for lung resection (usually a tumor) should be performed in the ambulatory setting. Use of the following criteria to select candidates for lung resection has reduced mortality for patients with COPD:

- *For pneumonectomy,* the major criteria for operability are FEV_1 2 L or more and FVC 50% of predicted or more. Patients with an FEV_1 below 2 L should have quantitative perfusion lung scanning to determine the FEV_1 that can be expected after pneumonectomy (e.g., if 30% of perfusion and ventilation goes to the affected lung, the patient's pulmonary function will be decreased by approximately 30% postoperatively). Those with a predicted postoperative FEV_1 as low as 0.8 to 1 L can undergo pneumonectomy, although their mortality risk is probably increased.
- Patients not meeting the criteria for pneumonectomy may tolerate lobectomy or segmental resection. Most patients with a preoperative FEV_1 1.5 L or more can tolerate a lobectomy. The patient may undergo resection of the segment or lobe if the predicted postoperative FEV_1 is greater than 0.8 to 1 L.

Other measures in preoperative planning for the patient with COPD undergoing pulmonary resection are similar to those described for such patients in the preceding section.

Asthma

Size of the Risk

Asthma affects approximately 3% of Americans, which makes it one of the most common pulmonary diseases (see Chapter 55). It is difficult to give a firm estimate of the operative risks posed by asthma because in most reports data on asthma are pooled with results for other types of obstructive airway disease. The most dangerous period for the asthmatic is not usually the period during general anesthesia because the anesthetic may be an effective bronchodilator, but the immediate postoperative period. The major risks are severe bronchospasm and inspissation of thick secretions.

Preoperative Planning

Office Evaluation. The asthmatic patient should have a comprehensive evaluation (Table 86.2) in the office before admission for surgery. Spirometry should be obtained at that time. This allows adequate time for changes in chronic management before admission. The patient should stop smoking 8 weeks before surgery.

Recommendations to the Surgeon. Spirometry (FEV_1 and FVC) should be performed in all asthmatic patients before the operation. Arterial blood gases should be measured in patients who are not in their stable baseline state or who have significant abnormalities in FEV_1. β_2-Sympathomimetics can be continued, as inhaled aerosols, until the induction of anesthesia and can be resumed in the recovery room. The serum concentration of aminophylline should be measured preoperatively because many patients who take aminophylline have subtherapeutic or toxic levels on standard dosages. Planning for the immediate preoperative period should include administration of oral bronchodilators on the morning of surgery and scheduling of surgery early in the day. In very severe asthmatic patients who are taking aminophylline, a constant infusion of aminophylline may be recommended for the preoperative period and for the period when the patient cannot take medicine by mouth; other patients are adequately treated by resuming aminophylline, intravenously, in the recovery room. Patients taking maintenance corticosteroids by aerosol or who have taken systemic corticosteroids for more than 2 weeks during the previous year should receive dosages of parenteral steroids sufficient to cover the stress of surgery (see below) (25).

PATIENTS WITH RENAL DISEASE

Size of the Risk

The size of the operative risk for patients with chronic renal disease depends on the severity of their disease (see Chapter 48). Overall, the surgical mortality after major surgery in patients with severe renal disease (i.e., creatinine clearance less than 10 to 15 mL/minute, including patients on dialysis) is approximately 2 to 4% when these cases are managed carefully. In patients not requiring dialysis, postoperative acute renal failure is the gravest complication (4).

The major complications associated with surgery in the patient with moderate to severe renal disease are electrolyte disturbances (especially acidosis and hyperkalemia), volume contraction, volume overload, toxicity caused by agents that are nephrotoxic or are excreted by the kidneys, and bleeding. Volume contraction, with the risk of ischemic cerebral, cardiac, or renal damage, is a particular risk in patients with the nephrotic syndrome; these patients usually have a slightly contracted intravascular volume at baseline and are at risk of hypovolemia if an effort is made to decrease their edema with potent diuretics preoperatively. Toxic renal damage may follow the use of two agents that are often used in the perioperative period: radiocontrast agents and aminoglycoside antibiotics.

Preoperative Planning

Office Evaluation

Before admission for surgery, patients with chronic renal failure should have the comprehensive evaluation outlined in Table 86.2, and current volume status should be documented. Radiocontrast studies should be avoided, if at all possible, in the preoperative workup of patients with significantly elevated serum creatinine concentrations or with other risk factors because the subsequent risk of acute renal failure is increased (4).

Recommendations to the Surgeon

The most important consideration in perioperative management of patients who do not require dialysis is avoidance of fluid imbalance. When the surgery carries a risk of significant volume shifts, Swan–Ganz catheterization should be considered to ensure close monitoring of the intravascular volume. Administration of drugs such as antihypertensives should follow the guidelines stated elsewhere in this chapter. Adjustments in the dosages of drugs should be appropriate for the patient's degree of renal insufficiency as outlined in Chapter 48 (3). The concentration of electrolytes and creatinine in the serum should be monitored carefully before and after surgery to detect, particularly, hyperkalemia and deterioration of renal function. Patients with renal failure often have a metabolic acidosis compensated by hyperventilation; postoperatively continued appropriate hyperventilation is necessary to avoid a potential precipitous fall in arterial pH. Preoperative prophylactic dialysis is not generally recommended in the patient not already on chronic dialysis. Furthermore, patients with chronic anemia secondary to renal failure usually are well compensated and do not require preoperative transfusion unless they are symptomatic from the anemia or a large blood loss is expected during surgery.

In general, the nephrologist caring for patients on chronic dialysis should coordinate the medical management of these patients throughout the surgical episode. Although these patients have a very high postoperative complication rate (caused by hyperkalemia, bleeding, arteriovenous fistula thrombosis, pneumonia, wound infection, and arrhythmias), their risk of dying from surgery remains in the 2 to 4% range if complications are carefully managed (4).

PATIENTS WITH ENDOCRINE DISEASE
Diabetes Mellitus

Size of the Risk

Total surgical mortality for all diabetic patients is approximately 2 to 4%; less than 0.3% die as a result of poor control of their diabetes. Approximately 14% of diabetic patients have postoperative complications that may be related to diabetes, particularly wound infection.

Preoperative Planning

Office Evaluation. Each diabetic patient should have the comprehensive preoperative evaluation outlined in Table 86.2. Most diabetic patients can undergo outpatient surgery if their diabetes is stable, whether controlled by diet alone, oral agents, or insulin. Patients with insulin-dependent diabetes and some diabetic patients on oral agents should have the ability for home glucose monitoring for outpatient surgery, be responsible, and be compliant with their monitoring and insulin regimens. Relative contraindications to outpatient surgery include significantly uncontrolled diabetes, the occasionally extremely labile diabetic, and noncompliant diabetic patients requiring insulin.

Recommendations to the Surgeons. Measurement of fasting blood glucose electrolytes, BUN, and creatinine should be obtained at the time of the preoperative office evaluation. If the patient is monitoring home glucose measurements these should be reviewed, as well as any recent glycohemoglobin A-1-C measurements. The patient should be told to call if his or her home glucose measurements are higher or lower than predetermined values between the time of the office medical evaluation and surgery. The patient or nurse should do a bedside glucose determination on arrival at the hospital. The state of hydration should be determined to ensure that the diabetic is not significantly volume contracted. Elective surgery should not be undertaken until diabetes is at least reasonably controlled (fasting blood glucose at 250 mg/l00 mL or less).

The appropriate perioperative treatment of diabetes depends on the type of surgical procedure planned and the preadmission regimen, as summarized in Table 86.17.

Diabetic patients who are controlled by diet can be monitored with daily fasting blood glucose levels throughout the operative episode and treated with insulin if unacceptable rises in glucose occur.

Treatment of patients taking oral agents varies because they represent a heterogeneous group. Patients with mild elevations of glucose who are undergoing minor procedures that will allow them to eat the same day can take their hypoglycemic drug on the day *before* surgery and resume it when they begin eating on the day of surgery. An exception is the patient taking *chlorpropamide* (Diabinese), which should be with-

Table 86.17.   Management of Diabetes on Day of Surgery

Surgical Procedure	Treatment Required to Control Glucose Preoperatively		
	Diet Only	Oral Hypoglycemic Agent	Insulin
Minor	Observe	Withhold until after procedure	Withhold until after procedure or use "major" protocol
Major	Observe	Change to long-acting insulin (achieve control with insulin before operation)	*Preferred regimen:* One-half to two-thirds of total long-acting insulin dosage preoperatively; regular insulin only if needed
			or
			One-third of total long-acting insulin dosage preoperatively; one-third postoperatively; regular insulin only if needed
			or
			Continuous low-dose infusion of regular insulin
			or
			Regular insulin in each liter of dextrose 5% in water (D_5W)

held 2 to 3 days before surgery because of its long half-life. Although experience is limited, *metformin* should be withheld at least 48 hours before surgery and not restarted until the patient is stable and eating, except for minor procedures. Metformin should also be withheld for 48 hours before any radiocontrast x-ray that is part of the preoperative evaluation. It is especially important to withhold metformin in major procedures with the risk of hypotension or renal failure (e.g., vascular surgery) because of the risk of lactic acidosis. If the patient is to undergo a major procedure, oral agents should be discontinued because they have long half-lives, control is less predictable, and the drugs cannot be given parenterally. Therefore, such a patient should be switched to management by diet only or to insulin. Human insulin is preferred for the patient who has not taken insulin previously.

For the patient who is taking insulin before surgery, one of several strategies is recommended for the preoperative period (Table 86.17). Because of its simplicity and the small risk of hypoglycemia, the first regimen (giving one-half to two-thirds of the usual total daily dosage of long-acting insulin preoperatively) is preferred. Postoperative management is easiest with a single morning dose of long-acting insulin, with the dosage adjusted according to the metabolic status and calorie intake; supplemental regular insulin may be given as needed. Blood glucose measurement using a bedside technique is recommended; fasting glucose and electrolyte concentrations should be measured daily in the immediate postoperative period.

Adrenal Insufficiency and Chronic Steroid Therapy

Size of the Risk

It is generally agreed that patients who are currently taking a pharmacologic dosage of corticosteroids (more than the equivalent of 20 to 30 mg of hydrocortisone daily), have taken corticosteroids at a pharmacologic dosage for 2 or more weeks in the past year, or are receiving replacement dosages for adrenal insufficiency are at risk of developing adrenal insufficiency because of the stress of surgery.

Patients in each of these groups should therefore receive extra corticosteroids in the perioperative period (see Chapter 74 for additional details).

Preoperative Planning

Office Evaluation. These patients should have a comprehensive evaluation before admission (Table 86.2). For patients with adrenal insufficiency, the evaluation should include particular attention to factors that may reflect the adequacy of corticosteroid replacement (i.e., lying and standing blood pressure, concentration of serum urea nitrogen or serum creatinine, glucose, and electrolytes). Adrenocorticotropic hormone (ACTH) stimulation or insulin-hypoglycemia testing to determine the need for steroid coverage in patients who are no longer receiving steroids but who have received large dosages of steroids in the past is not recommended for routine use

because there is not adequate evidence that a normal response precludes the need for steroid coverage during surgery.

Recommendations to the Surgeon. The patient may receive the usual steroid dosage by mouth the day before surgery. On the day of surgery, hydrocortisone 100 mg should be administered intravenously at 6 AM; a second 100-mg dose should be given intravenously during surgery; then a 100-mg dose should be given intravenously every 6 hours for the first 24 hours after surgery, followed by 50 mg every 6 hours for the second 24 hours after surgery and 25 mg every 6 hours for the third 24-hour period. The patient may then return to the preoperative medical regimen.

There are two exceptions to these guidelines. First, the regimen is based on the assumption that there is no prolonged stress after surgery; if this occurs, higher dosages of corticosteroids must be continued for a longer time postoperatively. Second, for minor procedures patients may return to their usual dosage within 24 to 48 hours postoperatively. For outpatient surgery, equivalent dosages of oral prednisone may be given as an outpatient for the postoperative care (preoperative dosage should still be given intravenously).

Hypothyroidism

Size of the Risk

The major potential complications of surgery in hypothyroid patients are increased sensitivity to and prolonged half-life of anesthetic agents, hypoventilation and respiratory arrest in the immediate postoperative period, hyponatremia caused by decreased free water clearance, and myxedema coma. The risks of surgery in patients with mild to moderate hypothyroidism may be less than previously thought (22).

Preoperative Planning

Office Evaluation. Hypothyroid patients should be evaluated carefully before admission for surgery. The patient should have the comprehensive evaluation outlined in Table 86.2 and the serum thyroid-stimulating hormone (TSH) concentration should be checked (unless a value from the past 2 months is available) (see Chapter 73 for details).

Recommendations to the Surgeon. Specific recommendations for preoperative management depend on the *status of the patient's hypothyroidism.* Patients with previously known and adequately treated hypothyroidism can undergo surgery. The half-life of administered T_4 is about 7 days. Therefore, oral T_4 can usually be omitted on the day of surgery and resumed when the patient is able to take oral medication. The stress of major surgery or severe infection may accelerate the turnover of T_4, occasionally necessitating daily treatment with intravenous T_4 (50% of the oral dosage) in patients in either of these situations.

If the hypothyroidism has been effectively treated for a long period (as indicated by no or only minor symptoms or a normal or only a slightly increased

TSH), the patient can usually tolerate surgery and thyroid replacement can be adjusted postoperatively. For hypothyroid patients who have not been treated or who remain significantly hypothyroid because of inadequate replacement therapy, elective surgery should be postponed because of the risks listed above. Such patients should receive adequate thyroid replacement for a minimum of 1 to 2 months before elective surgery (4 to 6 months for patients with profound myxedema). Surgery required before this period in mild to moderately hypothyroid patients may be considered, especially if minor surgery under local anesthesia is being performed, if the patient can be started on a total replacement dosage immediately, and if there is prompt improvement in signs and symptoms of hypothyroidism (see Chapter 73 for additional details).

When a patient with previously undiagnosed hypothyroidism requires immediate major surgery, an endocrinologist should be consulted regarding perioperative treatment and monitoring.

Hyperthyroidism

Size of the Risk

The major risk of operation in patients with uncontrolled hyperthyroidism is *thyroid storm* (see Chapter 73). In one series, there were only 25 episodes of thyroid storm after 1383 operations on thyrotoxic patients (24). However, surgery accounts for up to one-third of the cases of thyroid storm reported.

Preoperative Planning

Office Evaluation. The patient with known hyperthyroidism should be reassessed clinically and with thyroid function tests before admission for surgery. In previously undiagnosed patients, the usual approach should be used in evaluation and management (see Chapter 73).

Recommendations to the Surgeon. The treatment of the hyperthyroid patient during surgery depends on the patient's current thyroid status. Patients previously diagnosed and adequately treated should take their current treatment until midnight the night before surgery and should resume treatment when they can take substances by mouth again. Patients with new, known, or recurrent hyperthyroidism who are not euthyroid should be brought to a euthyroid state with thyroid blocking agents or iodides (see Chapter 73). Ideally, surgery should be postponed for several months in these patients until a consistent euthyroid state is attained.

An endocrinologist should be consulted regarding the treatment and monitoring of any patient with uncontrolled hyperthyroidism who requires urgent surgery.

Obese Patients

Size of the Risk

Massive obesity significantly increases the mortality risk associated with surgery. In one study, for example, women undergoing surgery for adenocarcinoma of the uterus had a 20% operative mortality if they weighed more than 300 lb (136 kg), compared with a 1.5% mortality for obese women weighing between 200 and 240 lb (91 and 110 kg) (30). Less severe obesity probably does not increase mortality risks.

Moderate or massive obesity also increases the risk of a number of perioperative problems, including difficult intubation, difficulty in ventilating the patient during anesthesia, the need for a large amount of anesthesia during induction, potential delay in anesthesia washout because of slow release of anesthetic agents from adipose tissue, postoperative atelectasis and pneumonia, thromboembolism, difficult postoperative mobilization, nosocomial wound infection (particularly when there is increased moisture caused by pannus adjacent to the surgical incision), wound dehiscence, and late incisional hernia.

Preoperative Planning

Office Evaluation. For massively obese patients, a program of gradual weight reduction (see Chapter 76) should be planned, if practical, before any elective operation; this may require up to 6 months. When prompt surgery is needed, these patients should have a comprehensive evaluation (Table 86.2). In particular, these patients should be checked for uncontrolled diabetes mellitus and significant hypoventilation, two common complications of obesity that increase the risk of surgery. Either of these two problems should be managed preoperatively, as discussed above.

Recommendations to the Surgeon. Massively obese patients should be given preoperative instruction in deep breathing and in the use of the incentive spirometer or other devices designed to prevent pulmonary complications postoperatively. Other recommendations for perioperative management depend on obesity-associated conditions, such as diabetes, that the patient may have.

PATIENTS WITH GASTROINTESTINAL OR HEPATIC DISEASE
Peptic Ulcer Disease

Size of the Risk

Data are lacking on the risk and the management of surgery in patients with active peptic ulcer disease.

Preoperative Planning

Office Evaluation. Patients with active ulcer disease should have elective nonulcer surgery postponed until the ulcer heals. The average time required for the healing of uncomplicated ulcers is 4 to 6 weeks for duodenal ulcer and 6 weeks for gastric ulcer (see Chapter 37). There is no consistent relationship between disappearance of ulcer symptoms, ulcer healing, and recurrence. Therefore it is best to wait several weeks after all symptoms have disappeared and 6 weeks to 3 months from the beginning of an episode before admission for elective nonulcer surgery. If surgery cannot be deferred this long or if ulcer recurrence is suspected, endoscopy should be considered preoperatively. Before surgery, these patients should also have the comprehensive medical evaluation summarized in Table 86.2, and multiple stool samples should be checked to exclude active bleeding.

There are no empiric data to confirm these guidelines or to indicate whether surgery can be done safely as soon as an ulcer has healed (as shown by endoscopy). If urgent abdominal surgery must be performed in a patient with active ulcer disease, consideration should be given to whether surgical treatment is needed for the ulcer as well (see detailed discussion of indications for and types of surgery, Chapter 37).

Recommendations to the Surgeon. Patients with remote or inactive ulcer disease require no special therapy preoperatively or postoperatively.

Patients with recently active ulcer disease should continue their current therapy until midnight the day before surgery. Because H₂ blockers (cimetidine, ranitidine, famotidine) can be given intravenously, one of these should be used throughout the period when the patient cannot take medications by mouth; nasogastric suctioning may also be recommended during this period.

Hepatitis

Size of the Risk

General anesthesia and surgery during acute hepatitis are associated with a high mortality and morbidity (17). The major problem accounting for these risks is postoperative hepatic encephalopathy and its complications. The catabolic effects of surgery, hypotension during anesthesia, and hepatic toxicity from anesthetic agents are the principal factors that may precipitate hepatic encephalopathy.

Preoperative Planning

Office Evaluation. Patients with a history of acute hepatitis should have a comprehensive evaluation (Table 86.2), and liver function tests (serum aminotransferases, bilirubin, alkaline phosphatase, albumin, and prothrombin time) should be obtained before admission for surgery. Serologic tests for hepatitis B antigen and hepatitis C antibody should also be performed (see Chapter 43).

Ideally, surgery should be postponed for a minimum of 6 to 12 months after all laboratory evidence of active liver disease has returned to normal. This cautious approach is advised because there is a risk of exacerbating hepatic injury if surgery is performed earlier. Only urgent, life-saving surgery should be performed during the acute phase of hepatitis, whatever its cause.

Recommendations to the Surgeon. Anticipation of postoperative complications (particularly bleeding and encephalopathy) is important in the patient with active hepatitis who must undergo surgery. For the patient with an abnormal prothrombin time (less than 50% of normal), fresh frozen plasma should be given throughout the immediate perioperative period. When immunologic tests or epidemiologic information indicates infectious hepatitis (see Chapter 43), the surgical team should be notified in order to minimize the risk of spreading infection.

Cirrhosis

Size of the Risk

Most quantitative data regarding the risks of surgery in the cirrhotic patient have been collected in trials of portal–systemic shunts; therefore, these data may not accurately reflect the risks of surgery unrelated to the liver. The most widely used measure of the mortality risk from shunt procedures is Child's index, which incorporates measurements of serum bilirubin, albumin, ascites, encephalopathy, and nutrition (Table 86.18). The perioperative complications encountered in these patients are those associated with chronic cirrhosis: encephalopathy, jaundice, gastrointestinal hemorrhage, infection, and hepatorenal syndrome.

Regional and spinal anesthesia do not entirely eliminate the risks of complications in cirrhotic patients. For example, increased morbidity and mortality caused by liver disease have been associated even with hernia repair under local anesthesia in some patients. The stress of the procedure itself, decreased hepatic blood flow, and complications such as hypotension and wound infection may worsen hepatic function, even in the absence of toxic general anesthetics.

Preoperative Planning

Office Evaluation. In addition to a comprehensive preoperative evaluation (Table 86.2), patients with cirrhosis should have liver function tests (serum transaminase, bilirubin, alkaline phosphatase, albumin, and prothrombin time). Liver biopsy is indicated in selected patients to establish the presence of cirrhosis, provide an additional indicator of the severity of liver damage, or exclude active hepatitis. Liver computerized tomography (CT) scan or sonogram is only occasionally needed to exclude other causes of hepatomegaly. In the history and physical examination, a careful search should be made for complications of cirrhosis, especially encephalopathy, bleeding, varices, and ascites.

The expected benefits of surgery must be weighed carefully against the risks in patients with cirrhosis. In general, risks are higher and only essential surgery should be performed. There are stable patients with mild cirrhosis, however, who have no ongoing injury (e.g., due to removal of a toxin or discontinuation of alcohol) and in whom standards may be liberalized.

Table 86.18. Child's Classification of Operative Mortality Risk in the Cirrhotic Patient

	Risk Group by Severity of Liver Disease		
	A (Minimal)	B (Moderate)	C (Advanced)
Bilirubin (mg/100 mL)	<2.0	2.0–3.0	>3.0
Serum albumin (g/100 mL)	>3.5	3.0–3.5	<3.0
Ascites	None	Controlled	Poorly controlled
Encephalopathy	None	Minimal	Coma
Nutrition	Excellent	Good	Poor ("wasted")
Operative mortality (%)	0	9	53

From Siefkin AD, Bolt RJ. Preoperative evaluation of the patient with gastrointestinal or liver disease. Med Clin North Am 63:1309, 1979.

Recommendations to the Surgeon. A number of precautions should be emphasized in the cirrhotic patient who does require surgery. Local (or, as a second choice, spinal) anesthesia may be safer than general anesthesia, although data are lacking. Therapy to prevent complications of liver disease, such as postoperative bleeding (fresh frozen plasma for the patient with an abnormal prothrombin time or partial thromboplastin time) and encephalopathy (see Chapter 43), should be established and maintained throughout the operative period, and the patient should be repeatedly checked for evidence of these two problems. The occasional patient who is taking chronic corticosteroid therapy for liver disease should have the steroid dosage increased during the perioperative period as described above.

PATIENTS WITH IATROGENIC IMPAIRMENT OF HEMOSTASIS

All anticoagulants and platelet inhibitors increase the risk of intraoperative and postoperative bleeding and should be discontinued before any type of surgery. Patients receiving drugs in these classes should have a comprehensive preoperative evaluation (Table 86.2) before admission for surgery, and an appropriate plan for perioperative management of anticoagulation should be communicated to the surgeon.

Coumarin Derivatives

On the basis of critical assessment of risks and benefits, less aggressive recommendations for the perioperative management of patients on oral anticoagulants have recently been revised (20).

Coumarin derivatives should be stopped 4 to 7 days before surgery according to a schedule determined by the patient's usual international normalized ratio (INR) and the INR desired during the perioperative period. In patients maintained at a higher INR, coumarin should be discontinued earlier. The INR should be measured the day before surgery. If the INR remains elevated, 1 mg of vitamin K_1 should be administered subcutaneously. Within 12 hours, this dose will usually normalize the INR of a patient who has been off coumarin for 4 to 7 days. The larger doses of oral vitamin K_1 previously recommended (e.g., 10 mg) are believed not to be necessary and to possibly cause a hypercoagulable state (20).

The authors of the recent review recommend preoperative use of intravenous heparin, as an inpatient or outpatient, while the INR is subtherapeutic only in patients at very high risk of thromboembolism, such as recent venous thromboembolism or arterial embolism (within 1 month). Postoperatively, intravenous heparin is also recommended in these high-risk patients and in patients who have had venous thromboembolism within the 3 months preceding surgery. An alternative to intravenous heparin preoperatively is subcutaneous low-molecular-weight heparin in therapeutic or prophylactic doses depending on the underlying diagnosis, although this is not yet an FDA-approved use for this drug. Intravenous heparin should be stopped about 6 hours before surgery. An INR and, if the patient is on heparin, partial thromboplastin time should be checked before surgery and be acceptable (20).

These recent recommendations for use of preoperative and postoperative heparin are much more limited than previous recommendations. Other authors recommend preoperative or postoperative intravenous heparin for other high-risk patients such as those with artificial mitral valves and multiple risks (e.g., artificial mitral valve, atrial fibrillation, and history of embolization).

Preoperative placement of a vena caval filter is an option in patients with recent venous thromboembolism or patients for whom the risk of bleeding on intravenous heparin is high (20).

Warfarin (Coumadin) ordinarily can be resumed 24 to 72 hours after surgery, at the preoperative dosage *if* all surgical bleeding is controlled; the INR usually reaches 2.0 after 3 days. Patients who have undergone intracranial, spinal, or ophthalmologic operations probably should not be anticoagulated for 48 hours to several weeks after surgery. For patients with a high risk of thromboembolism (see above), continuous-infusion heparin can be reinstituted 12 to 24 hours postoperatively without a bolus, if the surgeon is confident that hemostasis is ensured, and continued until full anticoagulation with warfarin has been reestablished (20).

Aspirin and Ticlopidine

Aspirin prolongs the bleeding time and may increase blood loss during and after operation in some patients. Generally, if aspirin is not being used as a critical therapy, it should be discontinued 1 week before surgery because aspirin continues to affect platelets for this period of time. Discontinuation of aspirin is particularly important before procedures for which hemostasis is critical, such as neurosurgical operations, or some ophthalmologic surgery.

Because *some NSAIDs other than aspirin* may impair platelet function in vitro, it is prudent to advise patients to discontinue NSAID use 1 week before surgery, especially surgery for which increased bleeding would be especially harmful (Table 86.4).

Ticlopidine (Ticlid), a platelet aggregation inhibitor, should be discontinued at least 2 weeks before surgery to ensure that the bleeding time is not prolonged in the perioperative period.

PATIENTS WITH A CHRONIC INFECTION

Two types of chronic bacterial infection pose risks to the patient and to others in the operating room and therefore require appropriate management before surgery: staphylococcal skin infections and pulmonary tuberculosis.

Skin Infections

Chronic bacterial skin infections (usually caused by staphylococci) pose a high risk for wound sepsis and may be the source of infections in other patients (18). Therefore they should be suppressed or eradicated before admission of the patient for an elective operation. Chapter 25 describes strategies for accomplishing this.

Tuberculosis

Active pulmonary tuberculosis poses a problem for the surgical patient because of the general debilitation it causes. It also creates the risk of infection for others in the operating room. Therefore adult patients with a history of unexplained chronic cough or a history of tuberculosis should be evaluated for active tuberculosis before admission for surgery. Patients with active pulmonary tuberculosis should be stable and have negative sputum cultures before admission for elective surgery. The ambulatory treatment of tuberculosis is described in Chapter 29.

Patients with HIV Infection

Acquired immunodeficiency syndrome (AIDS) poses many problems in preoperative evaluation that are beyond the scope of this book but are addressed elsewhere (see "General References," Chapter 34). Several important issues are summarized here.

The risk of transmission to health care workers is very small, but it does exist. Universal precautions are recommended in the care of all patients, not just known HIV-positive patients (see Table 34.17). Screening of all surgical patients for HIV infection is not currently recommended by expert consensus, but this issue continues to be controversial.

HIV-infected patients pose challenges in addition to the usual preoperative evaluation. Decision making is complicated by the wide spectrum of morbidity in HIV infection, ranging from the lack of symptoms in the recently infected patient to the debilitation in the preterminal patient. Decision making should balance the status and prognosis of the patient's HIV infection (asymptomatic, symptomatic), mean life expectancy, the patient's wishes, the increased risk for the specific operation posed by the HIV infection, and the indications for and expected benefit of the surgery during the patient's expected length of survival.

PATIENTS WITH NEUROPSYCHIATRIC DISEASE

Neuropsychiatric problems present ill-defined risks during surgery and the postsurgical period. The major concerns are worsening of mental status caused by both metabolic changes and psychologic stresses. The patient with psychiatric disease may decompensate postoperatively, making care difficult and jeopardizing wound healing.

Cerebrovascular Disease

Size of the Risk

Patients with recent strokes have a significant risk of worsening focal deficits during carotid artery surgery, but this risk cannot necessarily be extrapolated to other types of surgery. Patients with recent strokes (less than 6 weeks preoperatively) also have a risk of deterioration in their general mental status, regardless of the status of their focal deficits, if they undergo major surgery; however, firm data are lacking on the size of this risk.

Preoperative Planning

Patients with recent strokes should have a comprehensive preoperative evaluation (Table 86.2) emphasizing documentation of the preoperative neurologic impairment. The data regarding the course of the patient's stroke should be reviewed, and additional testing (see Chapter 83) should be performed if necessary to exclude a treatable cause.

No specific perioperative therapy for the patient with a stable completed stroke is needed. In general, it is prudent to delay elective, noncarotid surgery for at least 6 weeks after a completed stroke, although no firm data are available to support this practice.

Asymptomatic Cervical Bruit

Size of the Risk

Cervical bruits are present in approximately 4% of people over the age of 45. These bruits may be caused by a number of processes (see Chapter 83), including common or internal carotid stenosis. In the patient with an asymptomatic cervical bruit, there is slight or no increased risk of cerebrovascular accident during surgery (28).

Preoperative Planning

Apart from a careful history and physical examination to exclude evidence of a prior stroke or transient ischemic attack (TIA) related to the cervical bruit, no special approach is needed for these patients. Duplex carotid ultrasound can help establish whether the cervical bruit is caused by carotid stenosis and the degree of stenosis; its value has not been established for estimating risk of postoperative stroke. Hypotension and excessive neck manipulation should be avoided during surgery in patients known to have carotid bruits. The patient with a history of symptoms possibly related to the bruit should be evaluated as described in Chapter 83.

Data summarized in Chapter 83 show that patients with high-grade asymptomatic and symptomatic carotid stenosis have a lower long-term stroke rate if carotid endarterectomy is performed. When patients such as these require elective surgery for another condition, a decision must be made on which of two surgeries to do first.

Parkinson's Disease

Size of the Risk

The perioperative risks in patients with Parkinson's disease are caused by musculoskeletal rigidity, which may impair voluntary postoperative ventilation, mobilization, and swallowing. These patients are also subject to postoperative delirium. The rigidity of patients taking antiparkinson medication may worsen after the patient has missed one or more doses (see Chapter 82). Despite this potential problem, most patients with Parkinson's disease tolerate anesthesia and temporary omission of medications.

Preoperative Planning

The patient should have a comprehensive preoperative evaluation (Table 86.2), and the antiparkinsonian regimen should be tailored to provide the best possible relief of symptoms (see Chapter 82). For patients taking an anticholinergic agent, the drug may be continued until midnight before surgery and resumed when the patient is able to take oral medications. L-dopa or Sinemet (L-dopa/carbidopa) should be continued until induction of anesthesia, and the drug should be resumed as soon as possible after surgery. Postoperative physical therapy to maintain range of motion may help these patients until they are able to take oral medication. Parkinsonian patients should be observed for postoperative delirium and aspiration.

Dementia and Organic Brain Syndrome

Size of the Risk

Patients with dementia have an increased risk of mortality and morbidity during surgery. The increase in mortality is caused largely by lack of cooperation (e.g., with postoperative respiratory care). Much of the morbidity is related to the development of delirium caused by anesthesia, perioperative medications, and surgical stress. Because surgery is always a difficult process for a demented patient and because the degree of increased risk is ill defined, the potential benefits of surgery should be carefully reviewed before a final decision to operate is made.

Preoperative Planning

The patient should have a comprehensive evaluation (Table 86.2) before admission for surgery. The patient should be checked for metabolic abnormalities that may worsen cerebral function before admission, just before surgery, and throughout the postoperative period. Emphasis should be placed on detecting and correcting hypovolemia, electrolyte abnormalities, and hypoxia. Before major surgery it is advisable to document the patient's mental status formally (see "Mini-Mental Status Examination," Chapter 17) so that mental states after surgery can be compared with baseline status.

When demented patients undergo major procedures, constant observation is recommended for the first 24 to 48 hours after surgery.

Other Psychiatric Problems

Size of the Risk

The major problems associated with general surgery in psychiatric patients are lack of cooperation with postoperative care, postoperative psychosis, and interactions between psychotropic medications and anesthetic agents. The degree of cooperation that can be expected postoperatively can generally but not always be predicted on the basis of the patient's past behavior and preoperative mental status. Obtaining informed consent is also an issue.

Preoperative Planning

Office Evaluation. A careful history of the patient's past psychiatric illness should be obtained. The patient's mental status should be documented preoperatively (see Chapter 10) so that it can be compared with postoperative changes. A psychiatric consultation should be obtained in all patients with psychosis or other severe psychiatric problems. Additional issues that must be dealt with by the patient's personal physician and surgeon are the ability of the patient to give informed consent (see Chapter 10) and the effect of the patient's psychiatric state on the surgical evaluation (e.g., evaluating symptoms in a patient with one of the somatoform disorders, described in Chapter 12, or evaluating the need for cosmetic surgery).

Careful explanation of the operation is especially crucial to management of patients with psychiatric disorders or with anticipated stress reactions to surgery. The procedure should be explained in language the patient can understand. After the explanation, the patient should be asked to express any concerns about the planned surgery, and the patient's comprehension of the planned surgery should be assessed and documented. The need to ventilate about anxiety associated with disfiguring surgery (e.g., mastectomy, amputation) and with the fear of not waking up is particularly common in both anxiety-prone patients and those who are usually free of anxiety.

Patients with severe psychosis should be in a stable, manageable state before admission for elective surgery; this should be accomplished through close collaboration between the patient's primary physician, the surgeon, and a psychiatrist.

Patients with mild to moderate anxiety or depression can be managed by supportive counseling, use of support by family members, selective use of antidepressants or minor tranquilizers, and careful explanation of the procedure to the patient. These interventions should be initiated before hospital admission, not at the last minute before surgery.

Recommendations to the Surgeon. The principal recommendation for the perioperative period is that the patient's use of psychotropic drugs should be communicated to the anesthesiologist.

Neuroleptics and tricyclic antidepressants can interact with anesthetics to cause increased sedation, hypotension or hypertension, and arrhythmias. Small to moderate dosages of phenothiazines, haloperidol, and tricyclic antidepressants should be continued until about 12 hours before surgery. In the occasional patient taking a very high dosage of these agents, it is recommended that the drug be stopped about 24 hours before surgery, except in patients who have severely decompensated in the past when their medication has been changed.

The dosage of benzodiazepines does not need to be changed unless it is very high.

Lithium carbonate can prolong the action of muscle relaxants and cause myocardial depression and hypernatremia. Lithium should be discontinued 24 hours preoperatively; however, the anesthesiologist should be aware that it has been administered recently. A blood lithium level and electrolyte measurements should be obtained before surgery as a guideline. Additional information about lithium is in Chapter 15.

Monoamine oxidase inhibitor antidepressants can enhance the effect of sympathomimetic agents and sympathetic responses to anesthesia, and can decrease the rate of elimination of certain anesthetic agents. Because of these problems, monoamine oxidase inhibitors should be discontinued at least 2 weeks before surgery, and the anesthesiologist must be informed of their recent administration.

General References*

American College of Physicians. **Guidelines for assessing and managing the perioperative risk from coronary artery disease associated with major noncardiac surgery.** Ann Intern Med 127:309–312, 1997.
   Evidence-based clinical guidelines based on review of all literature from 1977 to 1996. Accompanying paper contains details and more than 200 references.

Caputo GM, Gross RG. Medical consultation on surgical services: an annotated bibliography. Ann Intern Med 118:290, 1993.

Gross RJ, Kammerer WS. Medical consultation on surgical services: an annotated bibliography. Ann Intern Med 95:523, 1981.
   Complementary annotated bibliographies.

Gross RJ, Caputo GC, eds. Medical consultation: the internist on surgical, obstetric, and psychiatric services. 3rd ed. Baltimore: Williams & Wilkins, 1998.
   A comprehensive multicontributor book, extensively referenced.

Specific References

1.   ACC/AHA Task Force. Guidelines for perioperative cardiovascular evaluation for noncardiac surgery. J Am Coll Cardiol 27:910–948, 1996.

2.   Babbott S, Gross RJ. Evaluation of the healthy patient and the ambulatory surgery patient. In: Gross RJ, Caputo GC, eds. Medical consultation: the internist on surgical, obstetric, and psychiatric services. 3rd ed. Baltimore: Williams & Wilkins, 1998;25–53.

3.   Bennett WM, Aronoff GR, Golper TA, et al. Drug prescribing in renal failure. Philadelphia: American College of Physicians, 1994.

4.   Briefel G, Turer P. Renal disease. In: Gross RJ, Caputo GC, eds. Medical consultation: the internist on surgical, obstetric, and psychiatric services. 3rd ed. Baltimore: Williams & Wilkins, 1998;207–295.

5.   Dajani AS, Taubert KA, Wilson W, et al. Prevention of bacterial endocarditis recommendations by the American Heart Association. JAMA 277:1794–1801, 1997.

6.   Detsky AS, Abrams HB, McLaughlin JR, et al. Predicting cardiac complications in patients undergoing non-cardiac surgery. J Gen Intern Med 1:211, 1986.

7.   Djokovic JL, Hedley-White J. Prediction of outcome of surgery and anesthesia in patients over 80. JAMA 242:2301, 1979.

8.   Eagle KA, Froehlich JB. Reducing cardiovascular risk in patients undergoing noncardiac surgery. N Engl J Med 335:1761–1762, 1996.

9.   Eagle KA, Coley CM, Newell JB, et al. Combining clinical and thallium data optimizes preoperative assessment of cardiac risk before major vascular surgery. Ann Intern Med 110:859–866, 1989.

10.   Falcone RA, Ziegelstein RC. Cardiovascular disease and hypertension. In: Gross RJ, Caputo GC, eds. Medical consultation: the internist on surgical, obstetric, and psychiatric services. 3rd ed. Baltimore: Williams & Wilkins, 1998;149–205.

11.   Gold BS, Kitz DS, Lecky JH, Neuhaus JM. Unanticipated admission to the hospital following ambulatory surgery. JAMA 262:3008, 1989.

12.   Goldman L. Supraventricular tachyarrhythmias in hospitalized adults after surgery. Chest 73:450, 1978.

13.   Goldman L, Caldera DL. Risks of general anesthesia and elective operation in the hypertensive patient. Anesthesiology 50:285, 1979.

14.   Goldman L, Caldera DL, Nussbaum SR, et al. Multifactorial index of cardiac risk in noncardiac surgical procedures. N Engl J Med 297:845, 1977.

15.   Goldman L, Caldera DL, Southwick FS, et al. Cardiac risk factors and complications in non-cardiac surgery. Medicine (Baltimore) 57:357, 1978.

16.   Gross RJ. Special topics. In: Gross RJ Caputo GC, eds. Medical consultation: the internist on surgical, obstetric, and psychiatric services. 3rd ed. Baltimore: Williams & Wilkins, 1997 (in press).

17.   Harville DD, Summerskill WHJ. Surgery in acute hepatitis. JAMA 184:257, 1963.

18.   Hiral D. Nasal *Staphylococcus aureus* and postoperative infection. Am Surg 46:310, 1980.

19.   Hosking MP, Warner MA, Lobdell CM, et al. Outcomes of surgery in patients 90 years of age and older. JAMA 261:1909, 1989.

20.   Kearon C, Hirsh J. Management of anticoagulation before and after elective surgery. N Engl J Med 336:1506–1511, 1997.

21.   Kroenke K, Lawrence VA, Theroux JF, Tuley MR. Operative risk in patients with severe obstructive pulmonary disease. Arch Intern Med 152:967, 1992.

22.   Ladenson PW, Levin AA, Ridgway EC, et al. Complications of surgery in hypothyroid patients. Am J Med 77:261, 1984.

23.   Lawrence VA, Page CP, Harris GD. Preoperative spirometry before abdominal operations: a critical appraisal of its predictive value. Arch Intern Med 149:280, 1989.

24.   McArthur JW, Rawson RW, Means JH, Cope O. Thyrotoxic crisis: an analysis of the thirty-six cases seen at the Massachusetts General Hospital during the past twenty-five years. JAMA 134:868, 1947.

25.   Oh SH, Patterson R. Surgery in corticosteroid-dependent asthmatics. J Allergy Clin Immunol 53:345, 1974.

26.   Rao Tadikonda LK, Jacobs K, El-Etr A. Reinfarction following anesthesia in patients with myocardial infarction. Anesthesiology 59:499, 1983.

27.   Roizen MF. Preoperative evaluation. In: Miller RD, ed. Anesthesia. 4th ed. New York: Churchill-Livingstone, 1994;1:827–882.

28.   Ropper AH, Wechsler LR, Wilson LS. Carotid bruit and the risk of stroke in elective surgery. N Engl J Med 307:1388, 1982.

29.   Rose EA, King TC. Understanding postoperative fatigue. Surg Gynecol Obstet 147:97, 1978.

30.   Strauss RJ, Wise L. Operative risks of obesity. Surg Gynecol Obstet 146:286, 1978.

31.   Tarhan S, Moffitt ED, Sessler AD, et al. Risk of anesthesia and surgery in patients with chronic bronchitis and chronic obstructive pulmonary disease. Surgery 74:720, 1973.

32.   Tisi GM. Preoperative evaluation of pulmonary function; validity, indications, and benefits. Am Rev Respir Dir 119:293, 1979.

33.   Vanzetto G, Machecourt J, Blendea D, et al. Additive value of thallium single-photon emission computed tomography myocardial imaging for prediction of perioperative events in clinically selected high cardiac risk patients having abdominal aortic surgery. Am J Cardiol 77:143–148, 1996.

---

*Bold print (general references) and bold numerals (specific references) denote published controlled clinical trials, meta-analyses, or consensus-based recommendations.

CHAPTER 87

Peripheral Vascular Disease and Arterial Aneurysms

CALVIN E. JONES, MD

The aging process is associated with the development of variable degrees of arterial disease. Longevity and quality of life may be improved by recognition, thorough evaluation, and appropriate therapy of peripheral arterial diseases. The purpose of this chapter is to provide guidelines for recognition and management of the more commonly encountered arterial problems of acute and chronic occlusive disease and abdominal and peripheral aneurysms.

ACUTE PERIPHERAL ARTERIAL OCCLUSION

Acute ischemia of the lower extremities demands immediate recognition and management in an effort to minimize morbidity, including limb loss, and death because irreversible changes such as muscle necrosis, extensive arterial thrombosis, and neurologic deficit may occur in the affected extremity as early as 4 to 6 hours after acute arterial occlusion.

The two major causes of acute arterial occlusion are cardioarterial embolism and in situ thrombosis. Surgical management of these two entities is different. Embolism demands immediate operation because preexisting collaterals are scanty. Thrombosis usually can be managed under less emergent conditions than embolus because preexisting collateral channels stimu-

lated by chronic underlying occlusive arterial disease provide marginal but adequate blood flow. Acute ischemia secondary to embolization involves the lower extremities in 75% of cases and is typically associated with atrial fibrillation or acute myocardial infarction (MI) with mural thrombosis. This problem can be managed expeditiously in the vast majority of patients by femoral embolectomy through a groin incision under local anesthesia. Management of ischemia secondary to thrombosis, usually seen in the absence of atrial fibrillation or acute MI, often requires complex vascular reconstructive surgical procedures that are best performed under elective conditions after adequate evaluation, which includes arteriography. However, when faced with a nonviable extremity, immediate operation for thrombosis, preceded by emergency angiography, is mandatory.

Newer techniques using thrombolytic therapy in carefully selected patients, followed by angioplasty, atherectomy, or endarterectomy, may salvage the thrombosed artery. These procedures are best accomplished early, but can be performed on a semiurgent basis up to 1 to 3 weeks after thrombosis.

More than 90% of the time, acute embolic occlusion may be distinguished from acute thrombotic occlusion on clinical grounds alone (see below). In instances in which doubt exists about the cause, especially in the absence of atrial fibrillation and recent MI, arteriography is essential to distinguish embolus from thrombosis (see "Laboratory and Radiographic Studies," below).

Causes

Most large arterial emboli originate in the heart. In a series of 338 patients, Fogarty and Buch (13) ascribed 94% of emboli to cardiac disease, mostly caused by atherosclerosis. Arrhythmias secondary to coronary insufficiency, recent MI with mural thrombosis, or old MI with ventricular aneurysm are risk factors for embolization. Rare sources include proximal arterial lesions such as aortic aneurysms or large ulcerative aortic plaques, which are commonly associated with arterioarterial *cholesterol microemboli* causing the blue toe syndrome (23). Left-atrial myxomas, debris from prosthetic heart valves, paradoxical emboli (venous clots passing through a congenital cardiac defect into the arterial circulation), and foreign body emboli have infrequently been associated with sudden arterial occlusion.

Although most acute arterial occlusions follow emboli, *in situ thrombosis* of an arteriosclerotic lesion accounts for approximately 25% of acute occlusive events. Such thrombotic complications are most likely to occur in segments of severe stenosis such as the aortic bifurcation, the iliac bifurcation, the common femoral bifurcation, and the superficial femoral artery just above the knee.

Upper-extremity ischemia is usually secondary to arterial embolism. Acute thrombosis virtually never causes ischemia in the upper extremity because chronic arteriosclerotic lesions are uncommon and collateralization is excellent. Thoracic outlet compression may rarely give rise to subclavian or axillary arterial thrombosis.

Concomitant problems such as hypovolemia from volume depletion or hemorrhage, congestive heart failure, polycythemia, or trauma all have profound influences on management.

Clinical Manifestations

Emboli lodge at arterial bifurcations, most often in the lower extremities (Fig. 87.1). Multiple emboli can result from a "shower discharge" of clots from the heart. Therefore, although the legs are affected most often, there may be symptoms and signs of ischemia elsewhere.

Clinical manifestations vary depending on the adequacy of preexisting collateral circulation and the site of occlusion. If preexisting collateral vessels, stimulated by underlying occlusive arterial disease, are present, acute ischemic symptoms may be mild. However, total arterial occlusion of a previously normal arterial tree causes severe symptoms. The cardinal features of acute ischemia include the six Ps of arterial occlusion: pulselessness, pallor, poikilothermia, pain, paralysis, and paresthesias. The latter three Ps reflect neurophysiologic sequelae of ischemia, and the former three result from mechanical occlusion of an artery. Three-quarters of patients complain of pain, but 20% note numbness as the first manifestation of sudden arterial occlusion. Initially, the pain may be mild, but as the ischemia progresses, pain worsens, only to subside later as anesthesia and paralysis develop.

Additional findings other than the six Ps include poor capillary filling and collapsed or severely sunken veins on the dorsum of the foot. Pedal edema, if present, is not a result of arterial occlusion, but it may be secondary to heart failure or pooling of blood in the extremities of patients who attempt to relieve ischemic pain by maintaining their legs in a dependent position for long periods.

Cardiac examination may reveal atrial fibrillation, a diastolic rumble or the opening snap of mitral stenosis,

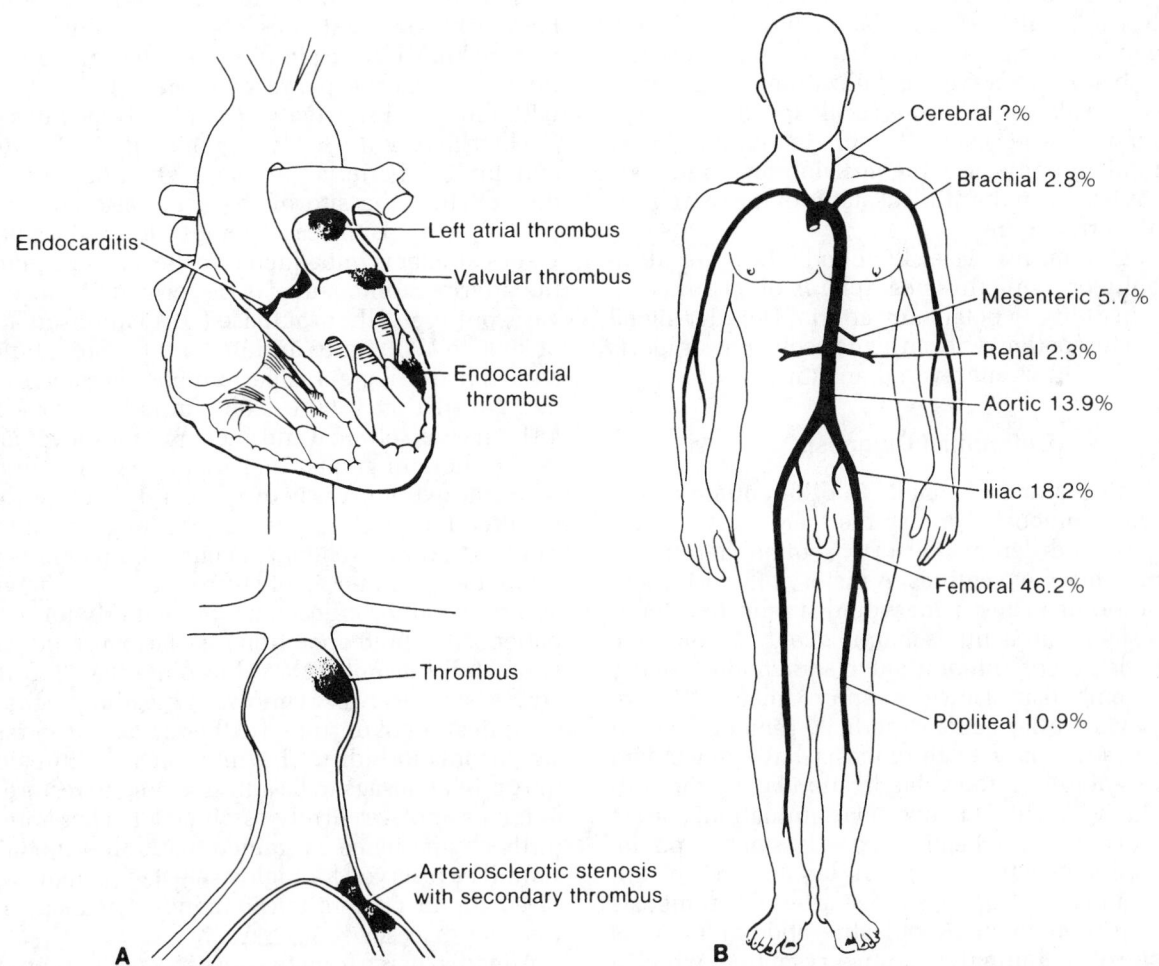

Figure 87.1. **A.** Sources of arterial emboli in 338 patients. More than 90% originate in the heart. **B.** Distribution of arterial emboli in the same group. More than 90% impact in the distal aorta or lower extremities. (Adapted from Rutherford RB, ed. Vascular surgery. 2nd ed. Philadelphia: WB Saunders, 1984.)

Labels in figure:
Endocarditis
Left atrial thrombus
Valvular thrombus
Endocardial thrombus
Thrombus
Arteriosclerotic stenosis with secondary thrombus
A

Cerebral ?%
Brachial 2.8%
Mesenteric 5.7%
Renal 2.3%
Aortic 13.9%
Iliac 18.2%
Femoral 46.2%
Popliteal 10.9%
B

or a gallop associated with congestive failure. A recent history of chest pain or electrocardiographic evidence of myocardial infarction implicates a cardiac origin of acute leg ischemia.

Laboratory and Radiographic Studies

Laboratory studies usually are not helpful in making the diagnosis of acute arterial ischemia of the lower extremities. Arterial blood gas measurements and pH should be obtained to serve as baseline studies for subsequent comparative measurement as well as to identify metabolic acidosis secondary to muscle ischemia. Hyperkalemia may be noted, particularly if advanced muscle ischemia has occurred. A roentgenogram of the chest may document cardiac enlargement or congestive heart failure. All of these studies should be obtained after the patient is hospitalized.

Arteriography in patients with acute ischemia is not performed routinely except in occasional instances of modest ischemia when it is needed to distinguish between thrombosis and embolus (see below). Evidence of generalized and severe arteriosclerosis, a tapered arterial occlusion, and well-developed collateral vessels suggest acute thrombosis. Normal-appearing arteries with scanty collateral circulation and an occlusion with an inverted meniscus configuration indicate embolic occlusion. However, embolization can occur in patients who also have chronic occlusive disease, and the diagnosis is occasionally still in question after angiography. In any case, the decision for immediate surgery is based on the clinical status of the extremity, not on the arteriogram.

Although noninvasive evaluation by Doppler ultrasonography or by plethysmography is often superfluous, the inability to obtain any arterial Doppler signal in the foot in a patient with an acute occlusion supports the decision for urgent revascularization.

Differential Diagnosis

Every effort should be made to differentiate embolism from thrombosis because the therapy of the two conditions is different. History is often helpful in separating these two entities. A history of intermittent claudication or of rest pain would implicate arterial thrombosis as the acute ischemic event. A complete lack of history of intermittent claudication usually indicates embolism. However, approximately 25% of patients who suffer acute superficial femoral arterial occlusion secondary to thrombosis have never had symptoms of intermittent claudication before the sudden occlusive event. On physical examination, classic findings of chronic ischemia such as loss of hair on the toes and dorsum of the foot and the leg, along with nail, skin, and muscle atrophy, suggest arterial thrombosis rather than embolism. A pulsatile abdominal mass diagnostic of abdominal aortic aneurysm from which a mural thrombus may have embolized to the distal arterial tree might be evident. Finally, if the acute ischemic episode involves only one leg, palpating the popliteal and femoral arteries may detect an aneurysm. If the contralateral vessel is vigorously pulsating and aneurysmal, a thrombosis of an aneurysm on the ipsilateral or symptomatic side may have occurred, especially if a nonpulsatile mass can be palpated.

An acute dissection of the thoracic and abdominal aorta may present as unilateral lower-extremity ischemia. Under these circumstances, patients relate a history of severe, searing, ripping thoracic back pain and may provide a history of long-standing hypertension. Also, among such patients a murmur of aortic insufficiency may be present and chest x-rays may reveal a widened mediastinal silhouette.

Treatment

Evaluation and therapy must proceed simultaneously in the management of acute arterial ischemia of the extremities. The cornerstone of early management is the immediate intravenous administration (in the physician's office) of 100 to 150 units of heparin sodium per kilogram of body weight and then urgent vascular surgery consultation. The introduction of the balloon-tipped embolectomy catheter by Fogarty et al. in 1963 revolutionized the management of acute embolic occlusion and converted a previously complex undertaking into a simple operative procedure that invariably can be performed under local anesthesia with improved survival and limb salvage rates (14).

There may be a role for the interventional radiologist and for intra-arterial infusion of *fibrinolytic* agents directly into the site of the acute arterial occlusion (22,38). If that is the case, a multiple-purpose polyethylene catheter is imbedded into the occluding clot after the arteriographic study is performed. Protocols may vary, but typically urokinase (UK) is infused at a rate of 3000 to 4000 units/minute for 30 to 60 minutes and a second arteriogram is performed. Therapy is continued with UK at 1000 to 2000 units/kg/hour for 24 to 48 hours with clinical and angiographic reevaluation at 8- to 12-hour intervals. Such therapy is contraindicated when the extremity is in dire jeopardy because the time required for lysis to occur may be longer than the safe interval before ischemia occurs. In patients whose limbs are not immediately threatened, this therapeutic approach can be efficacious, particularly for high-risk patients in whom operation may be contraindicated. It is generally accepted that clots older than 7 to 10 days are resistant to lysis. Untoward bleeding is the major complication of fibrinolytic therapy and may result in significant morbidity. The duration of the infusion and the optimal dosage to be administered to restore circulation are not yet firmly established. Therefore, until further experience is gained with this modality, it should be reserved for highly selected patients who are cared for in centers specializing in management of vascular disease.

After discharge from the hospital, patients are almost always maintained on therapeutic levels of oral anticoagulants for the rest of their lives (see Chapter 52). Furthermore, they must be evaluated several times a year in order to maintain optimal cardiac function and for continued evaluation of their peripheral circulation.

Results

Despite improved diagnosis, preoperative care, operative management, and postoperative support, mortality from acute lower-extremity ischemia continues to be discouraging. Before 1963 mortality after arterial embolectomy ranged between 34 and 63%. Mortality since 1963 has remained high and ranges between 10 and 40% (18,29,34). Virtually all deaths are related to complications of cardiovascular disease (15). Such findings reinforce the contention that recognition and correction of causes of embolism or thrombosis are an important aspect in the management of such patients.

The likelihood of successful limb salvage, which exceeds 95% in most series, is directly related to time between arterial occlusion and restoration of blood flow. Therefore, it is improbable that a 100% limb salvage rate will ever be achieved.

CHRONIC ARTERIAL OCCLUSIVE DISEASE

In contrast to the management of acute arterial occlusion, which requires emergent or urgent treatment, chronic arterial occlusive disease can usually be managed electively because of the presence of collateral channels that bypass slowly developing atherosclerotic lesions and maintain a viable extremity. A knowledge of the natural history of chronic arterial occlusive disease is necessary for the appropriate management of these patients.

Causes and Pathophysiology

Atherosclerosis is the cause of chronic arterial occlusive disease in most affected patients, and therefore signs and symptoms are unusual before the fifth decade. The disease process is adversely influenced by the presence of diabetes mellitus, hypertension, or hyperlipoproteinemia and by tobacco abuse, factors affecting blood viscosity such as polycythemia, and reduction in cardiac output. Furthermore, symptoms of arterial insufficiency of the legs are only regional manifestations of a generalized disease process that usually spares the upper extremities.

Although atherosclerosis is a generalized disease, it has a remarkably segmental distribution. Arteriosclerosis is prone to develop at major arterial bifurcations, in areas of arterial fixation, and at points of marked arterial angulation such as the aortic, common iliac, and common femoral artery bifurcations; the infrarenal aorta; and the distal superficial femoral artery as it enters Hunter's canal.

With gradual development of such lesions, the formation of collateral vessels compensates for segmental obstructive processes. In many instances collaterals are sufficient to provide adequate blood flow even during moderate exercise, so symptoms are minimal. However, as progressive main arterial involvement occurs, collateral channels may become ineffective or occluded, and ischemic symptoms progress from intermittent claudication to limiting claudication to rest pain and finally to tissue necrosis (see Chapter 88).

Diabetes mellitus (see Chapter 72) has a unique influence on the pathogenesis of atherosclerosis. Diabetic patients may manifest atherosclerosis of a more severe degree and at an earlier age than nondiabetic people. Furthermore, the distribution of the atherosclerotic process in the lower extremity of a diabetic typically involves the distal popliteal and tibial arteries and differs from the aortoiliac and femoral disease seen in the nondiabetic. Microangiopathy also affects peripheral nerves as well as nutrient vessels to skin and muscle and results in insensitivity, which compromises the natural protective mechanisms in the foot. Loss of normal sensation and inability to appreciate pain can result in the formation of an infected plantar ulcer of which the patient is unaware. Therefore, the feet of diabetic patients should be inspected every day. Diabetic neuropathy (see Chapter 72) also involves the sympathetic nervous system, and many of these patients have undergone autosympathectomy at the time they are initially seen by a clinician.

Thromboangiitis obliterans, or *Buerger's disease,* is a severe chronic panarteritis that leads to fibrosis and obliteration of small vessels at the tibial and pedal arterial levels. The arteries of the forearm and hand can be involved, and superficial phlebitis may be seen as well. Buerger's disease is an uncommon cause of lower-extremity arterial insufficiency in the United States. This entity affects young men in their twenties and thirties and is almost always associated with severe tobacco addiction. Successful management hinges on cessation of all forms of tobacco usage.

Natural History

Intermittent claudication reflects a fairly benign condition (3,18,20). Approximately one-third of patients improve, one-third remain stable and tolerate their symptoms, and one-third deteriorate and require revascularization. Relentless progression of the atherosclerotic process is unlikely in most nondiabetic patients, particularly if use of all tobacco products is discontinued. The risk of amputation is approximately 1% per year. On the other hand, patients with ischemic rest pain or gangrene are at very high risk for amputation if revascularization is not undertaken.

The overall 5- and 10-year survival rates among patients with intermittent claudication are approximately 70 and 40%, respectively, and the most common cause of death (75%) is coronary artery disease.

Clinical Manifestations

Symptoms of lower-extremity arterial occlusive disease range from mild muscular pain with exercise to severe rest pain, gangrene, and nonhealing ulceration. The distance a patient walks before developing claudication and the muscle groups involved (calf, thigh, buttock) should be documented. Men should be questioned specifically about impotence. Patients with ischemic rest pain when supine often note alleviation of their discomfort by dangling the involved leg over the side of a bed or by standing up, which indicates that blood flow is marginal and that gravity can increase flow slightly.

On *physical examination,* only a diminution in intensity of peripheral pulses may be noted in the mildest form of the disease. Complete vascular examination should routinely be performed, noting the status of all peripheral pulses, the presence or absence of bruits and peripheral aneurysms, and the blood pressure measurements in both upper extremities. Among patients with mild intermittent claudication, the skin, hair growth, and nails of the toes and feet may appear normal and faintly palpable dorsalis pedis and posterior tibial pulses could be present. However, with progressive arterial involvement trophic changes may occur with hair loss and the development of thin, parchmentlike skin. Lack of pulses below the inguinal ligaments, blanching and pallor with elevation of the extremity, and dependent rubor all indicate advanced ischemia. Gangrenous areas may be evident on the toes. The typical locations of ischemic ulcers are the calcaneus, the lateral malleolus, and the dorsum of the foot (see Chapter 88).

Laboratory and Radiographic Studies

The distribution and severity of peripheral arterial disease can be determined objectively by noninvasive Doppler flow studies. Doppler signals from the dorsalis pedis, posterior tibial, peroneal, or lateral tarsal arteries are located and a sphygmomanometer cuff is placed immediately above the malleoli and inflated to above systolic pressure to obliterate the Doppler signal. As the cuff is slowly deflated, Doppler signals return at the systolic opening pressure. The highest pressure recorded is compared with brachial arterial systolic pressure. A resting ankle/arm index of 1 or greater is normal. For patients with intermittent claudication the mean index is 0.59; for those with rest pain, 0.26; and for those with impending gangrene, 0.05 (40).

A Doppler study of lower-extremity blood flow, although important, is not necessarily required in evaluating all patients with lower-extremity arterial occlusive disease. However, noninvasive testing may be helpful in distinguishing vascular insufficiency from other causes of leg pain such as neurogenic claudication secondary to cauda equina compression from spinal stenosis. In the latter condition, Doppler ankle/arm indices are normal at rest and after exercise. (Doppler flow studies, with the patient at rest, are almost always sufficient to make the diagnosis of peripheral arterial occlusive disease. Rarely, the studies need to be repeated after exercise on a treadmill or even after simply walking the patient to the point of claudication.) Noninvasive studies can also document the efficacy of nonoperative therapy and determine whether deterioration of the circulation is progressive

(30). Also, comparison of preoperative and postoperative noninvasive data is useful in documenting the effectiveness of operative therapy.

The most important laboratory study, if it is determined the patient is a candidate for operation, is arteriography (see below). Although risks are very small in experienced hands, arteriography is used only when operation is indicated and agreed to by the patient.

Finally, laboratory studies may also reveal hyperglycemia or hyperlipidemia that requires appropriate management.

Treatment and Results

Treatment for arterial insufficiency of the legs may be either operative or nonoperative. Indications for operation are shown in Table 87.1. Patients should usually be managed nonoperatively unless one of these indications is present and medical management has failed (33). Knowing the natural history of the occlusive process aids significantly in determining whether the patient's symptoms warrant operative intervention in view of associated risk factors and life expectancy. Except for patients who are not considered operative candidates, ischemic rest pain, nonhealing ulcers, pregangrenous changes, and gangrene are unequivocal indications for expeditious revascularization.

General Measures

An itemized list of recommendations written in nontechnical language should be given to and carefully reviewed with the patient (Table 87.2). Meticulous skin hygiene and avoidance of injury to the foot, however slight, cannot be overemphasized. An otherwise asymptomatic ischemic foot becomes symptomatic when minimal trauma precipitates a nonhealing ulcer that may require revascularization. If the patient's feet are cold, particularly at night, a warm pair of socks or a muffler is advised but not the use of heating pads or hot water bottles, which may cause tissue breakdown and ulceration. Patients should inspect their feet every day and should bathe them at least once a day in lukewarm water and thereafter apply lanolin or hand cream to the skin to keep it soft and pliable, to avoid cracking and fissuring and subsequent skin breakdown. Diabetic patients with peripheral occlusive disease are at high risk of eventual foot amputation, and these protective measures are especially important for them. In addition, diabetic patients should be followed at least every 3 months by a podiatrist for trimming of calluses and nails and for close evaluation for early signs of infection or impending ulceration.

Other measures that significantly affect outcome

Table 87.1. Indications for Operation

Claudication that is intolerable in a good-risk patient
Ischemic rest pain
Impending gangrene
Nonhealing ulceration

Table 87.2. Advice that Should Be Given to Patients with Arterial Insufficiency

---

Quit smoking. Use *no* tobacco in *any* form.[a]
If overweight, lose weight.
Exercise (walk) to the point of discomfort at least 2 miles a day.
Keep feet very clean. Bathe at least daily in **lukewarm** water.
Gently apply lanolin or mild hand cream to feet after bathing.
Use a night light to avoid hitting toes or shins.
Wear clean, preferably cotton, socks daily (cotton does not retain moisture).
Avoid injury to feet. Wear properly fitting shoes to prevent calluses, corns, blisters. Avoid shoes made of synthetic material that does not "breathe." Wear slippers at night and use a night light after going to bed.
Place lamb's wool (available from pharmacies) between overriding toes.
Avoid extremes of temperature. Do no put feet in hot water or use heating pads on lower extremities. In cold weather, wear socks to bed to warm feet. Do not get feet cold or wet.
If feet hurt at night, raise head of bed 6–10 in. (15–25 cm) on blocks.
For any sudden change in symptoms such as prolonged pain, numbness or tingling, or inability to move foot or leg, consult your physician *immediately.*

---

[a]See Chapter 20 for ways to help patients to stop smoking.

include maintaining satisfactory cardiac function (see Chapter 61) and controlling diabetes mellitus. It is important that the patient be advised to exercise daily to stimulate the development of collateral channels. Exercise tolerance can be improved in up to two-thirds of patients. Cessation of the use of all tobacco products is of paramount importance. It must be emphasized to patients that smoking accelerates atherogenesis, causes relative tissue hypoxia because of carbon monoxide poisoning, and precipitates vasospasm in the important collateral vascular bed that may persist up to 1 hour after each cigarette. Patients must clearly understand that nicotine absorption occurs through the buccal mucosa with the use of chewing tobacco, pipes, cigars, and cigarettes, and does not require inhalation of smoke.

Management of coexistent hypertension is sometimes challenging and one often may have to settle for less than ideal blood pressure control because the symptoms of the arteriosclerotic occlusive process may worsen if the patient is returned to a poorly tolerated normotensive state. In patients taking antihypertensive drugs, it is important to check at each visit for orthostatic drops in blood pressure and to adjust the treatment regimen accordingly if orthostatic hypotension occurs (see Chapter 62).

Pharmacologic Management

There is little objective evidence to suggest that vasodilating drugs offer significant benefits to patients with symptomatic peripheral arterial insufficiency. Blood vessels in ischemic tissue beds are already maximally dilated. When systemic vessels are dilated by these drugs, thus increasing the vascular bed, blood flow to the involved extremity may actually decrease and vasodilators may have the paradoxical effect of exacerbating the ischemia. Therefore these drugs are

not recommended in the treatment of patients with occlusive vascular disease.

Similarly, although hospitalized patients are administered heparin acutely, long-term anticoagulation has not been shown to have any beneficial effect on retardation of atherosclerosis or the amelioration of symptoms and may pose significant hazards (see Chapter 52). Although platelet-inhibiting agents, specifically aspirin, have not been shown to be effective in the management of lower-extremity arterial occlusive disease, they are routinely used by most vascular surgeons (see Chapter 52).

Pentoxifylline (Trental) decreases blood viscosity by a direct effect on the red blood cell membrane and improves microcirculatory flow. It is a xanthine derivative whose precise mechanism of action is unknown. A randomized double-blind parallel group study of the efficacy of pentoxifylline in the treatment of intermittent claudication documented that statistically significant improvement in claudication distance was found in patients taking the drug (25,32). However, the degree of improvement was not enough to suggest that the drug would be effective without cessation of tobacco abuse and without a continued exercise program.

Pentoxifylline is available in 400-mg tablets, usually prescribed in a dosage of one tablet three times a day with meals. A positive effect, if it occurs, is seen within 1 to 2 months. The major side effects of the drug are nausea, dyspepsia, and dizziness, which often may be relieved by reducing the dosage to one tablet twice a day.

Operative Intervention

It is only upon failure of nonoperative therapy and among patients with clear indications for surgery that arteriographic studies are obtained. It must be understood that arteriography serves as a roadmap for the vascular surgeon when reconstructing the vascular tree. No characteristic arteriographic findings distinguish between patients with intermittent claudication, those with ischemic rest pain, and those with gangrene and ulceration. As a generalization, however, patients who have intermittent claudication usually have hemodynamically significant proximal arterial occlusive lesions affecting the iliofemoral or the femoral–popliteal system. Characteristically, such patients have reasonably good outflow with two or more tibial vessels patent. Patients with advanced ischemic changes are found to have diffuse multisegment involvement and none or only one patent tibial vessel in the lower leg or foot. However, overlapping between various groups is wide, and no single arteriographic finding consistently characterizes any one symptom complex.

Arteriography occasionally demonstrates a distribution of advanced arterial involvement without a reasonable runoff vessel for bypass. Under these circumstances, nonoperative therapy is all that may be offered and the patient should be warned that there is a real risk of subsequent amputation.

Indications for operation among patients with intermittent claudication relate mainly to the ability of the patient to tolerate the pain. Nonlimiting claudication and mild ischemic rest pain, controlled by non-narcotic analgesics, are not indications for operation, particularly in high-risk patients. A trial of conservative management is especially important if other risk factors, such as recent myocardial infarction, are present.

When it is determined that the condition of the patient warrants operative intervention and when arteriography documents adequate outflow vessels, a number of options for arterial reconstruction are open to the vascular surgeon, including autogenous vein or prosthetic graft bypass and endarterectomy. There is a definite preference for bypass rather than endarterectomy, which is rarely used today. Direct reconstructive procedures include aortofemoral bypass, femoral–popliteal bypass, and femoral–tibial bypass. Extra-anatomic reconstruction includes axillounifemoral bypass, axillobifemoral bypass, and femoral–femoral bypass.

The operative mortality rate for aortofemoral bypass grafting is approximately 5% with a patency rate of 80 to 90% at 5 years. Operative mortality for extra-anatomic reconstructions is slightly less than for aortofemoral bypass, but the outlook for graft patency is not as good. Operative mortality for autogenous vein femoral–popliteal and femoral–tibial bypass procedures ranges from 0.5 to 1% depending on the general condition of the patient. Five-year patency rates for such procedures vary between 60 and 70%, and it should be emphasized that patency varies directly with adequacy of the vein used and the extent of the disease in the vessel being reconstructed.

In general, in contrast to aneurysmal disease, arterial reconstruction for occlusive disease is palliative and does not significantly increase the patient's life expectancy because most patients have significant coincident coronary artery disease. However, the quality of life is vastly improved, particularly for those who would have undergone amputation if successful arterial reconstruction had not been feasible.

Patients with aortofemoral arterial occlusive disease without coincident coronary artery disease or diabetes mellitus have survival rates that equal those of the normal age- and sex-adjusted population. Observed differences in life expectancy between normal populations and those undergoing arterial reconstructive procedures usually result from the high prevalence of associated coronary artery disease and diabetes mellitus. It appears that the presence of coronary artery disease reduces life expectancy by approximately 10 years, and the presence of diabetes mellitus reduces life expectancy by an additional 15 years (26).

Balloon Angioplasty, Stents, and Laser and Mechanical Atherectomy

Since the mid-1970s, percutaneous transluminal arterial dilation (angioplasty) has been available as an alternative to surgical reconstruction for highly selected patients with arterial occlusive disease. Advan-

tages include lower morbidity, lower mortality, and possibly lower cost compared to arterial reconstruction. Patients who are not candidates for surgery, if subjected to percutaneous transluminal angioplasty, could conceivably require operation if complications occur following the percutaneous procedure. Therefore a cooperative approach between the interventional radiologist and the vascular surgeon is mandatory.

Most authors agree that the best results with percutaneous transluminal angioplasty are obtained in patients with short segment stenoses of the iliac arteries, in which success rates range from 76 to 93% at 1 year and from 66 to 92% at 2 years. The reported results of angioplasty for femoropopliteal disease range from 51 to 80% at 1 year and from 46 to 75% at 2 years. There is general agreement that results are less satisfactory if the arteriographic runoff is poor. In the properly selected patient the probability of early success of percutaneous transluminal angioplasty is high if the involved vessel is the iliac artery, there is a short segment of stenosis and not occlusion, and the runoff is good (24). Results are less satisfactory when multiple dilations are required. Results of angioplasty are improving with the advent of *metallic stents* placed at the time of initial balloon angioplasty, or at repeat angioplasty in the event of restenosis.

Patients with longer stenoses and total occlusions have less favorable outcomes, but in very poor-risk patients, angioplasty may be the only alternative to operative reconstruction. Occlusions less than 5 cm long and stenoses less than 10 cm long appear to be the outer limits for successful percutaneous transluminal angioplasty.

It is appealing to believe that percutaneous transluminal arterial dilation can be substituted for revascularization. This is a false assumption; the criteria for the use of this modality should be as rigid as those required for reconstructive surgery.

Laser atherectomy was introduced as an adjunct in the management of peripheral vascular disease (35). The laser was thought to be occasionally useful in developing a channel through an occlusion to allow passage of a balloon catheter for dilation (laser-assisted balloon angioplasty). At present the laser is rarely used, and all stenoses and most short occlusions can be treated with angioplasty and stenting without the need for laser atherectomy. In the case of long occlusions of the femoral artery, laser atherectomy resulted in a very high rate of recurrence stenosis (approximately 50% within 6 to 12 months). Therefore, with the advent of stents to complement angioplasty, a safe and efficacious therapy when indicated, the laser has essentially been relegated to experimental application.

Mechanical atherectomy devices, which use a cutting blade, are now limited to excision of intimal flaps after initial enthusiasm for widespread use.

Amputation

In debilitated patients with frank gangrene or unremitting ischemic rest pain in whom arterial reconstruction or transluminal angioplasty is not indicated or feasible, amputation is the only alternative. The goal of amputation is to relieve the patient of disabling pain, remove nonviable and potentially infected tissue, and select a level that will provide the greatest chance of healing with maximal prosthetic rehabilitation.

If the gangrenous process is dry and does not involve the great toe, autoamputation may be allowed to occur or formal surgical amputation may be performed. If pulses are palpable in the foot and the ischemic process affects the tips of the digits, primary healing usually occurs after toe amputation. Nonischemic neurotrophic ulcers on the plantar aspects of the foot in diabetic patients often heal if the head of the metatarsal is removed to relieve the pressure necrosis that occurs as a result of the diabetic neuropathy.

Mortality for amputation is directly related to the preoperative condition of the patient and to other complicating diseases. Mortality rates for amputations performed for occlusive arterial disease have been reported to be as high as 30%, with higher mortality rates recorded in the more proximal amputations.

After successful amputation, which includes primary healing that results in a stump amenable to prosthetic fitting, the most important aspect of therapy is rehabilitation. Prosthetic mobility requires almost twice as much energy with an above-knee amputation than with a below-knee amputation, and mobility is further inhibited by increased age, infirmity, obesity, and a poorly fitting prosthesis. It is difficult to predict successful rehabilitation in the atherosclerotic population, but cooperation between the surgeon and the rehabilitation team is pivotal to a satisfactory outcome.

ABDOMINAL AORTIC ANEURYSMS

Abdominal aortic aneurysm is the most common arterial aneurysm. It is encountered two to three times more often than the second most common type, the popliteal artery aneurysm. Abdominal aortic aneurysms have been found in almost 2% of consecutive postmortem studies (5).

Men are affected by aneurysmal disease 10 times more often than women. The occurrence of abdominal aortic aneurysms increases with age as well as in people who have a first-degree relative with an aneurysm (1,8,19).

Although it is not possible to implicate a single cause, most abdominal aortic aneurysms are arteriosclerotic in origin. Most are infrarenal and only approximately 5% encroach on visceral vessels, most commonly the renal arteries.

The *natural history* of untreated abdominal aortic aneurysms was unknown until the report of Estes (12) in 1950 that documented the grave consequences of this disease. Five-year survival of patients with untreated aneurysms is only about 20%. Within 5 years, 40 to 50% of patients with untreated abdominal aortic aneurysms die of rupture; 30% die of other causes, most notably myocardial infarction. Multiple groups have presented corroborating data emphasizing the improved life expectancy after surgical treatment of this condition (6,9,16,27,36) (see below).

Clinical Manifestations

History

The presentation of an abdominal aortic aneurysm depends on whether complications have occurred. More than 50% are asymptomatic when first discovered during routine examination by a physician, by the patient who complains of a second heart in the abdomen upon palpating a pulsatile epigastric mass, or serendipitously during radiographic or ultrasonographic abdominal studies in the pursuit of another diagnosis. The patient may complain of abdominal, flank, or back pain as the aneurysm expands and becomes symptomatic, a harbinger of rupture.

Rupture. Most aneurysms that rupture bleed into the retroperitoneal space, affording lifesaving tamponade. Under these circumstances, the patient presents with a history of syncope or of flank or back pain in a hypovolemic, but not necessarily hypotensive state. On the other hand, an uncontained intraperitoneal rupture of an abdominal aortic aneurysm typically presents with the patient in extremis secondary to blood loss and requires immediate operative intervention. Aneurysms may rupture into adjacent structures and cause large arteriovenous fistulae such as an aortocaval or aortorenal fistula with high-output cardiac failure, or into the gastrointestinal tract, usually the duodenum, causing an aortoenteric fistula with massive hematemesis or hematochezia.

Other complications. If aneurysms are large enough, they may compress adjacent structures such as the ureter, duodenum, vena cava, or vertebral column, with production of appropriate symptoms such as gastric outlet obstruction in patients with duodenal compression.

Dislodgment of laminated clots from the wall of the aneurysm occasionally may cause peripheral embolization to femoral, popliteal, or distal vessels. When emboli occur, patients may complain of symptoms of sudden leg ischemia as the first indication of an abdominal aortic aneurysm (see below). If embolic bits of debris are small and distal vessels are patent, small areas of tissue necrosis in the toes or skin or the lower extremities are seen. Aneurysms that rarely thrombose may present with acute bilateral lower-extremity ischemia.

Although the incidence of the various complications other than rupture is unknown, they do underscore the poor natural history of untreated abdominal aortic aneurysms. After seeking specific historical information regarding the aneurysm, the patient should be questioned about other symptoms so that an estimate of the extent of atherosclerotic involvement is obtained. This information often influences recommendations for or against surgical therapy (see Chapter 86). Symptoms of transient cerebral ischemia or previous stroke, angina pectoris or previous myocardial infarction, or cardiac decompensation such as significant severe shortness of breath, ankle edema, orthopnea, and paroxysmal nocturnal dyspnea are especially important in determining the risks in this group of patients.

Physical Examination

The diagnosis of abdominal aortic aneurysm by physical examination has been reported to be accurate in almost 90% of cases (9). As previously noted, most patients with asymptomatic aneurysms are discovered on routine physical examination to have an epigastric or left upper quadrant pulsatile mass. However, a pulsatile mass may not be palpable in obese patients or in those with very small aneurysms. Typically, asymptomatic aneurysms may be discovered when x-rays are obtained for other intra-abdominal conditions such as peptic ulcer or renal or colonic disease.

It is important to palpate the epigastrium because the bifurcation of the abdominal aorta is at the level of the umbilicus. Only rarely when palpating inferior to the umbilicus will one identify an abdominal aortic aneurysm unless both common iliac arteries are also aneurysmal. The laterally pulsatile nature of an aneurysm is a clue in differentiating it from the anteriorly transmitted aortic pulsation through viscera or from a mass overlying the aorta. Lesions confused with aneurysms include pancreatic pseudocyst, horseshoe kidneys, neoplasms of the stomach or transverse colon, and retroperitoneal soft tissue tumors. Often, a normal but prominently pulsatile abdominal aorta in a healthy person and an undilated but tortuous aorta in an elderly person may simulate an abdominal aortic aneurysm. In this circumstance, the pulsatile mass is felt to the left of the midline but not to the right. One should palpate the abdomen by approaching the midline both from the right and from the left to identify the laterally pulsatile characteristic of an aneurysm.

Risk of rupture correlates best with the size of the aneurysm as determined by ultrasonography and not by physical examination alone (see below).

One-quarter to one-third of patients have significant associated occlusive arterial disease as well as the abdominal aortic aneurysm, so a systematic evaluation should be performed. Systemic blood pressure should be measured in both arms. Carotid bruits can be detected by listening with the bell of the stethoscope over the carotid bifurcations at the angle of the mandible with the patient supine and holding his or her breath. Examination of the lower extremities should be directed to the character of the femoral, popliteal, and pedal pulses and to the presence or absence of femoral and popliteal bruits and aneurysms. In less than 10% of patients, there may be coexistent peripheral aneurysms involving the popliteal or femoral arteries.

Laboratory and Radiographic Studies

The presence or absence of an abdominal aortic aneurysm must be confirmed by ultrasonography. The

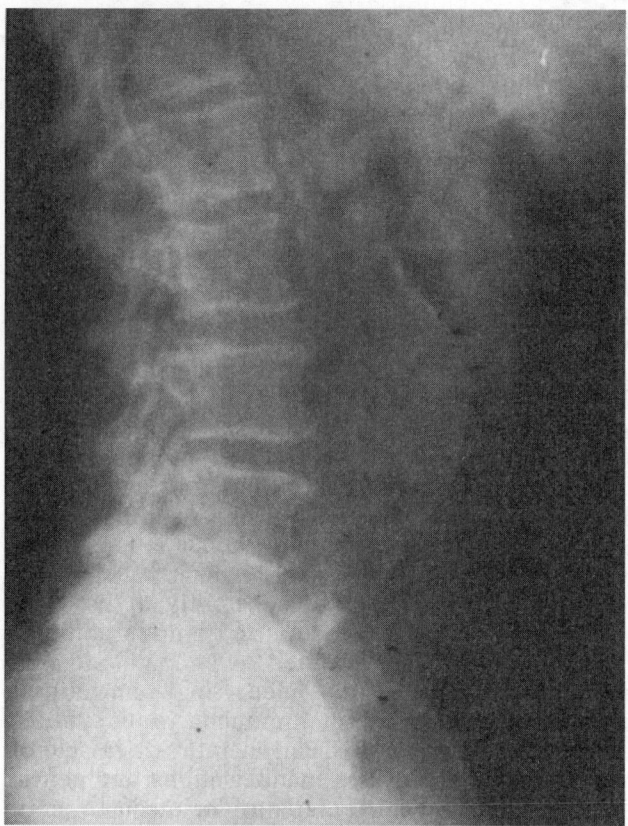

Figure 87.2. Cross-table lateral abdominal x-ray documenting calcified abdominal aortic aneurysm.

accuracy of ultrasonic diagnosis of abdominal aortic aneurysm approaches 98% (28,39). Anteroposterior and cross-table lateral plain x-rays of the abdomen also document abdominal aortic aneurysms in 70 to 80% of cases because the aneurysm wall is often calcified (Fig. 87.2). Ultrasonography is simple, safe, and cost-effective and is recommended as the method of choice for verifying or excluding abdominal aortic aneurysm as well as for serial follow-up every 6 months for patients being treated nonoperatively (17).

Computerized tomography (CT) and magnetic resonance imaging (MRI) are more expensive and should be used only as an adjunct to ultrasonography for confirming unusual situations such as a suspected leak in an otherwise stable patient, extent of visceral artery involvement, inflammatory change, or the presence and characteristics of horseshoe kidney. Generally, the cost of a CT scan is about double that of a sonogram. The MRI costs twice as much as the CT scan and rarely provides additional information.

Objective measurement of peripheral pulses in the lower extremities as well as baseline Doppler blood flow studies are of value during long-term follow-up. Because atherosclerotic disease is permanent and may be progressive, the patient is always followed on a yearly basis after convalescence from surgery.

Treatment and Results

Once the presence of an abdominal aortic aneurysm has been verified by ultrasound, a decision about therapy must be made. The risk of catastrophic rupture among patients with aneurysms greater than 6 cm in transverse diameter is so great that almost all such patients must be considered candidates for operation (Fig. 87.3). Aneurysms between 4 and 6 cm impose an intermediate risk of rupture of 10 to 30% within 2 to 3 years. When dealing with large aneurysms, even assuming an operative mortality rate of 13%, surgical therapy is clearly superior to nonsurgical therapy. Over

the last two decades, operative mortality has declined to 2 to 5% for elective aneurysmectomy (6,11). If operation is delayed until the aneurysm ruptures, operative mortality increases to a formidable 60 to 80%, particularly if the patient arrives at the hospital in hypovolemic shock. Even when such patients can be resuscitated adequately before operation, operative mortality remains approximately 50%. The case for elective resection is further reinforced by the fact that the mean total cost after elective aneurysmectomy is approximately one-half of that after rupture (31).

The natural history of abdominal aortic aneurysms dictates that even patients with small aneurysms should be treated surgically unless the risk is prohibitive (21). The classic study of Szilagyi et al. (37) comparing nonoperative with operative therapy is summarized in Figure 87.3. Even with the worst operative mortality (13%), survival after surgical management of small aneurysms is better than after nonsurgical management. As operative mortality declines, the disparity becomes greater. However, if a patient has significant life-limiting concurrent disease and a small asymptomatic abdominal aortic aneurysm, a close follow-up program can be instituted. Generally, aneurysms grow at an average rate of 0.4 cm/year (2), with a range of 0.24 cm to 0.9 cm/year (4,27); a 4-cm aneurysm can be predicted to attain 6 cm in 4 years (7). There are no reported cases of spontaneous regression.

Age in itself does not affect the risk of operation. Elective aneurysmectomy can be performed in a very elderly patient with an operative mortality rate comparable to a similar operation in younger patients, provided the patient is a satisfactory operative candidate. Furthermore, patients with major complications of their aneurysm (see above) do better than without surgical therapy (36). Therefore it is generally advised that aneurysmectomy be performed in all patients with a reasonable life expectancy who are judged to be able to tolerate the procedure with an operative mortality of less than 5%. Clearly, operation is mandatory for any patients who have complications of their aneurysms (see above). Endovascular stent-grafting of aortic aneurysms is an evolving technology under investigation that will replace operative intervention in selected cases.

Controversy exists regarding the routine use of preoperative aortography among patients with abdominal aortic aneurysms. Although some surgeons routinely recommend aortography, the majority use aortographic studies selectively. Under certain circumstances abdominal aortography is helpful and even mandatory. Indications for aortography include the possibility of anomalous renal or visceral vasculature or occlusive disease involving these same vessels that would alter the operative approach. It is important to determine the extent of reconstruction necessary so that the anomalous vessels are not violated and the occlusive lesions are addressed. Drug-resistant hypertension on a renovascular basis is an indication for aortography to document renal artery stenosis that can be corrected at

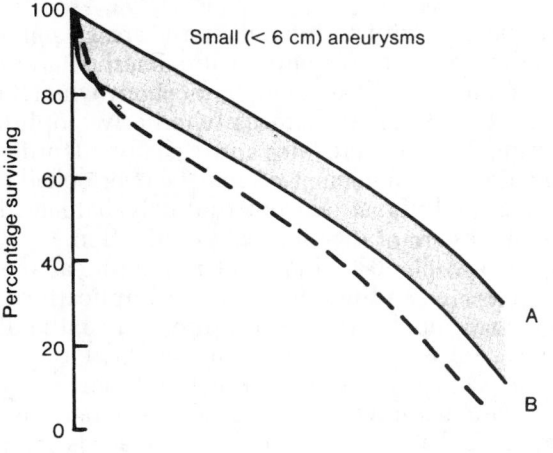

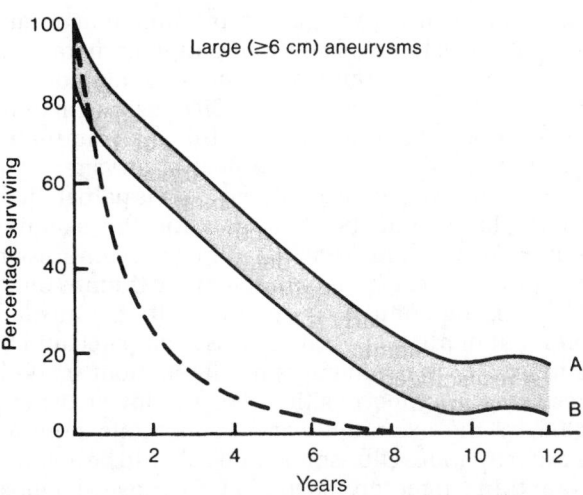

Figure 87.3. Survival curves for surgical and nonsurgical patients with large and small aortic aneurysms. The dashed lines represent survival rates in the nonsurgical groups; the bands, in the surgical groups. The top of the bands **(A)** assumed no operative mortality; the bottom **(B),** a 13% operative mortality. (Modified by Rutherford from data provided by Szilagyi.) Even with 13% operative mortality, surgical treatment is better than nonsurgical treatment. (Adapted from Rutherford RB, ed. Vascular surgery. 2nd ed. Philadelphia: WB Saunders, 1984.)

the time of abdominal aortic aneurysmectomy. Aortography is essential for delineation of the anomalous circulation of the rare horseshoe kidney initially detected by ultrasonography. Alternatively, spiral CT and three-dimensional reconstruction could be considered instead of aortography.

It is essential to inform the patient and family of various risks of operative versus nonoperative treatment. Equally important is explaining complications that may occur in the postoperative period. Although this is primarily the responsibility of the operating surgeon, it is appropriate for the primary physician to discuss with the patient what is likely to occur. The patient should know that a Dacron or polytetrafluoroethylene prosthesis will be used to replace the abdominal aorta and that such arterial grafts are very durable. Fortunately, complications are rare and include (but are not limited to) paraplegia from spinal cord ischemia, renal failure, amputation, graft infection, ischemic colitis, and aortoenteric fistula. It should be stressed to the patient and family that postoperative complications of abdominal aortic aneurysmectomy are magnified by the urgency of the operative procedure.

If operation is not recommended or accepted, patients should be evaluated every 3 to 6 months by interval history, physical examination, and ultrasonography. A patient with a rupturing or symptomatic aneurysm complains of steady dull abdominal, flank, or back pain. If such pain occurs or if a change in existing symptoms is noted in a patient being followed with an abdominal aortic aneurysm, the patient and family should be instructed to seek surgical attention promptly.

PERIPHERAL ARTERIAL ANEURYSMS

Peripheral arterial aneurysms may involve the carotid, subclavian, brachial, iliac, femoral, and popliteal arteries. More than 90% of peripheral aneurysms involve either popliteal or femoral arteries. Popliteal arterial aneurysms predominate. Tortuous vessels presenting as serpiginous pulsations under the skin may be mistaken for peripheral aneurysms. The most noted example of this is a tortuous subclavian or common carotid artery in an elderly, hypertensive patient that may be confused with a carotid or subclavian artery aneurysm.

Most peripheral arterial aneurysms are arteriosclerotic in origin; mycotic, traumatic, and syphilitic aneurysms are rare. Peripheral arteriosclerotic aneurysms are localized manifestations of a generalized disease process. This is underscored by noting that, among a group of 37 patients with common femoral aneurysms, 35 (95%) had another aneurysm elsewhere and 92% had associated aortoiliac aneurysms (10). Femoral aneurysms can be bilateral in up to 60% of cases. Similarly, among 36 patients with popliteal arterial aneurysms, almost 80% had an aneurysm elsewhere, two-thirds had aortoiliac aneurysms, and bilateral popliteal aneurysms occurred in 50% of these

patients (10). Therefore, when a peripheral aneurysm is found, the physician should be aware that they can be multiple and bilateral, and the popliteal, femoral, and aortoiliac areas should be carefully assessed by physical examination and ultrasonography.

Femoral and, particularly, popliteal arterial aneurysms are associated with a high incidence of distal thromboembolism and eventual limb loss. Untreated peripheral aneurysms may eventuate in limb loss approximately 75% of the time from either distal embolization or acute thrombosis. On the other hand, rupture with exsanguinating hemorrhage is not a major risk with femoral or popliteal arterial aneurysms.

Clinical Manifestations

Most patients with peripheral arterial aneurysms are elderly, and many are asymptomatic. Femoral arterial aneurysms are usually evident, particularly when they measure 4 or 5 cm in diameter. Similarly, popliteal aneurysms, if they are large, are easily identified. However, popliteal aneurysms may be overlooked because many clinicians do not routinely palpate the popliteal fossa during a physical examination.

Approximately 50% of femoral and popliteal aneurysms present with limb-threatening complications of thrombosis, embolization, or rupture. Hence, the discovery of an asymptomatic aneurysm in these anatomic areas is a clear indication for timely repair. Among patients in whom complications of peripheral aneurysms develop, successful limb salvage is significantly less likely, with an overall amputation rate of 25%, than among patients in whom prophylactic surgical therapy is offered for the asymptomatic aneurysm.

An enlarged artery with a very prominent femoral or popliteal pulse to physical examination is characteristic of a femoral or popliteal aneurysm and should be confirmed by ultrasonography. Diagnosis of femoral aneurysm is easily made on clinical examination alone, but the diagnosis of popliteal aneurysm may be more difficult. When the popliteal fossa is palpated, the patient's leg should be relaxed while the examiner passively flexes the knee with the fingers, compressing the popliteal artery in the fossa, and the thumbs on the patella, giving counter-compression. If an unusually prominent popliteal pulsatile mass is palpated and the examiner suspects aneurysm, the patient may be placed in the prone position and the lower leg supported by the examiner's arm to facilitate popliteal arterial palpation. Ultrasonography should be obtained for anything remotely suspicious because diagnosis and treatment before the occurrence of complications are exceedingly important. Occasionally, the only manifestations of a popliteal aneurysm are small punctate necrotic areas of skin over the anterior tibial region or small gangrenous areas of the tips of toes. This "blue toe syndrome" is a result of microemboli from the aneurysm that have showered to the periphery.

Once the diagnosis of a peripheral arterial aneurysm is made, the patient should be referred to a vascular surgeon. Arteriography is mandatory in order to confirm the anatomy and patency of the femoral–popliteal and tibial arteries when planning operative intervention.

Treatment and Results

Treatment of symptomatic peripheral aneurysms is indicated in all instances. Because the natural history is one of eventual limb loss, it is important to offer surgical therapy to maintain or improve quality of life by avoiding amputation. However, if patients have concurrent significant disease or are bedridden for other reasons, operation is not justified. Surgical correction includes replacement of femoral aneurysms with prosthetic or reversed autogenous saphenous vein grafts. Similarly, popliteal aneurysms are managed by bypassing the diseased segment with autogenous saphenous vein.

Operative mortality for management of peripheral aneurysms is approximately 1 to 3%. Limb salvage is obtained in more than 90% of cases and is related to the degree of arterial involvement peripheral to the aneurysm. In almost all series reporting repair of popliteal arterial aneurysms, amputations in the postoperative period have been associated with severe occlusive arterial disease manifested by gangrene and rest pain preoperatively.

General References

Boyd AM. The natural course of arteriosclerosis of the lower extremities. Angiology 11:10, 1960.
> This study of 1440 patients with intermittent claudication, carefully evaluated and followed over 15 years, for the first time documented the natural history of intermittent claudication. This study provides the control database against which results of surgical and nonsurgical therapy are judged.

Crawford ES, Saleh SA, Babb JW III, et al. Infrarenal abdominal aortic aneurysm: factors influencing survival after operation performed over a 25-year period. Ann Surg 193:699, 1981.
> Experience of an outstanding vascular surgical group that evaluated 920 consecutive patients operated on for abdominal aortic aneurysm. This paper is the gold standard against which the results of others are measured.

Dent TL, Lindenauer SM, Ernst CB, Fry WJ. Multiple arteriosclerotic arterial aneurysms. Arch Surg 105:338, 1972.
> Evaluation of 57 patients with peripheral aneurysms among 1488 with aneurysmal disease. Importance of coincidental multiple aneurysms when encountering patients with aneurysmal disease stresses the need for thorough vascular evaluation.

Ernst CB. Abdominal aortic aneurysm. N Engl J Med 328:1167, 1993.
> An excellent review.

Rutherford RB, ed. Vascular surgery. 3rd ed. Philadelphia: WB Saunders, 1989.
> The first comprehensive text of vascular surgery. Specific disease entities are extensively discussed, including nonoperative as well as operative aspects. Basic pathophysiologic concepts are lucidly presented. This work should be in the library of all interested in vascular diseases.

Wilt TJ. Clinical strategies in the diagnosis and management of lower extremity peripheral vascular disease. J Gen Intern Med 7:87, 1992.
> A well-referenced review.

Yao RST, Pearce WH, eds. Progress in vascular surgery. Stanford, CT: Appleton & Lange, 1997.
> Excellent review of emerging diagnostic and therapeutic modalities.

Specific References

1. Bengtsson H, Sonesson B, Lanne T, et al. Prevalence of abdominal aortic aneurysm in the offspring of patients dying from aneurysm rupture. Br J Surg 79:1142, 1992.
2. Bernstein EF, Dilley RB, Goldberger LE, et al. Growth rates of small abdominal aortic aneurysms. Surgery 80:765, 1976.
3. Boyd AM. The natural course of arteriosclerosis of the lower extremities. Angiology 11:10, 1960.
4. Brown PM, Patenden R, Gutelius JR. The selective management of small abdominal aortic aneurysms: the Kingston study. J Vasc Surg 15:21, 1992.
5. Carlsson J, Sternby NH. Aortic aneurysms. Acta Chir Scand 127:466, 1964.
6. Crawford ES, Saleh SA, Babb JW III, et al. Infrarenal abdominal aortic aneurysm; factors influencing survival after operation performed over a 25-year period. Ann Surg 193:699, 1981.
7. Cronenwett JL. Small asymptomatic abdominal aortic aneurysms. In: Decker BC, ed. Current therapy in vascular surgery. St. Louis: CV Mosby, 1987;107.
8. Darling RC III, Brewster DC, Darling RC, et al. Are familial abdominal aortic aneurysms different? J Vasc Surg 10:39, 1989.
9. DeBakey ME, Crawford ES, Cooley DA, Morris GC Jr. Aneurysm of the abdominal aorta; analysis of results of graft replacement therapy 1 to 11 years after operation. Ann Surg 160:622, 1964.
10. Dent TL, Lindenauer SM, Ernst CB, Fry WJ. Multiple arteriosclerotic arterial aneurysms. Arch Surg 105:338, 1972.
11. DeWeese JA, Blaisdell FW, Foster JH. Optimal resources for vascular surgery. Arch Surg 105:948, 1972.
12. Estes JE. Abdominal aortic aneurysm. A study of 102 cases. Circulation 2:258, 1950.
13. Fogarty TJ, Buch WS. The management of embolic and thrombotic arterial occlusion. In: Rutherford RB, ed. Vascular surgery. Philadelphia: WB Saunders, 1977;423.
14. Fogarty TJ, Cranley JJ, Krause RT, et al. A method for extraction of arterial emboli and thrombi. Surg Gynecol Obstet 116:241, 1963.
15. Fogarty TJ, Daily PO, Shumway NE, Krippaehne W. Experience with balloon catheter technique for arterial embolectomy. Am J Surg 122:231, 1971.
16. Foster JH, Bolasny BL, Gobbel WG Jr, Scott HW Jr. Comparative study of elective resection and expectant treatment of abdominal aortic aneurysm. Surg Gynecol Obstet 129:1, 1969.
17. Höjer J: Diagnosis of acute symptomatic aortic aneurysm: ultrasonography an important tool. J Intern Med 232:427, 1992.
18. Imparato AM, Kim G-E, Davidson T, Crowley JG. Intermittent claudication; its natural course. Surgery 78:795, 1975.
19. Johansen K, Koepsell T. Familial tendency for abdominal aortic aneurysms. JAMA 256:1934, 1986.
20. Juergens JC, Barker NW, Hines EA. Arteriosclerosis obliterans. Review of 520 cases with special reference to pathogenic and prognostic factors. Circulation 21:188, 1960.
21. Katz DA, Littenberg B, Cronenwett JL. Management of small abdominal aortic aneurysms. Early surgery vs watchful waiting. JAMA 268:2678, 1992.
22. Katzen BT, Edwards KC, Albert AS, VanBreda A. Low-dose direct fibrinolysis in peripheral vascular disease. J Vasc Surg 1:718, 1984.
23. Kempczinski RF. Lower extremity arterial emboli from ulcerating atherosclerotic plaques. JAMA 241:807, 1979.
24. Lally ME, Johnston KW, Andrews D. Percutaneous transluminal dilatation of peripheral arteries: an analysis of factors predicting early success. J Vasc Surg 1:704, 1984.
25. Lindgarde F, Jelnes R, Bjorkman H. Conservative drug treatment in patients with moderately severe chronic occlusive peripheral arterial disease. Circulation 80:1549, 1989.
26. Malone JM, Moore WS, Goldstone J. Life expectancy following aortofemoral arterial grafting. Surgery 81:551, 1977.
27. Nevitt MP, Ballard DJ, Hallett JW Jr. Prognosis of abdominal aortic aneurysms: a population-based study. N Engl J Med 321:1009, 1989.
28. Nusbaum JW, Freimans AK, Thomford NR. Echography in the diagnosis of abdominal aortic aneurysm. Arch Surg 102:385, 1971.

29. Panetta T, Thompson J, Talkington C, et al. Arterial embolectomy: a 34-year experience with 400 cases. Surg Clin North Am 66:339, 1986.

30. Palerito JS, Taylor KJ. Doppler color imaging. Peripheral arteries. Clin Diagn Ultrasound 27:97, 1992.

31. Pasch AR, Ricotta JJ, May AG. Abdominal aortic aneurysm: the case for elective resection. Circulation 70:I-1, 1984.

32. Porter SM, Baur EM. Pharmacologic treatment of intermittent claudication. Surgery 92:966, 1982.

33. Radack K, Wyderski RJ. Conservative management of intermittent claudication. Ann Intern Med 113:135, 1990.

34. Satiani B, Gross WS, Evans WE. Improved limb salvage after arterial embolectomy. Ann Surg 188:153, 1978.

35. Seeger JM, Abela GS, Silverman SH, et al. Initial results of laser recanalization in lower extremity arterial reconstruction. J Vasc Surg 9:10, 1989.

36. Szilagyi DE, Elliott JP, Smith RF. Clinical fate of the patient with asymptomatic abdominal aortic aneurysm and unfit for surgical treatment. Arch Surg 104:600, 1972.

37. Szilagyi DE, Smith R, DeRusso FJ, et al. Contribution of abdominal aortic aneurysmectomy to prolongation of life. Ann Surg 164:678, 1966.

38. Towne JB, Bandyk DF. Application of thrombolytic therapy in vascular occlusive disease. A surgical view. Am J Surg 154:548, 1987.

39. Winsberg G, Cole-Beuglet C, Mulder DS. Continuous ultrasound B scanning of abdominal aortic aneurysms. AJR 121:626, 1974.

40. Yao JST. Hemodynamic studies in peripheral arterial disease. Br J Surg 57:561, 1970.

C H A P T E R 88

Lower-Extremity Ulcers and Varicose Veins

ROBERT J. SPENCE, MD
CALVIN E. JONES, MD

LOWER-EXTREMITY ULCERS

Ulceration of a lower extremity, most often caused by either macrovascular or microvascular disease, is a common and important problem in ambulatory medical practice. Accurate diagnosis is based mainly on history and physical examination and is essential for appropriate treatment. Often the management of the various types of leg ulcers is completely different. Inappropriate therapy can lead to the loss of a toe or even a limb. Generally it is necessary to give detailed instructions to the patient and to have a great deal of patience. Patient compliance with treatment has been shown to be critical in the success of therapy and the prevention of recurrent ulceration (5).

History

A complete general medical history is extremely important. Illnesses such as arteriosclerotic vascular disease or hypertension, diabetes mellitus, sickle cell disease, and collagen–vascular disease may be associated with ulcers of the lower extremities. A history of corticosteroid therapy may explain failure of ulcers to heal. A history of drug abuse or a psychiatric history may be pertinent in the explanation of factitious ulcers.

Specific attention should be paid to duration of ulceration and previous attempts at therapy; symptoms of peripheral arteriosclerotic vascular disease, such as intermittent calf claudication, intermittent thigh or gluteal claudication, impotence, calf pain at rest, and feelings of coldness and tingling in the legs; a history of thrombophlebitis, ulceration, or injury to the lower extremities; a history of discomfort associated with footwear or of chronic swelling; and, if swelling has occurred, whether it has been alleviated by lying down.

Ischemic pain in the calf at rest is usually a symptom of advanced arteriosclerotic vascular disease, and it is characteristically alleviated if the patient dangles his or her feet over the edge of the bed, or sits in a chair, when awakened at night by ischemic pain. These symptoms must be differentiated from *nocturnal leg cramps* that occur in many people who have no evidence of peripheral vascular disease. Leg cramps are usually accompanied by palpable hardening of the calf muscles and involuntary muscle contraction of the flexor muscles of the toes. The cramps usually are relieved if the patient gets out of bed and walks around. Examination of the extremities in these patients (see below) is usually normal.

Physical Examination

A general physical examination of the patient is undertaken in conjunction with the examination of the lower extremities. The general examination should include a search particularly for abdominal aneurysm and other intra-abdominal masses, lymphatic masses in the groin, and signs of long-standing hypertension and cardiac disease. Needle tracks and brawny, indurated hands may indicate a history of drug abuse, as may skin ulcers in areas other than the lower extremities.

Examination of the Lower Extremities

Both lower extremities should be bared. Initial examination is performed while the patient is supine. Both legs are examined and compared. Particular points to be noted include *(a)* the presence of *pitting or nonpitting edema.* Pitting edema is a sign of chronic venous obstruction or of an acute inflammatory process. Nonpitting edema is a sign of lymphatic obstruction. If edema is present, it is important to note whether it is unilateral, and if it is bilateral, whether it is asymmetric or symmetric. Very firm, brawny edema suggests a very long-standing process; *(b)* the presence of *hemosiderin* deposited in the skin of the ankles (a sign of venous insufficiency); *(c)* the *general appearance* and quality of the skin, including hair growth (hair loss may signify arterial insufficiency); *(d)* evidence of *fungal infection* (scaling, apparently pruritic lesions); and *(e)* the *status of the nails* (deformity and hypertrophy are associated with arterial insufficiency).

After inspection of the feet and legs, a vascular examination of the lower extremities is conducted. Femoral, popliteal, dorsalis pedis, and posterior tibial pulses are palpated and graded. The *capillary refill time* after pressure on the toes with the legs elevated

45° is observed (normally less than 5 seconds). Auscultation from the midabdomen down to the popliteal regions is performed to detect bruits that are produced by narrowed atherosclerotic arteries. The temperature of the legs is felt with the dorsum of the hand, both descending from the thigh to the foot and comparing one side with the other. The patient is asked to sit up and to dangle his or her legs so that venous filling time and dependent rubor can be assessed. Evidence of *varicose veins* is best sought with the patient standing.

Inspection and Palpation of Ulcer or Ulcers

Ulcerated areas on the legs are often very tender; palpation, although necessary, should be done gently, with the gloved hand.

Site. An accurate description of the site of the ulcer, preferably with reference to some immovable anatomic landmark (e.g., the medial or the lateral malleolus) should be recorded.

Size. The size of the ulcer must be documented. The vertical and horizontal diameter in millimeters should be noted in the patient's record in a reproducible fashion. This measurement is particularly important for future reference when the progress of healing and the efficacy of treatment are assessed. Only by measuring in millimeters can the often subtle changes be appreciated in future evaluations.

General Character. It should be noted whether the ulcer is regular or irregular in outline. The edges should be examined to determine whether they are raised, heaped, everted, or flat, and whether they are undermined or there is any evidence of epithelial ingrowth from the edge of the ulcer toward the center (i.e., healing). The base should be examined to see whether it is clean or covered with exudate and to see the type of tissue of which it is constituted (e.g., clean fascia, granulation tissue, dirty exudate, debris). The vascularity of the base is the most critical characteristic to be noted when considering the potential of the ulcer for healing.

Tenderness. If the ulcer is tender, it should be determined whether it is very tender, such as in acute inflammation or ischemia, or only mildly tender, as in a neuropathy with loss of superficial sensation.

Changes in Adjoining Skin. It should be noted whether there are fluctuant areas of purulence near the ulcer, particularly on the sole of the foot; any callosities surrounding the ulcer; heavy deposition of pigment near the ulcer; or local edema.

When the examination of the ulcer is completed, the patient should stand, preferably on a stool, and face the examiner. Edema should now be looked for, as should the presence of varicose veins along the course of the short and long saphenous veins on the front and back of the legs (Fig. 88.1). In particular, the appearance of perforator varicosities (see "Physical Examination," under "Varicose Veins," below) should be noted, usually above the medial malleolus, and the relationship of these perforators to ulcerated areas should be sought.

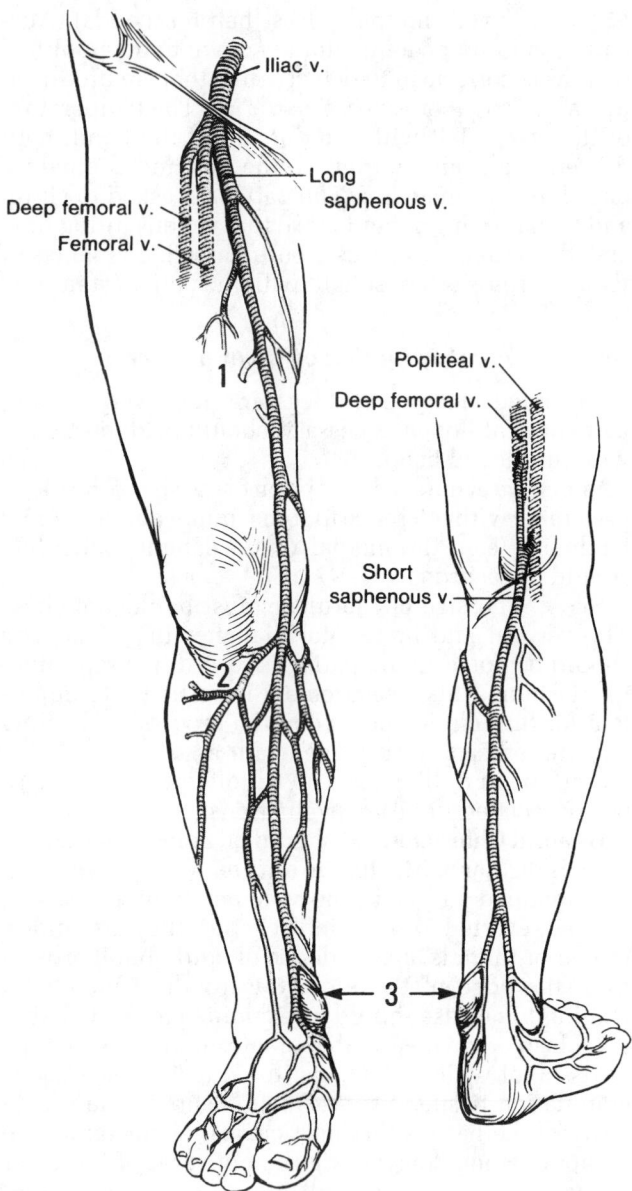

Figure 88.1. Venous circulation of the lower extremity. *1,* Hunter's canal perforator. *2,* Anterior communicating vein of the leg. *3,* Ankle perforators.

Types and Characteristics of Leg Ulcers

The principal characteristics of common ulcers are shown in Table 88.1.

Ulceration Associated with Venous Insufficiency

Chronic venous insufficiency is the most common cause of leg ulcers. The disorder probably follows deep venous thrombophlebitis with destruction of valves in the deep venous system and reversal of normal superficial-to-deep flow of blood in the perforating veins. The muscular action of the calf becomes ineffective, and blood flows to the superficial veins instead of in the usual centripetal direction through the deep venous system. Valves in the superficial (saphenous) system become incompetent, thereby raising the hydrostatic venous pressure at the ankle.

On a microcirculatory level, the old theory that stasis of venous blood was the cause of tissue hypoxia and necrosis has long been disproved; therefore, the term *stasis ulcer* is technically a misnomer. Browse and Burnand proposed the *fibrin cuff theory,* popular until recently, in which venous hypertension is postulated to distend the local capillary bed and widen the endothelial pores, allowing large molecules to escape. The most important of these molecules is assumed to be fibrinogen, which is believed to clot and form a fibrin cuff around the capillary. This cuff would be a barrier to the passage of oxygen and other nutrients leading to cell death and ulceration (1). More recent research suggests that venous hypertension leading to attachment and inappropriate activation of leukocytes in the cutaneous microcirculation with resultant endothelial injury is the more likely cause of ulceration associated with venous insufficiency. Although increased plasma fibrinogen and decreased fibrinolytic activity are present, there is also evidence of release of locally leukocyte-derived free radicals, proteolytic enzymes, cytokines, and other noxious mediators (2,13).

An important additional cause of recalcitrant venous ulcer is coexisting arterial disease seen in as many as 15 to 20% of patients (2). Often, minor trauma at the site is the initiating event in the process that culminates in an ulcer in a susceptible patient (see below).

The physical examination reveals edema, hemosiderin deposition, and ulceration, usually in line with the long saphenous vein, the short saphenous vein, or over a medial ankle perforator (Fig. 88.1). Arterial circulation in the leg may be entirely normal. Varicosities may or may not be present. The ulcer is usually fairly superficial and involves the skin, with irregular margins and with exudate covering the floor of the ulcer. The ulcer is usually movable with the skin and is tender. In grossly neglected cases, the ulceration may be massive and may involve most of the circumference of the leg. Occasionally, cellulitis may be evident, with erythema, tenderness, and fever secondary to superimposed bacterial infection (see Chapter 25).

Ulceration Associated with Arterial Insufficiency

Arterial insufficiency (see also Chapter 87) is the second most common cause of leg ulcers and, along with venous insufficiency, accounts for the great majority of leg ulcers. Ulcers associated with peripheral arterial occlusive disease usually begin with trauma and therefore appear at sites that are most subject to trauma (i.e., on toes, over the lateral or medial malleolus, at the base of the fifth metatarsal, at the head of the first metatarsal, on the heel or the ball of the foot, and in the distal pretibial region).

Ulcers secondary to occlusive arterial disease are characteristically painful, probably related to local inflammation and to ischemia. The foot may appear atrophic with shiny, fragile, transparent, hairless skin; the nails are often hypertrophied and deformed. Other hallmarks of arterial insufficiency (e.g., pulselessness and coolness) may be present. Because some patients are relieved of pain when they dangle the ulcerated leg, dependent edema may be present.

Dystrophic Ulcers

A neuropathic or dystrophic ulcer is usually associated with somatic or sympathetic neurologic dysfunction. The precise pathogenesis of these ulcers is unknown. Perhaps sympathetic dysfunction causes a reduction of arterial blood flow to local areas of skin that result in ulceration, or hypesthesia or anesthesia renders the patient more susceptible to trauma. Dystrophic ulcers are most commonly associated with peripheral neuropathies (see Chapter 84) and the neuropathies of congenital or acquired disease of the spinal cord, such as Friedreich's ataxia, syringomyelia, or multiple sclerosis. Peripheral neuropathies caused by vitamin deficiency or injuries may also result in ulcers. Ulceration almost always occurs in areas of pressure. The patient may complain of pain in the ulcer, but the ulcer is usually insensitive to light touch. There may be deformity in the foot associated with the neuropathy (*talipes calcaneovalgus* or *equinus,* deformities in which the anterior part of the foot is elevated and the heel is turned outward or in which the foot is plantar-flexed, respectively) or there may be a back deformity or surgical scar, as might occur in a patient with a meningomyelocele. Usually, neurologic examination of the lower extremity is abnormal, revealing decreased proprioception, decreased cutaneous sensation, and perhaps impaired movement. The ulcer may be undermined and there may be subcutaneous tracking of infected material into adjacent tissues that, on pressure, exude loculated pus from the undermined border of the ulcer. If the neuropathy is severe, the patient may be ambulating without pain, yet show advanced ulceration of the sole of the foot.

Posttraumatic Ulcers

Posttraumatic ulcers are common and usually are associated with impairment in nerve or vascular supply of the leg. Minor injury to the toe of a patient with arteriosclerotic occlusive vascular disease, or a leg injury in a patient with chronic venous insufficiency, may lead to ulceration. However, such ulcers may develop in the legs of otherwise healthy people, particularly after major injuries such as fractures that involve areas where vascular supply is normally marginal. The most susceptible site is the junction of the middle and lower third of the subcutaneous surface of the tibia. In this situation, most traumatic ulcers, even in healthy youngsters, heal with some difficulty, and in older patients and in those with even minimal arterial insufficiency, injury at this site resolves with great difficulty. Posttraumatic ulcers may be accompanied by problems of chronic infection and present with tenderness and local cellulitis.

Diabetic Ulcers

Diabetic ulcers have features of dystrophic, traumatic, and arterial ulcers because all three factors contribute to their development. The characteristic location of such an ulcer is in an area of pressure, such as a corn or a callosity (see Chapter 102). The ulcer is fairly insensitive, often heavily infected, with undermined edges and tracks under the plantar fascia or proximally on the dorsum of the foot. Although usually patients are aware that they are diabetic, some are not, and a thorough evaluation upon suspicion of diabetes is mandatory because control of the ulcer depends to a large extent on control of the diabetes. Radiologic examination is important because the bone underlying the ulcer may be the site of chronic osteomyelitis that necessitates surgical intervention (see example in Chapter 31, Fig. 31.1B).

Factitious Ulcers

Factitious ulcers are self-inflicted or self-maintained ulcers. Because they develop in the absence of any other local or systemic cause, diagnosis of factitious ulcers requires a high degree of suspicion. They most commonly occur in the legs of addicts who inject drugs into slightly varicose leg veins. The distribution of these ulcers is usually bizarre. They may be multiple and bilateral; if the history can be obtained, the diagnosis is easily made.

Factitious ulcers may also occur in patients with poor hygiene, psychiatric disorders, or disorders associated with pruritus, such as scabies, which has led to excoriation. The diagnosis should be suspected if the patient appears to derive some real or imaginary gain from having the ulcer. Any ulcer without a definite cause that fails to heal in an apparently healthy environment should lead to the suspicion that it is factitious.

Neoplastic Ulcers

Neoplastic ulcers of the leg are rare, but when they do occur, they are usually either basal cell or squamous cell carcinomas and have the usual characteristics of

Table 88.1 Characteristics of Common Leg Ulcers

Type of Ulcer	Usual Location	Edema	Pigmentation	Evidence of Arterial Insufficiency
Varicose	Medial leg	0 to +	0 to +	0
Stasis	Medial leg	++ to ++++	+++	0 to +
Arterial	Lateral leg, foot	0 to +	0	++++
Dystrophic	Sole, tip of toe	++	0	0
Traumatic	Midleg, toe	0	0	0 to ++++
Diabetic	Toes, dorsum, or foot	++	0	+ to +++
Factitious	Anywhere	+	0	0

these tumors (see Chapter 100). They have elevated or rolled edges, are anesthetic, and are usually attached to deeper tissue. *Marjolin's ulcer,* a rare form of squamous cell carcinoma that occurs in burn scars of long duration, also may be seen on the legs.

Hypertensive Ulcers

Another rare type of ulcer is associated with uncontrolled hypertension. It is thought that there is a progressive increase in the thickness of the arteriolar wall, decrease in the diameter of its lumen, progressive ischemia, and infarction of the skin (4). These ulcers are extremely painful and occur most often in women and on the posterolateral aspect of the leg and ankle. Ordinarily there is no evidence of peripheral arterial or venous disease.

Miscellaneous

Ulceration of the legs may occur in *sickle cell disease, polyarteritis nodosa* and other collagen diseases, and other systemic conditions (e.g., ulcerative colitis). In these instances, the diagnosis depends on making the diagnosis of the systemic disorder.

Corticosteroid therapy, particularly if it is long-standing, can lead to atrophy of the skin, increasing its fragility and susceptibility to injury. Furthermore, the impairment by corticosteroids of wound healing may prevent some ulcers from healing.

A toxic cause of skin ulceration is the *brown recluse spider bite,* common in the southeastern United States. The poison of the brown recluse spider contains a necrotizing enzyme that causes a rounded sloughing ulcer of approximately 3 to 4 cm with an indurated edge. The patient may not be aware of having been bitten by a spider. These ulcers are refractory to healing by use of conservative measures, and should be surgically excised and closed.

Cutaneous cytomegalovirus (CMV) infection has become more common in association with the increased incidence of acquired immune deficiency from human immunodeficiency virus (HIV) infection. CMV infection can cause lower-extremity ulceration.

In the tropics, ulceration of the foot and leg may occur from *local mycoses* such as *maduromycosis* and *cutaneous leishmaniasis;* these conditions should be kept in mind when a patient has returned from a tropical climate.

Laboratory Aids in Diagnosis

Bacteriology

Leg ulcers are often infected and almost invariably contaminated, usually with enteric organisms. Infections are particularly hazardous in diabetic patients and those with chronic arterial insufficiency. Cultures of the ulcer bed are useful, and cultures of obviously purulent ulcers are mandatory because antibiotic therapy is an important part of management, particularly when invasive infection is apparent (see Chapter 25). Viral culture of a small biopsy may be necessary to diagnose CMV-induced cutaneous ulceration. If fungal infection is suspected (unusual degree of scaling and excoriation), unless the physician is experienced in the scraping of lesions and the microscopic identification of fungi, dermatologic consultation is indicated.

Biopsy

Biopsy by a surgeon or a dermatologist is indicated if neoplastic or obscure fungal disease is suspected. Biopsy may be performed in the office under local anesthesia and should include a wedge-shaped section of the edge and floor of the ulcer. Any chronic ulcer that exists in a long-standing scar of any type should be biopsied to rule out squamous cell carcinoma. Sometimes only a biopsy of bone makes a definitive diagnosis of osteomyelitis that underlies a chronic ulcer.

Laboratory Tests for Systemic Disease

These tests are performed as dictated by the clinical diagnosis when the ulcer is suspected to be part of a systemic disorder (e.g., diabetes, polyarteritis nodosa, or sickle cell disease).

Noninvasive Vascular Testing

Noninvasive vascular testing is able to define the anatomy and function of the venous system of the lower extremities. Particularly in the case of persistent lower-extremity ulceration, noninvasive testing may be helpful in determining the cause and determining whether surgery might correct the venous problem and help heal the ulcer. When ulceration is noted in a patient with occlusive arterial disease, the patient should be referred to a vascular laboratory for testing. Noninvasive vascular testing is discussed more fully later in this chapter.

Natural History and Management

Generally, chronic ulcers develop initially from skin trauma, which may be exceedingly minor (3). However, the insult is compounded by a milieu of macrocirculatory or microcirculatory disease or other unfavorable local or systemic factors. Once the wound becomes inflamed, the local metabolic rate increases the demand for oxygen and nutrients, which leads to compromise and death of tissue when the demands are not met. The tissue then may become infected, resulting in more inflammation, propagating the cycle, making the ulcer enlarge and then become chronic. Treatment of the ulcer requires the breaking of this cycle.

Edema is commonly associated with lower-extremity ulcers, particularly those related to chronic venous disease. When present, it retards healing and reduces the skin resistance to trauma and subsequent infection. This makes the treatment of edema a very important component of ulcer therapy and prevention.

Chronic open wounds are all colonized by microorganisms to a greater or lesser extent. As long as an ulcer is an open wound, invasion by organisms is rare, and the threat of invasive infection and systemic toxicity is minimal. Furthermore, because the bacteria are on the surface of the wound rather than in the tissue, and the tissue in the base of the ulcer is often poorly vascularized, systemic antibiotics do not affect the surface flora significantly. Topical antibiotics are generally more appropriate for open wounds, and systemic antibiotics are reserved for evidence of invasive infections.

Pus under pressure (i.e., an abscess) greatly increases the risk of invasive infection. When a collection of loculated pus exists, it must be drained adequately. Eschars that overlie ulcers may hide such loculated pus and should generally be debrided. Wet eschars can simply be lifted with a tweezer and snipped. Dry eschars must be cut with a scissors or a scalpel along the plane of necrosis to avoid incising healthy tissue.

Most ulcers of the lower extremities can be treated on an ambulatory basis (5,7). However, the presence of one or both of the following may be an indication for hospitalization:

- The extent of the ulcer and the associated edema is so great that a period of absolute bed rest and elevation is required that is not possible outside the hospital.
- The appearance of invasive infection is heralded by cellulitis, lymphangitis, and systemic symptoms.

Ulceration Associated with Venous Insufficiency

Probably no other form of ulcer taxes the patient or the physician as much as that associated with chronic venous insufficiency (3,5). The mainstays of therapy are elimination of necrotic tissue and infection, cleansing of the ulcer bed to facilitate healthy tissue growth, and reduction of edema by elevation and compression. The patient should be at bed rest, and the ulcer should be treated with dressings and topical antibacterial agents if it is infected. Most of these ulcers heal by the use of nonoperative therapy.

The first step in managing these ulcers is to create an optimal environment. In the absence of other systemic factors, this step is primarily an attack on necrotic tissue, edema, and the bacterial colonization of the wound. Initial outpatient treatment consists of debridement of necrotic tissue and determination of the adequacy of arterial supply to the lower extremity in the office. Debridement can be performed safely using sharp scissors and forceps. Cutting within the necrotic tissue, leaving a thin layer above vascularized tissue, allows debridement without pain and bleeding. The residual necrotic layer resolves with adequate dressings, and wound and bacterial autolysis. Arterial inflow is adequate if bounding foot pulses are present, or the patient's ankle–brachial blood pressure index is greater than 0.8 (most accurately measured by a vascular laboratory).

Compression dressings can be used if arterial flow is adequate to reduce the edema, and should be worn whenever the extremity is dependent. Patients at home should be placed on bed rest with the extremity elevated. Wounds will not heal with contamination greater than 10^5 organisms per gram of tissue. After adequate bacteriologic cultures, a suitable topical antibacterial preparation such as silver sulfadiazine cream (e.g., Silvadene Cream 1%) or sodium oxychlorosene solution (Clorpactin 0.4% in water or isotonic saline) should be applied.

Invasive infection in the tissue surrounding the ulcer is uncommon, but should be suspected in ulcers in which an eschar trapped pus under pressure before debridement and in those that exhibit erythema, tenderness, and swelling locally. Invasive infection should be treated with an appropriate systemic antibiotic.

Recent studies suggest that systemic medical treatment with pentoxifylline may be given as adjunctive therapy. The drug is thought to reduce leukocyte activation and enhance fibrinolysis along with its well-recognized rheologic effects on blood and blood flow. Use of other systemic medications is less well established (2).

With intensive therapy, edema and bacterial overgrowth can be controlled in 48 to 72 hours. Thereafter, these optimal conditions must be maintained; healing is encouraged by the use of any one of several different dressings and techniques. Edema is kept to a minimum with leg elevation and compression bandages or stockings. Antibacterial dressings can be discontinued in favor of dressings more conducive to wound healing.

One of the following approaches can be used. (a) For *wet-to-dry dressing,* a sterile gauze pad moistened in normal saline (not soaking wet, as this can cause maceration) is secured over the ulcer (with a rolled bandage, not with an adhesive tape, which can damage the skin adjacent to an ulcer) and left to dry; necrotic tissue and other debris are removed when the dry dressing is removed, gently, at the end of each dressing interval. This procedure is appropriate early in ulcer management when there is substantial exudate and debris to remove, and there has been little healing. (b) Cleaner ulcers may have a similarly moistened dressing *(wet-to-wet dressing)* applied and then moistened again before removing. This results in somewhat less vigorous debridement, but protects the healing tissue of the ulcer. (c) The lower extremity may be wrapped with a zinc oxide–gelatin dressing (*Unna's boot,* Dome paste boot) that has long been used successfully in the treatment of leg ulcers. If used, it is imperative that it not be wrapped tightly and that it be placed smoothly from the metacarpal–phalangeal joints to just below the tibial tuberosity, including the heel. This can be done best by keeping the bandage roll on the surface of the leg as the leg is wrapped. Wrinkles, failure to wrap the heel, and too tight or too loose compression result in treatment failure, and can result in further ulcerations. The Unna's boot is then covered with an elastic (Ace) wrap for gentle compression. When first applied it should be removed within 48 hours to ascertain that the compression is adequate and that further problems are not being created. The bandage may then be reapplied and changed weekly, and healing usually results. An Unna's boot should not be applied if there is a suspicion of peripheral arterial disease because it could cause more ischemia. A similar type of dressing that has gained popularity is the *four-layer compression dressing.* This dressing works on a similar principle, but has an absorptive layer that may be useful, particularly for more exudative wounds. *(d)* When the ulcer is clean, or if it is quite shallow, a good alternative is a *hydrocolloid dressing* (e.g., Duoderm, Mitraflex) under an elastic bandage. This dressing does not disrupt the growth of healing tissue and allows healing in a moist environment (15). Small amounts of residual necrotic debris in the ulcer are removed by fibrinolytic action of the fluid that builds up under the dressing. It usually requires a change of dressing every 48 to 72 hours. However, it requires changing more frequently if the fluid that develops under the dressing strikes through (i.e., leaks out the side of the dressing).

Many new dressings are currently being evaluated in the treatment of lower-extremity ulcers. These include calcium alginate, hydrogels, and new types of debriding gauzes. Serial compression pumps to reduce edema are now available for home use. No conclusions can be drawn at this time regarding any outstanding efficacy of any of these new treatments.

Occasionally, diuretics may be helpful in managing edema even when no element of cardiac or renal failure exists. Elastic compression should always be used first to avoid the danger of volume depletion.

Ultimately, if edema and bacterial colonization can be controlled, the ulcer will usually heal, although several weeks to months may be required. After the healing, the patient must be advised to keep the leg elevated, if possible, when sitting down and to wear some form of elastic compression permanently, preferably a made-to-measure elastic support garment.

If the ulcer still fails to heal, skin grafting may be required along with venous ligation and stripping. This requires surgical consultation and hospitalization.

Ulceration Associated with Arterial Insufficiency

Arterial ulcers are very difficult to heal unless blood flow to the area can be improved. Therefore, if there is any suspicion of arterial insufficiency, the patient should be referred for noninvasive vascular testing and, possibly, surgical evaluation. If the patient's lesion is unsuitable for surgical correction, or if the patient has already had an operation but ulceration persists, the ulcer can sometimes be healed with painstaking debridements every 2 or 3 days. However, this treatment requires expertise; if doubt exists, surgical referral should be made.

A pair of sharp scissors or a scalpel is used to remove the dry eschar that covers the ulcer and to remove the necrotic edges of the ulcer carefully without causing bleeding (see above). Wet-to-wet dressings are then applied, using a topical antibiotic solution such as sodium oxychlorosene or polymyxin–bacitracin 5% aqueous suspension. The patient is instructed to apply the bandage wet in the morning and to remove it in the evening after wetting it again. This has the effect of debriding the ulcer and promoting wound healing, consisting of wound contraction and reepithelialization.

Very tenacious residual necrotic debris after sharp debridement may be removed with a short course of a *proteolytic enzyme* (e.g., Travase) applied three to four times a day followed by the application of a wet-to-dry dressing, or by hydrocolloid dressings. In conjunction with these measures, meticulously compulsive foot protection, soft footwear, elevation of the extremity, and avoidance of weight bearing are mandatory.

Dystrophic Ulcers

Dystrophic ulcers are a real threat to the limb because infection often advances unnoticed by the patient until there is considerable spread of pus under the eschar or in the tissue around the ulcer. Treatment consists of bed rest, relieving pressure on bony prominences frequently, appropriate antibiotic therapy as indicated after culture (see Chapter 25), debridement of necrotic skin edges (which can be done without anesthesia in the office; see above), and wet-to-wet dressings as described above.

Once the ulcer has been rendered clean by debridement and dressings, slow healing may progress, often over several months. In patients with dystrophic foot ulcers, total contact casting (see "Diabetic Ulcers," below) has been successful in relieving pressure on the ulcer and providing an environment conducive to healing. This technique has provided a new means of treating these patients while they remain ambulatory and has considerably reduced hospitalization rates for this condition.

Traumatic Ulcers

Traumatic ulcers usually heal by avoidance of weight bearing, elevation, topical antibiotic therapy when the ulcer is infected, and protection of the ulcer by dressings (see above). If no progress is made within 2 to 3 weeks, the patient should be seen by a surgeon for possible operative debridement and surgical closure of the wound.

Diabetic Ulcers

Infected diabetic ulcers impose such a serious risk of limb loss that most of these patients should be hospitalized. In the hospital, diabetes can be regulated more meticulously, any pockets of suppuration can be drained, proper debridement can be carried out, and bone biopsy can be done if osteomyelitis is suspected.

Once the ulcers are clean and uninfected, leg elevation and avoidance of pressure and shearing forces on the area of ulceration will allow healing. In patients with foot ulcers, *total contact casting* has been successful in alleviating these forces and in providing an optimal environment for healing while the patient remains ambulatory. The procedure involves the application of a plaster cast directly to the foot (without first wrapping the foot in gauze, as would be done for a fracture). The patient's weight is thereby distributed evenly over the entire foot, reducing pressure on the ulcer. Ordinarily, the cast is left in place for approximately a week. This technique is best provided by specialists experienced in its use because improper cast application can result in development of other skin problems or of worsening of the ulcer.

Factitious Ulcers

The key to the management of factitious ulcers is making the diagnosis. The diagnosis is made by maintaining a high degree of suspicion, particularly in ulcers that have no clear cause and occur in what appears to be an otherwise healthy environment. These ulcers usually heal if the cause can be found and controlled. An ulcer suspected of being a factitious ulcer can often be diagnosed and treated simultaneously by placing an occlusive dressing that prevents the patient from manipulating the ulcer. These patients must be carefully followed to monitor progress and to avoid the development of problems under the occlusive dressing.

Hypertensive Ulcers

Control of the patient's chronic hypertension and education regarding the importance of long-term control are the two keystones in the management of hypertensive ulcers. Otherwise, the management follows the general principles applied to venous stasis ulcers.

Chronic Ulcers Associated with Corticosteroid Treatment

Systemic corticosteroids have an inhibitory effect on wound healing that can be partially reversed by vitamin A. Ulcers that fail to heal in patients being treated with corticosteroids may be treated with vitamin A 25,000 units per day orally; ointments containing vitamin A (e.g., A and D Ointment) may be used alone or in combination (with silver sulfadiazine cream, for example) directly on the ulcer.

Neoplastic and Other Ulcers

Neoplastic and other unusual ulcers, such as that from the previously mentioned brown recluse spider bite, are a surgical problem; these patients should be referred promptly for consultation.

Growth Factor Therapy

Recent literature suggests that certain growth factors may be capable of reversing some or all of the adverse effects caused by some of the underlying local and systemic factors that contribute to lower-extremity ulcers. Specifically, *fibroblast growth factor* (FGF) and *transforming growth factor β* (TGF-β) seem to be most effective. Efforts to use this new form of therapy include wound healing centers, which use derivatives of the patient's blood, and the use of cultured or banked allograft skin in an attempt to apply growth factors to chronic ulcers. The use of synthetic or genetically engineered specific growth factors is still experimental but holds great promise for better therapy for lower-extremity ulcers in the near future.

Prevention and General Foot Care in Susceptible Patients

Foot and leg ulcers from any cause often recur after healing because, with the exception of varicose veins, factitious ulcers, and surgically corrected occlusive arterial disease, the underlying disease is difficult to reverse. It is therefore mandatory to be familiar with the principles of foot care, and patients must understand and carry out instructions aimed at minimizing exposure to trauma. Patients with peripheral arterial disease or diabetes should wear very comfortable footwear, even if it is not fashionable (see Chapter 102). The front of the shoe should be broad so that the toes can spread. Areas of pressure caused by foot deformities should be corrected by orthopedic shoes with appropriate fittings (e.g., insoles or metatarsal bars); patients with these problems should be referred to an orthopedic surgeon or podiatrist.

Patients should be instructed to keep their feet very clean (i.e., at least once-daily showers or footbaths in tepid water). Patients with impaired cutaneous sensation should use a mirror to examine the undersurface of their feet daily.

Nails should be carefully trimmed, preferably with clippers; under no circumstances should sharp scissors be used to trim the sides of nails because they may injure the delicate nail fold and become a portal of entry for infection. Patients can protect their toes during walking by inserting small, fluffy pieces of cotton wool between them. Lanolin or other emollient creams are useful in preventing cracking of hardened areas of skin and keeping the skin soft and supple. Patients should avoid extremes of temperature and should reduce exposure to trauma (e.g., a night light in the bedroom to avoid stubbing a toe). With attention to these small details, recurring trouble can often be prevented.

VARICOSE VEINS

Causes

Varicose (swollen) veins of the lower extremities are common; they affect women more often than men, and usually become symptomatic between the ages of 20 and 40. The prevalence of varicose veins varies widely, ranging from a low among women of lowland New Guinea of 0.1%, to a high among the women of South Wales of 50%. In the United States, varicose veins affect 19% of men and 36% of women.

Varicose veins are caused by an incompetence of the valves of the long or short saphenous veins (Fig. 88.1), permitting retrograde or downward flow of blood, or simply stagnation of the normal centripetal flow (8). In the perforator system, which is a system of veins communicating between the deep and the superficial veins, destruction of valves interferes with the unidirectional movement of blood from superficial to deep.

The disorder is aggravated, indeed may be caused, by conditions elevating intra-abdominal pressure, such as pregnancy, large intra-abdominal tumors, conditions causing chronic straining (e.g., prostatic obstruction, carcinoma of the sigmoid colon), and occasionally mechanical interference with venous return in the venous system itself, such as thrombosis of the pelvic veins.

Symptoms

The symptoms of uncomplicated varicose veins usually consist of heaviness and aching in the area of the veins or in the calves. The patient may complain of mild edema at the end of a long day's work. Occasionally, patients complain of varicose veins for cosmetic reasons and desire treatment. Patients with uncomplicated varicose veins do not complain of intermittent claudication or severe pain; in the presence of these symptoms, other causes must be carefully sought. Occasionally, thrombophlebitis supervenes in a varicose vein and causes severe pain; the vein is then palpable as an inflamed cord. After bed rest, elevation, application of local heat, and appropriate anti-inflammatory therapy (e.g., aspirin), the varix in the thrombosed vein disappears.

Physical Examination

It is useful to have some idea of the anatomy of the venous system of the leg (Fig. 88.1). This makes it possible to judge the patient's symptoms on the basis of an anatomic abnormality detected by physical examination. There are several types of varicose veins, which conform to the underlying anatomic arrangement of these veins.

Telangiectasia (Sunburst Varices)

These are not, in the true sense of the word, varicose veins but rather dilations of subcutaneous venous plexuses that have a spiderlike arrangement and an unsightly purple color. These veins are often the object of cosmetic complaints by patients. Otherwise, they are essentially asymptomatic.

Varicosities of Long Saphenous System

Varicosities of the long saphenous system are the most common type of varicose veins. The long saphenous vein begins anterior to the medial malleolus at the ankle, courses superficially to the medial side of the knee, and then curves upward to enter the deep system just below the inguinal ligament medial to the femoral artery. The vein has several tributaries in the calf and in the thigh that are superficial, and it is also joined by several perforating veins from the deep venous system; the valves at these junctions can become incompetent and lead to focal varicosities (Fig. 88.1). There are three or four consistent perforators: three above the medial malleolus at a distance separated by approximately 3 cm, and a fourth just above the knee joint. If varicosities appear in this situation, the perforator system is almost certainly incompetent. Varicosity of the long saphenous vein is clearly visible with the patient standing.

Varicosities of Short Saphenous System

The short saphenous vein arises behind the lateral malleolus and courses upward behind the calf to join the popliteal vein in the popliteal space (Fig. 88.1). Varicosities of this system are best seen with the patient standing with his or her back to the examiner.

Perforator Varicosities

As mentioned above, perforator incompetence is usually noticed in the long saphenous vein where the ankle perforators and the above-the-knee perforator join the vein; however, perforators join other superficial veins that, in turn, join the long and short saphenous system. Examination may reveal that there is no incompetence of the short or long saphenous veins, only of the perforators.

Clinical Testing to Determine Level of Incompetence

One or two easy clinical tests can be performed in the office that will aid in determination of the severity of the problem and selection of appropriate treatment.

Trendelenburg's Test

The patient lies supine and raises the affected leg to empty the veins. A venous tourniquet is applied just below the saphenous opening about 3 inches (7.7 cm) below the inguinal ligament and the patient then stands up. Constriction is released; if the saphenofemoral valve is incompetent, the veins will fill immediately from above; if not, the veins fill slowly from below. If the veins fill rapidly from above before the release of the tourniquet, this indicates an incompetent valve at the entry of the long saphenous vein into the femoral vein and signifies major long saphenous incompetence. This test is now repeated at successively lower levels in the leg so the location of incompetence may be mapped.

Perthes's Test

Perthes's test is a test for deep venous thrombosis in association with varicose veins. A tourniquet is lightly applied below the inguinal ligament, as in Trendelenburg's test, and the patient is instructed to walk in place. If varicose veins are accompanied by a thrombosed deep femoral system, the varicose veins become prominent after this exercise.

Noninvasive Vascular Testing

The advent of the modern vascular laboratory has revolutionized the evaluation of varicose veins. Any patient who, by physical examination, is suspected of having venous incompetence at the saphenous femoral junction should be referred to a noninvasive vascular laboratory for evaluation before treatment is planned.

Effective treatment of lower-extremity venous insufficiency is predicated on accurate localization of the problem. Various noninvasive vascular examinations and radiologic studies can be successfully used to define the anatomic extent of venous reflux (16). The utility and limitations of these modalities are based on the concept of systolic and diastolic closure of lower-extremity venous valves. Venous valves close in response to two distinct physiologic actions. Coaptation of valve cusps occurs during muscular contraction and subsequent forward (toward the heart) flow of blood (systolic closure). These valves include side branches and perforator veins. Diastolic closure occurs immediately following relaxation of muscular contraction when valves proximal to that contraction close to prevent reflux of blood.

Ambulatory venous pressure measurement is performed by cannulating a vein on the dorsum of the foot with a small gauge butterfly needle connected to a pressure transducer, amplifier, and recorder. Resting pressures are obtained with the patient standing still, supporting his or her weight on a frame. After the completion of 10 toe raises at one per second, another pressure reading is obtained. This is defined as the *ambulatory venous pressure* (AVP). The *pressure recovery time* (PRT) is the time for the pressure to return to the resting baseline pressure. In practice, measurement of the time to return to 90% of resting pressure provides a more reproducible PRT. Application of a 2.5-cm-wide pneumatic cuff or occlusive elastic tourniquet above and then below the knee permits segregation of the superficial venous system from the deep system. Obliteration of the saphenous system in this manner permits differentiation of the level of reflux. An AVP in excess of 45 mm Hg signifies venous incompetence, as does a PRT of less than 18 seconds. If the AVP and PRT remain abnormal after the segregation of the saphenous (superficial) system by tourniquets, deep venous and perforator involvement should be suspected (10,14).

Ambulatory venous pressure measurement is highly sensitive in the detection of venous reflux and is a direct measure of venous pressure. Limitations of this test include inconsistent reproducibility, patient discomfort, and lack of efficacy as a screening test.

The simplest noninvasive test for lower-extremity venous reflux is *continuous wave (CW) Doppler.* The examiner insonates the venous system with a Doppler probe and listens for venous reflux after provocative maneuvers, such as Valsalva maneuver or manual compression proximal to the transducer. The Valsalva maneuver and proximal compression normally result in the cessation of venous flow. The presence of venous signals during these maneuvers is indicative of venous reflux. CW Doppler samples any structure in the path of the emitted ultrasound and does not allow for discrimination of the vein being tested. Similarly, anatomic variations such as bifid veins will be unrecognized.

Photoplethysmography (PPG) can readily provide a noninvasive assessment of lower-extremity venous valvular function. PPG venous testing is performed with the patient in a sitting or standing position. A PPG diode that emits infrared light is placed superior to the medial malleolus (9). The amount of attenuation of the emitted and subsequently reflected light is related to numerous factors, which include the amount of blood in the tissues. Changes in the reflected light can be displayed qualitatively on a strip chart. After the establishment of a resting baseline recording, the lower extremity venous system is emptied by alternating plantar flexion and dorsiflexion of the foot or firm calf compressions. This results in a fall from the baseline on the strip chart. While the patient remains motionless, venous refill, which is displayed as a slow rise on the

chart, is recorded. The time from completion of venous emptying to return of PPG reading to baseline represents the *venous recovery time* (VRT). A VRT less than 23 seconds is considered abnormal. Similar to AVP testing, the saphenous system can be occluded with pneumatic cuffs or elastic tourniquets to permit differentiation of the level of disease. Normalization of a shortened VRT after application of an above-knee tourniquet demonstrates superficial venous incompetence. The deep/perforator system is considered involved if the VRT remains abnormal after constriction of the superficial veins.

Venous PPG has the advantage of being noninvasive and easily performed. Inconsistency of the effort of the patient to perform the necessary maneuvers and the inability to provide quantitative data are limitations of this modality. Similarly, PPG testing does not detect proximal valvular insufficiency in the presence of competent distal veins.

Vascular duplex scanning combines high-resolution ultrasonic imaging with pulsed-wave Doppler. This allows real-time visualization of vascular structures and precise placement of the Doppler sample. In addition to spectral waveforms, the Doppler information can be displayed in a color-coded format on the gray-scale image. The spectral waveforms and color coding obtained by Doppler depicts the velocity of the blood flow as defined by the Doppler equation. The Doppler-derived velocity is a vector that processes both magnitude and direction. Analysis of the Doppler data can therefore demonstrate the direction of blood flow relative to the transducer (14). The saphenofemoral and saphenopopliteal junctions can be imaged in the groin and popliteal space, respectively, and venous flow recorded by spectral analysis or color Doppler. Venous reflux in response to Valsalva maneuver or proximal limb compression can be observed as either waveforms that are inverted to the normal antegrade flow or color coding indicating retrograde flow. Duplex ultrasonography offers selective sampling of venous structures and precise localization of disease. A brief wisp of reflux is often observed following provocative maneuvers, and retrograde Doppler flow that lasts longer than 1 second is considered abnormal. The entire length of the deep and superficial systems can be interrogated. Careful duplex examination of the medial calf and thigh can demonstrate incompetent perforator veins. Not only is this diagnostic, but it can be used to localize and mark perforators for surgical ligation. Deep venous thrombosis can also be readily identified by this modality.

Venous duplex scanning must be performed by a skilled operator and requires expensive ultrasound equipment (14). However, its noninvasive nature makes it acceptable to patients. Duplex scanning correlates with AVP and can be used to quantitate the volume of reflux, which correlates with the degree of venous stasis skin changes (16).

Treatment

Depending on the patient's presentation, four options are available.

Observation

Observation is an acceptable option in patients with mild to moderate asymptomatic subcutaneous varices with no history of postural edema, superficial phlebitis, stasis dermatitis, or pain.

If the offending telangiectatic venous plexus is large enough to accommodate a 25-gauge needle, a sclerosing solution may be injected. The technique is described below. Other treatments such as freezing with carbon dioxide snow, cautery under local anesthesia, and even laser therapy have been advocated, but their use requires a great deal of skill, and unnecessary skin scarring may result that is, in the end, more unsightly than the original vein. Probably the safest treatment of this kind of vein is the use of masking cosmetic creams, together with reassurance.

Support Hose

Support hose maintain compression of subcutaneous varicose veins and prevent edema. Graduated compression hose in the 30- to 40-mm Hg range are available in most pharmacies in various ready-to-fit sizes including knee, thigh, and panty hose configurations. The patient should be measured and fit early in the morning before any edema has developed in order to obtain maximal therapeutic benefit from the compression hose. They should be worn continuously, removed at bedtime, and reapplied immediately upon arising in the morning.

Sclerotherapy

Sclerotherapy is efficacious for segmental subcutaneous varicose veins that are not associated with significant greater or lesser saphenous valvular incompetence, and for cosmetically unacceptable telangiectasia (17).

The procedure can easily be performed in the office by anyone skilled with a needle; however, the patient should be warned that several sittings may be required for complete elimination of the veins.

Technique. The patient stands with a tight tourniquet around the thigh, just enough to make the vein prominent. The area of the vein is lightly prepared with a suitable antiseptic, and 0.5 mL of sclerosing solution is injected by use of a 2-mL syringe, after initial aspiration to make sure the needle is in the vein. Immediately after the end of the injection, the needle is withdrawn and the vein is gently compressed with a 2- × 2-inch gauze for 3 minutes, after which the tourniquet is released and compression is continued for 2 minutes more. The patient wears an Ace bandage on the area for approximately 4 hours. The sclerosant produces an inflammatory reaction in the intima, which obliterates the vein. Failure to use a tourniquet may release an unnecessarily large amount of sclerosant into the major veins of the leg and cause undesirable thrombosis at distant sites. The patient should be warned that extravasation of the sclerosant is a possibility and may cause a small skin slough. Several commercially available sclerosant solutions, morrhuate sodium and sodium tetradecyl sulfate (Sotradecol), are suitable for injection.

Surgical Therapy

There is increasing interest among vascular surgeons in reconstructive rather than obliterative surgery for varicosities accompanied by valvular incompetence in the iliac, femoral, saphenofemoral, popliteal, and deep perforating veins that has caused greater and lesser saphenous insufficiency (18). The reconstructive approach may include various methods of direct and indirect valvuloplasty (11,12). Excision and stripping of a long and a short saphenous vein should be the last treatment option.

Symptomatic patients should be referred for surgical consultation. Attempts to inject and compress veins associated with clear-cut varicosities of the major superficial systems are doomed to failure without surgical intervention; nevertheless, injection or primary treatment of saphenous varicosities is preferred in some centers, mostly in Europe.

If an operation has been performed on the long or short saphenous system, there are often residual varicosities of a minor degree that require additional injection therapy, which may be performed in the office. The recurrence rate of major varicosities after operation is 10 to 20% in most large series.

Varicose veins should not be treated in patients who have an underlying cause associated with increased intra-abdominal pressure until the primary cause has been removed. However, the wearing of elastic stockings may give comfort during this time. Such stockings may be advisable for support in any patient with varicose veins in whom other treatment is undesirable or contraindicated. A further consideration in the selection of therapy is whether the patient has coronary artery disease; although veins that are severely varicose are not suitable for use in coronary bypass surgery, if patients have minimal varicose veins and may become candidates for a coronary artery bypass, these veins should be preserved, if possible, for potential use (6). Weight reduction in overweight patients is advisable for anyone with varicose veins, regardless of other modes of treatment.

General References

Barr DM. The Unna's boot as a treatment for venous ulcers. Nurse Prac 21:55, 1996.

Goldman MP, ed. Treatment of varicose and telangiectatic leg veins. St. Louis: CV Mosby, 1991.
> A superb compendium of office sclerotherapy.

Goldman MP, Bergan JJ. Ambulatory treatment of venous disease: an illustrative guide. St. Louis: CV Mosby, 1996.

Gottlob R, May R, eds. Venous valves. New York: Springer-Verlag, 1986.
> Discussion of morphology, function, radiology, and reconstructive surgery of venous valves.

Kistner RL. Veins and lymphatics. In: Hardy JD, ed. Textbook of surgery. Philadelphia: JB Lippincott, 1988.
> A good discussion of modern noninvasive vascular testing, as well as a discussion of surgical techniques available for the treatment of varicose veins.

Kominsky SJ. The ambulatory total contact cast. In: Frykberg RG, ed. The high-risk foot in diabetes mellitus. New York: Churchill Livingstone, 1991;449.

Ludbrook J. Primary great saphenous varicose veins revisited. World J Surg 10:954, 1986.

> An excellent overall review of the status of varicose vein therapy, and a discussion of theories of etiology.

Phillips TJ, Dover JS. Leg ulcers. J Am Acad Dermatol 26(6):965, 1991.

Rutherford RD, ed. Vascular surgery. 3rd ed. Philadelphia: WB Saunders, 1989.

> Several chapters of this excellent vascular surgery text are devoted to the diagnosis and treatment of lower-extremity venous disease.

Samitz MH. Ulcers. In: Samitz MH, ed. Cutaneous disorders of the lower extremities. Philadelphia: JB Lippincott, 1981;191.

Tam M, Moschella SL. Vascular skin ulcers of limbs. Cardiol Clin 9:555, 1991.

Tremblay S, Lewis EW, Allen PT. Selecting a treatment for primary varicose veins. Can Med Assoc J 133:20, 1985.

> A sensible discussion of options.

Trout A. Chronic skin ulcers. Emerg Med Clin North Am 10:823, 1992.

Walshe C. Living with a venous leg ulcer: a descriptive study of patients' experiences. J Adv Nursing 22:1092, 1995.

Specific References

1. Browse NL, Burnand KG. The cause of venous ulceration. Lancet 2:243, 1982.
2. Dormandy JA. Pharmacologic treatment of venous leg ulcers. J Cardiovasc Pharmacol 25(Suppl 2):S61, 1995.
3. Douglas WS, Simpson NB. Guidelines for the management of chronic venous leg ulceration. Report of a multidisciplinary workshop. Br J Dermatol 132:446, 1995.
4. Duncan HJ, Faris IB. Martorell's hypertensive ischemic leg ulcers are secondary to an increase in the local vascular resistance. J Vasc Surg 2:581, 1985.
5. Erickson CA, Lanza DJ, Karp DL, et al. Healing of venous ulcers in an ambulatory care program: the roles of chronic venous insufficiency and patient compliance. J Vasc Surg 22: 629, 1996.
6. Friedell ML, Samson RH, Cohen MJ, et al. High ligation of the greater saphenous vein for treatment of lower extremity varicosities: the fate of the vein and therapeutic results. Ann Vasc Surg 6:5, 1992.
7. Friedman SJ, Su WPD. Management of leg ulcers. Am Fam Physician 27:219, 1983.
8. Goldman MP, Fronek A. Anatomy and pathophysiology of varicose veins. J Dermatol Surg Oncol 15:138, 1989.
9. Nicolaides AN, Miles C. Photoplethysmography in the assessment of venous insufficiency. J Vasc Surg 5:405, 1987.
10. Nicolaides AN, Zukowski AJ. The value of dynamic venous pressure measurements. World J Surg 10:919, 1986.
11. O'Donnell TF, Mackey WC, Shepard AD, et al. Clinical, hemodynamic, and anatomic follow-up of direct venous reconstruction. Arch Surg 122:474, 1987.
12. Raju S, Fredericks R. Valve reconstruction procedures for nonobstructive venous insufficiency: rationale, techniques, and results in 107 procedures with two to eight-year follow-up. J Vasc Surg 154:189, 1987.
13. Smith PDC. The microcirculation in venous hypertension. Cardiovasc Res 32:789, 1996.
14. van Bemmelen PS, Bedford G, Beach K, Strandess, DE. Quantitative segmental evaluation of venous valvular reflux with duplex ultrasound scanning. J Vasc Surg 10:425, 1989.
15. van Rijswijk L, Brown D, Friedman S, et al. Multicenter clinical evaluation of a hydrocolloid dressing for leg ulcers. Cutis 35:173, 1985.
16. Vasdekis SN, Clarke H, Nicolaides AN. Quantification of venous reflux by means of duplex scanning. J Vasc Surg 10:670, 1989.
17. Weiss RA, Weiss MA, Goldman MP. Physicians' negative perception of sclerotherapy for venous disorders: review of a 7 year experience with modern sclerotherapy. South Med J 85:1101, 1992.
18. Wilson NM, Rutt DL, Browse NL. Repair and replacement of deep vein valves in the treatment of venous insufficiency. Br J Surg 78:388, 1991.

C H A P T E R 89

Diseases of the Breast

MICHAEL J. PURTELL, MD
LARRY WATERBURY, MD

One of every eight women in the United States will develop breast cancer. It is the second leading cause of cancer deaths among women, with 182,000 new cases seen each year and 44,000 deaths (50,52). Not surprisingly, the fear of breast cancer is prominent in the patient who has breast-related complaints, although most of these are secondary to benign causes. The primary care physician must have a rational approach to the diagnosis and treatment of breast complaints and breast masses. He or she carries out the screening program for cancer and supervises the patients' referral. If cancer is found, the primary physician is the one to whom the patient initially turns for information. A reassuring patient–doctor relationship is critical in dealing with this emotionally charged area of medicine.

NORMAL ANATOMY AND PHYSIOLOGY OF THE BREAST

The breast is a modified sweat gland. An extension of breast tissue reaches toward the axilla. There are 12 to 20 acini arranged like a bunch of grapes, with draining ducts emptying into openings on the nipple. These ducts are lined by two layers of epithelium, one of which serves as a basement membrane and source of epithelial cell reproduction. This "reverse layer" can proliferate in certain pathologic conditions. Surrounding each duct is a specialized periductal fibrous layer, which is under hormonal influence.

With each menstrual cycle, a fall in hormonal activity at the menses results in the desquamation of duct lining, which proliferates again at the cessation of menses. Increases in periductal vascularity and lymphocytic infiltration accompany this proliferation. During pregnancy the ducts and acini proliferate maximally, often never returning to normal in the postpartum period. In many parts of the breast, the glandular hypertrophy remains until it involutes at menopause. At that time there is a loss of parenchyma and an increase in fat, especially in the periductal region. The lobular anatomy slowly disappears. Variations in hormonal balance result in various benign pathologic conditions occurring during the active menstrual childbearing years and at menopause. It is important to realize that anatomic changes associated with normal hormonal fluctuations during a menstrual cycle do not occur to the same degree in all areas of the breast. This accounts for the asymmetric palpatory findings in the normal breast, which is often lumpy.

SCREENING PROCEDURES

Physical examination (see below) and mammography are useful screening procedures for the detection of breast masses (11,16,61,62). Mammographic techniques have improved considerably and the radiation exposure per examination has dropped to very low levels so that the risk of inducing breast cancer from routine screening mammography is almost negligible. Routine screening mammography in women over age 50 (but poorly studied over age 74) has been proven in controlled studies to decrease death from breast cancer (11,61). The American Cancer Society recommends yearly screening in this age group, although other studies show similar effectiveness with screening intervals of 2 to 3 years (61). All physicians should encourage routine physical examination and screening mammography in women over age 50. Although mammography is the more sensitive of the two screening procedures, physical examination is also important because up to 15% of palpable breast cancers are not visualized on mammography (36). Self-examination of the breast is often advocated but there is no evidence that it is effective (62) and certainly should not substitute for an examination by the physician and mammography.

Routine screening mammography in women under age 50 remains controversial except for women with increased risk by virtue of a previous breast cancer or a strong family history (4,11,12,16,19,36,65). The American Cancer Society and the American College of Radiology recommend baseline mammography between ages 35 and 40 and mammography yearly thereafter. Other organizations disagree. Both the American and Canadian Task Forces on periodic health examination do not recommend routine screening mammography before the age of 50 (11,36,46,65). In early 1997, the National Institutes of Health held a consensus conference devoted to breast cancer screening. It was concluded that there were not enough data to recommend routine mammographic screening for women under age 50. This statement stirred considerable public debate. The National Cancer Institute subsequently distanced itself from this conclusion and issued an independent recommendation for screening beginning at age 40. There are several reasons for this controversy: Although mammography can certainly identify non-palpable, highly curable breast cancers in young women, studies today have not demonstrated a convincing effect on survival in women under age 50. Many of the tumors found in the young are *in situ* cancers that may not become invasive for years, if ever. Of major concern is the lack of test specificity in young women, who often have dense breasts, complicating interpretation. This leads to a much higher benign to malignant biopsy ratio than that found in older women. In order to find cancer, lesions that are associated with cancer only 5% of the time or less are often biopsied (48). Thus, large numbers of normal women must undergo physical and psychologic trauma to find the occasional woman potentially benefited by the diagnosis of an early cancer. The recommendation for early follow-up of a suspicious lesion is potentially more harmful than biopsy. The impact of this frequent recommendation on a young woman (usually with no disease) is poorly studied but is likely to be profound, especially if she has problems with anxiety, depression, or somatization. Unfortunately, for the immediate future it will be up to the primary care physician and his or her anxious patient to sort through the complex scientific and political considerations.

Whatever decision the primary physician makes about the usefulness of screening mammography in the young woman, it is important that an office interview be scheduled for anyone contemplating screening. A woman needs to understand her likely experience when she goes for testing, particularly if it is her first mammogram. Patients should know that mammography may be uncomfortable because of the need for breast compression. The postmammography plan of communication should be worked out ahead of time to minimize the anxiety of waiting for a phone call. Young women in particular should understand the poor specificity of the test and the high likelihood of a recommendation for intervention (biopsy or early follow-up), especially with the first mammogram. The patient should know that if she receives that recommendation, in most instances, the chance of benign or no disease far outweighs the chance of cancer.

CLINICAL CHARACTERISTICS OF COMMON DISEASES OF THE BREAST
Benign Tumors

Fibroadenoma

Fibroadenoma is the most common cause of a unilateral discrete mass in the 15- to 35-year-old age group. The peak incidence is from 20 to 25 years of age. In 10 to 15% of cases, there are multiple tumors. Rapid growth seen during pregnancy, just before menopause, and in animals given estrogens all suggest that fibroadenomas are under hormonal control. The natural history of a fibroadenoma is that of a tumor growing rapidly in the pregnant patient and then growing old with the patient, perhaps calcifying in the postmenopausal woman.

A fibroadenoma has both fibrous and epithelial components. The tumor probably arises from terminal ducts and lobules, and the rare finding of lobular carcinoma rather than intraductal carcinoma within or in the vicinity of a fibroadenoma is consistent with such an origin.

The patient with a fibroadenoma usually complains only of the mass and denies pain, nipple discharge, or other breast changes. On physical examination, the lesion is usually firm, but not rock hard; it is smooth and well circumscribed, nontender, and easily movable. It often rolls about in the breast, mimicking a very large marble. In some adolescents giant fibroadenomas can be confused with virginal hypertrophy; however, they are usually more discrete than is diffuse hypertrophy. Mammography is often diagnostic, usually revealing a discrete, round, well-circumscribed lesion without associated calcium. In addition, a skilled cytopathologist can usually confirm the diagnosis with the sample from a fine-needle aspiration. However, because of the rare possibility of simultaneous lobular carcinoma or progression to cystosarcoma phylloides and the inability to definitely exclude carcinoma (present in 2 to 3% of cases), excisional biopsy sometimes may be recommended.

Cystosarcoma Phylloides

Cystosarcoma phylloides is a sarcomatous tumor of the breast that may arise from a fibroadenoma. The overgrowth of stroma mainly distinguishes it from a fibroadenoma. It has a malignancy rate of 20 to 30%, with 2 to 3% of cases having already metastasized at diagnosis. Benign tumors are treated with wide excision and malignant tumors by modified radical mastectomy.

Intraductal Papilloma

Intraductal papillomas often present with serosanguinous, spontaneous, recurrent, or persistent nipple discharge from a single duct. These small tumors are not palpable, but their location can usually be determined by applying pressure on various quadrants of the areolocutaneous margin and noting which quadrant produces the discharge. An intraductal papillary cancer is a possibility that must be excluded by excising a small, pie-shaped segment in the area producing the discharge.

Fibrocystic Disease

Fibrocystic changes of the breast are quite common and occur to some extent in most women. Because up to 90% of women have some degree of cysts and epithelial hyperplasia on biopsy or at autopsy, it may be reasonable to consider fibrocystic disease a normal variant rather than an actual pathologic entity (42). The patient with fibrocystic change usually complains of dull, aching pain in the area of most pronounced nodularity, and this pain is often more prominent just before the onset of menses. It is possible that much of the pain related to fibrocystic change is caused by cancer phobia, and it often lessens with a positive doctor–patient relationship. On physical examination the breast feels lumpy, with bilateral, diffuse, tender, easily movable ill-defined masses, usually in the upper outer quadrant of the breasts. At times, especially with a discrete cystic lesion, it is hard to distinguish cystic changes noted on examination or on a mammogram from cancer, making management of such cases difficult. Because of this uncertainty, many patients undergo at least one biopsy to rule out cancer. Most are benign (17). More than 95% of the time, the histology is either normal (70%) or shows only epithelial hyperplasia (25%). These findings are of little concern, and such patients are at low risk for developing breast cancer and do not require more vigilant follow-up than normal (17). In contrast, when hyperplasia with atypia is reported (3 to 4% of benign biopsies), this is significant, particularly if the mother or a sister of the patient has had breast cancer. In the absence of a positive family history, the finding of atypia increases the risk of the patient developing breast cancer fourfold, and in association with a positive family history this risk is increased nearly elevenfold (17). These patients do require careful follow-up with annual mammogram and biannual physical examinations, and in selected cases even prophylactic bilateral mastectomies may be considered.

Sometimes fibrocystic disease is associated with *duct ectasia,* usually heralded by spontaneous discharge of thick, gray-green fluid from multiple dilated ducts. At other times duct ectasia and discharge may be present in the absence of palpable fibrocystic lesions. In the first instance, a biopsy should be done to rule out carcinoma; in the second, the administration of estrogen may stop the discharge. If it does not, mammography should be performed and then a biopsy should be considered.

Premature Hyperplasia

A concentric unilateral swelling can occur beneath the nipple before puberty in girls. This commonly occurs during ages 7 to 9. The lump can be 1 to 2 cm in diameter and is usually nontender. Within a year, a contralateral lump appears and often both lumps remain static until puberty. A biopsy is contraindicated and is equivalent to total mastectomy.

Gynecomastia

The main differential in male breast masses lies between gynecomastia (see Chapter 77) and male breast cancer. The latter is rare, accounting for approximately 1% of all breast cancers. Although gynecomastia has many causes, its physical characteristics are usually unvaried. Gynecomastia presents as a breast mass beneath the areola, is usually slightly tender, and is easily movable. It is never associated with ulceration or nipple retraction. If gynecomastia is ruled out, a breast mass in a male should be examined by biopsy.

Cancer

The increased practice of routine screening for breast cancer by mammography, using sensitive equipment, has resulted in a change in the presentation of breast cancer. A large percentage (15 to 20%) now is detected by mammography alone without an associated palpable mass (36). The remaining breast cancers are found by the patient or the physician and 15% of these are clinically advanced. These advanced cases may be recognized by some of the following signs: skin changes (e.g., dimpling, peau d'orange, erythema), matted fixed axillary nodes, or a mass fixed to the chest wall. Less advanced cases may present with a painless, hard irregular mass, often (37%) located in the upper outer quadrant of the breast. These may be associated with subtle skin dimpling or nipple retraction. Palpable, movable axillary lymph nodes less than 2 cm in diameter about half of the time on biopsy are reactive only in patients with breast cancer, without tumor involvement.

EVALUATION OF A BREAST MASS
History: Risk Factors and Symptoms

The chance of a woman developing cancer increases with age (47,52). The risk to age 50 is approximately 2.5% and to age 70 is approximately 8% (and to age 110 approximately 12%). Many factors have been shown to alter these numbers (see below). Women are becoming increasingly sensitive to their high risk of developing breast cancer and are more aware of factors that may modulate their risk. (See Table 89.1.) Genetic testing for breast cancer susceptibility genes (BRCA1 and BRCA2) has now become commercially available. Woman with worrisome family histories (14) or those who have developed breast cancer when premenopausal may inquire about undergoing such testing. It

Table 89.1. Risk Factors for Carcinoma of the Breast

Factors	Relative Risk
Positive family history	1–5 (see text)
Early menarche and late menopause (cyclic ovarian activity greater than 40 years)	Slight
Nulliparity	Slight
Previous breast cancer	5
Benign disease of the breast	1–4 (see text)
Radiation	Dependent on dosage

falls upon the primary care physician to guide the patient in understanding her own risk and to counsel her whether her risk may justify such actions as prophylactic mastectomy or genetic testing (37). Individual factors are usually expressed as relative risk, or the increased risk when a factor is present relative to the risk when it is absent, all other factors being the same. Women sometimes incorrectly sum their various relative risks to achieve an overall estimated cumulative (absolute) risk that is several times higher than observed in epidemiologic studies. They also may fail to realize that their risk of dying of breast cancer is one-third of their chance of developing breast cancer (37). Probability curves have been developed to guide the physician in combining various risk factors to estimate a woman's chance of developing breast cancer over time and are available in recent publications (5,14,66). Genetic screening may be appropriate for women with a strong history (more then five relatives with a history of breast or ovarian cancer with onset less than 50) or a personal history of breast cancer under the age of 35, especially if they are of Jewish descent (29,33,39). It is recommended that these women receive expert genetic counseling before considering testing and that such testing be done in an academic center. Guidelines for such testing have been published by the American Society of Clinical Oncology (60).

In ascertaining a woman's risk, the menstrual and reproductive history is important (7). Early menarche and late menopause (i.e., prolonged duration of ovarian activity, greater than 40 years) are associated with a slightly increased risk of developing breast cancer, whereas menopause before age 35 (normal and surgical) reduces the risk. The risk of breast cancer is increased in nulliparous women, whereas a full-term pregnancy before age 18 offers some protective benefit. It appears unlikely that the use of oral contraceptives changes a woman's risk of breast cancer, but postmenopausal estrogen replacement therapy may increase that risk slightly (see Chapter 77). A family history of breast cancer is a major risk factor (2,3,55). The occurrence of breast cancer in a first-degree relative (sister or mother) increases a woman's probability of developing cancer twofold to fourfold. It is debatable to what extent this increase in risk depends on the relative having been premenopausal when diagnosed or having developed bilateral cancers. For instance, some reports estimate that the lifetime risk of developing breast cancer for a daughter or sister of a premenopausal woman with

bilateral disease is 50%, but that the risk is not increased if the relative was postmenopausal with unilateral disease (3). Others suggest that these estimates are too high or too low. It is important to assure patients that breast cancer in more distant relatives (e.g., aunts) has little or no effect on a woman's risk. The other major risk factor other than family history is a personal history of breast cancer, which increases the risk of contralateral breast cancer fivefold (49,53,67).

The patient should be questioned about the presence of other symptoms (pain, discharge) related to a breast mass, the duration of those symptoms if present, and whether the discovery of the mass or onset of the other symptoms was associated with changes in the menses, injury to the breast, pregnancy, or changes in medication.

After the presence of a mass, nipple discharge is the second most common sign of breast cancer. Nonlactational nipple discharge can be unilateral or bilateral, spontaneous or evoked only by pressure and massage, and persistent or recurrent. If the discharge is associated with a mass on physical examination, the mass should be the primary concern. Nipple discharge in women over 50 must be viewed with more suspicion than in younger women, regardless of its presentation. Discharge evoked only by trauma, massage, or pressure has no clinical importance. Spontaneous, recurrent, or persistent discharge from one or two ducts not associated with a mass requires surgical exploration of the duct to differentiate benign papilloma from intraductal papillary carcinoma. Both are possible without a presenting mass, and the character of the discharge is not helpful (see Chapters 74 and 77 for a discussion of galactorrhea).

Physical Examination

The patient should be seated undressed to the waist on an examining table. Inspection and palpation of the nodal drainage areas (supraclavicular and axillary) should be performed. Inspection and palpation of the nipples, areolae, and breasts are done next. While the patient is sitting, her arm on the side being examined can be raised by the physician to allow palpation high into the axilla. The examination should then be repeated with the patient in the supine position with her arm raised over her head so that the breast flattens on the chest wall. If the clinician cannot appreciate a mass noted by the patient, it is important to allow the patient sufficient time to find the lesion herself rather than to dismiss the complaint. If both the patient and the physician cannot locate the mass, the patient should be reassured that benign fibrous masses often disappear spontaneously, as do menstrual-related cysts.

Initial Management

The three most common masses found in the breast are fibroadenoma, fibrocystic changes, and carcinoma. Each of these common lesions has a peak incidence at different ages but there is considerable overlap. Because of this overlap and the inability of the physician from history, physical examination, or radiographic studies to make a diagnosis with certainty, a biopsy usually is the only definitive test to rule out carcinoma.

Ages 15 to 30

An easily movable, nontender, smooth, marblelike mass in a woman less than 30 years of age is most likely a fibroadenoma. The mass should be electively excised. This can be delayed up to several months if the mass is not growing rapidly and if there are no major risk factors (significant family history or prior breast cancer). A mammogram should not be routinely obtained in the evaluation of a discrete mass in this age group. The tissue is too dense to allow useful interpretation, and the radiation may slightly increase the risk for developing a neoplasm. Perhaps a patient with large breasts that are hard to examine, with persistent symptoms, or with a strong family history should have a mammogram.

Ages 30 to 50

A discrete mass noted during the reproductive years that feels cystic might be watched through one or two menstrual cycles. A sonogram can be useful in distinguishing a cystic from a solid mass. If the mass persists, a surgical consultation is probably necessary to allow histologic examination of the mass. A mammogram can be obtained before the consultation, especially if the patient has never had one. It should be noted that a persistent mass that is not seen on mammogram should not be ignored; 10 to 15% of palpable breast cancers are not seen on mammography (46).

Ages over 50

A patient with a suspicious mass should be referred for possible biopsy. A mammogram should be obtained to search for other areas of disease that also may need to be biopsied.

All Ages

The usual evaluation of a persistent palpable discrete breast mass involves histologic examination even if the mammogram is not suspicious. An exception is a cystic mass that disappears after aspiration or menstruation. If the mass is larger than 2 cm, an incisional biopsy is usually performed; otherwise it should be removed in toto. A *fine-needle aspiration* for cytology is often obtained first because it is easier and less traumatic than an open biopsy. Simultaneous biopsy, frozen section, histologic examination, and if malignant, immediate mastectomy should be considered only in special cases at the wish of the patient and only after detailed discussion. Waiting for permanent sections allows detailed examination of the tissue and certainty of the diagnosis. In addition, the treatment of primary breast cancer has undergone many changes in recent years, with several treatment options now available to the patient. The one-step approach deprives a patient of her right to a second opinion in regard to treatment options for her breast cancer.

Needle Aspiration of a Palpable Mass

In the past, aspiration was limited to nodules felt to be cystic, with sonography used to help distinguish cystic from solid lesions. More recently, aspiration by the surgeon of solid lesions to obtain material for cytologic examination has allowed the diagnosis of carcinoma to be made in the office and perhaps can spare some patients a surgical biopsy. In the case of the cystic lesion, if the mass does not completely disappear, or if the fluid is bloody or if the mass rapidly reoccurs, an open biopsy is necessary. (Cytologic examination of the fluid is usually of little use and need not be done routinely.) If the lesion disappears completely without recurrence, routine follow-up is sufficient. If the cytology of a needle aspiration of a solid lesion is negative, formal biopsy usually is required because false negatives are common.

Surgical Biopsy

The referring physician should not only inform the patient of the need for surgical consultation, but also explain clearly the reasons why it is needed and that a biopsy may be recommended by the surgeon. The patient should be encouraged to ask questions. The consultation is stressful and the patient is more likely to absorb information from her personal physician. In addition, the patient needs support from her personal physician and the reassurance of continued involvement in her care should a biopsy reveal cancer.

Preparation

Most biopsies can be carried out on an outpatient basis in an ambulatory surgery unit. Either local anesthesia with intravenous sedation (preferred) or general anesthesia can be used. The patient should not eat or drink after midnight on the night before the biopsy.

Operation

A 2.5- to 5.0-cm incision is used to allow an adequate biopsy that is cosmetically satisfactory. The incision site is selected very carefully to minimize the potential for disfigurement should cancer be found and should breast-conserving therapy subsequently be chosen. It should be explained to the patient that in addition to a possible residual mass, there is often a ridge of tissue secondary to sutures and scar remaining after the operation. Removal of a large mass might necessitate a small drain, which is withdrawn in the office 1 or 2 days after the biopsy.

If a mass is palpable, then the tissue of concern is easily located and biopsied. As noted previously, increasingly biopsies are being obtained for a mammographic lesion found in the absence of a palpable mass. In these instances the procedure is more complicated. Under mammographic guidance, a radiologist places thin needles or hooks into the breast, with the tips within a centimeter of the suspicious area on the mammogram. Methylene blue or some other color marker is then injected into the breast to mark visually the abnormal area of the breast noted on the mammogram. The patient then proceeds to the ambulatory surgery unit, where the surgeon excises the stained area. If the mammographic abnormality contains microcalcifications, the biopsy specimen is x-rayed to ensure that they have been removed with the biopsy. Several weeks after the biopsy the patient needs a mammogram to confirm that the suspicious area is no longer present. Many radiology departments now have the capacity to perform stereotactic core biopsies using specialized equipment that uses stereotactic mammography to guide an automatic biopsy gun equipped with a core biopsy needle. In experienced hands adequate tissue can be obtained nearly 100% of the time, with a diagnostic sensitivity of 95% or better (31,57). This greatly simplifies the diagnostic process and may allow a preliminary diagnosis to be made on the day of the procedure. However, because radiographic stereotactic biopsy shifts the diagnostic procedure from the surgeon to the radiologist, it must be clear to all whether the primary care physician or the radiologist is responsible for reporting the final results to the patient and arranging appropriate follow-up.

Follow-Up

Ecchymoses or hematoma (5% of the patients) and wound infection (1 to 2% of the patients) are the main complications of breast biopsy. A large hematoma may require evacuation, but this usually can be done in the office. Exercise and strenuous activities should be avoided for 7 to 10 days after a breast biopsy to guard against late bleeding. The long-term sequelae of breast biopsy are minimal; chronic scar formation may cause some difficulty with follow-up examinations and interpretation of mammograms. Detailed descriptions of the biopsy site should be noted in the chart by physicians on follow-up, and details of the biopsy should be conveyed to the radiologists reading future mammograms.

FOLLOW-UP MANAGEMENT OF A BENIGN BREAST MASS

Fibroadenoma

After excision of a fibroadenoma, the patient should have routine follow-up as defined by risk factors for carcinoma and age. The patient should be reassured that there is no increased risk of malignancy because of the fibroadenoma.

Fibrocystic Disease

If on histologic examination the epithelium is normal, no special follow-up is necessary for the patient with a benign biopsy. Even if proliferative epithelial changes are noted, the increased risk is so minimal (less than twofold) that again the patient should be reassured and no special follow-up is warranted. Only the finding of atypia, especially in a patient with a history

of breast cancer in a sibling or mother, requires special consideration. Without such a family history, monthly self-examinations of the breasts, a physical examination twice yearly, and an annual mammogram should suffice. With a positive family history the patient may consider the 40% lifetime risk of developing breast cancer sufficient to consider bilateral prophylactic simple mastectomy with reconstruction (17). Subcutaneous mastectomy with implants should not be considered as a compromise. The 15 to 20% of the breast that is left behind remains at risk.

As mentioned, the pain associated with fibrocystic changes is often ameliorated once a cancer has been excluded. If pain continues, the patient should be advised to wear a brassiere both day and night. A number of pharmacologic and dietary strategies are said to be effective in the management of painful fibrocystic changes (e.g., avoidance of caffeine), usually without adequate supporting evidence (41,56). However, danazol, a weak androgenic steroid, has been shown to decrease pain and nodularity in up to 70% of patients with fibrocystic changes when used in dosages of 100 to 400 mg a day for 4 to 6 months (8,43). Side effects are minor; weight gain, acne, and amenorrhea are the most common.

CANCER

If the biopsy reveals carcinoma, consultation with a medical oncologist and radiation oncologist should be considered. The treatment of breast cancer is complex and rapidly changing and involves the coordinated efforts of the surgeon, radiation oncologist, medical oncologist, and primary physician. The primary care physician may not be knowledgeable in all of the details of treatment, but the general concepts discussed below are important to understand because the patient will look to her physician for support and clarification as she struggles with difficult treatment decisions.

Staging

Several clinical staging systems have been devised for breast cancer, but none facilitates the management of individual patients. It is perhaps simplest to divide tumors into three main groups: *resectable* (tumors not fixed to the chest wall and not associated with fixed matted axillary nodes); *locally advanced*, *unresectable* (tumors fixed to the chest wall or associated with the presence of matted axillary nodes, or inflammatory skin changes, but without signs of metastases); and *metastatic tumors.*

In the absence of symptoms or physical findings, patients with resectable tumors require minimal further studies consisting of a chest x-ray and routine blood studies (including liver function tests and serum calcium) and, if not done before the biopsy, a mammogram to look for contralateral disease or multicentric lesions. In addition, the patient's history should be retaken to ensure that there are no musculoskeletal complaints suggestive of bony metastases. If there are, bone scan and local x-rays of the symptomatic region should be obtained. In general, liver and bone scans should not be obtained routinely because in the absence of symptoms, physical findings, or abnormal serum chemistries they are more likely to produce confusing false-positive results than to disclose unexpected metastases, especially with tumors less than 5 cm (10).

Surgery

Radical mastectomy, the standard for years, is no longer performed. The modified radical mastectomy (removal of the breast and the ipsilateral axillary lymph nodes), which preserves the pectoral muscles, is of equal efficacy but is less disfiguring, allows easier reconstruction, and only occasionally leads to clinically significant arm edema (24).

A *modified radical mastectomy* requires general anesthesia and a short period of hospitalization, usually no more than 2 to 5 days. Most patients are ambulatory and eating normally within 24 hours of the operation. Occasionally, patients may be discharged with drains, which are removed at the time of followup. Serous fluid may accumulate under the skin flaps even after the drains are removed and may require aspiration in the office. In the early postoperative period the patient may be inconvenienced with arm and shoulder discomfort but usually can use the arm normally within 2 to 3 weeks. Some patients may experience shoulder and arm pain for a much more extensive period. It is important for these patients to continue arm exercises as prescribed by the surgeon. In 10% of the patients, after modified radical mastectomy, lymphedema of the ipsilateral upper extremity develops. Usually swelling is minimal in the morning and increases during the day. Typically, the degree of swelling gradually becomes worse over several years. Management includes the following:

- Instruct the patient to sleep with the arm propped up on a pillow and to take special care not to sleep with the arm under her head.
- Minimize the amount of time that the arm is allowed to hang down (e.g., while sitting).
- Minimize trauma to the arm. This includes limiting the use of the affected arm for blood pressure determinations, phlebotomy, and insertion of intravenous catheters.
- Aggressively treat any infection of the arm. Patients should be instructed to see their physician as soon as signs or symptoms (erythema, swelling, or pain) of infection are noted, no matter how minimal. (Cellulitis is the major complication of lymphedema.)
- If the degree of swelling is unsightly or uncomfortable, the patient can be fitted with a Jobst sleeve (available at Jobst outlets in most cities) to be worn during waking hours. A trial with a lymphedema pump (a pneumatic sleeve, sold by medical supply houses, that applies intermittent compression to the affected arm) can be considered for severe, refractory cases. Severe lymph edema is managed with the help of a physical therapist.
- The physician should be attentive to sudden changes in the rate of edema formation, especially when it is associated with new arm pain. This may indicate recurrence of tumor in the axilla.

It is most important to be sensitive to cosmetic and emotional needs of the patient for what most patients consider disfiguring surgery. Most hospitals have a representative from the American Cancer Society Reach for Recovery program or someone serving a similar role who can assist in this regard, and this person should make contact with the patient in the perioperative period to offer help. Within 3 to 6 weeks of operation, most patients can be fitted with a breast form if skin healing is complete. These forms can be obtained in medical appliance stores.

Breast reconstruction after mastectomy should be discussed with the patient *before* the surgery to allow referral to a plastic surgeon *before* her scheduled mastectomy. The patient then can decide which of several reconstruction procedures she prefers and whether she would like reconstruction done simultaneously with the mastectomy or later. A common technique of breast reconstruction involves implantation of a tissue expander that is gradually inflated over several weeks to effect sufficient stretching of the chest tissues to allow the later insertion of a saline-filled implant after removal of the expander. Use of autologous tissue is gaining in popularity. Transrectus myocutaneous (TRAM) flap or the latissimus dorsi flap are most commonly used. Careful discussion of all the options with the plastic surgeon is critical for the patient's satisfaction with the surgical result.

Radiotherapy Combined with Surgery

Radiotherapy alone as treatment for primary breast cancer has not been systematically studied. The National Surgical Adjuvant Breast Project (NSABP) has established (for patients with resectable primary tumors 4 cm or less) that complete excision of the primary tumor (lumpectomy, usually with removal of lymph nodes, unless the tumor is only intraductal; see below) followed by breast irradiation five times a week for 5 weeks is as curative as a modified radical mastectomy (26). For larger lesions, the information is not as well established, but a certain number of these women, especially those with tumors less than 5 cm, might also be considered for excision and radiotherapy. The main considerations are cosmetic. These include the relative sizes of the tumor and the remaining breast and how close to the nipple complex the tumor lies. The larger the ratio of tumor size to uninvolved breast, the more likely a poor cosmetic result will occur because a larger percentage of the normal breast is exposed to radiation dosages that will lead to disfiguring fibrosis. Usually if tumors are close to or involve the nipple complex, a better cosmetic result is achieved after mastectomy and reconstruction than after lumpectomy and radiotherapy.

The main purpose of radiation after lumpectomy is to reduce the postlumpectomy local recurrence rate (42% following lumpectomy without radiation [26]), with little effect on overall survival. Even so, patients should be warned that there is a significant incidence of recurrent breast cancer in the irradiated breast, not only at the lumpectomy site, but also elsewhere in the breast (30). In most reported series this ranges around 20%, with recurrence up to two decades after lumpectomy, in contrast to a 2 to 9% local recurrence rate, with recurrence usually in the first 5 years after mastectomy (24,26,30,40). Fortunately, a local relapse after breast-conserving therapy does not appear to affect survival, unlike that after a mastectomy (26,40). Patients whose cancers recur after lumpectomy, whether previously irradiated or not, can undergo a salvage mastectomy and survive as long as patients initially treated with a modified radical mastectomy. However, any prior radiotherapy would make reconstruction more difficult in comparison to women choosing a modified mastectomy initially.

Of patients choosing lumpectomy and radiotherapy, over 80% are satisfied with the cosmetic results. The treatment is accompanied with minimal, if any, postoperative breast lymphedema or impaired wound healing. The irradiated breast atrophies over a number of months and may remain tender during this period. For some patients, reduction mammoplasty of the opposite breast may need to be considered.

In summary, for most patients with tumors less than 5 cm that can be completely excised without affecting the nipple/areolar complex when there is sufficient remaining breast tissue, there exists a choice between mastectomy and breast-conserving radiotherapy. All patients should have the choices well outlined and be given information that clearly describes the benefits and disadvantages of both treatment options.

Intraductal Carcinoma

With the increased use of mammography, up to 20% of all new breast cancers are noninvasive *intraductal lesions* (58). The optimal treatment for these lesions has not been precisely defined. Mastectomy is curative 99% of the time, but is probably overly aggressive treatment. However, a simple lumpectomy may not be sufficient. The NSABP has published the results of a study comparing local excision for patients with small (less than 2.5 cm) intraductal (noninvasive) carcinomas with or without breast irradiation (22). The results suggest that local excision for intraductal cancer without local radiation may prove to be unacceptable because of a high rate of relapse (16%) at or near the biopsy site. (Approximately half of the recurrences were invasive and radiotherapy appeared to reduce their incidence by 70%.) This conclusion is not universally accepted. It is unclear to what degree radio-

therapy prevented or merely delayed local recurrences. Other, albeit nonrandomized studies suggest that with careful patient selection a physician can identify women who may not need irradiation following removal of an intraductal lesion. The following features are associated with a better prognosis: completely excised, well-differentiated tumors without comedo necrosis, less than 25 mm in diameter; a tumor found incidentally or detected by mammographic microcalcifications; and a tumor that occurs in an older woman. The recurrence rate in such cases can be as low as 3% (38). Many believe that patients whose tumors have these characteristics may be cured by simple excision without irradiation.

Multimodality Treatment

Patients with locally advanced unresectable disease or with inflammatory disease should be considered for treatment with initial systemic chemotherapy followed by surgery if sufficient tumor reduction occurs or local irradiation, perhaps with further chemotherapy (34). For a select group, such an approach may allow long-term survival.

PROGNOSIS, FURTHER THERAPY, AND FOLLOW-UP

Prognosis

Current estimates of survival are based mainly on tumor size (27), whether the tumor is wholly intraductal (noninvasive), and the results of axillary node sampling. The cure rate with mastectomy approaches 100% for women whose tumor consists only of intraductal carcinoma. (Axillary node involvement occurs in less than 3% of these patients, so node resection gives little further information and may be omitted.)

A special case is *lobular carcinoma in situ* (LCIS). This diagnosis should more accurately be classified as a premalignant lesion and not considered a neoplasm. It should be viewed as a risk factor in a manner similar to the finding of hyperplasia with atypia on a biopsy. Although there continues to be some disagreement among experts about how significant a risk factor LCIS is, a reasonable estimate is that a woman with a finding of LCIS has a 15 to 30% lifetime risk of developing invasive cancer, or approximately 0.5 to 1% risk of cancer per year. It is important to realize that this risk applies to both breasts (as does any other risk factor). Recommendations vary for LCIS, but most recommend close mammographic follow-up with prophylactic bilateral mastectomies reserved for women psychologically unable to deal with their increased risk of breast cancer (35,54).

For women with invasive cancer, the status of the axillary lymph nodes is the best indicator of prognosis (Table 89.2) (6,20,24). Survival at 10 years is approximately 65% with no node involvement, 37% with one to three nodes, and 13% with four or more nodes involved (6,28). The size of the tumor is also important.

Table 89.2. Survival of Patients with Breast Cancer
Relative to Status of the Axillary Lymph Nodes

	Crude Survival (%)		5-Year Disease-Free Survival (%)
Status of Nodes	5-Year	10-Year	
All patients	63.5	45.9	60.3
Negative axillary lymph nodes	78.1	64.9	82.3
Positive axillary lymph nodes	46.5	24.9	34.9
1–3 positive axillary lymph nodes	62.2	37.5	50.0
≥4 positive axillary lymph nodes	32.0	13.4	21.1

From National Surgical Adjuvant Breast Project.

Patients with tumors larger than 5 cm do somewhat worse, especially if there are positive nodes; patients with tumors smaller than 1.0 cm (especially if less than 0.5 cm), with uninvolved nodes do better (1,27). Within these subgroups, patients whose tumor is rich in estrogen receptors (and progesterone receptors) do better than those whose tumors lack significant receptor levels (9,45). Patients whose tumors appear well differentiated to the pathologist appear to survive better than those whose tumors appear poorly differentiated. Tumors from individual patients are now routinely characterized by molecular biological analysis to assist in estimates of prognosis. Patients whose tumors show aneuploidy or more than 6 to 7% of their cells in S-phase (synthesizing DNA) appear to do worse than predicted by the current criteria of node status (13). DNA analysis for these parameters by flow cytometry is readily available through several commercial laboratories. Analysis for the increased presence and functioning of certain oncogenes (e.g., HER-2/Neu) in individual tumors is beginning to be considered for predicting survival and may be available commercially in the near future (59). The need to determine more accurately the prognosis of individual patients is important because prognostic category is the basis for patient selection for adjuvant therapy after the treatment of the primary tumor.

From the above discussion it is clear that axillary dissection serves only to obtain prognostic information and does not directly improve a patient's survival. Attempts have been made to determine the nodal status with a less invasive procedure than axillary dissection, thereby decreasing the risk of long-term adverse effects such as axillary nerve damage and arm swelling. Techniques are available to identify the single axillary node to which a particular woman's breast cancer would first metastasize. Removal and histologic examination of this sentinel node can then serve to ascertain what a woman's nodal status is. This procedure is not easily learned and is reliable only when performed by a well-trained, experienced surgeon. In addition, because no quantitative information is obtained, if decisions concerning adjuvant therapy are to be based not only on whether the nodes are positive but also on the number of positive nodes, examination of a single node would be inadequate (see below).

Adjuvant Therapy

Adjuvant systemic therapy decreases the predicted death rate by approximately 30% (18). Thus, the absolute degree of benefit from adjuvant therapy increases as the predicted prognosis worsens and conversely may be clinically insignificant in a woman whose cure rate with primary treatment alone is high. For example, a woman with one to three positive nodes has a 50% chance of her cancer returning. Adjuvant therapy can reduce this by 0.3 times 0.5, or 15%. However, a woman with a tumor less than 1.0 cm and no positive nodes has a cure rate of over 90%. In this case adjuvant therapy would improve her chances by only 0.3 times 0.1, or 3%. Most oncologists would urge adjuvant therapy in the former case, but be less enthusiastic in the latter. Consequently, in certain patients with poor prognoses, further treatment with chemotherapy or hormonal therapy is recommended by the medical or radiation oncologist in an attempt to improve disease-free survival and cure (see Chapter 8). Currently, patients are selected for various adjuvant therapy based on the number of axillary nodes involved, their menopausal status, and the estrogen receptor status of the tumor (18). Systemic chemotherapy is recommended to all premenopausal women with metastases to their axillary nodes. For patients opting for lumpectomy and radiotherapy, results seem to be better if the chemotherapy is sandwiched between the lumpectomy and the breast irradiation (51). Similarly, use of an antiestrogen, tamoxifen, is recommended for postmenopausal women with axillary node involvement if their tumors contain significant estrogen receptors. Tamoxifen may also be sufficient for premenopausal women if the tumor is estrogen receptor positive and especially if it is less than 2 cm in size. In addition, patients with four or more nodes involved with tumor might be candidates for postmastectomy chest wall irradiation because they are more at risk for local recurrences (34). Several adjuvant chemotherapeutic regimens are used. Among these, efficacy is probably equivalent but side effects and duration differ. High-dose chemotherapy with bone marrow or peripheral stem cell rescue is an option for patients with four or more nodes positive because their prognosis is poor. However, no study has conclusively shown that such therapy improves survival in this group more than conventional standard-dose chemotherapy, although the data for patients with 10 or more nodes positive are encouraging. Until such data are available, high-dose chemotherapy should be administered only within the controlled setting of a clinical trial. Combining chemotherapy with tamoxifen is sometimes advocated. For premenopausal patients, there are few data to support adding one to the other. In contrast, the postmenopausal patient with positive nodes whose tumor is estrogen receptor positive may obtain a small increase in survival (less than 8%) by the addition of chemotherapy to tamoxifen (25). Whether such treatment is warranted, given the additional toxicity, is for the individual patient to decide. Several large clinical trials further defining these issues have been completed and should be published in the next couple of years.

There are uncommon long-term side effects of adjuvant therapy but they must be recognized by the patient and the primary care physician. Chemotherapy may cause premature menopause and a slight increase in the incidence of second neoplasms, mainly hematologic. Radiotherapy may lead to darkened skin, pulmonary damage, or later solid neoplasms (but not breast cancer in the unaffected breast). In 20% of patients, tamoxifen may cause bothersome hot flashes that, if severe, can sometimes can be ameliorated with low-dose progesterone. There is an increased incidence of endometrial carcinomas in women treated with tamoxifen (annual rate of 1.7 per 1000, or an approximately twofold increased risk). Therefore all women taking tamoxifen should have annual gynecologic examinations and be instructed to report any spotting. More detailed follow-up, such as uterine sonograms, is probably unnecessary. Because of possible rare ocular effects, occasional eye examinations are also recommended. Abnormal liver function tests are occasionally observed, but it is unclear whether the drug can induce hepatoma in humans (as opposed to its effects in rats). Tamoxifen does seem to decrease the risk of developing cancer in the unaffected breast (21) and may have beneficial cardiovascular and bone-preserving effects in postmenopausal women.

The selection criteria for adjuvant systemic therapy are constantly being reexamined as new information is obtained. Based on studies (21,23,44) of the beneficial effects of systemic therapy on node-negative patients, the National Cancer Institute initially recommended that all premenopausal women with breast cancer receive adjuvant chemotherapy, independent of axillary node involvement, and that all postmenopausal women whose tumors contain estrogen receptors be given tamoxifen for 5 years or more (15). These criteria are now considered too broad and it is now believed that probably only tumors 1 cm or larger warrant adjuvant therapy (64). Recent data now suggest that the optimal duration of tamoxifen therapy is 5 years. Patients, especially those whose tumors are node negative, may paradoxically lose some of the benefit of tamoxifen if it is continued longer than 5 years.

Follow-Up

The patient with breast cancer is at a fivefold higher risk for development of cancer in the other breast (49,53,67). Consequently, she should be screened with routine mammography and physical examinations, as would any woman of moderately increased risk. Patients choosing lumpectomy and radiotherapy should have a biannual mammogram and careful examination of the irradiated breast every 3 months to look for a local, potentially curable recurrence. Patients who have had a mastectomy should have the scar examined at regular intervals because a small number (10%) of

patients with recurrences in the scar may be cured with local resection followed by radiotherapy.

At present there is little evidence to support the concept that the asymptomatic patient is benefited by prompt diagnosis and initiation of treatment of recurrent systemic metastases (32,63). No studies have demonstrated that monitoring patients with x-rays, liver function tests, or breast cancer markers at regular intervals improves survival or minimizes the morbidity of a relapse. This probably is because there is no curative salvage therapy. When these studies are normal, they serve to reassure the patient. However, when they are abnormal, they often initiate a series of difficult management issues that mainly provoke uncertainty in the physician and anxiety in the patient without clear benefit to either. Thus, follow-up plans can be individualized. Most women, when apprised of the lack of benefit from detailed laboratory and imaging follow-up, are comfortable doing without these studies (32).

Given the data suggesting that estrogen replacement is beneficial in ameliorating many postmenopausal changes, especially the development of osteoporosis, the primary care physician may well be asked about the risks of estrogen replacement therapy in the patient with a history of breast cancer. In the past the answer was simply that it is contraindicated. It now appears that this recommendation was not based on reliable data. In fact, it remains unknown what the effect of estrogen replacement will be on a woman's breast cancer. It may be that the risk is more theoretical than actual and this question is currently under investigation. Many oncologists feel that until further data are available, a physician could consider estrogen replacement in appropriate circumstances and with informed consent.

General References

Harris J, Morrow M, Norton L. Malignant tumors of the heart. In: DeVita VT Jr, Hellman S, Rosenberg SA, eds. Cancer: principles and practice of oncology. 4th ed. Philadelphia: Lippincott-Raven, 1997;1541.
    An in-depth chapter on breast cancer.
Harris JR, Lippman ME, Morrow M, Hillman S. Diseases of the breast. Philadelphia: Lippincott-Raven, 1996.
    An excellent and extensive reference.

Specific References

1. Adair F, Berg J, Joubert L, Robbins GF. Long-term followup of breast cancer patients: the 30-year report. Cancer 33:1145, 1974.
2. Adami H, Hansen J, Jung B, Rimsten A. Characteristics of familial breast cancer in Sweden: absence of relation to age and unilateral versus bilateral disease. Cancer 48:1688, 1981.
3. Anderson DE, Badzioch MD. Risk of familial breast cancer. Cancer 56:383, 1985.
4. Bailar JC. Mammography before age 50 years? JAMA 259:1548, 1988.
5. Benichou J, Gail MH, Mulvihill JJ. Graphs to estimate an individualized risk of breast cancer. J Clin Oncol 14:103, 1996.
6. Bonadonna G, Rossi A, Tancini G, et al. Adjuvant chemotherapy in breast cancer. Lancet 1:1157, 1983.
7. Brinton LA, Hoover R, Fraumeni JF. Reproductive factors in the aetiology of breast cancer. Br J Cancer 47:757, 1983.
8. Brookshaw JD. Danazol treatment of benign breast disease: a survey of U.S.A. multicenter studies. Postgrad Med J 55:52, 1979.

9. Butler JA, Bretsky S, Mendez-Botet C, Kinne DW. Estrogen receptor protein of breast cancer as a predictor of recurrence. Cancer 55:1178, 1985.

10. Caitto S, Pacini P, Azzini V, et al. Preoperative staging of primary breast cancer: a multicentric study. Cancer 61:1038, 1988.

11. Canadian Task Force on the Periodic Health Examination. 2. 1985 update. The periodic health examination. Can Med Assoc J 134:724, 1986.

12. Chu KC, Smart CR, Tarone RE. Analysis of breast cancer mortality and stage distribution by age for the Health Insurance Plan Clinical Trial. J Natl Cancer Inst 80:1125, 1988.

13. Clark GM, Dressler LG, Owens MA, et al. Prediction of relapse or survival in patients with node-negative breast cancer by DNA flow cytometry. N Engl J Med 320:627, 1989.

14. Claus EB, Risch N, Thompson WD. Autosomal dominant inheritance of early-onset breast cancer: implications for risk prediction. Cancer 73:643, 1994.

15. Clinical Alert. National Cancer Institute, May 1988.

16. Council on Scientific Affairs. Mammographic screening in asymptomatic women aged 40 years and older. JAMA 261:2535, 1989.

17. Dupont WD, Page DL. Risk factors for breast cancer in women with proliferative breast disease. N Engl J Med 312:146, 1985.

18. Early Breast Cancer Trialists' Collaborative Group. Systemic treatment of early breast cancer by hormonal, cytotoxic or immune therapy. Lancet 338:1, 71, 1992.

19. Eddy DM, Hasselblad V, McGivney W, Hender W. The value of mammography screening in women under age 50 years. JAMA 259:1512, 1988.

20. Fisher B, Bauer M, Wickerham L, et al. Relationship of number of positive axillary nodes to the prognosis of patient with primary breast cancer: an NSABP update. Cancer 52:1551, 1983.

21. Fisher B, Constantino J, Redmond C, et al. A randomized clinical trial evaluating tamoxifen in the treatment of patients with node-negative breast cancer who have estrogen-receptor–positive tumors. N Engl J Med 320:479, 1989.

22. Fisher B, Constantino J, Redmond C, et al. Lumpectomy compared with lumpectomy and radiation therapy for the treatment of intraductal breast cancer. N Engl J Med 328:1581, 1993.

23. Fisher B, Redmond C, Dimitrov NV, et al. A randomized clinical trial evaluating sequential methotrexate and fluorouracil in the treatment of patients with node-negative breast cancer who have estrogen-receptor–negative tumors. N Engl J Med 320:473, 1989.

24. Fisher B, Redmond C, Fisher ER, et al. Ten-year results of a randomized clinical trial comparing radical mastectomy and total mastectomy with or without radiation. N Engl J Med 312:674, 1985.

25. Fisher B, Redmond C, Legault-Poisson S, et al. Postoperative chemotherapy and tamoxifen compared with tamoxifen alone in the treatment of positive-node breast cancer patients aged 50 years and older with tumors responsive to tamoxifen: results from the National Surgical Adjuvant Breast and Bowel Project B-16. J Clin Oncol 8:1005 1992.

26. Fisher B, Redmond C, Poisson MD, et al. Eight-year results of a randomized clinical trial comparing total mastectomy and lumpectomy with or without irradiation in the treatment of breast cancer. N Engl J Med 320:822, 1989.

27. Fisher B, Slack NH, Bross IDJ. Cancer of the breast: size of neoplasm and prognosis. Cancer 24:1071, 1969.

28. Fisher B, Slack N, Katrych D, et al. Ten year follow-up results of patients with carcinoma of the breast in a cooperative clinical trial evaluating surgical adjuvant chemotherapy. Surg Gynecol Obstet 140:528, 1975.

29. FitzGerald MG, MacDonald DJ, Krainer M, et al. Germ-line BRCA1 mutations in Jewish and non-Jewish women with early-onset breast cancer. N Engl J Med 334:143, 1996.

30. Gage I, Recht A, Gelman R, et al. Long-term outcome following breast-conserving surgery and radiation therapy. Int J Radiat Oncol Biol Phys 33:245, 1995.

31. Gisvold JJ, Goellner JR, Grant CS, et al. Breast biopsy: a comparative study of stereotaxically guided core and excisional techniques. AJR 162:815, 1994.

32. GIVIO Investigators. Impact of follow-up testing on survival and health-related quality of life in breast cancer patients. A multicenter randomized controlled trial. JAMA 271:1587, 1994.

33. Greene MH. Genetics of breast cancer. Mayo Clin Proc 72:54, 1997.

34. Griem KL, Henderson IC, Gelman R, et al. The 5-year results of a randomized trial of adjuvant radiation therapy after chemotherapy in breast cancer treated with mastectomy. J Clin Oncol 5:1546, 1987.

35. Haagensen C, Lane N, Lattes R, Bodian C. Lobular neoplasia (so-called lobular carcinoma in situ) of the breast. Cancer 42:737, 1978.

36. Health and Public Policy Committee, American College of Physicians. The use of diagnostic tests for screening and evaluating breast lesions. Ann Intern Med 103:143, 1985.

37. Hoskins KF, Stopfer JE, Calzone KA, et al. Assessment and counseling for women with a family history of breast cancer. JAMA 272:577, 1995.

38. Lagios MD. Duct carcinoma in situ: pathology and treatment. Surg Clin North Am 40:853, 1990.

39. Langston AA, Malone KE, Thompson JD, et al. BRCA1 mutations in a population-based sample of young women with breast cancer. N Engl J Med 334:137, 1996.

40. Lichter A, Lippman M, Danforth D, et al. Mastectomy versus breast conserving therapy in the treatment of stage I and II carcinoma of the breast: a randomized trial at the National Cancer Institute. J Clin Oncol 10:976, 1992.

41. London RS, Sundaram GS, Goldstein PJ. Medical management of mammary dysplasia. Obstet Gynecol 59:519, 1982.

42. Love SM, Gelman SR, Silen W. Fibrocystic disease of the breast: a nondisease? N Engl J Med 307:1010, 1982.

43. Mansel RE, Wisbey JR, Hughes LE. Controlled trial of the antigonadotrophin danazol in painful nodular benign breast disease. Lancet 1:928, 1982.

44. Mansour EG, Gray R, Shatila AH, et al. Efficacy of adjuvant chemotherapy in high-risk node-negative breast cancer. N Engl J Med 320:485, 1989.

45. McGuire WL, Clark GM, Dressler LG, Owens MA. Role of steroid hormone receptors as prognostic factors in primary breast cancer. NCI Monogr 1:19, 1986.

46. Miller AB, Baines CJ, To T, Wall C. Canadian National Breast Screening Study: 1. Breast cancer detection and death rates among women aged 40 to 49 years. Can Med Assoc J 147:1459, 1992.

47. Miller BA, Feuer EJ, Hankey BF. Recent incidence trends for breast cancer in women and the relevance of early detection: an update. CA Cancer J Clin 43:27, 1993.

48. Moskowitz M. The predictive value of certain mammographic signs in screening for breast cancer. Cancer 51:1007, 1983.

49. Nielsen M, Christensen L, Andersen J. Contralateral cancerous breast lesions in women with clinical invasive breast carcinoma. Cancer 57:897, 1986.

50. Parker SL, Tong T, Bolden S, Wingo PA. Cancer statistics, 1997. CA Cancer J Clin 47:5, 1997.

51. Recht A, Come SE, Henderson IC, et al: The sequencing of chemotherapy and radiation therapy after conservative surgery for early-stage breast cancer. N Engl J Med 334:1356, 1996.

52. Ries LAG, Kosary CL, Hankey BF, et al. SEER cancer statistics review 1997–1993: tables and graphs. NIH pub. no. 96-2789. Bethesda, MD: National Cancer Institute, 1995.

53. Robbins GF, Berg JW. Bilateral primary breast cancers. Cancer 17:1501, 1964.

54. Rosen P, Lieberman P, Braum D, et al. Lobular carcinoma in situ of the breast. Am J Surg Pathol 2:225, 1978.

55. Sattin RW, Rubin GL, Webster LA, et al. Family history and the risk of breast cancer. JAMA 253:1908, 1985.

56. Schairer C, Rubin GL, Webster LA, et al. Methylxanthines and benign breast disease. Am J Epidemiol 124:603, 1986.

57. Schmidt RA. Stereotactic breast biopsy. CA Cancer J Clin 44:172, 1994.

58. Schnitt SJ, Silen W, Sadowsky NL, et al. Ductal carcinoma in situ (intraductal carcinoma) of the breast. N Engl J Med 318:898, 1988.

59. Slamon J, Godolphin W, Jones LA, et al. Studies of the HER-2/ neuproto-oncogene in human breast and ovarian cancer. Science 244:707, 1989.

60. Statement of the American Society of Clinical Oncology. Genetic testing for cancer susceptibility. J Clin Oncol 14:1730, 1996.

61. Tabor L, Gad A, Holmberg LH, et al. Reduction in mortality from breast cancer after mass screening with mammography: randomized trial from the Breast Cancer Screening Working Group of the Swedish National Board of Health and Welfare. Lancet 1:829, 1985.

62. Thomas DB, Gao DL, Self CG, et al. Randomized trial of breast self-examination in Shanghai: methodology and preliminarily results. J Natl Cancer Inst 89:355, 1997.

63. Tomin R, Donegan WL. Screening for recurrent breast cancer: its effectiveness and prognostic value. J Clin Oncol 5:62, 1987.

64. Treatment of early breast cancer. NIH Consensus Development Statement. JAMA 265:391, 1991.

65. U.S. Preventive Task Force. Recommendations for breast cancer screening. JAMA 257:2196, 1987.

66. Vogel VG. Assessing women's potential risk of developing breast cancer. Oncology 10:1451, 1996.

67. Webber BL, Heise H, Neifeld JP, Costa J. Risk of subsequent contralateral breast carcinoma in a population of patients with in-situ carcinoma. Cancer 47:2928, 1981.

C H A P T E R 90

Diseases of the Biliary Tract

ESTEBAN MEZEY, MD
JEFFREY S. BENDER, MD

Diseases of the biliary tract are commonly encountered in ambulatory practice. Many patients are discovered to have asymptomatic gallstones during the course of evaluation of another condition; others are found to have symptomatic chronic cholecystitis. Less commonly, patients present with an acute illness caused by acute cholecystitis or common bile duct obstruction. This chapter describes the cause, diagnosis, and treatment of these various conditions.

CHOLELITHIASIS

Epidemiology

Approximately 10% of the U.S. population has gallstones. In their lifetime, only 50% will ever be symptomatic, with 80% of them having chronic symptoms and 20% presenting with an acute illness. About 500,000 cholecystectomies are performed each year in the United States.

Ninety percent of gallstones found in patients in the United States are cholesterol gallstones; 10% are pigment (bilirubinate) stones. The prevalence of gallstones is greater in women than in men and increases with age. In the United States, 10 to 15% of men and 20 to 40% of women after age 60 are affected (8). The prevalence of cholesterol gallstones is particularly high in the Native Americans of the southwestern United States; for example, 70% of Pima women over age 25 have cholelithiasis (20).

Gallstone Formation

Bile is produced in the liver and excreted into the duodenum and contains bile acids (primarily cholic, deoxycholic, and chenodeoxycholic acid), phospholipids (primarily lecithin), and cholesterol. The solubility of cholesterol depends on its incorporation with bile and phospholipids into a micelle. In the intestinal tract, bile salts are necessary for the absorption of dietary fats; they solubilize fatty acids and monoglycerides into micellar solutions. The fatty acids are absorbed in the jejunum, whereas the bile salts are absorbed in the ileum and enter the enterohepatic circulation.

Three major types of gallstones form in human bile: cholesterol stones (more than 70% cholesterol), mixed stones (50 to 70% cholesterol), and pigment stones (12% cholesterol). These stones probably develop in three stages: first, the formation of a supersaturated bile; second, the crystallization or initiation of stone formation; and third, the growth of the stone to a certain detectable size before crystals in the bile are expelled into the intestine. It is likely, but not clearly established, that one of these stages is more important in the formation of certain types of stones than in others.

Cholesterol Stones

The hypersecretion of biliary cholesterol appears to be the real culprit in the pathogenesis of cholesterol stones, but this might not be true in all patients. Several mechanisms of increased cholesterol secretion have been identified (8). Cholesterol crystals form when the amount of cholesterol in bile exceeds the solubilizing properties of bile salts and phospholipid (supersaturated bile). The cholesterol crystals are caught in a film of mucin gel that lines the gallbladder and provides a nucleus for the formation of gallstones. Growth of these stones occurs, especially in a dyskinetic gallbladder, one in which contraction is impaired, as in diabetes mellitus and pregnancy. The mucin gel itself might decrease gallbladder motility and emptying.

Pigment Stones

Formation of pigment stones is probably initiated by supersaturation of unconjugated bilirubin in the gallbladder and common bile duct. Unconjugated bilirubin, like cholesterol, is insoluble in water. An increased concentration of unconjugated bilirubin in bile results either from its formation from conjugated bilirubin in the biliary tree through the action of a glucuronidase (perhaps of bacterial origin, in patients with infected bile, see below) or from increased production of unconjugated bilirubin by the liver (e.g., in patients with hemolytic anemia). A diseased gallbladder is probably not a factor in the formation of pigment stones.

Risk Factors

Because most patients with cholelithiasis are asymptomatic, it is difficult to evaluate risk factors precisely. Known risk factors for the development of cholesterol and pigment stones are listed in Table 90.1 (1).

Cholesterol Stones

The demography of cholesterol stones probably reflects both genetic predisposition and nongenetic ethnic characteristics. For example, it is known that obese people, and nonobese people who eat a high-calorie diet, secrete more cholesterol into their bile than does the average person. Therefore, populations in whom obesity is common (e.g., the Native Americans of the American Southwest) or who consume high-calorie diets (occidental societies in general) are more susceptible to cholelithiasis.

The reasons for the increasing incidence of gallstones in middle-aged and elderly people are unknown but may be related to the time that elapses between formation of supersaturated bile and formation of stones and between formation of stones and recognition of them.

The enhancement by estrogens of the secretion of cholesterol in bile is reflected in the higher prevalence of gallstones in women (between puberty and menopause) than in men (see above) and in women who take estrogenic preparations compared with women who do not (see Chapter 93).

Finally, there are a number of ways by which the concentration of bile acids in bile is reduced, favoring

---

Table 90.1.   Risk Factors for Gallstones

Cholesterol Stones
Demography: Northern Europe, North and South America more than the Orient; Native Americans; probably familial predisposition
Obesity
High-calorie diet
Drugs used in the treatment of hyperlipidemia; clofibrate, cholestyramine, and colestipol
Gastrointestinal disorders involving major malabsorption of bile acids; ileal disease, resection or bypass; cystic fibrosis, with pancreatic insufficiency
Female sex hormones: women more at risk than men, use of oral contraceptives and other estrogenic medications
Age, especially among men
Probable but not well established; pregnancy, diabetes mellitus, and polyunsaturated fats

Pigment Stones
Demography: oriental more than occidental; rural more than urban
Chronic hemolysis
Alcoholic cirrhosis
Biliary infection
Age

After Bennion LJ, Grundy SM. Risk factors for the development of cholelithiasis in man. N Engl J Med 299:1161, 1978.

the formation of gallstones: drugs used to treat hyperlipidemia, such as clofibrate, cholestyramine, and colestipol (see Chapter 75), decrease bile acid secretion, and certain disorders of the gastrointestinal tract (ileal resection, Crohn's disease of the ileum) reduce bile acid resorption.

Pigment Stones

The demography of pigment stones is entirely different from that of cholesterol stones. The propensity of oriental people to develop pigment stones is not entirely understood, but it may be attributable to the higher prevalence of bacterial infection of the bile (usually *Escherichia coli* infections), and of *Ascaris* infestation, in the Orient compared with the Occident. In the United States, patients with pigment gallstones do not usually have infected or infested bile. The recognized risk factors in the United States are hemolysis and alcoholic cirrhosis. Like cholesterol stones, pigment stones are more common with advancing age, but endogenous and exogenous estrogens and obesity have no influence on their development.

Natural History

Many attempts have been made to study the natural history of gallstones among the 2 to 3 million people in the United States known to harbor them. Of these people, 50% are asymptomatic, having had gallstones discovered incidentally on abdominal film (10 to 15% are radiopaque) or during celiotomy for treatment of another condition. The other 50% are symptomatic (i.e., gallstones are discovered during evaluation of the typical or atypical abdominal pain of acute or chronic cholecystitis; see below).

Approximately 18% of people with silent gallstones develop symptoms in 15 to 20 years, and 3% develop complications of biliary tract disease: acute cholecystitis, pancreatitis, or obstructive jaundice (5). The risk of developing complications is unrelated to the severity of symptoms but does increase with the length of time symptoms have been present. Most complications occur only among symptomatic patients. However, 20% of the time acute cholecystitis is the first indication of cholelithiasis. Complications, if they occur, are usually experienced within 5 years of the discovery of gallstones.

Causes of death related to cholelithiasis among patients not having cholecystectomy are acute cholecystitis, cholangitis with liver abscess, necrotizing pancreatitis, gallbladder carcinoma, and gallstone ileus with mechanical small bowel obstruction. In Lund's study of the natural history of cholelithiasis, 2.7% of the deaths among patients not operated on were attributed to gallbladder disease (11).

Asymptomatic Patients

It cannot be predicted on the basis of the size or number of stones or the sex or age of the patient which asymptomatic patients are likely to become symptomatic. Whether asymptomatic patients should undergo elective cholecystectomy, therefore, depends largely on the bias of the physician and the consulting surgeon. Approximately 18% of patients become symptomatic (see above), sometimes at a point in their lives when operation is more dangerous because of age, intercurrent illness, or the presence of acute cholecystitis. The risk of complications of cholelithiasis, other than acute cholecystitis, is negligible in the asymptomatic patient. Carcinoma of the gallbladder is more common among people with gallstones and the risk—0.3 to 1% over a lifetime—is approximately the same as the historic operative mortality from cholecystectomy. However, recent technologic changes have decreased the operative risk considerably. If the gallbladder is calcified, the risk of cancer is nearly 50%, however, and cholecystectomy should be performed. Likewise, prophylactic cholecystectomy is recommended for Native Americans with cholelithiasis, as they have a 3 to 5% risk of developing gallbladder cancer (10). Prophylactic cholecystectomy has also been recommended for children with gallstones, in whom symptoms almost always develop (16), and in patients with sickle cell anemia and cholelithiasis because the symptoms of either condition can easily be confused with the other. Otherwise, the consensus at this point is not to recommend elective cholecystectomy in the asymptomatic patient. The legitimacy of this same approach in the diabetic patient has been documented (3). This recommendation is unchanged even with the emergence of laparoscopic cholecystectomy and its attendant lower morbidity and shortened convalescence (see below).

CHOLECYSTITIS

The hallmark of cholecystitis is abdominal pain, often epigastric at onset, but localizing within a few hours to the right upper quadrant. The pain is characteristically but not always severe and unremitting, with only slight variations in intensity. Use of the term *biliary colic,* therefore, is not precise because colic is defined as pain that waxes and wanes. Some patients describe the pain as heavy and aching; others, as knifelike. Occasionally, it radiates into the right side of the back or, less often, into other parts of the abdomen. The pain, often accompanied by slight nausea, usually begins abruptly, within 1 to 3 hours of eating a meal. Patients may also complain of being awakened in the middle of the night. A typical attack subsides spontaneously within 2 to 3 hours. The frequency of such attacks is extremely variable, from every day to only once or twice a year.

A patient who presents with this history is very likely to have gallstones. However, the degree of inflammation of the gallbladder cannot be determined from the history. There may be gallstones without any inflammation at all; there may be acute inflammation; or there may be chronic inflammation with fibrosis. However, an attack lasting more than 6 hours generally heralds the onset of acute cholecystitis (i.e., acute inflammation). The severity of the symptoms and the presence or absence of signs of inflammation or biliary obstruction determine the physician's response (see below).

Acute Cholecystitis

Pathophysiology

More than 90% of the time, acute cholecystitis is caused by a gallstone that obstructs the cystic duct. Acute acalculous cholecystitis occurs primarily in patients who have sustained major trauma, including major operations. Inflammation of the gallbladder in early acute cholecystitis is probably caused by irritation by concentrated static bile. As the process progresses, the bile often becomes infected; bile cultures are positive in only 20 to 30% of patients during the first few days of an attack but, by 7 to 10 days, almost 80% of biliary cultures are positive. In certain patients (e.g., diabetics and patients with acalculous cholecystitis), mural ischemia might also play a role.

The difference between the presentation of acute and chronic cholecystitis (see below) is probably caused by the length of time the cystic duct has been totally obstructed and by the intensity of the inflammation.

Signs and Symptoms

The pain of classic acute cholecystitis is severe and persistent. It is usually accompanied by nausea and fever (99° to 102°F; 37° to 39°C) and, less often, by vomiting. Unless treated, the symptoms are likely to persist for up to a week.

The severity and persistence of the pain usually cause the patient to call or see his or her physician (see Chapter 36 for a general discussion of abdominal pain). On examination, the patient is restless. There is considerable right upper quadrant abdominal tenderness, associated with involuntary guarding of the abdominal wall. This guarding, indicative of early peritoneal inflammation, is particularly important to recognize. It is not a feature of less acute disease (see below). Murphy's sign, the sudden involuntary arrest of inspiration (because of pain) when the examiner palpates the right upper quadrant during inspiration, is caused by the abutment of the inflamed gallbladder against the examiner's fingers as it moves downward with expansion of the chest cavity. This sign is more often elicited after several days of inflammation. In one-third of patients, the gallbladder is palpable during an attack of acute cholecystitis if the right upper quadrant is probed very gently. Occasionally, patients are mildly jaundiced (see below).

Laboratory Tests

Leukocytosis (12,000 to 15,000 white blood cells/mm³) caused by a neutrophilic granulocytosis is common. Serum amylase activity may be increased in the absence of other evidence of acute pancreatitis. Often, serum aminotransferases (aspartate aminotransferase and alanine aminotransferase) are increased as well.

Twenty percent of patients have mild hyperbilirubinemia (less than 4 mg/100 mL).

Biliary scintigraphy is the test of choice in the diagnosis of acute cholecystitis. The imaging compounds are ^{99m}Tc-labeled derivatives of iminodiacetic acid (TcHIDA, PIPIDA, or DISIDA), which are concentrated in bile. The study requires injection of isotope intravenously and evaluation of uptake of the isotope by the gallbladder. If the cystic duct is obstructed, because of acute inflammation or because of a stone, uptake does not occur. The test takes 1 to 4 hours to complete. A positive study shows isotope in the biliary tree and in the duodenum but not in the gallbladder. A negative study shows isotope in the gallbladder as well. If isotope is not excreted, the test is uninterpretable, but if it is excreted, the sensitivity of the test is extremely high (essentially 100%). Specificity is also high (95%), but false-positive results may occur in patients with chronic cholecystitis or acute biliary obstruction caused by pancreatitis.

Differential Diagnosis

The differential diagnosis must include disorders that might cause severe right upper quadrant abdominal pain and, usually, leukocytosis and slightly abnormal hepatic function: acute pancreatitis, appendicitis, hepatitis, hepatic abscess, a perforated or penetrated peptic ulcer, acute pyelonephritis, myocardial infarction, and right lower lobe pneumonia or pleuritis. Because of the severity of the illness, these distinctions should be made in the hospital.

Treatment

The patient suspected of having acute cholecystitis should be hospitalized for observation, hydration, and further diagnostic procedures (see below and Chapter 36 for a discussion of these procedures as they pertain to ambulatory patients). If the pain is intolerable, the physician can administer a narcotic parenterally while arranging admission. The patient should be told that, in the hospital, intravenous rather than oral feeding will be given; that, if there is vomiting, a nasogastric tube will be passed; and that antibiotics will be administered. Because 30 to 40% of patients develop gangrenous or perforated gallbladders if cholecystectomy is delayed, urgent operation is generally indicated once the diagnosis is made, especially in the elderly (13,14), among whom rapid development of complications is more likely. A randomized prospective study that compared early and delayed cholecystectomy for acute cholecystitis concluded that the duration of hospitalization and the duration of disability were significantly reduced by early operation (7). The presence of emphysematous cholecystitis caused by gas-forming bacterial infection dictates emergency operation (air bubbles in the right upper quadrant on a plain film of the abdomen indicate the diagnosis).

A discussion of surgery of the biliary tract and of the results and complications of operations is provided below.

Chronic Cholecystitis

Pathophysiology

Symptomatic chronic cholecystitis is associated with gallstones more than 95% of the time; the remaining cases are caused by other diseases of the gallbladder, such as cholesterolosis (the appearance of macrophages laden with cholesterol crystals in the wall of the gallbladder, often without stones). Recurring attacks of mild acute cholecystitis cause eventual fibrosis, so the gallbladder empties poorly. The symptoms of chronic disease, like those of acute cholecystitis, are caused by obstruction by a gallstone of the cystic duct. In chronic recurrent cholecystitis, obstruction of the cystic duct is short (probably no more than a few hours) compared with the length of time of obstruction in acute cholecystitis, so inflammation is less intense. Chronicity of symptoms may also be related to gallbladder dyskinesia secondary to mural fibrosis.

Signs and Symptoms

Many patients who complain of biliary pain for the first time probably already have chronic gallbladder inflammation. The character and location of the pain are identical to those of acute cholecystitis. Pain is variably associated with nausea and, occasionally, vomiting. Unlike classic acute cholecystitis, fever is unusual with chronic disease. Typically, pain occurs after eating, begins 1 to 6 hours after a meal (see above), and lasts for 2 to 3 hours. Nonspecific symptoms—postprandial pain, bloating, belching, flatulence, so-called fatty food intolerance—thought by many to suggest gallbladder disease, are extremely common in the general population and therefore are not helpful diagnostically.

The patient with chronic cholecystitis usually seeks the physician less urgently than does the patient with acute cholecystitis. On examination during the attack, although there is tenderness to deep palpation in the right upper quadrant of the abdomen, there is no muscle guarding, as there is in patients with acute inflammation. Murphy's sign (see above) is absent, the gallbladder is rarely palpable, and jaundice usually is not present. Between attacks, there is no abdominal tenderness.

Laboratory Tests

The white blood count, serum amylase, serum aminotransferases, and serum bilirubin are usually normal.

Unlike patients with acute cholecystitis, patients with symptoms of chronic cholecystitis can be evaluated further in an ambulatory setting but some are hospitalized early in an attack because of an inability to distinguish it from an episode of acute cholecystitis. If a TcHIDA scan is obtained to help in making that distinction, it may be positive, even in patients with chronic cholecystitis, because of transient obstruction of the cystic duct.

Ultrasound.   Ultrasound has replaced oral chole-cystography (at approximately the same cost) as the principal test for the detection of gallstones. The advantages of ultrasound are that it exposes the patient to no radiation, it is much quicker (5 to 10 minutes), and it has no side effects. It is not influenced by associated gastrointestinal or hepatic disease. The detection rate for gallstones 3 mm or greater in diameter is 89 to 96% by ultrasound with 93 to 97% specificity (3 to 7% false positive) (2).

Oral Cholecystogram.   The oral cholecystogram (OCG) documents whether the gallbladder is functioning and whether radiolucent stones are present. Currently, it is obtained only if ultrasound is equivocal.

Patient Experience. To perform the test, the patient is given 3 g of iopanoic acid (Telepaque) in the evening after dinner and is instructed not to eat overnight; films of the abdomen are taken the following morning. If the gallbladder fails to visualize, the patient is given another 3 g of Telepaque and x-rays are repeated the following day. The patient should be warned that mild diarrhea may occur for up to a day after the ingestion of the Telepaque.

Approximately 75% of gallbladders are visible on the first dose, and another 15% become visible on the second dose. Although, as stated above, 10 to 15% of gallstones are radiopaque and can be seen on plain film, confirmation of their location in the gallbladder should be obtained by OCG. OCG is reliable only if the Telepaque is ingested at the proper time, retained in the gastrointestinal tract, absorbed from the small bowel, transported to the liver, esterified to glucuronide, and excreted by the liver into the bile. Therefore, gastrointestinal or hepatic disease may cause a false-positive study. However, the specificity of the test is high (4% false positive) if radiolucent stones are present in an opacified gallbladder or if the gallbladder fails to concentrate contrast material after the second Telepaque dose. The sensitivity of the test is lower (10% false negative), so OCG should be followed by sonography if the gallbladder is visualized and no stones are seen.

Computerized Tomography.   Computerized tomography (CT) accurately identifies gallstones 80% of the time. Currently, it has no advantages over (and costs about twice as much as) OCG and ultrasonography in the diagnosis of gallbladder disease. However, CT scans might be useful occasionally if both the oral cholecystogram and ultrasound are equivocal.

Upper Gastrointestinal Series.   Many patients are evaluated with an upper gastrointestinal (UGI) series in addition to an ultrasonogram, especially if symptoms are atypical of biliary tract disease. Max and Polk (12) reported 250 patients who underwent cholecystectomy, 145 of whom had an UGI and 105 of whom did not. Of the 145 patients selectively chosen for UGI, only 39 had positive findings. In only 7 of these patients was an associated gastroduodenal operation done at the time of cholecystectomy. Of these 7, only 3 patients had any new information added by UGI.

Based on these data, Max and Polk suggest guidelines for selectively choosing patients who might benefit from a UGI (Table 90.2).

Treatment

The treatment of choice for symptomatic chronic cholecystitis is elective cholecystectomy in patients who can tolerate an operation (see below). Medical therapies for cholelithiasis such as gallstone dissolution with ursodeoxycholic acid (Actigall) or gallstone lithotripsy are no longer used because of low effectiveness and high recurrence rates. These medical therapies became obsolete with the advent of laparoscopic cholecystectomy (see below). Risks of not treating patients with chronic cholecystitis include gangrene and perforation of the gallbladder, choledocholithiasis (see below), pancreatitis, and rarely, gallstone ileus (the obstruction of the small bowel by a large gallstone passed through an acute fistula that has formed between the gallbladder and the duodenum).

SYMPTOMATIC PATIENTS WHO HAVE NO DETECTABLE GALLSTONES

Adenomyomatosis of the Gallbladder

Adenomyomatosis of the gallbladder is often asymptomatic, but some patients have symptoms indistinguishable from those with chronic cholecystitis (18). The disease is caused by thickening of the gallbladder wall due to hyperplasia of the epithelium with the formation of glands and diverticula through the muscular wall. The diagnosis is often suspected during ultrasonography or cholecystography, but many cases are revealed by the pathologist after removal of the gallbladder. Adenomyomatosis is found in approximately 20% of patients who undergo cholecystectomy for biliary symptoms. It has been considered not to predispose to gallbladder cancer, but a report of a large number of cases from Japan shows a higher prevalence of gallbladder cancer in segmental adenomyomatosis, which is characterized by a concentric narrowing dividing the gallbladder into two segments (15). Cholecystectomy relieves the symptoms in most patients with symptomatic adenomyomatosis.

Table 90.2. Suggested Indications for Upper Gastrointestinal Series in Patients with Documented Biliary Tract Disease

Older patients (>50 yr)
Men
Previous gastroduodenal operations
Previously documented upper gastrointestinal disease
History of pancreatitis
History of presence of jaundice
Long atypical history

After Max MH, Polk HC. Routine preoperative upper gastrointestinal series (UGIS) in patients with biliary tract disease; a plea for more selectivity. Surgery 82:334, 1997.

Biliary Dyskinesia

Some patients with symptoms suggestive of gallstones have a normal abdominal sonogram, a normal OCG, and a normal abdominal CT scan. These patients may have *biliary dyskinesia,* a term used to denote abnormally decreased emptying of the gallbladder. The diagnosis is best made by cholecystokinin (Kinevac)-stimulated cholecystography with a ^{99m}Tc-iminodiacetic derivative (i.e., TcHIDA). Often, the patient's pain is reproduced after the Kinevac injection (it stimulates gallbladder contraction), and abnormally decreased emptying of the gallbladder can be documented as a markedly decreased ejection fraction (percentage of the isotope excreted) of less than 30% compared with a group of normal subjects. Such patients, if severely symptomatic, should be offered elective cholecystectomy, after which symptoms usually abate.

Biliary Sludge

In some symptomatic patients who have no gallstones detectable by the standard techniques, the gallbladder reflects, on ultrasonography, echoes now recognized to be characteristic of biliary sludge (8). *Biliary sludge* is a term applied to excessively viscous bile that contains cholesterol crystals, calcium bilirubinate granules, and mucin. In such patients duodenal drainage, ordinarily done by a consulting gastroenterologist, may prove useful in identifying the cholesterol crystals or the bilirubinate granules.

Patient Experience. The test is performed by having the patient swallow a plastic double-lumen tube, weighted at the end by a mercury-filled bag. There are holes in the tube above the bag. When the bag has passed into the second portion of the duodenum (documented by fluoroscopy), magnesium sulfate is injected into one lumen of the tube to stimulate contraction of the gallbladder. Duodenal contents are then aspirated and the sediment is separated by centrifugation and examined under a microscope. The patient's experience during this procedure is similar to that of patients undergoing upper endoscopy (see Chapter 36).

Biliary sludge may be a precursor of gallstones, but in a given patient the course is entirely unpredictable. Nevertheless, as with biliary dyskinesia, severely symptomatic patients with biliary sludge should be offered elective cholecystectomy.

CHOLEDOCHOLITHIASIS

Epidemiology

Common duct stones occur in approximately 15% of patients with chronic cholecystitis, either before or after cholecystectomy. The incidence increases with age and the length of time symptoms of gallbladder disease have been present. There are three categories of common duct stones: *(a)* concomitant gallbladder stones and common duct stones, *(b)* retained stones found in the common duct soon after cholecystectomy or common duct exploration, and *(c)* common duct stones identified long after cholecystectomy or common duct exploration. The incidence of common duct stones decreases exponentially in the first year after cholecystectomy only to rise again, reaching a peak at 3 years. In one study, 26% of symptomatic common duct stones occurred 10 or more years after cholecystectomy (21). Also, patients with congenital agenesis of the gallbladder have a 20% incidence of common duct stones. These observations support the concept that common duct stones originate in the gallbladder or in the intrahepatic or common bile ducts.

Signs and Symptoms

Approximately 6% of patients with common duct stones are asymptomatic. More typically, patients develop severe colicky right upper quadrant pain, often associated with jaundice, mild fever, and nausea and vomiting. The pain usually begins abruptly and lasts up to an hour. If nothing is done, attacks recur at variable periods. Eventually cholangitis develops, manifested by persistent malaise and anorexia and intermittent fever, chills, and jaundice, associated with persistently high serum alkaline phosphatase activity. Suppurative ascending cholangitis characterized by right upper quadrant pain, high fever, shaking chills, and jaundice (Charcot's triad) is life threatening and constitutes a surgical emergency.

Rarely, painless jaundice is the only presenting complaint of a patient with choledocholithiasis. In such a circumstance the diagnostic studies should be the same ones performed on the patient with more typical signs and symptoms (see below).

On physical examination, if the patient is asymptomatic, no abnormal signs are elicited. If the patient is symptomatic, right upper quadrant abdominal tenderness and muscle guarding are usually present, similar to the findings in patients with acute cholecystitis. The patient is usually mildly to moderately jaundiced.

Laboratory Tests

Because of the acute onset of symptoms and the severity of pain in patients with choledocholithiasis, laboratory studies in the ambulatory setting are usually not appropriate. If such studies are done, leukocytosis and increases in serum alkaline phosphatase activity, serum bilirubin, serum aminotransferase activity, and serum amylase activity are likely to be observed.

Treatment

If common duct stones are discovered during cholecystectomy, they are removed. If the patient presents to the physician with severe right upper quadrant pain, tenderness, guarding, or jaundice, hospitalization for further diagnostic studies and treatment should be arranged. If sonography or CT scanning shows a dilated biliary tree with probable distal obstruction, endo-

scopic retrograde cholangiopancreatography (ERCP) should be performed. Common duct stones must be removed, either by operation (see below) or, if possible, at the time of ERCP by endoscopic sphincterotomy. ERCP is performed only in the hospital, usually in the radiology department because fluoroscopy and x-rays of the cannulated duct are required. The patient experience during the procedure is essentially the same as it is during other kinds of upper endoscopy (see Chapter 36), except that ERCP usually lasts for 30 to 60 minutes and may be complicated 5 to 10% of the time by postendoscopic infection, especially if the common duct is manipulated, and by pancreatitis. In an 8-year follow-up of patients after endoscopic sphincterotomy, papillary stenosis or recurrent bile duct stones occurred in less than 5% of the cases (17).

Cholangitis

Bacterial infection of the biliary tree generally occurs in association with bile duct obstruction caused by choledocholithiasis, tumor, or biliary strictures. The principal symptoms are fever, chills, and abdominal pain. Jaundice is often but not invariably present. On examination, there is abdominal tenderness and often rebound tenderness. Abnormal laboratory tests include leukocytosis and elevations of the serum bilirubin and alkaline phosphatase activity. Serum aminotransferases may also be moderately elevated. Blood cultures are often positive. The patient may deteriorate rapidly and develop hypotension and changes in mental status. Hospitalization is mandatory for therapy with antibiotics, followed by appropriate relief of biliary obstruction either surgically, by endoscopic sphincterotomy, or by placement of a biliary stent.

Primary sclerosing cholangitis (9) is a chronic inflammation of unknown cause of intrahepatic and extrahepatic bile ducts that leads ultimately to fibrosis and cholestatic liver disease. Most patients are men. There is a very high correlation with concomitant inflammatory bowel disease, most commonly ulcerative colitis. The course of the cholangitis is unpredictable, but patients with advanced disease develop jaundice, right upper quadrant abdominal pain, fever, pruritus, and weight loss and ultimately die of hepatic failure. Diagnosis is made most easily by the demonstration of typical cholangiographic changes during ERCP. Adenocarcinoma of the bile ducts is a common complication that occurs in at least 9 to 15% of patients. No specific treatment influences the outcome of affected patients (including those with inflammatory bowel disease) with the exception of liver transplantation (see below).

BILIARY TRACT OPERATIONS

General physicians should be aware of the mechanics of biliary surgical procedures so that they can inform and reassure patients who are to be referred to a surgeon.

Cholecystectomy

Laparoscopic cholecystectomy has replaced open cholecystectomy as the procedure of choice for the removal of the gallbladder for cholelithiasis and for acute and chronic cholecystitis. Laparoscopic cholecystectomy is performed under general anesthesia. A pneumoperitoneum is established and a laparoscope and three additional cannulas are inserted through which instruments are placed to remove the gallbladder. Relative contraindications to laparoscopic cholecystectomy include a gangrenous or perforated gallbladder, peritonitis, cholangitis, previous upper abdominal surgery, and cirrhosis (4). Common duct stones are also a contraindication unless they can be extracted by endoscopic sphincterotomy before the cholecystectomy or unless the surgeon is experienced in laparoscopic common duct exploration. Laparoscopic cholecystectomy has the advantage over open cholecystectomy of a short hospital stay. In elective cases, the stay is approximately 24 hours, with a return to normal activity in 10 to 14 days. In one study, laparoscopic cholecystectomy needed to be converted to open cholecystectomy in only 4.7% of cases (19). The common reasons for conversion are severe scarring or acute inflammation that obscures the anatomy, adhesions related to prior surgery, aberrant anatomic features that make dissection difficult, and bile duct or bowel injuries during surgery. Common duct stones encountered during the procedure can sometimes be removed by choledochoscopy, but otherwise require common duct exploration after conversion to laparotomy. In a reported series, complications occurred in 5.1% of cases (19). The most common complication is wound infection in 1.1% of cases, followed by bile duct injury in 0.5% of cases. Other complications are prolonged ileus, bowel injury, and operative bleeding. Mortality in elective cases is less than 0.1%

Elective open cholecystectomy has a mortality rate of 0.3% or less. Urgent or emergency operation for acute cholecystitis has a mortality rate of up to 10% depending on whether common duct stones are present. The morbidity of cholecystectomy is primarily related to superficial wound infection (less than 5 to 7%). Wound infection is more common if the operation lasts longer than 2 hours, the patient is obese or diabetic, and the patient has acute rather than chronic cholecystitis. Other possible but rare (less than 1%) immediate complications of cholecystectomy are postoperative bleeding, postoperative bile leak, injury to biliary ducts (0.1%), and retained common duct stones.

Cholecystostomy

Cholecystostomy may be required in the patient who is critically ill from acute cholecystitis and who has associated severe cardiac, pulmonary, or renal disease that contraindicates the use of general anesthesia or of a prolonged operation. Another less often cited indication for cholecystostomy is inability to detect normal biliary anatomy because of a severe inflammatory process near the main bile ducts. Rather than risk possible injury to structures in the porta hepatis, a cholecystostomy may be performed.

A cholecystostomy can be done through a small incision in the right upper quadrant under local anesthesia. A large drainage tube is inserted into the gallbladder through a stab wound in the fundus. The tube is brought through the abdominal wall and allowed to drain freely. An attempt should be made to empty the gallbladder of stones before placing the tube. If a stone is impacted at the cystic duct, future cholecystectomy will be necessary or a mucous fistula will persist after the tube is removed. However, if all stones are removed, only 30 to 50% of patients will develop recurrent symptoms of cholelithiasis within 2 years after the tube is removed. The operative mortality is very high from cholecystostomy, not because of the operation, but because of the patient's critical condition.

Choledochotomy

Common duct exploration or choledochotomy, whether combined with cholecystectomy or as an isolated operation, has a higher morbidity and mortality rate than does simple cholecystectomy. The operation takes longer than cholecystectomy and patients are generally older, two factors important in determining morbidity and mortality. Generally the patient is hospitalized 3 to 5 days longer for common duct exploration than for cholecystectomy alone (see below). A drain (called a T-tube) is generally placed in the common duct at the time of operation. This is done to stent the repair and allow postoperative imaging to rule out retained stones or other technical problems.

COURSE AFTER OPEN BILIARY SURGERY
Normal Course

The patient is usually discharged 5 to 7 days after an uncomplicated biliary tract operation. Skin sutures will have been removed, and the patient will be allowed to bathe. Usually patients are requested to avoid driving and sexual relations for 1 week from the day of discharge. Patients are generally advised to avoid heavy (approximately 15 pounds [7 kg] or more) lifting for 4 to 6 weeks. The incidence of incisional hernia (see Chapter 91) is low after a right subcostal oblique incision and slightly higher with a vertical midline or paramedian incision. The patient returns to the surgeon's office for evaluation at 1 and 6 weeks after operation. The wound and the drain sites, if present, should be healed unless there has been wound infection. If a common duct exploration was performed, the T-tube is removed at the first visit. The patient should be able to resume an unrestricted regular diet within a few days of operation without difficulty. Stools should be at preoperative frequency and of normal color. Immediate weight loss of 10 to 20 pounds is normal, even in uncomplicated cases.

The patient should be expected to complain about pulling sensations in the area of the incision because the right rectus muscle has been divided and resutured.

Table 90.3. Frequency and Causes of PCS

	Bodvall and Oevergaard (1967)	Stefanini et al. (1974)	Hess (1977)	Brandstatter et al. (1976)
Number of patients with cholecystectomy	1930	800	919	—
PCS total	764 (40%)	249 (31%)	142 (26%)	—
Severe PCS	104 (5%)	32 (4%)	—	—
Cause				
Organic total	—	—	58%	66%
Organic biliary	9%	14%	4.5%	43%
Organic extrabiliary	—	—	53.5%	23%
Nonorganic total	—	—	42%	34%

Modified from Tondelli P, Gyr K, Stalder GA, Allgower M. The biliary tract. Part I. Cholecystectomy. Clin Gastroenterol 8:486, 1979.

If the subcostal incision was made close to the costal margin, the patient often complains also about discomfort on bending or sitting. The area just below a right subcostal incision is apt to be numb for several months because of interruption of a cutaneous sensory nerve to this area. Sensitivity does return, however, in most cases. It is not surprising to find patients gaining weight after cholecystectomy, especially if they had lost weight preoperatively.

Postcholecystectomy Syndrome

Approximately 90% of patients operated on for symptomatic biliary tract disease become asymptomatic or have trivial symptoms (e.g., occasional dyspepsia). The other 10% may continue to be symptomatic, either because they were treated for the wrong disease or because they have developed a postoperative complication. In the former category are patients who had gallstones but whose symptoms actually emanated from another disease (e.g., recurrent pancreatitis, peptic ulcer disease, angina, reflux esophagitis, or hiatus hernia).

Postoperative problems associated with the operation itself include retained common duct stones, an excessively long cystic duct remnant, and common duct injury with eventual bile duct stricture and recurrent cholangitis. Sphincter-of-Oddi dysfunction is being increasingly recognized as one of the treatable causes of postcholecystectomy syndrome. The diagnosis is made by showing a decrease in the emptying of the biliary tree by cholecystokinin cholecystography with ^{99m}Tc-iminodiacetic derivatives (see above) and by demonstrating an elevated sphincter pressure by manometry during ERCP. Sphincterotomy in patients with elevated sphincter pressure results in pain relief in more than 90% of cases (6).

Tondelli et al. (22) collated data from a number of series on the incidence and cause of the postcholecystectomy syndrome (PCS) (Table 90.3). Mild PCS refers to symptoms of dyspepsia, constipation, diarrhea, and intolerance to certain foods. Severe PCS refers to severe upper abdominal pain, cholangitis, or biliary fistula. Organic biliary etiologies include retained common duct stones, papillary stenosis, bile duct stricture, cystic duct remnant, chronic pancreatitis, or bile duct tumor. Organic extrabiliary etiologies include esophagitis, ulcer disease, pancreatitis, liver disease, heart disease, colon or urinary tract disease, and adhesions. Nonorganic disease includes irritable bowel syndrome and psychiatric or metabolic disease.

General References

Kaplowitz N. Liver and biliary diseases. 2nd ed. Baltimore: Williams & Wilkins, 1996.
> A comprehensive and current text.

Ransohoff DF, Gracie WA. Treatment of gallstones. Ann Intern Med 119:606–619, 1993.
> A comprehensive review of risks and benefits of therapy for patients with gallstones.

Specific References

1. Bennion LJ, Grundy SM. Risk factors for the development of cholelithiasis in man. N Engl J Med 299:1161–1167, 1978.
2. Ferruci T. Body ultrasonography. N Engl J Med 300:538–542, 590–602, 1979.
3. Friedman LS, Roberts MS, Brett AS, Marton KI. Management of asymptomatic gallstones in the diabetic patient. A decision analysis. Ann Intern Med 109:913–919, 1988.
4. Gadacz TR. Laparoscopy cholecystectomy. In: Cameron JL, ed. Current surgical therapy. 4th ed. St. Louis: CV Mosby, 1992; 330–334.
5. Gracie WA, Ransohoff DF. The natural history of silent gallstones. The innocent gallstone is not a myth. N Engl J Med 307:798–800, 1982.
6. Greenen JE, Hogan WJ, Dodds WJ, et al. The efficacy of endoscopic sphincterotomy after cholecystectomy in patients with sphincter-of-Oddi dysfunction. N Engl J Med 320:82–87, 1989.
7. Jarvinen HJ, Hastbacka J. Early cholecystectomy for acute cholecystitis: a prospective randomized study. Ann Surg 191: 501–505, 1980.
8. Johnston DE, Kaplan MM. Pathogenesis and treatment of gallstones. N Engl J Med 328:412–421, 1993.
9. Lee YM, Kaplan MM. Medical progress: primary sclerosing cholangitis. N Engl J Med 310:918–933, 1984.
10. Lowenfels AB, Lindstrom CG, Conway MJ, Hastings PR. Gallstones and risk of gallbladder cancer. J Natl Cancer Inst 75:77–80, 1985.
11. Lund J. Surgical indications in cholelithiasis; prophylactic cholecystectomy elucidated on the basis of long-term follow-up on 526 nonoperated cases. Ann Surg 151:153–162, 1960.
12. Max MH, Polk HC. Routine preoperative upper gastrointestinal series (UGIS) in patients with biliary tract disease: a plea for more selectivity. Surgery 82:334–341, 1977.
13. Morrow DJ, Thompson J, Wilson SE. Acute cholecystitis in the elderly, a surgical emergency. Arch Surg 113:1149–1152, 1978.
14. Mundth ED. Cholecystitis and diabetes mellitus. N Engl J Med 267:642–646, 1962.
15. Ootani T, Shirai Y, Tuskada K, Muto T. Relationship between gallbladder carcinoma and the segmental type of adenomyomatosis of the gallbladder. Cancer 69:2647–2652, 1992.

16. Pokorny WJ, Saleem M, O'Gorman RB, et al. Cholelithiasis and cholecystitis in childhood. Am J Surg 148:742, 1984.
17. Prat F, Malak NA, Pelletier G. Biliary symptoms and complications more than 8 years after endoscopic spichterotomy. Gastroenterology 110:894–899, 1996.
18. Ram MD, Midha D. Adenomyomatosis of the gallbladder. Surgery 78:224–229, 1975.
19. Southern Surgeons Club. A prospective analysis of 1518 laparoscopic cholecystectomies. N Engl J Med 324:1073–1078, 1991.
20. Thistle JL, Schoenfield LJ. Lithogenic bile among young Indian women: lithogenic potential decreased with chenodeoxycholic acid. N Engl J Med 284:177–181, 1971.
21. Thurston OG, McDougall RM. The effect of hepatic bile on retained common duct stones. Surg Gynecol Obstet 143:625–627, 1976.
22. Tondelli P, Gyr K, Stalder GA, Allgower M. The biliary tract. Part I. Cholecystectomy. Clin Gastroenterol 8:487–505, 1978.

C H A P T E R 91

Abdominal Hernias*

MARK D. DUNCAN, MD
JEFFREY S. BENDER, MD

DEFINITIONS

A hernia is a protrusion of a viscus or part of a viscus from its normal location in the body. Clinically, common hernias are protrusions of a part of an abdominal viscus through the abdominal wall. Depending on the site at which hernias occur, they are described as inguinal, femoral, umbilical, epigastric, and so on. The term *ventral hernia,* referring to an anterior abdominal wall hernia, is commonly used to denote an incisional hernia. A hernia is called *reducible* if its contents can be pushed back into the abdominal cavity, and *irreducible* or *incarcerated* if they cannot be pushed back. *Strangulation* of a hernia occurs when the blood supply to the herniated viscus is compromised. All strangulated hernias are incarcerated but incarcerated hernias may not be strangulated.

This chapter describes the more common types of hernias and discusses the role of the general physician in their diagnosis and treatment.

Michael E. Zenilman, MD, and Gardner W. Smith, MD, contributed to this chapter in the fourth edition.

HERNIAS OF THE GROIN

Inguinal Hernias

Inguinal hernias (Fig. 91.1) are classified as direct or indirect; more than two-thirds are indirect. *Direct hernias* are portions of the bowel or omentum that protrude directly through the floor of the inguinal canal to emerge through the external inguinal ring and protrude above the inguinal ligament (Fig. 91.2). *Indirect hernias* enter the inguinal canal through its internal ring, lateral to the inferior epigastric vessels, traverse the canal, and emerge also through the external inguinal ring (Fig. 91.2). Indirect hernias, as they get larger, have a propensity to extend into the scrotum.

Epidemiology and Causes

Inguinal hernia is a common problem in ambulatory practice and accounts for approximately 75% of all abdominal wall hernias. Approximately 85% of inguinal hernias occur in men. At some time in their lives, 5 to 10% of men in the United States develop an inguinal hernia. Even in women, inguinal hernia accounts for more than half of the abdominal hernias. Although femoral hernias (see below) are much more common in women than in men, the most common groin hernia in women is an indirect inguinal hernia. Less than 10% of inguinal hernias in adults are bilateral when the patient is first seen, but a hernia may occur on the opposite side at some time in the future. The chance of developing a contralateral inguinal hernia is the same regardless of the side affected first.

All *indirect inguinal hernias* are due to a congenital defect in which the processus vaginalis remains patent. The processus vaginalis is a tract lined with peritoneum that extends from the peritoneal cavity into the scrotum in the male. With time this tract may enlarge, and abdominal contents may herniate into it. Occasionally, only intra-abdominal fluid may gravitate into the scrotum, causing scrotal swelling when the patient is upright but draining back into the abdominal cavity when the patient is supine. Such a lesion is called a *communicating hydrocele* and is more commonly seen in children than in adults. The severity of the combination of this congenital abnormality and a predisposing acquired condition that increases intra-abdominal pressure (e.g., obesity, chronic obstructive airway disease, ascites, chronic constipation with straining at stool, prostatism with straining at urination, and hard physical labor) determines when an inguinal hernia develops.

Direct inguinal hernias are acquired lesions and are influenced not only by changes in intra-abdominal pressure but also by progressive attenuation of the inguinal structures as part of the normal aging process. Rarely, inherited defects in collagen synthesis (e.g., Marfan's syndrome) provide an obvious explanation for accelerated weakening of these structures.

Direct hernias are predominantly problems of middle-aged and elderly people. Indirect hernias, because they are associated with a congenital defect,

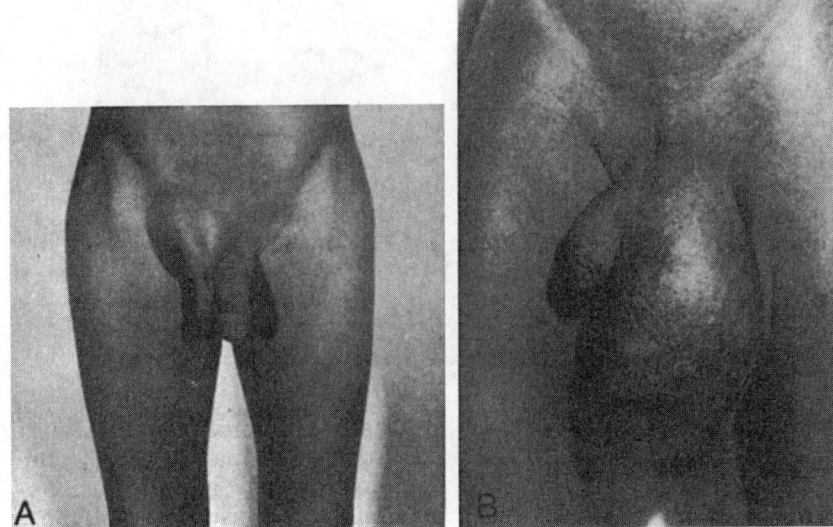

Figure 91.1. **A.** Right inguinal hernia in a young adult male. **B.** Left scrotal hernia. (From Zimmerman LM, Anson BJ. Anatomy and surgery of hernia. 2nd ed. Baltimore: Williams & Wilkins, 1967;152.)

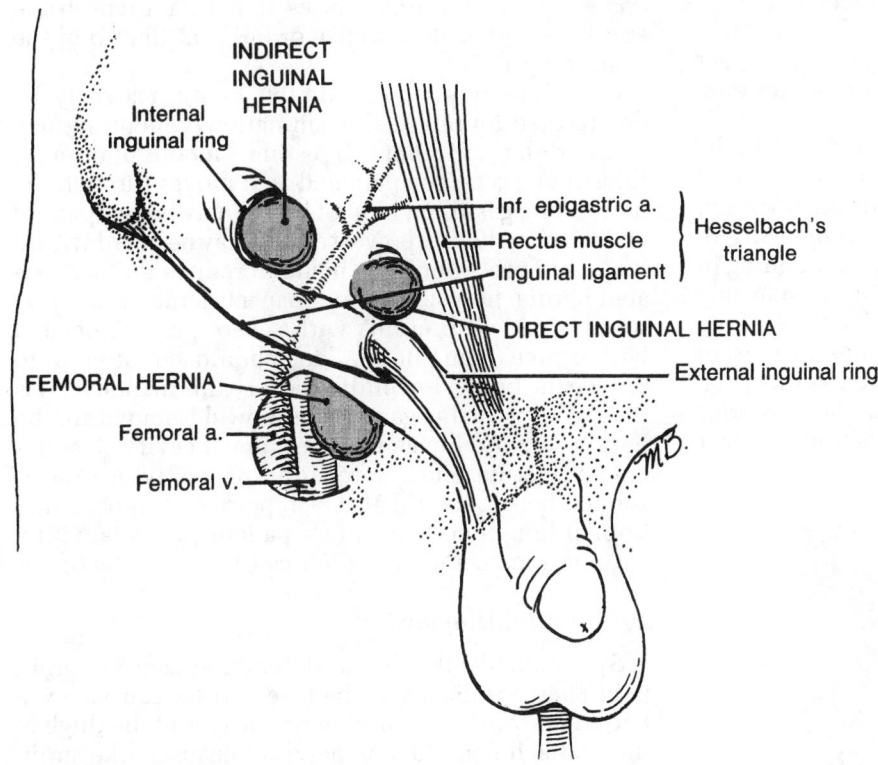

Figure 91.2. Artist's rendition of groin region illustrating indirect and direct inguinal hernias and femoral hernia. (Modified from Dunphy JE, Botsford TW. Physical examination of the surgical patient. 3rd ed. Philadelphia: WB Saunders, 1964;118.)

develop in younger people, but these also increase in incidence with advancing age and are about four to five times more common after age 50 than before.

History

Most patients complain of a dull ache in the groin and a bulge, either localized to the groin or extending into the scrotum (in women, the labia are the anatomic counterpart of the scrotum). Sometimes pain precedes discovery of the mass by some months (perhaps because, in early stages of herniation, the internal canal is stretched before omentum or bowel presents as a bulge

at the external inguinal ring). Occasionally, a patient recalls a short burning pain during straining, which represents the initial herniation. Often the patient or the physician notices the herniated mass, but no pain has been experienced. If the hernia becomes large enough, it may cause a dragging sensation when the patient walks. Small reducible indirect hernias may be noticed intermittently, at times of increased intra-abdominal pressure.

If a hernia incarcerates, it may become more painful, although many patients with chronically incarcerated hernias are pain free. Indirect hernias have an approximately 10% chance of incarcerating; direct hernias incarcerate only rarely. Essentially all strangulated hernias are symptomatic: The hernia becomes extremely painful and tender, and nausea, vomiting, abdominal distension, constipation, and fever (with leukocytosis) are common.

Physical Examination

The examination should first be performed while the patient is standing. An indirect hernia sometimes can be distinguished from a direct hernia by inspection: An indirect hernia, once it has entered the inguinal canal, presents as an elliptical swelling descending toward or even into the scrotum (Fig. 91.3). A direct hernia presents as an isolated oval swelling near the pubis; it rarely is found in the scrotum (Fig. 91.4). If the hernia is visible, an attempt should be made to push it back into the abdominal cavity. If the hernia cannot be reduced, the patient should be asked to lie down and another attempt should be made to reduce it. Approximately 10% of inguinal hernias are incarcerated when they are first diagnosed.

If the hernia is not visible, the physician's finger should be placed at the base of the scrotum and then gently advanced cephalad and laterally into the inguinal canal (Fig. 91.5). The external ring can be examined without causing the patient a great deal of discomfort. The size of the ring, in itself, does not predict the presence of a hernia or the propensity to develop one because the external ring is an opening in the aponeurosis of the external oblique muscle that does not contribute to the integrity of the floor of the inguinal canal. Further palpation identifies the crest of the pubic bone, the fibers of the external inguinal ring, the spermatic cord, and weakness in the posterior inguinal canal, if present. When the examining finger

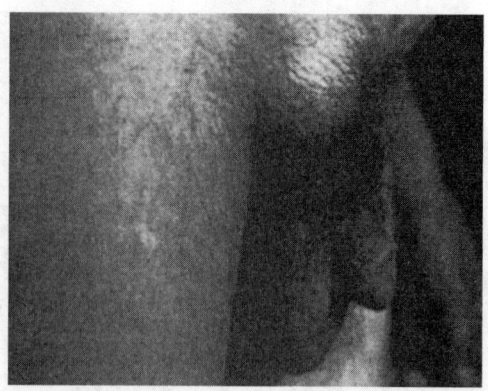

Figure 91.4. Direct inguinal hernia. Note medially situated globular swelling. (From Zimmerman LM, Anson BJ. Anatomy and surgery of hernia. 2nd ed. Baltimore: Williams & Wilkins, 1967;154.)

has been directed through the external ring, having the patient increase intra-abdominal pressure by coughing or straining causes a hernia to protrude and to be felt as an impulse or bulge at the tip of the examining finger.

Occasionally, contents of the hernia sac may be determined by physical examination: Omentum may feel nodular and pliant; intestine, smooth and tense. Intestinal gas can be palpated as it moves through the bowel, or a gas-filled loop of bowel may be tympanitic and on auscultation bowel sounds may be heard within it. An attempt should be made to reduce an incarcerated hernia; however, if one suspects strangulation, as when a patient presents with severe pain associated with a preexisting hernia, one should not attempt to reduce the hernia forcefully because this maneuver has the risk of reducing gangrenous bowel from within the hernia sac into the general peritoneal cavity. A strangulated hernia must be repaired promptly. An incarcerated hernia should also be repaired upon presentation, although occasionally a patient presents with a chronic incarceration, which can be fixed electively.

Differential Diagnosis

Symptomatically, the most common cause of groin pain that is mistakenly believed to be caused by a hernia is *strain of the adductor muscles* of the thigh at their attachment to the pelvis. Because, like groin hernia, the onset of this symptom is related to physical labor, both the patient and the physician are convinced that a hernia must be present. In the absence of appropriate physical findings, the temptation to explore the groin must be firmly resisted.

An incarcerated scrotal hernia must be distinguished from other scrotal lesions (Fig. 91.6). One of the most common of these is a *hydrocele,* a tense, slightly fluctuant mass that can be distinguished from a hernia or a solid mass by transillumination.

Another common scrotal mass is a *varicocele,* an enlarged venous plexus that on palpation feels soft and wormlike and extends from the testicle up toward the spermatic cord. It does not transilluminate and, when

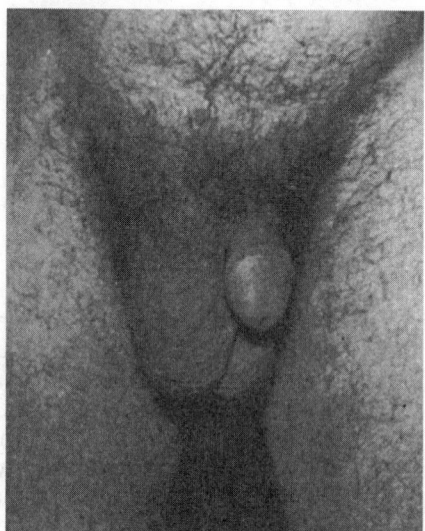

Figure 91.3. Indirect inguinal hernia. Swelling is oblique and cylindrical, and extends into the scrotum. (From Zimmerman LM, Anson BJ. Anatomy and surgery of hernia. 2nd ed. Baltimore: Williams & Wilkins, 1967;155.)

the patient lies down, it collapses. If a varicocele is of recent onset in the adult, occurs on the left, and does not disappear in the supine position, one must consider obstruction of the left spermatic vein (which enters the left renal vein) by a retroperitoneal neoplasm.

A *spermatocele* is a localized but vaguely circumscribed mass that also does not transilluminate and that persists when the patient lies down.

Apart from distinguishing a hernia from another kind of scrotal mass, an important component of the physical examination is the examination of the testicle and its surrounding structures. In that way epididymal cysts, epididymitis, orchitis, testicular torsion, and testicular tumors can be detected. *Epididymal cysts* may be in any portion of the epididymis and may be smooth or lobulated; some of them transilluminate; they are innocuous and require no treatment. *Epididymitis* presents as a tender, swollen epididymis. The inflammation, if untreated, may spread to the testicle (orchitis); see Chapter 27 for a discussion of this problem. Often, elevation and immobilization of the scrotum relieve the pain associated with an inflammatory process. In contrast, the pain produced by *torsion of the testicle* is unremitting. Sudden onset of testicular pain in an otherwise healthy person is characteristic of

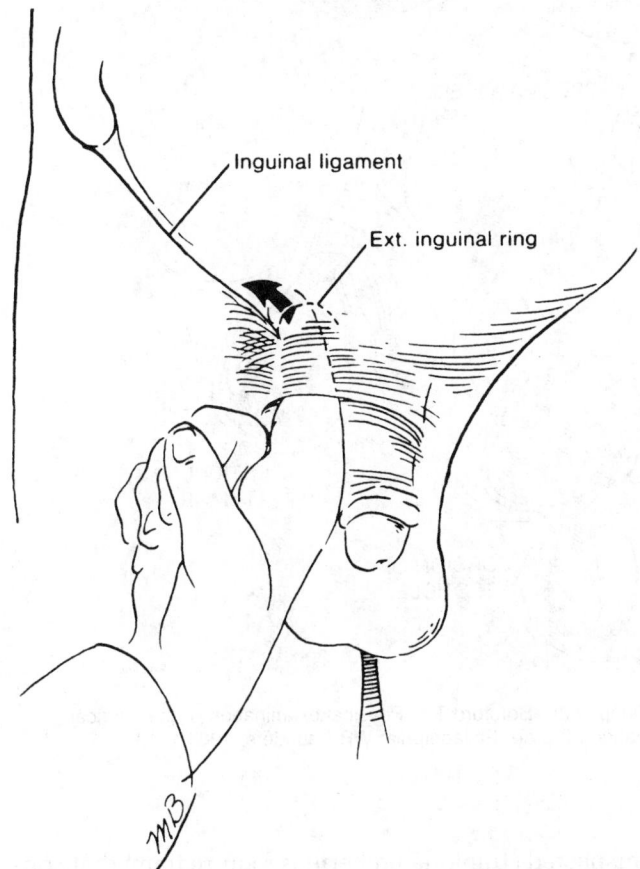

Figure 91.5. Examination of the inguinal canal. The examining finger gently invaginates the scrotum into the inguinal canal. (Modified from Dunphy JE, Botsford TW. Physical examination of the surgical patient. 3rd ed. Philadelphia: WB Saunders, 1964;116.)

this problem. On examination, the testicle is enlarged and exquisitely tender. The patient should be referred immediately to a general surgeon or urologist. *Testicular tumors* can involve the entire testicle or simply protrude as a small nodule from the testicular surface. These masses are more indurated than the common benign scrotal masses and usually lack the slight tenderness of the normal testicle. Patients with suspected tumors should be referred as soon as possible to a urologist.

Preoperative Evaluation of the Patient with a Hernia

When evaluating a patient with a hernia, it is important to consider whether coexistent disease has allowed the hernia to be manifest at that point in time. Focused questions in the medical history should include a specific inquiry about smoking, a history of a cough, difficulty urinating, or difficulty with bowel movements, including straining and constipation. A rectal examination, to assess for the presence of prostatic hypertrophy or a rectal mass, is an important part of the preoperative evaluation. The examiner should also ascertain whether ascites is present. Anything that increases intra-abdominal pressure will place tension on the endoabdominal fascia and may contribute to the development or presentation of hernia. A practitioner would not want to miss a diagnosis of lung cancer, prostate cancer, or colorectal cancer when referring a patient for hernia repair. Furthermore, attention to any predisposing causes of increased intra-abdominal pressure may limit the negative effect these conditions have on hernia recurrence rates.

Management

Almost all inguinal hernias should be repaired. Severe coexistent illness is the only real contraindication to herniorrhaphy (see Chapter 86 for a discussion of anesthesia/surgery risks in patients with coexistent medical conditions). Although no sense of urgency is associated with elective repair, it should be recognized that the risk of incarceration or of strangulation is much greater with indirect than with direct hernia. Accordingly, the repair of a direct hernia may be more confidently deferred, or even declined, in the face of a significant medical illness. Nonoperative therapy should be discouraged; the wearing of a truss is potentially dangerous and does not guarantee that a hernia will remain reduced. Also, the pressure of the truss on the margin of a large defect eventually leads to atrophy of the fascial and aponeurotic (broad tendinous) layers, causing the hernia to enlarge. Subsequent repair is more difficult and therefore carries a greater risk of recurrence.

Elective herniorrhaphy prevents acute incarceration (and strangulation) and the need to perform an emergency operation. If the hernia is chronically incarcerated and there are no symptoms of strangulation (strangulation is primarily a risk in acutely incarcerated, small indirect hernias), repair may still be scheduled electively. If the hernia has incarcerated acutely, the

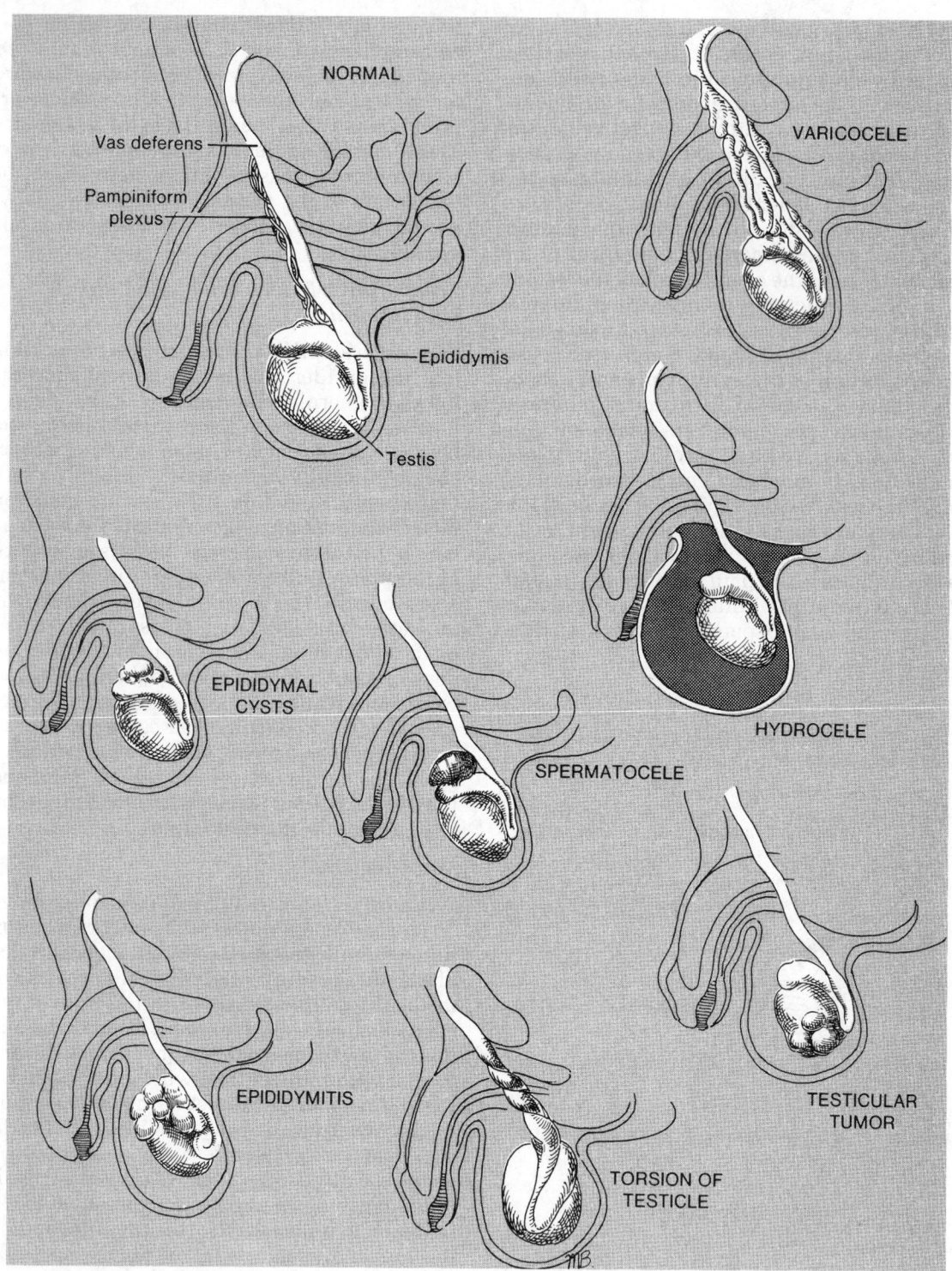

Figure 91.6. Lesions palpable in the scrotum. A correct diagnosis can usually be made if the normal anatomic relationships of the contents of the scrotum are borne in mind. (Modified from Dunphy JE, Botsford TW. Physical examination of the surgical patient. 3rd ed. Philadelphia: WB Saunders, 1964;111.)

patient must be hospitalized and attempts made to reduce the hernia before operation. Strangulated hernia is a true surgical emergency because delay in treatment can lead to gangrene of the intestine or omentum.

Suspected strangulated hernias require immediate operative intervention.

Bilateral hernias may be repaired at one operation or as staged procedures, depending on their size, the type of repair required, the age of the patient, and coexistent problems. If the patient is elderly, and the hernias are large and require complex repair, herniorrhaphies should be staged 4 to 6 weeks apart. Bilateral repairs of indirect inguinal hernias in children or young adults are routinely done at one operation.

Currently, most unilateral inguinal hernias are repaired through a 6- to 8-cm incision under local or regional anesthesia as outpatient procedures. Some surgeons routinely use prosthetic mesh during the repair. The patient is rarely uncomfortable during the operation. This approach leads to fewer postoperative complications, such as atelectasis and acute urinary retention, and also reduces the cost of hospitalization. Epidural, spinal, or general anesthesia is used in patients who cannot tolerate the procedure under local anesthesia, patients with large hernias requiring complex repair, or obese patients in whom repair of the hernia under local anesthesia is technically difficult. Bilateral inguinal herniorrhaphy may also require epidural, spinal, or general anesthesia. Repair of hernias in children is usually done under general anesthesia.

Laparoscopic Herniorrhaphy. Laparoscopic (or minimally invasive) surgery has gained popularity in the treatment of groin hernias. General anesthesia is required. A laparoscope and two or three instruments are introduced into the peritoneal cavity, usually through three separate 0.5 to 1.0-cm incisions rather than one long incision. Under direct visualization, indirect hernia sacs can be dissected and even large defects can be repaired using prosthetic mesh. Laparoscopic herniorrhaphy is an outpatient procedure. Reported advantages to the laparoscopic approach include lower levels of postoperative pain and shorter recuperative time than after the standard repairs. Several large studies document the safety of the procedure with good short-term follow-up. It is perhaps particularly suited to recurrent groin hernias or bilateral hernia repair. Disadvantages include the need for general anesthesia and a higher complication rate (10 to 17%) than for anterior repair (1 to 10%). Ilioinguinal neuralgia seems to occur more often following laparoscopic repair, but this may also be true of anterior repairs in which mesh is used. More significantly, clinical data regarding long-term recurrence rates are lacking. The cost of laparoscopic repair at this time is significantly higher than that of open repair. As surgeons' familiarity with the laparoscopic approach to the groin improves, complication rates should decrease; if long-term review validates low recurrence rates, the postoperative benefits of laparoscopic repair will make it attractive for selected patients with groin hernias. The predominant approach still remains the traditional open anterior repair.

Course and Recovery

No matter which anesthesia or technique is used, certain *complications of herniorrhaphy* are possible (in approximately 7% of patients): recurrence (the most common complication, see below), urinary retention, wound infection, hydrocele formation, femoral or ilioinguinal neuralgia, scrotal hematoma, and rarely, unilateral testicular atrophy. The general physician and the surgeon should discuss these complications with the patient before the operation and provide assurance that, except for recurrence of hernia, they are usually treatable or transient problems.

When patients are discharged from the hospital, they are ambulatory and usually require no more than codeine for relief of pain. Patients are admitted to the hospital only if urinary retention or another complication such as bleeding or hypotension occurs. Patients with preexisting medical illnesses, particularly cardiac disease, may be admitted as needed for medical management perioperatively. For the first week, the patient is advised to avoid lifting or straining and to use a stool softener and a mild laxative (see Chapter 39). The patient can return to light work (and light activity such as long walks) within another 2 weeks, but an occupation that requires heavy lifting or considerable exertion requires a total convalescence of about 4 to 6 weeks. Driving a car during the first 2 weeks should be discouraged, not because it is a form of strenuous activity, but because the patient, fearing pain or injury, may not step on the brake vigorously enough or soon enough in a crisis to avoid a collision. Sexual activity is permitted if it is not uncomfortable to the patient. Resumption of normal recreational and work activities requires common sense. Most patients are fully rehabilitated and working less than 1 month after herniorrhaphy. Because recurrence may be related to premature untoward exertion, patients must be cautioned to avoid strenuous activity for 6 weeks. However, most recurrences are caused by technical problems related to the hernia repair or wound infections.

Approximately 1 to 7% of indirect and 4 to 10% of direct inguinal hernias recur. More than 50% of the recurrences occur within 5 years of the initial repair. Unfortunately, the recurrence rate after repair of a recurrent hernia is very high, ranging from 5 to 35%. Most surgeons use mesh in repairing recurrent hernias. Apart from advising patients with a recurrent hernia that has been repaired to avoid straining and heavy lifting and to lose weight if they are obese, there is no special advice that these patients can be given.

Femoral Hernias

Epidemiology and Causes

A femoral hernia is a protrusion of omentum or bowel through the femoral canal (Fig. 91.2). It is the second most common type of abdominal hernia, accounting for 10% of all abdominal hernias. It is much more common in women than in men; 33% of abdominal hernias in women, but only 3% of abdominal hernias in men, are femoral hernias. The incidence increases with increasing age, presumably because of the degradation of collagen and attenuation of tissue that accompanies aging (see "Inguinal Hernias," above). It is likely, however, that a contributing cause of a femoral hernia is a congenitally large femoral ring. Preperitoneal fat, forced through the large ring, enlarges it further. Increased pressure produced by straining or pregnancy undoubtedly contributes to femoral herniation. Femoral hernias are bilateral in 15% or more of cases. The risk of incarceration, and particularly of strangulation, is especially high with this type of hernia.

History

The primary symptom of a femoral hernia is a bulge in the groin. A dull pain may be experienced, but less commonly than in patients with an inguinal hernia. Approximately 20% of femoral hernias incarcerate (twice the rate of indirect inguinal hernias). The symptoms of incarceration and strangulation are the same as they are in patients with inguinal hernias.

Physical Examination

A mass is often palpable, medial to the femoral vessels, and inferior to the inguinal ligament. The mass is usually reducible, and occasionally it is tender. Despite careful examination, the hernia often is difficult to detect, especially in obese women, even if it is incarcerated or strangulated. Therefore, women with signs and symptoms of unexplained intestinal obstruction should be examined carefully for evidence of a strangulated femoral hernia.

Differential Diagnosis

A femoral hernia must be distinguished from an enlarged lymph node, a lipoma, a saphenous varix, and a direct inguinal hernia. The first three of these possibilities are not reducible. A lymph node or lipoma may not transmit an impulse to the examiner's finger when the patient coughs. A saphenous varix may simulate a hernia impulse, however, because increased venous pressure induced by the Valsalva maneuver is transmitted to the varix. A lymph node or a lipoma is more movable than a hernia, and a varix can be collapsed by compression of the saphenous vein. The distinction between a femoral and other groin hernias sometimes can be made only at operation.

Management and Course

Femoral hernias should be repaired unless the patient is unable to tolerate an operation. The increased risk of incarceration and strangulation adds to the urgency of the recommendation. The operative and postoperative considerations of inguinal hernia (see above) apply to femoral hernias as well except that, for technical reasons, a larger proportion of these may have to be performed under spinal or general anesthesia, usually as outpatient procedures. Laparoscopy (see above) can also be used in femoral hernia repair. From 1 to 7% of femoral hernias recur and, like inguinal hernias, 5 to 35% of repaired recurrent hernias also recur.

INCISIONAL HERNIAS

An incisional hernia is the protrusion of omentum or bowel through a surgical incision. Unlike the other types of abdominal hernia, a congenital weakness of the abdominal wall does not contribute to the development of the hernia. Any abdominal incision may be the site of a hernia. The major risk factors leading to the development of an incisional hernia are poor surgical technique, wound infection, and obesity. With the increasing use of chronic ambulatory peritoneal dialysis to treat patients in chronic renal failure (see Chapter 48), it has become apparent that incisional hernias (as well as inguinal hernias) are particularly common in this group of patients.

The hernia usually presents as a bulge through the incision that may enlarge if neglected (Fig. 91.7) and may even lead to intestinal obstruction. It should be repaired soon after the diagnosis is made to avoid the development of a larger defect that will complicate repair and be more likely to recur. If possible, an obese patient should lose weight before the operation (see Chapter 76). In the presence of a previous incision and adhesions, these hernias should not be repaired laparoscopically.

UMBILICAL HERNIAS

An umbilical hernia is a protrusion of omentum or bowel through the umbilical ring. These hernias are probably due to congenital defects. Among adults, they appear most often in middle-aged multiparous women, in patients with cirrhosis of the liver and ascites, and in frail elderly people. They are also common in infants, especially African-American infants.

Most umbilical hernias are obvious as an enlargement of the umbilical ring with protrusion of intra-abdominal contents through it. However, a few patients complain only of vague intermittent pain and tenderness in the region of the umbilicus. On examination, a small defect is usually found that contains a small piece of omentum, preperitoneal fat, or a knuckle of bowel. If the patient is placed in the supine position and asked to raise his head and cough, the hernia can be palpated.

The most common complication of umbilical hernia is incarceration with or without strangulation. For that reason, unless the patient cannot tolerate an operation, all umbilical hernias in adults should be repaired. Morbidity and mortality from such an operation are much lower if it is performed electively rather than in response to acute incarceration or strangulation. The only exception to this recommendation is umbilical hernias in infants. These tend to close spontaneously as the child gets older and repair should be deferred until school age.

The procedure may be done under local anesthesia if the hernia is small; otherwise, general or spinal anesthesia should be used. The procedure does not require overnight hospitalization.

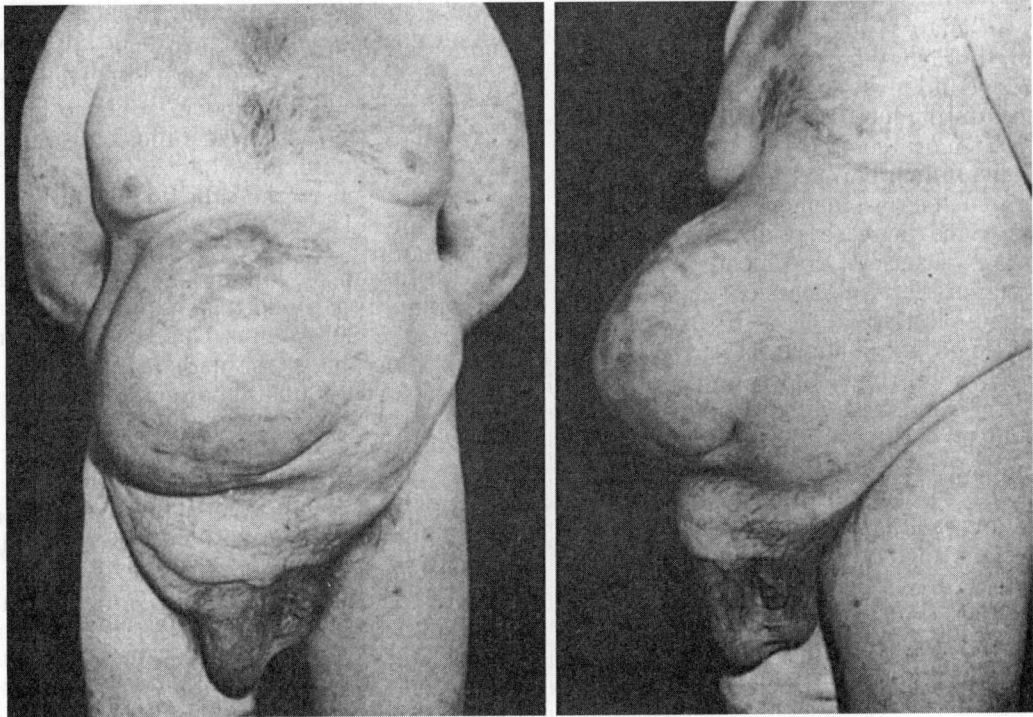

Figure 91.7. Large postoperative (ventral) hernia after cholecystectomy. (From Zimmerman LM, Anson BJ. Anatomy and surgery of hernia. 2nd ed. Baltimore: Williams & Wilkins, 1967;287.)

EPIGASTRIC HERNIAS

An epigastric hernia is a protrusion of fat or omentum through the linea alba between the umbilicus and the xiphoid cartilage. These hernias almost never contain a viscus. A congenital defect in the linea alba is probably the major disposing factor. Epigastric hernias most commonly appear between the ages of 20 and 50 and are three times more common in men than in women.

Most patients complain of a small painless subcutaneous mass, most often just to the left of the midline. Usually the hernia consists of preperitoneal fat or fat of the falciform ligament. Larger defects also contain omentum.

Complications are more common in patients with small hernias because these are more likely to incarcerate. When this happens, there is usually local pain and tenderness and, less often, deep epigastric pain, abdominal distension, and nausea and vomiting.

All epigastric hernias should be repaired, usually as outpatient procedures. The recurrence rate after epigastric herniorrhaphy is approximately 10% and usually can be attributed to failure to appreciate multiple defects in the linea alba at the time of the initial operation.

General References

Memon MA, Rice D, Donohue JH. Laparoscopic herniorrhaphy. J Am Coll Surg 184:325, 1997.
  Review of the experience with laparoscopic hernia repair.
Nyhus LM, Condon RE, eds. Hernia. Philadelphia: JB Lippincott, 1995.
  A definitive text.
Rutkow IM, ed. Hernia surgery. Surg Clin North Am 73(3), 1993.
  Fourteen articles on different aspects of hernias.

CHAPTER 92

Benign Conditions of the Anus and Rectum

GARDNER W. SMITH, MD

Anorectal disorders are often encountered in ambulatory practice. This chapter describes four particularly common problems: pruritus ani, anal fissure, hemorrhoidal disease, and perirectal abscess. Also included, because of their importance to the general physician, are somewhat less common problems such as proctalgia fugax and rectal prolapse. The final section addresses sexually transmitted diseases that affect the anus and rectum. Cutaneous disorders that involve the perianal area and perineum are discussed in Chapters 94 ("Nonmalignant Vulvovaginal and Cervical Disorders") and 100 ("Common Problems of the Skin"). Other conditions that may affect the rectum are discussed in Chapters 26 ("Acute Gastroenteritis and Associated Conditions") and 39 ("Constipation and Diarrhea").

PRURITUS ANI

Definition

Pruritus ani, a distressing perianal itch, is a common complaint, particularly among men. The symptom varies in intensity but is usually greatest at night. Often the itching abates spontaneously, only to recur after variable asymptomatic periods.

Causes

It is important to note that pruritus ani is a symptom, not a primary condition. Accordingly, although the cause is often unknown (50 to 75% of the time), the symptom may be a manifestation of many anorectal disorders (Table 92.1). In older adults, pruritus ani is associated with colorectal and anal neoplasia. Whatever the cause, the itching is often associated with moist macerated perianal skin, often complicated by excoriation and secondary infection. These changes may be caused by fecal contamination or excessive cleansing efforts, exacerbated by scratching.

Diagnosis

When a patient complains of perianal itching, specific historical information should be obtained and several observations should be made to aid in establishing a diagnosis.

History

Stress is often a contributing factor and a careful personal history may therefore be significant. A dietary history is also important because an excess intake of milk, coffee, tea, alcohol, cola, chocolate, tomato products, and spices may be associated with pruritus ani. Medications such as laxatives or colchicine, which cause gastrointestinal irritation, can be a cause of perianal itching, as is also true of certain oral antibiotics such as the tetracyclines. Chronic diarrhea may also be causative.

General Examination

The patient should be examined for the presence of a dermatologic problem such as psoriasis, scabies, or fungal infection (Table 92.1) that may be associated with pruritus ani. In addition, in women, a pelvic examination should be performed because of the occasional association of vaginal infection with pruritus ani (see Chapter 94).

With the patient in the lateral decubitus or the knee–chest position and with the buttocks separated, the perianal area is inspected. During the inspection the patient should be asked to strain, a maneuver that

Table 92.1.   Common Problems Associated with Pruritus Ani

Drugs
    Oral antibiotics (tetracycline)
    Colchicine
    Laxatives
Dermatologic disorders
    Psoriasis
    Atopic dermatitis
    Contact dermatitis
    Lichen planus
    Condylomata
    Venereal warts
    Herpes simplex
    Tumors
Diarrhea
Fissures
Fistulas
Infection
    Fungi and yeast (especially in diabetic patients) (see Chapter 100, "Common Problems of the Skin")
    Erythrasma
    Scabies (see Chapter 100, "Common Problems of the Skin")
    Pinworm (*Enterobius vermicularis*) infestation, more common in children
    Vaginal infections (see Chapter 94, "Nonmalignant Vulvovaginal and Cervical Disorders")
Obesity and excessive sweating
Poor anal hygiene
Rectal prolapse
Prolapsed hemorrhoids (most often hemorrhoids are not associated with pruritus and other causes should be sought)

may demonstrate prolapse or fecal or flatal incontinence, or an anal fissure.

If skin lesions are identified, appropriate evaluation (e.g., a KOH preparation) to establish a diagnosis (e.g., *Tinea* or *Candida*) should be done to initiate definitive therapy (see Chapter 100). In children up to age 14, and in adults who live in the same household with infected children, the evaluation should include several cellophane tape preparations in an attempt to demonstrate the ova of pinworms (see below).

Rectal Examination

Digital rectal examination should always be performed using a well-lubricated gloved finger. Evaluation must be gentle to avoid spasm of the anal sphincter, which precludes adequate examination. At initiation of the examination, the patient should be asked to bear down, which minimizes discomfort. Excessive pain or tenderness localized to a specific area should alert the physician to the possible presence of an anal fissure (see below). All structures of the anal canal within the reach of the finger should be assessed (the anus, distal rectum, prostate gland, and cervix).

Anoscopy

After rectal examination, and without laxative or enema preparation, an anoscopy (with the use of an instrument that permits a side or oblique view) should be performed. The usual disposable anoscope, although convenient, provides only a barely adequate

side view. A well-lubricated anoscope should be inserted gently, while the patient bears down, to minimize discomfort. The instrument should be inserted slowly as deeply as possible. Then, after removal of the obturator, the rectum should be inspected using adequate light. Visualization is possible only through the side or oblique aspect of the instrument as it is withdrawn gradually. It is important to avoid rotation of the anoscope, which is uncomfortable and may tear the anal mucosa. For adequate inspection of all quadrants of the anal canal, the instrument must be reinserted and withdrawn three or four times.

Cellophane Tape Examination for Pinworms

Cellophane tape examination is easily accomplished by the patient at home or by the physician in the office. Swabs are commercially available (Pinworm Diagnostic Tapes, Parke-Davis), but they are also easily made by folding clear cellophane tape, sticky side out, over a tongue blade. At night pinworms migrate from the anal canal to the perianal area, where they deposit eggs. Therefore the swab should be obtained upon arising, before a bowel movement and before the perianal area is cleansed. The swab is placed at the anal verge and then the tape is mounted onto a glass microscopic slide. A specimen obtained in this way keeps for several days. The slides should be examined under the low power (×10) objective of the microscope, searching for the typical ova of pinworm (Fig. 92.1).

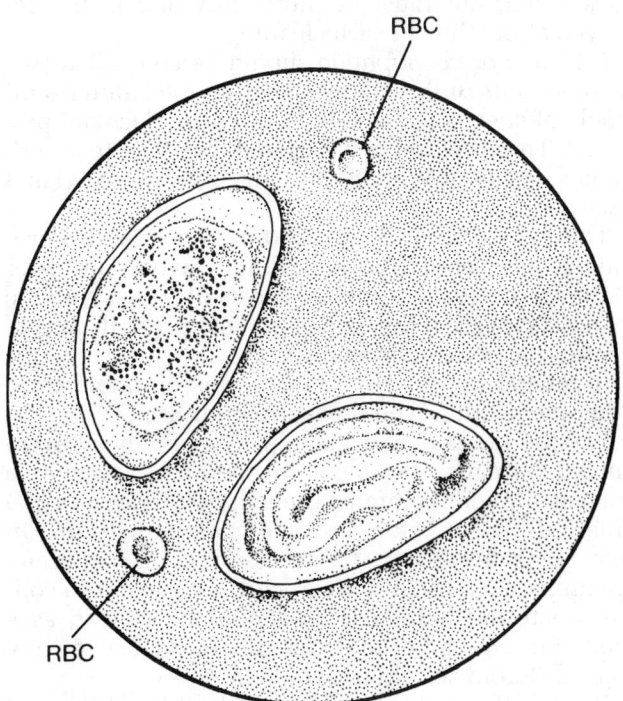

Figure 92.1.   Appearance of the eggs of *Enterobius vermicularis* (pinworm). The egg is approximately 20 to 50 m and typically has one flattened side.

Treatment

Most patients with pruritus ani can be diagnosed and treated adequately by the general physician. Even when the evaluation is inconclusive except for the identification of excoriation, symptoms can be controlled by simple measures.

Counseling concerning the factors responsible for pruritus ani should ensure a clear understanding of the potential role of stress, lifestyle, and diet.

Dietary change should eliminate potentially causative foods and beverages. It may take 2 weeks for the symptom to resolve after diet modification. It will recur within 48 hours of resuming the offending food.

Tepid sitz baths for 15 to 20 minutes provide excellent temporary relief (e.g., at bedtime). If possible, these should be used several times daily at the outset of symptoms.

Anal cleanliness and dryness are mandatory and must be gentle. Once or twice daily, and after each bowel movement, the perineal area should be cleansed with a plain mild soap such as Ivory and then rinsed with cotton swabs moistened with warm water. Glycerin–witch hazel wipes (Tucks) may be used unless they cause irritation or burning. After cleansing, the area should be thoroughly dried by blotting, not rubbing, with soft, white, nonperfumed toilet paper (colored or perfumed tissues, which are potentially allergenic or irritating, should be avoided). A handheld blow dryer is a useful alternative.

The perianal area must be kept dry at all times. This is best accomplished by the application of cornstarch powder or plain talc (Johnson's Baby Powder). A thick layer of zinc oxide or A and D Ointment may be substituted, but must be thoroughly and gently removed at the time of each cleaning.

Diarrhea or constipation should be controlled (see Chapter 39). Bulk laxatives such as Metamucil and stool softeners such as Colace or Peri-Colace are preferred. These are not irritating and they tend to absorb mucus, a possible irritant to the sensitive perianal tissue.

The patient should wear cotton underwear to provide better ventilation and should avoid polyester clothing. Prolonged sitting, especially on synthetic materials (e.g., vinyl seats), which prevent proper ventilation, should be avoided.

In general, the use of all other creams, ointments, and other medications should be discontinued.

For the occasional patient with symptoms severe enough to cause insomnia, an antipruritic sedative such as diphenhydramine (Benadryl) or trimeprazine (Temaril), taken before bedtime, may be helpful. On rare occasions it may be necessary to use minimal amounts of 0.5 or 1.0% hydrocortisone cream to control nocturnal itching. This should be viewed as a temporary measure, and the prolonged use of any topical steroid should be avoided.

If a specific problem is identified during the initial evaluation of a patient with pruritus ani (Table 92.1), it must be treated appropriately; see the chapters on dermatology (Chapter 100) and nonmalignant vulvo-vaginal disorders (Chapter 94) or the section on gastrointestinal problems (Section 4).

Referral

A patient with idiopathic pruritus ani that is not responsive to these therapies should be referred to a gastroenterologist. Further evaluation, especially in the older age group, should include the entire colon and rectum.

Enterobius vermicularis (Pinworms)

If *Enterobius vermicularis* is identified, all members of the household should be evaluated with the cellophane tape test. The ova are easily disseminated and survive in the environment for up to 3 weeks.

The drug of choice to eradicate this infestation is pyrantel pamoate (Pin-X). It is available as an oral suspension and is given as a single dose. An alternative drug, mebendazole (Vermox), is given as a single chewable tablet; it should not be used in infants or pregnant women. These agents approach 100% effectiveness in killing the worms, and symptoms usually subside within 48 hours. The patient is no longer infective once the deposited eggs are removed from the perianal area and clothing by cleaning. Both drugs are well tolerated but may cause mild, transient gastrointestinal distress. Pyrantel pamoate has been associated with transitory elevation of liver enzymes, and its use should be avoided in patients with known liver disease.

Clothing and bed linens should be laundered with detergent and hot water on the same day that oral treatment is given. All infected members of the household should be treated simultaneously. It should be understood that reinfection is common and that retreatment may be necessary.

ANAL FISSURE

Definition

An anal fissure is an acutely painful elliptical mucosal tear extending from the anal verge to the pectinate line (Fig. 92.2). It is most often located in the posterior midline of the anal canal, less commonly anteriorly. The inciting factor is usually trauma secondary to the passage of a large, hard stool or, less commonly, to anal intercourse. The underlying pathophysiology is diminished anodermal blood supply abetted by increased anal sphincter tone (7). The problem is a common one, occurring with equal frequency in men and women. Most patients and many physicians attribute the pain to hemorrhoids, which are not a cause of acute anal pain.

As an anal fissure becomes chronic it looks more like an ulcer crater, with raised edges, scarring, and the exposed external sphincter at the base. These changes are usually associated with a prominent posterior skin tag known as a sentinel pile. Occasionally, a chronic fissure, maybe in an atypical location, is caused by an

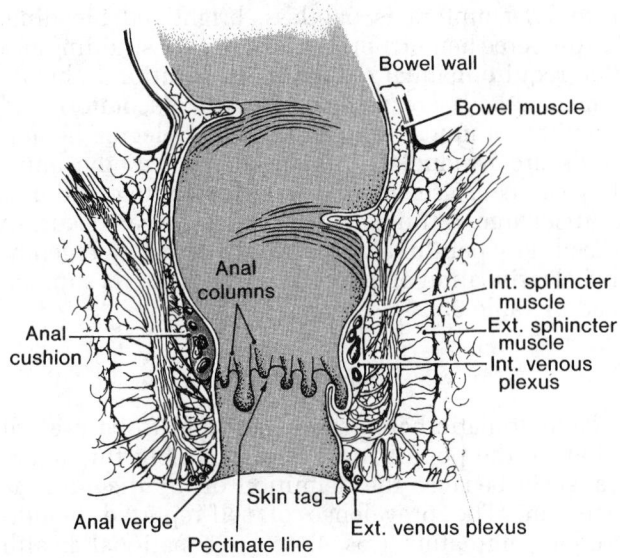

Figure 92.2. Important structures of the anal area.

inflammatory condition such as Crohn's disease, syphilis, gonorrhea, or tuberculosis; iatrogenic scarring from local surgery or irradiation; or anal cancer.

Diagnosis

An acute anal fissure presents with the sudden onset of sharp rectal pain that occurs during defecation and is followed by a dull aching discomfort that may persist for several hours. There may be associated minimal bright red bleeding, usually noticed just on the toilet tissue. Itching and mucus discharge can be additional complaints. The pain is so severe that patients avoid having a bowel movement, further aggravating the situation.

On examination, when the buttocks are gently retracted, most anal fissures can be readily visualized, usually at the posterior margin of the anal verge. It may help if the patient is asked to strain. With more chronic fissures, a posterior sentinel pile may be appreciated. If a fissure is suspected, the examination is facilitated by the preliminary application of 2% lidocaine gel on a cotton swab. Once an anal fissure is identified by inspection, generally no attempt should be made to perform a digital rectal examination or anoscopy until treatment has alleviated the symptoms.

Treatment

Many patients with an acute anal fissure can be made comfortable within a day or two, and cured within 3 weeks, by the use of conservative therapy. Stool softeners such as Colace or Peri-Colace, or a bulk laxative such as Metamucil, should be taken and cathartics should be avoided. A high-fiber diet is recommended, along with the consumption of eight glasses of water daily.

Anal discomfort is relieved by the use of sitz baths for 15 to 20 minutes two to three times per day and after each bowel movement, and by the use of topical agents or suppositories. Effective topical agents are Balneol, Anusol-HC cream, and Nupercainal cream. Anosol-HC suppositories are useful as well. Agents containing topical corticosteroids, such as Anusol-HC, should not be used for more than 2 to 3 weeks, but plain Anusol can then be substituted.

Recent evidence indicates that nitric oxide (NO) mediates relaxation of the internal anal sphincter. Therefore, NO donors such as nitroglycerin, isosorbide dinitrate, or glyceryl trinitrate might be effective in the treatment of anal fissures. Preliminary studies suggest that the topical use of these agents has resulted in early symptomatic relief, and in the cure of up to 80% of both acute and chronic anal fissures after 6 weeks of treatment (7). Recurrence rates are unknown. The major side effect has been headache. A similar effect has been achieved by the local injection of botulin toxin. It is conceivable that these approaches might obviate operation for at least some chronic fissures.

Once a fissure becomes chronic or if 6 weeks of conservative therapy has failed, the next step is surgical referral for a lateral anal sphincterotomy. This procedure is usually done on an ambulatory basis, often under local anesthesia. Postoperative complications, such as bleeding or abscess formation, occur in less than 5% of cases. There may be early problems with some degree of anal incontinence in up to 8% of cases, but this is a long-term problem in less than 1% of patients, and is usually confined to difficulty controlling flatus or liquid.

Pain relief is noted within 48 hours and the fissure is usually healed in 2 to 3 weeks. The recurrence rate is 1 to 2%, and 95% of patients have a lasting excellent or satisfactory result.

HEMORRHOIDAL DISEASE

Definition

A precise characterization of hemorrhoidal disease is impossible because, despite centuries of medical speculation, neither the pathogenesis nor the cause has ever been elucidated. Hemorrhoids are not varicosities of the rectal venous plexus. There are no certain data to prove any of the popular theories of causation such as a low-fiber diet, constipation, straining at stool, venous hypertension, obesity, certain occupations, genetic predisposition, and many others.

The currently popular theory associates hemorrhoids with distal displacement of the anal cushions. Anal cushions are part of the normal anatomy of the anal canal (Fig. 92.2). These cushions, which consist of hemorrhoidal venous and arterial plexuses, smooth muscle, and connective tissue, lie under the mucosa. The cushions apparently permit the passage of variable-sized stools without disruption of the rectal mucosa. Three cushions are usually found in the right anterior, right posterior, and left lateral portions of the anal canal (Fig. 92.3), the common locations of internal hemorrhoids. This theory is consistent with an

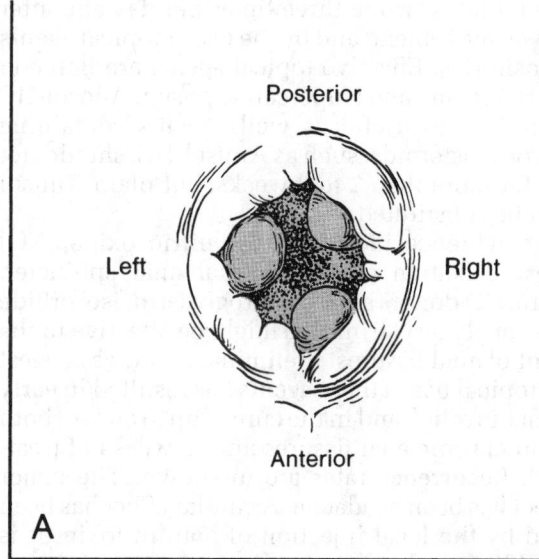

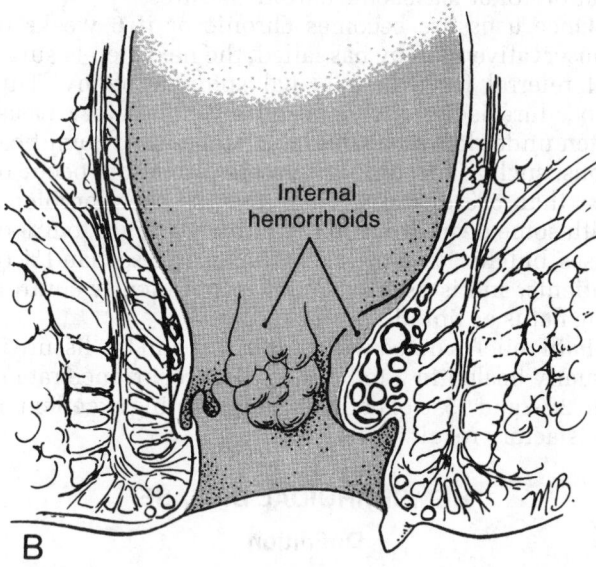

Figure 92.3. **A**. Common sites of hemorrhoids. **B**. Protrusion of anal cushions.

observed increase in hemorrhoidal disease in association with aging, groin hernias, and urogenital prolapse, all potentially caused by connective tissue degeneration.

Classification

Hemorrhoids are described as internal or external depending on whether they originate above or below the pectinate (dentate) line. External skin tags are commonly, and erroneously, referred to as hemorrhoids as well (Fig. 92.2). Internal hemorrhoids are graded based on the degree of prolapse. First-degree hemorrhoids project into the anal canal, but do not prolapse. Second-degree hemorrhoids prolapse with defecation and spontaneously reduce. At these stages

the only symptom is painless, bright red bleeding. Third-degree hemorrhoids protrude with straining and often require manual reduction. In addition to hematochezia, these are associated with discomfort and sometimes a mucus discharge. Fourth-degree hemorrhoids are irreducibly prolapsed through the anus. They can cause severe discomfort, bleeding, and mucus discharge. At this stage strangulation can occur, an exceedingly painful and potentially lethal emergency. This classification of hemorrhoidal disease is summarized in Table 92.2.

Epidemiology

Asymptomatic hemorrhoids are said to be present in half of the population over age 50, but this figure is suspect because the definition of the diagnosis is uncertain. The prevalence of self-reported hemorrhoidal complaints was 4.4% in a national health survey, but patients tend to attribute all anorectal symptoms to hemorrhoids (2). The prevalence is the same in both sexes, but women develop hemorrhoids earlier and men more commonly seek treatment.

Diagnosis

Symptoms

External hemorrhoids present with pain, often exquisite, as a result of thrombosis in the external venous plexus. There is a tender lump, and the pain is exacerbated by defecation.

Asymptomatic hemorrhoids noticed incidentally during an examination should not be considered a problem and should not be treated. The symptoms associated with internal hemorrhoids were summarized in the classification scheme presented above, and can be elaborated upon as follows.

Bleeding. Characteristically, the bleeding from

Table 92.2. Classification of Hemorrhoids

External skin tags: Small discrete skin tags arising from the anal verge.

External hemorrhoids: Hemorrhoids arising from the inferior hemorrhoidal plexus exterior to the anal verge, covered by pain-sensitive skin. Thrombosis may cause acute and sometimes severe discomfort.

Internal hemorrhoids: Hemorrhoids arising from the vascular cushions, normal structures, lying above the anal verge, covered by pain-insensitive mucosa. Internal hemorrhoids may be classified further.

   First-degree: Hemorrhoids bulging into the lumen of the anal canal that produce bleeding

   Second-degree: Hemorrhoids that prolapse during defecation but reduce spontaneously

   Third-degree: Prolapsed hemorrhoids that require manual reduction

   Fourth-degree: Hemorrhoids that are irreducibly prolapsed

Thrombosed internal hemorrhoids: An internal hemorrhoid may prolapse and strangulate, which leads to thrombosis, an excruciating painful condition. If swelling progresses, gangrene of the hemorrhoids with ulceration, local infection, or pyelphlebitis (septic phlebitis of the portal venous system) may result.

hemorrhoids is mild, intermittent, and bright red. Occasionally it may drip into the commode or be sustained. Massive hemorrhage is rare. Rectal bleeding should never be attributed to hemorrhoids unless all other causes can be ruled out.

Prolapse. Prolapse of internal hemorrhoids produces the sensation of fullness in the anal canal, especially after defecation. This discomfort affects 80% of patients with symptomatic hemorrhoids, but it is not true pain.

Pain. The acute pain attributed to internal hemorrhoids usually is caused by a fissure (see above). Pain caused by internal hemorrhoids indicates thrombosis or strangulation and mandates referral to a surgeon. Thrombosis and strangulation occur when fourth-degree hemorrhoids are trapped by congestion and spasm of the anal canal. If ulceration ensues, localized infection may result, which rarely may spread to the portal venous plexus, leading to potentially lethal pylephlebitis.

Examination

The patient is placed in the lateral decubitus or knee–chest position and the buttocks are gently separated. Skin tags are seen as soft painless excrescences just beyond the anal verge. A thrombosed external hemorrhoid presents in the anal canal as a firm tender mass with a bluish discoloration. Internal hemorrhoids can sometimes be visualized as well, especially if the patient strains.

Digital rectal examination is performed principally to rule out other anal and distal rectal disease. Nonvisible internal hemorrhoids are occasionally palpable.

Anoscopy is the definitive diagnostic procedure for internal hemorrhoids. It should be performed thoroughly and carefully, as described above for the diagnosis of pruritus ani, using a good side-viewing anoscope.

Sigmoidoscopy, using the flexible fiberoptic sigmoidoscope, should be performed on any patient over the age of 40 with the recent onset of bleeding from internal hemorrhoids. This is a part of the assessment of gastrointestinal bleeding, as discussed more fully in Chapter 38.

Differential Diagnosis

Several problems may be confused with hemorrhoidal disease: *Hypertrophied anal papilla* occurs along the pectinate (dentate) line (Fig. 92.2) in association with an anal fissure (see above), with Crohn's disease, or without obvious cause. These papillae usually are asymptomatic and require no therapy unless they have become particularly large, eroded, or infected, or unless they bleed. Hypertrophied anal papillae often have the appearance of a fibrous polyp and are easily differentiated from hemorrhoids by their location and consistency.

Rectal prolapse is more common in the elderly but can occur at any age. Prolapse is identified by the circumferential abnormal downward displacement, or herniation, of rectal mucosa or of the full thickness of the rectal wall. When mild, it is commonly mistaken for hemorrhoidal disease, and may respond to similar methods of treatment.

Protruding tumors such as rectal polyps, anal carcinoma, and even low-lying rectal carcinoma can be confused with hemorrhoids. If there is suspicion about the diagnosis, referral to a surgeon or a gastroenterologist for evaluation and biopsy is appropriate.

Course

Without treatment, symptoms of hemorrhoids usually resolve spontaneously or in response to self-treatment within several days to several weeks, even when thrombosis is present. However, most patients develop recurrent symptoms, although the intervals between symptoms may be long.

Treatment

The aim of treatment (8) is to relieve symptoms, and only symptomatic hemorrhoids need treatment. Therapy does not necessarily reduce venous bulges, although often they do regress. Most patients respond to conservative therapy.

Skin tags rarely need treatment. If they are sufficiently prominent to cause true discomfort, the patient can be referred for surgical excision.

Thrombosed external hemorrhoids are often acutely and severely painful and require surgical referral for management. If the patient presents more than 72 hours after the onset of pain, and as the acute symptom is subsiding, conservative measures usually resolve the problem. These consist of the approach used for the conservative treatment of symptomatic internal hemorrhoids. In addition, topical analgesics such as Nupercainal or 5% lidocaine ointment should be applied. If prolonged sitting is necessary, an inflatable ring is helpful.

Symptomatic internal hemorrhoids, even fourth-degree ones in the absence of severe symptoms, deserve a trial of conservative management. The first step is to avoid constipation and straining by giving a bulk laxative such as Metamucil and stool softeners such as Colace or Peri-Colace. In conjunction, the patient should eat a high-fiber diet with bran cereals and whole wheat bread and drink at least eight glasses of water daily.

Swelling and prolapse often respond to warm sitz baths taken twice daily and after each bowel movement.

Topical preparations may relieve discomfort, and putatively reduce swelling as well. Corticosteroid-containing preparations such as Anusol-HC and ProctoFoam-HC may be used initially, but their use should be discontinued after 2 or 3 weeks and the non–steroid-containing versions substituted. These preparations come as creams, foams, and suppositories. All three forms are beneficial, and their use depends on patient and physician preference.

Referral for Surgical Management

Patients should be referred to a surgeon for evaluation whenever there is doubt about the diagnosis, if the patient does not respond within 3 or 4 weeks to conservative therapy, if pain is severe (as may occur with thrombosis), or if there is evidence of strangulation, ulceration, or perianal infection. When uncomplicated hemorrhoids are recurrently symptomatic, the patient should be referred to a surgeon for definitive treatment.

The surgeon evaluates the patient, confirms the diagnosis, and then considers several therapeutic options that are not normally provided by general physicians.

External Hemorrhoids

The usual indication for the surgical treatment of external hemorrhoids is painful acute thrombosis, especially within 48 to 72 hours of onset. The procedure is surgical excision under local anesthesia on an ambulatory basis (the local anesthesia of choice for all anal and perianal procedures is bupivacaine 0.5% with epinephrine 1:200,000 and sodium bicarbonate). Incision and evacuation of the thrombus are not adequate treatment. The entire thrombosed portion of the external venous plexus should be excised along with a transverse elliptical wedge of overlying skin.

Sometimes external skin tags are sufficiently troublesome to warrant excision. This can be done as an office procedure under local anesthesia.

The remaining headings in this section on surgical management all refer to the treatment of symptomatic internal hemorrhoids.

Injection of Sclerosing Agents

The submucosal injection of a symptomatic hemorrhoid with several milliliters of a sclerosing solution causes fibrosis and retraction of the hemorrhoid. This procedure is excellent therapy for small bleeding internal hemorrhoids (first- or second-degree) (Table 92.2); it is simple, requires no anesthesia, and can easily be performed in the office in a few minutes. There may be a period of several days when the patient experiences a sensation of anal fullness. This symptom is usually well tolerated or is easily controlled by the use of sitz baths three to four times a day and by mild analgesics such as acetaminophen. After this procedure the patient usually requires no recovery period and can return to work immediately.

The physician performing this procedure must be experienced with its use. With the proper technique there are essentially no complications. If the solution is improperly injected, severe pain, necrosis, and rectal stenosis may occur. Injection of sclerosing agents generally provides temporary relief, but recurrence is common. The procedure may be repeated several times, but persistent recurrence should lead to the consideration of another mode of therapy. This approach is most useful for symptomatic first-degree hemorrhoids that are so small that there is insufficient tissue for rubber band ligation.

Rubber Band Ligation

Rubber band ligation of hemorrhoids is a simple office procedure that is the initial treatment of choice for most symptomatic internal hemorrhoids of all degrees except the fourth (Table 92.2) (4,5). The patient requires no special preparation and no anesthesia is necessary. Using an anoscope and a special instrument, one or two rubber bands are applied near the base of the hemorrhoids, and at least 0.5 cm above the pectinate line. No more than two hemorrhoids should be treated at a single session, but all of the hemorrhoids should be banded ultimately. Constriction by the rubber band results in ischemic necrosis of the hemorrhoid, which sloughs and is passed in the stool 5 to 10 days later, usually along with a small amount of blood. Complications are very rare, but delayed massive bleeding and pelvic cellulitis have occurred.

Usually, after rubber band ligation of hemorrhoids, the patient is not disabled and has only minimal discomfort characterized by a sensation of rectal fullness, a symptom that is usually well controlled by the use of sitz baths and mild oral analgesics such as acetaminophen. Aspirin and nonsteroidal anti-inflammatory analgesics should not be used because of the risk of delayed bleeding. If the discomfort is more severe, a mild relaxant such as diazepam (Valium) is helpful to relieve anal sphincter spasm. If the rubber band is improperly placed below the pectinate line, the patient will experience severe pain and the rubber band must be removed.

After rubber band ligation, the usual conservative measures for internal hemorrhoids should be practiced for 2 to 3 weeks until healing is complete. Further ligation is then performed if necessary. Banding provides good relief of hemorrhoidal disease approximately 70 to 90% of the time. Symptoms may recur in 15 to 45% of patients after anywhere from 18 months to 5 years.

Laser Therapy and Infrared Photocoagulation

Laser therapy and infrared photocoagulation are available as treatment modalities for first-, second-, and third-degree hemorrhoids (Table 92.2). Both require expensive equipment, and the CO_2 laser demands special expertise. Therefore neither modality is widely available.

Hemorrhoidectomy

Hemorrhoidectomy is indicated for large internal hemorrhoids when other forms of therapy have failed, for strangulated, ulcerated or gangrenous third- or fourth-degree hemorrhoids, and when symptomatic hemorrhoids are present in conjunction with other benign anorectal conditions (e.g., fistulas, fissures) that require surgery (7). The procedure is usually done under general or regional anesthesia, although local anesthesia is possible. Patient preparation consists of taking a laxative the evening before the operation. The purpose of the operation is to remove hemorrhoidal tissue and to appose the skin and mucous membrane. The operation has a reputation for severe postoperative pain. This problem can be greatly ameliorated by anal dilation to four fingers before the resection of the hemorrhoids. The postoperative discomfort is then controlled by sitz baths, stool softeners, oral analgesics, and a muscle relaxant such as diazepam (Valium). Topical nitroglycerin may also be beneficial. Most patients can go home within 24 hours.

Postoperative complications are urinary retention and bleeding. The former can be averted by adequate control of pain and muscle spasm. There is an incidence of significant bleeding of 1 to 2%, and infection is rare. Late complications of incontinence or of anal stenosis should occur in less than 1% of patients. The late recurrence rate is less than 5%.

Special Considerations

Because of an increased risk of complications associated with operative procedures in patients with severe congestive heart failure or debilitating disease, the treatment of hemorrhoids in these patients should be as conservative as possible. Patients who have cirrhosis present a special risk because of the frequent associa-

tion of hemostatic dysfunction. Hemorrhoidectomy should not be done in patients with Crohn's disease and should be done in patients with ulcerative colitis only when they are in remission. Immunocompromised patients should not undergo anorectal surgery.

Hemorrhoids are common in pregnancy and are best managed conservatively. They often resolve spontaneously after delivery. Occasionally, development of strangulated hemorrhoids requires surgical intervention during the pregnancy.

ANORECTAL ABSCESSES AND ANORECTAL FISTULAS

Definition

An anorectal abscess is an abscess involving the perineum and perianal structures. Abscesses are classified by their anatomic location (Fig. 92.4). Low intramuscular or perianal abscesses are located in the subcutaneous tissue immediately surrounding the anus, which is the site of 40 to 50% of all anorectal abscesses. An ischiorectal abscess is located in the ischiorectal fossa, a fat-filled space between the distal levator ani (external anal sphincter) and the ischial tuberosity, and accounts for 20 to 40% of anorectal abscesses. Intersphincteric, high intermuscular (postanal), and pelvirectal (supralevator) abscesses are far less common and account for approximately 10% of all

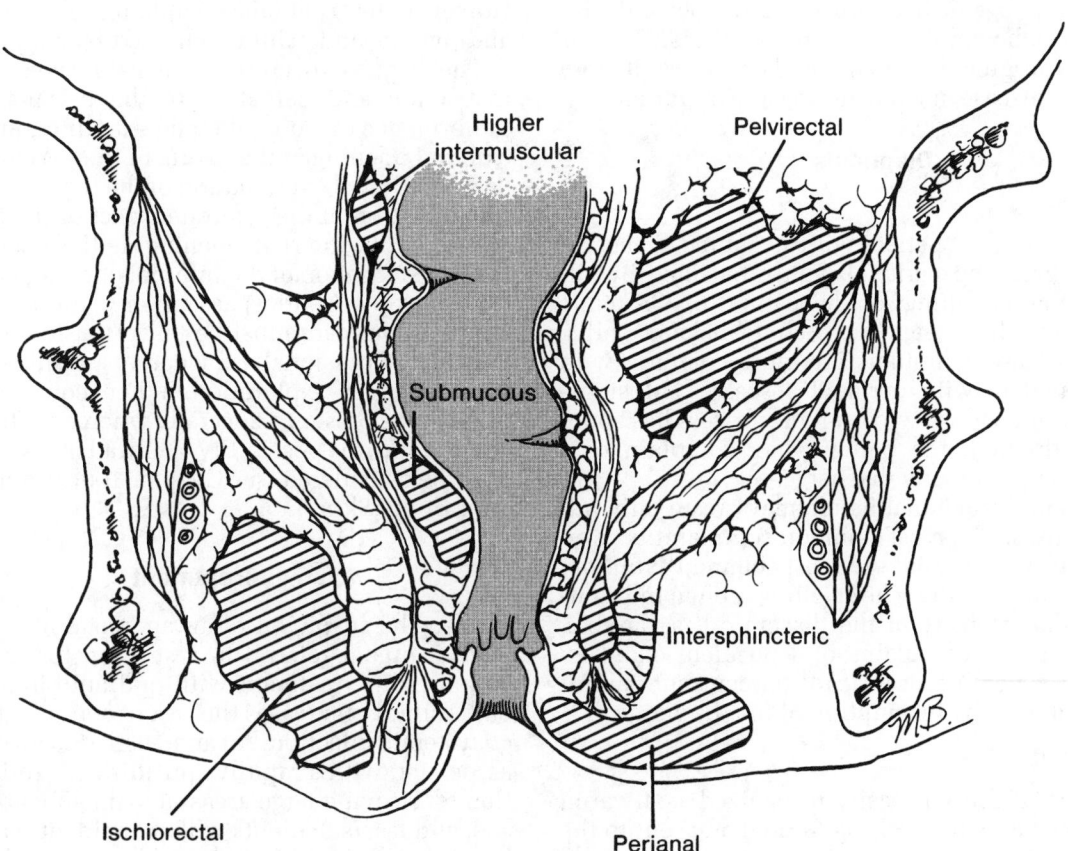

Figure 92.4.   Anatomic classification of common anorectal abscesses.

abscesses. Anorectal abscesses are common, and the general physician should be familiar with their presentation so that patients suspected of having this problem are promptly referred to a surgeon.

An *anorectal fistula (fistula-in-ano)* is a tract lined by granulation tissue having an internal opening in the anal canal and an external opening in the perianal skin. The internal opening is usually located in one of the anal crypts at the upper end of the anal canal just above the pectinate line (Fig. 92.2).

Causes

Anorectal abscesses are more common in men. Most are associated with cryptoglandular infection. Occasionally, anorectal abscesses occur in association with other anal and perianal disorders (Table 92.3). Anal glands, thought to be diverticula of the anal canal mucosa, are located circumferentially around the anus at the level of the pectinate line. Many of these glands pass through the internal sphincter into the intersphincteric space. They normally drain into the anal crypts (see above). Infection and abscess formation result when drainage of these glands is blocked. Bacterial cultures from the abscesses usually isolate a mixed flora.

Most anorectal fistulas result from abscess formation in the anal glands and drainage through the perianal skin. The incidence of fistula formation following the drainage of anorectal abscesses is 30 to 60%. Some fistulas are not pyogenic in origin and are associated with inflammatory bowel disease or tuberculosis. Fistulas that do not originate in anal glands may result from diverticular disease, neoplastic disease, or trauma.

Diagnosis

History

Most commonly, a patient with an anorectal abscess describes throbbing perianal pain intensified by sitting, walking, coughing, or defecating (9). Systemic symptoms may be present and include malaise, chills, and fever. These symptoms are more common with ischiorectal than with perianal abscesses. Most patients have some leukocytosis. If the abscess has spontaneously drained, the patient may complain of a mucopurulent or bloody discharge.

An uncomplicated anal fistula may create only minor complaints. The most common complaint is painful perianal swelling, but the most common symptom is discharge and soiling. The swelling is often intermittent, and the intensity of the discomfort is variable. Often the patient complains of a purulent anal discharge that, when it ceases, leads to recurrent painful swelling relieved by resumption of the discharge.

Examination

A perianal abscess is easily recognized as a warm, tender, subcutaneous swelling located adjacent to the anus. With an ischiorectal abscess there is often only

Table 92.3. Conditions that May Be Complicated by Anorectal Abscess and Fistula-in-Ano

Inflammatory bowel disease
Chronic infections (uncommon)
  Actinomycosis
  Tuberculosis
  Lymphogranuloma venereum
  Schistosomiasis (rare)
  Amebiasis (rare)
Infection anatomically adjacent to the rectal area and presenting as anorectal abscess or fistula-in-ano
  In women
    Pelvic inflammatory disease
    Bartholin gland abscess
  In men
    Infections of a Cowper gland (small periurethral glands)
    Pilonidal sinus (occasionally occurs in females)
Foreign body (e.g., an ingested bone or a penetrating wooden splinter)
Trauma
  Surgery (e.g., hemorrhoidectomy or prostatectomy)
  Radiation
  Laceration (e.g., from an enema)
Abnormalities of host defense (e.g., bone marrow aplasia, leukemia or lymphoma, diabetes mellitus)
Carcinoma of anus or rectum

tenderness and induration detected by pressure on the skin overlying the ischiorectal fossa or the lateral wall of the anal canal during a rectal examination. The high anorectal abscesses may present few or no findings on perianal inspection or even on rectal examination. However, these patients complain of severe rectal pain and pyrexia and exhibit a marked leukocytosis.

The diagnosis of an anorectal fistula is established by inspection and palpation of the perianal area and performance of a digital rectal examination. Often the external opening of the fistula in the perianal area can be seen. Digital examination of the rectum may enable identification of the indurated tract of the fistula as it passes to its internal opening at the pectinate line. Often the location of the internal opening is facilitated by anoscopy. Gentle passage of a probe may be attempted, but care must be taken not to create a false passage. Occasionally, accurate localization must await surgical exploration. When complex perineal infection is present, especially when no internal opening is found, the possibility of hidradenitis suppurativa must be considered (see Chapter 100, "Common Problems of the Skin").

Treatment

Even the suspicion of an anorectal abscess should lead to urgent referral to a surgeon for drainage (9). Temporizing treatment with oral antibiotics and sitz baths simply increases the risk of complications, such as systemic infection. An anorectal abscess may also be associated with a rapidly spreading necrotizing infection, destroying large areas of skin, subcutaneous tissue, and fascia. Patients with coincident diabetes mellitus are particularly vulnerable to complicated and extensive perirectal involvement. Finally, spontaneous rupture may occur either externally or internally, resulting in a complex fistula that is difficult to manage.

Preoperative broad-spectrum antibiotics need be given only to patients with anorectal abscesses who have valvular heart disease, diabetes, extensive inflammation or who are immunocompromised. Perianal abscesses may be drained under local anesthesia in the office or emergency room, but all other anorectal abscesses require regional or general anesthesia in the operating room. Following drainage, the patient should receive oral analgesics and stool softeners and be instructed to begin sitz baths three times a day.

Most fistulas require fistulotomy (9). The internal and external openings must both be carefully identified and the tract converted into an open wound, which heals by secondary intention. Complex chronic fistulae can present difficult technical problems, and other surgical options may have to be considered. The wounds that result from any of these options commonly take 6 to 12 weeks to heal. The most serious postoperative complication is anal incontinence, which occurs in 3 to 7% of cases. The recurrence rate, even for simple fistulas, is approximately 5%, and is higher for complex ones.

Some patients with fistula-in-ano may be treated nonsurgically, either because of a lack of symptoms or because of complicating factors such as acquired immunodeficiency syndrome (AIDS). If there is a history of inflammatory bowel disease, a gastroenterologist should also be consulted.

PROCTALGIA FUGAX

Occasionally, healthy young adults develop the sudden onset of severe rectal pain, variably intermittent and generally lasting less than 30 minutes to 1 hour: proctalgia fugax. It often awakens a patient at night. It is significantly more common in women than in men, and it can occur after sexual intercourse. The pain is described usually as a spasm or a cramp. The problem is not associated with systemic illness or other gastrointestinal diseases such as the irritable bowel syndrome, and the cause is uncertain. There is often an association with psychiatric disturbances. Proctalgia fugax was thought to result from spasm of a portion of the levator ani muscle, but recent studies suggest paroxysmal hyperkinesis of the smooth muscle of the internal anal sphincter (6). Patients with proctalgia fugax may obtain relief by taking a hot sitz bath or applying pressure in the perianal area near the site of the discomfort. There are no proven pharmacologic remedies for this affliction. However, if the attacks are severe and frequent, some patients may find relief by the use of sublingual or cutaneous nitrates. There is also the possibility that nifedipine, a calcium channel blocker, decreases the frequency and intensity of attacks, and that the inhalation of albuterol shortens the duration of pain. The problem usually persists for many years but then disappears in later life.

RECTAL PROLAPSE

Definition

Prolapse is a protrusion of the rectum through the anus. The protrusion may contain only mucosa, a mucosal prolapse, or it may contain all layers of the bowel wall, a full-thickness prolapse (procidentia). There can also be an internal prolapse, or internal rectal intussusception, which produces typical symptoms without any external protrusion. This is often associated with the solitary rectal ulcer syndrome.

Causes

Prolapse is more prevalent in women (approximately 80% of the cases), with a peak incidence between the ages of 60 and 80. In men the peak incidence occurs at about the age of 40. The exact pathogenic mechanism is not known. Multiple factors are associated with this disease. Weakening of the fascial attachments of the rectum, attenuated muscles in the perirectal area and pelvic diaphragm, straining caused by chronic constipation, and even congenital fascial defects all lead to the development of rectal prolapse. Prolapse is often observed after severe chronic diarrhea.

Prolapse also occurs commonly in children, usually under the age of 2 years. This is almost always a mucosal prolapse and conservative treatment usually suffices until the condition spontaneously resolves.

Diagnosis

History

Patients have variable symptoms, depending on the degree of prolapse. Initially, the protrusion occurs only with defecation, and the patient can easily reduce it manually. At this stage there may be no associated incontinence and the condition is sometimes mistaken for symptomatic internal hemorrhoids. The patient may complain of a sensation of displaced tissue at the time of a bowel movement, and there is often a feeling of incomplete evacuation. With progression of the problem, prolapse occurs with any straining and, eventually, simply with walking or even standing. At this stage incontinence is almost invariably a problem. With more profound prolapse the patient may complain of tenesmus and also develop a continuous mucous discharge. The prolapsed rectum may become excoriated and ulcerated, leading many patients to complain of bleeding. In association with an advanced degree of prolapse, the patient may also have urinary incontinence, and in females there may be associated uterine prolapse. Patients with increasing degrees of prolapse experience considerable embarrassment and consequently avoid social contact.

Examination

The physician can best recognize rectal prolapse by inspecting the anus when the patient strains in a squatting position or sitting on a commode. It is wise to anticipate incontinence with this maneuver. If the prolapse is full thickness (procidentia), concentric folds of the rectal mucosa are seen, whereas if there is only mucosal prolapse, only radial folds are seen. Digital examination almost always reveals a patulous and relaxed anal sphincter that often admits two to four fingers. Palpation of the protruding tissue between the examiner's finger provides the sensation of only mucosa in mucosal prolapse and a double layer of bowel wall in full-thickness prolapse. The rectal examination in patients with prolapse is usually associated with minimal if any discomfort.

Occasionally, prolapsed hemorrhoids may be confused with rectal prolapse, but the absence of concentric or radial folds of mucosa and the prominent location of prolapsed hemorrhoids in the left lateral, right anterior, or right posterior edges of the anus suggest the proper diagnosis (Fig. 92.3). On occasion, a prolapse may be associated with a rectal tumor. For that reason a flexible fiberoptic sigmoidoscopic examination should be performed on any patient with rectal prolapse. Other diagnostic studies are not usually required, but a defecatory videoproctogram (available in only a few centers) is useful, especially for identifying an associated rectocele or internal prolapse.

Treatment

When the prolapse is small and limited to the mucosa, the patient may benefit from taking stool softeners and using an irritant rectal suppository (see Chapter 39) to initiate defecation and thereby avoid straining at stool. If prolapse progresses despite this treatment, or if extensive mucosal prolapse is noted, it is appropriate to refer the patient to a surgeon. Redundant tissue may be treated either by rubber band ligation, as for internal hemorrhoids, or by sclerosis. Both procedures can usually be performed in the surgeon's office without anesthesia and are usually successful in preventing progressive degrees of rectal mucosal prolapse.

When procidentia (full-thickness prolapse) is present, only operative treatment is effective. Several procedures are available for the restoration of anal continence and reduction of prolapse. All these operations require hospitalization, and most require general anesthesia. One important factor to consider before operation is whether incontinence will be improved. If a full preoperative assessment of anorectal function leads the gastroenterologist and surgeon to believe that incontinence is likely to persist, the alternative of providing the patient with a permanent diverting colostomy must be considered.

Both abdominal and perineal operations are available for the treatment of complete procidentia. The perineal approaches have usually been reserved for very elderly or high-risk patients because of perceived less perfect results. However, recent publications indicate that these operations may be satisfactory (1).

Nonetheless, the most successful operative procedures for full-thickness rectal prolapse require an abdominal proctopexy, in which the rectum is secured to presacral fascia either by primary suture or by the use of synthetic mesh. This may or may not be accompanied by anterior resection of redundant sigmoid colon. Complications associated with the transabdominal surgical repair of prolapse are fecal impaction, presacral hemorrhage, stricture, infection, fistula formation, pelvic abscesses, and intestinal obstruction. The complication rate is 3 to 6%. However, fecal impaction can occur in up to 6 to 10% of the patients after abdominal proctopexy. The complication rate for perineal repairs is low, and fecal impaction is rare. However, anastomotic leak with pelvic abscess, pelvic hematoma, and anastomotic stricture can occur. The operative mortality rate for abdominal operations is less than 3%, and for perineal procedures less than 1%.

The long-term results are generally good, with recurrence rates in the range of 2 to 10% for the abdominal approaches and 10 to 30% for the perineal ones. However, of patients with preoperative fecal incontinence, 15 to 30% continue to have some degree of postoperative incontinence. This problem sometimes responds to biofeedback, ordinarily available only in specialized gastroenterology laboratories.

SEXUALLY TRANSMITTED DISEASE

Definition

In addition to the putatively more common sexually transmitted diseases such as gonorrhea and syphilis, proctitis characterized by rectal pain, tenesmus, and often anal discharge should raise suspicion of the so-called *gay bowel syndrome.* This syndrome and other anorectal diseases have become increasingly common as a consequence of the sexual practices of homosexual men such as anal receptive intercourse and anilingus. Homosexuality is not, by itself, a risk factor for proctitis. However, the tendency toward promiscuity, the lack of use of condoms, and the anonymity of multiple contacts lead to a high risk of developing the syndrome, which can also occur in women who engage in the same practices.

Causes

Gay bowel syndrome is a generic term that refers to numerous types of anal and rectal diseases seen in homosexual men. Although the problem is often a nonspecific inflammation caused by trauma, this form of proctitis can be caused by a variety of pathogens (bacteria, viruses, spirochetes, and parasites) (3). The nature and prevalence of a number of specific causes of perianal disease and proctitis in this population are listed in Table 92.4. It should be noted that lymphogranuloma venereum (LGV) is caused by specific immunotypes of *Chlamydia.* Condylomata acuminata associated with certain human papilloma virus (HPV) types are particularly prone to result in high-grade anal

Table 92.4. Sexually Transmitted Anorectal Diseases in Homosexual Men

Cause	Prevalence (%)
Bacterial	
Chlamydia trachomatis and lymphogranuloma venereum	15
Gonorrhea	45–55
Chancroid	5
Shigella	30–50
Granuloma inguinale	Uncommon
Viral	
Herpes simplex virus type 2	95
Condylomata acuminata	50–75
Molluscum contagiosum	Uncommon
Spirochetes	
Syphilis	Common
Protozoa	
Amebiasis	20–32
Giardiasis	4–18

dysplasia, and even invasive squamous carcinoma. This is a particular risk for human immunodeficiency virus (HIV)-positive patients.

Diagnosis

Perianal lesions are seen in association with condylomata acuminata, herpes simplex virus type 2 (HSV2), syphilis, chancroid, granuloma inguinale, and molluscum contagiosum. Perianal lesions in the form of abscesses, strictures, and fistulas are a late manifestation of LGV and granuloma inguinale.

Condylomata acuminata are recognized as a typical collection of venereal warts often extending within the anal canal. There is no specific diagnostic test. *HSV2* presents initially as perianal or anal canal vesicles, but these have usually ruptured and coalesced into ulcerations before the patient is seen. Precise diagnosis requires either a direct fluorescent monoclonal antibody technique or culture of the virus. A *perianal chancre* may suggest the diagnosis of primary syphilis, and the typical verrucous excrescence of a *condyloma latum,* although rare, is pathognomonic of primary or secondary syphilis. The diagnosis must be confirmed by dark-field examination for spirochetes. *Chancroid* is associated with anorectal ulcers and abscesses and the diagnosis is confirmed by culture. *Granuloma inguinale* is a chronic granuloma that eventually causes red, hard perianal masses. Biopsy is necessary for diagnosis. *Molluscum contagiosum* causes self-limited painless round umbilicated lesions that can be confused with cutaneous cryptococcosis in patients with AIDS.

Proctitis is a manifestation of gonorrhea, *Chlamydia* infection, HSV2, amebiasis, shigellosis, and occasionally rectal syphilis. All of these cause essentially similar and nonspecific symptoms of rectal discharge, pruritus, tenesmus, hematochezia, and constipation or diarrhea. Pain (odynochezia) is especially typical of

HSV2, *Chlamydia* infection, and chancroid and may also accompany syphilis. The proctitis of amebiasis has a rather typical appearance on sigmoidoscopy, but the symptoms are principally those of colitis, as is also true of shigellosis. Constitutional symptoms accompany HSV2 and consist of urinary retention, impotence, and unexplained but disabling dysesthesias of the perineum, buttocks, and posterior thighs. Inguinal adenopathy is a common finding in conjunction with syphilis, LGV, and HSV2.

Diagnosis of all of these lesions requires anoscopy and flexible sigmoidoscopy. Gonorrhea causes a nonspecific mucosal inflammation with erythema, friability, and an exudate. Gram's stain of the exudate reveals Gram-negative intracellular diplococci, and a culture is confirmatory. Luetic proctitis is also nonspecific, and the diagnosis is made by dark-field examination of the exudate and serologic tests for syphilis (see Chapter 30). Chlamydia causes only a nonspecific proctitis, but LGV causes linear and aphthous ulcers extending up from the rectum to the distal colon as well. Histologically as well as clinically, these findings resemble Crohn's disease, and the diagnosis of LGV requires culture of the organism, which commonly necessitates tissue culture inoculation. Rising acute convalescent antichlamydial serum antibody titers are confirmatory, but usually not manifest for 1 month. Although the warts of condylomata acuminata usually present in the perianal area, anoscopy is necessary to look for involvement of the anal canal. HSV2 also causes predominantly perianal lesions, but anoscopy and sigmoidoscopy should be performed because the anal canal can contain vesicular lesions or ulcers and the distal rectum may reveal proctitis with or without ulcers as well. Amebiasis often presents a characteristic sigmoidoscopic appearance of punched-out ulcers with a yellow base in addition to diffuse inflammation. The diagnosis is confirmed by stool examination for ova and parasites, as is also true for giardiasis. A positive stool culture makes the diagnosis of shigellosis, which shows proctitis with ulcerations on proctoscopy.

It should be emphasized that none of these lesions is likely to be recognized unless an appropriate history is obtained. These patients rarely volunteer information regarding their sexual practices, so the physician is obligated to ask the necessary questions or the diagnosis will be missed.

Treatment

Surgical referral is rarely appropriate for these diseases and, when surgery is required, evaluation by a gastroenterologist should precede any operative approach except in the case of condylomata acuminata. Indeed, for most of these lesions the differential diagnosis is sufficiently complex that gastroenterology consultation is usually appropriate. The exception is perhaps gonorrheal proctitis because the diagnosis, if suspected, is easily made and treatment is usually successful (see Chapters 27 and 94). Luetic proctitis is also easily treated (see Chapters 30 and 94).

Chlamydia infections (see Chapter 27) respond to doxycycline, azithromycin, ofloxacin, or erythromycin base. The duration and success of treatment depend first on a correct diagnosis (Crohn's disease does not respond to antibiotics), and second on the severity and duration of the infection. LGV may progress to abscess, fistula, and stricture formation and require surgical management, occasionally necessitating a colostomy.

Condylomata acuminata, if the lesions are small, may be treated by the topical application of podophyllin or bichloracetic acid (see Chapter 100). Larger warts require surgical treatment by a combination of excision and fulguration. The CO_2 laser is of no advantage in the treatment of these lesions. There is experimental interest in the use of an autologous vaccine and interferon, but there are no definitive clinical studies as yet. Recurrence is likely, whatever method is used (see also Chapter 94, "Nonmalignant Vulvovaginal and Cervical Disorders"). Molluscum contagiosum is a self-limited disease, but is also sometimes treated by local destruction to prevent spread.

There is no cure for HSV2, but the use of Acyclovir 200 to 400 mg by mouth daily for 10 days shortens the clinical course.

Amebiasis is treated with metronidazole and, usually, with diiodohydroxyquin as well (see Chapter 26). Metronidazole is also the therapy for giardiasis.

Chancroid responds to ceftriaxone, azithromycin, or erythromycin base. The drug therapy for shigellosis is ciprofloxacin or double-strength trimethoprim–sulfamethoxazole. Granuloma inguinale responds to doxycycline or streptomycin.

General References*

Corman ML. Colon and rectal surgery. 3rd ed. Philadelphia: JB Lippincott, 1993.
Fazio VW, Tjandra JJ. The management of perianal diseases. Adv Surg 29:59, 1996.
Janicke DM, Pundt MR. Anorectal disorders. Emerg Med Clin North Am 14:757, 1996.
Nagle D, Rolandelli RH. Primary care office management of perianal and anal disease. Prim Care 23:609, 1996.

Specific References

1. Agachan F, Pfiefer J, Joo JS, et al. Results of perineal procedures for the treatment of rectal prolapse. Am Surg 63:9, 1997.
2. Johanson JF, Sonnenberg A. The prevalence of hemorrhoids and chronic constipation. An epidemiologic study. Gastroenterology 98:380, 1990.
3. Modesto VL, Gottesman L. Sexually transmitted diseases and anal manifestations of AIDS. Surg Clin North Am 74:1433, 1994.
4. Murie AJ, Sim AJW, Mackenzie I. Rubber band ligation versus haemorrhoidectomy for prolapsing haemorrhoids: a long term prospective clinical trial. Br J Surg 69:536, 1982.
5. Nivatvongs S, Goldberg SM. An improved technique of rubber band ligation of hemorrhoids. Am J Surg 144:379, 1982.
6. Rao SS, Hatfield RA. Paroxysmal anal hyperkinesis: a characteristic feature of proctalgia fugax. Gut 39:609, 1996.
7. Schouten WR, Briel JW, Auwerda JJ, Boerma MO. Anal fissure: new concepts in pathogenesis and treatment. Scand J Gastroenterol Suppl 218:78, 1996.
8. Standards Practice Task Force, American Society of Colon and Rectal Surgeons. Practice parameters for the treatment of hemorrhoids. Dis Colon Rectum 36:1118, 1993.
9. Standards Practice Task Force, American Society of Colon and Rectal Surgeons. Practice parameters for treatment of fistula-in-ano: supporting documentation. Dis Colon Rectum 39:1363, 1996.

---

*Bold print (general references) and bold numerals (specific references) denote published controlled clinical trials, meta-analyses, or consensus-based recommendations.

Gynecologic Problems

SECTION 13

Gynecologic Problems

CHAPTER 93

Birth Control

JEFFREY M. SMITH, MD, MPH
GEORGE R. HUGGINS, MD

Contraception provides a woman and her partner with the ability to determine the number and timing of pregnancies. In general, avoidance of unwanted pregnancies and continued consistent use of a method should be considered issues that require ongoing management and consultation rather than an isolated decision.

There are many contraceptive methods (4). It is important to understand the benefits and limitations of all of them to be able to educate the patient fully about her options. The physician should be prepared to deal with patients who have varying knowledge and experience about contraception. Table 93.1 lists the percentage distribution of use of contraceptive methods by women using a method in the United States. This most recent data, from 1990, does not include percentage distribution for Norplant and Depo-Provera, each estimated to be less than 5%. In 1990, 59.3% of all women of reproductive age were using a contraceptive method.

The failure rates of various methods of contraception are shown in Table 93.2. The low and high rates among women in the United States refer to those who are less or more likely than average to use the method correctly and consistently. Clearly there is very little difference between the failure rates of some methods, whereas others show a considerable difference. This information should be used in helping educate the patient.

Once it is established that fertility regulation is desired by the patient, a careful medical history should be obtained, including information about past pregnancies, menstruation, smoking, and family history that might suggest a contraindication to her getting pregnant (see "Limitations," below). A physical examination with special emphasis on the pelvic examination is important. A cancer detection smear and, if indicated (e.g., in a patient with multiple sexual partners), a gonococcus culture and chlamydia smear (see Chapter 94) of the endocervix are suggested. After this evaluation, the physician and patient are ready to discuss the various contraceptive methods and develop a satisfactory plan.

However, a pelvic examination is not immediately necessary for the initiation or continuation of a hormonal method such as oral contraceptive pills and Depo-Provera. Although an annual pelvic examination is seen as a necessary step in the preventive health care of reproductive age women, the deferral of this examination should not preclude prescription of a safe contraceptive method and risk an unsafe or unwanted pregnancy.

CONTRACEPTION IN SPECIAL CIRCUMSTANCES

During the time leading up to the menopause, a woman's concern regarding unplanned pregnancy is heightened by abnormal menstrual cycles and episodes of amenorrhea. Although fertility declines with age, missing a period is disturbing to a woman in the perimenopause unless a very reliable method of contraception is being used.

The postpartum patient needs help in getting back on a contraceptive program, and usually her obstetrician has given her advice in this regard. Also, the patient wishing to use an intrauterine device (IUD) needs to wait for involution of the uterus—which usually occurs 4 to 6 weeks postpartum—and therefore is at risk for pregnancy until the IUD is inserted. The physiology of the female reproductive cycle, important to an understanding of the many contraceptive methods, is discussed in Chapter 77.

Occasionally, the physician is confronted with the

need to provide emergency contraception, as for example following sexual assault. This is discussed fully in Chapter 5.

ORAL CONTRACEPTIVES

Mechanism of Action

Oral contraceptives prevent ovulation by inhibition of gonadotropin-releasing factors in the hypothalamus. The principal effect of this inhibition appears to be suppression of the surge in activity of luteinizing hormone at midcycle, thereby removing a major stimulus to ovulation. In addition, oral contraceptives make cervical mucus more viscus and therefore less easily traversed by sperm. They also have a direct effect on endometrial development in high doses, making the

uterus less receptive to implantation of the fertilized ovum (9).

Preparations and Dosage Schedules

The combined oral contraceptive was first introduced for use in the United States in 1960. In the ensuing years, significant changes have been made in steroid dosages and some new steroids have been introduced. Since 1970, all new oral contraceptives introduced in the United States have contained ethinyl estradiol as their estrogen. Most oral contraceptives in current use contain levonorgestrel or norethindrone, but since 1992 two new progestins, norgestimate and desogestrel, have been introduced in the United States in an effort to decrease unwanted side effects.

There are three different modes of administration of oral contraceptive pills:

- Monophasic contain the same dosage of estrogen and progestin for 21 days each cycle.
- Multiphasic contain 1 to 2 levels of estrogen and 2 to 3 levels of progestin, which vary through the cycle.
- Progestin only (mini-pill) contain progestin only in a steady, continuous dosage.

Many currently available oral contraceptive preparations are listed in Table 93.3. The progestin-only preparations do not consistently inhibit ovulation, and unwanted pregnancy is three to five times more likely than with oral contraceptives that contain estrogen and progestogen. Therefore they should be prescribed only for patients who cannot be given estrogen (e.g., those

Table 93.1.   Contraceptive Use Among U.S. Women

Contraceptive	% U.S. Women Aged 15–60 in 1995
Oral contraceptive	26
Sterilization	24
Condom (male)	19
Withdrawal	6
Rhythm	3
Progestin injection	3
Diaphragm	2
Progestin implant	1
IUD	1
Others—each 1% or less[a]	15

Modified from Ortho Pharmaceutical Company 1995 - Annual Birth Control Study - OPC, Raritan NJ 08869-0602; phone: 800-682-6532.

[a]Includes douche, foam, cream/jelly alone, sponge, vaginal suppository, cervical cap, and female condom.

Table 93.2.   Summary of Methods of Contraception, Their Mechanism of Action, Failure Rate, and Major Adverse Effects

Method	Mechanism of Action	Failure Rate %[a] Low	Failure Rate %[a] High	Some Adverse Effects
No method		85	85	
Spermicide alone	Inactivation of sperm	21.6	25.6	Irritation can occur
Withdrawal		14.7	27.8	
Periodic abstinence	Avoidance of coitus during presumed fertile days	13.8	19.2	
Diaphragm or cervical cap with spermicide	Mechanical barrier to sperm; inactivation of sperm	12	38.9	Increased risk of urinary tract or vaginal infection
Condom	Mechanical barrier to sperm	9.8	18.5	Allergic reactions
Oral contraceptives		3.8	8.7	
Combined	Suppression of ovulation, changes in cervical mucus and endometrium			Estrogen-related risk of thromboembolism, stroke; myocardial infarction in older smokers; hypertension
Progestin only	Changes in cervical mucus and endometrium, possibly suppression of ovulation			Irregular, unpredictable bleeding in some

Intrauterine device
  Progesterone T
  Copper T 380A
	Inhibition of sperm migration, fertilization, or ovum transport	2.5	4.5	Pelvic inflammatory disease; uterine perforation; increase in menstrual blood loss with copper

Medroxyprogesterone (Depo-Provera)	Changes in cervical mucus and endometrium, suppression of ovulation	<1	<1	Menstrual irregularities; headache; weight gain
Levonorgestrel subdermal implants (Norplant)	Same as medroxyprogesterone acetate	<1	<1	Menstrual irregularities; headache; weight gain
Sterilization				
Vasectomy	Vas deferens occlusion	0.2	0.5	Surgical procedure
Tubal ligation	Fallopian tube occlusion	0.5	1.8	

Adapted from Choice of contraceptives. Med Lett Drugs Ther 34:111, 1992.

[a]Percentage accidental pregnancy during first year of use among women in the United States more likely (low failure rate) and less likely (high failure rate) than average to use the method correctly and consistently (Harlap S et al. Preventing pregnancy, protecting health. New York: Alan Guttmacher Inst, 1991;33).

Table 93.3.   Some Oral Contraceptives Available in the United States

Drug	Estrogen (µg)[a]	µg per Cycle	Progestin (mg)[b]	mg per Cycle
Combination				
Loestrin 1/20 21, 28 (Parke-Davis)	Ethinyl estradiol (20)	420	Norethindrone acetate (1)	21
Loestrin 1.5/30 21, 28 (Parke-Davis)	Ethinyl estradiol (30)	630	Norethindrone acetate (1.5)	31.5
Levlen 21, 28 (Berlex)	Ethinyl estradiol (30)	630	Levonorgestrel (0.15)	3.15
Nordette 21 (Wyeth-Ayerst)[c]	Ethinyl estradiol (30)	630	Levonorgestrel (0.15)	3.15
Lo/Ovral 21 (Wyeth-Ayerst)[c]	Ethinyl estradiol (30)	630	Norgestrel (0.3)	6.3
Desogen (Organon)	Ethinyl estradiol (30)	630	Desogestrel (0.15)	3.15
Ortho-Cept 21 (Ortho)[c]	Ethinyl estradiol (30)	630	Desogestrel (0.15)	3.15
Tri-Levlen 21, 18 (Berlex)	Ethinyl estradiol (30, 40)	680	Levonorgestrel (0.05, 0.075, 0.125)	1.925
Triphasil 21 (Wyeth-Ayerst)[c]	Ethinyl estradiol (30, 40)	680	Levonorgestrel (0.05, 0.075, 0.125)	1.925
Ortho Tri-Cyclene (Ortho)[c]	Ethinyl estradiol (35, 35, 35)	735	Norgestimate (0.18, 0.215, 0.25)	4.515
Ovcon 35 21, 28 (Mead Johnson)	Ethinyl estradiol (35)	735	Norethindrone (0.4)	8.4
Brevicon 21, 28 (Syntex)	Ethinyl estradiol (35)	735	Norethindrone (0.5)	10.5
Genora 0.5/35 21, 28 (Rugby)	Ethinyl estradiol (35)	735	Norethindrone (0.5)	10.5
Modicon 21 (Ortho)[c]	Ethinyl estradiol (35)	735	Norethindrone (0.5)	10.5
Nelova 0.5/35 21, 28 (Warner-Chilcott)[c]	Ethinyl estradiol (35)	735	Norethindrone (0.5)	10.5
Tri-Norinyl 21, 28 (Syntex)	Ethinyl estradiol (35, 35, 35)	735	Norethindrone (0.5, 1.0, 0.5)	15
Ortho-Novum 7/7/7 21 (Ortho)[c]	Ethinyl estradiol (35, 35, 35)	735	Norethindrone (0.5, 0.75, 1.0)	15.75
Nelova 10/11 21 (Warner-Chilcott)[c]	Ethinyl estradiol (35)	735	Norethindrone (0.5, 1.0)	16
Ortho-Novum 10/11 21 (Ortho)[c]	Ethinyl estradiol (35, 35)	735	Norethindrone (0.5, 1.0)	16
Janest-28 (Organon)	Ethinyl estradiol (35)	735	Norethindrone (1)	21
Genora 1/35 21, 28 (Rugby)	Ethinyl estradiol (35)	735	Norethindrone (1)	21
N.E.E. 1/35 21, 28 (Lexis)	Ethinyl estradiol (35)	735	Norethindrone (1)	21
Nelova 1/35 21 (Warner-Chilcott)[c]	Ethinyl estradiol (35)	735	Norethindrone (1)	21
Norethin 1/35E 21, 28 (Roberts)	Ethinyl estradiol (35)	735	Norethindrone (1)	21
Norinyl 1/35 21, 28 (Syntex)	Ethinyl estradiol (35)	735	Norethindrone (1)	21
Ortho-Novum 1/35 21 (Ortho)[c]	Ethinyl estradiol (35)	735	Norethindrone (1)	21
Ortho-Cyclen (Ortho)[c]	Ethinyl estradiol (35)	735	Norgestimate (0.25)	5.25
Demulen 1/35 21 (Searle)[c]	Ethinyl estradiol (35)	735	Ethynodiol diacetate (1)	21
Ovral (Wyeth-Ayerst)[c]	Ethinyl estradiol (50)	1050	Norgestrel (0.5)	10.5
Ovcon 50 21, 28 (Mead Johnson)	Ethinyl estradiol (50)	1050	Norethindrone (1)	21
Demulen 1/50 21 (Searle)[c]	Ethinyl estradiol (50)	1050	Ethynodiol diacetate (1)	21
N.E.E. 1/50 21, 28 (Lexis)	Mestranol (50)	1050	Norethindrone (1)	21
Genora 1/50 21, 28 (Rugby)	Mestranol (50)	1050	Norethindrone (1)	21
Nelova 1/50 21 (Warner-Chilcott)[c]	Mestranol (50)	1050	Norethindrone (1)	21
Norethin 1/50-M-21, 28 (Roberts)	Mestranol (50)	1050	Norethindrone (1)	21
Norinyl 1/50 21, 28 (Syntex)	Mestranol (50)	1050	Norethindrone (1)	21
Ortho-Novum 1/50 21 (Ortho)[c]	Mestranol (50)	1050	Norethindrone (1)	21
Progestin Only				
Ovrette (Wyeth-Ayerst)	None		Norgestrel (0.075)	2.1
Nor-QD (Syntex)	None		Norethindrone (0.35)	7.35
Microno (Ortho)	None		Norethindrone (0.35)	9.8

Adapted from Choice of contraceptives. Med Lett Drugs Ther 37:941, 1995.

[a]Ethinyl estradiol and mestranol are not equivalent on a milligram basis; the results of some studies indicate that 35 µg of ethinyl estradiol is equivalent to 50 µg of mestranol.

[b]Different progestins are not equivalent on a milligram basis.

[c]Also available in 28-day regimen.

Table 93.4.   Absolute Contraindications to Oral Contraceptives

Thrombophlebitis or thromboembolic disorders (current or remote)
Cerebral vascular or coronary artery disease (current or remote)
Known or suspected carcinoma of the breast
Known or suspected estrogen-dependent neoplasia
Undiagnosed, abnormal genital bleeding
Known or suspected pregnancy
Known or suspected liver failure

with a history of thromboembolism). Few patients are taking progestin-only preparations at present.

Absolute contraindications to oral contraceptives are listed in Table 93.4.

If oral contraception is selected, then the first choice should be a combination preparation containing 30 to 35 µg of estrogen and 1 mg or less of norethindrone.

Occasionally, it is necessary to change to a higher dosage of estrogen to control breakthrough bleeding (see below). However, preparations containing more than 35 µg of an estrogen should be used only for a short period of time (e.g., two or three menstrual cycles). If higher dosages seem necessary because there is no withdrawal bleeding or there continues to be breakthrough bleeding, consultation with an obstetrician–gynecologist is suggested.

To suppress ovulation and yet allow periodic bleeding, the combination tablet is taken every day for 3 weeks. The patient starts the medication by the fifth day of her cycle, counting the first day of menstrual bleeding as day 1. An alternative is to start on the first Sunday after the onset of a menstrual period. This latter practice allows the packaging of the tablets to provide for the user a minicalendar, which minimizes missing a dose. The tablets are arranged in circles or rows, making it easier to use them regularly. In the 28-day formulation, the last seven tablets have no hormonal effect and are there only to keep the patient on schedule and thereby improve compliance. The drop in hormone level after 21 days produces withdrawal bleeding just as it does in the normal menstrual cycle.

Postpartum women choosing an oral contraceptive should wait 3 weeks because of the theoretical increased risk of thromboembolism, but no longer than 4 to 6 weeks, at which time ovulation typically resumes. Breast-feeding women rarely need additional contraception for the first 6 months postpartum. However, combined oral contraceptives are usually avoided because they may decrease the quantity of breast milk. Patients who have had a spontaneous or therapeutic abortion may start taking the drug on the first Sunday following the event.

Noncontraceptive Benefits

In the past few years, oral contraceptives have been found to be associated with a significant number of beneficial side effects. These involve a decreased risk of benign breast tumors, functional ovarian cysts, pelvic inflammatory disease, endometrial carcinoma, and carcinoma of the ovary. Table 93.5 shows the estimated number of hospitalizations averted each year in the United States by oral contraceptive usage.

In the United States and other developed countries, a number of deaths are averted each year by the use of oral contraceptives because of their protective effect against ovarian and endometrial carcinoma. On balance, probably more deaths are averted than are caused by oral contraceptive use in developed countries. Of course, in developing countries where obstetric practices are primitive, many maternal deaths

Table 93.5. Noncontraceptive Health Benefits of Oral Contraceptives[a]

Disease	Rate of Hospitalizations Prevented per 1 Million Pill Users	Number of Hospitalizations Prevented	Number of Deaths Averted
Benign breast disease	235	20,000	
Ovarian retention cysts	35	3,000	
Iron deficiency anemia[b]	320	27,000	
Pelvic inflammatory disease (first episodes)			
Total episodes[b]	600	51,000	100
Hospitalizations	156	13,300	
Ectopic pregnancy	117	9,900	10
Endometrial cancer[c]	5	2,000	100
Ovarian cancer[c]	4	1,700	1,000

Adapted from Ory HW. The noncontraceptive health benefits from oral contraceptive use. Fam Plann Perspect 14:182, 1982.

[a]Rate of hospitalizations prevented and deaths averted annually by use of oral contraceptives, per 100,000 pill users, and estimated number of hospitalizations and deaths prevented annually, by specific disease in the United States. Except where noted, figures refer to hospitalizations prevented among the estimated 8.5 million current users of oral contraceptives in the United States.

[b]Episodes prevented regardless of whether hospitalization occurred.

[c]Based on an estimated 39 million U.S. women who have ever used oral contraceptives.

are averted by the avoidance of pregnancy with oral contraceptives.

Recognition of these noncontraceptive benefits of oral contraceptives helps place them in a much more positive perspective for patients and, indeed, puts the risk/benefit ratio of oral contraceptives in a more proper perspective.

Limitations

Thromboembolic Disease

In the late 1960s, the first epidemiologic studies conducted in Great Britain and the United States showed an increased risk of thromboembolic disorders and myocardial infarction among oral contraceptive users. It was quickly determined that the risk of thrombophlebitis and other vascular accidents was related to the dosage of estrogen, the age of the patient, and whether the patient was a smoker or nonsmoker (17,32). Decreasing the estrogen dosage in the oral contraceptives from 80 to 50 µg achieved approximately a 30% reduction in incidence of thromboembolic disease. A further reduction from 50 µg into the range of 30 to 35 µg further decreased the risk of venous thrombosis and other serious vascular complications.

However, the risk of thromboembolic disease must be kept in perspective. The general risk of thromboembolism in a nonpregnant woman of reproductive age is about 4 per 100,000. For women on oral contraceptive the risk is about 10 to 15 per 100,000. However for a woman who is pregnant the risk is 60 per 100,000 (23).

Approximately 10 million women in the United States use oral contraceptives. Cardiovascular problems, heart attack, stroke, thrombophlebitis, and pulmonary emboli are the main causes of serious morbidity and death associated with oral contraceptive use (13,20).

Age and smoking play significant roles in determining risk of serious cardiovascular events. An estimated 86% of deaths associated with oral contraceptive use result from a combination of smoking and pill use by women aged 35 and older (24). Because of the risk of thromboembolism, oral contraceptives should be discontinued 30 days before major surgery. They need not be discontinued before minor surgery (5).

Hypertension

With the older high-dose oral contraceptives, the risk of developing high blood pressure was approximately 7%. With the new low-dose preparations (under 50 µg of estrogen) evaluated in controlled studies, no significant hypertension resulting from the oral contraceptive has been identified. Therefore, if an oral contraceptive user develops hypertension, the hypertension should be promptly evaluated and not ascribed to contraceptive usage. Women with preexisting hypertension or a family or personal history of hypertension are probably no more likely to develop high blood pressure or worsening hypertension when they take low-dose oral contraceptive preparations. Hypertension that is controlled is not a contraindication to use of oral contraceptives.

Neoplasia

After nearly 35 years of contraceptive use, the data concerning the relationship between oral contraceptive use and neoplasia are mostly reassuring (Table 93.6).

There is a relationship between the long-term use of oral contraceptives and the development of benign hepatic neoplasia (10). These lesions are rare, and although the increased relative risk of developing one of these lesions in long-term users is high, the absolute incidence is very low. Long-term use of oral contraceptives has been associated with a significantly decreased incidence of endometrial and ovarian cancer (3,33). This protective effect of oral contraceptives appears to be directly related to the length of usage, and the protective effect is greater than 50% and appears to persist for more than 10 years after discontinuing oral contraceptives.

The data are inconclusive for malignant melanoma and cervical neoplasia. With regard to the development of cervical neoplasia, several recent studies show a slightly increased risk directly related to the length of oral contraceptive use (1,33). Nevertheless, no firm conclusions can be drawn at this time.

Similarly, data regarding breast cancer and oral contraceptive use are conflicting and no conclusions are currently possible (29). Although some data suggest that oral contraceptives may advance premenopausal breast cancer, this is a rare disease. Epidemiologic evidence reveals that if the association does indeed exist it is small (30). The incidence of benign breast tumors and fibrocystic disease is reduced by the administration of high-progestin-dose oral contraceptive hormones. Data on the newer low-dose progestin contraceptive pills are inconclusive (19).

Altered Metabolism of Glucose or Lipids

With the oral contraceptives that contain more than 50 µg of estrogen, abnormal glucose tolerance tests can be seen after 3 months of use. However, this reduction in glucose tolerance is not seen with the low-dose preparations. Also, the new triphasic and low-dose forms do not appear to alter the lipid profile even in long-term users, whereas the high-dose preparations (more than 50 µg of estrogen) adversely affect the lipid profile (16,27).

Gallbladder Disease

The incidence of symptomatic gallbladder disease increases twofold within the first 1 to 2 years of oral contraceptive use. An estrogen-associated increase in the concentration of cholesterol in the bile has been demonstrated in patients taking oral contraceptives and may be the pathogenetic mechanism.

Headaches

Some patients with a history of migraine headaches note a worsening of these headaches while taking oral

Table 93.6. Oral Contraceptives and Neoplasia Risk

	Increased	No Effect	Decreased	Inconclusive Information
Hepatocellular adenoma	X			
Cervical neoplasia				X
Endometrial cancer			X	
Ovarian cancer			X	
Breast cancer		X		
Pituitary adenoma		X		
Malignant melanoma				X

contraceptives. The development of severe recurrent headaches is a reason to recommend another contraceptive method.

Birth Defects

The suggestion that hormonal ingestion during the first 3 months of pregnancy may result in the subsequent development of birth defects is unlikely. Initial epidemiologic studies done in the 1960s and early 1970s seem to favor an association with some cardiovascular and limb defects. More recent studies tend to refute this association. There is no evidence that prior use of contraceptives has any effect on the development of any birth defect. Establishing a pregnancy within one to two cycles after discontinuation of oral contraceptives is not associated with a higher incidence of birth defects (6,18), so no period of protection with another contraceptive method is needed when pregnancy is desired.

Other Side Effects

In general, minor side effects occur early in the course of taking oral contraceptives and may be transient. Thorough education by the physician increases the likelihood that the patient will tolerate these effects and continue taking the medication.

Alopecia.   Alopecia is a rarely reported side effect (see Chapter 100). Most often it is transient; but if hair loss is reported for longer than 3 months, the drug should be discontinued and the patient should use some other form of contraception.

Nausea.   Nausea occurs in approximately 5% of patients, typically resolves within 3 months of initiating the method, and almost always can be eliminated by taking the contraceptive at bedtime.

Fatigue.   Increased fatigability is occasionally described by patients but usually is of short duration.

Change in Menstrual Flow.   The most typical pattern is a reduction in the amount and duration of menstrual flow. This usually is welcomed by the patient. On occasion, there is no bleeding; if the patient has taken the oral contraceptive regularly (so pregnancy is not likely), she can be advised to continue it for another cycle. If she is again amenorrheic, a pregnancy test (see below) should be done. If pregnancy is ruled out, the patient can either select another contraceptive method, be placed temporarily on a 50-mg estrogen pill, (which results in more menstrual bleeding), or be reassured that if she continues taking the method correctly she will remain amenorrheic.

Breakthrough Bleeding. Breakthrough bleeding is most common in the early cycles after initiation of an oral contraceptive. It is of no concern as long as the patient has not missed a dose. Failure to take daily doses increases the chance of breakthrough bleeding, particularly in the early part of the cycle. If a dose or two has been forgotten early in the cycle, the patient should catch up and continue the normal regimen together with temporary use of a barrier form of protection. If breakthrough bleeding continues for several cycles, referral to a gynecologist is indicated to rule out an organic cause and to consider using a higher dosage of estrogen.

Weight Gain. Approximately 5% of patients show some weight gain, sometimes associated with fluid retention (22).

Vaginitis. It has been difficult to document a close relationship between oral contraceptives and vaginitis. The hormones do alter the vaginal milieu, but vaginitis develops in only a small proportion of patients. Standard diagnostic methods and subsequent therapy (see Chapter 94) allows most patients to continue to use the oral contraceptive.

Skin Changes. Some patients, especially dark-skinned ones, note chloasma (yellowish-brown discoloration of the skin) and a change in hair texture. Chloasma is unlikely to resolve with continued administration of the oral contraceptive and is therefore a reason to discontinue it if the cosmetic effect is unacceptable.

Emotional Changes. Some women have become depressed while taking oral contraceptives. Therefore patients who have a history of depression should be followed especially carefully. If depression develops, the medication should be discontinued.

Effects on Laboratory Tests. Oral contraceptives can alter the results of a number of laboratory tests (11). The alterations reflect physiologic changes in the patient in most instances but rarely signify clinically significant disease.

Drug Interactions. Oral contraceptives may alter the effectiveness of a number of other drugs; conversely, a number of other drugs may alter the effectiveness of oral contraceptives. In general, concomitant use of antibiotics does not decrease oral contraceptive effectiveness. Physicians should investigate the possibility of drug interaction before prescribing any other medication to a patient using an oral contraceptive preparation. Table 93.7 lists drugs that may interact with oral contraceptives.

Patient Follow-Up. A patient taking oral contraceptives should see a physician once a year for a pelvic examination and a cervical smear for cytology (at an appropriate interval; see Chapter 95). Screening for sexually transmitted diseases (see Chapter 94) may need to be done if the patient is at risk. Oral contraceptives may be discontinued at any time if pregnancy is desired or another method of contraception is planned. The first few menstrual periods after withdrawal may be heavier than during the time oral contraceptives were used. There is no change in fertility after a course of oral contraceptives, regardless of duration of use. A pill-free or rest period is no longer advocated.

Table 93.7. Selected Drugs that May Interact with Oral Contraceptive Preparations (OCPs)

Drugs that may decrease the effectiveness of OCPs resulting in breakthrough bleeding, pregnancy, or both:
  Well-established, commonly occurring drug reactions
    Anticonvulsants: barbiturates, phenytoin (Dilantin), or primidone (Mysoline)
    Antimicrobial: Rifampicin
  Reported instances of possible drug interactions
    Antimicrobials
      Breakthrough bleeding only: Neomycin, Nitrofurantoin, phenoxymethylpenicillin (penicillin V)
      Breakthrough bleeding and pregnancy: Ampicillin, chloramphenicol, sulfamethoxypridaxine (Kynex, Midicel)
    Others: chlordiazepoxide (Librium), meprobamate, Phenacetin, and phenylbutazone (Butazolidin)
Drugs whose effectiveness may be altered by OCPs:
  Anticoagulants: The effect of anticoagulants may be reduced by the simultaneous administration of OCPs.
  Clofibrate (Atromid-S): Control of cholesterol and triglyceride levels may be lost when OCPs are simultaneously administered with clofibrate.
  Thyroid hormone in patients without functioning thyroid gland: Mostly a theoretical concern; however, there may be a need for an increased dosage of thyroid hormone in patients without a functioning thyroid gland.
  Tricyclic antidepressants: Higher dosages of estrogen may inhibit the effect of antidepressants, and tricyclic toxicity may be increased.
  Caffeine: There may be decreased metabolism of caffeine induced by OCPs. Patients who take large amounts of caffeine (e.g., 4–8 cups of coffee/day) should be cautioned regarding symptoms of caffeinism.

SUBDERMAL CONTRACEPTIVE

The Norplant subdermal contraceptive method consists of six Silastic capsules (Dow Corning, Midland, MI) each containing 36 mg of levonorgestrel (a progestin) in crystalline form. The capsules are 34 mm long and 2.4 mm in diameter. They are inserted subdermally in the inner aspect of the upper arm. They provide contraceptive protection for at least 5 years, with a first-year failure rate of only 0.2 pregnancies per 100 users (8). Pregnancy rates range from 0.5 to 1.1 for 100 woman-years for the remaining 4 years. This level of effectiveness is much higher than that of any other form of reversible contraception except Depo-Provera and is similar to that seen with first-year failure rates for surgical sterilization (Table 93.2). The system contains no estrogen and therefore is useful in some patients for whom combined oral contraceptives would be contraindicated. The system initially releases levonorgestrel at approximately the level seen with the mini-pill progestin-only oral medication (see above). Over the first 12 to 18 months, this level falls 50% and remains constant for the remainder of the 5 years. This level is about one-third that seen in patients taking low-dose combined oral contraceptives. Thus the Norplant system provides superior protection from pregnancy with no estrogen component and a substantially reduced level of progestin. Norplant prevents contraception through thickening of the cervical mucus, disordered maturation of the endometrial lining, and suppression of ovulation. Approximately 50% of patients after the first year resume normal ovulatory cycles. Therefore the main contraceptive effect is via the thickening of the cervical mucus.

Patient Experience. Worldwide Norplant insertions and removals are performed by nurses, general physicians, and obstetricians. The insertion is done in an office setting using only local anesthesia. Most insertions take 5 to 10 minutes. Removal takes somewhat longer and is likewise done under local anesthesia. Most patients report minimal or no discomfort with either insertion or removal when performed by someone experienced and skilled in these techniques.

Contraindications

Because Norplant contains no estrogen, there are few absolute contraindications. Pregnancy, active thromboembolic phenomena, undiagnosed genital bleeding, acute liver disease, and carcinoma of the breast constitute absolute contraindications. The system can be safely used by patients who have diabetes mellitus, hypertension, and migraine headaches. Effectiveness is lowered in patients taking barbiturates, phenytoin, carbamazepine, primidone, phenylbutazone, and rifampicin.

Side Effects

Change in the menstrual bleeding pattern is the most common side effect associated with Norplant use and patients should be prepared for this when choosing the method. The change in pattern is one of unpredictability. Some patients have prolonged spotting; others (10 to 15%) develop amenorrhea; only rarely do patients develop prolonged heavy bleeding. In some studies, up to 75% of women experience menstrual irregularities during the first year. Less common side effects are similar to those seen in oral contraceptive users. Less than 10% experience headaches, nervousness, dizziness, abdominal cramping, nausea, acne, and weight gain. Only rarely do patients complain of hair loss.

Removal

Following removal (see above for patient experience) of the Norplant, serum blood levels of contraceptive hormone fall to undetectable levels within 2 weeks. The return of fertility among those who discontinue Norplant is considered immediate.

INTRAMUSCULAR INJECTABLE CONTRACEPTIVE

Depo-medroxyprogesterone acetate (Depo-Provera, UpJohn, Kalamazoo, MI), a C-21-17 acetoxy progestogen that is similar to natural progesterone, has been in use in the United States since 1992. Prior issues and concerns regarding a relationship to breast cancer have been successfully resolved. Depo-Provera is administered as an intramuscular injection of 150 mg that provides contraceptive efficacy for at least 14 weeks. Administration every 12 weeks provides a margin of error should the patient fail to return at the exact appointed time. In this dosage the failure rate is comparable to that of Norplant (7). Despite a large worldwide experience with this form of contraception, there are no data on its use by self-injection; accordingly, it should be administered by a health professional.

Mode of Action

Like other progestin-only contraceptives and combination oral contraceptives, Depo-Provera acts by inhibiting ovulation, thickening cervical mucus, and altering the composition of the endometrium.

Side Effects

The most common side effect associated with Depo-Provera is a disruption in the menstrual pattern. This disruption is unpredictable and can range from prolonged periods of amenorrhea to episodes of heavy bleeding. Approximately 50% of women using Depo-Provera for 1 year develop amenorrhea, as compared with 10 to 15% of Norplant patients. Other side effects are similar to those seen with Norplant. Following discontinuation of Depo-Provera, patients wishing to achieve a pregnancy experience a temporary delay in return to fertility lasting as long as 4 to 9 months after the last injection. By 2 years postinjection, these patients have essentially achieved the same fertility as patients who discontinue other nonhormonal methods.

INTRAUTERINE DEVICE

The intrauterine device (IUD) is one of the most effective methods of contraception, although its exact mode of action is unknown. Pregnancy rates range from 1 to 3 per 100 women per year. The first modern IUDs appeared in the early 1960s and were made of a biologically inert plastic. The second-generation IUDs, copper- and progesterone-containing devices, have been available since the early 1970s (28).

During the late 1970s, serious concerns were raised regarding the safety of all IUDs. Studies showed a strong relationship between IUD use and the development of pelvic inflammatory disease. The Dalkon Shield specifically was removed from the market because of its link to spontaneous septic abortions and pelvic inflammatory disease. The clearly increased risk for infection with this product has been attributed to the multifilament (versus monofilament on other IUDs) tail (the string that hangs into the vagina), which seemed to act as a wick for bacteria. Because of the publicity from the Dalkon Shield, distribution of other devices was discontinued by the manufacturers because of low sales volume or concern regarding litigation costs. The ongoing concern over the relationship between IUD use and the development of pelvic inflammatory disease with resultant tubal infertility is valid. However, epidemiologic studies in the 1970s tended to overstate the risk of pelvic infection from IUD use. The reasons for this are as follows:

- In most early studies the control group included women who were using diaphragms and oral contraceptives. These are protective against pelvic inflammatory disease.
- The risks for specific IUDs were not analyzed separately. Dalkon Shield wearers, with substantially higher risk of infection, were included in most analyses.
- Most studies did not analyze for factors that significantly affect the risk of pelvic inflammatory disease, such as multiple sexual partners and previous history of pelvic infection.

Recent epidemiologic studies have adjusted the relative risks of tubal infertility by type of IUD used and number of sexual partners. They have shown that women who had only one sexual partner in their lifetime had no significantly increased risk of tubal infertility. However, women who had more than one sexual partner had a three to four times higher risk (2). At present, IUD use is recommended only for women who have had at least one child and who are in a mutually faithful monogamous relationship.

Types

Two types of IUDs are available in the United States: the progesterone-releasing (Progestasert) and the copper-bearing (ParaGard). The Progestasert is a plastic T-shaped device that contains a reservoir of 38 mg of progesterone in the vertical bar. This progesterone is released at a rate of 65 μg/day and exerts a local contraceptive effect. The progesterone reservoir is depleted after 12 months and the device must then be removed and replaced by a new one. A longer-lasting levonorgestrel-releasing IUD has been successfully tested but is not yet available. The ParaGard device has a body of polyethylene wound with copper wire and has a copper collar on each of its transverse arms but contains no hormone. Currently it is approved by the FDA for 10 years of continuous use. This is a major benefit when compared with the Progestasert system, which is approved for only 1 year of continuous use. Both devices have a *monofilament string* attached, which allows for surveillance and removal (see below).

Use and Insertion

If the physician is not experienced in IUD insertion, the patient should be referred to a gynecologist. The IUD is best inserted at the time of a menstrual period. This provides assurance that the patient is not pregnant, and it permits easier insertion of the device because the cervix is slightly dilated. The usual small amount of bleeding associated with insertion becomes a part of the normal menstrual flow. The patient thereafter usually notices some increased bleeding with her periods and possibly some increased cramping, which generally subsides within 3 months.

Patient Experience. Most often the patient experiences some cramps when the IUD is inserted. Administration of nonsteroidal analgesics before the insertion (e.g., ibuprofen 400 mg) affords some relief. These cramps usually subside in a few hours. Rarely they may be so severe as to necessitate removal of the device. If they persist beyond a few hours, this may be an indication that the device is not inserted properly, and the device should be removed. After insertion the patient can feel the string of the IUD, and by doing this after each menstrual period, can be assured that the device is in place.

Risks

Contraindications to the use of an IUD are shown in Table 93.8. The most commonly encountered serious side effect is the development of pelvic inflammatory disease. The patient must be instructed to report any fever, pelvic pain, or discomfort promptly. She must also report any missed menstrual periods because this mandates that she be evaluated for pregnancy. The patient who has missed a menstrual period must be evaluated also for ectopic pregnancy, as pregnancies with the IUD in place are more commonly ectopic. A patient who becomes pregnant with an IUD in place has a 5% risk of ectopic pregnancy and a 50% risk of spontaneous abortion. If the IUD string is visible, the spontaneous abortion rate can be reduced to approximately 25% by removal of the IUD. Uterine perforation, a rare complication, is most likely to occur at the time of insertion. Finally, the use of the intrauterine device by a young nulliparous patient who has multiple sex partners is associated with a significantly increased incidence of uterine infection.

Monitoring

There should be an annual follow-up that includes a review of any problems; a pelvic examination includ-

Table 93.8. Contraindications to Insertion of an IUD

Pregnancy or suspicion of pregnancy.
Abnormalities of the uterus resulting in distortion of the uterine cavity.
Acute, or history of, pelvic inflammatory disease.
Postpartum endometritis or infected abortion in the past 3 months.
Known or suspected uterine or cervical malignancy, including unresolved abnormal Pap smear.
Genital bleeding of unknown cause.
Untreated acute cervicitis until infection is controlled.
Wilson's disease (copper-containing IUDs).
Known allergy to copper.
History of ectopic pregnancy.
Patient or her partner has multiple sexual partners.
Conditions associated with increased susceptibility to infections with microorganisms. Such conditions include leukemia, diabetes, acquired immunodeficiency syndrome (AIDS), and those requiring chronic corticosteroid therapy.
Genital actinomycosis.
A previously inserted IUD that has not been removed.

ing a cervical cancer smear, a gonorrhea culture, and a chlamydia culture (if either is indicated); and detection of the device. The follow-up is best done by a gynecologist if the general physician is not experienced in examining patients with an IUD.

The IUD is easily removed by gentle traction on the string at or around the time of a menstrual period. Removal at this time allows the bleeding associated with removal to be part of the menstrual period. Also, it is easier to remove during menstruation than later in the cycle (see above).

As with other methods, if a patient terminates this form of contraception other than to attempt pregnancy, she will need help in choosing another form of contraception.

SPONGE

The sponge is a barrier contraceptive device. It is a small, donut-shaped, polyurethane plastic device filled with nonoxynol 9 (a spermicidal agent) that is placed high in the vagina before intercourse. If it is left in place longer than 24 hours, vaginal irritation and vaginitis may result and the rare occurrence of toxic shock syndrome has been reported with its use (see Chapter 94). The sponge is no longer available in the United States.

DIAPHRAGM

The diaphragm is a dome-shaped rubber device held open by a metallic band or spring. It is filled with a spermicidal cream or jelly before each use and placed in the vagina over the cervix to prevent sperm deposited during ejaculation from reaching the cervical os. As seen in Table 93.2, with typical use the failure rate is high, whereas correct or ideal usage results in a lower failure rate, as is true of all barrier methods.

The diaphragm is prescribed and fitted by a physician or an assistant. For better effectiveness, the patient should be asked to insert the diaphragm in the office and have the provider check its placement. The device fits between the posterior fornix and the symphysis. The largest device that is comfortable is the proper one to use. Manufacturers of diaphragms have excellent booklets that are useful in helping a patient acquire the skill necessary for comfortable use of this form of contraception.

The patient applies spermicidal jelly to the inside of the dome and inserts the diaphragm in the vagina as long as 4 hours before intercourse. She should check for position with her finger and allow the device to remain in place for at least 6 hours after coitus. If repeated intercourse occurs within 6 to 8 hours, additional jelly should be placed in the vagina first, without removal of the diaphragm.

With care a diaphragm should last 2 years. The patient will need a new fitting if she gains or loses significant weight, has a baby, or has pelvic surgery. *The cervical cap* has been approved for use by the FDA. Such devices come in several sizes and they must be fitted by a health professional to go over the cervix. Proper fitting can be accomplished in approximately 80% of women. The cap may be used with or without spermicide. The spermicide may increase slightly the contraceptive effect. Generally, the cap is about as effective as the diaphragm and can be left in place for up to 48 hours.

Benefits

The diaphragm is a low-cost device that has no major risks other than the higher risk of unwanted pregnancy compared with oral contraceptives or the IUD.

Limitations

Restrictions on the use of the diaphragm are sensitivity to the rubber or the spermicidal material. Alterations in pelvic shape may also preclude the proper fitting of the different diaphragms available. It is not suited for patients who will not or cannot touch their vagina, such as patients who are very obese or who have a musculoskeletal disorder.

Some women may report discomfort while the diaphragm is in place. This discomfort is most often related to a wrong design or to improper fitting, and reevaluation usually identifies the problem. A few patients develop recurrent cystitis with frequent diaphragm use.

CONDOM

The *male condom* is a latex rubber sheath that is placed over the erect penis. It is the only reversible effective male method of contraception except for coitus interruptus. Condoms properly used are an effective form of contraception, and their failure rate with experienced and strongly motivated couples is as low as 1 or 2 per 100 couple-years of exposure. However, rates during the first year of use or in less motivated couples may be considerably higher. Its effectiveness can be enhanced if it is combined with application of a spermicidal jelly or foam in the vagina. Some condoms are now being manufactured in containers with a spermicidal lubricant. The condom, when used properly, provides considerable protection against sexually transmitted diseases, including gonorrhea, herpes, chlamydia, and human immunodeficiency virus (HIV) infection (see Chapter 34). Its only side effect is a rare instance of sensitivity to the lubricating material or latex or skin irritation from friction.

The *female condom* is a disposable, prelubricated polyurethane sheath between two rings of differing sizes. One ring is placed in the vagina, as with the diaphragm, and the larger ring rests exteriorly on the vulva. Studies show that it is impenetrable to the passage of HIV as well as common sexually transmitted diseases. Expected pregnancy rates are comparable to those of the male condom (4,12).

VAGINAL SUPPOSITORIES, FOAM, OR JELLY

Vaginal suppositories, foam, and jelly contain a spermicidal material combined with cream, jelly, or foam. The material is inserted in the vagina at least 10 to 15 minutes before intercourse. The spermicidal material is dispersed in the vagina and over the cervix. This creates a barrier around the cervical os to prevent sperm from entering the intrauterine cavity. All of these forms of contraception may be obtained without prescription. They are especially useful when additional protection is desired at midcycle with the condom or to increase the effectiveness of the diaphragm when repeated intercourse occurs. The side effects are minor and are related to sensitivity to the spermicidal material.

RHYTHM

The human ovum probably is viable for only 12 to 24 hours after ovulation. Sperm retain the capability for fertilization for 48 hours, although this may be possible for up to 5 days. New information suggests that conception is most likely during a 6-day interval ending on the day of ovulation (34). The development of a method of contraception that avoids intercourse at the fertile time is logical. Three methods have been developed:

- The *calendar method* attempts to establish the portion of the cycle when intercourse is safe. The patient keeps a careful record for several months of the duration of each menstrual cycle beginning with the first day of bleeding. She then subtracts 18 days from the shortest cycle and 11 days from the longest cycle, which represents the beginning and the end of the fertile time. Intercourse is avoided during this fertile time. Obviously, the more regular she is, the shorter is this interval and the better the protection. For example, if the shortest cycle is 27 days and the longest is 33 days, then she is possibly fertile from day 9 until day 22, or an interval of 12 days. On the other hand, if she is regular and bleeds every 28 days, her fertile period is 7 days in duration, starting on day 10 of the menstrual cycle.
- The *basal body temperature method* takes advantage of the slight drop in body temperature associated with ovulation, followed by a rise in temperature of approximately 1°F (0.5°C). The woman takes her temperature each morning from day 3 of the cycle until it has remained elevated to a higher level than baseline for 72 hours; usually this temperature elevation is to approximately 98.6° to 99°F (36.8° to 37.2°C). This indicates that she is postovulatory and can resume coitus (the ovum must be fertilized within 24 to 48 hours).
- The *cervical mucus method* requires the patient to learn, over a number of cycles, the changes that indicate ovulation. She is taught to examine her cervical mucus for clarity. She learns to identify abdominal discomfort associated with ovulation and to use this information to avoid intercourse when

conception is possible. This method requires effort and regular cycles but has been used effectively by many women.

The *rhythm method* or *periodic abstinence* is the only method of birth control approved by religious organizations that oppose artificial contraceptive methods. The risk of pregnancy in women who use this method of contraception is high (Table 93.2).

STERILIZATION

Simple methods of permanent contraception are available to both men and women (14,31). At present in the United States sterilization is the most popular method of contraception in people over 30. The total number of sterilizations is rising, and at present the rate of elective sterilization is somewhat higher for women than men (26).

Patients considering sterilization need very careful education so that they understand its nature and risks. Informed consent is required for these procedures.

Vasectomy

Vasectomy, when properly performed, has a failure rate of 1/200 to 1/500. The complication rate is approximately 4/1000 and, for the most part, complications are minor. They include infection, hematoma, epididymitis, and granuloma formation. Long-term serious side effects have not been reported among the very large numbers of men who have had the procedure performed. There was a transient concern, now known to be unwarranted (21), that antibodies to sperm that develop in some men after vasectomy predispose to atherosclerosis. Before 1990, several studies examined the possible influence of vasectomy on the risk of developing prostate cancer. The results showed no statistically significant relationship. However, two studies published in early 1993 suggest that there is an increased risk of developing prostate cancer among men who have had a vasectomy. A consensus conference convened by the National Institutes of Health in March 1993 considered the currently available data. The consensus conference concluded that currently there are insufficient data to recommend changes in the current clinical practice concerning vasectomy (15).

Patient Experience. This procedure is done under local anesthesia in the urologist's office or outpatient surgical suite. There is minimal operative discomfort. Postoperatively mild discomfort is common but it is usually controlled with a mild analgesic, such as acetaminophen. Vigorous physical activity and sexual activity are restricted for 5 to 7 days until the wound has healed. Follow-up visits are necessary so that sperm counts can be performed. It usually requires 6 to 12 weeks or 20 ejaculations for the ejaculate to become free of sperm. Therefore another contraceptive method is necessary until aspermia is confirmed.

Reanastomosis of the vas deferens may be accomplished surgically and results in patency in approximately 60% of patients. Nevertheless, vasectomy should not be undertaken unless the patient genuinely wants permanent sterilization.

Tubal Ligation

Although recent information suggests that the failure rate for tubal ligation may be higher than expected, it remains among the best methods of long-term sterilization. Overall failure rates at 1 year are 5/1000 and at 10 years are approximately 18/1000 (25). The major complication rate is approximately 4/1000. The complications are bleeding, infection, and bowel, bladder, or uterine trauma.

Patient Experience. Laparoscopy or minilaparotomy is usually performed using general anesthesia in this country. Uncomplicated tubal ligation is generally performed as an outpatient procedure and is very well tolerated. Mild abdominal discomfort, when present, usually lasts only for a few days and rarely for a few weeks. Mild analgesics (e.g., acetaminophen) provide relief. The patient is usually able to return to her usual activities in 48 to 72 hours. Sterilization is immediate and intercourse is permitted as soon as the wound is no longer painful.

Tubal ligation is performed in the first half of the menstrual cycle before ovulation has occurred. This avoids the possibility of fertilization of an ovum occurring a day or two before the surgical procedure. If the woman is using effective contraception, tubal ligation may be performed at any time. Reanastomosis of the fallopian tubes can be accomplished surgically and results in a significant chance of fertility. The success of reanastomosis depends primarily on the type and extent of the initial ligation and is not related to the time between ligation and anastomosis. Nevertheless, a woman should not undergo tubal ligation unless she genuinely desires permanent sterilization.

The existence of a posttubal syndrome characterized by heavier menstrual bleeding and more pelvic pain than are found in the unsterilized populations has been questioned. After sterilization, most patients notice no significant change in symptoms associated with their menstrual periods.

DIAGNOSING PREGNANCY

Human chorionic gonadotropin is a glycoprotein hormone that is produced by the blastocyst and the placenta. Its secretion begins very early and can be detected in the maternal blood as early as 6 days after fertilization. In the past, a number of conditions could give rise to a false-positive result, such as the presence of foreign protein, cross-reaction with the luteinizing hormone (LH), follicular-stimulating hormone (FSH), and thyroid-stimulating hormone (TSH). The α subunit for human chorionic gonadotropin (HCG) is common to all of these hormones. However, the β subunit for HCG is unique, and the currently available pregnancy tests that use the monoclonal antibody methodology test only for the β subunit. A false-positive reaction,

even with home pregnancy detection kits, is extremely rare. There are four major types of pregnancy tests; are all very accurate and each has its own characteristics (see below). The Icon, an enzyme-linked immunoassay, is the most commonly used because of its simplicity, accuracy, and availability. Any physician who may be asked to diagnose pregnancy should have a rapid pregnancy diagnosing kit in the office. There is no clinical situation in which one of these tests has a distinct advantage over another.

Radioimmunoassay (Serum): Chorio Quant, Beta Tec, HCG Beta III

- Accurate (Close to 100% accuracy for positive result in normal pregnancy) when used at least 7 days after conception.
- No LH cross-reaction.
- Specific for HCG (detects βsubunit).
- Used for assessing abnormal pregnancy (ectopic, molar, threatened abortion).
- Requires that the specimen be sent to a laboratory, and the typical turnaround time is 1 day.

Enzyme-Linked Immunoassay (Urine or Serum): Icon, Confidot, Quest

- Accurate when used at least 12 days after conception.
- No LH cross-reaction.
- Specific for HCG (detects β subunit).
- Used for routine pregnancy confirmation.
- Easy to use and results are available in a few minutes.

Radioreceptorassay (Serum): Biocept-G

- Accurate when used at least 14 days after conception.
- LH cross-reaction possible.
- Used for early confirmation of normal pregnancy.
- Specimen usually is sent to a laboratory, and the turnaround time is typically 1 day.

Immunoassay (Urine or Serum): Neocept, Pregnosis

- Accurate when used at least 28 days after conception.
- LH cross-reaction possible.
- Used for routine pregnancy confirmation.
- Serum assay usually is sent to a laboratory, but this urine assay can be done in the office.

The biological half-life of HCG is approximately 1.5 days. The serum HCG becomes negative approximately 10 days after delivery, artificial termination of pregnancy, or spontaneous or therapeutic abortion, if all trophoblastic tissue is expelled.

The HCG test may remain positive for weeks to months if small foci of functioning trophoblastic tissue remain. This could be seen after incomplete abortion, persistent hydatidiform mole, and choriocarcinoma.

UNPLANNED PREGNANCY

All contraceptive methods are associated with some failures, which result in an *unplanned pregnancy.* Patients with such a pregnancy are faced with the difficult decision of whether to carry or to terminate the pregnancy. Estimates are that almost 50% of the approximately 4 million births in the United States in 1992 were unplanned. Currently, about 1.5 million *therapeutic abortions* are performed each year in the United States. The usual method of early termination of pregnancy in the United States is a surgical suction dilation and curettage performed in an outpatient center, free-standing clinic, or obstetrician's office, usually under local anesthesia. A new *antiprogesterone compound,* RU 486, is currently being used in several European countries for the medical termination of early pregnancy. This agent is now being tested in the United States.

General References*

Colditz GA. Oral contraceptive use and mortality during 12 years of follow-up: the nurses' health study. Ann Intern Med 120:821, 1994.
> A very large study showing that the long-term use of oral contraceptives is safe.

Hatcher RA, Guest F, Stewart F, et al. Contraception technology 1994–1996. 16th ed. New York: Irvington, 1994.
> A regularly updated text covering all aspects of contraception. It is highly recommended.

Speroff L, Darney PD. A clinical guide for contraception. Baltimore, MD: Williams & Wilkins, 1992.

Specific References

1. Brinton LA, Huggins GR, Lehman HF, et al. Long term use of oral contraceptives and risk of invasive cervical cancer. Int J Cancer 38: 339, 1986.
2. Burkman RT. The Woman's Health Study. Association between intrauterine device and pelvic inflammatory disease. Obstet Gynecol 57:269, 1981.
3. Centers for Disease Control. Cancer and steroid hormone study. Oral contraceptive use and ovarian cancer. JAMA 249:1596, 1983.
4. Choice of Contraceptives. Med Lett Drugs Ther 37:941, 1995.
5. Coagulation and thrombosis with OC use. physiology and clinical relevance. Dialogues in Contraception. Little Falls, NJ: Health Learning Systems, 1996.
6. Contraceptives and congenital anomalies: ACOG Committee Opinion: Committee on Gynecologic Practice. Number 124, July 1993. Int J Gynecol Obstet 42:316, 1993.
7. Cullins VE. Injectable and implantable contraceptives. Curr Opin Obstet Gynecol 4:536, 1992.
8. Cullins VE, Remsburg RE, Blumenthal PD, Huggins GR. Norplant: welcome new contraceptive option. Contemp Obstet Gynecol 37:46, 1992.
9. Durand JL, Bressler R. Clinical pharmacology of the steroidal oral contraceptives. Adv Intern Med 24:97, 1979.
10. Edmondson HA, Henderson B, Benton B. Liver-cell adenomas associated with use of oral contraceptives. N Engl J Med 294:470, 1976.
11. Effect of oral contraceptives in laboratory test results. Med Lett Drugs Ther 21:54, 1979.
12. The female condom. Med Lett Drugs Ther 35:123, 1993.
13. Hannaford PC, Croft PR, Kay CR. Oral contraception and stroke: evidence from the Royal College of General Practitioners' Oral Contraception Study. Stroke 25:935, 1994.
14. Hulka JF. Current status of elective sterilization in the United States. Fertil Steril 28:515, 1977.
15. Klitsch M. Vasectomy and prostate cancer: more questions than answers. Fam Plann Perspect 25:33, 1993.
16. Krauss RM, Burkman RT. The metabolic impact of oral contraceptives. Am J Obstet Gynecol 167:1177, 1992.
17. Layde PM, McCarthy PS, Lord JAH, Smith CFC. Incidence of arterial disease among oral contraceptive users: Royal College of General Practitioners Oral Contraceptive Study. J R Coll Gen Pract 33:75, 1983.
18. Linn S, Schoenbaum SC, Monson RR, et al. Lack of association between contraceptive usage and congenital malformation of offspring. Am J Obstet Gynecol 147:923, 1983.
19. LiVolsi VA, Stadel BV, Kelsey JL, et al. Fibrocystic breast disease in oral-contraceptive users. N Engl J Med 299:381, 1978.
20. Lowe GDO, Greer IA, Cooke TG, et al. Risk of and prophylaxis for venous thromboembolism in hospital patients. BMJ 305: 567, 1992.
21. Massey FJ Jr, Bernstein GS, O'Fallon WN, et al. Vasectomy and health. Results from a large cohort study. JAMA 252:1023, 1984.
22. Moore LL, Valuck R, McDougall C, Fink W. A comparative study of one-year weight gain among users of medroxyprogesterone acetate, levonorgestrel implants, and oral contraceptives. Contraception 52:215, 1995.
23. Nilsson S, Mellbin T, Hofvander Y, et al. Long-term follow-up of children breast-fed by mothers using oral contraceptives. Contraception, 34:443, 1986.
24. Ory HW, Forrest JD, Lincoln R. Making choices, evaluating health risks and benefits of birth control methods. New York: Alan Guttmacher Institute, 1983.
25. Peterson HB, Xia Z, Hughes JM, et al. The risk of pregnancy after tubal sterilization: findings from the U.S. Collaborative Review of Sterilization. Am J Obstet Gynecol 174:1161, 1996.
26. Peterson LS. Contraceptive use in the United States: 1982–90. Hyattsville, MD: US Department of Health and Human Services. Public Health Service. Centers for Disease Control and Prevention. National Center for Health Statistics, 1995.
27. Petitti DB, Sidney S, Bernstein A, et al. Stroke in users of low-dose oral contraceptives. N Engl J Med 335:8, 1996.
28. Population Information Program. Population reports: intrauterine devices. IUDs: a new look. Baltimore: Johns Hopkins University, Series B, No. 5, 1988.
29. Rosenberg L, Palmer JR, Clarke EA, Shapiro S. A case-control study of the risk of breast cancer in relation to oral contraceptive use. Am J Epidemiol 136:1437, 1992.
30. Schlesselman JJ. Net effect of oral contraceptive use on the risk of cancer in women in the United States. Obstet Gynecol 85:793, 1995.
31. Seiler JS. The evolution of tubal sterilization. Obstet Gynecol Surv 39:177, 1984.
32. Stadel BV. Oral contraceptives and cardiovascular disease (two parts). N Engl J Med 305:612, 672, 1981.
33. Trussell J, Stewart F, Potts M, et al. Should oral contraceptives be available without prescription? Am J Public Health 83:1094, 1993.
34. Wilcox AJ, Weinberg CR, Baird DD. Timing of sexual intercourse in relation to ovulation. N Engl J Med 333:1517–1521, 1995.

---

*Bold print (general references) and bold numerals (specific references) denote published controlled clinical trials, meta-analyses, or consensus-based recommendations.

CHAPTER 94

Nonmalignant Vulvovaginal and Cervical Disorders

VANESSA E. CULLINS, MD, MPH
GEORGE R. HUGGINS, MD

Vulvovaginal symptoms constitute a significant proportion of problems presented to the primary physician. The diagnosis and treatment of these disorders can be both satisfying and exasperating. Most diagnoses are readily made in one office visit. Treatment is usually easily rendered. However, the patient with recurrent or persistent symptoms presents special problems. Appropriate evaluation and treatment of both the easily treated patient and the patient with persistent symptoms require a knowledge of the anatomy, physiology, and pathology of the vulva and vagina.

ANATOMY AND PHYSIOLOGY

Vulva

The external genitalia of the female is denoted the vulva (Fig. 94.1). The vulva consists of the labia majora, labia minora, vestibule, clitoris, prepuce, and mons pubis.

The mons pubis (mons veneris) is a cushion of fat covered by stratified squamous skin and its appendages (hair follicles, sebaceous and apocrine sweat glands). The mons is located superior to the clitoris and encompasses the triangular-shaped hair-bearing tissue situated in front of the symphysis pubis. The labia majora are composed of longitudinal folds of fat and connective tissue corresponding to the dartos of the male scrotum. When the labia majora are parted, the vaginal vestibule is seen. The vestibule begins at the hymenal ring, extends outward to the labia minora, upward to the frenulum of the clitoris, and downward to include the posterior fourchette. The vaginal orifice (introitus) and urethral meatus open in the midline of the vestibule. Ducts of the Skene's glands (paraurethral glands), Bartholin's glands (major vestibular glands), and the minor vestibular glands also open in the vestibule. The hymen, a firm, often crescent-shaped membrane consisting of a double plate of stratified squamous epithelium, partially obscures the vaginal orifice (introitus) in virgins. Residual tags of the hymen, the carunculae hymenalis, are often noted at the inferior edges of the introitus. The fourchette, the most posterior boundary of the vestibule, is formed by the fusion of the inferior aspects of the labia majora. The clitoris, homolog of the penis, is located in the midline at the most superior aspect of the vestibule. The labia minora bifurcate anteriorly, forming the prepuce and frenulum of the clitoris.

Vulvar Glands

The major vestibular glands, or Bartholin's glands, are paired glands whose ducts exit at the introitus, above the fourchette at the 5 and 7 o'clock positions. The minor vestibular glands are numerous small glands whose ducts exit laterally to the hymenal ring. These small glands may extend superiorly to the region of the urethra. Ducts from the Skene's (paraurethral glands) open in the vestibule immediately beneath the urethral meatus.

Vagina

The vaginal canal extends from the vestibule to the uterine cervix. The vaginal wall consists of an outer fibrous layer, middle muscular layer, and inner epithelial layer composed of nonkeratinizing, stratified squamous cells. Glands are not present in the normal vagina.

When stimulated, the major nerve endings of the vagina cause the sensation of pain or light touch. Compared with the neural supply of the vulva, the vagina has few nerve endings. Therefore vaginal infections are often asymptomatic until the discharge comes in contact with the vulva. The squamous epithelium of the vagina is hormone dependent. In the absence of estrogen, the vaginal epithelium is thin and fragile and consists of undifferentiated basal and parabasal cells. Progesterone leads to a decrease in superficial cells and a relative increase in intermediate cells. Pregnancy, lactation, and oral contraceptives produce the progesterone-dominant state. Normal vaginal discharge is composed of transudation through the vaginal wall, secretions of Bartholin's and Skene's glands, desquamated vaginal epithelial cells, cervical mucus, endometrial fluid, tubal fluid, and leukocytes.

Bacteria normally present in the vagina include lactobacillus, *Staphylococcus epidermidis, Corynebacterium* species, nonhemolytic streptococci, diphtheroids, peptococci, peptostreptococci, *Bacteroides* species, and *Eubacterium* species (24,31). Yeast are normal inhabitants of the vagina (8,30,41). Presence of *Gardnerella vaginalis,* also a normal inhabitant of many women's vaginas, is not diagnostic of vaginal pathology (4,10).

Physiologic vaginal discharge (pH of 3.5 to 4.1) is not malodorous or associated with pruritus. It varies in amount, is white or mucoid in color, and typically has a floccular consistency. The amount and consistency of the discharge depend on several factors: hormonal profile, presence of menstrual flow, frequency of coitus, and use of antibiotics (14,25). The *saline wet slide preparation* of normal discharge shows rare leukocytes, variable numbers of mononuclear cells, large Gram-positive rods, and vaginal epithelial cells with distinct borders (Table 94.1).

VULVOVAGINITIS

Abnormal vaginal discharge with associated vulvar irritation is the hallmark of vulvovaginitis. The most common vulvovaginal problems are *Candida, Gardnerella,* and *Trichomonas* infections and atrophic vaginitis. Foreign bodies are a rare cause of vulvovaginitis in adults. Although not a cause of adult vaginitis, gonorrhea and chlamydial infections of the cervix may initially present as an abnormal discharge and therefore may be misinterpreted as a vulvovaginitis.

Candida

Candida (Table 94.1) is an extremely common cause of adult vulvovaginitis. Approximately 40% of women with vulvovaginitis are infected with *Candida albicans. C. albicans* is a yeast that has no true mycelial form, and for this reason infection should be called *candidiasis* rather than *moniliasis* (a common term used in older literature), which implies infection by a mycelial form. The presence of *Candida* within the vagina is not sufficient for the diagnosis of vulvovaginitis; up to 16% of nonpregnant, reproductive-aged women are normally colonized with the yeast (8,30). Therefore the physician should prescribe treatment only if the woman is symptomatic from vulvovaginal candidiasis; the presence of yeast in a Pap smear or other examination is not in itself an indication for treatment.

The change in *Candida* from normal flora to a pathogen occurs when the organisms proliferate to the point that the normal microbiological balance of the vagina is upset. Predisposing factors to infection include pregnancy, diabetes mellitus, immunosuppression, antibiotic or corticosteroid therapy, iron deficiency anemia, vaginal surgery, oral contraceptives, and infection with human immunodeficiency virus (HIV) (15,27,41). Skin conditions that predispose to *Candida* infection generally involve alterations of the barrier function of the skin through persistent moisture and development of maceration, as occurs with occlusive synthetic clothing. Candidal proliferation is associated with an increased estrogen milieu and an increase in vaginal pH.

Patients usually present with intense vulvar itching or burning associated with a thick, curdlike vaginal discharge. The vulva and vagina are typically inflamed. The vaginal mucosa may exhibit adherent white patches of exudate similar in appearance to oral thrush. Vulvar erosions with satellite pustules may be seen.

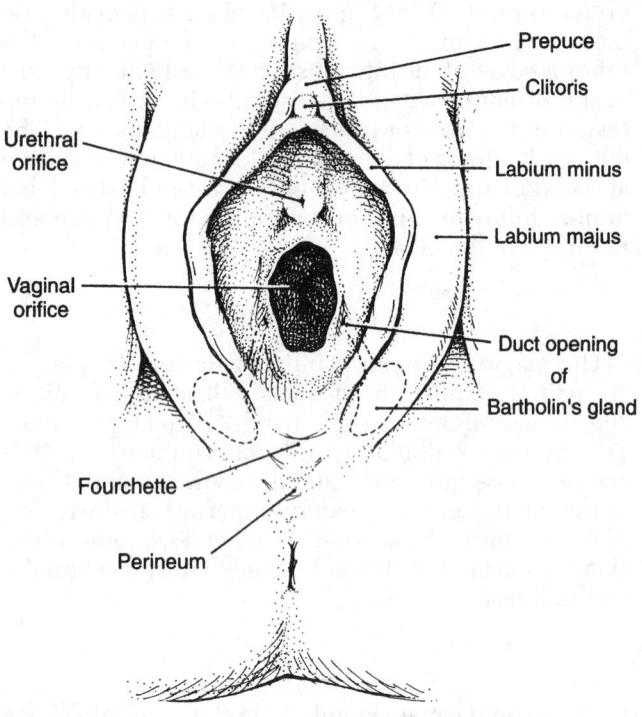

Urethral orifice

Vaginal orifice

Fourchette

Perineum

Prepuce

Clitoris

Labium minus

Labium majus

Duct opening of Bartholin's gland

Figure 94.1. Anatomy of the vulva.

Table 94.1.   Vaginal Discharge

	Physiologic	*Candida*	Bacterial Vaginosis	*Trichomonas*	Atrophic
Symptoms	None	Pruritus, burning	± Pruritus, burning	± Pruritus	± Vulvar, vaginal dryness
Malodor	None	Yeast smell	Fishy or musty	Variable	Variable
Increased mucosal erythema	None	Yes	±	Yes	±
Consistency	Floccular	Thick, curdlike	Thin, creamy	Copious, frothy	Mucoid, blood tinged
pH	3.5–4.1	3.5–4.5	5.0–6.0	6.0–7.0	As high as 7.0
Wet smear	Rare WBCs, large Gram-positive rods, squamous epithelial cells	Budding filaments, spores, pseudohyphae	Clue cells	Copious WBCs, trichomonads	Copious WBCs, parabasal and intermediate cells, paucity of superficial cells
KOH		Budding filaments, spores, pseudohyphae	Fishy odor, musty odor		
Treatment of choice (see text for dosages)	None	Imidazole or triazole derivative	Metronidazole or clindamycin	Metronidazole	Estrogen cream

The diagnosis is confirmed through examination of a slide preparation of a few drops of 20% potassium hydroxide placed over a few drops of vaginal secretions. The potassium hydroxide causes lysis of epithelial cells, leukocytes, and red blood cells. The resulting preparation is thus not obscured by cells that may overlie the fungus and prevent identification of budding filaments, pseudohyphae, or spores (Fig. 94.2).

Treatment

Candida vulvovaginitis may be treated either topically or orally. Usually the topical treatment is given first. Oral treatment is reserved for some recurrent infections (see below) or situations in which the patient cannot or will not apply the topical agent. Antifungal medications include imidazole derivatives, the Triazole derivative gentian violet, and the antifungal polyene macrolide antibiotic nystatin. The imidazole derivatives Triazoles and nystatin increase the permeability of the cell membrane of fungi. This alteration of permeability results in the loss of the selective barrier function of the cell membrane such that potassium and other cellular constituents are lost.

FDA-approved prescription treatment of vulvovaginal candidiasis includes an oral and a topical Triazole. The topical treatment, terconazole, provides antifungal activity against a broad spectrum of candidal strains, including *C. albicans, C. glabrata,* and *C. tropicalis* (6). Terconazole (Terazol) is prescribed as one 80-mg suppository or one applicator full of 0.4% cream intravaginally at bedtime for 3 days, or one applicator full of 0.8% cream intravaginally at bedtime for 7 days. The oral treatment, fluconazole (Diflucan) 150 mg in one dose, primarily has activity against *C. albicans.* Fluconazole may interact with antacids, anticholinergics, anticoagulants, astemizole, cimetidine, cyclosporine, digoxin, diuretics, isoniazid, loratadine, methylprednisolone, oral contraceptives, phenytoin, potassium, rifampin, sulfonylureas, and terfenadine. Although it is unlikely that one 150-mg dose will cause a serious adverse reaction, there is potential for arrhythmia when fluconazole is taken with a nonsedating antihistamine, or idiosyncratic liver dysfunction, which

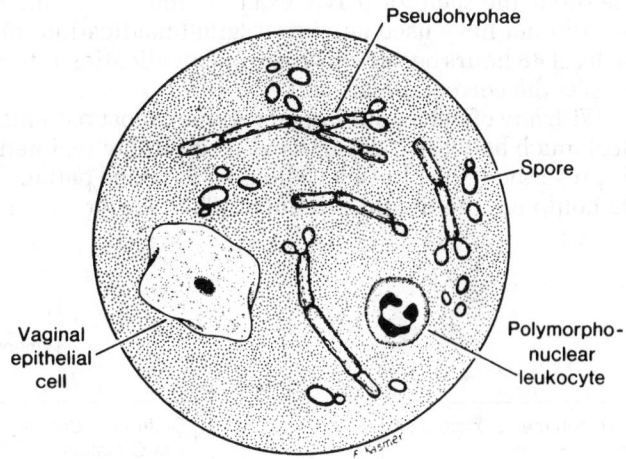

Figure 94.2.   KOH preparation showing yeast and pseudohyphae of candidiasis.

could be more serious when occurring in a patient with existing liver disease. The advantage of fluconazole is patient compliance, which must be weighed against its limited spectrum of activity, contraindication in pregnancy, and drug interaction and side effect potential. Fluconazole is probably best reserved for recurrent or persistent albicans vulvovaginitis.

A number of imidazoles that were originally available only by prescription are now available over the counter. Topical miconazole, clotrimazole, butoconazole, and tioconazole are available as nonprescription medications. These over-the-counter imidazoles are effective primarily against *C. albicans.* Although *C. albicans* is the most commonly isolated pathogen among women with vulvovaginal candidiasis, the number of nonalbicans strains has increased substantially over the last decade. Currently, up to 25% of candidal vulvovaginitis is caused by nonalbicans strains (18,22,40). Therefore it is prudent to prescribe a broad-spectrum antifungal when treating this vaginitis. Of particular note are studies that show enhanced in vitro or in vivo activity against *Candida* species with terconazole (Terazol), butoconazole (Femstat), and tioconazole (Vagistat) (1,6).

Many women seek advice about an abnormal discharge via telephone or often after attempting self-medication (Fig. 94.3). However, self-medication with over-the-counter antifungals is recommended only if

- The woman has had candidal vulvovaginitis previously diagnosed by a health care provider.
- Her symptoms are consistent with the previous infection.
- She does not have signs or symptoms suggestive of pregnancy, pelvic inflammatory disease, or other condition requiring physical evaluation.
- She agrees to be evaluated if there is no response in 3 days or no cure in 7 days.

If a pelvic examination is performed because of uncertainty of the diagnosis based on the telephone discussion, then certain precautions are necessary. Before being seen for pelvic examination, the woman should not have used any intravaginal medication for at least 48 hours because intravaginal medication often masks the correct diagnosis.

With any effective antifungal regimen, most patients feel much better in a day or two. If a multiday regimen is prescribed, the physician should encourage patients to complete the treatment course. The 7-day regimen described above is more effective during pregnancy, when the infection can be more resistant.

All patients should be advised that excess vaginal moisture and heat associated with nylon, other synthetic materials, and tight-fitting pants may increase susceptibility to candidiasis.

Resistant or Recurrent Candidiasis

Candida infections of the vagina may be persistent or become recurrent. Persistent vulvovaginal candidiasis is a consequence of inadequate treatment. Recurrent infections are caused by reinfection (i.e., reintroduction of the organism). The only method of distinguishing the two is by documenting eradication of the infection after a treatment course. This documentation in practice is not done commonly after an initial episode. However, when a second episode of *Candida* vulvovaginitis is experienced soon, the physician should see the patient in follow-up within 1 to 2 weeks to reexamine the patient and determine by a KOH preparation (see above) whether the organism has been eradicated. Persistent infection should be treated with a 7-day course of a broad-spectrum antifungal agent. Recurrent infection requires more intensive treatment and an investigation for potential sources of the organ-

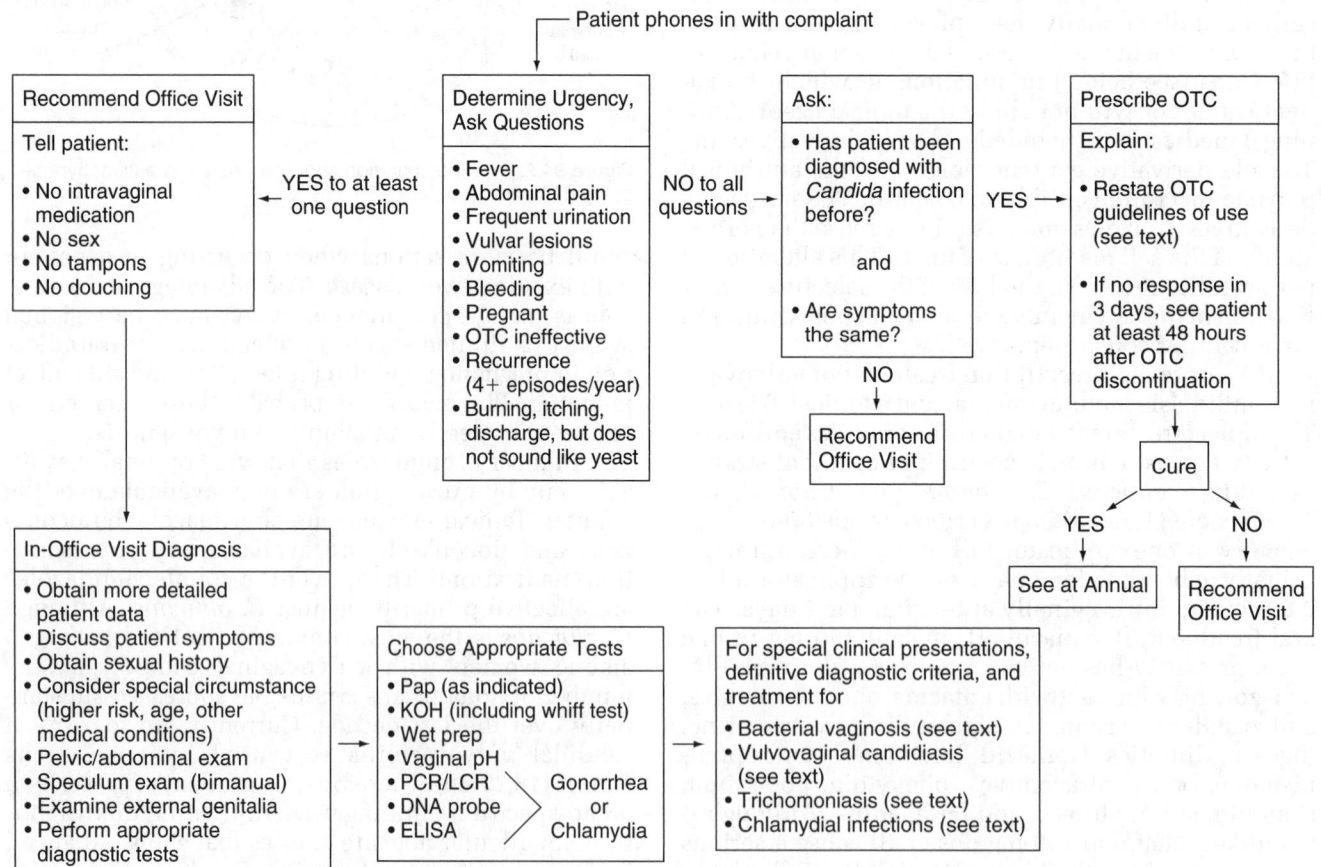

Figure 94.3. Telephone triage advice for patients with probable vulvovaginal candidiasis. (Modified from Vulvovaginitis: a practice protocol for the managed care clinician. National Association of Managed Care Physicians Roundtable Highlights 1:14, January 1996.)

ism. In certain instances the inherent properties of *Candida* may be the cause of recurrent infection. *Candida* possesses the ability to change its surface antigens (36). A change in antigenicity alters susceptibility to antifungals. Because each imidazole derivative has a distinct spectrum of activity against the various species of *Candida,* switching to a different imidazole derivative or Triazole may effect a cure. If that fails, referral to a gynecologist is appropriate for confirmation of the diagnosis and consideration of an alternative therapy such as gentian violet, nystatin, boric acid, or suppressive therapy.

Reinfection should prompt the physician to inquire regarding the patient's sexual practices and partner(s). Because the partners may be colonized, they should be empirically treated with an antifungal cream or fluconazole. If cream is chosen, the cream should be placed on the scrotum, penile glans, and shaft every night for 7 nights. *Candida* may also be transmitted during oral–genital contact. Therefore, if the patient's partner engages in cunnilingus, the partner should be treated with oral nystatin or fluconazole (150 mg as a single dose).

The gastrointestinal tract is a natural reservoir for *Candida.* Perineal contamination of the vulva through improper hygiene is thought to be another factor in the pathogenesis of recurrent infection. Therefore patients with recurrent infections should be instructed to wipe from front to back when bathing and after urination or defecation. For patients interested in home remedies, 8 oz of lactobacillus acidophilus yogurt eaten daily for 6 to 12 months may decrease recurrences. If recurrences continue, a gynecologist should be consulted. An additional consideration that may be suggested at this point is prolonged systemic antifungal therapy. Ketoconazole (Nizoral) 200-mg tablets two times a day orally for 2 weeks, followed by 100 mg (1/2 tablet) a day for 6 to 12 months or fluconazole (Diflucan) 150 mg orally once a month for 12 doses (i.e., 1 year). Neither ketoconazole nor fluconazole can be used in pregnancy. Current data do not support the use of oral nystatin to prevent recurrence (34).

If recurrences are related predictably to specific events, such as menses, a prophylactic topical antifungal (prescription or nonprescription) used once a day for 3 days may be preventive. Sometimes recurrences are related to coitus, and for women in whom coital events can be predicted, prophylactic therapy is helpful.

Patients who continue to have recurrent infections despite the institution of these measures should be evaluated for diabetes mellitus (see Chapter 72) and HIV infection (see Chapter 34). If these are absent, a gynecologist should be consulted. Some of these patients may be found to have a primary deficiency of cell-mediated immunity to *Candida* that often is temporary.

Bacterial Vaginosis

Bacterial vaginosis (BV) vulvovaginitis (*Gardnerella* vaginitis, nonspecific vaginitis, *Corynebacterium* vaginitis, anaerobic vaginosis, and *Haemophilus* vaginitis) (Table 94.1) is the second most common vulvovaginitis encountered in the United States.

In addition to *Gardnerella vaginalis,* an increased proportion of anaerobic bacteria such as *Bacteroides, Peptococcus,* and *Eubacterium* are recovered from the vaginas of symptomatic women (12,38,39). Like *Candida albicans,* most of these organisms are found in low concentrations in the vaginas of normal asymptomatic women (1,10,31).

Patients with bacterial vaginosis usually complain of thin, creamy malodorous vaginal discharge with accompanying vulvar itching or burning. The vaginal mucosa and vulva may be mildly inflamed. The odor of this infection is usually described as fishy or musty and is commonly noted after coitus, when the alkaline seminal fluid has caused the release of volatile fatty acids and amines.

The diagnosis is confirmed through examination of the saline wet preparation (see above), production of the characteristic odor, and determination of the vaginal pH. Using nitrazine paper, vaginal pH can be determined easily. Vaginal discharge of women with BV typically has a pH between 5.0 and 6.0. The saline wet preparation is significant for vaginal squamous cells covered with *Gardnerella vaginalis* and other bacteria ("clue cells") (Fig. 94.4). Leukocytes are generally not abundant unless a mixed infection is present. The addition of a 20% potassium hydroxide solution to the discharge causes the release of amines and volatile fatty acids that produce the fishy odor.

The diagnosis of BV vulvovaginitis is made when at least three of the following four criteria are met (2):

- Vaginal pH above 4.5
- Thin, homogeneous vaginal discharge of variable amount
- Fishy odor after the addition of 20% potassium hydroxide solution to the discharge (whiff test)
- Clue cells on saline wet preparation

Treatment

The treatment of choice for BV vaginitis is metronidazole (Flagyl, Protostat) 500 mg orally two times a day for 7 days, or 0.75% metronidazole gel (Metrogel) intravaginally two times a day for 5 days, or 2% clindamycin phosphate cream (Cleocin vaginal cream) intravaginally for 7 nights. Metronidazole is contraindicated in the first trimester of pregnancy. Because of the side effects that develop when the drug is taken with alcohol, its use should be avoided in anyone using alcohol or anyone suspected of having severe hepatic disease. Alternative regimens that may be tried if metronidazole is contraindicated are clindamycin 300 mg orally two times a day for 7 days, or 2% clindamycin phosphate cream (see above). Patients should be advised that the mineral oil in clindamycin cream may weaken condoms, diaphragms, and cervical caps. There is no role for sulfa-based vaginal cream or ampicillin in the treatment of bacterial vaginosis.

The role of sexual transmission in the acquisition of bacterial vaginitis has not been resolved completely.

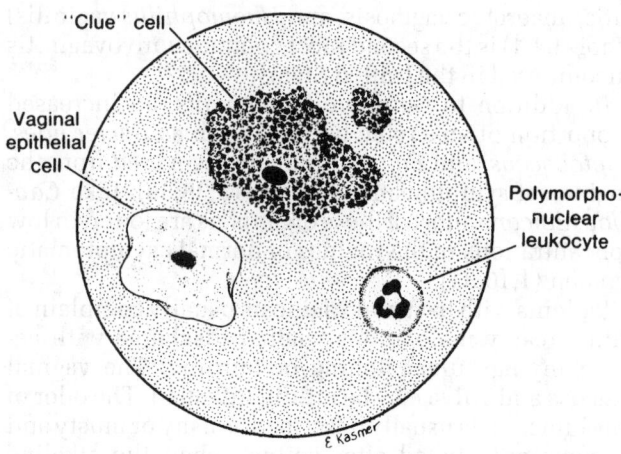

Figure 94.4. "Clue" cells.

Gardnerella vaginalis can be recovered in most male contacts of infected women, yet *Gardnerella* can be isolated from up to one-third of women who have never been sexually active. In addition, recurrence rates for the infection are the same for women whose partners harbor as for those whose partners do not harbor *Gardnerella vaginalis* (42). Because of the possible role of sexual transmission, condoms should be used during therapy. If the infection recurs, the patient's partner(s) should be treated.

Because of its association with preterm birth and posthysterectomy vaginal cuff cellulitis, BV should be treated in asymptomatic pregnant women or women who are soon to undergo hysterectomy (26).

Trichomonas

Trichomonas (Table 94.1) is a common sexually transmitted disease. It is caused by the motile, unipolar flagellated protozoan *Trichomonas vaginalis.* Aside from sexual transmission, the organism can be acquired through close contact with contaminated water or clothing.

Patients generally have a copious and often frothy vaginal discharge accompanied by vulvar pruritus. Additional symptoms include vaginal burning, vaginal spotting, and symptoms of urethral irritation: dysuria, frequency, and urgency. Pelvic discomfort may be experienced by some patients. Dyspareunia is common. On physical examination, variable amounts of vulvovaginal erythema may be seen. Typically, there is less erythema than is seen in *candida vulvovaginitis.* The vaginal mucosa or cervix may exhibit a characteristic strawberry appearance (reddish color with punctuation).

The diagnosis is established by assessing vaginal pH and examining the saline wet preparation (see above). The vaginal pH is generally between 6 and 7. On the saline preparation (Fig. 94.5), a multitude of polymorphonuclear leukocytes are seen. Among the white blood cells, trichomonads can be identified by the movement of their flagellae. It should be noted that cold

saline causes immobilization of the trichomonads. The solution should be at a comfortable room temperature. Atrophic vaginitis (see below) produces a discharge with a pH between 6 and 7 and copious white blood cells, but characteristically it does not contain mature squamous cells. Therefore the presence of discharge containing numerous white cells and mature squamous epithelial cells, with a pH between 6 and 7, is presumptive evidence of trichomonas vulvovaginitis.

Treatment

Treatment consists of a single 2-g dose of oral metronidazole (Flagyl, Protostat). Patients who do not respond to this therapy may be treated with metronidazole 500 mg two times per day for 7 days, or 2 g a day for 3 to 5 days. Patients not responding to either of these regimens should be referred to a gynecologist for evaluation and treatment, which is likely to be difficult. Metronidazole is contraindicated in the first trimester of pregnancy, and it should be used cautiously in patients with severe hepatic disease; when taken within 24 hours of alcohol consumption, metronidazole causes severe reactions similar to those when alcohol and disulfiram (Antabuse) are consumed together. In these situations or when there is an intolerance to systemic metronidazole, metronidazole gel twice a day for 7 days may be tried as an alternative. The sexual partner(s) should be similarly treated also, and it is usually pointless to attempt to recover the organism from the partner. Intercourse should be avoided or a condom used during treatment.

Atrophic Vaginitis

Atrophic vaginitis (Table 94.1) is a common disorder of postmenopausal women. Caused by estrogen deficiency, it may be seen in women who are postoophorectomy, have premature ovarian failure, or are breastfeeding. Rarely, premenarchal girls (i.e., having unestrogenized tissues) have atrophic vaginitis when an additional precipitant (e.g., wearing of occlusive clothing made of synthetic materials) is encountered.

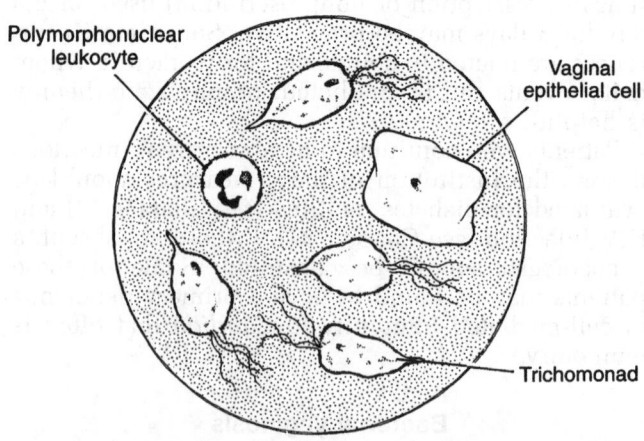

Figure 94.5. Saline preparation showing trichomonads.

Estrogen deficiency results in thinning and fragility of the vaginal and vulvar epithelium. Instead of the glycogen-rich superficial cells, the epithelium is composed primarily of parabasal and intermediate cells. This altered vaginal environment is associated with an elevation of pH to as high as 7.0. In this milieu, pathogenic bacteria may flourish. The patient may complain of a thin, blood-tinged vaginal discharge and vulvar and vaginal dryness. Some patients also note urinary incontinence (see Chapter 6).

Visual examination of the normal atrophic vagina reveals a pale vaginal mucosa with decreased or absent rugal folds. Vulvar examination demonstrates thin, often shiny skin with decreased subcutaneous tissue and variable loss of hair. In atrophic vaginitis, erythema and petechial hemorrhages may be superimposed on these findings.

Examination of a saline wet preparation (see above) of the discharge of women with atrophic vaginitis typically shows numerous leukocytes mixed with immature, intermediate, and parabasal epithelial cells. Microorganisms seen on the slide are generally secondary invaders of the inflamed mucosa. Often in the past, diagnosis was made by taking a smear of the vaginal wall and determining the maturation index; however, this test is no longer recommended because it has not proved to be reliable. Not all women with atrophy on vaginal examination have atrophic vaginitis. Treatment should be instituted only if symptoms are present and examination of the saline wet preparation reveals the findings described above.

Local rather than oral estrogen is the treatment of choice for atrophic vaginitis and other urogenital manifestations of estrogen deficiency (11,28). Optimally, patients with this disorder should be placed on an oral therapy for systemic estrogen replacement therapy benefits and topical therapy for expeditious relief from atrophic vaginitis. One-half to one applicator of estrogen cream every night for 1 to 2 weeks is followed by application every other night for 1 to 2 weeks. The medication can then generally be discontinued, and most patients have only infrequent symptoms (e.g., every 1 to 2 months), so an applicator full for 1 or 2 days when there are symptoms usually provides adequate control. Local therapy may also be achieved through the use of the FDA-approved estradiol vaginal drug (Estring). This ring is placed in the vagina and works continuously for 3 months (3,17). The ring does not require removal for intercourse. Absorption of estrogen to a level consistent with the early follicular phase of the female menstrual cycle may occur with topically applied preparations. Therefore, if administration of a topical estrogen is prolonged (e.g., daily or every other day for more than 1 year), the patient will be at risk for complications of continuous unopposed estrogen therapy (see Chapter 77), including uterine cancer (see Chapter 95). Such patients should be followed concomitantly by a gynecologist if the general physician is not experienced in screening for uterine cancer or so that a progestin can be prescribed (see Chapter 77). The physician should be certain that none of the contrain-

dications for estrogens (e.g., breast cancer) is present and that the same precautionary surveillance (e.g., for hypertension) is provided to the patient using long-term topical estrogen preparations.

Some patients cannot or will not use topical vaginal preparations and refuse long-term systemic hormonal replacement therapy. In this instance, oral conjugated estrogen (Premarin) 0.625 mg/day may be prescribed for 1 month. Occasionally a repeated course of oral estrogens is necessary if symptoms persist. When retreatment courses become frequent, it is necessary to provide close surveillance for the complications of estrogen therapy (see above and Chapter 77). Generally a gynecologist should be consulted to participate in the care of a patient with frequently recurrent attacks of atrophic vaginitis.

Cytolytic Vaginosis and Desquamative Inflammatory Vaginitis

Cytolytic vaginosis and *desquamative inflammatory vaginitis* are uncommonly recognized *vulvovaginitides*, which are often confused with other vaginal inflammatory conditions. Cytolytic vaginitis is caused by an overgrowth of long, serpiginous lactobacilli rod-shaped organisms, which causes shedding and cytolysis of vaginal epithelial cells. The vaginal discharge of cytolytic vaginosis usually increases during the luteal phase of the menstrual cycle and grossly resembles a candidal discharge; the discharge is thick and white, with an acidic pH. The patient usually experiences severe vulvar burning, dysuria, and dyspareunia. KOH preparation reveals an absence of fungi. The saline wet preparation reveals an abundance of lactobacilli, fragmented epithelial cells, and naked nuclei. Therapy has not been well established. Currently an intravaginal douche two to three times a week of 30 to 60 mg sodium bicarbonate in 1 L of warm water is recommended. Alternatively, the patient can take amoxicillin clavulanate (Augmentin) 500 mg three times a day for 7 days (5,19).

Desquamative inflammatory vaginitis (DIV) is a disorder of unknown cause usually characterized by copious vaginal discharge and epithelial cell exfoliation. Patients experience intense vulvar pain and burning, severe dyspareunia, and dysuria. The vulva and vagina are usually very inflamed, with various stages of denudation. The discharge is seropurulent, with a pH of 6.0 to 7.0. The characteristic violaceous papules and gingival and buccal mucosal lesions of lichen planus may be seen if the patient has the form of DIV associated with lichen planus (21,29). Saline wet preparation reveals parabasal cells, an absence of lactobacilli, a predominance of inflammatory cells, and fragmented epithelial cells. This entity is distinguished from atrophic vaginitis by nonresponse to topical estrogen. Treatment is with topical corticosteroids. One-half of a 25-mg rectal steroid suppository (Cort Dome) or one applicator of rectal hydrocortisone foam (Cortifoam) intravaginally should be used twice daily for 1 to 2 months, and can be reduced to once a day for an additional 2 months, followed by one- to three-times-a-week maintenance therapy. If the patient does not respond, a gynecologist or dermatologist should be consulted for confirmation of the diagnosis and consideration of additional treatments, including systemic corticosteroids or antibiotics (35).

Foreign Body

An occasional cause of vaginal discharge in adults is a foreign body. Lost tampons, forgotten diaphragms, and other smaller objects are easily found by examination. Symptoms improve after removal of the foreign body. Because secondary bacterial infection is also present, use of metronidazole, or clindamycin as prescribed for bacterial vaginosis, and a Providone (Betadine or Femidine) douche once daily for 3 to 4 days may accelerate healing.

GONOCOCCAL AND CHLAMYDIAL INFECTIONS

In the United States, gonococcal and chlamydial infections are the most common sexually transmitted diseases of the upper genital tract. These infections may initially present as an abnormal discharge that is the result of an associated cervicitis, not a vaginitis. However, the patient usually considers the discharge a sign of vaginal infection. Although a purulent discharge is classically associated with gonorrhea, a mucopurulent discharge is seen with chlamydia. For both infections, most patients do not recognize signs or symptoms until the disease affects the upper genital tract and causes pelvic inflammatory disease (PID).

Gonococcal Infection

In the United States, gonorrhea has always been considered the classic sexually transmitted disease. It is the entity with which other upper genital tract diseases are compared, and it is therefore important to understand this disease and its more common counterpart, chlamydial infection (see below).

Transmission of gonorrhea from infected men to uninfected women or men is efficient and occurs in up to 90% of exposures; transmission from infected women to uninfected men or women is less efficient. Risk of infection from the latter mode of transmission is approximately 20% per exposure (9). The diagnosis and management of gonorrhea in male patients are discussed in Chapter 27.

Infected patients may have no symptoms, symptoms of direct inoculation of organisms (cervical, rectal, or pharyngeal), or symptoms of local or distant spread of infection. The clinical manifestations of uncomplicated gonococcal infection include vaginal symptoms (purulent vaginal discharge, vaginal itching, dyspareunia, dysuria, vague lower abdominal pain), anorectal symptoms (pruritus, painful defecation, rectal fullness), and pharyngeal symptoms. Because the infection is initially asymptomatic, routine screening is important in women with multiple sexual partners or

with other sexually transmitted diseases. Symptoms generally occur once the organism has spread to the fallopian tubes and has initiated acute salpingitis or PID. Early consultation and prompt therapy significantly reduce the serious sequelae of PID (i.e., ectopic pregnancy and infertility). A single mild episode of acute salpingitis causes infertility in approximately 13% of patients and this complication rate increases to 75% after three or more bouts with PID (45).

PID usually begins shortly after a menstrual period (which may be altered) and is characterized by fever, nausea, abdominal pain, and marked tenderness of the pelvic organs to touch or motion. The adnexa may also be enlarged. The white blood cell count is usually elevated. The Centers for Disease Control and Prevention, in an attempt to reduce the number of unrecognized, untreated cases of PID, have simplified the minimum criteria necessary to initiate antibiotic treatment for probable PID. The minimum criteria are as follows:

- Lower abdominal tenderness
- Adnexal tenderness
- Cervical motion tenderness
- No evidence of competing diagnosis (e.g., ectopic pregnancy or appendicitis) (4a,32)

PID during pregnancy is rare. An obstetrician–gynecologist should be consulted promptly if this diagnosis is entertained during pregnancy.

The most common manifestation of disseminated gonorrhea is the *arthritis–dermatitis syndrome*. Symptoms and signs of this syndrome include polyarthralgia, tenosynovitis of elbows, wrists, or knees, purulent monoarthritis, and skin lesions. This syndrome usually develops 1 week or more after the initial infection.

Gram's stain of the cervical material is diagnostic when intracellular Gram-negative diplococci are identified. This finding may be used as a basis for diagnosis and treatment before the results of culture (requires special media, such as chocolate agar), DNA probe test, polymerase chain reaction, fluorescent antibody test, or enzyme immunoassay are available. However, such confirmation should be done and the results from any of these methods can usually be available within a day or two. Especially in women, Gram's stain alone is not a sensitive indicator of infections (9). A pharyngeal test is indicated in those who give a history of oral–genital sexual activity.

Management plans appropriate for the various forms of gonococcal infection and PID are summarized in Table 94.2. Follow-up tests to ensure that the treatment has been effective should be done approximately 3 weeks after the therapy is completed. Women receiving treatment for gonorrhea or PID should either abstain from sexual intercourse or ensure that their partners use condoms until completion of therapy. Furthermore, partners must be treated for presumed infection (see Chapter 27 for treatment of male partners).

Gonorrhea is a reportable disease; whenever gonorrhea is confirmed, the information concerning the

Table 94.2.   Management of Gonococcal and Chlamydial Infections

Uncomplicated Gonococcal Infection (asymptomatic, cervicovaginal, or anorectal symptoms; pharyngitis)
1. a. Ceftriaxone 125 mg IM once (or equivalent cephalosporin) or
    b. Spectinomycin 2.0 g IM (once) or
    c. Ciprofloxacin 500 mg orally (once) or ofloxacin 400 mg orally (once; contraindicated in pregnancy and in those 16 and younger) or
    d. Cefixime 400 mg orally (once) or
2. Treat for chlamydia with doxycycline, azithromycin or ofloxacin (see below).
3. Treat partner(s).
4. Report to local health department.

Chlamydia Cervicitis; Possible Gonorrhea/Chlamydia Infection (a common situation with manifestations of infection present but without culture confirmation)
1. a. Azithromycin 1 g orally once for treatment of uncomplicated chlamydial infection and ofloxacin 400 mg orally once for treatment of uncomplicated gonorrhea or
    b. Doxycycline 100 mg twice a day for 7 days or
    c. Ofloxacin 300 mg orally two times a day for 7 days.
2. Treat partner(s).

Pelvic Inflammatory Disease (gonorrhea, *Chlamydia,* or both may be the cause)
1. Ambulatory treatment
    a. Ceftriaxone 250 mg IM, one dose or cefoxitin 2 g IM, one dose with Probenecid 1 g orally plus doxycycline 100 mg orally twice a day for 14 days or
    b. Ofloxacin 400 mg orally two times a day for 14 days plus metronidazole 500 mg orally two times a day for 14 days.
    c. Contact or observation within 72 hours to ensure improvement.
2. Indications for hospitalization
    a. Diagnosis uncertain (to exclude appendicitis, ectopic pregnancy, nongonococcal pelvic inflammatory disease, pelvic abscess).
    b. Diagnosis is certain but patient is toxic or unable to follow ambulatory treatment reliably.
    c. Patient does not respond promptly to ambulatory treatment.
    d. Pregnancy.
3. Indications for parenteral therapy: same as indications for hospitalization plus
    a. When a pelvic abscess is present.
    b. Immunodeficiency.
4. Inpatient treatment or ambulatory parenteral treatment
    a. Cefoxitin 2 g IV every 6 hours or cefotetan 2 g IV every 12 hours and doxycycline 100 mg IV every 12 hours or
    b. Gentamicin 2.0 mg/kg as an initial dose followed by 1.5 mg/kg every 8 hours and clindamycin 900 mg IV every 8 hours.
    c. After hospital discharge or adequate clinical response from parenteral antibiotics, continue oral therapy with either doxycycline 100 mg twice a day or clindamycin 450 mg orally four times a day for at least 14 days total therapy.

Gonococcal/Arthritis–Dermatitis Syndrome (hospitalization is recommended)
1. a. Ceftriaxone 1.0 g IM or IV daily for at least 49 hours or ceftizoxime 1 g IV every 8 hours for at least 48 hours.
    b. For patients allergic to β-lactam drugs, spectinomycin 2 g IM, every 12 hours should be given.
    c. Patients may be discharged 48 hours after clinical improvement, with close follow-up (see 4 below).
2. When the infecting organism is proven to be penicillin-sensitive, parenteral treatment may be switched to ampicillin 1 g every 6 hours.
3. Treat for potential coexistent chlamydial infection (see above).
4. The patient should complete 7 days of antibiotic therapy with either cefixime 400 mg orally two times a day or ciprofloxacin 500 mg orally two times a day (contraindicated in pregnancy and in those age 16 or younger).

References 4a, 7, 23, and 43.
Note: Of the antibiotics listed above, use azithromycin, amoxicillin, gentamicin, clindamycin, spectinomycin, or cephalosporins in pregnant women.
Ceftriaxone is effective against penicillinase-producing *Neisseria gonorrhoeae* (as well as many other organisms).

patient should be reported to the local health department. Sexual partner(s) should be treated regardless of decision to test or test results.

Chlamydia Trachomatis Infection

In recent years the role of *Chlamydia trachomatis* in the production of genitourinary infections has been clarified (32,33). Chlamydia is felt to be the etiologic agent in a substantial number of cases of pelvic inflammatory disease. In the United States, chlamydial infections are more common than gonorrhea.

Genital tract chlamydial infection is more indolent than is gonorrhea, but symptoms are similar: lower abdominal pain, dysuria, mucopurulent discharge, and fever. On examination the cervix may be red, edematous, and friable. Typically, the cervical discharge is less profuse than it is in patients with gonorrhea.

Although the gold standard for chlamydia diagnosis is culture, newer laboratory procedures, ligase chain reaction (LCR) and polymerase chain reaction (PCR), are highly specific and sensitive for chlamydia. The physician should always use the one that is more available or less expensive. Culture is not ordinarily done because it is expensive and growth is slow. The fluorescent antibody staining technique, enzyme immunoassay, and DNA probe test (Microtrak, Chlamydiazyme, and Gen-Probe) are inexpensive and reliable and one of these tests is recommended to confirm chlamydial infection if either of the newest methods (LCR or PCR) is not available (44). For all these laboratory procedures, the manufacturer-designated cotton swab should be used when obtaining a sample of endocervical discharge.

In addition to using one of the office laboratory assays in patients suspected of having chlamydial infection, the primary physician should screen any woman who has been diagnosed with another sexually transmitted disease.

When chlamydial infection is suspected, azithromycin or doxycycline is the drug of choice (Table 94.2). Treatment should be initiated before the results of the diagnostic assays are available. As with gonorrhea, untreated chlamydia infections can progress to PID (see above).

In instances of uncomplicated pelvic inflammatory disease, the first line of treatment is a cephalosporin, such as cefoxitin or ceftriaxone, plus doxycycline (Table 94.2). PID is usually polymicrobial (13). This broad-spectrum antibiotic coverage is effective against chlamydia, gonorrhea, and anaerobes, the common organisms involved. Erythromycin, amoxicillin, or azithromycin should be used in the pregnant patient because of the effect of tetracycline on fetal development and the possible effect on maternal liver function. Because the male sexual partner is often infected as well, he should be treated (see Chapter 27). Women receiving treatment for chlamydia or PID should either abstain from intercourse or ensure that their partners use a condoms until completion of therapy.

VULVAR ULCERATIONS

Herpes Simplex

The most common cause of vulvar ulceration is herpes simplex, an enveloped DNA-containing virus specific for humans. Although both herpes simplex types I and II may cause genital ulceration, type II is implicated in most genital infections. This sexually transmitted disease is characterized by exacerbations and remissions that are independent of repeated exposure to the virus. Many cases of primary and some episodes of recurrent herpes are asymptomatic (1a). The virus exists in latent form in pelvic nerve ganglia and within autonomic nerves along the uterosacral ligaments. Factors influencing recurrence of the infection are not well understood. It is thought that recurrences are correlated with stress and the premenstrual period of the menstrual cycle. Fifty percent of women develop a recurrence within 6 months of the initial infection (1a,20).

When the infection is initially contracted, the patient may develop a prodromal illness characterized by fever, malaise, and lymphadenopathy. Rarely, meningitis or encephalitis can develop. Before lesions appear, paresthesias and burning may occur. The initial formation of vulvar vesicles may be asymptomatic. These vesicles typically measure 1 to 10 mm in diameter. They are most commonly located on the labia minora, labia majora, and around the clitoris in a clustered, linear, or serpiginous arrangement (Fig. 94.6) (16).

In the next stage of the process, the vesicles enlarge and rupture to form shallow, painful ulcerations. The ulcerations generally coalesce and are surrounded by an erythematous border.

Clinical suspicion of this diagnosis should be confirmed through a viral culture (requires a special viral

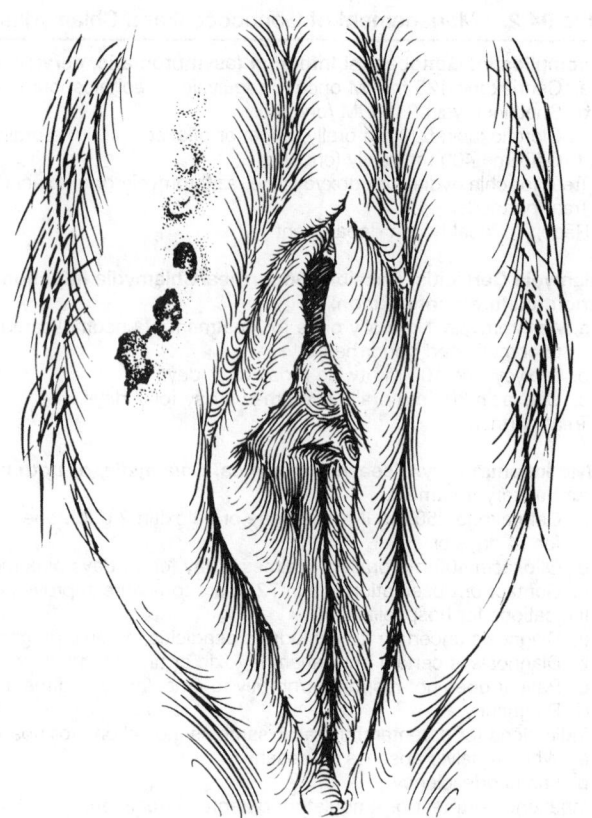

Figure 94.6.   Herpes simplex.

transport culture medium) available through the health department or with a direct fluorescent antibody test. The culture or antigen detection test should be prepared from fluid obtained from an unroofed vesicle or the base of an ulcer. Viral identification via culture (usually positive in 48 hours, but occasionally 7 days or longer is required) or antigen detection is most likely during the first 3 days of infection. Therefore, a negative test obtained after this period is not a guarantee of the absence of herpes. The measurement of titers of serum antibodies to herpes virus is not generally helpful in the diagnosis of herpetic infection because of lack of specificity of the finding. In the near future, type-specific herpes simplex hybridization (e.g., polymerase chain reaction) and type-specific serologic tests will be commercially available (1a).

Ulcerations in close proximity to the urethra may result in dysuria or urinary retention. Although the cervix and vagina are involved in more than 50% of cases, cervical and vaginal ulcerations may be asymptomatic because of the lack of free nerve endings in the vagina or cervix. With extensive cervical involvement, however, cervical motion tenderness may be elicited.

A honey-colored crust forms as the lesions heal. The ulcerations usually heal spontaneously in 1 to 3 weeks. Secondary bacterial invasion may prolong this healing process to 6 weeks or more. Usually, there is no permanent scarring.

The symptoms of recurrences are generally milder

than the initial attack. Of patients with symptomatic recurrent herpes, 85% experience a prodrome of itching, tingling, burning, or tenderness.

Treatment

Therapy for herpes is aimed at palliation of symptoms and slowing viral replication. As yet, there is no means to eradicate the latent virus.

The antiviral agent acyclovir (acyclic purine analog, Zovirax) may decrease the period of symptoms and viral shedding. It should be prescribed for primary attacks. The dosage of oral acyclovir depends on whether the treatment is for an initial attack or is being prescribed for recurrence or suppression. The *therapy for an initial attack* should be with one 200-mg capsule of acyclovir every 4 hours five times per day or 400 mg three times a day both for 7 to 10 days. The timing of therapy is shortened to 5 days for *recurrences*. In patients with a history of more than six recurrences a year, *suppressive therapy* should be prescribed. Acyclovir (400 mg orally two times a day) may be given (1a,4a). The dosage of acyclovir must be adjusted for patients with renal impairment. After 1 year of suppressive therapy, acyclovir should be discontinued to assess the frequency of recurrence. Safety of up to 6 years of suppressive therapy has been documented.

Other oral antiviral medications that may be used for initial, recurrent, or suppressive therapy include the following:

- *Initial:* Valacyclovir (Valtrex) 1000 mg two times a day or famciclovir (Famvir) 250 mg three times a day for 7 to 10 days
- *Recurrent:* Valacyclovir 500 mg two times a day for 5 days or famciclovir 125 mg two times a day for 5 days
- *Suppression:* Valacyclovir 1000 mg/day or famciclovir 250 mg two times a day (1a,4a)

Oral analgesics, topical anesthetics, compresses of Domeboro solution (over-the-counter), witch hazel pads (e.g., Tucks or generic), warm tea bag compresses, and sitz baths may alleviate symptoms. Ten percent povidone–iodine (e.g., Betadine) applied twice daily for several days inhibits secondary bacterial infection and promotes drying of the lesions. A patient who also has dysuria from the infection may benefit from phenazopyridine (Pyridium) 100 to 200 mg three to four times a day for 3 to 4 days. For any topical therapies, patients should be instructed to use a finger cot or rubber glove when touching unhealed lesions; this will prevent autoinoculation. Finally, although topical acyclovir has been used often in the past for symptomatic relief of recurrent herpetic infection, it has been shown to be ineffective and should not be used in this way (1a,4a,46).

Patients who experience a severe initial attack manifested by high fever, inability to void, meningitis, or encephalitis should be hospitalized for intravenous treatment with acyclovir. Vidarabine (Vira-A), another purine nucleoside analog, may be used in cases of herpetic encephalitis, or if intravenous acyclovir has been found to be ineffective. Either increased oral dosage or intravenous acyclovir is also indicated in the treatment of initial and recurrent herpes simplex infections in immunocompromised patients. Because asymptomatic disease is more prevalent than previously thought, condom use is recommended during all sexual exposures (4a).

Syphilis

Vulvar ulcerations can be seen in all stages of syphilis (see Chapter 30). The primary chancre appears approximately 3 weeks after the infection has been contracted. It is a single, hard, painless lesion with an ulcerated central core. Often, multiple lesions occur that are painful and soft because of secondary bacterial invasion. Chancres are commonly found on the labia or introitus. Dark-field examination of the base of the lesion reveals spirochetes *(Treponema pallidum)*. These initial lesions usually heal spontaneously in 1 to 6 weeks. Between 3 and 4 days after the appearance of the chancre, inguinal adenopathy develops. With time, these firm, nontender lymph nodes become bilateral.

Secondary syphilis develops 3 to 6 weeks after the chancre. Condyloma latum represent the classic vulvar, secondary syphilitic lesion. The plaques are multiple and commonly confluent. They are often grayish with a moist, necrotic appearance. The center of the lesion may be ulcerated. Other manifestations of secondary syphilis include malaise, flulike syndrome, arthralgias, maculopapular rash, and lymphadenopathy.

Treatment

Primary, secondary, and latent syphilis of less than 1 year's duration should be treated with 2.4 million units of benzathine penicillin G (1.2 million units in each buttock) (4a,37). Alternative therapy for those allergic to penicillin is doxycycline 100 mg two times a day or tetracycline 500 mg orally four times a day, both for 14 days. A less effective alternative is erythromycin 500 mg orally four times a day for 14 days (4a). Latent syphilis of more than 1 year's duration should be treated with 2.4 million units of benzathine penicillin G intramuscularly every week for 3 weeks for a total dosage of 7.2 million units. Alternative therapy includes doxycycline 100 mg orally two times a day for 4 weeks, or tetracycline 500 mg orally four times a day for 4 weeks (4a). Adequacy of treatment should be guided by the fall in Venereal Disease Research Laboratory (VDRL) or RPR (rapid plasma reagin) titers (see Chapter 30). HIV testing is indicated in anyone diagnosed as having syphilis (4b). All patients with latent syphilis (regardless of duration) should be evaluated for tertiary disease (see Chapter 30) (4a). See Chapter 30 for indications for cerebrospinal fluid examination of HIV-infected patients. Pregnant women with syphilis should be referred to an obstetrician for therapy. As with any sexually transmitted disease, partners must be treated.

Other Causes of Vulvar Ulcerations

Less common causes of vulvar ulceration include granuloma inguinale, lymphogranuloma venereum, chancroid, hidradenitis suppurativa, Behçet's disease, Crohn's disease, and tuberculosis. A synopsis of common findings, diagnosis, and treatment of vulvar ulcerations is found in Table 94.3. Any patient with an ulcer that is nonhealing, recurrent, or not easily diagnosed should be referred to a gynecologist or dermatologist.

MISCELLANEOUS LESIONS

Bartholin's Cyst/Abscess

Obstruction of the major duct of the Bartholin's gland (Fig. 94.1) (major vestibular gland) results in a Bartholin's cyst (Table 94.4). Infection and obstruction of the duct lead to a Bartholin's abscess. Most Bartholin's cysts occur because of mechanical blockage of the outflow of normal mucus secreted by the gland. If the cyst causes no symptoms and is only 1 to 2 cm in diameter, no treatment is necessary. Rapid enlargement, pain, hemorrhage, or secondary abscess formation requires the same therapy as a primary abscess; when a Bartholin's cyst or abscess is suspected to confirm the diagnosis and rule out carcinoma in an older woman and to initiate treatment, the gynecologist creates a fistula from the cyst or abscess to the vestibule by marsupialization, incision and drainage, or rarely, excision. A Bartholin's abscess harbors *Neisseria gonorrhoeae* in approximately 10% of cases. Therefore culture for *Neisseria gonorrhoeae* is indicated. Adequate drainage usually obviates systemic antibiotics. Sitz baths provide temporary symptomatic relief until drainage can be performed.

To drain a Bartholin's abscess,

1. Inject lidocaine in a vertical line over the most fluctuant area of the abscess at the medial aspect of the labia majora.
2. With a scalpel, incise the anesthetized area to the abscess cavity.
3. Drain all purulent material.
4. Break up loculation within the abscess cavity with a clamp.
5. Irrigate copiously with a 1:1 solution of physiological saline and hydrogen peroxide.
6. Pack the cavity with Nu Gauze or place a small catheter in the cavity.
7. Instruct the patient to take sitz baths three or four times a day.
8. Repeat irrigation and packing one or two times a week until the cavity has healed.

Condylomata Acuminata (Venereal Warts, Anogenital Warts, Genital Warts)

Condylomata acuminata is caused by human papilloma virus (HPV) and is transmitted sexually. This viral infection appears to be more prevalent now, and importantly, nonacuminata HPV types may be related to the subsequent development of cervical and vulvar dysplasia (see Chapter 95). Condyloma acuminata usually occurs during the reproductive years and is commonly seen in association with other vulvovaginal infections (including candidiasis, trichomoniasis, bacterial vaginosis, gonorrhea, or syphilis). It is common in pregnancy and has a more active course in pregnant women.

The patient most often complains of a new growth on her vulva, perineum, or anus, and there is often associated itching and a vaginal discharge. These symptoms may be part of an associated vaginal infection or may represent infection in the crevices of the wart. Often, there is a history of warts on the penis of the sexual partner, who should also be evaluated.

The examination is characteristic and is almost always diagnostic. A wart of 1 to 2 mm usually first appears on the labia, often about the posterior introitus, but then spreads, with discrete or congruent lesions appearing on the perineum, anus, vagina, and cervix. They may coalesce into a cauliflowerlike lesion that may become huge (Fig. 94.7). In the male, genital warts are often less conspicuous. Examination after swabbing the genitalia with a weak (e.g., 3%) acetic acid solution usually makes the lesions more visible.

Treatment

Two patient-applied therapies are FDA approved: Podofilox (Condylox) 0.5% solution or gel or Imiquimod (Aldara) 5% cream. Neither is proven safe in pregnancy. Patients must be shown how and where to apply the treatment. Podofilox is applied twice daily for 3 days and followed by 4 days of no therapy for a maximum of four cycles. Imiquimod is applied at bedtime three times a week for up to 16 weeks. Imiquimod must be washed off with soap and water within 10 hours of application.

Provider-administered treatment of the warts is accomplished by painting them carefully with a 10 to 25% tincture of podophyllum. This solution is irritating: It commonly causes transient discomfort and burns normal skin if applied to it. If such contamination does occur, the skin should be washed promptly with alcohol and then water. The podophyllum should be left on the warts for 8 to 12 hours and then removed with soap and water. During that time, the patient should not engage in sexual intercourse. The patient should be seen weekly for retreatment until healing occurs. If her sexual partner has warts, he should be treated also, and he should use a condom during intercourse until healing is complete.

If improvement has not occurred after the third treatment, the physician should switch to trichloroacetic acid (80 or 90%). The trichloroacetic acid is applied to the warts at weekly intervals. The solution should be applied only to the warts. A plain water and baking soda slurry is useful to neutralize the acid and remove any excess solution. Neither podophyllin nor trichloroacetic acid is suitable for eradication of large warts (greater than 2 to 2.5 cm) or warts on the cervix or vagina. Also, podophyllin has been reported to cause fetal abnormalities and should not be used during

Table 94.3. Causes of Vulvar Ulcerations

Disease Entity	Cause	Appearance	Transmission	Symptoms: Other Manifestations	Diagnosis	Treatment
Herpes simplex (see text)	Herpes simplex II Rarely herpes simplex I	Vulvar vesicle(s) Vulvar ulceration	Sexual	Fever, malaise, lymphadenopathy, burning, paresthesia, dysuria, urinary retention, painful ulcer	Viral culture or direct fluorescent antibody test	Acyclovir Palliative treatment of lesions
Herpes zoster	Varicella zoster	Ulceration following the distribution of dermatome	Previous varicella zoster infection	Fever, malaise, lymphadenopathy, painful ulcer	Distribution of lesions Viral culture or direct fluorescent antibody test	Acyclovir, valacyclovir, or famciclovir Palliative treatment of symptoms
Syphilis (see text and Chapter 30)	Treponema pallidum	Primary: Chancre (hard, painless lesions with central ulceration, lymphadenopathy) Secondary: Condyloma latum (multiple flat plaques, often confluent). Rash (esp. palm and soles, lymphadenopathy) Tertiary: Gummatous tumors or ulceration	Sexual	Secondary: Malaise, flu-like syndrome, arthralgias, lymphadenopathy Tertiary: CNS signs and symptoms	Positive FTA Rising VDRL or RPR titers	Benzathine penicillin G, tetracycline, or doxycycline
Granuloma inguinale	Calymmatobacterium granulomatis	Painless, erythematous nodule that ulcerates (ulcers have irregular borders with a granulation base). Lymphadenopathy latter stages (scarring and lymphedema)	Sexual	Nonhealing ulcer that becomes painful after secondary bacterial infection	Donovan bodies (macrophages containing intracytoplasmic pleomorphic rods) on tissue crush preparation or biopsy	Trimethoprim/sulfamethoxazole (Bactrim, Septra) or doxycycline, alternatively ciprofloxacin or erythromycin with addition of gentamycin if improvement is inadequate with either in a few days.
Lymphogranuloma venereum	Chlamydia trachomatis serotype L_1, L_2, or L_3	Vulvar papule that ulcerates in 4–6 wk; hallmark inguinal adenitis; nodes are unilateral and edematous; later bubo formation (enlarged matted nodes held together by inflammatory reaction); fistula formation, vulvar fenestration	Sexual	Fever, malaise, initially painless	Titer of at least 1:64 on LGV complement fixation test	Aspiration of fluctuant buboes Doxycycline Erythromycin Surgical reconstruction
Chancroid	Haemophilus ducreyi	Soft, painful, chancrelike ulcer	Sexual	Painful ulcer Inguinal adenopathy	Culturing is difficult; diagnosis of exclusion.	Azithromycin Ceftriaxone Erythromycin Ciprofloxacin
Hidradenitis suppurativa (see Chapters 25 and 100)	Inflammation/infection of apocrine sweat glands	Vulvar abscess formation with draining sinuses, scarring and induration; fistula formation	Nontransmittable	Pruritus, burning	Appearance Biopsy	Surgical excision Occasionally systemic antibiotics Rarely systemic or intralesional corticosteroids
Behçet's disease	? Autoimmune	Vulvar ulcerations with associated oral ulcerations and ocular inflammation	—	Arthritis, erthema nodosum, pyoderma, thrombophlebitis, acne, ulcerative colitis, neurologic symptoms	Diagnosis of exclusion	No definitive treatment High-dose oral contraceptives Intralesional corticosteroids Chlorambucil
Crohn's disease	Unknown	Linear ulcerations similar to a knife cut; draining sinuses; fistulous tracts	—	Oral ulcerations GI symptoms	Biopsy	Corticosteroids Sulfones Metronidazole Surgical reconstruction
Tuberculosis (see Chapter 29)	Mycobacterium tuberculosis	Painless ulceration	Airborne Primary inoculation		Biopsy, acid-fast cultures	Antituberculous therapy

Table 94.4. Common Nonmalignant Vulvar Lesions

Disease Entity	Cause	Appearance	Symptoms	Complications	Diagnosis	Treatment	Other
Bartholin's cyst	Obstruction of the duct of the gland	Discrete swelling of the inferior aspect of labium majus	None or vulvar pain caused by enlargement	Infection, hemorrhage into the cyst Carcinoma, if age ≥40	Visual inspection	None, unless symptomatic, infected, or hemorrhagic—then incision and drainage	
Bartholin's abscess	Infection and obstruction of the duct of the gland	Discrete swelling of the inferior aspect of the labium majus	Pain	Hemorrhage Carcinoma, if age ≥40	Visual inspection	Incision and drainage Marsupialization Rarely, excision	Culture for gonorrhea
Condylomata acuminata	Human papillomavirus	Single or multiple 2–3 mm diameter and 10–15 mm high, fine, fingerlike projections or flat-topped lesions; lesions may become confluent	Itching, vaginal discharge	Secondary ulceration and infection	Visual inspection, biopsy	10–25% podophyllum Trichloracetic acid Liquid nitrogen or nitrous oxide or interferon injection	5-Fluorourucil for intravaginal lesions Laser surgery, excision, or electrosesication Treat partner
Sebaceous cyst	Unknown	Discrete swelling, often 1 cm in diameter; firm, solid with a yellow color	Vulvar irritation caused by enlargement Pain, if infected	Infection	Visual appearance, biopsy	None Excision, if infected or bothersome	

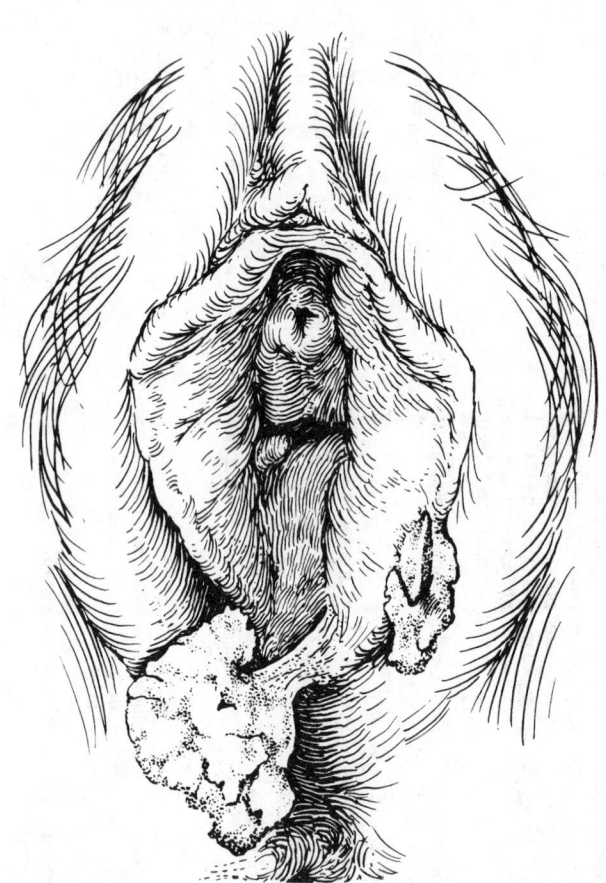

Figure 94.7. Condylomata acuminata.

pregnancy. In these instances and when complete eradication has not occurred after six treatments, referral to a dermatologist or a gynecologist is suggested for evaluation and consideration of treatment using other modalities such as cryosurgery, laser surgery, electro-

desiccation, simple surgical excision, or intralesional interferon injection (Alferon N injection).

Sebaceous Cyst (Epidermal, Keratinous, or Inclusion Cysts), Seborrheic Dermatitis

Sebaceous cyst and seborrheic dermatitis are discussed in Chapter 100.

Vulvar Papules

Folliculitis

Overgrowth of skin staphylococci and streptococci can result in vulvar folliculitis (Table 94.5). Predisposing factors for this disorder include immunosuppressive therapy, local trauma, poor hygiene, or occlusive (synthetic) clothing. Infection of the hair follicle is identified by erythematous papules or pustules with a central hair shaft. Treatment consists of cleansing the area with a germicidal soap (e.g., pHisoHex or Betadine). Warm sitz baths or compresses help relieve the discomfort. Gentamicin or Neosporin ointment may be prescribed to accelerate healing. If the lesions do not heal within 1 week, systemic dicloxacillin, cephalexin, or erythromycin should be prescribed. In a diabetic patient, the infection could become worse more rapidly, so a systemic and a topical antimicrobial agent are usually prescribed at the time of diagnosis.

Acrochordon

Acrochordons, commonly known as skin tags, are sessile or pedunculated fibroepithelial polyps. Acrochordons are benign and should be removed only if they are large or annoying to the patient. A gynecologist or dermatologist should be consulted or biopsy performed if there is doubt regarding the diagnosis.

Molluscum Contagiosum

Molluscum contagiosum is a benign lesion caused by a pox virus and is transmitted by close contact, including sexual intercourse. However, sexual intercourse is not necessary for transmission because the disease may be spread via fomites or autoinoculation. Although trunk, face, and extremity lesions are common among schoolchildren, the lesions of adults are generally located on the genitalia. The adult patient characteristically sees a physician because of a painless new growth in the vulva, perineal area, or thighs. The lesions have a typical appearance, permitting diagnosis by inspection in most instances (Fig. 94.8). The individual lesions are wartlike papules varying from 1 to 10 mm in size. They have a smooth surface and a central umbilical depression containing keratin. There may be multiple separate lesions or one large coalesced lesion. If there is any doubt about the diagnosis, the central cheeselike core may be expressed onto a slide and examined under a microscope using the low-power objective. Characteristic large inclusion bodies, which occupy most of the cytoplasm of the cells, are identified. Occasionally, the lesion resembles bacterial infection such as folliculitis or furunculosis, but in these instances the expression of pus versus a cheesy material from the lesion permits differentiation. If doubt remains regarding the diagnosis, the patient should be referred to a dermatologist or gynecologist for confirmation.

Because spontaneous resolution may take from months to years, treatment should be given. Therapy consists of scraping open the papule (with a scalpel blade), evacuating its contents, and curetting or cauterizing the base. Large lesions may need to be anesthetized with lidocaine injection before they are opened or curetted. The patient should be seen in approximately 1 week after the initial treatment for retreatment of any resistant or new lesions. Also, the patient should be evaluated for the presence of another sexually transmitted disease that may have been acquired simultaneously. Even if another sexually transmitted disease is not found, tests for chlamydia and gonococcal infection (see above) and a serologic test for syphilis should be obtained. The patient's sexual partner should be evaluated for lesions of molluscum contagiosum or evidence of another sexually transmitted disease. A condom should be used until the patient's lesions have healed.

Hypopigmented and Hyperpigmented Lesions of the Vulva

Hypopigmented and hyperpigmented lesions of the vulva may range from nonmalignant to malignant disorders. Differentiation of the various processes is difficult by inspection alone. Biopsy must be performed to determine the diagnosis. Referral to a gynecologist or dermatologist is recommended when any such lesion is identified (see Chapter 95).

Intertrigo

Intertrigo, an important and common disorder, is discussed in Chapter 100.

Contact Dermatitis (Reactive Dermatitis)

Contact dermatitis is discussed in Chapter 100.

Vulvodynia

Vulvodynia is a syndrome of unexplained vulvar pain. The syndrome is often accompanied by sexual dysfunction and psychological disability. Vulvodynia may respond to a tricyclic antidepressant or a serotonergic reuptake inhibitor. Most patients suffering from this syndrome require a multidisciplinary approach from the primary care physician, gynecologist, and psychiatrist or psychologist. Before the diagnosis of vulvodynia is made, other commonly misdiagnosed vulvar or vaginal conditions must be excluded. These conditions include vaginismus, cytolytic vaginosis, desquamative inflammatory vaginitis, pudendal neuralgia, vulvar dermatoses, vulvar allergic or reactive dermatitis, vulvar adenomas, and vulvar vestibulitis. If a woman continues to experience vulvar pain and burning despite treatment of recognized disorders, the physician should refer her to a gynecologist experienced in diagnosis and treatment of vulvovaginal disorders.

Table 94.5. Common Vulvar Papules

Disease Entity	Cause	Appearance	Symptoms	Diagnosis	Treatment
Folliculitis (see Chapter 25)	Staphylococcus or streptococcus	Erthematous papules or pustules with a central hair shaft	Asymptomatic Vulvar irritation or pain	Appearance	Germicidal soap, e.g., pHisoHex Sitz baths or warm compresses Rarely, gentamicin or Neosporin ointment Rarely, systemic dicloxacillin or erythromycin
Acrochordon	—	Soft, skin-colored, sessile or pedunculated tags of skin	Asymptomatic unless infarcted	Appearance; biopsy	No treatment or excision, electrocautery, laser, or cryotherapy
Molluscum contagiosum	Pox virus Possibly sexually transmitted	Wartlike papules 1–10 mm in size with a central umbilical depression		Appearance; biopsy	Scraping open the papule, evacuating the contents, and cauterizing or curetting the base

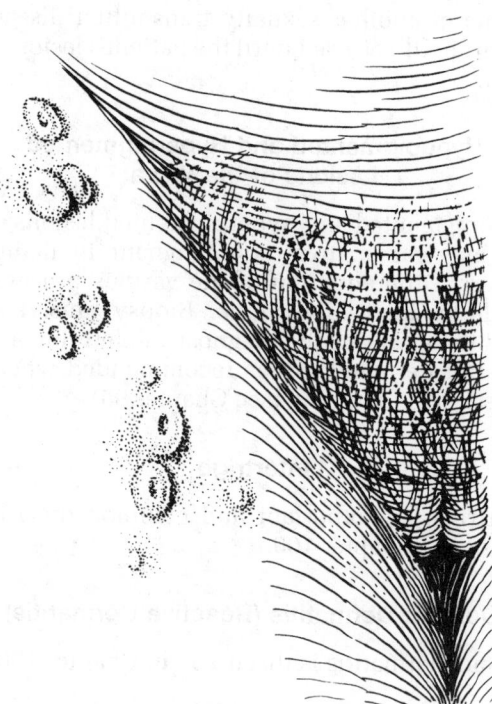

Figure 94.8. Molluscum contagiosum.

Tampon-Related Ulceration and Toxic Shock Syndrome

Repetitive tampon use during periods of diminished or absent menstrual flow may result in vaginal ulceration. Typically, patients with this problem develop intermenstrual bleeding or abnormal vaginal discharge. The ulcers are usually located in one of the vaginal fornices. They are superficial, erythematous, and 1 or 2 mm in diameter (often they are mistaken for herpes). The ulcers heal spontaneously in a few days if the tampon use is discontinued.

Toxic shock syndrome is caused by coagulase-positive *Staphylococcus aureus.* It is associated with fever greater than 102°F (39°C), severe headache, sore throat, vomiting, and diarrhea. Hypotension and shock may develop within 48 hours of the onset of the disorder. Other manifestations include palmar erythema, sunburnlike rash with skin desquamation, myalgias, and conjunctivitis.

Pelvic examination typically reveals a purulent vaginal discharge. The vaginal walls are usually inflamed and may be ulcerated. Bimanual examination does not usually reveal any abnormal tenderness.

If a tampon is present at the time of the examination, it should be removed and cultured. Testing for gonorrhea and chlamydia as described above should be done to rule out either infection, which may be occasionally associated with symptoms that mimic the toxic shock syndrome.

The vagina should then be thoroughly cleaned with Betadine. The patient should be hospitalized for intravenous therapy with a therapy effective against β-lactamase–resistant organism and supportive care.

Patients with toxic shock syndrome must be reported to the state health department as well as to the Centers for Disease Control and Prevention.

The patient should not use tampons for several subsequent menstrual cycles. In general, all patients using tampons should be encouraged to change them every 6 hours at least and to avoid tampons made of superabsorbent material (super tampons).

Pubic Lice

Pubic lice is discussed in Chapter 100.

Scabies

Scabies is discussed in Chapter 100.

Urethral Syndrome

Urethral syndrome is discussed in Chapter 27.

Psoriasis

Psoriasis is discussed in Chapter 100. The classic appearance of psoriasis is usually altered on the vulva. Because the vulva is moist, the psoriatic scale often may not be present, and psoriasis may appear as a nonspecific dermatitis. It is rare for a patient to have psoriasis only on the vulva, so a general dermatologic examination should be performed. Patients suspected of psoriasis on the vulva should be referred to a dermatologist or gynecologist for confirmation of the diagnosis.

PSYCHOSEXUAL ASPECTS OF VULVOVAGINAL COMPLAINTS

A physician should not suggest treatment for an organic vulvovaginal disorder unless its diagnosis is confirmed. The vulvovaginal region may be the focus of symptoms of a psychologic disorder. Alternatively, a woman with chronic vulvar pain (e.g., vulvodynia) who has received no relief may develop psychologic symptoms. A psychiatric diagnosis should be considered when the patient seeks repeated appointments and the physician finds no organic cause of the symptom. Psychologic support should be considered in any patient who experiences any form of chronic pain. The psychiatric section (Section 2) of this book deals in detail with diagnosis and management of specific sexual psychologic disorders (see Chapter 18) and other psychologic disorders, particularly somatoform disorders (see Chapter 12) that may present with symptoms related to sexual function.

General References*

Black MM, Mckay M, Braude P. Obstetric and gynecological dermatology. London: Mosby-Wolfe, 1995.

---

*Bold print (general references) and bold numerals (specific references) denote published controlled clinical trials, meta-analyses, or consensus-based recommendations.

An excellent text with color photographs of a large variety of vulvar lesions.

Briggs GG, Freeman RK, Yaffe SJ. Drugs in pregnancy and lactation. 4th ed. Baltimore: Williams & Wilkins, 1994.

A compendium of drugs with fetal and neonatal risk assessments for each drug.

Drugs for sexually transmitted diseases. Med Lett Drugs Ther 36:1, 1994.

Kaufman RH, Friedrich EG Jr, Gardner HL. Benign diseases of the vulva and vagina. 3rd ed. Chicago: Year Book, 1989.

Though dated, this text is the classic reference for disorders of the vulva and vagina.

Lynch PJ, Edwards L. Genital dermatology. New York: Churchill Livingstone, 1993.

Easy to read, with excellent photographs.

McCormack WM. Pelvic inflammatory disease. N Engl J Med 330: 115, 1994.

A thorough and well-referenced review.

Sobel JD. Vaginitis. N Engl J Med 337:1896, 1997.

An excellent review with good figures and summary tables covering all the common vaginitidies.

Tobin MJ. Vulvovaginal candidiasis: topical versus oral therapy. Am Fam Physician 54:1715, 1995.

Easy-to-read review of topical and systemic therapy.

Walker CK, Kahn JG, Washington AE, et al. Pelvic inflammatory disease: metaanalysis of antimicrobial regimen efficacy. J Infect Dis 168:969, 1993.

Appraisal of 21 studies of treatment between 1966 and 1992. Confirms antibiotic regimen choices described in the CDC guidelines.

Specific References

1. ACOG. Vaginitis. ACOG Tech Bull 226:1, 1996.
1a. American Medical Association. Genital herpes: a clinician's guide to diagnosis and treatment. Part I. In: Evans RM, Brakl MJ, eds. Chicago: AMA, 1997 (available by writing to the Division of CME, attention: Genital Herpes Education Program, AMA, 515 N. State Street, Chicago, IL 60610).
2. Amsel R, Totten PA, Spiegel CA, et al. Nonspecific vaginitis: diagnostic criteria and microbial and epidemiologic associations. Am J Med 74:14, 1983.
3. Bachmann G. The estradiol vaginal ring: a study of existing clinical data. Maturitas 22:S21, 1995.
4. Biswas MK. Bacterial vaginosis. Clin Obstet Gynecol 36:166–176, 1993.
4a. Centers for Disease Control and Prevention. 1997 sexually transmitted diseases treatment guidelines. MMWR 1–116, 1997.
5. Cibley LJ, Cibley LJ. Cytolytic vaginosis. Am J Obstet Gynecol 165:1245–1249, 1991.
6. Cooper CR, McGinnis R. In vitro susceptibility of clinical yeast isolates to fluconazole and terconazole. Am J Obstet Gynecol 175:1626, 1996.
7. Covino JM, Cummings M, Smith B, et al. Comparison of Ofloxacin and Ceftriaxone in treatment of uncomplicated gonorrhea caused by penicillinase-producing and non–penicillinase-producing stains. Antimicrob Agents Chemother 34:148, 1990.
8. Desmond FB, Eastcott DF, Anyon CP. A study of candida in one thousand and seven women. NZ Med J 73:9, 1971.
9. Duncan NC. Gonorrhea 1983. Dermatol Clin 1:43, 1983.
10. Dunkelberg WE, Hefner JD, Patow WE, et al. Hemophilus vaginalis among asymptomatic women. Obstet Gynecol 20:629, 1962.
11. Elia G, Bergman A. Estrogen effects on the urethra: beneficial effects in women with genuine stress incontinence. Obstet Gynecol Surv 48:509, 1993.
12. Erkkola R, Jarvomem H, Terho P, et al. Microbial flora in women showing symptoms of nonspecific vaginosis: applicability of KOH test for diagnosis. Scand J Infect Dis 40:59, 1983.
13. Eschenbach DA, Buchanan TM, Pollock HM, et al. Polymicrobial etiology of acute pelvic inflammatory disease. N Engl J Med 293:166, 1975.
14. Friedrich EG Jr. Vaginitis. Am J Obstet Gynecol 152:247, 1985.
15. Galask RP. Vaginal colonization by bacteria and yeast. Am J Obstet Gynecol 158:993, 1988.
16. Guinan ME, MacCalman J, Kern ER, et al. The course of untreated recurrent genital herpes simplex infection in 27 women. N Engl J Med 304:759, 1981.
17. Henriksson L, Stjernquist M, Boquist L, et al. A one-year multicenter study of efficacy and safety of a continuous, low-dose, estradiol-releasing vaginal ring (Estring) in postmenopausal women with symptoms and signs of urogenital aging. Am J Obstet Gynecol 174:85, 1996.
18. Horowitz BJ. Mycotic vulvovaginitis: a broad overview. Am J Obstet Gynecol 165:1188–1192, 1991.
19. Horowitz BJ, Mardh PA, Nagy E, Rank EL. Vaginal lactobacillosis. Am J Obstet Gynecol 170:857, 1994.
20. Kaufman RH, Faro S. Herpes genitalis: clinical features and treatment. Clin Obstet Gynecol 28:152, 1985.
21. Kaufman RH, Friedrich EG Jr, Gardner HL. Benign diseases of the vulva and vagina. 3rd ed. Chicago: Year Book, 1989.
22. Kent HL. Epidemiology of vaginitis. Am J Obstet Gynecol 165:1168–1176, 1991.
23. Landers DV, Wolner-Hanssen P, Paavonen J, et al. Combination antimicrobial therapy in the treatment of acute pelvic inflammatory disease. Am J Obstet Gynecol 164:849, 1991.
24. Larsen B, Galask RP. Vaginal microbial flora: practical and theoretic relevance. Obstet Gynecol 55:1005, 1980.
25. Leppaluoto P. The coitus-induced dynamics of vaginal bacteriology. J Repro Med 7:169, 1971.
26. McGregor JA, French JI, Parker R, et al. Prevention of premature birth by screening and treatment for common genital tract infections: results of a prospective controlled evaluation. Am J Obstet Gynecol 173:157–167, 1995.
27. McKay M. Cutaneous manifestations of candidiasis. Am J Obstet Gynecol 158:991, 1988.
28. Notelovitz M. Estrogen therapy in the management of problems associated with urogenital ageing: a simple diagnostic test and the effect of the route of hormone administration. Maturitas 22 Suppl:S31–S33, 1995.
29. Oates JK, Rowen D. Desquamative inflammatory vaginitis. A review. Genitourin Med 66:275–279, 1990.
30. Oriel JD, Partridge BM, Denny MJ, et al. Genital yeast infections. BMJ 4:761, 1972.
31. Paavonen J. Physiology and ecology of the vagina. Scand J Infect Dis 40(Suppl):31, 1983.
32. Rolfs RT. Think PID. New directions in prevention and management of pelvic inflammatory disease. Sex Transm Dis 18: 131, 1991.
33. Schachter J. Chlamydia infections. N Engl J Med 298:428, 490, 540, 1978.
34. Sobel JD. Pathogenesis and treatment of recurrent vulvovaginal candidiasis. Clin Infect Dis 14(Suppl 1):S148, 1992.
35. Sobel JD. Gynecology: desquamative inflammatory vaginitis: a new subgroup of purulent vaginitis responsive to topical 2% clindamycin therapy.
36. Soll DR. High-frequency switching in *Candida albicans* and its relations to vaginal candidiasis. Am J Obstet Gynecol 158:997, 1988.
37. Spence MR. The treatment of gonorrhea, syphilis, chancroid, lymphogranuloma venereum, and granuloma inguinale. Clin Obstet Gynecol 31:453, 1988.
38. Spiegel CA, Amsel R, Eschenbach D, et al. Anaerobic bacteria in nonspecific vaginitis. N Engl J Med 303:601, 1980.
39. Spiegel CA, Davick P, Totten PA, et al. *Gardnerella vaginalis* and anaerobic bacteria in the etiology of bacterial (nonspecific) vaginosis. Scand J Infect Dis 40(Suppl):41, 1983.
40. Spinillo A, Capuzzo E, Gulminetti R, et al: Prevalence of and risk factors for fungal vaginitis caused by non-albicans species. Am J Obstet Gynecol 176:138, 1997.
41. Syverson RE, Buckley H, Gibian J, et al. Cellular and humoral immune status in women with chronic candida vaginitis. Am J Obstet Gynecol 134:624, 1979.
42. Vontver LA, Eschenbach DA. The role of *Gardnerella vaginalis* in nonspecific vaginitis. Clin Obstet Gynecol 24:439, 1981.

43. Walters MD, Gibbs RS. A randomized comparison of gentamicin–clindamycin and cefoxitin–doxycycline in the treatment of acute pelvic inflammatory disease. Obstet Gynecol 75:867, 1990.
44. Watts DH, Eschenbach DA. Treatment of *Chlamydia, Mycoplasma,* and group B streptococcal infections. Clin Obstet Gynecol 31:435, 1988.
45. Westom L. Effect of acute pelvic inflammatory disease on fertility. Am J Obstet Gynecol 121:707, 1975.
46. Worrall G. Topical acyclovir for recurrent herpes labialis in primary care. Critical appraisal. Can Fam Physician 37:92–93, January 1991.

C H A P T E R 95

Early Detection of Gynecologic Malignancy*

JEFFREY M. SMITH, MD, MPH
GEORGE R. HUGGINS, MD

The female reproductive organs are common sites for the development of malignancy. Between 15 and 20% of cancers in women arise from the genital tract. Women who have gynecologic cancers discovered while it is still confined to the site of origin can expect a 60 to 90% 5-year survival rate. In contrast, more extensive cancers involving distant spread have a 5-year survival of 0 to 60% (11). If preinvasive lesions are detected and appropriate treatment is initiated, a 100% cure rate is expected. The vulva, vagina, and cervix all have well-characterized preinvasive lesions.

With the exception of the vulva and breast, the patient is unable to perform a satisfactory gynecologic self-screening examination. However, with the pelvic examination, all components of the genital system except the fallopian tubes may be inspected, palpated, and screened for cancer or its precursors.

---

*Preston M. Gazaway, MD, contributed to the previous editions of this chapter.

DETECTION OF VULVAR LESIONS

The vulvar skin is subject to disease similar to that of the skin elsewhere, but the prevalence of various conditions is modified in that the vulva is unexposed to solar radiation. The benign conditions are common, whereas the malignant conditions are uncommon, representing only approximately 4% of malignancies of the female genital tract. For example, squamous cell carcinoma comprises almost 85% of all vulvar cancers, followed by melanoma (5%) and sarcoma (2%). In contrast, basal cell cancer, common in sun-exposed skin, accounts for only 1.5% of vulvar malignancies.

Preinvasive lesions of the vulva are called *vulvar intraepithelial neoplasia* (VIN). *VIN* is the term now used to include diseases that were once called *Bowen's disease, erythroplasia of Queyrat, squamous cell carcinoma in situ, Paget's disease,* and *condyloma acuminata.* The average age of women with preinvasive lesions is between 40 and 50. Most women with invasive vulvar cancer are in their 60s and 70s, although it may occasionally develop in women under 40. This age differential supports the hypothesis that progression from preinvasive lesions to cancer of the vulva is an indolent process that takes several years. An increased risk of vulvar cancer is associated with a history of condyloma acuminata, increasing number of lifetime sexual partners, immunosuppression, and smoking.

The pathognomonic lesion of VIN is a papular or maculopapular lesion with a roughened surface; however, VIN may have many different guises and the lesions often appear to be well defined and innocent.

The lesions may vary from white to hyperpigmented. They may be sharply demarcated or generalized over the vulva and may even spread to adjacent regions. Some may resemble seborrheic keratoses, nevi, lentigo, intertrigo, condylomata acuminata, or condylomata lata. Because VIN and vulvar cancer can masquerade as many other disease entities, the diagnosis and definitive treatment are often delayed while treatment for an incorrectly diagnosed lesion is instituted.

Some women with vulvar cancer note symptoms for up to 16 months before seeking treatment. Furthermore, medical management may have been used for up to 12 months before the definitive diagnosis was made (8).

One should be suspicious when any lesion is seen, especially if the lesions are chronic and not immediately responsive to topical treatment. The most common symptom of vulvar neoplasia is itching, which occurs in 70% of patients. Other symptoms include ulceration, bleeding, pain, or the presence of a mass.

Unfortunately, a vulvar equivalent of the cervical Pap smear is not available; therefore the primary method of diagnosis of lesions is the early recognition and prompt referral to a gynecologist for diagnosis by biopsy.

The treatment of VIN depends on the extent of the lesion. If the vulvar lesions grossly appear to be *condyloma acuminata* and are not extensive, they may be treated empirically without biopsy (see Chapter 94 for illustration, Fig. 94.7, and details). If no decrement in size is apparent within 2 to 4 weeks, the suspected condylomata acuminata should be biopsied to confirm the diagnosis. The gynecologist and pathologist must be aware of prior treatment of the lesion because podophyllin and 5-fluorouracil (two common topical agents used in the treatment of condyloma acuminata) may cause abnormal mitoses and bizarre cells that cause an erroneous diagnosis to be made of advanced VIN or cancer.

Small lesions may be excised entirely. Laser vaporization, or skinning vulvectomy, is necessary for widespread disease.

Vulvar cancer may also masquerade as *vulvar leukoplakia, lichen sclerosus,* or *kraurosis vulvae.* Once these lesions are proven by biopsy, they may be treated safely by a generalist by the twice-weekly application of a topical androgen (usually 2% testosterone propionate ointment). This preparation is not commercially available as such but can be made up on request by a pharmacist. When it is used only twice weekly, side effects are minimal.

Prevention of advanced disease requires that the patient be taught to examine her vulva periodically by use of a mirror and to report any changes in the external genitalia. It is important that one examine the patient promptly if a change is noted and that a periodic examination, usually in conjunction with a routine gynecologic examination, be performed even when there are no complaints. Special sensitivity must be used in older women, who are often reluctant to complain of a vaginal or vulvar problem and who often are resistant to a screening vaginal examination.

DETECTION OF CERVICAL LESIONS

Epidemiology and Etiologic Factors

Invasive epithelial carcinoma of the cervix is the third most common malignancy of the reproductive organs behind endometrial and ovarian carcinoma (3). Approximately 13,500 new cases of cervical cancer are diagnosed annually, with approximately 6,000 annual deaths. Significant reduction in mortality and morbidity has been achieved by vigorous promotion and acceptance of the annual pelvic examination in combination with the cancer detection smear (Pap smear) (12). The incidence of cervical cancer has increased in younger women. In 1981, women younger than 50 years old accounted for 21% of all cervical cancer deaths. By 1987, this figure had risen to 27% (2). This increase in cervical cancer in this population parallels the increasingly early onset of sexual activity among women. In 1971, 28% of 15- to 19-year-old women had had sexual relations; however, in 1982, 42% of women in the same age group admitted to sexual activity (17).

The cause of cervical cancer is still not settled, but the *human papilloma virus* (HPV) is a significant etiologic agent. The virus is transmitted sexually, by autoinoculation from condylomata elsewhere on the body, or from mother to neonate. More than 60 strains

of HPV have been identified, at least 11 of which are tropic for the genital tract. HPV 6/11 is most often found in cervical condylomata and low-grade dysplasia. HPV 16 is found in approximately 55% of cervical cancers, HPV 18 is found in 15 to 20%, and HPV 31/33/35 are found occasionally (17). Women who become infected with HPV before age 25 are 40 times more likely to develop cervical cancer than those who are uninfected (5).

Infection with herpes simplex virus type 2 and with the Epstein–Barr virus correlates with the incidence of cervical cancer. However, the question remains whether these viruses are promoters, cocarcinogens, or solely an index of past sexual behavior. Decreased exposure to these agents through use of barrier contraception until a mutually monogamous relationship is established is a reasonable intervention.

Pap Smear

The mainstay of cervical cancer control is regular screening through Pap smears, with referral for colposcopy and biopsy whenever a significant abnormality is found. *Colposcopy* is an office procedure, done during a pelvic examination, that uses an instrument similar to a dissecting microscope. It illuminates and magnifies (×8 to ×10) the cervix, vagina, and vulva. The efficacy of the Pap smear as a screening tool has never been tested in a prospective blinded study. The typical false-negative rate for a Pap smear in most laboratories is 20%, but reports cite values from 3 to 60% (12). Despite this limitation, the widespread use of the Pap smear has been accompanied by a significant decrease in the incidence of invasive carcinoma of the cervix. Likewise, there has been a corresponding increase in the detection of preinvasive lesions (Fig. 95.1). The

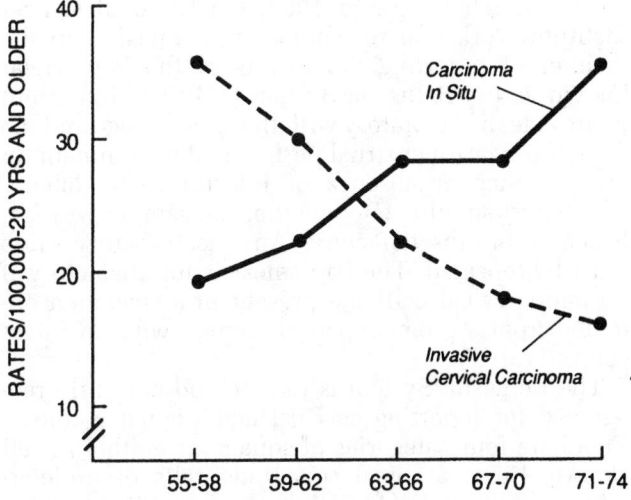

Figure 95.1. Average annual age-adjusted incidence rate trends for invasive carcinoma and carcinoma in situ of the cervix from the Toledo, Ohio area. (Redrawn from Kim K, Rigal RD, Patrick JR, et al. The changing trends of uterine cancer and cytology; a study of morbidity and mortality trends over a twenty year period. Cancer 42:2439, 1978.)

success of cytologic screening of the cervix has led many physicians to place an inordinate amount of faith in the Pap smear. It should never be considered a perfect diagnostic test. Any visible cervical lesions of uncertain origin may represent an early cancer, and patients with such lesions should be referred to a gynecologist for evaluation.

A screening Pap smear should not be obtained if a woman has douched or used vaginal medication or a tampon in the previous 24 hours. These activities may alter or remove cells completely and yield an erroneous interpretation. Lubricants may also interfere with cytologic interpretation. The speculum used in the examination should be unlubricated or, if necessary, lubricated only with water.

The most important area to be sampled is the squamocolumnar junction because most cervical neoplastic processes arise at this site. The anatomic relationship of this junction varies in the adolescent, the sexually active woman, and the postmenopausal woman (Fig. 95.2). Once the cervix is visualized, the cervical spatula should be placed firmly against the cervix and rotated at least 360°, preferably 720°, in a continuous unidirectional sweep. A plastic brush (Cytobrush, Milex) should be used to sample the endocervical canal. This increases the recovery of endocervical cells and decreases the number of inadequate Pap smears. Both specimens should then be smeared together onto a clean microscopic slide and immediately sprayed or immersed in fixative to prevent an air-drying artifact. An additional sample taken from the posterior vaginal fornix of perimenopausal or postmenopausal women may occasionally detect malignant cells that have exfoliated from the endometrium, fallopian tubes, or ovaries.

One should select a reputable cytology laboratory, use the proper fixative techniques required by the laboratory, and learn the reporting systems of the particular laboratory. In 1988, the National Cancer Institute Workshop recommended a revision in the manner of reporting the results of the Pap smear known as the Bethesda System (15). It is important to provide the laboratory with the patient's age and the date of her last menstrual period, and to comment on the presence or absence of infection. The laboratory report should state whether the sample was satisfactory or unsatisfactory. An unsatisfactory slide must be repeated. The Pap smear is unsatisfactory if no endocervical cells are present in a specimen obtained from a premenopausal woman with an intact cervix (12).

The Bethesda System is the method currently recognized for reporting cervical and vaginal cytology. There are four categories of squamous epithelial cell abnormalities: atypical squamous cells of undetermined significance (ASCUS; further qualified, see below), low-grade squamous intraepithelial lesion (LSIL), high-grade squamous intraepithelial lesion (HSIL), and squamous cell carcinoma. Patients with Pap smears showing HSIL or squamous carcinoma should be referred to a gynecologist for evaluation and

management. Some patients with LSIL who are reliable and free of risk factors can be followed because approximately 60% of LSILs regress spontaneously. These women need Pap smears every 4 to 6 months for 2 years. If repeat Pap smears show persistent abnormalities, the patient should be referred for colposcopy and biopsy.

Pap smears showing ASCUS are further qualified as reactive or suggestive of an intraepithelial lesion. Specific cervical or vaginal infections associated with an ASCUS-reactive report should be treated and the smear repeated in 3 months. A few weeks after treatment, 90% of smears with atypia secondary to chlamydia will revert to normal (14). ASCUS-favoring intraepithelial lesion Pap smears should be treated as LSIL Pap smears, with careful follow-up or colposcopy and biopsy, especially if risk factors are present or follow-up is questionable (13).

A consensus panel convened in 1988 made recommendations regarding frequency of cervical cancer screening (15). Annual screening should begin once a woman is 18 or becomes sexually active and should continue into the postmenopausal years. After a woman has had three consecutive annual Pap smears that are satisfactory and normal, the interval may be reduced to every 1 to 3 years, at the provider's discretion, depending on the presence of risk factors for cervical cancer. These include HPV infection, HIV infection, cigarette smoking, or multiple sexual partners. Additional risk factors for preinvasive lesions, which should be considered as well, include early age at first coitus, early age at first pregnancy, low socioeconomic status, and African-American or Hispanic race. Women married to men whose previous wives developed cervical cancer are at three times greater risk of developing cervical cancer themselves. Risk factors are listed in Table 95.1.

After a patient has undergone treatment for a preinvasive lesion there should be increased surveillance, preferably every 3 to 4 months, for 1 year. Cytologic smears may be performed yearly thereafter, if normal. Women who have undergone total hysterectomy (cervix removed) for malignant or premalignant disease should receive an annual smear from the vaginal apex to evaluate for local recurrence. The effectiveness of screening women whose hysterectomy was for benign indications has not been shown (7).

DETECTION OF ENDOMETRIAL CARCINOMA
Epidemiology and Etiologic Factors

An estimated 33,000 cancers of the endometrium are detected each year. This cancer accounts for 8% of all cancers in women and almost 50% of all new gynecologic cancers. Only 13% of cancer deaths result from endometrial carcinoma, approximately 4,000 annually, despite its high prevalence (3).

Unopposed estrogen stimulation has been firmly implicated in the genesis of this cancer, and several situations are associated with such exposure: Endog-

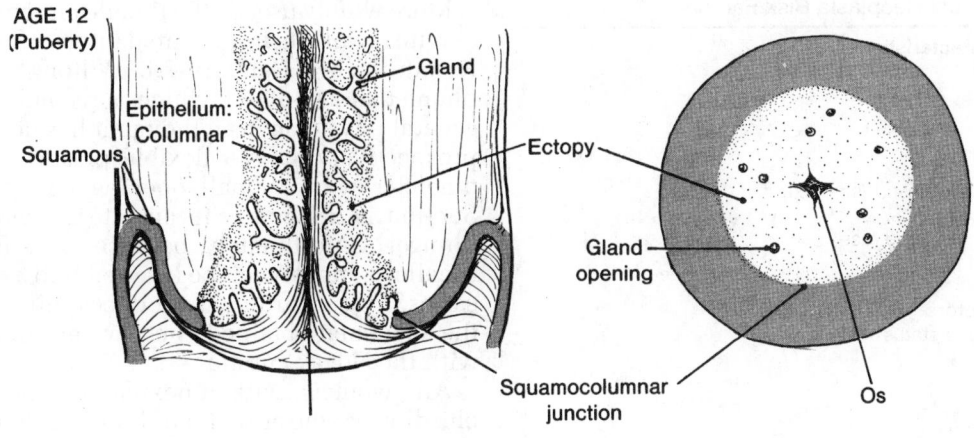

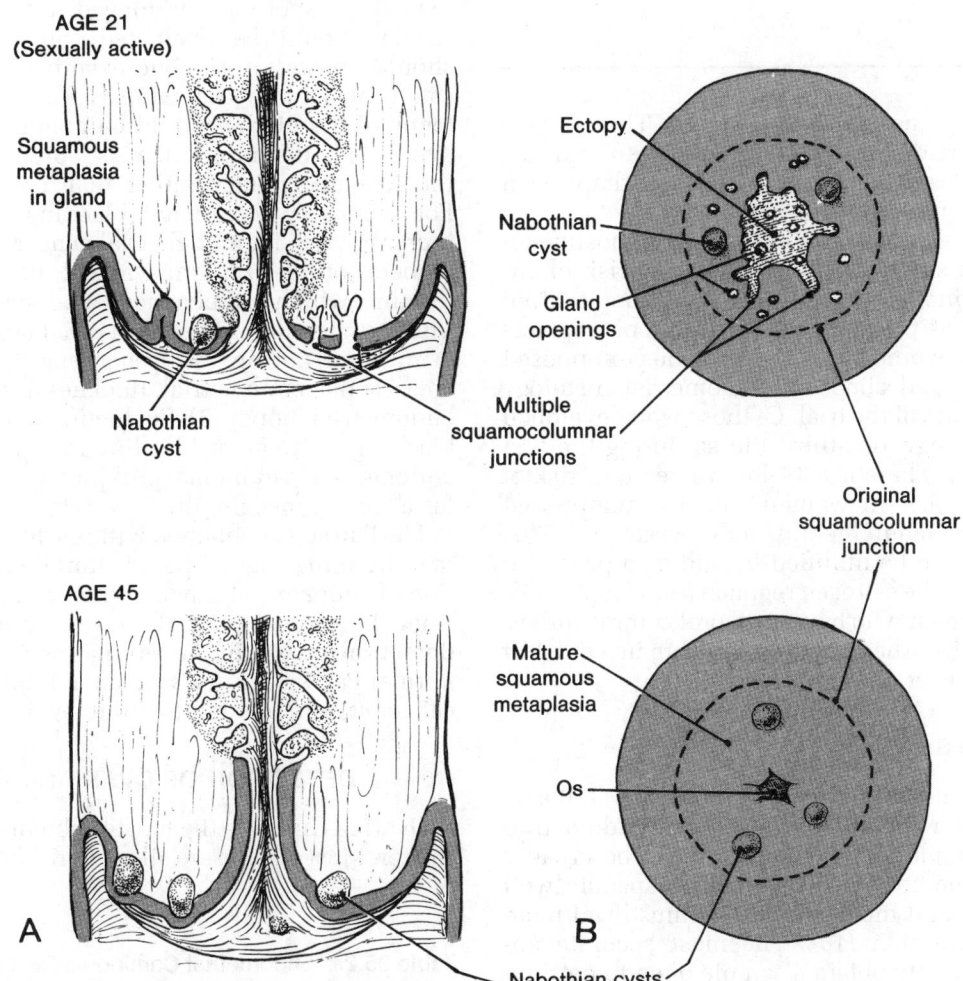

Figure 95.2.   The uterine cervix in women of various ages. **A.** Coronal section of the cervix and vaginal vault. **B.** Vaginal view of the cervix. (Redrawn from Briggs RM. Dysplasia and early neoplasia of the uterine cervix. A review. Obstet Gynecol Surv 34: 70, 1980.)

enous stimulation occurs in women who are anovulatory, such as patients with polycystic ovarian disease, diabetes mellitus, and extreme obesity. These women often have a history of infrequent menses and infertility. Factors that affect endometrial cancer risk are listed in Table 95.2.

Women who are extremely obese or who have diabetes mellitus metabolize sex steroids differently than

Table 95.1. Cervical Neoplasia Risk Factors

Epidemiologic Characteristics
Early intercourse
Multiple sex partners
Early marriage
Early childbearing
Prostitution
Male factors: high-risk consort (see text)
Low socioeconomic status
African-American or Hispanic race
Sexually transmitted infection

Other Potential Factors
Compromised immune status
Oral contraceptive use
Cigarette smoking
Prior radiation
Intrauterine DES exposure

Viral Relations
Papillomavirus
Herpesvirus
Cytomegalovirus

do women with normal body weight. There is increased conversion of androstenedione to estrone, which stimulates the endometrium and perhaps even predisposes them to cancer.

Long-term use of unopposed estrogen in postmenopausal women significantly increases the risk of endometrial carcinoma. In the PEPI Trial, a longitudinal study looking at postmenopausal hormone replacement, 62.2% of women taking continuous unopposed estrogen developed abnormal endometrial histology during the 3 years of the trial. Of those who developed abnormal histology, one-third did so during the first year of use (21). There is a 14-fold increase in risk of endometrial cancer in women who use unopposed estrogen replacement therapy for 7 years (9). This increased risk can be nullified by adding a progestin (e.g., Provera) to the estrogen regimen (see Chapter 77). In contrast, women who have used oral contraceptives and those who have had children have a reduced risk of endometrial cancer.

Screening Techniques

No population-based screening tools exist, but several methods for the early detection of endometrial cancer are suitable for office practice. To be broadly applied, such methods must be sensitive, specific, well tolerated, safe, and inexpensive, and must lead to an effective intervention (16). The most accurate approach is to directly obtain a sample of endometrium for histologic examination. The Novak curette is a 4-mm resterilizable metal cylinder with a serrated opening distal to its tip. The instrument is introduced into the endometrial cavity, and four quadrants of the uterus are scraped while suction is applied with a small syringe. The Vabra aspirator and Vakutage are similar instruments. All three of these instruments, when used by an experienced physician, yield a high correlation (80 to 95%) compared with material obtained from a dilation and curettage.

More widely used is the Pipelle endometrial suction curette (available from United International Marketing Resources, 475 Danbury Rd., Wilton, CT 06897; telephone 800-243-6608), which is recommended for the general physician even though it has not been studied prospectively. It is a flexible plastic tube 1 mm in diameter with a small opening near the blunt tip. Suction is applied with an integral movable plastic plunger. Unfortunately, because of its flexibility, the Pipelle cannot always be inserted into a stenotic cervical os. This instrument produces minimal pain, and the specimen obtained is equivalent to that obtained with the Novak curette.

All women with unexplained postmenopausal bleeding or who are at high risk for endometrial cancer should undergo an evaluation. Additionally, some premenopausal women over age 30 who have intermenstrual spotting, prolonged menses, or menorrhagia should be evaluated. Such an evaluation should consist of a pelvic examination and, if indicated, an endometrial biopsy. The size and consistency of the uterus should be noted. When observed over time, the rapid increase of uterine size may indicate malignancy rather than growth of fibroids. For women who are not bleeding but who are at increased risk for endometrial cancer (e.g., those with diabetes or obesity), transvaginal ultrasound may determine which women need endometrial sampling. Those with an endometrial thickness greater than 5 mm and not on estrogen replacement (which increases the endometrial thickness) should undergo endometrial biopsy (6). Evaluation of postmenopausal bleeding or irregular bleeding in a patient at risk for endometrial carcinoma is typically managed by referral to a gynecologist.

The Pap smear obtained without an additional specimen from the vaginal pool is unreliable for the detection of endometrial cancer. When a sample is obtained from the vaginal pool, the recovery of abnormal endometrial cells may be as high as 65%. However, a normal Pap smear in a woman at risk for endometrial cancer should not delay further evaluation.

DETECTION OF OVARIAN CANCER

Ovarian cancer is the most problematic gynecologic cancer. Most lesions are silent until they have reached

Table 95.2. Endometrial Carcinoma Risk Factors

Increased Risk	Diminished Risk
Unopposed menopausal estrogen	Ovulation
Replacement therapy	Progestin therapy
Menopause after 52 years	Combination oral contraceptives
Obesity	Menopause before 49 years
Nulliparity	Normal weight
Diabetes	Multiparity
Feminizing ovarian tumors	
Polycystic ovarina syndrome	
Tamoxifen therapy for breast cancer	

a size large enough to produce symptoms from the pressure of the mass. By this time, they have usually metastasized. The cure rate for advanced lesions is low. Annually approximately 20,500 new cases of ovarian cancer are discovered among American women, resulting in 12,500 deaths. They make up 4% of all cancers and 26% of gynecologic cancers. However, they account for 50% of deaths from gynecologic cancers (3). The cause of ovarian cancer is unknown, and little progress has been made in identifying the patient at risk, in early detection, or in improving the survival rate (18). This risk increases with increasing age and may affect 1 or 2% of women in their ninth decade. Factors that affect the risk of ovarian cancer are listed in Table 95.3.

The symptoms of ovarian cancer are nonspecific and are often ignored by both patient and physician until the tumor is far advanced. Most commonly, symptoms are referable to the gastrointestinal tract and consist of feelings of abdominal fullness, bloating, eructation, and pelvic pressure. Pain or constipation appears only very late. Abnormal uterine bleeding occurs only rarely in association with ovarian cancer.

The most common sign of ovarian cancer is an adnexal or abdominopelvic mass. The diagnostic evaluation of such a mass differs in each stage of a woman's life.

Although use of pelvic ultrasound and measurement of serum tumor markers (e.g., CA125) is becoming more widespread for screening for ovarian cancer, the efficacy of these tests has not been proven. Frequent false-positive test results and subsequent unnecessary intervention suggest the need for an improved screening protocol. Currently, the American College of Obstetrics and Gynecology does not recommend routine screening for ovarian cancer beyond yearly pelvic examinations. A randomized clinical trial addressing this issue is under way, sponsored by the National Cancer Institute (20).

Unfortunately, neither ultrasound nor computerized tomography (CT) of the abdomen and pelvis is able to indicate the malignant potential of ovarian masses. Nevertheless, these procedures are useful in determining the extent of the tumor. The determination of the concentration of tumor markers such as α fetoprotein, human chorionic gonadotropin, and carcinoembryonic antigen may be helpful in the evaluation of an ovarian mass and in following the course of the patient after treatment.

Premenarche Period

About two-thirds of ovarian tumors are benign in this age group. The most common tumors are a *benign cystic teratoma* (dermoid), a *benign simple cyst*, or a *cystadenoma.*

Malignant tumors in this age group arise from the germ cells or gonadal stromal cells in 80 to 90% cases (4). Generally no risk factors are elucidated. The most common presenting complaint is pain, which is caused by rapid tumor growth.

Table 95.3. Ovarian Carcinoma Risk Factors

Increased Risk	Decreased Risk
Older age	Multiparity
Late menopause	Oral contraceptive pills
Nulliparity	
Late childbearing	
Breast-feeding	
Personal or family history of breast cancer	

Reproductive Period

Most ovarian masses found during this period are functional cysts. The normal premenopausal ovary is $1.5 \times 3 \times 3.5$ cm. If ovulation fails to occur, a unilocular cyst is formed and may reach 10 cm in diameter. When ovulation does occur, a corpus luteum forms that may occasionally become enlarged because of internal hemorrhage. Both of these ovarian cysts are often detected because of the frequent evaluation by pelvic examination of women in this age group. These cysts usually resolve spontaneously within 2 to 4 weeks.

If the ovarian enlargement is persistent after 2 to 4 weeks and if it is demonstrated to be truly cystic by ultrasound, a period of suppressive therapy and observation is warranted. Oral contraceptive pills containing 35 to 50 µg of ethinyl estradiol (see Chapter 93) may be prescribed for 2 months to suppress gonadotropins. Estrogen blocks the pituitary gonadotrophins that are the stimulus for the formation and maintenance of ovarian cysts. When the ovarian cyst persists for longer than 60 days despite gonadotropin suppression, the diagnosis of ovarian neoplasia should be considered strongly and a gynecologist should be consulted.

Spanos found that 92% of persistent ovarian masses were neoplastic, although only 6.8% were malignant (19). Ultrasound is the best method to diagnose and monitor ovarian cysts. Any ovarian tumor that is irregular, septate, semisolid, solid, or greater than 8 cm in diameter upon ultrasound evaluation should be strongly suspected to be malignant. For women with those findings, prompt arrangements for gynecologic consultation should be made.

Perimenopausal and Menopausal Periods

During this era of a woman's life the incidence of ovarian cancer is highest. In the American population, the annual incidence increases from 15.7 per 100,000 for women aged 40 to 50 years to 35 per 100,000 after age 50. This dramatic increase in incidence has led some investigators to propose aggressive means to manage minimal ovarian enlargement.

In 1971, Barber proposed that any palpable ovary in a postmenopausal women was abnormal and required laparotomy. He called this the *postmenopausal palpable ovary (PMPO) syndrome* (1). However, in recent years experience has proved that although evaluation is essential, a more conservative approach to management of the PMPO syndrome is warranted. Less than 10% of patients with the PMPO syndrome have ovarian malignancies (10).

The only available method for screening for ovarian cancer is the periodic pelvic examination. Postmenopausal women should have periodic pelvic examination if there are no mitigating factors that preclude aggressive therapy, such as very advanced age, chronic illness, or disability.

General References*

American College of Physicians. Screening for ovarian cancer: recommendations and rationale. Ann Intern Med 121:141, 1994.
> A thoughtful statement concerning the ineffectiveness of ovarian cancer screening in most women.

Berek JS, Hacker NF. Practical gynecologic oncology. 2nd ed. Baltimore: Williams & Wilkins, 1993.

Herbst AL, Mishell DR Jr, Stenchever MA, Droegemueller W. Comprehensive gynecology. 2nd ed. St. Louis: CV Mosby, 1992.

Morow CP, Townsend DE. Synopsis of gynecologic oncology. New York: Wiley, 1987.

Specific References

1. Barber HRK, Graber EA. The PMPO syndrome (postmenopausal palpable ovary syndrome). Obstet Gynecol Surv 28:357, 1973.
2. Booth M, Beral V. Cervical cancer deaths in young women. Lancet 1:616, 1989.
3. Boring CC, Squires TS, Tong T. Cancer statistics, 1993. CA 43(1):7, 1993.
4. Breen JL, Marson WS. Ovarian tumors in children and adolescents. Clin Obstet Gynecol 20:607, 1977.
5. Butler EB, Stanbridge CM. Condylomatous lesions of the lower female genital tract. Clin Obstet Gynecol 11:171, 1984.

---

*Bold print (general references) and bold numerals (specific references) denote published controlled clinical trials, meta-analyses, or consensus-based recommendations.

6. Carter J, Carson LF, Byers L, et al. Transvaginal ultrasound in gynecologic oncology. Obstet Gynecol Surv 46:687, 1991.
7. Cervical cytology: evaluation and management of abnormalities. ACOG Technical Bulletin 183, 1993.
8. DiSilva PJ, Creasman WT, eds. Clinical gynecologic oncology. St. Louis: CV Mosby, 1989.
9. Ernster VI, Bush TL, Huggins GR, et al. Benefits and risks of menopausal estrogen and/or progestin hormone use. J Prevent Med 17:201, 1988.
10. Goldstein SR, Sulramanyan B, Snyder JR, et al. The postmenopausal cystic adnexal mass: the potential role of ultrasound in conservative management. Obstet Gynecol 73:8, 1989.
11. Kennedy AW, Flagg JS, Webster FD. Gynecologic cancer in the very elderly. Gynecol Oncol 32:49, 1989.
12. Koss LG. The Papanicolaou test for cervical cancer: a triumph and a tragedy. JAMA 261:737, 1989.
13. Kurman RJ, Henson DE, Herbst AL, et al. Interim guidelines for management of abnormal cervical cytology. JAMA 271:1866, 1994.
14. Mecsei R, Haugen OA, Halvorsen LE, Dalen A. Genital *Chlamydia trachomatis* infections in patients with abnormal cervical smears: effect of tetracycline on cell changes. Obstet Gynecol 73:317, 1989.
15. National Cancer Institute Workshop. The 1988 Bethesda system for reporting cervical/vaginal cytologic diagnoses. JAMA 262:7, 1989.
16. Pritchard KI. Screening for endometrial cancer. Is it effective? Ann Intern Med 110:177, 1989.
17. Richard RM. Typing HPV DNA gains clues for therapy. Contemp Ob/Gyn 31:4, 1988.
18. Smith LH, Oi RH. Detection of the patient at risk; clinical, radiological and cytological detection. Clin Obstet Gynecol 20:607, 1977.
19. Spanos WJ. Preoperative hormonal therapy of cystic adnexal masses. Am J Obstet Gynecol 116:551, 1973.
20. Westhoff C. Current status of screening for ovarian cancer. Gynecol Oncol 55:S34–S37, 1994.
21. Writing Group for the PEPI Trial. Effects of hormone replacement therapy on endometrial histology in postmenopausal women. JAMA 275:370, 1996.

Problems of the Eyes and Ears

SECTION

14

Problems of the Eyes and Ears

C H A P T E R   96

Hearing Loss and Associated Problems

JOHN K. NIPARKO, MD

In the United States, an estimated one in nine people develops a permanent hearing impairment that diminishes the ability to carry out everyday communication. Hearing loss is especially common in the elderly, who account for 40% of the hearing impaired. In fact, the only chronic disorders that are more prevalent are hypertension and arthritis. Many causes of hearing impairment are preventable. Early detection and intervention can often ameliorate an acquired hearing impairment.

When evaluating a patient with hearing loss, the diagnostic strategy should determine the mechanism of loss (conductive or sensorineural), the likely cause, and the need for referral to an otolaryngologist for further evaluation. This chapter includes a brief review of the anatomy and physiology of the auditory system that will help in understanding auditory pathology, and details strategies of diagnosis and early treatment.

EAR STRUCTURE AND FUNCTION

The *external ear* (Fig. 96.1) is composed of the auricle, the auditory meatus, and the external ear canal.

The outer portion of the canal is cartilaginous and is covered by thick skin that contains hair follicles and the cerumen-secreting glands; cerumen protects the epithelium and captures foreign particles entering the canal. The inner portion of the canal is bony and is covered by squamous epithelium without hair follicles or cerumen glands.

The *middle ear* (Fig. 96.1) consists of the tympanic membrane, the air space behind it, and the three linked ossicles: the malleus, incus, and stapes. The malleus is attached to the tympanic membrane and is linked to the stapes by the incus. The stapes makes contact with the inner ear via the stapes footplate at the oval window. The middle ear is lined with a mucus-secreting epithelium similar to that which lines the nose. The middle ear communicates with the nasopharynx via the eustachian tube and posteriorly with the mastoid air cells. Intermittent opening of the eustachian tube ensures equal pressure on either side of the tympanic membrane, which facilitates the transmission of sound from the tympanic membrane to the oval window.

The *inner ear* (Fig. 96.1) lies within the temporal bone of the lateral skull base and is encased in the compact otic capsule and is fluid filled. It consists of sensory organs for hearing *(cochlea)* and balance *(vestibular labyrinth)*. Nerves from the cochlea and vestibular labyrinth unite to form the eighth cranial nerve.

Cranial nerve VII (facial) traverses the temporal bone in close association with the middle and inner ear structures. For this reason, facial muscle paresis and paresthesias of the anterior two-thirds of the tongue and soft palate may manifest from pathologic processes of the middle and inner ear.

Sound is funneled through the auricle into the external ear canal, vibrating the tympanic membrane; the vibration is transferred across the ossicular chain. The large surface area of the vibrating tympanic membrane, and the lever action of the ossicles improve sound transmission to the inner ear, where vibrations of the stapes footplate create a fluid wave in the cochlea. This wave stimulates the hair cells that translate vibratory energy into action potentials that trigger auditory neurons.

DETERMINING SEVERITY AND MECHANISM OF HEARING LOSS

Regardless of the specific cause of hearing loss, the approximate severity of the impairment and the probable cause can often be determined in the office. This determination can be made from a combination of the history, the patient's ability to hear the spoken voice, and testing with a tuning fork.

Suggested Questions for History

To determine the likely cause of hearing loss, the following information should be acquired:

- Is one ear involved or both?
- Was the onset of hearing loss abrupt or gradual? Has

Figure 96.1. Normal structures of the ear.

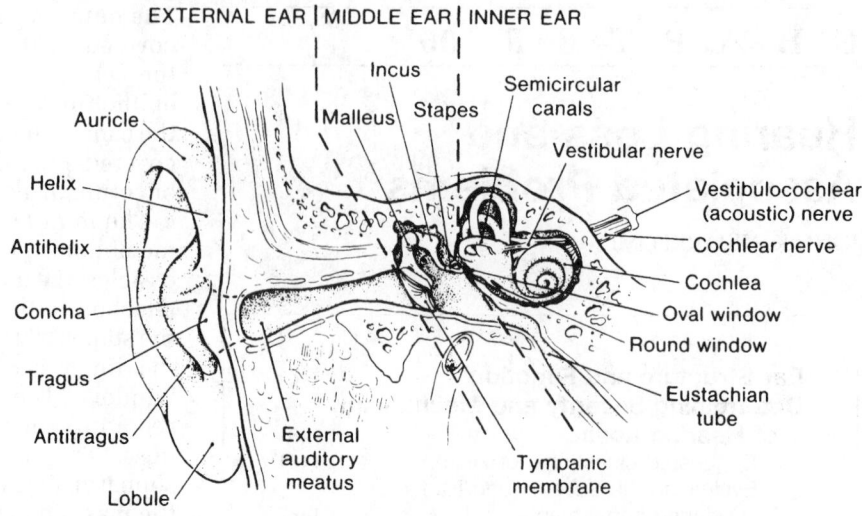

Table 96.1. A Practical Method for Approximating the Severity of Hearing Loss in the Office

Severity of Hearing Loss	Social Difficulty	Office Voice Test	Pure-Tone Audiogram
Normal hearing	None	18 ft or more using normal voice	No loss over 10 dB
Slight hearing loss	Long-distance speech	Not over 12 ft using normal voice	10–30 dB loss
Moderate hearing loss	Short-distance speech	Not over 3 ft using normal voice	Up to 60 dB loss
Severe hearing loss	All unamplified voices	Raised voice at meatus	Over 60 dB loss
Profound hearing loss	Voices never heard	All speech and sound	Over 90 dB loss

Adapted from Mawson SP. Disease of the ear. Baltimore: Williams & Wilkins, 1974.

it progressed rapidly? Has hearing acuity fluctuated?
- Does the patient have associated tinnitus, vertigo, otalgia, otorrhea, or facial weakness?
- Is there a family history of hearing loss?
- Has the patient a history of noise exposure?
- Are there related causes of hearing loss such as syphilis, diabetes mellitus, hypothyroidism, head trauma, or autoimmune disease?
- Has the patient been exposed to ototoxic agents such as aminoglycosides, diuretics, aspirin, or chemotherapeutic agents?

Evaluating the Severity and Range of Hearing Impairment

A practical method for evaluating the *severity of hearing impairment* includes a historical estimate of speech recognition impairment in noisy settings and an assessment of response to voice testing in the office; these two findings can be equated with various levels of abnormality in the audiogram (Table 96.1). *Slight* impairment indicates difficulty in hearing distant speech in noise (e.g., group meetings, social gatherings, or the theater). *Moderate impairment* includes some difficulty with short-distance speech and conversation. *Severe impairment* indicates no understanding of the conversational voice but understanding of the amplified voice. Amplification may be achieved by raising the voice or electronically by use of a hearing aid (see below). *Profound* (or total) impairment indicates inability to hear and understand the spoken voice despite maximal amplification. This also may be summarized

by recalling that a soft whisper is about 25 decibels (dB), a moderate whisper is about 40 dB, and conversational speech is about 60 dB. In the office, ambient sound can markedly affect the ability of a patient with hearing impairment to respond to this cursory assessment of audition. Therefore as quiet an environment as possible is advised.

In the patient with significant hearing impairment, the *frequency range* can be approximated in the office by testing recognition of words containing the sound "ah" (low frequency, vowel sound), such as *apple, hot dog,* and *airplane,* and the sounds "s" (high frequency, consonant), such as *ice cream, stairway, baseball,* and *sunset,* when these words are spoken in a medium voice about 2 feet behind the test ear, with the opposite ear covered.

Physical Findings

Otoscopy

Assessment of the External Canal and Tympanic Membrane. Complete inspection of the external ear canal and drum requires pulling the pinna in a posterosuperior direction to align the membranous and bony portions of the canal. The entire drum should be inspected (Fig. 96.2), particularly the posterosuperior aspect, where chronic inflammatory changes often occur. Cerumen accumulation in this region of the drum is unusual and may suggest an underlying problem (Fig. 96.3).

Membrane Mobility. During the otoscopic examination, it is important to assess tympanic membrane mobility with air insufflation. To do this, the examiner must seal the otoscope speculum tip with the ear canal. The absence of mobility suggests a pathologic condition such as negative pressure consequent to eustachian tube dysfunction, middle ear fluid, or a mass.

Preliminary Hearing Testing

Tuning Fork Tests

The mechanism of hearing loss can be classified as conductive or sensorineural through use of a 512-Hz tuning fork. Conductive losses result from external or middle ear disease, whereas sensorineural losses are caused by an inner ear or auditory neuronal problem.

Weber's Test.   For Weber's test, the tuning fork is held against a spot in the midline of the forehead and the patient is asked in which ear it sounds louder (Table 96.2). A unilateral conductive hearing loss with normal bilateral inner ear function produces a louder sound in the affected ear. A unilateral sensorineural hearing loss produces a louder sound in the normal ear.

Rinne's Test.   In the Rinne test, the vibrating tuning fork stem is placed against the mastoid bone and held in place until it becomes no longer audible, then it is held about an inch away from the external meatus (Table 96.2). Rinne's test can differentiate conductive from sensorineural hearing losses. Air conduction is perceived longer than bone conduction with normal hearing and with sensorineural hearing loss, whereas the reverse is true for conductive losses.

Speech Recognition Testing

In patients with sensorineural hearing loss, impaired understanding of speech may differentiate cochlear and neural (retrocochlear) deficits. In the latter condition, patients generally have a greater reduction of speech discrimination than do those who have cochlear disorders. Recruitment, a sense of ear discomfort with sudden increments in the loudness of a sound, is characteristic of cochlear dysfunction.

Audiometry

Whereas the office examination can only approximate the loss, audiometric evaluation establishes the precise level of hearing loss. Pure tone air conduction and bone conduction measurements are made for sounds of varying intensity (decibels) and frequency. Results are plotted on a graph called an audiogram in which the vertical axis shows the sounds heard in decibels and the horizontal axis shows the frequency of the stimulus in Hertz. Examples of audiograms showing normal hearing, conductive hearing loss, and sensorineural hearing loss are reproduced in Figure 96.4. Speech audiometry measures the subject's ability to hear and understand the spoken word.

Audiometry is performed by audiologists, some of whom have their offices in association with an otolaryngologist. Many, however, are independent. Patients can be referred directly to an audiologist from a primary care physician. The location of an accredited audiologist can be obtained by telephoning the action line of the American Speech-Language Association (ASHA) at 800-638-8255.

An audiogram is easily accomplished when proper testing facilities are available. The patient is comfortably seated in a soundproof room and is asked to record the sounds heard. A series of pure tones are presented to the patient. The procedure takes only about 20 to 30 minutes.

Small hand-held audioscopes, costing about $500, are available for use in the office by general physicians. These are useful as a rough screen of hearing impairment. Usually four pure tones are emitted in sequence. Because of masking effects, background noise can adversely affect a patient's ability to respond to test signals and the examining room must be quiet.

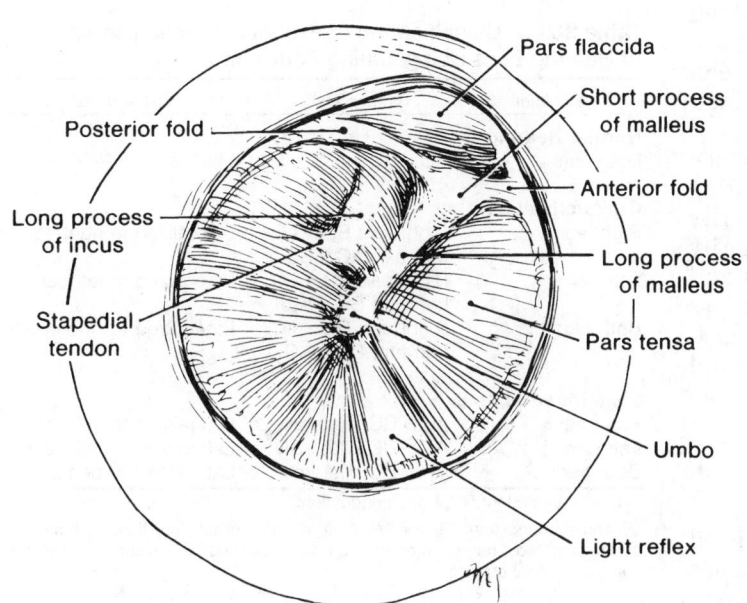

Figure 96.2.   Right tympanic membrane, showing important landmarks.

Pars flaccida

Short process of malleus

Posterior fold

Anterior fold

Long process of incus

Long process of malleus

Stapedial tendon

Pars tensa

Umbo

Light reflex

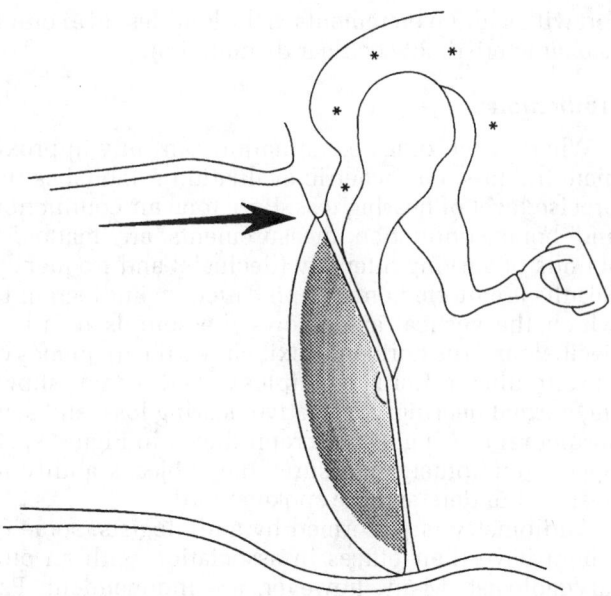

Figure 96.3. Cross-sectional drawing of middle ear depicted in Figure 96.1. Arrow indicates the region of the tympanic membrane that may develop a retraction. Retraction pockets may accumulate desquamated debris and extend into regions of the epitympanum depicted by asterisks.

The lowest audible intensity for normal ears is approximately 10 to 20 dB (Fig. 96.4). Conversational speech is typically delivered at 45 to 55 dB. The American Speech-Language and Hearing Association has categorized hearing loss as mild (26 to 40 dB), moderate (41 to 55 dB), moderately severe (56 to 70 dB), severe (71 to 90 dB), and profound (greater than 91 dB).

An *assisted listening device* can be valuable in conversing in the office with a patient who is hearing impaired. This device is simply a system of a microphone, amplifier, and earphones. It also reduces some of the background noise in the room and amplifies the examiner's spoken word. Such devices can be obtained in electronics stores or by ordering directly from a manufacturer (e.g., Pocketalker, Williams Sound, telephone 800-328-6190; or Chorus, Audiological Engineering Corp., 800-283-4601).

After this initial evaluation, the presence or absence of hearing loss should be established. If there is hearing loss, it should be determined whether it is primarily unilateral or bilateral and whether it is primarily sensorineural or conductive. Further assessment and care for patients with moderate or severe hearing loss usually requires the assistance of an otolaryngologist. An asymmetric hearing loss should prompt a referral for more sophisticated testing (see discussion of specific conditions below).

CAUSES OF HEARING LOSS: OVERVIEW

The major causes of hearing loss in adults are listed in Table 96.3. For each condition, the table indicates

mechanism, onset (rapid or gradual), and whether the condition is typically unilateral or bilateral. The guidelines that follow will enable the general physician to reach a working diagnosis in most instances and to choose between primary treatment and referral for care by a specialist.

Conditions of the External Ear

Cerumen Impaction

The patient usually complains of intermittent fullness and hearing impairment on the affected side and may give a history of episodes. These symptoms may increase after showering or swimming, as moisture occludes the ear canal, or with cotton-tipped swab use. Diagnosis is made by otoscopy.

Several precautions should be kept in mind in considering cerumen removal. An only hearing ear, a postsurgical ear, and an ear that is prone to infection should not be irrigated. If the cerumen appears to be soft, it may be removed by irrigation with use of a rubber-bulb syringe and warm tap water, directing the water upward and backward against the wall of the canal. If the cerumen is impacted and difficult to remove, a few drops of hydrogen peroxide (or carbamide peroxide, Debrox) should be instilled twice daily for 1 week before irrigation. Alternatively, a ceruminolytic agent (Cerumenex) may be used. In general, ceruminolytic agents should be used only in the office because casual use by the patient at home increases the risk of allergic dermatitis. With the patient's head tilted laterally at 45° angle, the ear is filled with ceruminolytic drops. A cotton plug is inserted for 15 to 20 minutes; the ear is then irrigated with lukewarm water and a soft rubber syringe. After irrigation, the tympanic membrane usually shows some injection around the handle of the malleus. Hearing impairment should be relieved after removal of cerumen. The occasional patient with an impaction

Table 96.2. Classification of Probable Mechanism of Hearing Loss Using Tuning Fork Tests

Classification	Rinne's Test	Weber's Test
Normal Hearing		
Both ears	AC > BC	Midline
Conductive Loss[a]		
Right ear	Right ear: BC > AC	Lateralized to right ear
	Left ear: AC > BC	
Left ear	Right ear: AC > BC	Lateralized to left ear
	Left ear: BC > AC	
Both ears	Right ear: BC > AC	Lateralized to poorer ear
	Left ear: BC > AC	
Sensorineural Loss		
Right ear	AC > BC bilaterally	Lateralized to left ear
Left ear	AC > BC bilaterally	Lateralized to right ear
Both ears	AC > BC bilaterally	Lateralized to better ear

AC, Air conduction; *BC*, bone conduction.
[a]Because sound transmission by air is much more efficient than by bone, air conduction may remain greater than bone conduction in early or minimal conductive hearing loss.

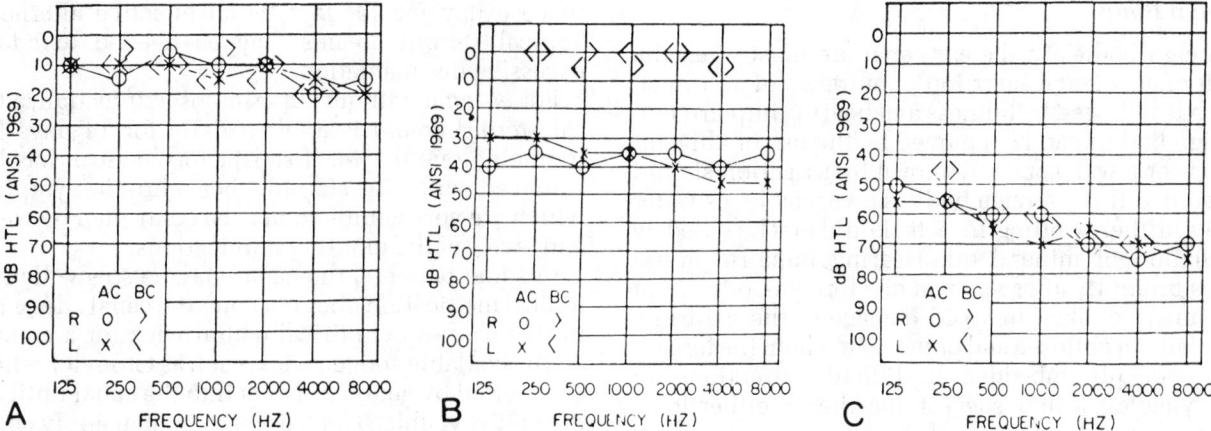

Figure 96.4. Examples of audiograms. **A.** Audiogram in a person with normal hearing. **B.** Bilateral conductive hearing loss (moderate). **C.** Bilateral sensorineural hearing loss (severe). (From Price L, Snider R. The geriatric patient: ear, nose and throat problems. In: Reichel W, ed. Clinical aspects of aging. Baltimore: Williams & Wilkins, 1978;489.)

Table 96.3.   Causes of Hearing Loss in Adults

Causes	Mechanism	Onset Rapid (Hours to Days) or Gradual (Months to Years)	Bilateral or Unilateral
External Auditory Canal			
Cerumen impaction	C	Either	Usually unilateral
Foreign body	C	Rapid	Unilateral
Otitis externa	C	Rapid	Unilateral
New growth	C	Gradual	Unilateral
Middle Ear			
Serous otitis media	C	Either	Either
Acute otitis media	C	Rapid	Unilateral
Barotrauma	C or SN	Rapid	Unilateral
Traumatic perforation of tympanic membrane	C	Rapid	Unilateral
Chronic otitis media	C	Gradual	Unilateral
Cholesteatoma	C or SN	Gradual	Either
Ossicular chain problem			
Adhesive otitis media	C	Gradual	Unilateral
Tympanosclerosis	C	Gradual	Either
Traumatic injury	C or SN	Rapid	Unilateral
Otosclerosis	C and/or SN	Gradual	Bilateral
New growths	C or SN	Gradual	Unilateral
Inner Ear			
Presbycusis	SN	Gradual	Bilateral
Acoustic trauma	SN	Gradual	Bilateral
Drug-induced	SN	Either	Bilateral
Ménière's syndrome	SN	Rapid	Usually unilateral
Central nervous system infection			
Meningitis	SN	Rapid	Either
Syphilis	SN	Either	Either
Tuberculosis	SN	Either	Either
Acoustic neuroma	SN	Gradual	Unilateral
Mumps	SN	Rapid	Unilateral
Atraumatic Sudden Sensorineural Hearing Loss	SN	Rapid	Unilateral

C, Conductive; *SN*, sensorineural.

may not respond to the usual measures described above and should be referred to an otolaryngologist.

An impaction often follows vigorous efforts by the patient to remove wax with a cotton-tipped swab. The patient should be reminded that ear wax is secreted to protect the lining of the canal and that the swab should be used only to remove cerumen in the outer portion of the canal, for cosmetic purposes.

Recurrent impactions are often caused by eczema of the skin of the external ear canal and may require regular irrigation and possibly topical therapy of the skin condition (see below).

Foreign Body

Foreign bodies in the ear canal are most often the result of accidental insertion or entrance of an insect, which is followed by fullness and hearing impairment. Foreign bodies can be removed by the use of alligator forceps or a wax spoon. Removal by irrigation should be avoided if the foreign body is a vegetable, as water causes further swelling. Insects should first be killed by instillation of mineral oil. Hearing impairment resolves promptly after removal of a foreign body. Great care must be taken to avoid damage to the eardrum, especially in children and patients in whom the foreign body is deeply imbedded. In difficult extractions, an otolaryngologist may suggest anesthesia, either local injection or general.

Otitis Externa (Swimmer's Ear)

Otitis externa is most common in the summer, when heat and moisture promote swelling and maceration of the stratum corneum of the skin. In the external canal, this process may at first cause pruritus. The patient may give a history of having scratched the ear for a few days before the onset of drainage and pain. The pain is aggravated by movement of the external ear and jaw motion. Hearing impairment occurs in patients with swelling or debris that occludes the canal. The characteristics of the skin of the canal and of the exudate may provide adequate clues to the cause, and cultures are needed only for patients who do not respond promptly to topical treatment. Copious or greenish exudate suggests *Pseudomonas,* the bacteria most often seen in otitis externa. Yellow crusting in the midst of a purulent exudate suggests *Staphylococcus aureus.* Canal skin that is scaling, cracked, and weeping indicates *secondary eczema.* Fluffy material resembling bread mold, varying in color from white to black, suggests a *fungal agent* (*Aspergillus* or *Candida*).

There are two general principles of treatment for all types of otitis externa: removal of all infected debris (with a suction cannula if available) and instillation of an appropriate topical antimicrobial (see below). Lavage with hydrogen peroxide, commonly done in the past, is not recommended because it may be irritating to the inflamed and sensitive tissues and it is not adequately cidal to microbes.

For *bacterial infections* the patient should instill an antimicrobial–corticosteroid combination (e.g., Cortisporin Otic Suspension, containing polymyxin B–neomycin–hydrocortisone, three or four drops three to four times daily for 5 to 7 days). Acetic acid preparations (white vinegar) either alone or with steroids have also been used with good results for acute otitis externa.

For *fungal infections,* the canal should be thoroughly cleaned out and a light dusting of sulfanilamide powder should be applied by the clinician. A dispenser containing sulfanilamide powder for this use can be obtained from any pharmacy. The fungal infection usually resolves after a single dusting with this powder. Clotrimazole (Lotrimin) 1% solution, three drops twice a day for 14 days, is an effective alternative. Topical steroid creams may be needed to address excessive desquamation.

For *eczema* without superimposed infection, a topical *steroid cream* is applied daily for 14 days (e.g., triamcinolone 0.1%). If satisfactory control has been achieved with the steroid, then chronic symptoms, which are very common, may be controlled by weekly and, eventually, monthly applications.

In some patients, the canal may be so swollen that topical medication does not enter the canal adequately. In this case, a cylindrical cotton wick (or a commercially available sponge wick, such as Oto-wick) should be inserted by gentle twisting into the canal until only the end is visible. The patient may then apply several drops of the medication to the wick three to four times daily, and the wick will carry it into the canal. The wick can usually be removed after 48 to 72 hours, and treatment can be continued as stated above.

Most episodes of otitis externa resolve completely after 5 to 7 days, and it is important to terminate topical treatment at this time. Topical medicines alter the canal environment and persistent treatment often leads to atopic or chemical dermatitis or fungal colonization. As a precaution against overtreatment, the prescription for eardrops should be nonrefillable, and only a small amount (10 mL) should be dispensed.

During treatment of otitis externa, moisture must be kept from entering the ear canal. During bathing, the ear should be plugged with cotton impregnated with petroleum jelly. To prevent recurrence, the patient should be warned against using cotton-tipped swabs. Hearing impairment caused by otitis externa should resolve promptly when swelling recedes.

In two situations, the patient with otitis externa requires prompt referral to an otolaryngologist: patients whose findings suggest *mastoiditis* (slow response of the otitis externa to treatment and tenderness over the mastoid process); and patients whose findings suggest *malignant otitis externa,* usually diabetic or immunologically impaired patients. This process is actually an osteitis of the bone underlying the external auditory canal, caused by *Pseudomonas.* The distinguishing features are fever, excruciating pain, and the presence of friable, reddish granulation tissue that fills a breach in the canal epithelium. Because of the propensity for rapid spread to contiguous structures, this condition is an emergency, requiring hospital admission for debridement and intravenous antibiotics.

New Growth

Malignancies of auricular and periauricular skin are both common and notoriously difficult to control (13), and any suspicion of a new growth should prompt urgent referral to an otolaryngologist. Cutaneous malignancies that commonly occur in these sites are *basal cell carcinomas,* with clinically indistinct borders, and *squamous cell carcinomas,* which often exhibit aggressive clinical characteristics. Moreover, multiple tissue planes and the topography of this region can confound cure. If diagnosed late, auricular and periauricular cutaneous malignancies often extend to involve the parotid gland, mastoid cortex, and external ear canal. The morbidity and mortality associated with such extensions underscore the importance of early complete initial removal of malignancies in this region.

Conditions of the Middle Ear

Conductive hearing loss is produced by conditions of the middle ear, tympanic membrane, and external ear canal. Most commonly, however, conductive hearing loss results from interference with the sound transformer mechanism of the tympanic membrane and middle ear ossicles. In addition to the history, the middle ear assessment includes otoscopic inspection for signs of acute inflammation (erythema, discharge, or bulging of the tympanic membrane), changes in the tympanic membrane not caused by acute inflammation (retraction, scarring, distortion of normal structures, perforation), cholesteatoma (squamous debris accumulation within the middle ear), and evidence of reduced middle ear aeration as indicated by diminished movement of the drum on pneumatic insufflation.

Serous Otitis Media

The patient usually complains of fullness and decreased hearing in one or both ears with minimal or no pain. There is often a history of recent viral upper respiratory infection, exacerbation of allergic or vasomotor rhinitis, or prior acute otitis media. Rarely, serous otitis media may be caused by nasopharyngeal carcinoma, and this possibility must be ruled out in adults with a new onset of serous otitis that does not resolve after appropriate management (see below). There is otoscopic evidence of eustachian tube closure and retraction of the tympanic membrane, failure of the membrane to move on pneumatic otoscopy (a crude test of eustachian tube patency, but not always abnormal in serous otitis), or a visible air–fluid level behind the membrane. Usually the tuning fork test reveals a conductive hearing loss (see above).

Medical management consists first of using systemic antibiotics for 10 days (4,16). Recommended regimens include erythromycin ethylsuccinate (e.g., 250 mg four times a day) and sulfisoxazole (e.g., Gantrisin 500 mg four times a day), trimethoprim–sulfamethoxazole (e.g., Septra, Bactrim, or generic twice a day), and amoxicillin (250 mg three times a day), either alone or combined with clavulanate. Topical decongestants in the form of nasal sprays or drops are often used to relieve eustachian tube obstruction. Nasal sprays containing the sympathomimetics may be obtained over the counter (e.g., Neo-Synephrine 0.25 or 0.50% spray or drops). The patient administers two puffs to each nostril, followed 5 to 10 minutes later by two more puffs, four times daily. After 3 to 4 days of topical treatment, rebound nasal mucosal hyperemia may occur. Therefore the patient should be instructed explicitly to discontinue spray (or drops) after 3 days. Systemic decongestants (e.g., pseudoephedrine) are probably not helpful (5). If a patient with serous otitis

media has a history of allergic rhinitis, an antihistamine or specific treatment for the condition may be helpful (see Chapter 23).

All patients should be reevaluated after 4 to 6 weeks. If conductive hearing loss persists beyond 6 weeks, the patient should be referred to an otolaryngologist, who will confirm and quantify the conductive hearing loss and check for other conditions that may be causing the hearing loss. Persistent effusion after 3 months of medical therapy is an indication for surgery, particularly when associated with hearing loss or tympanic membrane changes. Surgery consists of a myringotomy with or without a drainage stent. This procedure is usually done under local anesthesia in the office. The results are excellent but the patient must not get any moisture in the ear (e.g., avoid swimming) until healing is complete, which usually takes 6 to 18 months. A stent, if placed, typically falls out spontaneously in several months.

Acute Otitis Media

Patients with acute suppurative otitis media complain of marked pain in the ear and most give a history of a recent upper respiratory infection. Drainage of purulent material from the ear indicates probable tympanic membrane perforation or concomitant otitis externa. On examination, there is injection and loss of luster of the tympanic membrane, grayish-pink coloration of the entire membrane, and, eventually, bulging of the membrane and loss of landmarks. Some patients have a conductive hearing loss demonstrated by tuning fork tests (see above). There may be tenderness to palpation of the mastoid bone because the mucosa lining of the mastoid cells is continuous with that of the middle ear. Evidence of otitis externa is usually not present. The most common etiologic agents are *Streptococcus pneumoniae* (Pneumococcus), *Haemophilus influenzae, S. aureus,* and β-*hemolytic Streptococcus.* Although some cases are caused by viral pathogens, diagnosis of these cases is usually not practical and treatment should be the same for all patients with acute otitis media.

Medical treatment consists of systemic antimicrobials for 10 days. The antibiotic course should be completed to avoid recurrent or persistent infection and mastoiditis.

Amoxicillin, 500 mg three times daily for 10 days, remains the drug of first choice, although in some communities the prevalence of β-lactamase–producing bacteria may necessitate a different agent (e.g., amoxicillin–clavulanate [Augmentin 250/125 or 500/125 tablets] or cefaclor [Ceclor 250 or 500 mg Pulvules]). For penicillin-allergic patients, erythromycin (250 mg four times a day) or trimethoprim–sulfamethoxazole (e.g., Bactrim, Septra, or generic, two tablets two times a day) may be used. Aspirin, acetaminophen, or ibuprofen every 4 to 6 hours should be recommended for pain. If perforation with discharge occurs, Cortisporin otic suspension, four drops three times daily for 1 week, may be added to the treatment. If the tympanic membrane is bulging with pus and the patient describes severe pain or vertigo, myringotomy by an otolaryngologist is indicated to prevent extension of the infection and resultant complications.

Recovery from the pain of acute otitis media is usually prompt. Within 1 to 4 weeks, hearing impairment should resolve and the tympanic membrane assumes its normal appearance. Serous otitis may be present after other signs and symptoms of acute otitis have resolved.

In the patient who notes persistent otalgia, fever, or other signs of toxicity despite adequate antibiotics for 48 hours, subacute mastoiditis should be suspected, and prompt referral to an otolaryngologist is indicated. Facial nerve dysfunction and signs of central nervous system infection likewise require prompt evaluation and management. Failure of serous otitis to resolve, persistence of a tympanic membrane perforation, and significant persistent hearing loss after 4 to 6 weeks are also indications for referral.

Barotrauma

Barotrauma refers to symptoms and signs produced by a sudden pressure differential between the middle ear and the surrounding atmosphere. The patient gives a history of fullness, pain, and decreased hearing in one or both ears. This problem is most commonly associated with descents while flying or scuba diving. Otoscopic findings vary from mild tympanic membrane retraction to hemotympanum, with or without perforation. There may be conductive or neurosensory hearing loss. Any patient with moderate or severe unilateral hearing loss should be referred to an otolaryngologist because of the possibility of inner ear involvement. For patients with mild symptoms, topical or oral decongestants may alleviate symptoms. Prophylaxis against barotrauma consists of use of the Valsalva maneuver and chewing gum or swallowing during descent in airplanes, and management of allergic conditions involving the upper respiratory tract.

Temporal Bone Fractures

Traditional classification of the lateral skull base is based on the orientation of the fracture line in relation to the long axis of the temporal bone (petrous pyramid). Knowledge of the fracture line orientation predicts the extent of middle- and inner-ear damage and the pattern of cranial nerve injury. Eighty percent of temporal bone fractures are longitudinal, most often caused by blows to the lateral skull (12). The plane of fracture extends along the external ear canal to involve the ossicular chain (to produce a conductive hearing loss) and occasionally the facial nerve. Transverse temporal bone fractures extend perpendicularly to the long axis of the petrous pyramid, crossing the inner ear (to produce a sensorineural hearing loss) and often the facial nerve. Transverse fractures account for approximately 20% of temporal bone fractures. Evaluation of a temporal bone fracture requires a careful otoscopic and cranial nerve evaluation, supplemented by high-resolution computerized tomography (CT) scanning. Treatment is dictated by sequelae of the fracture.

Traumatic Perforation of Tympanic Membrane

A tympanic membrane perforation may be caused by a cotton-tipped swab or other object for removing wax, foreign bodies, forcefully directed water, and blast waves resulting from detonation of high explosives. Symptoms include decreased hearing, tinnitus, pain, and bleeding. Otoscopic examination reveals a perforation, commonly in the area of the pars tensa (Fig. 96.2). Air insufflation, which aids in the diagnosis, especially if a perforation is suspected but not seen, shows an immobile tympanic membrane.

The objective of treatment is the prevention of infection. Most linear tears and small perforations of the membrane heal spontaneously in several weeks. Large perforations may require grafting by an otolaryngologist. This procedure is usually done under general anesthesia as an outpatient procedure. A piece of temporal fascia is used for the patch. The results are highly successful with minimal postoperative discomfort. If there is a strong possibility that the middle ear has been contaminated at the time of injury, oral antibiotics (ampicillin or erythromycin 250 mg four times daily for 1 week) are indicated. Patients should prevent water or other contaminants from entering the ear by the insertion of a petroleum jelly-covered cotton plug. Swimming should be avoided altogether. Patients whose perforation was self-inflicted should be warned against future syringing and probing to remove cerumen.

After spontaneous closure or myringoplasty, the hearing loss caused by perforation usually resolves completely. Within a few months the perforation or surgical repair is no longer visible, although occasionally a thin area or a whitish scar remains. Tinnitus, sensorineural hearing loss, and vertigo are signs of inner ear injury and necessitate prompt referral to an otolaryngologist, who will evaluate the patient for a fistula, which requires prompt repair.

Chronic Otitis Media

Chronic otitis is present when a patient has otorrhea, either persistent or recurrent, and there is perforation of the tympanic membrane and usually some degree of conductive hearing loss. The management of this problem has two objectives: eradication of infection and restoration of hearing. When chronic otitis media is initially recognized, the patient should be referred to an otolaryngologist for evaluation (11).

Chronic otitis media can be divided into two major subgroups: inactive and active. The clinical characteristics of these two groups are summarized in Table 96.4. The fundamental difference in the active subgroup is the presence of, or potential for, bone destruction caused by invasion by squamous epithelium known as *cholesteatoma*. Cholesteatoma occurs when squamous epithelium of the auditory canal invades the middle ear through a preexisting perforation (acquired cholesteatoma). The cholesteatoma appears as a mass of keratinaceous debris that accumulates at the site of invasion of squamous epithelium. As the mass enlarges, it carries the potential to erode bone and promote fur-

Table 96.4. Chronic Otitis Media: Features Distinguishing Inactive and Active (Cholesteatoma) Forms

Feature	Inactive	Active (Cholesteatoma)
Discharge	Mucoid or muco-purulent	Purulent, foul
Location of pathology	Middle ear; eustachian tube	Middle ear, attic, antrum, any part of temporal bone
Tympanic membrane perforation	Pars tensa (central)[a]	Pars flaccida[a] of marginal
Middle ear mucosa	Mucous membrane	Stratified squamous epithelium
X-rays	Normal; clouding of mastoid cells	Underdevelopment of sclerosis of mastoid cells; bone destruction
Cholesteatoma formation	No	Yes
Bone erosion	No	Yes
Treatment of infection	Medical/surgical (surgery if the perforation fails to heal spontaneously)	Surgical

[a]See Figure 96.2.

ther infection. Facial paralysis caused by cranial nerve VII involvement, meningitis, and brain abscess may occur as a complication of active cholesteatoma.

The commonly performed surgical procedures for chronic otitis media are described below.

Simple mastoidectomy removes the mastoid cells and cholesteatoma, usually through a postauricular incision. The canal wall remains intact.

In *modified radical mastoidectomy,* the mastoid cells are exteriorized to form a common cavity with the external auditory canal, draining and eradicating infection caused by cholesteatoma.

In *myringoplasty,* the tympanic membrane perforation is closed by use of a tissue graft.

In *tympanoplasty,* the conductive mechanism, including tympanic membrane perforation and ossicular disruptions, is repaired.

These operative procedures are usually done as outpatient surgical procedures. General anesthesia is usually required for both types of mastoidectomy, whereas the plasty procedures can most often be done with only local anesthesia. There is moderate discomfort for 2 to 3 days. However, for 4 to 6 weeks after any of these procedures, the patient must avoid heavy lifting, strenuous exercise, or any similar activity that could result in a Valsalva maneuver, which results in the increase of air pressure in the middle ear and may disrupt the repair. The success rate of all these procedures is approximately 80%.

Complications of Otitis Media. Acute or chronic suppurative otitis media may become complicated by extension of infection beyond the confines of the middle ear into bone and other surrounding structures. These complicating infections are mastoiditis, facial nerve paralysis (caused by cranial nerve VII involvement), petrositis (inflammation of the petrous portion of the sphenoid with diplopia, pain around the eye, and

persistent otorrhea), labyrinthitis, brain abscess, extradural abscess, subdural abscess, lateral sinus thrombophlebitis, meningitis, and otitic hydrocephalus. Symptoms not attributable to the typical course of acute or chronic otitis media may signify the presence of one of these complications and require immediate referral and hospitalization.

Ossicular Chain Problems

The most common of these (adhesive otitis media and tympanosclerosis) occur as sequelae to otitis media. Others (ossicular injury or otosclerosis) may affect the ossicular chain in the absence of a history of or signs of prior otitis media. Ossicular chain problems may be recognized by demonstrating conductive hearing loss (usually chronic, either unilateral or bilateral). Changes of the tympanic membrane indicative of prior otitis media may or may not be present, depending on the problem (see above). In some conditions, otoscopy may even be diagnostic. Each of these conditions requires referral to an otolaryngologist for accurate diagnosis and consideration of surgical management.

Adhesive Otitis Media. There is a history of ear infection, and the tympanic membrane is retracted and atrophic in areas of healed perforations. The eardrum is usually draped over the promontory and incudostapedial complex. Adhesive otitis media is usually a late complication seen in patients with persistent middle ear inflammation. Hearing loss is usually mild, although some patients may require ossicular reconstruction or a hearing aid (see below).

Tympanosclerosis. There is a history of infection, often bilateral. There is usually, but not always, a tympanic membrane perforation, and discrete plaques of dense collagen with calcified hyaline may be seen in the middle ear. In selected patients tympanic membrane and ossicular reconstruction is necessary to improve hearing.

Traumatic Ossicular Injury. There is a history of trauma (e.g., temporal bone fracture and the causes of traumatic perforation listed above) followed by unilateral hearing loss, which may be conductive or mixed. A hemotympanum (blood behind the eardrum) is usually seen, although occasionally the tympanic membrane is normal. Hearing status after surgical exploration depends on the type of injury found at surgery.

Otosclerosis. Otosclerosis is a disease of the labyrinthine capsule in which spongelike bone is laid down, causing fixation of the stapes and conductive hearing loss, usually bilateral. The history discloses a slowly progressive hearing loss, usually in adults in their second or third decades, more commonly in females, and often accelerated by pregnancy. History is key in establishing the diagnosis because examination of the tympanic membrane is usually normal. This is the most common cause of progressive conductive hearing loss in young adults. The results of surgery, consisting of stapedectomy or stapedotomy and prosthetic replacement, are excellent.

New Growths of Middle Ear

A number of benign and malignant growths may be seen on inspection of the tympanic membrane of patients with progressive unilateral conductive hearing loss. Malignant tumors most commonly present with a history of chronic discharge, occasionally bloody.

CHRONIC SENSORINEURAL HEARING LOSS

Presbycusis

A certain degree of hearing loss, beginning in the high-frequency range, is universal among elderly people. Most do not complain of deafness, and often a family member is the first to notice the hearing deficit. Clearly, social and psychologic factors are important in determining the level of reported disability. For this reason, in the general population of elderly, in whom hearing loss is common, screening of asymptomatic patients using an office audiogram is not usually recommended because obtaining a hearing aid (see below), the usual prescription, is expensive and cumbersome and most patients will not use one until they have perceived their hearing problem and seek a remedy on their own.

When an older patient is first found to have moderate hearing loss, the patient and family should be counseled as outlined below, and the patient should be offered a referral for evaluation by an audiologist (see "Audiometry," above) or by an otolaryngologist (12).

Noise-Induced Hearing Loss

Noise-induced hearing loss is a form of sensorineural hearing loss commonly found in patients employed in high-noise industries or exposed to intense noise from power tools, firearms, and other sources (8). Loud rock music also may cause hearing loss, but because of the range of sound it is a slower process, often occurring 10 to 15 years after repeated exposure. Like presbycusis, it is initially a high-frequency hearing loss, eventually involving lower frequencies. Prophylaxis by wearing muffs and earplugs in high-noise settings and reducing noise levels are the best ways to prevent acoustic trauma. Established hearing loss caused by noise is usually irreversible, but progressive hearing loss can be prevented. Acute hearing loss caused by an acute episode of acoustic trauma, such as gunfire or cordless telephone ringer accidents (a loud sound or shock caused by electrical surge), is often reversible and referred to as a temporary threshold shift.

Drug-Induced Hearing Loss

A number of drugs may produce bilateral sensorineural hearing loss, and the patient's personal physician often is the first to learn of this problem (Table 96.5). For most of these drugs, ototoxicity is dose related; however, hearing impairment may occur even at therapeutic dosages. A mild hearing loss occurs in as many as 10% of patients whose serum levels of genta-

Table 96.5.   Drugs That May Cause Sensorineural Hearing Loss

Antibiotics	Diuretics
Streptomycin	Ethacrynic acid
Neomycin	Furosemide
Gentamycin	
Tobramycin	**Other Drugs**
Chloramphenicol	Salicylates
Vancomycin	Quinidine
	Quinine
	Cisplatin

micin and tobramycin are maintained within the therapeutic range (17).

The prognosis for drug-induced hearing loss varies according to the drug. Salicylates in high dosages and quinine usually produce temporary, high-frequency deafness, but permanent deafness has been reported in patients surviving salicylate poisoning and in infants of mothers who received quinine during pregnancy. Aminoglycoside ototoxicity may occur suddenly after a few doses, may be permanent, and may progress after discontinuation of the drug. Diuretic-induced ototoxicity may be seen after extremely high dosages, usually in patients with renal insufficiency. Its onset may be sudden, after intravenous (and rarely oral) administration, and the hearing deficit may be permanent.

Ménière's Syndrome

Ménière's syndrome is characterized by spells of a constellation of otologic symptoms. Symptoms are thought to be caused by endolymphatic hydrops manifested by excess fluid and pressure in the cochlea and vestibular labyrinth. Ménière's attacks consist of fluctuant hearing loss, roaring tinnitus, aural fullness, and spontaneous peripheral-pattern vertigo (see Chapter 81). However, in many instances the disorder produces a nonclassic array of symptoms. An attack may last for minutes to an hour, often with nystagmus present on physical examination. Between attacks, tinnitus and sensorineural hearing loss often persist. Symptoms are unilateral in 70 to 80% of cases (3). The hearing loss and vertiginous episodes may occur simultaneously, or in tandem. Vertigo may be accompanied by nausea and emesis. In severe episodes, other vagal symptoms may occur, including pallor and sweating and rarely bradycardia. Audiometry demonstrates sensorineural hearing loss, predominantly in lower frequencies in early stages of the disease.

The *differential diagnosis* of Ménière's syndrome includes a number of conditions that may also present with hearing loss and vertigo unrelated to position change: viral labyrinthitis, acoustic neurinoma, syphilitic vertigo, labyrinthine fistula, vestibular granuloma, temporal bone fracture, or multiple sclerosis (see Chapter 81 for details regarding vertigo).

Treatment. Patients with suspected Ménière's syndrome should be referred promptly to an otolaryngologist to confirm the diagnosis and initiate treatment.

Patients are treated empirically with diuretics, 25 to 50 mg of hydrochlorothiazide daily or its equivalent, with attention to avoid hypokalemia (see Chapter 46). The antihistamine meclizine can be tried in a dosage of 25 mg three to four times daily, but often this fails to prevent attacks of vertigo. For nausea, the patient should take the antiemetic prochlorperazine either as a 5- or 10-mg capsule four times daily, or as a 25-mg suppository twice daily. After the acute attack has subsided, the patient should continue diuretic treatment; after 1 year without recurrence, diuretic treatment can be discontinued. For the occasional patient with severe recurrent Ménière's syndrome refractory to medical treatment, several surgical procedures offer high response rates.

ACOUSTIC NEUROMA

Acoustic neuroma, an uncommon, benign tumor, usually arises from the vestibular fibers of nerve VIII. It grows slowly, expanding within the internal auditory meatus until it is large enough to extend into the posterior fossa and compress adjacent structures. Essentially all patients present with symptoms of eighth nerve impairment: unilateral hearing loss is found in the majority of patients and chronic, usually mild, positional vertigo or sense of imbalance occurs in many patients. Audiometry usually demonstrates significant sensorineural hearing loss with poor discrimination. Neurologic examination (see Chapter 78) shows involvement of the following neurologic structures, in decreasing order of frequency: cranial nerves V, VII, VI, and cerebellum (ataxia, with tendency to fall toward the side of the lesion). Referral to an otolaryngologist for evaluation is essential whenever unilateral sensorineural hearing loss is initially found. Diagnosis of acoustic neuroma is based on a characteristic audiogram and computed tomography scanning or magnetic resonance imaging (1). The results of surgical treatment generally permit the patient to resume usual activity, but often with permanent unilateral hearing loss (15). In a few patients with good hearing preoperatively, it may be possible to preserve hearing.

SUDDEN SENSORINEURAL HEARING LOSS

Sudden sensorineural hearing loss, usually unilateral, is an otologic emergency. The cause is often difficult to ascertain and may include viral cochleitis, arterial occlusion (especially in patients with other evidence of arterial occlusive disease, such as embolic transient ischemic attacks), inner ear fistula, autoimmune factors (10), sudden expansion of a cerebellopontine angle tumor (e.g., a meningioma or acoustic neuroma, discussed above), temporal bone fracture, and noise trauma. Symptoms, which occur over a matter of minutes to hours, include tinnitus or hearing loss. After prompt evaluation for conductive hearing loss (including simple cerumen impaction), these patients should be referred immediately for evaluation by an otolaryngologist. A number of empirical medical therapies (e.g., corticosteroids, vasodilators, membrane-

deforming agents, or anticoagulants) have been tried with varying success. For patients with suspected inner ear fistulas, surgical exploration may be necessary.

Most patients have permanent, severe unilateral hearing loss, and they and their families should be instructed about adequate noise protection for the only hearing ear, preferential seating for optimal use of the good ear, and precautions when driving to compensate for missed sound cues.

TINNITUS

Tinnitus ("ringing") is the perception of sounds in the absence of a normal sound stimulus. Intermittent tinnitus is common in the general population. Persistent tinnitus may be caused by a number of identifiable problems. Occasionally, tinnitus may be experienced only at night, in bed, when ambient noise is reduced.

Subjective Tinnitus

The term *subjective tinnitus* is used when the subject complains of noises that cannot be heard by the observer. Subjective tinnitus may be subdivided into two types.

Tympanic tinnitus usually arises as a result of a conductive lesion (all of the causes of conductive hearing loss). It is thought to be caused by removal of the normal masking effect of ambient noise, with emergence of otherwise subaudible tympanic, vascular, and muscular noises. The patient often describes the tinnitus as pulsating.

Petrous tinnitus is caused by conditions affecting the cochlea or eighth nerve that lead to sensorineural hearing loss. It is attributed to recognition of auditory stimuli produced by mechanical cochlear deformation or hyperirritability of the acoustic nerve. It may be intermittent or continuous with varying intensity.

After the patient's primary otologic problem has been defined, the most important requirement in helping the patient with tinnitus is reassurance because patients may believe that their tinnitus reflects a serious intracranial condition. Bedtime sedation to ensure adequate sleep is important. Some patients also find that the sound of an FM radio (FM delivers a broader range of frequencies, particularly in the higher spectrum than AM) helps them get to sleep by competing with the more distressing sounds caused by tinnitus. For patients with severe tinnitus, *masking treatment* (an apparatus that externally generates white noise and is available from an audiologist) may be helpful. The distressing nature of severe and chronic tinnitus has resulted in the development of tinnitus clinics and support groups in most large cities (9,14).

Objective Tinnitus

Objective tinnitus is a noise audible to the examiner and originates from the region of the patient's ear. Causes include aneurysm of the internal carotid artery, benign vascular tumors of the middle ear, temporomandibular joint instability, and myoclonus of the palatal muscles. These patients should be referred to an otolaryngologist for a diagnostic workup. Also, patients with tinnitus that lateralizes to one ear should also be referred for further evaluation.

DEALING WITH THE PATIENT WITH PERMANENT HEARING LOSS

Communication

Counseling of the family and others who speak to the patient with moderate to severe hearing loss should emphasize the following points.

Facilitate communication by consistently using the following adjuncts to speech: face patients, obtain their attention, use gestures, speak at a moderate pace and audibly, or move closer if the patient says that it helps.

Ensure adequate lighting (to aide in lip reading and facial expressions) and minimize background noise, which confuses sound perception.

Be patient and ask how you can facilitate communication.

For the patient with *profound* or *total hearing loss,* the principle governing all communication is that the message must be seen by the patient. Most patients let the physician know the mode of communication they prefer (lip reading or writing). Whenever there is any question about the effectiveness of lip reading, written exchange of information should be used. This can be facilitated by ensuring that paper and a pen or pencil are always available to the patient. Also, various devices are now available, although they are moderately expensive, that make it possible for totally deaf people to receive telephone calls (messages are entered by the sender in code on a touch-tone unit and displayed visually for the deaf receiver) and to follow television programs. Many people who are totally deaf at an early age learn sign language and programs for learning sign language are widely available. Valuable information to help people with any level of hearing impairment may be obtained from Self-Help for Hard of Hearing People, Inc. (SHHH), 7800 Wisconsin Ave., Bethesda, MD 20814, telephone 301-657-2248.

Hearing Aids

Hearing aids (miniature, battery-powered microphone–amplifier–loudspeaker units) can assist the patient with sensorineural hearing loss and patients with irreversible conductive loss (7). The currently available aids include in-the-ear, delicate, and behind-the-ear units. Older devices were incorporated into eyeglasses or carried in a pocket with a wire connection to the ear mold. Hearing aids can increase the intensity of a sound by up to 70 dB. Thus, a sound of about 60 dB (the level of average conversational speech) passing through an aid may enter the ear at a level of 130 dB. This represents the maximal usable gain of an aid because sounds above this level become painful.

Federal law now prevents the sale of hearing aids to people who have not been evaluated first by a physician. Only trial and adjustment determine whether a patient referred for a hearing aid will benefit. Medicare and other third-party insurers do not pay for hearing aids and they are expensive, typically costing $300 to $1,000. Most hearing aid dealers allow a 30-day trial period during which the patient pays a rental fee; some states require this by law. Currently, only a minority of people who would benefit from a hearing aid own one, usually because of the cost and the difficulty or embarrassment perceived in using it. Also, many who own units do not use them regularly because of difficulty in using them or the presence of irritating sounds, which often can be eliminated by adjustment of the device by an audiologist.

Patients may mention certain specific problems with the hearing aid to their personal physicians. There may be irritation of the conchal cartilage, infection in the external canal, or an increase in cerumen accumulation. In each of these situations, use of the aid should be evaluated by the fitting audiologist. A better fitting mold is needed to avoid recurrence in some patients. Others may do well by removing the aid periodically during the day.

For selected patients, implantable bone conduction aids and cochlear implants are now available (6). The cochlear implant is used in patients who are unable to derive significant benefit from the use of powerful hearing aids.

General References*

Cummings C, Fredrickson J, Harker L, Schuller D, eds. Otolaryngology: head and neck surgery. St. Louis: CV Mosby, 1992.

Jerger J, Chmiel R, Wilson N, Lachi R. Hearing impairment in older adults: new concepts. J Am Geriatr Soc 43:928, 1995.

Nadol JB. Hearing loss. N Engl J Med 329:1092, 1993.

Niparko J, Kemink J. Hearing loss: strategies in evaluation and management. Consultant 27:39, 1987.

Rosenfeld RM. **An evidence-based approach to treating otitis media.** Pediatr Clin North Am 43(6):1165, 1996.

Rosenfeld RM, Post JC. **Meta-analysis of antibiotics for the treatment of otitis media with effusion.** Otolaryngol Head Neck Surg 106(4): 378, 1992.

Specific References

1. Armington WG, Harnsberger HR, Smoker WR, Osborn AG. Normal and diseased acoustic pathway: evaluation with MR imaging. Radiology 167(2):509, 1988.

2. Backous D, Minor L, Niparko J. Trauma to the external auditory canal and temporal bone. Otolaryngol Clin North Am 29:5, 1996.

3. Balkany TJ, Kires B, Arenberg IK. Bilateral aspects of Ménière's disease. Otolaryngol Clin North Am 13:4, 1980.

4. Bluestone CD. Antimicrobial treatment of eustachian tube dysfunction for otitis media with effusion ("secretory" otitis media). Pediatr Ann 13:405, 1984.

5. Bluestone CD, Mandel EM, Cantekin EI, et al. Evaluation of decongestant antihistamine therapy for otitis media with effusion. Ann Otol Rhinol Laryngol 92(6):35, 1983.

6. Cohen N, Waltzman S. The Department of Veterans Affairs Cochlear Implant Study Group: a prospective, randomized study of cochlear implants. N Engl J Med 328:233, 1993.

7. Department of Health, Education and Welfare. A report on

---

*Bold print (general references) and bold numerals (specific references) denote published controlled clinical trials, meta-analyses, or consensus-based recommendations.

hearing aid health care. Washington, DC: US Government Printing Office, 1974.

8. Dobie RA. Noise-induced hearing loss: the family physician's role. Am Fam Physician 36(6):141, 1987.

9. Hawthorne MR, O'Connor S, Britten SR, Webber P. The management of a population of tinnitus sufferers in a specialized clinic: part I. Description of the clinic organization and the population seen. J Laryngol Otol 101(8):784, 1987.

10. Hughes GB, Barna BP, Kinney SE, et al. Clinical diagnosis of immune inner-ear disease. Laryngoscope 98(3):251, 1988.

11. Kemink J, Telian S, Niparko J. Evaluation and treatment of the draining ear. Modern Med 56:76, 1988.

12. Miller MH. Restoring hearing to the older patient: the physician's role. Geriatrics 41(12):75, 1986.

13. Niparko J, Swanson N, Baker S, et al. Local control of auricular and periauricular cutaneous carcinoma with Mohs surgery. Laryngoscope 100:1047, 1990.

14. O'Connor S, Hawthorne M, Britten SR, Webber P. The management of a population of tinnitus sufferers in a specialized clinic: part II. Identification of psychiatric morbidity in a population of tinnitus sufferers. J Laryngol Otol 101(8):791, 1987.

15. Ojemann RG, Montgomery WW, Weiss AD. Evaluation and surgical treatment of acoustic neuroma. N Engl J Med 287:895, 1972.

16. Paradise JL. Antimicrobial prophylaxis for recurrent acute otitis media. Ann Otol Rhinol Laryngol 90:53, 1984.

17. Smith CR, Lipsky JJ, Laskin OL, et al. Double-blind comparison of the nephrotoxicity and auditory toxicity of gentamycin and tobramycin. N Engl J Med 302:1106, 1980.

C H A P T E R 97

Common Problems Associated with Impaired Vision: Cataracts and Age-Related Macular Degeneration

ANDREW P. SCHACHAT, MD

CATARACTS

A cataract is an opacification of the lens of the eye. Approximately 95% of people over 60 years of age have some opacification of the lens, but most often these opacities are of no visual importance. A *significant cataract* results in interference with visual acuity. In the United States, cataracts are a common cause of diminished vision and may result in blindness. The incidence of diminished visual acuity from cataracts increases steadily after age 50, reaching nearly 50% of people over the age of 75. Cataracts are usually bilateral, and the progression is slow and may vary between eyes. The rate of progression is not individually predictable, and there is no treatment that retards the progression. When the cataract is advanced, the only therapy is surgery. A large clinical trial, the Age-Related Eye Disease Study, is investigating the role of vitamins in the progression of cataract and age-related macular degeneration. More than 4000 patients are enrolled, and as of 1998, there is 4 to 5 years of follow-up. However, results are not anticipated until the early 2000s.

Anatomy and Physiology

The lens is derived entirely from the evagination of surface ectoderm in the fetus. It is located immediately posterior to the iris and is suspended there by radially attached zonular fibers from the ciliary body (see Chapter 98, Fig. 98.1). It is a biconvex transparent structure with an elastic capsule whose shape is altered by ciliary body contraction, permitting images to be brought into sharp focus on the retina. The lens is acellular and avascular and lacks innervation. Nourishment is provided from the surrounding aqueous and vitreous humor, and metabolic byproducts are removed by diffusion into the aqueous humor. The continued transparency of the lens requires the active metabolism of the elastic capsular epithelium, so any insult to the epithelium may result in lenticular opacities. New lenticular fibers are produced throughout life, and because none are lost, increasing density of the fibers of the lens develops with age, which contributes to cataract formation as well.

Causes

There are many causes of cataracts (Table 97.1). Although senescent cataracts—the result of the aging process described above—account for the vast majority of cataracts, the general physician occasionally sees patients with congenital or traumatic lens opacities as well. The mechanism of opacification in all of these instances is thought to be direct trauma or interference with the metabolic activity of the capsular epithelium and with continued fiber production.

Many of these types of cataracts have a distinctive appearance. The ophthalmologist may therefore suggest to the general physician the possibility of an underlying disorder such as myotonic dystrophy (iridescent spots) or Wilson's disease (sunflower cataract). Steroid therapy and radiation treatment are associated with posterior subcapsular cataracts, although these may be idiopathic or related to numerous other conditions as well. Age-related cataract is significantly associated with dermatologic abnormalities and its treatment. Steroid use is particularly strongly associated (8).

Table 97.1. Causes of Cataracts

Congenital
  Autosomal-dominant inheritance (25% of congenital cataracts)
  Maternal malnutrition
  Maternal infections (rubella, syphilis)
  Maternal metabolic disease (e.g., diabetes mellitus)
  Maternal medication (corticosteroids)
  Prematurity
Traumatic
Senescent
Secondary
  Drug therapy (corticosteroids)
  Degenerative eye disease (sever myopia)
  Retinal dystrophy
  Essential iris atrophy
  Retinal detachment
  Glaucoma
  Intraocular neoplasia
  Ocular ischemia (e.g., Takayasu's disease)
Associated with metabolic disease
  Diabetes mellitus
  Wilson's disease
  Hypoparathyroidism

Symptoms and Examination

The primary symptom of cataract is impaired vision; usually patients describe a constant fog over the eye. They may also see rings or halos around lights and objects. Objects appear more blue and yellow in color. With immature cataract formation, distant vision often is impaired to a greater extent than is near vision.

The location of the cataract within the lens determines the extent of the visual loss. Central opacities cause noticeable loss of vision and a distinct glare when the patient is in bright light. Bright light constricts the pupil so that the dense portion of the lens occludes and diffuses light. Therefore the patient who has central opacities finds that his or her vision is better in low light when his pupil is widely dilated. In select cases, use of dilating drops (mydriatics) is helpful and delays the need for surgery. Because there may be contraindications to the use of mydriatics (e.g., narrow-angle glaucoma attacks may be precipitated), it is best to rely on an ophthalmologist to prescribe these. Peripheral opacities cause noticeable loss of vision only late in the development of the cataract.

Cataracts are easily identified by illuminating the lens with a slitlamp, but most general physicians find that they can see a cataract easily through a moderately plus lens (e.g., a +2 or +3 lens on the dial) of the direct ophthalmoscope. The lens appears cloudy. Similarly, a light from a small flashlight may be reflected off the opacity in the lens. Visual acuity should be tested in both eyes when cataracts are suspected. If the patient describes any visual symptoms or if the physician measures an impairment in visual acuity, the patient should be referred to an ophthalmologist. In adults, screening for cataracts is best done by a visual acuity examination with use of a Snellen chart. The *Snellen chart* is easy to use and the result is a ratio of the distance a patient stands from the chart to the distance that a subject with normal vision would stand to read the line of images in question. Therefore, 20/100 means that the patient is seeing clearly at 20 feet an image that a person with normal vision would see at 100 feet. It is critical to check separately the visual acuity of each eye with the other covered and with the patient using his or her glasses.

Cataract Surgery

Indications

Before surgery is indicated, optical manipulations such as mydriatics to help a patient see around a central cataract (discussed above) or new glasses for the progressive myopia associated with many nuclear cataracts may improve the vision of patients with cataracts. Also, visual aids, such as magnifying lenses and large-print materials, may be helpful (see "Advice for the Visually Impaired," below). The decision to remove a cataract is determined by the visual needs of the patient, the degree of the cataract, and the presence of any other ocular abnormalities. The ophthalmologist performs a complete ocular assessment before advising the patient about surgery.

Each patient must determine his or her own visual need based on daily activities. The ability to read, drive, cross streets safely, and perform a daily routine is clearly of prime importance. For example, a patient usually requires visual acuity of at least 20/40 in the better eye to operate a motor vehicle safely or to continue moderately active daily life. Blurred vision has an important impact on patients' functioning and well-being. The impact of blurred vision on role limitations caused by other health problems was significantly greater than the impact of hypertension, history of myocardial infarction, type 2 diabetes, indigestion, trouble urinating, or headache (4). Because the impact of blurred vision is so significant and the success rate for cataract surgery so high, it is not surprising how often the procedure is performed.

Surgery

Cataract surgery should be performed only after considerable deliberation because a number of complications might occur and vision after cataract extraction may still be a major problem (see below). For patients with other health problems, the general physician and the ophthalmologist should plan cataract surgery together. Cataract extraction is an elective procedure, and the patient should be in the best possible condition at the time of operation.

Approximately 600,000 cataract extractions are performed in the United States every year, and cataract surgery is the most common major surgical procedure performed in the elderly in this country. Surgery involves the removal of the opacified lens from the eye. The extraction may be intracapsular, involving complete removal of the lens, or extracapsular, leaving the posterior capsule of the lens intact. In the 1990s, the overwhelming majority of cataract surgeries are extracapsular. Microsurgical techniques have greatly improved the immediate outcome of surgery and have significantly shortened the period of disability. Extracapsular extraction is most commonly performed because it leaves the posterior capsule intact, permits easier lens implantation (see below), and is associated with fewer postoperative complications. A large randomized trial in India on thousands of patients recently confirmed that the extracapsular techniques is preferred. Both eyes usually require operation, but normally only one lens is extracted at a time so that the patient has vision in the nonoperated side when the eye that has been operated on is covered by a patch for a few days after surgery. Some surgeons attempt to avoid the use of a patch, and so called no-stitch surgery with very small incisions is in vogue. There is no proof that any particular extracapsular surgical approach is better than any other. For patients with bilateral cataracts, the second procedure is usually performed a few months after the first; once the visual result is known in the first eye, the patient and ophthalmologist again assess the visual needs, risks, benefits, and alternatives to surgery in the second eye.

Preoperative Evaluation.   The current standard of care is a history and physical examination, but few if any laboratory investigations are required. Health ser-

vice researchers are debating the extent of a preoperative evaluation. In the current climate of cost awareness, a minimalist approach is being phased in. The history should elicit clues about bleeding tendencies. If appropriate, aspirin should be discontinued for 7 to 14 days before the surgery, although some surgeons do not stop aspirin, given the low risk of bleeding with small incision surgery. The ability of the patient to lie flat should be assessed. Diabetes mellitus and hypertension, if present, should be controlled. A recent myocardial infarction (within 6 months) should delay surgery. A randomized trial, the PORT-II study, is comparing essentially no preoperative medical testing with standard (minimal) testing. The results of this study should be available in 1998 or 1999.

Patient Experience. Cataract surgery is performed most often by use of local anesthesia supplemented with intravenous analgesia and sedation. Surgery is normally performed on an outpatient basis. The patient experiences moderate discomfort, but this lasts only a day or so and is controlled with analgesics. A hyperosmotic agent (e.g., glycerin or mannitol) or local pressure may be used to dehydrate and soften the eye in preparation for surgery.

After discharge from the surgical unit a patient must restrict his or her activities for several weeks to minimize the frequency of complications, although with small incisions and the newest microsurgical techniques the rehabilitation period is becoming shorter. These restrictions are listed in Table 97.2 and are rather conservative. Many ophthalmologists are much more liberal. There are no permanent restrictions; however, caution with steps or when walking and working with machinery may be necessary if perception is seriously altered by use of aphakic spectacles (see below).

Complications

Complications occur in approximately 5% of patients who have had cataract extraction, and 1 of every 5000 eyes operated on is lost because of complications. Knowledge of the possible complications after cataract surgery aids the general physician in educating patients. Because of the potential for complications, the general physician must ensure that the patient keeps the scheduled postoperative appointments with the ophthalmologist.

Optometrists are allowed under Medicare to receive reimbursement for postoperative follow-up care. Although no data indicate that an ophthalmologist (as opposed to an optometrist) can do this better, it makes sense that follow-up during the postoperative period by the surgeon is preferable.

Inflammation and Infection.   All postoperative patients have some degree of traumatic intraocular inflammation. This is usually controlled effectively with topical corticosteroids. Bacterial intraocular infection, endophthalmitis, is a dangerous postoperative inflammation that must be recognized early before it devastates the eye. If a patient complains of decreased vision, pain, discharge, and redness, endophthalmitis may be present and the patient should be seen immediately by an ophthalmologist. Most infections occur within a few

Table 97.2. Temporary Restrictions After Cataract Surgery

Wear eye shield during sleep and wear glasses at other times; shields are usually worn for 1 month and then discontinued.

Minimize bending or stooping for 3 or 4 weeks.

Do not sleep on side of operated eye for 3 or 4 weeks.

Do not wash hair for 2 weeks.

No showers for 2 weeks, although a bath is allowed (but with assistance to prevent a fall).

No strenuous or excessive physical activity for 4 weeks and then only after approval of the ophthalmologist.

These are suggested to prevent inadvertent injury to the eye, diminish disruptive pressure on the wound, avoid sudden rise in ocular pressure, and diminish the chance of infection. These recommendations are conservative. The ophthalmologist may prefer a more liberal set.

days of surgery; however, an operated eye is predisposed to infection from systemic infection, so a patient with an acute red eye occurring at any time after eye surgery should be seen urgently by an ophthalmologist. Low-grade chronic inflammation is common after cataract surgery and resultant macular edema is one of the most common causes of postoperative visual loss.

Hemorrhage. The sudden occurrence of hemorrhage in the uveal tract (the iris, the ciliary body, and the choroid) can adversely influence the final visual outcome. Although this complication is usually seen intraoperatively, rarely it may occur postoperatively. The event is characterized by a usually painless but precipitous change in visual acuity. Postoperative hemorrhage from the iris or an inadequately closed corneoscleral wound is more common than is vitreous hemorrhage. In all instances of hemorrhage, urgent referral to an ophthalmologist is indicated. Although anticoagulation is not an absolute contraindication to cataract extraction, it does increase the risk of hemorrhage. For this reason, anticoagulants and antiplatelet agents such as aspirin are stopped, if possible, before and for 1 to 2 weeks after surgery.

Retinal Detachment. The incidence of retinal detachment after cataract surgery is approximately 1 to 3%. Retinal detachment is characterized by suddenly decreased visual acuity, flashes of light, and the development of floaters, veils, or curtains in the visual field. Patients with symptoms of retinal detachment should be seen immediately by an ophthalmologist so that surgical reattachment of the retina may be accomplished. The success of reattachment is good when the procedure is done expeditiously.

Glaucoma. This secondary form of glaucoma is caused by several factors that lead to true or functional angle closure: the effect of the proteolytic agent chymotrypsin on the angular structures at the time of intracapsular operation (rare today), scarring caused by postoperative inflammation, or the misdirection into and subsequent trapping of the aqueous in the vitreous gel (see Chapter 98, Fig. 98.1). Glaucoma may develop within a few days of surgery. Early glaucoma is usually transient, but it may become chronic. Glaucoma may appear as late as 1 to 2 years after surgery in 0.6 to 5% of patients depending on the type of surgery. The patient who has developed secondary glaucoma usu-

ally complains of redness, tenderness, and pain in the eye. Furthermore, if the patient has been fitted with a temporary spectacle, he or she notices a decrease in visual acuity caused by corneal edema. A postoperative patient suspected of having glaucoma should be seen immediately by an ophthalmologist. Additional information about glaucoma is provided in Chapter 98.

Delayed Opacification of the Posterior Capsule. Extracapsular extraction is performed more often than intracapsular extraction because it is associated with fewer complications. However, 20 to 50% of patients experience a gradual decrease in vision in the first few years after this technique because of opacification of the posterior lens capsule. This complication can now be treated effectively by a special laser instrument (yttrium–aluminum–garnet [YAG]) that opens the posterior capsule without the need for intraocular surgery. The procedure is painless and is performed in the office. However, it is performed only when the potential for visual improvement outweighs the risks, as retinal detachment and perhaps macular edema become somewhat more common (9). Clinical trials of an agent that may retard the development of opacification of the posterior capsule are under way.

Optical Correction After Cataract Extraction

The removal of a cataract improves light transmission to the retina, but vision remains blurred without corrective lenses. Three types of lenses are used: aphakic spectacles, contact lenses, and intraocular lenses. The last option is now the norm. Aphakic spectacles are discussed mainly for historical reasons. Contact lenses are used more than aphakic spectacles, but almost all patients, even children, are now candidates for intraocular lenses.

Aphakic spectacles are rarely used today. With aphakic spectacles there is a narrower field of vision, as well as considerable distortion of images, which appear rounded and three to five times larger than when the lens is present in the eye. Peripheral ring scotomata and loss of some depth perception also occur. Even modern aphakic spectacles are heavy and thick so that a patient often has considerable initial difficulty adjusting to them and needs support, understanding, and encouragement from family members. With experience, however, most patients can function acceptably and perform all of their necessary daily activities.

A unilateral cataract extraction results in a pronounced disparity in image size if an aphakic spectacle is used postoperatively; therefore, unilateral surgery is generally not advised unless the patient will be able to use a contact lens or is a candidate for an intraocular lens implantation (see below). Indeed, because intraocular lenses are used so often, unilateral cataracts are operated on much more often than they were in early decades; also, under certain circumstances monolenticular extraction may be indicated to permit the ophthalmologist to follow the course of these ocular diseases.

The use of *contact lenses* after cataract extraction

provides considerable improvement over spectacles. There is substantial distortion reduction and expansion of the field of vision. However, the patient must be motivated to use contact lenses, and this motivation must be considered before surgery is undertaken. Often elderly patients are concerned about being agile enough to insert contact lenses, although there are some long-wear lenses on the market. The patient must also be fitted with a pair of spectacles with one lens missing so that he or she can see well enough to place one contact lens. A regular set of aphakic spectacles is also necessary as a backup to the contact lens.

Because of the visual handicap experienced after cataract extraction, plastic *intraocular lenses* are inserted at the time of surgery in 95% or more of patients undergoing cataract extraction. They are even used successfully in developing countries. Long-term survival of these inert prostheses is very good. The insertion of intraocular implants adds a few minutes to the operative time beyond that required for lens extraction. If the eye is otherwise healthy, using this technique more than 90% of patients experience an improvement in vision to 20/40 or better. New multifocal lenses (to replace bifocals) are under investigation.

AGE-RELATED MACULAR DEGENERATION

Age-related macular degeneration (AMD) is the leading cause of severe visual loss in people over age 50. The macula is the central area of the retina used for fine focus such as reading. There is no universally agreed upon definition of age-related macular degeneration. It is characterized by the development of drusen, retinal pigment epithelial changes, and in some cases abnormal choroidal vessels and hemorrhage. Drusen are excrescences that develop along Bruch's membrane, which lies between the retina and choroid and appear, on ophthalmologic examination, as tiny discrete white or yellow deposits. They are at times difficult to visualize and the ophthalmoscope must be in sharp focus on the retina. Most patients over age 50 have a few drusen, and there is no consensus as to how many drusen and how extensive retinal pigment epithelial changes constitute age-related macular degeneration. Drusen formation alone almost never reduces visual acuity.

Epidemiology

The Framingham Eye Study found that age-related macular degeneration was present in one or both eyes of almost 6% of subjects age 52 or older (5). The prevalence is strongly age related. Comparable rates were found in the Health and Nutrition Examination Survey (HANES) (2). In the Beaver Dam Eye Study, approximately 30% of adults aged 75 or older have early AMD and another 28% will develop it over the next 5 years. Early signs are twice as common in women and patients with early AMD have significantly greater risk of developing advanced AMD (3). Risk factors that have been identified in some series include

hyperopia (far vision), decreased hand grip strength, light iris color, systemic hypertension, family history, cardiac hypertrophy, short height, history of previous lung infection, cigarette smoking, cardiovascular disease, chemical exposure, and sunlight exposure. The strength and validity of these associations are debated and at least two major epidemiologic studies investigating risk factors are currently close to completion.

Clinical Features

There are two major forms of macular degeneration. The nonneovascular or *atrophic form* is characterized simply by drusen formation and atrophic retinal pigment epithelial changes. It is the most common form of macular degeneration. The *neovascular or exudative form* of macular degeneration, in which subretinal choroidal neovascularization occurs, can lead to subretinal hemorrhage and fluid accumulation and, eventually, extensive scarring. Although it is the rarer form of macular degeneration, it accounts for the majority of visual loss seen in patients with macular degeneration.

Drusen may vary in distribution, number, size, and shape. They may or may not have pigmentary alterations around them. Small drusen are difficult to see with the direct ophthalmoscope, but larger or so-called soft drusen should be apparent (Figs. 97.1 and 97.2). Atrophy associated with age-related macular degeneration may represent true atrophy of retinal pigment epithelium or may simply represent loss of pigment from within retinal pigment epithelial cells. Clinically, the distinction is impossible to make (Fig. 97.3). When atrophy involves the macula (the aspect of the central retina that is temporal to and slightly below the optic disc), visual acuity is usually reduced.

Neovascular macular degeneration is characterized by the accumulation of fluid, hemorrhage, or lipid beneath or within the retina (Fig. 97.4). Accumulation of fluid beneath the retinal pigment epithelium may

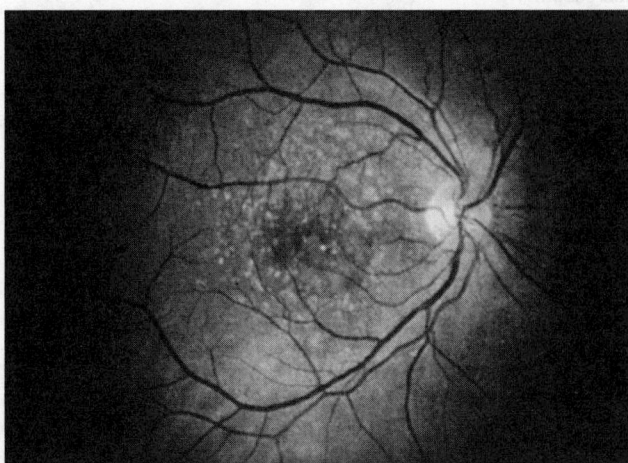

Figure 97.1. Hard drusen are the tiny dots in the central retina (macular area). They are minimally elevated and, when viewed in color, are yellow-white. The visual acuity is normal.

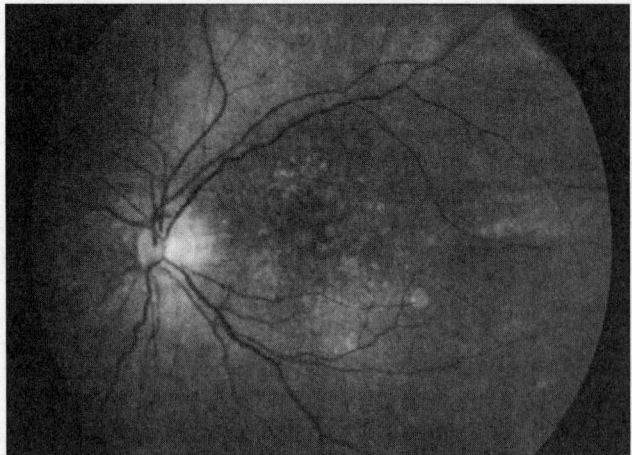

Figure 97.2. The larger blotches in the central retina are soft drusen. Patients with soft drusen are at increased risk of developing neovascular exudative macular degeneration. The visual acuity is normal.

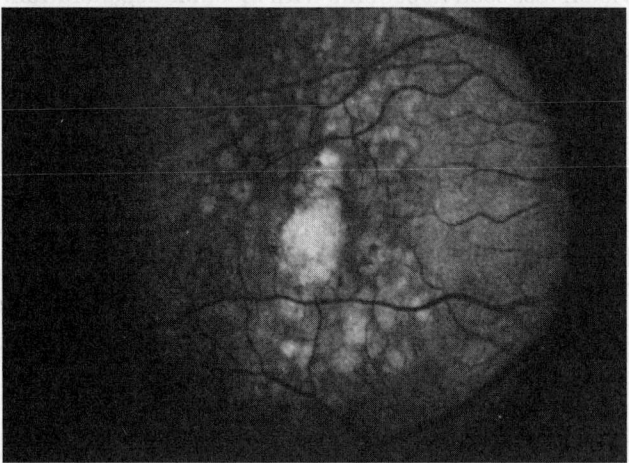

Figure 97.3. The patient with nonneovascular atrophic macular degeneration has hard and soft drusen. There is a zone of central atrophy, and if the center of the macula is involved, vision is usually decreased.

lead to pigment epithelial detachment. Choroidal neovascularization may grow through or actually cause breaks in Bruch's membrane. The new blood vessels beneath the retina are the cause of the hemorrhage and lipid accumulation (Fig. 97.5*A*). After the active phase, subretinal fibrosis or a so-called disciform scar is seen (Fig. 97.5B and C).

Although the subretinal new vessels are rarely directly visible, the technique of *fluorescein angiography* allows their diagnosis (Fig. 97.6). Intravenous fluorescein dye is injected in the antecubital fossa. Within 10 to 20 seconds, the dye can be photographed traversing vessels in the eye. The presence of increasing hyperfluorescence in certain patterns as the angiogram progresses is a marker for choroidal neovascularization. The interpretation of fluorescein angiograms is complex and requires the expertise of an ophthalmolo-

gist experienced in the procedure. For patients allergic to fluorescein, and perhaps in special situations, indocyanine green (ICG) angiography may be useful and is being used by some retina specialists. Because ICG contains iodine, the ophthalmologist may request that metformin be temporarily discontinued.

Natural History and Treatment

The natural history of bilateral drusen is uncertain. Patients who have exudative disease in one eye and drusen only in the second eye have a rate of 4 to 15% per year of the development of exudative disease in the previously uninvolved eye. In high-risk nonneovascular disease (numerous large drusen and pigment changes) if the fellow eye already has choroidal neovascularization, there is approximately a 50% or greater chance the second eye will be involved within 5 years. Patients with macular degeneration should be examined by an ophthalmologist at least annually or, in high-risk cases, perhaps twice annually.

Although numerous dietary and vitamin therapies have been recommended for patients with the atrophic form of the disease, no information is available at this time that substantiates these recommendations. The one investigator who has reported a benefit from oral zinc supplementation for macular degeneration concludes that because of the pilot nature of the study and the possible toxic effects of the drug, widespread use of zinc in patients with macular degeneration is not warranted (7). The Age-Related Eye Disease Study is investigating the role of vitamin supplementation over a 10-year period. Four thousand patients have been randomized and have reached 4 or 5 years of follow-up as of 1998. Results are not expected until the early 2000s.

Because chronic light toxicity may play a role in the pathogenesis of macular degeneration, avoidance of sunlight has been considered. One review (1) con-

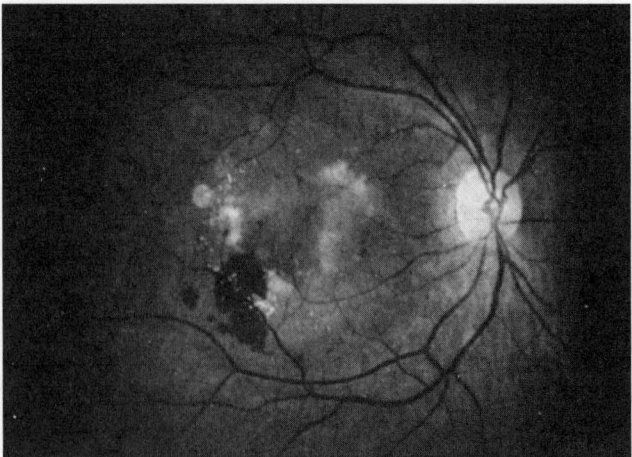

Figure 97.4. Neovascular macular degeneration. There is subretinal blood and lipid. Subretinal fluid can be seen on stereoscopic photographs (not shown). The patient has choroidal neovascularization.

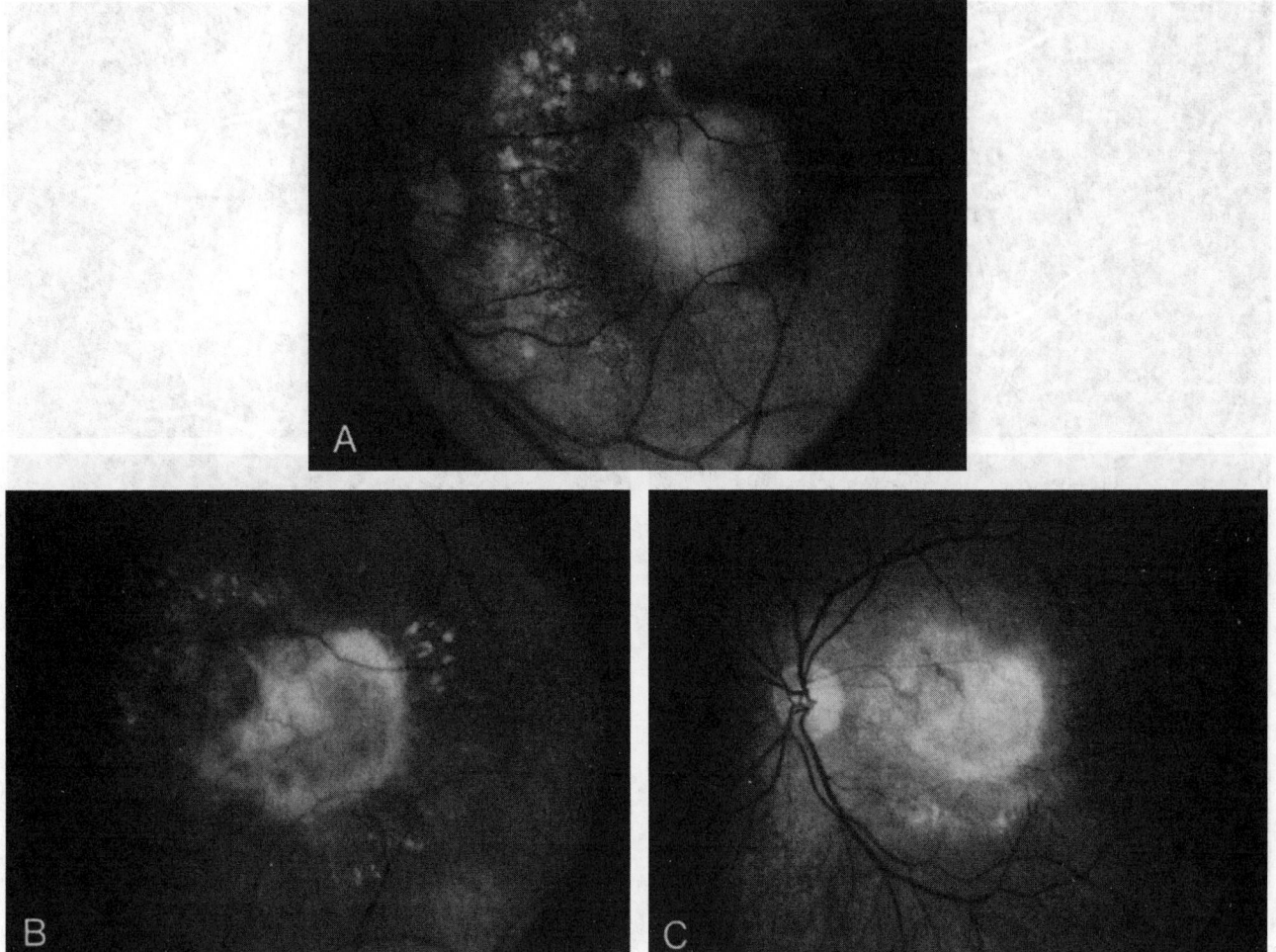

Figure 97.5. **A.** Neovascular macular degeneration characterized by blood, lipid, and subretinal fluid accumulation, all sequelae of choroidal neovascularization. **B.** Six months later the blood has resorbed, the lipid is less, and subretinal fibrosis is beginning. **C.** One year later, a disciform scar has formed.

cludes that no data exist to support the notion that any form of sunglasses can reduce chronic photic insult and thereby reduce a putative factor in the development of age-related macular degeneration. Nevertheless, the use of sunglasses is inexpensive and without side effects and therefore should not be discouraged.

There is a treatment for a small subgroup of patients with neovascular disease, but because the clinical features are subtle and the treatment is beyond the scope of general practice, referral to an ophthalmologist is indicated. The Macular Photocoagulation Study (MPS) compared the value of laser photocoagulation with no treatment for patients with well-defined choroidal neovascularization outside the center of the macular area. After 3.5 years' follow-up, 62% of untreated patients had a loss of six or more lines of vision on a Snellen chart, compared with 47% of treated patients. The difference is statistically significant (6). Subsequent investigations by the MPS investigators extended the treatment recommendations to include lesions closer to the center of the macula (juxtafoveal lesions) as well as lesions in the macular center (subfoveal lesions). A large randomized trial of interferon, a systemic agent with antiangiogenesis activity, showed no benefit. Other antiangiogenesis agents are under study. There are numerous reports concerning low-dose radiation therapy. Radiation has antiangiogenesis effects. The results are contradictory but the treatment is of doubtful benefit. Surgery to remove the abnormal blood vessels from beneath the retina is under investigation in a large prospective randomized trial (Subfoveal Surgery Trial, or SST) and results are expected shortly after the completion of the study in 1999 or 2000. A new low-energy laser combined with an intravenous photosensitizing agent is under study. Given the poor natural history, general physicians should encourage their patients with macular degeneration to seek active investigational protocols when appropriate.

ADVICE FOR THE VISUALLY IMPAIRED

When vision cannot be improved or maintained at an acceptable level, it is important for the physician to aid

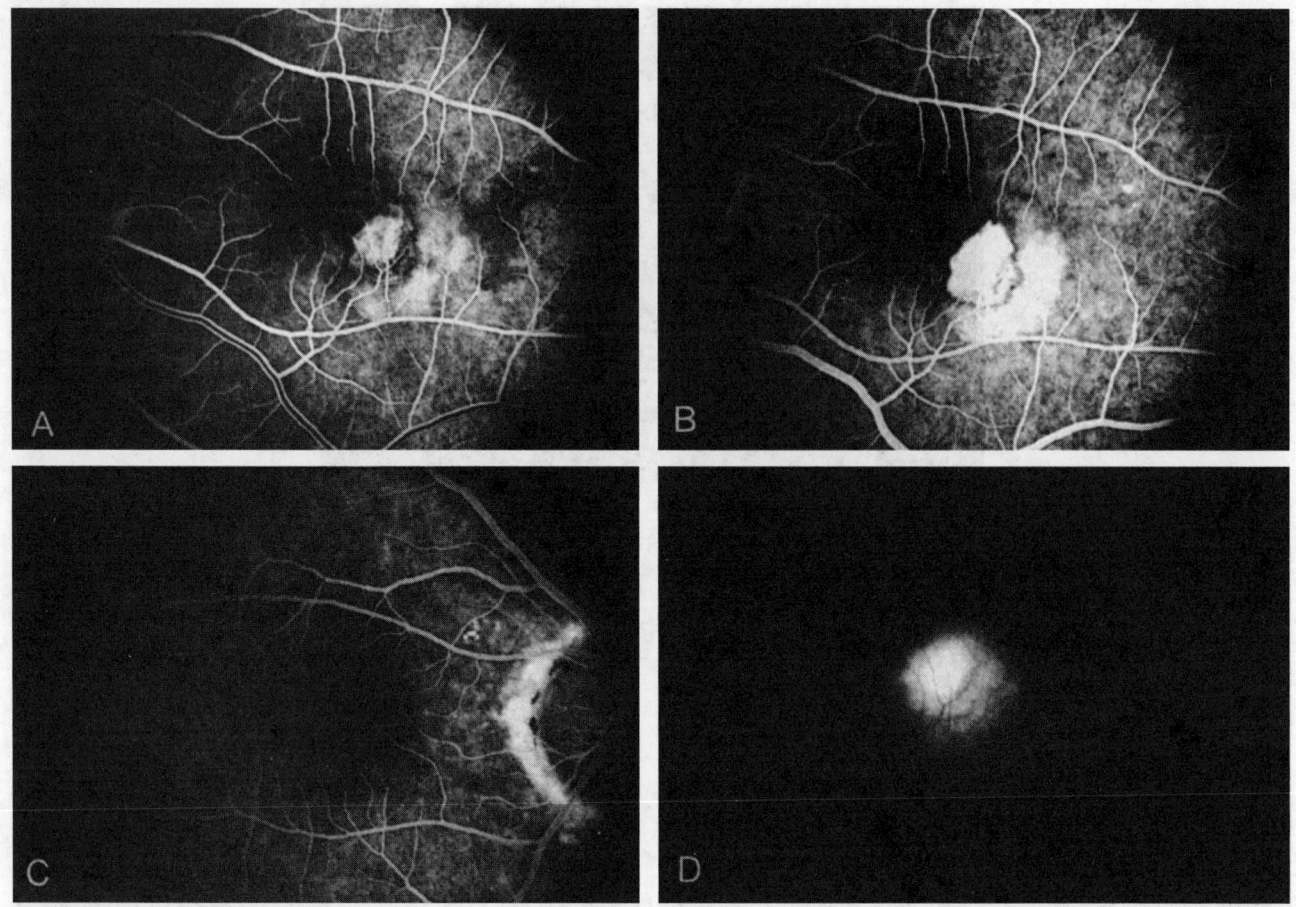

Figure 97.6. Fluorescein angiogram of choroidal neovascularization. **A.** In the early phase, 18 seconds after intravenous injection of dye, the fluorescein is seen filling retinal arteries and laminar venous filling is beginning. A zone of hyperfluorescence (brightness) is seen at the inferotemporal aspect of the macula. This is caused by dye leaking from abnormal choroidal vessels (choroidal neovascularization). **B.** The leaking increases 10 seconds later. **C.** For comparison, a view of the normal fellow eye illustrates a normal angiographic pattern. **D.** A late frame, taken approximately 10 minutes after the injection, shows continued leaking of dye from the choroidal new vessels.

the patient in finding resources that may provide some help in lessening the ever-increasing isolation and loss of mobility that result from blindness. Dr. DeWitt Stetten (see "General References") wrote an essay describing his experience with progressive blindness, outlining a number of useful aids that he identified. He describes the increasingly available large-print books, journals, and newsprint (e.g., *The New York Times*). Many books are available on tape from the *Talking Books Program* of the Library of Congress. Most local libraries can provide information on the availability of these tapes. Some journals may be obtained on tapes from *Recorded Periodicals* (919 Walnut St., Philadelphia, PA 19107). *Newsweek* magazine is available on disposable phonographic records (Newsweek, P.O. Box 6435, 1839 Frankfort Ave., Louisville, KY 40206). A variety of aids for the blind may be ordered from the catalog of SFB Products (Box 385, Wayne, PA 19087) or the Lighthouse low-vision products (36-20 Northern Blvd., Long Island City, NY 11101, telephone 800-453-4923). A portable cassette tape recorder designed for the blind can be purchased through the American Printing House for the Blind, Inc. (General Office, P.O. Box 6085, Louisville, KY 40206). Talking clocks and Braille timepieces may be very useful, and information concerning these and other aids are available from the National Institutes of Health (Volunteers for the Visually Handicapped, 4405 East–West Hwy., Bethesda, MD 20814). Several reading machines or magnifying devices are also available, although these are expensive (see Stetten, "General References").

Visual Foundation, Inc. (770 Center St., Newton, MA 02158) is a self-help organization developed by people with impaired vision. They have published a handbook, *Coping with Sight Loss*, that provides information for the visually impaired on visual aids, devices, recreation, tax benefits, reading materials, and referral sources. The handbook is published in large print and on cassette tapes and is a useful resource for the patient experiencing loss of vision as well as for physicians caring for these patients.

General References

Elman MJ, Fine SL. Exudative age-related macular degeneration. In: Ryan SJ, ed. Retina. 2nd ed. St. Louis: CV Mosby, 1994;1103–1141.

Jaffe NS, Jaffe MS, Jaffe GF. Cataract surgery and its complications. St. Louis: CV Mosby, 1990.

Liesegang TJ. Cataracts and cataract operation: two parts. Mayo Clin Proc 59:556, 622, 1984.

Sarks SH, Sarks JP. Age-related macular degeneration: atrophic form. In: Ryan SJ, ed. Retina. 2nd ed. St. Louis: CV Mosby, 1994;1071–1102.

Stark WJ, Woethen DM, Holladay JT, et al. The FDA report on intraocular lenses. Ophthalmology 90:311, 1983.
    The standard reference regarding intraocular lenses.

Stetten D Jr. Coping with blindness. N Engl J Med 305:458, 1981.
    A concise description of aids to help cope with blindness, written by Dr. Stetten as he experienced progressive vision loss.

Straatsma BR, Foos RY, Horwitz J, et al. Aging-related cataract: laboratory investigation and clinical management. Ann Intern Med 102:82, 1985.
    This UCLA conference reviews all aspects of senescent cataracts and contains superb color photographs of a variety of common cataract patterns.

Specific References

1. Bressler NM, Bressler SB, Fine SL. Age-related macular degeneration. Surv Ophthalmol 32:375, 1988.
2. Klein BE, Klein E. Cataracts and macular degeneration in older Americans. Arch Ophthalmol 100:571, 1982.
3. Klein R, Klein BEK, Jensen SC, Meuer SM. The five-year incidence and progression of age-related maculopathy. The Beaver Dam Eye Study. Ophthalmology 104:7, 1997.
4. Lee PL, Spritzer K, Hays R. The impact of blurred vision on functioning and well-being. Ophthalmology 104:390, 1997.
5. Leibowitz H, Krueger DE, Maudner LR, et al. The Framingham Eye Study Monograph. Surv Ophthalmol 24(Suppl):335, 1980.
6. Macular Photocoagulation Study Group. Argon laser photocoagulation for neovascular maculopathy: three-year results from randomized clinical trials. Arch Ophthalmol 104:694, 1986.
7. Newsome DA, Swartz M, Leone NC, et al. Oral zinc in macular degeneration. Arch Ophthalmol 106:192, 1988.
8. Phillips CI, Donnelly CA, Clayton RM, Cuthbert J. Skin disease and age-related cataract. Acta Derm Venereol (Stockholm) 76:314, 1996.
9. Tielsch JM, Legro MW, Cassard SD, Schein OD, et al. Risk factors for retinal detachment after cataract surgery. A population-based case-control study. Ophthalmology 103:1537, 1996.

C H A P T E R   98

Glaucoma

ANDREW P. SCHACHAT, MD

Anatomy and Physiology	1481
Types of Glaucoma	1482
Primary Open-Angle Glaucoma	1482
Primary Angle-Closure Glaucoma	1485

Glaucoma is a common disorder characterized by an increase in intraocular pressure sufficient to cause damage to the optic nerve. It is the second leading cause of blindness in the United States. Almost 2 million Americans have it, but only half know they have it. The glaucomas are classified into primary and secondary groups (Table 98.1). The primary group accounts for 95% of all patients with glaucoma in the United States.

Patients with glaucoma usually are followed by an ophthalmologist. However, the general physician needs to be familiar with the techniques of screening for and diagnosing glaucoma and with the long-term care of patients who have glaucoma.

ANATOMY AND PHYSIOLOGY

The *aqueous humor* helps maintain the shape of the eye and the correct relationship among the refractile elements of the eye; it also provides the nutrition of the avascular intraocular structures such as the lens (Fig. 98.1). There is continuous production and removal of the aqueous humor. In most cases of glaucoma, an obstruction to the outflow of aqueous humor appears to be the basis for the increased intraocular pressure.

The aqueous humor is a clear ultrafiltrate of the blood and occupies part of the posterior and anterior chambers of the eye. It is produced by the ciliary epithelium of the ciliary body, which is a portion of the uveal tract of the eye. It appears most likely that the aqueous is formed partially by secretion and partially by a process of ultrafiltration. At least two enzymes have been implicated in aqueous formation: sodium/potassium–activated ATPase and carbonic anhydrase. Antagonists of these enzymes appear to reduce the rate of aqueous formation and thereby lower intraocular pressure; however, the precise mechanism of action of these drugs is uncertain. Once produced, the aqueous humor circulates from the posterior chamber into the anterior chamber of the eye. The trabecular meshwork, an intricate system of connective tissue fibers, is located in the periphery of the anterior chamber. The aqueous percolates through this meshwork to be reunited with the venous blood via Schlemm's canal.

TYPES OF GLAUCOMA

Table 98.1 outlines the major types and causes of glaucoma. However, only primary open-angle glaucoma and primary angle-closure glaucoma are discussed in this chapter because they are the only types likely to be seen with any frequency by the general physician. Open-angle glaucoma takes its name from the normal-appearing anterior chamber angle, a contrast to the narrow angle of angle-closure glaucoma, as shown in Figure 98.2. General physicians may hear the term *normal-tension glaucoma* (NTG). NTG is basically open-angle glaucoma in patients who appear to have pressures in the normal range; the patients probably are more susceptible to damage than the general population.

Table 98.1.   Types of Glaucoma

Primary
Open-angle: 90% of patients
Angle-closure: 5% of patients
Congenital: infant and juvenile onset

Secondary
Open-angle: Results from topical or systemic steroids, ocular inflammation, or obstructed venous return from the eye (e.g., carotid cavernous sinus fistula)
Angle-closure: Results from trauma, neovascular change in the iris, ocular neoplasia, cataract surgery, and iris degeneration from various causes

Primary Open-Angle Glaucoma

Prevalence and Risk Factors

Primary open-angle glaucoma is by far the most common cause of glaucoma in the United States; the prevalence increases after the age of 40 years and approaches 3% of people over 75 years of age. Indeed, because open-angle glaucoma is so prevalent, is asymptomatic, and is treatable, open-angle glaucoma is the primary reason behind the recommendation for annual eye examination for people 65 years and older. Primary open-angle glaucoma causes 15 to 20% of all blindness in this country (see Chapter 97 for a discussion of blindness). Men and women are affected equally, but African Americans are affected at a higher frequency and at an earlier age, and open-angle glaucoma is the leading cause of blindness in African Americans. Open-angle glaucoma is familial, but the pattern of inheritance is not yet known with certainty. In patients who have a positive family history of glaucoma, there is an association between glaucoma and leukocyte antigen HLA-B12. It has been proposed that there is an association between open-angle glaucoma and both diabetes mellitus and elevated blood pressure, but these hypotheses are uncertain and more research is necessary to define such relationships. Patients who have high degrees of myopia (near vision) are often said to have a higher risk of open-angle glaucoma, but there remains uncertainty about this hypothesis as well. The glau-

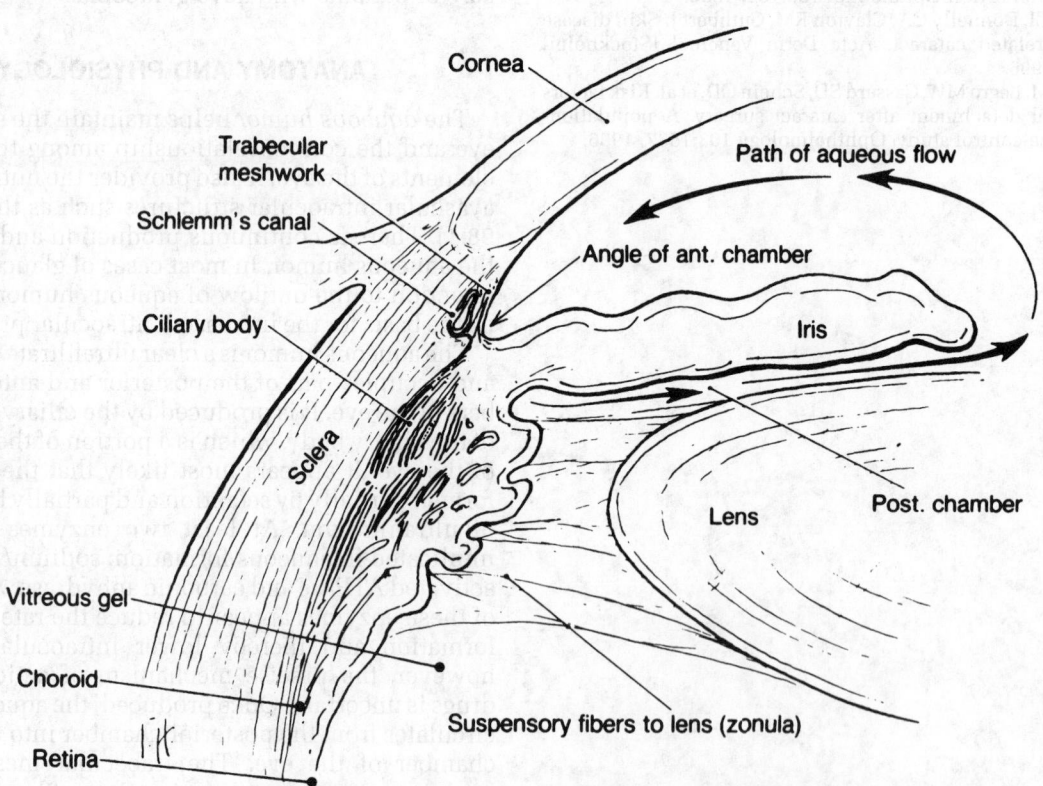

Figure 98.1.   Anatomy of the eye: cross-section of the cornea. (From Basmajian JV. Grant's method of anatomy. 8th ed. Baltimore: Williams & Wilkins, 1971;543.)

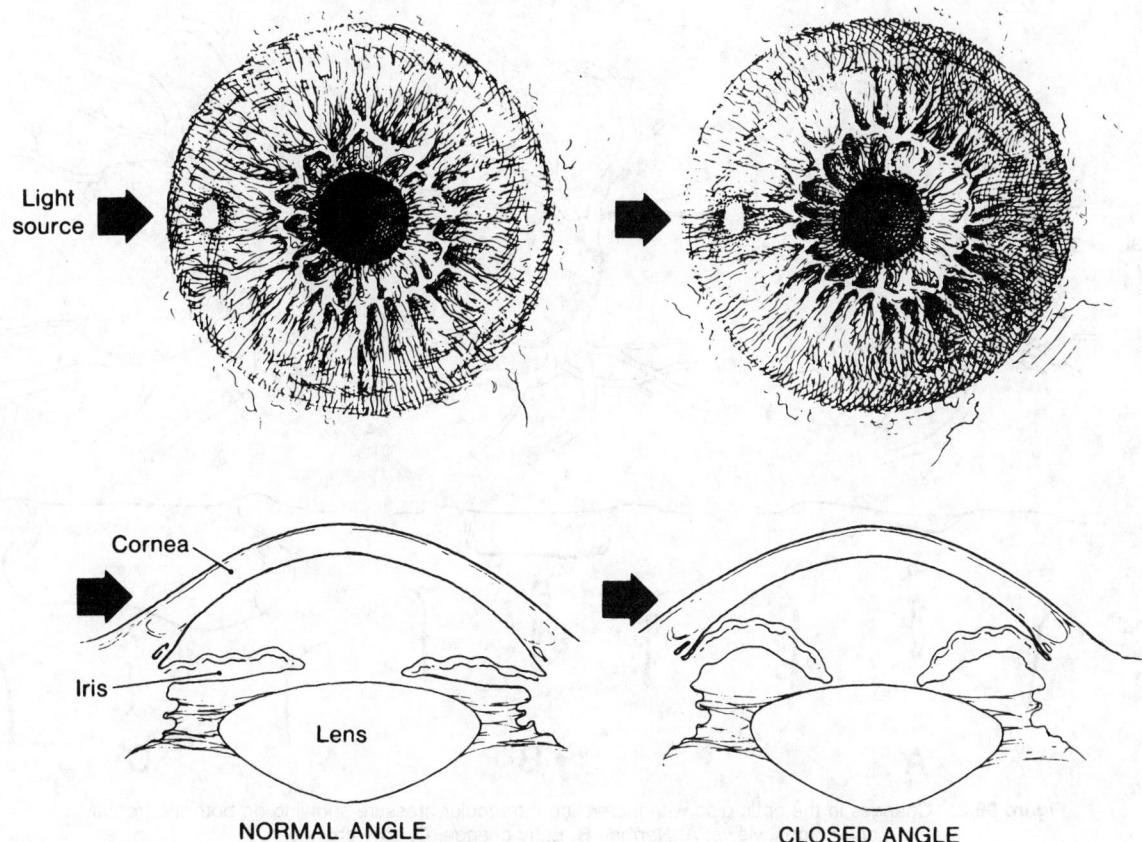

Figure 98.2. Illustration showing a shadow cast on the nasal side of the iris resultant from the bowed iris in angle-closure glaucoma. In open-angle glaucoma, the iris is not bowed, so the shadow is not cast.

coma risk may be increased with prolonged use of asthma inhalers (2).

Manifestations and Physical Examination

In primary open-angle glaucoma, elevated eye pressure appears to result from increased resistance in the trabecular meshwork to aqueous outflow. The elevation of the intraocular pressure is roughly related to the degree of obstruction. The disease is asymptomatic until its latest stages. When symptoms do occur, neural damage is present and may be substantial. Macular (central) vision and the ability to recognize forms on a vision test chart are preserved until very late. For this reason, testing of visual acuity is not a reliable method to screen for glaucoma. Occasionally, a patient with open-angle glaucoma may notice halos around lights and blurring of vision if there is a sudden rise in intraocular pressure, as might occur with rapid ingestion of a large quantity of fluid (e.g., 1 L). Patients with this history should be referred to an ophthalmologist. Patients with open-angle glaucoma rarely complain of headache that can be attributed to increased intraocular pressure.

The ocular pressure may be elevated for years before any change in the optic disc is noted. The change in the optic disc is revealed by increasing excavation of the central physiologic disc cup, visible on fundus-

copic examination (Fig. 98.3). This is most easily seen by use of the red filter of the direct ophthalmoscope. Over years the pink color of the disc fades and becomes pale, and vessels coursing over the disc show a sharp bend at the rim. Patients thought to have an enlarged optic cup should be referred to an ophthalmologist.

The general physician should assume that open-angle glaucoma has no symptoms until the patient is on the verge of blindness. Detection must be accomplished based on knowledge of risk factors (age, race, and family history) and examination findings. The diagnosis is then confirmed after referral to an ophthalmologist.

In evaluating the patient with increased intraocular pressure, the ophthalmologist performs tonometry to measure the eye pressure, gonioscopy (see below), funduscopy, and visual field examinations (see below). Characteristic visual field changes called nerve fiber bundle defects are seen in glaucoma.

Screening for Open-Angle Glaucoma

The ideal method for screening for primary open-angle glaucoma is controversial, and high false-positive and false-negative detection rates are the norm. Nevertheless, screening seems reasonable because the disease is silent until permanent ocular damage has occurred, screening is relatively simple in

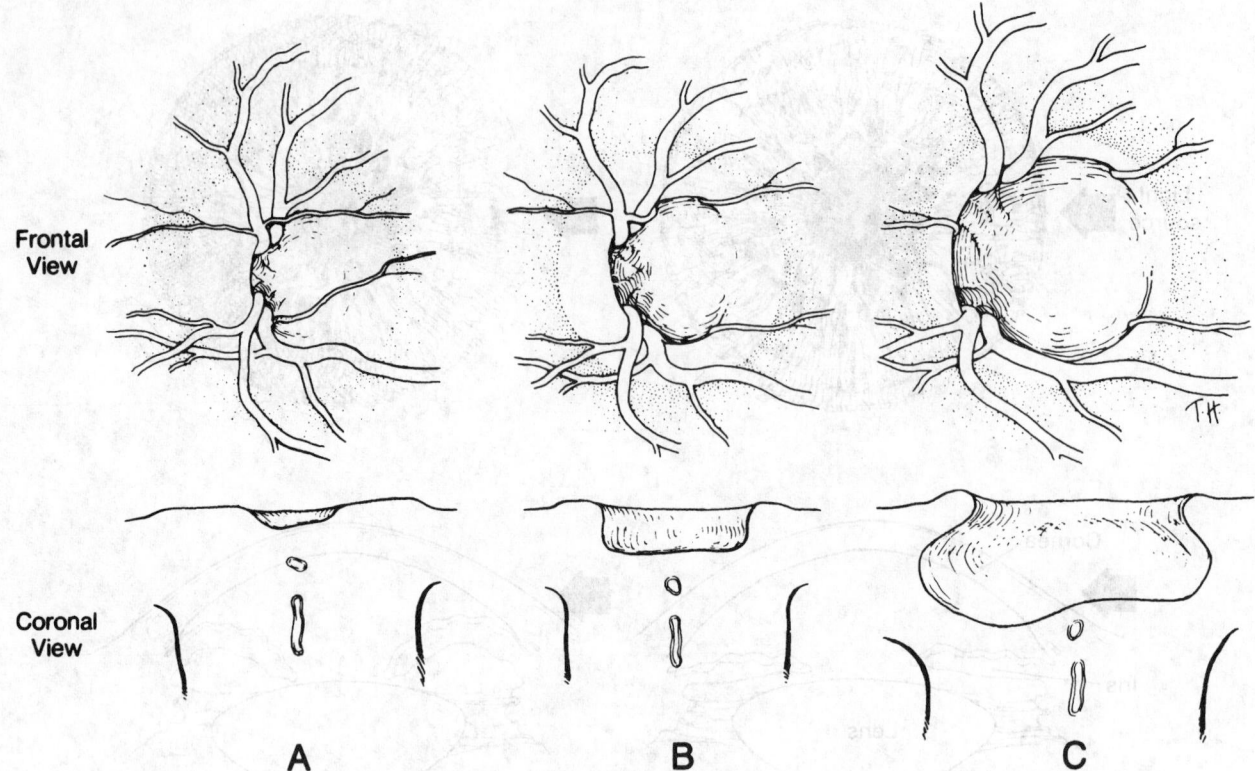

Figure 98.3. Changes in the optic disc with increasing intraocular pressure showing on both the frontal and coronal views: **A.** Normal. **B.** Early change. **C.** Late change.

experienced hands and without significant risk, treatment usually can prevent eye damage, and this form of glaucoma is common, especially in older patients.

Screening in theory could be accomplished in one or more of three ways: tonometry, funduscopic assessment of the optic cup through the dilated pupil, and visual field assessment. For years it has been recommended that primary care physicians screen high-risk patients for glaucoma by measuring eye pressure directly with a Schiötz tonometer. This approach is now believed to be too insensitive and nonspecific to be of value. Current thinking suggests that combinations of tests are needed to improve the sensitivity and specificity of glaucoma screening. Ophthalmologists generally do all three evaluations, but this is not practical for the general physician. For this reason, the report of the United States Preventive Services Task Force (see "General References") does not recommend the routine performance of tonometry by primary care physicians. Instead, primary care physicians are encouraged to advise patients aged 65 and older (those at high risk) to be referred to an eye specialist every year or two for glaucoma screening. African Americans should be referred at an earlier age, perhaps even age 40.

Patients referred to an ophthalmologist generally have an evaluation consisting of several observations: determination of the intraocular pressure by applanation tonometry, by use of a complex piece of equipment, and requiring only a drop of topical anesthetic; funduscopic assessment of the optic disc and retina

through the dilated pupil; visual field assessment, usually with a computerized perimeter; and gonioscopic examination, which permits the ophthalmologist to visualize the angle of the anterior chamber by using an instrument containing a contact lens and mirror. The patient usually experiences minimal or no discomfort during these procedures.

Approximately one-third of patients who on preliminary screening are found to have asymptomatic increased intraocular pressure are found after thorough evaluation to have glaucoma. Approximately 30% may be found not to have elevated pressures on reassessment, and about 25% have "ocular hypertension" without glaucoma. This latter group of patients, with elevated intraocular pressure but with normal-appearing optic discs and normal visual fields, should be followed yearly by the ophthalmologist; approximately 1% of these patients develop glaucoma each year. The rate is higher for those with a positive family history of glaucoma and for those with the highest pressures.

Treatment

When the ophthalmologist establishes the diagnosis of open-angle glaucoma, treatment based on the level of intraocular pressure, the degree of visual field loss, and the amount of optic nerve damage is prescribed. Although a definitive controlled study on the efficacy of therapy in the prevention of visual damage from glaucoma has not been done, the overwhelming consensus is that treatment to lower the ocular pressure is beneficial to the patient.

The treatment of open-angle glaucoma has been largely medical, with use of agents that facilitate the outflow (e.g., miotics) or reduce the amount of production (e.g., β-blockers and carbonic anhydrase inhibitors) of aqueous humor. Many ophthalmologists now are considering initial laser treatment (laser trabeculoplasty, see below) as a first option; drug side effects are avoided, the surgical side effects are minimal, and quality of life may be enhanced. Cost, compared to the ongoing cost of the drugs, is not significant. In England, initial surgery is often advised. Which first step is better is open to debate and a randomized trial comparing medical management with immediate surgery is under way.

The aim of therapy is to maintain the intraocular pressure at a level that does not lead to optic nerve damage. This target pressure is usually 20 mm Hg. Patients are usually prescribed a topical β-blocker and sometimes epinephrine or a mild miotic, such as carbachol or pilocarpine. The β-adrenergic receptor blocking agent timolol maleate (e.g., Timoptic Ophthalmic Solution) reduces ocular pressure and has the advantage of producing little or no effect on pupil size or visual acuity. For this reason, decreased, blurred, or impaired night vision is not the problem with timolol that it is with miotic agents. However, significant systemic effects of the timolol maleate, including the exacerbation of congestive heart failure, may occur. Newer, more selective β-blocking agents such as levobunolol hydrochloride ophthalmic solution (Betagan) appear to have fewer systemic effects and for this reason are preferable for someone starting this therapy.

Other agents, such as carbonic anhydrase inhibitors and stronger miotics, are added or replace the milder agents as necessary. Acetazolamide (Diamox) and methazolamide (Neptazane), carbonic anhydrase inhibitors, have proved clinically important in the treatment of glaucoma. A topical carbonic anhydrase inhibitor, dorzolamide (Trusopt), has been introduced, has fewer side effects, and lowers eye pressure almost as well (3). Many ophthalmologists are using the newest pharmacologic agents. Therefore more and more the general physician will find patients receiving new versions of older drugs. Examples are Timolol gel (Timoptic XE), a new long-acting topical nonselective β-adrenergic blocking agent; and latanoprost (Xalatan), a prostaglandin analog about as effective as Timolol. Because it works by a different mechanism (increasing uveoscleral outflow), latanoprost is often used in combination with other drops. (However, about 1 in 14 patients on latanoprost develops a gradual change in eye color.) Brimonidine tartrate (Alphagan), a new selective α_2-adrenergic agent, is used three times daily.

Often, early in the course treatment must be changed because drug tolerance is common and side effects may occur. Once the decreased ocular pressure has been attained, the ophthalmologist usually examines the patient approximately three times per year for assessment of visual fields, measurement of intraocular pressure, funduscopic examination, and gonioscopy.

Argon laser trabeculoplasty (ALT) may be used by the ophthalmologist to lower ocular pressure when medical therapy is unsatisfactory. This office procedure requires only topical anesthesia and can result in a significant reduction in ocular pressure in nearly two-thirds of patients. However, most patients continue to require the continued use of medications. The mechanism by which laser trabeculoplasty exerts its beneficial effects is uncertain. As noted above, ALT is used as an initial treatment option by more and more ophthalmologists (1).

Surgery in primary open-angle glaucoma is designed to construct outflow channels for the aqueous humor or, in the worst cases, to freeze the ciliary body and destroy the site of aqueous production. In the last few years, tremendous advances have been made in glaucoma filtering surgery. The major problem with the procedure, which makes a hole in the eye to allow aqueous drainage into the subconjunctival space, is the tendency for healing, which closes the hole in younger patients and certain other groups at high risk for filter failure. Antineoplastic agents are being used to retard healing, with an important increase in the success rate. There is concern about late infections in all patients who have had glaucoma filtering surgery, and late infections may be more common in so-called antimetabolite procedures. Topical intraoperative mitomycin C, 5FU, and other agents are being used. Currently, unless results from new trials recommend otherwise, surgical procedures are reserved for patients in whom medical management fails. Medications may still be required after surgery.

Monitoring

The primary physician should ensure that the patient with open-angle glaucoma is receiving regular ophthalmologic follow-up and should be alert to any side effects from the drugs prescribed by the ophthalmologist (Table 98.2).

There has been particular concern about systemic medications that have anticholinergic (atropinelike), adrenergic, vasodilator, or corticosteroid properties and that may adversely affect ocular pressure. However, few data contraindicate the use of these agents in patients with open-angle glaucoma. Only if an anticholinergic drug paralyzes accommodation (noticeable as blurriness when the eyes are used for close work, as in reading) should there be concern about it causing increased ocular pressure; in this situation the drug should be withdrawn, or if its use is mandatory, an ophthalmologist should be consulted. Systemic corticosteroids and, in particular, corticosteroids applied to the eye in the absence of intraocular inflammation may make the control of open-angle glaucoma more difficult. There is no evidence that vasodilator or adrenergic drugs affect the course of glaucoma.

Primary Angle-Closure Glaucoma

Although this form of glaucoma is far less common than open-angle glaucoma, it is important that the

Table 98.2.   Systemic Effects of Medications Used to Treat Glaucoma

Considerable absorption of drug may occur through the nasal mucosa via flow through the lacrimal duct.

β-Adrenergic Blocking Agents
Pulmonary: bronchospasm (the incidence is markedly decreased with highly selective β-blockers)
Cardiovascular: bradycardia, hypotension, decreased cardiac contractility
Central nervous system: fatigue, depression, memory loss

Miotics (e.g., Pilocarpine)
Refractive error, decreased night vision especially in those with cataracts, ciliary muscle spasms, ocular burning; long-acting agents such as phospholine iodide because of irreversible depletion of cholinesterase may make general anesthesia dangerous

Sympathomimetics
Increased respiratory rate, headache, tremor, tachycardia, arrhythmia

Carbonic Anhydrase Inhibitor
Malaise, fatigue, anorexia, depression, decreased libido, systemic acidosis (especially a risk in those with severe respiratory disease or those taking large dosages of salicylates), nausea, vomiting, diarrhea, alterations in taste of carbonated beverages

Developed from Everitt DE, Avorn J. Systemic effects of medication used to treat glaucoma. Ann Intern Med 112:120, 1990.

general physician be aware of it because an attack may be precipitated by the use of mydriatics; if this occurs, urgent recognition and treatment are mandatory to prevent damage to the eye. In addition, all too often, cases of angle-closure glaucoma are misdiagnosed as possible neurosurgical conditions (because of symptoms such as headaches, nausea and vomiting, and visual loss) so recognition of the condition is important. Patients often have a positive family history, and women are affected more than men.

The basic defect in primary angle-closure glaucoma is the inability of aqueous humor to reach the filtration apparatus. When the pupil is dilated halfway, the iris is bowed forward, which blocks the outflow of aqueous humor (Fig. 98.2). The primary sire of aqueous blockage is the iris-lens touch. The iris bows forward as the pressure rises and there is blockage of the trabecular meshwork by the peripheral iris.

Patients who have narrow anterior ocular chambers are predisposed to primary angle-closure glaucoma. Moreover, the lens may be of such size that there is encroachment of the aqueous-filtering trabecular meshwork. Patients with these predispositions often have acute attacks of increased intraocular pressure when the eye is dilated, occluding aqueous outflow, as might occur in the dark or when a mydriatic is placed in the eye for funduscopic examination.

Diagnosis

Early diagnosis of this problem is critical because blindness may ensue and virtually every case is surgically curable if diagnosed early enough. Cure is increasingly less likely if repeated attacks have occurred and have resulted in scarring of the trabecular mesh-

work at the angle of the anterior chamber. The acute attack usually is unilateral and may be precipitated by emotion (from associated pupillary dilation). The classic symptoms are episodes of ocular pain (usually located in the periocular or supraocular region), episodes of blurred vision, and seeing halos around lights at night. These symptoms occur because of corneal epithelial edema that has developed as a result of the increased intraocular pressure. Often patients find relief in well-lighted rooms or outdoors, where daylight causes constriction of the pupil and opening of the angle of the anterior chamber.

Examination during an acute attack usually reveals marked elevation of intraocular pressure, to 60 to 90 mm Hg. However, chronic obstruction may compromise the circulation of the ciliary body and result in a fall in aqueous production and subsequently a reduction in ocular pressure. However, there is considerable individual tolerance of the vascular supply of the ciliary body to the increased pressure.

In patients predisposed to angle-closure glaucoma, the anterior chamber is shallow. This may be seen by illuminating the eye with a flashlight from the side and showing a shadow resulting from the bowed iris over the nasal portion of the eye (Fig. 98.2). Examination of the anterior chamber angle with a gonioscopic lens may reveal scarring of the trabecular meshwork and peripheral anterior synechia. Corneal edema is present during an acute attack, and the anterior chamber may appear cloudy because of inflammation.

If the diagnosis of acute angle-closure glaucoma is suspected, a prompt referral to an ophthalmologist is indicated. The ophthalmologist will probably initiate treatment with immediate administration of acetazolamide (Diamox) 250 mg orally, and instillation of 2 drops of a miotic such as pilocarpine (Pilocar) 4% every 15 minutes. If it will take hours to reach an ophthalmologist, the primary care physician should initiate therapy. In severe cases, the ingestion of hyperosmotic glycerol—1 mL/kg mixed as a 50% solution with chilled juice—almost always interrupts an acute attack. Hyperosmotic agents such as glycerol or intravenous mannitol dehydrate the vitreous and lower eye pressure. Physicians who use mydriatics for funduscopic examination or patients who have narrow anterior ocular chambers and who do not have immediate access to an ophthalmologist may want to have an angle-closure kit consisting of pilocarpine (Pilocar, 4%), glycerol (glycerin, available as generic), and acetazolamide (Diamox) for use during an acute attack. Patients found to have a shallow anterior chamber even if they have not had a symptomatic attack of glaucoma should be referred to an ophthalmologist for evaluation, for education regarding specific manifestations of an acute attack, and for their initial treatment, usually prophylactic argon laser iridectomy.

Differential Diagnosis

The patient who has acute angle-closure glaucoma may come with an acute red eye to a general physician.

Initially the physician will want to differentiate angle-closure glaucoma from acute iritis, acute conjunctivitis, and iridocyclitis. Chapter 99 discusses this differential diagnosis.

Course Without Treatment

Severe attacks of angle-closure glaucoma may cause blindness in 2 to 3 days or less depending on the level of intraocular pressure and the sensitivity of the ciliary body and optic nerve to ischemia. In some instances, ciliary ischemia stops aqueous production before blindness occurs. However, repeated attacks are the rule, and these eventually result in scarring of the trabecular meshwork. The frequency and rapidity of recurrences are unpredictable. An examination between attacks usually reveals only a shallow anterior chamber (Fig. 98.2) and normal intraocular pressure. Peripheral anterior synechiae and segmental iris atrophy may be seen depending on the frequency and severity of previous attacks. A history of an acute attack, an actual acute attack, or the demonstration of a shallow anterior chamber should lead to prompt ophthalmologic consultation.

The treatment of primary angle-closure glaucoma is essentially surgical. If the diagnosis is made early enough in the course of the disease, a peripheral iridectomy can be done to prevent the attacks of increased intraocular pressure and the development of scarring. Laser peripheral iridectomy under topical anesthesia has little risk and results in cure in most cases. Surgical iridectomy may also be performed. The eye involved in an acute attack is operated on as soon as the attack is controlled (see above). Generally, the other eye is operated on prophylactically a week or so later. Follow-up care by the ophthalmologist after surgery is necessary. If pressure control has not been achieved, medical therapy (see above) may be necessary. However, this is unusual if surgery is performed early.

When the physician is aware that a patient has a narrow anterior chamber or is under treatment for angle-closure glaucoma, there should be concern about the use of certain medications. Systemic anticholinergics or adrenergic drugs may rarely precipitate an acute attack by causing dilation of the pupils. Corticosteroids or vasodilating drugs are not contraindicated in patients with angle-closure glaucoma.

General References

American Academy of Ophthalmology Preferred Practice Pattern Committee. Primary open angle glaucoma preferred practice pattern. San Francisco: American Academy of Ophthalmology, 1996.

Anderson DR. Automated static perimetry. St. Louis: CV Mosby, 1992.
> Explains the details of visual field testing.

Editorial. Intraocular pressure control in glaucoma. Lancet 2:81, 1984.
> A brief overview of current therapy of elevated intraocular pressure, with pertinent references.

Everitt DE, Avorn J. Systemic effects of medications used to treat glaucoma. Ann Intern Med 112:120, 1990.
> A brief review of the important systemic manifestations of topical and systemic drugs used to treat glaucoma.

Fraunfelder FT, Roy FN. Current ocular therapy. 4th ed. Philadelphia: WB Saunders, 1995.
> This text provides a brief review of many common eye problems. It gives excellent therapeutic guidelines and has some pertinent references.

Leske MC, Rosenthal J. Epidemiological aspects of open angle glaucoma. Am J Epidemiol 109:250, 1979.

Newell FW. Ophthalmology, principles and concepts. St. Louis: CV Mosby, 1996.

Quigley HA. Open-angle glaucoma. N Engl J Med 328:1097, 1993.

Remis LL, Epstein DL. Treatment of glaucoma. Annu Rev Med 35:195, 1984.

Shields MB. Textbook of glaucoma. 3rd ed. Baltimore: Williams & Wilkins, 1992.

Sommer A. Doyne lecture: glaucoma: facts and fancies. Eye 10:295, 1996.

U.S. Preventive Services Task Force. Screening for glaucoma. In: Guide to clinical preventive services. Baltimore: Williams & Wilkins, 1989;124.

Specific References

1. Committee on Ophthalmic Procedure Assessment, American Academy of Ophthalmology Board of Trustees. Laser trabeculoplasty for primary open angle glaucoma. Ophthalmol 103:1706, 1996.
2. Garbe E, LeLorier J, Boiuin JF, Suissa S. Inhaled and nasal glucocorticoids and the risks of ocular hypertension or open angle glaucoma. JAMA 277:722, 1997.
3. Maus TL, Larsson LI, McClaren JW, Brubaker RF. Comparison of dorzolamide and acetazolamide as suppressors of aqueous humor flow in humans. Arch Ophthalmol 115:45, 1997.

CHAPTER 99

The Red Eye

ANDREW P. SCHACHAT, MD

Red eye is common in an ambulatory practice. The problem is usually caused by an infection and most often is self-limited; however, there are serious considerations in the differential diagnosis that must be recognized so that an urgent ophthalmologic consultation can be obtained if necessary. This chapter provides a framework for the recognition of conditions that require consultation and provides a discussion of conditions that may be managed by the general physician. Figure 99.1 illustrates the important structures and landmarks of the external eye; Figure 98.1 shows the cross-sectional anatomy of the eye.

DIFFERENTIAL DIAGNOSIS

Conditions that Require Referral

Hyperacute conjunctivitis (see below), keratitis (corneal inflammation), iritis or uveitis (inflammation of the uveal tract), scleritis, and acute glaucoma are important vision-threatening conditions that cause a red eye; patients suspected of having one of these conditions should be referred to an ophthalmologist (Table 99.1).

Several important features of the history and physical examination (Table 99.2) show how this information may suggest a specific diagnosis. The patient should be asked specifically whether treatment for an ocular disorder has been given, whether pain in one or both eyes has been experienced, and whether there is visual loss or photophobia (light sensitivity). When the eyes are examined, it is essential to evaluate the following features: visual acuity, the nature of the discharge, the appearance of the cornea, the size and reactivity of the pupil, and the extent of the redness.

When evaluating the extent of redness, an attempt should be made to determine whether there is simply conjunctival injection or whether there is ciliary injection as well. The ciliary vessels run in the sclera beneath the conjunctiva. Ciliary injection usually causes a purplish or violaceous zone of injection around the cornea. Unlike the conjunctival vessels, ciliary vessels do not constrict after the administration of a weak solution of a mydriatic such as 2.5% phenylephrine (Neo-Synephrine). The conjunctival vessels move with the conjunctiva when the conjunctiva is touched with a cotton swab. Ciliary vessels do not. Glaucoma, keratitis, and scleritis are characterized in most cases by ciliary injection. In selected patients special tests, such as measurement of ocular tension or inspection of the eye after fluorescein staining, are necessary.

Specific Conditions

Acute glaucoma is discussed in Chapter 98.

Iritis may be caused by a specific problem such as trauma or infection, but often a specific cause cannot be identified. In this condition, failure to initiate proper treatment, which usually includes a dilating agent and corticosteroids, may result in permanent scarring that affects pupillary movement and in some cases may lead to secondary glaucoma.

Iritis can usually be recognized because it is a painful condition that characteristically is acute in onset and is associated with photophobia. Often vision is blurred as well. Occasionally, the pupil of the involved eye is small and fixed compared with the contralateral one. Typically the redness in iritis surrounds the cornea (so-called ciliary flush or injection). Patients suspected of having iritis should see an ophthalmologist urgently so that the diagnosis can be confirmed, the cause found, and treatment initiated.

Corneal injury is usually recognized easily because of intense pain localized to the cornea after an injury and because of identification of a corneal lesion. If the injury is secondary to minor trauma (corneal abrasion) from a foreign body, the foreign body should be removed and a patch placed over the eye for 24 hours; topical antiprostaglandins without patching are also considered (see "Foreign Body," below). On the other hand, if an extensive epithelial defect (as revealed by fluorescein staining) is present, urgent ophthalmologic referral is indicated.

Fluorescein staining is easily accomplished by moistening a sterile fluorescein strip in the lower conjunctival sac and waiting a moment for the fluorescein to diffuse into the tears. The epithelial defect stains a brilliant green. A penlight with a cobalt blue filter (e.g., Blu-Spot No. 2015, available from medical supply companies) is inexpensive and highlights fluorescein staining. Corneal ulcers also stain with fluorescein, but staining appears to be deeper, indicating subepithelial corneal involvement. Corneal ulceration can lead to blindness, and patients suspected of having this condition should see an ophthalmologist urgently.

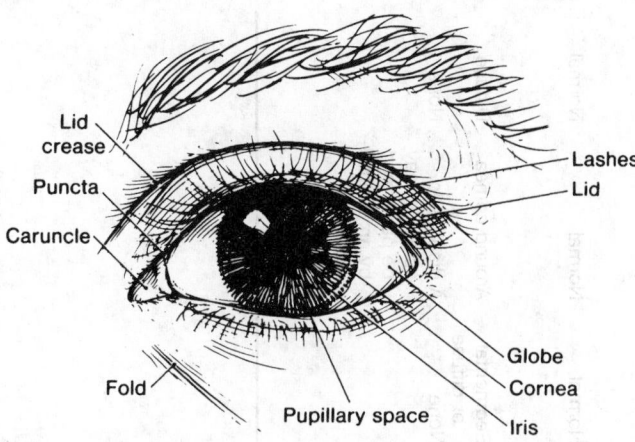

Figure 99.1. External landmarks of the eye.

Scleritis usually is seen in association with a systemic disorder (e.g., rheumatoid arthritis). Scleritis is often associated with iritis (see above). The patient usually complains of discomfort in the eye, and sometimes of severe pain, which is intensified if the eye is moved. The deep vessels of the sclera are dilated; this may be demonstrated by the instillation of a drop of phenylephrine (Neo-Synephrine) 2.5%, which constricts the superficial but not the deep vessels. However, mydriatics (e.g., Neo-Synephrine) should be avoided in patients with a history of narrow-angle glaucoma (see Chapter 98). The treatment of scleritis is usually complicated, and an ophthalmologist should be consulted urgently when scleritis is suspected.

Episcleritis is a common problem characterized by pain caused by a sharply localized area of inflammation of the superficial layer of the sclera. The cause is unknown, but it is occasionally associated with a systemic disorder such as rheumatoid arthritis or a specific infection such as herpes zoster or, rarely, tuberculosis. A few patients have an associated iritis (see above) that is usually mild. The palpebral conjunctiva (i.e., that lining the eyelid) is not involved and there is no discharge; these two observations help differentiate this problem from conjunctivitis. Episcleritis is short-lived but is often recurrent; for this reason, ophthalmologic consultation is indicated.

Hyperacute bacterial conjunctivitis (see below) is also a condition that should prompt urgent referral to an ophthalmologist.

Conditions that Usually Can Be Managed by the General Physician

Before making the decision to treat, a physician should ask the following:

- Has a thorough ocular examination been performed?
- Is there impaired vision and, if so, has an explanation for impaired visual acuity been identified?
- Is the natural history of the condition known or, if treatment is planned, is the usual response to treatment known?

- Has the appropriate follow-up arrangement been made to confirm that the condition is self-limited and improving and that referral to an ophthalmologist is not required?

Conjunctival infections, allergies, eyelid inflammation, and irritation are the most common causes of red or irritated eyes and are discussed in detail below. In many cases these problems can be managed without consulting an ophthalmologist.

CONJUNCTIVITIS

General Considerations

The diagnosis and management of conjunctivitis can be confusing, considering the variety of ocular infections. Most cases in adults are not emergencies, and, often, they are self-limited. However, conjunctivitis may lead to serious complications such as corneal scarring, lid damage, or, in cases in which the patient has had antecedent intraocular surgery, endophthalmitis.

Conjunctival Flora

Under normal conditions the conjunctival sac has a bacterial flora composed of several species. The most commonly encountered organism is *Staphylococcus albus,* followed by corynebacteria, *Staphylococcus aureus,* and *Streptococcus* species. Some normal patients harbor *Pseudomonas* species as well as fungi. This complex flora complicates the establishment of a specific cause in a patient with infectious conjunctivitis.

Presentation

Conjunctivitis is usually not painful, but often there is mild discomfort, burning, discharge, tearing, itching, and lid swelling. Vision is well preserved. Most often, infectious conjunctivitis is bilateral.

Laboratory Diagnosis

When there is doubt about the diagnosis, a simple culture or staining of the conjunctival material helps in

Table 99.1. Major Causes of a Red Eye

Conditions that Require Referral
Acute glaucoma
Acute iritis
Acute corneal tear or infection (keratitis)
Acute scleritis or episcleritis
Bacterial conjunctivitis (hyperacute)

Conditions that Usually Can Be Managed by the General Physician
Bacterial conjunctivitis (acute and chronic)
Viral conjunctivitis
Inclusion conjunctivitis
Allergic conjunctivitis
Chemical conjunctivitis
Foreign body
Subconjunctival hemorrhage

Table 99.2. Important Observations in Evaluation of a Patient with a Red Eye

	Glaucoma	Iritis	Corneal Injury	Scleritis	Episcleritis	Bacterial Conjunctivitis	Inclusion Conjunctivitis	Viral Conjunctivitis	Keratitis	Allergic Conjunctivitis
History of previous ocular disorder or condition predisposing to an ocular disorder	+/−	+/−	+	+	+	−	−	−	Often	Previous history of allergies
Pain[a]	+	+	+	+	+	Mild discomfort or burning	Mild discomfort or burning	Mild discomfort or burning		−
Visual acuity	Diminished and blurred	Blurred	Usually diminished	Normal	Normal	Normal	Occasionally blurred, if chronic	Normal	Diminished	Usually normal
Discharge	None	None	Usually none	None	None	Present: thick or thin	None or mucopurulent	Watery	Usually some	Mild or none
Appearance of cornea	May be hazy	Normal	May be streaky	Normal	Normal	Normal	Normal except if late when superior dots or streaking may be seen	Normal	Corneal opacity	Normal
Pupil	Often dilated, mid-dilated, or fixed	Small and different from opposite side	Normal	Normal	Normal	Normal	Normal	Normal	Normal	Normal
Redness	Around cornea	Around cornea	Localized or diffuse	Localized or diffuse	Localized	Diffuse	Diffuse (variable)	Segmental or diffuse	Around cornea	Diffuse
Selected evaluations	Ocular pressure[b] in eye is high (see Chapter 98)	Normal	Fluorescein stain[c] shows epithelial defect as brilliant green	A drop of Neo-Synephrine 2½ or 5% in conjunctiva will constrict superficial but not deep vessels (see the text)	None	None	None	None	A diagnostic scraping may be performed by an ophthalmologist	None

[a]Photophobia in addition to pain may be seen in varying degrees with nearly any of these conditions but its presence is neither universal nor diagnostic.

[b]Should not be measured if a discharge is present or a corneal ulceration is seen.

[c]Use individually packaged sterile fluorescein strips.

determining the cause and subsequent management of the condition. The eyes and conjunctivae are not sterile and organisms, even pathogens, may be cultured from normal subjects. A positive culture does not necessarily mean there is a clinical infection. Most often, however, an adequate diagnosis can be made from the appearance of the conjunctiva, and a culture is unnecessary. New immunologic tests are available and permit immediate diagnosis of some causes of infectious conjunctivitis, especially chlamydia. The availability of these tests varies from community to community. Therefore the general physician not familiar with their use should consult an ophthalmologist for a recommendation.

Culture

Specimens for culture should be obtained with a sterile cotton swab by everting the eyelid and wiping the conjunctival sac. This material should be obtained without topical anesthesia because the preservatives in the anesthetic solution inhibit the growth of organisms. The specimen must be transferred immediately into transport media or delivered immediately to the laboratory for culturing. When a culture is considered necessary, consideration should be given to culturing each eye separately, even if there is only monocular involvement, so that the apparently uninfected eye provides information about the nature of the normal flora.

Scraping

After culture, a topical anesthetic (e.g., Ophthaine) should be instilled, and scrapings of the conjunctiva, well away from the cornea, should be obtained. A sterile platinum spatula (available from medical supply stores) or the dull side of a sterile scalpel blade can be used to scrape the conjunctiva. The material obtained by this method is smeared on a glass slide and stained with Gram's stain or Giemsa stain. The appearance of the cells found in these scrapings is helpful in determining the diagnosis, so scraping is recommended in the evaluation of patients with conjunctivitis when the diagnosis is uncertain. Most general physicians prefer to consult an ophthalmologist in situations wherein scrapings are considered. The differential findings are discussed below and listed in Table 99.3.

Table 99.3. Diagnosis Based on Cells in Material Scraped from Conjunctiva

Cells	Significance
Polymorphonuclear leukocytes	Bacterial, fungal, chlamydial (inclusion conjunctivitis), trachoma, Stevens–Johnson syndrome
Mononuclear cells	Viral
Eosinophils	Allergy, ocular pemphigoid
Epithelial metaplasia (atypical, large cells)	*Chlamydia*, herpes simplex

Specific Types

Hyperacute Bacterial Conjunctivitis

The name of this condition reflects its onset and the very thick exudate associated with it (Fig. 99.2, Color Plate 1). Typically, the discharge is so copious that it accumulates in the lashes or runs down the patient's cheek. One eye is usually involved before the other, but within several days the second eye becomes involved through autoinoculation. The infection quickly involves the surrounding structures and is associated with aching discomfort, swelling of the lid, and tenderness of the eye. Enlarged preauricular lymph nodes are often present. Early in the infection the cornea is not involved, but as the conjunctival swelling and reaction increase, a peripheral corneal ring ulcer may develop because of compression of the peripheral corneal circulation.

Neisseria gonorrhoeae or *Neisseria meningitidis* is usually implicated in this infection. Inoculation is a result of spread by an inanimate object or substance or through autoinoculation from infected genitalia. The gonococcus has the ability to penetrate the intact corneal epithelium, so central corneal ulceration and endophthalmitis may also occur. Meningococcal conjunctivitis is indistinguishable from gonococcal conjunctivitis, although the former occurs more often in younger patients, may be bilateral at the onset, and can proceed to metastatic meningitis or meningococcemia.

Conjunctival scrapings reveal an overwhelming number of polymorphonuclear leukocytes and intracellular Gram-negative diplococci. Culture should be obtained on Thayer–Martin selective medium or should be sent to the laboratory on Transgrow medium. The differentiation between gonococcus and meningococcus requires special bacteriologic studies.

Therapy of hyperacute conjunctivitis must be prompt to avoid corneal damage or systemic spread and should include the administration of both systemic and topical antibiotics. Because of the seriousness of this condition, an ophthalmologist should be consulted immediately. Institution of appropriate antibiotics by the ophthalmologist should result in the disappearance of the discharge within 24 to 48 hours, although lid swelling and conjunctival reaction do not abate for several days. If a corneal ulcer occurs, it is slow to heal; if the cornea has been scarred, visual acuity may be affected. In rare cases endophthalmitis may occur, and blindness is possible.

Acute Bacterial Conjunctivitis

Acute bacterial conjunctivitis, like hyperacute bacterial conjunctivitis, has an abrupt onset but is characterized by a less thick, often mucopurulent discharge. This form of conjunctivitis is often called catarrh or *pink eye* (Fig. 99.3, Color Plate 1); it is seen at all ages and at any time of year. *Pink eye* is a nonspecific term applied to almost any minor infectious conjunctivitis, especially bacterial and viral forms. The most common cause of bacterial conjunctivitis is *S. aureus* infection. *Pneumococcus* and *Haemophilus* species also cause the problem, but infections with these organisms have a more restricted geographic distribution than do staphylococcal infections; pneumococcal infections occur primarily in the northern states during the colder months, and *Haemophilus infections* occur more commonly in the warmer regions of the United States throughout the year. Also, pneumococcal or *Haemophilus conjunctivitis* is more common in younger patients than is staphylococcal conjunctivitis. Rarely, other bacteria, such as *Moraxella lacunata, Escherichia coli,* or *Proteus* species, cause this form of conjunctivitis.

Patients complain of eye irritation and watering, and typically the eyelids stick together after sleep. The infection starts unilaterally, but very often, because of autoinoculation, the contralateral eye becomes involved in 1 or 2 days. Examination reveals hyperemia of the palpebral conjunctiva (i.e., the conjunctival side of the eyelid); bulbar conjunctival petechiae, characteristic of *Haemophilus* infection, may be seen.

Acute bacterial conjunctivitis is usually self-limited and generally lasts 7 to 14 days, although *Haemophilus* infections may last somewhat longer.

The diagnosis is suspected by the examination; however, whenever there is doubt, diagnosis should be confirmed by examination of the scrapings of the conjunctiva and by culturing the exudate.

Topical treatment usually results in the resolution of symptoms in a day or two. A number of topical antibiotics are available, and one should be used for 5 to 6 days. Sodium sulfacetamide (Sulamyd-10%)—either the solution (two drops in the eye every 3 hours while awake) or the ointment (a small amount applied to the lower conjunctival sac four times a day and at bedtime)—is generally satisfactory. If there is an allergy to sulfa drugs, a 1% chloramphenicol ointment (Chloromycetin ophthalmic ointment), four times a day and at bedtime, may be used. Also, cool compresses several times a day may provide comfort and diminish matting.

Chronic Bacterial Conjunctivitis

S. aureus causes most cases of chronic bacterial conjunctivitis, but occasionally it is caused by other agents, such as *Staphylococcus epidermidis, Moraxella lacunata, Corynebacterium diphtheriae,* or *Streptococcus pyogenes. S. aureus* colonizes the margin of the eyelid and the follicles containing the eyelashes. Both *S. aureus* and *S. epidermidis* elaborate an exotoxin that injures the conjunctiva and cornea, and this toxin is responsible for the chronic inflammation.

Patients with chronic bacterial conjunctivitis complain of a sensation of a foreign body in the eye as well as of redness and itching; often eyelids stick together after sleep. There is often a history of recurrent styes (see below) and loss of eyelashes. Examination shows erythema of the lid margin, and sometimes a minimal exudate is present. Occasionally, mucous strands may be found in the conjunctival fornices, and the eyelids may appear thickened and red (Fig. 99.4, Color Plate 1).

The lid margins, surrounding skin, conjunctiva, and cornea may be involved singly or collectively. The skin may also show changes of seborrheic dermatitis or it may be excoriated and macerated, especially at the lateral canthal margin. Crusting is noted at the bases of the eyelashes. The conjunctiva may show changes of papillary hyperplasia (multiple conjunctival mounds with a central single vessel). Corneal changes occur after months of inflammation and are manifest as fine, discrete peripheral defects. There may also be ulceration, clouding, and vascularization of the margins of the cornea.

The diagnosis is made by examination and, in cases in doubt, by scraping the conjunctivae as well as the margins of the eyelids and by culturing the exudate.

Usually, gentamicin or tobramycin solution or ointment (Garamycin or Tobrex ophthalmic drops or ointment), one or two drops or a small amount of ointment every 4 hours while awake, or erythromycin ointment (Ilotycin ophthalmic ointment), every 4 hours while awake, is effective. Treatment should be continued for 2 weeks. Daily cleansing of the eyelashes with a neutral soap (e.g., Johnson's Baby Shampoo) followed by the application of an antibiotic ointment (e.g., gentamicin, tobramycin, or erythromycin) to the eyelashes four times a day for several weeks reduces the bacterial count, cleanses the lids, and minimizes recurrences.

Viral Conjunctivitis

Viral conjunctivitis, also known as acute follicular conjunctivitis, is common. It is caused by a variety of agents. The onset is abrupt and unilateral, but contralateral involvement in a day or two from autoinoculation is common. Excessive tearing is often a major complaint, but there is no purulent discharge. The conjunctiva nearly always shows hyperemia, which may be diffuse or segmental (Fig. 99.5, Color Plate 1). Viral conjunctivitis may be accompanied by tender preauricular lymphadenopathy. Often, the lymphoid tissue of the eyelid becomes edematous in response to the infection and may appear as elevated palpebral as well as bulbar conjunctival lesions (Fig. 99.5, Color Plate 1). When there is doubt about the diagnosis, examination of the conjunctival scrapings shows mononuclear cells. Viral cultures are expensive but are used in special circumstances.

The disease is self-limited, lasting only a few days, and treatment is therefore supportive. Vasoconstrictive drops (two drops four times a day for a few days) containing naphazoline (e.g., over-the-counter agents Albalon, Naphcon-A, or Vasocon-A) are helpful in relieving conjunctival congestion and hyperemia, and cool compresses as needed also provide relief. Sulfacetamide (Sulamyd) or erythromycin (Ilotycin), as described above, may be used if symptoms have not been controlled in a few days with topical vasoconstrictive drops; in this instance bacterial conjunctivitis may have developed.

Rarely, corneal inflammation may develop and cause an opacity in the cornea. When corneal opacification is noted, an ophthalmologist should be consulted urgently because loss of vision may occur. Some types of viral conjunctivitis *(epidemic keratoconjunctivitis*

[EKC]) are highly contagious. The examiner should take care not to become infected or to infect other patients; all instruments should be cleansed and thorough hand washing is critical. The family should be instructed that disease transmission is via tear droplets, so towels and washcloths should not be shared. Because EKC is so contagious, the patient may be asked to stay away from school or certain jobs for up to 10 to 12 days. Making this decision should not be taken lightly, and referral to an ophthalmologist often is appropriate.

Inclusion Conjunctivitis (Inclusion Blennorrhea)

Inclusion conjunctivitis is common in sexually active young adults. The disease is caused by a species of *Chlamydia* and is a result of contamination of the eye from the urethra after a sexual contact.

The problem is usually characterized by the abrupt onset of ocular discomfort, with varying degrees of diffuse conjunctival hyperemia and sometimes mucopurulent discharge that may result in matting of the eyelashes. The eyelids appear swollen, and inspection of the palpebral conjunctiva, especially of the lower lid, shows many small follicles (raised pale mounds of varying size) (Fig. 99.6, Color Plate 1). Occasionally, preauricular lymphadenopathy develops. Without treatment, the disease becomes chronic and remitting and, in 2 or 3 weeks, a superficial corneal inflammation (keratitis) may appear. This may be identified with the naked eye as dots or cloudy streaks on the superior portion of the cornea. Also at this stage, there may be an associated iritis manifested by photophobia and blurring of vision.

This syndrome may occur in association with urethritis in men or with cervicitis and a vaginal discharge in women. Most often, however, there are no genitourinary symptoms, although *Chlamydia* species can be cultured from the urethra in men or the endocervical canal in women. The culture is time-consuming and expensive, however. Two highly specific and sensitive direct slide tests for the detection of *Chlamydia* (see Chapter 27) are increasingly available commercially, and these appear to be diagnostic in patients with conjunctivitis. In some cases, Reiter's syndrome is present (see Chapter 71).

The diagnosis is suggested by the history and appearance, but if there is doubt, it may be confirmed by the direct slide test of the conjunctiva or examination of the material obtained from conjunctival scraping. This material, when stained with Giemsa stain, shows large basophilic cytoplasmic inclusion bodies (Fig. 99.7, Color Plate 1). Gram's stain does not reveal these bodies but shows many polymorphonuclear leukocytes.

Therapy is effective but must be systemic. Oral tetracycline, 250 mg four times daily for 21 days, is the preferable regimen; when tetracycline cannot be given, good results are achieved with erythromycin, 250 mg four times a day for 21 days, or trimethoprim–sulfamethoxazole (e.g., Bactrim DS or Septra DS), 1 tablet twice a day for 21 days. It may take several months for the follicular hyperplasia to resolve, but the patient should experience symptomatic improvement within several days. The application of cool compresses for 20 minutes several times a day also provides comfort in the first few days of treatment. Because this disease is difficult to diagnose, referral to an ophthalmologist is appropriate.

Because the disease must be assumed to be sexually transmitted, the sexual partner should be similarly treated; other venereal diseases should be looked for, and the man should use a condom until therapy has been completed.

Allergic Conjunctivitis

Allergic conjunctivitis is a common and mild conjunctivitis often encountered in patients with allergic rhinitis (see Chapter 23). Often the patient describes a history of allergy to grasses, pollens, and other agents and usually complains of itching and tearing. Often, there is marked swelling of the conjunctiva (Fig. 99.8, Color Plate 1) and slight to moderate redness of the eye, and at times there is serous crusting in the morning.

When there is doubt about the diagnosis, conjunctival scrapings may be examined. A finding of many eosinophils is diagnostic. When conjunctivitis is associated with allergic rhinitis, it usually parallels the rhinitis in severity and duration. When it occurs as an isolated problem, it is short-lived and treatment is symptomatic. An over-the-counter topical astringent solution (e.g., Albalon, Naphcon-A, or Vasocon-A using 1 to 2 drops four times per day for a day or two) and cool compresses as needed are very effective. Occasionally, symptoms are severe, and oral antihistamines may relieve itching.

Corticosteroid eye drops (e.g., HMS Liquifilm or FMI Liquifilm) are very effective for this condition, but they must be used cautiously because their use is associated with corneal ulceration and perforation in the presence of herpes simplex infection, the development of fungal infection, and when used chronically, with the development in some patients of open-angle glaucoma and, rarely, cataract formation. For these reasons, topical corticosteroids are not recommended without at least a telephone consultation with an ophthalmologist.

Chemical Conjunctivitis

Many agents may enter the conjunctiva and produce inflammation. Irritation from such agents as smoke, smog, sprays, chlorinated water, hairspray, makeup, and industrial dust is common. The history of the exposure makes the diagnosis obvious. The patient should thoroughly rinse the conjunctival sac with water as soon as contamination with a chemical has occurred. The patient will also benefit from cool compresses for 15 to 20 minutes several times a day, and occasionally the use of an over-the-counter topical vasoconstrictor solution (Albalon, Naphcon-A, or Vasocon-A) is necessary.

In the case of an injury from an acid or alkali, serious permanent damage may occur and this problem is a true ophthalmologic emergency. Patients should be advised to irrigate the conjunctival sac with copious amounts of water and to see an ophthalmologist immediately. If the patient is seen by the primary care physician, irrigation should be repeated promptly and the patient should then be sent immediately to an ophthalmologist. Overirrigation may increase irritation slightly, but underirrigation may make blindness more likely. Therefore, when in doubt, one should always irrigate. Normal saline stings less than water, but one should use whatever is immediately available.

Foreign Body

Foreign bodies often lodge in the conjunctiva or cornea. Most often they can be visualized with the naked eye; if not, sterile fluorescein staining (see above) may outline an area of corneal epithelial damage. Foreign bodies may be removed by irrigation of the conjunctival sac with a sterile solution of physiological saline or eyewash. If they are not rinsed away, mechanical removal is indicated. This may be accomplished, when the object is in the cornea, by placing in the eye a drop of topical anesthetic (e.g., Ophthaine) and removing the foreign body with a sterile needle held carefully with the physician's arm braced. A cotton swab should not be used to remove a foreign body from the cornea because often it is irritating to the structure and thus delays healing. Most nonophthalmologists are reluctant to use a needle; therefore, most patients with corneal foreign bodies are referred. If the foreign body is not on the cornea, removal is easier and usually does not require anesthesia. After removal, it is wise to instill a drop of antibiotic (e.g., Sulamyd 10% or Bacitracin) and cover the eye with a patch for 24 hours. The eye patch should be applied tightly enough to prevent the eyelids from moving. If the patch falls off before the 24-hour period is up, the patient should not try to reapply it because often this may cause more irritation. Today, ophthalmologists are using patching for corneal abrasions less often. A topical antiprostaglandin such as Acular is used for a day or two for comfort.

If the offending material is a piece of metal, rust rings surrounding the area of the epithelial defect may be observed. These rings are not harmful in themselves and only the foreign body should be removed.

In any instance when the foreign body is not easily removed, or if symptoms persist beyond a day after removal of a foreign body, an ophthalmologist should see the patient urgently.

Subconjunctival Hemorrhage

Subconjunctival hemorrhage is a common condition that often is alarming to the patient. A small blood vessel ruptures in the conjunctival tissue after the patient coughs or strains, and a painless wedge-shaped hemorrhage develops. Often the patient has no memory of the coughing or straining, but incidentally notices the red eye. Occasionally, viral conjunctivitis may be manifested only by the appearance of a subconjunctival hemorrhage. Isolated subconjunctival hemorrhage requires no treatment and should resolve

within several days. If the problem becomes recurrent or multiple, an abnormality of hemostasis should be considered.

EYELID CONDITIONS

Several conditions that affect the eyelid are commonly seen in ambulatory practice, and these may mimic a red eye. These conditions are usually readily diagnosed by their appearance and may be treated easily without an ophthalmologic consultation.

Hordeolum

A hordeolum is a common infection in the glands of the eyelid caused by *S. aureus*. It is characterized by the sudden onset of localized pain, swelling, redness, and often purulent discharge. The infected gland may be a meibomian gland just under the conjunctival side of the eyelid, or an *internal hordeolum*. This infection may be large and may point to either the skin or the conjunctival side of the lid. Also, a smaller gland associated with an eyelash follicle under the skin side of the lid may be infected, in an *external hordeolum* or sty. A sty usually is smaller than an internal hordeolum and always points to the skin side of the lid.

Both types of hordeolum may be treated without obtaining a culture. Treatment is tripartite: Warm compresses should be applied for 15 to 20 minutes several times a day and provide comfort and establish drainage of the infected gland; the lid should be scrubbed with a gentle soap (e.g., Johnson's Baby Shampoo) each morning; and every 3 to 4 hours for a few days a topical antimicrobial agent, such as a sulfonamide (e.g., Sulamyd-10%) or gentamicin (Garamycin) or tobramycin (Tobrex), should be applied to prevent the development of an associated cellulitis or eye infection. If the hordeolum has not begun to respond to treatment in a day or two, it may need to be incised; referral to an ophthalmologist is usually indicated.

Blepharitis

Marginal blepharitis is a very common chronic bilateral inflammation of the lid margins usually associated with seborrhea or a contact dermatitis (e.g., from mascara). Marginal blepharitis is discussed in Chapter 100. Blepharitis also may be associated with chronic bacterial infection (see "Chronic Bacterial Conjunctivitis," above).

Chalazion

A chalazion is a lipogranulomatous inflammation of a meibomian gland secondary to chronic inflammation and it may follow a hordeolum. It presents as a swelling similar to an internal hordeolum (see above) except that it is chronic and usually does not manifest acute inflammation. The swelling may appear anywhere on the eyelid (although the upper lid is a more common location), and it usually points toward the conjunctival side. Usually a chalazion does not spontaneously resolve, and if the patient is symptomatic, referral to an ophthalmologist for excision is indicated.

General References

Fraunfelder FT. Drug induced ocular side effects and drug interactions. 4th ed. Philadelphia: Lea & Febiger, 1995.

A useful text that provides a resource for possible drug-induced eye problems, including conjunctivitis, iritis, cataracts, and many other problems.

Newell FW. Ophthalmology principles and concepts. 8th ed. St. Louis: CV Mosby, 1996.

A very well-written short textbook that provides an overview of many eye problems, including the differential diagnosis of the red eye and the different forms of conjunctivitis.

Schachat AP, Cruess AF. Ophthalmology. Baltimore: Williams & Wilkins, 1984.

This short paperback text provides a useful overview and general approach to many common problems, including the red eye.

Color Plate 1

Figure 99.2. Hyperacute bacterial conjunctivitis. Note the severe degree of infection, swelling, and pustular discharge.

Figure 99.3. Acute bacterial conjunctivitis. Note the severe erythema and edema.

Figure 99.4. Chronic bacterial conjunctivitis. **A.** Injected conjunctiva and erythema of lid margins. **B.** Telangiectasia of upper lid and debris in the lashes.

Figure 99.5. Viral conjunctivitis. Note the redness as well as the edema of the lid and conjunctiva.

Figure 99.6. Inclusion conjunctivitis. Note the redness as well as the edema of the lid and conjunctiva and many small follicles appearing as pale mounds.

Figure 99.7. Scraping of conjunctiva from a patient with inclusion conjunctivitis showing inclusion body *(arrow)* (Giemsa stain).

Figure 99.8. Allergic conjunctivitis. Note the conjunctival edema.

Color Plate 2

Figure 100.1. Fixed drug reactions. **A.** Back. Hyperpigmented macules with an erythematous halo (reaction during administration of the drug). **B.** Side of neck. Sharply circumscribed macular hyperpigmentation (persistent hyperpigmentation after withdrawal of the drug; absence of inflammation, i.e., erythema).

Figure 100.2. Multiple seborrheic keratoses (upper back). "Stuck-on," sharply circumscribed, tan to deep brown, finely papillated to verrucous flat-topped papules and plaques.

Figure 100.3. Atypical moles (dysplastic nevi). Multiple lesions, showing one to four of the ABCDs: asymmetry, border irregularity, color variegation, diameter 6 mm or greater.

Figure 100.4. Superficial spreading malignant melanoma.

Figure 100.5. Actinic keratosis, nose.

Figure 100.6. Basal cell carcinoma.

Figure 100.7. Squamous cell carcinoma.

Figure 100.9. Asteatotic dermatitis (upper back and arm). Reticulate erythema highlighting minute cracks in the skin, diffuse dryness (asteatosis), and scale.

Figure 100.10. Acute contact dermatitis from shoes.

Figure 100.19. Erythema multiforme (extensor arm). Erythematous macules with dusky central area ("target") with focal areas of fine scale.

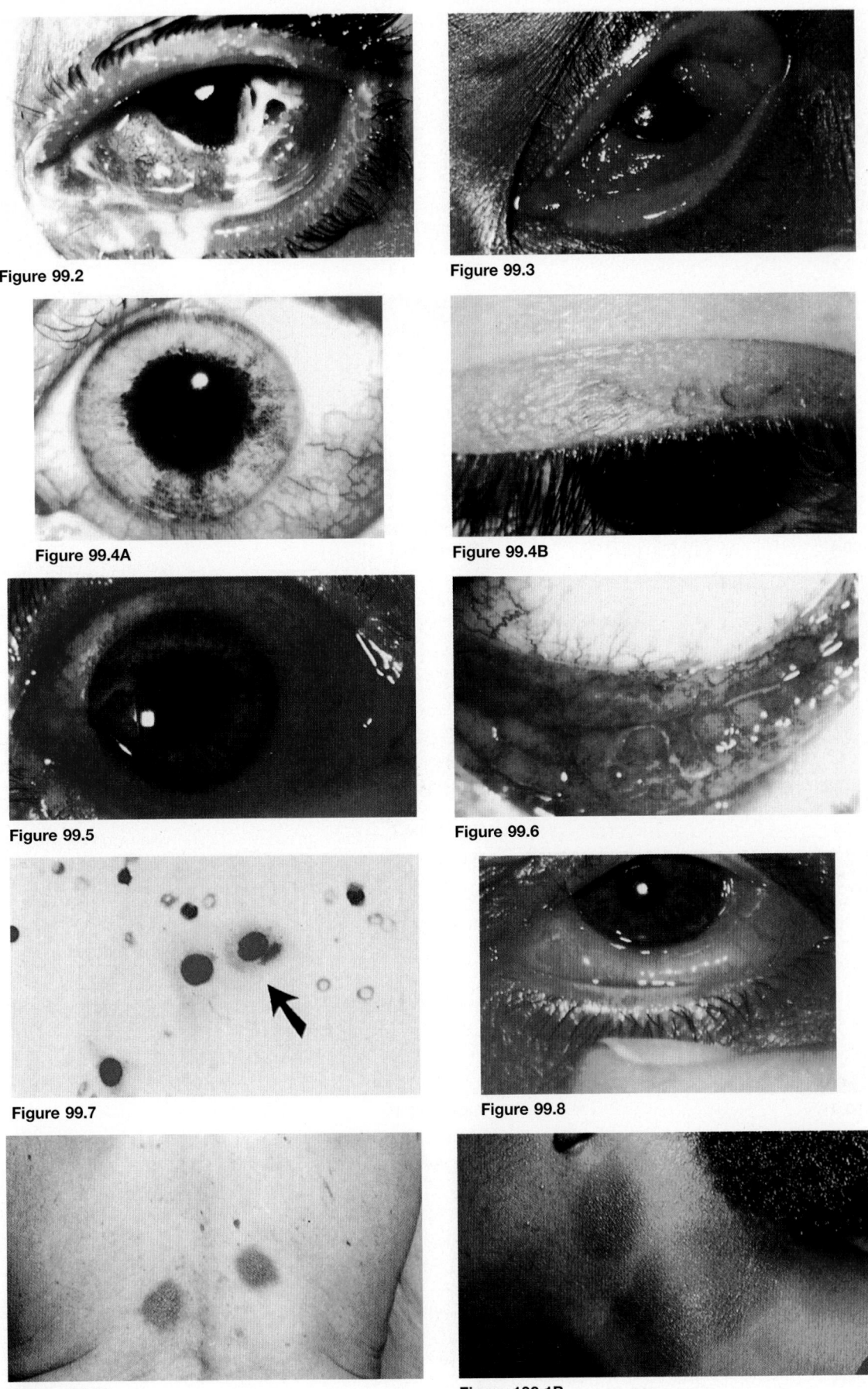

Figure 99.2

Figure 99.3

Figure 99.4A

Figure 99.4B

Figure 99.5

Figure 99.6

Figure 99.7

Figure 99.8

Figure 100.1A

Figure 100.1B

Color Plate 1

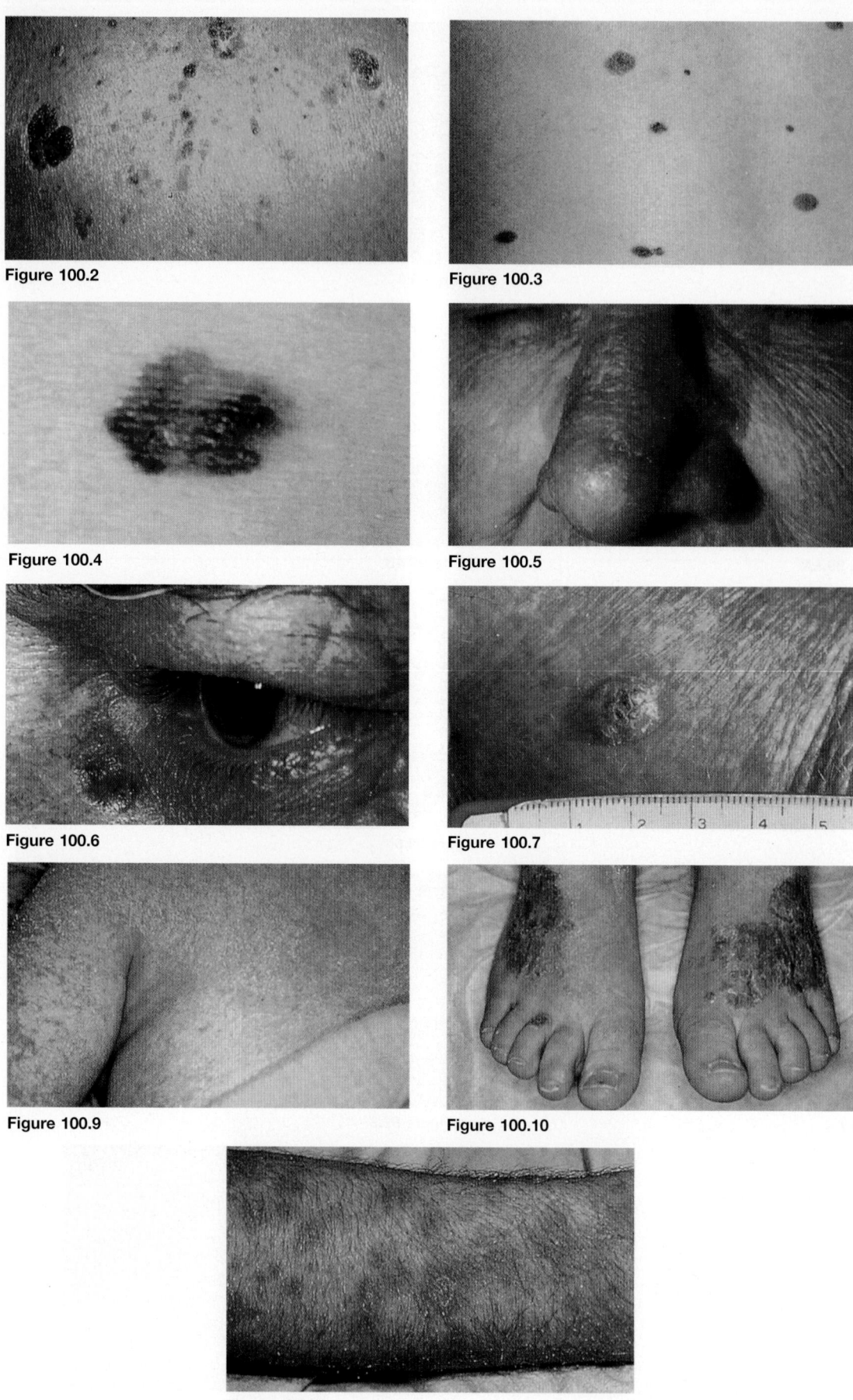

Figure 100.2

Figure 100.3

Figure 100.4

Figure 100.5

Figure 100.6

Figure 100.7

Figure 100.9

Figure 100.10

Figure 100.19

Color Plate 2

Miscellaneous Problems

C H A P T E R 100

Common Problems of the Skin

S. ELIZABETH WHITMORE, MD

EXAMINATION OF THE SKIN, GLOSSARY OF DERMATOLOGIC TERMS, AND TABLE OF SKIN DISORDERS

The primary goal of the skin examination is to determine the *morphology* (appearance) of the lesion and the extent of disease. The former allows the correct diagnosis to be made, and the latter aids in the determination of prognosis and treatment.

The examination should be directed at the lesion or eruption of concern, followed by a complete examination of the skin. This second step is important because it may reveal additional cutaneous findings helpful in diagnosis of the primary complaint or may expose a previously unrecognized skin disease. The complete skin examination is most easily done in a systematic fashion, starting at the top with the scalp, face, and oral mucosa and then moving first to the anterior then the posterior aspect of the body, including the external genital and body fold skin. Good lighting is essential and a magnifying lens may be helpful.

A few definitions make dermatologic diagnosis easier:

Atrophy: Thinning of the epidermis or dermis causing fine wrinkling or depression of the skin (e.g., discoid lupus erythematosus, steroid-induced atrophy, normal aging).

Bulla: A blister, similar to a vesicle but larger than 5 mm in diameter, filled with serous or serosanguinous fluid (e.g., friction blister, bullous pemphigoid).

Burrow: A linear, threadlike elevation of the skin, typically a few millimeters long (pathognomonic for scabies).

Comedone: A plugged pilosebaceous (or hair) follicle (e.g., a closed comedone, or whitehead, in acne).

Crust: Yellowish-brown sticky debris consisting of dried serum, scale, and usually bacteria (e.g., impetigo, impetiginized eczema).

Cyst: A circumscribed, firm, yet often slightly compressible, spherical lesion, fixed in the dermis (e.g., epidermal inclusion cyst).

Erosion: Loss of portion of the epidermis, nonscarring (e.g., candidiasis in the mammary crease with a moist surface, impetigo).

Excoriation: Same as an erosion, but a witnessed or historical self-inflicted removal of part or all of the epidermis.

Fissure: Vertical cut extending into the dermis (e.g., angular cheilitis [cracks at the angle of the mouth]) caused by *Candida,* salivary enzymes, or a vitamin deficiency.

Hive: See *Wheal.*

Hyperkeratotic: Heaped up or stacked scale (e.g., hypertrophic actinic keratosis, squamous cell carcinoma, wart).

Macule or *macular:* Flat color change (e.g., café-au-lait spot, junctional nevus ["flat brown mole"], freckle).

Morphology: Shape of the primary lesion (e.g., stellate, linear, round, or diffuse).

Nodule: A solid lesion up to 2 cm in diameter with an appreciable deep (dermal or subcutaneous) component (e.g., dermatofibroma, nodular melanoma, erythema nodosum, lipoma).

Papule: Elevated, often dome-shaped bump up to 10 mm in diameter, (e.g., intradermal nevus [skin-colored mole], molluscum contagiosum).

Plaque: A flat-topped, elevated area of skin, the surface area of which is much greater than the thickness (e.g., psoriasis, cutaneous T-cell lymphoma [mycosis fungoides]).

Pustule: Circumscribed lesion visibly filled with purulent material (e.g., folliculitis, acne pustule, pustular psoriasis).

Scale: Surface alteration resulting in a flaky surface, caused by abnormal proliferation or desquamation of the outermost epidermal layer, the stratum corneum (e.g., psoriasis, seborrheic dermatitis, tinea).

Sclerosis: Scarlike induration (e.g., systemic sclerosis, localized scleroderma [morphea]).

Secondary changes: Changes that occur as a result of the natural development or external manipulation of the primary lesion.

Telangiectasia: A dilated superficial capillary or venule; may be linear, spiderlike, or matlike (e.g., starburst leg telangiectasias, telangiectasias in a basal cell carcinoma or in an area of steroid- or lupus-induced atrophy).

Tumor: A large mass, greater than 2 cm in diameter, with significant thickness (more than several millimeters; e.g., neglected squamous cell carcinoma, cutaneous lymphoma).

Ulcer: Loss of skin extending into the dermis that always heals with scarring (any loss that penetrates the dermal–epidermal junction scars; e.g., venous stasis ulcer, pyoderma gangrenosum).

Urticarial: A localized area of edema and erythema, or wheal (e.g., urticaria, urticarial vasculitis, Sweet's syndrome [acute febrile neutrophilic dermatosis]).

Vesicle: A blister up to 5 mm in diameter filled with serous or serosanguinous fluid (e.g., herpes simplex infection, vesicular hand dermatitis).

Wheal or hive: An erythematous or blanched, edematous plaque with no surface change, present for no more than 24 hours.

Based on the morphology of the observed skin changes, a differential diagnosis or diagnosis of the skin lesion or eruption may be made, which may or may not require biopsy for confirmation. Table 100.1 provides a summary of selected disorders categorized by morphology and pathophysiology of disease. Practical advice about the diagnosis and management of these skin conditions is included in the table. Conditions that are common and those that are diagnostically or therapeutically complicated are discussed in detail in the text that follows.

NEVI AND MELANOMA
Dysplastic or Atypical Nevi

Atypical moles (or dysplastic nevi) affect 10 to 30% of the general population. They are acquired lesions that have clinical and histologic features that differ from typical common moles. *Typical moles or nevi are round,* tan to dark brown in color, sharply circumscribed (outlined), and present since childhood or early adulthood; the average adult has 20 typical nevi. On the other hand, *atypical moles or dysplastic nevi are larger* than usual moles, macular or papular, irregular or ill-defined, variegated in color (Fig. 100.3, Color Plate 2), and continue to appear after age 35. Because of these atypical features, biopsy may be required to exclude the possible diagnosis of melanoma.

Patients with few nonfamilial atypical moles and no personal history of melanoma are at increased risk for melanoma when compared with the general population; however, the relative risk is probably only two to eight times higher (57). These patients should be instructed to perform monthly self-examinations, looking for any change in appearance of a mole, and have physician skin examinations done every 6 to 12 months.

The *familial atypical mole and melanoma (FAMM) syndrome,* formerly called the dysplastic nevus syndrome, is associated with an extremely high risk of melanoma. Although the prevalence of this disease is not known precisely and is probably grossly underestimated, it has been said to affect at least 300,000 people. These individuals begin to develop atypical lesions at puberty and continue to develop new lesions throughout their lives. Patients with this syndrome may be identified by three criteria: a family history of melanoma in at least one first- or second-degree relative; many nevi, often more than 50, some or many of which are clinically atypical (see above) and show certain atypical features histologically. Patients with the FAMM syndrome have a lifetime risk of developing melanoma approaching 100%. Patients with sporadic atypical mole syndrome with a mole pattern similar to

Table 100.1.   Table of Selected Skin Disorders Based on Morphology

Disorder	Description	Common Presentation	Possible Systemic Associations	Risks	Recommendations	Differential Diagnosis	Key to Diagnosis
Hypopigmented and Depigmented Macules and Patches							
Vitiligo	Depigmented patches caused by melanocytes, probably immunologically mediated; favors periorificial and "tip" areas	New onset stark white skin around the eyes, lips, fingertips, and penis	Autoimmune thyroiditis, pernicious anemia, Addison's disease, diabetes melitus	Skin cancer	Sunscreens	Postinflammatory hypopigmentation, albinism, chemical leukoderma	Acquired depigmentation without a history of exposure to phenolic compounds, which may cause chemical leukoderma
Idiopathic guttate hypomelanosis "snowflakes"	Hypopigmented shiny 3- to 8-mm macules caused by defective melanocyte melanin production in older patients	Gradually increasing number of asymptomatic whitish macules on the pretibial and extensor arm surfaces	None	None	Sunscreens (lessen color contrast)	Vitiligo	Small macules of hypopigmentation on sun-damaged skin
Tinea versicolor	See text						
Halo nevus	Symmetric depigmented halo around a nevus	Small symmetric halo surrounding dome-shaped evenly pigmented brown papule	In patients with a history of melanoma, it may be an indication that metastatic melanoma has occurred	Misdiagnosis	If halo is not symmetric or nevus is abnormal, biopsy to rule out an abnormal nevus or melanoma	Melanoma with reaggression, dysplastic nevus	Symmetric mole with halo of depigmentation
Hyperpigmented Macules and Patches							
Junctional nevus	Evenly colored light to dark brown, sharply circumscribed, usually 1- to 6-mm macule, may develop from early childhood to early 30s; formed by nests of melanocytes at the dermal–epidermal junction	Multiple 2- to 6-mm sharply circumscribed, evenly pigmented brown macules, most of which are on the trunk	None	People with excessive numbers of nevi have an increased risk of melanoma, probably because of their greater melanocyte load (more than 40–50 nevi)	Monthly self-examinations; intermittent physican examination	Lentigo simplex, freckle	May be difficult to clinically distinguish between lentigo and freckles, however all are benign
Solar lentigo	"Liver spot"; brown, often asymmetric 2-mm to 2-cm macule occurring on a background of chronic sun-damaged skin	Multiple hyperpigmented 3- to 8-mm light to medium brown macules on the face and dorsal hands	None	None	Prevention: sunscreen use; elective treatment: liquid nitrogen cryosurgery, laser surgery, hydroquinone fading creams	Lentigo simplex, lentigo maligna	Homogenous pigmentation on background of sun-damaged skin

Continued

Table 100.1—*continued.* Table of Selected Skin Disorders Based on Morphology

Disorder	Description	Common Presentation	Possible Systemic Associations	Risks	Recommendations	Differential Diagnosis	Key to Diagnosis
Hyperpigmented Macules and Patches							
Café-au-lait spot	Evenly pigmented light to medium brown macule; present at birth, may develop in early childhood	Slowly expanding tan brown macule	*Neurofibromatosus (NF):* Presence of six café-au-lait spots greater than 1.5 cm is generally diagnostic NF; often have axillary freckling, too; may have tumors of the CNS, pheochromocytomas, etc. *Albright's syndrome:* Large, unilateral pigmented macule with an irregular border; have polyostotic fibrous dysplasia and precocious puberty (rarely seen in men) *Tuberous sclerosis:* May have café-au-lait spots; seizures, mental retardation (not all), and adenoma sebaceum (perinasal skin colored papules), also ash leaf macules (hypopigmented leaf-shaped macules)		Lightening or removal may be done with laser	Junctional nevus	No surface change (i.e., no epidermal change)
Melasma	Irregular tan to brown pigmentation variably present over the face; spares margins, favors cheeks and forehead; sun exposure, however minimal, is required for development	Patchy brown discoloration often on central forehead and cheeks	Exogenous and endogenous estrogen and sun exposure	N/A	Sunscreens and avoidance of sun exposure, hydroquinone fading creams, or laser therapy, electively	Hydroquinone induced in "pseudoochronosis"	Female, facial location, intensifies in the summer
Fixed drug eruption (Fig. 100.1, Color Plate 1)	Drug reaction that begins with 1 to several erythematous variable edematous, sometimes bullous, sharply circumscribed round to oval patches or plaques; resolve with a blue/brown macule; when offending drug is readministered, pigmented lesion becomes erythematous again	History of recurrent large red "hive" or blister after taking a drug, which resolves, leaving a dark mark	Caused most commonly by phenolphthalein (Phenomint and other laxatives), tetracycline, sulfonamides, quinine, quinidine, aspirin, codeine, chlordiazepoxide, acetaminophen, antiovulatory drugs, barbiturates, bismuth, gold, nystatin, and penicillins	*Note:* Fixed drug eruption may represent a localized erythema multiforme or toxic epidermal necrolysis; next dose of causative drug could cause either of these reactions.	Stop offending drug	Postinflammatory hyperpigmentation	Recurrent fixed nature on readministration of causative drug; sharply circumscribed

Xanthelasma	See Chapter 75					
Xanthoma	See Chapter 75					
Papules						
Warts, tumors	See text					
Moles	See text					
Compound nevus	Tan to dark brown, usually 2- to 8-mm dome-shaped soft to slightly firm papules, consisting of nests of melanocytes, both at the dermal epidermal junction and in the dermis	Brown "mole" that is becoming more elevated, lighter in color, and softer	None	Patient self-examinations for changes, as with all nevi	Melanoma, intradermal nevus, dermatofibroma, neurofibroma	Soft, circumscribed, symmetric, evenly colored papule
Intradermal nevus	Skin color to light brown, generally 2- to 8-mm fleshy papule; consists of nests of melanocytes confined to the dermis	Skin-colored papules that catch clothing	None	May be shaved or excised because they are in the way	Melanoma, intradermal nevus, dermatofibroma, neurofibroma	Soft, circumscribed, symmetric, evenly colored papule, usually skin colored
Seborrheic keratosis (Fig. 100.2, Color Plate 2)	"Stuck on" appearing yellowish-brown to black few mm to 1-cm plaque with a flat top; soft, friable, finely papulated surface; infrequently smooth surface with peppering of tiny white flecks of keratin within; begin occurring after age 20; caused by local proliferation of the epidermis, common in the elderly	Tan to dark brown finely populated "stuck on" flattened papules over the trunk	"Sudden" eruption of many seborrheic keratoses in association with a malignancy, most often with adenocarcinomas; typically run parallel course to malignancy	Liquid nitrogen cryosurgery or curettage may be used on pruritic or cosmetically bothersome lesions	Warts, squamous cell carcinoma, basal cell carcinoma, nevi	Characteristic "stuck on" appearance and age of the patient
Cherry angioma	Common red to maroon compressible 0.5- to 6-mm dome-shaped papules, favor trunk, common after age 30 or 40; formed by dilated capillaries; they are nonblanching	Multiple, barely visible red specks to 4-mm red dome-shaped papules	*Osler Weber Rendu* (hereditary hemorrhagic telangiectasia): autosomal dominant inheritance of punctate telangiectasias on the oral mucosa and fingers +/– AV malformations in the GI tract, lungs, and CNS *Crest:* Punctate and matlike telangiectasias on the face and fingers accompanied by sclerodactyly	Cauterize if desired for cosmesis	Hemangioma	Characteristic size and cherry red appearance

Continued

Table 100.1—continued.   Table of Selected Skin Disorders Based on Morphology

Disorder	Description	Possible Systemic Associations	Common Presentation	Risks	Recommendations	Differential Diagnosis	Key to Diagnosis
Papules							
Dermatofibroma	Benign, circumscribed, either flat or elevated 3- to 10-mm papules in the skin; feel like a "pea in the skin"; composed of fibroblasts, questionable reaction to earlier insect bite	*Lupus erythematosus* (LE): It has been reported that LE patients more often have multiple dermatofibromas	Small, brownish ill-defined macule with underlying papule	None	Excision possible, but leaves a scar	Nodular melanoma, nevus	Characteristic "pea-like" dermal papule
Condyloma acuminatum	See text and Chapter 94						
Molluscum contagiosum	See text and Chapter 94						
Basal cell carcinoma	See text						
Squamous cell carcinoma	See text						
Kaposi's sarcoma	See Chapter 34						
Plaques							
Psoriasis	See text						
Seborrheic dermatitis	See text						
Atopic dermatitis	See text						
Nummular dermatitis	See text						
Secondary syphilis	See Chapter 30						
Contact dermatitis	See text						
Tinea	See text						
Xanthoma	See Chapter 35						
Pityriasis rosea	Acute, self-limited eruption, typically lasting a few to several weeks, but occasionally several months; herald patch; initial lesion, oval 1–10 cm erythematous plaque with fine peripheral scale, usually on the chest, precedes by 7 to 14 days, the eruption of similar but smaller plaques in a "Christmas tree" pattern over the trunk; variable pruritic	None	1- to 3-cm oval plaque, followed by a shower of 25–100 similar 3- to 15-mm papules and plaques on the trunk, with the long axes of the lesions oriented along the skin lines	None	If pruritic, midpotency topical corticosteroids; if extremely pruritic, consider phototherapy	Secondary syphilis, tinea corporis, tinea versicolor, psoriasis; these should be considered initially and RPR checked; reassess patient if the rash lasts beyond 6 weeks	Herald patch, negative test for syphilis

Pityriasis alba	Possibly a very mild form of dermatitis, seen primarily in patients less than 20 years old, presenting with hypopigmented, sharply circumscribed, slightly scaly, 1-cm to several cm diameter macules or minimally elevated plaques, variably scattered over the face, trunk, and extremities; usually asymptomatic, occasionally pruritic; typically resolves spontaneously	Long history of asymptomatic scaly patches over the arms and legs	Possibly more common in patients with atopic dermatitis	None	Emollients, hydrocortisone; if disfiguring, phototherapy	Tinea versicolor, hypopigmented mycosis fungoides, sarcoidosis	Difficult to exclude other diagnoses without further evaluation (i.e., KOH +/- biopsy)
Mycosis fungoides	Epidemiographic cutaneous T-cell lymphoma most often affecting people over age 40, however, any age may be affected; lesions may be asymptomatic or pruritic; erythematous to violaceous or brawny patches, plaques, or tumors; morphology is usually oval or annular; however, may assume bizarre irregular shapes	Several-year history of scaly reddish plaques gradually increasing in number over the trunk	None	Although a systemic lymphoma, evidence of systemic involvement with simple testing is usually absent unless the disease progresses; more sensitive testing, such as Southern blot for T-cell receptor gene rearrangement on peripheral T cells and lymph nodes is often positive; unpredictable course; poor prognosis is associated with tumors, greater than 10% body surface area involvement, and lymphadenopathy	Treatment varies with the stage of the disease, age of patient; PUVA electron beam, topical nitrogen mustard, observation	Parapsoriasis, psoriasis, sarcoidosis, pityriasis alba	Biopsy; variable present lymphadenopathy

Continued

Table 100.1—*continued.*   Table of Selected Skin Disorders Based on Morphology

Disorder	Description	Common Presentation	Possible Systemic Associations	Risks	Recommendations	Differential Diagnosis	Key to Diagnosis
Nodules							
Erythema nodosum	Hypersensitivity reaction to some antigen, erythematous, tender nodules most often on the pretibial legs; develop in crops and involute over 2–3 weeks, resolve with a local bruise, never suppurate and drain; caused by a localized inflammatory infiltrate in the septum surrounding fat lobules	Acute onset of three erythematous nodules over the pretibial area associated with mild arthralgias in women on oral contraceptives	May be caused by any antigen, but more commonly reported associations include streptococcal infection, vaginal candidiasis, tuberculosis, coccidioidomycosis, histoplasmosis, lymphogranuloma venereum, *Yersinia* enterocolitica; noninfectious associations include sarcoilitis, inflammatory bowel disease, sulfonamides, barbiturates, various antibiotics, salicylates, oral contraceptives, and pregnancy	None	Workup to exclude possible causes; repeated review of all Rx and OTC medications, throat culture, ASO titer, chest x-ray, PPD; viral hepatitis (esp. C) screen; more extensive workup depending on clinical findings; if disease becomes chronic, search for "occult trigger antigen" again with dental films, sinus films, evaluation for gallbladder disease, etc.	Other forms of panniculitis	
Lipoma	Benign fatty tumor, most often solitary on the trunk; size is quite variable and may be many centimeters	Asymptomatic rubbery nodule, movable under the skin	None	None	Excision if desired	Cyst, neurofibroma	Soft nodule, freely movable under the skin
Ulcers							
Leg ulcers	See Chapters 87 and 88						

that of the FAMM syndrome also have a significantly increased risk of developing melanoma. All of these patients should perform monthly self-examinations, looking for any changes in the appearance of their moles. Additionally, they should be examined at 4- to 12-month intervals by a dermatologist so that appropriate biopsies or photographs can be taken. Patients should be counseled on self-examination and sun protection (avoidance of exposure during peak sun intensity hours [11 AM to 3 PM], use of sunscreen and protective clothing) because sun exposure increases the risk of malignancy (57). Also, it should be made clear that other family members may be similarly affected and advised of this because early detection saves lives.

Melanoma

Cutaneous malignant melanoma is the third most common type of skin cancer and the leading cause of death from skin disease (39,64,84). In the United States, melanoma is the seventh most common malignancy, being diagnosed in an estimated 38,300 people and causing related deaths in 7,300 people in 1996 (68). From 1973 to 1992, the rate of increase in incidence of melanoma has been 4% annually, exceeding similar rates for all other cancers in this country. Mortality has increased by 34%, making this the third highest increase among cancers (16). The estimated lifetime risk of an American developing invasive melanoma is 1 in 87; in white males, this figure rises to 1 in 70. Melanoma is the most common and second most common cancer in women 25 to 29 and 30 to 34 years of age, respectively (68). Unfortunately, public knowledge of melanoma is poor, as a recent survey has demonstrated that 50% of men and 35% of women were unfamiliar with the term *melanoma,* and only 31% of adults limit sun exposure, 28% use sunscreen routinely, and 28% wear protective clothing (85).

Although melanoma may occur in anyone, risk factors include moles or atypical moles and the FAMM syndrome (see above), personal or family history of melanoma, freckles, history of severe or frequent sunburns, inability to tan, light hair, and blue eyes. Although rare in African Americans, melanomas are more commonly found in acral locations in this population. Although the cause of melanoma is unknown, ultraviolet radiation is an important risk factor. People living closer to the equator, those having a history of blistering sunburns, and those with a history of basal or squamous cell carcinoma have a higher incidence of melanoma (46).

All pigmented lesions should be examined closely for one or more atypical features that may suggest melanoma. These include the *ABCDs: asymmetry, border irregularity, color variegation* (variable degrees of brown, tan, black, red, white, or blue), *and diameter greater than 6 mm.* Although some or all of these features may be present in a given melanoma, they may be absent. For instance, a nodular melanoma usually presents as a symmetric dome-shaped, deeply but

evenly pigmented, rapidly growing papule or nodule, exhibiting none of the ABCDs. For this reason, excisional biopsy of *changing* or *atypical* moles should generally be performed and ongoing surveillance of patients with many remaining moles or the sporadic or familial atypical mole syndrome by a dermatologist or practitioner skilled in the area should be recommended. Finally, patient education is of key importance with regard to the appearance of atypical moles and melanomas, monthly or bimonthly self-examination using the ABCDs, protection from the sun (sun avoidance, sunscreens, and protective clothing), and the possible familial link (i.e., patients should inform relatives of the possible genetic link and the need for skin examination).

There are four common subtypes of melanoma: superficial spreading, nodular, lentigo maligna, and acral lentiginous melanoma. Also, rarely seen and difficult to diagnose clinically is amelanotic melanoma or a melanoma lacking brown pigmentation, usually white, pink, or red. The characteristics of these are given in Table 100.2.

Fifty percent of *superficial spreading melanomas* arise from a preexisting nevus, typically showing radial (outward) growth for months to years. Clinical changes caused by this malignant transformation are generally seen as a change in size and color or border irregularity. With time, growth descends vertically from the epidermal–dermal junction and the surface becomes papular. This vertical growth creates the potential for metastasis. A superficial spreading melanoma is shown in Figure 100.4 (Color Plate 2).

Nodular melanoma usually does not manifest any of the ABCDs of atypical pigmented lesions because it has no radial but only a vertical growth phase. This type of melanoma is usually a dome-shaped or polypoid, symmetric, deeply pigmented papule. It may develop de novo or arise within a preexisting nevus. Unfortunately, a nodular melanoma tends to grow rapidly over weeks to months.

Lentigo maligna melanoma occurs on sun-damaged skin, most often the face. It arises from a preexisting lentigo maligna, which is a tan, brown, or brown/black, typically irregularly outlined macule on a sun-exposed site, usually present for many years. Lentigo maligna melanoma has a radial growth phase like that of superficial spreading melanoma and therefore commonly shows the ABCDs of atypical pigmented lesions.

Acral lentiginous melanoma occurs most often in African Americans and Asians on the palms, soles, or subungually. It usually displays some of the ABCDs of atypical pigmented lesions. Hutchinson's sign marked by pigment extending onto the skin of the nail fold in association with a subungual pigmented lesion is highly suggestive of melanoma, and biopsy is mandatory. Acral lentiginous melanomas typically have a poor prognosis because they are usually diagnosed late. Up to 50% of patients with acral lentiginous melanoma give a history of preceding trauma of the skin in the area of the lesion. This history and the mistaken acceptance by the physician that the pigment

Table 100.2. Features of the Subtypes of Melanoma

Melanoma Subtype[a]	Approximate Frequency (%)	Clinical Appearance	Location	Age Group Most Often Affected	Differential Diagnosis
Superficial spreading	70	Usually brown, but may be variably colored brown, black, blue, red, and white; flattish papule, plaque, or maculopapule, usually over 6 mm in diameter; usually showing 1 or more of the ABCDs (see text) of atypical moles and melanoma	Anywhere, often on the back in men and on the legs in women	30–40 yr	Nevus, seborrheic keratosis
Nodular	16	Colored as above or amelantoic, dome-shaped or polypoid papule or nodule; typically symmetric and uniform	Anywhere	40–50 yr	Nevus, thrombosed capillary hemangioma, pyogenic granuloma
Lentigo maligna	5	Tan or brown, less often black, blue, or red, irregular macule with focal surface elevation; later may develop distinct papules and nodules within	Face most often; other sun-exposed surfaces	50–70 yr	Solar lentigo (liver spots)
Acral lentiginous	<5	Similar in appearance to lentigo maligna melanoma; when it occurs as a pigmented streak in the nail with extension onto the nail fold skin, it is called Hutchinson sign (see text); seen most often in African Americans and Asians	Palms, soles, phalanges	All ages	Nevus, postinflammatory or drug-induced hyperpigmentation, fungal infection-induced nail dystrophy; pyogenic granuloma

[a]Other rare types combined make up less than 5% of melanoma.

change or nail dystrophy is the result of trauma often leads to a delay in diagnosis.

Because death caused by melanoma is preventable with early diagnosis, physical examination of all patients should include a thorough inspection of the skin. Similar to the recommended testicular self-examinations for men and breast self-examinations for women, patients should be instructed to periodically examine their skin thoroughly. Notably, most melanomas are self-discovered (53%) or detected by a family member (17%) (40). Information pamphlets prepared by the American Cancer Society are available through local chapters or the American Academy of Dermatology (approximately $15 per package of 50 pamphlets; Schaumburg, IL, 708-330-0230) and are helpful in educating patients about self-examination of the skin.

Patients with suspicious lesions should be referred to a dermatologist or surgeon for excisional biopsy without delay. In instances where full excision of the lesion is not possible because of anatomic location or size, an incisional biopsy of the most atypical and elevated area of the lesion should be performed. If the diagnosis of melanoma is confirmed histologically, reexcision with an appropriate margin of normal surrounding tissue, as dictated by the vertical thickness of the melanoma, is necessary (0.5 cm for melanoma in situ; 1 cm to 2 or 3 cm for invasive melanoma) (39).

Follow-up surveillance and testing in patients after melanoma excision is controversial; however, a recent nonconcurrent prospective study has addressed this issue: 261 patients having moderate or high risk for recurrent melanoma (thickness greater than 1.68 mm) were studied, undergoing examination monthly for 2 months, then bimonthly for the first year, and every 4 months and 6 months for the second and third years, respectively. Evaluation included history, physical examination, complete blood count, chemistry, and chest x-ray. Of these patients, 161 developed recurrent melanoma; 145 were fully evaluable. Recurrent disease most often occurred in the regional lymph nodes (45%) or skin (22%). Disease was detected by the patient or physician history (68%), physician examination (26%), and chest x-ray (6%), suggesting that routine blood testing is not necessary for follow-up surveillance, and chest x-ray yield is limited (91).

The prognosis for a patient after excision of a primary cutaneous melanoma depends on the thickness of the melanoma and whether there is evidence of spread to lymph nodes or distant metastases. The overall 5-year survival in patients without adenopathy or distant metastases (stage I disease) with tumor thickness less than 0.76 mm is 96 to 99%; thickness 0.76 to 1.50 mm, 87 to 94%; thickness 1.51 to 4.0 mm, 66 to 77%; and thickness greater than 4 mm, less than 50%. Women have a better prognosis. In one study of 371 patients without lymph node or distant metastases, female and male 5-year survival rates depending on tumor thickness were, respectively, 1 mm, 94 versus 80%; 2 mm, 91 versus 71%; 3 mm, 88 versus 62%; 4 mm, 85 versus 53%; 5 mm, 82 versus 44%; and 6 mm or greater, 79 versus 35% (36). In patients with metastases to the regional lymph nodes (stage II disease), the 5-year median survival is less than 30%. When distant metastases are present (stage III disease), the median survival is 6 months (39).

ACTINIC KERATOSIS, KERATOACANTHOMA, AND NONMELANOMA SKIN CANCERS

Actinic Keratosis

Actinic keratoses are sun induced precancers or focal areas of epidermal dysplasia (Table 100.3). Although occasionally seen in teenagers, they generally develop in the fourth or fifth decades of life in fair-skinned people with other evidence of sun damage, such as freckling or solar lentigo (liver spot) formation. Clinically, lesions appear as ill-defined erythematous, generally 2- to 8-mm, scaly macules or minimally elevated hyperkeratotic papules on sun-exposed sites (Fig. 100.5, Color Plate 2). They are most easily detected by gently running the fingertips over the area because they feel like islands of fine sandpaper. Although actinic keratoses represent precancers, few (less than 1%) actually progress to invasive SCC.

Patients with actinic keratoses should be treated with topical 5-fluorouracil cream (Fluoroplex, Efudex) or cryotherapy using liquid nitrogen to destroy the abnormal epidermis. With cryotherapy, the treated area may blister and crust and then heal in 1 to 2 weeks without scarring. However, postinflammatory hypopigmentation or depigmentation, leaving a whitish macule, is not uncommon. If the physician is unfamiliar with either of these forms of therapy, referral to a dermatologist is indicated. New lesions are likely to occur, and patients with actinic keratoses should be examined every 6 to 12 months.

Keratoacanthoma

Keratoacanthoma (KA) mimics squamous cell carcinoma both clinically and histologically. However, KA is believed to be a benign tumor that develops rapidly over several weeks, then spontaneously involutes. Most are 1 to 2 cm in diameter; however, lesions may be many centimeters and cause significant scarring.

KAs usually develop in elderly people on sun-exposed skin; they begin as small papules that rapidly enlarge and develop a central hyperkeratotic plug, appearing somewhat like a crater.

Because of their resemblance to carcinoma and their often scarring nature of these lesions, patients suspected of having them should undergo incisional or excisional biopsy.

Nonmelanoma Skin Cancers

The two most common nonmelanoma skin cancers (NMSCs) as well as most common cancers in humans, *basal* and *squamous cell carcinomas* make up 95% of the estimated 1 million skin cancers diagnosed in the

Table 100.3. Nonmelanoma Skin Cancers, Keratoacanthomas, Actinic Keratoses

Clinical Type	Presentation	Key Features	Differential Diagnosis
Actinic Keratosis			
Actinic keratosis	Erythematous, scaly to hyperkeratotic macule; ill-defined border; usually multiple; always on sun-damaged skin	Scaly, ill-defined lesion on sun-damaged skin	Bowen's disease, superficial BCC, SCC, dermatitis, tinea
Keratoacanthoma			
Keratoacanthoma	Firm to hard, volcanolike crater with a central keratin plug	Keratin-filled "crater"	SCC, prurigo nodularis
Basal Cell Carcinoma			
Nodule-ulcerative	Small, firm, waxy papule often with telangiectasias; may ulcerate, especially on the face	Waxy papule	Intradermal nevus, fibrous papule, folliculitis, seborrheid keratosis
Superficial	Erythematous, sharply circumscribed, scaly macule border or thin plaque with a thin thready border, especially on the trunk	Threadlike	Actinic keratosis, Bowen's disease, nummular dermatitis, contact dermatitis, tinea
Morpheaform	Spontaneous scarlike lesion; whitish yellow, smooth, shiny scar surface	"Spontaneous"	Scar, granuloma annulare, sarcoid, localized scleroderma
Pigmented	Blue, brown, or black waxy papule; mostly found in deeply pigmented Caucasian, Oriental, or African-American people	Pigmented waxy papule	Seborrheic keratosis, nevus, melanoma
Squamous Cell Carcinoma			
Common SCC	Firm to hard, erythematous, hyperkeratotic nodule, or ulcerated nodule; especially on the dorsal hands, forearms, and face	Firm/hard keratotic nodule	Keratoacanthoma, hypertrophic actinic keratosis, seborrheic keratosis, prurigo nodularis
Bowen's disease, SCC in situ	Erythematous, sharply circumscribed, scaly macule or thin papule	Circumscribed scaly erythema	Actinic keratosis, superficial BCC, dermatitis, tinea

BCC, Basal cell carcinoma; *SCC*, squamous cell carcinoma.

United States in 1996. The ratio of basal cell carcinoma (BCC) to squamous cell carcinoma (SCC) in the United States is approximately 4:1 (54,65).

The most important risk factors for these nonmelanoma skin cancers are cumulative sun exposure (for most Americans, 80% of the lifetime sun exposure occurs before age 18), fair skin color, and older age. Less well established and important risk factors for SCC include tobacco smoking and sunlamp or suntan parlor use (3).

Even though almost all NMSCs occur on sun-exposed surfaces, they may occur on covered sites such as the hair-bearing scalp or on the genitalia or lower extremities. The former is often associated with a childhood history of scalp irradiation for the treatment of tinea or a hemangioma, whereas the latter may be associated with chronic inflammation, as might be seen in a patient with hidradenitis suppurativa or a chronic leg ulcer.

Patients who have undergone organ transplants are also at increased risk for nonmelanoma skin cancers, probably caused by iatrogenic immune suppression (63). The frequency of SCCs in these patients may reach 30 to 40% 10 years after transplantation. This represents a 4- to 21-fold increase in frequency above the general population (31).

In certain disorders, patients have early onset of innumerable skin cancers. The most common of these is *basal cell nevus syndrome,* an autosomal-dominant inherited disorder in which patients develop palmar pits (icepicklike indentations), jaw cysts, and calcification of the falx cerebri, in combination with multiple BCCs, usually beginning in the teens or twenties. A mutation in the Patched (Ptc) gene on chromosome 9 is believed to be responsible for this syndrome as well as some sporadic BCCs (34). Another disorder, xeroderma pigmentosum, is an autosomal-recessive condition with childhood onset of SCCs, BCCs, and occasionally melanomas. Patients have a defect in excision or postreplication repair of ultraviolet radiation–induced DNA changes.

Basal Cell Carcinoma

Eighty percent of BCCs develop on the head and neck (65). Other more commonly affected sites include the upper trunk in both sexes, and the legs in women. Patients typically give a history of a new lesion or a lesion that repeatedly gets red, peels, or bleeds, then improves, only to repeat the cycle. Basal cell carcinoma may be divided into subtypes based on clinical morphology: *nodular ulcerative, superficial, morpheaform or sclerosing,* and *pigmented.*

Nodular ulcerative BCC accounts for approximately half of all cases of BCC. The lesion is initially a firm, superficial opalescent (shiny pinkish-white) papule with telangiectasias. As it enlarges and outgrows the blood supply, ulceration occurs forming the classic "rodent ulcer" (Fig. 100.6, Color Plate 2). Before ulceration, the differential diagnosis includes an intradermal nevus, fibrous papule, inflamed hair follicle, and seborrheic keratosis. Several points may help distinguish these entities: A nevus is soft and typically present for many years, an inflamed hair follicle should resolve in no longer than a few weeks from onset, and a seborrheic keratosis has a stuck-on appearance and a fine papulated or pebbly surface. If the diagnosis of BCC cannot be excluded clinically, biopsy must be performed. With regard to a suspected ulcerated BCC, in general, any lesion that has ulcerated spontaneously should be assumed to be a cancer until biopsy excludes this diagnosis.

Superficial BCC appears as a sharply circumscribed, erythematous, scaly, 3-mm to many centimeter macule or a slightly elevated plaque with a characteristic threadlike border. The differential diagnosis includes actinic keratosis, Bowen's disease (SCC in-situ), extramammary Paget's disease, dermatitis (nummular or contact), psoriasis, and tinea. These are discussed below and in Table 100.3.

Morpheaform or sclerotic BCC develops as a spontaneous, macular, slightly elevated or depressed scar. It has a white, faint pink, or yellow appearance, looking devoid of vessels and appendageal structures (hairs and sebaceous and eccrine glands). The differential diagnosis includes a traumatic or surgical scar, localized scleroderma (morphea), and less often, granuloma annulare and cutaneous sarcoidosis.

Pigmented BCCs are similar in appearance to nodular or superficial BCCs, but are pigmented. They occur most often on more deeply pigmented Caucasians, Asians, and African Americans. The differential diagnosis includes melanoma, seborrheic keratosis, and nevus.

Squamous Cell Carcinoma

SCC may develop de novo or may arise from an actinic keratosis (see above). It appears as a firm to hard, erythematous to brawny-violaceous nodule, often with central hyperkeratotic (heaped) scale or ulceration. The hyperkeratotic scale may form a horn (pointed surface protrusion). Figure 100.7 (Color Plate 2) shows an SCC. The differential diagnosis includes keratoacanthoma, wart, and seborrheic keratosis.

Pathogenesis of Nonmelanoma Skin Cancers

BCC and SCC are derived from keratinocytes; BCC specifically arises from basal keratinocytes of the epidermis and adnexa. It is believed that damage caused by ultraviolet B radiation (wavelengths 290 to 320 nm) to deoxyribonucleic acid (DNA) with the formation of pyrimidine dimers, inadequacy of DNA repair mechanisms, and suppression of the local immune surveillance system are all important in the development of nonmelanoma skin cancer.

Prognosis and Therapy of Nonmelanoma Skin Cancer

Although BCC rarely (less than 1 per 4000) metastasizes, SCC may do so in approximately 3% of patients. Rates are greatest for SCCs developing on the lips, in scar tissue, and in areas of chronic inflammation. Metastatic sites may include regional lymph nodes, liver, lung, bone, and brain. Metastatic SCC is associated with a 5-year survival rate between 14 and 39%.

People who have had one nonmelanoma skin cancer are at increased risk for future skin cancers. Within 5 years of one nonmelanoma skin cancer, a patient has a 50% chance of developing a second tumor (35). Additionally, people with previous BCC and SCC have a 17-fold increase risk of developing melanoma (46).

Suspected nonmelanoma skin cancer should be biopsied to confirm the diagnosis before definitive treatment. Treatment options for cancers include excisional therapy, *Mohs micrographic surgery* (a procedure in which the visible cancer is excised and the specimen immediately examined histologically to ensure that the margins are free of cancer; if cancer is still present, a deeper section is taken and examined; this is repeated until the resected tissue is free of cancer), electrodesiccation and curettage, cryosurgery, or radiation therapy. The treatment modality depends on the type of cancer (cell type, primary or recurrent), location, the patient's age and ability to tolerate a procedure, local availability of the procedure, and patient preference (65).

In patients who develop many cancers, such as those having organ transplants or with basal cell nevus syndrome or xeroderma pigmentosum (see above), chemoprophylaxis with retinoids may be considered. At appropriate dosages of isotretinoin, etretinate, or acitretin, patients seem to develop fewer cancers. Unfortunately, the retinoid must be continued indefinitely to maintain the protective effect. Retinoids have many potential side effects; in addition to being teratogenic and often causing elevation of lipids, they may cause tendon calcification and vertebral hyperostosis with chronic administration (9,62).

ACNE AND RELATED DISORDERS

Definition and Pathogenesis

Acne vulgaris is a chronic disorder of the pilosebaceous units (hair follicles and sebaceous glands), particularly those on the face, chest, and back, where the pilosebaceous units are most dense. *Four things must be present* for acne to develop: androgen-stimulated sebum production; *Propionibacterium acnes,* an anaerobic diphtheroid that constitutes most of the normal follicular flora and proliferates in response to increased sebum; altered keratinization and desquamation of the cells lining the follicles; and a host inflammatory response.

Sebum production is known to be greater in people with acne than in those without acne. It is stimulated by *androgens* (testosterone in males; primarily testosterone and dehydroepiandrosterone in females) and causes proliferation of the lipophilic *P. acnes. P. acnes* breaks sebum into glycerol and free fatty acids; the free fatty acids are believed to cause hyperkeratinization and *impaired desquamation* of the follicular epithelium, leading to *plugging and inflammation,* represented clinically by comedones and erythematous papules, respectively. *P. acnes* also causes inflammation directly, triggering the release of proteolytic enzymes, hyaluronidase, and neutrophil chemotactic factors. The resultant changes are seen as erythematous papules and pustules. If enough follicular damage occurs, the contents of the follicle spills out into the dermis, causing an exaggerated host response and an acne cyst (pseudocyst) (79).

Epidemiology

Acne is the most common skin disease in the United States. It affects at least 85% of the population between the ages of 12 and 25 (79), and often persists or recurs in the third, fourth, and fifth decades (38). Acne may contribute significantly to psychosocial problems such as clinical depression, anxiety, self-imposed isolation, and a negative body image. Successful acne treatment usually corrects or significantly improves these problems (26). Drugs associated with the development of acne are listed below (see "Drug Eruptions").

Clinical Presentation

The earliest changes in acne may be seen in the prepubescent years with the appearance of closed and open *comedones* (whiteheads and blackheads, respectively). As the disease progresses, *erythematous, follicular papules, pustules, and* sometimes *cysts* develop on the face and often the upper trunk. Patients may be asymptomatic or complain of itching and soreness; they may find it impossible to resist picking or excoriating the lesions.

Evaluation

Patients should be questioned regarding their past use of over-the-counter as well as prescription topical and systemic therapies to treat their acne because medications not previously tolerated or unsuccessful should be avoided. A general medication history should also be reviewed because patients may be on drugs that cause or aggravate acne (see "Drug Eruption," below). Such agents include hormonal contraceptives, which have progestins with stronger androgenic effects (e.g., levonorgestrel as in Norplant), corticosteroids, lithium, iodides, phenytoin, anabolic steroids, and high dosages of vitamins B_2 (riboflavin), B_6 (pyridoxine), and B_{12} (cyanocobalamin) (82).

The evaluation of patients with acne should include excluding possible androgen excess with a review of the menstrual and reproductive histories, and examination of the scalp for androgenic alopecia (see below) and the face and trunk for hirsutism. Abnormal findings warrant hormonal evaluation (23,44).

Therapy

Except for isotretinoin therapy (see below), treatment is intended to control the disease and is not curative (Table 100.4). All patients with acne should be instructed to use a gentle antibacterial soap, such as Lever 2000, Dial, or Almay, wash with nothing more harsh than the fingertips, avoid cosmetics containing

Table 100.4. Acne Therapy

Type of Acne	Clinical Appearance	General Hygiene	Initial Therapy	Reevaluate	Therapy if Not Responding[a]	Therapy Change if Responding Nicely
Comedonal acne	Open and closed comedones (blackheads and whiteheads)	*Gently* wash face with fingertips two times/day using soap. Avoid lotions or cosmetics containing oil.	Retin A 0.01% gel or 0.05% cream, pea-sized amount at bedtime	8 wk	Increase Retin A to two times/day or change to 0.025% gel or 0.1% cream at bedtime if tolerated.	No change.
Inflammatory acne	Comedones and inflammatory papules ± pustules	As above.	Retin A, as above; Benzoyl peroxide (BPO) gel every AM or as tolerated[b] *or* erythromycin 2% or clindamycin 1% solution or gel two times/day	8 wk	Add oral antibiotics; tetracycline 500 mg two times/day or erythromycin 333 mg three times/day. Next change to erythromycin or tetracycline, whichever was not used previously; if still no response after 8 wk, refer.	Decrease oral antibiotics by 1 tablet every 4–6 weeks; at dosage when flare occurs, increase 1 tablet and hold for several months; then reevaluate (goal of therapy is topical ongoing management until acne is "outgrown"). Unusually acne may extend into the latter decades.
a. Cystic alone or b. Scarring inflammatory acne[b]	a. As above plus cystic or nodular lesions b. Inflammatory acne with resultant scarring	As above.	Retin A and BPO or topical antibiotic,[c] plus oral antibiotics as above	8 wk	Accutane[d] (*cis*-retinoic acid) administered by a physician with experience using this teratogenic drug (see text).	

[a]If not responding, always review patient's regimen; may be noncompliant or just incorrectly using medications.

[b]BPOs, such as OTC Oxy or Rx Brevoxyl 4%, Benzac AC 5%, Desquam E 5%. The advantage of BPO over topical antibiotic is that BPOs are bacteriocidal and antibiotics are bacteriostatic for *Propionibacterium* acnes, so there is less chance for bacterial resistance. Patients should be instructed to use, as limited by irritation and excessive dryness (once-weekly application significantly reduces cutaneous *p. acnes* population).

[c]Topical erythromycin such as A/T/S or EryMax; clindamycin such as Cleocin T gel

[d]Scarring inflammatory acne is not an FDA-approved indication for Accutane; recommend referral to a dermatologist who is willing to treat such patients with Accutane to prevent further permanent, disfiguring scarring.

A good review of acne therapy is provided in Leyden JJ. Therapy for acne vulgaris. N Engl J Med 336:1156–1162, 1997.

oil, and confine moisturizing lotions to localized dry patches of skin. If there is evidence of picking characterized by excoriated papules, the patient must be taught not to manipulate acne lesions because doing so may cause scarring. Finally, adjunctive tanning treatment through natural sun exposure and ultraviolet light therapy, once thought to improve acne, only camouflages lesions and may result in photoaging and skin cancer in subsequent years.

Patients should understand that 6 to 8 weeks is usual before obvious improvement occurs with any treatment of acne. If there is no improvement after 2 to 3 months of treatment (see below), or if lesions are cystic or scarring, referral to a dermatologist is appropriate.

Comedonal Acne

Comedonal acne (see introductory glossary, above) is treated with a single comedolytic agent. These agents essentially unplug comedones by promoting normal desquamation of the follicular epithelium. Available products include salicylic acid (SalAc Wash, Neutrogena Acne Wash, both over-the-counter) and *trans*-retinoic acid (Retin-A, by prescription). If retinoic acid is used, 0.05% cream or 0.01% gel should be pre-scribed, reserving the more drying gel for patients with oilier skin or those living in more humid climates. Because of the vehicle (cream versus gel) effect, these different concentrations have similar therapeutic retinoid effects. A pea-sized volume of medication is spread evenly over the face and chest and twice this volume for the back, if needed. Warning must be given of expected mild peeling, redness, and possibly a flare of acne in the first 2 weeks of treatment. Patients may be advanced to 0.1% cream or 0.025% gel if the medication has been well tolerated on follow-up at 8 weeks.

Retin-A (like all retinoids, i.e., vitamin A and its natural and synthetic derivatives) is teratogenic. Even though systemic absorption with topical application is minimal, Retin-A is probably best avoided in patients who are or who are attempting to become pregnant or in women of reproductive age who are not using effective birth control.

Inflammatory Acne

Mild inflammatory acne consisting of comedones and erythematous papules with or without pustules (usually up to 15 papules) may be treated with a combination of a comedolytic agent (see above) and a topical antibacterial directed at *Propionibacterium acnes.* Appropriate antibacterial agents for this condition are topical benzoyl peroxide, which is bactericidal, or a bacteriostatic drug such as erythromycin or clindamycin. Benzoyl peroxide is a primary irritant, so low concentrations are best (2.5 to 4%) in all patients, except those with exceptionally excessive sebum, in whom a more concentrated gel (8 to 10%) is helpful because of its drying effect. Benzoyl peroxide as a leave-on gel or wash-off cleanser is available over the counter (e.g., Oxy Sensitive Skin Treatment 2.5% gel or Oxy 10 Acne Treatment 10% gel; Oxy Clean Moisturizing Face Wash or Medicated Cleansing Bar) and by prescription (e.g., Brevoxyl 4 or 8% Gel or Cleansing Lotion, Benzac AC 2.5 or 10% Gel). Daily or less frequent use as tolerated is recommended, being adjusted by the patient. Alternatively, topical erythromycin 2% (e.g., A/T/S, Em-Gel) or clindamycin 1% (e.g., Cleocin T Pledgets, Cleocin T Gel) may be used. Benzoyl peroxide and retinoic acid should not be used simultaneously because of resultant oxidation of retinoic acid; therefore one is used in the morning and the other at night. Topical antibiotics and retinoic acid may be applied together.

If inflammatory acne does not improve in 6 to 8 weeks of treatment, or if patients initially present with extensive or scarring inflammatory acne with depressed, irregular, or pitted scars, treatment should include an oral antibiotic, either tetracycline 500 mg two times a day (if nausea develops, 250 mg two times a day) or erythromycin 333 mg three times a day (if nausea develops, 250 mg two times a day). Oral antibiotics are always used in combination with topicals, in anticipation of tapering or discontinuing oral therapy after several weeks or months while continuing topicals alone (Table 100.4). Patients should be told that antibiotics only suppress and do not cure acne. Therefore, as long as a patient is still in his or her "acne years" (a very individualized time period), ongoing treatment is necessary. Patients on long-term oral or topical antibiotic therapy should be watched for the development of *Propionibacterium acnes antibiotic resistance,* characterized by worsening or suddenly unresponsive acne (20).

Cystic Acne

Cystic acne, characterized by deep-seated inflammatory nodules or cysts, should always be treated aggressively because it almost invariably causes scarring. If patients do not respond to oral antibiotics in combination with topical agents, a systemic synthetic retinoid, isotretinoin (13-*cis*-retinoic acid, Accutane), should be prescribed if there are no contraindications. Isotretinoin is curative in approximately 70% of patients, although the basis for this is unknown. Because of difficulties with side effects of this drug, it is best administered under the direction of a dermatologist. The greatest concern about isotretinoin is its teratogenic potential. It may produce fetal anomalies involving the central nervous system, heart, bones, and thymus in 30 to 40% of exposed fetuses. All women should be counseled to use two methods of contraception (see Chapter 93) simultaneously and, if these fail, an abortion should be recommended. If a patient is morally against abortion even in such instances of a medical indication, she should remain abstinent from sexual intercourse for the 20-week period of treatment, as well as for 1 month before and after treatment, or forgo isotretinoin therapy. The maker of isotretinoin (Roche Dermatologics) has developed a package of patient instructions and consent forms that are most important for both the physician and the patient to review (see below). The manufacturer of isotretinoin currently will also pay for initial patient consultation with a gynecologist to discuss birth control.

Some side effects with isotretinoin therapy are essentially inescapable. These include dry skin, nose, and eyes. Mild elevations of triglyceride, cholesterol, and liver enzymes are seen in approximately 25% of patients. Infrequent or unusual side effects include hair loss, musculoskeletal aches, *Staphylococcus aureus* folliculitis and ocular keratitis, reduced night vision, marked elevation of triglyceride with the potential for an associated acute pancreatitis, marked elevation of cholesterol and liver enzymes, leukopenia, and pseudotumor cerebri (52).

Patients are usually treated with a 1 mg/kg per day dosage of isotretinoin (Accutane 10-, 20-, or 40-mg capsules) for approximately 20 weeks. Before treatment and monthly until 1 month after completion of treatment, serum triglyceride, cholesterol, liver enzymes, and (for women of childbearing potential) serum HCG pregnancy tests should be monitored. If triglyceride levels double or triple, appropriate diet modification and complete alcohol avoidance should be instituted. If levels exceed 500, isotretinoin should generally be stopped and repeat testing performed. Minor elevations in liver enzymes require no action; however, when two- to threefold elevations occur, other causes of aminotransferase elevations should be excluded, and drug discontinuance or dosage reduction with close follow-up is indicated. Patients should be seen monthly to discuss and evaluate their progress, and for women, to review their two forms of birth control and to check a serum HCG. If this pregnancy test is found to be positive, the drug should be stopped immediately and consultation with a gynecologist should be obtained. Physicians prescribing isotretinoin should review the manufacturer's (Roche Laboratories) recommendations for prescribing, warnings, and precautions in the PDR. In addition, the manufacturer's free "Pregnancy Prevention Program for Women on Accutane" should be obtained (800-955-6611).

Acne Rosacea

Acne rosacea is a chronic inflammatory disorder favoring the central portion of the face. It occurs most commonly in fair-skinned Caucasians with blue eyes. Affected patients usually develop initial signs of the disease in their twenties or thirties with central facial erythema and telangiectasias and intermittent erythematous follicular papules and pustules. Intermittent flushing and edema are often present also. Rarely, patients may develop associated *rhinophyma;* this bulbous nose enlargement is seen more often in men than in women and is caused by hyperplasia of the sebaceous glands of the nasal skin. Rosacea does not cause comedones and therefore can be differentiated from acne. However, some patients have both rosacea and acne.

Rosacea may also involve the eyes, causing a mild inflammation of the lid margins manifest by mild erythema and a dry eye or foreign body sensation. Other slightly or somewhat less common changes include conjunctivitis, blepharitis, episcleritis, and recurrent chalazion and hordeolum (see Chapter 99). Less than 5% of patients with rosacea develop a painful and vision-threatening condition of the cornea, *rosacea keratitis.*

Although the cause of rosacea remains unknown, the condition is usually easily controlled with an antibiotic. Systemic treatment is similar to that for inflammatory acne (see above): tetracycline 500 mg orally two times a day or erythromycin 333 mg orally three times a day. If a good response is seen, the dosage of tetracycline is halved at 4-week intervals times two and stopped (erythromycin decreased by one-third and then one-half). If a flare occurs, the dosage is increased to the next higher dosage. Some patients can discontinue therapy after several months; however, most flare without some therapy. Because topical therapies are generally preferable, an alternative to systemic antibiotic therapy is topical metronidazole gel or cream (MetroGel, MetroCream) applied to the central face two times a day after washing. Patients who have very sensitive skin may not tolerate any topical products and should be treated with oral antibiotics initially until inflammation is controlled. Once it is controlled, MetroCream or MetroGel may be tolerated. Finally, one advantage of systemic therapy over topical skin therapy is that it also suppresses ocular rosacea.

Hidradenitis Suppurativa

Hidradenitis suppurativa is a disorder characterized by inflammation and occlusion of apocrine glands. It generally affects patients between the second and fifth decades. Sites where apocrine glands are normally present or ectopic apocrine glands are sporadically present are affected. These sites include the axillae, perineum, inguinal folds, pubic region, and often the umbilicus, breasts, postauricular area, scalp, and back. Affected areas are studded with large comedones, inflammatory papules, pustules, and cysts. Sinus tracts form when cysts rupture and drain serum, blood, or purulent material. Patients may also have cystic facial acne (see above) and scarring scalp folliculitis (see below).

Secondary complications of hidradenitis suppurativa may include secondary amyloidosis, anemia of chronic disease, depression, and occasionally, an associated sacroiliitis. Finally, patients are at risk for episodes of acute cellulitis and, over the years, squamous cell carcinoma in this chronically inflamed tissue.

The differential diagnosis of hidradenitis suppurativa includes recurrent bacterial folliculitis and furunculosis (see Chapter 25), scrofuloderma (*Mycobacterium tuberculosis* infection with an ulcerated draining lymph node), granuloma inguinale (*Calymmatobacterium granulomatis* sexually transmitted infection characterized by genital and inguinal sinuses and hypertrophic scars), lymphogranuloma venereum (see Chapter 94), Crohn's disease (see Chapter 39), and a pilonidal cyst. The diagnosis of hidradenitis suppurativa is made by recognizing comedones, which are not present in these other disorders. Skin biopsy (see below) may be required to exclude other diagnoses. If there is doubt about the diagnosis, referral to a dermatologist is recommended.

The pathogenesis of this disorder is not well understood. It is debated whether infection in these patients is a primary or secondary event. Treatment consists of short courses of antibiotics for acute flares of disease, with specific antibiotic therapy based on the results of culture and antibiotic sensitivity of discharge from draining lesions. Chronic ongoing therapy includes oral tetracycline or erythromycin for antiinflammatory and antibacterial effects, and topical benzoyl peroxide in a regimen similar to that used in acne (see above). Surgical therapy ranging from tract marsupialization to deep, wide excision is indicated in patients with severe unresponsive disease.

Miliaria

Miliaria is a disorder of sweat retention caused by occlusion of the ducts of the eccrine glands. Although it is not a follicular disorder, as are acne and folliculitis, it may mimic these disorders. Miliaria occurs most often in active people who are perspiring heavily and wearing occlusive clothing or those confined to bed, lying supine for extended periods (e.g., workers exposed to hot environmental temperatures wearing occlusive clothing, febrile patients lying supine in bed).

The eruption almost always occurs on the trunk. When the sweat duct is occluded very superficially, asymptomatic, noninflammatory 1- to 2-mm vesicles that easily rupture are seen in the upper central chest or back *(miliaria crystallina).* When the duct is occluded deeper in the skin, pruritic nonfollicular erythematous papules occur over the chest and back *(miliaria rubra).* Lesions may be few to many in number.

The differential diagnosis of miliaria rubra includes infectious and noninfectious folliculitis. These entities are distinguished by their involvement of hair follicles as opposed to eccrine ducts. Miliaria crystallina is unique in its appearance.

The treatment of miliaria includes providing a cool environment, eliminating occlusive clothing, and decreasing a patient's fever. Cool baths (see "Topical Therapeutics," below) and topical antipruritic lotions containing menthol or phenol (e.g., Sarna lotion) may reduce distressing pruritus.

DERMATITIS

Dermatitis, or *eczema,* is a nonspecific term indicating inflammatory changes of the skin. These changes always affect the epidermis, so skin surface change is seen. No matter what specific type of dermatitis is present (see below), acute, subacute, and chronic changes may be present. In *acute dermatitis,* changes consist of edema, papules, vesicles, serous discharge, crusting, scaling, and erythema. In *subacute dermatitis,* the lesions are erythematous and scaly, and may be edematous, but there is no serous discharge or crusting. In *chronic dermatitis,* the changes consist of a scaly thickening, giving a washboard or tree bark appearance called *lichenification.* The clinical appearance or phase (acute, subacute, chronic) of the dermatitis more accurately guides treatment than the specific type of dermatitis. Table 100.5 summarizes the features, treatment, and prognosis of all specific types of dermatitis, with the exception of perioral and intertriginous dermatitis (see below). The different types of dermatitis are categorized in several ways based on associated manifestations, as with atopic dermatitis; cause, as with contact dermatitis; morphology, as with nummular dermatitis; and location, as with hand dermatitis. Dermatitis may be caused by endogenous or exogenous factors or variable combinations of both.

Atopic Dermatitis

Atopic dermatitis is considered an endogenous dermatitis. Patients typically have associated allergic rhinitis or asthma and 70% give a family history of atopy. Often, various immunologic alterations, including elevated serum IgE levels, decreased delayed hypersensitivity responsiveness, decreased numbers of T-suppressor lymphocytes, increased percentage of B lymphocytes with surface-bound IgE-1, and decreased number or activity of natural killer lymphocytes may be seen. Not all patients with atopic dermatitis express these abnormalities, and their role in the development of atopic dermatitis is unclear. These studies should not be a part of the routine evaluation of a patient with atopic dermatitis.

Atopic dermatitis may be divided into subsets based on age of onset: infantile, childhood, and adult atopic dermatitis with onset between 2 months and 2 years, 2 years and adolescence, and adulthood, respectively. Areas of involvement are typically those that patients can scratch. Therefore, affected sites include the cheeks, extensor arms, and legs in infants, the flexural arms, legs, neck, wrists, and ankles in children, and these same sites and often also (or only) the hands or face in adults (Fig. 100.8). The morphology of the lesions varies, mostly based on the duration. *Acute lesions* consist of erythema, edema, papules, vesicles, erosions, crusts, and scale, whereas *chronic lesions* consist of scaly papules coalescing into lichenified plaques, often with focal excoriations and crusts.

Treatment depends on the patient's age and the location of the dermatitis. Generally, the face is treated with 1% hydrocortisone ointment or cream (both available without prescription) in all patients and, in children, hydrocortisone is also used on nonfacial sites. For more chronic lichenified lesions that are not on the face, midpotency (triamcinolone, betamethasone valerate) to high-potency (fluocinonide, betamethasone dipropionate) fluorinated corticosteroids are used. Care must be taken to avoid local (see "Topical Therapeutics," below) and systemic side effects. Corticosteroids applied to significant body surface areas may produce hypercortisolism and hypothalamic–pituitary–adrenal axis suppression. Topical corticosteroids should always be used in

Table 100.5. Summary of the Diagnostic, Therapeutic, and Prognostic Features of the Phases of Dermatitis

Phase	Typical Morphology	Primary Treatment of Dermatitis	Indicators of Colonization or Secondary Infection Requiring Therapy	Treatment of Infection	Second-Line Treatment for Unresponsive Dermatitis, or First-Line Treatment for Very Severe Dermatitis	General Prognosis
Acute dermatitis	Papules, papulovesicles, erythema, serous discharge, and crusting	Saline compresses four times/day, switching when dry to corticosteroid creams[a] two times/day (high potency) and emollients +/– antipruritics	Moderate to severe crusting representing impetiginization or erythema representing erysipelas or cellulitis	Oral antistaphylococcal antibiotics (dicloxacillin or cephalexin) except in cases of erysipelas or cellulitis, which typically require IV antibiotics (see Chapter 25)	Prednisone 0.7 to 1 mg/kg/day tapered over approximately 2 wk	Usually excellent
Subacute dermatitis	Erythema, edema, papules, and scale	Topical corticosteroid (high-potency) ointments[a] and emollients[b]	As above or numerous excoriations	As above	Phototherapy or photochemotherapy with UVB or PUVA, respectively	Usually good, but recurrences are not uncommon
Chronic dermatitis	Lichenified or thickened papules and plaques	As above	As above or nonhealing fissures	As above	As above	Treatment is difficult, recurrences very common

[a]Only low-potency corticosteroids should be used on the face; elsewhere, when using super-, high-, or mid-potency corticosteroids, side effects such as atrophy, telangiectasia, striae, or systemic absorption with hypercortisolism and hypothalamic–pituitary–adrenal axis suppression are possible.
[b]Corticosteroids and emollients are discussed in detail in the section entitled "Topical Therapeutics."

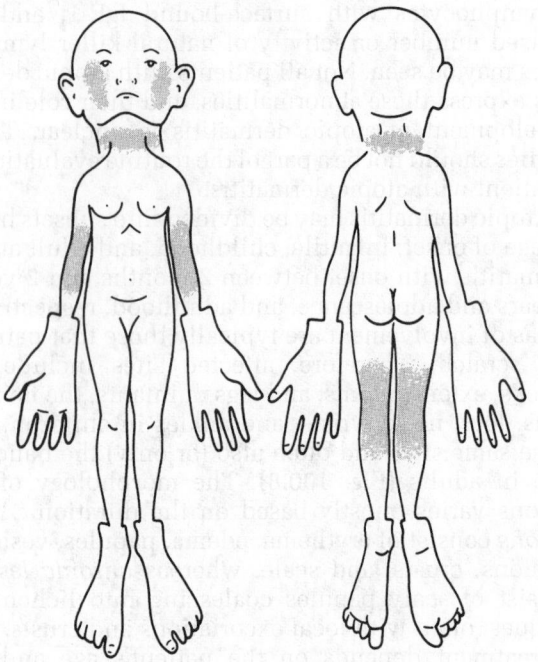

Figure 100.8. Lichenified pruritic areas in flexural regions and on the face are typical locations for adult atopic dermatitis.

combination with emollients (see "Topical Therapeutics," below) to protect, hydrate, and reduce pruritus of the skin. Use should be discontinued as soon as lesions are clear and should be restarted as needed. Some patients also require oral antibiotics for recurrent infection, or "dermatitis triggering" colonization with *Staphylococcus aureus.* For patients unresponsive to therapy, other therapies, including in-office phototherapy with ultraviolet-B (UVB) radiation or photochemotherapy with psoralen and ultraviolet-A (UVA) radiation, may be prescribed. Because systemic corticosteroid therapy is associated with numerous long-term unacceptable side effects, it should be avoided as a treatment for atopic dermatitis. Intended short courses of oral corticosteroids often lead to unintentional chronic therapy at the patient's request and persistence. Finally, external factors exacerbating the disease including irritants, harsh soaps, recurrent wetting and drying, and coarse fabrics should be avoided. Food allergies seem to be important in a small percentage of patients with infantile and childhood atopic dermatitis in whom avoidance may have a positive effect (74). In contrast, respiratory allergen desensitization does not alter the course of atopic dermatitis.

Nummular Dermatitis

Nummular dermatitis is an idiopathic dermatosis seen most often in adults. Lesions consist of pruritic, sharply circumscribed, variably sized (1 to 2 cm), vesicular (acute) to lichenified (chronic), erythematous plaques most often seen on the extremities. Lesions may be mistaken for tinea corporis and impetigo because of their annular shape. Tinea is distinguished by a positive potassium hydroxide (KOH) preparation and

impetigo has a more superficial scalded appearance or heavy honeycomblike surface crust (see below).

Treatment for nummular dermatitis is similar to that for atopic dermatitis (see above). Emollients in combination with fluorinated corticosteroids generally clear patients; after clearing, the topical corticosteroid should be tapered over 2 weeks (one application every other or every third day) to prevent recurrences (see "Topical Therapeutics," below). Patients with recalcitrant dermatitis are often noncompliant with their therapeutic regimen or instead have a secondary staphylococcal infection that requires treatment (Table 100.5).

Asteatotic Eczema

Asteatotic, xerotic, or *dry skin* eczema is most often seen in the wintertime in elderly people living in low-humidity areas. *Asteatosis* and *xerosis* simply mean dry skin without associated inflammation. The cause of asteatotic eczema is not fully understood. Diminished epidermal and sebaceous gland lipids appear to allow loss of normally retained water from the stratum corneum. Skin changes typically begin with dryness in the early fall, which then progress to patches of faint erythema appearing *cracked* or superficially fissured (Fig. 100.9, Color Plate 2). Patients complain of a stinging, tight feeling to their skin with or without associated pruritus. Treatment involves hydration of the skin with warm baths or showers using oilated soaps (e.g., Dove, Oilatum, or Aveeno Oilated Oatmeal Soap) followed by *patting dry,* leaving some moisture on the skin, the application of a midpotency corticosteroid ointment (not cream) to areas of erythema, and a *top coat* of an oil-based emollient to all skin areas (see "Topical Therapeutics," below). Hot showers, which *strip* natural body oils, harsh soaps (e.g., original Ivory, a pure soap with a very high pH), and stiff, large-fiber clothing (e.g., wool) should be avoided. When the eczema has cleared, only the topical corticosteroid is discontinued; all other measures must be continued throughout the cold, dry months to prevent recurrences.

Contact Dermatitis

Contact dermatitis may be either irritant or allergic. Irritant is the more common type of contact dermatitis. Irritant contact dermatitis may develop in anyone, whereas allergic contact dermatitis occurs only in people immunologically capable of recognizing and reacting to a particular allergen.

Irritant contact dermatitis to harsh chemicals (see Chapter 7) results in a scalded, erythematous, moist appearance of the skin with peeling back of the most superficial epidermis, leaving a lacy border. This is often caused by substances with extremes of pH, such as harsh alkaline cleansers and strong acid solutions. In contrast, mild irritants produce macular erythema that, with chronic exposure, may evolve into scaly plaques. With all forms of contact dermatitis, the eruption is limited to the area of contact. It is often the localized distribution and shape of the lesion that suggests the diagnosis (e.g., the forearm site of a solvent spill [irritant] or the earlobes bearing earrings [allergic]).

Allergic contact dermatitis is caused by a delayed hypersensitivity reaction. Initial sensitization takes place through cutaneous allergen exposure and requires approximately 1 week: A substance containing an allergen is applied to the skin; the allergen acts as a hapten, binding to a protein to form a complete allergen, which is processed by the Langerhans cell, the resident antigen-presenting cell in the epidermis. If sensitization occurs, the Langerhans cell moves into the dermis and through the lymphatics to the local lymph nodes, where it stimulates a lymphocyte clone that recognizes the antigen. If the substance is still in the skin 1 week after initial application (or upon subsequent reexposure), the Langerhans cells within the epidermis present the allergen to the memory T helper cells. These T cells secrete cytokines and other soluble mediators, which lead to recruitment of additional inflammatory cells (e.g., monocytes, neutrophils), resulting in the clinical picture of an acute dermatitis.

The most common cause of allergic contact dermatitis is a *plant dermatitis,* caused by the *Rhus* genus, which includes *poison ivy, oak, and sumac.* The oleoresin or oil within these plants is strongly allergenic. Typically, an acute vesiculobullous eruption develops in the areas of contact (Fig. 100.10, Color Plate 2). Because affected patients often note that new blisters continue to develop over many days, they often think that the rash is spreading, believing that blister fluid leakage causes spreading. This is incorrect. Once the allergen is flushed from the skin, spreading is impossible. The reason that new lesions may continue to develop for many days is because lesions take longer to evolve on skin where penetration is reduced or a lesser amount of oleoresin contact has occurred. Also, continued unintentional exposure to the resin, which may persist on clothing, tools, sports equipment, or the fur of pets may lead to "chronic poison ivy." Allergens other than Rhus are less common sensitizers and typically produce a less pronounced dermatitis with erythema, edema, and mild or no vesiculation. Such allergens include nickel (commonly found in costume jewelry); neomycin, benzocaine, and merthiolate in topical medicinals; fragrances and preservatives in cosmetics and personal products; and preservatives in ophthalmologic, otic, and dermatologic prescription and nonprescription medications. *Occupational exposures* may also cause allergic contact dermatitis (see Chapter 7). Common allergens include potassium dichromate in cement, dyes, or textiles; epoxy resins in adhesives, finishing products, and casings for electrical devices; rosin in adhesive materials; thiuram, mercaptobenzothiazole, and carbamates in rubber products; glyceryl monothioglycolate and paraphenylenediamine in hair wave and dye formulations; and acrylates in methylmethacrylate used in orthopedic surgery, dentistry, and nail sculpturing. *Allergic contact dermatitis* tends to appear suddenly after a history of many exposures

without reactions. Evaluation for possible allergic contact dermatitis requires a detailed history of personal product use, as well as occupational exposures, followed by patch testing with standardized common and suspected allergens to confirm the suspected diagnosis and identify the causative allergen.

The prevention of irritant and allergic contact dermatitis involves the recognition of irritants or allergens and elimination or minimization of exposure. Topical treatment is similar to that used for atopic dermatitis (see above and Table 100.5) with emollients in combination with mid- to high-potency topical corticosteroids (see "Topical Therapeutics," below). In cases of vesiculobullous dermatitis or dermatitis involving the face, hands, or genitalia, oral corticosteroids should be administered if no contraindications exist. Treatment should be approximately 0.7 mg of prednisone per kilogram of body weight, tapered over 2 weeks (e.g., 40 mg for 4 days, 30 mg for 5 days, and 20 mg for 5 days).

Contact Urticaria

Contact urticaria, although not a dermatitis, is a contact reaction. It may be caused by a nonimmunologic substance or may be a true IgE reaction to an allergen. The most common cause of contact urticaria is *latex protein* (13,86). This allergy is greatly increased in patients undergoing chronic intermittent bladder catheterization (particularly children) and, to a lesser extent, in health care workers, particularly those with an atopic diathesis who are exposed to latex repeatedly.

Affected patients develop hives in areas of contact with gloves. A common complaint is itching after wearing gloves for a few minutes. Identification of this allergy is important because latex exposure may cause not only localized urticaria, but also generalized urticaria and even anaphylaxis depending on how much histamine reaches the systemic circulation. Anaphylaxis is more likely to occur with mucosal or visceral latex contact. The diagnosis of latex contact urticaria is made by in vitro latex IgE RAST test or in vivo patch, prick, or scratch testing. The former is preferred, as in vivo testing may cause anaphylaxis. However, RAST testing sensitivity is not 100%; therefore, when allergy is strongly suspected and RAST testing is negative, referral to an allergist for skin testing is appropriate (13). Patients with latex contact urticaria should be counseled to avoid all latex items, including gloves, balloons, condoms, and medical devices such as latex tubing, dental dams, surgeon's latex gloves, and catheters. A Medic Alert bracelet and an epinephrine-containing autoinjector (Epi-Pen) should be prescribed for possible emergencies. Chapter 23 provides detailed information on the treatment of anaphylaxis.

Hand Dermatitis

Hand dermatitis is a very broad term encompassing such conditions as *primary dyshidrotic hand dermatitis* and several forms of dermatitis, including atopic hand dermatitis, nummular hand dermatitis (see above), and contact hand dermatitis (see above).

Dyshidrotic hand eczema is an idiopathic condition confined to the hands and has characteristic vesicles 1 to 2 mm in diameter, particularly located on the sides of the fingers and often over the palms. The lesions are intensely pruritic, and flares of disease tend to cycle over weeks to months. As vesicles resolve, there is focal desquamation and drying of the skin.

Although this disorder is called dyshidrotic, there is actually no consistently identified problem with hidrosis (sweating). If any suspicion of allergic contact dermatitis arises, patch testing should be done to exclude this diagnosis. Treatment should consist of emollients and topical corticosteroid ointments for flares of disease (see "Topical Therapeutics," below). Recalcitrant cases should be referred to a dermatologist for consideration of phototherapy or photochemotherapy.

Infectious Eczematoid Dermatitis

Infectious eczematoid dermatitis is a secondary change within a primary form of dermatitis. Patients become colonized and infected with *Staphylococcus aureus* and show extensive crusting and exudation within their background dermatitis. Treatment includes systemic antistaphylococcal antibiotics (e.g., dicloxacillin 250 to 500 mg four times a day, depending on the size of the patient and the severity of infection), as well as treatment of the primary dermatosis (see above) with soaks, topical corticosteroids, and emollients (see "Topical Therapeutics," below).

Perioral Dermatitis

Perioral and sometimes periorificial dermatitis is an eruption of minute papules and pustules on a background of erythema and scant scale in a perioral or periorificial (mouth, eyes, and nares) location. Although it may occur in the very young as well as in the elderly, it is most common in young women. Compared to acne, it is uncommon. It is differentiated from acne by the lack of comedones and by nonfollicular skin involvement and from contact dermatitis (see above) by the fact that it always spares the vermilion border, beginning 2 to 3 mm outside this border, and symptoms include burning and stinging as opposed to itching.

The cause of perioral dermatitis is not known, but it has been associated with topical and aerosolized inhaled fluorinated corticosteroids and fluorinated toothpastes. Initial treatment is similar to that used for acne rosacea (see above), but medications can usually be stopped in 4 to 8 weeks, often without a recurrence. Recurrences are treated similarly to the first episode.

Intertrigo (Intertriginous Dermatitis)

Intertrigo is a form of dermatitis that may occur in areas in which skin directly opposes skin, such as the inframammary creases, abdominal folds, inguinal folds, gluteal cleft, and angles of the mouth. Patients develop moist erythema and, at times, fissures and exudation. The affected areas burn, sting, and itch. Such skin changes provide a very hospitable environment for yeast and bacterial growth.

The differential diagnosis of intertrigo includes primary *Candida* infection, *seborrheic dermatitis*, and *psoriasis. Candida* infection is diagnosed with a KOH preparation (see below). Seborrheic dermatitis and psoriasis are usually diagnosed by identifying skin lesions elsewhere (see below). When intertrigo does not respond to therapy (see below), unusual diagnoses such as *Bowen's disease* (squamous cell carcinoma in situ), *Paget's disease,* and glucagonoma syndrome should be considered and a biopsy performed.

Therapy should be directed at keeping the areas of skin contact dry. Gauze may be placed between the folds where appropriate, and a powder (e.g., Zeasorb and Zeasorb-AF, which contains an antifungal agent) or plain talc should be applied frequently to dry the skin and reduce yeast colonization or infection. If obesity is the cause of the problem (e.g., abdominal or inguinal folds), weight reduction will help. A cool environment is also beneficial. In elderly edentulous patients with chronic fissures at the angles of the mouth, after appropriate treatment for possible oral candidiasis, collagen injections may be considered. Collagen is injected into the crease formed by the opposing folds of skin. Although collagen injections must be repeated every 6 to 12 months, they may still be worthwhile for this chronic and painful cracking.

Seborrheic Dermatitis

Seborrheic dermatitis is a common idiopathic papulosquamous dermatosis that is present in approximately 3 to 5% of the population. An inflammatory epidermal hyperproliferation affects the seborrheic areas of the body (areas more heavily populated with sebaceous glands) and therefore favors the scalp and facial hair-bearing areas, central face (glabellar area and nasal folds), ears, presternal chest, axillae, umbilicus, inguinal folds, gluteal cleft, and perianal skin (Fig. 100.11). Pruritus is variably present. *Dandruff,* a term commonly used synonymously with seborrheic dermatitis, is a similar but noninflammatory (nonerythematous) scaling of the skin in the seborrheic areas. The onset of seborrheic dermatitis is usually in early adulthood and the course is characterized by frequent spontaneous remissions and exacerbations.

Causes and Pathogenesis

Although the cause of seborrheic dermatitis is unknown, several observations have been made and hypotheses proposed over the years. An increase in the colonizing population of *Pityrosporum* (a lipophilic yeast normally present on the skin) may be found in some patients. It has therefore been suggested that the yeast stimulates an immune response and hence the clinical cutaneous inflammation. Furthermore, seborrheic dermatitis occurs with increased frequency and severity in patients infected with the human immunodeficiency virus (see Chapter 34) and in patients with

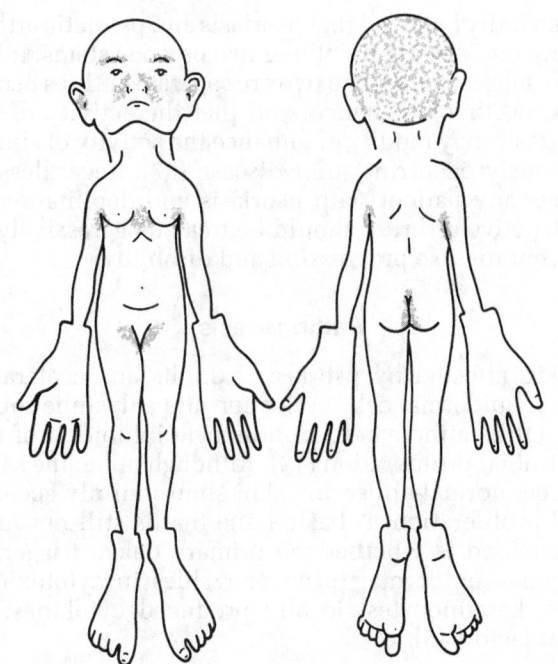

Figure 100.11. Usual location of erythema and scale in seborrheic dermatitis.

Parkinson's disease. It is speculated that *Pityrosporum* or other colonizing microbes may be involved in these patients. Other causative or contributory factors in seborrheic dermatitis have been proposed, including nutritional deficiencies and alterations caused by various neurologic disorders.

Treatment

Treatment is directed at decreasing epidermal hyperproliferation, inflammation, and *Pityrosporum* using tar shampoos, topical corticosteroids (cream for nonhairy areas and clear, nongreasy lotion or solution for hairy areas), and ketoconazole (or selenium sulfide) shampoos, respectively. For the scalp, a tar (e.g., Neutrogena T-Gel or Denorex) or a selenium sulfide shampoo (e.g., Head and Shoulders Intensive Formula or Selsun Blue) every other night for 1 month, then ongoing prophylactic use twice weekly, is usually effective. If this alone is not effective after 1 month, fluorinated corticosteroid solution (e.g., Cormax Scalp Application, Lidex Solution), two to three drops applied after shampooing to each quarter-sized affected area of the scalp may be added. Once control is obtained, the corticosteroid is discontinued and repeated for recurrences only. For facial and body seborrheic dermatitis, hydrocortisone 1% cream (solution for the beard, mustache, eyebrows, outer auditory canal) may be used up to two times a day to control redness and scaling. Alternatively, ketoconazole cream (e.g., Nizoral 2% cream) may be used twice daily in a similar fashion. However, unlike steroids, ketoconazole cream is continued after clearance to prevent recurrences.

PSORIASIS

Definition and Prevalence

Psoriasis is an idiopathic benign epidermal hyperproliferation that affects 2% of the population (5,25). It is believed to be of multifactorial inheritance, with multiple genetic and environmental factors required for expression. More than one-third of affected patients develop the disease before age 19, and the average age of onset is 27 years (33,90). Most patients who develop psoriasis have lifelong disease with periods of remission and exacerbation. Factors associated with exacerbation include sunlight deprivation, infections, certain drugs including lithium and antimalarials (see "Drug Eruption," below), local cutaneous trauma, alcohol ingestion, and physical and psychologic stress.

Psoriasis may have a significant negative impact on many important aspects of life. Unlike other chronic diseases that may be easily concealed from strangers, acquaintances, and friends, psoriasis may be blatantly obvious because of thickened crumbly nails, extensive hand involvement, and heavy scalp scale. Summertime clothing brings yet other areas of involvement to light. The effect of the disease on the quality of life in patients with psoriasis has been compared with patients having other chronic diseases. When asked how many years of life patients would be willing to give up or how willing they would be to risk their lives to be free of their disease, patients with moderate psoriasis respond similarly to patients having had a kidney transplant. Patients with severe psoriasis respond similarly to those undergoing hospital-based dialysis (5). Patients may also experience social rejection by people who believe that the disease is contagious or represents a manifestation of acquired immunodeficiency syndrome (AIDS). Beyond the negative psychosocial impact of psoriasis, patients may also be burdened economically because of physical and occupational disability caused by hand, foot, or generalized skin involvement or incapacitating psoriatic arthritis.

Clinical Presentation

Psoriasis may be divided into four major subtypes depending on the appearance of lesions: plaque, guttate, erythrodermic, or pustular. *Chronic plaque psoriasis* is the most common type of psoriasis. Patients exhibit one to many deeply erythematous, sharply demarcated, oval plaques several centimeters in diameter, with moderate to heavy silvery-white surface scale, commonly on the scalp and over one or more extensor joints. Intertriginous plaques may also be present in the axillary, inframammary, umbilical, abdominal, inguinal, gluteal, and popliteal fossae (Fig. 100.12). These fold area lesions have little or no scale and are moist and intensely erythematous. Patients who have numerous widespread plaques have *"generalized" plaque psoriasis.*

Guttate psoriasis is the next most common type of psoriasis. It is characterized by an acute, exanthemlike eruption of guttate (droplike) erythematous, scaly papules, generally 1 mm to 1 cm in diameter. Although

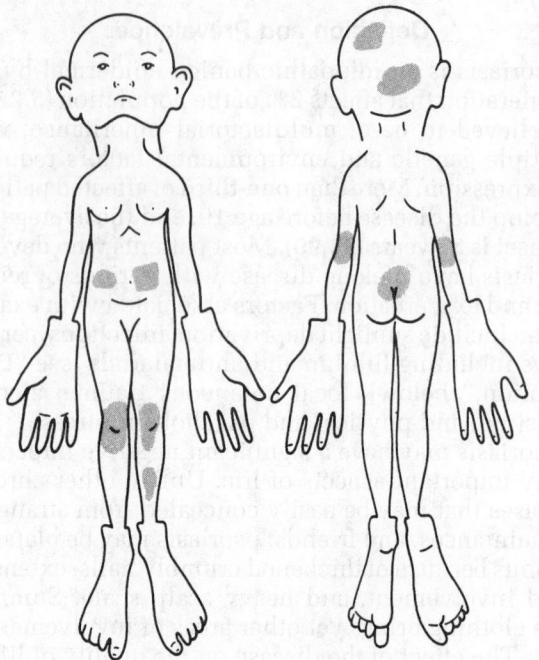

Figure 100.12. Psoriasis tends to be found on extensor surfaces and areas of repeated trauma, such as the waistline.

lesions are typically on the trunk and proximal extremities, the eruption may be widespread, involving the face, scalp, hands, and feet. Guttate psoriasis is often triggered by an infection, most often a streptococcal pharyngitis or a viral upper respiratory tract infection.

Erythrodermic psoriasis and *pustular psoriasis* are rare. In both types, a generalized exfoliative erythroderma (a scaly erythema) is present. In addition, in pustular psoriasis crops of tiny, superficial, nonfollicular pustules develop, coalesce into "lakes of pus," then desquamate in waves of lacy scale. Erythrodermic and pustular psoriasis are severe diseases, particularly in patients with other chronic illnesses. Potential complications include high-output congestive heart failure, sepsis, and vitamin and nutrient deficiencies caused by increased requirements and losses.

Although psoriasis presenting in one of these classic forms is usually easy to diagnose by clinical criteria alone, some patients have only one body plaque or patchy thick scalp scale. In some of these patients, clues to the diagnosis may be found in their nails. *Nail involvement* is present in 30% of patients. Although not pathognomonic, the most commonly noted changes are pitting (icepicklike depressions of the nail plate, Fig. 100.13), *onycholysis* (separation of the nail plate from the nail bed, with resultant white color caused by air between the plate and bed), and *subungual hyperkeratosis* (crumbly scale between the plate and bed).

Extracutaneous Disease

Arthritis has been estimated to affect less than 5% to nearly one-third of patients with psoriasis. Although it

is generally believed that psoriasis and psoriatic arthritis are one disease involving two organ systems, it has been suggested that the two are separate entities occurring together by chance, and that the activity of the psoriasis may modify or enhance the activity of simultaneously occurring joint disease (37). Regardless of cause, any patient with psoriasis and debilitating or destructive arthritis should be treated aggressively to prevent disease progression and disability.

Pathogenesis

Skin affected by psoriasis exhibits an accelerated rate of epidermal cell replication and a dysfunction of normal keratinocyte-to-keratinocyte inhibition of uncontrolled proliferation (42). Although not to the same degree, normal-appearing skin shows mildly accelerated proliferation. A basic issue that is still not fully understood is whether the primary defect triggering defective epidermal turnover resides in cytotoxic T cells, keratinocytes, locally produced cytokines, or other factors (5).

Treatment

Therapy for psoriasis depends on the degree of body surface area involvement and the clinical subtype of disease and prior response to therapy (25). One basic caveat should be noted: Systemic corticosteroids, which generally dramatically improve psoriasis, should never, or only with a rare exception, be administered because dosage tapering may precipitate erythrodermic or pustular psoriasis.

Localized chronic plaque psoriasis is treated with bland emollients, keratolytics (e.g., Lac-Hydrin lotion 12%, by prescription) and low- to midpotency topical corticosteroids (see "Topical Therapeutics," below), or a topical vitamin D derivative, calcipotriene (Dovonex ointment or cream), twice daily. A new topical syn-

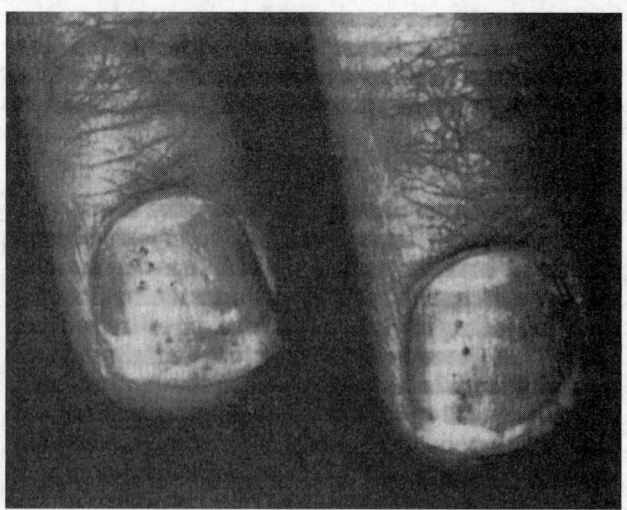

Figure 100.13. Minute pits are commonly seen on the surface of nails in patients with psoriasis.

thetic vitamin A derivative, tazarotene (Tazorac), 0.05 and 0.1% gel applied twice daily is now available. This treatment, topical vitamin D, and topical corticosteroids all appear to be of equal efficacy in clinical trials; however, in a given patient one treatment may be much more effective than another. Side effects common to topical corticosteroids include tachyphylaxis and atrophy, whereas those more common to calcipotriene and vitamin A derivatives include irritation and stinging.

Generalized plaque psoriasis is more difficult, timeconsuming, and expensive to treat with topical preparations. Also, widespread use of mid- to high-potency corticosteroids may produce an effect similar to systemic corticosteroid administration. Generalized plaque psoriasis is usually treated with phototherapy using ultraviolet B (UVB; UV radiation 290 to 320 nm wavelength) or photochemotherapy with the phototoxic agent 8-methoxypsoralen (Oxsoralen Ultra) orally in combination with controlled ultraviolet-A (UVA; UV radiation 320 to 400 nm wavelength) given in a phototherapy light box (psoralen + UVA = PUVA therapy). Patients are generally treated three times a week until clearance occurs, then either given maintenance light treatments (PUVA only; UVB maintenance cannot be used because of the risk of sunburn) or discontinued until the next flare of psoriasis occurs. A patient should never be given 8-methoxypsoralen to be used with natural sunlight or in a suntan parlor because severe burns and even death may occur. Also, selfadministered light treatment even without a phototoxic agent is best avoided because careful monitoring is not possible and severe burning may result. Over a long period, PUVA therapy increases a patient's risk of skin cancer. Therefore patients treated in this way should be followed indefinitely for the possible later development of skin cancer. Alternative therapies to phototherapy and photochemotherapy include methotrexate and etretinate (see below).

Guttate psoriasis, particularly with the initial episode, is usually very responsive to most treatments. Emollients, low-potency topical corticosteroids (see "Topical Therapeutics," below), and sunlight or in-office UVB phototherapy work well. In addition, because triggering infections may precipitate guttate psoriasis, an appropriate evaluation to exclude this possibility should be performed.

Erythrodermic and pustular psoriasis may cause severe and even life-threatening illness, particularly in elderly patients with cardiovascular disease. Depending on the severity of the psoriasis and underlying medical problems, patients may require hospitalization, bed rest, warm baths, bland emollients, and systemic therapy with etretinate (a synthetic retinoid), weekly low-dose methotrexate, or infrequently, cyclosporine. Often, patients have signs and symptoms identical to those seen with sepsis, with cyclic fevers up to 40°C and an increase in white blood cells (WBCs) up to 40,000 cells/mm^3 with neutrophilia, tachycardia, and orthostatic hypotension, so that possible sepsis must be excluded with blood cultures and other appro-

priate testing. The hemodynamic instability seen is caused by marked vasodilation and increased cardiac output, and is particularly problematic in the setting of preexistent cardiovascular disease. In addition, vitamin and nutrient deficiencies may result from the accelerated epidermal turnover rate. After all the acute cutaneous and systemic problems have been addressed and the patient's cutaneous disease is controlled, systemic therapy for psoriasis must be continued or PUVA substituted to prevent severe flares.

Patients receiving methotrexate, etretinate, or cyclosporine must be monitored closely. The most important side effects of methotrexate are acute cytopenias and chronic hepatitis and cirrhosis, whereas that of etretinate is mutagenesis. With chronic dosing, etretinate has a half-life of approximately 120 days and detectable drug and metabolites may be found in the fat for many years after treatment. For this reason, etretinate should not be used in women of childbearing potential. Etretinate may also induce hypertriglyceridemia and hypercholesterolemia, hepatitis, pseudotumor cerebri, bony hyperostosis, hair loss, fragile skin, painful palmar and plantar desquamation, and arthralgias. Cyclosporine has many notable side effects, including hypertension, decreased renal blood flow, glomerular and tubular toxicity, paresthesias, and anergy (8,21). Whether it is associated with an increased risk of cutaneous or lymphoproliferative malignancies in nontransplant patients is unclear (8,96).

ACANTHOSIS NIGRICANS

Acanthosis nigricans (AN) takes its name from its appearance: a hyperpigmented, velvety textural change of the skin over the base of the neck, extensor joints of the hands, and flexural surfaces. It may be seen in association with endocrine disorders (insulin resistance, diabetes mellitus, obesity, polycystic ovary disease, ovarian hyperthecosis, Cushing's disease, Addison's disease, acromegaly, hypothyroidism, and pineal hyperplasia or pinealoma) (67), various drugs and peptides (nicotinic acid, diethylstilbestrol, glucocorticoids, urogastrone, growth hormone, adrenocorticotropic hormone, and probably insulinlike growth factor and others) (67,69), and malignancies (most often gastric adenocarcinoma, but also hepatic, uterine, cervical, breast, and lung carcinoma, lymphoma, and rarely, other cancers). It has been noted that malignancy-associated AN usually occurs in patients over 40 years old and, in approximately 35% of such cases, affects the tongue and lips (11). AN may also be transmitted as an isolated benign autosomal-dominant trait or as part of various syndromes. In these instances, onset is in infancy or very early childhood.

AN associated with endocrinopathies appears to be more common than previously recognized. In a screen of over 1400 sixth- to eighth-grade children, AN was found in approximately 7%, being significantly overrepresented (13%) in the several hundred African Americans studied within this group (83). Testing in a subset of these children revealed a strong correlation between hyperinsulinemia and AN (83). Similar data in adults suggest that the presence of AN is a significant independent indicator of hyperinsulinemia (32). This association of AN and insulin resistance has been substantiated and further divided into type A (seen in girls and young women with hyperandrogenic features and often with polycystic ovary disease) and type B (seen in patients with autoimmune disorders characterized by insulin receptor autoantibodies). Clearly, the importance of recognizing AN lies in the evaluation it triggers for detection and treatment of an underlying condition. Cosmetically, AN may be treated with topical retinoic acid (tretinoin, Retin-A) (19), using the protocol described for comedonal acne (see above).

HAIR LOSS

To fully appreciate hair loss, normal hair growth must be considered. Hair growth is divided into different stages depending on whether it is active or inactive. These stages are *anagen* (the growing phase of hair, which may last up to 7 years), *catagen* (the transition or "apoptosis" phase, which may last days to weeks), and *telogen* (the resting phase just before hair shedding, which lasts 2 to 3 months). Hair loss or *alopecia* of the scalp is divided into *nonscarring* and *scarring* forms; nonscarring alopecia is far more common.

Nonscarring Alopecia Without Inflammation

Nonscarring alopecia is so designated because the affected hair follicles are not permanently lost or damaged. Noninflammatory, nonscarring alopecia (hair loss without any other changes such as erythema, scale, scarring) is characteristic of male or female pattern hair loss (also called androgenetic alopecia), alopecia areata (see below), telogen effluvium (see below), anagen effluvium (see below), and various systemic causes of diffuse hair thinning, including thyroid disease, systemic lupus erythematosus, and drug-induced hair loss.

Androgenetic alopecia is common in both men and women. Men differ in their pattern of hair loss. Typically men experience a frontal and vertex type of thinning, variably followed by confluence of these areas; women experience diffuse thinning over the crown. In both sexes, the onset of androgenetic alopecia may be as early as the late teens. Rarely, women show a male pattern of hair loss, and in these patients signs of virilization (e.g., facial hair growth, clitoral hypertrophy, deepening voice, and muscular body habitus) may be present. Appropriate evaluation should be performed to exclude hyperandrogenemia caused by adrenal hyperplasia, polycystic ovary disease, and various adrenal and ovarian tumors (see Chapter 77).

Treatment options in patients who desire more hair include oral finasteride (Propecia, 1-mg tablets) for men, and for both men and women, topical *minoxidil, hair transplants,* and various *hair prostheses* varying from woven-in individual hairs to full-scalp wigs. Each of these treatments has its disadvantages. Over-the-counter topical *minoxidil* 2% solution (Rogaine) produces significant hair growth in only approximately 20% of patients; however, a much higher percentage of patients probably have reduction in the rate of further hair loss. A new Rogaine Extra Strength for Men (minoxidil 5% solution) is now available and said to grow 45% more hair than the original Rogaine. Treatment with either must be ongoing to maintain hair growth or halt hair loss, and the cost of this treatment is approximately $30 per month (generic for the 2% is 50 to 67% of this price). Hair *transplants* are expensive and are associated with some discomfort, and once an initial transplant line has been started, patients generally feel compelled to continue with repeated hair transplants to avoid a very artificial-appearing frontal hairline with nothing behind it. Hair weaves in which natural or synthetic hair is woven into the patient's own hair must be repeated as the hair grows out, so they are expensive. Finally, although some people do very well with wigs, wigs may be uncomfortable, difficult to manage, and costly.

Telogen effluvium is a common disorder in which patients experience shedding of telogen hairs diffusely over the scalp. Telogen or resting hairs make up approximately 10 to 20% of the scalp hair, so hair loss is usually evident only to the patient, who notes massive amounts of hair coming out in his or her brush. Telogen effluvium may occur two to several months after such events as childbirth, general anesthesia, and catabolic states such as high fever for many days, rapid weight loss, and protein malnutrition. This form of alopecia is reversible once the precipitating factor is no longer present. However, several months elapse before this hair loss stops and new anagen hair growth is seen.

Numerous nonchemotherapeutic drugs are known to cause hair loss through a variety of mechanisms, primarily affecting telogen hairs (10 to 20% of the scalp hairs), therefore producing a chronic telogen effluvium that is usually appreciable only to the patient. The most common of these drugs are androgens, anticoagulants, anticonvulsants, and cholesterol-lowering agents. This hair loss is reversible with discontinuance of the causative medication.

Anagen effluvium may be caused by chemotherapeutic agents and ionizing irradiation. Patients have shedding of the actively growing hairs in the scalp, which constitute approximately 80% of the total scalp hair. Hairs are shed rapidly over a matter of days, and patients typically have no or only very sparse hairs left on the scalp (telogen hairs). As with telogen effluvium, this pattern of hair loss is reversible after the insult is removed, with the exception of ionizing irradiation, which may cause permanent hair loss.

Alopecia areata, typically presenting with one to a few coin-shaped areas of hair loss, is believed to be an immunologically mediated form of hair loss. Uncommonly, patients may have total scalp hair loss, called *alopecia totalis,* or total body hair loss, called *alopecia universalis.* Most patients with mild limited alopecia areata have full hair regrowth within 1 year without treatment; however, recurrences in the same or new sites are common. Patients with alopecia areata have an increased prevalence of autoimmune thyroid disease, pernicious anemia, and Addison's disease. Initial treatment of patients with alopecia areata usually consists of topical corticosteroid solutions (e.g., Cormax Topical Scalp Application or Lidex solution, three to four drops applied to each quarter-sized area, including 0.5 cm of surrounding normal scalp) or corticosteroid scalp injections. Other treatments (e.g., topical irritants, topical sensitizers, PUVA) seem to be helpful in some patients but, as with topical and intralesional corticosteroids, well-controlled studies demonstrating efficacy are limited or lacking.

Although other disorders may cause variable degrees of nonscarring alopecia, the alopecia is merely secondary to the primary process, as in tinea capitis (see below) and seborrheic dermatitis (see above).

Scarring Alopecia

Scarring alopecia is uncommon. It is characterized by hair loss with a scarred appearance of the scalp, notably lacking hair follicles. It is associated with a number of systemic disorders and primary cutaneous disorders. Associations have been made with discoid lupus erythematosus, scarring folliculitis (i.e., folliculitis decalvans), kerion formation in tinea infection (see below), scarring (cicatricial) pemphigoid, lichen planus (subtype, lichen planopilaris), and pseudopelade (idiopathic scarring alopecia).

These forms of scarring alopecia are irreversible in most instances because the hair follicles are scarred and incapable of producing new anagen hairs. Patients suspected of having scarring alopecia should be referred as early as possible to a dermatologist because certain treatments may prevent further permanent hair loss.

DERMATOPHYTE INFECTIONS

Dermatophyte infections are caused by fungi that penetrate only the surface stratum corneum of the skin, hair, and nails. The different types of infection (see below) are seen in various age groups, although all types can be seen in all ages. Symptoms of fungal infections, regardless of location, are usually those of pruritus, burning, or stinging. Transmission of infection may occur through direct contact; however, indirect transmission occurs more commonly with exposure to dermatophyte-laden bed linens, towels, and clothing, as well as baths, showers, pools, and gymnasium floors.

Potassium Hydroxide Wet Mount Preparation

Dermatophyte and yeast infections of the skin are diagnosed with microscopic examination of the skin surface scale or stratum corneum. For this examination, scale is scraped from the advancing margin of an active lesion using a number 15 surgical blade held at a slightly less than 90° angle to the skin surface. The scale is placed on a glass slide, one to two drops of potassium hydroxide (KOH) 20% added, and a coverslip applied. This is gently heated with a low flame, avoiding boiling, because this causes crystallization. With light microscopy, the slide is scanned with the 10× objective and then examined more closely with the 40× objective. Dermatophyte hyphae are seen as refractile, rod-shaped filaments of uniform width with characteristic branching (Fig. 100.14A). These hyphae traverse several normal cells and therefore can be distinguished from cell membranes. In contrast to dermatophytes, *Candida* and *Pityrosporum* appear as nonbranching hyphae and clusters of budding spores (Fig. 100.14B). At times, *Candida* may show branching hyphae.

Fungal Culture

When the diagnosis of a fungal infection is strongly suspected despite negative KOH preparation or when the identification of a dermatophyte is important, a fungal culture should be done. Depending on the site of suspected infection, scale is taken from the advancing margin of the skin lesion, under the nail, or the scalp.

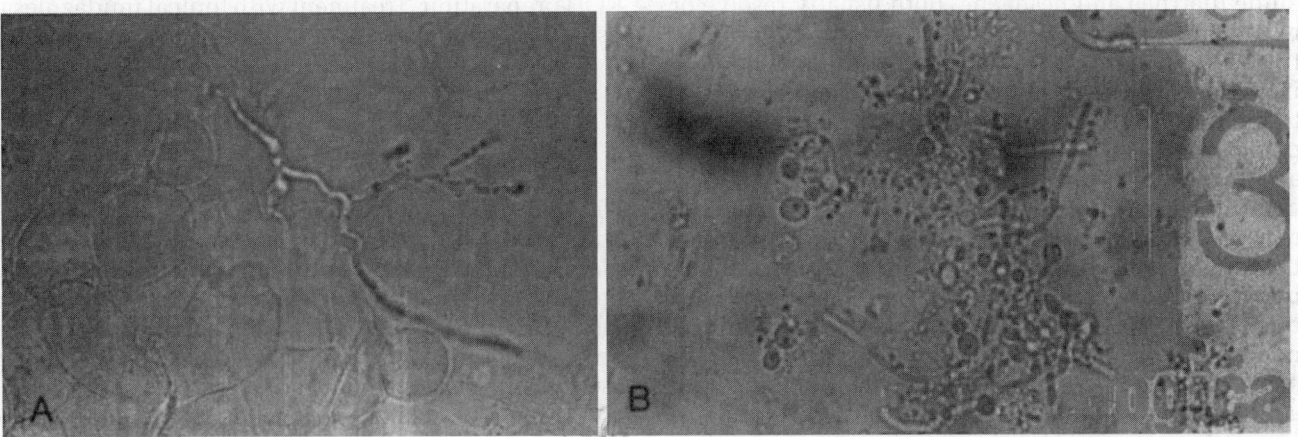

Figure 100.14. **A.** Hyphae of tinea (KOH preparation, ×400). **B.** Pseudohyphae of *Candida* (KOH preparation, ×400). (**B** courtesy of William G Merz, PhD.)

The latter sample should also include epilated hairs (four to six hairs removed with forceps; easily removed or broken "black dot" hairs, 1 to several millimeters long, are most desirable). Specimens are placed between two glass slides, taped together, and sent in a sterile urine cup to the laboratory for KOH preparation and fungal culture.

Tinea Capitis

Tinea capitis (scalp infection) is unusual in adults, being seen primarily in preadolescent children 4 to 12 years old. In the United States, tinea capitis is caused most often by *Trichophyton tonsurans.* Within areas of scalp scale and minimal to moderate erythema, broken-off hairs, 1 to 20 mm in length, are seen. The most severe complication of tinea capitis is *kerion formation,* in which boggy, inflammatory, pustular plaques of potentially scarring hair loss develop. If this is not treated early and aggressively with antifungals in combination with intralesional or oral corticosteroids, it generally causes permanent scarring in the scalp. When extensive, this may be a readily visible physical and cosmetic deformity. Tinea capitis is diagnosed with a positive KOH preparation or fungal culture. With a kerion, the KOH and fungal culture may be negative because of the intense host response. When the diagnosis of kerion is strongly suspected, treatment should be given as soon as possible in an attempt to prevent permanent disfigurement. This includes selenium sulfide shampoos (e.g., Selsun Blue, Head and Shoulders Intensive Formula) every one to few days to reduce spore shedding and oral griseofulvin to eradicate the fungus. Specifically formulated microsized or ultramicrosized griseofulvin is preferable to griseofulvin because absorption is better. Because these forms are not available in suspensions for young children, microsize griseofulvin capsules (Grisactin 250-mg capsules) may be opened and mixed with a food such as applesauce. Children are given 10 to 15 mg/kg per day with a meal in two divided doses for 6 weeks. Repeat culture is then done and treatment should be continued for 2 weeks after culture-negative scrapings are taken. More common side effects of griseofulvin include diarrhea and headache. Both usually resolve or become minimal after 1 week despite continued therapy. When this is not the case, dosage reduction or initiation of another antifungal (e.g., itraconazole or terbinafine (27)) should be substituted if not otherwise contraindicated. Because these drugs are not FDA approved for treatment of children, it is prudent to contact the drug manufacturer regarding the most recent studies of use and dosage in children. Additional potential side effects of griseofulvin include hypersensitivity reactions, *Candida* infections, and rare leukopenia and proteinuria. Finally, griseofulvin not only is teratogenic but also impairs absorption of birth control pills. Young women who are sexually active need to be made fully aware of this, and instructed on the use of two forms of birth control if they are or may become sexually active while taking griseofulvin. A pregnancy test (serum HCG) should be done before institution of therapy if there is any question of pregnancy. Monitoring laboratory tests are usually not done when griseofulvin is used for several weeks; however, when it is used for several months or more, it is recommended that CBC and liver enzymes be monitored every 3 months.

Tinea Faciei

Tinea faciei is often misdiagnosed as rosacea or cutaneous lupus because lesions tend not to be as sharp and annular as fungal infections elsewhere on the body. The picture is further confused by the fact that patients often note that lesions flare with sun exposure, suggesting possible diagnoses such as lupus erythematosus or acne rosacea. Lesions vary from erythematous, ill-defined, scaly plaques to the more typical fungal lesion morphology of sharply circumscribed plaques, leading edge scale, and central clearing. Diagnosis may be made with a positive KOH preparation; however, on the face false-negative KOH preparations are common and diagnosis may require culture or even biopsy. Treatment usually requires an oral antifungal (e.g., griseofulvin, itraconazole, fluconazole) because topical therapy often fails to clear this infection.

Tinea Corporis

Tinea corporis indicates a tinea infection outside areas such as the head, face, groin, hands, and feet. Classic lesions are annular (ringlike) plaques that show a delicate scale at the advancing margin. KOH preparation from these lesions is usually positive. Treatment consists of topical imidazole antifungals (see "Topical Therapeutics," below) applied twice a day for 4 to 6 weeks.

Tinea Cruris

Tinea cruris is predominantly seen in men. Lesions are semicircular, scaly plaques on the superior medial thighs, often extending into the perineal and inguinal areas. Diagnosis is made with performing a positive KOH preparation. Treatment with topical imidazoles is usually adequate (see "Topical Therapeutics," below).

Tinea Pedis

Tinea pedis is the most common dermatophyte infection, eventually affecting up to 80% of all men. Patients may have interdigital or plantar involvement with absent to intense erythema, scale, and focal maceration. Less commonly seen is inflammatory tinea pedis, represented by tense blisters. Occasionally, interdigital tinea pedis with interdigital fissures may provide a point of entry for *Streptococcus,* which may ascend and produce recurrent streptococcal cellulitis of the leg (78). Diagnosis is made by with a positive KOH preparation, and treatment may be initiated with topical imidazoles (see "Topical Therapeutics," below). Plantar tinea pedis is often refractory and requires oral therapy if complete clearance is the goal. However, often these patients are asymptomatic and therapy may not be necessary. In contrast, patients at risk for leg cellulitis (e.g., history of leg cellulitis, venous stasis, or deep or superficial venous thrombosis) should be treated aggressively in an attempt to clear interdigital tinea pedis to eliminate a potential portal of entry for *Streptococcus* (78).

Tinea Manuum

Tinea of the palmar skin is uncommon. When seen, it often manifests as "two feet, one hand" syndrome, with areas of involvement as the name implies. The palm shows diffuse, usually noninflammatory scaling and the KOH preparation is positive. Treatment typically requires systemic therapy, but topical imidazoles (see below, "Topical Therapeutics") may initially be tried for 6 to 8 weeks. If systemic therapy is unsuccessful or nail involvement is also present and clearance is desired, oral itraconazole or terbinafine may be prescribed (see below).

Tinea Unguium (Onychomycosis)

Dermatophyte toenail infections are common, whereas fingernail infection is less common. Although the incidence of tinea unguium is from 2 to 13% of the general population, the prevalence in the geriatric male population is much higher. Tinea unguium represents approximately 30% of all mycotic infections of the skin and nails (1). Changes include white discoloration, subungual crumbly debris, and thickening of the nails. Patients are typically asymptomatic unless the toenails become ingrown or secondary bacterial infection occurs. Treatment of these patients is notoriously difficult. Griseofulvin may be used, but long-term clearance rates are below 30% after a full year of therapy. When patients desire therapy and understand the expense, potential side effects, and required laboratory studies (see below), itraconazole (200 mg/day for 3 months or pulse dosing of 200 mg twice daily for 1 week *only* of each month, also for 3 months; capsules 100 mg) or terbinafine (250 mg/day) may be used. Cure rates several months after completion of the 3-month course of therapy vary from 50% to more than 70%. Because these drugs are retained in the nail for many months after drug discontinuance, patients are not evaluated for clearance until several months after completion of therapy. If they are still not clear, another 3-month course of therapy may be initialed. Both itraconazole and terbinafine may cause hepatotoxicity, so baseline and 4- to 6-week liver function studies should be performed. After completion of systemic therapy, ongoing topical prophylactic antifungal preparations will probably help prevent recurrences (e.g., Mycocide NS Solution, available without prescription; although controlled studies are lacking, Mycocide NS twice daily monotherapy for 1 year may clear nails). Finally, adjunctive cutting or sanding, filing, and aggressive brushing to physically reduce the amount of infected nail may be helpful. Toenail infections are also discussed in Chapter 102.

YEAST INFECTIONS

Candidiasis

Candida albicans and other *Candida* species are yeastlike fungi that most often cause superficial cutaneous infections; however, in immunocompromised patients *Candida* may cause systemic infections, including septicemia. *Candida* infection can affect all ages, but most often it is seen as a cause of a diaper rash in infants, summertime inframammary rash in women, vaginitis in premenopausal women (see Chapter 94), oral candidiasis in endogenously or exogenously immunosuppressed patients, and buttock and perineal rash in incontinent patients. The cutaneous changes are similar in most areas and appear as erythematous, slick, shiny patches with an irregular border of delicate scale and often satellite papules and pustules. The diagnosis can be confirmed with KOH preparation (see above). Oral candidiasis is described in Chapter 101.

Candidiasis may be treated with topical nystatin cream or an imidazole cream (see "Topical Therapeutics," below). Topicals are applied two times a day until complete clearing is seen, which generally occurs over 2 to 3 weeks. In nonresponsive recalcitrant eruptions (and when benefit outweighs risks), oral itraconazole or fluconazole for 10 to 14 days may be used. Because of the potential for rare severe hepatotoxicity with these drugs, infection should be proven with KOH or culture before treatment. Pretreatment liver function tests are prudent, particularly in patients with multiple medical problems. Also, patients should be instructed to report any signs or symptoms or hepatotoxicity during treatment. Topical nystatin powder or simple drying powders (e.g., plain talc) may be helpful in preventing recurrences (see "Topical Therapeutics," below).

Tinea Versicolor

Tinea versicolor is a chronic or chronically recurring superficial yeast infection of the skin caused by *Pityrosporum orbiculare,* also known as *Malassezia furfur.* Tinea versicolor is seen most often in patients in their teens and early twenties. It is more common in tropical climates and during the warm months in temperate climates.

Tinea versicolor appears as round to oval, scaly, hypopigmented, hyperpigmented, or erythematous patches that coalesce into large confluent lesions over the upper trunk and less often, on the face, scalp, genitalia, and proximal extremities. Although the infection is usually asymptomatic, some patients may have significant pruritus, particularly when perspiring heavily. Diagnosis is made with a positive KOH preparation (see above) showing pseudohyphae and spores (Fig. 100.15). Treatment should be initiated with topical ketoconazole 2% shampoo (Nizoral), selenium

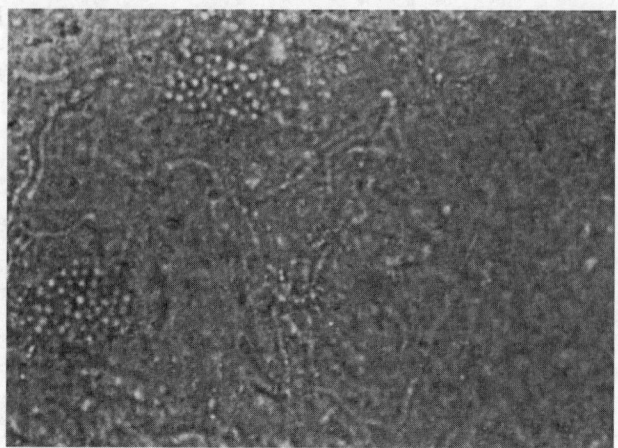

Figure 100.15. Short hyphae and spores of *Malassezia furfur* seen in tinea versicolor (KOH preparation, ×400).

sulfide 2.5% lotion (Selsun lotion; sulfur odor), or Head and Shoulders Intensive Formula Shampoo (selenium sulfide 1%; less odiferous) lathered and left on for 15 minutes. This is repeated each night for 2 weeks and then once monthly as prophylaxis. Recurrences are common and nightly treatment for 2 weeks should be repeated as needed.

In contrast to all the superficial fungal infections mentioned above, which involve only the epidermis, deep fungal infections involve the underlying dermis and usually result from distant organ infection (e.g., pulmonary) with secondary seeding of the skin. Some of the more common deep fungal infections are briefly summarized in Table 100.6.

LOCALIZED VIRAL INFECTIONS OF THE SKIN

Warts

Warts, also known as verrucae, are benign proliferations of the epidermis caused by human papilloma virus (HPV). Warts are most common in children, young adults, and immunocompromised patients. Three notable clinical features of all forms of warts are that they disrupt normal skin lines, often exhibit visible surface thrombosed capillaries appearing as pinpoint black dots, and appear on sites of contact, commonly at sites of trauma.

Common warts (verrucae vulgaris) may be noted initially as smooth, skin-colored, 1-mm papules that gradually enlarge to several millimeters with a rough, finely papulated or hyperkeratotic (warty) surface. Warts may coalesce to form large plaques. Common warts are most often found on the hands.

Flat warts (verrucae plana) are skin-colored to pink, flat-topped papules usually less than a few millimeters in diameter. They occur most commonly on the dorsal aspect of the hands, face, and in women, legs.

Genital warts (condylomata acuminata) begin as minute flat papules that often become verrucous, similar to common warts, variably present on the external genitalia, vagina, cervix, and anal canal. This HPV infection of the cervix and anorectal area (more commonly, but not exclusively, found in homosexual men) predisposes to intraepithelial neoplasia. Immunosuppressed renal transplant recipients also are predisposed to anal intraepithelial neoplasia when genital warts are present.

Plantar warts (verruca plantaris) appear as circumscribed, thickened, barely elevated papules with surface callous. Severe infection with the human papillomavirus on the foot may lead to warts covering the entire heel or plantar aspect of the foot. Plantar warts are often confused with corns or clavi (see below). Warts can be distinguished by paring the surface with a number 15 surgical blade because minute black dots (thrombosed capillaries) should become visible. In contrast, paring of corns reveals a central core that is easily removed with the paring blade.

Treatment

Two precepts should be remembered when treating warts: There are no guarantees in the success of any treatment, and the lesions themselves are benign and should not be treated with therapeutic modalities that could result in harm or scarring, such as ionizing irradiation, deep surgical excision (into the dermis), or deep destructive therapies.

Treatment of common, flat, and plantar warts is typically daily self-application of *topical 17% salicylic acid solution* (e.g., Occlusal or Duofilm) or a 40% salicylic acid patch (MediPlast) available over the counter. Before application, the wart may be soaked in warm water for several minutes, then painlessly filed to remove the macerated (white) surface with a nail file or pumice stone. If after 6 weeks of consistent therapy the wart is still present, weekly or biweekly *liquid nitrogen cryotherapy* may be started. Patients should be warned that although liquid nitrogen should not cause scarring, it may cause permanent depigmentation of the skin caused by greater sensitivity of melanocytes than keratinocytes to liquid nitrogen destruction. This is particularly important on the face and in more deeply pigmented people. A swab with additional tightly wrapped cotton (a quarter of a cotton ball) is dipped into a small amount of liquid nitrogen dispensed in a styrofoam cup. Excess liquid nitrogen is removed from the swab tip by holding the swab perpendicular to the floor and using a sharp downward motion and abrupt halt. The swab is then applied to the wart for 10 to 20 seconds, depending on the size and location. It should be remembered that treatment of a wart located on the lateral surfaces of the finger may freeze and damage the digital nerves; when treating a wart in this area, the skin should be tented upward by pinching the skin. A serous or blood blister may form in several hours to a few days. This is best left intact because satellite warts may occur if fluid containing HPV is allowed to seep onto the surrounding skin. Patients should schedule a follow-up appointment in 2 weeks, but cancel if the wart has disappeared by this time. If the wart is still present, treatments should be continued at 1- to 2-week intervals until resolution has occurred. If after 10 treatments the wart is still present, other treatment modalities should be considered, such as laser vaporization or curette and desiccation. The latter treatments may cause scarring and patients should be warned of this possibility.

Condylomata acuminata are usually first treated with *podophyllin 25% in tincture of benzoin* (Pod-Ben-25) applied weekly by the physician. This is the only form of therapy that does not work through gross destruction of the epidermis containing HPV; instead, it kills the virus by interfering with microtubule formation and therefore ribonucleic acid (RNA) synthesis. Podophyllin must be meticulously applied to the wart with a swab and allowed to dry. After the first application, the medication is washed off in 2 to 4 hours; with each subsequent application, this time is increased by 2 to 4 hours, up to 24 hours. Within several hours of application, patients usually experience stinging and burning. As local wart necrosis occurs, the discomfort may increase, particularly when the warts are large. The response of different patients is variable; some may clear with a few treatments, whereas others, particularly human immunodeficiency virus (HIV)-positive and transplant patients, may still not clear after many treatments.

An alternative to physician-applied podophyllin is a patient-applied podophyllin derivative, podofilox 0.5% (Condylox). The much lower concentration reduces side effects, but stinging, burning, and irritation are still common. Patients follow the package instruc-tions, applying the solution two times a day for 3 days, then resting for 4 days. This cycle is repeated up to four times and the patient then returns for examination to ensure that improvement or resolution has occurred. Additional cycles may be repeated if needed.

If podophyllin is ineffective, cryotherapy may be used in the same manner as outlined above for other warts. Additional alternative therapies include laser vaporization, curette and desiccation, and scalpel excision.

Molluscum Contagiosum

Molluscum contagiosum is common in young children and HIV-positive patients. Lesions are caused by the pox virus, a DNA virus. The lesions are umbilicated, skin-colored to whitish, 1- to 4-mm papules, typically on the neck, trunk, genital, and eyelid areas. The central umbilicated depression contains molluscum bodies, which are enlarged degrading keratinocytes, packed with viral material. The diagnosis may be made by obtaining a curette of the molluscum for KOH preparation (potassium hydroxide preparation, see above). With light microscopy, the round, homogeneous 25-μm molluscum bodies are easily seen.

When considering therapy, it should be remembered that infection is self-limited and in immunocompetent patients, the host eradicates the virus, although sometimes it takes years. Unfortunately, lesions may increase in number before this clearance. In children,

Table 100.6.   Selected Deep Fungal Infections

Fungus	Endemic Area in the United States/Source	Usual Site of Primary Infection/Associated Cutaneous Hypersensitivity Reactions	Primary Cutaneous Inoculation[a]	Cutaneous Lesions Caused by Organisms
Blastomyces dermatitidis	Mississippi River basin, Great Lakes region, Southeast United States/bird excreta, wood	Pulmonary/rare erythema nodosum	Rare	Present in 70%; centrifugally enlarging plaques with a verrucous, pustular border; also, pustular ulcerations, subcutaneous abscesses, widespread or acral pustules
Coccidioides immitis	Southwest United States/soil	Pulmonary/50% of symptomatic infections with toxic erythema: diffuse exanthum, erythema multiforme, erythema nodosum	Rare	Verrucous plaque or granulomatous nodule (especially face); also, papules, pustules, nodules, subcutaneous
Histoplasma capsulatum	Central and Southeast United States/bird and bat excreta, especially chicken coops	Pulmonary/rare erythema nodosum	Rare	Nasal or oral mucosal lesions in 50%; also, 6% with variable cutaneous lesions; ulcerating papules, nodules, plaques; ulcers, erythroderma[b]
Sporothrix schenckii	Ubiquitous, humidity favors growth/decaying vegetable matter, wood ("splinters")	Cutaneous (pulmonary possible)	Common	A papule that enlarges into an ulcerated nodule, usually with associated regional lymphangitis and lymphadenopathy
Cryptococcus neoformans	Ubiquitous/pigeon excreta, soil, some fruits	Pulmonary	Rare	Papules, pustules, ulcerating nodules, ulcers, abscesses, acreiform lesions, cellulitis, ecchymoses, vasculitis[b]
Candida albicans and *Candida tropicalis*	Ubiquitous	Oral mucosa then esophagus most likely	Rare	Erythematous to purpuric 0.5- to 1-cm papulonodules commonly on the trunk and proximal extremities, with associated fever and myalgia; also cellulitis, ecthyma gangrenosumlike eschar, nodular folliculitis and abscesses, purpura

[a]Nodule or chancriform ulcer with or without lymphangitis or lymphadenopathy.

[b]In HIV-infected patients, may develop molluscum contagiosum–like lesions.

simple, nonthreatening treatments are best. Simple scotch tape stripping (tape quickly and firmly applied and immediately removed a dozen times) once to twice daily for several weeks may suffice by unroofing the lesion and stimulating a host response caused by the mild local trauma. Alternatively, topical salicylic acid 17% preparations (as for warts; see above) or topical tretinoin (Retin-A 0.025% gel) applied directly to the lesion twice a day may be tried for 6 weeks. If lesions persist, either cryotherapy with liquid nitrogen (as for warts; see above), remembering that this could cause permanent depigmentation especially troublesome on the face in darker-skinned people, or curettage without anesthesia may be attempted.

HERPES INFECTION

Herpes Simplex

Herpes simplex virus (HSV) infection may be caused by HSV type I or II, typically with type I causing *herpes labialis* and type II causing *herpes genitalis.* A study of 500 randomly selected patients in a family medicine clinic found 56% seropositivity for HSV I, 23% seropositivity for HSV II, and 12% seropositivity for both HSV I and II, and 33% seronegativity (58). Infection results in a recurrent localized clustered (herpetic) blistering of the skin. After a primary infection has occurred, the virus remains dormant in the cranial nerve or dorsal root nerve ganglia innervating the region of cutaneous infection. Lesions may recur at any time, often being triggered by sun exposure, illness, menses, local trauma, and physical and psychologic stress. Transmission occurs through direct contact with an infected person actively shedding virus. The virus may live on fomites, but unlike HPV, HSV quickly dies on drying (30 minutes), making fomites transmission unlikely.

Primary herpes infection in the oral cavity causes the painful, febrile illness, acute herpetic gingivostomatitis (AHG) (see Chapter 101). After healing, the virus remains latent and subsequent reactivation causes herpes labialis, manifest as clustered vesicles on or about the lips. Notably, most patients with recurrent herpes labialis have no history of primary AHG or herpetic infection elsewhere, and therefore are presumed to have had an asymptomatic primary oral infection. Lesions heal in approximately 1 to 2 weeks, with a typical sequence of rupture, crusting, and desquamation. The lesions are infectious as long as the skin is not intact. The importance of asymptomatic viral shedding in viral transmission, as is known to occur with herpes genitalis and with exceptionally high frequency in patients with AIDS (60), is not known. Herpes genitalis, the most common cause of genital ulcers, is discussed fully in Chapter 94.

Herpes simplex infection may occur anywhere on the body; a common site in health care workers is on the finger *(herpetic whitlow),* acquired through exposure to a patient with active herpes infection. Viral transmission has been reported to occur through vinyl gloves, so health care workers are wise to double-glove when touching open herpes lesions.

Chronic herpetic infections in immunocompromised patients appear as chronic, punched-out ulcers that may be solitary or multiple. The expanded AIDS surveillance case definition for AIDS diagnosis (see Chapter 34) now includes a chronic herpes simplex ulcer present for 1 month or longer in an HIV-positive patient.

Fortunately, *cutaneous complications* of HSV infection are rare. These may include *cutaneous dissemination* in patients with generalized atopic dermatitis and recurrent erythema multiforme as a hypersensitivity response. A history of the latter is an indication for ongoing prophylactic antiviral therapy (see below, *erythema multiforme).* Potential ocular complications include *herpetic keratitis* (see Chapter 99), a primary or secondary infection that involves the cornea of the eye and is best managed emergently by an ophthalmologist because of the potential for permanent corneal scarring and loss of vision. The most common systemic complication of HSV probably relates to the recently recognized association of HSV I as the major etiologic agent in Bell's palsy (53). Other systemic complications that are fortunately unusual include acute ascending necrotizing myelopathy (94) and necrotizing lymphadenitis (15) associated with herpes genitalis and possibly recurrent lymphocytic meningitis (75,87). Although all of these require immediate diagnosis and treatment, the first of these is rapidly progressive and associated with a high mortality rate.

Treatment

A new antiviral topical has recently been released: penciclovir (Denavir cream), which is said to speed lesion healing when applied every 2 hours for 4 days. Herpes labialis, unlike recurrent herpes genitalis (discussed in Chapter 94), for which patients are often treated with chronic prophylactic (51) or self-initiated intermittent therapy (73), is generally not treated with systemic antiviral medication. Exceptions include patients with AIDS or other immunocompromised patients having chronic persistent infections and patients with secondary complications, as described above. The former, persistent HSV lesions in immunocompromised patients, often requires higher than usual dosages (2 to 4×) of oral or instead intravenous antiviral therapy. The latter problem of secondary cutaneous complications is generally prevented with intermittent antiviral therapy for recurrent HSV in patients with atopic dermatitis and ongoing prophylactic antiviral therapy in patients with recurrent HSV-associated erythema multiforme. Intermittent therapy should be initiated within 24 to 48 hours of new lesion onset and may include acyclovir (Zovirax) 200 mg five times a day, valacyclovir (Valtrex) 500 mg twice a day, or famciclovir (Famvir) 125 mg twice a day, each for 5 days. Prophylactic therapy may include acyclovir 400 mg twice a day. Of these three agents, valacyclovir tends to be least expensive (89).

Short courses (2 weeks) of prophylactic therapy may be useful in various settings. Prophylaxis should be given when HSV recurrences may complicate procedures, such as facial cutaneous surgeries, oral surgery, and dental work. Finally, prophylaxis is welcomed by patients when recurrences may be anticipated, such as skiing and beach vacations (oral antiviral as well as topical high SPF sunscreen), weddings, and other important events (70,92). The antiviral dosage must be reduced for patients with renal impairment (see Chapter 48).

Herpes Zoster (Shingles)

Herpes zoster represents a reactivation of the varicella–zoster virus. After initial varicella (chickenpox) infection, the virus resides in a dorsal root or cranial nerve ganglia. At any point thereafter, latent virus may be reactivated and produce multiple erythematous plaques surmounted by clustered vesicles, in a dermatomal or zosteriform distribution. In an immunocompetent patient, zoster evolves and resolves over 2 to 3 weeks. Lesions begin with vesicles that become turbid in 3 days, dry and crust in 7 to 10 days, and clear within 2 to 3 weeks. At the onset, new lesions may appear for up to 7 days. Herpes zoster affects a thoracic dermatome in 50%, a cervical dermatome in 20%, the trigeminal dermatome in 15%, and a lumbosacral dermatome in 10% of patients. Of patients with herpes zoster, 66% are over 50 years of age, and 10% are less than 20 years of age (59).

Often, patients who have herpes zoster develop a prodrome of pain in the affected dermatome. Occasionally, herpes zoster is misdiagnosed, for example, as pleurisy, myocardial infarction, cholecystitis, appendicitis, renal colic, or ruptured intervertebral disc. Rarely, patients may experience acute segmental neuralgia with a concurrent rise in varicella virus antibodies without developing skin lesions. This entity has been called zoster siné herpete (59).

The presumptive diagnosis of herpes zoster is made clinically. A *Tzanck smear* showing multinucleated giant cells (see below) confirms that the eruption is herpes zoster or herpes simplex and rules out other blistering disorders such as impetigo, erythema multiforme, and pemphigus. Herpes simplex can occur in a dermatomal pattern, so any case of "recurrent" herpes zoster should be cultured to exclude the possibility of recurrent dermatomal HSV infection because recurrent zoster raises the possibility of an associated illness causing immunosuppression, and should prompt further evaluation of immune function. A specimen for culture is obtained in a fashion similar to that used for Tzanck smear; the scraping is inoculated into a standard liquid viral culture medium. Treatment affects the course of disease only if initiated within 48 to 72 hours of onset. A 1-week course of an oral antiviral (e.g., acyclovir [Zovirax] 800 mg five times a day, valacyclovir [Valtrex] 1000 mg three times a day, famciclovir [Famvir] 500 mg three times a day) is used in immunocompetent patients. Acyclovir has been shown to reduce zoster-associated acute pain and new lesion formation, and both valacyclovir and famciclovir reduce acute pain and speed healing (48,88,89). Recently, wholesale price of treatment with valacyclovir is $97 versus $129 with either of the two other antivirals (89); this price is higher than that for *H. simplex* because of dosing differences. An important consideration in choosing an antiviral is the effect it may have on the frequency and duration of postherpetic neuralgia (defined below). Both valacyclovir and famciclovir appear to reduce the incidence and duration of postherpetic neuralgia (88,89). The clinician is left to decide about using antivirals based on the above facts and his or her judgment of the severity and location of the lesions. The utility of supplemental corticosteroids in the prevention of postherpetic neuralgia remains controversial (41,92,93,95) and therefore is not recommended until several prospective controlled trials demonstrate its clear effectiveness. Kost and Straus recently put forth a useful algorithm for treatment of acute herpes zoster and postherpetic neuralgia (41), although it has not yet been confirmed by others.

Supplemental therapy beyond antivirals is also important. Topical wet to damp dressings promote drying of the lesions and a topical antibacterial agent (e.g., Silvadene, bacitracin ointment) generously applied promotes healing, prevents secondary infection, and eases pain from air contact of the denuded skin. If acute neuralgia is present, nonsteroidal anti-inflammatory drugs (NSAIDs) (see Chapter 70 for full discussion) or narcotics may be needed but clearly must be used with caution, particularly in the elderly, in whom the incidence of side effects is high.

Postherpetic neuralgia or pain after the cutaneous lesions have resolved is most commonly seen in patients over 50 years. Treatment of this common problem may be difficult. However, some success has been reported with topical capsaicin cream (Zostrix 0.025% or generic and Zostrix HP 0.075%, no generic available, both available without prescription) applied four times a day. Capsaicin is derived from peppers. It depletes substance P in peripheral sensory neurons and may alleviate pain. Not infrequently there is a delay of several weeks before an effect is appreciated, so a therapeutic trial should be at least 1 month in length. Patients must be cautioned that about four applications are needed to fully deplete the substance contributing to pain (substance P), so the first three applications (when substance P is being released) produce local burning and stinging (like eating hot peppers), but with subsequent regular applications the pain should not recur because the substance P is prevented from reaccumulating. If patients use less frequent applications or skip a day, thereby allowing reaccumulation of substance P, reinitiation burns again for the first few applications. Patients should also be warned that capsaicin is expensive. Oral amitriptyline in dosages of 12.5 to 150 mg per day (47) may also decrease the discomfort of postherpetic neuralgia. Although postherpetic neuralgia most often remits spontaneously within 6 months, it may be chronic and referral to a pain specialist is appropriate.

Other potential complications of zoster are numerous (59,66). When the trigeminal dermatome is affected, involvement of the second branch may cause lesions of the eye, and such patients must be evaluated emergently by an ophthalmologist because keratitis, uveitis, secondary glaucoma, iridocyclitis, or rarely panophthalmitis may develop. *Ramsay–Hunt* syndrome is herpes zoster affecting the facial and auditory nerves, causing facial palsy with cutaneous zoster of the external ear or tympanic membrane and associated tinnitus, vertigo, or deafness. Motor paralysis occurs in 1 to 5% of patients. The incidence of motor involvement is probably understated because mild or partial deficits often go undetected. Paralysis usually begins within 2 weeks of the onset of the rash and involves the muscle groups corresponding to the affected dermatome. In most instances, total or functional recovery occurs spontaneously. Meningoencephalitis may develop with cranial nerve herpes zoster in immunocompromised patients, most often in association with cutaneous dissemination. *Granulomatous angiitis* of cerebral arteries is an unusual complication of ophthalmic zoster that may lead to a syndrome of delayed contralateral hemiplegia occurring weeks to months after the episode of zoster. Such patients are usually diagnosed as having a typical cerebrovascular accident, but arteriograms reveal segmental narrowing or occlusion of cerebral arteries ipsilateral to the site of the ophthalmic zoster. Disseminated herpes zoster is defined as more than 20 vesicles at a distance from the primary dermatome, and is seen almost exclusively in immunocompromised patients. Such patients should be hospitalized for urgent treatment with intravenous acyclovir. Approximately 10% of patients with disseminated cutaneous lesions develop widespread, often fatal visceral infection, particularly of the lungs, liver, and brain (66).

Tzanck Smear

The sensitivity of a *Tzanck smear* in detecting herpetic changes is greatest when a specimen is taken from the intact vesicle. A chosen vesicle is unroofed and the base is firmly scraped with a number 15 surgical blade and smeared onto a glass slide. When vesicles are not present, an early crusted papule is sampled by removing the surface crust and scraping the base. (Alternatively, a biopsy of this crusted lesion may be done; routine histology, ready 2 to 4 days later, should reveal multinucleated giant cells.) Immediate tissue smear staining is performed with the commercially available Tzanck stain (Dif-Quik Stain, Baxter Scientific Products, McGraw Park, IL), which is a three-step immediate stain. Alternatively, a Giemsa stain may be done by combining 0.5 mL water with 0.5 mL Giemsa tissue stain in a small syringe and flooding over the specimen, then thoroughly rinsing with tap water after 30 seconds. Although the slide may be viewed directly,

covering with mounting medium and a coverslip greatly improves resolution. The slide is searched for giant cells containing multiple syncytial nuclei (nuclei that mold together in a jigsaw puzzle–like fashion). A Tzanck smear is shown in Figure 100.16. The Tzanck smear preparation should be positive when performed on lesions of herpes simplex, varicella, and herpes zoster eruptions.

INFESTATIONS

Scabies

Human scabies is caused by infestation with the mite *Sarcoptes scabiei* var. *hominis.* Infestation causes an intense intractable pruritus that is classically most disturbing at night, when competing external stimuli are minimal. The signs and symptoms of scabies infestation are caused by the host's immune response to the mite and its eggs and feces. Generally, this response is delayed, so patients become itchy approximately 10 days to 2 weeks after exposure and infestation. Scabies is seen most often in children, and the pathognomonic lesions are burrows, which are threadlike linear ridges a few millimeters in length with a minute black dot at one end. Burrows occur most often on the hands, wrists, penis, nipples, axillae, and gluteal cleft (Fig. 100.17). Depending on the duration of infestation, patients may have few to innumerable scratches, excoriations, crusts, and eczematous papules and plaques. Less often, small nodules may develop, tending to favor the scrotum, axillae, and buttocks.

Scabies infestation is confirmed by identifying the burrowed mite, eggs, or feces in the superficial skin. This often can be done by scraping the black dot at one end of a burrow using a number 15 surgical blade. If a black dot is not seen, both ends of the burrow are scraped. The sample is put on a glass slide and one to two drops of mineral oil and a coverslip are applied in preparation for light microscopic viewing. The mite is

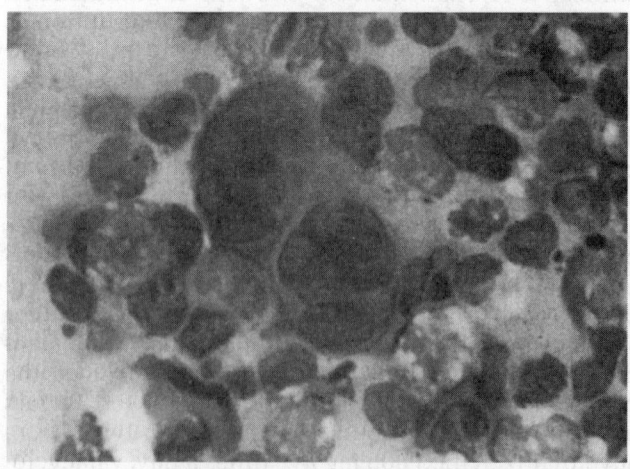

Figure 100.16. Tzanck smear; gentle scraping from the base of a vesicle and stained with Wright's or Giemsa stain. Multinucleated cells from herpes simplex are shown (×400).

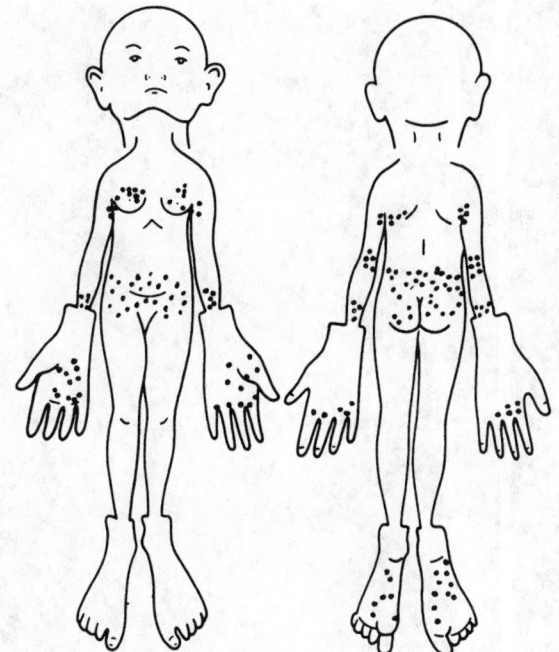

Figure 100.17.   Pruritic papules are most prevalent about the waist, pelvis, elbows, and hands and feet in scabies.

an approximately 0.2-mm hemispherical shape with eight short legs; eggs are smaller and oval in shape and feces are smaller yet round pellets.

Patients and family members should be treated with an overnight application of prescription lindane lotion (Kwell lotion, 30 g per single application, volume as dispensed) or permethrin cream (Elimite cream, 30 g per single application, 60-g tube). Either is applied from the neck down, using a toothbrush to get under the finger and toenails and showered off 8 to 12 hours later. Patients often require emollients and a midpotency corticosteroid (e.g., triamcinolone 0.1% ointment) after using the scabicides to suppress the "hyperreactivity" caused by the mites. Although both lindane and permethrin are neurotoxins, systemic absorption of lindane is greater (49) so it should be avoided in infants, pregnant and lactating women, patients with seizure disorders, and because of augmented absorption, patients with extensive secondary excoriations and dermatitis or with another widespread skin disease (e.g., generalized atopic dermatitis, widespread psoriasis). All bedclothing, linens, unwashed worn clothing, and stuffed animals should be washed and dried in a hot dryer because is it the dryer that kills the mite. Alternatively, the mites and eggs may be killed by placing the items in airtight plastic bags for 2 weeks.

A possible alternative treatment now available in this country (56) in patients resistant to topical scabicidal therapy is ivermectin (6-mg tablets). Although it is not FDA approved for this indication at present, a report of successful therapy using a one-time dose of 0.2 mg/kg (e.g., a one-time dose of two tablets for a 60-kg adult) is promising (50).

Pediculosis

Infestation with the human louse *(Pediculus humanus capitis* and *corporis, Phthirus pubis)* affects different areas of the body and is called *pediculosis capitis, corporis,* and *pubis. Pediculosis capitis* is most common in children. Patients with lice often have intense pruritus, scalp and posterior neck excoriations, and often secondary bacterial infection with pustules, crusting, and adenopathy. *Pediculosis corporis* is seen most often in patients exposed to others who, like themselves, cannot maintain good hygiene. *Pediculosis pubis* (pubic lice) is usually a sexually transmitted disorder.

Patients with pediculosis usually have nits firmly attached to head, body, or pubic hairs (Fig. 100.18). Nits are less than 1-mm-long "shells" that may or may not still contain an egg. Lice hatch from these eggs and are visible, being less than 2 mm long with three pairs of legs that terminate in sharp claws. They are found in the hair or adjacent skin and specifically in pediculosis corporis, in the seams of clothing. Treatment should be initiated with pyrethrin shampoo (e.g., RID, over-the-counter) or lindane shampoo (e.g., Kwell, by prescription) for pediculosis capitis and pubis and lindane lotion for pediculosis corporis. The shampoo is left on for 5 to 10 minutes and then washed off; the body lotion is left on overnight. Because no pediculicides are 100% ovicidal (61), nits that potentially contain living eggs and will remain attached to the hair after treatment must be removed with a fine-tooth comb after white vinegar is applied to the hair for 15 minutes. Close contacts should be treated in a similar fashion and bedclothing and linens and unwashed worn clothes should be washed and put through a hot dryer cycle to destroy the lice and eggs. Alternatively, these items may be sealed in an airtight plastic bag for 2 weeks.

AUTOIMMUNE BLISTERING DISORDERS

Primary bullous dermatoses associated with autoantibodies to various components of the epidermis (29) include bullous pemphigoid, pemphigus vulgaris, bullous lupus erythematosus, acquired epidermolysis bullosa acquisita, linear IgA bullous dermatosis, vancomycin and other drug-induced linear IgA dermatoses, and paraneoplastic pemphigus. Patients with these conditions have flaccid to tense bullae, with or without an erythematous, urticarial base distributed in a localized or generalized fashion on the skin and mucosal surfaces. Because some of these disorders may be associated with significant morbidity and mortality, patients suspected of having an autoimmune blistering disorder should undergo skin biopsy for routine histologic and special staining (direct immunofluorescence to identify the site of deposited immunoglobulin within the epidermis). Often very aggressive therapies, including prednisone, cytotoxic agents, or plasmapheresis, may be required. The various patterns of these disorders are briefly described below.

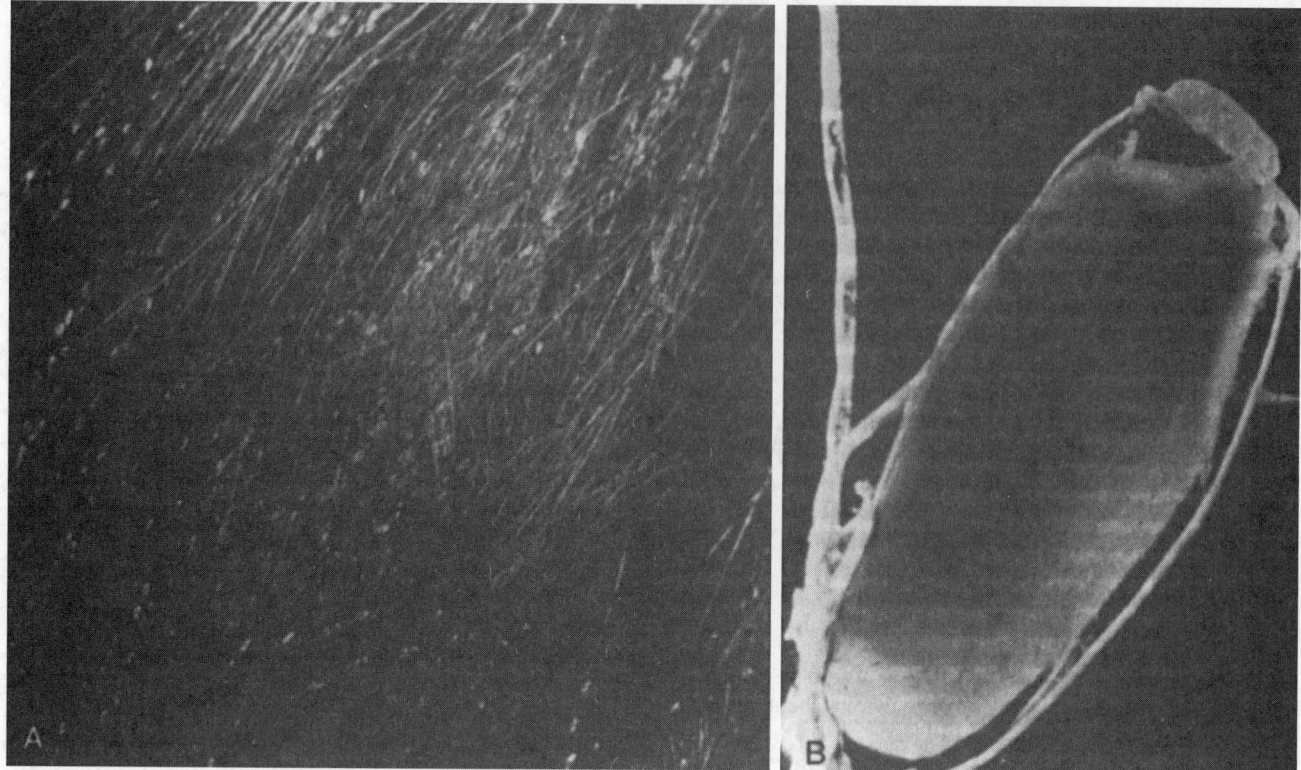

Figure 100.18. *Pediculus humanis* var. *Capitis* (head louse). **A.** Gross appearance of nits on the hair shaft. **B.** Microscopic appearance (×100). (**B** courtesy of Reed and Carnrick, Kenilworth, NJ.)

Bullous pemphigoid typically includes mild asymptomatic oral involvement and tense skin blisters; affected patients are usually over age 60. Herpes gestationis is similar to bullous pemphigoid, but it occurs in pregnant women or occasionally in women taking estrogens. *Pemphigus* (vulgaris) and *paraneoplastic* pemphigus (2) (reported associated neoplasms include lymphoma, chronic lymphocytic leukemia, poorly differentiated sarcoma, bronchogenic squamous cell carcinoma, and thymoma) are associated with extensive oral lesions, and in pemphigus, cutaneous blisters exhibit a positive *Nikolsky* sign (pressure applied to a blister causes the blister to enlarge by spreading outward into the adjacent skin). *Bullous lupus erythematosus* occurs in the setting of systemic lupus erythematosus. Vancomycin and other drug-induced linear IgA dermatoses appear similar to bullous pemphigoid but usually clear upon withdrawal of the causative drug.

DRUG ERUPTIONS

Numerous prescription and nonprescription medications may cause a wide array of cutaneous abnormalities (12) and aggravate preexisting dermatoses (Table 100.7). It has been estimated that in hospitalized patients, 2 to 3% have adverse cutaneous drug reactions and 2% of these reactions are severe, being associated with significant morbidity and potential mortality (7,72). General adverse drug events in hospitalized patients are associated with a 1.7- to 3.5-fold

increase in mortality rate, length of stay, and costs of hospitalization (18).

The common drug eruptions (e.g., exanthems), potentially life-threatening eruptions (72) (e.g., toxic epidermal necrolysis (71) and vasculitis), and poorly tolerated reactions (e.g., acne, alopecia, photosensitivity, psoriasis, and pigmentary changes) are discussed. A Medic Alert bracelet indicating the drug and type of reaction should be prescribed for all patients having severe drug eruptions.

Exanthems

The most commonly seen acute drug-induced eruption is a pruritic exanthem. This is usually macular and papular (morbilliform), but may be a purely macular erythema, exfoliative erythroderma, or scarlatiniform eruption. Although innumerable drugs may cause this eruption, the most commonly implicated drugs include penicillins and semisynthetic penicillins (43), cephalosporins, sulfonamides, quinidine, cimetidine, allopurinol, carbamazepine, phenytoin, isoniazid, and nitrofurantoin.

Eruptions may begin at any time, but usually occur at one of two periods of drug administration: after 2 to 3 days, or after 9 to 10 days. The early form is seen in patients who have previously been sensitized to the drug. With this prior sensitization, an exanthem may or may not have occurred, depending on the timing of sensitization and how soon the drug was stopped. The

Table 100.7. Adverse Cutaneous Drug Reactions and Some Common Causative Drugs

Acne (12, 82)
Androgenic hormones
Corticosteroids
Halogens (bromides, iodides)
Anticonvulsants
Tuberculostatic drugs
Lithium
Cyclosporin
Vitamin B_{12}
Oral contraceptives

Alopecia (12)
Cytostatic drugs
Anticoagulants
Androgenic hormones
Phenytoin
Cholesterol-lowering agents
Colchicine

Erythema Multiforme (and Toxic Epidermal Neurolysis; See Text) (12)
Sulfonamides
Penicillins
Nonsteroidal anti-inflammatory drugs
Anticonvulsants

Exanthematous Eruptions (See Text) (12)
Penicillins
Sulfonamides
Barbiturates
Phenytoin
Carbamazepine
Allopurinol
Gold salts
Phenothiazines

Fixed Drug Eruptions (one or more, 1–4 cm, asymmetrically distributed erythematous patches that resolve with hyperpigmentation and become acutely inflamed again with drug readiminstration) (12)
Phenolphthalein
Tetracyclines
Sulfonamides
Barbiturates
Penicillins

Nonpigmenting Fixed Drug Eruption (one or more, 1–4 cm, erythematous macules that fade completely and become acutely inflamed with drug readministration) (6, 81)
Acetaminophen
Pseudoephedrine
Radiocontrast media

Leukocytoclastic Vasculitis (12)
Sulfonamides
Phenytoin
Allopurinol

Papulosquamous Eruptions (psoriasislike eruptions or exacerbation of psoriasis) (22)
Antimalarials
Lithium
β-Blockers
ACE inhibitors
Sulfonamides

Lichen Planuslike Eruptions (22)
Gold
Captopril
Furosemide
β-Blockers
Quinidine
Quinine
Sulfonylureas
Thiazides

Pityriasis Rosea–Like Eruptions (See Table 100.1; Pityriasis Rosea) (22)
Barbiturates
Gold
Metronidazole
Bismuth
Captopril
Clonidine
Metoprolol

Photosensitivity (12)
Tetracycline
Demeclocycline
Doxycycline
Sulfonamides
Nonsteroidal anti-inflammatory drugs
Phenothiazines
Thiazide diuretics
Psoralens

Porphyria Cutanea Tarda (12)
Estrogens
Androgens
Alcohol
Antimalarials
Sulfonamides
Sulfonylureas
Rifampicin
Quinidine
Quinine

Porphyria Variegata (and Acute Intermittent Porphyria) (12)
Estrogens
Androgens
Alcohol
Antimalarials
Sulfonamides
Sulfonylureas
Barbiturates

Urticaria/Angioedema (30)
Opiates
Penicillins
Sulfonamides
Aspirin
Quinine
Nonsteroidal anti-inflammatory drugs
ACE inhibitors
Radiocontrast media
Hyperosmolar solutions
Amphetamines
Azodyes and benzoates in drugs

Eczematous Eruptions (12)
β-Blockers
Diuretics
Sulfonylureas
Phenothiazines
Penicillins
Sulfonamides

Pruritus (12)
Opiates
Aspirin
Antidepressants
Belladonna alkaloids
Barbiturates
CNS stimulants
Estrogens
Hepatotoxic drugs

more delayed reaction occurring 9 to 10 days after drug initiation occurs in patients not previously sensitized to the drug. Systemic manifestations of drug sensitivity such as associated fever, lymphadenopathy, and visceral hypersensitivity are usually absent. When visceral hypersensitivity occurs, it may involve the kidneys (see below), liver (hepatitis, cholestasis), and gastrointestinal tract (bleeding) (45,80). Systemic involvement is more common with certain drugs such as allopurinol (45), phenytoin (80), and isoniazid. Rarely, an exanthem may be complicated by the subsequent development of toxic epidermal necrolysis (see below).

With uncomplicated nonbullous cutaneous eruptions, the suspected causative drug should be stopped if possible, and topical treatment begun to reduce pruritus. Such treatment includes as often as desired application of bland topical over-the-counter preparations containing menthol or phenol such as Sarna or Sarna HC (with 1% hydrocortisone) lotion or Aveeno Anti-Itch cream. In contrast, systemic drug hypersensitivity syndromes require immediate intervention with prompt discontinuation of all suspected drugs and close observation.

Erythema Multiforme

Erythema multiforme (EM) is a mucocutaneous hypersensitivity syndrome caused most commonly by a drug or infection. It is divided into EM minor and EM major, depending on whether it affects one or more than one mucosal surface, respectively (17,55,71,72). Although the pathogenesis of EM is unknown, it is believed that infection or a drug leads to a cell-mediated cytotoxic reaction in the epidermis.

EM major, which accounts for approximately 20% of cases of EM, may cause morbidity and even mortality. It is associated with drugs more often than EM minor, but similar infections may cause both forms (see below). Patients usually have a prodrome of malaise, myalgia, fever, and sometimes upper respiratory symptoms. The eruption develops rapidly, is generally widespread, and involves at least two mucosal surfaces, usually the conjunctiva and the oral mucosa. Cutaneous lesions evolve quickly from macules into targetlike plaques with dusky centers (Fig. 100.19, Color Plate 2), often surmounted by blisters and often confluent over large areas. Usually the lips are covered with hemorrhagic crusts and the mucosa shows diffuse pseudomembranous denudation, and the eyes show conjunctival injection, erosions, or exudate. Less often the nasal, genital, esophageal, and rarely, the respiratory mucosae are involved.

The most common and significant acute complication of EM major is secondary bacterial infection and sepsis; the most devastating long-term complication is ocular scarring and vision loss. Patients with EM major must be hospitalized and, depending on the extent of disease, may benefit from care in a burn unit. Ophthalmologic consultation should be obtained and recommended eye care must be exemplary.

EM minor causes 80% of all cases of EM. It is seen in patients of all ages but is more common in those in their 20s and 30s. Most cases of EM minor are caused by a preceding HSV infection (55). Most patients with recurrent EM minor, even those without a history of HSV infection, have detectable HSV DNA in the lesions (10). Causes of EM minor other than herpes simplex infection include other viral infections, *Mycoplasma pneumoniae,* other bacterial infections, and drugs (most commonly sulfonamides, penicillins, NSAIDs, and anticonvulsants) (55).

EM minor begins with asymptomatic to tender, erythematous to violaceous macules that evolve into papules with an expanding border, leaving a nonblanchable, dusky, slightly depressed center, creating an iris or target lesion. Lesions may coalesce into plaques or become bullous *(bullous EM).* The eruption favors the palms and soles, dorsal hands and feet, and knees and elbows, but may be widely distributed. Approximately 20% of patients have mucosal lesions with mild to extensive flaccid bullae and deep erosions of the lips, buccal mucosa, and gingiva. EM is occasionally limited to the mouth without cutaneous lesions. Patients may have associated fever and malaise. If the diagnosis cannot be made on clinical grounds, skin biopsy should be done and will show necrotic keratinocytes, epidermal and dermal edema, and a mononuclear cell infiltrate. The treatment of EM minor involves identification of the causative drug or infection and withdrawal of any suspected offending drug. Although necessary, treatment of a causative infection does not change the course of the EM. For symptomatic relief, the oral lesions may be treated with an oral suspension containing diphenhydramine and antacid (e.g., Benadryl Elixir and Maalox in equal parts; swish for 1 minute and expectorate, four to six times per day), or sucralfate (e.g., Carafate 16 g [16 tabs] in 60 mL water; add to 180 mL 70% sorbitol; paint on erosions with finger as needed) in combination with 3% hydrogen peroxide washes (swish for 15 seconds and expectorate or swab with dental sponge four to six times per day). Topical anesthetics (Xylocaine gel) may be applied to individual painful lesions before meals. The use of systemic corticosteroids is still controversial; if used, corticosteroid therapy should be given early in the course of the disease because later use after the eruption has fully evolved would not be expected to alter the severity of EM and may increase the risk of secondary infection and impair healing. In cases of recurrent EM minor triggered by herpes simplex virus, prophylactic acyclovir should be given to prevent HSV recurrences (see "Herpes Simplex," above).

Toxic Epidermal Necrolysis

Toxic epidermal necrolysis (TEN) (72), fortunately uncommon, is associated with a 25% to more than 40% mortality rate (4,17,28,56). Because it has many features in common with EM major, these reactions are believed to represent a continuum of one disease. TEN is most often caused by drugs, especially sulfonamides, anticonvulsants, NSAIDs, allopurinol, colchicine, cephalosporins, quinolones, and aminopenicillins (71).

Similar to a sunburn, TEN typically begins with a diffuse, painful erythema, often first noted on the trunk. Rapidly, patchy, and then coalescing areas of dusky epidermal necrosis and skin sloughing develop. Oral and ocular manifestations are similar to the changes seen in EM major. Although the diagnosis is made presumptively and appropriate management initiated, biopsy should be done to confirm the diagnosis. This reveals epidermal necrosis with sloughing of the epidermis from the dermis and a sparse mononuclear perivascular dermal infiltrate.

Patients with TEN are critically ill and may develop a number of associated problems, including cytopenias, hepatitis, hypoalbuminemia, hypophosphatemia, and prerenal azotemia, disseminated intravascular coagulation, and pancreatitis (4,72).

Patients with TEN should be admitted urgently to a hospital and ideally to a burn unit (28). Urgent consultation with a dermatologist, burn specialist, and an ophthalmologist should be obtained. Acute mortality is most often caused by sepsis, whereas chronic morbidity is most often caused by cutaneous and ocular scarring, with the latter potentially leading to severe vision loss.

Nonspecific Eruptions Secondary to Drug Toxicity in the Elderly

Drug toxicity is an important cause of cutaneous eruptions in patients with declining renal or hepatic function, particularly when they are on multiple drugs that compete for hepatic metabolism or renal secretion (76). Such situations are typical of the elderly, who are most at risk for drug reactions in general (see Chapter 6). For example, in one study of 714 elderly patients, 25% of those over age 80 developed adverse drug reactions, compared with only 12% of those in their 40s (77).

Toxic drug eruptions may occur at any time while the patient is taking a drug. When the first eruption occurs months or even years after the start of a drug, a toxic drug reaction is often not considered. Such instances of toxicity after many months of drug administration may result in pruritus with an associated or resultant dermatitis and possibly exacerbation of previously existing skin diseases (e.g., psoriasis, atopic dermatitis) (24,76). Drug withdrawal in this situation usually leads to a slow improvement over several weeks. Toxic drug reactions should be considered in patients complaining of new, usually symmetric dermatoses or exacerbation of previously stable skin conditions, even if a patient has been on a drug for months or years. Whenever possible, such drugs should be eliminated or reduced in dosage (14,24,76).

PHOTOSENSITIVITY

Photosensitivity is an abnormal response to natural sunlight or artificial ultraviolet (UV) radiation or visible light exposure. It manifests as a diffuse macular erythema *(phototoxic reaction)* or a papular or papulovesicular erythema *(photoallergic reaction)* on the exposed surfaces. The phototoxic or sunburnlike reaction is caused by phototoxic drugs such as sulfonamides, quinolones, doxycycline, demeclocycline, phenothiazines, NSAIDs, porphyrin precursors, and psoralens. This is a non–immunologically mediated reaction that occurs in any patient who has a serum drug level that is high enough and sufficient ultraviolet A (UVA) radiation exposure (greater in tanning parlor lights than sunlight). Although any of these drugs may cause severe phototoxicity, notable frightening reports include a woman taking psoralen, exposing herself in a suntan parlor, and developing an ultimately fatal total body burn; and another woman given a fluoroquinolone, attending her usual suntan parlor session, and developing an extensive, severe blistering burn.

Sun-exposed site papular or papulovesicular erythema may represent a *drug-induced photoallergic eruption, polymorphous light eruption,* or *cutaneous lupus erythematosus.* The drug-induced photoallergic eruption is a cell-mediated immune reaction that most often is caused by thiazides, NSAIDs, especially piroxicam (Feldene), sulfonamides and sulfonylureas, oral contraceptives, and quinidine.

Polymorphous light eruption (PMLE) is a common idiopathic disorder in which patients typically develop a pruritic, papular eruption on the extensor arms and other sun-exposed sites, typically sparing the chronically sun-exposed ("hardened") face. The eruption typically occurs with each of the first several beach, pool, or picnic sun exposures in the late spring or summer months. After these two or three exposure-associated rashes, patients usually become "hardened," tan, and have no further problems until the next spring or summer.

When the diagnosis of photoallergic drug eruption or PMLE cannot be made based on the patient's appearance and clinical course (photoallergy should clear with drug withdrawal and PMLE should resolve with continued sun exposure), further evaluation for possible lupus erythematosus, including *skin biopsy,* should be done.

In all patients with photosensitive disorders, appropriate protective sun-blocking clothing and high sun protection factor (SPF), broad-spectrum sunscreens should be used. These eruptions are caused primarily by UVA radiation in the case of drug eruptions and ultraviolet B and UVA radiation in the case of PMLE and lupus erythematosus. Notably, UVA (but not UVB) passes through window glass and patients who are photosensitive or are on photosensitizing drugs should be made aware of this.

Sunscreens and Sunblocks

Sunscreens and sunblocks should be recommended not only for people with photosensitivity, but also for normal people spending time out of doors in sunny seasons. *Sunburns* (for which there is no effective treatment other than palliative oral analgesics and tepid baths) and suntanning should be discouraged because both UVB and UVA are known carcinogens.

Sunscreens contain chemicals that absorb UV radiation. Most of these products contain benzophenones or cinnamates that absorb UVB (290- to 320-nm wavelengths) and the shorter wavelengths of UVA (320 to 340 nm) very well, but are less effective in screening the longer wavelengths of UVA (340 to 400 nm), which are of key importance in causing drug phototoxicity and other photosensitivities. Some newer products, including Shade UVA Guard, contain Parsol 1789, which absorbs even long-wavelength UVA very well. Adverse reactions to any sunscreen may occur. These chemicals are altered by radiation, and this is believed to be the cause of burning and stinging that may occur with stronger sunscreens, particularly when used on the face. This seems most common in fair-skinned women using α-hydroxy acid or retinoic acid–based (Renova, Retin-A) facial creams. Alternative agents that block rather than absorb UV radiation (sunblocks) include plain zinc oxide (visibly white) and micronized zinc oxide and titanium dioxide (translucent when applied). Sunblocks tend to be less cosmetically acceptable because they have a chalky feel, but they effectively block both UVB and UVA.

Sunscreens and sunblocks are given a *sun protection factor* (SPF) rating, which is the ratio of time needed for UVB radiation to cause minimal erythema (redness) when using versus not using the sunscreen. In the laboratory, an SPF of 15 screens 92% of UVB, and an SPF of 30 screens 96% of UVB. However, most sunscreen users apply less than 50% of the amount of lotion needed for this protection, effectively turning an SPF 30 product into an SPF 15 product. For this reason, it is best to recommend an SPF 30 sunscreen, preferably waterproof. Alternatively, because sunscreens are expensive, sun protection can be provided with tight-weave clothing, hats, and avoidance of sunlight exposure during peak UVB radiation times (10 AM to 3 PM). Finally, because some people may obtain vitamin D from the sun instead of their daily diet or a vitamin tablet, the recommendation for sunscreens and sun avoidance should also include a recommendation for adequate daily vitamin D ingestion (e.g., two glasses of fortified milk or 400 IU/day, as found in a multiple vitamin).

TOPICAL THERAPEUTICS

Topical Corticosteroids

Topical corticosteroids are categorized based on the degree of vasoconstriction they produce upon application to the skin, with superpotent products producing the most vasoconstriction. Vasoconstriction correlates well not only with biologic activity and therapeutic efficacy, but also with undesirable side effects. These include local effects such as acne, rosacea, striae, atrophy (cigarette paper–like wrinkling of the skin), and increased risk of skin infection (especially fungal infection). In addition, systemic effects, as evidenced

by hypothalamic–pituitary–adrenal axis suppression, may occur with the use of potent corticosteroids over large areas.

It is best to become familiar with single corticosteroids of low, medium, high, and super potencies and use these agents appropriately. All topical corticosteroids except 0.5% and 1% hydrocortisone are by prescription only. Examples include the following:

- Low potency: hydrocortisone 1% or 2.5% (e.g., Hytone)
- Mid-potency: triamcinolone 0.1% (e.g., Kenalog) or fluocinolone acetonide 0.025% (e.g., Synalar)
- High potency: fluocinonide (e.g., Lidex)
- Super potency: clobetasol (e.g., Temovate)

Generally, only low-potency preparations should be used on the face and in areas of thin skin (i.e., folds, genitalia). Unless a drying effect is desired (e.g., a patient with an acne-prone face is being treated or treatment is in an environment that is excessively humid), ointments rather than creams should be prescribed. They should be applied sparingly to avoid a greasy or unpleasant feeling.

An accurate estimation of the amount of corticosteroid that is needed is important because of the cost of these preparations. Dermatoses are generally treated until they clear, and the application is repeated for recurrences. Acute and subacute dermatitis generally clear in 1 to 2 weeks; chronic dermatitis may require chronic intermittent therapy. One gram covers a 10 × 10 cm area. Two grams covers the hands, head, face, or anogenital area; 3 g covers the anterior or posterior trunk or an arm; 4 g covers a single lower extremity; and 30 g covers the entire skin surface. Therefore one should prescribe for a 1-week, two times a day application for treatment of each of these areas 30 g, 45 g, 60 g, and 420 g, respectively. Most corticosteroids come in 15-, 30-, 60-, and 120-g tubes. In addition, 1-pound jars of hydrocortisone or 0.1% triamcinolone cream or ointment may be requested.

Emollients (Skin Moisturizers)

Simplistically, emollients may be broken down into *oil in water* (mostly water), *water in oil* (mostly oil), and *oil* preparations. Because the purpose of emollients is to trap moisture after hydrating the skin with a warm bath or shower, the more occlusive the substance, the better. Unfortunately, not all patients are amenable to putting Vaseline jelly or Aquaphor ointment (oils) on their skin one or two times a day. A good compromise is Eucerin Original lotion (water in oil) or Eucerin Plus cream or lotion. Other good lighter oil-in-water moisturizers include Lubriderm, Moisturel, Curel, Wondra, and Keri lotions. New formulations (e.g., Lac-Hydrin V, Eucerin Plus, and AquaGlycolic lotions) contain α-hydroxy acids, which aid in normal desquamation of the skin, making it softer and smoother. Although they are useful and well liked by some patients, others who have more sensitive or very dry skin may experience stinging and develop an irritant contact dermatitis from the added α-hydroxy acid. Elderly patients with very dry skin should be warned about this potential problem.

Topical Antifungal Agents

Topical antifungal agents may be divided into *polyene antibiotics* such as nystatin (Mycostatin cream, ointment, and powder; all by prescription), use of which is limited to yeast; *imidazoles* such as clotrimazole (Mycelex OTC and Lotrimin AF cream, lotion, and solution, all over-the-counter), sulconazole (Exelderm 1% cream or solution, by prescription), and ketoconazole (Nizoral 2% cream or shampoo, by prescription), which are all fungistatic at low concentrations and fungicidal at high concentrations; and *allylamines* such as terbinafine (Lamisil, by prescription) or butenafine (Mentax, by prescription), which are fungicidals. Because clotrimazole is over-the-counter, it is less expensive than the other topical antifungals and provides an excellent first-line therapy. If treatment failure occurs, one of the prescription topicals may be prescribed.

All of these agents are available in creams; nystatin also is available as a solution and powder. Exelderm is available as a drying solution, and Nizoral is available as a shampoo. Creams are applied one or two times per day and should be continued for 2 weeks after clinical resolution of the infection, and as needed for recurrences. Exelderm solution is useful when a more drying effect is desired, as in interdigital tinea pedis. Nizoral shampoo is intended for treatment of scalp seborrheic dermatitis, but it may also be used for tinea versicolor. For the former, it is lathered on the scalp and rinsed after 3 minutes, two or three times per week; for the latter, it is lathered on the trunk from the neck to the waistline, left 15 minutes, then rinsed, daily for 10 to 14 days, and a single application is repeated every 1 to 2 weeks to prevent recurrences.

Compresses and Baths

Compresses are used to *dry* and *debride* localized areas of acute dermatitis, characterized by moist, erythematous, edematous papules, plaques, and vesicles or bullae with serous discharge; primary or secondary impetiginization, characterized by golden crusting; and primary or secondary ulceration. *Several solutions dry by precipitating protein* (Burow's aluminum acetate solution, 1:20 dilution; Domeboro aluminum sulfate and calcium acetate solution, 1:20 dilution; Aveeno Colloidal Oatmeal Packet). *Some act as germicidals* (silver nitrate 0.1 to 0.5% solution, acetic acid 1 to 5% solution). *All* (including saline made by adding 2 teaspoons salt per 1 L of water) *promote drying through evaporation and remove devitalized tissue* through physical softening, allowing mechanical removal upon lifting the damp (wet to wet or damp) or dry (wet to dry) dressing.

Compresses may be gauze or cotton sheeting. For the latter, a clean sheet should be cut and folded into six to eight layers to a size to approximate the area of affected skin. It is dipped into the soaking solution and wrung such that it is almost but not still dripping wet. It is placed on the site for 15 to 30 minutes, three or four times per day, and is rewetted every 15 minutes.

When more than one-third of the body surface area is affected by acute dermatitis or impetiginization, compresses are not only impractical but may cause hypothermia. For such patients, lukewarm *baths* are the treatment of choice. Evaporation is impeded with baths, and pruritus and inflammation are effectively reduced. Additives to bath water that may be used include Aveeno Oatmeal Packet, sodium bicarbonate (baking soda, 3 cups), hydrolyzed starch (Lint, 4 cups mixed with water in a large mixing bowl and then added to the bath water), and a mix of half of each of the bicarbonate and starch mixtures.

Baths are also useful for generalized dry, pruritic dermatoses such as atopic dermatitis, generalized psoriasis, morbilliform drug eruptions, and erythroderma. Instead of drying agents, oil (⅛ cup bath oil or Aveeno Oilated Oatmeal Packet) is added to the bath water to help trap moisture in the skin. Patients must be warned about oil making the bathtub slippery and should be advised to purchase secure bath mats for the tub and for the floor outside the tub. Unsteady or frail patients should not use bath oil. Baths should be taken three or four times a day for 20 minutes and a heavy moisturizer (e.g., Vaseline jelly, Aquaphor ointment, Eucerin Original Lotion) must be reapplied immediately after lightly patting dry, leaving some moisture on the skin.

SKIN BIOPSY

Skin biopsy for histologic examination of the skin is required to confirm the diagnosis of many skin conditions. It is a simple and invaluable tool, but it should be used with appropriate discrimination by people who have learned the technique from a skilled teacher. The technique cannot be learned from a book.

Types of biopsies that may be used include *punch, ellipse,* and *shave.* They may be *incisional* (sampling a portion of the lesion) or *excisional* (removing the entire lesion). For any of these procedures, the skin is prepared with a chlorhexidine or alcohol scrub and then anesthetized, usually with 1% lidocaine with epinephrine, 1:100,000 dilution, injected into the dermis and, if necessary, the fat. A punch biopsy is done with a penlike instrument with a circular cutting edge, available in diameters from 2 to 8 mm. It is placed on the lesion and rotated 180° clockwise and counterclockwise until a plug of tissue down to the fat is obtained. An ellipse is done with a number 15 surgical blade on a scalpel handle in the usual surgical fashion. A shave is a more superficial biopsy, usually of the epidermis and upper dermis, and may also be performed with a number 15 blade. The blade is held at an appropriate angle to sample the lesion at the desired depth. Both punch and ellipse biopsies are closed with nonabsorbable 4-0 to 6-0 nylon suture (dissolution of absorbable suture is too unpredictable and therefore is not used), which is removed in 5 to 14 days, depending on the location. The usually small amount of bleeding that occurs with a shave biopsy is easily controlled with a swab application of 20% aluminum chloride solution. Biopsy specimens are placed in formalin for routine histologic examination, in special transport media obtained from the dermatoimmunology laboratory for immunofluorescence study, and in saline-soaked gauze in a sterile container for culture. The latter must be immediately transported to the laboratory.

General References*

American Cancer Society, local chapters. An excellent resource for educational materials on skin cancer for physicians and patients.

Arnold HL Jr, Odom RB, James WD. Andrew's diseases of the skin: clinical dermatology. 8th ed. Philadelphia: WB Saunders, 1990.
A complete general reference text.

Fitzpatrick TP, Johnson RA, Wolff K, et al. Color atlas and synopsis of clinical dermatology. 3rd ed. New York: McGraw-Hill, 1996.
A brief, concise disease discussion, with excellent photographs.

Habib TP. Clinical dermatology, a color guide to diagnosis. 2nd ed. St. Louis: CV Mosby, 1990.
An excellent text of clinical diagnosis and therapy.

Specific References

1. André J, Achten G. Onychomycosis. Int J Dermatol 26:481, 1987.
2. Anhalt GA, Soo Chan K, Stanley JR, et al. Paraneoplastic pemphigus. N Engl J Med 323:1729, 1990.
3. Aubry F, MacGibbom B. Risk factors of squamous cell carcinoma of the skin. Cancer 55:907, 1985.
4. Avakian R, Flowers FP, Araujo OE, et al. Toxic epidermal necrolysis: a review. J Am Acad Dermatol 25:69, 1991.
5. Baughman RD. A 61-year-old man with psoriasis. JAMA 276:1421, 1996.
6. Benson PM, Giblin WJ, Douglas DM, et al. Transient nonpigmenting fixed drug eruption caused by radiopaque contrast media. J Am Acad Dermatol 23:379, 1990.
7. Bigby M, Jick S, Jick H, Arndt K. Drug-induced cutaneous reactions: a report from the Boston Collaborative Drug Surveillance Program on 15,438 Consecutive Patients, 1975–1982. JAMA 256:3358, 1986.
8. Bos JD. Use of cyclosporin A in psoriasis. Lancet 2:8678, 1989.
9. Bouwes Bavinck JN, Tieben LM, Van Der Woude FJ, et al. Prevention of skin cancer and reduction of keratotic skin lesions during acitretin therapy in renal transplant recipients: a double-blind, placebo-controlled study. J Clin Oncol 13:1933, 1995.
10. Brice SL, Krzemie ND, Weston WL, Huff JC. Detection of herpes simplex virus DNA in cutaneous lesions of erythema multiforme. J Invest Dermatol 93:183,1989.
11. Brown J, Winkelmann RK. Acanthosis nigricans: a study of 90 cases. Medicine (Baltimore) 47:33, 1986.
12. Bruinsma W. A guide to drug eruptions 1990–1995. 6th ed. Amsterdam: Free University Amsterdam, 1995.
13. Bubak ME, Reed CE, Fransway AF. Allergic reactions to latex among health-care workers. Mayo Clin Proc 67:1075, 1992.
14. Carrington PR, Sanusi ID, Zahradka S, Winder PR. Enalapril-associated erythema and vasculitis. Cutis 51:121, 1993.
15. Case records of the Massachusetts General Hospital Weekly Clinicopathological Exercises, Case 45-1994. N Engl J Med 331:1703, 1994.
16. Centers for Disease Control. Deaths from melanoma: United States, 1976–1992. MMWR 44:337, 343–347, 1995.
17. Chan HL, Stern RS, Arndt KA, et al. The incidence of erythema multiforme, Stevens–Johnson syndrome, and toxic epidermal necrolysis. Arch Dermatol 126:43, 1990.
18. Classen DC et al. Adverse drug events in hospitalized patients: excessive length of stay, extra costs, and attributable mortality. JAMA 277:301, 1997.
19. Darmstadt GL, Yokel BK, Horn TD. Treatment of acanthosis nigricans with tretinoin. Arch Dermatol 127:1139, 1991.
20. Eady EA, Jones CE, Tipper JL, Cove JH. Antibiotic resistant propionibacteria in acne: need for policies to modify antibiotic usage. BMJ 306:555, 1993.
21. Ellis CN, Fradin MS, Messana JM, et al. Cyclosporin for plaque type psoriasis. N Engl J Med 324:277, 1991.
22. Fox BJ, Odom RB. Papulosquamous diseases: a review. J Am Acad Dermatol 12:597, 1985.
23. Gidwani GP. Androgen assessment in hirsutism and alopecia. Cleve Clin J Med 57:292, 1990.
24. Gilleaudeau P, Vallat VP, Carter DM, Gottlieb AB. Angiotensin-converting enzyme inhibitors as possible exacerbating drugs in psoriasis. J Am Acad Dermatol 28:490, 1993.
25. Greaves MW, Weinstein GD. Treatment of psoriasis. N Engl J Med 332:581, 1995.
26. Gupta MA. Psychosocial correlates of acne vulgaris. Dermatol Q, Fall 1989.
27. Haroon TS, Hussain I, Aman S, et al. A randomized double-blind comparative study of terbinafine for 1, 2 and 4 weeks in tinea capitis. Br J Dermatol 135:86, 1996.
28. Heimbach DM, Engrav LH, Marvin JA, et al. Toxic epidermal necrolysis: a step forward in treatment. JAMA 257:2171, 1987.
29. Helm KF, Peters MS. Subspecialty clinics: dermatology. Immunodermatology update: the immunologically mediated vesiculobullous diseases. Mayo Clin Proc 66:187, 1991.
30. Horan RF. Urticaria and angioedema. Curr Challenge Dermatol 1:Winter, 1993.
31. Hoyo E, Kanitakis J, Euvrard S, Thivolet J. Proliferation characteristics of cutaneous squamous cell carcinomas developing in organ graft recipients. Arch Dermatol 129:324, 1993.
32. Hud JA Jr, Cohen JB, Wagner JM, Cruz PD. Prevalence and significance of acanthosis nigricans in an adult population. Arch Dermatol 128:941, 1992.
33. Hutton KP, Orenberg EK, Jacobs AH. Childhood psoriasis. Cutis 39:26, 1987.
34. Johnson RL et al. Human homology of patched, a candidate gene for the basal cell nevus syndrome. Science 272:1668, 1996.
35. Karagas MR, Stukel TA, Greenberg ER, et al. Risk of subsequent basal cell carcinomas and squamous cell carcinoma of the skin among patients without prior skin cancer. JAMA 267(24):3305, 1992.
36. Karakousis CP, Emrich LJ, Rao U. Tumor thickness and prognosis in clinical stage I malignant melanoma. Cancer 64:1432, 1989.
37. Katz A. Psoriasis and arthritis. Cutis 46:323, 1990.
38. Kligman AM. Postadolescent acne in women. Cutis 48:75, 1991.
39. Koh HK. Cutaneous melanoma. N Engl J Med 325:171, 1991.
40. Koh HK, Miller DR, Geller AC, et al. Who discovers melanoma. J Am Acad Dermatol 26:914, 1992.
41. Kost RG, Straus SE. Postherpetic neuralgia: pathogenesis, treatment, and prevention. N Engl J Med 335:32, 1996.
42. Lever WF. Histopathology of the skin. 7th ed. Philadelphia: JB Lippincott, 1990.
43. Lin R. A perspective on penicillin allergy. Ann Intern Med 152:930, 1992.
44. Lucky AW. Hormonal correlates of acne and hirsutism. In: Proceedings of a symposium, NICHD conference: androgens and women's health. Am J Med 98(1A)5A:89S, 1995.
45. Lupton GP, Odom RB. The allopurinol hypersensitivity syndrome. J Am Acad Dermatol 1:365, 1979.
46. Marghoob AA, Slade J, Salopek TG, et al. Basal cell and squamous cell carcinoma are important risk factors for cutaneous malignant melanoma. Cancer 75:707–714, 1995.
47. Max MB, Schafer SC, Culnane M, et al. Amitriptyline, but not lorazepam, relieves post-herpetic neuralgia. Neurology 38:1427, 1988.
48. McKendrick MW, McGill JI, White JE, Wood MJ. Oral acyclovir in acute herpes zoster. BMJ 293:1529, 1986.

---

*Bold print (general references) and bold numerals (specific references) denote published controlled clinical trials, meta-analyses, or consensus-based recommendations.

49. Meinking TL, Taplin D. Safety of permethrin versus lindane for the treatment of scabies. Arch Dermatol 132:959, 1996.
50. Meinking TL, Taplin D, Hermida JL, et al. The treatment of scabies with ivermectin. N Engl J Med 333:26, 1995.
51. Mertz GJ, Loveless MO, Levin MJ, et al. Oral famciclovir for suppression of recurrent genital herpes simplex virus infection in women: a multicenter, double-blind, placebo-controlled trial. Arch Intern Med 157:343, 1997.
52. Millan SB, Flowers FP, Sherertz EF. Isotretinoin. South Med J 80(4):494, 1987.
53. Murakami S, Mizobuchi M, Nakashiro Y, et al. Bell palsy and herpes simplex virus: identification of viral DNA in endoneurial fluid and muscle. Ann Intern Med 124:27, 1996.
54. National Melanoma/Skin Cancer Detection and Prevention Month, May 1996. JAMA 275:1537, 1996.
55. Nethercott JR, Choi BCK. Erythema multiforme; chart review of 123 hospitalized patients. Dermatologica 171:383, 1985.
56. Nightingale SL. From the Food and Drug Administration: ivermectin approved for strongyloidiasis and onchocerciasis. JAMA 277:703, 1997.
57. NIH Consensus Development Panel on Early Melanoma. Diagnosis and treatment of early melanoma. JAMA 268:1314, 1992.
58. Oliver L, Wald A, Kim M, et al. Seroprevalence of herpes simplex virus infection in a family medicine clinic. Arch Fam Med 4:228, 1995.
59. Oxman MN, Alani R. Varicella and herpes zoster. In: Fitzpatrick TB, Eisen AZ, Wolff K, et al, eds. Dermatology in general medicine. 4th ed. New York: McGraw-Hill, 1993;2543–2572.
60. Pannuti CS, Finck MC, Grimbaum RS, et al. Asymptomatic perianal shedding of herpes simplex virus in patients with acquired immunodeficiency syndrome. Arch Dermatol 133:180, 1997.
61. Parker J. Treatment of head lice (Letter to the Editor). N Engl J Med 336:735, 1997.
62. Peck GL, D'Giovanna JJ, Sarnoff DS, et al. Treatment and prevention of basal cell carcinoma with oral isotretinoin. J Am Acad Dermatol 19:176, 1988.
63. Penn I. Cancers of the anogenital region in renal transplant patients: analysis of 65 cases. Cancer 58:611, 1986.
64. Perniciaro C. Dermatopathologic variants of malignant melanoma. Mayo Clin Proc 72:273, 1997.
65. Preston DS, Stern RS. Nonmelanoma cancers of the skin. N Engl J Med 327(23):1649, 1992.
66. Ragozzino MW, Melton LJ III, Kurland LT, et al. Population-based study of herpes zoster and its sequelae. Medicine 61:310, 1982.
67. Rendon MI, Cruz PD Jr, Sontheimer RD, Bergstresser PR. Acanthosis nigricans: a cutaneous marker of tissue resistance to insulin. J Am Acad Dermatol 21:461, 1989.
68. Rigel DS, Friedman RJ, Kopf AW. The incidence of melanoma in the United States: issues as we approach the 21st century. J Am Acad Dermatol 341:839, 1996.
69. Rigel DS, Jacobs MI. Malignant acanthosis nigricans: a review. J Dermatol Surg Oncol 6:923, 1980.
70. Rooney JF, Strauss SE, Mannix ML, et al. Oral acyclovir to suppress frequently recurrent herpes labialis. Ann Intern Med 118:268, 1993.
71. Roujeau JC, Kelly JP, Naldi L, et al. Medication use and the risk of Stevens–Johnson syndrome or toxic epidermal necrolysis. N Engl J Med 333:1600, 1995.
72. Roujeau JC, Stern RS. Severe adverse cutaneous reactions to drugs. N Engl J Med 331:1272, 1994.
73. Sacks SI, Aoki FY, Diaz-Mitoma F, et al. Patient initiated twice daily oral famciclovir for early recurrent genital herpes: a randomized, double blind, multicenter trial. JAMA 276:44, 1996.
74. Sampson HA, Picasco MC, Caskil CC. Food hypersensitivity and atopic dermatitis: evaluation of 113 patients. J Pediatr 107:669, 1985.
75. Schlesinger Y, Tebas P, Gaudreault-Keener M, et al. Herpes simplex virus type 2 meningitis in the absence of genital lesions: improved recognition with use of the polymerase chain reaction. Clin Infect Dis 20:842, 1995.
76. Schmitt CL. Drug reactions in the elderly. Cutis 41:58, 1988.
77. Seidl LG, Thornton GF, Smith JW, Cluff LW. Studies on the epidemiology of adverse drug reactions: 111 reactions in patients on a general medical service. Bull Johns Hopkins Hosp 119:299, 1966.
78. Semel JD, Goldin H. Association of athlete's foot with cellulitis of the lower extremities: diagnostic value of bacterial cultures of ipsilateral interdigital space samples. Clin Infect Dis 23:1162, 1996.
79. Shalita AR, Pochi PE, Leyden JJ, et al. Acne therapy in the '90s. J Int Postgrad Med 4(1):1, 1991.
80. Shear NH, Spielberg SP. Anticonvulsant hypersensitivity syndrome. J Clin Invest 82:1826, 1988.
81. Shelley WB, Shelley ED. Nonpigmenting fixed drug eruption as a distinctive reaction pattern: examples caused by sensitivity to pseudoephedrine hydrochloride and tetrahydrozoline. J Am Acad Dermatol 17:403, 1987.
82. Sherertz EF. Acneiform eruption due to megadose vitamins B_6 and B_{12}. Cutis 48:119, 1991.
83. Stuart CA, Pate CJ, Peters EJ. Prevalence of acanthosis nigricans in an unselected population. Am J Med 87:269, 1989.
84. Su WPD. Malignant melanoma: basic approach to clinicopathologic correlation. Mayo Clin Proc 72:267, 1997.
85. Survey of knowledge and of awareness about melanoma: United States, 1995. JAMA 275:1537, 1996.
86. Sussman GL, Tarlo S, Dolovich J. The spectrum of IgE-moderated responses to latex. JAMA 265:2844, 1991.
87. Tedder DG et al. Herpes simplex virus infection as cause of benign recurrent lymphocytic meningitis. Ann Intern Med 121:334, 1994.
88. Tyring S, Barbarash RA, Nahlik JE, et al, and the Collaborative Famciclovir Herpes Zoster Study Group. Famciclovir for the treatment of acute herpes zoster: effects on acute disease and postherpetic neuralgia. A randomized, double-blind, placebo-controlled trial. Ann Intern Med 123:89, 1995.
89. Valacylovir. Med Lett 38(965):4, January 5, 1996.
90. Watson W, Cann HM, Farber EM, et al. The genetics of psoriasis. Arch Dermatol 105:197, 1972.
91. Weiss M, Loprinzi CL, Creagan ET, et al. Utility of follow-up tests for detecting recurrent disease in patients with malignant melanoma. JAMA 274:1703, 1995.
92. Whitley RJ, Gnann JW Jr. Acyclovir: a decade later. N Engl J Med 327:782, 1992.
93. Whitley RJ, Weiss H, Gnann JW, et al. Acyclovir with and without prednisone for the treatment of herpes zoster. A randomized, placebo-controlled trial. Ann Intern Med 125:376, 1996.
94. Wiley CA, VanPatten PD, Carpenter PM, et al. Acute ascending necrotizing myelopathy caused by herpes simplex virus type II. Neurology 37:1791, 1987.
95. Wood MJ, Johnson RW, McKendrick MW, et al. A randomized trial of acyclovir for 7 days or 21 days with and without prednisolone for treatment of acute herpes zoster. N Engl J Med 330:896, 1994.
96. Zacharie H, Kragballe K. Cyclosporin versus methotrexate toxicity in psoriasis. Lancet 335:924, 1990.

CHAPTER 101

Common Problems of the Teeth and Oral Cavity

DOUGLAS K. MACLEOD, DMD

The purpose of this chapter is twofold: to provide guidelines for recognizing, treating, and referring patients with acute dental and oral problems; and to increase awareness of chronic dental and oral problems that may require referral and treatment. These types of problems are often neglected by the patient because of fear or ignorance about possible corrective treatment, anticipated pain from the procedure, or the anticipated cost of treatment.

ORAL EXAMINATION

The systematic examination of the oral cavity should include lips, cheeks (buccal mucosa), hard and soft palate, salivary ducts (parotid duct orifice in the buccal mucosa opposite the upper second molars and submandibular duct orifice beside the lingual frenulum), tonsillar area, tongue, floor of the mouth, gingiva, and teeth, noting the normal structures and any deviations from normal.

A dental examination includes an evaluation of the number (20 in the primary dentition and 32 in the permanent dentition; Fig. 101.1), position, and arrangement of the teeth, and a check for caries (see below), erosions, abrasions, and fractures. It is important to examine the gingiva completely. The normal healthy gingiva is firm, pink, and nontender, and does not bleed on palpation or probing. The parts of a tooth and its adjacent structures are shown in Figure 101.2.

ACUTE DENTAL AND ORAL PROBLEMS
Toothaches (Pulpitis)

Presentation

Patients with toothache have a large carious lesion (see "Dental Caries," below), a large restoration (filling), or a combination of both. In the early stages, there is inflammation involving a portion of the pulp tissue (the central portion of the tooth, containing vital soft tissue; Fig. 101.2A).

There is severe pain in response to thermal stimuli, particularly cold, and this pain persists for longer than 15 seconds after the stimulus is removed. As the area of inflammation increases, the pain becomes more severe; it may radiate to the suborbital area, the side of the face, or the ear. When total necrosis of the pulp occurs, sensitivity to thermal stimuli is lost. If at this point the inflammatory exudate cannot escape into the oral cavity, the pressure is released via the root apex, and there is exquisite sensitivity to percussion of the crown of the tooth. The signs and symptoms of pulpitis may be confused with pericoronitis (painful wisdom teeth, see below) or periodontitis (see below), and without further diagnostic aids (i.e., dental x-rays) it may be difficult to differentiate between these conditions.

If pulpitis is not treated, complications may occur, ranging from a localized alveolar abscess (an abscess of the bony supporting structure of the teeth) to facial cellulitis. The rate and type complication depend on the location of the affected tooth, host resistance, and virulence of the bacteria present.

Treatment

Depending on the situation when the patient is seen, one has three options. For patients who are afebrile and have no extraoral swelling (swelling that produces facial asymmetry) or intraoral swelling (swelling that disrupts the supporting alveolar bone and soft tissue), analgesics (acetaminophen 650 mg or codeine 30 mg every 4 hours) and referral within 24 hours are indicated. When slight extraoral or intraoral swelling or a low-grade temperature elevation is present, antibiotics (penicillin V 250 mg or, for patients allergic to penicillin, erythromycin 250 mg every 6 hours) should be added, and the patient should be seen by a dentist within 12 to 24 hours. Patients with temperatures greater than 101°F (38.5°C) with intraoral or extraoral swelling causing facial asymmetry need immediate consultation and treatment by a dentist. Treatment of these types of problems varies from extraction of the affected tooth, root canal therapy (endodontics), or incision and drainage, to hospital admission for intravenous antibiotics for facial cellulitis.

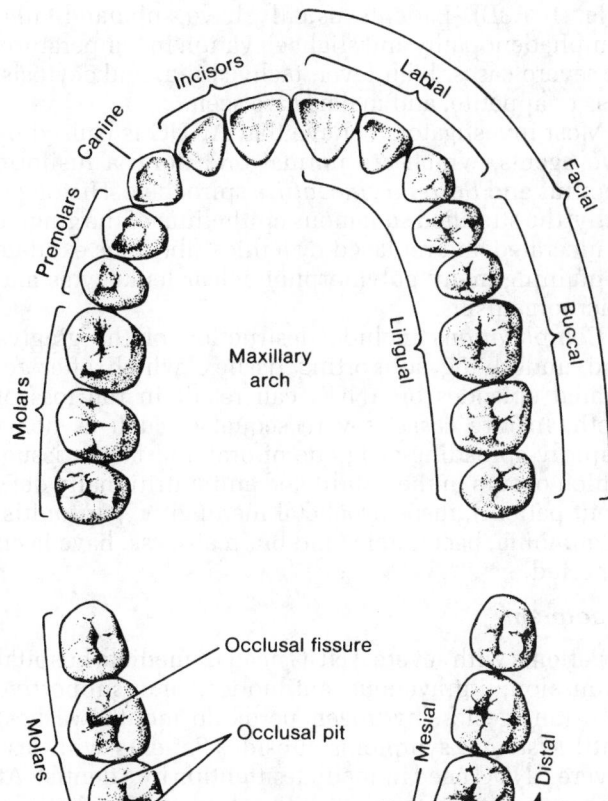

Figure 101.1. Permanent dentition.

Pericoronitis (Third Molar or Wisdom Tooth Pain)

Presentation

Pericoronitis is acute inflammation of the tissue around the crown of a partially erupted tooth. Patients with pericoronitis are usually between the ages of 15 and 25, although rarely the condition can be seen in older patients if they still have their third molars (see below), and they may give a history of subacute episodes of pain of the gingiva that partially covers the crown of an incompletely erupted tooth. The tooth most often affected is the mandibular third molar (wisdom tooth). The space between the crown of the tooth and the overlying gingival flap is an ideal area for the accumulation of food and bacteria; this leads to inflammation. The flap is traumatized by contact with the tooth in the opposing jaw, usually the maxillary third molar, and the inflammation is aggravated.

The patient describes pain that radiates to the ear, throat, and floor of the mouth. He or she complains of

a foul taste, and there is swelling of the affected area so that he cannot close the jaw properly. In severe cases, pain spreading to the oropharynx and base of the tongue makes it difficult to swallow. The gingival tissue is markedly red, swollen, and tender (Fig. 101.3A). Occasionally, tender lymphadenopathy and systemic manifestations (fever, leukocytosis, and malaise) are present. Peritonsillar abscess, cellulitis, and Ludwig's angina (cellulitis of the floor of the mouth) are possible complications.

Treatment

In afebrile patients, one needs only to make a dental referral and prescribe analgesics. Febrile patients should be treated with antibiotics (penicillin V 500 mg or, for patients allergic to penicillin, erythromycin 500 mg every 6 hours), moderate analgesics (acetaminophen 650 mg or codeine 30 mg every 4 to 6 hours), and chlorhexidine gluconate 0.12% oral rinse twice a day (Peridex or Periogard, by prescription); the rinse should be expectorated after use. All patients should be seen by a dentist within 24 hours. Depending on many factors, the dentist either excises or debrides the flap or removes the partially erupted lower tooth. The preferred treatment for third molars that are erupting in a position that produces poor occlusion is to remove the traumatizing maxillary third molar tooth and allow the infected flap to heal. The mandibular tooth is then removed 7 to 10 days later, after the acute infection has resolved. When pericoronitis involves eruption of

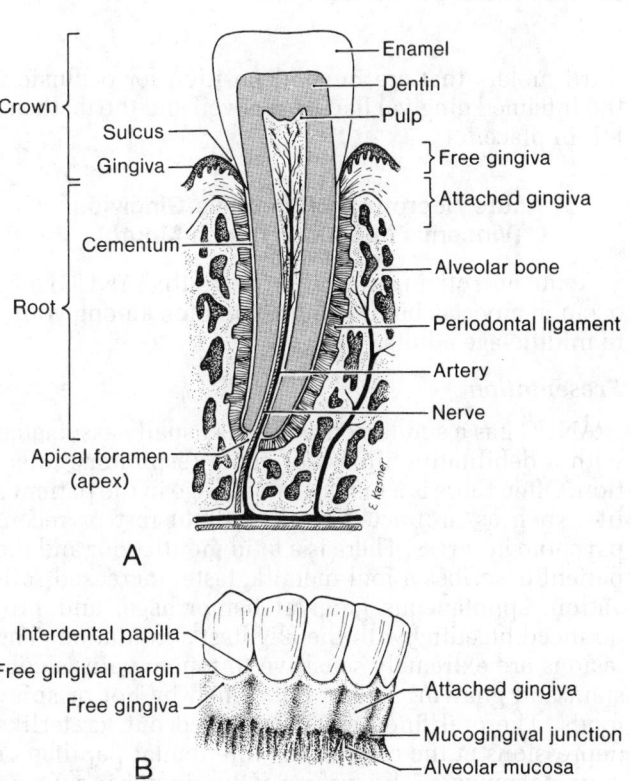

Figure 101.2. Structure of normal teeth and gingiva. **A.** A tooth and its parts. **B.** Teeth and gingiva.

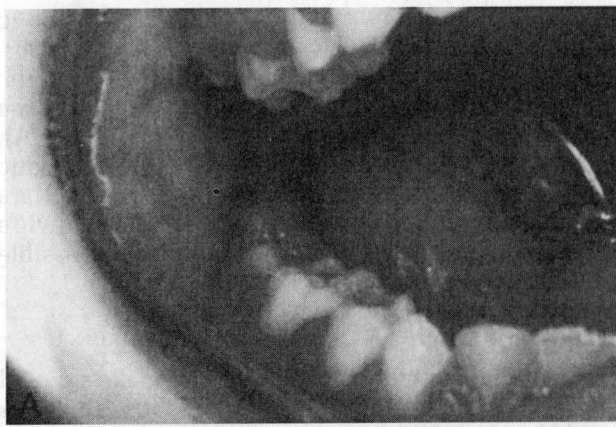
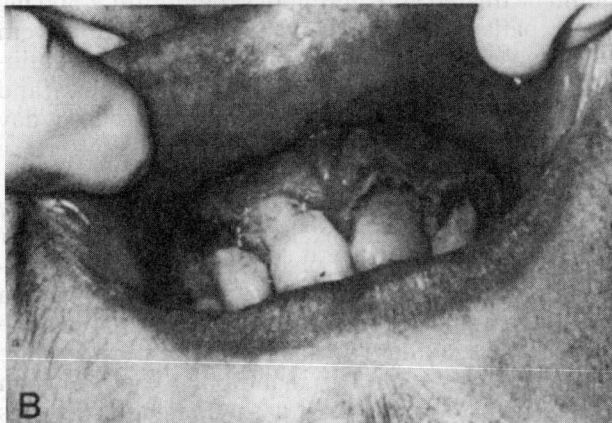

Figure 101.3. **A**. Pericoronitis of the mandibular third molar. **B**. Acute necrotizing ulcerative gingivitis.

third molars that are in good position for occlusion, the inflamed gingival flap is removed and the teeth are left in place.

Acute Necrotizing Ulcerative Gingivitis (Vincent's Infection, Trench Mouth)

Acute necrotizing ulcerative gingivitis (ANUG) may occur at any age, but it is more common among young to middle-age adults.

Presentation

ANUG has a sudden onset and is usually associated with a debilitating illness or acute respiratory infection. Often there is a history of a change in the patient's life, such as protracted work without rest or recent psychologic stress. There is a fetid mouth odor and the patient describes a foul metallic taste, increased salivation, spontaneous gingival hemorrhage, and pronounced bleeding with the slightest stimulation. The lesions are extremely sensitive to touch; pain is constant and gnawing and is intensified by hot or spicy foods. The oral findings are punched out, craterlike depressions at the crest of the interdental papillae or marginal gingiva. The surface of the gingiva is covered by gray pseudomembranous slough that is demarcated from the gingiva by a pronounced linear erythema

(Fig. 101.3B). Patients usually have submandibular lymphadenopathy and slight elevation in temperature; in severe cases, high fever, tachycardia, leukocytosis, loss of appetite, and malaise are seen.

Most investigators believe that ANUG is caused by two agents, which are normal oral flora: a fusiform bacillus and *Borrelia vincentii,* a spirochete. Histologically, the stratified squamous epithelium of the gingiva is ulcerated and replaced by a thick fibrinous exudate containing many polymorphonuclear leukocytes and microorganisms.

Complications include destruction of the gingiva and underlying supporting tissues, which after repeated episodes of ANUG can result in the loss of teeth. In rare cases, severe sequelae, such as noma (rapidly spreading gangrene of oral and facial tissue, which occurs in the debilitated and nutritionally deficient patient), fusospirochetal meningitis, peritonitis, pneumonia, bacteremia, and brain abscess, have been reported.

Treatment

Patients with severe ANUG need immediate hospital admission, intravenous antibiotics, and supportive care (analgesics, hydrogen peroxide mouth washes) until systemic symptoms subside. Patients with less severe ANUG need immediate attention by a dentist. At this visit, after treatment with a topical anesthetic, a cotton pellet and carbamide peroxide solution (an oxygenating and foaming agent, such as Gly Oxide) are used to remove the pseudomembrane and surface debris. Antimicrobials are usually prescribed for a few days by the dentist. After irrigation with warm water, the superficial calculus is removed. Patients are instructed to avoid tobacco and alcohol, to rinse with warm water and chlorhexidine gluconate 0.12% twice daily, and to confine toothbrushing to the removal of surface debris. When these instructions are followed after effective removal of all irritants by the dentist, a patient usually improves markedly within 5 days. If after the acute phase the patient does not continue periodic dental care, ANUG may recur and lead to eventual tooth loss.

Recurrent Aphthous Stomatitis

Aphthous ulcers, also called canker sores, occur at some time in 20 to 50% of the adult population, are slightly more common in females, have familial tendencies, and occur most often during the winter and spring (5). Recurrent aphthous stomatitis (RAS) was once thought to be a recurrent infection by the herpes simplex virus (HSV), but that is not the case; the cause of the condition is still unknown.

Presentation

Aphthous stomatitis is characterized by superficial ulcerations on the mucous membranes of the lips, cheek, tongue, floor of the mouth, palate, and gingiva. This condition begins with a prodromal burning 1 to 48 hours before the appearance of discrete vesicles, which are approximately 2 to 5 mm in diameter and are painful. After 2 days, they rupture and form saucerlike ulcers that consist of a red or grayish red central portion and an elevated rimlike periphery. There may be a single lesion or multiple ulcers.

The lesions heal spontaneously within 7 to 10 days. As a rule, the lesions are larger than those seen in acute herpetic gingivostomatitis (see below) and do not exhibit the diffuse gingival involvement or systemic symptoms seen in that condition.

RAS occurs in the following forms:

- *Occasional aphthae:* a single lesion, at intervals from months to years, that heals uneventfully
- *Acute multiple aphthae:* acute episode that persists for weeks, with lesions developing sequentially at different sites in the mouth, often associated with acute gastrointestinal disorders
- *Chronic recurrent aphthae:* one or more lesions always present for years

Treatment

Treatment of aphthae is symptomatic. A mouthwash containing equal parts of Benadryl suspension and Kaopectate (Benadryl 5 mg/mL mixed with an equal amount of Kaopectate, prepared by a pharmacist) is helpful in reducing the pain, as is viscous Xylocaine applied by cotton tip applicator to painful lesions. Another useful agent is Zilactin (available without prescription), a 7% tannic acid suspension that is applied four times a day for a few days (usually a minimum of 2 days is necessary). In more severe cases, tetracycline has been successful in decreasing pain and duration of the ulcers; the patient should be instructed to empty a 250-mg capsule in 50 mL of water and to use this as a rinse, which is then swallowed, three or four times a day for 5 to 7 days. The patient should be encouraged to take sufficient amounts of nonirritating liquids or soft food to maintain hydration and nutrition. Intake may be facilitated by using a straw to prevent contact with the painful ulcers.

Acute Herpetic Gingivostomatitis

Acute herpetic gingivostomatitis occurs most often in infants and children below the age of 6 years, and it is equally common in males and females. It is caused by HSV, and most oral infections are caused by HSV type 1. However, it also occurs in older patients, including (rarely) the elderly. Most adults have developed immunity to HSV as a result of childhood infection, usually inapparent. Although recurrent acute herpetic gingivostomatitis has been reported, it does not usually recur unless immunity has been altered by a debilitating systemic disease

Presentation

Acute herpetic gingivostomatitis appears as a diffuse, erythematous, shiny involvement of the gingiva and the adjacent oral mucosa, with varying degrees of edema and gingival bleeding. In the initial stage it is characterized by the presence of discrete spherical gray vesicles that may occur in the gingiva, labial and buccal mucosa, soft palate, pharynx, sublingual mucosa, and tongue. Within 24 hours the vesicles rupture and form small, painful ulcers with a red, elevated, halolike margin and a depressed yellowish or grayish white central portion. Regional lymphadenopathy, fever as high as 105°F (40.5°C), and generalized malaise are common. The course is limited to 7 to 10 days and the ulcers heal without scarring. It is differentiated from RAS (see above) by the diffuse gingival involvement and the systemic symptoms.

Treatment

The treatment is the same as that for RAS (see above). Antibacterial agents are not helpful, and corticosteroids are contraindicated. Idoxuridine has been used successfully in treating immunosuppressed patients with primary herpes infections, but because of toxicity its use should be limited to such patients, in consultation with a specialist in infectious disease. The role of oral acyclovir in herpetic gingivostomatitis is uncertain. Its use is probably warranted in the management of severe infection, although this should be done in consultation with an infectious disease specialist or a dentist (see Chapter 94 for a discussion of acyclovir).

Herpes Simplex Labialis

Recurrent herpes simplex infections of the lips or perioral area occur in 20 to 40% of the adult population. Evidence suggests that recurrent herpes is not a reinfection but a reactivation of virus that remains latent in the nerve tissue.

Presentation

The natural history of this problem has been well delineated. Most affected subjects have several episodes during an average year. In approximately 60% of episodes, there is prodromal tingling for a number of hours before the appearance of the first vesicles. Pain is moderate to severe during the first 24 hours after appearance of vesicles and then rapidly diminishes. After 48 hours, vesicles are usually replaced by ulcer crusts. The process usually resolves after 7 to 9 days, but lesions may persist as long as 2 weeks. The therapy of this condition is discussed in Chapter 100, "Common Problems of the Skin."

Sialadenitis

Presentation

Sialadenitis is an inflammation of the salivary gland. Patients with sialadenitis experience pain and enlargement of the affected gland. In bacterial sialadenitis, the pain and swelling are not related to eating. The overlying skin may be red and tense, and the affected gland yields a purulent discharge at the duct orifice. Bacterial sialadenitis is more common in children than in adults. Obstructive sialadenitis is more common than bacterial infection of the salivary glands and is associated with salivary stones or a mucous plug. It occurs most often in middle-age males. The involved gland is enlarged and painful, and the symptoms are more prominent before, during, and soon after eating. The submandibular gland is most often affected (75% of cases), whereas the parotid (20% of cases) and major sublingual glands (5% of cases) are less often involved. Mumps is more common in children but does occur in adults when it often is more severe. The parotid gland is swollen and tender, and there is usually no redness, heat, or discharge. Most often both parotids are involved and, often, other salivary glands. Systemic symptoms are common.

Treatment

Treatment of bacterial sialadenitis consists of heat application (external moist heat packs to the affected gland for 15 to 20 minutes and intraoral warm rinses), analgesics (acetaminophen 650 mg or codeine 30 mg every 4 to 6 hours), antibiotics (penicillin V 500 mg or, for patients allergic to penicillin, erythromycin 500 mg every 6 hours for 10 days), and a liquid diet for the first 2 to 3 days.

The management of obstructive sialadenitis is more complex. When this diagnosis is suspected, the patient should be referred to a dentist or otolaryngologist. In cases in which the stone is lodged in the duct, the acute phase is managed in the same manner as is bacterial sialadenitis, after which a sialogram is obtained to determine the extent of the problem. Surgical removal of the stone from the duct is eventually performed to prevent recurrence. In chronic obstructive sialadenitis, surgical excision of the gland is often necessary. The likelihood of recurrence after the first episode is unknown.

Temporomandibular Joint Pain

Several studies of healthy populations have shown that symptoms of temporomandibular joint (TMJ) disorders are present at some time in 25 to 50% of people but are not considered a serious problem by most patients (4). Most (70 to 90%) of patients who have these symptoms are women between the ages of 24 and 40. Multiple factors may lead to TMJ pain; there may be a history of stress, bruxism (grinding of teeth), external blows to the jaws, or whiplash injury. TMJ pain may be present at some point in 20% of patients with rheumatoid arthritis. Patients with osteoarthritis of other joints may complain of TMJ clicking and snapping, but pain is usually absent.

Presentation

TMJ disorders are characterized by pain and tenderness in the muscles of mastication and in the TMJ, by crepitus when the joint is moved, and by a decrease in range of motion. In some severe cases there is a noticeable incoordination on the opening and closing of the jaw. This appears as a unilateral shift of the chin upon opening or closing the mouth. Examination may show malocclusion caused by teeth that interfere with the normal movement of the mandible or tenderness of the muscles of mastication.

Treatment

Patients with acute TMJ pain should be managed with moderate analgesics (acetaminophen 650 mg or codeine 30 mg every 4 to 6 hours) and referral to a dentist within 24 to 48 hours to begin therapy. The dentist's goal is to make the patient aware of the cause of the problem through education. Depending on the severity of symptoms and the state of the patient's dentition, the dentist will prescribe one or a combination of the following: avoidance of excessive jaw motion, moist heat to affected muscles, soft diet, disengagement of upper and lower jaws with a night guard to separate the upper and lower teeth (a hard appliance constructed to fit the individual patient, which is quite costly), therapeutic exercises, and vapocoolant spray (ethyl chloride to decrease muscle pain). In atypical cases, trigger point injections of Xylocaine may be used to distinguish TMJ symptoms from trigeminal neuralgia (see Chapter 79). Once the acute episode has subsided (in about 7 to 14 days) the dentist can detect and eliminate any occlusal interferences and rule out any degenerative joint disease that may have predisposed the patient to TMJ symptoms. In the past, injections of sclerosing agents into the TMJ and condylectomy were tried, but with poor success.

In a 10-year study, 97 of 100 patients treated conservatively improved. Of these, 83 had permanent improvement. Of the 3 patients who had intractable, severe symptoms, 2 required prolonged psychotherapy and 1 developed systemic arteritis (1).

Local Alveolar Osteitis (Dry Socket)

Local alveolar osteitis (dry socket) is the most common complication of tooth extraction. It occurs in approximately 5% of all tooth extractions, but it is more common after the removal of an impacted third molar. This problem results from the loss of the blood clot located at the site of the extraction. Most often this occurs when the extraction has been difficult and has resulted in considerable trauma to the socket and gum.

Patients with this problem describe intense localized pain 2 or 3 days after an extraction. This pain is caused by irritation of the sensory nerves in the dry, exposed bony socket. There is often a foul odor emanating from the socket, but no suppuration is present.

One should control the pain the patient is experiencing with codeine 30 mg every 3 to 4 hours and acetaminophen 650 mg three to four times per day. The patient should be referred promptly to a dentist for irrigation and the placement of a dressing. The dentist needs to see the patient every day or two for approximately 10 days until the socket becomes reepithelialized. There are no long-term sequelae.

CHRONIC DENTAL AND ORAL PROBLEMS

Periodontal Disease (Pyorrhea)

Periodontal disease is a general term used to describe diseases that destroy the gingival and bony structures that support the teeth (Figs. 101.4 and 101.5). Periodontal disease is usually subdivided into *gingivitis* and *periodontitis*. The major difference between the two is that in periodontitis there is loss of the supporting bony apparatus of the teeth.

Two-thirds of young adults, 80% of middle-age adults, and 90% of people in the United States over 65 suffer from periodontal disease (8). Poor oral hygiene, which permits plaque to accumulate on the teeth, is the major etiologic factor. Most periodontal disease, and therefore most loss of teeth, is preventable. Prevention consists of routine plaque control (see below).

Relationship of Calcium Channel Blocking Drugs to Gingival Overgrowth

Calcium channel blocking drugs are widely used for management of cardiovascular conditions. Nifedipine is one of the most often prescribed drugs in this group and the first to be associated with gingival overgrowth. Most other calcium channel blocking agents have been associated with gingival enlargement, although not to the same degree as nifedipine. The onset of gingival enlargement usually appears within 2 months after initiation of nifedipine therapy and is most pronounced in the anterior facial gingiva. The tendency for overgrowth occurs in approximately 15 to 20% of patients and although it does not appear to be dose related, a decrease in enlargement after dosage reduction has been reported. The histologic, histochemical, and electron microscopic examinations of nifedipine-induced gingival enlargement closely resembles phenytoin- or cyclosporine-induced gingival overgrowth, suggesting that the pathogenic mechanism is similar. Chronic inflammation is always present and an association between plaque accumulation and drug-induced overgrowth has been documented. Meticulous plaque control does not usually cause remission or consistently stop recurrence after surgical removal. Whenever gingival overgrowth develops, an alternative to nifedipine should be considered. If a calcium channel blocking agent is essential for the patient, an agent other than a dihydrophyridine (examples of such agents that should be used in this situation are diltiazem, verapamil, or bepridil) should be used.

Patients who have had organ transplants may be taking cyclosporine, an immunosuppressant drug used extensively to suppress organ and bone marrow transplant rejection. The combination of cyclosporine and calcium channel blocking agents appears to have a synergistic effect on the gingiva. The hyperplasia produced is extreme and often recurs following surgical excision.

Gingivitis

Presentation. Gingivitis is usually seen in one of four forms: *acute,* a painful condition that has a rapid onset and is of short duration; *subacute,* which is less severe than the acute condition; *recurrent,* which reappears after being eliminated by treatment or after disappearing spontaneously; and *chronic,* the most common form, which has a slow onset, is of a long duration, and is usually painless unless complicated by acute exacerbations (Fig. 101.5).

The early signs of inflammation of the gingiva, which precede frank gingivitis, are increased gingival fluid secretion and bleeding from the gingival sulcus upon gentle probing. Healthy gingiva is usually coral pink, whereas in gingivitis the gingiva becomes bright red secondary to increased vascularity and a decrease in keratinization. These changes start in the interdental papillae and free gingiva and spread to the attached gingiva. Both acute and chronic forms produce changes in the normally firm, resilient consistency of the gingiva. In acute gingivitis the gingiva has a diffuse edematous appearance, whereas in the chronic form the tissue has a fibrous appearance that pits on pressure.

The development of gingivitis is a consequence of supragingival and subgingival plaque formation

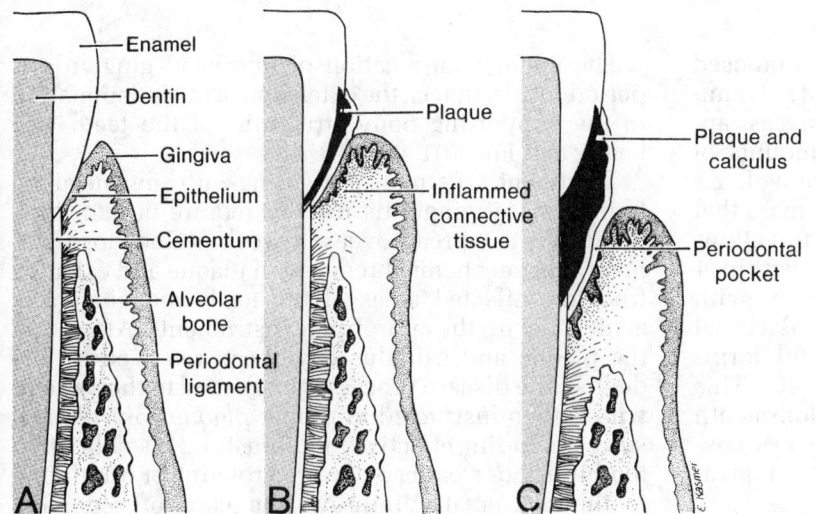

Figure 101.4. Dentogingival junction in health. **A.** Plaque free. **B.** Gingivitis resulting from plaque accumulation with inflammation of soft tissue. **C.** Periodontitis resulting from long-standing inflammation that has caused bone loss and tooth mobility.

Enamel
Dentin
Gingiva
Epithelium
Cementum
Alveolar bone
Periodontal ligament

Plaque
Inflamed connective tissue

Plaque and calculus
Periodontal pocket

Figure 101.5. Normal gingiva **(A)** and chronic periodontal inflammation **(B)** showing swelling, blunting of interdental papillae, erythema, and bleeding.

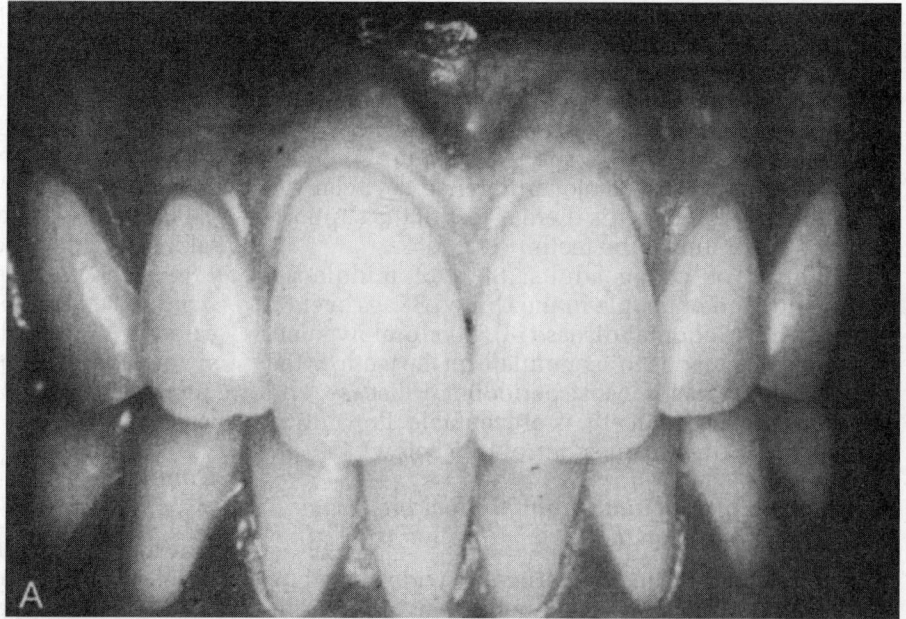
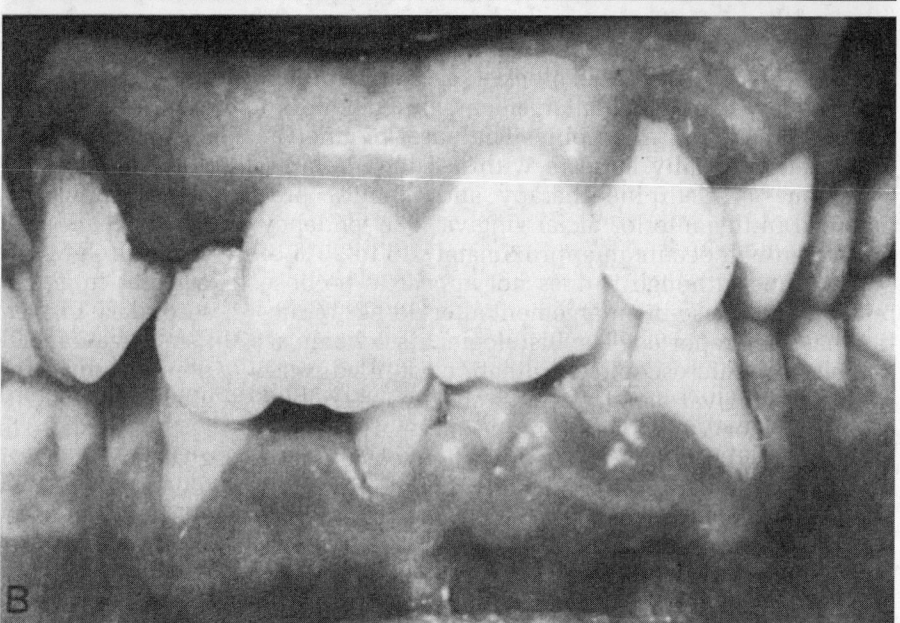

(Fig. 101.4). Plaque is a transparent deposit composed primarily of bacteria and their byproducts. Gram-positive filamentous rods, mainly *Actinomyces,* appear to be of major significance. Small amounts of plaque are not visible unless they are stained. As plaque accumulates, it becomes visible as a mass that varies in color from gray to yellowish gray to yellow. Measurable amounts of plaque may form within 1 hour after a thorough cleaning of the teeth, with maximal accumulation in 30 days or less. Bacterial plaque, if left undisturbed, mineralizes and forms calculus (tartar), as shown in Figure 101.4C. This process usually starts between the first and fourteenth day after plaque formation. Calculus is always covered by plaque. When calculus is present, the gingival tissues are unhealthy by definition.

The major complication of untreated gingivitis is periodontitis; that is, the extension of the inflammation to the supporting bony structures of the teeth (see below and Fig. 101.4C).

Treatment. Patients presenting with any one of the four forms of gingivitis usually require one to three dental visits (spread over a 4-week period) for treatment. The mechanical removal of plaque and calculus from the affected areas of the teeth and gingiva is achieved with the appropriate instruments. After all of the plaque and calculus have been removed by the dentist, the disease process is explained to the patient, who is then instructed in proper *plaque control measures,* including effective toothbrushing (a soft bristled toothbrush or a battery-powered rotating or oscillating toothbrush greatly improve the ease of removing plaque and facilitate cleansing of the gingiva and the teeth and should be recommended) and effective flossing (the floss should be rubbed vertically up and down three to five times in each interdental space, once daily). Maintenance of the disease-free state is possible only by continued effective plaque control measures by the patient and by professional cleaning every 6 to 12 months (to remove plaque and calculus that may be missed by brushing and flossing). Mouthwashes are available that help in the treatment of gingivitis (3). Chlorhexidine gluconate, 0.12% oral rinse twice daily (Peridex or Periogard available by prescription), has been shown to be microbicidal. The rinse should be expectorated after use. Complications are common and include a brown stain of the teeth, possible taste alterations, and increase in calculus formation. For these reasons a patient should not use the material without consulting a dentist.

Factors that usually result in recurrence are incomplete removal of plaque and calculus, inadequate plaque control because of insufficient patient instruction, premature dismissal of the patient before competence is demonstrated, and lack of patient cooperation.

Periodontitis

Presentation. A patient with periodontitis has red and bleeding gums and an unpleasant taste in his or her mouth, but is usually free of pain unless there is an acute infection superimposed on the underlying chronic process. The principal physical findings are the signs of inflammation of the gingiva described above and periodontal pockets around the teeth, from which pus may often be expressed upon gentle pressure. As periodontitis advances, the teeth loosen and spread apart, creating unattractive spaces and exposing the roots of the teeth as the bony support is lost. Mastication is impaired, and spontaneous pain and acute abscess may occur. The most important consequence of periodontitis is the destruction of the alveolar bone, which deprives the teeth of their support and is responsible for the loss of the teeth. The essential steps leading to destruction of bone are gingivitis, degeneration of collagen bundles of the periodontal ligament, and conversion of the shallow (3 mm or less) physiologic gingival sulcus to a deepened periodontal pocket (more than 3 mm). As this pocket deepens, more debris accumulates in it. Inflammation progresses further inward, and the gums recede permanently. The apically progressing inflammation eventually reaches the alveolar crest, and bone resorption begins. This process continues, resulting in continued destruction of the alveolar bone.

Treatment. Most patients with periodontitis can be treated effectively, provided that the diagnosis is made before a significant amount of supporting alveolar bone is lost. The aims of treatment are to preserve the teeth by eliminating the disease, restore effective function, and prevent recurrence. When treated in the early stages, the major consequence of periodontitis (loss of bone support for the teeth) can be prevented. If proper treatment is postponed, there may be insufficient bone support once treatment is undertaken, and

the natural teeth may eventually be lost. Some patients are not concerned with this problem but are ultimately disappointed when their dentures do not function efficiently.

Treatment of periodontitis is divided into two phases. Phase I is similar to the treatment of gingivitis described above; that is, removal of local irritant (plaque and calculus) and institution of effective plaque control (continual removal of the plaque). This treatment allows resolution of the inflammation. The success of this phase of therapy depends largely on the patient's ability to maintain plaque-free teeth (see "Acute Necrotizing Ulcerative Gingivitis," below). Phase II is the surgical phase, in which the goal is to improve the gingival architecture that remains despite the disease. Experience shows that patients have difficulty preventing inflammation in periodontal pockets greater than 5 mm. Surgical treatment is therefore designed to decrease the depths of the pockets.

Denture Problems

Twenty million American adults are missing all of their teeth. Of these, many have obtained dentures. In addition, many of the edentulous population have managed well without teeth, are content to remain as they are, and, regardless of the quality of dentures constructed, are unwilling or unable to adapt to using dentures.

Presentation

Often the physician is confronted with a patient who has had dentures for years, but upon specific questioning indicates that the dentures are not satisfactory. The most common denture problems are looseness and discomfort. If the patient is followed at least yearly by his or her dentist, the physician can generally assume that the present situation is the best that can be achieved. On the other hand, if the patient has tolerated the same set of loose or uncomfortable dentures without seeking help for a number of years, he or she should be encouraged to seek care promptly. Failure to remove dentures at night is the reason for denture problems in some patients. This practice can cause bony erosion with loss of conformity of the dentures to the supporting structures, mucosal ulceration, and oral candidiasis.

Treatment

Depending on the condition of the patient's oral cavity, the present dentures, and the edentulous ridges, a number of treatment modalities are available, including rebasing or relining the existing dentures (5 to 7 days), making a new set of dentures (2 to 5 weeks), and preprosthetic correction of soft and hard tissue (4 to 6 weeks healing), followed by relining, rebasing, or remaking of dentures. In recent years, there have been marked improvements in dental implants for patients who have had trouble using dentures (especially lower dentures). The placement of implants is expensive ($1200 to $1500 per implant, often with a reduction in price for multiple installations, and often five to six implants are used per arch) and time-consuming (2 to 3 months) and requires that new dentures be made after placement of implants. The implants function as a replacement for the teeth roots that the patient had previously lost through dental caries, periodontitis, or trauma. Most conservative dentists reserve implants for the patient missing at least all posterior teeth or all natural teeth.

Dental Caries

Dental caries is a disease of the calcified tissues of the teeth characterized by demineralization of the inorganic portion (enamel and dentin of the tooth; see Fig. 101.2A).

Dental caries is one of the most common diseases in humans. It affects all people regardless of race, location, or economic stratum, and it can occur at any age. Poor oral hygiene and a diet high in sugar promote caries, whereas routine oral hygiene and raw, coarse foods tend to reduce caries. Ingestion of fluorides in drinking water reduces susceptibility to caries. The form of the tooth affects caries; that is, the deep pits and fissures on molars and premolars especially predispose these teeth to the disorder.

Presentation

Dental caries usually presents as a nonpainful, white, brown, or black spot on the enamel of a tooth. The most common location is the biting surface in conjunction with the pits and fissures of the tooth. Other locations include the smooth surfaces where the teeth come into contact with each other. Without the aid of special equipment (x-rays and hand instruments) and expertise of dental personnel, the best indicator of dental caries is the presence of brown or black spots in areas associated with lost portions of the tooth.

When a caries progresses rapidly to involve the pulp, as in children, the term *acute caries* is used. Slowly progressing caries seen in adults is called chronic caries. Occasionally, a carious lesion may cease to progress (arrested caries). This is caused by breakage of enamel walls, thereby exposing the lesion to the cleaning action of the toothbrush, saliva, fluoride, and mastication. The term *recurrent caries* is used for carious lesions that begin around the margins of defective restorations.

A carious lesion usually develops after bacterial plaque (see above) forms on the tooth surface. The primary bacteria involved in this process are *Streptococcus mutans* and *Lactobacillus acidophilus*. These bacteria metabolize dietary fructose to produce lactic acid, which results in decalcification of the enamel. The rate of development of caries depends on the susceptibility of the enamel.

Treatment

The treatment for most carious lesions is their removal, followed by a restoration (filling) that replaces the lost portions of the tooth. The goals are to remove the lesion, protect the pulp from irritants, and restore the tooth to function. With the advent of enamel and dentin bonding agents, a sealant (a thin plastic layer of resin) can be placed over a noncarious tooth in the deep fissures to prevent dental caries. In cases when caries involves a tooth already significantly affected by periodontal disease, the tooth must be removed.

The major *complication* that results from delaying treatment is acute pulpitis and its complications (see above). In addition, delaying treatment may result in a more difficult restoration or possible loss of the involved tooth. In cases in which the existing decay process is very close to the pulp, the heat generated by the rotary instruments used to prepare the restoration may result in a transient pulpal inflammation. This inflammation results in a dull ache in the tooth for 2 to 3 days, which is usually relieved by aspirin. When the restoration process leaves only a paper-thin layer of dentin covering the pulp tissue, the transient pulpitis may be converted to acute pulpitis (irreversible), which then requires tooth extraction or root canal therapy for relief of pain. Root canal therapy consists of three parts: removal of the infected nerve tissue, debridement and preparation of the nerve canal space, and obturation (filling) of the canal space with a biologically inert material.

Angular Cheilosis

Presentation

Angular cheilosis is characterized by a feeling of dryness and a burning sensation at the corners of the mouth. The epithelium at the commissures appears wrinkled and macerated. In time, the wrinkles deepen to fissures that appear ulcerated but do not bleed, although a crust may form. These lesions stop at the junction of the mucous membranes. They show a tendency for spontaneous improvement; only rarely do the lesions completely disappear.

There are several causes for cheilosis. A number of microorganisms may cause it in otherwise healthy people: *Candida albicans,* staphylococci, and streptococci. In addition, angular cheilosis caused by overclosure of the jaws may be seen in edentulous patients. Overclosure causes a fold to be produced at the corners of the mouth in which saliva tends to collect, inviting the growth of microorganisms. Angular cheilosis is also seen in riboflavin deficiency, which usually occurs in patients with multiple vitamin deficiencies. The lips show fissures, painful cracks, and scaling; these changes become severe at the corners of the mouth and are similar in appearance to angular cheilosis caused by overclosure of the mandible.

Treatment

Edentulous patients troubled by angular cheilosis should be referred to a dentist, who will evaluate them for mandibular overclosure, because correction of this problem (making or remaking of dentures) may lead to remission. Treatment is otherwise symptomatic and consists of applying petrolatum-containing ointment (e.g., Vaseline, Chapstick) to the scaling area to minimize discomfort.

Thrush (Oral Candidiasis)

Presentation

The typical lesions of oral candidiasis are white, curdlike plaques on an erythematous mucosa (Fig. 101.6). These plaques are loosely attached and may be scraped off the oral mucosa. They begin as pinpoint spots. Involvement may include the corners of the mouth, as noted in the previous section. The tongue is often reddened, and the patient describes a burning sensation.

Thrush may occur chronically in patients with poor oral hygiene and poor nutrition. It may also be brought on or exacerbated by debilitating systemic illness, antibiotic therapy, impaired immune system, use of steroids or antimetabolites, or dental extraction. Thrush does not appear to be more common in diabetic patients. It is common in patients with human immunodeficiency virus (HIV) infection (see Chapter 34).

The white plaques of thrush may suggest hyperkeratosis or leukoplakia. In these instances, a scraping reveals hyphae and blastospores when the condition is candidiasis.

Treatment

The patient should be advised to use good oral hygiene practices. Specific treatment consists of nystatin oral suspension, 4 to 6 mL held in the mouth for several minutes before swallowing, four times daily. Thrush usually resolves entirely after 1 to 2 weeks of treatment. Treatment should be continued for several

days after visible lesions have disappeared. More intensive treatment is needed in patients with HIV infection (see Chapter 34).

Halitosis

Presentation

Halitosis is a foul or offensive odor emanating from the oral cavity. Mouth odors originate from local or remote sites. The local causes can be retention of odoriferous food particles on or between the teeth, ANUG (see above), caries, chronic periodontal disease, dentures, tobacco smoking, and healing of surgical or extraction wounds. Extraoral causes of halitosis include infection in adjacent structures (rhinitis, sinusitis, tonsillitis), pulmonary infections, alcoholic breath, the acetone odor of the diabetic, or the uremic breath associated with renal failure.

Treatment

Local causes of this condition are treated by improvement in oral hygiene and by specific treatment of the underlying conditions by a dentist. If these measures are unsuccessful, pleasant-smelling mouthwashes or breath fresheners used frequently (every 2 to 4 hours) may greatly reduce the problem. Halitosis caused by remote factors may be masked with mouthwashes and fresheners until the remote problem has been resolved.

Xerostomia (Dry Mouth)

Presentation

Xerostomia, or dry mouth, results from a partial or complete lack of saliva. This defect results in cracking of the lips, difficulty in swallowing, or changes in the tongue texture. The patient often increases liquid consumption in order to eliminate the dryness. Xerostomia may be a secondary complication of salivary gland disease (e.g., Sjögren's syndrome) or radiation treatment, but medication is the most common cause. Anticholinergic, decongestant, and antihistamine drugs are the most common offenders.

The loss of saliva results in a loss of the protective coating of the mucous membranes of the oral cavity. Infections, severe dental caries, and problems with dentures very commonly result from the loss of saliva.

Treatment

Treatment of xerostomia is symptomatic. Patients should be referred to a dentist for a complete dental evaluation and to eliminate any caries and for instruction in the use of daily topical fluoride to help prevent recurrence of caries. The dryness may be lessened if the patient regularly irrigates the mouth with topical methylcellulose, glycerin, or a saliva substitute (Glandosane, Oralube, MOI STIR, Salive Substitute [Roxane Laboratories] or Xerolube, all available without prescription). The saliva substitutes also decrease the risk of caries because they contain sodium fluoride.

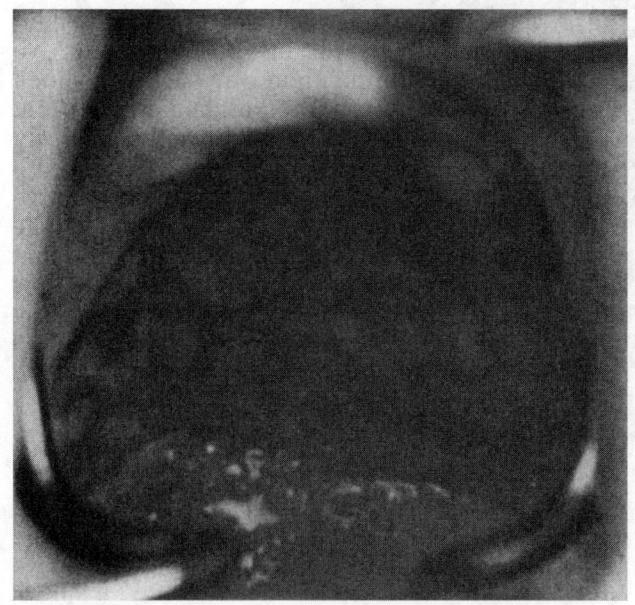

Figure 101.6.   Candidiasis (thrush) of the hard palate.

Common Tongue Conditions

Geographic Tongue

Benign migratory glossitis, or geographic tongue, is an asymptomatic inflammatory condition consisting of multiple areas of desquamation of the filiform papillae of the tongue in an irregular pattern (Fig. 101.7A). The central portion of an affected area is usually denuded, and the border may be outlined by a thin, yellowish white line or band. The fungiform papillae persist in the desquamated area as small, elevated red dots. The areas of desquamation remain for a short time in one location, then heal and reappear in other locations. The condition may persist for weeks or months and then regress, only to recur at a later date. Women are affected twice as often as men, and there is no racial difference. Because the cause is unknown and the condition is benign, management consists of reassurance. Large doses of vitamins are not effective.

Hairy Tongue

Hairy tongue is a condition characterized by hypertrophy of the filiform papillae of the tongue caused by the lack of normal desquamation of the keratin layer (Fig. 101.7B). This results in a thick, matted layer on the dorsum of the tongue. The color of the papillae varies from yellowish white to brown or even black depending on their staining by extrinsic factors (tobacco, foods, or medications). The hypertrophied tissue may touch the palate and produce gagging in some patients. Most patients with hairy tongue are heavy smokers, but the cause is unknown. Treatment of this benign condition consists of brushing the tongue with a tongue blade or toothbrush to promote desquamation and remove debris.

Median Rhomboid Glossitis

Median rhomboid glossitis is a congenital abnormality of the tongue that appears clinically as an ovoid-,

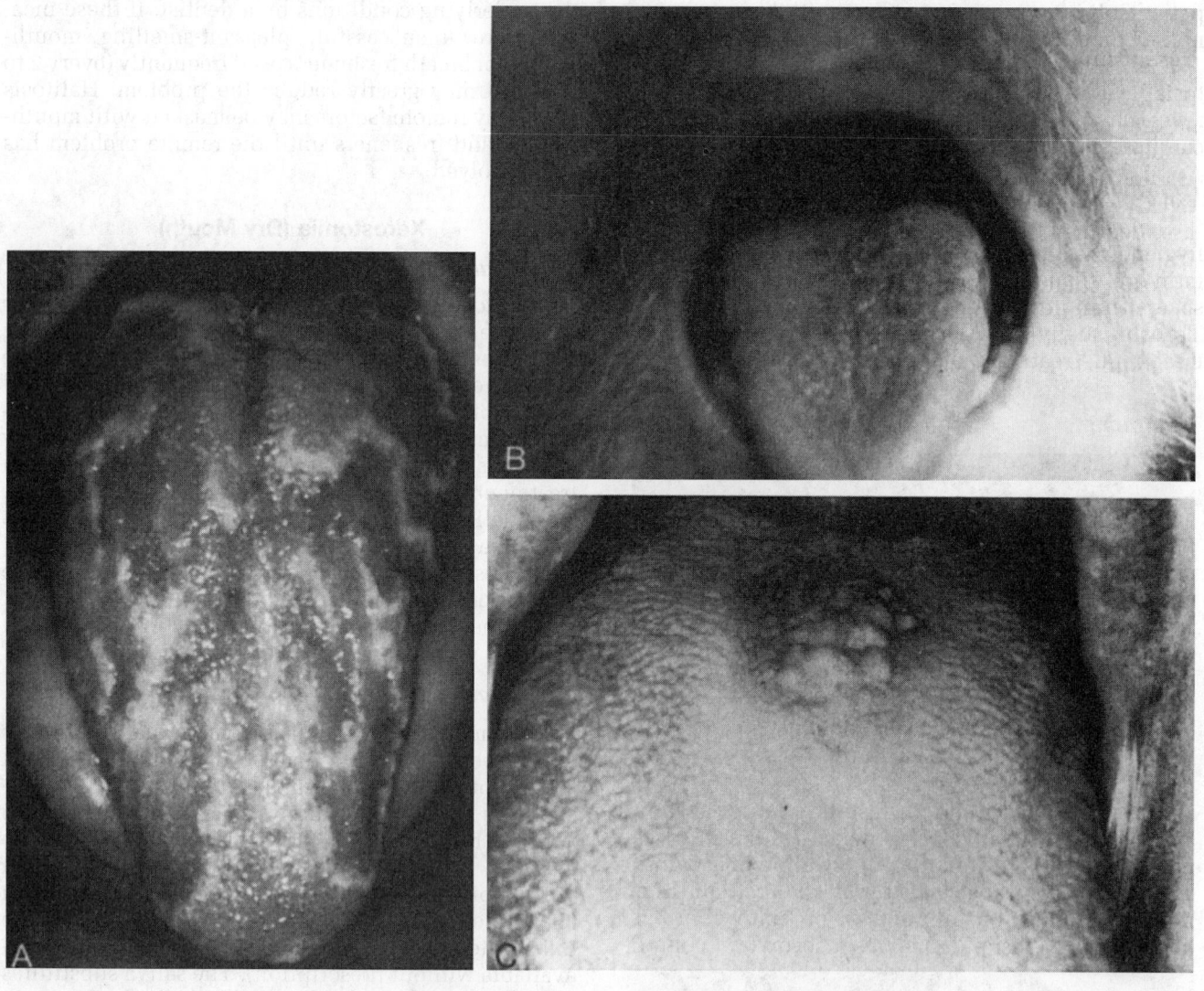

Figure 101.7. Common benign problems of the tongue. **A**. Geographic tongue. **B**. Hairy tongue. **C**. Median rhomboid glossitis.

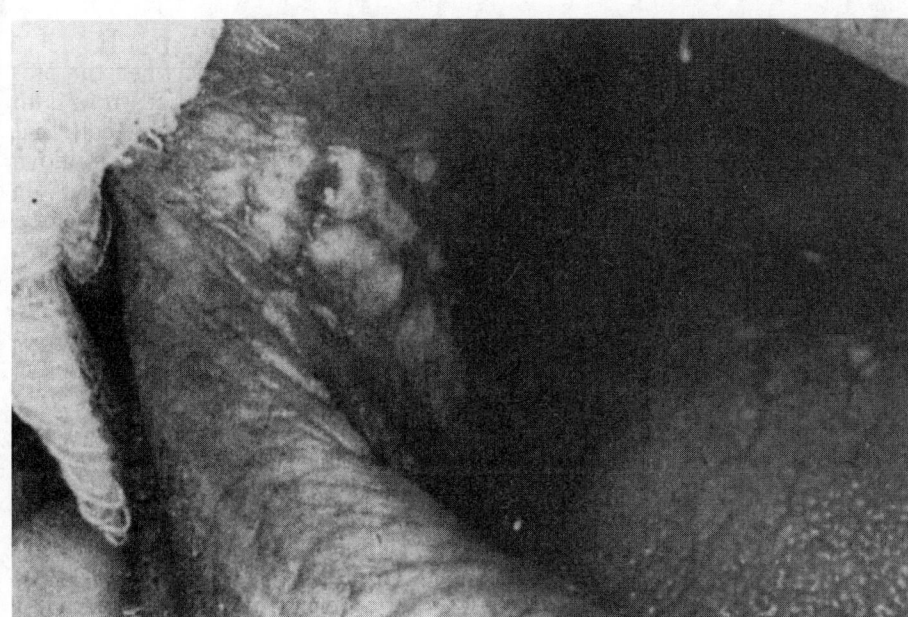

Figure 101.8. Leukoplakia showing early changes of epidermoid carcinoma.

diamond-, or rhomboid-shaped reddish patch on the dorsal surface of the tongue. On examination, there is a slightly raised or flat area that is distinctive because there are no filiform papillae (Fig. 101.7C). Despite its name, this abnormality is not inflammatory; it is caused by failure of the tuberculum impar to retract before fusion of the lateral halves of the tongue, so that a structure free of papillae is interposed. The prevalence of the abnormality is less than 1%, and there are no sex or racial differences. The only clinical significance of this innocuous condition is that it is occasionally mistaken for a carcinoma; differentiation from cancer is aided by the presence of the lesion since childhood and the fact that a carcinoma rarely develops on the dorsum of the tongue. If the physician is unsure of the diagnosis, the patient should be referred to a dentist.

Leukoplakia and Erythroplakia

Presentation

Leukoplakia and erythroplakia are asymptomatic conditions of the oral mucosa that may become malignant.

Leukoplakia varies in appearance from a grayish white, flattened, scaly lesion to a thick, irregularly shaped plaque (Fig. 101.8). Histologically, there is hyperkeratosis, acanthosis, and some degree of dyskeratosis. It is commonly associated with underlying inflammation caused by a chronic irritant (tobacco, alcohol, poorly constructed dentures). Leukoplakia may be found anywhere in the oral cavity, but most often it is found in the buccal mucosa, followed, in descending order, by the alveolar mucosa, tongue, lip, hard and soft palates, floor of the mouth, and gingiva.

Erythroplakia refers to a lesion that is velvety red in appearance, small (2 cm or less), and with or without a hyperkeratotic component. It is found in the floor of the mouth, soft palate, and ventrolateral border of the tongue.

The significance of these lesions has been delineated in a longitudinal study of mucosal lesions (7). Of 200 white lesions examined by biopsy, only 4 were malignant. In the same study, an erythroplastic component was present in 90% of the 158 asymptomatic squamous cell carcinomas that were found, suggesting, but not proving, that erythroplakia may be an important precursor of squamous cell cancer.

Treatment

It is impossible to determine which lesion showing leukoplakia or erythroplakia will undergo malignant transformation. Discontinuance of chronic irritants is recommended, followed by a 14-day observation period to allow inflammatory lesions to heal. If the lesion persists, referral to a dental surgeon for a biopsy and regular follow-up surveillance, even if the lesion is benign, are indicated. The biopsy procedure is as simple as having a restoration (filling) or a tooth extraction.

Other conditions that may resemble leukoplakia or erythroplakia are lichen planus, chemical burns, candidiasis (thrush), psoriasis, lupus erythematosus, and syphilitic mucous patches. Each of these has characteristic histologic features.

Squamous Cell Carcinoma

More than 90% of all malignant tumors of the oral cavity are squamous cell carcinomas. They are four times more common in men than women and are most common after the fourth decade. In the United States, oral cancer is the eighth most common form of cancer in men and the twelfth in women. Fifteen thousand

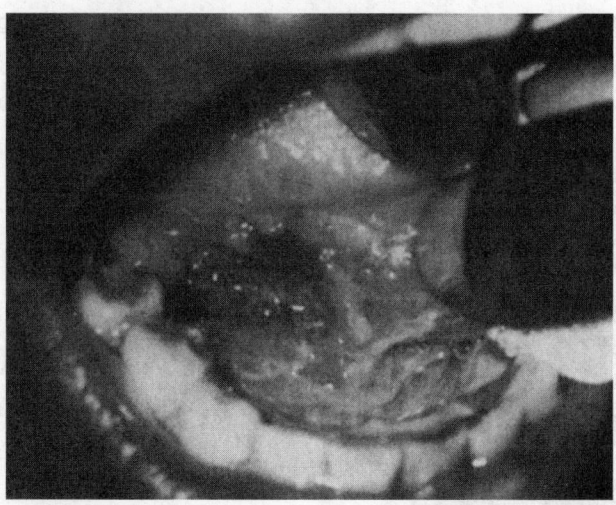

Figure 101.9.   Squamous cell carcinoma of the floor of the mouth.

new cases are found each year, and about 7500 patients die of this disease annually. Of lip carcinomas, 95% occur on the lower lip and appear as an ulcer, wart, sore, or scale (6). This lesion is more common in fair-skinned patients. Of the intraoral carcinomas, 50% occur on the tongue (usually the ventrolateral border; Fig. 101.9) and 16% on the floor of the mouth; the remaining 34% are equally distributed between the gingival mucosa, palate, and buccal mucosa. Sixty percent of intraoral carcinomas present as ulcers, 30% as growths, and the remaining 10% as white lesions or other abnormalities of the mucosa (2). Carcinoma of the tongue and floor of the mouth metastasizes early and carries a poor prognosis.

The cause of oral carcinoma is unknown. Ill-fitting dentures, actinic radiation, tobacco, jagged teeth, syphilitic glossitis, and alcoholism are believed to be risk factors.

Presentation and Evaluation

Patients usually give a history of knowledge of the lesion for 6 to 18 months when they first present; for many reasons they have not sought evaluation. All patients with suspicious lesions should be referred promptly to a dental surgeon for biopsy. Biopsy is a simple procedure, not very different from having a restoration or tooth extraction; usually it is done under local anesthesia.

Treatment

Definitive surgery is a team effort between the otolaryngologist and the dentist. The dentist's role is to evaluate, for long-term prognosis, any of the teeth that are not to be removed in the surgical field and to remove any of these teeth that are affected with untreatable periodontitis; this is done to avoid osteoradionecrosis, a condition seen in the postradiation patient in whom the socket of an extracted tooth fails to heal as the result of diminished blood supply. Lip tumors have the highest success rate (10-year cure rate between 80 and 92%), whereas only one-fifth of patients with tongue cancer live longer than 5 years.

General References

Cummings CW, ed. Otolaryngology: head and neck surgery. 2nd ed. St. Louis: CV Mosby, 1993.
> Volume 2, edited by David E. Schuller, contains several excellent chapters on the oral cavity and the diseases affecting it. There are many excellent color photographs of clinically common lesions.
Epstein JB, Stevensen Moore P, Scally C. Management of xerostomia. J Can Dent Assoc 58(2):140, 1992.
Friedman MH, Weisberg J. Temporomandibular joint disorders. Lombard, IL: Quint, 1985.
McDowell JD, Kassebaum DK. Diagnosing and treating halitosis. J Can Dent Assoc 124:55, 1993.
Thaller SR, Montgomery WW, eds. Guide to dental problems for physicians and surgeons. Baltimore: Williams & Wilkins, 1988.
Williams RC. Periodontal disease. N Engl J Med 322:373, 1990.
Wood NK, Goaz PW. Differential diagnosis of oral lesions. 5th ed. St. Louis: CV Mosby, 1996.

Specific References

1. Apfelberg DB, Lavey E, Janetos G, et al. Temporomandibular joint disease: results of a ten year study. Postgrad Med 65:167, 1979.
2. Bhaskar SN. Synopsis of oral pathology. 4th ed. St. Louis: CV Mosby, 1973;463.
3. Briner WW, Grossman E, Buckner RY, et al. Effect of chlorhexidine gluconate mouth rinse on plaque bacteria. J Periodontal Res 21(Suppl 16):44, 1986.
4. Franks AS. The social character of temporomandibular joint dysfunction. Dent Pract Dent Rec 15:94, 1964.
5. Graykowski EA, Barile MF, Lee WB, Stanley HR Jr. Recurrent aphthous stomatitis: clinical, therapeutic, histopathologic, and hypersensitivity aspects. JAMA 196:637, 1966.
6. Loesch WJ. Periodontal disease as a risk factor for heart disease. Compendium 15:976, 1994.
7. Mashberg A, Morrissey JB, Garfinkel L. A study of the appearance of early asymptomatic oral squamous cell carcinoma. Cancer (Philadelphia) 32:1436, 1973.
8. U.S. Department of Health, Education and Welfare, Public Health Service. Research explores pyorrhea and other gum diseases: periodontal disease (PHS Publication 1482). Washington, DC: US Government Printing Office, 1970.

C H A P T E R   102

Common Problems of the Feet

BRUCE S. LEBOWITZ, DPM

The general physician is often called on to treat patients who complain of problems with their feet. Although disorders of the feet are not life threatening, they should not be taken lightly. Any patient with a painful foot attests that the pain takes the joy out of living.

STRUCTURE AND FUNCTION

The abnormal foot cannot be understood unless the structure of the foot and its function during gait are understood.

Normal Gait

The bones and joints of the feet facilitate walking and running in an upright position (Fig. 102.1). The foot and leg function together to allow a smooth, even transfer of weight as one extremity moves ahead of the other. During gait, the foot first adjusts to a variable terrain and then acts to propel the body's weight forward.

In the *first stage of gait*, the heel strikes the ground and body weight begins to move distally over the lateral aspect of the foot. The foot is in a pronated position, meaning that the arch is flattened. In effect, the foot resembles a loose bag of bones during this stage, permitting it to adapt to the terrain and to act as a shock absorber when body weight strikes the ground.

In the *second stage of gait,* as weight moves distally to the ball of the foot and the body is propelled forward, the foot must convert to a rigid lever. This conversion, or supination, takes place in the subtalar and midtarsal joints. Supination serves to heighten the arch, pushing the bones and joints of the foot together rigidly enough to propel body weight forward efficiently.

For the lower extremity to function normally, certain structural criteria must be met; if they are not met, compensation occurs. Ideally, the leg should be in a plane perpendicular to the foot and ground, as in a stick figure drawing. The forefoot should be in a plane parallel to the rear foot, but various congenital factors may act to prevent this normal angulation. Varus (toward the midline or inverted) or valgus (away from the midline or everted) positions of the forefoot or hindfoot are the most common of these congenital factors.

Excessive Pronation

Excessive pronation (pronation extended through too much of the gait cycle) is the most common compensating mechanism when structural abnormalities are present. When the foot remains pronated during gait and does not resupinate in time, or at all, the condition known as *flatfoot* exists. The degree of this flatfoot position reflects the degree of pronation that is present. A number of problems may evolve from excessive pronation during gait, including bunions, calluses, and hammertoes. As pointed out in the discussion that follows, assessment of the mechanical basis for the condition is important in planning appropriate treatment for it.

Shoes

Shoes clearly play a role in the way feet function. Shoes protect feet from the elements, cushion the effect of walking on hard, flat surfaces, and provide some support to the bones and ligaments. Unfortunately, many people favor short, narrow shoes, high heels, and pointed toes. Obviously, squeezing a basically rectangular foot into a triangular shoe with the heels elevated from 2 to 5 inches creates significant stress for the foot. Most of the disorders of the foot discussed in this chapter are intensified by these demands of fashion.

Most people, in fitting themselves for shoes, do not take into account the variations in their foot size throughout the day and the variation in shoe size from manufacturer to manufacturer. Therefore the following advice is often helpful: Buy shoes in the late afternoon when any swelling that might occur is already present; lightweight shoes are preferable to heavy ones; and

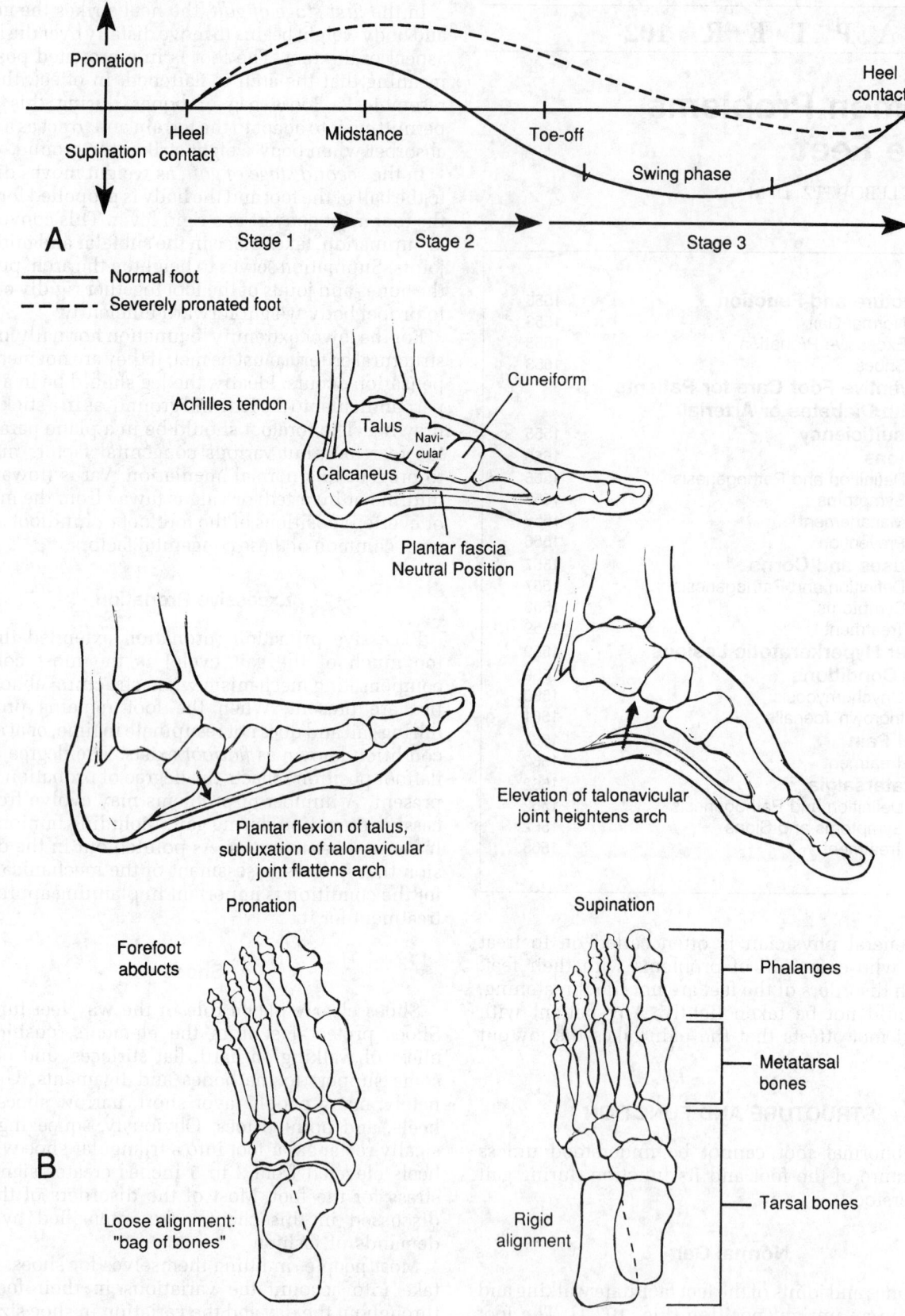

Figure 102.1. **A.** Schematic representation of the gait cycle for a normal foot and for a foot with excessive pronation. **B.** Sche-matic illustration of foot structure during pronation and supination during gait cycle.

leather, because it is more porous, is preferable to synthetic materials in shoe construction.

Interest in shoes appropriate to sports, especially jogging and running, has escalated in recent years. Sneakers or running shoes should be well fitted and firm enough to prevent excessive splaying of the foot during activity. For shock absorption, the shoes should have studded soles, and there should be a raised, resilient heel wedge. The midsole should be flexible to help prevent Achilles tendon stress, and there should be a well-molded Achilles pad to prevent irritation of the tendon. The tongue should be well padded to prevent irritation of the dorsum of the foot. These features are illustrated in Figure 102.2.

It is a misconception that wearing sneakers excessively harms the feet. Actually, the better running shoes available today are so supportive and so well padded that they may be recommended to patients for numerous painful foot conditions. For example, highly arched feet (which are supinated and may pronate only slightly) lack shock-absorbing qualities; constant impact on the ground can cause severe metatarsal, heel, and arch pain. For patients with this condition, the support and resiliency provided by a modern running shoe are ideal. Likewise, a flat or pronated foot may be very well supported by the built-in arch supports of well-made running shoes.

Running magnifies the problems associated with excessive pronation, and the long-term management of this condition requires the selection of shoes that provide good support. The use of well-designed running shoes is important in preventing most exercise-related injuries of the lower extremity, as explained in Chapter 67, "Exercise-Related Musculoskeletal Problems."

PREVENTIVE FOOT CARE FOR PATIENTS WITH DIABETES OR ARTERIAL INSUFFICIENCY

To understand the need for professional diabetic foot care, one must consider the special devastating effect diabetes mellitus has on the feet.

The most important podiatric problem of diabetes is

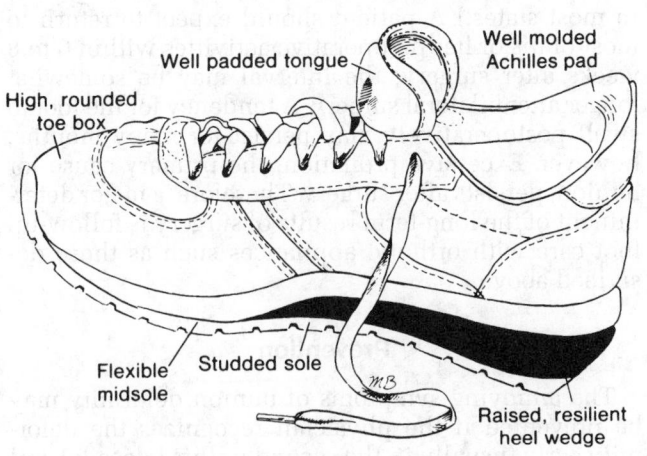

Figure 102.2.   Features of a well-designed running shoe.

High, rounded toe box

Well padded tongue

Well molded Achilles pad

Flexible midsole

Studded sole

Raised, resilient heel wedge

neuropathy (see Chapter 72, "Diabetes Mellitus"). Sensory neuropathy may cause burning and sometimes unbearable pain in the feet and legs, especially at night. At the same time, sensory neuropathy lessens the ability of the patient to interpret and respond to painful stimuli. A foreign body that is not felt, or a thick corn or callus not treated, can result in irritation of the tissues with complicating infection.

In addition, motor neuropathy causes wasting of the small muscles of the foot. Without the intrinsic muscles helping to stabilize the motions of the toes and metatarsal phalangeal joints, the tendency to form severe hammertoe and callus is greatly increased. The mechanical forces on the toes and metatarsals are increased as the ability to sense pain is reduced.

Sympathetic neuropathy leads to excessively dry skin and the feet of a diabetic patient are often anhidrotic and at risk for secondary infection.

In addition to neuropathy, the diabetic foot is affected by vascular disease. Vascular disease also occurs in many independent of diabetes mellitus, and the same issues apply. Arteriosclerosis is accelerated in the diabetic patient. The changes that are often seen lead to claudication and rest pain. Diabetic small vessel disease affects the nourishment of tissues, accounting for the finding of normal pedal arterial pulses and yet severely dysvascular digits that sometimes require amputation.

Prevention and early detection of problems on the surface of the foot are particularly important in patients with these conditions (see Chapter 87, "Peripheral Vascular Disease and Arterial Aneurysms," and Chapter 88, "Lower Extremity Ulcers and Varicose Veins"). This requires periodic examination by the physician or nurse and routine examination by the patient. The single most important advice that can be impressed upon the patient is to look at his or her feet every day. When obesity or lack of visual acuity is a problem, someone else should examine the patient's feet every day. Irritations, abrasions, and calluses that usually produce pain must be identified visually when there are sensory abnormalities in the feet. Advice about selection of shoe gear (see above) should be provided routinely to patients with diabetes and vascular insufficiency. Following these procedures minimizes the risk of serious foot ulcers and infections.

These patients should also be advised not to use over-the-counter remedies for corns and ingrown toenails. Such commercial preparations include acids and tanning agents that can seriously injure the tender skin of these patients. Normal toenails should be allowed to grow past the end of the fleshy part of the toe; thick nails are best trimmed by a podiatrist, as are corns and calluses (see below). Soft cotton should be worn between toes that tend to rub each other, and talcum powder should be used to prevent interdigital moisture and maceration. Lanolin should be applied to dry and thickened skin to prevent fissuring, especially common in the heels of diabetic patients with anhidrosis from sympathetic neuropathy.

A final note on prevention: Patients should be encouraged to shake out their shoes before putting them on as a simple, obvious way to prevent foreign body penetration.

BUNIONS

Definition and Pathogenesis

Bunion (literally *turnip*) is a term used to describe the collective deformities of the first metatarsophalangeal joint (Fig. 102.3). These deformities include enlargement of the medial, medial–dorsal, or dorsal aspect of the first metatarsophalangeal joint and lateral deviation of the great toe. The enlargement of the joint may consist of bone or soft tissue or a combination of the two.

For many years, tight-fitting shoes were mistakenly considered to be the cause of bunions. It is known now that, although the pressure of tight shoes on an existing bunion can certainly result in pain that calls attention to the problem, bunions are not caused by poorly fitted shoes. The chief cause of the deformity is a hypermobile first metatarsal bone, most often related to excessive pronation (see above). The first metatarsal and great toe, which help propel body weight forward, should be stable during the final stage of gait when a tight, rigid bony structure is needed. The intrinsic and extrinsic musculature should help to hold the metatarsal tight at this point. When there is excessive pronation, the entire foot remains loose and unstable. One result of such laxity in this stage of gait is hypermobility of the first metatarsal and buckling of the first toe; intrinsic and extrinsic muscles cause the first metatarsal to deviate medially and the great toe to deviate laterally. The combined deformity is called *hallux abducto valgus*. Eventually, arthritic hypertrophy of the head of the first metatarsal bone develops.

Symptoms

The presenting complaint of a patient with a bunion is pain localized to the first metatarsophalangeal joint. Pressure of the shoe on the enlarged metatarsal head, with or without pressure on adventitious bursa, can cause pain that is severe and even disabling; pain can also result from the joint motion itself. Often, crepitus can be felt within the joint. Sometimes the patient seeks help not because of pain, but because he or she is unable to wear shoes as a result of the deformity.

In evaluating a patient, the physician must be certain that the symptoms are a result of the bunion alone. Gout (see Chapter 69) may not only produce acute pain in the first metatarsophalangeal joint but may also aggravate a chronically painful joint. Therefore gout should always be considered, especially in patients with bilateral bunion deformity and acute nonarticular pain in a foot.

Management

Acute symptoms caused by a bunion should be managed with rest, elimination of pressure on the bunion, soaks in warm water, and systemic anti-inflammatory medication such as naproxen (Naprosyn) 250 to 500 mg every 8 to 12 hours or piroxicam (Feldene) 10 to 20 mg every 24 hours; aspirin 600 mg every 4 to 6 hours may also be used, but the onset of action is slower. After the acute symptoms have subsided, the patient should be started on a program of long-term management.

Conservative long-term management of a bunion involves accommodating the deformity and attempting to arrest its progress. This is achieved by the use of molds and protective shields (Fig. 102.3B and C). A mold, usually called an arch support, may be made from various types of materials to accommodate the plantar aspect of the foot. Protective shields are made of latex rubber.

Full foot molds or protective shields made by a podiatrist from a plaster impression are preferable to commercially made devices found in pharmacies and shoe stores. Commercial devices are manufactured to fit average shoe and foot sizes and do not take into account the shape of the individual patient's foot. The mold should be in place during the fitting of all new shoes. Occasionally, if the mold makes conventional shoes too tight, a specially built shoe, called an extra depth-inlay shoe, may be used. These enlarged shoes have a removable insole, for which one may substitute the patient's mold. The mold and shoes should minimize pressures against the bunion. In addition, the mold acts to reduce excessive pronation, thereby reducing the deforming forces in the forefoot.

Patients whose symptoms are not adequately controlled with conservative measures should be considered for surgery. The surgical management of a bunion must be individually planned for each patient and, in fact, for each foot, to correct the specific deformity. Correction might involve resection of the bony protuberance of the first metatarsal head only. In occasional patients with severe degenerative joint disease, surgical management involves removal of all or part of the joint and insertion of a Silastic joint replacement (Fig. 102.3D). Depending on locale, referral for surgical correction of a bunion may be made to a general, orthopedic, or podiatric surgeon. (This surgery, like most podiatric surgery, is done on an ambulatory basis in most states.) A patient should expect to return to most of his or her preoperative activities within 6 to 8 weeks after surgery; the interval may be somewhat longer after bilateral surgery. A tendency for the foot to swell postoperatively may persist for many months, however. Excessive pronation, the primary cause for bunion, persists after surgery. Therefore, a major determinant of the long-term results of surgery is follow-up foot care with orthotic appliances such as those described above.

Prevention

The annoying symptoms of bunion deformity may be prevented if the physician recognizes the deformity early (usually in the second or third decade) and refers the patient for conservative management by a podiatrist.

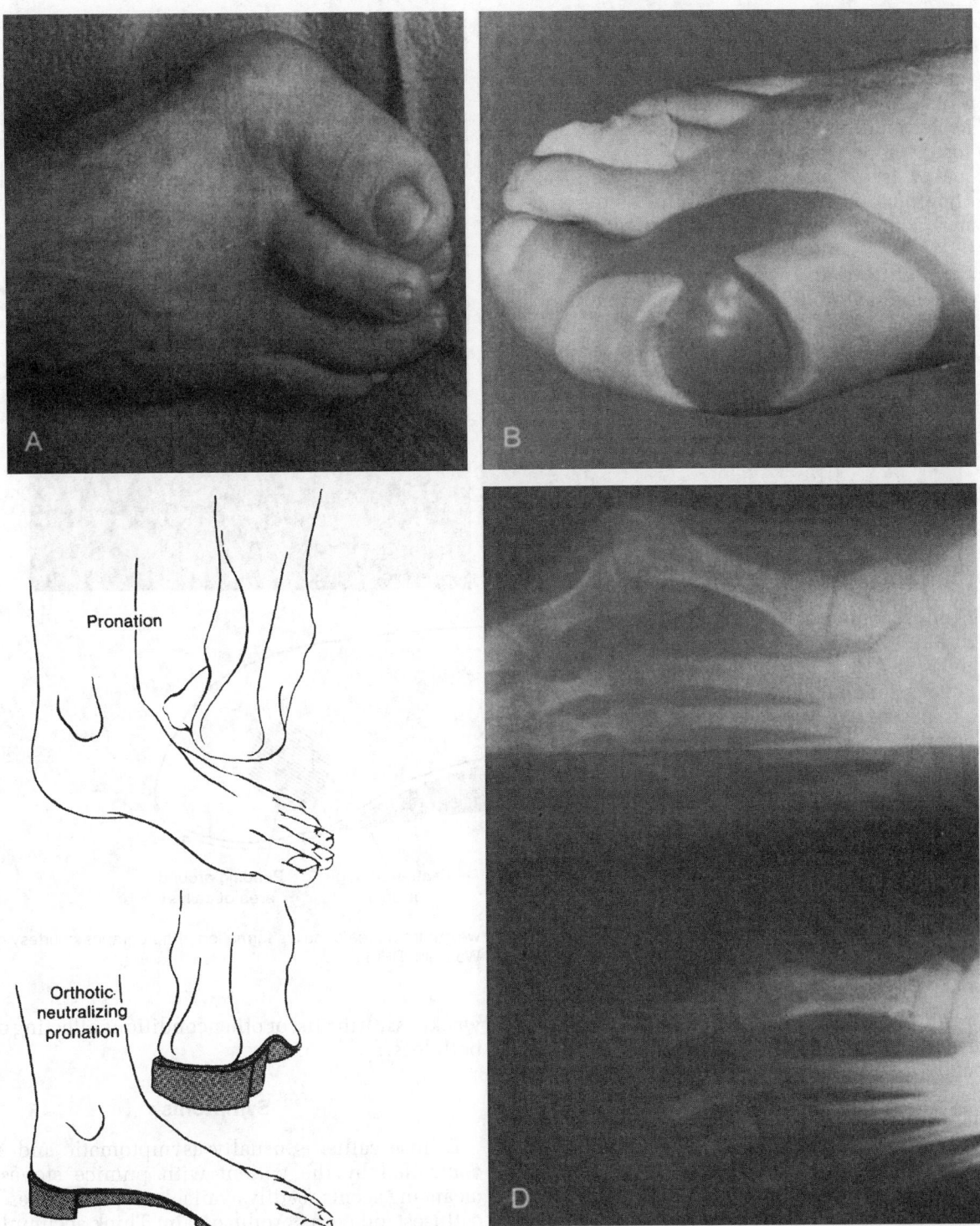

Figure 102.3.   Bunions: appearance, orthotic compensation, and surgical repair. **A.** Bunion deformity. **B.** Bunion protected by latex shield. **C.** Leather orthotic arch support. **D.** Bunion deformity shown radiologically before and after surgical correction.

CALLUSES AND CORNS

Definition and Pathogenesis

A *callus* is a thickening of the epidermis as a result of chronic intermittent trauma (Fig. 102.4). When there is intermittent irritation of an area of skin, the initial response is vasodilation; this is followed by increased production of corneum and hyperkeratosis. This process is normal and protective to skin and underlying tissue. When the process continues until there is buildup of excessive or highly concentrated

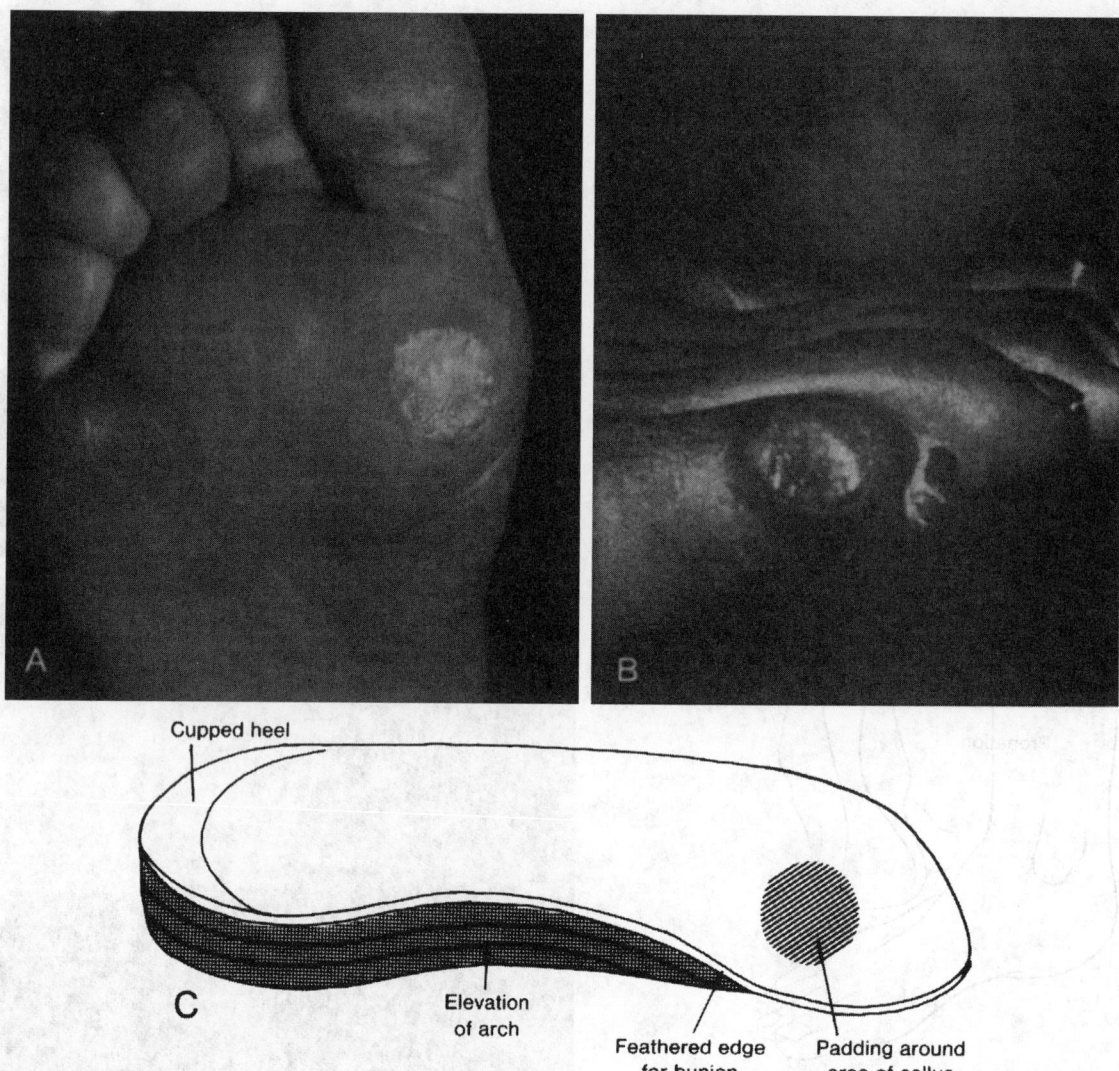

Figure 102.4. Calluses and corns. **A.** Typical plantar callus. **B.** Corn on the fifth digit. **C.** Orthotic device designed to shift weight from area of callus formation. (Photographs courtesy of Max Weisfeld, DPM.)

callus, resulting in a corn, problems may develop. Skin lines may remain visible in callused tissue, but they usually do not pass through the highly concentrated center of a corn. Corns are most often located overlying the proximal interphalangeal joints of the lesser toes and centrally within plantar calluses. A number of processes not related to chronic trauma can produce focal calluses as well, namely *verruca plantaris* (plantar wart), *foreign body granuloma,* and *porokeratosis plantaris discreta.* These lesions are discussed below.

The primary cause for most symptomatic calluses is excessive pronation (see above), not restrictive shoes or walking on unyielding surfaces. During excessive pronation, the long flexor and extensor tendons pull on the distal phalanges, the toes appear to hammer, and a retrograde force pushes down on the metatarsal heads, increasing pressure on the plantar skin. Other conditions that may promote this increased pressure are excessive supination (highly arched foot) and imbalance of the peroneal and tibial muscles caused by

weakness, arthritis, or other conditions affecting one or both legs.

Symptoms

Diffuse callus is usually asymptomatic and easily controlled by the patient with pumice stones and cleansing agents readily available in pharmacies. Both calluses and corns produce pain. Thick accumulation of callus tends to cause a burning sensation in the foot. A corn located within a plantar callus gives the sensation of walking on a sharp pebble. Corns that occur dorsolaterally on fifth toes (Fig. 102.4B) often cause exquisite pain, especially with tight-fitting shoes. Such corns often have adventitious bursae associated with them and may produce symptoms of both bursitis and the discomfort of the corn pressing down on subcutaneous tissues.

Although corns and calluses can cause discomfort for the average person, they can cause serious morbidity in a diabetic patient (see above). A discrete lesion on the foot produces constant pressure on the underlying dermis. In a diabetic patient, this pressure often results in local breakdown of tissues, ulceration, and infection. Diabetic patients have the additional medical and mechanical problem of neurotrophic joints. In patients with the tendency to develop hammertoe and plantar-flexed metatarsal heads, these changes (and the calluses and corns that accompany them) may be accelerated by the loss of normal proprioception and pain sensation of a neurotrophic joint.

Corns and calluses can be a serious problem also for patients with conditions other than diabetes that impair arterial circulation to the lower extremities (see Chapter 87).

Treatment

Treatment of corns and calluses depends on the location, severity, and type of lesion and on the physical condition of the patient.

The physician occasionally sees patients who complain of severely painful corns and calluses. Dramatic relief may be obtained from the simple debridement of these painful lesions, using a sterile number 10 or 15 scalpel blade. If the blade is kept nearly parallel to the skin, injury to the underlying healthy dermis can be avoided. There is no need to debride the entire callus; any reduction in the thickness of the lesion brings relief to the patient.

Conservative long-term management of corns and calluses in the feet of otherwise healthy people requires control of the source of the problem, namely excessive pronation. If excessive pronation is neutralized with orthotic devices (see above), foot function is improved, pathologic forces are decreased, and lesions may regress. Lesions that have been present for a year or longer usually indicate that there also has developed structural changes in the bones and joints, with secondary histopathologic changes in the skin.

For patients whose symptoms are not controlled with conservative treatment, surgery may be helpful. A number of surgical procedures may be used to realign metatarsal heads or reduce hammertoe deformities. Often it is necessary to combine the surgical reconstruction of affected areas with control of pronation in order to achieve lasting resolution of symptoms. This may mean 6 to 8 weeks of convalescence (i.e., no weight bearing for several days, then progression to partial and then full weight bearing, usually by 6 weeks) after foot surgery and the continued use of orthotics in shoes. The result is greater foot health and comfort.

For the patient with diabetes or peripheral vascular disease, conservative treatment involves frequent debridement of the hyperkeratotic areas, padding for protection, and the fabrication of molds (by a podiatrist or orthopedist) to shift weight away from problem areas and accommodate deformities (Fig. 102.4C). Extra-depth shoes are often prescribed in conjunction with such appliances. When refractory infection or ulceration occurs despite conservative management, surgical procedures may be performed to eliminate a bony prominence. Surgery may rehabilitate a bedridden patient or obviate future amputation. Management requires close collaboration between the patient's physician and the consultant.

OTHER HYPERKERATOTIC LESIONS

Other discrete hyperkeratotic lesions commonly found on the foot include verruca plantaris, porokeratosis plantaris discreta, and foreign body granuloma.

Verruca plantaris, or *plantar warts,* occur on the plantar aspect of the foot, usually on weight-bearing surfaces (Fig. 102.5A). They are discussed also in Chapter 100, "Common Problems of the Skin," but a brief account is provided here because of the importance of differentiating them from corns, calluses, and other hyperkeratotic lesions. Plantar warts can be asymptomatic or extremely painful. They are caused by a papilloma virus for which there is no specific treatment or prevention. Because they are benign and often resolve spontaneously, aggressive or untried therapies should be avoided.

The appearance of a verrucous lesion is illustrated in Figure 102.5A. They may vary in size from 1 mm to 1 cm. The lesions can be differentiated from hyperkeratotic corns in several ways: Warts usually have rough surfaces, are painful with the application of surface and lateral pressure, and bleed upon debriding because of their capillary supply; corns are usually smooth surfaced, most painful with surface pressure, and do not bleed upon debridement. The treatment is best directed by a podiatrist because it is essential to destroy the wart without producing a scar, which itself may be permanently painful. The treatment of warts in general is described in Chapter 100.

A *porokeratotic lesion* is a circumscribed, discrete hyperkeratotic lesion on the plantar aspect of the foot that develops as a result of keratin occluding a sweat duct in the skin (Fig. 102.5B). The obstruction and resultant backup create a reaction in the skin similar to a deep, large corn. This lesion need not be under a weight-bearing surface. It is usually painful, and after debridement there is characteristically even more distress. Treatment by the dermatologist or podiatrist is usually by local curettage.

Foreign bodies in the plantar surface of the foot can generate a local inflammatory reaction and thus create a hyperkeratotic lesion. One of the most common offending substances is hair (animal or human). For example, a dog hair, trapped in a carpet long enough to have dried out, can penetrate the skin rather easily. This lesion, although grossly resembling a simple callus, has a small aperture (entry wound) near the center, seen upon examination with a magnifying glass. The local reaction may or may not include infection. Treatment is simple excision of the foreign body.

NAIL CONDITIONS

Only two nail conditions are commonly brought to medical attention: onychomycosis (fungal infection) and ingrown toenails, with or without concomitant inflammation (paronychia).

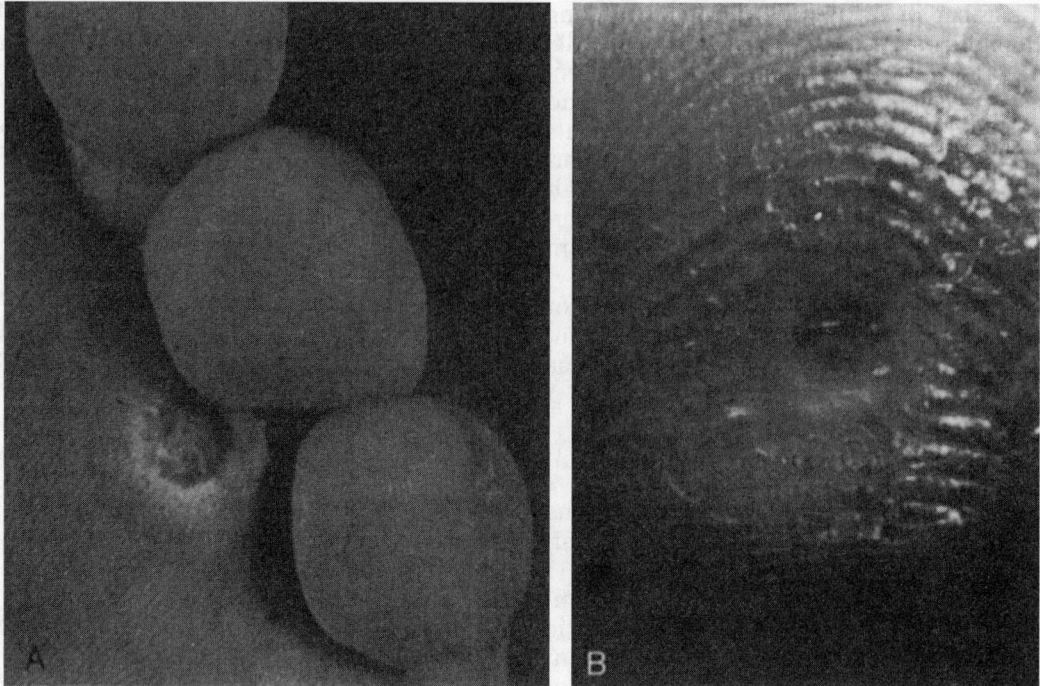

Figure 102.5.   Hyperkeratotic lesions not caused by chronic trauma. **A.** Plantar wart. **B.** Porokeratosis on plantar surface. (Photographs courtesy of Max Weisfeld, DPM.)

Onychomycosis

Causes and Findings

The typical fungal infection of a toenail begins distally at the tip of the toe and moves proximally, subungually, and through the nail plate itself (Fig. 102.6). Etiologic agents are *Trichophyton mentagrophytes, Trichophyton rubrum,* or *Candida albicans.* The fungus produces yellowish discoloration and longitudinal striations in the nails and in the epidermis; the accompanying local inflammatory reaction stimulates hyperkeratosis under the nail. This hyperkeratotic accumulation tends to lift the nail up from the epidermis, facilitating further progression of the fungus. Eventually, the nail becomes mottled brownish yellow, thickened, and powdery. Usually these infections are asymptomatic; patients are most concerned about the appearance of their nails, the possibility of spread of infection, and sometimes the inability to wear shoes when severe thickening of the nail plate is present.

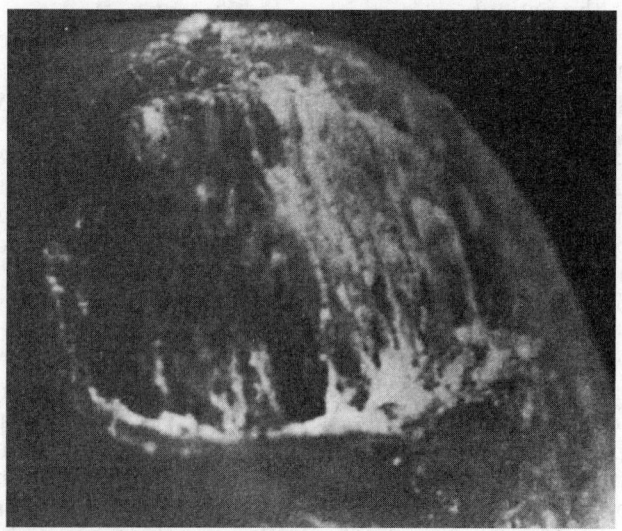

Figure 102.6.   Myotic toenail.

Treatment

Fungus infections of toenails are difficult to eradicate medically. No topical medications have been shown to be effective. Oral medications are available to treat and resolve onychomycosis. Itraconazole is effective against dermatophytes such as *T. rubrum* and nondermatophytes such as yeasts and molds. Terbinafine is effective against most dermatophytes. Because not all dystrophic toenails are mycotic, treatment should be based on the results of nail fungal cultures. Both drugs are taken orally once a day for 3 months: terbinafine (Lamisil 250 mg) and itraconazole (Sporanox 200 mg). Potentially severe drug interactions occur with itraconazole and both medications warrant monitoring of white blood cell counts and liver enzymes at baseline and in 6 weeks.

When nail thickening is regarded as a problem by the patient, the process can be controlled by regular and thorough debridement. The debridement of mycotic or otherwise thickened toenails is a process generally performed by podiatrists. The debridement first involves soaking of the feet and cutting of the nails by heavy-duty cutters. Finally, the nails are thoroughly filed down with an electrically powered, diamond-studded burr. These drills are fitted with vacuum extraction systems to protect the patient and podiatrist from breathing in the nail dust.

Another treatment is permanent removal of the nail, including matrixectomy. Because toenails serve no useful function, their absence causes no functional impairment. However, surgical correction should be reserved for patients whose nails are painful or for whom the appearance of the feet is a significant factor. The most common type of surgical correction of toenails performed by dermatologists, podiatrists, or surgeons is nail excision, followed by chemical destruction of matrix tissue and nail bed with 88% phenol. After a sterile dressing is applied to the toe, the patient may continue normal activities. The patient needs only to change bandages and soak the feet daily until healing is complete in 2 to 3 weeks. Skin formerly below the nail plate thickens. Anyone can disguise the fact that their nails have been removed by applying nail polish to this thickened skin.

Ingrown Toenails

Causes and Findings

Ingrown toenail, a painful condition in which the medial or lateral border of a toenail penetrates the flesh, is a common problem (Fig. 102.7). Ingrown toenails have been attributed to factors such as improper trimming, heredity, bony pathology, improper shoe fit, tight

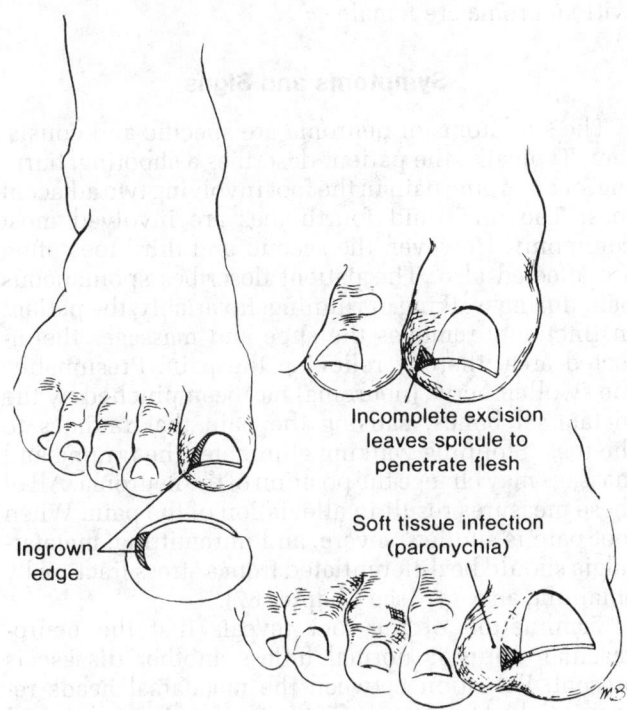

Incomplete excision leaves spicule to penetrate flesh

Soft tissue infection (paronychia)

Ingrown edge

Figure 102.7. Schematic illustration of an ingrown toenail and complications that may occur.

socks, obesity, and trauma. However, there is no clear-cut cause, and there are probably many contributing causes. The great toe is the one almost always involved, and the problem can be identified by inspection and by finding point tenderness upon pressing the margin of the toenail.

Treatment

There is a popular misconception that cutting a V in the center of a toenail causes the lateral borders to grow toward the center, thereby relieving the ingrown condition. This belief has no basis in fact because the nail plate is merely hornified keratin: nonliving, fixed tissue in which growth no longer occurs.

Initial treatment of ingrown toenail depends on whether the patient's toe is infected (paronychia) or is chronically painful but not infected when the patient seeks care. The patient with an ingrown toenail often seeks help after attempting to excise the offending edge of toenail with whatever instruments are available; most of the nail edge may be removed in this way by the patient, but a small, sharp piece of nail usually remains that pierces the skin with each step and promotes infection; the toe becomes red, swollen, and exquisitely tender. The most vigorous soaking and the use of local and systemic antibiotics will not arrest such an infection as long as a nail spicule continues to penetrate the flesh. Therefore the patient should be referred to a dermatologist, podiatrist, or surgeon for excision of the offending border of the nail; this procedure is done under local anesthesia and is curative. However, approximately 10% of patients have a recurrence, usually within 1 year. Systemic antimicrobials are rarely necessary. Definitive treatment of the ingrown nail itself varies according to the condition and needs of the patient.

For otherwise healthy patients, the procedure described above for removal of the entire toenail and for matrix destruction can also be used to eradicate permanently an ingrown border. After local anesthesia (obtained by injecting the base of the toe to create a full block, injecting a field on the medial surface from dorsal to lateral and on the lateral surface from dorsal to lateral), the offending edge of toenail is excised, then phenol and alcohol are applied to cauterize the matrix tissue. This procedure, followed by complete healing in 2 to 3 weeks, usually eliminates permanently this painful and sometimes dangerous condition.

Treatment of diabetic patients and patients with arterial insufficiency must be conservative because wound healing may be poor after surgical removal of the nail. In these patients, frequent and thorough debridement of ingrown borders is effective and safe. Treatment by a podiatrist or other practitioner who is skilled in this procedure may be needed every 3 to 4 weeks to prevent complicating soft tissue infection.

HEEL PAIN

Heel pain is a common complaint. The most common pattern is pain that is localized to the medial plantar aspect of the heel. (Heel pain localized to the posterior aspect of the foot, the heel cord, is discussed in Chapter 67; and heel pain as a manifestation of the tarsal tunnel syndrome is discussed in Chapter 84.) Characteristically, the first step in the morning is particularly painful. After 5 to 10 minutes of walking the pain eases, but during the course of the day's activities it becomes progressively worse. The reason that these symptoms appear, disappear, and reappear is not understood.

Examination of the foot reveals a tender area of the heel approximately 4.5 cm from the posterior margin of the plantar surface, corresponding to the medial condyle of the calcaneus. X-rays often reveal a calcaneal exostosis or spur at the point of tenderness (Fig. 102.8). These spurs are commonly found on x-rays of asymptomatic heels, and they are not the cause of pain in symptomatic heels. Because the attachment of the plantar fascia coincides with the point of greatest tenderness, it is believed that pain is caused by *plantar fasciitis*. One can picture the plantar fascia as an extension of the Achilles tendon, with the calcaneus acting as a fulcrum between fascia and tendon (Fig. 102.1B). Any condition that increases stress on the Achilles tendon may also stress the plantar fascia, such as overuse in running or jogging (especially with shoes having inflexible midsoles), excessive pronation (see above), or a sudden change to flat shoes after wearing high heels for prolonged periods. Heel pain may also be a manifestation of gout or Reiter's syndrome, and these diagnoses should always be considered when evaluating such a patient (see Chapters 69 and 71).

Treatment

Treatment should be aimed at both the local inflammatory process and the underlying mechanical problem. Initial treatment includes using an oral anti-inflammatory medication (see Chapter 70), resting, and

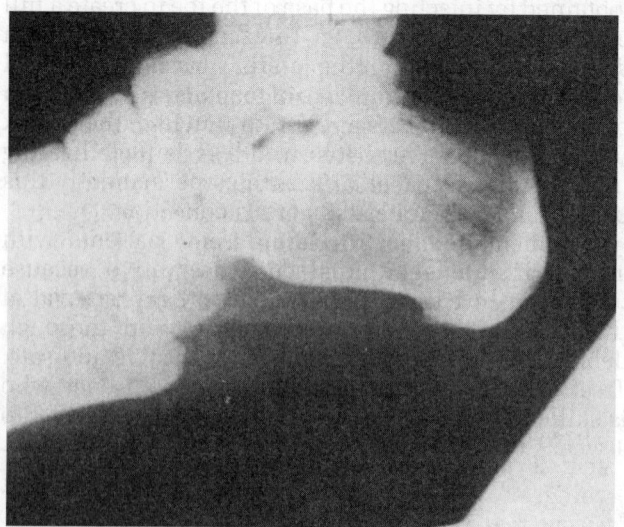

Figure 102.8. Radiologic view of a calcaneal exostosis (spur). (Photograph courtesy of Max Weisfeld, DPM.)

soaking in warm water. An injection (using a 25-gauge 1-inch needle) of a corticosteroid and lidocaine (approximately 0.5 to 1 mL of suspension of a corticosteroid diluted with 1 to 2 mL of 1 to 2% lidocaine) into the tender area from the medial aspect of the heel usually brings dramatic relief from pain that has not responded to other measures (see also Table 66.4).

Recurrent symptoms can be prevented by having the patient use a quarter-inch felt heel pad. When this is inserted into the shoes, it decreases tension on the Achilles tendon, so tension on the plantar fascia is also reduced. The increased angulation of the foot shifts weight away from the heel to the forefoot. Felt, rather than foam, which is too compressible, is available from medical and surgical supply houses. When a simple heel pad is not sufficient, consultation with an orthopedist or podiatrist is indicated. The consultant fabricates an appropriate orthotic to minimize pronation, raise the heel, and protect the painful area. Rarely, a painful heel requires surgical fasciotomy and removal of the spur.

METATARSALGIA

Definition and Pathogenesis

Metatarsalgia is pain in the forefoot. The most common condition causing metatarsalgia is *Morton's neuroma*. This is a condition in which two interdigital plantar nerves between adjacent toes become compressed, inflamed, and ultimately painful. The compression of these nerves is enhanced by elevating the heel and compressing the forefoot. Therefore women's fashionable high-heeled, pointed toe shoes are associated with this condition. In fact, 80 to 90% of patients with neuroma are female.

Symptoms and Signs

The symptoms of neuroma are specific and consistent. Typically, the patient describes a shooting, burning, or cramping pain in the foot involving two adjacent toes. The third and fourth toes are involved most commonly. However, the second and third toes often are affected also. The patient describes spontaneous pain during walking or running. Invariably, the patient instinctively removes the shoe and massages the affected area, thereby relieving the pain. Presumably, the swollen nerve (neuroma) has been pinched by the metatarsal bones, causing the pain that radiates to the toes. Stopping walking eliminates the trauma and massage may change the position of the neuroma. All of these measures result in alleviation of the pain. When foot pain is sudden, severe, and unremitting, metatarsalgia should be differentiated from a stress fracture by obtaining an x-ray (see Chapter 67).

Examination of the foot reveals that the neurovascular status is normal unless another disease is present. Palpation between the metatarsal heads reveals marked tenderness. If the forefoot is compressed while the web space is palpated, the area may be exquisitely tender.

Treatment

The most effective treatment for metatarsalgia is the wearing of low, flat, wide, soft leather shoes. Corticosteroid (lidocaine) injections into the web space and reaching the plantar surface (0.5 mL of deposteroid with 1 mL of lidocaine using a 25-gauge 1-inch needle) may provide temporary relief. Nonsteroidal antiinflammatory drugs are ineffective. Orthotics are helpful; however, if the patient is willing to wear wide enough shoes to accommodate them, the condition usually resolves, even without the orthotic. Surgical excision is successful in 80 to 90% of cases and is indicated if symptoms persist. For patients undergoing surgery, a recovery period of 4 to 6 weeks is necessary before they can return to full activity and wear their usual shoes.

Metatarsalgia not caused by neuroma is more difficult to characterize, evaluate, and treat. Nonneuritic metatarsal pain may occur anywhere in the forefoot with or without radiation and be exacerbated by high-heeled or, at times, low-heeled shoes. Palpation often reveals pain directly on a metatarsal head rather than between them. Rest, the application of ice, and elevation of the foot may help some patients but most require referral to a podiatrist for padding, orthotics, or other treatment.

General References

Alexander I. The foot exam and diagnosis. Philadelphia: Churchill Livingstone, 1997.
> Paperback book covering multiple foot issues aimed at the primary care physician.

Kozak GP. Management of diabetic foot problems. Philadelphia: WB Saunders, 1995.

Lemont H. Common foot disorders. In: Berkow R, ed. The Merck manual. 16th ed. Rahway, NJ: Merck, Sharp & Dohme, 1992.

Levin ME, O'Neal LW, ed. The diabetic foot. 4th ed. St. Louis: CV Mosby, 1988.
> The most highly regarded resource for the care of the diabetic foot.

McGlamry ED, Banks AS, Downey MS, eds. Comprehensive textbook of foot surgery. 2nd ed. Baltimore: Williams & Wilkins, 1992.
> This two-volume text covers all aspects of foot care, including medical and surgical treatments.

Robbins J, ed. Primary podiatric medicine. Philadelphia: WB Saunders, 1994.
> Intensive evaluation and management of foot diseases aimed at the specialist, but very readable.

INDEX

Page numbers followed by *t* and *f* indicate tables and figures, respectively.